AMERICAN COLLEGE OF SURGEONS

ACS SURGERY

Principles & Practice

2003

AMERICAN COLLEGE OF SURGEONS

ACS SURGERY

Principles & Practice

2003

DOUGLAS W. WILMORE, M.D., F.A.C.S.
Frank Sawyer Professor of Surgery,
Harvard Medical School
EDITORIAL CHAIRMAN

LAURENCE Y. CHEUNG, M.D., F.A.C.S.
Professor and Chairman, Department of Surgery,
University of Kansas School of Medicine
EDITOR

ALDEN H. HARKEN, M.D., F.A.C.S.
Professor, Department of Surgery,
University of Colorado Health Sciences Center
EDITOR

JAMES W. HOLCROFT, M.D., F.A.C.S.
Professor, Department of Surgery,
University of California, Davis,
School of Medicine
EDITOR

JONATHAN L. MEAKINS, M.D., D.Sc., F.R.C.S.(C), F.A.C.S.
Nuffield Professor of Surgery,
University of Oxford
EDITOR

NATHANIEL J. SOPER, M.D., F.A.C.S.
Professor, Department of Surgery,
Washington University School of Medicine
EDITOR

www.acssurgery.com

Library of Congress has cataloged the first edition of this work as follows:

Library of Congress Cataloging-in-Publication Data

ACS surgery: principles and practice / Douglas W. Wilmore ... [et al.], editor.
    p. ; cm.
  Includes bibliographical references and index.
  ISBN 0-9703902-1-1 (2002)—ISBN 0-9703902-4-6 (2003) (alk. paper)
   1. Therapeutics, Surgical. 2. Surgery. I. Wilmore, Douglas W. (Douglas Wayne), date.
 II. American College of Surgeons.
  [DNLM: 1. Surgical Procedures, Operative—methods. 2. Perioperative Care—methods.
WA 300 G775c 2000]
 RD49 .A275 2001
 617′.9—dc21

                                          2001026575

Vice President and Publisher	Nancy E. Chorpenning
Director, Electronic Publishing	Liz Pope
Managing Editor	Richard P. Lindsey
Senior Copy Editor	John J. Anello
Production Editor	Dave Terry
Art and Design Editor	Elizabeth Klarfeld
Electronic Composition	Diane Joiner, Jennifer Smith
Manufacturing Producer	Kelly Mercado
Indexer	Julia Brooks Figures

Printed in the United States of America.

Published by WebMD Inc.

WebMD Professional Publishing
WebMD Inc.
224 West 30th Street
New York, NY 10001

ACS Surgery: Principles and Practice 2003 is sponsored by the American College of Surgeons and written by individuals who are recognized experts. The text represents the authors' approaches to clinical problems and to other important issues in surgical practice. It should be used as a general reference with other sources in the formation of an integrated care plan.

The authors, editors, and publisher have conscientiously and carefully tried to ensure that recommended measures and drug dosages in these pages are accurate and conform to the standards that prevailed at the time of publication. The reader is advised, however, to check the product information sheet accompanying each drug to be familiar with any changes in the dosage schedule or in the contraindications. This advice should be taken with particular seriousness if the agent to be administered is a new one or one that is infrequently used. *ACS Surgery: Principles and Practice 2003* describes basic principles of diagnosis and therapy. Because of the uniqueness of each patient and the need to take into account a number of concurrent considerations, however, this information should be used by physicians only as a general guide to clinical decision making.

To better care for all surgical patients

CONTENTS

III   TRAUMA AND THERMAL INJURY

VI SPECIAL PERIOPERATIVE PROBLEMS

VII   CARE IN THE ICU

VIII   POSTOPERATIVE MANAGEMENT

CONTRIBUTORS

ELIAS J. ANAISSIE, M.D. Professor of Medicine, University of Arkansas for Medical Sciences, and Director, Supportive Care, Myeloma Institute for Research and Treatment, Arkansas Cancer Research Center at the University of Arkansas for Medical Sciences

MAHA F. ANSARA, M.D. Fellow, Endocrinology and Metabolism, Division of Endocrinology, Diabetes and Metabolism, New Hanover Regional Medical Center, Wilmington, North Carolina

FRANK R. ARKO, M.D. Assistant Professor, Stanford University, and Director, Endovascular Surgery, Stanford University Medical Center

WALID S. ARNAOUT, M.D., F.A.C.S. Associate Director, Center for Liver Diseases and Transplantation, Cedars-Sinai Medical Center, Los Angeles

JYOTI ARYA, M.D. Assistant Professor, Department of Surgery, University of Colorado School of Medicine

ALAN N. BARKUN, M.D. Associate Professor, Department of Medicine, McGill University Faculty of Medicine, and Director, Division of Gastroenterology, McGill University Health Centre

JEFFREY S. BARKUN, M.D., F.A.C.S. Associate Professor, Department of Surgery, McGill University Faculty of Medicine

ROBERT H. BARTLETT, M.D., F.A.C.S. Professor, Department of Surgery, University of Michigan Medical School, and Director, Critical Care and Surgery Intensive Care Unit, University of Michigan Hospital

STEPHEN T. BARTLETT, M.D., F.A.C.S. Head, Division of Transplantation, Department of Surgery, University of Maryland School of Medicine

FELIX D. BATTISTELLA, M.D., F.A.C.S. Associate Professor, Department of Surgery, University of California, Davis, School of Medicine, and Staff Physician, University of California, Davis, Medical Center

ROBERT W. BEART, JR., M.D., F.A.C.S. Costello Professor of Surgery, Keck School of Medicine of the University of Southern California, and Surgeon, University of Southern California/Kenneth Norris Cancer Center and Hospital

RAMON BERGUER, M.D., F.A.C.S. Staff Surgeon, VA Northern California Healthcare System

CLAUDIA BERMAN, M.D. Professor, Department of Radiology, University of South Florida College of Medicine, and Director, Nuclear Medicine, H. Lee Moffitt Cancer Center and Research Institute

PALMER Q. BESSEY, M.D., F.A.C.S. Professor, Department of Surgery, Weill Medical College of Cornell University, and Associate Director, William Randolph Hearst Burn Center, New York Presbyterian Hospital–Cornell Medical Center

A. GRISWOLD BEVIN, M.D. Professor Emeritus, Department of Plastic Surgery, University of North Carolina at Chapel Hill School of Medicine

ALBAIR B. BISHARA, M.D. Postdoctoral Fellow, Department of Surgery, University of Arkansas College of Medicine, Little Rock

F. WILLIAM BLAISDELL, M.D., F.A.C.S. Professor and Chairman, Department of Surgery, University of California, Davis, School of Medicine, and Chief of Surgical Services, Department of Surgery, Mather Veterans Affairs Hospital, Mather, California

LESLIE H. BLUMGART, M.D., F.A.C.S., F.R.C.S. Professor of Surgery, Weill Medical College of Cornell University; and Chief, Hepatobiliary Service, and Enid A. Haupt Chair in Surgery, Memorial Sloan-Kettering Cancer Center

DAVID C. BROOKS, M.D., F.A.C.S. Associate Professor of Surgery, Harvard Medical School, and Director of Minimally Invasive Surgery, Brigham and Women's Hospital

JON M. BURCH, M.D., F.A.C.S. Professor, Department of Surgery, University of Colorado Health Sciences Center, and Chief, Department of General and Vascular Surgery, Denver Health Medical Center

BRUCE A. CAIRNS, M.D. Assistant Professor, Department of Surgery, University of North Carolina at Chapel Hill School of Medicine; Director of Research, North Carolina Jaycee Burn Center; and Attending Surgeon, Department of Surgery, University of North Carolina Hospitals

JOHN L. CAMERON, M.D., F.A.C.S. Professor and Chairman, Department of Surgery, Johns Hopkins University School of Medicine, and Professor and Chairman, Department of Surgery, Johns Hopkins Hospital

DAVID W. CHANG, M.D. Fellow in Critical Care, Brigham and Women's Hospital

LAURENCE Y. CHEUNG, M.D., F.A.C.S. Professor and Chairman, Department of Surgery, University of Kansas School of Medicine, and Chief of Surgery, Department of Surgical Services, University of Kansas Hospital, Kansas City

NICOLAS V. CHRISTOU, M.D., Ph.D., F.A.C.S. Professor, Department of Surgery, McGill University Faculty of Medicine, and Head, Division of General Surgery, McGill University Health Centre

CLAUDIO S. CINÀ, M.D., Sp. Chir. (It.), M.Sc., F.R.S.C.(C) Assistant Professor, Department of Surgery and Department of Clinical Epidemiology and Biostatistics, McMaster University Faculty of Health Sciences, and Staff Surgeon, Division of Vascular Surgery, Department of Surgery, Victoria Medical Centre

ORLO H. CLARK, M.D., F.A.C.S. Professor, Department of Surgery, University of California, San Francisco, School of Medicine, and Chief, Department of Surgery, Mount Zion Medical Center of UC-San Francisco

CATHERINE M. CLASE, M.B., B.Chir., M.Sc., F.R.C.P.(C) Associate Professor, McMaster University Faculty of Health Sciences, and Medical Director, Chronic Renal Insufficiency Program, St. Joseph's Healthcare

ZANE COHEN, M.D., F.A.C.S. Professor, Department of Surgery, University of Toronto Faculty of Medicine, and Surgeon-in-Chief, Mount Sinai Hospital, Toronto

ARNOLD G. CORAN, M.D., F.A.C.S. Professor of Surgery and Head of Section of Pediatric Surgery, University of Michigan Medical School; and Surgeon-in Chief and Head of Section of Pediatric Surgery, C.S. Mott Children's Hospital, University of Michigan Health System

CHARLES COX, M.D., F.A.C.S. Professor of Surgery and Director, Comprehensive Breast Cancer Program, University of Salt Lake; and Director, Comprehensive Breast Cancer Program, H. Lee Moffitt Cancer Center and Research Institute

PHILIP E. CRYER, M.D. Professor of Medicine, Washington University School of Medicine, and Barnes-Jewish Hospital

JOHN M. DALY, M.D., F.A.C.S. Lewis Atterbury Stimson Professor and Chairman, Department of Surgery, Weill Medical College of Cornell University, and Surgeon-in-Chief, New York Presbyterian Hospital-Cornell Medical Center

JOHN MIHRAN DAVIS, M.D., F.A.C.S. Professor, Department of Surgery, Robert Wood Johnson Medical School, and Site Program Director, Jersey Shore Medical Center

ROMANO DELCORE, M.D., F.A.C.S. Professor, Department of Surgery, University of Kansas School of Medicine, and Medical Director, Department of Surgery, University of Kansas Medical Center

E. PATCHEN DELLINGER, M.D., F.A.C.S. Professor and Vice Chairman, Department of Surgery, University of Washington School of Medicine, and Chief, Division of Surgery, and Associate Medical Director, University of Washington Medical Center

ERIC J. DEMARIA, M.D., F.A.C.S. Professor, Department of General Surgery, Virginia Commonwealth University Medical College of Virginia

ACHILLES A. DEMETRIOU, M.D., Ph.D., F.A.C.S. Professor and Vice Chairman, Department of Surgery, UCLA School of Medicine, and Chairman, Department of Surgery, Cedars-Sinai Medical Center

ROBERT H. DEMLING, M.D., F.A.C.S. Professor, Department of Surgery, Harvard Medical School, and Director, Burn Center, Brigham and Women's Hospital

JOSEPH J. DISA, M.D., F.A.C.S. Assistant Professor, Department of Plastic and Reconstructive Surgery, Weill Medical College of Cornell University, and Assistant Attending Surgeon, Plastic and Reconstructive Surgery Service, Memorial Sloan-Kettering Cancer Center

BRIAN J. EASTRIDGE, M.D., F.A.C.S. Assistant Professor, Department of Surgery, University of Texas Southwestern Medical School

DAVID C. EVANS, M.D., F.A.C.S. Assistant Professor, Department of Surgery, McGill University Faculty of Medicine, and Director, Trauma Unit, Montreal General Hospital

ALICIA FANNING, M.D. Laparoscopic/Endoscopic Fellow, Cleveland Clinic Foundation

SAMIR M. FAKHRY, M.D., F.A.C.S. Clinical Professor, Department of Surgery, Georgetown University School of Medicine, and Chief of Trauma Services and Associate Chair for Research and Education, Department of Surgery, Inova Fairfax Hospital

LIANE S. FELDMAN, M.D. Assistant Professor, Department of Surgery, McGill University Faculty of Medicine, and Staff, Departments of Videoendoscopic Surgery and Surgery, McGill University Hospital Centre

DAVID V. FELICIANO, M.D., F.A.C.S. Professor, Department of Surgery, Emory University School of Medicine, and Chief of Surgery, Grady Memorial Hospital, Atlanta

F. MICHAEL FERRANTE, M.D. Professor of Clinical Anesthesiology and Medicine, Department of Anesthesiology, David Geffen School of Medicine, University of California, Los Angeles, and Director of Pain Medicine, UCLA Medical Center

RICHARD J. FINLEY, M.D., F.A.C.S. Professor and Head, Division of Thoracic Surgery, Department of Surgery, University of British Columbia Faculty of Medicine

PIERO M. FISICHELLA, M.D. Fellow in Gastrointestinal Surgery, University of California, San Francisco, School of Medicine

RAJA M. FLORES, M.D. Department of Surgery, Memorial Sloan-Kettering Cancer Center

YUMAN FONG, M.D., F.A.C.S. Professor of Surgery, Weill Medical College of Cornell University, and Murray F. Brennan Chair in Surgery, Memorial Sloan-Kettering Cancer Center

GERALD M. FRIED, M.D., F.A.C.S. Professor of Surgery, Division of General Surgery, McGill University Faculty of Medicine, and Senior Surgeon, McGill University Health Centre

DONALD E. FRY, M.D., F.A.C.S. Professor and Chairman, Department of Surgery, University of New Mexico School of Medicine, and Chief of Surgery, University of New Mexico Hospital

MICHEL GAGNER, M.D., F.A.C.S. Professor of Surgery, Mt. Sinai School of Medicine, and Chief, Division of Laparoscopic Surgery, Mt. Sinai Hospital, New York

ROSEMARY GIULIANO, A.R.N.P. Associate Director of Clinical Research, Advanced Registered Nurse Practitioner, Lakeland Regional Cancer Center

FRANK GLASS, M.D. Associate Professor, Departments of Medicine and Pathology, H. Lee Moffitt Cancer Center and Research Institute, University of South Florida College of Medicine

ROBERT C. GOSSELIN, M.T. Coagulation Specialist, University of California, Davis, Medical Center

VIVIENNE M. GOUGH, M.B., Ch.B. Senior House Officer in Vascular Surgery, Wythenshawe Hospital, Manchester, England

VALERIE J. HALPIN, M.D. Resident, Department of Surgery, Washington University School of Medicine

ALDEN H. HARKEN, M.D., F.A.C.S. Professor, Department of Surgery, University of Colorado Health Sciences Center

HERBERT B. HECHTMAN, M.D., F.A.C.S. Professor, Department of Surgery, Harvard Medical School, and Surgeon Emeritus, Brigham and Women's Hospital

W. SCOTT HELTON, M.D., F.A.C.S. Professor and Chief, Division of General Surgery, Department of Surgery, University of Illinois College of Medicine

DAVID A. HIDALGO, M.D., F.A.C.S. Associate Professor, Department of Surgery, Weill Medical College of Cornell University, and Associate Professor, Division of Plastic and Reconstructive Surgery, Manhattan Eye, Ear, and Throat Hospital

ASHER HIRSHBERG, M.D. Associate Professor, Department of Surgery, Baylor College of Medicine; and Director of Vascular Surgery and Chief, Blue Surgery Service, Ben Taub General Hospital

HUNG S. HO, M.D., F.A.C.S. Associate Professor, Division of Gastrointestinal and Laparoscopic Surgery, Department of Surgery, University of California, Davis, School of Medicine, and Medical Director and Attending Staff, Section of Gastrointestinal and Laparoscopic Surgery, Department of Surgery, University of California, Davis, Medical Center

JAMES W. HOLCROFT, M.D., F.A.C.S. Professor, Department of Surgery, University of California, Davis, School of Medicine

RICHARD J. HOWARD, M.D., Ph.D., F.A.C.S. Robert H. and Kathleen M. Axline Professor of Surgery, Department of Surgery, University of Florida College of Medicine, and Director, Transplantation Program, Shands Hospital

STEPHEN C. JACOBS, M.D., F.A.C.S. Professor of Urology, University of Maryland Medical Center, and Head, Division of Urology, University of Maryland Medical Systems

JENNIFER W. JANELLE, M.D. Clinical Assistant Professor, University of Florida College of Medicine, and Epidemiologist, Shands Hospital

DENISE JOFFE, M.D. Cardiovascular Anesthesiologist, Children's Hospital of Pittsburgh

GREGG H. JOSSART, M.D., F.A.C.S. Director of Minimal Invasive Surgery, California Pacific Medical Center, San Francisco

HENRIK KEHLET, Prof. M.D., Ph.D. Professor of Surgery, Department of Surgical Gastroenterology, and Chief Surgeon, Hvidovre University Hospital

KEITH A. KELLY, M.D., F.A.C.S. Professor Emeritus, Department of Surgery, Mayo Medical School, and Consultant in Research, Mayo Clinic Arizona

JAMES P. KENNEDY, M.D. Assistant Professor, Division of Clinical Orthopedic Surgery, Department of Surgery, Northeastern Ohio Universities College of Medicine

MARK KIRK, M.D. Assistant Professor, Department of Emergency Medicine, University of Virginia, and Director, Medical Toxicology Fellowship, University of Virginia Health Center

DENNIS R. KLASSEN, M.D. Fellow, Laparoscopic and Minimally Invasive Surgery, McGill University Faculty of Medicine, and Fellow, Laparoscopic and Minimally Invasive Surgery, Montreal General Hospital

IRA J. KODNER, M.D., F.A.C.S. Solon and Bettie Gershman Professor, Division of Colon and Rectal Surgery, Department of Surgery, Washington University School of Medicine, and Colon and Rectal Surgeon, Department of Surgery, Barnes-Jewish Hospital

CONSTANTINOS KYRIAKIDES, M.D. Senior Clinical Vascular Fellow, Regional Vascular Unit, St. Mary's Hospital, London, England

RENE LAFRENIERE, M.D., C.M., F.A.C.S. Professor and Head, Department of Surgery, University of Calgary Faculty of Medicine; and Regional Clinical Department Head of Surgery, Calgary Regional Health Authority, Calgary, Alberta

BERNARD LANGER, M.D., F.R.C.S.(C), F.A.C.S. Professor, Department of Surgery, University of Toronto Faculty of Medicine, and Senior Staff Surgeon, Toronto General Hospital

W. THOMAS LAWRENCE, M.D., F.A.C.S. Professor and Chairman, Section of Plastic Surgery, Department of Surgery, University of Kansas School of Medicine, and Chief, Department of Plastic Surgery, Kansas University Medical Center

ANNA M. LEDGERWOOD, M.D., F.A.C.S. Professor, Department of Surgery, Wayne State University School of Medicine, and General Surgeon, Detroit Receiving Hospital

JAMES T. LEE, M.D., Ph.D., F.A.C.S. Professor, Department of Surgery, University of Minnesota Medical School

RONALD T. LEWIS, M.B.B.S., M.Sc., F.R.C.S.(C), F.A.C.S. Associate Professor, Department of Surgery, University of Ottowa Faculty of Medicine, and Vascular Surgeon, Ottowa Hospital

KEITH D. LILLEMOE, M.D., F.A.C.S. Professor and Vice-Chairman, Department of Surgery, Johns Hopkins University School of Medicine

JOSEPH LOCICERO III, M.D., F.A.C.S. Professor and Chair of Surgery, Finch University of Health Sciences at the Chicago Medical School, and Chair of Surgery, Mt. Sinai Hospital

STEVEN R. LOWENSTEIN, M.D., M.P.H. Associate Professor of Surgery, Medicine, and Preventive Medicine and Biometrics, University of Colorado School of Medicine, and Associate Director, Emergency Department, University of Colorado Hospital

STEPHEN F. LOWRY, M.D., F.A.C.S. Professor and Chairman, Department of Surgery, University of Medicine and Dentistry of New Jersey Robert Wood Johnson Medical School

CHARLES E. LUCAS, M.D., F.A.C.S. Professor, Department of Surgery, Wayne State University School of Medicine, and Senior Staff Attending Surgeon, Detroit Receiving Hospital and Harper University Hospital

JOSEPH MAMAZZA, M.D. Assistant Professor, Department of Surgery, University of Toronto Faculty of Medicine; Medical Director of Minimal Access Therapeutics, and Director of Minimally Invasive Surgery, St. Michael's Hospital

JOHN C. MARSHALL, M.D., F.R.C.S.(C), F.A.C.S. Professor, Department of Surgery, University of Toronto Faculty of Medicine, and Attending Surgeon, Toronto General Hospital University Health Network

JOHN A. MARX, M.D. Clinical Professor, Department of Emergency Medicine, University of North Carolina at Chapel Hill School of Medicine; and Chairman and Chief, Department of Emergency Medicine, Carolinas Medical Center, Charlotte, North Carolina

BYRON J. MASTERSON, M.D., F.A.C.S. J. Wayne Reitz Professor of Gynecologic Surgery and Chairman Emeritus, University of Florida College of Medicine, Gainesville; and Professor, School of Public Health, University of South Florida (courtesy), Tampa

KENNETH L. MATTOX, M.D., F.A.C.S. Professor and Vice Chairman, Division of Thoracic Surgery, Department of Surgery, Baylor College of Medicine, and Chief of Staff and Chief of Surgery, Ben Taub General Hospital, Houston

JACK W. MCANINCH, M.D., F.A.C.S. Professor, Department of Urology, University of California, San Francisco, School of Medicine, and Chief, Department of Urology, San Francisco General Hospital

JACQUELINE C. MCCLARAN, M.D. Assistant Medical Director, John Radcliffe Trust, University of Oxford

DANIEL P. MCKELLAR, M.D., F.A.C.S. Associate Clinical Professor, Department of Surgery, Wright State University School of Medicine

JONATHAN L. MEAKINS, M.D., D.Sc., F.R.C.S.(C), F.A.C.S. Nuffield Professor of Surgery, University of Oxford

JANE MESSINA, M.D. Associate Professor of Pathology and Medicine, University of South Florida College of Medicine; Staff Dermatopathologist, University of South Florida Medical Clinic; Pathologist Member, Cutaneous Oncology Program, and Program Director, Pathology Residency, H. Lee Moffit Cancer Center

ANTHONY A. MEYER, M.D., Ph.D., F.A.C.S. Roscoe B. G. Cowter Distinguished Professor and Chair, Department of Surgery, University of North Carolina School of Medicine; Director, Critical Care Service for Surgery; Program Director, General Surgery Residency Program; and Assistant Director, North Carolina Jaycee Burn Center

RUSTY MILHOAN, M.D., F.A.C.S. Trauma Surgeon, Department of Trauma Services, Christus St. Elizabeth Hospital, Beaumont, Texas

CHARLES M. MILLER, M.D., F.A.C.S. Alfred and Florence Gross Professor of Surgery, Mt. Sinai School of Medicine of the City University of New York, and Director, Recanati-Miller Transplantation Institute, Mount Sinai Medical Center, New York City

BERNARD MONTREUIL, M.D. Assistant Professor, Division of Vascular Surgery, Department of Surgery, Royal Victoria Hospital, Montreal

ERNEST E. MOORE, M.D., F.A.C.S. Professor and Vice Chairman, Department of Surgery, University of Colorado Health Sciences Center, and Chief, Department of Surgery, Denver Health Medical Center

FREDERICK A. MOORE, M.D., F.A.C.S. Professor and Vice Chairman, Department of Surgery, University of Texas Medical School at Houston; Chief, Department of General Surgery, Trauma, and Critical Care, and Medical Director, Memorial Hermann Hospital

WESLEY S. MOORE, M.D., F.A.C.S. Professor, Division of Vascular Surgery, Department of Surgery, David Geffen School of Medicine, University of California, Los Angeles, and Vascular Surgeon, UCLA Medical Center

LAURIE MORRISON, M.D. Clinical Assistant Professor, Indiana University School of Medicine, and Staff Physician, Department of Surgery, Bloomington Hospital

J. PAUL MUIZELAAR, M.D., Ph.D. Professor and Chairman, Department of Neurological Surgery, University of California, Davis, School of Medicine

LENA M. NAPOLITANO, M.D., F.A.C.S. Associate Professor, Department of Surgery, University of Maryland Medical System, and Director of Surgical Critical Care, Surgical Care Center, VA Maryland Health Care System, Baltimore

AVERY B. NATHENS, M.D., Ph.D., M.P.H., F.A.C.S. Assistant Professor of Surgery, University of Washington; Director of Acute Care Section, Harborview Injury Prevention and Research Center; and Director of Surgical Critical Care Services, Harborview Medical Center

RONALD LEE NICHOLS, M.D., M.S., F.A.C.S. William Henderson Professor, Department of Surgery, Tulane University School of Medicine, and Professor of Surgery, Tulane Health Sciences Center

CARL NOHR, M.D., Ph.D., F.R.C.S.(C), F.A.C.S. Chief, Palliser Health Authority, Alberta, Canada

JEFFREY A. NORTON, M.D., F.A.C.S. Professor and Vice Chair, Department of Surgery, University of California, San Francisco, School of Medicine, and Chief of Surgical Service, San Francisco VA Medical Center

JOHN T. OWINGS, M.D., F.A.C.S. Associate Professor, Department of Surgery, University of California, Davis, School of Medicine, and Attending Physician, Department of Surgery, University of California, Davis, Medical Center

CHERIE P. PARUNGO, M.D. Department of Surgery, Brigham and Women's Hospital

MARCO G. PATTI, M.D., F.A.C.S. Associate Professor, Department of Surgery, University of California, San Francisco, School of Medicine, and Director, University of California Swallowing Center, Moffit-Long Hospital

WILLIAM C. PEVEC, M.D., F.A.C.S. Associate Professor of Vascular Surgery, Department of Surgery, University of California, Davis, School of Medicine, and Associate Professor of Clinical Surgery, University of California, Davis, Health System

JEFFREY L. PONSKY, M.D., F.A.C.S. Professor of Surgery, Cleveland Clinic Health Sciences Center of the Ohio State University, and Director, Section of Endoscopic Surgery, Department of General Surgery, Cleveland Clinic Foundation

ERIC C. POULIN, M.D., M.Sc. Professor, Department of Surgery, University of Toronto Faculty of Medicine, and Surgeon-in-Chief, St. Michael's Hospital

EDWARD J. QUEBBEMAN, M.D., Ph.D., F.A.C.S. Professor, Department of Surgery, Medical College of Wisconsin, and Surgical Oncologist, Froedtert Memorial Lutheran Hospital

THERESA M. QUINN, M.D. Assistant Professor, Division of Laparoscopic Surgery, Department of Surgery, Mt. Sinai Medical Center, New York

BABAK N. RAD, M.D. Fellow in Colorectal Surgery, Keck School of Medicine, University of Southern California

ALEKSANDAR RADAN, M.D., B.Sc., B.F.A. General Surgery Resident, Department of Surgery, McMaster University Faculty of Health Sciences

FELIX T. RAPAPORT, M.D. Distinguished Professor (Emeritus), Department of Surgery, State University of New York at Stony Brook School of Medicine; Senior Attending Surgeon (Emeritus), University Hospital at Stony Brook; and Editor-in-Chief, *Transplantation Proceedings* (deceased)

RICHARD B. REILING, M.D., F.A.C.S. Clinical Professor of Surgery, Wright State University School of Medicine, and Vice President for Cancer Services, Grant/Riverside Methodist Hospitals, Columbus, Ohio

H. DAVID REINES, M.D., F.A.C.S. Professor of Surgery, Georgetown University School of Medicine, and Vice Chair of Surgery, Inova Fairfax Hospital

DOUGLAS REINTGEN, M.D., F.A.C.S. Professor, Department of Surgery, University of South Florida College of Medicine, and Program Leader, Department of Cutaneous Oncology, H. Lee Moffitt Cancer Center and Research Institute

ROBERT S. RHODES, M.D., F.A.C.S. Associate Executive Director, American Board of Surgeons

CHARLES L. RICE, M.D., F.A.C.S. Professor, Departments of Surgery and Physiology and Biophysics, University of Illinois at Chicago College of Medicine, and Vice Chancellor for Health Affairs, University of Illinois Medical Center at Chicago

ROLANDO H. ROLANDELLI, M.D., F.A.C.S. Professor, Department of Surgery, Temple University School of Medicine, and Chief of General Surgery, Temple University Hospital

JOHN L. ROMBEAU, M.D., F.A.C.S. Professor, Division of Colorectal Surgery, Department of Surgery, University of Pennsylvania School of Medicine, and Staff Colorectal Surgeon, Division of Gastrointestinal Surgery, Department of Surgery, Hospital of the University of Pennsylvania

BARRY J. ROSEMAN, M.D. Roseman and Budayr, M.D., P.C., Maryville, Tennessee

LAWRENCE ROSENBERG, M.D., Ph.D., F.A.C.S. Professor of Surgery and Medicine and Director, Division of Surgical Research, McGill University Faculty of Medicine; and Senior Surgeon, McGill University Health Centre

DANIEL ROSENTHAL, M.D., F.A.C.S. Clinical Professor, Department of Surgery, University of Texas Medical School at San Antonio, and Uniformed Services University of the Health Sciences School of Medicine, Bethesda

M. JOYCE ROSENTHAL, R.N., M.S., C.E.T.N. Gastrointestinal Nurse, Baptist Medical Center, San Antonio

ORI D. ROTSTEIN, M.D., M.Sc., F.R.C.S.(C), F.A.C.S. Professor, Department of Surgery, University of Toronto Faculty of Medicine, and Head, Division of General Surgery, Toronto General Hospital, University Health Network

GRACE S. ROZYCKI, M.D., F.A.C.S. Associate Professor, Department of Surgery, Emory University School of Medicine, and Director of Trauma/Surgical Critical Care, Grady Memorial Hospital

FRANCESCO RUBINO, M.D. Research Fellow, Division of Laparoscopic Surgery, Mt. Sinai Medical Center, New York

VALERIE W. RUSCH, M.D., F.A.C.S. Professor, Department of Surgery, Weill Medical College of Cornell University, and William G. Cahan Chair of Surgery and Chief of Thoracic Surgery, Memorial Sloan-Kettering Cancer Center

EDMUND J. RUTHERFORD, M.D., F.A.C.S. Associate Professor, Department of Surgery, University of North Carolina at Chapel Hill School of Medicine, and Chief of Surgical Critical Care, UNC Hospitals

JOHN L. SAWYERS, M.D., F.A.C.S. John Clinton Foshee Distinguished Professor (Emeritus), Department of Surgery, Vanderbilt University School of Medicine, and Director, Section of Surgical Sciences (Emeritus), Vanderbilt University Hospital

DAVID W. SCHARP, M.D., F.A.C.S. Chief Scientific Officer, Novocell, Inc., Irvine, California

CHRISTOPHER M. SCHLACHTA, M.D., F.A.C.S. Lecturer and General Surgeon, Department of Surgery, University of Toronto Faculty of Medicine

RICHARD T. SCHLINKERT, M.D., F.A.C.S. Professor, Department of Surgery, Mayo Graduate School of Medicine, and General Surgeon, Department of Surgery, Mayo Clinic Scottsdale

THEODORE R. SCHROCK, M.D., F.A.C.S. Chairman, Associate Dean for Clinical Services, and J. Englebert Dunphy Professor, Department of Surgery, University of California, San Francisco, School of Medicine

ALAN E. SEYFER, M.D., F.A.C.S. Professor of Surgery, Anatomy, and Cell/Developmental Biology, Division of Plastic and Reconstructive Surgery, Oregon Health Sciences University; and Staff Surgeon, Department of Plastic Surgery, Doernbecher Children's Hospital

GEORGE F. SHELDON, M.D., F.A.C.S. Professor of Surgery and Social Medicine, University of North Carolina at Chapel Hill School of Medicine

THOMAS M. SINCLAIR, M.D., C.M., F.R.C.S., F.A.C.S. Attending Plastic Surgeon, Department of Surgery, Mineral Springs Hospital, Banff, Alberta

BARBARA L. SMITH, M.D., Ph.D., F.A.C.S. Assistant Professor, Department of Surgery, Harvard Medical School, and Co-Director, Gillette Center for Women's Cancers, Massachusetts General Hospital

R. JOHN SOLARO, Ph.D. Distinguished University Professor and Head, Department of Physiology and Biophysics, University of Illinois at Chicago College of Medicine

JOSEPH S. SOLOMKIN, M.D., F.A.C.S. Professor, Department of Surgery, University of Cincinnati College of Medicine, and Director of Research, Department of Surgery, University of Cincinnati Medical Center

WILEY W. SOUBA, M.D., Sc.D., F.A.C.S. John A. and Marian T. Waldhaun Professor of Surgery, and Chair, Department of Surgery, Penn State College of Medicine, and Surgeon-in-Chief, Milton S. Hershey Medical Center

CYNTHIA SPRY, R.N., M.S.N. International Clinical Consultant, Advanced Sterilization Products

RENAE E. STAFFORD, M.D. Assistant Professor of Surgery, Division of Trauma and Critical Care, Medical College of Wisconsin, and Staff Physician, Department of Surgery, Froedtert Memorial Lutheran Hospital

THOMAS E. STARZL, M.D., Ph.D., F.A.C.S. Professor, Department of Surgery, and Director, Thomas E. Starzl Transplantation Institute, University of Pittsburgh School of Medicine

HARVEY J. SUGERMAN, M.D., F.A.C.S. David M. Hume Professor of Surgery, Virginia Commonwealth University School of Medicine, and Chief, General Surgery Division, Medical College of Virginia Hospitals

WILLIAM D. SUGGS, M.D., F.A.C.S. Associate Professor, Department of Surgery, Albert Einstein College of Medicine of Yeshiva University, and Attending Surgeon, Montefiore Medical Center

BARRY SULLIVAN, M.D. Assistant Professor, Department of Surgery, University of British Columbia, and Surgeon, St. Paul's Hospital, Vancouver, British Columbia

BRYCE R. TAYLOR, M.D., F.A.C.S. Professor and Associate Chair, Division of General Surgery, Department of Surgery, University of Toronto Faculty of Medicine; and Surgeon-in-Chief and Director of Surgical Services, University Health Network

ERWIN R. THAL, M.D., F.A.C.S. Professor, Department of Surgery, University of Texas Southwestern Medical Center, Dallas

SETH THALLER, M.D., F.A.C.S. Professor and Chief, Department of Plastic Surgery, University of Miami School of Medicine

KIMBERLY J. VAN ZEE, M.D., F.A.C.S. Assistant Professor, Department of Surgery, Weill Medical College of Cornell University, and Assistant Attending Surgeon, Breast Service, Memorial Sloan-Kettering Cancer Center

FRANK J. VEITH, M.D., F.A.C.S. Professor and Vice Chairman, Department of Surgery, Albert Einstein College of Medicine of Yeshiva University, and The William J. von Liebig Chair in Vascular Surgery, Montefiore Medical Center

GEORGE E. WANTZ, M.D. Clinical Professor of Surgery, Cornell University Medical College (deceased)

JAMES M. WATTERS, M.D., F.A.C.S. Professor, Department of Surgery, University of Ottawa Faculty of Medicine, and Attending Surgeon, Department of Surgery, Ottawa Hospital-Civic Campus

HUNTER WESSELLS, M.D., F.A.C.S. Associate Professor, Department of Urology, University of Washington School of Medicine, and Chief of Urology, Harborview Medical Center

MARVIN J. WEXLER, M.D., F.A.C.S. Professor, Departments of Surgery and Oncology, McGill University Faculty of Medicine, and Senior Surgeon, Department of Surgery, Royal Victoria Hospital, Montreal

H. BRUCE WILLIAMS, M.D. Professor, Department of Surgery, McGill University Faculty of Medicine, and Surgeon-in-Chief, Department of Surgery, Montreal Children's Hospital

KAREN STANLEY WILLIAMS, M.D. Chief, Anesthesia and Surgical Services, Warren G. Magnuson Clinical Center, National Institutes of Health

DOUGLAS W. WILMORE, M.D., F.A.C.S. Frank Sawyer Professor, Department of Surgery, Harvard Medical School, and Senior Staff Surgeon, Department of Surgery, Brigham and Women's Hospital

DAVID H. WISNER, M.D., F.A.C.S.   Professor and Chief, Division of Trauma Surgery, Department of Surgery, University of California, Davis, School of Medicine

JOHN YEE, M.D.   Assistant Professor, Division of Thoracic Surgery, Department of Surgery, University of Michigan Medical School

CHRISTOPHER K. ZARINS, M.D., F.A.C.S.   Chidester Professor of Surgery, Stanford University School of Medicine, and Chief, Division of Vascular Surgery, Stanford University Medical Center

MARIKE ZWIENENBERG-LEE, M.D.   Research Fellow, Department of Neurological Surgery, University of California, Davis, School of Medicine

PREFACE

Welcome to *ACS Surgery: Principles and Practice.*

The primary aim of this book is to apply the best current thinking to the practice of modern surgery, in the hope of encouraging more effective surgical decision making. To this end, we adopt a problem-oriented approach throughout the book, incorporating the best information available (ideally in the form of randomized prospective trials or meta-analyses of multiple studies) into practical clinical recommendations.

Today, practicing surgeons are expected to be highly efficient yet adaptable, capable of providing high-quality, cost-effective care in a wide variety of clinical situations. Such efficiency requires rapid integration of new information into surgical practice so that the range of possible approaches to specific clinical problems can be thoroughly and intelligently evaluated. Accordingly, it is vital that surgeons have ready access to an information system that provides the best medical information in the context of clinical care. This focus on self-education based on new evidence represents a paradigm shift from the usual approach of surgical training, which is based primarily on teaching traditions of practice. Evidence-based surgical care affects all aspects of what we do, from discussing the options available for treating a patient with carcinoma of the breast to the postoperative use of nasogastric tubes, drains, and urinary catheters. We strongly believe that moving toward this new paradigm is no mere academic exercise but a critical step along a path leading to improved surgical care.

In keeping with its editorial goals, the structure of this publication is unlike that of the usual encyclopedic surgical text. The chapters are sequenced in a precise order, starting with surgical emergencies and moving to topics on elective surgical care. Each of the chapters that cover a topic related to perioperative care begins with an algorithm that graphically depicts the decision-making process for the given problem. Each node on the algorithm refers to a specific section in the text, which provides more details to facilitate and deepen understanding of the decision under consideration. The chapter often also includes a discussion section, which explores basic science concepts and new theories as they apply to the field. Thus, the reader can explore the subject at any of several levels, depending on interest and time available.

Those chapters that discuss operative procedures [*see V Operative Management*] are also problem oriented, albeit from a different perspective. They typically begin with brief descriptions of indications and preoperative preparation. The experts who write these sections then break each operation down into its key steps, highlighting potential problem areas and providing strategies for preventing or controlling them. New contributions to this section since the last version include chapters on laparoscopic adrenalectomy, laparoscopic donor nephrectomy, open hepatic resection, open esophagectomy (as a complement to the chapter on minimally invasive esophageal procedures), and peripheral arterial bypass (expanding the coverage of vascular procedures). More procedure chapters are planned for the future.

This information is available not only in book form but also on the Internet (www.acssurgery.com) and on CD-ROM. These electronic modes of transmitting information allow surgeons the kind of flexibility that a lengthy paper volume typically cannot: the material can be consulted at home, in the office, or in the hospital, and access to most of the references can be rapidly obtained via an Internet link to MEDLINE. *ACS Surgery* on the Web is unique in terms of surgical information in that it is immediately available to subscribers in any corner of the world where an Internet connection is available. Between the publication of the premiere hardcover version of *ACS Surgery* in 2002 and the publication of this 2003 volume, about 40% of the material in the text was updated. In addition, new information continues to be inserted into the Internet version at monthly intervals. This process provides the surgeon with a constant stream of contemporary information, accompanied by a CME program on the Web that will satisfy most current licensing requirements.

A cardinal virtue of this continuing update approach is that it allows us to keep pace with changing times by closely tracking developments in surgical care. For example, what was once a single chapter on perioperative care has now been divided into three chapters to better reflect the current state of practice. One chapter addresses assessment of patients for outpatient surgery, the second discusses issues related to fast track surgery (i.e., major operations that require only 1 or 2 days of hospitalization), and the third describes the traditional hospital care needed for patients undergoing major operations who have comorbidities or complications and for whom neither outpatient surgery nor fast track surgery is appropriate. Preoperative assessment, postoperative care, and discharge planning in elective settings vary depending on the surgical site and the operative plan, and separate decision-making approaches are outlined for these discrete situations.

This 2003 volume also features a new chapter on risk assessment. Our cardiac surgical colleagues have advanced their field by developing programs that preoperatively predict outcome. General surgeons need to develop similar data so that they can advise patients appropriately regarding their level of risk and make responsible judgments regarding the use of expensive hospital resources. This chapter provides the most current data available on risk assessment and outcome prediction in general surgical patients.

The original impetus for what became *ACS Surgery* was the perception by the Pre and Post Operative Committee of the American College of Surgeons in the early 1980s that traditional publishing methods were less and less able to keep up with the pace of medical advances. That perception eventually resulted first in an updatable loose-leaf, then in a CD-ROM, and finally, with the fall 2002 publication of *ACS Surgery* on the Web and in print, in the first (and so far only) online general surgical textbook. The name *ACS Surgery* reflects the commitment made by the College to provide contemporary information to surgeons in practice to enhance their efficiency and optimize patient care.

The contents of this book reflect the contributions of numerous authors who have provided the authoritative manuscripts under the thoughtful leadership of a superb Editorial Board: Laurence Y. Cheung, M.D., F.A.C.S., Alden H. Harken, M.D., F.A.C.S., James W. Holcroft, M.D., F.A.C.S., Jonathan L. Meakins, M.D., F.A.C.S., and Nathaniel J. Soper, M.D., F.A.C.S. The Editors have shown uncommon dedication to this project, and this 2003 volume represents the capstone of their years of hard work.

Like *ACS Surgery* itself, the Editorial Board continues to evolve, with the goal of ensuring that the most contemporary thinking on surgical problems continues to be presented to surgeons. As of 2003, the Editorial Board passes the torch to a new generation of surgical leaders: Mitchell P. Fink, M.D., F.A.C.S., Gregory J. Jurkovich, M.D., F.A.C.S., William H. Pearce, M.D., F.A.C.S., Larry R. Kaiser, M.D., F.A.C.S., John H. Pemberton, M.D., F.A.C.S., Nathaniel J. Soper, M.D., F.A.C.S., and Wiley W. Souba, M.D., Sc.D., F.A.C.S. We look forward to the evolution of this leadership group and to the new directions in which they will eventually take *ACS Surgery*.

Drs. Cheung, Harken, Holcroft, and Meakins join our Council of Founding Editors, so that we may continue to take advantage of their advice and insights. Speaking both professionally and personally, I am grateful for the long-standing commitment of the original Editorial Board, and I am proud to have worked alongside them on *ACS Surgery*.

We hope that *ACS Surgery: Principles and Practice* provides the basis for better care for all surgical patients.

Douglas W. Wilmore, M.D., F.A.C.S.

The surgical patient

Patient presents with nontraumatic condition (Section II)

- Neck mass
- Asymptomatic carotid bruit
- Breast complaints
- Abdominal pain or mass
- Jaundice
- Intestinal obstruction
- Upper or lower GI bleeding
- Skin lesions
- Soft tissue infection

Patient is in need of resuscitation (Section I)

- CPR and correction of dysrhythmias
- Resuscitation for trauma and thermal injury
- Management of shock, bleeding, electrolyte abnormalities, and acid-base disorders
- Acute wound care
- Management of altered consciousness (coma, seizures, drugs, etc.)

Patient presents with trauma or thermal injury (Section III)

- ED evaluation
- Injuries to CNS, face and jaw, neck, and chest
- Injuries to abdomen
- Injuries to GU tract
- Injuries to extremities
- Burns
- Miscellaneous thermal injuries

Patient is evaluated in preparation for surgical treatment (Section IV)

- Preoperative assessment
- Cardiac risk evaluation
- Prophylaxis of postoperative infection
- Choice of surgical approach (in-hospital, fast track, or outpatient)

Special perioperative problems are addressed (Section VI)

- Pulmonary problems
- Thromboembolism
- Endocrine problems
- Obesity
- Immunosuppression
- Age
- Pregnancy
- Infection

Patient undergoes operation (Section V)

Patient receives postoperative care (Section VIII)

- General postoperative management
- Pain control
- Stomal care
- Burn rehabilitation

Patient is managed in the ICU (Section VII)

- Cardiopulmonary monitoring and support
- Management of individual or multiple organ dysfunction
- Management of metabolic derangement
- Nutritional support
- Control of fever or hypothermia
- Modulation of systemic inflammatory response

I RESUSCITATION

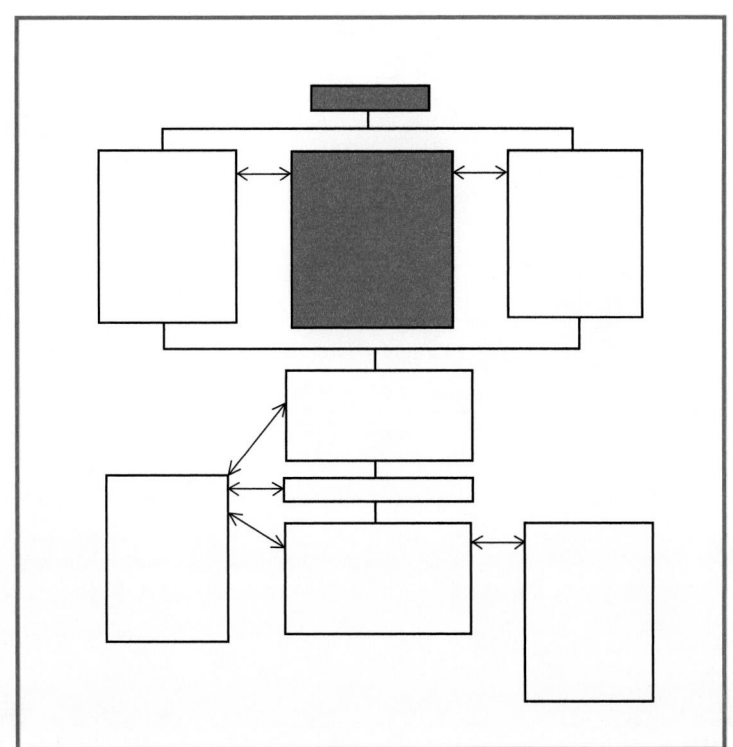

1 INITIAL EMERGENCY MANAGEMENT OF NONINJURED PATIENTS: CARDIOPULMONARY RESUSCITATION AND CORRECTION OF ACUTE DYSRHYTHMIAS

Steven R. Lowenstein, M.D., M.P.H., and Alden H. Harken, M.D.

Management of Cardiac Arrest and Acute Dysrhythmia

Cardiopulmonary arrest is the sudden cessation of breathing and circulation in a patient who is not expected to die. Victims are unresponsive, and their skin is ashen and mottled. Respirations are agonal or absent, and no pulses are present in the large arteries. The success of cardiopulmonary resuscitation (CPR) is directly related to how soon it is begun.

The approach to the patient in cardiac arrest must be organized, vigorous, and bold. First, verify the patency of the airway. Second, assure adequacy of the breathing effort. Third, restore the circulatory bed. The ABCs—*A*irway, *B*reathing, and *C*irculation—apply not only to resuscitation of victims of full cardiopulmonary arrest but also to resuscitation of all sick or injured patients. The ABCs have stood the test of time as the most basic mnemonic in all of medicine.

There are two important exceptions to the orderly rule of the ABCs. The first applies to the patient in a monitored setting who experiences sudden ventricular fibrillation (VF). On discovery of VF, immediate electrical defibrillation takes precedence over airway management, pharmacologic therapy, and CPR.

The second exception applies to the trauma patient in cardiac arrest [see I:2 Trauma Resuscitation]. In these patients, the cause of cardiac arrest is usually exsanguination or a critical thoracic injury (e.g., cardiac tamponade, tension pneumothorax, or flail chest). In trauma patients, the head tilt [see Basic Life Support, below] should not be used to open the airway if there is suspicion of cervical spine injury. There is also no evidence that external chest compressions are effective in traumatic (hypovolemic) cardiac arrest[1]; instead, restoration of circulating blood volume and a resuscitative thoracotomy are urgently needed. In what follows, we consider only the resuscitation of noninjured patients.

Basic Life Support

Basic life support (BLS) consists of placing the victim on his or her back, opening the airway, performing mouth-to-mouth breathing, and initiating rhythmic chest compressions. Each of these sequential BLS steps has been delineated in the guidelines of the American Heart Association (AHA).[2] Each of the ABC steps should begin with an assessment phase—verify unresponsiveness, evaluate airway patency, assess breathing—before active

intervention. Unfortunately, BLS provides suboptimal blood flow to the heart, brain, and other vital tissues, and it cannot reverse cardiac arrhythmias. BLS only buys time. Advanced life support (ALS) provides the definitive treatment [see Advanced Life Support, *below*]. ALS includes defibrillation, tracheal intubation, drug and fluid therapy, and various procedures (e.g., external or internal pacemaker placement, pericardiocentesis, tube thoracostomy, and open thoracotomy).

INITIAL STEPS

Verify cardiopulmonary arrest Shout at or gently shake the victim to determine unresponsiveness. Next, to establish the absence of functional ventilation, listen and feel for airway movement at the nose and mouth, and look

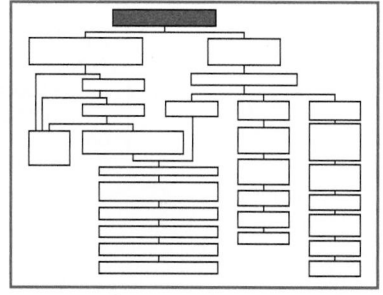

for movement of the thoracic cage. If the patient is unresponsive and if breathing is absent or agonal, CPR must be initiated. It is not necessary to check pupils, pulses, or heart sounds.

Call for help and position the patient If the patient is outside the hospital, activate the emergency medical services (EMS) system. Place the victim supine on a hard surface (floor or backboard). If trauma is likely, take precautions to minimize motion of the cervical spine: hold the head in a neutral position, and then logroll the victim to the supine position, conveying the head, the neck, and the torso as a single unit [see I:2 Trauma Resuscitation].

THE ABCS

Airway

Basic life support begins with relief of airway obstruction. The most common cause of airway obstruction in unconscious humans is the tongue, which falls backward against the posterior pharyngeal wall. In addition, during labored breathing, negative pressure is generated in the hypopharynx; the tongue and

Management of Cardiac Arrest

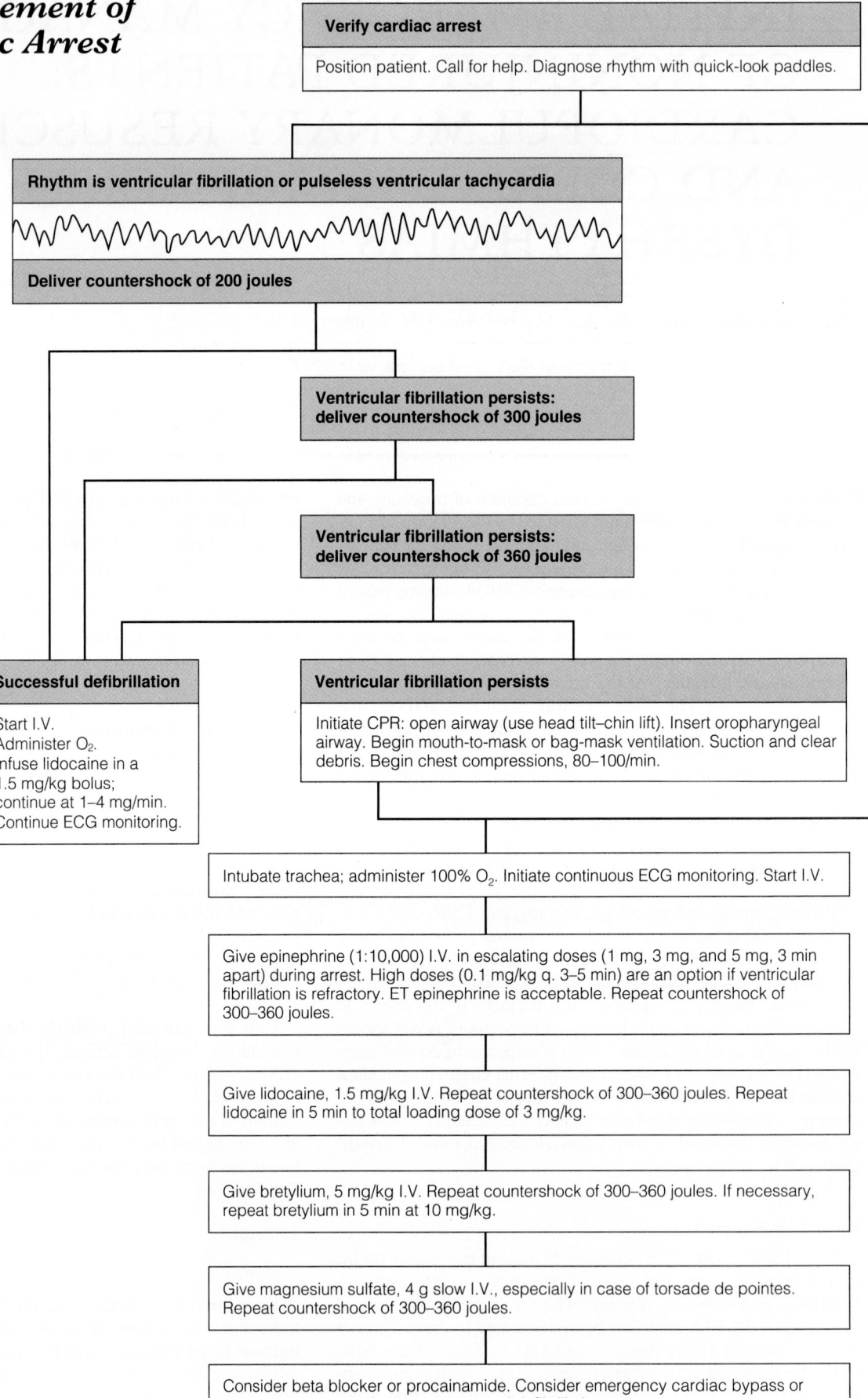

Verify cardiac arrest

Position patient. Call for help. Diagnose rhythm with quick-look paddles.

Rhythm is ventricular fibrillation or pulseless ventricular tachycardia

Deliver countershock of 200 joules

Ventricular fibrillation persists: deliver countershock of 300 joules

Ventricular fibrillation persists: deliver countershock of 360 joules

Successful defibrillation

Start I.V.
Administer O$_2$.
Infuse lidocaine in a
1.5 mg/kg bolus;
continue at 1–4 mg/min.
Continue ECG monitoring.

Ventricular fibrillation persists

Initiate CPR: open airway (use head tilt–chin lift). Insert oropharyngeal airway. Begin mouth-to-mask or bag-mask ventilation. Suction and clear debris. Begin chest compressions, 80–100/min.

Intubate trachea; administer 100% O$_2$. Initiate continuous ECG monitoring. Start I.V.

Give epinephrine (1:10,000) I.V. in escalating doses (1 mg, 3 mg, and 5 mg, 3 min apart) during arrest. High doses (0.1 mg/kg q. 3–5 min) are an option if ventricular fibrillation is refractory. ET epinephrine is acceptable. Repeat countershock of 300–360 joules.

Give lidocaine, 1.5 mg/kg I.V. Repeat countershock of 300–360 joules. Repeat lidocaine in 5 min to total loading dose of 3 mg/kg.

Give bretylium, 5 mg/kg I.V. Repeat countershock of 300–360 joules. If necessary, repeat bretylium in 5 min at 10 mg/kg.

Give magnesium sulfate, 4 g slow I.V., especially in case of torsade de pointes. Repeat countershock of 300–360 joules.

Consider beta blocker or procainamide. Consider emergency cardiac bypass or thoracotomy, open-chest massage, and defibrillation.

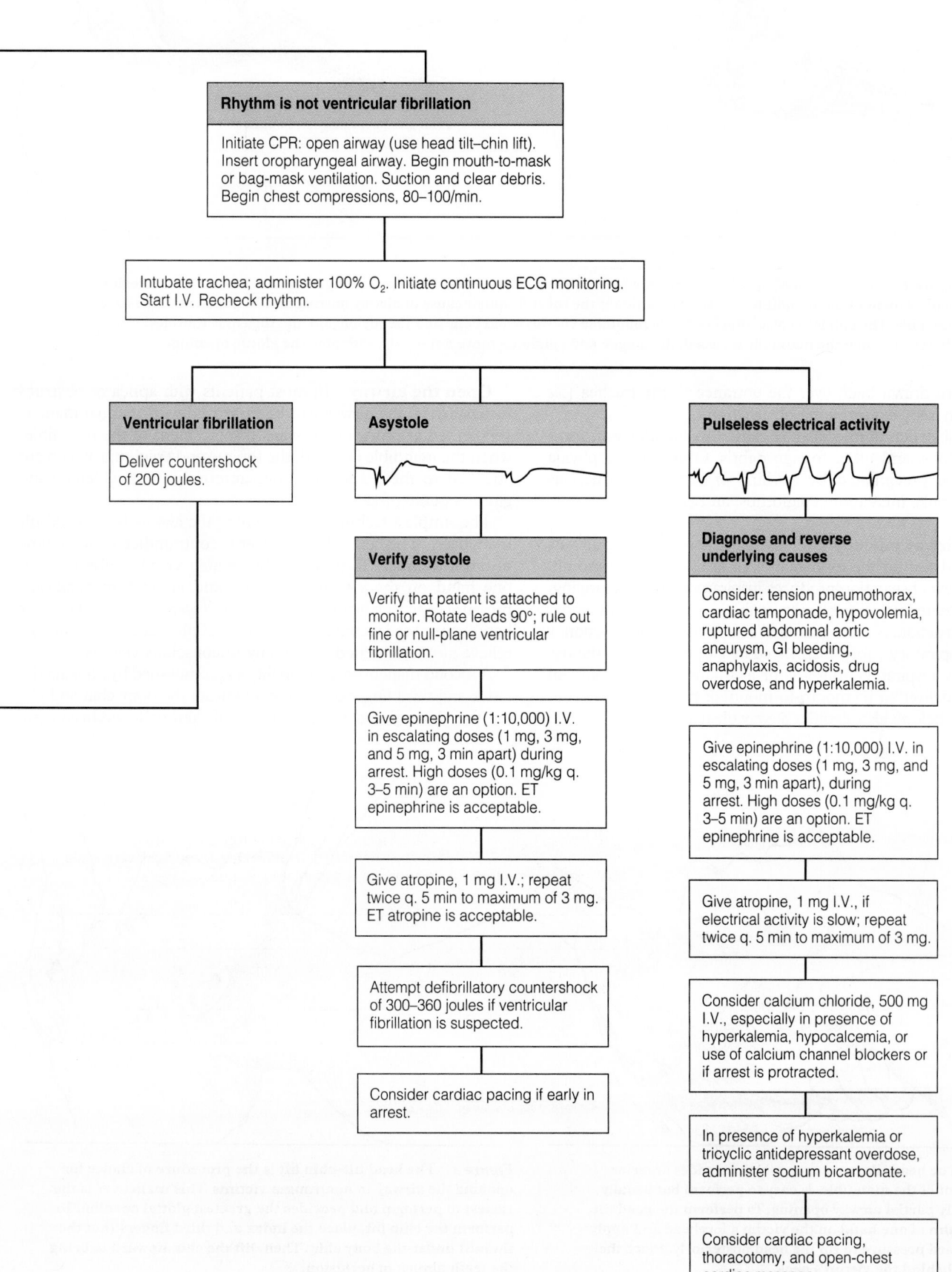

Rhythm is not ventricular fibrillation

Initiate CPR: open airway (use head tilt–chin lift). Insert oropharyngeal airway. Begin mouth-to-mask or bag-mask ventilation. Suction and clear debris. Begin chest compressions, 80–100/min.

Intubate trachea; administer 100% O₂. Initiate continuous ECG monitoring. Start I.V. Recheck rhythm.

Ventricular fibrillation

Deliver countershock of 200 joules.

Asystole

Verify asystole

Verify that patient is attached to monitor. Rotate leads 90°; rule out fine or null-plane ventricular fibrillation.

Give epinephrine (1:10,000) I.V. in escalating doses (1 mg, 3 mg, and 5 mg, 3 min apart) during arrest. High doses (0.1 mg/kg q. 3–5 min) are an option. ET epinephrine is acceptable.

Give atropine, 1 mg I.V.; repeat twice q. 5 min to maximum of 3 mg. ET atropine is acceptable.

Attempt defibrillatory countershock of 300–360 joules if ventricular fibrillation is suspected.

Consider cardiac pacing if early in arrest.

Pulseless electrical activity

Diagnose and reverse underlying causes

Consider: tension pneumothorax, cardiac tamponade, hypovolemia, ruptured abdominal aortic aneurysm, GI bleeding, anaphylaxis, acidosis, drug overdose, and hyperkalemia.

Give epinephrine (1:10,000) I.V. in escalating doses (1 mg, 3 mg, and 5 mg, 3 min apart), during arrest. High doses (0.1 mg/kg q. 3–5 min) are an option. ET epinephrine is acceptable.

Give atropine, 1 mg I.V., if electrical activity is slow; repeat twice q. 5 min to maximum of 3 mg.

Consider calcium chloride, 500 mg I.V., especially in presence of hyperkalemia, hypocalcemia, or use of calcium channel blockers or if arrest is protracted.

In presence of hyperkalemia or tricyclic antidepressant overdose, administer sodium bicarbonate.

Consider cardiac pacing, thoracotomy, and open-chest cardiac massage.

Figure 1 In unconscious, apneic patients, the patency of the airway may be improved by maneuvers that cause anterior displacement of the mandible. The tongue, which is the most frequent cause of airway obstruction, is attached to the lower mandible. The epiglottis also attaches to the mandible via the hyoid bone and the mylohyoid and digastric muscles. Therefore, when the mandible is raised, the tongue and epiglottis move anteriorly, widening the glottic opening.

epiglottis are drawn back over the entrance to the trachea [*see Figure 1*], thereby exacerbating obstruction.[3]

Glottal obstruction may also be caused by blood, teeth, vomitus, secretions, and other foreign debris. Obstructive asphyxia may also be precipitated by swelling of laryngeal tissues, as occurs in smoke inhalation, epiglottitis, and anaphylaxis.

Verify airway patency To assess the patency of the airway, listen to and feel for the exchange of air at the nose and mouth. Partial airflow obstruction produces inspiratory stridor. Gurgling, choking, hoarseness, and difficulty with speech also signify upper airway obstruction. Another cardinal sign of airway obstruction is extreme respiratory effort, manifested by gasping breaths, the use of accessory respiratory muscles, or a strained, weak cough. An inability to deliver air by mouth-to-mouth or bag-valve-mask ventilation (see below) also signifies airway obstruction.

Open the airway In most patients with apnea or obstructive asphyxia, the airway can be improved with manual maneuvers aimed at providing forward displacement of the mandible: when the mandible is raised, the tongue and epiglottis, which are attached to the mandible, move anteriorly, thus widening the glottic opening [*see Figure 1*].[3]

The simplest technique for opening the airway is the head tilt maneuver. (The head tilt maneuver is contraindicated in victims of blunt trauma.) To perform this maneuver, place the palm of one hand on the victim's forehead and apply firm backward pressure to tip the head posteriorly [*see Figure 2*]. Place the other hand behind the victim's neck. The head tilt maneuver alone can relieve glottal obstruction in many unconscious victims.[2]

A second maneuver, the chin lift, is accomplished by hooking the index and third finger of one hand beneath the bony chin and lifting the chin upward to bring the teeth almost to occlusion [*see*

Figure 2 The head tilt maneuver, which provides anterior displacement of the mandible, is easy to perform but usually provides only partial airway opening. To perform the head tilt, place the palm of one hand on the victim's forehead and apply firm backward pressure to tip the head posteriorly. Place the other hand behind the victim's neck.

Figure 3 The head tilt–chin lift is the procedure of choice for opening the airway in nontrauma victims. This maneuver is the easiest to perform and provides the greatest glottal opening. To perform the chin lift, place the index and third fingers (not the thumb) under the bony chin. Then, lift the chin upward to bring the teeth almost to occlusion.

Figure 4 The jaw thrust is an effective, although technically difficult, airway opening procedure. To perform it, grasp the angles of the lower jaw and lift, using both hands, to bring the mandible anteriorly to the maximal prognathic position. The jaw thrust without a head tilt is the procedure of choice in trauma victims.

Figure 3].[2] The combined head tilt–chin lift maneuver is the easiest, least fatiguing airway maneuver to perform. It also provides the greatest forward displacement of the mandible, the greatest relief of glottal obstruction, and the largest tidal volumes during rescue breathing.

The jaw thrust is also an effective technique for improving patency of the airway. To perform the jaw thrust, grasp the angles of the lower jaw and lift, using both hands, to bring the mandible anteriorly to the maximal prognathic position [*see Figure 4*]. The combined head tilt–jaw thrust maneuver provides satisfactory airway patency, although it is more difficult and tiring to perform.

Check for resumption of spontaneous respirations Once the head, neck, and jaw are optimally positioned, check for spontaneous ventilation. Some patients who have suffered obstructive asphyxia may resume breathing.

Improving airway patency The oropharyngeal tube is a useful adjunct to improve airway patency in unconscious patients [*see Figure 5*]. It is a plastic, semicircular device that lifts the base

of the tongue off the posterior pharynx. When the tube is well into the patient's mouth, rotate it 180° into its proper position. The oropharyngeal tube should not be inserted in conscious patients, because it provokes laryngospasm, gagging, vomiting, and aspiration. Patients with intact gag reflexes will better tolerate a rubber nasopharyngeal (trumpet) airway [*see Figure 6*].

Breathing

Perform mouth-to-mouth breathing To perform rescue breathing, gently pinch the victim's nose closed, inhale deeply, seal your lips around and over the victim's mouth, and deliver two slow rescue breaths. Each inflation should last 1.5 to 2.0 seconds, and there should be time for full deflation after each breath. An adequate tidal volume is about 800 ml, or just enough to make the chest rise visibly. The mouth-to-nose technique is preferable if trismus precludes mouth-to-mouth ventilation.

The fraction of inspired oxygen (F_IO_2) in a rescuer's exhaled air is 0.16, a value sufficient to meet a victim's needs.[4] Still, mouth-to-mouth breathing is not a perfect form of airway management. Air leaks at the victim's face often lead to inadequate lung inflation, atelectasis, arteriovenous shunting, and hypoxemia. The chief hazard of artificial ventilation is gastric insufflation followed by regurgitation and aspiration. Gastric insufflation is more likely if quick breaths are delivered at a high peak inspiratory pressure (PIP).[5] An excessive PIP overcomes the opening pressure of the lower esophageal sphincter. In simulated models of CPR, as much as 75% of each mouth-to-mouth breath enters the stomach, not the lungs.[5] Furthermore, as lung compliance declines during cardiopulmonary arrest, the chance of inflating the stomach instead of the lungs increases.

Three strategies are available to reduce the risk of gastric inflation and regurgitation.[5] First, maintain proper head position and airway patency. Second, perform rescue breathing slowly, allowing full exhalation between breaths. Third, employ the Sellick maneuver: pressure applied to the cricoid cartilage reduces the risk of gastric inflation and emesis during CPR [*see Figure 7*].[5]

Performing direct mouth-to-mouth resuscitation may expose rescuers to saliva, blood, and other body fluids, increasing the risk that rescuers will acquire hepatitis, tuberculosis, herpes simplex virus, HIV infection. The probability that a rescuer will acquire an infection after CPR is minimal. Although cases of tuberculosis and

Figure 5 The oropharyngeal airway is inserted into the posterior pharynx in unconscious patients to relieve obstruction of the airway. This plastic device is inserted in an inverted position and then rotated 180°. Once properly positioned, the oropharyngeal airway lifts the base of the tongue, thus improving airway patency.

Figure 6 **In conscious patients, the oropharyngeal airway is often poorly tolerated and frequently produces laryngospasm, coughing, vomiting, and aspiration. The rubber nasopharyngeal (trumpet) airway (shown here) is a better choice for conscious patients with an intact gag reflex.**

herpesvirus transmission have been reported, cases of HIV and hepatitis transmission have not.[2] Nevertheless, universal blood and body fluid precautions [*see VI:19 Viral Infection*] should be observed during all phases of CPR. Goggles, gowns, and latex gloves should be worn. Rescuers should perform mouth-to-mouth breathing with the assistance of a protective face shield or mask, preferably one that has a one-way valve to divert expired air away from the rescuer.[2]

Circulation

Verify pulselessness After opening the airway and delivering the first two rescue breaths, check for a carotid arterial pulse. If none is present, circulatory arrest is confirmed, and chest compressions must begin at once. If pulses are present, continue

airway support and artificial ventilation, using slow breaths (1.5 to 2.0 seconds each), 12 times a minute.[5]

Provide external chest compression Rhythmic, manual chest compressions provide some blood flow to the brain and heart as a result of a global rise in intrathoracic pressure (the thoracic pump), direct compression of the heart (the cardiac pump), or both.[6]

To perform chest compressions, place the heels (not the fingers) of the hands on the lower half of the sternum; place one hand atop the other [*see Figure 8*]. With each compression, depress the sternum 1.5 to 2.0 inches, keeping the elbows locked. The rate of compressions should be 80 to 100/min. The duration and vigor of chest compressions are also important; maximal coronary blood flow is achieved if the compression downstroke is forceful and brief.[7] The time allowed for chest compression should equal, but not exceed, the time allowed for release.

Avoid the ribs and the xiphoid process during chest compressions. Errant or overvigorous chest thrusts increase the incidence of abdominal visceral trauma, rib fractures, mediastinal bleeding, hemopericardium, hemopneumothorax, and other complications. About 40% of CPR recipients suffer at least one CPR-related complication.[8,9]

Advanced Life Support

Under the best circumstances, CPR provides only 25% of the prearrest cardiac output. Although peak systolic blood pressures of 60 mm Hg are often achieved, diastolic pressures seldom exceed 20 mm Hg. Blood flow to the brain is only 15% of normal, and coronary arterial blood flow is essentially zero.[6,10]

ADJUNCTS TO ASSIST VENTILATION

Bag-Valve-Mask Devices

The resuscitation bag is self-inflating and attaches via a non-rebreathing valve to a clear mask [*see Figure 9*]. This device can

Thyroid Cartilage

Cricoid Cartilage

Cervical Vertebra

Trachea

Esophagus

Figure 7 **During assisted ventilation in unintubated patients, gastric insufflation, vomiting, and aspiration are constant hazards. The risk of aspiration is reduced if digital pressure is applied to the cricoid cartilage. This simple procedure (the Sellick maneuver) should be employed during bag-valve-mask and mouth-to-mask ventilation.**

deliver adequate oxygenation and tidal volume if properly used. An oropharyngeal airway must be in place, the victim's head extended, and the jaw elevated to support the airway. The bag is compressed evenly and forcefully while a patent airway and a leakproof seal are maintained. The bag is attached to a long-tubing reservoir with a capacity that equals or exceeds the tidal volume of the bag. High-flow oxygen is delivered to the reservoir at a flow rate that meets or exceeds the patient's minute ventilation. With proper technique, adequate tidal volumes and an F_IO_2 of at least 0.75 can be achieved.

TRACHEAL INTUBATION

Intubation provides better tidal volumes and better oxygenation than mouth-to-mouth or mouth-to-mask breathing and is the only reliable protection against aspiration of gastric contents. A secure endotracheal tube also provides a conduit to evacuate secretions and a route to administer first-line resuscitation drugs.

The decision to secure an airway can be made by rapid evaluation of five parameters: (1) airway patency, (2) adequacy of ventilation, (3) adequacy of oxygenation, (4) level of consciousness, and (5) overall patient condition. Virtually all patients with cardiopulmonary arrest who cannot be immediately resuscitated by an electrical countershock [see Treatment of Ventricular Fibrillation, Electrical Defibrillation, below] will require intubation. The trachea can be intubated by the oral, the nasal, or the transcricoid route, but with the exception of patients who have suffered foreign-body aspiration and upper airway obstruction, all noninjured cardiac arrest victims should be intubated by the oral route.

Orotracheal Intubation

Preparation Success in intubation is dependent on steps taken before the endotracheal tube is touched. First, assemble all essential equipment: suction apparatus, a working laryngoscope blade and handle, and an endotracheal tube of the correct size (for adults, 7.5 to 8.5 mm in internal diameter or, more roughly, about the diameter of the patient's thumbnail). Second, preoxygenate the patient by mouth-to-mask or bag-valve-mask ventilation. Third, place the patient in the so-called sniffing position. Hyperextension of the neck is not desirable. Instead, flex the lower cervical vertebral segments in relation to the trunk and extend the head only at the atlanto-occipital joint. More simply, (1) keep the plane of the patient's face parallel to the floor, (2) leave the shoulders on the stretcher, (3) elevate the occiput anteriorly to shoulder level on a pillow or towel, and then (4) extend the head at the atlanto-occipital joint. This pose brings the trachea, larynx, pharynx, and mouth (as well as the eye of the rescuer) into alignment.

Intubation Intubation requires a good view of the larynx. Begin the intubation process with the laryngoscope in the left hand and a suction catheter, not an endotracheal tube, in the right hand. Clear away secretions, vomitus, and blood. Only then, after the larynx is clearly visualized, exchange the suction tube for the ET tube and insert the ET tube.

Figure 8 **The proper hand position for external chest compression is the lower end of the sternum (*a*). Avoid the ribs and the xiphoid process to reduce the risk of thoracic or abdominal visceral injury. To perform chest compressions, place the heel of one hand on the lower half of the sternum, with the long axis of the hand along the long axis of the victim's sternum (*b*). Place the second hand on top of the first (*c*). With the elbows locked, begin forceful, rhythmic chest compressions at a rate of 80 to 100/min.**

Figure 9 **The resuscitation bag-valve-mask device is difficult to use because it requires simultaneous maintenance of a leakproof seal of the mask and face, elevation of the jaw, extension of the victim's head, and forceful squeezing of the ventilation bag. High-flow oxygen must also be delivered to the attached oxygen reservoir. With proper technique, an adequate minute ventilation and an F_IO_2 of at least 0.75 can be achieved.**

Proper use of the laryngoscope is essential. Insert the blade into the right side of the mouth, and sweep the tongue away to the left. Once the epiglottis is visualized, lift it anteriorly. Do not insert the blade too far. Do not cock the blade back against the teeth (the incisors will break, but the larynx will never be seen). Lift the laryngoscope handle anteriorly in the same direction in which it is being pointed—that is, at a 90° angle to the blade.

If no portion of the glottis can be visualized, do not insert the ET tube. Return to mask ventilation, which is always preferable to gastric ventilation via an errant ET tube. Successful placement of an ET tube must be confirmed by both auscultation of the chest and chest x-ray.

Treatment of Ventricular Fibrillation

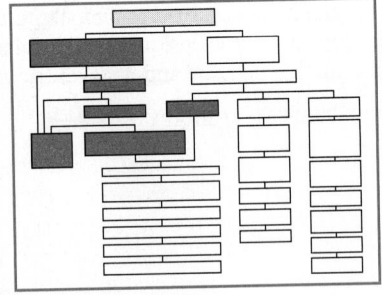

In all patients with sudden collapse, the quick-look paddles should be applied immediately to determine the electrical rhythm. Ventricular fibrillation is easily recognized on the electrocardiogram by its rapid, undulating, chaotic waves.

Successful treatment of VF depends on three factors: the speed of the initial defibrillation attempt, meticulous technique, and the use of epinephrine to augment coronary arterial perfusion.

ELECTRICAL DEFIBRILLATION

If VF is present, the treatment of choice is electrical counter-shock, administered without delay. The first shock should be at 200 joules. This energy will defibrillate most adults, regardless of weight or body habitus. Higher energy levels are injurious and self-defeating, resulting in more myocardial damage, a higher incidence of postshock arrhythmias, and a lower rate of survival.[11] If the initial shock fails, a second should be administered immediately at 300 joules. The third attempt, if needed, should be at 360 joules. The first three defibrillatory shocks must be performed expeditiously, without any pause for BLS, airway management, or drugs.[12] Mortality increases by 10% for each minute that the first countershock is delayed.[13]

Although time is the most critical determinant of the success of defibrillation, technique is also important. Success depends on correct paddle placement, firm paddle pressure, and the use of a low-resistance conducting gel [*see Figure 10*]. Defibrillation during the exhalation phase of ventilation and delivery of two or three countershocks in rapid succession will lower transthoracic impedance and facilitate defibrillation.[11,14]

If the initial three defibrillatory shocks fail, CPR must be initiated. The airway and an intravenous line should be secured, and pharmacologic therapy should be started.

EPINEPHRINE

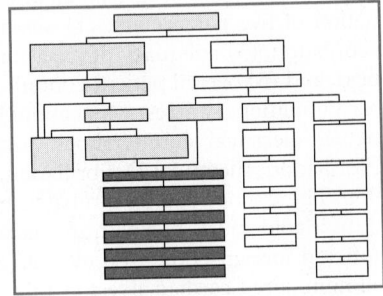

If the first three attempts at defibrillation fail, the first drug administered should be epinephrine (1 mg I.V. or 3 mg endotracheally in a 1:10,000 dilution). By means of its alpha-adrenergic (pressor) properties, epinephrine augments aortic diastolic blood pressure and increases perfusion to the heart.[15] It may not coarsen the fibrillatory waves or enhance electrical defibrillation per se, but it is critical to restoring a pulsatile rhythm, especially after a delayed defibrillation.[6,16]

After administration of epinephrine, defibrillation (at a maximal output of 360 joules) should be attempted. If VF persists, check paddle placement and technique, and verify the placement of the endotracheal tube and the adequacy of ventilation. Epinephrine administration must be repeated every 3 to 5 minutes. Epinephrine has proven merit in resuscitation. One acceptable regimen is to administer escalating doses of epinephrine (1 mg, 3 mg, and 5 mg) 3 minutes apart, continued at 5 mg every 5 minutes thereafter [*see Table 1 and* Discussion, Drug Therapy, *below*].

ANTIDYSRHYTHMIC DRUGS

If VF is resistant to electrical countershock and epinephrine, a loading dose of lidocaine (1.5 mg/kg) should be administered. This lidocaine dose should be repeated in 5 minutes to a total loading dose of 3 mg/kg. Only bolus therapy is indicated in cardiac arrest. A single endotracheal dose (3 mg/kg) may also be effective.

Bretylium should be given if lidocaine fails (earlier use of bretylium has been recommended if VF is caused by hypothermia). The combination of lidocaine and bretylium may act synergistically to prevent the recurrence of VF.[17] Initiate treatment with 5 mg/kg by intravenous push. An additional bolus (10 mg/kg) may be given in 5 minutes.

Lidocaine, bretylium, and procainamide are recommended in refractory VF because they are familiar, fast-acting drugs. All three agents have proven efficacy in suppressing ventricular ectopic activity in ischemic hearts. However, no clinical study has demonstrated that these agents are helpful in VF patients. In fact, lidocaine may increase the energy requirement for electrical defibrillation.[17,18] In one randomized prehospital trial of VF

Figure 10 **Proper electrode placement is essential to promote defibrillation. The apical paddle should be placed just lateral to the left nipple in the midaxillary line; the other paddle should be placed beneath the right clavicle, just to the right of the upper sternum. The two paddles should be well separated. Myocardial current flow and defibrillation are enhanced if firm paddle pressure and a conducting gel are used and if defibrillation is performed during the exhalation phase of the respiratory cycle.**

patients, administration of lidocaine resulted in an increase in the incidence of postcountershock bradyasystolic rhythms.[19]

After successful defibrillation, the myocardium remains electrically unstable and prone to refibrillation. Therefore, all patients should be treated with full loading doses and an I.V. infusion of lidocaine. If the patient proves refractory to lidocaine during the resuscitation, an infusion of procainamide or bretylium is indicated.

OTHER ANTIFIBRILLATORY AGENTS

In cases of refractory VF, it may also be helpful to administer magnesium sulfate, 4 g over a period of 1 minute, particularly to patients receiving digitalis or diuretics. In one retrospective report, amiodarone was administered intravenously to 14 patients who were in prolonged arrest from ventricular tachycardia (VT) or VF. Eleven of the 14 were successfully resuscitated, and eight survived to hospital discharge.[20]

Table 1   Epinephrine Dosing

Standard first dose
  1 mg I.V. push every 3–5 min
Escalating dose*
  1 mg, then 3 mg, then 5 mg I.V. push, administered 3 min apart
  5 mg every 3–5 min thereafter
High dose†
  0.1 mg/kg every 5 min

*Use if standard first dose fails.

†Optional—recommended before countershock when ventricular fibrillation is prolonged or refractory.

Treatment of Asystole

Whenever a flat-line or low-amplitude electrocardiogram is recorded, it is important to confirm the absence of cardiac activity. First, verify the absence of pulses; then, check for technical failures, such as a low battery or loose or disconnected monitor leads.[21] Third, rotate the monitoring leads 90° to detect a null-plane episode of VF. Defibrillation should be attempted only if the rhythm is unclear or if it appears to be fine VF.[14,21] In fine VF, pretreatment with a high dose of epinephrine (5 mg) is indicated before a countershock is administered [*see Table 1*]. Fine VF usually signals a long elapsed arrest time and a poorly perfused heart.

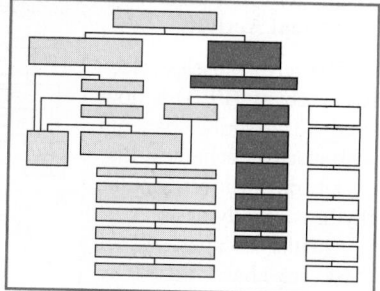

PHARMACOLOGIC THERAPY

Asystole is an ominous condition. The pharmacologic management of asystole consists of a two-pronged attack. First, administer epinephrine. Epinephrine acts via its vasoconstrictive action, not its inotropic action, to increase diastolic blood pressure (thus enhancing coronary perfusion), increase venous return, augment cardiac output during chest compression, and increase perfusion to the heart and brain.[6,22,23] The goal is to evoke good, coarse VF that should be responsive to cardioversion.

Epinephrine should be administered by the intravenous route in rapidly escalating or high doses [*see Table 1*]. Endotracheal administration is acceptable, but intracardiac injections should be utilized only if no other route of drug administration is available.

The second prong of antiasystole therapy is atropine, a parasympatholytic drug. Administer 1 mg intravenously (or 2 mg intratracheally), and repeat every 5 minutes to a maximum dosage of 3 mg. In theory, high levels of parasympathetic tone may accompany or cause cardiopulmonary arrest. Acidosis, hypoxia, and manipulation of the oropharynx during assisted ventilation or endotracheal intubation may add to parasympathetic overactivity.

Some patients with bradyasystole may respond favorably to intravenous administration of aminophylline, even after oxygenation, epinephrine, and atropine therapies have failed.[24] Aminophylline may act by blocking the effects of adenosine, an endogenous nucleoside that inhibits supraventricular activity, pacemaker activity, and atrioventricular conduction.

ELECTRICAL THERAPY

Electrical defibrillation is often employed to treat asystole. Occasionally, fine VF may masquerade as asystole, especially if it is of low amplitude or if the polarity of the fibrillatory waves is at right angles to the monitoring lead.[25] According to careful studies of prehospital cardiac arrest, however, the frequency with which VF masquerades as a flat-line electrocardiogram is low. More commonly, so-called reversible asystole is actually caused by technical failures, such as a faulty battery, a loose lead, or a disconnected monitor; these technical problems must always be addressed before defibrillation is attempted.[21]

Pacemaker therapy, when applied late in the resuscitation effort, is seldom effective. Electrical capture is common, but mechanical activity is rare and survival is nil. Transcutaneous (external) pacing may be slightly more efficacious if initiated early for postdefibrillation asystole and heart block,[26] and it is considerably more expeditious than internal pacing.

Treatment of Pulseless Electrical Activity

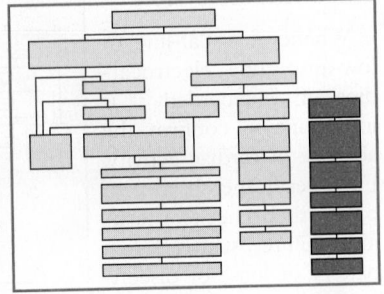

The term pulseless electrical activity (PEA) is now used to describe patients with electromechanical dissociation, idioventricular rhythms, bradyasystole, or ventricular escapes. All of these are characterized by organized electrocardiographic activity without effective myocardial contractions. In PEA, although some synchronous myocardial contractions (demonstrable only by central aortic pressure measurements or by echocardiography) may occur,[26,27] peripheral perfusion and effective cardiac output have ceased. PEA is the proximate cause of death in the majority of delayed or difficult resuscitations.

To manage PEA, first search for reversible causes [see Table 2]. PEA may signal absolute or relative hypovolemia. Causes include gastrointestinal hemorrhage, rupture of an abdominal aortic aneurysm, the septic response, and anaphylaxis. These disorders are characterized by flat jugular veins and a rapid, narrow-complex ECG rhythm (sinus tachycardia). Tension pneumothorax, pulmonary embolus, cardiac tamponade, and acute prosthetic valve dysfunction, which present mechanical barriers to ventricular filling, are also important reversible causes of PEA. In these disorders, cardiac filling is reduced but jugular venous pressure is paradoxically elevated because intrathoracic pressure is high. One robust clue to the presence of a treatable form of PEA is the finding of a rapid, narrow-complex rhythm (sinus tachycardia) on the ECG.[28]

Therefore, to treat PEA, first reverse nonmyocardial causes, such as hypovolemia, cardiac tamponade, and pneumothorax. Empirically administer normal saline or lactated Ringer's solution. If anaphylaxis is a likely cause of the PEA (e.g., if cardiac arrest has occurred after contrast administration in the radiology suite), administer epinephrine and a volume expander. Empirical chest tube placement or pericardiocentesis may be warranted in difficult PEA resuscitations [see I:2 Trauma Resuscitation]. If hyperkalemia is suspected, administer calcium chloride (500 mg I.V.) and sodium bicarbonate (1 mg/kg I.V.).

Drug overdoses and toxic exposures may also incite PEA. Many toxic overdoses have specific, lifesaving antidotes. Carbon monoxide poisoning occurs with exposure to smoke or inhalation of the exhaust from incomplete combustion; high-flow oxygen is the cornerstone of treatment. Cyanide is another by-product of combustion; the antidote is intravenous sodium nitrite and sodium thiosulfate. Tricyclic antidepressants act as type Ia antiarrhythmic agents, slowing cardiac conduction and provoking hypotension, seizures, and ventricular arrhythmias; management of these complications requires vigorous alkalinization and seizure control. Quinidine and procainamide may be proarrhythmic even at therapeutic levels; they prolong the QT interval and may induce torsade de pointes, the treatment of which includes cardioversion followed by magnesium and ventricular pacing. Other common drug overdoses that cause PEA include overdose of beta blockers, calcium channel blockers, and digitalis. Calcium channel blocker and beta-blocker overdoses necessitate atropine, pressor agents, intravenous calcium, glucagon, pacing, or, in desperate cases, cardiopulmonary bypass. Digitalis overdose is treated with digoxin-specific antibodies.

The only hope in refractory PEA is to restore coronary perfusion; therefore, the treatment of choice is epinephrine in rapidly escalating or high doses [see Table 1]. Other alpha-adrenergic drugs

Table 2 Reversible Causes of Pulseless Electromechanical Activity

Etiology	History and Physical Findings	Jugular Venous Pressure	ECG Findings	Treatment
Tension pneumothorax	History of asthma, mechanical ventilation, or trauma Decreased breath sounds Cyanosis Deviated trachea Resistance to ventilation Rib fractures Subcutaneous emphysema	Elevated	Narrow complex Rapid heart rate Right axis deviation	Chest tube
Pulmonary embolus	Acute pulmonary hypertension Risk factor for thromboembolism	Elevated	Narrow complex Rapid heart rate Right axis deviation	Thoracotomy or thrombolytic therapy
Cardiac tamponade	History of malignancy or recent myocardial infarction Aortic dissection Trauma	Elevated	Narrow or wide complex Reduced voltage Electrical alternans	Pericardiocentesis
GI bleeding	Evidence of bleeding	Nonelevated	Narrow complex Rapid heart rate	Blood and volume expansion
Ruptured abdominal aneurysm	Back or abdominal pain Abdominal pulsatile mass or distention	Nonelevated	Narrow complex Rapid heart rate	Volume expansion, MAST suit, operation
Anaphylaxis	Arrest after drug or contrast administration Urticaria, thick tongue, angioedema Stridor or wheezing	Nonelevated	Narrow complex Rapid heart rate	Epinephrine Volume expansion
Hyperkalemia	Renal failure, dialysis fistula Diabetes or severe acidosis Chemotherapy (cell lysis)	Nonelevated	Wide, slow complex Absent P waves	Calcium and sodium bicarbonate Insulin and glucose

(e.g., methoxamine) may also exert a salutary effect; in canine models of PEA, epinephrine and other alpha-adrenergic catecholamines augment diastolic blood pressure, coronary arterial blood flow, and myocardial contractility and lead to improved survival.[29]

There is no other pharmacologic antidote for PEA. Oxygenation and ventilation should be optimized. Atropine should be administered if the rate is slow. Sodium bicarbonate should be used with restraint, if at all, because it generates new CO_2 and leads to intracellular acidosis. In the heart, intracellular acidosis worsens the contractile state and may contribute to refractory PEA.

Prevention of In-Hospital Cardiac Arrest

Even expeditious treatment of cardiopulmonary arrest is not always successful, and for all patients, an ounce of prevention may offer more hope than a pound of cure. Although the incidence of preventable or iatrogenic cardiac arrest cannot be known, it is certain that errors of omission and commission occur.

Anesthetic and sedating agents are responsible for a small number of inpatient cardiac arrests.[30] Suppressive drugs and iatrogenic hypoventilation—especially in emergency cases—are usually responsible. In almost every case, progressive bradycardia is a harbinger of trouble, and its significance must be appreciated. Dyspnea, tachypnea, and sudden changes in mental status (acute confusion) are the most frequent signals.[31,32]

Resuscitation: Summary

In addition to time, only four ingredients are critical to resuscitation: (1) prompt, proper BLS, (2) rapid defibrillation, (3) airway management, and (4) epinephrine, if needed. Epinephrine is the vasopressor agent of choice in cardiopulmonary resuscitation. Epinephrine augments peripheral vascular tone, increases stroke volume during CPR, optimizes arteriovenous pressure gradients, and improves regional blood flow to the heart and brain. Epinephrine and other alpha agonists have proved efficacious in resuscitation, regardless of the electrocardiographic pattern.

Management of Acute Dysrhythmia Arising after Resuscitation

After successful CPR, the most common hemodynamically destabilizing problem is an abnormal heart rhythm. In what follows, we outline the approach to a resuscitated patient with an apparent acute cardiac dysrhythmia [see Figure 11].

The purpose of the heart's electrical activity is to induce mechanical activity. Abnormal electrical activity (arrhythmia or dysrhythmia) that occurs in the absence of hemodynamic compromise should be examined and treated with forbearance because therapy itself poses some hazards: all antidysrhythmic agents except oxygen are negatively inotropic. Thus, there are four questions that should be asked in the evaluation of a patient who appears to exhibit an acute cardiac dysrhythmia:

1. Does the patient actually have a cardiac dysrhythmia?
2. Does the patient require therapy (i.e., is the patient sufficiently stable that treatment is NOT indicated)?
3. How soon should therapy be started?
4. Which therapy is the safest and most effective?

PATIENT IS HEMODYNAMICALLY UNSTABLE

The choice of therapy is determined by the stability of the patient and the origin of the dysrhythmia. An electrocardiogram is required. All hemodynamically unstable patients who have a dysrhythmia other than asystole should be treated immediately by cardioversion (see below); treatment of asystole has already been examined [see Treatment of Asystole, above].

The two primary goals in the management of an acute dysrhythmia are to control the ventricular rate and to maintain a normal sinus rhythm. However, hemodynamic instability in a patient who has a ventricular rate between 60 and 100 beats/min is almost certainly not the result of a cardiac rhythm disturbance. Furthermore, heart rates in excess of 100 beats/min do not necessarily require therapy. Most patients can remain hemodynamically stable—and, in fact, increase their cardiac output—while increasing their heart rate up to 220 beats/min minus their age. In addition, it is not critical to reestablish normal sinus rhythm in all cases.[33] In a young, healthy patient with a normal heart, the so-called atrial kick adds almost nothing to cardiac output.[34] If normal sinus rhythm is abolished and atrial fibrillation is electrically induced in such patients, the ventricles and the rest of the cardiovascular system compensate almost immediately to prevent a fall in cardiac output.[35] On the other hand, loss of synchronous atrial activity in patients with end-stage cardiac decompensation may decrease cardiac output by as much as 40%[36]; such a degree of end-stage cardiac compromise, however, is rare.

Cardioversion

Cardioversion delivers sufficient electrical energy to the precordium (or directly to the heart) to depolarize cells, even those in a relatively refractory state. Cardioversion attempts to impose an electrical organization on the heart, the theory being that after depolarization, all the myocardial cells will repolarize simultaneously and continue to beat synchronously thereafter [see Sidebar The Intracardiac Cardioverter Defibrillator].

Certain precautions are necessary with cardioversion. It is of no use in patients who are in asystole or who have fine VF, because there is no cardiac activity to organize. Supraventricular dysrhythmias such as atrial flutter can be converted by using extremely low energies (e.g., ≤ 5 joules), but such low energies should not be employed in emergency situations. When an unstable patient is treated, it is critical to use an energy level that will work. For a hemodynamically unstable patient, the initial cardioverting energy should be 100 joules; if the dysrhythmia is not abolished, the voltage should be increased rapidly (to a maximum of 360 joules).

PATIENT IS HEMODYNAMICALLY STABLE

Ventricular Rate Is Slow

If the patient is bradycardic before or after cardioversion, atropine should be administered in a 0.5 mg I.V. push. This dose may be repeated at 2-minute intervals. Because the effects of atropine are transient, a temporary internal or external pacemaker should be used to maintain the heart rate [see Sidebar Troubleshooting a Pacemaker].

Ventricular Rate Is Fast

If a patient is hemodynamically stable, a full 12-lead electrocardiogram should be obtained; a long rhythm strip should be obtained as well. The best ECG lead to use for evaluating acute dysrhythmias is one that has good-voltage QRS complexes and maximal P waves, if the latter are present.

Electrocardiography A cardiac impulse produces a positive, or upward, deflection on the monitor or oscilloscope as it

Figure 11 Shown is an algorithm for the management of postresuscitation acute dysrhythmia.

approaches an ECG electrode and a negative, or downward, deflection as it moves away from the electrode. The important factor in dysrhythmia recognition, however, is not the direction of the impulse but its duration. Normal conduction velocity is fast: an impulse is transmitted by healthy Purkinje fibers at a rate of 2 to 3 m/sec.[35] Hence, when an impulse that arises in the atrium (supraventricular) is transmitted via the atrioventricular (AV) node to the high-velocity Purkinje system, the entire ventricle is electrically activated in 0.08 second. An impulse that is generated at an ectopic ventricular site, however, cannot access the high-velocity Purkinje fibers as rapidly as a normal impulse, and ventricular activation is delayed. The QRS complex arising from an ectopic ventricular focus is therefore wider, signifying aberrant ventricular conduction.

Because dysrhythmias of supraventricular origin typically display a narrow QRS complex, the width of the QRS can generally be used to distinguish dysrhythmias of ventricular origin from those of supraventricular origin [see Figure 12]. A wide QRS, however, may also be produced by an impulse that originates in the atrium and is aberrantly conducted to or through the ventricles (supraventricular rhythm with aberrancy). Such rhythms do not pose a serious problem, however, because they are relatively uncommon (the incidence is approximately 10%); more important,

the patient will never suffer if all dysrhythmias with a wide QRS [see Figure 13] are treated as if they were of ventricular origin.

When the ventricular rate is fast and the QRS is narrow, the 12-lead ECG should be searched for P waves, which indicate the presence of atrial activity. If P waves are absent and the QRS complexes are irregular [see Figure 14], the patient probably has atrial fibrillation. It is not, however, crucial to know this; the focus again should be on the width of the QRS complex. Verapamil should be administered to control the ventricular rate (mix 10 mg of verapamil in 10 ml of saline; give 1 mg/min until the ventricular rate slows). A patient with a wide-complex tachycardia is treated by cardioversion (see above) accompanied by administration of lidocaine, 100 mg I.V., whereas a patient with a narrow-complex tachycardia is treated with verapamil.[35,37] Therefore, it is not necessary to identify the specific type of dysrhythmia to treat it effectively.

Verapamil acts by producing profound AV nodal blockade (see below); however, it is also a peripheral vasodilator. Moderate to profound systemic hypotension can be anticipated until the patient converts to sinus rhythm.

Much has been written about the risks of using verapamil in patients who are already receiving beta blockers. Abrupt and com-

The Intracardiac Cardioverter Defibrillator

Over 30 years ago, Michel Mirowski developed the first automatic intracardiac cardioverter defibrillator (ICD), a device that detects dangerous tachyarrhythmias and delivers a cardioverting shock.[130] In the intervening time, it has become abundantly clear that some of the 400,000 Americans who die "suddenly" of tachyarrhythmias each year could have been identified as high risk, although they could not have been saved by pharmacologic or surgical treatment. For these patients, an ICD can be lifesaving.[131]

The ICD identifies dangerous rhythm patterns by means of two algorithms. The first of these algorithms analyzes the patient's heart rate. The patient's maximum attainable sinus rate must be determined by exercise testing before the device is implanted; the ICD is then programmed to detect heart rates above this value. (The ICD can be externally programmed to detect rates between 155 and 200 beats/min.[132])

Using rate criteria alone, however, the ICD cannot discriminate between sinus tachycardia and ventricular or supraventricular tachycardia. Inappropriate shocks are the Achilles heel of the ICD: almost one third of patients experience at least one inappropriate shock annually, when the device detects an episode of sinus tachycardia in which the rate exceeds the threshold programmed earlier. The ICD misinterprets the event as ventricular tachycardia and delivers a shock to the hemodynamically stable patient.[133] Patients liken this to being punched hard in the chest. Although rarely of electrophysiologic significance, an inappropriate shock can be psychologically crippling.[134]

Although computer circuitry is facile and rapid, an ICD recognizes patterns poorly. Fine (or even coarse) VF may not exhibit enough positive spikes to be recognized as a tachyarrhythmia by the ICD. A second algorithm (the probability density function algorithm) was developed to analyze electrophysiologic data and improve the specificity of the ICD's sensing circuitry. A unique feature of ventricular fibrillation is the virtual absence of isoelectric time. Conversely, during sinus tachycardia and supraventricular tachycardia, the ECG is at the isoelectric baseline much of the time. The probability density function algorithm enables the ICD to determine the proportion of time that the ECG is spending at the isoelectric baseline and thereby to detect ventricular fibrillation.

The ICD typically requires more than 5 seconds to appreciate ventricular tachycardia or fibrillation. It then charges its energy storage capacitors for 15 seconds and delivers a 30-joule cardioverting shock. If necessary, the device will deliver a second, third, fourth, and fifth countershock. If the rhythm disorder persists after the fifth countershock, the device will not recycle.

ICD systems are not complex. The device consists of a battery, which is heavy (though newer batteries are becoming lighter), and circuitry, which is light, with a total weight of less than 100 g. Most implanted defibrillators are currently placed without a thoracotomy. A sensing and defibrillating lead system (14 French) is inserted percutaneously via the subclavian vein into right ventricular–right atrial position. The distal electrode tip senses ventricular fibrillation and tachycardia. The cardioverting energy is then discharged between a coil electrode on the diaphragmatic surface of the right ventricle and another coil electrode positioned in the superior vena cava.

It is now clear that ICDs really do work and are capable of extending life. The most effective predictor of outcome in patients with ICDs is the severity of heart failure.[135] The ICD does not prevent malignant arrhythmias: it is, in essence, a safety net that cardioverts ventricular tachycardia or VF when it occurs. Therefore, it must still be used in conjunction with antidysrhythmic drugs.[136,137]

It is easy for a surgeon to become spooked by an ICD. The most effective strategy for managing a patient with an ICD is simply to ignore the ICD. If such a patient is being transported to the OR, however, the device should be inactivated before the electrocautery is used: the ICD will misinterpret the cautery current as VF and respond by delivering a shock to the patient.

The aura of mystery surrounding the ICD may be instantly eliminated by turning off the device (see below). Once the ICD is inactivated, the patient can be treated as any other patient would be. If external cardioversion is indicated, the ICD can be disregarded; external cardioversion will not harm or activate it.

How to Turn the ICD Off

1. If you can find the industry representative to program the device to remain off, do so. Then treat the patient exactly as you would if the ICD were not present.
2. If you cannot find the representative or the situation is urgent:
   a. Palpate the ICD generator, which is typically implanted in the left subcostal region.
   b. Place a heavy pacemaker (or, better yet, an ICD magnet) over the upper corner of the device, toward the patient's left shoulder. Older devices used to emit a soft beep (synchronous with the heartbeat) in response to a magnet when they were active. Unfortunately, that feature has since been engineered out, and newer ICDs are silent.
   c. Tape the magnet in place over the upper border of the device. As long as the magnet is in place, the ICD is off and the electrocautery can be used safely.

plete AV block rarely occurs. In the vast majority of patients, however, the risk of persistent supraventricular tachycardia is greater than the risk of third-degree heart block. Previous beta blockade should not be considered a contraindication to the use of verapamil. Some clinicians may prefer to use adenosine.

Adenosine (see below) produces conduction delay in the AV node and deserves recognition as a second very good (albeit transiently effective) option for treatment of paroxysmal narrow-complex tachycardia or for diagnosis of supraventricular tachycardia with aberrancy (including Wolff-Parkinson-White syndrome). Adenosine is given in a 6 mg I.V. push, followed 2 minutes later by a 12 mg I.V. push and, after another 2 minutes, by a final 12 mg I.V. push over 2 seconds.[34,38]

Patients receiving adenosine complain of a frightening feeling of breathlessness and pressure that is not angina or dyspnea. This feeling typically resolves within 30 seconds. Facial flushing is also common. Unlike verapamil, adenosine is associated with hypotension in fewer than 1% of patients. Transient atrial or ventricular ectopy, with varying degrees of AV block, occurs in more than half of patients. None of the side effects of adenosine necessitate therapy. Compared with verapamil, adenosine has certain advantages. Adenosine's rapid onset and short-duration AV nodal blockade permit diagnostic probing of questionable wide-complex tachycardias, and its side effects are trivial and self-limited. On the other hand, the profound neuroendocrine and electrolyte perturbations that provoked the dysrhythmias in the first place—perturbations that are very common in the surgical intensive care unit—are likely to persist, and the rhythm disorder typically recurs. If adenosine works, the longer-acting verapamil should also work.

Verapamil Both the sinoatrial (SA) node and the AV node are activated by the movement of calcium through the so-called slow calcium channels.[39] Verapamil, a calcium channel blocker, is the most powerful agent currently available for blocking the transmission of impulses across the AV node. A supraventricular dysrhythmia produces an acceleration in the ventricular rate because impulses generated by an ectopic source above the AV node are transmitted too rapidly to the ventricle [see Figure 15]. Verapamil produces a pharmacologic blockade of the AV node, reducing the number of impulses reaching the ventricles and thereby controlling the ventricular rate.

Adenosine Adenosine is an endogenous nucleoside that has differential antidysrhythmic effects in both supraventricular and ventricular tissue. The real appeal of adenosine as a therapeutic

Patient with pacemaker experiences palpitations or presyncope

Obtain 30-second rhythm strip to assess pacing and sensing functions.

All wide (paced) QRS complexes are preceded by pacemaker artifacts

Pacing function is normal.

Heart rate is adequate, and no pacemaker artifacts are visible

Place magnet over pacemaker to inactivate sensing circuit and convert to fixed-rate mode.

Some or all pacemaker artifacts are not followed by wide (paced) QRS complexes

Ventricular pacing threshold is higher than pacemaker output.

No pacemaker artifacts are visible with magnet

Pacemaker battery is dead.

Pacemaker artifacts that appear at appropriate distances from prior QRS complexes (i.e., outside refractory period) provoke paced QRS

Sensing and pacing functions are normal.

Pacemaker artifacts that appear at appropriate distances from prior QRS complexes (i.e., outside refractory period) *do not* provoke paced QRS

Consider two possibilities:
• Adequate pacemaker output may not be reaching an excitable portion of the ventricle, or
• Ventricular pacing threshold is higher than pacemaker output.

Troubleshooting a Pacemaker

Few industries have benefited more from the United States space program than has the cardiac pacemaker industry. Much of the microcircuitry developed for the space shuttle is directly applicable to pacemakers. Yet the array of programmable parameters that has become standard in most implanted pacemakers, while providing therapeutic flexibility to electrophysiologists, can be intimidating to the mere mortal surgeon. The purpose of this discussion is to delineate simple methods for identifying problems with the two dominant pacemaker functions: pacing and sensing (see above and right).

Any of the following situations might prompt evaluation of pacemaker function: (1) the patient informs you that he or she has a pacemaker, (2) you note a pacemaker bulge in the pectoral area, (3) a chest x-ray reveals a pacemaker with a wire descending onto the diaphragmatic surface of the right ventricle, or (4) a patient with an implanted pacemaker notes symptoms of palpitations or presyncope. At this point, you need to obtain a 30-second rhythm strip to determine whether the pacemaker can capture the patient's ventricle—that is, whether the pacemaker emits an impulse that stimulates the ventricle to depolarize.

(continued)

Obtain drug history to rule out an increase in ventricular threshold caused by antidysrhythmic agents.

Obtain chest x-ray to determine whether endocardial lead has been fractured or dislodged.

Endocardial lead is intact and in good anatomic position

Reprogram pacemaker to higher output.

All pacemaker artifacts are followed by a paced beat

Intermittent capture persists

Relocate endocardial lead to lower threshold site.

---

and diagnostic tool is that it depresses automaticity and conduction within the SA and AV nodes.[40] Two clinically relevant types of adenosine receptors are present in cardiac tissue: (1) A_1 receptors, which are present on AV nodal tissue and cardiomyocytes and promote AV block and bradycardia, and (2) A_2 receptors, which reside on vascular endothelial and smooth muscle cells and mediate coronary vasodilatation. A_3 receptors are present in the myocardium, and selective activation of these has a cardioprotective effect; however, these receptors are not important in antidysrhythmic therapy.[41]

Adenosine and acetylcholine exhibit identical cardiac effects and share similar receptor-effector coupling systems. Adenosine and acetylcholine provide an opposing balance to the sympathetic neurotransmitters norepinephrine and epinephrine. Thus,

predictably, the adenosine antagonists caffeine, theophylline, and aminophylline provoke tachycardia and ectopy.

Because of the rapid intravascular metabolism of adenosine (half-life, 6 seconds), an intravenous bolus of adenosine (6 mg or 100 µg/kg) produces a negligible effect on systemic blood pressure, as confirmed by multiple clinical studies. Thus, adenosine is safe, but its effects are transient.

Adenosine is useful in blocking AV nodal conduction. Intracardiac recordings exhibit prolongation of the A-H interval with no alteration in conduction distal to the His bundle and on into the ventricular myocardium (the His-Purkinje system is unaffected).

In more than 90% of cases, adenosine is effective in terminating supraventricular tachycardia. Interestingly, adenosine was as

Troubleshooting a Pacemaker *(continued)*

Ventricular Capture

a

Note the pacemaker artifact (↑) that precedes each wide QRS complex in rhythm strip *a*, above. The QRS complex is wide because ventricular activation does not originate from the AV node, and ventricular conduction is therefore aberrant. At this point, you know that your patient is pacing, and you can determine the pacing rate. You do not, however, know the pacing threshold (i.e., the minimum voltage required for ventricular capture) or the safety margin between pacemaker output and pacing threshold. At this moment (and presumably yesterday and tomorrow), this pacemaker is appropriately discharging its most important function—pacing the heart and maintaining an adequate rate.

Ventricular Sensing

b

In rhythm strip *b*, above, normal P waves are followed by regular QRS complexes, and no pacemaker artifacts are evident. It is most likely that this patient's pacemaker has been programmed to fire at a paced rate that is slower than this patient's intrinsic heart rate, and the pacemaker is thus appropriately sensing each QRS complex. It is unlikely but possible, however, that the pacemaker is not sensing appropriately. Instead, one of the following problems may be occurring: (1) the pacemaker battery is dead, which is unlikely unless the battery was implanted more than 5 years ago, (2) the intracardiac electrode has been fractured, which is also unlikely, because current leads are remarkably durable, (3) the intracardiac electrode has been dislodged (this is an uncommon late problem that typically results in pacemaker artifacts unrelated to each QRS complex), or (4) the patient is taking an antidysrhythmic drug that has profoundly depressed ventricular excitability below threshold level for capture (this problem is very rare and can be excluded by taking a drug history). It is overwhelmingly likely, therefore, that rhythm strip *b* simply demonstrates that the pacemaker is sensing appropriately.

Assessing Ventricular Capture When the Spontaneous Heart Rate Is High

Typically, by the time you see the syncopal patient in the emergency department or recovery room, the patient is sufficiently excited that his or her heart rate has recovered, and the rhythm strip will look like rhythm strip *b*. In a patient in whom heart rate is adequate and no pacemaker artifacts are visible, it is necessary to override the pacemaker's sensing circuit to determine whether the pacemaker is capable of emitting a pacing impulse that will capture the ventricle. The pacemaker's sensing circuit may be inactivated by placing a magnet over the pacemaker. Alternatively, the pacemaker may be reprogrammed to a paced rate that is faster than the patient's intrinsic heart rate. In this fashion, capture may easily be assessed. (Unfortunately, the programmers are expensive and are therefore often locked in some inaccessible closet. Programmers have great theoretical value but very little practical value to the surgeon.)

c

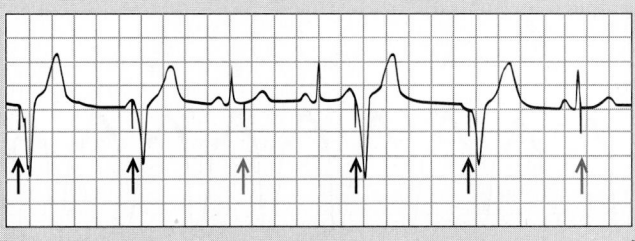

|←—————————————————— Magnet ——————————————————→|

In rhythm strip *c*, above, a magnet has converted the patient's pacemaker from the demand mode to the fixed-rate mode. The pacemaker artifacts that precede the wide (paced) QRS complexes in this rhythm strip (black arrows) show that the pacing function of this pacemaker is intact. Occasionally, a pacemaker artifact occurs during the electrical refractory period that immediately follows the QRS complex (red arrows). Pacing during the refractory period will not result in ventricular capture. Pacing during the refractory period should not result in ventricular capture and must not be interpreted as intermittent capture. In a patient whose pacemaker seems to be sensing appropriately (as in rhythm strip *b*), the magnet permits assessment of ventricular capture. Rhythm strip *c* demonstrates normal ventricular capture in the presence of a magnet.

Some or All Pacemaker Artifacts Are Not Followed by Wide QRS Complexes

If a pacemaker impulse that occurs outside the refractory period is not followed by a wide QRS complex, two possibilities should be considered. First, an adequate pacemaker impulse may not be reaching an excitable portion of the ventricle because of fracture or dislodgment of the endocardial lead. This problem can usually be identified by a chest x-ray. Second, if the chest x-ray shows that the lead is intact and in good anatomic position, the pacemaker output is not sufficient to reach the pacing threshold. Occasionally, this problem is caused by fibrosis at the endocardial electrode tip. If the pacemaker can be reprogrammed to a higher output, the capture problem should resolve. Otherwise, the lead must be repositioned to a site at which the pacing threshold is lower.

Occasional Pacemaker Artifacts Closely Follow a Spontaneous QRS Complex

If the patient's rhythm strip looks like rhythm strip *c, in the absence of a magnet*, the pacemaker is not sensing properly. In the demand mode, most pacemakers require at least a 2.5 mV signal to suppress output. Thus, if the pacemaker emits stimuli in spite of a normal spontaneous heart rate, an adequate QRS signal either is not being sensed (the lead tip may be lodged at the site of a prior myocardial infarction or scar) or is not being transmitted to the pacemaker (because of lead fracture or dislodgment).

effective at terminating atrioventricular reentry (85%) as at terminating atrioventricular node reentry (86%).[40] Because of adenosine's short half-life, however, the supraventricular dysrhythmia is likely to recur within 2 minutes in up to one third of patients. Thus, adenosine is diagnostically valuable in discriminating supraventricular from ventricular dysrhythmias. Continuous (therapeutic) infusion of adenosine (150 to 300 µg/kg/min) is rational from a physiologic standpoint but is frighteningly expensive. The transient (and safe) characteristics of adenosine permit its diagnostic use [*see Figure 11*]. If the QRS width is confusing and it is therefore uncertain whether the rhythm disorder is supraventricular (QRS < 0.08 second) or ventricular (QRS > 0.08 second),

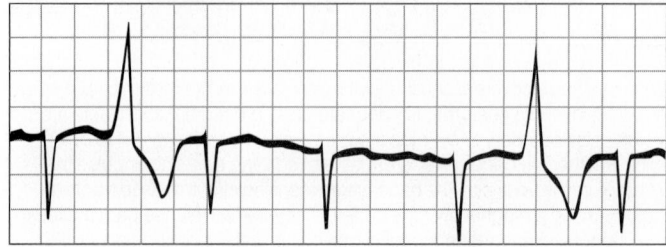

Figure 12 This tracing depicts frequent ventricular ectopic depolarizations interspersed among depolarizations from a supraventricular source. Note that the QRS depolarizations of supraventricular origin are narrow, whereas the QRS complexes of ectopic ventricular origin are wide.

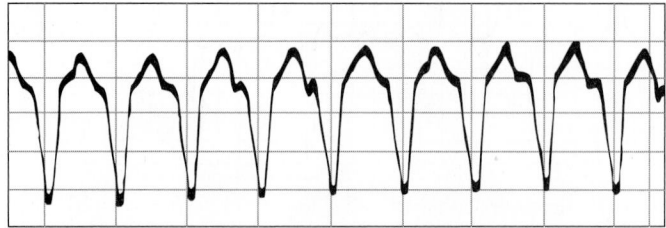

Figure 13 In a wide-complex tachycardia, each impulse is conducted aberrantly through the ventricles. The QRS complex is therefore prolonged to more than 0.08 second and occupies more than two small boxes on the ECG tracing.

Figure 14 P waves are absent and the QRS complexes are narrow and irregular in this ECG tracing from a patient with atrial fibrillation.

Figure 15 In a narrow-complex tachycardia, the entire ventricle is activated in less than 0.08 second. Presumably, the impulse originated at a supraventricular source and accessed the ventricle via the high-velocity Purkinje system.

adenosine (6 mg I.V. bolus) may be infused and repeated if necessary. If the dysrhythmia breaks, that means it was supraventricular. If it does not break, proceed to cardioversion (see above).

Several clinical studies have compared adenosine with verapamil for therapeutic AV nodal blockade, with predictable results. Both agents block the AV node and control the ventricular rate: cumulative efficacy with either agent is more than 90%. Postconversion dysrhythmias in the two groups were similar. Spontaneous reinitiation of supraventricular dysrhythmias occurs more frequently with adenosine, whereas systemic hypotension is more commonly

associated with verapamil (at least until the dysrhythmia breaks). Thus, for help in seconds (approximately 20 seconds), use adenosine (6 mg I.V. bolus, may be repeated); for help in minutes (3 to 5 minutes), use verapamil (1 mg/min I.V. up to 10 mg); and for help in hours, infuse digoxin, 0.5 mg I.V. Although digitalis effectively blocks the AV node, it should be remembered that digitalis actually increases automaticity and excitability in both the atrium and the ventricle. The calcium channel blockers are superior to digoxin in controlling the ventricular rate.[39]

The adverse effects of adenosine, like the beneficial effects, are transient.[40] Facial flushing, chest pressure (adenosine has been implicated in the sensation of angina), and transient third-degree heart block are very common. Significant side effects are rare. Nebulized adenosine can cause bronchoconstriction, especially in asthmatic patients. Bronchoconstriction has not been reported after intravenous administration of adenosine.

Magnesium Magnesium is the second most abundant cation in man. It is involved in many enzymatic reactions that influence the production and utilization of cellular energy. Abnormalities in electrolyte homeostasis (potassium and calcium in particular) are associated with a robust increase in cardiac myocellular excitability and automaticity, especially when these abnormalities are concurrent with myocardial ischemia.[42] Multiple clinical studies confirm the efficacy of intravenous magnesium infusion even in the absence of objective hypomagnesemia.[43,44] Magnesium appears to be uniquely beneficial in the setting of digitalis toxicity and acute myocardial ischemia. Intravenous magnesium appears to help even when the measured serum values are normal. No one knows the mechanism. When confronted with a patient exhibiting either supraventricular or ventricular ectopy, it is safe (and often effective) to administer magnesium chloride at a dosage of 7 g or 100 mg/kg I.V. over 1 to 3 hours. It is not necessary to measure the serum magnesium concentration first; the serum value will not influence therapy.

Amiodarone Amiodarone is a potent inhibitor of alpha- and beta-adrenergic stimulation with a half-life of 1 month. It prolongs the myocardial action potential and refractory period and delays both sinus node function and AV conduction.

Although the primary effect of amiodarone is to slow down cardiac activity (actually, amiodarone exhibits electrophysiologic characteristics of all four antiarrhythmic classes [*see* Discussion, Drug Therapy, *below*]),[45] it must have additional therapeutic efficacy. It reduces transmural proarrhythmic heterogeneity (which predisposes to arrhythmias) in the human heart[46] [*see* Discussion, Reentrant Dysrhythmias, *below*]. Intravenous amiodarone has also proved effective against refractory ventricular tachycardia and VF. In one randomized trial,[44] I.V. amiodarone brought about a significant improvement in survival compared with placebo in patients suffering out-of-hospital cardiac arrest.

Intravenous amiodarone was approved in the United States for use against malignant ventricular tachyarrhythmias in 1995. Rates of effective suppression for ventricular arrhythmias have been reported to be as high as 91% in uncontrolled trials.[47] Although this gratifyingly effective agent is available and works well, it has significant side effects. In trials of low-dose amiodarone (200 mg/day), thyroid, neurologic, cutaneous, ocular, bradycardic, and hypotensive problems were statistically more frequent; interestingly, pulmonary fibrosis was not.[48] The recommended dosages for adults are as follows: loading dose, 150 mg I.V. over 10 minutes; maintenance infusion, 0.5 mg/min; and oral dose, 200 to 400 mg/day (after loading).

Cardiac Dysrhythmias during Pregnancy

Fortunately, cardiac dysrhythmias are not frequent in young women of childbearing age. When rhythm problems do occur, they tend not to be hemodynamically destabilizing. The most commonly used obstetric drug with electrophysiologic side effects is magnesium.[49] When magnesium is infused intravenously into the mother, the fetus may exhibit a dose-dependent bradycardia and a progressive decrease in healthy heart rate variability.[50,51] Antidysrhythmic (indeed, any) drugs should be avoided during the first trimester of pregnancy, although most antidysrhythmic agents carry relatively little risk.[49] Quinidine, procainamide, lidocaine, digoxin, adenosine, and beta blockers all have a long record of safety during pregnancy. Flecainide has proved to be effective in treating fetal supraventricular tachycardia complicated by hydrops. Phenytoin and amiodarone have been associated with congenital abnormalities.[49]

The important point is that if the mother is unstable, direct current cardioversion is safe and effective.

Proarrhythmia with Antidysrhythmic Drugs

Proarrhythmic manifestations have been linked primarily to agents that prolong repolarization. Early afterdepolarizations (see below) associated with agents that retard repolarization or an increase in spatial and temporal dispersion of repolarization are the putative mechanisms of proarrhythmia.[52]

The class III antidysrhythmic agents have traditionally been the agents most likely to cause dysrhythmias.[52] The best way of preventing dysrhythmias, however, is to follow the general policy of not using drugs at all if they are not needed.[53]

Discussion

In the fifth century B.C., the Greek poet Pindar admonished all physicians: "Thou shall treat and thou shall not kill, but do not attempt to return a dead soul to life."[54] Fortunately, no one listened to the poet then, and no one is listening now. Since Biblical times, humans have sought to reanimate the dead, mixing science, prayer, alchemy, and the magic arts. Today, CPR is the cornerstone of resuscitation and is practiced by millions of health professionals and laypersons in communities throughout the world.

In recent years, investigators have made fundamental new discoveries in CPR. A mechanism of blood flow that contradicts the conventional notion of cardiac massage has been identified. Some apocryphal drugs, including calcium and isoproterenol (and, in some circles, sodium bicarbonate), have finally been abandoned. One old technique, open-chest cardiac massage, has resurfaced and appears promising. Controversies have arisen at every turn.

What has prompted the renaissance of interest and research in resuscitation? Primarily, it has been the observation that the majority of cardiac arrest victims do not survive. Only 15% of patients with prehospital cardiopulmonary arrest survive to hospital discharge.[55] Much higher survival rates (30% to 50%) have been reported in some urban communities, but only if (1) the arrest is witnessed, (2) a bystander administers CPR, (3) the initial rhythm is ventricular fibrillation, (4) BLS is provided within 4 minutes, and (5) definitive ALS is provided within 8 minutes of arrest.[55]

Among long-term survivors of prehospital arrest, permanent neurologic impairment is all too common. At least 20% of prehospital victims who are resuscitated and admitted to hospitals never regain consciousness. Permanent brain dysfunction occurs in one half of all long-term survivors.[56] To promote resuscitation with preservation of intellect and independence, the new field of cardiopulmonary-cerebral resuscitation (CPCR) has evolved.

Sudden, unexpected cardiac arrests are also common in the hospital setting. In fact, in teaching hospitals, resuscitation is attempted on 1% of patients admitted and on 30% of patients who die.[57] Although response times are short, resuscitation equipment is at hand, and the bystanders are physicians and nurses, success rates for resuscitation in general hospitals are low: 50% of patients remain alive for 1 hour or longer, but only 10% survive to discharge.[57] For those patients who do survive cardiac arrest and resuscitation efforts, however, the long-term outcome is favorable. Most survivors walk out of the hospital and return to their homes,[58] and 6 months later, 80% of those who returned home are still alive and well. When longevity, independence, and mental fitness are considered, the majority of patients who survive resuscitation have an excellent prognosis. In one study, 21 (55%) of 38 patients who survived for 6 months or longer said that they would choose to undergo cardiopulmonary resuscitation again.[55,58]

Most patients who experience in-hospital cardiac arrest have critical circulatory, respiratory, malignant, or neurologic disorders, which may explain their poor survival rate. Indeed, azotemia, cancer, sepsis, hypotension, and a homebound lifestyle have all been shown to predict a poor outcome. In the absence of a witness[57] or in the presence of a rhythm other than VF or VT,[59] resuscitation is likely to be unsuccessful. Advanced age does not appear to be an independent predictor of poor outcome when comorbidity and illness severity are controlled for[58,60]; thus, CPR is not precluded in elderly patients. Nevertheless, most chronically ill elderly patients will not survive resuscitation in the hospital.[57,61] When a patient is both elderly and irreversibly ill, the physician and the patient or family should give careful consideration to the hazards (and the probable futility) of CPR.[62]

Circulatory Physiology during CPR

CARDIAC PUMP

Kouwenhoven and coworkers first suggested that during CPR the heart is squeezed like a pump between the sternum and the spine.[63] According to this theory, each downstroke on the chest results in a systole, during which the left ventricle is compressed and blood is propelled into the arterial circulation. Because the cardiac valves operate in only one direction, anterograde blood flow is assured. The relaxation phase of CPR (diastole) also mimics the natural circulation. As the sternum recoils to its normal position, intracardiac pressures fall, the atrioventricular valves open, and blood is drawn into the heart from the lungs and the venae cavae.

During the intercompression interval, a small inflow of air occurs from the trachea. However, because this flow is insufficient for ventilation, positive pressure ventilation must be applied. The cardiac pump concept is the basis for the current standards of CPR: ventilation and compression are alternated so that inflation of the lungs will not impede direct massage of the heart.

THORACIC PUMP

Many physiologists now favor a different mechanism of blood flow during CPR: the thoracic pump. According to this theory, external chest compression does not massage the heart; instead, each deflection of the sternum generates an abrupt increase in intrathoracic pressure, which in turn propels blood into the arterial tree.[6] The increase in pressure is uniform in all hollow viscera of the thorax, including the four chambers of the heart, the intrathoracic aorta, and the great veins. The mitral and tricuspid valves are rendered incompetent, and no atrioventricular or ventriculoaortic pressure gradients are established. While the extrathoracic jugular veins collapse during thoracic compression, the thick-walled carotid arteries remain patent and receive the forward spurt of blood. Thus, in contrast to the cardiac pump, the thoracic pump generates forward blood flow because of an arteriovenous pressure gradient established outside, not within, the chest. According to the thoracic pump concept, the heart is a passive conduit, not a pump, during CPR.

The relative contributions of the cardiac and thoracic pumps remain unsettled.[64] Each mechanism probably contributes to systemic perfusion, depending on the configuration and stiffness of the chest wall, the presence or absence of cardiac enlargement, and the method of CPR.[6] In an individual patient, there may even be variations in the mechanism of blood flow. Cardiac compressions may predominate early in the resuscitation effort, especially at the points of maximal sternal deflection and minimal lung inflation. In any case, whether the cardiac or thoracic pump is operative, the blood flow generated increases with the depth, force, and rate of chest compressions.

LIMITED VITAL ORGAN PERFUSION DURING CPR

Blood flow during CPR can barely sustain life. When standard CPR is applied to the patient in cardiac arrest, the cardiac output is only 25% of normal.[6,10,16] Although the peak systolic blood pressure at the downstroke of the chest compression may reach 60 mm Hg, the diastolic blood pressure is less than 20 mm Hg.

Cerebral cortical flow seldom exceeds 15% of prearrest values. Standard CPR does not sustain cerebral oxygenation, pupillary reactivity, or electroencephalographic activity during prolonged resuscitation.[10]

The situation in the coronary circulation is even more precarious. During conventional CPR, blood flow in the coronary vascular bed falls to 5% of normal.[10] In fact, reverse coronary flow has been observed. Indeed, the thoracic pump provides no mechanism at all for blood flow to the heart. In the cardiac arrest victim, the sole determinant of coronary blood flow is the coronary perfusion pressure (i.e., aortic diastolic pressure minus right atrial diastolic pressure). Both components of this equation lie within the thorax and increase and decrease together during CPR. In addition, unlike the cerebral vascular bed, the coronary venous circulation has no one-way valves to protect it from pressure increases. Therefore, the essential problem with CPR is that it raises arterial pressure and venous pressure to virtually the same degree, generating no gradient for coronary blood flow at all.

MEASURES OF EFFECTIVE CPR

Traditionally, clinicians have judged the effectiveness of CPR by the strength of the victim's pulses and the size of the pupils. Near-normal blood gas levels have also been considered a favorable sign. However, none of these parameters actually correlates with vital organ perfusion or with success of resuscitation.[65] Instead, the best predictors of outcome are hemodynamic measures: the success of resuscitation correlates most closely with the coronary perfusion gradient (i.e., aortic blood pressure minus right atrial pressure) during the release phase (diastole) of CPR.[6,16] In prolonged CPR, neurologic recovery and long-term survival are possible only if certain critical hemodynamic thresholds are met or exceeded: aortic diastolic (coronary perfusion) blood pressure must equal 30 mm Hg; calculated coronary perfusion gradient, 20 mm Hg; and myocardial blood flow, 20 ml/min/100 g (about 30% of baseline). These requisite hemodynamic parameters are highly correlated with one another and with survival. A cerebrocortical blood flow of 20 ml/min/100 g (20% of the prearrest level) is essential for neurologic recovery. None of these critical indices can be achieved by conventional CPR alone.

NEW CPR TECHNIQUES

Volume Loading during CPR

For many years, dextrose and water at a keep-open rate has been considered the appropriate fluid for CPR. Now, however, volume expansion may be more appropriate. Volume infusion is helpful in some cases of PEA, especially those caused by blood loss, systemic inflammatory response syndrome, anaphylaxis, pericardial tamponade, pulmonary embolus, and tension pneumothorax. In one porcine model of PEA, prearrest volume expansion with a crystalloid-hydroxyethyl starch mixture improved survival.[66] Expansion of the central circulatory volume is a logical adjunct to improve cardiac output and vital organ perfusion during CPR.

Interposed Abdominal Compression CPR

A more promising modification of CPR is the technique of manual interposed abdominal compression (IAC-CPR). In IAC-CPR, a third rescuer is recruited whose role is to apply pressure to the midabdomen during the release phase (i.e., diastole) of the chest compression-relaxation cycle. Otherwise, standard CPR is administered by using alternating ventilation and compression. Like an intra-aortic balloon pump, IAC-CPR augments aortic diastolic blood pressure and improves cerebral and myocardial perfusion. As noted earlier, coronary flow and survival are closely related to the central arteriovenous pressure difference during the release phase of CPR.

Active Compression-Decompression CPR

Early clinical studies suggested that active compression-decompression CPR (ACD-CPR) might outperform standard CPR. In one study of 10 patients in whom standard advanced life-support interventions had failed, institution of ACD-CPR resulted in immediate augmentation of cardiac output and coronary arterial perfusion.[67] A randomized clinical trial of 62 patients on a hospital ward demonstrated the superiority of ACD-CPR over standard CPR.[68] Short-term survival (24 hours) was 45% in the ACD-CPR group, compared with only 9% in the standard-CPR group. Neurologic recovery was higher in the ACD-CPR group as well. ACD-CPR may also improve ventilation. In contrast, Schwab and colleagues found no improvement in outcome with ACD-CPR in a large out-of-hospital trial.[69]

CURRENT-BASED DEFIBRILLATION

Rapid electrical defibrillation is the key to resuscitation success. One promising new technique is current-based defibrillation, which imposes an electrical current on the heart that is strong enough to interrupt the VF reentry circuit. The optimal current for successful defibrillation is about 30 to 40 amperes. Today, operators of defibrillators do not select the current needed; rather, they select the total energy dose, measured in joules.

However, selection of a standard energy dose fails to take into account that the flow of current is determined not only by the energy dose but also by the patient's transthoracic impedance (measured in ohms).[70] Transthoracic impedance varies from case to case because of differences in paddle pressure, patient size, chest wall configuration, conducting gels, lung inflation, and previous countershocks. The average transthoracic impedance in humans is about 70 ohms; however, impedance varies widely among cardiac arrest patients—from 15 to 150 ohms. If a patient's transthoracic impedance is high, the standard energy dose of 200 joules may deliver insufficient current. In a patient with low transthoracic resistance, this energy dose may be too high, provoking postcountershock bradyasystole.

Drug Therapy

AGENTS USED IN RESUSCITATION

Physicians have traditionally practiced resuscitation with "the empiricism of a grandmother's cooking,"[71] mixing sodium bicarbonate, calcium, and inotropes "according to taste." In truth, only one class of drugs—the alpha-adrenergic agonists—has proved effective in CPR.

Epinephrine and Other Alpha Agonists

In 1906, Crile and Dolley recognized that "the basic problem in resuscitation is to secure by means of some infusion a coronary [perfusion] pressure amounting to 30 to 40 mm Hg."[72] Of course, the aortic diastolic blood pressure is the driving force for coronary perfusion; indeed, in 1963, Redding and Pearson demonstrated experimentally that an aortic diastolic blood pressure of 40 mm Hg was a prerequisite for resuscitability.[73] Subsequent investigations have indicated that it is virtually impossible to attain this level of aortic blood pressure by external chest compression alone. Epinephrine is an essential adjunct.[15]

Alpha-adrenergic (pressor) agents cause venoconstriction, thus augmenting stroke volume during chest compression. Alpha-adrenergic agents also improve regional blood flow during CPR by inducing a selective increase in noncerebral and noncoronary vascular tone.[22] For example, epinephrine augments cerebrocortical blood flow by vasoconstricting peripheral arterial beds, by preventing or reversing carotid artery collapse at the thoracic outlet, and by constricting the extracerebral carotid artery,[22] thereby reducing blood flow to the tongue and facial musculature. Epinephrine and phenylephrine administration leads to improved cerebral cortical blood flow and neurologic recovery after CPR.[22,74]

Epinephrine also has a positive effect on the aortic diastolic (coronary perfusion) blood pressure. The myocardial perfusion pressure increases after epinephrine infusion because this drug augments aortic diastolic blood pressure without substantially increasing the right atrial pressure.[10]

Resuscitation is critically dependent on alpha-adrenergic tone no matter what the arrest rhythm. In prolonged ventricular fibrillation, successful electrical reversion to a pulsatile rhythm is enhanced by administration of epinephrine. This enhances defibrillation not by coarsening the fibrillatory waves (a beta-adrenergic effect) but by augmenting myocardial perfusion. Isoproterenol, a pure beta-adrenergic agonist, increases the frequency and amplitude of the fibrillatory waves; there is no proof that this coarser fibrillatory pattern is more easily cardioverted, but it certainly seems to suggest a more favorable outcome. Isoproterenol may even be detrimental: its unopposed beta-adrenergic activity causes peripheral vasodilatation, increases intraventricular pressures, reduces

subendocardial blood flow, increases oxygen demand, and is detrimental to the CPR effect. Indeed, isoproterenol is no longer recommended in any cardiac arrest situation.

Alpha agonists are also critical in the treatment of asystole. When epinephrine is administered to asystolic animals, it is the alpha-adrenergic (pressor) action, not the beta-adrenergic (inotropic-chronotropic) action, that facilitates the return of a spontaneous rhythm.[73] In asphyxiated dogs, asystole may be reverted with equal success by using epinephrine, phenylephrine, metaraminol, or methoxamine.

Although the catecholamine of choice for resuscitation in all forms of cardiac arrest is epinephrine (a balanced alpha- and beta-adrenergic drug), preliminary studies suggested that the use of pure alpha-adrenergic agonists, such as methoxamine or phenylephrine, might be preferable. The standard dose of epinephrine in cardiac resuscitation has long been 1 mg, but this dose has no clinical or experimental basis. In fact, in the landmark animal studies of epinephrine performed over 90 years ago, 1 mg was a homeopathic dose.[29,72] Adequate coronary perfusion pressure is achieved in dogs only with the administration of 0.05 to 0.20 mg/kg—the equivalent of 3.5 to 14.0 mg every 5 minutes in a 70 kg human. Recent experimental and clinical studies have demonstrated that only these larger doses of epinephrine will consistently produce coronary perfusion pressures that exceed the threshold required for return of spontaneous circulation.[16]

Investigators have attempted to determine whether high-dose epinephrine is beneficial in cardiac arrest patients. In one large prehospital trial, patients who received a high dose (15 mg) of epinephrine had a higher return of spontaneous pulse and a higher hospital admission rate than patients who received a standard dose (1 mg).[75] However, survival to hospital discharge was not improved. In a large out-of-hospital study, high-dose epinephrine (0.2 mg/kg) did not increase the return of spontaneous pulse, number of hospital admissions, consciousness at hospital discharge, or overall survival.[76] A randomized trial comparing epinephrine doses of 1 mg and 7 mg for both in-hospital and out-of-hospital cardiac arrests found that the use of high-dose epinephrine did not improve 1-hour survival, survival to discharge, or neurologic recovery.[77]

Human and animal studies of epinephrine have consistently demonstrated that a moderate dose (5 mg) of epinephrine is superior to the standard dose (1 mg) in augmenting myocardial perfusion.[16] However, it remains unclear whether moderate-dose and high-dose epinephrine enhance long-term survival or neurologic recovery. In addition, high doses of epinephrine may increase cardiac metabolic demand during VF and may even cause recurrent or refractory VF. Therefore, an escalating dosing regimen is advised [see Table 1]. The first dose of epinephrine should be 1 mg, but if this is ineffective, the dose should be increased after 3 minutes to 3 mg, and then, after 3 additional minutes, to 5 mg; a dose of 5 mg should then be repeated every 3 to 5 minutes.

Calcium

Calcium excites the myocardium and has long been advocated as a first-line panacea in all forms of cardiac arrest. Indeed, in the spontaneously beating heart, calcium augments contractile force, facilitates excitation-contraction coupling, and stimulates impulse formation and conduction.[78,79] Unfortunately, the arrested heart, unlike the beating heart, does not respond to infusions of calcium. In clinical trials, calcium has not been effective in patients with PEA, asystole, or VF.[79]

Calcium can also have pernicious effects. After injection of standard doses of calcium, dangerously high serum levels of calcium are frequently observed.[80] Rapid boluses can cause sinus arrest, suppression of normal automaticity, provocation of ventricular ectopy, and cerebrovascular spasm.[80] Hypercalcemia is particularly dangerous in patients receiving digitalis.

Calcium should not be administered routinely in cardiac arrest. With delayed or prolonged resuscitation, however, administration of calcium chloride may be helpful. Investigators have documented a time-dependent state of ionized hypocalcemia that may impede resuscitation.[81,82] Calcium should be administered if hyperkalemia is suspected (e.g., when cardiac arrest occurs in renal failure), if hypocalcemia is suspected, or if patients are receiving calcium channel blockers. Today, there is greater interest in treatment with calcium blockers than in treatment with calcium to promote tissue salvage and to aid in resuscitation.[79,83]

Sodium Bicarbonate

Acidemia is inevitable during prolonged cardiopulmonary arrest. Inadequate ventilation leads to carbon dioxide accumulation. CO_2 then passes readily across biologic membranes into cells. The result is a fall in pH in the cytosol, as predicted by the Henderson-Hasselbalch equation [see I:7 Life-Threatening Acid-Base Disorders]. Metabolic acidosis also occurs during protracted arrest, even if CPR is effective. The critical reduction in delivery of oxygen to tissues leads to anaerobic metabolism and lactic acidosis [see I:7 Life-Threatening Acid-Base Disorders].

Unmitigated acidosis exerts noxious effects on circulation.[84] Acidosis increases pulmonary vascular resistance but causes a loss of vasomotor tone in the peripheral arterial circulation. It causes arteriolar dilatation but venous constriction, leading to capillary stasis. Acidosis attenuates both the vascular and the cardiac responses to circulating adrenergic amines while enhancing the effects of vagal stimulation. Thus, acidosis leads to reduced chronotropy, inotropy, and vascular tone and predisposes to cardiovascular collapse. In addition, a fall in pH is associated with ventricular irritability and a lower threshold for VF.

It is actually the intracellular pH that matters. Therefore, respiratory acidosis is the more critical cause of myocardial dysfunction during cardiopulmonary arrest.[85] Myocardial contractile function is exquisitely sensitive to increases and decreases in arterial carbon dioxide tension because CO_2 enters cells so readily. As intracellular pH falls, myocardial contractile function declines. Thus, hypercapnia and intracellular acidosis are potent negative inotropes that can cause refractory PEA.[64]

The primary treatment of the acidemia that results from cardiac arrest is adequate ventilation, which ensures removal of CO_2. In clinical and animal studies, survival and correction of the pH correlate most closely with adequacy of ventilation.[86]

Traditionally, bicarbonate has also been administered to cardiac arrest victims to correct the base deficit associated with metabolic acidosis. In the myocardium, intracellular hypercapnia is a powerful negative inotrope (see above). In the globally ischemic heart, excessive sodium bicarbonate administration may cause contractile failure, refractory PEA, and a failed resuscitation effort (but only in the absence of adequate ventilation).[85] The second hazard of sodium bicarbonate administration is its hypertonicity. Each 50 mEq ampule of sodium bicarbonate contains 2,000 mOsm of the agent. This hypertonicity reduces aortic vasomotor tone, which, in turn, lowers the coronary arterial perfusion pressure. When coronary perfusion falls, a successful return of a perfusing rhythm is unlikely regardless of the pH achieved. Coronary blood flow—not arterial pH—is the critical factor that determines the success or failure of CPR.[87] No clinical or animal studies have documented that sodium bicarbonate helps in resuscitation ex-

cept in cases of hyperkalemia and of tricyclic antidepressant overdose.[88] There is no evidence that administration of sodium bicarbonate helps manage the pH, improves the rate of defibrillation, or aids resuscitation.

Monitoring pH and Cardiac Output during Resuscitation

Measurements of arterial blood gases are usually considered the best guides for managing acid-base disturbances, and in most clinical circumstances, arterial and venous measurements of pH and carbon dioxide tension (PCO_2) are roughly equivalent.[89] However, cardiopulmonary arrest may be an exception: a striking discordance between venous and arterial blood gas measurements has been uncovered.[85,90] During the initial minutes of cardiac resuscitation, marked mixed venous hypercapnia and acidosis occur routinely. Venous hypercapnia and acidosis probably reflect the production of lactic acid in underperfused tissues and the subsequent generation of new CO_2 as the anaerobically produced lactic acid is buffered by sodium bicarbonate. Venous hypercapnia also reflects venous pooling and impaired pulmonary excretion of CO_2, as a consequence of the drastic fall in cardiac output.

It is interesting to note that the mixed venous hypercapnia and acidosis are selective; that is, they are usually not reflected in the arterial blood. Arterial blood gases often reveal a low PCO_2 and alkalosis if lung ventilation is adequate. Researchers have found venous-arterial PCO_2 gradients of greater than 60 mm Hg.[85]

Arteriovenous differences in pH and PCO_2 may have clinical importance in CPR. Mixed venous blood, with its high PCO_2 and low pH, may reflect tissue hypoperfusion more accurately. Venous pH is also more predictive of the outcome of CPR because it is a marker of both circulatory and ventilatory adequacy. Administration of sodium bicarbonate in an effort to maintain normal arterial blood gases may exacerbate the disparity between arterial and venous pH and PCO_2 in the absence of adequate ventilation.[90]

End-tidal CO_2 monitoring The best and least invasive monitor of the efficacy of CPR is the expired CO_2 concentration because it is an indicator of circulatory delivery of CO_2 to the lung. The end-tidal CO_2 concentration rises and falls with pulmonary blood flow and therefore with cardiac output. End-tidal CO_2 monitoring (also known as capnography) provides continuous measurements of the blood flow generated during CPR, and its utilization correlates directly with increased coronary perfusion and survival.[91] Because end-tidal CO_2 varies not only with pulmonary perfusion but also with alveolar ventilation, sodium bicarbonate load, and carbon dioxide production,[92] it may provide a superb minute-by-minute window on the arrest victim's circulatory function, ventilation, and metabolism. Monitoring the end-tidal CO_2 at the bedside is almost as easy as palpating the carotid pulse; furthermore, the end-tidal CO_2 is a far more accurate measure of blood flow and the efficacy of CPR.

Median-frequency analysis of VF During prolonged VF, myocardial work and oxygen demand continue at nearly the same level as they do during sinus rhythm. Because myocardial blood flow is nil, myocardial oxygen, glucose, and high-energy phosphate stores are rapidly depleted and intracellular lactic acidosis becomes pronounced.[93,94] After a long period of VF, the fibrillatory waveform becomes less coarse. This pattern, often called fine VF, has long been recognized as a marker of a long arrest time[95] and a predictor of a poor outcome. The amplitude of the fibrillatory waves declines linearly as time elapses and signals that the heart is desperately underperfused.

Computer-assisted analyses of the fibrillatory waves have led to useful insights regarding VF. The median frequency of the ECG signals during VF is now recognized as a better marker of downtime and the adequacy of myocardial perfusion.[96] The median frequency of VF correlates with myocardial perfusion and appears to predict accurately the success or failure of electrical defibrillation. The median frequency of the VF tracing can be measured in seconds and may therefore serve as a valuable guide to the timing of defibrillation and the optimal dosing of epinephrine.[97]

Drug Administration: Peripheral, Central, Tracheal, or Cardiac?

A lifeline is essential in CPR. The safest and most expedient access to the circulation is generally considered to be a peripheral antecubital vein. However, medications reach the arterial circulation faster if injected into the internal jugular or subclavian vein. Central venous injections also result in higher peak arterial concentrations.[98] Therefore, central drug administration is recommended. A supradiaphragmatic (subclavian or internal jugular) vein should be cannulated because perfusion to, and drug absorption from, the lower extremities and subdiaphragmatic torso are markedly impaired during CPR.[99] After delivery of each drug, a 20 to 30 ml bolus of fluid should be given to speed delivery to the central circulation.[2]

If vascular access is not feasible, an endotracheal tube provides a satisfactory route for administration of some first-line resuscitation drugs. Most lipophilic drugs, including epinephrine, atropine, lidocaine, diazepam, and naloxone, can be administered by this route. Sodium bicarbonate, calcium, and vasopressors should not be administered intratracheally, because excessive volumes, tissue necrosis, and inactivation of surfactant result. Drug administration by endotracheal (ET) tube takes advantage of the relatively high blood flow to the lungs and the vast (70 m^2) absorptive area of the alveolar-capillary membrane.[100,101]

The pharmacokinetics of endotracheal drugs is best understood in the case of epinephrine. Its absorption is very rapid: peak drug levels and physiologic responses are detected 15 and 120 seconds after injection. Administration into the lungs also provides a beneficial depot effect: 5 minutes after injection of epinephrine, 80% of the initial blood level is still present in circulation. However, the peak blood concentration of epinephrine after ET administration is only 10% of that achieved with an equal I.V. dose.[100,101]

The method of ET drug injection is simple. About 2.5 times the standard I.V. dose (epinephrine, 2 to 5 mg; atropine, 3 mg; lidocaine, 3 mg/kg) should be administered after dilution in 10 ml of distilled water or saline. Shallow instillation is ineffective; the drug must be injected forcibly into a catheter that is placed beyond the distal end of the endotracheal tube and disseminated into the alveolar space by forced manual hyperventilation.[102] The efficacy and risks of endotracheal administration of drugs in patients with parenchymal lung disease are not known.

An alternative route to venous access, used primarily for children, is the tibial bone marrow. A large-bore needle can be inserted directly into the medullary cavity of the tibia in a matter of seconds.[103,104]

ANTIDYSRHYTHMIC AGENTS

Verapamil, lidocaine, and adenosine are the only drugs of value for the acute treatment of cardiac dysrhythmias. Because patients may already be taking oral agents for chronic dysrhythmias, however, it is important to be aware of the actions and side effects of these drugs when treating an individual with an acute dysrhythmia. Antidysrhythmic drugs have been classified on the basis of

their dominant electrophysiologic effect[105]; this classification has been reviewed and placed in a clinical context.[37] Adenosine has a unique receptor that modulates cyclic adenosine monophosphate (cAMP), resulting in cholinergic activity. It is not similar to other antidysrhythmic agents and is therefore unclassified.

Class I Agents (Membrane Active)

Class I agents are fast sodium channel blockers. All class I agents—which include lidocaine, procainamide, quinidine, and disopyramide—are local anesthetics. These agents block the fast inward sodium current and thereby decrease both the amplitude of the action potential, or phase 0 depolarization (see below), and conduction velocity. These agents also depress the rate of spontaneous phase 4 depolarization, or automaticity, and thus are useful for abolishing premature ventricular contractions (PVCs); class I agents are sometimes termed PVC killers.

Because these agents slow the conduction velocity, they can predispose to reentrant cardiac dysrhythmias in some patients.[52,53]

Class II Agents (Beta Blockers)

Class II agents are beta blockers and include such drugs as propranolol. Sympathetic hyperactivity, marked by increased release of catecholamines, is one of the major causes of cardiac dysrhythmias that result from increased automaticity.[52,53,106] Beta-adrenergic blockade has produced a decrease in such automatic dysrhythmias under both clinical and experimental conditions.[106]

Class III Agents (to Prolong Repolarization)

Class III agents, such as bretylium, act directly on the myocardial cell membrane to delay phases 2 and 3 of repolarization and thereby prolong refractoriness. Bretylium is effective in terminating reentrant dysrhythmias because it prolongs the refractory period of the ectopic focus to the point where this region is still unexcitable when an impulse returns to reenter the circuit.[33,34] Bretylium apparently has no effect on either automaticity or conduction velocity.[107]

Class IV Agents (Calcium Channel Blockers)

Class IV agents, of which verapamil is the most effective, block the movement of calcium across the slow calcium channels but have virtually no effect on the so-called fast sodium channels.[105] Because both the SA node and the AV node are composed of slow-response fibers that are activated by the movement of calcium ions across the slow channels, the class IV agents are particularly effective in preventing unwanted supraventricular impulses from reaching the ventricles. Verapamil decreases the conduction velocity through the AV node and increases the refractory period of the AV node.

Class V Agents (Unclassified)

The vagus nerve innervates the SA node, the atria, and the AV node, but it has almost no influence over the His-Purkinje system or ventricular muscle. At therapeutic levels, digitalis has an antidysrhythmic action that is mediated almost exclusively via the vagus nerve. Toxic doses of digitalis, however, may produce an increased automaticity characterized by multifocal premature ventricular depolarizations [*see* Pathophysiology of Cardiac Dysrhythmias, *below*]. Caution must be observed in digitalizing a patient who is prone to atrial dysrhythmias, because digitalis increases atrial excitability and hence increases the risk of atrial ectopy. Because digitalis also induces AV nodal blockade mediated by the vagus nerve, however, any atrial dysrhythmias produced by digitalization will be less clinically significant.[108,109]

Cellular Electrophysiology

Electromechanical activity of all muscle, including the heart, is determined by the concentration and flow of ions, particularly calcium, potassium, and sodium. Knowledge of cardiac electrophysiology can serve as a conceptual framework on which to build a rational therapeutic program. Direct observation of cellular electrical activity using a glass microelectrode reveals that the cell membrane is semipermeable: it permits easy passage of cations such as sodium, potassium, and calcium but provides a barrier to anions such as proteins. Negatively charged intracellular proteins that cannot cross the cell membrane create a transmembrane potential in which the interior of the cell is negatively charged relative to the exterior. The membrane potential of a cell, E_K, is proportional to the difference between the logarithms of the intracellular potassium concentration, $[K]_i$, and the extracellular potassium concentration, $[K]_o$:

$$E_K = c(\log [K]_i - \log [K]_o)$$

The proportionality constant, c, varies with temperature, but at 37° C it is –60 mV. Thus, under physiologic conditions,

$$E_K = -60 \text{ mV} \times \log \frac{[K]_i}{[K]_o}$$

This relation, termed the Nernst equation, can be used to calculate the myocardial cell membrane potential if the potassium concentrations are known. For example, if the potassium concentration is normal—that is, 150 mEq/L intracellularly and 3.8 mEq/L extracellularly—then the membrane potential is

$$E_K = -60 \text{ mV} \times \log \frac{150}{3.8}$$

$$E_K = -90 \text{ mV}$$

If, however, the serum potassium concentration rises to 6.0 mEq/L, then the membrane potential also changes:

$$E_K = -60 \text{ mV} \times \log \frac{150}{6.0}$$

$$E_K = -80 \text{ mV}$$

Thus, the resting membrane potential is determined primarily by the concentration gradient for potassium across the cell membrane. The transmembrane potential can be calculated if the transmembrane potassium concentrations are measured with a glass microelectrode. Under clinical conditions, however, only the serum potassium level can be measured. This value does not provide an adequate guide to the transmembrane electrical voltage, because many physiologic factors are capable of altering the intracellular potassium concentration.[43] Such factors include electrolyte and acid-base balance, the level of osmotic and metabolic activity, and the serum levels of glucose and insulin.

Any factor that causes osmotic movement of water into the cell will produce a decrease in the intracellular potassium concentration. The transmembrane gradients of sodium and calcium are maintained by energy-requiring pumps in the cell membrane. When these pumps are inactivated, as during myocardial ischemia,[42] sodium and calcium can leak into the cell. If, as often occurs, sodium leaks into the cell faster than potassium leaks out, water will be drawn in, producing myocardial edema. Tissue acidosis can also alter the transmembrane potassium gradient. In acidosis, hydrogen ions can leak into the cell in exchange for potassium, thereby decreasing the intracellular potassium concentration and increasing the membrane potential. Variations in glucose transport can also affect the potassium gradient. Under the influence of insulin and epinephrine, glucose may move across the membrane into the myocardial cell, drawing in water by osmosis. The decline in intracellular potassium concentrations stimulates the sodium pump to exchange extracellular potassium for intracellular sodium. Concurrent administration of glucose and insulin is the standard method for treating hyperkalemia because it shifts potassium from the extracellular fluid into the cells.

ACTION POTENTIAL GENERATION

Stimulation of either cardiac muscle or skeletal muscle produces an action potential. Unlike a skeletal muscle action potential, which lasts only several milliseconds, a cardiac action potential may persist for as long as several hundred milliseconds.[110] The standard Purkinje, or ventricular muscle, action potential has five discernible phases [see Figure 16].

Phase 4

In phase 4, the resting membrane potential, or the diastolic potential, of the cell is generated by active metabolic processes that produce substantial transmembrane potassium and sodium gradients. An energy-dependent sodium-potassium pump counteracts a significant influx of sodium and efflux of potassium in the resting cell to maintain this resting membrane potential. As noted, when the extracellular potassium concentration rises from a typical value of 3.8 mEq/L to 6.0 mEq/L, the resting membrane potential increases from –90 mV to –80 mV. This effect would tend to increase automaticity, but it is superseded by the effect of hyperkalemia on the sodium current. A rise in the extracellular potassium level progressively impairs the flux of sodium through sodium-specific channels, leading to an overall decrease in myocardial excitability.

Phase 0

During phase 0, an electrical stimulus causes the sodium-specific fast channels and the calcium-specific slow channels to open, usually for no longer than one millisecond. As positive ions rush in, depolarization occurs as the membrane potential rises to threshold, or –60 mV, and an action potential is generated [see Figure 16]. Under normal physiologic conditions, the stimulus that produces an action potential is electrical, but any stimulus—electrical, physical (such as a precordial thump), or chemical—that depolarizes a membrane to threshold can generate an action potential. There are various abnormalities that can cause the resting membrane potential to move toward threshold. For example, conditions that produce a decrease in energy supply (or, alternatively, an increase in energy demand) will have this effect because energy is required to maintain the potassium and sodium gradients across the resting membrane. Under such conditions, automaticity is enhanced because lesser stimuli can achieve the threshold potential, and the cardiac muscle is said to be hyperexcitable, or irritable.

Phases 1 and 2

Phase 1 is characterized by repolarization to the plateau phase, or phase 2. During phase 2, the slow calcium channels as well as the fast sodium channels are activated, and the membrane potential remains relatively constant for as long as 100 milliseconds.[80] The long duration of this plateau phase is the most dramatic difference that is observed between an action potential in cardiac

Figure 16 **The standard Purkinje (or ventricular muscle) action potential has five distinct phases: phase 0, rapid depolarization; phase 1, early repolarization; phase 2, plateau; phase 3, rapid repolarization; and phase 4, diastole.**

muscle and one in skeletal muscle. During this interval, termed the effective refractory period, the myocardium is relatively refractory to excitation.

Phase 3

During phase 3, potassium channels reopen to promote efflux of potassium from the cell. Rapid repolarization ensues, and the resting membrane potential is reestablished at –90 mV.

Spontaneous Phase 4 Depolarization

Unlike ordinary atrial and ventricular muscle, the Purkinje fibers do not have a stable phase 4 diastolic potential [*see Figure 17*]. Instead, these fibers undergo continuous depolarization during diastole as a result of deactivation of the potassium efflux current.[80,111] If the Purkinje fibers reach the threshold voltage, they will fire an action potential. Under normal conditions, however, the SA and AV nodes exhibit faster diastolic depolarization and reach threshold sooner than the Purkinje fibers. Because the cardiac impulse in the SA node normally reaches threshold first, the SA node typically assumes the pacemaker function of the heart. Premature ventricular contractions develop when a hyperexcitable cell or fiber in ventricular myocardium undergoes rapid diastolic depolarization and reaches threshold before the cells in the SA node. This cell or fiber then assumes the pacemaker function of the heart for that beat. The PVCs that result from such ventricular ectopy can be abolished by overdrive pacing. In this manner, a mechanical pacemaker is used to pace the heart at a rate faster than that of the PVC (i.e., the RR interval is shorter). The artificial device thereby assumes the pacemaker function and regularizes the heart rate, producing a beneficial cosmetic effect on the ECG without altering the hyperexcitability of the diseased cell.

Pathophysiology of Cardiac Dysrhythmias

All dysrhythmias are caused by enhanced automaticity, reentry, or a combination of these two mechanisms.

AUTOMATIC DYSRHYTHMIAS

Any area of myocardial tissue that independently depolarizes, reaches threshold, and fires is termed automatic, and the electrical impulse that activates the adjacent myocardium generates an automatic rhythm. Acute dysrhythmias tend to be automatic; such automatic dysrhythmias are frequently seen in patients in emergency rooms and coronary care units and in patients undergoing operation. Five major clinical phenomena that tend to increase automaticity have been identified: local myocardial hypoxia, hypokalemia, hypercalcemia, increased catecholamine levels, and digitalis administration.

Local Myocardial Hypoxia

Energy-dependent cell membrane pumps maintain the resting membrane potential, and when oxygen supply to myocardial tissue is inadequate because of ischemia, the pumps fail to function properly. Consequently, the potassium gradient declines, and the membrane potential drifts closer toward threshold. Small membrane potential fluctuations or stimuli of less than normal magnitude are then sufficient to bump the membrane potential up to threshold and initiate an action potential. Ventricular muscle cells, not only those cells in specialized conduction tissue, can spontaneously generate electrical fluctuations, or oscillations, in membrane potential [*see* Slow Afterdepolarizations, *below*]. If the resting membrane potential is initially closer to normal because of local myocardial hypoxia, then these spontaneous oscillations are more likely to achieve threshold and fire an action potential.[112]

Hypokalemia

Extracellular hypokalemia increases the resting membrane potential, drawing it further away from threshold and producing hyperpolarization. This effect tends to decrease tissue excitability or automaticity.[112,113] Hypokalemia, however, also increases the size of the sodium channels, thereby promoting more rapid influx of sodium during phase 0. Because the net result of hypokalemia is increased automaticity, the effect of hypokalemia on sodium influx appears to override its effect on membrane hyperpolarization. Hypokalemia is one of the most easily treated (and overtreated) forms of hyperexcitability.

Hypercalcemia

Calcium is a potent inotropic agent, mediating the interaction between actin and myosin that produces muscle contraction.[80]

Figure 17 **In normal cardiac Purkinje fibers, the membrane potential does not remain flat during phase 4 but instead rises gradually. This spontaneous phase 4 depolarization is the result of a resting potassium current.**

High extracellular calcium levels may cause myocardial work to exceed the energy supply and thus impair the function of the membrane pump. As a result, the resting membrane potential drifts up toward threshold, enhancing automaticity. Excess calcium also appears to promote spontaneous oscillations in membrane potential [see Slow Afterdepolarizations, below].[114] Because of calcium's inotropic effect, such oscillations are accompanied by muscle activity.

Elevated Catecholamine Levels

Increased catecholamine levels also appear to predispose to automaticity, as evidenced by a significant increase in the incidence of multiple premature ventricular contractions reported in patients who have been infused with high doses of catecholamines, such as epinephrine or dopamine. Catecholamines increase both heart rate and contractility. As with hypercalcemia, elevated catecholamine levels may increase cardiac work beyond the limits of energy supply and cause the membrane potential to move closer to threshold. This effect on the energy-dependent membrane pumps has been observed in isolated preparations of Purkinje muscle fibers. The addition of catecholamines to preparations of Purkinje muscle fibers has decreased the outward potassium current to the point that the resting membrane potential was shifted as much as 25 mV toward depolarization, enhancing automaticity.[80,111] In addition to affecting the operation of the membrane pumps, catecholamines can also produce large spontaneous oscillations in membrane voltage.[80,114] Catecholamines are elaborated endogenously; a patient who is in pain, for example, may be releasing large amounts of epinephrine into his or her own circulation. In such cases, morphine can be used effectively as an antidysrhythmic agent.[115]

Drugs

Digitalis is the prototypical cardiac stimulant. Typically, any agent other than oxygen that causes the heart to pump harder and faster also increases cardiac excitability. Digitalis toxicity can produce diffuse myocardial hyperexcitability, manifested by automatic ventricular ectopy. In this condition, the cardiac impulse originates from multiple sites in the ventricle. In patients with ventricular ectopy caused by digitalis intoxication, the QRS complex has an altered morphology, and multifocal PVCs are apparent on the ECG—the classic multifocal ectopy of digitalis toxicity [see Figure 18].[116-118]

Figure 18 ECG demonstrates multifocal PVCs, indicating a diffuse hyperexcitability of the ventricles. Such hyperexcitability may arise from a metabolic abnormality such as hypokalemia or a pharmacologic cause such as digitalis toxicity.

REENTRANT DYSRHYTHMIAS

In the normally functioning heart, the rich cell-cell conduction pathways promote uniform activation of the atria or ventricles in waves. Because activation occurs by means of large electrical wave fronts and because all cardiac tissue has a long refractory period, it is highly unlikely that any cells remain excitable at the completion of each beat. However, disorders such as myocardial ischemia, fibrosis, and necrosis slow electrical conduction and also produce nonconductive areas that interrupt the normal electrical wavefront.[119] These conditions set up one of the requirements for reentry: areas of differential myocardial repolarization.[120]

A circuit whose length exceeds the length of the reentrant impulse circuit is required for the initiation of reentry of continuous conduction; such a circuit may develop because of anatomic or physiologic heterogeneity in myocardial tissue.[119,120] Slow conduction, a shortened refractory period, and anatomic heterogeneity all favor reentry [see Figure 19]. The circuit wavelength of an impulse is the product of the conduction velocity and the duration of the longest refractory period in the circuit.[121] For example, for normal myocardium, the conduction velocity is 200 cm/sec and the refractory period is 0.4 second; therefore, the circuit length for a normally conducted myocardial impulse would have to be 80 cm. Because the reentrant circuit would have to be extraordinarily tortuous to encompass 80 cm, it

Figure 19 Schematic diagram portrays a conceptual framework for understanding the generation of reentrant dysrhythmias. In normal conduction (a), as in sinus rhythm or ventricular pacing, an impulse is propagated along two different anatomic pathways and is extinguished at the bottom. In b, one pathway has a region of slow conduction (red area), which results in a rate-dependent block. In c, the impulse is also blocked in the right limb (red area), but it travels over the alternative pathway sufficiently slowly (zigzag line) for the origin to be able to repolarize before the initial impulse returns; the conducted impulse then depolarizes the origin and reenters the circuit.

Figure 20 In electrophysiologic testing, the electrical complexes are spread out to facilitate the recognition of ventricular electrical morphology. In panel *a,* critically timed paced stimuli capture one ventricle, but when pacing is stopped, the rhythm reverts to sinus rhythm. In panel *b,* critically timed paced stimuli achieve rate-dependent block in one arm of a reentrant circuit. When the activation wave front returns to the origin, this tissue is no longer refractory and undergoes depolarization. With reexcitation, the conditions for reentry are met, and the impulse continues after pacing stops.

would appear that concomitant slow conduction is essentially mandatory to shorten the circuit wavelength and permit initiation of a reentrant dysrhythmia. Regions such as the AV and SA nodes normally exhibit slow conduction, and therefore, any disturbance that produces minor additional slowing in these areas predisposes to reentry. It has also been suggested that extreme anatomic heterogeneity might permit microreentry.[120] For example, a tortuous path over stunned, slowly conducting ventricular muscle in an individual with heterogeneous myocardial infarction might achieve the prerequisites for reentry.

In vitro studies have investigated physiologic factors that might produce changes in conduction and excitability that predispose to reentrant dysrhythmias. For example, abnormal conduction has been observed in a Purkinje network subjected to local changes in potassium concentration.[110,115] The decrease in conduction velocity can vary in different areas of the Purkinje network, leading to functional conduction block.[112,113] In T- or X-shaped Purkinje preparations, the impulses were observed either to summate electrically or, conversely, to inhibit each other when they arrived at the same junction simultaneously. It is difficult to study the cardiac microenvironment in living animals or humans, but in these studies,[122] the Purkinje network was subjected to potassium fluctuations that certainly occur during induced cardioplegia and that may well exist in cases of myocardial ischemia that lead to the formation of necrotic areas adjacent to healthy cells.

Electrophysiologic testing with programmed stimulation in a patient with a history of cardiac dysrhythmias can reveal whether latent substrates of reentry are present. Because organized ventricular reentry does not occur in normal myocardium, all reentrant dysrhythmias, whether they are induced or spontaneous, are pathologic. Rapidly paced stimuli may provoke a decrease in action potential duration and shorten refractoriness in myocardium in which the conduction velocity has already been reduced. Critically timed premature paced stimuli may then penetrate selective zones of myocardium, leading to a reentrant dysrhythmia

[*see Figure 20*].[123] A ventricular tachydysrhythmia that can be induced by programmed stimulation carries an ominous prognosis unless it can be abolished by pharmacotherapy or operation.[123]

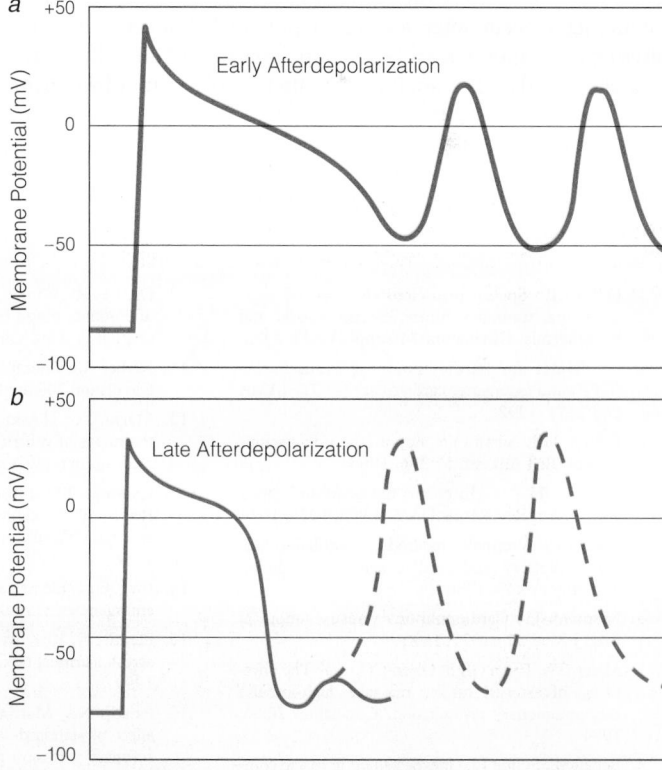

Figure 21 Membrane oscillatory instability may be manifested by either (*a*) early afterdepolarizations or (*b*) late afterdepolarizations. If the late afterdepolarizations achieve the threshold voltage, they can fire an action potential (dotted lines).

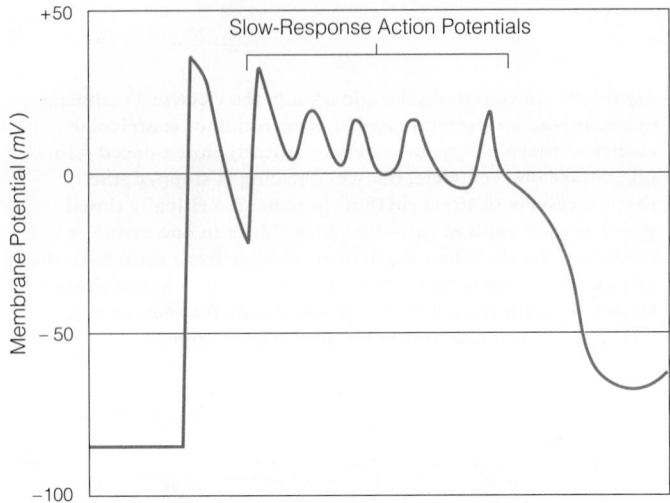

Figure 22 **Early afterdepolarizations may lead to slow-response action potentials. If any of these potentials reach threshold, they may lead to either organized electrical activity (premature ventricular depolarization) or disorganized electrical activity (fibrillation).**

SLOW AFTERDEPOLARIZATIONS

Damaged atrial and ventricular muscle exhibits resting membrane potential instability.[124] The oscillations in membrane potential may at times be large enough to raise the membrane voltage to threshold level and fire. The phenomenon of oscillatory instability, which was first recognized in the 1940s,[125] is now thought to play an important role in the genesis of cardiac dysrhythmias. Injury,[124] elevated calcium levels,[110] digitalis,[116,117] and catecholamines all promote membrane oscillatory instability, which may be manifested as either early or late afterdepolarizations. Both phenomena occur after an action potential; however, an early afterdepolarization occurs before repolarization of the cell, whereas a late afterdepolarization occurs after repolarization [*see Figure 21*]. Both early and late afterdepolarizations may be followed by extreme membrane oscillatory instability that leads to slow-response action potentials [*see Figure 22*]. If any of these slow potentials reach threshold, they may result in either organized electrical activity (premature ventricular depolarization) or disorganized electrical activity (fibrillation).

The recognition of slow potentials, depressed fast responses, and very slow conduction was originally based on in vitro studies of cardiac tissue.[126] For example, bathing superfused Purkinje fibers in a solution with a high potassium concentration inactivates the fast sodium channels and markedly alters normal phase 0 depolarization. Under such circumstances, slow potentials that were less than 80 mV in amplitude, that depolarized at a rate of 1 to 2 V/sec, and that lasted for up to 1 second were observed.[115,126] The amplitude and the overshoot of these slow potentials could be magnified by increasing the extracellular calcium concentration and could be abolished by adding manganese, an agent that blocks the slow calcium channels. These results suggested that the slow potentials were mediated by the slow calcium channels rather than by the fast sodium channels responsible for routine phase 0 depolarization. Although extraordinary nonphysiologic conditions are employed to induce such slow potentials in the laboratory, the myocardial microenvironment during the peri-infarction and postinfarction periods as well as after cardioplegia may well be bizarre. For example, even after extensive myocardial infarction, there are often healthy Purkinje fibers overlying areas of damaged, ischemic myocardium.[127] Slow conduction and slow potentials are characteristic of stunned myocardium.[128,129]

Slow potentials have been incriminated in the generation of reentrant dysrhythmias for three reasons: (1) because they are caused by an active calcium influx that produces 40 to 80 mV depolarizations, they may be conducted long distances; (2) because the conduction velocity may be 1,000 times slower than normal, the circuit wavelength is reduced accordingly; and (3) because slow potentials leave a long refractory wake, they set up zones of functional conduction block.[128,129]

References

1. Ornato JP: Special resuscitation situations: near drowning, traumatic injury, electric shock, and hypothermia. Circulation 74(suppl IV):23, 1986

2. Guidelines for cardiopulmonary resuscitation (CPR) and emergency cardiac care (ECC). JAMA 268:2171, 1992

3. Boidin MP: Airway patency in the unconscious patient. Br J Anaesth 57:306, 1985

4. Comroe JH: ". . . In comes the good air" (pts 1 and 2). Am Rev Respir Dis 119:803, 1025, 1979

5. Melker RJ: Alternative methods of ventilation during respiratory and cardiac arrest. Circulation 74(suppl IV):63, 1986

6. Niemann JT: Cardiopulmonary resuscitation. N Engl J Med 327:1075, 1992

7. Maier GW, Tyson GS Jr, Olsen CO, et al: The physiology of external cardiac massage: high-impulse cardiopulmonary resuscitation. Circulation 70:86, 1984

8. Bedell SE, Fulton EJ: Unexpected findings and complications at autopsy after cardiopulmonary resuscitation (CPR). Arch Intern Med 146:1725, 1986

9. Powner DJ, Holcombe PA, Mello LA: Cardiopulmonary resuscitation–related injuries. Crit Care Med 12:54, 1984

10. Ditchey RV, Winkler JV, Rhodes CA: Relative lack of coronary blood flow during closed-chest resuscitation in dogs. Circulation 66:297, 1982

11. Kerber RE: Energy requirements for defibrillation. Circulation 74(suppl IV):117, 1986

12. Martin TG, Hawkins NS, Weigel JA, et al: Initial treatment of ventricular fibrillation: defibrillation or drug therapy. Am J Emerg Med 6:113, 1988

13. Cummins RO: From concept to standard-of-care? Review of the clinical experience with automated external defibrillators. Ann Emerg Med 18:1269, 1989

14. Ewy GA: Electrical therapy for cardiovascular emergencies. Circulation 74(suppl IV):111, 1986

15. Paradis N, Koscove EM: Epinephrine in cardiac arrest: a critical review. Ann Emerg Med 19:1288, 1990

16. Paradis NA, Martin GB, Rosenberg J, et al: The effect of standard- and high-dose epinephrine on coronary perfusion pressure during prolonged cardiopulmonary resuscitation. JAMA 265:1139, 1991

17. Jaffe AS: The use of antiarrhythmics in advanced cardiac life support. Ann Emerg Med 22:307, 1991

18. Wesely RC, Resh W, Zimmerman D: Reconsiderations of the routine and preferential use of lidocaine in the emergent treatment of ventricular arrhythmias. Crit Care Med 19:1439, 1991

19. Weaver WD, Fahrenbruch CE, Johnson DD, et al: Effect of epinephrine and lidocaine therapy on outcome after cardiac arrest due to ventricular fibrillation. Circulation 82:2027, 1990

20. Williams ML, Woelfel A, Cascio WE, et al: Intravenous amiodarone during prolonged resuscitation from cardiac arrest. Ann Intern Med 110:839, 1989

21. Cummins RO, Austin D Jr: The frequency of 'occult' ventricular fibrillation masquerading as a flat line in prehospital cardiac arrest. Ann Emerg Med 17:813, 1988

22. Koehler RC, Michael JR, Guerci AD, et al: Beneficial effect of epinephrine infusion on cerebral and myocardial blood flows during CPR. Ann Emerg Med 14:744, 1985

23. Paradis NA, Martin GB, Rivers EP, et al: Coronary perfusion pressure and the return of spontaneous circulation in human cardiopulmonary resuscitation. JAMA 263:1106, 1990

24. Bertolet BD, McMurtrie EB, Hill JA, et al: Theophylline for the treatment of atrioventricular block after myocardial infarction. Ann Intern Med 123:509, 1995

25. Ewy GA: Ventricular fibrillation masquerading as asystole. Ann Emerg Med 13:811, 1984

26. Cummins RO, Graves JR, Larsen MP, et al: Out-of-hospital transcutaneous pacing by emergency medical technicians in patients with asystolic cardiac arrest. N Engl J Med 328:1377, 1993

27. Bocka JJ, Overton DT, Hauser A: Electromechanical dissociation in human beings: an echocardiographic evaluation. Ann Emerg Med 17:450, 1988

28. Paradis NA, Martin GB, Goetting MG, et al: Aortic pressure during human cardiac arrest: identification of pseudo-electromechanical dissociation. Chest 101:123, 1992

29. Brown CG, Werman HA: Adrenergic agonists during cardiopulmonary resuscitation. Resuscitation 19:1, 1990

30. Keenan RL, Boyan CP: Cardiac arrest due to anesthesia: a study of incidence and causes. JAMA 253:2373, 1985

31. Bedell SE, Deitz DC, Leeman D, et al: Incidence and characteristics of preventable iatrogenic cardiac arrests. JAMA 265:2815, 1991

32. Franklin C, Mathew J: Developing strategies to prevent inhospital cardiac arrest: analyzing responses of physicians and nurses in the hours before the event. Crit Care Med 22:244, 1994

33. Cannom DS, Prystowsky EN: Management of ventricular arrhythmias: detection, drugs and devices. JAMA 281:172, 1999

34. Reiffel JA: Selecting an antiarrhythmic agent for atrial fibrillation should be a patient-specific, data-driven decision. Am J Cardiol 82:72N, 1998

35. Harken AH, Honigman B, VanWay CW III: Cardiac dysrhythmias in the acute setting: recognition and treatment or anyone can treat cardiac dysrhythmias. J Emerg Med 5:129, 1987

36. Raichlen JS, Campbell FW, Edie RN, et al: Effect of the site of placement of temporary epicardial pacemakers on ventricular function in patients undergoing cardiac surgery. Circulation 70:I, 1984

37. Sarubbi B, Ducceschi V, D'Andrea A, et al: Atrial fibrillation: what are the effects of drug therapy on the effectiveness and complications of electrical cardioversion? Can J Cardiol 14:1267, 1998

38. Bigger JT Jr: Epidemiological and mechanistic studies of atrial fibrillation as a basis for treatment strategies. Circulation 98:943, 1998

39. Botto GL, Bonini W, Broffoni T: Modulation of ventricular rate in permanent atrial fibrillation: randomized, crossover study of the effects of slow-release formulations of gallopamil, diltiazem, or verapamil. Clin Cardiol 11:837, 1998

40. Glatter KA, Cheng J, Dorostkar P, et al: Electrophysiologic effects of adenosine in patients with supraventricular tachycardia. Circulation 99:1034, 1999

41. Tracy WR, Magee W, Masamune H, et al: Selective activation of adenosine A3 receptors with N6-(C3-chlorobenzyl)-5'-N-methylcarboxamideoadenosine (CB-MECA) provides cardioprotection via KATP channel activation. Cardiovasc Res 40:138, 1998

42. Zumino AP, Baiardi G, Schanne OF, et al: Differential electrophysiologic effects of global and regional ischemia and reperfusion in perfused rat hearts. Effects of Mg^{2+} concentration. Mol Cell Biochem 186:79, 1998

43. Siddiqui MN, Zafar H, Alvi R, et al: Hypomagnesaemia in postoperative patients: an important contributing factor in postoperative mortality. Int J Clin Pract 52:265, 1998

44. Hobbs WJ, Fitchet A, Cotter L: Atrial arrhythmias after cardiac surgery. N Engl J Med 337:860, 1997

45. Gonzalez ER, Kannewurf BS, Ornato JP: Intravenous amiodarone for ventricular arrhythmias: overview and clinical use. Resuscitation 39:33, 1998

46. Drouin E, Lande G, Charpentier F: Amiodarone reduces transmural heterogeneity of repolarization in the human heart. J Am Coll Cardiol 32:1063, 1998

47. Kowey PR, Marinchak RA, Rials SJ, et al: Intravenous amiodarone. J Am Coll Cardiol 29:1190, 1997

48. Vorperian VR, Havighurst TC, Miller S, et al: Adverse effects of low-dose amiodarone: a meta-analysis. J Am Coll Cardiol 30:791, 1997

49. Joglar JA, Page RL: Treatment of cardiac arrhythmias during pregnancy: safety considerations. Drug Saf 20:85, 1999

50. Cardosi RJ, Chez RA: Magnesium sulfate, maternal hypothermia, and fetal bradycardia with loss of heart rate variability. Obstet Gynecol 92:691, 1998

51. Hamersley SL, Landy HJ, O'Sullivan MJ: Fetal bradycardia secondary to magnesium sulfate therapy for preterm labor. A case report. J Reprod Med 43:206, 1998

52. Hohnloser SH: Proarrhythmia with class III antiarrhythmic drugs: types, risks, and management. Am J Cardiol 80:82G, 1997

53. Sager PT: New advances in class III antiarrhythmic drug therapy. Curr Opin Cardiol 14:15, 1999

54. Negovsky VA: Reanimatology today: some scientific and philosophic considerations. Crit Care Med 10:130, 1982

55. Cummins RO, Eisenberg MS: Prehospital cardiopulmonary resuscitation: is it effective? JAMA 253:2408, 1985

56. Eisenberg MS, Bergner L, Hallstrom A: Survivors of out-of-hospital cardiac arrest: morbidity and long-term survival. Am J Emerg Med 2:189, 1984

57. Taffet GE, Teasdale TA, Luchi RJ: In-hospital cardiopulmonary resuscitation. JAMA 260:2069, 1988

58. Lowenstein SR, Sabyan EM, Lassen CF, et al: Benefits of training physicians in advanced cardiac life support. Chest 89:512, 1986

59. Skovron ML, Goldberg E, Suljaga-Petchel K: Factors predicting survival for six months after cardiopulmonary resuscitation: multivariate analysis of a prospective study. Mt Sinai J Med 52:271, 1985

60. Office of Technology Assessment: Life-sustaining technologies in the elderly. OTA-BA-306. US Congress, 1987, p 167

61. Murphy DJ, Murray AM, Robinson BE, et al: Outcomes of cardiopulmonary resuscitation in the elderly. Ann Intern Med 111:199, 1989

62. Schiedermayer DL: The decision to forgo CPR in the elderly patient. JAMA 260:2096, 1988

63. Kouwenhoven WB, Jude JR, Knickerbocker GG: Closed-chest cardiac massage. JAMA 173:1064, 1960

64. Chandra NC: Mechanisms of blood flow during CPR. Ann Emerg Med 22:281, 1993

65. Steen-Hansen JE, Hansen NN, Vaagenes P, et al: Pupil size and light reactivity during cardiopulmonary resuscitation: a clinical study. Crit Care Med 16:69, 1988

66. Grundler W, Weil MH, Rackow EC: Effects of volume expansion on reversal of electromechanical dissociation. Chest 86:282, 1984

67. Cohen TJ, Tucker KJ, Lurie KG, et al: Active compression-decompression: a new method of cardiopulmonary resuscitation. Cardiopulmonary Resuscitation Working Group. JAMA 267:2916, 1992

68. Cohen TJ, Goldner BG, Maccaro PC, et al: A comparison of active compression-decompression cardiopulmonary resuscitation with standard cardiopulmonary resuscitation for cardiac arrests occurring in the hospital. N Engl J Med 329:1918, 1993

69. Schwab TM, Callaham ML, Madsen CD, et al: A randomized clinical trial of active compression-decompression CPR vs standard CPR in out-of-hospital cardiac arrest in two cities. JAMA 273:1261, 1995

70. Kerber RE: Electrical treatment of cardiac arrhythmias: defibrillation and cardioversion. Ann Emerg Med 22:296, 1993

71. Greenberg MI: Drug selection and delivery in cardiopulmonary resuscitation. Am J Emerg Med 2:457, 1984

72. Crile G, Dolley DH: Experimental resuscitation of dogs killed by anesthetics and asphyxia. J Exp Med 6:713, 1906

73. Redding JS, Pearson JW: Evaluation of drugs for cardiac resuscitation. Anesthesiology 24:203, 1963

74. Brown CG, Werman HA, Davis EA, et al: The effect of high-dose phenylephrine versus epinephrine on regional cerebral blood flow during CPR. Ann Emerg Med 16:743, 1987

75. Callaham M, Madsen CD, Barton CW, et al: A randomized clinical trial of high-dose epinephrine and norepinephrine vs standard-dose epinephrine in prehospital cardiac arrest. JAMA 268:2667, 1992

76. Brown CG, Martin DR, Pepe PE, et al: A comparison of standard-dose and high-dose epinephrine in cardiac arrest outside the hospital. Multicenter High-Dose Epinephrine Study Group. N Engl J Med 327:1051, 1992

77. Stiell IG, Hebert PC, Weitzman BN, et al: High-dose epinephrine in adult cardiac arrest. N Engl J Med 327:1045, 1992

78. Hughes WG, Ruedy JR: Should calcium be used in cardiac arrest? Am J Med 81:285, 1986

79. Thompson BM, Steuven HS, Tonsfeldt DJ, et al: Calcium: limited indications, some danger. Circulation 74(suppl IV):90, 1986

80. Meldrum DR, Cleveland JC Jr, Rowland RT, et al: Cardiac surgical implications of calcium dyshomeostasis in the heart. Ann Thorac Surg 61:1273, 1996

81. Urban P, Scheidegger D, Buchmann B, et al: Cardiac arrest and blood ionized calcium levels. Ann Intern Med 109:110, 1988

82. Katz AM: Is calcium beneficial or deleterious in patients with cardiac arrest? Ann Intern Med 109:91, 1988

83. White BC, Winegar CD, Wilson RF, et al: Possible role of calcium blockers in cerebral resuscitation: a review of the literature and synthesis for future studies. Crit Care Med 11:202, 1983

84. Narins RG, Cohen JJ: Bicarbonate therapy for organic acidosis: the case for its continued use. Ann Intern Med 106:615, 1987

85. Weil MH, Rackow EC, Trevino R, et al: Difference in acid-base state between venous and arterial blood during cardiopulmonary resuscitation. N Engl J Med 315:153, 1986

86. Bishop RL, Weisfeldt ML: Sodium bicarbonate administration during cardiac arrest: effect on arterial pH, P_{CO_2} and osmolality. JAMA 235:506, 1976

87. Weisfeldt ML, Guerci AD: Sodium bicarbonate in CPR. JAMA 266:2129, 1991

88. Planta M, Bar-Joseph G, Wiklund L, et al: Pathophysiologic and therapeutic implications of acid-base changes during CPR. Ann Emerg Med 22:404, 1993

89. Relman AS: "Blood gases": arterial or venous? (editorial). N Engl J Med 315:188, 1986

90. Adrogue HJ, Rashad MN, Gorin AB, et al: Assessing acid-base status in circulatory failure: differences between arterial and central venous blood. N Engl J Med 320:1312, 1989

91. Gudipati CV, Weil MH, Bisera J, et al: Expired carbon dioxide: a noninvasive monitor of cardiopulmonary resuscitation. Circulation 77:234, 1988

92. Falk JL, Rackow EC, Weil MH: End-tidal carbon dioxide concentration during cardiopulmonary resuscitation. N Engl J Med 318:607, 1988

93. Kern KB, Garewal HS, Sanders AB, et al: Depletion of myocardial adenosine triphosphate during prolonged untreated ventricular fibrillation: effect on defibrillation success. Resuscitation 20:221, 1990

94. Neumar RW, Brown CG, Van Ligten P, et al: Estimation of myocardial ischemic injury during ventricular fibrillation with total circulatory arrest using high-energy phosphates and lactate as metabolic markers. Ann Emerg Med 20:222, 1991

95. Weaver WD, Cobb LA, Dennis D, et al: Amplitude of ventricular fibrillation waveform and outcome after cardiac arrest. Ann Intern Med 102:53, 1985

96. Brown CG, Griffith RF, Van Ligten P, et al: Median frequency—a new parameter for predicting defibrillation success rate. Ann Emerg Med 20:787, 1991

97. Brown CG, Dzwonczyk R, Martin DR: Physiologic measurement of the ventricular fibrillation ECG signal: estimating the duration of ventricular fibrillation. Ann Emerg Med 22:70, 1993

98. Talit U, Braun S, Halkin H, et al: Pharmacokinetic differences between peripheral and central drug administration during cardiopulmonary resuscitation. J Am Coll Cardiol 6:1073, 1985

99. Emerman CL, Bellon EM, Lukens TW, et al: A prospective study of femoral versus subclavian vein catheterization during cardiac arrest. Ann Emerg Med 19:26, 1990

100. Greenberg MI, Roberts JR, Baskin SI, et al: The use of endotracheal medication in cardiac emergencies. Emergency Medicine Annual 2:91, 1983

101. Hasegawa EA: The endotracheal use of emergency drugs. Heart Lung 15:60, 1986

102. Gonzalez ER: Pharmacologic controversies in CPR. Ann Emerg Med 22:317, 1993

103. Rosetti VA, Thompson BM, Miller J, et al: Intraosseous infusion: an alternative route of pediatric intravascular access. Ann Emerg Med 14:885, 1985

104. Iserson KV, Criss E: Intraosseous infusions: a usable technique. Am J Emerg Med 4:540, 1986

105. The Sicilian gambit: a new approach to the classification of antiarrhythmic drugs based on their actions on arrhythmogenic mechanisms. Task Force of the Working Group on Arrhythmias of the European Society of Cardiology. Circulation 84:1831, 1991

106. Brodsky MA, Orlov MV, Allen BJ, et al: Clinical assessment of adrenergic tone and responsiveness to beta-blocker therapy in patients with symptomatic ventricular tachycardia and no apparent structural heart disease. Am Heart J 131:51, 1996

107. Kowey PR, Marinchak RA, Rials SJ, et al: Pharmacologic and pharmacokinetic profile of class III antiarrhythmic drugs. Am J Cardiol 80:16G, 1997

108. Stafford RS, Robson DC, Misra B, et al: Rate controls and sinus rhythm maintenance in atrial fibrillation: national trends in medication use, 1980-1996. Arch Intern Med 158:2144, 1998

109. Van Gelder IC, Brugemann J, Crijns HJ: Current treatment recommendations in antiarrhythmic therapy. Drugs 55:331, 1998

110. Uchida T, Yashima M, Gotoh M, et al: Mechanism of acceleration of functional reentry in the ventricle: effects of ATP-sensitive potassium channel opener. Circulation 99:704, 1999

111. Cleveland JC Jr, Meldrum DR, Rowland RT, et al: Optimal myocardial preservation: cooling, cardioplegia, and conditioning. Ann Thorac Surg 61:760, 1996

112. Janse MJ: Why does atrial fibrillation occur? Eur Heart J 18(suppl C):C12, 1997

113. Yue L, Feng J, Gaspo R, et al: Ionic remodeling underlying action potential changes in a canine model of atrial fibrillation. Circ Res 81:512, 1997

114. Priebe L, Beuckelmann DJ: Simulation study of cellular electric properties in heart failure. Circ Res 82:1206, 1998

115. Levi AJ, Dalton GR, Hancox JC, et al: Role of intracellular sodium overload in the genesis of cardiac arrhythmias. J Cardiovasc Electrophysiol 8:700, 1997

116. Riaz K, Forker AD: Digoxin use in congestive heart failure. Current status. Drugs 55:747, 1998

117. Reddy S, Benatar D, Gheorghiade M: Update on digoxin and other oral positive inotropic agents for chronic heart failure. Curr Opin Cardiol 12:233, 1997

118. Umans VA, Cornel JH, Hic C: Digoxin in patients with heart failure. N Engl J Med 337:129, 1997

119. Patterson E, Kalcich M, Scherlag BJ: Phase 1B ventricular arrhythmia in the dog: localized reentry with the mid-myocardium. J Interv Card Electrophysiol 2:145, 1998

120. Boineau JP, Cox JL: Slow ventricular activation in acute myocardial infarction: source of reentrant premature ventricular contractions. Circulation 48:702, 1973

121. Swynghedaauw B: Molecular mechanisms of myocardial remodeling. Physiol Rev 79:215, 1999

122. Koning MMG, Gho BCG, Klaarwater EV, et al: Rapid ventricular pacing produces myocardial protection by nonischemic activation of K+-ATP channels. Circulation 93:178, 1996

123. Kastor JA, Horowitz LN, Harken AH, et al: Clinical electrophysiology of ventricular tachycardia. N Engl J Med 304:1004, 1981

124. Yamabe H, Okumura K, Misumi I, et al: Role of bipolar electrogram polarity mapping in localizing recurrent conduction in the isthmus early and late

after ablation of atrial flutter. J Am Coll Cardiol 33:39, 1999

125. Bozler E: The initiation of the cardiac impulse. Am J Physiol 138:273, 1943

126. Carmeliet EE, Vereecke J: Adrenaline and the plateau phase of the cardiac action potential. Pflugers Arch 313:303, 1969

127. Friedman P, Stewarts J, Fenoglio J: Survival of subendocardial Purkinje fibers after extensive myocardial infarction in dogs. Circ Res 33:597, 1973

128. Masui A, Tamura K, Tarumi N, et al: Resolution of late potentials with improvement of left ventricular systolic pressure in patients with first myocardial infarction. Clin Cardiol 20:466, 1997

129. Ferrari R, Pepi P, Ferrari F, et al: Metabolic derangement in ischemic heart disease and its therapeutic control. Am J Cardiol 82:2K, 1998

130. Pires LA, Lehmann MH, Steinman RT, et al: Sudden death in implantable cardioverter-defibrillator recipients: clinical context, arrhythmic events and device responses. J Am Coll Cardiol 33:24, 1999

131. Yee R, Connolly SJ, Gillis AM: Appropriate use of the implantable cardioverter defibrillator: a Canadian perspective. Canadian Working Group on Cardiac Pacing. Pacing Clin Electrophysiol 22:1, 1999

132. Swygman CA, Homoud MK, Link MS, et al: Technologic advances in implantable cardioverter defibrillators. Curr Opin Cardiol 14:9, 1999

133. Grimm W, Menz V, Hoffmann J, et al: Complications of third generation implantable cardioverter defibrillator therapy. Pacing Clin Electrophysiol 22:201, 1999

134. Pauli P, Wiedemann G, Dengler W, et al: Anxiety in patients with an automatic implantable cardioverter defibrillator: what differentiates them from panic patients? Psychosom Med 61:69, 1999

135. Anvari A, Gottsauner-Wolf M, Turel Z, et al: Predictors of outcome in patients with implantable cardioverter defibrillators. Cardiology 90:180, 1998

136. Movsowitz C, Marchlinski FE: Interactions between implantable cardioverter-defibrillators and class III agents. Am J Cardiol 82:41I, 1998

137. Dorian P, Newman D, Greene M: Implantable defibrillators and/or amiodarone: alternatives or complementary therapies. Int J Clin Pract 52:425, 1998

Acknowledgment

Figures 1 through 10   Carol Donner.

2 TRAUMA RESUSCITATION

Frederick A. Moore, M.D., and Ernest E. Moore, M.D.

Initial Approach to the Critically Injured Patient

Salvage of the critically injured is optimized by a coordinated team effort in an organized trauma system. Management of life-threatening injuries must be decided according to physiologic necessity for survival; that is, active efforts to support airway, breathing, and circulation (the ABCs) are usually initiated before specific diagnosis. This chapter presents a systematic approach to severely injured patients within the so-called golden hour. The discussion is divided into prehospital care and emergency department management; the ED component is further divided into (1) primary survey and initial resuscitation, (2) evaluation, with continuation of resuscitation, and (3) secondary survey and definitive diagnosis.

Prehospital Care

Resuscitation and evaluation of trauma patients begin at the injury site. Prehospital care and hospital destination are much different from those of the medical arrest victim. Whereas provision of advanced cardiac life support (ACLS) at the scene clearly improves survival for the medical patient,[1] the goal in trauma is to get the *right patient to the right hospital at the right time*. First responders (typically, firefighters and police) provide rapid basic trauma life support (BTLS) and are followed by paramedics and flight nurses with advanced skills. Medical control is ensured by preestablished field protocols, radio communication with a base hospital physician, and subsequent trip audits. Management priorities of BTLS on the scene are to (1) assess and control the scene for the safety of the patient and the prehospital care provider, (2) tamponade external hemorrhage with direct pressure, (3) protect the spine after blunt trauma, (4) supplement inspired oxygen, (5) extricate the patient, and (6) stabilize long bone fractures. Active airway support is a major asset of advanced trauma life support (ATLS) in prehospital systems, achieved with skilled paramedics under close medical control.[2] However, the value of intravenous fluid administration in such systems remains controversial.[3-5] The heart of the controversy is whether it is preferable (1) to give fluids until a normal blood pressure is reached, thus causing hemodilution and disruption of early hemostatic clots, or (2) to withhold resuscitation, thus prolonging cellular shock, which may become irreversible by the time operative control is accomplished. The compromise between these two approaches is moderate volume loading.[5-8]

Application of the pneumatic antishock garment (PASG) is warranted for active hemorrhage caused by major pelvic fractures and may be appropriate for profound shock if transport time is expected to exceed 30 minutes.[6,9,10] In any situation, implementation of

ATLS depends on the expertise of field personnel, the patient's condition, and the distance to the hospital.[11-13]

Prehospital trauma scores have been devised to identify critically injured trauma victims, who represent about 10% to 15% of all injured patients. When it is geographically and logistically feasible, critically injured patients should be taken directly to a designated level I facility (i.e., an Urban Regional Trauma Center) or to a level II facility (i.e., a Rural Regional Trauma Center). The currently available field trauma scores, however, are imperfect for identifying critically injured patients.[14] A 25% over-triage is probably necessary to capture most of the patients with life-threatening injury. Advance transmission of key patient information to the receiving trauma center facilitates organization of the trauma team and ensures availability of ancillary services.

Emergency Department Management

Initial ED management of seriously injured patients requires simultaneous treatment and evaluation. Rapid assessment of vital function is done while an empirical sequence of lifesaving therapeutic and diagnostic procedures is initiated.[15] The ultimate goal is to establish adequate oxygen delivery to the vital organs. This is accomplished by first progressing through the ABCs: airway control with cervical spine precautions—along with assisted breathing, ventilation, and occasional empirical tube thoracostomy to relieve a pneumothorax—maximizes oxygen delivery to the alveoli. Support of circulation (tamponade of external bleeding and fluid administration via large-bore I.V. catheters) is required to restore effective blood volume, thus enhancing myocardial performance and oxygen delivery to the tissues.

PRIMARY SURVEY AND INITIAL RESUSCITATION

Airway/Breathing

After blunt trauma, airway control should proceed on the assumption that an unstable cervical spine fracture exists; thus, hyperextension of the neck must be avoided. Airway management in the seriously injured victim can usually be accomplished with simple techniques, but occasionally, it can be extremely challenging. Evaluation begins by asking the patient a question such as "How are you?" A response given in a normal voice indicates that the airway is not in immediate jeopardy; a breathless, hoarse response or no response at all indicates that the airway may be compromised.

Initial Approach to the Critically Injured Patient

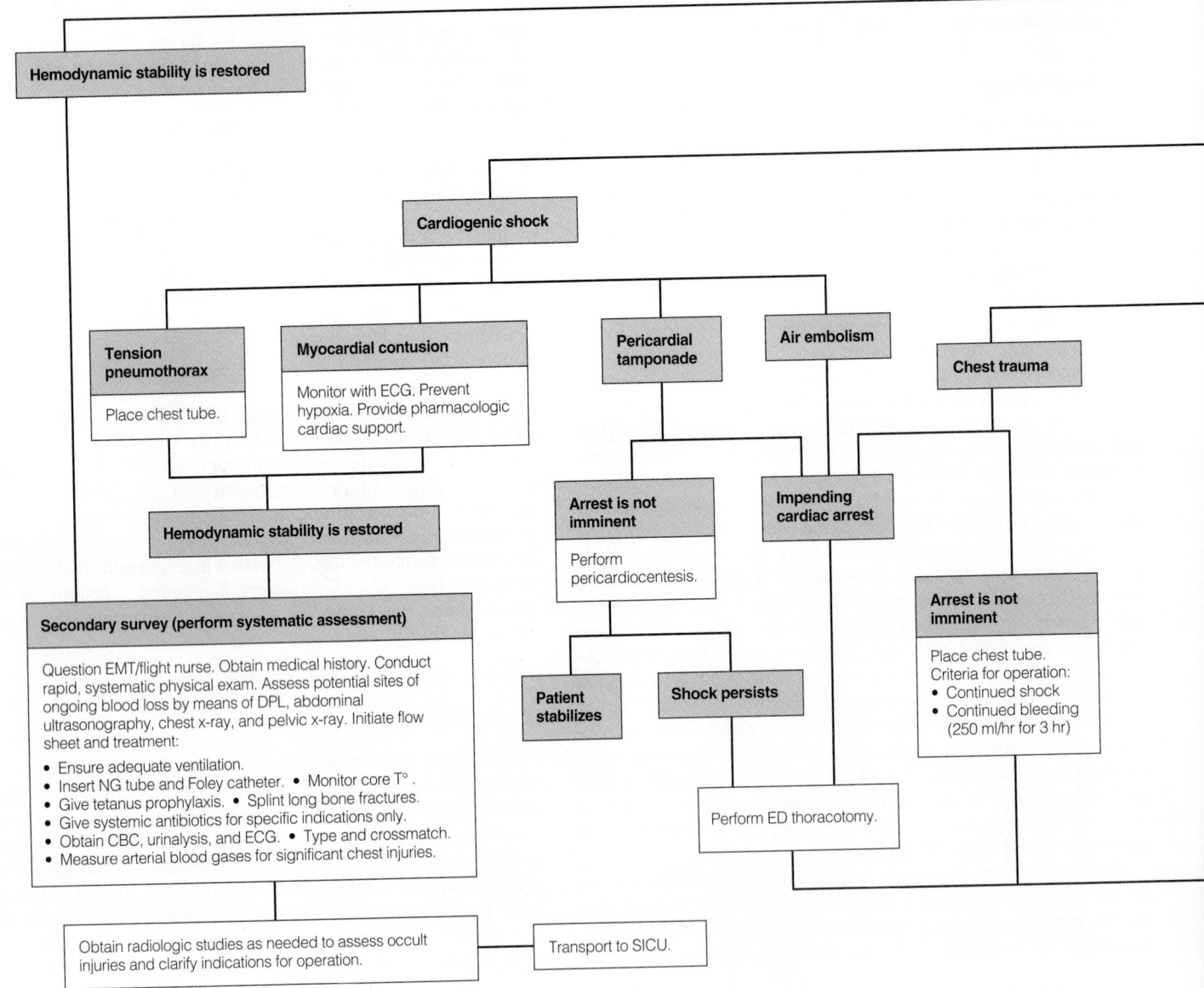

Communicate with base hospital

Field triage: Level I, II, or III facility
Assemble trauma team:
- Trauma surgeon
- ED physician
- Surgical specialist
- Radiology technicians
- Nurses
- Respiratory technicians

Ensure ancillary services:
- OR
- CT scanning
- Blood bank
- Interventional radiology

Hemodynamic stability is restored

Cardiogenic shock

Tension pneumothorax

Place chest tube.

Myocardial contusion

Monitor with ECG. Prevent hypoxia. Provide pharmacologic cardiac support.

Pericardial tamponade

Air embolism

Chest trauma

Hemodynamic stability is restored

Arrest is not imminent

Perform pericardiocentesis.

Impending cardiac arrest

Arrest is not imminent

Place chest tube.
Criteria for operation:
- Continued shock
- Continued bleeding (250 ml/hr for 3 hr)

Secondary survey (perform systematic assessment)

Question EMT/flight nurse. Obtain medical history. Conduct rapid, systematic physical exam. Assess potential sites of ongoing blood loss by means of DPL, abdominal ultrasonography, chest x-ray, and pelvic x-ray. Initiate flow sheet and treatment:

- Ensure adequate ventilation.
- Insert NG tube and Foley catheter. • Monitor core T° .
- Give tetanus prophylaxis. • Splint long bone fractures.
- Give systemic antibiotics for specific indications only.
- Obtain CBC, urinalysis, and ECG. • Type and crossmatch.
- Measure arterial blood gases for significant chest injuries.

Patient stabilizes

Shock persists

Perform ED thoracotomy.

Obtain radiologic studies as needed to assess occult injuries and clarify indications for operation.

Transport to SICU.

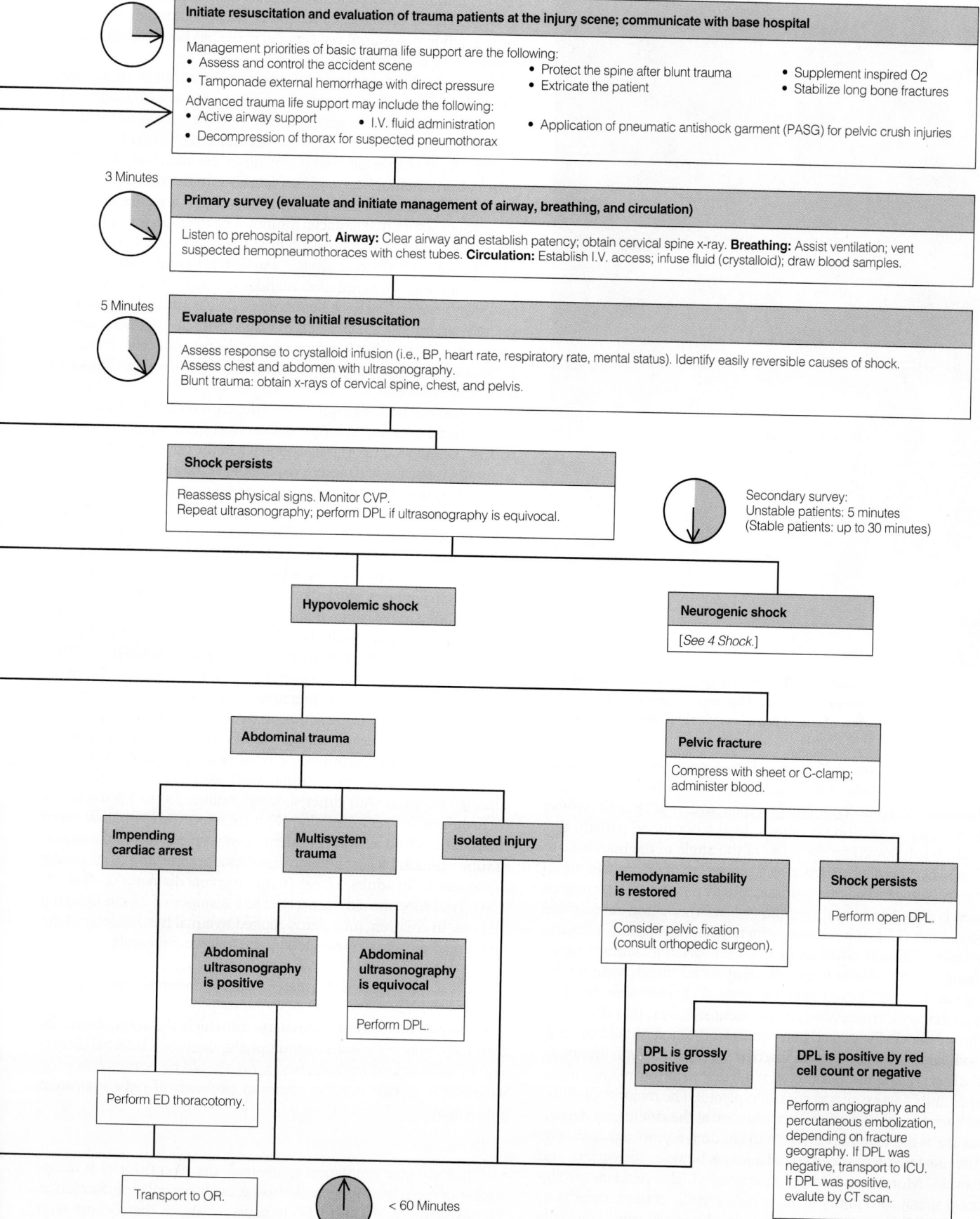

Urban: < 15 minutes
(Rural: > 30 minutes)

Initiate resuscitation and evaluation of trauma patients at the injury scene; communicate with base hospital

Management priorities of basic trauma life support are the following:
• Assess and control the accident scene   • Protect the spine after blunt trauma   • Supplement inspired O2
• Tamponade external hemorrhage with direct pressure   • Extricate the patient   • Stabilize long bone fractures
Advanced trauma life support may include the following:
• Active airway support   • I.V. fluid administration   • Application of pneumatic antishock garment (PASG) for pelvic crush injuries
• Decompression of thorax for suspected pneumothorax

3 Minutes

Primary survey (evaluate and initiate management of airway, breathing, and circulation)

Listen to prehospital report. **Airway:** Clear airway and establish patency; obtain cervical spine x-ray. **Breathing:** Assist ventilation; vent suspected hemopneumothoraces with chest tubes. **Circulation:** Establish I.V. access; infuse fluid (crystalloid); draw blood samples.

5 Minutes

Evaluate response to initial resuscitation

Assess response to crystalloid infusion (i.e., BP, heart rate, respiratory rate, mental status). Identify easily reversible causes of shock.
Assess chest and abdomen with ultrasonography.
Blunt trauma: obtain x-rays of cervical spine, chest, and pelvis.

Shock persists

Reassess physical signs. Monitor CVP.
Repeat ultrasonography; perform DPL if ultrasonography is equivocal.

Secondary survey:
Unstable patients: 5 minutes
(Stable patients: up to 30 minutes)

Hypovolemic shock

Neurogenic shock

[*See 4 Shock.*]

Abdominal trauma

Pelvic fracture

Compress with sheet or C-clamp;
administer blood.

Impending cardiac arrest

Multisystem trauma

Isolated injury

Hemodynamic stability is restored

Consider pelvic fixation
(consult orthopedic surgeon).

Shock persists

Perform open DPL.

Abdominal ultrasonography is positive

Abdominal ultrasonography is equivocal

Perform DPL.

DPL is grossly positive

DPL is positive by red cell count or negative

Perform angiography and
percutaneous embolization,
depending on fracture
geography. If DPL was
negative, transport to ICU.
If DPL was positive,
evalute by CT scan.

Perform ED thoracotomy.

Transport to OR.

< 60 Minutes

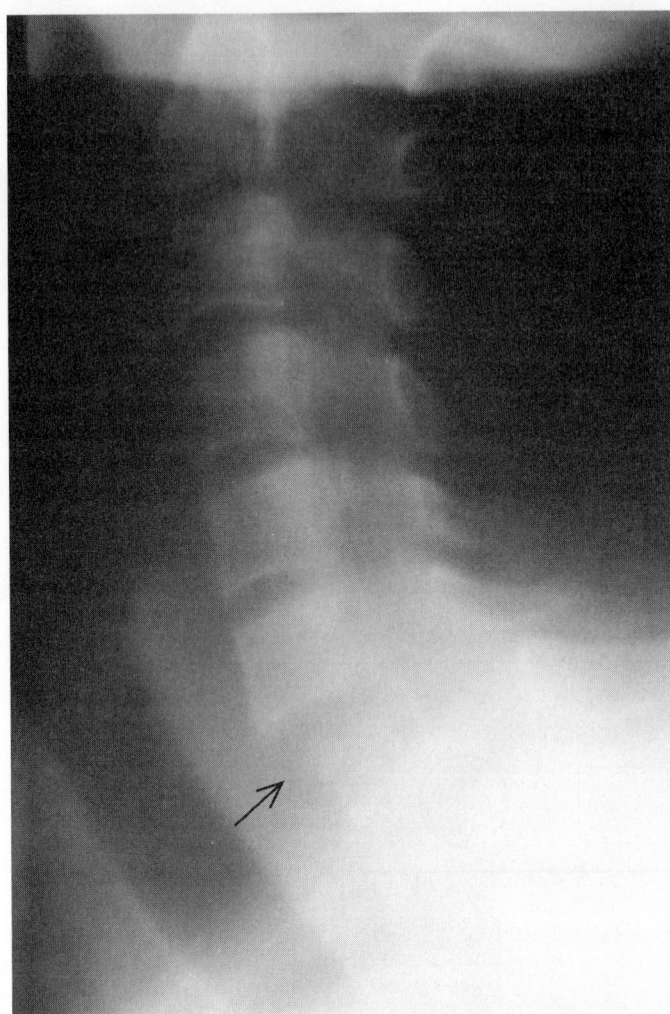

Figure 1 **The cross-table lateral cervical spine x-ray is integral to acute airway management decisions. The most frequent mistake is inadequate visualization of the seventh cervical vertebra (arrow).**

Airway obstruction and hypoventilation are the most likely causes of respiratory failure. The critical decision is whether active airway intervention is needed. The first maneuver is to clear the airway of debris and to suction secretions. In the obtunded patient, this procedure is followed by elevation of the angle of the mandible to alleviate pharyngeal obstruction and placement of an oropharyngeal or nasopharyngeal tube to maintain airway patency. Supplemental oxygen is given via a nasal cannula (6 L/min) or a non-rebreathing oxygen mask (12 L/min). Airway patency does not ensure adequate ventilation. Clinical evidence of hypoventilation includes poor air exchange at the nose and mouth, diminished breath sounds, and decreased chest wall excursion; the most likely causes are head injury, spinal cord transection, hemopneumothorax, flail chest, and profound shock. Suspected hemopneumothoraces should be vented with large-bore chest tubes inserted via the midlateral thorax.

Early cervical spine assessment is integral to airway management. The timing of active airway control is pivotal. The majority of significant spinal injuries in adults arriving alive at the emergency department are at the C5 to C7 levels.[16] In children 8 years old or younger, the most frequent site of spinal injury is between the occiput and C3 level.[17] Moreover, children experience a higher incidence of significant spinal cord injury without radiographic abnormalities (i.e., the SCIWORA syndrome).[18] A fractured cervical spine is usually tender to direct palpation in alert patients, but pain may be masked by distracting injuries.[19] A good-quality cross-table lateral cervical spine (CTLCS) x-ray will delineate 98% of unstable fractures [*see Figure 1*]. In high-risk patients, initial airway management is based on the CTLCS film and clinical judgment,[20] although a cervical collar is left in place until the cervical spine has been radiologically evaluated for bony integrity.

Ideally, after blunt trauma or transcervical gunshot wounds, intubation should be deferred until CTLCS films are available, although neurologic injury from a gunshot wound to the neck is virtually always complete at the time of injury. Bag-mask ventilation is an effective temporizing measure, but it consumes the attention of a skilled trauma team member, it may insufflate air into the stomach, it is resisted by spontaneously breathing patients, and it is ineffective in the presence of severe maxillofacial trauma. The decision for urgent airway control is clinical; there is no time to obtain a confirmatory arterial blood gas (ABG) analysis.[21] Persistent airway obstruction or signs of inadequate ventilation mandate prompt intervention. Patients with expanding neck hematomas, deteriorating vital signs, or severe head trauma are also best managed with an aggressive airway approach. On the other hand, in equivocal situations (e.g., increased P_aCO_2 or base deficit despite a satisfactory S_aO_2), an ABG analysis may be decisive.

The best method of airway control depends on (1) the presence of maxillofacial trauma, (2) suspected cervical spine injury, (3) overall patient condition, and (4) the experience of the physician. Patients in respiratory distress with severe maxillofacial trauma warrant operative intervention. Cricothyrotomy is the preferred approach in adults and has virtually replaced tracheostomy in the ED [*see Figure 2*]; the rare exceptions are in patients with direct laryngeal trauma or complete tracheal disruption. Percutaneous transtracheal ventilation may be safer than both of these surgical procedures for temporary airway management, particularly in children.[22] Nasotracheal intubation is the airway route of choice in nonapneic patients with potential cervical injury in the field but is rarely employed in the ED. The current standard approach is rapid sequence intubation (RSI) of the trachea orally with inline immobilization.[23,24] Our RSI guidelines include nine steps: (1) preparation of equipment and supplies; (2) preoxygenation; (3) sedation to decrease anxiety; (4) premedication to mitigate the negative effects of intubation (e.g., a defasciculating dose of pancuronium or lidocaine for patients with head injuries to prevent increased intracranial pressure); (5) cricoid pressure; (6) paralysis with either succinylcholine, 1.0 to 1.5 mg/kg, or rocuronium, 0.5 to 1.2 mg/kg; (7) intubation with visualization of the vocal cords to permit confident airway access; (8) confirmation of tube position by auscultation and capnography; and (9) securing of the airway. In adults, a large (8 mm internal diameter) cuffed endotracheal tube should be inserted to a distance of 23 cm from the incisors. In children, tube size is gauged to equal the diameter of the little finger or may be estimated by the following formula:

$$\frac{age + 16}{4} = \text{internal diameter (mm) of endotracheal tube}$$

The proper depth (in centimeters) to which the tube should be inserted can be estimated by multiplying the tube's internal diameter (in millimeters) by 3. A chest x-ray should be obtained as soon as possible to rule out the common problem of right mainstem intubation.

Circulation

Once alveolar ventilation is ensured, the next priority is to optimize oxygen delivery by maximizing cardiovascular performance. Hypovolemia is the most likely cause of shock that occurs after the patient receives an injury [*see I:4 Shock*]; therefore, treatment is

Figure 2 depicts cricothyrotomy technique.

Figure 2 **Technique for cricothyrotomy is illustrated here. The larynx is stabilized with one hand, and a 2 cm vertical incision is made over the cricothyroid space. The cricothyroid membrane is palpated and incised horizontally. A Trosseau dilator is inserted and spread vertically for visualization of the subglottic space (left). A tracheal hook is used to retract the inferior border of the thyroid cartilage as a tracheostomy tube with a 6 mm internal diameter is inserted into the trachea (right).**

initiated with crystalloid infusion via large-bore I.V. cannulas, and external hemorrhage is controlled by manual compression. If the PASG has been applied in the field, it should not be removed until effective volume restitution has been achieved. Of special concern are cases in which the PASG has been applied to manage otherwise uncontrollable lower-extremity hemorrhage. In such cases, with effective volume loading, bleeding may become profuse. Application of the PASG in the ED should be reserved for the control of bleeding from major pelvic fractures—if used at all. In fact, wrapping the pelvis with a sheet in the ED is now preferred for initial mechanical stabilization of major pelvic fractures.

The size, number, and sites of I.V. catheters depend on the degree of shock and on estimates of the severity of the injury. If the patient arrives in shock or has obvious multiple injuries, a short 14 French catheter should be placed in each antecubital vein. When vascular collapse precludes peripheral percutaneous access, saphenous vein cutdown at the ankle is preferred [*see Figure 3*] because the site is distant from sites of other resuscitative efforts, the vein will easily accept a large catheter, and the only adjacent structure is a trivial branch of the saphenous nerve. An acceptable alternative is intubation of the femoral vein at the groin by means of the Seldinger technique. Intraosseous infusion through a cannula placed in the medullary cavity of a long bone is a safe and efficacious method for emergency vascular access in infants and children 6 years old or younger. This procedure is typically performed in the anteromedial aspect of the tibial plateau in an uninjured extremity; the distal femur, the distal tibia, and the sternum are other potential sites. Intraosseous infusion gen-

erally allows administration of sufficient fluid to facilitate subsequent cannulation of the venous circulation.[25] With establishment of the first intravenous line, blood should be drawn for hematocrit, white blood cell count, amylase level, electrolyte concentrations, blood-group typing, coagulation profile, and toxicology screen as indicated.

EVALUATION AND CONTINUED RESUSCITATION

Systemic blood pressure, heart rate, respiratory rate, and the patient's general appearance are most helpful in judging the degree of acute blood loss and in assessing the response to initial crystalloid resuscitation. As a general rule, the carotid pulse is palpable at a systolic blood pressure of 60 mm Hg, the femoral pulse at 70 mm Hg, and the radial pulse at 80 mm Hg. In patients with hypovolemic shock, crystalloid loading is initiated with ongoing monitoring of vital signs. Studies from Houston, however, emphasize that in patients with free intraperitoneal or intrathoracic bleeding, overzealous fluid administration before definitive vascular control is achieved may increase blood loss.[3] Consequently, such patients should be promptly transported to the operating room without aggressive efforts to normalize vital signs. It is important to note that acute massive blood loss may paradoxically trigger a vagal-mediated

Figure 3 Saphenous vein cutdown is indicated when vascular collapse precludes peripheral access. The greater saphenous vein lies superficial to the anterior periosteum at the medial malleolus. A transverse skin incision is made one fingerbreadth superior and anterior to the malleolus. A hemostat is inserted and brought across the anteromedial aspect of the tibia. The only structures that should be included under the hemostat are the saphenous vein and a trivial branch of the saphenous nerve.

bradycardia, and therefore, the traditional inverse correlation of increasing heart rate and reduced effective blood volume may not occur in the early resuscitation period.[26] When crystalloid infusion exceeds 50 ml/kg, blood should be administered[27]; type-specific whole blood is rarely associated with complications and should be available within 20 minutes. If type-specific blood is not available, reconstituted O-negative packed red blood cells may be used. Micropore filters are not used in blood infusion lines in hemodynamically unstable patients, because they impede infusion capabilities.[28] In the future, hemoglobin-based blood substitutes may become available that would obviate the need for crossmatching and filtration. Electrocardiographic monitoring, serial measurement of vital signs, rapid physical examination, rectal temperature reading, and initiation of a flow sheet complete the initial assessment of the patient.

The next step is to evaluate the response to resuscitation. In patients with persistent shock, chest x-rays [see Figure 4], pelvic x-rays, and thoracic and abdominal ultrasonography are performed early in the resuscitation to identify occult sources of hemorrhage.[29,30]

Persistent shock may be hypovolemic, cardiogenic, or neurogenic [see I:4 Shock]. Measurement of central venous pressure (CVP) may aid in differentiating between these types of shock. With hypovolemic shock, the CVP is generally less than 5 mm Hg, whereas in clinically significant cardiogenic shock, the CVP usually exceeds 20 mm Hg. Unfortunately, the CVP may be falsely elevated because of rapid volume infusion, hyperventilation, patient straining, a malfunctioning catheter, or improper location of the catheter tip.

The differential diagnosis of traumatic cardiogenic shock consists basically of (1) tension pneumothorax, (2) pericardial tamponade, (3) myocardial contusion, and (4) air embolism. Except for refractory shock, telltale physical signs are frequently hard to discern in a noisy ED, especially when compounded by persistent hypovolemia. Timely diagnosis requires a high index of suspicion. Tension pneumothorax, the most common etiology, is often confirmed with emergency chest tube placement [see Figure 5]. In traumatic pericardial tamponade, the classic signs of tamponade, termed Beck's triad (hypotension, muffled heart sounds, and jugular venous distention), are frequently absent, and pulsus paradoxus is rarely detectable. With

Figure 4 ED chest x-ray shows a massive hemothorax. If the chest tube fails to evacuate the blood, this is a so-called caked hemothorax, which is an indication for emergency thoracostomy in the OR.

the wider use of ultrasonography by trauma surgeons, ED echocardiography should be the first test employed in patients with a high-risk penetrating wound, clinical signs of tamponade, and persistent central venous hypertension.[31,32] With documented pericardial blood on echocardiography and persistent tachycardia, pericardiocentesis should be performed even in the presence of normal systolic blood pressure to relieve any ongoing subendocardial ischemia [*see Figure 6*]. Patients who have persistent signs of pericardial tamponade despite a negative echocardiogram or pericardiocentesis should be transported to the OR for a subxiphoid pericardial window. It is important to remember that results of pericardial aspiration for acute hemopericardium are falsely negative in 15% of patients because the blood in the pericardial sac is clotted and cannot be aspirated. If the patient is in extremis, ED thoracotomy should be performed promptly [*see Figure 7*].[33] Myocardial contusion should be suspected in a patient with unexplained cardiogenic shock or arrhythmia. ECG changes are usually nonspecific.[34,35] Fundamental measures include correction of acidosis, hypoxia, and electrolyte abnormalities; judicious administration of fluid; and pharmacologic suppression of life-threatening arrhythmias. Air embolism into the left atrium from a pulmonary laceration is probably more common than is recognized[36]; typically, hemodynamic instability occurs after positive pressure ventilation is initiated, forcing

Figure 5 In acute trauma, a tube thoracostomy is performed through the fourth or fifth interspace at the midaxillary line, well above the diaphragm (*a*). A short subcutaneous tunnel is fashioned over the superior edge of the rib, and the overlying fascia and intercostal muscle are divided sharply. The pleural space is entered by bluntly perforating the pleura with a Kelly clamp (*b*). A gloved finger is then inserted to confirm penetration of the thoracic cavity and to free up intrapleural adhesions (*c*). A large-bore tube (36 French) is directed posteriorly toward the pleural apex; the proximal port must be well inside the chest (*d*). The tube is then secured to the chest wall with No. 5 braided polyethylene suture and connected to a standard collection apparatus.

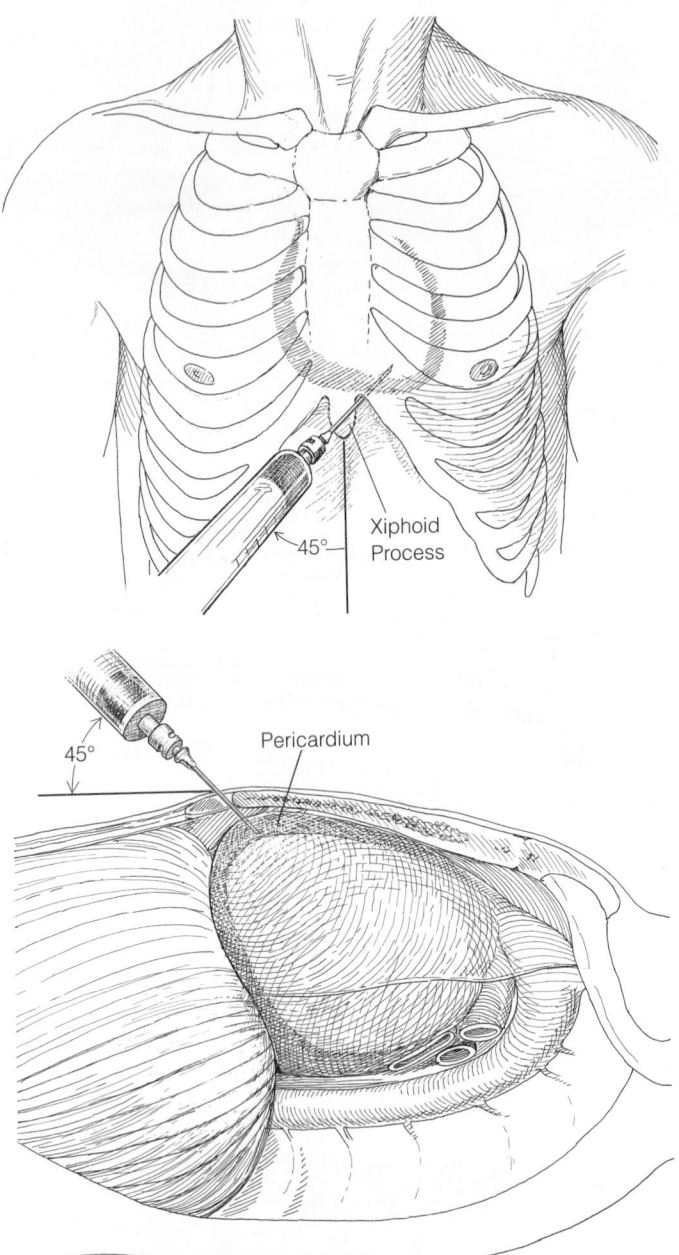

Figure 6 For pericardiocentesis, an 18-gauge spinal needle is inserted at the left xiphoid-costal junction and inserted toward the inferior tip of the left scapula (angled 45° to the patient's right and 45° from the chest wall). The needle is advanced until blood or air is encountered; a "pop" may be appreciated as the needle tip traverses the pericardium. If air is withdrawn, the needle tip should be directed more toward the patient's midline. If blood is withdrawn, 50 ml should be aspirated and injected onto a sheet so that it can be inspected for clots. As a rule, intraventricular blood will clot, whereas defibrinated pericardial blood will not clot.

air from the injured lung into the open pulmonary veins and ultimately into the coronary arteries. ED thoracotomy is essential for pulmonary hilar cross-clamping, air aspiration from the left ventricle, and cardiac massage. The patient is then transferred to the OR for definitive management of the pulmonary lesion before the hilar clamp is released.

ED thoracotomy is an integral part of the initial management of the patient who arrives in extremis and deteriorates to imminent cardiac arrest [*see Figures 7 and 8*].[33] The physiologic rationale is to minimize the time of profound shock; ED thoracotomy permits (1) release of pericardial tamponade, (2) control of intrathoracic blood loss, (3) internal cardiac massage, and (4) cross-clamping of the descending thoracic aorta to enhance coronary and cerebral perfusion as well as to reduce subdiaphragmatic bleeding. Internal cardiac massage should be done bimanually; otherwise, a forceful thumb may rupture the relatively thin right ventricle as it becomes distended. Simple ventricular lacerations are repaired with pledgeted horizontal mattress sutures, whereas atrial injuries are controlled with a partially occluding vascular clamp and repaired with a running suture [*see Figure 8*].

SECONDARY SURVEY AND
DEFINITIVE DIAGNOSIS

After immediate physiologic demands have been addressed, acutely injured patients can usually be rendered hemodynamically stable, and the secondary survey phase can begin. In this phase, the goal is to complete a systematic assessment to identify all potentially life-threatening injuries. Such assessment is crucial to allow proper triage from the ED to the OR, the CT scanning suite, the interventional suite, or the ICU. Mechanism of injury, severity of shock, and response to resuscitation will dictate the time expended. Details of the patient's medical history as well as those related to the injury are critical. The prehospital emergency medical technicians can provide important details and should be questioned before they leave the ED. A minimal review of the patient's medical history should include preexisting medical illness, current medications and when they were most recently ingested, allergies, tetanus immunization, and time of last meal. A rapid but systematic physical examination is done, literally from head to toe. Patients must be completely disrobed and, once spinal injury is excluded, rolled side to side so that the back and flanks can be inspected. Rectal examination for blood and sphincter tone, inspection of the perineum and axillae, and assessment of neurologic function and peripheral pulses are essential.

A good-quality lateral cervical spine x-ray should be obtained as soon as possible after blunt trauma. Until the x-ray is available and all seven cervical vertebral bodies are clearly visualized, the neck is rigidly immobilized. Splinting of long bone fractures minimizes pain, blood loss, and soft tissue damage. Insertion of a nasogastric tube serves to decompress the stomach and reduce the risk of pulmonary aspiration, but because maxillofacial injury may provide a pathway into the cranial vault,[37] the tube should be placed orally when there are midfacial fractures. Blood in the gastric aspirate may be the only sign of an otherwise occult injury of the stomach and duodenum. A Foley catheter empties the bladder, may disclose hematuria, and permits the physician to monitor urinary output, but it should not be inserted until abdominal ultrasonography is completed. Urine volume is a sensitive index of tissue perfusion. The trauma victim is uniquely susceptible to hypothermia; a rectal temperature probe is therefore essential in patients who have been exposed to a cold environment or who require massive volume replacement. A core temperature reading lower than 32° C (89.6° F) should be confirmed with an esophageal probe, and rewarming measures appropriate for the degree of hypothermia should be initiated [*see VII:10 Fever, Hyperpyrexia, and Hypothermia*].[38-40] Tetanus prophylaxis is routine. Systemic antibiotics should be withheld until a specific indication arises. Minimal laboratory tests for trauma include a complete blood count and urinalysis. An electrocardiogram is obtained after blunt chest trauma, and an ABG analysis is done in select patients to confirm adequate ventilation and metabolic balance. The size of the base deficit can be a useful measure of the depth of hemorrhagic shock.[41] In any patient with evidence of hypovolemia, a blood sample should be sent for blood-group typing.

All potential sites of ongoing blood loss should be evaluated in the hypovolemic patient. A chest x-ray is the most reliable screening test for intrathoracic bleeding; it also confirms the location of endotracheal, nasogastric, and thoracostomy tubes as well as the central venous catheter. Pleural fluid can be difficult to appreciate on a supine chest x-ray; 1 L of blood may produce only a hazy appearance in a hemithorax. Hemothoraces should be drained promptly by tube thoracostomy [see Figure 5]. Continued bleeding must be monitored carefully by means of chest tube output, serial chest films to detect retained intrapleural blood, and vital signs. Abrupt cessation of chest tube output may be deceptive; if hypotension persists or recurs, a second chest tube should be inserted and another chest x-ray should be obtained. The inability to clear the thorax with chest tubes (so-called caked hemothorax [see Figure 4]) is an indication for prompt thoracotomy.

Abdominal examination is notoriously misleading in detecting acute hemoperitoneum.[42] The peritoneal cavity may sequester up to 3,000 ml of blood with only minimal abdominal distention. Laparotomy is clearly indicated for gunshot wounds with violation of the peritoneum[43] or in patients with overt peritonitis after a stab wound or blunt trauma. After blunt trauma, however, head injury or intoxication frequently alters the patient's response to acute injury, and pain from associated fractures may overshadow peritoneal irritation secondary to bleeding. Ultrasonography is the most rapid method of identifying free blood, but it may yield false negative results in as many as 5% to 10% of patients on initial examination. Diagnostic peritoneal lavage (DPL) [see Figure 9] is the most expedient and reliable method of identifying significant intraperitoneal hemorrhage; in patients with life-threatening bleeding, sensitivity approaches 100%. Paradoxically, because of its extreme sensitivity in identifying blood, DPL lacks specificity for determining the need for laparotomy in stable patients.[44,45] A grossly positive aspirate (> 10 ml of blood) mandates emergency laparotomy in cases of penetrating wounds and in cases of blunt trauma with hemodynamic instability. A red blood cell count higher than 100,000/mm³ in a patient with penetrating trauma is an indication for semiemergent celiotomy, whereas a red blood cell count exceeding 50,000/mm³ in a patient with blunt trauma

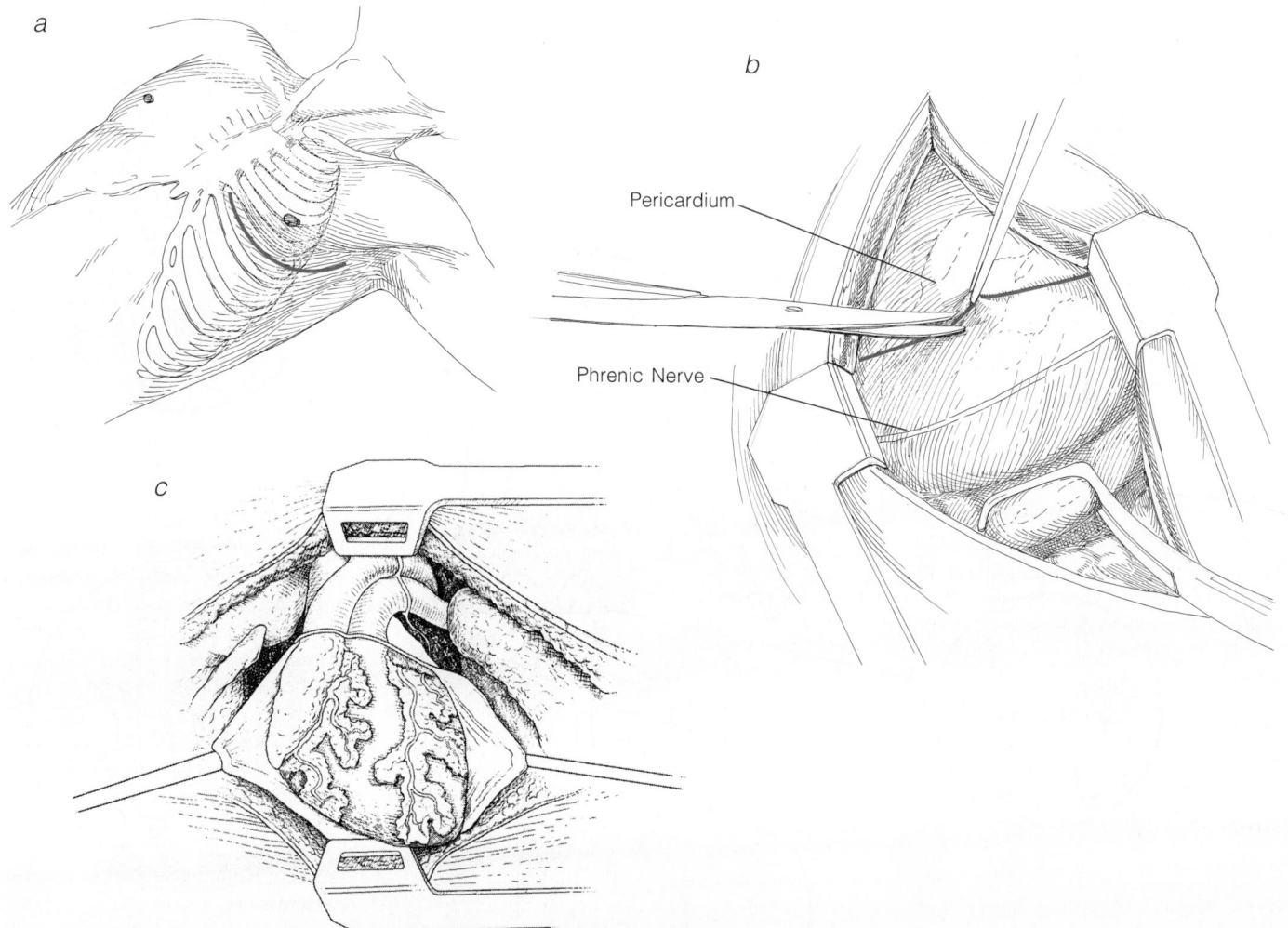

Figure 7   (*a*) **A left anterolateral thoracotomy is performed through the fifth intercostal space. (*b*) The lung is reflected superomedially, and a Satinsky vascular clamp is placed on the descending thoracic aorta. A pericardiotomy is performed with scissors anterior to the phrenic nerve. (*c*) A so-called butterfly extension across the sternum creates a bilateral anterolateral thoracotomy, providing access to both thoracic cavities and to the pulmonary hila, heart, and proximal great vessels.**

warrants further evaluation by computed tomography of the abdomen. Furthermore, in the setting of both blunt trauma and penetrating trauma, elevation in the peritoneal lavage white blood cell count, the amylase level, and the alkaline phosphatase concentration may identify hollow viscus injury; threshold levels, however, have not been determined.[46-48] In penetrating wounds to the lower chest, the red blood cell count threshold for abdominal exploration is lowered to 10,000/mm³ because isolated diaphragmatic perforations may not bleed.[49] An intermediate red blood cell count of 1,000 to 10,000/mm³ warrants further definitive evaluation by thoracoscopy.[49,50] Because DPL does not sample the retroperitoneum, triple-contrast CT scanning may be of help in cases of high-risk penetrating wounds to the back or the flank.[51,52] Most injuries to retroperitoneal hollow viscera, however, are identified on the basis of extraluminal gas or fluid rather than contrast extravasation.

Assessment of bony stability by physical examination and plain films of the pelvis is crucial for the early identification of major pelvic fractures. Life-threatening hemorrhage occurs most commonly with fracture patterns involving the posterior columns [see Figure 10].[53,54] Appropriate initial management includes vigorous blood volume replacement and mechanical support of the pelvis [see Figure 11]. Most patients can be rendered hemodynamically stable and are potential candidates for external skeletal fixation if the fracture geography is appropriate.[55,56] The unstable patient with a clearly positive ultrasonogram should undergo laparotomy because of a high probability of major hepatic, splenic, or mesenteric bleeding.[57] Conversely, the hemodynamically unstable patient in whom the ultrasonogram is normal and DPL yields confirmatory negative results should undergo prompt pelvic arteriography for selective embolization.[58]

The length of time expended in the ED, the decision for urgent operation, and the need for special radiologic studies are critical triage decisions that must take into account the mechanism of injury, the response to resuscitation, and the availability of a staffed OR. A patient in refractory shock with a central abdominal gunshot wound, for example, should be assigned by triage to the OR in a matter of minutes, whereas a far more complex decision is required in the case of a motor vehicle accident victim with altered mental status, a widened mediastinum on chest x-ray, and a positive ultrasonogram. If the latter patient is hemodynamically unstable, laparotomy should be performed first because intraperitoneal bleeding is the most likely cause of persistent shock. If this patient is hemodynamically stable, however, CT scanning and aortography should be performed first because the results of these procedures facilitate a multiteam approach and allow prioritizing of operative needs.[59,60]

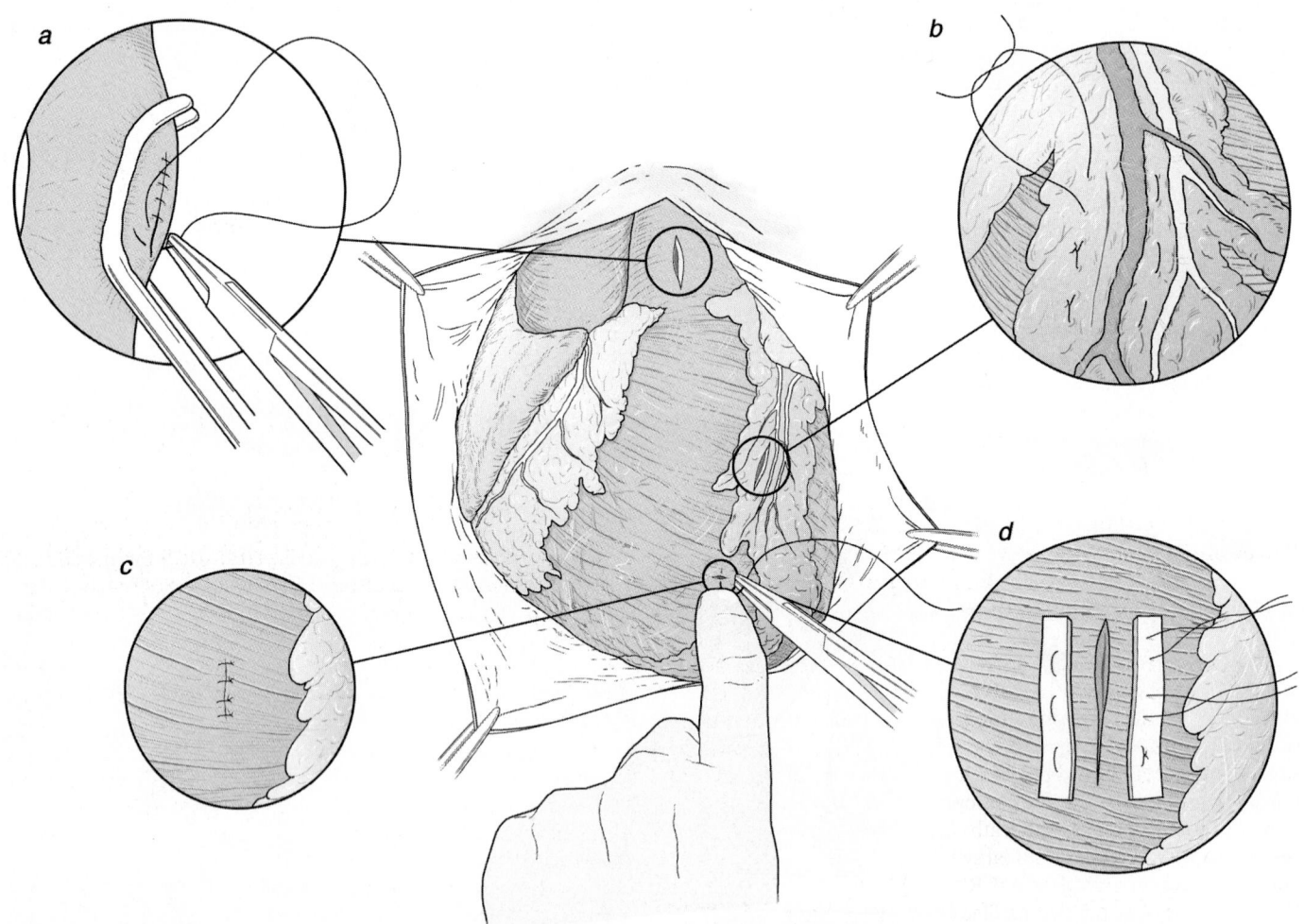

Figure 8   (*a*) **A Satinsky vascular clamp is used to control arterial and major vessel injuries while they are closed with a running suture. (*b*) For wounds close to coronary arteries, horizontal mattress sutures should be used to exclude the arteries. (*c*) Small wounds to the thick left ventricle can be closed with interrupted simple sutures. (*d*) Larger wounds should be closed using pledgets.**

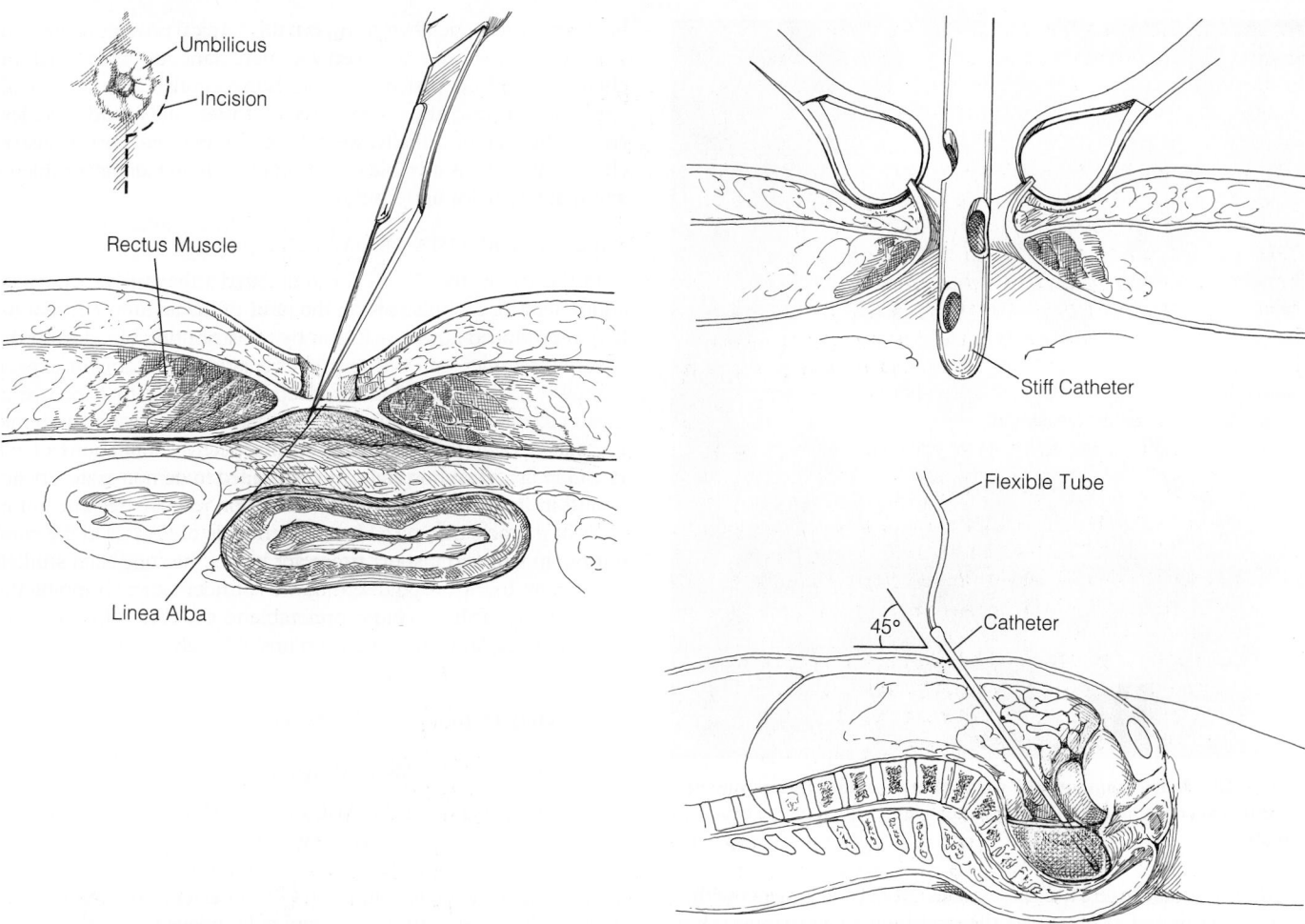

Figure 9 Illustrated here is the semiopen technique for peritoneal lavage. A 3 to 4 cm incision is made over the infraumbilical ring, and the linea alba is incised vertically for 1 cm. The fascial edges are grasped with towel clips and elevated. A standard peritoneal dialysis catheter is introduced into the peritoneum at a 45° angle and then advanced into the pelvis without use of the trocar. If 10 ml of gross blood is aspirated, the study is considered to be positive. Otherwise, 1 L of normal saline (10 ml/kg for children) is infused. The lavage fluid is retrieved by gravity siphonage; the empty saline bag is dropped to the floor. A 50 ml sample of the fluid is submitted for laboratory analysis.

Discussion

Prehospital Care

ADVANCED TRAUMA LIFE SUPPORT

The principles of initial assessment and management in ACLS and ATLS are based on the ABCs—airway maintenance, breathing, and circulation. In both settings, upper airway control and assisted ventilation are imperative for optimizing alveolar oxygen tension. With respect to circulation, however, the protocols diverge markedly because of differing pathophysiology.

It is estimated that 60% of deaths caused by coronary artery disease occur within 1 hour of initial symptoms, usually before the patient can receive medical care.[61] Rhythm disturbance is the most frequent cause of death after cardiac arrest; there is only a 6-minute period until irreversible cerebral damage occurs.[62] Temporary artificial circulation in these normovolemic patients can be achieved by closed-chest compression. The technique is simple and effective and requires no special equipment. However, arrhythmias, the most common cause of preventable death, become refractory if pharma-

cologic or electrical treatment is delayed.[63] ECG monitoring and venous access allow the necessary interventions to be initiated effectively in the field, and indeed, ACLS results in a fivefold reduction in the incidence of cardiac arrest en route to the hospital. In contrast, the major reversible threat to life for the severely injured patient is persistent hemorrhage, which requires hospital facilities for effective treatment.

Sophistication of emergency medical services has dramatically expanded the scope of prehospital care. Qualified paramedics using ACLS skills have produced dramatic improvement in survival of acute myocardial infarction by treating arrhythmias in the field.[64] Unquestionably, these efforts also improve trauma resuscitation, but the extent of prehospital ATLS remains a highly controversial issue. Advocates of the so-called scope-and-run philosophy argue that field stabilization is detrimental because it delays definitive care. However, in systems with rigorous medical control, the addition of advanced techniques (e.g., endotracheal intubation, I.V. access, and fluid administration) adds less than 10 minutes to the on-scene time.[2] In the Denver Emergency Medical Service system, para-

Figure 10 Pelvic angiography with selective embolization may be an integral component in the early management of a pelvic crush injury.

medics routinely insert I.V. catheters in critically ill patients within 1.0 to 1.5 minutes.[65] Moreover, the availability of hypertonic saline solution and human polymerized hemoglobin for prehospital fluid resuscitation may provide an undisputed physiologic rationale for establishing I.V. access at the scene.[66-71] Clearly, the relative benefits of paramedic intervention depend on mechanism of injury, patient status, and availability of a trauma center. An efficient prehospital care system should be tailored to the community's needs, providing well-thought-out protocols, appropriate field personnel, and active medical control. Unfortunately, a paradox exists: ATLS skills are needed most in sparsely populated rural areas where transport time exceeds 30 minutes, but the limited volume of trauma precludes the experience necessary to maintain this expertise.

AIRWAY MANAGEMENT

The principles of initial resuscitation are governed by physiologic rationale. The goal is to reestablish adequate oxygen delivery to vital organs. Efforts to improve tissue perfusion will be unproductive unless the oxygen content of the circulating blood is sufficient. Airway patency and maintenance of adequate ventilation are thus the initial priorities. Current policy dictates that emergency airway control after blunt vehicular trauma be performed with the assumption that an unstable cervical spine fracture exists until such injuries are excluded radiologically; however, this policy does not preclude RSI.[72] Cervical neck injury has been documented in 25% of accidental fatalities[73] and in 60% of fatalities in which the patient had sustained head trauma,[74] but the incidence of truly occult unstable cervical fractures in neurologically intact survivors of vehicular trauma is unknown. The current recommendation of orotracheal intubation with in-line manual stabilization of the head and neck has proved safe in clinical series to date. For patients with extensive maxillofacial trauma that precludes oral intubation, the traditional alternative

has been to do a cricothyrotomy, but this surgical procedure has definite risks. The success achieved with percutaneous dilatational tracheostomy in ICU patients[75] suggests that similar approaches with percutaneous cricothyrotomy may be easier and would pose less risk to the patient. Finally, we believe that percutaneous transtracheal ventilation is a viable option in challenging airway problems and that it remains underutilized.[22]

PNEUMATIC ANTISHOCK GARMENT

In the 1970s, the PASG was mandated as essential prehospital equipment for ambulances on the basis of the assumption that inflation produced autotransfusion by redistributing blood from the lower extremities into the central circulation. Subsequent experimental work challenged this concept and showed that the rise in mean arterial pressure is merely the result of an elevated systemic vascular resistance.[76] Randomized prospective evaluations of the PASG in urban prehospital care have failed to demonstrate a benefit and in fact suggest that PASG inflation may be detrimental in cases of thoracic trauma.[6] However, the role of PASGs in the rural setting, in which transport times are longer, has not been studied adequately. In the hospital setting, we consider either wrapping the pelvis or use of the C clamp preferable to the PASG for management of unrelenting bleeding from unstable pelvic fractures.

Emergency Department Management

AIRWAY, BREATHING, AND CIRCULATION

The primary goal of the ABCs is to establish adequate oxygen delivery to vital organs so as to give the physician time to identify and treat immediately life-threatening injuries. Oxygen delivery is the product of cardiac output (CO) and arterial oxygen content (C_aO_2). By convention, CO is generally indexed to body surface area and expressed as cardiac index (CI), which when multiplied by C_aO_2 yields an oxygen delivery index (DO_2). Normal DO_2 is roughly 500 ml/min/m²; it will increase by as much as 30% in response to injury. C_aO_2 and DO_2 are calculated as follows:

$$C_aO_2 \text{ (ml/dl)} = [\text{Hb}] \text{ (g/dl)} \times 1.38 \times S_aO_2 \text{ (\%)} +$$
$$[P_aO_2 \text{ (mm Hg)} \times 0.003]$$
$$DO_2 \text{ (ml/min/m}^2) = \text{CI (L/min/m)} \times C_aO_2 \text{ (ml/dl)} \times 10$$

where [Hb] is the hemoglobin concentration, S_aO_2 is oxyhemoglobin saturation, P_aO_2 is arterial oxygen tension, and 0.003 is the solubility of O_2 in blood.

S_aO_2 is the first important variable to consider. Given the low solubility of oxygen in plasma, the level of P_aO_2 is only important insofar as it relates to S_aO_2. A review of the oxyhemoglobin dissociation curve [*see I:7 Life-Threatening Acid-Base Disorders*] makes it clear why pushing P_aO_2 to levels higher than 100 mm Hg will not affect S_aO_2 appreciably and thus will have little impact on DO_2. During initial resuscitation, a high fraction of inspired oxygen (F_IO_2) is administered, and pulse oximetry is used to assess S_aO_2. As a rule, a low S_aO_2 is easily treated by increasing the F_IO_2 further. Intubated patients who do not respond when the F_IO_2 is increased to 100% can be treated with low levels of positive end-expiratory pressure (PEEP) once adequate volume status is ensured.

The second important variable is the hemoglobin concentration. The initial hemoglobin level is notoriously misleading because the patients have not yet been volume loaded and because there has not been sufficient time for substantial flux of interstitial fluid into the intravascular space. The initial hemoglobin level is also problematic because of the lag time before the results come back from the laborato-

Figure 11 **Shown is the wrapping technique currently used for mechanical support of the pelvis.**

ry. Once recognized, a low hemoglobin level is easily treated with blood transfusion. Given the concerns just mentioned, however, early blood transfusion should be empirically administered in patients who arrive in severe class IV hemorrhagic shock or who have injuries associated with significant bleeding (e.g., vertical shear pelvic fracture or bilateral femur fractures), especially if they are elderly.

CO is the third important variable to consider. Unfortunately, it is difficult to monitor CO in the ED. Decreased preload is by far the most likely problem; consequently, empirical volume loading is recommended. When the patient is unresponsive, a central venous pressure reading can be helpful in differentiating persistent hypovolemia from cardiogenic shock. There is evidence to suggest that noninvasive monitoring of subcutaneous tissue perfusion status may be a valuable adjunct in assessing the adequacy of DO_2.[77]

BLOOD VOLUME RESTITUTION

During profound shock, fluid is lost from the intravascular as well as interstitial space because of sodium flux into the cellular compartment.[78] Crystalloid solutions, which rapidly equilibrate with the total extracellular space, are preferred.[79] Most authorities agree that albumin or artificial plasma expanders are no more effective in restoring tissue perfusion when adequate sodium is provided.[80,81] Moreover, they are costly and may aggravate posttraumatic compli-

cations. The type of crystalloid fluid used for initial volume replacement is of less importance. Lactated Ringer solution is theoretically preferred to normal saline because it provides a better buffer for metabolic acidosis of protracted shock.[82,83] The role of hypertonic saline continues to be investigated. There is some evidence to suggest that hypertonic saline may attenuate neutrophil-mediated injury.[84,85] Acute whole blood loss can be replaced initially with crystalloid because (1) this solution repletes the total extracellular space, (2) hemodilution enhances perfusion by means of reduced blood viscosity, and (3) increased CO and peripheral oxygen extraction provide adequate tissue oxygenation.[86] There is, of course, a limit to these compensatory mechanisms. With massive hemorrhage, the crystalloid replacement for blood may approach a ratio of 8 : 1 because of a progressive fall in plasma oncotic pressure and intracellular sequestration of sodium.[87] In general, blood should be added to fluid resuscitation when crystalloid infusion exceeds 50 ml/kg.[27,88] Diagnosis and management of shock, as well as the pathophysiology of the various shock states, is discussed in detail elsewhere [*see I:4 Shock*].

Fully crossmatched blood is rarely available for emergency trauma resuscitation. Uncrossmatched type-specific whole blood or packed red blood cells can be safely administered[89,90] and are available in most hospitals within 20 minutes. If type-specific blood is unavailable, reconstituted O-negative packed red blood cells should be used. Type O-negative blood has no cellular antigens; therefore, the risk of major hemolytic reactions caused by patient antibodies attacking donor antigens is minimal. However, O-negative whole blood, the universal donor, is not considered safe, because its plasma contains anti-A and anti-B antibodies.[91] When O-negative packed cells are unavailable, the O-positive packed red blood cells may be used. The patient will become sensitized to the Rh factor, but this is significant only in women of childbearing age.

A 1994 clinical trial found that for hypotensive patients with penetrating torso injuries, survival improved when fluid resuscitation was delayed until surgical intervention had controlled the source of hemorrhage.[3] A subsequent subset analysis revealed that survival was improved only in patients who had sustained cardiac injuries and not in patients who had sustained major vascular, abdominal solid organ, and noncardiac thoracic injuries.[92] Although this clinical trial had some methodologic flaws, it is important for the appropriate emphasis it placed on source control of hemorrhage as an imperative priority. Whether resuscitation should be totally withheld until control of hemorrhage is achieved is doubtful; such an approach is clearly not the current standard of care.[15]

Animal studies using the traditional controlled hemorrhagic shock models have shown that if shock is allowed to persist for several hours, an irreversible shock state occurs from which the animals cannot be resuscitated.[93] On the other hand, more recent animal studies using uncontrolled hemorrhagic shock models with graded resuscitation have found that moderately resuscitated animals survive better than animals who receive either less aggressive or more aggressive resuscitation. A systolic pressure of 90 mm Hg may be acceptable, but the overriding priority must be timely surgical intervention. What this means in blunt trauma is not clear. If a non–head-injured patient arrives in class IV shock with a positive abdominal ultrasonogram, operative control of bleeding is the overriding priority. However, the possibility of a serious associated head injury frequently exists. The surgeon cannot determine whether the low Glasgow Coma Scale score is attributable to cerebral hypoperfusion or to intracranial pathology. If the brain is indeed injured, decreased perfusion pressure can produce secondary brain injury and worsen outcome.[94] Moreover, prehospital extrication and initial ED assessment times are longer with blunt trauma, and definitive con-

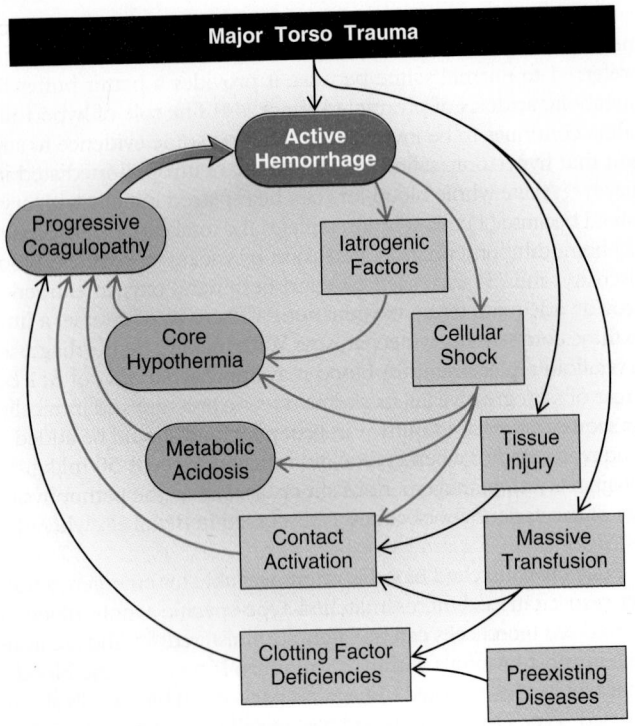

Major Torso Trauma

Active Hemorrhage

Progressive Coagulopathy

Iatrogenic Factors

Core Hypothermia

Cellular Shock

Metabolic Acidosis

Tissue Injury

Contact Activation

Massive Transfusion

Clotting Factor Deficiencies

Preexisting Diseases

Figure 12 **Illustrated is the so-called bloody vicious cycle. This syndrome has a multifactorial pathogenesis, with the usual manifestations including coagulopathy, hypothermia, and metabolic acidosis.**[118]

trol of bleeding may take hours to orchestrate. Finally, for blunt trauma patients who survive early prolonged hypoperfusion, soft tissue injury combined with severe shock contributes to a high incidence of late multiple organ failure.[95]

Diverse clinical experience has substantiated the feasibility of autotransfusion, and in trauma, there has been increasing enthusiasm for its use in the ED as well as in the OR.[96] Autotransfusion clearly eliminates the infectious, allergic, and incompatibility problems of stored blood, an important concern because of the acquired immunodeficiency syndrome (AIDS). However, when large amounts of unprocessed collected blood are reinfused, a consumptive coagulopathy and platelet dysfunction occur.[97] These risks may outweigh the benefits of autotransfusion in the critically injured patient who has multiple potential bleeding sites.

Much attention has been directed toward production of a red blood cell substitute. Fluosol-DA, a perfluorocarbon, appeared promising,[98] but clinical trials failed to demonstrate an advantage over standard lactated Ringer solution, and animal studies clearly established an immunologic penalty.[99] Consequently, Fluosol-DA failed to receive the approval of the Food and Drug Administration. In contrast, progress has been made with hemoglobin-based blood substitutes, although tetrameric hemoglobin has been problematic.[71,100] Experience with human polymerized hemoglobin as a blood substitute after major surgical procedures suggests that this agent may be available for trauma resuscitation in the near future. Transfusion considerations are discussed in detail elsewhere [*see I:5 Bleeding and Transfusion*].

EMERGENCY DEPARTMENT THORACOTOMY

ED thoracotomy is an integral part of the initial management of trauma patients who arrive in extremis.[33,101] With insufficient blood volume, open cardiac massage is superior to closed-chest compression in maintaining systemic blood flow[102]; coronary and

cerebral perfusion is maintained at adequate levels for up to 30 minutes. Adjunctive thoracic aorta occlusion enhances both coronary and cerebral perfusion by maintaining aortic diastolic pressure and by increasing carotid systolic pressure. Aortic cross-clamping also decreases subdiaphragmatic bleeding in the event of associated abdominal injury.[103,104] These benefits are obtained at the expense of increased myocardial oxygen demand and a lack of perfusion to the lower torso. Irreversible cardiovascular collapse and splanchnic dysfunction occur with prolonged cross-clamping times. Clinical experience suggests that 30 minutes is the limit for prevention of serious ischemic sequelae. The possibility of patient salvage is largely determined by the mechanism of injury as well as the patient's condition at the time of thoracotomy. Success approaches 50% in patients arriving with profound shock from a penetrating cardiac wound and 20% for all penetrating wounds. On the other hand, patient outcome is dismal when ED thoracotomy is performed for blunt trauma; it is now considered futile in patients lacking cardiac activity. Adding laparotomy in the ED for definitive control of abdominal hemorrhage has not improved outcome.[105]

PHYSIOLOGIC MONITORING

It is imperative that the critically injured patient undergo early hemodynamic monitoring and assessment of oxygen transport. The adequacy of resuscitation is initially determined by blood pressure, pulse rate, and general patient appearance. Once these factors have stabilized, urine output (> 0.5 ml/kg/hr in adults) is used to gauge additional fluid requirements. All major trauma patients should have continuous ECG and pulse oximetry monitoring. In addition, core temperature should be monitored with a rectal temperature probe capable of recording temperatures lower than 32° C (89.6° F). Atrial and ventricular arrhythmias from cardiac contusion or ischemia may require therapy. A data flow sheet for physiologic indices, laboratory test results, and fluid administration allows quick analysis of trends, but isolated points may be misleading. Measurement of central venous pressure is helpful in differentiating persistent hypovolemia from cardiogenic shock [*see I:4 Shock*], but several conditions can produce a false elevation of the CVP. Although arterial lines and pulmonary arterial catheters are of limited use in ED trauma management, they are important in the radiology suite, particularly if the patient requires beta blockade for a suspected torn aorta.[60] End-tidal CO_2 monitoring should be available for patients undergoing emergency endotracheal intubation.

COAGULOPATHY

The most devastating complication of massive blood and fluid resuscitation is a bleeding diathesis. Paradoxically, although clotting is accelerated at the capillary level because of shock and tissue damage,[106] the circulating blood becomes hypocoagulable.[107,108] The pathogenesis of bloody vicious cycle is complex [*see Figure 12*]. Factors predictive of a severe coagulopathic state (i.e., prothrombin time [PT] > 2 times normal and partial thromboplastin time [PTT] > 2 times normal) include (1) massive rapid blood transfusion (10 units/4 hr), (2) persistent cellular shock (oxygen consumption index < 110 ml/min/m^2, lactate concentration > 5 mmol/L), (3) progressive metabolic acidosis (pH < 7.20, base deficit > 14 mEq/L), and (4) refractory core hypothermia (< 34° C).[109] The extent of tissue disruption (as quantitated by the Injury Severity Score) is not a strong independent risk factor; however, it clearly is a facilitating event.

Stored blood is deficient in factors V and VIII and platelets and replete with fibrin split products and vasoactive substances. Timely administration of fresh frozen plasma and platelets will minimize the risk of coagulopathy after massive transfusion [*see I:5 Bleeding*] *and Transfusion*]. Although blood components are not usually indicated in the early resuscitation phase, they may be appropriate in patients with massive hemorrhage caused by pelvic fracture.

Germane to the initial period of massive blood transfusion are the potential complications of hypocalcemia, acidosis, and hypothermia. Hypocalcemia caused by citrate binding of ionized calcium does not occur until the blood transfusion rate exceeds 100 ml/min (1 U/5 min). Decreased serum levels of ionized calcium depress myocardial function before impairing coagulation.[110,111] Calcium gluconate (10 mg/kg I.V.) should be reserved for cases in which there is ECG evidence of ST interval prolongation or, rarely, for cases of unexplained hypotension during massive transfusion. Moderate hypothermia (< 32° C) causes platelet sequestration and inhibits the release of platelet factors that are important in the intrinsic clotting pathway.[39] In addition, moderate hypothermia has consistently been associated with poor outcome in trauma patients.[112] Core temperature often falls insidiously because of exposure at the scene and in the ED and because of administration of resuscitation fluids stored at ambient temperature. The first step is to prevent further heat loss by covering the body (including the head) and infusing warm blood and fluid. Another simple technique is to heat and aerosolize ventilator gases. Active external rewarming with heating blankets and increased room temperature should also be used. However, it is important to note that the above techniques are not very effective in reversing established hypothermia. In this setting, lavage of the abdominal or chest cavities can increase core temperature at a rate of 1° to 2° C an hour. Recently, Gentilello and others have introduced relatively simple extracorporeal techniques that can increase core temperature at a rate of 2° to 5° C an hour.[113] Whether these rapid rewarming techniques improve patient outcome is currently being investigated.

The use of bicarbonate in the treatment of systemic acidosis remains controversial. Moderate acidosis (pH < 7.20) impairs coagulation,[114] myocardial contractility,[115] and oxidative metabolism.[116] Acidosis in the trauma patient is caused primarily by a rise in lactic acid production secondary to tissue hypoxia and will usually resolve when the volume deficit has been corrected [*see I:7 Life-Threatening Acid-Base Disorders*]. Administration of sodium bicarbonate may cause a leftward shift of the oxyhemoglobin dissociation curve, reducing tissue oxygen extraction, and it may worsen intracellular acidosis caused by carbon dioxide production.[117] Bicarbonate infusion, therefore, should be limited to persons with protracted shock. Patients in shock should be ventilated on 100% oxygen; thus, blood gases obtained from a central venous line are clinically useful in the assessment of acid-base status. Blood gases should be corrected for core body temperature; pH should be increased by 0.15 for every 1° C drop below normal.

References

1. Eisenberg MS, Bergner L, Hallstrom A: Cardiac resuscitation in the community: importance of rapid provision and implications for program planning. JAMA 241:1905, 1979

2. Copass MK, Oreskovich MR, Baldergroen MR, et al: Prehospital cardiopulmonary resuscitation of the critically injured patient. Am J Surg 148:20, 1984

3. Bickell WH, Wall MJ Jr, Pepe PE, et al: Immediate versus delayed fluid resuscitation for hypotensive patients with penetrating torso injuries. N Engl J Med 331:1105, 1994

4. Soucy DM, Rude M, Hsrg WC, et al: The effects of varying fluid volume and rate of resuscitation during uncontrolled hemorrhage. J Trauma 46:209, 1999

5. Burris D, Rhee P, Kaufman C, et al: Controlled resuscitation for uncontrolled hemorrhagic shock. J Trauma 46:216, 1999

6. Mattox KL, Bickell WH, Pepe PE, et al: Prospective randomized evaluation of antishock MAST in posttraumatic hypotension. J Trauma 26:779, 1986

7. Capone AC, Safar P, Stezoski W, et al: Improved outcome with fluid restriction in treatment of uncontrolled hemorrhagic shock. J Am Coll Surg 180:49, 1995

8. Kowalenko T, Stern S, Dronen S, et al: Improved outcome with hypotensive resuscitation of uncontrolled hemorrhagic shock in a swine model. J Trauma 33:349, 1992

9. Cayten CG, Berendt BM, Byrne DW, et al: A study of pneumatic antishock garments in severely hypotensive trauma patients. J Trauma 34:728, 1993

10. Domerer RM, O'Conner, Delbridge TR, et al: National Association of EMS Physicians, Position Paper: Use of the pneumatic anti-shock garment (PASG). Prehosp Emerg Care 1:32, 1997

11. Aprahamian C, Thompson BM, Towne JB, et al: The effects of a paramedic system on mortality of major open intra-abdominal vascular trauma. J Trauma 23:687, 1983

12. Jacobs LM, Sinclair A, Beiser A, et al: Prehospital advanced life support: benefits in trauma. J Trauma 24:8, 1984

13. Pons PT, Honigman B, Moore EE, et al: Prehospital advanced trauma life support for critical penetrating wounds to the thorax and abdomen. J Trauma 25:828, 1985

14. Hoyt DB, Mikulaschek AW, Winchel RJ: Trauma triage and interhospital transfer. Trauma, 4th ed. Mattox KL, Feliciano DV, Moore EE, Eds. McGraw-Hill, New York, 2000

15. Committee on Trauma, American College of Surgeons: Advanced Trauma Life Support Manual. American College of Surgeons, Chicago, 1981

16. Ducker TB, Russo GL, Bellegarrique R, et al: Complete sensorimotor paralysis after cord injury: mortality, recovery, and therapeutic implications. J Trauma 19:837, 1979

17. Bohn D, Armstrong D, Becker L, et al: Cervical spine injuries in children. J Trauma 30:463, 1990

18. Pang D, Pollack IF: Spinal cord injury without radiographic abnormality in children—the SCIWORA syndrome. J Trauma 29:654, 1989

19. Roth BJ, Martin RR: Roentgenographic evaluation of the cervical spine: a selective approach. Arch Surg 129:643, 1994

20. Shaffer MA, Doris PE: Limitation of the cross table lateral view in detecting cervical spine injuries: a retrospective analysis. Ann Emerg Med 10:508, 1981

21. Robinson RJS, Mulder DS: Airway control. Trauma, 4th ed. Mattox KL, Feliciano DV, Moore EE, Eds. McGraw-Hill, New York, 2000

22. Jorden RC, Moore EE, Marx JA, et al: A comparison of PTV and endotracheal ventilation in an acute trauma model. J Trauma 25:978, 1985

23. Norwood S, Myers MB, Butler TJ: The safety of emergency neuromuscular blockade and orotracheal intubation in the acutely injured trauma patient. J Am Coll Surg 179:646, 1994

24. Vijayakumar E, Bosscher H: The use of neuromuscular blocking agents in the Emergency Department to facilitate tracheal intubation in the trauma patient: help or hindrance? J Crit Care 13:1, 1998

25. Sawyer RW, Bodai BI, Blaisdell FW, et al: The current status of intraosseous infusion. J Am Coll Surg 179:353, 1994

26. Vayer JS, Henderson JV, Bellamy RF, et al: Absence of a tachycardic response to shock in penetrating intraperitoneal injury. Ann Emerg Med 17:227, 1988

27. Rush BF Jr, Richardson JD, Bosomworth P, et al: Limitations of blood replacement with electrolyte solutions: a controlled clinical study. Arch Surg 98:49, 1969

28. Durtschi MB, Haisch CE, Reynolds L, et al: Effect of micropore filtration on pulmonary function after massive transfusion. Am J Surg 138:8, 1979

29. Rozycki GS, Ochsner MG, Jaffin JH, et al: Prospective evaluation of surgeon's use of ultrasound in the evaluation of trauma patients. J Trauma 34:516, 1993

30. Rozycki GS, Feliciano DV, Ochsner MG, et al: The role of ultrasound in patients with possible penetrating cardiac wounds: a prospective multicenter study. J Trauma 46:543, 1999

31. Breaux EP, Dupont JB Jr, Albert HM, et al: Cardiac tamponade following penetrating mediastinal injuries: improved survival with early pericardiocentesis. J Trauma 19:361, 1979

32. Plummer D, Brunette D, Asinger R, et al: Emergency department echocardiography improves outcome in penetrating cardiac injury. Ann Emerg Med 21:709, 1992

33. Biffl WL, Moore EE, Harken AH: Emergency department thoracotomy. Trauma, 4th ed. Mattox KL, Feliciano DV, Moore EE, Eds. McGraw-Hill, New York, 2000

34. Biffl WL, Moore FA, Moore EE, et al: Cardiac enzymes are irrelevant in the patient with suspected myocardial contusion. Am J Surg 169:523, 1994

35. Illig KA, Swierzewski MJ, Feliciano DV, et al: A rational screening and treatment strategy based on the electrocardiogram alone for suspected cardiac contusion. Am J Surg 162:537, 1991

36. King MW, Aitchison JM, Nel JP: Fatal air embolism following penetrating lung trauma: an autopsy study. J Trauma 24:753, 1981

37. Fremstad JD, Martin SH: Lethal complication from insertion of nasogastric tube after severe basilar skull fracture. J Trauma 18:820, 1978

38. Gentilello LM: Temperature-associated injuries and syndromes. Trauma, 4th ed. Mattox KL, Feliciano DV, Moore EE, Eds. McGraw-Hill, New York, 2000

39. Patt A, McCroskey BL, Moore EE: Hypothermia induced coagulopathies in trauma. Surg Clin North Am 68:775, 1988

40. Reed RL II, Bracey AW Jr, Hudson JD, et al: Hypothermia and blood coagulation: dissociation between enzyme activity and clotting factor levels. Circ Shock 32:141, 1990

41. Davis JW, Kaups KL: Base deficit in the elderly: a marker of severe injury and death. J Trauma 45:873, 1998

42. Thompson JS, Moore EE, Van Duzer-Moore S, et al: The evolution of abdominal stab wound management. J Trauma 20:478, 1980

43. Moore EE, Moore JB, Van Duzer-Moore S, et al: Mandatory laparotomy for gunshot wounds penetrating the abdomen. Am J Surg 140:847, 1980

44. Marx JA, Moore EE, Jorden RC, et al: Limitations of computed tomography in the evaluation of acute abdominal trauma: a prospective comparison with diagnostic peritoneal lavage. J Trauma 25:933, 1985

45. Fabian TC, Mangiante EC, White TJ, et al: A prospective study of 91 patients undergoing both computed tomography and peritoneal lavage following blunt abdominal trauma. J Trauma 26:602, 1986

46. Feliciano DV, Bitondo-Dyer CG: Vagaries of the lavage white blood cell count in evaluating abdominal stab wounds. Am J Surg 168:680, 1994

47. Jacobs DG, Angus A, Rodriguez A, et al: Peritoneal lavage white count: a reassessment. J Trauma 30:607, 1990

48. McAnena OJ, Marx JA, Moore EE: Peritoneal lavage enzyme determinations following blunt and penetrating abdominal trauma. J Trauma 31:1161, 1991

49. Moore JB, Moore EE, Thompson JS: Abdominal injuries associated with penetrating trauma in the lower chest. Am J Surg 140:724, 1980

50. Uribe RA, Pachon CE, Frame SB, et al: A prospective evaluation of thoracoscopy for the diagnosis of penetrating thoracoabdominal trauma. J Trauma 37:650, 1994

51. McAllister E, Perez M, Albrink MH, et al: Is triple contrast computed tomographic scanning useful in the selective management of stab wounds to the back? J Trauma 37:401, 1994

52. Easter DW, Shackford SR, Mattrey RF: A prospective, randomized comparison of computed tomography with conventional diagnostic methods in the evaluation of penetrating injuries to the back and flank. Arch Surg 126:1115, 1991

53. Burgess AR, Eastridge BJ, Young JWR, et al: Pelvic ring disruptions: effective classification system and treatment protocols. J Trauma 30:848, 1990

54. Cryer HM, Miller FB, Evers BM, et al: Pelvic fracture classification: correlation with hemorrhage. J Trauma 28:973, 1988

55. Latenser BA, Gentilello LM, Tarver AA, et al: Improved outcome with early fixation of skeletally unstable pelvic fractures. J Trauma 31:28, 1991

56. Riemer BL, Butterfield SL, Diamond DL, et al: Acute mortality associated with injuries to the pelvic ring: the role of early patient mobilization and external fixation. J Trauma 35:671, 1993

57. Moreno C, Moore EE, Rosenberger A, et al: Hemorrhage associated with major pelvic fracture: a multi-specialty challenge. J Trauma 26:987, 1986

58. Panetta T, Sclafani SJA, Goldstein AS, et al: Percutaneous transcatheter embolization for massive bleeding from pelvic fractures. J Trauma 25:1021, 1985

59. Harris JH, Horowitz DR, Zelitt DL: Unenhanced dynamic mediastinal computed tomography in the selection of patients requiring aortography for detection of acute traumatic aortic injury. Emerg Radiol 2:67, 1995

60. Fabian TC, Davis KA, Gavant ML, et al: Prospective study of blunt aortic injury: helical CT is diagnostic and antihypertensive therapy reduces rupture. Ann Surg 227:666, 1998

61. Lombardi G, Gallagher EJ, Gennis P: Outcome of out-of-hospital cardiac arrest in New York City. JAMA 271:678, 1994

62. Messer JV: Management of emergencies: XIV. Cardiac arrest. N Engl J Med 275:35, 1966

63. Roth R, Stewart RD, Rogers K, et al: Out-of-hospital cardiac arrest: factors associated with survival. Ann Emerg Med 13:237, 1984

64. DeBard ML: Cardiopulmonary resuscitation: analysis of six years' experience and review of the literature. Ann Emerg Med 10:408, 1981

65. Pons PT, Moore EE, Cusick JM, et al: Prehospital venous access in an urban paramedic system: a prospective on-scene analysis. J Trauma 28:1460, 1988

66. Kramer GC, Perron PR, Lindsey DC, et al: Small-volume resuscitation with hypertonic saline dextran solution. Surgery 100:239, 1986

67. Mattox KL, Maningas PA, Moore EE, et al: Prehospital hypertonic saline/dextran infusion for post-traumatic hypotension. Ann Surg 213:482, 1991

68. Younes RN, Aun F, Accioly CQ, et al: Hypertonic solutions in the treatment of hypovolemic shock: a prospective, randomized study in patients admitted to the emergency room. Surgery 111:380, 1992

69. Vassar MJ, Fischer RP, O'Brien PE, et al: A multicenter trial for resuscitation of injured patients with 7.5% sodium chloride. Arch Surg 128:1003, 1993

70. Shackford SR, Schmoker JD, Zhuang J: The effect of hypertonic resuscitation on pial arteriolar tone after brain injury and shock. J Trauma 37:899, 1994

71. Gould SA, Moore EE, Holt D, et al: The first randomized trial of human polymerized hemoglobin as a blood substitute in acute trauma and emergency surgery. J Am Coll Surg 187:113, 1998

72. Aprahamian C, Thompson BM, Finger WA, et al: Experimental cervical spine injury model: evaluation of airway management and splinting techniques. Ann Emerg Med 13:584, 1984

73. Bucholz RW, Burkhead WZ, Graham W, et al: Occult cervical spine injuries in fatal traffic accidents. J Trauma 19:768, 1979

74. Davis D, Bohlman H, Walker AE, et al: The pathological findings in fatal craniospinal injuries. J Neurosurg 34:603, 1971

75. Moore FA, Haenel JB, Moore EE, et al: Percutaneous tracheostomy/gastrostomy in brain-injured patients: a minimally invasive alternative. J Trauma 33:435, 1992

76. Gaffney FA, Thal ER, Taylor WF, et al: Hemodynamic effects of medical anti-shock trousers (MAST garment). J Trauma 21:931, 1981

77. McKinley BA, Marvin RG, Cocanour CS, et al: Tissue hemoglobin O_2 saturation during resuscitation of traumatic shock monitored using near infrared spectometry. J Trauma 48:637, 2000

78. Shires GT, Cunningham JN, Backer CR, et al: Alterations in cellular membrane function during hemorrhagic shock in primates. Ann Surg 176:288, 1972

79. Shires GT, Canizaro PC: Fluid resuscitation in the severely injured. Surg Clin North Am 53:1341, 1973

80. Cochrane Injuries Group Albumin Reviewers: Human albumin administration in critically ill patients: systematic review of randomised controlled trials. BMJ 317:235, 1998

81. Choi PT-L, Yip G, Quinonez LF, et al: Crystalloids vs. colloids in fluid resuscitation: a systematic review. Crit Care Med 27:200, 1999

82. Trinkle JK, Rush BF, Eiseman B: Metabolism of lactate following major blood loss. Surgery 63:782, 1968

83. Healey MA, Davis RE, Liu FC, et al: Lactated Ringer's is superior to normal saline in a model of massive hemorrhage and resuscitation. J Trauma 45:894, 1998

84. Ciesla DJ, Moore EE, Gonzalez R, et al: Hypertonic saline inhibits neutrophil (PMN) priming via attenuation of p38 MAPK signaling. Shock 14:265, 2000

85. Rhee P, Wang D, Ruff P, et al: Human neutrophil activation and increased adhesion by various resuscitation fluids. Crit Care Med 28:74, 2000

86. Moore FD, Dagher FJ, Boyden CM, et al: Hemorrhage in normal man: I. Distribution and dispersal of saline infusions following acute blood loss: clinical kinetics of blood volume support. Ann Surg 163:485, 1966

87. Cervera AL, Moss G: Progressive hypovolemia leading to shock after continuous hemorrhage and 3:1 crystalloid replacement. Am J Surg 129:670, 1975

88. Mann DV, Robinson MK, Rounds JD, et al: Superiority of blood over saline resuscitation from hemorrhagic shock: a ^{31}P magnetic resonance spectroscopy study. Ann Surg 226:653, 1997

89. Blumberg N, Bove JR: Un–cross-matched blood for emergency transfusion: one year's experience in a civilian setting. JAMA 240:2057, 1978

90. Gervin AS, Fischer RP: Resuscitation of trauma patients with type-specific uncrossmatched blood. J Trauma 24:327, 1984

91. Barnes A Jr, Allen TE: Transfusions subsequent to administration of universal donor blood in Vietnam. JAMA 203:695, 1968

92. Wall MJ, Granchi T, Liscum K, et al: Delayed versus immediate resuscitation in patients with penetrating trauma: subgroup analysis. J Trauma 39:173, 1995

93. Wiggers CJ: Physiology of Shock. Commonwealth Publications, New York, 1950

94. Rosner MJ, Daughton S: Cerebral perfusion pressure management in head injury. J Trauma 30:933, 1990

95. Sauaia AJ, Moore FA, Moore EE, et al: Multiple organ failure can be predicted as early as 12 hrs postinjury. J Trauma 45:291, 1998

96. Jurkovich GJ, Moore EE, Medina G: Auto-transfusion in trauma: a pragmatic analysis. Am J Surg 148:782, 1984

97. Silva R, Moore EE, Bar-Or D, et al: The risk:benefit of autotransfusion—comparison to banked blood in a canine model. J Trauma 24:557, 1984

98. Tremper KK, Friedman AE, Levine EM, et al: The preoperative treatment of severely anemic patients with a perfluorochemical oxygen-transport fluid, Fluosol-DA. N Engl J Med 314:1653, 1986

99. Gould SA, Rosen AL, Lakshman RS, et al: Fluosol-DA as a red-cell substitute in acute anemia. N Engl J Med 314:1653, 1986

100. Sloan EP, Koenigsberg M, et al: Diaspirin cross-linked hemoglobin (DCLHb) in the treatment of severe traumatic hemorrhagic shock: a randomized controlled efficacy trial. JAMA 282:1857, 1999

101. Rhee PM, Acosta J, Bridgeman A, et al: Survival after emergency department thoracotomy: review of published data from the past 25 years. J Am Coll Surg 190:288, 2000

102. Sanders AB, Kern KB, Ewy GA, et al: Improved resuscitation from cardiac arrest with open-chest massage. Ann Emerg Med 13:672, 1984

103. Ledgerwood AM, Kazmers M, Lucas CE: The role of thoracic aortic occlusion for massive hemoperitoneum. J Trauma 16:610, 1976

104. Millikan JS, Moore EE: Outcome of resuscitative thoracotomy and descending aortic occlusion performed in the operating room. J Trauma 24:387, 1984

105. Mattox KL, Allen MK, Feliciano DV: Laparotomy in the emergency department. JACEP 8:180, 1979

106. Hardaway RM, Chun B, Rutherford RB: Coagulation in shock in various species including man. Acta Chir Scand 130:157, 1965

107. Collins JA: Problems associated with the massive transfusion of stored blood. Surgery 75:274, 1974

108. Miller RD, Robbins TO, Tong MJ, et al: Coagulation defects associated with massive blood transfusions. Ann Surg 174:794, 1971

109. Cosgriff N, Moore EE, Sauaia A, et al: Predicting life-threatening coagulopathy in the massively transfused trauma patient: hypothermia and acidoses revisited. J Trauma 42:857, 1997

110. Stulz PM, Scheidegger D, Drop LJ, et al: Ventricular pump performance during hypocalcemia: clinical and experimental studies. J Thorac Cardiovasc Surg 78: 185, 1979

111. Trunkey D, Carpenter MA, Holcroft J: Calcium flux during hemorrhagic shock in baboons. J Trauma 16: 633, 1976

112. Jurkovich GJ, Greiser WB, Luterman A, et al: Hypothermia in trauma victims: an ominous predictor of survival. J Trauma 27:1019, 1987

113. Gentilello LM, Jurkovich GJ, Maier R, et al: Is hypothermia in the victim of major trauma protective or harmful? a randomized prospective study. Ann Surg 226:439, 1997

114. Dunn EL, Moore EE, Breslich DJ, et al: Acidosis-induced coagulopathy. Forum on Fundamental Surgical Problems 30:471, 1979

115. Clowes GHA Jr, Sabga GH, Konitaxis A, et al: Effects of acidosis on cardiovascular function in surgical patients. Ann Surg 154:524, 1961

116. Fry DE, Ratcliffe DJ, Yates JR: The effects of acidosis on canine hepatic and renal oxidative phosphorylation. Surgery 88:269, 1980

117. Douglas ME, Downs JB, Mantini EL, et al: Alteration of oxygen tension and oxyhemoglobin saturation: a hazard of sodium bicarbonate administration. Arch Surg 114:326, 1979

118. Moore EE: Thomas G. Orr Memorial Lecture. Staged laparotomy for the hypothermia, acidosis, and coagulopathy syndrome. Am J Surg 172:405, 1996

Acknowledgments

Figures 2 and 6   Carol Donner, revised by Tom Moore.

Figures 3, 5, 7a, 7b, and 9   Carol Donner.

Figures 7c, 8, and 11   Tom Moore.

Figure 12   Seward Hung.

3 BURN CARE IN THE IMMEDIATE RESUSCITATION PERIOD

Robert H. Demling, M.D.

Approach to the Burn Patient in the First 24 Hours

Neutralization of the Source of the Burn

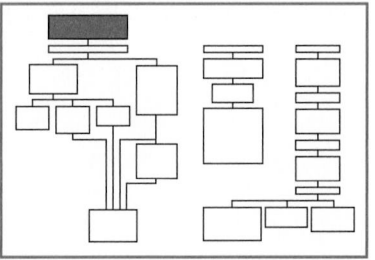

CLOTHING

The first objective is to stop the burning process because the deeper the burn, the greater the potential for mortality and morbidity. With chemical burns, chemicals can remain in fabric and on skin for long periods. With a flame or scald burn, clothing can retain heat for a considerable time. Rapid removal of clothing is thus essential. Clothes are often still smoldering when the patient arrives at the emergency room. If clothing is burned or melted into the tissues, the surrounding fabric can be cut off. Adherent clothing can be removed after admission, when further wound cleaning and debridement are performed.

CHEMICAL BURNS

Removal of the chemical is urgent. Acid burns should be irrigated for up to 60 minutes with warm tap water. For burns resulting from alkali contact, lavage for at least 60 minutes may be beneficial [see Table 1]. If necessary, particles of corrosive powders should be surgically removed before the wound is irrigated. The skin burn itself is not the only concern, because the absorption of certain chemicals can lead to systemic toxicities such as neurologic dysfunction, red cell hemolysis, and liver and kidney failure.

It is important to avoid severe hypothermia during irrigation because hypothermia results in significant morbidity. Therefore, once the burn source is removed, the patient should be covered with clean, dry dressings or sheets.

Establishment of Airway and Adequate Ventilation

DIAGNOSIS AND TREATMENT OF CARBON MONOXIDE TOXICITY

Carbon monoxide toxicity is one of the leading causes of death associated with fires. As oxygen is being consumed in the process of combustion, CO is being released. Carbon monoxide is rapidly transported across the alveolar membrane and preferentially binds to hemoglobin in place of oxygen to form carboxyhemoglobin (COHb). In addition, CO causes the oxyhemoglobin dissociation curve to shift to the left, thereby impairing oxygen unloading at the tissue level; this shift results in a substantial reduction in oxygen delivery, given that 98% of the oxygen supplied to the tissues comes bound to hemoglobin. With prolonged exposure, CO can saturate the cell, binding to cytochrome oxidase and thereby further impairing mitochondrial function and adenosine triphosphate (ATP) production.

Patients who were injured in a closed space or who have inhalation injuries should be suspected of inhaling CO [see Table 2]. CO toxicity is determined by a high index of suspicion and by measuring the COHb level. Persistent metabolic acidosis in a patient with adequate volume resuscitation and adequate cardiac output indicates persistent impairment of oxygen utilization and delivery by CO or hydrocyanide. The chemical alteration of hemoglobin or of the cytochrome system by CO will not affect the amount of oxygen dissolved in plasma, and arterial oxygen tension (P_aO_2) will thus remain relatively normal. However, the measured oxygen saturation of hemoglobin will be markedly decreased relative to the oxygen tension.

Treatment of CO toxicity consists of promptly displacing CO from hemoglobin by administering 90% to 100% oxygen until the COHb level is less than 7%. If 20% oxygen is administered, the half-life of COHb is about 90 minutes; if concentrated high-flow oxygen is administered, the half-life is 20 to 30 minutes. The concentration of COHb is thus reduced by approximately 50% every 20 to 30 minutes if an oxygen concentration of 90% to 100% is used. Hyperbaric oxygen (2 to 3 atm) yields even more rapid displacement, particularly from the cell cytochrome system, and can be used to treat severe CO toxicity (i.e., a CO level > 50% or an elevated CO level that does not respond to standard oxygen therapy).

DIAGNOSIS AND TREATMENT OF CYANIDE TOXICITY

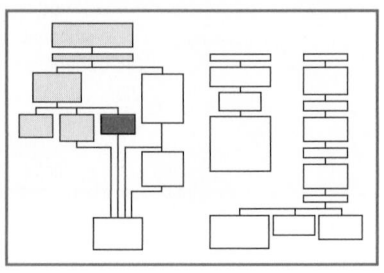

Hydrocyanide, the gaseous form of cyanide, is a well-recognized cause of fire-associated morbidity and mortality, particularly when synthetics such as polyurethane are burned. Although cyanide can be absorbed through the GI tract or through skin, it is most dangerous when aerosolized and inhaled because it is absorbed especially rapidly through the respiratory tract. Once absorbed, cyanide binds to the cytochrome system, thereby inhibiting cell metabolism and ATP production. All cells, and hepatocytes in particular, have a detoxifying system in which the enzyme rhodenase converts hydrocyanide to thiocyanate, which is then excreted in the urine. If, however, a large amount of cyanide is absorbed, this protective system can be overwhelmed, especially in the face of hypovolemia, which hinders metabolism and clearance of cyanide.

The diagnosis of cyanide toxicity is made on the basis of the history and a high index of suspicion and is confirmed by the presence of elevated blood cyanide levels (normal, < 0.1 mg/L; values higher than 1 mg/L are usually lethal). Treatment begins with volume replenishment. From 10 to 20 ml of a 3% sodium nitrite solution is then given over a period of 10 minutes; methemoglobin is produced as the cyanide is detoxified. Finally, 50 ml of a 25% solution of sodium thiosulfate is given; this converts the cyanide to sodium thiocyanate, which is excreted in the urine.

DIAGNOSIS OF THE PRESENCE AND EXTENT OF INHALATION INJURY

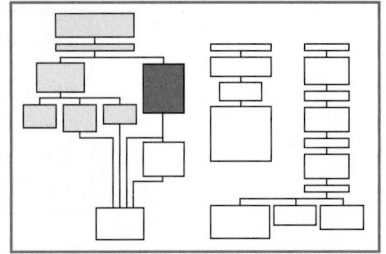

Inhalation injury, a complex and deadly disease process, occurs when the heat and toxins in smoke make contact with airway mucosa and alveoli. The degree of injury depends on the composition of the smoke, which varies according to its source. Heat affects primarily the supraglottic area and causes edema and upper airway obstruction, whereas the gas and particle components of the smoke affect primarily the airway mucosa and cause the actual chemical burn. The initial smoke injury occurs shortly after exposure, but the ensuing intense inflammatory reaction evolves over a period of hours to days [see Figure 1]. The degree of mucosal damage can range from simple erythema and irritation to complete mucosal sloughing that leads to distal airway obstruction and subsequently to atelectasis and increased shunting. Alveolar instability can also occur as a result of direct surfactant denaturation. Alveolar edema is a late finding.

Table 1 Chemical Burns

Agent	Pathophysiology	Treatment
Acids	Acids cause deep skin burns through tissue desiccation and protein denaturation; with concentrated acids, injury may extend well below skin. Acids such as H_2SO_4, HCl, and HNO_3 cause local damage. Burned area is tan to gray in appearance; extreme pain is a common finding. *Hydrofluoric acid:* Hydrofluoric acid causes a deep skin burn that may be extensive. It also exerts systemic effects, which are attributable to hypocalcemia resulting from the formation of a Ca^{2+}-F^- complex.	Perform vigorous water lavage for as long as 60 min after injury; use warm water with extensive exposure to prevent hypothermia. Assume that the burn will be much deeper than initial appearance indicates. Apply standard fluid resuscitation principles. *Hydrofluoric acid:* Perform vigorous water lavage. Inject calcium gluconate locally, and apply 2.5% calcium gluconate gel topically; end point of calcium gluconate administration is relief of pain. Monitor plasma calcium levels, and replace calcium deficits if necessary.
Alkalies	Alkalies cause deep skin burns through tissue desiccation and protein denaturation resulting from chemical reaction with hydrated tissue. Alkali burns tend to be worse than acid burns, but alkalies tend not to be absorbed systemically and thus rarely exert systemic effects. The burned area is tan to gray; extreme pain is a characteristic finding.	Perform vigorous water lavage for at least 60 min after injury—longer for lye burns—and take pains to prevent hypothermia. Assume that the burn will increase in depth. Apply standard fluid resuscitation principles.
Gasoline	Gasoline immersion produces both superficial skin injury and systemic injury (resulting from absorption of hydrocarbons). The systemic injury comprises the following: *Renal injury:* lipid degenerative changes to proximal tubules *Pulmonary injury:* surfactant denaturation, atelectasis, lipoid pneumonia *CNS injury:* edema producing seizures or coma *Hepatic injury:* lipid degenerative changes, hepatitis Burned area is erythematous in appearance.	Immerse injured area in water. Aggressively maintain hydration and pulmonary support, and provide general critical care support.
Phenol	Phenol produces both a partial-thickness burn and systemic injury (resulting from absorption), which is directly proportional to amount of skin exposed. The systemic injury comprises the following: *Renal injury:* direct glomerular and tubular damage as well as indirect damage from precipitated hemoglobin *Hematologic injury:* red cell hemolysis *CNS injury:* seizures or coma *Hepatic injury:* centrolobular necrosis Burned area is dull tan to gray in appearance.	Spray or pour large amounts of water on burned surface. Do not swab or use small amounts of water; these actions serve only to increase surface area of exposure. After lavage, quickly wipe skin with polyethylene or propylene glycol. To minimize hemoglobin precipitation, keep urine alkaline by administering bicarbonate. Maintain optimal hydration and blood volume to support injured kidney and any other injured organs.
Tar	Hot tar causes a superficial to deep skin burn, depending on the temperature of the tar when it contacts the skin. As a rule, there is no systemic absorption.	Remove tar to allow burn wound management. Bacitracin ointment and Neosporin (polymyxin B–bacitracin–neomycin) ointment contain the emulsifier Tween-80, which is very useful for dissolving tar. Apply the ointment and wash it off several times a day until tar is removed. Avoid hydrocarbon solvents. Perform general mechanical debridement if desired.

Patient presents with burn

Neutralize the burn source: remove clothing and chemicals.
Irrigate acid and alkali burns.
Continue wet dressings only in 2° burns < 15% TBS.
Avoid hypothermia at all times.

1. Establish and maintain airway and adequate ventilation

- **Patient is conscious,**
- **No airway or ventilation problems,**
  and
- **No deep facial burn**

Give 100% O_2 by mask.
Obtain blood gases, COHb levels, cyanide levels.

One of the following is present:
- **Unconsciousness**
- **Deep facial burn**
- **Hypoventilation**
- **Hypoxia on mask O_2**

Secure airway (use tube ≥ 7 mm).
Diagnose and treat ↑COHb.
Begin CPAP or PEEP at 5 cm H_2O; ↑ to maintain O_2 sat. > 90%.
Assess lower airways.
Obtain baseline chest x-ray.

COHb is normal

Give O_2 to maintain O_2 sat. > 90%.
Monitor for pulmonary problems.

COHb ↑

Give O_2 until COHb < 7%.
If COHb > 40%, intubate and use PEEP.
Reserve hyperbaria for most severe cases.

Cyanide ↑

Give sodium nitrite, followed by sodium thiosulfate.

Ventilation is inadequate

Consider bronchodilators for airway spasm.

Chest wall burn present?
- Circumferential 3°: perform escharotomy
- Noncircumferential: monitor closely; perform escharotomy on symptoms of restriction

Begin standard Rx for smoke exposure

Maintain
- Aggressive pulmonary toilet
- Close monitoring of gas exchange
- Controlled fluid Rx
- Airway assessment

Do not use prophylactic corticosteroids.

Approach to the Burn Patient in the First 24 Hours

2. Establish and maintain adequate circulation

Burns > 20% TBS

Begin administration of lactated Ringer solution

Estimate initial rate according to % TBS burned and weight.

Maintain
- BP > 90 mm Hg systolic
- Urine output 0.5–1.0 ml/kg/hr
- Pulse < 130 beats/min
- T° ≥ 37° C

Modify protocol in the presence of massive burns, inhalation injury, or shock and in elderly patients

Include hypertonic lactated saline (first 8–10 hr) or colloid.

Consider inotrope if fluid alone is inadequate (low-dose dopamine is first choice).

Use pulse oximeter (ideal for measuring O_2 sat.).

Add arterial line to monitor BP and blood gases.

Monitor cardiac output, PAWP, mixed venous P_{O_2} with pulmonary arterial line in the presence of
- heart disease, or
- persistent hemodynamic instability, or
- inotrope administration.

3. Initiate wound management

Determine extent of injury

Estimate depth.

Estimate area, using Rule of Nines.

Consider risk factors: age, inhalation injury, trauma, concomitant illness.

Follow ACS guidelines for tetanus prophylaxis

Maintain perfusion

Elevate burned extremities.

Remove constricting items.

Monitor distal perfusion; perform escharotomy if necessary.

Control pain with frequent small doses of I.V. narcotics

Clean the wound

Use chlorhexidine in warm solution.

Avoid body immersion.

Debride loose tissue and dirt; spare large blisters, hands, and feet.

Dress the wound

Superficial 2° burn

Face or neck: Apply bacitracin t.i.d. No dressing.

Extremities or flat surfaces: Temporary skin substitute or grease gauze dressing. Second choice: topical antibiotics.

Perineum or buttocks; gross contamination anywhere: Silver sulfadiazine b.i.d. with or without dressings.

Medium to deep 2° burn

Apply silver sulfadiazine, with dressings in most areas.

Change b.i.d. or t.i.d.

3° burn

Dressings preferred in most areas.

Uninfected wound: Use silver sulfadiazine b.i.d.

Infected wound: Use mafenide b.i.d.

Table 2 Symptoms of Carbon Monoxide Intoxication

Carboxyhemoglobin Level (%)	Symptoms
0–15	None
15–20	Headache, confusion
20–40	Disorientation, fatigue, nausea, visual impairment
40–60	Hallucination, combativeness, coma, shock
60+	Death

Inhalation injury should be suspected in (1) individuals who were injured in a closed space; (2) patients with extensive burns or with burns of the face; (3) patients who were unconscious at the time of injury; (4) patients with singed nasal hairs, hoarseness, or wheezing; and (5) patients who are coughing up carbonaceous sputum.

Pulmonary injury is known to result in substantially increased late burn mortality and morbidity as well as increased early fluid requirements and metabolic demands. Early intubation and positive pressure ventilation have been reported to improve outcome. The mode of ventilation used depends on the specific physiologic problem present; different modes may become necessary as the disease changes over time.

Pulmonary changes can be classified according to cause: thermal injury (heat) or chemical injury (incomplete products of combustion).

Thermal Injury

A number of techniques have been used to assess the degree of supraglottic injury and to determine the need for endotracheal intubation. Fiberoptic bronchoscopy or laryngoscopy will reveal physical evidence of mucosal injury. Spirometry detects early obstructive patterns in the airways, but reliable data can be obtained only in a cooperative patient without severe facial burns. Because the injury process is progressive during the first 18 to 24 hours, none of these tests accurately predicts the severity of subsequent airway compromise; serial studies must be performed.

Chemical Injury

Diagnosis of chemical injury is complicated by the fact that facial burns or other signs evident in heat injury may be absent; indeed, the patient may not have been exposed to heat. Fiberoptic bronchoscopy detects the reddened, sometimes ulcerated mucosa that indicates the presence—but not the severity—of chemical injury. Ventilation-perfusion lung scans using xenon-133 reportedly detect early changes in the small airways, as do analyses of flow-volume curves and a simple 1-second forced expiratory volume (FEV_1). Preexisting lung disease, however, will alter the interpretation of findings. Measurement of lung water is of minimal benefit because major changes in water content usually occur only in an alveolar injury in which early respiratory failure is prominent. Initial chest x-ray, blood gas levels, and physical examination results are frequently normal.

INTUBATION

Endotracheal intubation is indicated for (1) deep facial burns—especially of the lips, the mouth, the neck, or the oropharynx—because subsequent edema will impair airway patency; (2) cases of smoke inhalation in which heat or chemical burns to the airway have been demonstrated by laryngoscopy or bronchoscopy; and (3) massive body burns, especially in the presence of circumferential chest burns, because ventilatory support is needed.

With deep burns of the face, the mouth, or the neck, the airway can be compromised by anatomic distortion and compression from the burn-edema process. Edema-induced distortion peaks at 18 to 24 hours after a burn; both airway patency and the ability to clear secretions are impaired. As edema increases, it becomes much more difficult to secure an airway. Endotracheal intubation is thus preferably performed on admission, before severe edema develops. A patient with inhalation injury can be closely monitored for upper airway obstruction without a tube, preferably with the head elevated at 30°, only if intubation will be technically possible later. However, if anatomic distortion from face and neck burns is increasing to a point where safe intubation might soon be precluded, the procedure is carried out immediately. Tracheostomy through burned tissue is contraindicated because the risk of infection, both in the wound and in the airway, is substantially increased.

Heat injury usually heals in a matter of a few days to a week, as the mucosal edema resolves and the relatively superficial mucosal injury heals.

Positive end-expiratory pressure (PEEP) is frequently necessary to keep the edematous airways open and to maintain an adequate functional residual capacity; it is also often used in the early management of severe CO toxicity (COHb > 40%). Prophylactic endotracheal intubation and PEEP have been reported to decrease deaths from early pulmonary complications after severe burns and smoke inhalation. A large enough tube (i.e., approximately 7.5 mm internal diameter in adults) should be used because very thick secretions develop as the lung injury becomes manifest, and changing tubes in the presence of edema is very dangerous. Therefore, although the nasotracheal route may be more comfortable for the patient, the choice of a route of placement must be based on the tube size required.

Figure 1 **The view through a fiberoptic bronchoscope shows erythema and edema of the larynx 18 hours after a burn.**

INITIATION OF AGGRESSIVE PULMONARY SUPPORT

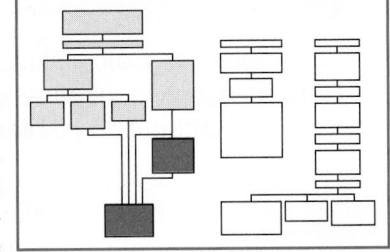

Continuous administration of humidified oxygen is indicated to maintain adequate oxygen delivery as well as to assist in the clearance of secretions. If the patient's hemodynamic condition will tolerate it, elevation of the head and chest by 20° to 30° is helpful in reducing neck and chest wall edema. The early addition of bronchodilators, usually by aerosol, is especially advantageous in managing the bronchospasm seen after chemical injury. The beta$_2$-adrenergic agent metaproterenol (via nebulizer) is an effective bronchodilator. Intravenous aminophylline, although helpful, is frequently limited in its use because of the tachycardia seen in the early postburn period. Intravenous steroids have not been found to decrease the degree of injury; however, aerosolized steroid preparations identical to those used in asthma patients can decrease airway hyperreactivity, which is often a major problem in patients with smoke inhalation injury and which may not be responsive to aerosolized beta agonists. On the other hand, intravenous steroids have been successful in attenuating obliterative bronchiolitis, an uncommon but uniformly fatal late complication of severe smoke inhalation injury. Prophylactic antibiotics are not indicated to prevent a lung infection after smoke injury.

Close monitoring of the adequacy of gas exchange by serial blood gas determination is necessary, particularly during the early evolution of complications from the inhalation injury. An indwelling arterial line is indicated in the presence of severe injuries. When placement of such a line is not possible, a pulse oximeter is very useful if an unburned finger or earlobe is available. The pulse oximeter reads arterial oxygen saturation by means of a photosensor, which detects the color of the blood flowing beneath the probe.

Chest Wall Escharotomy

A full-thickness burn of the anterior and lateral chest wall can lead to severe restriction of chest wall motion as edema develops beneath the nonviable tissue (eschar), even in the absence of a completely circumferential burn. Chest wall escharotomy is required to relieve the restriction; the incision must penetrate completely through the eschar so that the subeschar space can expand and decrease tissue pressure. In a full-thickness burn, nerve endings are destroyed along with the entire epidermis and dermis. Analgesics are thus usually not necessary for escharotomy. The escharotomy incisions are placed along the anterior axillary lines, with bilateral incisions connected by a subcostal incision [see Figure 2 and Initiation of Wound Management, Subeschar Edema

in Extremities, below]. Occasionally, another incision from the suprasternal notch to the xiphoid process is needed. Bleeding can usually be managed by pressure and occasional use of the electrocautery unit.

Restoration and Maintenance of Hemodynamic Stability

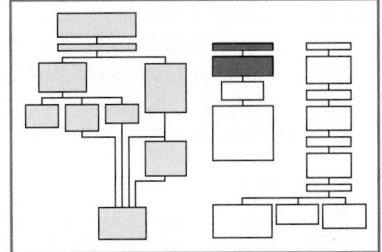

ESTIMATION OF BURN SIZE

Fluid requirements depend on the size of the burn. A simple determination of the burn surface area can be made using the Rule of Nines: each arm is considered to be 9% of total body surface (TBS), each leg 18%, the anterior trunk 18%, the posterior trunk 18%, and the head 9% [see Figure 3]. In small children, the determination must be modified because the head approaches 18% of TBS.

INTRAVENOUS ACCESS

A peripheral venous catheter through unburned tissue is the preferred route for fluid administration. A central venous line or pulmonary arterial line is only occasionally needed to monitor the patient during the initial resuscitation period and is removed as soon as it is no longer needed. These lines are usually required only in elderly patients or in patients who have severe heart disease. An extremely high complication rate reportedly accompanies the use of central catheters in burn patients because of infection and embolic episodes related to a hypercoagulable state. Because of the high infection rate, an intravenous catheter should not be placed through burn tissue unless every other possible route has been ruled out. A line that is dedicated to total parenteral nutrition should be completely isolated from the burn wound and cared for by covering the entrance site with an occlusive dressing [see III:13 Burn Care after the First Postburn Week].

Figure 2 The red lines on the illustrated human figure represent guidelines for the placement of escharotomy incisions.

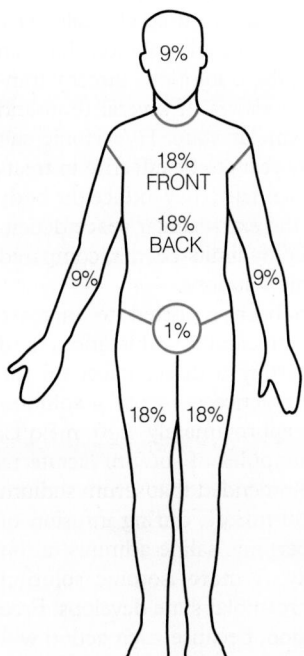

Figure 3 The size of a burn can be estimated by means of the Rule of Nines, which assigns percentages of total body surface to the head, the extremities, and the front and back of the torso.

RESUSCITATION FLUIDS

In general, fluids containing salt in quantities at least isotonic with plasma are appropriate for use in resuscitation after burn injury if given in sufficient amounts. These fluids should be free of glucose because burn patients exhibit early glucose intolerance as a result of the early release of catecholamines and other stress hormones. The oral route can be used in the case of smaller burns, but intestinal ileus frequently occurs after deep burns in excess of 20% of total body surface. A number of intravenous fluids, including colloids, are used to decrease edema in unburned tissues and to maintain a higher blood volume.

Crystalloid

Crystalloid—in particular, lactated Ringer solution, with a sodium concentration of 130 mEq/L—is the most popular resuscitation fluid in the United States. The loss of large quantities of sodium and water from the vascular space into the burn wound is well described. Isotonic crystalloid, if given in sufficient amounts, can restore cardiac output toward normal in most patients, the exceptions being patients who are extremely young or extremely old, those whose burns are massive, and those with superimposed inhalation injury. Lactated Ringer solution is preferred to normal saline because of its physiologic pH of 6.5 versus saline's pH of 5.0. Because isotonic salt solutions generate no differential in osmotic pressure between plasma and interstitial spaces, the entire extracellular space must be expanded to replace intravascular losses.

The amount of isotonic crystalloid required in the first 24 hours is based primarily on the calculated deficit of sodium from the extracellular space. This amount has been estimated to be 0.5 to 0.6 mEq sodium/kg/% TBS burned, which is equal to 4 ml/kg/% TBS burned of lactated Ringer solution. The quantity of crystalloid needed is also determined by measuring the parameters used to monitor resuscitation. In most burn centers, a urine output of 0.5 ml/kg/hr is considered an indication of adequate perfusion. The patient will require about 3 to 5 ml/kg/% TBS burned in the first 24 hours; about half of this amount is given in the first 8 hours [see Table 3].

Sodium is apparently the key element in crystalloid infusion; water is primarily the solvent. Solutions with increased sodium concentration therefore have a theoretical advantage because less water is infused. The hypertonic salt solutions used clinically have an osmolarity of 400 to 600 mOsm/L (isotonic solutions have an osmolarity of 280 to 300 mOsm/L); these solutions thereby transiently generate potential osmotic pressures of several thousand mm Hg relative to the normal isosmolar state. Hypertonic salt solutions have been known for many years to be effective in treating shock states, including burns. Essentially, they induce the body to borrow intracellular water to fill the extracellular space deficit. Infusion of hypertonic solutions thereby limits edema, compared with treatment by infusion of isotonic solutions.

Hypertonic solutions have also been reported to increase myocardial contractility, produce precapillary dilatation, and decrease vascular resistance by exerting a direct effect on the capillary smooth muscle. Current practice is to use a solution with a sodium concentration of approximately 240 mEq/L, which is prepared by adding two ampules of sodium lactate to each liter of normal saline. It is recommended that serum sodium levels not be allowed to exceed 160 mEq/L during infusion of the solution. Complications of hypertonic saline administration relate primarily to hyperosmolarity. A more isotonic solution should be given if an excessive hyperosmolar state develops. Free water cannot be given during infusion, because such action will simply lead to a more isotonic solution and in turn no decrease

---

Table 3 **Calculations to Determine Resuscitation Requirements in a Young Patient without an Inhalation Injury**

The patient is a 35-year-old male. His weight is 70 kg. His burns cover 50% TBS, most of which are second degree.

Recommendations:

3–4 ml lactated Ringer solution/kg body weight/% TBS burned
Administer 1/2 the required volume in the first 8 hr after the burn.
Administer 1/2 the required volume during the next 16 hr.

Calculation:

4 ml × 70 kg × 50% TBS burned = 14,000 ml/24 hr

Give

7,000 ml during the first 8 hr (875 ml/hr)
7,000 ml during the next 16 hr (435 ml/hr)

Monitor

Blood pressure (systolic > 90 mm Hg; mean > 80 mm Hg)
Pulse (< 120 beats/min)
Urine output (30–50 ml/hr)
Arterial blood gases (PO_2 > 90 mm Hg)
pH (> 7.35)

Adjust fluid administration in response to circulatory requirements:

Diminish fluid administration if hemodynamic stability is achieved at these infusion rates

or

Add colloid if adequate hemodynamic stability is not achieved at 4 ml/kg/% TBS burned.

---

in total administered fluid. Increased water retention is likely to occur with the institution of hypotonic solutions beginning on postburn day 2, at least until isotonicity results.

Colloids

Unburned tissue appears to regain normal permeability very soon after injury. Because hypoproteinemia may accentuate edema in uninjured tissues, protein restoration should begin 8 to 12 hours after a burn if nonburn edema and total fluid requirements are to be minimized. This method is particularly advantageous in patients who have massive burns and in elderly patients.

The amount of protein to be infused remains undefined. Many investigators have arbitrarily used between 0.5 and 1.0 ml/kg/% TBS burned during the first 24 hours. The amount depends on the magnitude of the injury and on the degree of hemodynamic instability. The protein should be infused at a constant rate [see Adjustment of Infusion Rate, below]; pulsed infusion will transiently increase pressure and increase the rate of edema formation.

If early administration of colloids is required because hemodynamic instability persists despite the infusion of large quantities of crystalloid (about 4 ml/kg/% TBS burned), nonprotein colloids are more economical. Although the weight of dextran 70 (70 kd) is almost identical to that of albumin, dextran's molecular size is considerably larger because of its branched configuration. A standard 6% solution of dextran 70 exerts an oncotic pressure more than twice that generated by a 6% albumin solution. This property makes the compound advantageous as a volume expander. Dextran 40 (40 kd) in a 10% solution, infused at about 2 ml/kg/hr, is an even more potent volume expander because it generates a colloid osmotic pressure six to eight times that of a protein of comparable weight. To prevent platelet deficits, the total dose of dextran 70 during any 24-hour period should not exceed 33 ml/kg; the total dose of dextran 40 should not exceed 15 ml/kg during any 24-hour period. Therefore, these preparations are usually used in the early resuscitation period and are replaced by protein in the later resuscitation period. The use of the hapten PROMIT—a 1 kd dextran—before the administration of the dextran solution essentially precludes allergic reactions to the dextran molecule.

Hetastarch, a 6% starch solution, has colloid properties very similar to those of a 6% protein solution and generates a comparable oncotic pressure. Hetastarch molecules are much larger than those of most dextrans, and vascular clearance is therefore much slower. This solution is being used with increasing frequency as a volume expander.

Blood

Because there is no actual early red cell deficit with a burn alone, blood replacement is usually not needed during this period unless severe hemolysis occurs. Occasionally, however, blood can be a very useful volume expander to restore cardiac output if perfusion is not adequately maintained by other resuscitation fluids.

ADJUSTMENT OF INFUSION RATE

Fluids should be infused at a constant rate because rapid fluid challenge transiently increases pressure above the level required for adequate perfusion and contributes to edema formation. Fluid requirements in the first 6 to 8 hours after a burn will clearly exceed those in the subsequent 18 hours because the largest fluid shifts occur early. Approximately half of the total amount of fluid required in the first 24 hours will be given in the first 8 hours. During those first 8 hours, once a fluid infusion rate is reached at which adequate perfusion is maintained, only minor changes should be made so as to avoid large hemodynamic fluctuations. Beginning 8 to 10 hours after a burn, when fluid requirements begin to diminish, an attempt should be made to decrease the infusion rate gradually and to determine the smallest amount of fluid or fluids necessary to maintain adequate perfusion. The rate required in the 12- to 24-hour period must usually deliver around 50% to 60% of the initial requirements. Fluid requirements during the first 24 hours usually range from 3 to 4 ml/kg/% TBS burned, depending on the type of fluid, the patient's age, and the presence of other injuries [see Table 3].

HEMODYNAMIC PARAMETERS TO MONITOR

Perfusion-Related Parameters

The adequacy of perfusion is difficult to assess after major burns. Burn injury leads to increased tissue demand for oxygen, but at the same time, the body's ability to increase oxygen delivery is impaired by capillary leakage into the burn. Inhalation injury places additional fluid requirements and metabolic demands on burn patients. The increased hemodynamic instability seen in burn patients is probably attributable to activation of systemic inflammation by the burn as well as to airway injury. Infusion of larger amounts of resuscitation fluid may be necessary; however, this may lead to additional edema, which also results in complications. The best approach is to rely on repeated clinical assessments based on sound physiologic principles. Monitoring the following parameters can facilitate the assessment and improvement of perfusion.

Mean arterial pressure The increased sympathetic tone characteristic of the early postburn period makes arterial pressure an insensitive measure of volume status; however, minimal perfusion pressure (mean, > 90 mm Hg) must be maintained, which means that blood pressure must be monitored. In each patient, however, the precise blood pressure required to maintain adequate organ perfusion and tissue oxygenation becomes evident only in the process of observing the patient's response to fluid infusion.

If the patient is hemodynamically unstable, if the extremities are burned to such an extent that a sphygmomanometer cannot be used, or if frequent measurement of not only P_aO_2 but also pH and arterial carbon dioxide tension (P_aCO_2) is required, insertion of an arterial catheter may be necessary. The catheter should be placed through unburned skin and should be removed as soon as possible. A pulse oximeter can provide continuous readings of oxygen saturation and has the additional benefit of being noninvasive.

Pulse rate Tachycardia is inevitable in the early postburn period, given the development of hypovolemia and the release of catecholamines as a result of tissue trauma and pain. The degree of tachycardia can be a useful indicator of the adequacy of volume replacement, except in elderly patients or in patients with preexisting heart disease, whose heart rate cannot increase in proportion to the stimulus. In most patients, a pulse rate lower than 120 beats/min usually indicates adequate volume, whereas a pulse rate higher than 130 beats/min usually indicates that more fluid is needed. This guideline assumes that the pulse rate response corresponds to the other monitors of perfusion being used. Sometimes, the pulse rate does not follow the other indicators of impaired perfusion, in which case it becomes less useful for monitoring purposes. A case in point is a burn patient who is taking a beta blocker.

Pulmonary arterial wedge pressure In most young patients, even those with massive burns, it is not necessary to measure pulmonary arterial wedge pressure (PAWP) in the course of initial resuscitation: the risks associated with inserting a pulmonary arterial catheter may well exceed any benefits to be gained with respect to assessing adequacy of perfusion. Like central venous pressure, PAWP is usually normal to low (6 to 10 mm Hg) in the early postburn period, even when perfusion is adequate. Hypoperfusion is almost always attributable to hypovolemia; other well-recognized causes are (1) impaired left ventricular function resulting from impaired left ventricular filling (as with high mean airway pressure or pneumothorax) and (2) a marked increase in afterload resulting from high levels of circulating vasoconstrictors. There are three main patient groups in whom measurement of PAWP may be beneficial: (1) elderly patients who have deep burns covering more than 30% of TBS or who have suffered substantial smoke inhalation injury, (2) patients with preexisting heart disease who have massive burns or substantial smoke inhalation injury, and (3) young patients with massive burns who are not maintaining adequate perfusion despite fluid intake well in excess of predicted requirements.

Cardiac output and mixed venous oxygen tension The primary objective of fluid management is maintenance of adequate delivery of oxygen to tissues. Direct measurement of cardiac output (usually expressed as cardiac index) facilitates this task. In an uninjured person, a cardiac index of 2.5 L/min/m² or higher would be considered normal. In an injured person, however, such a value would not necessarily be indicative of adequate oxygen delivery, because injured tissue requires more oxygen than normal tissue does. Monitoring of mixed venous oxygen tension ($P_{mv}O_2$) can be of great assistance in this situation. A $P_{mv}O_2$ higher than 35 mm Hg indicates that oxygen delivery is adequate, a $P_{mv}O_2$ between 30 and 35 mm Hg indicates that oxygen delivery is marginal, and a $P_{mv}O_2$ lower than 30 mm Hg indicates that oxygen delivery is inadequate.

Arterial blood gas values Whether P_aO_2 and P_aCO_2 must be monitored depends on the percentage of TBS burned and on the risk of respiratory abnormalities (particularly in patients with a history of smoke exposure). Pulse oximetry is useful for measuring P_aO_2. Measurement of pH and evaluation of acid-base balance are also extremely useful in the assessment of tissue oxygenation. A base deficit during the early postburn phase usually reflects impaired tissue oxygenation caused by hypovolemia or by carbon monoxide or hydrocyanide toxicity [see I:7 Life-Threatening Acid-Base Abnormalities].

Blood lactate concentration A normal blood lactate concentration does not indicate that perfusion is optimal; it only indicates that anaerobic metabolism is not taking place. A high lactate concentration, on the other hand, reflects severe hypoperfusion.

Urine output Urine output via a Foley catheter is a valuable indicator of adequate renal blood flow if the urine is nonglycosuric and if output has not been increased by administration of solutes (e.g., mannitol or dextran). An output of 0.5 ml/kg/hr in adults or 1.0 ml/kg/hr in children is adequate. Antidiuretic hormone and aldosterone are automatically released in response to the burn stress; therefore, a urine output greater than 0.5 to 1.0 ml/kg/hr may necessitate a rate of fluid infusion far higher than that necessary to maintain perfusion, and excess edema will result.

Other Parameters

Serum creatinine and blood urea nitrogen concentration Baseline values for serum creatinine and blood urea nitrogen may help rule out intrinsic renal disease, which impairs the reliability of urine output as an index of perfusion.

Body weight and temperature Obtaining a baseline body weight as early as possible after the burn will facilitate assessment of fluid balance. The preburn weight should be used to determine nutrition needs and drug dosages.

Body temperature should be obtained as well. Hypothermia is a major complication of burns; it is controlled by warming the environment. Hyperthermia can also occur as a result of early pyrogen release and can alter vital signs to be misleadingly suggestive of profound hypovolemia; it should be treated with antipyrogens.

Electrocardiographic status Arrhythmias are not common in young patients with burns as long as oxygenation is adequate, but they become a major concern in patients older than 45 years as a result of the stress response to the burn. Because arrhythmias may be the first clues to the presence of hypoxia and electrolyte or acid-base abnormalities, continuous electrocardiographic monitoring is required during the early postburn period.

Intake and output What goes in and what comes out should be carefully tabulated. Intake will far exceed output during the early postburn period as edema develops.

Hematocrit and hemoglobin concentration Although it is helpful to monitor the hematocrit and the hemoglobin concentration, changes in these values may not accurately reflect changes in blood volume. The rate of plasma loss often exceeds the rate of whole blood loss, which means that the hematocrit may be normal even in the face of severe volume depletion; consequently, blood loss (e.g., from escharotomies, line placement, internal bleeding, or fractures) can easily be underestimated. If, however, the hematocrit declines in the absence of hemolysis, this is a clear indication that there is a significant source of blood loss somewhere. After large burns, normalization of blood volume is almost impossible until 24 to 48 hours after the burn.

White blood cell count The initial white blood cell count may be high, normal, or low, depending on the magnitude of the stress response and the degree of white cell sequestration into the burn. The absolute value is not a particularly useful parameter during the early postburn period.

Blood glucose level The increased release of catecholamines in burn patients often leads to hyperglycemia. In elderly and diabetic patients, insulin may be required; some glucose should be infused at this time as well. Infants are prone to hypoglycemia as a result of decreased glucose stores.

Electrolyte status Because most of the fluid lost initially is plasma rather than whole blood, concentrations of sodium, chloride, and potassium remain relatively constant despite hypovolemia; variations in these values are mainly a function of the type of resuscitation fluid used. The potassium concentration will rise if severe hemolysis has occurred or if renal impairment is present. The HCO_3^- concentration varies according to perfusion status and acid-base balance.

Plasma protein and myoglobin levels A marked decrease in the plasma protein level occurs soon after a burn, with the greater part of the decrease coming in the first 4 to 6 hours. Not much can be done about this change until about 10 to 12 hours after the burn, given the rapid fluid and protein shifts. The plasma albumin level should be maintained above 2.5 g/dl.

In patients with very deep burns, especially if the burns are electrical in origin, the plasma myoglobin level should be measured. Myoglobin released from deeply injured muscles will affect renal function. This problem can be largely prevented by maintaining a higher than normal urine output.

Prothrombin time, partial thromboplastin time, and platelet count Initial values for prothrombin time and partial thromboplastin time and an initial platelet count are useful for determining whether administration of coagulation factors will be necessary. In the first 36 hours after the burn, coagulation factors and platelets are rarely needed unless a prolonged shock state has initiated disseminated intravascular coagulation or unless the patient has preexisting hepatic or hematologic disease.

INOTROPIC SUPPORT

Inotropic support in the first 24 hours is indicated if inadequate perfusion persists despite vigorous fluid resuscitation. This situation is most common in the elderly burn patient. If improved renal blood flow is the major goal, low-dose dopamine (1 to 4 µg/kg/min) is preferred. Moderate-dose dopamine (5 to 10 µg/kg/min) or dobutamine will increase contractility and improve cardiac output. Dobutamine results in less tachycardia. Digoxin is not recommended in the immediate postburn period, because the rapid fluid shifts during this period can lead to digitalis toxicity; in addition, digoxin is generally a less potent inotropic agent than dopamine or dobutamine.

DIURETICS

Diuretics are rarely indicated in the first 24 hours of resuscitation. The exceptions are when hemoglobinuria or myoglobinuria is present, as may occur after electrical injuries.

Initiation of Wound Management

COOLING THE WOUND

Cooling will increase heat loss, and neutralizing the heat source is a primary goal of initial management. Immediate cooling of the burn also decreases edema, apparently by stabilizing skin mast cells and thereby preventing histamine release. This effect, however, is short-lived. After the first 30 minutes, the benefit of cooling with water at a temperature of approximately 20° C is principally that of pain relief in superficially burned tissues. Prolonged cooling for pain relief is indicated only in second-degree burns covering less than 15% of TBS. Ice should never be used directly on the skin, because a freezing injury can result.

After a deep burn, the normal protective mechanism of skin vasoconstriction is absent. The barrier to water loss by evaporation—and hence the barrier to heat loss—is markedly impaired, an extremely important problem to recognize in the resuscitation period. Body heat is lost 25 times more quickly in water (wet dressings or hydrotherapy) than in air because of increased heat conductivity in water. Once hypothermia develops, rewarming is extremely slow, and decreased body temperature may affect cardiac output and perfusion of vital organs.

ASSESSMENT OF BURN DEPTH

At this point, more precise assessments of burn size and depth are needed to determine the manner of burn care and the need for transfer to a burn facility [see Figure 4 and Table 4]. The size of second- and third-degree burns must be determined in relation to total body surface [see Figure 3].

Burn depth is classified by degree of injury. Unfortunately, clinical assessment of the depth of anything more serious than a superficial second-degree burn is difficult at admission. Moreover, deeper burns tend to increase in depth over a period of hours to days as the injured but viable tissue eventually becomes nonviable, usually as a result of a low-flow state (initially) or inflammation (in the later stages). A number of techniques for clinical determination of burn depth have been employed; all have met with some success, but none have been widely adopted.

First-Degree Burns

A first-degree burn involves only the thinner outer epidermis layer and is characterized by erythema and mild discomfort. Tissue damage is minimal, and protective functions of the skin are intact. Pain, the chief symptom, usually resolves in 48 to 72 hours, and healing takes place uneventfully. The pain is probably caused by local vasodilator prostaglandin production. In 5 to 10 days, the damaged epithelium peels off in small scales, leaving no residual

Figure 4 **Illustrated here are the depths to which skin damage extends with burns of varying degrees.**

scarring. The most common causes of first-degree burns are overexposure to sunlight and brief scalding by hot liquids.

Second-Degree Burns

Second-degree burns [see Figure 5] are those in which the entire epidermis and variable portions of the dermis have been destroyed by heat. A superficial second-degree burn involves heat injury to the upper third of the dermis. The microvessels perfusing this area are injured, and permeability is increased, with the result that large amounts of plasma leak into the interstitium. This fluid in turn lifts the thin, heat-destroyed epidermis, forming blisters. Despite the

Table 4   Physical Characteristics of Burns

Cause	Appearance	Depth	Pain
Hot liquids			
Short exposure	Wet; pink; blisters	2°	Severe
Long exposure	Wet; dark red	2°–3°	Minimal
Flames			
Flash exposure	Wet; pink; blisters	2°	Severe
Direct contact	Dry, white, and waxy; leathery brown or black	3°	Minimal
Chemicals			
Acid, alkalies	Light brown to light gray	2° (converts to 3°)	Severe

loss of the entire basal layer of the epidermis, a superficial second-degree burn will heal in 7 to 14 days owing to repopulation by the epithelial cells that line the hair follicles, sweat glands, and other skin appendages anchored deep in the dermis. Minimal scarring occurs because the wound closes rapidly; consequently, inflammation, which stimulates excessive collagen deposition, is short-lived. A deep dermal second-degree burn extends well into the dermal layer; fewer viable epidermal cells remain. Epithelialization is extremely slow, sometimes requiring months. Blister formation is not characteristically seen: because the layer of dead tissue is thick and adherent to underlying dermal collagen, it cannot be readily lifted off the surface. Exceptions occur in very young or very old patients, who have a very thin dermis. The surface of the wound is usually red, with some evidence of plasma leakage from remaining intact blood vessels. Blood supply to the burned tissue is marginal; thus, there is a high probability that tissue damage will deepen with time. Pain is present but to a lesser degree than in more superficial burns. Fluid losses and the metabolic effects of deep dermal burns are basically the same as those seen with third-degree burns. Dense scarring usually results if skin grafts are not performed.

Third-Degree Burns

In a full or third-degree burn [see Figure 6], the entire epidermis and dermis are destroyed; no residual epidermal cells remain to repopulate or epithelialize. Areas of the wound not closed by wound contraction will require skin grafting. Characteristically, avascular burned tissue has the waxy white color typical of any avascular tissue. If the burn extends into the fat or if contact with a flame source has been prolonged, the leathery brown or black color typical of charred tissue is seen. The most common cause of third-degree burns is a short exposure to a very high temperature, such as direct contact with a flame. However, prolonged contact with only moderately hot liquids (e.g., water at 125° F), as seen with intentional scalding, can result in a third-degree burn. Prolonged contact with hot liquid that leads to a third-degree burn will also lead to red cell hemolysis and release of myoglobin from underlying muscle, resulting in a red pigment deposition in the wound. The red-pigmented wound can be mistaken for viable dermis; the same appearance in a flame burn would represent only a deep second-degree injury. Therefore, a dark-red appearance in a scald burn may actually represent a full-thickness injury. The microvessels are not immediately thrombosed in second-degree injury and therefore continue to leak plasma for days. In full-thickness flame burns, however, injured capillaries are usually immediately occluded by thrombosis. The absence of pain sensation in full-thickness burns is the result of heat destruction of nerve endings. This sensory deficit distinguishes a third-degree burn from a partial-thickness injury.

Full-thickness chemical burns are light gray to brown in appearance. Pain is usually extreme because retained chemicals prolong the burning process; these retained chemicals commonly convert partial burns to full-thickness burns.

In the early postburn period (24 to 72 hours after the burn), a zone of ischemia is usually present below the dead tissue and above the deeper living tissue. The vasculature to this area has been injured. Some vessels are thrombosed; others are patent but have endothelial cell damage. The marginally viable tissue can readily convert to eschar if blood flow is further decreased because of local mediator release or infection. A deep second-degree burn—in which healing is still possible—can therefore progress to a third-degree burn. Wound conversion is prevented or minimized with prompt, adequate resuscitation.

Figure 5 **Immediately after injury, a second-degree burn typically has a wet, reddish appearance.**

PAIN MEDICATION

Pain medication is necessary for partial-thickness burns, particularly when the wounds are cleaned. Pain control should be initiated before aggressive wound manipulation because it is important to minimize the subsequent stress response. With minor burns, oral or intramuscular narcotics may be adequate if given about 30 minutes before wound care. For major burns [see Table 5], intravenous narcotics in small doses are appropriate; erratic absorption from the gastrointestinal tract, skin, and muscles makes these routes of administration both ineffective and dangerous.

REMOVAL OF FOREIGN BODIES AND LOOSE NONVIABLE TISSUE

When a patent airway, breathing, and circulation are ensured, the wound can be debrided and cleaned. Soot and dirt are best removed with a mild dilute detergent such as a chlorhexidine product. Gross debris, loose sloughed skin, or skin overlying broken blisters should be gently removed with forceps and scissors. Rough scrubbing should be avoided to prevent further harm to the injured tissues. Ground-in dirt will gradually work its way to the surface with daily dressing changes. The surrounding skin should be

Figure 6 **Shown is a full-thickness burn of the hand that actually extends below the dermis into subdermal tissue.**

Table 5 Classification of Severity of Burn Injury

Critical burns
2° burns involving > 30% TBS
3° burns involving > 10% TBS
Any burns complicated by respiratory tract injury, fractures, or involvement of critical areas (i.e., face, hands, feet, perineum)
High-voltage electrical burns
Lesser burns in patients with significant preexisting disease

Moderate burns
2° burns involving 15%–20% TBS (if critical areas are not involved)
3° burns involving 2%–10% TBS (if critical areas are not involved)

Minor burns
2° burns involving < 15% TBS (if critical areas are not involved)
3° burns involving < 2% TBS (if critical areas are not involved)

---

shaved to facilitate local wound care. Large intact blisters can be left in place for 48 hours, reducing discomfort and the risk of underlying dermal desiccation.

If a hydrotherapy tank is to be used at this time for wound cleaning, the patient must be hemodynamically stable because good hemodynamic monitoring will be impossible during the procedure. Sequential cleaning of the various burned areas at bedside allows continuous monitoring and minimizes hypothermia and is thus a safer approach. A warm environment during burn care, preferably 30° to 35° C (86° to 95° F), is necessary to avoid heat loss.

Tar burns present unique problems. Tar removal is particularly difficult because the heat of the tar (150° to 200° C) usually results in a deep burn, and the rapid cooling leads to adherence to the skin. Tar can be gently removed without further tissue damage by means of repeated applications of petroleum-based ointments (such as Neosporin), which also contain surface-active emulsifying agents that dissolve the tar and make it easier to remove.

TETANUS PROPHYLAXIS

As with any large wound, the risk of tetanus must be minimized by using standard measures [see I:8 Acute Wound Care].

PROPHYLACTIC ANTIBIOTICS

Numerous studies have demonstrated that prophylactic systemic antibiotics do not decrease wound infection rates in either minor or major burns. The blood supply to the relatively avascular deep burn is insufficient to provide adequate tissue antibiotic levels. In addition, any open wound will become colonized with bacteria. The only exception to the dictum against prophylactic systemic antibiotics would be prophylaxis against β-hemolytic streptococcus with low-dose penicillin, particularly if the patient is at high risk for infection with this organism (i.e., if the patient is a carrier or was recently exposed).

EARLY INFECTION CONTROL: TOPICAL ANTIBIOTICS AND SKIN SUBSTITUTES

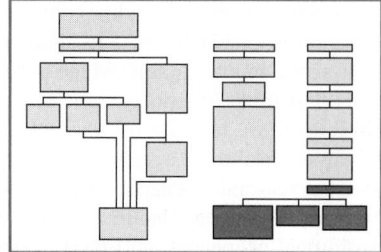

Topical Antibiotics

Because topical antibiotics decrease the rate of wound healing (in particular, the rate of epithelialization) as compared with biologic dressings or other forms of temporary skin substitutes, these agents are most useful for deep burns with eschar present and are less useful for most superficial burns or clean, healing burns. Topical agents are applied to the wound, which is then covered with dressings or left open to the environment. Both techniques are used, but the closed dressing technique is employed more because pain, heat, and fluid loss are decreased if dressings are applied. In addition, residual dermis is less likely to desiccate under a dressing.

The deep burn must be protected from early bacterial invasion, which can rapidly convert the wound to a still deeper injury. Topical antibiotics that are sufficiently water soluble to penetrate the burn eschar will temporarily control bacterial growth in the wound [see Table 6]. The half-life of the currently available topical agents is only a few hours; therefore, the agent must be applied at least twice daily to achieve a reasonable level of antibacterial protection.

Silver sulfadiazine (Silvadene) is the most commonly used topical agent because it has good antibacterial properties and because fewer complications are associated with its use. This agent, however, penetrates thick eschar less readily than some other agents and is therefore better used to prevent infection than to treat an established infection. Antibacterial properties are primarily directed against gram-negative organisms, with some antifungal effects. The primary complication of silver sulfadiazine is leukopenia as a result of transient bone marrow suppression. A white blood cell count of 2,000 to 3,000/mm^3 can be seen after application is begun. The effect is transient; the white cell count returns toward normal after several days, even if the agent is continued.

Mafenide (Sulfamylon) is the most effective agent in its ability to penetrate burn eschar. It also has the most potent antibacterial

---

Table 6 Topical Antibiotic Agents

Agent	Antimicrobial Spectrum	Eschar Penetration	Local Tissue Toxicity	Systemic Toxicity	Pain on Application	Occlusive Dressings
10% Mafenide (Sulfamylon)	Broad*	Excellent	Moderate	Acidosis; carbonic anhydrase inhibition	Yes	Unnecessary
1% Silver sulfadiazine (Silvadene)	Broad	Good	Low	Transient leukopenia	Minimal	Preferred
0.1% Gentamicin sulfate ointment	Broad†	Fair	Low	? Renal toxicity; ? ototoxicity	Minimal	Preferred
0.5% Povidone-iodine (Betadine)	Broad	Fair	Low	Renal, CNS, and iodine toxicity	Yes	Preferred
Bacitracin ointment	Gram-positive organisms	Surface only	Low	Renal toxicity	No	Optional

*Most potent of the topical agents. †Has no antifungal properties.

properties and is particularly effective against gram-negative organisms. The agent has some antifungal properties as well. However, mafenide, as a carbonic anhydrase inhibitor, can potentiate pulmonary insufficiency and metabolic acidosis; hence, it also produces the most significant complications. In addition, application is painful in many cases. This agent is used primarily as a second line of defense or as a primary treatment for small, infected wounds.

Povidone-iodine (Betadine) ointment is usually used only on relatively thin eschar because its tissue penetration is not very good. The active agent is iodine, which is quite effective against both bacteria and fungi. Agents such as gentamicin and bacitracin can be used for more selective infections [see Table 6], but systemic toxicity can occur if these agents are used over large open wounds. Bacitracin is reasonably effective against wound colonization with gram-positive organisms. Bacitracin and gentamicin, however, have no antifungal properties, and prolonged use on an open wound can precipitate fungal growth.

Temporary Skin Substitutes

A number of temporary skin substitutes have been developed to improve healing of partial-thickness wounds as well as to protect clean, excised wounds when autografts are not performed immediately. Skin substitutes allow excision of burned tissue even if insufficient skin is available for autograft, permitting more rapid removal of devitalized tissue. The properties required of a temporary skin substitute have been well defined. Most important, it must adhere to the wound to maximize the epithelialization rate and minimize inflammation and fibrosis.

There are two types of temporary skin: biologic and synthetic. Biologic dressings are from previously living tissue, including amniotic membranes, xenografts, and allografts (or cadaver skin), although the last is only of limited availability and is used primarily to cover excised wounds. A number of synthetic skin substitutes have been developed that have the advantages of ready availability, long shelf life, and minimal risk of disease transmission.

SUBESCHAR EDEMA IN EXTREMITIES

The increased pressure that accompanies the development of subeschar edema is of particular concern in extremities with circumferential burns. In such cases, if the increasing pressure cannot be dissipated, a decrease in venous outflow results; this effect speeds the rate of edema formation and further elevates tissue pressure until there is marked impairment of arterial blood flow to the tissues distal to the obstruction.

Immediate elevation of the burned extremity decreases the magnitude of tissue edema. Perfusion is best monitored by the Doppler flowmeter or by assessment of capillary refill. Immediate escharotomy is indicated [see Figure 2] if there is a decrease in pulsatile flow beyond the burn.

Transfer to Specialized Burn Facility

Patients whose burns are critical [see Table 5] should be transferred to specialized burn facilities as early as possible after their injury, once the initial assessment and resuscitation have begun. Moderate burns necessitate hospitalization but may be manageable outside a burn facility if a local surgeon with an interest or expertise in burns will accept responsibility for the patient's care. Minor burns may be manageable on an outpatient basis.

A major reason for the impressive progress made in the field of burn therapy has been the expansion of the concept of specialized centers for burns. There are now more than 150 burn units in the United States as compared with a mere dozen 30 years ago. About 21,000 burn patients—approximately one third of all hospitalized burn patients—are treated yearly in these 1,700 specialized burn care beds. The centralization of patients has made possible not only improved care but also multidisciplinary research.

Recommended Reading

Barillo D, Goode R, Esch V: Cyanide poisoning in victims of fire: analysis of 364 cases and review of the literature. J Burn Care Rehabil 15:46, 1994

Crapo R: Causes of respiratory injury. Respiratory Injury: Smoke Inhalation and Burns. Haponik E, Munster A, Eds. McGraw-Hill Book Co, New York, 1990, p 47

Crum RL: Cardiovascular and neurohumoral responses following burn injury. Arch Surg 125:1065, 1990

Deitch E: The management of burns. N Engl J Med 323: 1249, 1990

Demling R: Fluid resuscitation. The Art and Science of Burn Care. Boswick J, Ed. Aspen, Rockville, Maryland, 1982, p 189

Demling R: Smoke inhalation injury. New Horizons in Critical Care. Demling R, Ed. Williams & Wilkins, Baltimore, 1993, p 422

Demling R, Knox J, Youn Y, et al: Oxygen consumption early post burn becomes oxygen dependent with the addition of smoke inhalation injury. J Trauma 32:593, 1992

Fitzpatrick J, Cioffi W: Diagnosis and treatment of inhalation injury. Total Burn Care. Herndon D, Ed. WB Saunders Co, Philadelphia, 1996, p 174

Fratianno R, Brandt C: Improved survival of adults with extensive burns. J Burn Care Rehabil 18:347, 1997

Heimbach D: Burn depth. World J Surg 16:10, 1992

Jeng J, Lee K, Jordan M: Serum lactate and base deficit suggest inadequate resuscitation of patients with burn injury. J Burn Care Rehabil 18:402, 1997

Masanes M, Legendre C: Fiberoptic bronchoscopy for the early diagnosis of subglottal inhalation injury: comparative value in the assessment of prognosis. J Trauma 36:59, 1994

Pruitt B: The evolutionary development of biologic dressings and skin substitutes. J Burn Care Rehabil 18:52, 1997

Scheulen JJ, Munster AM: The Parkland formula in patients with burns and inhalation injury. J Trauma 22:869, 1982

Silverman S, Purdue G, Hunt J, et al: Cyanide toxicity in burned patients. J Trauma 28:171, 1988

Vinus B, Matsuda T, Coprizo JB, et al: Prophylactic intubation and continuous positive airway pressure in the management of inhalation injury in burn victims. Crit Care Med 9:519, 1981

Youn Y, LaLonde C, Demling R: Oxidants and pathophysiology of burn and smoke inhalation injury. Free Radic Biol Med 12:409, 1992

Acknowledgment

Figures 2 through 4 Carol Donner.

4 SHOCK

James W. Holcroft, M.D.

Approach to the Treatment of Shock

Classification of Shock

Shock may be defined as a state in which either (1) the cardiovascular system lacks adequate power for perfusion of the peripheral tissues or (2) there is adequate power for perfusion, but only at the cost of excessive and inefficient use of oxygen by the heart, which renders the heart vulnerable to ischemia. The first type of shock is commonly termed decompensated shock; the second, compensated shock.

Shock, whether decompensated or compensated, can be classified into five categories according to the physiologic derangement that is the primary cause of the shock state: (1) extracardiac compressive/obstructive shock, (2) hypovolemic shock, (3) inflammatory shock, (4) neurogenic shock, and (5) cardiogenic shock [*see Tables 1 and 2*]. Frequently, this classification is a non-exclusive one—that is, a given clinical condition (e.g., tension pneumothorax) might cause shock by several mechanisms. Nonetheless, a physiologic classification of shock that emphasizes a single primary cause is frequently helpful in the initial stages of treatment.

In extracardiac compressive shock, forces external to the heart compress the thin-walled chambers of the heart (the atria and right ventricle) and the great veins (both systemic and pulmonary) as they enter the heart, thus decreasing ventricular end-diastolic volumes. In extracardiac obstructive shock, the heart fails because it encounters excessive hindrance during contraction or because the extrapericardial veins returning blood to the heart become compressed. Many of the conditions associated with excessive hindrance to contraction also compress the great systemic and pulmonary veins.

In hypovolemic shock, small ventricular end-diastolic volumes lead to inefficient or inadequate cardiac production of power.

Inflammatory shock arises from the release of inflammatory and coagulatory mediators. It can be caused by ischemia-reperfusion injuries, trauma, or infection (in which case it is sometimes referred to as septic shock). Inflammatory shock is also known as distributive shock because the abnormalities in some cases derive partly from increased blood flow to the skin or stagnation of blood in dilated peripheral venules and small veins.

Inflammatory and coagulatory mediators cause inflammatory shock via three main mechanisms: (1) disruption of the microvascular endothelium, both at the inflammatory site and distally, (2) dilation of the microvasculature, both locally and distally, and (3) depression of the myocardium. The result is plasma loss into the interstitium, which produces a hypovolemic state, distant organ failure, and cardiac insufficiency or inadequacy. If the predominant feature of the shock state is loss of plasma volume into the interstitium through a permeable microvasculature, the patient's skin will be cool and clammy (hence the terms cold septic shock and cold inflammatory shock). If blood volume has been restored or the predominant feature of the shock state is cutaneous vasodilatation, the skin will be flushed and warm (hence the term warm inflammatory shock).

The causes of inflammatory shock are all associated with the presence of large amounts of infected or traumatized tissue in proximity to a robust blood supply and drainage. An avascular infection (e.g., a contained abscess) will not cause inflammatory shock, because the inflammatory mediators do not have access to the circulation; however, an uncontained abscess (e.g., a ruptured appendiceal abscess or a surgically drained subphrenic abscess) can cause inflammatory shock because the mediators that spill out of the abscess are picked up by the vasculature in the surrounding tissue. In like manner, dry gangrene, because of its poor vascular supply, will not cause inflammatory shock, whereas wet gangrene can.

Neurogenic shock arises from loss of autonomic innervation of the vasculature and, in some cases, of the heart. Causes include spinal cord injury, regional anesthesia, administration of drugs that block the adrenergic nervous system (including some systemically administered anesthetic agents), certain neurologic disorders, and fainting. Loss of arteriolar tone leads to hypotension; loss of venular and small venous tone leads to pooling of blood in the denervated parts of the body. If the blockade is generalized or at a high enough level, the denervation can also decrease myocardial contractility and heart rate.

In cardiogenic shock, the heart itself, through an intrinsic abnormality, is incapable of efficiently pushing its contained blood into the vasculature with adequate power.

Recognition of Shock

The presence of a shock state is typically signaled by one or more characteristic clinical markers [*see Table 3*].

HYPOTENSION

A low blood pressure is a specific sign of shock but not a sensitive one. A very low blood pressure (≤ 89 mm Hg) almost always indicates some form of shock. Postural falls in blood pressure can also be a helpful signal: a sustained (> 30 seconds) systolic pressure drop greater than 10 mm Hg in a patient who has arisen from a supine position to an upright one is abnormal and frequently is an indication of underlying shock.

The absence of hypotension does not, however, rule out shock. Adrenergic discharge and the release of circulating and locally produced vasoconstrictors during shock often sustain blood pressure despite volume depletion or depressed myocardial contractility. Furthermore, how hypotension should be defined in a particular case depends on the patient's usual blood pressure, which may not be known to the physician. For instance, in a patient with severe preexisting hypertension, a systolic pressure of 120 mm Hg might reflect shock. Thus, hypotension—either supine or postural—can strongly suggest the diagnosis of shock, but normotension in a patient suspected of being in shock means nothing.

Approach to the Treatment of Shock

Patient shows signs of possible shock

Characteristic signs include
- Hypotension
- Tachycardia or bradycardia
- Tachypnea
- Cutaneous hypoperfusion
- Mental abnormalities
- Oliguria
- Myocardial ischemia
- Metabolic acidemia
- Hypoxemia

Shock resolves

Extracardiac compressive/obstructive shock

Compression or obstruction of the heart or great vessels, as an immediately life-threatening condition (see above), should already have been treated. However, periodic reassessment during workup is appropriate because this type of shock can develop secondary to another process.

Hypovolemic shock

Control bleeding.
Obtain vascular access, and infuse NS or lactated Ringer solution (to 60 ml/kg or more).
If [Hb] ≤ 9 g/dl, consider giving RBCs. [Hb] should be ≥ 7 g/dl in young healthy patients with controlled bleeding, up to ≥ 11 g/dl in other patients.
Treat pain, hypothermia, acidemia, and coagulopathy.

Inflammatory shock

Obtain vascular access, and infuse fluids as necessary to replenish volume.
Give RBCs as for hypovolemic shock.
Treat pain, hypothermia, and acidemia.
Once resuscitation is well under way, search for and treat underlying inflammatory cause of shock.

Shock resolves

Periphery is priority

Goals: SV 60–100 ml, MAP 90 mm Hg, HR 60–100/min, filling pressures in midteens.

Treatment measures:
- Infuse fluids to ensure generous end-diastolic volumes.
- Increase contractility as needed with dobutamine (5–15 μg/kg/min) and milrinone (50 μg, then 0.375–0.75 μg/kg/min).
- If absolutely necessary to increase BP, give a vasoconstrictor—dopamine (2–20 μg/kg/min) if HR ≤ 90/min, norepinephrine (4–12 μg/kg/min) if HR > 90/min.

Periphery and heart are equal priorities

Goals: SV 55–85 ml, MAP 80 mm Hg, HR 60–90/min, filling pressures in low teens.

Treatment measures:
- Give fluids or initiate diuresis so that the smaller of the two end-diastolic volumes is slightly greater than normal.
- Cautiously increase contractility as necessary with dobutamine (5–15 μg/kg/min) and milrinone (50 μg, then 0.375–0.75 μg/kg/min).
- If absolutely necessary, give a vasoconstrictor—dopamine (2–20 μg/kg/min) if HR ≤ 70/min, norepinephrine (4–12 μg/kg/min) if HR > 70/min.
- For HR ≥ 110/min, initiate beta blockade with esmolol (500 μg/kg, then 50 μg/kg/min), followed by metoprolol (5–10 mg q. 6 hr).

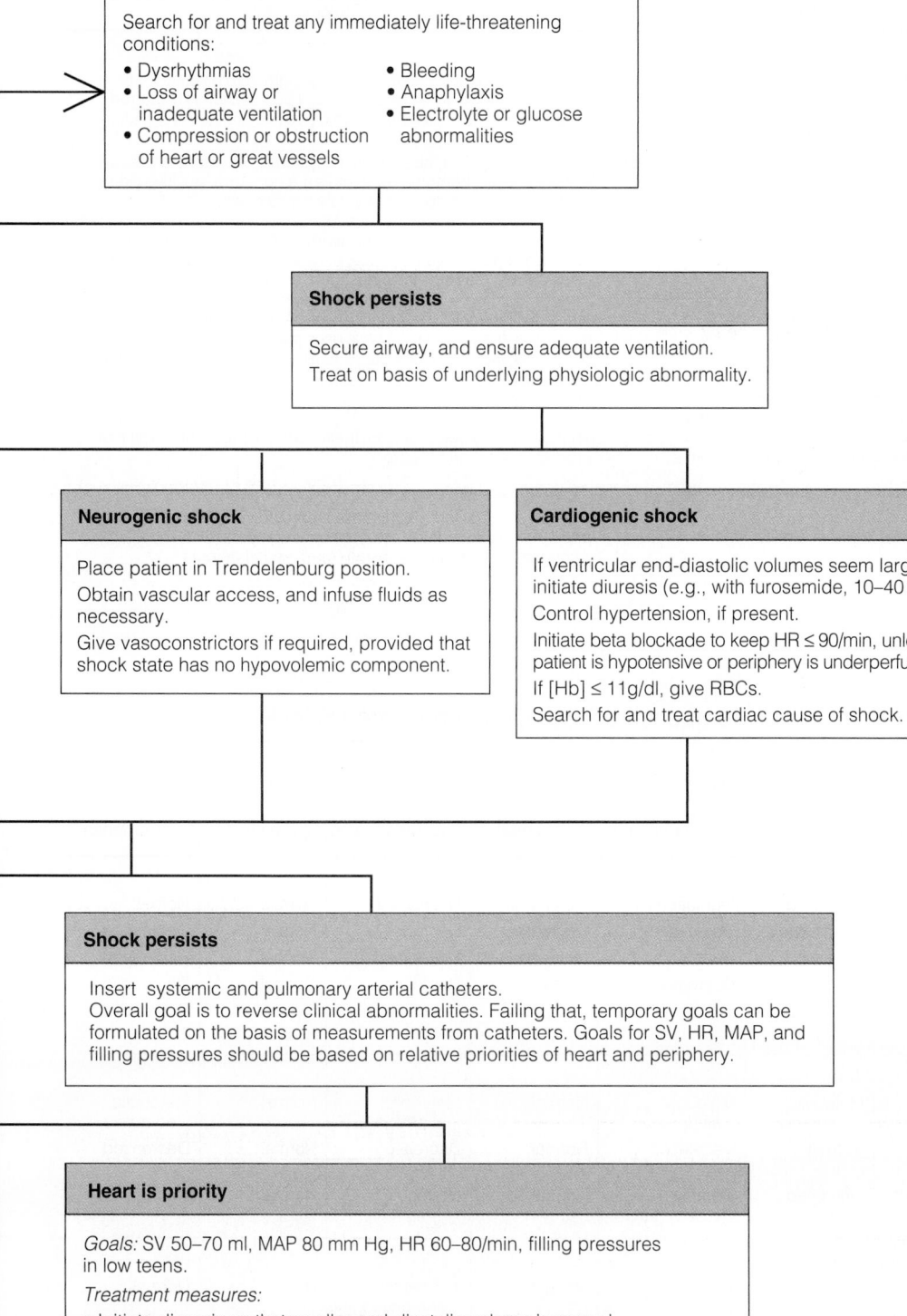

Search for and treat any immediately life-threatening
conditions:
- Dysrhythmias
- Loss of airway or
  inadequate ventilation
- Compression or obstruction
  of heart or great vessels
- Bleeding
- Anaphylaxis
- Electrolyte or glucose
  abnormalities

Shock persists

Secure airway, and ensure adequate ventilation.
Treat on basis of underlying physiologic abnormality.

Neurogenic shock

Place patient in Trendelenburg position.
Obtain vascular access, and infuse fluids as
necessary.
Give vasoconstrictors if required, provided that
shock state has no hypovolemic component.

Cardiogenic shock

If ventricular end-diastolic volumes seem large,
initiate diuresis (e.g., with furosemide, 10–40 mg).
Control hypertension, if present.
Initiate beta blockade to keep HR ≤ 90/min, unless
patient is hypotensive or periphery is underperfused.
If [Hb] ≤ 11g/dl, give RBCs.
Search for and treat cardiac cause of shock.

Shock persists

Insert systemic and pulmonary arterial catheters.
Overall goal is to reverse clinical abnormalities. Failing that, temporary goals can be
formulated on the basis of measurements from catheters. Goals for SV, HR, MAP, and
filling pressures should be based on relative priorities of heart and periphery.

Heart is priority

Goals: SV 50–70 ml, MAP 80 mm Hg, HR 60–80/min, filling pressures
in low teens.
Treatment measures:
- Initiate diuresis so that smaller end-diastolic volume is normal
  or (if necessary for adequate SV and filling pressures) slightly larger.
- Control BP with nitroprusside (0.5–10 μg/kg/min), nitroglycerin
  (5–200 μg/min), or ACE inhibitors (e.g., enalaprilat, 1.25–5 mg q. 6 hr).
  as needed.
- Initiate beta blockade to keep HR ≤ 90/min.
- Obtain coronary arteriogram and initiate cardiac catheterization as needed.
- Intervene with coronary angioplasty, balloon pump, or cardiac surgery
  as indicated.

Table 1   Pathophysiologic Classification of Shock

Type of Shock	Abnormality	Causes
Extracardiac Compressive	Compression of the thin-walled chambers of the heart—the atria and the right ventricle—and compression of the great veins entering the heart	Pericardial tamponade, elevated diaphragm from pregnancy or abdominal bleeding or intestinal distention or ascites, ruptured diaphragm, tension pneumothorax, positive pressure ventilation with large tidal volumes
Obstructive	Excessive hindrance to ventricular emptying imposed by cardiac valvular stenosis or excessive vascular stiffness or resistance	Pulmonary embolism, air embolism, systemic hypertension, tension pneumothorax, hemothorax, ruptured diaphragm, positive pressure ventilation, aortic or pulmonary valvular stenosis
Hypovolemic	Depletion of vascular volume	Bleeding, protracted vomiting or diarrhea, fluid sequestration in obstructed gut or injured tissue, excessive use of diuretics, adrenal insufficiency, diabetes insipidus, dehydration, anaphylaxis
Inflammatory (formerly known as septic or traumatic shock)	Complex response associated with the systemic inflammatory and coagulative reaction to infected or injured tissues	Pneumonia, peritonitis, cholangitis, pyelonephritis, soft tissue infection, meningitis, mediastinitis, crush injuries, major fractures, high-velocity penetrating wounds, major burns, retained necrotic tissue, pancreatitis, anaphylaxis
Neurogenic	Pooling of blood in autonomically denervated venules and small veins; hypotension arising from denervated arterioles and sometimes from a denervated heart	Spinal cord injury, regional anesthetic, administration of drugs that produce autonomic blockade
Cardiogenic	Decreased myocardial contractility	Bradyarrhythmias, tachyarrhythmias, cardiac valvular insufficiency, papillary muscle rupture, myocardiopathy, myocarditis, myocardial ischemia, myocardial contusion (rare), septal defects

Table 2   Clinical Features of Compensated and Decompensated Shock

Parameter	Hypovolemic Shock		Inflammatory Shock		Neurogenic Shock		Left-Sided Cardiogenic Shock	
	Compensated	Decompensated	Compensated	Decompensated	Compensated	Decompensated	Compensated	Decompensated
Cardiovascular								
Heart rate	Increased	Variable	Increased	Increased	Increased	Decreased	Normal	Normal
BP	Normal	Decreased	Decreased	Decreased	Decreased	Decreased	Normal	Decreased
Cardiac output	Normal	Decreased	Increased	Normal	Increased	Decreased	Normal	Decreased
Power	Normal	Decreased	Normal	Decreased	Normal	Decreased	Normal	Decreased
Cardiac efficiency*	Decreased	Decreased	Decreased	Decreased	Decreased	Decreased	Decreased	Decreased
Metabolic								
Acid-base status	Normal	Metabolic acidemia	Metabolic acidemia	Metabolic acidemia	Normal	Metabolic acidemia	Normal	Metabolic acidemia
O_2 consumption	Normal	Decreased	Normal	Decreased	Normal	Decreased	Normal	Decreased
Glucose concentration	Moderately increased	Moderately increased	Increased	Variable	Normal	Normal	Normal	Normal
Clinical								
Temperature	Normal	Normal to decreased	Increased	Variable	Normal	Normal to decreased	Normal	Normal
Respiratory rate	Increased	Increased	Increased	Increased	Normal	Variable	Normal	Increased
Skin	Pale, cool	Pale, cool, clammy	Pink, warm	Pale, cool, clammy	Pink, warm in denervated areas	Pink, warm in denervated areas	Normal	Pale, cool, clammy
Neurologic state	Anxious	Anxious, confused, combative, obtunded	Anxious	Obtunded	Anxious; lower body paralyzed	Anxious; upper and lower body paralyzed	Normal	Anxious
Urine output	Decreased	Minimal	Decreased	Minimal	Decreased	Minimal	Decreased	Minimal

*Cardiovascular power divided by myocardial O_2 requirements.

TACHYCARDIA OR BRADYCARDIA

The pulse rate—perhaps the most evident of all the physical findings in clinical medicine—can increase in shock; such an increase is frequently cited as a cardinal feature of shock. When tachycardia is present, the possibility of shock should be considered; however, the absence of tachycardia should not be taken as a sign that the patient is not in shock. In extreme cases of shock, the pulse rate eventually falls to 0/min. Even in less extreme cases, the pulse rate may slow down, presumably to allow added time both for ventricular filling and for coronary perfusion of the myocardium as well as to reduce myocardial oxygen requirements. Thus, a normal or even a slow heart rate does not rule out shock and may even be an indication of a decompensated shock state.[1-3]

TACHYPNEA

A rapid respiratory rate may be a response to a metabolic acidemia, which is a typical finding with decompensated shock of any cause.

CUTANEOUS HYPOPERFUSION

Poor skin perfusion is often the first sign of shock. In all types of shock other than warm inflammatory shock and neurogenic shock, adrenergic discharge and the release of vasopressin and angiotensin II constrict the arterioles, venules, and small veins throughout the body. This constriction compensates for what otherwise could be profound hypotension. Cutaneous vasoconstriction produces the most sensitive sign of shock: the pale, cool, and clammy skin of someone exhibiting the fight-or-flight reaction. This sign is not specific for shock—it can also be the result of hypothermia, for example—but when it is seen in conjunction with collapsed and constricted subcutaneous veins in a patient with suspected hypovolemic or decompensated inflammatory shock, it establishes the diagnosis.

MENTAL ABNORMALITIES

Patients in severe decompensated shock frequently exhibit mental abnormalities, which can range from anxiousness to agitation to indifference to obtundation. These findings are not sensitive—indeed, they develop only in the late stages of shock—nor are they specific. They are, however, a strong warning to the physician that something must be done quickly. The body protects the brain at all costs; if blood supply to the brain is becoming inadequate, there usually is little time left.

OLIGURIA

Whenever the diagnosis of shock is being entertained, a Foley catheter should be placed. In many cases of compensated shock and in all cases of decompensated shock (except those in which shock results from inappropriate diuresis involving either a previously administered drug or ingestion of ethanol), urine output falls off. Oliguria is one of the most sensitive and specific of all the signs of shock.

MYOCARDIAL ISCHEMIA

An electrocardiogram, which should be obtained promptly whenever a patient is suspected of being in shock, may show signs of ischemia. The ischemia may be caused either by a primary myocardial problem or by a secondary extracardiac problem (e.g., hypotension resulting from hemorrhage or excess hindrance to ventricular contraction resulting from pulmonary embolism). In either case, the presence of myocardial ischemia, like the presence of mental abnormalities, should prompt quick action.

METABOLIC ACIDEMIA

Metabolic acidemia, as a sign of shock, may be manifested by an increased respiratory rate, but analysis of blood gases is usually re-

Table 3 Clinical Markers of Possible Shock State

Clinical Marker	Value or Findings Indicative of Shock
Systolic blood pressure	
Adult	≤ 110 mm Hg
Schoolchild	≤ 100 mm Hg
Preschool child	≤ 90 mm Hg
Infant	≤ 80 mm Hg
Sinus tachycardia	
Adult	≥ 90 beats/min
Schoolchild	≥ 120 beats/min
Preschool child	≥ 140 beats/min
Infant	≥ 160 beats/min
Cutaneous vasoconstriction	Pale, cool, clammy skin with constricted subcutaneous veins
Mental changes	Anxiousness, agitation, indifference, lethargy, obtundation
Urine output	
Adult	≤ 0.5 ml·kg⁻¹·hr⁻¹
Child	≤ 1.0 ml·kg⁻¹·hr⁻¹
Infant	≤ 2.0 ml·kg⁻¹·hr⁻¹
Myocardial ischemia or failure	Chest pain, third heart sound, pulmonary edema, abnormal ECG
Metabolic acidemia	$[HCO_3^-] \leq 21$ mEq/L Base deficit ≥ 3 mEq/L
Hypoxemia (on room air)	
0–50 yr	≤ 90 mm Hg
51–70 yr	≤ 80 mm Hg
≥ 71 yr	≤ 70 mm Hg

quired for confirmation. The acidemia may take the form of either a low calculated bicarbonate level or a base deficit.[4] Some patients in the early stages of shock—even severe shock—are not acidemic. If flow is sufficiently reduced, the anaerobic products of metabolism will be confined to the periphery; they may not be washed into the central circulation until some degree of resuscitation has taken place. Systemic arterial acidemia may become evident only after the diagnosis has been made and treatment initiated.

HYPOXEMIA

Systemic arterial hypoxemia is a common sign of shock. Low flow results in marked desaturation of blood leaving the metabolizing peripheral tissues and entering the pulmonary artery. If pulmonary function is compromised to any significant degree, as is often the case with shock, the markedly desaturated pulmonary arterial blood becomes only partially saturated as it passes through the lungs.

Identification and Treatment of Immediately Life-Threatening Conditions

If the patient shows signs of possible shock, the next step is to search for and treat any conditions that could kill the patient immediately. Such conditions include dysrhythmias, loss of airway or inadequate ventilation, extracardiac compression of the heart or obstruction of the vasculature, bleeding, and certain life-threatening medical conditions (e.g., anaphylaxis and highly abnormal electrolyte concentrations).

DYSRHYTHMIAS

Given that an electrocardiogram should be obtained promptly in any patient suspected of being in shock, any dysrhythmias present will usually be recognized at an early point. An agonal patient with a dysrhythmia should undergo cardioversion, ideally even before the airway is secured and before I.V. access is obtained. Cardioversion, when successful, can restore a moribund patient with ventricular fibrillation, ventricular tachycardia, or atrial fibrillation to life with full neurologic recovery. It is of no value for a patient in asystole; however, the possibility of fully resuscitating a patient in ventricular standstill is so remote that it usually makes little difference what mode of therapy is attempted or whether therapy is attempted at all.

A nonagonal patient should be treated in accordance with standard resuscitation routines [see I:1 Initial Emergency Management of Noninjured Patients: Cardiopulmonary Resuscitation and Correction of Acute Dysrhythmias].

LOSS OF AIRWAY OR INADEQUATE VENTILATION

If a patient can talk in a full voice without undue effort, the airway can be assumed to be intact; if not, the possibility of airway compromise must be considered. Airway compromise has a number of possible causes, ranging from loss of protective reflexes to mechanical obstruction. Sometimes, a jaw thrust is all that is needed for the physician to make the diagnosis and treat the problem.[5] In cases of profound shock, however, a definitive airway, such as that gained by inserting an oral endotracheal tube, becomes necessary. A definitive airway allows the physician to proceed with other lifesaving measures. If, after initial resuscitation, shock resolves and the patient regains consciousness and begins to struggle against intubation, the tube may be removed.

Of all the conditions that can render ventilation inadequate, tension pneumothorax is the most deadly. The most common causes of tension pneumothorax are trauma and therapeutic interventions by medical personnel (e.g., central venous punctures and positive pressure ventilation). Characteristic signs include decreased or absent breath sounds on the involved side, a hyperresonant hemithorax, and, if the patient is normovolemic, distended neck veins. (A tracheal shift—a commonly described feature in patients with tension pneumothoraces—is hard to detect and, in my experience, rarely helpful in making the diagnosis.) Treatment consists of needle decompression or tube thoracostomy.

Institution of mechanical ventilation does not guarantee that the patient will be adequately ventilated. The ventilator may malfunction, or the endotracheal tube may be misplaced or obstructed. If the chest wall does not rise with inspiration, mechanical ventilation should be promptly discontinued, and ventilation with an Ambu bag should be initiated at an inspired oxygen fraction (F_IO_2) of 1.0. If increasing abdominal distention is apparent, the possibility of esophageal intubation or displacement of the endotracheal tube into the hypopharynx should be considered. Treatment consists of reintubation. If breath sounds are absent on the left, right mainstem bronchial intubation should be considered. Treatment consists of partial withdrawal of the tube. Endotracheal tubes can become obstructed with clotted blood or inspissated secretions. Treatment consists of suctioning. Bleeding in the tracheobronchial tree (from injuries or from friable bronchial mucosa or tumor tissue) can eliminate ventilation from the lung segment supplied by the injured or

obstructed bronchus and flood the initially uninjured lung with blood. If the bleeding is thought to be coming from the left lung, the endotracheal tube should be advanced into the right mainstem bronchus. Bleeding from the right lung can be more problematic because selective left mainstem intubation may be impossible. Prompt control of bleeding can sometimes be obtained via endobronchial or open surgical intervention; both interventions also may be needed either for acute control or for definitive management of bleeding from the left lung.

Massive hemothoraces with collapse and compression of the lung should be treated with tube thoracostomy and, if necessary, surgical intervention. A massive left-side air leak from trauma or a ruptured bleb can be treated by advancing the endotracheal tube into the right mainstem bronchus. A massive right-side air leak usually necessitates surgical intervention, as does any leak that does not close quickly.

COMPRESSION OR OBSTRUCTION OF THE HEART OR THE GREAT VESSELS

Acute pericardial tamponade is usually manifested by muffled heart tones and occasionally by an exaggerated (> 10 mm Hg) decrease in systolic blood pressure on spontaneous breathing. If the patient is not hypovolemic, the neck veins are typically distended. Treatment consists of needle decompression or surgical creation of a pericardial window. Chronic tamponade can also produce shock but often does not give rise to the findings characteristic of acute tamponade; it is treated in the same way.

Diaphragmatic rupture and the ensuing intrusion of abdominal viscera into the chest can compress the heart, the great veins, and the extracardiac pulmonary vasculature, as can an intact but elevated diaphragm. Such compression can become a major problem if the patient is also hypovolemic. Treatment of a ruptured hemidiaphragm consists of operative reduction and repair; treatment of gut distention, decompression; treatment of bleeding, vascular control; and treatment of ascites, paracentesis of small amounts of fluid (just enough to lower intra-abdominal pressure).[6] Late-term pregnant women should be turned onto the left side so as to relieve compression of the right common iliac vein and the inferior vena cava.

Positive pressure ventilation can compress the heart, the great veins, and the vasculature in the pulmonary parenchyma.[7-11] In cases of suspected shock, tidal volumes should be kept small (≤ 7 ml/kg ideal body weight); inspiratory times should be short (≤ 1 second); end-expiratory pressure should be set at 0; and the initial respiratory rate should be kept low to minimize the total time spent in inspiration. Oxygenation can be maintained by using a high F_IO_2 (initially, 1.0). When blood gas analysis becomes available, the respiratory rate should be adjusted to prevent respiratory acidemia, and the inspired oxygen concentration should be decreased, provided that arterial saturation remains above 95%. When the patient is more stable, arterial saturation can be kept at a slightly lower level (≥ 92%); however, in the acute setting, it should be kept higher to buffer unanticipated decreases in oxygenation.

Besides compromising ventilation, tension pneumothoraces can compress the heart, the great systemic and pulmonary veins as they enter the atria, and the extracardiac pulmonary vasculature. Massive hemothoraces can exert similar effects. These conditions are treated as previously described [see Loss of Airway or Inadequate Ventilation, above].

Intravascular obstruction from a pulmonary thromboembolism or air embolism can kill quickly. Treatment of massive thromboembolism consists of prompt administration of fibrinolytics or heparin [see VI:2 Thromboembolic Problems], followed, in many cases, by pulmonary arteriography and further lytic therapy. Right-side air embolism can arise from penetrating injuries to large veins in the upper part of the body or from a percutaneous puncture with a large-bore needle if air is allowed access to the venous system while the patient takes a deep breath, especially if the patient is upright. Right-side air embolism can also arise as a complication of insufflation of gas into the peritoneal cavity during laparoscopy. Initial treatment consists of elimination of the source of air. Air that forms an air trap in the outflow tract of the right ventricle can sometimes be translocated to the apex of the ventricle by placing the patient in the Trendelenburg position with the left side down. Treatment consists of administration of 100% oxygen to wash out any residual nitrogen, followed by attempts to aspirate the air with a long central venous catheter. Coronary air embolism can occur whenever a patient with a penetrating injury to the lung parenchyma, either from trauma or from a needle puncture, is placed on positive pressure ventilation. The positive airway pressure can push air from an injured bronchus into an adjacent injured pulmonary vein, thereby allowing the air access to the left ventricle, the coronary arteries, and the brain. The diagnosis is usually made when a patient at risk goes into arrest shortly after initiation of positive pressure ventilation. Coronary air embolism is treated by giving 100% oxygen, opening the chest on the side with the suspected pulmonary penetration, and cross-clamping the hilum of the lung. The heart is then massaged while the descending thoracic aorta is compressed, and vasoconstrictors are administered.

BLEEDING

Bleeding should be controlled by any means necessary. Bleeding from an easily accessible site in an extremity, for instance, may be readily controlled with compression, whereas bleeding from an injury to the suprarenal aorta calls for meticulous exposure and control. Fracture-dislocations should be reduced if possible or, if not immediately reduced, immobilized.

ACUTE MEDICAL CONDITIONS

Anaphylaxis and life-threatening abnormalities in electrolyte or glucose concentrations usually are not recognized in the initial stages of shock management, but once they come to light, they should be treated promptly.

Treatment of Shock on the Basis of the Underlying Physiologic Abnormality

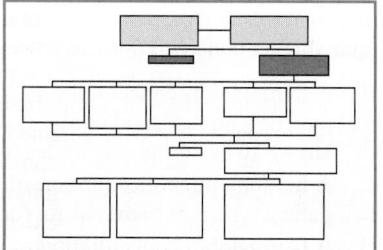

If shock persists after immediately life-threatening conditions have been treated, the next step in management is to categorize the shock state on the basis of the underlying physiologic abnormality and to initiate treatment accordingly.

As a rule, all that is needed to make this preliminary classification is the history, the physical examination, a chest x-ray, an electrocardiogram, and, in some cases, a complete blood count, electrolyte concentrations, a glucose level, and an arterial blood gas analysis. The classification is seldom neat: more than one cause of cardiovascular inadequacy is usually present, as when a patient with a myocardial infarction (MI) requires ventilation or when a patient with a ruptured abdominal aortic aneurysm has a distended abdomen. Nevertheless, such categorization is useful, in that it focuses the physician's attention on the primary problem, the cause of the persistent shock state.

First, the airway should be secured (if it has not been secured al-

ready), and supplemental oxygen should be given via a mask or a nasal cannula. The patient should be intubated, and ventilatory support should be provided if needed. The F_IO_2 should be 1.0 initially. Tidal volumes should be kept small (approximately 7 ml/kg ideal body weight) to minimize overdistention of alveoli and compression of the pulmonary vasculature and the heart. No end-expiratory pressure should be used initially. Inspiratory times should be kept short (≤ 1 second), and the respiratory rate should be kept as slow as possible. These measures will minimize ventilation-induced obstruction of the pulmonary vasculature and compression of the vena cavae and the heart—hemodynamic consequences that can be fatal, especially when superimposed on preexisting shock.

EXTRACARDIAC COMPRESSIVE/OBSTRUCTIVE SHOCK

As a condition that can kill quickly, extracardiac compressive/obstructive shock should already have been treated [see Compression or Obstruction of the Heart or the Great Vessels, above]. It is wise, however, to keep these two causes of shock in mind as workup proceeds: they often develop secondarily, as when tension pneumothorax develops in a mechanically ventilated patient who is being worked up or treated for some nonpulmonary problem.

HYPOVOLEMIC SHOCK

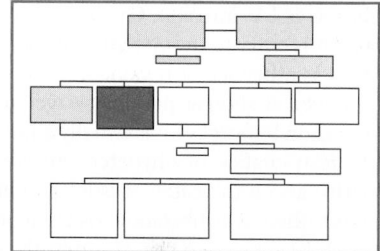

Treatment of Underlying Cause

At first glance, it might seem obvious that treatment of the underlying causes of shock should have the highest of priorities. This is indeed the case for hypovolemic shock caused by hemorrhage: it makes no sense to pour fluid and blood into a patient while controllable bleeding continues unchecked. For other types of shock, however, it is better to postpone treatment of the underlying causes until after the patient has been adequately resuscitated [see Inflammatory Shock, below].

Vascular Access

Simultaneously with efforts to control the underlying cause of hypovolemic shock, vascular access should be obtained, if it has not been already. If possible, superficial veins in the upper extremities should be cannulated with two large-bore catheters. If this is impossible, cutdowns may be performed on an antecubital or a basilic vein in the upper extremity, a cephalic vein at the shoulder, an external jugular vein at the base of the neck, or a saphenous vein at the ankle or in the groin.

Cutdowns in the upper extremity cause little morbidity but can take time to perform because upper-extremity veins are most likely to be thrombosed from earlier use. Morbidity is also low with the cephalic veins and the external jugular veins; however, exposure is sometimes difficult because of either the overlying fascia (in the case of the cephalic veins) or the overlying muscle (in the case of the external jugular veins). The saphenous vein at the ankle is readily exposed, large, and easy to cannulate. It cannot be used if there is extensive trauma to the extremity: if the cannula is left in place at the ankle for more than 24 hours, it is likely to cause superficial thrombophlebitis. The saphenous vein in the groin is harder to expose, but it too is large and easy to cannulate. If the cannula is left in place in the groin for more than 24 hours, there is a substantial chance that it will cause iliofemoral thrombophlebitis, which can lead to massive and possibly disabling edema in the involved extremity. Therapeutic anticoagulation is required in patients who may be at high risk for bleeding.

Percutaneous cannulation of the internal jugular vein provides not only access for infusion of fluids and drugs but also a port for central venous monitoring. In hypovolemic patients, this vein is usually collapsed, and puncture of the adjacent common carotid artery becomes a possibility; if puncture does occur, it may be difficult to recognize. The pulsatility of blood drawn from an arterial catheter may not be apparent; desaturated arterial blood may take on the appearance of a venous aspirate.

Percutaneous puncture of the subclavian vein provides large-bore access and monitoring capability; however, it may be difficult to accomplish in a hypovolemic patient. Pneumothorax may result, but it is usually easy to treat if recognized early. Puncture of the subclavian artery with decompression into the pleural cavity (a nontamponading space) can be fatal, especially in a patient made vulnerable by coexisting shock.

Percutaneous puncture of the common femoral vein is among the easiest of all techniques for venous access and provides large-bore monitoring capability. Because the femoral artery is immediately adjacent to the vein, unintentional puncture of the artery is common under urgent conditions. If the patient is in extremis, the artery should be cannulated. Intra-arterial infusion of fluids is as effective as I.V. infusion. Great care must be taken to ensure that no air gains entry to the system, and the catheter should be removed as soon as other access is gained. A femoral venous catheter should be removed as soon as possible as well. Percutaneous puncture of the common femoral vein is usually a fallback approach. If it is used in the resuscitation of a hypercoagulable shock patient (the usual scenario) and if the catheter is left in place for more than even a few hours, there is a substantial risk of iliofemoral deep vein thrombosis or even septic deep vein thrombosis—a potentially fatal complication in a critically ill patient.

In pediatric patients, intraosseous access has become a useful means of gaining vascular access under difficult conditions. On rare occasions, this approach may be used in young adults.[12,13]

The first attempts at obtaining vascular access should be made in the upper extremities with a percutaneous technique. If these attempts fail, the physician should fall back on a technique with which he or she is comfortable. There is no single best approach.

Fluid Administration

Once vascular access is obtained, a 20 ml/kg bolus of normal saline should be infused. If the patient is in profound shock, the fluid bolus should be given within 5 minutes if possible; if the situation is less urgent, it may be given over a period of 15 minutes or so. If shock does not resolve, two more boluses should be given.

I consider normal saline the fluid of choice for initial resuscitation in most patients. Its sodium concentration (154 mmol/L) is close to that of normal serum. Its chloride concentration (also 154 mmol/L) can induce hyperchloremic metabolic acidemia, but this state seems not to be harmful to the patient; if it is not severe, it may even augment myocardial contractility. The slight hyperosmolality of the solution may yield a modest increase in contractility as well. If the patient has severe metabolic acidemia with a chloride concentration exceeding 115 mmol/L, lactated or acetated Ringer solution is used. Both the lactate and the acetate accept a proton to form an organic acid, which is converted in the liver to carbon dioxide and water. As long

as hepatic function and pulmonary function are adequate, which is usually the case, the result of this process is buffering of the acidemia that can accompany the shock state. Both of these solutions, however, are hyponatremic and hypoosmotic; the latter is a potential problem in patients at risk for increased intracranial pressure.

Solutions containing glucose should not be used in the initial resuscitation of a patient in shock unless the patient is known to be hypoglycemic. Most patients in shock, in fact, are hyperglycemic as a result of high plasma levels of epinephrine and cortisol.[14] Excessively high plasma glucose concentrations can induce an inappropriate diuresis.

Hypertonic saline solutions containing up to 7.5% sodium chloride (compared with 0.9% for normal saline) show promise for resuscitating patients in situations where large-volume resuscitation with isotonic solutions is impossible (e.g., battle, events involving mass casualties, and prehospital trauma care). Hypertonic solutions provide far more blood volume expansion than isotonic solutions do. They also have advantages in treating hypotensive patients with head injuries. These solutions are approved for use and are commercially available in Brazil (the country where the idea originated), Chile, Argentina, and Europe; they are not currently approved for use in the United States.[15-21]

Albumin-containing solutions should not be given in the acute phase of shock resuscitation except perhaps in unusual circumstances—for example, when only small amounts of resuscitative fluids can be given because of logistical problems, such as those encountered with mass casualties or under battlefield conditions. Initially, protein- or colloid-containing solutions achieve greater plasma volume expansion than crystalloid solutions, but the data from randomized trials with albumin convincingly demonstrate that long-term survival is no better and possibly worse if albumin is used in a setting where large-volume crystalloid can be given instead.[22] The reasons for the poorer survival rates are not entirely clear, but it may be that administration of albumin under conditions of increased microvascular permeability results in accumulation of excessive amounts of albumin in the interstitium. Once in the interstitium, albumin, unlike water and other smaller molecules, can regain access to the plasma space only via lymphatic drainage. If lymphatic drainage capacity is exceeded, persistent postoperative edema may result.

Blood should be given to ensure that the hemoglobin concentration is at least 7 g/dl, if not substantially higher. Certain patients require higher concentrations, as reflected in the following guidelines:

1. A hemoglobin concentration of 7 g/dl is adequate in a young patient who has good coronary arteries and whose bleeding is known to be completely under control.[23]

2. A hemoglobin concentration of 8 g/dl is adequate in a young patient who is at slight risk for further bleeding.

3. A hemoglobin concentration of 9 g/dl is required if the risk of bleeding is substantial.

4. A hemoglobin concentration of 10 g/dl should be the goal if there is any possibility of coronary artery disease, even in the absence of ongoing myocardial ischemia. (The heart is a working muscle, even when the body is at rest, and uses much of the oxygen delivered to it by the coronary arteries. Obstruction of the arteries proximal to the working muscle can lead to usage of all the oxygen carried in the blood. Accordingly, it is crucial to maintain an adequate hemoglobin concentration in this setting. Provided that the arteries are not obstructed, the other organs in the resting body are not susceptible, because they use only a fraction of the oxygen delivered to them.)

5. A hemoglobin concentration of 11 g/dl should be maintained if the heart shows any signs of ongoing myocardial ischemia.

In an emergency, O-negative red blood cells reconstituted with normal saline may be given. If the patient can wait a few more minutes, type-specific blood may be given so as to conserve the blood bank's supply of O-negative blood. Whole blood can be administered more quickly than packed red blood cells, but use of packed cells has the advantage of conserving the blood bank's supply of fresh frozen plasma. Filtering reduces the amount of particulate material administered with the blood but may also reduce the rate at which blood can be administered.

The use of blood substitutes for resuscitation is an attractive option from a conceptual perspective. To date, however, clinical trials using these agents in this setting have yielded disappointing results.[24,25]

Treatment of Pain, Hypothermia, Acidemia, and Coagulopathy

Once blood volume has been at least partially replenished, pain may be treated with small I.V. doses of narcotics. Pain relief can decrease the stress response associated with shock and perhaps diminish the severity of its late sequelae; however, narcotics can also decrease tone in the venules and small veins, thereby exacerbating the shock state. Accordingly, it is vital to keep doses small, to titrate the dosage carefully, and to be ready to reverse the effect with a narcotic antagonist if necessary. Sometimes, a drop in blood pressure after administration of a narcotic can even be a good thing if it alerts the physician to an underlying hypovolemia that should be treated more aggressively.

If hypothermia is present initially, it should be corrected; if it is not present initially, it should not be allowed to develop. Hypothermia slows metabolic processes. In some situations (e.g., cold-water drowning), this may be beneficial to a degree. In the majority of cases, however, it is better for the patient to have a normal body temperature, normal myocardial contractility, and intact coagulatory and immune function. The patient must be unclothed during the initial evaluation, but after that, he or she should be covered, especially the head (a potential source of major heat loss). The room should be kept warm, and any fluids administered should be prewarmed either in an oven or with heating devices.

A low arterial pH should be brought up to a 7.20 by means of either modest degrees of hyperventilation or administration of bicarbonate. Attempts to achieve higher values, at least in the initial shock setting, are probably counterproductive. As noted [see Fluid Administration, above], moderate acidemia may enhance myocardial contractility and immune function. Ideally, acidemia is corrected by treating the underlying cause of shock. Administration of bicarbonate should be kept to a minimum.

Coagulopathy should be treated with fresh frozen plasma and platelets [see I:5 Bleeding and Transfusion]. The decision to use these components should be based on observation of bleeding and clotting in the patient, not on laboratory measurements of coagulation or platelet counts, which can be normal even during exsanguination.

INFLAMMATORY SHOCK

For the most part, initial treatment of inflammatory shock is similar to that of hypovolemic shock because the most pronounced feature of inflammatory shock is loss of plasma into the interstitium through a permeable microvasculature, leading to depletion of vascular volume. The main difference between treatment of hypovolemic shock and treatment of inflammatory shock has to do with when the underlying cause of the shock state should be treated. With hemorrhagic shock, the first priority is control of bleeding. With inflammatory shock, the first priority is replenishment of vascular volume, and definitive treatment (e.g., debridement of dead tissue, drainage of pus, or diversion of the GI tract) should be postponed until the patient is at least partially resuscitated. Such definitive procedures can impose a major physiologic burden on the patient; thus, it is usually best to wait until the patient can withstand the operative insult.

Other potential differences between treatment of inflammatory shock and treatment of hypovolemic shock have to do with the replenishment of depleted compensatory factors and with the use of blockers of inflammatory mediators. A 2001 study suggested that infusion of activated protein C might well be lifesaving for some patients with the septic response.[26] To date, however, studies using blockers of inflammatory mediators to treat inflammatory shock have yielded disappointing results.[27,28]

NEUROGENIC SHOCK

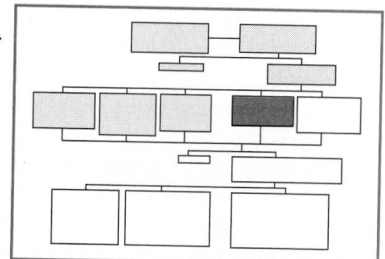

Initial management of neurogenic shock is similar to that of hypovolemic shock, with two exceptions. First, patients in neurogenic shock often benefit from being placed in the Trendelenburg position. Autonomic denervation of the systemic venules and small veins leads to pooling of blood in these capacitance vessels. The Trendelenburg position causes this blood to be translocated to the vascular structures in the chest, including the heart, thereby helping to restore ventricular end-diastolic volumes. Patients with other forms of shock, however, derive no benefit from the Trendelenburg position. In hypovolemic shock, for example, the systemic venules and small veins are already depleted of their blood, as a consequence of both volume loss and adrenergic constriction of the vessel walls. Thus, no blood can be translocated. Furthermore, the left ventricle must pump its blood uphill to perfuse the abdominal viscera and the lower extremities, and the increased work can exhaust an overworked heart.[29]

Second, patients in neurogenic shock often benefit from the use of vasoconstrictors. Vasoconstrictors play no role in the initial management of hypovolemic or inflammatory shock. In these forms of shock, fluid replenishment is a crucial initial measure, and constrictors can be deadly in these settings because they can shut off residual flow to organs already rendered ischemic by depletion of the vascular volume. In neurogenic shock, however, the arterioles are fully dilated in the denervated parts of the body, and this dilatation can lead to central hypotension and inadequate perfusion of the brain and heart. Vasoconstrictors constrict the denervated arterioles, thereby helping to restore central pressures. They also constrict denervated systemic venules and small veins, thereby helping to restore ventricular end-diastolic volumes.

If the heart rate is slow, as it may be if denervation extends high enough to block the sympathetic nerves going to the heart, dopamine (2 to 20 μg/kg/min) may be used. If the heart rate is rapid, norepinephrine or phenylephrine is a good choice. Norepinephrine is given by continuous infusion at a dosage of 4 to 12 μg/min; phenylephrine is initially given at a dosage of 100 to 180 μg/min, which is then decreased to 40 to 60 μg/min.

The danger in giving a vasoconstrictor to a patient in neurogenic shock is that the underlying cause of shock may also have caused occult bleeding. Thus, the vasoconstrictor may maintain the blood pressure, reassuring the physician while the patient bleeds to death. Vasoconstrictors should be used in patients in neurogenic shock only after it has been established that the shock state has no hypovolemic component.

CARDIOGENIC SHOCK

In most cases of cardiogenic shock, management begins with diuresis rather than fluid administration. Furosemide (10 to 40 mg I.V. over a period of 2 to 5 minutes) is a good first choice. If the patient

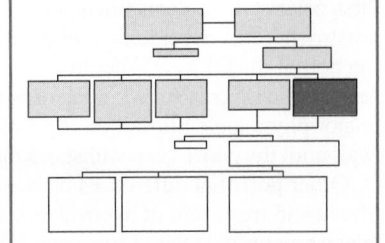

has been receiving furosemide for an extended period, high dosages may be necessary, or spironolactone (25 to 200 mg orally) may have to be added.

Hypertension, if present, may be treated in several ways, depending on the conditions observed. Morphine sulfate (1 to 6 mg I.V. every 1 to 4 hours) is a good first choice if the patient is in pain from an MI and if the physical examination and the chest x-ray indicate pulmonary edema. Nitroglycerine is a good choice if the patient is experiencing angina. It should initially be given I.V. at a dosage of 5 μg/min, which may then be raised in increments of 5 μg/min every 5 minutes. When the dosage reaches 20 μg/min, it may then be raised in increments of 10 μg/min to a maximum dosage of 200 μg/min. Nitroprusside is effective under any conditions. It should initially be given at a dosage of 0.5 μg/kg/min, which may then be raised in increments of 0.5 μg/kg/min to a maximum dosage of 3 μg/kg/min. An angiotensin-converting enzyme (ACE) inhibitor (e.g., enalaprilat, 1.25 to 5.0 mg every 6 hours) is a good choice if the patient's renal function is not compromised and if time is not critical. Sometimes, all of these drugs can be used.

As a rule, hydralazine should not be used; it can increase the heart rate and can markedly increase myocardial oxygen requirements. Calcium channel blockers should be given only after other approaches have failed; they can reduce myocardial oxygen requirements but at the cost of a substantially decreased cardiac output. Nitroprusside and ACE inhibitors generally do not reduce cardiac output, nor, in patients with large ventricular end-diastolic volumes, do morphine and nitroglycerine.

Beta blockade can be extremely effective in controlling blood pressure in a hypertensive patient and heart rate in any patient. Esmolol, a short-acting agent, is the best first choice. A loading dose of 500 μg/kg is given, followed by infusion at a rate of 50 μg/kg/min. If it proves necessary to increase the dosage, another 500 μg/kg loading dose is given, and the infusion rate is raised to 100 μg/kg/min. If the patient responds well to this regimen, he or she should be switched from esmolol to the long-acting agent metoprolol (5 to 15 mg every 6 hours).

Beta blockers can reduce cardiac output, but they also markedly reduce myocardial oxygen requirements by decreasing heart rate, blood pressure, stroke volume, and myocardial contractility. These agents should not be given to patients who are hypotensive or show signs of marked peripheral hypoperfusion, but they should be given to all other patients in whom myocardial ischemia is a possibility.

In many patients with acute myocardial ischemia and shock, all of the aforementioned treatments should be employed, with the addition of heparin anticoagulation and emergency coronary angiography. The mortality associated with cardiogenic shock in a patient with an acute MI is extremely high. Accordingly, every effort should be made to find a correctable lesion and treat it with coronary angioplasty, stenting, or surgical revascularization. If necessary, an intra-aortic balloon pump may be placed once angiography, angioplasty, and stenting have been completed or in preparation for surgical correction of ischemia.

The hemoglobin concentration in patients with cardiogenic shock should be maintained at a generous level (i.e., about 11 g/dl).

Treatment of Shock That Persists Despite Initial Management

INVASIVE MONITORING

In most cases of shock, regardless of category, the initial approach just described leads to resolution

of all the clinical abnormalities. Some patients, however, do not respond to these treatment measures. In my view, invasive monitoring is warranted for these unresponsive patients.

Invasive monitoring permits direct assessment of patients' thermodynamic needs, thus allowing the physician to deal with the most difficult problem in managing unresponsive shock patients—namely, how to balance the metabolic needs of the noncardiac tissues against the demands made on a potentially ischemic myocardium. Almost all interventions that increase perfusion of the peripheral tissues also increase myocardial oxygen requirements, and almost all interventions that decrease myocardial oxygen requirements also decrease perfusion of noncardiac tissues [see Sidebar Thermodynamic Concepts of Clinical Relevance to Shock].[30,31]

GOALS OF RESUSCITATION

The primary goal of shock management is to correct the clinical abnormalities that led to the diagnosis in the first place. The secondary goal is to enable the patient to generate adequate blood pressure and cardiac output—that is, adequate power [see Table 4]—for perfusion of the tissues without overburdening the heart.

Determining what constitutes adequate blood pressure can be difficult at times. The pressure must be, at the very least, high enough to perfuse the brain, an organ that has a very active metabolic rate and very little vascular tone. Drops in blood pressure put the brain at risk because, unlike all the other organs in the body, it is unable to vasodilate in response to falling perfusion pressure. In an alert patient, determining adequate blood pressure is not difficult. In an obtunded patient, an arbitrary value must be assigned; a reasonable systolic pressure might be 90 mm Hg in a younger patient and somewhat higher in an older patient. Carotid stenosis necessitates a higher pressure, and stenoses in any of the arteries supplying actively metabolizing organs call for higher central pressures.

Although, under ordinary circumstances, all noncerebral organs have some tonic contracture of the arterioles that allows vasodilatation if pressure falls, the arterioles in an organ made ischemic by proximal obstruction and active metabolism are maximally dilated; the organ therefore becomes vulnerable to hypotension. The classic example of this phenomenon is the heart in a patient with coronary disease, but the same mechanism comes into play in the gut in a patient with mesenteric arterial occlusive disease, in the kidney in a patient with renal artery stenosis, in the spinal cord in a patient with obstructed intercostal arteries, and in the extremities in a patient with peripheral arterial disease.

In sum, the only way of setting the goal for adequate blood pressure is to combine clinical judgment with assessment of the patient's response to treatment. If a given blood pressure is associated with an altered level of consciousness, myocardial ischemia, oliguria, or any other sign suggesting inadequate flow, it must be increased.

Although there is general agreement on how to set goals for adequate blood pressure, there is little agreement on how to set goals for optimum cardiac output. One approach is to attempt to determine whether the patient's oxygen consumption (measured with a pulmonary arterial catheter and based in part on measurements of cardiac output) is dependent on oxygen delivery (the product of cardiac output, hemoglobin concentration, and arterial oxygen saturation). At very low levels of oxygen delivery, there is no question that oxygen consumption must decrease.[32] At excessively high levels, however, oxygen consumption may continue to rise if oxygen delivery is increased by the administration of inotropes. These agents usually have beta-adrenergic effects and can increase peripheral oxygen metabolism; they also increase myocardial oxygen requirements. Thus, the act of increasing delivery can increase peripheral consumption.

Another approach is to maintain all patients at very high levels of oxygen delivery without making any attempt to see if there is a correlation between delivery and peripheral consumption. This proposed approach was examined in randomized trials in critically ill patients, which found that maintaining supranormal levels of oxygen delivery was of no benefit.[33-36]

A third approach is to use mixed venous oxygen saturation (also measured with a pulmonary arterial catheter) as a primary end point in resuscitation. This approach has the advantage of simplicity and is certainly useful with some forms of shock (e.g., hypovolemic

Table 4 Different Forms of Power Generated in the Cardiovascular System

Form of Power	Formula
Power delivered into aortic root each minute	SV·HR·LVESP
Power generated by left atrium	SV·HR·LAP
Power generated by left ventricle	SV·HR·(LVESP−LAP)
Mean power delivered into aortic root	SV·HR·MAP
Oscillatory power delivered into aortic root	SV·HR·(LVESP−MAP)
Power used to perfuse peripheral tissues	SV·HR·(MAP−RAP)
Power used to fill right atrium	SV·HR·RAP

Note: see VII:1 Cardiopulmonary Monitoring.
HR—heart rate   LAP— mean left atrial pressure   LVESP—left ventricular end-systolic pressure   MAP—mean arterial pressure (equivalent to mean aortic root pressure)   RAP—mean right atrial pressure   SV—stroke volume

shock). Many patients in inflammatory shock, however, have quite high mixed venous oxygen saturations, partly because of peripheral shunting through the cutaneous vasculature and partly because of functional shunting by cells that cannot metabolize the oxygen presented to them. In these patients, a high mixed venous oxygen saturation might even indicate a severe metabolic derangement rather than resolution of shock.[34]

Yet another resuscitation approach is to avoid using any direct measurement of cardiovascular adequacy and to use other end points of resuscitation instead. Perhaps the most attractive such end point is gastric mucosal pH. In many forms of shock, the gut is quickly made ischemic; conceivably, if the gut mucosa can be shown to be well perfused, one can assume that the rest of the body is also well perfused. Further trials are necessary to ascertain whether gastric mucosal pH can be used in lieu of detailed measurements of cardiac performance.[37]

Thermodynamic principles may also be employed to set resuscitation end points. Such an approach implies that cardiac output itself should be used in conjunction with blood pressure to assess adequacy of resuscitation. Recent work by Chang and associates suggests that a normal cardiac output is probably an adequate one.[38,39] One might wish to aim for slightly supranormal values in patients with major injuries or overwhelming infections, but excessively high values should rarely be necessary.

To define what a normal cardiac output is, one must take some account of patient size, expressed in terms either of body weight (ideal, current, or premorbid) or of body surface area (which in turn is calculated in part on the basis of weight). I prefer to use ideal body weight in the calculations rather than current body weight or premorbid weight. Ideal body weight is calculated on the basis of the patient's height, with adjustments made for age, on the assumption that ideal weight in an unconditioned older individual decreases by 10% each decade after 50 years of age. The age adjustment can have a substantial effect on the calculation. For example, a patient who is 80 years old—not an uncommon age for an ICU patient today—might have had an ideal body weight of 70 kg at age 50. At 80 years of age, if the patient is not in good condition, ideal body weight will have fallen to 51 kg. This makes a significant difference in terms of target cardiac output: whereas a cardiac output of 7 L/min might have been required when the patient was 50 years old, an output of 5 L/min is probably more than adequate 30 years later. Finally, the choice of a goal for cardiac output is sometimes facilitated by trial and error. For example, if a supranormal cardiac output causes an abnormality (e.g., metabolic acidemia) to resolve when a normal output did not, then an effort should be made to keep the output high for a while.

Thermodynamic Concepts of Clinical Relevance to Shock

In my view, treatment of shock is best approached with an eye to the thermodynamics of cardiovascular function. Thermodynamics is the scientific discipline developed in the 19th century to explain the generation and transfer of energy, including power and heat, between systems. For the purposes of this chapter, an exhaustive familiarity with thermodynamic principles is unnecessary; however, there are a few thermodynamic concepts of direct clinical relevance that are worth outlining here. These concepts become increasingly pertinent as one moves from easily managed patients to more challenging ones.

A key concept is that of power. Power, in thermodynamic terms, is flow multiplied by pressure [see Table 4]. In the case of the heart, the power generated by the left atrium and the left ventricle (and consequently the power delivered into the aortic root) is approximately equal to cardiac output multiplied by left ventricular end-systolic pressure (LVESP):

Power into aortic root = SV·HR·LVESP

where cardiac output is expressed as the product of stroke volume (SV) and heart rate (HR).

The main challenge in treating the patient in shock is to balance the needs of the peripheral circulation against the demands made on the heart. Left ventricular oxygen requirements are directly proportional to left ventricular power: doubling power doubles oxygen requirements. The significance of this relation in the management of shock will be apparent from an examination of the formulas for left ventricular power and power for peripheral tissue perfusion:

Left ventricular power = SV·HR·(LVESP-LAP)

Power for peripheral perfusion = SV·HR·(MAP-RAP)

where LAP is mean left atrial pressure, MAP is mean arterial pressure (which is equivalent to mean aortic root pressure), and RAP is mean right atrial pressure.

From these formulas, it is clear that any therapy that increases SV or HR will increase both power for peripheral perfusion and left ventricular power (and thus left ventricular oxygen requirements). Any therapy that increases MAP will increase power for peripheral perfusion and usually will increase ventricular oxygen requirements because LVESP generally rises when MAP rises. Finally, any therapy that decreases RAP will increase power for peripheral perfusion and usually will increase left ventricular oxygen requirements because LAP generally falls when RAP falls. Thus, in increasing power for perfusion of the peripheral tissues, one almost always increases left ventricular oxygen requirements as well. In other words, there is no thermodynamic free lunch.

Thus, the end points of shock management are for the most part clinical end points—namely, reversal of cutaneous signs of shock, hypotension, mental abnormalities, myocardial ischemia, metabolic acidemia, hypoxemia, and heart rate abnormalities. If these end points cannot be reached initially, the goal should then be to reach thermodynamic end points—that is, adequate pressures and adequate flow (power [see Table 4])—while trying to minimize myocardial oxygen requirements. This is the main challenge in resuscitating a patient from shock. As a rule, increasing the heart rate, end-diastolic volumes, contractility, and the hindrance against which the ventricles contract (up to a limit) all increase the power output of the heart; they also all increase myocardiac oxygen requirements. Incorporating a thermodynamic perspective into management brings this problem into the open.

Depending on the resuscitative priorities in a given patient, one of the following three hemodynamic goals is generally appropriate:

1. Increased provision of nutrients to noncardiac tissues along with robust amounts of energy, even though production of that energy by the heart puts a strain on the myocardium.
2. Decreased demands on the heart, even though, as a consequence, less energy will be available for perfusion of noncardiac tissues.
3. A balance between (1) and (2), aimed at achieving the most efficient possible production of energy by the heart while admitting the possibility that a compromise between the two might end up achieving neither.

An example of a patient for whom the first goal might be appropriate is a young trauma patient with a robust myocardium but extensive noncardiac injuries. The second goal might be appropriate for a patient with an uncomplicated MI. The third goal might be appropriate for a patient with known coronary artery disease who has just undergone resection of a ruptured abdominal aortic aneurysm.

ASSESSMENT OF RELATIVE PRIORITIES OF PERIPHERY AND HEART

The next task in the management of unresponsive shock states is to determine whether priority should be given to the needs of the periphery or to those of the heart. The difficulty here is that many of the patients who have reached this stage of treatment—that is, in whom initial therapeutic measures have been unsuccessful—have both cardiac and noncardiac problems. Management of these patients is a challenge.

Periphery Is Priority

Fluid administration and assessment of ventricular end-diastolic volumes If priority is given to the periphery, the patient will probably require fluids. As a starting point, the goal should be to achieve a pulmonary arterial wedge pressure in the midteens (assuming that the patient is being mechanically ventilated). As therapy progresses and as more measurements are made, this goal may have to be modified. The ultimate goal, however, is not to produce any specific wedge pressure but rather to produce generous right and left ventricular end-diastolic volumes.[40] To estimate these volumes, it is necessary to synthesize several pieces of information.

Intracavitary right atrial pressure (a commonly measured value obtained via the proximal port of a pulmonary arterial catheter)

yields a good estimate of intracavitary right ventricular end-diastolic pressure. Pulmonary arterial wedge pressure is equivalent to intracavitary left atrial pressure (which, in the absence of mitral valvular stenosis, is the same as left ventricular end-diastolic pressure) if there is an open column of blood when the balloon is inflated between the end of the catheter and the left atrium. This open communication between the catheter tip and the atrium is usually present because the catheter, once inserted, is directed by flow into the well-perfused parts of the pulmonary vasculature. On occasion, however, the catheter ends up in a poorly perfused part of the lung (zone I), in which case it measures intra-alveolar pressure instead of left atrial pressure. This malpositioning is usually signaled by excessive swings in wedge pressure that coincide with the cycling of the ventilator. In theory, inaccuracies can creep into pressure measurements if there is robust collateral flow around the vasculature occluded by the balloon, as with the bronchial circulation. In practice, however, this is seldom a problem.

Given acceptably accurate intracavitary end-diastolic pressure values, the challenge is to extrapolate from these values to reasonably good estimates of ventricular end-diastolic volume. There is not a simple proportional correspondence between pressure and volume, because volume depends not only on pressure but also on the stiffness of the ventricle during diastole and on the stiffness of the structures surrounding the heart.[41-43]

In a patient breathing spontaneously, a right atrial pressure of 2 to 5 mm Hg measured with respect to atmosphere with the transducer zeroed at the midaxillary line is generally sufficient to generate an adequate right ventricular end-diastolic volume. For the left ventricle, a wedge pressure of 5 to 8 mm Hg usually suffices. In a patient with compression of the heart as a result of inflation of the lungs by positive pressure ventilation, an intracavitary right atrial (or right ventricular end-diastolic) pressure of 9 to 12 mm Hg is usually necessary for a normal right ventricular end-diastolic volume; a wedge pressure of 12 to 15 mm Hg is usually necessary for a normal left ventricular end-diastolic volume.

These values work for patients with essentially normal lungs; however, most patients on mechanical ventilators do not have normal lungs. In such patients, the lungs can form a stiff compartment around the heart that does not give when the heart is pushed into the compartment by an elevated diaphragm. To complicate matters further, the diastolic stiffness of the ventricular musculature is increased in many critically ill patients, and the intracavitary pressures must overcome this added stiffness as well. On occasion, right and left intracavitary ventricular end-diastolic pressures exceeding 20 mm Hg are necessary to produce normal end-diastolic volumes.

The estimates of end-diastolic pressure can sometimes be confirmed by increasing the filling pressures of the heart with a fluid bolus and assessing the cardiovascular response. Increases in stroke volume, especially if associated with increases in pulmonary and systemic arterial pressures, suggest that the initial end-diastolic volumes were too small and that more fluid is needed. In other cases, initial end-diastolic volumes might have been unnecessarily large. If so, a diuretic can be given. If stroke volumes and blood pressures do not decrease, further diuresis is indicated.

Right ventricular end-diastolic volume can be measured directly by means of a pulmonary arterial catheter equipped with a fast-response thermistor. These catheters are more expensive than those not so equipped, but they can be helpful in complicated cases.[44] Left ventricular end-diastolic volume can be measured directly with transesophageal echocardiography in difficult cases (e.g., a patient with an elevated diaphragm).

If measurements are available from only one ventricle, the physician can cautiously use this information to estimate the corresponding values from the other, keeping in mind that in many critically ill patients, there is a marked discrepancy between right and left ventricular end-diastolic volumes. The general finding from studies comparing right ventricular end-diastolic volumes (measured with a fast thermistor) and left ventricular end-diastolic volumes (measured with transesophageal echocardiography) is that right ventricular values are frequently larger than left ventricular values in patients in inflammatory shock, sometimes by a factor of 3.[45] In patients with left-sided congestive heart failure, however, left ventricular end-diastolic volumes can be substantially larger than right. Thus, knowing the volume of one chamber does not necessarily mean that one knows the volume of the other, but the clinical scenario can provide some guidance.

Inotropes   Inotropes such as dobutamine (5 to 15 μg/kg/min) and milrinone (50 μg, then 0.375 to 0.75 μg/kg/min) can be given freely. They will increase myocardial oxygen requirements, but this is not a problem in a patient with a strong heart. The only limitation on use of the inotropes is the development of a tachycardia. If the heart rate begins to exceed 100 beats/min, the dosage should be reduced.

Vasoconstrictors   There are only three indications for administration of vasoconstrictors to patients in whom the primary concern is perfusion of the periphery: (1) profound hypotension in a patient who is in neurogenic shock; (2) hypotension so severe that cerebral or spinal cord perfusion is thought to be inadequate on the basis of either neurologic symptoms (if the patient is neurologically intact) or cerebral perfusion pressure (if the patient is not neurologically intact); and (3) hypotension in a patient who has critical stenosis in the cerebral, coronary, mesenteric, or renal arteries or in the arteries supplying the spinal cord or who has a severely ischemic extremity. For virtually all other patients whose main problem is inadequate perfusion of the periphery, fluids and, occasionally, inotropes are enough.

If a vasoconstrictor is indicated, dopamine may be given if the initial heart rate is 90 beats/min or slower. The heart rate should not be driven above 100 beat/min. Norepinephrine may be given if the initial heart rate exceeds 90 beats/min.

Periphery and Heart Are Equal Priorities

Fluid management in patients who have both inadequate peripheral perfusion and marginal myocardial reserve must be finely tuned. Every effort should be made to estimate the ventricular

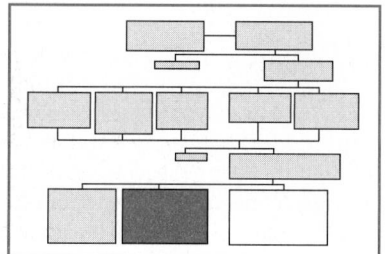

end-diastolic volumes accurately. Excessively large end-diastolic volumes will increase myocardial oxygen requirements unnecessarily, and inadequate end-diastolic volumes will make it impossible for the ventricles to produce adequate pressure and stroke volumes. In some patients, diuresis is indicated; in others, administration of fluids. Frequently, trial and error will be necessary.

If pressures and stroke volumes are still inadequate after fluids have been replenished, inotropes should be tried. These agents must be used with some caution because they will increase myocardial oxygen requirements.

Vasoconstrictors should be used only as previously discussed [*see* Periphery Is Priority, *above*]. Dopamine may be given if the initial heart rate is 70 beats/min or slower. The heart rate should not be driven above 90 beats/min. Norepinephrine may be given if the heart rate exceeds 70 beats/min.

Beta blockade is frequently necessary when the heart rate exceeds 90 beats/min. Maintenance of a slow heart rate is the single most important factor in minimizing myocardial oxygen requirements, but it usually can be achieved only at the cost of decreasing pressures and stroke volumes. Esmolol is a good first choice because it is quickly reversible; metoprolol may be given later if it is clear that beta blockade was needed and the patient is stable.

Heart Is Priority

If the priority is the heart and there is comparatively little reason for concern about noncardiac tissues, treatment is usually straightforward, though the results may be less than might be hoped for. The treatment ap-

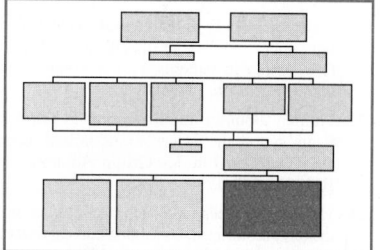

proach should be patterned on that for cardiogenic shock (see above). Invasive monitoring allows precise measurements that can be useful, particularly during diuresis. The goal of diuresis is to produce normal ventricular end-diastolic volumes so as to minimize myocardial oxygen requirements. Often, this proves impossible. Larger end-diastolic volumes are necessary to make up for poor contractility. Invasive monitoring helps the physician strike the necessary balance. Vasoconstrictors and inotropes should not be used, because they will increase myocardial oxygen requirements. If blood pressure or stroke volumes become inadequate, the therapeutic approach should be changed to take the needs of the periphery into account as described earlier [*see* Periphery and Heart Are Equal Priorities, *above*].

References

1. Demetriades D, Chan LS, Bhasin P, et al: Relative bradycardia in patients with traumatic hypotension. J Trauma 45:534, 1998

2. Little RA: 1988 Fitts Lecture: heart rate changes after haemorrhage and injury—a reappraisal. J Trauma 29:903, 1989

3. Shenkin HA, Cheney RH, Govons SR, et al: On the diagnosis of hemorrhage in man: a study of volunteers bled large amounts. Am J Med Sci 208:421, 1944

4. Gore DC, Ferrando A, Barnett J, et al: Influence of glucose kinetics on plasma lactate concentration and energy expenditure in severely burned patients. J Trauma 49:673, 2000

5. Gausche M, Lewis RJ, Stratton SJ, et al: Effect of out-of-hospital pediatric endotracheal intubation on survival and neurological outcome: a controlled clinical trial. JAMA 283:783, 2000

6. Chang MC, Miller PR, D'Agostino R, et al: Effects of abdominal decompression on cardiopulmonary function and visceral perfusion in patients with intra-abdominal hypertension. J Trauma 44:440, 1998

7. Ventilation with lower tidal volumes as compared with traditional tidal volumes for acute lung injury and the acute respiratory distress syndrome. Acute Respiratory Distress Syndrome Network. N Engl J Med 342:1301, 2000

8. Amato MBP, Barbas CSV, Medeiros DM, et al: Effect of a protective-ventilation strategy on mortality in the acute respiratory distress syndrome. N Engl J Med 338:347, 1998

9. Bulger EM, Jurkovich GJ, Gentilello LM, et al: Current clinical options for the treatment and management of acute respiratory distress syndrome. J Trauma 48:562, 2000

10. Ranieri VM, Suter PM, Tortorella C, et al: Effect of mechanical ventilation on inflammatory mediators in patients with acute respiratory distress syndrome: a randomized controlled trial. JAMA 282:54, 1999

11. Rankin JS, Olsen CO, Arentzen CE, et al: The effects

of airway pressure on cardiac function in intact dogs and man. Circulation 66:108, 1982

12. Sawyer RW, Bodai BI, Blaisdell FW, et al: The current status of intraosseous infusion. J Am Coll Surg 179: 353, 1994

13. Waisman M, Waisman D: Bone marrow infusion in adults. J Trauma 42:288, 1997

14. Wilmore DW: Metabolic response to severe surgical illness: overview. World J Surg 24:705, 2000

15. Angle N, Hoyt DB, Coimbra R, et al: Hypertonic saline resuscitation diminishes lung injury by suppressing neutrophil activation after hemorrhagic shock. Shock 9:164, 1998

16. Ciesla DJ, Moore EE, Zallen G, et al: Hypertonic saline attenuation of polymorphonuclear neutrophil cytotoxicity: timing is everything. J Trauma 48:388, 2000

17. Ho HS, Liu H, Cala PM, et al: Hypertonic perfusion inhibits intracellular Na and Ca accumulation in hypoxic myocardium. Am J Physiol Cell Physiol 278: C953, 2000

18. Rotstein OD: Novel strategies for immunomodulation after trauma: revisiting hypertonic saline as a resuscitation strategy for hemorrhagic shock. J Trauma 49:580, 2000

19. Vassar MJ, Fischer RP, O'Brien PE, et al: A multicenter trial for resuscitation of injured patients with 7.5% sodium chloride. Arch Surg 128:1003, 1993

20. Velasco IT, Pontieri V, Rocha e Silva M, et al: Hyperosmotic NaCl and severe hemorrhagic shock. Am J Physiol 239:H664, 1980

21. Wade CE, Grady JJ, Kramer GC, et al: Individual patient cohort analysis of the efficacy of hypertonic saline/dextran in patients with traumatic brain injury and hypotension. J Trauma 42:S61, 1997

22. Human albumin administration in critically ill patients: systematic review of randomised controlled trials. Cochrane Injuries Group Albumin Reviewers. BMJ 317:235, 1998

23. Hébert PC, Wells G, Blajchman MA, et al: A multicenter, randomized, controlled clinical trial of transfusion requirements in critical care. N Engl J Med 340: 409, 1999

24. Cohn SM: Surgical research review: blood substitutes in surgery. Surgery 127:599, 2000

25. Sloan EP, Koenigsberg M, Gens D, et al: Diaspirin cross-linked hemoglobin (DCLHb) in the treatment of severe traumatic hemorrhagic shock: a randomized controlled efficacy trial. JAMA 282:1857, 1999

26. Bernard GR, Vincent JL, Laterre PF, et al: Efficacy and safety of recombinant human activated protein C for severe sepsis. N Engl J Med 344:699, 2001

27. Angus DC, Birmingham MC, Balk RA, et al: E5 murine monoclonal antiendotoxin antibody in gram-negative sepsis: a randomized controlled trial. JAMA 283:1723, 2000

28. Ketoconazole for early treatment of acute lung injury and acute respiratory distress syndrome: a randomized controlled trial. ARDS Network Authors. JAMA 283: 1995, 2000

29. Sibbald WJ, Paterson NAM, Holliday RL, et al: The Trendelenburg position: hemodynamic effects in hypotensive and normotensive patients. Crit Care Med 7:218, 1979

30. McDonald's Blood Flow in Arteries: Theoretical, Experimental and Clinical Principles, 4th ed. Nichols WW, O'Rourke MF, Eds. Arnold and Oxford University Press, London and New York, 1998

31. Suga H: Ventricular energetics. Physiol Rev 70:247, 1990

32. Cain SM: Oxygen delivery and uptake in dogs during anemic and hypoxic hypoxia. J Appl Physiol 42:228, 1977

33. Durham RM, Neunaber K, Mazuski JE, et al: The use of oxygen consumption and delivery as endpoints for resuscitation in critically ill patients. J Trauma 41:32, 1996

34. Gattinoni L, Brazzi L, Pelosi P, et al: A trial of goal-oriented hemodynamic therapy in critically ill patients. N Engl J Med 333:1025, 1995

35. Hayes MA, Timmins AC, Yau EHS, et al: Elevation of systemic oxygen delivery in the treatment of critically ill patients. N Engl J Med 330:1717, 1994

36. Velmahos GC, Demetriades D, Shoemaker WC, et al: Endpoints of resuscitation of critically injured patients: normal or supranormal? A prospective randomized trial. Ann Surg 232:409, 2000

37. Ivatury RR, Simon RJ, Islam S, et al: A prospective randomized study of end points of resuscitation after major trauma: global oxygen transport indices versus organ-specific gastric mucosal pH. J Am Coll Surg 183:145, 1996

38. Chang MC, Meredith JW, Kincaid EH, et al: Maintaining survivors' values of left ventricular power output during shock resuscitation: a prospective pilot study. J Trauma 49:26, 2000

39. Chang MC, Mondy JS, Meredith JW, et al: Redefining cardiovascular performance during resuscitation: ventricular stroke work, power, and the pressure-volume diagram. J Trauma 45:470, 1998

40. Miller PR, Meredith JW, Chang MC: Randomized, prospective comparison of increased preload versus inotropes in the resuscitation of trauma patients: effects on cardiopulmonary function and visceral perfusion. J Trauma 44:107, 1998

41. Grossman W: Diastolic dysfunction in congestive heart failure. N Engl J Med 325:1557, 1991

42. Hess OM, Osakada G, Lavelle JF, et al: Diastolic myocardial wall stiffness and ventricular relaxation during partial and complete coronary occlusions in the conscious dog. Circ Res 52:387, 1983

43. Isoyama S, Apstein CS, Wexler LF, et al: Acute decrease in left ventricular diastolic chamber distensibility during simulated angina in isolated hearts. Circ Res 61:925, 1987

44. Chang MC, Blinman TA, Rutherford EJ, et al: Preload assessment in trauma patients during large volume shock resuscitation. Arch Surg 131:728, 1996

45. Kraut EJ, Owings JT, Anderson JT, et al: Right ventricular volumes overestimate left ventricular preload in critically ill patients. J Trauma 42:839, 1997

46. Perdue PW, Balser JR, Lipsett PA, et al: "Renal dose" dopamine in surgical patients: dogma or science? Ann Surg 227:470, 1998

5 BLEEDING AND TRANSFUSION

John T. Owings, M.D., and Robert C. Gosselin, M.T.

Approach to the Patient with Ongoing Bleeding

A surgeon is often the first person to be called when a patient experiences ongoing bleeding. To treat such a patient appropriately, the surgeon must identify the cause or source of the bleeding. Causes fall into two main categories: (1) conditions leading to loss of vascular integrity, as in a postoperative patient with an unligated vessel that is bleeding or a trauma patient with a ruptured spleen, and (2) conditions leading to derangement of the hemostatic process. In this chapter, we focus on the latter category, which includes a broad spectrum of conditions ranging from aspirin-induced platelet dysfunction to von Willebrand disease (vWD) to disseminated intravascular coagulation (DIC) and even to hemophilia.

Coagulopathies are varied in their causes, treatments, and prognoses. Our aim is not to obviate the hematologic tests required for identification of rare congenital or acquired clotting abnormalities but to outline effective management approaches to the coagulopathies surgeons see most frequently. The vast majority of these coagulopathies can be diagnosed by means of a brief patient and family history, a review of medications, physical examination, and laboratory studies—in particular, activated partial thromboplastin time (aPTT), prothrombin time (PT, commonly expressed as an international normalized ratio [INR]), complete blood count (CBC), and D-dimer assay.

Exclusion of Technical Causes of Bleeding

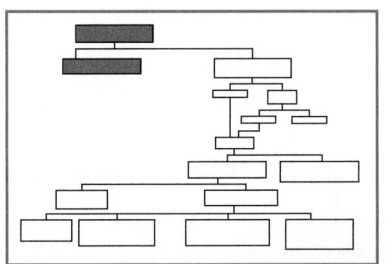

It is critical for the surgeon to recognize that the most common causes of postoperative bleeding are technical: an unligated vessel or an unrecognized injury is much more likely to be the cause of a falling hematocrit than either a drug effect or an endogenous hemostatic defect. Furthermore, if an unligated vessel is treated as though it were an endogenous hemostatic defect (i.e., with transfusions), the outcome is likely to be disastrous. For these reasons, in all cases of ongoing bleeding, the first consideration must always be to exclude a surgically correctable cause.

Ongoing bleeding may be surprisingly difficult to diagnose. Healthy young patients can usually maintain a normal blood pressure until their blood loss exceeds 40% of their blood volume (roughly 2 L). If the bleeding is from a laceration to an extremity, it will be obvious; however, if the bleeding is occurring internally (e.g., from a ruptured spleen or an intraluminal GI source), there may be few physiologic signs [*see I:4 Shock*]. For the purposes of the ensuing discussion, we assume that bleeding is known to have occurred or to be occurring.

Even when a technical cause of bleeding has seemingly been excluded, the possibility often must be reconsidered periodically throughout assessment. Patients who are either unresuscitated or underresuscitated undergo vasospasm, which may cause tamponade of the bleeding point.[1] As resuscitation proceeds, the catecholamine-induced vasospasm subsides and the bleeding may recur. For this reason, constant reassessment of the possibility of a technical cause of bleeding is appropriate. Only when the surgeon is confident that a missed injury or unligated vessel is not the cause of the bleeding should other potential causes be investigated.

Initial Assessment of Potential Coagulopathy

The first step in assessment of a patient with a potential coagulopathy is to draw a blood sample. The blood should be distributed into a tube containing ethylenediaminetetraacetic acid (EDTA) (for a CBC) and a citrated tube (for coagulation analysis).

At the same time, the patient's temperature should be noted. Because coagulation is a chemical reaction, it slows with increasing cold.[2] Thus, a patient with a temperature lower than 35° C (95° F) clots more slowly and less efficiently than one with a temperature of 37° C (98.6° F).[3] The resulting coagulatory abnormality is what is known as a hypothermic coagulopathy. Upon receipt of the drawn specimen, the laboratory warms the sample to 37° C to run the coagulation assays (aPTT and INR). In a patient with a purely hypothermic coagulopathy, this step results in normal coagulation parameters. Hypothermic patients should be actively rewarmed.[4] Typically, such patients cease to bleed after rewarming, and no further treatment is required. If the patient is normothermic and exhibits normal coagulation values but bleeding continues, attention should again be focused on the possibility of an unligated bleeding vessel or an uncontrolled occult bleeding source (e.g., the GI tract).

Ongoing bleeding in conjunction with abnormal coagulation parameters may have any of several underlying causes. In this setting, one of the most useful pieces of information to obtain is a personal and family history. A patient who has had dental extractions without major problems or who had a normal adolescence without any history of bleeding dyscrasias is very unlikely to have a congenital or hereditary bleeding disorder.[5] If there is a personal or family history of a specific bleeding disorder, appropriate steps should be taken to diagnose and treat the disorder [*see* Discussion, Bleeding Disorders, *below*].

Patient experiences ongoing bleeding

First, consider possible technical cause (unligated vessel after operation or unrecognized injury).

Patient has unligated vessel or unrecognized injury

Control bleeding vessel.

Approach to Patient with Ongoing Bleeding

Patient has family history of bleeding disorder

Initiate directed testing and therapy.

Patient has normal INR and aPTT

Consider platelet dysfunction.
Give platelets and initiate directed therapy.

Patient has normal INR and prolonged aPTT

Consider drug effects (heparin, lepirudin), acquired factor deficiency, and vWD.
Give protamine (to reverse heprin), replace factors, or initiate directed therapy for vWD.

No technical cause of bleeding is apparent

Draw blood for laboratory tests.
Check T°.

T° is normal

T° is low

Warm patient.

Bleeding continues

Bleeding stops

Assess platelet status and
coagulation parameters.

Platelet status or coagulation parameters are abnormal

Look for family history of specific bleeding disorder.

Platelet status and coagulation parameters are normal

DIC is not present.
Reconsider possibility of unligated vessel [*see above, left*].

Patient has no family history of bleeding disorder

Continue evaluation guided by laboratory test results.

Patient has increased INR and normal aPTT

Consider drug effects (warfarin), hepatic failure, and
malnutrition.
Give I.V. vitamin K or FFP as appropriate; treat cirrhosis-related
variceal bleeding surgically.

Patient has increased INR and prolonged aPTT

If D-dimer level is elevated, assume DIC and
treat accordingly.
If D-dimer level is normal, consider end-stage
renal disease and multifactor deficiency.
Give FFP, and initiate directed therapy.

Measurement of Coagulation Parameters

NORMAL INR, NORMAL aPTT

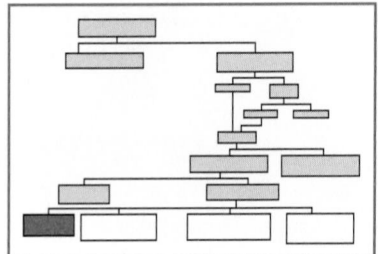

Patients with a normal INR and aPTT who exhibit ongoing bleeding may have impaired platelet activity. Inadequate platelet activity is frequently manifested as persistent oozing from wound edges or as low-volume bleeding. Such bleeding is rarely the cause of exsanguinating hemorrhage, though it may be life-threatening on occasion, depending on its location (e.g., the head or the pericardium). Inadequate platelet activity may be attributable either to an insufficient number of platelets or to platelet dysfunction. In the absence of a major surgical insult, a platelet count of 20,000/mm³ or higher is usually adequate for normal coagulation.[6,7] There is some disagreement regarding the absolute level to which the platelet count must fall before platelet transfusion is justified in the absence of active bleeding. Patients undergoing procedures in which even capillary oozing is potentially life-threatening (e.g., craniotomy) should be maintained at a higher platelet count (i.e., > 20,000/mm³). Patients without ongoing bleeding who are not specifically at increased risk for major complications from low-volume bleeding may be safely watched with platelet counts lower than 20,000/mm³.

Oozing in a patient who has an adequate platelet count and normal coagulation parameters may be a signal of platelet dysfunction. The now-routine administration of aspirin to reduce the risk of myocardial infarction and stroke has led to a rise in the incidence of aspirin-induced platelet dysfunction. Aspirin causes irreversible platelet dysfunction through the cyclo-oxygenase pathway; the effect of aspirin can thus be expected to last for approximately 10 days. The platelet dysfunction caused by other nonsteroidal anti-inflammatory drugs (e.g., ibuprofen) is reversible and consequently does not last as long as that caused by aspirin. Newer platelet-blocking agents have been found to be effective in improving outcome after coronary angioplasty.[8] These drugs function predominantly by blocking the platelet surface receptor glycoprotein (GP) IIb-IIIa, which binds platelets to fibrinogen.

In patients with platelet dysfunction caused by an inhibitor of platelet function, such as an elevated blood urea nitrogen (BUN) level, 1-desamino-8-D-arginine vasopressin (DDAVP) is capable of partially reversing the dysfunction.[9] DDAVP has also been successful in partially reversing aspirin-induced platelet dysfunction.

Less common causes of bleeding in patients with a normal INR and a normal aPTT include factor XIII deficiency, hypofibrinogenemia or dysfibrinogenemia, and derangements in the fibrinolytic pathway [see Discussion, Mechanics of Hemostasis, below].

NORMAL INR, PROLONGED aPTT

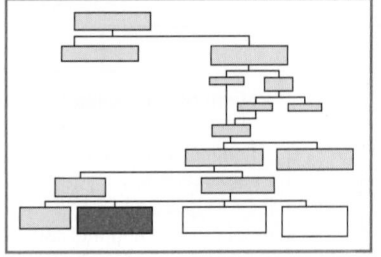

Patients with a normal INR and an abnormal aPTT are likely to have a drug-induced coagulation defect. The agent most commonly responsible is unfractionated heparin. Reversal of the heparin effect, if desired, can be accomplished by administering protamine sulfate. Protamine should be given with caution, however, because it has been reported to induce a hy-

percoagulable state.[10] It is likely that many of the thrombotic complications are related to simple reversal of a needed anticoagulant state. Protamine should also be used with caution in diabetic patients. These persons sometimes become sensitized to impurities in protamine through their exposure to similar impurities in insulin, and this sensitization may result in an anaphylactic reaction.

It should be remembered that the aPTT does not accurately measure the anticoagulant activity of low-molecular-weight heparins. Because such heparins exert the greater proportion of their anticoagulant effect by potentiating antithrombin to inactivate factor Xa rather than factor IIa, an assay that measures anti-Xa activity is needed to measure the anticoagulant effect. This effect, however, like that of unfractionated heparin, is reversible by protamine. A crucial point is that the administration of fresh frozen plasma (FFP) will not correct the anticoagulant effect of either unfractionated heparin or low-molecular-weight heparins. In fact, given that plasma contains antithrombin and that both unfractionated heparin and low-molecular-weight heparins act by potentiating antithrombin, administration of FFP could actually enhance the heparins' anticoagulant effect.

A variety of direct thrombin inhibitors (e.g., hirulog and lepirudin) are currently available in Europe, Asia, and North America.[11] Many of them cause prolongation of the aPTT. One disadvantage shared by most of the direct thrombin inhibitors is that the effects are not reversible; if thrombin inhibition is no longer wanted, FFP must be given to correct the aPTT. Because the inhibitor that is circulating but not bound at the time of FFP administration will bind the prothrombin in the FFP, the amount of FFP required to correct the aPTT may be greater than would be needed with a simple factor deficiency.

von Willebrand disease is frequently, though not always, associated with a slight prolongation of the aPTT. Its clinical expression is variable. Confirmation of the diagnosis can be obtained by testing for circulating factor levels. Platelet function analysis will also show abnormal function. Correction is accomplished by administering directed therapy (von Willebrand factor [vWF]) [see Discussion, Bleeding Disorders, below], DDAVP, or cryoprecipitate.

Hemophilia may either cause spontaneous bleeding or lead to prolonged bleeding after a surgical or traumatic insult. As noted, hemophilia is rare in the absence of a personal or family history of the disorder. The most common forms of hemophilia involve deficiencies of factors VIII, IX, and XI (hemophilia A, hemophilia B, and hemophilia C, respectively). In contrast to depletion of natural anticoagulants such as antithrombin and protein C [see VI:2 Thromboembolic Problems], depletion of procoagulant factors rarely gives rise to significant manifestations until it is relatively severe. Typically, no laboratory abnormalities result from depletion of procoagulant factors until factor activity levels fall below 40% of normal, and clinical abnormalities are frequently absent even when factor activity levels fall to only 10% of normal. This tolerance for subcritical degrees of depletion is a reflection of the built-in redundancies in the procoagulant pathways.

If hemophilia is suspected, specific factor analysis is indicated. Appropriate therapy involves administering the deficient factor or factors [see Table 1]. Hemophiliac patients who have undergone extensive transfusion therapy may pose a particular challenge: massive transfusions frequently lead to the development of antibodies that make subsequent transfusion or even directed therapy impossible. Accordingly, several alternatives to transfusion or directed factor therapy (e.g., recombinant activated factor VII) have been developed for use in this population.

Table 1 Preparations Used in Directed Therapy for Hemophilia

Product (Manufacturer)	Origin	Factors Contained		
		Factor VIII	Factor IX	vWF
Alphanate (Alpha Therapeutic)	Plasma	Yes	—	Yes
Monarc-M (American Red Cross)	Plasma	Yes	—	Yes
Hemofil M (Baxter Healthcare)	Plasma	Yes	—	Yes
Humate-P (Centeon)	Plasma	Yes	—	Yes
Koāte-HP (Bayer)	Plasma	Yes	—	Yes
Monoclate-P (Centeon)	Plasma	Yes	—	Yes
Recombinate (Baxter Healthcare)	Recombinant	Yes	—	—
Kogenate (Bayer)	Recombinant	Yes	—	—
Bioclate (Baxter Healthcare), Helixate (Centeon)	Recombinant	Yes	—	—
Hyate:C (Speywood)	Porcine plasma	Yes	—	—
Autoplex T (prothrombin complex concentrate) (NABI)	Plasma	—	Yes	—
Feiba VH Immuno (prothrombin complex concentrate) (Immuno-US)	Plasma	—	Yes	—
Mononine (Centeon)	Plasma	—	Yes	—
AlphaNine-SD (Alpha Therapeutic)	Plasma	—	Yes	—
Bebulin VH Immuno (Immuno-US)	Plasma	—	Yes	—
Proplex T (Baxter Healthcare)	Plasma	—	Yes	—
Konȳne 80 (Bayer)	Plasma	—	Yes	—
Profilnine SD (Alpha Therapeutic)	Plasma	—	Yes	—
BeneFix (Genetics Institute)	Recombinant	—	Yes	—
Novo Seven (Novo Nordisk)	Recombinant	Yes	Yes	—

INCREASED INR, NORMAL aPTT

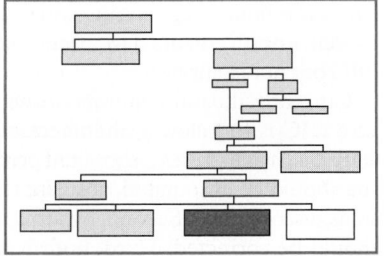

An increased INR in association with a normal aPTT is a more ominous finding in a patient with a coagulopathy. Any of a number of causes, all centering on factor deficiency, may be responsible.

Cirrhosis is arguably the most serious of the causes of an elevated INR. It is a major problem not so much because of the coagulopathy itself but because of the associated deficits in wound healing and immune function that result from the synthetic dysfunction and the loss of reticuloendothelial function. In all cases, factor replacement should be instituted with FFP. If the bleeding is a manifestation of the cirrhosis (as in variceal bleeding), emergency portal decompression should be accomplished before the coagulopathy worsens. Management of cirrhotic patients who have sustained injuries is particularly troublesome because such patients are at disproportionately high risk for subdural hematoma. The reason this risk is so high is that in addition to their pathologic autoanticoagulation, these patients often have some degree of cerebral atrophy as a result of one of the more frequent causes of cirrhosis—namely, alcoholism. As a result, the bridging intracranial veins are more vulnerable to tears and more likely to bleed. Modest elevations of the INR in patients who are not actively bleeding, have not recently undergone operation, and are not specifically at increased risk for life-threatening hemorrhage may be observed without correction.

An elevated INR with a normal aPTT may also be a consequence of warfarin administration. Such a coagulopathy is the result of a pure factor deficiency, and its degree is proportional to the prolongation of the INR. Because warfarin acts by disrupting vitamin K metabolism, the coagulopathy may be corrected by giving vitamin K [*see Table 2*].[12] If the patient is actively bleeding, vitamin K should still be given, but the primary corrective measure should be to administer FFP in an amount proportional to the patient's size and the relative increase in the INR. The INR should subsequently be rechecked to ensure that replacement therapy is adequate. Vitamin K replacement therapy has two main potential drawbacks: (1) if the patient is to be reanticoagulated with warfarin in the near future, dosing will be difficult because the patient will exhibit resistance to warfarin for a variable period; and (2) anaphylactic reactions have been reported when vitamin K is given I.V.

Table 2 Management of the Patient with an Increased INR[12]

Indication	Recommended Treatment
INR above therapeutic range but < 5.0	If no bleeding is present or surgery is indicated, lower or hold next dose
INR > 5.0 but < 9.0	
Patient has no significant bleeding	In the absence of additional risk factors for bleeding, withhold next 1–2 doses; alternatively, withhold next dose and give vitamin K, 1.0–2.5 mg (oral route is acceptable)
Rapid reduction of INR is required	Give vitamin K, 2.0–4.0 mg p.o.; expected reduction of INR should occur within 24 hr
INR > 9.0	
Patient has no significant bleeding	Give vitamin K, 3.0–5.0 mg p.o.; expected reduction of INR should occur within 24 hr
Patient has serious bleeding or is overly anticoagulated (INR > 20.0)	Give vitamin K, 10 mg I.V., and FFP; further vitamin K supplementation may be required every 12 hr
Patient has life-threatening bleeding or is seriously overanticoagulated	Prothrombin complexes may be indicated, along with vitamin K, 10 mg I.V.

INCREASED INR, PROLONGED aPTT

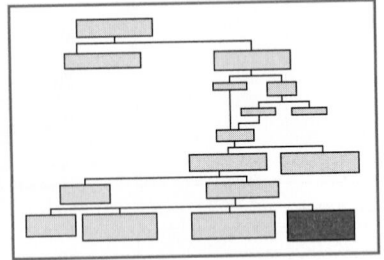

Increases in both the INR and the aPTT may be the most problematic finding of all. When both assays show increases, the patient is likely to have multiple factor deficiencies; possible causes include DIC, severe hemodilution, and renal failure with severe nephrotic syndrome. However, when dramatic elevations of the aPTT and the INR are observed in a seemingly asymptomatic patient, the problem may lie not in the patient's condition but in the laboratory analysis. If the tube in which the blood sample was placed for these tests was not adequately filled, the results of the coagulation assays may be inaccurate. In such cases, the blood sample should be redrawn and the tests repeated.

Hemodilution and nephrotic syndrome result in a coagulopathy that is attributable to decreased concentration of coagulation proteins. Dilutional coagulopathy may occur when a patient who is given a large volume of packed red blood cell (RBC) units is not also given coagulation factors.[13] Because of the tremendous redundancy of the hemostatic process, pure dilutional coagulopathy is rare. It is considered an unlikely diagnosis until after one full blood volume has been replaced (as when a patient requires 10 units of packed RBCs to maintain a stable hematocrit). Nephrotic syndrome is associated with loss of protein (coagulation proteins as well as other body proteins) from the kidneys.

Both hemodilution and nephrotic syndrome should be distinguished from DIC (which is a consumptive rather than a dilutional process[14]), though on occasion this distinction is a difficult one to make. A blood sample should be sent for D-dimer assay. If the D-dimer level is low (< 1,000 ng/ml), DIC is unlikely; if it is very high (> 2,000 ng/ml) and there is no other clear explanation (e.g., a complex unstable pelvic fracture), the diagnosis of DIC rather than dilution should be made. Treatment of dilutional coagulopathy should be directed at replacement of lost factors. FFP should be given first, followed by cryoprecipitate, calcium, and platelets. Transfusion

should be continued until the coagulation parameters are corrected and the bleeding stops.

DIC is a diffuse, disorganized activation of the clotting cascade within the vascular space. It may result either from intravascular presentation of an overwhelming clotting stimulus (e.g., massive crush injury or transfusion reaction) or from presentation of a moderate clotting stimulus in the context of shock. Different degrees of severity have been described. In the mildest form of DIC, acceleration of the clotting cascade is seen, and microthrombi are formed in the vascular space but are cleared effectively. Thus, mild DIC may be little more than an acceleration of the clotting cascade that escapes recognition. In the moderate form of DIC, the microthrombi are ineffectively lysed and cause occlusion of the microcirculation. This process is clinically manifested in the lungs as the acute respiratory distress syndrome (ARDS), in the kidneys as renal failure, and in the liver as hepatic failure.

Neither mild DIC nor moderate DIC is what surgeons traditionally think of as DIC. Severe DIC arises when congestion of the microvasculature with thrombi occurs, resulting in large-scale activation of the fibrinolytic system to restore circulation. This fibrinolytic activity results in breakdown of clot at previously hemostatic sites of microscopic injury (e.g., endothelial damage) and macroscopic injury (e.g., I.V. catheter sites, fractures, or surgical wounds). Bleeding and reexposure to tissue factor stimulate activation of factor VII with increased coagulation activity; thus, microthrombi are formed, and the vicious circle continues. The ultimate manifestation of severe DIC is bleeding from (1) fibrinolysis and (2) depletion (consumption) of coagulation factors.

Several scoring systems have been devised to assess the severity of DIC. These scoring systems are most useful for distinguishing DIC from other causes of coagulopathy (e.g., hypothermia, dilution, or drug effects) [see Table 3].[15]

DIC is a diagnosis of exclusion, largely because none of the various treatment strategies tried to date have been particularly successful. Heparin has been given in large doses in an attempt to break the cycle by stopping the clotting, thus allowing clotting factor levels to return to normal. Antifibrinolytic agents (e.g., ε-aminocaproic acid) have also been tried in an attempt to reduce fibrinolytic activity and thus slow the bleeding that stimulates subsequent clot formation. Antithrombotics (e.g., antithrombin and protein C) have been used as well; improvements have been noted in laboratory measures of DIC but not in survival.

Currently, the most appropriate way of treating a patient with severe DIC is to follow a multifaceted approach. First, the clotting stimulus, if still present, should be removed: dead or devitalized tissue should be amputated, abscesses drained, and suspect transfusions discontinued. Second, hypothermia, of any degree of severity, should be corrected. Third, both blood loss (as measured by the hematocrit) and clotting factor deficits (as measured by the INR) should be aggressively corrected (with blood and plasma, respec-

Table 3 Coagulopathy (DIC) Score

Score	INR (sec)	aPTT (sec)	Platelets (1,000/mm³)	Fibrinogen (mg/dl)	D-dimer (ng/ml)
0	< 1.2	< 34	> 150	> 200	< 1,000
1	> 1.2	> 34	< 150	< 200	< 2,000
2	> 1.4	> 39	< 100	< 150	< 4,000
3	> 1.6	> 54	< 60	< 100	> 4,000

DIC—disseminated intravascular coagulopathy   INR—international normalized ratio   aPTT—activated partial thromboplastin tively). This supportive approach is only modestly successful. For certain groups of patients in whom DIC develops (e.g., those who have sustained head injuries), mortality approaches 100%. This alarmingly high death rate is probably related more to the underlying pathology than to the hematologic derangement.

An increased INR with a prolonged aPTT may also be caused by various isolated factor deficiencies of the common pathway. Congenital deficiencies of factors X, V, and prothrombin are very rare. Acquired factor V deficiencies have been observed in patients with autoimmune disorders. Acquired hypoprothrombinemia has been documented in a small percentage of patients with lupus anticoagulants who exhibit abnormal bleeding. Factor X deficiencies have been noted in patients with amyloidosis.

Stabilized warfarin therapy will increase both the INR and the aPTT. Several current rodenticides (e.g., brodifacoum) exert the same effect on these parameters that warfarin does; however, because they have a considerably longer half-life than warfarin, the reversal of the anticoagulation effect with vitamin K or FFP may be correspondingly longer.[16] Animal venoms may also increase the INR and the aPTT.

Management of Anemia and Indications for Transfusion

Treatment of anemia has changed substantially since the early 1990s. Blood cell transfusions have been shown to have significant immunosuppressive potential, and transmission of fatal diseases through the blood supply has been extensively documented. Moreover, at least one large trial found that using a restrictive RBC transfusion protocol in place of a more traditional one improved survival.[17] These findings have led to a paradigm shift with respect to RBC transfusion: whereas the traditional view was that anemia by itself was a sufficient indication for transfusion, the current consensus is that a second indication must be present in addition to a decreased hemoglobin concentration.

The decision whether to transfuse should be based on the patient's current or predicted need for additional oxygen-carrying capacity [see Figure 1]. A major component of this decision is to determine as promptly as possible whether the patient is in a steady state with respect to hemoglobin supply (in which case transfusions are less likely to be needed) or not (in which case transfusions are usually indicated). Thus, there is no specific hemoglobin concentration or hematocrit (i.e., transfusion trigger) at which all patients should receive transfusions.

There are two large groups of patients who should be managed more aggressively than the general patient population with respect to RBC transfusion. Patients who are either actively bleeding or at high risk for active bleeding and patients who have significant coronary artery disease (CAD) should receive transfusions according to a more liberal protocol than that applied to other patients.

ACTIVE BLEEDING

Patients who are actively bleeding (e.g., those with GI hemorrhage) should receive transfusions up to a level sufficient to keep up with blood loss. Coagulation factors must also be replaced as necessary [see Measurement of Coagulation Parameters, Increased INR, Prolonged aPTT, above]. Patients at high risk for active bleeding (e.g., from massive liver injury) should receive transfusions up to a level at which, if bleeding occurs or recurs, enough reserve oxygen-carrying capacity is afforded to allow diagnosis and correction of the hemorrhage without significant compromise of oxygen delivery. In cases of major injury, we advocate a target hematocrit of 30%; however, this is not a fixed value but a rule-of-thumb figure

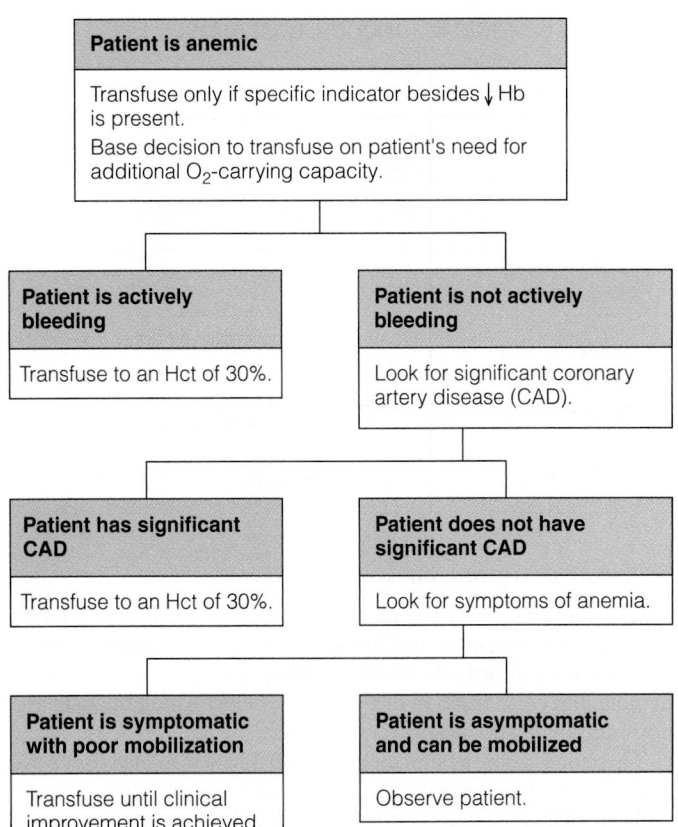

Figure 1 Algorithm depicts decision-making process for transfusion in anemic patients.

that may be increased or decreased as appropriate, depending on the individual patient's reserves and the individual surgical team's ability to diagnose and correct the underlying problem.

SIGNIFICANT CORONARY ARTERY DISEASE

Although no studies have conclusively shown that patients with significant CAD benefit from increased RBC mass, there is also no published evidence to support a restrictive transfusion policy.[17] The major trials that found most patients to benefit from a restrictive transfusion policy specifically excluded CAD patients out of concern that adverse cardiovascular events (e.g., myocardial infarction and cerebrovascular accidents) might increase in frequency at lower hematocrits. Studies evaluating the potential benefit of a more aggressive transfusion policy (i.e., to hematocrits > 30%) failed to show any benefit. Consequently, a target hematocrit of 30% is generally considered appropriate for patients with significant CAD.

SYMPTOMATIC ANEMIA

An additional indication for transfusion is oxygen-carrying capacity that is insufficient to support necessary activities (e.g., wound healing, mobilization, and physical therapy). Typical manifestations are light-headedness, tachycardia, and tachypnea either during the activity in question or at rest. Clearly, some degree of tachycardia is to be expected in any patient who has undergone a major operation or sustained a serious injury. The key point with respect to symptomatic anemia is that patients who have physiologically compensated for anemia must be distinguished from those whose health or recovery is compromised by anemia, and only the latter group should receive transfusions.

Table 4 Blood Substitutes[76]

Product (Manufacturer)	Source
PHP (Apex Bioscience)	Pyridoxylated human hemoglobin conjugated to polyoxyethylene
PEG-hemoglobin (Enzon)	Bovine hemoglobin conjugated to polyethylene glycol
PolyHeme (Northfield Laboratories)	Glutaraldehyde-polymerized pyridoxylated human hemoglobin
Hemopure (Biopure)	Glutaraldehyde-polymerized bovine hemoglobin
Hemolink (Hemosol)	Oxidized raffinose–crosslinked human hemoglobin from expired stored blood
Oxygent (Alliance Pharmaceutical)	Emulsified perflubron

OBSERVATION OF ANEMIA

It has become standard practice to observe patients with low hemoglobin concentrations that in the past would have triggered transfusion. The data currently available support this approach down to a hemoglobin concentration of 6 to 7 g/dl; below 6 g/dl, the data are not sufficient to support observation alone.

There does come a hemoglobin level below which life is not possible. Certain religions prohibit blood transfusion even when death is the probable or certain consequence. Such prohibitions have challenged the medical community to find techniques for supporting life at lower and lower hemoglobin concentrations. In addition, they have helped to define the limits beyond which a restrictive transfusion protocol may be fatal.

When RBC transfusion is not possible (whether for cultural reasons or because compatible blood is unavailable), there are a number of temporizing measures that can be used to support life. If oxygen-carrying capacity cannot be increased, one option is simply to decrease oxygen demand. Oxygen demand is directly proportional to metabolic activity; that is, as metabolic rate increases, so too does oxygen demand. Once unnecessary activity (e.g., assuming an upright posture or walking) has been eliminated, respiration becomes an activity that requires a significant amount of energy. Mechanical ventilation reduces the work of breathing and with it the oxygen requirements of the respiratory muscles. Even with full mechanical ventilation, however, most patients continue to initiate breaths on their own. This energy-requiring activity can be eliminated by administering a neuromuscular blocking agent, which dramatically reduces oxygen demand in essentially all skeletal muscle. The metabolic rate can be further reduced by inducing hypothermia. This measure should be used with caution, however, because hypothermia in the absence of neuromuscular blockade results in uncontrollable shivering, which actually increases the metabolic rate. In addition, trials addressing the use of hypothermia in head injury patients to reduce cerebral oxygen demand reported increased infection rates in the hypothermic groups.

A completely different approach to the issue of the unacceptability or unavailability of RBC transfusion involves the use of RBC substitutes to augment oxygen-carrying capacity. A variety of different substitutes are currently under investigation [*see Table 4*].[18] None have been approved for routine use by the United States Food and Drug Administration, but several have demonstrated promise in clinical trials. Without modification, the hemoglobin molecule is nephrotoxic. Accordingly, virtually all of the products now being studied depend on techniques for making an acellular hemoglobin molecule nontoxic for I.V. administration.

Acellular blood substitutes clearly possess a number of advantages, including greatly increased shelf life, reduced risk of viral transmission, availability that is not limited by donor supply, reduced or eliminated risk of incompatibility reactions, and—potentially, at least—reduced cultural and religious objections.[19] To what extent this approach is suited to the treatment of anemia in surgical patients should be clarified when the results of the trials now under way are published.[18]

Discussion

Mechanics of Hemostasis

Hemostasis is the term for the process by which cellular and plasma components interact in response to vessel injury in order to maintain vascular integrity and promote wound healing. The initial response to vascular injury (primary hemostasis) involves the recruitment and activation of platelets, which then adhere to the site of injury. Subsequently, plasma proteins, in concert with cellular components, begin to generate thrombin, which causes further activation of platelets and converts fibrinogen to fibrin monomers that polymerize into a fibrin clot. The final step is the release of plasminogen activators that induce clot lysis and tissue repair.

The cellular components of hemostasis include endothelium, white blood cells (WBCs), RBCs, and platelets. The plasma components include a number of procoagulant and regulatory proteins that, once activated, can accelerate or downregulate thrombin formation or clot lysis to facilitate wound healing. In normal individuals, these hemostatic components are in a regulatory balance; thus, any abnormality involving one or more of these components can result in a pathologic state, whether of uncontrolled clot formation (thrombosis) or of excessive bleeding (hemorrhage). These pathologies can result from either hereditary defects of protein synthesis or acquired deficiencies attributable to metabolic causes.

CELLULAR COMPONENTS

Endothelium

The endothelium has both procoagulant and anticoagulant properties. When vascular injury occurs, the endothelium serves as a nidus for recruitment of platelets, adhesion of platelets to the endothelial surface, platelet aggregation, migration of platelets across the endothelial surface, generation of fibrin, and expression of adhesion molecule receptors (E-selectin and P-selectin). Exposure of collagen fibrils and release of vWF from the Weibel-Palade bodies cause platelets to adhere to the cellular surface of the endothelium. The presence of interleukin-1β (IL-1β), tissue necrosis factor (TNF), interferon-8 (IFN-8), and thrombin promotes expression of tissue factor (TF) on the endothelium.[20,21] TF activates factors X and VII, and these activated factors generate additional thrombin, which increases both fibrin formation and platelet aggregation.

The endothelium also acts in numerous ways to downregulate coagulation.[22] Heparan sulfate and thrombomodulin are both downregulators of thrombin formation. In the presence of thrombin, the endothelium responds by (1) releasing thrombomodulin, which forms a complex with thrombin to activate protein C; (2) producing endothelium-derived relaxing factor (i.e., nitric oxide[23]) and prostacyclin, which have vasodilating and platelet aggregation–inhibiting effects, respectively; and (3) releasing tissue plasminogen activator (t-PA) or urokinase-type plasminogen activator (u-PA), either of which converts the zymogen plasminogen to an active form (i.e., plasmin) that degrades fibrin and fibrinogen.[20,24] Heparan sulfate, on the endothelium wall, forms a complex with plasma antithrombin to neutralize thrombin. The endothelium is also the source of tissue factor pathway inhibitor (TFPI), which downregulates TF-VIIa-Xa complexes.

Erythrocytes and Leukocytes

The nonplatelet cellular components of blood play indirect roles in hemostasis. RBCs contain thromboplastins that are potent stimulators of various procoagulant proteins. In addition, the concentration of RBCs within the bloodstream (expressed as the hematocrit) assists in primary hemostasis by physically forcing the platelets toward the endothelial surfaces. When the RBC count is low enough, the absence of this force results in inadequate endothelium-platelet interaction and a bleeding diathesis.

Leukocytes have several functions in the hemostatic process. The interaction between the adhesion molecules expressed on both leukocytes and endothelium results in cytokine production, initiation of inflammatory responses, and degradation of extracellular matrix to facilitate tissue healing. In the presence of thrombin, monocytes express TF, which is an integral procoagulant for thrombin generation. Neutrophils and activated monocytes bind to stimulated platelets and endothelial cells that express P-selectin. Adhesion and rolling of neutrophils, mediated by fibrinogen and selectins on the endothelium, appear to facilitate vessel integrity but may also lead to inflammatory responses.[25,26] Lymphocytes also adhere to endothelium via adhesion molecule receptors and appear to be responsible for cytokine production and inflammatory responses.

Platelets

The roles platelets play in hemostasis and subsequent fibrin formation rest on providing a phospholipid surface for localizing procoagulant activation. Activation of platelets by agonists such as adenosine triphosphate (ATP), adenosine diphosphate (ADP), epinephrine, thromboxane A_2, collagen, and thrombin causes platelets to undergo morphologic changes and degranulation. Degranulation of platelets results in the release of procoagulants that promote further platelet adhesion and aggregation (e.g., thrombospondin, vWF, fibrinogen, ADP, and ATP), vasodilation (e.g., serotonin), and surface expression of P-selectin, which induces cellular adhesion. Platelet degranulation also results in the release of β-thromboglobulin, platelet factor 4 (which has antiheparin properties), various growth factors, coagulation procoagulants, and calcium as well as the formation of platelet microparticles. Plasminogen activator inhibitor–I (PAI-I) released from degranulated platelets neutralizes the fibrinolytic pathway by forming a complex with t-PA.

Upon exposure to vascular injury, platelets adhere to the exposed endothelium via binding of vWF to the GPIb-IX-V complex.[27] Conformational changes in the GPIIb-IIIa complex on the activated platelet surface enhance fibrinogen binding, which results in platelet-to-platelet interaction (i.e., aggregation). The phospholipid surface of the platelet membranes anchors activated IXa-VIIIa and Xa-Va complexes, thereby localizing thrombin generation.[28]

PLASMA COMPONENTS

Procoagulants

Traditional diagrams of the coagulation cascade depict two distinct pathways for thrombin generation: the intrinsic pathway and the extrinsic pathway. The premise for the distinction between the two is that the intrinsic pathway requires no extravascular source for initiation, whereas the extrinsic pathway requires an extravascular component (i.e., TF). This traditional depiction is useful in interpreting coagulation tests, but it is not an accurate reflection of the hemostatic process in vivo. Accordingly, our focus is not on this standard view but rather on the roles contact factors (within the intrinsic cascade) and TF play in coagulation. As noted, circulating plasma vWF is necessary for normal adhesion of platelets to the endothelium. Plasma vWF also serves as the carrier protein for factor VIII, preventing its neutralization by the protein C regulatory pathway.

Even in patients in whom laboratory tests strongly suggest a severe clotting abnormality (i.e., the aPTT is markedly prolonged), contact factors do not play a significant role in the generation of thrombin. However, contact factor activation does appear to play secondary roles that are essential to normal hemostasis and tissue repair. Factor XII, prekallikrein, and high-molecular-weight kininogen are bound to the endothelium to activate the bradykinin (BK) pathway. The BK pathway exerts profibrinolytic effects by stimulating endothelial release of plasminogen activators. It also stimulates endothelial production of nitric oxide and prostacyclin, which play vital regulatory roles in vasodilation and regulation of platelet activation.[29]

The key initiator of plasma procoagulant formation is the expression of TF on cell surfaces.[21,30] TF activates factor VII and binds with it to form the TF-VIIa complex, which activates factors X and IX. Factor Xa also enhances its own production by activating factor IX, which in turn activates factor X to form factor Xa. Factor Xa also produces minimal amounts of thrombin by cleaving the prothrombin molecule. The thrombin generated from this process cleaves the coagulation cofactors V and VIII to enhance production of the factor complexes IX-VIIIa (intrinsic tenase) and Xa-Va (prothrombinase), which catalyze conversion of prothrombin to thrombin [see Figure 2].[31]

Thrombin has numerous functions, including prothrombotic and regulatory functions. Its procoagulant properties include cleaving fibrinogen, activating the coagulation cofactors V and VIII, inducing platelet aggregation, inducing expression of TF on cell surfaces, and activating factor XIII. In cleaving fibrinogen, thrombin causes the release of fibrinopeptides A and B (fibrin monomer). The fibrin monomer undergoes conformational changes that expose the α and β chains of the molecule, which then polymerize with other fibrin monomers to form a fibrin mesh. Activated factor XIII cross-links the polymerized fibrin (between the α chains and the γ chains) to stabilize the fibrin clot and delay fibrinolysis.

Fibrin(ogen)olysis

Plasminogen is the primary fibrinolytic zymogen that circulates in plasma. In the presence of t-PA or u-PA (released from the endothelium), plasminogen is converted to the active form, plasmin. Plasmin cleaves fibrin (or fibrinogen) between the molecule's D and E domains, causing the formation of X, Y, D, and E fragments. The secondary function of the fibrinolytic pathway is the activation by u-PA of matrix metalloproteinases that degrade the extracellular matrix.[32]

Regulatory Factors

In persons with normal coagulation status, downregulation of hemostasis occurs simultaneously with the production of procoagulants (e.g., activated plasma factors, stimulated endothelium, and stimulated platelets). In addition to their procoagulant activity, both thrombin and contact factors stimulate downregulation of the coagulation process. Thrombin forms a complex with endothelium-bound thrombomodulin to activate protein C, which inhibits factors Va and VIIIa. The thrombin-thrombomodulin complex also regu-

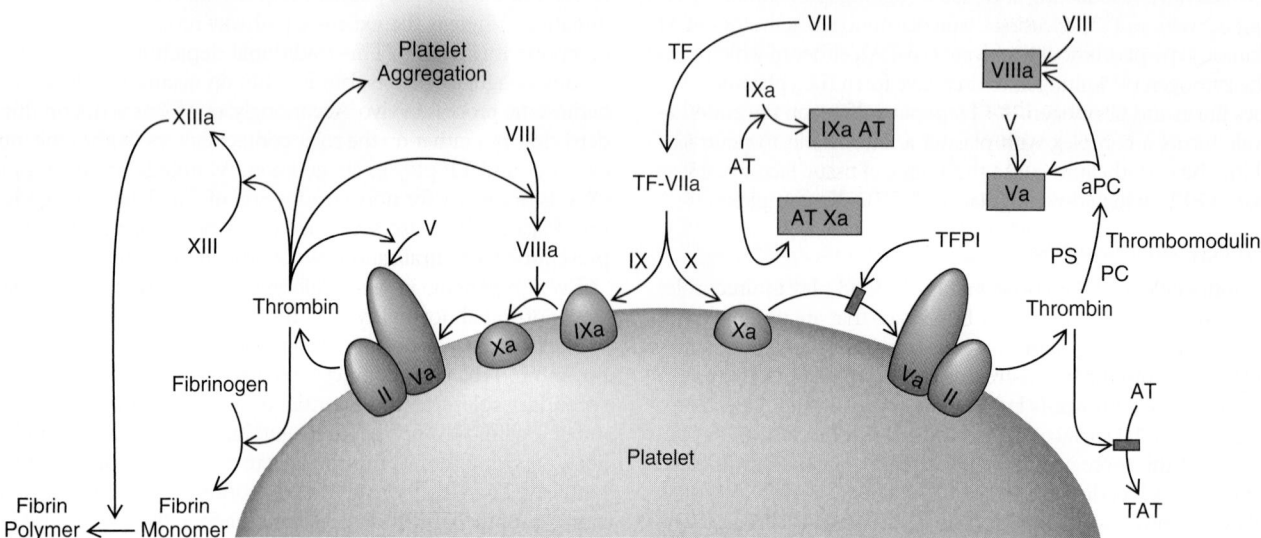

Figure 2 Shown is a schematic representation of the procoagulant pathways.

lates the fibrinolytic pathway by activating a circulating plasma protein known as thrombin-activatable fibrinolysis inhibitor (TAFI), which appears to suppress conversion of plasminogen to plasmin.[33] Contact factors are known to be required for normal surface-dependent fibrinolysis, and there is some evidence that contact factor deficiencies can lead to thromboembolism. Another plasma protein responsible for regulation of fibrinolysis is α_2-antiplasmin, which binds to circulating and bound plasmin to limit breakdown of fibrin.

Circulating downregulating proteins include antithrombin (a serine protease inhibitor of activated factors—especially factors IXa, Xa, and XIa—and thrombin[31]), proteins C and S (regulators of factors VIIIa and Va[34]), C1 inhibitor (a regulator of factor XIa), TFPI (a regulator of the TF-VIIa-Xa complex[35]), and α_2-macroglobulin (a thrombin inhibitor—the primary thrombin inhibitor in neonates[36]). Limitation of platelet activation occurs secondarily as a result of decreased levels of circulating agonists and endothelial release of prostacyclin [see Figure 2].

Bleeding Disorders

INHERITED COAGULOPATHIES

Numerous congenital abnormalities of the coagulation system have been identified. In particular, various abnormalities involving plasma proteins (e.g., hemophilia and vWD), platelet receptors (e.g., Glanzmann thrombasthenia and Bernard-Soulier syndrome), and endothelium (e.g., telangiectasia) have been described in detail. For the sake of brevity, we will refer to abnormal protein synthesis resulting in a dysfunctional coagulation protein as a defect and to abnormal protein synthesis resulting in decreased protein production as a deficiency.

Most of the coagulation defects associated with endothelium are closely related to thrombosis or atherosclerosis. Defects or deficiencies of thrombomodulin, TFPI, and t-PA, albeit rare, are associated with thrombosis.[37,38] Vascular defects (e.g., hemorrhagic telangiectasias) may carry an increased risk of bleeding as a consequence of dysfunctional fibrinolysis, concomitant platelet dysfunction, or coagulation factor deficiencies.[39]

Defects or deficiencies of RBCs and WBCs have other primary clinical manifestations that are not related to hemostasis. Alterations in the physical properties of blood (e.g., decreased blood flow from increased viscosity, polycythemia vera, leukocytosis, and

sickle-cell anemia) have been reported to lead to thrombosis, but usually not to major bleeding.

Inherited platelet membrane receptor defects are relatively common. Of these, vWD is the one that most frequently causes bleeding.[40] The condition is characterized by vWF abnormalities, which may take three forms: vWF may be present in a reduced concentration (type I vWD), dysfunctional (type II vWD), or absent altogether (type III). Diagnosis of vWD is based on a combination of the patient history (e.g., previous mucosal bleeding) and laboratory parameters [see Laboratory Assessment of Bleeding, below]. It is necessary to identify the correct type or subtype of vWD: some treatments (e.g., DDAVP) are contraindicated in patients with type IIb vWD.[41]

Less common receptor defects include Glanzmann thrombasthenia (a defect in the GPIIb-IIIa complex), Bernard-Soulier syndrome (a defect in the GPIb-IX complex), and Scott syndrome (a defect in the platelet's activated surface that promotes thrombin formation); other agonist receptors on the platelet membrane may be affected as well.[42,43] Intracellular platelet defects are relatively rare but do occur; examples are gray platelet syndromes (e.g., alpha granule defects), Hermansky-Pudlak syndrome, dense granule defects, Wiskott-Aldrich syndrome, and various defects in intracellular production and signaling (involving defects of cyclooxygenase synthase and phospholipase C, respectively).[43]

Numerous pathologic states are also associated with deficiencies or defects of plasma procoagulants. Inherited sex-linked deficiencies of factor VIII (i.e., hemophilia A) and factor IX (i.e., hemophilia B and Christmas disease) are relatively common.[44-46] The clinical presentations of hemophilia A and hemophilia B are similar: hemarthroses are the most common clinical manifestations, ultimately leading to degenerative joint deformities. Spontaneous bleeding may also occur, resulting in intracranial hemorrhage, large hematomas in the muscles of extremities, hematuria, and GI bleeding. Factor XI deficiency is relatively common in Jewish persons but rarely results in spontaneous bleeding.[47,48] Such deficiency may result in bleeding after oral operations and trauma; however, there are a number of major procedures (e.g., cardiac bypass surgery) that do not result in postoperative bleeding in this population.[49]

Inherited deficiencies of the other coagulation factors are very rare. Factor XIII deficiencies result in delayed postoperative or posttraumatic bleeding. Congenital deficiencies of factor V, factor VII, factor X, prothrombin, and fibrinogen may become apparent in the neonatal period (presenting, for example, as umbilical stump bleeding); later in life, they result in clinical presentations such as epistaxis, intracranial bleeding, GI bleeding, deep and superficial bruising, and menorrhagia.

Defects or deficiencies in the fibrinolytic pathway are also rare and are most commonly associated with thromboembolic events. α_2-Antiplasmin deficiencies and primary fibrin(ogen)olysis are rare congenital coagulopathies with clinical presentations similar to those of factor deficiencies. In primary fibrin(ogen)olysis, failure of regulation of t-PA and u-PA leads to increases in circulating plasmin levels, which result in rapid degradation of clot and fibrinogen.[50,51]

ACQUIRED COAGULOPATHIES

A wide range of clinical conditions may cause deficiencies of the primary, secondary, or fibrinolytic pathways. Acquired coagulopathies are very common, and most do not result in spontaneous bleeding. (DIC is an exception [see below].)

As noted, coagulopathies related to the endothelium are primarily associated with thrombosis rather than bleeding. There are a number of disorders that may cause vascular injury, including sickle-cell anemia, hemolytic-uremic syndrome, and thrombotic thrombocytopenic purpura.

Acquired platelet abnormalities, both qualitative (i.e., dysfunction) and quantitative (i.e., decreases in absolute numbers), are common occurrences. Many acquired thrombocytopathies are attributable to either foods (e.g., fish oils, chocolate, red wine, garlic, and herbs) or drugs (e.g., aspirin, ibuprofen, other nonsteroidal anti-inflammatory drugs, ticlopidine, various antibiotics, certain antihistamines, and phenytoin).[52-56] Direct anti–platelet receptor drugs (e.g., abciximab and eptifibatide) block the GPIIb-IIIa complex, thereby preventing platelet aggregation.[57] Thrombocytopenia can be primary or secondary to a number of clinical conditions. Primary bone disorders (e.g., myelodysplastic or myelophthisic syndromes) and spontaneous bleeding may arise when platelet counts fall below 10,000/mm³. Thrombocytopenia can be associated with immune causes (e.g., immune thrombocytopenic purpura or thrombotic thrombocytopenic purpura) or can occur secondary to administration of drugs (e.g., heparin). Acquired platelet dysfunction (e.g., acquired vWD) that is not related to dietary or pharmacologic causes has been observed in patients with immune disorders or cancer.

Acquired plasma factor deficiencies are common as well. Patients with severe renal disease typically exhibit platelet dysfunction (from excessive amounts of uremic metabolites), factor deficiencies associated with impaired synthesis or protein loss (as with increased urinary excretion), or thrombocytopenia (from diminished thrombopoietin production).[58,59] Patients with severe hepatic disease commonly have impairment of coagulation factor synthesis, increases in circulating levels of paraproteins, and splenic sequestration of platelets.

Hemodilution from massive RBC transfusions can occur if more than 10 packed RBC units are given within a short period without plasma supplementation. Immunologic reactions to ABO/Rh mismatches can induce immune-mediated hypercoagulation. Acquired multifactorial deficiencies associated with extracorporeal circuits (e.g., cardiopulmonary bypass, hemodialysis, and continuous venovenous dialysis) can arise as a consequence of hemodilution of circuit priming fluid or activation of procoagulants after exposure to thrombogenic surfaces.[60-62] Thrombocytopenia can result from platelet destruction and activation caused by circuit membrane exposure, or it can be secondary to the presence of heparin antibody.

Animal venoms can be either procoagulant or prothrombotic. The majority of the poisonous snakes in the United States (rattlesnakes in particular) have venom that works by activating prothrom-

bin, but cross-breeding has produced a number of new venoms with different hemostatic consequences. The clinical presentation of coagulopathies associated with snakebites generally mimics that of consumptive coagulopathies.[63]

Drug-induced factor deficiencies are common, particularly as a result of anticoagulant therapy. The most commonly used anticoagulants are heparin and warfarin. Heparin does not cause a factor deficiency; rather, it accelerates production of antithrombin, which inhibits factor IXa, factor Xa, and thrombin, thereby prolonging clot formation. Warfarin reduces procoagulant potential by inhibiting vitamin K synthesis, thereby reducing carboxylation of factor VII, factor IX, factor X, prothrombin, and proteins C and S. Newer drugs that may also cause factor deficiencies include direct thrombin inhibitors (e.g., lepirudin and hirulog[64]) and fibrinogen-degrading drugs (e.g., ancrod[65]).

Isolated acquired factor deficiencies are relatively rare. Clinically, they present in exactly the same way as inherited factor deficiencies, except that there is no history of earlier bleeding. In most cases, there is a secondary disease (e.g., lymphoma or an autoimmune disorder) that results in the development of antibody to a procoagulant (e.g., factor V, factor VIII, factor IX, vWF, prothrombin, or fibrinogen).[66-68]

Disseminated Intravascular Coagulation

DIC is a complex coagulation process that involves activation of the coagulation system with resultant activation of the fibrinolytic pathway and deposition of fibrin; the eventual consequence is the multiple organ dysfunction syndrome (MODS).[69] The activation occurs at all levels (platelets, endothelium, and procoagulants), but it is not known whether this process is initiated by a local stimulus or a systemic one. It is crucial to emphasize that DIC is an acquired disorder that occurs secondary to an underlying clinical event (e.g., a complicated birth, severe gram-negative infection, shock, major head injury, polytrauma, severe burns, or cancer. As noted [see Measurement of Coagulation Parameters, Increased INR, Prolonged aPTT, *above*], there is some controversy regarding the best approach to therapy, but there is no doubt that treating the underlying cause of DIC is paramount to patient recovery.

DIC is not always clinically evident: low-grade DIC may lack clinical symptoms altogether and manifest itself only through laboratory abnormalities, even when thrombin generation and fibrin deposition are occurring. In an attempt to facilitate recognition of DIC, the disorder has been divided into three phases, distinguished on the basis of clinical and laboratory evidence. In phase I DIC, there are no clinical symptoms, and the routine screening tests (i.e., INR, aPTT, fibrinogen level, and platelet count) are within normal limits.[70] Secondary testing (i.e., measurement of antithrombin, prothrombin fragment, thrombin-antithrombin complex, and soluble fibrin levels) may reveal subtle changes indicative of thrombin generation. In phase II DIC, there are usually clinical signs of bleeding around wounds, suture sites, I.V. sites, or venous puncture sites, and decreased function is noted in specific organs (e.g., lung, liver, and kidneys). The INR is increased, the aPTT is prolonged, and the fibrinogen level and platelet count are decreased or decreasing. Other markers of thrombin generation and fibrinolysis (e.g., D-dimer level) show sizable elevations. In phase III DIC, MODS is observed, the INR and the aPTT are markedly increased, and fibrinogen and D-dimer levels are markedly depressed. A peripheral blood smear would show large numbers of schistocytes, indicating RBC shearing resulting from fibrin deposition.

The activation of the coagulation system seen in DIC appears to be primarily caused by TF. The brain, the placenta, and solid tumors are all rich sources of TF. Gram-negative endotoxins also in-

Figure 3 **Algorithm depicts use of coagulation parameters in assessment of coagulopathies.**

duce TF expression. The exposure of TF on cellular surfaces causes activation of factors VII and IX, which ultimately leads to thrombin generation. Circulating thrombin is rapidly cleared by antithrombin. Moreover, the coagulation pathway is downregulated by activated protein C and protein S. However, constant exposure of TF (as a result of underlying disorders) results in constant generation of thrombin, and these regulator proteins are rapidly consumed. TAFI and PAI also contribute to fibrin deposition by restricting fibrinolysis and subsequent fibrin degradation and clearance. Finally, it is likely that release of cytokines (e.g., IL-6, IL-10, and TNF) may play some role in causing the sequelae of DIC by modulating or activating the coagulation pathway.

Laboratory Assessment of Bleeding

Laboratory testing is an integral part of the diagnostic algorithm used in assessing the bleeding patient. It may not be prudent to wait for laboratory values before beginning treatment of acute bleeding,

but it is imperative that blood samples for coagulation testing be drawn before therapy. The development of microprocessor technology has made it possible to perform diagnostic laboratory testing outside the confines of the clinical laboratory (so-called near-care testing). Whether near-care testing or clinical laboratory testing is employed, it is important to recognize that valuable as such testing is, it does not provide all of the needed diagnostic information.

In particular, the value of a careful patient history must not be underestimated. Previous bleeding events and a familial history of bleeding are both suggestive of a congenital coagulopathy. A thorough medication inventory is necessary to assess the possible impact of drugs on laboratory and clinical presentations. In the patient history query, it is advisable to ask explicitly about nonprescription drugs—using expressions such as "over-the-counter drugs," "cold medicines," and "Pepto-Bismol"—because unless specifically reminded, patients tend to equate the term medications with prescription drugs. If this is not done, many drugs that are capable of influencing hemostasis in vivo and in vitro (e.g., salicylates, cold and allergy medicines, and herbal supplements) may be missed. Mucosal and superficial bleeding is suggestive of platelet abnormalities, and deep bleeding is suggestive of factor deficiency.

It is important to be clear on the limitations of coagulation testing. At present, there are no laboratory or ex vivo methods capable of directly measuring the physiologic properties of the endothelium. Indirect assessments of endothelial damage can be obtained by

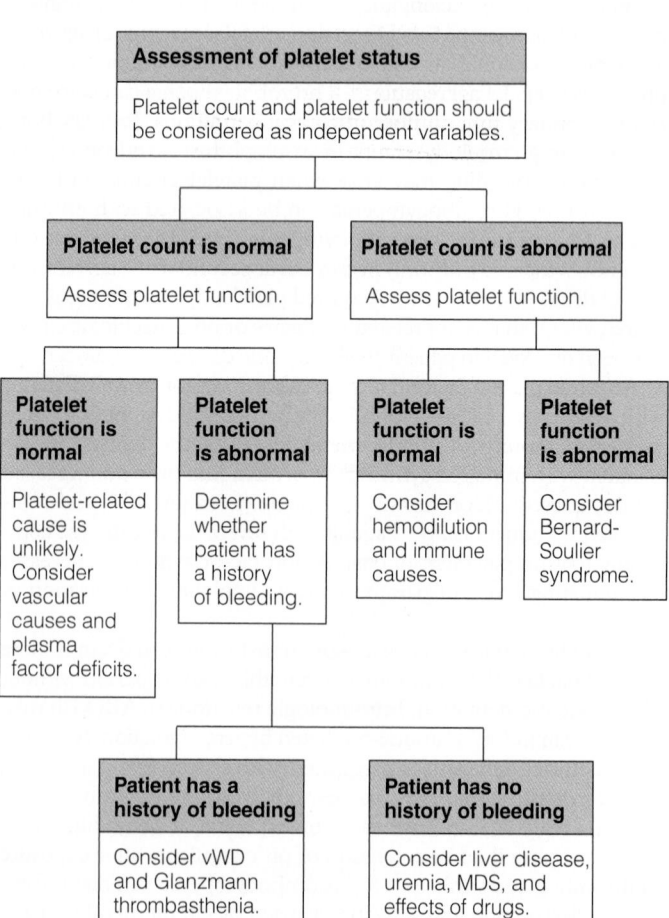

Figure 4 **Algorithm depicts use of platelet count and platelet functional status in assessment of coagulopathies.**

Table 5 Tests of Platelet Function

Product (Manufacturer)	Method
PFA-100 (Dade Behring)	Measures time required to occlude aperture after exposure to platelet agonists at shear rates
hemoSTATUS (Medtronic)	Measures activated clotting time; platelet-activating factor is the platelet agonist
AggreStat (Centocor)	Measures changes in voltage (impedance) after addition of platelet agonist
Thromboelastograph (Haemascope)	Measures changes in the viscoelastic properties of clotting blood induced by a rotating piston
Sonoclot Analyzer (Sienco)	Measures changes in the viscoelastic properties of clotting blood induced by a vibrating probe
Clot Signature Analyzer (Xylum)	Measures changes in platelet function at shear rates
Ultegra Analyzer (Accumetrics)	Used primarily for measuring the effect of platelet glycoprotein blockers (e.g., abciximab and eptifibatide); thrombin receptor activator peptide is the agonist

measuring levels of several laboratory parameters (e.g., vWF, the soluble cytokines endothelian-1 and E-selectin, and thrombomodulin), but such measurements have no clinical utility in the assessment of a bleeding patient.

Another issue is that of bias resulting from technical factors. PT (i.e., INR) and aPTT testing involves adding activators, phospholipids, and calcium to plasma in a test tube (or the equivalent) and determining the time to clot formation. Time to clot formation is a relative value, in that it is compared with the time in a normal population. A perturbation within the coagulation cascade, an excess of calcium, or poor sampling techniques (e.g., inadequately filled coagulation tubes, excessive tourniquet time, and clotted or activated samples) can bias the results. Hemolysis from the drawing of blood can also bias results via the effects of thromboplastins released from RBC membranes to initiate the coagulation process. In addition, many coagulation factors are highly labile, and failure to process and run coagulation samples immediately can bias test results.

Finally, not all coagulation tests are functionally equivalent: different laboratory methods may yield differing results.[71] Coagulation reagents have been manufactured in such a way as to ensure that the coagulation screening tests are sensitive to factor VIII and IX deficiencies and the effects of anticoagulation with warfarin or heparin. Thus, a normal aPTT in a patient with an abnormal INR may not exclude the possibility of common pathway deficiencies (e.g., deficiencies of factors X, V, and II), and most current methods of determining the INR and the aPTT do not detect low fibrinogen levels. The approach we use assumes that the methods used to assess INR and aPTT can discriminate normal factor activity levels from abnormal levels (< 0.4 IU/ml).

The CBC (including platelet count and differential count), the INR, and the aPTT tests should be the primary laboratory tests for differentiating coagulopathies [see Figure 3].

Platelet count and platelet function should be considered as independent values [see Figure 4]. Patients with congenital thrombocytopathies often have normal platelet counts; therefore, assessment of platelet function is required as well. Historically, the bleeding time has been used to assess platelet function. This test is grossly inadequate, in that it may yield normal results in as many as 50% of patients with congenital thrombocytopathies.[72,73] Numerous rapid tests of platelet function are currently available that can be used to screen for platelet defects; these tests can and should be included in the diagnostic approach to the bleeding patient [see Table 5].[73-75]

References

1. Bickell WH, Wall MJ Jr, Pepe PE, et al: Immediate versus delayed fluid resuscitation for hypotensive patients with penetrating torso injuries. N Engl J Med 331: 1105, 1994

2. Gubler KD, Gentilello LM, Hassantash SA, et al: The impact of hypothermia on dilutional coagulopathy. J Trauma 36:847, 1994

3. Watts DD, Trask A, Soeken K, et al: Hypothermic coagulopathy in trauma: effect of varying levels of hypothermia on enzyme speed, platelet function, and fibrinolytic activity. J Trauma 44:846, 1998

4. Gentilello LM, Jurkovich GJ, Stark MS, et al: Is hypothermia in the victim of major trauma protective or harmful? A randomized, prospective study. Ann Surg 226:439, 1997

5. Rapaport SI: Blood coagulation and its alterations in hemorrhagic and thrombotic disorders. West J Med 158:153, 1993

6. Practice guidelines for blood component therapy: a report by the American Society of Anesthesiologists Task Force on Blood Component Therapy. Anesthesiology 84:732, 1996

7. Heckman KD, Weiner GJ, Davis CS, et al: Randomized study of prophylactic platelet transfusion threshold during induction therapy for adult acute leukemia: 10,000/μL versus 20,000/μL. J Clin Oncol 15:1143, 1997

8. Dyke CM, Bhatia D, Lorenz TJ, et al: Immediate coronary artery bypass surgery after platelet inhibition with eptifibatide: results from PURSUIT. Platelet Glycoprotein IIb/IIIa in Unstable Angina: Receptor Suppression Using Integrelin Therapy. Ann Thorac Surg 70:866, 2000

9. Despotis GJ, Levine V, Saleem R, et al: Use of point-of-care test in identification of patients who can benefit from desmopressin during cardiac surgery: a randomised controlled trial. Lancet 354:106, 1999

10. Levy JH, Schwieger IM, Zaidan JR, et al: Evaluation of patients at risk for protamine reactions. J Thorac Cardiovasc Surg 98:200, 1989

11. Fenton JW 2nd, Ofosu FA, Brezniak DV, et al: Thrombin and antithrombotics. Semin Thromb Hemost 24:87, 1998

12. Hirsh J, Dalen JE, Anderson DR, et al: Oral anticoagulants: mechanism of action, clinical effectiveness, and optimal therapeutic range. Chest 114(5 suppl):445S, 1998

13. Murray DJ, Pennell BJ, Weinstein SL, et al: Packed red cells in acute blood loss: dilutional coagulopathy as a cause of surgical bleeding. Anesth Analg 80:336, 1995

14. Holcroft JW, Blaisdell FW, Trunkey DD, et al: Intravascular coagulation and pulmonary edema in the septic baboon. J Surg Res 22:209, 1977

15. Owings JT, Bagley M, Gosselin R, et al: Effect of critical injury on plasma antithrombin activity: low antithrombin levels are associated with thromboembolic complications. J Trauma 41:396, 1996

16. Weitzel JN, Sadowski JA, Furie BC, et al: Surreptitious ingestion of a long-acting vitamin K antagonist/rodenticide, brodifacoum: clinical and metabolic studies of three cases. Blood 76:2555, 1990

17. Hébert PC, Wells G, Blajchman MA, et al: A multicenter, randomized, controlled clinical trial of transfusion requirements in critical care. Transfusion Requirements in Critical Care Investigators, Canadian Critical Care Trials Group. N Engl J Med 340:409, 1999

18. Maxwell RA, Gibson JB, Fabian TC, et al: Resuscitation of severe chest trauma with four different hemoglobin-based oxygen-carrying solutions. J Trauma 49:200, 2000

19. Creteur J, Sibbald W, Vincent JL: Hemoglobin solutions—not just red blood cell substitutes. Crit Care Med 28:3025, 2000

20. Mantovani A, Sozzani S, Vecchi A, et al: Cytokine activation of endothelial cells: new molecules for an old paradigm. Thromb Haemost 78:406, 1997

21. Edington TS, Mackman N, Brand K, et al: The structural biology of expression and function of tissue factor. Thromb Haemost 66:67, 1991

22. Vane JR, Anggard EE, Botting RM: Regulatory function of the vascular endothelium. N Engl J Med 323:27, 1990

23. Ignarro LJ, Buga GM, Wood KS, et al: Endothelium-derived relaxing factor produced and released from artery and vein is nitric oxide. Proc Natl Acad Sci 84:9265, 1987

24. ten Cate JW, van der Poll T, Levi M, et al: Cytokines:

triggers of clinical thrombotic disease. Thromb Haemost 78:415, 1997

25. Cerletti C, Evangelista V, de Gaetano G: P-selectin-β2-integrin crosstalk: a molecular mechanism for polymorphonuclear leukocyte recruitment at the site of vascular damage. Thromb Haemost 82:787, 1999

26. Brunetti M, Martelli N, Manarini S, et al: Polymorphonuclear apoptosis is inhibited by platelet mediated-released mediators, role of TGFβ-1. Thromb Haemost 84:478, 2000

27. Stel HV, Sakariassen KS, de Groot PG, et al: Von-Willebrand factor in the vessel wall mediates platelet adherence. Blood 65:85, 1985

28. Michelson AD, Barnard MR: Thrombin-induced changes in platelet membrane glycoproteins Ib, IX, and IIb-IIIa complex. Blood 70:1673, 1987

29. Motta G, Rojkjaer R, Hasan AA, et al: High molecular weight kininogen regulates prekallikrein assembly and activation on endothelial cells: a novel mechanism for contact activation. Blood 91:516, 1998

30. Osterud B, Rappaport SI: Activation of factor IX by the reaction product of tissue factor and factor VII: additional pathway for initiating blood coagulation. Proc Natl Acad Sci USA 74:5260, 1997

31. Mann KG: Biochemistry and physiology of blood coagulation. Thromb Haemost 82:165, 1999

32. Collen D, Lijnen HR: Basic and clinical aspects of fibrinolysis and thrombolysis. Blood 78:3114, 1991

33. Chetaille P, Alessi MC, Kouassi D, et al: Plasma TAFI antigen variations in healthy subjects. Thromb Haemost 83:902, 2000

34. Esmon CT, Owen WG: Identification of an endothelial cell cofactor for thrombin-catalyzed activation of protein C. Proc Natl Acad Sci USA 78:2249, 1981

35. Broze GJ, Warren LA, Novotny WF, et al: The lipoprotein-associated coagulation inhibitor that inhibits factor Xa: insight into its possible mechanism of action. Blood 71:335, 1988

36. Schmidt B, Mitchell L, Ofosu FA, et al: Alpha-2-macroglobulin is an important progressive inhibitor of thrombin in neonatal and infant plasma. Thromb Haemost 62:1074, 1989

37. Juhan-Vague I, Valadier J, Alessi MC, et al: Deficient tPA release and elevated PA inhibitor levels on patients with spontaneous recurrent DVT. Thromb Haemost 57:67, 1987

38. Korninger C, Lechner K, Niessner H, et al: Impaired fibrinolytic capacity predisposes for recurrence of venous thrombosis. Thromb Haemost 52:127, 1984

39. Shovlin CL: Molecular defects in rare bleeding disorders: hereditary hemorrhagic telangiectasia. Thromb Haemost 78:145, 1997

40. Sadler JE, Mannucci PM, Berntop E, et al: Impact, diagnosis, and treatment of von Willebrand's disease. Thromb Haemost 84:160, 2000

41. Mannucci PM: Desmopressin: a nontransfusional form of treatment for congenital and acquired bleeding disorders. Blood 72:1449, 1988

42. Weiss HJ: Congenital disorders of platelet function. Semin Thromb Hemost 17:228, 1980

43. Nurden AT: Inherited abnormalities of platelets. Thromb Haemost 82:468, 1999

44. Ljung RC: Prenatal diagnosis of haemophilia. Haemophilia 5:84, 1999

45. Lillicrap D: Molecular diagnosis of inherited bleeding disorders and thrombophilia. Semin Hematol 36:340, 1999

46. Cawthern KM, van't Veer C, Lock JB, et al: Blood coagulation in hemophilia A and hemophilia C. Blood 91:4581, 1998

47. Rodriguez-Merchan EC: Common orthopaedic problems in haemophilia. Haemophilia 5[suppl 1]:53, 1999

48. Mannucci PM, Tuddenbam EG: The hemophilias: progress and problems. Semin Hematol 36[4 suppl 7]:104, 1999

49. Bolton-Maggs PH: The management of factor XI deficiency. Haemophilia 4:683, 1998

50. Minowa H, Takahashi Y, Tanaka T, et al: Four cases of bleeding diathesis in children due to congenital plasminogen activator inhibitor-1 deficiency. Haemostasis 29:286, 1999

51. Lind B, Thorsen S: A novel missense mutation in the human plasmin inhibitor (alpha2-antiplasmin) gene associated with a bleeding tendency. Br J Haematol 107:317, 1999

52. Turpeinen AM, Mutanen M: Similar effects of diets high in oleic or linoleic acids on coagulation and fibrinolytic factors in healthy humans. Nutr Metab Cardiovasc Dis 9(2):65, 1999

53. Li D, Sinclair A, Mann N, et al: The association of diet and thrombotic risk factors in healthy male vegetarians and meat-eaters. Eur J Clin Nutr 53:612, 1999

54. Temme EH, Mensink RP, Hornstra G: Effects of diets enriched in lauric, palmitic or oleic acids on blood coagulation and fibrinolysis. Thromb Haemost 81:259, 1999

55. Rein D, Paglieroni T, Wun T, et al: Cocoa inhibits platelet activation and function. Am J Clin Nutr 72:30, 2000

56. Rein D, Paglieroni T, Wun T, et al: Cocoa and wine polyphenols modulate platelet activation and function. J Nutr 130:2120S, 2000

57. Bhatt DL, Topol EJ: Current role of platelet glycoprotein IIb/IIIa inhibitors in acute coronary syndromes. JAMA 284:1549, 2000

58. Humphries JE: Transfusion therapy in acquired coagulopathies. Hematol Oncol Clin North Am 8:1181, 1994

59. Zachee P, Vermylen J, Boogaerts MA: Hematologic aspects of end-stage renal failure. Ann Hematol 69:33, 1994

60. Peek GJ, Firmin RK: The inflammatory and coagulative response to prolonged extracorporeal membrane oxygenation. ASAIO J 45:250, 1999

61. Hobisch-Hagen P, Wirleitner B, Mair J, et al: Consequences of acute normovolaemic haemodilution on haemostasis during major orthopaedic surgery. Br J Anaesth 82:503, 1999

62. Konrad C, Markl T, Schuepfer G, et al: The effects of in vitro hemodilution with gelatin, hydroxyethyl starch, and lactated Ringer's solution on markers of coagulation: an analysis using SONOCLOT. Anesth Analg 88:483, 1999

63. Boyer LV, Seifert SA, Clark RF, et al: Recurrent and persistent coagulopathy following pit viper envenomation. Arch Intern Med 159:706, 1999

64. Eriksson BI, Kalebo P, Ekman S, et al: Direct thrombin inhibition with rec-hirudin CGP 39393 as prophylaxis of thromboembolic complications after total hip replacement. Thromb Haemost 72:227, 1994

65. Sherman DG, Atkinson RP, Chippendale T, et al: Intravenous ancrod for treatment of acute ischemic stroke: the STAT study: a randomized controlled trial. Stroke Treatment with Ancrod Trial. JAMA 282:2395, 2000

66. Oleksowicz L, Bhagwati N, DeLeon-Fernandez M: Deficient activity of von Willebrand's factor-cleaving protease in patients with disseminated malignancies. Cancer Res 59:2244, 1999

67. Francis JL, Biggerstaff J, Amirkhosravi A: Hemostasis and malignancy. Semin Thromb Hemost 24:93, 1998

68. Amirkhosravi M, Francis JL: Coagulation activation by MC28 fibrosarcoma cells facilitates lung tumor formation. Thromb Haemost 73:59, 1995

69. Williams EC, Moshen DF: Disseminated intravascular coagulation. Hematology: Basic Principles and Practice. Hoffman R, Benz EJ Sr, Shattil SJ, et al, Eds. Churchill-Livingstone, New York, 1995, p 1758

70. Muller-Berghaus G, ten Cate H, Levi M: Disseminated intravascular coagulation: clinical spectrum and established as well as new diagnostic approaches. Thromb Haemost 82:706, 1999

71. Lawrie AS, Kitchen S, Purdy G, et al: Assessment of Actin FS and Actin FSL sensitivity to specific clotting factor deficiencies. Clin Lab Haematol 20:179, 1998

72. Lind SE: The bleeding time does not predict surgical bleeding. Blood 77:2547, 1991

73. Mammen EF, Comp PC, Gosselin R, et al: PFA-100™ System: A new method for assessment of platelet dysfunction. Semin Thromb Hemost 24:195, 1998

74. Speiss BD: Coagulation function in the operating room. Anesth Clin North Am 8:481, 1990

75. LeForce WR, Bruno DS, Kanot WP, et al: Evaluation of the Sonoclot analyzer for the measurement of platelet function in whole blood. Am Clin Lab Sci 22:30, 1992

76. Winslow RM: Blood substitutes. Adv Drug Deliv Rev 40:131, 2000

Acknowledgments

Figures 1, 3, and 4   Marcia Kammerer.

Figure 2   Seward Hung.

6 LIFE-THREATENING ELECTROLYTE ABNORMALITIES

Kimberly J. Van Zee, M.D., and Stephen F. Lowry, M.D.

Evaluation and Treatment of Electrolyte Emergencies

Assessment of Volume Status

Proper management of any life-threatening electrolyte abnormality must include the clinical assessment of extracellular fluid (ECF) volume status. Because no simple specific laboratory test is sufficient

for accurate determination of intravascular and interstitial fluid volume, clinical assessment aimed at detecting signs and symptoms of deficits or excesses of body fluid is necessary. Such assessment should include historical information that might bear on the pathogenesis of these volume changes.

EVALUATION AND TREATMENT OF
EXTRACELLULAR FLUID VOLUME DEFICITS

Deficits in ECF volume may adversely affect cardiovascular function, central nervous system function, and metabolic and temperature regulation, as well as induce more subtle changes in peripheral muscle function. Moderate decreases in ECF volume lead to orthostatic hypotension and associated tachycardia with evidence of reduced venous filling; drowsiness and a mild decrease in body temperature may result as well. Such decreases in ECF volume are also associated with a small, soft tongue and reduced skin turgor. More severe volume deficits eventually lead to stupor or coma, with reduced deep tendon reflexes and muscle atony. These deficits also result in hypotension and reduced pulse pressure with cutaneous lividity. A marked decrease in body temperature to 34° to 36° C (93° to 97° F) may also be observed.

ECF volume depletion results from loss of both sodium and water, not necessarily in the same proportion. In surgical patients, sodium is often lost in acute or chronic losses of gastrointestinal fluids. Postoperatively or after injury, fluid sequestration, or so-called third spacing, often causes subtle deficits in isotonic fluid volume.[1,2] In addition, preexisting renal or adrenal disease or previous administration of diuretics may lead to excess sodium loss in urine and thereby cause volume deficiencies.

Severe ECF volume deficits must be corrected as quickly as possible. Initially, until further abnormalities of electrolyte or acid-base status are identified, fluid should be replaced through

the administration of a physiologic salt solution. In some patients, except for those with symptomatic hypernatremia, it may be preferable to begin fluid volume resuscitation with normal saline until adequate renal function and urine output can be established. Hemodynamically stable patients should initially receive 100 to 200 ml. Unstable patients can receive initial boluses of up to 500 ml according to need. There is no standard formula for calculating the amount of saline required to correct ECF volume depletion. Consequently, the adequacy of repletion must be clinically assessed. Blood pressure, pulse, urine output, and hematocrit should be monitored during the initial phases of this resuscitation. If further abnormalities of electrolyte status are discovered, management should be continued (see below).

EVALUATION AND TREATMENT OF
EXTRACELLULAR FLUID VOLUME EXCESS

Extracellular fluid volume excess may be associated with both systemic and organ-specific findings. Unless ECF excess is associated with other problems related to oxygen transport, however, it does not give rise to specific central nervous system signs of fluid volume excess. On the other hand, moderate ECF excess yields several significant cardiovascular findings, including higher pulse pressure, evidence of venous distention, and, possibly, congestive heart failure. More severe ECF excess results in pulmonary edema. Pitting edema may occur even with moderate ECF excess, and in more extreme cases, there is associated vomiting and diarrhea as intestinal edema progresses.

Acute volume excess usually results from acute or chronic renal or cardiovascular failure and occasionally from underlying liver disease. In surgical patients, volume excess from organ failure may be compounded by administration of too much fluid or failure to recognize fluid mobilization postoperatively.

Whatever the underlying cause, water intake should be restricted in patients with evidence of ECF volume excess. Fluid replacement should be the minimal daily requirement of approximately 500 ml, with additions to replace significant extraneous losses or to maintain hemodynamic stability. Further measures, such as administration of diuretics or inotropic cardiac agents or, in extreme cases, the use of dialysis, may be necessary to reduce fluid volume successfully. In such circumstances, serial determinations of electrolytes, particularly potassium, should be performed because changes in electrolyte status will inevitably influence subsequent therapeutic efforts.

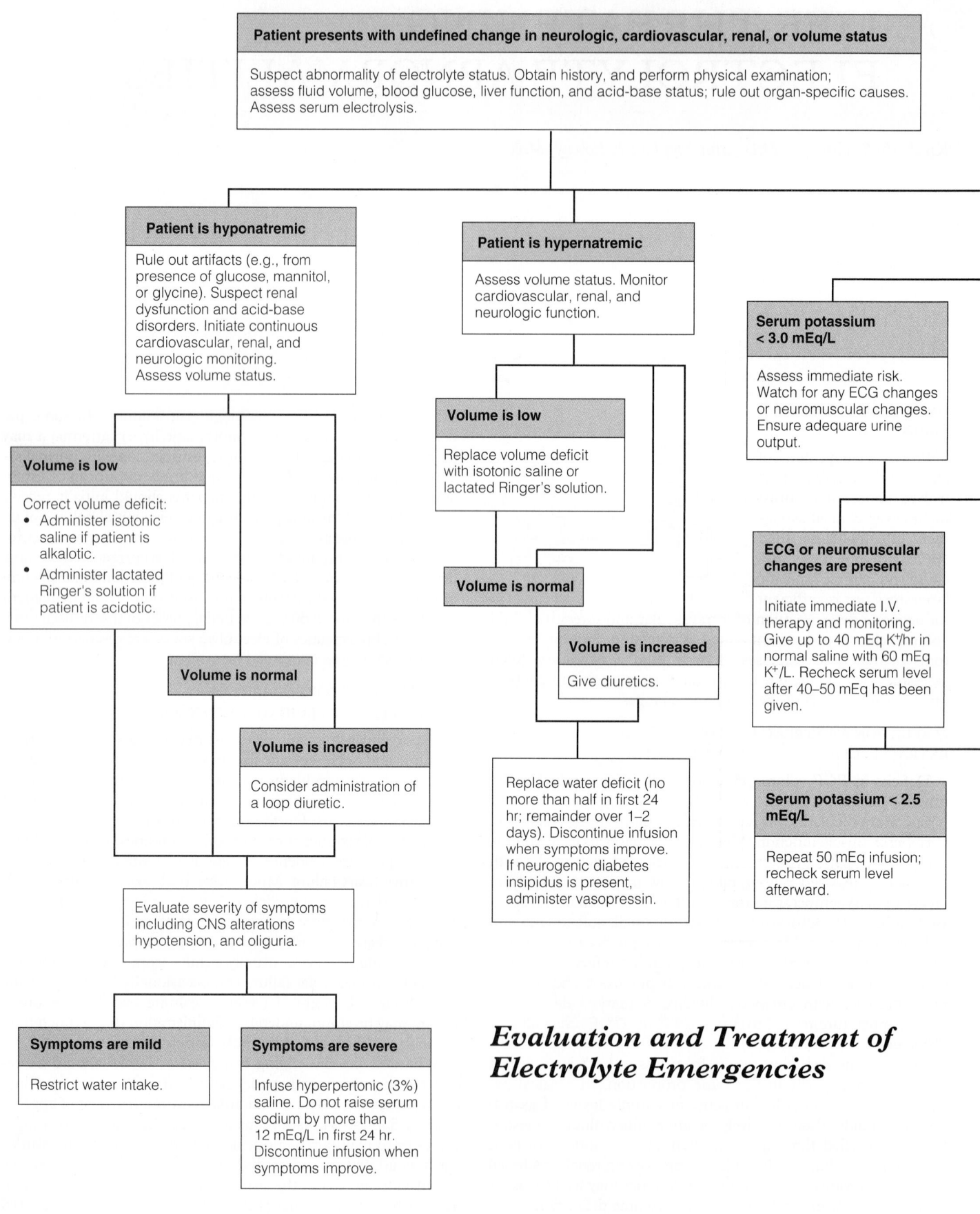

Patient presents with undefined change in neurologic, cardiovascular, renal, or volume status

Suspect abnormality of electrolyte status. Obtain history, and perform physical examination; assess fluid volume, blood glucose, liver function, and acid-base status; rule out organ-specific causes. Assess serum electrolysis.

Patient is hyponatremic

Rule out artifacts (e.g., from presence of glucose, mannitol, or glycine). Suspect renal dysfunction and acid-base disorders. Initiate continuous cardiovascular, renal, and neurologic monitoring. Assess volume status.

Patient is hypernatremic

Assess volume status. Monitor cardiovascular, renal, and neurologic function.

Serum potassium < 3.0 mEq/L

Assess immediate risk. Watch for any ECG changes or neuromuscular changes. Ensure adequare urine output.

Volume is low

Correct volume deficit:
- Administer isotonic saline if patient is alkalotic.
- Administer lactated Ringer's solution if patient is acidotic.

Volume is low

Replace volume deficit with isotonic saline or lactated Ringer's solution.

ECG or neuromuscular changes are present

Initiate immediate I.V. therapy and monitoring. Give up to 40 mEq K+/hr in normal saline with 60 mEq K+/L. Recheck serum level after 40–50 mEq has been given.

Volume is normal

Volume is normal

Volume is increased

Consider administration of a loop diuretic.

Volume is increased

Give diuretics.

Serum potassium < 2.5 mEq/L

Repeat 50 mEq infusion; recheck serum level afterward.

Evaluate severity of symptoms including CNS alterations hypotension, and oliguria.

Replace water deficit (no more than half in first 24 hr; remainder over 1–2 days). Discontinue infusion when symptoms improve. If neurogenic diabetes insipidus is present, administer vasopressin.

Symptoms are mild

Restrict water intake.

Symptoms are severe

Infuse hyperpertonic (3%) saline. Do not raise serum sodium by more than 12 mEq/L in first 24 hr. Discontinue infusion when symptoms improve.

Evaluation and Treatment of Electrolyte Emergencies

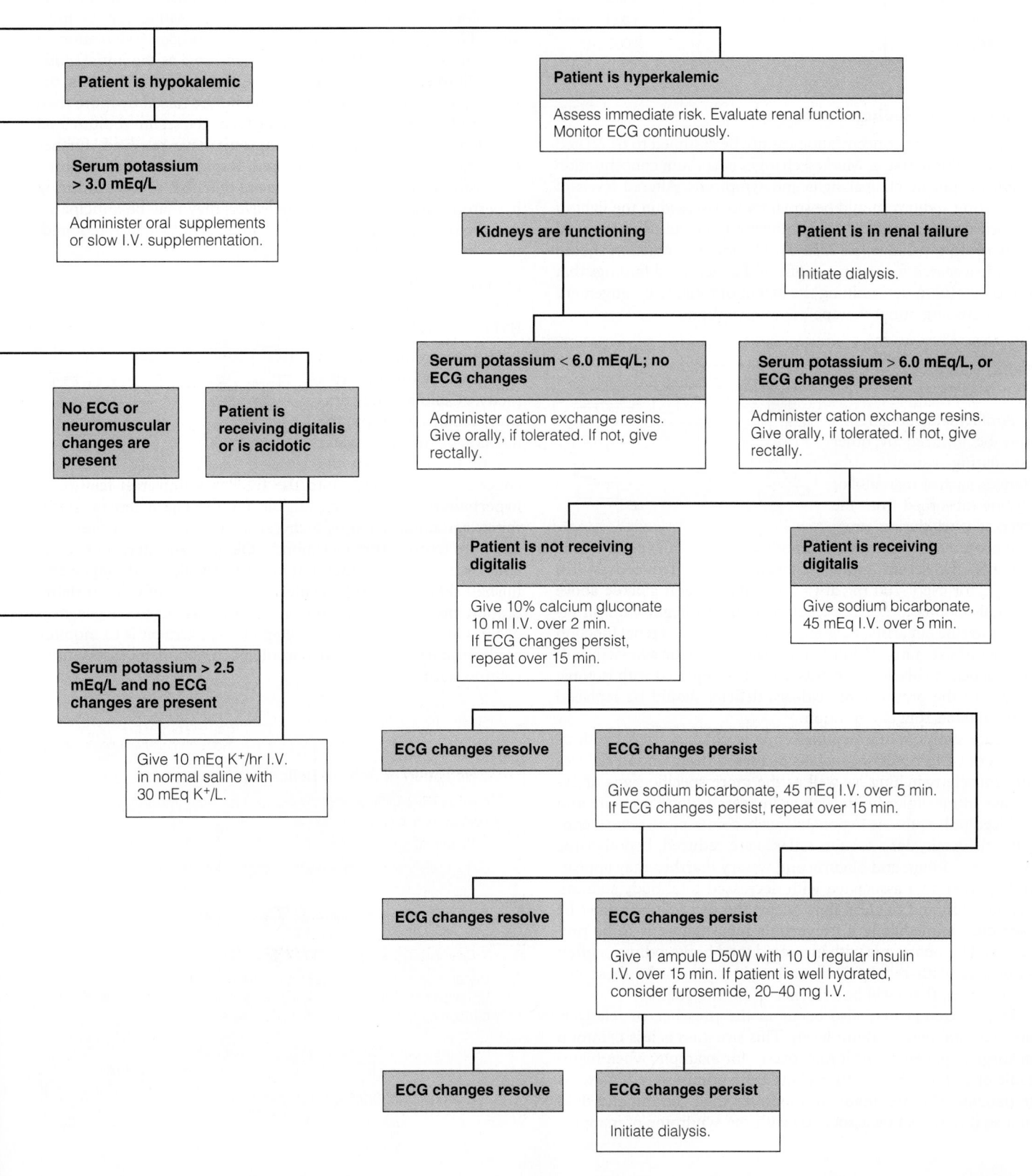

Patient is hypokalemic

Serum potassium > 3.0 mEq/L

Administer oral supplements or slow I.V. supplementation.

No ECG or neuromuscular changes are present

Patient is receiving digitalis or is acidotic

Serum potassium > 2.5 mEq/L and no ECG changes are present

Give 10 mEq K$^+$/hr I.V. in normal saline with 30 mEq K$^+$/L.

Patient is hyperkalemic

Assess immediate risk. Evaluate renal function. Monitor ECG continuously.

Kidneys are functioning

Patient is in renal failure

Initiate dialysis.

Serum potassium < 6.0 mEq/L; no ECG changes

Administer cation exchange resins. Give orally, if tolerated. If not, give rectally.

Serum potassium > 6.0 mEq/L, or ECG changes present

Administer cation exchange resins. Give orally, if tolerated. If not, give rectally.

Patient is not receiving digitalis

Give 10% calcium gluconate 10 ml I.V. over 2 min. If ECG changes persist, repeat over 15 min.

Patient is receiving digitalis

Give sodium bicarbonate, 45 mEq I.V. over 5 min.

ECG changes resolve

ECG changes persist

Give sodium bicarbonate, 45 mEq I.V. over 5 min. If ECG changes persist, repeat over 15 min.

ECG changes resolve

ECG changes persist

Give 1 ampule D50W with 10 U regular insulin I.V. over 15 min. If patient is well hydrated, consider furosemide, 20–40 mg I.V.

ECG changes resolve

ECG changes persist

Initiate dialysis.

Table 1 Approximate Values for Serum and Total Body Electrolytes

Electrolyte	Serum Level (mEq/L)	Total Body Level (mEq)
Sodium	136–145	3,000
Potassium	3.5–5.0	3,400
Calcium	4.4–5.2	50,000
Magnesium	1.5–2.5	2,000

Assessment of Sodium Status

Serum sodium concentration cannot be assumed to be related to ECF volume status. Marked changes in sodium concentration result in specific clinical signs and symptoms. Altered levels of circulating sodium should be sought and assessed in the light of historical and clinical evidence indicating the status of the total body sodium balance [*see Table 1*]. The initial evaluation should include a search for organ-specific and generalized findings that can be useful in determining the extent of tonicity derangement and in guiding initial therapeutic interventions.

EVALUATION AND TREATMENT OF HYPONATREMIA

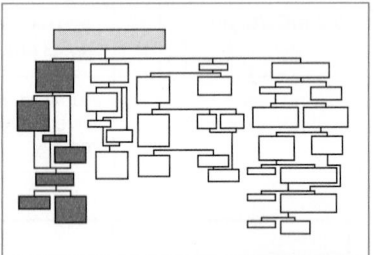

Artifactual hyponatremia may be induced by other circulating osmotic substances, such as mannitol or glycine (absorbed from the irrigant used during prostate procedures) or, most commonly, glucose. In hyperglycemic patients, the serum sodium concentration is reduced by 1.6 mEq/L for every 100 mg/dl (5.5 mmol/L) rise in glucose above normal. Evaluation of hyponatremia should begin with an attempt to rule out artifacts, along with assessment of renal function and acid-base status. Volume status should also be assessed. Volume deficits in alkalotic patients should be replaced with isotonic saline. In the presence of acidosis, deficits should be replaced with lactated Ringer's solution.

Acute symptomatic hyponatremia is characterized by alterations of CNS function, such as increased deep tendon reflexes and muscle twitching, as well as the more specific signs of excessive intracellular fluid, such as increased blood pressure and reduced pulse rate. As hyponatremia becomes more severe, convulsions occur, deep tendon reflexes are reduced, hypothermia becomes evident, and oliguria and watery diarrhea may appear. In hyponatremia associated with decreased total body sodium, hypotension and oliguria may occur; these conditions must be corrected immediately if irreversible renal failure is to be prevented. Hyponatremia with increased total body sodium is often associated with renal failure and with cirrhosis. In these circumstances, there will be evidence of pitting edema.[3]

Hyponatremia may also occur in the presence of relatively normal total body sodium levels. This situation is less common in surgical patients, but it may occur, for example, when hypotonic or sodium-free solutions have been administered in excess to patients who are unable to modulate their sodium and fluid intake; it may also be associated with the syndrome of inappropriate secretion of antidiuretic hormone (SIADH), which is characterized by impaired excretion of renal free water. In patients with this syndrome, urine is excessively concentrated (osmolarity > 100 mOsm/L), and high urinary sodium concentrations occur.[4] Hyponatremia caused by SIADH or administration of excess free water is treated by free water restriction.

If hyponatremia gives rise to serious side effects that warrant emergency treatment (e.g., coma, seizures, myoclonus, or focal neurologic deficits), infusion of hypertonic saline may be initiated. The estimated sodium deficit [*see Sidebar* Calculation of Sodium Deficit and Replacement] can serve as the initial guide for sodium replacement. To avoid neurologic complications, the serum sodium concentration should not be raised by more than 12 mEq/L during the first 24 hours. Once the serum sodium level is 120 mEq/L or higher or symptoms have resolved, further correction generally is not required. Rapid extracellular volume expansion and pulmonary edema are potential problems during hypertonic volume infusions; however, they may be anticipated and avoided through careful monitoring. If treatment is required, loop diuretics are effective.

EVALUATION AND TREATMENT OF HYPERNATREMIA

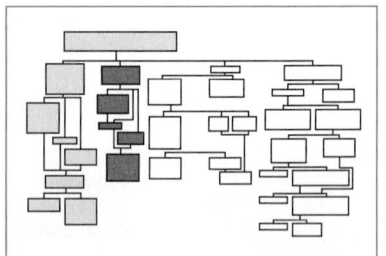

Hypernatremia is always associated with hypertonicity. Cellular dehydration resulting from the movement of free water out of the cell down the concentration gradient into the ECF is a universal feature of hypernatremia and is responsible for the characteristic signs: thirst, agitation, lethargy, tachycardia, reduced blood pressure, and core temperature elevation.[5,6] Oliguria and dry, sticky mucous membranes are often found, and a swollen, red tongue and flushed skin may also be evident. As this state of cellular dehydration progresses, delirium and cardiovascular collapse may occur. Consequently, the first step in management is to monitor cardiovascular, renal, and neurologic function to assess fluid volume status.

Calculation of Sodium Deficit and Replacement

Normal serum Na+ (mEq/L) – actual serum Na+ (mEq/L) = sodium deficit (mEq/L)

    Example: 140 – 110 = 30

0.6 x body weight (kg) = normal body water volume (L)

    Example: 0.6 x 60 = 36

Normal body water volume (L) x sodium deficit (mEq/L) = estimated body Na+ deficit (mEq)

    Example: 36 x 30 = 1,080

Because a 3.0 percent hypertonic saline solution contains 0.5 mEq sodium/ml, the volume of solution needed for sodium replacement can be calculated as follows:

$$\frac{\text{Estimated body Na+ deficit (mEq)}}{0.5} = \text{necessary volume of 3.0 percent saline (ml)}$$

    Example: 1,080/0.5 = 2,160

Hypernatremia may occur in conjunction with hypovolemia, isovolemia, or hypervolemia. Careful clinical evaluation of ECF volume is therefore essential. In hypernatremia associated with hypovolemia, there is generally a total body sodium deficit. This condition may occur in patients with excessive GI losses (from nasogastric suction, severe diarrhea, or vomiting), renal losses (from osmotic diuresis caused by hyperglycemia, hyperalimentation, or diuretic administration), cutaneous losses (from burns, hyperthermia, or excessive sweating), or peritoneal losses (from peritonitis or peritoneal dialysis). It should be treated by administering isotonic saline or lactated Ringer's solution.

Hypernatremia may also result from the administration of hypertonic saline (e.g., solutions containing sodium bicarbonate), hyperaldosteronism, or Cushing's syndrome. In hypernatremic patients who are hypervolemic, diuretics and water replacement are indicated.

Neurogenic diabetes insipidus (DI) is a not uncommon cause of hypernatremia in the ICU. In this condition, total body sodium is often normal, but a relative state of pure water deficit exists. The diagnosis of DI is suggested by polyuria and a urine osmolarity lower than 200 mOsm/L. Treatment comprises administration of vasopressin and replacement of free water.

Water deficits can be calculated as follows:

$$\text{Normal body water (L)} = 0.6 \times \text{body weight (kg)}$$

$$\text{Current body water (L)} = \frac{\text{normal serum Na}^+\text{ (mEq/L)} \times \text{normal body water (L)}}{\text{measured serum Na}^+\text{ (mEq/L)}}$$

$$\text{Body water deficit (L)} = \text{normal body water (L)} - \text{current body water (L)}$$

An amount equal to one half of the calculated water deficit should be administered over the first 24 hours; the remaining deficit should be corrected over the next one to two days. More rapid correction of the hypernatremia may result in lethargy or convulsions secondary to cerebral edema.

Assessment of Potassium Status

Because 98 percent of potassium is intracellular and only two percent is extracellular, a shift of a small amount of potassium into or out of the intracellular compartment can result in a dramatic change in the serum potassium concentration. The resultant alteration of the potassium gradient across the cell membrane causes neuromuscular dysfunction, especially in cardiac tissue, with potentially grave consequences. The distribution of potassium is affected by a number of factors, including acid-base balance, hormone levels, body fluid tonicity, the actions of pharmacological agents, and changes in body cell mass.[7]

EVALUATION AND TREATMENT OF HYPOKALEMIA

Hypokalemia may result from inadequate intake of potassium, excessive renal or GI losses, or redistribution of normal body

stores.[8] Management of hypokalemia includes an assessment of immediate risk and is based on monitoring changes in neuromuscular activity (e.g., weakness or hyporeflexia) as well as on monitoring electrocardiographic changes. Evidence of neuromuscular changes or of progressive ECG changes (frequent premature ventricular contractions → flat or inverted T waves → U waves → depressed ST segments → prolonged PR intervals → tall P waves → widened QRS complexes) is an indication for immediate intravenous therapy.[5] In patients with severe hypokalemia, cautious administration of up to 40 mEq/hr of potassium may be undertaken but only with continuous electrocardiographic monitoring and close physician supervision. Any potassium infusion at rates greater than 10 mEq/hr should be administered into a central vein to avoid inadvertent formation of a potassium bolus, which could result in myocardial depression. Even in the absence of clinical and electrocardiographic evidence of impending severe hypokalemic complications, patients who are receiving digitalis or who have concurrent metabolic acidosis should also receive immediate intravenous potassium supplementation. In the latter cases, administration of up to 10 mEq/hr may be cautiously undertaken. For patients whose serum potassium level is 3 mEq/L or greater, either oral supplementation or slow intravenous potassium supplementation is appropriate. Patients who present with simultaneous hypokalemia and hypomagnesemia will require magnesium replacement before abnormalities in potassium levels can be fully corrected.

EVALUATION AND TREATMENT OF HYPERKALEMIA

The classic signs of hyperkalemia are progressive electrocardiographic changes: tall peaked T waves → widened QRS complexes → depressed ST segments → decreased amplitude of R waves → prolonged PR interval → diminished P waves → widened QRS complex with prolongation of the QT interval, resulting in a sine wave pattern → diastolic arrest.[5] These changes are usually seen when the potassium level is 6.0 to 6.5 mEq/L or higher but may also occur with potassium levels between 5.0 and 6.0 mEq/L.

Treatment of hyperkalemia consists of taking immediate measures to reduce the serum potassium level, withholding any exogenous potassium, limiting severe catabolism, and correcting renal failure. As with hypokalemia, the immediate risk must be assessed; in addition, the adequacy of renal function must be established, and continuous ECG monitoring must be initiated. If the kidneys are functioning but the serum potassium level is higher than 6 mEq/L or electrocardiographic changes are present, patients not receiving digitalis therapy may undergo intravenous calcium gluconate infusion (90 mg of elemental calcium in a 10 ml ampule, given over two minutes). The calcium antagonizes the membrane effects of hyperkalemia in a matter of minutes and has a duration of action of about one hour. The next step is sodium bicarbonate (45 mEq I.V. over five minutes). Bicarbonate causes potassium to shift into the intracellular space within 15 to 30 minutes and has a duration of action of about one to two hours. Patients who are taking digitalis should not receive intravenous calcium. Instead, they should initially receive sodium bicarbonate (45 mEq over five minutes).

If ECG changes persist, the following additional approaches may be tried: (1) administration of glucose and insulin (one ampule of 50 percent dextrose in water and 10 units of regular insulin), which also shifts potassium into cells within 15 to 30 minutes and has a duration of action of two to four hours, and (2) administration of furosemide (20 to 40 mg I.V.), which increases renal excretion of potassium within about 15 to 30 minutes in well-hydrated patients with functioning kidneys. Cation exchange resins, given by either the oral or the rectal route, should be administered simultaneously with this immediate intravenous therapy in patients with life-threatening hyperkalemia or as a means of primary therapy in patients with less severe hyperkalemia. Patients who show evidence of impaired renal function or who respond inadequately to the measures just described should be prepared to undergo dialysis immediately.

Assessment of Calcium Status

Calcium is present in the plasma in two forms: either bound to protein or as a positively charged ion. The degree to which calcium is bound is influenced by the amount of protein present in the plasma. Several corrective calculations have been suggested to determine the true total calcium in the presence of low levels of serum proteins. The following is one such calculation:

$$\text{Corrected calcium (mg/dl)} = \text{measured calcium} + [(4 - \text{albumin [g/dl]}) \times 0.8]$$

A simpler way of determining true total calcium is to assume that every 1 g/dl decrease in serum albumin falsely lowers the serum calcium by 1 mg/dl. Serum calcium can also be markedly altered by the degree of acid-base abnormality. In severe alkalosis, the ionic calcium level can be lowered and hypocalcemic symptoms precipitated, even if the patient has a normal or low normal total calcium. Similarly, hyperventilation alkalosis can lower the ionic calcium and precipitate symptoms. In much the same way, renal tubular acidosis can lead to elevated serum calcium levels.

EVALUATION AND TREATMENT OF HYPERCALCEMIA

Because calcium is ubiquitous in the body, symptoms and signs of hypercalcemia are widespread and often nonspecific, and their etiology is frequently unclear [see Table 2]. The common gastrointestinal symptoms are early, nonspecific, and often vague. Increased gastric acid secretion and pancreatitis are much more often noted in patients whose elevated calcium levels result from primary hyperparathyroidism. There is considerable controversy regarding this point, however, and the true prevalence of hyperparathyroidism as an etiology is still unknown. The neuromuscular symptoms are widespread and, like the GI symptoms, nonspecific; they usually consist of depression, fatigue, lethargy, and clouding of consciousness. Profound muscle weakness, usually of proximal muscle type, may be followed by stupor and even by irreversible coma in late or unrecognized states. Characteristic electroencephalographic abnormalities have been described.[9,10]

The major renal symptom of hypercalcemia is a reversible renal tubular defect in the ability to concentrate urine that mimics the manifestations of diabetes insipidus, resulting in some degree of total body water deficit and sodium deficit in

---

Table 2 Causes of Hypercalcemia

Primary hyperparathyroidism

Malignancy
  With bone metastasis
  Without bone metastasis

Drugs
  Thiazide or other diuretics
  Vitamins A and D
  Calcium carbonate

Granulomatous diseases
  Wegener's granulomatosis
  Sarcoid

Metabolic disorders
  Paget's disease
  Osteoporosis
  Familial hypercalcemic hypocalciuria
  Thyrotoxicosis
  Renal tubular acidosis

Other
  Pheochromocytoma

---

most patients. Dehydration decreases the glomerular filtration rate, thereby exacerbating the renal damage and bringing about a progressive increase in hypercalcemia, which leads to further renal failure.

In patients with primary hyperparathyroidism and prolonged urinary loss of calcium, nephrocalcinosis or renal stones are common; however, renal stones are relatively rare in patients with primary hypercalcemia of malignancy.

The cardiovascular symptoms of hypercalcemia are related to the major role calcium plays in neurotransmission. Acute hypercalcemia can actually slow the heart rate and shorten the ventricular systole. In moderate hypercalcemia, the QT interval is shortened, whereas in severe hypercalcemia (calcium levels > 16 mg/dl), the QT interval lengthens. Digitalis must be used cautiously in patients with hypercalcemia.

Severe hypercalcemia is a medical emergency and requires hospitalization and aggressive treatment. Although the definitive treatment of acute hypercalcemic crisis in patients with primary hyperparathyroidism is surgical, calcium levels should, if possible, be reduced before exploration is begun. The patient must be monitored so that fluid balance and central venous pressure may be accurately determined. Foley catheterization is usually required to assess renal function and volume status. As acute treatment progresses, the etiology of the hypercalcemia should be actively investigated [see Figure 1].

The first step is rehydration with normal saline solution. In mild to moderate cases, the usual amount infused is 3 to 5 L/day, but in severe cases, as much as 10 L/day may be required. These larger amounts should be accompanied by administration of furosemide, beginning with a dose of 40 mg, followed by dosages of 40 to 80 mg every two to four hours. Ethacrynic acid is acceptable as an alternative diuretic, but the thiazides are not. In addition to serum calcium levels, serum sodium, potassium,

Figure 1 **Illustrated is an algorithm for management of hypercalcemia.**

and magnesium levels must be monitored constantly to ensure that major deficits of these electrolytes do not result in a parallel metabolic derangement.

If hydration in conjunction with furosemide fails, or if hypercalcemia is life threatening, calcitonin should be used. Calcitonin acts by inhibiting bone resorption and increasing renal excretion of calcium and is the most rapidly acting anti-calcemic agent available (onset of action, two hours; duration of action, six to eight hours). The recommended dosage is 4 IU/kg administered subcutaneously or intramuscularly every 12 hours. Skin testing with 1 unit (0.1 ml of a 1:10 dilution of calcitonin) administered subcutaneously should precede administration to exclude any allergy.

Because calcitonin alone is a relatively weak agent, additional therapeutic measures should be considered. The bisphosphonates (especially pamidronate and clodronate) are well tolerated and quite effective: they are capable of normalizing calcium levels in 70 to 100 percent of patients within seven days. They act by inhibiting osteoclast function and have an onset of action of approximately two days and a duration of action of approximately one week.[11]

Plicamycin (25 µg/kg over four to six hours) has a more rapid onset of action than the bisphosphonates (about 12 hours) but is more toxic, causing renal and hepatic dysfunction, thrombocytopenia, and nausea. If it is given at intervals of several days, these adverse effects are infrequent. The use of this cytotoxic antibiotic has decreased as other, less toxic drugs have become available.

Gallium nitrate is a relatively new agent that acts by inhibiting bone absorption. Its onset and duration of action are similar to those of the bisphosphonates and substantially slower than those of calcitonin. Gallium nitrate is administered as a continuous intravenous infusion (200 mg/m²/day for five days). Although it is more effective than calcitonin,[12] it has significant nephrotoxicity. Clinical experience with this agent is still limited.

Corticosteroids may be useful as adjunctive therapy for hypercalcemia associated with lymphomas, multiple myeloma, non–parathyroid hormone–secreting tumors that are metastatic to bone, Addison's disease, granulomatous diseases, and vitamin D intoxication. Hydrocortisone, 100 mg intravenously every six to eight hours for 24 hours, followed by prednisone, 10 to 30 mg/day orally, is the preferred regimen. Steroids have a slow onset of action (several days); however, if no effect is seen in one week, they should be rapidly tapered and discontinued.

Administration of inorganic phosphates causes a rise in the serum phosphorus level, which leads to a fall in the serum calcium level, regardless of the cause of the hypercalcemia. Intravenous administration of phosphates, though effective, can result in serious complications, such as hypotension, myocardial infarction, acute renal failure, and ectopic calcifications. Phosphate therapy is justified only when other treatments are ineffective and its use would be lifesaving. The safest use for orally administered phosphates is in the treatment of mild to moderate hypercalcemia in a patient with a low serum phosphate level; however, careful monitoring of renal function and serum electrolytes is still necessary.

In patients with either mild hypercalcemia or stable, asymptomatic hypercalcemia, the most important task is the elucida-

Table 3 Differential Diagnosis of Hypercalcemia

SYMPTOMS AND SIGNS

	Malignancy	Primary Hyperparathyroidism
History	Known malignancy / Known bone metastases / Weight loss	No malignancy / No bone metastases / No weight loss
Serum Ca²⁺	Abrupt rise / Usually > 12 mg/dl / No renal stones	Long-standing slow rise / Often < 12 mg/dl / Nephrocalcinosis

INVESTIGATIONS

	Malignancy	Primary Hyperparathyroidism
Serum Ca²⁺	Recent abrupt elevation	Long-standing slow elevation
Serum PO_4^*	Normal	Low
Serum Cl⁻	Normal	Elevated
Cl⁻ to PO_4 ratio	> 33	< 33
Serum parathyroid hormone	Normal	Elevated
Urinary Ca²⁺	Normal or elevated	Elevated
Urinary cAMP	Normal	Elevated
Serum bicarbonate	Normal	Low
Alkaline PO_4^*	Normal or elevated	Normal or elevated
Bone scan	Isolated sites of increased uptake; metastatic disease	Diffuse, increased uptake

*PO_4 stands for $H_2PO_4^-$, HPO_4^{2-}, and PO_4^{3-}.

Patient is hypocalcemic (serum calcium < 8.0–8.5 mg/dl [~2 mmol/L])

Patient is symptomatic

Patient is asymptomatic

Symptoms are severe (e.g., carpopedal spasm or tetany)

Emergency I.V. treatment is required: 20 ml 10% calcium gluconate over 20 min, then 15 mg/kg calcium gluconate q. 6 hr.
Reassure patient to minimize respiratory alkalosis associated with hyperventilation.

Symptoms are mild (e.g., perioral or extremity paresthesias)

Initiate nonurgent oral treatment: 15 ml calcium glubionate q.i.d. and 0.25 µg 1,25–$(OH)_2$ vitamin D t.i.d.

Seek cause of hypocalcemia

If calcium replacement does not reverse symptoms of hypocalcemia, consider magnesium deficiency.

Exclude or, if present, correct:
• Nutritional deficiency • Hypoalbuminemia
• Excess hydration • Hyponatremia
Measure serum phosphate.

Serum phosphate is high (> 5 mg/dl)

Suspect hypoparathyroidism as cause of hypocalcemia. Origin of hypoparathyroidism may be previous thyroid or parathyroid operation, idiopathic, or autoimmune.

Serum phosphate is normal or low

Suspect bone disease (postparathyroidectomy hungry bone syndrome) as cause of hypocalcemia.

Figure 2 **Illustrated is an algorithm for management of hypocalcemia.**

tion of the etiology. The essential distinction that must be made is between hypercalcemia of parathyroid origin and hypercalcemia that is caused by malignant disease [*see Table 3*]. Other conditions rarely progress to major life-threatening hypercalcemia.

EVALUATION AND TREATMENT OF HYPOCALCEMIA

Biochemical hypocalcemia is usually defined as a serum calcium level below the lower limit of normal in the laboratory—usually 8.0 to 8.5 mg/dl (2.0 to 2.1 mmol/L). In asymptomatic patients, no immediate therapy is required other than a search for the cause of the hypocalcemia. In symptomatic patients who have perioral or extremity paresthesias, treatment can be initiated on a nonurgent basis with oral medication. In patients with more severe symptoms, particularly those of carpopedal spasm and tetany, emergency intravenous treatment is required. Not the least important part of this urgent treatment is reassurance of the patient; reassurance serves to diminish hyperventilation

and the accompanying respiratory alkalosis, which merely compounds the hypocalcemia [*see Figure 2*].

Ten milliliters of a 10 percent calcium gluconate solution contains 93 mg (4.6 mEq) of elemental calcium. Ten milliliters of a 10 percent calcium chloride solution contains 273 mg of elemental calcium (14 mEq). The calcium chloride solution thus has a greater osmolarity (2.04 mOsm/ml) than the calcium gluconate solution (0.7 mOsm/ml), which makes it potentially more irritating to the vein on infusion. The 15 mg/kg of calcium gluconate can be given as five ampules in 1,000 ml at 100 ml/hr. In oral replacement, 5 ml of a calcium glubionate preparation has 115 mg of elemental calcium, which is equivalent to 1.2 g of calcium gluconate. Calciferol, which contains 1,25-dihydroxy-vitamin D, has a brief half-life of three to six hours and can be given in a dosage of 0.25 µg three or four times a day.

Mild biochemical hypocalcemia is more common in hospitalized patients who are severely malnourished and have been rigorously treated with intravenous fluids. It is rarely symptomatic,

Table 4 Causes of Hypocalcemia

Thyroidectomy or parathyroidectomy
Idiopathic autoimmune hypoparathyroidism
Pseudohypoparathyroidism
Acute pancreatitis
Dilutional or nutritional deficiency
Severe magnesium depletion
Drugs
Chronic vitamin D deficiency
Multiple transfusions
Chronic renal failure

although the serum calcium can occasionally fall to very low levels. Low levels of serum albumin may exacerbate the hypocalcemia. For practical purposes, a 1 g/dl fall in serum albumin can cause the total serum calcium to fall by 1 mg/dl. Treatment in this case should be directed at restoring the overall biochemical imbalances, along with meeting the nutritional needs of the patient.

There are numerous possible causes of hypocalcemia [*see Table 4*]. The more acute problems are those that occur after thyroid or parathyroid operations. Patients who have undergone a total thyroidectomy have postoperative hypocalcemic symptoms that can be highly dramatic. Similarly, patients who have undergone a parathyroidectomy, in which all parathyroid tissue has been damaged or removed, can experience profound hypocalcemia.

Profound hypocalcemia is more commonly seen in patients who are undergoing a reoperation for parathyroid disease and in whom the amount of parathyroid tissue previously removed is unknown. These patients often have severe and long-standing hyperparathyroidism, along with the significant bone disease associated with it. Hypocalcemia can be compounded by two conditions: (1) hypoparathyroidism and (2) so-called hungry bones. Differentiation between these two entities is best achieved by measuring the serum phosphate levels. In hypoparathyroid patients, the serum phosphate level will rise, often to 6 mg/dl, whereas in patients with severe bone disease, the serum phosphate will remain low, despite the low calcium level. If symptoms attributed to hypocalcemia are not reversed by calcium replacement, magnesium deficiency should always be considered because it is a not uncommon cause of inability to restore serum calcium levels to normal.

Assessment of Magnesium Status

EVALUATION AND TREATMENT OF HYPOMAGNESEMIA

An estimated six to twelve percent of ambulatory and hospitalized patients are hypomagnesemic [*see Figure 3*]. Because

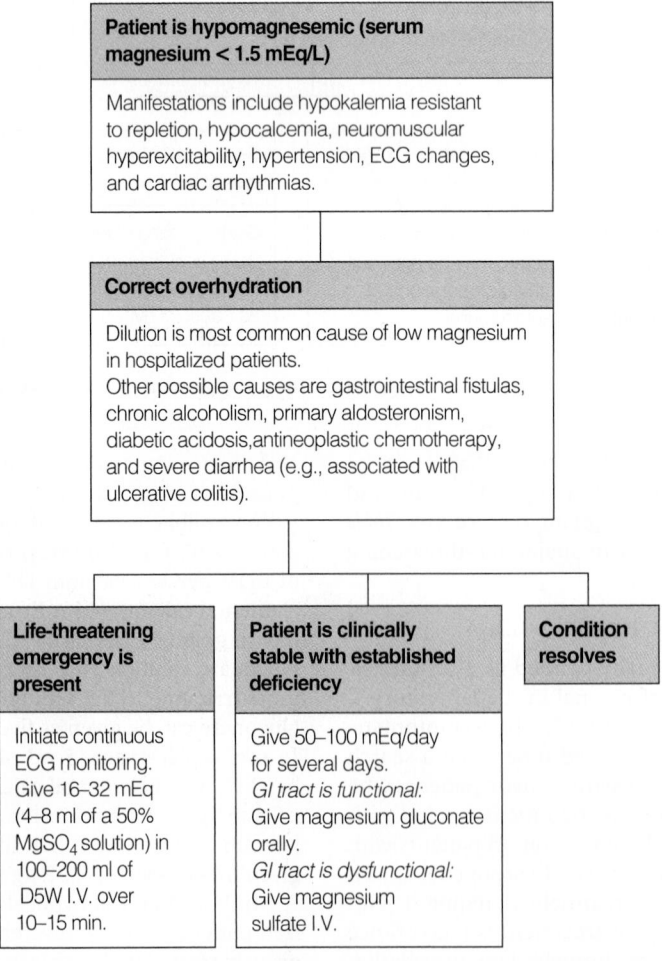

Figure 3 **Presented here are guidelines for management of hypomagnesemia.**

magnesium is not included in the usual panel of electrolytes, disorders of magnesium are often overlooked. The daily requirement for magnesium is about 10 to 30 mEq, and inadequate magnesium intake for as short a period as one week can result in hypomagnesemia. Vigilance and appropriate replacement can decrease the incidence of complications.

Common causes of hypomagnesemia in hospitalized patients include dilution, GI fistulas, diarrhea, prolonged bowel rest, alcoholism, diabetic ketoacidosis, primary aldosteronism, and excessive urinary losses resulting from chemotherapy (especially with cisplatin). Manifestations of magnesium deficiency include hypokalemia that is resistant to repletion, hypocalcemia, neuromuscular hyperexcitability, hypertension, ECG changes, and cardiac arrhythmias.[13]

In a life-threatening emergency, such as severe hypomagnesemia that is causing seizures, cardiac arrhythmias, or neuromuscular excitability, large doses of magnesium should be administered. In conjunction with continuous ECG monitoring, 16 to 32 mEq (4 to 8 ml of a 50 percent $MgSO_4$ solution) in 100 to 200 ml of five percent dextrose in water should be infused intravenously over 10 to 15 minutes.

In clinically stable patients with an established magnesium deficiency, it may be necessary to give 50 to 100 mEq/day for several days to replenish body stores. Patients at high risk for magnesium deficiency include those who are on bowel rest, those who are receiving total parenteral nutrition, and those who have chronic diarrhea or fistulas. Magnesium should be given intravenously (in a dose of 10 to 50 mEq) to patients with dysfunctional GI tracts; patients with functional GI tracts can receive magnesium orally. Although a 500 mg magnesium gluconate tablet supplies only 2.4 mEq of elemental magnesium (compared with 122.4 mEq from 15 g of $MgSO_4$ powder), it is much better tolerated than magnesium sulfate, which commonly causes diarrhea and abdominal cramps.

EVALUATION AND TREATMENT OF HYPERMAGNESEMIA

Hypermagnesemia is much less common than hypomagnesemia: it is seen only in renal insufficiency. In patients with renal failure who are on a normal diet and are taking no magnesium-containing supplements, serum magnesium levels will stabilize at about 2.5 mEq/L. If, however, magnesium-containing supplements (e.g., antacids) are being administered, plasma concentrations can reach 4 to 6 mEq/L, a level at which signs and symptoms of toxicity often begin to appear. At a serum magnesium level of 4 mEq/L, the most common symptoms are drowsiness, lethargy, diaphoresis, nausea, and vomiting. At higher levels, hyporeflexia and abnormal cardiac conduction are seen. As serum magnesium levels approach 10 mEq/L, respiratory paralysis, narcosis, hypotension, and even complete heart block may occur.[14]

Treatment consists of immediate withholding of all exogenous magnesium, hydration, and intravenous administration of calcium, starting with 90 to 180 mg (10 to 20 ml of a 10 percent calcium gluconate solution) over five to 10 minutes. The calcium will immediately reverse the effects of magnesium toxicity, but the effect is transient. Dialysis may be required to sustain a decrease in magnesium levels in patients with severe hypermagnesemia.

Discussion

Physiology of Body Fluids

Knowledge of the extent and composition of various body fluid compartments is a necessary basis for rational treatment of pathophysiological changes in electrolyte and water balance. Total body water generally constitutes between 50 and 70 percent of total body weight; however, it can be radically altered by a number of variables, including age, sex, and organ-specific or systemic disease. For example, in young men, total body water accounts for 60 percent of body weight, whereas in young women, it accounts for 50 percent. As a percentage of total body weight, total body water decreases steadily and significantly with age, eventually reaching a low of approximately 52 percent in men and 47 percent women. The percentage of total body weight accounted for by water is also higher in thin subjects than in obese ones and higher in infants than in adults.

The body water is divided into three functional compartments. The first, the intracellular compartment, accounts for 30 to 40 percent of body weight. Extracellular fluid represents approximately 20 percent of body weight; it can be further subdivided into intravascular fluid, or plasma (accounting for five percent of body weight), which makes up the second compartment, and interstitial, or extravascular, extracellular fluid (accounting for 15 percent of body weight), which makes up the third compartment.

INTRACELLULAR AND EXTRACELLULAR FLUID

Isotopic and biopsy studies of the intracellular compartment have yielded accurate measurements of the composition of intracellular fluid [see Figure 4]. In addition to water, its major constituents are potassium and magnesium, which are the principal cations, and phosphates and proteins, which are the principal anions.

The interstitial fluid has two main components, one of which equilibrates rather rapidly (functional) and the other relatively slowly (nonfunctional). The second component includes connective tissue water as well as what is termed transcellular water, which includes cerebrospinal fluid and joint fluids. This nonfunctional component of the interstitial fluid represents only a minor portion (10 percent) of the interstitial fluid volume and is not the same as the additional nonfunctional extracellular fluid, commonly referred to as third space, that is found after burns, soft tissue injuries, or surgery. In normal extracellular fluid, sodium is the predominant cation, and chloride and bicarbonate are the principal anions [see Figure 4]. The plasma compartment has a higher protein content; consequently, the total concentration of cations is higher and the concentration of inorganic anions somewhat lower than in the interstitial compartment. For clinical purposes, however, the concentration and composition of the plasma and the interstitial compartment can be considered to be equivalent.

Figure 4   **This schematic diagram represents the composition of plasma, interstitial fluid, and intracellular fluid.**[17]

OSMOTIC PRESSURE

The activity of electrolytes within a compartment depends on (1) the number of particles present per unit volume (mmol/L), (2) the number of electric charges per unit volume (mEq/L), and (3) the number of osmotically active particles or ions per unit volume (mOsm/L). The molar expression of a substance is commonly encountered, but this definition gives no information about the number of osmotically active particles in solution or about the electric charge present in solution. The electrolytes of the body are customarily expressed in terms of their chemical combining power or equivalents. Within any compartment, the number of equivalents of anions must balance the number of equivalents of cations.

The number of osmotically active particles within any given compartment is between 290 and 310 mOsm/L. Protein dissolved in the plasma compartment is responsible for the effective osmotic pressure between the plasma and the interstitial compartment, commonly referred to as the colloid oncotic pressure. Differences in ionic composition between the intracellular and extracellular fluid compartments are maintained by the cell wall, which functions as a semipermeable membrane. The effective osmotic pressure between the extracellular and intracellular fluid compartments is altered in proportion to the levels of substances that do not freely traverse the cell membrane. Sodium, which is the principal cation of the extracellular fluid, accounts for most of the osmotic pressure of the interstitial fluid. Other substances that do not penetrate the cell membrane freely, such as glucose, can also increase the effective osmotic pressure.

The effective osmotic pressure in the two compartments must be maintained. Because the cell membrane is completely perme-able to water, any condition that alters the effective osmotic pressure in either the intracellular or the extracellular compartment will result in redistribution of water. For example, an increase in serum sodium concentration will result in increased extracellular fluid volume, with a net transfer of water from intracellular to extracellular fluid. This transfer of water continues until the osmotic pressure between the two compartments is equalized. On the other hand, a reduction in serum sodium will result in a net transfer of water from the extracellular to the intracellular fluid compartment, whereas isosmotic depletion of the extracellular fluid, which does not change the concentration of ions, causes no transfer of water between compartments. Thus, the intracellular fluid is affected by losses that involve a change in the concentration or composition of the extracellular fluid, but it is affected little, if at all, by losses involving isotonic volume.

Pathophysiological Body Fluid Changes

Disorders of fluid and electrolyte balance may be generally classified into three categories: volume disturbances, concentration disturbances, and composition disturbances. Although these disturbances may be interrelated, and any or all of them may occur in clinically complex patterns, for purposes of management and interpretation of data, each one should be analyzed as a separate entity. Changes in volume are most readily identified as loss of isotonic saline solution from the extracellular fluid space. If the osmolarity in the intracellular and extracellular spaces remains unchanged, net transfer of fluid from the intracellular space to the depleted extracellular space is unlikely. If, however, water alone is added to or lost from the extracellular

Table 5 Normal Volume and Composition of Gastrointestinal Secretions

Secretion	Volume (L/day)	Concentration (mEq/L)			
		Na$^+$	K$^+$	Cl$^-$	HCO$_3^-$
Saliva	≈1	20–80	10–20	20–40	20–160
Gastric juice	1–2	20–100	5–10	120–160	—
Bile	≈1	150–250	5–10	40–60	20–60
Pancreatic juice	1–2	120	5–10	10–60	80–120
Succus entericus	1–2	140	5	variable	variable

fluid or the concentration of osmotically active particles changes, water will pass between the intracellular and extracellular spaces and so return the osmolarity to normal. The extracellular concentration of most ions—except for sodium, which is the dominant extracellular ion—can change without significantly affecting the total osmolarity. Such changes, commonly referred to as compositional changes, are infrequent when the kidneys are functioning normally.

VOLUME DISTURBANCES

Extracellular Fluid Volume Depletion

ECF volume depletion results from loss of both sodium and water, but the two constituents may be lost in differing proportions. For instance, the sodium content of gastrointestinal secretions varies widely throughout the GI tract; the precise amounts of sodium and water lost are governed by the source of the loss [see Table 5]. If the loss is isonatremic, the tonicity of the ECF is relatively unaffected and the intracellular volume will not change. If, however, as is common, water loss exceeds sodium loss (as in sweating, hyperventilation, nasogastric suction, and severe diarrhea), hypernatremia results, leading to increased ECF osmolarity and shifting of intracellular water to the extracellular compartment. By contrast, hyponatremia may result if excessive administration of fluid lowers the ECF sodium concentration below the normal level. Measurement of serum sodium only determines the concentration of sodium with respect to water: it provides no information about the absolute quantities of either substance present in the body.

Among the extrarenal causes of extracellular fluid volume depletion is volume depletion caused by losses of gastrointestinal fluid. Sequestration of fluid after injury may also result in significant extracellular fluid volume depletion if not enough of the lost fluid is replaced or if inappropriately concentrated solutions are administered. Preexisting renal or adrenal disease or previous administration of diuretics may lead to excess sodium loss in urine.

The aim of management is to restore reduced ECF volume by administering solutions designed to replace both the lost fluid and the lost electrolytes. Several different saline solutions can be used [see Table 6]. There is no standard formula for calculating the amount of saline required to correct ECF volume depletion. Consequently, the adequacy of repletion must be assessed clinically through physical signs, renal function, and hematocrit.

Extracellular Fluid Volume Excess

In surgical patients, ECF volume excess is usually iatrogenic or secondary to renal disease. It can be aggravated by coexisting conditions, such as congestive heart failure, nephrosis, cirrhosis, and conditions associated with hypoalbuminemia. These latter conditions are thought to result in a reduction of the effective arterial volume, leading to renal salt and water retention.

Table 6 Electrolyte Content of Parenteral Fluids (mEq/L)

Solution	Cations					Anions		
	Na$^+$	K$^+$	Ca^{2+}	Mg^{2+}	NH$_4^+$	Cl$^-$	HCO$_3^-$	HPO$_4^-$
Extracellular fluid	142	4	5	3	0.3	103	27	3
Lactated Ringer's solution	130	4	2.7			109	28*	
0.9% sodium chloride (saline)	154					154		
M/6 sodium lactate	167						167*	
M (molar) sodium lactate	1,000						1,000*	
3% sodium chloride	513					513		
5% sodium chloride	855					855		
0.9% ammonium chloride					168	168		

*Present in solution as lactate, which is converted to bicarbonate.

ABNORMALITIES OF SODIUM CONCENTRATION

Hyponatremia

Hyponatremia may be defined as a lower than normal concentration of sodium in the serum. Serum osmolarity is reduced. Because concentration is a measure not of total sodium but of the ratio of sodium to water, the presence of hyponatremia does not necessarily imply a deficit of body sodium; in fact, hyponatremia is often associated with an excess of total body salt (as in the edema-forming state). Consequently, an estimate of the total body sodium balance is necessary for the proper interpretation of an abnormality of serum sodium.

When there is no loss of sodium without water, hyponatremia is the net result of loss of isotonic or hypotonic fluid that is replaced by water without salt. In such circumstances, the administration of an isotonic saline solution is the treatment of choice because volume depletion is more threatening than hypotonicity, and water diuresis may be restored when volume depletion is corrected.

Water intoxication, which is usually caused by administration of water to patients unable to manifest a water diuresis (e.g., those who have just undergone operation or who have renal insufficiency), is usually managed by restriction of water intake. Administration of hypertonic saline may be indicated in those rare cases in which hyponatremia is severe and symptomatic. In such circumstances, administration of hypertonic saline solution should be used only to increase the serum sodium concentration to the point where clinical symptoms are resolved; it should not be used to restore serum sodium concentration to normal. This potentially dangerous mode of therapy can result in severe circulatory overload and therefore should be performed only in certain rare situations in which severe symptoms, such as delirium, exist. Careful physiologic monitoring is essential.

A state of severe hyponatremia that has been associated with SIADH may occur in a variety of disorders, most often in lesions of the pulmonary or central nervous system. The hyponatremia initially is a result of water retention but then is complicated by urinary loss of sodium. The essential criteria for diagnosis of this syndrome are (1) hyponatremia, (2) urine that is hypertonic to plasma at all times, even during water administration, (3) inappropriately large amounts of urinary sodium, even after water loading, (4) no renal or adrenal cause for this constellation of abnormalities, and (5) disappearance of all abnormalities after adequate restriction of water intake.

Both hyperglycemia and hyperlipidemia may increase extracellular osmolarity, thereby causing water to move from the intracellular to the extracellular compartment. As a result, the tonicity of extracellular fluid is underestimated; in general, however, no immediate therapy is required other than that aimed at rectifying the underlying metabolic disorder.

Hypernatremia

Hypernatremia leads to increased tonicity (osmolarity) and may result from either loss of water or gain of sodium. When hypernatremia is from loss of water, both intracellular and extracellular fluid compartments are diminished in volume; when it is from gain of sodium, extracellular fluid volume is increased, and intracellular fluid volume is decreased.

Hypernatremia most often occurs in patients unable to obtain free water. This inability may be the result of insufficient water intake, as in coma, vomiting, hypothalamic lesions, excessive sweating, hyperpnea, diarrhea, and polyuria of renal or extrarenal origin (e.g., diabetes insipidus or mellitus or administration of osmotic diuretics). Hypernatremia caused by pure salt gain is uncommon and usually iatrogenic but may be chronic in hyperaldosteronism and Cushing's syndrome.

Although urine volume is usually diminished and specific gravity increased during hypernatremia, the hematocrit may not be increased because of proportionate loss of plasma and red blood cell water. The change in ECF volume may be small unless water depletion is severe. The resulting loss of intracellular fluid volume leads to diminished skin turgor as well as to changes in pressure and in pressure regulation.

The usual treatment for hypernatremia is administration of solute-free water. The amount of water required is calculated according to the equation supplied earlier [see Assessment of Sodium Status, above].

Mixed Volume and Concentration Changes

The clinical picture associated with combined fluid and concentration abnormalities tends to be a composite of the signs and symptoms associated with each state. One of the more common mixed abnormalities is the combination of extracellular fluid deficit and hyponatremia. In surgical patients, this problem frequently occurs during the postoperative period, when lost gastrointestinal fluids are replaced with hypotonic or solute-free solutions. Extracellular fluid excess combined with hypernatremia is also seen in surgical patients, typically as a result of prolonged administration of excessive quantities of sodium salts and restricted water intake, as when pure water losses (such as insensible loss of water from skin and lungs) are replaced with sodium-containing solutions only. In patients with renal insufficiency and an associated inability to generate a water diuresis, excessive administration of water or hypotonic salt solutions may

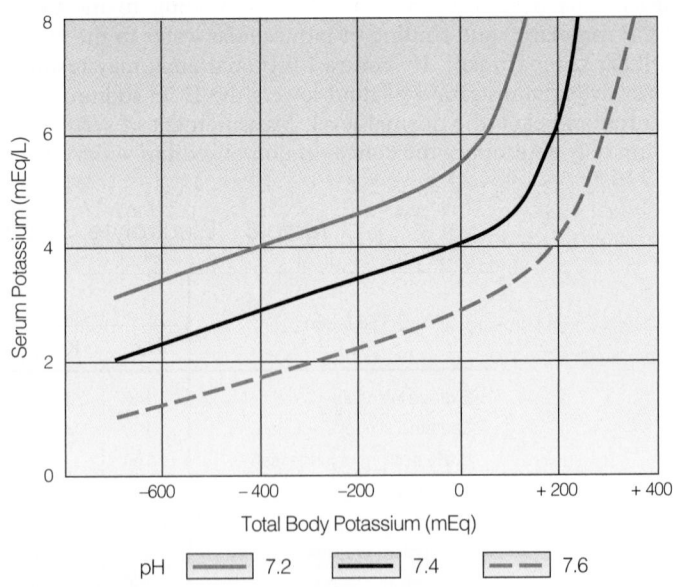

Figure 5 Serum potassium concentrations reflect total body potassium concentrations, as illustrated here. The effect of arterial pH on their relation is also shown.[18]

induce extracellular fluid volume excess in combination with hyponatremia.

ABNORMALITIES OF POTASSIUM CONCENTRATION

Body Balance

Urinary correction accounts for the majority of potassium lost from the body. The kidneys, which are responsible for regulating body potassium balance, are able to increase excretion in response to high potassium intake; however, they are less able to adjust to very low levels of potassium intake. There are no major renal conservation mechanisms for potassium, as there are for sodium; consequently, 5 to 10 mEq of potassium continues to appear in the urine even after a prolonged period of potassium-free intake.

On the whole, even though ECF contains only about two percent of total body potassium, the serum potassium concentration reflects the total body potassium content. Therefore, when total body potassium is elevated, serum concentration is high as well; when total body potassium is low, serum levels are also reduced [see Figure 5].

The distribution of potassium between intracellular and extracellular compartments can be influenced by many pathophysiological conditions. Large quantities of intracellular potassium may be released into the extracellular space as a consequence of severe injury, surgical stress, or acidosis or during catabolic states. In these conditions, there may be a significant rise in serum potassium if oliguric or anuric renal failure is present, but life-threatening hyperkalemia is rarely encountered when renal function is normal.

Hypokalemia

Reductions in serum potassium may result either from loss of potassium from the body or from a shift of potassium in the cells. Potassium deficiency in the surgical patient is commonly the result of excess losses; for practical purposes, the only potassium deficiencies caused by movement from serum to cells result from insulin use, respiratory alkalosis, or athletic training. Diarrhea, intestinal or biliary fistulas, ureteroenterostomy, vomiting, and nasogastric suction can all cause significant potassium losses from the gastrointestinal tract. Losses associated with vomiting or nasogastric suction may induce a potassium deficit greater than can be explained by the loss of potassium in fluids; such a deficit usually results from the enhanced urinary excretion of potassium that is associated with alkalosis and ECF volume contraction. Common causes of urinary loss of potassium include renal tubular disorders, osmotic diuresis, diuretic or corticosteroid therapies, Cushing's syndrome, hyperaldosteronism, and Bartter's syndrome. Reductions in circulating potassium level may also result from intracellular potassium shift resulting from administration of alkali or from parenteral administration of glucose or insulin without adequate potassium supplementation.

Although a mild depression in serum potassium may not be a life-threatening emergency, a risk assessment is essential in any patient with a serum potassium level of less than 3 mEq/L. A variety of oral supplementations providing potassium are available, including potassium chloride, which may be administered diluted in juice. Other potassium formulations, including potassium gluconate and potassium bicarbonate, are also available for oral administration and can be administered to patients whose serum chloride is normal. When hypokalemic alkalosis is present, however, potassium chloride is preferable because the chloride component is necessary for correction of the alkalosis and the associated chloride deficit.

Intravenous administration of potassium must always be undertaken with great caution and in conjunction with intensive monitoring. Rates of administration higher than 10 mEq/hr are seldom indicated except when signs of impending neuromuscular or cardiovascular collapse are present.

When there is evidence of potassium loss through gastrointestinal fluids, fluid replacement can be initiated, with the composition of the fluid to be determined by the level of the loss [see Table 5]. In such conditions, it is safe to replace the entire amount that it is anticipated will be lost because patients with normal renal function can easily handle any excess.

Hyperkalemia

Hyperkalemia invariably results from decreased renal excretion of potassium caused by intrinsic dysfunction or secondary to rapid release of potassium from cells after massive cellular injury or transcellular shifts related to a fall in blood pH. Artifactual elevations of serum potassium concentration may occur in association with an elevated platelet count or in conjunction with hemolysis or prolonged refrigeration of blood samples.

Hyperkalemia may be treated by measures that counteract the effects of potassium, those that force cellular entry of potassium, or those that actually remove potassium from the body. The urgency of the situation should be assessed on the basis both of the serum potassium concentration and of any ECG changes that are observed.

CALCIUM METABOLISM

Calcium is a key electrolyte in numerous body functions. The normal daily dietary intake of calcium is about 1,000 mg, and the overall net absorption is about 100 mg. Secretion into the intestine is variable but usually is about 300 mg; about 40 percent of what is ingested is absorbed [see Table 7].

Table 7 Calcium Metabolism

Total Body Calcium	
Exchangeable bone pool	4 g
Stable bone pool	1,000 g
Intracellular fluid	11 g
Extracellular fluid	0.9 g
GI tract	1.5 g
Calcium Lost Daily	
Feces	1 g
Urine	100 mg
Skin	30–100 mg
Calcium Exchanged Daily	
Bone	500 mg
GI tract	1 g
Glomerular filtrate	10 g

The greater part of the roughly 1,000 mg of calcium distributed throughout the extracellular fluid is exchanged with bone. This exchange is both rapid and slow. The exchangeable bone pool is approximately 4 g, and the stable bone pool is approximately 1,000 g. From 300 to 500 mg of calcium is exchanged with bone each day; accretion depends on the age of the patient. About 10,000 mg of calcium is exchanged daily by glomerular filtration, which means that the entire supply of extracellular fluid is exchanged 40 to 50 times every 24 hours. Virtually all excreted calcium is reabsorbed in the kidney; only 100 mg is excreted daily in the urine, and only 900 to 1,000 mg in the feces. Even in severe hypercalcemia, urinary excretion of calcium barely reaches 500 mg/day. This fact partially explains why in hypercalcemic states urinary excretion of calcium cannot compensate for the excess mobilization of bone calcium.

Plasma and blood levels remain stable within narrow limits, and disturbances of these levels can cause numerous abnormalities of function. The primary causes of disturbed calcium metabolism resulting in hypercalcemia are primary hyperparathyroidism and malignancy. In five to 10 percent of all cases of malignancy, elevated calcium levels will develop at some time in the course of the illness. Hypercalcemia is linked with a number of different neoplasms, the most common of which are breast cancer, renal cell cancer, lung cancer, and multiple myeloma. Primary hyperparathyroidism is common, occurring in up to 1,000 to 2,000 of the general population. There are numerous other causes of hypercalcemia, but they neither are as common as hyperparathyroidism or malignancy nor cause such severe hypercalcemia. Hyperparathyroidism and malignancy can coexist: of 100 patients with proven primary hyperparathyroidism in a cancer hospital, 34 (34 percent) also had a malignant disorder, whereas of 180 patients with proven primary hyperparathyroidism at an adjacent general hospital, 17 (nine percent) had a malignant disorder within a similar interval.[15] One review of patients with breast malignancy suggests that the prevalence of hyperparathyroidism in these patients is similar to that in the general population.[16]

MAGNESIUM METABOLISM

The total body content of magnesium is approximately 2,000 mEq. More than half of this amount is contained in bone; the remainder is distributed intracellularly. Only one percent is in the ECF, which means that the rate of magnesium loss must be slow because the exchangeable pool is turning over slowly. Normal intake is approximately 20 mEq/day; the majority is excreted in feces, and a lesser amount is excreted in urine. Virtually all absorbed magnesium is excreted by the kidneys. Magnesium plays a major role in intracellular enzyme function. The homeostatic mechanism by which it is controlled is not well understood, but it is known to involve parathyroid hormone. Urine has a strong tendency to retain magnesium, and normally functioning kidneys protect against excessive losses by this route.

References

1. Shires GT, Williams J, Brown F: Acute changes in extracellular fluids associated with major surgical procedures. Ann Surg 154:803, 1961

2. Wright HK, Gann DS: Correction of defect in free water excretion in postoperative patients by extracellular fluid volume expansion. Ann Surg 158:70, 1963

3. Schrier RW, Anderson RJ: Renal sodium excretion, edematous disorders, and diuretic use. Renal and Electrolyte Disorders, 2nd ed. Schrier RW, Ed. Little, Brown & Co, Boston, 1980

4. Goldberg M: Hyponatremia. Med Clin North Am 65:251, 1981

5. Van Zee KJ, Barie PS, Lowry SF: Electrolyte disorders. Current Surgical Therapy, 4th ed. Cameron JL, Ed. Mosby–Year Book, St Louis, 1992, p 1005

6. Feig PU, McCurdy DK: The hypertonic state. N Engl J Med 297:1444, 1977

7. Cox M: Potassium homeostasis. Med Clin North Am 65:363, 1981

8. Knochel JP: Etiologies and management of potassium deficiency. Hosp Pract 22:153, 1987

9. Allen EM, Singer FR, Melamed D: Electroencephalographic abnormalities in hypercalcemia. Neurology 20:15, 1970

10. Moure JMB: The electroencephalogram in hypercalcemia. Arch Neurol 17:34, 1967

11. Bilezikian JP: Management of acute hypercalcemia. N Engl J Med 326:1196, 1992

12. Warrell RP, Israel R, Frisone M, et al: Gallium nitrate for acute treatment of cancer-related hypercalcemia: a randomized, double-blind comparison to calcitonin. Ann Intern Med 108:669, 1988

13. England MR, Gordon G, Salem M, et al: Magnesium administration and dysrhythmias after cardiac surgery: a placebo-controlled, double-blind, randomized trial. JAMA 268:2395, 1992

14. Agus ZS, Massry SG: Hypomagnesemia and hypermagnesemia. Maxwell & Kleeman's Clinical Disorders of Fluid and Electrolyte Metabolism, 5th ed. Narins RG, Ed. McGraw-Hill, New York, 1994, p 1099

15. Farr HW: Hyperparathyroidism and cancer. CA Cancer J Clin 26:66, 1976

16. Axelrod DM, Bockman RS, Wong GY, et al: Distinguishing features of primary hyperparathyroidism in breast cancer patients. Cancer 60:1620, 1987

17. Shires GT, Canizaro PC, Lowry SF: Fluid, electrolyte, and nutritional management of the surgical patient. Principles of Surgery, 4th ed. Schwartz SI, Shires GT, Spencer FC, et al, Eds. McGraw-Hill Book Co, New York, 1984, p 45

18. Taggart DD: Fluid and electrolyte disturbances. Manual of Medical Therapeutics, 20th ed. Rosenfeld MG, Ed. Little, Brown & Co, Boston, 1971

Acknowledgments

Figures 1 through 3   Talar Agasyan.

Figures 4 and 5   Al Miller.

7 LIFE-THREATENING ACID-BASE DISORDERS

Lena M. Napolitano, M.D., and Anthony A. Meyer, M.D., Ph.D.

Evaluation of Acid-Base Imbalance

Normal acid-base balance is maintained via complex interactions among the cardiovascular, renal, pulmonary, gastrointestinal, and hepatic systems. Perturbations in one or more of these systems result in the many different disorders of acid-base metabolism. These disorders vary with respect to cause, severity of presentation, and management. For all of them, however, the fundamental goal of management is to reestablish acid-base homeostasis.

Given that acid-base disorders are very common in critically ill patients, a working knowledge of these conditions is essential for any physician who treats such patients. Early diagnosis and early therapeutic intervention may prevent serious complications. In what follows, we place special emphasis on those acid-base disorders that are common in surgical patients and on those that are potentially life-threatening.

Definitions and Measurement Issues

Arterial pH is very tightly regulated and is normally maintained between 7.35 and 7.45. Because mixed venous carbon dioxide tension ($P_{mv}CO_2$) is higher than arterial carbon dioxide tension (P_aCO_2) as a result of production of CO_2 by tissues, venous pH is usually slightly lower than arterial pH. Consequently, acid-base balance can be more accurately determined by using arterial blood samples, which is therefore highly recommended.

The following definitions will be used throughout the chapter:

- Acidemia: a blood pH value lower than 7.35.
- Alkalemia: a blood pH value higher than 7.45.
- Acidosis: a physiologic process that causes acidemia if not compensated.
- Alkalosis: a physiologic process that causes alkalemia if not compensated.

TEMPERATURE CORRECTION FOR ARTERIAL BLOOD SAMPLES

It is known that temperature variation alters measured blood gas values in vitro, thereby changing measured pH in a linear fashion.[1] Although arterial blood samples are drawn at the patient's body temperature, which may be lower or higher than normal, they are always warmed or cooled to 37° C before undergoing analysis for measurement of pH, P_aCO_2, and arterial oxygen tension (P_aO_2). The numbers obtained, therefore, reflect what pH, P_aCO_2, and P_aO_2 would be if the patient's temperature were 37° C, not necessarily what they are at the patient's actual body temperature.

Temperature correction is the process by which mathematical adjustments based on the patient's true body temperature at the time of blood sampling are applied to the arterial blood gas values obtained at 37° C to make these values a more accurate reflection of the true in vivo values. There is considerable controversy regarding whether such temperature correction is necessary; it is not clear whether it has any real impact on either clinical interpretation or the choice of therapeutic intervention.[2,3] In our view, uncorrected arterial blood gas values provide the most useful information for assessment and management of acid-base disturbances in hypothermic patients; corrected values have little clinical relevance. In most cases, therefore, temperature correction of arterial blood samples for acid-base analysis is unnecessary.[4]

MEASURED VERSUS CALCULATED BICARBONATE CONCENTRATION

In the evaluation of acid-base balance, it is extremely important to consider the bicarbonate concentration. The bicarbonate concentration in serum or arterial blood can be either measured directly or calculated by means of the Henderson-Hasselbalch equation:

$$pH = pK_a + \log \frac{[HCO_3^-]}{[H_2CO_3]}$$

As a rule, the carbonic acid (H_2CO_3) concentration is not measured directly in clinical laboratories, but it can be approximated by multiplying P_aCO_2 by the CO_2 solubility coefficient, for which the generally accepted value is 0.0301 at physiologic pH.

In most cases, calculated values for the bicarbonate concentration are roughly equivalent to measured values. Sometimes, however, they differ by as much as 7 to 8 mEq/L. When this occurs, the measured bicarbonate concentration is considered correct: the CO_2 solubility coefficients used in the Henderson-Hasselbalch equation may change in patients with acute acid-base disorders, and such change renders calculated bicarbonate concentrations less accurate. For this reason, assessment of acid-base homeostasis should make use of the bicarbonate value that is directly measured in the serum electrolyte panel, not the calculated value that is derived from arterial blood gas analysis.

Primary versus Mixed Acid-Base Disturbances

The primary acid-base disturbances are metabolic acidosis, respiratory acidosis, metabolic alkalosis, and respiratory alkalosis. When one of these primary acid-base disturbances is present and chemical buffering is unable to prevent a change in pH, the body initiates compensatory responses in an attempt to maintain electrical neutrality. These compensatory responses are dependent on the renal sys-

Patient has acid-base imbalance

Metabolic acidosis (pH < 7.35, P_aco_2 < 40 mm Hg)

Condition is life-threatening (pH < 7.2)

Correct hypoxemia, hypovolemia, and hypoperfusion.

Initiate fluid resuscitation.

Consider placing a central venous or pulmonary arterial catheter.

Consider HCO_3^- therapy to raise pH to ≥ 7.2.

Condition is not life-threatening

Identify and treat cause of acidosis

Calculate anion gap:
Anion gap = $[Na^+] - ([Cl^-] + [HCO_3^-])$

Anion gap is increased

Possible causes include
• Lactic acidosis
• Diabetic ketoacidosis
• Alcoholic ketoacidosis
• Renal failure
• Ingestion of toxins
• Rhabdomyolysis

Anion gap is normal

Possible causes include
• Excessive HCO_3^- loss
    Diarrhea
    Enteric fistulas
    Ureterosigmoidostomy
    Renal tubular acidosis
    Carbonic anhydrase
        inhibitors (e.g.,
        acetazolamide)
• Hypoaldosteronism
• Addison's disease
• Excessive acid
    administration

Respiratory acidosis (pH < 7.35, P_aco_2 < 40 mm Hg)

Condition is life-threatening (pH < 7.2, P_aco_2 > 60 mm Hg, or patient has respiratory distress or is unresponsive)

Perform emergency endotracheal intubation and institute mechanical ventilation.

Condition is not life-threatening

Determine whether there is a history of pulmonary disease or chronic hypercapnia.

Identify and treat cause of acidosis

Airway obstruction

Possible causes include
• Laryngospasm
• Foreign body
• External compression
• Sleep apnea

For laryngospasm, correct the cause and give racemic epinephrine.

For external compression, correct problem surgically.

Pulmonary disease

Conditions that may be present include
• Asthma exacerbation
• COPD
• Pneumonia
• Empyema
• Pulmonary edema
• ARDS
• Pneumothorax
• Hemothorax

For asthma, give bronchodilators and consider high-dose steroid therapy if pulmonary inflammation is present

Respiratory muscle weakness

Possible causes include
• Hypokalemia
• Hypophosphatemia
• Neuromuscular blockade
• Aminoglycosides
• Muscular and neurologic disorders

Correct electrolyte abnormalities and provide nutritional support.

Reverse neuromuscular blockade.

Depressed respiratory drive

Possible causes include
• Drugs
• CNS pathology
• Primary idiopathic alveolar hypoventilation

Reverse effects of narcotics or sedatives. Avoid excessive O_2 therapy.

Metabolic alkalosis (pH > 7.45, P_aco_2 > 35 mm Hg)

Respiratory alkalosis (pH > 7.45, P_aco_2 < 35 mm Hg)

Condition is life-threatening (pH > 7.6, [HCO₃⁻] > 40 mEq/L)

Condition is not life-threatening

Consider administering acetazolamide, 250–500 mg I.V.

If this is ineffective, calculate chloride deficit: Cl⁻ deficit = 0.2 L/kg x weight (kg) × (103 – [Cl⁻]) [mEq/L]).

Administer exogenous acid (0.1N HCl solution) at a rate no faster than 2 mEq/kg/hr or 125 ml/hr.

Condition is life-threatening (pH > 7.6, P_aco_2 < 20 mm Hg, or cardiac arrhythmias are present)

Condition is not life-threatening

Consider emergency intubation and mechanical ventilation.

Identify and treat cause of alkalosis

Identify and treat cause of alkalosis

Obtain spot measurement of urine [Cl⁻].

Central causes

Possible causes include
- Anxiety
- Pain
- Hypoxemia
- Sepsis
- Intracranial pathology
- Hepatic encephalopathy

Consider anxiolytic therapy, supplemental O_2, pain medication, and treatment of infection.

For possible intracranial pathology, perform CT scan of the head.

[Cl⁻] > 10 mEq/L

Alkalosis is saline-responsive. Possible causes include
- Gastric drainage
- GI loss of HCl via vomiting
- Diuretic therapy
- Overshoot from alkalinizing therapy
- Excess acetate in parenteral nutrition solutions

Restore fluid volume with normal saline.

Correct hypokalemia with KCl.

Give H_2 receptor blockers to decrease H^+ secretion.

Consider discontinuing diuretics.

Pulmonary causes

Possible causes include
- Asthma
- Pneumonia
- Pulmonary embolism
- Congestive heart failure
- Atelectasis
- Pneumothorax

Treat underlying pulmonary disorder.

[Cl⁻] > 20 mEq/L

Alkalosis is saline-unresponsive. Possible causes include
- Mineralocorticoid excess
- Primary aldosteronism
- Cushing's syndrome
- Hypokalemia
- Hypomagnesemia
- Hypophosphatemia

Correct electrolyte abnormalities.

Remove mineralocorticoid source or block action of mineralocorticoid with spironolactone or amiloride.

Iatrogenic causes

Possible causes include
- Inappropriate ventilator management
- Drugs

Adjust mechanical ventilation.

Discontinue drug responsible for alkalosis; if this is not possible, adjust dose.

Evaluation of Acid-Base Imbalance

Table 1   Expected Compensation for Primary Acid-Base Disorders[31,32]

Disorder	Primary Event*	Compensation	Rate of Compensation
Metabolic acidosis	$\downarrow [HCO_3^-]$	$\downarrow P_aCO_2$	For 1 mEq/L $\downarrow [HCO_3^-]$, $P_aCO_2 \downarrow$ 1–1.5 mm Hg
Metabolic alkalosis	$\uparrow [HCO_3^-]$	$\uparrow P_aCO_2$	For 1 mEq/L $\uparrow [HCO_3^-]$, $P_aCO_2 \uparrow$ 0.5–1 mm Hg
Respiratory acidosis Acute (< 12–24 hr) Chronic (3–5 days)	 $\uparrow P_aCO_2$ $\uparrow P_aCO_2$	 $\uparrow [HCO_3^-]$ $\uparrow\uparrow [HCO_3^-]$	 For 10 mm Hg $\uparrow P_aCO_2$, $[HCO_3^-] \uparrow$ 1 mEq/L For 10 mm Hg $\uparrow P_aCO_2$, $[HCO_3^-] \uparrow$ 4 mEq/L
Respiratory alkalosis Acute (< 12 hr) Chronic (1–2 days)	 $\downarrow P_aCO_2$ $\downarrow P_aCO_2$	 $\downarrow [HCO_3^-]$ $\downarrow\downarrow [HCO_3^-]$	 For 10 mm Hg $\downarrow P_aCO_2$, $[HCO_3^-] \downarrow$ 1–3 mEq/L For 10 mm Hg $\downarrow P_aCO_2$, $[HCO_3^-] \downarrow$ 2–5 mEq/L

*Normal serum $[HCO_3^-]$ is 24 mEq/L; normal P_aCO_2 is 40 mm Hg.

tem and the pulmonary system. Primary metabolic disorders evoke compensatory respiratory changes, whereas primary respiratory disorders evoke compensatory metabolic changes. For instance, metabolic acidosis, which is characterized by a decreased blood bicarbonate concentration, initiates compensatory hyperventilation, which decreases P_aCO_2. Similarly, respiratory acidosis, which is characterized by increased P_aCO_2, initiates a renal compensatory change that raises the blood bicarbonate concentration. Whether renal or respiratory, these compensatory responses act in essentially the same way: they attempt to counteract the change in pH by reversing the change in the ratio of P_aCO_2 to $[HCO_3^-]$.

The compensatory metabolic and respiratory changes that occur in response to primary acid-base disorders are quite predictable. When the individual patient's compensatory responses fall outside the usual range [*see Table 1*], there are two main possibilities: either not enough time has passed for compensation to occur or the patient has a mixed acid-base disorder—that is, a combination of primary acid-base disorders (e.g., respiratory acidosis and metabolic alkalosis in a patient with chronic obstructive pulmonary disease [COPD] who is receiving diuretics).

Metabolic Acidosis

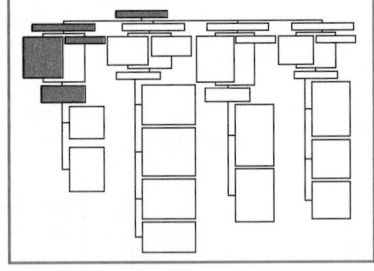

Of the primary acid-base disorders, metabolic acidosis is the one that is most often life-threatening in surgical patients. It is characterized by a loss of bicarbonate or an accumulation of fixed acids, either of which can lead to a decrease in pH.

In surgical patients, life-threatening metabolic acidosis is most often the result of inadequate oxygen delivery as a consequence of inadequate perfusion from hypovolemia or blood loss. Treatment must therefore be directed at restoration of perfusion and correction of the underlying disorder whenever possible. Restoration of perfusion is accomplished by means of fluid resuscitation with crystalloid, colloid, or blood products, depending on the patient's clinical condition. If the patient is healthy, intravascular volume resuscitation can be guided by simple measures of urine output. If, however, the patient has cardiac disease or other medical problems, such as respiratory insufficiency or renal insufficiency, placement of a pulmonary artery catheter to guide resuscitation should be considered. Severe metabolic acidosis can also be caused by inadequate oxygen delivery resulting from hypoxemia, anemia, or inadequate cardiac output, especially in critically ill patients.

It is rarely necessary to administer sodium bicarbonate to patients with acute metabolic acidosis, provided that aggressive fluid resuscitation and treatment of underlying disorders are initiated promptly. Experimental studies have documented that cardiac function and catecholamine responsiveness are unaffected as long as pH remains at or above 7.2. In addition, metabolic acidosis causes the oxyhemoglobin dissociation curve to shift to the right, thereby augmenting oxygen delivery [*see Figure 1*]. Consequently, we do not recommend bicarbonate treatment for clinically stable patients with metabolic acidosis and a pH of 7.2 or higher.

Once blood pH falls below 7.2, however, the risk of cardiac dysfunction and arrhythmias is increased, and life-threatening problems may occur suddenly. When metabolic acidosis is life-threatening secondary to impairment of cardiac function, judicious administration of sodium bicarbonate may be required. It is important, however, to titrate bicarbonate therapy very carefully to prevent iatrogenic metabolic alkalosis. Iatrogenic metabolic alkalosis may be difficult to correct and may impair oxygen delivery to the tissues by decreasing cardiac contractility and shifting the oxyhemoglobin dissociation curve to the left [*see Figure 1*], thereby causing hemoglobin to bind oxygen more avidly. In addition, the bicarbonate ad-

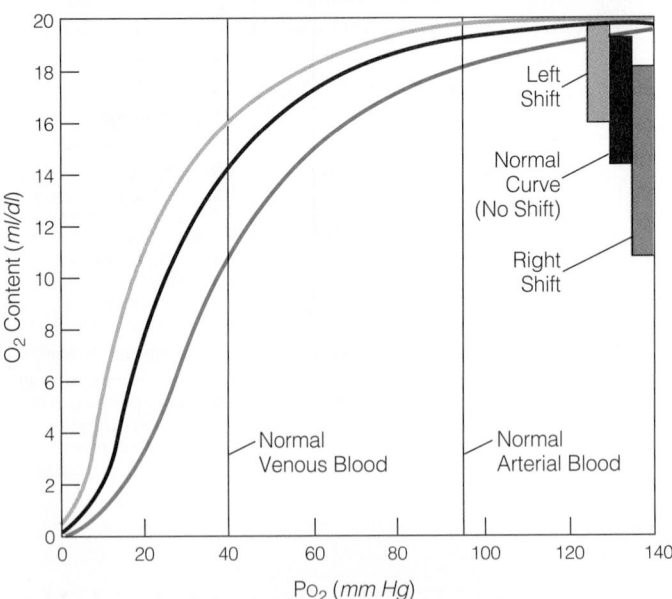

Figure 1   Depicted is the oxyhemoglobin dissociation curve. Shifting this curve to the left (light-red line and bar) or the right (dark-red line and bar) affects the amount of oxygen available for extraction by tissues.

ministered constitutes an excess alkali load that must be excreted by the body.

Metabolic acidosis can be divided into two broad categories on the basis of whether the anion gap is increased or normal. The anion gap is the difference between measured cations and measured anions in serum. This difference does not reflect a true disparity between positive and negative charges, given that serum actually is electrically neutral when all serum cations and anions are measured. Rather, the anion gap is a measurement artifact resulting from the fact that only certain cations and anions (Na^+, K^+, Cl^-, and HCO_3^-) are routinely measured. The anion gap is usually calculated by subtracting the serum chloride and bicarbonate concentrations from the serum sodium concentration:

$$Anion\ gap = [Na^+] - ([Cl^-] + [HCO_3^-])$$

The normal range for the anion gap is 8 to 12 mEq/L.

INCREASED ANION GAP

Metabolic acidosis with an increased anion gap is secondary to the addition of endogenous or exogenous acid. There are numerous possible causes. When it has been determined that an increased anion gap metabolic acidosis is present, there are 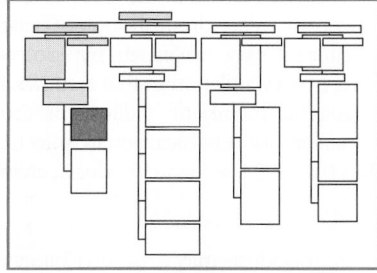 specific laboratory values the surgeon should consider obtaining: arterial or mixed venous lactate concentrations, serum and urine ketone levels, blood glucose levels, serum potassium concentrations, blood urea nitrogen (BUN) and serum creatinine concentrations, and blood alcohol levels. Serum and urine toxic drug screens should be considered as well. Blood creatine kinase levels and urine myoglobin concentrations should be measured if rhabdomyolysis is a possibility. Other values that are useful in the assessment of increased anion gap metabolic acidosis are methanol and ethylene glycol levels and serum osmolality. The results of these laboratory tests should help determine the cause of the acidosis. If, however, a patient appears underperfused and the increased anion gap metabolic acidosis improves with therapy, further workup usually is not necessary.

Lactic Acidosis

Inadequate tissue perfusion leads to inadequate aerobic metabolism at the cellular level and triggers anaerobic metabolism, which results in the production of lactic acid and an increased anion gap metabolic acidosis [see Discussion, *below*]. The right shift in the oxyhemoglobin dissociation curve facilitates the release of oxygen to the tissues as a protective mechanism. When tissue oxygenation is restored to normal through resuscitation and improvement of oxygen delivery, the lactic acid that has accumulated as a result of anaerobic metabolism is rapidly metabolized to bicarbonate by the liver and the kidneys, and the metabolic acidosis resolves.

Tissue hypoperfusion is the most common cause of lactic acidosis in critically ill patients. Prolonged hypoperfusion leads to tissue hypoxia and cellular acidosis and can trigger a cascade of events that leads to irreversible damage and cell death unless oxygen delivery is promptly reestablished [see Figure 2]. Consequently, the most important treatment priority in these patients is to restore tissue perfusion rapidly by improving oxygen delivery and limiting oxygen consumption as much as possible. Oxygen delivery may be improved by increasing cardiac output (through volume resuscitation or inotropic support), increasing the hemoglobin concentration (through trans-

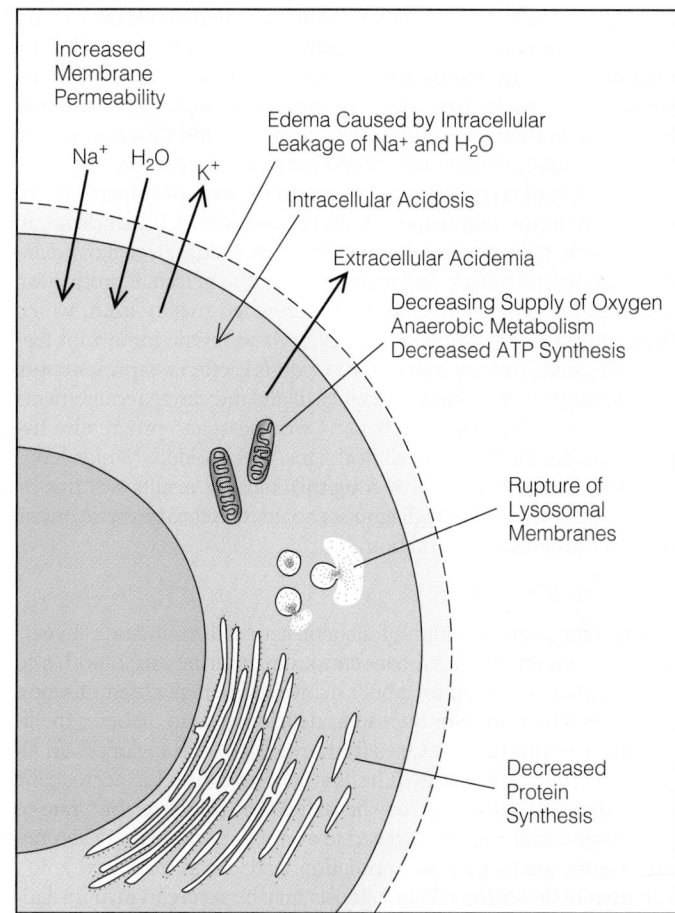

Figure 2   **Energy pathways are affected by cellular changes that are associated with hypoxia. Decreased production of adenosine triphosphate (ATP) and loss of cellular integrity result.**[29]

fusion of red blood cells), or increasing arterial oxygen saturation. Oxygen consumption may be decreased by administering sedatives judiciously, eliminating fever and shivering, or instituting mechanical ventilation in patients with increased work of breathing [see VII:1 *Cardiopulmonary Monitoring*].

The morbidity and mortality associated with lactic acidosis are related to the severity of the acidosis and the response of the underlying disorder to treatment. Severe, acute lactic acidosis is associated with a low survival rate; the survival rate is inversely correlated with the blood lactate concentration. Bicarbonate therapy may actually increase morbidity and mortality in patients with severe, life-threatening acidosis; however, judicious use of such therapy to raise pH to 7.2 or higher may still be prudent, especially in patients with myocardial dysfunction. Administration of dichloroacetate (DCA), which enhances cardiac output and promotes oxidation of pyruvate and lactate by stimulating pyruvate dehydrogenase activity, may eventually prove to be an important therapeutic modality for patients with severe, unremitting lactic acidosis.[5,6]

In the absence of renal or hepatic insufficiency, blood lactate concentrations can help quantitate the degree of tissue hypoxia present or the extent to which perfusion is inadequate. They can also be useful in monitoring the patient's response to therapeutic interventions, such as fluid resuscitation, transfusion, or augmentation of cardiac output. Only values obtained from arterial or mixed venous blood samples should be relied on, however. Peripheral venous lactate concentrations reflect regional, rather than systemic, perfusion and lactate metabolism; arterial lactate concentrations, on the other hand, reflect the net effect of lactate production and hepatic clearance, and mixed venous concentrations correlate very well with arterial lactate measurements. In addition, the specimen should be quickly transported on ice to the laboratory for immediate analysis because red blood cells continue to produce lactate in vitro and thus may generate a spurious elevation in the blood lactate concentration.

If the patient is receiving a continuous infusion of epinephrine or nitroprusside, discontinuation should be considered. Either drug can cause lactic acidosis, epinephrine by stimulating glycogen breakdown in skeletal muscle and increasing the rate of lactate production and nitroprusside by releasing cyanide when metabolized, which then can uncouple oxidative phosphorylation. One important feature of cyanide toxicity is that lactic acidosis is often not present until the late stages of the illness. Tolerance of and increasing requirements for nitroprusside, headache, nausea, weakness, and progressive hypotension are the common clinical signs. Whole blood cyanide levels can be measured (normal < 5 μg/ml), but the results will not be available immediately; the diagnosis should therefore be made on the basis of the clinical presentation.

Diabetic Ketoacidosis

The typical presentation of diabetic ketoacidosis includes hyperglycemia, elevated ketone concentrations in urine and blood, and an increased anion gap metabolic acidosis. When glucose utilization is impaired by fasting or by insulin deficiency, as in diabetes mellitus, the liver produces ketones from free fatty acids to supply an alternative source of energy. The first ketone formed is acetoacetic acid, which subsequently may be reduced to β-hydroxybutyrate or nonenzymatically decarboxylated to acetone. Because these ketones are organic acids, their accumulation leads to an increased anion gap metabolic acidosis. Ketoacidosis may be severe in insulin-deficient patients with diabetes mellitus; insulin deficiency impairs ketone utilization as well as glucose utilization, and it promotes lipolysis, which causes more free fatty acids to be delivered to the liver and converted into keto acids.

The test that is used to measure keto acids in blood and urine—the nitroprusside test—is not entirely accurate: it may underestimate the degree of ketoacidosis or even fail to detect it in severe cases. The reason is that the nitroprusside test detects only acetoacetate and acetone, not β-hydroxybutyrate, which is the most prevalent keto acid in all types of ketoacidosis. A simple way of compensating for this flaw is to add a few drops of hydrogen peroxide to a urine sample. The hydrogen peroxide nonenzymatically converts the β-hydroxybutyrate to acetoacetate, which is detectable by the nitroprusside test.[7]

The aim of therapy for diabetic ketoacidosis is to correct hypovolemia, hyperglycemia, ketoacidosis, and potassium and phosphorus depletion. Because insulin deficiency is responsible for many of these abnormalities, insulin administration is extremely important. Exogenous insulin administration helps correct the hyperglycemia, reduces ketoacidosis by increasing peripheral ketone utilization, and limits further ketone production by decreasing the rate of lipolysis and decreasing glucagon secretion. Initially, regular insulin is administered as an intravenous bolus; it has a half-life of only 4 to 5 minutes and is completely cleared from plasma within 30 minutes. Subsequently, regular insulin is administered by continuous intravenous infusion so that the amount of insulin required to lower the plasma glucose concentration into the normal range can be accurately determined. Regular insulin should not be administered to critically ill patients by the subcutaneous route. Absorption may be erratic if this is done, especially in patients who require vigorous volume resuscitation and in whom anasarca may develop.

Fluid resuscitation corrects the hypovolemia present in diabetic ketoacidosis. Fluid resuscitation also helps correct hyperglycemia and ketoacidosis by virtue of its dilutional effect, and it leads to improved renal function and thus improved renal glucose clearance. Serum creatinine concentrations are often falsely elevated in patients with diabetic ketoacidosis because acetoacetate can be mismeasured as creatinine.

Potassium replacement is necessary in all patients with diabetic ketoacidosis, even though serum potassium concentrations may be normal or high initially. These deceptive findings reflect the movement of potassium from the cells into the extracellular space secondary to insulin deficiency and hyperglycemia. Continuous ECG monitoring is necessary in all cases as well: the acid-base and potassium imbalances place these patients at risk for severe cardiac dysrhythmias.

Phosphate depletion is also a common finding in patients with diabetic ketoacidosis. Routine phosphate replacement is not recommended, however: two clinical studies have documented that it has no effect on morbidity or outcome, does not accelerate correction of electrolyte abnormalities, and may induce hyperphosphatemia or hypocalcemia.[8-10] Phosphate therapy is therefore reserved for patients with severe (serum phosphate < 1.0 mEq/dl) or symptomatic hypophosphatemia. Administration of bicarbonate should also be avoided because it may exacerbate hyperosmolality and hypokalemia, prolong hyperventilation so that respiratory alkalosis develops, and cause iatrogenic metabolic alkalosis as the keto acids are metabolized. Small amounts of bicarbonate may be indicated when arterial pH is less than 7.2 [see Lactic Acidosis, above].

Alcoholic Ketoacidosis

Ketoacidosis may arise after binge drinking or sudden abstinence on the part of an alcoholic, usually in association with low food intake or vomiting. Alcoholic ketoacidosis results from the interplay among the effects of ethanol, starvation, and volume depletion. Alcoholic ketoacidosis can be differentiated from diabetic ketoacidosis by the absence of significant hyperglycemia. Perhaps surprisingly, serum ethanol concentrations may be low in patients with alcoholic ketoacidosis; this condition usually occurs with abstinence or 1 to 3 days after heavy drinking, by which time the ethanol has undergone oxidation by the liver. Serum ketone levels may be low as well. The ratio of β-hydroxybutyrate to acetoacetate is higher in patients with alcoholic ketoacidosis than in those with diabetic ketoacidosis because of the NADH production consequent to the oxidation of alcohol. As a result, the nitroprusside test, being unable to measure β-hydroxybutyrate [see Diabetic Ketoacidosis, above], typically yields a weakly positive or even a negative reaction. Patients who have alcoholic ketoacidosis often respond dramatically to fluid resuscitation and usually do not require bicarbonate therapy. Infusion of glucose decreases keto acid formation in the liver, and infusion of saline promotes renal clearance of keto acids.

Acute and Chronic Renal Failure

Increased anion gap metabolic acidosis occurs in renal failure as a consequence of decreased renal ammoniagenesis and decreased excretion of titratable acids. Patients with advanced renal failure cannot excrete the fixed acids (phosphate, sulfates, and other organic acids) generated as by-products of the body's normal metabolic processes, and the accumulation of these acids leads to the increased anion gap metabolic acidosis. For metabolic acidosis caused by chronic renal failure, treatment is rarely required; for severe metabolic acidosis caused by acute renal failure, supplemental bicarbonate therapy may be necessary.

Ingestion of Toxins

Salicylate Salicylate intoxication may give rise to an increased anion gap metabolic acidosis as a result of the accumulation of salicylate anion and other organic anions, such as lactate and keto anions. Salicylates also uncouple oxidative phosphorylation, thereby increasing the production of organic acids and CO_2. The diagnosis of salicylate intoxication should be considered in any patient who has an increased anion gap metabolic acidosis of unknown origin. Chemical determination of blood salicylate levels establishes the diagnosis: levels higher than 30 mg/dl are considered above the therapeutic limit. Therapy is instituted immediately. The first step is to ensure that the airway is open and that oxygenation and ventilation are adequate. Correction of fluid deficits is mandatory. Gastric lavage and administration of charcoal are then undertaken to prevent further absorption of salicylates from the GI tract.

In systemic acidemia, the nonionized form of salicylate (the form that enters the cells) becomes more prevalent, which means that tissue uptake is increased. In addition, the nonionized species is reabsorbed in the renal tubules, whereas the ionized form is not, which means that renal excretion of salicylates is lower than normal. Immediate correction of systemic acidemia is therefore of utmost importance. Respiratory acidosis (which may also be present in salicylate intoxication as a result of hypoventilation) is corrected by mechanical ventilation, and metabolic acidosis is corrected by the administration of bicarbonate until a mild systemic alkalemia (pH = 7.46 to 7.49) is achieved. Urinary alkalinization also prevents tubular reabsorption and promotes effective renal excretion of the salicylates. Dialysis is reserved for patients who have renal dysfunction or life-threatening complications.

Methanol and ethylene glycol Ketoacidosis may occur in adult alcoholics as a result of methanol or ethylene glycol ingestion. Both drugs are consumed as cheap alternatives to ethanol. Methanol is used in industry and is being studied as an energy source; ethylene glycol is found in antifreeze solutions. Methanol and ethylene glycol are rapidly converted to toxic metabolites (formic acid and glycolic acid, respectively) in the liver, and even small amounts of these metabolites may be lethal. In determining whether ethanol, methanol, or ethylene glycol is responsible for an increased anion gap metabolic acidosis, it may be helpful to calculate the serum osmolal gap, which is the difference between measured serum osmolality and calculated serum osmolality. Calculated serum osmolality is derived by using three variables: sodium ion concentration, BUN, and glucose concentration. If ethanol is present and the blood ethanol concentration is available, a fourth expression (ethanol [mg/dl]/4.6) should be added to the calculation.

$$\text{Calculated serum osmolality (mOsm/L)} =$$
$$2[Na^+]\,(mEq/L) + \frac{BUN\,(mg/dl)}{2.8} + \frac{glucose\,(mg/dl)}{18}$$

Normally, the serum osmolal gap is less than 10 mOsm/L. An increased osmolal gap indicates the presence in plasma of an osmotically active substance that normally is absent. The substances that most frequently cause an increased osmolal gap are ethanol, ketones, lactate, mannitol, methanol, and ethylene glycol.

Therapy for methanol or ethylene glycol ingestion should be instituted immediately and should include gastric lavage, administration of activated charcoal (to remove unabsorbed toxin), intravenous infusion of ethanol (to competitively inhibit metabolism of methanol or ethylene glycol to their toxic metabolites), and, in life-threatening situations, hemodialysis.

Paraldehyde Paraldehyde has been used clinically as a sedative and an anticonvulsant; currently, however, it is rarely given. Paraldehyde intoxication is associated with an increased anion gap meta-

bolic acidosis, hyperkalemia, and leukocytosis. The increased anion gap acidosis is likely to be secondary to increased concentrations of β-hydroxybutyrate, which means that the nitroprusside test commonly yields negative results in these patients. Treatment should include intravenous hydration to correct fluid deficits, correction of systemic acidemia with bicarbonate administration, and emergency dialysis if acute renal failure is present or other life-threatening complications exist.

Rhabdomyolysis

Rhabdomyolysis—extensive muscle breakdown caused by myonecrosis—may also cause an increased anion gap metabolic acidosis. The acidosis results from the accumulation of organic acids and may worsen if acute myoglobinuric renal failure develops. Measurement of serum concentrations of creatine kinase or aldolase (an enzyme confined to skeletal muscle) and urine concentrations of myoglobin may facilitate diagnosis. Fluid resuscitation should be begun immediately; early aggressive management may prevent acute renal failure and ensure a favorable prognosis.

NORMAL ANION GAP

When a surgical patient has a metabolic acidosis but the calculated anion gap is within normal limits (8 to 12 mEq/L), the most likely cause is the loss of excess bicarbonate via the GI tract. Other possible causes must also be considered, however.

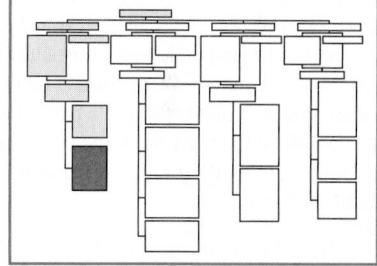

Excessive Bicarbonate Loss

Metabolic acidosis associated with a normal anion gap is characterized by impairment of bicarbonate buffering. In surgical patients, this is commonly secondary to loss of bicarbonate from the GI tract. Intestinal fluids, including pancreatic and biliary secretions, are relatively alkaline. Consequently, any process that causes the loss of such fluids (e.g., diarrhea, a villous adenoma, or the removal of pancreatic, biliary, or intestinal secretions via tube drainage or fistulas) can lead to a normal anion gap metabolic acidosis. When bicarbonate is lost in urine or stool, there is a compensatory increase in chloride, so that the anion gap remains normal. Another possible initiating process is occult laxative use, which should be considered in any patient with a hyperchloremic metabolic acidosis of unknown etiology.

Ureterosigmoidostomy can also lead to a hyperchloremic metabolic acidosis through two mechanisms: (1) chloride entering the colon from the urine is exchanged with bicarbonate, so that an increased amount of bicarbonate is lost, and (2) the colon reabsorbs NH_4^+, which is derived from urine and from colonic bacteria, and NH_4^+ is metabolized in the liver to NH_3 and H^+. The development of the ureteroileostomy procedure has minimized these complications.

Renal tubular acidosis is another possible cause of normal anion gap acidosis in surgical patients. Normally, about 50 to 100 mEq of acid is generated each day by tissue catabolism; in critically ill patients, this value may be significantly higher. Renal tubular cells excrete H^+ into the urine, thereby triggering the production of bicarbonate, which is then secreted back into the blood. Failure of this normal mechanism leads to renal tubular acidosis. There are several different forms of renal tubular acidosis, depending on which part of the nephron is abnormal. The urinary anion gap is useful in the assessment of renal tubular acidosis. It is calculated by subtracting the urine chloride concentration from the sum of the urine sodium concentration and the urine potassium concentration:

$$\text{Urinary anion gap} = ([Na^+] + [K^+]) - [Cl^-]$$

The urinary anion gap can be used to identify defects in renal tubular acidification in patients with normal anion gap metabolic acidosis. When this value is considered in tandem with urinary pH, it is possible to determine whether the likely cause of the acidosis is excessive gastrointestinal bicarbonate losses or defective renal tubular acidification [see Table 2]. Basically, the urinary anion gap serves as a crude index of urinary ammonium excretion, thereby reflecting, in part, net acid excretion.

The antifungal agent amphotericin B has also been reported to result in renal tubular acidosis, probably by altering the extent to which the membrane of the distal nephron is permeable to hydrogen and potassium ions. In general, the renal tubular acidosis tends to be mild and does not necessitate withdrawal of amphotericin B. Enteral potassium and bicarbonate supplements are useful for maintaining normal serum electrolyte concentrations.

The administration of carbonic anhydrase inhibitors (such as acetazolamide) can also lead to the development of hyperchloremic normal anion gap acidosis in critically ill patients by impairing proximal bicarbonate reabsorption. The clinical presentation of this acidosis can be indistinguishable from that of renal tubular acidosis. Patients should be asked if they routinely take carbonic anhydrase inhibitors (e.g., for glaucoma), and these agents should be used with caution in the ICU.

Hypoaldosteronism and Addison's Disease

Hypoaldosteronism may be an important pathogenetic factor in the acidification defect noted in patients with hyperkalemic distal renal tubular acidosis, which is also known as type IV renal tubular acidosis. Aldosterone deficiency causes a reduction in net acid secretion in the distal nephron. Other disorders that are associated with mineralocorticoid deficiency, including Addison's disease, may also lead to the development of renal tubular acidosis.

Excessive Acid Administration

The administration of ammonium chloride, the transfusion of massive amounts of blood preserved with citrate, and high-volume resuscitation with normal saline can all present the body with an excessively large acid load. Excessive acid administration can lead to the accumulation of inorganic acids and consequently to the development of a hyperchloremic normal anion gap metabolic acidosis. When high-volume crystalloid resuscitation is required in a surgical patient (e.g., after trauma), lactated Ringer's solution is preferred to normal saline for resuscitation: the higher chloride content of normal saline may contribute to the development of a hyperchloremic normal anion gap metabolic acidosis.

Table 2 Use of Urinary Anion Gap and Urinary pH in Differential Diagnosis of Normal Anion Gap Metabolic Acidosis[33,34]

Urinary Anion Gap	Urinary pH	Diagnosis
Negative	< 5.5	Normal
Positive	> 5.5	Renal tubular acidosis
Negative	> 5.5	Diarrhea or enteric fistula

Respiratory Acidosis

ACUTE

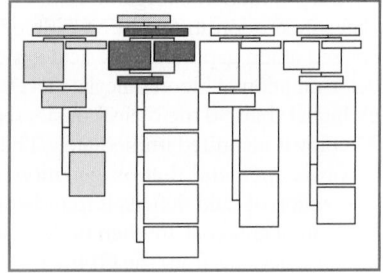

Acute respiratory acidosis is caused by alveolar hypoventilation, which results in retention of CO_2 and an acute increase in P_aCO_2 (hypercapnia) and ultimately may lead to acute respiratory failure. The body's compensatory response to acute respiratory acidosis is renal retention of bicarbonate: the plasma bicarbonate concentration rises by an average of 1 mEq/L for every 10 mm Hg increase in P_aCO_2. Because the renal response takes time to develop, the cell buffers, particularly hemoglobin and proteins, constitute the only protection against acute hypercapnia.

Acute respiratory acidosis also depresses myocardial function. Many studies have documented that increased P_aCO_2 (as in respiratory acidosis) impairs myocardial contractility to a greater degree than decreased bicarbonate concentration (as in metabolic acidosis).[11,12] This finding is related to the observation that intracellular pH changes more quickly in response to extracellular respiratory acidosis than in response to metabolic acidosis.[13,14]

Respiratory acidosis should be considered potentially life-threatening in patients who appear to be in respiratory distress, are unresponsive or have altered mental status (CO_2 narcosis), or exhibit acute changes in arterial pH (to < 7.2) or P_aCO_2 (to > 60 mm Hg). Emergency endotracheal intubation and mechanical ventilatory support are indicated for these patients. Once this treatment has been implemented, it is imperative to determine the underlying cause of the acute respiratory acidosis and to initiate appropriate treatment.

If acute respiratory acidosis is identified, the patient is stable, and emergency intubation is not indicated, it is important to identify the cause, institute appropriate treatment, and determine whether there is any history of pulmonary disease (e.g., COPD or asthma) or chronic hypercapnia. The major objectives in the treatment of acute respiratory acidosis, regardless of the specific cause, are correction of hypoxia and correction of hypercapnia. Initial treatment involves administering supplemental oxygen, correcting anemia, attempting to correct reversible problems such as sedative or narcotic overdose, improving pulmonary function and tissue oxygenation, and, if other treatments fail, initiating mechanical ventilation. Bicarbonate therapy should not be administered to patients who have a pure respiratory acidosis: it will only increase the body's carbon dioxide load.

There are four main causes of the alveolar hypoventilation that underlies acute respiratory acidosis: (1) airway obstruction, (2) pulmonary diseases that affect alveolar-capillary gas exchange, (3) weakened respiratory muscles, and (4) depressed respiratory drive.

Airway Obstruction

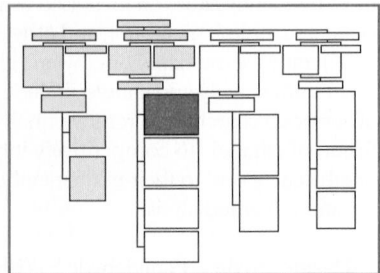

Airway obstruction can lead to acute severe respiratory acidosis. If the obstruction is caused by laryngospasm, the preferred treatment is correction of the specific cause of the laryngospasm (e.g., removal of a foreign body) or administration of racemic epinephrine. Slight positive pressure bag-valve-mask ventilation and steroid administration may also be helpful in some instances. Airway obstruction may also be caused by external compression (for example, from head and neck tumors, a large thyroid gland, or excess pharyngeal tissue, as in the sleep apnea syndrome). In most cases, external causes of airway obstruction leading to respiratory acidosis must be corrected surgically.

Pulmonary Diseases

A variety of pulmonary diseases, including asthma, pneumonia, pulmonary edema, acute respiratory distress syndrome (ARDS), acute lung injury, and aspiration pneumonia, can lead to acute respiratory acidosis. All of them induce some degree of ventilation-perfusion mismatch. Structural causes of acute CO_2 retention leading to respiratory acidosis include pneumothorax, hemothorax, empyema, and severe chest wall injury with underlying pulmonary contusions.

Asthma exacerbation and COPD are the two most common causes of acute respiratory acidosis. In the initial stages of an asthma exacerbation, respiratory alkalosis is often present because bronchospasm-induced hypoxia causes patients to hyperventilate. During more sustained episodes of bronchospasm, respiratory muscle fatigue eventually develops, and patients are unable to sustain hyperventilation. A normocapnic state ensues, followed by hypercapnic respiratory acidosis, which is a harbinger of impending respiratory failure in patients who have severe reactive small airway disease. The presence of acute respiratory acidosis in patients who have asthma is therefore indicative of a poor prognosis and suggests that intubation and mechanical ventilation are likely to be necessary.

In addition to general treatment measures for acute respiratory acidosis (see above), aggressive treatment of respiratory acidosis caused by asthma includes administering inhaled and parenteral bronchodilators (e.g., beta-adrenergic agents, theophylline, and, in children and young adults, epinephrine). Inhaled steroids and high-dose parenteral steroids should be considered in patients with associated pulmonary inflammation. Magnesium sulfate (a smooth muscle relaxant) may be helpful in the treatment of severe asthma.

Respiratory Muscle Weakness

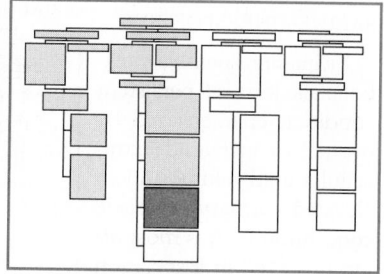

Various disorders that affect the respiratory muscles and the chest wall can also cause acute respiratory acidosis. Both hypokalemia and hypophosphatemia are known to weaken respiratory muscles; aggressive replacement therapy should be instituted if either abnormality is identified. The administration of aminoglycosides is associated with renal potassium and magnesium wasting and may lead to severe hypokalemia. Myopathy secondary to hypokalemia can be rapidly reversed by the administration of large quantities of potassium. Serum potassium and phosphate levels should be monitored in critically ill patients, especially when active weaning from mechanical ventilatory support is being considered.

Neuromuscular blockade induces respiratory muscle weakness, especially when it is prolonged. There have been numerous reports of persistent paralysis in critically ill patients after the administration of neuromuscular blocking agents.[15] Consequently, these agents should not be used unless absolutely required. If they are required,

the patient should be monitored with a peripheral nerve stimulator to ensure that the dosage is appropriate.

Certain muscular and neurologic disorders (e.g., myasthenia gravis, multiple sclerosis, Guillain-Barré syndrome, amyotrophic lateral sclerosis, and muscular dystrophy) can affect respiratory muscles and thus lead to acute respiratory acidosis, as can some spinal column abnormalities (e.g., kyphoscoliosis). In patients with these disorders, treatment centers on preventing any electrolyte abnormalities that might further impair respiratory muscle function, providing ongoing medical therapy for the underlying disorders, attempting to prevent pulmonary infection, and providing nutritional support to keep muscle function from degenerating further.

Depressed Respiratory Drive

The central nervous system controls the rate of pulmonary CO_2 excretion (and thus whole body CO_2 balance) through both voluntary and involuntary modulations of the frequency and depth of respiration. Accordingly, drugs that inhibit the medullary respiratory centers (e.g., sedatives, general anesthetics, and narcotics) may induce acute respiratory acidosis by causing primary failure in the drive to ventilation; care should be taken when these drugs are given to critically ill patients. Depressed respiratory drive can also be a long-term sequela of a cerebrovascular accident or cerebral trauma, and patients with respiratory acidosis should be evaluated for possible intracranial pathology.

Primary idiopathic alveolar hypoventilation is another possible cause of acute respiratory acidosis secondary to depressed respiratory drive. In this disorder, the respiratory centers lack normal responsiveness to hypercapnia, and this lack results in hypoventilation. Primary idiopathic alveolar hypoventilation can also occur in patients with chronic respiratory acidosis who have pulmonary diseases that cause CO_2 retention, and excessive oxygen therapy may exacerbate respiratory failure in patients with COPD. Hypnotic or sedative drugs should be administered with great caution to these patients, who are particularly susceptible to further respiratory depression.

CHRONIC

Chronic respiratory acidosis differs from acute respiratory acidosis primarily with respect to the duration of CO_2 retention. Chronic CO_2 retention can occur secondary to the same mechanisms that produce the initial hypercapnia that results in acute respiratory acidosis: chronic airway obstruction, depression of respiratory drive, respiratory muscle weakness, and pulmonary diseases that interfere with the efficient exchange of CO_2 or cause persistent ventilation-perfusion mismatch.

The body's compensatory response to chronic respiratory acidosis differs from its response to acute respiratory acidosis: the plasma bicarbonate concentration rises by approximately 4 mEq/L for every 10 mm Hg increase in P_aCO_2 [see Table 1]. The persistent elevation in P_aCO_2 stimulates renal secretion of H^+ over a period of 3 to 5 days, resulting in the addition of bicarbonate to the extracellular fluid. The efficiency of this renal compensation is such that the associated changes in arterial pH are relatively small; this means that P_aCO_2 can rise to much higher levels in patients with chronic respiratory acidosis than in those with acute hypercapnia.

Treatment of chronic respiratory acidosis also differs from that of acute respiratory acidosis. Extensive efforts should be made to avoid having to institute intubation and mechanical ventilation because patients with chronic respiratory acidosis are often difficult to wean. Excessive supplemental oxygen therapy should be avoided because it may suppress spontaneous respiratory efforts. Aggressive supportive therapy is indicated, including treatment of any underlying pulmonary infections, treatment of associated congestive heart failure, administration of oral or inhaled bronchodilators, prevention of associated acid-base abnormalities (e.g., metabolic alkalosis resulting from diuretic therapy), and, possibly, pharmacologic stimulation of respiration.

Metabolic Alkalosis

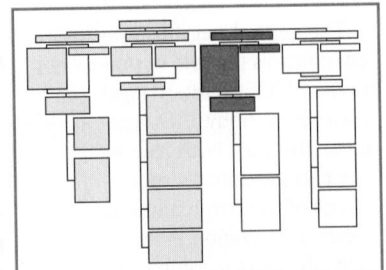

Metabolic alkalosis results from any pathophysiologic process that causes the loss of H^+, the addition of bicarbonate, or the loss of extracellular fluid (which leads to alkalemia because this fluid contains more chloride than bicarbonate). When metabolic alkalosis is potentially life-threatening (pH > 7.6 or $[HCO_3^-]$ > 40 mEq/L), administration of the carbonic anhydrase inhibitor acetazolamide should be considered; however, this agent is associated with renal loss of potassium, which must be anticipated and managed appropriately. If acetazolamide is not effective or the metabolic alkalosis worsens, exogenous acid, in the form of a 0.1N solution of hydrochloric acid (100 mEq/L), should be administered through a central venous catheter. The amount of exogenous acid to be given should be determined on the basis of the calculated chloride deficit, which is derived as follows:

$$\text{Calculated Cl}^- \text{ deficit} = 0.2 \text{ L/kg} \times \text{weight (kg)}$$
$$\times (103 - [\text{Cl}^-] \text{ [mEq/L]})$$

Arterial blood gases must be monitored frequently to ensure that only the amount necessary is given; overshoot can cause metabolic acidosis.

A number of complications are commonly associated with metabolic alkalosis. In critically ill patients, metabolic alkalosis may lead to supraventricular or ventricular arrhythmias that are refractory to medical therapy until the metabolic alkalosis has been corrected and normal acid-base balance restored. Moreover, metabolic alkalosis can induce a reduction in cardiac output and cause the oxyhemoglobin dissociation curve to shift to the left, thereby diminishing oxygen delivery to the tissues. Alkalosis may also stimulate glycolysis, thereby increasing oxygen consumption at a time when oxygen delivery is already impaired. Furthermore, the respiratory compensation for metabolic alkalosis is hypoventilation with CO_2 retention (secondary hypercapnia), which may lead to hypoxemia; these conditions may produce further impairment of tissue oxygenation. An additional problem is that this respiratory compensation may hinder weaning from mechanical ventilation. Aggressive efforts must be made to correct the underlying disorder that caused the metabolic alkalosis before weaning from mechanical ventilation can be resumed.

Severe alkalemia (pH > 7.6) may cause neuromuscular abnormalities in critically ill patients, including mental confusion, stupor, lethargy, muscle weakness and cramping and, possibly, seizures. The mechanism by which alkalemia causes these neuromuscular abnormalities is not fully understood; it may be related to reduced plasma ionized calcium concentrations resulting from increased binding of calcium to plasma proteins.

A useful first step in determining the cause of metabolic alkalosis is a spot measurement of the urine chloride concentration. If the urine chloride concentration is lower than 10 mEq/L, the metabolic alkalosis is likely to be saline-responsive; if it is higher than 20 mEq/L, the metabolic alkalosis is saline-unresponsive and may be more difficult to treat.

SALINE-RESPONSIVE

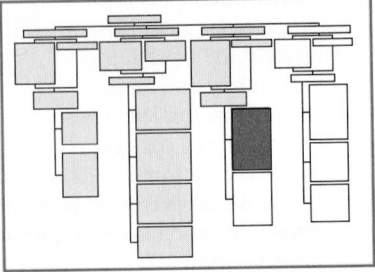

Two of the most common causes of saline-responsive metabolic alkalosis in surgical patients are continuous gastric aspiration and gastrointestinal loss of hydrochloric acid secondary to vomiting. The severity of the alkalosis depends on the magnitude and duration of the acid losses, the extent of volume depletion, and the severity of potassium depletion.

Initial therapy involves restoring extracellular fluid volume by infusing normal saline, correcting hypokalemia by administering potassium chloride, and monitoring the patient closely for possible associated complications. Because the serum potassium concentrations may not reflect the full extent of total body potassium deficiency, potassium replacement should be aggressive; the goal should be to achieve serum levels of 4.5 to 5.5 mEq/L. The administration of an H_2 receptor antagonist (e.g., cimetidine or ranitidine) may help attenuate further loss of H^+ from the GI tract.

Long-term administration of thiazide or loop diuretics is also a common cause of saline-responsive metabolic alkalosis in surgical patients. The degree of metabolic alkalosis caused by diuretic administration is directly correlated with the degree of volume depletion. Ideally, diuretic therapy should be discontinued and the lost potassium and chloride should be replaced; however, this is not always possible. If diuretic therapy must be continued, the potassium and chloride deficits must be corrected. The use of potassium-sparing diuretics may also be considered for patients who require long-term diuretic therapy.

Iatrogenic causes of metabolic alkalosis include the overenthusiastic application of exogenous alkali therapy [see Metabolic Acidosis, above] and the provision of excess acetate in parenteral nutrition solutions.

SALINE-UNRESPONSIVE

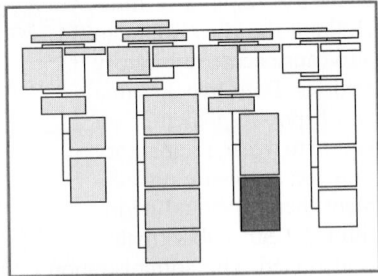

Saline-unresponsive metabolic alkalosis is a persistent condition characterized by normal or increased extracellular fluid volume and an elevated urinary chloride concentration. It is most often observed in association with mineralocorticoid excess, and it is resistant to sodium chloride therapy.

Primary aldosteronism is a common cause of saline-unresponsive metabolic alkalosis: the aldosterone excess enhances acid secretion in the distal nephron and results in a metabolic alkalosis. The clinical presentation includes arterial hypertension and hypokalemia as well as metabolic alkalosis. Cushing's syndrome may also be associated with metabolic alkalosis: cortisol possesses some intrinsic mineralocorticoid activity, and consequently, cortisol excess mimics some of the physiologic effects of aldosterone excess.

Treatment of saline-unresponsive metabolic alkalosis involves correcting the electrolyte deficiencies and removing the source of the mineralocorticoid excess. If surgical removal of the mineralocorticoid source is not possible, the action of the mineralocorticoid can be blocked by means of spironolactone or amiloride.

Respiratory Alkalosis

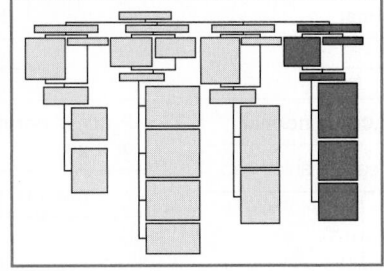

Care must be taken at all times in surgical patients to avoid hyperventilation and respiratory alkalosis so as not to impair tissue oxygenation. In this patient population, respiratory alkalosis is most often attributable to early sepsis or early ARDS. Mild respiratory alkalosis may result from pain or anxiety and subsequent hyperventilation. In addition, iatrogenic respiratory alkalosis secondary to excessive ventilation is quite common and is often overlooked. Overventilation can lead to decreased oxygen delivery by shifting the oxyhemoglobin dissociation curve to the left.

If respiratory alkalosis is potentially life-threatening (pH > 7.6, P_aCO_2 < 20 mm Hg, or cardiac arrhythmias are present), emergency intubation and mechanical ventilation must be considered. If respiratory alkalosis is not life-threatening, management should focus on identifying and correcting the underlying disorder that caused it.

Central causes of respiratory alkalosis include hyperventilation resulting from anxiety, hypoxemia, pain, or sepsis. Anxiolytic therapy, supplemental oxygen, pain medication, and treatment of infections, respectively, are appropriate for this group of patients. Intracranial pathology (e.g., CNS infection, tumor, or trauma) can also cause hyperventilation and thus respiratory alkalosis. A computed tomography scan of the head is the most reliable diagnostic test for determining whether such pathology is a possible cause of the respiratory alkalosis.

Pulmonary causes of respiratory alkalosis include those diseases that affect the alveolar-capillary membrane, hindering gas exchange, creating a ventilation-perfusion mismatch, and eventually leading to hypoxia. The body's response to hypoxia is hyperventilation, which results in respiratory alkalosis. The pulmonary diseases that are most often responsible for respiratory alkalosis in surgical patients are asthma, pneumonia, pulmonary embolism, congestive heart failure, atelectasis, and pneumothorax.

Iatrogenic causes of respiratory alkalosis are mainly related to inappropriate management of mechanical ventilation. Various drugs can also cause iatrogenic respiratory alkalosis. Discontinuation of the medication is the optimal therapy. If the medication is necessary, adjustment of the dose may be helpful.

Mixed Acid-Base Disorders

The mixed acid-base disorders fall into two main categories [see Table 3]. In additive combinations, the pH deviations are in the same direction, whereas in counterbalancing combinations, the pH deviations are in opposite directions. Depending on the precise combination present, a mixed acid-base disorder can result in normal arterial pH, acidemia, or alkalemia [see Figure 3].

The patients at highest risk for life-threatening complications associated with mixed acid-base disorders are those who have additive combinations. For example, a patient who has severe diabetic ketoacidosis (primary metabolic acidosis) and who subsequently experiences acute respiratory failure (primary respiratory acidosis) may have life-threatening acidemia, which would necessitate emergency intubation and mechanical ventilation for immediate correction of the primary respiratory acidosis as well as continued treatment for diabetic ketoacidosis. Similarly, a patient who has a contraction alkalosis resulting from excessive diuretic therapy (primary metabolic alkalosis) and who subsequently requires mechanical ventilation for respiratory failure and is erroneously overventilated (primary respiratory alkalosis) may have life-threatening alkalemia.

Interpretation and diagnosis of complex mixed acid-base disorders can be quite difficult, often involving numerous calculations.

Table 3 Classification of Mixed Acid-Base Disorders[35]

Additive Combinations	Causes	Counterbalancing Combinations	Causes
Respiratory acidosis and metabolic acidosis	Cardiopulmonary arrest Pulmonary edema Chronic lung disease with hypoxia Hypokalemic myopathy plus metabolic acidosis Severe phosphorus depletion Poisoning—drug toxicity (ethanol, methanol, or ethylene glycol)	Respiratory acidosis and metabolic alkalosis	Excess diuresis in chronic lung disease Severe potassium depletion
Respiratory alkalosis and metabolic alkalosis	Severe trauma Blood transfusion Pregnancy Respirator-induced	Respiratory alkalosis and metabolic acidosis	Aspirin intoxication Advanced liver disease Pulmonary-renal syndromes
Mixed elevated anion gap and normal anion gap metabolic acidosis (high anion gap metabolic acidosis with excessive decrease in [HCO$_3^-$]: change in [HCO$_3^-$] > change in anion gap)	Renal-related causes Early chronic renal failure Uremic acidosis with proximal or distal renal tubular acidosis Diabetes mellitus Diarrhea Hypoaldosteronism Repair phase of diabetic ketoacidosis Lactic acidosis complicating diarrhea or other causes of normal anion gap metabolic acidosis	Metabolic acidosis and metabolic alkalosis (high anion gap with less than equimolar reduction in serum [HCO$_3^-$]: change in [HCO$_3^-$] < change in anion gap)	Renal-related causes Uremic vomiting Alkali therapy in uremia Transfusion alkalosis Aluminum hydroxide (Amphojel) plus sodium polystyrene sulfonate (Kayexalate) Diuretic administration Diabetes mellitus Diabetic ketoacidosis and vomiting NaHCO$_3^-$ therapy for diabetic ketoacidosis Lactic acidosis when complicated by various causes of metabolic alkalosis

Figure 3 **Patients with mixed acid-base disorders can have normal arterial pH (*a*), acidemia (*b*), or alkalemia (*c*), depending on the precise combination of disorders present.[30] Shown are algorithms that may facilitate the evaluation of such disorders.**

Automatic computer interpretation of acid-base disturbances was initiated in the late 1960s; however, the systems that were developed were highly complex, and few were implemented in clinical practice.[16-18] In the early 1990s, a computer system was designed to help clinicians interpret complex acid-base disturbances on the basis of numerical laboratory measurements.[19] In accuracy, versatility, and clinical utility, this system compared favorably with a medical expert; moreover, it saved time by performing all necessary calculations. Sim-

ilar computer programs have been put into routine practice in a number of ICUs and are now commercially available. It is of the utmost importance that the data and conclusions generated by computer systems such as this be used in tandem with the clinical findings obtained by examining the patient. The integration of computer system analysis with clinical examination may result in the timely diagnosis of complex mixed acid-base disturbances and allow earlier initiation of appropriate therapy, especially in life-threatening situations.

Discussion

Biochemical Basis of Lactic Acidosis

Lactic acidosis results from excessive production or impaired degradation of lactic acid or from a combination of the two. In virtually all cells, the formation of pyruvate in the cytosol by anaerobic glycolysis is the first step in glucose metabolism. Pyruvate then enters the cellular mitochondria, where it is metabolized to NADH via the citric acid (Krebs) cycle:

$$\text{Pyruvate} + \text{coenzyme A} + \text{NAD}^+ \rightarrow$$
$$\text{acetyl coenzyme A} + CO_2 + \text{NADH}$$

Oxidative phosphorylation then results in the production of adenosine triphosphate (ATP). This aerobic metabolism is a highly efficient process: 36 mol of ATP is produced for each 1 mol of glucose consumed.

When oxygen is not available at the cellular level, pyruvate is metabolized to lactate by the enzyme lactate dehydrogenase (LDH):

$$\text{Pyruvate} + \text{NADH} + \text{H}^+ \xrightarrow{\text{LDH}} \text{lactate} + \text{NAD}^+$$

Compared with the aerobic pathway, the anaerobic pathway is very inefficient, producing only 2 mol of ATP for every 1 mol of glucose that is converted to lactate.

Most of the lactate produced by the body is cleared by the liver; a lesser amount is cleared by the kidney. The heart, the liver, and the kidneys are capable of converting lactate to pyruvate and then converting pyruvate to CO_2 and ATP via aerobic metabolism. In addition, the liver and the kidneys are able to produce glucose from lactate via gluconeogenesis. From a quantitative viewpoint, gluconeogenesis is the most important process for removing lactate from the blood. The continuous cyclic flow of lactate from peripheral tissues (e.g., skeletal muscle, which is the main source of lactate) to the liver, where it is converted to glucose, and back to the peripheral tissues is known as the Cori cycle. The Cori cycle ensures a continuous supply of glucose to the tissues that have an absolute requirement for glucose, namely, the brain, erythrocytes, and the medullae of the kidneys. When hepatic or renal insufficiency develops in critically ill patients, lactate clearance is altered as a result, and blood lactate concentrations thus become a less accurate indicator of the extent of tissue hypoxia present.

Patients with lactic acidosis were initially classified by Huckabee[20] into two groups on the basis of whether the ratio of lactate to pyruvate was normal (10:1) or increased. A revised classification formulated by Cohen and Woods[21] divided patients into two categories on the basis of whether tissue hypoxia was apparent (type A) or not (type B); these categories were then broken down into subcategories [see Table 4]. The fundamental point made by this classification is that the determination of whether lactic acidosis is caused by tissue hypoxia or not is important for initiating appropriate treatment. The various causes of lactic acidosis have been reviewed more extensively elsewhere.[22]

Therapy for Lactic Acidosis: Alkalinizing Agents and Dichloroacetate

Alkalinizing agents have been given to patients who have lactic acidosis with the aim of reducing the excess acid load and treating its associated adverse effects. In 1992, the National Conference on Cardiopulmonary Resuscitation established current guidelines, according to which the routine use of sodium bicarbonate is no longer recommended.[23] Occasionally, however, patients with severe lactic acidosis still require alkalinizing agents; accordingly, clinicians must be familiar with the indications for the use of these agents and knowledgeable about potential complications.

Parenteral bicarbonate therapy can induce a hyperosmolar state and may further increase lactate production by increasing phosphofructokinase activity and accelerating glycolysis. In addition, it can lead to so-called overshoot alkalosis. The increase in arterial pH associated with bicarbonate administration may increase the affinity of hemoglobin for oxygen, thereby impairing tissue oxygen delivery and worsening tissue hypoxia. Experimental studies have shown that mortality after bicarbonate therapy is not significantly lower than mortality after saline administration, and clinical studies have confirmed these findings. Therefore, bicarbonate administration may have no real advantages as a treatment modality.

Other alkalinizing agents, such as Carbicarb (an equimolar solution of sodium bicarbonate and sodium carbonate) and tris-hydroxymethyl aminomethane (THAM), have been studied. Because of the substitution of carbonate for bicarbonate, Carbicarb tends to cause less production of CO_2, and it is better than bicarbonate at raising serum pH without increasing the serum lactate concentration.[24] THAM has vasodilatory properties that lead to decreased peripheral vascular resistance, an effect that is potentially detrimental in many patients. At present, there is little clinical experience with these agents; further study is required.

DCA is receiving increased attention as a potential adjunctive treatment of lactic acidosis.[25] By inhibiting the action of a protein kinase that inactivates the enzyme pyruvate dehydrogenase, DCA brings about enhanced metabolism of pyruvate and hence lactate. DCA may also have a direct inotropic effect on myocardium: studies have demonstrated improvements in cardiac output and blood pressure that do not appear to be related to changes in extracellular pH. These effects may result in improved oxygen delivery, thereby decreasing lactate production. Clinical trials using DCA have demonstrated overall improvements in blood lactate concentration, pH, cardiac output, and blood pressure; however, follow-up studies have documented no improvement in clinical outcome.[5,26] It has also been documented that DCA alleviates lactic acidosis during liver transplantation. Two clinical studies concluded that DCA, 40 to 80 mg/kg, safely and effectively attenuated lactic acid accumulation, moderated acidosis, decreased

Table 4 Classification of Lactic Acidosis[21]

Tissue Hypoxia	Type	Cause
Apparent	A	Severe hypoxia, asthma, or CO poisoning; severe anemia; hypovolemic shock, hemorrhage, hypotension, or cardiac arrest; congestive heart failure or pulmonary edema; cardiogenic shock
Not apparent	B1	Acquired disease: diabetes mellitus, hepatic failure, Reye's syndrome, sepsis, malignancies, alcoholic ketoacidosis, renal failure, pancreatitis, systemic inflammatory response syndrome
	B2	Drugs or toxins: ethanol, ethylene glycol, methanol, sodium nitroprusside, acetaminophen, salicylates, epinephrine, norepinephrine, isoniazid, streptozocin, nalidixic acid
	B3	Congenital disorders: glucose-6-phosphatase deficiency, fructose-1,6-diphosphatase deficiency, pyruvate dehydrogenase deficiency, pyruvate carboxylase deficiency

NaHCO$_3$ requirements, and reduced the incidence of hypernatremia during orthotopic liver transplantation.[27,28]

Although the findings from preliminary clinical study of DCA are promising, it appears that for the time being, use of this agent should be reserved for patients with type B lactic acidosis (i.e., lactic acidosis associated with adequate oxygen delivery). Primary therapy for type A lactic acidosis involves attempting to restore tissue oxygen delivery by administering appropriate fluid resuscitation therapy, providing inotropic support, and, if necessary, transfusing blood or giving supplemental oxygen.

References

1. Rosenthal TB: The effects of temperature on the pH of the blood and plasma in vitro. J Biol Chem 173:25, 1948

2. Ream AK, Reitz BA, Silverberg G: Temperature correction of pCO$_2$ and pH in estimating acid-base status: an example of the emperor's new clothes? Anesthesiology 56:41, 1982

3. Hansen JE, Sue DY: Should blood gas measurements be corrected for the patient's temperature? N Engl J Med 303:341, 1980

4. Delaney KA, Howland MA, Vassallo S, et al: Assessment of acid-base disturbances in hypothermia and their physiologic consequences. Ann Emerg Med 18: 72, 1989

5. Narins RG, Cohen JJ: Bicarbonate therapy for organic acidosis: the case for its continued use. Ann Intern Med 106:615, 1987

6. Stacpoole PW, Lorenz AC, Thomas RG, et al: Dichloroacetate in the treatment of lactic acidosis. Ann Intern Med 108:58, 1988

7. Narins RG, Jones ER, Stom MC, et al: Diagnostic strategies in disorders of fluid, electrolyte and acid-base homeostasis. Am J Med 72:496, 1982

8. Keller U, Berger W: Prevention of hypophosphatemia by phosphate infusion during treatment of diabetic ketoacidosis and hyperosmolar coma. Diabetes 29:87, 1980

9. Wilson HK, Kever SP, Lea AS, et al: Phosphate therapy in diabetic ketoacidosis. Arch Intern Med 142:527, 1982

10. Winter RJ, Harris CJ, Phillips LS, et al: Diabetic ketoacidosis: induction of hypocalcemia and hypomagnesemia by phosphate therapy. Am J Med 67:897, 1979

11. Cingolani HE, Mattiaze AR, Blesa ES, et al: Contractility in isolated mammalian heart muscle after acid-base changes. Circ Res 26:269, 1970

12. Pannier JL, Leusen I: Contraction characteristics of papillary muscle during changes in acid-base composition of the bathing fluid. Arch Int Physiol Biochim 76:624, 1968

13. Cingolani HE, Blesa ES, Gonzalez NC, et al: Extracellular vs. intracellular pH as a determinant of myocardial contractility. Life Sci 8:775, 1969

14. Poole-Wilson PA, Cameron IR: A comparison of the control of intracellular pH in cardiac and skeletal muscle. Clin Sci 44:15P, 1973

15. Hoyt JW: Neuromuscular blockade in critical care. New Horizons 2:1, 1994

16. Cohen ML: A computer program for the interpretation of blood gas analysis. Comp Biomed Res 2:549, 1969

17. Bleich HL: The computer as a consultant. N Engl J Med 284:141, 1971

18. Bleich HL: Computer-based consultation: electrolyte and acid-base disorders. Am J Med 53:285, 1972

19. Pince H, Verberckmoes R, Willems JL: Computer aided interpretation of acid-base disorders. Int J Biomed Comput 25:177, 1990

20. Huckabee WE: Abnormal resting blood lactate: II. Lactic acidosis. Am J Med 30:840, 1961

21. Cohen RD, Woods HF: Clinical and Biochemical Aspects of Lactic Acidosis. Blackwell, Oxford, 1976

22. Vary TC, Siegel JH, Rivkind A: Clinical and therapeutic significance of metabolic patterns of lactic acidosis. Perspectives in Critical Care 1:85, 1988

23. Emergency Cardiac Care Committee and Subcommittees, American Heart Association: Standards and guidelines for cardiopulmonary resuscitation and emergency cardiac care. JAMA 268:2171, 1992

24. Sun JH, Filley GF, Hord K, et al: Carbicarb: an effective substitute for NaHCO$^-$ for the treatment of acidosis. Surgery 102:835, 1987

25. Stacpoole PW, Henderson GN, Yan Z, et al: Clinical pharmacology and toxicology of dichloroacetate. Environ Health Perspect 106(suppl 4):989, 1998

26. Stacpoole PW, Harman EM, Curry SH, et al: Treatment of lactic acidosis with dichloroacetate. N Engl J Med 309:390, 1983

27. Shangraw RE, Rabkin JM, Lopaschuk GD: Hepatic pyruvate dehydrogenase activity in humans: effect of cirrhosis, transplantation and dichloroacetate. Am J Physiol 274:G569, 1998

28. Shangraw RE, Winter R, Hromco J, et al: Amelioration of lactic acidosis with dichloroacetate during liver transplantation in humans. Anesthesiology 81:1127, 1994

29. Arturson G, de Verdier C-H: Respiratory functions of blood. Surgical Physiology. Burke JF, Ed. WB Saunders Co, Philadelphia, 1983, p 451

30. Walmsley RN, White GH: A Guide to Diagnostic Clinical Chemistry. Blackwell Scientific, Melbourne, 1983, p 114

31. Brewer ED: Disorders of acid-base balance. Pediatr Clin North Am 37:429, 1990

32. Bernards WC, Kirby RR: Acid-base chemistry and physiology. Critical Care, 2nd ed. Civetta JM, Taylor RW, Kirby RR, Eds. JB Lippincott Co, Philadelphia, 1992, p 343

33. Battle DC, Hizon M, Cohen E, et al: The use of the urinary anion gap in the diagnosis of hyperchloremic metabolic acidosis. N Engl J Med 318:594, 1988

34. Marino PL: The ICU Book. Williams & Wilkins, Baltimore, 1998

35. Riley LJ, Ilson BE, Narins RG: Acute metabolic acid-base disorders. Crit Care Clin 5:699, 1987

Reviews

Brenner M, Welliver J: Pulmonary and acid-base assessment. Nurs Clin North Am 25:761, 1990

Clinical Disorders of Fluid and Electrolyte Metabolism, 4th ed. Maxwell MH, Kleeman CR, Narins RG, Eds. McGraw-Hill Book Co, New York, 1987

Fluids and Electrolytes, 2nd ed. Kokko JP, Tannen RL, Eds. WB Saunders Co, Philadelphia, 1990

Kruse JA, Carlson RW: Lactate metabolism. Crit Care Clin 5:725, 1990

Rose BD: Clinical Physiology of Acid-Base and Electrolyte Disorders, 2nd ed. McGraw-Hill Book Co, New York, 1984

Walmsley RN, Guerin MD: Disorders of Fluid and Electrolyte Balance. John Wright & Sons Ltd, Bristol, 1984

Acknowledgments

Figure 1   Albert Miller.
Figure 2   Seward Hung.
Figure 3   Talar Agasyan.

8 ACUTE WOUND CARE

W. Thomas Lawrence, M.D., A. Griswold Bevin, M.D., and George F. Sheldon, M.D.

Approach to Acute Wound Management

When a patient presents with an acute wound, the priorities are a careful, complete history and a thorough physical examination. Most cutaneous wounds are obvious and easily diagnosed but are not life threatening.

However, the wounded patient may also have less apparent problems that are potentially lethal and demand immediate attention. The management of such potentially life-endangering problems takes precedence over wound management.

After more urgent problems have been ruled out or corrected, wound management can be addressed. Information about the time and mechanism of injury must be obtained. The patient should be asked about a coagulopathy and about conditions (e.g., diabetes, immune disorders, renal disease, hepatic dysfunction, and malignancies), practices (e.g., smoking), and medications (e.g., corticosteroids or chemotherapeutic agents) that could interfere with healing. The patient's nutritional status must be assessed, and the patient must be checked for signs of arterial or venous insufficiency in the wounded area.

The wound must then be carefully examined. Active hemorrhage must be noted. Wounded tissue must be assessed for viability, and foreign bodies must be sought. The possibility of damage to nerves, ducts, muscles, or bones in proximity to the injury must be assessed. X-rays and a careful motor and sensory examination may be required to rule out such coexistent injuries. It may be necessary to probe such ducts as the parotid or the lacrimal duct to assess them for injury. The patient's tetanus immunization status should be considered [*see* Tetanus Prophylaxis, *below*]. Antirabies treatment should be considered for patients who have been bitten by wild animals such as skunks, raccoons, foxes, and bats [*see II:11 Soft Tissue Infection and VI:19 Viral Infection*].

Tetanus Prophylaxis

With any wound, it is important to consider the status of the patient's tetanus immunization.[1] The effectiveness of antibiotics for the prophylaxis of tetanus is uncertain.[2] Large, deep

wounds with devitalized tissue are especially prone to tetanus infection and are defined as tetanus prone[3] [*see Tables 1 and 2*]. There is no one characteristic that defines a wound as tetanus prone: instead, wounds are considered tetanus prone if they have

a significant number of the characteristics considered to define this state.

For non–tetanus-prone wounds, tetanus immune globulin (human) (TIG) is never indicated. If a patient with a non–tetanus-prone wound was never completely immunized or has not received a tetanus booster dose within the past 10 years, a booster dose of tetanus and diphtheria toxoids adsorbed (Td) is required. For a patient who has been previously immunized and has received a tetanus booster within the past 10 years, no further treatment is required.

For a patient with a tetanus-prone wound who has been completely immunized and has received a booster dose within the past 5 years, no treatment is indicated. If a previously immunized patient with a tetanus-prone wound has not been immunized within the past 5 years, a booster Td dose is administered. If a patient with a tetanus-prone wound either was not immunized or was incompletely immunized, TIG is given along with a dose of Td.

Antibiotic Prophylaxis

Prophylactic antibiotics are not indicated for most wounds. They are, however, indicated for contaminated wounds in immunocompromised or diabetic patients. They are also indi-

cated for patients with extensive injuries to the central area of the face, to prevent spread of infection through the venous system to the meninges; for patients with valvular disease, to prevent endocarditis; and for patients with prostheses, to limit the chance of bacterial seeding of the prosthesis. Lymphedematous extremities

Table 1 Wound Classification[3]

Clinical Features	Tetanus-Prone Wounds	Non–Tetanus-Prone Wounds
Age of wound	> 6 hr	≤ 6 hr
Configuration	Stellate wound, avulsion, abrasion	Linear wound
Depth	> 1 cm	≤ 1 cm
Mechanism of injury	Missile, crush, burn, frostbite	Sharp surface (e.g., knife or glass)
Signs of infection	Present	Absent
Devitalized tissue	Present	Absent
Contaminants (e.g., dirt, feces, soil, or saliva)	Present	Absent

Obtain history and perform physical examination

Life-threatening conditions take priority over wound care.

Consider prophylaxis against tetanus or rabies, or both

Consider antibiotic therapy for contaminated wounds in immunocompromised patients for cellulitis around the wound, for human-bite wounds, for abscesses of the central area of the face, for patients with valvular heart disease or prostheses, for stool-contaminated wounds, and for wounds in lymphedematous extremities

Determine timing of wound closure

Small or superficial wound that will heal secondarily within 2 weeks

Example:
    Puncture wounds
    Superficial abrasions

Secondary healing:
Clean and dress the wound and allow it to heal.

Fresh, acute wound with viable wound margins, limited bacterial contamination, and no unusual problems with foreign bodies or hemorrhage

Examples:
    Dog-bite wounds
    Kitchen-knife wounds
    Surgical wounds

Primary closure:
Proceed immediately to consideration of method of wound closure.

Determine method of wound closure

Choices:
    Direct approximation
    Skin graft
    Flap (local or distant)

Simplest method possible in a given situation is preferred.

Provide general or local anesthesia as needed; prepare wound for closure.

Wound with edges in proximity

Close wound by direct approximation.
Consider use of drains.

Wound edges cannot be approximated; wound contains no denuded bones, cartilage, nerve, or tendon; and a skin graft is cosmetically and functionally acceptable

Apply a skin graft.

Wound edges cannot be approximated, and a skin graft is not possible or desirable

Utilize a flap for wound closure.
Consider use of drains.

Approach to Acute Wound Management

Acute wound with uncontrollable hemorrhage	Acute wound with questionably viable tissue or extreme contamination with foreign bodies	Acute or neglected wound with excessive bacterial contamination

Example:
    Wound in a hemophiliac
 	
Tertiary closure:
Pack or wrap wound tightly until bleeding is controlled; then proceed with closure.
	Examples:
	    Wounds with embedded road tar
	    Wounds with severely contused tissue
	
	Tertiary closure:
	Proceed with debridement of foreign bodies and necrotic tissue, and initiate dressing changes until wound is clean; then proceed with closure.
		Example:
		    Human-bite wounds
		
		Tertiary closure:
		Debride and irrigate wound and initiate dressing changes with antibacterial cream until bacterial count is < 10^5/g tissue; then proceed with closure.

are particularly prone to cellulitis, and antibiotics are indicated when such extremities are wounded. Stool-contaminated wounds and human-bite wounds are considered infected from the moment of infliction and must be treated with antibiotics [*see II:11 Soft Tissue Infection*].[4,5] As a rule, dog-bite wounds are less severely contaminated with bacteria; however, a 1994 meta-analysis suggested that prophylactic antibiotics are probably beneficial in this setting.[6] In addition, antibiotic prophylaxis is often indicated for wounds with extensive amounts of devitalized tissue (e.g., farm injuries).

When antibiotic prophylaxis is called for, the agent or agents to be used should be selected on the basis of the bacterial species believed to be present. *Staphylococcus aureus*, α-hemolytic streptococci, *Eikenella corrodens*, *Haemophilus* species, and anaerobes are often cultured from human-bite wounds.[4,5] To cover these species, a broad-spectrum antibiotic or combination of antibiotics should be administered; amoxicillin-clavulanate, a β-lactamase inhibitor, is a common choice.

Pasteurella multocida is the most common infecting organism in cat-bite wounds. *P. multocida* is also common in dog-bite wounds, though α-hemolytic streptococci and *S. aureus* are frequently isolated as well.[6,7] For cat-bite wounds, penicillin alone usually suffices, whereas for dog-bite wounds, a broad-spectrum agent (e.g., penicillin-clavulanate) is preferable. Mutilating injuries that are caused by farm equipment are often contaminated with a mixture of gram-positive organisms and gram-negative organisms, though not always excessively so.[8] When antibiotics are indicated for such injuries, broad-spectrum coverage is appropriate.

The anatomic location of a wound may also suggest whether oral flora, fecal flora, or some less aggressive bacterial contaminant is likely to be present. A Gram stain can provide an early clue to the type of bacteria present as well. The choice of prophylactic antibiotic to be given is ultimately based on the clinician's best judgment regarding which agent or combination of agents will cover the pathogens likely to be present in the wound on the basis of the information available.

Antibiotics are clearly indicated if cellulitis is present when an injured patient is first seen. The presence of infection suggests that there has been a significant delay between wounding and presentation for treatment. Routine soft tissue infections are usually caused by staphylococci or streptococci, and gram-positive coverage is generally indicated. The presence of crepitus or a foul smell suggests a possible anaerobic infection. Initial antibiotic choices are made empirically; more specific antibiotic treatment can be instituted when the results of bacterial culture and sensitivity studies become available.

Timing of Wound Closure

The goal of acute wound management should be a closed, healing wound. The first issue to address is the timing of closure. The choices are (1) primary closure, that is, to close the wound at the time of initial presentation; (2) secondary closure, that is, to allow the wound to heal on its own; and (3) tertiary closure, that is, to close the wound after a period of secondary healing. The proper choice depends on how the following questions are answered:

1. Must the wound be closed, or will secondary healing produce an acceptable result?
2. If closure is required,
   a. Can hemorrhage be easily controlled?
   b. Can all necrotic material and foreign bodies be clearly identified and excised?
   c. Is excessive bacterial contamination present?

Normal healing can proceed only if tissues are viable, the wound contains no foreign bodies, and tissues are free of excessive bacterial contamination.

SMALL OR SUPERFICIAL WOUNDS

Superficial wounds involving only the epidermis and a portion of the dermis will frequently heal secondarily within 1 to 2 weeks. In such wounds, the functional and aesthetic results of secondary healing are generally as good as or better than those obtained by primary or tertiary closure. For puncture wounds, secondary healing is preferred because it diminishes the likelihood of infection and produces an aesthetically acceptable scar. For wounds on concave surfaces such as the medial canthal region and the nasolabial region, secondary healing generally yields excellent aesthetic results.[9]

ACUTE WOUNDS WITHOUT BACTERIAL CONTAMINATION, FOREIGN BODIES, OR NECROTIC TISSUE

If wound closure is required, primary closure is preferred if it is feasible: it eliminates the need for extensive wound care; the wound reaches its final, healed state more quickly; and it minimizes patient discomfort. However, a wound with foreign bodies or necrotic tissue that cannot be removed by irrigation or debridement, or a wound with excessive bacterial contamination, should not be closed primarily (see below), nor should wounds in which hemostasis is incomplete. Hematomas,[10] necrotic tissue,[11] and foreign bodies[12] promote the growth of bacteria and provide a mechanical barrier between healing tissues.

Table 2 Immunization Schedule*

History of Tetanus Immunization (Doses)	Tetanus-Prone Wounds		Non–Tetanus-Prone Wounds	
	Td[†]	TIG	Td[†]	TIG
Unknown or < 3	Yes	Yes	Yes	No
3 or more	No[‡]	No	No[§]	No

Note: The only contraindication to tetanus and diphtheria toxoids for the wounded patient is a history of neurologic or severe hypersensitivity reaction to a previous dose. Local side effects alone do not preclude continued use. If a systemic reaction is suspected to represent allergic hypersensitivity, postpone immunization until appropriate skin testing is performed. If a contraindication to a tetanus toxoid–containing preparation exists, consider passive immunization against tetanus for a tetanus-prone wound.

*Modified from the recommendations of the Centers for Disease Control and Prevention.

†For children younger than 7 yr, diphtheria and tetanus toxoids and pertussis vaccine adsorbed (or diphtheria and tetanus toxoids adsorbed, if pertussis vaccine is contraindicated) is preferable to tetanus toxoid alone. For persons 7 yr of age and older, Td is preferable to tetanus toxoid alone.

‡Yes, if more than 5 yr since last dose.

§Yes, if more than 10 yr since last dose.

Td—tetanus and diphtheria toxoids adsorbed (for adult use)

TIG—tetanus immune globulin (human)

ACUTE WOUNDS WITH EXCESSIVE BLEEDING

Hemorrhage can be readily controlled in most wounds with pressure, cauterization, or ligation. Occasionally, as with a patient with a bleeding diathesis, primary wound closure is precluded by inadequate hemostasis. In such cases, the wound should be packed or wrapped tightly and elevated if the anatomic site of the wound allows. The wound should then be re-examined within 24 hours to determine whether hemostasis is sufficient to allow safe closure. If bleeding within a wound occurs after closure, the course of action depends on the size of the resulting hematoma. Small hematomas, which will be resorbed, can be ignored. Larger hematomas, which provide a significant barrier to healing, require drainage.

ACUTE WOUNDS WITH FOREIGN BODIES OR NECROTIC TISSUE

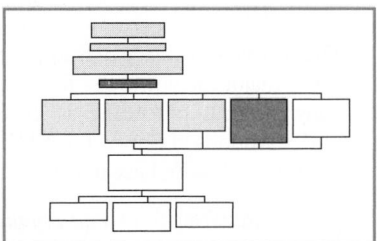

Foreign Bodies

Most foreign bodies can be easily removed from wounds manually or debrided surgically. Patients injured in motorcycle accidents, however, frequently slide along asphalt pavements for long distances at high speeds, with the result that many small fragments of asphalt become embedded in and beneath the skin. Exploding gunpowder also causes many small pieces of foreign material to be embedded within the skin. These foreign bodies are often difficult to extract, but they should be removed as soon as possible after the injury. High-pressure irrigation with saline will remove many foreign bodies. Surgical debridement or vigorous scrubbing with a wire brush may be required for the removal of more firmly embedded foreign material. If too much time elapses between injury and treatment, the embedded material is gradually covered and encapsulated by advancing epithelium and thereby becomes sealed within the dermis. In such instances, surgical dermabrasion is necessary for the removal of the foreign material.[13,14]

Foreign materials such as paint, oil, and grease are sometimes inadvertently injected subcutaneously under pressure (600 to 12,000 psi) by the spray guns used for painting, automotive body work, or industrial purposes.[15,16] On initial examination, the injury may appear deceptively benign in that a punctate entry wound draining foreign material is often the only sign of injury other than edema. Nevertheless, these wounds must be treated aggressively if extensive tissue loss is to be avoided. With some injected materials, radiographs are useful for demonstrating the extent of distribution. The involved area, which is frequently the hand, should be incised, and as much of the foreign material as possible should be surgically debrided (preferably, if the hand is involved, by a surgeon who specializes in hand injuries). Because the foreign material is often widely distributed in the soft tissues, extensive incisions may be necessary. Antibiotics and tetanus prophylaxis are also recommended. The ultimate prognosis is at least partially determined by the type of material injected: paint is associated with a particularly poor prognosis, whereas water is associated with a good one.[17] Early aggressive therapy does not rule out the possibility of amputation, especially if the injected material is notably caustic.

High-velocity missiles such as bullets are rendered sterile by the explosion required for their propulsion; therefore, deeply embedded bullets can often be left safely where they have lodged. Center-fire rifle bullets and .44 magnum pistol bullets carry a large amount of kinetic energy and can produce extensive tissue damage. Wounds created by such high-velocity missiles may have to be debrided to permit excision of necrotic tissue. The mechanism of injury may suggest the possibility of a foreign body within the wound that is not immediately apparent. If a radiopaque material, such as metal or leaded glass, is being looked for, radiographs may detect its presence. For less opaque materials, xeroradiography, magnified radiographs, and computed tomographic scans are sometimes diagnostically useful.[18]

Identification and Debridement of Necrotic Tissue

The necrotic tissue in most wounds can be identified and surgically debrided at initial presentation. In some wounds, there may be a significant amount of tissue of questionable viability. If the amount of questionable material precludes acute debridement, dressing changes may be initiated. When all tissue has been identified as viable or necrotic, and when the necrotic tissue has been debrided surgically or by means of dressing changes, the wound can be closed.

Sometimes, a flap of tissue may be of questionable viability. Signs that suggest whether tissue is viable include color, bright-red arteriolar bleeding, and blanching on pressure followed by capillary refill. A flap can also be evaluated acutely by administering up to 15 mg/kg of fluorescein intravenously and observing the flap for fluorescence under an ultraviolet lamp after 10 to 15 minutes have elapsed.[19] Viable tissue fluoresces. Flap tissue that is thought to be devascularized, on the basis of physical examination or fluorescein examination, should be debrided. If the viability of a segment of tissue is in doubt, it may be sewn back in its anatomic location and allowed to define itself as viable or nonviable over time.

In burn wounds, it is impossible to assess the extent of final tissue damage at presentation because the injury can worsen during the first few days after the burn.[20] Closure of the burn wound is often delayed until the depth of the injury can be more precisely defined [see III:13 Burn Care after the First Postburn Week].

Another type of wound in which the severity of the injury may not be readily apparent is the crush injury. With a crush injury, there may not be an external laceration, even though tissue damage may be extensive. The primary concern is whether muscle damage in the fascial compartments is severe enough to induce swelling sufficient to compromise the vascularity of the muscle. If pulses are diminished or paresthesias are developing, the pressure within the fascial compartment is clearly excessive, and fasciotomies are indicated. In less clear-cut cases, intracompartmental pressures may be assessed by percutaneous placement of catheters or wicks into the fascial compartments. The catheters or wicks are attached to pressure monitors or transducers. An intracompartmental pressure greater than 40 mm Hg indicates that capillary filling pressure has been exceeded and muscle perfusion is compromised. The fascial compartment must then be released to prevent ischemic muscle damage; the fasciotomies must be performed on an emergency basis. If the degree of damage is not severe enough to necessitate fasciotomy, the injured part should be elevated and dressed in a mildly compressive dressing to limit edema formation. If there is muscle damage, the possibility of crush syndrome with renal damage caused by rhabdomyolysis must be considered. If myoglobin is found in the urine, diuresis should be induced, and the urine should be alkalinized.

ACUTE OR NEGLECTED WOUNDS WITH BACTERIAL CONTAMINATION

An infected wound is defined as one with bacterial concentrations greater than 10^5 organisms/g tissue.[21,22] β-Hemolytic streptococci are an exception to this rule and can produce clinical infections in lower concentrations.[23] It is often difficult to assess the degree of bacterial contamination of a wound solely through visual inspection. Ideally, quantitative cultures are ordered so that precise information about the type and numbers of bacteria present can be obtained. The rapid slide technique typically yields bacterial counts within 1 hour.[24] If this information cannot be obtained, the clinician must rely on more empirical information.

The age of the wound is one factor correlated with the degree of bacterial contamination. The initial 6 to 8 hours after wounding has been referred to as the golden period because closure can usually be accomplished safely during this period. In a clinical study in a civilian setting, most wounds less than 5 to 6 hours old were contaminated with fewer than 10^5 bacteria/g tissue and therefore could be safely closed primarily.[25] Experimental data suggest that bacteria trapped within the fibrinous exudate that forms over a wound's surface cause the infections seen in wounds closed after 6 to 8 hours.[26,27] The bacteria proliferate after wounding and generally take 6 to 8 hours to reach levels of 10^5/g tissue. The longer wounds remain open, the greater the likelihood that they will become infected.[25]

The location of the injury is also significant. Lacerations of the face, which has an abundant blood supply, are more likely to resist bacterial proliferation (and to do so for a longer time) than injuries to less adequately perfused areas, such as the lower extremities.[28] Immune status is also important. A wound is less likely to become infected in a young, healthy person than in an elderly, debilitated patient or a person receiving immunosuppressive medication.[29]

The mechanism of injury can suggest whether a wound may become infected and what species of bacteria are most likely to be present in the wound [see Antibiotic Prophylaxis, above]. Wounds with a high degree of bacterial contamination (e.g., human-bite wounds) generally should not be closed.

An infected wound can sometimes be excised to produce a fresh, less contaminated wound. A 1997 study of human facial bites reported successful wound closure when extensive debridement was performed before closure and patients were treated with antibiotics for 1 week.[30] An alternative approach to a contaminated wound is to close it over a drain and administer topical and systemic antibiotics; this approach has yielded low infection rates in some series.[31,32]

In situations in which the nature of the injury precludes complete wound excision or in which there is cellulitis of surrounding tissues, dressing changes should be initiated. The use of certain topical agents will lead to a decreased bacterial count. Silver sulfadiazine (Silvadene) is used frequently because its antibacterial spectrum is broad, it is comfortable for the patient, and it does not commonly lead to metabolic problems such as those seen with other agents, such as mafenide (Sulfamylon) or silver nitrate.[33,34] Silver sulfadiazine may also optimize the rate of epithelialization.[35] Parenteral antibiotics are not useful for killing bacteria in the wound itself, because they do not penetrate the wound directly.[36] In experiments on animals, parenteral antibiotics have proved useful for controlling bacteria within wounds when used in conjunction with proteolytic enzymes such as Travase.[26,37] This combination of treatments has not been widely used clinically.

Once bacterial control has been accomplished, the wound can be closed. In one series, tertiary closure was successful in more than 90% of cases when bacterial counts in tissue had diminished to less than 10^5/g.[38]

An alternative to either primary closure or dressing changes in these patients is delayed primary closure, a technique developed empirically during wartime.[39] Saline-soaked gauze is packed into the wound at the time of injury, and the wound is reexamined after several days. If the wound appears clean, the wound edges are then approximated. If the wound appears to be contaminated at follow-up, dressing changes are instituted. This approach limits the infection rate in potentially contaminated wounds.

When infection develops after closure of a wound, treatment involves removal of some or all of the sutures and initiation of dressing changes, often with use of topical antibacterials [see Dressings, below]. Any cellulitis surrounding the wound is treated with systemic antibiotics [see II:11 Soft Tissue Infection].

Surgical Wounds

The American College of Surgeons has divided operative wounds into four major categories [see Table 3]. The likelihood of infection after any surgical procedure is correlated with the category of wound.[40] Wounds in classes I and II have low infection rates, whereas wounds in class IV have infection rates as high as 40%.

Wounds Resulting from Wild-Animal Bites: Special Considerations

Rabies prophylaxis must be considered for bite wounds from high-risk wild animals such as skunks, raccoons, foxes, coyotes, and bats.[41] Rabies is generally not a risk in bite wounds from rodents, rabbits, pets, and domestic animals unless the animal is acting unusually aggressive and is salivating excessively. If there is any possibility that the biting animal has rabies and the animal is available, it should be watched for symptoms of rabies for 10 days. If the biting animal can be killed and examined, rabies can be confirmed or excluded by means of an immunofluorescent antibody study of its brain. If rabies is confirmed or if the biting animal is not available for examination and rabies is suspected, the patient should be treated with both rabies immune globulin and human diploid cell vaccine. Specific schedules for administration appear elsewhere [see II:11 Soft Tissue Infection].

With snakebite wounds, the possibility of envenomation must be considered. The poisonous snakes native to the United States are coral snakes and three species of pit vipers—namely, rattlesnakes, copperheads, and water moccasins.[42-44] The pit vipers can be identi-

Table 3 Classification and Infection Rates of Operative Wounds

Classification	Infection Rate (%)	Wound Characteristics
Clean (class I)	1.5–5.1	Atraumatic, uninfected; no entry of GU, GI, or respiratory tract
Clean-contaminated (class II)	7.7–10.8	Minor breaks in sterile technique; entry of GU, GI, or respiratory tract without significant spillage
Contaminated (class III)	15.2–16.3	Traumatic wounds; gross spillage from GI tract; entry into infected tissue, bone, urine, or bile
Dirty (class IV)	28.0–40.0	Drainage of abscess; debridement of soft tissue infection

fied by the pit between the eye and nostril on each side of the head, the vertical elliptic pupils, the triangular shape of the head, the single row of caudal plates, and the characteristic fang marks they inflict when they bite. Coral snakes have rounder heads and eyes and lack fangs; they are identified by their characteristic color pattern, consisting of red, yellow, and black vertical bands. Patients bitten by any of the pit vipers must be examined for massive swelling and pain, which, along with fang marks, suggest envenomation. The pain and swelling generally develop within 30 minutes of the bite, although they may take up to 4 hours to become manifest. Secondary local signs, such as erythema, petechiae, ecchymoses, and bullae, sometimes appear; if envenomation is extensive, systemic signs, such as disseminated intravascular coagulation (DIC), bleeding, shock, acute respiratory distress syndrome, and renal failure, may also be seen. Patients bitten by coral snakes, on the other hand, show no obvious local signs when envenomation has occurred. Consequently, the physician must look for systemic signs, such as paresthesias, increased salivation, fasciculations of the tongue, dysphagia, difficulty in speaking, visual disturbances, respiratory distress, convulsions, and shock. These symptoms may not develop until several hours after the bite.

No local care is necessary for coral snake bite wounds; however, a variety of techniques have been used for local care of pit viper bite wounds. Some groups have advocated surgical approaches, such as early incision with suction and wound excision, whereas others have suggested topical application of ice or use of tourniquets to limit the spread of venom. None of these treatments have been shown to provide a definite benefit. At present, topical application of ice is discouraged because it is more likely to lead to secondary injuries than to benefit the patient. Tight tourniquets cannot be left in place for long periods without risking damage to the extremity; however, loose tourniquets that slow lymphatic drainage may be of some value. Excision of the bite wound may be effective if it is performed within 1 to 2 hours of injury. To reduce the incidence of unintentional injuries, excision should be performed only by persons with medical training.

Antivenin is indicated if pain and swelling are substantial enough to suggest extensive envenomation. It should be administered only if it is clearly necessary because it is of equine origin and frequently produces serum sickness. Antivenin is almost never required for copperhead bites but is more commonly needed for rattlesnake bites.[45] When indicated, it should be administered as soon as possible because it is less effective when given after signs of envenomation have become severe.

Whenever there is any suggestion of envenomation, a battery of tests, including hematocrit, fibrinogen level, coagulation studies, platelet count, urinalysis, and serum chemistry values, should be performed. These tests should be repeated every 8 to 24 hours to evaluate any venom-induced changes. With severe envenomation, decreased fibrinogen levels, coagulopathies, and bleeding may be seen, as may myoglobinuria.

Envenomation is also a consideration with the bites of brown recluse spiders and black widow spiders.[44] The brown recluse spider has a violin-shaped mark on its dorsum; is found in dark, dry places; and is nocturnal. The symptoms of the bite may range from minor irritation to extreme tenderness associated with edema and erythema; the tenderness, erythema, and edema generally do not develop until 2 to 8 hours after the bite. In more severe cases, tissue necrosis can develop in as little as 12 hours, although more often the area of necrosis does not demarcate itself for weeks. Severe systemic reactions, including hemolysis and DIC, have been reported. The tissue necrosis resulting from the bite of the brown recluse can be minimized by the use of dapsone.[46] The black widow often has a red hourglass mark on its abdomen and lives in dark, dry, protected

areas.[44] The venom is a neurotoxin that produces severe local pain. Neurologic signs usually develop within 15 minutes and consist of muscle pain and cramps starting in the vicinity of the bite. The abdominal muscles frequently become involved. Other symptoms that may develop are vomiting, tremors, increased salivation, paresthesias, hyperreflexia, and, with severe envenomation, shock. In sensitive individuals, paralysis, hemolysis, renal failure, or coma may be seen. Treatment of black widow envenomation includes parenteral 10% calcium gluconate, parenteral methocarbamol, and one dose of parenteral antivenin.

Method of Wound Closure

When a wound is ready to be closed, the appropriate type of wound closure must be chosen. The types of wound closure are (1) direct approximation, (2) skin graft (autograft), (3)

local flap, and (4) distant flap. In general, the simplest method possible in a given situation is preferred.

DIRECT WOUND APPROXIMATION

The most common surgical problem is the deep, relatively acute traumatic or surgical wound that is suitable for primary closure by direct approximation of the edges of the wound. In this setting, the goal is to provide the best possible chance for uncomplicated healing.

Adequate general or local anesthesia is an extremely important first step. If local anesthesia is indicated, as for small traumatic injuries, 0.5% or 1.0% lidocaine (Xylocaine) is generally injected directly into the wounded tissues. Although other local anesthetic agents can be used, lidocaine is the most popular choice because it acts quickly, it rarely provokes allergic reactions, and it provides local anesthesia for the 1 to 2 hours required for most wound closures. Epinephrine in a dilution of 1:100,000 or 1:200,000 is often used in combination with the lidocaine. Epinephrine prolongs the effectiveness of the anesthetic, increases the anesthetic dose that can be safely used, and aids hemostasis.[47] Lower concentrations of epinephrine can be effective, but it becomes unstable if stored for long periods at low concentrations. Traditionally, epinephrine has not been used in the fingers and toes out of concern that it might induce vasospasm, which could result in loss of one or more digits. In the first half of 2001, this guideline was questioned by a prospective study in which a series of digital blocks with epinephrine resulted in no reported morbidity.[48] In reviewing the literature, the authors of the study could not identify a single case in which local anesthesia alone resulted in digital loss. An experimental study from 1985 suggested that the use of epinephrine is associated with a higher incidence of infection[49]; however, this association has not been noted clinically.

The maximum safe doses of lidocaine traditionally cited are 4 mg/kg without epinephrine and 7 mg/kg with epinephrine. The upper limit of the maximum safe dose has been questioned. During liposuction procedures, up to 35 mg/kg of lidocaine has been administered in a 0.1% solution containing epinephrine in a 1:1,000,000 dilution without reaching toxic drug levels.[50,51] Given that some of the anesthetic is aspirated in the course of a liposuction procedure, caution should be exercised in extrapolating this finding to other types of procedures. The pain involved in injecting the local anesthetic can be minimized by using a small-caliber needle, warming the drug, injecting the drug slowly, using the subcutaneous rather than the intradermal route (even though the rate of onset is thereby slowed),[52] providing counterirritation, and buffering the agent with sodium bicarbonate to limit its acidity.[53]

Topical local anesthetics have been gaining in popularity. TAC (a solution of 0.5% tetracaine, 1:2,000 adrenaline [epinephrine], and 11.8% cocaine) has been demonstrated to be as effective as injectable anesthetics when applied topically to an open wound, especially in the face or scalp.[54,55] Concerns have been expressed about the possible toxicity of the cocaine, and efforts have been made to identify alternative topical agents. Topical 5% lidocaine with 1:2,000 epinephrine,[56] topical 4% lidocaine with 0.1% epinephrine and 0.5% tetracaine,[57] 0.48% bupivicaine with 1:26,000 norepinephrine,[58] and 3.56% prilocaine with 0.10% phenylephrine[59] have all been demonstrated to be equivalent to TAC. EMLA (a eutectic mixture of lidocaine and prilocaine) has been used to induce local anesthesia in intact skin, often before venous cannulation,[60] and it has been evaluated in open wounds as well.[61] EMLA is a more effective local anesthetic than TAC for open wounds of the lower extremity. To induce sufficient anesthesia to be useful, however, EMLA must be in contact with the skin for 1 to 2 hours.

Hair may be clipped to facilitate exposure and wound closure, if necessary. Close shaving should be avoided, however, because it potentiates wound infections.[62] Clipping of eyebrows should also be avoided because they may not grow back.

The next step is to irrigate the wound with a high-pressure (≥ 8 psi) spray to decrease the number of bacteria in the wound.[63-65] A pressurized irrigation device is preferred, but if none is available, high-pressure irrigation may be performed by using (1) a 30 to 50 ml syringe and a 19-gauge needle or catheter or (2) a flexible bag of intravenous 0.9% saline attached to tubing and a 19-gauge catheter with a pressure device.[63] Low-pressure irrigation and scrubbing of the wound with a saline-soaked sponge have not been demonstrated to decrease the incidence of wound infections.[65,66] Irrigants that have been demonstrated to be nontoxic to tissues include 0.9% saline[67] and Pluronic F-68,[68,69] though lactated Ringer solution is also acceptable. Pluronic F-68 has surfactant properties that improve wound cleansing without damaging tissues. Antibiotics are sometimes added to irrigation solutions to increase their effectiveness at killing bacteria. Solutions of 1% neomycin sulfate and 2% kanamycin sulfate, which do not kill fibroblasts in culture,[70] have limited toxicity to tissues. There is some evidence[71] that antibiotic supplements are more effective than saline solution in decreasing bacterial counts in contaminated wounds.

There are a number of solutions that should never be placed on a wound. Povidone-iodine scrub and soaps containing hexachlorophene are especially damaging to normal tissues.[67,72,73] Chlorhexidine, which is found in various brands of soaps, has also been demonstrated to impede the healing process.[74,75] Alcohol is toxic to tissues and should not be placed in wounds.[76] A 0.5% solution of sodium hypochlorite (Dakin solution) has been demonstrated to be toxic to fibroblasts, to impair neutrophil function, and to slow epithelialization in open wounds.[70,77] A 0.25% solution of acetic acid has been demonstrated to kill fibroblasts in culture and to slow epithelialization in open wounds.[70] Hydrogen peroxide has been shown to kill fibroblasts in culture and to cause histologic damage to tissues.[67,70] Even standard hand soap can induce some tissue damage that is visible on histologic examination.[67,76] The dictum "Don't put in a wound what you wouldn't put in your eye" is a valid guideline.[78]

After adequate anesthesia has been achieved, hair has been clipped, and the wound has been irrigated, the tissue surrounding the wound is prepared with an antibacterial solution such as povidone-iodine,[79,80] and a sterile field is created by using sterile drapes. Skin preparation limits contamination of the wound by bacteria from adjacent skin. The wound is surgically debrided of any foreign bodies or necrotic material to limit the chances of postoperative infection.[81] If the wound edges are beveled and adequate local tissue is available, the wound edges should be excised by means of incisions perpendicular to the skin.

Although wound closure can usually proceed in a straightforward manner, special caution is necessary in certain situations. When a wound crosses tissues with different characteristics, such as at the vermilion border of the lip, at the eyebrow, or at the hairline of the scalp, great care must be taken to align the damaged structures accurately. Injured nerves or ducts should generally be repaired at the time of wound closure. In acute wounds, it is generally best to avoid more complex tissue rearrangements such as a Z-plasty or W-plasty. Actual reconstructive surgery in the face of trauma is rarely indicated [see V:30 Plastic Surgical Reconstruction]. Direct approximation of wounds does not always produce a uniform or aesthetically desirable result, particularly in extensive wounds, wounds lying outside normal skin folds or creases, wounds in children older than 2 years, wounds in the sternal and deltoid regions, U-shaped wounds, wounds with beveled edges, or wounds in regions of thick oily skin, such as the tip of the nose, where scars are often less acceptable. Wounds heal optimally when two perpendicular, well-vascularized wound edges are approximated in a tension-free manner.

An ideal method of wound closure would support the wound until it had nearly reached full strength (i.e., about 6 weeks), would not induce inflammation, would not induce ischemia, would not penetrate the epidermis and predispose to additional scars, and would not interfere with the healing process in any way. No existing method of wound closure accomplishes all of these goals: some sort of compromise is virtually always necessary.

Materials for Wound Closure

Materials available for wound closure are sutures, staples, tapes, and tissue adhesives. Of these, sutures are most commonly used. Absorbable sutures, such as those made of plain or chromic catgut, polyglactin 910 (Vicryl), polyglycolic acid (Dexon), polyglyconate (Maxon), or polydioxanone (PDS), are generally used for dermis, fat, muscle, or superficial fascia. Nonabsorbable sutures, such as those made of nylon, Ethibond, or polypropylene (Prolene), are most commonly used either for the skin (in which case they are removed) or for deeper structures that require prolonged wound support, such as the fascia of the abdominal wall or tendons.

The suture should be as small in diameter as possible while still being able to maintain approximation. The decision to remove skin sutures or staples involves balancing of optimal cosmesis with the need for wound support. Optimal cosmesis demands early removal of sutures, before inflammation can develop and before epithelialization can occur along the suture tracts. An epithelialized tract will develop around a suture or staple that remains in the skin for more than 7 to 10 days; after removal of the stitch, the tract will be replaced by an unwanted scar.[82] On the other hand, it takes a number of weeks for the wound to gain significant tensile strength, and early removal of wound support can lead to dehiscence of wounds subject to substantial tension. Wounds on the face and wounds along skin tension lines (e.g., incisions for thyroidectomy) are subject to limited tension, and sutures can be removed from these areas relatively early. Sutures are generally removed at day 4 or 5 from the face and generally by day 7 from other areas where skin tension is limited.

Sutures should remain longer in wounds subject to a greater amount of stress, such as wounds in the lower extremities and wounds closed under tension. Sutures also remain longer in wounds in persons with healing limitations, such as malnutrition. Less aesthetically pleasing consequences may have to be accepted in these cases.

One way of sustaining skin wound support while avoiding unwanted scars from skin sutures is to use buried dermal sutures. Synthetic materials, such as Vicryl, Dexon, PDS, or Maxon, are preferable to chromic or plain catgut because the former are absorbed by simple hydrolysis with little inflammatory response, whereas the latter provoke an active cellular inflammatory response that slows the healing process. Buried dermal sutures are often used in conjunction with either tapes (e.g., SteriStrips) or fine epidermal sutures to aid in precise epidermal alignment.

Closure with staples is more rapid than suture closure, although approximation may not be as precise.[83] Tape is easy to apply, is comfortable for the patient, and leaves no marks on the skin.[84-86] However, patients may inadvertently remove tapes, and approximation is less precise with tapes alone than with sutures. Furthermore, wound edema tends to cause inversion of taped wound edges. Supplemental dermal sutures can enhance the precision of the closure achieved with staples or tapes.

Cyanoacrylate tissue adhesives, used by surgeons for over 30 years, are strong, reasonably flexible, and biocompatible. When these compounds first became available, isobutyl cyanoacrylate and trifluoropropyl cyanoacrylate were placed between wound edges to hold them together. Adhesives used in this way created a mechanical barrier to healing and increased wound inflammation and infection rates. This use of cyanoacrylate tissue adhesives was abandoned relatively quickly.[87] Since then, cyanoacrylates have been applied topically to intact skin at the edge of wounds to hold injured surfaces together. Contact with open wounds is carefully avoided to limit toxicity. Hystoacryl Blue (n-butyl-2-cyanoacrylate) has been used extensively with good clinical results.[88] It creates limited wound strength during the first day after injury and should not be used in wounds subject to stress.[89]

Octylcyanoacrylate is stronger than Hystoacryl Blue. A prospective, randomized trial in Canada[90] compared octylcyanoacrylate to sutures for wound closure. There were few cases of dehiscence, and the aesthetic results of wounds assessed 3 months after closure were similar to those obtained with sutures. As would be expected, octylcyanoacrylate closures were faster for the surgeon and less painful to the patient. Octylcyanoacrylate was not used in deep wounds that penetrated fascia, and the authors also specifically recommended against its use on the hands and over joints where either washing or repetitive motion might lead to premature removal of the adhesive.[90]

Fibrin glue has been utilized to improve the adherence and take of skin grafts[91,92]; it has also been used with a limited number of sutures to close wounds subjected to limited tension (e.g., blepharoplasty incisions[93]) and to curtail seroma formation under flaps.[94] Although fibrin glue is helpful in these settings, it is not strong enough to be usable alone for the closure of wounds subject to even limited tension. Autologous fibrin can be produced from plasma, though the process is sufficiently laborious to discourage routine use. Homologous fibrin has been available in Europe for some time. As a result of its superb safety record, homologous fibrin has been approved by the Food and Drug Administration for general use in the United States.

The old surgical principle that dead space should be closed or obliterated seems to call for the closure of subcutaneous tissues. However, studies in both laboratory animals and humans have demonstrated that multiple layers of closure contribute to an increased incidence of infection.[95,96] Therefore, sutures should be avoided whenever possible in subcutaneous fat, which cannot hold them.

Deeper fascial layers that contribute to the structural integrity of areas such as the abdomen or the chest should be closed as a separate layer to prevent hernias or other structural deformities.

If there appears to be a potential risk of fluid collecting in an unclosed subcutaneous space, drains are a more suitable alternative than subcutaneous stitches. In addition to preventing the accumulation of blood or serum in the wound, suction drains also aid in the approximation of tissues. They are particularly useful in aiding tissue approximation under flaps. Most drains—especially those made of silicone rubber—are relatively inert. However, all drains tend to potentiate bacterial infections and should be removed from a wound as soon as possible.[97]

Drains can usually be safely removed when drainage reaches levels of 25 to 50 ml/day. If a seroma develops after drain removal, intermittent sterile aspirations followed by application of a compressive dressing are indicated. In the unusual case in which drainage is persistent and refractory to intermittent aspirations, a drain may be reintroduced. In unusual cases with prolonged drainage, drains have been left in place for weeks to avoid the development of a seroma.[98]

Occasionally, despite a surgeon's best efforts, a closed wound will dehisce. Dehiscence usually results from tension combined with local and systemic factors. Local factors include poor surgical technique and tissue damage by trauma, prior surgery, or radiation—or, in the case of the abdomen, increased intra-abdominal pressure. Systemic factors include malnutrition, obesity, and concurrent use of medications such as steroids or chemotherapeutic agents. If the dehiscence is noted within 6 to 8 hours and it involves only skin and superficial tissues, the wound can be reclosed or, alternatively, allowed to heal secondarily with dressing changes. Dehiscence of deeper structures such as the abdominal fascia can be a more serious problem. Fascial dehiscence in the abdomen is often heralded by serosanguineous discharge between sutures on days 5 to 8. Fascial separation of less than a few centimeters can be treated expectantly; if the dehiscence is larger, reoperation for fascial reclosure should be performed if the patient's condition permits.

SKIN GRAFTS

If a wound can be directly approximated without excessive tension or distortion of normal structures, that is almost always the method of choice. If a wound is so extensive that direct approximation is impossible, skin grafts should be considered [see V:30 Plastic Surgical Reconstruction]. However, skin grafts cannot be used to close injuries that involve bone denuded of periosteum, cartilage denuded of perichondrium, tendon denuded of paratenon, and nerve denuded of perineurium. Skin grafts will not heal over large areas (> 1.0 to 1.5 cm^2) of denuded bone, cartilage, nerve, or tendon, because these structures are relatively, if not totally, avascular, and blood vessels are not present to revascularize the graft. For such wounds, flaps must be considered (see below).

Skin grafts vary in thickness, from very thin split-thickness grafts that incorporate the epidermis and only a small portion of the dermis to full-thickness grafts that incorporate the entire dermis. (There are further variations within these two classifications.) The nature of the graft affects how readily the graft takes. Thin full-thickness skin grafts from areas such as the eyelid, the retroauricular area, or the medial surface of the upper arm take more reliably than thicker ones from other areas. Similarly, thin split-thickness grafts take more reliably than thicker ones. Grafts that incorporate most or all of the dermis maximally inhibit wound contraction. The ability to inhibit wound contraction is not dependent on the absolute thickness of the graft; rather, it is related to the amount of deeper dermis the graft contains.[99]

Skin grafting produces a second wound at the donor site. All donor sites for full-thickness grafts must be closed independently either by direct wound approximation or by application of an additional graft. Donor sites for split-thickness grafts generally heal secondarily. Donor sites for thicker grafts tend to heal more slowly; donor sites for very thick split-thickness grafts may require grafting for adequate closure.

Skin grafts can be meshed and expanded like a pantograph. This technique increases the area that can be covered and facilitates drainage of fluid through the resulting interstices. Meshed grafts conform well to irregular surfaces. However, the aesthetic result of a meshed graft is usually less satisfactory than that of an intact, unmeshed skin graft, especially if the meshed graft is expanded widely. Wound contraction is increased with an expanded meshed skin graft, which can be a problem around flexion and extension creases near joints.

A suitable donor site should provide a good color match for the wounded tissue and be as inconspicuous as possible.[100] Because humans are relatively symmetrical, the ideal graft tissue in terms of color and texture match is tissue from the contralateral structure. However, this type of graft is often impractical because the donor site is frequently too conspicuous. In general, skin anywhere above the clavicles resembles facial skin; the retroauricular and supraclavicular regions and the scalp are relatively inconspicuous donor sites for facial wounds. The buttocks and upper thighs are preferred donor sites for wounds of the trunk or the extremities.

Grafts will not take if bacterial contamination is excessive,[101] if a seroma or hematoma develops between the graft and the wound site, or if shearing occurs between the graft and the wound site. Infected wounds and wounds in which bleeding is inadequately controlled should not be grafted. Compressive, immobilizing dressing techniques and elevation can help prevent shearing and limit seroma formation. A graft must be protected to some extent until it reaches maturity, usually 6 months after placement.[102] Such measures are especially important for lower-extremity grafts, which may be more susceptible to trauma and dependent edema.

The color of grafted skin generally changes after transfer and is usually darker than it appeared in situ.[103] Hair is transferred only with full-thickness or very thick split-thickness skin grafts. In thicker split-thickness skin grafts, sebaceous activity is lost initially but resumes within 3 months. In the interim, the graft must be lubricated with skin creams. Sensibility in skin grafts is more like that of the recipient site than that of the area from which the graft was taken.[104] Perspiration returns with sensibility, and its pattern also is determined by that of the recipient site.[104] Full-thickness skin grafts have normal growth potential when they are placed during the early years of life, but the growth of split-thickness skin grafts is limited.[105] Skin grafts can be remarkably durable after complete healing and can be used effectively even on the soles of the feet.

FLAPS

Like skin grafts, flaps allow coverage of a wound that cannot be satisfactorily closed primarily; again, the cost is a secondary wound at the donor site. Flaps can be used to close any uninfect-

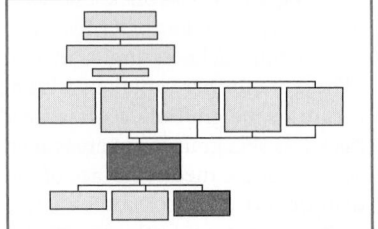

ed wound. They do not require as vascular a wound bed as grafts do, because they maintain their blood supply after transfer and do not depend on revascularization for survival. Flaps are indicated for wounds containing denuded bone, cartilage, tendon, or nerve that cannot be closed by direct approximation. Flaps may be used in some situations in which skin grafts are also a possible choice because they may provide tissue with desirable characteristics such as bulk or a more natural appearance. Flaps that include bone or muscle may also be indicated for functional purposes. Any flap creates at least some functional or aesthetic deficit, a consideration when deciding what type of flap should be used. When feasible, use of local flaps is generally preferred because they usually require a less complex operation and because local tissue is generally the most natural-looking substitute for the wounded tissue. Sometimes, however, specific tissue requirements mandate use of distant flaps.

A flap can be classified as either random or axial. A random flap is supplied with blood from the subdermal plexus but has no specific blood vessel supplying it. An axial flap must be supplied by a specific, predictable blood vessel. Generally, a flap that includes large amounts of tissue or specialized tissue such as muscle or bone is constructed as an axial flap. The most complex distant flap is an axial one that requires microvascular anastomoses of the primary blood vessels of the flap to appropriate recipient vessels in surrounding tissue [see V:30 Plastic Surgical Reconstruction].

The blood supply to the flap must not be impaired by poor design, kinking of the vascular pedicle, pressure from an ill-placed dressing, poor patient positioning, or hematoma formation. Drains are frequently placed under flaps both to encourage tissue approximation and to prevent collection of blood and serum under the flap. Flaps will retain their color, texture, hair-bearing characteristics, and sebaceous activity regardless of the recipient site. Sensibility and perspiration return to some extent between 6 weeks and 3 months after flap transfer. With certain axial flaps, sensibility and other neural functions are preserved from the outset. In children, flaps are also durable and have normal growth potential.

Dressings

Different types of dressings perform different functions. Therefore, for any wound, the purpose a dressing is to serve must be carefully considered before the dressing is applied.

Partial-thickness injuries, such as abrasions and skin graft donor sites, heal primarily by epithelialization and are best treated with dressings that maintain a warm, moist environment.[106,107] A variety of dressings can accomplish this goal, including biologic dressings (e.g., allograft,[108] amnion,[109] or xenograft[110]), synthetic biologic dressings (e.g., Biobrane[111]), hydrogel dressings, and dressings of semipermeable or nonpermeable membranes (e.g., Op-Site or Duoderm).[107] These dressings need not be changed as long as they remain adherent. Small, superficial wounds also heal readily when dressed with Xeroform or Scarlet Red; these dressings are often changed with greater regularity.[112] The traditional approach to partial-thickness injuries has been to apply gauze, often impregnated with a petrolatum-based antimicrobial such as bismuth tribromophenate (Xeroform), and to allow it to dry. Heat lamps have been used to accelerate the drying process. With this method, the gauze provides a matrix that facilitates scab formation.

A scab, which consists of dried fibrin, blood cells, and wound exudate, will protect a wound and limit desiccation and bacterial invasion. Epithelial cells advancing beneath a scab, however, must debride the scab-wound interface enzymatically to migrate across the wound surface beneath the scab.[113] Epithelialization is therefore slower under a scab than it would be under an occlusive dressing. Thus, wounds covered with a scab tend to cause the patient more discomfort than wounds covered with occlusive dressings as well.

For wounds containing necrotic tissue, foreign bodies, or other debris, wet-to-dry dressings are preferred. In this approach, saline-soaked, wide-meshed gauze dressings are applied, allowed to dry, and then changed every 4 to 6 hours. Granulation tissue (including necrotic tissue and other debris) and wound exudate become incorporated within the wide-meshed gauze; thus, a debriding effect is produced when the gauze is removed.[114,115] The disadvantage of this type of dressing is that some viable cells are damaged by the debridement process. Wet-to-wet dressing changes, in which the saline is not allowed to dry, minimize tissue damage but do not produce as much debridement. Enzymatic agents (e.g., Travase, Santyl, and Accuzyme) can debride wounds effectively and are a reasonable alternative to wet-to-dry or wet-to-wet dressings for wounds containing necrotic tissue.[116]

Virtually any type of dressing change will lower the bacterial count in infected wounds; however, application of antibacterial agents, which directly affect the infecting bacteria, generally decreases the bacterial count more quickly than other dressing-change regimens. Silver sulfadiazine is frequently used because in addition to its broad antibacterial spectrum and low incidence of side effects, it has the secondary benefits of maintaining the wound in a moist state and speeding epithelialization.[33]

For wounds with exposed tendons or nerves, it is particularly important to maintain a moist environment to prevent desiccation of the exposed vital structures. Although the biologic and membrane dressings mentioned accomplish this, they are difficult to use on deep or irregular wounds and wounds with a great deal of drainage. Consequently, wet-to-wet dressings or dressings including creams that contain agents such as silver sulfadiazine are often used.

For sutured wounds, the purpose of a dressing is to prevent bacterial contamination, protect the wound from trauma, manage any drainage, and facilitate epithelialization. One approach is to use a dressing with multiple layers, each of which serves a different purpose. The contact layer immediately adjacent to the wound must be sterile and nontoxic. An ideal contact layer does not stick to the

wound or absorb fluid but instead facilitates drainage through itself to the overlying layers of the dressing. Materials with these characteristics include Xeroflo, a fine-meshed gauze impregnated with a hydrophilic substance, and N-terface, a synthetic fine-meshed gauze. The dressing layer directly over the contact layer should be absorptive and capable of conveying exudate or transudate away from the wound surface. Wide-meshed gauze facilitates capillary action and drainage.[117] Such absorptive layers must not be allowed to become soaked, because if they do, exudate collects on the wound surface, and maceration and bacterial contamination may occur. The outermost dressing layer is a binding layer, the purpose of which is to fix the dressing in place. Tape is most commonly used as a binding layer, though elastic wraps or other materials may sometimes be used instead.

With sutured wounds, dressings are required only until drainage from the wound ceases. With nondraining wounds, dressings may be removed after 48 hours, by which time epithelial cells will have sealed the superficial layers of the wound. An alternative method of treating minimally draining incisional wounds is to apply an antibacterial ointment. Such ointments are occlusive and maintain a sterile, moist environment for the 48 hours required for epithelialization.

Some physicians use occlusive dressings for incisional wounds. These dressings, as mentioned, create a warm, moist, sterile environment that is optimal for epithelialization. Some of these are transparent, allowing observation of the wound. The disadvantage of most of these dressings is their limited absorptive capacity, allowing drainage from the wound to collect under the dressing.

In certain small wounds in areas that are difficult to dress, such as the scalp, it may be reasonable to forgo a synthetic dressing and simply allow a scab to form on the wound surface.

Some novel approaches to wound management have been developed since the latter part of the 1990s. One such approach involves the use of skin substitutes, such as Alloderm, Integra, and Apligraf. Alloderm and Integra contain only dermal elements, whereas Apligraf and others contain cellular components, including epithelium. The cellular elements most likely do not remain in the wound for long, but they are thought to provide cytokines that may stimulate the healing process in the short term.

Discussion

Physiology of Wound Healing

Phylogenetically, humans have lost the ability of many lower animals, such as planaria and salamanders, to regenerate specialized structures in most of their tissues. Although the wound-healing process differs slightly from tissue to tissue, the process is similar throughout the body. The result in almost all tissues is scar, the so-called glue that repairs injuries. The goal of acute wound management is to facilitate the body's innate tendency to heal so that a strong but minimally apparent scar results. Generally, however, the normal wound-healing process cannot be accelerated.

The physiology of wound healing is usually described in phases [see Figure 1]. Although each of these phases will be discussed as a separate entity, the phases blend without distinct boundaries.

HEMOSTASIS

Most wounds extend into the dermis, injuring blood vessels and resulting in bleeding. This process stimulates vasoconstriction in the injured vessels, mediated by epinephrine from the peripheral circu-

lation and norepinephrine from the sympathetic nervous system. Prostaglandins, such as prostaglandin $F_{2\alpha}$ ($PGF_{2\alpha}$), and thromboxane A_2 are also involved. As the vessels contract, platelets adhere to the collagen exposed by damage to the blood vessel endothelium and form a plug. Platelet aggregation during the hemostatic process results in the release of cytokines and other proteins from the alpha granules of the cytoplasm of platelet cells. These cytokines include platelet-derived growth factor (PDGF), transforming growth factor–β (TGF-β), transforming growth factor–α (TGF-α), basic fibroblast growth factor (bFGF, also called fibroblast growth factor 2 [FGF2]), platelet-derived epidermal growth factor (PD-EGF), and platelet-derived endothelial cell growth factor (PD-ECGF). Some of these cytokines have direct effects early in the healing process, and others are bound locally and play critical roles in later aspects of healing.

The extrinsic coagulation cascade is stimulated by a tissue factor released from the injured tissues and is essential for clot formation. The intrinsic cascade is triggered by exposure to factor XII and is

INFLAMMATORY PHASE

Serum and Fibrin
Platelets
Polymorphonucleocyte
Thrombosed Vessel

MIGRATORY PHASE

Scab
Advancing Epithelial Cells
Capillary Bud
Macrophage
Fibroblast

PROLIFERATIVE PHASE

Regenerating Epithelium
New Capillary Loop
Macrophage
Fibroblasts

LATE PHASE: SCAR REMODELING

Healed Epithelium
New Blood Vessel
Collagen Fibers

Figure 1 Depicted are the phases of wound healing. In the early phases (top, left), platelets adhere to collagen exposed by damage to blood vessels to form a plug. The intrinsic and extrinsic coagulation cascades generate fibrin, which combines with platelets to form a clot in the injured area. Initial local vasoconstriction is followed by vasodilatation mediated by histamine, PGE_2, PGI_2, serotonin, and kinins. Neutrophils are the predominant inflammatory cells (a polymorphonucleocyte is shown here). In the migratory phase (top, right), fibrin and fibronectin are the primary components of the provisional wound matrix. Additional inflammatory cells, as well as fibroblasts and other mesenchymal cells, migrate into the wound area. Gradually, macrophages replace neutrophils as the predominant inflammatory cells. Angiogenic factors induce the development of new blood vessels as capillaries. Epithelial cells advance across the wound area from the basal layer of the epidermis. The fibrin-platelet clot may dehydrate to form a scab. In the proliferative phase (bottom, left), the advancing epithelial cells have covered the wound area. New capillaries form. The wound's strength grows as a result of steadily increasing production of collagen and glycosaminoglycans by fibroblasts. Collagen replaces fibrin. Myofibroblasts induce wound contraction. In the late phase (bottom, right), scar remodeling occurs. The overall level of collagen in the wound plateaus; old collagen is broken down as new collagen is produced. The number of cross-links between collagen molecules increases, and the new collagen fibers are aligned so as to provide a gradual increase in wound tensile strength. New capillaries combine to form larger vessels. The epithelium is healed, although it never quite regains its normal architecture.

not essential. Both coagulation cascades generate fibrin, which acts with platelets to form a clot in the injured area [*see I:5 Bleeding and Transfusion*]. In a large wound, the superficial portion of this clot may dehydrate over time to produce a scab.

In addition to contributing to hemostasis, fibrin is the primary component of the provisional matrix that forms in the wound during early healing. Fibrin becomes coated with vitronectin from the serum and fibronectin derived from both serum and aggregating platelets. Fibronectins are a class of glycoproteins that facilitate the attachment of migrating fibroblasts as well as other cell types to the fibrin lattice.[118] By influencing cellular attachment, fibronectin is a key modulator of the migration of various cell types in the wound.[119,120] In addition, the fibrin-fibronectin lattice binds various cytokines released at the time of injury and serves as a reservoir for these factors in the later stages of healing.[121]

INFLAMMATION

Tissue damage at the site of injury stimulates the inflammatory response. This response is most prominent during the first 24 hours after a wound is sustained. In clean wounds, signs of inflammation dissipate relatively quickly, and few if any inflammatory cells are seen after 5 to 7 days. In contaminated wounds, inflammation may persist for a prolonged period. The signs of inflammation, originally described by Hunter in 1794, include erythema, edema, heat, and pain.

The signs of inflammation are generated primarily by changes in the 20 to 30 μm diameter venules on the distal side of the capillary bed. In the first 5 to 10 minutes after wounding, the skin blanches as a result of the vasoconstriction that contributes to hemostasis. The initial vasoconstriction is followed by vasodilatation, which generates the characteristic erythema. The vasodilatation is mediated by (1) vasodilator prostaglandins such as PGE_2 and prostacyclin, released by injured cells; (2) histamine, released by mast cells and possibly by platelets to a lesser degree; (3) serotonin, also released by mast cells;

(4) kinins, the release of which is stimulated by the coagulation cascade; and possibly by other factors as well. As the blood vessels dilate, the endothelial cells lining the microvenules tend to contract and separate from one another, resulting in increased vascular permeability. Serum migrates into the extravascular space, giving rise to edema. Inflammatory cells initially adhere loosely to endothelial cells lining the capillaries and roll along the endothelial surface of the vessels. The inflammatory cells eventually adhere to the vessel wall, in a process mediated by the β2 class of integrins, and subsequently transmigrate into the extravascular space.[122] Chemoattractants stimulate the migration of inflammatory cells to the injured area. As monocytes migrate from the capillaries into the extravascular space, they transform into macrophages in a process mediated by serum factors and fibronectin.[123-125] After migration, the inflammatory cells must be activated before they can perform their biologic functions.

Neutrophils are the predominant inflammatory cell in the wound during the 2 to 3 days after wounding, but macrophages eventually become the predominant inflammatory cell in the wound. Because monocytes are present in the serum in much lower numbers than neutrophils, it is not unexpected that they are rarely seen in the wound area initially. After appearing in the wound, both neutrophils and macrophages engulf damaged tissue, digesting them in lysosomes. After neutrophils phagocytose damaged material, they cease to function and often release lysosomal contents, which can contribute to tissue damage and a prolonged inflammatory response. Inflammatory cells and liquefied tissue are the constituents of pus, which may or may not be sterile, depending on whether bacteria are present. Unlike neutrophils, macrophages survive after phagocytosing bacteria or damaged material. The shift in predominant inflammatory cell type within the wound from neutrophils to macrophages is at least in part due to macrophages' extended life span. Macrophage-specific chemoattractants may also selectively attract macrophages into the wound.

In addition to phagocytosis, macrophages are capable of secreting matrix metalloproteinases (MMPs) that break down damaged tis-

Table 4 Involvement of Cytokines in Wound-Healing Functions

Wound-Healing Function	Cytokines Involved
Neutrophil chemotaxis	PDGF IL-1
Macrophage chemotaxis	PDGF TGF-β IL-1
Fibroblast chemotaxis	EGF PDGF TGF-β
Fibroblast mitogenesis	EGF PDGF IGF TGF-β TGF-α IL-1 TNF-α
Angiogenesis, endothelial cell chemotaxis, mitogenesis	EGF Acidic and basic FGF (FGF1 and FGF2) TGF-β TGF-α TNF-α VEGF PD-ECGF
Epithelialization	EGF Basic FGF (FGF2) TGF-β TGF-α KGF IGF
Collagen synthesis	EGF Basic FGF (FGF2) PDGF TGF-β IL-1 TNF-α
Fibronectin synthesis	Basic FGF (FGF2) PDGF TGF-β EGF
Proteoglycan synthesis	Basic FGF (FGF2) PDGF TGF-β IL-1
Wound contraction	Basic FGF (FGF2) TGF-β
Scar remodeling, collagenase stimulation	EGF PDGF TGF-β IL-1 TNF-α

EGF—epidermal growth factor FGF—fibroblast growth factor IGF—insulinlike growth factor IL-1—interleukin-1 KGF—keratinocyte growth factor PD-ECGF—platelet-derived endothelial cell growth factor PDGF—platelet-derived growth factor TGF—transforming growth factor TNF—tumor necrosis factor VEGF—vascular endothelial growth factor

Table 5 Cell Sources of Cytokines

Cell Type	Cytokines
Platelet	EGF PDGF TGF-β TGF-α
Macrophage	FGF PDGF TGF-β TGF-α IL-1 TNF-α IGF-1
Lymphocyte	TGF-β IL-2
Endothelial cell	FGF PDGF
Epithelial cell	TGF-α PDGF TGF-β
Smooth muscle cell	PDGF

sue; they are also a primary source of cytokines that mediate other aspects of the healing process. Experimental studies have demonstrated that neutrophils are not essential to normal healing,[126] whereas macrophages are necessary.[127] These additional macrophage functions—especially their role as a cytokine source—most likely are what make them essential.

MIGRATORY PHASE

Many substances attract fibroblasts and other mesenchymal cells into the wound during the migratory phase, including many of the cytokines[118,128-130] [see Table 4]. It is not known which of them are most active biologically at different points after wounding. The fibroblasts migrate along the scaffold of fibrin and fibronectin, as mentioned. This migration involves the upregulation of integrin receptor sites on the cell membranes, which allows the cells to bind at different sites in the matrix and pull themselves through the scaffold. Migration through the provisional matrix is also facilitated by synthesis of MMPs, which help cleave a path for the cells. Additional cytokines stimulate the proliferation of mesenchymal cells important in the wound-healing process once these cells have been attracted into the wound area[131,132] [see Table 4].

Angiogenesis

Angiogenesis is also initiated in the migratory phase during the first 2 or 3 days after wounding. Before revascularization of the injured area, the wound microenvironment is hypoxic and is characterized by high lactic acid levels and a low pH. Angiogenic factors stimulate the process of neovascularization. Some of the more potent angiogenic factors are derived from platelets and macrophages[133,134] [see Tables 4 and 5]. New vessels develop from existing vessels as capillaries. The capillaries grow from the edges of the wound toward areas of inadequate perfusion within the provisional wound matrix, where lactate levels are increased and tissue oxygen tension is low. The generation of new vessels involves both migration and proliferation of cells. Both cellular activities are modulated by the angiogenic cytokines. A key aspect of endothelial cell migration is the upregulation of the α-β_3 integrin binding domain that facilitates the binding of the endothelial cells to the matrix. Migrating endothelial cells produce plasminogen activator, which catalyzes the breakdown of fibrin, as well as MMPs, which help create paths through the matrix for the developing blood vessels. When the budding capillaries meet other developing capillaries, they join and blood flow is initiated. As the wounded area becomes more vascularized, the capillaries consolidate to form larger blood vessels.

Epithelialization

Epithelialization of skin involves the migration of cells from the basal layer of the epidermis across the denuded wound area.[135] This migratory process begins approximately 24 hours after wounding. The migrating cells develop bands 40 to 80 Å wide that can be seen with electron microscopy and stained with antiactin antibodies. About 48 hours after wounding, the basal epidermal cells at the wound edge enlarge and begin to proliferate, producing more migratory cells. If the normal basement membrane is intact, the cells simply migrate over it; if it is not, they migrate over the provisional fibrin-fibronectin matrix.[136] As migration is initiated, desmosomes that link epithelial cells together and hemidesmosomes that link the cells to the basement membrane disappear.[137] Migrating cells express integrins on their cell membranes that facilitate migration. As they migrate, they secrete additional proteins that become part of the new basement membrane, including tenascin,[138] vitronectin, and collagen types I and V. In addition, they generate MMPs to facilitate migration, as noted.

When epithelial cells migrating from two areas meet, contact inhibition prevents further migration. The cells making up the epithelial monolayer then differentiate into basal cells and divide, eventually yielding a neoepidermis consisting of multiple cell layers. Epithelialization progresses both from wound edges and from epithelial appendages. Epithelial advancement is facilitated by adequate debridement and decreased bacterial counts, as well as by the flattening of rete pegs in the dermis adjacent to the wound area. The epithelium never returns to its previous state. The new epidermis at the edge of the wound remains somewhat hyperplastic and thickened, whereas the epidermis over the remainder of the wound is thinner and more fragile than normal. True rete pegs do not form in the healed area.

PROLIFERATIVE PHASE AND COLLAGEN SYNTHESIS

The proliferative phase of wound healing usually begins approximately 5 days after wounding. During this phase, the fibroblasts that have migrated into the wound begin to synthesize proteoglycans and collagen, and the wound gains strength. Until this point, fibrin has provided most of the wound's strength. Although a small amount of collagen is synthesized during the first 5 days of the healing process,[139] the rate of collagen synthesis increases greatly after the fifth day. Wound collagen content continually increases for 3 weeks, at which point it begins to plateau.[140]

Although there are at least 18 types of collagen, the ones of primary importance in skin are type I, which makes up 80% to 90% of the collagen in skin, and type III, which makes up the remaining 10% to 20%. A higher percentage of type III collagen is seen in embryologic skin and in early wound healing. A critical aspect of collagen synthesis is the hydroxylation of lysine and proline moieties within the collagen molecule. This process requires specific enzymes as well as oxygen, vitamin C, α-ketoglutarate, and ferrous iron, which function as cofactors. Hydroxyproline, which is found almost exclusively in collagen, serves as a marker of the quantity of collagen in tissue. Hydroxylysine is required for covalent cross-link formation between collagen molecules, which contributes greatly to wound strength. Deficiencies in oxygen or vitamin C or the suppression of enzymatic activity by corticosteroids may lead to underhydroxylated collagen incapable of generating strong crosslinks. Underhydroxylated collagen is easily broken down. After collagen molecules are synthesized by fibroblasts, they are released into the extracellular space. There, after enzymatic modification, they align

Figure 2 The tensile strength of skin wounds begins to increase gradually about 3 weeks after wounding. The collagen elaborated early in the healing process is replaced by stronger collagen that is aligned along the lines of stress in the tissue. Closer bonding and a greater number of cross-links between fibers augment the wound's tensile strength. The process of collagen replacement and scar remodeling continues for years.[248]

themselves into fibrils and fibers that give the wound strength. Initially, the collagen molecules are held together by electrostatic cross-links as fibrils form. These cross-links are subsequently replaced by more stable covalent bonds. The covalent bonds form between lysine and lysine, between lysine and hydroxylysine, and between hydroxylysine and hydroxylysine[141]; the strongest cross-links form between hydroxylysine and hydroxylysine.

Proteoglycans, also synthesized during the proliferative phase of healing, consist of a protein core linked to one or more glycosaminoglycans. Dermatan sulfate, heparin, heparan sulfate, keratan sulfate, and hyaluronic acid are the more common proteoglycans. The biologic effects of proteoglycans are less well understood than those of collagen. They generally anchor specific proteins in certain locations and affect the biologic activity of target proteins. Heparin is an important cofactor of bFGF during angiogenesis. Other proteoglycans most likely facilitate the alignment of collagen molecules into fibrils and fibers.

Wound Contraction

Collagen has no contractile properties, and its synthesis is not required for wound contraction. During the proliferative phase, myofibroblasts appear in the wound and probably contribute to its contraction.[142] Myofibroblasts are unique cells that resemble normal fibroblasts and may be derived from them. They have convoluted nuclei, vigorous rough endoplasmic reticula, and microfilament bundles 60 to 80 Å in diameter. These microfilaments can be stained with antiactin and antimyosin antibodies. Many authorities believe that the myofibroblasts pull the wound together from the edges of the wound; however, others believe, on the basis of observations in collagen lattices, that it is the fibroblasts within the center of the wound that generate the force of wound contraction. To date, this issue has not been resolved. TGF-β is a potent stimulant of wound contraction in experimental models.[143]

The wound edges are pulled together at a rate of 0.60 to 0.75 mm/day. The rate of contraction varies with tissue laxity. Contraction is greatest in anatomic sites where there is redundant tissue. Wound contraction generally continues most actively for 12 to 15 days or until wound edges meet.

LATE PHASE: SCAR REMODELING

Approximately 3 weeks after wounding, scar remodeling becomes the predominant feature of the healing process. Collagen synthesis is downregulated, and the wound becomes less cellular as apoptosis occurs. During this phase, there is continual turnover of collagen molecules as old collagen is broken down and new collagen is synthesized along lines of stress.[144,145] Collagen breakdown is mediated by several MMPs, found in scar tissue as well as in normal connective tissues.[146] At least 25 MMPs that affect different substrates have been identified. The more common of these include MMP-1 (collagenase-1), MMP-2 (gelatinase A), and MMP-3 (stromelysin-1). The activity of these collagenolytic enzymes is modulated by several tissue inhibitors of metalloproteinases (TIMPs). During this phase, there is little net change in total wound collagen,[144] but the number of cross-links between collagen strands increases.

The realigned, highly cross-linked collagen is much stronger than the collagen produced during the earlier phases of healing. The result is a steady, gradual growth in wound tensile strength that continues for 6 to 12 months after wounding [see Figure 2]. Scar tissue never reaches the tensile strength of unwounded tissue, however. The rate of gain in tensile strength begins to plateau at 6 weeks after injury. The common clinical recommendation that patients avoid heavy lifting or straining for 6 weeks after laparotomy, her-

nia repair, or many orthopedic procedures is based on the time required for increased tensile strength.

Role of Cytokines in Wound Healing

Wounding stimulates specific cellular activities in a consistent manner that is reproducible from wound to wound. Many, if not all, of these cellular activities appear to be mediated by cytokines. The predictability with which cellular activities start and stop after wounding suggests that the cytokines mediating them are released in a closely regulated fashion; however, the details of this process have not yet been elucidated.

Numerous cytokines are known to be capable of mediating the major biologic activities involved in wound healing [see Table 4]. Most of these activities can be mediated by more than one factor, and researchers have not yet been able to determine which factors are the most important stimulants of wound-healing functions in vivo. One possible explanation for the duplication in mediating functions is that factors with similar activities may act at different times in the course of the wound-healing process.

Cytokines are produced by platelets, macrophages, lymphocytes, endothelial cells, epithelial cells, and smooth muscle cells [see Table 5]. Some cytokines, such as PDGF, are produced by several cell types,[147-150] whereas others, such as interleukin-2 (IL-2), are produced by only one cell type.[151,152] The cell of origin is a key variable that determines the time at which a factor will be present after wounding. Platelets, for example, release PDGF,[147] TGF-β,[153] and epidermal growth factor (EGF),[154] and it would be expected that these cytokines would be found in a wound soon after injury. Factors produced by several different cell types at different times may be released by individual cell types at different times. For example, PDGF[148,149] and TGF-β,[155] which are produced by both platelets and macrophages, might be released by platelets soon after wounding and by macrophages at a later stage in the healing process.

The names of cytokines are frequently misleading. In many cases, they derive from the first known cell of origin or from the first function discovered (or hypothesized) for the factor. As a result, a polyfunctional factor may have a name implying that it has only one function, a factor produced by multiple cell types may have a name suggesting that it is produced by a single cell type, or a factor's name may lay claim to a capability that the factor does not have. For example, TGF-β received its name because it was originally believed to be capable of transforming normal cells into malignant ones. Although it is now known that TGF-β does not have this capability, the name has not been altered.

Cytokines are also a promising tool in the biologic modification of the wound-healing process. Early experimental work was done with small quantities of factors extracted from biologic sources (e.g., platelets). Currently, recombinant technology can provide

Table 6 Factors Impairing Wound Healing

Local	Systemic
Infection	Malnutrition
Foreign bodies	Cancer
Ischemia/hypoxia	Diabetes mellitus
Venous insufficiency	Uremia
Toxins (e.g., spider venom)	Jaundice
Previous trauma	Old age
Radiation	Systemic corticosteroids
Cigarette smoking	Chemotherapeutic agents
	Alcoholism

large quantities of highly purified material that can be used clinically. It has been experimentally demonstrated that many of the cytokines are capable of accelerating wound healing in normal and healing-impaired models. TGF-β has markedly increased wound-breaking strength in incisional wounds in rats soon after wounding.[156] bFGF has increased the strength of incisional wounds when injected on day 3 after wounding.[157] EGF has accelerated the closure of partial-thickness wounds in pigs when applied topically,[158] and it has accelerated collagen accumulation in a wound chamber model.[159] PDGF has accelerated healing in incisional wounds in rats when administered in a slow-release vehicle at the time of wounding.[160] Cytokines have also been observed to reverse healing deficits produced by diabetes,[161] steroids,[162] doxorubicin,[163] and radiation[164] in experimental models.

The positive results of these experimental studies encouraged the use of cytokines in clinical trials in humans. In an early human study, EGF accelerated the healing of skin graft donor sites.[165] In another study, it was applied topically to chronic nonhealing wounds in an uncontrolled group of patients and was considered to contribute to improved healing in the majority.[166] Autogenous platelet extracts have been used on chronic nonhealing wounds as well, with good results.[167] In a better-controlled study, recombinant human PDGF-bb accelerated healing when applied topically to pressure sores in a randomized, double-blind, placebo-controlled fashion.[168] In another carefully controlled, randomized, prospective study, bFGF was also demonstrated to be efficacious as a topical wound-healing supplement for pressure sores.[169] PDGF-bb has been demonstrated to be efficacious and has been approved for use on diabetic ulcers.[170] It is being marketed as becaplermin (Regranex).

It is not known which factors will be most effective as healing adjuvants in either normal or impaired healing states. It would seem logical that addition of a combination of factors in a sequence mimicking that characteristic of normal healing would produce optimal effects when healing is unimpaired. When healing is impaired, it would seem logical to augment the quantity of whatever factors are lacking or present at reduced levels. However, much work remains to be done—first, to determine which factors are most critical in normal states and, second, to determine which factors are lacking in impaired states so that the best use can be made of the recombinant factors now available.

Physiology of Skin Graft Healing

Although the physiology of skin graft healing is similar to that of open wound healing, differences arise because the wound is covered by the graft and because the graft has its own intrinsic architectural nature. Initially, fibrin holds the graft on the recipient site. The strength of attachment increases rapidly for the first 8 hours after graft placement, after which the rate of increase tapers off slightly.[171] For the first 48 hours, the graft survives by serum imbibition[172]: plasmalike fluid is absorbed by the graft, which increases in weight by up to 30% during this period. The absorbed fluid supports only minimal metabolic activities and maintains cellular viability until revascularization occurs. After approximately 48 hours, new blood vessels begin to grow into the graft from the recipient site.[173] It is not known whether a new vascular network grows within the graft or whether vessels from the recipient site simply connect with existing vessels in the graft. Skin graft revascularization probably involves a combination of these two processes.[174] Blood flow in the graft reaches nearly normal levels approximately 7 days after grafting. The vascular system continues to mature, with smaller vessels merging into larger ones. By 21

days after grafting, the graft's vascular supply appears nearly normal on dye injection studies.[173]

Lymphatic channels begin to develop 4 to 5 days after grafting, and the lymphatic system gradually matures until it, too, is nearly normal after 21 days.[175] Epithelial cells and fibroblasts remain dormant for 3 days after placement of a skin graft and subsequently proliferate.[176] The epithelium remains hyperplastic for 6 weeks.[177] By 7 to 8 days after grafting, fibroblasts are more plentiful in the graft than in the surrounding skin, and new collagen is being synthesized.[176,177] Collagenolytic activity develops simultaneously and actually exceeds collagen synthesis for 2 weeks, leading to a net loss in graft collagen. However, during the third week after grafting, the net amount of collagen starts to increase as the rate of collagen synthesis begins to exceed the rate of collagenolysis. Active collagen synthesis continues for at least 20 weeks.[102]

Disturbances of Wound Healing

Healing does not always occur in a straightforward, undisturbed fashion. Both local and systemic factors can interfere with healing. Local factors include infection, foreign bodies, tissue hypoxia, venous insufficiency, local toxins, mechanical trauma, irradiation, and cigarette smoking. Systemic factors include malnutrition, cancer, diabetes mellitus, uremia, jaundice, old age, corticosteroids, chemotherapeutic agents, and alcoholism. Several of these local and systemic factors [see Table 6] will be discussed in more detail.

LOCAL FACTORS

Infection

The body maintains a symbiotic relationship with bacteria. Normal dry skin contains up to 1,000 bacteria/g,[4] and saliva contains 100 million bacteria/ml.[178] The bacterial population is kept in control by several mechanisms. Invasion is mechanically limited by an intact stratum corneum in the skin and intact oral mucosa.[5] Sebaceous secretions contain bactericidal and fungicidal fatty acids that modulate bacterial proliferation.[179] Edema dilutes these fatty acids, making edematous areas more infection prone. Lysozymes in skin hydrolyze bacterial cell membranes, further limiting bacterial proliferation.[180] The immune system augments local barriers to infection.

Infection occurs when the number or virulence of bacteria exceeds the ability of local tissue defenses to control them. Generally, as mentioned, infection exists when bacteria have proliferated to levels beyond 10^5 organisms/g tissue (β-hemolytic streptococci being the only exception). At this level, bacteria overwhelm host defenses and proliferate in an uncontrolled fashion. This number was defined by studies performed at the United States Army Institute of Surgical Research and elsewhere.[21,181-183] Local factors such as impaired circulation or radiation injury increase the risk of infection. Systemic diseases such as diabetes, AIDS, uremia, and cancer also increase the susceptibility to wound infection.

Hypoxia and Smoking

Delivery of oxygen to healing tissues is critical for prompt wound repair. Oxygen is necessary for cellular respiration as well as for hydroxylation of proline and lysine residues. Adequate tissue oxygenation requires an adequate circulating blood volume,[184] adequate cardiac function, and adequate local vasculature. Vascular disorders may be systemic, as in peripheral vascular disease, or localized, caused by scarring from trauma or prior surgery. Wound healing in ischemic extremities is directly correlated with transcutaneous oxygen tension.[185] Hyperbaric oxygen has been used in the treatment of many types of wounds in which tissue hypoxia may impair healing. Anemia, however, is not associated with impaired healing unless the anemia is severe enough to limit circulating blood volume.[186]

Smoking can impair tissue oxygenation. Smoking stimulates vasoconstriction acutely and contributes to the development of atherosclerosis and vascular disease over time.[187-189] Approximately 3% to 6% of cigarette smoke is carbon monoxide, which binds to hemoglobin, producing carboxyhemoglobin. Smokers have carboxyhemoglobin levels between 1% and 20%.[190] Carboxyhemoglobin limits the oxygen-carrying capacity of the blood, increases platelet adhesives,[191] and produces endothelial changes.[192,193]

Irradiation

Irradiation damages the DNA of cells in exposed areas. Some cells die, and others are rendered incapable of undergoing mitosis. When radiation is administered therapeutically, doses are fractionated and tangential fields are used to limit damage to normal cells while maximizing damage to tumor cells. Despite such techniques, normal cells are damaged by irradiation.

Radiation therapy initially produces inflammation and desquamation in a dose-dependent fashion.[194] After a course of irradiation, healing ensues if surrounding normal tissues have not been irreparably damaged. Additional cells must migrate into the treated area for adequate healing to occur. Fibroblasts migrating into irradiated tissue are often abnormal because of irradiation. These cells are characterized by multiple vacuoles, irregular rough endoplasmic reticulum, degenerating mitochondria, and cytoplasmic crystalline inclusion bodies. Increased levels of inflammatory mediators contribute to an abnormal healing response. Collagen is synthesized to an abnormal degree in irradiated tissue, causing characteristic fibrosis. The media of dermal blood vessels in irradiated areas thickens and some blood vessels become occluded, resulting in a decrease in the total number of blood vessels. Superficial telangiectasias may be seen. The epidermis becomes thinned, and changes in pigmentation often develop. Irradiated skin is dry because of damage to sebaceous and sweat glands, and it has little hair. The epidermal basement membrane is abnormal, and nuclear atypia is common in keratinocytes.

Abnormal healing is predictable after wounding of previously irradiated tissue. Decreased vascularity and increased fibrosis limit the ability of platelets and inflammatory cells to gain access to wounds in the area. The quantity of cytokines released is therefore limited in wounds in irradiated tissue. This relative cytokine deficiency causes impairment of virtually all cellular aspects of healing. Damaged fibroblasts and keratinocytes in the area may not respond normally to wound-healing stimulants. In addition, irradiated tissue is predisposed to infection, which can further slow the healing process.

Clinically, impaired healing is manifest by a higher rate of complications when an operation is performed on irradiated tissue.[195] Vitamin A has been used to reverse the healing impairment caused by radiation therapy.[196] Difficult wounds in irradiated tissue can often be managed surgically by bringing a new blood supply to the area with flaps from nonirradiated areas.

SYSTEMIC FACTORS

Malnutrition

Adequate amounts of protein, carbohydrates, fatty acids, vitamins, and other nutrients are required for wounds to heal. Malnutrition frequently contributes to suboptimal healing.[197] In experimental studies,[198] a loss of 15% to 20% of lean body mass has been associated with a decrease in wound-breaking strength and a decrease in colonic bursting pressure. Hypoproteinemia inhibits proper wound healing by limiting the supply of critical amino acids required for synthesis of collagen and other proteins. Collagen synthesis essentially stops in the absence of protein intake,[199] resulting in impaired healing.[200,201] Arginine and glutamine appear to be particularly important amino acids. Cystine residues are found along the nonhelical peptide chain associated with procollagen; in the absence of these cystine residues, proper alignment of peptide chains into a triple helix is inhibited.[202]

Carbohydrates and fats provide energy for healing, and wound healing slows when carbohydrate or fat stores are limited. As an alternative energy source, protein is broken down instead of contributing primarily to tissue growth.[203] Fatty acids are also vital components of cell membranes.

Several vitamins are essential for normal healing. As mentioned, vitamin C is a necessary cofactor for hydroxylation of lysine and proline during collagen synthesis. The ability of fibroblasts to produce new, strongly cross-linked collagen is diminished if vitamin C is deficient. Clinically, existing scars dissolve because collagenolytic activity continues without adequate compensatory collagen synthesis, and new wounds fail to heal. Vitamin C deficiency is also associated with impaired resistance to infection.[203] Because vitamin A is essential for normal epithelialization, proteoglycan synthesis, and normal immune function,[204-206] healing is impaired when vitamin A is deficient. Thiamine deficiency has also been associated with impaired healing.[207] Vitamin D, required for normal calcium metabolism, is needed for bone healing. Exogenous vitamin E impairs wound healing in rats, most likely by influencing the inflammatory response in a corticosteroid-like manner.[208]

The minerals necessary for normal healing include the trace element zinc, a necessary cofactor for DNA polymerase and reverse transcriptase. Because zinc deficiency can result in an inhibition of cellular proliferation and deficient granulation tissue formation[209] and healing,[210] zinc replacement should be given if a deficiency is diagnosed. Pharmacologic overdosing with zinc does not accelerate wound healing and can have detrimental effects.[210]

Correction of generalized malnutrition requires refeeding. The amount of food ingested in the immediate preoperative period may have a greater influence than the overall degree of malnutrition, possibly by inducing positive nitrogen balance.[211] A prospective, randomized study of patients undergoing total parenteral nutrition prior to surgery demonstrated a significant reduction in postoperative morbidity and mortality.[212]

Cancer

Impaired wound healing associated with cancer has been demonstrated experimentally[213] and is often noted clinically. Cancer-bearing hosts may have impaired healing for a variety of reasons. Cancer-induced cachexia, manifest as weight loss, anorexia, and asthenia, significantly limits healing. Cachexia is a result of either decreased caloric intake, increased energy expenditure, or both.

Decreased oral intake may be due to anorexia or mechanical factors. Anorexia is mediated through as yet imperfectly defined circulating factors. Changes in taste perception, hypothalamic function, and tryptophan metabolism may contribute to anorexia. Tumors in the gastrointestinal tract can produce obstruction and generate fistulae that limit nutrient absorption. Other cancers generate peptides such as gastrin and vasoactive intestinal polypeptide (VIP) that alter transit times and interfere with absorption of nutrients.

Cancers alter host metabolism in dysfunctional ways as well. Glucose turnover may be increased, sometimes leading to glucose intolerance. The effect of increased glucose use is higher energy needs.[214] Protein catabolism may be accelerated. Protein breakdown in muscle is increased, as is hepatic utilization of amino acids. Such changes in protein metabolism produce a net loss of plasma protein. Unlike malnourished patients, cancer patients may not be able to alter their metabolism to rely on fat for most energy needs. In tumor-bearing animals, fat accumulates, while other, more vital tissues are broken down for energy. In addition, vitamin C may be taken up preferentially by some tumors, limiting availability of the vitamin for hydroxylation of proline and lysine moieties in collagen. All of these metabolic changes contribute to a negative energy balance and inefficient energy use.

Cancer patients may be relatively anergic, most likely because of abnormal inflammatory cell activity. Macrophages do not migrate or function normally in cancer patients. Inflammatory cell dysfunction may limit the availability of cytokines required for healing and may also predispose to infection.

Impaired healing must be anticipated in cancer patients because of the many alterations in metabolism and immune function. It has been suggested that vitamin A can improve healing in tumor-bearing mice,[215] but this effect has not been demonstrated in humans.

Old Age

The elderly heal less efficiently than younger persons. DuNuoy and Carrell,[216] who studied patients injured during World War I, demonstrated that wounds in 20-year-old patients contracted more rapidly than those in 30-year-old patients. In a blister epithelialization model,[217] younger patients also healed more rapidly than older patients. Another study[218] found that wound disruption occurred with less force in the elderly.

Diabetes

Diabetes mellitus is also associated with impaired healing. In a prospective study of 23,649 surgical wounds,[219] the risk of infection was five times greater in diabetic patients than in nondiabetic patients. This impairment has been demonstrated experimentally in several models.[220-222] A major contributor to this phenomenon is the impaired inflammatory response associated with hyperglycemia. Diabetes is associated with impaired granulocyte chemotaxis,[223] phagocytic function,[224-226] and humoral and cellular immunity. In addition, diabetes is associated with a microangiopathy that can limit blood supply to the healing wound, particularly in older diabetic patients.[227] Diabetic neuropathy impairs sensation, classically in a stocking or glove nerve distribution in extremities. Although this neuropathy does not limit healing directly, it can diminish an individual's ability to protect himself or herself from trauma. The diabetes-induced impairment in healing may be reduced by tight control of blood sugar levels with insulin.[228-230]

Uremia

Uremia has been associated with impaired healing, partially as a direct effect of urea and partially as the result of coexisting malnutrition. This healing impairment has been demonstrated experimentally in both incisional skin wounds and intestinal anastomoses in rats[231] and in an implantable Gore-Tex wound-healing model in humans.[232] This impairment may be ameliorated by regular dialysis.

Alcoholism

In mice chronically fed alcohol, cellular ingrowth and collagen accumulation were diminished in a sponge model.[233]

Steroids and Immunosuppression

Adrenocortical steroids inhibit all aspects of healing. In incisional wounds, steroids slow the development of breaking strength[234]; in open wounds healing secondarily, they impede wound contraction[235,236] and epithelialization.

This impaired healing results from derangements in cellular function induced by steroids. A primary feature of wounds in steroid-treated individuals is a deficiency in inflammatory cell function. As discussed, inflammatory cells, particularly macrophages, mediate essentially all aspects of healing through cytokines. By diminishing the supply of cytokines, steroids and other immunosuppressive agents profoundly impair all aspects of healing. Macrophage migration, fibroblast proliferation, collagen accumulation, and angiogenesis are among the processes diminished by steroid administration. Sandberg[237] demonstrated that the effects of steroids on healing are most pronounced when the drug is administered several days before or after wounding.

All aspects of steroid-induced healing impairment other than wound contraction can be reversed by supplemental vitamin A. The recommended dose is 25,000 IU/day. Topical vitamin A has also been found effective for open wounds.[238] Anabolic steroids and growth hormone–releasing factor have also reversed steroid-induced healing impairments.

Chemotherapeutic Agents

Chemotherapeutic agents impair healing primarily through inhibition of cellular proliferation. Many agents have been examined in experimental models, and virtually all agents impair healing.[239] Nitrogen mustard, cyclophosphamide, methotrexate, BCNU (carmustine), and doxorubicin are the most damaging to the healing process. Most chemotherapeutic regimens use a combination of agents, compounding their deleterious effects. Clinical trials with chemotherapeutic agents have not been associated with as high an incidence of complications as might be anticipated from experimental evidence. The timing of drug administration as well as the doses utilized may explain this apparent contradiction. Doxorubicin, for example, is a more potent inhibitor of wound healing when delivered preoperatively than postoperatively.[240]

Jaundice and Liver Failure

Liver dysfunction most likely impairs healing through the direct effect of hyperbilirubinemia and through metabolic impairments, such as hypoalbuminemia and hypoprothrombinemia, that develop when the synthetic functions of the liver are impaired. The effect of obstructive jaundice on wound healing has been examined experimentally by several investigators. Bayer and Ellis[241] demonstrated decreased wound-breaking strength in abdominal wounds in rats with obstructive jaundice. In jaundiced animals with gastric wounds, angiogenesis was subjectively diminished, but wound-breaking strength was normal. Arnaud and coworkers[242] demonstrated impaired healing with obstructive jaundice,[242] but Greaney and associates[243] could not duplicate their results in a similar model. Greaney did show diminished collagen accumulation, however, in the wounds of jaundiced animals. In humans, Ellis and Heddle[244] noted an increased incidence of wound dehiscence and hernias in patients undergoing surgery for relief of obstructive jaundice, although others have disagreed.

Clinicians must be aware of both local and systemic factors that can influence healing in an individual patient and take appropriate measures, whenever possible, to improve chances for optimal healing.

HYPERTROPHIC SCARS AND KELOIDS

The events involved in normal healing begin and end in a controlled fashion, producing flat, unobtrusive scars. Healing is a biologic process, and as with all biologic processes, it may occur to a greater or lesser degree. Disturbances that diminish healing have already been discussed. Excessive healing can result in a raised, thickened scar with both functional and cosmetic complications. If the scar is confined to the margins of the original wound, it is called a hypertrophic scar.[245] Keloids extend beyond the confines of the original injury, so that the original wound often can no longer be distinguished.

Certain patients and certain wounds are at higher risk for abnormal scarring. Dark-skinned persons and patients between the ages of 2 and 40 are at higher risk for the development of hypertrophic scars or keloids. Wounds in the presternal or deltoid area, wounds that cross skin tension lines, and wounds in thicker skin have a greater tendency to heal with a thickened scar. Some parts of the body, such as the genitalia, the eyelids, the palms of the hands, and the soles of the feet, almost never develop abnormal scars.

Certain patient and wound characteristics increase the relative likelihood of developing a hypertrophic scar as opposed to a keloid.[246] Keloids are more likely than hypertrophic scars to be familial. Hypertrophic scars are more likely to be seen in light-skinned people; both hypertrophic scars and keloids occur more frequently in dark-skinned people. Hypertrophic scars generally develop soon after injury, whereas keloids may develop up to a year after an injury. Hypertrophic scars may subside in time, whereas keloids rarely do. Hypertrophic scars are more likely to be associated with a contracture across a joint surface.

Keloids and hypertrophic scars result from a net increase in the quantity of collagen synthesized by fibroblasts in the wound area. The fibroblasts within keloids may be different in terms of their biologic responsiveness from those within normal dermis. Although many theories have been suggested, the etiology of keloids and hypertrophic scars is unknown. Treatment of hypertrophic scars and keloids has included surgical excision, steroid injection, pressure garments, topical Silastic gel, radiation therapy, and combinations of these approaches. The absence of a uniform treatment program accurately suggests that no specific treatment is predictably effective for these lesions.[247]

References

1. Committee on Trauma, American College of Surgeons: Early Care of the Injured Patient, 3rd ed. Walt AJ, Peltier LF, Pruitt BA Jr, et al, Eds. WB Saunders Co, Philadelphia, 1982, p 69

2. Grossman JAI, Adams JP, Kunec J: Prophylactic antibiotics in simple hand lacerations. JAMA 245:1055, 1981

3. Committee on Trauma, American College of Surgeons: A Guide to Prophylaxis against Tetanus in Wound Management, 1984 Revision. The American College of Surgeons, Chicago, 1984

4. Peeples C, Bowick JA Jr, Scott FA: Wounds of the hand contaminated by human or animal saliva. J Trauma 20:383, 1980

5. Edlich RF, Rodeheaver GT, Morgan RF, et al: Principles of emergency wound management. Ann Emerg Med 17:1284, 1988

6. Cummings P: Antibodies to prevent infection in patients with dog bite wounds: a meta-analysis of randomized trials. Ann Emerg Med 23:536, 1994

7. Brook I: Human and animal bite infections. J Fam Pract 28:713, 1989

8. Fitzgerald RH Jr, Cooney WP III, Washington JA II, et al: Bacterial colonization of mutilating hand injuries and its treatment. J Hand Surg [Am] 2:85, 1977

9. Zitelli JA: Wound healing by secondary intention: a cosmetic appraisal. J Am Acad Dermatol 9:407, 1983

10. Krizek TJ, Davis JH: The role of the red cell in subcutaneous infection. J Trauma 5:85, 1965

11. Howe CW: Experimental studies on determinants of wound infection. Surg Gynecol Obstet 123:507, 1966

12. Elek SD: Experimental staphylococcal infections in the skin of man. Ann NY Acad Sci 65:85, 1956

13. Iverson PC: Surgical removal of traumatic tattoos of the face. Plast Reconstr Surg 2:427, 1947

14. Agris J: Traumatic tattooing. J Trauma 16:798, 1976

15. Gelberman RH, Posch JL, Jurist JM: High-pressure injection injuries of the hand. J Bone Joint Surg [Am] 57:935, 1975

16. Mrvos RM, Dean BS, Krenzelok EP: High pressure injection injuries: a serious occupational hazard. J Toxicol Clin Toxicol 25:297, 1987

17. Weltmer JB Jr, Pack LL: High-pressure water-gun injection injuries to the extremities: a report of six cases. J Bone Joint Surg [Am] 70:1221, 1988

18. Lammers RL: Soft tissue foreign bodies. Ann Emerg Med 17:1336, 1988

19. Myers MB: Prediction of skin sloughs at the time of operation with the use of fluorescein dye. Surgery 51:158, 1962

20. Hinshaw JR: Progressive changes in the depth of burns. Arch Surg 87:993, 1963

21. Teplitz C, Davis D, Mason AD, et al: Pseudomonas burn wound sepsis: I. Pathogenesis of experimental burn wound sepsis. J Surg Res 4:200, 1964

22. Shuck JM, Moncreif JA: The management of burns: I. General considerations and the Sulfamylon method. Current Problems in Surgery. Year Book Medical Publishers, Inc, Chicago, 1969

23. Robson MC, Heggers JP: Surgical infection: II. The beta-hemolytic streptococcus. J Surg Res 9:289, 1969

24. Heggers JP, Robson MC, Ristroph JD: A rapid method of performing quantitative wound cultures. Milit Med 134:666, 1969

25. Robson MC, Duke WF, Krizek TJ: Rapid bacterial screening in the treatment of civilian wounds. J Surg Res 14:426, 1973

26. Rodeheaver GT, Rye DR, Rust R, et al: Mechanisms by which proteolytic enzymes prolong the golden period of antibiotic action. Am J Surg 136:379, 1978

27. Edlich RF, Smith OT, Edgerton MT: Resistance of the surgical wound to antimicrobial prophylaxis and its mechanism of development. Am J Surg 126:583, 1973

28. Kanthak FF, Dubrul EL: The immediate repair of war wound of the face. Plast Reconstr Surg 2:110, 1947

29. Ad Hoc Committee of the Committee on Trauma, Division of Medical Sciences, National Academy of Sciences–National Research Council: Postoperative wound infections: the influence of ultraviolet radiation of the operating room and of various other features. Ann Surg 160(suppl 1):1, 1964

30. Donkor P, Bankas DO: A study of primary closure of human bite injuries to the face. J Oral Maxillofac Surg 55:479, 1997

31. McIlrath DC, van Heerden JA, Edis AJ, et al: Closure of abdominal incisions with subcutaneous catheters. Surgery 60:411, 1976

32. Zelko JR, Moore EE: Primary closure of the contaminated wound: closed suction wound catheter. Am J Surg 142:704, 1981

33. Kucan JO, Robson MC, Heggers JP, et al: Comparison of silver sulfadiazine, povidone-iodine and physiologic saline in the treatment of chronic pressure ulcers. J Am Geriatr Soc 24:232, 1981

34. Moncrief JA: Topical therapy for control of bacteria in the burn wound. World J Surg 2:151, 1978

35. Geronemus RG, Mertz PM, Eaglstein WH: Wound healing: the effects of topical antimicrobial agents. Arch Dermatol 115:1311, 1979

36. Robson MC, Edstrom LE, Krizek TJ, et al: The efficacy of systemic antibiotics in the treatment of granulating wounds. J Surg Res 16:299, 1974

37. Rodeheaver G, Edgerton MT, Elliott MB, et al: Proteolytic enzymes as adjuncts to antibiotic prophylaxis of surgical wounds. Am J Surg 127:564, 1974

38. Robson MC, Heggers JP: Delayed wound closure based on bacterial counts. J Surg Oncol 2:379, 1970

39. Hepburn HH: Delayed primary suture of wounds. Br Med J 1:181, 1919

40. Cruise PJE, Foord R: The epidemiology of wound infection: a 10-year prospective study of 62,939 wounds. Surg Clin North Am 60:27, 1980

41. Klein M: Nondomestic mammalian bites. Am Fam Physician 32:137, 1985

42. Kurecki BA 3rd, Brownlee HJ Jr: Venomous snakebites in the United States. J Fam Pract 25:386, 1987

43. Sprenger TR, Bailey WJ: Snakebite treatment in the United States. Int J Dermatol 25:479, 1986

44. Pennell TC, Babu S-S, Meredith JW: The management of snake and spider bites in the southeastern United States. Am Surg 53:198, 1987

45. Lawrence WT, Giannopoulos A, Hansen A: Pit viper bites: rational management in locales in which copperheads and cottonmouths predominate. Ann Plast Surg 36:276, 1996

46. Rees RS, Altenbern P, Lynch JB, et al: Brown recluse spider bites: a comparison of early surgical excision versus dapsone and delayed surgical excision. Ann Surg 202:659, 1985

47. Siegel RJ, Vistnes LM, Iverson RE: Effective hemostasis with less epinephrine: an experimental and clinical study. Plast Reconstr Surg 51:129, 1973

48. Wilhelmi BJ, Blackwell SJ, Miller JH, et al: Do not use epinephrine in digital blocks: myth or truth? Plast Reconstr Surg 107:293, 2001

49. Tran D-T, Miller SH, Buck DS, et al: Potentiation of infection by epinephrine. Plast Reconstr Surg 76:933, 1985

50. Klein JA: Tumescent technique for local anesthesia improves safety in large-volume liposuction. Plast Reconstr Surg 92:1085, 1993

51. Samdal F, Amland PF, Bugge JF: Plasma lidocaine levels during suction-assisted lipectomy using large doses of dilute lidocaine with epinephrine. Plast Reconstr Surg 93:1217, 1994

52. Arndt KA, Burton C, Noe JM: Minimizing the pain of local anesthesia. Plast Reconstr Surg 72:676, 1983

53. Christoph RA, Buchanan L, Begalla K, et al: Pain reduction in local anesthesia administration through pH buffering. Ann Emerg Med 17:117, 1988

54. Anderson AB, Colecchi C, Baronoski R, et al: Local anesthesia in pediatric patients: topical TAC versus lidocaine. Ann Emerg Med 19:519, 1990

55. Hegenbarth MA, Allen MF, Hawk WH, et al: Comparison of topical tetracaine, adrenaline, and cocaine anesthesia with lidocaine infiltration for repair of lacerations in children. Ann Emerg Med 19:63, 1990

56. Blackburn PA, Butler KH, Hughes MJ, et al: Comparison of tetracaine-adrenaline-cocaine (TAC) with topical lidocaine-epinephrine (TLE): efficacy and cost. Am J Emerg Med 13:315, 1995

57. Schilling CG, Bank DE, Borchert BA, et al: Tetracaine, epinephrine (adrenalin) and cocaine (TAC) versus lidocaine, epinephrine and tetracaine (LET) for anesthesia of lacerations in children. Ann Emerg Med 25:203, 1995

58. Smith GA, Strausbaugh SD, Harbeck-Weber C, et al: Comparison of topical anesthetics without cocaine to tetracaine-adrenaline-cocaine and lidocaine infiltration during repair of lacerations: bupivicaine-norepinephrine is an effective topical anesthetic agent. Pediatrics 97:301, 1996

59. Smith GA, Strausbaugh SD, Harbeck-Weber C, et al: Prilocaine-phenylephrine and bupivicainephenylephrine topical anesthetics compared with tetracaine-adrenaline-cocaine during repair of lacerations. Am J Emerg Med 16:121, 1998

60. Lander J, Hodgins M, Nazarali S, et al: Determinants of success and failure of EMLA. Pain 64:89, 1996

61. Zempsky WT, Karasic RB: EMLA versus TAC for topical anesthesia of extremity wounds in children. Ann Emerg Med 30:163, 1997

62. Alexander JW, Fischer JE, Boyajian M, et al: The influence of hair-removal methods on wound infections. Arch Surg 118:347, 1983

63. Madden H, Edlich RF, Schauerhamer R, et al: Application of principles of fluid dynamics to surgical wound irrigation. Current Topics in Surgical Research 3:85, 1971

64. Gross A, Cutright DE, Bhaskar SN: Effectiveness of pulsating water jet lavage in treatment of contaminated crushed wounds. Am J Surg 124:373, 1972

65. Hamer ML, Robson MC, Krizek TJ, et al: Quantitative bacterial analysis of comparative wound irrigations. Ann Surg 181:819, 1975

66. Schauerhamer RA, Edlich RF, Panek P, et al: Studies in the management of the contaminated wound: VII. Susceptibility of surgical wounds to postoperative surface contamination. Am J Surg 122:74, 1971

67. Branemark PI, Albrektsson B, Lindstrom J, et al: Local tissue effects of wound disinfectants. Acta Chir Scand 357(suppl):166, 1966

68. Rodeheaver GT, Smith SL, Thacker JG, et al: Mechanical cleansing of contaminated wounds with a surfactant. Am J Surg 129:241, 1975

69. Rodeheaver G, Turnbull V, Edgerton MT, et al: Pharmacokinetics of a new skin cleanser. Am J Surg 132:67, 1976

70. Lineaweaver W, Howard R, Soucy D, et al: Topical antimicrobial toxicity. Arch Surg 120:267, 1985

71. Dirschl DR, Wilson FC: Topical antibiotic irrigation in the prophylaxis of operative wound infections in orthopedic surgery. Ortho Clin North Am 22:419, 1991

72. Rodeheaver G, Bellamy W, Kody M, et al: Bactericidal activity and toxicity of iodine-containing solutions in wounds. Arch Surg 117:181, 1982

73. Custer J, Edlich RF, Prusak M, et al: Studies in the management of the contaminated wound: V. An assessment of the effectiveness of pHisoHex and beta-dine surgical scrub solutions. Am J Surg 121:572, 1971

74. Mobacken H, Wengstrom C: Interference with healing of rat skin incisions treated with chlorhexidine. Acta Derm Venereol (Stockh) 54:29, 1974

75. Saatman RA, Carlton WW, Hubben K, et al: A wound healing study of chlorhexidine digluconate in guinea pigs. Fundam Appl Toxicol 6:1, 1986

76. Branemark PI, Ekholm R: Tissue injury caused by wound disinfectants. J Bone Joint Surg [Am] 49:48, 1967

77. Kozol RA, Gillies C, Elgebaly SA: Effects of sodium hypochlorite (Dakin's solution) on cells of the wound module. Arch Surg 123:420, 1988

78. Rodeheaver G: Controversies in wound management. Wounds 1:19, 1989

79. Lowbury EJL, Lilly HA, Bull JP: Methods for disinfection of hands and operation sites. Br Med J 2:531, 1964

80. Saggers BA, Stewart GT: Polyvinyl-pyrrolidone-iodine: an assessment of antibacterial activity. J Hyg (Camb) 62:509, 1964

81. Haury B, Rodeheaver G, Vensko J, et al: Debridement: an essential component of traumatic wound care. Am J Surg 135:238, 1978

82. Ordman LJ, Gillman T: Studies in the healing of cutaneous wounds: II. The healing of epidermal, appendageal, and dermal injuries inflicted by suture needles and by suture material in the skin of pigs. Arch Surg 93:883, 1966

83. George TK, Simpson DC: Skin wound closure with staples in the accident and emergency department. J R Coll Surg Edinb 30:54, 1985

84. Golden T: Non-irritating, multipurpose surgical adhesive tape. Am J Surg 100:789, 1960

85. Golden T, Levy AH, O'Connor WT: Primary healing of skin wounds and incisions with a threadless suture. Am J Surg 104:603, 1962

86. Conolly WB, Hunt TK, Zederfeldt B, et al: Clinical comparison of surgical wounds closed by suture and adhesive tapes. Am J Surg 117:318, 1969

87. Edlich RF, Prusak M, Panek P, et al: Studies in the management of the contaminated wound: VIII. Assessment of tissue adhesives for repair of contaminated tissue. Am J Surg 122:394, 1971

88. Mizrahi S, Bicke A, Ben-Layisfh E: Use of tissue adhesives in the repair of lacerations in children. J Ped Surg 23:312, 1988

89. Yaron M, Halperin M, Huffler W, et al: Efficacy of tissue glue for laceration repair in an animal model. Acad Emerg Med 2:259, 1995

90. Quinn J, Wells G, Sutcliffe T, et al: A randomized trial comparing octylcyanoacrylate tissue adhesive and sutures in the management of lacerations. JAMA 277:1527, 1997

91. Saltz R, Sierra D, Feldman D, et al: Experimental and clinical applications of fibrin glue. Plast Reconstr Surg 88:1005, 1991

92. Jabs AD Jr, Wider TM, DeBellis J, et al: The effect of fibrin glue on skin grafts in infected sites. Plast Reconstr Surg 89:268, 1992

93. Mandel MA: Minimal suture blepharoplasty: closure of incisions with autologous fibrin glue. Aesthetic Plast Surg 16:269, 1992

94. Ersek RA, Schade K: Subcutaneous pseudobursa secondary to suction and surgery. Plast Reconstr Surg 85:442, 1991

95. Ferguson DJ: Clinical application of experimental relations between technique and wound infection. Surgery 63:377, 1968

96. DeHoll D, Rodeheaver G, Edgerton MT, et al: Potentiation of infection by suture closure of dead space. Am J Surg 127:716, 1974

97. Magee C, Rodeheaver GT, Golden GT, et al: Potentiation of wound infection by surgical drains. Am J Surg 131:547, 1976

98. Taldych L, Donegan WL: Postmastectomy seroma and wound drainage. Surg Gynecol Obstet 165:483, 1987

99. Rudolph R: The effect of skin graft preparation on wound contraction. Surg Gynecol Obstet 142:49, 1976

100. Edgerton MT, Hansen FC: Matching facial color with split thickness skin grafts from adjacent areas. Plast Reconstr Surg 25:455, 1960

101. Krizek TJ, Robson MC, Kho E: Bacterial growth and skin graft survival. Forum on Fundamental Surgical Problems 18:518, 1967

102. Klein L, Rudolph R: 3 H-Collagen turnover in skin grafts. Surg Gynecol Obstet 135:49, 1972

103. Mir y Mir L: The problem of pigmentation in the cutaneous graft. Br J Plast Surg 14:303, 1961

104. Ponten B: Grafted skin—observations on innervation and other qualities. Acta Chir Scand 257(suppl):1, 1960

105. Baran NK, Horton CE: Growth of skin grafts, flaps, and scars in young minipigs. Plast Reconstr Surg 50:487, 1972

106. Gimbel NS, Farris W: Skin grafting: the influence of surface temperature on the epithelialization rate of split thickness skin donor sites. Arch Surg 92:554, 1966

107. Alvarez OM, Mertz PM, Eaglstein WH: The effect of occlusive dressings on collagen synthesis and re-epithelialization in superficial wounds. J Surg Res 35:142, 1983

108. Shuck JM, Pruitt BA, Moncrief JA: Homograft skin for wound coverage: a study of versatility. Arch Surg 98:472, 1969

109. Robson MC, Krizek TJ, Koss N, et al: Amniotic membranes as a temporary wound dressing. Surg Gynecol Obstet 136:904, 1973

110. Bromberg BE, Song IC, Mohn MP: The use of pig skin as a temporary biologic dressing. Plast Reconstr Surg 36:80, 1965

111. Woodruff EA: Biobrane, a biosynthetic skin prosthesis. Burn Wound Coverings. Wise DL, Ed. CRC Press, New York, 1984

112. Salomon JC, Diegelman RF, Cohen IK: Effect of dressings on donor site epithelialization. Forum on Fundamental Surgical Problems 25:516, 1974

113. Winter GD, Scales JT: Effect of air drying and dressings on the surface of a wound. Nature 197:91, 1963

114. Noe JM, Kalish S: The problem of adherence in dressed wounds. Surg Gynecol Obstet 147:185, 1978

115. Noe JM, Kalish S: Wound Care. Chesebrough Pond's, Greenwich, Connecticut, 1976

116. Varma AO, Bugatch E, German FM: Debridement of dermal ulcers with collagenase. Surg Gynecol Obstet 136:281, 1973

117. Noe JM, Kalish S: The mechanism of capillarity in surgical dressings. Surg Gynecol Obstet 143:454, 1976

118. Grinnell F, Billingham RE, Burgess L: Distribution of fibronectin during wound healing in vivo. J Invest Dermatol 76:181, 1981

119. Clark RAF, Folkvord JM, Wertz RL: Fibronectin as well as other extracellular matrix proteins mediate human keratinocyte adherence. J Invest Dermatol 84:378, 1985

120. Grinnell F: Fibronectin and wound healing. J Cell Biochem 25:107, 1984

121. Wysocki AB, Grinnell F: Fibronectin profiles in normal and chronic wound fluid. Lab Invest 63:825, 1990

122. Ley K: Leukocyte adhesion to vascular endothelium. J Reconstr Microsurg 8:495, 1992

123. Newman SL, Henson JE, Henson PM: Phagocytosis of senescent neutrophils by human monocyte-derived macrophages and rabbit inflammatory macrophages. J Exp Med 156:430, 1982

124. Proveddini DM, Deftos LJ, Manolagas SC: 1,25-Dihydroxyvitamin D3 promotes in vitro morphologic and enzymatic changes in normal human

monocytes consistent with their differentiation into macrophages. Bone 7:23, 1986

125. Wright SD, Meyer BC: Fibronectin receptor of human macrophages recognizes sequence Arg-Gly-Asp-Ser. J Exp Med 162:762, 1985

126. Simpson DM, Ross R: Effects of heterologous anti-neutrophil serum in guinea pigs: hematologic and ultrastructural observations. Am J Pathol 65:79, 1971

127. Leibovich SJ, Ross R: The role of the macrophage in wound repair: a study with hydrocortisone and anti-macrophage serum. Am J Pathol 78:71, 1975

128. Seppa H, Grotendorst G, Seppa S, et al: Platelet-derived growth factor is chemotactic for fibroblasts. J Cell Biol 92:584, 1982

129. Gauss-Miller V, Kleinman H, Martin GR, et al: Role of attachment factors and attractants in fibroblast chemotaxis. J Lab Clin Med 96:1071, 1980

130. Grotendorst GR, Chang T, Seppa HEJ, et al: Platelet-derived growth factor is a chemoattractant for vascular smooth muscle cells. J Cell Physiol 113:261, 1982

131. Stiles CF, Capone GT, Scher CD, et al: Dual control of cell growth by somatomedins and platelet-derived growth factor. Proc Natl Acad Sci USA 76:1279, 1979

132. Leibovich SJ, Ross R: A macrophage-dependent factor that stimulates the proliferation of fibroblasts in vitro. Am J Pathol 84:501, 1976

133. Thakral KK, Goodson WH III, Hunt TK: Stimulation of wound blood vessel growth by wound macrophages. J Surg Res 26:430, 1979

134. Knighton DR, Hunt TK, Thakral KK, et al: Role of platelets and fibrin in the healing sequence: an in vivo study of angiogenesis and collagen synthesis. Ann Surg 196:379, 1982

135. Van Winkle W Jr: The epithelium in wound healing. Surg Gynecol Obstet 127:1089, 1968

136. Clark RAF, Lanigan JM, DellaPelle P, et al: Fibronectin and fibrin provide a provisional matrix for epidermal cell migration during wound reepithelialization. J Invest Dermatol 70:264, 1982

137. Gipson IK, Spurr-Michaud SJ, Tisdale AS: Hemidesmosomes and anchoring fibril collagen appear synchronously during development and wound healing. Dev Biol 126:253, 1988

138. Mackie EH, Halfter W, Liverani D: Induction of tenascin in healing wounds. J Cell Biol 107:2757, 1988

139. Cohen IK, Moore CD, Diegelman RF: Onset and localization of collagen synthesis during wound healing in open rat skin wounds. Proc Soc Exp Biol Med 160:458, 1979

140. Peacock EE Jr: Wound Repair, 3rd ed. WB Saunders Co, Philadelphia, 1984

141. Veis A, Averey J: Modes of intermolecular crosslinking in mature and insoluble collagen. J Biol Chem 240:3899, 1965

142. Rudolph R, Guber S, Suzuki M, et al: The life cycle of the myofibroblast. Surg Gynecol Obstet 145:389, 1977

143. Montesano R, Orci L: Transforming growth factor beta stimulates collagen-matrix contraction by fibroblasts: Implications for wound healing. Proc Natl Acad Sci USA 85:4894, 1988

144. Madden JW, Peacock EE Jr: Studies on the biology of collagen during wound healing: III. Dynamic metabolism of scar collagen and remodelling of dermal wounds. Ann Surg 174:511, 1971

145. Forrester JC, Zederfeldt BH, Hayes TL, et al: Wolff's law in relation to the healing skin wound. J Trauma 10:770, 1970

146. Riley WB Jr, Peacock EE Jr: Identification, distribution and significance of a collagenolytic enzyme in human tissue. Proc Soc Biol Med 214:207, 1967

147. Witte LD, Kaplan KL, Nossel HL, et al: Studies of the release from human platelets of the growth factor for cultured human arterial smooth muscle cells. Circ Res 42:402, 1978

148. Martinet Y, Bitterman PB, Mornex JF, et al: Activated human monocytes express the c-sis proto-oncogene and release a mediator showing PDGF-like activity. Nature 319:158, 1986

149. Shimokado K, Raines EW, Madtes DK, et al: A significant part of macrophage-derived growth factor consists of at least two forms of PDGF. Cell 43:277, 1985

150. Walker LN, Bowen-Pope DF, Ross R, et al: Production of platelet-derived growth factor-like molecules by cultured arterial smooth muscle cells accompanies proliferation after arterial injury. Proc Natl Acad Sci USA 83:7311, 1986

151. Barbul A, Knud-Hansen J, Wasserkrug HL, et al: Interleukin 2 enhances wound healing in rats. J Surg Res 40:315, 1986

152. DeCunzo LP, MacKenzie JW, Marafino BJ Jr, et al: The effect of interleukin-2 administration on wound healing in Adriamycin-treated rats. J Surg Res 49:419, 1990

153. Assoian RK, Komoriya A, Meyers CA, et al: Transforming growth factor-β in human platelets: identification of a major storage site, purification, and characterization. J Biol Chem 258:7155, 1983

154. Pesonen K, Viinikka L, Myllyla G, et al: Characterization of material with epidermal growth factor immunoreactivity in human serum and platelets. J Clin Endocrinol Metab 68:486, 1989

155. Assoian RK, Fleurdelys BE, Stevenson HC, et al: Expression and secretion of type β transforming growth factor by activated human macrophages. Proc Natl Acad Sci USA 84:6020, 1987

156. Mustoe TA, Pierce GF, Thomason A, et al: Accelerated healing of incisional wounds in rats induced by transforming growth factor-β. Science 237:1333, 1987

157. McGee GS, Davidson JM, Buckley A, et al: Recombinant basic fibroblast growth factor accelerates wound healing. J Surg Res 45:145, 1988

158. Brown GL, Curtsinger L III, Brightwell JR, et al: Enhancement of epidermal regeneration by biosynthetic epidermal growth factor. J Exp Med 163:1319, 1986

159. Laato M, Niinikoski J, Lebel L, et al: Stimulation of wound healing by epidermal growth factor: a dose-dependent effect. Ann Surg 203:379, 1986

160. Pierce GF, Mustoe TA, Senior RM, et al: In vivo incisional wound healing augmented by platelet-derived growth factor and recombinant c-sis gene homodimeric proteins. J Exp Med 167:974, 1988

161. Tsuboi R, Rifkin DB: Recombinant basic fibroblast growth factor stimulates wound healing in healing-impaired db/db mice. J Exp Med 172:245, 1990

162. Pierce GF, Mustoe TA, Lingelbach J, et al: Transforming growth factor-β reverses the glucocorticoid-induced wound-healing deficit in rats: possible regulation in macrophages by platelet-derived growth factor. Proc Natl Acad Sci USA 86:2229, 1989

163. Curtsinger LJ, Pietsch JD, Brown GL, et al: Reversal of Adriamycin-impaired wound healing by transforming growth factor-beta. Surg Gynecol Obstet 168:517, 1989

164. Mustoe TA, Purdy J, Gramates P, et al: Reversal of impaired wound healing in irradiated rats by platelet-derived growth factor-BB. Am J Surg 158:345, 1989

165. Brown GL, Nanney LB, Griffen J, et al: Enhancement of wound healing by topical treatment with epidermal growth factor. N Engl J Med 321:76, 1989

166. Brown GL, Curtsinger L, Jurkiewicz MJ, et al: Stimulation of healing of chronic wounds by epidermal growth factor. Plast Reconstr Surg 88:189, 1991

167. Knighton DR, Ciresi K, Fiegel VD, et al: Stimulation of repair in chronic, nonhealing, cutaneous ulcers using platelet-derived wound healing formula. Surg Gynecol Obstet 170:56, 1990

168. Robson MC, Phillips LG, Thomason A, et al: Recombinant human platelet-derived growth factor-BB for the treatment of chronic pressure ulcers. Ann Plast Surg 29:193, 1992

169. Robson MC, Phillips LG, Lawrence WT, et al: The safety and effect of topically applied recombinant basic fibroblast growth factor on the healing of chronic pressure sores. Ann Surg 216:401, 1992

170. Steed DL, Diabetic Ulcer Study Group: Clinical evaluation of recombinant human platelet derived growth factor for the treatment of lower extremity diabetic ulcers. J Vasc Surg 21:71, 1995

171. Polk HC: Adherence of thin skin grafts. Forum on Fundamental Surgical Problems 17:487, 1966

172. Converse JM, Uhlschmid GK, Ballantyne DL Jr: "Plasmatic circulation" in skin grafts: the phase of serum imbibition. Plast Reconstr Surg 43:495, 1969

173. Marckmann A: Autologous skin grafts in the rat: vital microscopic studies of the microcirculation. Angiology 17:475, 1966

174. Smahel J: The healing of skin grafts. Clin Plast Surg 4:409, 1977

175. Psillakis JM: Lymphatic vascularization of skin grafts. Plast Reconstr Surg 43:287, 1969

176. Converse JM, Ballantyne DL: Distribution of diphosphopyridine nucleotide diaphorase in rat skin autografts and homografts. Plast Reconstr Surg 30:415, 1962

177. Hinshaw JR, Miller ER: Histology of healing split-thickness, full-thickness autogenous skin grafts and donor sites. Arch Surg 91:658, 1965

178. Kligman AM: The bacteriology of normal skin. Skin Bacteria and Their Role in Infection. Wolcott BW, Rund DA, Eds. McGraw-Hill, New York, 1965, p 13

179. Ricketts CR, Squire JR, Topley E: Human skin lipids with particular reference to the self sterilising power of the skin. Clin Sci 10:89, 1951

180. Heggers JP: Natural host defense mechanisms. Clin Plast Surg 6:505, 1979

181. Lindberg RB, Moncrief JA, Switzer WE, et al: The successful control of burn wound sepsis. J Trauma 5:601, 1965

182. Kass EH: Asymptomatic infections of the urinary tract. Trans Assoc Am Physicians 69:56, 1956

183. Bendy RH, Nuccio PA, Wolfe E, et al.: Relationship of quantitative bacterial counts to healing of decubiti: effect of gentamicin. Antimicrob Agents Chemother 4:147, 1964

184. Hunt TK, Zederfeldt BH, Goldstick TK, et al: Tissue oxygen tensions during controlled hemorrhage. Surg Forum 18:3, 1967

185. Hauser CJ: Tissue salvage by mapping of skin transcutaneous oxygen tension index. Arch Surg 122:1128, 1987

186. Heughan C, Grislis G, Hunt TK: The effect of anemia on wound healing. Ann Surg 179:163, 1974

187. Roth GJ, McDonald JB, Sheard C: The effect of cigarettes and of intravenous injections of nicotine on the electrocardiogram, basal metabolic rate, cutaneous temperature, blood pressure, and pulse rate of normal persons. JAMA 125:761, 1944

188. Bruce JW, Miller JR, Hooker DR: The effect of smoking upon the blood pressures and upon the volume of the hand. Am J Physiol 24:104, 1909

189. Wright IS, Moffat D: The effects of tobacco on the peripheral vascular system. JAMA 103:318, 1934

190. Sackett DL, Gibson RW, Bross IDJ, et al: Relation between aortic atherosclerosis and the use of cigarettes and alcohol: an autopsy study. N Engl J Med 279:1413, 1968

191. Birnstingl MA, Brinson K, Chakrabarti R: The effect of short-term exposure to carbon monoxide on platelet stickiness. Br J Surg 58:837, 1971

192. Astrup P, Kjeldsen K: Carbon monoxide, smoking and atherosclerosis. Med Clin North Am 58:323, 1973

193. Kjeldsen K, Astrup P, Wanstrup J: Ultra-structural intimal changes in the rabbit aorta after a moderate

carbon monoxide exposure. Atherosclerosis 16:67, 1972

194. Fajardo LF, Berthong M: Radiation injury in surgical pathology. Part III. Salivary glands, pancreas and skin. Am J Surg Pathol 5:279, 1981

195. Rudolph R: Complications of surgery for radiotherapy skin damage. Plast Reconstr Surg 70:179, 1982

196. Levenson SM, Gruber CA, Rettura G, et al: Supplemental vitamin A prevents the acute radiation-induced defect in wound healing. Ann Surg 200:494, 1984

197. Howes EL, Briggs H, Shea R, et al: Effect of complete and partial starvation on the rate of fibroplasia in the healing wound. Arch Surg 27:846, 1933

198. Ward MW, Danzi M, Lewin MR, et al: The effects of subclinical malnutrition and refeeding on the healing of experimental colonic anastomoses. Br J Surg 69:308, 1982

199. Haydock DA, Hill GL: Impaired wound healing in surgical patients with varying degrees of malnutrition. JPEN J Parenter Enteral Nutr 10:550, 1986

200. Thompson WD, Ravdin IS, Frank IL: Effect of hypoproteinemia on wound disruption. Arch Surg 36:500, 1938

201. Devereux DF, Thistlewaite PA, Thibault LF, et al: Effect of tumor bearing and protein depletion on wound breaking strength in the rat. J Surg Res 27:233, 1979

202. Williamson MB, Fromm HJ: Effect of cystine and methionine on healing of experimental wounds. Proc Soc Exp Biol Med 80:623, 1957

203. Levenson SM, Seifter E: Dysnutrition, wound healing, and resistance to infection. Clin Plast Surg 4:375, 1977

204. Freiman M, Seifter E, Connerton C, et al: Vitamin A deficiency and surgical stress. Surg Forum 21:81, 1970

205. Shapiro SS, Mott DJ: Modulation of glycosaminoglycan synthesis by retinoids. Ann NY Acad Sci 359:306, 1981

206. Cohen BE, Till G, Cullen PR, et al: Reversal of postoperative immunosuppression in man by vitamin A. Surg Gynecol Obstet 149:658, 1979

207. Alvarez OM, Gilbreath RL: Effect of dietary thiamine on intermolecular collagen crosslinking during wound repair: a mechanical and biochemical assessment. J Trauma 22:20, 1982

208. Ehrlich HP, Tarver H, Hunt TK: Inhibitory effects of vitamin E on collagen synthesis and wound repair. Ann Surg 175:235, 1972

209. Fernandez-Madrid F, Prasad AS, Oberleas D: Effect of zinc deficiency on nucleic acids, collagen, and noncollagenous protein of the connective tissue. J Lab Clin Med 82:951, 1973

210. Haley JV: Zinc sulfate and wound healing. J Surg Res 27:168, 1979

211. Windsor JA, Knight GS, Hill GL: Wound healing response in surgical patients: recent food intake is more important than nutritional status. Br J Surg 75:135, 1988

212. Muller JM, Brenner U, Dienst C, et al: Preoperative parenteral nutrition in patients with gastrointestinal carcinomas. Lancet 1:68, 1982

213. Lawrence WT, Norton JA, Harvey AK, et al: Wound healing in sarcoma-bearing rats: tumor effects on cutaneous and deep wounds. J Surg Oncol 35:7, 1987

214. Chlebowski RT, Heber D: Metabolic abnormalities in cancer patients: carbohydrate metabolism. Surg Clin North Am 66:957, 1986

215. Weingweg J, Levenson SM, Rettura G, et al: Supplemental vitamin A prevents the tumor-induced defect in wound healing. Ann Surg 211:269, 1990

216. DuNuoy P, Carrell A: Cicatrization of wounds. J Exp Biol 34:339, 1921

217. Grove GL: Age-related differences in healing of superficial skin wounds in humans. Arch Dermatol Res 272:381, 1982

218. Sandblom P, Peterson P, Muren A: Determination of the tensile strength of the healing wound as a clinical test. Acta Chir Scand 105:252, 1953

219. Cruse PJE, Foord RA: A prospective study of 23,649 surgical wounds. Arch Surg 107:206, 1973

220. Goodson WH, Hunt TK: Studies of wound healing in experimental diabetes mellitus. J Surg Res 22:221, 1977

221. Prakash A, Pandit PN, Sharma LK: Studies in wound healing in experimental diabetes. Int Surg 59:25, 1974

222. Arquilla ER, Weringer EJ, Nakajo M: Wound healing: a model for the study of diabetic microangiopathy. Diabetes 25(suppl 2):811, 1976

223. Mowat AG, Baum J: Chemotaxis of polymorphonuclear leukocytes from patients with diabetes mellitus. N Engl J Med 284:621, 1971

224. Bybee JD, Rogers DE: The phagocytic activity of polymorphonuclear leukocytes obtained from patients with diabetes mellitus. J Lab Clin Med 64:1, 1964

225. Nolan CM, Beaty HN, Bagdade JD: Further characterization of the impaired bactericidal function of granulocytes in patients with poorly controlled diabetes. Diabetes 27:889, 1978

226. Bagdade JD, Root RK, Bugler RJ: Impaired leukocyte function in patients with poorly controlled diabetes. Diabetes 23:9, 1974

227. Duncan HJ, Faris IB: Skin vascular resistance and skin perfusion pressure as predictors of healing of ischemic lesions of the lower limb: influences of diabetes mellitus, hypertension, and age. Surgery 99:432, 1986

228. Gottrup F, Andreassen TT: Healing of incisional wounds in stomach and duodenum: the influence of experimental diabetes. J Surg Res 31:61, 1981

229. Weringer EJ, Kelso JM, Tamai IY, et al: Effects of insulin on wound healing in diabetic mice. Acta Endocrinol 99:101, 1982

230. Yue DK, McLennan S, Marsh M, et al: Effects of experimental diabetes, uremia, and malnutrition on wound healing. Diabetes 36:295, 1987

231. Colin JF, Elliot P, Ellis H: The effect of uremia upon wound healing: an experimental study. Br J Surg

66:793, 1979

232. Goodson WH III, Lindenfield SM, Omachi RS, et al: Chronic uremia causes poor healing. Surg Forum 33:54, 1982

233. Benveniste K, Thut P: The effect of chronic alcoholism on wound healing. Proc Soc Exp Biol Med 166:568, 1981

234. Howes EL, Plotz CM, Blunt JW, et al: Retardation of wound healing by cortisone. Surgery 28:177, 1950

235. Hunt TK, Ehrlich HP, Garcia JA, et al: The effect of vitamin A on reversing the inhibitory effect of cortisone on the healing of open wounds in animals. Ann Surg 170:633, 1969

236. Stephens FO, Dunphy JE, Hunt TK: Effect of delayed administration of corticosteroids on wound contraction. Ann Surg 173:214, 1971

237. Sandberg N: Time relationship between administration of cortisone and wound healing in rats. Acta Clin Scand 127:446, 1964

238. Hunt TK, Ehrlich HP, Garcia JA, et al: Effects of vitamin A on reversing the inhibitory effects of cortisone on healing of open wounds in animals and man. Ann Surg 170:633, 1969

239. Shamberger RC, Devereux DF, Brennan MF: The effect of chemotherapeutic agents on wound healing. Int Adv Surg Oncol 4:15, 1981

240. Lawrence WT, Talbot TL, Norton JA: Preoperative or postoperative doxorubicin hydrochloride (Adriamycin): which is better for wound healing? Surgery 100:9, 1986

241. Bayer I, Ellis HL: Jaundice and wound healing: an experimental study. Br J Surg 63:392, 1976

242. Arnaud J-P, Humbert W, Eloy M-R, et al: Effect of obstructive jaundice on wound healing. Am J Surg 141:593, 1981

243. Greaney MG, Van Noort R, Smythe A, et al: Does obstructive jaundice adversely affect wound healing? Br J Surg 66:478, 1979

244. Ellis H, Heddle R: Does the peritoneum need to be closed at laparotomy? Br J Surg 64:733, 1977

245. Peacock EE Jr, Madden JW, Trier WC: Biologic basis for the treatment of keloids and hypertrophic scars. South Med J 63:755, 1970

246. Brody GS, Peng STJ, Landel RF: The etiology of hypertrophic scar contracture: another view. Plast Reconstr Surg 67:673, 1981

247. Lawrence WT: In search of the optimal treatment of keloids: report of a series and a review of the literature. Ann Plast Surg 27:164, 1991

248. Levenson SM, Greever EF, Crowley LV, et al: The healing of rat skin wounds. Ann Surg 161:293, 1965

Acknowledgments

Figure 1   Carol Donner.

Figure 2   Janet Betries.

9 COMA, SEIZURES, COGNITIVE IMPAIRMENT, AND BRAIN DEATH

Marike Zwienenberg-Lee, M.D., and J. Paul Muizelaar, M.D., Ph.D.

Management of the Patient with Altered Consciousness

Every clinician will at some point encounter a patient who is in an altered state of consciousness. Altered consciousness is not a disease per se but rather a symptom of some underlying process. It is variable in degree, ranging from mere confusion to deep coma.

Consciousness depends on both the reticular activating system (RAS), which is responsible for general alertness, and the cerebral cortex, which is responsible for the quality of behavior. The integrity of the cerebral hemispheres, the RAS, and the connections between them is essential for the maintenance of conscious behavior.

Coma is thought to result from a lesion to the hemispheres, the RAS, or both and may be caused by structural or toxic metabolic abnormalities. Specific causes of coma are numerous and include alcohol and drug intoxication, epilepsy, infection, uremia and other metabolic disorders, head injury, cerebral tumors, hypothermia, psychiatric disorders, and stroke and other vascular diseases. Accordingly, the management of coma is complex. In what follows, we discuss the various underlying causes of coma and provide general and specific guidelines.

Loss of consciousness associated with seizure activity is thought to result from a global disturbance of electrochemical activity that involves both hemispheres. Brain death represents the extreme end of the spectrum of altered consciousness and results when the loss of cerebral and brain-stem function is irreversible. Management of seizures and determination of brain death are discussed separately from management of coma.

Cognitive impairment is common in surgical patients, particularly in those who undergo major surgical procedures. The degree and nature of impairment are dependent on the underlying disease and the presence of precipitating factors, which may range from communication deficits, anxiety, and sleep deprivation to drug withdrawal, metabolic disturbances, and infection. Cornerstones of management include identification and alleviation of risk factors as well as recognition of frequent causes of cognitive impairment, such as delirium, depression, and dementia.

Often, little information is available about the circumstances leading to the disturbance in consciousness or about the patient's medical history. It is therefore essential that the surgeon follow a systematic management approach that quickly establishes the etiology and prevents unnecessary delay in initiating appropriate treatment.

Initial Management of the Comatose Patient

Initial management of the comatose patient is aimed at stabilization of the patient's condition and prevention of further central nervous system damage. The immediately occurring damage that is preventable results from cerebral hypoxia, ischemia, and low blood glucose levels. Therefore, initial evaluation and treatment of the comatose patient must be carried out simultaneously: the airway (A), breathing (B), and circulation (C) must be assessed and controlled, and hypoglycemia must be excluded or corrected. Attention should then be directed toward treatment of specific causes of coma, such as seizures, drug or alcohol overdose, head injury, or infection. Specific questions regarding medical history, recent changes in behavior, use of medications or drugs, recent trauma, and history of seizures must be asked so that the events leading to coma can be reconstructed. If the cause of coma remains elusive, the physical and neurologic examinations may yield clues that clarify the underlying etiology. In addition, laboratory tests and diagnostic imaging methods, such as computed tomography and magnetic resonance imaging, can provide important information for establishing a diagnosis and instituting proper treatment.

AIRWAY

To ensure adequate oxygenation and ventilation, the patient's airway must be cleared of all foreign material, the patency of the airway must be verified, and oxygen must be administered. The spontaneous rate and rhythm of respiration should be noted before they are obscured by therapeutic measures. The respiratory pattern is a good indicator of the depth of depression and the etiology of the coma [see Physical and Neurologic Examinations, *below*].

BREATHING

An oropharyngeal or nasopharyngeal airway may suffice in unresponsive patients who are breathing normally; however, endotracheal intubation is indicated in patients who are dyspneic, hypoventilating, or vomiting uncontrollably. Hyperventilation with a bag

Patient is in state of altered consciousness

Patient is in coma

Coma is defined as a sleeplike state of continuous unarousable unresponsiveness in which there is no spontaneous activity.

Ensure adequate ventilation and circulatory support. Obtain specimens for laboratory screening:
- CBC
- Serum electrolytes
- BUN
- Creatinine
- Glucose
- Liver function tests
- Osmolarity
- Toxic screen

Administer glucose and thiamine

Assess glucose level by bedside technique. If level is low or not immediately obtainable, give 50 mg of 50% glucose solution I.V. immediately. Before glucose administration, give 50–100 mg of thiamine I.V., followed by 100 mg I.M. daily for 3 days.

Manage intoxication

Provide early intubation and respiratory support; maintain normal BP. Perform gastric lavage if
- Ingestion occurred within 4 hr (or within 10 hr for salicylates), or
- Patient has been in shock, or
- Time of ingestion is not known.

Excretion of toxins can be facilitated with catharsis, diuresis, dialysis, or charcoal hemoperfusion. Give antidotes (if known).

Perform basic physical and neurologic examinations

Physical: Search for signs of trauma, systemic illness, infection, or drug ingestion.
Neurologic: Ascertain cause of coma and site of impairment. Differentiate between anatomic and structural lesions:
- Presence of lateralizing signs suggests structural lesion.
- Presence of pupillary light response is an important feature of metabolic coma, except in cases of drug ingestion or prolonged anoxia.
- Absence of pulillary response to light suggests structural lesion.
- Decorticate posturing suggests structural lesion; decerebrate rigidity may be caused by structural or metabolic coma (posturing has little diagnostic value after the acute phase of the coma).
If structural coma is suspected, the clinical diagnosis may be confirmed by appropriate imaging studies (CT or MRI).

Patient has seizure

Seizure is self-limited

Emergency treatment is not required.

Tonic-clonic seizure persists

Treat status epilepticus:
- Obtain quick history and perform physical examination while assistant draws blood and inserts venous line.
- Perform bedside blood glucose determination. If glucose < 60 mg/dl or not immediately available, infuse dextrose (50 ml of 50% solution for adults and 1–2 ml/kg of 25% solution for children).
- Give adult patients 100 mg thiamine I.V.
- Correct hyponatremia with 3% NaCl solution in slow I.V. infusion.
- Give calcium (1–2 ampules of calcium gluconate for 5–10 min) if necessary.
Administer anticonvulsants in the following sequence:
- Phenytoin
- Benzodiazepines
- Phenobarbital
Last resort: general anesthesia or pentobarbital-induced coma

Metabolic coma

Restore acid-base balance.
Restore electrolyte balance.
Restore normal body temperature.

Treat underlying conditions:
- Hypoxia
- Hypoglycemia or hyperglycemia
- Infection
- Overdose
- Specific disease process

Structural coma

Treat structural lesions. Determine severity of symptoms and rapidity of their evolution as soon as possible.
If patient is stable, obtain CT scan or MRI urgently: perform contrast study (CT or MRI) if structural lesion is suspected on the basis of noncontrast studies. If patient is deeply comatose or symptoms are evolving rapidly, treat elevated ICP urgently:
- Hyperventilate patient to P_aco_2 of 25–30 mm Hg.
- Give osmotic diuretics (e.g., 0.25 –1.5 g/kg of 20% mannitol solution I.V.).
- If patient does not have severe intracranial hypertension, consider elevating head of bed 30°–50°.
- If patient does not respond to hyperventilation or mannitol, consider barbiturate administration or, if possible, ventriculostomy.

Other causes of coma and similar syndromes

Alternative causes of coma and coma-resembling states include hypothermia, psychiatric disorders, persistant vegetative states, and locked-in syndrome.
Treat causative conditions as appropriate.

Patient is cognitively impaired

Eliminate or mitigate known risk factors for cognitive impairment.

Institute general supportive measures and perioperative precautions.

Treat causative conditions:
- Delirium
- Dementia
- Depression
- Head injury
- Side effects of drugs

Patient is suspected of being brain-dead

Document the presence of a potential cause of brain death. CT suffices in most cases; perform CSF examination if a definite diagnosis cannot be made.

Rule out complicating medical conditions and drug intoxication or poisoning.

Ensure that core T° ≥ is 32° C.

Initial conditions for brain death are met

Test for three cardinal features of brain death.
- Coma or unresponsiveness
- Absence of brain-stem reflexes
- Apnea (via apnea test)

Order confirmatory tests if (1) clinical criteria cannot be evaluated reliably or (2) the country, locality, or institution requires such confirmation.

Initial conditions for brain death are not met

Reevaluate patient.

Management of the Patient with Altered Consciousness

and mask and 100% oxygen should be performed before intubation to ensure adequate oxygenation during the procedure. If there is any possibility of a cervical spine injury, intubation should be delayed until fracture can be ruled out radiographically. If, however, the patient's condition is such that delay is inadvisable, intubation should be done without manipulation of the spine. In patients with head injury who are at risk for basilar skull fractures, the oropharyngeal route is preferred for intubation. In these patients, an aggressive approach to early intubation is usually indicated because hypoxia aggravates brain injury. In the Traumatic Coma Data Bank study, mortality was almost twice as high among hypoxic patients as among nonhypoxic patients (50% versus 27%).[1] It should be noted, however, that hypoxia alone adds little to mortality; it is the combination of ischemia and hypoxia that appears to be responsible for the increase in mortality.

CIRCULATION

Because substrate delivery to the brain is dependent on the cardiovascular system, circulation must be vigorously supported. A large-bore I.V. or central venous catheter is inserted, and blood volume is replenished with fluids or volume expanders. Solutions that contain free water (e.g., 5% dextrose in water) should be avoided, particularly in patients with head injury, because they may exacerbate brain edema. Vasoactive agents are infused if necessary. An electrocardiographic monitor is placed, and cardiac rate and rhythm are recorded. When vasopressor therapy is instituted, insertion of a pulmonary catheter is recommended in elderly patients or in patients with current or past cardiopulmonary disease. In patients suffering from head injury, hypotension and shock rarely result from a cerebral lesion; their presence should alert the physician to seek a source of extracorporeal or intracorporeal hemorrhage. However, when hypertension is present in these patients, it should be left untreated because it is likely to be an adaptive response (i.e., part of the Cushing response) of the brain to the increase in intracranial pressure (ICP) [see III:2 Injuries to the Central Nervous System].

LABORATORY SCREENING

As soon as the venous line is in place, blood specimens are obtained for laboratory screening. The following tests and measurements should be performed:

1. Complete blood count.
2. Serum electrolyte (Na, K, Cl, CO_2, Ca, PO_4) levels.
3. Blood urea nitrogen level.
4. Creatinine level.
5. Glucose level.
6. Liver function tests.
7. Osmolarity.
8. Toxic screen (including drugs and alcohol).

GLUCOSE ADMINISTRATION

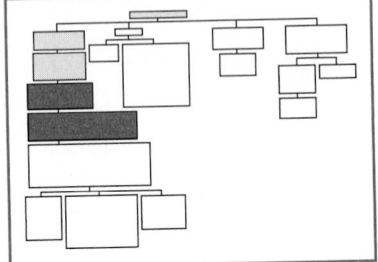

Glucose is the basic substrate for cerebral metabolism. Even a transient decrease in oxidative metabolism of glucose may lead to an abrupt disruption of brain function. Blood glucose levels should be assessed by means of a rapid bedside technique and verified in the laboratory. If the bedside determination yields a low value (< 40 to 60 mg/dl) or cannot be done immediately, 50 mg of a 50% glucose solution is administered I.V., even if laboratory verification of the blood glucose

level is not yet available. The risk of hypoglycemic cerebral damage outweighs the risk of temporary worsening of the rare case of hyperosmolar coma. Many patients admitted to the emergency ward while in coma are chronic alcoholics or malnourished and thus are prone to Wernicke encephalopathy, which is caused by thiamine deficiency and can be precipitated by a large glucose load. To prevent acute symptomatic thiamine deficiency, 50 to 100 mg of thiamine should be given I.V. to all patients before glucose is administered. Afterward, 100 mg is given I.M. every day for 3 days.

Physical and Neurologic Examinations

When the necessary resuscitative measures have been initiated, the next step is to perform basic physical and neurologic examinations. These examinations should be brief yet sufficiently thorough to yield the key information required for further evaluation and treatment. The physical examination should focus on signs of trauma, chronic disease (e.g., alcoholism or renal failure), infection, or self-administration of drugs. The neurologic examination should focus on diagnosing those conditions that call for rapid treatment, such as the following:

1. Lateralizing signs in trauma patients.
2. Signs of an increase in ICP.
3. Meningism.
4. Seizures.

LEVEL OF CONSCIOUSNESS

The patient's level of consciousness is assessed by means of the Glasgow Coma Scale (GCS), which is widely accepted as the standard method [see III:2 Injuries to the Central Nervous System]. The GCS consists of three components: eye opening (E), motor function (M), and verbal response (V) [see Table 1]. The score on each component is assessed by recording the response of the patient to verbal or noxious stimuli, such as pressure on the supraorbital notch or compression of the distal interphalangeal joints; the total GCS score is the sum of the scores of these three components [see Table 1]. The maximum GCS score is 15, and the minimum score is 3. Coma is usually defined as a GCS score of 9 or less.

A persistent misconception about the GCS, which results from equating abnormal flexion with so-called decorticate rigidity and extensor response with so-called decerebrate rigidity, is that the type of motor response corresponds to the level of the lesion. In this view, decorticate rigidity would indicate a lesion affecting the hemispheres or the diencephalon, and decerebrate rigidity would suggest a lesion affecting the midbrain or the brain stem, as shown in the Sherrington preparations.[2,3] It is now clear, however, that in patients with head injury, decerebrate motor posturing and prolonged coma are not associated with brain-stem dysfunction but rather with dysfunction of the hemispheres.[4] Therefore, we prefer to use the terms abnormal flexion and extension or flexor and extensor posturing instead of the terms decorticate and decerebrate rigidity.

LOCALIZING OR LATERALIZING SIGNS

The presence of localizing or lateralizing signs suggests that the underlying abnormality of coma is structural (i.e., caused by a focal lesion) rather than metabolic. Rapid radiologic evaluation (CT scan) is essential in these cases, particularly in patients with head injuries who may harbor an expanding intracranial hematoma, for which

Table 1 Glasgow Coma Scale[80]

Test	Response	Score
Eye opening (E)	Spontaneous	4
	To verbal command	3
	To pain	2
	None	1
Best motor response (arm) (M)	Obedience to verbal command	6
	Localization of painful stimulus	5
	Flexion withdrawal response to pain	4
	Abnormal flexion response to pain (decorticate rigidity)	3
	Extension response to pain (decerebrate rigidity)	2
	None	1
Best verbal response (V)	Oriented conversation	5
	Disoriented conversation	4
	Inappropriate words	3
	Incomprehensible sounds	2
	None	1
	Total (E + M + V)	3–15

rapid surgical intervention is indicated. Patients are observed for asymmetrical movements of the extremities, which may occur spontaneously or in response to noxious stimuli. They are also evaluated for asymmetry of tone and reflexes, with special attention paid to such signs as unilateral flaccidity, spasticity, clonus, or Babinski signs. Most comatose patients, however, will have bilateral Babinski signs regardless of the cause of their condition.

PUPILLARY SIZE AND RESPONSE

The pathways involved in the pupillary response to light are relatively resistant to most metabolic causes of coma; unless the patient is under the influence of certain drugs, this response is preserved until the near-terminal stages of metabolic coma. Consequently, the presence or absence of the pupillary light reflex is the most useful single sign for distinguishing metabolic causes of coma from structural causes. Both the size of the pupil and its direct and consensual response to light should be noted.

Bilateral reactive constricted pupils are most often seen in patients in metabolic coma. Pinpoint pupils are indicative of either a pontine lesion or an overdose of narcotics; the latter is more likely if the pupillary constriction is reversed when naloxone is administered. Fixed dilated pupils can be the result of an intrinsic midbrain lesion or, more commonly, damage to the parasympathetic fibers accompanying the third nerve in its intracranial course. Unilateral pupillary dilatation usually indicates an ipsilateral mass and is typically a sign of uncal herniation when associated with contralateral hemiplegia. Rarely, unilateral pupillary dilatation is associated with ipsilateral hemiplegia as a result of a mass that compresses the cerebral peduncle of the midbrain against the opposite tentorial margin (Kernohan's notch). Bilateral fixed dilated pupils indicate severe midbrain damage, usually from transtentorial herniation. Fixed midposition pupils are the result of injury at the midbrain level, which impairs both sympathetic (dilatation) and parasympathetic (constriction) outflow.

It has been suggested that a decrease in brain-stem blood flow, rather than direct mechanical compression of the third cranial nerve, may be a cause of mydriasis after severe head injury.[5] The investigators measured cerebral blood flow (CBF) in the brain stems of 162 patients with severe head injury and correlated these findings with pupillary response. Brain-stem blood flow was significantly lower in patients with bilateral nonreactive pupils than in patients with responsive pupils, indicating that decreased pupillary reactivity may be the result of brain-stem ischemia. This hypothesis is supported by a subsequent study documenting significantly decreased brain-stem CBF and absent pupillary response in the presence of transtentorial herniation, both of which findings were reversed after administration of hypertonic saline.[6]

EYE MOVEMENTS

Eye movements are of major importance in the physical diagnosis of coma because they involve pathways that stretch through a large part of the brain and the brain stem. In conscious patients, eye movements are either voluntary—that is, controlled by the hemispheres—or dictated by superimposed involuntary brain-stem reflexes (which in turn are influenced by afferent impulses from the labyrinth and the vestibular nuclei). In deeply comatose patients, spontaneous eye movements are usually absent; however, they may occur even in the absence of functioning frontal or occipital cortices, in which case they generally take the form of conjugate horizontal roving. This movement indicates that the midbrain and the pontine tegmentum are spared. Ocular bobbing, a brisk downward and slow upward conjugate motion of the globes, is an indication of bilateral pontine damage. Conjugate lateral deviation of the eyes suggests the presence of either an ipsilateral hemispheric lesion or a contralateral pontine lesion. Seizures may cause sustained eye deviation, in which the eyes look away from the seizure focus and exhibit rhythmic, jerky movements in the direction of the deviation.

In drowsy patients, divergence of eye positions in the horizontal plane is normal; it disappears when consciousness returns or the coma deepens. An adducted eye signals sixth-nerve palsy or pontine damage. Unilateral or bilateral sixth-nerve palsy may be associated with increased ICP. An abducted eye signals third-nerve palsy. Skew deviation, in which the eyes are not in the same horizontal plane, is usually the result of pontine or cerebellar damage.

BRAIN-STEM REFLEXES

If spontaneous eye movements are absent, the integrity of the brain stem can be assessed by means of the so-called doll's-eyes maneuver or the caloric test. These tests are based on the observation that brain-stem reflexes become hyperactive when they are released from hemispheric inhibitory influences, as in coma or sleep. The anatomic pathways involved in these brain-stem reflexes arise from the upper cervical spinal cord and the medulla (the sources of vestibular and proprioceptive input from head turning) and from the inner ear via the vestibular and sixth nerves. The fibers then pass through the contralateral medial longitudinal fasciculus to the level of the third nerve in the midbrain.

The doll's-eyes maneuver tests the oculocephalic reflex. When coma is caused by hemispheric disease and the brain stem is intact, the doll's-eyes maneuver yields horizontal conjugate deviation of the eye in the direction opposite the direction of rotation, flexion, or extension; thus, the gaze remains stationary as the head is turned. When the brain stem is dysfunctional, there is no such deviation of the eyes; thus, the gaze does not remain stationary but moves as the head is turned. The connection between the vestibular nuclei and the third, fourth, and sixth cranial nerves, which is termed the medial longitudinal fasciculus, is interrupted. As a result, the oculocephalic reflexes are impaired, so that patients with bilateral lesions are unable to maintain a stationary gaze as the head is turned and those with unilateral lesions are unable to turn their gaze toward the side on which the lesion is located.

The caloric test is used to evaluate the oculovestibular reflex. It yields much the same information as the doll's-eyes maneuver; however, it is a stronger stimulus to reflex eye movements and therefore should be performed only if the doll's-eyes maneuver yields negative results. The patient's head is elevated 30°, and the external auditory canal is irrigated with 20 to 50 ml of ice water. The ice-water injection generates convection currents in the endolymph of the labyrinth that inhibit the normal spontaneous firing of the vestibular nerve. If the coma is caused by hemispheric disease and the brain stem is intact, the normal response is sustained conjugate deviation of the eyes toward the side of the irrigated ear. Structural brain-stem lesions may abolish these responses, as may an overdose of a sedative, a hypnotic, or phenytoin. Disconjugate ocular deviation suggests the presence of either a unilateral brain-stem lesion or a metabolic depression of the brain-stem pathways. Failure of one or both eyes to adduct indicates that the lesion is located in the medial longitudinal fasciculus or the third cranial nerve. Failure to abduct signals a sixth-nerve lesion.

Other brain-stem reflexes are the corneal reflex and the gag reflex. The corneal reflex is mediated by the fifth and seventh cranial nerves and is elicited by briefly striking the corneal surface with a piece of cotton wool twisted to a point. Both eyes should blink quickly in response to this stimulus. Bilateral absence of the corneal reflex usually suggests a deep coma, and unilateral absence of the reflex indicates an ipsilateral lesion. The gag reflex is elicited by stimulating the back of the throat or by passing a suction tube down the endotracheal tube while the patient is intubated. In unconscious patients who are at risk for aspiration, this reflex should be elicited only when the airway is protected (i.e., when the endotracheal cuff is inflated). The sensory stimulus is relayed via the ninth cranial nerve, but the 10th cranial nerve mediates the resulting palatal movement. A depressed or absent gag reflex usually indicates significant brain-stem pathology.

RESPIRATION

Respiration is dependent on neural influences arising from nearly every level of the brain, from the forebrain to the upper cervical spinal cord. Oxygenation and acid-base balance are primarily regulated in the lower brain stem. If the function of the hemispheres or the thalamus is structurally or metabolically impaired, the respiratory response to carbon dioxide is reset, so that a higher level of carbon dioxide is required to trigger the respiratory drive. The resulting respiratory pattern, known as Cheyne-Stokes respiration, is characterized by periods of increasing hyperventilation alternating with apnea in a crescendo-decrescendo fashion. If more caudal regions at the level of the midbrain and the upper pons are injured, central neurogenic hyperventilation may result. This pattern of respiration, characterized by hyperventilation with forced and prolonged inspiration and expiration, is commonly seen in metabolic disorders such as hypoxia. In the lower brain stem, if the lower pons or the medulla is injured, any of several respiratory patterns may occur. Apneusis, a pattern in which long inspiration is followed by a pause lasting a few seconds and then by normal expiration, results from pontine lesions and occasionally from metabolic suppression. Cluster breathing, a pattern in which breaths are irregular and fall into groups, is associated with lower pontine lesions. Atactic breathing, characterized by irregular respiratory rate and amplitude, with gasps held in inspiration intermingling with periods of apnea, is associated with lower medullary lesions and may be indicative of a terminal respiratory pattern in severely brain-damaged patients.

Other patterns of respiration, such as slow and shallow but regular breathing, are suggestive of metabolic or drug-induced depression. Kussmaul respiration, a pattern of rapid, deep breathing that is also known as air hunger, occurs with metabolic acidosis.

ELEVATED INTRACRANIAL PRESSURE

An increase in ICP occurs when an increase in the volume of one of the three components of the intracranial cavity (i.e., blood, cerebrospinal fluid, and brain parenchyma) cannot be compensated for by a similar decrease in the volume of one of the other components.[7,8] Causes of increased intracranial volume include intracranial hematoma, hydrocephalus, tumor, vascular congestion, and cerebral edema. Cerebral edema is a nonspecific accompaniment of many disorders, such as head injury, tumor, stroke, and infection. Cerebral edema and increased ICP are particularly common after severe head injury and are important determinants of the prognosis of these patients[9-11] [see III:2 Injuries to the Central Nervous System]. Signs and symptoms of rising ICP include increasing arterial blood pressure, slowing of the pulse rate, and slowing or periodic respiration. This so-called Cushing response has been related to brain-stem ischemia; however, brain-stem blood flow is not always decreased in the presence of a Cushing response.[12] Papilledema caused by raised ICP takes several weeks to develop and is usually not a presenting symptom in patients with rapidly rising ICP.

MENINGISM

Meningism, or neck stiffness, occurs when the meninges are irritated by inflammation (as in meningitis) or the presence of blood (as in subarachnoid hemorrhage). In addition to nuchal rigidity, signs of meningeal irritation include a positive Kernig sign (elicited by flexing the thigh to 90° with the knee bent and then straightening the knee; the sign is positive when this maneuver causes pain in the hamstrings) and a positive Brudzinski sign (elicited by flexing the neck in a supine patient, which results in involuntary flexion of the hip).

Differential Diagnosis of Coma: Metabolic, Structural, and Other Causes

The differential diagnosis of coma is complex. It is essential to differentiate coma of metabolic origin from coma caused by structural lesions. In addition, both of these varieties of coma must be distinguished from psychogenic and other causes of coma and similar states, such as a persistent vegetative state and locked-in syndrome. Each of these types of coma has a characteristic clinical presentation and evolution [see Table 2].

TOXIC METABOLIC COMA

General Considerations

Toxic metabolic coma results from derangement of metabolism, alteration in resting membrane potentials, or suppression of neurotransmission in the cerebral cortex or the brain stem. Both exogenous toxins, such as sedatives and alcohol, and endogenous toxins, such as those produced in the course of uremia and hepatic failure, may suppress metabolic and electrical processing in the brain. Hypoxia and hypoglycemia lead to acute deficiencies of metabolic substrates. Acid-base and electrolyte imbalance suppress neuronal excitability, as do osmolarity abnormalities. Metabolic causes of coma usually cannot be demonstrated by means of radiography; however, signs of cerebral edema or increased ICP may be apparent on CT scan.

The hallmark of metabolic coma is that it is difficult to attribute neurologic signs to a restricted region because not all levels of the CNS are depressed concurrently and equally; for example, pupillary responses may be normal, and consciousness and respiration may be suppressed. The preservation of the pupillary light reflex even in the presence of signs of lower brain injury is an important feature distinguishing metabolic from structural coma. This rule does not, however, hold true for patients who have ingested drugs or sustained anoxic damage. The ingestion of narcotics results in reactive pinpoint pupils; the ingestion of the anticholinergic agents atropine and scopolamine gives rise to fixed fully dilated pupils; and the ingestion of glutethimide yields moderately dilated pupils that are unequal in size and frequently fixed. Severe anoxia may lead to bilateral fixed dilated pupils. Profound barbiturate poisoning or hypothermia may cause pupils to be both fixed and dilated. Although asymmetry of motor function is rare in metabolic coma, it does occur, often fluctuating from side to side. Abnormal motor signs such as tremor, myoclonus, and asterixis are characteristic of a metabolic derangement.

Specific Causes

Hypoglycemic coma Hypoglycemic coma is a serious complication of long-term insulin use, with a single episode occurring in at least one third of these patients at some point in their lives.[13] Tremor, tachycardia, sweating, blurring of vision, confusion, irritability, and abnormal behavior may precede the loss of consciousness, but in patients who are long-term insulin users, the premonitory symptoms may be absent and these patients may slip into a coma without any warning.

Diabetic ketoacidosis Diabetic ketoacidosis is a metabolic acidosis that develops in diabetic patients as a result of raised levels of circulating ketone bodies.[13] It is a severe complication of uncontrolled diabetes that requires emergency treatment. Initially, these patients present with severe dehydration, compensatory hyperventilation (Kussmaul respiration), vomiting, depression of consciousness, and sometimes abdominal pain. Coma is not common.

Uncontrolled hyperglycemia Nonketotic hyperosmolar coma results when uncontrolled hyperglycemia leads to dehydration and increased osmolality.[13] In this type of uncontrolled hyperglycemia, endogenous insulin secretion is still sufficient (and thus peripheral lipolysis and hepatic ketogenesis are inhibited), but hepatic glucose production, which is less sensitive to insulin control, is unrestrained. Patients with this disorder typically are in middle or later life and have been previously diagnosed with mild diabetes or have undiagnosed diabetes. Initial symptoms are profound dehydration and a decreased level of consciousness. The condition may be precipitated by an underlying infection or, in older patients, by vascular disease.

Hepatic and renal failure Hepatic encephalopathy may occur in the setting of acute fulminant hepatitis, in which there is no history of liver disease, or after rapidly progressive chronic liver disease.[14] The exact cause of the encephalopathy is not known, but possible factors include the release of toxins from the damaged liver, failure to detoxify metabolic products, and alterations in cerebral neurotransmitters caused by amino acid imbalances. Initial symptoms include slowness of mentation and affect, fluctuant mild confusion, reversed sleep rhythm, slurred speech, alternating euphoria and depression, and untidiness. Additional clues to underlying liver disease include fetor hepaticus, flapping tremor (asterixis), and constructional apraxia. A progressive deterioration in mental status and behavior usually follows, leading eventually to coma. In the early stages of coma, patients hyperventilate and their pupils react sluggishly to light. There is a general muscle hypertonia, and a grasp reflex may be elicited. Deeper coma develops rapidly if no treatment is instituted, and extensor posturing, loss of oculovestibular reflexes, hypotension, cardiac arrhythmias, and respiratory arrest occur.

Untreated acute and chronic renal failure may lead to uremic encephalopathy, which is associated with a progressive decrease in the

Table 2 **Etiology of Coma**

Causes of structural coma	Tumor
	Vascular
	   Cerebrovascular accident
	   Subarachnoid hemorrhage
	   Arteriovenous malformation
	   Global ischemia (vasospasm)
	Trauma
	   Intracranial hematoma
	   Multiple contusions
	   Diffuse axonal injury
	Infection
	   Cerebral abscess
	   Meningoencephalitis

Causes of toxic metabolic coma	Hypoxia Hypercarbia Hypoglycemia Hepatic failure Renal failure Electrolyte disorders Endocrine abnormalities Poisons Drugs
Other causes of coma	Hypothermia Hypotension and shock Psychiatric disorders

level of consciousness, hyperventilation, asterixis, myoclonic jerking, tetany, and convulsions.[15] Higher mental functions are affected first, followed by motor symptoms. The onset of uremic encephalopathy depends on both the severity of the uremia and its rate of onset; rapid onset is associated with early CNS manifestations.

Electrolyte disturbances Coma can result from disturbances in sodium, potassium, and magnesium homeostasis.[16] Hyponatremia (e.g., from renal or GI sodium loss) may cause coma when the plasma sodium concentration falls below 110 to 115 mmol/L, particularly when the fall is rapid. Hypernatremia occurs in a hyperosmolar nonketotic coma. The level of consciousness falls and convulsions develop when the plasma sodium concentration rises above 155 to 160 mmol/L. Hypokalemia usually does not produce a frank coma, but rather a decrease in the level of consciousness. Death in these patients is caused by ventricular tachycardia. Both hypomagnesemia (e.g., from severe vomiting and diarrhea) and hypermagnesemia (e.g., from renal failure) can produce coma. Increased irritability, hallucinations, convulsions, myoclonus, and chorea usually precede hypomagnesemia, whereas hypermagnesemia is preceded by increased lethargy and generalized weakness. Death in patients with hypermagnesemia results from respiratory paralysis.

STRUCTURAL COMA

General Considerations

Structural brain lesions produce coma either by destroying the brain parenchyma or by causing shifting or herniation of the brain within the rigid confines of the tentorium and skull [see Discussion, Pathophysiology of Coma, Herniation Syndromes, *below*]. Supratentorial lesions produce coma by causing a caudal shift of the cerebral contents beyond the confines of the tentorium, which results in compression of the brain stem and dysfunction of the ascending RAS. Infratentorial lesions produce coma by compressing the brain stem from either inside (i.e., intrinsic brain-stem lesions) or outside (i.e., cerebellar lesions).

As mentioned previously, the hallmark of a structural lesion underlying coma is the presence of localizing signs. In addition, unilateral pupillary abnormalities and unilaterally absent brain-stem reflexes are highly suggestive of an anatomic lesion. Some structural lesions (e.g., aneurysmal subarachnoid hemorrhage) often have a typical clinical presentation, and this may aid in the differential diagnosis. Specific structural causes of coma and their clinical presentation are discussed below.

Specific Causes

Cerebral tumor Coma is usually not the presenting symptom in patients with brain tumors. In most patients with cerebral tumors, a progressive neurologic deficit or focal seizure activity precedes the onset of coma, and their presence is an important clue in the differential diagnosis. Headache is also a common presenting symptom and is present in approximately 50% of patients with primary brain tumors or metastatic lesions. The classic headache associated with a brain tumor is described as being worse in the morning; exacerbated by coughing, straining, or bending forward; and accompanied by nausea and vomiting, which often afford relief for the patient. However, this classic pattern occurs only in a subset of patients. In a study of 111 patients with brain tumors, investigators showed that 77% of the patients had headaches that were similar to tension headaches, 9% had headaches that were migrainelike, and only 8% had the typical headache symptoms of a brain tumor.[17]

Signs and symptoms of supratentorial tumors include those caused by raised ICP (e.g., mass effect of the tumor or blockage of CSF drainage), focal deficits (e.g., destruction of the brain parenchyma; compression of the parenchyma by edema, mass, or hemorrhage; and compression of the cranial nerves), headache, seizures, mental status changes, transient ischemic attack symptoms (caused by vessel occlusion or hemorrhage into the tumor), and, in the case of pituitary tumors, endocrine symptoms and visual impairment. Patients with infratentorial tumors usually do not present with seizures, because such seizures are thought to arise from irritation of the cerebral cortex. Signs and symptoms of these lesions include headache, nausea, vomiting, papilledema, gait disturbances, vertigo, diplopia, and cranial nerve abnormalities and nystagmus when there is brain-stem involvement.

Stroke Stroke is categorized as cerebral infarction (thromboembolic or ischemic stroke), which signifies ischemic brain damage, or cerebral hemorrhage (hemorrhagic stroke), in which damage to the brain mainly consists of vascular rupture and extravasation of blood into the brain parenchyma. The hallmark of both types of stroke is the abrupt onset of a focal neurologic deficit. Whereas brain-stem infarcts can result in an immediate coma, ischemic stroke usually does not produce coma as a predominant symptom. In most cases, coma develops later, when edema develops in and around the infarct or when hemorrhagic conversion of the infarct results in the development of a massive hematoma that produces brain herniation.

In intracerebral hemorrhage (ICH), loss of consciousness is a prominent feature. The hallmarks of ICH are a rapidly developing neurologic deficit, vomiting, and a fluctuating level of consciousness. Coma usually indicates a large lobar or ganglionic hemorrhage (> 60 ml),[18] and coma is thought to result either from direct destruction or from herniation caused by the mass effect of the hemorrhage.

Both hemorrhagic and thromboembolic stroke predominantly affect the elderly. Diabetes, atherosclerosis, cardiac disease, hypertension, vasculitis, and hematologic disorders are important risk factors for ischemic stroke. The main causes of ICH include hyper-

tension, arteriovenous (AV) malformations, ruptured aneurysms, arteriopathies, tumors, coagulation or clotting disorders, venous or dural sinus thrombosis, abuse of drugs (e.g., cocaine or amphetamines), eclampsia, postsurgical complications (e.g., repair of congenital heart defects in children, hyperemia after carotid endarterectomy, or repair of AV malformation), and infection. Whether hypertension actually causes ICH is still subject to debate because 66% of patients older than 65 years are hypertensive, and the observed hypertension associated with ICH may in fact be part of the physiologic Cushing response and not a preexisting condition.[19]

Aneurysmal subarachnoid hemorrhage Subarachnoid hemorrhage (SAH) refers to bleeding within the subarachnoid space rather than the brain parenchyma and is the result of either a ruptured aneurysm (aneurysmal SAH) or a severe head injury (traumatic SAH). Aneurysmal SAH occurs most frequently in the fourth to sixth decades of life. The classic manifestations of aneurysmal SAH are headache of sudden onset (commonly described as the most severe headache ever experienced), a variable period of consciousness, meningism, photophobia, vomiting, and focal signs. The clinical severity of SAH is graded by using the Hunt and Hess Scale [see Table 3][20] or the World Federation of Neurological Surgeons Scale [see Table 4].[21]

Delayed cerebral ischemia or vasospasm is responsible for considerable morbidity and mortality and is an important cause of impaired consciousness and coma in patients with aneurysmal SAH. Vasospasm has a typical pattern of development. It generally occurs between day 5 and day 14 after aneurysmal SAH, with a peak incidence between day 7 and day 10. Clinical signs and symptoms include an insidious decrease in the level of consciousness and fluctuating neurologic signs. The diagnosis is confirmed by means of transcranial Doppler ultrasonography or cerebral angiography.

Table 3 Hunt and Hess Classification of Subarachnoid Hemorrhage[20]

Score*	Definition
0	Unruptured aneurysm
1	Asymptomatic; or mild headache and slight nuchal rigidity
1a	No acute meningeal/brain reaction, but with fixed neurologic deficit
2	Moderate to severe headache and nuchal rigidity; or CNS palsy (e.g., III, IV)
3	Lethargy or confusion; mild focal deficit
4	Stupor; moderate to severe hemiparesis
5	Deep coma, extensor posturing, moribund appearance

*Add one grade for serious systemic disease (e.g., hypertension, diabetes mellitus, severe atherosclerosis, chronic obstructive pulmonary disease) or severe vasospasm on arteriography.

Table 4 World Federation of Neurological Surgeons Committee on Universal Subarachnoid Hemorrhage Grading Scale[21]

Grade	GCS Score	Motor Deficit
I	15	Absent
II	13–14	Absent
III	13–14	Present
IV	7–12	Present or absent
V	3–6	Present or absent

GCS—Glasgow Coma Scale

Traumatic SAH is a common phenomenon in patients with severe head injuries. The diagnosis is made by means of CT. In a study from the National Institutes of Health Traumatic Coma Data Bank, traumatic SAH was identified in 39% of 753 patients with severe head injury.[22] Clinically, traumatic SAH is associated with signs and symptoms of vasospasm that are similar to those occurring with aneurysmal SAH. Vasospasm affects between 25% and 40% of patients with severe head injuries,[23] and the presence of traumatic SAH appears to be related to an unfavorable outcome.

Meningoencephalitis and cerebral abscess   Bacteria, viruses, spirochetes, and fungi may infect the meninges and the subarachnoid space. In most cases, infection of the CNS results from an infection that originates somewhere else. For example, meningococcal meningitis is often a complication of meningococcal bacteremia; tuberculous meningitis is the result of breakdown of a tuberculous lesion or miliary tuberculosis; and herpes zoster, listeriosis, and cryptococcal meningitis are opportunistic CNS infections that typically occur with debilitating disease or altered immune status. After neurosurgery, gram-negative aerobic bacilli usually cause meningitis. Signs and symptoms of meningoencephalitis include fever, headache, raised ICP, meningism, photophobia, seizures, and focal signs. A depressed level of consciousness, sometimes progressing to a frank coma, is a relatively common clinical manifestation of CNS infection. About 50% of patients with acute meningitis have a depressed level of consciousness.[24] The exact mechanism behind depressed levels of consciousness in CNS infection is unknown. A direct effect of the organism or its toxins on the brain parenchyma has been suggested, but disturbance of the cerebral microcirculation and occlusion of the larger vessels through either vessel wall thickening or vasospasm have also been suggested.[25]

Cerebral abscesses commonly produce focal signs or seizures but may lead to brain herniation and coma when they expand. In the classic case, the presentation is acute, with fever followed by confusion and the development of focal signs over the course of days; however, a cerebral abscess may also develop gradually, without overt disease. Cerebral abscesses may be associated with sinusitis, otitis, cranial trauma, or disseminated infection.

Head injury   Head injury is discussed in more detail elsewhere [see III:2 Injuries to the Central Nervous System].

OTHER CAUSES OF COMA AND COMA-RESEMBLING SYNDROMES

Hypothermia

Hypothermia occurs when the body's core temperature is 35° C or lower. It can result from exposure (i.e., from cold stress exceeding the body's maximum heat production), exhaustion (i.e., from depletion of the body's available energy sources), or failure of central temperature regulation (mainly in elderly patients and newborns). Loss of consciousness by itself may result in hypothermia. Consciousness decreases when the core body temperature is at or below 32° C and progresses to coma with further temperature decline. Metabolic processes slow, and for each 1° C decrease in body temperature, CBF diminishes by about 6%. At 28° C, the metabolic rate is 50% of normal, and below 25° C, asystole and death occur. At this point, cerebral autoregulation fails, and CBF follows the systemic blood pressure in a pressure-passive manner.[26]

Psychiatric Disorders

Psychogenic coma is an uncommon cause of unresponsiveness. It may be observed in patients with psychiatric disorders such as conversion reactions, catatonic schizophrenia, severe psychotic depres-

sion, or frank malingering. In most cases, the physical examination reveals normal tone and reflexes, as well as normal oculocephalic and oculovestibular reflexes. Occasionally, EEG is necessary to demonstrate a normal waking pattern.

Persistent Vegetative State

A vegetative state is a syndrome of diffuse cortical damage in which brain-stem activity is preserved. Consequently, eye opening and muscle movements are observed, but there is no voluntary control of the movements. A vegetative state is usually a long-term and often a permanent state associated with injuries such as head trauma and global ischemia.

Locked-in Syndrome

The locked-in syndrome is a state in which quadriplegia and paralysis of the lower cranial nerves are present but the level of consciousness is normal. This syndrome is rare and usually results from thrombosis of the basilar artery, which is attributed to a variety of causes. Patients can communicate only by eye movements (e.g., blinking). Long-term survival is uncommon but has been reported.[27]

Radiologic Imaging

Radiologic imaging modalities depict the anatomic configuration of intracranial structures and play a crucial role in the evaluation of comatose patients, particularly when an adequate history cannot be obtained and the physical examination is inconclusive. They can be used to confirm or exclude the presence of clinically suspected abnormalities or, in some instances, to make a specific diagnosis, thereby greatly expediting treatment or intervention.

TYPES OF IMAGING MODALITIES

Plain Skull Radiography

Plain skull radiography is particularly useful in the evaluation of patients with head injuries. Bullets and bullet fragments can be easily detected, and the points of entry and exit can generally be determined with this method. In patients with closed head injuries, plain skull radiography is used to detect fractures of the cranial vault and base. It is important to obtain a skull radiograph in patients with head injuries because the presence of a fracture is related to intracranial hematoma and thus is an indication of the severity of head injury [see Table 5].

Computed Tomography and Magnetic Resonance Imaging

Both CT and MRI provide detailed information on brain anatomy, including the configuration and size of the ventricular chambers; the presence of midline displacements; the presence of subfalcial, transtentorial, or uncal herniations; and the position of vascular structures. CT is usually the first investigation performed in comatose patients. Compared with MRI, CT takes less time for a complete investigation, and the CT unit is much easier to access. These are significant advantages of CT in comatose patients, who are usually monitored with multiple electronic devices—a practice that, by itself, limits the use of MRI because of the effect of the magnetic field on these devices. In addition, CT is better at imaging bony structures than MRI is, it is an excellent method of demonstrating ICH, and it offers the best resolution for demonstrating SAH. MRI, however, offers the advantage of imaging in multiple planes, which allows accurate anatomic visualization of the lesion. Furthermore, it is more sensitive than CT in detecting intracranial abnormalities and thus is better able to find small lesions. In addition, the absence of bony artifacts makes MRI more useful for imaging lesions in the

Table 5 Relation between Presence of Skull Fracture and Intracranial Hematoma in Patients with Severe, Moderate, and Minor Head Injury[124]

Severity	Hematoma on CT	No Hematoma on CT	Total
Severe (GCS 8)			
Fracture	74 (44%)	94 (56%)	168
No fracture	43 (32%)*	91 (68%)	134
Moderate (GCS 9–12)			
Fracture	49 (29%)	118 (71%)	167
No fracture	25 (8%)†	299 (92%)	324
Minor (GCS 13–15)			
Fracture	42 (10%)	391 (90%)	433
No fracture	27 (1%)‡	2,549 (99%)	2,576
Total	260	3,542	3,802

*$P < 0.05$. †$P < 0.001$. ‡$P < 0.0001$.
GCS—Glasgow Coma Scale

posterior and temporal fossae. Overall, CT is preferred for initial evaluation of comatose patients. MRI should be reserved for patients who require less monitoring, who are able to remain still for prolonged examination, and in whom CT has not been beneficial or is inconclusive.

RADIOLOGIC DIAGNOSIS OF SPECIFIC CAUSES OF COMA

Cerebral Tumor

CT (with and without injection of contrast) is a useful and quick first investigation for detecting a tumor. It demonstrates mass effect, edema, calcifications, and accompanying disorders that may necessitate rapid intervention (e.g., hydrocephalus). Low-grade gliomas show a decreased density on CT scans that does not enhance with contrast. The surrounding edema is minimal. Calcifications may be present, particularly in certain subtypes (e.g., oligodendrogliomas). High-grade gliomas are usually large and enhance intensely after contrast administration [*see Figure 1*]. In most cases, the enhancement is irregular. A central area of low density may also be present, indicating necrosis. High-grade gliomas are usually surrounded by marked cerebral edema and compression of the ipsilateral ventricle by a hemispheric mass; alternatively, the surrounding edema may result in obstructive hydrocephalus with dilatation of the contralateral ventricle.

On MRI, low-grade gliomas may present as abnormal areas of decreased T_1 signal (spin-lattice or longitudinal relaxation time) and increased T_2 signal (spin-spin or transverse relaxation time), even in the absence of CT evidence of a tumor. High-grade gliomas characteristically have a low signal intensity on T_1-weighted images and a high signal on T_2-weighted images. Gadolinium enhancement is more likely to occur in high-grade gliomas. Metastatic lesions have a variable intensity on T_2-weighted images, and they commonly enhance with gadolinium. Meningiomas are hypointense to isointense on T_1 and hyperintense to isointense on T_2, and they enhance strongly with contrast. Nerve sheath tumors are isointense or hypointense on T_1 and hyperintense on T_2 and enhance intensely with contrast. Pituitary tumors are best visualized on T_1-weighted imaging. They are hypointense lesions within the intermediate intensity of the anterior lobe. Lymphomas are usually hypointense to isointense on T_1-weighted images and isointense to hyperintense on T_2-weighted images. These tumors enhance after I.V. injection of gadolinium.

Stroke

CT abnormalities can be detected a few hours after an ischemic stroke. In patients with a middle cerebral artery (MCA) stroke, CT findings include effacement of the sulci, loss of distinction of the caudate nucleus and lentiform nucleus, and loss of the insular ribbon. The hyperdense MCA sign, which is caused by the clot in the artery, is present in almost 50% of patients when a CT scan is performed within the first 2 hours.[28,29] The characteristic triangle-shaped hypodensity usually develops fully within 3 days, and the mass effect, caused by cerebral swelling as well as petechial hemorrhages and indicating hemorrhagic conversion, may be seen at this time. The likelihood of edema increases with the size of MCA infarcts; if the infarct size, as determined on CT scan within 5 hours after the insult, is larger than 50% of the MCA territory, significant edema develops in 85% of patients.[30]

Figure 1 Characteristic appearance of butterfly glioma is apparent on coronal T_1-weighted MRI. The tumor mass extends to the contralateral side across the corpus callosum.

Table 6 Fisher CT Classification of Subarachnoid Hemorrhage[31]

| Grade | Amount of Blood on CT | No. of Patients | Angiographic Vasospasm | | DIND |
			Slight	Severe	
1	No SAH detected	11	2	2	0
2	Diffuse or vertical layers* < 1 mm	7	3	0	0
3	Localized clot and/or vertical layer > 1 mm	24	1	23	23
4	Intracerebral or intraventricular clot with diffuse or no SAH	5	2	0	0

*Vertical layers refer to blood within the vertical subarachnoid spaces, including the interhemispheric fissure, insular cistern, and ambient cistern.
DIND—delayed ischemic neurologic deficit   SAH—subarachnoid hemorrhage

Supratentorial, cerebellar, and brain-stem hemorrhages appear as hyperdense lesions on CT scan. Putaminal hemorrhages may extend into the thalamus and enter the ventricular system. Caudate hemorrhage may be difficult to detect because the ventricular extension may predominate. Lobar hematomas on CT scan may show compression of the sulci, midline shift, and compression of the lateral ventricle. MRI is a useful test for excluding metastasis, occult vascular malformations, previous hemorrhages associated with amyloid angiopathy, or cerebral venous thrombosis that is not detected with CT.

Cerebellar hematomas may cause significant compression and obliteration of the basal cisterns, resulting in CSF obstruction and hydrocephalus; these signs, together with the size of the hematoma,

Figure 2 **Cerebral angiography shows a large right middle cerebral artery aneurysm.**

are important determinants of further management. In patients with pontine hemorrhage, massive hemorrhages are most frequent, but small ones occur as well.

Subarachnoid Hemorrhage

Aneurysmal SAH is classified according to the Fisher CT classification, which relates severity of bleeding to prognosis [*see Table 6*].[31] The sensitivity of CT scanning for detecting SAH is very high, approximately 95%.[32,33] In many cases, there is a slight preponderance of blood deposited in the area of the ruptured aneurysm, which may aid in determining the location of the aneurysm or the location of multiple intracranial aneurysms. Cerebral angiography [*see Figure 2*] is the gold standard for evaluating the size and location of the aneurysm, though newer methods (e.g., MR angiography and CT angiography) are being used increasingly.[34-38]

Lumbar puncture is never the first choice of investigation for confirming a diagnosis of SAH. As noted, a mass lesion in the posterior fossa may closely mimic the signs and symptoms of SAH, and patients are at considerable risk for herniation if a lumbar puncture is performed. A CT scan usually yields the diagnosis, and a lumbar puncture is rarely necessary. If SAH is suspected and CT is not available, it is safer to transport the patient to a facility where CT scanning is available, particularly when the patient is rapidly deteriorating.[33] Lumbar puncture, however, must be used when the CT scan is negative and there is even a slight suspicion of aneurysmal SAH.

Meningoencephalitis and Cerebral Abscess

Other than diffuse basal dural enhancement on MRI, meningoencephalitis usually does not produce specific signs on CT or MRI. A CT scan is indicated in comatose patients, however, to rule out complications of meningitis such as hydrocephalus, subdural empyema, and abscess. On CT, a cerebral abscess appears as a smooth thin-walled lesion with a low-density center that enhances brightly after administration of contrast. In some cases, it is difficult to distinguish between a tumor and an abscess on CT, and stereotactic biopsy is essential to confirm the diagnosis [*see Figure 3*]. Diffusion-weighed MRI also may be useful in these cases.[39] MRI can show intracranial abscesses with a much greater resolution than CT scanning can, and it is excellent for detecting cerebritis and abscesses that are undetectable or uncertain on CT.[40]

Head Injury

Fractures of the cranial vault and base are sometimes difficult to detect, particularly by the inexperienced investigator. Depressed and linear fractures are the most common types [*see Figure 4*]. Types of ICH that are often seen after head injury and that can be detected with CT include contusions and epidural, subdural, subarachnoid, and intraparenchymal hemorrhages. An epidural hematoma

Figure 3   MRI reveals a cerebral abscess. Axial T₁-weighted image with gadolinium contrast medium shows multiloculated, brightly enhancing mass. Signal intensity is low at the abscess wall. There is significant surrounding edema and mass effect, which results in effacement of the ipsilateral occipital horn of the left lateral ventricle. Local involvement of the meninges is indicated by enhancement of the overlying meninges.

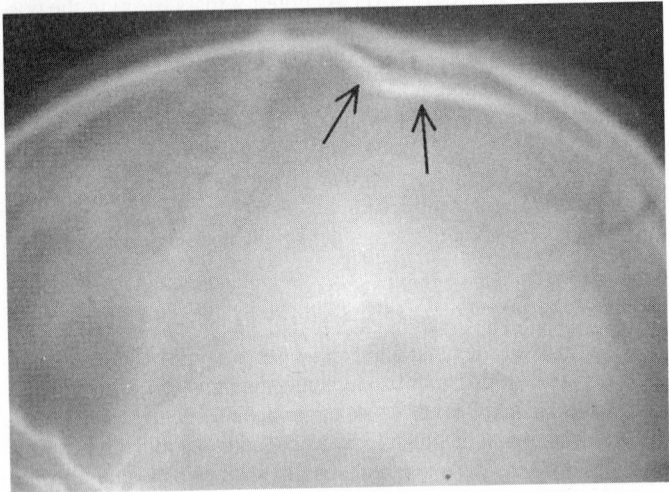

Figure 4   Conventional lateral radiograph shows a skull fracture.

characteristically appears as a biconvex hyperdense lesion [*see Figure 5*]. Epidural hematomas have been classified into three types on the basis of CT scan criteria.[41] Type I (acute) hematomas are characterized by a lucent swirl (unclotted blood) in a dense hematoma. Some investigators call these hematomas hyperacute extradural hematomas. Type II (subacute) hematomas appear as solid clots. Type III (chronic) hematomas appear as mixed-density or lucent hematomas with a contrast-enhanced membrane.

Subdural hematomas appear as convex-concave lesions on CT [*see Figure 6a, b*]. In many cases, subdural hemorrhage is accompanied by SAH, indicating severe injury.[42] The complex of subdural hematoma and adjacent contusion in the brain is sometimes referred to as a burst lobe. Acute subdural hematomas are hyperdense with

respect to the adjacent brain, subacute hematomas are hyperdense to isodense, and chronic hematomas [*see Figure 6c*] are hypodense.

Intraparenchymal lesions appear as an area of increased density on CT scans [*see Figure 7*]. The hematomas are usually associated with extensive lobar contusions, from which they are indistinguishable in many cases.[43,44] The amount of blood in a lesion determines whether the lesion is classified as a hematoma or a contusion. If blood accounts for at least two thirds of the lesion, the lesion is classified as an intracerebral hematoma. The remaining lesions are described as disrupted tissue with areas of microscopic hemorrhage.[45] A hemorrhagic mass should be considered an intracerebral hematoma when there is a homogeneous collection of blood with relatively well-defined margins. Multiple intracerebral hematomas are found in approximately 20% of cases.[46]

Contusions, appearing as small hyperdense lesions on CT, usually have a characteristic distribution, affecting the frontal poles, the orbital gyri, the cortex above and below the sylvian fissures, the temporal poles, and the lateral and inferior aspects of the temporal lobes. Over time, significant swelling may accompany these lesions, appearing as hypodense areas around the contusion.

Diffuse axonal injury is characterized by the presence of punctate hemorrhages or so-called Strich hemorrhages and indicates severe head injury.[47] Strich hemorrhages are most commonly found in the corpus callosum, the walls of the third ventricle (hypothalamus, columns of the fornix, and anterior commissure), the internal capsule, the basal ganglia, the dorsolateral brain stem, and the superior cerebellar peduncles.

Midline shift and compression of the subarachnoid space are parameters indicating the extent of mass expansion or cerebral swelling. The National Institutes of Health Traumatic Coma Data Bank introduced a classification of head injury based on initial CT findings [*see Table 7*].[48] This classification is commonly used in clinical trials investigating new treatments for severe head injury. Eisenberg and colleagues have shown a correlation between some of the CT scan characteristics after severe head injury (i.e., compression of the basal cisterns, the presence of SAH, and midline shift) and the frequency of raised ICP, mortality, and other outcomes.[22]

Figure 5   CT scan shows acute epidural hematoma. Note the characteristic biconvex hyperdense lesion.

Figure 6 **Shown are three examples of subdural hematoma: (*a*) hyperacute subdural hematoma (note that there is only a slight difference in density between the convex-concave hematoma and the brain parenchyma; the hematoma causes significant midline shift and ipsilateral brain compression), (*b*) acute subdural hematoma, and (*c*) chronic subdural hematoma after surgical evacuation.**

Treatment of Coma

METABOLIC COMA

Management of Intoxication

Many comatose patients who are seen in the emergency ward are suffering from an overdose of alcohol, narcotics, sedatives, or a combination thereof. Most of these drugs induce respiratory and cardiovascular depression, which is a major cause of mortality in comatose patients. Anticipation and early treatment of these complications may alleviate their effects.

Early intubation, respiratory support, and maintenance of normal blood pressure are essential. Gastric lavage is effective when ingestion of a drug is discovered no more than 4 hours after the event, except in the case of salicylates, which may be removed in substantial amounts as long as 10 hours after ingestion. As a rule, little is gained by performing gastric lavage more than 4 hours after ingestion, unless the patient has been in shock and consequently manifests delayed gastric emptying and slowed absorption. In comatose or uncooperative patients, however, it is rarely possible to determine the exact time of ingestion; thus, gastric lavage is almost always indicated.

Patients are intubated with a cuffed endotracheal tube (to protect the airway from aspirated gastric contents) and then positioned on their left side (to allow pooling of the gastric contents) with the head down. Lavage is then performed with copious amounts of fluid until the return is clear. After evacuation, a slurry of 10 g of activated charcoal in 30 to 50 ml is instilled in the stomach via a nasogastric

Figure 7 **CT scan shows intracerebral hematoma resulting from a cranial gunshot wound.**

Table 7   Classification of Head Injury Based on Initial CT Findings

Category	Definition
Diffuse injury I	No visible intracranial pathology on CT scan
Diffuse injury II	Cisterns present with midline shift of 0–5 mm and/or the following: Lesion densities present No high- or mixed-density lesion > 25 ml May include bone fragments and foreign bodies
Diffuse injury III (swelling)	Cisterns compressed or absent, with midline shift of 0–5 mm; no high- or mixed-density lesion > 25 ml
Diffuse injury IV	Midline shift > 5 mm; no high- or mixed-density lesion > 25 ml
Evacuated mass lesion	Any lesion surgically evacuated
Nonevacuated mass lesion	High- or mixed-density lesion > 25 ml, not surgically evacuated

tube. After lavage, cathartic agents may be used to shorten the transit time through the GI tract and thus to decrease absorption of the ingested material. Diuresis (saline, ionized, or osmotic), dialysis, and charcoal hemoperfusion all facilitate the excretion of toxins. Specific antidotes exist for several common intoxicants; however, these antidotes are beyond the scope of the present discussion [*see I:10 Substance Abuse*].

Hypoglycemic Coma

Initial treatment of hypoglycemic coma is discussed elsewhere [*see* Initial Management of the Comatose Patient, *above*]. In addition, treatment consists of prevention, in the form of education in the use of insulin and encouragement of patients to carry glucose tablets or sweets with them at all times. A supply of glucagon (1 g I.M.) that can be administered by relatives may also be stored at home.

Diabetic Ketotic Coma

Treatment must be initiated as soon as possible because these patients often present with profound dehydration. Key points in the management of diabetic ketoacidosis include the following:

1. Replace fluid losses (the average fluid loss is approximately 7 L).
2. Replace electrolytes and monitor potassium carefully.
3. Restore acid-base balance (with bicarbonate infusion only in severe cases).
4. Replace insulin deficiency (4 to 6 U/hr).
5. Replace energy losses (dextrose infusion with insulin cover until the patient can eat).
6. Look for an underlying cause (infection is common).

Hyperglycemic Hyperosmolar Nonketotic Coma

Management of hyperosmolar nonketotic coma does not differ from that of diabetic ketotic coma; however, meticulous rehydration should be performed, particularly because many patients with this condition are elderly.

STRUCTURAL COMA

Cerebral Tumor

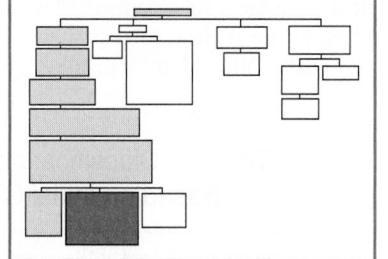

Management of brain tumors consists of surgery, radiotherapy, and other adjuvant treatments (e.g., chemotherapy). Ultimately, treatment of these lesions depends on both tumor characteristics (e.g., localization, malignancy, tumor spread, and associated edema) and patient characteristics (e.g., age, medical history, and personal beliefs). An in-depth discussion of the diverse treatment strategies, however, is beyond the scope of this chapter.

In the comatose patient, two interventions deserve particular consideration. First, to reduce cerebral edema, patients should be started on glucocorticosteroid therapy (e.g., dexamethasone), particularly when signs of elevated ICP are present. Second, coexisting hydrocephalus may be alleviated by the insertion of a ventricular catheter.

Stroke

In patients with thromboembolic stroke, coma is usually caused by brain swelling. Cerebral edema occurs in approximately 10% to 20% of patients with MCA stroke and in almost 100% of those with complete MCA occlusion.[49,50] It typically occurs after 2 to 7 days and is characterized by a gradual deterioration, though the lev-

el of consciousness may fluctuate in some patients. Measurement of ICP is indicated because it has been shown that ICP may predict the ultimate outcome of these patients[49] and thus can serve as a guide for patient management.[51] Administration of mannitol is initially selected to treat an increase in ICP. Acute episodes of impending herniation may be treated with hyperventilation if mannitol fails, and further clinical deterioration can be followed by decompressive surgery if the patient has no other significant disease and is relatively young. In addition, a ventriculostomy can be placed if significant contralateral hydrocephalus is present.

In patients with nondominant ischemic stroke, including comatose patients and patients with a fixed dilated pupil, decompressive surgery has been successful, though it has not been tested in a randomized clinical trial.[52-57] Moreover, it should be noted that although mortality may decrease substantially with decompressive surgery, it may not be desirable to salvage those patients who may end up with a severe disability or in a vegetative state. In a recent study of 32 surgically treated patients, mortality decreased by 35% in comparison with historic controls, but one in four patients experienced severe disability.[55]

Treatment of so-called supratentorial hypertensive intraparenchymal hemorrhage is still subject to considerable debate. No uniform treatment guidelines are available, and there is very little clinical evidence to support either a surgical or a conservative medical approach. In two randomized trials, no significant differences in outcome were found between surgical and medical management.[58,59] Stereotactic aspiration of the clot has achieved some degree of success, but to date, no comparative studies have been published.[60,61]

Subarachnoid Hemorrhage

Treatment of a ruptured aneurysm consists of either surgical clipping or endovascular treatment, depending on the location, size, and shape of the aneurysm and the age, clinical condition, and past medical history of the patient. Ideally, patients are treated within 48 hours of hemorrhage because the risk of rebleeding is highest early after the initial bleeding episode. The estimated frequency of repeat bleeding in untreated patients is 4% on day 1 and 1.5% from day 2 to day 14. Overall, 15% to 20% of patients experience repeat bleeding within 14 days, and 50% within 6 months; thereafter, the risk is 3% per year, with an annual mortality of 2%.[62,63] An advantage of clipping or coiling the aneurysm is that it allows the institution of so-called triple-H therapy (i.e., therapy for hypertension, hypervolemia, and hemodilution) and transluminal balloon angioplasty in the case of vasospasm. In a subset of patients (i.e., those with poor neurologic condition or those who present with symptomatic vasospasm), surgical treatment may be postponed, or the aneurysm may be treated by means of endovascular techniques.

Cerebral vasospasm is initially treated with ample fluid replacement and discontinuance of any antihypertensive or diuretic agents. When necessary, triple-H therapy and transluminal balloon angioplasty to dilate the vasospastic vessels are instituted.[64,65] Prevention of vasospasm by means of prophylactic transluminal balloon angioplasty is currently under investigation.[66]

Meningoencephalitis and Cerebral Abscess

If there is a strong suspicion of bacterial meningitis, I.V. antibiotics should be started immediately because this condition can be rapidly fatal. If there is a delay in obtaining the CSF, one should start treatment blind. Antibiotic selection depends on the initial expectation of the organism most likely to be involved, the results of Gram stain of the CSF, and the drug's ability to penetrate the CNS. Neurosurgical consultation is obtained in the case of a suspected cerebral abscess or hydrocephalus, both of which may require emergency drainage. Subdural empyema is a rare complication of meningitis that usually requires drainage. In the case of diffuse cerebral edema, management and monitoring of ICP are indicated.

Treatment of a cerebral abscess consists of identification of the bacterial organisms, institution of antibiotic therapy, and drainage or excision of the abscess through a craniotomy or bur hole.[67-70] Repeated aspiration of the abscess may be necessary. Surgical excision is considered if there is persistent reaccumulation of the abscess, if the abscess is in an accessible site or is located in the cerebellum, or if there is a well-formed fibrous capsule that fails to collapse despite repeated aspiration.

Head Injury

The main goal in the management of head injury is the prevention of secondary injury. Treatment of such injuries is addressed more fully elsewhere [see III:2 Injuries to the Central Nervous System].

OTHER CAUSES OF COMA

Hypothermia

Early intubation and respiratory support facilitate oxygenation and rewarming. In the case of circulatory arrest, for every decrease of 1° C in body temperature, the time during which there is hope for recovery without cardiopulmonary resuscitation can be doubled (this applies only to patients with primary hypothermia, not to those who are hypothermic because of cardiac arrest). Hypothermia can cause considerable coagulation disturbances, which predispose the patient to bleeding. To detect these abnormalities, the physician should perform clotting tests at the patient's core body temperature rather than at 37° C.

External or surface rewarming by covering the patient, by conducting treatment in a warm room, and by giving warmed I.V. fluids and warmed humidified oxygen is indicated in patients with a core body temperature higher than 30° C. In patients with a core body temperature below 30° C, surface rewarming is contraindicated. In these patients, surface rewarming could cause shunting of the blood to the dilated skin vessels, thereby exacerbating hypotension and further decreasing the core temperature, both of which predispose these patients to ventricular fibrillation. Active core rewarming is therefore instituted in these patients, which consists of delivering warmed humidified gases and parenteral fluids, performing peritoneal dialysis (4 to 8 L/hr at a temperature of 37° to 42° C), circulating water at 42° C through a closed irrigation system inserted into the esophagus or stomach (3 L/hr), or performing hemodialysis with the blood flowing past a dialysis solution warmed to 40° C. Considerations in the management of hypothermia are discussed more fully elsewhere [see VII:10 Fever, Hyperpyrexia, and Hypothermia].[71-77]

Seizures

Seizures or epileptic attacks are episodes of transient disturbance of electrochemical activity within the brain, expressed as abnormal motor, sensory, or psychological behavior. Epilepsy is defined as a condition characterized by recurrent

Table 8 Classification of Epilepsy

Generalized: bilaterally symmetrical; no local onset; loss of consciousness from onset
  Generalized tonic-clonic: idiopathic, no anatomic abnormality
  Absence (petit mal seizure): impaired consciousness with mild or no motor involvement
  Bilateral myoclonus: syndrome of three seizure types, including myoclonic jerks, generalized tonic-clonic seizures, and absence
  Infants and children: infantile spasms, atonic seizures, and tonic seizures

Partial: focal from onset
  Simple (usually no loss of consciousness)
  Complex (any alteration of consciousness, automatisms)
  Partial with secondary generalization

Unclassified epileptic seizures

unprovoked seizures. Traditionally, epileptic attacks are classified into three main groups [see Table 8]. Partial (focal) seizures are often associated with a structural abnormality, such as a scar, a tumor, or an AV malformation. Generalized seizures are a result of diffuse neuronal hyperactivity; there is usually no identifiable structural abnormality. Seizures that induce loss of consciousness may involve both cerebral hemispheres and may either be generalized from onset (primary generalized seizures) or begin focally and then spread to involve both hemispheres (secondary generalized seizures).

Several systemic and neurologic diseases can give rise to seizures. Head trauma, cerebrovascular disease, and CNS infections are common causes, as are metabolic imbalances such as hypoglycemia, hypoxia, hyponatremia, hypernatremia, hypocalcemia, and hypomagnesemia. In addition, hypothermia can induce seizures. Drugs and toxins, such as methylxanthines, tricyclic antidepressants, phenothiazine, cocaine, and local anesthetics (e.g., lidocaine), can lead to seizures. Withdrawal of a drug—particularly of a barbiturate, alcohol, or a hypnotic—can cause seizures if too abrupt.

Generalized tonic-clonic seizures are characterized by sudden loss of consciousness associated with tonic-clonic movements. There is no preceding aura, but occasionally, there may be preictal irritability or a rising epigastric sensation. During the seizure, the patient falls to the ground, sometimes with a cry; tongue biting and loss of sphincter control are often noted. After an initial period of tonic rigidity and short-lived apnea, clonic jerking of the neck, trunk, and extremities ensues. The clonic jerking gives way to flaccid relaxation accompanied by labored breathing, pallor, and hypersalivation. Consciousness, lost at the beginning of the seizure, is gradually regained, but postictal confusion and drowsiness may last for hours. Grand mal seizures may predispose the patient to serious bodily injuries, such as vertebral compression fractures, cerebral trauma, and drowning.

Status epilepticus occurs when the seizures follow one another without recovery of consciousness between episodes. Specifically, it is defined as more than 30 minutes of convulsive activity or repeated convulsions over the course of 30 minutes without return of consciousness in between. This arbitrary definition is related to the onset of cerebral metabolic and systemic consequences of prolonged seizure activity [see Discussion, Cellular, Metabolic, and Systemic Effects of Status Epilepticus, below]. Withdrawal of antiepileptic drugs is the most common cause of status epilepticus among patients with epilepsy. Status epilepticus can be classified into convulsive status epilepticus and nonconvulsive status epilepticus. Tonic-clonic status epilepticus is the most feared complication of epilepsy and is potentially lethal. The death rate approaches 60% in untreated patients; even with skilled management, the death rate is 10%.[78] In what follows, we focus on management of tonic-clonic status epilepticus.

MANAGEMENT OF STATUS EPILEPTICUS

General Management of Seizures

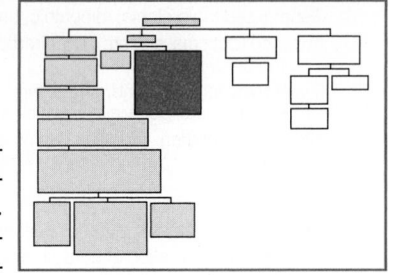

Most seizures are self-limited and therefore rarely require emergency treatment. When a seizure does not resolve quickly and spontaneously, treatment must be rapid and efficient. The primary goals of treatment are (1) to ensure adequate ventilation so as to prevent hypoxia and (2) to prevent complications such as aspiration and physical injuries. A quick history and physical examination are performed in an attempt to determine the underlying cause of the seizure, while an assistant begins drawing blood and inserting a venous line. Blood specimens are obtained for measurement of anticonvulsant drug levels, biochemical tests, a hemogram, and assessment of arterial blood gas pressures. Blood glucose level is determined by means of rapid bedside techniques; if it cannot be estimated immediately or is estimated to be lower than 60 mg/dl, dextrose is infused (50 ml of a 50% solution for adults and 1 to 2 ml/kg of a 25% solution for children). Adult patients are also given 100 mg of thiamine I.V. as a safeguard against an exacerbation of Wernicke encephalopathy, which is a relatively common disease among patients with status epilepticus. Thiamine is always given before dextrose is administered.

Patients with hyponatremia, whose condition may be associated with compulsive water drinking, fluid overload, or the syndrome of inappropriate antidiuretic hormone secretion, are given a hypertonic (3%) solution of sodium chloride by slow I.V. infusion. Half the calculated sodium deficit is administered, which is usually sufficient to stop seizures; the remaining deficit can be corrected by fluid restriction and diuresis. Excessively rapid correction of hyponatremia may result in cardiovascular overload or central pontine myelinosis. Patients with a recent history of thyroid or parathyroid surgery as well as a prolonged QT interval on the ECG should immediately be given I.V. calcium—1 to 2 ampules of calcium gluconate for 5 to 10 minutes—even if confirmatory laboratory results are not yet available. Because oxygenation, blood pressure, acid-base balance, and blood glucose may all be disturbed by prolonged convulsions, supportive medical care is just as important as anticonvulsant drug therapy.

Pharmacotherapy for Status Epilepticus

The three main drugs or drug classes used in the treatment of status epilepticus are the benzodiazepines, phenytoin, and the barbiturates. Usually a benzodiazepine is administered first, followed immediately by a loading dose of phenytoin. Benzodiazepines exert their effect by enhancing γ-aminobutyric acid (GABA) inhibition, whereas phenytoin interferes with sodium entry into the cell [see Discussion, below]. Among the benzodiazepines, lorazepam is the preferred drug. Because diazepam is redistributed rapidly in fatty tissue, seizures may recur within 10 to 20 minutes. Furthermore, diazepam appears to be less effective in aborting status epilepticus. A 1995 study showed that lorazepam aborted status epilepticus in 97% of cases and diazepam in only 68%.[79] A side effect of benzodiazepines is respiratory depression, which occurs in approximately 12% of patients. Lorazepam appears to cause less respiratory depression than diazepam. In adults, lorazepam is given I.V. in a dosage of 4 mg over 2 minutes; the dose may be repeated after 5 min-

utes. In pediatric patients, a dose of 0.1 mg/kg is used, up to a maximum of 5 to 6 mg.

In adult patients who are not already taking phenytoin, the loading dose is 20 mg/kg, infused at a maximum rate of 50 mg/min. In patients taking phenytoin, 0.74 mg/kg is given to raise the level by 1 μg/ml. If the phenytoin level is unknown, a loading dose of 500 mg is given. In pediatric patients, the loading dose is 20 mg/kg infused at a rate of 1 to 3 mg/kg/min.

If the seizures continue, the initial strategy is to give additional doses of phenytoin (5 mg/kg each, to a maximum of 30 mg/kg). Thereafter, phenobarbital is loaded (20 mg/kg in adults, to a maximum of 100 mg/minute; 5 to 10 mg/kg in pediatric patients every 20 to 30 minutes, to a maximum of 30 to 40 mg/kg), or diazepam is given (100 mg/500 ml drip at 40 ml/min). As a last resort, general anesthesia is instituted, usually with pentobarbital. EEG monitoring should be performed in these patients, and pentobarbital should be titrated until burst-suppression occurs. In addition, blood pressure should be monitored closely because hypotension may occur.

Cognitive Impairment

Cognitive functions include consciousness; attention; orientation to time, place, and person; immediate, recent, and remote memory; abstraction; language; praxis; and visuomotor ability. Cognitive impairment is a common consequence of coma, particularly in patients with structural lesions. It may also follow status epilepticus, though more likely as a result of underlying brain abnormalities than of status epilepticus itself.[80]

In surgical settings, however, cognitive impairment is most common in patients who undergo major operations. It is often the result of delirium but may also be associated with dementia, amnestic disorders, depression, and various other mental disorders. In addition, several drugs may cause cognitive impairment, especially when administered in combination. Early detection is important because patients with cognitive deficits have higher rates of perioperative morbidity and mortality, longer hospital stays, and higher rates of institutionalization than patients with normal cognitive function do.

PERIOPERATIVE CARE: RISK FACTORS AND PREVENTIVE MEASURES

Certain factors increase the risk that cognitive impairment will develop in a surgical patient [see Table 9].[81,82] It is important to iden-

---

Table 9 Risk Factors and Exacerbating Factors for Cognitive Impairment

Risk factors	Exacerbating factors
Age > 60 yr	Unfamiliar environment
Addiction to alcohol, narcotics, or both	Communication deficits
Cerebral damage or disease	Sensory deprivation or overload
Cardiac, renal, or hepatic disease	Sleep deprivation
Visual or auditory impairment	Immobilization
Preoperative depression	Anxiety
History of delirium or functional psychosis	Pain
Family history of psychosis	

Table 10 Precipitating Medical and Surgical Causes of Delirium

Drug intoxication
Alcohol, anesthesia, antianxiety agents, anticholinergics, anticonvulsants, antidepressants, antihistamines, antihypertensives, antiparkinsonian agents, cimetidine, clonidine, digitalis, insulin, lithium, neuroleptics, opiates, salicylates, sedative-hypnotics

Drug withdrawal
Alcohol, antianxiety agents, sedative-hypnotics

Metabolic disturbances
Electrolyte, fluid, or acid-base imbalance; endocrine disorders; hepatic or renal failure; hypoglycemia; hypothermia; hypoxia; paraneoplasm

Acute cerebral disorders
Edema, encephalitis, epilepsy, fat emboli, primary or metastatic neoplasm, stroke, transient ischemic attack, vasculitis

Infections
Bacterial endocarditis, meningitis, pneumonia, septicemia, urinary tract infection

Hemodynamic disturbances
Anemia, arrhythmia, congestive heart failure, hypertensive encephalopathy, hypotension, hypovolemia, myocardial infarction, orthostatic hypotension

Respiratory disorders
Pulmonary embolus

Nutritional and vitamin deficiency

Trauma
Burns, fractures, head injury

tify and, when possible, reduce these risk factors by adopting the following measures:

1. Simplify drug regimens.
2. Taper and discontinue unnecessary medications. Obtain psychiatric consultation for patients receiving monoamine oxidase (MAO) inhibitors to determine whether the drug can be discontinued 2 weeks before operation.
3. Ensure therapeutic blood levels of drugs such as digitalis, anticonvulsants, and lithium. Lithium should be discontinued 1 to 2 days before operation.
4. For patients dependent on alcohol, analgesics, or anxiolytic-sedatives, stabilize drug intake, make proper substitutions, or, if time permits, gradually withdraw the agent.
5. Ensure nutritional, thiamine, and multivitamin supplementation in alcoholic patients and in malnourished elderly patients.
6. Review the management of the patient's existing medical and psychiatric disorders and obtain early consultation to provide optimal preoperative management.
7. Correct visual and auditory deficits if possible.

In addition, general supportive measures should be instituted as early as possible, and factors that exacerbate cognitive impairment should be mitigated [*see Table 9*]. Patients with cognitive impairment should be further evaluated for suicidal intent and behavior. If the patient is at risk of suicide or exhibits dangerous behavior (e.g., wandering, falling, or acting aggressively), psychiatric consultation should be obtained immediately, the physical environment should be secured, and a sitter should be present when family and staff are absent. Pharmacologic management may be necessary and is usual-

ly preferable to physical restraints, which can increase agitation, decrease mobility, and damage soft tissue.

Meticulous intraoperative care can prevent or diminish postoperative delirium in high-risk and cognitively impaired patients. The following precautionary measures are recommended:

1. If the patient has received an MAO inhibitor within 2 weeks of operation, monitor blood pressure levels carefully. If hypotension develops, treat with a direct-acting sympathomimetic such as phenylephrine.[83]
2. Plan anesthesia and surgical interventions so as to minimize operative time, hypotension, tissue damage, and the use of psychoactive drugs.
3. Avoid premedication with highly anticholinergic drugs (e.g., scopolamine or atropine).
4. Schedule the operation to minimize waiting time, anxiety, and fasting.
5. Maintain normal body temperature, especially in an elderly patient.
6. Carefully monitor hemodynamic, cardiac, and metabolic functions.
7. Ensure that orienting procedures and the use of glasses and hearing aids are resumed in the recovery room.

In the postoperative period, measures to prevent medical and surgical causes of delirium include the following:

1. Administer essential medications, sufficient calories, and detoxification agents parenterally until oral intake can be resumed.
2. Avoid excessive analgesic administration or routine use of long-acting benzodiazepines (e.g., diazepam or flurazepam).
3. Initiate early and vigorous treatment of metabolic imbalances, infection, hemodynamic disturbances, respiratory failure, and trauma (e.g., from falls or bedsores).
4. Reduce factors that contribute to cognitive impairment by continuing the supportive measures that were initiated before the operation.
5. Preserve maximum possible visual input in eye-surgery patients; enhance tactile and auditory clues.
6. Encourage all patients to become mobile and to resume autonomous functioning as soon as physical and cognitive abilities permit.

DIAGNOSIS AND MANAGEMENT OF FREQUENT CAUSES OF COGNITIVE IMPAIRMENT

The Mini-Mental State Examination and the Confusion Assessment Method are useful, rapid tests for evaluating cognitive functions,[84-87] though their sensitivity largely depends on the experience and background of the investigator.[88] These tests should be repeated daily in patients with cognitive impairment and in high-risk patients. The most frequent causes of cognitive impairment are delirium, dementia, depression, head injury, and pharmacotherapy.

Delirium

An obvious deterioration in cognitive ability, behavior, or mood during the first week after operation is usually caused by delirium and signals the presence of potentially life-threatening disorders [*see Table 10*]. Delirium is a transient mental disorder characterized by acute onset of global impairment of cognitive functions and widespread disturbance of cerebral metabolism. Delirium may arise immediately after the operation but typically follows after an interval of several days. Early manifestations include restlessness, irritability, insomnia, lethargy, kinesthetic sensations, vivid and frightening dreams, illusions, difficulty in thinking, and thickening or slurring of speech. As

---

Table 11   DSM-IV Diagnostic Criteria for Delirium

Disturbance of consciousness (i.e., reduced clarity of awareness of environment) with reduced ability to focus or sustain or shift attention

Change in cognition (e.g., memory deficit, disorientation, language disturbance) or the development of a perceptual disturbance that is not better accounted for by a preexisting, established, or evolving dementia

Development of the disturbance over a short time (usually hours to days) and fluctuation during the course of the day

Evidence from the history, physical examination, or laboratory findings that the disturbance is caused by a general medical condition, substance intoxication, substance withdrawal, or more than one such cause

DSM-IV—Diagnostic and Statistical Manual of Mental Disorders, 4th edition.

Table 12   Laboratory Studies to Investigate Delirium

Routine procedures
  Complete blood count
  Blood chemistry tests for electrolytes; calcium, phosphate, and glucose; blood urea nitrogen; liver enzymes
  Urinalysis
  Erythrocyte sedimentation rate
  Serologic test for syphilis
  Chest x-ray
  Electrocardiogram

Special procedures
  Blood chemistry tests for creatinine, magnesium, vitamin B_{12}, folate, thyroxine, ammonia, serum proteins, osmolality, arterial blood gases, cortisol
  Test for levels of medications in the blood
  Blood and urine toxicology screens
  Blood cultures
  HIV antibody test
  Lupus erythematosus preparation and antinuclear antibody test
  Urine tests for osmolality, porphobilinogen, 5-hydroxyindoleacetic acid
  CSF examination for cells, protein, glucose, culture, viral serology, pressure
  Cranial CT scan or MRI
  Electroencephalogram

---

the syndrome progresses, fluctuations in attention, perception, orientation, language, and intellectual functioning may become apparent. Sleep becomes fragmented, and day and night cycles may be reversed. Urinary incontinence, loss of motor coordination, focal neurologic signs, nystagmus, and various types of tremor may also be noted. Bilateral asterixis and multifocal myoclonus are highly suggestive of delirium. Current diagnostic criteria for delirium are given in the fourth edition of the *Diagnostic and Statistical Manual of Mental Disorders* (*DSM-IV*) [see Table 11].

When delirium is suspected on clinical grounds, appropriate laboratory studies should be performed to help identify precipitating organic causes [see Table 12]. Management of delirium includes treatment of precipitating factors [see Table 9], control of exacerbating factors [see Table 9], continuation of prophylactic measures, and management of agitation (see below).

Dementia

Dementia is a clinical syndrome that usually occurs in the elderly [see VI:7 The Elderly Surgical Patient]. Dementia has a protracted course that is characterized by loss of cognitive abilities, disorganization of personality, and decreased ability to perform activities of daily living. Consciousness is usually not disturbed, unless delirium is present. Dementia can be totally reversed in 10% to 15% of patients if detected early and treated appropriately, and it can be arrested or at least partially improved in 25% to 30%.[89,90] Of the many disorders that cause dementia [see Table 13], Alzheimer disease and vascular diseases (multi-infarct dementia) are most commonly implicated, accounting for, respectively, 40% to 60% and 10% to 25% of all cases.[89,90] The diagnosis of Alzheimer disease is based on the presence of a progressive dementia of insidious onset with prominent aphasia, apraxia, and cognitive impairment, but with relatively intact motor functions until the final stages of the disease.[91] A family history of the disease may be present. The diagnosis of vascular dementia is suggested by a sudden onset, a stepwise deteriorating course, focal neurologic signs and symptoms, and evidence of significant cerebrovascular disease from the history, clinical examination, or laboratory tests. Other causes of dementia are excluded by the history, clinical examination, and laboratory results.[90,92] *DSM-IV* also lists criteria for dementia [see Table 14], and recommended investigations for suspected dementia are similar to those outlined previously [see Table 12]. In addition, psychological tests may be helpful in certain cases.[89,93,94]

Management of dementia includes treating underlying causes and superimposed delirium or coexisting depression, minimizing exacerbating factors for cognitive impairment [see Table 9], and alleviating common manifestations of dementia (e.g., intellectual impairment, depression, insomnia, wandering, agitation, immobility, motor instability, incontinence, iatrogenic conditions, and family

---

Table 13   Causes of Dementia

Degenerative
  Senile dementia, Alzheimer disease, Pick disease, Huntington chorea, Parkinson disease, Creutzfeldt-Jakob disease, normal-pressure hydrocephalus, multiple sclerosis

Intracranial space-occupying lesions
  Tumor, subdural hematoma

Trauma
  Single severe head injury, repeated head injury (e.g., in boxers, football players)

Infections and related conditions
  Encephalitis, neurosyphilis, cerebral sarcoidosis

Vascular
  Multi-infarct dementia, occlusion of the carotid artery, cranial arteritis

Metabolic
  Sustained uremia, liver failure, remote effects of carcinoma or lymphoma, renal dialysis

Toxic
  Alcohol, poisoning with heavy metals (e.g., lead, arsenic, thallium)

Anoxia
  Anemia, postanesthesia, carbon monoxide, cardiac arrest, chronic respiratory failure

Vitamin deficiency
  Sustained lack of vitamin B_{12}, folic acid, thiamine

Table 14 DSM-IV Diagnostic Criteria for Dementia

Development of multiple cognitive deficits

Impaired memory (new and previously learned information)

One or more of the following: aphasia, apraxia, agnosia, and disturbed executive functioning (planning, organizing, sequencing, abstracting)

Each of the above cognitive deficits must cause significant social or occupational impairment and represent a significant decline from previous functioning

Deficits do not occur exclusively during the course of delirium

Additional criteria are required for diagnosis of one of the following dementia types

Dementia of Alzheimer type

Gradual onset and continuing cognitive decline; cognitive deficits resulting from other CNS conditions, systemic conditions, or substance-induced conditions not better accounted for by other axis I disorders

Vascular dementia

Focal signs and symptoms or laboratory evidence of cerebrovascular disases that are judged to be etiologically related

Dementia resulting from other general medical conditions

Evidence that the disturbance is a direct physiologic consequence of a general medical disorder (to be coded on axis III)

Substance-induced persistent dementia

Deficits present beyond the usual duration of substance intoxication or withdrawal. Evidence that deficits are etiologically related to the persisting effects of substance use.

Dementia resulting from multiple etiologies

Evidence that the disturbance has more than one cause

DSM–IV—Diagnostic and Statistical Manual of Mental Disorders, 4th edition.

---

burden). Specific patient management and pharmacologic interventions are discussed elsewhere.[95-102]

Depression

Features that suggest a depressive disorder underlying cognitive impairment include a history of affective disorder in the patient or the family, a clearly depressed mood, and an atypical recent history of cognitive deficit.[103-105] Depression may also be the result of a general medical condition or an underlying organic cause; in addition, medications, substance abuse, endocrinopathies, malignant disorders, head injury, infectious disorders, and metabolic disorders should always be considered. Furthermore, the depressive episode may continue even after the precipitating organic factor has been removed and may require the same treatment as a major depressive episode. *DSM-IV* outlines the criteria for a major depressive episode [see Table 15].

If the patient is currently depressed and is already receiving a maintenance regimen of antidepressants, the dose should be increased every 2 to 5 days until the maximum daily dose is reached, intolerable side effects occur, or a clinical response is achieved. If the patient is starting antidepressant therapy and there is no history of a good response to any particular drug in either the patient or the family, the treatment of choice should be a tricyclic antidepressant (TCA) with minimal anticholinergic properties (e.g., desipramine) or a selective serotonin reuptake inhibitor (SSRI) (e.g., fluoxetine or sertraline). In elderly patients, it is wise to initiate therapy with a low dose and to increase the dose gradually while watching for adverse effects, such as delirium or orthostatic hypotension with a TCA and nausea, anxiety, insomnia, or headache with an SSRI.[106-108]

A combined antidepressant-neuroleptic regimen or electroconvulsive therapy may be indicated in delusional patients. Electroconvulsive therapy is also indicated for severely depressed patients at risk of suicide or rapid physical decline. Depressed patients with a personal or family history of hypomania may need additional medication with lithium or anticonvulsant agents (i.e., carbamazepine or valproate). In these last three groups of patients, psychiatric consultation is advisable.

Head Injury

Cognitive impairment is common after severe head injury. The extent of cognitive impairment is not always clearly reflected in the Glasgow Outcome Scale (GOS) [see Table 16], however, which is one of the most popular scales used to assess outcome after head injury.[109,110] Many patients cannot function normally months or years after severe traumatic brain injury; common cognitive deficits include memory and behavior disturbances. In the group of patients with so-called GOS good recovery, a substantial number of patients undergo personality changes that interfere with their personal lives and careers.[111-113] In a study of 82 patients with severe head injury, the investigators monitored GOS scores and psychosocial reintegration (defined in terms of employment, interpersonal relationships, social contacts, and leisure interests) for 6 years after injury.[114] Of the 82 patients, 76% were classified as having poor or substantially limited reintegration; among the patients with favorable GOS scores (i.e., good recovery or moderate disability), only 50% were found to have good reintegration.

The severity of cognitive impairment is related to the severity of the initial injury (as reflected in the GCS), the time between injury and hospital admission, the type of brain lesion, the duration of coma, and the extent of posttraumatic amnesia.[115,116] In a study of 117 patients with severe head injuries, neuropsychological sequelae were ascertained from two examinations in 30 of the conscious survivors within the first year after injury and were related to CT examinations. CT findings included diffuse axonal injury, diffuse swelling,

---

Table 15 DSM-IV Diagnostic Criteria for Major Depressive Episodes

At least five of the following symptoms have been present during the same 2-week period and represent a change from previous functioning

and

either symptom 1 or 2 is present

and

symptoms are not caused by a general medical condition or by mood-incongruent delusions or hallucinations.

1. Depressed mood
2. Markedly diminished interest or pleasure
3. Significant gain or loss of weight or appetite
4. Insomnia or hypersomnia
5. Psychomotor agitation or retardation
6. Fatigue or loss of energy
7. Feelings of worthlessness or excessive or inappropriate guilt
8. Diminished ability to think, concentrate, or make decisions
9. Recurrent thoughts of death or suicide, suicide attempt, or suicide plan

Symptoms do not meet criteria for a mixed (with manic features) episode.

Symptoms cause clinically significant distress or impairment of functioning.

Symptoms do not result from a substance (e.g., drug or abuse of medication) or a general medical condition.

Symptoms are not explained by bereavement.

DSM–IV—Diagnostic and Statistical Manual of Mental Disorders, 4th edition.

Table 16 Glasgow Outcome Scale[110]

Description	Score
Good recovery	5
Moderate disability	4
Severe disability	3
Vegetative state	2
Death	1

and focal injuries. Neuropsychological outcome varied with the type of CT lesion and the function measured. Overall differences in memory and learning were found among the three categories of CT lesions, whereas differences in intelligence and visuomotor functions were not significant. Levels of memory, learning, and visuomotor speed were higher after diffuse swelling injuries, but less improvement was noted. Greater improvements in memory, learning, and visuomotor speed occurred after diffuse axonal injury. After focal injuries, visuomotor speed improved, but recall and learning did not.[117]

Cognitive Side Effects of Pharmacologic Therapy

Cognitive side effects may be produced by a variety of medications from multiple drug classes. As noted, multidrug pharmacotherapy is an important cause of cognitive impairment, and drug regimens should be carefully evaluated, particularly in elderly patients. Impaired renal and hepatic function and the use of medications that interfere with hepatic and renal drug excretion may predispose patients to untoward effects. Elderly patients are more susceptible to cognitive side effects because of age-related alterations in pharmacokinetics, increased use of medications, and an increased incidence of premorbid cognitive impairment. Cognitive impairment in demented patients may be exacerbated by medications, and dementia increases the risk of delirium by twofold to threefold.[118] A comprehensive review of the cognitive side effects of pharmacotherapy together with an excellent source of references is available elsewhere.[119]

MANAGEMENT OF AGITATION

Agitation is frequently seen in patients with cognitive impairment and may present as increased psychomotor activity, often accompanied by wandering, shouting, and verbal or physical aggression. Management includes treatment of underlying disorders and intervention to reduce symptoms. The first steps in management consist of removing any obvious causes of the behavior, orienting the patient, increasing levels of safe activity, and improving pain control, any or all of which may suffice. If these measures are inadequate or the situation becomes life-threatening, psychopharmacologic management is indicated.

In several delirium syndromes, an antipsychotic drug is not the treatment of choice. In anticholinergic delirium, anticholinergic drugs are discontinued and supportive care is provided. If the delirium is life-threatening (i.e., associated with coma, seizures, or cardiac arrhythmias), parenteral physostigmine may reverse the danger. Because of its side effects, however, this drug should be used with caution.[120] For hepatic encephalopathy, a short-acting benzodiazepine that requires little hepatic degradation is preferred (e.g., oral oxazepam 15 to 30 mg every 6 hours as required). For delirium caused by alcohol or benzodiazepine withdrawal, benzodiazepines are preferred to antipsychotics, which are epileptogenic and may cause akathisia (motor restlessness). For alcohol withdrawal, 50 to 100 mg of thiamine should also be administered.[121] In emergency situations, 50 mg of chlordiazepoxide, 10 mg of diazepam, or 2 mg of lorazepam may be given slowly I.V. every 1 or 2 hours until control is established. Alternatively, 4 mg of lorazepam may be given I.M. In less urgent situations, 25 to 50 mg of chlordiazepoxide given I.M. or orally four times a day will suffice. As soon as the patient's condition is stable, the dosage can be tapered at a daily rate of about one tenth to one quarter of the initial dose. Fuller descriptions of the management of alcohol, benzodiazepine, barbiturate, and other sedative-hypnotic withdrawal syndromes are available elsewhere [*see I:10 Substance Abuse*].

Haloperidol is the drug of choice for most other causes of agitation, particularly if patients display psychosis, aggression, or both. Haloperidol is relatively free from anticholinergic, autonomic, and drug-interaction effects. Side effects of the drug include extrapyramidal syndromes (i.e., Parkinson-like symptoms, akathisia, dyskinesia, or dystonia) and neuroleptic malignant syndrome, which is a rare but life-threatening complication. Brief treatment, however, does not usually cause severe side effects.

Mild forms of agitation are managed with haloperidol dosages of 2 to 15 mg orally twice a day. In elderly patients, 0.5 to 3 mg/day is usually sufficient. In emergency situations, haloperidol should be administered I.V. in a dose of 1 to 5 mg, and the dose should be increased by 5 to 10 mg/hour until an effective dose is achieved. Use of single doses of 30 mg and maximum daily doses of 100 mg has been reported.[121] For refractory cases, 1 to 4 mg of I.V. lorazepam may be added. Once improvement occurs, the regimen may be continued via the I.M. or oral route. In less urgent situations, severely agitated patients will usually respond to haloperidol, 2 to 10 mg/hr I.M., up to a daily dose of 10 to 60 mg (one third of this dose in the elderly). Supplementary parenteral dosages of 2 to 10 mg/hr may be administered. When the patient's behavior is controlled, haloperidol should be continued orally; if no supplementary doses are necessary, the dosage should be decreased by one quarter each day until discontinuance.

For delirium, the total duration of treatment with haloperidol is usually 3 to 5 days. For agitation associated with psychoses, longer

Figure 8 Algorithm depicts the procedure for the apnea test in brain death.[124]

treatment is usually required and psychiatric follow-up is advisable. Patients who cannot tolerate or fail to respond to haloperidol may respond to a phenothiazine antipsychotic such as chlorpromazine (25 to 50 mg I.M. every hour, followed by 25 to 100 mg orally every 4 to 6 hours). Side effects of chlorpromazine include hypotension, drowsiness, cardiac arrhythmias, seizures, respiratory depression, and coma.

Brain Death

The term brain death implies irreversible cessation of activity in the cerebrum and brain stem. Brain death is frequently a consequence of severe head injury, (re)rupture of a cerebral aneurysm, or ICH[122,123]; less commonly, it is a consequence of fulminant encephalitis, bacterial meningitis, or anoxic-ischemic encephalopathy. A qualified physician should determine the occurrence of brain death, but legal requirements are different in various states and countries. Areas of concern include recognition of conditions that may mimic brain death, the procedure for the apnea test, indications for confirmatory tests, and management of physiologic changes associated with brain death. In addition, early identification of potential donor candidates is important, though selection of these candidates can proceed only after the clinical diagnosis of brain death has been established and family members have given their consent.

GUIDELINES FOR THE DETERMINATION OF BRAIN DEATH

The guidelines for determining brain death in adults and children have been published elsewhere[124]; accordingly, we provide here only a brief summary of the procedures involved. In most cases, the differences in the criteria for brain death from one state or country to another have to do with the type and number of confirmatory tests (see below) that are needed. The clinical diagnosis of brain death requires the following:

1. The presence of a cause that is compatible with brain death.
2. The absence of complicating medical conditions that may confound clinical assessment.
3. The absence of drug intoxication or poisoning.
4. A core temperature of at least 32° C.

In most patients, a CT scan will document an abnormality that is compatible with brain death. In patients with normal CT scans, the diagnosis should be reconsidered, unless there is a high certainty about the mechanism that has led to brain death (e.g., ischemic-anoxic brain death caused by cardiac arrest or asphyxia). CSF examination is indicated if a definite diagnosis cannot be made. Severe electrolyte, acid-base, and endocrine disturbances should be excluded, and a drug screen may be helpful to detect a specific drug or poison. In the presence of barbiturates, the diagnosis of brain death can likely be made when the levels are subtherapeutic; however, supportive data for this approach are available only for pediatric patients.[125] The core temperature should be at least 32° C because brain-stem reflexes are absent below 27° C.

If these conditions are met, clinical testing should follow. Three cardinal features of brain death are evaluated, as follows:

1. Coma or unresponsiveness.
2. Absence of brain-stem reflexes.
3. Apnea.

Coma or unresponsiveness is evaluated by assessing the motor response to painful stimuli, such as either supraorbital pressure or nail-bed pressure; this response should be absent. Pitfalls include the observation of spontaneous spinal motor responses (Lazarus sign), which may occur during pain stimuli, during the apnea test, and after recent administration of neuromuscular blocking agents. In the latter case, examination with a bedside nerve stimulator is required (so-called train-of-four monitoring). In a brain-dead patient, the pupils are typically in the middle position (4 to 6 mm) and fixed, although dilated pupils may be observed as well. Many drugs affect pupil size, but the light reflex usually remains intact. Topical ocular instillation of drugs, trauma to the cornea or the bulbus oculi, preexisting anatomic abnormalities, and previous surgical procedures should all be considered in the evaluation of the pupils and the pupillary response. The oculocephalic and caloric responses are then tested; these too should be absent. The caloric response can be diminished or abolished by a variety of drugs, including sedatives, TCAs, anticholinergics, antiepileptics, and chemotherapeutics. In addition, clotted blood or cerumen may occlude the external auditory canal, and fracture of the petrous bone may result in unilateral absence of a response. Finally, the corneal, pharyngeal, and tracheal reflexes are tested, all of which should be absent.

If all brain-stem reflexes are absent, the apnea test is performed [see Figure 8].[126] To minimize confounding factors, such as marked hypotension, severe cardiac dysrhythmias, and desaturations, the following precautions are taken[125]:

1. Core temperature must be 36° C or higher (rewarm the patient if temperature is lower).
2. Systolic BP must be 90 mm Hg or higher (use dopamine if BP is lower).
3. Fluid balance must be positive for 6 hours or longer (use vasopressin if this cannot be accomplished).
4. Arterial PCO_2 must be 40 mm Hg or higher (decrease minute ventilation if PCO_2 is lower).

Table 17   Guidelines for the Determination of Brain Death in Children

Historical criteria

Determination of the proximate cause of coma

Absence of remediable or reversible conditions such as toxins, drugs (sedatives, hypnotics, paralytics), metabolic disorders, surgically correctable conditions, hypotension, and hypothermia

Physical examination criteria

Coexisting coma and apnea (standardized apnea test)

Absence of brain-stem function

Absence of hypothermia or hypotension

Flaccid tone or absence of spontaneous or induced movements (except spinal cord events)

Consistent examination findings throughout observation and testing periods

Observation periods and laboratory testing

7 days to 2 months: two clinical examinations and apnea tests and two EEGs at least 48 hr apart

2 to 12 months: two clinical examinations and apnea tests and two EEGs at least 24 hr apart*

> 12 months: two clinical examinations and apnea tests at least 12 hr apart†

*Repeat examination and EEG are obviated by the absence of flow on cerebral angiogram.
†If hypoxic-ischemic encephalopathy is suspected, the observation period should be extended to 24 hr. Laboratory testing is not required if there is absence of a remediable or reversible condition.

5. Arterial PO_2 must be 200 mm Hg or higher (inspired oxygen fraction = 1.0 for 10 minutes).

CONFIRMATORY TESTS

Brain death is essentially a clinical diagnosis; it may be repeated after 6 hours to establish the final diagnosis. In most cases, this clinical diagnosis is sufficient; however, in cases in which the specific components of clinical testing cannot be evaluated reliably (e.g., as a result of drug intoxication, altered metabolic status, shock, or hypothermia), confirmatory tests may be indicated. Moreover, some countries require such confirmation by law, and many hospitals have their own policies for determining brain death. Generally accepted tests include EEG, cerebral angiography, single-photon emission CT, and, more recently, transcranial Doppler ultrasonography. In our experience, angiography not only is the most reliable and rapid way of establishing brain death but also occasionally shows that the cerebral circulation is normal and that further therapeutic efforts (such as hemicraniectomy) are justified. The tests are particularly important when organ and tissue donation are under consideration.

DETERMINATION OF BRAIN DEATH IN CHILDREN

Finally, a word is reserved for the determination of brain death in children. In children younger than 5 years, caution is indicated in applying the neurologic criteria for brain death. In comparison with adult brains, the brains of infants and young children have an increased resistance to cerebral damage that makes it easier for them to recover substantial functions, even after exhibiting unresponsiveness for longer than is possible in adults. Guidelines for the determination of brain death in children are available [see Table 17], but clear recommendations are lacking.[124,127,128]

Discussion

Pathophysiology of Coma

The pathophysiologic basis of coma is either a structural disruption of crucial areas in the cerebral hemispheres or brain stem (structural coma) or a diffuse depression of cerebral metabolism (metabolic coma). Cerebral metabolism is described in greater detail elsewhere [see III:2 Injuries to the Central Nervous Sysytem]. Key variables for understanding the pathophysiology of coma include ICP, mean arterial pressure (MAP), cerebral perfusion pressure (CPP) (defined as MAP minus ICP), CBF (derived from CPP via the Poiseuille equation), the global arterial–jugular venous oxygen difference (A-VDO_2), and the cerebral metabolic rate of oxygen ($CMRO_2$) (derived via the Fick equation, CBF times A-VDO_2).

Because 95% of the energy in the normal brain is generated by oxidative metabolism, $CMRO_2$ is considered a sensitive measure of cerebral metabolism. Metabolic causes of coma predominantly interfere with $CMRO_2$, whereas structural causes of coma may interfere with both $CMRO_2$ and the supply of substrates. In patients with head injury, the observed depression in $CMRO_2$ has been related to impairment of mitochondrial function and consequently to depression of oxidative ATP generation.[129]

The resting CBF is approximately 55 ml/100 g/min, which is adequate for meeting normal metabolic demands and includes a modest safety margin to accommodate most physiologic changes. Between a CBF of 55 ml/100g/min and one of 25 ml/100 g/min, increased oxygen extraction compensates for the decrease in CBF, and $CMRO_2$ can be maintained. When the mean CBF drops below 25 ml/100 g/min, slowing of brain electrical activity is apparent on EEG, and a progressive depression of consciousness occurs clinically. This represents a stage of reversible brain dysfunction. Below a CBF of 18 ml/100 g/min, however, ATP generation is insufficient to support $CMRO_2$. Consequently, arrest of the sodium-potassium pump occurs, leading to membrane failure, cell swelling, and irreversible brain dysfunction. The resulting cell damage depends on both the duration and the amount of CBF depression.[130] In most circumstances, structural lesions affect CBF by their effect on the CPP.

Because CPP is defined as MAP minus ICP, it follows that CPP can be decreased by severe hypotension, which is a common complication in structural lesions such as head injuries, or by raised ICP, which may accompany any type of intracranial lesion.

As mentioned before, ICP is the product of a constantly changing interplay between CSF volume, brain tissue volume, and cerebral blood volume (CBV). These three compartments are enclosed within a rigid cranium, which implies that if ICP is to remain constant, any volume gained (e.g., from tumor, hematoma, or abscess) must be balanced by volume lost. In the presence of a cerebral mass, ICP can be maintained initially because CSF is displaced to the spinal compartment. At a certain volume, however, this compensatory mechanism is exhausted, and ICP rises rapidly [see Figure 9]. The resulting pressure-volume curve is exponential in shape; in other words, a relatively small increase in volume may cause only a small rise in ICP at the flat portion of the curve but a large increase in ICP at the steep portion. A small increase in volume (such as results from CO_2 retention [see below] or obstruction of venous outflow) can prove fatal to a patient with an elevated ICP.

Manipulation of CBV is an artificial method of compensating for raised ICP. CBV is determined by the total diameter of the vascular bed, and changes in diameter thus affect CBV. The cerebral vessels are sensitive to changes in the pH of the CSF and thus respond to changes in the partial pressure of CO_2 with caliber adjustments. CO_2 can be regulated by adjusting ventilatory settings, and hyperventilation (i.e., induction of hypocapnia) to induce vasoconstriction is a useful method to manage acute episodes of raised ICP. For long-term treatment of ICP, however, hyperventilation is not recommended [see III:2 Injuries to the Central Nervous System].

Translocation of different parts of the brain produces specific herniation syndromes that have characteristic clinical presentations and temporal profiles. Brain herniation occurs in five major patterns.[1]

HERNIATION SYNDROMES

Subfalcial (Cingulate) Herniation

Mass lesions in the anterior or middle fossa may result in herniation of the cingulate gyrus under the free edge of the falx cerebri. Usually, patients with this condition are asymptomatic. If the herniation is severe, however, the pericallosal arteries may be compressed, resulting in unilateral or bilateral frontal infarcts in their region of distribution. Clinically, this may result in paresis of one or both legs.

Lateral (Uncal) Tentorial Herniation

Uncal herniation is caused by mass lesions in the lateral middle fossa or temporal lobe, which displace the medial edge of the uncus and hippocampal gyrus medially over the ipsilateral edge of the tentorium cerebelli. The uncus and the hippocampus thus herniate in the space between the midbrain and the tentorial edge, resulting in compression of the midbrain from side to side and elongation of its anteroposterior diameter. The ipsilateral cerebral peduncle and the

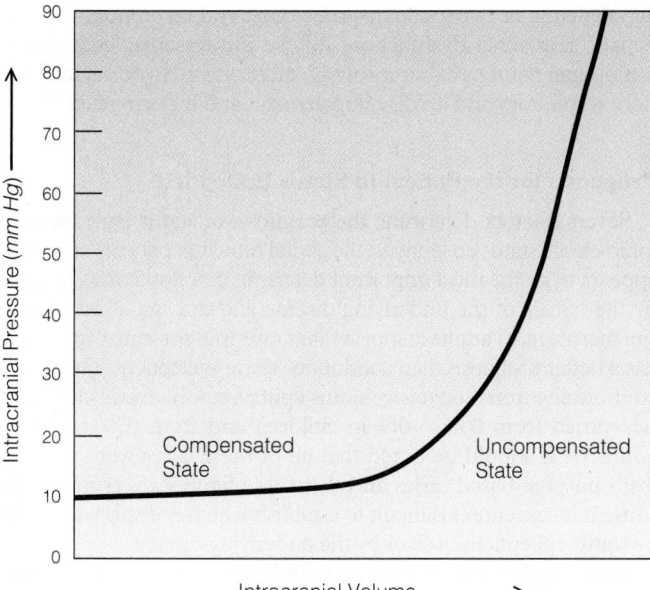

Figure 9 **Depicted is the relation between ICP and intracranial volume.**

oculomotor nerve are compressed, resulting in the classic syndrome of uncal herniation, which consists of contralateral hemiparesis, decreased consciousness (possibly caused by distortion or deafferentiation of the upper part of the RAS), and ipsilateral pupillary dilatation. In some cases, the herniation may cause compression of the contralateral cerebral peduncle against the tentorium, resulting in ipsilateral hemiparesis (Kernohan's notch). In these cases, the contralateral oculomotor nerve may also be stretched.

As uncal herniation progresses, it becomes clinically indistinguishable from central herniation. Early recognition of uncal herniation is important because deterioration may proceed rapidly once signs of herniation and brain-stem compression appear. In its initial stages, uncal herniation is fully reversible; however, as it evolves, neurologic recovery becomes progressively less likely.

Posterior (Tectal) Herniation

Posterior or tectal herniation may occur in patients who have purely frontal or occipital lesions or have bilateral lesions such as a bilateral chronic subdural hematoma. Under these circumstances, the medial temporal structures do not herniate between the tentorium and midbrain; instead, they herniate posteriorly or on both sides, thereby compressing the quadrigeminal plate at the level of the superior colliculi. Clinically, this results in findings resembling Parinaud syndrome. The patient has bilateral ptosis and an upward gaze paralysis in the presence of initially preserved pupillary response.

Central (Axial) Herniation

Central or axial herniation is defined as a downward shift of the entire brain stem toward the foramen magnum. Because of the downward herniation, the brain stem is elongated in its anteroposterior diameter, and stretching may occur in the central perforating branches of the basilar artery. This stretching is thought to produce ischemia and hemorrhage, although hemorrhage occasionally results from reversal of the displacement by operative decompression. Impaired consciousness has been related to this axial displacement. The Cushing response (arterial hypertension, bradycardia, and respiratory irregularity) has also been related to brain-stem ischemia.

Brain-stem blood flow is not always decreased in the presence of a Cushing response, however, and variant Cushing responses (e.g., hypotension) exist.[12,131]

The first clinical signs are reduced consciousness; symmetrical, small, reactive pupils; paresis of the upward gaze; signs of bilateral corticospinal tract dysfunction; and periodic breathing (Cheyne-Stokes respiration). As herniation progresses, flexor and eventually extensor posturing occurs, the pupils become fixed and dilated or remain in midposition, and hyperpnea results. At later stages, the lower pons and upper medulla are affected; this is characterized by fixed midposition pupils, limb flaccidity, bilateral Babinski responses, abolished oculovestibular reflexes, and shallow, regular breathing, often at an increased rate. Finally, medullary dysfunction occurs; patients display slow, irregular respiration interrupted by deep sighs and gasps. All reflexes disappear and the pupils become widely dilated.

Tonsillar Herniation

Prolapse of the cerebral tonsils through the foramen magnum can occur with either supratentorial or infratentorial masses or with a generalized increase in ICP. Tonsillar herniation causes obliteration of the cisterna magna and compression of the medulla oblongata, the latter resulting in apnea. The shape and size of the tentorial opening determine whether signs of tentorial or tonsillar herniation predominate with supratentorial mass lesions. When the opening is small, major symptoms are usually tentorial in nature; however, when the opening is large, tonsillar herniation may follow without any preceding signs of tentorial herniation.

Prognosis for the Comatose Patient

Even when optimal treatment is provided, the overall prognosis for the comatose patient is poor. Only about 40% of patients who are unconscious as a result of head trauma make a satisfactory recovery. In nontraumatic coma, the outcome is worse. In a study of 596 patients who were admitted for cardiac arrest (31%), cerebral infarction (36%), or ICH (36%), follow-up at 2 months showed that 69% had died, 20% survived with severe disability, 8% survived without severe disability, and 3% survived with unknown functional status.[132]

Outcome depends primarily on the etiology and the duration of coma, the initial clinical signs of neurologic damage, and the general medical condition and age of the patient. In patients with head injury, a motor score of 3 on admission, episodes of hypoxia ($PO_2 < 60$ mm Hg), hypotension (systolic blood pressure < 90 mm Hg), and raised ICP are important prognosticators of poor outcome.[133] Coma caused by depressant drug poisoning carries the most favorable prognosis if treated early: overall mortality is 1% to 5%.[134,135] Hypoxic-ischemic coma carries the worst prognosis: overall mortality is as high as 54%.[135,136] Most patients who recover from drug overdose suffer no residual brain damage, even after prolonged coma, whereas in one study, more than 50% of patients with hypoxic-ischemic coma who survived for at least 2 weeks remained comatose and suffered permanent brain damage.[135]

Cellular, Metabolic, and Systemic Effects of Status Epilepticus

The events that initiate status epilepticus are not known. The presence of an abnormally prolonged seizure has been attributed to excessive excitation, a failure of inhibition, or a combination of the two. However, relatively little is known about the cellular and molecular changes within a neuronal network that are responsible for persistent seizure activity. Excitation is a glutamate-dependent process and is initiated when the neurotransmitter glutamate binds to postsynaptic N-methyl-D-aspartate (NMDA) and non-NMDA glutamate receptors.[137] Initially, only non-NMDA channels are activated, resulting in the influx of sodium and depolarization. Ion flow through NMDA channels is blocked because of the presence of magnesium in the ion channel and because of GABA-mediated inhibitory mechanisms. In status epilepticus, however, GABA-mediated inhibition is suppressed, resulting in depolarization of the NMDA receptor, removal of magnesium from the ion channel, and influx of calcium, followed by further depolarization and intracellular calcium accumulation. Cell death after status epilepticus has been attributed to increased calcium accumulation, initiation of cell swelling, and calcium-mediated cell destruction.[138]

The effects of status epilepticus on cerebral metabolism and circulation can be divided into two phases, whereby the transition from phase 1 to phase 2 typically occurs at 30 to 60 minutes of continuous seizure activity.[138] In phase 1, an increase in CBF compensates for the increase in cerebral metabolic activity caused by the seizures, and the delivery of oxygen and glucose is maintained. In phase 2, the physiologic compensation mechanism (i.e., cerebral autoregulation) begins to fail because CBF is no longer sufficient to support the high metabolic demands of the epileptic tissue, and ischemia ensues.[139-141] Ischemia is further precipitated by systemic hypotension, which almost invariably occurs in phase 2 and which is in turn greatly exacerbated by I.V. antiepileptic drug therapy, particularly when these drugs are infused quickly. ICP can rise exponentially in late status epilepticus, and this rise, combined with hypotension, results in a decrease in CPP, which further compromises the cerebral circulation.

Other general metabolic and systemic effects of status epilepticus occurring in phase 1 include autonomic changes such as tachycardia, cardiac dysrhythmias, hypertension, apnea, pupillary enlargement, hypersecretion, sweating, incontinence, hyperglycemia, and lactic acidosis. In phase 2, changes include hypoglycemia, hyponatremia, hypokalemia or hyperkalemia, metabolic and respiratory acidosis, hepatic and renal dysfunction, diffuse intravascular coagulation, multiorgan failure, rhabdomyolysis, leukocytosis, hypoxia, hypotension, respiratory and cardiac impairment, and hyperpyrexia.[138]

Prognosis for the Patient in Status Epilepticus

Several factors determine the prognosis of status epilepticus. In tonic-clonic status epilepticus, the actual time that patients are seizing appears to be the most important determinant of outcome, followed by the nature of the underlying disease and the age of the patient. Furthermore, in adults it appears that intermittent status epilepticus has a better prognosis than continuous status epilepticus. The reported mortality from convulsive status epilepticus in several clinical series varied from 0% to 6% in children and from 0% to 10% in adults.[142] It should be noted that all of these cases were retrieved from hospital-based series and that these figures are estimates because it is sometimes difficult to establish whether death was caused by status epilepticus itself or by the underlying disease.

Status epilepticus in patients with head injury may represent a significant contribution to poor outcome, but sufficient clinical data are unavailable. Seizure prophylaxis is recommended in patients with head injuries, but no guidelines are currently available to indicate who should receive it (i.e., patients with severe head injuries only or those with moderate head injuries as well). In a recent study of 94 patients with moderate to severe head injuries who underwent continuous EEG monitoring, seizure activity was demonstrated in 22% of patients despite phenytoin prophylaxis. Six of them displayed status epilepticus, all of whom subsequently died; these results indicate that continuous evaluation for seizures or status epilepticus should be seriously considered in these patients, together with aggressive intervention.[143]

References

1. Miller J, Becker D: Pathophysiology of head injury. Neurological Surgery, 2nd ed. Youmans J, Ed. WB Saunders Co, Philadelphia, 1982, p 1896
2. Denny-Brown D: Selected Writings of Sir Charles Sherrington. Oxford University Press, Oxford, 1979
3. Eccles J, Gibson W: Sherrington, His Life and Thought. Springer International, Berlin, 1979
4. Greenberg RP, Stablein DM, Becker DP: Noninvasive localization of brain-stem lesions in the cat with multimodality evoked potentials: correlation with human head-injury data. J Neurosurg 54:740, 1981
5. Ritter AM, Muizelaar JP, Barnes T, et al: Brain stem blood flow, pupillary response, and outcome in patients with severe head injuries. Neurosurgery 44:941, 1999
6. Qureshi A, Wilson D, Traystman R: Treatment of elevated intracranial pressure in experimental intracerebral hemorrhage: comparison between mannitol and hypertonic saline. Neurosurgery 44:1055, 1999
7. Kellie G: On death from cold, and on congestions of the brain. An account of the appearances observed in the dissection of two of three individuals presumed to have perished in the storm of 3rd November 1821; with some reflections on the pathology of the brain. Trans Med Chir Soc Edinburgh 1:84, 1824
8. Monro A: Observations on the Structure and Function of the Nervous System. Creech and Johnson, Edinburgh, 1783
9. Chesnut RM, Marshall LF: Management of head injury. Treatment of abnormal intracranial pressure. Neurosurg Clin N Am 2:267, 1991
10. Eisenberg HM, Frankowski RF, Contant CF, et al: High-dose barbiturate control of elevated intracra-nial pressure in patients with severe head injury. J Neurosurg 69:15, 1988
11. Miller JD, Becker DP, Ward JD, et al: Significance of intracranial hypertension in severe head injury. J Neurosurg 47:503, 1977
12. Rowan JO, Teasdale G: Brain stem blood flow during raised intracranial pressure. Acta Neurol Scand Suppl 64:520, 1977
13. Souhami R, Moxham J: Textbook of Medicine. Churchill Livingstone, Edinburgh, 1990, p 747
14. Souhami R, Moxham J: Textbook of Medicine. Churchill Livingstone, Edinburgh, 1990, p 971
15. Souhami R, Moxham J: Textbook of Medicine. Churchill Livingstone, Edinburgh, 1990, p 806
16. Souhami R, Moxham J: Textbook of Medicine. Churchill Livingstone, Edinburgh, 1990, p 968
17. Forsyth PA, Posner JB: Headaches in patients with brain tumors: a study of 111 patients. Neurology 43:1678, 1993
18. Ropper A, Gress D: Computerized tomography and clinical features of large cerebral hemorrhages. Cerebrovasc Dis 1:38, 1991
19. Brott T, Thalinger K, Hertzberg V: Hypertension as a risk factor for spontaneous intracerebral hemorrhage. Stroke 17:1078, 1986
20. Hunt WE, Hess RM: Surgical risk as related to time of intervention in the repair of intracranial aneurysms. J Neurosurg 28:14, 1968
21. Drake C: Report of World Federation of Neurological Surgeons Committee on a universal subarachnoid hemorrhage grading scale. J Neurosurg 68:985, 1988
22. Eisenberg HM, Gary HE Jr, Aldrich EF, et al: Initial CT findings in 753 patients with severe head injury. A report from the NIH Traumatic Coma Data Bank. J Neurosurg 73:688, 1990
23. Martin NA, Doberstein C, Alexander M, et al: Post-traumatic cerebral arterial spasm. J Neurotrauma 12:897, 1995
24. Romer F: Difficulties in the diagnosis of acute bacterial meningitis: evaluation of antibiotic pretreatment and causes of admission to the hospital. Lancet 2:345, 1977
25. Bolton C: Infections of the central nervous system. Coma and Impaired Consciousness. Young G, Ropper A, Bolton C, Eds. McGraw-Hill Book Co, New York, 1998, p 228
26. Young G: Impaired consciousness and disorders of temperature. Coma and Impaired Consciousness. Young G, Ropper A, Bolton C, Eds. McGraw-Hill Book Co, New York, 1998, p 213
27. Katz RT, Haig AJ, Clark BB, et al: Long-term survival, prognosis, and life-care planning for 29 patients with chronic locked-in syndrome. Arch Phys Med Rehabil 73:403, 1992
28. Tomsick TA, Brott TG, Chambers AA, et al: Hyperdense middle cerebral artery sign on CT: efficacy in detecting middle cerebral artery thrombosis. AJNR Am J Neuroradiol 11:473, 1990
29. Tomsick T, Brott T, Barsan W, et al: Thrombus localization with emergency cerebral CT. AJNR Am J Neuroradiol 13:257, 1992
30. Wijdicks E: The Clinical Practice of Critical Care Neurology. Lippincott-Raven, Philadelphia, 1997, p 193

31. Fisher CM, Kistler JP, Davis JM: Relation of cerebral vasospasm to subarachnoid hemorrhage visualized by computerized tomographic scanning. Neurosurgery 6:1, 1980

32. Brouwers PJ, Wijdicks EF, Van Gijn J: Infarction after aneurysm rupture does not depend on distribution or clearance rate of blood. Stroke 23:374, 1992

33. Hillman J: Should computed tomography scanning replace lumbar puncture in the diagnostic process in suspected subarachnoid hemorrhage? Surg Neurol 26:547, 1986

34. Hashimoto H, Iida J, Hironaka Y, et al: Use of spiral computerized tomography angiography in patients with subarachnoid hemorrhage in whom subtraction angiography did not reveal cerebral aneurysms. J Neurosurg 92:278, 2000

35. Strayle-Batra M, Skalej M, Wakhloo AK, et al: Three-dimensional spiral CT angiography in the detection of cerebral aneurysm. Acta Radiol 39:233, 1998

36. Velthuis BK, Rinkel GJ, Ramos LM, et al: Subarachnoid hemorrhage: aneurysm detection and preoperative evaluation with CT angiography. Radiology 208:423, 1998

37. Harrison MJ, Johnson BA, Gardner GM, et al: Preliminary results on the management of unruptured intracranial aneurysms with magnetic resonance angiography and computed tomographic angiography. Neurosurgery 40:947, discussion 955, 1997

38. Wardlaw JM, White PM: The detection and management of unruptured intracranial aneurysms. Brain 123:205, 2000

39. Desprechins B, Stadnik T, Koerts G, et al: Use of diffusion-weighted MR imaging in differential diagnosis between intracerebral necrotic tumors and cerebral abscesses [see comments]. AJNR Am J Neuroradiol 20:1252, 1999

40. Miller ES, Dias PS, Uttley D: CT scanning in the management of intracranial abscess: a review of 100 cases. Br J Neurosurg 2:439, 1988

41. Zimmerman RA, Bilaniuk LT: Computed tomographic staging of traumatic epidural bleeding. Radiology 144:809, 1982

42. Gennarelli TA, Thibault LE: Biomechanics of acute subdural hematoma. J Trauma 22:680, 1982

43. Gudeman SK, Kishore PR, Miller JD, et al: The genesis and significance of delayed traumatic intracerebral hematoma. Neurosurgery 5:309, 1979

44. Ribas G, Jane J: Traumatic contusions and intracerebral hematomas. Central Nervous System Trauma Status Report 1991. J Neurotrauma 9[suppl 1]: S265, 1992

45. Becker D, Doberstein C, Hovda D: Craniocerebral Trauma: Mechanisms, Management, and the Cellular Response to Injury. Current Concepts. The Upjohn Co, Kalamazoo, Michigan, 1994

46. Chesnut R, Servadei F: Surgical treatment of post-traumatic mass lesions. Traumatic Brain Injury. Marion D, Ed. Thieme Medical Publishers, New York, 1999, p 81

47. Strich S: Shearing of nerve fibers as a cause of brain damage due to head injury: a pathological study of twenty cases. Lancet 2:443, 1961

48. Marshall LF, Marshall SB, Klauber MR, et al: The diagnosis of head injury requires a classification based on computed axial tomography. J Neurotrauma 9(suppl 1):S287, 1992

49. Ropper AH, Shafran B: Brain edema after stroke. Clinical syndrome and intracranial pressure. Arch Neurol 41:26, 1984

50. Shaw C, Alvord E, Berry R: Swelling of the brain following ischemic infarction with arterial occlusion. Arch Neurol 1:161, 1959

51. Schwab S, Aschoff A, Spranger M, et al: The value of intracranial pressure monitoring in acute hemispheric stroke. Neurology 47:393, 1996

52. Doerfler A, Forsting M, Reith W, et al: Decompressive craniectomy in a rat model of "malignant" cerebral hemispheric stroke: experimental support for an aggressive therapeutic approach. J Neurosurg 85:853, 1996

53. Forsting M, Reith W, Scheabitz WR, et al: Decompressive craniectomy for cerebral infarction: an experimental study in rats. Stroke 26:259, 1995

54. Rabb CH: Surgical treatment strategies in ischemic stroke. Neuroimaging Clin N Am 9:527, 1999

55. Rieke K, Schwab S, Krieger D, et al: Decompressive surgery in space-occupying hemispheric infarction: results of an open, prospective trial. Crit Care Med 23:1576, 1995

56. Sakai K, Iwahashi K, Terada K, et al: Outcome after external decompression for massive cerebral infarction. Neurol Med Chir (Tokyo) 38:131, 1998

57. Schwab S, Steiner T, Aschoff A, et al: Early hemicraniectomy in patients with complete middle cerebral artery infarction. Stroke 29:1888, 1998

58. McKissock W, Richardson A, Taylor J: Primary intracerebral hemorrhage: a controlled trial of surgical and conservative treatment in 180 unselected cases. Lancet 2:221, 1961

59. Juvela S, Heiskanen O, Poranen A, et al: The treatment of spontaneous intracerebral hemorrhage: a prospective randomized trial of surgical and conservative treatment. J Neurosurg 70:755, 1989

60. Kandel EI, Peresedov VV: Stereotaxic evacuation of spontaneous intracerebral hematomas. J Neurosurg 62:206, 1985

61. Kanno T, Nagata J, Nonomura K, et al: New approaches in the treatment of hypertensive intracerebral hemorrhage. Stroke 24(12 suppl):I96, 1993

62. Winn HR, Richardson AE, Jane JA: The long-term prognosis in untreated cerebral aneurysms: I. The incidence of late hemorrhage in cerebral aneurysm: a 10-year evaluation of 364 patients. Ann Neurol 1:358, 1977

63. Winn HR, Richardson AE, O'Brien W, et al: The long-term prognosis in untreated cerebral aneurysms: II. Late morbidity and mortality. Ann Neurol 4:418, 1978

64. Dorsch NW: Cerebral arterial spasm—a clinical review. Br J Neurosurg 9:403, 1995

65. Levy ML, Giannotta SL: Induced hypertension and hypervolemia for treatment of cerebral vasospasm. Neurosurg Clin North Am 1:357, 1990

66. Muizelaar JP, Zwienenberg M, Rudisill NA, et al: The prophylactic use of transluminal balloon angioplasty in patients with Fisher grade 3 subarachnoid hemorrhage: a pilot study. J Neurosurg 91:51, 1999

67. Dyste GN, Hitchon PW, Menezes AH, et al: Stereotaxic surgery in the treatment of multiple brain abscesses. J Neurosurg 69:188, 1988

68. Kala M: Aspiration or extirpation in cerebral abscess surgery? Neurosurg Rev 16:121, 1993

69. Mampalam TJ, Rosenblum ML: Trends in the management of bacterial brain abscesses: a review of 102 cases over 17 years. Neurosurgery 23:451, 1988

70. Tekkeok IH, Erbengi A: Management of brain abscess in children: review of 130 cases over a period of 21 years. Childs Nerv Syst 8:411, 1992

71. Ballester JM, Harchelroad FP: Hypothermia: an easy-to-miss, dangerous disorder in winter weather. Geriatrics 54:51, 1999

72. Gentilello LM: Advances in the management of hypothermia. Surg Clin N Am 75:243, 1995

73. Goodlock JL: Methods of rewarming the hypothermic patient in the accident and emergency department. Accid Emerg Nurs 3:114, 1995

74. Haskell RM, Boruta B, Rotondo MF, et al: Hypothermia. AACN Clinical Issues 8:368, 1997

75. Kofstad J: Blood gases and hypothermia: some theoretical and practical considerations. Scand J Clin Lab Invest Suppl 224:21, 1996

76. Lloyd EL: Accidental hypothermia. Resuscitation 32:111, 1996

77. McGowan J: Management of hypothermia in adults. Nursing Crit Care 4:59, 1999

78. Patten J: Attacks of Altered Consciousness, 2nd ed. Springer-Verlag, Berlin, 1996

79. Appleton R, Sweeney A, Choonara I, et al: Lorazepam versus diazepam in the acute treatment of epileptic seizures and status epilepticus. Dev Med Child Neurol 37:682, 1995

80. Dodrill CB, Wilensky AJ: Intellectual impairment as an outcome of status epilepticus. Neurology 40 (suppl 2):23, 1990

81. Lipowski Z: Delirium in surgery: historical introduction. Delirium: Acute Brain Failure in Man. Charles C Thomas, Springfield, Illinois, 1980, p 213

82. Fisher B, Gilchrist D: Postoperative delirium in the elderly. Ann R Coll Phys Surg Canada 26:358, 1993

83. El-Ganzouri A, Ivankovich A, Braverman B, et al: Monoamine oxidase inhibitors: should they be discontinued preoperatively? Anesth Analg 64:592, 1985

84. Grigoletto F, Zappalaa G, Anderson DW, et al: Norms for the Mini-Mental State Examination in a healthy population. Neurology 53:315, 1999

85. McDowell I, Kristjansson B, Hill GB, et al: Community screening for dementia: the Mini-Mental State Exam (MMSE) and Modified Mini-Mental State Exam (3MS) compared. J Clin Epidemiol 50:377, 1997

86. Rapp CG, Wakefield B, Kundrat M, et al: Acute confusion assessment instruments: clinical versus research usability. Appl Nurs Res 13:37, 2000

87. Wind AW, Schellevis FG, Van Staveren G, et al: Limitations of the Mini-Mental State Examination in diagnosing dementia in general practice. Int J Geriatr Psychiatry 12:101, 1997

88. Rolfson DB, McElhaney JE, Jhangri GS, et al: Validity of the confusion assessment method in detecting postoperative delirium in the elderly. Int Psychogeriatrics 11:431, 1999

89. Spar JE: Dementia in the aged. Psychiatr Clin N Am 5:67, 1982

90. Kaplan H, Sadock B, Grebb J: Dementia. Synopsis of Psychiatry. Williams & Wilkins, Baltimore, 1994, p 345

91. McKhann G, Drachman D, Folstein M, et al: Clinical diagnosis of Alzheimer's disease: report of the NINCDS-ADRDA Work Group under the auspices of Department of Health and Human Services Task Force on Alzheimer's Disease. Neurology 34:939, 1984

92. Cummings J: Neuropsychiatric aspects of Alzheimer's disease and other dementing illnesses. Textbook of Neuropsychiatry. Yudofsky S, Hales R, Eds. American Psychiatric Association, Washington, DC, 1992, p 605

93. McEvoy J: Organic brain syndromes. Ann Intern Med 95:212, 1981

94. Wells C: Organic syndromes: dementia. Comprehensive Textbook of Psychiatry. Kaplan H, Sadock B, Eds. William & Wilkins, Baltimore, 1985, p 851

95. Daly MP: Diagnosis and management of Alzheimer disease. J Am Board Fam Pract 12:375, 1999

96. Davis RE, Emmerling MR, Jaen JC, et al: Therapeutic intervention in dementia. Crit Rev Neurobiol 7:41, 1993

97. Diaz Brinton R, Yamazaki RS: Advances and challenges in the prevention and treatment of Alzheimer's disease. Pharm Res 15:386, 1998

98. Flint AJ, van Reekum R: The pharmacologic treatment of Alzheimer's disease: a guide for the general psychiatrist. Can J Psychiatry 43:689, 1998

99. Foy JM, Starr JM: Assessment and treatment of dementia in medical patients. Psychother Psychosom 69:59, 2000

100. Nyenhuis DL, Gorelick PB: Vascular dementia: a contemporary review of epidemiology, diagnosis, prevention, and treatment. J Am Geriatr Soc 46:1437, 1998

101. Rabins PV: Developing treatment guidelines for Alz-

heimer's disease and other dementias. J Clin Psychiatry 59(suppl 11):17, 1998

102. Scheltens P, van Gool WA: Emerging treatments in dementia. Eur Neurol 38:184, 1997

103. Sadavoy J: A review of pseudodementia. Mod Med Canada 39:319, 1984

104. Wells C: Pseudodementia. Am J Psychiatry 136:895, 1979

105. Yesavage J: Differential diagnosis between depression and dementia. Am J Med 94(suppl 5a):23s, 1993

106. Touringny-Rivard M: Treatment of depression in the elderly. Med North Am 1:56, 1986

107. Jenike M: Treatment of affective illness in the elderly with drugs and electroconvulsive therapy. Geriatr Psychiatry Neurol 22:77, 1989

108. Rosenberg D, Wright B, Gerson S: Depression in the elderly. Dementia 3:157, 1992

109. Jennett B, Snoek J, Bond MR, et al: Disability after severe head injury: observations on the use of the Glasgow Outcome Scale. J Neurol Neurosurg Psychiatry 44:285, 1981

110. Teasdale GM, Pettigrew LE, Wilson JT, et al: Analyzing outcome of treatment of severe head injury: a review and update on advancing the use of the Glasgow Outcome Scale. J Neurotrauma 15:587, 1998

111. Blyth B: The outcome of severe head injuries. N Z Med J 93:267, 1981

112. Gensemer IB, McMurry FG, Walker JC, et al: Behavioral consequences of trauma. J Trauma 28:44, 1988

113. Gensemer IB, Smith JL, Walker JC, et al: Psychological consequences of blunt head trauma and relation to other indices of severity of injury. Ann Emerg Med 18:9, 1989

114. Tate RL, Broe GA, Lulham JM: Impairment after severe blunt head injury: the results from a consecutive series of 100 patients. Acta Neurol Scand 79:97, 1989

115. Dikmen S, Temkin N, McLean A, et al: Memory and head injury severity. J Neurol Neurosurg Psychiatry 50:1613, 1987

116. Paniak CE, Shore DL, Rourke BP: Recovery of memory after severe closed head injury: dissociations in recovery of memory parameters and predictors of outcome. J Clin Exp Neuropsychol 11:631, 1989

117. Uzzell BP, Dolinskas CA, Wiser RF, et al: Influence of lesions detected by computed tomography on outcome and neuropsychological recovery after severe head injury. Neurosurgery 20:396, 1987

118. Francis J: Delirium in older patients. J Am Geriatr Soc 40:829, 1992

119. Meador KJ: Cognitive side effects of medications. Neurol Clin 16:141, 1998

120. Burns MJ, Linden CU, Grandins A, et al: A comparison of physostigmine and benzodiazepines for the treatment of anticholinergic poisoning. Ann Emerg Med 35:374, 2000

121. Tesar GE, Murray GB, Cassem NH: Use of high-dose intravenous haloperidol in the treatment of agitated cardiac patients. J Clin Psychopharmacol 5:344, 1985

122. Black PM: Brain death (pt 1). N Engl J Med 299:338, 1978

123. Black PM: Brain death (pt 2). N Engl J Med 299:393, 1978

124. Report of Special Task Force: Guidelines for the determination of brain death in children. Pediatrics 80:298, 1987

125. LaMancusa J, Cooper R, Vieth R, et al: The effects of the falling therapeutic and subtherapeutic barbiturate blood levels on electrocerebral silence in clinically brain-dead children. Clin Electroencephalogr 22:112, 1991

126. Wijdicks E: Precautions for the apnea test in brain death. Neurology of Critical Illness. FA Davis Co, Philadelphia, 1995, p 329

127. Lynch J, Eldadah MK: Brain-death criteria currently used by pediatric intensivists. Clin Pediatr 31:457, 1992

128. Mejia RE, Pollack MM: Variability in brain death determination practices in children [see comments]. JAMA 274:550, 1995

129. Verweij BH, Muizelaar JP, Vinas FC, et al: Mitochondrial dysfunction after experimental and human brain injury and its possible reversal with a selective N-type calcium channel antagonist (SNX-111). Neurol Res 19:334, 1997

130. Jones T: Thresholds of focal cerebral ischemia in awake monkeys. J Neurosurg 54:773, 1981

131. Marshiman L: Cushing's variant response (acute hypotension) after subarachnoid hemorrhage. Association with moderate intracranial hypertension and subacute cardiovascular collapse. Stroke 28:1445, 1997

132. Hamel MB, Goldman L, Teno J, et al: Identification of comatose patients at high risk for death or severe disability. SUPPORT Investigators. Understand Prognoses and Preferences for Outcomes and Risks of Treatments. JAMA 273:1842, 1995

133. Combes P, Fauvage B, Colonna M, et al: Severe head injuries: an outcome prediction and survival analysis. Intensive Care Med 22:1391, 1996

134. Ghodse A: Deliberate self-poisoning: a study in London casualty departments. Br Med J 1:805, 1977

135. Sacco RL, VanGool R, Mohr JP, et al: Nontraumatic coma. Glasgow Coma Score and coma etiology as predictors of 2-week outcome. Arch Neurol 47:1181, 1990

136. Bertini G, Margheri M, Giglioli C, et al: Prognostic significance of early clinical manifestations in post-anoxic coma: a retrospective study of 58 patients resuscitated after prehospital cardiac arrest. Crit Care Med 17:627, 1989

137. Fountain N, Bleck T: Mechanism of action of drugs for status epilepticus. Epilepsy Quarterly, winter 1996

138. Shorvon S: Status Epilepticus: Its Clinical Features and Treatment in Children and Adults. Cambridge University Press, Cambridge, 1994, p 54

139. Meldrum B: Metabolic factors during prolonged seizures and their relation to cell death. Status Epilepticus. Mechanisms of Brain Damage and Treatment, Vol 34. Delgado-Escueta A, Wasterlain C, Treiman D, et al, Eds. Raven Press, New York, 1986, p 261

140. Franck G, Sadzot B, Salmon F, et al: Regional cerebral blood flow and metabolic rates in human focal epilepsy and status epilepticus. Basic Mechanisms of the Epilepsies: Molecular and Cellular Approaches, Vol 44. Delgado-Escueta A Jr., Woodbury D, Porter R, Eds. Raven Press, New York, 1986, p 935

141. Siesjo B, Wieloch T: Epileptic brain damage: pathophysiology and neurochemical pathology. Basic Mechanisms of the Epilepsies: Molecular and Cellular Approaches, Vol 44. Delgado-Escueta A Jr., Woodbury D, Porter R, Eds. Raven Press, New York, 1986, p 813

142. Shorvon S: Status Epilepticus: Its Clinical Features and Treatment in Children and Adults. Cambridge University Press, Cambridge, 1994, p 296

143. Vespa P, Prins M, Ronne-Engstrom E, et al: Increase in extracellular glutamate caused by reduced cerebral perfusion pressure and seizures after human traumatic brain injury: a microdialysis study. J Neurosurg 89:971, 1998

Acknowledgments

Portions of this chapter are adapted from material contained in two chapters previously published in *Scientific American® Surgery*: "Coma, Seizures, and Brain Death," by Ehud Arbit, M.D., and George Krol, M.D., and "Cognitive and Sensory Deficits," by Richard Monks, M.D.

10 SUBSTANCE ABUSE

John A. Marx, M.D., and Mark Kirk, M.D.

The Substance Abuser in the Emergency Department

Substance abuse may take the form of acute toxic exposure, chronic use, withdrawal, or a combination thereof; each form in itself poses a significant threat. Furthermore, substance abuse and abstinence may mask or masquerade as clinical features of surgical disease, thereby greatly complicating management. Four classes of abused substances will be considered in some detail: narcotics, stimulants, hallucinogens, and alcohols. Other classes of substances (e.g., sedative-hypnotics) are abused as well, but we consider these four classes to comprise the substances of greatest concern for practicing surgeons. Acute exposure, chronic use, and withdrawal will be separately addressed.

Resuscitation

The first priority is establishment of a patent airway. Because drug toxicity produces obtundation and loss of airway-protective reflexes, aspiration is a common complication. Aspiration pneumonitis carries increased risks of prolonged ventilatory support, pneumonia, prolonged hypoxic states, and progression to acute respiratory distress syndrome.

Left lateral decubitus positioning helps prevent aspiration in patients who are obtunded and do not have a protective endotracheal tube in position. Vomitus in the airway should be suctioned. Proper head positioning and use of oral airway equipment may be sufficient to keep the upper airway unobstructed. The need for endotracheal intubation is determined clinically. Indications include inability to protect the airway, hypoxemia despite supplemental oxygen administration, significant hypercapnia, and severe respiratory distress. The presence or absence of the gag reflex is not a reliable indicator of need.

Any abnormality in one or more vital signs warrants insertion of an intravenous catheter. In acute overdose, even if vital signs do not appear abnormal, intravenous access should routinely be obtained and maintained, together with cardiac monitoring (see below), until it is clear that the responsible substance or substances are benign or that the patient's clinical course has progressed to the point where intravenous access is no longer needed. Standard routes for intravenous access may not exist in the chronic intravenous drug abuser. These patients can often direct the clinician to the most viable venous

alternative. Central venous lines and extremity cutdowns may be necessary.

Continuous cardiac monitoring and pulse oximetry are appropriate in patients with or at risk for alterations in vital signs, respiratory failure, seizures, or acidosis. Appropriate measures should be taken to manage hypoxemia, hypotension, hypertension, and acid-base abnormalities, as well as their precipitating factors.

Urgent Syndromes

There are three common urgent syndromes associated with substance abuse that warrant discussion. These three syndromes are coma or altered mental status, seizures, and severe agitation [*see I:9 Coma, Seizures, Cognitive Impairment, and Brain Death*]. For each of these three syndromes, there is a wide spectrum of possible causes

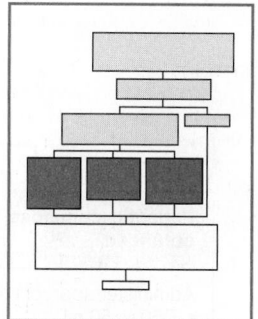

to be identified and managed, both within and outside the category of toxic exposure.

COMA AND ALTERED MENTAL STATUS

Depressed mental status, including coma, can result from high doses of ethanol, narcotics, or sedative-hypnotics. It is an unusual presentation for Wernicke-Korsakoff syndrome, a nutritional complication of chronic ethanol abuse and poor diet. Complications of poisoning, as opposed to direct toxic effects causing altered mental status, include the following: anoxic brain injury, cerebral hemorrhage, cerebral infarction, central nervous system infections, and septic emboli. The depth of coma can be appraised with brain stem reflex testing. Prolonged coma or waxing-and-waning states of consciousness are seen with some toxins. Coma with fixed, dilated pupils and an isoelectric electroencephalogram can mimic brain death.[1]

Antidotes

Dextrose One ampule (50 ml = 25 g dextrose) of 50 percent dextrose in water (D50W) should immediately be given intravenously when delirium, obtundation, or coma is present and when hypoglycemia (blood glucose < 60 mg/dl) is confirmed by rapid bedside testing (e.g., Dextrostix). If rapid bedside testing is unavailable, patients with altered mentation or coma but without focal neurologic findings should be treat-

The Substance Abuser in the Emergency Department

Patient presents with symptoms and signs of substance abuse

Symptoms and signs include
- Unusual or bizarre behavior
- Lethargy, confusion
- Pressure-dependent ecchymoses, bullae, necrotic areas
- Cyanosis
- Hypotension
- Altered respiration
- Track marks
- ↑ or ↓ T°
- Mydriasis, miosis, horizontal or vertical nystagmus
- Peculiar odors
- Tachyarrhythmias

Suggestive clinical scenarios include
- Trauma
- Near-drownings, fires
- Domestic violence, suicide attempts, homicide
- Reckless driving, single-car accidents

Assess airway and ventilatory status and vital signs

If airway is inadequate: place obtunded patients in left lateral decubitus position; suction vomitus; place ET tube if necessary.

Vital signs are abnormal, or acute overdose is present

Establish I.V. access.

Monitor via continuous ECG or pulse oximetry.

Correct hypoxemia, hypotension, hypertension, and acid-base abnormalities.

Manage any urgent syndromes present.

Vital signs are normal, and acute overdose is absent

Patient is comatose, delirious, or obtunded

Administer appropriate antidotes:
- D50W, 50 ml
- Naloxone, 2 mg I.V., repeated q. 2–3 min to total of 10 mg as necessary (ineffective against ethanol-induced coma)
- Thiamine, 50–100 mg by I.V. bolus, for suspected chronic alcoholism, poor diet, or Wernicke-Korsakoff syndrome

Patient has seizures

Protect patient from injury.
Administer anticonvulsants:
- Diazepam, 5 mg I.V. q. 5 min as needed, or lorazepam, 1–2 mg I.V. q. 5 min as needed to total of 10–12 mg
- Phenobarbital, 10–20 mg/kg for status epilepticus

Patient is severely agitated

Rule out hypoxemia, closed head injury, pain, and respiratory distress.

Use physical restraints as necessary. If patient is violent, sedate with haloperidol, 5–10 mg I.V. q. 10 min as needed. Give benzodiazepines for stimulant- or withdrawal-induced agitation once patient's violent behavior is controlled.

Continue evaluation and consider perioperative needs

If possible, obtain history, focusing on
- Course of symptoms and signs
- Amount, route, and time of exposure
- Bizarre or violent behavior
- Trauma
- Accidents
- Other medications or drugs

Perform detailed physical exam to rule out traumatic, metabolic, and endocrine causes.

Order lab tests (serum electrolytes, blood gases, skeletal muscle enzymes, renal function, x-rays, ECG) as necessary on the basis of clinical findings. Qualitative and quantitative toxicologic analyses are often of limited utility.

Consider gut decontamination (lavage or charcoal therapy).

Preoperative considerations: need for and risks of anesthesia; universal HIV precautions
Postoperative considerations: pain control (narcotic addicts may require large doses); possible withdrawal syndromes

Initiate specific management

ed empirically. Hemiplegia is present in most patients with cerebral ischemia but in only 2.5 percent of patients with hypoglycemia. If empirical glucose administration is withheld from this subset of patients until glucose levels can be measured, the adverse effects of hyperglycemia after cerebral ischemia can be prevented.[2] Substance abuse–related causes of hypoglycemia include poor nutrition, liver failure, and alcohol-induced hypoglycemia in chronic alcoholics, as well as systemic infection in intravenous drug abusers.

Naloxone Naloxone is a pure opioid antagonist with a therapeutic half-life of 30 to 60 minutes for reversal of respiratory depression. It is indicated in any patient with depressed mentation or coma and is effective against both natural and synthetic opioids. The standard dose of naloxone is 2 mg I.V. for adults and for children weighing more than 20 kg, with onset of action in one to three minutes. For children weighing less than 20 kg, 0.1 to 0.2 mg/kg should be given. These doses can be repeated up to a total dose of 10 mg when the response is only partial or when opioids known to be less susceptible to naloxone (e.g., propoxyphene, diphenoxylate, pentazocine, or butorphanol) are suspected.[2] If necessary, naloxone can be administered via subcutaneous, intramuscular, or intralingual routes or via an endotracheal tube. There are no well-documented adverse consequences of naloxone administration, with the exception of opioid withdrawal in narcotic-dependent patients. If narcotic addiction is known or suspected, a lower dose (0.1 to 0.2 mg) may be used to prevent violent withdrawal and can be titrated to the cessation of respiratory and CNS depression. The need to protect the airway with suction or endotracheal intubation should be anticipated because withdrawal may precipitate vomiting without arousal. A patient suspected of narcotic overdose who responds to naloxone must be observed for at least two hours after the last dose of naloxone has been administered.

Flumazenil Flumazenil is a pure competitive benzodiazepine antagonist. It is safe and effective for the reversal of benzodiazepine-induced sedation in short diagnostic or surgical procedures. However, securing the airway should take precedence over the reversal of benzodiazepine-induced respiratory and CNS depression. Because the half-life of this agent is 30 to 80 minutes (much shorter than that of virtually all benzodiazepines currently used), resedation is likely after its administration. Because flumazenil can precipitate severe benzodiazepine withdrawal or seizures and dysrhythmias from coingestants (e.g., cyclic antidepressants),[3] it should not be used in patients with mixed or unknown overdoses.

Thiamine Thiamine is a water-soluble vitamin whose absence causes Wernicke-Korsakoff syndrome. It should be administered to patients who are chronic ethanol abusers, have a poor diet, or are suspected of having Wernicke-Korsakoff syndrome. Specific indications include lethargy, confusion, bradycardia, hypotension, and hypothermia of unknown cause. Thiamine can be safely administered in doses of 50 to 100 mg by I.V. bolus.[4] A 50 mg dose of thiamine is frequently part of intravenous multivitamin preparations.

SEIZURES

Toxin-caused seizures are grand mal unless there is preex-

isting focal CNS pathology. They can be direct sequelae of acute narcotic and stimulant use or hyperadrenergic events attributed to ethanol and sedative-hypnotic withdrawal. Hypoxemia caused by airway compromise, hypoventilation, or respiratory complications should be considered.

Management of seizures includes avoidance of physical injury to the patient and, when required, intervention to protect the airway. Because most grand mal seizures are brief and self-limited, immediate pharmacological intervention is rarely necessary. For persistent seizures, the first-line medication is a benzodiazepine administered intravenously (e.g., diazepam, 5 mg every five minutes in adults and 0.1 to 0.3 mg/kg every five minutes in children, or lorazepam, 1 to 2 mg every five minutes up to 10 to 12 mg in adults and 0.05 to 0.10 mg/kg in children). If there is an ongoing risk of seizure, phenobarbital, 10 to 20 mg/kg I.V., should be administered. Phenytoin has no role in emergent treatment of toxin-induced seizures. Elimination of the substance or condition that precipitated the seizure (e.g., a toxin or hypoxemia) should be undertaken simultaneously with these measures.

SEVERE AGITATION

Causes of combativeness should be sought, including respiratory distress, closed head injury, and significant pain. Irritability and agitation should be interpreted as hypoxemia until this is ruled out. When violent behavior endangers the patient and staff or hinders urgent management, application of physical restraints and judicious sedation are indicated. To gain control of agitated patients who could harm the staff or themselves, intravenous haloperidol or droperidol (5 to 10 mg I.V. initially, then every 10 minutes as needed) is effective within 10 minutes.[5] These agents do not cause cardiorespiratory deterioration, lower the seizure threshold, or interfere with neurosurgical assessment. Use of opioids, barbiturates, or benzodiazepines to sedate combative patients can lead to depressed circulatory and respiratory function and can exacerbate acute toxic effects if the abused substance is from the same pharmaceutical class. Once the patient is under control, however, benzodiazepines are the most beneficial agents for treatment of agitation, seizures, hyperthermia, and hyperdynamic states caused by stimulants (e.g., cocaine) and by sedative-hypnotic withdrawal.

Patient Evaluation

HISTORY

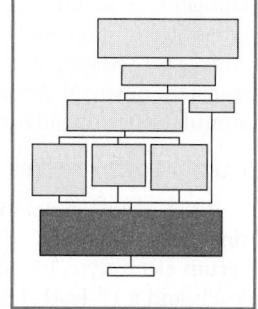

The patient, the family, friends, and paramedics can all provide useful data regarding the current presentation, patterns of substance abuse, and associated medical complications. It is helpful to determine when, in what quantity, and by what route the patient was exposed to the substance; whether additional substances were involved; what symptoms occurred and how they developed over time; and what medications the patient is taking. In addition, certain clinical scenarios should prompt concern. Unexpected or bizarre patterns of behavior suggest drug toxicity. Substance abuse is frequently involved in domestic violence, suicide, and homicide and commonly plays a role in near-drownings and fires.[6] Virtually all forms of penetrating and blunt trauma are strongly associated with substance abuse.[7] Reckless driving and single-car accidents, especially late at night and early in the morning, are particularly suggestive.[8]

PHYSICAL EXAMINATION

Characteristic clinical findings are often produced by specific classes of drugs (e.g., narcotics, sympathomimetics, and anticholinergics).[9] It is imperative, however, to perform a complete detailed examination to differentiate substance abuse from traumatic, metabolic, and endocrine causes.

Initial inspection may reveal odors peculiar to the alcohols or toluene. Cyanosis is most likely to be the result of hypoventilation or aspiration (associated with ethanol, narcotics, or sedative-hypnotics), but noncardiogenic pulmonary edema (associated with narcotics) may be responsible. Pressure-dependent ecchymoses, bullae, and necrotic areas, especially in users of long-acting sedative-hypnotics, can be mistaken for thermal burns. These necrotic areas can signal underlying muscle injury (rhabdomyolysis) and possibly compartment syndrome. Fresh and old track marks are typically present in narcotic and stimulant abusers.

Altered vital signs are a particularly helpful clue. Hypotension and depressed ventilation are most often associated with brain stem depression secondary to abuse of ethanol, narcotics, or sedative-hypnotics. Rapid respirations and tachyarrhythmias can be either direct effects of stimulants and hallucinogens or manifestations of the excitatory state induced by ethanol and sedative-hypnotic withdrawal. Deep, rapid breathing (Kussmaul's respiration) is a respiratory compensation for the acidemia caused by alcoholic ketoacidosis and toluene abuse. Hypothermia is a frequent finding in ethanol and sedative-hypnotic overdose. Temperature elevation can result either from the hypermetabolic state induced by acute stimulant use or from withdrawal from ethanol or sedative-hypnotics.

Mydriasis is characteristic of sympathomimetic effects (such as those that result from cocaine or amphetamine overdose or withdrawal from depressants); miosis is a very common sign of narcotic overdose. Horizontal and, less commonly, vertical nystagmus are prevalent in severe ethanol intoxication but are also frequently associated with barbiturate and other sedative-hypnotic intoxication. Psychotic behavior and hallucinatory behavior are usual after acute and chronic exposure to hallucinogens or stimulants and in the course of abstinence from ethanol. Lethargy and confusion are common in ethanol, narcotic, and sedative-hypnotic intoxication; they are also typical transient postictal symptoms, suggesting a seizure provoked by stimulant use or sedative withdrawal.

LABORATORY STUDIES

Basic diagnostic testing of poisoned patients relies on routine determinations of end-organ toxicity. Measurement of serum electrolyte, blood urea nitrogen, creatinine, and glucose levels and a 12-lead electrocardiogram are helpful in the detection of metabolic acidosis, electrolyte abnormalities, and cardiotoxic effects (e.g., sodium channel blockade).[9] Additional laboratory studies are tailored to the patient's clinical presentation and differential diagnosis. Detection of urine heme in the absence of microscopic hematuria suggests rhabdomyolysis and calls for evaluation of skeletal muscle enzymes and renal function. Rhabdomyolysis may result in acute renal failure and electrolyte abnormalities, including hyperkalemia, hypocalcemia, and hyperphosphatemia. Clinical findings will determine the need for arterial blood gas analysis or chest radiography.

Certain caveats apply to toxicologic diagnostics. First, data from qualitative toxicologic screening rarely alter decisions about the clinical management of poisoned patients.[10] Second, toxicologic analyses vary tremendously in availability, sensitivity, and specificity. Third, detection of drugs in the urine merely confirms drug exposure: it does not confirm that the clinical findings at that moment are related to drug exposure.[11] Finally, because most emergency drug screens can detect only eight to 10 common drugs, a negative screen does not rule out poisoning as the cause of a patient's illness.

Quantitative levels of specific agents (e.g., ethanol, isopropyl, ethylene glycol, methanol, or acetaminophen) are sometimes clinically useful. A comprehensive drug screen may identify substance abuse that necessitates chemical-dependency intervention, exposure to stimulants in patients who present with new-onset seizures or ischemic chest pain, or the presence of unsuspected drugs in patients with unexplained critical illness.

Prevention of Drug Absorption and Enhancement of Drug Elimination

PREVENTING ABSORPTION

The goal of gut decontamination is to prevent further absorption of toxin. The primary variables influencing gut decontamination are the interval between ingestion and intervention, the presence of coingestants, and gastric emptying time. Administration of activated charcoal is safe and adequate treatment in the majority of overdose cases.

Several large studies have failed to show that gastric emptying (provoked by syrup of ipecac or gastric lavage) plus activated charcoal has any clinical advantages over activated charcoal alone.[12] Ipecac has no role in emergency department management.

Gastric lavage is useful only in patients seen soon after ingestion of life-threatening substances. If gastric lavage is deemed necessary, it should be viewed as a specific technique with expected complications. Protection of the airway takes precedence over performance of gastric lavage. Any patient with lost or depressed airway reflexes or a decreasing level of consciousness should receive endotracheal intubation before the procedure. The patient is placed in Trendelenburg's position with the left side down. A large-bore (No. 32 to 40) orogastric tube is inserted, and small aliquots of 200 to 500 ml of tap water or saline are administered until the recovered lavage solution is clear or a maximum of 2 L has been given. Complications of lavage include posterior pharyngeal and esophageal injury, pneumothorax, and pulmonary aspiration.

Activated charcoal has a large surface area that absorbs many toxins. Charcoal should be given orally as quickly as possible after clinically indicated airway management and orogastric lavage. The usual dose is 25 to 50 g, although larger amounts may be indicated in special circumstances. Multiple doses of activated charcoal can enhance elimination of drugs with enteroenteric and intrahepatic circulation.[13]

Whole bowel irrigation may be indicated for toxins that are

poorly absorbed by charcoal and for cases of body stuffing and body packing. In body stuffing, substance abusers use the stomach, the rectum, the vagina, or an ear to hide illegal substances from authorities attempting to apprehend them. Body packing, a technique employed by drug smugglers, involves swallowing of large quantities of latex-wrapped drug. A ruptured packet or condom could rapidly be fatal. The preferred treatment includes multiple doses of activated charcoal and bowel cleansing with polyethylene glycol solution (e.g., 20 ml/min of GoLYTELY up to a total of 4 L or until diarrhea is clear of particulate matter).

Induced emesis, gastric lavage, and the removal of packets by endoscopy or laparotomy have been utilized.[14] Any procedure to remove packets should consider the risk of their rupture and prepare for possible rapid systemic absorption of drug. The main objective of any procedure is to protect the patient from harm, not to collect evidence for the police. Careful observation is required until all packets pass, although it may be difficult to determine when this occurs.[15]

Cathartics such as sorbitol and magnesium citrate have no proven efficacy, are not risk free, and should be reserved for special indications.

ENHANCEMENT OF ELIMINATION

Altering urine pH can enhance renal elimination of certain drugs. For example, alkaline diuresis promotes more rapid clearance of phenobarbital, yet it has not been shown to alter clinical outcome. Acid diuresis is no longer recommended for phencyclidine or amphetamine overdose, because the yield of pH manipulation is low and rhabdomyolysis is frequent. In such circumstances, acid diuresis can exacerbate renal tubular damage.

Hemodialysis and hemoperfusion enhance the elimination of a limited number of substances but are of unproven clinical benefit for most drugs of abuse.

Perioperative Considerations

Toxic exposure and withdrawal syndromes can complicate the management of patients undergoing operation. The concerns specific to each toxic syndrome must be considered. In addition, there are several general issues that are germane: anesthesia, universal human immunodeficiency virus (HIV) precautions, and pain control.

The effectiveness and hazards of anesthesia in substance abuse patients depend on the responsible substance, the anesthetic, and the physiologic status of the patient. Before anesthesia is administered, hypoxemia and profound acidemia must be resolved. A full stomach should be anticipated. Chronic abuse (e.g., of narcotics) may impair the effectiveness of an anesthetic agent and result in high tolerance. Chronic barbiturate and ethanol use may speed metabolism of certain liver-dependent anesthetics. Conversely, liver metabolism may be adversely affected by cirrhosis caused by chronic ethanol abuse. Renal excretion of anesthetics is compromised by renal failure resulting from sustained hypotension or rhabdomyolysis. Synergistic actions of toxins and anesthetics are predictable, and care should be taken to prevent unwitting anesthetic overdose. Chronic alcoholics receiving disulfiram are at increased risk for unexpectedly deep anesthesia when thiopental is used.[16] Patients who have taken an overdose of a sympa-

thomimetic (e.g., an amphetamine or cocaine) are more likely to sustain arrhythmias when volatile anesthetics are used; enflurane exerts this effect more strongly than isoflurane, and halothane more strongly still.

Health care personnel must be steadfast in their use of universal precautions to help prevent transmission of HIV and various forms of viral hepatitis known to be exceptionally prevalent in the substance abuse population [see VI:19 Viral Infection].

Patients who are chronically dependent on narcotics may require unusually high dosages of analgesics in the postoperative period. The physician's qualitative assessment of a patient's pain can be quite inaccurate. Knowledge of a patient's recent history of narcotic use (including both type and amount) will help the physician provide adequate pain relief [see VIII:2 Postoperative Pain].

Narcotics

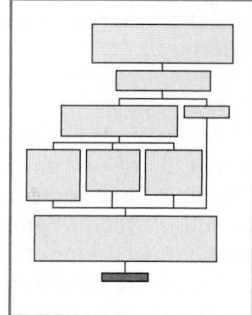

Narcotics (also known as opioids) are a class of drugs that are principally used in medical practice for the purposes of analgesia. Besides the natural opiates (e.g., opium, morphine, and codeine), there are numerous synthetic derivatives (e.g., heroin, meperidine, fentanyl, methadone, and pentazocine).

ACUTE EXPOSURE

The narcotics are readily absorbed by intravenous, intradermal, inhalational, nasal, or oral routes. Manifestations of narcosis can be observed within 10 minutes of intravenous administration, 30 minutes of intramuscular administration, and 90 minutes of oral or subcutaneous administration. With certain compounds (e.g., diphenoxylate and loperamide), the onset of toxicity is delayed. Duration of action varies with the substance, the route of administration, and the adequacy of hepatic degradation but is usually less than eight hours. Typical clinical findings in an overdose include respiratory depression, a decreased level of consciousness, and miosis. Bradycardia, hypotension, and hypothermia may occur. Meperidine and propoxyphene can cause seizures. Cardiac dysrhythmias may occur with propoxyphene.

Noncardiogenic pulmonary edema is a complication of profound narcosis and is particularly associated with I.V. heroin use.[17] It is usually seen early but may occur as late as 12 hours after exposure. Pathogenesis is attributed to hypoxemia and increased capillary permeability. Other complications of overdosage include aspiration pneumonitis, anoxic encephalopathy, rhabdomyolysis, and compartment syndrome.

Narcotic poisoning is a clinical diagnosis. Acute narcotic overdose does not alter routine laboratory test results. Qualitative toxicologic screens confirm exposure; quantitative testing is not clinically useful. Arterial blood gas analysis, chest x-rays, measurement of creatine kinase levels, and urine screening for myoglobin are indicated in severe cases.

Management

Supportive care is the mainstay of therapy, with particular attention to active airway management. Because vomiting is common, an endotracheal tube should usually be inserted and well secured before naloxone is administered. Naloxone is a pure competitive antagonist at the opioid receptors.[18] The onset of action of naloxone occurs one to three minutes after administration, with maximum effect in five to 10 minutes [see Urgent Syndromes, above]. With some opioids, higher doses (up to 10 mg) are required for a reversal response. Gut decontamination may be helpful if the ingestion is recent, but no form of elimination enhancement is indicated. Noncardiogenic pulmonary edema is treated by optimizing oxygen delivery. Positive end-expiratory pressure may be necessary.

Prescription analgesic medications are often opioids in combination with other drugs, such as acetaminophen or salicylates. In an overdose, the toxic effects of the coingestant must be taken into account. Abusers may use combinations, such as heroin and cocaine (a so-called speedball). Reversal of the opioid effect may allow the coingestant to have predominant toxic effects.

CHRONIC USE

A variety of infectious complications ensue from contaminated drugs or unsterile intravenous injection practices.[19] These include bacterial endocarditis, extremity abscesses and cellulitis, wound botulism, diskitis, and septic emboli. Acute and chronic forms of hepatitis, especially hepatitis B, and HIV infection are extremely prevalent in this population.[20]

The clinical presentation (e.g., fever or signs of endocarditis) dictates the cultures and serologic analyses that should be requested. Empirical laboratory studies are not indicated.

Management

Management of infectious and other complications is directed by clinical need and the laboratory results.

WITHDRAWAL

The time course of abstinence withdrawal depends on the particular narcotic abused.[21] With short-acting drugs (e.g., meperidine and hydromorphone), the syndrome begins within three to six hours and lasts four to five days. With less potent drugs (e.g., codeine and propoxyphene) or longer-acting drugs (e.g., methadone), it begins within 24 hours and lasts two to four days. Manifestations include yawning, lacrimation, rhinorrhea, restlessness, gooseflesh, aching, cramps, nausea, vomiting, and diarrhea. Fever and hypertension may be present. These symptoms and signs progress to a peak and then subside over a period of hours to days.

Naloxone administration can provoke intense withdrawal that begins within five minutes, peaks in 30 minutes, and lasts one to two hours, regardless of the opioid involved. Longer-acting opioid antagonists (e.g., nalmefene and naltrexone) can precipitate withdrawal that will persist for many hours.

Attention to electrolyte levels may be necessary if gastrointestinal losses are marked.

Management

The opiate abstinence syndrome may be ameliorated with clonidine, a central alpha$_2$ agonist. A 0.2 mg oral dose is given initially, followed by 0.1 to 0.2 mg every eight hours.[22] Methadone, a long-acting opioid, is an alternative treatment for detoxification. The administration of other drugs for re-

ducing anxiety (e.g., benzodiazepines), abdominal cramps (e.g., anticholinergics), or nausea (e.g., prochlorperazine) may be considered.

Stimulants

The stimulants commonly abused include cocaine, amphetamines, and amphetamine-like drugs. Stimulants cause catecholamine excess, both within the CNS and peripherally. Clinically, all stimulant intoxications are similar. CNS excitation causes agitation and seizures; cardiovascular provocation causes tachycardia and hypertension. Hyperthermia can be severe.

COCAINE

Users snort cocaine as a powder; smoke it as an alkaloid (crack) or, less frequently, as a coca paste; and administer it intravenously. Recently, much attention has focused on the combination of cocaine and ethanol. A metabolite of this combination (cocaethylene) can be more toxic to the heart than cocaine alone.

Acute Exposure

Cocaine is a sympathomimetic agent and a CNS stimulant. Mild intoxication produces minimal alteration of vital signs. Changes in mental status include euphoria, excitement, and irritability. Mydriasis may be seen. Hypertension, hyperthermia, tachycardia, and agitation predominate in overdose. A single generalized seizure or status epilepticus can occur. Cerebral hemorrhage and ischemic strokes have been reported.[23] In extreme cases, coma, hypotension, severe metabolic acidosis, hyperkalemia, hyperthermia, and wide QRS complex dysrhythmias can lead to rapid death. Chest pain after cocaine use is a particular clinical dilemma. The pronounced Valsalva maneuver associated with smoking cocaine can result in pneumothorax or pneumomediastinum.[24] CNS stimulation produces severe anxiety, which may contribute to atypical chest pain. Myocardial infarction has been reported in patients with and without preexisting coronary artery disease. The myocardium becomes ischemic because cocaine constricts coronary arteries, forms thrombi, and accelerates atherosclerosis.[25,26] Acute aortic dissection can also occur. Ischemic infarction of the skin, bowel, kidneys, and muscle have all resulted from intense vasoconstriction attributable to cocaine.

Cocaine can be detected in the blood for a very short time after exposure, but a metabolite (benzoylecgonine) can be detected in urine for 48 to 72 hours. Adrenergic excess from cocaine causes leukocytosis, hypokalemia, metabolic acidosis, and hyperglycemia. Serum creatine kinase levels should be monitored because cocaine-induced muscle injury can result in acute renal failure from myoglobinuria.

Management Beyond good supportive care, therapy to inhibit excess adrenergic stimulation may be necessary. Benzodiazepines are most effective in inhibiting CNS stimulation and can attenuate cardiovascular stimulation both centrally and peripherally. Beta blockers, which have been associated with worsening clinical outcome, should be avoided. Wide QRS complex arrhythmias should be treated with intravenous sodium bicarbonate. Severe hypertension is managed with benzodiazepines and, if necessary, nitroprusside, phentolamine, or nifedipine. A patient who is seizing should receive benzodiazepines and, if necessary, phenobarbital. If hyperthermia is present, benzodiazepines and aggressive external cooling are indicated. For myocardial ischemia and myocardial infarction, generous benzodiazepine therapy is necessary in addition to the usual measures. Thrombolytics have been used successfully in patients with acute myocardial infarction caused by cocaine.[26]

Decontamination should be considered only in cases of recent exposure to large doses, such as those that result from packet breakage inside the body. Emesis, lavage, and attempts at endoscopic removal can result in the sudden release of large amounts of cocaine, with severe consequences, including death.

Chronic Use

Chronic insufflation of cocaine can lead to rhinitis and nasal erosions and perforations. A variety of psychiatric disorders may be present, including euphoria, dysphoria, and psychosis. Complications of parenteral drug abuse should be anticipated.

Withdrawal

During withdrawal, chronic cocaine users may experience depression, tiredness, nausea, and vomiting with abstinence. A severe withdrawal syndrome is highly unusual.

AMPHETAMINES

Acute Exposure

Amphetamine, its isomers (dextroamphetamine and methamphetamine), and numerous analogues are all available for misuse (for weight loss, prolonged wakefulness, and enhanced athletic performance) and abuse. Patients may be exposed by the oral, inhalational, subcutaneous, or intravenous route. The duration of clinical effect, regardless of the route of exposure, is typically long, ranging from six hours to several days.

Acute amphetamine overdose manifests itself via stimulation of the cardiovascular and central nervous systems. Mild toxic effects include restlessness, insomnia, irritability, nausea and vomiting, flushing, diaphoresis, mydriasis, and combativeness. Moderate toxic effects include chest pain, vomiting and abdominal pain with hypertension, tachycardia, tachypnea, mild temperature elevation, profuse diaphoresis, and hallucinations. Indicators of severe overdose include more marked alterations in vital signs, such as hyperpyrexia and severe hypotension or hypertension, cardiac arrhythmias, seizures, focal neurologic signs, and coma.

Acute complications are cardiovascular (myocardial infarction and dysrhythmias), cerebrovascular (intracranial hemorrhage and vasospasm), hyperthermic (hypermetabolic state and status epilepticus), renal (myoglobinuric renal failure), neurologic (amphetamine psychosis, with paranoia and hallucinations), and peripheral vascular (infectious and vasospastic complications of injection).

Qualitative analysis can confirm amphetamine exposure; quantitative analysis is not clinically useful. Leukocytosis with no other apparent cause is frequent after amphetamine use. Hypokalemia, hyperglycemia, and a mild metabolic acidosis may be seen. It may be necessary to evaluate cardiac and skeletal muscle enzyme activity as well as the effect of rhabdomyolysis on electrolyte concentrations, renal function, and coagulation. CT of the head, which is indicated for severe headache, meningismus, or localizing CNS findings, may reveal intracerebral, subdural, or subarachnoid hemorrhage. Cerebral angiography may demonstrate characteristic beading of small-caliber arteries.[27]

Management Management should focus on life-threatening cardiovascular and cerebrovascular complications of acute amphetamine overdose. Benzodiazepines are the treatment of choice to decrease CNS stimulation and centrally mediated cardiovascular stimulation. Acute severe hypertension that is unresponsive to benzodiazepines can be treated with nitroprusside, phentolamine, or calcium channel blockers. Seizures should be managed with parenteral benzodiazepines and phenobarbital. Patients in status epilepticus who do not respond to these measures may have to be intubated and paralyzed to prevent hyperthermia, profound acidemia, and rhabdomyolysis. Agitation and combativeness can be treated with either benzodiazepines or haloperidol. Haloperidol and appropriate physical restraints are indicated for patients with amphetamine psychosis. Activated charcoal therapy is indicated for acute ingestions. Alteration of pH to enhance elimination is contraindicated, and hemodialysis and hemoperfusion are not useful.

Chronic Use

Chronic amphetamine abusers may present with complaints of insomnia, weight loss, depression, hypertension, or toxic psychosis. Patients who use these drugs by parenteral means are subject to infectious and extremity complications similar to those found in narcotic abusers.

Toxicologic analysis can reveal the source of the patient's concerns. Other laboratory studies are generally unhelpful.

Management Clinical need is sufficient to guide management of chronic abusers; therapy is directed at the clinical signs and symptoms.

Withdrawal

Abstinence after chronic use of amphetamines is characterized by depression, anxiety, sleep disturbance, abdominal pain, myalgia, and voracious appetite. These manifestations typically last three to six days and are not life threatening. Seizures should not be anticipated.

Hallucinogens

The hallucinogens include the psychedelics (lysergic acid diethylamide [LSD], mescaline, and psilocybin), phencyclidine (PCP), and marijuana. Of these, the first two are the most germane to surgical practice.

LSD

Acute Exposure

LSD is the prototypical psychedelic. It occurs naturally as an ergot alkaloid, but far more of it is manufactured than is found in nature. LSD has no medical uses in the United States. It is ingested as capsules, tablets, or a solution on blotting paper, sugar cubes, or gelatin; it is rarely taken intravenously or by insufflation. Unlike opioids, amphetamines, and cocaine, which are associated with repetitive, sustained patterns of abuse, LSD is used only intermittently. It is well absorbed from the gastrointestinal tract; the clinical effect begins to be noticeable 30 to 90 minutes after ingestion, peaks in three to five hours, and lasts eight to 12 hours.

Typical physiologic alterations include mild increases in pulse, temperature, respiratory rate, and pupil size. Nausea, vomiting, weakness, ataxia, and modest increases in salivation and lacrimation may occur. CNS manifestations predominate among the clinical effects.[28] Behavior is unpredictable and ranges from passive and reserved to hostile and threatening. Although LSD experiences are intended to be pleasurable, they often are not. Acute panic reactions are the most commonly seen complications. Acute toxic psychosis with distorted perceptions and hallucinations is also common. Orientation is usually preserved, but judgment is grossly impaired. Impaired judgment, coupled with depressive reactions, may prompt unintentional self-destructive behavior, such as attempting to fly.

Flashbacks involving visual, time, and body image distortion can follow LSD use. These may be precipitated by physiologic or emotional stresses. Flashbacks occurring more than six months after use of the drug are seen predominantly in patients with obsessive and schizoid personalities.

Rare but severe complications of LSD use include seizures and coma. Vasospasm and angiitis may cause focal neurologic deficits. Massive overdoses and violent hyperactivity may result in pronounced temperature elevations, rhabdomyolysis, and metabolic acidosis.[29]

LSD can be detected in urine to verify exposure. Urine should be routinely screened for myoglobin in patients with a history of seizures or prolonged hyperactivity.

Management Seizure, coma, and rhabdomyolysis are rare with LSD use. If these life-threatening manifestations occur, the usual measures are indicated. Gut decontamination is usually futile. Panic attacks respond best to reduction of sensory stimuli and constant reassurance. Physical restraints or administration of benzodiazepines or haloperidol may be required for panic and psychotic reactions. Use of phenothiazines as neuroleptics may be unsafe and should be avoided.

Withdrawal

No abstinence syndrome for LSD has been reported.

PCP

Acute Exposure

PCP was discovered in 1957 and was briefly used for anesthesia in humans and animals. Currently, it is classified as a dissociative anesthetic, but it has no medical uses. PCP is well absorbed by all routes. Most users either sprinkle PCP powder onto a marijuana or tobacco cigarette or dip the cigarette into a liquid form of the drug. Some snort or ingest PCP, but the development of clinical toxicity is more difficult to predict when these methods are adopted.

Symptoms and signs of PCP intoxication include increased heart rate and blood pressure, nystagmus (horizontal, vertical, or rotatory), miosis, markedly diminished ability to feel pain and temperature, ataxia, increased muscle tone, and slurred speech.[30] The patient's behavior can be lethargic, bizarre, agitated, euphoric, or violent. These changes usually last six hours after exposure but occasionally last as long as 24 hours. Toxic psychosis is heralded by delusions, hallucinations, depersonalization, and disorganized thoughts and can last four hours to seven days (average, one to two days). The combination of psychosis and lack of pain sensation can lead to violent and combative acts of extraordinary proportions.

Medical complications include acute hypertension, hyperpyrexia, seizures, and rhabdomyolysis with renal failure.[31] Severe trauma is common. Drowning and other types of accidental death, violent suicide, and homicide are well known to occur in this population.

Toxicology screens can detect the presence of PCP in urine. Quantitative blood analysis is poorly correlated with toxic patterns.

Management Respiratory depression, seizures, and coma are treated in the standard fashion. Gut decontamination is usually ineffective; in addition, it is generally difficult to perform, given the patient's pattern of behavior. Urinary acidification is dangerous in patients with PCP intoxication. Although urinary acidification enhances urinary excretion of PCP, its effect on clinical outcome is unclear, and it may exacerbate renal injury resulting from rhabdomyolysis.[31]

Supportive care and pharmacological therapy may be required for patients with hypertension, hyperthermia, and rhabdomyolysis. Typically, the greatest problem encountered by medical staff is control of the violent patient. Outbreaks are unpredictable, and the patient's strength can be superhuman. A coordinated effort must be made by all available personnel to ensure the safety of the patient and the staff. Liberal use of benzodiazepines, butyrophenones (haloperidol or droperidol), or both may be necessary.

Chronic Use

Chronic use of PCP is associated with memory deficits, emotional lability, social isolation, and, in rare instances, organic brain syndrome.

Withdrawal

No severe physical reactions occur in withdrawal, but depression, anxiety, and fatigue may be seen for weeks to months after the initiation of abstinence.

Alcohols

Alcohol exists in many forms and remains an immensely popular and exceedingly prevalent drug throughout the world. The pathology it creates or contributes to is exceptionally varied and frequently serious, and no organ system is unaffected. Moreover, alcohol is the leading cause of morbidity and mortality as well as the principal risk factor for unintentional and intentional injuries in the United States.[6]

ACUTE EXPOSURE

Clinical Findings

Ethanol is rapidly absorbed in the stomach and the proximal small bowel. Blood concentration peaks 30 to 120 minutes after ingestion. Alcohol is primarily metabolized in the liver by alcohol dehydrogenase; chronic alcoholics have auxiliary degradative enzyme systems. The hourly rate of metabolism ranges from 15 to 20 mg/dl in the nonalcoholic to 40 mg/dl in chronic alcoholics.

At low concentrations, ethanol impairs higher cortical function, and at high concentrations, it can inhibit brain stem function. The primary manifestations of ethanol intoxication reflect its cerebellar effects; thus, dysarthria, nystagmus, and gait disturbance are prominent. Prediction of serum ethanol levels according to clinical presentation demands careful scrutiny of the patient's history, his or her experience with drinking, and the examination findings. Whereas inexperienced drinkers may be grossly ataxic and stuporous at blood ethanol levels of 100 mg/dl, chronic alcoholics are often alert and conversant at levels in excess of 500 mg/dl.

Acute ethanol intoxication may cause delayed or erroneous diagnosis in patients with concomitant disorders.[7] It is imperative to perform a careful initial examination and serial evaluations in acutely intoxicated patients. The differential diagnosis of altered mentation in cases of suspected ethanol intoxication is broad. Closed head injury is exceedingly common in intoxicated patients. Metabolic conditions, including alcohol-induced hypoglycemia, hepatic encephalopathy, the presence of other alcohols or drugs, the presence of disulfiram alone or in combination with ethanol, and hypothermia are frequently seen as well. Infections are more common in chronic alcoholics, and particular attention should be given to the possibility of CNS infections and aspiration or bacterial pneumonia. Most alcohol-related causes of abnormal mentation are neurologic; these include the postictal state that follows an alcohol withdrawal seizure, alcohol withdrawal itself, and Wernicke-Korsakoff syndrome.

Alcohol-induced hypoglycemia is a common disorder ascribed to impaired gluconeogenesis and inadequate glycogen stores. Chronic alcoholics, binge drinkers, and children (because of their marginal glycogen stores) are at the greatest risk.[32] Hypoglycemia may occur during intoxication or as much as six to 20 hours after the last drink. Its onset is insidious, and the clinical picture is dominated by neuroglycopenia rather than catecholamine response. Lethargy and obtundation proceed to seizures and coma. Focal neurologic signs are frequently seen in adults, and seizures are common in children.[33]

Nonethanol alcohols (e.g., methanol, ethylene glycol, and isopropyl alcohol) are consumed either accidentally or deliberately and are both common and readily available.[34] Methanol is found in windshield-washer cleaner, gas-line antifreeze, and shellacs. Symptoms appear 40 minutes to 72 hours after ingestion. Nausea, vomiting, abdominal pain, and tenderness may be accompanied by gastrointestinal bleeding. Ophthalmologic abnormalities include blurred vision and "spots" or "snow" before the eyes, optic disk hyperemia, and retinal edema; permanent blindness may result. Methanol may also cause lethargy, confusion, and, in severe cases, seizures and coma. High anion gap metabolic acidosis occurs as a result of the toxic metabolic product formic acid. Ethylene glycol is most often used in radiator antifreeze and windshield deicer. Its clinical course proceeds through three stages: stage 1—metabolic acidosis and CNS depression, including seizures and coma, are seen in the first 30 minutes to 12 hours after ingestion; stage 2—in severe cases, cardiopulmonary findings, including pulmonary edema, cardiomegaly, and cardiovascular collapse,

occur 12 to 36 hours after ingestion; and stage 3—acute renal failure becomes apparent 48 to 72 hours after exposure. Isopropyl alcohol (also termed rubbing alcohol) is found in numerous home products. The manifestations of isopropyl alcohol intoxication are very similar to those of acute ethanol intoxication; however, at the same dosage, isopropyl alcohol produces more profound clinical intoxication than ethanol. Isopropyl alcohol is metabolized partly to acetone, resulting in ketosis without acidosis.[35]

Disulfiram, a drug that is widely prescribed for the treatment of chronic alcoholism, can itself cause psychosis, delirium, and seizures in rare cases. Ingestion of alcohol by a patient on long-term disulfiram therapy can cause the disulfiram-ethanol reaction (DER), which can be severe and sometimes fatal.[36] Chronic disulfiram users who ingest alcohol will experience clinical symptoms that appear within five to 15 minutes, peak within 20 to 30 minutes, and usually dissipate within two to four hours. Because disulfiram has a long elimination half-life, the DER can occur in patients who stopped taking disulfiram as long as two weeks before ingesting alcohol. Patients who have taken their first dose of disulfiram and then ingest alcohol may not show symptoms for eight to 12 hours. Characteristic features of the DER include facial and truncal skin flushing, headache, nausea, and vomiting; more serious reactions include severe dyspnea, chest pain, and shock.

Laboratory Studies

Quantitative assessment of ethanol can be accomplished by analysis of blood or alveolar air. Most laboratories test for ethanol only, although some routinely screen for ethanol, methanol, and isopropyl alcohol. Ethylene glycol is analyzed by different methods and should be requested separately when indicated. The Breathalyzer provides reasonably accurate measurements of ethanol in the blood, but it has two drawbacks: first, inadequate ventilation can render levels falsely low, and second, the device measures all alcohols but cannot distinguish one from another. Saliva test strips show good correlation with serum measurements but only at low concentrations of ethanol.[37]

Mandatory serum glucose analysis in the intoxicated patient is unnecessarily expensive. Alcohol-induced hypoglycemia can be easily and rapidly detected by bedside determinations.

Obtaining quantitative measurements of nonethanol alcohols facilitates management. When serum levels are not available, they can be estimated on the basis of the osmolar gap (measured osmolality minus calculated osmolality). Ancillary tests in poisonings by nonethanol alcohols include serum electrolyte concentrations, arterial blood gas values, assessment of renal function, and urinalysis.

Management

Patients with suspected ethanol intoxication in whom other causes for altered mentation have been excluded by clinical or laboratory means should be observed and examined repeatedly. Airway patency and ventilation should be assured. Extremely obtunded patients should be placed in the left lateral decubitus position to prevent aspiration. In the presence of craniofacial trauma, cervical spine immobilization and appropriate x-rays are indicated. Intravenous access is helpful and allows administration of 50 mg of thiamine as prophylaxis against Wernicke-Korsakoff syndrome. The welfare of the patient should be safeguarded with physical restraints and haloperidol when necessary. Intoxicated patients should remain under close observation until clinical sobriety has been attained. Gut decontamination is rarely effective.[38] Hemodialysis has rarely been used and is not clinically useful.

Patients with alcohol-induced hypoglycemia should immediately be given one or two ampules of D50W, followed by 1 to 2 L of D5W or D10W over a period of six to 10 hours. Their return to a normal diet should be assured before they are discharged.

Treatment for nonethanol alcohol poisoning is determined by the substance ingested, the time of ingestion, and the clinical and laboratory findings. Isopropyl alcohol intoxication can be handled in much the same way as ethanol intoxication. Methanol and ethylene glycol are relatively nontoxic in themselves; it is their by-products that are dangerous. Prevention of metabolism to harmful by-products is accomplished by means of intravenous ethanol administration and, when required, hemodialysis.[39]

Patients with severe DER must be monitored. Hypotension is managed by infusing crystalloid. Pressors are rarely required.

CHRONIC USE

Clinical Findings

The effects of chronic ethanol abuse are myriad. Physical findings include spider telangiectasis, jaundice, caput medusae, palmar erythema, ascites, and generalized wasting. Acute, subacute, and chronic myopathies of cardiac and skeletal muscle occur. Atrial dysrhythmias are common during intoxication and withdrawal. Numerous diseases of the gastrointestinal and biliary systems follow prolonged use. The incidence of gastrointestinal hemorrhage caused by gastritis, peptic ulcer, Mallory-Weiss tears, and esophageal varices is increased in patients with cirrhosis. Abdominal pain and tenderness can be caused by alcoholic hepatitis and acute or chronic pancreatitis.

The hematologic manifestations of alcoholism are caused by the direct actions of alcohol, nutritional deficiency, and liver involvement. Each of the three major hematopoietic cell lines is affected.[40] Megaloblastic anemia is extremely common. Hypersplenism, sideroblastic changes, and iron deficiency contribute to the development of anemia. Leukopenia occurs in three to eight percent of alcoholics, most often affecting the granulocytic line. Thrombocytopenia is found in as many as 40 percent of alcoholics and is caused by decreased production, folate deficiency, and hypersplenism. Levels below 20,000/mm^3 are rarely seen. Because the liver is the site of production of all coagulation factors except factor VIII, alcohol-related liver disease leads to synthetic incompetence of these factors and resultant abnormalities in prothrombin time, partial thromboplastin time, and thrombin time.[41]

The neurologic consequences of chronic alcoholism are the most frequently seen and the most devastating.[42] Peripheral neuropathy is frequent. Cerebellar dysfunction is common and can be profound. Cortical atrophy and loss of higher function are well documented. Wernicke-Korsakoff syndrome is caused by thiamine deficiency and, in the United States, is seen almost exclusively in chronic alcoholics with poor diet. In this syndrome, ophthalmoplegia, gait disturbance, and mental sta-

tus changes tend to develop over a period of several days to weeks.[43] Generally, all three are found, although the mental changes may lag behind the others by days to weeks. Ocular changes include horizontal and vertical nystagmus and ophthalmoplegia. Bilateral abducens nerve palsy is virtually pathognomonic of the disease. Gait and stance ataxia are nonspecific findings and generally are not accompanied by tremor, appendicular ataxia, or a cerebellar speech pattern. Abnormal mentation usually presents as mild delirium, disorientation, and apathy. Full Korsakoff's syndrome, characterized by anterograde and retrograde amnesia with the former dominating, often follows. Unusual presentations of Wernicke-Korsakoff syndrome include coma, hypothermia, and hypotension.

Laboratory Studies

Hematologic, chemical, and radiographic examinations are based on the clinical presentation. Diagnosis of Wernicke-Korsakoff syndrome is entirely clinical. Specialized assays to detect chronic alcoholism exist, but they are never available without delay and are no substitute for clinical judgment.

Management

Abstinence stabilizes and improves most chronic-use conditions. If Wernicke-Korsakoff syndrome is suspected, 100 mg of thiamine should be given intravenously at the outset and each day until the patient returns to a normal diet.[44] Magnesium, a necessary cofactor for thiamine, is frequently depleted in chronic alcoholics and must be replenished if thiamine therapy is to be effective.

WITHDRAWAL

Clinical Findings

The manifestations of abstinence from ethanol typically depend on the habitual dose and chronicity of use, but there is wide interindividual variation. Patients with a history of withdrawal are likely to experience similar manifestations with subsequent periods of abstinence. Generally, four to five weeks of daily and significant ethanol ingestion is required to produce significant withdrawal, although as little as five days may be sufficient. Alcohol withdrawal can be divided into five syndromes: (1) minor withdrawal, (2) alcoholic hallucinosis, (3) alcohol withdrawal seizures, (4) delirium tremens, and (5) alcoholic ketoacidosis, a frequent metabolic complication of the withdrawal period. These syndromes frequently merge and share features. They do not necessarily progress in any particular order.

Minor withdrawal   The minor withdrawal syndrome begins six to eight hours after the cessation of alcohol use, peaks in 24 to 36 hours, and may persist as long as 10 to 14 days. Patients with the minor withdrawal syndrome are hyperalert and anorectic, with nausea and vomiting, and may show mild tachycardia, hypertension, hyperreflexia, and tremor on examination.

Alcoholic hallucinosis   Alcoholic hallucinations occur six to 96 hours after the beginning of abstinence and usually peak at 12 to 48 hours. Hallucinations are typically visual (as opposed to the auditory hallucinations associated with schizophrenia), and the images tend to be frightening to the patient. The duration of illness is generally two to three days.

Alcohol withdrawal seizures The majority of alcohol withdrawal seizures occur between six and 48 hours after discontinuance of ethanol, with the peak incidence coming between 13 and 24 hours; virtually all seizures occur within 96 hours.[45] Withdrawal seizures occur singly in about 50 percent of patients and in groups of two to six in the remainder. Status epilepticus is rare. When multiple seizures do occur, they tend to cluster within a 12-hour period in 95 percent of patients. Alcohol withdrawal seizure tends to be grand mal and self-limited; however, the high prevalence of prior closed head injury in chronic alcoholics explains why focal seizures are seen in as many as 40 percent of cases. Other features of withdrawal, including autonomic hyperactivity, hallucinosis, and tremor, may or may not be seen.

Delirium tremens Delirium tremens usually appears 72 to 96 hours after cessation of drinking and lasts one to three days. It is the most dramatic and serious form of alcohol withdrawal and is characterized by profound confusion, disorientation, delusions, vivid hallucinations, tremor, agitation, insomnia, and psychomotor, speech, and autonomic hyperactivity.[46] The most distinguishing features are hypersympathetic symptoms with tachycardia, hypertension, fever, mydriasis, and profuse diaphoresis. Cardiovascular collapse may occur. Associated illnesses (particularly pneumonia, pancreatitis, and hepatitis) are common and often contribute to the cause of death.

Alcoholic ketoacidosis Alcoholic ketoacidosis is typically seen after a long drinking binge followed by several days of abstinence, anorexia, nausea, and vomiting.[47] Examination may reveal signs of hypovolemia, tachycardia, and Kussmaul's respiration if acidemia is severe. Abdominal pain is a typical symptom, and tenderness is common. In extreme cases, rebound and guarding can be severe enough to mimic the signs of an acute abdomen. Sensorium is usually normal.

Laboratory Studies

Patients with alcoholic ketoacidosis exhibit a high anion gap metabolic acidosis caused by the production of ketoacids.[48] Because metabolic alkalosis secondary to vomiting and respiratory alkalosis secondary to alcohol withdrawal often coexist, the pH in these patients is extremely variable. Serum glucose levels should be normal or low (the opposite of the situation with diabetic ketoacidosis). Hypokalemia and hypophosphatemia are frequent. Ketoacids are detectable in the serum or urine; however, it must be remembered that routine ketoacid measurements are not sensitive to β-hydroxybutyric acid, the predominant ketoacid species in this disorder.

For the other alcohol withdrawal syndromes, laboratory studies are of negligible diagnostic value. Fluid and electrolyte deficits may be severe in patients with delirium tremens or alcoholic ketoacidosis.

Management

The goals of treatment are to prevent progression of withdrawal, to alleviate symptoms, and to recognize and treat underlying disorders.[49] A variety of drugs may be administered, of which the benzodiazepines are the most widely used.[50] In mild cases of withdrawal, oral delivery may suffice. In severe cases, intravenous administration permits immediate loading and titration of the sedative. Intramuscular administration is contraindicated because of poor and variable absorption and the risk of hematoma or abscess formation in compromised alcoholics. None of the benzodiazepines has demonstrated clear superiority in the treatment of alcohol withdrawal; however, oxazepam and lorazepam are less dependent on hepatic function and may be preferred when severe hepatic dysfunction exists. The dosages required are widely variable and should be governed by the clinical presentation and the response to therapy. Continued observation for persistent or worsening manifestations is required in all patients.[51] Deterioration despite benzodiazepine therapy may necessitate careful management in an ICU.

Antipsychotics may be required for management of hallucinosis or combativeness. Beta blockers, barbiturates, paraldehyde, and chloral hydrate have no advantages over the benzodiazepines for treatment of withdrawal.

Patients who respond to pharmacological intervention and who do not require admission for alcohol withdrawal or other illnesses are best referred to a detoxification facility, where their withdrawal can be carefully observed until it is complete and symptoms have abated entirely.

Minor withdrawal Supportive therapy, including two days of oral administration of benzodiazepines or beta blockers, is sufficient.

Alcoholic hallucinosis Alcoholic hallucinosis is distinguished from delirium tremens by the absence of autonomic hyperactivity. Haloperidol is appropriate.

Alcohol withdrawal seizures The first time a patient presents with alcohol withdrawal seizure, a diagnostic workup, including serum chemistries, computed tomography of the head, and electroencephalography, should be performed.[52] As many as 10 percent of patients with alcohol withdrawal seizures have focal CNS pathology that necessitates additional diagnostic or therapeutic efforts. Repeat presentations for suspected alcohol withdrawal seizure call for careful examination and exclusion of traumatic, infectious, and metabolic causes, but further workup is not necessary. Because withdrawal seizures are usually self-limited, there is no need for acute pharmacotherapy (e.g., with diazepam). Long-term outpatient antiepileptic therapy should not be initiated unless a structural focus has been identified.[53] Prophylaxis against withdrawal seizures (e.g., clorazepate, 15 mg, or lorazepam, 1 to 2 mg, twice daily for three days) during abstinence is probably warranted, particularly in patients who have a history of withdrawal seizures.[54]

Delirium tremens Patients with delirium tremens require continuous intensive care monitoring, crystalloid therapy for volume deficits, cooling measures for hypothermia, physical restraints, and parenteral benzodiazepines. Benzodiazepines should be administered intravenously to produce a state of calm; tremendous dosages, titrated over five- to 15-minute intervals, may be necessary. These patients have vivid and threatening hallucinations, and their behavior is unpredictable. Thus, physical restraints must be maintained until calm is ensured. Serious coexisting medical conditions are common.

Alcoholic ketoacidosis I.V. fluids with dextrose should be given at a minimum rate of 125 ml/hr. Potassium and phosphate are often required. Sodium bicarbonate administration is rarely necessary, and insulin is not indicated. The condition generally resolves within eight to 12 hours.

Consultation and Referral

Early consultation with a toxicologist or regional poison center is appropriate. Patients with acute or chronic conditions related to substance abuse should ultimately be referred to counselors, psychiatrists, and centers expert in the medical and psychosocial complications of alcoholism. Family members and friends are often unwitting codependents and can benefit from similar referrals.

References

1. Powner D: Drug-associated isoelectric EEGs: a hazard in brain death certification. JAMA 236:1123, 1976

2. Hoffman RS, Goldfrank LR: The poisoned patient with altered consciousness: controversies in the use of a 'coma cocktail.' JAMA 274:562, 1995

3. Spivey WH, Roberts JR, Derlet RW: A clinical trial of escalating doses of flumazenil for reversal of suspected benzodiazepine overdose in the emergency department. Ann Emerg Med 22:1813, 1993

4. Frommer DA, Marx J: Wernicke's encephalopathy (letter). N Engl J Med 313:638, 1985

5. Silverstein SC, Frommer DA, Marx JA, et al: The safety and efficacy of parenteral haloperidol for the combative patient: a prospective study (abstr). Ann Emerg Med 15:636, 1986

6. Seventh Special Report to Congress on Alcohol and Health. National Institute on Alcohol Abuse and Alcoholism. US Department of Health and Human Services. Rockville, Maryland, 1990

7. Marx JA: Alcohol and trauma. Emerg Med Clin North Am 8:929, 1990

8. Alcohol as a risk factor for injuries—United States. MMWR 32:61, 1983

9. Kulig K: Initial management of ingestions of toxic substances. N Engl J Med 326:1677, 1992

10. Wiltbank TB, Sine HE, Brody BB: Are emergency toxicology measurements really used? Clin Chem 20:116, 1974

11. Brett AS: Implications of discordance between clinical impression and toxicology analysis in drug overdose. Arch Intern Med 148:437, 1988

12. Kulig K, Bar-Or D, Cantrill SV, et al: Management of acutely poisoned patients without gastric emptying. Ann Emerg Med 14:562, 1985

13. Pond SM, Olson KR, Osterloh JD, et al: Randomized study of the treatment of phenobarbital overdose with repeated doses of activated charcoal. JAMA 251:3104, 1984

14. Utecht MJ, Stone AF, McCarron MM: Heroin body packers. J Emerg Med 11:33, 1983

15. Marc B, Baud FJ, Maison P, et al: Cardiac monitoring during medical management of cocaine body packers. Clin Tox 30:387, 1992

16. Eneanya DI, Bianchine JR, Duran DO, et al: The actions of metabolic rate of disulfiram. Annu Rev Pharmacol Toxicol 21:575, 1981

17. Duberstein JL, Kaufman DM: A clinical study of an epidemic of heroin intoxication and heroin-induced pulmonary edema. Am J Med 51:704, 1971

18. Ford M, Hoffman R, Goldfrank L: Opioids and designer drugs. Emerg Med Clin North Am 8:495, 1990

19. Cherubin CE, Sapira JD: The medical complications of drug addiction and the medical assessment of the intravenous drug user: 25 years later. Ann Intern Med 119:1017, 1993

20. Friedland GH, Harris C, Butkus-Small C, et al: Intravenous drug abusers and the acquired immunodeficiency syndrome (AIDS). Arch Intern Med 145:1413, 1985

21. Freitas PM: Narcotic withdrawal in the emergency department. Am J Emerg Med 3:456, 1985

22. Holman PW: Clonidine and naloxone in ultrashort opiate detoxification. Clin Pharm 4:100, 1985

23. Brody SL, Slovis CM, Wrenn KD: Cocaine-related medical problems: consecutive series of 233 patients. Am J Med 88:325, 1990

24. Shesser R, Davis C, Edelstein S: Pneumomediastinum and pneumothorax after inhaling alkaloidal cocaine. Ann Emerg Med 10:213, 1981

25. Hollander JE, Hoffman RS, Gennis P, et al: Prospective multicenter evaluation of cocaine-associated chest pain. Acad Emerg Med 1:330, 1994

26. Hollander JE: The management of cocaine-associated myocardial ischemia. N Engl J Med 333:1267, 1995

27. Rumbaugh CL, Bergeron RT, Fang HC, et al: Cerebral angiographic changes in the drug abuse patient. Radiology 101:335, 1971

28. Kulig K: Emergency aspects of drug abuse. Emerg Med Clin North Am 8:551, 1990

29. Klock JC, Boerner U, Becker CE: Coma, hyperthermia and bleeding associated with massive LSD overdose: a report of eight cases. West J Med 120:183, 1974

30. Baldridge EB, Bessen HA: Phencyclidine. Emerg Med Clin North Am 8:541, 1990

31. McCarron MM, Schulze BW, Thompson GA, et al: Acute phencyclidine intoxication: clinical patterns, complications, and treatment. Ann Emerg Med 10:290, 1981

32. Sporer KA, Ernst AA, Conte R, et al: The incidence of ethanol-induced hypoglycemia. Am J Emerg Med 10:403, 1992

33. Madison LL: Ethanol-induced hypoglycemia. Advances in Metabolic Disorders 3:85, 1968

34. Kulig K, Duffy JP, Lenden CH, et al: Toxic effects of methanol, ethylene glycol and isopropyl alcohol. Topics in Emergency Medicine 6:14, 1984

35. Marx JA, Duffens K: Response to E. Otten's letter (ketoacidosis and isopropyl alcohol). J Emerg Med 6:342, 1988

36. Brewer C: Recent developments in disulfiram treatment. Alcohol 28:383, 1993

37. Bates ME, Brick J, White HR: The correspondence between saliva and breath estimates of blood alcohol concentration: advantages and limitations of the saliva method. J Stud Alcohol 54:17, 1993

38. Pollack CV Jr, Jorden RC, Carlton FB, et al: Gastric emptying in the acutely inebriated patient. J Emerg Med 10:1, 1992

39. Christiansson LK, Kaspersson KE, Kulling PE: Treatment of severe ethylene glycol intoxication with continuous arteriovenous hemofiltration dialysis. J Toxicol Clin Toxicol 33:267, 1995

40. Eichner ER, Hillman RS: The evolution of anemia in alcoholic patients. Am J Med 50:218, 1971

41. Cowan DH: Effect of alcoholism on hemostasis. Semin Hematol 17:137, 1980

42. Diamond I, Messing RO: Neurologic effects of alcoholism. West J Med 161:279, 1994

43. Victor M, Adams RD, Collins GH: The Wernicke-Korsakoff Syndrome. FA Davis Co, Philadelphia, 1971

44. Frommer D, Kulig K, Marx J, et al: Tricyclic antidepressant overdose patients managed in an emergency department observation unit. Presented to the III World Congress of the World Federation of Associations of Clinical Toxicology and Poison Control Centres and the XII International Congress of the European Association of Poison Control Centres, Brussels, Belgium, August 1986

45. Victor M, Brausch C: The role of abstinence in the genesis of alcoholic epilepsy. Epilepsia 8:1, 1967

46. Schuckit MA, Tipp JE, Reich T, et al: The histories of withdrawal convulsions and delirium tremens in 1648 alcohol dependent subjects. Addiction 90:1335, 1995

47. Duffens K, Marx JA: Alcohol ketoacidosis—a review. J Emerg Med 5:399, 1987

48. Wrenn KD, Slovis CM, Minion GE, et al: The syndrome of alcoholic ketoacidosis. Am J Med 91:119, 1991

49. Saitz R, Mayo-Smith MF, Roberts MS, et al: Individualized treatment for alcohol withdrawal: a randomized double-blind controlled trial. JAMA 272:519, 1994

50. Hoey LL, Nahum A, Vance-Bryan K: A retrospective review and assessment of benzodiazepines in the treatment of alcohol withdrawal in hospitalized patients. Ann Med 26:101, 1994

51. Lohr RH: Treatment of alcohol withdrawal in hospitalized patients. Mayo Clin Proc 70:777, 1995

52. Earnest MP, Feldman H, Marx JA, et al: Intracranial lesions shown by CT scans in 259 cases of first alcohol-related seizures. Neurology 38:1561, 1988

53. Chance JF: Emergency department treatment of alcohol withdrawal seizures with phenytoin. Ann Emerg Med 20:520, 1991

54. Marx JA, Berner J, Bar-Or D, et al: Prophylaxis of alcohol withdrawal seizures: a prospective study (abstr). Ann Emerg Med 15:637, 1986

II COMMON PRESENTING PROBLEMS

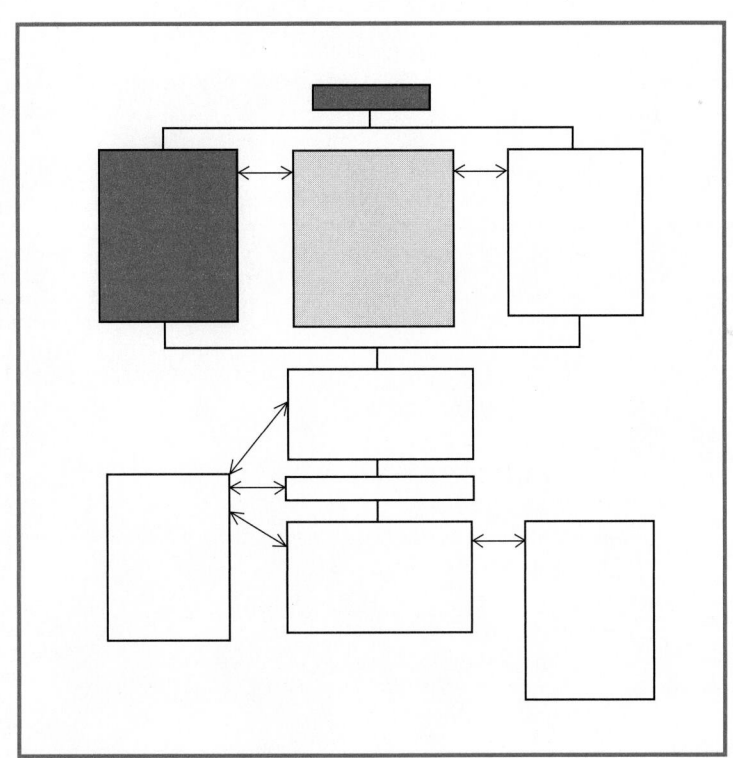

1 NECK MASS

Barry J. Roseman, M.D., and Orlo H. Clark, M.D.

Assessment of a Neck Mass

History

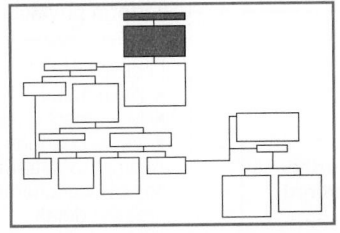

The evaluation of any neck mass begins with a careful history. The history should be taken with the differential diagnosis in mind [*see Table 1*] because directed questions can narrow down the diagnostic possibilities and focus subsequent investigations. For example, in younger patients, one would tend to look for congenital lesions, whereas in older adults, the first concern would always be neoplasia.

The duration and growth rate of the mass should be determined: malignant lesions are far more likely to exhibit rapid growth than benign ones, which may grow and shrink. Next, the location of the mass in the neck should be determined. This is particularly important for differentiating congenital masses from neoplastic or inflammatory ones because each type usually occurs consistently in particular locations. In addition, the location of a neoplasm is both diagnostically and prognostically significant. The possibility that the mass reflects an infectious or inflammatory process should also be assessed. One should check for evidence of infection or inflammation (e.g., fever, pain, or tenderness); a recent history of tuberculosis, sarcoidosis, or fungal infection; the presence of dental problems; and a history of trauma to the head and neck. Masses that appear inflamed or infected are far more likely to be benign.

Finally, factors suggestive of cancer should be sought: a previous malignancy elsewhere in the head and neck (e.g., a skin lesion or a head and neck tumor); night sweats (suggestive of lymphoma); excessive exposure to the sun (a risk factor for skin cancer); smoking or excessive alcohol consumption (risk factors for squamous cell carcinoma of the head and neck); nasal obstruction or bleeding, otalgia, odynophagia, dysphagia, or hoarseness (suggestive of a malignancy in the upper aerodigestive tract); or exposure to low-dose therapeutic radiation (a risk factor for thyroid cancer).

Physical Examination

Examination of the head and neck is challenging in that much of the area to be examined is not easily visualized. Patience and practice are necessary to master the special instruments and techniques of examination. A head and neck examination is usually performed with the patient sitting in front of the physician. Constant repositioning of the head is

Table 1 Etiology of Neck Mass

Inflammatory and infectious disorders	Acute lymphadenitis (bacterial or viral infection)
	Subcutaneous abscess (carbuncle)
	Infectious mononucleosis
	Cat-scratch fever
	AIDS
	Tuberculous lymphadenitis (scrofula)
	Fungal lymphadenitis (actinomycosis)
	Sarcoidosis
Congenital cystic lesions	Thyroglossal duct cyst
	Branchial cleft cyst
	Cystic hygroma (lymphangioma)
	Vascular malformation (hemangioma)
	Laryngocele
Benign neoplasms	Salivary gland tumor
	Thyroid nodules or goiter
	Soft tissue tumor (lipoma, sebaceous cyst)
	Chemodectoma (carotid body tumor)
	Neurogenic tumor (neurofibroma, neurilemoma)
	Laryngeal tumor (chondroma)
Malignant neoplasms	*Primary*
	Salivary gland tumor
	Thyroid cancer
	Upper aerodigestive tract cancer
	Soft tissue sarcoma
	Skin cancer (melanoma, squamous cell carcinoma, and basal cell carcinoma)
	Lymphoma
	Metastatic
	Upper aerodigestive tract cancer
	Skin cancer (melanoma, squamous cell carcinoma)
	Salivary gland tumor
	Thyroid cancer
	Adenocarcinoma (breast, GI tract, GU tract, lung)
	Unknown primary

Assessment of a Neck Mass

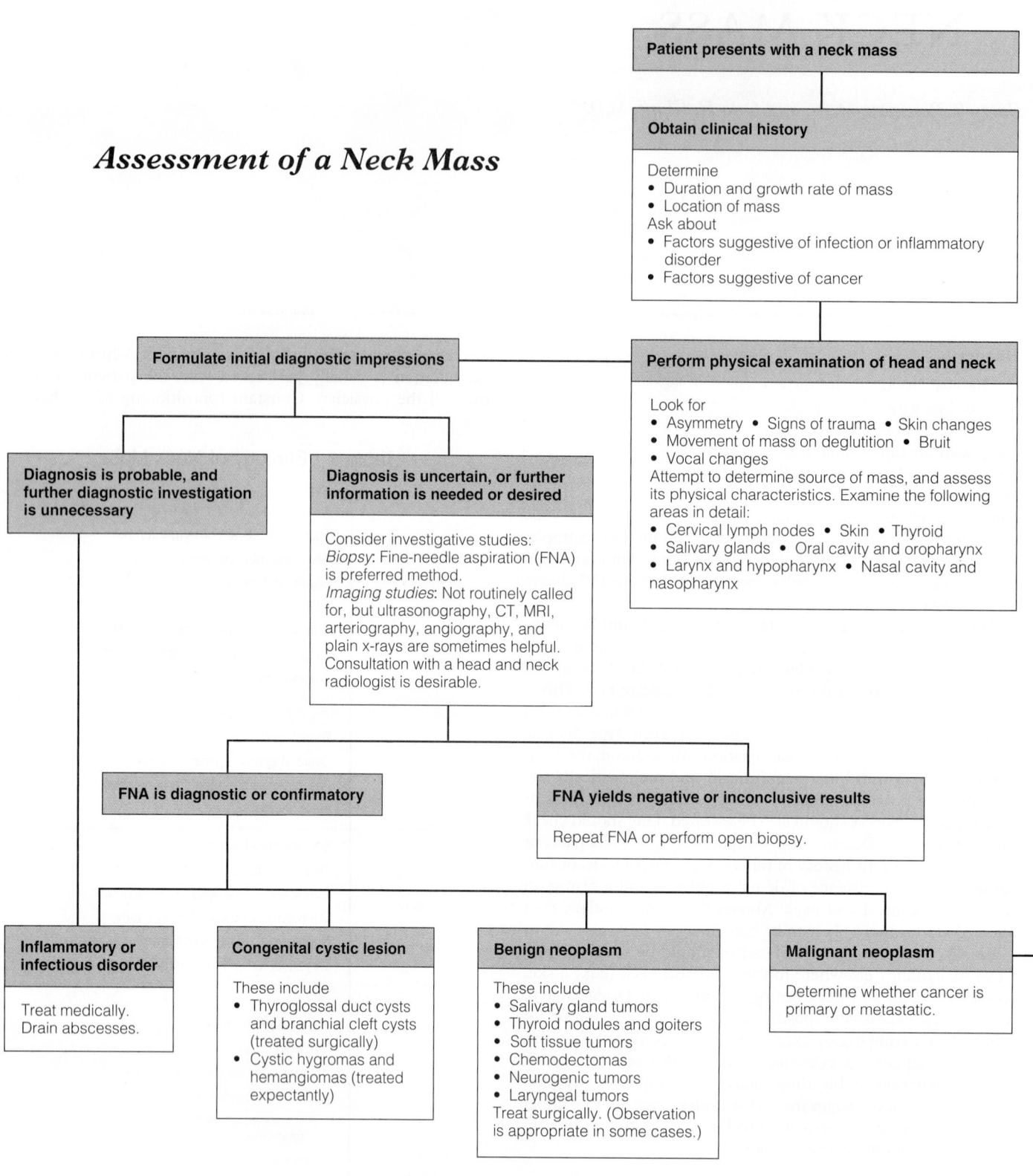

Patient presents with a neck mass

Obtain clinical history

Determine
- Duration and growth rate of mass
- Location of mass

Ask about
- Factors suggestive of infection or inflammatory disorder
- Factors suggestive of cancer

Perform physical examination of head and neck

Look for
- Asymmetry • Signs of trauma • Skin changes
- Movement of mass on deglutition • Bruit
- Vocal changes

Attempt to determine source of mass, and assess its physical characteristics. Examine the following areas in detail:
- Cervical lymph nodes • Skin • Thyroid
- Salivary glands • Oral cavity and oropharynx
- Larynx and hypopharynx • Nasal cavity and nasopharynx

Formulate initial diagnostic impressions

Diagnosis is probable, and further diagnostic investigation is unnecessary

Diagnosis is uncertain, or further information is needed or desired

Consider investigative studies:
Biopsy: Fine-needle aspiration (FNA) is preferred method.
Imaging studies: Not routinely called for, but ultrasonography, CT, MRI, arteriography, angiography, and plain x-rays are sometimes helpful. Consultation with a head and neck radiologist is desirable.

FNA is diagnostic or confirmatory

FNA yields negative or inconclusive results

Repeat FNA or perform open biopsy.

Inflammatory or infectious disorder

Treat medically.
Drain abscesses.

Congenital cystic lesion

These include
- Thyroglossal duct cysts and branchial cleft cysts (treated surgically)
- Cystic hygromas and hemangiomas (treated expectantly)

Benign neoplasm

These include
- Salivary gland tumors
- Thyroid nodules and goiters
- Soft tissue tumors
- Chemodectomas
- Neurogenic tumors
- Laryngeal tumors

Treat surgically. (Observation is appropriate in some cases.)

Malignant neoplasm

Determine whether cancer is primary or metastatic.

Primary neoplasm

These include
- Lymphoma • Thyroid cancer • Upper aerodigestive tract cancer • Soft tissue sarcoma
- Skin cancer

Treat with surgery, radiation therapy, and/or chemotherapy, as appropriate.

Metastatic tumor

Primary is known

Metastatic squamous cell carcinoma: Perform selective neck dissection, and consider adjuvant radiation therapy.
Metastatic adenocarcinoma: Perform neck dissection (selective or other), and consider adjuvant radiation therapy.
Metastatic melanoma: Perform full-thickness excision and SLN biopsy; if there are positive SLNs or lymph nodes are palpable, perform modified neck dissection.

Primary is unknown

Evaluate nasopharynx, larynx, esophagus, hypopharynx, and tracheobronchial tree endoscopically.
Biopsy nasopharynx, tonsils, and hypopharynx.
Perform unilateral neck dissection followed by irradiation of neck, entire pharynx, and nasopharynx.

necessary to obtain adequate visualization of the various areas. Gloves must be worn during the examination, particularly if the mucous membranes are to be examined. Good illumination is essential. The time-honored but cumbersome head mirror has been largely supplanted by the headlight (usually a high-intensity halogen lamp). Fiberoptic endoscopy with a flexible laryngoscope and a nasopharyngoscope has become a common component of the physical examination for evaluating the larynx, the nasopharynx, and the paranasal sinuses, especially when these areas cannot be adequately visualized with more standard techniques.

The examination should begin with inspection for asymmetry, signs of trauma, and skin changes. One should ask the patient to swallow to see if the mass moves with deglutition. Palpation should be done both from the front and from behind. Auscultation is performed to detect audible bruits. One should also ask about the patient's voice, changes in which may suggest either a laryngeal tumor or recurrent nerve dysfunction from locally invasive thyroid cancer.

During the physical examination, one should be thinking about the following questions: What structure is the neck mass arising from? Is it a lymph node? Is the mass arising from a normally occurring structure, such as the thyroid gland, a nerve, a blood vessel, or a muscle? Or is it arising from an abnormal structure, such as a laryngocele, a branchial cleft cyst, or a cystic hygroma? Is the mass soft, fluctuant, easily mobile, well-encapsulated, and smooth? Or is it firm, poorly mobile, and fixed to surrounding structures? Does it pulsate? Is there a bruit? Does it appear to be superficial, or is it deeper in the neck? Is it attached to the skin? Is it tender?

The following areas of the head and neck are examined in some detail.

CERVICAL LYMPH NODES

Enlarged lymph nodes are by far the most common neck masses encountered. The cervical lymphatic system consists of interconnected groups or chains of nodes that parallel the major neurovascular structures in the head and neck. The skin and mucosal surfaces of the head and neck all have specific and predictable nodes associated with them. The classification of cervical lymph nodes has been standardized to comprise six levels [see Table 2 and Figure 1]. Accurate determination of lymph node level on physical examination and in surgical specimens not only helps establish a common language among clinicians but also permits comparison of data among different institutions.

The location, size, and consistency of lymph nodes furnish valuable clues to the nature of the primary disease. Other physical characteristics of the adenopathy should be noted as well, including the number of lymph nodes affected, their mobility, their degree of fixation, and their relation to surrounding anatomic structures. One can often establish a tentative diagnosis on the basis of these findings alone. For example, soft or tender nodes are more likely to derive from an inflammatory or infectious condition, whereas hard, fixed, painless nodes are more likely to represent metastatic cancer. Multiple regions of enlarged lymph nodes are usually a sign of systemic disease (e.g., lymphoma, tuberculosis, or infectious mononucleosis), whereas solitary nodes are more often due to malignancy. Firm, rubbery nodes are typical of lymphoma. Low cervical nodes are more likely to contain metastases from a primary source other than the head and neck, whereas upper cervical nodes are more likely to contain metastases from the head and neck.

The submental and submandibular nodes (level I) are palpated bimanually. Metastases to level I are commonly from the lips, the oral cavity, or the facial skin. The three levels of internal jugular chain nodes (levels II, III, and IV) are best examined by gently rolling the sternocleidomastoid muscle between the thumb and the index finger. Level II and level III lymph nodes are common sites for lymph node metastases from primary cancers of the oropharynx, the larynx, and the hypopharynx. Metastases in level IV lymph nodes can arise from cancers of the upper aerodigestive tract, from cancers of the thyroid gland, or from cancers arising below the clavicle (Virchow's node). The nodes in the posterior triangle (level V) are all palpated. Nodal metastases in this region can arise from nasopharyngeal and thyroid cancers as well as from squamous cell carcinoma or melanoma of the posterior scalp and the pinna of the ear. The tracheoesophageal groove nodes (level VI) are then palpated.

SKIN

Careful examination of the scalp, the ears, the face, and the neck will identify potentially malignant skin lesions, which may give rise to lymph node metastases.

THYROID GLAND

The thyroid gland is first observed as the patient swallows; it is then palpated and its size and consistency assessed with an eye to determining whether it is smooth, diffusely enlarged, or nodular and whether one nodule or several are present. If it is unclear whether the mass is truly thyroid, one can clarify the point by asking the patient to swallow and watching to see whether the mass moves. Signs of superior mediastinal syndrome (e.g., cervical venous engorgement and facial edema) suggest retrosternal extension of a thyroid goiter. The larynx and trachea are examined, with special attention to the cricothyroid membrane, over which Delphian nodes can be palpated. These nodes can be a harbinger of thyroid or laryngeal cancer.

MAJOR SALIVARY GLANDS

Examination of the paired parotid and submandibular glands involves not only palpation of the neck but also an intraoral examination to inspect the duct openings. The submandibular glands are best assessed by bimanual palpation, with one finger in the mouth and one in the neck. They are normally lower and more prominent in older patients. The parotid glands are often palpable in the neck, though the deep lobe cannot always be assessed. A mass in the region of the tail of the parotid must be

Table 2 Classification of Cervical Lymph Nodes

Level	Nodes
I	Submental nodes Submandibular nodes
II	Upper internal jugular chain nodes
III	Middle internal jugular chain nodes
IV	Lower internal jugular chain nodes
V	Spinal accessory nodes Transverse cervical nodes
VI	Tracheoesophageal groove nodes

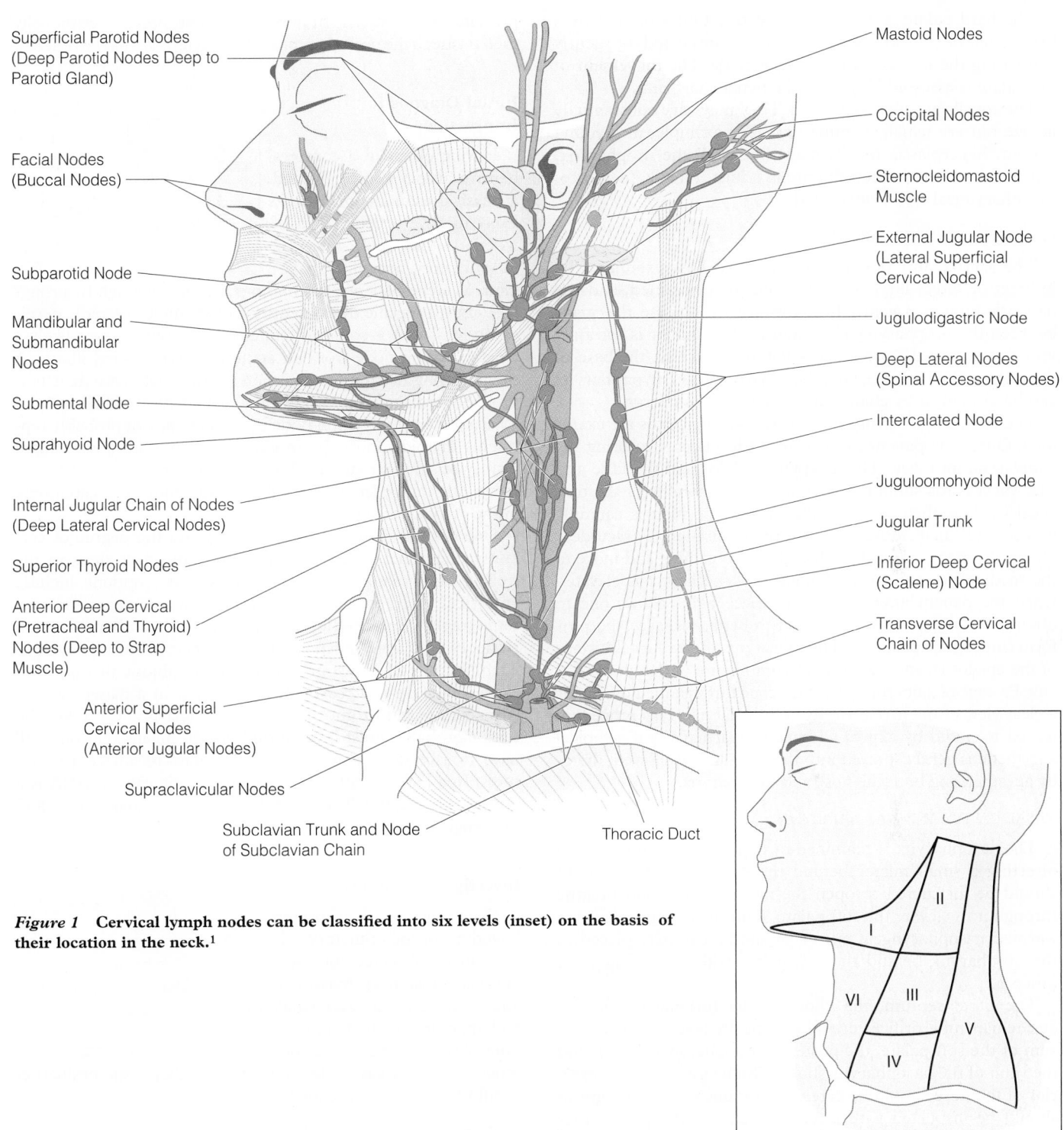

Figure 1 Cervical lymph nodes can be classified into six levels (inset) on the basis of their location in the neck.[1]

distinguished from enlarged level II jugular nodes. The oropharynx is inspected for distortion of the lateral walls. The parotid (Stensen's) duct may be found opening into the buccal mucosa, opposite the second upper molar.

ORAL CAVITY AND OROPHARYNX

The lips should be inspected and palpated. Dentures should be removed before the mouth is examined. The buccal mucosa, the teeth, and the gingiva are then inspected. The patient should be asked to elevate the tongue so that the floor of the mouth can be examined and bimanual inspection performed. The tongue should be inspected both in its normal position in the mouth and during protrusion.

Most of the oropharyngeal contents are easily visualized if the tongue is depressed. Only the anterior two thirds of the tongue is clearly visible on examination, however. The base of the tongue is best visualized by using a mirror. In most persons, the tongue base can be palpated, at the cost of some discomfort to the patient. The ventral surface of the tongue must also be carefully inspected and palpated.

The hard palate is examined by gently tilting the patient's head backward, and the soft palate is inspected by gently depressing the tongue with a tongue blade. The movement of the palate is assessed by having the patient say "ahh."

The tonsils are then examined. They may vary substantially in size but are usually symmetrical. For example, in a young patient, hyperplastic tonsils may almost fill the oropharynx, but this is an uncommon finding in adults. Finally, the posterior pharyngeal wall is inspected.

LARYNX AND HYPOPHARYNX

The larynx and the hypopharynx are best examined by indirect or direct laryngoscopy. A mirror is warmed, and the patient's tongue is gently held forward to increase the space between the oropharyngeal structures. The mirror is carefully introduced into the oropharynx without touching the base of the tongue. The oropharynx, the larynx, and the hypopharynx can be visualized by changing the angle of the mirror.

The lingual and laryngeal surfaces of the epiglottis are examined. Often, the patient must be asked to phonate to bring the endolarynx into view. The aryepiglottic folds and the false and true vocal cords should be identified. The mobility of the true vocal cords is then assessed: their resting position is carefully noted, and their movement during inspiration is recorded. Normally, the vocal cords abduct during breathing and move to the median position during phonation. The larynx is elevated when the patient attempts to say "eeeee"; this allows one to observe vocal cord movement and to better visualize the piriform sinuses, the postcricoid hypopharynx, the laryngeal surface of the epiglottis, and the anterior commissure of the glottic larynx. Passage of a fiberoptic laryngoscope through the nose yields a clear view of the hypopharynx and the larynx. This procedure is well tolerated by almost all patients, particularly if a topical anesthetic is gently sprayed into the nose and swallowed, thereby anesthetizing both the nose and the pharynx.

NASAL CAVITY AND NASOPHARYNX

The nasopharynx is examined by depressing the tongue and inserting a small mirror behind the soft palate. The patient should be instructed to open the mouth widely and breathe through it to elevate the soft palate. With the patient relaxed, a warmed nasopharyngeal mirror should be carefully placed in the oropharynx behind the soft palate without touching the mucosa.

The nasal septum, the choanae, the turbinates, and the eustachian tube orifices are systematically assessed. The dorsum of the soft palate, the posterior nasopharyngeal wall, and the vault of the nasopharynx should also be assessed. The exterior of the nose should be carefully examined, and the septum should be inspected with a nasal speculum. Polyps or other neoplasms can be mistaken for turbinates.

Careful evaluation of the cranial nerves is essential, as is examination of the eyes (including assessment of ocular movement and visual activity), the external ear, and the tympanic membrane.

ADDITIONAL AREAS

The remainder of the physical examination is also important, particularly as regards the identification of a possible source of metastases to the neck. Other sets of lymph nodes—especially axillary and inguinal nodes—are examined for enlargement or tenderness. Women should undergo complete pelvic and rectal examinations. Men should undergo rectal, testicular, and prostate examinations; tumors from these organs occasionally metastasize to the neck. Appropriate blood tests should be ordered.

Initial Diagnostic Impressions

Having obtained a comprehensive history and performed a physical examination, one is likely to have a better idea of whether the neck mass is inflammatory, benign, or malignant. In some patients, the findings are clear enough to strongly suggest a specific disease entity. For example, a rapidly developing mass that is soft and tender to palpation is most likely a reactive lymph node from an acute bacterial or viral illness. A slow-growing facial mass associated with facial nerve deficits is probably a malignant parotid tumor. A thyroid nodule with an adjacent abnormal lymph node in a young patient probably represents thyroid cancer. In an elderly patient with a substantial history of smoking and alcohol use, a neck mass may well be a metastatic tumor (most likely from a squamous cell carcinoma in the aerodigestive tract).

One's initial diagnostic impressions and the degree of certainty one attaches to them determine the next steps in the workup and management of a neck mass; options include empirical therapy, ultrasonographic scanning, computed tomography, fine-needle aspiration (FNA), and observation alone. For example, in a patient with suspected bacterial lymphadenitis from an oral source, empirical antibiotic therapy with close follow-up is a reasonable approach. In a patient with a suspected parotid tumor, the best first test is a CT scan: the tumor probably must be removed, which means that one will have to ascertain the relation of the mass to adjacent structures. In a patient with suspected metastatic cancer, FNA is a sensible choice: it will confirm the presence of malignancy and may suggest a source of the primary cancer.

Investigative Studies

Neck masses of suspected infectious or inflammatory origin can be observed for short periods. Most neck masses in adults, however, are abnormal, and they are often manifestations of serious underlying conditions. In most cases, therefore, further diagnostic evaluation should be rigorously pursued.

BIOPSY

Whether or not the history and the physical examination strongly suggest a specific diagnosis, the information obtained by sampling tissue from the neck mass is often highly useful. In many cases, biopsy establishes the diagnosis; at the least, it may reduce the diagnostic possibilities. At present, the preferred method of obtaining material from a neck mass is FNA. FNA is the most important initial invasive diagnostic procedure in this setting. It is generally well tolerated and can usually be performed without local anesthesia. Although FNA is, on the whole, both safe and accurate, it is not completely free of potential problems (e.g., bleeding): it should therefore be done only if the results are likely to influence treatment.

FNA reliably distinguishes cystic from solid lesions and can often diagnose malignancy. It has in fact become the standard for making treatment decisions in patients with thyroid nodules and for confirming the clinical suspicion of a cystic lesion. FNA is also useful in patients with a known distant malignancy in whom confirmation of metastases is needed for staging and for planning therapy, as well as in patients with a primary tumor of the head and neck who are not candidates for operation but in whom a tissue diagnosis is necessary for appropriate nonsurgical therapy to be initiated. In addition, FNA is helpful in dealing with overly anxious patients in whom the clinical index of suspicion for a neoplasm is low and the head and neck examination is negative: negative biopsy results tend to reassure these patients and allow the surgeon time to follow the mass more confidently. (Of course, negative FNA results should not be considered the end point of any search and do not rule out cancer.)

Several studies have shown FNA to be approximately 90% accurate in establishing a definitive diagnosis. Lateral cystic neck masses that collapse on aspiration usually represent hygromas, branchial cleft cysts, or cystic degeneration of a metastatic papillary thyroid cancer. Fluid from these masses is sent for cytologic examination. If a palpable mass remains after cyst aspiration, a biopsy of the solid component should be done; the morphology of the cells will be better preserved.

If an extensive physical examination has been completed and the FNA is not diagnostic, one may have to perform an open biopsy to obtain a specimen for histologic sections and microbiologic studies. It is estimated that open biopsy eventually proves necessary in about 10% of patients with a malignant mass. In an open biopsy, it is important to orient skin incisions within the boundaries of a neck dissection; the incisions can then, if necessary, be extended for definitive therapy or reexcised if reoperation subsequently proves necessary. Crossing incisions should never be situated over vessels.

A suspected lymphoma constitutes a special situation. FNA alone is often incapable of determining the precise histologic subtype. Lymphoproliferative disease usually calls for open biopsy, frozen-section confirmation, and submission of fresh tissue to the pathologist. The intact node is placed in normal saline and sent directly to the pathologist for analysis of cellular content and nodal architecture and identification of lymphocyte markers. If infection is suspected, portions of the excised tissue are also sent for bacterial, fungal, mycobacterial, and viral cultures.

IMAGING STUDIES

Diagnostic imaging should be used selectively in the evaluation of a neck mass; imaging studies should be performed only if the results are likely to affect subsequent therapy. Such studies often supply useful information about the location and characteristics of the mass and its relation to adjacent structures. Diagnostic imaging is particularly useful when a biopsy has been performed and a malignant tumor identified. In such cases, these studies can help establish the extent of local disease and the presence or absence of metastases.

Ultrasonography reliably differentiates solid masses from cystic ones and is especially useful in assessing congenital and developmental cysts. It is a valuable noninvasive technique for vascular lesions and clearly delineates thyroid and parathyroid abnormalities. CT is also useful for differentiating cysts from solid lesions and for determining whether a mass is within or outside a gland or nodal chain. In addition, CT scanning can delineate small tongue-base or tonsillar tumors that have a min-imal mucosal component. MRI provides much the same information as CT. T_2-weighted gadolinium-enhanced scans are particularly useful for delineating the invasion of soft tissue by tumor: endocrine tumors are often enhanced on such scans. Arteriography is useful mainly for evaluating vascular lesions and tumors fixed to the carotid artery. Angiography is helpful for evaluating the vascularity of a mass, its specific blood supply, or the status of the carotid artery, but it provides very little information about the physical characteristics of the mass. Plain radiographs of the neck are rarely helpful in differentiating neck masses, but a chest x-ray can often confirm a diagnosis (e.g., in patients with lymphoma, sarcoidosis, or metastatic lung cancer). A chest x-ray is required in any patient with a new diagnosis of cancer to determine if pulmonary metastases are present. It is also an important component of preoperative evaluation for any patient older than 40 years who requires an operation.

It is important to communicate with the radiologist: an experienced head and neck radiologist may be able to offer valuable guidance in choosing the best diagnostic test in a specific clinical scenario. Furthermore, providing the radiologist with a detailed clinical history facilitates interpretation of the images.

Management of Specific Disorders

INFLAMMATORY AND INFECTIOUS DISORDERS

Acute infection of the neck (cervical adenitis) is most often the result of dental infection, tonsillitis, pharyngitis, viral upper respiratory tract infection, or skin infection. Lymph node enlargement is a frequent finding that may reflect any of a number of infectious disorders. The most common cause of this symptom is an acute infection of the mouth or pharynx. In this situation, the enlarged lymph nodes are usually just posterior and inferior to the angle of the mandible. Signs of acute infection (e.g., fever, malaise, and a sore mouth or throat) are usually present. A constitutional reaction, tenderness of the cervical mass, and the presence of an obvious infectious source confirm the diagnosis. Treatment should be directed toward the primary disease and should include a monospot test for infectious mononucleosis.

Neck masses may also derive from subcutaneous abscesses, infected sebaceous or inclusion cysts, or multiloculated carbuncles (most often occurring in the back of the neck in a patient with diabetes mellitus). The physical characteristics of abscesses make recognition of these problems relatively straightforward.

On occasion, primary head and neck bacterial infections can lead to infection of the fascial spaces of the neck. A high index of suspicion is required: such infections are sometimes difficult to diagnose. Aggressive treatment with antibiotics and drainage of closed spaces is indicated to prevent overwhelming fasciitis.

Various chronic infections (e.g., tuberculosis, fungal lymphadenitis, syphilis, cat-scratch fever, and AIDS) may also involve cervical lymph nodes. Certain chronic inflammatory disorders (e.g., sarcoidosis) may present with cervical lymphadenopathy as well. Because of the chronic lymph node involvement, these conditions are easily confused with neoplasms, especially lymphomas. Biopsy is occasionally necessary; however, skin tests and serologic studies are often more useful for establishing a diagnosis. Treatment of these conditions is primarily medical; surgery is reserved for complications.

CONGENITAL CYSTIC LESIONS

Thyroglossal Duct Cysts

Thyroglossal duct cysts are remnants of the tract along which the thyroid gland descended into the neck from the foramen cecum [see Figure 2]. They account for about 70% of all congenital abnormalities of the neck. Thyroglossal duct cysts may be found in patients of any age but are most common in the first decade of life. They may take the form of a lone cyst, a cyst with a sinus tract, or a solid core of thyroid tissue. They may be so small as to be barely perceptible, as large as a grapefruit, or anything in between. Thyroglossal duct cysts are almost always found in the midline, at or below the level of the hyoid bone; however, they may be situated anywhere from the base of the tongue to the suprasternal notch. They occasionally present slightly lateral to the midline and are sometimes associated with an external fistula to the skin of the anterior neck. They are often ballotable and can usually be moved slightly from side to side but not up or down; however, they do move up and down when patients swallow or protrude the tongue.

Thyroglossal duct cysts must be differentiated from dermoid cysts, lymphadenomegaly in the anterior jugular chain, and cutaneous lesions (e.g., lipomas and sebaceous cysts). Operative treatment is almost always required, not only because of cosmetic considerations but also because of the high incidence of recurrent infection, including abscess formation. About 1% of thyroglossal duct cysts contain cancer; papillary cancer is the neoplasm most commonly encountered, followed by squamous cell carcinoma.

Branchial Cleft Cysts

Branchial cleft cysts are vestigial remnants of the fetal branchial apparatus from which all neck structures are derived. Early in embryonic development, there are five branchial arches and four grooves (or clefts) between them. The internal tract or opening of a branchial cleft cyst is situated at the embryologic derivative of the corresponding pharyngeal groove, such as the tonsil (second arch) or the piriform sinus (third and fourth arches). The second arch is the most common area of origin for such cysts. The position of the cyst tract is also determined by the embryologic relation of its arch to the derivatives of the arches on either side of it.

The majority of branchial cleft cysts (those that develop from the second, third, and fourth arches) tend to present as a bulge along the anterior border of the sternocleidomastoid muscle, with or without a sinus tract. Branchial cleft cysts may become symptomatic at any age, but most are diagnosed in the first two decades of life. They often present as a smooth, painless, slowly enlarging mass in the lateral neck. Frequently, there is a history of fluctuating size and intermittent tenderness. The diagnosis is more obvious when there is an external fistulous tract and there is a history of intermittent discharge. Infection of the cyst may be the reason for the first symptoms.

Treatment consists of complete surgical removal of the cyst and the sinus tract. Any infection or inflammation should be treated and allowed to resolve before the cyst and the tract are removed.

Cystic Hygromas (Lymphangiomas)

A cystic hygroma is a lymphangioma that arises from vestigial lymph channels in the neck. Almost always, this condition is first noted by the second year of life; on rare occasions, it is first diagnosed in adulthood. A cystic hygroma may present as a relatively simple thin-walled cyst in the floor of the mouth or may involve all the tissues from the floor of the mouth to the mediastinum. About 80% of the time, there is only a painless cyst in the posterior cervical triangle or in the supraclavicular area. A cystic hygroma can also occur, however, at the root of the neck, in the angle of the jaw (where it may involve the parotid gland), and in the midline (where it may involve the tongue, the floor of the mouth, or the larynx).

The typical clinical picture is of a diffuse, soft, doughy, irregular mass that is readily transilluminated. Cystic hygromas look and feel somewhat like lipomas but have less well defined margins. Aspiration of cystic hygromas yields straw-colored fluid. They may be confused with angiomas (which are compressible), pneumatoceles from the apex of the lung, or aneurysms. They can be distinguished from vascular lesions by means of arteriography. On occasion, a cystic hygroma grows suddenly as a result of an upper respiratory tract infection, infection of the hygroma itself, or hemorrhage into the tissues. If the mass becomes large enough, it can compress the trachea or hinder swallowing.

In the absence of pressure symptoms (i.e., obstruction of the airway or interference with swallowing) or gross deformity, cystic hygromas may be treated expectantly. They tend to regress spontaneously; if they do not, complete surgical excision is indicated. Excision can be difficult because of the numerous satellite extensions that often surround the main mass and because of the association of the tumor with vital structures such as the cranial nerves. Recurrences are common; staged resections for complete excision are often necessary.

Vascular Malformation (Hemangiomas)

Hemangiomas are usually considered congenital because they either are present at birth or appear within the first year of life. A number of characteristic findings—bluish-purple coloration, increased warmth, compressibility followed by refilling, bruit, and thrill—distinguish them from other head and neck masses. Angiography is diagnostic but is rarely indicated.

Given that most of these congenital lesions resolve spontaneously, the treatment approach of choice is observation alone unless there is rapid growth, thrombocytopenia, or involvement of vital structures.

BENIGN NEOPLASMS

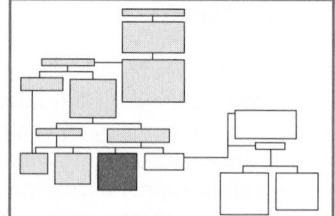

Salivary Gland Tumors

The possibility of a salivary gland neoplasm must be considered whenever an enlarging solid mass lies in front of and below the ear, at the angle of the mandible, or in the submandibular triangle. Benign salivary gland lesions are often asymptomatic; malignant ones are often associated with seventh cranial nerve symptoms or skin fixation. Diagnostic radiographic studies (CT or MRI) indicate whether the mass is salivary in origin but do not help classify it histologically. The diagnostic test of preference is open biopsy in the form of complete submandibular gland removal or superficial parotidectomy.

With any mass in or around the ear, one should be prepared to remove the superficial lobes of the parotid, the deep lobes, or both and to perform a careful facial nerve dissection. Any less complete approach reduces the chances of a cure: there is

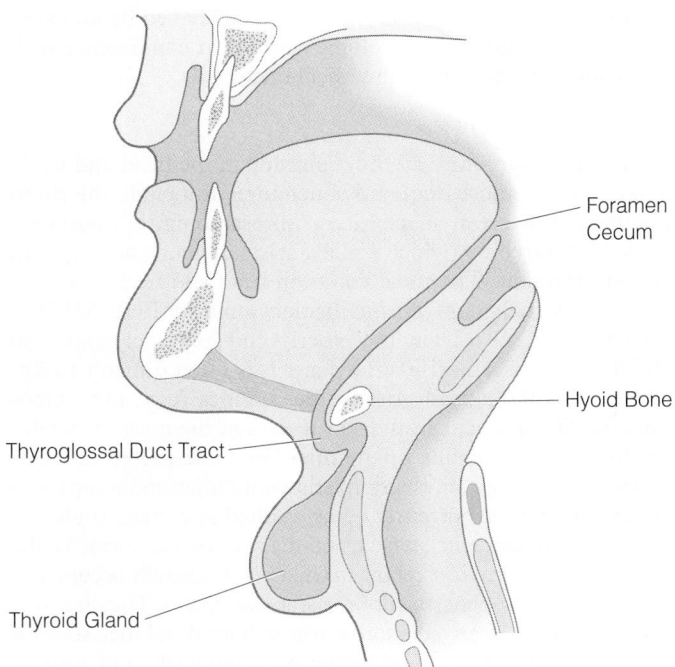

Figure 2 Shown is the course of the thyroglossal duct tract from its origin in the area of the foramen cecum to the pyramidal lobe of the thyroid gland.[2] In the operative treatment of a thyroglossal duct cyst, the central portion of the hyoid bone must be removed to ensure complete removal of the tract and to prevent recurrence.

Foramen Cecum

Hyoid Bone

Thyroglossal Duct Tract

Thyroid Gland

a high risk of implantation and seeding of malignant tumors. Benign mixed tumors make up two thirds of all salivary tumors; these must also be completely removed because recurrence is common after incomplete resection.

Benign Thyroid Nodules and Nodular Goiters

Thyroid disease is a relatively common cause of neck masses: in the United States, about 4% of women and 2% of men have a palpable thyroid nodule. Patients should be questioned about local symptoms (pain, dysphagia, pressure, hoarseness, or a change in the voice), about the duration of the nodule, and about systemic symptoms (from hyperthyroidism, hypothyroidism, or any other illness). Although most nodules are benign, malignancy is a significant concern. Nodules in children, young men, pregnant women, or persons with a history of radiation exposure or a family history of thyroid cancer are more likely to be malignant. Nodules that are truly solitary, feel firm or hard on examination, are growing rapidly, or are nonfunctional on scans are more likely to be malignant.

If physical examination suggests a discrete thyroid nodule, FNA should be done to ascertain whether malignancy is present within the nodule. If malignancy is confirmed or suspected, surgery is indicated. If the nodule is histologically benign or disappears with aspiration, thyroid suppression and observation are often sufficient. FNA often yields unrepresentative results in patients with a history of radiation exposure, in whom there is approximately a 40% chance that one of the nodules present contains cancer.

Surgery for thyroid nodules involves excisional biopsy consisting of at least total lobectomy; enucleation is almost never indicated. The surgical approach of choice for most patients with Graves disease or multinodular goiter is subtotal thyroidectomy or total lobectomy on one side and subtotal lobectomy on the other (Dunhill's operation). Treatment of thyroid cancer is discussed elsewhere [*see* Primary Malignant Neoplasms, Thyroid Cancer, *below*].

Soft Tissue Tumors (Lipomas, Sebaceous Cysts)

Superficial intracutaneous or subcutaneous masses may be sebaceous (or epidermal inclusion) cysts or lipomas. Final diagnosis and treatment usually involves simple surgical excision, often done as an office procedure with local anesthesia.

Chemodectomas (Carotid Body Tumors)

Carotid body tumors belong to a group of tumors known as chemodectomas (or, alternatively, as glomus tumors or nonchromaffin paragangliomas), which derive from the chemoreceptive tissue of the head and neck. In the head and neck, chemodectomas most often arise from the tympanic bodies in the middle ear, the glomus jugulare at the skull base, the vagal body near the skull base along the inferior ganglion of the vagus, and the carotid body at the carotid bifurcation. They are occasionally familial and sometimes occur bilaterally.

A carotid body tumor presents as a firm, round, slowly growing mass at the carotid bifurcation. Occasionally, a bruit is present. The tumor cannot be separated from the carotid artery by palpation and can usually be moved laterally and medially but not in a cephalocaudal plane. The differential diagnosis includes a carotid aneurysm, a branchial cleft cyst, a neurogenic tumor, and nodal metastases fixed to the carotid sheath. The diagnosis is made by means of CT scanning or arteriography, which demonstrate a characteristic highly vascular mass at the carotid bifurcation. Neurofibromas tend to displace, encircle, or compress a portion of the carotid artery system, events that are readily demonstrated by carotid angiography.

Biopsy should be avoided. Chemodectomas are sometimes malignant and should therefore be removed in most cases to prevent subsequent growth and pressure symptoms. Fortunately, even malignant chemodectomas are usually low grade; long-term results after removal are excellent on the whole. Some experience with vascular surgery is desirable: bleeding may occur, and clamping of the carotid artery may result in a stroke. Expectant treatment may be indicated in older or debilitated individuals. Radiotherapy may be appropriate for patients with unresectable tumors.

Neurogenic Tumors (Neurofibromas, Neurilemomas)

The large number of nerves in the head and neck renders the area susceptible to neurogenic tumors. The most common of such tumors, neurilemomas (schwannomas) and neurofibromas, arise from the neurilemma and usually present as painless, slowly growing masses in the lateral neck. Neurilemomas can be differentiated from neurofibromas only by means of histologic examination.

Given the potential these tumors possess for malignant degeneration and slow but progressive growth, surgical resection is indicated. This may include resection of the involved nerves, particularly with neurofibromas, which tend to be more invasive and less encapsulated than neurilemomas.

Laryngeal Tumors

In rare cases, a chondroma may arise from the thyroid cartilage or the cricoid cartilage. It is firmly fixed to the cartilage and may present as a mass in the neck or as the cause of a progressively compromised airway. Surgical excision is indicated.

PRIMARY MALIGNANT NEOPLASMS

Lymphomas

Cervical adenopathy is one of the most common presenting symptoms in patients with Hodgkin and non-Hodgkin lymphoma. The nodes tend to be softer, smoother, more elastic, and more mobile than nodes containing metastatic carcinoma would be. Rapid growth is not unusual, particularly in non-Hodgkin lymphoma. Involvement of extranodal sites, particularly Waldeyer's tonsillar ring, is often seen in patients with non-Hodgkin lymphoma; enlargement of these sites may provide a clue to the diagnosis. The diagnosis is confirmed via excisional biopsy of an intact lymph node. As noted, the precise histologic subtype usually cannot be determined by FNA alone; open biopsy must be done, and fresh tissue must be submitted for surface marker and electron microscopic studies.

Lymphoma is treated by means of radiation therapy, chemotherapy, or both, depending on the disease's pathologic type and clinical stage.

Thyroid Cancer

The approach to suspected thyroid cancer differs in some respects from the approach to benign thyroid disease. The operation of choice for papillary thyroid cancer that is occult (< 1 cm in diameter) and confined to the thyroid gland and for minimally invasive follicular thyroid cancer (i.e., with only capsular invasion) is thyroid lobectomy; the prognosis is excellent. The procedure of choice for papillary, follicular, Hürthle cell, and medullary thyroid cancer is total or near-total thyroidectomy (when it can be done safely) [see V:1 Thyroid and Parathyroid Procedures]. Patients who present with thyroid nodules and have a history of radiation exposure or a family history of thyroid cancer should also undergo total or near-total thyroidectomy because about 40% of them will have at least one focus of papillary thyroid cancer. Total thyroidectomy decreases recurrence and permits the use of iodine-131 (^{131}I) to scan for and treat residual disease; it also makes serum thyroglobulin and calcitonin assays more sensitive for diagnosing recurrent or persistent differentiated thyroid tumors of follicular or parafollicular cell origin.

Patients with medullary thyroid cancer should undergo meticulous elective (prophylactic) or therapeutic central neck dissection. They should be screened for *ret* proto-oncogene mutations on chromosome 10. Therapeutic modified neck dissection is indicated for all patients with thyroid cancer and palpable nodes laterally. Prophylactic modified neck dissection is indicated for patients with medullary thyroid cancer and either primary tumors larger than 1.5 cm or evidence of central neck node involvement.

Patients with anaplastic thyroid cancer are probably best treated with a combination of chemotherapy and radiation therapy, in conjunction with the removal of as much of the neoplasm as can safely be excised. Most patients with thyroid lymphoma should receive chemotherapy, radiation therapy, or both.

Upper Aerodigestive Tract Cancer

Deciding on the optimal therapeutic approach to tumors of the aerodigestive tract (i.e., surgery, radiation therapy, or some combination of the two) generally requires expertise beyond that of most general surgeons. Therefore, cancers involving the nose, the paranasal sinuses, the nasopharynx, the floor of the mouth, the tongue, the palate, the tonsils, the piriform sinus,

the hypopharynx, or the larynx are best managed by an experienced head and neck oncologic surgeon in conjunction with a radiation therapist and a medical oncologist.

Soft Tissue Sarcomas

Malignant sarcomas are not common in the head and neck. The sarcomas most frequently encountered include the rhabdomyosarcoma seen in children, fibrosarcoma, liposarcoma, osteogenic sarcoma (which usually arises in young adults), and chondrosarcoma. The most common head and neck sarcoma, however, is malignant fibrous histiocytoma (MFH). MFH is seen most frequently in the elderly and extremely rarely in children, but it can arise at any age. It is often difficult to differentiate pathologically from other entities (e.g., fibrosarcoma). MFH can occur in the soft tissues of the neck or involve the bone of the maxilla or the mandible. The preferred treatment is wide surgical resection; adjuvant radiation therapy and chemotherapy are currently being studied in clinical trials.

Rhabdomyosarcoma, usually of the embryonic form, is the most common form of sarcoma in children. It generally occurs near the orbit, the nasopharynx, or the paranasal sinuses. The diagnosis is confirmed by biopsy. A thorough search for distal metastases is made before treatment—consisting of a combination of surgical resection, radiation therapy, and chemotherapy—is begun.

Skin Cancer

Basal cell carcinomas are the most common of the skin malignancies [see II:10 Skin Lesions]. These lesions arise in areas that have been extensively exposed to sunlight (e.g., the nose, the forehead, the cheeks, and the ears). Treatment consists of local resection with adequate clear margins. Metastases are rare, and the prognosis is excellent. Inadequately excised and neglected basal cell carcinomas may ultimately spread to regional lymph nodes and can cause extensive local destruction of soft tissue and bone. For example, basal cell carcinoma of the medial canthus may invade the orbit, the ethmoid sinus, and even the brain. Periauricular basal cell carcinoma can spread across the cartilage of the ear canal or into the parotid gland.

Squamous cell carcinoma also arises in areas associated with extensive sunlight exposure; the lower lip and the pinna are the most common sites. Unlike basal cell carcinoma, however, squamous cell carcinoma tends to metastasize regionally and distally. This tumor must also be excised with an adequate margin.

Melanoma is classified on the basis of size, location, depth of invasion, and histologic subtype, although the prognosis is closely related to the thickness of the tumor [see Metastatic Tumors, Metastatic Melanomas, below]. In addition to the typical pigmented, irregularly shaped skin lesions [see II:10 Skin Lesions], malignant melanoma may also arise on the mucous membranes of the nose or the throat, on the hard palate, or on the buccal mucosa. The treatment of choice is wide surgical resection. Radiation therapy, chemotherapy, and immunotherapy may also be considered.

METASTATIC TUMORS

Any surgeon who is managing patients with head and neck cancers must have a thorough understanding of neck dissections and should have sufficient training and experience to perform these operations in the appropriate clinical circumstances.

Types of Neck Dissections

There are two classification systems for neck dissections. The first is based on the indications and goals of surgery. An *elective* (or *prophylactic*) neck dissection is done when the neck is clinically negative (that is, when no abnormal lymph nodes are palpable or visible on radiographic imaging). A *therapeutic* neck dissection is done to remove all palpable and occult disease in patients with suspicious lymph nodes discovered via physical examination or CT scanning.

The second system is based on the extent and type of dissection. *Comprehensive* neck dissections include the classic radical neck dissection as well as the modified radical (or functional) neck dissection [*see Figure 3*]. In a radical neck dissection, the sternocleidomastoid muscle, the internal and external jugular veins, the spinal accessory nerve, and the submaxillary gland are removed, along with all lymph node–bearing tissues. The modified radical or functional neck dissection is a modification of the radical neck dissection in which the lymphatic tissue from these areas is removed but the functional structures are preserved. *Selective* neck dissections involve the removal of specific levels of lymph nodes [*see Figure 1*]. The rationale for selective dissections is that several head and neck cancers consistently metastasize to specific localized lymph node regions. The following are examples of selective neck dissections: suprahyoid neck dissection (levels I and II); supraomohyoid neck dissection (levels I, II, and III); lateral neck dissection (levels II, III, and IV); and posterolateral neck dissection (levels II, III, IV, and V).

Metastatic Squamous Cell Carcinomas

The basic principle in the management of metastatic squamous cell carcinoma is to treat all regional lymph node groups at highest risk for metastases by means of surgery or radiation therapy, depending on the clinical circumstances. Selective lymph node dissection can be performed along with wide excision of the primary tumor at the time of initial operation. For example, carcinomas of the oral cavity are treated with supra-omohyoid neck dissection, and carcinomas of the oropharynx, the hypopharynx, and the larynx are treated with lateral neck dissection. If extranodal extension or the presence of multiple levels of positive nodes is confirmed by the pathologic findings, the patient should receive adjuvant bilateral neck radiation for 4 to 6 weeks after operation.

Metastatic Adenocarcinomas

Adenocarcinoma in a cervical node most frequently represents a metastasis from the thyroid gland, the salivary glands, or the GI tract. The primary tumor must therefore be sought through endoscopic and radiologic study of the bronchopulmonary tract, the GI tract, the genitourinary tract, the salivary glands, and the thyroid gland. Other possible primary malignancies to be considered include breast and pelvic tumors in women and prostate cancer in men.

If the primary site is controlled and the patient is potentially curable or if the primary site is not found and the neck disease is the only established site of malignancy, neck dissection is the appropriate treatment. Postoperative adjuvant radiation may also be considered. If the patient has thyroid cancer and palpable nodes, lateral neck dissection and ipsilateral central neck dissection are recommended.

Overall survival is low—about 20% at 2 years and 9% at 5 years—except for patients with papillary or follicular thyroid cancer, who have a good prognosis. Two factors associated with a better prognosis are unilateral neck involvement and limitation of disease to lymph nodes above the cricoid cartilage.

Metastatic Melanomas

If the patient has a thin melanoma (Breslow thickness < 1 mm; Clark level I, II, or III), full-thickness excision with 1 cm margins should be done. Intermediate-thickness melanomas (Breslow thickness 1 to 4 mm; Clark level IV) are also staged with lymphatic mapping and sentinel lymph node (SLN) biopsy [*see V:3 Lymphatic Mapping and Sentinel Lymph Node Biopsy*]. All patients with intermediate-thickness melanomas and multiple positive SLNs and all melanoma patients with palpable lymph nodes should undergo modified neck dissection for adequate local disease control. Because these tumors may metastasize to nodes in the parotid region, superficial parotidectomy is often included in the neck dissection, particularly in the case of melanoma located on the upper face or the anterior scalp. Consultation with a medical oncologist is indicated for all patients with intermediate-thickness or thick (Breslow thickness > 4 mm; Clark level IV or V) melanomas; immunotherapy or chemotherapy may be considered. Radiation therapy is often considered in patients with extensive local or nodal disease.

Metastases from an Unknown Primary Malignancy

Management of patients with an unknown primary malignancy is challenging for the surgeon. It is helpful to know that when cervical lymph nodes are found to contain metastatic squamous cell carcinoma, the primary tumor is in the head and neck about 90% of the time. Typically, such patients are found to have squamous cell carcinoma on the basis of FNA of an abnormal cervical lymph node; this finding calls for an exhaustive review of systems as well as a detailed physical examination of the head and neck.

If no primary tumor is identified, the patient should undergo endoscopic evaluation of the nasopharynx, the hypopharynx, the esophagus, the larynx, and the tracheobronchial tree under gen-

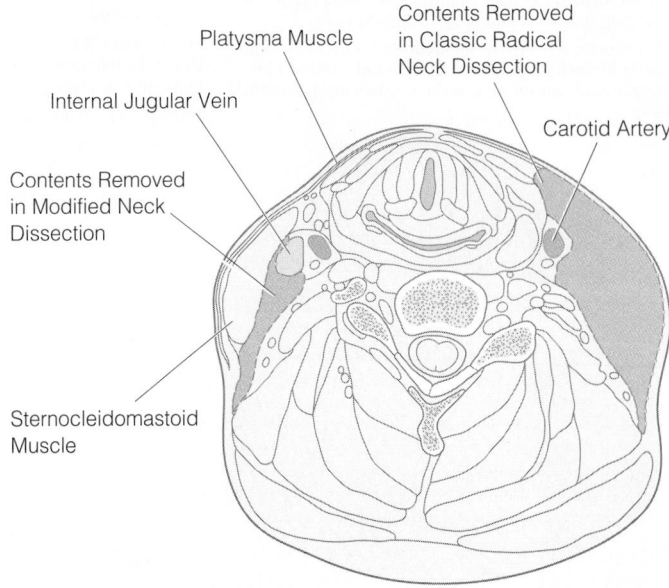

Figure 3 Cross section of the neck shows the structures removed in a classic radical neck dissection (right) and in a modified radical neck dissection (left).[3]

eral anesthesia. Biopsies of the nasopharynx, the tonsils, and the hypopharynx often identify the site of origin (although there is some debate on this point). If the biopsies do not reveal a primary source of cancer, the preferred treatment is unilateral neck dissection, followed by radiation therapy directed toward the neck, the entire pharynx, and the nasopharynx. In 15% to 20% of cases, the primary cancer is ultimately detected. Overall 5-year survival in such cases ranges from 25% to 50%.

If a malignant melanoma is found in a cervical lymph node but no primary tumor is evident, the patient should be asked about previous skin lesions, and a thorough repeat head and neck examination should be done, with particular attention to the scalp, the nose, the oral cavities, and the sinuses. An ophthalmologic exam-

ination is also required. If physical examination and radiographic studies find no evidence of metastases, modified neck dissection should be performed on the involved side.

Metastatic adenocarcinoma in a cervical lymph node with no known primary tumor is discussed elsewhere [see Metastatic Adenocarcinomas, above]. The most common primary sites in the head and neck are the salivary glands and the thyroid gland. The possibility of an isolated metastasis from the breast, the GI tract, or the genitourinary tract must also be rigorously investigated. If no primary site is identified, the patient should be considered for protocol-based chemotherapy and radiation therapy, directed according to what the primary site is most likely to be in that patient.

References

1. Fabian RL: Benign and malignant diseases of the head and neck. Current Practice of Surgery. Levine BA, Copeland EM III, Howard RJ, et al, Eds. Churchill Livingstone, New York, 1993, vol 2, sect VII, chap 1

2. Cohen JI: Benign neck masses. Boie's Fundamentals of Otolaryngology: A Textbook of Ear, Nose and Throat Disease, 6th ed. Adams GL, Boie LR Jr, Hilger PA, Eds. WB Saunders Co, Philadelphia, 1989

3. Coleman JJ III, Sultan MR: Tumors of the head and neck. Principles of Surgery, 6th ed. Schwartz SI, Shires GT, Spencer FC, Eds. McGraw-Hill Book Co, New York, 1994, p 595

Recommended Reading

Beenken SW, Maddox WA, Urist MM: Workup of a patient with a mass in the neck. Adv Surg 28:371, 1995

Byers RM: Neck dissection: concepts, controversies and technique. Semin Surg Oncol 7:9, 1991

Chandler JR, Mitchell B: Branchial cleft cysts, sinuses and fistulas. Otolaryngol Clin North Am 14:175, 1981

Clark O, Duh QY: Textbook of Endocrine Surgery. WB Saunders Co, Philadelphia, 1997

Clark OH, Noguchi S: Thyroid Cancer Diagnosis and Treatment. Quality Medical Publishing, St Louis, 2000

Davidson BJ, Spiro RH, Patel S, et al: Cervical metastases of occult origin: the impact of combined modality therapy. Am J Surg 168:195, 1994

Delbridge L, Guinea AL, Reeve TS: Total thyroidectomy for bilateral benign multinodular goiter: effect of changing practice. Arch Surg 134:1385, 1999

Hainsworth JD: Poorly differentiated carcinoma and poorly differentiated adenocarcinoma of unknown primary tumor site of the neck. Semin Oncol 20:279, 1993

Hoffman HT, Karnell LH, Funk GF, et al: The National Cancer Database report on cancer of the head and neck. Arch Otolaryngol Head Neck Surg 124:951, 1998

Jossart GH, Clark OH: Well-differentiated thyroid cancer. Curr Probl Surg 31:933, 1994

Lee NK, Byers RM, Abbruzzese JL, et al: Metastatic adenocarcinoma to the neck from an unknown primary source. Am J Surg 162:306, 1991

McGuirt WF: Diagnosis and management of masses in the neck, with special emphasis on metastatic disease. Oncology 4:85, 1990

Moley JF, De Beneditti MK: Patterns of nodal metastases in palpable medullary thyroid carcinoma: recommendations for extent of node dissection. Ann Surg 225:880, 1999

Montgomery WW: Surgery of the neck. Surgery of the Upper Respiratory System, 2nd ed. Lea & Febiger, Philadelphia, 1989, p 83

Nguyen TD, Malissard L, Theobald S, et al: Advanced carcinoma of the larynx: results of surgery and radiotherapy without induction chemotherapy (1980–1985): a multivariate analysis. Int J Radiat Oncol Biol Phys 36:1013, 1996

Shah JP, Medina JE, Shaha AR, et al: Cervical lymph node metastasis. Curr Probl Surg 30:1,1993

Spiro RH: Management of malignant tumor of the salivary glands. Oncology 12:671, 1998

Van den Brekel MW, Castelijns JA: Surgery of lymph nodes in the neck. Semin Roentgenol 35:42, 2000

Wu HS, Young MT, Ituarte P, et al: Death from thyroid cancer of follicular cell origin. J Am Coll Surg 191:600, 2000

Acknowledgment

Figures 1 through 3   Tom Moore.

2 ASYMPTOMATIC CAROTID BRUIT

Claudio S. Cinà, M.D., Sp.Chir. (It.), M.Sc., Catherine M. Clase, M.B., B.Chir., M.Sc., and Aleksandar Radan, M.D., B.Sc., B.F.A.

Assessment of Asymptomatic Carotid Bruit

The term bruit refers to any noise detected on auscultation in the neck. The conventional method of auscultation is to use the bell of the stethoscope and listen over an area extending from the upper end of the thyroid cartilage to just below the angle of the jaw.[1-3] The principal reason why bruits in the neck are matters of some concern is that they may reflect underlying occlusive carotid artery disease, which carries an increased risk of stroke.

In what follows, we outline a problem-oriented approach to the workup of patients found to have cervical bruits at the time of routine or focused vascular examination.

Clinical Assessment

CAROTID BRUITS VERSUS OTHER CERVICAL SOUNDS

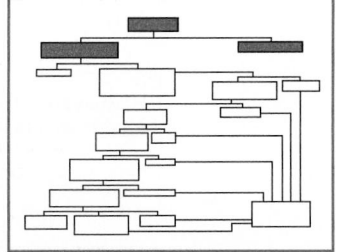

Clinical assessment begins with evaluation of the character of the bruit and examination of the precordium and the cervical structures. Carotid bruits must be distinguished from other sounds heard in the neck. Venous hums are relatively common, being reported in 27% of young adults.[4] They tend to have a diastolic component, are louder when the patient sits or turns the head away from the side of auscultation, and disappear when the patient lies down or when the Valsalva maneuver is performed.[4] Ejection systolic murmurs of cardiac origin may radiate into the neck, but generally, they are bilateral, are louder within the chest, and are less audible distally in the neck[5]; the same is true of bruits arising in other intrathoracic vessels.[6,7] No definitive clinical sign has yet been identified that clearly differentiates bruits from transmitted cardiac murmurs. On occasion, a bruit may be heard over the thyroid gland; however, this finding is extremely rare and is usually accompanied by thyromegaly and other features of autoimmune thyroid disease.[5] In dialysis patients, a bruit may be generated by the increased flow resulting from the creation of an arteriovenous fistula in the forearm.[8]

SYMPTOMATIC VERSUS ASYMPTOMATIC CAROTID BRUITS

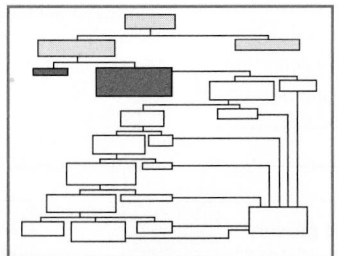

Transient ischemic attacks (TIAs) are defined as brief episodes of focal loss of brain function that can usually be localized to a specific portion of the brain supplied by a single vascular system.[9] By arbitrary convention, such an ischemic episode is considered a TIA if it lasts less than 24 hours; a similar episode, in the absence of evidence of trauma or hemorrhage, is considered an ischemic stroke if it lasts more than 24

hours or causes death.[9] Amaurosis fugax is a transient (< 24 hours) loss of vision in one eye or a portion of the visual field.[9] If a patient with a carotid bruit has a history of any of these conditions in the ipsilateral eye or brain, then the bruit is regarded as neurologically symptomatic, and the relevant question at that point is whether the patient has significant carotid stenosis and may be a candidate for carotid endarterectomy on that basis. Given the substantial differences between the management of patients with symptomatic bruits and those with asymptomatic bruits, the distinction between these two patient groups is crucial.

The history is of critical importance in the diagnosis of TIA because most TIAs last less than 4 hours,[10] which means that patients typically are not seen by physicians during the period of neurologic deficit.[11] Patients should be specifically asked about transient focal problems with vision, language, facial paresis, dysarthria, and arm or leg numbness or weakness. A 1984 study reported good interobserver agreement ($\kappa = 0.65$) [see Table 1] between clinicians diagnosing previous ischemic episodes.[12] Assigning a probable neurologic territory to a TIA or stroke, however, proved more difficult: for TIAs, the interobserver agreement between two independent neurologists asked to distinguish between carotid and vertebrobasilar events was relatively poor ($\kappa = 0.31$).[12] There is some evidence that using a standardized protocol for the diagnosis of previous ischemic episodes might improve this low interobserver agreement (e.g., to $\kappa = 0.65$[12] or $\kappa = 0.77$[13]). Similar difficulties attend diagnosis of stroke by means of history and physical examination.[14]

Many patients with a possible TIA or stroke will have undergone neurologic imaging. Such imaging is unhelpful if it yields negative results; however, in some cases, it reveals the presence of an infarct, thereby confirming the ischemic nature of the event and establish-

Table 1 Quantification of Interobserver Agreement*

$\kappa^\dagger$	Strength of Agreement
≤ 0.2	Poor
$> 0.2, \leq 0.4$	Fair
$> 0.4, \leq 0.6$	Moderate
$> 0.6, \leq 0.8$	Good
$> 0.8, \leq 1$	Very good

*Reliability (how closely an assessment agrees with another similar assessment on a second occasion or by a second observer) and validity (how closely the assessment agrees with another criterion or a gold standard) are the key properties of any assessment. When agreement between two observers is poor, the assessment in question, whether it is a physical finding, a clinical diagnosis, or an interpretation of a diagnostic test, is lacking in reliability; if more reliable methods are available, they should be considered instead. In clinical medicine, however, more reliable methods are not always available. When this is the case, the physician must use a relatively unreliable assessment as the best available alternative, while remaining aware of its limitations.[118]

$^\dagger\kappa$ is a statistical measure used to quantify agreement between two or more observers. It takes a value between 0 and 1, where 0 represents agreement no better than that expected by chance alone and 1 represents perfect agreement.[118]

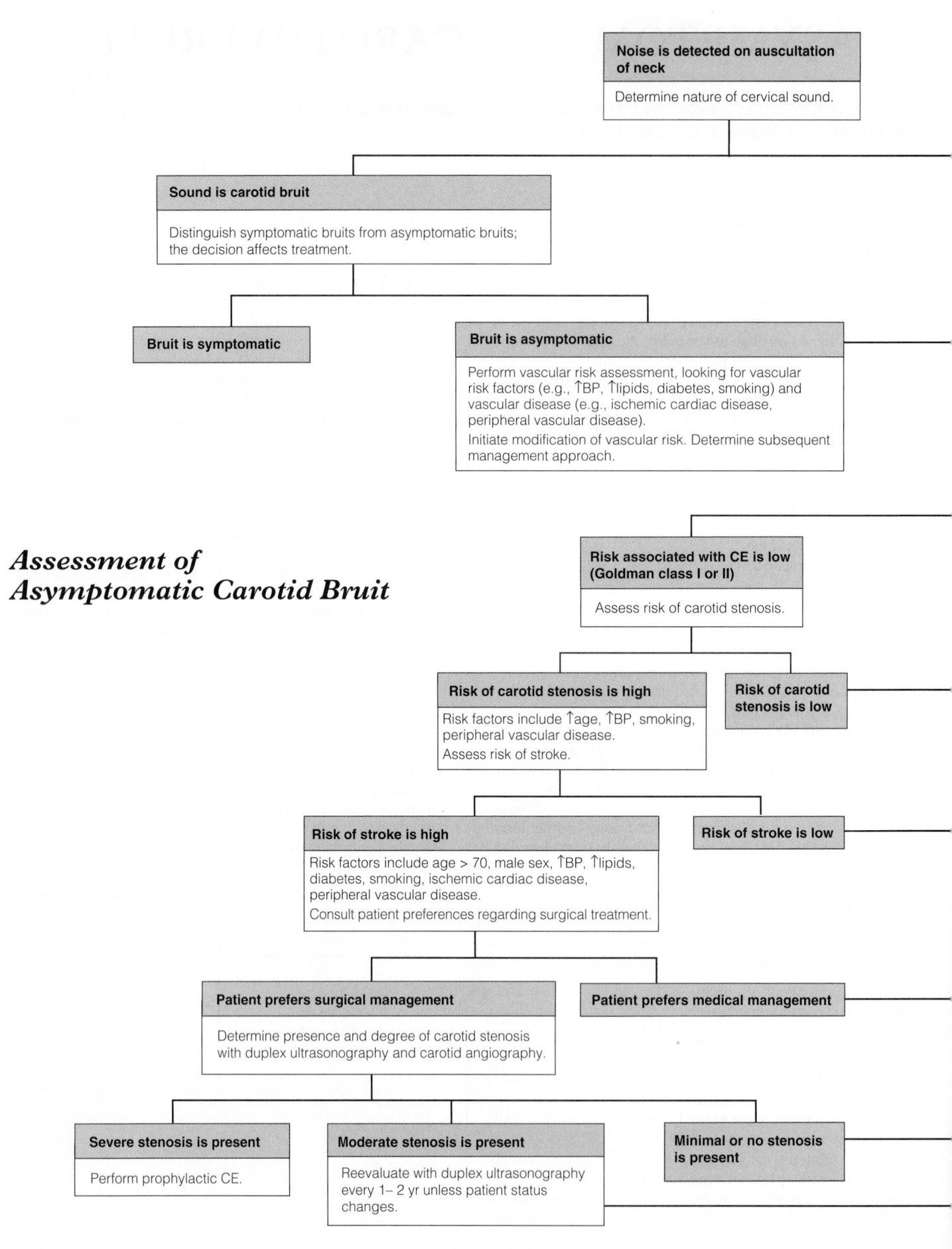

Noise is detected on auscultation of neck

Determine nature of cervical sound.

Sound is carotid bruit

Distinguish symptomatic bruits from asymptomatic bruits; the decision affects treatment.

Bruit is symptomatic

Bruit is asymptomatic

Perform vascular risk assessment, looking for vascular risk factors (e.g., ↑BP, ↑lipids, diabetes, smoking) and vascular disease (e.g., ischemic cardiac disease, peripheral vascular disease).

Initiate modification of vascular risk. Determine subsequent management approach.

Assessment of Asymptomatic Carotid Bruit

Risk associated with CE is low (Goldman class I or II)

Assess risk of carotid stenosis.

Risk of carotid stenosis is high

Risk factors include ↑age, ↑BP, smoking, peripheral vascular disease.
Assess risk of stroke.

Risk of carotid stenosis is low

Risk of stroke is high

Risk factors include age > 70, male sex, ↑BP, ↑lipids, diabetes, smoking, ischemic cardiac disease, peripheral vascular disease.
Consult patient preferences regarding surgical treatment.

Risk of stroke is low

Patient prefers surgical management

Determine presence and degree of carotid stenosis with duplex ultrasonography and carotid angiography.

Patient prefers medical management

Severe stenosis is present

Perform prophylactic CE.

Moderate stenosis is present

Reevaluate with duplex ultrasonography every 1– 2 yr unless patient status changes.

Minimal or no stenosis is present

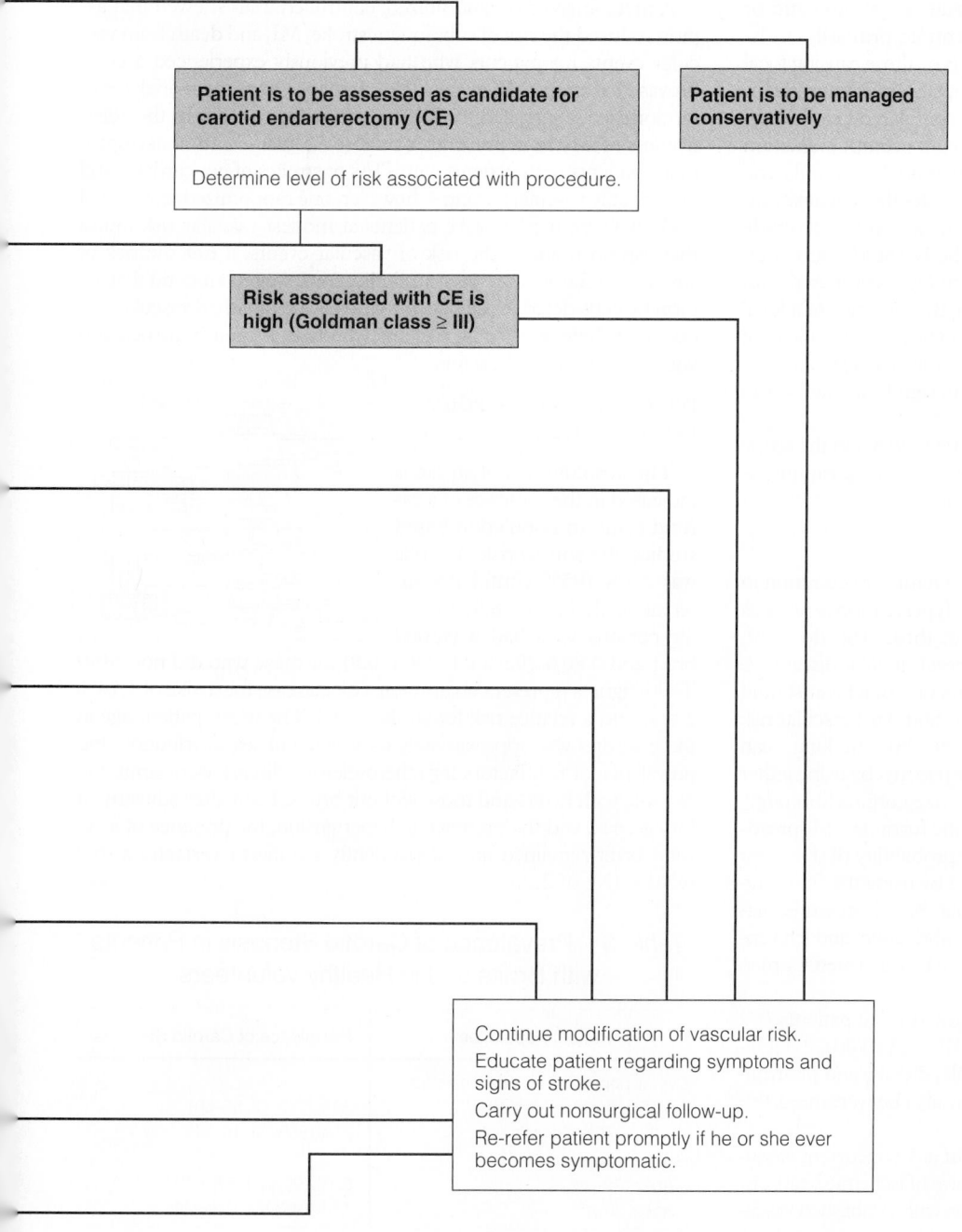

Sound is venous hum, radiating cardiac murmur or intrathoracic bruit, or thyroid bruit

Patient is to be assessed as candidate for carotid endarterectomy (CE)

Determine level of risk associated with procedure.

Patient is to be managed conservatively

Risk associated with CE is high (Goldman class ≥ III)

Continue modification of vascular risk.

Educate patient regarding symptoms and signs of stroke.

Carry out nonsurgical follow-up.

Re-refer patient promptly if he or she ever becomes symptomatic.

ing its location. For a bruit to be regarded as symptomatic on the basis of imaging studies, at least one infarct must be seen in the appropriate ipsilateral anterior vasculature.

It is evident that distinguishing between symptomatic and asymptomatic bruits on clinical grounds may be difficult; nonetheless, it is worthwhile to make the effort because the risk of stroke in the asymptomatic population is quite different from that in the symptomatic population. For example, whereas the Asymptomatic Carotid Atherosclerosis Study (ACAS), which included patients believed on clinical grounds to be neurologically asymptomatic, reported an overall stroke rate of 6.2% at 2.7 years in its medically managed group,[15] the North American Symptomatic Carotid Endarterectomy Trial (NASCET), which included patients assessed as neurologically symptomatic (i.e., with a history of amaurosis fugax, TIA, or minor stroke), reported a stroke rate of 26% at 3 years in its medically managed group.[16]

In determining whether a unilateral bruit is symptomatic or asymptomatic, the physician should concentrate primarily on ischemic deficits in the ipsilateral hemisphere (i.e., those causing focal contralateral motor or sensory deficits) and ipsilateral amaurosis fugax. However, symptoms referable to the contralateral carotid artery, even if no bruit is heard on that side, might prompt evaluation of the patient for symptomatic carotid stenosis on the contralateral side. The absence of a bruit by no means excludes the diagnosis: carotid bruits are absent in 20% to 35% of patients with high-grade stenosis of the internal carotid artery.[17] In the NASCET subgroup in which the physical finding of a carotid bruit was compared with angiographic imaging of the carotid system, the presence of a focal ipsilateral carotid bruit had a sensitivity of 63% and a specificity of 61% for high-grade (70% to 99%) stenosis; the absence of a bruit did not significantly change the probability of significant stenosis in this population (pretest 52%, posttest 40%).[18]

Workup of patients with symptomatic bruits is beyond the scope of this chapter. Accordingly, the ensuing discussion focuses on assessment of patients with asymptomatic bruits.

VASCULAR RISK ASSESSMENT

Vascular diseases and other vascular risk factors are common in patients with asymptomatic carotid bruits. Hypertension is twice as common in patients who have bruits as in those who do not[19]; smoking, ischemic heart disease, and peripheral vascular disease are also more prevalent.[20,21] Consequently, detection of a bruit should prompt a thorough vascular risk assessment. Standard vascular risk factors—hypertension, hyperlipidemia, diabetes, and smoking—can be integrated into risk profiles for particular patients by using either the New Zealand risk tables (http://www.nzgg.org.nz/library/gl_complete/bloodpressure/appendix.cfm) or the formula and spreadsheets provided by Anderson et al.[22,23] The probability of stroke for various follow-up periods may be quantified by using the Framingham stroke-risk profile.[24] From age, systolic blood pressure, diabetes, smoking, cardiovascular disease, atrial fibrillation, and left ventricular hypertrophy, probability of stroke may be calculated for men and women according to a point system.[24]

Smoking cessation should be recommended to all patients,[25-27] and hypertension should be controlled (BP < 140/90).[28-31] Depending on a patient's individual risk profile, dietary and pharmacologic management of hyperlipidemia may also be warranted.[32-34] Diabetic control should be optimized.[35,36]

Patients should be asked specifically about any concurrent vascular disease—in particular, symptoms suggestive of ischemic heart disease or of claudication or rest pain. In patients with established vascular disease, the risk that future vascular events (e.g., coronary-related death, myocardial infarction [MI], new angina, stroke, TIA, new con-

Table 2 Annual Risk of Stroke

Patient Population	Annual Risk of Stroke
Population without bruits, age > 60 yr[19,43,44]	0.86% (95% CI, 0.8–0.9)
Population with bruits, age > 60 yr[19,20,43]	2.1% (95% CI, 0.6–8.5)
Male population without bruits, age > 60 yr[19,24]	0.9% (95% CI, 0.1–3.0)
Male population with bruits, age > 60 yr[19]	8.0% (95% CI, 0.2–38.0)
Female population without bruits, age > 60 yr[24]	2.0% (95% CI, 0.8–4.2)
Female population with bruits, age > 60 yr[19]	2.4% (95% CI, 0.7–5.5)

gestive heart failure, or peripheral vascular syndrome) will occur in the next 5 years is greater than 20%.[22,37] In such patients, consultation of formulas or tables is unnecessary, and all modifiable risk factors should be aggressively managed (target BP < 140/90; target ratio of total cholesterol to high-density lipoprotein [HDL] cholesterol < 4).[22]

A meta-analysis of randomized, controlled trials showed that aspirin reduced the risk of subsequent stroke, MI, and death from vascular events for patients who had previously experienced a cerebrovascular event, MI, or unstable angina.[38] Other meta-analyses of randomized, controlled trials[39,40] were unable to confirm the effectiveness of aspirin in preventing cerebrovascular events in asymptomatic patients or in patients with TIAs or strokes of noncardiac (and presumably vascular) origin[41]; however, one randomized, controlled trial involving hypertensive patients at modest vascular risk found that aspirin reduced the risk of vascular events, if not the risk of stroke.[42] In the absence of contraindications, we recommend that aspirin be considered for all patients who have established vascular disease elsewhere and for all patients who have a bruit in association with any vascular risk factors.

INDICATIONS FOR SURGICAL INTERVENTION

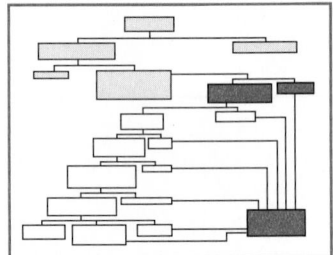

The absolute risk of stroke is increased in the presence of a carotid bruit. In population-based studies, the annual risk of stroke was 2.1% (95% confidence interval [CI], 0.6 to 8.5)[19,20,43,44] for persons who had a carotid bruit and 0.86% (95% CI, 0.8 to 0.9) for those who did not.[19,43,44] These figures represent an absolute risk increase for stroke of 1.24% a year and a relative risk for stroke of 2.4. The mean patient age in these studies was approximately 65 years, and sex distribution and prevalence of risk factors for atherosclerotic disease were similar in patients with bruits and those without bruits. Even after adjustment for age, sex, and the presence of hypertension, the presence of a carotid bruit remained an independently significant variable, with a relative risk of 2.0.[19]

Table 3 Prevalence of Carotid Stenosis in Patients with Bruits and in Healthy Volunteers

Patient Population	Prevalence of Carotid Stenosis
Overall population with cervical bruits	
> 35% stenosis[20,56-58,119]	58% (95% CI, 55–60)
>60%–75% stenosis[56-58]	21% (95% CI, 18–24)
Healthy volunteers*	
Age > 70 yr[89]	5.1% (95% CI, 2.6–9.0)
Age ≤ 70 yr[89]	1.5% (95% CI, 0.2–5.3)

*In healthy volunteers, the incidence of asymptomatic carotid stenosis is significantly correlated with age ($P < 0.01$) and with the presence of hypertension ($P < 0.005$).

Table 4 Necessary Criteria for Offering an Interventional Approach to Selected Patients with Carotid Bruits

Center-specific criteria
Either
DUS is documented to have a > 90% PPV for stenosis > 50% on angiography and is used alone
or
DUS has a lower PPV and is used as a screening test only, and angiography in patients with cerebrovascular disease has a documented complication (stroke or death) rate of around 1%
Surgeon-specific criterion
Perioperative rate of stroke or death is < 3% for carotid endarterectomy

DUS—duplex ultrasonography   PPV—positive predictive value

Given the low absolute risk of stroke in asymptomatic patients with bruits [*see Table 2*], the low prevalence of surgically relevant stenosis in patients with bruits [*see Table 3*], and the small (and only marginally statistically significant) absolute benefit of carotid endarterectomy in patients with asymptomatic stenosis,[45,46] we and others[47-51] do not believe that further investigation with a view to carotid endarterectomy is mandatory in the asymptomatic population. Many surgeons may prefer to manage these patients conservatively, reevaluating them promptly if they become symptomatic [*see Discussion, below*]. Other surgeons may wish to pursue a more interventional strategy with selected patients, in which case further evaluation with an eye to surgical treatment depends on the presence of the following key findings in a given patient: (1) low risk associated with carotid endarterectomy, (2) relatively high risk of carotid stenosis, and (3) high risk of stroke if carotid stenosis is documented. In addition, the patient's preferences should be consulted: no patient should be subjected to further evaluation who is not prepared to undergo surgical treatment if such management is recommended. Patients who, on the basis of any of these criteria, are not suitable candidates for intervention will not benefit from imaging studies and should be managed medically.

Finally, surgeons and centers who are contemplating offering prophylactic carotid endarterectomy for asymptomatic stenosis should be able to document that their rates of stroke or perioperative death for this procedure are lower than 3% [*see Table 4*]. When complication rates exceed this threshold, the value of carotid endarterectomy becomes negligible, and surgeons may find themselves doing more harm than good.[45,46]

Low Risk Associated with Carotid Endarterectomy

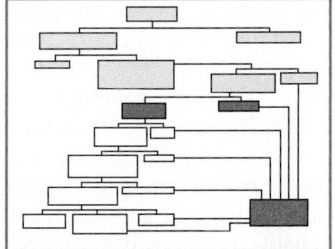

In NASCET and ACAS, patients were excluded if they had coexisting medical disease likely to produce significant mortality and morbidity (e.g., cardiac valvular or rhythm disorders, uncontrolled hypertension or diabetes, unstable angina pectoris, or MI in the previous 4 months)[16]; accordingly, the results of these trials are not generalizable to patients who have such conditions. Further evidence for the impact of operative risk on outcomes is provided by a retrospective review of 562 patients who underwent carotid endarterectomy for symptomatic and asymptomatic disease in a large community hospital.[52] For patients in Goldman class I or II,[53] the overall rate of death or

nonfatal MI was 2% (95% CI, 1.1 to 3.9), whereas for patients in class III or IV, the corresponding figure was 21% (95% CI, 9.2 to 39.9) [*see Table 5*]. Given that 50 prophylactic carotid endarterectomies would have to be performed to prevent one stroke over the subsequent 3-year period (i.e., the number needed to treat [NNT] is 50), it is clearly unacceptable to perform this procedure in a population facing a 21% incidence of MI or death, in which for every 5 patients undergoing the operation, one would experience an MI or die (i.e., the number needed to harm [NNH] is only 5). Further consideration of prophylactic carotid endarterectomy in patients for whom the procedure carries a high risk is not warranted.

High Risk of Carotid Stenosis

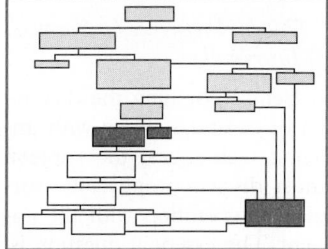

Cohort[45,54-60] and population-based[19,61,62] studies suggest that patients with asymptomatic carotid bruits are more likely to have significant carotid stenosis if they are older, are hypertensive, smoke, or have advanced peripheral vascular disease. In one study, hemodynamically significant stenosis (i.e., > 50%) was found by means of ultrasonography in 32% of patients scheduled to undergo peripheral vascular procedures but in only 6.8% of those scheduled to undergo coronary artery bypass grafting (CABG).[63] (All figures for degree of stenosis in this chapter are determined according to the formula used in NASCET [*see Table 6 and Figure 1*].)

Further consideration of carotid endarterectomy may be warranted in patients with vascular risk factors or known peripheral vascular disease; in the absence of these findings, the risk of significant carotid stenosis is low. Further evaluation is unnecessary for patients who are younger, do not smoke, are not hypertensive or diabetic, and are not known to have peripheral vascular disease.

High Risk of Stroke

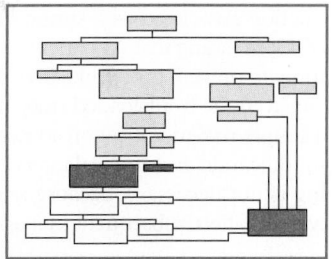

Within the group of patients with asymptomatic carotid stenosis, there is only limited direct evidence for the existence of subgroups of patients at higher risk for stroke. Men seem to be at higher risk for stroke than women are: in the medical arm of ACAS, the incidence of stroke or death at 2.7 years was 7.0% (95% CI, 4.9 to 9.4) for men and 4.9% (95% CI, 2.7 to 8.0) for women. Gender-related differences aside, however, identification of other subgroups at higher risk relies on extrapolation of data from other populations at risk for artery-to-artery embolism. Data from NASCET indicate that for symptomatic patients with greater than 70% carotid stenosis, the presence of a higher number of identifiable clinical risk factors (age > 70 years; male sex; systolic or diastolic hypertension; the occurrence of a cerebrovascular event within the preceding 31 days; the occurrence of a more serious cerebrovascular event, namely, stroke rather than a TIA or amaurosis fugax; smoking; MI; congestive heart failure; diabetes; intermittent claudication; or hyperlipidemia) was associated with a higher annual stroke risk. For patients with zero to three risk factors, the annual stroke risk was 6.6%; for those with four or five, 9.2%; and for those with six or more, 15.8%. Data from the same study indicate that among patients with a contralateral asymptomatic stenosed carotid artery, patients with zero to three risk factors have an annual stroke risk of 1.4% in the territory of the asymptomatic stenosis; those with four or five, 2.8%; and those with six or more, 3.8%.[64]

Obesity is another risk factor for stroke.[49,50] Some 60% of patients who experience a stroke before 65 years of age have a body mass index greater than 24 kg/m[2].[49] This finding, in conjunction with a history of smoking, was found to predict 60% of strokes in men in this age group.[50]

Patients with carotid bruits who do not have significant systemic risk factors or other vascular disease are at low absolute risk for stroke and are unlikely to benefit from carotid endarterectomy; hence, further investigation is not warranted.[5,18,49] Patients with numerous (i.e., six or more) clinical risk factors [see Table 7] are at relatively high risk for stroke, and it is in this population that most of the benefit from carotid endarterectomy is likely to be concentrated.

Patient Preference for Surgical Intervention

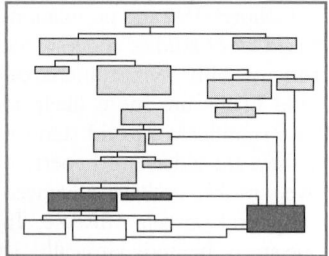

Before pursuing the diagnosis of carotid stenosis with imaging techniques, the surgeon must discuss prophylactic surgical intervention with the patient. The essential question is, if significant stenosis is documented, will the patient wish to undergo carotid endarterectomy? It should be remembered that at this point in the workup, we are considering only those patients (1) for whom the cardiac risk associated with the procedure is acceptably low and (2) who are considered to be at relatively high risk for stroke if carotid stenosis is demonstrated.

Patients should be informed that if they are found to have significant carotid stenosis, their risk of stroke is 6.3% over the ensuing 2.7 years if they do not undergo operation and 4.0% over the same period if they do.[15] They should also be informed that these figures take into account a 3% risk of perioperative stroke or death (2.7% risk of stroke and 0.3% risk of death).[15] The 2.3% absolute risk reduction associated with surgical treatment translates into an NNT of 43, meaning that 43 patients would have to undergo endarterectomy to prevent one stroke over the next 2.7 years.

Given the front-loaded risks of surgery, some patients will prefer a simple risk-modification strategy to a strategy including both risk modification and surgical intervention. In such cases, carotid imaging is not necessary, because knowledge of the degree of stenosis will not affect subsequent management.

Diagnosis of Asymptomatic Carotid Stenosis

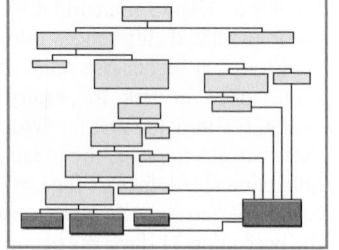

The purpose of investigation of asymptomatic neck bruits is to identify persons with significant carotid stenosis who are at increased risk for cerebrovascular disease[65,66] and who are likely to benefit from carotid endarterectomy. In the absence of other significant findings, cervical bruits are not sufficiently predictive of significant carotid stenosis or ischemic stroke to be useful in selecting candidates for noninvasive imaging.[51] Noninvasive testing is a reasonable step in patients with the characteristics listed above, but routine screening of all patients with asymptomatic carotid bruits is not warranted.[51]

DUPLEX ULTRASONOGRAPHY

Duplex ultrasonography (DUS) should be performed bilaterally. A meta-analysis conducted in 1995 found that for detecting greater

Table 5 Cardiac Risk Assessment*

Parameter	Weighted Score on Cardiac Risk Index		
	Goldman	Detsky	Eagle
Age > 70 yr	5	5	1
MI			1
< 6 mo	10	10	
> 6 mo		5	
Angina			1
Class III		10	
Class IV		20	
Unstable		10	
Diabetes			1
Operation			
Emergency	4	10	
Aortic, abdominal, or thoracic	3		
CHF	11		1
< 1 wk		10	
> 1 wk		5	
ECG			
Rhythm other than sinus	7	5	
> 5 PVCs/min	7	5	
Poor medical status†	3	5	

Risk of Perioperative Cardiac Events

Low	0–12 (class I, II)	0–15	0
Intermediate	13–25 (class III)	16–30	1–2
High	> 25 (class IV)	> 30	≥ 3

*The Goldman cardiac risk index[53] is a multifactorial index of cardiac risk in patients undergoing noncardiac surgery. Modifications have been proposed by Detsky,[121-123] who included angina and institution-specific perioperative cardiac event rates in the model. The Eagle index[124-126] is another risk index based on five clinical variables. Despite the lack of consensus regarding the relative merits of these tools for preoperative cardiac risk assessment, stratification of patients into risk categories is helpful in assessing the risk and benefits of a procedure such as carotid endarterectomy.
†P_aO_2 < 60 mm Hg; P_aCO_2 > 50 mm Hg; K^+ < 3 mmol/L; serum HCO_3 < 20 mmol/L; serum urea > 18 mmol/L; creatinine > 260 µmol/L; abnormal ALT; signs of chronic liver disease; bedridden from cardiac causes.
CHF—congestive heart failure   MI—myocardial infarction   PVC—premature ventricular contraction

than 50% stenosis (determined by means of angiography, the gold standard), DUS had a sensitivity of 91% (95% CI, 89 to 94) and a specificity of 93% (95% CI, 88 to 95).[67] Given a disease prevalence of approximately 41% in patients referred for DUS, these findings translate into a positive predictive value of 90% and an accuracy of 92%.[67] A subsequent prospective study of patients (both symptomatic and asymptomatic) in whom carotid endarterectomy was being considered reported a sensitivity of 100% and a specificity of 98% for greater than 60% stenosis, with a positive predictive value of 99%.[68]

At centers where DUS has been internally validated in comparison with angiography and where this level of performance has been documented, the surgeons may choose to proceed to surgery without angiography.[68-70] At centers where DUS is less reliable, however, it should be regarded as a screening test, and angiography should be performed when DUS suggests greater than 50% stenosis.

CAROTID ANGIOGRAPHY

As an invasive procedure, carotid angiography carries a significant risk of morbidity and mortality. All centers performing carotid angiography for cerebrovascular disease should audit their stroke rates

Table 6 Conversion between Different Methods of Measuring Degree of Carotid Stenosis

Method	Severity of Disease				
	Minimal	Moderate		Severe	Occlusion
ECST*	24%–57%	58%–69%	70%–81%	82%–99%	100%
NASCET	0%–29%	30%–49%	50%–69%	70%–99%	100%
CC method†	35%–56%	57%–61%	62%–80%	81%–99%	100%

*Conversion from ECST to NASCET was done according to the following formula: ECST % stenosis = 0.6(NASCET % stenosis) + 40.[127]
†The relation of the NASCET method to the CC method is linear, with a ratio of 0.62 between the distal internal carotid diameter and the common carotid diameter.[117]

periodically. Since 1990, four prospective studies[71-74] have addressed the question of the risks associated with angiography in patients with atherosclerotic cerebrovascular disease. When the data from these studies were pooled, the risk of permanent neurologic deficit or death was 1.1% (95% CI, 0.6 to 2.0).[75] In ACAS, the 1.2% of patients in the intervention arm who experienced stroke or died after angiography accounted for 40% of the strokes and deaths attributable to surgical intervention.[15] Angiographic complication rates significantly worse than these will adversely impact the risk-benefit ratio associated with surgical intervention. Centers that consistently record relatively high angiographic complication rates should not offer evaluation for and surgical treatment of asymptomatic carotid disease.

Carotid Endarterectomy

At this point in management, it is reasonable to offer surgical treatment of asymptomatic disease to patients with greater than 50% stenosis. ACAS[15] and two meta-analyses[45,46] that included other trials of surgical therapy for asymptomatic carotid stenosis documented a small and marginally statistically significant benefit from prophylactic carotid endarterectomy in asymptomatic patients with greater than 50% to 60% carotid stenosis. Because the absolute benefit is small, we do not consider it obligatory to pursue the diagnosis or to follow an invasive strategy in patients identified solely on the basis of an asymptomatic bruit; however, patients possessing all the characteristics listed earlier [*see* Indications for Surgical Intervention, *above*] probably constitute a group that is particularly able to benefit from surgical intervention. Patients with higher degrees of stenosis are at higher risk for stroke and are therefore most likely to benefit.[76-79]

The degree of stenosis and the presence or absence of plaque ulceration may modify the final decision for or against operative management [*see* Discussion, Subgroup Analyses for Potential High-Risk Factors, *below*].

Technical details of carotid endarterectomy are discussed elsewhere [*see V:23 Carotid Arterial Procedures*].

Patient Education

All patients with asymptomatic carotid bruits, whether they are undergoing prophylactic endarterectomy or not, should be carefully advised regarding the symptoms and signs of stroke, TIAs, and amaurosis fugax and should be strongly encouraged to seek urgent medical attention if such problems arise. Patients who experience one of these untoward events should undergo full reevaluation for stroke risk factors (e.g., hypertension, hyperlipidemia, diabetes, smoking, and atrial fibrillation); in the absence of atrial fibrillation (which should prompt consideration of prophylactic anticoagulation[80-82]), a change in antiplatelet therapy should be considered. Both ticlopidine[83] and clopidogrel[84,85] are more effective than aspirin in preventing stroke. (Ticlopidine is associated with reversible but severe neu-

tropenia in fewer than 1% of cases; accordingly, monitoring for this complication is indicated.)

If a patient who is a surgical candidate experiences a TIA or stroke as a result of an ischemic event in the carotid region in the absence of atrial fibrillation, he or she must be promptly referred back to the vascular surgeon. This possibility should be clearly explained to patients once the initial evaluation is complete and they have been referred back to their primary care physicians. Patients referred back to a vascular surgeon under these circumstances should then be regarded as having symptomatic carotid disease. A subgroup analysis of patients with symptomatic stenosis reported that carotid endarterectomy performed soon after a nondisabling stroke was not associated with a significantly higher operative complication rate than endarterectomy performed 30 days or longer after a stroke.[75,86] Performing endarterectomy early reduces the risk period for recurrent stroke and may therefore increase the potential benefit of the intervention; the usual approach is to perform the procedure within a week or two of a patient's first neurologic event.[86]

Management of cardiovascular risk factors and concurrent vascular disease should continue. In the absence of concurrent vascular disease, patients may be referred back to the family practitioner, internist, or cardiologist in place of specific surgical follow-up.

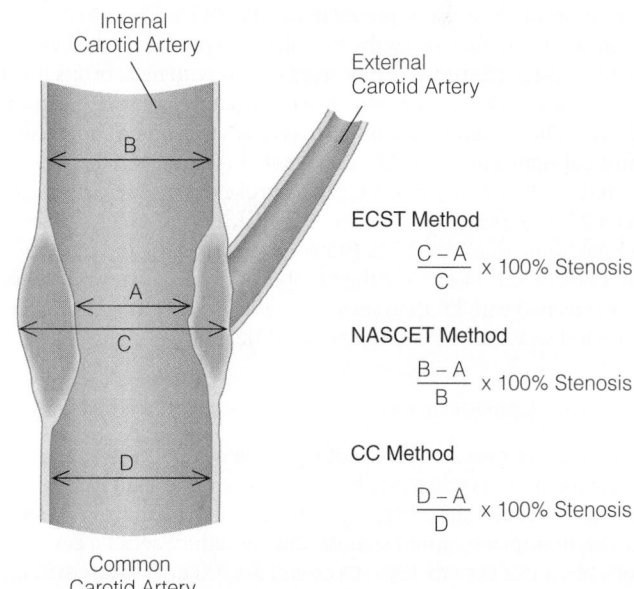

Figure 1 **Carotid angiography remains the gold standard for determining the extent of carotid arterial disease. Several methods of reporting angiographically defined stenosis have been described in the literature.[115] The most commonly used methods are those adopted by the NASCET and ECST investigators, though the so-called common carotid (CC) method has its advocates as well.[116,117]**

Table 7 Risk Factors for Stroke[128,129]

Age > 70 yr	Smoking (or history of smoking)
Male sex	> 80% carotid stenosis
Hypertension*	Presence of ulceration
Hyperlipidemia	Ischemic heart disease†
Diabetes	Peripheral vascular disease

*Defined as systolic BP > 160 mm Hg or diastolic BP > 90 mm Hg.
†MI or CHF.

Follow-up of Patients with Lower-Grade Stenosis

Carotid stenosis progresses in about one quarter of patients with asymptomatic carotid stenosis monitored with DUS over a 2-year period.[87] In a population of asymptomatic patients with bruits who were referred to a vascular laboratory, 282 stenotic carotid arteries (average stenosis, 50%) were followed for 38 ± 18 months. Progression of stenosis, defined as an increase in degree of stenosis to 80% or beyond, occurred in 17% of arteries, and 2% became completely occluded. Progression was associated with an increase in stroke risk of 4.9% at 1 year, 16.7% at 3 years, and 26.5% at 5 years. In comparison, the estimated stroke risk in an asymptomatic population of patients with 50% to 79% stenosis was 0.85%, 3.6%, and 5.4% for the same three periods ($P = 0.001$).[76]

Although carotid stenosis, once identified, tends to progress over time,[20,54,76,88] the data are currently insufficient to permit recommendation of routine ultrasonographic or other surveillance for all patients with neck bruits outside a research setting. In our view, reevaluation every 1 to 2 years with noninvasive diagnostic tests is a reasonable approach to patients (1) who are already known to have greater than 50% stenosis, (2) who do not undergo surgery, and (3) who are at high risk for stroke, are surgical candidates, and are not averse to surgery.

Discussion

Epidemiology

In cross-sectional and population-based studies, the overall prevalence of greater than 75% carotid stenosis has been low. A 1992 study reported a 2.3% prevalence in men and a 1.1% prevalence in women; there was a significant ($P < 0.0001$) increase with age with each decade from 65 years to beyond 85 years, but there were no significant differences between men and women.[62] In the Framingham study population, the incidence of greater than 50% stenosis was 8% (95% CI, 6.5 to 9.8).[61] In a study of healthy volunteers, the incidence of greater than 50% stenosis was 5.1% (95% CI, 2.6 to 9.0) in patients 70 years of age or older and 1.5% (95% CI, 0.2 to 5.3) in younger patients.[89]

The pooled risk of greater than 60% to 75% stenosis in patients with carotid bruits referred for noninvasive vascular evaluation at an average age of 65 years is reported to be 21% (95% CI, 18 to 24),[56-58] which is three to four times the prevalence expected on the basis of population-based studies. Thus, five persons with neck bruits must be screened to detect one patient with moderate to severe carotid stenosis. The absolute benefit of surgery is small and of borderline statistical significance. In ACAS, as noted (see above), the relative risk reduction for an ipsilateral major stroke or perioperative death over a 2.7-year period was 36.5% (95% CI, 27.5 to 47.1), the absolute risk reduction was 2.3% (95% CI, 0.2 to 7.0), and the NNT was 43 (95% CI, 14 to 500); the number of patients that would have to be screened with DUS to prevent one stroke over a 3-year follow-up period was 250 (95% CI, 70 to 2,500).

Economic Considerations

A cogent argument in favor of pursuing a surgical strategy in at least some patients was made by a 1997 economic analysis,[90] which demonstrated that although prophylactic endarterectomy in patients with asymptomatic carotid stenosis did not reduce societal costs appreciably, it was nonetheless, at a cost of $8,000/quality-adjusted life year (QALY), within the range of many interventions considered by society to be cost-effective. It should be pointed out, however, that this economic analysis addressed only carotid endarterectomy in patients with identified carotid stenosis, not screening strategies for patients with bruits, and consequently did not consider costs associated with investigation and follow-up to the point of recommendation for or against carotid endarterectomy in the broader group of patients with bruits. These costs would alter the economic analysis substantially, and if they are included, it is far from clear whether the resulting overall cost/QALY would still be acceptable. To date, no trial or economic analysis of a screening strategy has been published.

Screening Issues

For the reasons previously discussed, we do not feel justified in recommending routine screening for patients with asymptomatic carotid bruits. Given the available evidence, we believe that such patients may reasonably be managed in either of two ways. One choice is simply to conclude that screening patients with carotid bruits as possible candidates for carotid endarterectomy has not been proved to be a useful intervention and to concentrate instead on general vascular risk reduction. The other, which is appropriate in centers where noninvasive or invasive diagnostic tests reach acceptable standards with an acceptable degree of risk and where the procedure is done by surgeons whose documented perioperative stroke and death rates are less than 3%, is to take a selective approach that addresses various issues related to stroke risk, cardiac risk, and patient preferences before noninvasive tests are ordered.

Subgroup Analyses for Potential High-Risk Factors

Given the small absolute risk reduction reported by ACAS[15] and by the two meta-analyses of all asymptomatic carotid stenosis trials,[45,46] it would be useful to be able to identify one or more high-risk groups within the broader group of patients identified as having stenosis.

SEX

ACAS included a subgroup analysis addressing the effect of sex on ability to benefit from surgery: the absolute reduction in the risk of perioperative stroke or death or ipsilateral stroke at 2.7 years was 3.6% (95% CI, 1.1 to 9.9) for men and 0.5% (95% CI, 0.01 to 2.7) for women.

DEGREE OF STENOSIS

In asymptomatic patients stratified according to their ultrasonographically determined degree of stenosis, the risk of stroke is low both for patients with less than 30% stenosis (4% cumulative event rate at 3 years) and for those with 30% to 74% stenosis (9% cumulative event rate at 3 years); it is highest for those with greater than 75% stenosis (21% cumulative event rate at 3 years).[20] The European Carotid Surgery Trialists (ECST) study,[47] using angiographic data from the asymptomatic carotid arteries of 2,295 patients, reported that the Kaplan-Meyer estimate of stroke risk at 3 years was only 2% and remained low (< 2%) when patients with less than 79% stenosis were considered; stroke risk increased to 9.8% for patients with 70% to 79% stenosis and to 14.4% for those with 80% to 99% stenosis. In a population of patients referred to a vascular laboratory with asymptomatic carotid stenosis on DUS who were followed for a mean of 38 months, the incidence of stroke was 2.1% in patients with 50% to 79% stenosis and 10.4% in those with greater than 80% stenosis.[76]

In ACAS, there were too few strokes to permit subgroup analysis of the effect of degree of stenosis on ability to benefit from carotid endarterectomy. In both ECST[79] and NASCET,[75,77,78,91] however, higher degrees of stenosis in symptomatic patients were consistently observed to be associated with higher stroke risk as well as with greater ability to benefit from surgical treatment [see Table 8].

PLAQUE ULCERATION AND PLAQUE STRUCTURE

At present, there are no subgroup analyses examining the effect of plaque ulceration on the ability of asymptomatic patients to benefit from surgical treatment. In NASCET, however, when symptomatic patients with 70% to 99% stenosis were considered, those with angiographic evidence of plaque ulceration were at higher risk for stroke than those without ulceration[92] and derived greater benefit from surgery.[75] Angiography had a sensitivity of 46% and a specificity of 74% in the detection of ulcerated plaques, with a positive predictive value of 72%.[93] A 1994 study reported that when ulceration was detected with B-mode imaging in patients with asymptomatic carotid stenosis, the incidence of silent cerebral infarction detected by magnetic resonance imaging was 75%, compared with an incidence of 25% when ulceration was absent.[94]

It has also been suggested that carotid plaques of differing structures may have differing embolic potentials.[95] DUS can distinguish between fibrous plaques (which are highly echogenic) and plaques with high concentrations of lipid and necrotic material (which are echolucent). Echolucent plaques are more frequently associated with neurologic symptoms and computed tomography–proven cerebral infarction.[95-97] Interobserver reliability for plaque echostructure, however, seems to be highly variable, ranging from good ($\kappa = 0.79$) for greater than 70% stenosis[95] to average ($\kappa = 0.51$) for greater than 40% stenosis[98] to poor ($\kappa = 0.29$) for greater than 80% stenosis.[99] A 1994 report found no correlation between the presence or type of symptoms and plaque structure as determined by DUS.[100] The true importance of carotid plaque echomorphology and surface characteristics as predictors of cerebrovascular events remains to be defined.

CONTRALATERAL DISEASE

It has been suggested that the presence of contralateral carotid disease is a risk factor for future cerebrovascular events. In NASCET patients with greater than 70% stenosis,[101] contralateral occlusion significantly increased the benefit of surgery with respect to the incidence of stroke or death, but contralateral high-grade stenosis did not.[75]

ASYMPTOMATIC CEREBRAL INFARCTION

The presence of areas of asymptomatic cerebral infarction ipsilateral to the area of carotid stenosis on head CT may identify patients who would benefit from surgery.[102] In asymptomatic patients with carotid stenosis, the incidence of silent strokes demonstrated by CT has been reported to be 10% in patients with 35% to 50% stenosis on DUS, 17% in those with 50% to 75% stenosis, and 30% in those with greater than 75% stenosis.[103] The incidence of silent cerebral infarctions demonstrated by MRI in the same type of population has been reported to be 42%, increasing to 75% for greater than 50% stenosis.[94] Use of CT and MRI of the brain in risk stratification of patients with asymptomatic carotid stenosis is controversial and currently is not advised.

CONCLUSIONS

Although only limited data on patients with asymptomatic stenosis are available, we believe that consideration of sex, degree of stenosis, and possibly the presence of plaque ulceration may be helpful in making the final decision on whether to offer carotid endarterectomy to these patients; at present, plaque morphology is insufficiently reliable to be a useful guide to clinical management.

Special Situations

RESTENOSIS OR PREVIOUS CAROTID SURGERY

Patients who have previously undergone carotid surgery have been excluded from most studies of asymptomatic patients; when they have been included in trials addressing symptomatic stenosis, they have experienced increased rates of perioperative complications.[16,50] Patients in whom restenosis occurs after an earlier carotid endarterectomy should be advised against surgery while they remain asymptomatic.[15] It is therefore unnecessary to follow patients with ultrasonography after carotid endarterectomy if no symptoms develop.

PREOPERATIVE ASSESSMENT FOR CORONARY ARTERY BYPASS GRAFTING

Some 20% to 30% of patients undergoing assessment for CABG are found to have carotid bruits,[49,104] and 5% to 20% have greater than 50% stenosis on DUS[105-107] or ocular plethysmography.[108] In asymptomatic patients with carotid stenosis who are undergoing CABG, there is no direct evidence favoring prophylactic carotid endarterectomy either before or in conjunction with CABG. Cohort studies including symptomatic and asymptomatic carotid ste-

Table 8   Effectiveness of Surgery by Degree of Stenosis in Patients with Symptomatic Carotid Stenosis[75]

Degree of Stenosis	Relative Risk Reduction or Increase	Absolute Risk Reduction or Increase	Number Needed to Treat or Harm
70%–99%	RRR, 48% (95% CI, 27–63)	ARR, 6.7% (95% CI, 3.2–10)	NNT, 15 (95% CI, 10–31)
50%–69%	RRR, 27% (95% CI, 5–44)	ARR, 4.7% (95% CI, 0.8–8.7)	NNT, 21 (95% CI, 11–125)
≤ 49%	RRI, 20% (95% CI, 0–44)	ARI, 2.2% (95% CI, 0–4.4)	NNH, 45 (95% CI, 22–∞)

ARI—absolute risk increase   ARR—absolute risk reduction   NNH—number needed to harm   NNT—number needed to treat
RRI—relative risk increase   RRR—relative risk reduction

nosis indicate that patients undergoing CABG and carotid endarterectomy in the same operation have a stroke rate of 6% (95% CI, 4.6 to 7.8), an MI rate of 4.6% (95% CI, 3.1 to 6.5), and a mortality of 4.7% (95% CI, 3.4 to 6.4).[109] For cohorts in which carotid endarterectomy was performed before CABG, the stroke rate is 3.2% (95% CI, 2.1 to 4.5), the MI rate is 5.2% (95% CI, 3.6 to 6.9)—a nonsignificant increase—and the mortality is 4.7% (95% CI, 3.4 to 6.4).[109] For cohorts in which CABG was done first and carotid stenosis was treated on its own after the cardiac procedure, the stroke rate is 3.5% (95% CI, 1.0 to 9.0), the MI rate is 2% (95% CI, 0.2 to 6.0), and the mortality is 0.8% (95% CI, 0.02 to 4.8).[110-112]

We recommend against a combined surgical approach in patients with asymptomatic carotid stenosis. Given the equivalent stroke rate and the lower MI rate and mortality, we believe that the preferred strategy in patients with bruits is first to proceed with CABG if indicated and then to determine whether the patient should be further evaluated as a candidate for carotid endarterectomy in the same manner as other elective patients would be.

Effect of Center-Specific Variations on Risk-to-Benefit Ratio

In ACAS, 1.2% of the overall 2.7% perioperative stroke rate was accounted for by strokes occurring after angiography. Centers where ultrasonography has been documented to have high predictive values may avoid this risk by proceeding directly from ultrasonography to surgery. If these complications had been avoided in ACAS, the absolute risk reduction would have been more substantial: 3.43% (95% CI, 1.1 to 9.9), corresponding to an NNT of 29 (95% CI, 1 to 80). The true perioperative combined stroke and death rate achieved in this study was 1.5%, a result that is definitive of excellence in the surgical management of carotid endarterectomy and that constitutes a useful quality assurance measure for centers and individual surgeons.

Issues for the Future

It is possible, perhaps likely, that in the future, magnetic resonance angiography[67] and three-dimensional CT angiography,[113,114] together with DUS, will replace angiography as preferred imaging methods for diagnosing internal carotid artery stenosis. As for surgical treatment and screening, further data on patients with asymptomatic carotid stenosis are necessary before definitive recommendations can be made. The Asymptomatic Carotid Surgery Trial (ACST), a large study currently under way in Europe, will be completed in the next few years; it is to be hoped that this trial will provide these additional data.

References

1. Chambers BR, Norris JW: Clinical significance of asymptomatic neck bruits. Neurology 35:742, 1985

2. Harrison MJ: Cervical bruits and asymptomatic carotid stenosis. Br J Hosp Med 32:80, 1984

3. Ratcheson RA: Clinical diagnosis of atherosclerotic carotid artery disease. Clin Neurosurg 29:464, 1982

4. Jones FL: Frequency, characteristics and importance of the cervical venous hum in adults. N Engl J Med 267:658, 1962

5. Sauve JS, Laupacis A, Ostbye T, et al: Does this patient have a clinically important carotid bruit? JAMA 270:2843, 1993

6. Caplan LR: Carotid artery disease. N Engl J Med 315:886, 1986

7. Thompson JE, Patman RD, Talkington CM: Asymptomatic carotid bruit: long term outcome of patients having endarterectomy compared with unoperated controls. Ann Surg 188:308, 1978

8. Messert B, Marra TR, Zerofsky RA: Supraclavicular and carotid bruits in hemodialysis patients. Ann Neurol 2:535, 1977

9. National Institute of Neurological Disorders and Stroke: Special Report from the National Institute of Neurological Disorders and Stroke. Classification of Cerebrovascular Diseases III. Stroke 21:637, 1990

10. Werdelin L, Juhler M: The course of transient ischemic attacks. Neurology 38:677, 1988

11. Albers GW, Hart RG, Lutsep HL, et al: AHA Scientific Statement. Supplement to the guidelines for the management of transient ischemic attacks: a statement from the Ad Hoc Committee on Guidelines for the Management of Transient Ischemic Attacks, Stroke Council, American Heart Association. Stroke 30:2502, 1999

12. Kraaijeveld CL, van Gijn J, Schouten HJ, et al: Interobserver agreement for the diagnosis of transient ischemic attacks. Stroke 15:723, 1984

13. Koudstaal PJ, van Gijn J, Staal A, et al: Diagnosis of transient ischemic attacks: improvement of interobserver agreement by a check-list in ordinary language. Stroke 17:723, 1986

14. von Arbin M, Britton M, de Faire U, et al: Validation of admission criteria to a stroke unit. J Chronic Dis 33:215, 1980

15. Toole JF, Baker WH, Castaldo JE, et al: Endarterectomy for asymptomatic carotid artery stenosis. JAMA 273:1421, 1995

16. North American Symptomatic Carotid Endarterectomy Trial Collaborators (NASCET): Beneficial effect of carotid endarterectomy in symptomatic patients with high-grade carotid stenosis. N Engl J Med 325:445, 1991

17. Davies KN, Humphrey PRD: Do carotid bruits predict disease of the internal carotid arteries? Postgrad Med J 70:433, 1994

18. Sauve JS, Thorpe KE, Sackett DL, et al: Can bruits distinguish high-grade from moderate symptomatic carotid stenosis? The North American Symptomatic Carotid Endarterectomy Trial. Ann Intern Med 120:633, 1994

19. Heyman A, Wilkinson WE, Heyden S, et al: Risk of stroke in asymptomatic persons with cervical arterial bruits: a population study in Evans County, Georgia. N Engl J Med 302:838, 1980

20. Chambers BR, Norris JW: Outcome in patients with asymptomatic neck bruits. N Engl J Med 315:860, 1986

21. Meissner I, Wiebers DO, Whisnant JP, et al: The natural history of asymptomatic carotid artery occlusive lesions. JAMA 258:2704, 1987

22. Anderson KM, Odell PM, Wilson PW, et al: Cardiovascular disease risk profiles. Am Heart J 121(1 pt 2): 293, 1991

23. Anderson KM, Wilson PW, Odell PM, et al: An updated coronary risk profile: a statement for health professionals. Circulation 83:356, 1991

24. Wolf PA, D'Agostino RB, Belanger AJ, et al: Probability of stroke: a risk profile from the Framingham Study. Stroke 22:312, 1991

25. Wolf PA, D'Agostino RB, Kannel WB, et al: Cigarette smoking as a risk factor for stroke. The Framingham Study. JAMA 259:1025, 1988

26. Wannamethee SG, Shaper AG, Whincup PH, et al: Smoking cessation and the risk of stroke in middle-aged men. JAMA 274:155, 1995

27. Shinton R, Beevers G: Meta-analysis of relation between cigarette smoking and stroke. BMJ 298:789, 1989

28. Prevention of stroke by antihypertensive drug treatment in older persons with isolated systolic hypertension: final results of the Systolic Hypertension in the Elderly Program (SHEP). SHEP Cooperative Research Group. JAMA 265:3255, 1991

29. Sutton-Tyrrell K, Alcorn HG, Herzog H, et al: Morbidity, mortality, and antihypertensive treatment effects by extent of atherosclerosis in older adults with isolated systolic hypertension. Stroke 26:1319, 1995

30. Sutton-Tyrrell K, Wolfson SK Jr, Kuller LH: Blood pressure treatment slows the progression of carotid stenosis in patients with isolated systolic hypertension. Stroke 25:44, 1994

31. Collins R, Peto R, MacMahon S, et al: Blood pressure, stroke, and coronary heart disease. Part 2, Short-term reductions in blood pressure: overview of randomised drug trials in their epidemiological context. Lancet 335:827, 1990

32. Randomised trial of cholesterol lowering in 4444 patients with coronary heart disease: the Scandinavian Simvastatin Survival Study (4S). Lancet 344:1383, 1994

33. Furberg CD: Lipid-lowering trials: results and limitations. Am Heart J 128(6 pt 2):1304, 1994

34. Furberg CD, Adams HP Jr, Applegate WB, et al: Effect of lovastatin on early carotid atherosclerosis and cardiovascular events. Asymptomatic Carotid Artery Progression Study (ACAPS) Research Group. Circulation 90:1679, 1994

35. The effect of intensive treatment of diabetes on the development and progression of long-term complications in insulin-dependent diabetes mellitus. The Diabetes Control and Complications Trial Research Group. N Engl J Med 329:977, 1993

36. Intensive blood-glucose control with sulphonyl-ureas or insulin compared with conventional treatment and risk of complications in patients with type 2 diabetes (UKPDS 33). UK Prospective Diabetes Study (UKPDS) Group [published erratum appears in Lancet 354:602, 1999]. Lancet 352:837, 1998

37. Anderson KM, Wilson PW, Odell PM, et al: An updated coronary risk profile: a statement for health professionals. Circulation 83:356, 1991

38. Collaborative overview of randomised trials of antiplatelet therapy—I. Prevention of death, myocardial infarction, and stroke by prolonged antiplatelet therapy in various categories of patients. Antiplatelet Trialists' Collaboration [published erratum appears in BMJ 308:1540, 1994]. BMJ 308:81, 1994

39. Hart RG, Halperin JL, McBride R, et al: Aspirin for the primary prevention of stroke and other major vascular events: meta-analysis and hypotheses. Arch Neurol 57:326, 2000

40. Kronmal RA, Hart RG, Manolio TA, et al: Aspirin use and incident stroke in the cardiovascular health study. CHS Collaborative Research Group. Stroke 29:887, 1998

41. Barnett HJM, Eliasziw M, Meldrum HE: Drugs and surgery in the prevention of ischemic stroke. N Engl J Med 332:238, 1995

42. Hansson L, Zanchetti A, Carruthers SG, et al: Effects of intensive blood-pressure lowering and low-dose aspirin in patients with hypertension: principal results of the Hypertension Optimal Treatment (HOT) randomised trial. HOT Study Group. Lancet 351:1755, 1988

43. Wiebers DO, Whisnant JP, Sandok BA, et al: Prospective comparison of a cohort with asymptomatic carotid bruit and a population-based cohort without carotid bruit. Stroke 21:984, 1990

44. Shorr RI, Johnson KC, Wan JY, et al: The prognostic significance of asymptomatic carotid bruits in the elderly. J Gen Intern Med 13:86, 1998

45. Benavente OR, Moher D, Pham B: Carotid endarterectomy for asymptomatic carotid stenosis: a meta-analysis. BMJ 317:1477, 1998

46. Chambers BR, You RX, Donnan GA: Carotid endarterectomy for asymptomatic carotid stenosis. Cochrane Database Syst Rev (2):CD001923, 2000

47. European Carotid Surgery Trialists' Collaborative Group: Risk of stroke in the distribution of an asymptomatic carotid artery. Lancet 345:209, 1995

48. Gorelick PB: Carotid endarterectomy: where do we draw the line? (editorial) Stroke 30:1745, 1999

49. Gorelick PB, Sacco RL, Smith DB, et al: Prevention of a first stroke: a review of guidelines and a multidisciplinary consensus statement from the National Stroke Association. JAMA 281:1112, 1999

50. Feinberg RW: Primary and secondary stroke prevention. Curr Opin Neurol 9:46, 1996

51. Lee TT, Solomon NA, Heidenreich PA, et al: Cost-effectiveness of screening for carotid stenosis in asymptomatic persons. Ann Intern Med 126:337, 1997

52. Musser DJ, Nicholas GG, Reed JF III: Death and adverse cardiac events after carotid endarterectomy. J Vasc Surg 19:615, 1994

53. Goldman L, Caldera DL, Nussbaum SR, et al: Multifactorial index of cardiac risk in noncardiac surgical procedures. N Engl J Med 297:845, 1977

54. Roederer GO, Langlois YE, Jager KA, et al: The natural history of carotid arterial disease in asymptomatic patients with cervical bruits. Stroke 15:605, 1984

55. Fowl RJ, Marsh JG, Love M, et al: Prevalence of hemodynamically significant stenosis of the carotid artery in an asymptomatic veteran population. Surg Gynecol Obstet 172:13, 1991

56. Zhu CZ, Norris JW: Role of carotid stenosis in ischemic stroke. Stroke 21:1131, 1990

57. AbuRahma AF, Robinson PA: Prospective clinico-pathophysiologic follow-up study of asymptomatic neck bruit. Am Surg 56:108, 1990

58. Lusiani L, Visonà A, Castellani V, et al: Prevalence of atherosclerotic lesions at the carotid bifurcation in patients with asymptomatic bruits: an echo-Doppler (duplex) study. Angiology 36:235, 1985

59. Kartchner MM, McRae LP: Noninvasive evaluation and management of the "asymptomatic" carotid bruit. Surgery 82:840, 1977

60. Clagett GP, Youkey JR, Brigham RA, et al: Asymptomatic cervical bruit and abnormal ocular pneumoplethysmography: a prospective study comparing two approaches to management. Surgery 96:823, 1984

61. Wilson PWF, Hoeg JM, D'Agostino RB, et al: Cumulative effects of high cholesterol levels, high blood pressure, and cigarette smoking on carotid stenosis. N Engl J Med 337:516, 1997

62. O'Leary DH, Polak JF, Kronmal RA, et al: Distribution and correlates of sonographically detected carotid artery disease in the Cardiovascular Health Study. The CHS Collaborative Research Group. Stroke 23:1752, 1992

63. Hennerici M, Aulich A, Sandmann W, et al: Incidence of asymptomatic extracranial arterial disease. Stroke 12:750, 1981

64. Barnett HJ, Eliasziw M, Meldrum HE, et al: Do the facts and figures warrant a 10-fold increase in the performance of carotid endarterectomy on asymptomatic patients? Neurology 46:603, 1996

65. Warlow C: Endarterectomy for asymptomatic carotid stenosis? Lancet 345:1254, 1995

66. Amarenco P, Cohen A, Tzourio C, et al: Atherosclerotic disease of the aortic arch and the risk of ischemic stroke. N Engl J Med 331:1474, 1994

67. Blakeley DD, Oddone EZ, Hasselblad V, et al: Noninvasive carotid artery testing: a meta-analytic review. Ann Intern Med 122:360, 1997

68. Ballotta E, DaGiau G, Abbruzzese E, et al: Carotid endarterectomy without angiography: can clinical evaluation and duplex ultrasonographic scanning alone replace traditional arteriography for carotid surgery workup? A prospective study. Surgery 126:20, 1999

69. Wolf RK, Williams EL II, Kistler PC: Transbrachial balloon catheter tamponade of ruptured abdominal aortic aneurysms without fluoroscopic control. Surg Gynecol Obstet 164:463, 1987

70. Baird RN: Should carotid endarterectomy be purchased? treatment avoids much morbidity. BMJ 310:316, 1995

71. Hankey GJ, Warlow CP, Molyneux AJ: Complications of cerebral angiography for patients with mild carotid territory ischaemia being considered for carotid endarterectomy. J Neurol Neurosurg Psychiatry 53:542, 1990

72. Heiserman JE, Dean BL, Hodak JA, et al: Neurologic complications of cerebral angiography. AJNR Am J Neuroradiol 15:1401, 1994

73. Davies KN, Humphrey PR: Complications of cerebral angiography in patients with symptomatic carotid territory ischaemia screened by carotid ultrasound. J Neurol Neurosurg Psychiatry 56:967, 1993

74. Grzyska J, Freitag J, Zeumer H: Selective cerebral intraarterial DSA: Complication rate and control of risk factors. Neuroradiology 32:296, 1990

75. Cinà CS, Clase CM, Haynes RB: Refining indications for carotid endarterectomy in patients with symptomatic carotid stenosis: a systematic review. J Vasc Surg 30:606, 1999

76. Rockman CB, Riles TS, Lamparello PJ, et al: Natural history and management of the asymptomatic, moderately stenotic internal carotid artery. J Vasc Surg 25:423, 1997

77. Cina CS, Clase CM, Haynes RB: Carotid endarterectomy for symptomatic carotid stenosis. Cochrane Database Syst Rev (2):CD001081, 2000

78. Rothwell PM, Slattery J, Warlow CP: Clinical and angiographic predictors of stroke and death from carotid endarterectomy: systematic review. BMJ 315:1571, 1997

79. European Carotid Surgery Trialists' Collaborative Group: Randomized trial of endarterectomy for recently symptomatic carotid stenosis: final results of the MRC European Carotid Surgery Trial. Lancet 351:1379, 1998

80. Stroke Prevention in Atrial Fibrillation Study: Final results. Circulation 84:527, 1991

81. Warfarin versus aspirin for prevention of thromboembolism in atrial fibrillation: Stroke Prevention in Atrial Fibrillation II Study. Lancet 343:687, 1994

82. Go AS, Hylek EM, Phillips KA, et al: Implications of stroke risk criteria on the anticoagulation decision in nonvalvular atrial fibrillation: the Anticoagulation and Risk Factors in Atrial Fibrillation (ATRIA) study. Circulation 102:11, 2000

83. Hass WK, Easton JD, Adams HP Jr, et al: A randomized trial comparing ticlopidine hydrochloride with aspirin for the prevention of stroke in high-risk patients. Ticlopidine Aspirin Stroke Study Group. N Engl J Med 321:501, 1989

84. Creager MA: Results of the CAPRIE trial: efficacy and safety of clopidogrel. Clopidogrel versus aspirin in patients at risk of ischaemic events. Vasc Med 3:257, 1998

85. A randomised, blinded trial of clopidogrel versus aspirin in patients at risk of ischaemic events (CAPRIE). CAPRIE Steering Committee. Lancet 348:1329, 1996

86. Gasecki AP, Ferguson GG, Eliasziw M, et al: Early endarterectomy for severe carotid artery stenosis after a nondisabling stroke: results from the North American Symptomatic Carotid Endarterectomy Trial. J Vasc Surg 20:288, 1994

87. Bornstein NM, Chadwick LG, Norris JW: The value of carotid Doppler ultrasound in asymptomatic extracranial arterial disease. Can J Neurol Sci 15:378, 1988

88. Bornstein NM, Norris JW: Management of patients with asymptomatic neck bruits and carotid stenosis. Neurol Clin 10:269, 1992

89. Colgan MP, Strode GR, Sommer JD, et al: Prevalence of asymptomatic carotid disease: results of duplex scanning in 348 unselected volunteers. J Vasc Surg 8:674, 1988

90. Cronenwett JL, Birkmeyer JD, Nackman GB, et al: Cost-effectiveness of carotid endarterectomy in asymptomatic patients. J Vasc Surg 25:298, 1997

91. Barnett HJ, Taylor DW, Eliasziw M, et al: Benefit of carotid endarterectomy in patients with symptomatic moderate or severe stenosis. North American Symptomatic Carotid Endarterectomy Trial Collaborators (NASCET). N Engl J Med 339:1415, 1998

92. Eliasziw M, Streifler JY, Fox AJ, et al: Significance of plaque ulceration in symptomatic patients with high-grade carotid stenosis. North American Symptomatic Carotid Endarterectomy Trial. Stroke 25:304, 1994

93. Streifler JY, Eliasziw M, Fox AJ, et al: Angiographic detection of carotid plaque ulceration. comparison with surgical observations in a multicenter study. North American Symptomatic Carotid Endarterectomy Trial. Stroke 25:1130, 1994

94. Hougaku H, Matsumoto M, Handa N, et al: Asymptomatic carotid lesions and silent cerebral infarction. Stroke 25:566, 1994

95. Sabetai MM, Tegos TJ, Nicolaides AN, et al: Hemispheric symptoms and carotid plaque echomorphology. J Vasc Surg 31(1 pt 1):39, 2000

96. Meairs S, Hennerici M: Four-dimensional ultrasonographic characterization of plaque surface motion in patients with symptomatic and asymptomatic carotid artery stenosis. Stroke 30:1807, 1999

97. Kessler C, von Maravic M, Bruckmann H, et al: Ultrasound for the assessment of the embolic risk of carotid plaques. Acta Neurol Scand 92:231, 1995

98. de Bray JM, Baud JM, Delanoy P, et al: Reproducibility in ultrasonic characterization of carotid plaques. Cerebrovasc Dis 8:273, 1998

99. Albers GW: Expanding the window for thrombolytic therapy in acute stroke: the potential role of acute MRI for patient selection. Stroke 30:2230, 1999

100. Hill SL, Donato AT: Ability of the carotid duplex scan to predict stenosis, symptoms, and plaque structure. Surgery 116:914, 1994

101. Gasecki AP, Eliasziw M, Ferguson GG, et al: Long-term prognosis and effect of endarterectomy in pa-

tients with symptomatic severe carotid stenosis and contralateral carotid stenosis or occlusion: results from nascet. North American Symptomatic Carotid Endarterectomy Trial (NASCET) group. J Neurosurg 83:778, 1995

102. Findlay JM, Tucker WS, Ferguson GG, et al: Guidelines for the use of carotid endarterectomy: current recommendations from the Canadian Neurosurgical Society. Can Med Assoc J 157:653, 1997

103. Norris JW, Zhu CZ: Silent stroke and carotid stenosis. Stroke 23:483, 1992

104. Halliday AW, Thomas D, Mansfield A: The Asymptomatic Carotid Surgery Trial (ACST): rationale and design. Steering Committee. Eur J Vasc Surg 8:703, 1994

105. Ricotta JJ, O'Brien MS, DeWeese JA: Carotid endarterectomy for non-hemispheric ischaemia: long-term follow-up. Cardiovasc Surg 2:561, 1994

106. Faggioli GL, Curl GR, Ricotta JJ: The role of carotid screening before coronary artery bypass. J Vasc Surg 12:724, 1990

107. Courbier R, Jausseran JM, Poyen V: Current status of vascular grafting in supraaortic trunks. Personal experience. Int Surgery 73:210, 1988

108. Pillai L, Gutierrez IZ, Curl GR, et al: Evaluation and treatment of carotid stenosis in open-heart surgery patients. J Surg Res 57:312, 1994

109. Borger MA, Fremes SE, Weisel RD, et al: Coronary bypass and carotid endarterectomy: does a combined approach increase risk? A metaanalysis. Ann Thorac Surg 68:14, 1999

110. Rosenthal D, Caudill DR, Lamis PA, et al: Carotid and coronary arterial disease: a rational approach. Am Surg 50:233, 1984

111. Newman DC, Hicks RG, Horton DA: Coexistent carotid and coronary arterial disease. Outcome in 50 cases and method of management. J Cardiovasc Surg (Torino) 28:599, 1987

112. Ennix CL Jr, Lawrie GM, Morris GC Jr, et al: Improved results of carotid endarterectomy in patients with symptomatic coronary disease: an analysis of 1,546 consecutive carotid operations. Stroke 10:122, 1979

113. Sameshima T, Miyao J, Oda T, et al: [Effects of allopurinol on renal damage following renal ischemia.] Masui—Japan J Anesthesiol 44:349, 1995

114. Cinat ME, Pham H, Vo D, et al: Improved imaging of carotid artery bifurcation using helical computed tomographic angiography. Ann Vasc Surg 13:178, 1999

115. Fox AJ: How to measure carotid stenosis (editorial). Radiology 186:316, 1993

116. Rothwell PM, Gibson RJ, Slattery J, et al: Equivalence of measurements of carotid stenosis: a comparison of three methods on 1001 angiograms. European Carotid Surgery Trialists' collaborative group. Stroke 25:2435, 1994

117. Eliasziw M, Smith RF, Singh N, et al: Further comments on the measurement of carotid stenosis from angiograms. North American Symptomatic Carotid Endarterectomy Trial (NASCET) group. Stroke 25:2445, 1994

118. Landis R, Koch G: The measurement of observer agreement for categorical data. Biometrics 33:159, 1997

119. Floriani M, Giulini SM, Anzola GP, et al: Predictive value of cervical bruit for the detection of obstructive lesions of the internal carotid artery: data from 2000 patients. Ital J Neurol Sci 10:321, 1989

120. Thiele BL, Jones AM, Hobson RW, et al: Standards in noninvasive cerebrovascular testing. Report from the Committee on Standards for Noninvasive Vascular Testing of the Joint Council of the Society for Vascular Surgery and the North American Chapter of the International Society for Cardiovascular Surgery. J Vasc Surg 15:495, 1992

121. Detsky AS, Abrams HB, Forbath N, et al: Cardiac assessment for patients undergoing noncardiac surgery. Arch Intern Med 146:2131, 1986

122. Detsky AS, Abrams HB, McLaughlin JR, et al: Predicting cardiac complications in patients undergoing non-cardiac surgery. J Gen Intern Med 1 (July–August):211, 1986

123. Wong T, Detsky AS: Preoperative cardiac risk assessment for patients having peripheral vascular srugery. Ann Intern Med 116:743, 1992

124. Eagle K, Brundage B, Chaitman B, et al: Guidelines for perioperative cardiovascular evaluation for noncardiac surgery: report of the American College of Cardiology/American Heart Association Task Force on Practice Guidelines (Committee on Perioperative Cardiovascular Evaluation for Noncardiac Surgery). J Am Coll Cardiol 27:910, 1996

125. Eagle K, Froelich J: Reducing cardiovascular risk in patients undergoing noncardiac surgery (editorial). N Engl J Med 335:1761, 1996

126. Eagle KA, Coley CM, Newell JB, et al: Combining clinical and thallium data optimizes preoperative assessment of cardiac risk before major vascular surgery. Ann Intern Med 110:859, 1989

127. Rothwell PM, Gibson RJ, Slattery J, et al: Prognostic value and reproducibility of measurements of carotid stenosis: a comparison of three methods on 1001 angiograms. European Carotid Surgery Trialists' collaborative group. Stroke 25:2440, 1994

128. NASCET: Clinical alert: benefit of carotid endarterectomy for patients with high-grade stenosis of the internal carotid artery. national institute of neurological disorders and stroke stroke and trauma division. North American Symptomatic Carotid Endarterectomy Trial (NASCET) investigators. Stroke 22:816, 1991

129. NASCET: North American Symptomatic Carotid Endarterectomy Trial. Methods, patient characteristics, and progress. Stroke 22:711, 1991

Acknowledgment

Figure 1 Laurie Grace.

3 BREAST COMPLAINTS

Barbara L. Smith, M.D., Ph.D., and Wiley W. Souba, M.D., Sc.D.

Assessment and Management of Breast Complaints

One of every two women will consult her physician about a breast disorder at some point in her life. Although breast cancer is the most common malignancy of women in the United States, most breast disorders are nonmalignant: it is estimated that 80% to 90% of clinical presentations related to the breast are caused by benign disease. (The true incidence of benign diseases of the breast is difficult to estimate because of the blurred distinction between true breast disease and physiologic breast symptoms such as nodularity, lumpiness, and tenderness.) Because breast disorders are so common, it is important for the practicing general surgeon to be knowledgeable about the workup, diagnosis, and management of breast complaints.

Common Presenting Symptoms of Breast Disease

Most of the breast problems surgeons encounter in routine practice fall into six general categories, which are associated with varying degrees of risk for breast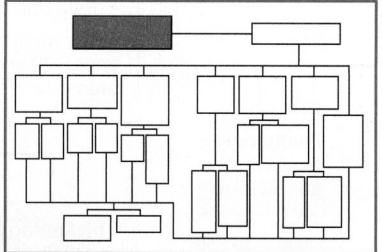
cancer [*see Table 1*]. Some presentations, such as a dominant mass in a postmenopausal woman, are clearly suggestive of malignancy, and their workup is relatively straightforward. Others, such as a tender thickening in a premenopausal woman, usually reflect benign disease. It is important to recognize, however, that any of these presenting symptoms can be associated with a malignancy, and thus all of them warrant a complete evaluation. In fact, it is the evaluation of the usually benign symptoms that places the greatest demands on the physician's clinical judgment. When such symptoms are the main presenting complaint of a breast cancer, their apparently benign nature may be misleadingly reassuring and delay the diagnosis of malignancy.

Risk Factors for Breast Cancer

The central task facing a physician examining a patient with a breast complaint is to determine whether the abnormality is benign or malignant. To this end, knowledge of the main risk factors for breast cancer is essential: prompt identification of the patients at highest risk for malignancy allows the physician to take an appropriately vigorous approach from the beginning of the diagnostic workup.

Various factors that place women at increased risk for breast carcinoma have been identified[1] [*see Table 2*]. These risk factors include increasing age; mutations in breast cancer risk genes (including *BRCA1* and *BRCA2, PTEN,* and *p53*) and other factors related to a family history of breast cancer[2]; hormonal and reproductive factors, including early menarche, late menopause, nulliparity, the absence

of lactation, and the use of exogenous hormones[1,3-9]; environmental factors, including diet and the lifestyle characteristic of developed Western nations[10-12]; certain pathologic findings within breast tissue, including previous breast cancer and various premalignant lesions[13-15]; and certain nonbreast malignancies, including ovarian and endometrial carcinomas. There are also a number of molecular markers that can be correlated with prognosis.

Recognition of risk factors facilitates appropriate screening and clinical management of the individual patient. It is important to recognize, however, that in many women in whom breast cancer develops, known risk factors for breast carcinoma are entirely absent. The absence of these risk factors should not prevent full evaluation or biopsy of a suspicious breast lesion.

Workup of the Patient with a Breast Complaint

Evaluation of any breast problem should include a detailed history of the presenting complaint, previous breast problems, and any risk factors for breast carcinoma;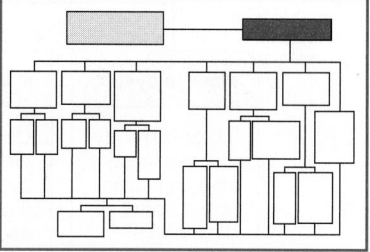
a thorough physical examination of the breasts; appropriate imaging studies; and evaluation of the patient's general medical condition. Particular attention must be paid to any findings that increase the suspicion of malignancy.

HISTORY

The patient should be asked to describe when and how the problem was first identified. Changes in the size or tenderness of any palpable abnormalities since their initial discovery should be recorded, with particular attention paid to any changes that occurred during the menstrual cycle. Previous breast problems or breast operations should be documented, and pathology reports from any such operations should be obtained. All imaging studies or medical evaluations that have already been performed should be reviewed.

Next, those portions of the medical history that bear on the risk of breast cancer should be explored in detail. Age at menarche and either the date of the last menstrual period or, if applicable, age at menopause should be recorded. Parity, age at the first term pregnancy, and duration of lactation should be determined. Any use of exogenous hormones should be recorded, including use of oral contraceptives (with years of use before the first term pregnancy recorded separately), use of postmenopausal estrogen replacement therapy, and use of any other hormones as part of a fertility program or for other purposes.

In addition, any history of breast cancer in family members, up to and including third-degree relatives, should be detailed, and age

Assessment and Management of Breast Complaints

Patient presents with breast complaint

The most common presenting problems are
- Palpable mass • Normal physical examination with abnormal mammogram
- Vague thickening or nodularity • Nipple discharge • Breast pain
- Breast infection or inflammation

Evaluate likelihood that lesion reflects cancer [*see Table 1*], and be aware of patient risk factors for cancer [*see Table 2*].

Palpable mass

Factors increasing suspicion of malignancy:
- Skin dimpling
- Palpable axillary nodes
- Mass with irregular borders
- Increasing age

Determine whether mass is cystic or solid.

Abnormal mammogram after normal breast examination

Factors increasing suspicion of malignancy:
- Previous normal mammogram
- Localized soft tissue mass
- Stellate-appearing lesion
- Clustered microcalcifications

Vague thickening or nodularity

Factors increasing suspicion of malignancy:
- Skin changes
- Asymmetry between right and left breast
- No generic hormonal changes (e.g., pregnancy, beginning or ceasing contraception)
- Palpable axillary nodes

Order mammogram if patient is > 35 yr or > 30 yr with a family history of breast cancer.

Mass is cystic

If fluid is bloody or mass remains after aspiration, obtain tissue diagnosis. If not, follow up as for a simple cyst.

Mass is solid

Obtain tissue diagnosis by means of fine-needle aspiration, core-needle, or open surgical biopsy.

Mammogram is suspicious

Perform biopsy (open or stereotactic or ultrasound-guided core-needle).

Mammogram is not suspicious

Follow up with mammograms every 6 mo for 2 yr.

Thickening is suspicious

Perform open biopsy (FNA is not appropriate).

Thickening is not suspicious

Reexamine patient after 2 menstrual cycles.

If area resolves, provide routine follow-up. If lesion persists or worsens, perform open biopsy.

Malignancy is present

Perform clinical staging.

Consider treatment options.

Initiate definitive therapy for breast cancer.

No malignancy is present

Continue routine screening, as appropriate for patient's age.

Work up patient:
- History, with particular attention to risk factors for breast cancer
- Physical examination
- Imaging studies (e.g., mammography)

Initiate evaluation of specific breast problem.

Nipple discharge

Factors increasing suspicion of malignancy:
- Bloody discharge
- Unilateral discharge
- Palpable mass (see facing page)
- Abnormal mammogram (see facing page)

Breast pain

Factors increasing suspicion of malignancy:
- Abnormal skin changes
- Noncyclic pain

Order mammogram if pain is noncyclic and patient is > 35 yr or > 30 yr with a family history of breast cancer.

Breast infection or inflammation

Factors increasing suspicion of malignancy:
- No elevation of white blood cell count
- No response to antibiotics
- Symptoms not associated with lactation

High-risk patients without symptons

Perform risk assessment (e.g., using Gail or Claus model).

Consider genetic testing for risk gene mutations.

Discuss risk with patient.

Select treatment option:
1. Close surveillance
2. Prophylactic mastectomy
3. Chemoprevention with tamoxifen or participation in chemoprevention trial

Mammogram is abnormal, or palpable mass is detected

Work up as indicated for palpable mass or abnormal mammogram.

Mammogram is normal, and physical examination yields normal results

Offer comfort, reassure, and perform follow-up examination in 2 mo.
If pain resolves or there is still no palpable abnormality, reassure further and follow up routinely. If there is a palpable abnormality, obtain tissue diagnosis.

Discharge is suspicious

Order mammogram. Perform biopsy of any lesions found.
If a single duct is the source of the pathologic discharge, excise duct. If source of discharge can only be localized to a quadrant, excise ducts in that quadrant.

Discharge is not suspicious (physiologic discharge or galactorrhea)

If discharge is physiologic, reassure patient; no further treatment is needed.
If galactorrhea is present, initiate appropriate workup (serum prolactin levels, thyroid function tests, and MRI if necessary).

Patient is lactating

Give oral antibiotics to cover gram-positive cocci, use warm soaks, and attempt to keep breast emptied.

If abscess forms, incise and drain.

Patient is not lactating

Incise and drain any abscesses, and give antibiotics to cover skin organisms (including anaerobes).

If there is no response to short course of antibiotics, rule out inflammatory carcinoma; perform biopsy, including skin. If infection is chronic, excise subareolar duct complex.

207

Table 1   Common Presenting Symptoms of
Breast Disease

Symptom	Likelihood of Malignancy	Risk of Missed Malignancy
Palpable mass	Highest	Lowest
Abnormal mammogram with normal breast examination	↑	
Vague thickening or nodularity		
Nipple discharge		
Breast pain		↓
Breast infection	Lowest	Highest

at diagnosis should be recorded. Similarly, any family history of ovarian cancer or other cancers (particularly those that developed when the relative was young) should be recorded, along with age at diagnosis. Any personal history of cancer should be recorded, with particular attention paid to breast, ovarian, and endometrial cancers. Previous exposure to radiation, especially in the area of the chest wall, should be noted.

Finally, as with any surgical patient, an overview of the general medical history should be obtained that includes current medications, allergies, tobacco and alcohol use, previous surgical procedures, medical problems, and a brief social history.

PHYSICAL EXAMINATION

First, as the patient sits with her hands behind her head and her elbows back, the breasts should be inspected for asymmetry, dimpling of the skin, erythema, or edema. Each breast should then be carefully palpated from the clavicle to below the inframammary fold and from the sternum to the posterior axillary line, with pains taken to include the subareolar area. This is done with the patient both supine and sitting. If an abnormal area is identified, its size, contour, texture, tenderness, and position should be described; a diagram of the lesion is extremely useful for future reference.

Table 2   Risk Factors for Breast Cancer

Increasing age
White race
Age at menarche ≤ 11 years
Age at menopause ≥ 55 years
Nulliparity
Age at first pregnancy ≥ 30 years
Absence of history of lactation
? Prolonged use of oral contraceptives before first pregnancy
Use of postmenopausal estrogen replacement, especially if prolonged
Use of other hormones, fertility regimens, or diethylstilbestrol
Mutations in breast cancer risk genes, including *BRCA1* and *BRCA2*, *PTEN*, and *p53*
Family history of breast cancer: multiple affected relatives, early onset, bilaterality
Family history of ovarian cancer: multiple affected relatives, early onset
Pathologic findings that indicate increased risk (e.g., atypical hyperplasia, lobular carcinoma in situ, proliferative fibrocystic disease)
Previous breast cancer
Previous breast problems
Previous breast operations
Previous exposure to radiation

Next, the nipples and areolae are inspected for skin breakdown and squeezed gently to check for discharge. The number and position of any ducts from which discharge is obtained should be recorded, and the color of the discharge (milky, green, yellow, clear, brown, or bloody) and its consistency (watery, sticky, or thick) should be noted. Discharge on one side calls for a careful search for discharge on the other side because unilateral, single-duct discharge is much more suspicious than bilateral, multiple-duct discharge. Any discharge obtained should be tested for occult blood. Cytologic study of nipple discharge generally is not indicated: it adds expense and rarely contributes significantly to the decision whether biopsy is needed.

Finally, the axillary and supraclavicular nodes are examined bilaterally. If enlarged nodes are discovered, their size, mobility, and number should be recorded. Any matting of nodes or fixation of nodes to the chest walls should also be recorded. Tenderness of enlarged nodes may suggest a reactive process and should therefore be recorded as well.

IMAGING STUDIES

Mammography

According to current recommendations, a baseline screening mammogram need not be performed until 40 (or possibly, as some suggest, until 50[16]) years of age; however, it is reasonable to perform a mammogram to rule out synchronous, nonpalpable lesions whenever a woman older than 35 years presents with a palpable breast mass or other specific symptoms. Approximately 4% to 5% of breast cancers occur in women younger than 40 years, and about 25% occur in women younger than 50 years.[17,18] On the other hand, mammography fails to detect 10% to 15% of all palpable malignant lesions, and its sensitivity is particularly decreased in women with lobular carcinoma or radiographically dense breast tissue. It must therefore be emphasized that a negative mammogram should not influence the decision to perform a biopsy of a clinically palpable lesion. The purpose of mammography is to look for synchronous lesions or nonpalpable calcifications surrounding the palpable abnormality, not to determine whether to perform a biopsy of the palpable lesion.

Ultrasonography

The main value of ultrasonography is in distinguishing cystic from solid lesions. If the lesion is palpable, this distinction is best made by direct needle aspiration, which is both diagnostic and therapeutic; if the lesion is not palpable, ultrasonography can determine whether the lesion is cystic and thus potentially eliminate the need for additional workup or treatment. Ultrasonography has not proved useful for screening: it fails to detect calcifications, misses a large number of malignancies, and identifies a great deal of normal breast texture as potential nodules. It is useful, however, for directing fine-needle or core-needle biopsy of the lesions that it does visualize: it permits real-time manipulation of the needle and direct confirmation of the position of the needle within the lesion. The use of advanced ultrasound technology for diagnostic purposes in the breast is currently being explored.

Magnetic Resonance Imaging

Magnetic resonance imaging after injection of gadolinium contrast enhances many malignant lesions in relation to normal breast parenchyma. Although some benign lesions (e.g., fibroadenomas) are also enhanced by gadolinium, the contrast agent appears to enhance malignant lesions more rapidly and often to a greater extent.

The sensitivity and specificity of MRI in distinguishing benign from malignant lesions are still being assessed. The main approved use of MRI in breast disease is for identification of leaks in silicone breast implants, because MRI can detect the ruptured silicone membrane within the silicone gel. MRI is also useful in identifying occult primary tumors in women who have palpable axillary nodes but no palpable or mammographically identified primary breast lesion. MRI appears to be effective for assessing the extent of vaguely defined tumors, identifying unsuspected multifocal disease, and helping identify patients who are not eligible for breast-conserving surgery. In addition, it appears that MRI can distinguish between a locally recurrent tumor and surgical scarring or radiation change after lumpectomy and radiation, although the technology may not provide reliable readings until 18 months or more after surgery or the completion of radiation therapy. The utility of MRI for screening of young high-risk women with mammographically dense breast tissue is being explored.

Nuclear medicine studies such as sestamibi scintimammography and positron emission tomography (PET) scanning remain primarily investigational tools. There is currently no role for thermography or xerography in the evaluation of breast problems.

Management of Specific Breast Problems

PALPABLE MASS

The workup and management of a discrete breast mass are governed by the age of the patient, the physical characteristics of the palpable lesion, and the patient's medical history.[19] The likelihood of malignancy is 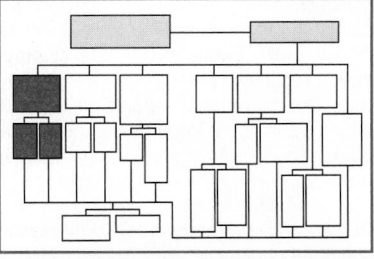 greater when the patient is 40 years of age or older, when the mass has irregular borders, or when skin dimpling or enlarged axillary nodes are present. A prebiopsy mammogram is indicated for women older than 35 years and for those younger than 35 years who have a strong family history of premenopausal breast cancer.

It is important to determine whether the mass is solid or cystic. Cysts are almost always benign; usually, aspiration is all that is required. Solid masses are more likely to be cancerous; a tissue diagnosis must be obtained to rule out malignancy. Clinical examination is not accurate in distinguishing cysts from a solid mass. In one study, only 58% of 66 palpable cysts were correctly identified on physical examination.[20]

Cystic Masses

If it is suspected that a palpable mass is a cyst, the suspicion should generally be confirmed by aspiration, even if ultrasound examination has already shown the mass to be a simple cyst. Aspiration verifies that the palpable mass corresponds to the lesion seen on ultrasonography; it also permits more thorough examination of the surrounding breast tissue. If the cyst fluid is bloody or a mass remains after aspiration, there is a significant chance of malignancy, and the aspirate should be sent for cytologic analysis.[21] At this point, excisional biopsy is generally indicated [see V:2 Breast Procedures], even if the cytologic analysis reveals no malignancy. If the cyst fluid is not bloody and no mass remains after aspiration, there is little chance of malignancy, and the aspirate need not be sent for cytologic analysis.[22,23] In one study, there were no malignancies in 6,747 nonbloody cyst aspirates.[24]

If a cyst is aspirated without having been demonstrated to be a simple cyst by ultrasonography, the patient should be reexamined in 4 to 8 weeks. Fewer than 20% of simple cysts recur after a single as-

piration, and fewer than 9% recur after two or three aspirations.[25] If a cyst recurs rapidly after aspiration, it should be reaspirated and its contents sent for cytologic analysis. If the results of the analysis are suspicious or if the cyst recurs yet again, an excisional biopsy should be performed. If, however, a new cyst appears in a different area of breast tissue, this additional workup is not required, and the new cyst should be evaluated as a new problem. Additional cysts may be expected to occur in more than 50% of patients.[26]

Solid Masses

If a discrete mass in the breast is believed to be solid, either on the basis of ultrasonographic findings or because attempts at aspiration yield no fluid, a tissue diagnosis is necessary to rule out malignancy. Physical examination alone is insufficient: it correctly identifies masses as malignant in only 60% to 85% of cases.[27,28] Furthermore, experienced examiners often disagree on whether biopsy is needed for a particular lesion: in one study, four surgeons unanimously agreed on the necessity of biopsy for only 11 (73%) of 15 palpable masses that were later shown by biopsy to be malignant. Tissue diagnosis may be accomplished by fine-needle aspiration (FNA) biopsy, core-needle biopsy, or open surgical biopsy [see Sidebar Breast Biopsy and V:2 Breast Procedures].

Phyllodes tumors The phyllodes tumor, a mesenchymal tumor limited to mammary tissue, is a rare condition. The tumor is typically smooth, round, firm, well defined, and mobile and causes no pain. It has no pathognomonic mammographic or ultrasonographic features and is difficult, if not impossible, to distinguish from a fibroadenoma on physical examination or radiologic evaluation unless it is quite large. Palpable axillary lymph nodes are encountered in 20% of patients with phyllodes tumors, but histologic evidence of malignancy is encountered in fewer than 5% of axillary lymph node dissections for clinically positive nodes. The remainder of the nodes are enlarged as a result of necrosis of the primary tumor.

Tumors are classified as low, intermediate, or high grade on the basis of five criteria: stromal cellularity, stromal atypia, the microscopic appearance of the tumor margin (infiltrating, effacing, or bulging), mitoses per 10 high-power fields, and the macroscopic size of the tumor. Structural[29] and cytogenetic[30] studies of constituent cells have demonstrated similarities between fibroadenomas and phyllodes tumors, and there is evidence[31] that certain fibroadenomas develop into phyllodes tumors. FNA is usually nondiagnostic, primarily because of the difficulty of obtaining adequate numbers of stromal cells for cytogenic analysis.[32] Although phyllodes tumors have minimal metastatic potential, they have a proclivity for local recurrence and should be excised with a 1 cm margin. Local recurrence has been correlated with excision margins but not with tumor grade or size.[33]

The diagnosis of phyllodes tumor should be considered in all patients with a history of a firm, rounded, well-circumscribed, solid (i.e., noncystic) lesion in the breast. Simple excisional biopsy should be performed if aspiration fails to return cyst fluid or if ultrasonography demonstrates a solid lesion. Because phyllodes tumors mimic fibroadenomas, they are often enucleated or excised with a close margin. If a 1 cm margin is not obtained after examination of the permanent section, the patient should undergo reexcision to obtain wider margins. Otherwise, a recurrence rate of 15% to 20% can be expected. If a simple excision cannot be accomplished without gross cosmetic deformity or if the tumor burden is too large, a simple mastectomy may be performed. Axillary lymph node dissection should be reserved for clinically palpable nodes. Radiation therapy may have a role in patients with chest wall invasion. Chemotherapy, which is reserved for patients with metastatic disease, is based on guidelines for the treatment of sarcomas, rather than breast adenocarcinomas.

Breast Biopsy

Techniques

FINE-NEEDLE ASPIRATION BIOPSY

Fine-needle aspiration (FNA) biopsy with a 22- to 25-gauge needle may be performed with minimal patient discomfort when a palpable mass is identified on physical examination; mammographically or ultrasonographically guided FNA biopsy may also be performed when a nonpalpable lesion is identified. The false negative rate with FNA biopsy ranges from 1% to 35% for palpable lesions[28,110] and may be as high as 68% for nonpalpable lesions.[111] The false positive rate generally ranges from 1% to 2%.[28,109] Nonspecific findings, such as normal or fibrocystic breast tissue, or any atypical findings on cytologic analysis should be evaluated further, usually by means of open surgical biopsy.

CORE-NEEDLE BIOPSY

A second nonsurgical form of breast biopsy is core-needle biopsy. This technique is more uncomfortable for the patient than FNA biopsy because a much larger needle is used and a small nick must be made in the skin. Core-needle biopsy obtains an 11- to 14-gauge cylinder of tissue from the mass being sampled, and the tissue is analyzed by conventional pathology rather than cytology.[112] Core-needle biopsy may be guided by palpation for palpable lesions or by stereotactic mammography or ultrasonography for nonpalpable lesions. As with FNA biopsy, the false positive rate is very low. False negative rates are lower than for FNA biopsy[111-113] but higher with needles smaller than 14 gauge,[112] with freehand rather than image-guided biopsy, and with less experienced operators.

The finding of atypical ductal hyperplasia (ADH) or any equivocal diagnosis with core-needle biopsy necessitates open surgical biopsy to rule out malignancy. A significant number of open biopsies find ductal carcinoma in situ (DCIS) after an initial core-needle biopsy indicates ADH. Core-needle biopsy findings that appear to contradict clinical or mammographic findings should be viewed with suspicion and followed with open surgical biopsy.

The use of core-needle biopsy instead of needle-localized open surgical biopsy for diagnosis of breast cancer can reduce the number of surgical procedures and the cost of diagnosis. In one series,[113] an average of 1.25 open surgical procedures were required for diagnosis of a nonpalpable breast malignancy by core-needle biopsy, compared with an average of nearly two surgical procedures per malignancy when open surgical biopsy was used for diagnosis.

OPEN BIOPSY

Open surgical biopsy remains the gold standard for diagnosis of breast lesions. It has a major advantage over FNA biopsy and core-needle biopsy in that it removes the lesion, thus allowing a more complete pathologic analysis, including analysis of the margins and the extent of intraductal disease in malignant lesions. However, open surgical biopsy costs more, takes more time, and causes more patient discomfort than either FNA or core-needle biopsy.

With palpable lesions, the surgeon should attempt to excise the lesion along with a narrow rim of normal-appearing breast tissue. Because most breast masses prove to be benign, it is important to avoid unnecessary distortion of the breast. With nonpalpable lesions, preoperative wire local-ization is performed to direct the surgeon to the appropriate area. The surgeon then removes tissue around the wire in such a way as to include the lesion along with a rim of normal-appearing breast tissue. A radiograph of the specimen should be obtained before the patient leaves the operating room to confirm that the lesion is contained within the specimen.

Most biopsies, including needle-localized biopsies of nonpalpable lesions, are now performed with the patient under local anesthesia or local anesthesia with sedation; general anesthesia is reserved for special circumstances, such as cases in which multiple biopsies are necessary. The approach to surgical biopsy that once was standard—general anesthesia, frozen section diagnosis, and immediate definitive cancer surgery—has largely been abandoned. In addition to the logistical difficulties this approach poses for both patients and surgeons, it is clear that performing definitive surgery on the same day as biopsy does not improve survival or reduce the incidence of metastasis. Now that multiple treatment options are available for women with breast cancer, a staged approach that allows ample time for discussion of treatment options and decision making after a diagnosis of malignancy is preferred.

Analysis of Tissue

In addition to routine histologic analysis, a number of tests that provide prognostic or therapeutic information are now routinely performed on malignant breast tissue.

HORMONE RECEPTOR LEVELS

Determination of estrogen and progesterone receptor levels in breast carcinomas is essential because these levels predict response to hormone therapy. Furthermore, some studies suggest that patients with estrogen receptor–positive tumors have a better prognosis than patients with estrogen receptor–negative tumors. Receptor levels may be determined by using a competitive binding assay to measure cytosol receptor levels or by performing an immunohistochemical assay in which a monoclonal antibody binds to the receptor.

OTHER MOLECULAR MARKERS AND PROGNOSTIC FACTORS

A number of molecular markers have been identified that may eventually play a role in treating or determining the prognosis for patients with breast cancer. The true clinical value of these markers remains to be determined, but several of them have already been analyzed with the aim of assessing their relevance to the management of breast cancer.[114] At present, the marker with the greatest clinical relevance is HER-2-*neu,* a transmembrane protein thought to be involved in the control of cell growth. The overexpression of HER-2-*neu* appears to be an independent predictor of poor prognosis in breast cancer patients[115,116] and may be a predictor of a favorable response to chemotherapy in node-positive breast cancer patients.[117,118] Antibodies to HER-2-*neu* are available and are being evaluated in the treatment of breast cancers.

The density of neovascularization and the occurrence of cathepsin D, *myc, ras,* and *p53* have been measured in breast tumor specimens[114]; however, these studies are investigational, and their impact on clinical practice remains to be determined. Measurements of **S**-phase fraction and the proliferation marker Ki-67, used to estimate the growth rate of malignant tumors, may not be independent prognostic factors. The DNA content of tumor cells, measured by flow cytometry, does not appear to correlate well with prognosis.

ABNORMAL MAMMOGRAM WITH NORMAL FINDINGS ON PHYSICAL EXAMINATION

Routine mammographic screening has led to increased identification of nonpalpable lesions. The American College of Surgeons Commission on Cancer found that an abnormal screening mammogram was one of the presenting complaints for 56.1% of breast cancers in 1990, compared with 29.6% in 1983.[17] For two thirds of the cancers detected mammographi-cally in 1990, an abnormal mammogram was the only abnormal finding.

Most mammographic abnormalities, however, are not associated with malignancy. In the United States, only 15% to 30% of mammographic lesions for which biopsy is recommended prove to be malignant.[34] Mammographic screening also identifies a number of abnormalities that are less suspicious for malignancy—so-called probably benign lesions. These lesions may be safely followed with mammograms at short intervals (e.g., every 6 months for 2 years), with biopsy reserved for lesions that become more suspicious during follow-up.[35-37] The decision whether to follow or to excise a particular mammographic lesion is based on (1) the mammographic appearance of the lesion, (2) assessment of the patient's risk factors for carcinoma, and (3) the patient's preferences.

In general, whenever the radiologist states that a lesion identified on mammography is suspicious, a tissue diagnosis should be obtained by means of either open needle-localized biopsy or mammographically guided stereotactic core-needle biopsy [see V:2 Breast Procedures]. Findings especially suggestive of malignancy include the presence of a localized soft tissue mass within the breast that either is new or has changed in size or appearance, architectural distortion with irregular borders producing a stellate-appearing lesion, and clustered microcalcifications, with or without a new or changed mass or architectural distortion.

VAGUE THICKENING OR NODULARITY

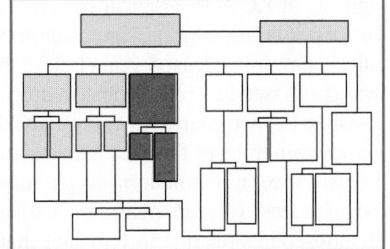

Normal breast texture is often heterogeneous, particularly in premenopausal women. Consequently, vague thickenings or areas of nodularity are frequently found in the breast, sometimes associated with tenderness and sometimes not. These areas must be distinguished from true masses.

In clinical practice, the first step in evaluating a nodular area is to compare it with the corresponding area of the opposite breast. Symmetrical areas of thickening—for example, in the upper outer quadrant of both breasts—are rarely pathologic, particularly those that are tender. These areas often represent fibrocystic changes and may resolve spontaneously. Asymmetrical areas of vague thickening in premenopausal women should be reexamined after one or two menstrual cycles. If the asymmetrical thickening resolves, it was probably caused by a benign process. If the asymmetrical thickening persists, however, the possibility of malignancy is increased, and biopsy should be performed to rule out malignancy. For any woman older than 35 years who has not had a mammogram in the past 6 months, a mammogram should be ordered at this point to rule out synchronous lesions. The value of a negative FNA biopsy in the presence of a vague thickening rather than a discrete mass is questionable. Open biopsy is generally required for adequate sampling.

NIPPLE DISCHARGE

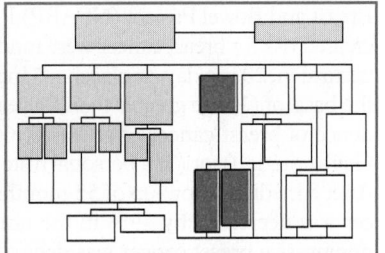

Nipple discharge may be classified as physiologic discharge, pathologic discharge, or galactorrhea. In most instances, it is physiologic—that is, bilateral, nonspontaneous, and arising from multiple ducts. The discharge is usually yellow to green and may be evoked by certain drugs, such as estrogen or tranquilizers, or by sexual stimulation. If physical examination and mammography do not identify a pathologic entity, the patient may be reassured that the discharge is benign, in which case no treatment or additional evaluation is necessary.

Pathologic discharge is spontaneous and is usually unilateral and localized to a single duct. It may be serous, bloody, or brownish. Although the most common causes of bloody nipple discharge are benign intraductal papillomas and duct ectasia, the presence of red blood cells and clusters of ductal cells may suggest malignancy.[38,39] The likelihood of malignancy is increased when the discharge arises in a postmenopausal woman. The workup should include mammography, careful physical examination, and biopsies of any lesions

found. Ductography is rarely useful: it almost never eliminates the need for a surgical procedure and rarely, if ever, changes the extent of the surgical procedure that is required. If a single duct can be identified as the source of the pathologic discharge, it should be excised flush with the nipple; if only the quadrant of the duct can be identified, excision of the major ducts in that quadrant is the procedure of choice [see V:2 Breast Procedures].[40,41]

Galactorrhea is a bilateral discharge that is milky, contains fat, and arises from multiple ducts. As many as one third of women with galactorrhea have pituitary tumors; this is especially likely if they are also amenorrheic. Other causes of galactorrhea are hypothyroidism, chest wall trauma, and certain drugs. The evaluation of galactorrhea includes measurement of serum prolactin levels and thyroid function tests. If the prolactin level is elevated, a magnetic resonance imaging scan of the head, with particular attention to the sella turcica, should be obtained.

BREAST PAIN

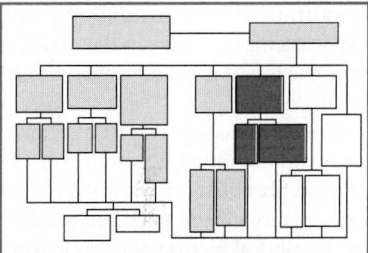

Breast pain, or mastalgia, is one of the most common breast symptoms for which patients consult physicians. At present, the causes of breast pain are poorly understood. Given that it is usually cyclic and typically resolves at menopause, there is reason to believe that it may be of hormonal origin. Several studies, however, have shown no differences in circulating estrogen levels between women with mastalgia and pain-free control subjects. It has been postulated that in women with breast pain, progesterone levels may be decreased or prolactin release may be increased in response to thyrotropin-releasing factor hormone.[42] Although histologic findings consistent with cysts, apocrine metaplasia, and ductal hyperplasia have been noted in the breasts of women with mastalgia, there is no convincing evidence that any of these pathologic changes actually cause breast pain.

In the examination of the patient with breast pain, it is worthwhile to attempt to differentiate between cyclic and noncyclic breast pain and to rule out causes of pain that do not arise from the breast itself. Cyclic breast pain generally is most severe shortly before the menses and is relieved with their onset. Noncyclic pain, on the other hand, bears no relation to the menstrual cycle. Both types of pain may be either intermittent or continuous and may be described by the patient as burning. Mammography and physical examination usually yield normal results in patients with breast pain. The likelihood of malignancy is increased when a patient with mastalgia is postmenopausal and not taking estrogens or when the pain is associated with skin changes or palpable abnormalities; however, these situations are uncommon.

For most women with breast pain, treatment consists of relieving symptoms and reassuring the patient that the workup has not identified an underlying breast carcinoma or another serious disorder. Nonsteroidal anti-inflammatory drugs and supportive bras are helpful. Elimination of caffeine, reduction of salt intake, and the use of diuretics, although generally harmless, have not been proved to be beneficial. Evening primrose oil, taken orally, has been reported to produce significant or complete pain relief in about 50% of women with cyclic mastalgia.[43]

For the rare patients who have severe pain that does not respond to conservative measures, administration of hormones or drugs may be appropriate. Danazol has been successful against breast pain and should be considered the first-line agent, although its androgenic effects may be troubling to many women.[44,45] Bromocriptine (a prolactin antagonist) and tamoxifen have also been used to treat mastalgia.[46,47] Pharmacotherapy for mastalgia is contraindicated in patients who are trying to become pregnant.

BREAST INFECTION OR INFLAMMATION

Infections of the breast fall into two general categories: (1) lactational infections and (2) chronic subareolar infections associated with duct ectasia. These benign infections must be distinguished from inflammatory carcinoma.

Both cellulitis and abscesses may occur in lactating women, often during weaning or at other times when engorgement occurs. In the early stages, infections are treated by giving oral antibiotics that cover gram-positive cocci, applying warm packs to the breast, and actively attempting to keep the breast emptied. Weaning is not necessary: the infant is not adversely affected by nursing from the infected breast.[48,49]

Once a breast abscess forms, however, surgical drainage is necessary, and the infant generally must be weaned. Because of the network of fibrous septa within the breast, breast abscesses in lactating women rarely form fluctuant masses.[48] The diagnosis is established by the clinical picture of fever, leukocytosis, and exquisite point tenderness in the breast. General anesthesia is almost always required for drainage of these abscesses, because of the tenderness of the affected area and the amount of manipulation necessary to break up the loculated abscess cavity adequately. The cavity should be packed open, as with any abscess.

Nonlactational infections of the breast often present as chronic relapsing infections of the subareolar ducts associated with periductal mastitis or duct ectasia. These infections usually involve multiple organisms, including skin anaerobes.[50,51] Retraction or inversion of the nipple, subareolar masses, recurrent periareolar abscesses, or a chronic fistula to the periareolar skin may result,[41,52] as may palpable masses and mammographic changes that mimic carcinoma. In the acute phase of infection, treatment entails incision, drainage, and administration of antibiotics that cover skin organisms, including anaerobes. In cases of repeated infection, the entire subareolar duct complex should be excised after the acute infection has completely resolved, with antibiotic coverage provided during the perioperative period. The necessity of drain placement is debated. Even after wide excision of the subareolar duct complex and intravenous antibiotic coverage, infections recur in some patients; these can be treated by excising the nipple and the areola.[40,53]

HIGH-RISK PATIENTS PRESENTING FOR SCREENING

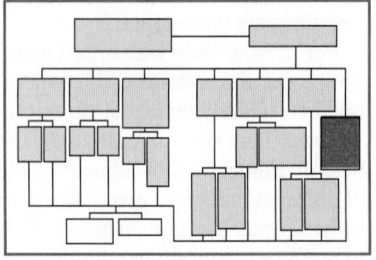

On the basis of established risk factors [see Risk Factors for Breast Cancer, *above, and Table 2*], certain asymptomatic women can be determined to be at increased risk for the development of breast cancer. The risk can be assessed by genetic testing for mutations in breast cancer risk genes or by the use of mathematical models to estimate risk. The Gail model,[54] which relies on data from the Breast Cancer Detection Demonstration Project, and the Claus model,[55] which relies on data from the Cancer and Steroid Hormone Project, are two of the tools that have

been used to make this determination. At present, there are three treatment options for women at high risk for breast cancer: (1) close surveillance, (2) prophylactic mastectomy, and (3) chemoprevention with tamoxifen or other agents in the setting of a clinical trial. Although most women at high risk choose the option of close surveillance, the growing body of data on chemoprevention and prophylactic mastectomy may increase selection of the other two options.

For women with a previous diagnosis of breast cancer, surveillance protocols are described elsewhere [see Management of the Patient with Breast Cancer, Follow-up after Treatment, *below*]. For women with lobular carcinoma in situ (LCIS) or a family history of breast carcinoma, surveillance should include twice-yearly physical examinations. Mammography should be performed annually after the diagnosis of LCIS or atypical hyperplasia. For women with a family history of breast cancer, mammography should be performed annually, beginning at least 5 years before the earliest age at which cancer was diagnosed in a relative and in any case no later than the age of 35 years.[56] For women who carry *BRCA1* or *BRCA2* mutations and other women from families with an autosomal dominant pattern of breast cancer transmission, annual mammographic screening should begin at least 10 years before the earliest age at which the cancer was diagnosed in a relative and no later than 25 years of age.[56]

Long-term results of prophylactic mastectomy in high-risk women[57] indicate that breast cancer risk was reduced by at least 90% in women at high or very high risk who underwent this procedure, compared with women who did not, with risk predicted by the Gail model.[54] Mathematical modeling suggests that prophylactic mastectomy could translate into improved survival for women at very high risk if it confers a 90% reduction in risk.[58]

Chemoprevention may be defined as the use of nutrients or pharmacologic agents to augment physiologic mechanisms that protect against the development of malignancy. Chemopreventive strategies are designed either to block the initiation of the carcinogenic process or to prevent (or reverse) the progression of the premalignant cell to an invasive cancer.[59] Chemoprevention began with the development of the antiestrogen tamoxifen. Whereas the efficacy of tamoxifen in estrogen receptor (ER)–positive breast cancer patients has been recognized for some time, its chemopreventive potential has only recently been established.

The first—and still the most extensive—study to be published on breast cancer chemoprevention was the National Surgical Adjuvant Breast and Bowel Project (NSABP) P-1 trial, in which women at increased risk for breast cancer were randomly assigned to receive either tamoxifen, 20 mg/day, or placebo.[60] Increased risk was determined on the basis of (1) age greater than 60 years, (2) a 5-year predicted incidence of breast cancer of at least 1.66% (determined according to Gail's criteria[54]), or (3) a personal history of lobular carcinoma in situ. After a median follow-up of 55 months, the overall risk of breast cancer was decreased by 49% in the tamoxifen group, and the risk of noninvasive breast cancer was decreased by 50%. The reduction in breast cancer risk was limited to ER-positive breast cancers. Several adverse side effects were noted in the tamoxifen group, the most worrisome of which were a threefold increase in the incidence of endometrial cancer, a higher incidence of deep vein thrombosis and pulmonary embolism, and a higher incidence of stroke. Although two subsequent trials, one from the United Kingdom[61] and one from Italy,[62] did not confirm these findings, the FDA found the results of the NSABP P-1 trial to be compelling enough to warrant approval of tamoxifen as a chemopreventive agent in high-risk women. As of June 2002, a fourth randomized trial of tamoxifen chemoprevention, the International Breast Cancer Intervention Study, is still in progress.

Concerns about the side effects of tamoxifen have generated growing interest in the use of selective estrogen receptor modulators (SERMs) as chemopreventive agents.[63] It appears possible that such so-called designer estrogens may have fewer side effects than tamoxifen while reducing the rate of new breast cancers and lowering the incidence of osteoporosis and cardiovascular disease. One of the SERMs, raloxifene, has been approved by the FDA for the treatment of postmenopausal osteoporosis and is known also to exert beneficial effects on lipid profiles. Unlike tamoxifen, raloxifene appears not to have stimulatory effects on the endometrium.[63] Moreover, the Multiple Outcomes of Raloxifene Evaluation (MORE) trial found that fewer breast cancers were noted in women treated with raloxifene than would have been expected without such treatment.[64]

On the basis of findings from osteoporosis trials, the NSABP incorporated raloxifene into an extensive multi-institutional chemoprevention trial that began enrolling patients in 1999. The Study of Tamoxifen and Raloxifene (STAR) trial is a randomized, double-blind trial whose purpose is to compare the effectiveness of raloxifene with that of tamoxifen in postmenopausal women at increased risk for breast cancer. Entry criteria are similar to those for the NSABP P-1 study. A total of 22,000 postmenopausal high-risk women will be randomly assigned to receive either tamoxifen, 20 mg/day orally, or raloxifene, 60 mg/day orally, for 5 years.

There are a number of newer agents that may possess some capacity for breast cancer chemoprevention. Aromatase inhibitors, which have been used as second-line therapies after tamoxifen in cases of advanced breast cancer, may exert chemopreventive effects by inhibiting parent estrogens and their catechol metabolites, thereby preventing cancer initation.[65] In addition, gonadotropin-releasing hormone agonists, monoterpenes, isoflavones, retinoids, rexinoids, vitamin D derivatives, and inhibitors of tyrosine kinase are all undergoing evaluation in clinical or preclinical studies with a view to assessing their potential chemopreventive activity.[66] Whether any of these compounds will play a clinically useful role in preventing breast cancer remains to be seen.

Management of the Patient with Breast Cancer

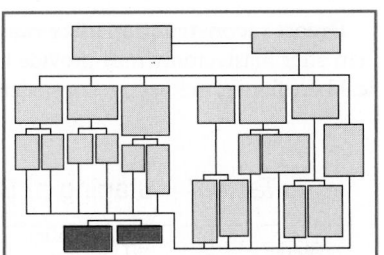

STAGING

In patients with newly diagnosed breast cancer, it is important to determine the overall extent of disease before embarking on definitive therapy. This process, referred to as clinical staging, includes (1) physical examination to identify any areas of palpable disease in the breasts or the axillary and supraclavicular nodes, along with a detailed clinical history to identify symptoms that may suggest metastatic disease; (2) imaging studies, including mammography, chest x-ray, and, sometimes, bone scans or CT scans of the chest, the abdomen, or the head; and (3) laboratory studies, including a complete blood count (CBC) and liver function tests. Several clinical staging systems for breast cancer are currently in use [see Tables 3 and 4].

The extent of preoperative staging should be guided by the size and other characteristics of the primary tumor and by the patient's history and physical examination. For patients with early-stage cancer and a low probability of metastatic disease, extensive testing adds cost without offering much benefit and should therefore be discouraged. For patients with stage I or II disease, a CBC, liver function tests, and a chest x-ray should be performed before defini-

tive surgical therapy is initiated, and imaging studies should be reserved for patients who have abnormal test results or clinical symptoms that suggest metastatic disease (e.g., bone pain). For patients with higher-stage disease at presentation, the use of additional staging studies should be guided by the patient's clinical situation.

TREATMENT OPTIONS

Mastectomy versus Limited Surgery

Clinical trials in the 1970s and 1980s clearly demonstrated that in eligible women with stage I and II breast carcinoma, limited surgery—consisting of lumpectomy or quadrantectomy, axillary dissection, and radiation—yielded overall survival rates that were equivalent to those achieved with radical or modified radical mastectomy.[67-70] Certain categories of patients are now widely considered to be eligible for breast conservation and radiation therapy [see Table 5]: not only are long-term survival rates after breast conservation with limited surgery identical to those achieved with mastectomy in these groups, but local recurrence rates are low as well (5% to 10%). Approximately two thirds of all women with breast cancer are eligible for breast conservation. Nevertheless, many eligible women in the United States are still treated with mastectomy.[71-75] When a patient is eligible for limited surgery, the decision between mastectomy and breast conservation with radiation therapy is made on the basis of patient and physician preference, access or lack of access to radiation therapy, and the presence or absence of contraindications to breast conservation.

Contraindications to breast conservation There remain patients for whom mastectomy is still clearly the treatment of choice. These patients fall into four broad categories: (1) those in whom radiation therapy is contraindicated, (2) those in whom lumpectomy would have an unacceptable cosmetic result, (3) those for whom local recurrence is a concern, and (4) those high-risk patients in whom surgical prophylaxis is appropriate [see Management of Specific Breast Problems, High-Risk Patients Presenting for Screening, above].

Radiation therapy may be contraindicated for any of several reasons. Some patients choose not to undergo radiation therapy, either because it is inconvenient or because they are concerned about potential complications (including the induction of second malignancies). Some patients simply do not have access to radiation therapy, either because they live in a rural area or because they have physical conditions that make daily trips for therapy cumbersome. Other patients have medical or psychiatric disorders that would make it extremely difficult for them to comply with the daily treatment schedule. Still others have specific medical contraindications to radiation therapy, including pregnancy, collagen vascular disease, or previous irradiation of the chest wall (as in a woman with a local recurrence of a breast carcinoma that was treated with radiation therapy). Although there are some clinical data supporting the use of repeat local excision without further irradiation to treat local recurrence after radiation therapy, most authorities favor mastectomy.[76,77]

When resection of the primary tumor to clean margins would render the appearance of the remaining breast tissue cosmetically unacceptable, mastectomy with immediate reconstruction may be preferable. This is likely to be the case, for example, in patients with large primary tumors relative to their breast size: resection of the primary tumor would remove a substantial portion of the breast tissue. Another example is patients with multiple primary tumors, who would have not only an increased risk of local recurrence but also poor cosmetic results after multiple wide excisions. Patients with superficial central lesions, including Paget disease, are eligible for wide excision (including the nipple and areola) followed by radi-

Table 3 TNM Clinical Classification of Breast Cancer[119]

Tumor (T)

TX	Primary tumor cannot be assessed
T0	No evidence of primary tumor
Tis	Carcinoma in situ: intraductal carcinoma, lobular carcinoma in situ, or Paget disease of the nipple with no invasive tumor
T1	Tumor ≤ 2 cm in greatest dimension
	T1mic: Microinvasion ≤ 0.1 cm
	T1a: Tumor > 0.1 cm and ≤ 0.5 cm
	T1b: Tumor > 0.5 cm and ≤ 1.0 cm
	T1c: Tumor > 1 cm and ≤ 2 cm
T2	Tumor > 2 cm and ≤ 5 cm in greatest dimension
T3	Tumor > 5 cm in greatest dimension
T4	Tumor of any size; direct extension to chest wall or skin
T4a	Extension to chest wall
T4b	Edema (including *peau d'orange*) or ulceration of the skin of the breast or satellite skin nodules confined to the same breast
T4c	Both T4a and T4b
T4d	Inflammatory carcinoma

Nodes (N)

NX	Regional lymph nodes cannot be assessed (e.g., previously removed)
N0	No regional lymph node metastases
N1	Metastasis to movable ipsilateral axillary node(s)
N2	Metastasis to ipsilateral axillary node(s) fixed to one another or other structures
N3	Metastasis to ipsilateral internal mammary lymph node(s)

Metastasis (M)

MX	Presence of distant metastasis cannot be assessed
M0	No distant metastases
M1	Distant metastasis, including metastasis to ipsilateral supraclavicular lymph node(s)

ation therapy, provided that clean margins are obtained. The survival and local recurrence rates in these patients are equivalent to those in other groups of patients undergoing lumpectomy and radiation.[78-80] In many cases, the cosmetic results of this procedure are preferable to those of immediate reconstruction, and there is always the option to reconstruct the nipple and areola later.

Patients who are at high risk for local recurrence often choose mastectomy as primary therapy. Features of primary tumors that are associated with higher local recurrence rates after limited surgery and radiation include gross residual disease after lumpectomy, multiple primary tumors within the breast, an extensive intraductal component, large tumor size, lymphatic vessel invasion, and lobular histologic findings.

In practice, obtaining clean margins is probably the most critical factor in decreasing the risk of local recurrence. The difficulty of obtaining microscopically clean margins in tumors with an extensive intraductal component and in lobular carcinomas may account for the higher local recurrence rates sometimes seen with these tumors. Histologic analysis of mastectomy specimens from patients with tumors with an extensive intraductal component has shown a high rate of multifocality within ipsilateral breast tissue; this residual disease is thought to be the nidus for local recurrence.[81]

The long-term benefits of choosing mastectomy to reduce local recurrences are not clear. Whereas the appearance of distant metastases typically heralds incurable and ultimately fatal disease, local recurrence after breast conservation appears to have little, if any, impact on overall survival. Prospective, randomized trials have had difficulty showing a statistically significant reduction in survival in women who have had a local recurrence after limited surgery and radiation. It has been suggested that additional follow-up may eventually confirm reduced survival in some patients with local recurrences.[82] Still, most of the evidence suggests that local recurrences are not the source of subsequent distant metastases. It is worthwhile to keep in mind, however, that even if mastectomy to prevent local recurrence does not actually improve survival, it may nevertheless provide significant benefit by reducing patient anxiety, the amount of follow-up testing required, and the need for subsequent treatment.

Options for axillary staging Axillary node status is one of the most powerful predictors of prognosis in breast cancer. Staging of the axilla, generally via a level I or II axillary dissection, has been a standard component of breast cancer surgery. Decisions about systemic and radiation therapy are often made on the basis of the number of axillary nodes involved by metastatic disease. The value of axillary dissection has been questioned, however, because of the increased use of systemic therapy even for many node-negative breast cancers as well as the morbidity associated with axillary dissection, including pain, reduced arm mobility, and the risk of lymphedema.

As an alternative to axillary dissection, sentinel lymph node (SLN) biopsy [*see V:3 Lymphatic Mapping and Sentinel Lymph Node Biopsy*] has become increasingly popular as a way of assessing axillary node status with less morbidity.[83,84] The technique is technically demanding, however, and discussion continues as to the most appropriate way of implementing this approach in general practice.[85] SLN biopsy identifies an increased number of patients with micrometastases, with some identified by immunohistochemical staining alone. Treatment of patients with only micrometastases to axillary nodes remains a topic of debate, to be addressed in an ongoing clinical trial of SLN biopsy by the American College of Surgeons Oncology Group.

Breast reconstruction after mastectomy Breast reconstruction after mastectomy may provide both cosmetic and psychological benefits. In the past, reconstruction was generally delayed for

Table 4 Staging of Breast Cancer[119]

Stage	T	N	M
Stage 0	Tis	N0	M0
Stage I	T1	N0	M0
Stage IIA	T0	N1	M0
	T1	N1	M0
	T2	N0	M0
Stage IIB	T2	N1	M0
	T3	N0	M0
Stage IIIA	T0	N2	M0
	T1	N2	M0
	T2	N2	M0
	T3	N1, N2	M0
Stage IIIB	T4	Any N	M0
	Any T	N3	M0
Stage IV	Any T	Any N	M1

1 to 2 years after mastectomy; now, it is most often performed immediately after mastectomy.[17] This change has not been shown to have any serious adverse effects: it has not significantly increased recurrence or shortened survival, nor has it significantly delayed the detection of local recurrence or the administration of adjuvant chemotherapy.[86] Reconstruction options [see V:2 Breast Procedures] include the placement of subpectoral saline implants (either immediately or after tissue expansion), latissimus dorsi myocutaneous flap reconstruction, and transverse rectus abdominis muscle myocutaneous flap reconstruction. Free flaps may also be employed under special circumstances.

Radiation Therapy

Current radiation therapy regimens consist of the delivery of approximately 5,000 cGy to the whole breast at a dosage of approximately 200 cGy/day, along with, in most cases, the delivery of an additional 1,000 to 1,500 cGy to the tumor bed, again at a dosage of 200 cGy/day. Axillary node fields are not irradiated unless there is evidence that the patient is at high risk for axillary relapse—namely, multiple (generally more than four) positive lymph nodes, extranodal extension of tumor, or bulky axillary disease (i.e., palpable nodes several centimeters in diameter). Because the combination of surgical therapy and radiation therapy increases the risk of lymphedema of the arm, it is appropriate only when there is sufficient risk of axillary relapse to justify the increased complication rate. As a rule, supraclavicular node fields are irradiated only in patients with multiple positive axillary nodes, who are at increased risk for supraclavicular disease. The internal mammary nodes are seldom irradiated prophylactically.

Postmastectomy radiation therapy involves the delivery of radiation to the chest wall after mastectomy; it is mainly reserved for patients with T3 or T4 primary tumors or multiple positive lymph nodes. Such therapy is recommended particularly when there are multiple positive axillary lymph nodes: significant axillary disease predicts higher rates of chest wall recurrence after mastectomy. Two series[87,88] have suggested that postmastectomy radiation therapy significantly improves survival in premenopausal women with any positive axillary nodes.

Irradiation of the breast or chest wall is generally well tolerated: most women experience only minor side effects, such as transient skin erythema, mild skin desquamation, and mild fatigue. Because a small amount of lung volume is included in the irradiated fields, there is usually a clinically insignificant but measurable reduction in pulmonary function. In addition, because the heart receives some radiation when the left breast or left chest wall is treated, there may be a slightly increased risk of future myocardial infarction. There is also a 1% to 2% chance that the radiation will induce a second malignancy (sarcoma, leukemia, or a second breast carcinoma). These radiation-induced malignancies appear after a long lag time, generally 7 to 15 years or longer.

Systemic Drug and Hormone Therapy

Despite the success of surgical treatment and radiation therapy in achieving local control of breast cancer, distant metastases still develop in many patients. Various drugs and hormones have therefore been used to treat both measurable and occult metastatic disease. It became clear in early trials that multiple-agent (or combination) chemotherapy was superior to single-agent chemotherapy.[89,90] It also became clear that chemotherapy and hormone therapy were limited in their ability to control large tumor masses, although on occasion, patients with large tumor masses showed dramatic partial responses or even complete responses to therapy.

Table 5 Determinants of Patient Eligibility for Lumpectomy and Radiation Therapy

Primary tumor ≤ 5 cm (may be larger in selected cases)
Tumor of lobular or ductal histology
Any location of primary within breast if lumpectomy to clean margins (including central lesions) will yield acceptable cosmetic results
Clinically suspicious but mobile axillary nodes
Tumor either positive or negative for estrogen and progesterone receptors
Any patient age

With the goal of eradicating breast cancer metastases while they are still microscopic, systemic therapy is now administered in a so-called adjuvant setting—that is, when there is no evidence of distant metastases but there is sufficient suspicion that metastasis may have occurred. Until the late 1980s, adjuvant chemotherapy was given primarily to women who had axillary node metastases but no other evidence of disease.[89,91,92] In node-positive premenopausal women, adjuvant chemotherapy appeared to be significantly more beneficial than adjuvant hormone therapy. In node-positive postmenopausal women, on the other hand, hormone therapy appeared to be as beneficial as chemotherapy and less toxic.[91]

This approach to adjuvant systemic therapy changed in 1988, when the National Cancer Institute issued a clinical alert stating that there was sufficient evidence of benefit to allow recommendation of adjuvant chemotherapy or hormone therapy for even node-negative breast cancer patients.[93] By that time, a number of studies had shown that adjuvant chemotherapy could improve survival in node-negative breast cancer patients.[92-95] A consensus conference of experts in the field suggested that such therapy be reserved for node-negative women with primary tumors larger than 1 cm in diameter.[96] In 1992, a meta-analysis that reviewed the treatment of 75,000 women in 133 randomized clinical trials of adjuvant therapy for breast cancer concluded that in node-negative premenopausal women, overall long-term survival was 20% to 30% higher in those who received chemotherapy than in those who did not.[97] This benefit also appeared to extend to postmenopausal women between 50 and 60 years of age. A 1998 overview of the use of adjuvant tamoxifen in randomized trials[98] demonstrated that in women with ER-positive tumors, those given tamoxifen for 5 years had a 47% reduction in tumor recurrence and a 26% reduction in mortality, compared with those women who were given placebo. In this analysis, the effects of tamoxifen on recurrence and survival were independent of age and menopausal status. Tamoxifen did not appear to improve survival, however, in women with ER-negative tumors. These results, together with data on the efficacy of tamoxifen for chemoprevention, have led to increased use of tamoxifen for premenopausal women and for women with small tumors.

TREATMENT OF NONINVASIVE CANCER

Ductal Carcinoma in Situ

Before mammographic screening was widely practiced, ductal carcinoma in situ (DCIS) was generally identified either as a palpable lesion (usually with comedo histology) or as an incidental finding on a biopsy performed for another lesion. With the increasing use of mammography, DCIS is accounting for a growing proportion of breast cancer cases. The diagnosis of DCIS is now made in 6.6% of all needle-localized breast biopsies and 1.4% of breast bi-

Figure 1   **Algorithm illustrates the approach to managing ductal carcinoma in situ.**

opsies for palpable lesions. About 30% of all mammographically detected malignancies are DCIS.[14]

It was recognized early on that DCIS had a very favorable prognosis compared with other forms of breast cancer: long-term survival approached 100% after treatment with mastectomy. Axillary lymph nodes were positive in only 1% to 2% of patients, most of whom had large or palpable lesions or comedo histology. The prognosis for DCIS continues to be very favorable in relation to that for invasive breast cancers. In theory, there is no potential for metastatic disease with a purely in situ lesion. In practice, however, axillary node metastases continue to be found in 1% to 2% of patients thought to have pure DCIS, presumably arising from a small area of invasion that was missed on pathologic evaluation.

DCIS is believed to be a true anatomic precursor of invasive breast cancer. There are at least two lines of evidence that support this conclusion. First, when DCIS is treated with biopsy alone (usually because it was missed on the initial biopsy and not found until subsequent review), invasive carcinoma develops in 25% to 50% of patients at the site of the initial biopsy; all these tumors appear within 10 years and are of ductal histology. Second, when DCIS recurs locally after breast conservation, invasive ductal carcinoma appears in about 50% of patients. The true relationship between DCIS and invasive ductal carcinoma awaits a better understanding of the molecular biology of breast cancer development.

The consequence of the view that DCIS is a precursor of invasive cancer is that treatment is required once the diagnosis is made. Treatment options for DCIS are similar to those for invasive breast cancer [*see Figure 1*]; however, it should be remembered that although the risk of local recurrence is greater after breast conservation for DCIS than after mastectomy, the likelihood of metastatic disease is very small. Wide excision to microscopically clean margins fol-

lowed by radiation therapy has become an accepted alternative to mastectomy. Smaller areas of DCIS, particularly of low to intermediate nuclear grade, are increasingly treated with wide excision without radiation.[99] If clean margins cannot be obtained or if the cosmetic result is expected to be poor after excision to clean margins, mastectomy should be performed. The NSABP B-17 study,[100] which examined the role of radiation in the treatment of DCIS, found that the addition of radiation therapy to wide excision reduced the recurrence rate at 43 months after operation by approximately half, from 16.4% with wide excision alone to 7.0% with wide excision and radiation. The report also suggested that the addition of radiation therapy may reduce the incidence of invasive recurrences.

Most patients in whom DCIS is identified mammographically can choose between mastectomy and wide excision with or without radiation, either of which yields excellent long-term survival. Given the lack of any significant difference in survival between the two options, the patient must weigh her feelings about the risk of a local, possibly invasive, recurrence after breast conservation against her feelings about the cosmetic and psychological effects of mastectomy. Mastectomy remains a reasonable treatment even for patients with very small DCIS lesions if the primary concern is to maximize local control of the cancer. Breast reconstruction after mastectomy for DCIS is an option that is open to most such patients.

Axillary dissection is not usually performed in conjunction with lumpectomy for DCIS, because the probability of positive nodes is low: it increases morbidity and expense while providing little prognostic information. On the other hand, low axillary dissection is often included in mastectomy for DCIS: a level I axillary dissection adds little morbidity to a mastectomy, and many surgeons believe that dissection must be carried into the low axilla to ensure that the entire axillary tail of the breast is removed.

In some patients with areas of mammographically detected DCIS lesions measuring less than 2.5 cm in diameter, it may be possible to omit radiation therapy, particularly if the lesions do not have comedo histology. Omission of radiation therapy is a complex decision that should be based on the individual patient's histology, the presence or absence of other risk factors, the presence or absence of contraindications to radiation therapy, and the degree to which the patient is willing to accept a higher local recurrence rate. This option is probably best pursued in the context of a clinical trial.

There are certain patients with DCIS for whom mastectomy remains the preferred treatment, such as those who have lesions larger than 5 cm in diameter. Some surgeons would also include those who have comedo lesions larger than 2.5 cm and those who present with palpable DCIS in this category. In these patients, the local recurrence rate after breast conservation, even in conjunction with radiation therapy, remains high. As many as half of these recurrences will contain invasive cancer with metastatic potential. These also are the DCIS patients who are at highest risk for positive axillary nodes. For this reason, an axillary node sampling is often performed in conjunction with the mastectomy.

Lobular Carcinoma in Situ

LCIS, also referred to as lobular neoplasia,[101] does not have the same clinical implications as DCIS, invasive ductal carcinoma, or invasive lobular carcinoma. It is now generally accepted that LCIS is a predictor of increased risk of subsequent invasive breast carcinoma rather than a marker of the site at which the subsequent carcinoma will arise.[13,14] Most of the carcinomas that develop after a biopsy showing LCIS are of ductal histology.[102-104] The increased risk of subsequent carcinoma is equally distributed between the biopsied breast and the contralateral breast and is thought to be between 20% and 25% in patients with LCIS and no other risk factors; it may be additive with other risk factors [see Risk Factors for Breast Cancer, *above*]. Because the two breasts are at equal risk for future carcinoma, unilateral mastectomy is inappropriate. Appropriate treatment options include (1) careful observation coupled with physical examination two or three times annually and mammograms annually, (2) prophylactic bilateral simple mastectomies with or without reconstruction, and (3) chemoprevention with tamoxifen or participation in chemoprevention trials with other agents. Most patients choose the first option, but there are some patients for whom prophylactic mastectomy is still preferable, either because of patient anxiety or because of concurrent risk factors.[105]

Management of tumors that contain LCIS mixed with invasive carcinoma of either lobular or ductal histology is dictated primarily by the features of the invasive carcinoma. Staging is not affected by the presence of LCIS.

TREATMENT OF INVASIVE CANCER

Although the optimal treatment regimen for breast cancer continues to be the subject of active investigation, there is at least a par-

Figure 2 **Algorithm illustrates the approach to managing early-stage invasive breast cancer.**

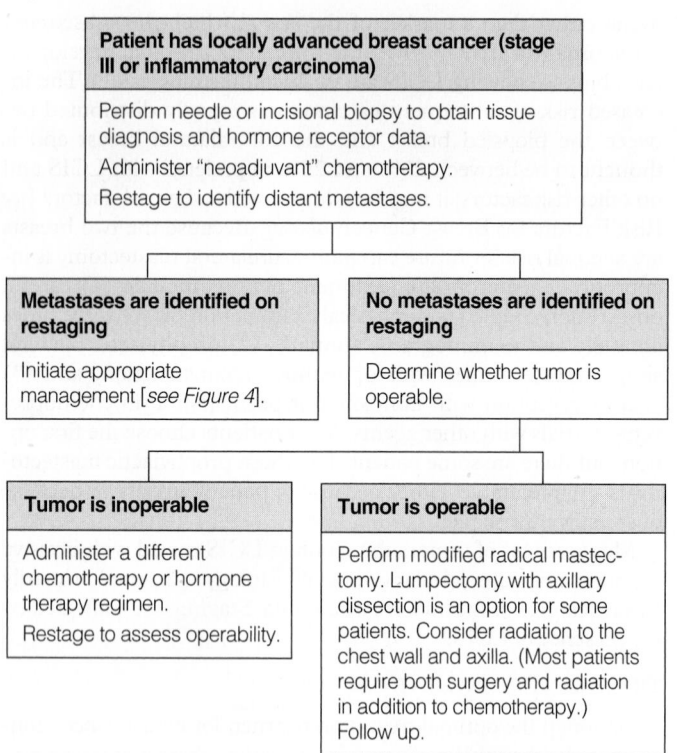

Figure 3 Algorithm illustrates the approach to managing locally advanced breast cancer.

tial consensus regarding current treatment options for the various stages of breast cancer.

Early-Stage Invasive Cancer

Local treatment In patients with stage I or II breast cancer, lumpectomy to microscopically clean margins combined with axillary dissection and radiation therapy [*see Figure 2*] appears to yield approximately the same long-term survival rates as mastectomy. Patients undergoing lumpectomy and radiation are, however, at risk for local recurrence in the treated breast as well as for the development of a new primary tumor in the remaining breast tissue. Local recurrences can generally be managed with mastectomy; overall survival is equivalent to that of women who underwent mastectomy at the time of initial diagnosis. There may, however, be a significant cost to the patient in terms of anxiety about recurrence, as well as the morbidity and potential mortality associated with undergoing a second surgical procedure.

On the other hand, patients who choose mastectomy as their initial surgical treatment face the psychological consequences of losing a breast. Although they are at lower risk for local recurrence than patients who choose lumpectomy, axillary node dissection, and radiation, their overall survival does not seem to be significantly improved. Each physician and each patient must weigh the inconvenience and potential complications of radiation therapy and the risk of local recurrence against the value of breast preservation, keeping in mind that the choice between procedures appears to have no significant effect on survival.

Adjuvant therapy It is generally agreed that adjuvant chemotherapy, adjuvant hormone therapy, or both should be considered for all women with tumors larger than 1 cm in diameter, even those with negative axillary lymph nodes.[96,97] For patients with tumors that have a very favorable prognosis (i.e., that are smaller than 1 cm or have a fa-

vorable histology), the potential benefits of adjuvant therapy are probably outweighed by its risks. Tamoxifen therapy is now being reconsidered for women with such low-risk tumors, given the data on the efficacy of this agent for both treatment and prevention of breast cancers.[98] In premenopausal women, adjuvant therapy should consist of combination chemotherapy, with hormone therapy reserved for clinical trials; in postmenopausal women, hormone therapy (generally consisting of tamoxifen, 10 mg twice daily) is the first-line treatment. Currently, however, the idea that menopause should be an absolute cutoff point for consideration of chemotherapy is being reassessed. For healthy postmenopausal women, particularly those between 50 and 60 years of age, the decision between hormone therapy and chemotherapy plus hormone therapy is made on an individual basis and takes into account the woman's overall health and the specifics of her tumor.

In cases of node-positive disease, combination chemotherapy is used for premenopausal women and for healthy postmenopausal women up to 60 years of age or even older. Hormone therapy is generally the treatment of choice in postmenopausal women who are older than 60 years and in poor health, particularly those with ER-positive tumors. There is currently renewed interest in other hormonal manipulations, such as oophorectomy and chemical castration, for premenopausal women who are at high risk for metastatic disease.[106]

Locally Advanced Cancer

Patients with locally advanced breast cancer include those with primary tumors larger than 5 cm (particularly those with palpable axillary lymph nodes), those with fixed or matted N2 axillary nodes, and those with inflammatory breast carcinoma. These patients are at high risk for systemic disease as well as for local failure after standard local therapy. Current practice is to administer multimodality therapy, with chemotherapy as the first treatment modality [*see Figure 3*]. This so-called neoadjuvant chemotherapy often has the effect of downstaging local disease, in some cases making inoperable tumors amenable to surgical resection. Patients are treated with FNA, core-needle, or open incisional biopsy to obtain a tissue diagnosis, hormone receptor data, and HER-2/*neu* status; they then undergo careful restaging after systemic therapy to identify any distant metastases. If the tumor responds to chemotherapy, the patient may then undergo radiation therapy, surgery, or both. Most patients require all three modalities for optimum local and systemic control.

The optimum treatment of patients with stage IIIa breast cancer remains controversial. Some practitioners favor neoadjuvant chemotherapy, whereas others favor surgery followed by chemotherapy and radiation therapy. The choice of surgical procedure for women with locally advanced breast cancer is also controversial. Whereas many surgeons favor mastectomy for all tumors larger than 5 cm, others offer wide excision with axillary dissection to patients in whom excision to clean margins will leave a cosmetically acceptable breast.

Stage IV Cancer

Patients who have distant metastases, whether at their initial presentation or after previous treatment for an earlier-stage breast cancer, are rarely cured. Before treatment begins, a tissue diagnosis consistent with breast cancer must be obtained from the primary lesion (at the initial presentation of the disease) or from a metastasis (if there is any doubt about the metastatic nature of the lesion or the source of the metastatic disease). Any tissue samples obtained should be sent for estrogen and progesterone receptor assays.

The usual first-line treatment for metastatic breast cancer is cytotoxic chemotherapy or hormone therapy [*see Figure 4*]. Radiation therapy may be used to relieve pain from bone metastases or to avert a pathologic fracture at a site of metastatic disease. There is also occasionally a role for so-called toilet mastectomy for patients who have metastatic disease and a locally advanced and ulcerated primary tumor if the condition of the primary tumor prevents the administration of needed chemotherapy.

Treatment for stage IV breast cancer should be on protocol whenever possible. For patients who are ineligible for therapy on protocol, palliative chemotherapy or hormone therapy may be the best treatment option.

FOLLOW-UP AFTER TREATMENT

Patients who have been treated for breast cancer remain at risk for both the recurrence of their original tumor and the development of a new primary breast cancer. The rate of recurrence of breast cancer is nearly linear over the first 10 years after treatment. After the first decade, recurrence becomes less likely, but it continues at a significant rate through the second decade and beyond. In patients who have undergone limited surgery and radiation therapy, radiation-induced breast and chest wall malignancies begin to appear 7 or more years after treatment and continue to appear for at least 20 years after treatment.

Follow-up of breast cancer patients thus includes screening of the breasts and nodal areas for locoregional recurrence or a new primary tumor by means of physical examination and mammography. There is no general agreement on the optimum intervals for follow-up. For patients treated with breast conservation, annual mammography is appropriate, beginning after any acute radiation reaction has resolved (generally 6 to 9 months after completion of radiation therapy). For patients treated with mastectomy, mammography should be continued on an annual basis for the contralateral breast. Physical examination and review of symptoms are generally performed at 3- to 6-month intervals for the first 5 years after completion of therapy, although these intervals have not yet been tested in a prospective fashion.

Although there has been little debate about the value of early detection of a local recurrence within the treated breast or of a new primary tumor in either breast, there has been a great deal of debate about the value of early detection of metastatic disease. Two prospective, randomized trials addressed this issue. In one, a group of breast cancer patients was intensively followed with blood tests every 3 months along with chest x-rays, bone scans, and liver ultrasonography annually.[107] There was no difference in survival or quality of life between this group and the control group, and metastatic disease was diagnosed, on average, less than 1 month earlier in the intensively followed group than in the control group. In the second study, a group of breast cancer patients received chest x-rays and bone scans every 6 months for 5 years.[108] Pulmonary and bone metastases were detected significantly earlier in this group than in the control group, but there was no improvement in survival. This study demonstrated that early detection of metastatic disease could be achieved with short-interval screening, but given current therapeutic options, early detection had no beneficial effect on survival. Both studies concluded that at present, there is no role for routine imaging studies in the follow-up of breast cancer patients and that imaging studies should be ordered only as prompted by clinical findings.

FUTURE DIRECTIONS IN TREATMENT

Efforts continue to be made to minimize the number and extent of invasive treatments for breast cancer without compromising survival or local control. Trials are now under way whose aim is to explore the need for radiation therapy for tumors in elderly women or tumors consisting of pure DCIS. The need for axillary dissection has been questioned, and the idea that features of the primary tumor rather than axillary node status should be

used to determine the prognosis and the need for adjuvant therapy is being discussed. Trials of SLN biopsy are under way.

Many current trials of chemotherapy for breast cancer focus on increasing the efficacy of treatment through dose intensification. Very high dose chemotherapy in conjunction with administration of growth factor or autologous bone marrow transplantation is being assessed in the hope that higher doses of chemotherapy will improve response rates and duration of response.

The early results from studies of bone marrow transplantation have been somewhat disappointing: median survival is prolonged by only 7 to 10 months beyond what is achievable with more standard chemotherapy.[109] There is, however, a small but significant group of long-term survivors who remain free of disease for more than 5 years after undergoing bone marrow transplantation to treat breast cancer with 10 or more positive lymph nodes at initial presentation.[108] Trials of improved bone marrow transplantation regimens continue in the hope that the toxicity and cost of the treatment can be reduced and the number of long-term survivors increased.

Immune therapy using antibodies to HER-2/*neu* protein, alone or in conjunction with chemotherapy, is being evaluated for tumors that overexpress the oncogene HER-2/*neu*. At present, there is no definitive evidence that the biologic therapies and immune therapies now available are of significant value in the treatment of breast cancer. These types of therapy continue to be actively explored.

Even more exciting than the prospect of improved therapy is the concept of chemoprevention—that is, the use of pharmacologic, hormonal, or other interventions to prevent the development or progression of a malignancy. Positive results of trials using tamoxifen for chemoprevention have raised hopes that many breast cancers can be prevented and have increased interest in identifying additional agents that can reduce breast cancer risk with minimal side effects. These results underscore the importance of understanding risk factors for breast cancer, including gene mutations, to better identify women who might benefit from chemoprevention.

MULTIDISCIPLINARY BREAST CANCER CARE

Care of even the earliest breast cancers now routinely entails consultation with and treatment by several specialists, including surgeons, radiation oncologists, medical oncologists, radiologists, and pathologists. The selection and timing of individual treatments are determined by this team of physicians in consultation with the patient. This process is greatly simplified when the physicians concerned are able

Figure 4 **Algorithm illustrates the approach to managing stage IV breast cancer.**

to coordinate their visits with the patient, thereby both saving time for the patient and facilitating decision making among the various specialists. A number of centers have established multidisciplinary breast centers that allow a patient to see all the specialists in a single visit while also allowing the physicians to consult with each other in reviewing the clinical data, imaging studies, and pathology and determining treatment options.

Patient education is also becoming more and more critical in the management of breast cancer. Patients are increasingly being asked to participate in decision making, and as hospital stays for breast cancer treatments become shorter, they are also being asked to participate more actively in their own care. To participate effectively, patients must be educated about the advantages and disadvantages of the various aspects of cancer management. The shifting of a larger proportion of cancer care to the outpatient setting also necessitates the use of other support services, such as visiting nurses, social workers, and outpatient infusion services. How best to coordinate these complex services while maintaining a focus on the problems and needs of the individual patient remains one of the major challenges faced by physicians caring for patients with breast cancer.

References

1. Henderson IC: Risk factors for breast cancer development. Cancer 71(suppl):2127, 1993
2. Slattery ML, Kerber RA: A comprehensive evaluation of family history and breast cancer risk. JAMA 270:1563, 1993
3. Newcomb PA, Storer BE, Longnecker MP, et al: Lactation and a reduced risk of premenopausal breast cancer. N Engl J Med 330:81, 1994
4. Marchant DJ: Estrogen-replacement therapy after breast cancer: risk versus benefits. Cancer 71(suppl): 2169, 1993
5. Squitieri R, Tartter PI, Ahmed S, et al: Carcinoma of the breast in postmenopausal hormone user and non-user control groups. J Am Coll Surg 178:167, 1994
6. Steinberg KK, Thacker SB, Smith SJ, et al: A meta-analysis of the effect of estrogen replacement therapy. JAMA 265:1985, 1991
7. Wingo PA, Lee NC, Ory H, et al: Age specific differences in the relationship between oral contraceptive use and breast cancer. Obstet Gynecol 78:161, 1991
8. Colditz GA, Stampfer MJ, Willett WC: Prospective study of estrogen replacement therapy and risk of breast cancer in post-menopausal women. JAMA 264:2648, 1990
9. Dupont WD, Page DL: Menopausal estrogen-replacement therapy and breast cancer. Arch Intern Med 151:67, 1991
10. Hunter DJ, Manson JE, Colditz GA, et al: A prospective study of the intake of vitamins C, E, and A and the risk of breast cancer. N Engl J Med 329:234, 1993
11. Willett WC, Hunter DJ, Stampfer MJ, et al: Dietary fat and fiber in relation to risk of breast cancer: an 8-year follow-up. JAMA 268:2037, 1992
12. Armstrong B, Doll R: Environmental factors and cancer incidence and mortality in different countries, with special reference to dietary practices. Int J Cancer 15:617, 1975
13. Page DL, Jensen RA: Evaluation and management of high risk and premalignant lesions of the breast. World J Surg 18:32, 1994
14. Frykberg ER, Bland KI: Management of in situ and minimally invasive breast carcinoma. World J Surg 18:45, 1994
15. Jacobs TJ, Byrne C, Colditz G, et al: Radial scars in benign breast-biopsy specimens and the risk of breast cancer. N Engl J Med 340:430, 1999
16. Fletcher SW, Black W, Harris R, et al: Report of the International Workshop on Screening for Breast Cancer. J Natl Cancer Inst 85:1644, 1989
17. Osteen RT, Cady B, Chmiel JS, et al: 1991 national survey of carcinoma of the breast by the Commission on Cancer. J Am Coll Surg 178:213, 1994
18. Surveillance, Epidemiology, and End Results: Incidence and Mortality Data, 1973-1977. DHEW Publ No. (NIH)81-2330. Public Health Service, Bethesda, Maryland, 1981
19. Donegan WL: Evaluation of a palpable breast mass. N Engl J Med 327:937, 1992
20. Rosner D, Blaird D: What ultrasonography can tell in breast masses that mammography and physical examination cannot. J Surg Oncol 28:308, 1985
21. Hamed H, Coady A, Chaudary MA, et al: Follow-up of patients with aspirated breast cysts is necessary. Arch Surg 124:253, 1989
22. Cowen PN, Benson GA: Cytological study of fluid from benign breast cysts. Br J Surg 66:209, 1979
23. Sartorius O, Smith H, Morris P, et al: Cytologic evaluation of breast fluid in the detection of breast disease. J Natl Cancer Inst 59:1073, 1977
24. Ciatto S, Cariaggi P, Bulgaresi P: The value of routine cytologic examination of breast cyst fluids. Acta Cytol 31:301, 1987
25. Leis HP Jr: Gross breast cysts: significance and management. Contemp Surg 39(2):13, 1991
26. Hughes LE, Bundred NJ: Breast macrocysts. World J Surg 13:711, 1989
27. Boyd NF, Sutherland HJ, Fish EB, et al: Prospective evaluation of physical examination of the breast. Am J Surg 142:331, 1981
28. Layfield LJ, Glasgow BJ, Cramer H: Fine-needle aspiration in the management of breast masses. Pathol Annu 24:23, 1989
29. Silverman JS, Tameness A: Mammary fibroadenoma and some phyllodes tumor stroma are composed of CD34+ fibroblasts and factor XIIIa+ dendrophages. Histopathology 29:411, 1996
30. Dietrich CU: Karyotypic changes in phyllodes tumors of the breast. Cancer Genet Cytogenet 78:200, 1994
31. Noguchi S, Yokouchi H, Aihara T, et al: Progression of fibroadenoma to phyllodes tumor demonstrated by clonal analysis. Cancer 76:1779, 1995
32. Shimizu K: Cytologic evaluation of phyllodes tumors as compared to fibroadenomas of breast. Acta Cytol 38:891, 1994
33. Mangi AA, Smith BL, Gadd MA, et al: Surgical management of phyllodes tumors. Arch Surg 134:487, 1999
34. Hall FM, Storella JM, Silverstone DZ, et al: Nonpalpable breast lesions: recommendations for biopsy based on suspicion of carcinoma at mammography. Radiology 167:353, 1988
35. Sickles EA: Periodic mammographic follow-up of probably benign lesions: results in 3,184 consecutive cases. Radiology 179:463, 1991
36. Wolfe JN, Buck KA, Salane M, et al: Xeroradiography of the breast: overview of 21,057 consecutive cases. Radiology 165:305, 1987
37. Helvie MA, Pennes DR, Rebner M, et al: Mammographic follow-up of low-suspicion lesions: compliance rate and diagnostic yield. Radiology 178:155, 1991
38. Takeda T, Suzuki M, Sato Y, et al: Cytologic studies of nipple discharge. Acta Cytol 26:35, 1982
39. Chaudary M, Millis R, Davies G, et al: Nipple discharge: the diagnostic value of testing for occult blood. Ann Surg 196:651, 1982
40. Urban JA: Excision of the major duct system of the breast. Cancer 16:516, 1963
41. Passaro ME, Broughan TA, Sebek BA, et al: Lactiferous fistula. J Am Coll Surg 178:29, 1994
42. Watt-Boolsen S, Eskildsen P, Blaehr H: Release of prolactin, thyrotropin and growth hormone in women with cyclical mastalgia and fibrocystic disease of the breast. Cancer 56:500, 1985
43. Pashby NL, Mansel RE, Hughes LE, et al: A clinical trial of evening primrose oil in mastalgia. Br J Surg 68:801, 1981
44. Baker H, Snedecor P: Clinical trial of danazol for benign breast disease. Am Surg 45:727, 1979
45. Lauersen N, Wilson K: The effect of danazol in the treatment of chronic cystic mastitis. Obstet Gynecol 48:93, 1976
46. Mansel R, Preece P, Hughes L: A double blind trial of the prolactin inhibitor bromocriptine in painful benign breast disease. Br J Surg 65:724, 1978
47. Fentiman I, Caleffi M, Brame K, et al: Double-blind controlled trial of tamoxifen therapy for mastalgia. Lancet 1:287, 1986
48. Benson EA: Management of breast abscesses. World J Surg 13:753, 1989
49. Niebyl JR, Spence MR, Parmley TH: Sporadic (nonepidemic) puerperal mastitis. J Reprod Med 20:97, 1978
50. Brook I: Microbiology of non-puerperal breast abscesses. J Infect Dis 157:377, 1988
51. Walker AP, Edmiston CE, Krepel CJ, et al: A prospective study of the microflora of nonpuerperal breast abscess. Arch Surg 123:908, 1988
52. Smith BL: Duct ectasia, periductal mastitis, and breast infections. Breast Diseases. Harris JR, Hellman S, Henderson IC, et al, Eds. JB Lippincott Co, Philadelphia, 1991, p 38
53. Hadfield J: Excision of the major duct system for benign disease of the breast. Br J Surg 47:472, 1960
54. Gail MG, Brinton LA, Byar DP, et al: Projecting individualized probabilities of developing breast cancer for white females who are being examined annually. J Natl Cancer Inst 81:1879, 1989
55. Claus EB, Risch N, Thompson WD: Autosomal dominant inheritance of early-onset breast cancer: implications for risk prediction. Cancer 73:643, 1994
56. Lynch HT, Marcus JN, Watson P, et al: Familial breast cancer, family cancer syndromes and predisposition to breast neoplasia. The Breast: Comprehensive Management of Benign and Malignant Diseases. Bland KI, Copeland EM, Eds. WB Saunders Co, Philadelphia, 1991, p 262
57. Hartmann LC, Schaid DJ, Woods JE, et al: Efficacy of bilateral prophylactic mastectomy in women with a family history of breast cancer. N Engl J Med 340: 77, 1999

58. Schrag D, Kuntz KM, Garber JE, et al: Decision analysis—effects of prophylactic mastectomy and oophorectomy on life expectancy among women with BRCA1 or BRCA2 mutations. N Engl J Med 336:1465, 1997

59. Zujewski J: Selective estrogen receptor modulators (SERMS) and retinoids in breast cancer chemoprevention. Environ Mol Mutagen 39:264, 2002

60. Fisher B, Costantino JP, Wickerham DL, et al: Tamoxifen for prevention of breast cancer: report of the National Surgical Adjuvant Breast and Bowel Project P-1 Study. J Natl Cancer Inst 90:1371, 1998

61. Powles T, Eeles R, Ashley S, et al: Interim analysis of the incidence of breast cancer in the Royal Marsden Hospital tamoxifen randomised chemoprevention trial. Lancet 352:98, 1998

62. Veronesi U, Maisonneuve P, Costs A, et al: Prevention of breast cancer with tamoxifen: preliminary findings from the Italian randomised trial among hysterectomised women. Lancet 352:93, 1998

63. Dalton R, Kallab A: Chemoprevention of breast cancer. South Med J 94:7, 2001

64. Cummings S, Eckert S, Kreuger K, et al: The effect of raloxifene on risk of breast cancer in postmenopausal women: results from the MORE randomized trial. Multiple Outcomes of Raloxifene Evaluation. JAMA 281:2189, 1999

65. Goss P, Strasser K: Chemoprevention with aromatase inhibitors—trial strategies. J Steroid Biochem Mol Biol 79:143, 2001

66. Fabian CJ: Breast cancer chemoprevention: beyond tamoxifen. Breast Cancer Res 3:99, 2001

67. Veronesi U, Banfi A, DelVecchio M, et al: Comparison of Halstead mastectomy with quadrantectomy, axillary dissection and radiotherapy in early breast cancer: long term results. Eur J Cancer Clin Oncol 22:1085, 1986

68. Sarrazin D, Le M, Rouesse J, et al: Conservative treatment versus mastectomy in breast cancer tumors with macroscopic diameter of 20 millimeters or less: the experience of the Institut Gustave Roussy. Cancer 53:1209, 1984

69. Fisher B, Bauer M, Margolese R, et al: Five-year results of a randomized clinical trial comparing total mastectomy and segmental mastectomy with or without radiation in the treatment of breast cancer. N Engl J Med 312:665, 1985

70. Fisher B, Redmond C, Poisson R, et al: Eight year results of a randomized clinical trial comparing total mastectomy and lumpectomy with or without irradiation in the treatment of breast cancer. N Engl J Med 320:822, 1989

71. Farrow DC, Hunt WC, Samot JM: Geographic variation in the treatment of localized breast cancer. N Engl J Med 326:1097, 1992

72. Nattinger AB, Gottlieb MS, Veum J, et al: Geographic variation in the use of breast-conserving treatment for breast cancer. N Engl J Med 326:1102, 1992

73. Osteen RT, Steele GD, Menck HR, et al: Regional differences in surgical management of breast cancer. Cancer 42:39, 1992

74. Lazovich D, White E, Thomas DB, et al: Underutilization of breast conserving surgery and radiation therapy among women with stage I or II breast cancer. JAMA 266:3433, 1991

75. Lee-Feldstein A, Anton-Culver H, Feldstein PJ: Treatment differences and other prognostic factors related to breast cancer survival: delivery systems and medical outcomes. JAMA 271:1163, 1994

76. Kurtz JM, Spitalier JM, Almaric R, et al: Results of wide excision for local recurrence after breast-conserving therapy. Cancer 61:1969, 1989

77. Haffty GB, Goldberg NB, Rose M, et al: Conservative surgery with radiation therapy in clinical stage I and II breast cancer: results of a 20 year experience. Arch Surg 124:1266, 1989

78. Harris JR, Hellman S, Kinne DW: Limited surgery and radiotherapy for early breast cancer. N Engl J Med 313:1365, 1985

79. Clarke DH, Le M, Sarrazin D, et al: Analysis of local regional relapses in patients with early breast cancers treated by excision and radiotherapy: experience of the Institut Gustave Roussy. Int J Radiat Oncol Biol Phys 11:137, 1985

80. Fisher B, Wolmark N: Limited surgical management for primary breast cancer: a commentary on the NSABP reports. World J Surg 9:682, 1985

81. Holland R, Connolly JL, Gelman R, et al: The presence of an extensive intraductal component following a limited excision correlates with prominent residual disease in the remainder of the breast. J Clin Oncol 8:113, 1990

82. Harris JR, Osteen RT: Patients with early breast cancer benefit from effective axillary treatment. Breast Cancer Res Treat 5:17, 1985

83. Krag D, Weaver D, Ashikaga T, et al: The sentinel node in breast cancer: a multicenter validation study. N Engl J Med 339:941, 1998

84. Giuliano AE, Jones RC, Brennan MM, et al: Sentinel lymphadenectomy in breast cancer. J Clin Oncol 15:2345, 1997

85. McMasters KM, Giuliano AE, Ross MI, et al: Sentinel-lymph node biopsy for breast cancer—not yet the standard of care. N Engl J Med 339:990, 1998

86. Eberlein TJ, Crespo LD, Smith BL, et al: Prospective evaluation of immediate reconstruction following mastectomy. Ann Surg 218:29, 1993

87. Overgaard M, Hansen PS, Overgaard J, et al: Postoperative radiotherapy in high-risk premenopausal women with breast cancer who receive adjuvant chemotherapy. N Engl J Med 337:949, 1997

88. Ragaz J, Jackson SM, Le N, et al: Adjuvant radiotherapy and chemotherapy in node-positive premenopausal women with breast cancer. N Engl J Med 337:956, 1997

89. Bonadonna G, Valagussa P, Tancini G, et al: Current status of Milan adjuvant chemotherapy trials for node-positive and node-negative breast cancer. J Natl Cancer Inst Monogr 1:45, 1986

90. Fisher B, Redmond C, Fisher E, et al: Systemic adjuvant therapy in treatment of primary operable breast cancer: NSABP experience. J Natl Cancer Inst Monogr 1:35, 1986

91. Consensus Conference: Adjuvant chemotherapy for breast cancer. JAMA 254:3461, 1985

92. Fisher B, Costantino J, Redmond C, et al: A randomized trial evaluating tamoxifen in the treatment of patients with node-negative breast cancer who have estrogen-receptor-positive tumors. N Engl J Med 320:479, 1989

93. Clinical Alert from the National Cancer Institute. Department of Human Services, National Cancer Institute, National Institutes of Health, May 16, 1988

94. Fisher B, Redmond C, Dimitrov NV, et al: A randomized clinical trial evaluating sequential methotrexate and fluorouracil in the treatment of patients with node-negative breast cancer who have estrogen-receptor-negative tumors. N Engl J Med 320:473, 1989

95. Mansour EG, Gray R, Shatila NH, et al: Efficacy of adjuvant chemotherapy in high-risk node-negative breast cancer. N Engl J Med 320:485, 1989

96. NIH Consensus Conference: Treatment of early-stage breast cancer. JAMA 265:391, 1991

97. Early Breast Cancer Trialists' Collaborative Group: Systemic treatment of early breast cancer by hormonal, cytotoxic, or immune therapy: 133 randomised trials involving 31,000 recurrences and 24,000 deaths among 75,000 women. Lancet 339:71, 1992

98. Tamoxifen for early breast cancer: an overview of the randomised trials. Early Breast Cancer Trialists' Collaborative Group. Lancet 351:1451, 1998

99. Silverstein MJ, Lagios MD, Groshen S, et al: The influence of margin width on local control of ductal carcinoma in situ of the breast. N Engl J Med 340:1455, 1999

100. Fisher B, Costantino J, Redmond C, et al: Lumpectomy compared with lumpectomy and radiation therapy for the treatment of intraductal breast cancer.

N Engl J Med 328:1581, 1993

101. Haagensen CD, Lane N, Lattes R, et al: Lobular neoplasia (so-called lobular carcinoma in situ) of the breast. Cancer 42:737, 1978

102. Rosen PP: Lobular carcinoma in situ and intraductal carcinoma of the breast. Monogr Pathol 25:59, 1984

103. Rosen PP, Kosloff C, Lieberman PH, et al: Lobular carcinoma in situ of the breast: detailed analysis of 99 patients with average follow-up of 24 years. Am J Surg Pathol 2:225, 1978

104. Fisher ER, Fisher B: Lobular carcinoma of the breast: an overview. Ann Surg 185:377, 1977

105. Kinne D: Clinical management of lobular carcinoma in situ. Breast Diseases. Harris JR, Hellman S, Henderson IC, et al, Eds. JB Lippincott Co, Philadelphia, 1991, p 239

106. Scottish Cancer Trials Breast Group: Adjuvant ovarian ablation versus CMF chemotherapy in premenopausal women with pathological stage II breast carcinoma: the Scottish trial. Lancet 341:1293, 1993

107. GIVIO Investigators: Impact of follow-up testing on survival and health-related quality of life in breast cancer patients. JAMA 271:1587, 1994

108. Del Turco MR, Palli D, Cariddi A, et al: National Research Council Project on Breast Cancer Follow-up. Intensive diagnostic follow-up after treatment of primary breast cancer: a randomized trial. JAMA 271:1593, 1994

109. Peters WP: High-dose chemotherapy and autologous bone marrow support for breast cancer. Important Advances in Oncology. DeVita VT Jr, Hellman S, Rosenberg SA, Eds. JB Lippincott Co, Philadelphia, 1991, p 135

110. Hammond S, Keyhani-Rofagha S, O'Toole RV: Statistical analysis of fine needle aspiration cytology of the breast: a review of 678 cases plus 4,265 cases from the literature. Acta Cytol 31:276, 1987

111. Dowlatshahi KD, Yaremko ML, Kluskens LF, et al: Nonpalpable breast lesions: findings of stereotaxic needle-core biopsy and fine-needle aspiration cytology. Radiology 181:745, 1991

112. Ballo MS, Sneige N: Can core needle biopsy replace fine needle aspiration cytology in the diagnosis of palpable breast carcinoma: a comparative study of 124 women. Cancer 78:773, 1996

113. Smith DN, Christian R, Meyer JE: Large-core needle biopsy of nonpalpable breast cancers: the impact on subsequent surgical excisions. Arch Surg 132:256, 1997

114. El-Ashry D, Lippman ME: Molecular biology of breast carcinoma. World J Surg 18:12, 1994

115. Slamon DJ, Godolphin W, Jones LA, et al: Studies of the HER-2/neu proto-oncogene in human breast and ovarian cancer. Science 244:707, 1989

116. Gusterson BA, Gelber RD, Goldhirsch A, et al: Prognostic importance of c-erbB-2 expression in breast cancer: International (Ludwig) Breast Cancer Study Group. J Clin Oncol 10:1049, 1992

117. Perren TJ: C-erbB-2 oncogene as a prognostic marker in breast cancer (editorial). Br J Cancer 63:328, 1991

118. Gullick WJ, Love SB, Wright C, et al: C-erbB-2 protein overexpression in breast cancer is a risk factor in patients with involved and uninvolved lymph nodes. Br J Cancer 63:434, 1991

119. American Joint Committee on Cancer: AJCC Cancer Staging Manual, 5th ed. Lippincott-Raven Publishers, Philadelphia, 1997, p 171

Acknowledgments

Figure 1   Marcia Kammerer.

Figures 2 through 4   Talar Agasyan.

4 ACUTE ABDOMINAL PAIN

Romano Delcore, M.D., and Laurence Y. Cheung, M.D.

Assessment of Acute Abdominal Pain

The term acute abdominal pain generally refers to previously undiagnosed pain that arises suddenly and is of less than 7 days' (usually less than 48 hours') duration.[1] It may be caused by a great variety of intraperitoneal disorders, many of which call for surgical treatment, as well as many extraperitoneal disorders,[2] which typically do not call for surgical treatment [*see* Tentative Differential Diagnosis, *below*]. Abdominal pain that persists for 6 hours or longer is usually caused by disorders of surgical significance.[3] The primary goal in the management of patients with acute abdominal pain is to determine whether operative intervention is necessary and, if so, when the operation should be performed. Often, this determination is easy to make; on occasion, however, the evaluation of patients with acute abdominal pain can be one of the most difficult challenges in clinical surgery. It is essential to keep in mind that most (at least two thirds) of the patients who present with acute abdominal pain have disorders for which surgical intervention is not required.[2,4,5]

Making the correct decision regarding whether to operate on a patient with acute abdominal pain requires sound surgical judgment. The decision must be based on a detailed medical and surgical clinical history as well as a meticulous physical examination. These, in turn, must be based on experience, a thorough knowledge of the anatomy and physiology of the peritoneal cavity, and a clear understanding of the pathologic processes that occur within the abdomen. Much has been written about the diagnosis of acute abdominal pain since 1921, when Sir Zachary Cope first published his now classic paper.[3] Although the basic approach to assessment of acute abdominal pain remains much the same today, the introduction of new diagnostic technologies and better resuscitation methods, coupled with an aging population (in the United States and other developed countries) and new disease processes, necessitates periodic revision of the traditional approach as well as constant broadening of the differential diagnosis. For example, with the proliferation of less invasive surgery, the use of laparoscopy has expanded far beyond its initial application to cholecystectomy. Emergency laparoscopy has become more widely accepted in the treatment of acute surgical diseases (e.g., acute appendicitis and perforated peptic ulcer) as general surgeons gain competence in its use. Diagnostic laparoscopy has also proved valuable in the assessment of acute abdominal pain (see below).

Historically, diagnosis of the causes of acute abdominal pain has been based largely on pattern recognition, in which clinicians attempt to match new cases to preexisting stereotypes (so-called classic presentations) of various diseases. Certainly, knowledge of these classic presentations is basic to successful diagnosis, but it is crucial to remember that at least one third of patients with acute abdominal pain exhibit atypical features that render pattern recognition unreliable.[4,6,7]

Clinical History

A careful and methodical clinical history should be obtained that includes the mode of onset, duration, frequency, character, location, chronology, radiation, and intensity of the pain, as well as the presence or absence of any aggravating or alleviating factors and associated symptoms. Often, such a history is more valuable than any single laboratory or x-ray finding and determines the course of subsequent evaluation and management. Unfortunately, when the ability of clinicians to take an organized and accurate history has been studied, the results have been disappointing.[7] For this reason, the use of standardized history and physical forms, with or without the aid of diagnostic computer programs, has been recommended.

Computer-aided diagnosis has been extensively studied in England.[8-11] In these studies, physicians collected clinical data on structured data sheets and entered the information into a computer running a diagnostic program; the computer, which contained a large clinical database, then generated diagnostic probabilities. One such study demonstrated that integration of computer-aided diagnosis into the management of 16,737 patients with acute abdominal pain yielded a 20% improvement in diagnostic accuracy.[8] This improvement resulted in statistically significant reductions in inappropriate admissions, negative laparotomies, serious management errors (e.g., failure to operate on patients who require surgery), and length of hospital stay, as well as statistically significant increases in the number of patients who were immediately discharged home without adverse effects and the promptness with which those requiring surgery underwent operation. Although these impressive results are undoubtedly attributable to more than one cause, it is certain that the required use of a structured data sheet to record the patient's history for computer analysis played a crucial role. In fact, when the data sheets were used without the computer, diagnostic accuracy and overall decision making were still significantly improved.

There now appears to be more than sufficient evidence to support the routine use of structured data sheets in the initial stages of obtaining a history from a patient with acute abdominal pain.[9-11] An example of such a data sheet is the pain chart developed by the World Organization of Gastroenterology (OMGE) [*see Figure 1*]. The components of this data sheet represent the consensus of the more than 2,000 surgeons worldwide who contributed to its development and have used it to collect

ABDOMINAL PAIN CHART

NAME _____ REG. NUMBER _____

MALE _____ FEMALE _____ AGE _____ FORM FILLED BY _____

MODE OF ARRIVAL _____ DATE _____ TIME _____

PAIN

Site of Pain

At Onset

At Present

Radiation

Aggravating Factors
movement
coughing
respiration
food
other
none

Relieving Factors
lying still
vomiting
antacids
food
other
none

Progression of Pain
better
same
worse

Duration

Type
intermittent
steady
colicky

Severity
moderate
severe

HISTORY

Nausea
yes   no

Vomiting
yes   no

Anorexia
yes   no

Indigestion
yes   no

Jaundice
yes   no

Bowels
normal
constipation
diarrhea
blood
mucus

Micturition
normal
frequency
dysuria
dark
hematuria

Previous Similar Pain
yes   no

Previous Abdominal Surgery
yes   no

Drugs for Abdominal Pain
yes   no

Female-LMP
pregnant
vaginal discharge
dizzy/faint

EXAMINATION

Temp.   Pulse
BP

Mood
normal
upset
anxious

Color
normal
pale
flushed
jaundiced
cyanotic

Intestinal Movement
normal
poor/nil
peristalsis

Scars
yes   no

Distention
yes   no

Location of Tenderness

Rebound
yes   no

Guarding
yes   no

Rigidity
yes   no

Mass
yes   no

Murphy's Sign Present
yes   no

Bowel Sounds
normal
absent
increased

Rectal-Vaginal Tenderness
left
right
general
mass
none

Initial Diagnosis & Plan

Results
amylase
blood count (WBC)
urine
x-ray

other

Diagnosis & Plan after Investigation

(time   )

Discharge Diagnosis

History and examination of other systems on separate case notes.

Figure 1 Shown is a data sheet modified from the abdominal pain chart developed by the OMGE.[13]

Assessment of Acute Abdominal Pain

Patient presents with acute abdominal pain

Obtain clinical history

Assess mode of onset, duration, frequency, character, location, chronology, radiation, and intensity of pain.
Look for aggravating or alleviating factors and associated symptoms.
Use structured data sheets if possible.

Generate working diagnosis

Proceed with subsequent management on the basis of the working diagnosis.
Reevaluate patient repeatedly. If patient does not respond to treatment as expected, reassess working diagnosis and return to differential diagnosis.

Perform basic investigative studies

Laboratory: complete blood count, hematocrit, electrolytes, creatinine, blood urea nitrogen, glucose, liver function tests, amylase, lipase, urinalysis, pregnancy test, ECG (if patient is elderly or has atherosclerosis).

Radiologic: Plain abdominal films (upright and supine) and chest radiographs.
(Note: These studies are rarely diagnostic by themselves; their purpose is primarily confirmatory.)

Patient requires immediate laparotomy

Conditions necessitating immediate laparotomy include ruptured abdominal aortic or visceral aneurysm, ruptured ectopic pregnancy, spontaneous hepatic or splenic rupture, major blunt or penetrating abdominal trauma, and hemoperitoneum from various causes.
Severe hemodynamic instability is the essential indication.

Patient has suspected surgical abdomen

Determine whether urgent laparotomy is necessary.

Patient requires urgent laparotomy or laparoscopy

Conditions necessitating urgent laparotomy include perforated hollow viscus, appendicitis, Meckel diverticulitis, strangulated hernia, mesenteric ischemia, and ectopic pregnancy (unruptured).

Laparoscopy is recommended for acute appendicitis and perforated ulcers (provided that surgeon has sufficient experience and competence with the technique).

Patient should be hospitalized and observed

Observe patient carefully, and reevaluate condition periodically.

Consider additional investigative studies (e.g., CT, ultrasonography, diagnostic peritoneal lavage, radionuclide imaging, angiography, MRI, and GI endoscopy).

Diagnostic laparoscopy is recommended if pain persists after a period of observation.

Patient requires early laparotomy or laparoscopy

Early laparotomy or laparoscopy is reserved for patients whose conditions are unlikely to become life threatening if operation is delayed for 24–48 hr (e.g., those with uncomplicated intestinal obstruction, uncomplicated acute cholecystitis, uncomplicated acute diverticulitis, or nonstrangulated incarcerated hernia).

Patient is candidate for elective laparotomy or laparoscopy

Elective laparotomy or laparoscopy is reserved for patients who are highly likely to respond to conservative medical management or whose conditions are highly unlikely to become life threatening during prolonged evaluation (e.g., those with IBD, peptic ulcer disease, pancreatitis, or endometriosis).

Diagnosis is uncertain, or patient has suspected nonsurgical abdomen

Reevaluate patient as appropriate
(see facing page).

Generate tentative differential diagnosis

Remember that the majority of patients will turn out to have nonsurgical diagnoses.
Take into account effects of age and gender on diagnostic possibilities.

Perform physical examination

Evaluate general appearance and ability to answer questions; estimate degree of obvious pain; note position in bed; identify area of maximal pain; look for extra-abdominal causes of pain and signs of systemic illness.
Perform systematic abdominal examination: (1) inspection, (2) auscultation, (3) percussion, (4) palpation.
Perform rectal, genital, and pelvic examinations.

Diagnosis is uncertain

Determine whether patient should be hospitalized or can be managed as an outpatient.

Patient has suspected nonsurgical abdomen

Nonsurgical conditions causing acute abdominal pain include both extraperitoneal [see Table 2] and intraperitoneal disorders.

Patient should be hospitalized and observed

Provide narcotic analgesia as appropriate.
Observe patient carefully, and reevaluate condition periodically.
Consider additional investigative studies. CT and ultrasonography may be especially useful.

Patient can be evaluated in outpatient setting

Patient should be hospitalized and observed

Provide narcotic analgesia as appropriate.
Observe patient carefully, and reevaluate condition periodically.
Consider additional investigative studies.

Diagnosis is uncertain or patient has suspected surgical abdomen

Reevaluate patient as appropriate (see above, left, and facing page).

Diagnosis is nonsurgical

Refer patient for medical management.

Patient has suspected surgical abdomen

Reevaluate patient as appropriate (see facing page).

Diagnosis is uncertain, or patient has suspected nonsurgical abdomen

Reevaluate patient as appropriate (see above, right, and facing page).

information for the Research Committee of the OMGE and other groups studying acute abdominal pain.[12,13] Given that the data sheet is by no means exhaustive, individual surgeons may want to add to it; however, they would be well advised not to omit any of the symptoms and signs on the data sheet from their routine examination of patients with acute abdominal pain.[14]

When the surgeon obtains a complete clinical history with an open mind, the patient often provides important clues to the correct diagnosis. Patients should be allowed to relate the history in their own words, and examiners should refrain from suggesting specific symptoms, except as a last resort. Any questions that must be asked should be open-ended—for example, "What happens when you eat?" rather than "Does eating make the pain worse?" Leading questions should be avoided. When a leading question must be asked, it should be posed first as a negative question (i.e., one that calls for an answer in the negative), since a negative answer to a question is more likely to be honest and accurate. For example, if peritoneal inflammation is suspected, the question asked should be "Does coughing make the pain better?" rather than "Does coughing make the pain worse?"

The mode of onset of abdominal pain may help the examiner determine the severity of the underlying disease. Pain that has a sudden onset suggests an intra-abdominal catastrophe, such as a ruptured abdominal aortic aneurysm, a perforated viscus, or a ruptured ectopic pregnancy. Rapidly progressive pain that becomes intensely centered in a well-defined area within a period of a few minutes to an hour or two suggests a condition such as acute cholecystitis or pancreatitis. Pain that has a gradual onset over several hours, usually beginning as slight or vague discomfort and slowly progressing to steady and more localized pain, suggests a subacute process and is characteristic of peritoneal inflammation. Numerous disorders may be associated with this mode of onset, including acute appendicitis, diverticulitis, pelvic inflammatory disease (PID), and intestinal obstruction.

Pain can be either intermittent or continuous. Intermittent or cramping pain (colic) is pain that occurs for a short period (a few minutes), followed by longer periods (a few minutes to one-half hour) of complete remission during which there is no pain at all. Intermittent pain is characteristic of obstruction of a hollow viscus and results from vigorous peristalsis in the wall of the viscus proximal to the site of obstruction. This pain is perceived as deep in the abdomen and is poorly localized. The patient is restless, may writhe about incessantly in an effort to find a comfortable position, and often presses on the abdominal wall in an attempt to alleviate the pain. Whereas the intermittent pain associated with intestinal obstruction (typically described as gripping and mounting) is usually severe but bearable, the pain associated with obstruction of small conduits (e.g., the biliary tract, the ureters, and the uterine tubes) often becomes unbearable. Obstruction of the gallbladder or bile ducts gives rise to a type of pain often referred to as biliary colic; however, this term is a misnomer, in that biliary pain is usually constant because of the lack of a strong muscular coat in the biliary tree and the absence of regular peristalsis.

Continuous or constant pain is pain that is present for hours or days without any period of complete relief; it is more common than intermittent pain. Continuous pain is usually indicative of peritoneal inflammation or ischemia. It may be of steady intensity throughout, or it may be associated with intermittent pain. For example, the typical colicky pain associated with simple intestinal obstruction changes when strangulation occurs, becoming continuous pain that persists between episodes or waves of cramping pain.

Certain types of pain are generally held to be typical of certain pathologic states—for example, the general burning pain of a perforated gastric ulcer, the tearing pain of a dissecting aneurysm, and the gripping pain of intestinal obstruction. However, the character of the pain is not always a reliable clue to its cause.

For several reasons—atypical pain patterns, dual innervation by visceral and somatic afferents, normal variations in organ position, and widely diverse underlying pathologic states—the location of abdominal pain is only a rough guide to diagnosis. It is nevertheless true that in most disorders, the pain tends to occur in characteristic locations, such as the right upper quadrant (cholecystitis), the right lower quadrant (appendicitis), the epigastrium (pancreatitis), or the left lower quadrant (sigmoid diverticulitis) [see Figure 2]. It is important to determine the location of the pain at onset because this may differ from the location at the time of presentation (so-called shifting pain). In fact, the chronological sequence of events in the patient's history is often more important for diagnosis than the location of the pain alone. For example, the classic pain of appendicitis begins in the periumbilical region and settles in the right lower quadrant. A similar shift in location can occur when escaping gastroduodenal contents from a perforated ulcer pool in the right lower quadrant.

It is also important to take into account radiation or referral of the pain, which tends to occur in characteristic patterns [see Figure 3]. For example, biliary pain is referred to the right subscapular area, and the boring pain of pancreatitis typically radiates straight through to the back. The more severe the pain is, the more likely it is to be referred.

The intensity or severity of the pain is related to the magnitude of the underlying insult. It is important to distinguish between the intensity of the pain and the patient's reaction to it because there appear to be significant individual differences with respect to tolerance of and reaction to pain. Pain that is intense enough to awaken the patient from sleep usually indicates a significant underlying organic cause. Past episodes of pain and factors that aggravate or relieve the pain often provide useful diagnostic clues. For example, pain caused by peritonitis tends to be exacerbated by motion, deep breathing, coughing, or sneezing, and patients with peritonitis tend to lie quietly in bed and avoid any movement. The typical pain of acute pancreatitis is exacerbated by lying down and relieved by sitting up. Pain that is relieved by eating or taking antacids suggests duodenal ulcer disease, whereas diffuse abdominal pain that appears 30 minutes to 1 hour after meals suggests intestinal angina.

Associated gastrointestinal symptoms, such as nausea, vomiting, anorexia, diarrhea, and constipation, often accompany abdominal pain; however, these symptoms are nonspecific and therefore may not be of great value in the differential diagnosis. Vomiting in particular is common: when sufficiently stimulated by pain impulses traveling via secondary visceral afferent fibers, the medullary vomiting centers activate efferent fibers and cause reflex vomiting. Once again, the chronology of events is important, in that pain often precedes vomiting in patients with conditions necessitating operation, whereas the opposite is usually the case in patients with medical (i.e., nonsurgical) conditions.[4,6] This is particularly true for patients with acute appendicitis, in whom pain almost always precedes vomiting by several hours. Similarly, constipation may result from a reflex paralytic ileus when sufficiently stimulated visceral afferent fibers activate efferent sympathetic fibers (splanchnic nerves) to

a

b

EPIGASTRIC REGION
Peptic Ulcer
Gastritis
Pancreatitis
Duodenitis
Gastroenteritis
Early Appendicitis
Mesenteric Adenitis
Mesenteric Thrombosis
Intestinal Obstruction
Inflammatory Bowel Disease
Aneurysm

UMBILICAL REGION
Early Appendicitis
Gastroenteritis
Pancreatitis
Hernia
Mesenteric Adenitis
Mesenteric Thrombosis
Intestinal Obstruction
Inflammatory Bowel Disease
Aneurysm

DIFFUSE
Peritonitis
Early Appendicitis
Pancreatitis
Leukemia
Sickle Cell Crisis
Gastroenteritis
Mesenteric Adenitis
Mesenteric Thrombosis
Intestinal Obstruction
Inflammatory Bowel
  Disease
Aneurysm
Metabolic Causes
Toxic Causes

HYPOGASTRIC REGION
Cystitis
Diverticulitis
Appendicitis
Prostatism
Salpingitis
Hernia
Ovarian Cyst/Torsion
Endometriosis
Ectopic Pregnancy
Nephrolithiasis
Intestinal Obstruction
Inflammatory Bowel Disease
Abdominal Wall Hematoma

c

RIGHT UPPER QUADRANT
Cholecystitis
Choledocholithiasis
Hepatitis
Hepatic Abscess
Hepatomegaly from
Congestive Heart Failure
Peptic Ulcer
Pancreatitis
Retrocecal Appendicitis
Pyelonephritis
Nephrolithiasis
Herpes Zoster
Myocardial Ischemia
Pericarditis
Pneumonia
Empyema
Gastritis
Duodenitis
Intestinal Obstruction
Inflammatory Bowel Disease

LEFT UPPER QUADRANT
Gastritis
Pancreatitis
Splenic Enlargement
Splenic Rupture
Splenic Infarction
Splenic Aneurysm
Pyelonephritis
Nephrolithiasis
Herpes Zoster
Myocardial Ischemia
Pneumonia
Empyema
Diverticulitis
Intestinal Obstruction
Inflammatory Bowel Disease

RIGHT LOWER QUADRANT
Appendicitis
Intestinal Obstruction
Inflammatory Bowel Disease
Mesenteric Adenitis
Diverticulitis
Cholecystitis
Perforated Ulcer
Leaking Aneurysm
Abdominal Wall Hematoma
Ectopic Pregnancy
Ovarian Cyst/Torsion
Salpingitis
Mittelschmerz
Endometriosis
Ureteral Calculi
Pyelonephritis
Nephrolithiasis
Seminal Vesiculitis
Psoas Abscess
Hernia

LEFT LOWER QUADRANT
Diverticulitis
Intestinal Obstruction
Inflammatory Bowel Disease
Appendicitis
Leaking Aneurysm
Abdominal Wall Hematoma
Ectopic Pregnancy
Mittelschmerz
Ovarian Cyst/Torsion
Salpingitis
Endometriosis
Ureteral Calculi
Pyelonephritis
Nephrolithiasis
Seminal Vesiculitis
Psoas Abscess
Hernia

Figure 2 **In most disorders that give rise to acute abdominal pain, the pain tends to occur in specific locations.**

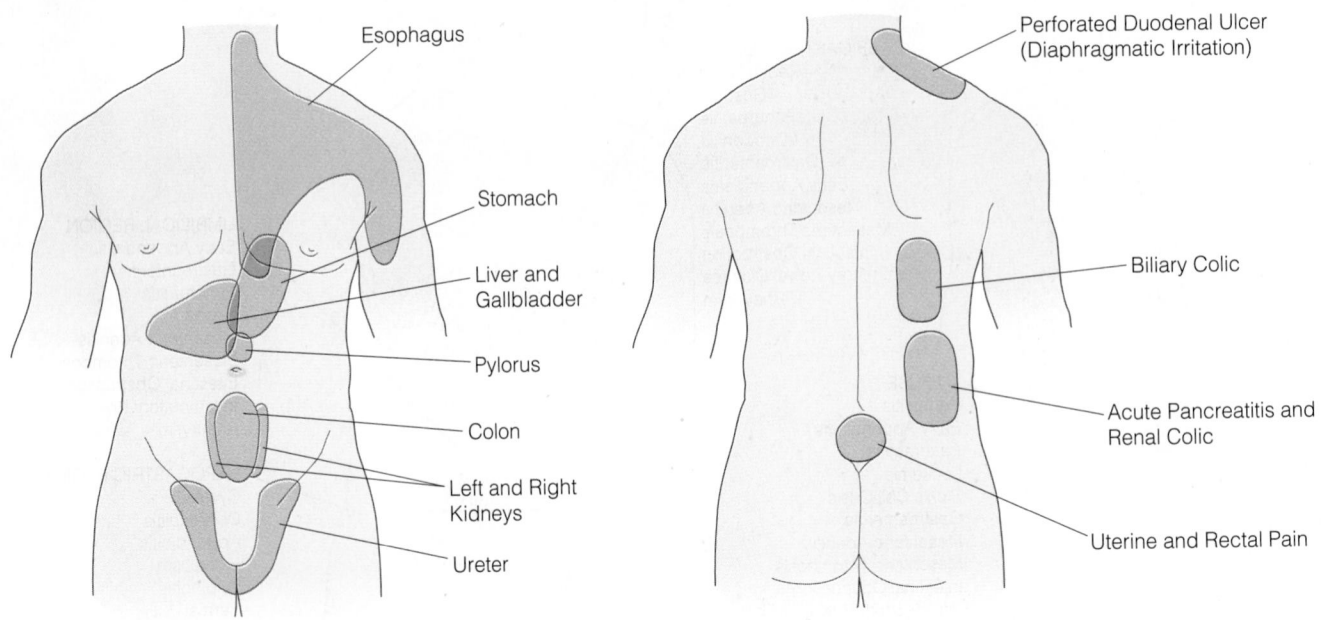

Figure 3 **Pain of abdominal origin tends to be referred in characteristic patterns.**[43] **The more severe the pain is, the more likely it is to be referred. Shown are anterior (left) and posterior (right) areas of referred pain.**

reduce intestinal peristalsis. Diarrhea is characteristic of gastroenteritis but may also accompany incomplete intestinal obstruction. More significant is a history of obstipation, because if it can be definitely established that a patient with acute abdominal pain has not passed gas or stool for 24 to 48 hours, it is certain that some degree of intestinal obstruction is present. Other associated symptoms that should be noted include jaundice, melena, hematochezia, hematemesis, and hematuria. These symptoms are much more specific than the ones just discussed and can be extremely valuable in the differential diagnosis. Most conditions that cause acute abdominal pain of surgical significance are associated with some degree of fever. Fever suggests an inflammatory process; however, it is usually low grade and often absent altogether, particularly in elderly and immunocompromised patients. The combination of a high fever with chills and rigors indicates bacteremia, and concomitant changes in mental status (e.g., agitation, disorientation, and lethargy) suggest impending septic shock.

A history of trauma (even if the patient considers the traumatic event trivial) should be actively sought in all cases of unexplained acute abdominal pain; such a history may not be readily volunteered (as is often the case with trauma resulting from domestic violence). With female patients, it is essential to obtain a detailed gynecologic history that includes the timing of symptoms within the menstrual cycle, the date of the last menses, previous and current use of contraception, any abnormal vaginal bleeding or discharge, an obstetric history, and any risk factors for ectopic pregnancy (e.g., PID, use of an intrauterine device, or previous ectopic or tubal surgery).

A complete history of previous medical conditions must be obtained because associated diseases of the cardiac, pulmonary, and renal systems may give rise to acute abdominal symptoms and may also significantly affect the morbidity and mortality associated with surgical intervention. Weight changes, past illnesses, recent travel, environmental exposure to toxins or infectious agents, and medications used should also be investigated. A history of previous abdominal operations should be obtained but should not be relied on too heavily in the absence of operative reports. A careful family history is important for detection of hereditary disorders that may

cause acute abdominal pain. A detailed social history should also be obtained that includes tobacco, alcohol, or illicit drug use as well as a sexual history.

Tentative Differential Diagnosis

Once the patient's history has been obtained, the examiner should generate a tentative differential diagnosis and carry out the physical examination in 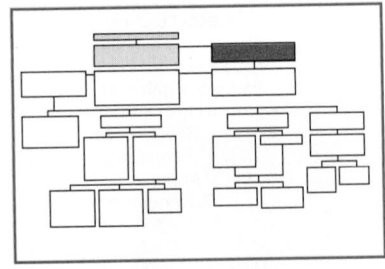 search of specific signs or findings that either rule out or confirm the diagnostic possibilities. Given that the list of conditions that can cause acute abdominal pain is almost endless [*see Tables 1 and 2*], there is no substitute for some general knowledge of what the most common causes of acute abdominal pain are and how age, gender, and geography may affect the likelihood that any of these potential causes is present.

Ambulatory patients with acute abdominal pain as a chief complaint constitute 2% to 3% of all patients in an office practice and 5% to 10% of all patients seen in the emergency department.[4,13,15] At least two thirds of these patients have disorders that do not call for surgical intervention.[2,4,5] Although acute abdominal pain is the most common surgical emergency and most non–trauma-related surgical admissions (and 1% of all hospital admissions) are accounted for by patients complaining of abdominal pain, little information is available regarding the clinical spectrum of disease in these patients.[16] Nevertheless, detailed epidemiologic information can be an invaluable asset in the diagnosis and treatment of acute abdominal pain.

The most extensive information available comes from the ongoing survey begun in 1977 by the Research Committee of the OMGE. As of the last progress report on this survey, which was published in 1988,[12] more than 200 physicians at 26 centers in 17 countries had accumulated data on 10,320 patients with acute

Table 1 Intraperitoneal Causes of Acute Abdominal Pain[44]

Inflammatory
  Peritoneal
    Chemical and nonbacterial peritonitis
      Perforated peptic ulcer/biliary tree,
        pancreatitis, ruptured ovarian cyst,
        mittelschmerz
    Bacterial peritonitis
      Primary peritonitis
        Pneumococcal, streptococcal,
          tuberculous
        Spontaneous bacterial peritonitis
      Perforated hollow viscus
        Esophagus, stomach, duodenum, small
          intestine, bile duct, gallbladder, colon,
          urinary bladder
  Hollow visceral
    Appendicitis
    Cholecystitis
    Peptic ulcer
    Gastroenteritis
    Gastritis
    Duodenitis
    Inflammatory bowel disease
    Meckel diverticulitis
    Colitis (bacterial, amebic)
    Diverticulitis
  Solid visceral
    Pancreatitis
    Hepatitis

Pancreatic abscess
Hepatic abscess
Splenic abscess
Mesenteric
  Lymphadenitis (bacterial, viral)
  Epiploic appendagitis
Pelvic
  Pelvic inflammatory disease (salpingitis)
  Tubo-ovarian abscess
  Endometritis

Mechanical (obstruction, acute distention)
  Hollow visceral
    Intestinal obstruction
      Adhesions, hernias, neoplasms, volvulus
      Intussusception, gallstone ileus, foreign
        bodies
      Bezoars, parasites
    Biliary obstruction
      Calculi, neoplasms, choledochal cyst,
        hemobilia
  Solid visceral
    Acute splenomegaly
    Acute hepatomegaly (congestive heart
      failure, Budd-Chiari syndrome)
  Mesenteric
    Omental torsion
  Pelvic
    Ovarian cyst

Torsion or degeneration of fibroid
Ectopic pregnancy

Hemoperitoneum
  Ruptured hepatic neoplasm
  Spontaneous splenic rupture
  Ruptured mesentery
  Ruptured uterus
  Ruptured graafian follicle
  Ruptured ectopic pregnancy
  Ruptured aortic or visceral aneurysm

Ischemic
  Mesenteric thrombosis
  Hepatic infarction (toxemia, purpura)
  Splenic infarction
  Omental ischemia
  Strangulated hernia

Neoplastic
  Primary or metastatic intraperitoneal
    neoplasms

Traumatic
  Blunt trauma
  Penetrating trauma
  Iatrogenic trauma
  Domestic violence

Miscellaneous
  Endometriosis

abdominal pain [see Table 3]. The most common diagnosis in these patients was nonspecific abdominal pain (NSAP)—that is, the retrospective diagnosis of exclusion in which no cause for the pain can be identified.[17,18] Nonspecific abdominal pain accounted for 34% of all patients seen; the four most common diagnoses accounted for more than 75%. The most common surgical diagnosis was acute appendicitis, followed by acute cholecystitis, small bowel obstruction, and gynecologic disorders. Relatively few patients had perforated peptic ulcer, a finding that confirms the recent downward trend in the incidence of this condition. Cancer was found to be a significant cause of acute abdominal pain. There was little variation in the geographic distribution of surgical causes of acute abdominal pain (i.e., conditions necessitating operation) among developed countries. In patients who required operation, the most common causes were acute appendicitis (42.6%), acute cholecystitis (14.7%), small bowel obstruction (6.2%), perforated peptic ulcer (3.7%), and acute pancreatitis (4.5%).[12]

The finding that NSAP is the most common diagnosis in patients with acute abdominal pain has been confirmed by several other clinical studies[4,5,16,19]; the finding that acute appendicitis, cholecystitis, and intestinal obstruction are the three most common diagnoses in patients with acute abdominal pain who require operation has also been amply confirmed[1,4,5,16,19] [see Table 3].

The data described so far provide a comprehensive picture of the most likely diagnoses for patients with acute abdominal pain in many centers around the world; however, this picture does not take into account the effect of age on the relative likelihood of the various potential diagnoses. It is well known that the disease spectrum of acute abdominal pain is different in different age groups, especially in the very old and the very young.[20] This variation is apparent

when the 10,320 patients from the OMGE study are segregated by age[21] [see Table 4]. In patients 50 years of age or older, cholecystitis was more common than either NSAP or acute appendicitis, and small bowel obstruction, diverticular disease, and pancreatitis were all approximately five times more common than in patients younger than 50 years. Hernias were also a much more common problem in older patients. In the entire group of patients, only one of every 10 instances of intestinal obstruction was attributable to a hernia, whereas in patients 50 years of age or older, one of every three instances was caused by an undiagnosed hernia. Cancer was 40 times more likely to be the cause of acute abdominal pain in patients 50 years of age or older; vascular diseases (including myocardial infarction, mesenteric ischemia, and ruptured abdominal aortic aneurysm) were 25 times more common in patients 50 years of age or older and 100 times more common in patients older than 70 years. What is more, outcome was clearly related to age: mortality was significantly higher in patients older than 70 years (5%) than in those younger than 50 years (less than 1%). Whereas the peak incidence of acute abdominal pain occurred in patients in their teens and 20s, the great majority of deaths occurred in patients older than 70 years.[22]

Further analysis of the data from the OMGE survey also makes it clear that the disease spectrum in children is different from that in adults: well over 90% of cases of acute abdominal pain in children are diagnosed as either acute appendicitis (32%) or nonspecific abdominal pain (62%).[22] Similar age-related differences in the spectrum of disease have been confirmed by other studies,[16] as have various gender-related differences.

Knowledge of the most common causes of acute abdominal pain and familiarity with the special circumstances that make particular causes more likely than others allow the surgeon to play the odds.[14] As has often been said, common things are common—or, to put it another way, most people get what most people get.

Physical Examination

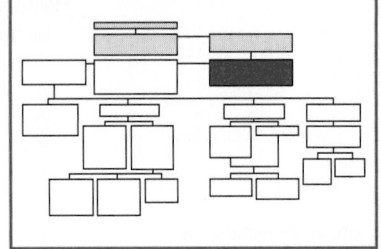

In physical examination, as in history taking, there is no substitute for organization and patience; the amount of information that can be obtained is directly proportional to the gentleness and thoroughness of the examiner. The physical examination begins with a brief but thorough evaluation of the patient's general appearance and ability to answer questions. The degree of obvious pain should be estimated. The patient's position in bed should be noted: as an example, a patient who lies motionless with flexed hips and knees is more likely to have generalized peritonitis, whereas a restless patient who writhes about in bed is more likely to have colicky pain, which suggests different diagnoses. The area of maximal pain should be identified before the physical examination is begun.

The examiner can easily do this by simply asking the patient to cough and then to point with one finger to the area of maximal pain. This allows the examiner to avoid the area in the early stages of the examination and to confirm it at a later stage without causing the patient unnecessary discomfort in the meantime.

A complete physical examination should be performed and extra-abdominal causes of pain and signs of systemic illness should be sought before attention is directed to the patient's abdomen. Systemic signs of shock, such as diaphoresis, pallor, hypothermia, tachypnea, tachycardia with orthostasis, and frank hypotension, usually accompany a rapidly progressive or advanced intra-abdominal condition and, in the absence of extra-abdominal causes, are an indication for immediate laparotomy. The absence of any alteration in vital signs, however, does not necessarily exclude a serious intra-abdominal process.

The surgeon then begins the abdominal examination. This is done with the patient resting in a comfortable supine position. The examination should include inspection, auscultation, percussion, and palpation of all areas of the abdomen, the flanks, and the groin (including all hernia orifices) in addition to rectal and genital examinations (and, in female patients, a full gynecologic examination). A systematic approach is crucial: an examiner who methodically follows a set pattern of abdominal examination every time will be rewarded more frequently than one who improvises haphazardly with each patient.

Table 2 Extraperitoneal Causes of Acute Abdominal Pain

Genitourinary
Pyelonephritis
Perinephric abscess
Renal infarct
Nephrolithiasis
Ureteral obstruction (lithiasis, tumor)
Acute cystitis
Prostatitis
Seminal vesiculitis
Epididymitis
Orchitis
Testicular torsion
Dysmenorrhea
Threatened abortion

Pulmonary
Pneumonia
Empyema
Pulmonary embolus
Pulmonary infarction
Pneumothorax

Cardiac
Myocardial ischemia
Myocardial infarction
Acute rheumatic fever
Acute pericarditis

Metabolic
Acute intermittent porphyria
Familial Mediterranean fever
Hypolipoproteinemia
Hemochromatosis
Hereditary angioneurotic edema

Endocrine
Diabetic ketoacidosis
Hyperparathyroidism (hypercalcemia)
Acute adrenal insufficiency (Addisonian crisis)
Hyperthyroidism or hypothyroidism

Musculoskeletal
Rectus sheath hematoma
Arthritis/diskitis of thoracolumbar spine

Neurogenic
Herpes zoster
Tabes dorsalis
Nerve root compression
Spinal cord tumors
Osteomyelitis of the spine
Abdominal epilepsy
Abdominal migraine
Multiple sclerosis

Inflammatory
Schönlein-Henoch purpura
Systemic lupus erythematosus
Polyarteritis nodosa
Dermatomyositis
Scleroderma

Infectious
Bacterial
Parasitic (malaria)
Viral (measles, mumps, infectious mononucleosis)
Rickettsial (Rocky Mountain spotted fever)

Hematologic
Sickle cell crisis
Acute leukemia
Acute hemolytic states
Coagulopathies
Pernicious anemia
Other dyscrasias

Vascular
Vasculitis
Periarteritis

Toxins
Bacterial toxins (tetanus, staphylococcus)
Insect venom (black widow spider)
Animal venom
Heavy metals (lead, arsenic, mercury)
Poisonous mushrooms
Drugs
Withdrawal from narcotics

Retroperitoneal
Retroperitoneal hemorrhage (spontaneous adrenal hemorrhage)
Psoas abscess

Psychogenic
Hypochondriasis
Somatization disorders

Factitious
Munchausen syndrome
Malingering

Table 3 Frequency of Specific Diagnoses in Patients with Acute Abdominal Pain

Diagnosis	Frequency in Individual Studies (% of Patients)					
	OMGE[12] (N = 10,320)	Wilson[19] (N = 1,196)	Irvin[16] (N = 1,190)	Brewer[4] (N = 1,000)	de Dombal[1] (N = 552)	Hawthorn[5] (N = 496)
Nonspecific abdominal pain	34.0	45.6	34.9	41.3	50.5	36.0
Acute appendicitis	28.1	15.6	16.8	4.3	26.3	14.9
Acute cholecystitis	9.7	5.8	5.1	2.5	7.6	5.9
Small bowel obstruction	4.1	2.6	14.8	2.5	3.6	8.6
Acute gynecologic disease	4.0	4.0	1.1	8.5	—	—
Acute pancreatitis	2.9	1.3	2.4	—	2.9	2.1
Urologic disorders	2.9	4.7	5.9	11.4	—	12.8
Perforated peptic ulcer	2.5	2.3	2.5	2.0	3.1	—
Cancer	1.5	—	3.0	—	—	—
Diverticular disease	1.5	1.1	3.9	—	2.0	3.0
Dyspepsia	1.4	7.6	1.4	1.4	—	—
Gastroenteritis	—	—	0.3	6.9	—	5.1
Inflammatory bowel disease	—	—	0.8	—	—	2.1
Mesenteric adenitis	—	3.6	—	—	—	1.5
Gastritis	—	2.1	—	1.4	—	—
Constipation	—	2.4	—	2.3	—	—
Amebic hepatic abscess	1.2	—	1.9	—	—	—
Miscellaneous	6.3	1.3	5.2	15.5	4.0	8.0

The first step in the abdominal examination is careful inspection of the anterior and posterior abdominal walls, the flanks, the perineum, and the genitalia for previous surgical scars (possible adhesions), hernias (incarceration or strangulation), distention (intestinal obstruction), obvious masses (distended gallbladder, abscesses, or tumors), ecchymosis or abrasions (trauma), striae (pregnancy or ascites), everted umbilicus (increased intra-abdominal pressure), visible pulsations (aneurysm), visible peristalsis (obstruction), limitation of movement of the abdominal wall with ventilatory movements (peritonitis), or engorged veins (portal hypertension).

The next step in the abdominal examination is auscultation. Although it is important to note the presence (or absence) of bowel sounds and their quality, auscultation is probably the least rewarding aspect of the physical examination. Severe intra-abdominal conditions, even intra-abdominal catastrophes, may occur in patients with normal bowel sounds, and patients with silent abdomens may have no significant intra-abdominal pathology at all. In general, however, the absence of bowel sounds indicates a paralytic ileus; hyperactive or hypoactive bowel sounds often are variations of normal activity; and high-pitched bowel sounds with splashes, tinkles (echoing as in a large cavern), or rushes (prolonged, loud gurgles) indicate mechanical bowel obstruction.

The third step is percussion to search for any areas of dullness, fluid collections, sections of gas-filled bowel, or pockets of free air under the abdominal wall. Tympany may be present in patients with bowel obstruction or hollow viscus perforation. Percussion can be useful as a way of estimating organ size and of determining the presence of ascites (signaled by a fluid wave or shifting dullness). It is most useful, however, as a means of demonstrating peritoneal irritation (rebound tenderness). The customary technique is to dig the fingers deep into the patient's abdomen and then let go abruptly. This technique is a time-honored one, but it is painful and often misleads the examiner into assuming that an acute process is present when none exists. Gentle percussion over the four quadrants of the abdomen is much better tolerated by the patient; in addition, it is much more accurate in demonstrating rebound tenderness.

The last step, palpation, is the most informative aspect of the physical examination. Palpation of the abdomen must be done very gently to avoid causing additional pain early in the examination. It should begin as far as possible from the area of maximal pain and then should gradually advance toward this area, which should be the last to be palpated. The examiner should place the entire hand on the patient's abdomen with the fingers together and extended, applying pressure with the pulps (not the tips) of the fingers by flexing the wrists and the metacarpophalangeal joints. It is essential to determine whether true involuntary muscle guarding (muscle spasm) is present. This determination is made by means of gentle palpation over the abdominal wall while the patient takes a long, deep breath. If guarding is voluntary, the underlying muscle immediately relaxes under the gentle pressure of the palpating hand. If, however, the patient has true involuntary guarding, the muscle remains in spasm (i.e., taut and rigid) throughout the respiratory cycle (so-called boardlike abdomen). True involuntary guarding is indicative of localized or generalized peritonitis. It must be remembered that muscle rigidity is relative: for example, muscle guarding may be less pronounced or absent in debilitated and elderly patients who have poor abdominal musculature. In addition, the evaluation of muscle guarding is dependent on the patient's cooperation.

Palpation is also useful for determining the extent and severity of the patient's tenderness. Diffuse tenderness indicates generalized peritoneal inflammation. Mild diffuse tenderness without guarding usually indicates gastroenteritis or some other inflammatory intestinal process without peritoneal inflammation. Localized tenderness suggests an early stage of disease with limited peritoneal inflammation.

Careful palpation can elicit several specific signs [see Table 5]—such as the Rovsing sign (associated with acute appendicitis) and the Murphy sign (acute cholecystitis)—that are indicative of localized peritoneal inflammation. Similarly, specific maneuvers can elicit signs of localized peritoneal irritation, such as the psoas sign (associated with retrocecal appendicitis), the obturator sign (pelvic appendicitis), and the Kehr sign (diaphragmatic irritation). One very important maneuver is the Carnett test, in which the patient elevates his or her head off the bed, thus tensing the abdominal muscles. Tenderness to palpation persists when the pain is caused by abdominal wall conditions (e.g., rectal sheath hematoma) but decreases or disappears when the pain is caused by intraperitoneal conditions (the Carnett sign).

Rectal, genital, and (in women) pelvic examinations are an essential part of the evaluation in all patients with acute abdominal pain. The rectal examination should include evaluation of sphincter tone, tenderness (localized versus diffuse), and prostate size and tenderness, as well as a search for the presence of hemorrhoids, masses, fecal impaction, foreign bodies, and gross or occult blood. The genital examination should search for adenopathy, masses, discoloration, edema, and crepitus. The pelvic examination in women should check for vaginal discharge or bleeding, cervical discharge or bleeding, cervical mobility and tenderness, uterine tenderness, uterine size, and adnexal tenderness or masses. Although a carefully performed pelvic examination can be invaluable in differentiating nonsurgical conditions (e.g., PID) from conditions necessitating prompt operation (e.g., acute appendicitis), the possibility that a surgical condition is present should not be prematurely dismissed solely on the basis of a finding of tenderness on pelvic or rectal examination.

Basic Investigative Studies

Although laboratory and radiologic studies rarely, if ever, establish a definitive diagnosis by themselves, they are often useful for confirming the diagnosis suggested by the history and the physical examination.

LABORATORY STUDIES

In all except extremely hemodynamically unstable patients, a complete blood count, blood chemistries, and a urinalysis are routinely obtained. The hematocrit is important in that it allows the surgeon to detect significant changes in plasma volume (e.g., dehydration caused by vomiting, diarrhea, or fluid loss into the peritoneum or the intestinal lumen), preexisting anemia, or bleeding. An elevated white blood cell count is indicative of an inflammatory process and is a particularly helpful finding if associated with a marked left shift; however, the presence or absence of leukocytosis should never be the single deciding factor as to whether the patient should undergo an operation. A low white blood cell count may be a feature of viral infections, gastroenteritis, or NSAP.

Serum electrolyte, blood urea nitrogen, and creatinine concentrations are useful in determining the nature and extent of fluid losses. Blood glucose and other blood chemistries may also be helpful. Liver function tests (serum bilirubin, alkaline phosphatase, and transaminase levels) are mandatory when abdominal pain is suspected to be hepatobiliary in origin. Similarly, amylase and lipase determinations are mandatory when pancreatitis is suspected, although it must be remembered that amylase levels may be low or normal in patients with pancreatitis and may be markedly elevated in patients with other conditions (e.g., intestinal obstruction, mesenteric thrombosis, and perforated ulcer).

Urinalysis may reveal red blood cells (suggestive of renal or ureteral calculi), white blood cells (urinary tract infection or inflammatory processes adjacent to the ureters, such as retrocecal appendicitis), increased specific gravity (dehydration), glucose, ketones (diabetes), or bilirubin (hepatitis). A pregnancy test should be considered in any woman of childbearing age with acute abdominal pain.

An electrocardiogram is mandatory in elderly patients and in patients with a history of atherosclerotic heart disease. Abdominal pain may be a manifestation of myocardial disease, and the physiologic stress of acute abdominal pain can increase myocardial oxygen demands and induce ischemia in patients with coronary artery disease.

RADIOLOGIC STUDIES

In most patients with acute abdominal pain, initial radiologic evaluation should include plain films of the abdomen in the

Table 4 Frequency of Specific Diagnoses in Younger and Older Patients with Acute Abdominal Pain in the OMGE Study[12,21]

Diagnosis	Frequency (% of Patients)	
	Age < 50 Yr (N = 6,317)	Age ≥ 50 Yr (N = 2,406)
Nonspecific abdominal pain	39.5	15.7
Appendicitis	32.0	15.2
Cholecystitis	6.3	20.9
Obstruction	2.5	12.3
Pancreatitis	1.6	7.3
Diverticular disease	< 0.1	5.5
Cancer	< 0.1	4.1
Hernia	< 0.1	3.1
Vascular disease	< 0.1	2.3

Table 5 Common Abdominal Signs and Findings Noted on Physical Examination[7]

Sign or Finding	Description	Associated Clinical Condition(s)
Aaron sign	Referred pain or feeling of distress in epigastrium or precordial region on continued firm pressure over the McBurney point	Acute appendicitis
Ballance sign	Presence of dull percussion note in both flanks, constant on left side but shifting with change of position on right side	Ruptured spleen
Bassler sign	Sharp pain elicited by pinching appendix between thumb of examiner and iliacus muscle	Chronic appendicitis
Beevor sign	Upward movement of umbilicus	Paralysis of lower portions of rectus abdominis muscles
Blumberg sign	Transient abdominal wall rebound tenderness	Peritoneal inflammation
Carnett sign	Disappearance of abdominal tenderness when anterior abdominal muscles are contracted	Abdominal pain of intra-abdominal origin
Chandelier sign	Intense lower abdominal and pelvic pain on manipulation of cervix	Pelvic inflammatory disease
Charcot sign	Intermittent right upper quadrant abdominal pain, jaundice, and fever	Choledocholithiasis
Chaussier sign	Severe epigastric pain in gravid female	Prodrome of eclampsia
Claybrook sign	Transmission of breath and heart sounds through abdominal wall	Ruptured abdominal viscus
Courvoisier sign	Palpable, nontender gallbladder in presence of clinical jaundice	Periampullary neoplasm
Cruveilhier sign	Varicose veins radiating from umbilicus (*caput medusae*)	Portal hypertension
Cullen sign	Periumbilical darkening of skin from blood	Hemoperitoneum (especially in ruptured ectopic pregnancy)
Cutaneous hyperesthesia	Increased abdominal wall sensation to light touch	Parietal peritoneal inflammation secondary to inflammatory intra-abdominal pathology
Dance sign	Slight retraction in area of right iliac fossa	Intussusception
Danforth sign	Shoulder pain on inspiration	Hemoperitoneum (especially in ruptured ectopic pregnancy)
Direct abdominal wall tenderness	—	Localized inflammation of abdominal wall, peritoneum, or an intra-abdominal viscus
Fothergill sign	Abdominal wall mass that does not cross midline and remains palpable when rectus muscle is tense	Rectus muscle hematoma

(continued)

supine and standing positions and chest radiographs.[23] If the patient is unable to stand, a left lateral decubitus radiograph should be obtained. Like the basic laboratory studies (see above), these plain radiographs may help confirm diagnoses suggested by the history and the physical examination, such as pneumonia (signaled by pulmonary infiltrates); intestinal obstruction (air-fluid levels and dilated loops of bowel); intestinal perforation (pneumoperitoneum); biliary, renal, or ureteral calculi (abnormal calcifications); appendicitis (fecalith); incarcerated hernia (bowel protruding beyond the confines of the peritoneal cavity); mesenteric infarction (air in the portal vein); chronic pancreatitis (pancreatic calcifications); acute pancreatitis (the so-called colon cutoff sign); visceral aneurysms (calcified rim); retroperitoneal hematoma or abscess (obliteration of the psoas shadow); and ischemic colitis (so-called thumbprinting on the colonic wall).

A prospective study published in 1999 evaluated the utility of routine plain abdominal radiographs in the management of adult patients with acute right lower quadrant abdominal pain.[24] The results seem to demonstrate that indiscriminate use of such radiographs in this patient subset is not helpful but that discriminating use in selected patients with clinically suspected small bowel obstruction or urinary symptoms may be worthwhile. Admittedly, plain abdominal radiographs cost relatively little; still, refraining from

routinely obtaining them in all patients with suspected acute appendicitis would help reduce the cost of medical care appreciably.

Working Diagnosis

Ideally, the tentative differential diagnosis list generated after the clinical history was obtained should be narrowed down to a working diagnosis by the physical examination and the information provided by the basic laboratory and radiologic studies. Once this working diagnosis has been established, subsequent management depends on the accepted treatment for the particular condition believed to be present. In general, the course of management follows four basic pathways (see below), depending on whether the patient (1) is in need of immediate laparotomy, (2) is believed to have an underlying surgical condition, (3) has an uncertain diagnosis, or (4) is believed to have an underlying nonsurgical condition.

It must be emphasized that the patient must be constantly reevaluated (preferably by the same examiner) even after the working diagnosis has been established. If the patient does not

Table 5 *(continued)*

Sign or Finding	Description	Associated Clinical Condition(s)
Grey Turner sign	Local areas of discoloration around umbilicus and flanks	Acute hemorrhagic pancreatitis
Iliopsoas sign	Elevation and extension of leg against pressure of examiner's hand causes pain	Appendicitis (retrocecal) or an inflammatory mass in contact with psoas
Kehr sign	Left shoulder pain when patient is supine or in the Trendelenburg position (pain may occur spontaneously or after application of pressure to left subcostal region)	Hemoperitoneum (especially ruptured spleen)
Kustner sign	Palpable mass anterior to uterus	Dermoid cyst of ovary
Mannkopf sign	Acceleration of pulse when a painful point is pressed on by examiner	Absent in factitious abdominal pain
McClintock sign	Heart rate > 100 beats/min 1 hr post partum	Postpartum hemorrhage
Murphy sign	Palpation of right upper abdominal quadrant during deep inspiration results in right upper quadrant abdominal pain	Acute cholecystitis
Obturator sign	Flexion of right thigh at right angles to trunk and external rotation of same leg in supine position result in hypogastric pain	Appendicitis (pelvic appendix); pelvic abscess; an inflammatory mass in contact with muscle
Puddle sign	Alteration in intensity of transmitted sound in intra-abdominal cavity secondary to percussion when patient is positioned on all fours and stethoscope is gradually moved toward flank opposite percussion	Free peritoneal fluid
Ransohoff sign	Yellow pigmentation in umbilical region	Ruptured common bile duct
Rovsing sign	Pain referred to the McBurney point on application of pressure to descending colon	Acute appendicitis
Subcutaneous crepitance	Palpable crepitus in abdominal wall	Subcutaneous emphysema or gas gangrene
Summer sign	Increased abdominal muscle tone on exceedingly gentle palpation of right or left iliac fossa	Early appendicitis; nephrolithiasis; ureterolithiasis; ovarian torsion
Ten Horn sign	Pain caused by gentle traction on right spermatic cord	Acute appendicitis
Toma sign	Right-sided tympany and left-sided dullness in supine position as a result of peritoneal inflammation and subsequent mesenteric contraction of intestine to right side of abdominal cavity	Inflammatory ascites

respond to treatment as expected, the working diagnosis must be reassessed and the possibility that another condition exists must be immediately entertained and investigated by returning to the differential diagnosis list.

Indications for Immediate Laparotomy

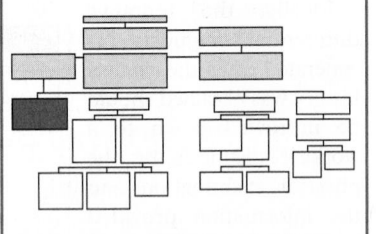

A systematic approach to patients with acute abdominal pain is essential because in some patients, action must be taken immediately and there is not enough time for an exhaustive evaluation. As outlined (see above), such an approach should include a brief initial assessment, a complete clinical history, a thorough physical examination, and basic laboratory and radiologic studies. These steps can usually be completed in less than 1 hour and should be insisted on in the evaluation of most patients.

There are, in fact, very few abdominal crises that mandate immediate operation, and even with these conditions, it is still necessary to spend a few minutes on assessing the seriousness of the problem and establishing a probable diagnosis. Among the most common of the abdominal catastrophes that necessitate immedi-

ate operation are ruptured abdominal aortic or visceral aneurysms, ruptured ectopic pregnancies, and spontaneous hepatic or splenic ruptures. The relative rarity of such conditions notwithstanding, it must always be remembered that patients with acute abdominal pain may have a progressive underlying intra-abdominal disorder causing the acute pain and that unnecessary delays in diagnosis and treatment can adversely affect outcome, often with catastrophic consequences.

When immediate operation is not called for, the physician must decide whether urgent or nonurgent but early operation is necessary, whether additional tests are required before a decision can be made, whether the patient should be admitted to the hospital for careful observation, or whether nonsurgical treatment is indicated [*see* Suspected Surgical Abdomen, Uncertain Diagnosis, *and* Suspected Nonsurgical Abdomen, *below*].

Suspected Surgical Abdomen

INDICATIONS FOR URGENT LAPAROTOMY OR LAPAROSCOPY

Once a definitive diagnosis has been made, it is easy to decide whether a patient should undergo operation. On occasion, however, a patient must be operated on before a precise diagnosis is reached. In contemporary clinical practice, the misuse or abuse of available technology frequently undermines the importance of sound surgical judgment at the bedside: in particular, too many patients with obvious surgical abdomens are subjected to time-consuming imaging studies before surgical consultation is obtained. *It cannot be emphasized too strongly that although diagnostic accuracy is intellectually satisfying and undoubtedly important, the primary goal in the management of patients with acute abdominal pain is not to arrive at an exact clinicopathologic diagnosis but rather to determine which patients require immediate or urgent surgical intervention.* Indications for immediate laparotomy (see above) are essentially limited to severe hemodynamic instability. Indications for urgent laparotomy are somewhat more numerous.

Urgent laparotomy implies operation within 1 to 2 hours of the patient's arrival; thus, there is usually sufficient time for adequate resuscitation, with proper rehydration and restoration of vital organ function, before the procedure. Indications for urgent laparotomy may be encountered during the physical examination, may be revealed by the basic laboratory and radiologic studies, or may not become apparent until other investigative studies are performed. Involuntary guarding or rigidity during the physical examination, particularly if spreading, is a strong indication for urgent laparotomy. Other indications include increasing severe localized tenderness, progressive tense distention, physical signs of sepsis (e.g., high fever, tachycardia, hypotension, and mental status changes), and physical signs of ischemia (e.g., fever and tachycardia). Basic laboratory and radiologic indications for urgent laparotomy include pneumoperitoneum, massive or progressive intestinal distention, signs of sepsis (e.g., marked or rising leukocytosis, increasing glucose intolerance, and acidosis), and signs of continued hemorrhage (e.g., a falling hematocrit). Additional findings that constitute indications for urgent laparotomy include free extravasation of radiologic contrast material, mesenteric occlusion on angiography, endoscopically uncontrollable bleeding, and positive results from peritoneal lavage (i.e., the presence of blood, pus, bile, urine, or gastrointestinal contents). Acute appendicitis, perforated hollow viscera, and strangulated hernias are examples of common conditions that necessitate urgent laparotomy.

Several studies from the 1990s suggest that laparoscopy is the procedure of choice when the primary clinical diagnosis is acute appendicitis or perforated peptic ulcer.[25-30] In a prospective, randomized trial,[26] Hansen and associates reported that laparoscopic appendectomy is as safe as open appendectomy. Although laparoscopic appendectomy requires a longer operating time (63 minutes versus 40 minutes), it has two advantages: the surgical site infection rate is lower, and patients return to normal activities earlier. Accordingly, we recommend laparoscopic appendectomy as a worthwhile alternative for patients with a clinical diagnosis of acute appendicitis. It has also been shown that diagnostic laparoscopy through the right lower abdominal incision is very helpful in establishing the correct diagnosis in patients who are operated on for suspected acute appendicitis but in whom the appendix is grossly normal.[27]

Laparoscopic treatment of perforated peptic ulcers—either with an omental patch or with sutures[28-30]—is becoming more popular as surgeons gain experience and competence with the technique. Compared with open approaches, laparoscopic repair results in reduced wound pain and respiratory complications as well as earlier return to normal activities.

HOSPITALIZATION AND ACTIVE OBSERVATION

Numerous studies have shown that of all patients admitted for acute abdominal pain, only a minority require immediate or urgent operation.[2,4,5] It is therefore cost-effective as well as prudent to adopt a system of evaluation that allows for thought and investigation before definitive treatment in all patients with acute abdominal pain except those identified early on as needing immediate or urgent laparotomy. The traditional wisdom is that spending time on observation opens the door for complications (e.g., perforating appendicitis, intestinal perforation associated with bowel obstruction, or strangulation of an incarcerated hernia); however, careful clinical trials evaluating active in-hospital observation of patients with acute abdominal pain of uncertain origin have demonstrated that such observation is safe, is not accompanied by an increased incidence of complications, and results in fewer negative laparotomies.[31]

After the initial assessment has been completed, narcotic analgesia for pain relief should not be withheld.[32,33] In appropriately titrated doses, analgesics neither obscure important physical findings nor mask their subsequent development. In fact, some physical signs may be more easily identified after adequate pain relief.[34,35] Severe pain that persists in spite of adequate doses of narcotics suggests a serious condition that is likely to call for operative intervention.[33]

Active observation allows the surgeon to identify most of the patients whose acute abdominal pain is caused by NSAP or various specific nonsurgical conditions. It must be emphasized that active observation means something more than simply admitting the patient to the hospital: it implies an active process of thoughtful, discriminating, and meticulous reevaluation of the patient (preferably by the same examiner) at intervals ranging from minutes to a few hours, to be complemented by appropriately timed additional investigative studies.

Additional investigative studies beyond the basic ones already mentioned should be obtained only if the results are likely to alter or improve patient management significantly. Furthermore, the invasiveness, morbidity, and cost-effectiveness of each additional test must be carefully weighed. More liberal use of supplemental studies is justified in those patients in whom the history and physical findings tend to be less reliable (e.g., the very young, the elderly, the critically ill, or the immunocompromised).

Supplemental studies that may be considered include computed tomography, ultrasonography, diagnostic peritoneal lavage, radionuclide imaging, angiography, magnetic resonance imaging, gastrointestinal endoscopy [*see V:6 Gastrointestinal Endoscopy*], and diagnostic laparoscopy. Diagnostic laparoscopy has been recommended when surgical disease is suspected but its probability is not high enough to warrant open laparotomy.[36] It is particularly valuable in young women of childbearing age, in whom gynecologic disorders frequently mimic acute appendicitis.[37] A report by Chung and coworkers showed that diagnostic laparoscopy had the same diagnostic yield as open laparotomy in 55 patients with acute abdomen[38]; 34 (62%) of these patients were safely managed with laparoscopy alone, with no increase in morbidity and with a shorter average hospital stay. Diagnostic laparoscopy has also been shown to be useful in the assessment of acute abdominal pain in ICU patients[39] and patients with AIDS.[40]

INDICATIONS FOR EARLY OR ELECTIVE LAPAROTOMY OR LAPAROSCOPY

Early laparotomy or laparoscopy (within 24 to 48 hours of the initial evaluation) is reserved for patients whose conditions are not likely to become life threatening if operation is delayed to permit further resuscitation or additional investigative studies. It is often possible to perform early laparotomy or laparoscopy in patients with uncomplicated acute cholecystitis or diverticulitis and those with nonstrangulated incarcerated hernias, thereby preventing the increased patient risk that always accompanies unplanned emergency operations as well as avoiding the logistical impediments to unscheduled surgical procedures in the middle of the night or on weekends or holidays. Similarly, patients with simple uncomplicated intestinal obstructions often benefit from several hours of nasogastric tube decompression and fluid and electrolyte resuscitation.

Elective laparotomy or laparoscopy is reserved for patients whose condition is highly likely to respond to conservative medical management or highly unlikely to become life threatening during prolonged periods (several days or even weeks) of diagnostic evaluation.

Uncertain Diagnosis

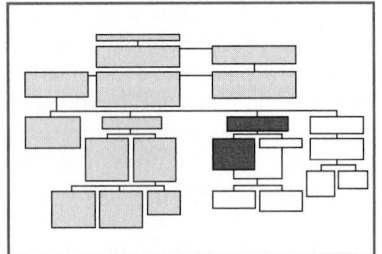

HOSPITALIZATION AND ACTIVE OBSERVATION

If the diagnosis is unclear, the surgeon's task is to determine whether hospitalization and active observation are necessary or whether outpatient evaluation is an option. All patients with acute abdominal pain and evidence of extracellular fluid deficits, electrolyte imbalances, or sepsis must be hospitalized. Furthermore, any patient with unexplained abdominal symptoms whose condition has not improved within 24 hours of the initial evaluation should be hospitalized.[41]

Supplemental studies are often required for further evaluation and complete workup of patients with uncertain diagnoses and for the exclusion of many medical conditions that do not call for operation. When the diagnosis is not obvious from the history and the physical examination, apparent on the plain radiographs, or suggested by the basic laboratory studies, ultrasonography and CT, both of which are now widely available, should be considered. CT is more useful in the early evaluation of patients with acute abdominal pain because it is not operator dependent, is not hampered by the presence of overlying gas (which transmits sound waves poorly and interferes with ultrasonography), and can be performed rapidly (a complete scan of the abdomen and pelvis takes less than 15 minutes). Although watchful observation with ongoing reexamination is a time-honored approach to the patient with acute abdominal pain of uncertain origin, excessive reliance on this practice or on esoteric physical diagnosis maneuvers (which most medical students have witnessed in awe at one time or another) suggests that the surgeon is unaware of how valuable, rapid, and accurate a CT scan can be in the early diagnosis of these patients.

Diagnostic peritoneal lavage, although most useful in the evaluation of blunt abdominal trauma, may be particularly helpful in obtunded or critically ill patients, whose condition is difficult to assess by means of history taking and physical examination.[42]

OUTPATIENT EVALUATION

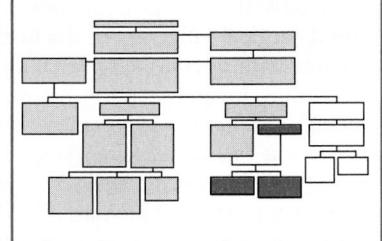

The epidemiology of acute abdominal pain is such that for every patient who requires hospitalization, there are at least two or three others who have self-limiting conditions for which neither operation nor hospitalization is necessary. Much or all of the evaluation of such patients, as well as any treatment that may be needed, can now be completed in the outpatient department. To treat acute abdominal pain cost-effectively and efficiently, the surgeon must be able not only to identify patients who need immediate or urgent laparotomy or laparoscopy but also to reliably identify those whose condition does not present a serious risk and who therefore can be managed without hospitalization. The reliability and intelligence of the patient, the proximity and availability of medical facilities, and the availability of responsible adults to observe and assist the patient at home are factors that should be carefully considered before the decision is made to evaluate or treat individuals with acute abdominal pain as outpatients.

Suspected Nonsurgical Abdomen

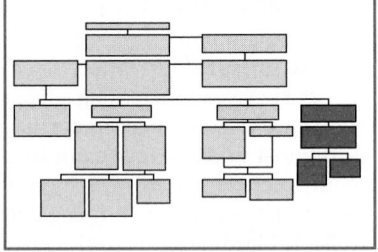

There are numerous disorders that cause acute abdominal pain but do not call for surgical intervention. These nonsurgical conditions are often extremely difficult to differentiate from surgical conditions that present with almost indistinguishable characteristics.[2] For example, the acute abdominal pain of lead poisoning or acute porphyria is difficult to differentiate from the intermittent pain of intestinal obstruction, in that marked hyperperistalsis is the hallmark of both. The pain of acute hypolipoproteinemia may be accompanied by pancreatitis, which, if not recognized, can lead to unnecessary laparotomy. Similarly, acute and prostrating abdominal pain accompanied by rigidity of the abdominal wall and a low hematocrit may lead to unnecessary urgent laparotomy in patients with sickle cell anemia crises. To further complicate the clinical picture, cholelithiasis is also often found in patients with sickle cell anemia.

In addition to numerous extraperitoneal disorders [see Table 2], nonsurgical causes of acute abdominal pain include a wide variety of intraperitoneal disorders, such as acute gastroenteritis (from enteric bacterial, viral, parasitic, or fungal infection), acute gastritis, acute duodenitis, hepatitis, mesenteric adenitis, salpingitis, Fitz-Hugh–Curtis syndrome, mittelschmerz, ovarian cyst, endometritis, endometriosis, threatened abortion, spontaneous bacterial peritonitis, and tuberculous peritonitis. Acute abdominal pain in immunosuppressed patients or patients with AIDS is now encountered with increasing frequency and can be caused by a number of unusual conditions (e.g., cytomegalovirus enterocolitis, opportunistic infections, lymphoma, and Kaposi sarcoma) as well as by the more usual ones.

As noted [see Tentative Differential Diagnosis, above], most patients with acute abdominal pain presenting to the office or the emergency department have an underlying nonsurgical condition and do not require operation.[2,4,5] Again, the single most common diagnosis in these patients is NSAP.[5,12,16-19] Although the natural history of NSAP has been well documented (harmless abdominal pain that is relieved in a few days without any treatment), there have been no prospective studies detailing the symptomatology and physical findings associated with this disorder. Furthermore, it remains unclear whether NSAP is in fact a single disease entity or is simply the presenting symptom complex for many different minor and self-limited conditions.[18] A complete clinical history and physical examination, coupled with careful in-hospital observation and a high index of suspicion, will in most cases prevent unnecessary laparotomy in patients with nonsurgical causes of acute abdominal pain. On rare occasions, diagnostic laparoscopy may be employed to prevent unnecessary laparotomy.

Conclusion

In the management of patients with acute abdominal pain, it occasionally happens that even with the aid of considerable clinical acumen and liberal use of diagnostic tests, the surgeon cannot readily determine whether a patient requires operation. In such cases, laparotomy or diagnostic laparoscopy may constitute the definitive, as well as the safest, approach to the evaluation of acute abdominal pain.

References

1. de Dombal FT: Diagnosis of Acute Abdominal Pain, 2nd ed. Churchill Livingstone, London, 1991

2. Purcell TB: Nonsurgical and extraperitoneal causes of abdominal pain. Emerg Med Clin North Am 7:721, 1989

3. Silen W: Cope's Early Diagnosis of the Acute Abdomen, 17th ed. Oxford University Press, New York, 1990

4. Brewer RJ, Golden GT, Hitch DC, et al: Abdominal pain: an analysis of 1,000 consecutive cases in a university hospital emergency room. Am J Surg 131: 219, 1976

5. Hawthorn IE: Abdominal pain as a cause of acute admission to hospital. J R Coll Surg Edinb 37:389, 1992

6. Staniland JR, Ditchburn J, de Dombal FT: Clinical presentation of acute abdomen: study of 600 patients. Br Med J 3:393, 1972

7. Hickey MS, Kiernan GJ, Weaver KE: Evaluation of abdominal pain. Emerg Med Clin North Am 7:437, 1989

8. Adams ID, Chan M, Clifford PC, et al: Computer aided diagnosis of acute abdominal pain: a multicentre study. Br Med J 293:800, 1986

9. Paterson-Brown S, Vipond MN: Modern aids to clinical decision-making in the acute abdomen. Br J Surg 77:13, 1990

10. Wellwood J, Johannessen S, Spiegelhalter DJ: How does computer-aided diagnosis improve the management of acute abdominal pain? Ann R Coll Surg Engl 74:40, 1992

11. de Dombal FT: Computers, diagnoses and patients with acute abdominal pain. Arch Emerg Med 9:267, 1992

12. de Dombal FT: The OMGE acute abdominal pain survey. Progress Report, 1986. Scand J Gastroenterol 144(suppl):35, 1988

13. American College of Emergency Physicians: Clinical policy for the initial approach to patients presenting with a chief complaint of nontraumatic acute abdominal pain. Ann Emerg Med 23:906, 1994

14. de Dombal FT: Surgical Decision Making in Practice: Acute Abdominal Pain. Butterworth-Heinemann Ltd, Oxford, 1993, p 65

15. Walters DT, Wendel HF: Abdominal pain. Prim Care 13:3, 1986

16. Irvin TT: Abdominal pain: a surgical audit of 1190 emergency admissions. Br J Surg 76:1121, 1989

17. Jess P, Bjerregaard B, Brynitz S, et al: Prognosis of acute nonspecific abdominal pain: a prospective study. Am J Surg 144:338, 1982

18. Gray DW, Collin J: Non-specific abdominal pain as a cause of acute admission to hospital. Br J Surg 74: 239, 1987

19. Wilson DH, Wilson PD, Walmsley RG, et al: Diagnosis of acute abdominal pain in the accident and emergency department. Br J Surg 64:249, 1977

20. Bender JS: Approach to the acute abdomen. Med Clin North Am 73:1413, 1989

21. Telfer S, Fenyo G, Holt PR, et al: Acute abdominal pain in patients over 50 years of age. Scand J Gastroenterol. Suppl 144:47, 1988

22. Dickson JAS, Jones A, Telfer S, et al: Acute abdominal pain in children. Progress Report, 1986. Scand J Gastroenterol. Suppl 144:43, 1988

23. Plewa MC: Emergency abdominal radiography. Emerg Med Clin North Am 9:827, 1991

24. Boleslawski E, Panis Y, Benoist S, et al: Plain abdominal radiography as a routine procedure for acute abdominal pain of the right lower quadrant: prospective evaluation. World J Surg 23:262, 1999

25. Fritts LL, Orlando R: Laparoscopic appendectomy: a safety and cost analysis. Arch Surg 128:521, 1993

26. Hansen JB, Smithers BM, Schache D, et al: Laparoscopic versus open appendectomy: prospective randomized trial. World J Surg 20:17, 1996

27. Schrenk P, Rieger R, Shamiyeh A, et al: Diagnostic laparoscopy through the right lower abdominal incision following open appendectomy. Surg Endosc 13: 133, 1999

28. Matsuda M, Nishiyama M, Hanai T, et al: Laparoscopic omental patch repair for the perforated peptic ulcer. Ann Surg 221:236, 1995

29. Tate JJ, Dawson JW, Lau WY, et al: Sutureless laparoscopic treatment of perforated duodenal ulcer. Br J Surg 80:235, 1993

30. Darzi A, Cheshire NJ, Somers SS, et al: Laparoscopic omental patch repair of perforated duodenal ulcer with an automated stapler. Br J Surg 80:1552, 1993

31. Thomson HJ, Jones PF: Active observation in acute abdominal pain. Am J Surg 152:522, 1986

32. Zoltie N, Cust MP: Analgesia in the acute abdomen. Ann R Coll Surg Engl 68:209, 1986

33. Boey JH: The acute abdomen. Current Surgical Diagnosis and Treatment, 10th ed. Way LW, Ed. Appleton & Lange, Norwalk, Connecticut, 1994, p 441

34. Cuschieri A: The acute abdomen and disorders of the peritoneal cavity. Essential Surgical Practice. Cuschieri A, Giles GT, Moosa AR, Eds. Wright PSG, Bristol, 1982, p 885

35. Attard AR, Corlett MJ, Kidner NJ, et al: Safety of early pain relief for acute abdominal pain. BMJ 305:554, 1992

36. Salky BA, Edye MB: The role of laparoscopy in the diagnosis and treatment of abdominal pain syndromes. Surg Endosc 12: 911, 1998

37. Borgstein PJ, Gordijn RV, Eijsbouts QA, et al: Acute appendicitis—a clear-cut case in men, a guessing game in young women: a prospective study on the role of laparoscopy. Surg Endosc 11:923, 1997

38. Chung RS, Diaz JJ, Chari V: Efficacy of routine laparoscopy for the acute abdomen. Surg Endosc 12:219, 1998

39. Orlando R, Crowell KL: Laparoscopy in the critically ill. Surg Endosc 11:1072, 1997

40. Box JC, Duncan T, Ramshaw B, et al: Laparoscopy in the evaluation and treatment of patients with AIDS and acute abdominal complaints. Surg Endosc 11: 1026, 1997

41. Hobsley M: An approach to the acute abdomen. Pathways in Surgical Management, 2nd ed. Edward Arnold Ltd, London, 1986

42. Larson FA, Haller CC, Delcore R, et al: Diagnostic peritoneal lavage in acute peritonitis. Am J Surg 164: 449, 1992

43. Cheung LY, Ballinger WF: Manifestations and diagnosis of gastrointestinal diseases. Hardy's Textbook of Surgery. Hardy JD, Ed. JB Lippincott Co, Philadelphia, 1983, p 445

44. McFadden DW, Zinner MJ: Manifestations of gastrointestinal disease. Principles of Surgery, 6th ed. Schwartz SI, Shires GT, Spencer FC, Eds. McGraw-Hill, New York, 1994, p 1015

Acknowledgment

Figures 2 and 3   Tom Moore.

5 ABDOMINAL MASS

Romano Delcore, M.D., and Laurence Y. Cheung, M.D.

Evaluation of Abdominal Masses

Abdominal masses are mentioned in some of the earliest known medical writings. The Papyrus Ebers (ca. 1500 B.C.) discusses the differential diagnosis of abdominal masses and describes methods of abdominal examination by palpation.[1] In his *Book of Prognostics* (ca. 400 B.C.), Hippocrates discussed the prognostic significance of abdominal masses:

> That state of the hypochondrium is best when it is free from pain, soft, and of equal size on the right side and the left. But if inflamed, or painful, or distended; or when the right and left sides are of disproportionate sizes; all these appearances are to be dreaded.... Such swellings as are soft, free from pain, and yield to the finger, occasion more protracted crises, and are less dangerous than the others.... Such, then, as are painful, hard, and large, indicate danger of speedy death.[2]

The term abdominal mass generally refers to a palpable mass that is anterior to the paraspinous muscles and is located anywhere between the costal margins, the iliac crests, and the pubic symphysis. An abdominal mass may be noticed initially by the patient or may be discovered by the surgeon as a new finding. In either case, the mass may have been present for days, months, or even years and may be caused by any of a great variety of intra-abdominal, pelvic, or retroperitoneal disorders as well as by any of numerous different abdominal wall lesions.

Occasionally, after examining a patient with an abdominal mass, the surgeon is so certain about the diagnosis that no further investigation is necessary and appropriate management for the condition can be instituted immediately. Conditions that often can be readily diagnosed in this fashion include obesity, ascites, pregnancy, abdominal wall hernias, sebaceous cysts, and lipomas. It must be remembered, however, that even when an experienced clinician is convinced of the presence of a mass, it is still possible that no abnormality exists. In one study, 22% of patients thought to have a palpable mass on the basis of physical examination proved not to have any abnormalities on further investigation.[3]

Most often, the surgeon is confronted with a diagnostic challenge, in which assessing the origin and character of the abdominal mass proves difficult, time consuming, and expensive. This challenge involves not only establishing the correct diagnosis but also determining whether this can be accomplished without operative intervention. Making the correct decision regarding whether to operate on a patient with an abdominal mass requires sound surgical judgment. The decision must be based on a detailed medical and surgical history as well as on a meticulous physical examination. These, in turn, must be guided by experience; a thorough knowledge of the anatomy and physiology of the abdominal wall, abdominal cavity, and retroperitoneum; and a clear understanding of the physiologic and pathologic processes within and around the abdomen. The arrival of new diseases, coupled with the continuous development of new diagnostic technologies, calls for constant broadening of the differential diagnosis and periodic revision of established approaches to the evaluation of abdominal masses.

Clinical History

A careful and methodical clinical history should be obtained that includes the mode of onset, duration, character, location, and chronology of the abdominal mass as well as the presence or absence of any associated symptoms. When the surgeon obtains an unhurried and complete clinical history, the patient often provides all the information needed for making the correct diagnosis. In addition, such a history is often more valuable than any single laboratory or radiologic finding and determines the course of subsequent evaluation and management. Patients should be allowed to relate the history in their own words, and examiners should refrain from suggesting specific chronologies or symptoms except as a last resort. Any questions that must be asked should be open-ended—for example, "When did you first notice a mass?" rather than "Did you just notice the mass?" Leading questions should be avoided. When a leading question must be asked, it should be posed first as a negative question (i.e., one that calls for an answer in the negative), since a negative answer to a question is more likely to be honest and accurate.

Various GI symptoms (e.g., nausea, vomiting, anorexia, diarrhea, constipation, and a decrease in stool caliber) often accompany an abdominal mass. These symptoms are nonspecific but may still be of some value in the differential diagnosis. Other associated symptoms that should be noted are jaundice, melena, hematochezia, hematemesis, hematuria, and menorrhagia. These symptoms are more specific and can be very valuable in the differential diagnosis. Urinary hesitancy or urgency in the presence of a lower abdominal mass may suggest bladder distention secondary to urethral obstruction or urinary retention caused by anticholinergic medications (e.g., phenothiazines). A female patient with a pelvic mass should be asked for a detailed gynecologic history that includes the timing of symptoms within the menstrual cycle, the date of the last menses, previous and current use of contraception, any abnormal vaginal bleeding or discharge, and a complete obstetric history. All patients with abdominal masses should also be asked about previous injuries, however minor: even a traumatic event the patient considers trivial can be diagnostically significant.

A complete history of previous medical conditions must be obtained because associated diseases may give rise to abdominal masses and may also significantly affect morbidity and mortality from subsequent surgical intervention. Weight changes suggesting carcinoma, past illnesses, previous abdominal operations, and recent travel (raising the possibility of amebic abscess or parasitic cyst) should also be investigated. A careful family history is important for detection of hereditary disorders that may cause abdominal masses.

Tentative Differential Diagnosis

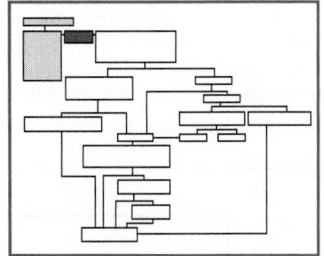

Once the history has been obtained, the examiner should generate a tentative differential diagnosis and carry out the physical examination in search of specific signs or findings that either confirm or rule out the diagnostic possibilities. Failure to include a broad array of possibilities in the tentative differential diagnosis is a common and often costly mistake. For example, when urinary retention is not considered as part of the early differential diagnosis of a large lower abdominal mass, the patient may undergo needlessly extensive and expensive evaluations.

In the light of the large number of conditions that can give rise to an abdominal mass, the task of arriving at a specific diagnosis can appear overwhelming. To lessen the difficulty of this task, it would be invaluable to have some general knowledge of what the most common causes of abdominal masses are as well as how age, gender, associated symptoms, and geography may affect the likelihood that any of these potential causes is present. Unfortunately, abdominal masses as such usually are not coded in the medical record; rather, specific diseases or definitive diagnoses are coded. Consequently, the true incidence of abdominal mass remains unknown, nor is there much information in the literature regarding the relative frequency with which specific diseases present with an abdominal mass.[4] As of early 1999, only two series had been published that provided a differential diagnosis of abdominal masses based on statistical analysis and relative frequency.[1,5] These two series have now been rendered hopelessly outdated by modern medical practice and the advent of newer diagnostic and therapeutic modalities. Nevertheless, knowledge of the most common disease processes associated with abdominal masses and familiarity with the characteristic signs and symptoms that accompany the most common causes of this presenting symptom can greatly facilitate and shorten the evaluation of patients presenting with abdominal masses.

Physical Examination

In physical examination, as in history taking, there is no substitute for organization and patience; the amount of information that can be obtained is directly proportional to the gentleness and thoroughness of the examiner. As in the evaluation of the acute abdomen [see II:4 Acute Abdominal Pain], the physical examination begins with a brief but thorough evaluation of the patient's general appearance. Any obvious pain or

associated discomfort should be noted. A complete physical examination should be performed, and possible extra-abdominal causes of the mass as well as signs of systemic illness should be sought before attention is directed to the mass. Systemic signs of shock, such as tachycardia, tachypnea, diaphoresis, pallor, orthostasis, and frank hypotension, usually accompany a rapidly progressive or advanced condition and are an indication for immediate resuscitation and laparotomy. Abdominal masses that may occur in association with systemic signs of shock and that must be recognized as soon as possible include abdominal aortic and other visceral aneurysms, hepatic and splenic subcapsular hematomas, blood-filled pancreatic pseudocysts, and empyema of the gallbladder with associated ascending cholangitis. The abdominal examination should include inspection, auscultation, palpation, and percussion, generally in that order; these maneuvers are described in more detail elsewhere [see II:4 Acute Abdominal Pain].

Inspection of the abdomen may reveal either generalized enlargement or distention of the entire abdomen or the presence of one or more discrete masses of varying sizes. Conditions that may give rise to generalized abdominal distention include obesity, tympanites or meteorism (swelling of the abdomen caused by gas within the intestine or peritoneal cavity), ascites, pregnancy, fecal impaction, and neoplasm. An easy way of remembering these conditions is to use the so-called six Fs mnemonic device: Fat, Fluid, Flatus, Fetus, Feces, and Fatal growths.[6-8]

The most common cause of transient generalized enlargement of the abdomen is intestinal gas or bloating. Gaseous distention may appear or disappear in minutes to hours and is usually accompanied by discomfort. Percussion of the abdomen elicits tympany. Because aerophagia and certain foods are common causes of gaseous distention, the differential diagnosis necessitates a detailed dietary history. Intestinal ileus and intestinal obstruction (in particular, distal obstruction) can present with generalized abdominal enlargement resulting from gaseous distention.

The most common cause of chronic abdominal enlargement is obesity. This condition is usually readily apparent on inspection and is confirmed on examination by the greatly increased skinfold thickness of the abdominal wall. When obesity results from adipose tissue in the mesentery, the omentum, and the extraperitoneal layer, the diagnosis may not be so readily apparent. In general, obesity makes evaluation of discrete abdominal masses by means of physical examination much more difficult, to the point where masses of remarkable size can be missed by even the most careful examiner. Massive enlargement of a single organ (e.g., the liver, the spleen, or the kidneys) or a large fluid-filled cyst can also cause generalized abdominal enlargement, as can accumulation of ascitic fluid in the peritoneal cavity. A common and often overlooked cause of an abdominal mass, particularly in elderly or institutionalized patients, is fecal impaction. Removal of the impaction causes the mass to disappear.

A distended urinary bladder may extend up to the level of the umbilicus; it is usually in the midline, and because of its extreme size, it is commonly mistaken for an abdominal mass. The swelling is fluctuant and resolves with catheterization. In cases of acute gastric dilatation, the distended stomach may also occasionally be large enough to all but fill the abdomen. Decompression with a nasogastric tube leads to complete resolution.

When the mass is discrete rather than generalized, the examiner should note whether it moves with respiration; such movement suggests that the mass is associated with a mobile organ in the abdominal cavity rather than located in the retroperitoneum

Evaluation of Abdominal Masses

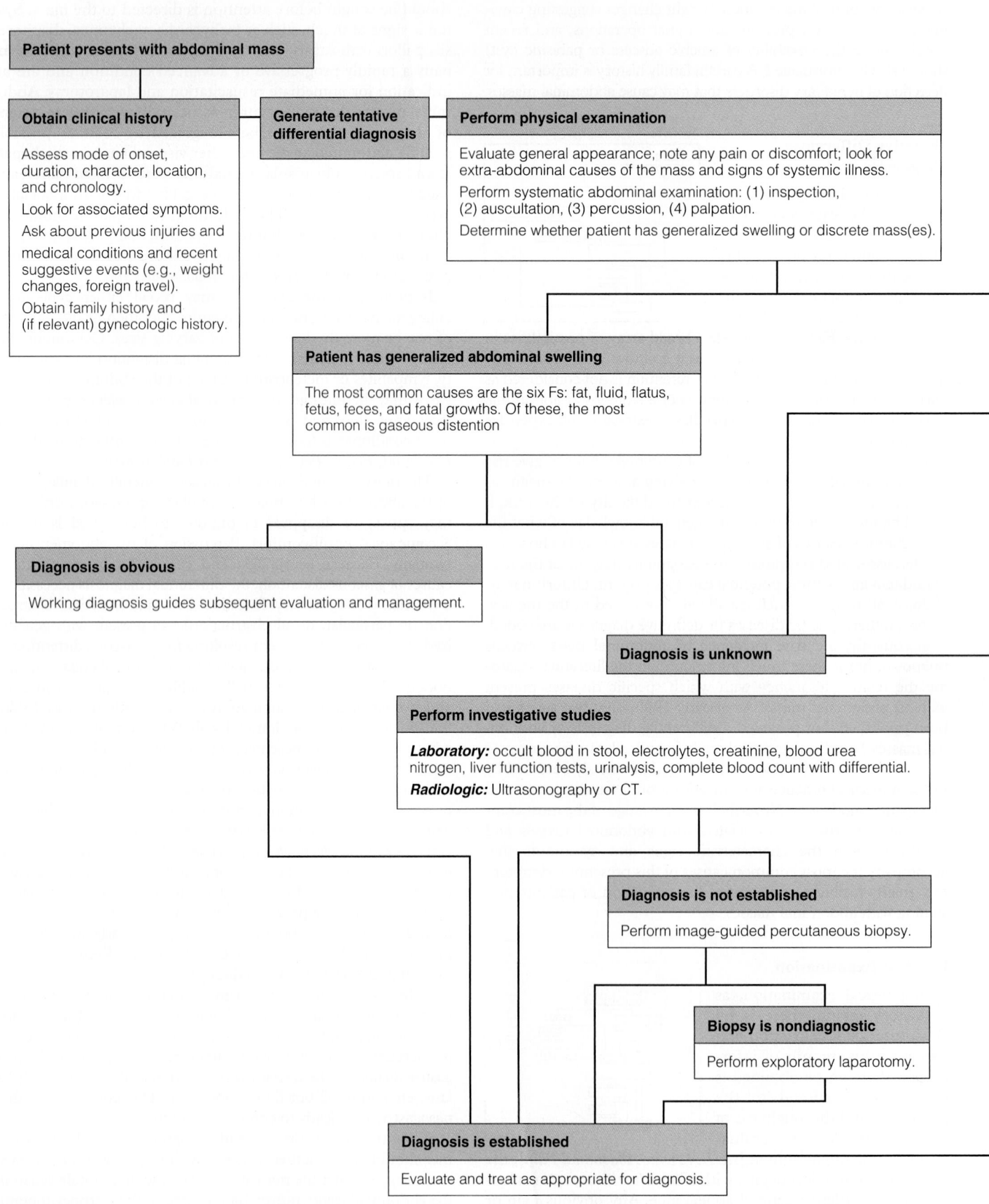

Patient presents with abdominal mass

Obtain clinical history

Assess mode of onset, duration, character, location, and chronology.

Look for associated symptoms.

Ask about previous injuries and medical conditions and recent suggestive events (e.g., weight changes, foreign travel).

Obtain family history and (if relevant) gynecologic history.

Generate tentative differential diagnosis

Perform physical examination

Evaluate general appearance; note any pain or discomfort; look for extra-abdominal causes of the mass and signs of systemic illness.

Perform systematic abdominal examination: (1) inspection, (2) auscultation, (3) percussion, (4) palpation.

Determine whether patient has generalized swelling or discrete mass(es).

Patient has generalized abdominal swelling

The most common causes are the six Fs: fat, fluid, flatus, fetus, feces, and fatal growths. Of these, the most common is gaseous distention

Diagnosis is obvious

Working diagnosis guides subsequent evaluation and management.

Diagnosis is unknown

Perform investigative studies

Laboratory: occult blood in stool, electrolytes, creatinine, blood urea nitrogen, liver function tests, urinalysis, complete blood count with differential.
Radiologic: Ultrasonography or CT.

Diagnosis is not established

Perform image-guided percutaneous biopsy.

Biopsy is nondiagnostic

Perform exploratory laparotomy.

Diagnosis is established

Evaluate and treat as appropriate for diagnosis.

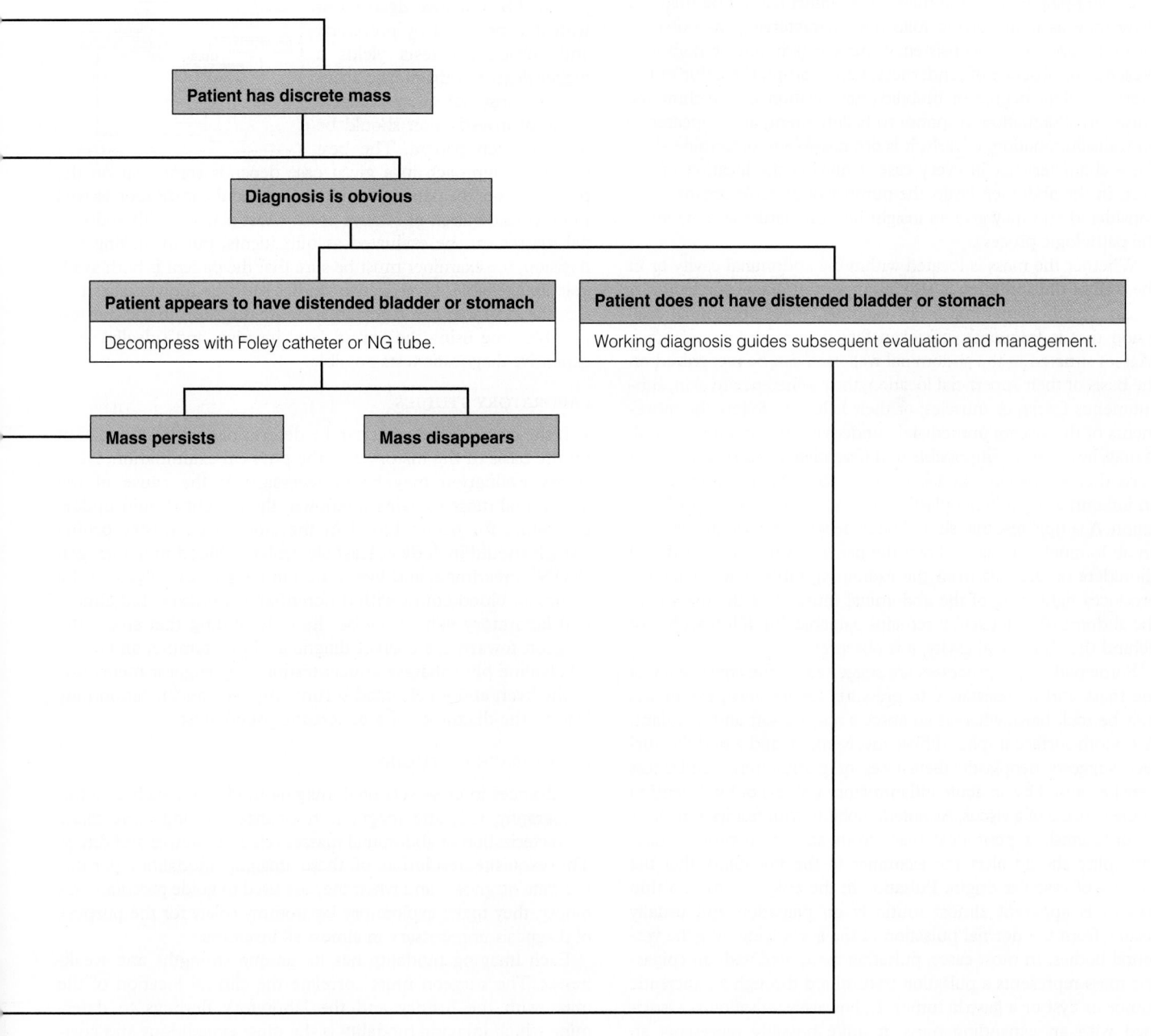

Patient has discrete mass

Diagnosis is obvious

Patient appears to have distended bladder or stomach

Decompress with Foley catheter or NG tube.

Patient does not have distended bladder or stomach

Working diagnosis guides subsequent evaluation and management.

Mass persists

Mass disappears

or attached to the abdominal wall. Inspection should be followed by auscultation, before percussion and palpation stimulate the abdominal viscera to abnormal activity that may obscure vascular bruits.

The examination begins with light palpation of the entire abdomen, which may reveal regions of tenderness and increased resistance that should be examined later in detail. Light palpation can determine only the presence of a mass and its location; further information must be sought through deep palpation, which is done to confirm the findings from inspection and light palpation and to search for previously unsuspected masses. Frequently, a mass that is not visible on inspection is easily felt on palpation. Normal structures felt during palpation must not be confused with abdominal masses. Prominent segments of the abdominal wall musculature, the abdominal aorta, and the sacral promontory may be mistaken for abdominal masses on a cursory examination. Masses must also be distinguished from muscle spasms.

During palpation of the mass, every effort should be made to determine as many of the following characteristics as possible: location, size, shape, consistency, surface (smooth or nodular), presence or absence of tenderness, temperature, the color of the overlying skin, degree of mobility, any fixation or attachments, pulsatility, fluctuation, response to ballottement, and appearance on transillumination. Clearly, it is not possible to determine all of these characteristics in every case. Knowing the location of the mass in the abdomen limits the number of possible organs to be considered and may give an insight into the nature and extent of the pathologic process.

Whether the mass is located within the abdominal cavity or in the wall of the abdomen is also an important diagnostic factor. A rectus sheath hematoma is an example of an abdominal wall lesion that is frequently mistaken for an intra-abdominal mass. Masses situated in the abdominal wall itself can be recognized on the basis of their superficial location; their adherence to skin, subcutaneous fascia, or muscles; or their failure to follow the movements of the viscera immediately underlying the abdominal wall. It may, however, be impossible to differentiate an intra-abdominal mass that has become attached to the abdominal wall (as either an inflammatory or a neoplastic process) from an abdominal wall lesion. A simple test that should be done with any patient who has an abdominal mass is to direct the patient to raise the head and shoulders or the legs from the examining table. This maneuver produces tightening of the abdominal muscles. If the mass is in the abdominal wall itself, it remains palpable, but if it is within or behind the abdominal cavity, it is obscured.

Some pathologic processes are suggested by the consistency of the mass and its resistance to pressure: for instance, carcinoma may be rock-hard, whereas an abscess may be soft and fluctuant. A smooth surface implies diffuse involvement, and a nodular surface suggests neoplastic metastases or granulomas. Tenderness may be caused by an acute inflammatory process or by distention of the capsule of a viscus. As noted, mobility with respiration tends to distinguish a peritoneal mass from an extraperitoneal one. Pulsatility should alert the examiner to the possibility that the mass is of vascular origin. Pulsation in the epigastrium of a thin patient is apparent almost routinely on palpation and usually results from the normal pulsation of the aorta lying over the vertebral bodies. In most cases, pulsation associated with an epigastric mass represents a pulsation transmitted through a pancreatic tumor or cyst or a gastric tumor. If, however, pulsation is associated with an expanding mass, it quite possibly represents an abdominal aortic aneurysm. Fluctuation may indicate a cyst, a pseudocyst, a hematoma, or an abscess.

Working Diagnosis

The tentative differential diagnosis list that is generated after the clinical history has been obtained can often be narrowed down to a working diagnosis on the basis of the physical examination. Once a working diagnosis has been established, subsequent management depends on the accepted methods of evaluation and treatment for the particular condition believed to be present. In a number of cases, however, the diagnosis remains unknown even after the physical examination. When this is the case, investigative studies are required. Often, basic investigative studies (e.g., laboratory testing, ultrasonography, or CT) are sufficient to establish the diagnosis. Occasionally, they are not, and further investigative studies are needed.

Investigative Studies

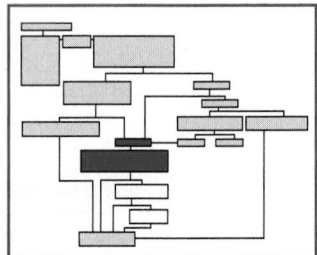

Integrating the information provided by one investigative test with that provided by preceding and subsequent tests yields a higher degree of diagnostic accuracy. Clearly, not every available mode of investigation should be used in each patient. The best evaluative approach in a given case depends somewhat on the preferences of the patient, the physician, and the institution as well as on consideration of relative costs. Most patients with abdominal masses can be evaluated as outpatients, but in making this decision, the examiner must be sure that the patient is both available and reliable. Investigative studies must be individualized so that the examiner can reach an accurate diagnosis in the shortest possible time using the fewest, least invasive, and (ideally) least expensive diagnostic tests possible.

LABORATORY STUDIES

If the cause of the mass can be determined without question on the basis of the history and the physical examination, laboratory evaluation may be unnecessary. If the cause of the abdominal mass remains unknown, the patient should undergo testing for occult blood in the stool, a chemistry profile (which should include at least electrolytes, blood urea nitrogen [BUN], creatinine, and liver function tests), a urinalysis, and a complete blood count with differential. An unexpected abnormal laboratory value may be the only finding that steers the surgeon toward the correct diagnosis. For example, an elevated alkaline phosphatase concentration may suggest metastasis to the liver, and an elevated serum amylase concentration may lead to the diagnosis of a pancreatic pseudocyst.

RADIOGRAPHIC STUDIES

Advances in cross-sectional imaging modalities, such as ultrasonography, CT, and magnetic resonance imaging, have made characterization of abdominal masses relatively simple and direct. The exquisite resolution of these imaging modalities permits accurate diagnosis, and when they are used to guide percutaneous biopsy, they make exploratory laparotomy solely for the purpose of diagnosis unnecessary in almost all instances.[9]

Each imaging modality has its unique strengths and weaknesses. The surgeon must correlate the clinical location of the mass with the history and the laboratory findings to determine which imaging modality is the most expeditious and cost-effective in a given instance. Of the currently available imaging procedures, ultrasonography [see V:4 Ultrasonography: Surgical

a

b

c

Figure 1 **A 51-year-old patient presented with a palpable abdominal mass. (*a*) A transverse ultrasonogram showed a complex, multiply septated peritoneal cyst. A normal transverse ultrasonogram of the same region (*b*) is provided for purposes of comparison. (*c*) A longitudinal ultrasonogram of the same patient shows the cyst from a different viewpoint.**

Applications] is the least expensive, the least invasive, and the most readily available. Proper interpretation of ultrasonograms is highly dependent on the skill and experience of the ultrasonographer; however, even examiners who lack great expertise with this modality generally are still able to obtain most of the information they need to evaluate an abdominal mass. The essential information available from the ultrasonogram includes where the mass is anatomically located, whether it is solid or cystic, and on what surrounding structures it impinges [*see Figure 1*]. Once this information is obtained, further imaging procedures are often unnecessary.

Plain Abdominal Radiographs

The plain abdominal radiograph (kidneys-ureters-bladder [KUB]) usually reveals only nonspecific and indirect evidence of a mass, such as alteration in the size or density of an organ or displacement of normal structures or fat planes. Occasionally, however, this low-cost technique can make specific diagnoses, such as a calcified aortic aneurysm, acute gastric distention, fecal impaction, or an enlarged porcelain gallbladder.

Conventional Barium Studies

At one time, barium studies were the best noninvasive method for evaluating abdominal masses. The advent of cross-sectional imaging has relegated barium studies to an adjunctive role in the evaluation of upper abdominal and midabdominal masses because unless a mass arises directly from the alimentary tract, barium studies yield only indirect signs of its presence. Barium studies still play an important role in the evaluation of adult patients with lower abdominal masses whose history suggests GI pathology (e.g., anemia and weight loss, suggesting a colonic neoplasm, or fever and leukocytosis, suggesting a diverticular inflammatory mass).

Excretory Urography

Excretory urography is not recommended as an initial examination in the evaluation of abdominal masses, because unless the mass originates directly from the kidney or bladder, this technique yields only indirect signs, such as displacement or obstruction of the kidney, the ureter, or the bladder.

Angiography

Cross-sectional imaging modalities have relegated arteriography and venography to secondary roles in the evaluation of abdominal masses. The major role of these techniques is to provide a vascular road map for the surgeon before operation.

Radionucleotide Scanning

Cross-sectional imaging has essentially eliminated the use of radionucleotide studies in the evaluation of abdominal masses.

Magnetic Resonance Imaging

MRI can display abdominal masses directly and is excellent at discriminating varying degrees of density in soft tissue. Because MRI is not as widely available as ultrasonography or CT and because its cost-effectiveness in relation to these modalities has not been demonstrated, MRI is not used as a primary imaging modality for abdominal masses.

Ultrasonography

Ultrasonography has several advantages in the evaluation of abdominal masses: widespread availability, speed, absence of ionizing radiation, portability, low cost, and the ability to document a

a
b

Figure 2 **A 58-year-old male patient presented with a palpable, visible (*a*) abdominal mass. (*b*) A CT scan showed a mass arising from the omentum. An omental leiomyosarcoma was surgically resected.**

mass's size, consistency, and (usually) origin in real time.[10,11] In addition, the necessary equipment can be transported to the patient's bedside, and the test requires no patient preparation and only minimal patient cooperation.

Ultrasonography can readily differentiate solid from cystic masses, but its ability to visualize the abdominal cavity is limited by the acoustic barriers presented by intestinal gas and bone, which prevent the evaluation of underlying structures. Another limitation is that spatial resolution decreases as depth of penetration increases [*see V:4 Ultrasonography: Surgical Applications*]. For these reasons, ultrasonography is most effective in regions where an acoustic window exists, such as the right upper quadrant, the pelvis, and the left upper quadrant.

The principal disadvantage of ultrasonography is its dependence on the technical proficiency of the operator. Because ultrasonography is so operator dependent, it is quite possible that in the hands of an inexperienced ultrasonographer, it can contribute to misdiagnosis. The experience level of the ultrasonographer must always be taken into account when ultrasonography is used in the evaluation of an abdominal mass.

Computed Tomography

Currently, CT is the most efficient imaging modality available for the evaluation of abdominal masses[3,9,12]: it has excellent spatial resolution and exquisite density discrimination, and it provides cross-sectional images that are unaffected by bowel gas, bone, excessive abdominal fat, or unusually large body size [*see Figures 2 and 3*]. CT yields excellent visualization of vascular structures and can assess the vascularity of an abdominal mass after intravenous administration of contrast material. It routinely visualizes retroperitoneal and abdominal wall structures and perfectly displays the peritoneal compartments, clearly defining tissue planes and illustrating relations between masses and adjacent organs and structures.[13-15] If, however, the bowel is not opacified, the accuracy of CT in evaluating abdominal masses is significantly reduced because unopacified intestinal loops can simulate a mass or an abscess.

When the examiner suspects that an abdominal mass is neoplastic, CT is the initial imaging procedure of choice because in addition to imaging the mass itself directly, CT provides invaluable information for staging purposes (e.g., evidence of contiguous spread or the presence of distant metastases).

a
b

Figure 3 **A 49-year-old female patient presented with an abdominal mass. (*a*) A CT scan reveals a uterine fibroid presenting as a pelvic mass. A normal CT of the same region (*b*) is provided for purposes of comparison.**

BIOPSY

Image-Guided Percutaneous Biopsy

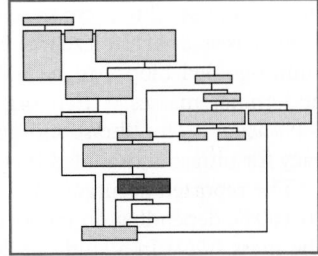

The value of image-guided percutaneous biopsy in the evaluation of abdominal masses is now firmly established.[16,17] Recent improvements in imaging techniques (in particular, developments in high-resolution cross-sectional imaging), advances in cytologic methods (in terms of both performance technique and interpretation of findings) that permit accurate evaluation of minute quantities of aspirated material, and the availability of fine flexible needles for obtaining tissue specimens have all contributed to the rapid growth in the use of this diagnostic method.[18]

Both ultrasonography and CT can be used to guide percutaneous needle insertion.[19-23] The choice between the two depends on several factors, including how large the mass is, where it is, whether it is better visualized with one imaging modality than with the other, and which modality is more readily available. With many masses, either ultrasound guidance or CT guidance will yield good results; in these cases, the choice depends largely on the personal preference and experience of the radiologist performing the biopsy. MRI can also be used to guide needle biopsy, but it has not yet been thoroughly evaluated against ultrasonography and CT in this role.

Traditionally, ultrasound guidance has been used for biopsy of large, superficial, and cystic masses. Currently, however, because of improvements in instrumentation and biopsy techniques, ultrasonography can also accurately guide biopsy of small, deep, and solid masses. The greatest advantage ultrasonography possesses as a guidance modality is that it enables real-time visualization of the needle tip as it passes through tissue planes into the mass. This real-time visualization allows the examiner to place the needle with considerable precision and to avoid important intervening structures. Another advantage ultrasonography has is that it facilitates angled approaches to the mass, in that it is capable of providing guidance in multiple transverse, longitudinal, or oblique planes. In addition, color flow Doppler imaging can identify blood vessels in and around a mass and can prevent complications by helping the examiner to avoid any vascular structures lying in the path of the needle. Theoretically, any mass that is well visualized on an ultrasonogram is amenable to ultrasound-guided biopsy; in practice, however, this technique probably is still best suited to masses located superficially or at moderate depth in thin or average-sized patients.

CT is well established as an accurate guidance method for percutaneous biopsy of most regions of the body. In the abdomen, CT provides excellent spatial resolution of all structures between the skin and the lesion, regardless of how large the patient is or how deep the mass is. Its only limitation is that it does not provide continuous visualization of the needle during insertion and biopsy. In most cases, however, the direction and depth of the needle can be established reliably with CT guidance [*see Figure 4*]; substantial repositioning of the needle is rarely necessary.

Numerous different needles of varying caliber, length, and tip design have been used for percutaneous image-guided biopsy. They can be grouped into two general categories: small caliber (20 to 25 gauge) and large caliber (14 to 19 gauge). Small-caliber needles are employed primarily to obtain specimens for cytologic analysis but may also be employed to obtain small pieces of tissue for histologic examination. Their flexible shafts permit movement of the needle during respiration and minimize the risk of tissue or

Figure 4 **A 51-year-old female patient presented with a palpable abdominal mass. (*a*) A CT scan located a suspicious lesion. A normal CT scan of the same region (*b*) is provided for purposes of comparison. (IVC—inferior vena cava) (*c*) A CT-guided needle biopsy was performed, and the results indicated that the lesion was a gastric leiomyosarcoma.**

organ laceration and damage from tearing. The main advantage of these smaller needles is that biopsies of masses situated behind loops of bowel can be done with minimal risk of infection. Large-caliber needles are employed to obtain greater amounts of material for histologic as well as cytologic analysis.

The following three events are relative contraindications to percutaneous biopsy:

1. Uncorrectable coagulopathy. Although postbiopsy embolization of the needle tract is capable of controlling hemorrhage in patients with uncorrectable coagulopathy, special expertise and equipment are required.
2. Absence of a safe biopsy route. When the location of the mass necessitates that the biopsy path extend through a large blood vessel, the stomach, or an intestinal loop, the potential for hemorrhage or infection increases; however, neither potential complication is a contraindication if a small-caliber needle is used. Biopsies done through collections of ascitic fluid have also proved safe.
3. Lack of cooperation on the part of the patient. An uncooperative patient's uncontrolled motion during needle placement can substantially increase the risk of tissue laceration and hemorrhage; in such cases, sedation or anesthesia may be necessary.

The safety of image-guided percutaneous biopsy is well attested.[18,24] Several large multi-institutional reviews have reported mortalities ranging from 0.008% to 0.031% and major complication rates ranging from 0.05% to 0.18%.[25-27] A review of 11,700 patients who underwent percutaneous abdominal biopsy with 20- to 23-gauge needles between 1969 and 1982 found a total complication rate of only 0.05% and a mortality of only 0.008%.[25] Another study, involving 63,180 patients, demonstrated a complication rate of 0.16%.[28] A single-institution review of 8,000 ultrasound-guided needle biopsies done with both large- and small-caliber needles reported similar results: a mortality of 0.038% and a major complication rate of 0.187%.[29] A prospective study of 3,393 biopsies (1,825 ultrasound-guided and 1,568 CT-guided) showed a mortality of 0.06% and a complication rate of 0.34% (0.3% for ultrasound-guided biopsies and 0.5% for CT-guided biopsies).[24]

Of the major complications, hemorrhage is the most commonly reported. Other major complications reported are pneumothorax, pancreatitis, bile leakage, peritonitis, and needle-track seeding. Although needle-track seeding is an important theoretical consideration when a mass seems likely to be of malignant neoplastic origin, it remains an exceedingly rare complication: fewer than 100 cases have been reported in the literature, for an estimated frequency of only 0.005%.[28,30,31] Because seeding is so rare, it should affect the decision to perform percutaneous biopsy only when the surgeon is convinced the lesion is amenable to curative surgical resection. Most cases of needle-track seeding have occurred after biopsy of a pancreatic carcinoma; however, it has also been reported after biopsy of hepatic and retroperitoneal lesions. There is some evidence to suggest that with masses in solid organs, using large-caliber needles or cutting needles does not lead to a significantly higher complication rate than fine-needle aspiration biopsy does, provided that there is a direct path to the mass.[24,32,33]

The reported accuracy of ultrasound-guided biopsy ranges from 66% to 97%, depending on the location, size, and histologic origin of the mass.[24] In one series of ultrasound-guided biopsies of 126 consecutive small (< 3 cm) solid masses in various anatomic locations and of various histologic types, the overall accuracy of biopsy was 91%.[34] Results improved as the size of the mass increased, rising from 79% in masses 1 cm or less in diameter to

98% in masses 2 to 3 cm in diameter. The accuracy of biopsy for hepatic masses of any size was 96%.[34] Another report found ultrasound-guided biopsy to be 91% accurate for small (< 2.5 cm) abdominal masses.[35] Two organ-specific reviews demonstrated 94% accuracy for ultrasound-guided liver biopsy[36] and 95% accuracy for ultrasound-guided biopsy of pancreatic masses.[37]

The reported accuracy of CT-guided biopsy ranges from 80% to 100%, depending on the location, size, and histologic origin of the mass.[21,22,33] In a study of 200 consecutive CT-guided needle biopsies, the overall accuracy for all sites was 95%. Accuracy of diagnosis was very high for hepatic (99%) and renal (100%) biopsies and for characterization of fluid collections (100%) but somewhat lower for retroperitoneal (87.5%) and pancreatic (82%) biopsies.[21] In a prospective study of 1,000 consecutive CT-guided biopsies, the procedure was 91.8% sensitive and 98.9% specific.[33]

Laparoscopic Biopsy

Even though laparoscopy provides excellent visualization of the inside of the abdominal cavity and now plays an important role in the staging of some abdominal neoplasms, its role in the evaluation of abdominal masses is limited.[38] Laparoscopic biopsy specimens are best obtained under direct vision with a biopsy needle introduced at an independent site rather than with a biopsy forceps: forceps biopsy usually produces superficial, small, squeezed, and distorted specimens. Although percutaneous biopsies of this type can be especially useful when bleeding from the biopsy site is a concern, image-guided percutaneous biopsy usually offers a more expedient, less invasive, cheaper, and often safer means of obtaining the diagnosis. More important, in the presence of adhesions, laparoscopic biopsy is much less effective and typically fails to make a diagnosis altogether unless the mass is clearly visible on the anterior surface of the viscera.

Exploratory Laparotomy

Despite recent advances in diagnostic imaging and laparoscopic procedures, it still occasionally proves necessary to perform an exploratory laparotomy for the sole purpose of establishing a diagnosis in the patient with an abdominal mass. It is essential 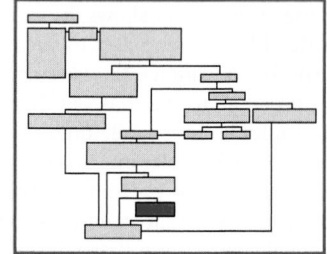 to keep in mind, however, that many patients with abdominal masses have disorders for which operative intervention is not required. In addition, although exploratory laparotomy can yield crucial information and may be, in a sense, the "ultimate diagnostic test" (as some have referred to it), it is not infallible. Errors in the intra-abdominal surgical diagnosis of abdominal masses can and do occur. For example, in six instances observed during an 18-month period at a single institution, exploratory laparotomy failed to reveal abdominal masses that had already been demonstrated by preoperative evaluation and were subsequently confirmed during the postoperative period.[39]

Conclusion

Management of the patient with an abdominal mass ultimately depends on the accurate tissue diagnosis established by microscopic examination of histologic specimens obtained from the mass. To obtain an adequate tissue sample safely, without subjecting the patient to an otherwise unnecessary laparotomy, remains the surgeon's primary responsibility.

References

1. Butler DB, Bargen JA: Abdominal masses. Gastroenterology 19:1, 1951

2. Hippocrates: The Book of Prognostics, part 7. The Internet Classics Archives, http://classics.mit.edu/Hippocrates/prognost.7.7.html

3. Dixon AK, Kingham JGC, Fry IK, et al: Computed tomography in patients with an abdominal mass: effective and efficient? A controlled trial. Lancet 1:1199, 1981

4. Cassidy D: Abdominal mass. The Clinical Practice of Emergency Medicine, 2nd ed. Harwood-Nuss AL, Linden CH, Luten RC, et al, Eds. Lippincott-Raven, Philadelphia, 1996, p 133

5. Cabot RC: Differential Diagnosis, Presented Through an Analysis of 317 Cases, 2nd ed. WB Saunders Co, Philadelphia, 1915, vol 2, p 709

6. Schaffner F: Abdominal enlargement and masses. Gastroenterology. Haubrich WS, Schaffner F, Berk JE, Eds. WB Saunders Co, Philadelphia, 1998, p 138

7. Morales TG, Fennerty MB: Abdominal distention. Clinical Medicine, 2nd ed. Greene HL, Fincher RME, Johnson WP, et al, Eds. Mosby–Year Book, St. Louis, 1996, p 290

8. DeGowin EL, DeGowin RL: Bedside Diagnostic Examination. Macmillan Publishing Co, New York, 1976, p 471

9. Gore RM: Palpable abdominal masses. Diagnostic Imaging: An Algorithmic Approach. Eisenberg RL, Ed. JB Lippincott Co, Philadelphia, 1988, p 214

10. Aspelin P, Hildell J, Karlsson S, et al: Ultrasonic evaluation of palpable abdominal masses. Acta Chir Scand 156:501, 1980

11. Barker CS, Lindsell DRM: Ultrasound of the palpable abdominal mass. Clin Radiol 41:98, 1990

12. Williams MP, Scott IHK, Dixon AK: Computed tomography in 101 patients with a palpable abdominal mass. Clin Radiol 35:293, 1984

13. Engel IA, Auh YH, Rubenstein WA, et al: Large posterior abdominal masses: computed tomographic localization. Radiology 149:203, 1983

14. Pistolesi GF, Procacci C, Caudana R, et al: C.T. criteria of the differential diagnosis in primary retroperitoneal masses. Eur J Radiol 4:127, 1984

15. Pandolfo I, Blandino A, Gaeta M, et al: CT findings in palpable lesions of the anterior abdominal wall. J Comput Assist Tomogr 10:629, 1986

16. Gazelle GS, Haaga JR: Guided percutaneous biopsy of intraabdominal lesions. AJR Am J Radiol 153:929, 1989

17. Welch TJ, Reading CC: Imaging-guided biopsy. Mayo Clin Proc 64:1295, 1989

18. Grainger RG, Allison D: Interventional radiology. Diagnostic Radiology: A Textbook of Medical Imaging. Grainger RG, Allison D, Eds. Churchill Livingstone, New York, 1997, p 2485

19. Staab EV, Jaques PF, Partain CL: Percutaneous biopsy in the management of solid intra-abdominal masses of unknown etiology. Radiol Clin North Am 17:435, 1979

20. Ennis MG, MacErlean DP: Percutaneous aspiration biopsy of abdomen and retroperitoneum. Clin Radiol 31:611, 1980

21. Sundaram M, Wolverson MK, Heiberg E, et al: Utility of CT-guided abdominal aspiration procedures. AJR Am J Radiol 139:1111, 1982

22. Smith C, Butler JA: Efficacy of directed percutaneous fine-needle aspiration cytology in the diagnosis of intra-abdominal masses. Arch Surg 123:820, 1988

23. Jaeger HJ, MacFie J, Mitchell CJ, et al: Diagnosis of abdominal masses with percutaneous biopsy guided by ultrasound. Br Med J 301:1188, 1990

24. Rumack CM, Wilson SR, Charboneau JW: Ultrasound-guided biopsy and drainage of the abdomen and pelvis. Diagnostic Ultrasound. Rumack CM, Wilson SR, Charboneau JW, Eds. Mosby–Year Book, New York, 1998, p 600

25. Livraghi R, Damascelli B, Lombardi C, et al: Risk in fine needle abdominal biopsy. J Clin Ultrasound 11:77, 1983

26. Fornari F, Civardi G, Cavanna L, et al: Complications of ultrasonically guided fine needle abdominal biopsy: results of a multi-centre Italian study and a review of the literature (The Cooperative Italian Study Group). Scand J Gastroenterol 24:949, 1989

27. Smith EH: Complications of percutaneous abdominal fine needle biopsy. Review Radiology 178:253, 1991

28. Smith EH: The hazards of fine needle aspiration biopsy. Ultrasound Med Biol 10:629, 1984

29. Nolsoe C, Nielsen L, Torp-Pedersen S, et al: Major complications and deaths due to interventional ultrasonography: a review of 8000 cases. J Clin Ultrasound 18:179, 1990

30. Engzell U, Esposti PL, Rubio C, et al: Investigation on tumour spread in connection with aspiration biopsy. Acta Radiol Ther Phys Biol 10:385, 1971

31. Smith FP, Macdonald JS, Schein PS, et al: Cutaneous seeding of pancreatic cancer by skinny-needle aspiration biopsy. Arch Intern Med 140:855, 1980

32. Martino CR, Haaga JR, Bryan PJ, et al: CT-guided liver biopsies: eight years' experience. Radiology 152:755, 1984

33. Welch TJ, Sheedy PF, Johnson CD, et al: CT-guided biopsy: prospective analysis of 1,000 procedures. Radiology 171:493, 1989

34. Reading CC, Charboneau JW, James EM, et al: Sonographically guided percutaneous biopsy of small (3 cm or less) masses. AJR Am J Radiol 151:189, 1988

35. Downey DB, Wilson SR: Ultrasonographically guided biopsy of small intra-abdominal masses. Can Assoc Radiol J 44:350, 1993

36. Buscarini L, Fornari F, Bolondi L, et al: Ultrasound-guided fine-needle biopsy of focal liver lesions: technique, diagnostic accuracy and complications: a retrospective study on 2091 biopsies. J Hepatol 11:344, 1990

37. Brandt KR, Charboneau JW, Stephens DH, et al: CT- and US-guided biopsy of the pancreas. Radiology 187:99, 1993

38. Sackier JM, Berci G, Paz-Partlow M: Elective diagnostic laparoscopy. Am J Surg 161:326, 1991

39. Harbin WP, Wittenberg J, Ferrucci JT, et al: Fallibility of exploratory laparotomy in detection of hepatic and retroperitoneal masses. AJR Am J Roentgenol 135:115, 1980

6 JAUNDICE

Jeffrey S. Barkun, M.D., and Alan N. Barkun, M.D.

Approach to the Jaundiced Patient

The term jaundice refers to the yellowish discoloration of skin, sclerae, and mucous membranes that results from excessive deposition of bilirubin in tissues. It usually is unmistakable but on occasion may manifest itself subtly. It is generally held that jaundice develops when serum bilirubin levels rise above 34.2 μmol/L (2 mg/dl)[1]; however, the appearance of jaundice also depends on whether it is conjugated or unconjugated bilirubin that is elevated and on how long the episode of jaundice lasts.

In what follows, we outline a problem-based approach to the jaundiced patient that involves assessing the incremental information provided by successive clinical and laboratory investigations as well as the information obtained by means of modern imaging modalities. We also propose a classification of jaundice that stresses the therapeutic options most pertinent to surgeons. We have not attempted a detailed review of bilirubin metabolism and the various pediatric disorders that cause jaundice; such issues are beyond the scope of this chapter. Finally, we emphasize that modern decision making in the approach to the jaundiced patient includes not only careful evaluation of anatomic issues but also close attention to patient morbidity and quality-of-life concerns, as well as a focus on working up the patient in a cost-effective fashion. For optimal treatment, in our view, an integrated approach that involves the surgeon, the gastroenterologist, and the radiologist is essential.

Clinical Assessment

When a patient presents with a skin discoloration suggestive of jaundice, the first step is to confirm that icterus is indeed present. To this end, the mucous membranes of the mouth, the palms, the soles, and the sclerae should be examined in natural light. Because such areas are protected from the sun, photodegradation of bile is minimized; thus, the yellowish discoloration of elastic tissues may be more easily detected. Occasionally, deposition of a yellowish pigment on skin may mimic jaundice but may in fact be related to the consumption of large quantities of food containing lycopene or carotene or drugs such as rifampin or quinacrine. In these cases, the skin is usually the only site of coloration, and careful inspection of sclerae and mucous membranes generally reveals no icteric pigmentation. In certain cultures, long-term application of tea bags to the eyes may lead to a brownish discoloration of the sclerae that can mimic jaundice.[2]

DIRECT VERSUS INDIRECT HYPERBILIRUBINEMIA

Once the presence of jaundice has been confirmed, further clinical assessment determines whether the hyperbilirubinemia is predominantly direct or indirect. This distinction is based on the division of bilirubin into conjugated and unconjugated fractions, which are also known, respectively, as direct and indirect fractions on the basis of their behavior in the van den Bergh (diazo) reaction.[3] If the patient has normal-colored urine and stools, unconjugated bilirubin [*see Sidebar* Unconjugated (Indirect) Bilirubin] is predominant [*see Table 1*]. If the patient has dark urine, pale stools, or any other signs or symptoms of a cholestatic syndrome (see below), the serum bilirubin fractionation usually indicates that conjugated bilirubin is

---

Unconjugated (Indirect) Bilirubin

The breakdown of heme leads to the production of unconjugated bilirubin, which is water insoluble, is tightly bound to albumin, and does not pass into the urine. Excessive production of unconjugated bilirubin typically follows an episode of hemolysis. In the absence of concomitant liver disease or biliary obstruction, the liver can usually handle the extra bilirubin, and only a modest rise in serum levels is observed. There is a substantial increase in bile pigment excretion, leading to large quantities of stercobilinogen in the stool. A patient with hemolysis may therefore be slightly jaundiced with normal-colored urine and stools. Blood tests reveal that 60% to 85% of bilirubin is indirect.[105]

Possible causes of indirect hyperbilirubinemia include a variety of disorders that result in significant hemolysis or ineffective erythropoiesis. The diagnosis of indirect hyperbilirubinemia attributable to hemolysis is confirmed by an elevated serum lactate dehydrogenase (LDH) level, a decreased serum haptoglobin level, and evidence of hemolysis on microscopic examination of the blood smear.

Disorders associated with defects in hepatic bilirubin uptake or conjugation can also produce unconjugated hyperbilirubinemia. The most common of these, Gilbert syndrome, is a benign condition affecting up to 7% of the general population.[106,107] It is not a single disease but a heterogeneous group of disorders, all of which are characterized by a homozygosity for a defect in the promoter controlling the transcription of the UDP glucuronyl transferase I gene.[108] The consequent impairment of bilirubin glucuronidation presents as a mild unconjugated hyperbilirubinemia. The elevated bilirubin level is usually detected on routine blood testing, and affected patients may report that their skin turns yellow when they are fatigued or at stressful times (e.g., after missing meals, after vomiting, or in the presence of an infection). Other causes of an unconjugated hyperbilirubinemia are beyond the scope of this chapter.

<table>
<tr><td colspan="2">Table 1 Causes of Unconjugated Hyperbilirubinemia</td></tr>
</table>

Increased RBC breakdown
  Acute hemolysis
  Chronic hemolytic disorders
  Large hematoma resorption, multiple blood transfusions
  Gilbert syndrome

Decreased hepatic bilirubin conjugation
  Gilbert syndrome
  Crigler-Najjar syndrome types I and II
  Familial unconjugated hyperbilirubinemia

---

predominant. Rarely, the clinical picture may be secondary to a massive increase in both direct and indirect bilirubin production after the latter has overcome the ability of the hepatocytes to secrete conjugated bilirubin.

It is nearly always possible to distinguish between direct and indirect hyperbilirubinemia on clinical grounds alone.[4] Our emphasis here is on direct hyperbilirubinemia, which is the type that is more relevant to general surgeons.

Cholestatic Syndrome

The term cholestasis refers to decreased delivery of bilirubin into the intestine (and subsequent accumulation in the hepatocytes and in blood), irrespective of the underlying cause. When cholestasis is mild, it may not be associated with clinical jaundice. As it worsens, a conjugated hyperbilirubinemia develops that presents as jaundice. The conjugated hyperbilirubinemia may derive either from a defect in hepatocellular function (hepatic jaundice, also referred to as nonobstructive or medical jaundice) or from a blockage somewhere in the biliary tree (posthepatic jaundice, also referred to as obstructive or surgical jaundice). In this chapter, we refer to hepatic and posthepatic causes of jaundice, reserving the term cholestasis for the specific clinical syndrome that is attributable to a chronic lack of delivery of bile into the intestine. This syndrome is characterized by signs and symptoms that are related either to the conjugated hyperbilirubinemia or to chronic malabsorption of fat-soluble vitamins (i.e., vitamins A, D, E, and K): jaundice, dark urine, pale stools, pruritus, bruising, steatorrhea, night blindness, osteomalacia, and neuromuscular weakness.[5]

HEPATIC VERSUS POSTHEPATIC JAUNDICE

Once the presence of direct hyperbilirubinemia is confirmed, the next step is to determine whether the jaundice is hepatic or posthepatic. A number of authors have studied the reliability of clinical assessment for making this determination.[6-17] The sensitivities of history, physical examination, and blood tests alone range from 70% to 95%,[6-11] whereas the specificities are approximately 75%.[10,11] The overall accuracy of clinical assessment of hepatic and posthepatic causes of jaundice ranges from 87% to 97%.[8,12] Clinically, hepatic jaundice is most often signaled by acute hepatitis, a history of alcohol abuse, or physical findings reflecting cirrhosis or portal hypertension[13]; posthepatic jaundice is most often signaled by abdominal pain, rigors, itching, or a palpable liver more than 2 cm below the costal margin.[14]

By using discriminant analysis in a pediatric patient population, two investigators[15] were able to isolate three biochemical tests that differentiated between biliary atresia and intrahepatic cholestasis with an accuracy of 95%: total serum bilirubin concentration, alkaline phosphatase level, and γ-glutamyl-transpeptidase level. Serum transaminase levels added no independent information of significance to the model. Another multivariate analysis model[16] demonstrated that patients with posthepatic jaundice were younger, had a longer history of jaundice, were more likely to present with fever, and had greater elevations of serum protein concentrations and shorter coagulation times than patients with hepatic jaundice. This model, however, despite its 96% sensitivity (greater than that of any single radiologic diagnostic modality), could not accurately predict the level of a biliary obstruction. Other investigators[8,12,13] have reported similar findings, and most agree that strategies that omit ultrasonography are clearly inferior.[17]

In summary, a clinical approach supported by simple biochemical evaluation displays good predictive ability to distinguish hepatic from posthepatic jaundice; however, a clinical approach alone does not accurately identify the level of biliary obstruction in a patient with posthepatic jaundice.

The remainder of this chapter focuses primarily on management of posthepatic jaundice; hepatic jaundice is less often seen and dealt with by general surgeons [*see Table 2 and Sidebar Hepatic Jaundice*].

Imaging

Once the history has been obtained and bedside and laboratory assessments have been completed, the next step is imaging, the goals of which are (1) to confirm the presence of an extrahepatic obstruction (i.e., to verify that the jaundice is indeed posthepatic rather than hepatic), (2) to determine the level of the obstruction, (3) to identify the specific cause of the obstruction, and (4) to provide complementary information relating to the underlying diagnosis (e.g., staging information in cases of malignancy).

Of the many imaging methods available today, the gold standard for defining the level of a biliary obstruction before operation in a jaundiced patient remains direct cholangiography, which can be performed either via endoscopic retrograde cholangiopancreatography (ERCP) [*see V:6 Gastrointestinal Endoscopy*] or via percutaneous transhepatic cholangiography (PTC). Unlike other imaging modalities, direct cholangiography poses significant risks to the patient: there is a 4% to 7% incidence of pancreatitis or cholangitis after ERCP[18,19] and a 4% incidence of bile leakage, cholangitis, or bleeding after PTC.[20] There are also several risks that are particular to the manipulation of an obstructed biliary system (see below). For these reasons and because both modalities have therapeutic capability, it is important to gather as much imaging information as possible on the likely cause of the jaundice before performing ERCP or PTC. We have found the following approach to be an efficacious, cost-effective,[21] and safe way of obtaining such

Approach to the Jaundiced Patient

Patient has confirmed hepatic jaundice

[*See Sidebar* Hepatic Jaundice.]

Patient has presumed posthepatic jaundice

Obtain ultrasonogram to confirm posthepatic jaundice and identify level of biliary obstruction.

In some unusual clinical situations, ultrasonography may not detect the posthepatic cause of jaundice, and HIDA scanning, ERCP, PTC, or repeat ultrasonography may be necessary. If all these situations are ruled out, seek a hepatic cause and consider liver biopsy.

Patient has confirmed posthepatic jaundice

Proceed according to clinical scenario present.

Suspected cholangitis

Choledocholithiasis is the most likely diagnosis.

Resuscitate, correct any coagulopathy, and give appropriate antibiotics.

Perform ERCP for definitive diagnosis and treatment. If ERCP cannot be done, consider transhepatic drainage or surgery.

Suspected choledocholithiasis

Perform preoperative MRCP or ERCP and laparoscopic cholecystectomy.

Alternatively, perform laparoscopic cholecystectomy with intraoperative cholangiography.

Patient presents with skin discoloration suggestive of jaundice

Perform clinical assessment

Perform physical exam and obtain history.

Confirm icterus by examining oral mucous membranes, palms, soles, and sclerae in natural light.

Distinguish indirect (unconjugated) from direct (conjugated) hyperbilirubinemia:

- Normal-colored urine and stools suggest indirect hyperbilirubinemia
- Dark urine, pale stools, and signs or symptoms of a cholestatic syndrome suggest direct hyperbilirubinemia

Measure total serum bilirubin and percentage of conjugated bilirubin.

Patient has indirect hyperbilirubinemia

[*See Sidebar* Unconjugated (Indirect) Bilirubin.]

Patient has direct hyperbilirubinemia

Distinguish hepatic ("medical") jaundice from posthepatic ("surgical") jaundice.

- Acute hepatitis, alcohol abuse, and physical evidence of cirrhosis or portal hypertension suggest hepatic jaundice
- Abdominal pain, rigors, itching, and a palpable liver > 2 cm below costal margin suggest posthepatic jaundice

Patient has presumed hepatic jaundice

[*See Sidebar* Hepatic Jaundice.]

Suspected lesion other than choledocholithiasis

The most common single cause is pancreatic cancer; many of the other possible causes also involve malignancy.

Perform spiral CT or MRI with MRCP to diagnose lesion and assess resectability.

Consider EUS for distal-third obstruction.

Perform Doppler ultrasonography to stage lesion further; CT angiography or MRA may be considered if ultrasonogram is abnormal.

Perform MRCP to assess intrahepatic biliary system in patients with middle-third or upper-third obstruction.

Lesion appears unresectable, and surgical palliation is not indicated

Treat with ERCP or PTC and drainage. For advanced malignant disease, supportive care alone may be indicated.

Lesion appears resectable, or surgical palliation is indicated

Treat with surgical bypass or resection as appropriate for level of obstruction.

Perform laparoscopy to confirm resectability before laparotomy.

Upper-third obstruction

Palliation: bypass with left (segment III) hepaticojejunostomy.

Resection for cure: resection of tumor, possibly with hepatectomy or segmentectomy, and reconstruction with hepaticojejunostomy or cholangiojejunostomy.

Middle-third obstruction

Palliation: bypass with hepaticojejunostomy.

Resection for cure: resection of tumor and reconstruction with hepaticojejunostomy.

Lower-third obstruction

Palliation: bypass with Roux-en-Y choledochojejunostomy.

Resection for cure: resection of tumor with pancreaticoduodenectomy or local ampullary excision.

Table 2 Causes of Hepatic Jaundice[113]

Hepatitis
  Viral
  Autoimmune
  Alcoholic
Drugs and hormones
Diseases of intrahepatic bile ducts
Liver infiltration and storage disorders
Systemic infections
Total parenteral nutrition
Postoperative intrahepatic cholestasis
Cholestasis of pregnancy
Benign recurrent intrahepatic cholestasis
Infantile cholestatic syndromes
Inherited metabolic defects
No identifiable cause (idiopathic hepatic jaundice)

information in a patient with presumed posthepatic jaundice.

The presence of ductal dilatation of the intrahepatic or extrahepatic biliary system confirms that a posthepatic cause is responsible for the jaundice. Ultrasonography detects ductal dilatation with an accuracy of 95%, although results are to some extent operator-dependent.[22] If ultrasonography does not reveal bile duct dilatation, it is unlikely that an obstructing lesion is present. In some cases, although ductal dilatation is absent, other ultrasonographic findings may still point to a specific hepatic cause of jaundice (e.g., multiple liver metastases, cirrhosis, or infiltration of the liver by tumor).

There are a few specific instances in which ultrasonography may fail to detect a posthepatic cause of jaundice. For instance, very early in the course of an obstructive process, not enough time may have elapsed for biliary dilatation to occur. In this setting, a hepato-iminodiacetic acid (HIDA) scan may help identify bile duct blockage.[23] The yield from this test is highest when the serum bilirubin level is lower than 100 µmol/L, and it diminishes as the serum bilirubin level rises.[1] Occasionally, the intrahepatic biliary tree is unable to dilate; possible causes of such inability include extensive hepatic fibrosis, cirrhosis, sclerosing cholangitis, and recent liver transplantation. If one of these diagnoses is suspected, either ERCP or PTC will eventually be required to confirm the diagnosis of biliary obstruction. Occasionally, the biliary tree dilatation may be intermittent; possible causes of this condition include choledocholithiasis and some biliary tumors. In a patient with gallstones, transient liver test abnormalities by themselves may suggest an intermediate to high likelihood of common bile duct (CBD) stones, even if there is no biliary ductal dilatation.[24,25] If one of these diagnoses is suspected, ultrasonography may be repeated after a short period of observation (when clinically applicable); biliary ductal dilatation then generally becomes apparent. If all of these unusual clinical situations have been ruled out, a hepatic cause for the jaundice should be sought [*see Table 2*] and a liver biopsy considered.[26,27]

Besides being able to identify the presence of extrahepatic ductal obstruction with a high degree of reliability, ultrasonography can accurately determine the level of the obstruction in 90% of cases.[28] For example, a dilated gallbladder suggests

Hepatic Jaundice

Hepatic jaundice may be either acute or chronic and may be caused by a variety of conditions [*see Table 2*].

Acute hepatic jaundice may arise de novo or in the setting of ongoing liver disease. Historical clues may suggest a particular cause, such as medications or viral hepatitis. Physical examination usually reveals little; however, an enlarged liver is sometimes palpated. In the presence of preexisting chronic liver disease, bedside stigmata (e.g., ascites, spider nevi, caput medusae, palmar erythema, gynecomastia, or Dupuytren contracture) may be present. Although specific therapies exist for certain clinical problems (e.g., acetylcysteine for acetaminophen ingestion and penicillin plus silibinin for *Amanita phalloides* poisoning), treatment in most cases remains supportive. Patients in whom encephalopathy develops within 2 to 8 weeks of the onset of jaundice are usually classified as having fulminant hepatic failure [*see VII:6 Hepatic Failure*]. Evidence of encephalopathy, renal failure, or a severe coagulopathy is predictive of poor outcome in this setting.[109] The most common causes of fulminant hepatic failure are viral hepatitis and drug toxicity. The mortality from fulminant hepatic failure remains high even though liver transplantation has favorably affected the prognosis.[110]

In cases of chronic hepatic jaundice, the patient may have chronic hepatitis or cholestasis, with or without cirrhosis. The cause usually is determined on the basis of the history in conjunction with the results of serology, biochemistry, and, occasionally, histology. Causes include viral infection, drug-induced chronic hepatitis, autoimmune liver disease, genetic disorders (e.g., Wilson disease and α_1-antitrypsin deficiency), chronic cholestatic disorders, alcoholic liver disease, and steatohepatitis.[111] Physical examination reveals the stigmata of chronic liver disease and occasionally suggests a specific cause (e.g., Kayser-Fleischer rings on slit-lamp examination in Wilson disease).

Treatment, once again, is usually supportive, depending on the clinical presentation; whether more specific therapy is needed and what form it takes depend on the cause of liver disease. Although physiologic tests have been developed to quantify hepatic reserve, the most widely used and best-validated prognostic index remains the Child-Pugh classification (see below), which correlates with individual survival and has been shown to predict operative risk.[112] Liver transplantation is the treatment of choice in most cases of end-stage liver disease.

The Child-Pugh Classification[112]
Numerical Score (*points*)

Variable	1	2	3
Encephalopathy	Nil (0)	Slight to moderate (1, 2)	Moderate to severe (3–5)
Ascites	Nil	Slight	Moderate to severe
Bilirubin, mg/dl (µmol/L*)	< 2 (< 34)	2–3 (34–51)	> 3 (> 51)
Albumin, g/dl (g/L*)	> 3.5 (> 35)	2.8–3.5 (28–35)	< 2.8 (< 28)
Prothrombin index	> 70%	40%–70%	< 40%

Modified Child's risk grade (depending on total score): 5 or 6 points, grade A; 7 to 9 points, grade B; 10 to 15 points, grade C.
*Système International d'Unités, or SI units.

that the obstruction is probably located in the middle third or the distal third of the CBD.

Some centers prefer CT to ultrasonography as the initial imaging modality,[29] but we, like a number of other authors,[30] find ultrasonography to be the most expedient, most readily available, least invasive, and most economical imaging method for differentiating between hepatic and posthepatic causes of jaundice as well as for suggesting the level of obstruction.[31] Traditional imaging techniques, such as oral or intravenous cholangiography, have a negligible role to play in this setting because of their very poor accuracy and safety, especially in jaundiced patients.

Magnetic resonance cholangiopancreatography (MRCP) [see Figure 1] and endoscopic ultrasonography (EUS) have been used to visualize the biliary and pancreatic trees in a variety of populations of patients with obstructive jaundice,[32-36] and experience with these newer imaging modalities is accumulating rapidly. Compared with direct cholangiography, both MRCP and EUS appear to be excellent at diagnosing biliary obstruction and establishing its location and nature.[37,38] MRCP exhibits more modest detection rates when diagnosing small CBD stones.[39] Helical, or spiral, CT scanning is also useful in diagnosing biliary obstruction and determining its cause, though concomitant oral or I.V. cholangiography is required to detect choledocholithiasis.[40,41]

In addition to their ability to detect choledocholithiasis, spiral CT, EUS, and MRCP in combination with abdominal magnetic resonance imaging (e.g., of the pancreas) are very useful in diagnosing and staging biliopancreatic tumors.[42-44] Cytology specimens are readily obtained via fine-needle aspiration (FNA) during CT or EUS.[43]

It is our current practice to employ these modalities as second-line tests after the initial abdominal ultrasonographic examination. We favor EUS for periampullary pathologic conditions and MRI with MRCP for more proximal diseases of the biliary tree.

In making the choice among the various available second-line tests, cost-effectiveness becomes an important consideration. Several of these imaging modalities, individually or in combination with others, have been evaluated for their cost-effectiveness in the workup of patients with obstructive jaundice. Unfortunately, the reports published to date have been flawed, suffering either from limited assumptions (when the methodology involved decision modeling) or from the lack of an effectiveness-type design (when the methodology involved allocation of patients).

Workup and Management of Posthepatic Jaundice

Once ultrasonography has confirmed that ductal obstruction is present, there are three possible clinical scenarios: suspected cholangitis, suspected choledocholithiasis without cholangitis, and a suspected lesion other than choledocholithiasis. The direction of the subsequent workup depends on which of the three appears most likely.

SUSPECTED CHOLANGITIS

If a jaundiced patient exhibits a clinical picture compatible with acute suppurative cholangitis (Charcot's triad or Raynaud's pentad), the most likely diagnosis is choledocholithiasis. After

a

b

Figure 1 ERCP (*a*) and corresponding MRCP (*b*) demonstrate the presence of a stone in the distal CBD.

appropriate resuscitation, correction of any coagulopathies present, and administration of antibiotics, ERCP is indicated for diagnosis and treatment.[45] If ERCP is unavailable or is not feasible (e.g., because of previous Roux-en-Y reconstruction), transhepatic drainage or surgery may be necessary. It is important to emphasize here that the mainstay of treatment of severe cholangitis is not just the administration of appropriate antibiotics but rather the establishment of adequate biliary drainage.

SUSPECTED CHOLEDOCHOLITHIASIS WITHOUT CHOLANGITIS

Choledocholithiasis is the most common cause of biliary obstruction[13,14] and should be strongly suspected if the jaundice is episodic or painful or if ultrasonography has demonstrated the presence of gallstones or bile duct stones. Patients with suspected choledocholithiasis should be referred for laparoscopic cholecystectomy with either preoperative ERCP or intraoperative cholangiography [see V:12 Laparoscopic Cholecystectomy]. We favor preoperative ERCP in this setting of jaundice because its diagnostic yield is high,[46] it allows confirmation of the diagnosis preoperatively (thus obviating intraoperative surprises), and it is capable of clearing the CBD of stones in 95% of cases. Decision analyses appear to confirm the utility of this strategy when laparoscopic CBD exploration is not an option.[47-50] Many authors, however, favor a fully laparoscopic approach, in which choledocholithiasis is detected in the OR by means of intraoperative cholangiography[51,52] or ultrasonography[53-55] and laparoscopic biliary clearance is performed when choledocholithiasis is confirmed. Given that both the ERCP approach and the fully laparoscopic approach have advantages and limitations, one may reasonably maintain that the optimal approach in a particular setting should be dictated by local expertise.

SUSPECTED LESION OTHER THAN CHOLEDOCHOLITHIASIS

If no gallstones are identified, if the clinical presentation is less acute (e.g., constant abdominal or back pain), or if there are associated constitutional symptoms (e.g., weight loss, fatigue, and long-standing anorexia), the presence of a lesion other than choledocholithiasis should be suspected. In such cases, another imaging modality besides the ultrasonography already performed must be considered before the decision is made to proceed to cholangiography or operation.

Possible causes of posthepatic obstruction (other than choledocholithiasis) may be classified into three categories depending on the location of the obstructing lesion (as suggested by the pattern of gallbladder and biliary tree dilatation on the ultrasonogram): the upper third of the biliary tree, the middle third, or the lower (distal) third [see Table 3]. Once it has been determined that choledocholithias is unlikely, the most common cause of such obstruction is pancreatic cancer.[13,14] In adults, many of the other possible causes also involve malignant processes. Consequently, the next step in the workup of the patient is typically the assessment of resectability and operability [see V:11 Biliary Tract Procedures].

Diagnosis and Assessment of Resectability

Because surgery is the only chance for definitive treatment of a biliary or pancreatic malignancy, it is important not to deny a patient this chance. Assessment of the resectability of a

---

Table 3   Causes of Posthepatic Jaundice

Upper-third obstruction
  Polycystic liver disease
  Caroli disease
  Hepatocellular carcinoma
  Oriental cholangiohepatitis
  Hepatic arterial thrombosis (e.g., after liver transplantation or chemotherapy)
  Hemobilia (e.g., after biliary manipulation)
  Iatrogenic bile duct injury (e.g., after laparoscopic cholecystectomy)
  Cholangiocarcinoma (Klatskin tumor)
  Sclerosing cholangitis
  Papillomas of the bile duct

Middle-third obstruction
  Cholangiocarcinoma
  Sclerosing cholangitis
  Papillomas of the bile duct
  Gallbladder cancer
  Choledochal cyst
  Intrabiliary parasites
  Mirizzi syndrome
  Extrinsic nodal compression (e.g., from breast cancer or lymphoma)
  Iatrogenic bile duct injury (e.g., after open cholecystectomy)
  Cystic fibrosis
  Benign idiopathic bile duct stricture

Lower-third obstruction
  Cholangiocarcinoma
  Sclerosing cholangitis
  Papillomas of the bile duct
  Pancreatic tumors
  Ampullary tumors
  Chronic pancreatitis
  Sphincter of Oddi dysfunction
  Papillary stenosis
  Duodenal diverticula
  Penetrating duodenal ulcer
  Retroduodenal adenopathy (e.g., lymphoma, carcinoid)

---

tumor usually hinges on whether the superior mesenteric vein, the portal vein, the superior mesenteric artery, and the porta hepatis are free of tumor and on whether there is evidence of significant local adenopathy or extrapancreatic extension of tumor. Unfortunately, the majority of lesions will be clearly unresectable, either because of tumor extension or because of the presence of hepatic or peritoneal metastases.

Many imaging modalities are currently being used to determine resectability, and several of these have been established as effective alternatives to direct cholangiography because they involve little if any morbidity. Their accuracy varies according to the underlying pathology and the expertise of the user. They have been studied mostly with respect to the staging and diagnosis of pancreatic, periampullary, and biliary hilar cancers.

For determining resectability and staging lesions before operation, we rely mainly on spiral CT, which allows good definition of the nature and extent of the lesion. At present, this modality is thought to be superior for the diagnosis and staging of lesions such as pancreatic cancer.[42,56-58] Spiral CT exhibits a high negative predictive value and has a false positive rate of less than

10%; its sensitivity is optimal for pancreatic lesions larger than 1.5 cm in diameter. The presence of ascites, liver metastases, lymph nodes larger than 2 cm in diameter, and invasion into adjacent organs are all signs of advanced disease.[59] On the basis of these criteria, spiral CT can predict that a lesion will not be resectable with an accuracy approaching 95%; however, as many as 33% of tumors that appear to be resectable on CT are found to be unresectable at operation.[57,58] Occasionally, spiral CT does not yield sufficient information, and as a result, supplementary imaging studies are required.

MRI has also been shown to be helpful in determining the nature of the malignant obstruction, and MRI-based staging, along with MRCP, can further dictate the subsequent choice of therapy.[59-62] MRI may be particularly useful for following up patients in whom clip artifacts interfere with a CT image.[59] It also appears to be successful in detecting cholangiocarcinoma spreading along the proximal biliary tree.[63]

Only in a few very rare instances is traditional angiography used to assess resectability or stage a hepatobiliary or pancreatic neoplasm. Increasingly, it is being replaced by CT angiography or duplex Doppler ultrasonography, which can confirm the presence of flow in the hepatic arterial or portal venous systems and occasionally can demonstrate invasion of these vessels by tumor.[64] Magnetic resonance angiography (MRA) has also been used with excellent results. As yet, none of these noninvasive modalities has been shown to be clearly superior to any of the others.[65]

EUS appears to be a highly promising modality, particularly with respect to assessment of the resectability of pancreatic tumors.[43,66,67] In a large study comprising 232 patients, EUS was found to be superior to CT and to standard ultrasonography in detecting venous and gastric invasion by cancers measuring 3 cm or less in diameter.[68] In another large series, it was reported to be more accurate than CT in the comparative staging of pancreatic and ampullary cancers.[69] EUS is also useful for identifying small (< 2 cm) pancreatic tumors, which may be suspected in a patient with an obstruction of the distal third of the bile duct and whose CT scan is normal.[67] An additional benefit is that one can perform guided FNA at the time of EUS. Furthermore, EUS is currently the dominant technique for staging ampullary tumors.[70]

At this point in the evaluation, patients can be referred for direct cholangiography (usually ERCP) to better delineate the proximal biliary anatomy (for upper-third lesions) or to clarify a still-unclear diagnosis. There is, however, a growing body of evidence suggesting that in patients with either pancreatic[71,72] or hepatic[73] malignancies, routine preoperative direct cholangiography with decompression may be associated with a higher incidence of postoperative complications when tumor resection is ultimately carried out.

If a biliary stricture is detected at cholangiography, brush cytology or biopsy is mandatory. Biliary cytology, however, has been disappointing, particularly at ERCP: diagnostic accuracy ranges from 40% to 85%,[74,75] mostly because the negative predictive value is poor. Accuracy improves with multiple sampling and when a biliary rather than a pancreatic malignancy is detected. In addition, biopsy tends to be more accurate than brush cytology.[74]

If a pancreatic tumor is suspected, percutaneous FNA cytology may be helpful; the yield is best for larger tumors. Direct FNA of the lesion at EUS is also an increasingly attractive option. In the case of potentially resectable lesions, however, this measure adds very little to the decision-making process.

The limited data currently available suggest that assays of tumor markers in serum and pancreatic fluid are useful, particularly for cystic lesions of the pancreas.[76]

Nonoperative Management: Drainage and Cholangiography

In the majority of patients with malignant obstructions, treatment is palliative rather than curative. It is therefore especially important to recognize and minimize the iatrogenic risks related to the manipulation of an obstructed biliary system; this is why staging and cholangiography are currently being performed with less invasive methods.

Cholangiography and decompression of obstructed biliary system As a rule, we favor ERCP, although PTC may be preferable for obstructions near the hepatic duct bifurcation. Whichever imaging modality is used, the following four principles apply.

1. In the absence of preexisting or concomitant hepatocellular dysfunction, drainage of one half of the liver is generally sufficient for resolution of jaundice.
2. Because of its external diameter, a transhepatic drain, once inserted, does not necessarily permit equal drainage of all segments of the liver, particularly if there are a number of intrahepatic ductal stenoses. Accordingly, some patients with conditions such as sclerosing cholangitis or a growing tumor may experience persistent sepsis from an infected excluded liver segment even when the prosthesis is patent [*see Figure 2*]. An excluded segment may even be responsible for severe persistent pruritus.
3. Any attempt at opacifying an obstructed biliary tree introduces a significant risk of subsequent cholangitis, even when appropriate antibiotic prophylaxis is provided. Accordingly, when one elects to perform direct cholangiography, there should be a plan for biliary drainage either at the time of ERCP or PTC or soon thereafter.
4. Even though jaundice is believed to be associated with multiple adverse systemic effects (e.g., renal failure, sepsis, and impaired wound healing),[77,78] routine preoperative drainage of an obstructed biliary system does not benefit patients who will soon undergo operative correction.[79,80] In fact, as noted (see above), routine preoperative drainage of subsequently resected hepatic or pancreatic malignancies may be deleterious.

When direct cholangiography is ordered, it should be thought of as more than just a diagnostic test: it is the ideal setting for cytology, biopsy, or even drainage of the obstructed bile duct via a sphincterotomy, a nasobiliary tube, or a catheter or stent. Accordingly, it is essential that the surgeon, the gastroenterologist, and the radiologist discuss the possible need for drainage well before it is required. Early, open communication among all the members of the treating team is a hallmark of the modern management of biliary obstruction.

Palliation in patients with advanced malignant disease
When a patient has advanced malignant disease, drainage of the biliary system for palliation is not routinely indicated,

a

b

c

Figure 2   **ERCP (*a*) demonstrates missing liver segments. Transhepatic cholangiography (*b*) of segment VI reveals excluded liver ductal system. MRCP (*c*) shows the excluded liver segments as well as the biliary system, which still communicates with the common hepatic duct.**

because the risk of complications related to the procedure may outweigh the potential benefit. Indeed, the best treatment for a patient with asymptomatic obstructive jaundice and liver metastases may be supportive care alone.[81] Biliary decompression is indicated if cholangitis or severe pruritus that interferes with quality of life is present.

We, like others,[21] consider a stent placed with ERCP to be the palliative modality of choice for advanced disease, although upper-third lesions may be managed most easily through the initial placement of an internal/external catheter at the time of PTC. Metal expandable stents remain patent longer than large conventional plastic stents,[82,83] but the high price of the metal stents has kept them from being widely used, and their overall cost-effectiveness has yet to be clearly demonstrated. Whether plastic biliary stents should be replaced prophylactically or only after obstruction has occurred remains controversial; however, results from a randomized trial favor the former approach.[84]

Randomized controlled trials suggest that surgical biliary bypass should be reserved for patients who are expected to survive for prolonged periods because bypass is associated with more prolonged palliation at the cost of greater initial morbidity.[85]

The role of prophylactic gastric drainage at the time of operative biliary drainage remains controversial.[86] However, jaundiced patients with unresectable lesions who also present with duodenal or jejunal obstruction should be referred for gastrojejunostomy at the time of biliary bypass surgery. There is evidence to suggest that when a pancreatic malignancy is present, intraoperative celiac ganglion injection should be performed for either prophylactic or therapeutic pain control.[87]

Operative Management at Specific Sites: Bypass and Resection

Surgical treatment of tumors causing biliary obstruction is determined primarily by the level of the biliary obstruction. There is a growing body of evidence

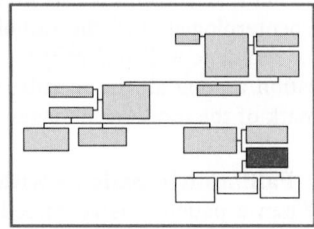

indicating that modern surgical approaches are resulting in lower postoperative morbidity and, possibly, improved 5-year survival[88]; however, the prognosis is still uniformly poor, except for patients with ampullary tumors. In fact, the surgical procedure rarely proves curative, even after meticulous preoperative patient selection.

The first step toward potential resection of a jaundice-causing cancer should be laparoscopy to determine resectability and to prevent the hospital stay and prolonged convalescence associated with an unnecessary laparotomy. Laparoscopy is used mostly to detect peritoneal carcinomatosis, liver metastases, malignant ascites, and gross hilar adenopathy.[89,90] In a trial involving 115 patients with potentially resectable peripancreatic tumors, full laparoscopic staging could be performed in 94%, and the overall resectability rate was 76%.[89] In several studies, a combined approach including both laparoscopy and laparoscopic ultrasonography was associated with shorter hospital stays and lower costs.[90-92] The main limitation of such an approach appears to be that it does not accurately detect the spread of tumors to lymph nodes or the vascular system.[92]

Once laparoscopy confirms that there is no obvious advanced disease, the patient should undergo a full laparotomy, usually in the same setting but occasionally in a different operative session.

In what follows, only the general principles of resection or bypass at each level of obstruction are discussed; operative technical details are addressed elsewhere [*see V:11 Biliary Tract Procedures*]. Our preferred method of biliary anastomosis, for either reconstruction or bypass, involves the fashioning of a Roux-en-Y loop, followed by a mucosa-to-mucosa anastomosis. In all cases, a cholecystectomy is performed to facilitate access to the biliary tree.

Upper-third obstruction

Palliation. In the absence of liver compromise, drainage of one half of the liver usually leads to clearance of jaundice.[93] Because the left hepatic duct has a long extrahepatic segment that makes it more accessible, the preferred bypass technique for an obstructing upper-third lesion is a left (or segment III) hepaticojejunostomy. This operation has superseded the Longmire procedure because it does not involve formal resection of liver parenchyma. Laparoscopic bypass techniques that make use of segment III have been developed, but their performance has yet to be formally assessed.[94,95]

Resection for cure. The hilar plate is taken down to lengthen the hepatic duct segment available for subsequent anastomosis. Often, a formal hepatectomy or segmentectomy is required to ensure an adequate margin of resection. If the resection must be carried out proximal to the hepatic duct bifurcation, several cholangiojejunostomies will have to be done to anastomose individual hepatic biliary branches. Frozen section examination of the proximal and distal resection margins is important because of the propensity of tumors such as cholangiocarcinoma to spread in a submucosal or perineural plane.

The results of aggressive hilar tumor resections that included as much liver tissue as was necessary to obtain a negative margin appear to justify this approach.[96] In cases of left hepatic involvement, resection of the caudate lobe (segment I) is indicated as well.[97]

Middle-third obstruction

Palliation. Surgical bypass of middle-third lesions is technically simpler because a hepaticojejunostomy can often be performed distal to the hepatic duct bifurcation, which means that exposure of the hilar plate or the intrahepatic ducts is unnecessary.

Resection for cure. Discrete tumors in this part of the bile duct, though uncommon, are usually quite amenable to resection along with the lymphatic chains in the porta hepatis. Resection of an early gallbladder cancer may, on occasion, necessitate the concomitant resection of segment V, although the value of resecting this segment prophylactically has not been conclusively demonstrated. Sometimes, jaundice from a suspected middle-third lesion is in fact caused by a case of Mirizzi syndrome [*see Figure 3*]. In such cases, a gallstone is responsible for extrinsic obstruction of the CBD, either by causing inflammation of the gallbladder wall or via direct impingement. Proper treatment of this syndrome may involve hepaticojejunostomy in addition to cholecystectomy if a cholecystocholedochal fistula is present.[98]

Lower-third obstruction

Palliation. The preferred bypass technique for lower-third lesions is a Roux-en-Y choledochojejunostomy. Cholecystojejunostomy carries a higher risk of complications and subsequent development of jaundice[99]; this remains

true even when it is performed laparoscopically.[94] Occasionally, it may be done as a temporizing measure before a more definitive procedure in the context of an upcoming transfer to a specialized center.

Resection for cure. Occasionally, an impacted CBD stone at the duodenal ampulla mimics a tumor and is not clearly identified

preoperatively. In this situation, intraoperative choledochoscopy before resection helps confirm the diagnosis and may even permit removal of the stone. Because of the growing use of EUS and MRCP, such a situation is increasingly uncommon. Resection of a lower-third lesion usually involves a pancreaticoduodenectomy [*see V:13 Pancreatic Procedures*], although local ampullary resection may be an acceptable alternative for a small adenoma of the ampulla; local duodenal resection with removal of the head of the pancreas has also been described. For optimal results, pancreaticoduodenectomy is best performed in specialized centers.[100]

It has been suggested that postoperative adjuvant therapy may improve the prognosis after resection of a pancreatic adenocarcinoma,[88] but this debate falls outside the scope of our discussion.

Postoperative Jaundice

A clinical scenario of particular pertinence to surgeons that we have not yet addressed is the development of jaundice in the postoperative setting.

Jaundice develops in approximately 1% of all surgical patients after operation.[101] When jaundice occurs after a hepatobiliary procedure, it may be attributable to specific biliary causes, such

Figure 3 **ERCP demonstrates extrinsic compression of the common hepatic duct by a stone in Hartmann's pouch. A biliary stent has been inserted for drainage.**

as retained CBD stones, postoperative biliary leakage (through reabsorption of bile leaking into the peritoneum) [*see Figure 4*], injury to the CBD, and the subsequent development of biliary strictures. In most instances, however, the jaundice derives from a combination of disease processes, and only rarely is invasive testing or active treatment required.[102]

A diagnostic approach similar to the one outlined earlier (see above) is applicable to postoperative jaundice; however, another useful approach is to consider the possible causes in the light of the time interval between the operation and the subsequent development of jaundice.

- Jaundice may develop within 48 hours of the operation; this is most often the result of the breakdown of red blood cells, occurring in the context of multiple blood transfusions (particularly with stored blood), the resorption of a large hematoma, or a transfusion reaction. Hemolysis may also develop in a patient with a known underlying hemolytic anemia and may be precipitated by the administration of specific drugs (e.g., sulfa drugs in a patient who has glucose-6-phosphate dehydrogenase deficiency).[103] Cardiopulmonary bypass or the insertion of a prosthetic valve may be associated with the development of early postoperative jaundice as well. Gilbert syndrome [*see Sidebar* Hepatic Jaundice] may first manifest itself early in the postoperative period. Occasionally, a mild conjugated hyperbilirubinemia may be related to Dubin-Johnson syndrome, which is an inherited disorder of bilirubin metabolism. This condition is usually self-limited and is characterized by the presence of a melaninlike pigment in the liver.

- Intraoperative hypotension or hypoxemia or the early development of heart failure can lead to conjugated hyperbilirubinemia within 5 to 10 days after operation. The hyperbilirubinemia may be associated with other end-organ damage (e.g., acute tubular necrosis). In fact, any impairment of renal function causes a decrease in bilirubin excretion and can be responsible for a mild hyperbilirubinemia.

- Jaundice may develop 7 to 10 days after operation in association with a medication-induced hepatitis attributable to an anesthetic agent. This syndrome has an estimated incidence of one in 10,000 after an initial exposure.[103] More commonly, the jaundice is related to the administration of antibiotics or other medications used in the perioperative setting.[103]

- After the first week, jaundice associated with intrahepatic cholestasis is often a manifestation of a septic response and usually presents in the setting of overt infection, particularly in patients with multiple organ dysfunction syndrome. Gram-negative sepsis from an intra-abdominal source is typical; if it persists, the outcome is likely to be poor. Jaundice may occur in as many as 30% of patients receiving total parenteral nutrition (TPN). It may be attributable to steatosis, particularly with formulas containing large amounts of carbohydrates. In addition, decreased export of bilirubin from the hepatocytes may lead to cholestasis, the severity of which appears to be related to the duration of TPN administration. Acalculous cholecystitis or even ductal obstruction may develop as a result of sludge in the gall-

Figure 4 **Jaundice has occurred after laparoscopic cholecystectomy as a result of bile leakage from a distal biliary tributary. A stent has been inserted to decrease bile duct luminal pressure and foster spontaneous resolution.**

bladder and the CBD. An elevated postoperative bilirubin level at any time may also result from unsuspected hepatic or posthepatic causes (e.g., occult cirrhosis, choledocholithiasis, or cholecystitis). A rare cause of postoperative jaundice is the development of thyrotoxicosis. Another entity to consider (as a diagnosis of exclusion) is so-called benign postoperative cholestasis, a primarily cholestatic, self-limited process with no clearly demonstrable cause that typically arises within 2 to 10 days after operation. Benign postoperative cholestasis may be attributable to a combination of mechanisms, including an increased pigment load, impaired liver function resulting from hypoxemia and hypotension, and decreased renal bilirubin excretion caused by varying degrees of tubular necrosis.[104] The predominantly conjugated hyperbilirubinemia may reach 40 mg/dl and remain elevated for as long as 3 weeks.[103] This is a diagnosis of exclusion.

- In the late postoperative period, the development of non-A, non-B, non-C viral hepatitis after transfusion of blood products will usually occur within 5 to 12 weeks of operation.

References

1. Schiff L: Jaundice: a clinical approach. Diseases of the Liver, 7th ed. Schiff L, Schiff ER, Eds. JB Lippincott Co, Philadelphia, 1993, p 334

2. Jabbari M: Personal communication

3. Scharschmidt BF, Gollan JL: Current concepts of bilirubin metabolism and hereditary hyperbilirubinemia. Progress in Liver Diseases. Popper H, Schaffner F, Eds. Grune & Stratton, New York, 1979, p 187

4. Frank BB: Clinical evaluation of jaundice: a guideline of the Patient Care Committee of the American Gastroenterological Association. JAMA 262:3031, 1989

5. Schiff's Diseases of the Liver, 8th ed. Schiff ER, Sorrell MF, Maddrey WC, Eds. Lippincott-Raven, Philadelphia, 1999, p 119

6. Lindberg G, Björkman A, Helmers C: A description of diagnostic strategies in jaundice. Scand J Gastroenterol 18:257, 1983

7. Lumeng L, Snodgrass PJ, Swonder JW: Final report of a blinded prospective study comparing current non-invasive approaches in the differential diagnosis of medical and surgical jaundice. Gastroenterology 78:1312, 1980

8. Martin W, Apostolakos PC, Roazen H: Clinical versus actuarial prediction in the differential diagnosis of jaundice. Am J Med Sci 240:571, 1960

9. Matzen P, Malchow-Möller A, Hilden J, et al: Differential diagnosis of jaundice: a pocket diagnostic chart. Liver 4:360, 1984

10. O'Connor K, Snodgrass PJ, Swonder JE, et al: A blinded prospective study comparing four current non-invasive approaches in the differential diagnosis of medical versus surgical jaundice. Gastroenterology 84:1498, 1983

11. Schenker S, Balint J, Schiff L: Differential diagnosis of jaundice: report of a prospective study of 61 proved cases. Am J Dig Dis 7:449, 1962

12. Theodossi A, Spiegelhalter D, Portmann B, et al: The value of clinical, biochemical, ultrasound and liver biopsy data in assessing patients with liver disease. Liver 3:315, 1983

13. Pasanen PA, Pikkarainen P, Alhava E, et al: The value of clinical assessment in the diagnosis of icterus and cholestasis. Ital J Gastroenterol Hepatol 24:313, 1992

14. Theodossi A: The value of symptoms and signs in the assessment of jaundiced patients. Clin Gastroenterol 14:545, 1985

15. Fung KP, Lau SP: Differentiation between extrahepatic and intrahepatic cholestasis by discriminant analysis. J Paediatr Child Health 26:132, 1990

16. Pasanen PA, Pikkarainen P, Alhava E, et al: Evaluation of a computer-based diagnostic score system in the diagnosis of jaundice and cholestasis. Scand J Gastroenterol 28:732, 1993

17. Malchow-Möller A, Gronvall S, Hilden J, et al: Ultrasound examination in jaundiced patients: is computer-assisted preclassification helpful? J Hepatol 12:321, 1991

18. Loperfido S, Angelini G, Benedetti G, et al: Major early complications from diagnostic and therapeutic ERCP: a prospective multicenter study. Gastrointest Endosc 48:1, 1998

19. Freeman ML, DiSario JA, Nelson DB, et al: Risk factors for post-ERCP pancreatitis: a prospective, multicenter study. Gastrointest Endosc 54:425, 2001

20. Lillemoe KD: Surgical treatment of biliary tract infections. Am Surg 66:138, 2000

21. Rossi LR, Traverso W, Pimentel F: Malignant obstructive jaundice: evaluation and management. Surg Clin North Am 76:63, 1996

22. Taylor KJW, Rosenfield A: Grey-scale ultrasonography in the differential diagnosis of jaundice. Arch Surg 112:820, 1977

23. Kaplun L, Weissman HS, Rosenblatt RR, et al: The early diagnosis of common bile duct obstruction using cholescintigraphy. JAMA 254:2431, 1985

24. Abboud PA, Malet PF, Berlin JA, et al: Predictors of common bile duct stones prior to cholecystectomy: a meta-analysis. Gastrointest Endosc 44:450, 1996

25. Roston AD, Jacobson IM: Evaluation of the pattern of liver tests and yield of cholangiography in symptomatic choledocholithiasis: a prospective study. Gastrointest Endosc 45:394, 1997

26. Richter JM, Silverstein MD, Schapiro R: Suspected obstructive jaundice: a decision analysis of diagnostic strategies. Ann Intern Med 99:46, 1983

27. Bravo AA, Sheth SG, Chopra S: Liver biopsy. N Engl J Med 344:495, 2001

28. Blackbourne LH, Earnhardt RC, Sistrom CL, et al: The sensitivity and role of ultrasound in the evaluation of biliary obstruction. Am Surg 60:683, 1994

29. Sherlock S: Ultrasound (US), computerized axial tomography (CT) and magnetic resonance imaging (MRI). Diseases of the Liver and Biliary System 5:70, 1989

30. Cosgrove DO: Ultrasound in surgery of the liver and biliary tract. Surgery of the Liver and Biliary Tract, 2nd ed, Vol 1. Blumgart LH, Ed. New York, Churchill Livingstone, 1994, p 189

31. Lindsell DRM: Ultrasound imaging of pancreas and biliary tract. Lancet 335:390, 1990

32. Gillams A, Gardener J, Richards R, et al: Three-dimensional computed tomography cholangiography: a new technique for biliary tract imaging. Br J Radiol 67:445, 1994

33. Low RN, Sigeti JS, Francis IR, et al: Evaluation of malignant biliary obstruction: efficacy of fast multiplanar spoiled gradient-recalled MR imaging vs spin-echo MR imaging, CT, and cholangiography. AJR Am J Roentgenol 162:315, 1994

34. Amouyal P, Amouyal G, Levy P, et al: Diagnosis of choledocholithiasis by endoscopic ultrasonography. Gastroenterology 106:1062, 1994

35. Guibaud L, Bret PM, Reinhold C, et al: Bile duct obstruction and choledocholithiasis: diagnosis with MR cholangiography. Radiology 197:109, 1995

36. Ishizaki Y, Wakayama T, Okada Y, et al: MR cholangiography for evaluation of obstructed jaundice. Am J Gastroenterol 88:2072, 1993

37. Bardou M, Romagnuolo J, Barkun AN, et al: Magnetic resonance cholangiopancreatography, a new gold standard for pancreatico-biliary disease? a systematic review of literature. Can J Gastroenterol (in press)

38. Mallery S, Van Dam J: Current status of diagnostic and therapeutic endoscopic ultrasonography. Radiol Clin North Am 39:449, 2001

39. Sugiyama M, Atomi Y, Hachiya J: Magnetic resonance cholangiography using half-Fourier acquisition for diagnosing choledocholithiasis. Am J Gastroenterol 93:1886, 1998

40. Soto JA, Alvarez O, Munera F, et al: Diagnosing bile duct stones: comparison of unenhanced helical CT, oral contrast-enhanced CT cholangiography, and MR cholangiography. AJR Am J Roentgenol 175:1127, 2000

41. Soto JA, Velez SM, Guzman J: Choledocholithiasis: diagnosis with oral-contrast-enhanced CT cholangiography. AJR Am J Roentgenol 172:943, 1999

42. Freeny PC: Computed tomography in the diagnosis and staging of cholangiocarcinoma and pancreatic carcinoma. Ann Oncol 10(suppl 4):12, 1999

43. Hawes RH, Xiong Q, Waxman I, et al: A multispecialty approach to the diagnosis and management of pancreatic cancer. Am J Gastroenterol 95:17, 2000

44. Megibow AJ, Lavelle MT, Rofsky NM: MR imaging of the pancreas. Surg Clin North Am 81:307, 2001

45. Lai EC, Mok FP, Tan ES, et al: Endoscopic biliary drainage for severe acute cholangitis. N Engl J Med 326:1582, 1992

46. Barkun JS, Fried GM, Barkun AN, et al: Cholecystectomy without operative cholangiography: implications for bile duct injury and common bile duct stones. Ann Surg 218:371, 1993

47. Sahai AV, Mauldin PD, Marsi V, et al: Bile duct stones and laparoscopic cholecystectomy: a decision analysis to assess the roles of intraoperative cholangiography, EUS, and ERCP. Gastrointest Endosc 49(3 pt 1):334, 1999

48. Abraham N, Barkun AN, Barkun JS, et al: What is the optimal management of patients with suspected choledocholithiasis in the era of laparoscopic cholecystectomy? a decision analysis. Gastroenterology 116:G0012, 1999

49. Erickson RA, Carlson B: The role of endoscopic retrograde cholangiopancreatography in patients with laparoscopic cholecystectomies. Gastroenterology 109:252, 1995

50. Urbach DR, Khajanchee YS, Jobe BA, et al: Cost-effective management of common bile duct stones: a decision analysis of the use of endoscopic retrograde cholangiopancreatography (ERCP), intraoperative cholangiography, and laparoscopic bile duct exploration. Surg Endosc 15:4, 2001

51. Memon MA, Hassaballa H, Memon MI: Laparoscopic common bile duct exploration: the past, the present, and the future. Am J Surg 179:309, 2000

52. Crawford DL, Phillips EH: Laparoscopic common bile duct exploration. World J Surg 23:343, 1999

53. Falcone RA Jr, Fegelman EJ, Nussbaum MS, et al: A prospective comparison of laparoscopic ultrasound vs intraoperative cholangiogram during laparoscopic cholecystectomy. Surg Endosc 13:784, 1999

54. Thompson DM, Arregui ME, Tetik C, et al: A comparison of laparoscopic ultrasound with digital fluorocholangiography for detecting choledocholithiasis during laparoscopic cholecystectomy. Surg Endosc 12:929, 1998

55. Wu JS, Dunnegan DL, Soper NJ: The utility of intracorporeal ultrasonography for screening of the bile duct during laparoscopic cholecystectomy. J Gastrointest Surg 2:50, 1998

56. Freeny PC, Traverso LW, Ryan JA: Diagnosis and staging of pancreatic adenocarcinoma with dynamic computed tomography. Am J Surg 165:600, 1993

57. Freeny PC, Marks WM, Ryan JA, et al: Pancreatic ductal adenocarcinoma: diagnosis and staging with dynamic CT. Radiology 166:125, 1988

58. Moosa AR, Gamagami RA: Diagnosis and staging of pancreatic neoplasms. Surg Clin North Am 75:871, 1995

59. Megibow AJ, Zhou XH, Rotterdam H, et al: Pancreatic carcinoma: CT vs MR imaging in the evaluation of resectability. Radiology 195:327, 1995

60. Hann LE, Winston CB, Brown KT, et al: Diagnostic imaging approaches and relationship to hepatobiliary cancer staging and therapy. Semin Surg Oncol 19:94, 2000

61. Zidi SH, Prat F, Le Guen O, et al: Performance characteristics of magnetic resonance cholangiography in the staging of malignant hilar strictures. Gut 46:103, 2000

62. Kim MJ, Mitchell DG, Ito K, et al: Biliary dilatation: differentiation of benign from malignant causes--value of adding conventional MR imaging to MR cholangiopancreatography. Radiology 214:173, 2000

63. Georgopoulos SK, Schwartz LH, Jarnagin WR, et al: Comparison of magnetic resonance and endoscopic retrograde cholangiopancreatography in malignant pancreaticobiliary obstruction. Arch Surg 134:1002, 1999

64. Smits NJ, Reeders JW: Current applicability of duplex Doppler ultrasonography in pancreatic head and biliary malignancies. Baillieres Clin Gastroenterol 9:153, 1995

65. Arslan A, Buanes T, Geitung JT: Pancreatic carcinoma: MR, MR angiography and dynamic helical CT in the evaluation of vascular invasion. Eur J Radiol 38:151, 2001

66. Giovannini M, Seitz JF: Endoscopic ultrasonography with a linear-type echoendoscope in the evaluation of 94 patients with pancreatobiliary disease. Endoscopy 26:579, 1994

67. Snady H, Cooperman A, Siegel J: Endoscopic ultrasonography compared with computed tomography and E.R.C.P. in patients with obstructive jaundice or small peri-pancreatic mass. Gastrointest Endoscopy 38:27, 1992

68. Nakaizumi A, Uehara H, Iishi H, et al: Endoscopic ultrasonography in diagnosis and staging of pancreatic cancer. Dig Dis Sci 40:696, 1995

69. Bakkevold KE, Arnesjo B, Kambestad B: Carcinoma of the pancreas and papilla of Vater—assessment of resectability and factors influencing resectability in stage I carcinomas: a prospective multicentre trial in 472 patients. Eur J Surg Oncol 18:494, 1992

70. Cannon ME, Carpenter SL, Elta GH, et al: EUS compared with CT, magnetic resonance imaging, and angiography and the influence of biliary stenting on staging accuracy of ampullary neoplasms. Gastrointest Endosc 50:27, 1999

71. Povoski SP, Karpeh MS Jr, Conlon KC, et al: Preoperative biliary drainage: impact on intraoperative bile cultures and infectious morbidity and mortality after pancreaticoduodenectomy. J Gastrointest Surg 3:496, 1999

72. Sohn TA, Yeo CJ, Cameron JL, et al: Do preoperative biliary stents increase postpancreaticoduodenectomy complications? J Gastrointest Surg 4:258, 2000

73. Jarnagin WR, Bodniewicz J, Dougherty E, et al: A prospective analysis of staging laparoscopy in patients with primary and secondary hepatobiliary malignancies. J Gastrointest Surg 4:34, 2000

74. Davidson BR: Progress in determining the nature of biliary strictures. Gut 34:725, 1993

75. Hawes RH: Endoscopy and non-calculus biliary obstruction. Annuals of Gastrointestinal Endoscopy, 8th ed. Cotton PB, Tytgat GNJ, Williams CB, Eds. Current Science, England, 1995, p 101

76. Fernandez Del Castillo C, Warshaw AL: Cystic tumors of the pancreas. Surg Clin North Am 75:1001, 1995

77. Rege RV: Adverse effects of biliary obstruction: implications for treatment of patients with obstructive jaundice. AJR Am J Roentgenol 164:287, 1995

78. Grande L, Garcia-Valdecasas JC, Fuster J, et al: Obstructive jaundice and wound healing. Br J Surg 77:440, 1990

79. Pitt HA, Gomes AS, Lois JF: Does preoperative percutaneous biliary drainage reduce operative risk or increase hospital cost? Ann Surg 201:545, 1985

80. McPherson GA, Benjamin IS, Hodgson HJ, et al: Preoperative percutaneous transhepatic biliary drainage: results of a controlled trial. Br J Surg 71:371, 1984

81. Abraham N, Barkun J, Barkun AN, et al: Clinical risk factors of plastic biliary stent obstruction: a prospective trial. Am J Gastroenterol 95:2471, 2000

82. Knyrim K, Wagner HJ, Pausch J, et al: A prospective, randomized controlled trial of metal stents for malignant obstruction of the common bile duct. Endoscopy 25:207, 1993

83. Davids P, Groen A, Rauws E, et al: Randomized trial of self-expanding metal stents versus polyethylene stents for distal malignant biliary obstruction. Lancet 340:1488, 1992

84. Prat F, Chapat O, Ducot B, et al: A randomized trial of endoscopic drainage methods for inoperable malignant strictures of the common bile duct. Gastrointest Endosc 47:1, 1998

85. Smith AC, Dowsett JF, Russell RC, et al: Randomized trial of endoscopic stenting vs surgical bypass in malignant low bile duct obstruction. Lancet 344:1655, 1994

86. Lillemoe KD, Sauter P, Pitt HA, et al: Current status of surgical palliation of periampullary carcinoma. Surg Gynecol Obstet 176:1, 1993

87. Lillemoe KD, Cameron JL, Kaufman HS, et al: Chemical splanchnicectomy in patients with unresectable pancreatic cancer: a prospective randomized trial. Ann Surg 217:447, 1993

88. Lillemoe KD, Cameron JL, Yeo CJ, et al: Pancreaticoduodenectomy: does it have a role in the palliation of pancreatic cancer? Ann Surg 223:718, 1996

89. Conlon KC, Dougherty E, Klimstra DS, et al: The value of minimal access surgery in the staging of patients with potentially resectable pancreatic malignancy. Ann Surg 223:134, 1996

90. John TG, Greig JD, Carter DC, et al: Carcinoma of the pancreatic head and periampullary region: tumor staging with laparoscopy and laparoscopic ultrasonography. Ann Surg 221:156, 1995

91. Hunerbein M, Rau B, Schlag PM: Laparoscopic ultrasound for staging of upper gastrointestinal tumours. Eur J Surg Oncol 21:50, 1995

92. Jarnagin WR, Bodniewicz J, Dougherty E, et al: A prospective analysis of staging laparoscopy in patients with primary and secondary hepatobiliary malignancies. J Gastrointest Surg 4:34, 2000

93. Baer HU, Rhyner M, Stain SC, et al: The effect of communication between the right and left liver on the outcome of surgical drainage from jaundice due to malignant obstruction at the hilus of the liver. HPB Surg 8:27, 1994

94. Gagner M: Personal communication

95. Scott-Conner CE: Laparoscopic biliary bypass for inoperable pancreatic cancer. Semin Laparosc Surg 5:185, 1998

96. Chamberlain RS, Blumgart LH: Hilar cholangiocarcinoma: a review and commentary. Ann Surg Oncol 7:55, 2000

97. Ogura Y, Kawarada Y: Surgical strategies for carcinoma of the hepatic duct confluence. Br J Surg 85:20, 1998

98. Baer HU, Matthews JB, Schweizer WP, et al: Management of the Mirizzi syndrome and the surgical implications of cholecystocholedochal fistula. Br J Surg 77:743, 1990

99. Sarfeh MG, Rypins EB, Jakowatz JG, et al: A prospective, randomized clinical investigation of cholecystoenterostomy and choledochoenterostomy. Am J Surg 155:411, 1988

100. Lieberman MD, Kilburn H, Lindsey M, et al: Relation of perioperative deaths to hospital volume among patients undergoing pancreatic resection for malignancy. Ann Surg 222:638, 1995

101. Lamont JT, Isselbacher KJ: Current concepts of postoperative hepatic dysfunction. Conn Med 39:461, 1975

102. Matlof DS, Kaplan MM: Postoperative jaundice. Orthop Clin North Am 9:799, 1978

103. Moody FG, Potts JR III: Postoperative jaundice. Diseases of the Liver, 7th ed. Schiff L, Schiff ER, Eds. JB Lippincott Co, Philadelphia, 1993, p 370

104. Isselbacher KJ: Bilirubin metabolism and hyperbilirubinemia. Harrison's Principles of Internal Medicine, 12th ed. Wilson JD, Braunwald E, Isselbacher KJ, et al, Eds. McGraw-Hill, New York, 1991, p 1320

105. Watson CJ: Prognosis and treatment of hepatic insufficiency. Ann Intern Med 31:405, 1959

106. Sherlock S: Jaundice. Diseases of the Liver and Biliary System, 8th ed. Sherlock S, Ed. Blackwell Scientific Publications, Oxford, 1989, p 230

107. Gollan JL, Keefe EB, Scharschmidt BF: Cholestasis and hyperbilirubinemia. Current Hepatology, Vol I. Gitnick G, Ed. Houghton Mifflin, Boston, 1980, p 277

108. Bosma PJ, Chowdhury JR, Bakker C, et al: The genetic basis of the reduced expression of bilirubin UCP-glucuronosyltransferase 1 in Gilbert's syndrome. N Engl J Med 333:1171, 1995

109. O'Grady JG, Portmann B, Williams R: Fulminant hepatic failure. Diseases of the Liver, 7th ed. Schiff L, Schiff ER, Eds. JB Lippincott Co, Philadelphia, 1993, p 1077

110. Bismuth H, Samuel D, Castaing D, et al: Orthotopic liver transplantation in fulminant and subfulminant hepatitis. Ann Surg 222:109, 1995

111. Boyer JL, Reuben A: Chronic hepatitis. Diseases of the Liver, 7th ed. Schiff L, Schiff ER, Eds. JB Lippincott Co, Philadelphia, 1993, p 586

112. Pugh RN, Murray-Lyon IM, Dawson JL, et al: Transection of the esophagus for bleeding esophageal varices. Br J Surg 60:646, 1973

113. Fallon MB, Anderson JM, Boyer JL: Intrahepatic cholestasis. Diseases of the Liver, 7th ed. Schiff L, Schiff ER, Eds. JB Lippincott Co, Philadelphia, 1993, p 343

Acknowledgment

Figure 2c From *MRI of the Abdomen and Pelvis: A Text-Atlas*, by R. C. Semelka, S. M. Asher, and C. Reinhold. John Wiley and Sons, New York, 1997. Used with permission.

7 INTESTINAL OBSTRUCTION

W. Scott Helton, M.D.

Assessment of Intestinal Obstruction

Intestinal obstruction is a common medical problem and accounts for a large percentage of surgical admissions for acute abdominal pain [*see II:4 Acute Abdominal Pain*].[1] It develops when air and secretions are prevented from passing aborally as a result of either intrinsic or extrinsic compression (i.e., mechanical obstruction) or gastrointestinal paralysis (i.e., nonmechanical obstruction in the form of ileus or pseudo-obstruction). Small intestinal ileus is the most common form of intestinal obstruction; it occurs after most abdominal operations and is a common response to acute extra-abdominal medical conditions and intra-abdominal inflammatory conditions [*see Table 1*]. Mechanical small bowel obstruction is somewhat less common; such obstruction is secondary to intra-abdominal adhesions, hernias, or cancer in about 90% of cases [*see Table 2*]. Mechanical colonic obstruction accounts for only 10% to 15% of all cases of mechanical obstruction and most often develops in response to obstructing carcinoma, diverticulitis, or volvulus [*see Table 3*]. Acute colonic pseudo-obstruction occurs most frequently in the postoperative period or in response to another acute medical illness.

In what follows, several different methods of classifying mechanical obstruction are used: acute versus chronic, partial versus complete, simple versus closed-loop, and gangrenous versus nongangrenous. The importance of these classifications is that the natural history of the condition, its response to treatment, and the associated morbidity and mortality all vary according to which type of obstruction is present.

When chyme and gas can traverse the point of obstruction, obstruction is partial; when this is not the case, obstruction is complete. When the bowel is occluded at a single point along the intestinal tract, leading to intestinal dilatation, hypersecretion, and bacterial overgrowth proximal to the obstruction and decompression distal to the obstruction, simple obstruction is present. When a segment of bowel is occluded at two points along its course by a single constrictive lesion that occludes both the proximal and the distal end of the intestinal loop as well as traps the bowel's mesentery, closed-loop obstruction is present. When the blood supply to a closed-loop segment of bowel becomes compromised, leading to ischemia and eventually to bowel wall necrosis and perforation, strangulation is present. The most common causes of simple obstruction are intra-abdominal adhesions, tumors, and strictures; the most common causes of closed-loop obstruction are hernias, adhesions, and volvulus.

One of the most difficult tasks in general surgery is deciding when to operate on a patient with intestinal obstruction. The purpose of the following discussion is to outline a safe, efficient, and cost-effective stepwise approach to making this often diffi-cult decision and to optimizing the management of patients with this problem. Absolutes are few and far between: treatment must always be highly individualized. Consequently, the following recommendations are intended only as guidelines, not as surgical dicta.

History and Clinical Setting

When a patient complains of acute obstipation, abdominal pain and distention, nausea, and vomiting, the probability that either mechanical bowel obstruction or ileus is present is very high.[2] Mechanical obstruction can often be distinguished from ileus or pseudo-obstruction on the basis of the location, character, and severity of abdominal pain. Pain from mechanical obstruction is usually located in the middle of the abdomen, whereas pain from ileus and pseudo-obstruction is diffuse. Pain from ileus is usually mild, and pain from obstruction is typically more severe. In general, pain increases in severity and depth over time as obstruction progresses; however, in mechanical obstruction, pain severity may decrease over time as a result of bowel fatigue and atony. The periodicity of pain can help localize the level of obstruction: pain from proximal intestinal obstruction has a short periodicity (3 to 4 minutes), and distal small bowel or colonic pain has longer intervals (15 to 20 minutes) between episodes of nausea, cramping, and vomiting.

Abdominal distention, nausea, and vomiting usually develop after pain has already been felt for some time. The patient should be asked what degree of abdominal distention is present and whether there has been a sudden or rapid change. Distention developing over many weeks suggests a chronic process or progressive partial obstruction. Massive abdominal distention coupled with minimal crampy pain, nausea, and vomiting suggests long-standing intermittent mechanical obstruction or some form of chronic intestinal pseudo-obstruction. The combination of a gradual change in bowel habits, progressive abdominal distention, early satiety, mild crampy pain after meals, and weight loss also suggests chronic partial mechanical bowel obstruction. If the patient has undergone evaluation for similar symptoms before, any previous abdominal radiographs or contrast studies should be reviewed. The patient should be asked when flatus was last passed: failure to pass flatus may signal a transition from partial to complete bowel obstruction. Patients with an intestinal

Signs and symptoms of intestinal obstruction

Signs and symptoms include abdominal pain or distention, nausea, vomiting, and obstipation.

Clinical history

Assess character, severity, location, and periodicity of pain.

Assess degree of abdominal distention, and ask about any sudden or rapid changes.

Ask about changes in bowel habits, weight loss, and last passage of flatus.

Ask about (1) previous obstruction, (2) previous abdominal or pelvic procedures, (3) abdominal cancer, (4) intra-abdominal inflammation.

Consider clinical setting: ask about medical conditions or metabolic derangements, exposure to radiation, all medications. Immediate postoperative state is special situation.

Mechanical obstruction

Determine whether obstruction is complete or partial.

Nonmechanical obstruction

Classification of obstruction

The most useful distinction is mechanical vs. nonmechanical.

Terminally ill patients: consider no treatment other than comfort measures and hospice care.

Ileus

[*See Figure 12.*]

Pseudo-obstruction

[*See Figure 13.*]

Complete obstruction

Operate immediately.

Partial obstruction

Look for associated factors that may necessitate immediate operation.

Immediate operation indicated

Indications include peritonitis, incarcerated hernia, suspected or confirmed strangulation, pneumatosis cystoides intestinalis, sigmoid volvulus with systemic toxicity or peritoneal irritation, small bowel volvulus, colonic volvulus above sigmoid, and fecal impaction.

Operate immediately.

Assessment of Intestinal Obstruction

Urgent operation

Indications include
- Lack of response to 24–48 hr of nonoperative therapy (increasing abdominal pain, distention, or tenderness; NG aspirate changing from nonfeculent to feculent; ↑ proximal small bowel distention with ↓ distal gas).
- Early technical complications of operation (abscess, phlegmon, hematoma, hernia, intussusception, anastomotic obstruction).

Physical exam and resuscitate as necessary

Develop gestalt of patient's illness, and assess patient's vital signs, hydration, and cardiopulmonary system.

Place NG tube, Foley catheter, and I.V. line immediately. Assess volume and character of NG aspirate, and measure urine output.

Replace lost fluid with isotonic saline or lactated Ringer solution. Look for signs of abscess, pneumonia, or myocardial infarction, and be alert for dyspnea, labored breathing, or jaundice.

Perform systematic abdominal examination: observation → auscultation → palpation and percussion. Look for abdominal masses, tenderness, incisions, and hernias; assess bowel sounds; examine rectum for masses, fecal impaction, and occult blood.

Investigative studies

Obtain chest x-rays and abdominal films.

If uncertainty about presence or nature of colonic obstruction remains, perform sigmoidoscopy and barium enema examination.

Measure serum electrolytes and creatinine, determine hematocrit, and order coagulation profile. If ileus is suspected, measure serum magnesium and calcium and order urinalysis.

Perform CT (with oral or I.V. contrast agents), abdominal ultrasonography, or both.

Immediate operation not indicated

Manage initially with nonoperative measures.

Reassess patient every 4 hours.

For partial obstruction, consider administering oral diatrizoate meglumine.

Look for changes in pain, abdominal findings, and volume and character of NG aspirate.

Repeat abdominal x-rays, and look for changes in gas distribution, pneumatosis cystoides intestinalis, and free intraperitoneal air.

Classify patient's condition as improved, unchanged, or worse.

Decide whether operative treatment is necessary and, if so, whether it should be done on urgent or elective basis.

Arrival of contrast agent in right colon within 24 hr is highly predictive of successful resolution of adhesive obstruction without operation.

No operation

Conditions that typically resolve with nonoperative therapy include adhesive obstruction (unless it does not improve in 12 hr), early postoperative obstruction (unless it does not improve in 2 wk), and various inflammatory conditions (IBD, radiation enteritis, diverticulitis, acute Crohn disease).

Elective operation

Indications include nontoxic, nontender sigmoid volvulus with sigmoidoscopically managed obstruction; recurrent adhesive or stricture-related small bowel obstruction; partial colonic obstruction unresponsive to 24 hr of nonoperative therapy; development and resolution of small bowel obstruction in patient who has never undergone abdominal operation.

Table 1 Causes of Ileus

Intra-abdominal causes
Intraperitoneal problems
  Peritonitis or abscess
  Inflammatory condition
    Mechanical: operation, foreign body
    Chemical: gastric juice, bile, blood
    Autoimmune: serositis, vasculitis
  Intestinal ischemia: arterial or venous, sickle-cell disease
Retroperitoneal problems
  Pancreatitis
  Retroperitoneal hematoma
  Spine fracture
  Aortic operation
  Renal colic
  Pyelonephritis
  Metastasis

Extra-abdominal causes
Thoracic problems
  Myocardial infarction
  Pneumonia
  Congestive heart failure
  Rib fractures
Metabolic abnormalities
  Electrolyte imbalance (e.g., hypokalemia)
  Sepsis
  Lead poisoning
  Porphyria
  Hypothyroidism
  Hypoparathyroidism
  Uremia
Medicines
  Opiates
  Anticholinergics
  Alpha agonists
  Antihistamines
  Catecholamines
Spinal cord injury or operations
Head, thoracic, or retroperitoneal trauma
Chemotherapy, radiation therapy

read the operative report, which can provide a great deal of helpful information (e.g., description of adhesions, assessment of their severity, and evaluation of intra-abdominal pathology and anatomy). If abdominal cancer was present, one should find out what operation was performed and attempt to determine the likelihood of intra-abdominal recurrence.

The clinical setting often provides clues to the cause and type of bowel obstruction. In hospitalized patients, there is likely to be an associated medical condition or metabolic derangement that led to obstruction. A thorough review of the patient's medical history and hospital course should be undertaken to identify precipitating events that could have led to intestinal obstipation. One should ask the patient about any previous abdominal irradiation and should note and take into account all medications the patient is taking, especially anticoagulants and agents with anticholinergic side effects. Patients who are receiving chemotherapy or have undergone abdominal radiation therapy are prone to ileus. Severe infection, fluid and electrolyte imbalances, narcotic and anticholinergic medications, and intra-abdominal inflammation of any origin may be implicated. Acute massive abdominal distention in a hospitalized patient usually results from acute gastric distention, small bowel ileus, or acute colonic pseudo-obstruction. Excessive anticoagulation can lead to retroperitoneal, intra-abdominal, or intramural hematoma that can cause mechanical obstruction or ileus. Finally, there are specific problems that tend to arise in the postoperative period; these are discussed more fully elsewhere [see Urgent Operation, Early Postoperative Technical Complications, and No Operation, Early Postoperative Obstruction, below].

Table 2 Causes of Small Bowel Obstruction in Adults

Extrinsic causes
Adhesions*
Hernias (external, internal, incisional)*
Metastatic cancer*
Volvulus
Intra-abdominal abscess
Intra-abdominal hematoma
Pancreatic pseudocyst
Intra-abdominal drains
Tight fascial opening at stoma

Intraluminal causes
Tumors*
Gallstones
Foreign body
Worms
Bezoars

Intramural abnormalities
Tumors
Strictures
Hematoma
Intussusception
Regional enteritis
Radiation enteritis

*Approximately 85% of all small bowel obstructions are secondary to adhesions, hernias, or tumors.

stoma (ileostomy or colostomy) who present with signs and symptoms of obstruction often report abdominal distention and pain after a sudden change in stomal output of stool, liquid, or air.

The patient should also be asked about (1) previous episodes of bowel obstruction, (2) previous abdominal or pelvic operations, (3) a history of abdominal cancer, and (4) a history of intra-abdominal inflammation (e.g., inflammatory bowel disease, cholecystitis, pancreatitis, pelvic inflammatory disease, or abdominal trauma). Any of these factors increases the chance that the obstruction is secondary to an adhesion or recurrent cancer. Obstructive symptoms that come and go suddenly over several days in a patient older than 65 years should increase the index of suspicion for gallstone ileus.[3] If the patient has experienced episodes of obstruction before, one should ask about the etiology and the response to treatment. If the patient has ever undergone an abdominal operation, one should try to obtain and

Table 3 Causes of Colonic Obstruction

Common causes
Cancer (primary, anastomotic, metastatic)
Volvulus
Diverticulitis
Pseudo-obstruction
Hernia
Anastomotic stricture

Unusual causes
Intussusception
Fecal impaction
Strictures (from one of the following)
    Inflammatory bowel disease
    Endometriosis
    Radiation therapy
    Ischemia
Foreign body
Extrinsic compression by a mass
    Pancreatic pseudocyst
    Hematoma
    Metastasis
    Primary tumors

Physical Examination and Resuscitation

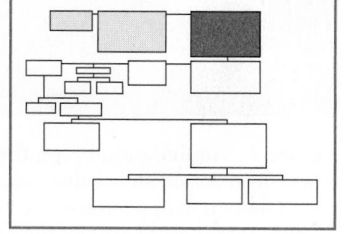

The initial steps in the physical examination are (1) developing a gestalt of the patient's illness and (2) assessing the patient's vital signs, hydration status, and cardiopulmonary system. A nasogastric tube, a Foley catheter, and an I.V. line are placed immediately while the physical examination is in progress. The volume and character of the gastric aspirate and urine are noted. A clear, gastric effluent is suggestive of gastric outlet obstruction. A bilious, nonfeculent aspirate is a typical sign of medial to proximal small bowel obstruction or colonic obstruction with a competent ileocecal valve. A feculent aspirate is a typical sign of distal small bowel obstruction. Volume replacement, if necessary, is initiated with isotonic saline solution or lactated Ringer solution. Urine output must be adequate (at least 0.5 ml/kg/hr) before the patient can be taken to the OR; supplemental potassium chloride (40 mEq/L) is administered once this is achieved.

Fever may be present, suggesting that the obstruction may be a manifestation of an intra-abdominal abscess. Signs of pneumonia or myocardial infarction should be sought: these conditions, like intestinal obstruction, can have upper abdominal pain, distention, nausea, and vomiting as presenting symptoms. Dyspnea and labored breathing may occur secondary to severe abdominal distention or pain, in which case immediate relief should be provided by placing the patient in the lateral decubitus position and offering narcotics as soon as the initial physical examination is performed. Jaundice raises the possibility of gallstone ileus or metastatic cancer.

Examination of the abdomen proceeds in an orderly manner from observation to auscultation to palpation and percussion. The patient is placed in the supine position with the legs flexed

at the hip to decrease tension on the rectus muscles. The degree of abdominal distention observed varies, depending on the level of obstruction: proximal obstructions may cause little or no distention. Abdominal scars should be noted. Abdominal asymmetry or a protruding mass suggests an underlying malignancy, an abscess, or closed-loop obstruction. The abdominal wall should be observed for evidence of peristaltic waves, which are indicative of acute small bowel obstruction.

Auscultation should be performed for at least 3 to 4 minutes to determine the presence and quality of bowel sounds. High-pitched bowel tones, tingles, and rushes are suggestive of an obstructive process, especially when temporally associated with waves of crampy pain, nausea, or vomiting. The absence of bowel tones is typical of intestinal paralysis but may also indicate intestinal fatigue from long-standing obstruction, closed-loop obstruction, or pseudo-obstruction.

Approximately 70% of patients with bowel obstruction have symmetric tenderness, whereas fewer than 50% have rebound tenderness, guarding, or rigidity.[2] The traditional teaching is that localized tenderness and guarding indicate underlying strangulated bowel; however, prospective studies have demonstrated that these physical findings are neither specific nor sensitive for detecting underlying strangulation[4] or even obstruction.[2] Nevertheless, most surgeons still believe that guarding, rebound tenderness, and localized tenderness reflect underlying strangulation and therefore are indications for operation. Patients with ileus tend to have generalized abdominal tenderness that cannot be distinguished from the tenderness of mechanical obstruction. Gentle percussion is performed over all quadrants of the abdomen to search for areas of dullness (suggestive of an underlying mass), tympany (suggestive of underlying distended bowel), and peritoneal irritation.

A thorough search is made for inguinal, femoral, umbilical, and incisional hernias. The rectum is examined for masses, fecal impaction, and occult blood. If the patient has an ileostomy or a colostomy, the stoma is examined digitally to make sure that there is no obstruction at the level of the fascia.

Investigative Studies

IMAGING STUDIES

One should obtain a chest x-ray in all patients with bowel obstruction to exclude a pneumonic process and to look for subdiaphragmatic air. In most cases, supine, upright, or lateral decubitus films of the abdomen can distinguish the type of obstruction present (mechanical or nonmechanical, partial or complete) and establish the location of the obstruction (stomach, small bowel, or colon). A useful technique for evaluating abdominal radiographs is to look systematically for intestinal gas along the normal route of the GI tract, beginning at the stomach, continuing through the small bowel, and, finally, following the course of the colon to the rectum. The following questions should be kept in mind as this is done.

- Are there abnormally dilated loops of bowel, signs of small bowel dilatation, or air-fluid levels?

- Are air-fluid levels and bowel loops in the same place on supine and upright films?

- Is there gas throughout the entire length of the colon (suggestive of ileus or partial mechanical obstruction)?

- Is there a paucity of distal colonic gas or an abrupt cutoff of colonic gas with proximal colonic distention and air-fluid levels (suggestive of complete or near-complete colonic obstruction)?

- Is there evidence of strangulation (e.g., thickened small bowel loops, mucosal thumb printing, pneumatosis cystoides intestinalis, or free peritoneal air)?

- Is there massive distention of the colon, especially of the cecum or sigmoid (suggestive of either volvulus or pseudo-obstruction)?

- Are there any biliary or renal calculi, and is there any air in the biliary tree (suggestive of gallstone ileus[5] or a renal stone that could be causing ileus)?

It is important to be able to distinguish between small and large bowel gas. Gas in a distended small bowel outlines the valvulae conniventes, which traverse the entire diameter of the bowel lumen [see Figure 1]. Gas in a distended colon, on the other hand, outlines the colonic haustral markings, which cross only part of the bowel lumen and typically interdigitate [see Figures 2 and 3]. Distended small bowel loops usually occupy the central abdomen [see Figure 1], whereas distended large bowel loops are typically seen around the periphery [see Figure 2]. In patients with ileus, distention usually extends uniformly throughout the stomach, the small bowel, and the colon [see Figure 3], and air-fluid levels may be found in the colon and the small intestine.

Patients with gastric outlet obstruction or gastric atony typically have a giant gastric bubble if no nasogastric tube has been placed, with little or no air in the small bowel or the colon. Patients with mechanical small bowel obstruction usually have multiple air-fluid levels, with distended bowel loops of varying sizes arranged in an inverted U configuration [see Figure 4]. A dilated loop of small bowel appearing in the same location on supine and upright films suggests obstruction of a fixed segment of bowel by an adhesion [see Figures 1 and 4]. Small bowel obstruction is often accompanied by a paucity of gas in the colon. The complete absence of colonic gas is strongly suggestive of complete small bowel obstruction; however, the presence of colonic gas does not exclude complete small bowel obstruction, in that there may have been unevacuated gas distal to a point of complete obstruction before the radiograph was taken. On the other hand, if repeat radiographs demonstrate decreased or absent colonic or rectal gas in a patient with small bowel obstruction who previously had more colonic or rectal gas, it is probable that partial obstruction has become complete, and immediate operation is almost always indicated. High-grade obstruction of the colon with an incompetent ileocecal valve may manifest itself as distended small bowel loops with air-fluid levels, thereby mimicking small bowel obstruction. Hence, it is sometimes necessary to perform a barium enema to exclude colonic obstruction.

Massive gaseous distention of the colon is usually secondary to distal colonic or rectal obstruction, volvulus, or pseudo-obstruction [see Figures 2, 5a, 5b, 6a, 6b, and 7]. There are well-defined radiographic criteria that are highly sensitive and specific for sigmoid volvulus.[5] If there is any uncertainty regarding the presence, type, or level of colonic obstruction, immediate sigmoidoscopy followed by barium enema is diagnostic.

LABORATORY STUDIES

Serum electrolyte concentrations, the hematocrit, the serum creatinine concentration, and the coagulation profile (prothrombin time [or international normalized ratio—INR] and platelet count) are helpful in determining the severity of volume

Figure 1 Supine radiograph from a patient with complete small bowel obstruction shows distended small bowel loops in the central abdomen with prominent valvulae conniventes (small white arrow). Bowel wall between the loops is thickened and edematous (large white arrow). No air is seen in the colon or the rectum. Note the presence of an isolated small bowel loop in the right lower quadrant (black arrow), which is seen fixed in the same location on upright films, as shown in Figure 4.

depletion and guiding resuscitative efforts. If ileus is suspected, serum magnesium and calcium levels should be measured, and urinalysis should be done to check for hematuria.

Determination of Need for Operation and Classification of Obstruction

The combination of a thorough history, a carefully performed physical examination, and correctly interpreted abdominal radiographs usually allows one to identify the type

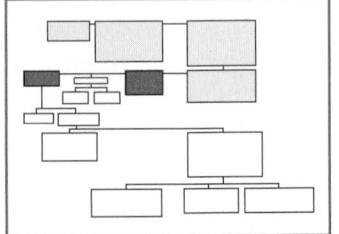

of bowel obstruction present and to decide whether a patient requires immediate, urgent, or delayed operation [see Table 4] or can safely be treated initially with nonoperative measures. To this end, it is particularly important and useful to stratify patients into those with mechanical obstruction and those with nonmechanical obstruction. In patients with mechanical bowel obstruction,

Figure 2 **Radiograph from a patient with acute colonic pseudo-obstruction shows a dilated colon with haustral markings (white arrow) and edematous small bowel loops (black arrow). Air extends down to the distal sigmoid. This picture is also consistent with rectal obstruction, which could have been excluded by rigid sigmoidoscopy.**

Figure 3 **Radiograph from a patient with postoperative ileus shows massive gastric distention (A), distended small bowel loops (B), air throughout the colon, mild dilatation of the sigmoid colon (C) with air mixed with stool, and a haustral fold in the apex of the sigmoid colon (D).**

an effort should be made to determine whether the obstruction is complete or partial. Except for a few clinical situations, patients with complete bowel obstruction require immediate operation; conversely, patients with partial bowel obstruction rarely do. Finally, an effort should be made to establish the level and cause of obstruction because these factors often help guide therapy and affect the probability of success in response to specific therapeutic intervention. Patients with nonmechanical obstruction, which derives from ileus or pseudo-obstruction [*see* Ileus and Pseudo-obstruction, *below*], do not require immediate operation.

ADJUNCTIVE TESTS FOR EQUIVOCAL SITUATIONS

Sigmoidoscopy

When one is uncertain whether the obstruction is mechanical or not on the basis of the information in hand, additional diagnostic measures are immediately indicated. When large amounts of colonic air extend down to the rectum, flexible or rigid sigmoidoscopy will readily exclude a rectal or distal sigmoid obstruction. If sigmoidoscopy yields normal findings and partial colonic obstruction is the most likely diagnosis, a barium enema with

Figure 4 **Upright radiograph from the same patient as the supine radiograph in Figure 1 shows multiple air-fluid levels of varying size arranged in inverted U's. In the right lower pelvis, a loop of small bowel is seen in exactly the same location as on the supine abdominal film (black arrow), a finding suggestive of adhesive obstruction.**

water-soluble contrast material should immediately be performed.[6] Abdominal ultrasonography, though not as definitive as a contrast examination, is also able to diagnose suspected colonic obstruction in 85% of patients.[7]

Ultrasonography and CT Scanning

Abdominal radiographs can be entirely normal in patients with complete, closed-loop, or strangulation obstruction.[8] Therefore, if the patient's clinical profile and the results of physical examination are consistent with intestinal obstruction despite normal abdominal radiographs, abdominal ultrasonography or CT scanning should be performed immediately.[8-15] Both of these imaging modalities are highly sensitive and specific for intestinal obstruction when performed properly and interpreted by experienced clinicians. Two prospective clinical trials found ultrasonography to be as sensitive as and more specific than abdominal radiography in diagnosing intestinal obstruction.[16,17] Both ultrasonography and CT are capable of detecting the cause of the obstruction as well as the presence of closed-loop or strangulation obstruction.[7,9,14,15,18-21] Sonographic criteria have been established for small bowel and colonic obstruction[7,18,19]: (1) simultaneous observation of distended and collapsed bowel segments, (2) free peritoneal fluid, (3) inspissated intestinal contents, (4) paradoxical pendulating peristalsis, (5) highly reflective fluid within the bowel lumen, (6) bowel wall edema between serosa and mucosa, and (7) a fixed mass of aperistaltic, fluid-filled, dilated intestinal loops. One group of authors has recommended that when abdominal radiographs are inconclusive or normal in patients with suspected colonic obstruction, ultrasonography, rather than CT or barium enema, should be the next diagnostic step.[7] Ultrasonography is well suited to critically ill patients: because it can be performed at the bedside, the risk associated with transport to the radiology suite is avoided. Given that ultrasonography is relatively inexpensive, is easy and quick to perform, and often can provide a great deal of information about the location, nature, and severity of the obstruction, it should be employed early on in the evaluation of all patients with intestinal obstruction.[16]

Several authors have recommended that patients with suspected small bowel obstruction and equivocal plain abdominal films undergo CT scanning before a small bowel contrast series is ordered.[10-13] CT scanning has several advantages over a small bowel contrast examination in this setting: (1) it can ascertain the level of obstruction, (2) it can assess the severity of the obstruction and determine its cause, and (3) it can detect closed-loop obstruction and early strangulation [*see Figures 8, 9, 10, and 11*]. CT can also detect inflammatory or neoplastic processes both outside and inside the peritoneal cavity and can visualize small amounts of intraperitoneal air or pneumatosis cystoides intestinalis not seen on conventional films [*see Figure 10*]. Prospective studies have demonstrated that the accuracy of CT in diagnosing bowel obstruction is higher than 95% and its sensitivity and specificity are each higher than 94%.[20,21] When CT scanning is nondiagnostic in a patient with suspected bowel obstruction, a small bowel follow-through examination with dilute barium is often useful.[13]

Figure 5 (*a*) **Radiograph from a patient with massive sigmoid volvulus shows a distended ahaustral sigmoid loop (white arrow), inferior convergence of the walls of the sigmoid loop to the left of the midline, and approximation of the medial walls of the sigmoid loop as a summation line (black arrow). (*b*) Barium enema of the colon shows a tapered obstruction at the rectosigmoid junction with a typical bird's-beak deformity (black arrow).**

a

b

Figure 6 (*a*) **Radiograph from a patient with cecal volvulus shows a dilated cecum with no air distally in the colorectum. Convergence of the medial walls of the loop (black arrow) points to the right, a typical finding in cecal volvulus. (*b*) Barium examination demonstrates a bird's-beak deformity tapering at the point of volvulus (large white arrow). Note walls of dilated cecum (small white arrows).**

Contrast Studies

Enteroclysis (direct injection of $BaSO_4$ into the small bowel) is generally considered the most sensitive method of distinguishing between ileus and partial mechanical small bowel obstruction: it has a diagnostic sensitivity of 87% for adhesive obstruction.[22,23] Many surgeons are concerned that injection of barium might cause partial obstruction to progress to complete obstruction; however, there is no evidence that this ever occurs, and one therefore should not refrain from using barium to diagnose partial small bowel obstruction.[24-27] If complete obstruction is identified, the patient should undergo immediate operation. If partial obstruction is identified in either the small or the large bowel, the patient is treated accordingly. If (1) mechanical obstruction is not identified and (2) a point of obstruction, as evidenced by the finding of both dilated and decompressed intestinal loops, cannot be identified through abdominal ultrasonography, CT scanning, or both, then the diagnosis is almost certainly ileus, in which case one's attention is directed toward identifying and correcting the underlying precipitating cause [*see Table 1 and* Mechanical Obstruction, No Operation, Adhesive Partial Small Bowel Obstruction, *below*].

Mechanical Obstruction

TERMINAL ILLNESS

Patients with a terminal illness (e.g., AIDS or advanced carcinomatosis) to whom surgical treatment offers little hope of improved quality or duration of life may choose not to undergo operative intervention for acute bowel obstruction. These patients should be offered comfort measures, including continuous morphine infusion, rehydration, and administration of antisecretory agents.[28-30] In some of these patients, endoscopic deployment of plastic stents may relieve high-grade partial obstruction, thus rendering laparotomy unnecessary.[31,32] Patients who do not wish to die of malignant bowel obstruction in a hospital should be offered hospice care or home visiting nurse services with continuous octreotide infusion, I.V. rehydration and gastrostomy decompression.[33,34] Two prospective, randomized clinical trials demonstrated that octreotide significantly attenuated the severity of nausea and vomiting and the degree of subjective discomfort in patients with inoperable obstruction and permitted the discontinuation of nasogastric tube decompression.[29,30] When long-term gastric decompression is required for palliation in a terminally ill patient, percutaneous endoscopic gastrostomy or jejunostomy should be considered [*see V:6 Gastrointestinal Endoscopy*].[35] It is essential to always pay attention to quality-of-life issues and to the patient's potential interest in pursuing nonoperative forms of palliation. For many terminally ill or incurable patients with bowel obstruction, the most humane and sensible treatment comprises nothing more than instituting palliative measures such as those described.

IMMEDIATE OPERATION

All patients with complete bowel obstruction, whether of the small intestine or the large, should undergo immediate operation unless extraordinary circumstances (e.g., diffuse carcinomatosis, terminal illness, or sigmoid volvulus that responds

to sigmoidoscopic decompression) are present. If one attempts to manage complete intestinal obstruction nonoperatively, one risks delaying definitive treatment of patients with intestinal ischemia and subjecting them to significantly increased morbidity and mortality should perforation or severe infection develop.[4,36]

Immediate operation is also indicated when bowel obstruction is associated with peritonitis; incarcerated strangulated hernias; suspected or confirmed strangulation; pneumatosis cystoides intestinalis; sigmoid volvulus accompanied by systemic toxicity or peritoneal irritation; colonic volvulus above the sigmoid colon; or fecal impaction. These conditions will not resolve without operation and are associated with increased morbidity, mortality, and cost if diagnosis and treatment are delayed. The only time one would not operate immediately on any patient with one of these diagnoses is when the patient requires cardiopulmonary stabilization, additional resuscitation, or both. Whenever there is any doubt as to the presence of any of these conditions, additional diagnostic tests (e.g., ultrasonography, CT, or contrast studies) are indicated to confirm or exclude them.

Strangulation and Closed-Loop Obstruction

Morbidity and mortality from intestinal obstruction vary significantly and depend primarily on the presence of strangulation and subsequent infection. Strangulation obstruction occurs in approximately 10% of all patients with small intestinal obstruction. It carries a mortality of 10% to 37%, whereas simple obstruction carries a mortality of less than 5%.[4,24,37,38] Early recognition and immediate operative treatment of strangulation obstruction are the only current means of decreasing this mortality. Strangulation obstruction occurs most frequently in patients with incarcerated hernias, closed-loop obstruction, volvulus, or complete bowel obstruction; hence, identification of any of these specific causes of obstruction is an important and clear indication for immediate operation. Radiographic evidence of pneumatosis cystoides intestinalis or free intraperitoneal air in a patient with a clinical picture of bowel obstruction is indicative of strangulation, perforation, or both and constitutes an indication for operation. High-quality abdominal CT with I.V. contrast can detect advanced strangulation as well as identify early, reversible strangulation [see Figure 11].[12,14,15]

Abdominal ultrasonography can also identify edematous, hemorrhagic loops of intestine. Accordingly, whenever one is concerned about possible strangulation or closed-loop obstruction but is not yet committed to taking the patient immediately to the OR, an ultrasonogram or a CT scan should be obtained. In fact, given that ultrasonography and CT are the only well-established means of diagnosing strangulation obstruction short of exploratory laparotomy or laparoscopy, an argument can be made that one or the other should be performed in all patients who have been admitted to the hospital with bowel obstruction and are initially being treated nonoperatively.

Many surgeons base the decision whether to operate on patients with bowel obstruction on the presence or absence of the so-called classic signs of strangulation obstruction—continuous abdominal pain, fever, tachycardia, peritoneal signs, and leukocytosis—and on their clinical experience. Unfortunately, these classically taught signs, even in conjunction with abdominal x-rays and clinical judgment, are incapable of reliably detecting closed-loop or gangrenous bowel obstruction.[4,24,36,39] In fact, one prospective clinical trial concluded that the five classic signs of strangulation obstruction and experienced clinical judgment were not sensitive for, specific for, or predictive of strangulation[4]: in more than 50% of the patients who had intestinal strangulation, the condition was not recognized preoperatively. Such findings suggest that early nonoperative recognition of intestinal strangulation is not feasible without ultrasonography or CT.

Incarcerated or Strangulated Hernias

A hernia that is incarcerated, tender, erythematous, warm, or edematous is an indication for immediate operation. Primary or incisional hernias may not be palpable in obese patients, in which case ultrasonography or CT scanning should be performed.

Nonsigmoid Volvulus and Sigmoid Volvulus with Systemic Toxicity or Peritoneal Signs

All intestinal volvuli are closed-loop obstructions and thus carry a high risk of intestinal strangulation, infarction, and perforation. Patients typically present with acute, colicky abdominal pain, massive distention, nausea, and vomiting. Sigmoid volvulus is the most common form of colonic volvulus, followed by cecal volvulus. Abdominal radiographs are fairly diagnostic for colonic volvulus [see Figures 5a, 5b, 6a, and 6b]. In contrast, small bowel volvulus may not be visualized on plain radiographs, because the closed loop fills completely with fluid and no air-fluid level can be seen. Small bowel volvulus is readily detected by ultrasonography or CT scanning; one or both of these procedures should be performed in patients presenting with signs and symptoms of bowel obstruction and normal abdominal radiographs. Small bowel volvulus is an indication for immediate operation.

If one observes signs of systemic toxicity, a bloody rectal discharge, fever, leukocytosis, or peritoneal irritation in a patient with sigmoid volvulus, the patient should undergo immediate operation; if all of these signs are absent, the patient should undergo sigmoidoscopy. When there are no signs of peritonitis or generalized toxicity, sigmoidoscopic decompression is safe and effective in more than 95% of patients with sigmoid volvulus.[40] If mucosal gangrene or a bloody effluent is noted at the time of sigmoidoscopy, immediate operative intervention is nec-

---

Table 4 Guidelines for Operative and Nonoperative Therapy

Situations necessitating emergent operation
Incarcerated, strangulated hernias
Peritonitis
Pneumatosis cystoides intestinalis
Pneumoperitoneum
Suspected or proven intestinal strangulation
Closed-loop obstruction
Nonsigmoid colonic volvulus
Sigmoid volvulus associated with toxicity or peritoneal signs
Complete bowel obstruction

Situations necessitating urgent operation
Progressive bowel obstruction at any time after nonoperative measures are started
Failure to improve with conservative therapy within 24–48 hr
Early postoperative technical complications

Situations in which delayed operation is usually safe
Immediate postoperative obstruction
Sigmoid volvulus successfully decompressed by sigmoidoscopy
Acute exacerbation of Crohn disease, diverticulitis, or radiation enteritis
Chronic, recurrent partial obstruction
Gastric outlet obstruction
Postoperative adhesions
Resolved partial colonic obstruction

Figure 7 Shown is a radiograph from a patient with complete colonic obstruction from an obstructing carcinoma in the descending left colon with proximal air-fluid levels. The absence of air distally in the rectum or the sigmoid is suggestive of complete obstruction. The ileocecal valve is competent, and thus, there is no small bowel air.

essary even in the absence of any clinical signs or symptoms of strangulation. After sigmoidoscopy, the patient can undergo

elective bowel preparation and a single-stage sigmoid resection before being discharged from the hospital. If, however, clinical toxicity, a bloody rectal discharge, fever, or peritoneal irritation arises at any time after sigmoidoscopic decompression while the patient is being prepared for elective operation, immediate operation is indicated.

Patients with volvulus proximal to the sigmoid colon should undergo immediate operation regardless of whether peritoneal irritation is present. The incidence of strangulation infarction is high in such patients, and nonoperative therapy often fails. If the diagnosis of nonsigmoid colonic volvulus is in doubt, a barium enema is indicated to exclude colonic pseudo-obstruction.

Fecal Impaction

Complete colonic obstruction secondary to fecal impaction in the rectum can sometimes be successfully relieved through disimpaction at the bedside; however, this can be difficult and extremely uncomfortable for the patient. The most expeditious and successful method of relieving the obstruction is to disimpact the patient while he or she is under general or spinal anesthesia.

URGENT OPERATION

Lack of Response to Nonoperative Therapy within 24 to 48 Hours

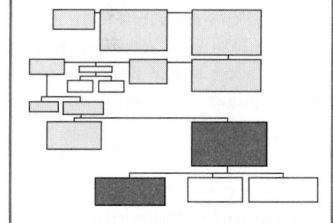

It is usually safe to manage partial bowel obstruction initially by nonoperative means: a nihil per os (NPO) regimen, nasogastric decompression, analgesics, and octreotide. Such therapy is successful in most cases, especially if the cause of

Figure 8 CT scan from a patient with partial small bowel obstruction shows distended, fluid-filled loops of small bowel with air-fluid levels, hyperemia, and bowel wall thickening (large white arrow). Note the discrepancy in caliber between dilated small bowel and decompressed small bowel (dashed white arrow) and the stranding (small black arrow) in the small bowel mesentery. Air in a decompressed descending colon (large black arrow) is indicative of partial obstruction.

Figure 9 CT scan from a patient with adhesive partial small bowel obstruction shows massively dilated small intestine (black arrow) proximal to a thick adhesive band (large white arrow) and decompressed small bowel distal to the adhesion (dashed white arrow). The patient was operated on because of the low probability that this obstruction would resolve with conservative management.

Figure 10 CT scan from a patient with partial small bowel obstruction from cancer shows distended small bowel (dashed white arrows) proximal to a mass (small white arrow). There is air in the cecum (black arrow), the transverse colon, and the descending colon (large white arrow). The small bowel is maximally dilated, with hyperemic, edematous bowel wall (B) just proximal to an obstructing recurrent colon carcinoma. Even though plain radiographs showed partial small bowel obstruction, this CT scan led to early operation because continued nonoperative management would not resolve the problem.

obstruction is from postoperative adhesions, but there is always the risk that complete bowel obstruction or strangulation already exists but is undetected. Furthermore, there is the risk that while the patient is being observed, partial obstruction will progress to complete obstruction or strangulation and perforation will develop. It is therefore crucial to be alert to changes in the patient's condition.

Repeated examination of the abdomen by the same clinician is the most sensitive way of detecting progressive obstruction. Examinations should be performed no less frequently than every 3 hours. If abdominal pain, tenderness, or distention increases or the gastric aspirate changes from nonfeculent to feculent, abdominal exploration is usually indicated. Abdominal radiographs should be repeated every 6 hours after nasogastric decompression and reviewed by the surgeon who is following the patient. If proximal small bowel distention increases or distal intestinal gas decreases, nonoperative therapy is less likely to be successful; in these circumstances, early operative intervention should be seriously considered. Conversely, if the patient's condition appears stable or improved and x-rays indicate that the obstruction either has resolved somewhat or at least is no worse, it is generally safe to continue nonoperative care for another 12 to 24 hours. If the clinical picture is stable after 24 hours of observation, one must decide whether to operate or to continue nonoperative therapy. One's clinical judgment and experience, coupled with a thorough and accurate assessment of the patient's underlying diagnosis and clinical condition, have traditionally been the most reliable guides for making this decision. Currently, however, it appears that the decision whether to operate can be made more cost-effectively and reliably on the basis of CT scans and contrast studies [*see* No Operation, Adhesive Partial Small Bowel Obstruction, *below*].

Early Postoperative Technical Complications

When normal bowel function initially returns after an abdominal operation but then is replaced by a clinical picture suggestive of early postoperative mechanical obstruction, the explanation may be a technical complication of the operation (e.g., phlegmon, abscess, intussusception, a narrow anastomosis, an internal hernia, or obstruction at the level of a stoma). An early, aggressive diagnostic workup should be performed to identify or exclude these problems because they are unlikely to respond to nasogastric decompression or other forms of conservative management. It is critical to know exactly what was done within the abdomen in the course of the operation. To this end, one should try to speak directly with the operating surgeon rather than attempt to deduce the needed information from the operative report.

If the patient had peritonitis or a colonic anastomosis at the initial operation, one should order a CT scan to look for an intra-abdominal abscess. An abscess or a phlegmon at the site of an anastomosis is usually secondary to anastomotic leakage and is an indication for reoperation. CT scanning can also identify intra-abdominal hematomas, which should be evacuated through early reoperation. In patients recovering from a proctectomy, herniation of the small bowel through a defect in the pelvic floor is a common cause of intestinal obstruction. Oral contrast studies can help identify patients with an internal hernia, intussusception, or anastomotic obstruction and should be performed after the CT scan. A retrograde barium examination should be performed in patients thought to have a problem related to a stoma or an intestinal anastomosis. When none of the above factors appears to be the cause of the postoperative obstruction, it is reasonable for the surgeon to assume that the obstruction is secondary to postoperative adhesions, which are best treated conservatively (see below).

Figure 11 Early closed-loop small bowel obstruction CT scan from a patient with early closed-loop obstruction of the small intestine shows markedly edematous, hyperemic small bowel, a finding indicative of early strangulation (white arrow). The patient had minimal symptoms, and there was air in the transverse colon and the descending colon (a finding indicative of partial small bowel obstruction); however, the finding of gangrenous, nonperforated small bowel on this CT scan led to early operation.

NO OPERATION

In selected patients, nonoperative management of partial small bowel obstruction is highly successful and carries an acceptably low mortality. Such patients include those whose partial obstruction is secondary to intra-abdominal adhesions,

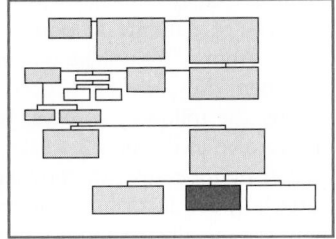

occurs in the immediate postoperative period, or derives from an inflammatory condition (e.g., inflammatory bowel disease, radiation enteritis, or diverticulitis).

Adhesive Partial Small Bowel Obstruction

Adhesive partial small bowel obstruction is treated initially with nasogastric decompression, I.V. rehydration, and analgesia. Parenteral nutrition should be begun if one believes that oral or enteral nutrition will not be adequate within 5 days. Nonoperative therapy leads to resolution of adhesive partial obstruction in as many as 90% of patients.[41] Some studies suggest that the nature of the previous abdominal operation or the type of adhesions present may influence the probability that the obstruction will not respond to medical therapy.[42] Operations associated with a lower likelihood of response to medical therapy include those performed through a midline incision; those involving the aorta, the colon, the rectum, the appendix, or the pelvic adnexa; and those done to relieve previous carcinomatous obstruction. Matted adhesions, which are more common in patients who have undergone midline incisions or colorectal procedures, are less amenable to conservative management than a simple obstructive band is.[42] In the context of this kind of operative history, strong consideration should be given to surgical intervention if the obstruction does not resolve within 24 hours—unless comorbid medical conditions tip the risk-benefit balance in the direction of nonoperative therapy.

There is an ongoing debate regarding how long patients with partial adhesive obstruction should be treated conservatively. After 48 hours of nonoperative management, the risk of complications increases substantially, and the probability that the obstruction will resolve diminishes.[38] Generally, if the obstruction is going to resolve with nonoperative therapy, there will be a fairly prompt response within the first 8 to 12 hours. Therefore, if a patient's condition has deteriorated or has not significantly improved by 12 hours after the operation, exploratory laparotomy is advisable. During this observation period, the patient must be constantly reevaluated, ideally by the same examiner. Analgesics can be safely administered, and repeat abdominal examinations should be performed at 3-hour intervals when the influence of narcotics has waned. Repeat abdominal x-rays should be obtained no later than 6 hours after nasogastric decompression, and the pattern of gas distribution should be compared with that seen on the admission films. A decrease in intestinal gas distal to a point of obstruction coupled with an increase in proximal dilatation suggests that the obstruction is worsening; conversely, a decrease in intestinal distention coupled with the appearance of more gas distally in the colon suggests that the obstruction is being reduced. The degree of abdominal distention, the passage of flatus, and the nature of the nasogastric aspirate should be evaluated periodically. If abdominal distention does not decrease or the gastric aspirate changes from bilious to feculent, the patient should be operated on.

Experimental and clinical studies suggest that patients undergoing nonoperative treatment for bowel obstruction may benefit from the administration of somatostatin analogues as a result of the potent effects these substances exert on intestinal sodium, chloride, and water absorption.[43] In one study, animals with either complete or closed-loop partial small bowel obstruction were given either long-acting somatostatin or saline; the treatment group had significantly less intestinal distention, less infarction, and longer survival than the control group.[43,44] In a prospective, randomized clinical trial evaluating the use of somatostatin in patients who had complete small bowel obstruction without clinical or radiologic evidence of strangulation, the treatment group was less likely to need operation, had less proximal intestinal distention, and exhibited decreased mucosal necrosis proximal to the point of obstruction.[45] In other trials, long-acting somatostatin analogues and other nonsecretagogues significantly decreased the amount of gastric contents aspirated and alleviated the symptoms of intestinal obstruction in terminally ill patients with nonoperable malignant disease.[28,29,33-35]

It should be possible to determine with a high degree of accuracy and safety which patients will require operation for adhesive small bowel obstruction within 24 hours of admission to the hospital. As a rule, patients with closed loop or complete bowel obstruction, who require immediate or urgent operation, can be readily identified by means of abdominal CT scanning.[11-13] For the remaining patients, who have some degree of partial obstruction, it is possible to make highly accurate predictions regarding whether conservative management will succeed or fail by recording the arrival of contrast material (either a water-soluble agent or a mixed barium preparation) in the right colon within a defined period of time.[13,26,46,47] One prospective study evaluated the arrival of diatrizoate meglumine–diatrizoate sodium in the colon within 24 hours as a predictor of successful nonoperative treatment and found this measure to have a sensitivity of 98%, a specificity of 100%, an accuracy of 99%, a positive predictive value of 100%, and a negative predictive value of 96%.[48] Other studies have used shorter arrival times (as early as 4 or 8 hours), with comparable results.[13,47,49]

Several prospective randomized clinical trials have addressed the issue of whether administration of contrast material can itself be therapeutic with respect to resolving adhesive small bowel obstruction. Two such studies examined small bowel follow-through with barium, either alone or mixed with diatrizoate meglumine.[26,27] Both found that the intervals between admission and operation were shorter for patients randomized to the contrast arm than for those in the control group but that contrast examination did not lead to more expeditious resolution of obstruction. Both studies also demonstrated that barium could be administered to patients with small bowel obstruction safely and without complications.

Two prospective, randomized trials investigated the effects of administering water-soluble hyperosmolar contrast agents to patients with small bowel obstruction.[46,50] In one study, administration of diatrizoate meglumine (1,900 mOsm/L) promoted resolution of adhesive partial obstruction and shortened hospital stay but had no effect on whether laparotomy was required.[46] The mean interval between operation and the first stool was 23.3 hours in the control group and 6.2 hours in the trial group ($P < 0.00001$). Ten (21%) of the 48 obstructive episodes in the control group necessitated operation, compared with six (10%) of the 59 in the trial group ($P = 0.12$). The mean hospital stay for patients who responded to conservative treatment was 4.4 days in the control group and 2.2 days in the trial group ($P < 0.00001$). No contrast-related complications were observed. This study demonstrated that oral administration of diatrizoate meglumine was safe in patients with partial adhesive obstruction, facilitated early identification of patients who required operation, and shortened hospital stay. In the second study, administration of a different water-soluble hyperosmolar contrast agent, ioxitalamate meglumine (1,500 mOsm/L), had no therapeutic effect on patients with partial small bowel obstruction.[50] Again, no contrast-related complications were observed. The disparate results of these two clinical trials notwithstanding, the significant treatment effect reported in the first trial and the absence of any deleterious consequences in either one constitute sufficient evidence to support the administration of 100 ml of diatrizoate meglumine to patients with adhesive partial small bowel obstruction.

By accelerating the resolution of partial small bowel obstruction and ileus, administration of water-soluble contrast agents can shorten the expected hospital stay and thereby also reduce the cost of care. Thus, it is reasonable that the first step in managing suspected partial small bowel obstruction from adhesions or postoperative ileus is to administer water-soluble contrast material intragastrically. If bowel function does not return within 24 hours, then the obstruction is less likely to resolve with nonoperative therapy, and early operation, especially when performed laparoscopically, may be the best option for shortening hospital stay. If ileus persists after intragastric administration of the contrast material and mechanical obstruction is excluded, then continued observation is warranted, with close attention paid to factors that may be causing the ileus. Prospective trials will be necessary to assess this potentially cost-effective strategy.

Laparoscopic adhesiolysis Laparoscopic or laparoscopic-assisted lysis of adhesions relieves bowel obstruction in more than 50% of patients and is associated with lower morbidity, earlier return of bowel function, quicker resumption of normal diet, and a shorter hospital stay than open operative lysis of adhesions.[51-54] A 2000 study found that despite a reduction in median length of stay (from 8 days to 3), patients treated laparoscopically were at increased risk for early unplanned reoperation.[54] Nevertheless, the preponderance of the published experience with laparoscopic adhesiolysis in patients with small bowel obstruction suggests that a minimal-access approach should be employed before laparotomy. If such an approach fails to identify and relieve an obvious point of obstruction or if adhesiolysis is inadequate or unsafe, conversion to an open approach is indicated.

Early Postoperative Obstruction

Early postoperative mechanical small bowel obstruction is often difficult to diagnose because it gives rise to many of the same signs and symptoms as postoperative ileus: obstipation, distention, nausea, vomiting, abdominal pain, and altered bowel sounds. In most cases, there are roentgenographic signs indicative of small bowel obstruction rather than ileus; however, in some cases, abdominal x-rays fail to diagnose the obstruction.[55] Traditionally, when plain radiographs are equivocal, an upper GI barium study with follow-through views is the next test performed to distinguish ileus from partial or complete small bowel obstruction[56]; however, such studies may yield the wrong diagnosis in as many as 30% of cases.[22,55,57] A number of authorities believe that abdominal ultrasonography is excellent at distinguishing postoperative ileus from mechanical obstruction and recommend that it be done before any contrast study.[19]

Early postoperative obstruction is caused by adhesions in about 90% of patients.[55,58] When there are no signs of toxicity and no acute abdominal signs, such obstruction can usually be managed safely with nasogastric decompression.[55,57,58] As many as 75% of patients respond to nasogastric suction within 2 weeks. About 70% of the patients who respond to nonoperative treatment do so within 1 week, and an additional 25% respond during the following 7 days. If postoperative obstruction does not resolve in the first 2 weeks, it is unlikely to do so with continued nonoperative therapy, and reoperation is probably indicated[55,58]; about 25% of patients whose postoperative obstruction was initially treated nonoperatively eventually require reoperation. An exception to this guideline arises in patients known to have severe dense adhesions (sometimes referred to as obliterative peritonitis) in response to multiple sequential laparotomies. These patients may have a combination of mechanical obstruction and diffuse small bowel and colonic ileus. The risk of closed-loop obstruction, volvulus, or strangulation in this group of patients is low. Repeat laparotomies and attempts to lyse adhesions may lead to complications, the development of enterocutaneous fistulae, or exacerbation of the adhesions. Often, the best approach to managing these patients is observation for prolonged periods (i.e., months). Total parenteral nutrition (TPN) is indicated in these patients. The addition of octreotide to the TPN solution may be helpful.

Because the risk of intestinal strangulation in patients with postoperative adhesive obstruction is extremely low (< 1%),[55,59] one can generally treat these patients nonoperatively for longer periods. In fact, the conservative approach is often the wise one: reoperation may do more harm than good (e.g., by causing enterotomies and inducing denser adhesions). The traditional indications for operation in patients with early postoperative obstruction include (1) deteriorating clinical status, (2) worsening obstructive symptoms, and (3) failure to respond to nonoperative management within 2 weeks. With the rising cost of hospitalization, it might in fact be more cost-effective to reoperate on patients who have persistent obstruction after 7 days. This speculation would have to be tested by a well-organized cost-benefit study conducted in a prospective fashion.

Long intestinal tubes have no beneficial role in the management of postoperative bowel obstruction; in fact, some authorities have reported that the use of such tubes increases morbidity.[24,38,39] One prospective randomized clinical trial compared the utility of long intestinal tubes with that of nasogastric tubes for the resolution of small bowel obstruction.[60] There were no differences between the two groups with respect to the percentage of patients who were able to avoid operation, the incidence of complications, the time between admission and operation, or the duration of postoperative ileus.

Inflammatory Conditions

Partial bowel obstruction secondary to inflammatory bowel disease, radiation enteritis, or diverticulitis usually resolves with nonoperative therapy. Bowel obstruction accompanying an acute exacerbation of Crohn disease usually resolves with nasogastric suction, I.V. antibiotics, and anti-inflammatory agents. If, however, CT scanning detects intra-abdominal abscess, there is evidence of a chronic stricture, or the patient exhibits persistent obstructive symptoms, operation may be necessary. Similarly, bowel obstruction arising from acute enteritis caused by radiation exposure or chemotherapy usually resolves with supportive care. Chronic radiation-induced strictures are problematic; astute clinical judgment must be exercised to determine when operative treatment is the best option.

Patients with acute diverticulitis typically present with a history of altered bowel movements, fever, leukocytosis, localized pain, tenderness, and guarding in the left lower quadrant of the abdomen. Approximately 20% of patients with colonic diverticulitis also present with signs and symptoms of partial colonic obstruction. A CT scan should be obtained early in all patients with diverticulitis to ascertain whether there is a pericolic abscess that could be drained percutaneously.[61] Partial colonic obstruction in these patients usually resolves with antibiotic therapy, an NPO regimen, and nasogastric decompression. If obstructive symptoms persist for more than 7 days or if obstructive symptoms from a documented stricture recur, operation is indicated.

ELECTIVE OPERATION

Nontoxic, Nontender Sigmoid Volvulus

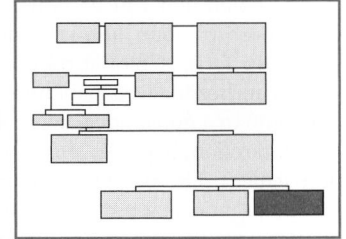

Patients with nontoxic, nontender sigmoid volvulus whose bowel obstruction is initially treated successfully with sigmoidoscopic decompression are at risk for recurrent colonic obstruction. Accordingly, these patients should undergo elective sigmoid resection after complete bowel preparation.

Recurrent Adhesive or Stricture-Related Partial Small Bowel Obstruction

Many patients whose adhesive bowel obstruction resolves experience no further obstructive episodes. If a patient does present with recurrent obstruction from presumed adhesions, either a contrast examination of the bowel or CT scanning is indicated to determine whether there is a surgically correctable point of stenosis. A strong argument can be made that non–high-risk patients should undergo elective operation after presenting with their second episode of mechanical obstruction. Similarly, patients with recurrent obstruction from strictures of any sort should undergo elective operation, given that these lesions are unlikely to resolve.

Partial Colonic Obstruction

The most common causes of partial colonic obstruction are colon cancer, strictures, and diverticulitis. Cancer and strictures usually must be managed surgically because they generally go on to cause obstruction later. Strictures from ischemia or endometriosis usually call for elective colonic resection. Inflammatory strictures from diverticulitis may resolve; however, if obstructive symptoms persist or if barium enema examination continues to yield evidence of colonic narrowing, elective resection is warranted.

When abdominal x-rays suggest distal colonic obstruction, digital examination and rigid sigmoidoscopy are performed to exclude fecal impaction, tumors, strictures, and sigmoid volvulus. If obstruction is proximal to the sigmoidoscope, barium contrast examination is indicated. If barium examination does not demonstrate mechanical obstruction, a presumptive diagnosis of colonic pseudo-obstruction is made.

The morbidity and mortality associated with elective colorectal procedures are significantly lower than those associated with emergency colonic surgery. Furthermore, immediate operation for left-side colonic obstruction almost always necessitates the creation of a diverting colostomy. If a colostomy takedown subsequently proves necessary, the overall cost of caring for the patient will be significantly higher than it would have been had a single-stage procedure been performed. For these reasons, one

should initially treat patients with partial colonic obstruction with nasogastric suction, enemas, and I.V. rehydration in the hope that the obstruction will resolve and that the patient thus can undergo mechanical and antibiotic bowel preparation and a single-stage procedure comprising resection and primary anastomosis. Patients who do not respond to nonoperative measures within 24 hours should undergo operation within 12 hours with the aim of preventing perforation.

In patients with partially obstructing rectal or distal sigmoid tumors or strictures that can be traversed with a radiologic guide wire, balloon dilatation can be performed and a self-expanding stent deployed.[32,62-65] Clinical improvement and resolution of obstruction occur in more than 90% of patients within 96 hours.[32,64] With restoration of the bowel lumen, patients can be prepared for elective surgery, can be spared the creation of a diverting colostomy, and can avoid the extra expense and morbidity associated with the performance of two operations.[64,65] This approach is also highly successful as primary therapy for bowel obstruction in patients who are not surgical candidates.[32] In patients with large, fixed rectal masses, one should obtain CT scans of the pelvis to assess the extent of the tumor. Transrectal laser fulguration and endoluminal stenting are palliative options for restoring bowel lumen patency that may be considered for patients with nonresectable recurrent rectal cancer or radiation strictures in whom operative risk is prohibitively high.

Bowel Obstruction without Previous Abdominal Operation

When partial small bowel obstruction develops and resolves in a patient who has not previously undergone an abdominal operation, one should perform a diagnostic workup to identify the cause of the obstruction; there may be an underlying condition that is likely to cause recurrent obstruction (e.g., an internal hernia, a tumor, malrotation, or metastatic cancer). The first diagnostic test to be ordered should be a CT scan, followed by an upper GI barium study with follow-through views and a barium enema.[66] If a pathologic lesion is identified, elective operation is indicated. An argument can be made that no additional diagnostic tests should be performed in these patients and that diagnostic laparoscopy should be performed instead to enable laparoscopic surgery in case a cause of obstruction is identified that can be treated with a minimally invasive procedure. If no cause of obstruction is found at laparoscopy, open laparotomy is performed.

Nonmechanical Obstruction

ILEUS

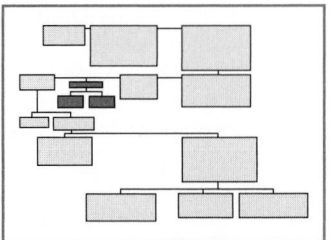

Ileus, or intestinal paralysis, is most common after abdominal operations but can also occur in response to any acute medical condition or metabolic derangement [see Table 1]. The pathophysiologic mechanisms that cause ileus are incompletely understood but appear to involve disruption of normal neurohumoral responses.[67] Ileus may be classified into two broad categories: postoperative ileus and ileus without antecedent abdominal operation. Postoperative ileus is manifested by atony of the stomach, the small intestine, and the colon and usually resolves spontaneously within a few days as normal bowel motility returns. Typically, the small bowel regains its motility within 24 hours of operation, followed 3 to 4 days later by the stomach and the colon. Initial therapy of ileus is directed at identifying and correcting the presumed cause [*see Figure 12*]. If the patient experiences abdominal distention, abdominal pain, nausea, or vomiting, then nasogastric decompression, placement of a Foley catheter, and I.V. rehydration are indicated. In postoperative patients, it is best not to use strong narcotics for analgesia and instead to rely on epidural anesthesia and non-steroidal anti-inflammatory drugs. When ileus develops in patients who have not recently undergone an operation, a thorough history, a careful physical examination, and well-chosen laboratory tests are necessary to identify the possible causes.

When ileus persists for what is, in one's best clinical judgment, an inordinate length of time for the operation performed (typically, longer than 3 to 4 days), the possibility of partial mechanical obstruction, possibly associated with an intra-abdominal abscess or another source of infection, must be considered. If an abscess is suspected, an abdominal CT scan should be obtained. Abdominal ultrasonography has been reported to distinguish postoperative ileus from mechanical obstruction reliably.[19] A small bowel contrast examination with barium identifies partial mechanical small bowel obstruction in about 75% of patients.[22,24] CT scanning distinguishes ileus from obstruction in about 80% of patients.

Intragastric administration of a water-soluble contrast agent has recently shown great potential in the treatment of ileus.[68,69] In one study, administration of 120 ml of diatrizoate meglumine or diatrizoate sodium via nasogastric tube to 40 adults with postoperative small bowel ileus led to restored intestinal motility within 6 hours in all 40, allowing them to resume oral alimentation within 24 hours.[68] Given these results, a prospective, randomized trial that addresses cost-management end points is warranted.

PSEUDO-OBSTRUCTION

Pseudo-obstruction [*see Figure 13*] can exist in the small bowel or the colon and can be either acute or chronic. Acute colonic pseudo-obstruction, also known as Ogilvie syndrome, is the most common form. Colonic pseudo-obstruction occurs most commonly in hospitalized patients in the postoperative period or in response to a nonsurgical acute illness (e.g., pneumonia, myocardial infarction, hypoxia, shock, intestinal ischemia, or electrolyte imbalance). The pathophysiologic mechanisms underlying idiopathic pseudo-obstruction appear to be related to an imbalance in the parasympathetic and sympathetic influences on colonic motility. The presenting symptoms of acute colonic pseudo-obstruction are massive dilatation of the colon (with the cecum more dilated than the distal colon), crampy pain, nausea, and

Figure 12 **Shown is an algorithm outlining an approach to management of ileus.**

Figure 13 **Shown is an algorithm outlining an approach to management of pseudo-obstruction.**

vomiting.[70] If peritoneal irritation or systemic toxicity is present, immediate laparotomy is indicated; if not, treatment involves nasogastric decompression, placement of a rectal tube, tap-water enemas, correction of any underlying metabolic disturbances, and avoidance of narcotic and anticholinergic medications. With conservative management, acute colonic pseudo-obstruction resolves within 4 days in more than 80% of cases.[71] Colonoscopy was previously the method of choice for decompression in this setting.[72] More recently, however, it has been shown that I.V. administration of neostigmine, 2.5 mg over 2 to 3 minutes, leads to prompt resolution of acute colonic pseudo-obstruction within

minutes in nearly all cases.[73,74] Now that this previously difficult and potentially lethal problem can readily be treated pharmacologically, one should reserve colonoscopic decompression and surgical intervention for cases in which pharmacologic measures fail.

Chronic intestinal pseudo-obstruction is a rare acquired disorder that is caused by various diseases involving gastrointestinal smooth muscle, the enteric nervous system, or the extrinsic autonomic nerve supply to the gut.[75] These disorders are treated with an NPO regimen, home TPN, and octreotide. Patients with chronic intestinal pseudo-obstruction should be followed closely for long periods and should undergo repeat contrast studies: there are times when a condition will develop that can cause mechanical obstruction and that may be surgically correctable.[76,77]

Cost Considerations

Cost considerations are exerting an ever-growing influence on surgical care in general and on the decision whether to operate in particular. A large percentage of the high total cost of caring for patients with ileus or mechanical intestinal obstruction is accounted for by the cost of hospitalization or need for laparotomy.

Strategies for reducing the overall cost of managing patients with bowel obstruction may take several forms: the development of diagnostic and therapeutic methods that lead to more rapid diagnosis and resolution of ileus and partial small bowel obstruction; the development of techniques for rapid identification of patients with complete or closed-loop obstruction and early reversible strangulation, which would permit earlier operative intervention and thereby reduce the incidence of complications; the development of therapeutic approaches that prevent postoperative ileus; and the development of methods for preventing intra-abdominal adhesions, which would significantly reduce the overall incidence of bowel obstruction.

From a management viewpoint, if a specific diagnostic test, medication, or approach (e.g., laparoscopy) costs less than a day of hospitalization does, it immediately becomes cost-effective if it reduces complications and shortens length of stay by 1 day. Intragastric administration of a water-soluble contrast agent to relieve small bowel ileus or partial adhesive obstruction is an example of an innovative, cost-effective therapeutic strategy. Diagnostic laparoscopy, abdominal ultrasonography, and CT scanning have all been successfully used to make earlier definitive management decisions and to prevent gangrenous obstruction. Laparoscopic adhesiolysis also leads to earlier hospital discharge. On the basis of the collective experience reported in a substantial number of studies (see above), a logical proposal for cost-effective management of patients with bowel obstruction would be to perform ultrasonography or abdominal CT scanning immediately after initial resuscitation, then to perform laparoscopic surgery on those patients in whom the contrast agent does not arrive in the right colon within 24 hours. However, prospective, randomized clinical trials are needed to evaluate the cost-effectiveness of this and other newer management strategies.

References

1. Irvin T: Abdominal pain: a surgical audit of 1190 emergency admissions. Br J Surg 76:1121, 1989

2. Eskelinen M, Ikonen J, Lipponen P: Contributions of history-taking, physical examination, and computer assistance to diagnosis of acute small-bowel obstruction: a prospective study of 1333 patients with acute abdominal pain. Scand J Gastroenterol 29:715, 1994

3. Reisner R, Cohen J: Gallstone ileus: a review of 1001 reported cases. Am Surg 60:441, 1994

4. Sarr M, Bulkley G, Zuidema G: Preoperative recognition of intestinal strangulation obstruction: prospective evaluation of diagnostic capability. Am J Surg 145:176, 1983

5. Burrell H, Baker D, Wardrop P, et al: Significant plain film findings in sigmoid volvulus. Clin Radiol 49:317, 1994

6. Fatarr S, Schulman A: Small bowel obstruction masking synchronous large bowel obstruction: a need for emergency barium enema. AJR Am J Roentgenol 140:1159, 1983

7. Lim J, Ko Y, Lee D, et al: Determining the site and causes of colonic obstruction with sonography. AJR Am J Roentgenol 163:113, 1994

8. Gough I: Strangulating adhesive small bowel obstruction with normal radiographs. Br J Surg 65:431, 1978

9. Ko Y, Lim J, Le D, et al: Small bowel obstruction: sonographic evaluation. Radiology 188:649, 1993

10. Balthazar E: For suspected small-bowel obstruction and an equivocal plain film, should we perform CT or a small-bowel series? AJR Am J Roentgenol 163:1260, 1994

11. Daneshmand S, Hedley C, Stain S: The utility and reliability of computed tomography scan in the diagnosis of small bowel obstruction. Am Surg 65:922, 1999

12. Donckier V, Closset J, Van Gansbeke D, et al: Contribution of computed tomography to decision making in the management of adhesive small bowel obstruction. Br J Surg 85:1071, 1998

13. Peck J, Milleson T, Phelan J: The role of computed tomography with contrast and small bowel follow-through in management of small bowel obstruction. Am J Surg 177:375, 1999

14. Zalcman M, Sy M, Donckier V, et al: Helical CT signs in the diagnosis of intestinal ischemia in small-bowel obstruction. AJR Am J Roentgenol 175:1601, 2000

15. Ha H: CT in the early detection of strangulation in intestinal obstruction. Semin Ultrasound CT MRI 16:141, 1995

16. Ogata M, Mateer J, Condon R: Prospective evaluation of abdominal sonography for the diagnosis of bowel obstruction. Ann Surg 223:237, 1996

17. Grunshaw N, Renwick IG, Scarisbrick G, et al: Prospective evaluation of ultrasound in distal ileal and colonic obstruction. Clin Radiol 55:356, 2000

18. Meiser G, Meissner K: Intermittent incomplete intestinal obstruction: a frequently mistaken identity. Ultrasonographic diagnosis and management. Surg Endosc 3:46, 1989

19. Meiser G, Meissner K: Ileus and intestinal obstruction—ultrasonographic findings as a guideline to therapy. Hepatogastroenterology 34:194, 1987

20. Megibow A: Bowel obstruction: evaluation with CT. Radiol Clin North Am 32:861, 1994

21. Balthazar E: CT of small-bowel obstruction. AJR Am J Roentgenol 162:255, 1994

22. Dunn JT, Halls JM, Berne TV: Roentgenographic contrast studies in acute small-bowel obstruction. Arch Surg 119:1305, 1984

23. Caroline DF, Herlinger H, Laufer I, et al: Small bowel enema in the diagnosis of adhesive obstructions. AJR Am J Roentgenol 142:1133, 1984

24. Brolin R: Partial small bowel obstruction. Surgery 95:145, 1984

25. Maglinte D, Peterson D, Vahey T, et al: Enteroclysis in partial small bowel obstruction. Am J Surg 147:325, 1984

26. Anderson C, Humphry W: Contrast radiography in small bowel obstruction: a prospective randomized trial. Mil Med 162:749, 1997

27. Fevang BT, Jensen D, Fevang J, et al: Upper gastrointestinal contrast study in the management of small bowel obstruction—a prospective randomised study. Eur J Surg 166:39, 2000

28. Muir J, von Gunten C: Antisecretory agents in gastrointestinal obstruction. Clin Geriatr Med 16:327, 2000

29. Mercadante S, Ripamonti C, Casuccio A, et al: Comparison of octreotide and hyoscine butylbromide in controlling gastrointestinal symptoms due to malignant inoperable bowel obstruction. Support Care Cancer 8:188, 2000

30. Ripamonti C, Mercadante S, Groff L, et al: Role of octreotide, scopolamine butylbromide, and hydration in symptom control of patients with inoperable bowel obstruction and nasogastric tubes: a prospective randomized trial. J Pain Symptom Manage 19:23, 2000

31. Matsushita M, Hajiro K, Takukawa H, et al: Plastic prosthesis in the palliation of small bowel stenosis secondary to recurrent gastric cancer: initial cost savings. Gastrointest Endosc 52:571, 2000

32. de Gregorio MA, Mainar A, Tejero E, et al: Acute colorectal obstruction: stent placement for palliative treatment—results of a multicenter study. Radiology 209:117, 1998

33. Khoo D, Hall E, Motson R, et al: Palliation of malignant intestinal obstruction using octreotide. Eur J Cancer 30A:28, 1994

34. Stiefel F, Morant R: Vapreotide, a new somatostatin analogue in the palliative management of obstructive ileus in advanced cancer. Support Care Cancer 1:57, 1993

35. Scheidbach H, Horbach T, Groitl H, et al: Percutaneous endoscopic gastrostomy/jejunostomy (PEG/PEJ) for decompression in the upper gastrointestinal tract. Initial experience with palliative treatment of gastrointestinal obstruction in terminally ill patients with advanced carcinoma. Surg Endosc 13:1103, 1999

36. Silen W, Hein MF, Goldman L: Strangulation obstruction of the small intestine. Arch Surg 85:137, 1962

37. Laws H, Aldrete J: Small bowel obstruction: a review of 465 cases. South Med J 69:733, 1976

38. Sosa J, Gardner B: Management of patients diagnosed as acute intestinal obstruction secondary to adhesions. Am Surg 59:125, 1993

39. Snyder EN, McCranie D: Closed loop obstruction of the small bowel. Am J Surg 111:398, 1966

40. Mangiante E, Croce M, Fabian T, et al: Sigmoid volvulus: a four-decade experience. Am Surg 55:41, 1989

41. Bizer L, Liebling R, Delany H, et al: Small bowel obstruction: the role of non-operative treatment in simple intestinal obstruction and predictive criteria for strangulation obstruction. Surgery 89:407, 1981

42. Miller G, Boman J, Shrier I, et al: Natural history of patients with adhesive small bowel obstruction. Br J Surg 87:1240, 2000

43. Mulvihill S, Pappas T, Fonkalsrud Z, et al: The effect of somatostatin on experimental intestinal obstruction. Ann Surg 207:169, 1988

44. Gittes G, Nelson M, Debas H, et al: Improvement in survival of mice with proximal small bowel obstruction treated with octreotide. Am J Surg 163:231, 1992

45. Bastounis E, Hadjinikolaou L, Ioannou N, et al: Somatostatin as adjuvant therapy in the management of obstructive ileus. Hepatogastroenterology 36:538, 1989

46. Assalia A, Schein M, Kopelman D, et al: Therapeutic effect of oral Gastrografin in adhesive, partial small-bowel obstruction: a prospective randomized trial. Surgery 115:433, 1994

47. Blackmon S, Lucius C, Wilson JP, et al: The use of water-soluble contrast in evaluating clinically equivocal small bowel obstruction. Am Surg 66:238, 2000

48. Chen SC, Chang KJ, Lee PH, et al: Oral urografin in postoperative small bowel obstruction. World J Surg 23:1051, 1999

49. Chen SC, Lin FY, Lee PH, et al: Water-soluble contrast study predicts the need for early surgery in adhesive small bowel obstruction. Br J Surg 85:1692, 1998

50. Feigin E, Seror D, Szold A, et al: Water-soluble contrast material has no therapeutic effect on postoperative small-bowel obstruction: results of a prospective, randomized clinical trial. Am J Surg 171:227, 1996

51. Leon EL, Metzger A, Tsiotos GG, et al: Laparoscopic management of small bowel obstruction: indications and outcome. J Gastrointest Surg 2:132, 1998

52. Strickland P, Lourie DJ, Suddleson EA, et al: Is laparoscopy safe and effective for treatment of acute small-bowel obstruction? Surg Endosc 13:695, 1999

53. Suter M, Zermatten P, Halkic N, et al: Laparoscopic management of mechanical small bowel obstruction; are there predictors of success or failure? Surg Endosc 14:478, 2000

54. Bailey IS, Rhodes M, O'Rourke N, et al: Laparoscopic management of acute small bowel obstruction. Br J Surg 85:84, 1998

55. Pickleman J, Lee R: The management of patients with suspected early postoperative small bowel obstruction. Ann Surg 212:216, 1989

56. Brolin R: The role of gastrointestinal tube decompression in the treatment of mechanical intestinal obstruction. Am Surg 49:131, 1983

57. Quatromoni J, Rosoff L, Halls J, et al: Early postoperative small bowel obstruction. Ann Surg 191:72, 1980

58. Stewart R, Page C, Brender J, et al: The incidence and risk of early postoperative small bowel obstruction. Am J Surg 154:643, 1987

59. Spears H, Petrelli N, Herrera L, et al: Treatment of small bowel obstruction after colorectal carcinoma. Am J Surg 155:383, 1988

60. Fleshner PR, Siegman MG, Slater GI, et al: A prospective, randomized trial of short versus long tubes in adhesive small-bowel obstruction. Am J Surg 170:366, 1995

61. Hulnick D, Megibow A, Balthazar E, et al: Computed tomography in the evaluation of diverticulitis. Radiology 152:491, 1984

62. Tejero E, Mainar A, Fernández L, et al: New procedure for the treatment of colorectal neoplastic obstructions. Dis Colon Rectum 37:1158, 1994

63. Itabashi M, Hamano K, Kameoka S, et al: Self-expanding stainless steel stent application in rectosigmoid stricture. Dis Colon Rectum 36:508, 1993

64. Binkert C, Ledermann H, Jost R, et al: Acute colonic obstruction: clinical aspects and cost-effectiveness of preoperative and palliative treatment with self-expanding metallic stents—a preliminary report. Radiology 206:199, 1998

65. Mainar A, DeGregorio Ariza MA, Tejero E, et al: Acute colorectal obstruction: treatment with self-expandable metallic stents before scheduled surgery—results of a multicenter study. Radiology 210:65, 1999

66. Stelmach W, Cass A: Small bowel obstructions: the case for investigation for occult large bowel carcinoma. Aust NZ J Surg 59:181, 1989

67. Fromm D: Ileus and obstruction. Surgery: Scientific Principles and Practice. Greenfield LJ, Mulholland MW, Oldham KT, et al, Eds. JB Lippincott Co, Philadelphia, 1993, p 731

68. Watkins D, Robertson C: Water-soluble radiocontrast material in the treatment of the postoperative ileus. Am J Obstet Gynecol 152:450, 1985

69. Zer M, Kanzenelson D, Feigenberg Z, et al: The value of Gastrografin in the differential diagnosis of paralytic ileus and mechanical obstruction. Dis Colon Rectum 20:573, 1977

70. Vanek V, Al-Salti M: Acute pseudo-obstruction of the colon (Ogilvie's syndrome): an analysis of 400 cases. Dis Colon Rectum 29:203, 1986

71. Sloyer A, Panella V, Demas B: Ogilvie's syndrome: successful management with colonoscopy. Dig Dis Sci 33:1391, 1988

72. Nakhgevany KB: Colonoscopic decompression of the colon in patients with Ogilvie's syndrome. Am J Surg 148:317, 1984

73. Hutchinson R, Griffiths C: Acute colonic pseudo-obstruction: a pharmacological approach. Ann R Coll Surg Engl 74:364, 1992

74. Ponec RJ, Saunders MD, Kimmey MB: Neostigmine for the treatment of acute colonic pseudo-obstruction. N Engl J Med 341:137, 1999

75. Faulk D, Anuras S, Christensen J: Chronic intestinal pseudo-obstruction. Gastroenterology 74:922, 1978

76. Schuffler M, Deitch E: Chronic idiopathic intestinal pseudo-obstruction: a surgical approach. Ann Surg 192:752, 1980

77. Knoll RF Jr, Schuffler MD, Helton WS: Small bowel resection for relief of chronic intestinal pseudo-obstruction. Am J Gastroenterol 90:1142, 1995

Acknowledgment

Figures 12 and 13 Marcia Kammerer.

8 UPPER GASTROINTESTINAL BLEEDING

Richard T. Schlinkert, M.D., and Keith A. Kelly, M.D.

Assessment and Management of Upper Gastrointestinal Bleeding

The most common causes of upper gastrointestinal bleeding are chronic duodenal ulcers, chronic gastric ulcers, esophageal varices, gastric varices, Mallory-Weiss tears, acute hemorrhagic gastritis, and gastric neoplasms [*see* Management of Specific Sources of Upper GI Bleeding, *below*]. Less common causes include various other gastrointestinal conditions as well as certain hepatobiliary and pancreatic disorders.

Presentation and Initial Management

INITIAL ASSESSMENT AND MANAGEMENT

Upper gastrointestinal hemorrhage may present as severe bleeding with hematemesis, hematochezia, and hypotension; as gradual bleeding with melena; or as occult bleeding detected by positive tests for blood in the stool. The initial steps in the evaluation of patients with upper GI bleeding are based on the perceived rate of bleeding and the degree of hemodynamic stability. Hemodynamically stable patients who show no evidence of active bleeding or comorbidities and in whom endoscopic findings are favorable may be treated on an outpatient basis, whereas patients who show evidence of serious bleeding should be managed aggressively and hospitalized.

The airway, breathing, and circulation should be rapidly assessed, and the examiner should note whether the patient has a history of or currently exhibits hematemesis, melena, or hematochezia. Blood should be drawn for a complete blood count, blood chemistries (including tests of liver function and renal function), and measurement of the prothrombin time (PT) and the partial thromboplastin time (PTT). Blood should be sent to the blood bank for typing and crossmatching.

If the patient is stable and shows no evidence of recent or active hemorrhage, the surgeon may proceed with the workup.

If, however, the patient is stable but shows evidence of recent or active bleeding, a large-bore intravenous line should be placed before workup is begun; the presence of the line ensures immediate I.V. access should the patient subsequently become unstable.

If the patient is unstable, resuscitation should be begun immediately.

RESUSCITATION

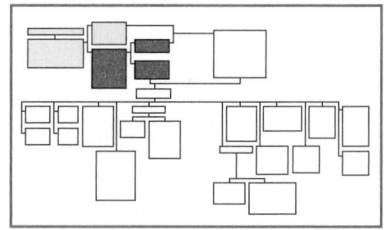

Resuscitation of an unstable patient is begun by establishing a secure airway and ensuring adequate ventilation. Oxygen should be given as necessary, either by mask or by endotracheal tube and ventilator. A large-bore I.V. line should then be placed, through which lactated Ringer solution should be infused at a rate high enough to maintain tissue perfusion. A urinary catheter should be inserted and urine output monitored. Blood should be given as necessary, and any coagulopathies should be corrected if possible. It is all too easy to forget these basic steps in a desire to evaluate and manage massive GI hemorrhage.

If the patient remains unstable and continues to bleed despite supportive measures, he or she should be taken to the operating room for intraoperative diagnosis. The abdomen should be opened through an upper midline incision, and an anterior gastrotomy should be performed. If inspection does not reveal the source of the bleeding or if bleeding is observed beyond the pylorus, a duodenotomy is made, with care taken to preserve the pylorus if possible. Bleeding from the proximal stomach may be difficult to verify, but it should be actively sought if no other bleeding site is identified.

Workup

HISTORY

Only after the initial measures to protect the airway and stabilize the patient have been completed should an attempt be made to establish the cause of the bleeding. The history should focus on known causes of upper GI bleeding (e.g., ulcers, recent trauma or stress, liver disease, varices, alcoholism, and vomiting) and on the possible use of medications that interfere with coagulation (e.g., aspirin, nonsteroidal anti-inflammatory drugs [NSAIDs], and dipyridamole) or alter hemodynamics (e.g., beta blockers and antihypertensive agents). The cardiac history is particularly important for assessing the patient's ability to withstand varying degrees of anemia.

PHYSICAL EXAMINATION

The physical examination is seldom of much help in determining the exact site of bleeding, but it may reveal jaundice, ascites, or other signs of hepatic disease; a tumor mass; or a bruit from an abdominal vascular lesion.

NASOGASTRIC ASPIRATION

The next step is nasogastric aspiration. A bloody aspirate is an indication for esophagogastroduodenoscopy (EGD), as is a clear, nonbilious aspirate if a bleeding site distal to the pylorus has not been excluded. If the aspirate is clear and bile-stained, the source of the bleeding is unlikely to be the stomach, the duodenum, the liver, the biliary tree, or the pancreas. Nonetheless, if subsequent evaluation of the lower GI tract for the source of the bleeding is unrewarding, an upper GI site that had stopped bleeding when the nasogastric tube was passed or that was distal to the ligament of Treitz should still be considered.

UPPER GI ENDOSCOPY (ESOPHAGOGASTRODUODENOSCOPY)

EGD [see V:6 Gastrointestinal Endoscopy] almost always reveals the source of upper GI bleeding; its utility and accuracy have been well documented in the literature. This procedure requires considerable skill: identification of bleeding sites in a blood-filled stomach is far from easy. Hematemesis is an indication for emergent EGD, usually within 1 hour of presentation. If the rate of bleeding is high, saline lavage may be performed to clear the stomach of blood and clots. If the rate of bleeding is moderate or low, as is often the case in patients with melena, urgent EGD is indicated.

EGD is not only an excellent diagnostic tool but also a valuable therapeutic modality. Indeed, most upper GI hemorrhages may be controlled endoscopically, though the degree of success to be expected in individual cases varies according to the expertise of the endoscopist and the specific cause of the bleeding. Therapeutic endoscopic maneuvers include injection, thermal coagulation, and mechanical occlusion of bleeding sites. The choice of therapy depends on the cause, the site, and the rate of bleeding.

OTHER TESTS

If endoscopic examination reveals no lesions in the stomach or the duodenum and bleeding has ceased, enteroclysis (direct introduction of $BaSO_4$ into the small bowel) and roentgenography of the duodenum and the jejunum should be done next. This is probably a more sensitive radiologic test than a standard small bowel roentgenogram. Nonetheless, the absence of a lesion on this test does not rule out the small bowel as the source of the hemorrhage; not uncommonly, the x-ray is negative when a bleeding small bowel lesion is present.

Tagged red cell scans may confirm the presence of an active bleeding site; however, scans are fairly nonspecific with respect to determining the anatomic location of the bleeding. Arteriography may demonstrate that a lesion is present, but it cannot reliably identify a bleeding site unless the bleeding is brisk (> 1 ml/min). Occasionally, arteriography reveals the cause of the bleeding even if the bleeding has stopped.

When a patient has recurrent bleeding that is believed to originate in the small bowel, intraoperative endoscopic exploration may prove useful. Before the small bowel is manipulated, a pediatric colonoscope is introduced either orally or through a distal jejunal enterotomy; the latter method allows easier viewing of the entire small bowel. The mucosal detail is examined as the surgeon guides the scope through the small bowel. The bowel must be handled gently to avoid a mucosal injury, which could mimic a significant lesion.

These tests, in conjunction with EGD, should allow the surgeon to establish the cause of upper GI bleeding at least 90% of the time.

Management of Specific Sources of Upper GI Bleeding

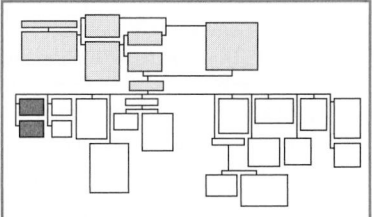

CHRONIC DUODENAL ULCER

The development of effective medical regimens for controlling uncomplicated duodenal ulcers has led to a drastic reduction in the number of elective surgical procedures performed for this purpose. Nevertheless, the incidence of bleeding from duodenal ulcers that is severe enough to necessitate emergency endoscopic or operative intervention has not decreased.

Once EGD has demonstrated that a duodenal ulcer is the source of the bleeding, the first question that must be addressed is whether active bleeding is present. If it is, an attempt should be made to control the hemorrhage endoscopically [see Figure 1]. Because ongoing blood loss eventually leads to coagulopathies, the surgeon must exercise good judgment in deciding how long to pursue endoscopic treatment before concluding that such treatment has failed and that surgical treatment is necessary. In general, substantial bleeding (four to six units or more) that is not easily controlled endoscopically is an indication for immediate surgical intervention. Likewise, ongoing hemorrhage in a hemodynamically unstable patient (especially an elderly one) calls for immediate surgical therapy.

If bleeding is controlled endoscopically, then an H_2 receptor blocker should be given intravenously. In addition, antibiotic therapy directed against Helicobacter pylori (e.g., a 14-day course of metronidazole, 500 mg p.o., t.i.d.; omeprazole, 20 mg p.o., b.i.d.; and clarithromycin, 500 mg p.o., b.i.d.) should be considered if the organism is present; such therapy has been shown to decrease rebleeding rates after antacid medication has been stopped. Food need not be withheld unless the likelihood of rebleeding is high, in which case operation or repeat endoscopy would be necessary. Resumption of oral feeding does not appear to affect rebleeding rates. Early oral intake also allows earlier initiation of therapy with a proton pump inhibitor.

If bleeding continues despite medical and endoscopic therapy, it should be managed surgically. In addition, certain patients whose bleeding was controlled endoscopically—such as those with a visible gastroduodenal artery and a clot in the base of the ulcer, those who experience rebleeding despite medical and endoscopic therapy, and those with giant ulcers—should be strongly considered for surgical therapy.

At operation, an upper midline incision is made. The duodenum is mobilized and an anterior longitudinal duodenotomy performed over the site of the ulcer. The bleeding vessel, which is usually on the posterior wall of the first portion of the duodenum, is ligated with nonabsorbable sutures at sites proximal and distal to the bleeding point. A third stitch is placed posterior to the bleeding vessel. Pains must be taken to avoid injury to the common bile duct during the placement of these sutures. The duodenotomy is then closed.

Assessment and Management of Upper Gastrointestinal Bleeding

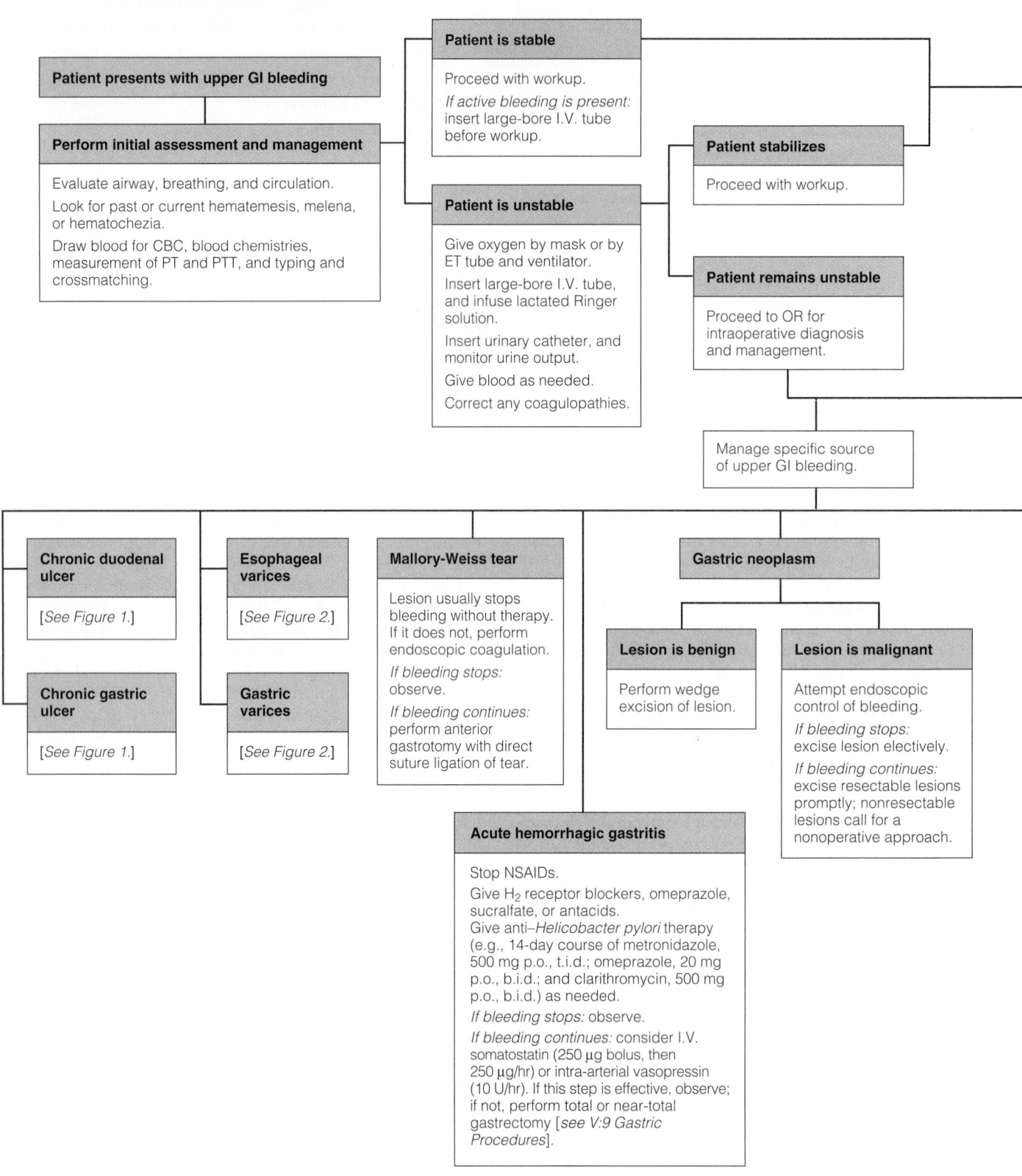

Patient presents with upper GI bleeding

Perform initial assessment and management

Evaluate airway, breathing, and circulation.

Look for past or current hematemesis, melena, or hematochezia.

Draw blood for CBC, blood chemistries, measurement of PT and PTT, and typing and crossmatching.

Patient is stable

Proceed with workup.

If active bleeding is present: insert large-bore I.V. tube before workup.

Patient is unstable

Give oxygen by mask or by ET tube and ventilator.

Insert large-bore I.V. tube, and infuse lactated Ringer solution.

Insert urinary catheter, and monitor urine output.

Give blood as needed.

Correct any coagulopathies.

Patient stabilizes

Proceed with workup.

Patient remains unstable

Proceed to OR for intraoperative diagnosis and management.

Manage specific source of upper GI bleeding.

Chronic duodenal ulcer

[See Figure 1.]

Chronic gastric ulcer

[See Figure 1.]

Esophageal varices

[See Figure 2.]

Gastric varices

[See Figure 2.]

Mallory-Weiss tear

Lesion usually stops bleeding without therapy. If it does not, perform endoscopic coagulation.

If bleeding stops: observe.

If bleeding continues: perform anterior gastrotomy with direct suture ligation of tear.

Gastric neoplasm

Lesion is benign

Perform wedge excision of lesion.

Lesion is malignant

Attempt endoscopic control of bleeding.

If bleeding stops: excise lesion electively.

If bleeding continues: excise resectable lesions promptly; nonresectable lesions call for a nonoperative approach.

Acute hemorrhagic gastritis

Stop NSAIDs.

Give H$_2$ receptor blockers, omeprazole, sucralfate, or antacids.

Give anti–*Helicobacter pylori* therapy (e.g., 14-day course of metronidazole, 500 mg p.o., t.i.d.; omeprazole, 20 mg p.o., b.i.d.; and clarithromycin, 500 mg p.o., b.i.d.) as needed.

If bleeding stops: observe.

If bleeding continues: consider I.V. somatostatin (250 μg bolus, then 250 μg/hr) or intra-arterial vasopressin (10 U/hr). If this step is effective, observe; if not, perform total or near-total gastrectomy [*see V:9 Gastric Procedures*].

Work up patient

Obtain history, focusing on known causes of upper GI bleeding and suspect medications.

Perform physical examination.

Perform NG aspiration.

Perform esophagogastroduodenoscopy [*see V:6 Gastrointestinal Endoscopy*].

Use other tests as appropriate:
- tagged red cell scans
- arteriography
- roentgenography with $BaSO_4$
- intraoperative endoscopic exploration

Dieulafoy lesion

Attempt endoscopic control of bleeding.

If bleeding stops: observe.

If bleeding continues: ligate or excise vessel.

Hemosuccus pancreaticus

Perform distal pancreatectomy [*see V:13 Pancreatic Procedures*], including excision of pseudocyst and ligation of bleeding vessel.

Vascular ectases

Attempt endoscopic control of bleeding.

Consider I.V. somatostatin (250 μg bolus, then 250 μg/hr).

If bleeding stops: observe.

If bleeding continues: resect lesion.

Jejunal ulcer

Manage underlying causes if known (e.g., medications, infections, or gastrinomas).

If bleeding stops: observe.

If bleeding continues: excise bleeding segment of jejunum.

Esophageal hiatal hernia

Hemobilia

Perform arteriographic embolization of affected portion of liver.

Other options are hepatic artery ligation and hepatic resection.

Aortoenteric fistula

Resect aortic graft.

Close enteric site of fistula.

Place extra-anatomic or in situ arterial graft.

Duodenal or jejunal diverticula

Excise lesion, with or without the aid of intraoperative endoscopy.

Paraesophageal hernia

Repair surgically (either via open laparotomy or via minimally invasive approach) [*see V:7 Open Esophageal Procedures and V:8 Minimally Invasive Esophageal Procedures*].

Sliding hernia

Give antacids and, if applicable, anti–*H. pylori* therapy.

If bleeding stops: continue medical therapy.

If bleeding continues: perform Nissen fundoplication [*see V:7 Open Esophageal Procedures and V:8 Minimally Invasive Esophageal Procedures*].

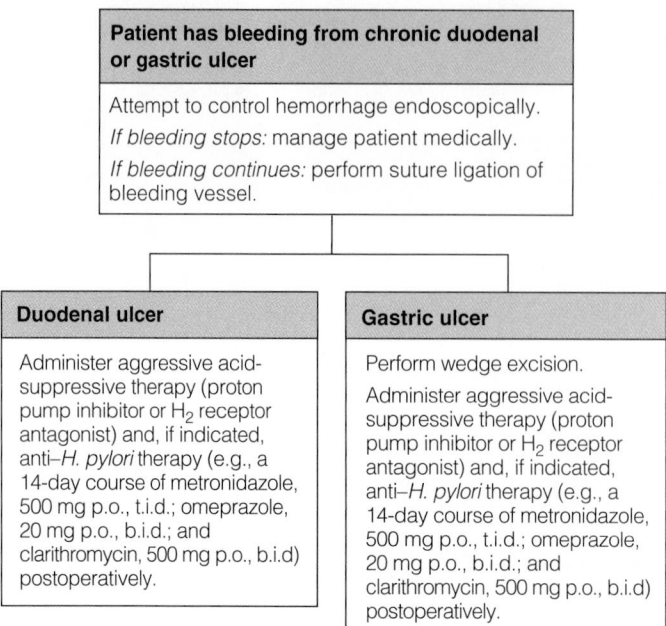

Figure 1 **Shown is an algorithm for management of bleeding from chronic duodenal or gastric ulcers.**

The role of vagotomy in the management of bleeding duodenal ulcers has been called into question. Previously, proximal gastric vagotomy was recommended for stable patients. It was considered preferable to truncal vagotomy because it is less likely to result in gastric atony, alkaline reflux gastritis, dumping, and diarrhea. In unstable patients, truncal vagotomy was typically performed in conjunction with pyloroplasty [*see* V:9 *Gastric Procedures*]. Frozen section to confirm the presence of nerve tissue is helpful for ensuring that the vagotomy is complete.

The recommendation for truncal vagotomy was based on data from studies done before proton pump inhibitor and anti–*H. pylori* therapy came into use. Subsequent studies that evaluated rebleeding rates with current medical regimens, however, demonstrated much lower rebleeding rates. Furthermore, it seems probable that long-term proton pump inhibitor therapy (e.g., omeprazole, 20 mg p.o., q.d.)—the medical equivalent of vagotomy—in conjunction with eradication of *H. pylori* and avoidance of NSAIDs, should decrease rebleeding rates significantly. Therefore, one may consider an alternative treatment approach in patients who had not been receiving ulcer therapy before the bleeding began—namely, ligation of the bleeding vessel, postoperative administration of H_2 receptor blockers, and anti–*H. pylori* therapy. This approach avoids the complications associated with truncal vagotomy.

CHRONIC GASTRIC ULCER

Initially, bleeding from a chronic gastric ulcer is managed in much the same way as that from a chronic duodenal ulcer (i.e., endoscopically) [*see Figure 1*]. To prevent aggravation of the bleeding, early biopsy generally is not recommended; repeat endoscopy and biopsy are done at a later date. Emergent surgical indications for gastric ulcers are the same as those for duodenal ulcers. In addition, if a gastric ulcer does not resolve after 6 weeks of medical therapy, surgical excision is often indicated.

In stable patients, surgical management of a nonhealing chronic gastric ulcer generally consists of a hemigastrectomy that includes the ulcer site; if the ulcer is located more proximally, wedge excision of the ulcer, antrectomy, and gastroduodenostomy or gastrojejunostomy are done [*see* V:9 *Gastric Procedures*]. Excision of the ulcer should be immediately followed by frozen section to rule out cancer. There is no need for a vagotomy in these instances. In unstable patients, hemigastrectomy should probably be avoided because of the increased morbidity and mortality that can follow it. Wedge excision can be combined with either truncal vagotomy and pyloroplasty or aggressive acid suppressive therapy (proton pump inhibitors or H_2 receptor antagonists), followed by anti–*H. pylori* treatment.

ESOPHAGEAL VARICES

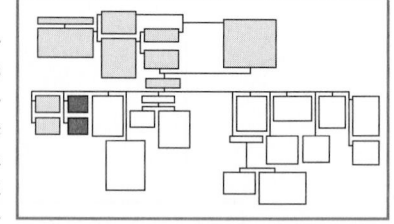

The value of endoscopy in the diagnosis and management of variceal bleeding cannot be overemphasized. Even in patients with known varices, the site of bleeding is frequently nonvariceal; endoscopy is therefore essential. If bleeding varices are identified, rubber banding or intravariceal sclerotherapy with 1.5% sodium tetradecyl sulfate is performed [*see Figure 2*]. If these measures do not control the hemorrhage, balloon tamponade is indicated. Patients who are to undergo this procedure should have an endotracheal tube in place. The tube we prefer to use for balloon tamponade is the four-port Minnesota tube, although the Sengstaken-Blakemore tube is also acceptable. The Minnesota tube has a gastric balloon, an esophageal balloon, and aspiration ports for the esophagus and the stomach. The gastric balloon is inflated first and placed on traction. If the bleeding is not controlled, the esophageal balloon is then

Figure 2 **Shown is an algorithm for management of bleeding from esophageal or gastric varices.**

inflated. The pressure in the balloons should be released in 24 to 48 hours to prevent necrosis of the esophageal or the gastric wall. Successful balloon tamponade is followed by endoscopic variceal injection or variceal banding.

I.V. somatostatin (250 μg bolus, followed by infusion of 250 μg/hr) should be administered in conjunction with the above-mentioned steps. Vasopressin (10 U/hr) may also be given; however, it causes diffuse vasoconstriction, and nitroglycerin is required to alleviate cardiac side effects. Somatostatin has proved superior to placebo in controlling variceal hemorrhage when used in conjunction with endoscopic sclerotherapy. It is as effective as vasopressin while giving rise to fewer side effects. Octreotide shares many of the properties of somatostatin but perhaps not all. Both agents decrease secretion of gastric acid and pepsin; to date, however, the decreased gastric blood flow observed with somato-

statin administration has not been reported with octreotide administration. Nevertheless, some clinicians elect to use octreotide (25 to 50 μg/hr) in place of I.V. somatostatin.

Multiple prospective, randomized trials have shown that propranolol (40 mg b.i.d., p.o.) decreases the incidence of first-time variceal bleeding as well as the incidence of recurrent variceal bleeding. Propranolol should not be used during active bleeding but should be started once bleeding stops.

After the acute variceal bleeding has been controlled, any remaining varices should be subjected to injection sclerotherapy or banding at 2-week intervals until they too are obliterated.

The main indications for surgical intervention in patients with bleeding esophageal varices are uncontrolled hemorrhage and persistent rebleeding despite endoscopic and medical therapy. When surgical intervention is planned, it is essential to determine whether the patient is a transplant candidate. If so, operation should be avoided and bleeding managed by decompressing the portal venous system with a transjugular intrahepatic portosystemic shunt (TIPS). TIPS yields excellent short-term results with respect to stopping bleeding and providing time to locate a liver suitable for transplantation; however, it has not been shown to have the capacity to control hemorrhage by itself over the long term. Thus, its use in patients who are not transplant candidates is questionable.

If the patient is not a transplant candidate and is not actively bleeding, a distal splenorenal shunt is preferable. Arteriograms with views of the portal vein and the left renal vein are obtained. Alternatively, computed tomographic angiography with three-dimensional reconstruction may be performed. If the venous anatomy is suitable—that is, if the diameter of the splenic vein is greater than 0.75 cm (preferably greater than 1.0 cm) and the vein is within one vertebral body of the renal vein on venography—a distal splenorenal shunting procedure should be feasible. If the venous anatomy is not suitable, then esophageal transection, a mesocaval venous graft, or a portacaval shunt is required.

In the emergency setting, we prefer a central portacaval shunt, usually in a side-to-side fashion. Esophageal transection is also a reasonable choice. This procedure is associated with a lower incidence of encephalopathy than a portacaval shunting procedure; however, it is associated with higher rates of rebleeding (particularly late rebleeding), and it can be difficult to perform when active bleeding is present. Suture ligation of the bleeding varices with devascularization (the Segura procedure) should also be considered.

In general, prognosis is related to the underlying liver disease. For example, patients with varices that are secondary to chronic extrahepatic portal venous or splenic venous occlusion generally have a much better prognosis than those whose portal hypertension is secondary to hepatic parenchymal causes. The severity of the cirrhosis also determines short-term and long-term survival and may influence the decision whether to perform a shunting procedure.

Varices in children are generally secondary to portal vein thrombosis. A conservative, nonoperative approach is preferred. If operation is required, either a portacaval shunt, a distal splenorenal shunt, or a devascularization procedure is performed. In children or adults with varices that are secondary to splenic vein thrombosis (sinistral portal hypertension), a splenectomy is usually curative.

GASTRIC VARICES

Gastric varices are managed in much the same way as esophageal varices [see Figure 2], though they are less amenable to sclerotherapy. The surgical options are the same, except that esophageal transection is not a good choice. If bleeding from gastric varices is not controlled by sclerotherapy, suture ligation is indicated.

MALLORY-WEISS TEARS

Mallory-Weiss tears are linear tears at the esophagogastric junction that are usually caused by vomiting. Any patient who presents with vomiting that initially was not

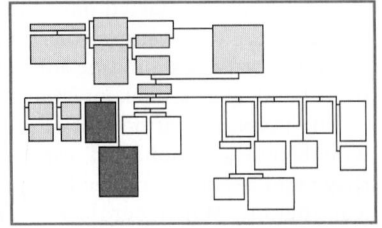

bloody but later turns so should be suspected of having a Mallory-Weiss tear. As a rule, these lesions stop bleeding without therapy. If bleeding is substantial or persistent, however, endoscopic coagulation may be necessary. In rare instances, the tear will have to be oversewn at operation. This is accomplished via an anterior gastrotomy and direct suture ligation of the tear.

ACUTE HEMORRHAGIC GASTRITIS

Bleeding from gastritis is virtually always managed medically with H_2 receptor blockers, omeprazole, sucralfate, or antacids (either alone or in combination), along with antibiotics if H. pylori is present. Somatostatin may be beneficial. Sometimes, administration of vasopressin via the left gastric artery is needed to control bleeding. In rare cases, total or near-total gastrectomy [see V:9 Gastric Procedures] is required; however, the mortality associated with this operation in this setting is high. Stress ulcer prophylaxis in severely ill or traumatized patients is essential to prevent this problem. The gastric pH should be kept as close to neutral as possible. If the gastritis is relatively mild, a biopsy specimen should be obtained and tested for H. pylori. Treatment consists of acid reduction and anti–H. pylori therapy.

NEOPLASMS

Benign tumors of the upper GI tract (e.g., leiomyomas, hamartomas, and hemangiomas) bleed at times. Wedge excision of the offending lesion is the procedure of choice.

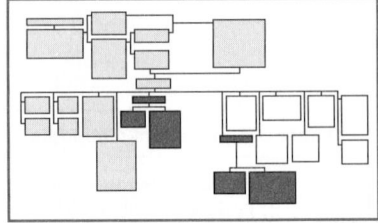

Bleeding from malignant neoplasms, whether early stage or late stage, generally can be controlled initially by endoscopic means; however, rebleeding rates are high. If the lesion is resectable, it should be excised promptly once the patient is stable and any coagulopathies have been corrected. If disease is advanced, however, surgical options are limited, and a nonoperative approach, though necessarily imperfect, is preferable.

ESOPHAGEAL HIATAL HERNIA

Not infrequently, the source of chronic enteric blood loss is an esophageal hiatal hernia. Major bleeding is rare in this condition but may occur as a result of linear erosions at the level of the diaphragm (Cameron lesions), gastritis within the hernia, or torsion of a paraesophageal hernia. Endoscopy is generally diagnostic, though the sources of chronic blood loss are not always obvious. Recognition that the bleeding derives from a Cameron lesion should incline the surgeon toward operative intervention: this lesion is usually mechanically induced and therefore tends to be less responsive to antacid therapy.

Chronic bleeding from a sliding esophageal hiatal hernia should be treated initially with a proton pump inhibitor; anti–H. pylori therapy should be added if biopsy shows this organism to be present. Operation (i.e., laparoscopic Nissen fundoplication [see V:8 Minimally Invasive Esophageal Procedures]) should be considered for fit patients who have complications associated with their hiatal hernia. A para-esophageal hernia should be repaired surgically. This repair may be performed via either a laparoscopic or an open approach; neither has yet been shown to be clearly superior.

DIEULAFOY LESION

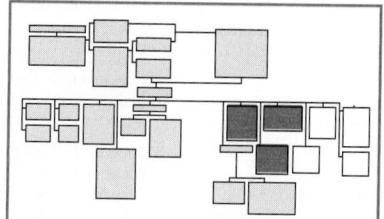

Dieulafoy lesion (also referred to as exulceratio simplex) is the rupturing of a 1 to 3 mm bleeding vessel through the gastric mucosa (usually in the proximal stomach) without surrounding ulceration. This lesion tends to be found high on the lesser curvature, but it can also occur in other locations. Histologic studies have not revealed any intrinsic abnormalities either of the mucosa or of the vessel.

Initial treatment consists of either coagulation of the bleeding vessel with a heater probe or mechanical control with clips or rubber bands; local injection of epinephrine may help control acute hemorrhage while this is being done. In skilled hands, endoscopic therapy has a 95% success rate, and long-term control is excellent. If endoscopic therapy fails, surgical options, including ligation or excision of the vessel involved, come into play. Arteriographic embolization may be employed in patients who are too ill to tolerate surgical intervention.

HEMOBILIA

Hemobilia should be suspected in all patients who present with the classic triad of epigastric and right upper quadrant pain, GI bleeding, and jaundice; however, only about 40% of patients with hemobilia present with the entire triad. Endoscopy demonstrating blood coming from the ampulla of Vater points to a source in the biliary tree or the pancreas (hemosuccus pancreaticus).

Arteriography may provide the definitive diagnosis: a bleeding tumor, a ruptured artery from trauma, or another cause. Arteriographic embolization of the affected portion of the liver is the preferred treatment option; hepatic artery ligation (selective if possible) or hepatic resection may be required.

HEMOSUCCUS PANCREATICUS

Bleeding into the pancreatic duct, generally from erosion of a pancreatic pseudocyst into the splenic artery, is signaled by upper abdominal pain followed by hematochezia. If endoscopy is performed when hematochezia is present, the bleeding site may not be seen; however, if endoscopy is performed when pain is first noted, blood may be seen coming from the ampulla of Vater. The combination of significant GI bleeding, abdominal pain, a history of alcohol abuse or pancreatitis, and hyperamylasemia should suggest the diagnosis. Distal pancreatectomy [see V:13 Pancreatic Procedures], including excision of the pseudocyst and ligation of the splenic artery, is the preferred treatment and generally leads to cure.

AORTOENTERIC FISTULA

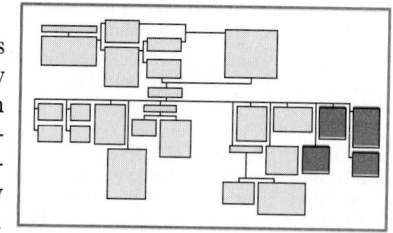

Aortoenteric fistulas may occur spontaneously as a result of rupture of an aortic aneurysm or perforation of a duodenal lesion; more often, they arise after aortic surgery. A common initial manifestation of an aortoenteric fistula is a small herald bleed that is followed a few days later by a massive hemorrhage. Patients often present with the triad of GI hemorrhage, a pulsatile mass, and infection; however, not all of these symptoms are invariably present. A high index of suspicion facilitates diagnosis. Endoscopy may show an aortic graft eroding into the enteric lumen, but this is an uncommon finding. CT scanning is the procedure of choice for diagnosis. The finding of air around the aorta or the aortic graft is diagnostic and is an indication for emergency exploration. The preferred surgical treatment is resection of the graft with extra-abdominal bypass. Some authorities, however, advocate resection of the graft with in situ graft replacement.

VASCULAR ECTASES

Vascular ectases (also referred to as vascular dysplasia, angiodysplasia, angiomata, telangiectasia, and arteriovenous malformations) may bleed briskly. As a rule, gastric lesions are readily identified and the bleeding controlled by endoscopic means. Lesions that continue to bleed, either acutely or chronically, despite endoscopic measures should be excised. Some patients have multiple and extensive lesions that necessitate resection of large portions of the stomach or the small intestine. Pharmacotherapy and hormonal therapy have been tried; the results have been mixed.

DUODENAL AND JEJUNAL DIVERTICULA

Duodenal and jejunal diverticula are rare causes of upper GI bleeding. Accurate identification of a bleeding site within a given diverticulum is difficult, but an attempt should be made to accomplish this by means of peroral enteroscopy. Excision is the preferred treatment. Great care must be taken in the treatment of duodenal diverticula in the region of the ampulla of Vater to ensure that the pancreatic duct and the bile ducts are not injured during excision.

JEJUNAL ULCER

Ulcerations of the jejunum are also rare. They may be secondary to medication, infection, a gastrinoma, or idiopathic causes. Offending medications should be stopped, infections should be treated, and gastrinomas should be excised. If these measures do not control the hemorrhage, the bleeding segment of the jejunum should be excised.

Recommended Reading

PROSPECTIVE, RANDOMIZED,
CONTROLLED TRIALS

Avgerinos A, Nevens F, Raptis S, et al: Early administration of somatostatin and efficacy of sclerotherapy in acute oesophageal variceal bleeds: the European Acute Bleeding Oesophageal Variceal Episodes (ABOVE) randomised trial. Lancet 350:1495, 1997

Cello JP, Grendell JH, Crass RA, et al: Endoscopic sclerotherapy versus portacaval shunt in patients with severe cirrhosis and variceal hemorrhage. N Engl J Med 311:1589, 1984

Clark AW, Westaby D, Silk DBA, et al: Prospective controlled trial of injection sclerotherapy in patients with cirrhosis and recent variceal hemorrhage. Lancet 2:552, 1980

Conn HO, Grace ND, Bosch J, et al: Propranolol in the prevention of the first hemorrhage from esophagogastric varices: a multicenter, randomized clinical trial. Hepatology 13:902, 1991

Garcia-Pagan JC, Feu F, Bosch J, et al: Propranolol compared with propranolol plus isosorbide-5-mononitrate for portal hypertension in cirrhosis: a randomized controlled study. Ann Intern Med 114:869, 1991

Graham DY, Hepps KS, Ramirez FC, et al: Treatment of

Helicobacter pylori reduces the rate of rebleeding in peptic ulcer disease. Scand J Gastroenterol 28:939, 1993

Gregory PB: Prophylactic sclerotherapy for esophageal varices in men with alcoholic liver disease: a randomized, single-blind, multicenter trial. N Engl J Med 324:1779, 1991

Groszmann RJ, Bosch J, Grace ND, et al: Hemodynamic events in a prospective randomized trial of propranolol versus placebo in the prevention of a first variceal hemorrhage. Gastroenterology 99:1401, 1990

Hartigan PM, Gebhard RL, Gregory PB: Sclerotherapy for actively bleeding esophageal varices in male alcoholics with cirrhosis. Gastrointest Endosc 46:1, 1997

Krejs GJ, Little KH, Westergaard H, et al: Laser photocoagulation for the treatment of acute peptic-ulcer bleeding: a randomized controlled clinical trial. N Engl J Med 316:1618, 1987

Laine L: Multipolar electrocoagulation versus injection therapy in the treatment of bleeding peptic ulcers: a prospective, randomized trial. Gastroenterology 99:1303, 1990

Laine L, Cohen H, Brodhead J, et al: Prospective evaluation of immediate versus delayed refeeding and prognostic value of endoscopy in patients with upper gastrointestinal hemorrhage. Gastroenterology 102:314, 1992

Metz CA, Livingston DH, Smith JS, et al: Impact of multiple risk factors and ranitidine prophylaxis on the development of stress-related upper gastrointestinal bleeding: a prospective, multicenter, double-blind, randomized trial. Crit Care Med 21:1844, 1993

Pascal JP, Cales P: Propranolol in the prevention of first upper gastrointestinal tract hemorrhage in patients with cirrhosis of the liver and esophageal varices. N Engl J Med 317:856, 1987

Saeed ZA, Winchester CB, Michaletz PA, et al: A scoring system to predict rebleeding after endoscopic therapy of nonvariceal upper gastrointestinal hemorrhage, with a comparison of heat probe and ethanol injection. Am J Gastroenterol 88:1842, 1993

Vinel JP, Lamouliatte H, Cales P, et al: Propranolol reduces the rebleeding rate during endoscopic sclerotherapy before variceal obliteration. Gastroenterology 102:1760, 1992

Warren WD, Henderson JM, Millikan WJ, et al: Distal splenorenal shunt versus endoscopic sclerotherapy for long-term management of variceal bleeding: preliminary report of a prospective, randomized trial. Ann Surg 203:454, 1986

META-ANALYSES

Cook DJ, Guyatt GH, Salena BJ, et al: Endoscopic therapy for acute nonvariceal upper gastrointestinal hemorrhage: a meta-analysis. Gastroenterology 102:139, 1992

Poynard T, Cales P, Pasta L, et al: Beta-adrenergic-antagonist drugs in the prevention of gastrointestinal bleeding in patients with cirrhosis and esophageal varices. N Engl J Med 324:1532, 1991

Tryba M: Prophylaxis of stress ulcer bleeding: a meta-analysis. J Clin Gastroenterol 13(suppl 2):S44, 1991

PROSPECTIVE STUDIES

Barkun AN, Cockeram AW, Plourde V, et al: Review article: acid suppression in non-variceal acute upper gastrointestinal bleeding. Aliment Pharmacol Ther 13:1565, 1999

Branicki FJ, Coleman SY, Pritchett CJ, et al: Emergency surgical treatment for nonvariceal bleeding of the upper part of the gastrointestinal tract. Surg Gynecol Obstet 172:113, 1991

Cebollero-Santamaria F, Smith J, Gioe S, et al: Selective outpatient management of upper gastrointestinal bleeding in the elderly. Am J Gastroenteral 94:1242, 1999

Gostout CJ, Wang KK, Ahlquist DA, et al: Acute gastrointestinal bleeding: experience of a specialized management team. J Clin Gastroenterol 14:260, 1992

Hunt PS, Fracs MS, Korman MG, et al: An 8-year prospective experience with balloon tamponade in emergency control of bleeding esophageal varices. Dig Dis Sci 27:413, 1982

Loftus EV, Alexander GL, Ahlquist DA, et al: Endoscopic treatment of major bleeding from advanced gastroduodenal malignant lesions. Mayo Clin Proc 69:736, 1994

Rockey DC, Cello JP: Evaluation of the gastrointestinal tract in patients with iron-deficiency anemia. N Engl J Med 329:1691, 1993

Terblanche J, Northoever JMA, Bornman P, et al: A prospective evaluation of injection sclerotherapy in the treatment of acute bleeding from esophageal varices. Surgery 85:239, 1979

Wilcox CM, Alexander LN, Straub RF, et al: A prospective endoscopic evaluation of the causes of upper GI hemorrhage in alcoholics: a focus on alcoholic gastropathy. Am J Gastroenteral 91:1343, 1996

Zuckerman G, Benitez J: A prospective study of bidirectional endoscopy (colonoscopy and upper endoscopy) in the evaluation of patients with occult gastrointestinal bleeding. Am J Gastroenterol 87:62, 1992

RETROSPECTIVE STUDIES

Corley DA, Stefan AM, Wolf M, et al: Early indicators of prognosis in upper gastrointestinal hemorrhage. Am J Gastroenterol 93:336, 1998

Cotton PB, Rosenberg MT, Waldram RPL, et al: Early endoscopy of oesophagus, stomach, and duodenal bulb in patients with haematemesis and melaena. Br Med J 2:505, 1973

Dempsey DT, Burke DR, Reilly RS, et al: Angiography in poor-risk patients with massive nonvariceal upper gastrointestinal bleeding. Am J Surg 159:282, 1990

Fox JG, Hunt PS: Management of acute bleeding gastric malignancy. Aust NZ J Surg 63:462, 1993

Gaisford WD: Endoscopic electrohemostasis of active upper gastrointestinal bleeding. Am J Surg 137:47, 1979

Henriksson AE, Svensson J-O: Upper gastrointestinal bleeding (with special reference to blood transfusion). Eur J Surg 157:193, 1991

Himal HS, Perrault C, Mzabi R: Upper gastrointestinal hemorrhage: aggressive management decreases mortality. Surgery 84:448, 1978

Jacobson AR, Cerqueira MD: Prognostic significance of late imaging results in technetium-99m-labeled red blood cell gastrointestinal bleeding studies with early negative images. J Nucl Med 33:202, 1992

Jim G, Rikkers LF: Cause and management of upper gastrointestinal bleeding after distal splenorenal shunt. Surgery 112:719, 1992

Kaye GL, McCormick A, Siringo S, et al: Bleeding from staple line erosion after esophageal transection: effect of omeprazole. Hepatology 15:1031, 1992

Kollef MH, O'Brien JD, Zuckerman GR, et al: Bleed: a classification tool to predict outcomes in patients with acute upper and lower gastrointestinal hemorrhage. Crit Care Med 25:1125, 1997

Liebler JM, Benner K, Putnam T, et al: Respiratory complications in critically ill medical patients with acute upper gastrointestinal bleeding. Crit Care Med 19:1152, 1991

Lipper B, Simon D, Cerrone F: Pulmonary aspiration during emergency endoscopy in patients with upper gastrointestinal hemorrhage. Crit Care Med 19:330, 1991

Miller AR, Farnell MB, Kelly KA, et al: The impact of therapeutic endoscopy on the treatment of bleeding duodenal ulcers, 1980–90. World J Surg 19:89, 1995

Norton ID, Petersen BT, Sorbi D, et al: Management and long-term prognosis of Dieulafoy lesion. Gastrointest Endosc 50:762, 1999

Sakorafas GH, Sarr MG, Farley DR: Hemosuccus pancreaticus complicating chronic pancreatitis: an obscure cause of upper gastrointestinal bleeding. Langenbeck Arch Surg 385:124, 2000

Sugawa C, Benishek D, Walt AJ: Mallory-Weiss syndrome: a study of 224 patients. Am J Surg 145:30, 1983

Sugawa C, Steffes CP, Nakamura R, et al: Upper gastrointestinal bleeding in an urban hospital: etiology, recurrence, and prognosis. Ann Surg 212:521, 1990

Wilairatana S, Sriussadaporn S, Tanphaiphat C: A review of 1338 patients with acute upper gastrointestinal bleeding at Chulalongkorn University Hospital, Bangkok. Gastroenterologia Japonica 26:58, 1991

Reviews

De Franchis R: Emerging strategies in the management of upper gastrointestinal bleeding. Digestion 60(suppl 3):17, 1999

Groszmann RJ, Grace ND: Complications of portal hypertension: esophagogastric varices and ascites. Gastroenterol Clin North Am 21:103, 1992

Jenkins SA: Drug therapy for non-variceal upper gastrointestinal bleeding. Digestion 60(suppl 3):39, 1999

Kankaria AG, Fleischer DE: The critical care management of nonvariceal upper gastrointestinal bleeding. Crit Care Clin 11:347, 1995

Katz PO, Salas L: Less frequent causes of upper gastrointestinal bleeding. Gastroenterol Clin North Am 22:875, 1993

Montgomery RS, Wilson SE: Surgical management of gastrointestinal fistulas. Surg Clin North Am 76:1148, 1996

Savides TJ, Jensen DM: Therapeutic endoscopy for nonvariceal upper gastrointestinal bleeding. Gastroenterol Clin North Am 29:465, 2000

Weiner FR, Simon DM: Gastric vascular ectases. Gastrointest Endosc Clin North Am 6:681, 1996

Zoller WG, Gross M: Beta-blockers for prophylaxis of bleeding from esophageal varices in cirrhotic portal hypertension: review of the literature. Eur J Med Res 1:407, 1995/96

9 LOWER GASTROINTESTINAL BLEEDING

Michael Rosen, M.D., and Jeffrey L. Ponsky, M.D.

Approach to Lower GI Bleeding

Lower gastrointestinal bleeding is defined as abnormal hemorrhage into the lumen of the bowel from a source distal to the ligament of Treitz. In the majority of cases, lower GI bleeding derives from the colon; however, the small bowel is identified as the source of bleeding in as many as one third of cases,[1,2] and the upper GI tract is identified as the source in as many as 11% of patients presenting with bright red blood per rectum.[3]

Lower GI bleeding is more common in men than in women. The incidence rises steeply with advancing age, exhibiting a greater than 200-fold increase from the third decade of life to the ninth. This increase is largely attributable to the various colonic disorders commonly associated with aging (e.g., diverticulosis and angiodysplasia).[4-6] The exact incidence of lower GI bleeding is not known, because there is no standardized technique for localizing it. Several investigators, however, estimate the incidence to be in the range of 20 to 27 cases per 100,000 adults.[4,7] A 1997 survey of GI bleeding from the American College of Gastroenterology found that lower GI hemorrhage accounted for 24% of all GI bleeding events.[8] Another study published the same year found that 0.7% of 17,941 discharges from a Veterans Affairs Hospital were for patients who had had lower GI bleeding.[9]

The basic components of management are (1) initial hemodynamic stabilization, (2) localization of the bleeding site, and (3) site-specific therapeutic intervention. There are many conditions that can cause lower GI hemorrhage [*see* Discussion, Etiology of Lower GI Bleeding, *below*]; accordingly, successful localization depends on timely and appropriate use of a variety of diagnostic tests. Despite the abundance of diagnostic modalities available, attempts to localize the source of the hemorrhage fail in as many as 8% to 12% of patients.[10,11] Once the bleeding site is localized, the appropriate therapeutic intervention must be carried out as expeditiously as possible.

Lower GI bleeding can be acute and life-threatening, chronic, or even occult. In what follows, we focus on severe, life-threatening hematochezia, reviewing the wide array of possible causes of lower GI bleeding and outlining the diagnostic and therapeutic modalities available for treating this difficult clinical problem.

Initial Evaluation and Resuscitation

Initial evaluation of a patient with lower GI bleeding should include a focused history and physical examination, to be carried out simultaneously with resuscitation. Of particular importance in

taking the history is to ascertain the nature and duration of the bleeding, including stool color and frequency. The patient should also be asked about any associated symptoms of potential significance (e.g., abdominal pain, changes in bowel habits, fever, urgency, tenesmus, or weight loss) as well as about relevant past medical events (e.g., previous GI bleeding episodes, injuries, surgical procedures, peptic ulcer disease, inflammatory bowel disease, and exposure to abdominal or pelvic radiation). Any complicating comorbid conditions (e.g., heart or liver disease and clotting disorders) should be investigated. A comprehensive review of medications—in particular, nonsteroidal anti-inflammatory drugs (NSAIDs) and anticoagulants—is mandatory.[12]

The physical examination should include determination of postural vital signs so that intravascular volume status can be accurately estimated. A drop in the orthostatic blood pressure greater than 10 mm Hg or an increase in the pulse rate greater than 10 beats/min indicates that more than 800 ml of blood (> 15% of the total circulating blood volume) has been lost. Marked tachycardia and tachypnea in association with hypotension and depressed mental status indicates that more than 1,500 ml of blood (> 30% of the total circulating blood volume) has been lost.[13] A complete abdominal examination, including digital rectal examination and anoscopy, should be performed.

Laboratory evaluation should include a complete blood count, measurement of serum electrolyte concentrations, a coagulation profile (prothrombin time and partial thromboplastin time) [*see* I:5 Bleeding and Transfusion], and typing and crossmatching.

A nasogastric tube should be placed for gastric lavage. If lavage yields positive results (i.e., the aspirate contains gross blood or so-called coffee grounds), esophagogastroduodenoscopy (EGD) is indicated [*see* V:6 Gastrointestinal Endoscopy]. An aspirate that contains copious amounts of bile is strongly suggestive of a lower GI source of bleeding, and the workup proceeds accordingly [*see* Diagnostic Testing, *below*]. The choice is less clear-cut with a clear aspirate. In the absence of bile, such an aspirate cannot rule out a duodenal source for the bleeding. Accordingly, there is some degree of latitude for clinical judgment: depending on the overall clinical picture, the surgeon may choose either to perform EGD to rule out a duodenal bleeding source or to proceed with colonoscopy on the assumption that the source of the bleeding is in the lower GI tract.

Resuscitative efforts should begin immediately, with the aim of maintaining the patient in a euvolemic state. Two large-bore peripheral intravenous catheters should be inserted and isotonic I.V. fluid administered. A Foley catheter should be placed to facilitate monitoring of intravascular volume status. Whether

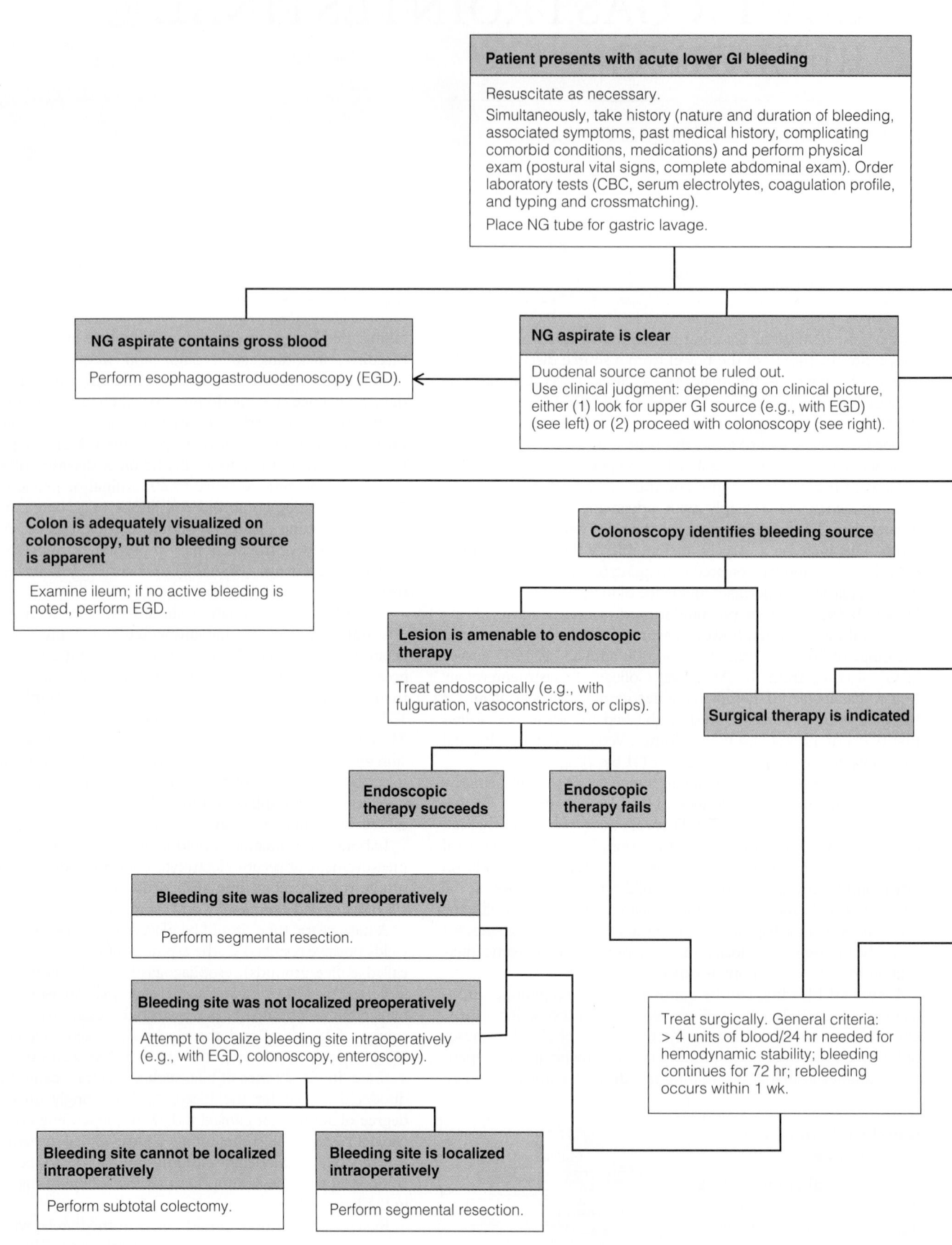

Patient presents with acute lower GI bleeding

Resuscitate as necessary.

Simultaneously, take history (nature and duration of bleeding, associated symptoms, past medical history, complicating comorbid conditions, medications) and perform physical exam (postural vital signs, complete abdominal exam). Order laboratory tests (CBC, serum electrolytes, coagulation profile, and typing and crossmatching).

Place NG tube for gastric lavage.

NG aspirate contains gross blood

Perform esophagogastroduodenoscopy (EGD).

NG aspirate is clear

Duodenal source cannot be ruled out.
Use clinical judgment: depending on clinical picture, either (1) look for upper GI source (e.g., with EGD) (see left) or (2) proceed with colonoscopy (see right).

Colon is adequately visualized on colonoscopy, but no bleeding source is apparent

Examine ileum; if no active bleeding is noted, perform EGD.

Colonoscopy identifies bleeding source

Lesion is amenable to endoscopic therapy

Treat endoscopically (e.g., with fulguration, vasoconstrictors, or clips).

Surgical therapy is indicated

Endoscopic therapy succeeds

Endoscopic therapy fails

Bleeding site was localized preoperatively

Perform segmental resection.

Bleeding site was not localized preoperatively

Attempt to localize bleeding site intraoperatively (e.g., with EGD, colonoscopy, enteroscopy).

Treat surgically. General criteria: > 4 units of blood/24 hr needed for hemodynamic stability; bleeding continues for 72 hr; rebleeding occurs within 1 wk.

Bleeding site cannot be localized intraoperatively

Perform subtotal colectomy.

Bleeding site is localized intraoperatively

Perform segmental resection.

Approach to Lower GI Bleeding

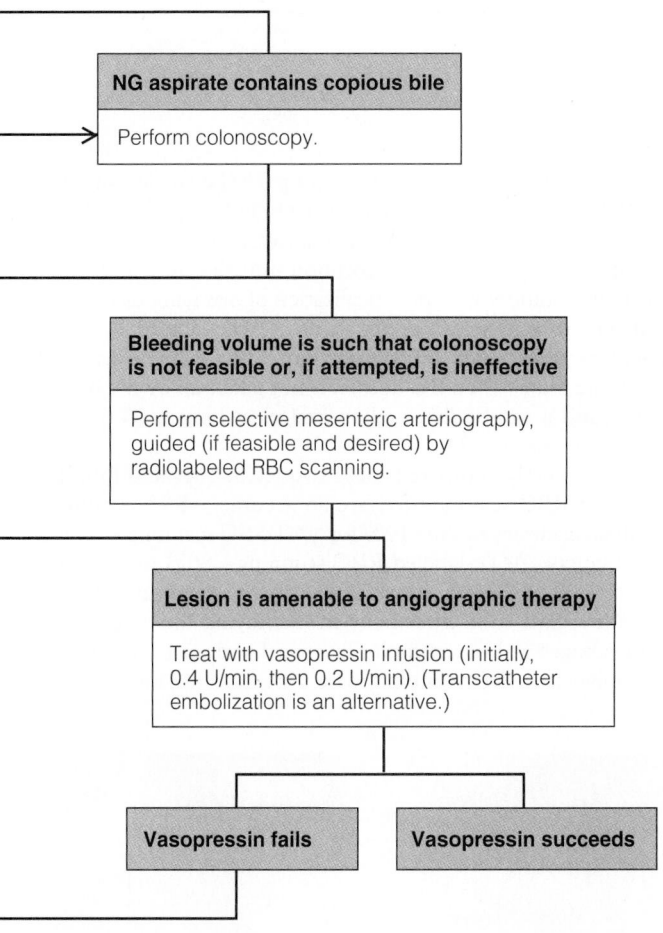

NG aspirate contains copious bile

Perform colonoscopy.

Bleeding volume is such that colonoscopy is not feasible or, if attempted, is ineffective

Perform selective mesenteric arteriography, guided (if feasible and desired) by radiolabeled RBC scanning.

Lesion is amenable to angiographic therapy

Treat with vasopressin infusion (initially, 0.4 U/min, then 0.2 U/min). (Transcatheter embolization is an alternative.)

Vasopressin fails

Vasopressin succeeds

and in what form to administer blood products is determined on an individual basis, with appropriate weight given to the presence or absence of comorbid conditions, the rate of blood loss, and the degree of hemodynamic stability. Severe hemodynamic instability may necessitate monitoring in the intensive care unit.

Diagnostic Testing

A number of diagnostic techniques are available for determining the source of lower GI hemorrhage, the most useful of which are colonoscopy [*see V:6 Gastrointestinal Endoscopy*], radionuclide scanning, and angiography (in the form of selective mesenteric arteriography). The goal of these tests is accurate localization of the site of bleeding so that definitive therapy can be properly directed. Which diagnostic test is chosen for a specific patient depends on several factors, including the hemodynamic stability of the patient, the bleeding rate, the comorbid conditions present, and the local expertise available at the physician's hospital.

COLONOSCOPY

Several large series that evaluated the diagnostic utility of colonoscopy in patients with lower GI bleeding found this modality to be moderately to highly accurate, with overall diagnostic yields ranging from 53% to 97% [*see Table 1*].[3,14-19] Those studies that reported

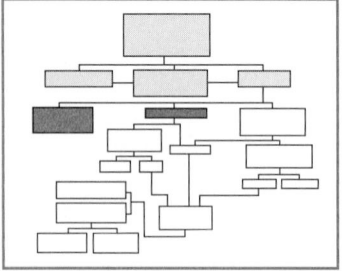

morbidity found colonoscopy to be safe as well, with an average complication rate of 0.5%. Colonoscopy has both a higher diagnostic yield and a lower complication rate than arteriography in this setting and thus would appear to be a more attractive initial test in most circumstances.[3,20] An argument has been made—one with which we agree—that colonoscopy should be considered the procedure of choice for structural evaluation of lower GI bleeding and that arteriography should be reserved for patients with massive, ongoing bleeding in whom endoscopy is not feasible or colonoscopy fails to reveal the source of the hemorrhage.[12]

The merits of colonic purging have been extensively debated in the literature.[3,15,21] Although no firm conclusion has been reached, we feel that adequate colonic purging can improve both the diagnostic yield and the safety of colonoscopy. Given the absence of any definitive data suggesting that colonic purging either reactivates or increases bleeding,[12] it is our practice to administer an oral purge after the patient has been adequately resuscitated.

If the entire colon has been adequately visualized and no source for the bleeding has been identified, the ileum should be intubated; fresh blood in this region suggests a possible small bowel source. If no active bleeding is observed in the ileum, upper GI endoscopy should be performed to rule out an upper GI bleeding site.

RADIOLABELED RED BLOOD
CELL SCANNING

Radionuclide scanning is highly sensitive for lower GI hemorrhage: it is capable of detecting bleeding at rates as slow as 0.1 to 0.4 ml/min.[22] Two imaging tracers, both labeled with technetium-99m (^{99m}Tc), are currently avail-

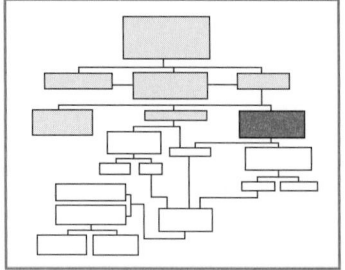

Table 1 Diagnostic Accuracy of Colonoscopy in Localizing Source of Lower GI Hemorrhage

Study	No. of Patients	Diagnostic Yield (%)
Richter[14]	78	70 (90%)
Jensen[3]	80	68 (85%)
Rossini[15]	409	311 (76%)
Geller[16]	524	280 (53%)
Goenka[17]	166	141 (85%)
Ohyama[18]	345	307 (89%)
Chaudhry[19]	85	82 (97%)
Total	1,687	1,259 (75%)

able for radionuclide scanning in this setting: ^{99m}Tc-labeled sulfur colloid (^{99m}Tc-SC) and ^{99m}Tc-labeled red blood cells. ^{99m}Tc-SC requires no preparation time and can be injected immediately into the patient; however, its rapid absorption into the liver and the spleen can often hinder accurate localization of overlying bleeding sites.[9] At our institution, we prefer to use ^{99m}Tc-labeled RBCs. This agent requires some preparation time, but it has a much longer half-life than ^{99m}Tc-SC does, it is not taken up by the liver and spleen, and it can be detected on images as long as 24 to 48 hours after injection [*see Figure 1*].[23,24]

One study directly compared these two techniques and found ^{99m}Tc-labeled RBC scanning to have an accuracy of 93%, compared with an accuracy of only 12% for ^{99m}Tc-SC scanning.[25] The high sensitivity of ^{99m}Tc-labeled RBC scanning—80% to 98%—is well attested, but there is considerable disagreement in the literature with regard to its specificity in identifying the anatomic site of bleeding.[26-31] For example, on one hand, a 1996 study found radiolabeled RBC scanning to be 97% accurate for localiz-

Figure 1 ^{99m}Technetium-labeled RBC scan demonstrates collection of tracer at hepatic flexure.

Figure 2 Angiographic study documents extravasation of contrast into small bowel.

ing bleeding in 37 patients undergoing surgical resection[27]; on the other hand, a 1990 study reported a 42% rate of incorrect resection when surgical therapy was based solely on this modality.[28]

To date, no prospective randomized trials have compared radionuclide scanning with colonoscopy as the initial diagnostic procedure for patients with lower GI hemorrhage. In our view, however, given that radionuclide scanning, unlike colonoscopy and angiography, has no therapeutic intervention capabilities, its best use is in patients with non–life-threatening lower GI bleeding as a prelude and a guide to mesenteric angiography after active hemorrhage has been confirmed.

ANGIOGRAPHY

Selective Mesenteric Arteriography

Selective mesenteric arteriography is somewhat less sensitive than radionuclide scanning for lower GI hemorrhage: bleeding

Figure 3 Intraoperative examination of bowel is aided by injection of methlyene blue dye, which facilitates localization of bleeding site and thereby helps direct surgical resection.

Table 2 Diagnostic Accuracy of Mesenteric Angiography in Localizing Source of Lower GI Hemorrhage

Study	No. of Patients	No. of Positive Angiograms (%)
Pennoyer[35]	131	37 (28%)
Ng[29]	49	22 (45%)
Rantis[36]	30	8 (27%)
Leitman[37]	68	27 (40%)
Casarella[38]	69	46 (67%)
Colacchio[39]	98	40 (41%)
Total	445	180 (40%)

must be occurring at a rate of at least 1.0 to 1.5 ml/min to be detectable with this test.[32] The procedure involves percutaneous placement of a transfemoral arterial catheter for evaluation of the superior mesenteric, inferior mesenteric, and celiac arteries. A positive test result is defined as extravasation of contrast into the lumen of the bowel [*see Figure 2*]. Once the bleeding vessel has been localized angiographically, the area must be marked so that it can be successfully identified intraoperatively; this is commonly accomplished by infusing methylene blue into the bleeding artery [*see Figure 3*].[33,34]

In several large series [*see Table 2*], the overall diagnostic yield of arteriography ranged from 27% to 67%.[29,35-39] The complication rate for arteriography performed for lower GI bleeding ranges from 2% to 4%.[2,39] Reported complications include contrast allergy, renal failure, bleeding from arterial puncture, and embolism from dislodged thrombus.[12]

Unlike radionuclide scanning, arteriography provides several therapeutic options, including vasopressin infusion and embolization of bleeding vessels. Nonetheless, given that arteriography has a lower diagnostic yield and a higher complication rate than colonoscopy does, it is reasonable to attempt colonoscopy first in patients with lower GI hemorrhage and to reserve angiography for patients in whom the volume of bleeding is such that colonoscopy would be neither safe nor accurate.

Provocative Angiography for Continued Obscure Bleeding

In a minority of patients, obscure bleeding persists despite negative findings from endoscopy, mesenteric arteriography, and radiolabeled RBC scanning. This obscure bleeding presents a considerable diagnostic challenge, which some investigators have proposed addressing by means of so-called provocative angiography.[40,41] Provocative angiography involves the use of short-acting anticoagulant agents (unfractionated heparin, vasodilators, thrombolytics, or combinations thereof) in association with angiography. Once the bleeding point has been localized, methylene blue is injected and the patient is immediately brought to the OR for surgical treatment. To date, unfortunately, little has been published on this technique, but it does appear to be a promising approach to this difficult problem.

Therapeutic Intervention

Although in the majority of cases, lower GI bleeding stops spontaneously, in a significant number of cases, hemorrhage continues and necessitates therapeutic intervention. Treatment options include endoscopic therapy, angiographic therapy, and surgical resection.

ENDOSCOPIC THERAPY

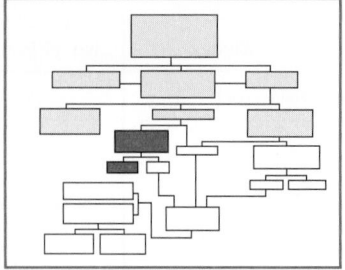

When colonoscopy identifies a bleeding source, endoscopic treatment may be an option [see V:6 Gastrointestinal Endoscopy]. Endoscopic modalities used to treat lower GI bleeding include use of thermal contact probes,[42,43] laser photocoagulation,[44] electrocauterization,[45] injection of vasoconstrictors, application of metallic clips,[46] and injection sclerotherapy.[47] The choice of a specific modality often depends on the nature of the offending lesion and on the expertise and resources available locally. A 1995 survey of members of the American College of Gastroenterology found that endoscopic therapy was used in 27% of patients presenting with lower GI bleeding.[8]

Diverticular hemorrhage can be difficult to treat endoscopically because of the high bleeding rate and the location of the bleeding point within the diverticulum. In 2000, one group of investigators reported their experience with endoscopic therapy for severe hematochezia and diverticulosis in a prospective series of 121 patients.[48] In this series, none of the patients treated endoscopically with epinephrine injections, bipolar coagulation, or both required surgery and none experienced recurrent bleeding episodes. A 2001 study from another group, however, reported high rates of recurrent bleeding episodes in both the early and the late posttreatment periods.[49] In the absence of prospective, randomized trials, it is difficult to draw definitive conclusions about the utility of endoscopic therapy in treating diverticular hemorrhage.

Angiodysplasias resulting in GI hemorrhage typically are amenable to endoscopic treatment. That these lesions are frequently found in the right colon makes perforation a concern; this complication is reported in approximately 2% of patients.[50] Good success rates have been reported with both injection and thermal methods.[51] In one series, endoscopic fulguration was successful in 87% of patients, and no rebleeding episodes occurred over a 1- to 7-year follow-up period.[51] Bleeding from multiple telangiectatic lesions in the distal colon resulting from radiation injury can be treated with thermal contact probes, lasers, or noncontact devices such as the argon plasma coagulator.[52]

Postpolypectomy hemorrhage can often be successfully treated by endoscopic means. Methods used include simple resnaring of the stalk while pressure is maintained[53]; electrocauterization, with or without epinephrine injection; endoscopic band ligation; and placement of metallic clips. For patients whose bleeding is attributable to benign anorectal causes, endoscopic therapy may include epinephrine injection, sclerosant injection, or band ligation of internal hemorrhoids.[54]

ANGIOGRAPHIC THERAPY

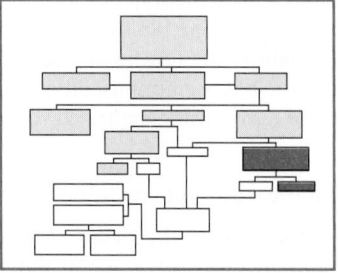

Diagnostic use of angiography in patients with lower GI bleeding can often be followed by angiographic therapy. The two main angiographic treatment options are intra-arterial injection of vasopressin and transcatheter embolization.

Vasopressin acts to control bleeding by causing arteriolar vasoconstriction and bowel wall contraction.[9] Once the bleeding site has been localized angiographically, the catheter is positioned in the main trunk of the vessel. Infusion of vasopressin is initiated at a rate of 0.2 U/min and can be increased to a rate of 0.4 U/min. Within 20 to 30 minutes, another angiogram is performed to determine whether the bleeding has ceased. If the bleeding is under control, the catheter is left in place and vasopressin is continuously infused for 6 to 12 hours. If the bleeding continues to be controlled, infusion is continued for an additional 6 to 12 hours at 50% of the previous rate. Finally, vasopressin infusion is replaced by continuous saline infusion, and if bleeding does not recur, the catheter is removed.[55,56]

The vasoconstrictive action of vasopressin can have deleterious systemic side effects, including myocardial ischemia, peripheral ischemia, hypertension, dysrhythmias, mesenteric thrombosis, intestinal infarction, and death.[9,37] Occasionally, simultaneous I.V. administration of nitroglycerine is necessary to counteract these systemic effects. The reported success rate of vasopressin in controlling lower GI bleeding ranges from 60% to 100%, and the incidence of major complications ranges from 10% to 20%.[57-60] Rebleeding rates as high as 50% have been reported.[59,60]

An alternative for patients with coronary vascular disease, severe peripheral vascular disease, or other comorbidities that prevent safe administration of vasopressin is transcatheter embolization. In this technique, a catheter is superselectively placed into the identified bleeding vessel and an embolizing agent (e.g., a gelatin sponge, a microcoil, polyvinyl alcohol particles, or a balloon) is injected. Several small series found this technique to be 90% to 100% successful at stopping bleeding.[61-64] Equally impressive was the finding that the rebleeding rates in these series were 0%. The complication rates of this procedure are generally reasonable as well; however, intestinal infarction has been reported.[37,65]

SURGICAL THERAPY

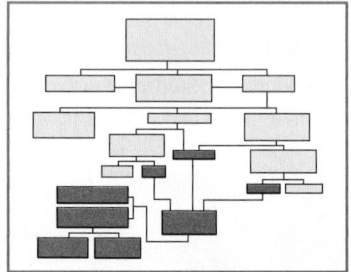

Although there are no absolute criteria for surgery, there are several factors— including hemodynamic status, associated comorbidities, transfusion requirements, and persistent bleeding—that are instrumental in making an appropriate and timely decision whether to operate. In general, patients who require more than 4 units of blood in a 24-hour period to remain hemodynamically stable, whose bleeding has not stopped after 72 hours, or who experience rebleeding within 1 week of an initial episode should undergo surgery.[9]

If the patient's hemodynamic status permits, surgical treatment should be undertaken after accurate localization of the bleeding site. When possible, directed segmental resection is the procedure of choice: it is associated with rebleeding rates ranging from 0% to 14% and mortalities ranging from 0% to 13%.[10,37,66] Blind segmental colectomy should never be performed: it is associated with rebleeding rates as high as 75% and mortalities as high as 50%.[67] If hemodynamic compromise and ongoing hemorrhage make it necessary to perform surgical exploration before the bleeding site can be localized, every effort should be made to identify the source of bleeding intraoperatively before embarking on resection. Intraoperative options for bleeding site localization include colonoscopy (to allow for this option, patients should always be placed in the lithotomy position), EGD, and transoral passage of a pediatric colonoscope for enteroscopy with simultaneous intraperitoneal assistance for small bowel manipulation.[9] If the bleeding site still cannot be accurately localized, subtotal colectomy is the procedure of choice. This procedure is associated with mortalities ranging from 5% to 33%,[68,69] which underscores the importance of accurate preoperative localization of bleeding before surgical intervention.

Discussion

Etiology of Lower GI Bleeding

As noted, lower GI bleeding has a wide array of possible causes [see Table 3].[9,70] Of these, diverticular disease is the most common, accounting for 30% to 40% of all cases.[21,71] Arteriovenous malformations (AVMs), though extensively described in the literature, are considerably less common causes, accounting for 1% to 4% of cases.[72-74] Other significant causative conditions are inflammatory bowel disease (IBD), benign and malignant neoplasms, ischemia, infectious colitis, anorectal disease, coagulopathy, use of NSAIDs, radiation proctitis, AIDS, and small bowel disorders.

DIVERTICULAR DISEASE

The reported prevalence of colonic diverticulosis in Western societies is 37% to 45%.[75] The vast majority of colonic diverticula are actually false diverticula (pseudodiverticula) that contain only serosa and mucosa. They occur at weak points in the colonic wall where the vasa recta penetrate the muscularis to supply the mucosa[9]; as the diverticulum expands, these vessels are displaced. A 1976 anatomical study of colonic specimens from patients with diverticular bleeding used angiography to demonstrate that in all cases, the vasa recta overlying the diverticulum ruptured into the lumen of the diverticulum, not into the peritoneum [see Figure 4].[76]

It has been estimated that approximately 17% of patients with colonic diverticulosis experience bleeding, which may range from minor to severe and life-threatening.[77] As many as 80% to 85% of diverticular hemorrhages stop spontaneously.[78] In one series, surgery was unlikely to be necessary if fewer than 4 units of packed RBCs were transfused in a 24-hour period, whereas 60% of patients receiving more than 4 units of packed RBCs in a 24-hour period required surgical intervention.[79] The risk of a second bleeding episode is approximately 25%.[3] Semielective surgical therapy is usually offered after a second diverticular bleeding episode because once a second such episode has occurred, the risk that a third will follow exceeds 50%.[80] In a series of 83 conservatively managed cases of diverticular disease, the predicted yearly recurrence rates were 9% at 1 year, 10% at 2 years, 19% at 3 years, and 25% at 4 years.[4]

COLITIS

The broad term colitis includes IBD, infectious colitis, radiation colitis, and idiopathic ulcers. IBD, in turn, includes Crohn disease and ulcerative colitis. Patients with IBD usually present with bloody diarrhea that is not life-threatening; however, 6% to 10% of patients with ulcerative colitis have lower GI bleeding severe enough to necessitate emergency surgical resection,[81,82] and 0.6% to 1.3% of patients with Crohn disease have acute life-threatening lower GI bleeding.[81,83] In one review, 50% of patients with intestinal hemorrhage from IBD experienced spontaneous cessation of bleeding.[81] Approximately 35% of patients whose bleeding stops without intervention will have another bleeding episode. Because of this high recurrence rate, semielective surgery is recommended after the first episode of severe GI bleeding secondary to IBD.

Colitis caused by various infectious agents (e.g., *Salmonella typhi*,[84,85] *Escherichia coli* O157:H7,[86] *Clostridium difficile*,[87] and cytomegalovirus[88]) can result in severe lower GI bleeding, but this is a relatively rare occurrence.

Table 3 Common Causes of Lower GI Hemorrhage

Cause of Bleeding	Frequency
Diverticulosis	17%–40%
Arteriovenous malformation	2%–30%
Colitis	9%–21%
Neoplasia (including postpolypectomy bleeding)	7%–33%
Benign anorectal disease	4%–10%
Upper GI source	0%–11%
Small bowel source	2%–9%

Figure 4 **Shown is the appearance of a bleeding diverticulum on colonoscopy.**

Increasing use of radiation therapy to treat pelvic malignancies has led to a corresponding increase in the incidence of chronic radiation proctitis.[89] Radiation therapy damages bowel mucosa, resulting in the formation of vascular telangiectases that are prone to bleeding.[90] From 1% to 5% of cases of acute lower GI bleeding from radiation-induced proctocolitis are severe enough to necessitate hospitalization.[4,15] In a survey of patients with prostate cancer who underwent pelvic irradiation, 5% of the subjects reported hematochezia daily.[91] Initial therapy for clinically significant hematochezia related to radiation proctitis should include some form of endoscopic treatment (e.g., argon beam coagulation). Surgery should be reserved for unstoppable hemorrhage or other major complications, such as fistulas and strictures.[89]

NEOPLASIA

Significant GI bleeding from colorectal neoplasia accounts for 7% to 33% of cases of severe lower GI hemorrhage.[3,15,21,37,92] Such bleeding is believed to result from erosions on the luminal surface.[93] One report identified ulcerated cancers as the cause in 21% of cases of hematochezia.[15] Adenomatous polyps are implicated in 5% to 11% of cases of acute lower GI bleeding.[7,8,15,94,95] Lower GI hemorrhage, either immediate or delayed, is the most common reported complication after endoscopic polypectomy, occurring in 0.2% to 6% of cases.[3,4,96,97] Immediate postpolypectomy bleeding is believed to result from incomplete coagulation of the stalk before transection.[53] Delayed bleeding has been reported as long as 15 days after polypectomy and is thought to be secondary to sloughing of the coagulum; it is less common than immediate bleeding, occurring in only 0.3% of cases.[15,53]

COAGULOPATHY

Lower GI bleeding can be a presenting symptom both for patients with iatrogenic coagulopathy from heparin or warfarin therapy and for patients with a hematologic coagulopathy from thrombocytopenia. It is unclear, however, whether severe coagulopathy leads to spontaneous hemorrhage or whether it predisposes to bleeding from an existing lesion.[98,99] In an early series of leukemic patients with thrombocytopenia and severe GI hemorrhage, 50% of bleeding patients had platelet counts lower than 20,000/mm^3 without any identifiable mucosal lesions; furthermore, when the platelet count rose above 20,000/mm^3, the incidence of bleeding decreased to 0.8%.[98] The investigator concluded that severe thrombocytopenia led to spontaneous GI hemorrhage. Other investigators subsequently challenged this conclusion, arguing that spontaneous bleeding from coagulopathy is in fact rare.[100,101] In one report, the distribution of pathologic lesions in patients with GI bleeding who were taking heparin or warfarin was essentially equivalent to that in the general population.[100] Regardless of what the precise relation between coagulopathy and GI hemorrhage may be, a thorough investigation for an anatomic lesion is imperative in the workup of patients with lower GI bleeding even in the face of coagulopathy or thrombocytopenia.

BENIGN ANORECTAL DISEASE

Hemorrhoids, ulcer/fissure disease, and fistula in ano must not be overlooked as causes of GI hemorrhage: in one review comprising almost 18,000 cases of lower GI bleeding, 11% were attributable to anorectal pathology.[72] It is crucial to remember that identification of a benign anorectal lesion does not eliminate the possibility of a more proximal cause of hemorrhage. In general, patients with hemorrhoids identified on physical exam-

Figure 5 Shown is the appearance of an arteriovenous malformation on colonoscopy.

ination should still undergo thorough endoscopic evaluation of the colon to rule out other pathologic conditions.

Portal hypertension, congestive heart failure, and splenic vein thrombosis can cause colonic or anorectal varices, which can result in massive lower GI hemorrhage.[102] The reported incidence of anorectal varices in patients with portal hypertension ranges from 78% to 89%.[103-105] If local measures fail to control hemorrhage, some form of portosystemic shunting is indicated.

COLONIC ARTERIOVENOUS MALFORMATIONS

The term arteriovenous malformation includes vascular ectasias, angiomas, and angiodysplasias. AVMs are ectatic blood vessels seen in the mucosa and submucosa of the GI tract. They are degenerative lesions of the GI tract, occurring more frequently with advancing age.[9] In autopsy series, the reported incidence of colonic AVMs is 1% to 2%.[106] In patients older than 50 years, the incidence of colonic AVMs is estimated to range from 2% to 30%.[107-110] In healthy asymptomatic adults, the prevalence is estimated to be approximately 0.8%.[111]

Colonic AVMs are believed to derive from chronic colonic wall muscle contraction, which leads to chronic partial obstruction of the submucosal veins, causing the vessels to become dilated and tortuous. This process eventually renders the precapillary sphincters incompetent, resulting in direct arterial-venous communication.[112,113] Colonic AVMs are most commonly found in the cecum.[10] They have been associated with several systemic diseases, including atherosclerotic cardiovascular disease, aortic stenosis, chronic renal disease, collagen vascular disease, von Willebrand disease, chronic obstructive pulmonary disease, and cirrhosis of the liver; to date, however, no definite causal relationship to any of these conditions has been established.[6,23,45,114]

The diagnosis of a colonic AVM is made at the time of angiography or colonoscopy. During angiography, visualization of ectatic, slow-emptying veins, vascular tufts, or early-filling veins establishes the diagnosis.[115] During endoscopy, angiodysplasias appear as red, flat lesions about 2 to 10 mm in diameter, sometimes accompanied by a feeding vessel [*see Figure 5*].[6,42,45,111]

Figure 6 **Shown are intraoperative specimens of small-bowel tumors causing lower GI hemorrhage.**

Typically, the bleeding caused by colonic AVMs is chronic, slow, and intermittent.[9] Although these lesions can cause severe lower GI hemorrhage, they are a relatively uncommon cause: in most large series, they account for only about 2% of cases of acute bleeding.[74,108] The bleeding stops spontaneously in 85% to 90% of cases,[10] but it recurs in 25% to 85%.[116] Accordingly, definitive surgical or colonoscopic treatment should be rendered once the lesion has been identified.

COLONIC ISCHEMIA

Acute lower GI bleeding can also be a presenting symptom of colonic ischemia. In several large series, colonic ischemia accounted for 3% to 9% of cases of acute lower GI hemorrhage.[4,8,15,94,117] Other vascular diseases reported as potential causes are polyarteritis nodosa, Wegener granulomatosis, and rheumatoid vasculitis.[118,119] The resultant vasculitis can cause ulceration, necrosis, and ultimately hemorrhage.[120]

SMALL INTESTINAL SOURCES

Small intestinal sources account for 0.7% to 9% of cases of acute lower GI bleeding.[3,4,121-123] About 70% to 80% of cases of small bowel hemorrhage are attributable to AVMs[124]; other, less common causes are jejunoileal diverticula, Meckel's diverticulum,[125] neoplasia, regional enteritis, and aortoenteric fistulas [*see Figure 6*].[92,126,127] Accurate localization of a bleeding site in the small intestine can be highly challenging: the length and the free intraperitoneal position of the small bowel make endoscopic examination difficult, and the nature of the overlying loops makes angiographic localization imprecise. For these reasons, the small intestine is usually left for last in the attempt to localize the source of lower GI bleeding and is examined only after sources in the colon, the upper GI tract, and the anorectum have been ruled out.[9]

AIDS

The etiology of lower GI bleeding in patients with AIDS differs from that in the general population.[93] In AIDS patients, lower GI bleeding is caused predominantly by conditions related to the underlying HIV infection. Cytomegalovirus colitis is the most common cause of such bleeding in this population, occurring in 39% of cases.[128] AIDS patients with hemorrhoids or anal fissures often experience significant bleeding as a result of HIV-induced thrombocytopenia.[128] A 1998 study reported that in 23% of AIDS patients hospitalized for lower GI bleeding, benign anorectal disease was the cause.[129] Other significant causes of lower GI hemorrhage in this population are colonic histoplasmosis, Kaposi sarcoma of the colon, and bacterial colitis.[129,130]

NSAIDS

The association between NSAID use and upper GI hemorrhage is well known.[131] Current data suggest that NSAIDs have a toxic effect on colonic mucosa as well.[132] An epidemiologic study estimated the incidence of NSAID-associated large-bowel bleeding to be 7/100,000.[133] A retrospective review found that patients who had experienced lower GI bleeding were twice as likely to have taken NSAIDs as those who had not.[134] NSAIDs have also been linked to diverticular hemorrhage: in one study, 92% of patients with diverticular bleeding were taking NSAIDs.[71] Although the exact mechanism of NSAID-induced colonic injury is unknown, however, heightened clinical awareness of this potential cause of lower GI bleeding is warranted.[93]

References

1. Briley CA, Jackson DC, Johnsrude IS, et al: Acute gastrointestinal hemorrhage of small-bowel origin. Radiology 136:317, 1980

2. Koval G, Benner KG, Rosch J, et al: Aggressive angiographic diagnosis in acute lower gastrointestinal hemorrhage. Dig Dis Sci 32:248, 1987

3. Jensen DM, Machicado GA: Diagnosis and treat-

ment of severe hematochezia: the role of urgent colonoscopy after purge. Gastroenterology 95:1569, 1988

4. Longstreth GF: Epidemiology and outcome of patients hospitalized with acute lower gastrointestinal hemorrhage: a population-based study. Am J Gastroenterol 92:419, 1997

5. McGuire H: Bleeding colonic diverticula: a reappraisal of natural history and management. Ann Surg 220:653, 1994

6. Foutch PG: Angiodysplasia of the gastrointestinal tract. Am J Gastroenterol 88:807, 1993

7. Bramely P, Masson J, McKnight G, et al: The role of an open-access bleeding unit in the manage-

ment of colonic hemorrhage. A 2 year prospective study. Scand J Gastroenterol 31:764, 1996

8. Peura DA, Lanza FL, Gostout CJ, et al: The American College of Gastroenterology Bleeding Registry: preliminary findings. Am J Gastroenterol 92:924, 1997

9. Vernava AM, Moore BA, Longo WE, et al: Lower gastrointestinal bleeding. Dis Colon Rectum 40:846, 1997

10. Boley SJ, DiBiase A, Brandt LJ, et al: Lower intestinal bleeding in the elderly. Am J Surg 137:57, 1979

11. Caos A, Benner K, Manier J, et al: Colonoscopy after Golytely preparation in acute rectal bleeding. J Clin Gastroenterol 8:46, 1986

12. Zuccaro G Jr: Management of the adult patient with acute lower gastrointestinal bleeding. American College of Gastroenterology. Practice Parameters Committee. Am J Gastroenterol 93:1202, 1998

13. Committee on Trauma ACS: Advanced Trauma Life Support, 5th ed. American College of Surgeons, Chicago, 1993, p 84

14. Richter JM, Christensen MR, Kaplan LM, et al: Effectiveness of current technology in the diagnosis and management of lower gastrointestinal hemorrhage. Gastrointest Endosc 41:93, 1995

15. Rossini FP, Ferrari A, Spandre M, et al: Emergency colonoscopy. World J Surg 13:190, 1989

16. Geller AJ, Mayoral W, Balm R, et al: Colonoscopy in acute lower gastrointestinal bleeding (abstract). Gastrointest Endosc 45:AB107, 1997

17. Goenka MK, Kochhar R, Mehta SK: Spectrum of lower gastrointestinal hemorrhage: an endoscopic study of 166 patients. Indian J Gastroenterol 12:129, 1993

18. Ohyama T, Sakurai Y, Ito M, et al: Analysis of urgent colonoscopy for lower gastrointestinal tract bleeding. Digestion 61:189, 2000

19. Chaudhry V, Hyser MJ, Gracias VH, et al: Colonoscopy: the initial test for acute lower gastrointestinal bleeding. Am Surg 64:723, 1998

20. Cohn SM, Moller BA, Zieg PM, et al: Angiography for preoperative evaluation in patients with lower gastrointestinal bleeding: are the benefits worth the risks? Arch Surg 133:50, 1998

21. Caos A, Benner KG, Manier J, et al: Colonoscopy after Golytely preparation in acute rectal bleeding. J Clin Gastroenterol 8:46, 1986

22. Alavi A, Dann RW, Baum S, et al: Scintigraphic detection of acute gastrointestinal bleeding. Radiology 124:753, 1977

23. Gupta N, Longo W, Vernava A: Angiodysplasia of the lower gastrointestinal tract: an entity readily diagnosed by colonoscopy and primarily managed nonoperatively. Dis Colon Rectum 38:979, 1995

24. McKusick KA, Froelich J, Callahan RJ, et al: 99mTc red blood cells for detection of gastrointestinal bleeding: experience with 80 patients. AJR Am J Roentgenol 137:1113, 1981

25. Bunker SR, Lull RJ, Hattner RS, et al: The ideal radiotracer in gastrointestinal bleeding detection. AJR Am J Roentgenol 138:982, 1982

26. Kester RR, Welch JP, Sziklas JP: The 99mTc-labeled RBC scan: a diagnostic method for lower gastrointestinal bleeding. Dis Colon Rectum 27:47, 1984

27. Suzman MS, Talmor M, Jennis R, et al: Accurate localization and surgical management of active lower gastrointestinal hemorrhage with technetium-labeled erythrocyte scintigraphy. Ann Surg 224:29, 1996

28. Hunter JM, Pezim ME: Limited value of technetium 99m-labeled red cell scintigraphy in localization of lower gastrointestinal bleeding. Am J Surg 159:504, 1990

29. Ng D, Opelka F, Beck D, et al: Predictive value of technetium Tc 99m labeled red blood cell scintigraphy for positive angiogram in massive lower gastrointestinal hemorrhage. Dis Colon Rectum 40:471, 1997

30. Wadwa KS, Kalloo AN: Bleeding scans in patients with lower gastrointestinal bleeding of undetermined cause: are they useful? [abstract]. Gastrointest Endosc 45:AB120, 1997

31. Prakash C, Sreenarasimhaih J, Royal H, et al: A varied diagnostic approach to acute lower gastrointestinal bleeding [abstract]. Am J Gastroenterol 92:1685, 1997

32. Baum S, Athanasoulis CA, Waltman AC: Angiographic diagnosis and control of large-bowel bleeding. Dis Colon Rectum 17:447, 1974

33. Athanasoulis CA, Moncure AC, Greenfield AJ, et al: Intraoperative localization of small bowel bleeding sites with combined use of angiographic methods and methylene blue injection. Surgery 87:77, 1980

34. Schrodt JF, Bradford WR: Presurgical angiographic localization of small bowel bleeding site with methylene blue injection. J Ky Med Assoc 94:192, 1996

35. Pennoyer WP, Vignati PV, Cohen JL: Management of angiogram positive lower gastrointestinal hemorrhage: long term follow-up of non-operative treatments. Int J Colorectal Dis 11:279, 1996

36. Rantis PC, Harford FJ, Wagner RH, et al: Technetium-labelled red blood cell scintigraphy: is it useful in acute lower gastrointestinal bleeding? Int J Colorectal Dis 10:210, 1995

37. Leitman IM, Paull DE, Shires GT 3rd: Evaluation and management of massive lower gastrointestinal hemorrhage. Ann Surg 209:175, 1989

38. Casarella WJ, Galloway SJ, Taxin RN: Lower gastrointestinal tract hemorrhage: new concepts based on arteriography. AJR Am J Roentgenol 121:357, 1974

39. Colacchio TA, Forde KA, Patsos TJ, et al: Impact of modern diagnostic methods on the management of active rectal bleeding: ten year experience. Am J Surg 143:607, 1982

40. Bloomfeld RS, Smith TP, Schneider AM, et al: Provocative angiography in patients with gastrointestinal hemorrhage of obscure origin. Am J Gastroenterol 95:2807, 2000

41. Shetzline MA, Suhocki P, Dash R, et al: Provocative angiography in obscure gastrointestinal bleeding. South Med J 93:1205, 2000

42. Krevsky B: Detection and treatment of angiodysplasia. Gastrointest Endosc 7:509, 1997

43. Foutch PG: Colonic angiodysplasia. Gastroenterologist 5:148, 1997

44. Rutgeerts P, Van Gompel F, Geboes K, et al: Long term results of treatment of vascular malformations of the gastrointestinal tract by neodymium Yag laser photocoagulation. Gut 26:586, 1985

45. Rogers BH: Endoscopic diagnosis and therapy of mucosal vascular abnormalities of the gastrointestinal tract occurring in elderly patients and associated with cardiac, vascular, and pulmonary disease. Gastrointest Endosc 26:134, 1980

46. Binmoeller KF, Thonke F, Soehendra N: Endoscopic hemoclip treatment for gastrointestinal bleeding. Endoscopy 25:167, 1993

47. Jaspersen D, Korner T, Schorr W, et al: Diagnosis and treatment control of bleeding intestinal angiodysplasias with an endoscopic Doppler device. Bildgebung 62:14, 1995

48. Jensen DM, Machicado GA, Jutabha R, et al: Urgent colonoscopy for the diagnosis and treatment of severe diverticular hemorrhage. N Engl J Med 342:78, 2000

49. Bloomfeld RS, Rockey DC, Shetzline MA: Endoscopic therapy of acute diverticular hemorrhage. Am J Gastroenterol 96:2367, 2001

50. Naveau S, Aubert A, Poynard T, et al: Long-term results of treatment of vascular malformations of the gastrointestinal tract by neodymium YAG laser photocoagulation. Dig Dis Sci 35:821, 1990

51. Santos JC, Aprilli F, Guimaraes AS, et al: Angiodysplasia of the colon: endoscopic diagnosis and treatment. Br J Surg 75:256, 1988

52. Eisen GM, Dominitz JA, Faigel DO, et al: An annotated algorithmic approach to upper gastrointestinal bleeding. Gastrointest Endosc 53:853, 2001

53. Habr-Gama A, Waye J: Complications and hazards of gastrointestinal endoscopy. World J Surg 13:193, 1989

54. Trowers E, Ganga U, Hodges D: Endoscopic hemorrhoidal ligation: preliminary clinical experience. Gastrointest Endosc 48:49, 1998

55. Athanasoulis CA, Baum S, Rosch J, et al: Mesenteric arterial infusions of vasopressin for hemorrhage from colonic diverticulosis. Am J Surg 129:212, 1975

56. Rahn NH 3rd, Tishler JM, Han SY, et al: Diagnostic and interventional angiography in acute gastrointestinal hemorrhage. Radiology 143:361, 1982

57. Levinson SL, Powell DW, Callahan WT, et al: A current approach to rectal bleeding. J Clin Gastroenterol 3(suppl 1):9, 1981

58. Lichtiger S, Karnbluth A, Salomon P, et al: Lower gastrointestinal bleeding. Gastrointestinal Emergencies. Taylor MB, Gollan JL, Peppercorn MA, et al, Eds. Baltimore, Williams & Wilkins, 1992, p 358

59. Clark RA, Colley DP, Eggers FM: Acute arterial gastrointestinal hemorrhage: efficacy of transcatheter control. AJR Am J Roentgenol 136:1185, 1981

60. Browder W, Cerise EJ, Litwin MS: Impact of emergency angiography in massive lower gastrointestinal bleeding. Ann Surg 204:530, 1986

61. Matolo NM, Link DP: Selective embolization for control of gastrointestinal hemorrhage. Am J Surg 138:840, 1979

62. Encarnacion CE, Kadir S, Beam CA, et al: Gastrointestinal bleeding: treatment with gastrointestinal arterial embolization. Radiology 183:505, 1992

63. Bookstein JJ, Chlosta EM, Foley D, et al: Transcatheter hemostasis of gastrointestinal bleeding using modified autogenous clot. Radiology 113:277, 1974

64. Peck DJ, McLoughlin RF, Hughson MN, et al: Percutaneous embolotherapy of lower gastrointestinal hemorrhage. J Vasc Interv Radiol 9:747, 1998

65. Gomes AS, Lois JF, McCoy RD: Angiographic treatment of gastrointestinal hemorrhage: comparison of vasopressin infusion and embolization. AJR Am J Roentgenol 146:1031, 1986

66. Wright HK, Pelliccia O, Higgins EF, et al: Controlled, semielective, segmental resection for massive colonic hemorrhage. Am J Surg 139:535, 1980

67. Eaton AC: Emergency surgery for acute colonic haemorrhage—a retrospective study. Br J Surg 68:109, 1981

68. McGuire HH, Haynes BW: Massive hemorrhage for diverticulosis of the colon: guidelines for therapy based on bleeding patterns observed in fifty cases. Ann Surg 175:847, 1972

69. Setya V, Singer JA, Minken SL: Subtotal colectomy as a last resort for unrelenting, unlocalized, lower gastrointestinal bleeding: experience with 12 cases. Am Surg 58:295, 1992

70. Jensen DM, Machicado GA: Colonoscopy for diagnosis and treatment of severe lower gastrointestinal bleeding: routine outcomes and cost

analysis. Gastrointest Endosc Clin N Am 7:477, 1997

71. Foutch PG: Diverticular bleeding: are non-steroidal anti-inflammatory drugs risk factors for hemorrhage and can colonoscopy predict outcome for patients? Am J Gastroenterol 90:1779, 1995

72. Vernava A, Longo W, Virgo K, et al: A nationwide study of the incidence and etiology of lower gastrointestinal bleeding. Surg Res Commun 18:113, 1996

73. Heer M, Ammann R, Buhler H: Die klinische Bedeutung der Angiodysplasien im Kolon. Schweiz Med Wochenschr 114:1416, 1984

74. Sebastian JJ, Lucia F, Botella MT, et al: Angiodisplasia gastrointestinal difusa asociada a cirrosis hepática criptogenética y coagulopatia que simulaba una enfermedad de von Willebrand. Rev Esp Enferm Dig 88:631, 1996

75. Hughes L: Postmortem survey of diverticular disease of the colon. Gut 10:336, 1969

76. Meyers MA, Alonso DR, Gray GF, et al: Pathogenesis of bleeding colonic diverticulosis. Gastroenterology 71:577, 1976

77. Rushford A: The significance of bleeding as a symptom in diverticulitis. J R Soc Med 49:577, 1956

78. Bokhari M, Vernava AM, Ure T, et al: Diverticular hemorrhage in the elderly—is it well tolerated? Dis Colon Rectum 39:191, 1996

79. McGuire HH: Bleeding colonic diverticula: a reappraisal of natural history and management. Ann Surg 220:653, 1994

80. Luk GD, Bynum TE, Hendrix TR: Gastric aspiration in localization of gastrointestinal hemorrhage. JAMA 241:576, 1979

81. Robert JR, Sachar DB, Greenstein AJ: Severe gastrointestinal hemorrhage in Crohn's disease. Ann Surg 213:207, 1991

82. Binder S, Miller H, Deterling R: Emergency and urgent operations for ulcerative colitis. Arch Surg 110:281, 1975

83. Cirocco WC, Reilly JC, Rusin LC: Life-threatening hemorrhage and exsanguination from Crohn's disease: report of four cases. Dis Colon Rectum 38:85, 1995

84. Reyes E, Hernandez J, Gonzalez A: Typhoid colitis with massive lower gastrointestinal bleeding: an unexpected behavior of Salmonella typhi. Dis Colon Rectum 29:511, 1986

85. Maguire TM, Wensel RH, Malcolm N, et al: Massive gastrointestinal hemorrhage cecal ulcers and salmonella colitis. J Clin Gastroenterol 7:249, 1985

86. Cohen M, Fianella R: Hemorrhagic colitis associated with Escherichia coli O157:H7. Adv Intern Med 37:173, 1992

87. Gould O, Khawaja FI, Rosenthal W: Antibiotic associated hemorrhagic colitis. Am J Gastroenterol 77:491, 1982

88. Escudero-Faber A, Cummings OW, Kirklin J, et al: Cytomegalovirus colitis presenting as hematochezia and requiring resection. Arch Surg 127:102, 1992

89. Tagkalidis PP, Tjandra JJ: Chronic radiation proctitis. Aust NZ J Surg 71:230, 2001

90. Den Harog Jager F, Van Haastert M, Batterman J, et al: The endoscopic spectrum of late radiation damage of the rectosigmoid colon. Endoscopy 17:214, 1985

91. Crook J, Esche J, Futter N: Effect of pelvic radiotherapy for prostate cancer on bowel, bladder, and sexual function: the patient's perspective. Urology 47:387, 1996

92. Ellis DJ, Reinus JF: Lower intestinal hemorrhage. Crit Care Clin 11:369, 1995

93. Zuckerman GR, Prakash C: Acute lower intestinal bleeding. Part II: etiology, therapy, and outcomes. Gastrointest Endosc 49:228, 1999

94. Wagner HE, Stain SC, Gilg M, et al: Systematic assessment of massive bleeding of the lower part of the gastrointestinal tract. Surg Gynecol Obstet 175:445, 1992

95. Makela JT, Kiviniemi H, Laitinen S, et al: Diagnosis and treatment of acute lower gastrointestinal bleeding. Scand J Gastroenterol 28:1062, 1993

96. Greenen J, Schmitt M, Wu W: Major complications of colonoscopy: bleeding and perforation. Am J Dig Dis 20:231, 1975

97. Macrae JF, Tan K, Williams C: Towards safer colonoscopy: a report on the complications of 5000 diagnostic or therapeutic colonoscopies. Gut 24:376, 1983

98. Gaydos L, Freireich J, Mantel N: The quantitative relationship between platelet count and hemorrhage in patients with acute leukemia. N Engl J Med 266:905, 1962

99. Wilkson J, Nour-Edlin F, Israels M, et al: Hemophilic syndromes: a survey of 267 patients. Lancet 2:947, 1961

100. Coon J, Willis JP: Hemorrhagic complications of anticoagulant therapy. Arch Intern Med 133:386, 1974

101. Mittal R, Spero JA, Lewis JH, et al: Patterns of gastrointestinal hemorrhage in hemophilia. Gastroenterology 88:515, 1985

102. Cappel M, Price J: Characterization of the syndrome of small and large intestinal variceal bleeding. Dig Dis Sci 32:422, 1987

103. Strong J: Colonic, anorectal and peristomal varices. Semin Colon Rectal Surg 5:50, 1994

104. Chawla Y, Dilawari J: Anorectal varices—their frequency in cirrhotic and non-cirrhotic portal hypertension. Gut 32:309, 1991

105. Goenka MK, Kochhar R, Nagi B, et al: Rectosigmoid varices and other mucosal changes in patients with portal hypertension. Am J Gastroenterol 86:1185, 1991

106. Baer JW, Ryan S: Analysis of cecal vasculature in the search for vascular malformations. Am J Roentgenol 126:394, 1976

107. Danesh BJ, Spiliadis C, Williams CB, et al: Angiodysplasia—an uncommon cause of colonic bleeding: colonoscopic evaluation of 1,050 patients with rectal bleeding and anaemia. Int J Colorectal Dis 2:218, 1987

108. Heer M, Sulser H, Hany A: Angiodysplasia of the colon: an expression of occlusive vascular disease. Hepatogastroenterology 34:127, 1987

109. Richter JM, Hedberg SE, Athanasoulis CA, et al: Angiodysplasia: clinical presentation and colonoscopic diagnosis. Dig Dis Sci 29:481, 1984

110. Zuckerman G, Benitez J: A prospective study of bidirectional endoscopy (colonoscopy and upper endoscopy) in the evaluation of patients with occult gastrointestinal bleeding. Am J Gastroenterol 87:62, 1992

111. Foutch PG, Rex DK, Lieberman D: Prevalance and natural history of colonic angiodysplasias among healthy asymptomatic adults. Am J Gastroenterol 90:564, 1995

112. Boley SJ, Sammartano R, Adams A, et al: On the nature and etiology of vascular ectasias of the colon: degenerative lesions of aging. Gastroenterology 72:650, 1977

113. Mitsudo SM, Boley SJ, Brandt LJ, et al: Vascular ectasias of the right colon in the elderly: a distinct pathologic entity. Hum Pathol 10:585, 1979

114. Imperiale TF, Ransohoff DF: Aortic stenosis, idiopathic gastrointestinal bleeding, and angiodysplasia: is there an association? A methodologic critique of the literature. Gastroenterology 95:1670, 1988

115. Boley SJ, Sprayragen S, Sammartano R, et al: The pathophysiologic basis for the angiographic signs of vascular ectasias of the colon. Radiology 125:615, 1977

116. Helmrich GA, Stallworth JR, Brown JJ: Angiodysplasia: characterization, diagnosis, and advances in treatment. South Med J 83:1450, 1990

117. Bramley PN, Masson JW, McKnight G, et al: The role of an open-access bleeding unit in the management of colonic haemorrhage: a 2-year prospective study. Scand J Gastroenterol 31:764, 1996

118. Moses FM: Gastrointestinal bleeding and the athlete. Am J Gastroenterol 88:1157, 1993

119. Burt R, Berenson M, Samuelson C, et al: Rheumatoid vasculitis of the colon presenting as pancolitis. Dig Dis Sci 28:183, 1983

120. Sokol R, Farrell M, McAdams A: An unusual presentation of Wegener's granulomatosis mimicking inflammatory bowel disease. Gastroenterology 87:426, 1984

121. Klinvimol T, Ho YH, Parry BR, et al: Small bowel causes of per rectum haemorrhage. Ann Acad Med Singapore 23:866, 1994

122. Gilmore PR: Angiodysplasia of the upper gastrointestinal tract. J Clin Gastroenterol 10:386, 1988

123. Netterville R, Hardy J, Martin R: Small bowel hemorrhage. Ann Surg 167:949, 1968

124. Lewis B, Waye J: Bleeding from the small intestine. Gastrointestinal Bleeding. Sugawa C, Schuman BM, Lucas CE, Eds. Igaku-Shoin, New York, 1992, p 178

125. Lu CL, Chen CY, Chiu ST, et al: Adult intussuscepted Meckel's diverticulum presenting mainly lower gastrointestinal bleeding. J Gastroenterol Hepatol 16:478, 2001

126. Longo WE, Vernava AM 3rd: Clinical implications of jejunoileal diverticular disease. Dis Colon Rectum 35:381, 1992

127. Buchman TG, Bulkley GB: Current management of patients with lower gastrointestinal bleeding. Surg Clin North Am 67:651, 1987

128. Chalasani N, Wilcox CM: Gastrointestinal hemorrhage in patients with AIDS. AIDS Patient Care STDS 13:343, 1999

129. Chalasani N, Wilcox CM: Etiology and outcome of lower gastrointestinal bleeding in patients with AIDS. Am J Gastroenterol 93:175, 1998

130. Becherer PR, Sokol-Anderson M, Joist JH, et al: Gastrointestinal histoplasmosis presenting as hematochezia in human immunodeficiency virus–infected hemophilic patients. Am J Hematol 47:229, 1994

131. Allison M, Howatson A, Torrance C, et al: Gastrointestinal damage associated with the use of nonsteroidal antiinflammatory drugs. N Engl J Med 327:749, 1992

132. Davies NM: Toxicity of nonsteroidal anti-inflammatory drugs in the large intestine. Dis Colon Rectum 38:1311, 1995

133. Langman MJ, Morgan LR, Worral J: Use of anti-inflammatory drugs by patients admitted with small or large bowel perforations and hemorrhage. BMJ 290:347, 1985

134. Holt S, Rigoglioso V, Sidhu M, et al: Nonsteroidal antiinflammatory drugs and lower gastrointestinal bleeding. Dig Dis Sci 38:1619, 1993

10 SKIN LESIONS

Alan E. Seyfer, M.D.

Assessment and Management of Skin Lesions

The clinical assessment and treatment of skin lesions can be challenging, since some skin lesions are capricious in their biologic behavior. History is of great importance. Recent changes in the appearance of a lesion usually indicate active growth, which increases the chance that the lesion is malignant. Likewise, a history of chronic sun exposure—particularly in a patient who has a fair complexion—multiplies the patient's risk of malignancy. Certain congenital lesions must also be viewed with suspicion, even though the incidence of malignancy in such lesions can be extremely variable. Any history that departs from the natural history of a simple nevus should raise suspicion of malignancy. In general, nevus tissue becomes apparent at 4 or 5 years of age. Nevi often darken with puberty and pregnancy and fade in the seventh to eighth decades of life. Malignancies usually differ from the characteristic clinical pattern of a simple nevus.

Nonsuspicious Lesions

In general, lesions are nonsuspicious if they remain stable and uniform in their physical characteristics (e.g., size, shape, color, profile, and texture). Non-suspicious lesions may be safely monitored conservatively, especially if they are located in regions easily visible to the patient. Excisional biopsy is warranted if 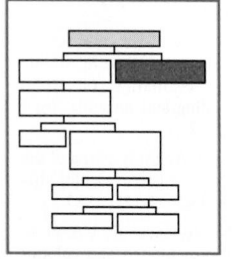 the lesions change in size, shape, color, profile, or texture. Cosmesis is always a subjective and relative indication for excision.

Suspicious Lesions

Changes and irregularities in the physical characteristics of a skin lesion (e.g., size, shape, color, profile, and texture) are important in helping determine whether the lesion is suspicious. For example, an irregular physical pattern, large size (1 to 2 cm or larger), 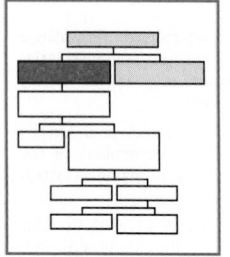 or unfavorable location (e.g., on skin that is unprotected from sun exposure) places the lesion in the suspicious category and is a relative indication for performing an excisional biopsy.

If the lesion is suspicious, a biopsy is warranted. If the suspicious area is small, it should be completely excised with a 1 to 4 mm margin, depending on the clinical characteristics. The important principle is to include a margin of normal skin around the lesion. This helps the patholo-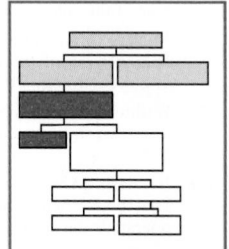gist and may include occult areas of importance. Shave biopsies should never be performed, because the depth of the lesion is of great diagnostic importance, and lesion depth is destroyed by this technique. To provide a complete specimen for study, my preference is to include a full thickness of the dermis with subcutaneous fat. As noted above, a small margin of normal skin is helpful to the pathologist [see Surgical Technique, Excisional Biopsy, *below*].

If the lesion is found to be benign, further treatment is unwarranted. If the lesion proves to be malignant, further excision with an appropriate margin is usually necessary, and staging of the tumor becomes important (see below). Presentation of the biopsy to the tumor board is of great value both clinically and medicolegally. In cases of melanoma or other so-called liquid tumors that shed their cells readily in all tissue, ancillary treatment (e.g., with perfusion therapy, radiation therapy, or chemotherapy) may be reasonable before reexcision with wider margins.

CLINICAL STAGING OF MALIGNANCY

If a malignancy is suspected, regional node status is important, and the nodes that drain the region should be thoroughly examined. If nodes are palpable and the lesion proves to be a malignancy, a regional node dissection or sampling is necessary to stage the patient's tumor and plan for further treatment. 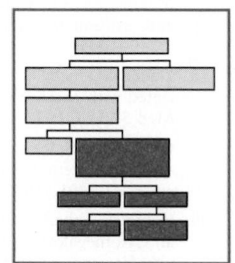 Likewise, a node dissection may be therapeutic and may contribute to local control of the lesion. If the nodes are positive, it is reasonable to consider adjuvant therapy or ancillary treatment. If the nodes are negative microscopically, it is reasonable to follow the patient with serial examinations. Again, an interdisciplinary tumor board will assist in making the appropriate management decision once a malignancy is confirmed by biopsy.

A staging approach that is being increasingly widely used in certain patient groups is lymphatic mapping and sentinel lymph node (SLN) biopsy [see Discussion, Malignant Melanoma, Melanoma Staging, *below*].

Assessment and Management
of Skin Lesions

Determine whether skin lesion is suspicious for malignancy

Obtain history and examine the patient's skin lesion.

Lesion suspicious

Changes and irregularities in physical characteristics, history of chronic sun exposure, unfavorable location, and presence of certain congenital lesions (e.g., dysplastic nevi) all raise suspicion of malignancy.

Lesion nonsuspicious

The lesion is stable and uniform in its physical characteristics (e.g., size, shape, color, profile, texture). Monitor conservatively. Patient may choose elective excision for cosmesis.

Perform excisional biopsy

Suspicious lesion should be completely excised with a 1–4 mm margin (depending on clinical characteristics), including the full thickness of the dermis with subcutaneous fat. Shave biopsies should *never* be performed on suspicious lesions.

Lesion benign

No further treatment is necessary.

Lesion malignant

Present biopsy to tumor board. If tumor is melanoma or other so-called liquid tumor, consider ancillary treatment (e.g., perfusion therapy, radiation therapy, chemotherapy) before reexcision.

Perform reexcision with appropriate margin and assess regional node status.

Consider lymphatic mapping and SLN biopsy as staging option for melanoma, squamous cell carcinoma, and Meckel cell carcinoma [*see V:3 Lymphatic Mapping and Sentinel Lymph Node Biopsy*].

Nodes nonpalpable

Follow clinically.

Nodes palpable

Perform appropriate regional node dissection.

Nodes negative

Follow clinically.

Nodes positive

Consider ancillary treatment (e.g., perfusion therapy, radiation therapy, chemotherapy).

Discussion

Nonmelanoma skin cancers are the most common cancers in the United States, accounting for about 35% of all cancers diagnosed every year.[1,2] Nonmelanoma skin cancers can be capricious, and it may be difficult to assess their biologic behavior from their appearance alone. Certainly, it is possible for a benign-looking papule to exhibit aggressive biologic behavior. Melanomas, at the more malignant end of the spectrum, can metastasize early and even present initially with cerebral metastasis.

Sun exposure with actinic changes in the skin is a predisposing factor for skin cancers of all types.[3-5] Fair-skinned persons lacking protective pigmentation are at much higher risk for the development of skin cancers.[6] Failure of the immunologic surveillance system, decreased cell-mediated immunity, and use of immunosuppressive agents have all been implicated as factors that may influence a patient's predisposition to malignant skin lesions.[7,8]

Basal Cell Carcinoma

Basal cell carcinomas originate in the pluripotential epithelial cells of the epidermis and skin adnexa.[1] These tumors tend to be characterized by slow growth and progressive morbidity by local extension. Their viability seems to depend on attachment to the dermis, and systemic metastases are therefore rare. However, certain types of basal cell carcinoma may be extremely aggressive, resulting in morbidity, mutilation, and death by local extension. This is particularly true of midface and sclerosing basal cell cancers.

Clinically, there are several types of basal cell carcinomas [*see Figure 1*]. The most common is the nodular type, which begins as a flesh-colored, raised, telangiectatic lesion that may be difficult to distinguish from a common nevus.[9] The nodular lesion is rounded in appearance during its early phase and characteristically assumes a raised rim with a craterlike central region, often

with scaling of superficial skin cells at its center [*see Figure 1a*]. Perhaps the most dangerous type is the sclerosing, or morpheaform, basal cell carcinoma—a light, plaquelike lesion that can resemble a stellate scar [*see Figure 1b*]. Morpheaform basal cell carcinomas tend to be locally invasive, with multiple cancer projections, resembling tentacles, that penetrate toward the deep portions of the tissue. Therefore, it is possible—even likely—that tumor will be left behind after an excisional biopsy of the lesion.[10] Such tumors can also ulcerate and resemble pigmented melanomas [*see Figure 1c*].

The distribution of basal cell cancers is strongly weighted toward the midface, cheek, and ear regions.[11] Treatment is usually surgical, with removal of a rim of normal skin around the lesion. Morpheaform basal cell cancers should be treated with a wider margin of excision, and careful attention should be paid to the margins to confirm clearance of tumor cells. In most cases, closure can be accomplished by wide undermining of the skin and fat and direct closure. Otherwise, a skin graft is a useful alternative.

Radiation therapy for basal cell carcinomas claims an overall cure rate of over 90%.[12] This therapy can be offered to each patient, but the repeated treatments require multiple visits. Radiation therapy is a safe, noninvasive form of treatment that can be an attractive alternative for patients who are, for whatever reasons, considered bad candidates for surgical extirpation. Radiation is a particularly attractive alternative for the treatment of lesions in areas that are difficult to reconstruct, such as the medial canthal margin of the eyelids, certain external ear lesions, and the nostril rim.

Another therapeutic option is Mohs' micrographic surgical operation. Frederic Mohs, a general surgeon, developed the technique for lesions like basal cell carcinomas without metastatic potential that were of full thickness and involved the skin and the mucous membranes of the nose.[13] Perhaps the best indi-

a *b* *c*

Figure 1   (*a*) A pearly luster and telangiectasias are evident in this typical basal cell carcinoma on the cheek of a 43-year-old man. (*b*) This sclerosing (morpheaform) basal cell carcinoma on the nose of a 55-year-old man was found to be deeply invasive and exhibited multidirectional growth. (*c*) This basal cell carcinoma on the lower leg of a 91-year-old woman showed ulceration and pigmentation similar to that of a melanoma.

Figure 2 (*a*) This squamous cell carcinoma on the lip of a 70-year-old man was related to sun exposure; the patient was a nonsmoker. (*b*) This squamous cell carcinoma involving the thumb and index finger of a 72-year-old man, a retired dentist, was related to exposure to occupational hazards; he had subjected these digits to repeated radiation exposures by holding dental x-rays against his patients' teeth. (*c*) The 61-year-old man who had this indolent, slow-growing squamous cell carcinoma on the hand also had a synchronous penile erythroplasia of Queyrat (localized)—a squamous cell carcinoma in situ; there was no evidence of metastasis from either lesion. (*d*) This squamous cell carcinoma on the helix of the external ear in a 73-year-old man can be seen extending to the scalp.

cation for the Mohs procedure is recurrent basal cell carcinomas, especially those of the morpheaform type. The Mohs technique usually incorporates wide enough margins to ensure a reasonable cure rate. The Mohs technique may also be appropriate for microcystic adnexal carcinoma and dermatofibrosarcoma protuberans.[14] The drawbacks to the Mohs procedure are that it requires a considerable amount of time, exposure, and expense but has a cure rate similar to that of simple surgical excision.

Squamous Cell Carcinoma

Like basal cell cancers, squamous cell cancers are associated with actinic solar damage but may also arise out of old scars, radiation-damaged skin, or chronic, open wounds[15] [*see Figure 2*]. Chronic inflammation and irritation appear to be the common denominators. The biologic activity of squamous cell cancers is aggressive in comparison with that of basal cell cancers; fortunately, they are less common. Persons of fair complexion are at increased risk; all skin cancers are more likely to develop in sun-exposed regions[16] [*see Figure 2a*]. Certain occupational hazards have been associated with an increased risk for squamous cell cancer, including those experienced by dental personnel who habitually expose their hands to x-ray energy and technicians who paint radium watch dials [*see Figure 2b*].

Histologically, squamous cell lesions are characterized by masses of squamous epithelium that invade downward through the dermis in a palisade arrangement. The degree of epithelial differentiation determines the grade of the tumor. This grade is measured as a ratio of atypical cells to normal cells. In higher grades of tumor (i.e., those with a high degree of biologic aggressiveness), differentiation and keratinization are greatly diminished.[1] Anaplastic (i.e., undifferentiated) tumors may require further characterization. The presence of cytokeratin antibodies (indicative of squamous cells) or antibody to S100 protein (which may identify melanocytes, indicative of melanoma) may also help in assessing the more anaplastic tumors. Immunoperoxidase staining may help distinguish between the desmoplastic variety of melanoma and certain squamous cell cancers.[1,17] Differentiation of a squamous cell cancer, depth of invasion, and the presence of perineural invasion correlate with biologic aggressiveness.[1]

Clinically, the lesion may appear as a gradually enlarging, nonhealing, nontender sore [see Figure 2c], or it may present as an actinic patch—typically on the cheek or the external ear [see Figure 2d]. Tumors that arise in old scars or open wounds are characteristically aggressive. Squamous cell carcinomas that develop from Marjolin's ulcer (which arises in burn scars and open wounds such as osteomyelitis drainage sites) are characterized by extreme aggressiveness after surgical resection; this aggressive behavior may be attributable to the relatively immunologically privileged status of the tumors before extirpation. Surgical excision seems to activate certain lesions. Although the lesion may have remained indolent for many years, tumor recurrence and metastasis are common after treatment.[18,19]

Certain areas of the body are especially prone to early metastases and have a higher risk of regional nodal metastases. For example, squamous cell cancers of the scalp, nose, and extremities seem to metastasize early. Regional metastases are associated with a poorer prognosis.[1,20]

Bowen disease, a carcinoma in situ, presents as a red patch or plaque with small areas of crusting. The recommended treatment is wide-margin (0.5 to 1.0 cm) surgical excision.[16]

Malignant Melanoma

Although the clinical course of malignant melanoma is characteristically unpredictable, treatment strategies for primary lesions and nodal drainage systems can be developed with the assistance of some important prognostic markers: the thickness of the lesion (Breslow thickness) and the depth of

tissue invasion (Clark level)[21] [see Melanoma Staging, below]. Melanomas tend to grow both vertically and radially; those that have a rapid onset in the vertical phase present as thicker lesions and have a worse prognosis.[22]

Over the past 40 years, the incidence of melanoma has increased; it is now the most rapidly increasing cancer among white males and the fourth most rapidly increasing cancer among white females.[23] Despite the poor prognosis associated with melanoma, survival after therapy has improved over the past 50 years. Some innovative and exciting immunotherapeutic strategies have been attempted, but the viable treatment options remain exclusively surgical.

As with other dermal neoplasms, a positive correlation is seen between sun exposure and the incidence of malignant melanoma. Some 98% of melanomas occur in whites, and within this population, the lighter-skinned persons are most at risk. Painful, blistering sunburns, early childhood exposure,[24] and sun-induced freckling are associated with a two to three times higher risk of cutaneous melanoma.[25]

DIFFERENTIAL CHARACTERISTICS OF BENIGN NEVI AND MALIGNANT MELANOMA

Unfortunately, the clinical presentation of malignant and benign pigmented lesions can be quite similar [see Figure 3]. However, certain differences do exist that can be helpful in making the distinction. For example, benign lesions tend to be less than 1 cm in diameter and have regular borders, a homogeneous color, and a smooth texture. Malignant lesions, on the other hand, are often larger, exhibit variable pigmentation and irregular borders, and are less orderly in their presentation.

Benign Nevi

Benign nevi, the most common pigmented lesions, are divided into three major histologic groups: (1) junctional, (2) compound, and (3) dermal. This classification, though arbitrary, refers to characteristic features of acquired melanocytic nevi.

Junctional nevi are the earliest stage of intraepidermal proliferation, the stage in which cells form nests along the dermal-

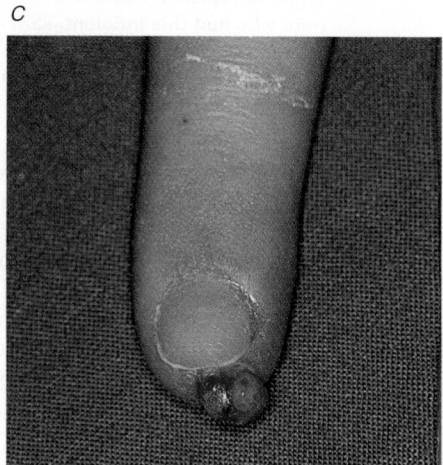

Figure 3 (a) Benign keratoacanthoma, such as this one on the hand of a 67-year-old man, is a rapidly growing lesion that can be mistaken for a malignancy. (b) This dark lesion on the distal ulnar area of a 31-year-old man, a posttraumatic arteriovenous fistula, is similar in appearance to a pigmented dermal lesion. (c) This rapidly growing pyogenic granuloma on the index finger of a 24-year-old woman developed after a small skin wound; microscopically, the lesion represents granulation tissue.

a

b

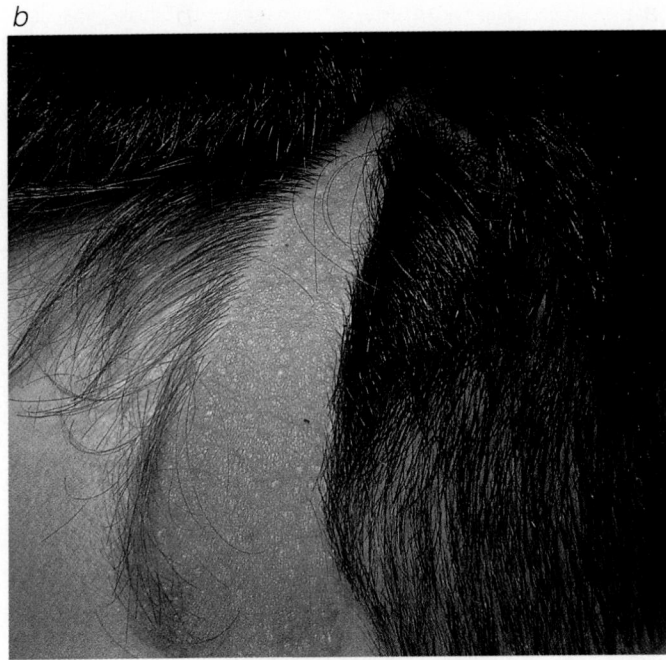

Figure 4 (*a*) **This nevus on the thigh of an infant is problematic because of its congenital nature. (*b*) This sebaceous nevus, or Jadassohn-Tièche nevus, involving the temporal scalp in a 19-year-old white man may undergo malignant change.**

epidermal junction. These lesions are relatively sessile and have a homogeneous, brownish pigmentation. Junctional nevi are characteristically smooth and have round or oval borders. They usually appear after 3 years of age and before adolescence, darken with the onset of puberty or pregnancy, and gradually fade in color and decrease in height in the later years of life. Compound nevi have junctional as well as dermal components. Dermal nevi are slightly raised, homogeneous in pigmentation, and well circumscribed, but they are confined to the dermis histologically.[26] Any lesion that tends to drift from this natural history should be regarded with suspicion, especially in the years after adolescence [*see Figure 4*].

Certain lesions, including dysplastic nevi, have a higher risk for malignant transformation.[27] The familial dysplastic nevus syndrome is characterized by an autosomal dominant pattern and a unique histologic appearance. Dysplastic nevi are typically larger than ordinary nevi, and significantly, their borders and color are irregular. Over time, dysplastic nevi progress to melanoma.

Malignant Melanoma

Malignant melanoma is characterized by radial and vertical growth phases.[21,22,26] During the radial growth phase, melanocytes within the epidermis and papillary dermis grow in all directions. The result is slow radial enlargement of the lesion. Vertical growth, which usually follows the radial growth phase, consists of growth perpendicular to the direction of growth that occurred in the radial phase. This pattern is characterized by deep invasion and subsequent development of metastases.

Three types of melanoma are clinically distinguishable [*see Figure 5*]. Superficial spreading melanoma is the most common type of melanoma, and it may arise in a preexisting nevus. The less common nodular melanoma usually exhibits more rapid and aggressive growth. Nodular melanoma is not usually associated with preexisting nevi, is more common in males, has

a higher incidence in middle age, and typically presents over the trunk, head, and neck.[26] Lentigo malignant melanoma represents only 7% to 8% of all melanomas.[28,29] It presents in older patients and tends to be indolent. Lentigo malignant melanoma was originally described by Hutchinson in 1894, and although it has been termed Hutchinson's freckle—a name that implies benignity—the lesion does have clear malignant potential.

MELANOMA STAGING

The most common criteria for the staging of melanomas are the classification systems formulated by Clark and Breslow.

Clark categorized tumors according to their level of invasion into five separate regions [*see Figure 6*]. Clark level I, in which the tumor involves the epidermis, is essentially carcinoma in situ. Level II indicates extension of the tumor into the papillary dermis. Level III signifies a spreading of tumor cells along the papillary-reticular dermal interface. Level IV indicates invasion into the reticular dermis. Level V indicates extension into the subcutaneous tissue. According to Clark's criteria, survival decreases as the depth of invasion increases.[30]

Clark's dermal layers may be cumbersome, but the Breslow thickness provides comparable therapeutic and prognostic discrimination. Breslow classified the level of invasion by using an ocular micrometer to measure from the granular layer in the epidermis to the deepest point of invasion in the dermis. Under Breslow's criteria, thin melanomas invade 0.75 mm or less into the dermis (stage IA, T1). Intermediate-thickness melanomas invade 0.76 to 3.99 mm; these are further subdivided into thin intermediate melanomas of 0.76 to 1.49 mm (stage IB, T2), intermediate intermediate melanomas of 1.5 to 2.49 mm (stage IIA, T3a), and thick intermediate melanomas of 2.5 mm to 3.99 mm (stage IIA, T3b). Thick melanomas invade 4.0 mm and deeper (stage IIB, T4).[31]

It is important to note that any suspicious lesion should initially be removed by means of a full-thickness excisional biop-

a

b

c

d

e

f

Figure 5 (*a*) This melanoma, on the sole of the foot of a 47-year-old black woman, shows irregularities in shape, contour, and pigmentation. (*b*) A so-called halo effect is visible along the left margin of this melanoma on the upper back of a 33-year-old white woman; irregularities in shape, contour, and pigmentation are also evident. (*c*) This melanoma of the postauricular scalp in a 56-year-old man exhibited ulceration and new growth (*d*) over the lower portion of the lesion 2 weeks later. (*e*) This melanoma on the thigh of a 31-year-old woman shows a slightly umbilicated center, irregular shape, and nonhomogeneous coloration. (*f*) This melanoma of the lower eyelid in another patient is visible as the darkly pigmented area just below the eyelashes.

Figure 6 Clark categorized skin tumors according to their level of invasion. Tumors of level I involve the epidermis and are essentially carcinoma in situ. In level II, the tumor has extended into the papillary dermis. Tumor cells at level III are spread along the papillary-reticular dermal interface. Invasion into the reticular dermis occurs at level IV. Level V tumors extend into the subcutaneous tissue. In general, survival decreases as the depth of invasion increases.

CLARK'S LEVELS

Epidermis

Papillary Dermis

Reticular Dermis

Subcutaneous Fat

sy. This diagnostic excisional biopsy may be close, encompassing as little as a 1 mm margin of normal skin. Sharp dissection into and including a portion of subcutaneous fat will enable accurate histologic (depth and levels) staging. Shave biopsies must always be condemned because depth cannot be assessed.

Lymphatic Mapping and Sentinel Lymph Node Biopsy

Technological advances have made it possible for surgeons to identify the general characteristics of lymphatic flow and intercept early metastatic tissue by performing lymphatic mapping and SLN biopsy. The rationale, techniques, and indications for this valuable procedure are discussed more fully elsewhere [*see V:3 Lymphatic Mapping and Sentinel Lymph Node Biopsy*], with particular reference to its use in patients with breast cancer or melanoma. In our unit, we now routinely employ lymphatic mapping and SLN biopsy for biopsy-proven melanomas, squamous cell carcinomas (especially large neurotropic ones), and Merkel cell carcinomas. Our usual practice is to use a combination of isosulfan blue dye and unfiltered technetium-labeled sulfur colloid.

TREATMENT

Effective treatment of melanoma remains exclusively surgical. Initial complete excision is the therapeutic goal. Thin melanomas can be safely excised with surgical margins of only 1 cm.[32,33] However, the appropriate margins for excision of intermediate-thickness lesions remain a matter of controversy.

The benefit of prophylactic regional node dissections in patients with intermediate-thickness lesions and nonpalpable nodes is also controversial. Prospective, randomized trials and a mathematical model indicate no survival benefit with elective lymph node dissection compared with subsequent so-called therapeutic regional lymphadenectomy only when nodes become palpable.[34,35] Intraoperative lymphatic mapping and selective lymphadenectomy may be warranted in a case-specific approach.[36]

Patients with intermediate-thickness tumors (between 0.76 and 3.99 mm) may benefit if an elective regional lymph node dissection (of nonpalpable nodes) is included in their initial surgical management. Benefit has also been shown with the use of elective regional lymph node dissection for the treatment of thick melanomas (4 mm and greater) and thin intermediate melanomas (between 0.76 mm and 1.49 mm) in men.[37] However, a clear understanding of the influence of other important factors, such as previous treatment, age, presence of comorbid disease, and location of the primary lesion, awaits the results of ongoing trials. In addition to providing local control, removal of lymph nodes may find its greatest utility in accurate pathologic staging.[38-40] Many aspects of this therapeutic approach remain controversial.[41]

Patients who have N1 or N2 regional node involvement traditionally have an unfavorable outcome but may benefit from isolated limb perfusion or limb infusion. Several investigators have reported increased survival rates in such patients with the use of isolated limb perfusion.[42] Perfusion with tumor necrosis factor–α appears to yield high local response rates, but the associated toxicity is high.[43] Intralesional immunotherapy, local radiation therapy, and systemic chemotherapy are options for the control of recurrent local lesions.[21] Unfortunately, regional disease develops within 3 years in all patients with thick melanomas (4 mm and greater) and stage IIIA disease, and distant metastases develop within 5 years in more than 60% of these patients.[30,31,37]

Although one might expect that patients with malignancies that have a high incidence of systemic involvement might benefit from adjuvant therapy, none has been proved to be uniformly effective. Allogeneic tumor vaccines (comprising a mixture of different tumor antigens) and other immunostimulation strategies are being studied in clinical trials.[21]

Trials of newer agents for the treatment of stage IV melanoma (involving distant metastases) have been disappointing. Studies of interleukin-2 (IL-2) immunotherapy for metastatic disease, both alone and with lymphokine-activated killer cells (LAK cells, or lymphocytes grown in IL-2), show potential rewards. IL-2 appears to have a 10% to 25% response rate in metastatic melanoma. Unfortunately, fewer than 50% of the responses are complete, and most are of limited duration. IL-2 is currently approved only for the treatment of renal cell cancer. IL-2 and other cytokines in combination with chemotherapeutic agents have generally shown little increase in benefit while carrying higher toxicity. IL-12, a macrophage-derived cytokine, enhances cellular immunity and may soon enter clinical trials.[21,44,45]

Certain melanoma surface antigens may be common to other tumors and may be recognized in an HLA class I molecule–restricted fashion. Melanoma patients who are HLA A1 positive (26% of all whites) and whose tumors contain *MAGE-1* (a tumor gene found in melanoma and other human tumors) could be immunized against their tumors with cytotoxic T cells sensitized to the melanoma cell surface antigen or against *MAGE-1* alone. Vaccinia recognizance (viral) vectors incorporating this *MAGE-1* gene are already being prepared for clinical trials.[21]

Surgical Technique

EXCISIONAL BIOPSY

The biopsy can often be performed in the clinic operating room with the patient under local anesthesia. Care should be taken to avoid injecting the lesion itself because the resulting bleeding may distort the histologic fixation of the specimen. A field block is usually sufficient.

Attention to proper surgical technique will prevent the spread of cancer cells and allow the pathologist sufficient tissue to make an accurate diagnosis. For the histologic diagnosis and staging of all skin lesions, the surgeon should submit at least a full-thickness portion of the lesion and preferably perform an excisional biopsy. With a larger tumor, it is important to incorporate a representative portion of the lesion with 1 mm of normal skin at the margin so that the pathologist can examine the skin adjacent to the neoplasm. Diagnostic biopsies should not be allowed to be damaged by electrocauterization. It is important to orient and mark the specimen properly so that the adequacy of the margins can be studied in relation to the overall anatomy.

Thus, the initial biopsy should include at least 1 mm of normal skin, and the surgeon should take care to perform a full-thickness excision into the fat. The tissue is gently retracted as the incision is continued around the lesion. Before the lesion is removed from the field, an orientation suture is placed. My preference is to make a small drawing on the pathology sheet, indicating where the suture is located in relation to the site on the body from which the lesion came. For example, a suture is placed at 12 o'clock, a small drawing is made of the patient's hand or face, and the specimen is sketched on the drawing itself. This allows the pathologist to identify and localize any margin that exhibits microscopic involvement with tumor cells. Similarly, excision of a segment of subcutaneous fat allows the pathologist to assess depth of invasion.

SUPERFICIAL AND RADICAL GROIN DISSECTIONS

The inguinal nodes drain the anterior and inferior abdominal wall, the perineum, the genitalia, the hips, the buttocks, and the thighs. A superficial groin dissection removes the inguinal nodes, whereas a radical dissection additionally incorporates the iliac and obturator nodes. Palpable nodes can be marked on the patient before operation. Photography can be very helpful for both orientation and documentation.

In cases of skin lesions overlying the anteromedial portion of the thigh, the primary excision can often incorporate an in-continuity groin dissection that is designed to eradicate the primary tumor along with the lymphatic drainage system.[46] As a general principle, the skin lesion, the subcutaneous fat, the lymphatic tissue, and the investing fascia are removed as a unit.

Technique

The patient is usually placed in a supine position on the operating table, with the hip slightly abducted and supported by a pillow and with the hip and knee slightly flexed. A Foley catheter is inserted, the patient is prepared and draped, and the drapes are stapled in position.

A wide ellipse (4 cm margin) incorporating the skin lesion is marked. The femoral artery is palpated and marked, and a diagonally oriented skin incision is planned. The incision will course from the region of the anterosuperior iliac spine, caudally over the central groin region, and through the femoral trigone, terminating at midthigh level on the anteromedial surface of the thigh. This incision interferes least with the musculocutaneous and cutaneous vascular territories of the skin, usually avoids ischemia to the skin, and promotes subsequent healing. The incision is made with a scalpel, and the electrocautery is employed sparingly. The initial incision should include the skin and subcutaneous fat and continue down through the deep investing fascia overlying the muscle. The dissection proceeds downward in a caudal direction, incorporating the fascia and exposing the inguinal ligament, the deep fascia, and the femoral vessels. Fat and nodal tissue are dissected off the external oblique aponeurosis, the spermatic cord, and the inguinal ligament [see Figure 7]. The superficial fascia over the vessels is removed, together with the fat and the contents of the femoral trigone, proceeding from lateral to medial. The femoral vessels and the femoral nerve are left undisturbed, and the dissection proceeds to the fossa ovalis femoris. The great saphenous vein is incorporated into the specimen, ligated by a suture at its junction with the femoral vein [see Figure 7]. The fascia is removed from the sartorius muscle, the adductor muscle

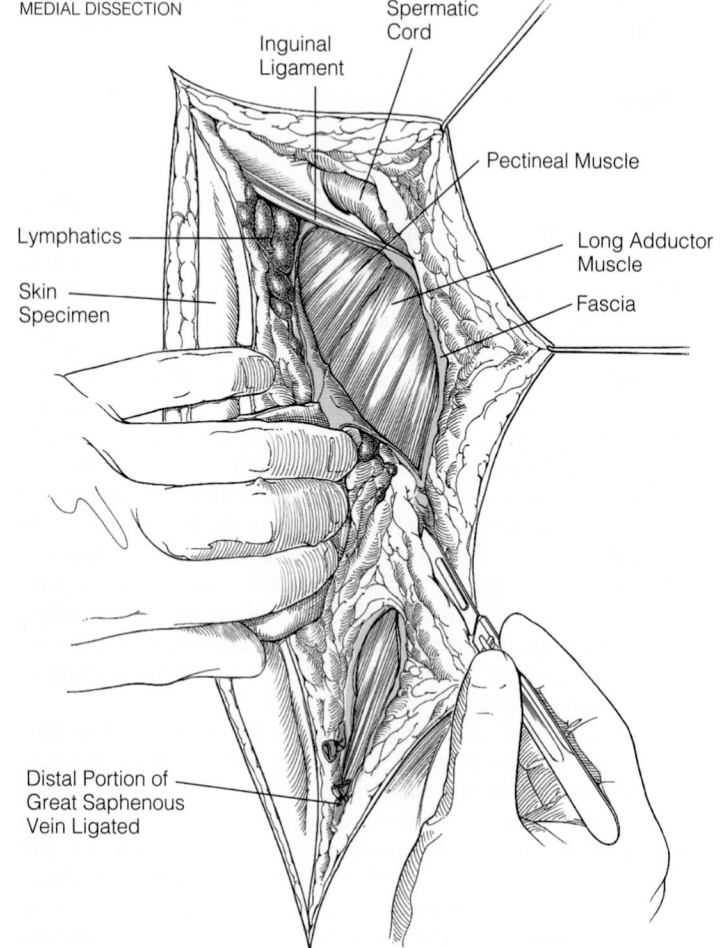

MEDIAL DISSECTION

Inguinal Ligament

Spermatic Cord

Pectineal Muscle

Long Adductor Muscle

Fascia

Lymphatics

Skin Specimen

Distal Portion of Great Saphenous Vein Ligated

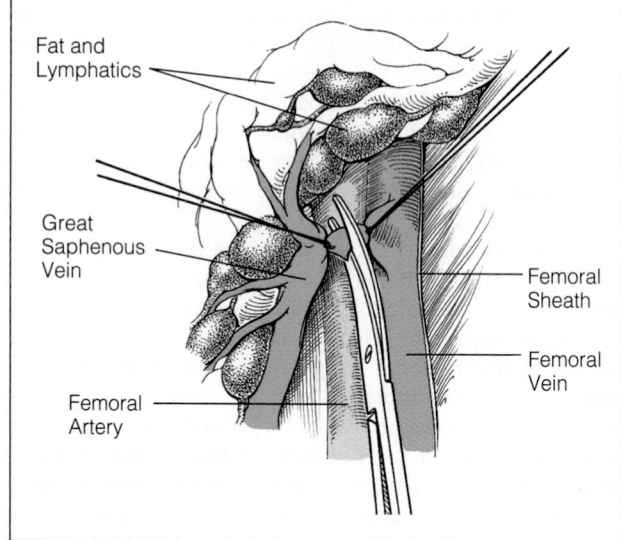

Fat and Lymphatics

Great Saphenous Vein

Femoral Artery

Femoral Sheath

Femoral Vein

Figure 7 In a superficial groin dissection, the incision is deepened to include the deep muscular fascia. The great saphenous vein is ligated and divided (inset).

Figure 8 **As the superficial groin dissection proceeds, the investing fascia overlying the femoral nerve and vessels is removed.**

Specimen Retracted

Inguinal Ligament

Lymphatics Continue under Inguinal Ligament Medial to Femoral Vein

Great Saphenous Vein Stump

Pectineal Muscle

Femoral Sheath Being Entered

Fascia

LATERAL DISSECTION

Iliopsoas Muscle through Fascia

Fascia

Branch of Femoral Nerve

Sartorius Muscle

Figure 9 **The superficial groin dissection is continued at the same level on the lateral side.**

group, and the rectus femoris, with all lymphatic tissue included in the surgical specimen [*see Figures 8 and 9*]. The dissection proceeds medially to the medial aspect of the femoral trigone. This completes the superficial portion of the groin dissection.

If the surgeon decides to perform a radical (ilioinguinal) node dissection, the incision is extended through the inguinal ligament, beginning medial to the anterosuperior iliac spine and continuing to a point approximately 2 cm lateral to the femoral artery. The inguinal canal is further exposed by releasing the internal oblique abdominal muscle, the transversus abdominis, and the fascia transversalis and dissecting into the retroperitoneal space. The deep circumflex iliac vessels are ligated, and blunt finger dissection separates the peritoneum from the preperitoneal fat and nodes.

Retractors are inserted to widen the retroperitoneal space, and the peritoneum and the abdominal viscera are retracted medially. The chain of lymph nodes, areolar tissue, and adventitial tissues along the external iliac vessels is dissected; the dissection proceeds proximally to the origins of the internal iliac vessels and incorporates the nodes overlying the obturator foramen by removing the internal obturator fascia. The deep epigastric vessels are usually ligated at their origins from the external iliac artery and vein. The lymph node–bearing specimen is then removed as a unit, oriented, and labeled appropriately with sutures. The inguinal canal is reconstructed to prevent a hernia, and the sartorius muscle is mobilized to the midportion of the wound to cover the femoral vessels. The skin and the subcutaneous tissues are then closed in layers over a soft suction drain.

References

1. Cottel WI: Skin tumors: basal cell and squamous cell carcinoma. Selected Readings in Plastic Surgery 7(6):1, 1992

2. Silverberg E, Lubera J: Cancer statistics. CA Cancer J Clin 39:3, 1989

3. Cancer of the Skin. Friedman RJ, Rigel DS, Kopf AW, et al, Eds. WB Saunders Co, Philadelphia, 1991

4. Koh HK, Kligler BE, Lew RA: Sunlight and cutaneous malignant melanoma: evidence for and against causation. Photochem Photobiol 51:765, 1990

5. Green HA, Drake L: Aging, sun damage, and sunscreens. Clin Plast Surg 20:1, 1993

6. Urbach F: Geographic distribution of skin cancer. J Surg Oncol 3:219, 1971

7. Dellon AL: Host-tumor relationship in basal cell and squamous cell cancer of the skin. Plast Reconstr Surg 62:37, 1978

8. Marshall V: Premalignant and malignant skin tumors in immunosuppressed patients. Transplantation 17: 272, 1974

9. Wade TR, Ackerman AB: The many faces of basal cell carcinoma. J Dermatol Surg Oncol 4:23, 1978

10. Salasche SJ, Amonette RA: Morpheaform basal cell epitheliomas: a study of subclinical extension in a series of 51 cases. J Dermatol Surg Oncol 7:387, 1981

11. Shanoff LB, Spira M, Hardy SB: Basal cell carcinoma: a statistical approach to rational management. Plast Reconstr Surg 39:619, 1967

12. Bart RS, Kopf AW, Peratos MA: X-ray therapy of skin cancer: evaluation of a "standardized" method for treating basal cell carcinoma. Fifth National Cancer Conference. JB Lippincott, Philadelphia, 1970, p 559

13. Mohs FE: Chemosurgery: microscopically controlled methods of cancer excision. Arch Surg 42:279, 1941

14. Robinson JK: Mohs micrographic surgery. Clin Plast Surg 20:149, 1993

15. Brownstein MH, Rabinowitz AD: The precursors of cutaneous squamous cell carcinoma. Int J Dermatol 18:1, 1979

16. Albricht SM: Treatment of malignant cutaneous tumors. Clin Plast Surg 20:167, 1993

17. Kohn H, Baumal R, From L: Role of immunohistochemistry in the diagnosis of undifferentiated tumors involving the skin. J Am Acad Dermatol 14:1063, 1986

18. Bostwick J, Pendergrast J, Vasconez L: Marjolin's ulcer: an immunologically privileged tumor? Plast Reconstr Surg 57:66, 1976

19. Traves N, Pack GT: The development of cancer in burn scars: analysis and report of 34 cases. Surg Gynecol Obstet 51:749, 1930

20. Ames FC, Hickey RC: Metastasis from squamous cell skin cancer of the extremities. South Med J 75: 920, 1982

21. Vetto J: Advances in the Therapy of Malignant Melanoma (monograph). Department of Surgery, Oregon Health Sciences University, Portland, Oregon, 1994

22. Morton DL, Dartyan DG, Wanek LA, et al: Multivariate analysis of the relationship between survival and the microstage of primary melanoma by Clark level and Breslow thickness. Cancer 71:3737, 1993

23. Koh HK: Cutaneous melanoma. N Engl J Med 325: 171, 1991

24. Armstrong BK: Epidemiology of malignant melanoma: intermittent or total accumulated exposure to the sun. J Dermatol Surg Oncol 14:835, 1988

25. Lew RA, Saber AJ, Cook N, et al: Sun exposure habits in patients with cutaneous melanoma: a case control study. J Dermatol Surg Oncol 9:981, 1983

26. Evans GR, Manson PN: Review and current perspectives of cutaneous malignant melanoma. J Am Coll Surg 178:523, 1994

27. Anderson RG: Skin tumors II: melanoma. Selected Readings in Plastic Surgery 7(7):1, 1992

28. Mihm MC, Clark WH, From L: The clinical diagnosis, classification, and histogenic concepts of the early stages of cutaneous melanoma. N Engl J Med 284: 1078, 1971

29. Friedman RJ, Rigel DS, Silverman MK, et al: Malignant melanoma in the 1990's: the continued importance of early detection and the role of physician examinations and self-examination of the skin. CA Cancer J Clin 41:201, 1991

30. Clark WH, From L, Bernardino EA, et al: The histogenesis and biologic behavior of primary human malignant melanomas of the skin. Cancer Res 29:705, 1969

31. Breslow A: Thickness, cross-sectional areas and depth of invasion in the prognosis of cutaneous melanoma. Ann Surg 172:902, 1970

32. Balch CM, Murad TM, Soong S, et al: Tumor thickness as a guide to surgical management of clinical stage I melanoma patients. Cancer 43:883, 1979

33. Veronisi U, Cascinelli N, Adamus J, et al: Thin stage I primary cutaneous malignant melanoma: comparison of excision with margins of 1 or 3 cm. N Engl J Med 318:1159, 1988

34. Sim FH, Taylor WF, Prichard DC, et al: Lymphadenectomy in the management of stage I malignant melanoma: a prospective randomized study. Mayo Clin Proc 61:697, 1986

35. Veronesi U, Adamus J, Bandiera DC, et al: Delayed regional lymph node dissection in stage I melanoma of the skin and lower extremities. Cancer 49:2420, 1982

36. Morton DL, Wen DR, Wong JH, et al: Technical details of intraoperative lymphatic mapping for early stage melanoma. Arch Surg 127:392, 1992

37. Balch CM, Soong SJ, Milton GW, et al: A comparison of prognostic factors and surgical results in 1,786 patients with localized (stage I) melanoma treated in Alabama, USA, and New South Wales, Australia. Ann Surg 196:677, 1982

38. Crowley NJ: The case against elective lymphadenectomy. Surg Oncol Clin North Am 1:223, 1992

39. Coates AS, Ingvar CI, Petersen-Schaefer K, et al: Elective lymph node dissection in patients with primary melanoma of the trunk and limbs treated at the Sydney melanoma unit from 1960 to 1991. J Am Coll Surg 180:402, 1995

40. Krag DN, Meijer SJ, Weaver DL, et al: Minimal-access surgery for staging of malignant melanoma. Arch Surg 130:654, 1995

41. Vetto J: Elective lymph node dissection for intermediate thickness melanoma: does it have a future? Clin Oncol Alert 11:6, 1996

42. Hartley JW, Fletcher WS: Improved survival of patients with stage II melanoma of the extremity using hyperthermic isolation perfusion with 1-phenylalanine mustard. J Surg Oncol 36:170, 1987

43. Lienard D, Lejeune FJ, Ewalenko P: In transit metastases of malignant melanoma treated by high dose rTNF-α in combination with interferon-gamma and melphalan isolation perfusion. World J Surg 16:234, 1992

44. Rosenberg SA, Lotze MT, Yang JC, et al: Prospective trial of high-dose interleukin-2 alone or in conjunction with lymphokine-activated killer cells for the treatment of patients with advanced cancer. J Natl Cancer Inst 85:622, 1993

45. Nastala CL, Edington HD, Storkus WJ, et al: Recombinant interleukin-12 (r-mil-12) mediates regression of both subcutaneous and metastatic murine tumors. Surg Forum 44:518, 1993

46. Karakousis CP: Technique of lymphadenectomy for melanoma. Surg Oncol Clin North Am 1:157, 1992

Recommended Reading

Cancer Facts and Figures—2001. American Cancer Society, New York, 2001

Hallock GG, Lutz DA: A prospective study of the accuracy of the surgeon's diagnosis and significance of positive margins in nonmelanoma skin cancers. Plast Reconstr Surg 107:942, 2001

Mathes SJ, Eriksson E, McGrath MH, et al: Management of cutaneous malignancies. Contemp Surg 49:307, 1996

Acknowledgments

Figures 7 through 9   Susan E. Brust, C.M.I.

The author is grateful to John Vetto, M.D., and Paul Manson, M.D., for their suggestions in the preparation of this chapter.

11 SOFT TISSUE INFECTION

Ronald T. Lewis, M.B.B.S., M.Sc.

Approach to the Patient with Soft Tissue Infection

The key to successful treatment of soft tissue infection is early recognition of infections that require prompt surgical drainage and debridement. It is convenient to classify lesions into those that are focal, such as cutaneous abscesses and pyoderma gangrenosum, and those that are diffuse and often require emergency treatment, such as cellulitis and necrotizing cellulitic infections. (There are also certain miscellaneous conditions, such as bite wound infections and purpura fulminans, that do not fit neatly into either category; these conditions are considered separately.) Many lesions appear deceptively innocent at first and are mistaken for nonspecific inflammation. To prompt recognition and effective treatment of any lesion, the answers to five questions should be sought:

1. Is infection present?
2. Is there an underlying systemic condition present that favors infection?
3. Should antibiotics be given?
4. Which antibiotics are most appropriate?
5. Is surgical treatment required?

Focal Inflammation

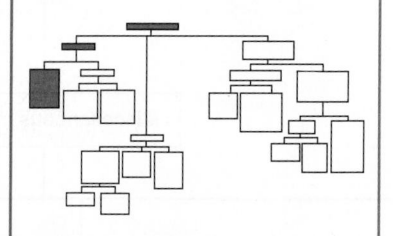

The history together with the clinical appearance of a focal lesion will indicate whether it is a minor, confined cutaneous abscess or a more serious, spreading focal lesion such as pyoderma gangrenosum. Cutaneous abscesses are very common and are readily recognized. Pyoderma gangrenosum, on the other hand, is a rare condition.

CONFINED CUTANEOUS ABSCESS

A cutaneous abscess is a walled-off collection of pus that presents as a painful fluctuant mass, usually with surrounding erythema and firm granulation tissue. It is treated by incision and drainage. Gram stain and culture of the pus are not done routinely, because antibiotics are not generally given. Antibiotics may be helpful, however, in immunocompromised patients and in patients with abscesses of the central area of the face. In such cases, the findings on Gram stain suggest appropriate antibiotic therapy. Gram-positive cocci in clusters indicate *Staphylococcus aureus,* which may be treated with an oral semisynthetic penicillin (e.g., cloxacillin, 0.5 to 1.0 g every 6 hours for 5 to 7 days). Mixed gram-positive and gram-negative bacilli represent an infection by aerobic and anaerobic organisms that can be treated with an oral cephalosporin (e.g., cephalexin, 0.5 g every 6 hours for 5 to 7 days). Occasionally, white blood cells but no organisms are seen. This finding confirms a sterile abscess, for which antibiotics are not needed.

SPREADING FOCAL LESION

Classic Pyoderma Gangrenosum

Classic pyoderma gangrenosum is characterized by a painful, raised pustular lesion that progresses to spreading ulceration with a typical necrotic center, bluish undermined edges, and surrounding erythema [*see Figure 1*].[1] It occurs either singly or in groups, most often on the legs. The lesions may localize at sites of minor trauma (so-called pathergy). Fever, malaise, myalgias, and arthralgias are common. A biopsy is usually performed to rule out disorders that produce similar lesions: ischemic ulceration, vasculitis of periarteritis nodosa, and chronic bacterial, mycobacterial, or fungal disorders. Massive neutrophil infiltration and necrosis of the epidermis are typical. In contrast with vasculitis, only minor vessel wall infiltration is present with pyoderma gangrenosum. Underlying disease, often parainflammatory or hemoproliferative, is present in 60% to 80% of cases.[2] The most common concomitant conditions are inflammatory bowel disease (especially ulcerative colitis),[1] polyarthritis,[3] monoclonal gammopathy,[4] and malignant hematologic neoplasms (especially leukemia).[5] Four variants have been identified: peristomal (seen, for example, in Crohn disease); vulvar or penoscrotal, simulating the lesions of Behçet disease; oral (peristomatitis vegetans); and bullous. The skin le-

Figure 1 **In this photograph of an advanced pyoderma gangrenosum lesion, the darker area surrounding the necrotic center corresponds to the violaceous zone of intense erythema.**

311

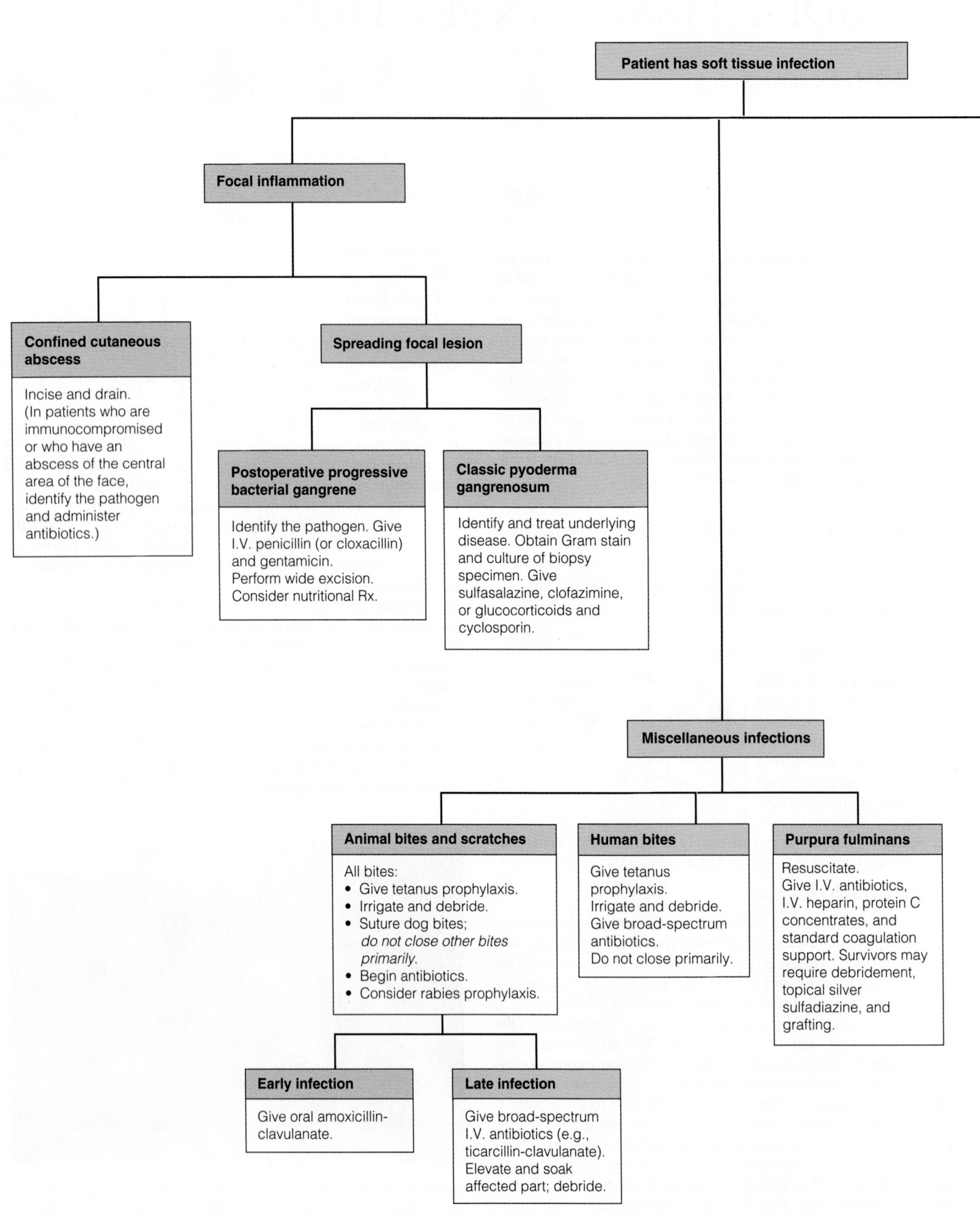

Patient has soft tissue infection

Focal inflammation

Confined cutaneous abscess

Incise and drain.
(In patients who are immunocompromised or who have an abscess of the central area of the face, identify the pathogen and administer antibiotics.)

Spreading focal lesion

Postoperative progressive bacterial gangrene

Identify the pathogen. Give I.V. penicillin (or cloxacillin) and gentamicin.
Perform wide excision.
Consider nutritional Rx.

Classic pyoderma gangrenosum

Identify and treat underlying disease. Obtain Gram stain and culture of biopsy specimen. Give sulfasalazine, clofazimine, or glucocorticoids and cyclosporin.

Miscellaneous infections

Animal bites and scratches

All bites:
• Give tetanus prophylaxis.
• Irrigate and debride.
• Suture dog bites; *do not close other bites primarily.*
• Begin antibiotics.
• Consider rabies prophylaxis.

Human bites

Give tetanus prophylaxis.
Irrigate and debride.
Give broad-spectrum antibiotics.
Do not close primarily.

Purpura fulminans

Resuscitate.
Give I.V. antibiotics, I.V. heparin, protein C concentrates, and standard coagulation support. Survivors may require debridement, topical silver sulfadiazine, and grafting.

Early infection

Give oral amoxicillin-clavulanate.

Late infection

Give broad-spectrum I.V. antibiotics (e.g., ticarcillin-clavulanate). Elevate and soak affected part; debride.

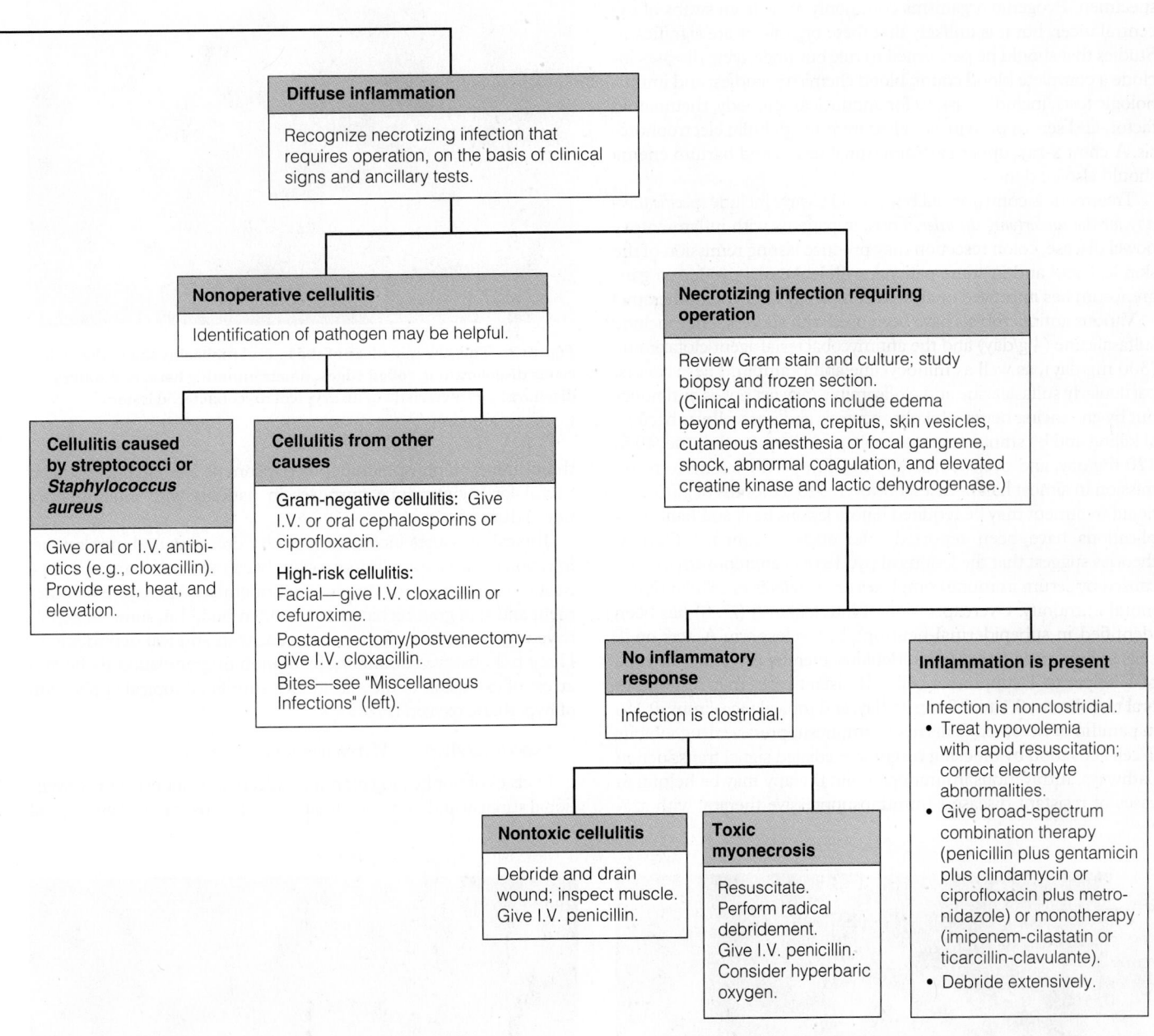

Diffuse inflammation

Recognize necrotizing infection that requires operation, on the basis of clinical signs and ancillary tests.

Nonoperative cellulitis

Identification of pathogen may be helpful.

Cellulitis caused by streptococci or *Staphylococcus aureus*

Give oral or I.V. antibiotics (e.g., cloxacillin). Provide rest, heat, and elevation.

Cellulitis from other causes

Gram-negative cellulitis: Give I.V. or oral cephalosporins or ciprofloxacin.

High-risk cellulitis:
Facial—give I.V. cloxacillin or cefuroxime.
Postadenectomy/postvenectomy—give I.V. cloxacillin.
Bites—see "Miscellaneous Infections" (left).

Necrotizing infection requiring operation

Review Gram stain and culture; study biopsy and frozen section.
(Clinical indications include edema beyond erythema, crepitus, skin vesicles, cutaneous anesthesia or focal gangrene, shock, abnormal coagulation, and elevated creatine kinase and lactic dehydrogenase.)

No inflammatory response

Infection is clostridial.

Nontoxic cellulitis

Debride and drain wound; inspect muscle. Give I.V. penicillin.

Toxic myonecrosis

Resuscitate.
Perform radical debridement.
Give I.V. penicillin.
Consider hyperbaric oxygen.

Inflammation is present

Infection is nonclostridial.
• Treat hypovolemia with rapid resuscitation; correct electrolyte abnormalities.
• Give broad-spectrum combination therapy (penicillin plus gentamicin plus clindamycin or ciprofloxacin plus metronidazole) or monotherapy (imipenem-cilastatin or ticarcillin-clavulante).
• Debride extensively.

Approach to the Patient with Soft Tissue Infection

sion seen in leukemia is typically the bullous variant: it remains superficial and exhibits more subdued colors than the classic lesion. About 30% of cases are idiopathic and remain so on follow-up of more than 2 years.[6]

Investigations should include Gram stain and culture of a biopsy specimen. Pyogenic organisms commonly grow from swabs of the central ulcer, but it is unlikely that these organisms are significant. Studies that should be performed to rule out underlying diseases include a complete blood count; blood chemistry studies; and immunologic tests, including assays for antinuclear antibody, rheumatoid factor, and serum protein as well as immunoglobulin electrophoresis. A chest x-ray, upper gastrointestinal series, and barium enema should also be done.

Treatment is controversial but should always include *specific therapy for the underlying disorder.* Thus, in patients with inflammatory bowel disease, colon resection may produce lasting remission of the skin lesions,[2] and in some patients with leukemia, pyoderma gangrenosum has improved or cleared completely after chemotherapy.[5]

Various antimicrobials have been used with success. They include sulfasalazine (4 g/day) and the antimycobacterial agent clofazimine (300 mg/day), as well as minocycline and rifampin. These agents, particularly sulfasalazine and clofazimine, may act not as antibiotics but by enhancing neutrophil phagocytosis and intracellular bacterial killing and by stimulating macrophage activity. Prednisone, 40 to 120 mg/day, and cyclosporin A, 5 mg/day, produce long-term remission in almost half of cases; however, 3 to 6 months of glucocorticoid treatment may be required before lesions heal, and fatal complications have been reported after such treatment.[3] Current theories suggest that the lesions of pyoderma gangrenosum may be caused by serum immune complexes or by defects in cellular or humoral immunity. Overexpression of interleukin-8 (IL-8) has been identified in subepidermal neutrophils. Cyclosporin A acts on T cells to limit production of interleukins, thereby reversing the ratio of T helper to T suppressor cells.[7] Resistant cases may respond to oral tacrolimus, 0.1 to 0.3 mg/kg/day, and topical tacrolimus, 0.1% in paraffin or beeswax.[8] This new immunosuppressive drug inhibits T-cell activation by blocking receptor-mediated signal transduction pathways. Intravenous immunoglobulin therapy may be helpful in cases of resistant disease.[9] Immunosuppressive therapy with aza-

Figure 2   **This chronic ulcer of the lateral malleolus shows the violaceous discoloration, rolled edges, nongranulating base, and watery discharge characteristic of an atypical mycobacterial lesion.**

thioprine, cyclophosphamide, or dapsone is less effective[10] but is useful for maintenance purposes in patients with inflammatory bowel disease.

Topical measures include wet-to-dry dressings and intralesional injection or surface application of antibacterials and immune agents. Saline compresses provide some debridement. Aggressive debridement and skin grafting have been condemned,[2] but some workers[11] have reported dramatic improvement with surgical debridement. Heng has observed abundant formation of granulation tissue and arrest of extension of ulceration by a simplified topical application of hyperbaric oxygen (HBO).[12]

Superficial Atypical Mycobacterial Lesions

In cases of nonhealing extremity ulcers unresponsive to conventional surgical and antibiotic treatment, the possibility of an atypical

Figure 3   **Progressive bacterial gangrene has developed in the decubitus ulcer shown at left. The edge of the necrotic lesion shows the three characteristic zones of necrosis, discoloration, and erythema (right).**

Figure 4 **Progressive bacterial gangrene developed in this patient's abdominal wall after cesarean section. In photograph at top, the lesion has been partially excised; extension of necrosis is evident. The lesion was widely excised (center). Extension of necrosis into the flank necessitated further excision and skin grafting (bottom); skin grafts done earlier on the central lesion are healing.**

mycobacterial infection should be considered. Although rare, indolent mycobacterial lesions that closely resemble pyoderma gangrenosum have been observed. In one study, infected ulcers in four steroid-dependent patients yielded atypical mycobacteria upon culture of the excised tissue. Two ulcers contained *Mycobacterium smegmatis*, which rarely causes disease in humans; the third, *M. kansasii;* and the fourth, *M. chelonei.*[13] The lesions presented as chronic ulcerations with violaceous edges, rolled margins, a nongranulating base, and watery discharge [*see Figure 2*]. In three of the four patients, wide local excision and intravenous antibiotic therapy followed by oral antibiotic therapy were required for successful treatment. One patient was treated successfully with debridement and oral antibiotic therapy.

Because experience in treating these ulcers has been limited, the best antibiotic therapy is uncertain. *M. kansasii* is usually sensitive to rifampin, isoniazid, and ethambutol; and *M. chelonei* is sensitive to amikacin, cefoxitin, tetracycline, and erythromycin. All three species respond well to cefoxitin (1 g every 6 hours) or to quinolones (e.g., ciprofloxacin, 0.4 g every 12 hours); accordingly, these agents should be prescribed.

Postoperative Progressive Bacterial Gangrene

The postoperative progressive bacterial gangrene of Meleney[14] is considered to be a variant of classic pyoderma gangrenosum.[11] The lesion appears 2 weeks or more after accidental trauma or after operative management of purulent peritoneal or pleural infection; it is characterized by wound edema, redness, and tenderness that progress to the three characteristic zones of pyoderma gangrenosum: a necrotic center, bluish undermined edges, and surrounding erythema [*see Figure 3*]. Fever, muscle wasting, and toxicity are often present. A swab taken from the central necrotic area usually yields hemolytic *S. aureus* on culture; later in the course of the illness, it may show gram-negative bacilli. Needle aspirate from the outer zone may grow microaerophilic nonhemolytic streptococci.

Broad-spectrum parenteral antibiotics should be started promptly and are useful in reducing systemic toxicity. Penicillin, 1 to 2 million units I.V. every 6 hours, along with gentamicin, 1.5 mg/kg every 8 hours, may be given, but if *S. aureus* is found on Gram stain, cloxacillin, 1 to 2 g every 6 hours, is substituted for penicillin. Antibiotic therapy is followed by wide excision of the skin lesion [*see Figure 4*]. The wound is left open to granulate, and skin grafts are applied later. Researchers found that HBO reduced the extent of excision required,[15,16] but the value of HBO therapy is controversial in this and other necrotizing soft tissue infections [*see Diffuse Inflammation, Inflammatory Response Is Absent (Clostridial Infection), below*]. Because these patients have marked systemic manifestations and significant muscle wasting, supportive nutritional therapy may be of benefit [*see VII:9 Nutritional Support*].

Diffuse Inflammation

NECROTIZING INFECTION REQUIRING OPERATION

In managing diffuse inflammatory lesions, it is crucial to recognize necrotizing infections promptly because they require surgical debridement. To spot a necrotizing infection, one must know the clinical setting in which it often occurs and must identify cer-

Figure 5 **Edema extending beyond the area of erythema is a marker of necrotizing soft tissue infection.**

Figure 6 **In this patient with necrotizing fasciitis, edema is present without skin vesicles, and there is necrosis of the deep layer of the superficial fascia.**

Figure 7 **Skin vesicles such as those on this patient's finger are seen early in streptococcal gangrene.**

tain clinical clues. In some cases, ancillary studies may help finalize the diagnosis. Necrotizing infections usually occur in patients with impaired host defense mechanisms, such as the elderly, those receiving immunosuppressive therapy, or those with an underlying systemic illness, such as cancer, chronic renal failure, chronic alcoholism, diabetes mellitus, or peripheral vascular disease. When cellulitis occurs in these patients, a necrotizing infection should be suspected. The initiating factor for necrotizing infections is often surprisingly minor, perhaps because of the poor host resistance. For example, necrotizing infections can occur in areas of blunt soft tissue contusion associated with a distant focus of infection.[17]

Important early clinical markers of necrotizing soft tissue infection include edema beyond the area of erythema, crepitus, and skin vesicles [*see Figures 5 through 7*]. The lymphangitis and lymphadenitis commonly seen in patients with nonoperative cellulitis are absent. In later stages of infection, cutaneous anesthesia, focal skin gangrene, shock, and impaired blood coagulation may occur.

Useful ancillary studies include soft tissue x-rays and blood chemistry studies. X-ray examination of the affected area may disclose soft tissue gas in patients in whom crepitus is not present on palpation [*see Figure 8*].[18] In addition, elevated blood levels of the muscle proteins creatine kinase and lactate dehydrogenase may suggest skeletal muscle breakdown.[19] Isoenzyme analysis may confirm the origin of these elevated enzymes.

Even in the initial absence of such clinical markers, a necrotizing infection should be suspected when cellulitis is refractory to appropriate antibiotic treatment. This is a signal to explore the wound.[20-23] On exploration, the diagnosis is almost always confirmed by the presence of gray necrotic fascia with little free pus and by easy dissection and undermining of the wound. Thrombosed blood vessels may also be seen. Incisional biopsies and frozen sections are favored for rapid diagnosis of necrotizing fasciitis.[24] The histologic criteria for diagnosis are the following:

1. Necrosis of the superficial fascia.
2. Infiltration of the dermis and of the fascia by polymorphic neutrophils.
3. Thrombosis of subcutaneous arteries and veins.
4. Angiitis and fibrinoid necrosis of arterial and venous walls.
5. Presence of microorganisms in the fascia and dermis on Gram stain.
6. Absence of muscle involvement.

In practice, the diagnosis of necrotizing infection is usually confirmed by the gross findings on surgical exploration. Histologic studies are not required for the initial diagnosis, although they are helpful in defining the cause of the infection [*see Inflammatory Response Is Absent (Clostridial Infection), below*].

Serial measurements of muscle compartment pressure have been used to confirm the need for operation.[19] Normal recumbent muscle compartment pressures are 0 to 8 mm Hg; pressures above 30 mm Hg are abnormal.[25]

Inflammatory Response Is Absent (Clostridial Infection)

On Gram stain or frozen section, histotoxic clostridial infection yields gram-positive rods without white blood cells [*see Figure 9*], whereas nonclostridial soft

Figure 8 **In some patients with necrotizing soft tissue infection, air may be seen in the soft tissues on x-ray even in the absence of crepitus.**

Figure 10 **In necrotizing fasciitis, an inflammatory response is present.**

Figure 11 **Bronzing of the skin occurs early in gas gangrene. Skin vesicles, as seen on this patient with advanced gas gangrene, occur later.**

tissue infection is associated with a significant number of white blood cells in the wound [*see Figure 10*].[26] Clostridial infection may present as a nontoxic cellulitis or toxic myonecrosis. Clostridial cellulitis develops 3 to 5 days after a wound is sustained. It is characterized by pain, a foul-smelling seropurulent discharge, skin vesicles that are small and flat, and limited systemic toxicity. Although pain may be severe, it does not compare to that experienced by patients with clostridial myonecrosis. Crepitus may be present. Effective treatment includes debridement and drainage of the wound and inspection of muscle to ensure that it is intact. Intravenous penicillin

Figure 9 **In clostridial myonecrosis, there is no inflammatory response.**

(6 to 12 million U/day for 7 to 10 days) decreases toxemia and limits the spread of infection.

Clostridial myonecrosis, also known as gas gangrene, occurs most commonly in the extremities of injured young men, in the abdominal wall of older men, and in the extremities of elderly patients with diabetes and peripheral arterial occlusive disease. The hallmarks of this infection are severe wound pain, marked swelling, and systemic toxicity. Hemolysis and coagulopathies are common. There may be a watery wound discharge with a musty odor, and a bronzing of the skin may occur. Skin vesicles, cutaneous gangrene, and crepitus, which may occur early in clostridial cellulitis, are late signs in myonecrosis [*see Figure 11*]. Resuscitation with I.V. fluids is required [*see I:4 Shock*], and administration of I.V. penicillin (12 million U/day) is helpful, but radical surgical debridement is the mainstay of treatment.

The use of HBO in clostridial myonecrosis remains controversial; it inhibits production of exotoxins but does not neutralize those already present. However, edema is reduced, progression of necrosis may be halted,[27] and tissue may be spared.[28,29] It has been suggested that mortality may be decreased by HBO,[28,30] but no comparative controlled studies exist. HBO may be a useful adjunct, but it is not a substitute for surgical treatment and must not be allowed to delay surgical debridement.

Inflammatory Response Is Present (Nonclostridial Infection)

The nonclostridial diffuse necrotizing soft tissue infections seen most often are hemolytic streptococcal gangrene [*see Figure 7*], necrotizing fasciitis with or without streptococcal toxic-shock syndrome (TSS), gram-negative synergistic necrotizing cellulitis, and idiopathic scrotal gangrene. Much confusion has arisen from reports that merge these syndromes under the single name of necrotizing fasciitis; in fact, they are multiple entities requiring a common initial approach.[26] The specific final diagnosis can be made only in retrospect. Although this diagnosis is valuable for fine-tuning therapy, it is not required for effective empirical initial treatment. Factors that increase mortality include delay in making the diagnosis, immunocompromise, shock and organ failure, a polymicrobial flora, and disease of the trunk rather than of the extremities. The principles of treatment are rapid resuscitation of the hypovolemia and correction of the electrolyte abnormalities [*see I:4 Shock and I:6 Life-Threatening Electrolyte Abnormalities*], administration of broad-spectrum antibiotics, extensive surgical debridement of all necrotic tissue, and supportive care.

Broad-spectrum antibiotics are usually given initially to cover the variety of organisms that may cause similar syndromes. Combination therapy may be used, such as penicillin (6 to 12 million U/day) with gentamicin (1.5 mg/kg every 8 hours) and clindamycin (600 mg every 6 hours) or ciprofloxacin (400 mg every 12 hours) with metronidazole (500 mg every 8 hours). Alternatively, monotherapy that is effective against gram-negative bacilli, streptococci, and anaerobes may be given, such as imipenem-cilastatin (0.5 to 1.0 g I.V. every 6 hours) or ticarcillin-clavulanate (3.1 g I.V. every 6 hours). Later, when pathogens are identified in blood or tissue, antibiotic therapy should be tailored to the organisms identified.

The initial surgical debridement of the wound should be aggressive. The wound should be incised, and the necrotic tissue should be excised. Wherever possible, however, viable skin should be preserved, and skin incisions should be placed so as to minimize devascularization. The deep fascia should be incised to allow inspection of the muscle. Finally, the wound should be packed open. Further debridement of the wound is the rule and should be performed 24 to 48 hours after the initial debridement. The extent of further debridement depends on the findings during operation and on the evolving clinical syndrome.

Adjunctive fasciotomy has been recommended.[19] Temporary dressings with amniotic membrane[31] or porcine xenografts[32] may be helpful in minimizing colonization of debrided wounds and may promote the growth of granulation tissue, allowing early initiation of split-thickness skin grafts. In immunocompromised patients with perineal gangrene, a diverting colostomy[33] established early in treatment minimizes further contamination of the wound.

Supportive care includes nutritional therapy[21,34] [*see VII:9 Nutritional Support*] and the use of low-dose subcutaneous heparin in order to reduce the risk of venous thrombosis.[35] HBO is the approach favored by some researchers[19,36] but not by others.[21,37,38]

NONOPERATIVE CELLULITIS

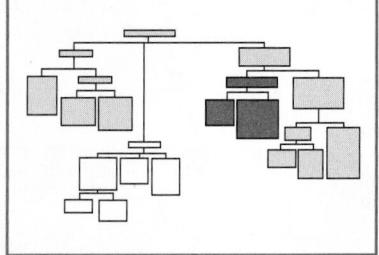

In the absence of clinical clues or histologic findings indicating necrotizing infection, diffuse inflammation is probably simple nonoperative cellulitis. The classic lesion is a warm, erythematous, edematous, painful spreading inflammation of the skin with nonelevated, poorly defined, advancing margins. Lymphangitis and lymphadenitis are often present in nonoperative cellulitis but not in necrotizing infection requiring operation [*see Figure 12*].

The identification of pathogens involved is not essential but may be helpful. If a primary lesion is found, swabs taken from it give the highest yields of positive cultures.[39] Needle aspiration of the advancing edge of cellulitis,[40] preferably without preliminary saline injection, yields positive cultures in only 20% to 40% of cases.[39,41,42] Blood cultures are positive in only 2% of cases, and false positive results are twice as common. Therefore, routine blood cultures are not cost-effective; however, blood cultures may be of value in cases where cellulitis of abrupt onset occurs in conjunction with high fever (> 38.4° C [101.1° F]), leukocytosis (> 13,500/mm^3), or immunodeficiency.[43] Serologic tests are of limited value.[44]

Most cellulitis is caused by group A streptococci (occasionally by groups B, C, D, and G) or by *S. aureus*. Oral or intravenous antibiotics are the primary treatment. Because streptococcal and staphylococcal cellulitis often cannot be differentiated clinically, a semisynthetic penicillin is commonly used, such as cloxacillin (4 to 6 g/day). Nonspecific measures such as rest, elevation, and warm compresses are also helpful.

Although cellulitis in adults is rarely caused by organisms other than streptococci or *S. aureus,* gram-negative cellulitis and high-risk cellulitis are nonetheless important variants. Gram-negative bacilli, particularly *Proteus mirabilis* and *Klebsiella* species, may cause cellulitis in immunocompromised patients and in patients with underlying disease (e.g., cirrhosis and congestive heart failure). Fever is often absent, but the white blood cell count is typically higher than 13,500/mm^3, and severe edema of the dermal papillae produces characteristic subepidermal vesicles or hemorrhagic bullae.[45] Similarly, cellulitis may develop in a laceration that has been exposed to soil or to water infested with *Aeromonas* species. These conditions all require broad-spectrum antibiotic therapy,[44] such as cefazolin or ce-

Figure 12 **Lymphangitis, as illustrated here, is commonly associated with nonoperative cellulitis but not with necrotizing infection requiring operation.**

Figure 13 **In this patient with late-stage erysipelas, bullae and induration of the cheeks are present along with well-demarcated erythema on the forehead.**

Figure 14 **This child has *Haemophilus influenzae* type b cellulitis of the right cheek.**

foxitin, 4 to 6 g/day in divided doses; oral ciprofloxacin, 500 mg twice daily; or oral cephalexin, 2 to 4 g/day.

High-risk cellulitis is often caused by unusual organisms. It occurs in critical locations, such as the face and the extremities (especially the hand), that are particularly vulnerable to serious complications. The term high-risk cellulitis includes several distinct conditions, namely, facial cellulitis, postadenectomy and postvenectomy cellulitis, and cellulitis after animal or human bites.

Facial cellulitis may be odontogenic, originating from the teeth and gums in older children, but most cases are nonodontogenic and occur in the upper face of infants and younger children. The best examples of facial cellulitis are erysipelas, *Haemophilus influenzae* type b (Hib) cellulitis, and orbital cellulitis. In erysipelas, a streptococcal upper respiratory infection invades the dermis and epidermis and produces a *peau d'orange* of the cheek [*see Figure 13*]. It responds to penicillin G, 1 million units I.V. four times daily. Hib cellulitis (now uncommon with the widespread use of *H. influenzae* vaccine) gives the cheek a bluish, bruised appearance [*see Figure 14*]. It is accompanied by severe respiratory infection, fever, leukocytosis, and Hib bacteremia.[46] A similar disorder occasionally occurs in adults.[47] Traditionally, ampicillin, 2 to 3 g/day I.V. in divided

doses, has been used for treatment, but currently, cefuroxime, 125 mg I.V. twice daily, is preferred. Orbital and periorbital cellulitis are characterized by pain, erythema, and swelling of the eyelids. Periorbital infections are common in children after minor trauma. Orbital cellulitis is a rare complication of acute sinusitis. The Chandler classification describes five stages of orbital cellulitis, determined on the basis of clinical findings and CT scanning: preseptal, postseptal, subperiosteal abscess, orbital abscess, and meningitis or brain abscess.[48] *S. aureus*, streptococci, and, occasionally, gram-negative aerobes are the usual causative organisms; accordingly, broad-spectrum antibiotics are the preferred agents. When an abscess is present, prompt orbital exploration and decompression are indicated if 36 hours of I.V. antibiotic therapy yields no improvement or if visual acuity or globe motion becomes impaired.[49]

Recurrent cellulitis may develop after adenectomy and in lymphedematous limbs after venectomy. Fever, toxic reactions, and chills are common. Non–group A streptococci (especially groups B, C, and G) are the usual causative organisms[50]; cloxacillin, 1 g I.V. every 4 to 6 hours, is the standard treatment. Similar syndromes related to lymphatic insufficiency have been reported in the breast after breast conservation therapy for carcinoma[51] and in the buttock after hip surgery.[52] In the former instance, *S. epidermidis*, *Streptococcus agalactiae*, and group B streptococci were incriminated. Initial treatment consists of oral cloxacillin or cephalexin, 500 mg to 1 g every 6 to 8 hours; if the infection does not respond to this regimen, specific therapy based on Gram staining or culture may be required. Patients with cellulitis of the buttock after hip surgery have been followed for several years, and no evidence of infection of the prosthetic implant has been found.

Animal and human bites may be complicated by severe infection, especially when they occur on the hands; they are discussed in more detail elsewhere (see below). Another high-risk infection of the hand is erysipeloid, in which cellulitis caused by a gram-positive rod, *Erysipelothrix rhusiopathae*, produces a purple-red infection of the finger or hand in fishers or butchers[53] [*see Figure 15*]. On rare occasions, erysipeloid is complicated by bacteremia or endocarditis. If the lesion is not recognized, diagnosis can be difficult, in that the organism lies deep in the skin and is hard to culture. A new PCR assay developed for diagnosis of swine erysipeloid has now been successfully applied in a human.[53] Erysipeloid responds to oral or parenteral penicillins (e.g., cloxacillin, 1 g every 6 hours).

Miscellaneous Infections

Of the miscellaneous soft tissue infections, only the common wound infections that occur after human and animal bites as well as the rare condition purpura fulminans are considered here. Established infection is more likely to occur when animal bites and scratches are seen late. When bites are seen early, infection is usually mild and responds well to treatment, which includes cleansing, tetanus prophylaxis [*see I:8 Acute Wound Care*], rabies prophylaxis (see below), administration of antibiotics (see below), and surgical debridement.

INFECTION AFTER ANIMAL BITES

From 80% to 90% of reported animal bites are caused by dogs, 10% to 20% by cats, and 1% to 2% by nondomestic animals. About 50% of animal bites are trivial; 1% to 2% necessitate hospitaliza-

Figure 15   **Characteristic of erysipeloid is an indolent, purple, non-purulent swelling of the finger.**

tion.[54] Washing with soap and water is effective immediately after a bite; later, high-pressure jet irrigation with saline is best. Fresh puncture wounds should be cleansed but not irrigated, because irrigation may compound tissue injury. Older puncture wounds should be opened to allow irrigation. Local anesthetics should be infiltrated to facilitate cleansing and debridement. When seen early, dog bites may be debrided and closed; infection is unlikely provided that appropriate antibiotics are also given. Cat bites and monkey bites are better debrided and left open, except when they occur on the face. Infected wounds and wounds that are older than 24 hours should be left open. Tetanus prophylaxis is given by intramuscular injection [*see I:8 Acute Wound Care*].

Another important consideration is rabies prophylaxis. Rabies is a viral infection transmitted in the saliva of infected animals. The virus enters the central nervous system of the host and results in encephalomyelitis that is nearly always fatal. Rabies prophylaxis is always indicated for bites by carnivorous wild animals (in particular, skunks, raccoons, foxes, and coyotes) and by bats but not for bites by a domestic animal unless the animal is thought to be rabid or unless it becomes rabid while confined. Prophylaxis is almost never indicated after bites by rodents such as mice, rats, or squirrels. In animal studies, wound cleansing and irrigation with virucidal agents such as povidone-iodine lowers the incidence of rabies markedly. Three rabies vaccines of comparable immunogenicity are available for commercial use: human diploid cell vaccine (HDCV); rabies vaccine adsorbed (RVA), and purified chick embryo vaccine (PCEC). Antibodies develop within 7 to 10 days of immunization; thus, passive protection with human rabies immune globulin (RIG) (half-life, 21 days) is also required.[54,55] Previously nonimmunized persons should receive five 1.0 ml doses of HDCV, RVA, or PCEC by intramuscular injection in the deltoid on days 0, 3, 7, 14, and 28. The recommended dose of human RIG is 20 IU/kg on day 0 or up to day 8; half of the dose should be infiltrated in the area of the wound, and the remainder should be given by intramuscular injection. The animal involved must be observed for rabies. A domestic animal should be confined for 10 days and killed only if it becomes rabid. A wild, stray, or unwanted animal—especially one that is behaving erratically—should be killed immediately, and its brain should be tested for evidence of rabies by means of immunofluorescence techniques.

About 85% of reported animal bites harbor pathogens, and

about 15% to 20% of dog bites and 50% to 60% of cat bites become infected. The most common pathogens in animal bites are *Pasteurella multocida, S. aureus,* and viridans streptococci.[54] Infections that occur within 24 hours of a bite are usually caused by *P. multocida* and deserve special attention. This gram-negative coccobacillus occurs in the mouths of up to 54% of dogs and 70% of cats and is the most common source of infection in wounds from domestic animal bites and scratches.[56] Typically, it causes infection within 12 to 18 hours, with marked local pain and tenderness. A serosanguineous discharge, low-grade fever, and regional adenopathy are less common. Infections that develop later are most often caused by *S. aureus* and viridans streptococci.

The ideal antibiotic for outpatient treatment of domestic animal bites is amoxicillin-clavulanate, 500 mg amoxicillin with 125 mg potassium clavulanate, given for 5 to 7 days. For inpatient treatment of infected bites, ampicillin-sulbactam, 3 g I.V. every 6 hours, or ticarcillin-clavulanate, 3.1 g every 6 hours for 7 days, is best. For patients allergic to penicillin, either (1) trimethoprim-sulfamethoxazole plus clindamycin or (2) cefuroxime axetil or cefuroxime sodium plus metronidazole is recommended. Elevation of the affected part is also helpful. Obvious pus must be drained and necrotic tissue debrided; however, unnecessary surgical treatment can cause marked disability.

INFECTION AFTER HUMAN BITES

Human bites are rarely seen before infection is established,[54] and they therefore require more vigorous treatment than do animal bites. The minimum treatment of those presenting

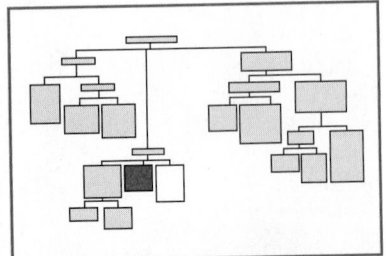

early includes tetanus prophylaxis [*see I:8 Acute Wound Care*], high-pressure saline irrigation, broad-spectrum antibiotics, and local debridement without closure of the wounds. The severely infected wound must be treated in the hospital. Wide debridement is necessary, and broad-spectrum parenteral antibiotics are given. The largest percentage of human bite wound infections are attributable to anaerobic bacteria (50%), including *Bacteroides* species (40%); however, viridans streptococci (25%), *S. aureus* (25%), *Eikenella corrodens* (15%), and others are also common pathogens. Appropriate antibiotic therapy consists of cefoxitin, 2 g every 8 hours, ceftriaxone, 2 g every 24 hours, or ticarcillin-clavulanate, 3.1 g every 6 hours for 7 to 10 days. Bites to a clenched fist in which tendon sheaths and joint spaces are entered typically are seen late and often are severely infected at presentation. *E. corrodens* is often isolated from these wounds. Since *E. corrodens* is not sensitive to erythromycin, patients who are allergic to penicillin should receive a cephalosporin instead.

Transmission of HIV and hepatitis B is an additional concern. Transmission of HIV through a human bite is extremely unlikely because proteolytic enzymes in the saliva usually inactivate the virus; consequently, postexposure HIV prophylaxis is not recommended. Hepatitis B, on the other hand, may be transmitted through mucosal contact with blood or saliva from actively infected subjects. A hepatitis B surface antigen (HbsAg)–positive person who bites another person and breaks the skin may transmit the virus; likewise, a seronegative person who bites an HBsAg-positive subject and breaks the skin may acquire the virus. Accordingly, hepatitis B immunoglobulin should be given to all nonimmunized exposed persons.

PURPURA FULMINANS

Purpura fulminans is a rare, life-threatening condition associated with meningococcal or pneumococcal bacteremia. The clinical picture consists of bacteremia, shock, and disseminated intravascular coagulation

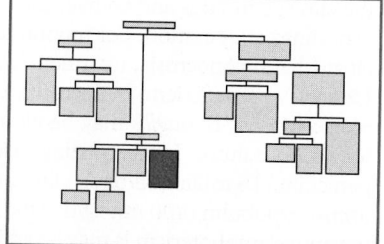

(DIC) causing symmetrical purpura in the skin and subcutaneous tissues of the distal extremities or the face.[57] Treatment includes immediate resuscitation for shock and sepsis and correction of the coagulation defects.[57] Complete volume replacement to establish a normal urine output, cardiotonic drugs, and specific antibiotic therapy are required. Heparin is advised for DIC. The heparin is given by continuous drip in sufficient dosage to maintain the activated partial thromboplastin time at twice the normal value; standard coagulation support is provided to keep the platelet count above 50,000/

mm³ and the serum fibrinogen level above 2.0 g/L. DIC is known to be associated with a profound decrease in protein C levels; consequently, administration of protein C concentrates early in the course of DIC plays a central role in current therapy. Protein C concentrates are given first in a 10 IU/kg test dose, then in a 100 IU/kg bolus, and finally in a continuous infusion at a rate of 10 to 15 IU/kg/ hour to keep the protein C level between 80 and 120 IU/ml. Antithrombin III is administered when the plasma level falls to 35 IU/ml, below which point heparin is ineffective as an anticoagulant. A 25 IU/kg bolus is given every 6 hours while plasma levels are being monitored. Usually, this approach leads to reversal of DIC within 5 days. Protein C therapy is then withdrawn gradually over a period of 2 days while heparin infusion is maintained at 5 to 10 IU/kg/hour.

If the patient survives the first few days, organ failure is the main problem. Surgical treatment is seldom required early in the course of the disease. The initial mortality is 40%, but some patients who survive may need amputation; others require debridement, topical silver sulfadiazine dressing, and skin grafts.

Discussion

Recognizing the Disorder

In the management of soft tissue infection, success depends on early recognition and prompt treatment of the disorder. The primary treatment is often surgical operation, chosen empirically. When antibiotics are indicated, the initial selection of an antibiotic is also largely empirical. The first goal, then, is not to find the precise diagnosis but to decide whether the condition requires operation. This approach holds for focal lesions, for which diagnosis is easy and treatment of the usual cutaneous abscess is simple. It also holds for diffuse lesions, but the diagnosis of necrotizing infection is often difficult, and the management is challenging.

Value of Classification Systems

Although several classification systems for necrotizing soft tissue infections have been proposed, most are impractical, and some contribute to the confusion that surrounds these disorders. A practical classification system for diffuse necrotizing soft tissue infection is based on the clinical presentation, the anatomic site of primary tissue involvement, and the microbiology of the causative organisms [see Table 1]. These factors determine the course of the various clinical syndromes and are sufficiently predictable to influence the plan of treatment after the initial empirical approach.

Role of Operation

Operation is often the main treatment of soft tissue infection. Furthermore, in necrotizing infection, operation must be performed early to limit tissue damage. The extent of surgical debridement depends on operative findings and cannot be predicted before operation. Therefore, it is more important to recognize that operation is required than to identify exactly which procedure will be done. Incision and drainage suffice for cutaneous abscesses. Various modifications, such as primary closure,[58] excision, and marsupialization, have been shown to be effective and are well known to most surgeons, although they are practiced infrequently. These methods, compared with incision and drainage, result in shorter healing times but are

associated with a higher rate of recurrence.[59,60] The role of operation in pyoderma gangrenosum is controversial,[2,10] but wide excision is generally required in the postoperative progressive bacterial gangrene of Meleney. In diffuse necrotizing infection, the wound is explored, by incision if necessary, to confirm the diagnosis. In necrotizing fasciitis, debridement of necrotic superficial fascia may create large, randomly based skin flaps that are poorly perfused. Some researchers have advocated preoperative planning of incisions by means of digital dermofluorometry.[61] Incision along a line joining the points of least fluorescence produces skin flaps with well-perfused bases. Thus, mutilation and disability are minimized.

In treating diffuse necrotizing soft tissue infections, reoperation is almost always required to inspect and debride the wound. The extent of debridement depends on the specific clinical syndrome,

Table 1 Classification and Characteristics of Diffuse Necrotizing Infections

Type	Characteristics
Clostridial	
Necrotizing cellulitis	Early local signs, moderate pain, and involvement of superficial tissue (skin and subcutaneous tissue)
Myonecrosis	Early systemic signs, severe pain, and involvement of deeper layers of tissue (primarily muscle)
Nonclostridial	
Monomicrobial necrotizing cellulitis Streptococcal gangrene *Vibrio* necrotizing infections	Rapid onset (1 to 3 days), single causative organism, and involvement of superficial tissue (skin and subcutaneous tissue)
Necrotizing fasciitis Classic bacteria Phycomycotic	Slower onset (4 to 7 days), bacterial synergy, some anaerobic activity, and involvement of deeper layers of tissue (Scarpa's fascia)
Synergistic necrotizing cellulitis caused by gram-negative bacteria	Slowest onset (5 to 10 days), bacterial synergy, greatest anaerobic activity, and involvement of deepest layers of tissue (deep fascia and possibly muscle)

which should be identifiable 24 to 48 hours after initial treatment on the basis of clinical, operative, and microbiological findings. Thus, in monomicrobial necrotizing cellulitis, only focal patchy areas of necrotic skin and subcutaneous tissue need to be excised. In necrotizing fasciitis, the superficial fascia requires further excision, whereas in synergistic necrotizing cellulitis and in clostridial myonecrosis, further debridement of muscle is required, and amputation of part or all of an extremity may be necessary.

Roles of Antibiotics and Pathogen Identification

Antibiotics play a limited role in treating focal soft tissue infection. They are not indicated in otherwise healthy patients with cutaneous abscesses.[62] In about 25% of patients,[63] however, systemic antibiotics are required because of the severity of associated systemic infection, because the patient is immunodeficient, or because a significant infection occurs in the central area of the face and carries a risk of cavernous sinus infection and thrombosis. The choice of antibiotics depends on the bacteria present. The anatomic site of the lesion, the duration of illness, the findings on Gram staining of specimens obtained by drainage or tissue aspiration, the odor of the pus, and the previous medical condition of the patient all provide clues to the likely pathogens.

Anaerobes are dominant in the perineum and rare on the hand. Swabs from cutaneous abscesses often initially yield *S. epidermidis* and streptococci; later, *S. aureus* may appear.[64] Pus that is foul smelling suggests anaerobic bacteria; *Clostridium* species, when present, cause a mousy odor. An abdominal wall abscess after bowel surgery may originate from an intestinal fistula. Gram stains obtained in these situations closely reflect the results of subsequent cultures.[63]

Only 4% of cutaneous abscesses are sterile. One third yield single isolates, usually *S. aureus* or occasionally *P. mirabilis;* the remainder yield a polymicrobial flora that includes many anaerobes.[63] *Bacteroides* species are the most common anaerobes. *B. melaninogenicus* and *B. ureolyticus* occur more frequently than *B. fragilis;* anaerobic gram-positive cocci occur less often, and *Clostridium* species are rare.

In patients with pyoderma gangrenosum, the significance of the pathogens obtained on primary lesion culture and needle aspirate culture is uncertain. A link between the pyogenic organisms found in the central lesion and the progressive destructive process of the skin has been proposed,[1] but this suggestion has not been substantiated, and the organisms are widely regarded as being merely opportunistic. The choice of antibiotics in classic pyoderma gangrenosum is not dictated by the pathogens identified. In his review of the postoperative variant of pyoderma gangrenosum, Meleney reported that when microaerophilic *Streptococcus* organisms and *S. aureus* were injected together into an experimental animal, cutaneous gangrene developed.[14] Injection of a pure culture of either organism failed to produce the skin lesion. These experiments confirmed the role of bacterial synergy in causing the clinical lesion. Gram-negative bacilli are sometimes found in the central area. Although the lesion must be excised for cure, broad-spectrum antibiotics are usually given empirically before surgery.

In diffuse necrotizing fasciitis, the initial antibiotic therapy is given empirically to manage the usual causative organisms. The best approaches are (1) combination therapy with I.V. penicillin, gentamicin, and clindamycin or with ciprofloxacin and metronidazole or (2) monotherapy with I.V. imipenem-cilastatin or ticarcillin-clavulanate [*see* Diffuse Inflammation, Inflammatory Response Is Present (Nonclostridial Infection), *above*]. Within 48 hours, the precise syndrome, whether clostridial or nonclostridial, may be defined by the results of Gram stain and culture of the tissue from the wound, by the clinical findings and course, and by the anatomic and pathologic findings at operation. For monomicrobial necrotizing cellulitis or clostridial myonecrosis, treatment with penicillin (6 to 12 million U/day I.V.) is sufficient. In necrotizing fasciitis, use of antibiotics directed against *B. fragilis* may be eliminated if this organism is not found on culture. In necrotizing fasciitis with streptococcal TSS, penicillin (18 million U/day), clindamycin (2.7 g/day), and human immunoglobulin (400 mg/kg/day for 5 days) are recommended. Intravenous amphotericin B may be added if hyphae on Gram stain or histologic section suggest necrotizing fasciitis of phycomycotic origin. The initial broad-spectrum antibiotic therapy should be maintained if muscle necrosis and the presence of aerobic and anaerobic gram-negative bacilli, including *B. fragilis,* suggest synergistic necrotizing cellulitis caused by gram-negative bacteria.

In patients with nonoperative cellulitis, systemic antibiotics are the main mode of therapy. There is no indication for autogenous vaccine therapy or for operation, both of which were popular many years ago.[65] The choice of antibiotic is based on the knowledge that cellulitis is usually caused by group A streptococci or by *S. aureus.* A semisynthetic penicillin covers both organisms adequately. Significant improvement can be observed within 48 hours.

The causative bacteria in the usual case of cellulitis are not as predictable as in specifically identified conditions such as erysipelas, but there are three lines of evidence that suggest the role of streptococci and staphylococci. First, the role of streptococci in spontaneous cellulitis occurring in the lymphedematous extremity of the dog has been documented.[66] Second, a rising titer of antistreptolysins and antifibrinolysins has been demonstrated in patients recovering from acute attacks of recurrent tropical lymphangitis[67]; these titers fall again over time. Third, in the few cases in which pus is present, streptococci and staphylococci are often cultured from patients with cellulitis.[41,68] Thus, the usual case of cellulitis may be treated without identification of the pathogen. Moreover, attempts to find bacteria by means of needle aspiration culture, blood culture, or even tissue biopsy culture are often unrewarding.[39]

Although clinical evaluation for the presence of infection is fairly accurate in most instances, it lacks specificity for a variety of disorders within the spectrum of extremity infection. Accordingly, to identify necrosis of soft tissue or infections in bone—complications that may jeopardize the integrity of the limb—further evaluation is useful. For years, plain roentgenograms and scintigrams have been used to define musculoskeletal infection. Currently, however, magnetic resonance imaging with I.V. gadolinium contrast is becoming the preferred modality for evaluating and diagnosing complicated extremity infections because it accurately depicts the degree to which bone and soft tissue are involved and identifies areas of necrosis.[68] Thus, MRI yields superior anatomic delineation of the extent of infection; furthermore, visualization of the bone marrow and definition of bony changes such as cortical destruction allow sensitive detection of osteomyelitis. These findings may be the stimulus for prolonged antibiotic therapy or for surgical intervention.

Traditionally, severe and high-risk cellulitis have been treated in the hospital setting, both to ensure access to surgical debridement when necessary and to facilitate I.V. administration of antibiotics. Often, such treatment has necessitated prolonged hospital stays. With the technology and the antibiotics currently available, however, it is usually possible to discharge patients early and to offer them outpatient parenteral antibiotic therapy (OPAT) or conversion to oral antibiotic therapy. This change in practice derives from (1) the evolution of safe techniques of central venous access for outpatient use, (2) the development of effective antibiotics with long half-lives for daily or twice-daily administration, and (3) the development of antibiotics of such high bioavailability when taken orally that oral regimens match the effectiveness of parenteral regimens. In the United States, skin and soft tissue infection is now the most common indication for referral for outpatient antibiotic therapy.

The vascular access modalities currently in use include peripherally inserted central catheters (PICCs), tunneled central catheters, and implanted ports. Of these, implanted ports are the least likely to become infected, but PICCs are now the most widely used because they are safe and easy to insert and use and because they have proved dependable and durable for prolonged antibiotic administration both in and outside the hospital setting.[69] The delivery systems used with these catheters include (1) slow I.V. injection (so-called I.V. push), which is suitable for time-dependent antibiotics (e.g., cephalosporins) but not for antibiotics that must be given over longer periods of time for reasons of safety and that depend on peak levels or prolonged persistent effects for efficacy (e.g., aminoglycosides and antifungals); (2) minibag and tubing systems that are used with rate-controlling roller clamps to generate a premixed diluted drip; and (3) a variety of portable electronic pumps and specialized tubing that are simple to use but expensive.

A number of antibiotics with long half-lives (e.g., ceftriaxone) have been developed that may be given once daily and are ideal for OPAT. One study of children with preseptal orbital cellulitis concluded that the maximum time for resolution of inflammatory signs was 36 hours, after which time transition to oral antibiotic therapy was appropriate.[70] Other antibiotics (e.g., cefazolin) that are given twice daily, either alone or with probenecid, have also been shown to be effective for home parenteral treatment of moderate and severe cellulitis. In one prospective trial of 61 such episodes of cellulitis, 88% of patients were cured, all peak antibiotic concentrations were higher than 40 μg/ml, and all trough concentrations were above the minimum inhibitory concentration for the expected pathogens.[71]

Antibiotics that possess high bioavailability after oral administration (e.g., quinolones) have greatly facilitated oral therapy for moderate to severe cellulitis. Quinolones are effective against moderate wound infections[72]; combined with single-dose or short-term parenteral antibiotics, they may also be used to treat more severe infections. Oral semisynthetic penicillins and first- or second-generation cephalosporins have long been used alone to treat mild infections or to complete the treatment of moderate cellulitis. Current data suggest that compared with other antibiotics, cephalexin may have a relatively high failure rate (40%) in treating uncomplicated cellulitis and that concomitant acid-suppressive therapy may explain this failure in part.[73]

Pathogenesis of Necrotizing Infections

The pathogenesis of the necrotizing soft tissue infections has been well discussed in the literature,[37,74,75] particularly the pathogenesis of clostridial infections. However, what causes a necrotizing infection rather than nonoperative cellulitis to develop is poorly understood, and even less is known about why a particular type of necrotizing infection occurs. The following are the four known pathogenetic factors in necrotizing soft tissue infections:

1. An anaerobic wound environment.
2. The presence of toxic lytic enzymes.
3. Bacterial synergy.
4. Thrombosis of nutrient blood vessels to skin and subcutaneous tissue.

CLOSTRIDIAL NECROTIZING INFECTIONS

The role of clostridia in producing gas gangrene has been well studied. Six species of clostridia have been reported to cause gas

gangrene in humans: *C. perfringens, C. novyi, C. septicum, C. histolyticum, C. bifermentans,* and *C. fallax. C. perfringens* accounts for more than 80% of cases, *C. novyi* for 30% to 60%, and *C. septicum* for 5% to 20%. About 30% of trauma wounds are contaminated by *C. perfringens,*[74] but in only a few does gas gangrene develop. A fall in redox potential in contaminated puncture wounds or in limbs with ischemic muscle allows the spores to be converted to the vegetative, toxic form. The isolation of clostridia from the wound does not, however, establish the diagnosis of gas gangrene. Simple contamination and clostridial cellulitis must be differentiated from gas gangrene. The diagnosis is clinical.[75] Acceptable criteria for the diagnosis of gas gangrene are the presence of necrotic tissue with seropurulent exudate, gas bubbling from the wound or wound crepitus, and recovery of *C. perfringens* or gram-positive bacilli without spores from a symptomatic patient. In clostridial cellulitis, local signs of infection, including pus formation, predominate over systemic findings.

The hallmarks of gas gangrene—liquefaction of muscle fiber and systemic toxicity—are caused by the exotoxins of clostridia. *C. perfringens* produces at least 12 well-described exotoxins in infected wounds; *C. novyi,* eight; and *C. septicum,* four. The best known of these exotoxins is the α-toxin, lecithinase. It destroys cell membranes, alters capillary permeability, causes hemolysis, and is highly lethal. The θ-toxin causes hemolysis and necrosis and is cardiotoxic; the κ-toxin, a collagenase, lyses protein; the ν-toxin, a hyaluronidase, acts as a spreading factor; the μ-toxin affects cell DNA; and neuraminidase destroys immunologic receptors on erythrocytes. Prominent systemic signs of gas gangrene are apathy, tachycardia out of proportion to increased body temperature, and cardiovascular collapse. Renal failure resulting from the combined effects of cardiovascular collapse and hemolysis is the most common complication.

NONCLOSTRIDIAL NECROTIZING INFECTIONS

The four pathogenetic factors in necrotizing infections (i.e., an anaerobic wound environment, the presence of toxic lytic enzymes, bacterial synergy, and thrombosis of nutrient blood vessels supplying skin and subcutaneous tissue) are less well understood in nonclostridial than in clostridial infections. However, although the mechanisms of action of these factors are not well understood, their roles in infection are known. An anaerobic wound environment facilitates bacterial synergy, especially between aerobic and anaerobic bacteria, and may also explain why radiographs show subcutaneous gas in the wound in 90% of cases [*see* Gas in the Wound, *below*].[34] Local findings in the wound, such as skin necrosis, are caused by the action of lytic enzymes and by the thrombosis of nutrient blood vessels to the skin.

The range of clinical presentations of the nonclostridial necrotizing infections has changed since the original description of streptococcal gangrene by Meleney in 1924[76] and now includes necrotizing fasciitis and necrotizing fasciitis with TSS. These changes may be related to differences in pathogenesis.

Streptococcal Gangrene

Meleney emphasized the rapid development of streptococcal gangrene: the initial erythema appears within 24 hours and is associated with fever and toxicity; in 48 hours, blue-purple discoloration, blisters, and bullae appear; and by day 4 or 5, the purple patches become gangrenous[76] [*see* Table 2]. McCafferty attributed this rapid spread to proteolytic enzymes activated by streptokinase or staphylokinase. Skin necrosis appears early because of thrombosis of subcutaneous blood vessels [*see Figure 7*].[77]

Necrotizing Fasciitis

Necrotizing fasciitis was recognized in the 1950s.[78] It differs from

Table 2 Changes in Characteristics of Nonclostridial Necrotizing Soft Tissue Infections

Factor	Streptococcal Gangrene	Necrotizing Fasciitis	Necrotizing Fasciitis with Group A Streptococcal Toxic-Shock Syndrome
Historical description	Meleney (1924)[76]	Wilson (1952)[78]	Greenberg (1983)[87]
Patients	Healthy, minor trauma	Multiple medical problems	Healthy, minor trauma Elderly with diabetes
Bacteria	Hemolytic streptococci	Mixed organisms	Group A streptococci
Pathogenesis	Lytic toxins	Bacterial synergy plus lytic toxins	Toxins Virulence (because of superantigens, M proteins, or susceptibility)
Symptoms	Erythema within 24 hr Blisters Gangrene within 4–5 days	Pain Erythema Blisters in the second week	Pain Edema Fever Shock Organ failure
Mortality	20% (preantibiotic era)	20%	20%–60%

streptococcal gangrene in the preponderance of systemic over local findings and in the slower onset of symptoms [see Table 2]. No clear explanation is available for these differences. Although few toxic lytic enzymes have been identified during pathogenesis, clinical and experimental evidence of their role in necrotizing fasciitis is available. Meade and Mueller found in 1968 that a collagenase elaborated by *Pseudomonas* species causes the rapid progression of necrosis in the subcutaneous tissue and along the superficial fascia.[79] More recently, Talkington and coworkers found that necrotizing tissue lesions in streptococcal necrotizing fasciitis are associated with a protease elaborated by the bacteria.[80] Thrombosis of nutrient blood vessels occurs late and may also cause skin necrosis. Barker and coworkers reported that the incidence of thrombosis of nutrient blood vessels is higher in patients with acute skin necrosis than in those with subacute cases.[81]

There are two main bacteriologic types of necrotizing fasciitis.[82] Most cases are type I, in which synergy occurs between Enterobacteriaceae or non–group A β-hemolytic streptococci and anaerobic cocci or penicillin-sensitive *Bacteroides* organisms. Type II cases are far less frequent and include group A streptococci either alone or with staphylococci. The clinical features in patients with type I or type II bacteriologies are indistinguishable. The hemolytic streptococcus seen in necrotizing fasciitis may be a different strain from that which produces hemolytic streptococcal gangrene: Meleney noted that different strains of hemolytic streptococcus injected under the skin of rabbits caused different outcomes.[76]

Bacterial synergy is the rule in the pathogenesis of necrotizing fasciitis. Using an animal model, Seal and Kingston[83] studied the role of bacterial synergy and lytic toxin in promoting both local progression and systemic toxicity in necrotizing fasciitis. Intradermal injection of group A β-hemolytic streptococci produced spreading infection and toxicity in 12% of animals. However, when cultures of *S. aureus* were coinjected with β-hemolytic streptococci, spreading infection occurred in 50% of cases; and when the α-lysin of *S. aureus* was coinjected with β-hemolytic streptococci, spreading lesions occurred in 75%. The predominantly anaerobic wound environment in necrotizing fasciitis and gram-negative synergistic necrotizing cellulitis facilitates the bacterial synergy between aerobic and anaerobic bacteria that is important in the pathogenesis of these syndromes.

Necrotizing soft tissue infection caused by halophilic noncholera marine *Vibrio* bacteria has been described.[84] Such infection occurs in minor wounds that have been exposed to seawater or in puncture wounds or small lacerations sustained when the patient is cleaning seafood. The clinical presentation is similar to the presentations of other types of monomicrobial necrotizing cellulitis and is more like that of hemolytic streptococcal gangrene than that of necrotizing fasciitis, which has a slower course. The onset is abrupt and is marked by swelling, erythema, and toxemia. *V. vulnificus, V. parahaemolyticus,* and *V. alginolyticus* are the usual bacteria. The mechanism of pathogenicity is not well understood, but *V. vulnificus* can cause transmural acute necrotizing vasculitis, which leads to thrombosis of subcutaneous blood vessels.

A variant form of necrotizing fasciitis caused by phycomycoses has been described.[85,86] As in other forms of necrotizing fasciitis, the clinical presentation of this form is insidious. The main causative organisms are *Rhizopus arrhizus, Mucor* species, and *Absidia* species. Phycomycotic necrotizing fasciitis can be identified promptly only by histologic examination of the infected tissue. The recommended therapeutic measures are urgent radical excision and I.V. amphotericin B.

Necrotizing Fasciitis with Streptococcal Toxic-Shock Syndrome

Since the 1980s, a marked increase in cases of streptococcal TSS—highly invasive group A streptococcal soft tissue infections largely associated with shock and organ failure—has been noted.[87] Streptococcal TSS is still uncommon (approximately 10 to 20 cases per 100,000 persons), but the increase may be accurately described as epidemic. However, this does not mean that widespread dissemination of infection by these so-called flesh-eating bacteria is imminent. The characteristics of streptococcal gangrene, necrotizing fasciitis, and necrotizing fasciitis with streptococcal TSS differ [see Table 2].

The pathogenesis of group A streptococcal TSS is particularly interesting—especially the roles exotoxins play in producing shock and in enhancing virulence of the bacteria. Streptococcal pyrogenic exotoxins (SPEs), produced by specific strains of *S. pyogenes,* are responsible for the characteristic fever, shock, and tissue injury of streptococcal TSS. SPE-A is associated with most cases of streptococcal TSS in the United States, whereas SPE-B and SPE-C are more prevalent causes in Europe and Canada. Some workers have shown that SPE-A and SPE-B cause monocytes to produce monokines, especially tumor necrosis factor–α (TNF-α), a prominent mediator of fever, shock, and tissue injury; IL-1β; and IL-6. Other

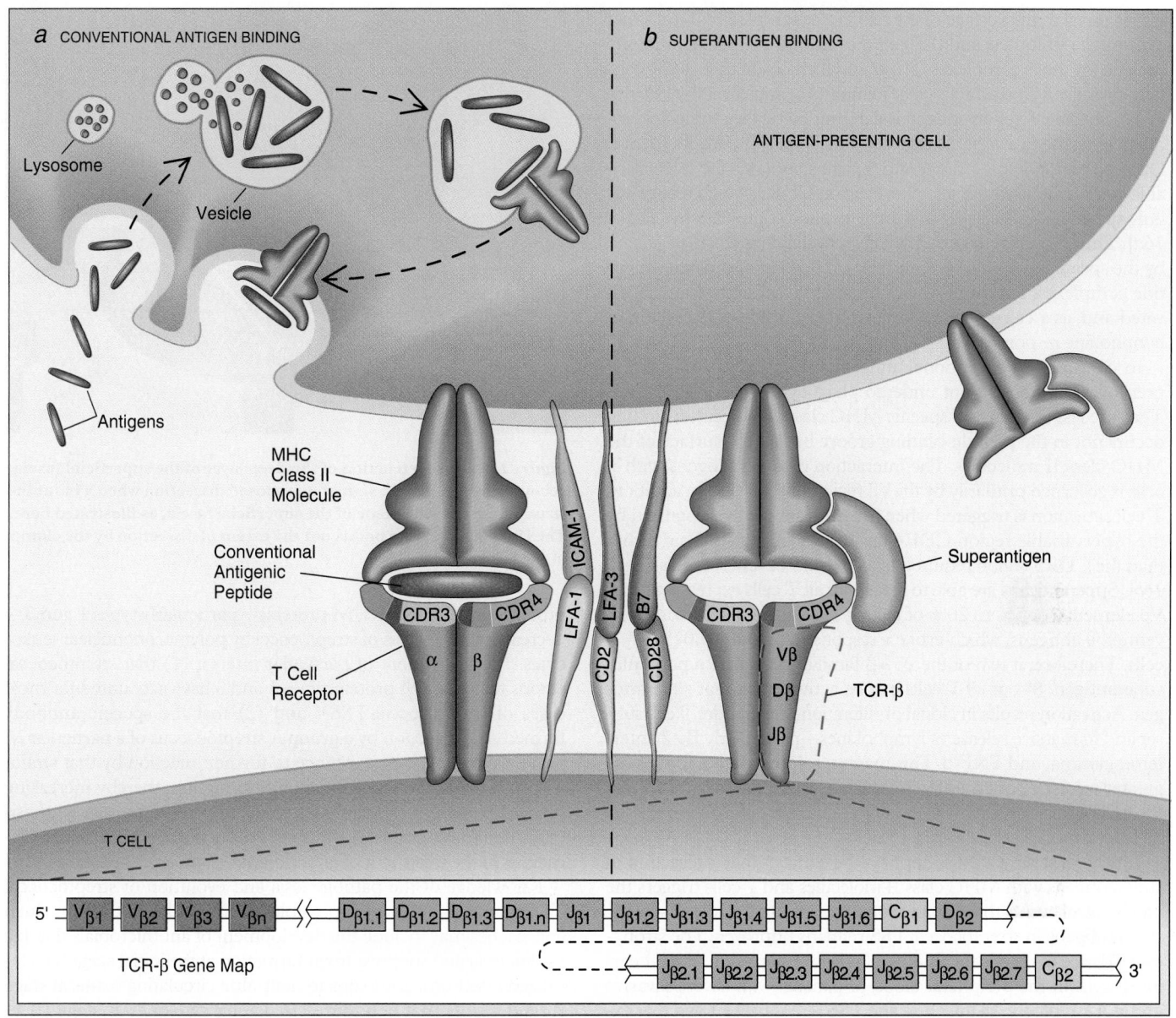

Figure 16 **Superantigens differ from conventional antigens in how they bind to and interact with T cells. A conventional antigen (*a*) is phagocytosed by an antigen-presenting cell (APC) and processed into an antigenic peptide in a lysosomal compartment. The processed peptide passes to a vesicle, where it binds to a major histocompatibility complex (MHC) class II molecule at the molecule's peptide-binding groove. The resultant MHC class II molecule–peptide complex travels to the surface of the APC to be sampled by T cells, whose specificity for the peptide is determined by the amino acid sequences of the five variable regions of the T cell receptor (TCR): the Vβ, Vα, Jβ, Jα, and Dβ segments. As a result, a conventional antigen is likely to be recognized by approximately 0.01% of T cells.**

Superantigens (*b*), by contrast, are not phagocytosed and are far less restricted to specific molecules. For example, binding occurs not in the peptide-binding groove of the MHC class II molecule but on the molecule's surface. Interaction between the MHC class II molecule–superantigen complex and the T cell is governed primarily by a single variable region of the TCR—the Vβ segment. The T cell is activated when the superantigen is recognized by the hypervariable complementarity-determining region CDR4 on the side of the Vβ chain rather than the CDR3 region employed by conventional antigens. Thus, superantigens are able to react with all T cells that have the same TCR-β chain, or between 5% and 20% of resting T cells.

exotoxins, such as streptolysin O, are also potent inducers of TNF-α and IL-1β. Peptidoglycan and lipotechoic acid also cause TNF-α release by monocytes. These mechanisms, added to the effects of the SPEs, result in shock.

Some investigators have tried to account for the increased virulence of group A streptococci in streptococcal TSS and for the dramatic morbidity of the syndrome by proposing that the SPEs also act as superantigens, which differ from conventional antigens in their interactions with T cells.

Conventional antigens interact with T cells in three phases: internalization and preprocessing (i.e., phagocytosis), binding, and T cell activation [*see Figure 16a*]. In phase 1—phagocytosis—antigens are internalized by monocytes and other antigen-presenting cells (APCs) and are processed into small peptide antigen determinants in the lysosomes. In phase 2, binding occurs: the peptides pass into special vesicles, where they form complexes with major histocompatibility complex (MHC) class II molecules at the molecules' peptide-binding groove. In phase 3, the MHC class II molecule–peptide complexes travel to the surface of the APC to be sampled by T cells that express the unique α and β T cell receptor (TCR) chains that are specific for those complexes. The α and β chains of each TCR contain constant (C), variable (V), joining (J), and diversity (D) regions. Specificity for an antigen is determined by the amino acid sequences of the five variable regions of the TCR: Vβ, Vα, Jβ, Jα, and Dβ. The region joining the α and β chains contains the hypervariable complementarity-determining region CDR3, which recognizes only specific MHC class II molecule–peptide complexes [*see Figure 16a*]. Thus, T cell activation by conventional antigens is restricted by the specificity of the TCR and the MHC class II molecule–peptide complexes. This limits the number of T cells that can be activated and, as a consequence, limits the magnitude of the resultant lymphokine response.

In contrast to conventional antigens, superantigens require no preprocessing and do not undergo phagocytosis [*see Figure 16b*]. They are less restricted to specific MHC class II molecules; binding occurs not in the peptide-binding groove but on the surface of the MHC class II molecules. The interaction of superantigens with T cells is governed primarily by the Vβ region of the TCR. In addition, T cell activation is triggered when the superantigen is recognized by the hypervariable region CDR4 on the side of the Vβ chain rather than the CDR3 region required by conventional antigens [*see Figure 16b*]. Superantigens are able to react with all T cells expressing those Vβ elements, or 5% to 20% of resting T cells, compared with conventional antigens, which evoke a response from only 0.01% of T cells. Therefore, if two of the 25 Vβ families recognize a particular superantigen, 8% of all T cells can be activated by that superantigen. Activation results in clonal proliferation of the entire T cell subset and in massive release of lymphokines—particularly IL-2, interferon gamma, and TNF-β. This massive response accounts for the greater virulence of group A streptococci in streptococcal TSS, for the extent and severity of the systemic manifestations, and for the increased mortality of the syndrome.

Although several studies support the concept that interaction of superantigens with MHC class II molecules and T cells triggers the biochemical events that initiate clonal expansion, the role of specific superantigens in streptococcal TSS remains unproven. The strongest evidence to date is the finding of selective depletion of Vβ-bearing T cells in the peripheral blood of patients with severe invasive group A streptococcal infection and TSS.[88] It is well known that exposure of T cells to superantigens can result either in proliferation or in deletion of target T cell subsets. When a superantigen, such as staphylococcal enterotoxin A (SEA), is injected into mice, an initial marked increase is seen in the number of circulating SEA-specific Vβ-bearing T cells for 4 days, after which a second phase ensues in which those T cells are deleted by the induction of anergy and programmed cell death, or apoptosis, and their numbers fall to very low levels for 1 to 4 months.[89] Other studies suggest that the amount of superantigen may determine whether T cell expansion or deletion occurs.[90] The activation of T cells by superantigens is facilitated by APC costimulatory molecules, such as B7 and intracellular adhesion molecule–1, and their respective ligands on the T cell, CD28 and leukocyte function–associated antigen–1. T cell–superantigen interaction may bring the costimulatory molecules and ligands closer together, allowing better transduction of the signals that direct T cell activation and proliferation. In the absence of costimulatory molecules, interaction of the TCR and superantigen may induce T cell anergy. On the other hand, when the interaction is primed by TNF-α or interferon gamma, preactivated T cells may undergo apoptosis and selective deletion when reexposed to a superantigen.

A further mechanism contributing to the syndrome of streptococcal TSS is an increased susceptibility to infection induced by M

Figure 17 **The destruction of the deep layer of the superficial fascia accounts for the classic sign of unopposed dissection when a blunt instrument probes the plane of the superficial fascia, as illustrated here. The right-hand clamp points out the extent of dissection by the clamp in the left hand.**

proteins on streptococci. M proteins—particularly types 1 and 3—decrease phagocytosis of streptococci by polymorphonuclear leukocytes.[91] It is therefore of particular interest (1) that streptococcal strains that carry M protein types 1 and 3 have accounted for most cases of streptococcal TSS[92] and (2) that the specific antibody formed after infection by a group A streptococcus of a particular M protein type provides resistance to further infection by that strain. M proteins also enhance exotoxin production, thereby increasing tissue destruction. Clindamycin, which impairs M protein synthesis (and therefore suppresses exotoxin production), is particularly efficacious in the treatment of experimental *S. pyogenes* infections.

Knowledge of the pathogenesis and evolution of streptococcal TSS may suggest specific possible future modes of therapy. Such approaches may include the development of antimicrobials that kill the bacteria and suppress toxin formation at the initial stage (i.e., localized infection), antitoxins to neutralize circulating toxins at stage II, and agents that neutralize circulating cytokines at stage III to control the syndrome and prevent progression to the multiple organ dysfunction syndrome of stage IV. Takei and coworkers have shown that human immunoglobulin contains antibodies that inhibit activation of T cells by staphylococcal toxin superantigens in cases of staphylococcal TSS.[93]

Streptococcal Myositis

Neither muscle nor deep fascia is involved in hemolytic streptococcal gangrene or in necrotizing fasciitis. The term fasciitis refers to the constant involvement of the deep layer of superficial fascia.[78] The destruction of this layer accounts for the classic sign of unopposed dissection when a blunt instrument probes the plane of the superficial fascia [*see Figure 17*].[23] An interesting variant with muscle involvement is streptococcal myositis, which has been differentiated from gas gangrene.[94] Most patients present with bacteremia and severe pain, but crepitus or gas in the tissues is unusual.[95] In streptococcal myositis, a group A hemolytic streptococcus is associated with anaerobic streptococci, *S. aureus,* or gram-negative bacilli. The muscle is inflamed but shows no evidence of the necrosis typical of gas gangrene.

Myositis may also occur as one element of necrotizing fasciitis with streptococcal TSS.[95] This so-called gangrenous streptococcal

Figure 18 **Fournier's gangrene of the scrotum is shown in this photograph.**

myositis is similar to clostridial myonecrosis in abruptness of onset, severity of pain, and high mortality, but it differs in the absence of underlying disease or of recent trauma and in the lack of crepitus or gas in the tissues. It has been suggested that the bacteria reach the muscle by hematogenous dissemination; a prodromal viral myositis may predispose the involved muscle to localization of coincident streptococcal infection.

Gram-Negative Synergistic Necrotizing Cellulitis

True muscle necrosis also occurs in synergistic necrotizing cellulitis caused by gram-negative bacteria. In this condition, the slow onset of disease, the deep anatomic location, and the anaerobic environment favoring bacterial synergy produce more extensive tissue necrosis than is generally seen in monomicrobial necrotizing cellulitis or in necrotizing fasciitis.[96] Although the perineal form of synergistic necrotizing cellulitis caused by gram-negative bacteria has been called Fournier's gangrene,[97] it is quite different from the idiopathic scrotal gangrene described by Fournier [*see Figure 18*].[98,99] Indeed, the parallel between idiopathic scrotal gangrene and so-called Fournier's gangrene is similar to the parallel between hemolytic streptococcal gangrene and necrotizing fasciitis. Synergistic necrotizing cellulitis is caused by synergy between anaerobic and aerobic gram-negative bacteria—usually *B. fragilis* or peptostreptococci and Enterobacteriaciae. Thus, it is polymicrobial from the outset. In addition, unlike idiopathic scrotal gangrene, perineal synergistic necrotizing cellulitis caused by gram-negative bacteria may extend onto the abdominal wall, necessitating extensive and repeated debridement [*see Figures 19 and 20*].

Idiopathic Scrotal Gangrene

Idiopathic scrotal gangrene[98,99] is characterized by sudden onset of fever, rapid progressive gangrene of the scrotal skin within 24 to 30 hours, and quick separation of the slough from the testes. The main causative organisms are anaerobic streptococci,[100] but secondary overgrowth of gram-negative bacilli may occur later.[101] The tissue loss is more superficial than that which occurs in Fournier's gangrene. Prompt and repeated surgical debridement reduces mortality. The wound granulates rapidly, and skin grafting may be performed later.

Gas in the Wound

Gas in the wound is an ominous sign to most physicians, perhaps because of its association with gas gangrene.[102,103] The significance of gas in the wound, however, depends on its source.

Figure 19 **Patients with synergistic necrotizing cellulitis caused by gram-negative bacteria may have necrotizing infection of the buttock (left). A perineal form is also seen (right).**

Figure 20 Synergistic necrotizing cellulitis caused by gram-negative bacteria on the anterior abdominal wall followed laparotomy for perforated carcinoma of the cecum in this patient. Ecchymosis and vesicles were present in the groin and anterior abdominal wall (left). Retroperitoneal dissection of infection and ecchymosis of the perianal region and scrotum are evident (center). Wide excision of the anterior abdominal wall revealed normal muscle in the flank but necrotic rectus abdominis and inguinal muscles in the lower abdomen (right).

Gas found in the wound may result from installation, leakage, or formation de novo. Installed gas is that left in the tissues in the course of tissue manipulation. It is characterized by the absence of other symptoms or signs and by gradual decrease in quantity over time.

Gas leakage into the tissues is characterized by a history of a predisposing event. It may occur after trauma—surgical or accidental—or after the violent retching and vomiting associated with spontaneous rupture of the esophagus. Air leakage from the esophagus, trachea, or lungs may follow blunt or penetrating trauma, and subcutaneous emphysema may follow tracheostomy or the insertion of a chest tube into the pleural space.

Gas formed in the tissues is truly spontaneous. It implies an anaerobic environment in which aerobic bacteria such as *E. coli*, *Klebsiella*, *Enterobacter*, or *Pseudomonas* or anaerobic bacteria such as peptostreptococci or *Bacteroides* species can produce gas. Usually, hydrogen and nitrogen are formed by processes of denitrification, fermentation, and deamination.[104] The volume of gas formed is quite variable. In some conditions, particularly synergistic necrotizing cellulitis caused by gram-negative bacteria, large volumes of gas may form, which dissect well beyond the area of infection. This occurrence, however, does not imply the need to excise or debride tissues beyond the area of infection. Simple incision will confirm that these tissues are not infected [*see Figure 21*].

Diagnosis and management of the patient with formed gas in the tissues is the same as that of the patient with a diffuse soft tissue infection. A search for telltale clinical features of necrotizing infection is combined with ancillary investigation—soft tissue x-ray, needle aspiration and Gram stain, blood culture, and serum muscle enzyme assay. The finding of gas within the muscle on x-ray is a telling sign of myonecrosis [*see Figure 22*].

Bite Wounds

Interesting differences between animal- and human-bite wounds should be noted because they affect management. Domestic animal bites and scratches occur far more often than human bites, but they are less serious. Only about half of all dog bites even receive medical attention. Human bites are more serious, in part because they usually present later, when infection is well established. In addition, the human oral cavity has a huge diversity of aerobic and anaerobic bac-

Figure 21 Exploratory incision must often be made to detect the presence of gas in the tissues beyond the area of necrosis.

Figure 22 **Gas seen within the muscle on x-ray is a telling sign of myonecrosis.**

teria. All human-bite wounds should be considered infected; therefore, they call for a broader spectrum of antibiotic coverage and wider debridement than animal bites. Above all, the wounds must not be closed primarily. Of all animal wounds, dog bites have the lowest risk of infection. They may be debrided and closed primarily, provided antibiotics are given.[105]

Finally, the special risk of rabies after animal bites often raises questions about the need for prophylaxis. The risk of rabies depends on the species of animal involved, the circumstances of the bite, and the type of exposure. Bites by wild carnivorous animals involved in unprovoked attacks carry the highest risk. The HDCV is more immunogenic and better tolerated than the duck embryo vaccine used formerly. Pregnancy is not a contraindication to the use of HDCV. Patients with a history of hypersensitivity, however, should be given HDCV with caution: antihistamines may be used, epinephrine should be close at hand, and the patient should be observed carefully.

Pathogenesis of Purpura Fulminans

The pathogenesis of purpura fulminans is interesting but controversial. The earmarks of acute purpura fulminans, typically associated with meningococcemia, are purpuric skin and severe acute DIC. The skin changes differ from those characteristic of simple hemorrhage in that the lesions are raised, indurated, and circumferential and tend to coalesce, blister, and break. These changes are due to rapidly progressive microvascular thrombosis in the dermis, resulting in perivascular hemorrhage and necrosis with minimal inflammation. Acute purpura fulminans closely resembles the Shwartzman reaction, induced in experimental animals by two I.V. injections of endotoxin 12 to 24 hours apart.[106] Endotoxin damages endothelial cells and activates the Hageman factor (factor XII), thereby initiating intravascular thrombosis and causing ischemia, vessel wall damage, and bleeding.[107]

Endotoxin-induced microvascular thrombosis is also associated with severe DIC, which is particularly interesting because of the related profound and disproportionate fall in plasma concentration of protein C and the recently defined central role of protein C administration in therapy. Protein C is a vitamin K–dependent glycoprotein that acts as a natural anticoagulant. It combines with thrombomodulin and small amounts of thrombin on the endothelial surface to form activated protein C (APC), which with cofactor protein S blocks further generation of thrombin by inhibiting factors Va and VIIIa. Factor VIIIa normally activates factor X and acts in conjunction with factors Va and Xa in the prothrombinase complex that generates thrombin from prothrombin. By limiting thrombin generation, APC limits fibrin formation; moreover, by promoting fibrinolysis, it limits fibrin accumulation.

In meningococcemia, induced microvascular thrombosis initiates a vicious circle that triggers disproportionate consumption of protein C and produces severe DIC. The endotoxemia also promotes release of TNF-α and IL-1, resulting in elevated levels of plasminogen activator inhibitor–1, which blocks fibrinolysis. In addition, TNF-α increases vascular permeability and white blood cell trapping.[108] Through its anticoagulant and fibrinolytic actions, administered protein C decreases microvascular thrombosis. This effect is critical in preventing organ failure and digital gangrene.[108] Administered protein C is also anti-inflammatory because APC blocks release of TNF-α and IL-1. Steroid therapy has also been suggested for this condition but should not be used because the Shwartzman reaction can be primed with cortisone.[109]

Chronic purpura fulminans is seen only in children. It presents many days after a febrile illness, usually a viral upper respiratory tract infection. Antigen-antibody complexes are deposited in the skin and lead to patches of skin necrosis.

References

1. Brunsting LA, Goeckerm WH, O'Leary PA: Pyoderma (echthyma) gangrenosum: clinical and experimental observations in five cases occurring in adults. Archives of Dermatology and Syphilology 22:655, 1930
2. Newell LM, Malkinson FD: Commentary: pyoderma gangrenosum. Arch Dermatol 118:769, 1982
3. Holt PJA, Davies MG, Saunders KC, et al: Pyoderma gangrenosum. Medicine (Baltimore) 59:114, 1980
4. van der Sluis I: Two cases of pyoderma (ecthyma) gangraenosum associated with the presence of an abnormal serum protein (β2 A-paraprotein). Dermatologica 132:409, 1966
5. Perry HO, Winkelmann RK: Bullous pyoderma gangrenosum and leukemia. Arch Dermatol 106:901, 1972
6. von den Driesch P: Pyoderma gangrenosum: a report of 44 cases with follow-up. Br J Dermatol 137:1000, 1997
7. Hughes JR, Smith E, Berry H, et al: Pyoderma gangrenosum in a patient with rheumatoid arthritis responding to treatment with cyclosporin A. Br J Rheumatol 33:680, 1994
8. Jolles S, Niclasse S, Benson E: Combination of oral and topical tacrolimus in therapy-resistant pyoderma gangrenosum. Br J Dermatol 140:564, 1999
9. Dirschka T, Kastner U, Behrens S, et al: Successful treatment of pyoderma gangrenosum with intravenous human immunoglobulin. J Am Acad Dermatol 39:789, 1998
10. Read AE: Pyoderma gangrenosum (editorial). Q J Med 55:99, 1985
11. Lewis SJ, Poh-Fitzpatrick MB, Walther RR: Atypical pyoderma gangrenosum with leukemia. JAMA 239:935, 1978
12. Heng MCY: Hyperbaric oxygen therapy for pyoderma gangrenosum. Aust NZ J Med 14:618, 1984
13. Plaus WJ, Hermann G: The surgical management of superficial infections caused by atypical mycobacteria. Surgery 110:99, 1991
14. Brewer GE, Meleney FL: Progressive gangrenous infection of the skin and subcutaneous tissues, following operation for acute perforative appendicitis. Ann Surg 84:438, 1926
15. Grainger RW, MacKenzie DA, McLachlin AD: Progressive bacterial synergistic gangrene: chronic undermining ulcer of Meleney. Can J Surg 10:439, 1967
16. Ledingham IMcA, Tehrani MA: Diagnosis, clinical course and treatment of acute dermal gangrene. Br J Surg 62:364, 1975
17. Svensson LG, Brookstone AJ, Wellsted M: Necrotizing fasciitis in contused areas. J Trauma 25:260, 1985

18. Fisher JR, Conway MJ, Takeshita RT, et al: Necrotizing fasciitis: importance of roentgenographic studies for soft-tissue gas. JAMA 241:803, 1979

19. Aitken DR, Mackett MCT, Smith LL: The changing pattern of hemolytic streptococcal gangrene. Arch Surg 117:561, 1982

20. Baxter CR: Surgical management of soft tissue infections. Surg Clin North Am 52:1483, 1972

21. Kaiser RE, Cerra FB: Progressive necrotizing surgical infections—a unified approach. J Trauma 21:349, 1981

22. Freischlag JA, Ajalat G, Busuttil RW: Treatment of necrotizing soft tissue infections: the need for a new approach. Am J Surg 149:751, 1985

23. Miller JD: The importance of early diagnosis and surgical treatment of necrotizing fasciitis. Surg Gynecol Obstet 157:197, 1983

24. Stamenkovic I, Lew PD: Early recognition of potentially fatal necrotizing fasciitis: the use of frozen-section biopsy. N Engl J Med 310:1689, 1984

25. Mubarak SJ, Hargens AR, Owen CA, et al: The wick catheter technique for measurement of intramuscular pressure: a new research and clinical tool. J Bone Joint Surg [Am] 58A:1016, 1976

26. Dellinger EP: Severe necrotizing soft-tissue infections: multiple disease entities requiring a common approach. JAMA 246:1717, 1981

27. Shupak A, Halpern P, Ziser A, et al: Hyperbaric oxygen therapy for gas gangrene casualties in the Lebanon War, 1982. Isr J Med Sci 20:323, 1984

28. Hitchcock CR, Demello FJ, Haglin JJ: Gangrene infection: new approaches to an old disease. Surg Clin North Am 55:1403, 1975

29. Hill GB, Osterhout S: Experimental effects of hyperbaric oxygen on selected clostridial species: II. In-vivo studies in mice. J Infect Dis 125:26, 1972

30. Heimbach RD, Boerema I, Brummelkamp WH, et al: Current therapy of gas gangrene. Hyperbaric Oxygen Therapy. Davis JC, Hunt TK, Eds. Undersea Medical Society, Inc, Bethesda, Maryland, 1977, p 153

31. Zarutskie P, Silverberg F: Amniotic membranes as a temporary wound dressing in necrotizing fasciitis. Obstet Gynecol 64:284, 1984

32. Sutton GP, Smirz LR, Clark DH, et al: Group B streptococcal necrotizing fasciitis arising from an episiotomy. Obstet Gynecol 66:733, 1985

33. Hiatt JR, Kuchenbecker SL, Winston DJ: Perineal gangrene in the patient with granulocytopenia: the importance of early diverting colostomy. Surgery 100:912, 1986

34. Majeski JA, Alexander JW: Early diagnosis, nutritional support, and immediate extensive debridement improve survival in necrotizing fasciitis. Am J Surg 145:784, 1983

35. Hammar H, Wanger L: Erysipelas and necrotizing fasciitis. Br J Dermatol 96:409, 1977

36. Gozal D, Ziser A, Shupak A, et al: Necrotizing fasciitis. Arch Surg 121:233, 1986

37. Tehrani MA, Ledingham IMcA: Necrotizing fasciitis. Postgrad Med J 53:237, 1977

38. Barzilai A, Zaaroor M, Toledano C: Necrotizing fasciitis: early awareness and principles of treatment. Isr J Med Sci 21:127, 1985

39. Hook EW III, Hooton TM, Horton CA, et al: Microbiologic evaluation of cutaneous cellulitis in adults. Arch Intern Med 146:295, 1986

40. Uman SJ, Kunin CM: Needle aspiration in the diagnosis of soft tissue infections. Arch Intern Med 135:959, 1975

41. Ginsberg MB: Cellulitis: analysis of 101 cases and review of the literature. South Med J 74:530, 1981

42. Leppard BJ, Seal DV, Colman G, et al: The value of bacteriology and serology in the diagnosis of cellulitis and erysipelas. Br J Dermatol 112:559, 1985

43. Perl B, Gottehrer NP, Schlesinger Y, et al: Cost-effectiveness of blood cultures for adult patients with cellulitis. Clin Infect Dis 29:1483, 1999

44. Slutkin G, Marzouk J, Dall L, et al: Comparison of cefonicid and cefazolin for treatment of soft-tissue infections. Rev Infect Dis 6(suppl 4):S853, 1984

45. Yoon TY, Jung SK, Chang SH: Cellulitis due to *Escherichia coli* in three immunocompromised subjects. Br J Dermatol 139:885, 1998

46. Fleisher G, Heeger P, Topf P: *Hemophilus influenzae* cellulitis. Am J Emerg Med 3:274, 1983

47. Drapkin MS, Wilson ME, Shrager SM, et al: Bacteremic *Hemophilus influenzae* type B cellulitis in the adult. Am J Med 63:449, 1977

48. Chandler JR, Langenbrunner DJ, Stevens ER: The pathogenesis of orbital complications in acute sinusitis. Laryngoscope 80:1414, 1970

49. Goodwin WJ Jr, Weinshall M, Chandler JR: The role of high resolution computerized tomography and standardized ultrasound in the evaluation of orbital cellulitis. Laryngoscope 92:729, 1982

50. Baddour LM, Bisno AL: Non-group A beta-hemolytic streptococcal cellulitis: association with venous and lymphatic compromise. Am J Med 79:155, 1985

51. Mertz KB, Baddour LM, Bell JL: Breast cellulitis following breast conservation therapy: a novel complication of medical progress. Clin Infect Dis 26:481, 1998

52. Studer-Sachsenberg EM, Ruffieux PH, Saurat J-H: Cellulitis after hip surgery: long term follow-up of seven cases. Br J Dermatol 137:133, 1997

53. Brooke CJ, Riley TV: Erysipelothrix rhusiopathiae: bacteriology, epidemiology and clinical manifestations of an occupational pathogen. J Med Microbiol 48:789, 1999

54. Fleisher GR: The management of bite wounds. N Engl J Med 340:138, 1999

55. Advisory Committee on Immunization Practices: Human rabies prevention—United States 1999. Recommendations of the Advisory Committee on Immunization Practices. MMWR 48:1, 1999

56. Francis DP, Holmes MA, Brandon G: *Pasteurella multocida*: infections after domestic animal bites and scratches. JAMA 233:42, 1975

57. Smith OP, White B: Infectious purpura fulminans: diagnosis and treatment. Br J Haematol 104:202, 1999

58. Ellis M: Incision and primary suture of abscesses of the anal region. Proc R Soc Med 53:652, 1960

59. Macfie J, Harvey J: The treatment of acute superficial abscesses: a prospective clinical trial. Br J Surg 64:264, 1977

60. Sorensen C, Hjortrup A, Moesgaard F, et al: Linear incision and curettage vs deroofing and drainage in subcutaneous abscess: a randomized clinical trial. Acta Chir Scand 153:659, 1987

61. Bongard FS, Elings VB, Markison RE: New uses of fluorescence in the surgical management of necrotizing soft tissue infection. Am J Surg 150:281, 1985

62. Llera JL, Levy RC: Treatment of cutaneous abscess: a double-blind clinical study. Ann Emerg Med 14:15, 1985

63. Becker LE, Tschen E: Common bacterial infections of the skin. Primary Care 10:397, 1983

64. Meislin HW, Lerner SA, Graves MH, et al: Cutaneous abscesses: anaerobic and aerobic bacteriology and outpatient management. Ann Intern Med 87:145, 1977

65. Hughes B: The treatment of cellulitis with special reference to the hand and arm. Practitioner 89:142, 1912

66. Drinker CK, Field ME, Ward HK, et al: Increased susceptibility to local infection following blockage of lymph drainage. Am J Physiol 112:74, 1935

67. Morales-Otero P, Pomales-Lebrón A: The development of antistreptolysins and antifibrinolysins following acute attacks of recurrent tropical lymphangitis. Trans R Soc Trop Med Hyg 30:191, 1936

68. Towers JD: The use of intravenous contrast in MRI of extremity infection. Semin Ultrasound CT MR 18:269, 1997

69. Brown JM: An overview of vascular access for the alternate care setting. Infusion 1:11, 1995

70. Blumer J, O'Brien C, Lemon E, et al: Skin and soft tissue infections: pharmacologic approaches. Pediatr Infect Dis 4:336, 1985

71. Leder K, Turnidge JD, Grayson ML: Home-based treatment of cellulitis with twice-daily cefazolin. Med J Australia 169:519, 1998

72. Lipsky BA, Miller B, Schwartz R, et al: Sparfloxacin versus ciprofloxacin for the treatment of community-acquired complicated skin and skin-structure infections. Clin Therapeutics 21:675, 1999

73. Madaras-Kelly KJ, Arbogast R, Jue S: Increased therapeutic failure for cephalexin versus comparator antibiotics in the treatment of uncomplicated outpatient cellulitis. Pharmacotherapy 20:199, 2000

74. Altemeier WA, Fullen WD: Prevention and treatment of gas gangrene. JAMA 217:806, 1971

75. MacLennan JD: The histotoxic clostridial infections of man. Bact Review 26:177, 1962

76. Meleney FL: Hemolytic streptococcus gangrene. Arch Surg 9:317, 1924

77. McCafferty EL, Lyons C: Suppurative fasciitis as the essential feature of hemolytic streptococcus gangrene. Surgery 24:438, 1948

78. Wilson B: Necrotizing fasciitis. Am Surg 18:416, 1952

79. Meade JW, Mueller CB: Necrotizing infections of subcutaneous tissue and fascia. Ann Surg 168:274, 1968

80. Talkington DF, Schwartz B, Black CM, et al: Association of phenotypic and genotypic characteristics of invasive *Streptococcus pyogenes* isolates with clinical components of streptococcal toxic shock syndrome. Infect Immun 61:3369, 1993

81. Barker FG, Leppard BJ, Seal DV: Streptococcal necrotizing fasciitis: comparison between histological and clinical features. J Clin Pathol 40:335, 1987

82. Giuliano A, Lewis F, Hadley K, et al: Bacteriology of necrotizing fasciitis. Am J Surg 134:52, 1977

83. Seal DV, Kingston D: Streptococcal necrotizing fasciitis: development of an animal model to study its pathogenesis. Br J Exp Pathol 69:813, 1988

84. Howard RJ, Pesa ME, Brennaman BH, et al: Necrotizing soft tissue infections caused by marine vibrios. Surgery 98:126, 1985

85. Wilson CB, Siber GR, O'Brien TF, et al: Phycomycotic gangrenous cellulitis. Arch Surg 111:532, 1976

86. Patino JF, Castro D, Valencia A, et al: Necrotizing soft-tissue lesions after a volcanic cataclysm. World J Surg 15:240, 1991

87. Greenberg RN, Willoughby BG, Kennedy DJ, et al: Hypocalcemia and "toxic" syndrome associated with streptococcal fasciitis. South Med J 76:916, 1983

88. Watanabe-Ohnishi R, Low DE, McGeer A, et al: Selective depletion of Vβ-bearing T cells in patients with severe invasive group A streptococcal disease and streptococcal toxic shock syndrome: implications for a novel superantigen. J Infect Dis 171:74, 1995

89. Kawabe Y, Ochi A: Selective anergy of Vβ8+, CD4+ T cells in *Staphylococcus* enterotoxin B–primed mice. J Exp Med 172:1065, 1990

90. McCormack JE, Callahan JE, Kappler J, et al: Profound depletion of mature T cells in vivo by chronic exposure to exogenous superantigen. J Immunol 150:3785, 1993

91. Lancefield RC: Current knowledge of type-specific M antigens of group A streptococci. J Immunol 89:307, 1962

92. Schwartz B, Facklam RR, Brieman RF: Changing epidemiology of group A streptococcal infection in the USA. Lancet 336:1167, 1990

93. Takei S, Arora YK, Walker SM: Intravenous immunoglobulin contains specific antibodies inhibitory to activation of T cells by staphylococcal toxin superantigens. J Clin Invest 91:602, 1993

94. MacLennan JD: Streptococcal infection of muscle. Lancet 1:582, 1943

95. Yoder EL, Mendez J, Khatib R: Spontaneous gangrenous myositis induced by *Streptococcus pyogenes*: case report and review of the literature. Rev Infect Dis 9:382, 1987

96. Stone HH, Martin JD Jr: Synergistic necrotizing cellulitis. Ann Surg 129:702, 1972

97. Rouse TM, Malangoni MA, Schulte WJ: Necrotizing fasciitis: a preventable disaster. Surgery 92:765, 1982

98. Fournier JA: Gangrène foudroyante de la verge. La Semaine Médicale 3:345, 1883

99. Rudolf R, Soloway M, DePalma RG, et al: Fournier's syndrome: synergistic gangrene of the scrotum. Am J Surg 129:591, 1975

100. Coenen H, Przedborski J: Die gangrän des penis und scrotums. Beitrage zur Klinischen Chirurgie 75:136, 1911

101. Slater DN, Smith GT, Mundy K: Diabetes mellitus with ketoacidosis presenting as Fournier's gangrene. J R Soc Med 75:530, 1982

102. MacLennan JD: Anaerobic infections of war wounds in the Middle East. Lancet 2:63, 1943

103. Altemeier WA, Culbertson WR: Acute non-clostridial crepitant cellulitis. Surg Gynecol Obstet 87:207, 1948

104. Van Beek A, Zook E, Yaw P, et al: Nonclostridial gas-forming infections: a collective review and report of seven cases. Arch Surg 108:552, 1974

105. Zook EG, Miller M, Van Beek AL, et al: Successful treatment protocol for canine fang injuries. J Trauma 20:243, 1980

106. Good RA, Thomas L: Studies on the generalized Shwartzman reaction: IV. Prevention of the local and generalized Shwartzman reactions with heparin. J Exp Med 97:871, 1953

107. Silbart S, Oppenheim W: Purpura fulminans: medical, surgical and rehabilitative considerations. Clin Orthop 193:206, 1985

108. Smith OP, White B, Vaughan D, et al: Use of protein C concentrate, heparin and haemofiltration in meningococcus induced purpura fulminans. Lancet 350: 1590, 1997

109. Thomas L, Good RA: The effect of cortisone on the Shwartzman reaction: the production of lesions resembling the dermal and generalized Shwartzman reactions by a single injection of bacterial toxin in cortisone-treated rabbits. J Exp Med 95:409, 1952

Acknowledgments

Figure 1 Wolfin/Medichrome.

Figure 2 From "The Surgical Management of Superficial Infection Caused by Atypical Mycobacteria," by W. J. Plaus and G. Hermann, in *Surgery* 110:99, 1991.

Figures 5 through 8, 21, and 22 Courtesy of Jonathan L. Meakins, M.D., Royal Victoria Hospital, Montreal.

Figures 9 and 10 Courtesy of E. Patchen Dellinger, M.D., Harborview Medical Center, Seattle.

Figures 13 and 15 From *Infectious Diseases Illustrated*, by Harold Lambert and W. Edmund Farrar. Gower Medical Publishing Ltd., London, 1981.

Figure 14 From *Color Atlas of Paediatric Dermatology*, by Julian Verbow and Neil Morley. MTP Press, Lancaster, England, 1983.

Figure 16 Dimitry Schidlovsky.

Figure 17 Courtesy of Charles R. Baxter, M.D., University of Texas Health Science Center at Dallas.

Figures 18 and 19 From *A Visual Exploration of Anaerobic Infections*, by Charles A. Kallick. Merck-Frosst Canada, Inc., Kirkland, Quebec, 1978.

III TRAUMA AND THERMAL INJURY

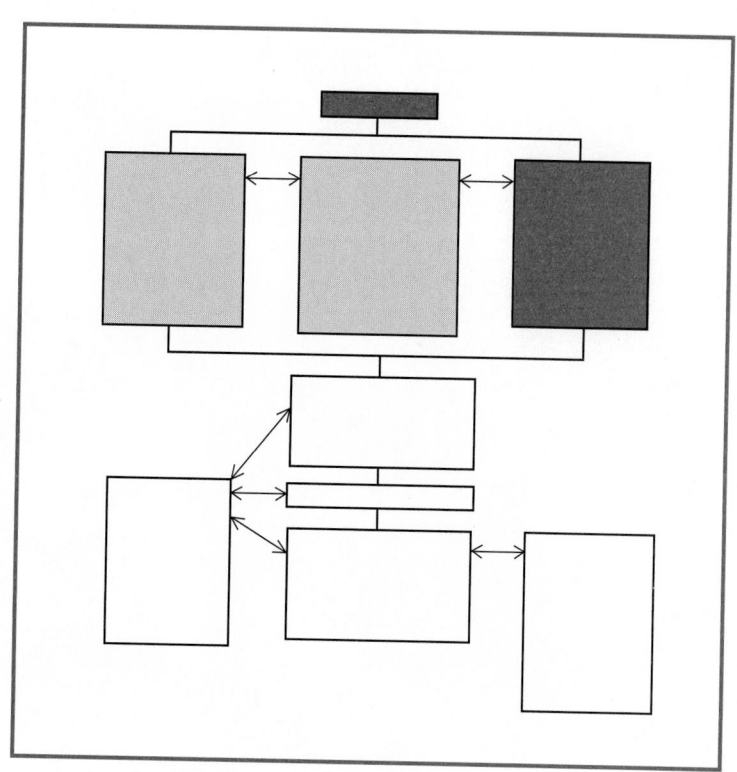

EMERGENCY DEPARTMENT EVALUATION OF THE PATIENT WITH MULTIPLE INJURIES

Felix D. Battistella, M.D.

Approach to the Multiply Injured Patient in the Emergency Department

Morbidity and mortality resulting from trauma can be minimized if evaluation of the acutely injured patient proceeds logically and efficiently. Given the rapid deterioration that can occur as injuries progress, trauma systems should be geared to expedite the initial evaluation, resuscitation, and treatment of multiply injured patients. Preestablished management strategies and protocols can be useful in organizing and coordinating the efforts of the trauma team.

The algorithms presented in the discussion that follows suggest strategies for the early management of trauma victims. They may not anticipate all possible scenarios, but they should at least provide a framework that facilitates the rapid decision making needed to get patients from the emergency department to the operating suite. These algorithms may have to be modified to some extent to take account of differences in local resources and expertise or the introduction of new technologies; however, the basic principles they embody are unlikely to be superseded for some time yet.

The approaches outlined in this chapter were developed according to two main premises:

1. The goal of trauma care should be to minimize preventable morbidity and mortality for all trauma victims. To this end, trauma care providers should place the same emphasis on identifying occult injuries in minimally injured patients as on treating patients with catastrophic injury.
2. Prioritization of diagnostic and therapeutic maneuvers is crucial for optimizing outcome after critical injury. Treatment priority is determined by the severity of the injury, its rate of progression, and its complexity. Easily correctable, rapidly progressive, life-threatening injuries should be addressed first; complex or slowly progressive injuries should receive a lower priority. Once a correctable life-threatening injury is identified, the trauma team should focus its efforts on stabilizing this condition before looking for additional life-threatening injuries that may not be apparent.

Initial evaluation and treatment of trauma victims are governed by the mechanism of injury (i.e., penetrating or blunt) and by the patient's hemodynamic status. Evaluation and treatment priorities for penetrating injury differ from those for blunt trauma because the two mechanisms give rise to different patterns of injury: penetrating trauma typically results in a localized injury, whereas blunt trauma frequently results in multiple injuries that involve several body regions. Furthermore, within each class of injury, evaluation and treatment priorities for hypotensive patients differ from those for hemodynamically stable patients. Whenever hemodynamic instability is present, its cause must be identified and corrected promptly to increase the patient's chance for survival. At my institution, hemodynamic instability is defined as either a systolic blood pressure lower than 90 mm Hg or a documented decrease of more than 30 mm Hg in systolic blood pressure. Admittedly, hemodynamic stability is a relative term, in that most patients, especially young ones, can compensate for hypovolemia and maintain a normal blood pressure even in the face of significant ongoing hemorrhage; nevertheless, even though blood pressure is not a sensitive detector of early shock, it is still a useful guide in the emergency department because it can be obtained promptly and frequently. Regardless of the patient's blood pressure, the evaluation and treatment of all injured patients should proceed without undue delay because ongoing bleeding can be occult.

I begin with guidelines for managing trauma patients who present in cardiac arrest. The subsequent guidelines for penetrating and blunt trauma patients who are not in cardiac arrest are based on the assumption that the ABCs of trauma and the primary survey have been completed [*see I:2 Trauma Resuscitation*]. Penetrating injuries are addressed according to their primary location—neck, chest, thoracoabdominal region, or extremities.

The neck is defined as the region below the mastoid process and above the clavicles; the chest, as the area below the clavicles but above the mamillary line; the thoracoabdominal region, as the area between the mamillary line and the inguinal ligaments; and the extremities, as the area distal to the deltopectoral groove or distal to the inguinal ligaments. Penetrating injuries that span more than one of these body regions require the surgeon to prioritize initial evaluation and treatment on the basis of the physical findings. Because blunt injuries typically involve more than one body region, they are addressed according to the patient's hemodynamic status. Finally, specific injuries or findings that are associated with blunt injury (e.g., potential cervical spine injury, wide mediastinum, and hematuria) are discussed.

Approach to the Multiply Injured Patient in the Emergency Department

Multiply injured patient presents to ED

Patient is in cardiopulmonary arrest

Determine mechanism of injury.

Penetrating injury

[*See Figure 1.*]

Blunt injury

[*See Figure 2.*]

Patient is not in cardiopulmonary arrest

Determine mechanism of injury.

Penetrating injury

Determine primary location of injury.

Blunt injury

Assess hemodynamic status.

Injury is primarily to neck

[*See Figure 3.*]

Injury is primarily thoracoabdominal

Patient is unstable

[*See Figure 6.*]

Patient is stable

[*See Figure 7.*]

Injury is primarily to chest

Patient is unstable

[*See Figure 4.*]

Patient is stable

[*See Figure 5.*]

Injury is primarily to extremity

[*See Figure 8.*]

Patient is unstable

[*See Figure 9.*]

Patient is stable

Obtain chest x-ray.

Patient has evidence of acute injury on chest x-ray

[*See Figure 10.*]

Patient has no evidence of acute injury on chest x-ray

[*See Figure 11.*]

Traumatic Cardiopulmonary Arrest

Survival after traumatic cardiopulmonary arrest is substantially influenced by mechanism of injury: the prognosis is dismal when cardiopulmonary arrest is attributable to blunt trauma and somewhat better when it is attributable to penetrating trauma.[1,2] The main reason for this divergence in outcomes is that cardiopulmonary arrest in a blunt trauma patient may be secondary to any of a number of causes, most of which are quite difficult to reverse rapidly (e.g., brain injury, high spinal cord injury, proximal aortic disruption, and exsanguination from a variety of injuries). The best survival rates after traumatic cardiopulmonary arrest are reported in patients with stab wounds to the heart, in whom the cardiac arrest is attributable to cardiac tamponade. In patients with cardiac tamponade, the heart often can be resuscitated simply by decompressing the pericardium [see I:2 Trauma Resuscitation].

It follows, then, that management of a patient in traumatic cardiac arrest after penetrating injury should be much more aggressive than that of a patient in cardiac arrest after blunt injury.

PENETRATING TRAUMA

Even given the generally better prognosis associated with cardiac arrest after penetrating trauma, resuscitation is futile if cardiopulmonary arrest has persisted for a prolonged period [see Figure 1]. If no signs of life (e.g., spontaneous respirations, a pulse, or spontaneous movement) are observed by medical personnel at the scene or in transport and the ECG in the emergency department shows anything but a narrow complex sinus rhythm, the victim should be pronounced dead on arrival. If the history is unclear or signs of life are observed, the patient should undergo an emergency room thoracotomy without delay. If the wound is to the chest, the injured side should be opened first. The incision can be extended across the sternum if necessary.

The pericardium should be opened and the heart inspected. Any pericardial blood should be evacuated and the heart massaged. When a central pulmonary injury is present, the hilum should be cross-clamped to control hemorrhage and prevent air embolization. If the surgeon believes the central pulmonary injury to be correctable, resuscitation should proceed and the patient should be taken to the operating room for definitive repair.

If no intrathoracic injury is identified, efforts should be focused on reestablishing spontaneous cardiac activity. If this cannot be accomplished by giving intravenous fluids and providing cardiac support, resuscitation may be terminated and the patient pronounced dead. If spontaneous cardiac activity is restored, the patient should be taken to the OR, where the injuries should be dealt with as expeditiously as possible. Bleeding vessels should be ligated rather than reconstructed, and treatment of intra-abdominal injuries should be limited to control of hemorrhage. Reoperation for definitive treatment of abdominal injuries should be scheduled in the next 24 to 48 hours once the coagulopathy is reversed and the patient is hemodynamically stable.

BLUNT TRAUMA

Given the extremely poor survival rate for patients in cardiac arrest as a result of blunt trauma, resuscitative efforts should focus on the relatively few patients in this group whose arrest was witnessed in the ED or who present with a normal sinus rhythm [see Figure 2]. The electrical activity of the heart is a useful guide to the potential benefit to be derived from continued resuscitative efforts.[3] If the victim has no cardiac activity or exhibits an agonal rhythm or a wide-complex rhythm, no further resuscitative efforts are warranted, and the patient

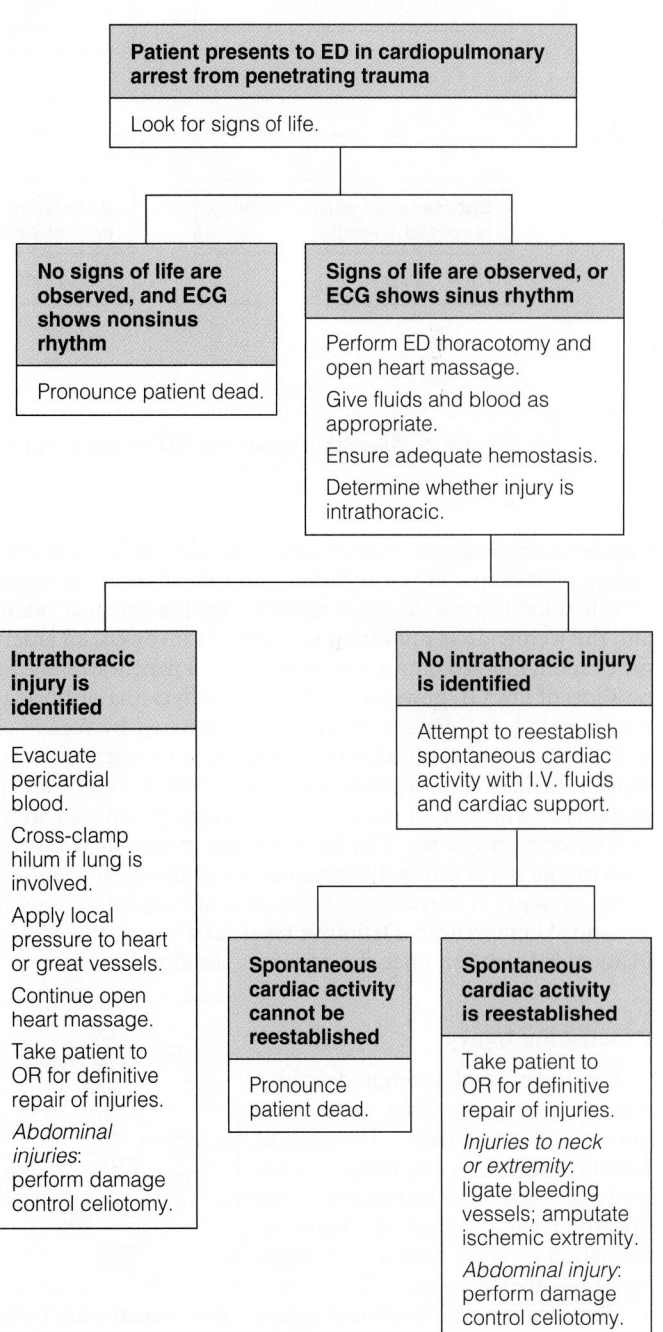

Figure 1 Algorithm illustrates ED evaluation of a penetrating trauma victim in cardiopulmonary arrest.

Patient presents to ED in cardiopulmonary arrest from penetrating trauma

Look for signs of life.

No signs of life are observed, and ECG shows nonsinus rhythm

Pronounce patient dead.

Signs of life are observed, or ECG shows sinus rhythm

Perform ED thoracotomy and open heart massage.

Give fluids and blood as appropriate.

Ensure adequate hemostasis.

Determine whether injury is intrathoracic.

Intrathoracic injury is identified

Evacuate pericardial blood.

Cross-clamp hilum if lung is involved.

Apply local pressure to heart or great vessels.

Continue open heart massage.

Take patient to OR for definitive repair of injuries.

Abdominal injuries: perform damage control celiotomy.

No intrathoracic injury is identified

Attempt to reestablish spontaneous cardiac activity with I.V. fluids and cardiac support.

Spontaneous cardiac activity cannot be reestablished

Pronounce patient dead.

Spontaneous cardiac activity is reestablished

Take patient to OR for definitive repair of injuries.

Injuries to neck or extremity: ligate bleeding vessels; amputate ischemic extremity.

Abdominal injury: perform damage control celiotomy.

Patient presents to ED in cardiopulmonary arrest from blunt trauma

Assess cardiac electrical activity.

Patient exhibits no cardiac activity or an agonal or wide-complex rhythm

Pronounce patient dead.

Patient exhibits ventricular tachycardia or fibrillation

Resuscitate patient with defibrillation and medical management.

Patient exhibits normal sinus rhythm, or arrest occurred in ED

Perform ED thoracotomy and open heart massage.

Give fluids as appropriate.

Spontaneous cardiac activity is reestablished

[*See Figure 7.*]

Spontaneous cardiac activity cannot be reestablished

Pronounce patient dead.

Spontaneous cardiac activity is reestablished

Take patient to OR.

Control hemorrhage.

Repair injuries definitively at planned reoperation.

Figure 2 Algorithm illustrates ED evaluation of a blunt trauma victim in cardiopulmonary arrest.

should be pronounced dead on arrival. In view of the probable failure of attempts at resuscitation, the risk of potential exposure to blood-borne diseases incurred by the medical team, and the tremendous utilization of resources involved, an emergency room thoracotomy is not warranted in a patient who shows no signs of life.[4] If, however, ventricular tachycardia or fibrillation is noted, the patient should be resuscitated by means of defibrillation and medical management A more aggressive approach (including emergency room thoracotomy) can be taken in patients who have a normal sinus rhythm or whose condition deteriorates in the ED; however, the prognosis is dismal even in this select group. In those rare cases in which adequate blood pressure is reestablished, the goal of surgical therapy is to control hemorrhage. Definitive repair can be completed in a planned reoperation once the patient is stabilized.

Penetrating Injury

The benefits of prompt definitive treatment of penetrating injury have been well documented.[5-7] The goals of initial resuscitation are, first, to rapidly identify patients who require urgent operation and, second, to obtain information that is critical for intraoperative management.

Identification of intrapleural injuries after penetrating torso wounds should be a priority [see I:2 *Trauma Resuscitation*]. Chest x-ray is an invaluable screening modality for such injuries. If a hemothorax or a pneumothorax is clinically obvious, a thoracostomy tube should be inserted before a chest x-ray is obtained, especially if the patient is hemodynamically unstable. In all other patients, a chest x-ray should be obtained immediately. Chest x-rays are helpful in most gunshot wound victims, even if the wound site is some distance from the thorax, because the path of the bullet is often unknown.

Factors affecting the management of penetrating injuries include the hemodynamic stability of the patient, the location of the wound, and the weapon used. Which diagnostic tests are performed and how quickly evaluation proceeds are determined primarily by the hemodynamic stability of the patient.

NECK

Although the airway is always a priority in critically injured patients, it is a particular concern in a patient with a penetrating neck wound because of the potential for compromise resulting from an expanding hematoma or edema associated with the injury. Accordingly, the airway should be monitored frequently during diagnostic procedures. A chest x-ray should be obtained early in the course of resuscitation to rule out intrathoracic injury [see Figure 3]. If an intrathoracic injury is identified, it should be evaluated and treated as outlined elsewhere [see Chest, *below*].

ED management of a hemodynamically unstable patient with a penetrating neck injury should be limited to applying local pressure, establishing intravenous access, and obtaining a chest x-ray. Exploration and definitive management of the injury in the operating suite should follow as soon as possible. The results of the neurologic examination done at the time of presentation should be documented because asymmetric neurologic findings may influence whether a carotid artery injury is repaired or ligated.[8]

In the past, evaluation and management of stable patients with neck injuries that penetrated the platysma depended on the location of the injury: injuries to zones I and III were evaluated roentgenographically, whereas injuries to zone II were an indication for mandatory exploration. Currently, however, thanks to the increased availability and improved safety of arteriography, the selective exploration strategy is favored for eval-

Figure 3 **Algorithm illustrates ED evaluation of a patient with penetrating injury to the neck.**

uating stable patients with penetrating neck injuries. Patients who have an obvious injury to a vascular or visceral structure (manifested by hypovolemic shock, pulsatile bleeding, airway compromise, or subcutaneous air in the neck) should undergo prompt exploration and treatment. Stable patients who do not have an obvious injury can be evaluated by means of urgent arteriography to exclude vascular injury. If arteriography identifies an injury, the patient should undergo exploration and treatment in the OR without further delay; if the arteriogram is normal, the airway and the esophagus should be evaluated endoscopically and roentgenographically.

Whenever a neck injury penetrates the platysma, evaluation of the carotid arteries is indicated; however, whether evaluation of the larynx and the trachea or of the pharynx and the esophagus is also indicated depends on the patient's symptoms and physical findings. Patients with difficulty in swallowing, voice changes, stridor, difficulty in breathing, or anterior neck pain should undergo both laryngotracheal and pharyngoesophageal evaluation. Direct laryngoscopy is the best means of evaluating the larynx and the trachea, and esophagography is the best means of evaluating the pharynx and the esophagus. Esophagoscopy can be performed either as an alternative or as an adjunct to esophagography. Individually, both esophagoscopy and esophagography have false negative rates of 10 to 15 percent, but when the two are combined, their sensitivity for detecting esophageal injuries rises to nearly 100 percent.[9,10] Delayed recognition and treatment of pharyngoesophageal injuries can lead to significant increases in morbidity and mortality; a high index of suspicion and early evaluation allow prompt identification of injuries and minimize morbidity.

If the platysma is intact or diagnostic tests yield negative results, the patient can simply be given local wound care and then discharged.

CHEST

Insertion of a therapeutic and diagnostic thoracostomy tube should be a priority in a hemodynamically unstable patient with a penetrating chest injury [*see Figure 4*]. This should be done before a chest x-ray is obtained so that adequate lung reexpansion can be ensured and any hemothorax present drained.

Urgent thoracotomy is indicated when the initial chest tube output is greater than 20 ml/kg or when subsequent chest tube output is greater than 2 ml/kg/hr for two consecutive hours. Patients with large undrained hemothoraces should also undergo early thoracotomy, especially if they are hemodynamically compromised. Thoracotomy is best done through an anterolateral incision with the patient supine; this approach permits simultaneous abdominal exploration if a diaphragmatic or intra-abdominal injury is found. Injuries to the esophagus, the descending thoracic aorta, and the distal airway are difficult to treat through an anterolateral exposure; if these structures are injured, a temporary closure can be performed once the bleeding is controlled, and the patient can then be repositioned for a formal posterolateral thoracotomy to treat the injuries.

An unstable patient who remains hypotensive but whose chest tube output and x-ray findings do not meet the criteria for urgent thoracotomy should undergo urgent celiotomy to exclude an intra-abdominal source of bleeding. If the injury is close to the heart, a pericardial window should be created at

Figure 4 Algorithm illustrates ED evaluation of an unstable patient with penetrating injury to the chest.

the time of laparotomy to rule out cardiac injury. A spinal cord injury should be suspected in a persistently hypotensive patient who exhibits no evidence of significant intra-abdominal or intrapericardial injury.

Most penetrating injuries to the chest can be managed simply by placing a chest tube in the affected hemithorax [see Figure 5]. Thoracotomy is indicated in a hemodynamically stable patient if there is evidence of significant bleeding (i.e., substantial chest tube output or a large clotted hemothorax), a tracheobronchial injury, a cardiovascular injury, or an esophageal injury. Exploration of the chest for a large hemothorax (evidenced by an initial chest tube output greater than 20 ml/kg, a subsequent chest tube output greater than 2 ml/kg/hr for two consecutive hours, or a cumulative 12-hour chest tube output greater than 30 ml/kg) can be performed through a posterolateral thoracotomy once intra-abdominal injury has been excluded.

A patient with a large air leak, massive subcutaneous or mediastinal emphysema, or a persistent pneumothorax should be evaluated via bronchoscopy to rule out tracheobronchial injury. Injuries to the intrathoracic trachea, the carina tracheae, or the right mainstem bronchus are best approached through a right anterolateral thoracotomy; injuries to the left mainstem bronchus are best approached through a left posterolateral thoracotomy.

A patient who is hemodynamically stable and does not require thoracotomy for hemorrhage or tracheobronchial injury should be evaluated for possible cardiac or vascular injury via echocardiography and arteriography if the injury is close to the heart or a great vessel. Most such injuries are associated with significant hemodynamic instability as a result of hemorrhage or pericardial tamponade; however, in rare cases, injuries to the heart or the great vessels may be occult. Echocardiographic evidence of pericardial fluid in a patient with a penetrating injury close to the heart is an indication for further

evaluation via a subxiphoid pericardial window.[11] If a hemopericardium is confirmed, the pericardial blood may be evacuated and the cardiac injury treated through a median sternotomy. Arteriography may reveal pseudoaneurysms, arteriovenous fistulas, or intimal flaps in stable patients with wounds close to great vessels. Injuries to the innominate artery or the common carotid arteries may be exposed via a median sternotomy; injuries to the proximal left subclavian artery should be exposed via an anterolateral thoracotomy for proximal control. The distal subclavian vessels can be exposed by resecting the medial third of the clavicle.

A patient who has a stab wound to the chest that is not close to the heart or a great vessel and whose chest x-ray is normal should be observed in the ED. A repeat chest x-ray should be obtained six hours after the injury; if this too is normal and examination reveals no worrisome findings, the patient can be discharged home.[12,13]

THORACOABDOMINAL REGION

Priorities in the management of a hypotensive patient with a penetrating thoracoabdominal injury include adequate intravenous access, insertion of a thoracostomy tube to decompress any hemothorax or pneumothorax, and urgent celiotomy [see Figure 6]. A chest x-ray should be obtained before operation to identify any intrathoracic injury. If the wound is close to the heart, a pericardial window should be created through a midline celiotomy to exclude cardiac injury. If a hemopericardium is identified, the injury may be exposed through a median sternotomy. If a significant lung injury is suspected, exposure is best obtained through a transverse thoracosternotomy.

If hemodynamic instability persists after intraperitoneal hemorrhage has been controlled, continuing intrathoracic hemorrhage must be excluded. Pleural bleeding should be quantified to determine whether a thoracotomy is necessary (see below). A repeat chest x-ray should be obtained to determine whether an undrained hemothorax is present. In the absence of a hemothorax or a tension pneumothorax that would account for the persistent hypotension, neurogenic shock from spinal cord injury must be excluded.

The mechanism of injury (gunshot wound versus stab wound) determines the initial evaluation priorities for a stable patient with a penetrating thoracoabdominal injury [see Figure 7]. A patient with a thoracoabdominal gunshot wound is highly likely to harbor an intra-abdominal injury and therefore should undergo urgent celiotomy. Substantial intra-abdominal injury may occur even in a patient who appears to be hemodynamically stable; prompt identification and definitive treatment are essential for minimizing morbidity. Preoperative diagnostic tests should be limited to routine blood and urine tests and a chest x-ray. An abdominal x-ray may be helpful in determining the path of the bullet and should be obtained if the patient is not in distress. Celiotomy can be avoided if the injury is obviously superficial or tangential and involves only the abdominal wall. Diagnostic laparoscopy or diagnostic peritoneal lavage may be helpful in a patient with a tangential wound in whom peritoneal penetration cannot be excluded by physical examination. If there are signs of peritonitis, however, celiotomy should not be delayed, even if the wound appears to be superficial.

Management of a thoracoabdominal stab wound in a stable patient varies according to the location of the wound and the

Figure 5 **Algorithm illustrates ED evaluation of a stable patient with penetrating injury to the chest.**

physical findings. If there is evidence of peritoneal penetration (e.g., omental herniation, evisceration, or obvious peritoneal irritation manifested by guarding and rebound tenderness), the patient should undergo urgent celiotomy. The preoperative workup should be similar to that for a stable gunshot wound victim. If peritoneal penetration is not obvious, the wound should be explored locally to determine whether the superficial fascia has been violated. If no fascial penetration has occurred, the patient can be discharged after receiving local wound care; if the fascia has been penetrated, further investigation is required to determine whether peritoneal penetration has occurred. Diagnostic laparoscopy or diagnostic peritoneal lavage can be performed to determine which patients require celiotomy to treat intra-abdominal injury. When diagnostic peritoneal lavage is used in this setting, a red blood cell count higher than 1,000/mm³ should be considered positive.[14] Diagnostic laparoscopy, though useful for identifying peritoneal penetration, is not a sensitive detector of bowel injuries.[15-18]

EXTREMITIES

Evaluation and treatment of a hypotensive patient with an isolated penetrating injury to an extremity involve essentially the same steps as evaluation and treatment of a hemodynamically unstable patient with a penetrating neck injury: local pressure to control hemorrhage, intravenous access for resuscitation, and prompt exploration and definitive treatment of the injury [see Figure 8].

Figure 6   **Algorithm illustrates ED evaluation of an unstable patient with penetrating injury to the thoracoabdominal region.**

Management of a stable patient with a penetrating injury to an extremity depends on the pulses distal to the injury. If distal pulses are absent, the patient should undergo exploration in the OR to identify any arterial injury present. Early exploration and repair of an arterial injury minimize ischemic time and subsequent reperfusion injury. If an arterial injury is not readily identified at exploration, an intraoperative arteriogram may be obtained to exclude thrombosis.

If distal pulses are normal and there is a penetrating injury close to an artery, the patient should undergo arterial duplex evaluation to exclude vascular injury.[19-21] I recommend duplex evaluation of all extremity gunshot wounds because of the possibility of stretch injuries to the artery as a result of the tremendous energy dispersed in the tissues. If the vascular examination is not suggestive of arterial injury, duplex evaluation is not urgent; instead, the patient can be observed and duplex evaluation performed once the resources are available (within 12 to 24 hours).

Distal vascular pulses should be monitored during the observation period; if distal pulses are lost, the patient should undergo prompt exploration of the affected artery. Any arterial injury identified by duplex evaluation should be confirmed and further defined by arteriography unless there is evidence of arterial occlusion, in which case the affected artery should be explored and repaired.

X-rays of the injured extremity should be obtained to exclude associated fractures and to localize any retained foreign bodies. If not all of the bullets can be accounted for, intravascular embolization should be suspected and the patient evaluated via multiple x-rays or fluoroscopy.

Figure 7 **Algorithm illustrates ED evaluation of a stable patient with penetrating injury to the thoracoabdominal region.**

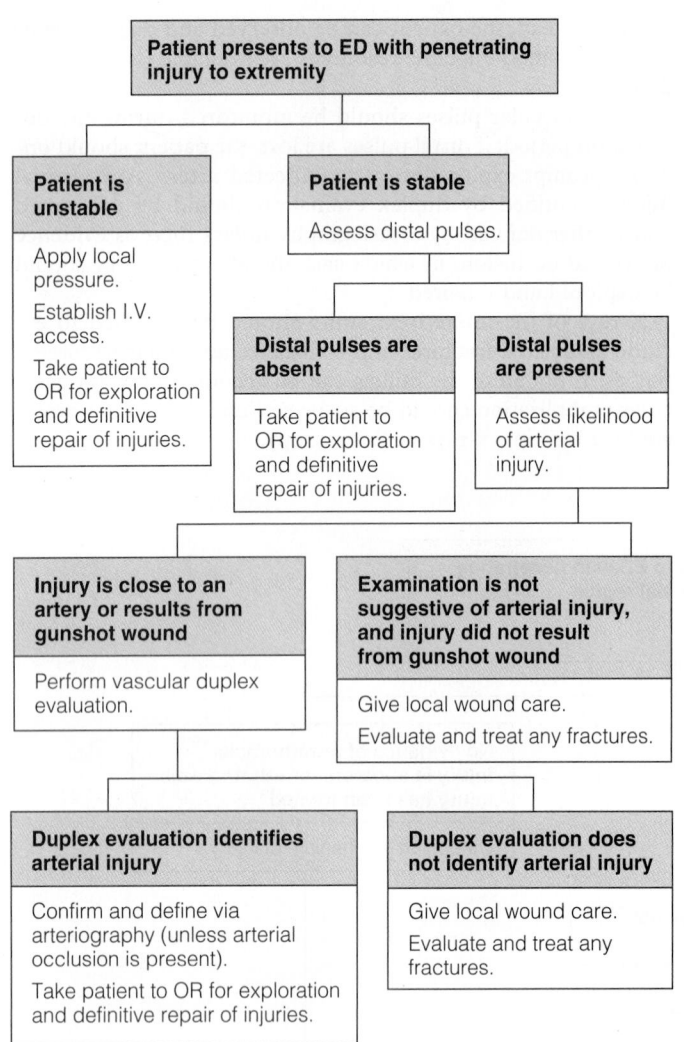

Figure 8 **Algorithm illustrates ED evaluation of a patient with penetrating injury to an extremity.**

Blunt Injury

Because blunt trauma typically involves multiple body regions, evaluation is directed primarily by the hemodynamic stability of the patient rather than by the location of the main injury. Extensive ED evaluation may be appropriate for a stable patient; however, a hypotensive patient should undergo an abbreviated evaluation, rapid resuscitation, and, if indicated, urgent oper-

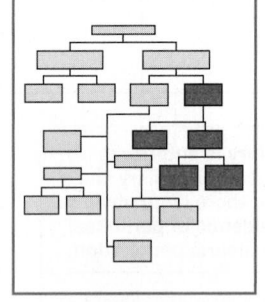

ative intervention, with assessment of non–life-threatening injuries left until after the patient has been stabilized.

Like the discussion of penetrating trauma (see above), the ensuing discussion is based on the assumption that the initial ABCs of trauma resuscitation have been addressed [*see I:2 Trauma Resuscitation*].

UNSTABLE PATIENT

Once the airway has been established, evaluation of the chest and prompt decompression of any hemothorax or pneu-

mothorax are priorities in a hypotensive blunt trauma victim [*see Figure 9*]. A chest tube should be inserted if breath sounds are diminished, the chest wall is grossly unstable, or subcutaneous emphysema is present. A chest x-ray should be obtained after the chest tube has been inserted to ensure proper placement and adequate decompression. In a patient without clinical signs of a hemothorax or a pneumothorax, a chest film should be obtained early in the initial evaluation period to detect occult thoracic injuries. If the patient's vital signs normalize after tube thoracoscopy, evaluation proceeds according to the specific injuries identified [*see Stable Patient, below*]. If the patient remains hemodynamically compromised, an urgent celiotomy should be performed to diagnose and treat any intra-abdominal injury.

When an urgent celiotomy is indicated, further evaluation is directed by the operative findings and the patient's response to the resuscitative efforts. If the intra-abdominal findings account for the patient's hemodynamic instability and the patient stabilizes after treatment, evaluation proceeds as dictated by the physical and laboratory findings. A damage control laparotomy should be performed in patients with continued hemodynamic instability and ongoing coagulopathy.[22] Non–life-threatening intra-abdominal injuries can be treated definitively at the time of reoperation. If the abdominal exploration reveals uncontrolled hemorrhage from a massive liver injury, the bleeding should be controlled and the patient transferred to the intensive care unit [*see III:7 Injuries to the Liver, Biliary Tract, Spleen, and Diaphragm*]. Further workup for associated injuries should proceed only after the coagulopathy has resolved and the patient's hemodynamic status has been stabilized.

If the intra-abdominal findings do not account for the patient's persistent hypotension, both chest cavities should be vented (if this has not already been done) and a pericardial window created. The presence of a hemopericardium signals a cardiac injury. Blunt cardiac rupture is associated with a high mortality; however, prompt identification and treatment can increase the chances that the patient will survive this devastating injury.[23]

If laparotomy reveals a large pelvic hematoma, the stability of the pelvis should be reassessed. If the pelvic ring is disrupted and unstable, the pelvis should be stabilized by rigid fixation. This will control bleeding in most patients with unstable pelvic fractures. If pelvic bleeding continues after reduction and fixation of the fracture, it can be treated with angiographic embolization; however, in my experience, this is rarely required once the bones are stabilized. The hemodynamic instability and coagulopathy associated with massive blood loss should be corrected in the ICU before the patient is subjected to further diagnostic tests.

The indications for thoracotomy after blunt trauma are similar to those for penetrating injuries: an initial chest tube output greater than 20 ml/kg or a subsequent chest tube output greater than 2 ml/kg/hr for two consecutive hours. Although thoracic exploration can be performed through an anterolateral incision with the patient supine, pulmonary and posterior mediastinal injuries are best exposed through a posterolateral thoracotomy. Thus, once the intra-abdominal injuries have been corrected and the patient's condition is sufficiently stable, he or she can be moved to the lateral decubitus position for a posterolateral thoracotomy.

Figure 9 **Algorithm illustrates ED evaluation of an unstable blunt trauma patient.**

Hypotension after blunt trauma should not be automatically ascribed to a head injury; instead, it should be assumed to result from hemorrhage. Hypotension associated with a head injury indicates brain stem involvement from direct trauma or herniation, either of which portends a hopeless prognosis. To assume that hypotension is the result of a head injury may delay prompt identification and treatment of hemorrhagic shock caused by a condition that may be easily manageable (e.g., a ruptured spleen). Thus, central nervous system injuries should be considered as causes of hypotension only after intra-abdominal and intrathoracic bleeding have been excluded.

STABLE PATIENT

Evaluation of a stable blunt trauma patient should proceed in the same rapid and efficient manner as evaluation of an unstable patient. Clearly, obvious peritonitis is an indication for prompt celiotomy. The real challenge in managing stable blunt trauma patients, particularly those who appear minimal-

ly injured, is to identify occult injuries, especially intra-abdominal injuries that may not be obvious at the time of initial presentation.

A chest x-ray early in the course of resuscitation provides information that is critical to the decision-making process [see Figure 10]. If a diaphragmatic hernia is identified, urgent celiotomy is indicated and further evaluation for intra-abdominal injury is unnecessary. If, however, a hemothorax large enough to warrant immediate thoracic exploration is identified [see Unstable Patient, above], diagnostic peritoneal lavage should be performed in the OR before thoracotomy. If the lavage fluid contains gross blood, celiotomy should precede thoracotomy. Once the abdominal bleeding is controlled, thoracic exploration can be performed through an anterolateral thoracotomy with the patient supine, or the patient can be repositioned for a posterolateral thoracotomy. If the lavage fluid is not bloody, the patient should be placed in the lateral decubitus position for a posterolateral thoracotomy.

Figure 10 Algorithm illustrates ED evaluation of a stable blunt trauma patient with obvious injury.

A patient with a large air leak in the chest tube or massive subcutaneous or mediastinal emphysema should undergo bronchoscopy so that the tracheobronchial tree can be evaluated. If there is evidence of a tracheobronchial injury, the patient should undergo diagnostic peritoneal lavage before thoracotomy. Again, if the aspirate is bloody, abdominal exploration and control of bleeding should precede thoracotomy. In a patient with a large air leak caused by a tracheobronchial injury, ventilation can often be facilitated by advancing the endotracheal tube into the unaffected bronchus at the time of diagnostic bronchoscopy. The evaluation for other non–life-threatening injuries can be completed once thoracic and abdominal hemorrhage are controlled and major airway injuries are repaired.

Evaluation of the abdomen in a stable patient without intrathoracic injury or in a patient whose thoracic injury has been treated depends on the patient's neurologic status [see Figure 11]. If the patient is awake and alert, observation with serial abdominal examinations and serial blood counts is appropriate. If there is a significant associated injury (i.e., one with an abdominal injury severity [AIS] score >2),[24] such as an extremity fracture, a rib fracture, a pelvic fracture, or a head injury, the patient should be admitted to the hospital for observation.

If peritonitis develops during the observation period, celiotomy is indicated for evaluation and treatment of the intra-abdominal injury. If the patient will require prolonged surgery for associated injuries, the abdomen should be assessed preoperatively by means of CT scanning, ultrasonography, or diagnostic peritoneal lavage. If abdominal examinations yield normal results but blood counts drop significantly (i.e., the hematocrit falls by more than six percent), either CT scanning or ultrasonography is indicated to rule out occult intra-abdominal hemorrhage. If abdominal examinations continue to reveal no significant abnormalities and blood counts remain stable, the patient can be discharged after 24 hours of observation.

Evaluation of the abdomen in an obtunded or comatose patient is complicated by the unreliability of the abdominal examination. The combination of an abdominal injury that necessitates therapeutic laparotomy with a head injury that necessitates craniotomy is a rare occurrence; however, a small number of patients who have both intracranial and intra-abdominal injuries may benefit from simultaneous abdominal and cranial procedures.[25] A comatose patient should be evaluated with early diagnostic peritoneal lavage or abdominal ultrasonography in the ED to facilitate triage.[26-28] If the lavage fluid is not grossly bloody or there is no free abdominal fluid on ultrasonography, an urgent CT scan of the head should be performed. If there is gross blood in the aspirate or free abdominal fluid is apparent on ultrasonography, further steps are determined by the results of the neurologic examination. Because of the strong correlation between lateralizing motor deficits and intracranial hemorrhage that necessitates craniotomy, patients with asymmetric motor deficits should undergo a CT scan of the head before celiotomy even if there is evidence of intra-abdominal injury, provided that the patient remains hemodynamically stable. If the patient becomes hemodynamically unstable during evaluation, CT scanning should be omitted and an urgent celiotomy performed to control hemorrhage; evaluation of the brain can proceed once

bleeding is controlled. The celiotomy may lead to short delays in the evaluation of the head injury; however, because hemorrhagic shock is detrimental to the injured brain as well as the rest of the patient, control of bleeding benefits both peripheral and central nervous perfusion. A patient with a nonfocal neurologic examination and evidence of intra-abdominal hemorrhage should undergo celiotomy, followed by an urgent CT scan of the head. Mannitol infusion can be used empirically to treat suspected high intracranial pressure in patients requiring urgent laparotomy or thoracotomy for hemostasis.

Evaluation of Specific Findings after Blunt Trauma

Physical examination and roentgenography will identify specific worrisome findings that call for further evaluation [see Figure 12]. When and how these findings are investigated depends on the stability of the patient, the need for surgical intervention to treat abdominal or thoracic hemorrhage, and the combination of injuries present. The trauma surgeon must prioritize the evaluation of specific findings according to the relative likelihood that a poor outcome will ensue if diagnosis is delayed. In what follows, these findings are addressed in decreasing order of urgency.

Loss of consciousness Once hemodynamic stability has been established, assessment for neurologic injury should be a priority. Whenever there has been a loss of consciousness or the neurologic examination reveals abnormalities, a CT scan of the head should be obtained.[29,30] The incidence of significant intracranial injury in patients with minor neurologic abnormalities is low; however, if an injury is missed, the potential for a poor clinical outcome is great.

A high index of suspicion is required for the diagnosis of blunt carotid artery injuries. Any patient who exhibits evidence of major cervical trauma or transient neurologic findings (e.g., hemiplegia or hemiparesis) may have a blunt carotid artery injury and should be evaluated with carotid artery duplex evaluation or arteriography.[31]

Wide mediastinum Traumatic pseudoaneurysms of the aorta should be suspected in victims of accidents involving rapid deceleration. Although x-ray findings (e.g., a depressed left mainstem bronchus, apical capping, a deviated trachea, or a deviated esophagus visualized with a nasogastric tube) may be suggestive, the mechanism of injury and the mediastinal silhouette are the two most sensitive markers for an injured thoracic aorta.[32] Evaluation of a wide mediastinum should proceed promptly once intra-abdominal hemorrhage has been controlled.

Aortography remains the gold standard for evaluating the aorta. Transesophageal echocardiography has been proposed as a screening tool; however, its sensitivity in identifying aortic injuries remains to be established.[33] Computed tomography of the chest is neither specific nor sensitive for traumatic aortic pseudoaneurysms and should not be relied on to exclude the diagnosis.[34]

Pulseless extremity The absence of distal pulses in a fractured or dislocated extremity demands urgent attention once life-threatening thoracoabdominal and head injuries have been addressed. Fractures and dislocations should be reduced promptly. If pulses return and are symmetric, no further eval-

Figure 11 **Algorithm illustrates ED evaluation of a stable blunt trauma patient without obvious injury.**

uation is necessary; however, the patient should be monitored for the development of compartment syndrome. If vascular injury is suspected because of a weak, asymmetric pulse or if a knee dislocation is present, the artery in question should be examined with either vascular duplex evaluation or arteriography. The pulseless extremity is best evaluated in the OR. An on-table arteriogram should suffice to localize the area of injury. The vessels can then be explored and repaired prompt-

ly, and the time to reperfusion of the extremity can thereby be minimized.

Cervical spine injury Cervical spine injury is present in fewer than five percent of cases of blunt trauma.[35] Nevertheless, all patients should be screened for cervical spine injury because of the potentially devastating consequences if an injury is missed. Every patient with known or suspected

Blunt trauma patient is or has been rendered hemodynamically stable

Specific worrisome findings are identified that call for further evaluation. Prioritize evaluation of these according to likelihood of poor outcome if left untreated.

History of loss of consciousness or Glasgow Coma Scale score < 14

Obtain CT scan of head. If results are abnormal, obtain neurosurgical consultation.

If there is evidence of major cervical trauma or transient neurologic findings, perform carotid artery duplex evaluation or arteriography.

Rapid deceleration injury with or without wide mediastinum

Evaluate aorta with aortography, and repair any aortic injury.

Pulseless extremity

Reduce any fractures.

Pulses do not return

Take patient to OR for arteriography and surgical exploration and treatment once more urgent injuries are stabilized.

Pulses return but are asymmetric, or knee dislocation is present

Assess suspected damaged vessel with vascular duplex evaluation or, if duplex is abnormal or unavailable, arteriography.

Pulses return and are symmetric

Observe patient.

Possible spinal injury

Physical examination is unreliable, patient has multiple injuries, patient complains of neck pain, or cervical tenderness is noted

Maintain patient in strict spinal precautions.
Obtain cervical spine x-rays.

Physical examination is reliable, and there are no distracting injuries, no complaints of neck pain, and no cervical tenderness

Clear patient clinically without x-rays.

Long bone fracture, pelvic fracture, or hip dislocation

Reduce dislocations and fracture-dislocations as soon as possible.
Once life-threatening injuries have been treated, obtain x-rays of proximal and distal joints and stabilize pelvic and long bone fractures.
Obtain early orthopedic consultation.

Hematuria

Adult patient has gross hematuria or microscopic hematuria with hypotension, or juvenile patient has any kind of hematuria

Obtain abdominal CT scan and cystogram.
Male patient with gross hematuria: obtain retrograde urethrogram.

Adult patient has microscopic hematuria without hypotension

No further evaluation is necessary unless renal pedicle disruption is likely.

Figure 12   **Algorithm illustrates evaluation of specific findings associated with blunt trauma after hemodynamic stability has been established.**

injury to the spine should be maintained in strict spinal precautions throughout assessment and resuscitation until the spine can be thoroughly evaluated. If the physical examination is reliable (i.e., if the patient is awake and alert and is not under the influence of alcohol or drugs) and there are no distracting injuries, no complaints of neck pain, and no tenderness on examination, the patient can be cleared clinically without roentgenography.[36] In all other cases, cervical spine x-rays should be obtained as soon as feasible; however, treatment of life-threatening injuries (including endotracheal intubation) should not be delayed to obtain the x-rays. An orotracheal airway can be secured safely in patients with a suspected cervical spine injury by maintaining the head and neck in a neutral position (in-line stabilization).[37]

Early mobilization in critically injured patients is important for facilitating adequate pulmonary hygiene and minimizing thrombotic complications. The spine should be evaluated and cleared within 24 hours of injury to permit early mobilization. Flexion-extension views should be obtained in patients with significant cervical spine tenderness, even if there is no evidence of bone injury, to determine whether there is any ligamentous injury. The thoracic, lumbar, and sacral regions of the spine should be evaluated in patients who complain of back pain or have neurologic deficits and in all patients whose physical examination is unreliable.

Extremity fractures or dislocations Early definitive fixation of long bone fractures is essential for minimizing morbidity and mortality from multiple trauma and should be performed as soon as torso and head injuries have been assessed and treated. Gross pelvic instability, long bone deformities, and open fractures should be identified during the primary and secondary surveys of a multiply injured patient. Dislocations and fracture-dislocations should be reduced as soon as possible to minimize the morbidity associated with compromised blood flow distal to the dislocation. Long bone fractures should be splinted to reduce tissue trauma as soon as the patient's condition permits. Broad-spectrum antibiotics should be administered if open fractures are present. A pelvic x-ray should be obtained early in the evaluation of a multiply injured trauma patient to identify occult fractures and to plan definitive fixation of the unstable pelvis. X-rays of extremities, including a joint above and a joint below the suspected fracture, should be obtained once life-threatening injuries have been treated.

Hematuria In a patient with life-threatening injuries, the kidneys and the intraperitoneal portion of the bladder can be assessed at the time of celiotomy. Patients with nonexpanding and nonpulsatile perinephric hematomas that are contained by Gerota's fascia should not undergo exploration, because most of these renal injuries go on to heal spontaneously and exploration of the hematoma results in a higher rate of nephrectomy. If the patient is found to have an expanding or uncontained hematoma, the kidney should be explored. Vascular control should be obtained centrally before the kidney is exposed.[38] Renal salvage should be considered if the patient's overall condition permits (i.e., if the patient is hemodynamically stable and disseminated intravascular coagulation is absent). Management of the renal injury depends on the patient's overall condition, the nature of the renal injury itself, and the status of the contralateral kidney. If the renal injury is complex and nephrectomy is contemplated, contralateral renal function may be assessed intraoperatively with an on-table one-shot excretory nephrogram. Alternatively, the ureter of the damaged kidney may be temporarily and atraumatically clamped. The anesthesiologist may then administer a vial of methylene blue intravenously. The appearance of blue urine in the tube draining the bladder confirms that the contralateral kidney is functional.

Whenever hematuria, including microscopic hematuria, is noted in a hypotensive patient, evaluation is indicated.[39] Evaluation may proceed as soon as life-threatening injuries have been treated and hemodynamic stability has been restored.

Any patient with gross hematuria should be evaluated for possible renal, bladder, and (if male) urethral injuries.[39] If the patient is stable, CT is the best method for evaluating the kidneys.[40] An abdominal CT scan with intravenous contrast material provides useful information about renal perfusion, the size and nature of any perinephric hematoma, and the integrity of the kidneys, as well as about possible associated occult intra-abdominal injuries. In some cases, CT may also provide information about bladder injuries.[41,42] At present, however, cystography remains the study of choice for evaluation of the bladder.

In a male patient with gross hematuria, a retrograde urethrogram should be obtained to exclude urethral injury. This is especially important if there is blood at the meatus, the prostate gland is high-riding and mobile, or passage of the Foley catheter is difficult. In women, the urethra is shorter and better protected and thus is rarely injured.

Patients with microscopic hematuria but no history of hypotension need not undergo further evaluation unless there is a high index of suspicion for renal pedicle disruption on the basis of the mechanism of injury.

References

1. Durham LA 3d, Richardson RJ, Wall MJ Jr, et al: Emergency center thoracotomy: impact of prehospital resuscitation. J Trauma 32:775, 1992

2. Lorenz HP, Steinmetz B, Lieberman J, et al: Emergency thoracotomy: survival correlates with physiologic status. J Trauma 32:780, 1992

3. Harnar TJ, Oreskovich MR, Copass MK, et al: Role of emergency thoracotomy in the resuscitation of moribund trauma victims: 100 consecutive cases. Am J Surg 142:96, 1981

4. Rosemurgy AS, Norris PA, Olson SM, et al: Prehospital traumatic cardiac arrest: the cost of futility. J Trauma 35:468, 1993

5. Lerer LB, Knottenbelt JD: Preventable mortality following sharp penetrating chest trauma. J Trauma 37:9, 1994

6. Ivatury RR, Nallathambi MN, Roberge RJ, et al: Penetrating thoracic injuries: in-field stabilization vs. prompt transport. J Trauma 27:1066, 1987

7. Pepe PE, Wyatt CH, Bickell WH, et al: The relationship between total prehospital time and outcome in hypotensive victims of penetrating injuries. Ann Emerg Med 16:293, 1987

8. Richardson R, Obeid FN, Richardson JD, et al: Neurologic consequences of cerebrovascular injury. J Trauma 32:755, 1992

9. Weigelt JA, Thal ER, Snyder WH 3d, et al: Diagnosis of penetrating cervical esophageal injuries. Am J Surg 154:619, 1987

10. Noyes LD, McSwain NE Jr, Markowitz IP: Pan-

endoscopy with arteriography versus mandatory exploration of penetrating wounds of the neck. Ann Surg 204:21, 1986

11. Meyer DM, Jessen ME, Grayburn PA: Use of echocardiography to detect occult cardiac injury after penetrating thoracic trauma: a prospective study. J Trauma 39:902, 1995

12. Ordog GJ, Balasubramanium S, Wasserberger J: Outpatient management of 357 gunshot wounds to the chest. J Trauma 23:832, 1983

13. Weigelt JA, Aurbakken CM, Meier DE, et al: Management of asymptomatic patients following stab wounds to the chest. J Trauma 22:291, 1982

14. Oreskovich MR, Carrico CJ: Stab wounds of the anterior abdomen: analysis of a management plan using local wound exploration and quantitative peritoneal lavage. Ann Surg 198:411, 1993

15. Fabian TC, Croce MA, Stewart RM, et al: A prospective analysis of diagnostic laparoscopy in trauma. Ann Surg 217:557 (discussion, 564), 1993

16. Rossi P, Mullins D, Thal E: Role of laparoscopy in the evaluation of abdominal trauma. Am J Surg 166:707, 1993

17. Ivatury RR, Simon RJ, Stahl WM: A critical evaluation of laparoscopy in penetrating abdominal trauma. J Trauma 34:822, 1993

18. Fabian TC, Croce MA, Stewart RM, et al: A prospective analysis of diagnostic laparoscopy in trauma. Ann Surg 217:557, 1993

19. Bynoe RP, Miles WS, Bell RM, et al: Noninvasive diagnosis of vascular trauma by duplex ultrasonography. J Vasc Surg 14:346, 1991

20. Fry WR, Smith RS, Sayers DV, et al: The success of duplex ultrasonographic scanning in diagnosis of extremity vascular proximity trauma. Arch Surg 128:1368, 1993

21. Knudson MM, Lewis FR, Atkinson K, et al: The role of duplex ultrasound arterial imaging in patients with penetrating extremity trauma. Arch Surg 128:1033, 1993

22. Rotondo MF, Schwab CW, McGonigal MD, et al: "Damage control": an approach for improved survival in exsanguinating penetrating abdominal injury. J Trauma 35:375, 1993

23. Leavitt BJ, Meyer JA, Morton JR, et al: Survival following nonpenetrating traumatic rupture of cardiac chambers. Ann Thorac Surg 44:532, 1987

24. Association for the Advancement of Automotive Medicine: The abbreviated injury scale. Association for the Advancement of Automotive Medicine, Des Plaines, Illinois, 1990

25. Wisner DH, Victor NS, Holcroft J: Priorities in the management of multiple trauma: intracranial versus intra-abdominal injury. J Trauma 35:271, 1993

26. Rozycki GS, Ochsner MG, Schmidt JA, et al: A prospective study of surgeon-performed ultrasound as the primary adjuvant modality for injured patient assessment. J Trauma 39:492, 1995

27. Bolton JW, Bynoe RP, Lazar HL, et al: Two-dimensional echocardiography in the evaluation of penetrating intrapericardial injuries. Ann Thorac Surg 56:506, 1993

28. Rozycki GS, Ochsner MG, Jaffin JH, et al: Prospective evaluation of surgeons' use of ultrasound in the evaluation of trauma patients. J Trauma 34:516, 1993

29. Moran SG, McCarthy MC, Uddin DE, et al: Predictors of positive CT scans in the trauma patient with minor head injury. Am Surg 60:533, 1994

30. Shackford SR, Wald SL, Ross SE, et al: The clinical utility of computed tomographic scanning and neurologic examination in the management of patients with minor head injuries. J Trauma 33:385, 1992

31. Cogbill TH, Moore EE, Meissner M, et al: The spectrum of blunt injury to the carotid artery: a multicenter perspective. J Trauma 37:473, 1994

32. Kirsh MM, Behrendt DM, Orringer MB, et al: The treatment of acute traumatic rupture of the aorta: a 10-year experience. Ann Surg 184:308, 1976

33. Smith MD, Cassidy JM, Souther S, et al: Transesophageal echocardiography in the diagnosis of traumatic rupture of the aorta. N Engl J Med 332:356, 1995

34. Durham RM, Zuckerman D, Wolverson M, et al: Computed tomography as a screening exam in patients with suspected blunt aortic injury. Ann Surg 220:699, 1994

35. Soicher E, Demetriades D: Cervical spine injuries in patients with head injuries. Br J Surg 78:1013, 1991

36. Roberge RJ, Wears RC, Kelly M, et al: Selective application of cervical spine radiography in alert victims of blunt trauma: a prospective study. J Trauma 28:784, 1988

37. Rhee KJ, Green W, Holcroft JW, et al: Oral intubation in the multiply injured patient: the risk of exacerbating spinal cord damage. Ann Emerg Med 19:511, 1990

38. Carroll PR, Klosterman P, McAninch JW: Early vascular control for renal trauma: a critical review. J Urol 141:826, 1989

39. Nicolaisen GS, McAninch JW, Marshall GA, et al: Renal trauma: re-evaluation of the indications for radiographic assessment. J Urol 133:183, 1985

40. Herschorn S, Radomski SB, Shoskes DA, et al: Evaluation and treatment of blunt renal trauma. J Urol 146:274, 1991

41. Kane NM, Francis IR, Ellis JH: The value of CT in the detection of bladder and posterior urethral injuries. Am J Roentgenology 153:1243, 1989

42. Horstman WG, McClennan BL, Heiken JP: Comparison of computed tomography and conventional cystography for detection of traumatic bladder rupture. Urol Radiol 12:188, 1991

Acknowledgment

Figures 1 through 12   Marcia Kammerer.

2 INJURIES TO THE CENTRAL NERVOUS SYSTEM

Marike Zwienenberg-Lee, M.D., and J. Paul Muizelaar, M.D., Ph.D.

Approach to Injuries to the Head and Spinal Cord

It is estimated that each year, two million patients present to physicians with a primary or secondary diagnosis of head injury. Of these patients, approximately 400,000 are admitted and 70,000 die, most of traumatic brain injury. Thus, brain injury can be considered epidemic. Neurosurgeons, who number 4,000 in the United States, are probably best trained to manage patients with severe head injuries, but the initial resuscitation and stabilization is usually performed by emergency department physicians, general surgeons, and trauma surgeons. These professionals are the ones who can make a difference for patients: recent insights into the pathophysiology of traumatic brain injury indicate that treatment during the first few hours is critical and often determines outcome.

Nonetheless, the role of surgeons immediately after resuscitation and in the ensuing days is not to be underestimated. Patients with multiple system injuries often receive care in surgical intensive care units under the supervision of a general surgeon. Less than optimal management at an early stage will have a greater impact because of the larger number of patients involved, but less than optimal management at a later stage, even in a mildly injured patient, will have a much more dramatic impact. Initial recovery, followed by relentless decline attributable to insufficient cerebral perfusion, is not an expected outcome. Although we cannot promote healing of the brain with pharmacologic means, we can prevent secondary injury to the brain by ensuring adequate cerebral circulation and oxygenation.

The reported incidence of spinal cord injury in the United States ranges from 29 to 53 per million.[1-3] About 50% of the injuries are related to motor vehicle accidents, 15% to 20% to falls, 15% to 20% to interpersonal violence, and the remaining 15% to 20% to sports and recreational activity. In general, the group at highest risk is between 16 and 30 years of age, not unlike the group at highest risk for head injuries. Most of those injured are males: several studies report that the percentage is approximately 75%.[4] Between 45% and 50% of patients with spinal cord injury have associated injuries that seriously affect their prognosis.[5]

The cervical spine is most often involved in spinal cord injury. The major study of trauma outcome, conducted from 1982 to 1989, revealed that the cervical spinal cord was involved in 55% of cases, the thoracic spinal cord in 30% of cases, and the lumbar spinal cord in 15% of cases of acute injury.[6] In an analysis of 358 patients with spinal cord injury, 78% of the 71 cases of thoracic injury were accompanied by complete neurologic injury; 60% of the 202 cases of cervical injury and 65% of the 85 cases of thoracolumbar injury were accompanied by complete neurologic injury.[7] Average direct costs of spinal cord injury (including hospitalization, rehabilitation, residence modification, and long-term care) are tremendous. In 1992, it was estimated that lifetime costs (in 1989 dollars) were $210,379 for a paraplegic and $571,854 for a quadriplegic.[8]

Initial resuscitation and evaluation of injured patients are discussed more fully elsewhere [*see I:2 Trauma Resuscitation and III:1 Emergency Department Evaluation of the Patient with Multiple Injuries*]. In this chapter, we outline approaches to the management of severe head injury and acute spinal cord injury. In addition, we address the pathophysiology of such injuries to provide the reader with the understanding required for making appropriate decisions about diagnosis and treatment of injured patients [*see Discussion, below*].

Head Injury

EMERGENCY DEPARTMENT MANAGEMENT

Because hypoxia and hypotension interfere with cerebral oxygenation, complete and rapid physiologic resuscitation is the first priority for patients with head injuries. A large study from the Traumatic Coma Data Bank demonstrated that a single observation of systolic blood pressure below 90 mm Hg in the field or hypoxia (arterial oxygen tension [P_aO_2] below 60 mm Hg) was a major predictor of poor outcome.[9] A multidisciplinary team should provide the patient with an adequate airway and ventilation (intubation, ventilation, and detection of hemothorax or pneumothorax) and restore and maintain hemodynamic stability (with adequate fluid replacement and detection and treatment of any bleeding), all according to the principles developed by the Advanced Trauma Life Support system.[10] The ABCs of emergency care (airway, breathing, and circulation) take precedence, irrespective of neurologic injuries. The initial neurologic assessment, which does not take more than 10 seconds, consists of rating the patient on the Glasgow Coma Scale (GCS) [*see Table 1*] and assessing the width and reactivity of the pupils. Although the same assessment is made after resuscitation as a guide for prognosis and therapy, it should also be made (and recorded) before resuscitation to permit evaluation of the effect of resuscitative measures and differentiation between primary and secondary neurologic injury.

Early orotracheal intubation and ventilation, if not performed in the field, is recommended for patients with a GCS score of 8 or lower or a motor score of 4 or lower. Other indications for immediate intubation are loss of protective laryngeal reflexes and ventilatory insufficiency (indicated by measurement of blood gases), including hypoxemia (P_aO_2 < 60 mm Hg), hypercarbia (arterial carbon dioxide tension [P_aCO_2] > 45 mm Hg), spontaneous hyperventilation (causing P_aCO_2 < 26 mm Hg), and respiratory arrhythmia. Indications for intubation before transport are deteriorating consciousness (even if the patient is not in a coma), bilateral fractured mandible, copious bleeding into the mouth (as occurs with fracture of the base of the skull), and seizures. An intubated patient must also be ventilated ($P_aCO_2 \approx 35$ mm Hg).

Table 1 Glasgow Coma Scale

Test	Response	Score
Eye opening (E)	Spontaneous	4
	To verbal command	3
	To pain	2
	None	1
Best motor response (arm) (M)	Obedience to verbal command	6
	Localization of painful stimulus	5
	Flexion withdrawal response to pain	4
	Abnormal flexion response to pain (decorticate rigidity)	3
	Extension response to pain (decerebrate rigidity)	2
	None	1
Best verbal response (V)	Oriented conversation	5
	Disoriented conversation	4
	Inappropriate words	3
	Incomprehensible sounds	2
	None	1
	Total (E + M + V)	3–15

Fluid replacement should be performed with isotonic solutions such as lactated Ringer's solution, normal saline, or packed red blood cells when appropriate. The patient should be examined rapidly and thoroughly for any concomitant life-threatening injuries.

Patients with spinal cord injury above T5 and vasogenic spinal shock may have severe hypotension, which should be treated vigorously; induction of mild hypertension or application of pneumatic antishock trousers may be necessary. Intracranial hypertension should be suspected if there is rapid neurologic deterioration. Clinical evidence of intracranial hypertension, manifest by signs of herniation, includes unilateral or bilateral dilatation of the pupils, asymmetrical pupillary reactivity, and motor posturing.

Intracranial hypertension should be treated aggressively. Hyperventilation, which does not interfere with volume resuscitation and results in rapid reduction of intracranial pressure (ICP), should be established immediately in cases of pupillary abnormalities. Recent research has shown that unilateral or bilateral pupillary abnormalities do not result from compression of the third cranial nerves, as previously thought, but from compression of the brain stem, with resulting brain stem ischemia.[11] Therefore, administration of mannitol is effective because it not only decreases ICP but also increases cerebral blood flow (CBF) through modulation of viscosity. Because mannitol is not used to dehydrate the body, all fluid losses through diuresis must be replaced immediately or even preventively, especially in patients suffering shock as a result of blood loss. Although arterial hypertension occurring after a severe head injury may reflect intracranial hypertension (Cushing's phenomenon), especially when accompanied by bradycardia, it should not be treated, because it may be the sole mechanism permitting the brain to maintain perfusion despite increasing intracranial pressure.

In the absence of signs of herniation, sedation should be used when indicated for safe and efficient transport of the patient. Transport of the patient should be kept to a minimum because it is often accompanied by secondary insults (e.g., hypoxia or hypotension). Pharmacologic paralysis, which interferes with neurologic examination, should be used only if sedation alone is inadequate for safe and effective transport and resuscitation of the patient. When phar-

macologic paralysis is used, short-acting agents are preferred. Prophylactic hyperventilation, which may exacerbate early ischemia, is not recommended for these patients. A guide to the resuscitation and initial treatment of patients with severe head injuries will assist in management [see Figure 1].

Minimal radiologic evaluation consists of a lateral cervical spine film or a swimmer's view [see Spinal Cord Injury, below]. After hemodynamic stability is achieved, unenhanced CT of the head should be used for all patients with persistent impairment of consciousness.

Operative Management

Rapid evacuation of mass lesions decreases intracranial pressure and consequently improves cerebral perfusion pressure (CPP) and CBF. Schroder and colleagues[12] have demonstrated reversal of ischemia soon after removal of a subdural hematoma. Subdural hematomas require emergent evacuation by a neurosurgeon; evacuation performed within 4 hours of injury has been shown to result in a better outcome.

Figure 1 **Shown is an algorithm for initial management of the patient with a severe head injury.**

An epidural hematoma, which is a life-threatening neurosurgical emergency, should be evacuated urgently. In cases of temporal fracture and rapid clinical deterioration, a temporal craniectomy can be performed. If there is no temporal fracture, an unenhanced CT scan should be obtained to avoid searching for a lesion with multiple bur holes. In cases of progressive deterioration, moderate hyperventilation ($P_aCO_2 \approx 30$) should be initiated and mannitol (1 g/kg) given while the patient is being readied for surgery.

Posterior fossa hematomas, which are rare, also require urgent evacuation, because obstructive hydrocephalus and brain stem compression can result in rapid neurologic deterioration. An intracerebral hematoma causing a midline shift larger than 5 mm is an indication for operative treatment, but surgery can usually be delayed for a few hours.

ICU MANAGEMENT

A GCS score of 8 or lower after resuscitation is an indication for admission to a neurosurgical ICU. Although the focus of ICU management is prevention of secondary injury and maintenance of adequate cerebral oxygenation, admission to an ICU does not eliminate the occurrence of secondary insults.[13] In a series of 124 patients admitted to a neurosurgical ICU, more than one episode of hypotension occurred in 73% of all patients, and more than one episode of hypoxia occurred in 40%.[14] Kirkpatrick and coworkers[15] performed online monitoring of CPP, jugular venous saturation, local CBF, and local tissue oxygenation in 14 patients who had sustained a severe head injury; 37% of the episodes involving decreased CBF, CPP, and saturation were related to clinical and nursing procedures.

Monitoring

A variety of bedside devices are available for monitoring of ICP, local CBF, and local and global cerebral oxygenation.[13,15,16] Aside from monitors for ICP and jugular venous oxygen saturation, most of these devices are experimental.

Intracranial pressure Monitoring of ICP has never been subjected to a prospective, randomized clinical trial designed to assess its efficacy in improving patient outcome. Nevertheless, many clinical studies indicate that ICP monitoring is useful for early detection of intracranial mass lesions; that it allows calculation of CPP, an important clinical indicator of CBF; that it limits the indiscriminate use of potentially harmful therapies for control of ICP; that it helps determine prognosis; and that it may improve outcome. ICP monitoring is indicated in patients with a GCS score of 3 to 7 after resuscitation or a GCS score of 8 to 12 and an abnormal CT scan at the time of admission. In patients with a GCS score of 8 to 9 and a normal CT scan, ICP monitoring is indicated if the patient is older than 40 years, has a systolic BP below 90 mm Hg, and exhibits unilateral or bilateral motor posturing.[16]

Jugular bulb oximetry CBF is an important determinant of neurologic outcome, and the arterial–jugular venous oxygen difference (A-VDo$_2$) is an important parameter of the adequacy of CBF. Monitoring of therapy by measuring CBF and A-VDo$_2$ would be ideal, but there is no practical way of doing this directly and continuously.

An estimate of global A-VDo$_2$ can be obtained from simultaneous monitoring of arterial oxygen saturation (S_aO_2) and jugular venous oxygen saturation ($S_{jv}O_2$). Jugular venous oxygen saturation is monitored by percutaneous retrograde insertion of a fiberoptic catheter in the internal jugular vein, with the tip of the catheter located in the jugular bulb. The catheter is usually inserted into the jugular vein with the dominant cerebral venous drainage (the right jugular vein in 80% to 90% of the population), but some prefer to insert the catheter at the site of most significant brain damage.

A-VDo$_2$ is calculated according to the following formula:

$$A\text{-}VDo_2 = (S_aO_2 - S_{jv}O_2) \times 1.34 \times Hb + [(P_aO_2 - P_{jv}O_2) \times 0.0031]$$

The contribution of the variables within the brackets, which is small, is usually ignored for practical purposes. Because calculation of A-VDo$_2$ requires the drawing of blood samples, it can be done only intermittently.

For continuous monitoring, $S_{jv}O_2$, the result of arterial oxygen input and cerebral extraction, is used. In normal individuals, $S_{jv}O_2$ ranges from 50% to 70%.[17] If $S_{jv}O_2$ values below 50% last for more than 15 minutes, they are considered desaturations, resulting either from insufficient arterial oxygenation (S_aO_2) or oxygen-carrying capacity (Hb concentration) or, when arterial saturation and oxygen-carrying capacity are normal, from inadequate CBF. Gopinath and colleagues[18] [see Table 2] described a relation between the occurrence of desaturations and neurologic outcome in patients with severe head injuries. Without desaturation, mortality was 16%; with one documented desaturation, 42%; and with multiple desaturations, 70%. High $S_{jv}O_2$ values indicate low oxygen extraction, which is the case when the cerebral metabolic rate of oxygen (CMRo$_2$) is low.

The limitations of jugular bulb oximetry should be kept in mind when $S_{jv}O_2$ values are interpreted.[19,20] Because $S_{jv}O_2$ represents global oxygenation, regional ischemia may go undetected if the ischemic region is too small to be represented in the total hemispheric $S_{jv}O_2$ value. Ischemia may also occur in a part of the brain being drained by the opposite jugular vein. In addition, extracerebral veins drain into the internal jugular vein approximately 2 cm below the jugular bulb. With low flow values, significant extracerebral contamination may occur, resulting in deceptively high $S_{jv}O_2$ values. Finally, artifactual readings are often encountered as a result of reduced light intensity when the catheter lodges against the vessel wall. With a new type of catheter, however, the number of artifacts appears to be much lower.

Management of Cerebral Perfusion Pressure

The rationale behind CPP therapy is expressed in Poiseuille's law [see Discussion, Pathophysiology, below]. Although the effect of CPP therapy has not been investigated in a randomized, controlled clinical trial, several studies suggest that a CPP of 70 to 80 mm Hg may be the clinical threshold below which mortality and morbidity increase.[21,22] CPP therapy involves manipulation of both arterial BP and ICP, but its objective is the reduction of ICP. If ICP reduction does not achieve a CPP of 70 mm Hg, arterial

Table 2 Jugular Desaturation* and Outcome in 116 Patients with Severe Head Injuries[18]

Jugular Desaturations (No.)	Outcome		
	Good Recovery/ Moderate Disability (%)	Severe Disability/ Vegetative (%)	Deceased (%)
0	45	39	16
1	26	32	42
>1	10	20	70

*Defined as jugular venous oxygen saturation < 50% for longer than 15 min.

hypertension is instituted. Mean arterial BP should be raised first by achieving good volume status: ample fluids, including albumin (25 to 30 ml/hr), are administered to maintain central venous pressure at 5 to 10 mm Hg. A pulmonary arterial catheter is suggested for patients older than 50 years and for individuals with known cardiac disease, multiple trauma (particularly chest or abdominal injuries), or a need for vasopressors or high-dose barbiturates. Pulmonary arterial wedge pressure (PAWP) should be maintained between 10 and 14 mm Hg. If necessary, an alpha-adrenergic drug (e.g., phenylephrine, 80 mg in 250 or 500 ml of normal saline) can be combined with the fluids.

Management of Intracranial Pressure

Because ICP is a determinant of CPP, treatment of ICP inevitably affects CPP. Because the goal is maintenance or improvement of CBF, measures for treating ICP should be evaluated in the light of their effect on CBF. It is not possible to establish an arbitrary threshold for treatment of elevated ICP that would be applicable in all situations. Any interpretation of ICP must be combined with assessment of clinical features and evaluation of CT scan findings because it is possible to have transtentorial herniation with an ICP of 20 mm Hg in the presence of a mass lesion. Conversely, with diffuse brain swelling, adequate CPP can be maintained despite an ICP as high as 30 mm Hg. As a general rule, ICP values between 20 and 25 mm Hg indicate that therapy should be initiated.

The recommended regimen for treatment of ICP starts with drainage of CSF through a ventriculostomy-ICP catheter and continues with sedation of the patient with morphine sulfate or propofol, administration of mannitol, paralysis of the patient with pancuronium or vecuronium, initiation of hyperventilation, and induction of a coma with pentobarbital or etomidate.

Although drainage of CSF has no documented deleterious side effects, concern is occasionally expressed that it may aggravate brain shift. Therefore, only a minimal amount should be drained to decrease the ICP below 20 mm Hg. Sedation with morphine sulfate, 4 mg I.V., is standard treatment. Muscular paralysis, which is used by many clinicians, has been shown to increase the risk of respiratory complications.

Mannitol is usually administered in I.V. boluses of 0.25 to 1 g/kg over 10 to 15 minutes until ICP is controlled or serum osmolality reaches 320 mOsm/L. Because volume depletion is an important side effect of mannitol therapy, urine losses should be replaced.

As mentioned, hyperventilation reduces ICP (by vasoconstriction) and CBF, which may be at ischemic levels in certain parts of the brain. Therefore, hyperventilation ($P_aCO_2 < 30$) should not be instituted prophylactically. If P_aCO_2 must be reduced to extremely low levels, hyperventilation can be combined with mannitol, improving CBF by reducing blood viscosity. Jugular bulb oximetry is recommended in these situations because it will determine how much the cerebral blood flow can be constricted.

Hemoglobin, Hematocrit, and Blood Viscosity

To ensure optimal cerebral oxygenation, CPP, hemoglobin concentration, and oxygen saturation should be optimized; vessel diameter should be maximized; and viscosity should be in the low range. The hematocrit and viscosity are inversely related, and a balance must be established to ensure optimal oxygenation. If the hematocrit is too high, viscosity increases; if the hematocrit is too low, the oxygen-carrying capacity of blood decreases. Maintaining the hematocrit between 0.30 and 0.35 is recommended: below 0.30, the oxygen-carrying capacity falls without a significant change in viscosity, and above 0.35, the viscosity increases out of proportion to the oxygen-carrying capacity.

Brain Protection

When oxygen delivery cannot be sufficiently improved, the brain can be protected by decreasing $CMRo_2$. Barbiturates appear to protect the brain and lower ICP through several mechanisms, including alteration of vascular tone, suppression of metabolism, and inhibition of free radical lipid peroxidation. The most important effect may involve coupling of CBF to regional metabolic demands, so that the lower the metabolic requirements, the lower the CBF and the related cerebral blood volume (CBV), with subsequent beneficial effects on ICP and global cerebral perfusion. Barbiturate therapy (usually pentobarbital to a blood level of 4 mg/L) is instituted when other measures to control ICP fail. Marshall and associates,[23] in a series of 25 patients with an ICP higher than 40 mm Hg, reported that barbiturates not only controlled ICP but also improved outcome. Of the patients whose ICP was controlled, 50% had a good recovery; in the patients whose ICP was not controlled by barbiturates, 83% died. Prophylactic barbiturate therapy failed to improve neurologic outcome.[24] Of the barbiturate-treated patients, 54% were hypotensive, compared with 7% of the control subjects,[24] but this trial was conducted before the present emphasis on maintaining CPP was recognized.

Etomidate, a rapidly acting agent with hypnotic properties similar to those of barbiturates, has fewer adverse effects on systemic BP or ICP. However, it suppresses adrenocortical function, and its solvent, propylene glycol, can cause renal insufficiency.[25]

Propofol is a sedative hypnotic with a rapid onset and a short duration of action.[26,27] It depresses $CMRo_2$, but not as effectively as barbiturates and etomidate. Studies of patients with head injuries have demonstrated that ICP decreases with administration of propofol, but systemic BP usually decreases as well, resulting in a net decrease in CPP. Blood lactate levels do not increase when propofol is administered, indicating that cerebral oxygenation is adequate. Propofol is being used with increasing frequency in neurosurgical ICUs, mainly because its short half-life allows accurate neurologic examination minutes after discontinuance of its use. If propofol is used, correction of hypovolemia is recommended to prevent hypotension associated with bolus injection. Finally, because of its preservative-free, lipid-base vehicle, there is an increased risk of bacterial or fungal infection, and the high caloric content (1 kcal/ml) may be problematic during a prolonged infusion.

Hypothermia produces a balanced reduction in energy production and utilization, decreasing $CMRo_2$ and CBF proportionally. Current protocols for hypothermia include cooling to 32° to 33° C (89.6° to 91.4° F) within 6 hours of injury and maintenance of this temperature for 24 to 48 hours. Two pilot clinical trials showed improvement in neurologic outcome.[28,29] Hypothermia to 33° C has also been shown to be effective for refractory high intracranial pressure and for improved outcome under those conditions. Side effects of hypothermia are cardiac arrhythmias and coagulation disorders, reported after cooling to 32° to 33° C. Another drawback of hypothermia is that it is difficult to detect infection because of the lack of warning signs (e.g, spiking and elevated temperature). Finally, hypothermia requires specialized equipment (rotor beds with cooling control) as well as personnel to induce and maintain the condition.

Spinal Cord Injury

DIAGNOSIS AND INITIAL MANAGEMENT

In the field, all patients with significant trauma, any trauma patients who lose consciousness, and any patients suffering minor trauma who have complaints referable to the spine or spinal cord should be treated as if they had a spinal cord injury until proven otherwise [see Figure 2]. If cardiopulmonary resuscitation is necessary, it takes precedence. The objectives are to maintain adequate oxygenation and maintain blood pressure by administering fluids and vasopressors (avoiding phenylephrine) and placing the patient in military antishock trousers (MAST). The main concerns of management in the field are immobilization before and during extrication from a vehicle (or removal from the scene of another type of accident) and immobilization during transport to prevent active or passive movement of the spine. Subsequently, the patient may require a rigid Philadelphia collar, support from sandbags and straps, a spine board, or a log-roll for turning. A brief motor examination may detect possible deficits.

Patient has apparent spinal cord injury

(In the field, all patients with significant trauma, any trauma patient who loses consciousness, and any patient with minor trauma who has complaints referable to the spine or the spinal cord should be treated as having spinal cord injury until proven otherwise.)

Resuscitate according to ATLS principles.

Immobilize spine, and use spine board, cervical orthosis, sandbags, straps, log-roll, and tape on forehead as necessary.

Perform trauma evaluation.

Perform emergency diagnostic or therapeutic procedures as indicated.

Maintain oxygenation; intubate and ventilate as needed.

Maintain systolic BP > 90 mm Hg with volume replacement (isotonic fluids), MAST, vasopressors (dopamine, 2–10 μg/kg/min) and, if bradycardia (< 45 beats/min) occurs, atropine, 0.5–1.0 mg I.V.

Place NG tube to prevent vomiting and aspiration.

Place Foley catheter to prevent urinary retention.

Normalize T°.

Perform detailed neurologic examination.

Evalute axial skeleton, and obtain x-rays of spine.

Cervical spine: lateral view showing craniocervical and C7–T1 junctions, followed by AP and odontoid views.

Thoracic and lumbosacral spine: AP and lateral views.

Urgent MRI is indicated if (1) there is an incomplete lesion with normal alignment, (2) deterioration occurs, (3) fracture level ≠ deficit level, or (4) a bony injury cannot be identified.

X-rays are clear; patient is alert, neurologically intact, and free of spinal pain or tenderness; and results of neurologic examination are normal

Discontinue immobilization of spine.

X-rays are clear; patient has impaired consciousness, is not neurologically intact, has spinal pain or tenderness, or has abnormal neurologic examination

Continue immobilization of spine.

Obtain specialist evaluation.

X-rays show evidence of fracture/dislocation

Obtain specialist evaluation.

Figure 2 **Shown is an algorithm for management of the patient with an acute spinal cord injury.**

When the patient arrives at the hospital, care should be taken to provide adequate oxygenation, prevent hypotension, and maintain immobilization. Patients with an injury above C4, who may have respiratory paralysis, may need ventilatory assistance. Lesions above T5 may be accompanied by loss of sympathetic tone and consequently by significant venous pooling and arterial hypotension. Because paralytic ileus is common, usually lasting several days, a nasogastric tube should be placed to prevent vomiting and aspiration. Because urinary retention is common, a Foley catheter should be inserted. Vasomotor paralysis may cause poikilothermy (uncontrolled temperature regulation), which should be treated with cooling blankets when necessary.

A detailed neurologic examination should ascertain whether the injury is complete or incomplete and at what level of the spinal cord the injury has occurred. If possible, a history should be taken to determine the mechanism of injury (e.g., hyperflexion, extension, axial loading, or rotation). There exists a protocol for sensory and motor examination of patients with spinal cord injuries, developed by the American Spinal Injury Association, that is precise and relatively easy to follow [see Figure 3].

Spinal shock, which occurs during major injury to the spinal cord, consists of loss of motor, sensory, and autonomic function. The motor component may consist of paralysis, flaccidity, and areflexia. The sensory component may involve both spinothalamic and dorsal column sensory function, and the autonomic component may include systemic hypotension, bradycardia, skin hyperemia, and warmth. Although the cause of spinal shock is unknown, it may be related to a disturbance in impulse conduction caused by a reversible imbalance of electrolytes or neurotransmitters. Usually, motor and sensory symptoms of spinal shock last 1 hour or less; longer-lasting deficits should be attributed to pathologic changes in the cord. Autonomic symptoms, however, may persist for days to months.

All patients with possible spine injuries should be examined radiologically. Roentgenography of the cervical spine, while the patient is in a rigid collar, should include a lateral view showing both the craniocervical and the C7-T1 junction. If the lateral view is obtained and the patient is coherent and has no neck tenderness or neurologic deficit, the collar can be removed for anteroposterior and odontoid views. If the lower cervical spine or the cervical-thoracic junction (or both) are not well visualized, a lateral view with caudal traction on the arms, or a swimmer's view, should be obtained. If the spine is still not visualized or if there is neurologic deficit, a CT scan should be obtained through the poorly visualized levels.

Anteroposterior and lateral views of thoracic and lumbosacral vertebrae should be obtained for all trauma patients who were thrown from a vehicle or fell more than 6 ft to the ground, complain of back pain, are unconscious, cannot reliably describe back pain or have altered mental status preventing adequate examination, or have an unknown mechanism of injury or other injuries that suggest the possibility of spinal injury.

Indications for an urgent MRI include the following: an incomplete lesion with normal alignment (to rule out the possibility that soft tissue is compressing the spinal cord); deterioration (worsening deficit or rising level); a fracture level different from the level of deficit; and the inability to identify a bony injury (to rule out the possibilities of soft tissue compression, disk herniation, or hematoma that would necessitate surgery).

In approximately 10% to 15% of adults and 40% of children with injury to the cervical spinal cord, no radiologic abnormalities are evident in plain, flexion, and extension films. Many patients have reversible incomplete cord lesions, but more severe lesions

STANDARD NEUROLOGICAL CLASSIFICATION OF SPINAL CORD INJURY

Figure 3 Shown is a form developed by the American Spinal Injury Association to record the principal information about motor, sensory, and sphincter function required for accurate neurologic classification of spinal cord injury. For the motor examination, 10 key muscles are tested (left). For the sensory examination, 28 key dermatomes are tested (right).

are observed in elderly people. Explanations for this phenomenon include spontaneous reduction of a subluxation, hyperextension injury, and disk prolapse. With MRI, T_2 (spin-spin)-weighted images may show increased signal within the spinal cord parenchyma.

TREATMENT

Traction

The objectives of craniocervical traction are to reduce fracture-dislocations, to maintain normal alignment or immobility of the cervical spine, to prevent further injury, to decompress the spinal cord and roots, and to facilitate bone healing. A common technique is placement of Gardner-Wells tongs.

Pharmacologic Treatment

A variety of drugs are known to interfere with the processes of secondary injury. The challenge is to identify the most effective treatment or combination of treatments with the fewest severe side effects, a challenge requiring many experiments for each treatment tested. Methylprednisolone, thought to act by scavenging free rad-

icals, has been reported to be neuroprotective in spinal cord injury.[30,31] Patients treated with methylprednisolone within 8 hours of injury exhibited significant improvements in both motor and sensory function compared with patients treated with naloxone or placebo, regardless of whether the injury was complete. After 1 year of follow-up, the advantage was still evident in patients treated with methylprednisolone, but this improvement in outcome was not seen in patients treated more than 8 hours after injury. The regimen studied comprised a 30 mg/kg bolus followed by 5.4 mg/kg/hr for 23 hours. Many centers use methylprednisolone, administered within 8 hours of injury.

The calcium channel blocker nimodipine causes significant increases in blood flow in the spinal cord,[32,33] but the dosage necessary to exert this effect is accompanied by significant systemic hypotension. In a prospective, placebo-controlled, double-blind study, a significant improvement in neurologic outcome was seen in patients treated with GM_1 ganglioside.[34] However, because of the small sample size (34 patients), certain aspects of spinal cord injury or treatment that might have affected outcome were not analyzed in detail. The third National Acute Spinal Cord Injury Study (NASCIS), initiated in 1991, compared methylprednisolone given for either 24 or 48 hours with tirilazad mesylate (an oxygen and lipid radical scavenger).[35] Methylprednisolone was administered in a bolus of 30 mg/kg within 8 hours of injury. Patients receiving methylprednisolone for 48 hours exhibited significant improvement in motor function compared with patients treated with the same agent for 24 hours after injury; however, the patients treated for 48 hours suffered from more severe sepsis and pneumonia. Overall, mortality was identical in the two groups receiving methylprednisolone. Motor function after 6 months in patients treated with tirilazad was similar to that of patients treated with methylprednisolone for 24 hours. On the basis of these findings, the authors suggested that methylprednisolone therapy started within 3 hours of injury should be continued for 24 hours, whereas methylprednisolone treatment started 3 to 8 hours after injury should be continued for 48 hours.

Surgical Treatment

The role of neurosurgery in the treatment of spinal fractures and spinal cord injury is controversial. There is considerable disagreement as to whether surgery should be performed, what type of surgery should be done, and when should it be done. The primary goal of treatment is to restore spinal stability, provide for early mobilization and rehabilitation, and maximize neurologic recovery.

There is general agreement among physicians that early immobilization and early stabilization of fractures and dislocations of the spine are necessary. The single widely accepted indication for early surgical treatment is ongoing neurologic deterioration in the presence of spinal canal compromise from bone and disk fragments, hematoma, or unreduced subluxation. Surgical indications still under debate include incomplete spinal cord injury (with persistent spinal cord deformity) and complete spinal cord injury with the possibility of some neurologic recovery.

Early surgical intervention has been associated with an increased risk of systemic complications (especially pulmonary) and neurologic deterioration. Marshall and coworkers[36] found that one third of all cases of neurologic deterioration could be attributed directly to surgical intervention; 4 of 26 patients who underwent spinal surgery within 5 days deteriorated, while none of the patients treated after 5 days had any neurologic sequelae.

Other studies, however, have not found an increased risk of deterioration with early intervention. Wilberger[37] studied 110 patients with cervical spinal cord injury, of whom 88 underwent surgery for spinal stabilization; in the 39 patients treated within 24 hours, the incidence of systemic complications was reduced by 50% compared with the incidence in the 49 patients treated 24 hours to 3 weeks after injury. In addition, the incidence of neurologic deterioration was 0% in the early-stabilization group versus 2.5% in the late-stabilization group. Data from the NASCIS II study showed improved outcome in patients undergoing surgery within 24 hours of injury compared with patients treated after 200 hours, but the difference was not statistically significant.[38] To date, there is no clear evidence that early surgical intervention improves outcome.

Diagnosis and Treatment of Specific Fractures and Dislocations

Cervical spine Injuries to the cervical spine include atlas fractures, axis fractures, fractures of the lower cervical spine, and atlanto-occipital and atlantoaxial dislocations. Atlanto-occipital dislocations are rare, occurring in approximately 1% of the patients with injury to the cervical spine. Most of these patients die immediately after trauma because of brain stem injury and respiratory arrest. Treatment, which is controversial, consists of either operative fusion or 4 to 6 months of immobilization in a Halo brace. Atlantoaxial dislocations, which are often fatal and therefore seldom encountered in clinical practice, are usually associated with an odontoid fracture. Because of severe ligamentous injury, these lesions are unstable.

Atlas (Jefferson) fractures, which represent 5% to 10% of all cervical spine fractures, result from axial load. Because of the large diameter of the spinal canal and the tendency of fragments to move outward, these fractures usually are not accompanied by significant neurologic injury, but 40% of patients with an atlas fracture have another cervical fracture (e.g., a fracture through both C1 arches). Treatment requires rigid immobilization in a Halo vest.

Axis fractures account for 10% to 20% of all cervical spine fractures in adults and 70% of cervical fractures in children. Odontoid fractures are the most common (60%). Fractures of the tip of the odontoid process (avulsion fracture, type I) are uncommon and unstable and may require surgical fusion. Fractures of the neck (type II) or at the junction of the odontoid process and the axis (type III) are more common (65% to 80% and 20% to 35%, respectively); they call for Halo-vest immobilization when the dislocation is less than 6 mm and open reduction and internal fixation when the dislocation is greater than 6 mm. Traumatic spondylolisthesis, or hangman's fracture, accounts for approximately 20% of C2 fractures. Injury usually results from axial compression in combination with hyperextension of the occipito-atlanto-axial complex on the lower spine, resulting in bilateral fracture of the pars interarticularis. Fractures affecting the ring of the axis without C2-C3 angulation are stable and can be treated with immobilization in a Philadelphia collar or a sterno-occipito-mandibular immobilizer (SOMI) brace. Halo-vest immobilization is recommended in unreliable patients or patients with both C1 and C2 fractures. The average healing time is 11.5 weeks.

Approximately 80% of all fractures of the lower cervical spine are produced by indirect forces. The vertebra most commonly involved is C5, and dislocations are most frequent at the C5-C6 level. The following injury mechanisms are observed: flexion and distraction (approximately 40% of cases), flexion and compression (22%), vertical compression (8%), extension and compression (24%), extension and distraction (6%), and lateral flexion (3%).

Flexion and distraction injuries usually result from a blow to the occiput from below. The initial disruption is within the posterior ligamentous complex, leading to facet dislocation and abnormally large divergence of the spinous processes. Unilateral facet dislocation and facet interlocking result when a rotatory component is involved. Bilateral facet dislocation with anterior translation of the superior vertebra results from severe hyperflexion. Cord and root involvement vary with the degree of luxation and translation: 50% of patients with unilateral facet dislocation present with moderate cord and root injury, and 90% of patients with bilateral facet dislocation and a full translation of the vertebral body have neurologic deficits, predominantly a complete cord lesion. Teardrop fractures (a bone chip just beyond the anterior inferior edge of the vertebral body) result from severe hyperflexion injury, and the fractured vertebra is usually displaced posteriorly on the vertebra below; these patients are often quadriplegic. Flexion and extension x-rays should be obtained to evaluate ligamentous injury.

Flexion and compression injuries, usually observed at C4-C5 and C5-C6 levels, usually result from a blow to the back of the head. The effect on the anterior vertebral body varies from a moderate rounding or loss of anterior height to a wedge shape with an oblique fracture from the anterior surface to the inferior subchondral plate. Approximately 50% of patients with the latter type of injury have a neurologic deficit. More severe injuries are accompanied by translation of the inferior posterior margin of the vertebral body into the neural canal. About 75% of pa-

ANTERIOR | MIDDLE | POSTERIOR

Anterior Longitudinal Ligament

Posterior Longitudinal Ligament

Intertransverse Ligament

Interspinal Ligament

Supraspinal Ligament

Figure 4 **Illustrated is the three-column concept for assessment of spinal stability. If two or more columns are destroyed or nonfunctional, instability is likely.**

tients have neurologic involvement. Translations of more than 3 mm result in a complete spinal cord lesion in most cases.

Extension and compression injuries are usually caused by a blow to the forehead and result in fractures of the posterior complex. About 40% of patients with unilateral vertebral arch fractures (articular process, pedicle, or lamina) have a neurologic deficit, predominantly a radiculopathy. Bilaminar fractures are accompanied by a complete cord lesion in 40% of cases. Bilateral vertebral arch fractures with complete anterior translation of the vertebral body present with radiculopathy (30%), central cord syndrome (30%), or incomplete cord lesion (30%). In Allen's series,[39] no complete cord lesions were observed with this type of injury.

Treatment of injuries to the lower cervical spine has not been standardized. As a general rule, severe ligament involvement and severe vertical compression require surgical intervention. Severely comminuted vertebral body fractures may also require surgery because of the high risk of progressive kyphosis. In the series reported by Lind and Nordwall,[40] 87% of patients with distractive flexion injury and 88% of those with compressive flexion injury healed with Halo-vest immobilization.

Thoracolumbar spine Approximately 64% of fractures of the spine occur at the T12-L1 junction, and 70% of these fractures are unaccompanied by immediate neurologic injury. Evaluation according to Denis' three-column principle[41] [*see Figure 4*] is useful for determining whether a fracture is stable, although the precise definition of stability remains controversial. Fractures of the thoracic spine (T1–T10) are more stable because of support from the surrounding rib cage and the strong costovertebral ligaments. When two of the three columns are affected, the fracture is considered unstable and generally requires surgical intervention. If there is no neurologic deficit, surgery can be performed by an orthopedic surgeon or a general surgeon, but if there is a neurologic deficit, a neurosurgeon should perform the operation. In general, the following conditions require surgical intervention: open lesions and dural lacerations, progressive neurologic deficit, marked and progressive angulation, and spinal instability.

The four major types of thoracolumbar spine injuries are compression fractures, burst fractures, seat belt fractures, and fracture-dislocations. These four types of fracture involve the anterior, middle, and posterior columns of the spine in different ways [*see Table 3*].

Minimal to moderate compression fractures with an intact posterior column can be treated with analgesics and bed rest. Ambulation should be started early, and depending on the degree of kyphosis, external immobilization (from a corset or a Boston brace) may or may not be indicated.

Severe compression injuries and seat-belt injuries should be treated with external immobilization in extension. If the loss of anterior height of the vertebral body exceeds 75%, there is an increased risk of progressive kyphosis. Occasionally, surgical intervention is required. An anterior injury is considered unstable if more than three elements in a row, or more than 50% of the height in a single element with angulation, is present.

Burst fractures are considered unstable even if there is no initial neurologic deficit. Early ambulation should be avoided because the axial loading may result in progressive collapse or angulation, with concomitant neurologic damage. Severe burst fractures with neurodeficit should be treated with surgical decompression and stabilization. L5 burst fractures are usually managed conservatively, because it is difficult for spinal instrumentation to maintain alignment at this level; if progressive deformity occurs, L4-S1 fixation is indicated.

Fracture-dislocations require surgical decompression and stabilization.

Table 3 Column Failure in the Four Types of Major Thoracolumbar Spinal Injury[41]

Fracture Type	Anterior Column	Middle Column	Posterior Column
Compression	Compression	Intact	Intact, or distraction if severe
Burst	Compression	Compression	Intact
Seat belt	Intact or mild compression of 10%–20% of anterior vertebral body	Distraction	Distraction
Fracture-dislocation	Compression, rotation, shear	Distraction, rotation, shear	Distraction, rotation, shear

Discussion

Pathophysiology

HEAD INJURY

Cerebral Metabolism

At 1,200 to 1,400 g, the brain accounts for only 2% to 3% of total body weight and does not do any mechanical work; yet it receives 15% to 20% of all cardiac output to meet its high metabolic demands. Of the total energy generated, 50% is used for interneuronal communication and the generation, release, and reuptake of neurotransmitters (synaptic activity), 25% is used for maintenance and restoration of ion gradients across the cell membrane, and the remaining 25% is used for molecular transport, biosynthesis, and other, as yet unidentified, processes.

Cell metabolism involves the consumption of adenosine triphosphate (ATP) during work and the ensuing consumption of metabolic substrates to resynthesize ATP from adenosine diphosphate (ADP). ATP is generated both in the cytosol (via glycolysis) and in the mitochondria (via oxidative phosphorylation). Glucose is the sole energy substrate, unless there is ketosis, and 95% of the energy requirement of the normal brain comes from aerobic conversion of glucose to water and CO_2. ATP generation is highly efficient. Glycolysis and subsequent oxidative phosphorylation result in the generation of 38 molecules of ATP for each molecule of glucose:

$$1 \text{ glucose} + 6 \text{ O}_2 + 38 \text{ ADP} + 38 \text{ P}_i \rightarrow 6 \text{ CO}_2 + 44 \text{ H}_2\text{O} + 38 \text{ ATP}$$

In the absence of oxygen, anaerobic glycolysis can proceed, but energy production is much less efficient. Two molecules of ATP and two molecules of lactate are generated for each molecule of glucose:

$$1 \text{ glucose} + 2 \text{ ADP} + 2 \text{ P}_i \rightarrow 2 \text{ lactate} + 2 \text{ ATP}$$

Regulation of Blood Flow

Because the reserves of glucose and glycogen within the astrocytes of the brain are limited and there is no significant storage capacity for oxygen, the brain depends on blood to supply the oxygen and glucose it requires. More specifically, substrate availability is determined by its concentration in blood, flow volume, and the rate of passage across the blood-brain barrier.

Under normal circumstances and with certain physiologic alterations, an adequate supply of substrates can be maintained by regulation of CBF. CBF increases with vasodilatation and decreases with vasoconstriction. Caliber changes take place mainly in cerebral resistance vessels (i.e., arterioles with a diameter of 300 μm down to 15 μm).[42,43] Control of CBF by influencing vessel caliber is commonly referred to as autoregulation of blood flow.

Metabolic autoregulation CBF is functionally coupled to cerebral metabolism, changing proportionally with increasing or decreasing regional or global metabolic demand. Thus, the brain precisely matches local CBF to local metabolic needs. Because 95% of the energy in the normal brain is generated by oxidative metabolism of glucose, CMR_{O_2} is considered to be a sensitive measure of cerebral metabolism. The relation between CBF and metabolism is expressed in the Fick equation:

$$CMR_{O_2} = CBF \times A\text{-}VD_{O_2}$$

CMR_{O_2}, expressed in milliliters per 100 g of brain tissue, is normally about 3.2 ml/100 g/min in awake adults.[17] The average CBF value for mixed cortical flow is 53 ml/100 g/min in a healthy adult. A-VD$_{O_2}$, a measure of cerebral oxygen extraction, can be calculated by subtracting the oxygen content of jugular venous blood (6.7 ml/dl) from that of arterial blood (13 ml/dl), resulting in a value of 6.3 ml/dl; this value can then be corrected for hemoglobin content according to the formula discussed earlier [see Head Injury, ICU Management, above]. Under conditions of increasing metabolic demand (increased CMR_{O_2}), such as seizures or fever, CBF increases proportionally, thus keeping A-VD$_{O_2}$ constant. With decreasing metabolism (anesthesia, deep coma), CBF decreases.

Pressure autoregulation Another important physiologic property of the cerebral circulation is maintenance of a constant supply of substrates at the level set by metabolism. According to Poiseuille's equation,

$$CBF = k \frac{CPP \times d^4}{8 \times l \times v}$$

in which d represents vessel diameter, l represents vessel length, and v represents blood viscosity, changes in CPP (e.g., arterial hypotension or increases in ICP) would be followed by changes in CBF, unless diameter regulation (so-called pressure autoregulation) takes place.[44] In humans, the limits of pressure autoregulation range from 40 to 150 mm Hg of perfusion pressure.

Viscosity autoregulation In accordance with Poiseuille's equation, CBF can vary with changes in the viscosity of blood. Blood viscosity changes with variations in hematocrit, γ-globulin, and fibrinogen components of plasma protein. Increased viscosity would increase cerebrovascular resistance ($8 \times l \times v/d^4$). By means of diameter adjustment (viscosity autoregulation), cerebrovascular resistance is decreased and CBF can be kept constant.[45]

CO_2 reactivity Vascular caliber and cerebral blood flow are also responsive to changes in arterial P_aCO_2. Cerebral blood flow changes 2% to 3% for each mm Hg in P_aCO_2 within the range of 20 to 60 mm Hg. Hypercarbia (hypoventilation) results in vasodilatation and higher CBF, and hypocarbia (hyperventilation) results in vasoconstriction and lower CBF. Autoregulation is a compensatory or adaptive response adjusting cerebral blood flow to metabolism; with CO_2 variation, vessel caliber changes and CBF follow passively. The vessels respond not to changes in P_aCO_2 but to the pH in the perivascular space. CO_2 can cross the blood-brain barrier freely, thus changing the pH, but over 20 to 24 hours, with a constant new level of P_aCO_2, the pH in blood and in the perivascular space returns to baseline, and the diameter of cerebral blood vessels also returns to baseline.[46] With CO_2 reactivity, changes in CBF are compensated for by changes in A-VD$_{O_2}$, so that a constant supply of substrates is maintained at the level set by metabolism (CMR_{O_2}). A constant A-VD$_{O_2}$ is a common feature of metabolic, pressure, and viscosity autoregulation; because CBF is tuned to metabolism ($CBF \approx CMR_{O_2}$), A-VD$_{O_2}$ can be kept constant.

Cerebral Circulation and Metabolism after Severe Head Injury

Arterial hypoxia and hypotension It is known from eyewitness reports of head injury and experimental studies immediately after the impact that arterial hypotension and interruption of normal respiration, sometimes with a period of prolonged apnea, are common findings. In the days after a head injury, there are many occasions and opportunities for hypoxic and hypotensive insults. Studies have identified hypotension (systolic BP below 90 mm Hg) and hypoxia (P_aO_2 below 60 mm Hg) as major determinants of poor outcome.[9,14,47]

The effect of hypotension on the brain depends on the status of autoregulation. If autoregulation is defective, decreased blood pressure leads directly and linearly to a decrease in CBF. If autoregulation is intact, arterial hypotension can lead to a considerable increase in ICP, which interferes with CBF by decreasing perfusion pressure.

Raised intracranial pressure According to the Monro-Kellie doctrine,[48,49] ICP is governed by three factors within the confines of the skull: brain parenchyma plus cytotoxic edema; CSF plus vasogenic edema; and CBV. When the volume in one compartment increases, ICP increases unless there is a compensatory decrease in volume in the other compartments. The relation between intracranial volume and ICP is expressed in the pressure-volume index (PVI).[50] PVI is defined by the volume that must be added to or withdrawn from the craniospinal axis to raise or decrease ICP 10-fold:

$$PVI = \frac{\Delta V}{\log ICP_i / ICP_o}$$

where ΔV represents the change in volume, ICP_o represents ICP before the volume change, and ICP_i represents ICP after the volume change. PVI is thus a measure for the compliance ($\Delta V/\Delta P$) or tightness of the brain. Under normal circumstances, PVI is 26 ± 4 ml; 26 ml of volume will raise ICP from 1 to 10 mm Hg, but the same volume will also raise ICP from 10 to 100 mm Hg. Conversely, a change in volume of only 6.4 ml is necessary to increase intracranial pressure from 10 mm Hg (normal) to the treatment threshold of 20 mm Hg. Thus, small changes in volume have a relatively large effect on ICP.

Apart from mass lesions, intracranial pressure typically increases after severe head injury because of cerebral edema. Initial compensation is by displacement of CSF from the cranium, which is visualized in a CT scan of the head as small ventricles and basal cisterns. Subsequent compensation would be by a decrease in CBV, which can be accomplished by means of vasoconstriction.

Relation between vessel diameter, cerebral blood volume, and intracranial pressure The total diameter of the cerebrovascular bed determines CBV. Cerebral veins contain most of the total blood volume, but their diameter and, thus, their volume are relatively constant. Approximately 20 ml of blood (i.e., one third of total CBV) is located in the cerebral resistance vessels (which range in diameter from 300 μm down to 15 μm).[51] Because most autoregulatory and CO_2-dependent variations in diameter take place in these vessels, cerebral blood volume is determined mainly by their diameter. Typically, the diameter ranges from 80% to 160% of baseline, resulting in volume changes between 64% and 256% of baseline. With a baseline value of 20 ml in the resistance vessels, CBV will range from 13 ml (maximal vasoconstriction) to 51 ml (maximal vasodilatation). Given a pressure-volume index of 26, change from maximal vasoconstriction to maximal vasodilatation will be accompanied by an almost 29-fold change in ICP.

Cerebral blood volume, intracranial pressure, and cerebral blood flow CBF and CBV are governed by vascular di-

ameter. Thus, depending on other parameters influencing CBF (such as mean arterial BP, ICP, and blood viscosity), changes in vascular caliber also affect CBF.

Hypocarbia reduces ICP by means of vasoconstriction, consequently improving CPP. However, net CBF is decreased because in Poiseuille's equation, vessel diameter is carried to the fourth power. A randomized clinical trial has shown that preventive hyperventilation retards clinical improvement after severe head injury, perhaps through reduction of CBF to ischemic levels.[52] However, its rapid effect on ICP is of great advantage in cases of acute neurologic deterioration (e.g., in the presence of an expanding mass lesion before evacuation can take place) and should be reserved for these situations.

There are two methods of reducing ICP by means of vasoconstriction without affecting CBF. The first is to reduce blood viscosity. As can be deduced from Poiseuille's equation, decreasing the blood viscosity will, by itself, lead to vasoconstriction, provided that viscosity autoregulation is intact. With impaired autoregulation, decreased viscosity will result in an increase in CBF but no decrease in ICP. However, this effect can be used to maintain CBF under vasoconstriction with hypocarbia. The effect of mannitol on ICP is thought to be mediated in part by lowering blood viscosity.[53,54]

The second method of reducing ICP without affecting CBF is to increase CPP, which can be done by raising blood pressure. Again, with intact autoregulation, an increase in CPP will lead to vasoconstriction, with net CBF remaining constant. With impaired autoregulation, CBF will follow CPP passively, and maintenance of normal blood pressure may be indicated in these cases. More important, however, is the avoidance of hypotension under these circumstances; the effect of CPP therapy may be attributable in part simply to prevention of hypotension.[21,55]

Cerebral ischemia Cerebral ischemia, defined as CBF that is inadequate to meet the metabolic demands of the brain, is an important mechanism of secondary injury in patients with severe head injury, and the adequacy of CBF has been associated with neurologic outcome. In autopsy findings from patients dying after severe head injury, histologic damage indicative of cerebral ischemia was seen in 80% of cases.[56] Bouma and associates[57] found ischemia (CBF < 18 ml/dl with abnormally high A-VDO$_2$ values) in 20% to 33% of patients with severe head injuries within 4 to 12 hours of injury, and the ischemia was associated with a poor prognosis. Of the intracranial lesions, acute subdural hematoma and diffuse cerebral swelling were most often associated with ischemia.

The relation between cerebral metabolism and CBF is expressed in the Fick equation [*see* Metabolic Autoregulation, *above*]. The normal brain tends to keep A-VDO$_2$ constant and to react to changes in metabolism with adjustments in blood flow. When CBF decreases in response to metabolism (as with hyperventilation or decreasing CPP with impaired autoregulation), oxygen supply is maintained by increasing oxygen extraction (i.e., A-VDO$_2$ increases). Increasing A-VDO$_2$ is thus a sensitive marker of insufficient cerebral perfusion. However, oxygen extraction is limited, and this limit is reached when A-VDO$_2$ is doubled (13.2 ml/dl). Consequently, any further reduction in CBF results in neuronal dysfunction (i.e., CMRO$_2$ decreases). Because 50% of the energy is used for synaptic activity, a reversible and functional loss is usually observed first. Further decline, however, will result in ion pump failure, loss of membrane integrity, consequent cell swelling (cytotoxic edema), and cell death (irreversible infarction). The occurrence of irreversible infarction depends on both the level and the duration of ischemia. When cerebral blood flow decreases to approximately 18 ml/100 g/min for more than 4 hours, it reaches the threshold for irreversible infarction.[58]

Maintenance or improvement of CBF is thus essential to the treatment of severe head injury, and A-VDO$_2$ is a sensitive marker of the adequacy of therapy. When therapeutic measures fail to sustain CBF, CMRO$_2$ can be decreased to reinstate the match between CBF and metabolism. CNS suppression can be obtained with the administration of hypnotic agents (e.g., barbiturates or propofol) or the induction of hypothermia. Decreasing cell metabolism will result in reduced production of CO$_2$, lactic acid, or both and (with blood vessels almost always remaining responsive to perivascular pH changes) in vasoconstriction accompanied by reductions in both CBF and ICP. The relations between CMRO$_2$, CBF, CBV, CPP, and A-VDO$_2$ are complicated. An overview is available elsewhere[59] [see Table 4].

Altered cerebral metabolism Anaerobic metabolism of glucose to the end product lactate is characteristic of cerebral hypoxia/ischemia.[60] Increased lactate production, hyperglycolysis, and low tissue glucose levels have been observed after severe head injury, suggesting an increased turnover of glucose by the anaerobic glycolytic pathway. Increased lactate levels have also been found in the presence of preserved CBF,[61,62] suggesting impairment not only of oxygen delivery but also of oxidative metabolism (i.e., of mitochondrial function). Recent findings in animals and humans indicate that mitochondrial function is impaired after severe head injury, which may explain poor outcomes despite adequate CBF levels; ATP generation by anaerobic glycolysis is usually insufficient to maintain the metabolic activity of the brain.[63,64] In part, however, such poor outcomes may be attributable to the effects of lactate production (acidosis), because high lactate and hydrogen ion levels interfere with the functional recovery of tissue.

SPINAL CORD INJURY

Spinal cord injury is often viewed as an all-or-nothing event that is irreversible from the moment of injury. By this view, spinal cord injury is classified as either incomplete or complete. This dichotomy is not absolute, however, because some functional recovery occurs even after severe spinal cord injury. The Second National Acute Spinal Cord Injury Study revealed that patients with so-called complete loss of neurologic function recovered on average 8% of the function they had lost, and patients with an incomplete injury recovered 59% of what they had lost.[65] An injury classified as complete does not necessarily involve loss of all connections. Several studies have demonstrated that many patients with a clinically complete lesion show evidence of residual connection.[66] A certain number of intact connections is probably necessary for functional recovery. The determinants of functional outcome are complex, however, and probably include not only the extent of axonal loss but also the level of dysfunction of the surviving axons and the plasticity of the spinal cord.

Animal studies have found that a small number of axons may be sufficient to support functional recovery.[67-69] Animals recover evoked potentials and the ability to walk with as few as 10% of their spinal axons. Nerve sprouting, one of the mechanisms of plasticity, allows a few nerves to carry out the function of many. Finally, animal studies have also shown that many of the axons surviving traumatic injury are dysfunctional and that many of the axons had lost part or all of their myelin sheath, which is the structural component that improves the reliability and speed of conduction. 4-Aminopyridine, an axon-excitatory drug used for the treatment of multiple sclerosis, has significantly improved

Table 4 Changes in CBF, CBV, ICP, and A-VDO$_2$ Associated with Primary Reduction of Selected Variables[59]

Variable Reduced	CBF	CBV (ICP)	A-VDO$_2$
CMRO$_2$	↓	↓	—
CPP (autoregulation intact)	—	↑	—
CPP (autoregulation defective)	↓	↓	↑
Blood viscosity (autoregulation intact)	—	↓	—
Blood viscosity (autoregulation defective)	↑	—	↓
P$_a$CO$_2$	↓	↓	↑
Conductance vessel diameter (vasospasm above ischemia threshold)	↓	↑	↑

A-VDO$_2$—arteriovenous oxygen content difference CBF—cerebral blood flow CBV—cerebral blood volume CMRO$_2$—cerebral metabolic rate of oxygen CPP—cerebral perfusion pressure ICP—intracranial pressure P$_a$CO$_2$—arterial carbon dioxide tension

conduction in animals and humans with spinal cord injury.[70-72] Unfortunately, the drug must be given continuously to support axon function, and this is not feasible in humans because of its side effects (seizures, tachycardia, and hyperthermia).

Injury initiates complex responses in the body and the spinal cord. Ischemia is a prominent feature of events occurring after spinal cord injury.[73,74] Within 2 hours of a spinal cord injury, there is a significant reduction in spinal cord blood flow. It is unclear whether this is mechanically or biochemically induced. Like the brain, the spinal cord possesses autoregulatory capacity (pressure autoregulation). When this autoregulation is impaired, blood flow becomes dependent on systemic blood pressure. In a patient with multiple injuries or vasogenic spinal shock (a lesion above T5) complicating the spinal cord injury, severe systemic hypotension may exacerbate the effects of spinal cord injury.

Edema, another prominent feature of spinal cord injury, tends to develop first at the injured site, subsequently spreading to adjacent and sometimes distant segments. The relation between spreading edema and potential worsening of neurologic function is poorly understood. The inflammatory response to injury ideally cleans up cellular debris and repairs tissue. This response is accompanied, however, by the release of toxic substances, which cause further tissue damage, or secondary injury. Processes resulting in secondary injury involve generation of free radicals, excessive calcium influx and excitotoxicity, the release of eicosanoids and cytokines, and programmed cell death.

Conclusion

Mortality has decreased considerably in patients with severe head injury. In the patients we have studied, mortality has decreased from approximately 40% to 45% in the decade between 1975 and 1984 to 25% to 30% at present, with a further downward trend evident. Increased recognition of the mechanism of secondary brain injury as well as avoidance of secondary insults by optimizing cerebral perfusion and oxygenation are probably responsible for most of the improvement in outcome. Pharmacologic brain protection and attempts to intervene in the damaging cascade of biochemical events occurring after injury have shown some beneficial effects in phase II trials, but no compound has clearly shown efficacy when tested in multicenter phase II clinical trials. Targeted strategies or combinations of drugs, based on pathophysiologic concepts, are expected to provide the major break-through in research on treatment of head injury.

The results in patients with acute spinal cord injury are not spectacular. Methylprednisolone has provided a modest improvement in outcome, suggesting that pharmacologic intervention can curtail damage from ongoing biochemical cascades in central nervous system injuries. As in research on head injuries, better insight into pathophysiology is a major focus. Early stabilization and multidisciplinary care, which can prevent some of the systemic and neurologic complications of spinal cord injury, can improve outcome.

References

1. Fine P, Kuhlemeier K, DeVivo M, et al: Spinal cord injury: an epidemiological perspective. Paraplegia 17: 237, 1979

2. Kalsbeek W, McLaurin R, Harris B, et al: The National Head and Spinal Cord Injury Survey: major findings. J Neurosurg 53:S19, 1982

3. Kraus J, Franti C, Riggins R, et al: Incidence of traumatic spinal cord lesions. J Chron Dis 28:471, 1975

4. Kraus J: Epidemiological aspects of acute spinal cord injury: review of incidence, prevalence, causes and outcome. Central Nervous System Trauma Status Report, 1985. Becker D, Poulishock J, Eds. National Institute of Neurological and Communicative Disorders and Stroke, Bethesda, Maryland, 1985, p 313

5. Factsheet No. 2: Spinal cord injury statistical information. National Spinal Cord Injury Association, Woburn, Massachusetts, 1992

6. Burney R, Maio R, Maynard F, et al: Incidence, characteristics, and outcome of spinal cord injury at trauma centers in North America. Arch Surg 128:596, 1992

7. Tator C: Spine-spinal cord relationships in spinal cord trauma. Clin Neurosurg 30:479, 1983

8. Gibson C: An overview of spinal cord injury. Phys Med Rehab Clin North Am 3:699, 1992

9. Chesnut RM, Marshall SB, Piek J, et al: Early and late systemic hypotension as a frequent and fundamental source of cerebral ischemia following severe brain injury in the Traumatic Coma Data Bank. Acta Neurochir Suppl (Wien) 59:121, 1993

10. American College of Surgeons Committee on Trauma: Advanced Life Support Course for Physicians, Instructor Manual, 2nd ed. American College of Surgeons, Chicago, 1985

11. Ritter AM, Muizelaar J, Barnes T, et al: Brain stem blood flow, pupillary response and outcome in patients with severe head injures. Neurosurgery 44:941, 1999

12. Schroder M, Muizelaar J, Kuta A: Documented reversal of global ischemia immediately after removal of a subdural hematoma: report of two cases. J Neurosurg 80:324, 1994

13. Andrews P, Piper I, Dearden N, et al: Secondary insults during intrahospital transport of head injured patients. Lancet 335:327, 1990

14. Jones P, Andrews P, Midgley S: Measuring the burden of secondary insults in head-injured patients during intensive care. J Neurosurg Anesthesiol 6:4, 1994

15. Kirkpatrick P, Smielewski P, Czosnyka M, et al: Near-infrared spectroscopy use in patients with severe head injury. J Neurosurg 83:963, 1995

16. Kanter M, Narayan R: Management of head injury: intracranial pressure monitoring. Neurosurg Clin North Am 2:257, 1991

17. Gibbs E, Lennox W, Nims L, et al: Arterial and cerebral venous blood: arteriovenous differences in man. J Biol Chem 144:325, 1942

18. Gopinath S, Robertson C, Contant C, et al: Jugular venous desaturation and outcome after severe head injury. J Neurol Neurosurg Psychiatry 57:171, 1994

19. Robertson C, Gopinath SP, Goodman J, et al: S$_{jv}$O$_2$ monitoring in head-injured patients. J Neurotrauma 12:891, 1995

20. Stochetti N, Paparella A, Bridelli F, et al: Cerebral venous oxygen saturation studied with bilateral samples in the internal jugular veins. Neurosurgery 34:38, 1994

21. Rosner M, Rosner S, Johnson A: Cerebral perfusion pressure: management protocol and clinical results. J Neurosurg 83:949, 1995

22. McGraw C: A cerebral perfusion pressure greater than 80 mm Hg is more beneficial. Springer-Verlag, Berlin, 1989

23. Marshall L, Smith R, Shapiro H: The outcome with aggressive treatment in severe head injuries, part II: acute and chronic barbiturate administration in the management of head injury. J Neurosurg 50:26, 1979

24. Ward J, Becker D, Miller JD, et al: Failure of prophylactic barbiturate coma in the treatment of severe head injury. J Neurosurg 62:383, 1985

25. Levy M, Aranda M, Zelman V, et al: Propylene glycol toxicity following continuous etomidate infusion for the control of refractory cerebral edema. Neurosurgery 37:363, 1995

26. Pinaud M, Lelasque J, Chetanneau A, et al: Effects of Diprivan on cerebral blood flow, intracranial pressure and cerebral metabolism in head-injured patients. Annales Françaises d'Anesthésie et de Réanimation 10:2, 1991

27. Bullock R, Stewart L, Rafferty C, et al: Continuous monitoring of jugular bulb oxygen saturation and the effect of drugs acting on cerebral metabolism. Acta Neurochir (Wien) 59:113, 1993

28. Clifton G, Allen S, Barrodale P, et al: A phase II study of moderate hypothermia in severe brain injury. J Neurotrauma 10:263, 1993

29. Marion D, Obrist W, Carlier P, et al: The use of moderate therapeutic hypothermia for patients with severe head injuries: a preliminary report. J Neurosurg 79: 354, 1993

30. Bracken M, Shepard M, Collins W, et al: A randomized controlled trial of methylprednisolone or naloxone in the treatment of acute spinal cord injury. N Engl J Med 322:1405, 1990

31. Bracken M, Shepard M, Collins W, et al: Methylprednisolone or naloxone treatment after acute spinal cord injury: 1-year follow-up data. J Neurosurg 76:23, 1992

32. Guha A, Tator C, Piper I, et al: Increase in rat spinal cord blood flow with the calcium channel blocker nimodipine. J Neurosurg 63:250, 1985

33. Guha A, Tator C, Smith C, et al: Improvement in posttraumatic spinal cord blood flow with a combination of a calcium channel blocker and a vasopressor. J Trauma 29:1440, 1989

34. Geisler F: GM-1 ganglioside and motor recovery following human spinal cord injury. J Emerg Med 11(SII):49, 1993

35. Bracken M, Shepard M, Holford T, et al: Administration of methylprednisolone for 24 or 48 hours or tirilazad mesylate for 48 hours in the treatment of acute spinal cord injury: results of the Third National Acute Spinal Cord Injury Randomized Controlled Trial. National Acute Spinal Cord Injury Study. JAMA 227:1597, 1997

36. Marshall L, Knowlton S, Garfan S, et al: Deterioration following spinal cord injury: a multi-center study. J Neurosurg 66:400, 1987

37. Wilberger J: Advances in the diagnosis and management of spinal cord trauma. J Neurotrauma 8:75, 1992

38. Wilberger J, Duh M: Surgical treatment of spinal cord injury—the NASCIS II experience. Presented at the annual meeting of the AANS, Boston, Massachusetts, April 1993

39. Allen BL Jr: Recognition of injuries to the lower cervical spine. The Cervical Spine, 2nd ed. The Cervical Spine Research Society, Ed. JB Lippincott Co, Philadelphia, 1989, p 286

40. Lind BL, Nordwall A: Halo-vest treatment of unstable traumatic cervical spine injuries. Spine 13:425, 1988

41. Denis F: The three column spine and its significance in the classification of acute thoracolumbar spinal injuries. Spine 8:817, 1983

42. Kontos H, Raper A, Patterson J: Analysis of vasoreactivity of local pH, pCO$_2$, and bicarbonate on pial vessels. Stroke 8:358, 1977

43. Kontos H, Wei E, Navari R, et al: Responses of cerebral arteries and arterioles to acute hypotension and hypertension. Am J Physiol 234:H371, 1978

44. McHenry LC Jr, West JW, Cooper ES: Cerebral autoregulation in man. Stroke 5:695, 1974

45. Muizelaar J, Wei E, Kontos H, et al: Cerebral blood flow is regulated by changes in blood pressure and in blood viscosity alike. Stroke 17:44, 1986

46. Muizelaar J, Poel H, Li Z, et al: Pial arteriolar vessel diameter and CO$_2$ reactivity during prolonged hyperventilation in the rabbit. J Neurosurg 69:923, 1988

47. Chesnut R, Marshall L, Klauber MR, et al: The role of secondary brain injury in determining outcome after severe head injury. J Trauma 34:216, 1993

48. Monro A: Observations on the structure and function of the nervous system. Creech and Johnson, Edinburgh, 1783

49. Kellie G: On death from cold, and on congestions of the brain: an account of the appearances observed in the dissection of two of three individuals presumed to have perished in the storm of 3rd November 1821; with some reflections on the pathology of the brain. Trans Med Chir Soc Edinburgh 84-169, 1824

50. Marmarou A, Shulman K, Rosende R: A nonlinear analysis of the cerebral spinal fluid system and intracranial pressure dynamics. J Neurosurg 48:332, 1978

51. Muizelaar JP: Cerebral Blood Flow, Cerebral Blood Volume, and Cerebral Metabolism after Severe Head Injury. WB Saunders Co, Philadelphia, 1989

52. Muizelaar JP, Marmarou A, Ward JD, et al: Adverse effects of prolonged hyperventilation in patients with severe head injury: a randomized clinical trial. J Neurosurg 75:731, 1991

53. Muizelaar JP, Wei EP, Kontos H, et al: Mannitol causes compensatory cerebral vasoconstriction and vasodilation in response to blood viscosity changes. J Neurosurg 59:822, 1983

54. Muizelaar JP, Lutz HI, Becker D: Effect of mannitol on ICP and CBF and correlation with pressure autoregulation in severely head-injured patients. J Neurosurg 61:700, 1984

55. Rosner M, Daughton S: Cerebral perfusion management in head injury. J Trauma 30:933, 1990

56. Adams J, Di G: The Pathology of Blunt Head Injury. Heinemann, London, 1972

57. Bouma G, Muizelaar JP, Choi S, et al: Cerebral circulation and metabolism after severe traumatic brain injury: the elusive role of ischemia. J Neurosurg 75: 685, 1991

58. Jones T, Morawetz R, Crowell R, et al: Thresholds of

focal cerebral ischemia in awake monkeys. J Neurosurg 54:773, 1981

59. Muizelaar JP, Schroder M: Overview of monitoring of cerebral blood flow and metabolism after severe head injury. Can J Neurol Sci 21:S6, 1994

60. Hochachka P, Mommsen T: Protons and anaerobiosis. Science 219:1391, 1983

61. Andersen B, Marmarou A: Functional compartmentalization of energy production in neural tissue. Brain Res 585:190, 1992

62. Inao S, Marmarou A, Clarke G, et al: Production and clearance of lactate from brain tissue, CSF and serum following experimental brain injury. J Neurosurg 69:736, 1988

63. Verweij B, Muizelaar J: Mitochondrial dysfunction after experimental and human brain injury and its possible reversal with a selective N-type calcium channel antagonist (SNX-111). Neurol Res 19:334, 1997

64. Xiong Y, Gu Q, Peterson P, et al: Mitochondrial dysfunction and calcium perturbation induced by traumatic brain injury. J Neurotrauma 14:23, 1997

65. Young W, Bracken M: The second National Acute Spinal Cord Injury Study. J Neurotrauma 9:S429, 1992

66. Dimitrijevic M, Dimitrijevic M, Faganel J, et al: Residual Motor Functions in Spinal Cord Injury. Raven Press, New York, 1988

67. Blight A, Young W: Central axons in injured cat spinal cord recover electrophysiological function following remyelination by Schwann cells. J Neurol Sci 91:15, 1989

68. Blight A, Decrescito V: Morphometric analysis of experimental spinal cord injury in the cat: the relation of injury intensity to survival of myelinated axons. Neuroscience 19:321, 1986

69. Blight A, Young W: Axonal morphometric correlates of evoked potentials in experimental spinal cord injury. Humana Press, New York, 1990

70. Blight A, Gruner J: Augmentation by 4-aminopyridine of vestibulospinal free fall responses in chronic phases of traumatic spinal cord injury in dogs: a phase I clinical trial. J Neurol Sci 82:155, 1987

71. Hayes K, Blight A, Potter P, et al: Preclinical trial of 4-aminopyridine in patients with chronic spinal cord injury. Paraplegia 31:216, 1993

72. Hayes K, Potter P, Wolfe D, et al: 4-aminopyridine-sensitive neurologic deficits in patients with spinal cord injury. J Neurotrauma 11:433, 1994

73. Sandler A, Tator C: Review of the effects of spinal trauma on vessels and blood flow in the spinal cord. J Neurosurg 45:638, 1972

74. Young W: Blood flow, metabolic and neurophysiologic mechanisms in spinal cord injury. Central Nervous System Trauma Status Report, 1985. Becker D, Poulishock J, Eds. National Institute of Neurological and Communicative Disorders and Stroke, Bethesda, Maryland, 1985

Acknowledgments

Figure 3   Reprinted courtesy of the American Spinal Injury Association, Chicago, Illinois.
Figure 4   Susan Brust, C.M.I.

3 INJURIES TO THE FACE AND JAW

Seth Thaller, M.D., and F. William Blaisdell, M.D.

Assessment and Management of Maxillofacial Injuries

Tremendous progress has been made in the management of patients with facial injuries. Reconstructive surgeons are treating an increasing number of challenging facial injuries because of excellent advances in the transportation of trauma victims and the regionalization of care in trauma centers. Although severe facial injuries are often associated with devastating cosmetic and functional defects, reconstructive surgeons are achieving better long-term surgical results and are able to repair certain injuries that were once considered nonreconstructible by employing craniofacial surgical techniques developed through the pioneering efforts of Dr. Paul Tessier, of Paris. These techniques include widespread subperiosteal exposure, rigid internal fixation with miniature plates and screws, and widespread primary bone grafting.

Initial Survey

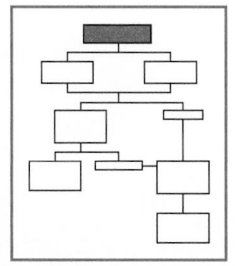

Maxillofacial injuries are secondary to either blunt or penetrating trauma. Motor vehicle accidents remain the most common cause of facial injuries characterized by bony comminution and distraction. However, penetrating injuries, such as knife wounds, can cause extensive soft tissue injuries to skin and underlying nerves, blood vessels, parotid structures, and other structures of the upper aerodigestive system. Gunshot wounds can cause devastating injuries that necessitate extensive flap reconstruction to provide satisfactory soft tissue coverage of the underlying bone.

On initial assessment, the physician must always pay special attention to correcting the most life-threatening problems, including an obstructed airway, bleeding, and shock [*see I:2 Trauma Resuscitation, I:4 Shock, and I:5 Bleeding and Transfusion*]. Patients with facial injuries often have multisystem involvement; priorities in the evaluation and treatment of associated significant injuries are discussed elsewhere [*see III:1 Emergency Department Evaluation of the Patient with Multiple Injuries*]. After establishing that the patient is stable, the examiner should quickly make note of lacerations and contusions, extensive bony disruptions, loss of vision, malocclusion, trismus, and bleeding.

In the evaluation of facial injuries, a quick analysis of occlusion provides extremely important diagnostic information that serves as the foundation for future fracture repair. Angle's clas-sification of malocclusion, which is more than 100 years old, remains one of the most commonly used systems. The maxillomandibular relation is determined by the position of the mesiobuccal cusp of the maxillary first molar in relation to the buccal groove of the mandibular first molar. Angle's class I, or neutroclusion, exists when the permanent maxillary first molar is ideally positioned—that is, the buccal cusp of the maxillary first molar and the mesiobuccal groove of the mandibular first molar occlude, resulting in a normal anteroposterior relation of the maxillary and mandibular dentition. Angle's class II, or distoclusion, exists when the maxillary first molar is mesial (i.e., toward the midline) to the corresponding mandibular first molar. Angle's class III, or mesioclusion, exists when the mandibular first molar is mesial to the maxillary first molar.

AIRWAY ASSESSMENT

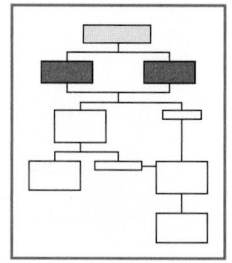

Facial bone fractures, bleeding, loose dentition, debris, and laryngeal injuries can contribute to airway compromise. Accordingly, whenever there is any evidence of maxillofacial injuries, it is essential to monitor the airway status carefully. If the patient is conscious, alert, and breathing at a rate of less than 20 respirations/min, without excessive airway secretions or excessive hemorrhage, it can be assumed that the patient has an adequate airway.

In a comatose patient with compromised vital reflexes (i.e., gag, cough, and swallow), an endotracheal tube must be inserted immediately to prevent aspiration. In the presence of nasopharyngeal bleeding, major maxillofacial injuries, or cerebrospinal fluid leakage, nasal intubation should be avoided because of the potential for intracranial contamination. If there is a possible fracture of the cribriform plate, either an orotracheal tube should be placed or a cricothyrotomy should be performed. In an agitated or restless patient, only a single attempt should be made at inserting an endotracheal or nasotracheal tube; if the attempt is unsuccessful, an emergency cricothyrotomy should be performed [*see I:2 Trauma Resuscitation*]. In slightly more elective circumstances, a deliberate tracheotomy may be the optimal means of ensuring an adequate airway. Cricothyrotomy and tracheotomy must never be taken lightly, because they can lead to significant complications. In addition, because newer treatment modalities using rigid fixation decrease the time required for extensive maxillo-

Assessment and Management of Maxillofacial Injuries

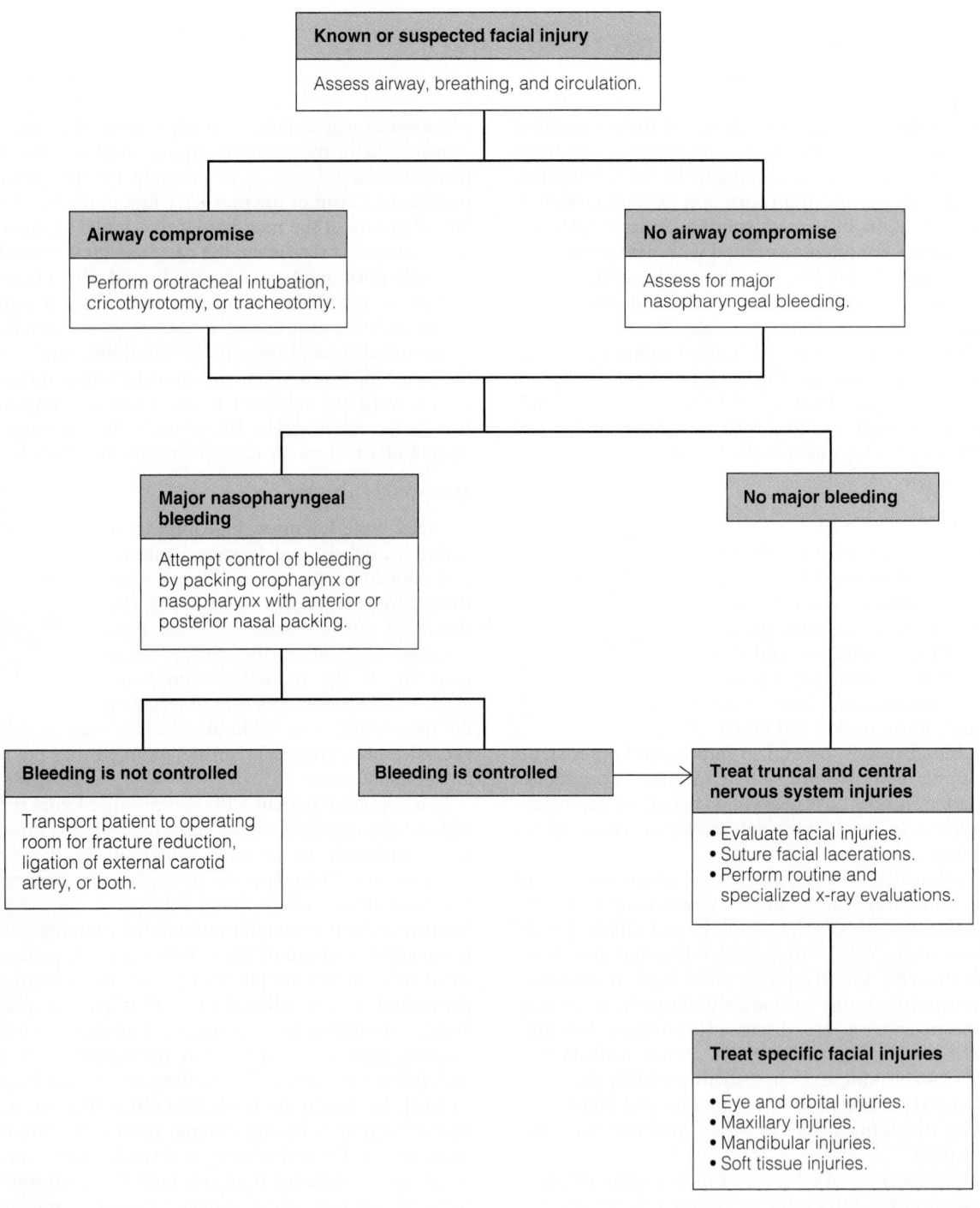

Known or suspected facial injury

Assess airway, breathing, and circulation.

Airway compromise

Perform orotracheal intubation, cricothyrotomy, or tracheotomy.

No airway compromise

Assess for major nasopharyngeal bleeding.

Major nasopharyngeal bleeding

Attempt control of bleeding by packing oropharynx or nasopharynx with anterior or posterior nasal packing.

No major bleeding

Bleeding is not controlled

Transport patient to operating room for fracture reduction, ligation of external carotid artery, or both.

Bleeding is controlled

Treat truncal and central nervous system injuries

- Evaluate facial injuries.
- Suture facial lacerations.
- Perform routine and specialized x-ray evaluations.

Treat specific facial injuries

- Eye and orbital injuries.
- Maxillary injuries.
- Mandibular injuries.
- Soft tissue injuries.

mandibular fixation, more conservative methods of airway control are often indicated.

If the respiratory rate is higher than 25/min or if there is evidence that the airway is obstructed or compromised, the patient should be carefully monitored. When the respiratory rate increases to 30/min or higher, an immediate assessment of arterial blood gases should be made under close observation. A respiratory rate higher than 35/min is an indication for both intubation and respiratory support unless the cause of the rapid rate can be identified and immediately reversed.

MAXILLOFACIAL BLEEDING

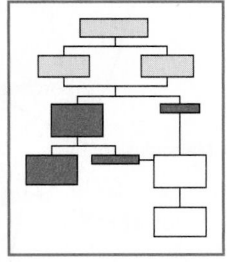

Once the airway has been satisfactorily stabilized, the next priority is to manage maxillofacial bleeding. There is a misconception that patients do not bleed profusely from facial injuries and that facial bleeding can be controlled easily.[1] Unfortunately, this is not necessarily always the case. In addition, because facial injuries themselves can be so striking, associated significant hemorrhage can often be overlooked or underestimated. Firm compression with moist sponges will temporarily stop most arterial and venous bleeding. Careful application of digital pressure or definitive ligation of the bleeding point can often control external bleeding. These procedures are best performed in the operating room, with the patient under general anesthesia.

If the source of hemorrhage is in the depths of a narrow laceration, bleeding can be controlled temporarily by packing. Blind clamping or suture ligation can damage important underlying facial structures, particularly branches of the facial nerve; therefore, such procedures must be avoided. Insertion of an anterior pack moistened with 1:10,000 epinephrine may be used to control nasal bleeding. However, persistent nasopharyngeal hemorrhage will necessitate either placement of a posterior pack or ligation of the internal maxillary artery or the external carotid artery.

In major maxillofacial injuries with extensive pharyngeal bleeding, immediate airway access is mandatory, either with an endotracheal tube or by cricothyrotomy. Once airway control has been achieved, the patient should be brought to the operating room for reduction of gross bony injuries, which will often stop uncontrollable hemorrhage. In those rare instances when maxillofacial injuries are associated with serious and uncontrollable hemorrhage, it may be necessary to obtain access to the external carotid artery for ligation of the major trunk or a branch if either is the source of bleeding [see III:4 Injuries to the Neck].

Definitive Evaluation

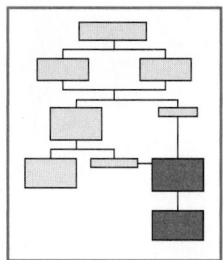

When there is no associated airway compromise, facial injuries are a lower priority than potential thoracic, abdominal, or head injuries [see III:1 Emergency Department Evaluation of the Patient with Multiple Injuries]. In fact, in the absence of airway compromise and severe hemorrhage, definitive diagnostic evaluation and management of maxillofacial injuries can be delayed until the more life-threatening injuries have been stabilized and treated.

EXAMINATION

Like any other anatomic region, the face must be examined in an orderly fashion, with careful attention paid to gross asymmetry, paralysis, weakness, eye movements, occlusal discrepancies, and ecchymosis. Areas of hypesthesia or anesthesia should be noted. Special attention should be directed toward bimanual palpation of bony prominences within the craniofacial region to look for crepitus, tenderness, irregularities, and step-offs. Palpation should start with the frontal bones and lateral and inferior orbital rims.

The zygomatic arch should be palpated for evidence of depression, and the region of the malar eminence should be evaluated for recession [see Figures 1 through 4]. Fracture of the

Figure 1 Broken nose.

Figure 2 Fractured zygoma.

Figure 3 **Infraorbital fracture.**

Figure 4 **Fractured mandible.**

zygomatic complex is often identified with an inferiorly displaced lateral canthus, paresthesias of the infraorbital nerve, visual impairment, displacement of the globe, or trismus secondary to impingement of the zygomatic arch on the coronoid process or temporal muscle.

Orbital evaluation is key to the assessment of facial injuries. The nasolacrimal duct should be inspected, and the distance between the medial canthi should be measured for the presence of telecanthus. (The normal intercanthal distance in the average adult is less than 35 mm.) Pupils should be checked for reactivity, and extraocular muscle motion should be assessed. Diplopia secondary to extraocular muscle entrapment should be determined. The position of the globe should also be assessed; orbital floor fractures may cause enophthalmos and severe swelling, and a blow-in type fracture may result in exophthalmos. A visual acuity test must be performed before any surgical intervention for correction of facial fractures. An ophthalmologic consultation is essential if there is any evidence of ocular damage, such as lens displacement, hyphema, retinal detachment, acute visual impairment, or global disruption.

Next, the nose should be gently palpated. Any depression, abnormal motion, or deviation of the nasal bones and cartilages should be noted. The nasal cavity should be examined specifically for the presence of septal deviation, septal hematoma, or leakage of cerebrospinal fluid. A septal hematoma can be ruled out by aspiration with an 18-gauge or 20-gauge needle and syringe; if bleeding is present, an incision and drainage and placement of a drain are necessary. If left untreated, a septal hematoma may lead to the development of a saddle-nose deformity. Flattening of the face, or dish-face deformity, is characteristic of midfacial fractures.

Mobility of the maxilla is determined by placing one hand over the bridge of the nose while the other grasps the palate and upper dentition and moves the maxilla anteriorly and posteriorly, checking for separation of the midfacial structures. The mandible should be palpated carefully with both hands to locate any intraoral mucosal lacerations or lesions. Bimanual

palpation of the mandible is accomplished by placing the thumbs over the molar occlusal surfaces and the index fingers externally over the inferior border of the mandible and torquing the bone to check for movement. Any missing or mobile teeth must be recorded. The floor of the mouth should also be examined with bimanual palpation.

The ears should be examined for evidence of lacerations or contusions of the external auditory canal that may be caused by condylar neck fractures. A simple diagnostic method is to insert the fingertip into the external auditory canal on one side; if no movement can be determined with mandibular excursion, a diagnosis of condylar fracture can be made.

FACIAL X-RAYS

A spectrum of available radiologic modalities plays a significant role in the diagnosis and treatment of facial injuries. Appropriate studies are mandatory. In addition, x-rays provide an excellent permanent record for medicolegal purposes. The initial x-rays of patients in the emergency room (the first level for assessment and clarification of maxillofacial injuries) should be performed using conventional films and should consist of a cervical spine series (with all the cervical vertebrae adequately visualized), skull x-rays, and facial x-rays, including the anteroposterior, lateral, Waters, Towne, submentovertex, panorex, and mandibular views. More definitive x-rays can be obtained later for complete evaluation of specific injuries. The Caldwell view defines the orbital walls and the frontal sinus structures. The Waters view is important for determining the bony continuity of the orbit, nose, zygoma, and lateral portion of the maxilla. The lateral skull view is helpful for evaluation of frontal sinus fractures. Oblique views of the orbit are excellent for demonstrating the apex and the medial, lateral, and orbital walls.

The lateral oblique and modified Towne views are used to evaluate the mandible. The lateral oblique is the most common and useful view and provides evaluation of the body, angle of the body, and the ascending ramus. A posteroanterior view is helpful in assessing the symphyseal and body regions as well as the condylar and coronoid processes. Panoramic x-rays are the best screening views for assessing mandibular fractures, especially within the condyles. Associated injuries to the dentition and supporting structures may necessitate dental spot films for more specific information.

OTHER STUDIES

Computed tomographic scanning can be of great value in diagnosing the more complex traumatic injuries, such as craniomaxillofacial injuries and associated central nervous system injuries. Computed tomography is used to evaluate most critically injured patients with craniocerebral trauma, and the studies can easily be extended to include the patient's facial skeleton with little additional risk. Both 3 mm axial and coronal CT cuts of the facial skeleton should be obtained, especially for examination of the orbit. A lateral oblique scan through the midportion of the globe provides additional information regarding the bony architecture of the orbit. This information can be reformatted, and three-dimensional reconstructions can be made for further evaluation. Magnetic resonance imaging is proving to be of benefit in assessing both bony and soft tissue injuries. Arteriography may be needed to evaluate the source of a hemorrhage or to rule out major vascular injuries.

Treatment of Soft Tissue Injuries

Soft tissue injuries are most often the result of penetrating trauma but can also be the result of blunt trauma [see Treatment of Maxillofacial Fractures, below]. Any patients who need general anesthesia, such as a child or a patient with extensive complex lacerations involving deeper structures, should be treated in the operating room after appropriate evaluation of their overall status. Soft tissue injuries can involve nerves, parotid ducts, lacrimal ducts, and other critical facial structures. Abrasions must be thoroughly cleaned, and lacerations should be irrigated with normal saline and conservatively debrided as necessary. With deeply embedded foreign material, debridement and irrigation must be particularly meticulous and extensive to prevent residual cosmetic deformities. Dermabrasion is especially good for large involved areas. Most facial lacerations can be closed primarily with standard suturing procedures [see I:8 Acute Wound Care]. Antibiotic coverage is left to individual preferences; however, 24 hours of prophylactic perioperative antibiotic coverage with a cephalosporin is strongly recommended. The examiner must always consider the possibility of underlying injuries, and careful palpation and visualization of important underlying structures should be part of the definitive wound evaluation and treatment.

Local anesthetic agents used in the head and neck region should always contain epinephrine for hemostasis. To decrease pain and discomfort, the local anesthetic should be administered through the margins of the wound rather than through the surrounding skin. Regional nerve blocks are preferred for suture closure of lacerations involving the forehead, cheeks, lips, and chin. The forehead can be blocked by local infiltration of the supraorbital nerve, which is located just superior to the eyebrow. The upper lip, side of the nose, and adjacent skin can be blocked by anesthetizing the infraorbital nerve. Injection of the mental nerve, located between the first and second bicuspids, will anesthetize the lower lip and surrounding chin. Regional blocks also provide the advantage of minimizing tis-

sue damage to already traumatized skin and lead to less scar formation.

NERVE INJURIES

The facial nerve is the nerve most vulnerable to maxillofacial trauma, and its function must be thoroughly evaluated before the administration of any local anesthetic. In addition, facial nerve injuries result in the most serious functional disabilities and aesthetic defects. Sensory nerves, such as the infraorbital and supraorbital nerves, can also be involved in traumatic injures; however, the associated hypesthesia causes only minimal long-term disability.

Whenever the posterior half of the parotid gland suffers a deep laceration, it should be assumed that a major branch of the facial nerve has been divided, and the face should be carefully examined. If there is a clean, sharp division of one of the five major trunks or of the proximal main nerve trunk, it can be repaired immediately with microanastomotic techniques. If there is substantial nerve loss, the nerve ends should be identified and appropriately tagged for future nerve grafting. If a nerve laceration occurs anterior to the region of the lateral canthus, nerve repair is generally unnecessary because there is sufficient crossover from the opposite side. Peripheral branch injury is manifest by inability to raise the eyebrow (frontal branch), inability to close the eyelids (malar), smoothness of the cheek (infraorbital), inability to smile (buccal), and inability to frown (marginal mandibular).

PAROTID DUCT INJURIES

The parotid duct is located between the parotid gland and the oral mucosa, opening opposite the second upper molar. Any deep laceration of the anterior parotid gland can damage this duct. If there is a possibility that the parotid duct is injured, the orifice of Stensen's duct should be probed. Should the probe enter the wound, division of the duct is verified. The proximal cut end of the duct can be located by expressing saliva from the gland. A catheter should then be passed through Stensen's duct and through the area of laceration, and the duct should be repaired over the catheter [see Figure 5].

LACRIMAL DUCT INJURIES

Whenever there is a laceration involving the medial canthal region, a lacrimal duct injury should be assumed. Acute reconstruction of the lacrimal duct is controversial. If both ends of the duct can be easily discerned, the severed ends should be realigned, splinted internally, and repaired. This procedure is best accomplished over a fine Silastic rod. Dissection to locate the residual parts of the duct should be delicate and meticulous, because traumatic dissection can aggravate the injury and result in further permanent damage.

SCALP INJURIES

When scalp injuries are repaired, extensive shaving is unnecessary. Scalp injuries can be associated with profuse bleeding because of the scalp's extensive vascular supply. To obtain adequate control of hemorrhage from the wound margins, closure can be achieved in a single layer with a running, locking 3-0 chromic suture on a large cutting needle. Associated underlying skull fractures are always a possibility, and the skull should be palpated and inspected through any full-thickness scalp wound.

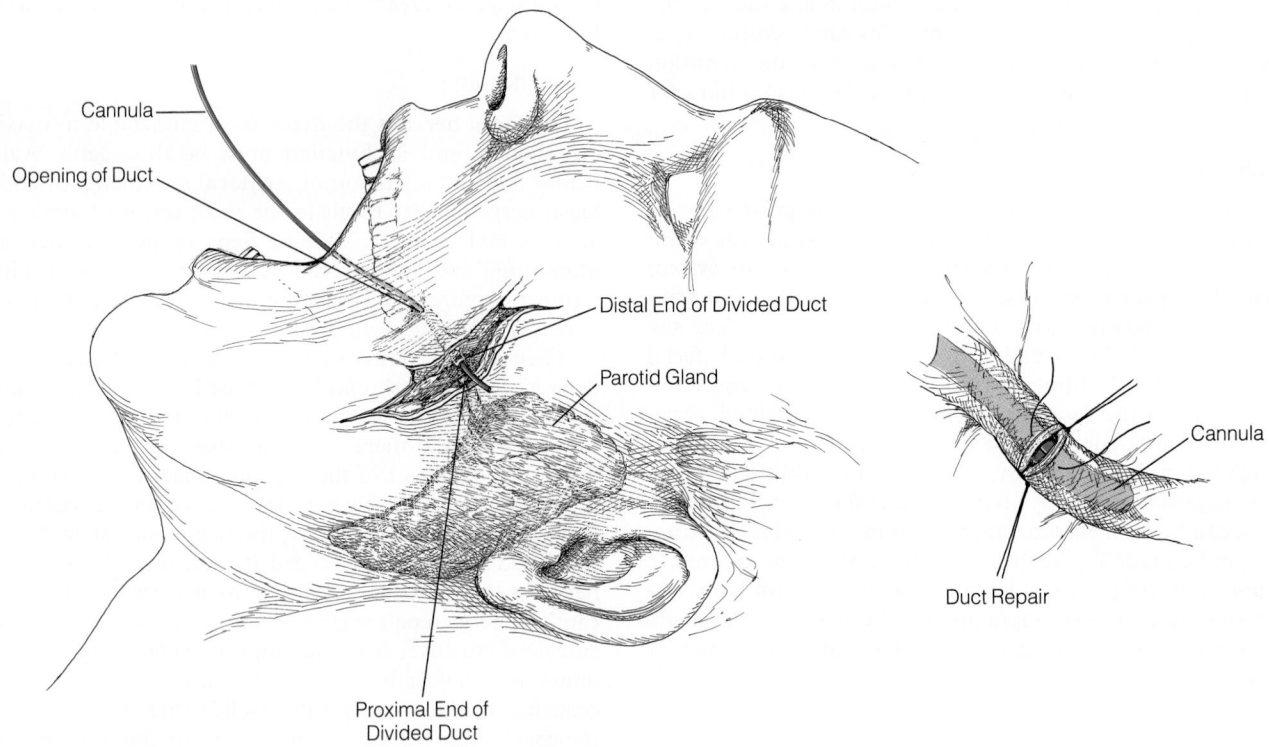

Figure 5 Injuries to the parotid duct are repaired by passing a catheter through Stensen's duct and through the area of laceration and then repairing the parotid duct over the catheter.

EYELID INJURIES

If the patient reports excessive eye pain, the initial examiner must always first rule out an associated ocular injury. In addition, when faced with through-and-through lid lacerations, the examiner must perform a very careful eye examination. Lacerations of the eyelid should be meticulously repaired by approximation of the margins of the lid defect, followed by closure of the laceration in three layers. The conjunctiva may be left unsutured if good apposition can be obtained by closing the tarsal plate and the pretarsal muscles that occupy the middle layer, which is preferably closed with fine absorbable sutures. Fine nonabsorbable skin sutures are employed to close the final layer. All skin sutures should be removed within 48 hours. When there is extensive tissue loss, it may be necessary to use plastic techniques to mobilize sufficient conjunctiva for closure.

EYEBROW INJURIES

For optimal cosmetic results, the eyebrows should be closed meticulously in layers with careful alignment of the eyebrow margins. Lacerations passing through the eyebrow should not be shaved; leaving them intact facilitates good plastic closure. Because the hairs of the eyebrow run obliquely to the surface of the skin, any incision for debridement should follow the line of the eyebrows to avoid further loss of hair.

EXTERNAL-EAR INJURIES

If avulsions of the ear are properly repaired, the chances are good that they will heal because of the highly vascular pedicle. Circulation is maintained if even a small pedicle is present.

Repair of ear wounds should be done in three layers by using fine nonabsorbable sutures to approximate the cartilage and the skin. If the ear is completely detached, the cartilage should be preserved within a subcutaneous pocket in the mastoid region for future reconstruction.

Hematomas can occur secondary to the shearing of the vascular mucoperichondrium from the underlying cartilage. These must be evacuated early, and a conforming pressure dressing should be placed to maintain the normal ear contour.

NASAL INJURIES

Through-and-through lacerations of the nose and near-avulsion injuries are cosmetic problems. Because the nose is extremely vascular, repair of these injuries should be especially meticulous and done in layers. The cartilage and skin should be aligned with fine nonabsorbable interrupted sutures. Absorbable sutures should be employed for repair of the mucosa. Key cosmetic points (i.e., epidermal-mucosal junctions, nasal fold junctions, or critical angles in jagged lacerations) should be sutured first to ensure that no deformity results.

LIP INJURIES

If the margin of the lip has been divided, the vermilion border should be carefully identified and tattooed, and the first sutures should be placed to approximate this critical margin. A common problem in the treatment of lip injuries is that it may become more difficult to identify landmarks when they are obliterated by local anesthetic injections or associated edema.

Treatment of Maxillofacial Fractures

Management of maxillofacial fractures can be extremely challenging. The common maxillofacial fractures include nasal, mandibular, orbital, zygomatic complex, sinus (e.g., maxillary, sphenoid, ethmoid, and frontal), and maxillary fractures (e.g., Le Fort I, II, or III). Management of these fractures often requires sophisticated specialty treatment involving plastic surgeons, ophthalmologists, neurosurgeons, otolaryngologists, or a combination of these.[2-7]

FRONTAL SINUS FRACTURES

The frontal sinus region is prone to injury because of its prominent location and relatively thin anterior bony wall.[8,9] Injuries to the frontal sinus area require comprehensive treatment, often with a team approach. The key to treatment lies in determining the status of the nasofrontal ducts.[10,11] Patients with such injuries also require careful, regular, long-term follow-up care because potentially life-threatening complications, such as meningitis, osteomyelitis, and mucopyocele, may develop.[12-15]

NASAL AND NASO-ORBITO-ETHMOIDAL FRACTURES

The nasal bone is the most commonly fractured facial bone.[16] Before any treatment is embarked on, it is always helpful to have the patient provide a preinjury photo of himself or herself so that it can be determined whether the nasal deformity is from the acute episode.[17] If a patient is seen almost immediately after injury and the associated swelling and ecchymosis are minimal, closed reduction can be performed at once. Nasal bone fractures can be reduced simply by inserting a scalpel handle or large hemostat into the nostril; the fracture segments can then be elevated and relocated. Usually, the nasal cavity is packed with petroleum jelly gauze to maintain alignment of the fracture and nasal septum, and a malleable splint is taped over the nose to provide counterpressure and assist in maintaining alignment. Packing is removed within 48 hours. However, treatment is generally not urgent and, depending on the individual situation, may be delayed for 7 to 10 days.

Naso-orbito-ethmoidal fractures generally occur secondary to direct force applied over the nasal bridge, resulting in posterior displacement of bony structures and involvement of the medial canthus, lacrimal duct, canaliculi, and sac.[18] Repair of naso-orbito-ethmoidal fractures can be extremely challenging because of the number of important structures involved and their extensive comminution.[19] Satisfactory surgical management should be conducted through a coronal approach, thereby permitting precise three-dimensional reduction and stabilization and extensive primary bone grafting for replacement augmentation.[20] If there is associated CSF rhinorrhea, neurosurgical assistance should be obtained and early fracture reduction done.

ORBITAL FRACTURES

Orbital fractures can occur as isolated events or as a component of more extensive injuries. Orbital fractures, such as lacrimal duct lacerations and injuries to the globe, require highly specialized management with the aid of an ophthalmologist. Naso-orbital fractures with telecanthus should be treated with open reduction and fixation, as should all displaced fractures of the orbital rim and floor.[21,22]

ZYGOMATIC FRACTURES

The zygoma is a tetrapod structure that forms the malar prominence and the inferior and lateral aspects of the orbit. Fractures of the zygomatic complex should be repaired to prevent the development of serious aesthetic and functional deformities. Satisfactory stabilization requires three-point fixation achieved through incisions placed within the regions of the upper and lower lids and the upper buccal sulcus.[23]

MAXILLARY FRACTURES

In 1901, maxillary fractures were classified by René Le Fort into three types.[24] Although the Le Fort classification system remains entrenched in the literature and serves as a basis for both communication and description, it is rare that patients exhibit pure Le Fort fracture patterns. Instead, trauma sur-

Figure 6 **Le Fort I fractures (black line) affect the upper jaw alone. In Le Fort II fractures (red line), the upper jaw and the central portion of the face are separated from the skull.**

Figure 7 **In Le Fort III fractures, all of the facial bones are separated from the skull.**

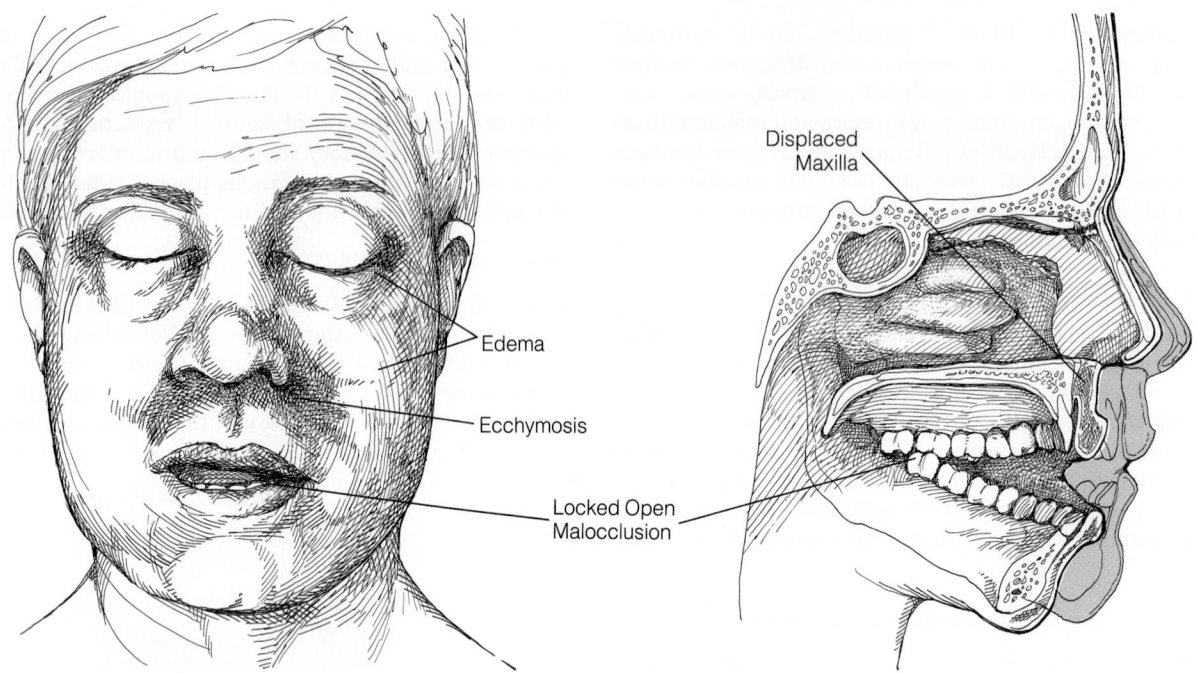

Figure 8   **Findings in patients with Le Fort III maxillary fractures immediately after injury, before obliterative edema develops.**

geons are generally challenged by severe bony comminution and distraction.

Le Fort I, or lower maxillary fractures, are the simplest type of maxillary fracture, consisting of horizontal detachment of the tooth-bearing segment of the maxilla at the level of the nasal floor [*see Figure 6*]. Le Fort II, or central or pyramidal fractures, pass through the central portion of the face, which includes the right and left maxillae, the medial aspect of the antra, the infraorbital rim, the orbital floor, and the nasal bones. Le Fort III, or craniofacial disjunction, is characterized by complete separation of all facial structures from the cranium [*see Figures 7 and 8*]. Le Fort III fractures pass through the upper portions of the orbits as well as through both zygomas.

All Le Fort fractures require highly specialized treatment that involves the use of craniofacial techniques, consisting of exploration and visualization of the entire fracture pattern, precise reduction, and rigid stabilization of bony segments.

MANDIBULAR FRACTURES

Diagnosis of mandibular fractures can usually be made on physical examination. Common findings include malocclusion, intraoral lacerations, and mobility at the fracture site. Radiographs are useful for planning treatment. Fractures of the mandible rarely involve the midline or symphyseal region. Most often, fractures will pass through areas of weakness, including the parasymphyseal region and the angle or neck of the condyle [*see Figure 9*]. The fracture pattern is usually determined by the site and mechanism of injury. Because of the mandible's architectural arrangement, more than one half of mandibular fractures involve multiple sites.

Mandibular fractures are not an emergency, but early defin-

itive treatment results in a decreased number of complications. Preinjury occlusal relations remain the keystone to treatment. Mandibular fractures can be repaired by closed reduction with maxillomandibular fixation or by open reduction and fixation with wire osteosynthesis. However, newer techniques with rigid internal fixation with miniature plates and screws have attained widespread popularity because of increased patient comfort.[25-31] In cooperative patients, a nondisplaced fracture can sometimes be handled conservatively with a dental soft diet and serial x-rays.

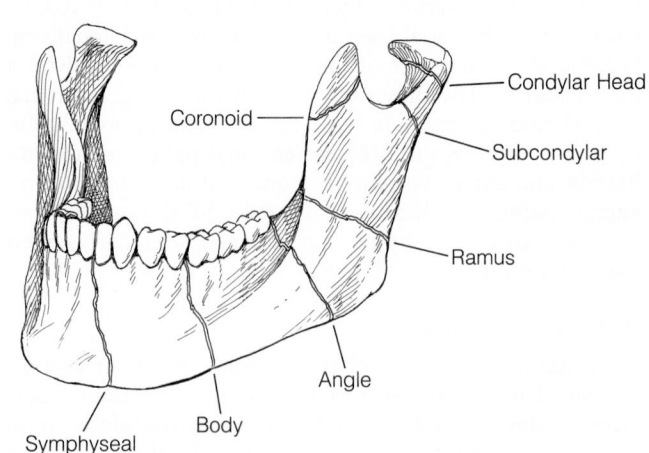

Figure 9   **Mandibular fractures.**

Discussion

Because the face is so thoroughly exposed, it is one of the most frequently injured areas of the body. Facial injuries can occur under a variety of circumstances, such as automobile accidents, altercations, or falls; more specifically, these injuries can be the results of bites, fires, explosions, lacerations, and contact with sharp or blunt objects. In automobile accidents, shards of glass may penetrate the wound, and these shards may not be radiopaque. If abrasions are present, note should be made of the abrading agent, whether it be grease, particles of dirt, gravel from a highway, or other contaminants. Underlying bony injury may or may not be obvious near the wounds. Because such injuries can expose the patient to tetanus or other anaerobic infections, antitetanic agents should be administered as part of the treatment regimen [see I:8 Acute Wound Care]. If treatment is delayed for any reason, a systemic prophylactic antibiotic should be administered. Minor lacerations of the face caused by domestic assaults or household accidents can be adequately treated in the emergency department under local anesthesia [see I:8 Acute Wound Care]. Lacerations that are contaminated are often best treated in the operating room with the patient under general anesthesia.

Only as much hair should be removed as is necessary for adequate assessment of the wound or for effective suturing. Eyebrows are best left unshaved to facilitate cosmetic repair. Local anesthesia should be induced, and abrasions should be scrubbed with a stiff brush until every particle of dirt is removed. If the dirt is deeply embedded, some tissue may have to be excised; this step can often be accomplished through the use of a fine curette or the point of a No. 11 blade. If dirt is not removed initially, it may be extremely difficult to remove later, and permanent tattooing may result.

Any dead or devitalized tissue should be excised, but there is no place for radical debridement of facial wounds. Tissue can survive on small pedicles. Full-thickness skin loss can be replaced with a free graft, which provides a better cosmetic match than a split-thickness skin graft [see V:30 Plastic Surgical Reconstruction]. If the wound is so ragged that it cannot be approximated, careful squaring of the edges may be advisable to facilitate a cosmetic closure. Dead or devitalized subcutaneous tissue should be removed conservatively.

Most facial wounds can be closed by simple suturing. Although the deadline for closure of wounds to other sites is usually 6 to 8 hours, facial wounds, unless heavily contaminated, can be closed as long as 24 hours after injury, particularly if meticulous attention is paid to procedural details. Such details include irrigation of the wound, removal of all foreign bodies, excision of devitalized tissue, and accurate approximation of tissue, with minimal dead space and no tension.

If the wound cannot be closed within the first 24 hours, delayed primary closure may be undertaken after 48 hours. In this event, the patient should be given systemic antibiotics, and the wound should be kept moist and protected as much as possible in the interval before closure. For best cosmetic results, the wound should be closed in multiple layers.

Sutures made of fine monofilament nylon, such as 6-0, are ideal for approximating the skin because they are nonreactive. The sutures should be applied loosely so that they do not strangulate tissue.

Key anatomic points should be identified and tattooed, mucosal edges should be approximated, and irregular margins of the skin should be excised and squared to provide the best possible fit. Margins of damaged structures, such as the nose or the ear, should be defined, and the critical margins should be determined and approximated initially. While the wound is being closed, all dead space in the wound should be obliterated and the edges everted. If the needle is passed through the skin at right angles, the edges of the skin will abut and eversion will occur. If, however, the needle is passed through the skin edge obliquely, inversion will result, and healing will be compromised. Subcutaneous or subcuticular sutures should be placed in such a way as to allow the skin edges to be approximated with minimal tension. If this procedure is done, through-and-through sutures can be removed in 3 days, and no marks will be left on the skin.

Any skin defects that require closure should be closed by grafting. No facial wound should be allowed to heal by granulation, because this would lead to excessive scarring. Instead, a temporary cover in the form of a skin graft should be provided to minimize scar formation; any deformity that results from the graft can be repaired at a later date [see V:30 Plastic Surgical Reconstruction].

The more complex of the maxillofacial fractures, such as major maxillary fractures, orbital fractures, malar fractures, and mandibular fractures [see Treatment of Maxillofacial Fractures, above], must be treated with specialty techniques; therefore, corresponding specialty consultation must be sought. However, in treating these fractures and soft tissue injuries [see Treatment of Soft Tissue Injuries, above], the priorities are to ensure adequacy of the airway and to control immediate bleeding. Once these aims have been achieved, none of the defects described, except for facial lacerations, require emergency treatment; they can be repaired days to even months later, if necessary, without jeopardizing a good cosmetic result.

References

1. Thaller S, Beal S: Maxillofacial trauma: a potentially fatal injury. Ann Plast Surg 27:281, 1991

2. Tung TC, Tseng WS, Chen CT, et al: Acute life-threatening injuries in facial fractures: a review of 1025 patients. J Trauma 49:420, 2000

3. Girotto JA, Gamble WB, Robertson B, et al: Blindness after reduction of facial fractures. Plast Reconstr Surg 104:875, 1999

4. Manson PN, Clark N, Robertson B, et al: Subunit principles in midface fractures: the importance of sagittal buttresses, soft tissue reductions, and sequencing treatment of segmental fractures. Plast Reconstr Surg 104:875, 1999

5. Gruss JS, Whelan MF, Rand RP, et al: Lessons learnt from the management of 1500 complex facial fractures. Ann Acad Med Singapore 28:677, 1999

6. McDonald WS, Thaller SR: Priorities in the treatment of facial fractures for the millennium. J Craniofac Surg 11:97, 2000

7. Mauriello JA, Lee HJ, Nguyen L: CT of soft tissue injury and orbital fractures. Radiol Clin North Am 37:241, 1999

8. Stanley R: Management of frontal sinus fractures. Facial Plast Surg 5:231, 1988

9. Stanley R: Fractures of the frontal sinus. Clin Plast Surg 16:115, 1989

10. Wolfe SA, Johnson P: Frontal sinus injuries: primary care and management of late complications. Plast Reconstr Surg 82:781, 1988

11. Luce E: Frontal sinus fractures: guidelines to management. Plast Reconstr Surg 80:500, 1987

12. Wilson B, Davidson B, Corey J, et al: Comparison of complications following frontal sinus fractures managed with exploration with or without obliteration over 10 years. Laryngoscope 98:516, 1988

13. Shockley W, Stucker F, White L, et al: Frontal sinus fractures: some problems and some solutions. Laryngoscope 98:18, 1988

14. Wallis A, Donald P: Frontal sinus fractures: a review of 72 cases. Laryngoscope 98:593, 1988

15. Rohrich R, Hollier L: Management of frontal sinus fractures. Clin Plast Surg 19:219, 1992

16. Spira M, Hardy S: Management of the injured nose. Tex Med 67:72, 1971

17. Rohrich RJ, Adams WP: Nasal fracture management: minimizing secondary nasal deformities. Plast Reconstr Surg 106:266, 2000

18. Gruss J: Naso-ethmoid-orbital fractures: classification and role of primary bone grafting. Plast Reconstr Surg 75:303, 1985

19. Gruss J, Pollock R, Phillips J, et al: Combined injuries of the cranium and face. Br J Plast Surg 42:385, 1989

20. Manson P, Crawley W, Yaremchuk M, et al: Midface fractures: advantages of immediate extended open reduction and bone grafting. Plast Reconstr Surg 76:1, 1985

21. Koutroupas S, Meyerhoff W: Surgical treatment of orbital floor fractures. Arch Otolaryngol 108:184, 1982

22. Antonyshyn O, Gruss J, Galbraith D, et al: Complex orbital fractures: a critical analysis of immediate bone reconstruction. Ann Plast Surg 22:220, 1989

23. Covington DS, Wainwright DJ, Teichgraeber JF, et al: Changing patterns in the epidemiology of treatment of zygoma fractures: 10-year review. J Trauma 37:243, 1994

24. Le Fort R: Etude expérimentale sur les fractures de la mâchoire supérieure. Rev Chir 23:208, 1901

25. Pogrel M: Compression osteosynthesis in mandibular fractures. Int J Oral Maxillofac Surg 15:521, 1986

26. El-Degwi A, Mathog R: Mandible fractures: economic considerations. Otolaryngol Head Neck Surg 108:213, 1993

27. Eid K, Lynch D, Whitaker L: Mandibular fractures: the problem patient. J Trauma 16:658, 1976

28. Thaller S, Reavie D, Daniller A: Rigid internal fixation with miniplates and screws: a cost-effective technique for treating mandible fractures? Ann Plast Surg 24:469, 1990

29. Bayles SW, Abramson PJ, McMahon SJ, et al: Mandibular fracture and associated cervical spine fracture, a rare and predictable injury: protocol for cervical spine evaluation and review of 1382 cases. Arch Otolaryngol Head Neck Surg 123:1304, 1997

30. Chu L, Gussack GS, Muller T: A treatment protocol for mandible fractures. J Trauma 36:48, 1994

31. Troulis MJ, Kaban LB: Endoscopic approach to the ramus/condyle unit: clinical applications. J Oral Maxillofac Surg 59:503, 2001

Acknowledgment

Figures 1 through 9   Carol Donner.

4 INJURIES TO THE NECK

David Wisner, M.D., and F. William Blaisdell, M.D.

Assessment and Management of Neck Injuries

Injuries to the neck can be secondary to both blunt and penetrating trauma. Most blunt injuries to the neck are managed nonoperatively; the initial diagnosis and treatment of these injuries in the emergency department setting are discussed elsewhere [*see III:1 Emergency Department Evaluation of the Patient with Multiple Injuries*]. Occasionally, blunt trauma to the neck causes injury to the 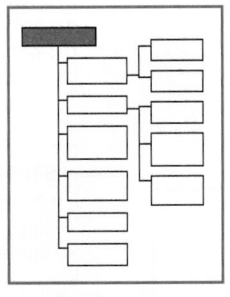 airway, the carotid artery system, or the vertebral artery system. Blunt airway injuries are sometimes surgical emergencies; the approach to these injuries is similar to that of penetrating injuries [*see* Airway Compromise *and* Isolated Laryngotracheal Injuries, *below*]. Blunt arterial injuries are almost always discovered by angiography and are usually treated nonoperatively. In the rare instance of a patient who undergoes operative treatment for a blunt injury to carotid or vertebral arteries, the operative and postoperative principles for penetrating arterial injuries should be applied [*see* Injuries to the Carotid Arteries, Jugular Veins, Pharynx, and Esophagus, *below*].

Patients with penetrating wounds of the neck can be loosely categorized into the following six groups according to the location and nature of the wound:

1. Patients with emergency or impending airway compromise.
2. Patients with an isolated injury to the larynx or trachea.
3. Patients with suspected or known injuries to the carotid arteries, jugular veins, pharynx, or esophagus.
4. Patients with wounds at the base of the neck (particularly when intrathoracic injury is suspected).
5. Patients with known injury to the vertebral arteries.
6. Patients with obviously superficial wounds of the neck.

Division of patients into these groups, though somewhat arbitrary, helps in choosing an incision and the initial operative priorities at exploration.

Airway Compromise

Some patients will present with emergency or impending airway compromise. The initial priority should be to ensure an adequate airway. In some patients, this requires orotracheal intubation. In other patients, a surgical airway must be created by means of either cricothyrotomy (in emergency cases) or tracheotomy (in less extreme cases).

CRICOTHYROTOMY

In true emergency situations, a cricothyrotomy should be done. The landmarks of the superior (notched) and inferior borders of the thyroid and the cricoid cartilage should be palpated. For this, it is helpful to stand on the patient's right side (for a right-handed surgeon) and to stabilize the cartilaginous framework by holding the thyroid cartilage in place with the left hand. A transverse incision should be made at the level of the cricothyroid membrane and developed rapidly through the subcutaneous tissue [*see I:2 Trauma Resuscitation*]. As with any transversely oriented incision of the anterior neck, the anterior jugular veins are at risk for injury. If such injury occurs, the damaged veins are best controlled with suture ligation after an airway is obtained. In true emergency circumstances when the exact site of injury is unknown, a vertical rather than transverse incision should be used to allow access to as much of the anterior surface of the airway as possible and to decrease the chance of injury to the anterior jugular veins.

After the skin and subcutaneous tissue have been divided, an incision should be made through the cricothyroid membrane. This is most rapidly done with a No. 11 knife blade. It is important to avoid pushing the knife blade too far and causing injury to the posterior wall of the airway or to the posteriorly located hypopharynx and esophagus. After the incision has been made, the opening should be enlarged by placing the knife handle in the incision and twisting it 90°. At this point, an indwelling endotracheal airway should be placed and secured. In most adults, a No. 6 airway is the largest that can be inserted; a No. 4 or larger airway is adequate for initial placement. Any incisional bleeding from the anterior jugular vein or other vessels should be controlled. Cricothyrotomies should be converted to tracheotomies within 48 to 72 hours as long as the patient's general condition permits [*see* Discussion, Conversion of Cricothyrotomy to Tracheotomy, *below*].

TRACHEOTOMY

In some instances, airway compromise may not be extreme but a surgical airway may still be necessary for safety or subsequent management of a laryngeal injury. In such circumstances, a tracheotomy rather than a cricothyrotomy should be done, because cricothyrotomy is more likely than tracheotomy to make definitive treatment more difficult.

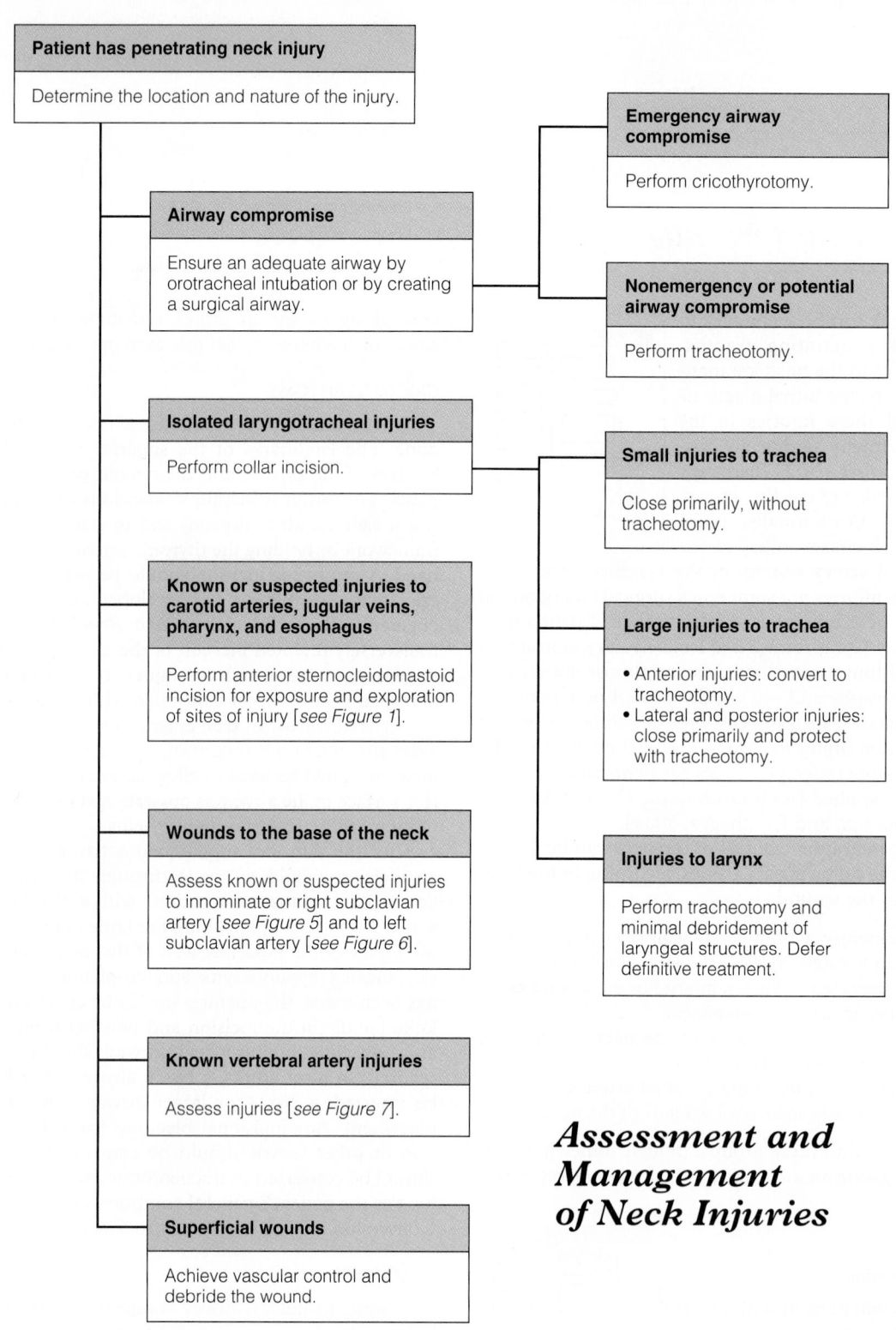

Patient has penetrating neck injury

Determine the location and nature of the injury.

Airway compromise

Ensure an adequate airway by orotracheal intubation or by creating a surgical airway.

Emergency airway compromise

Perform cricothyrotomy.

Nonemergency or potential airway compromise

Perform tracheotomy.

Isolated laryngotracheal injuries

Perform collar incision.

Small injuries to trachea

Close primarily, without tracheotomy.

Large injuries to trachea

- Anterior injuries: convert to tracheotomy.
- Lateral and posterior injuries: close primarily and protect with tracheotomy.

Known or suspected injuries to carotid arteries, jugular veins, pharynx, and esophagus

Perform anterior sternocleidomastoid incision for exposure and exploration of sites of injury [*see Figure 1*].

Injuries to larynx

Perform tracheotomy and minimal debridement of laryngeal structures. Defer definitive treatment.

Wounds to the base of the neck

Assess known or suspected injuries to innominate or right subclavian artery [*see Figure 5*] and to left subclavian artery [*see Figure 6*].

Known vertebral artery injuries

Assess injuries [*see Figure 7*].

Assessment and Management of Neck Injuries

Superficial wounds

Achieve vascular control and debride the wound.

376

The initial approach for emergency tracheotomy is similar to that for cricothyrotomy, the difference being that a so-called collar incision is made at a point one to two finger-breadths inferior to the level of the cricothyroid membrane. The incision should be wide enough to provide rapid exposure and should extend as far as the anterior border of the sternocleidomastoid bilaterally. Anteriorly located injuries at the level of the cricoid or trachea may already have a hole in the airway. In such cases, if the need for a surgical airway is immediate, the wound should be enlarged and used as a route of access to the airway.

On rare occasion, the injury is in the distal cervical or proximal intrathoracic trachea. In such circumstances, access to the trachea may not be possible through a cervical incision alone. Median sternotomy and lateral retraction of the innominate artery and left internal carotid artery allow exposure of the anterior surface of the trachea at the thoracic inlet. Right thoracotomy provides access to the more distal intrathoracic trachea.

Isolated Laryngotracheal Injuries

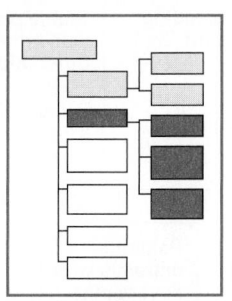

Most commonly, the presence of an isolated laryngotracheal injury is not recognized preoperatively. On occasion, however, isolated injuries to the larynx and trachea are recognized preoperatively on the basis of a suspicious history and the results of diagnostic studies, such as laryngoscopy and bronchoscopy.

Injuries to the larynx should be treated initially with a collar incision for the creation of a surgical airway [see Airway Compromise, Tracheotomy, above]; however, definitive treatment should be deferred. Minimal debridement of laryngeal structures should be carried out during the initial operative procedure. Injuries to the larynx should be handled on a semielective basis by otolaryngologists with expertise in laryngeal repair and reconstruction. Further investigation of the larynx, including laryngeal x-rays, laryngoscopy, and computed tomographic scanning, may be necessary.

Small injuries of the trachea can be repaired primarily without tracheotomy. Absorbable 3-0 or 4-0 sutures should be placed transversely, if possible, and should include tracheal rings above and below the site of injury. Large anterior defects should be converted to a tracheotomy, whereas defects to the lateral or posterior aspects of the trachea should be closed primarily and protected with a tracheotomy. Tension can be relieved from a repair by mobilizing the trachea proximally and distally. During this mobilization, the recurrent laryngeal nerves are subject to injury if the dissection is carried into the tracheoesophageal groove. Laryngotracheal injuries do not require routine drainage unless there is an associated injury to the pharynx or esophagus [see Injuries to the Carotid Arteries, Jugular Veins, Pharynx, and Esophagus, below].

If a large segment of trachea has been destroyed, primary anastomosis can be accomplished for defects up to five or six tracheal rings in length. Anastomosis requires mobilization of the intrathoracic trachea inferiorly and the laryngeal complex superiorly and is best done electively.[1,2]

Patients with laryngeal injuries should be watched carefully in the postoperative period for signs of mediastinitis, which may be from persistent airway leak or a missed pharyngo-esophageal injury. The chest x-ray should also be checked for pneumomediastinum as a sign of continued airway leakage, particularly in patients who remain on positive pressure ventilation.

Injuries to the Carotid Arteries, Jugular Veins, Pharynx, and Esophagus

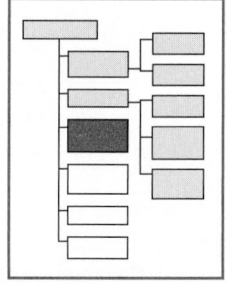

Probably the most common situation in penetrating cervical trauma is the patient with underlying structural injuries, the precise location and nature of which are unknown. Patients with known injuries to the carotid arteries, jugular veins, pharynx, and esophagus are less common. An anterior sternocleidomastoid incision provides good access to these areas and should be employed because of its relative ease and versatility.

STERNOCLEIDOMASTOID INCISION

If the location of underlying neck injuries is either unknown or confirmed by preoperative studies to be in the carotid arteries, the jugular veins, the pharynx, or the esophagus, an incision along the anterior border of the sternocleidomastoid muscle should be used [see Figure 1]. The sternocleidomastoid incision is particularly important in patients with true emergency conditions, such as external bleeding, focal neurologic deficits, coma, and an expanding neck hematoma. When bilateral exploration is necessary, separate sternocleidomastoid incisions should be done.

The use of an incision along the anterior border of the sternocleidomastoid muscle has several important advantages [see Figure 2]. For example, the incision can be lengthened to provide more extensive proximal or distal exposure. If a superior extension to below the earlobe is necessary, the incision should be curved posteriorly to avoid injury to the marginal mandibular branch of the facial nerve. Another advantage of the sternocleidomastoid incision is that it provides exposure of the carotid sheath, the pharynx, and the cervical esophagus.

Operative Technique

The patient should be supine with the head turned away from the side of exploration and the neck extended. In this regard, it is helpful to clear the cervical spine before operation. If both sides of the neck require exploration, the head should be left in the midposition, facing up. The entire neck and the appropriate side of the face and head should be prepped. The anterior chest should also be included in the preparation in case a median sternotomy is necessary for proximal control [see Exploration and Exposure, Arteries and Veins, below]. The patient should be draped in such a way as to leave the lateral neck as the primary field while the chest is kept easily accessible. The lateral chin and tip of the earlobe should also be kept in the field to provide landmarks. If the possibility exists that the injury is to the distal subclavian artery or the axillary artery, the patient's arm should be draped in a way that allows it to be manipulated.

The skin incision should be carried through the dermis and the platysma. After the platysma is divided in the direction of the incision, the investing fascia overlying the anterior border of the sternocleidomastoid muscle is incised, and the muscle is retracted laterally and posteriorly to expose the carotid sheath.

Known or suspected injuries to carotid arteries, jugular veins, pharynx, and esophagus

Perform anterior sternocleidomastoid incision for exposure and exploration of sites of injury.

Carotid artery injuries

Jugular vein injuries

Pharyngoesophageal injuries

Repair injuries and drain for approximately 1 wk. Institute antibiotic therapy for oral flora (several postoperative doses).

Common carotid and external carotid arteries

Internal carotid artery

Small injuries

Repair vein.

Large injuries

Simple injuries *or* complex injuries in a stable patient with no other severe injuries

Repair artery.

Complex injuries *or* injuries in a highly unstable patient with other severe injuries

Ligate artery.

Minimal or no back-bleeding is present

Ligate artery.

Back-bleeding is present

Stable patient with minimal other injuries

Repair vein surgically.

Unstable patient with severe other injuries

Ligate vein.

Stable patient with minimal other injuries

Repair artery.

Patient in extremis with severe other injuries

Ligate artery.

Figure 1 **This algorithm depicts the management of known or suspected injuries to the carotid arteries, jugular veins, pharynx, and esophagus.**

It is often necessary to divide a venous branch that connects the external jugular vein posterolaterally to the anterior jugular vein anteromedially. This vein lies in a plane immediately deep to the platysma.

Exploration and Exposure

When possible, proximal and distal control should be obtained before exploration of a carotid artery injury. In practice, obtaining proximal control before entering a perivascular hematoma is all that is absolutely necessary. Distal bleeding can be controlled with digital pressure while the dissection of the injured vessel is completed. Although it is often difficult to obtain control before addressing the area of injury, proximal and distal control of the vessel should be obtained at some point before any attempts at definitive repair. For injuries near the carotid bifurcation, it is necessary to control the common, internal, and external carotid arteries as well as the proximal branches of the external carotid artery.

Arteries and veins The initial exploration should attempt to rule out arterial or venous injury, unless an overt airway injury is present and requires immediate attention [*see* Airway Compromise, *above*]. If the airway is patent, the location of the carotid artery can then be confirmed by the presence of a pulse. It is often necessary to retract the jugular vein posterolaterally to provide adequate arterial exposure [*see Figure 3*]. Jugular vein retraction is facilitated by division of the facial vein, which is superficial to the carotid bifurcation. The

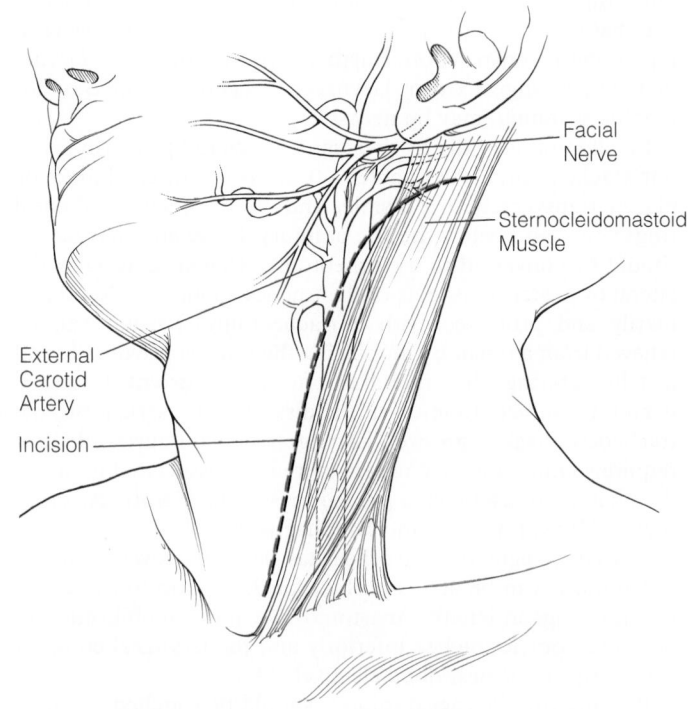

Facial Nerve

Sternocleidomastoid Muscle

External Carotid Artery

Incision

Figure 2 **In general, exposure of structures in the anterior areas of the neck is best done through an incision oriented along the anterior border of the sternocleidomastoid muscle.**

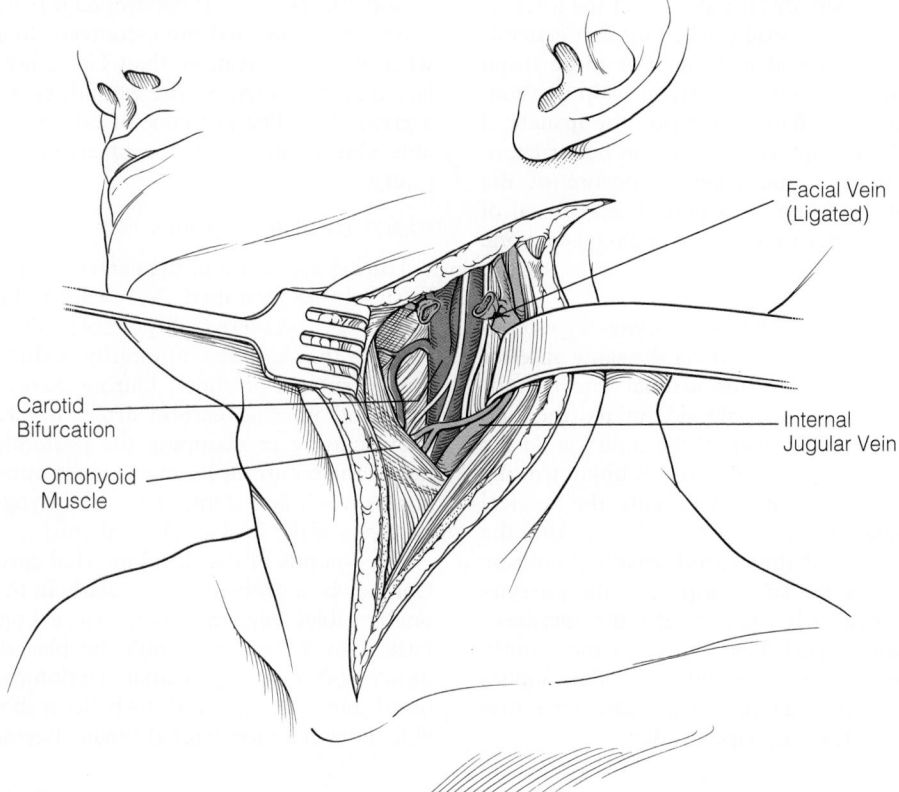

Figure 3 **After a plane along the anterior border of the sternocleidomastoid muscle has been developed, dissection is carried down to the level of the carotid sheath. Suture ligation of the facial vein facilitates this dissection. Lateral retraction of the internal jugular vein improves exposure of the carotid bifurcation.**

severed ends of the facial vein should be suture-ligated to ensure that the ties will not come off with increased intravenous pressure in the postoperative period—for example, secondary to a cough or a Valsalva maneuver.

Exposure of the proximal common carotid artery at the base of the neck is easier after division of the omohyoid muscle at the point where its superior and inferior bellies are joined. Division of the omohyoid muscle results in minimal functional deficit postoperatively. For proximal control of the common carotid artery, it may be necessary to enter the chest via median sternotomy. To minimize blood loss, the decision to do a sternotomy should be made without undue delay. Control of the proximal right common carotid artery via this route is relatively easy and is accomplished by first obtaining control of the innominate artery and then dissecting distally. Proximal control of the left common carotid artery via median sternotomy is more difficult, because its origin from the aortic arch is more posterior than the origin of the innominate artery.

Exposure of the distal internal carotid artery can be very difficult, particularly if there is an injury in that location. As dissection is carried distally on the internal carotid artery, a number of important structures should be identified and protected [see Figure 4]. The hypoglossal nerve is usually encountered within several centimeters of the carotid bifurcation and should be dissected free of the internal carotid and retracted upward. This is facilitated by division of the occipital artery, which crosses superficial to the hypoglossal nerve on its course

from the external carotid artery toward the occiput. It is also helpful to divide the ansa cervicalis branches that run inferiorly from the hypoglossal nerve to supply the muscles of the neck. Injury to the hypoglossal nerve results in impaired motor function of the tongue and can lead to dysarthria and dysphagia. Injury to or sectioning of the ansa cervicalis causes little or no morbidity.

Further distal exposure of the internal carotid artery may require unilateral mandibular subluxation or division of the ascending ramus of the mandible.[3,4] Such maneuvers are somewhat easier when the patient is nasotracheally intubated. They increase the size of the small area immediately behind the condyle and allow for easier division of the stylohyoid ligament and the styloglossus and stylopharyngeus muscles. These three structures can be divided together adjacent to their common origin at the styloid process. If this is done, care should be taken to preserve the facial nerve, which lies superficial to these muscles. The underlying glossopharyngeal nerve, which lies deep to these muscles and superficial to the internal carotid artery, should also be protected. Injury to the facial nerve results in loss of function of the muscles of facial expression. If the glossopharyngeal nerve is injured, loss of motor and sensory supply to parts of the tongue and pharynx increases the risk of aspiration.

Once the muscles originating from the styloid process have been divided, the styloid process itself can be resected to gain a further short distance of distal exposure. In very rare instances, it may prove useful to remove portions of the mastoid bone to provide even more distal exposure of the internal carotid artery as it enters the carotid canal. This can generally be accomplished via a cervical incision. For more distal lesions, it is necessary to place a posterolateral scalp incision, reflect a medially based scalp flap, and divide the ipsilateral external auditory canal. This approach results in better exposure of the mastoid process and allows exposure of the intrapetrous portion of the internal carotid after removal of the overlying bone of the mastoid with a high-speed bone drill.

Pharynx and esophagus   The oropharynx, hypopharynx, and cervical esophagus are exposed via the same anterior sternocleidomastoid incision used for arterial and venous injuries. If the patient has a known right-side injury, the incision should be made in the right neck. If the injury is on the patient's left side or if the exact site of injury is unknown, the exposure should be made from the left because the cervical esophagus is located slightly to the left of the midline. After the initial incision, the contents of the carotid sheath should be retracted laterally, exposing the lateral aspect of the pharynx and esophagus. This maneuver is made easier if the anesthesiologist places a large esophageal dilator through the mouth. The dilator makes identification of the otherwise flat esophagus easier, and the colored tubing of the dilator can sometimes be seen through defects in the esophageal wall.[5]

Sometimes, a pharyngoesophageal injury is suspected but cannot be confirmed preoperatively. In such cases—especially when the injury is more than 1 or 2 hours old—salivary amylase may be present in the wound, giving the surgeon's gloves a greasy feel. The presence of salivary amylase can be a valuable clue to the existence of an otherwise unknown occult injury.

CAROTID ARTERY INJURIES

During dissection of the external carotid artery, the branches should be identified. They can be ligated if necessary but should be preserved if possible (this usually depends on whether they can be temporarily occluded with vessel loops, a looped suture, or clips). During dissection around the common and internal carotid arteries, care should be taken to avoid cutting or clamping the posterolaterally located vagus nerve; the recurrent laryngeal nerve runs with the vagus nerve at this level, and damage to the laryngeal nerve can lead to paralysis of the ipsilateral vocal cord.

For wounds of the distal internal carotid artery, distal control may be a problem, particularly in the presence of vigorous ongoing bleeding, in which case a Fogarty balloon catheter (size 3 to 5 French) should be placed through the area of injury or through a proximal arteriotomy. The catheter should be advanced distally, and the balloon should be inflated to provide a dry field for arterial repair. Repair can be done around

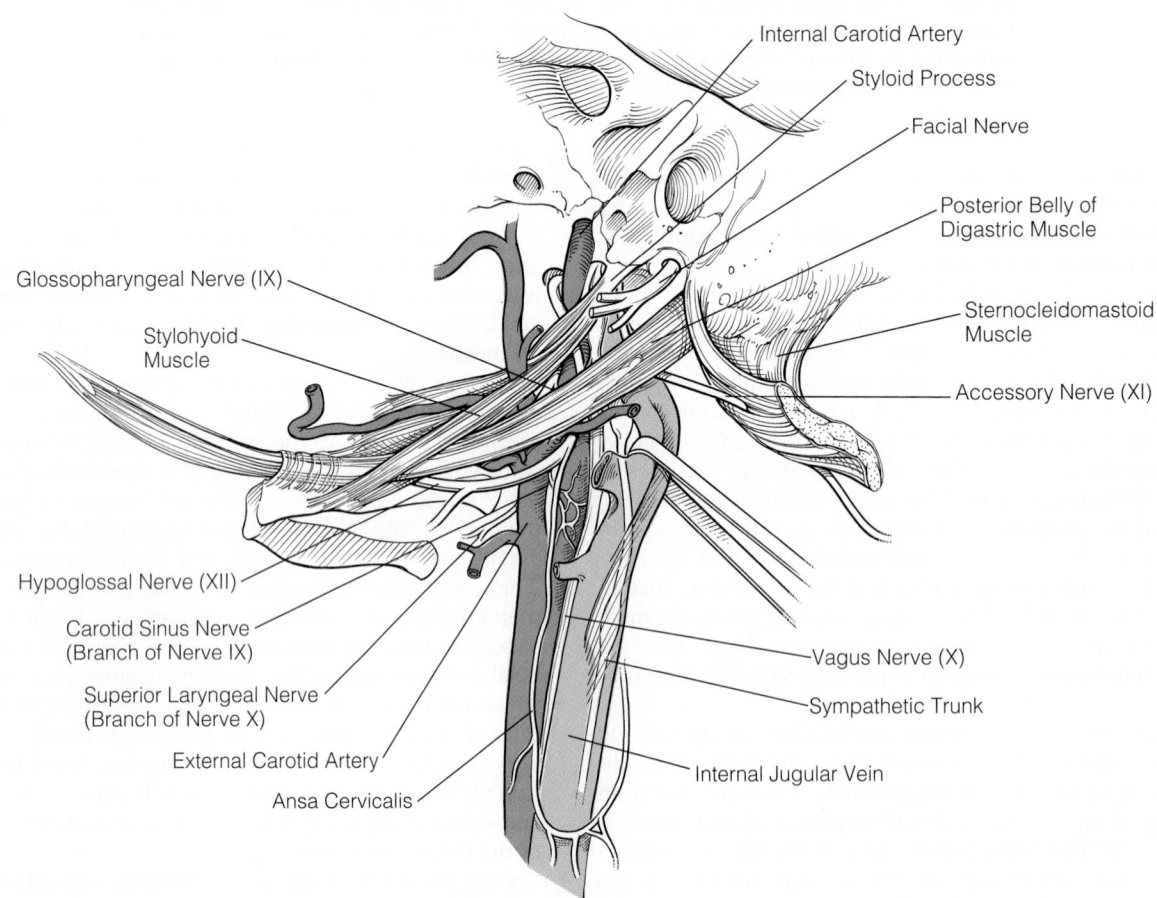

Figure 4   **During distal dissection of the internal and external carotid arteries, a number of important structures are encountered, including the hypoglossal nerve and the occipital artery.**

the catheter; the balloon is deflated near the conclusion of the repair, and the catheter is removed before the final several sutures are tied.

If associated injuries allow, a 5,000 to 10,000 unit bolus of heparin should be given before any of the arteries in the neck are occluded. Because they have no branches, the common and internal carotid arteries can be safely mobilized for some distance from the injury to ensure a tension-free repair.

Management of common or external carotid artery injuries is governed by the extent of injury and the overall status of the patient. Small, simple injuries should be repaired. Complex injuries should be repaired in stable patients and treated with ligation in patients with severe hemodynamic instability or major associated injuries.

Initial management of injuries to the internal carotid artery depends on a determination of the amount of back-bleeding from the artery distal to the site of injury.[6,7] If back-bleeding is minimal or absent, the artery should be ligated. If significant back-bleeding is present, the overall status of the patient and the nature of the associated injuries should be taken into account [see Discussion, Repair versus Ligation of Carotid Arteries, below]. If the patient is hemodynamically stable and has minimal or moderate associated injuries, the internal carotid artery should be repaired. If the patient is hemodynamically unstable or has devastating associated injuries, the internal carotid artery should be ligated even when back-bleeding is present.

If a carotid artery injury involves minimal loss of vascular wall, primary repair is straightforward and can be done with either a running or interrupted technique; interrupted sutures will not purse-string the vessel. In younger patients who are still growing, interrupted sutures should be used to prevent later stenosis. As in elective vascular surgery, nonabsorbable sutures should be used; the carotid arteries generally require a 5-0, 6-0, or 7-0 monofilament suture, depending on the location of the injury and the type of suture material employed.

Defects longer than 1 to 2 cm should not be repaired primarily, because this will place excessive tension on the repair. For large defects limited to one surface of the vessel, a patch repair should be done. Either a venous patch or a synthetic patch can be used; when available, a venous patch is preferred for better long-term patency and to avoid placing a foreign body in a potentially contaminated wound.[8] Saphenous vein from the groin is preferable for patches because of its durability; a saphenous vein from the ankle is easiest to harvest when time is of the essence.[9] Although the jugular vein is in the operative field and can be easily harvested, it is better not to interfere with venous outflow in a neck in which the arterial inflow is to undergo repair; in addition, the jugular vein is very thin and difficult to handle.

For repairs near the carotid bifurcation, an alternative to venous patches and synthetic patches is the use of the proximal external carotid artery. This approach is especially appropriate when the origin of the external carotid artery is itself involved in the area of injury. If the injury is to the proximal internal carotid artery and the origin of the external carotid artery is free of injury, it is better to leave the external carotid artery patent and to use a venous patch or a synthetic patch instead; if the repair fails, the external carotid artery provides collateral distribution to the internal carotid artery via the ophthalmic artery.

Repair of circumferential loss of the common or internal carotid arteries is difficult. In this circumstance, if the defect is too long for primary anastomosis and the patient's general and neurologic condition permits, an interposition graft should be done. As with patch grafts, either venous or synthetic material can be used. As for patch grafts, saphenous vein from the groin is generally the donor material of first choice because of its strength. The saphenous vein from the groin is also well suited for reconstruction of the common carotid artery.

Completion angiography should be done after interposition graft placements and complex repairs of the common or internal carotid arteries. In general, patients with carotid artery injuries should be admitted postoperatively to an intensive care unit. ICU observation need not be prolonged but should be continued for at least 12 to 24 hours postoperatively. In the early postoperative period, the patient should be observed for bleeding or for the development of a neck hematoma; large postoperative hematomas may compromise the airway. If the patient develops a tense hematoma postoperatively, the neck should be reexplored.

Labile blood pressure—particularly in patients with extensive dissection around the carotid bifurcation—is another potential postoperative problem. It is related to manipulation of the carotid body, and control may require pharmacologic intervention. Labile blood pressure is usually self-limiting and disappears over the first 1 to 3 days after operation, but it is another reason why patients with carotid artery repairs should be monitored initially in the ICU.

Antibiotics should be administered to cover common skin flora and should generally be continued only for one or two postoperative doses.

JUGULAR VEIN INJURIES

Any of the veins in the neck can be ligated when necessary. An exception to this rule is the rare instance when both internal jugular veins have been injured, in which case an attempt should be made to repair one of the veins, if possible. However, even in such cases, bilateral internal jugular ligation, if necessary, is usually tolerated. It is particularly important to use suture ligatures rather than simple ligatures on the cut ends of the internal jugular vein.

If the injury to the internal jugular is simple, the vein should be repaired. Large jugular vein injuries should be repaired only if the patient's general condition and associated injuries allow; if the patient is hemodynamically unstable or has severe associated injuries, large jugular vein injuries should be treated with ligation.

It is not always necessary to completely encircle the jugular vein proximal and distal to the site of injury; pressure with a finger or sponge stick will sometimes control bleeding while simple lateral venorrhaphy is done. In the case of more elaborate repairs, it is better either to encircle and occlude the proximal and distal vein or to place a side-biting vascular clamp for control during repair. Nonabsorbable 4-0 or 5-0 sutures should be used.

PHARYNGOESOPHAGEAL INJURIES

Either one-layer or two-layer repair of the pharynx and esophagus is acceptable, for which 3-0 or 4-0 absorbable sutures should be used. Attempts should be made to repair nearly all injuries, even when they are severe or are found on a delayed basis. In extreme cases of very large injuries or very delayed operative intervention, it may be necessary simply to drain the neck widely and turn the injury into a cervical esophagostomy. Esophageal diversion with distal esophageal ligation is rarely necessary in patients with isolated cervical esophageal injuries, except in cases when the injury is very low in the neck or in the thoracic esophagus.

Pharyngoesophageal injuries should be drained; either closed or Penrose drainage can be used. The drains should be left in place for approximately 1 week, at which time a radiographic contrast study should be obtained to determine whether the repair is competent. If the contrast study is negative for extravasation and the patient's general status permits, feeding can begin. If the feedings are well tolerated, the drains can be removed.[10]

Patients with pharyngoesophageal injuries should receive antibiotics appropriate for oral flora for several postoperative doses. If the repair is inadequate or breaks down, the resultant fistula will often heal with nonoperative management, provided that drainage is adequate. A high index of suspicion for mediastinitis should be maintained; the prevertebral space provides a ready route of access from the pharynx and cervical esophagus into the mediastinum. Therefore, missed or inadequately drained injuries may result in profound infection and a septic response.

Wounds at the Base of the Neck

Patients with wounds at the base of the neck should be identified early—particularly when an intrathoracic injury is suspected—so that the appropriate incision and operative approach can be undertaken.

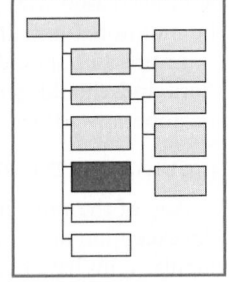

A median sternotomy should be done for (1) patients with injuries at the base of the right neck and (2) patients in whom the superior mediastinum is the most likely site of injury and the most likely arterial injuries are to either the innominate artery or the right subclavian artery[11,12] [see Figure 5]. Exposure of injuries to the proximal left subclavian artery is extremely difficult via sternotomy because of the artery's posterior location; in patients with such injuries, a left thoracotomy is needed [see Figure 6]. If a left thoracotomy is necessary, it is helpful to bump up the patient's left hip and shoulder to position the left chest 20° to 30° anteriorly. The head should be turned to the right, and the left arm should be prepped to the elbow and draped in such a way as to allow it free movement. Moving the arm is helpful in cases in which proximal exposure and control are done through the chest and distal exposure and control are done through a supraclavicular incision. It also allows for improved exposure of the axillary artery if necessary.

In stable patients with angiographically diagnosed injuries to either subclavian artery, a supraclavicular approach alone can be used, thereby eliminating the need for initial entry into the chest. Because proximal control may not be feasible via this limited incision, the patient should still be positioned, prepped, and draped so that sternotomy or thoracotomy is possible. If the injury is on the right side of the neck and proximal control is not possible, a median sternotomy should be done. If the injury is on the left side of the neck and proximal control is not possible, a left thoracotomy should be performed.

If a median sternotomy has been done for exposure of an innominate artery or right subclavian artery injury, it may prove necessary to extend the incision into the right neck to obtain adequate distal control and exposure. Either a right supraclavicular or an anterior sternocleidomastoid extension can be used. Although both are easily accomplished, the anterior sternocleidomastoid extension is the more versatile of the two. If a left thoracotomy is done for proximal control and exposure of the left subclavian artery, the distal subclavian artery should be exposed via a left supraclavicular incision. Improved exposure of the left subclavian artery at the thoracic outlet can be obtained either by resection of the medial one third to one half of the left clavicle or by a socalled trapdoor incision.[13] The trapdoor incision consists of a superior sternotomy and connection of the medial aspects of the thoracotomy and supraclavicular incisions. We find the trapdoor approach somewhat limited and cumbersome and prefer clavicular resection. Medial clavicular resection is accomplished by encircling the midclavicle in the subperiosteal plane via the supraclavicular incision. A Gigli wire saw is then passed around the clavicle, and the clavicle is divided. The medial aspect of the divided bone is then grasped with a bone hook or a Kocher clamp, and the dissection is carried medially in the subperiosteal plane to the sternoclavicular joint, which is disarticulated. If necessary, this dissection and resection can be accomplished in a matter of a few minutes.

After adequate exposure and control of innominate or subclavian artery injuries have been obtained, further management is determined by the nature of the injury and the status of the patient. Small injuries should always be repaired. Large injuries are not often seen, because they are usually incompatible with survival to a point where medical attention is available. Nonetheless, such injuries do occur, and their management is influenced by the status of the patient. Attempts at repair should be made for most such injuries, but in highly unstable patients, the artery should be ligated. However, arterial ligation is sometimes associated with severe morbidity, and it should be avoided if possible.

The wall of the subclavian artery is thin, and extra care should be taken in dissecting around it. Primary repair should be done with either interrupted or running nonabsorbable 4-0 or 5-0 sutures, laterally placed. Because of its location and the large number of branches, the subclavian artery is difficult to mobilize extensively. None of the branches are vital, however, and all can be divided as necessary to gain mobility. The vertebral artery should be preserved if possible, because in rare instances, ligation of the artery can lead to cerebral ischemia. Even with division of arterial branches, only short segments of the artery can be removed without the need for an interposition graft to prevent an anastomosis under tension. Saphenous vein is usually too small to be used as a graft, even when it is harvested from the groin. Accordingly, a synthetic graft is usually the better choice. Infections in this location are rare, even when the graft is placed in a contaminated field.[14]

Complex injuries of the innominate and subclavian veins should be treated with suture ligation, particularly when the patient has severe associated injuries. Simple injuries can be treated with lateral venorrhaphy. Depending on the circumstances, formal control of the proximal and distal vein can first be obtained, or pressure can be applied proximally and distally to provide for a bloodless field during repair. Another alternative for control of bleeding during venous repair is the use of a side-biting vascular clamp.

Some patients with injuries to the subclavian artery or subclavian vein require dissection of the supraclavicular area. The supraclavicular fat pad contains a large number of lymph nodes and lymphatic channels, and dissection of the fat pad can result in considerable weeping of lymphatic fluid; these wounds should therefore be drained. Either a closed or an open drain can be used, and the drain should be brought out through a separate stab wound near the incision. After a left-sided procedure, persistent milky drainage via either drains or the wound suggests injury to the thoracic duct and may necessitate repeat operative intervention if it persists.

Elevation or paralysis of the hemidiaphragm ipsilateral to the side of dissection can indicate injury to the phrenic nerve, which courses in the field of dissection on the anterior surface of the anterior scalene muscle.

Known Vertebral Artery Injuries

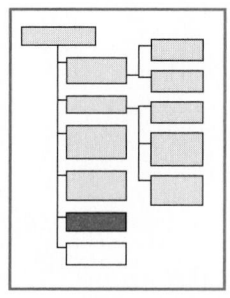

On occasion, patients who present with penetrating cervical wounds and are hemodynamically and neurologically stable are demonstrated on angiographic workup to have an injury to the vertebral artery. In rarer instances, the location of an injury in the posterior triangle of the neck and the presence of ongoing hemorrhage may also indicate the high likelihood of an injury to the distal vertebral artery [see Figure 7].

Most vertebral artery injuries occur in stable patients and are discovered on angiography. Because operative attempts at ligation are associated with blood loss that can be problematic, an alternative approach utilizing angiographic embolization has been developed.[15] In most cases of injury to the distal vertebral artery, the angiographic approach is preferred if available [see Discussion, Angiographic Embolization of Distal

Known or suspected injuries to innominate or right subclavian artery
Assess patient's hemodynamic stability.

Unstable patient with proximal injury
Perform median sternotomy, extending incision as needed.

Stable patient with distal injury
Perform right supraclavicular incision.

Small injury, patient stabilizes
Repair artery.

Large injury

Stable patient
Repair artery.

Highly unstable patient
Ligate artery.

Proximal control is possible

Proximal control is not possible
Perform median sternotomy, extending incision as needed.

Patient remains stable
Repair artery.

Patient becomes highly unstable and injury is devastating
Ligate artery.

Patient remains stable
Repair artery.

Large injury

Patient remains stable
Repair artery.

Patient becomes highly unstable
Ligate artery.

Figure 5 This algorithm depicts the management of wounds to the base of the neck causing known or suspected injuries to the innominate artery or the right subclavian artery.

Figure 6 This algorithm depicts the management of wounds to the base of the neck causing known or suspected injuries to the left subclavian artery.

Vertebral Artery Injuries, *below*]. If angiographic expertise is not available and the patient is stable enough for transfer, it is preferable to send the patient to a center with angiographic embolization capability if at all possible. In urgent circumstances, an angiographic approach is not practical. In such situations, the direct surgical approach is necessary.[16,17]

EXPOSURE AND EXPLORATION

In the rare case of a patient who presents with active, severe bleeding and in whom the most likely source of bleeding is the distal vertebral artery, exposure of the vertebral artery should be obtained by means of an anterior sternocleidomastoid incision [*see* Injuries to the Carotid Arteries, Jugular Veins, Pharynx, and Esophagus, *above*]. This approach can be used for exposure of both the proximal and the distal vertebral artery. The incision is developed down to the level of the carotid sheath. The lateral margin of the internal jugular vein is developed sharply, and the internal jugular vein and other contents of the sheath are retracted medially. After retraction of the carotid sheath, the plane just superficial to the prevertebral muscles is encountered. The ganglia of the cervical sympathetic chain are located here and should be protected, though this is not always possible in emergency circumstances. The anterior longitudinal ligament is located deep in the medial aspect of the wound and should be incised longitudinally. The ligament, the underlying periosteum, and the overlying longus colli and

longissimus capitis should be mobilized laterally with a periosteal elevator [*see Figure 8*]. The elevation should be carried laterally along the lateral margin of the bodies of the cervical vertebrae and along the anterior aspect of the transverse processes of the cervical vertebrae. To avoid injury to the laterally and posteriorly placed cervical nerve roots, the dissection should not be extended laterally beyond the tips of the transverse processes.

After the anterior aspects of the transverse processes of the cervical vertebrae have been exposed, they can be removed with a small rongeur. This should be done distal to the area of injury only; proximal ligation of the vertebral artery can be done in its more easily exposed proximal portion. Although the vertebral artery is also accessible in the spaces between the transverse processes, there are a number of venous branches in these regions, and it is therefore safer to approach the artery within the confines of the bony foramina.

The third and most distal portion of the vertebral artery can be approached most easily between the atlas and the axis. The segment of the artery between the transverse processes of these two vertebrae is longer and more exposed than the segments between the other cervical vertebrae and is therefore, in theory, somewhat easier to expose. In practice, rapid exposure of this portion of the vertebral artery can be very difficult, particularly in an actively bleeding patient. As with exposures to the second portion of the vertebral artery, lesions requiring this

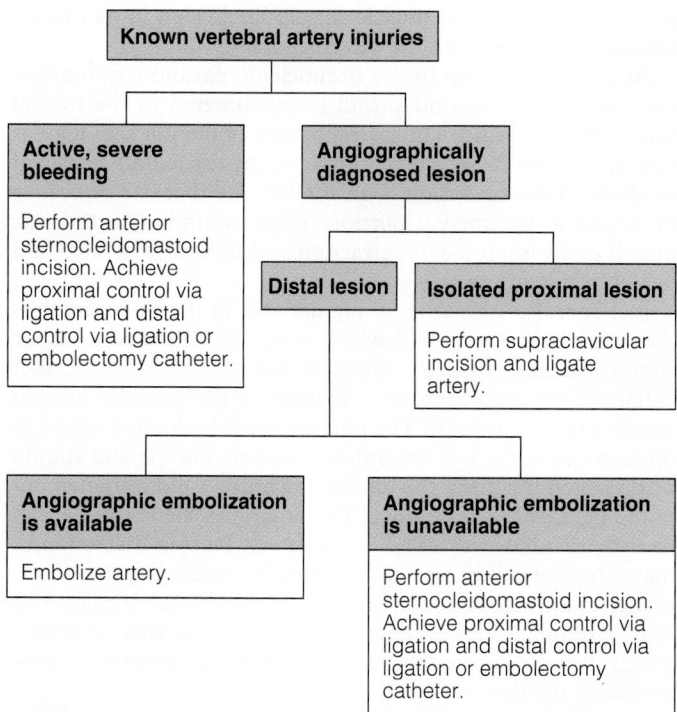

Figure 7 boxes:

Known vertebral artery injuries

Active, severe bleeding
Perform anterior sternocleidomastoid incision. Achieve proximal control via ligation and distal control via ligation or embolectomy catheter.

Angiographically diagnosed lesion

Distal lesion

Isolated proximal lesion
Perform supraclavicular incision and ligate artery.

Angiographic embolization is available
Embolize artery.

Angiographic embolization is unavailable
Perform anterior sternocleidomastoid incision. Achieve proximal control via ligation and distal control via ligation or embolectomy catheter.

Figure 7 **This algorithm depicts the management of known injuries to the vertebral artery, which are most often discovered by angiography.**

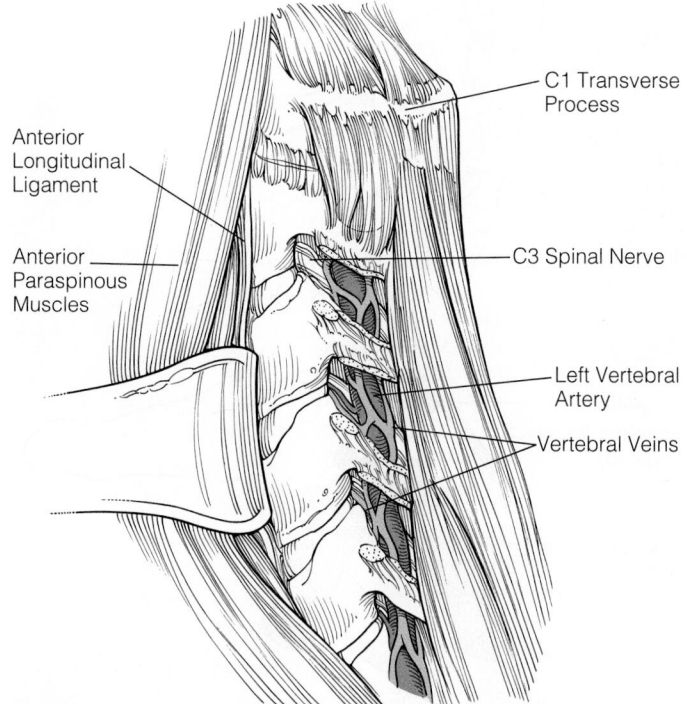

Anterior Longitudinal Ligament

Anterior Paraspinous Muscles

C1 Transverse Process

C3 Spinal Nerve

Left Vertebral Artery

Vertebral Veins

Figure 8 **Throughout most of their course, the vertebral artery and the vertebral veins are surrounded by the transverse processes of the cervical vertebrae. Exposure of this portion of the vertebral artery is best done with lateral mobilization of the longus colli and longissimus capitis.**

exposure are best treated with angiographic embolization if such expertise is available. If angiographic embolization is not an option, however, a surgical approach may be necessary.[18]

The standard anterior sternocleidomastoid incision is used but is carried superiorly with a curved extension to just below the tip of the ear. Once the plane is developed along the anterior border, the sternocleidomastoid muscle should be divided near its origin at the mastoid process. The spinal accessory nerve, which enters the sternocleidomastoid 2 to 3 cm below the tip of the mastoid, should be dissected free of the muscle and mobilized anteriorly. After division of the sternocleidomastoid muscle and anterior retraction of the spinal accessory nerve, the transverse process of the atlas is palpable and the prevertebral fascia is visible in the depths of the wound. The fascia should be incised in a line with the spinal accessory nerve, and the laterally placed levator scapulae and splenius cervicis should be divided as close to the transverse process of the atlas as possible [*see Figure 9*]. The anterior ramus of the nerve root of C2 is closely associated with the anterior edge of the levator scapulae and should be protected. After division of the levator scapulae and splenius cervicis, the distal vertebral artery is visible in the medial aspect of the wound. Venous branches associated with the vertebral artery are most likely to be located near the transverse processes; therefore, ligation should be preferentially directed to the middle of the interspace between the transverse processes.

Exposure of the proximal vertebral artery at the base of the neck can also be achieved via an incision along the anterior border of the sternocleidomastoid muscle. Initial exposure is identical to that used for exposure of the carotid arteries [*see Injuries to the Carotid Arteries, Jugular Veins, Pharynx, and Esophagus, above*]. At the level of the carotid sheath, however, dissection is carried lateral to the internal jugular vein, which is retracted medially to expose the supraclavicular fat pad. The proximal vertebral artery can then be controlled after dissection deep to the fat pad as described for the supraclavicular approach to isolated proximal vertebral artery injuries (see below).

TREATMENT

As opposed to injuries of the carotid arteries, in which either repair or ligation is an option, injuries to the vertebral arteries should always be treated with interruption of flow by surgical or other means. Proximal ligation should usually be done at the origin of the vertebral artery, because the approach to the artery at this point is easier than the approaches to the more distal segments. The artery should be suture-ligated as close to its origin as possible so as not to create a thrombogenic blind pouch off the subclavian artery. Distal ligation can be accomplished by first exposing the artery (see above) and then ligating with ligatures, suture ligatures, or surgical clips. The use of clips minimizes dissection around the artery, which, in turn, decreases the likelihood of further injury to surrounding veins.

In emergency circumstances, a useful technique is to surgically approach the proximal artery at the base of the neck and pass a thrombectomy catheter distally to the site of injury [*see Figure 10*]. First, the proximal vertebral artery is exposed and ligated at its origin. The thrombectomy catheter is then passed distally via an arteriotomy. The catheter balloon is inflated, and the wound is checked to determine whether bleeding has been controlled. If bleeding has been controlled, the distal end of the catheter is left in place, and the proximal end is brought

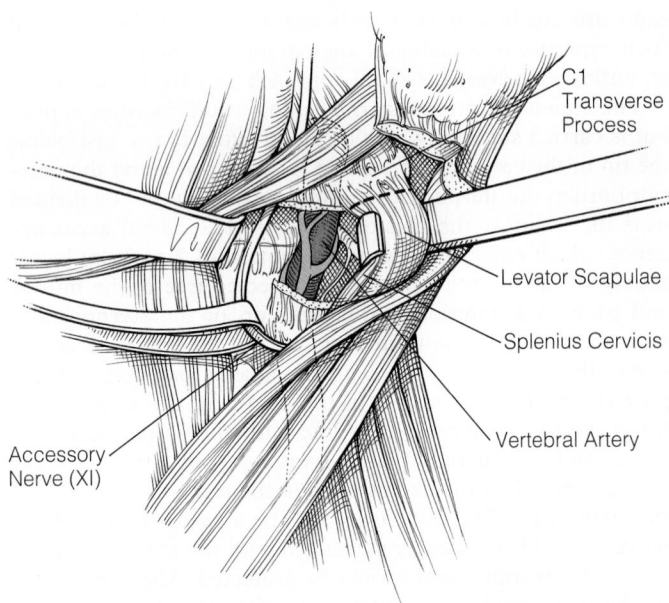

Figure 9   **Exposure of the distal vertebral artery is done via an incision along the anterior border of the sternocleidomastoid muscle. The sternocleidomastoid muscle is then divided near its origin at the mastoid process. The spinal accessory nerve is mobilized anteriorly. The vertebral artery is accessible after division of the levator scapulae and splenius cervicis.**

out through the wound. The catheter is left in situ for approximately 48 hours, at which time the balloon is deflated and the wound is again checked for bleeding. If there is no bleeding for 4 to 6 hours, the catheter can be withdrawn. If the use of a thrombectomy catheter is unsuccessful, a direct surgical approach to the second or third portion of the artery is necessary. However, one of the potential disadvantages of adopting a surgical approach is that proximal ligation of the vertebral artery precludes angiographic embolization except via the contralateral vertebral artery. Embolization via the contralateral vertebral artery is extremely difficult and may result in ischemia or uncontrolled embolization.

If the injury is known by preoperative angiography to be isolated to the first portion of the vertebral artery, both proximal and distal ligation may be possible via a supraclavicular incision [see Figure 11]. The patient is positioned with the head turned away from the side of injury, and the chest and ipsilateral neck are prepared and draped. Preparation and draping include the chest so that a left thoracotomy can be done later if necessary for proximal control of the left subclavian artery. In such cases, it is helpful to bump the patient up on the left so that an anterolateral thoracotomy incision can be carried further posteriorly.

The supraclavicular incision should be made approximately one fingerbreadth superior to the clavicle and should extend medially to the midpoint of the sternocleidomastoid insertion and laterally to the juncture of the middle and lateral thirds of the clavicle. The skin, subcutaneous tissue, and platysma should be incised. The external jugular vein, if in the operating field, should be suture-ligated. The clavicular head of the sternocleidomastoid muscle is encountered next, and its lateral aspect should be divided with the electrocautery at its insertion on the clavicle. The muscle is then retracted superiorly and medially. In the plane deep to the sternocleidomastoid

muscle, the omohyoid muscle should be divided in its middle tendinous portion with the electrocautery.

At a level just deep to the sternocleidomastoid and omohyoid muscles, the carotid sheath is encountered in the medial aspect of the wound. The lateral border of the internal jugular vein should be dissected free of adjacent tissue and retracted medially. If the operation is on the left, the thoracic duct may be found in the medial portion of the wound. The thoracic duct is easily injured with retraction and should be divided and ligated if it is in the way.

Just lateral to the internal jugular vein at the same depth is the supraclavicular fat pad, which should be dissected from the supraclavicular fossa in which it lies. Exposure is further enhanced by dissection and division of the laterally located anterior scalene muscle. The phrenic nerve is closely applied to the anterior surface of the anterior scalene muscle and should be dissected free from the underlying muscle and retracted out of the field with a vessel loop. The anterior scalene muscle can then be divided with the electrocautery. During dissection of the supraclavicular fat pad, it may be necessary to divide branches of the thyrocervical and costocervical trunks. The most prominent of these branches is the inferior thyroid artery, which stems from the thyrocervical trunk and courses medially toward the thyroid.

After the supraclavicular fat pad has been dissected, the proximal portion of the vertebral artery is reached. The vertebral vein usually lies slightly superficial and medial to the ver-

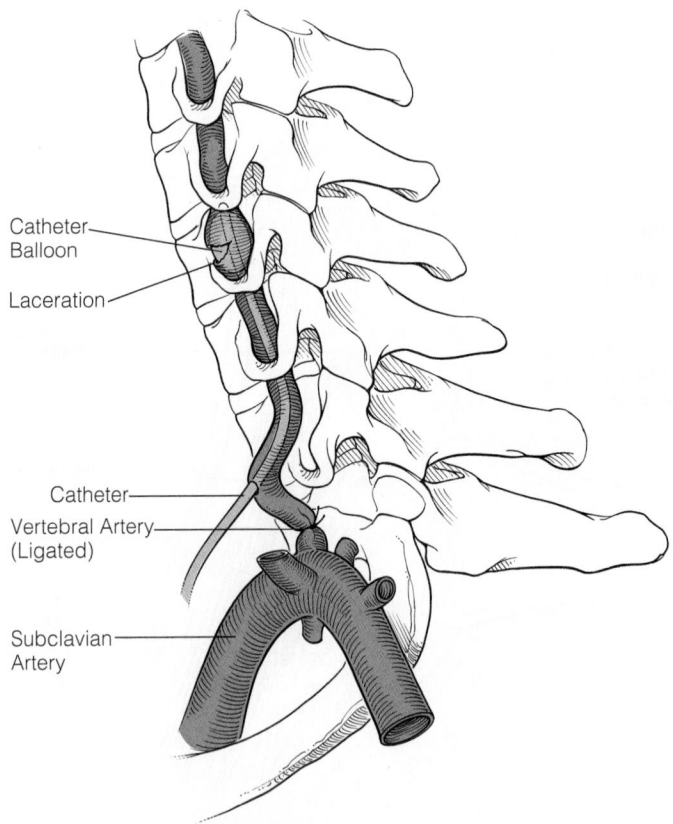

Figure 10   **Bleeding from vertebral artery injuries located within the transverse process of the cervical vertebrae can sometimes be controlled by exposing the proximal vertebral artery at the base of the neck, passing a thrombectomy catheter distally, and inflating the balloon at the site of injury.**

Figure 11 **The proximal vertebral artery can be approached via a supraclavicular incision. Dissection of the supraclavicular fat pad reveals the underlying vertebral artery where it diverges from the subclavian artery. During dissection, care should be taken to avoid injuring the phrenic nerve.**

tebral artery. It should be divided and suture-ligated for better exposure. Care should be taken not to retract too vigorously on the vertebral vein before suture ligation to avoid its avulsion from the subclavian vein. At the depth of the vertebral artery, the white, cordlike elements of the brachial plexus are often visible in the superolateral aspect of the wound. If possible, traction should not be placed on the brachial plexus, and use of the electrocautery around the plexus should be minimized. After exposure, the proximal vertebral artery should be ligated both proximal and distal to the site of injury. No attempts at repair should be made.

Angiographic embolization, the preferred treatment of angiographically diagnosed injuries of the distal vertebral artery, depends on the availability of equipment and expertise with the procedure [*see* Discussion, Angiographic Embolization of Distal Vertebral Artery Injuries, *below*]. Stable patients with angiographically documented injuries to the distal vertebral artery should be transferred to the closest center with cerebral embolization capability. If angiographic embolization is not available, exposure and ligation should be carried out as described above.

In cases where angiographic embolization of the vertebral artery has been employed, a postprocedure angiogram should be done several days to weeks after the procedure to ensure

that the artery remains occluded and that no arteriovenous fistula has developed between the injured vertebral artery and the surrounding venous plexus. Duplex scanning has also been used to a limited extent for follow-up screening. It can be used as an alternative to angiography, but its sensitivity relative to angiography is not yet proved.

Superficial Wounds

Some wounds are obviously superficial on the initial physical examination. Most commonly, these wounds are slash wounds caused by a knife or other sharp object as opposed to being true stab wounds. Rapid exposure and vascular control are sometimes easily accomplished through these wounds. In such circumstances, the surgical procedure 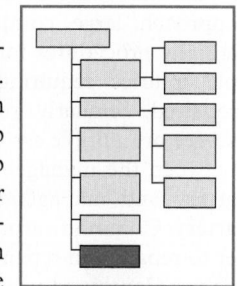 consists of debridement of the neck wound, and deep dissection is not necessary. If greater access and control are needed to rule out further injuries or for definitive repair, a standard anterior sternocleidomastoid incision should be done [*see* Injuries to the Carotid Arteries, Jugular Veins, Pharynx, and Esophagus, *above*].

Discussion

Repair versus Ligation of Carotid Arteries

Simple injuries to the external carotid artery should be repaired, whereas complex injuries should be ligated.

Injuries to the common carotid artery and internal carotid artery are more problematic. If the injury is simple and there is no suggestion that flow in the vessel has been interrupted, repair should always be undertaken. An example of such an injury is a simple stab wound of part of the circumference of the artery with an associated pseudoaneurysm and good distal flow. In this circumstance, lateral repair can be done quickly and easily with a short cross-clamp time. After control of the vessel proximally and distally, a check should be made for back-bleeding. If the back-bleeding from the distal circulation is brisk, as it usually is, repair can be done safely.

If an injury to the common carotid artery or internal carotid artery has interrupted flow in the vessel, repair creates a theoretical disadvantage. Interruption of flow may lead to focal brain ischemia and partial disruption of the blood-brain barrier. Sudden restoration of blood flow may cause hemorrhage in the area of the ischemia and worsen the extent of brain injury; an anemic, or white, infarct of the brain may be converted to a hemorrhagic, or red, infarct. Whether this pathophysiology is important after traumatic injury is unclear and controversial.

Deciding whether to repair or ligate when flow has been interrupted is often difficult.[6,7] One approach is to base the decision on the patient's preoperative neurologic status. If there is no neurologic deficit, it is presumed that there are no areas of brain ischemia and that repair is safe. Conversely, a focal neurologic deficit is presumed to be related to ischemia, and in such cases, the risk of worsening the patient's neurologic status with restoration of blood flow is increased. Even though this approach is rational, it is not applicable in cases in which a detailed neurologic examination before surgery is not possible. Furthermore, this approach may be applicable only to patients in coma or with severe neurologic deficits. There are indications that milder neurologic deficits respond favorably to revascularization.

Yet another approach is to gauge the appropriateness of repair according to the nature of the injury itself. In this approach, large, complicated injuries requiring involved and lengthy procedures for repair should be ligated, whereas simple injuries requiring only simple and quick repairs are repaired. Similarly, repair is not indicated in patients with severe or multiple associated injuries. There is also a difference between the management of injuries of the common carotid artery and management of injuries of the internal carotid artery. Common carotid injuries are more accessible and easier to repair, and repair is generally associated with a good outcome. Continued prograde flow in the internal carotid artery is more likely after injury to the common carotid artery than to the internal carotid artery because of the possibility of collateral flow via the external carotid artery.

A reasonable way to deal with repair dilemmas is to make the decision on the basis of distal back-bleeding. Interruption of blood flow to the brain is tolerated only for a short time, and restoration of flow is unlikely to be accomplished quickly enough to improve outcome. It is therefore logical to base the decision about revascularization on the state of back-

bleeding from the internal carotid artery. If back-bleeding is brisk, the patient is presumed to have good collateral flow, and the chances that there is an area of ischemia are low. Repair rather than ligation is safe in such circumstances. If internal carotid artery back-bleeding is minimal or absent, an ischemic infarct is more likely and restitution of arterial inflow is more dangerous. A corollary to this reasoning is that if back-bleeding is poor, a clot distal to the area of injury may be present, and return of flow with repair may dislodge the clot distally.

Nonoperative Management and Stenting of Carotid Artery Injuries

It is now well accepted that certain minimal injuries to the vasculature of the extremities (e.g., small pseudoaneurysms and endothelial injuries) do not always have to be repaired if they do not compromise distal flow and that such injuries usually heal over time without sequelae. It has been hypothesized that minimal injuries to the carotid vasculature can be approached in a similar fashion. The consequences of distal embolization or pseudoaneurysm rupture in the carotid circulation make such an approach somewhat risky; further experience with nonoperative management is necessary before this approach can be accepted for routine use with small carotid artery injuries.[19,20]

Another relatively new approach to carotid artery injuries is intraluminal stenting.[21-23] This approach is now commonly used for aneurysms of the thoracic and abdominal aorta and is also employed for more distal peripheral vascular lesions. On rare occasions, it has also been applied in the management of traumatic injuries to the thoracic aorta and selected injuries to the peripheral and the visceral vasculature. Not surprisingly, stenting has also been used for the management of carotid artery injuries, particularly injuries to the distal internal carotid artery that are not easily approached surgically. At present, however, only limited data on this approach are available, and the long-term results of carotid stenting are not yet known. It is possible that once more experience with intraluminal stenting has been amassed, it will become an accepted part of the armamentarium for managing carotid injuries. Given that most minor injuries seem to heal well with nonoperative management and that major injuries of the proximal carotid system are relatively easy to approach surgically and often call for emergency surgical repair, the most likely niche for carotid stenting after injury is in treating medium to large lesions of the distal internal carotid artery.

Angiographic Embolization of Distal Vertebral Artery Injuries

Most patients with vertebral artery injuries are stable without external bleeding, and the injury is discovered by angiography. A number of series have now been reported in which such lesions have been successfully treated with angiographic embolization. Given the difficulties of surgical exposure, lesions of the distal vertebral artery should be treated angiographically when the patient's general condition permits and when the necessary expertise is available.[15] If the patient is bleeding profusely, such an approach is not possible, and a rapid surgical approach should be done, with ligation of the proximal vertebral artery and an attempt at thrombectomy catheter control or packing of the wound until an angiographic approach can be attempted. If this is unsuccessful, the lesion should be approached directly [see Known Vertebral Artery Injuries, above].

If a patient with a distal vertebral artery lesion is stable—particularly when the lesion is otherwise silent and has been detected angiographically—an attempt should be made at angiographic embolization if the necessary expertise is available. If the patient is stable, transfer to the nearest center with cerebral angiographic embolization capability is appropriate. Embolization is done via the ipsilateral proximal vertebral artery. Detachable balloons or coils can be used.

Conversion of Cricothyrotomy to Tracheotomy

Cricothyrotomy is typically reserved for life-threatening airway compromise when the need for a rapid surgical airway is paramount [see Airway Compromise, above, and I:2 Trauma Resuscitation]. Tracheotomy is preferred if time and a lesser degree of urgency permit. Similarly, in the postoperative period, tracheotomy is preferred to cricothyrotomy. Traditional thinking, initially promulgated by Chevalier Jackson in 1921, is that cricothyrotomy is more likely than tracheotomy to result in airway stricture or damage to more proximal structures in the larynx. On the basis of this rationale, cricothyrotomies are converted to tracheotomies on a semielective basis within 24 to 48 hours of admission if the patient's general condition permits.[24,25]

Evidence to support a policy of routine conversion is mixed. Several series document a low but increased incidence of complications to the larynx and trachea from prolonged maintenance of cricothyrotomies. Even though incidence is low, the complications can be severe and may require extensive reconstructive procedures. Conversely, studies of cardiac patients undergoing routine cricothyrotomy do not demonstrate a significant increase in the incidence of airway complications. Cricothyrotomy is sometimes favored over tracheotomy in these patients because of concerns about the proximity of tracheotomy wounds to the patient's sternotomy incision. The results of studies of routine cardiac patients may be different from results of studies showing an increase in complications after cricothyrotomy, in that cardiac patients were intubated for shorter periods.

There have been no studies documenting a high incidence of complications in trauma patients who have undergone emergency cricothyrotomy and have remained intubated via the cricothyrotomy for longer than 2 or 3 days. Because complications are potentially so devastating, however, emergency cricothyrotomies should be converted to tracheotomy within 1 to 2 days of admission in stable patients. Assuming a stable patient, the risks of conversion are minimal, and conversion is justified to avoid the possibility of future complications.

References

1. Fuhrman GM, Steig FH III, Buerk CA: Blunt laryngeal trauma: classification and management protocol. J Trauma 30:87, 1990

2. Symbas IN, Hatcher CR Jr, Boehm GAW: Acute penetrating tracheal trauma. Ann Thorac Surg 22:473, 1976

3. Dossa C, Shepard AD, Wolford DG, et al: Distal internal carotid exposure: a simplified technique for temporary mandibular subluxation. J Vasc Surg 12:319, 1990

4. Fisher DF Jr, Clagett GP, Parker JI, et al: Mandibular subluxation for high carotid exposure. J Vasc Surg 1:727, 1984

5. Beal SL, Pottmeyer EW, Spisso JM: Esophageal perforation following external blunt trauma. J Trauma 28:1425, 1988

6. Fabian TC, George SM Jr, Croce MA, et al: Carotid artery trauma: management based on mechanism of injury. J Trauma 30:953, 1990

7. Richardson R, Obeid FN, Richardson JD, et al: Neurologic consequences of cerebrovascular injury. J Trauma 32:755, 1992

8. Feliciano DV, Mattox KL, Graham JM, et al: Five-year experience with PTFE grafts in vascular wounds. J Trauma 25:71, 1985

9. Archie JP Jr, Green JJ Jr: Saphenous vein rupture pressure, rupture stress, and carotid endarterectomy vein patch reconstruction. Surgery 107:389, 1990

10. Winter RP, Weigelt JA: Cervical esophageal trauma: incidence and cause of esophageal fistulas. Arch Surg 125:849, 1990

11. Aboujoud MS, Obeid FN, Horst HM, et al: Arterial injuries of the thoracic outlet: a ten-year experience. Am Surg 59:590, 1993

12. Rich NM, Baugh JH, Hughes CW: Acute arterial injuries in Vietnam: 1,000 cases. J Trauma 10:359, 1970

13. Wood VE: The results of total claviculectomy. Clin Orthop 207:186, 1986

14. McCready RA, Procter CD, Hyde GL: Subclavian-axillary vascular trauma. J Vasc Surg 3:24, 1986

15. Higashida RT, Halbach VV, Tsai FY, et al: Interventional neurovascular treatment of traumatic carotid and vertebral artery lesions: results in 234 cases. AJR Am J Roentgenol 153:577, 1989

16. Hatzitheofilou C, Demetriades D, Melissas J, et al: Surgical approaches to vertebral artery injuries. Br J Surg 75:234, 1988

17. Reid JD, Weigelt JA: Forty-three cases of vertebral artery trauma. J Trauma 28:1007, 1988

18. Blickenstaff KL, Weaver FA, Yellin AE, et al: Trends in the management of traumatic vertebral artery injuries. Am J Surg 158:101, 1989

19. Demetriades D, Asensio JA, Velmahos G, et al: Complex problems in penetrating neck trauma. Surg Clin North Am 76:661, 1996

20. Panetta TF, Sales CM, Marin ML, et al: Natural history, duplex characteristics, and histopathologic correlation of arterial injuries in a canine model. J Vasc Surg 16:867, 1992

21. Gomez CR, May AD, Terry JB, et al: Endovascular therapy of traumatic injuries of the extracranial cerebral arteries. Crit Care Clin 15:789, 1999

22. Kerby JD, May AD, Gomez CR, et al: Treatment of bilateral blunt carotid injury using percutaneous angioplasty and stenting: case report and review of the literature. J Trauma 49:784, 2000

23. Liu AY, Paulsen RD, Marcellus ML, et al: Long-term outcomes after carotid stent placement for treatment of carotid artery dissection. Neurosurgery 45:1368, 1999

24. Esses BA, Jafek BW: Cricothyroidotomy: a decade of experience in Denver. Ann Otol Rhinol Laryngol 96:519, 1987

25. Milner SM, Bennett JDC: Review article: emergency cricothyrotomy. J Laryngol Otol 105:883, 1991

Reviews

Surgical Anatomy, 6th ed. Anson B, McVay CB, Eds. WB Saunders Co, Philadelphia, 1984
Anatomic Exposures in Vascular Surgery. Wind G, Valentine R, Eds. Williams & Wilkins, Baltimore, 1991

Acknowledgments

Figure 1   Marcia Kammerer.
Figures 2 through 4   Susan E. Brust, C.M.I.
Figures 5 through 7   Marcia Kammerer.
Figures 8 through 11   Susan E. Brust, C.M.I.

5 INJURIES TO THE CHEST

Kenneth L. Mattox, M.D., and Asher Hirshberg, M.D.

Choice of Incision

The operative approach to thoracic trauma is determined primarily by the hemodynamic stability of the injured patient. As a general rule, anterolateral thoracotomy is the incision of choice in the unstable patient. This incision allows rapid access to the visceral content of the hemithorax, does not require special positioning, and does not interfere with access to other visceral compartments. The incision may also be rapidly extended across the sternum to the contralateral hemithorax. In the stable patient, thoracotomy follows a diagnostic workup with precise delineation of the injury, and thus, the incision can be targeted on the injured structure. The choice of thoracotomy incision in stable patients with bleeding into the pleural cavity or the airway is determined by the location of the injury. In patients with blunt or penetrating trauma to the right lower chest, bleeding is usually from an injured liver, and therefore, the initial approach is via a midline laparotomy. The right chest is entered only if laparotomy fails to reveal the source of bleeding. Injuries above the right nipple line and to any part of the left chest are approached through an anterolateral thoracotomy on the injured side.

Penetrating wounds to the base of the neck present special access problems. Injuries to the base of the right neck or those bleeding into the right pleural cavity are approached by median sternotomy. However, the first part of the left subclavian artery is intrapleural and posterior, and the appropriate incision for proximal control of this vessel is a left anterolateral thoracotomy in the third or fourth intercostal space. This incision is used for thoracic inlet injuries bleeding into the left pleura or for presumed left subclavian artery laceration. The more lateral parts of both subclavian arteries are approached through a supraclavicular incision, and exposure can be facilitated by removal of the medial third of the clavicle. An important operative adjunct is the insertion of a Foley balloon catheter into the missile tract to achieve temporary hemostasis by inflating the balloon while access and direct control are obtained.

The initial incision chosen for access to an actively bleeding thoracic inlet injury may prove inadequate and is immediately extended if necessary. A median sternotomy can be extended along the border of the sternocleidomastoid muscle or along the clavicle to improve access to the carotid or subclavian arteries. A so-called trapdoor incision is created by extending the median sternotomy into an anterolateral thoracotomy in conjunction with a supraclavicular incision. This incision is useful for proximal left carotid injuries and for obtaining control of the proximal left subclavian artery if the initial incision was a median sternotomy.

The choice of thoracotomy incision in stable patients hinges on precise delineation of the injured structures. The heart, ascending aorta, arch, and thoracic inlet vessels are approached via a median sternotomy. A posterolateral thoracotomy is indicated for injuries to the descending aorta, esophagus, lung, and bronchus.

Resuscitative Thoracotomy

The incision for resuscitative thoracotomy is made immediately beneath the nipple in men or beneath the manually retracted breast in women. It extends from the sternum medially as far lateral as possible. The incision is rapidly performed with a knife, and heavy scissors are used to cut the intercostal muscles. Time is not wasted on skin preparation, wound hemostasis, or identification of the severed internal mammary artery. A chest wall retractor is inserted with the handle away from the sternum and facing the axilla.

The subsequent operative maneuvers depend on the clinical circumstances. If a tamponade is suspected, the pericardial sac is opened longitudinally—anterior and parallel to the phrenic nerve—up to the aortic root superiorly and the diaphragm inferiorly. The heart is manually delivered into the left hemithorax and carefully examined for injuries. External visualization of the intact pericardium is misleading and should never be relied upon to exclude a tamponade. Attempts to repair cardiac lacerations in the suboptimal technical circumstances of the emergency room are frequently futile. Evacuation of blood and temporary control of the lacerations by digital pressure, a Foley catheter, or a skin stapler will allow transfer of the patient to the operating room for definitive repair under optimal conditions.

The descending thoracic aorta should be clamped to maintain cerebral and coronary perfusion in the agonal patient; clamping is also an important adjunct to open cardiac massage. This maneuver involves manual upward traction of the left lung, division of the inferior pulmonary ligament, incision of the mediastinal pleura, and just enough blunt finger dissection around the aorta to accommodate an aortic clamp. Digital aortic occlusion may be a safer and less traumatic alternative when visualization of the area is not optimal. When hemorrhage arises from the pulmonary hilum or parenchyma and when coronary air embolism is suspected, the pulmonary hilum is clamped. This maneuver also requires mobilization of the inferior pulmonary ligament.

As a general rule, the injured hemithorax is entered first. However, when it becomes apparent that the patient's agonal state is not explained by the findings in the open hemithorax, the incision should rapidly be extended across the sternum into the other hemithorax. This is particularly true for a right-sided thoracotomy, which does not provide access to the heart and the descending thoracic aorta. Extension of a left thoracotomy to the right hemithorax is done in the fourth intercostal space to facilitate access to the innominate artery. The resulting clam shell incision provides excellent access to all thoracic viscera (except the posterior mediastinal structures), albeit at the price of increased morbidity.

The technical keys to resuscitative thoracotomy are speed in entering the chest and avoiding complex repairs or maneuvers until the patient is in the operating room, where definitive repair of injuries is accomplished. The major pitfalls are iatrogenic injuries to the phrenic nerve or heart during pericardiotomy, avulsion of an intercostal artery, or esophageal perforation during attempted aortic clamping. Care should be taken to avoid laceration of the inferior pulmonary vein during division of the inferior pulmonary ligament. The transected internal mammary artery should be identified and ligated before closure.

Cardiac Trauma

SIMPLE INJURIES

Repair of simple anterolateral cardiac lacerations is a straightforward matter. The major determinants of a successful outcome in these cases are timely diagnosis and swift thoracotomy. The laceration itself is repaired either by simple or pledgeted monofilament suture. The most common site of myocardial disruption from blunt trauma is the right atrium, usually at the atriocaval junction. Atrial lacerations can sometimes be controlled with a partially occluding clamp to facilitate the repair.

COMPLEX INJURIES

Several factors may complicate the cardiorrhaphy [see Figure 1]. Injuries to the right side of the heart may not be accessible via a left thoracotomy and, thus, may require transsternal extension. Multiple holes or lacerations may require temporary control using digital

pressure, an occluding balloon catheter, or a skin stapler. Lacerations involving a coronary artery present a special problem. Ligation of a distal coronary artery is rarely associated with significant arrhythmias or infarction, whereas proximal coronary lacerations should be repaired. When the cardiac perforation is in close proximity to a coronary artery, horizontal mattress sutures passed beneath the artery help avoid inadvertent interruption of the vessel [see Figure 2].

Temporary inflow occlusion is a key maneuver in difficult situations, such as posterior lacerations or injuries to the intrapericardial great vessels. Both venae cavae are rapidly clamped, and the heart is allowed to empty. This results in a temporarily dry operative field, which may be just enough for several quick critical stitches. Large posterior atrial lacerations can sometimes be repaired from within the heart by atriotomy combined with inflow occlusion. Cardiopulmonary bypass is always a theoretical possibility but rarely a practical option in the acute situation.

Figure 1   Algorithm illustrates evaluation and treatment of a patient with hemopericardium or suspected injury to the heart.

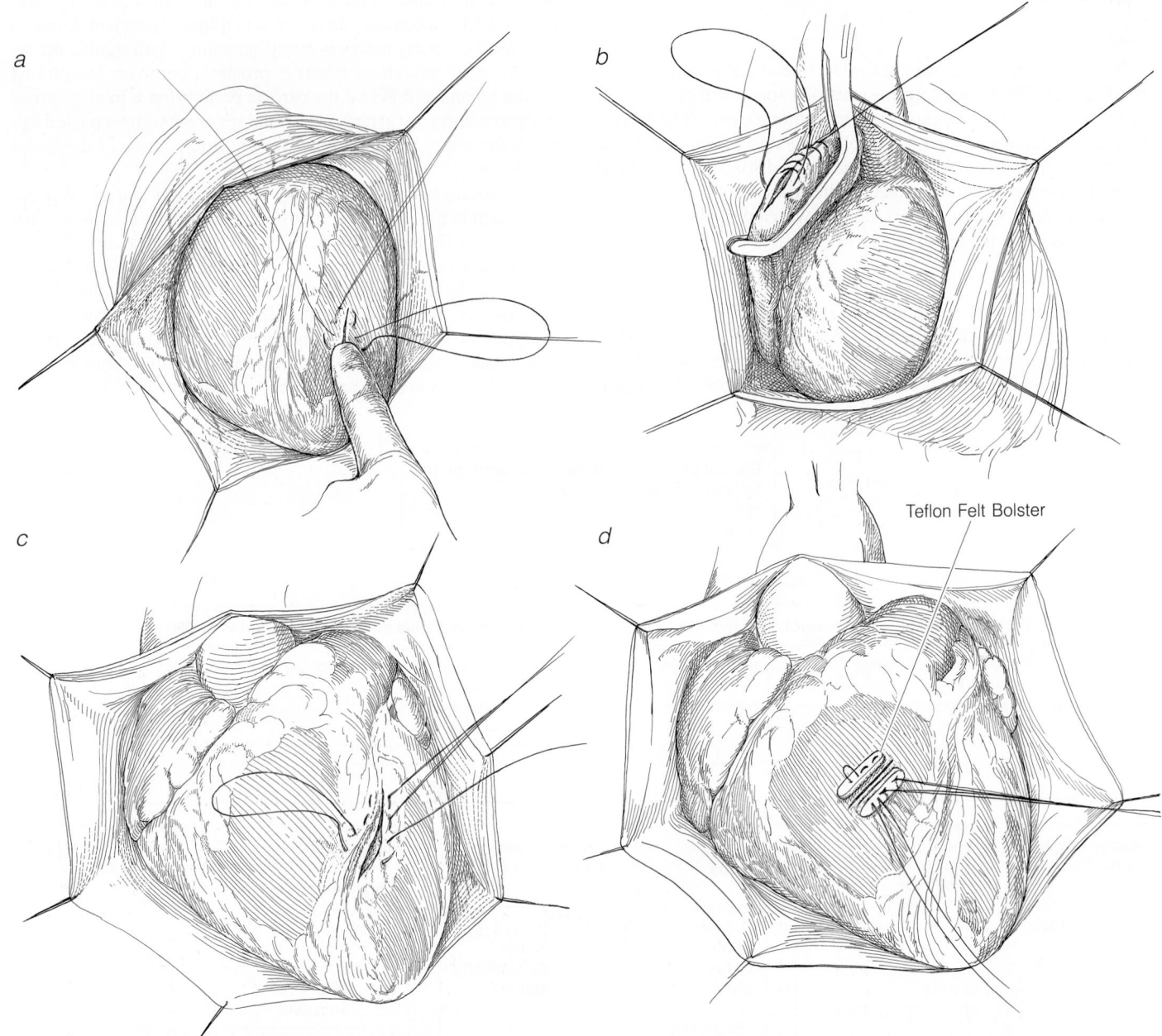

Figure 2 **Penetrating injuries to a cardiac chamber can usually be temporarily occluded with the tip of a finger (a); a Satinsky clamp can sometimes be used to control an atrial lesion (b). If the wound is close to a coronary artery, care must be taken not to obliterate the vessel during repair. Passing horizontal mattress sutures beneath the vasculature will allow closure of the cardiac laceration and avoid ligation of the artery (c). Injuries can sometimes be repaired with a simple running suture but are usually best handled with interrupted mattress sutures. Teflon pledgets or strips may be used if there is surrounding contusion or if the injury is to a ventricle (d). It is best to use cardiovascular suture material, but absorbable sutures may be used if cardiovascular material is not readily available.**

SPECIAL CONSIDERATIONS

Missile emboli to the heart can be caused by migration of air and particles from the peripheral venous injury site. Almost all such bullets will become embedded within the right ventricular trabeculations. Left in place, such a missile embolism can cause arrhythmias, further embolization to pulmonary arteries, endocarditis, and interference with tricuspid valve function. Such emboli have been removed by use of interventional radiologic techniques, cardiopulmonary bypass and right atriotomy, and entrapment and simple re-

moval via a right ventriculotomy without cardiopulmonary bypass.

The diagnosis of coronary air embolism is made intraoperatively when air bubbles are noted in the coronary arteries. This calls for immediate hilar clamping of the injured lung in conjunction with venting of air from the left side of the heart and ascending aorta by a needle inserted into the most ventral aspect of these structures. Manual occlusion of the aortic root is then accomplished by placing the fingers of the left hand into the transverse sinus and compressing the aorta between the thumb and the forefinger. The heart is massaged for several beats to drive the air through the coronary microcirculation. Once cardiac activity is reestablished, the left chambers are vented again to remove any residual air. The lung injury that allowed air entry into the pulmonary venous circulation must be addressed.

Aortic Injuries

Traumatic rupture of the descending thoracic aorta creates a contained hematoma, which allows precise angiographic definition of the injury before operative repair [see Figure 3]. The descending aorta is approached through a left posterolateral thoracotomy in the fourth intercostal space. The standard repair technique is direct repair with or without interposition graft placement using proximal and distal control (clamp repair). Only one lung is anesthetized, if possible. After entry into the left chest, the first operative target is the left subclavian artery, which is encircled using careful blunt dissection. Next, the mediastinal pleura overlying the distal descending aorta is incised and the aorta is encircled and prepared for clamping with special care taken to avoid damage to intercostal vessels. The critical maneuver during dissection is developing the correct plane around the aortic arch between the subclavian and the left carotid arteries in preparation for proximal clamping. The pleura between the vagus and the phrenic nerve is sharply incised, and a plane is de-veloped between the left (or main) pulmonary artery and the under-surface of the aortic arch. This is done with a combination of blunt and sharp dissection and may be especially difficult in elderly pa-tients, who often have tough fibrous periaortic tissue at this loca-tion. A large curved clamp is used to encircle the aortic arch, and the dissection is limited to the minimum necessary for safe passage of an umbilical tape and subsequent cross-clamping. Before clamp-ing the aorta, the surgeon may elect to use a temporary passive shunt, pharmacological control of central hypertension, or a pump-assist device [see Figure 4].

The aortic arch, subclavian artery, and distal aorta are then clamped, in this sequence, and the hematoma is entered. The later-al aspect of the aortic wall is carefully incised longitudinally for a distance of no more than 2 cm, a vein retractor is inserted, and the damage to the aortic wall is evaluated. This small incision is subse-quently extended, as dictated by the operative findings, and a deci-sion is made for primary repair or graft insertion. The aortic inci-sion should be carefully tailored to both the extent of damage and the selected repair technique. Similarly, debridement of the injured wall should be careful and conservative, especially if primary repair seems possible. Direct repair is accomplished with a 4-0 Prolene suture. Graft interposition is accomplished in a standard end-to-end fashion by using a soft woven graft and taking care not to enter

Figure 3 Algorithm illustrates evaluation and treatment of a patient with a thoracic aortic injury.

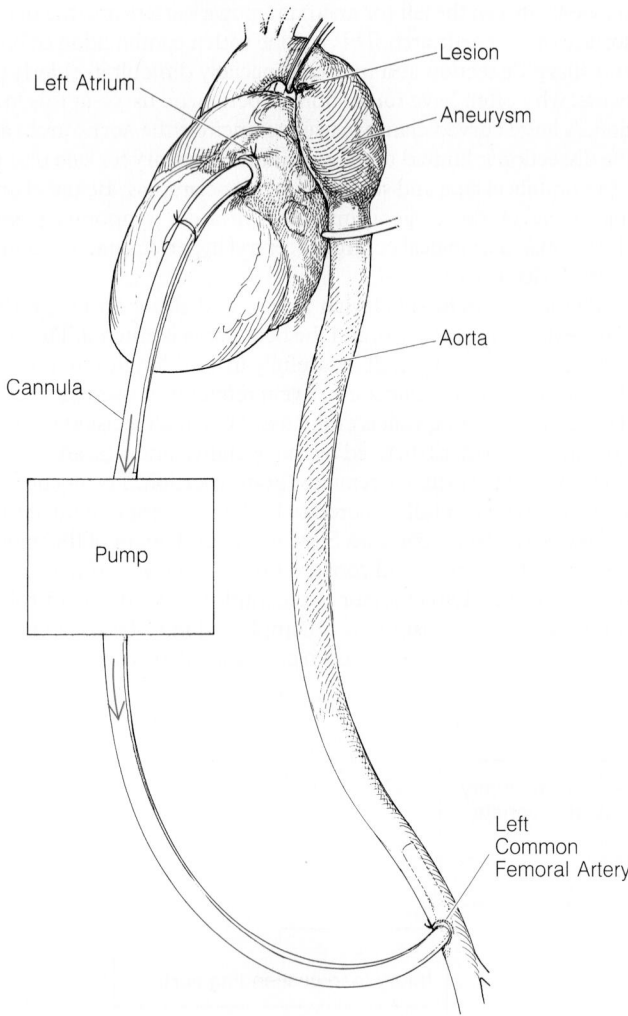

Left Atrium
Lesion
Aneurysm
Aorta
Cannula
Pump
Left Common Femoral Artery

Figure 4 Illustrated is a bypass from the left atrium to the left common femoral artery during operation for a transected descending thoracic aorta. This maneuver permits decompression of upper body hypertension, complete perfusion of the viscera, and some perfusion of the spinal cord. Once the transected area has been dissected out, the clamps should be placed as close as possible to the damaged area to allow maximal perfusion of the collateral circulation.

the esophagus with the posterior bites. After completion of the proximal anastomosis, the clamp should not be moved to the graft, particularly in young adults, because the aorta of young persons is relatively friable and should not be subjected to excessive tension. Aortic declamping is a critical maneuver that should be accomplished slowly and only after the nitroprusside infusion used to control central hypertension has been discontinued.

Thoracic Outlet Injuries

The second most common blunt thoracic vascular injury is a tear at the origin of the innominate artery off the aortic arch. This injury is repaired by following the bypass and exclusion principle, thus avoiding the need for cardiopulmonary bypass, shunts, or heparinization. After precise angiographic definition of the injury, access is obtained via a median sternotomy. The ascending aorta is exposed inside the pericardium. The distal innominate, right

subclavian, and right carotid arteries are dissected out and encircled preparatory to clamping, with care taken to avoid the hematoma itself. With a partially occluding (Satinsky) clamp on the ascending aorta, a 12 mm knitted Dacron graft is sewn to the normal ascending aorta in an end-to-side fashion, away from the injury. Occasionally, the innominate vein is ligated to optimize exposure. A second, partially occluding clamp is placed on the aortic arch at the origin of the innominate artery, with special care taken not to accidentally occlude the left carotid artery origin. The distal innominate artery or its branches are then clamped, and the distal anastomosis is completed. Only then is the hematoma entered and the injury oversewn by placing a row of pledgeted sutures on the aortic arch.

Penetrating injuries to the innominate vessels and proximal carotid arteries produce a mediastinal hematoma and, sometimes, torrential hemorrhage, which can be temporarily controlled either digitally or by placing a balloon catheter in the missile tract before obtaining access. The cardinal technical principle in the management of these injuries is never to enter a contained or partially contained mediastinal hematoma without prior proximal and distal control. Proximal control of these vessels can be obtained from within the pericardium, where the anatomy is not obscured by the hematoma. During dissection within the hematoma, the technical key is identification of the innominate vein, which may be ligated and divided with impunity if needed.

Injuries to the distal subclavian vessels can often be approached via a limited supraclavicular incision, but the safest approach, especially in the presence of active bleeding, is a more extensive incision. The medial third of the clavicle is rapidly resected by early subperiosteal division of the bone, grasping it with a towel clip and lifting it out of its bed. The subclavian artery is a very friable vessel, and limited resection of the injured segment with interposition of a graft (preferably one made of knitted Dacron) is a safer option than extensive mobilization and attempted end-to-end anastomosis.

Major Airway Disruption

The precise location of major airway injury is determined by bronchoscopy, and the operative approach is planned accordingly. Use of a double-lumen endotracheal tube is an important adjunct. The thoracic trachea and the right mainstem bronchus are approached via a right posterolateral thoracotomy, and the left mainstem bronchus is approached through a similar incision on the left. The anterior and left lateral aspects of the mediastinal trachea can also be approached through a median sternotomy. More than 80 percent of blunt tracheobronchial disruptions occur within 2 cm from the carina [*see Figure 5*].

The underlying technical principle in the management of airway injuries is to achieve primary repair with precise mucosa-to-mucosa apposition of the lacerated edges using interrupted absorbable sutures. Small tracheal wounds with well-opposed edges and no tissue loss can be managed conservatively by tracheal intubation and inflation of the balloon distal to the laceration. Large tracheobronchial wounds are managed by conservative debridement and airtight single-layer closure of the defect. Lacerations of the distal airways resulting in a large air leak or bleeding into the airway are managed by resection of the injured lung parenchyma.

Pulmonary Lacerations

Bleeding pulmonary lacerations can be either oversewn or resected [*see Figure 6*]. A continuous over-and-over Prolene suture

Figure 5 These x-rays are of a patient who was involved in a high-speed motor vehicle accident. His initial blood pressure was 90/60 mm Hg, and he was in respiratory distress. The initial chest x-ray (left) shows a right pneumothorax and a left hemothorax with pulmonary contusion. There is significant subcutaneous and mediastinal air. After bilateral tube thoracostomies, the chest x-ray shows persistent right pneumothorax (right); there was also a significant air leak through the chest tube. Bronchoscopy revealed disruption of the right mainstem bronchus, which was repaired.

controls bleeding from small or shallow lacerations, whereas deeper wounds require resection of the injured parenchyma. As a general rule, parenchymal resections for trauma are not anatomic. Rapid and simple resection of the injured lung tissue is usually accomplished using a wide linear stapler (TA-90), which is positioned just proximal to the injured segment, closed, and fired across. The tissue distal to the stapled line is then amputated, and the stapler is opened. Any residual bleeding or air leak from the stapled line is then oversewn with a Prolene suture.

Deep through-and-through injuries to the lung that do not involve hilar structures present a special technical problem because simple closure of the entry and exit wounds is inadequate. These injuries are managed by pulmonary tractotomy between two aortic clamps. The bridge of tissue between the clamps is cut, thus opening the tract and allowing selective suture-ligation of bleeders and air leaks. The tract is carefully inspected to ensure that no major vascular or bronchial injury is present that would require a formal resection. The lung tissue held by the aortic clamps is then oversewn with continuous Prolene suture, and the tractotomy is left open.

Central lung injuries are the source of exsanguinating hemorrhage, as well as air embolism. The key operative maneuver in the management of these injuries is early hilar clamping. The inferior pulmonary ligament is rapidly divided, and the entire hilum is clamped with a large vascular clamp, incorporating the pulmonary artery, both pulmonary veins, and the mainstem bronchus. The next step is a meticulous evaluation of the injuries to determine the method of definitive repair (i.e., vascular repair or pulmonary resection). If the vascular injury is immediately below the hilar clamp

and the patient's hemodynamic status allows, the pulmonary vessels can be individually isolated and controlled from within the pericardium to facilitate exposure and repair of the injury. Isolated vascular injuries can theoretically be repaired, but in practice, these wounds are often associated with extensive parenchymal destruc-

Figure 6 Algorithm illustrates evaluation and treatment of a patient with penetrations or lacerations of the lung.

tion and massive blood loss. Under these circumstances, rapid resection of the lobe or the entire lung is the only practical option.

Esophageal Injuries

Injuries to the upper thoracic esophagus are approached via a right posterolateral thoracotomy, and similar injuries to the lower esophagus are best approached through the same incision on the left side. Anterolateral thoracotomy provides suboptimal exposure of these injuries. The thoracic esophagus is totally inaccessible when the chest is entered through a median sternotomy.

The key consideration in esophageal repair is timing. An early perforation (less than 12 hours old) is associated with minimal spillage into the adjacent mediastinum and is, therefore, amenable to primary repair. Late perforations are associated with a marked inflammatory response in the esophageal wall and surrounding mediastinum, thus making primary repair unsafe or technically impossible. Under these circumstances, excision and diversion are the only options. While a 12- to 16-hour delay usually serves as the dividing line between early and late injuries, the final decision depends more on the amount of local inflammation and the feasibility of a sound closure than on arbitrary time limits.

Repair of an esophageal perforation is done in one or two layers, with the aim of obtaining a tension-free, watertight closure. It is important to maintain the suture line in a transverse orientation to avoid narrowing the repaired segment. The repair is buttressed with nontraumatized adjacent tissue, such as a small intercostal muscle flap, a tongue of parietal pleura, or the fundus of the stomach (by means of a Thal patch or a Nissen fundoplication). Wide mediastinal drainage with a large Argyle tube completes the repair.

Delayed operation for esophageal perforation employs the principles of proximal diversion and wide drainage to effectively control an inflamed and friable esophageal wall that does not hold sutures [see Figure 7]. The noninflamed intact esophagus above and below the injured segment is mobilized, encircled, and stapled with a linear stapler, and the area is widely drained. This step is then followed by laparotomy with construction of a gastrostomy and a feeding jejunostomy. The final step is the creation of a loop cervical esophagostomy into the left neck. Total exclusion and diversion as described above will later require esophageal resection and reconstruction using colon interposition. Thus, when the local situation allows and repair of the perforation is technically feasible, a less radical technical solution should be considered. The perforation may be repaired and temporarily excluded in continuity by means of Teflon band closure of the gastroesophageal junction in conjunction with a lateral cervical esophagostomy. The decision to repair or exclude an esophageal injury is not based solely on the length of delay and the local inflammatory response. Even with early perforations, it is safer to exclude the esophageal injury when it is extensive or in the presence of other serious associated injuries.

Chest Wall Injuries

The source of bleeding in the patient with ongoing hemorrhage into the pleural cavity is usually a lacerated intercostal artery. The keys to successful control of chest wall bleeders are adequate exposure and ligation of the bleeding intercostal vessel on both sides of the injury; each intercostal artery has a bidirectional blood supply. Occasionally, the bleeding vessel cannot be directly controlled because of extensive surrounding soft tissue destruction. Temporary effective packing of the area may be the only feasible technical so-

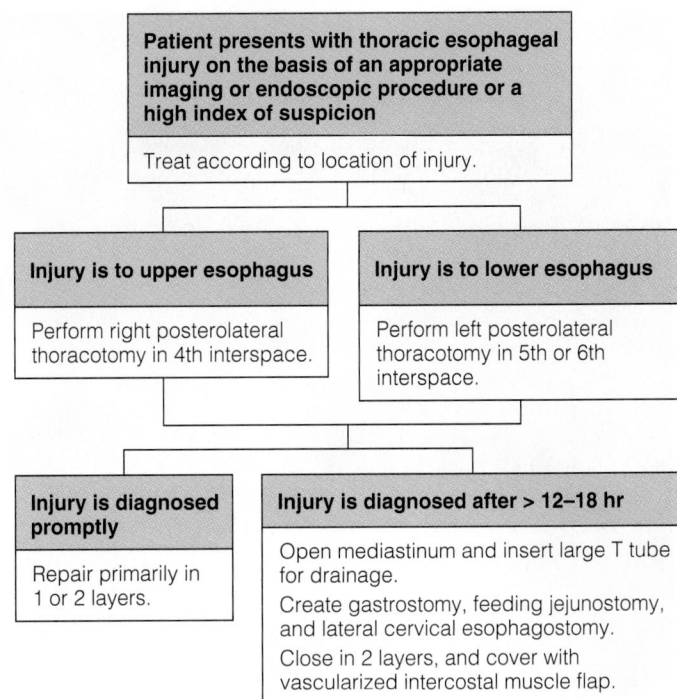

Figure 7 **Algorithm illustrates evaluation and treatment of a patient with thoracic esophageal injury.**

lution, especially in the presence of other life-threatening visceral injuries that demand immediate attention.

Massive chest wall defects are uncommon and are usually associated with extensive underlying visceral damage. Chest wall reconstruction is a low priority under these circumstances and is accomplished after the patient is stabilized. A myocutaneous flap based on the latissimus dorsi or on the pectoralis major muscle is the surgical solution for these wounds.

Surgical reduction and stabilization of the fractured sternum is indicated only when the fracture interferes with cardiac or pulmonary function or when the fractured segments override and may produce a painful pseudoarthrosis. It is important to remember that a sternal fracture is often a marker of underlying visceral damage, which is the first priority.

Special Operative Considerations

Thoracic injuries involving more than one truncal visceral compartment present unique operative problems. Transmediastinal penetrations are serious injuries for which the diagnostic and operative approaches have to be individualized. Whenever a transmediastinal penetration is suspected on the basis of the chest x-ray, the missile trajectory, or the clinical circumstances, injury to all three mediastinal components (i.e., heart, great vessels, and esophagus) must be ruled out. In hemodynamically unstable patients, this is done during operative exploration, but it should be remembered that an esophageal injury cannot be ruled out through a median sternotomy and thus requires either a different incision or esophagoscopy. Penetrating great vessel injuries cause massive hemorrhage and immediately become the focus of clinical attention. On the other hand, cardiac wounds do not always present with a dramatic clinical picture and may be missed even during surgical exploration if the pericardium is not opened.

Thoracoabdominal injury is another type of trauma involving more than one truncal visceral compartment. Diaphragmatic lacerations discovered at celiotomy are repaired from within the abdomen after reduction of any herniated viscera. While the diaphragmatic injury itself can be repaired from the chest as well, a laparotomy will be required to explore the abdominal cavity. Before transabdominal repair, the diaphragmatic laceration can be enlarged to enable limited visualization of the pleural space and lung on the injured side. The presence of blood in the pericardial space can be ruled out by performing a transabdominal subxiphoid pericardiotomy. However, this limited exposure does not allow any further interventions if blood is found in the pericardial cavity, so an immediate left anterolateral thoracotomy is indicated.

The reduction and repair of a chronic traumatic diaphragmatic hernia is undertaken from the chest through a posterolateral thoracotomy. This route is preferred because over time, dense adhesions surround the herniated abdominal viscera and make transabdominal reduction and repair technically difficult or even impossible.

Damage Control Tactics

Rapid emergency surgical techniques are employed to abbreviate the operative procedure in the critically injured patient who is rapidly approaching his or her physiologic limits. The hypothermic and coagulopathic patient is a poor candidate for lengthy formal procedures, and temporary or unorthodox technical solutions to control bleeding, air leak, and spillage are often employed in these patients. Formal anatomic repair either is postponed until after restitution of the patient's physiologic reserves postoperatively or is not performed at all.

Stapled lobectomy and pneumonectomy provide a rapid technical solution to exsanguinating hemorrhage from central lung injuries. The technique involves firing a wide linear stapler across the entire bronchovascular pedicle and subsequently oversewing any residual bleeding from the stump with a continuous Prolene suture. Pulmonary tractotomy and selective ligation is another useful damage-control technique. Pulmonary tractotomy is accomplished by placing two vascular clamps completely through a penetrating injury (ignoring anatomic lobar planes) and cutting between the clamps. Vascular control is achieved at the base of the tract, and a running suture line or linear staples are placed beneath each clamp for rapid control of bleeding and air leaks. Patients tolerate such techniques with virtually no postoperative sequelae.

Under emergency conditions, the subclavian and innominate arteries are sometimes ligated and not reconstructed. Rather, coagulopathic bleeding from soft tissue damage to the chest wall is packed, and the perforated esophagus is excluded by ligation of the esophagus above and below the injured segment with cotton tapes.

If reoperation is planned for definitive repair of the injuries, formal chest closure is not undertaken, because it is time consuming and unnecessary. Only the skin is closed, with a row of towel clips 1 to 2 cm apart or a running heavy nylon suture.

General Postoperative Concerns

The three major concerns in the immediate postoperative management of the critical patient with thoracic trauma are oxygenation, hypothermia, and bleeding. The combination of pulmonary trauma, massive bleeding, and aggressive preoperative and intraoperative fluid administration translates into compromised oxygen delivery. Early insertion of a pulmonary artery catheter is the key to maintaining adequate oxygenation under these circumstances. The physiologic insight provided by the pulmonary artery catheter allows tailored support of the preload, cardiac contractility, and afterload, as well as optimization of positive end-expiratory pressure (PEEP) and fraction of inspired oxygen (F_IO_2). Every attempt is made to avoid fluid overload, because the posttraumatic lung exhibits a marked degree of capillary leakage, and thus, fluid overload is immediately translated into interstitial pulmonary congestion and adversely affects oxygenation.

All critically injured patients are hypothermic, and rapid reversal of hypothermia is an urgent concern in an injured patient. Heat loss is especially severe in patients who underwent thoracotomy in conjunction with laparotomy and in patients who underwent prolonged operative procedures. In the intensive care unit, the patient is meticulously protected from additional conductive heat loss and undergoes aggressive active external rewarming. All intravenous fluids and blood components are warmed before they are administered. Extracorporeal rewarming may be indicated in selected patients.

Bleeding is the third urgent concern in the immediate postoperative period. Massive transfusion and hypothermia contribute to the development of coagulopathy, which is clinically apparent by continuous oozing of blood into the chest tubes and from the surgical incisions. This coagulopathy is managed by rewarming the patient and by empirical administration of fresh frozen plasma and platelets, because coagulation studies are unreliable in hypothermic patients. Continuous bleeding from the operated hemithorax raises the question of reoperation. As a general rule, the first priority is always to correct hypothermia and coagulopathy, and reoperation can be considered later.

A specific consideration in the postoperative patient operated on for a chest injury is that the cause of a sudden deterioration in oxygenation or hemodynamic collapse can often be found in the operated hemithorax. Tension pneumothorax, cardiac tamponade, and systemic air embolism are three mechanisms of sudden cardiovascular collapse that require immediate surgical action. If the patient has also had a laparotomy, a sudden deterioration in oxygenation, coupled with excessive inspiratory pressures, decreasing urinary output, and increased intra-abdominal pressure, should lead the surgeon to suspect the presence of the abdominal compartment syndrome, and immediate decompression should be performed.

Misleading chest tube output is a major pitfall in the postoperative patient. Chest tubes often become clogged, are misplaced, or are incorrectly connected to the underwater seal and suction system. Whenever the chest tube output becomes a cause for concern, the tube and its connections should be examined closely for evidence of clogging, kinking, and misplacement. A chest x-ray should be obtained and the tube exchanged if it is felt that the tube is not functioning properly. A chest tube is removed when it is no longer functioning for the purpose of its insertion. In the ventilated postoperative patient, a functioning chest tube is retained until the patient is weaned from positive pressure ventilation.

The possibility of a missed injury should be considered when there is any deviation from the expected course of recovery in the postoperative patient. Unexplained bleeding and unexpected sepsis are the two most common manifestations that should prompt a diligent search for a missed injury. The two most common sites for missed thoracic injuries are the chest wall vessels (intercostal and internal mammary arteries) and the heart. Both require urgent reoperation. Missed esophageal perforations are uncommon but devastating, and management is by proximal diversion, drainage of the perforation, distal drainage of GI contents via a large tube gastrostomy, and feeding tube jejunostomy. Total esophageal diversion is no longer considered an option.

Reoperation for thoracic trauma may be either planned or unplanned. Planned reoperation is performed in patients who underwent a damage control procedure and subsequent stabilization in the intensive care unit. The aim of this reoperation is to perform definitive repairs and formal chest closure. It is undertaken only after correction of hypothermia and coagulopathy and after oxygen delivery has been optimized. Unplanned procedures are usually performed for bleeding and may need to be undertaken in the surgical intensive care unit in a rapidly deteriorating patient. There are no firm quantitative guidelines to urgent reoperation, but reoperation should be considered in any patient whose postoperative bleeding markedly exceeds the surgeon's expectations. This decision should always be made by the surgeon who performed the initial thoracotomy.

Specific Postoperative Problems

PULMONARY COMPLICATIONS

Persistent Air Leak

Patients on sustained PEEP or with elevated ventilatory pressures may have a persistent and at times large-volume air leak. Often, increasing the negative pressure on the pleural space produces parietal and visceral pleura apposition that results in a decreased air leak. However, increased negative pressure may sometimes increase the air leak and create hypoxemia. On rare occasions, operative repair of a large torn lung or of a missed injury to a major bronchus is required. Operative repair should be undertaken only after the patient is off PEEP and has normal ventilatory pressures.

Retained Clotted Hemothorax

Unevacuated or retained clotted hemothorax is an indication for early evacuation, often by thoracoscopy and occasionally by thoracotomy. Use of thrombolytics and conservative treatment results in prolonged hospitalization and increased infectious complications.

Effusion and Empyema

Effusion and empyema may occur because of undrained pleural fluid, undetected esophageal or pulmonary leakage, or sympathetic reaction to subdiaphragmatic conditions. Both effusion and empyema require early detection and drainage.

Systemic Air Embolism

Systemic air embolism can occur with pulmonary parenchymal injury and increased intrabronchial pressure, creating a bronchopulmonary venous fistula. Sudden cerebral or cardiac insufficiency may be the initial sentinel clue that air has embolized to the coronary or cerebral vessels. Immediate prevention of further embolization of air with possible removal of the intravascular air is a therapeutic goal. Mortality associated with this complication is high.

CARDIAC COMPLICATIONS

Intracardiac Shunts

Left-to-right intracardiac shunts, which are manifested by continuous murmurs, are often found postoperatively. Detection may be aided by color Doppler imaging. Depending on the size of the fistula, closure of the fistula may be required by operative or transvascular interventional techniques.

Cardiac Herniation

Cardiac herniation can occur postoperatively in patients with a pericardium that has been only partially incised or incompletely repaired. It usually occurs when a patient is lying on the left side, and it is manifested by sudden hypotension and distended neck veins. Cardiac herniation is often reversible if the patient lies with the right side down. Such cases require either pericardiorrhaphy or wider pericardectomy.

Pericardial Effusion

Pericardial effusion is a rare but real entity that occurs after pericardiotomy or cardiorrhaphy. Such effusion may be sympathetic, chylous, reactive, or infectious. Diagnosis is made via echocardiography or a pericardial window. Such effusion may be part of a postpericardiotomy syndrome in some patients.

COMPLICATIONS OF THE GREAT VESSELS

Paraplegia

The dreaded complication of thoracic aortic surgery, paraplegia is the result of spinal cord ischemia, and there is currently no universally recognized preventive measure to reduce its incidence. Although ischemic myelopathy is most often apparent immediately after operation, it may occur as long as five days after surgery, suggesting other etiologies, such as spinal compartment syndrome and reperfusion injury.

False Aneurysms

False aneurysms occur at the site of undetected arterial injury or at vascular anastomotic sites. Some surgeons have recommended postoperative arteriograms in thoracic vascular reconstructions to establish a baseline study, whereas others obtain vascular images only when routine radiographs or symptoms suggest a posttraumatic false aneurysm. Delayed thoracic posttraumatic aneurysms frequently appear weeks or months after the injury rather than in the intensive care unit. Depending on the location of the aneurysm, direct surgical repair is indicated. Stenting of both arteriovenous fistulae and traumatic false aneurysms with intraluminal stents is a modern therapeutic option.

Arteriovenous Fistula

Arteriovenous fistula can occur in many thoracic locations, including the intercostal vessels, aorta to pulmonary artery, or pulmonary artery to pulmonary vein. The location of the last fistula listed may be the pulmonary parenchyma. Diagnosis is by arteriography, and treatment is by vascular reconstruction, occasionally after pulmonary resection.

ESOPHAGEAL, TRACHEAL, AND DIAPHRAGMATIC COMPLICATIONS

Esophageal Repair Breakdown

Penetrating injury to the thoracic esophagus repaired via an anterior thoracic incision has a 50 percent breakdown rate. Thus, it is recommended that a contrast esophagogram be performed in every patient who underwent an esophageal repair before resumption of oral food intake. When esophageal injury is discovered, it is best repaired via a posterior approach. Late esophageal leaks are handled as outlined earlier in this chapter.

Stenosis

Tracheal or bronchial stenosis can occur either from a missed injury, a constricted repair, or a buildup of granulation tissue around suture material at the site of a bronchial or tracheal repair. Suture line granuloma is less common when absorbable suture material is used. When braided or polypropylene suture materials are used, the externally placed knots are often discovered to be intraluminal at later bronchoscopy.

Posttraumatic Diaphragmatic Hernia

Acute diaphragmatic herniation is rare, because the appearance of this condition is usually delayed for months or years. Diagnosis is aided by gastric or colonic contrast studies. A posttraumatic diaphragmatic hernia is repaired via a thoracic incision, as opposed to acute herniations, which are approached via a laparotomy incision.

COMPLICATIONS OF THE CHEST WALL

Chylothorax

An uncommon but real occurrence, chylothorax usually becomes manifest on postinjury days 3 to 7. Conservative therapy involves either intravenous alimentation or enteral feedings with medium-chain triglycerides. To assist in the localization of persistent chylous leaks, preoperative or intraoperative gastrointestinal olive oil can be administered.

Causalgia

Posttraumatic causalgia, or reflex sympathetic dystrophy, may be caused by a partial injury to a peripheral nerve. Causalgia is also common after a so-called trap-door thoracotomy and is occasionally seen when a median sternotomy is opened very widely. Management is conservative and is based on response to physical therapy and stellate ganglion blocks. Occasionally, dorsal sympathectomy is required.

Radicular Pain

Intercostal radicular pain is common after a lateral thoracotomy. Frequently controlled by analgesics and intercostal nerve blocks initially, chronic pain of this etiology can be disabling. Use of permanent suture material for pericostal sutures during rib reapproximation contributes to radicular pain as the intercostal nerve becomes entrapped. Symptoms may be lessened by permanent intercostal nerve ablation.

Costal Chondritis

Thoracoabdominal incisions across the chondral border in trauma patients lead to a significant rate of chronic chondritis. This painful condition may be due to devascularization of the cartilaginous structures as a result of necrosis or infection. Such conditions are best treated by placement of a muscle flap into the adequately debrided area.

Recommended Reading

CHOICE OF INCISION

Mattox KL: Thoracic injury requiring surgery. World J Surg 7:47, 1982

Mattox KL: Indications for thoracotomy: deciding to operate. Surg Clin North Am 69:47, 1989

Pickard LR, Mattox KL: Thoracic trauma and indications for thoracotomy. Trauma. Mattox KL, Moore EE, Feliciano DV, Eds. Appleton & Lange, Norwalk, Connecticut, 1988, p 315

RESUSCITATIVE THORACOTOMY

Champion HR, Sykes L: Emergency room thoracotomy. Trauma Surgery, Part 1, 4th ed. Champion HR, Robbs JV, Trunkey DD, Eds. Butterworth & Co, London, 1989, p 70

Feliciano DV, Bitondo CG, Cruse PA, et al: Liberal use of emergency center thoracotomy. Am J Surg 152:654, 1986

Shannon FL, Moore EE, Moore JB: Emergency department thoracotomy. Trauma. Mattox KL, Moore EE, Feliciano DV, Eds. Appleton & Lange, Norwalk, Connecticut, 1988, p 175

CARDIAC INJURIES

Mattox KL, Beal AC Jr, Jordan GL Jr, et al: Cardiorrhaphy in the emergency center. J Thorac Cardiovasc Surg 68:886, 1974

Mitchell ME, Muakkassa FF, Poole GV, et al: Surgical approach of choice for penetrating cardiac wounds. J Trauma 34:17, 1993

Symbas PN: Cardiothoracic trauma. WB Saunders Co, Philadelphia, 1989, p 300

AORTIC INJURIES

Mattox KL, Holzman M, Pickard LR, et al: Clamp-repair: a safe technique for treatment of blunt injury to the descending thoracic aorta. Ann Thorac Surg 40:456, 1985

Mattox KL, Wall MJ Jr, Hirshberg A: Traumatic aneurysm of the thoracic aorta. Aneurysms—New Findings and Treatments. Yao JST, Pearce WH, Eds. Appleton & Lange, Norwalk, Connecticut, 1994, p 207

Mattox KL: Red River Anthology. J Trauma 42:353, 1997

von Oppell UO, Dunne TT, De Groot MK, et al: Traumatic aortic rupture: twenty-year metaanalysis of mortality and risk of paraplegia. Ann Thorac Surg 58:585, 1994

THE EXTRAPERICARDIAL VESSELS

Brawley RK, Murray GF, Crisler C, et al: Management of wounds of the innominate, subclavian and axillary blood vessels. Surg Gynecol Obstet 148:1130, 1970

Graham JM, Feliciano DV, Mattox KL: Management of subclavian vascular injuries. J Trauma 20:537, 1980

Johnston RH, Wall MJ Jr, Mattox KL: Innominate artery trauma: a thirty year experience. J Vasc Surg 17:134, 1993

MAJOR AIRWAY DISRUPTION

Symbas PN: Cardiothoracic trauma. Curr Probl Surg 28:747, 1991

Urschel HC, Razzuk MA: Management of acute traumatic injuries of tracheobronchial tree. Surg Gynecol Obstet 136:113, 1973

PULMONARY LACERATIONS

Wall MJ Jr, Hirshberg A, Mattox KL: Pulmonary tractotomy with selective vascular ligation for penetrating injuries to the lung. Am J Surg 168:665, 1994

Weincek RG Jr, Wilson RF: Central lung injuries: a need for early vascular control. J Trauma 28:1418, 1988

ESOPHAGEAL INJURIES

Cheadle W, Richardson JD: Options in management of trauma to the esophagus. Surg Gynecol Obstet 155:380, 1982

Defore WW Jr, Mattox KL, Hansen HA, et al: Surgical management of penetrating injuries of the esophagus. Am J Surg 134:734, 1977

CHEST WALL

Pate JW: Chest wall injuries. Surg Clin North Am 69:59, 1989

DAMAGE CONTROL TACTICS

Hirshberg A, Wall MJ Jr, Mattox KL: Planned reoperation for trauma: a two year experience with 124 consecutive patients. J Trauma 37:365, 1994

GENERAL POSTOPERATIVE CONCERNS

Hirshberg A, Wall MJ Jr, Ramchandani MK, et al: Reoperation for bleeding in trauma. Arch Surg 128:1163, 1993

Acknowledgments

Figures 1, 3, 6, and 7   Marcia Kammerer.
Figures 2 and 4   Carol Donner.

6 OPERATIVE EXPOSURE OF ABDOMINAL INJURIES AND CLOSURE OF THE ABDOMEN

Erwin R. Thal, M.D., Brian J. Eastridge, M.D., and Rusty Milhoan, M.D.

Management of abdominal trauma has changed significantly since the beginning of the 1990s. In part, the change is attributable to improvements in the available diagnostic studies and to the advent of nonoperative therapeutic approaches. Those patients who require operative intervention for treatment of abdominal injuries often present a major challenge to the surgical team. Although each such patient is unique, we believe that the application of a standard operative approach is nonetheless necessary to optimize patient care and to minimize the risk of missing injuries. The primary objective of this operative approach is the expeditious prioritization and treatment of injuries. To this end, all surgeons treating injured patients should have a general routine to follow and should be familiar with a variety of exposures and techniques that may be used to carry out this routine. Adequate exposure, rapid assessment, and sound clinical judgment are essential ingredients of the care of patients with abdominal injuries.

Patient Preparation

Before the celiotomy is begun, the patient must be adequately prepared. All contingencies must be planned for in advance. A nasogastric tube and a Foley catheter should be inserted, and a single dose of a broad-spectrum antibiotic should be given before the initial incision is made. With the patient positioned on the operating table, skin preparation is performed in such a way as to include the anterior chest as well as the abdomen; one thus has virtually immediate access to the chest in the event that a thoracic injury is discovered or thoracic vascular control is required. In addition, skin preparation should be extended over the anterior thighs in case distal vascular control is warranted or a vascular reconstruction conduit is needed. All exposed areas of the body that were not prepared must be covered to optimize thermoregulation. Drapes should be placed widely to allow easy access to all potential injuries.

Resuscitation, including the use of blood and blood products, should be continued as the patient is prepared. Both rapid volume infusion systems and cell saver systems are useful adjuncts in this setting. Room temperature must be controlled to minimize loss of heat from the patient during the operation.

Incision and Initial Exploration

CHOICE OF INCISION

A midline incision is the most expedient choice for opening the abdomen. It has several key advantages: it allows the abdominal cavity to be accessed easily and quickly, it provides good exposure (including exposure of the pelvis), and it can be extended into a median sternotomy or into either thoracic cavity if necessary. Its main disadvantage is the occasional difficulty that may be encountered in exploring the deep recesses of the upper quadrants.

Patients who have had previous midline incisions may be more challenging to operate on, depending on the extent to which intraperitoneal adhesions are present. Accordingly, alternative incisions may be considered. For example, a chevron incision or a transverse incision might allow better visualization of viscera adhering to a previous midline wound and thus might tend to protect them better from iatrogenic injury; however, these incisions are associated with certain disadvantages, in particular the need to divide the large rectus abdominis muscle, the restricted exposure provided, the additional time needed to close the incision, and the inherent limitations on extension of the incision if the need arises. Consequently, chevron and transverse incisions are rarely used and seldom recommended in this setting.

There are additional alternative incisions, such as paramedian, subcostal, retroperitoneal, and flank incisions, but they are not recommended, because they generally do not provide adequate exposure for assessment and treatment of abdominal injuries.

INITIAL EXPLORATION

Once the peritoneal cavity has been entered, initial exploration should proceed in an orderly manner so as to minimize hemorrhage and contamination and facilitate the identification of injuries. There may be an incipient drop in blood pressure when the abdomen is opened. The abdominal organs are eviscerated, and any gross blood, clotted or nonclotted, is evacuated. Laparotomy pads are then used for rapid packing of all four quadrants of the abdomen. When bleeding is under control, anesthesia is allowed to catch up with the resuscitation efforts before abdominal exploration is continued.

Once hemodynamic stability has been achieved, the peritoneal portion of the initial exploration is begun. If there is no discrete site of hemorrhage, the temporary packs are carefully removed, except for those around the solid viscera. The enteric viscera are inspected in an orderly fashion. The anterior aspect of the stomach is inspected from the esophagogastric junction to the pylorus. If there is a high index of suspicion, on the basis of the mechanism of injury or the presence of hematoma or soilage in the lesser sac, the gastrocolic omentum is opened to permit inspection of the posterior aspect of the stomach; this exposure also facilitates examination of the body of the pancreas. Exploration then continues distally. If duodenal or pancreatic injury is suspected, the Kocher maneuver is performed to mobilize the duodenum and the head of the pancreas fully. Once the duodenum has been visualized, the small bowel is inspected from the ligament of Treitz to the ileocecal valve. Careful consideration should be given to the possibility of mesenteric vascular injury, which is often manifested as a mesenteric hematoma. Next, the colon is inspected from the cecum to the peritoneal reflection over the rectum. If there are injuries or missile tracts in proximity to a portion of the ascending or descending colon, the colon must be mobilized by incising the peritoneal reflection (the white line of Toldt) so as to permit inspection of the posterior wall of the bowel as well. Finally, attention is turned toward evaluation of the solid viscera. The laparotomy pads are removed, and the liver and the spleen are visualized to ascertain whether any injury is present.

Once the peritoneal survey has been completed, the retroperitoneum is inspected for potential injury. Retroperitoneal hematomas are classified according to their location: zone 1 is the central portion of the retroperitoneum, zone 2 comprises the two lateral portions, and zone 3 is the pelvic portion [see Figure 1]. The decision whether to explore a retroperitoneal hematoma is based on its location and on the mechanism of injury [see Priorities in Management, Repair of Retroperitoneal Injuries, below]. The retroperitoneum is also evaluated with an eye to identifying any occult injuries to organs such as the pancreas, the duodenum, the posterior colon, the kidneys, and vascular structures. The initial exploration concludes with a brief pelvic survey undertaken to exclude injury to the rectum or the distal genitourinary tract (including the urinary bladder).

Operative Exposure

In what follows, we focus on exposure of specific organs and vessels in patients with abdominal injuries. Definitive repair of such injuries is addressed in more detail elsewhere [see III:7 In-

Figure 1 Shown are the anatomic zones of the retroperitoneum: zone 1 (central), zone 2 (flank), and zone 3 (pelvic).

juries to the Liver, Biliary Tract, Spleen, and Diaphragm; III:8 Injuries to the Stomach, Duodenum, Pancreas, Small Bowel, Colon, and Rectum; and III:9 Injuries to the Great Vessels of the Abdomen].

AORTA

Control of the aorta can be achieved at several different levels, depending on the site of injury. The supraceliac aorta can be exposed by incising the gastrohepatic ligament, retracting the left lobe of the liver cephalad, and retracting the stomach caudad. The esophagus and the periesophageal soft tissue are then mobilized laterally to permit identification of the abdominal aorta at the diaphragmatic hiatus, at which point the vessel can be clamped or compressed. The exposure this method gives is limited with respect to vascular access for definitive repair. Better exposure of the supraceliac aorta can be obtained by means of left medial visceral rotation [see Figure 2]. To reflect the left-sided viscera, the splenorenal ligament is mobilized with a combination of blunt and sharp dissection. The peritoneal reflection is incised, and the incision is extended down the left paracolic gutter to the level of the distal sigmoid colon. With the aid of blunt dissection, the left-sided viscera are gently mobilized to the right in a plane anterior to Gerota's fascia. This technique permits exploration of the entire length of the abdominal aorta as well as the origin of the celiac axis, the origin of the superior mesenteric artery, the left iliac system, and the origin of the right common iliac artery. In addition, it facilitates control of the left renal pedicle before exploration of a left-sided hematoma within Gerota's fascia.

If only distal access to the aorta is necessary, the vessel can be approached transperitoneally. The small bowel is retracted to the right, the transverse colon is retracted cephalad, and the descending colon is retracted to the left. The peritoneum is incised over the aorta, and the third and fourth portions of the duodenum are mobilized cephalad. The proximal limit of this dissection extends to the level of the left renal vein, which can, if necessary, be divided to provide access to the suprarenal aorta. If the left renal vein is ligated, care should be taken to place the ligature close to the vena cava so as to spare important venous collaterals. A somewhat more limited dissection may suffice to expose the distal infrarenal aorta; the exposure can subsequently be extended distally to expose both iliac vessels.

VENA CAVA

Access to the suprahepatic vena cava can be gained by incising the central tendon of the diaphragm or by performing a median sternotomy and opening the pericardium. The infrahepatic inferior vena cava can be exposed by means of right medial visceral rotation [see Figure 3] in much the same way as the aorta is exposed by means of left medial visceral rotation [see Aorta, above]. The right colon is mobilized by taking down the hepatic flexure and incising the peritoneal reflection within the right paracolic gutter. The colon, again, is reflected medially toward the aorta in a plane anterior to Gerota's fascia with the aid of blunt dissection. If additional exposure is necessary, the inferior margin of the peritoneal incision can be extended to the root of the mesentery and even beyond by sacrificing the inferior mesenteric vein. This exposure allows visualization of both the aorta below the origin of the superior mesenteric artery and the vena cava below the third portion of the duodenum. The portion of the inferior vena cava immediately below the liver can be exposed by performing the Kocher maneuver [see Figure 4] with subsequent medial mobilization of the duodenum and head of the pancreas.

Figure 2 **Left medial visceral rotation is performed to provide exposure of the entire length of the abdominal aorta, the left renal vasculature, the origins of the mesenteric arteries, and the common iliac bifurcation.**

Figure 3 **Right medial visceral rotation is performed to provide exposure of the inferior vena cava, the infrarenal abdominal aorta and iliac vessels, and the right renovascular pedicle.**

This right medial visceral exposure facilitates identification of the right renovascular pedicle for control before exploration of a right-sided perinephric hematoma.

PANCREAS

Intraoperative evidence of a central hematoma, peripancreatic edema, or bile staining in the retroperitoneum or the lesser sac raises the possibility of pancreatic injury. The contents of the lesser sac can be seen through the gastrohepatic ligament by direct inspection or by division of the ligament, or they can be visualized by dividing and ligating two or three gastroepiploic arcades of the gastrocolic ligament. If it proves necessary to explore the pancreas, the stomach is separated from the transverse colon by completing the division of the gastrocolic ligament. A Kocher maneuver is performed to reflect the second, third, and fourth portions of the duodenum medially, along with the head of the pancreas. This exposure allows inspection of the anterior and posterior surfaces of the head of the pancreas as well as the uncinate process. If injury to the body or tail of the pancreas is suspected, the splenorenal and splenocolic ligaments are incised. At this point, the spleen and, subsequently, the pancreas can be mobilized medially to a position near the level of the superior mesenteric vessels, and the anterior and posterior aspects of the body and tail can be examined.

DUODENUM AND BILIARY TRACT

The pancreatic head and the duodenum can be adequately exposed by means of the Kocher maneuver (see above). This technique is also used when injury to the distal extrahepatic biliary system is suspected. The proximal extrahepatic biliary tree is visualized by using the Kocher maneuver in combination with local exploration of the porta hepatis.

Priorities in Management

HEMORRHAGE CONTROL

If the patient remains hemodynamically unstable as a result of persistent hemorrhage, the initial and primary focus of the exploration becomes control of bleeding. There are several techniques by which hemostasis may be established. One is repeat packing of the specific bleeding site with laparotomy pads. The importance of adequate packing to the control of hemorrhage cannot be overestimated. Packing is effective as a temporizing measure until more definitive vascular control can be achieved or until a coagulopathy has been corrected.

If persistent hemorrhage is anticipated, proximal and distal control of the injured vessel is obtained by means of the exposure techniques already discussed [see Operative Exposure, above]. Given the potential for exsanguinating hemorrhage, one must be ready to gain control over aortic inflow at the diaphragmatic hiatus or to control the descending aorta in the chest via a left lateral thoracotomy. Effective aortic control may be obtained through digital compression of the vessel at the hiatus; subsequently, a padded Richardson retractor or an aortic compressor may be used to occlude the vessel. If prolonged occlusion of arterial inflow is necessary, an atraumatic vascular clamp may be applied at the hiatus. Injuries to the proximal abdominal aorta often necessitate control of the vessel within the chest.

In patients with parenchymal injury to the solid viscera, control of vascular inflow is crucial as both a diagnostic and a therapeutic maneuver. Control of the splenic hilum effectively stops splenic hemorrhage. Likewise, use of the Pringle maneuver [see III:7 Injuries to the Liver, Biliary Tract, Spleen, and Diaphragm] to control the vessels in the porta hepatis (the hepatic artery and the portal vein) is useful for determining the source of perihepatic hemorrhage. The Pringle maneuver is performed by compressing the portal structures digitally. If bleeding is diminished as a result, control of portal inflow can be maintained by means of an atraumatic vascular clamp or a Rumel tourniquet; however, if significant hemorrhage persists, one must consider the possibility of an injury to the retrohepatic vena cava.

In patients who have a retrohepatic vena caval injury, hepatic exclusion may be necessary for vascular control before definitive repair. This is accomplished by first gaining control of the inferior vena cava both above and below the liver. Control of the inferior vena cava above the liver is obtained by performing a median sternotomy and a pericardiotomy and occluding the vessel within the pericardium. Control of the inferior vena cava below the liver is accomplished by means of right medial visceral rotation in conjunction with the Kocher maneuver. Rumel tourniquets are applied to the vena cava above and below the liver. A monofilament purse-string suture is placed in the right atrial appendage. Extra side holes are cut in the middle portion of a 36 French chest tube. The right atrial appendage is opened, and the chest tube is passed down through the inferior vena cava and positioned so that all of the distal shunt holes are inferior to the Rumel tourniquet below the liver and the proximal shunt holes are superior to the Rumel tourniquet above the liver [see Figure 5]. The tourniquets are then secured around the tube. As an alternative, an endotracheal tube with extra proximal side holes may be used as a shunt. Control of venous inflow below the liver is obtained by inflating the balloon. It is important not to transect the insufflation channel while cutting the side holes. When this type of system is employed, adapters can be used to infuse fluid and blood directly into the right atrium.

Another technique for controlling retrohepatic hemorrhage is occlusion of the inferior vena cava both above and below the liver. This technique often results in significant hemodynamic instability, especially in volume-depleted patients; however, it may be tolerated by patients whose volume status is good. Complete hepatic exclusion involves both atriocaval shunting or clamping of the inferior vena cava and control of hepatic arterial and portal venous inflow.

CONTROL OF CONTAMINATION

Once hemorrhage has been controlled, the next priority is control of contamination. Small enterotomies may be temporarily closed with Babcock clamps while awaiting definitive repair; alternatively, they may be temporarily closed with a continuous suture to prevent ongoing spillage. When multiple enterotomies are present, suture closure is probably preferable to obviate the placement of multiple clamps within the operative field. If the patient has several holes in the bowel that are all in close proximity, the best way of containing the luminal contents is to apply atraumatic clamps at both the proximal end and the distal end of the injury site. If placing bowel clamps is not feasible or the clamps get in the way, a stapling device can be used to control an enteric leak. Once the spillage is controlled, all gross foreign material should be removed from the peritoneal cavity.

VASCULAR REPAIR

After the patient has been stabilized and hemorrhage and bowel contamination have been controlled, attention is directed to defini-

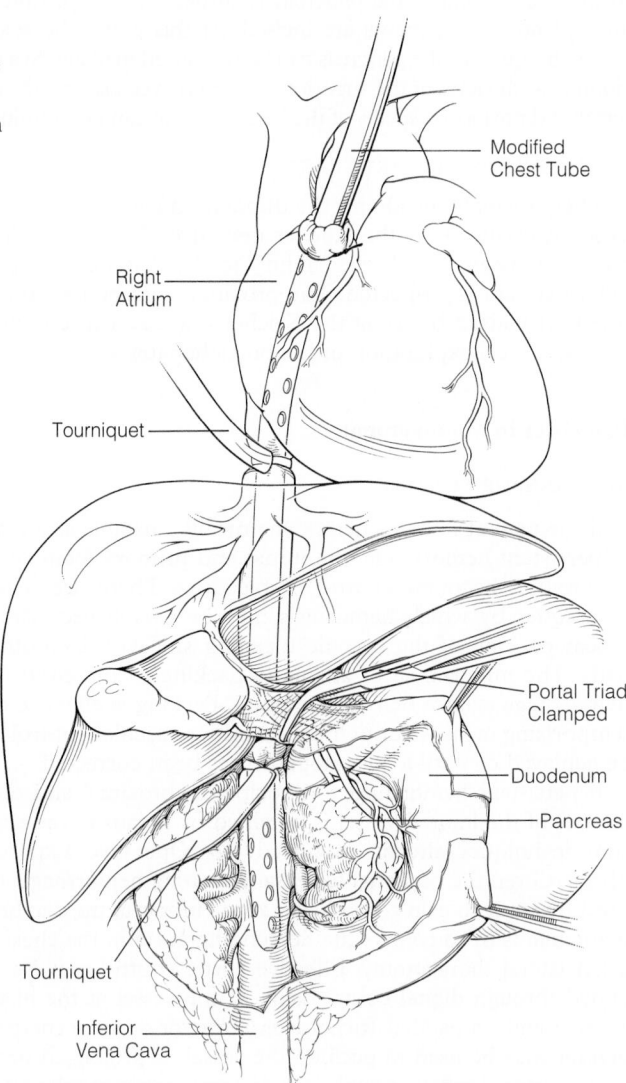

Figure 4 The Kocher maneuver reflects the duodenum and the pancreatic head from the retroperitoneum, allowing access to the infrahepatic inferior vena cava as well as to the distal common bile duct, the duodenum, and the pancreatic head.

tive vascular repair. Control of the injured vessel, both proximally and distally, is obtained if this has not already been done. The vascular injury is identified and adequately debrided, and continuity is reestablished. If the vascular injury is not amenable to ligation or primary repair, autogenous tissue is procured and used as either a patch or an interposition graft. If no suitable autogenous tissue is available, synthetic material must be considered for use as a vascular conduit. In cases of aortic or iliac arterial injury, primary ligation with subsequent extra-anatomic bypass is an acceptable alternative.

REPAIR OF DAMAGED OR DEVITALIZED BOWEL

The next priority is repair of enteric injuries. Because of the large size of the stomach and its rich vascularity, most gastric wounds can be repaired primarily. In general, small-bowel injuries that involve less than 50% of the circumference after debridement can be repaired primarily with either a one-layer or a two-layer closure. As a rule, single-layer closure is preferred because it is less likely to compromise the lumen of the bowel. If multiple enterotomies or large areas of devitalized tissue in close proximity are present, segmental enterectomy with primary anastomosis is a more prudent option. The entero-enterostomy can be performed as either a hand-sewn or a stapled anastomosis; the latter tends to be more expeditious. Solitary injuries to the colon that do not have to be resected and are not associated with shock, massive blood transfusion, or significant contamination can be repaired primarily. Large or multiple injuries located in the right colon are best managed with a right hemicolectomy followed by primary ileocolic anastomosis. Multiple or large injuries in the left colon are best treated with resection followed by proximal diversion and distal limb exteriorization. If distal diversion is impossible because of inadequate

Figure 5 Control of a retrohepatic vena caval injury is facilitated by the atriocaval shunt technique, in which a chest tube or an endotracheal tube with extra side holes cut in it is passed caudad through the right atrial appendage beyond the level of the inferior vena caval injury. Tourniquets are placed on the inferior vena cava above and below the liver, and the portal triad is clamped.

Figure 6 Retention sutures may be used to bolster fascial closure in wounds at high risk for breakdown. (*a*) Sutures are placed in the subfascial plane. (*b*) The defect is approximated, and the sutures are tied over skin bridges.

length, a Hartmann procedure can be performed. When significant left colon injury occurs in association with shock or gross contamination, proximal diversion should be considered.

REPAIR OF RETROPERITONEAL INJURIES

Once injuries within the peritoneal cavity have been addressed, the retroperitoneum should be inspected again, with particular attention paid to the possibility of hematoma expansion. Zonal distribution and mechanism of injury are the two important determinants governing the decision whether to explore a retroperitoneal hematoma. All zone 1 hematomas should be explored regardless of the mechanism: they signal possible aortic, vena caval, duodenal, or pancreatic injury. Zone 2 and 3 hematomas should be explored if the patient sustained a penetrating injury. Generally, except for expanding zone 2 hematomas, zone 2 and 3 hematomas need not be explored in cases of blunt trauma. Even in blunt trauma patients with pelvic fractures, zone 3 hematomas are not explored if one is certain that there is no injury to the dis-

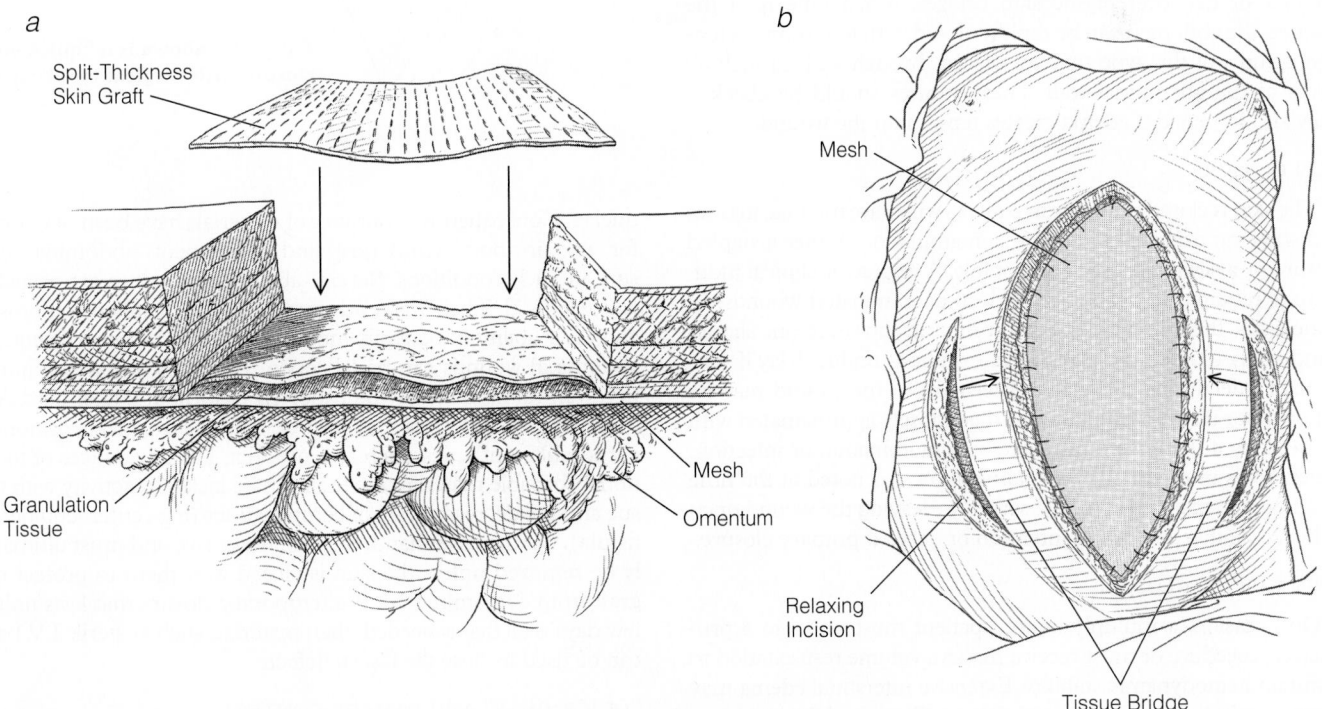

Figure 7 Mesh may be used for temporary or permanent abdominal closure in patients at risk for increased abdominal pressure. (*a*) Mesh is sutured into the fascial plane. (*b*) The abdominal defect is closed with mesh.

tal aorta or the iliac vessels. Before exploration of retroperitoneal hematomas, it is important to gain proximal vascular control to minimize hemorrhage once the retroperitoneal tamponade effect is lost. Vascular injuries discovered at this juncture should be repaired as discussed earlier (see above). Injuries to retroperitoneal organs (e.g., kidneys, pancreas, or adrenals) may be treated with debridement or resection with drainage as indicated.

Closure

GENERAL TECHNIQUE

Once the abdominal exploration has been completed, the abdomen should be copiously irrigated with a balanced salt solution. Generally, the optimal closure technique is chosen on the basis of five main considerations: the amount of blood lost, the volume of fluid received, the degree of contamination present, the patient's nutritional status, and the patient's overall stability. In some cases, the speed with which a closure can be performed may be the determining factor. Every effort should be made to close the fascia primarily. There are several methods that can be used to accomplish this. The most commonly used technique involves placement of a continuous monofilament suture. The major benefit of this type of closure is that it can be done relatively quickly. Alternatively, the fascia can be closed with interrupted sutures. There is no difference between the two techniques with respect to the rate of fascial dehiscence; however, the extent of the dehiscence is generally more limited with the interrupted suture method. Whichever method is used, the most important technical point is the necessity of avoiding excessive tension on the tissue.

Large monofilament sutures placed at intervals within the standard closure can serve as retention sutures [see Figure 6]. These sutures are used to support standard closure methods in patients who are at increased risk for fascial dehiscence and wound breakdown. They can be tied over bolsters fashioned from a red rubber catheter or tied over plastic skin bridges. When time is of the essence, the abdomen can be rapidly closed with four or five retention sutures of this type that are placed through and through all layers of the abdominal wall. These sutures should be checked daily and loosened if edema creates tension on the wound.

SKIN CLOSURE

The skin is closed primarily in patients who have minimal injuries and show no evidence of enteric contamination. Either a stapled closure or a sewn closure is acceptable. A degree of clinical judgment is required in dealing with clean-contaminated wounds. In some cases, the skin may be closed primarily; however, one should stand ready to open the wound again without undue delay if subsequent infection is suspected. Alternatively, the wound may be left open for three to five days and then loosely approximated with Steri-Strips if there is no evidence of contamination or infection. When gross intraperitoneal contamination was noted at the time of celiotomy, the patient is best served by leaving the wound open to heal by either secondary intention or delayed primary closure.

OPEN FASCIAL CLOSURE

On occasion, a multiply injured patient must undergo a protracted procedure or must receive massive volume resuscitation to maintain hemodynamic stability. Extensive interstitial edema may occur, precluding primary fascial closure. Closure of the abdomen in these circumstances may result in compromise of respiratory function or increased intra-abdominal pressure and its attendant se-

Figure 8 Shown is a "quick out" closure with surgical towel clips.

quelae. Consequently, a number of materials have been developed for use in both temporary and permanent abdominal closure in such conditions. Several absorbable meshes are available [see Figure 7]. Their main advantages are their inherent porosity and their ability to be easily incorporated into tissue. Subsequent abdominal wounds can be left open to heal by secondary intention; ventral hernias may be expected to form at a later date. Abdominal fascial defects may also be closed with sheets of nonincorporable synthetics, such as Gore-Tex. The advantages of these nonabsorbable materials are their innate lack of reactivity with tissue and the decreased rate of complications (e.g., enterocutaneous fistula). On the other hand, they are expensive and must ultimately be removed unless the skin is closed over them to protect the graft from contamination. If a temporary closure that lasts only a few days is all that is needed, then materials such as sterile I.V. bags can be used to close the fascial defect.

"QUICK OUTS" AND DAMAGE CONTROL

In grossly unstable or coagulopathic patients in whom surgical bleeding and contamination have been controlled, rapid abdominal closure may be necessary with the proviso that further exploration will be required. The basic objectives of the closure techniques used in these situations are control of peritoneal contamination and maintenance of intra-abdominal tamponade. One example of such a "quick out" is the use of towel clips to approximate skin [see Figure 8] in conjunction with a bioocclusive dressing for control of contamination. Another technique involves placement of a sterile plastic barrier within the fascial defect, followed by insertion of several closed suction drains over which open laparotomy pads are placed. Subsequently, an adherent bioocclusive sheet is draped over the abdominal wall to minimize thermal and insensible water losses.

Recommended Reading

Blaisdell FW, Trunkey DD: Abdominal Trauma. Thieme Medical Publishers, New York, 1993

Donovan AJ: Trauma Surgery. Mosby–Year Book Co, St Louis, 1994

Greenfield LJ: Complications in Surgery and Trauma. JB Lippincott Co, Grand Rapids, Michigan, 1990

Ivatury RR, Cayten CG: The Textbook of Penetrating Trauma. Williams & Wilkins, Baltimore, 1996

Mattox KL: Complications of Trauma. Churchill Livingstone, New York, 1994

Mattox KL, Feliciano DV, Moore EE: Trauma, 4th ed. Appleton & Lange, Stamford, Connecticut, 1998

Maull KI, Rodriguez A, Wiles CE: Complications in Trauma and Critical Care. WB Saunders Co, Philadelphia, 1996

Thal ER, Weigelt JA, Carrico CJ: Operative Trauma Management: An Atlas, 2nd ed. McGraw-Hill, New York, 2002

Acknowledgments

Figures 1, 4, and 5   Susan Brust, C.M.I.
Figures 2 and 3   Carol Donner.
Figures 6 through 8   Tom Moore. Adapted from *Operative Trauma Management: An Atlas*, by C. J. Carrico, E. R. Thal, and J. A. Weigelt. Appleton & Lange, Stamford, Connecticut, 1998.

7 INJURIES TO THE LIVER, BILIARY TRACT, SPLEEN, AND DIAPHRAGM

Jon M. Burch, M.D., and Ernest E. Moore, M.D.

Assessment and Management of Injuries to the Liver, Biliary Tract, Spleen, and Diaphragm

Injuries to the Liver

ASSESSMENT

The initial step in the management of penetrating abdominal injuries and of blunt abdominal injuries in cases when nonoperative treatment is contraindicated or has failed is exploratory laparotomy [*see III:6 Operative Exposure of Abdominal Injuries and Closure of the Abdomen*].

Visualization of the right lobe of the liver is hindered by the lobe's posterior attachments and by the right lower costal margin. Exposure of the right lobe is facilitated by elevating the right costal margin with a large Richardson retractor. Further exposure can be achieved with mobilization, which requires division of the right triangular and coronary ligaments. In dividing the superior coronary ligament, care must be taken not to injure the lateral wall of the right hepatic vein; in dividing the inferior coronary ligament, care must be taken not to injure the right adrenal gland (which is vulnerable because it lies directly beneath the peritoneal reflection) or the retrohepatic vena cava. When the ligaments have been divided, the right lobe of the liver can be rotated medially into the surgical field. Mobilization of the left lobe poses no unusual problems other than the risk of injury to the left hepatic vein, the left inferior phrenic vein, and the retrohepatic vena cava.

If optimal exposure of the junction of the hepatic veins and the retrohepatic vena cava is necessary, the midline abdominal incision can be extended by means of a median sternotomy. The pericardium and the diaphragm can then be divided toward the center of the inferior vena cava. This combination of incisions provides superb exposure of the hepatic veins and the retrohepatic vena cava while avoiding injury to the phrenic nerves.

The American Association for the Surgery of Trauma's Committee on Organ Injury Scaling has developed a grading system for classifying injuries to the liver [*see Table 1 and Figure 1*].[1] Hepatic injuries are graded on a scale of I to VI, with I representing superficial lacerations and small subcapsular hematomas and VI representing avulsion of the liver from the vena cava. Isolated injuries that are not extensive (grades I to III) often require little or no treatment; however, extensive parenchymal injuries and those involving the juxtahepatic veins (grades IV and V) may require complex maneuvers for successful treatment, and hepatic avulsion (grade VI) is lethal.

Clamping of the hepatic pedicle—the Pringle maneuver—is a helpful technique for evaluating grade IV and V hepatic injuries [*see Figure 2*]. This maneuver allows one to distinguish between hemorrhage from branches of the hepatic artery or the portal vein, which ceases when the clamp is applied, and hemorrhage from the hepatic veins or the retrohepatic vena cava, which does not. When performing the Pringle maneuver, we prefer to tear the lesser omentum manually and place the clamp from the left side while guiding the posterior blade of the clamp through the foramen of Winslow with the aid of the left index finger. The advantages of this approach are the avoidance of injury to the structures within the hepatic pedicle, the assurance that the clamp will be properly placed the first time, and the inclusion of a replacing or accessory left hepatic artery between the blades of the clamp.

MANAGEMENT OF INJURIES

Techniques for Temporary Control of Hemorrhage

Temporary control of hemorrhage is essential for two reasons. First, during treatment of a major hepatic injury, ongoing hemorrhage may pose an immediate threat to the patient's life, and temporary control gives the anesthesiologist time to restore the circulating volume before further blood loss occurs. Second, multiple bleeding sites are common with both blunt and penetrating trauma, and if the liver is not the highest priority, temporary control of hepatic bleeding allows repair of other injuries without unnecessary blood loss. The most useful techniques for the temporary control of hepatic hemorrhage are manual compression, perihepatic packing, and the Pringle maneuver.

Periodic manual compression with the addition of laparotomy pads is useful in the treatment of complex hepatic injuries to provide time for resuscitation [*see Figure 3*].[2-4]

Perihepatic packing with carefully placed laparotomy pads is capable of controlling hemorrhage from almost all hepatic injuries.[5-9] The right costal margin is elevated, and the pads are strategically placed over and around the bleeding site [*see Figure 4*]. Additional pads may be placed between the liver and the diaphragm and between the liver and the anterior chest wall until the bleeding has been controlled. Ten to 15 pads may be required to control the hemorrhage from an extensive right lobar injury. Packing is not as effective for injuries of the left lobe, because with the abdomen open, there is insufficient abdominal and thoracic wall anterior to the left lobe to provide adequate compression. Fortunately, hemorrhage from the left lobe can be controlled by dividing the left triangular and coronary ligaments and compress-

Table 1   AAST Organ Injury Scales for Liver, Biliary Tract, Diaphragm, and Spleen

Injured Structure	AAST Grade	Characteristics of Injury	AIS-90 Score
Liver*	I	Hematoma: subcapsular, nonexpanding, < 10% surface area	2
		Laceration: capsular tear, nonbleeding, < 1 cm parenchymal depth	2
	II	Hematoma: subcapsular, nonexpanding, 10%–50% surface area; intraparenchymal, nonexpanding, < 10 cm in diameter	2
		Laceration: capsular tear, active bleeding, 1–3 cm parenchymal depth, < 10 cm in length	2
	III	Hematoma: subcapsular, > 50% surface area, expanding; ruptured subcapsular hematoma with active bleeding; intraparenchymal, > 10 cm or expanding	3
		Laceration: > 3 cm parenchymal depth	3
	IV	Hematoma: ruptured intraparenchymal hematoma with active bleeding	4
		Laceration: parenchymal disruption involving 25%–75% of hepatic lobe or 1–3 Couinaud's segments within a single lobe	4
	V	Laceration: parenchymal disruption involving > 75% of hepatic lobe or > 3 Couinaud's segments within a single lobe	5
		Vascular: juxtahepatic venous injuries (i.e., injuries to retrohepatic vena cava or central major hepatic veins)	5
	VI	Vascular: hepatic avulsion	5
Extrahepatic biliary tree*	I	Gallbladder contusion/hematoma	2
		Portal triad contusion	2
	II	Partial gallbladder avulsion from liver bed; cystic duct intact	2
		Laceration or perforation of gallbladder	2
	III	Complete gallbladder avulsion from liver bed	3
		Cystic duct laceration	3
	IV	Partial or complete right or left hepatic duct laceration	3
		Partial common hepatic duct or common bile duct laceration (< 50%)	3
	V	> 50% transection of common hepatic duct or common bile duct	3–4
		Combined right and left hepatic duct injuries	3–4
		Intraduodenal or intrapancreatic bile duct injuries	3–4
Diaphragm†	I	Contusion	2
	II	Laceration < 2 cm	3
	III	Laceration 2–10 cm	3
	IV	Laceration > 10 cm, with tissue loss < 25 cm²	3
	V	Laceration with tissue loss > 25 cm²	3
Spleen*	I	Hematoma: subcapsular, nonexpanding, < 10% surface area	2
		Laceration: capsular tear, nonbleeding, < 1 cm parenchymal depth	2
	II	Hematoma: subcapsular, nonexpanding, 10%–50% surface area; intraparenchymal, nonexpanding, < 5 cm in diameter	2
		Laceration: capsular tear, active bleeding, 1–3 cm parenchymal depth, not involving a trabecular vessel	2
	III	Hematoma: subcapsular, > 50% surface area or expanding; ruptured subcapsular hematoma with active bleeding; intraparenchymal, > 5 cm or expanding	3
		Laceration: > 3 cm parenchymal depth or involving trabecular vessels	3
	IV	Hematoma: ruptured intraparenchymal hematoma with active bleeding	4
		Laceration: laceration involving segmental or hilar vessels producing major devascularization (> 25% of spleen)	4
	V	Laceration: completely shattered spleen	5
		Vascular: hilar vascular injury that devascularizes spleen	5

*Advance one grade for multiple injuries, up to grade III.
†Advance one grade for bilateral injuries, up to grade III.
AAST—American Association for the Surgery of Trauma

Figure 1   **Shown is an algorithm for the treatment of hepatic injuries.**

ing the lobe between the hands. Two complications may be encountered with the packing of hepatic injuries. First, tight packing compresses the inferior vena cava, decreases venous return, and reduces left ventricular filling; hypovolemic patients may not tolerate the resultant decrease in cardiac output. Second, perihepatic packing forces the right diaphragm superiorly and impairs its motion; this may lead to increased airway pressures and decreased tidal volume. Careful consideration of the patient's condition is necessary to determine whether the risk of these complications outweighs the risk of additional blood loss.

The Pringle maneuver is often used as an adjunct to packing for the temporary control of hemorrhage.[3] Over the years, the length of time for which surgeons believe a Pringle maneuver can be maintained without causing irreversible ischemic damage to the liver has increased. Several authors have documented the maintenance of a Pringle maneuver for longer than 1 hour in patients with complex injuries, without appreciable hepatic damage.[4,10] When a life-threatening hepatic injury is encountered on entry into the abdomen, the Pringle maneuver should be performed immediately and perihepatic packs placed. This combination of techniques should eliminate all hepatopetal blood flow and control retrograde venous bleeding.

Another technique for temporary control of hepatic hemorrhage is the application of a tourniquet or a liver clamp.[11] Once the bleeding lobe is mobilized, a 2.5 cm Penrose drain is wrapped around the liver near the anatomic division between the left lobe and the right. The drain is stretched until hemorrhage ceases, and tension is maintained by clamping the drain. Unfortunately, tourniquets are difficult to use: they tend to slip off or tear through the parenchyma if placed over an injured area. An alternative is the use of a liver clamp; however, the application of such devices is hindered by the variability in the size and shape of the liver.

Juxtahepatic venous injuries are technically challenging and often lethal. Complex procedures may be required for temporary control of these large veins. Of these procedures, the most important are hepatic vascular isolation with clamps, placement of the atriocaval shunt, and use of the Moore-Pilcher balloon.

Hepatic vascular isolation is accomplished by executing a Pringle maneuver, clamping the aorta at the diaphragm, and clamping the suprarenal and suprahepatic vena cava.[12] In patients scheduled for elective procedures, this technique has enjoyed nearly uniform success, but in trauma patients, the results have been disappointing. The relative ineffectiveness of hepatic vascular isolation with clamps in this setting is presumably due to the inability of a patient

Figure 2 **The Pringle maneuver controls arterial and portal vein hemorrhage from the liver. Any hemorrhage that continues must come from the hepatic veins.**

in shock to tolerate an acute reduction in left ventricular filling pressure; on occasion, sudden death has occurred on placement of the venous clamps.[13] If, however, a trauma patient requiring hepatic vascular isolation has been maintained in a relatively normal physiologic condition, it is reasonable to consider this method.

A new approach to exposure of complex injuries to the retrohepatic vena cava and the hepatic veins has recently been developed.[14] Vascular isolation of the liver is achieved by means of the clamping technique, and the suprahepatic vena cava is divided between vascular clamps. The liver and the suprahepatic vena cava are then rotated anteriorly to provide direct access to the posterior aspect of the retrohepatic vena cava. Anterior injuries of the large veins are repaired through an incision in the posterior aspect of the retrohepatic vena cava.

The atriocaval shunt was designed to achieve hepatic vascular isolation while still permitting some venous blood from below the diaphragm to flow through the shunt into the right atrium.[4] After a few early successes, the initial enthusiasm for the atriocaval shunt declined as high mortalities associated with its use began to be reported.[15-20] Surgeons' lack of familiarity with the technique; manipulation of a cold, acidotic heart; and poor patient selection have all contributed to the poor overall results.[13] A variation on the original atriocaval shunt has been described in which a 9 mm endotracheal tube is substituted for the usual large chest tube [*see Figure 5*].[21] The balloon of the endotracheal tube makes it unnecessary to surround the suprarenal vena cava with an umbilical tape. This minor change eliminates one of the most difficult maneuvers required for the original shunt procedure: because hemorrhage must be controlled by posterior pressure on the liver during the insertion of the shunt, access to the suprarenal vena cava is severely restricted, and thus, surrounding this vessel with an umbilical tape is almost impossible. A side hole must be cut in the

tube to allow blood to enter the right atrium. Care must be taken to avoid damage to the integral inflation channel for the balloon.

An alternative to the atriocaval shunt is the Moore-Pilcher balloon.[22] This device is inserted through the femoral vein and advanced into the retrohepatic vena cava. When the balloon is properly positioned and inflated, it occludes the hepatic veins and the vena cava, thus achieving vascular isolation. The catheter itself is hollow, and appropriately placed holes below the balloon permit blood to flow into the right atrium, in much the same way as the atriocaval shunt. At present, the survival rate for patients with juxtahepatic venous injuries who are treated with this device is similar to that for patients treated with the atriocaval shunt.[18]

Surgeons who attempt hepatic vascular isolation should be aware that none of these techniques provide complete hemostasis. Drainage from the right adrenal vein and the inferior phrenic veins and persistent hepatopetal flow resulting from unrecognized replacing or accessory left hepatic arteries contribute to this problem. The relatively small volume of blood that continues to flow after vascular isolation is readily removed by means of suction.

An adjunct to vascular isolation with clamps is venovenous bypass. This technique provides vascular decompression for the small bowel and maintains high cardiac filling pressures, which are often necessary. Venovenous bypass is accomplished by placing catheters in the inferior vena cava via the femoral vein and in the superior mesenteric vein via the inferior mesenteric vein. A centrifugal pump withdraws blood from these veins and pumps it into the superior vena cava through a third catheter placed in the jugular vein.

Techniques for Definitive Management of Injuries

Techniques available for the definitive management of hepatic injuries range from manual compression to hepatic transplantation. Grade I or II lacerations of the hepatic parenchyma can generally be controlled with manual compression. If these injuries do not respond to manual compression, they can often be controlled with topical hemostatic measures.

Figure 3 **Manual compression of large hepatic injuries temporarily controls blood loss in hypovolemic patients until the circulating blood volume can be restored.**

Figure 4 **Perihepatic packing is often effective in managing extensive parenchymal injuries. It has also been successfully employed for grade V juxtahepatic venous injuries.**

The simplest of these measures is electrocauterization, which can often control small bleeding vessels near the surface of the liver (though the machine's power output may have to be increased). Bleeding from raw surfaces of the liver that does not respond to the electrocautery may respond to the argon beam coagulator. This device imparts less heat to the surrounding hepatic tissue and creates a more consistent eschar, which enhances hemostasis. Also useful in similar situations is microcrystalline collagen in the powdered form. The powder is placed on a clean 10 × 10 cm sponge and applied directly to the oozing surface, with pressure maintained on the sponge for 5 to 10 minutes. Thrombin can also be applied topically to minor bleeding injuries by saturating either a gelatin foam sponge or a microcrystalline collagen pad and pressing it to the bleeding site.

Fibrin glue has been used in treating both superficial and deep lacerations and appears to be the most effective topical agent. It can also be injected deep into bleeding gunshot and stab wound tracts to prevent extensive dissection and blood loss. Fibrin glue is made by mixing concentrated human fibrinogen (cryoprecipitate) with a solution containing bovine thrombin and calcium. Because a coagulum forms quickly, the fibrinogen and the thrombin-calcium solution are placed in separate syringes joined with a Y connector, so that they are not mixed until immediately before application. Spray-on applicators have also been used. Topical hemostasis with fibrin glue became very popular after the publication of reports of large series of patients with serious hepatic injuries that were successfully managed with this material.[2,23,24] The initial enthusiasm, however, was tempered by subsequent reports of fatal anaphylactic reactions and hypotension temporally related to the application of fibrin glue.[25,26] The current role of this agent in the treatment of hepatic injuries remains to be defined.[27]

Although some grade III and IV lacerations respond to topical measures, many do not. In these instances, one option is to suture the hepatic parenchyma. Although this hemostatic technique has been maligned as a cause of hepatic necrosis, it still is frequently used.[3,4,10,17,28,29] Suturing of the hepatic parenchyma is often employed to control persistently bleeding lacerations less than 3 cm in depth; it is also an appropriate alternative for deeper lacerations if the patient cannot tolerate the further hemorrhage associated with hepatotomy and selective ligation. If, however, the capsule of the liver has been stripped away by the injury, this technique is far less effective.

The preferred suture material is 0 or 2-0 chromic catgut attached to a large, blunt-tipped, curved needle; the large diameter prevents the suture from pulling through Glisson's capsule. For shallow lacerations, a simple continuous suture may be used to approximate the edges of the laceration. For deeper lacerations, interrupted horizontal mattress sutures may be placed parallel to the edges. When tying sutures, one may be sure that adequate tension has been achieved when hemorrhage ceases or the liver blanches around the suture.

Most sources of venous hemorrhage can be managed with parenchymal sutures. Even injuries to the retrohepatic vena cava and the hepatic veins have been successfully tamponaded by

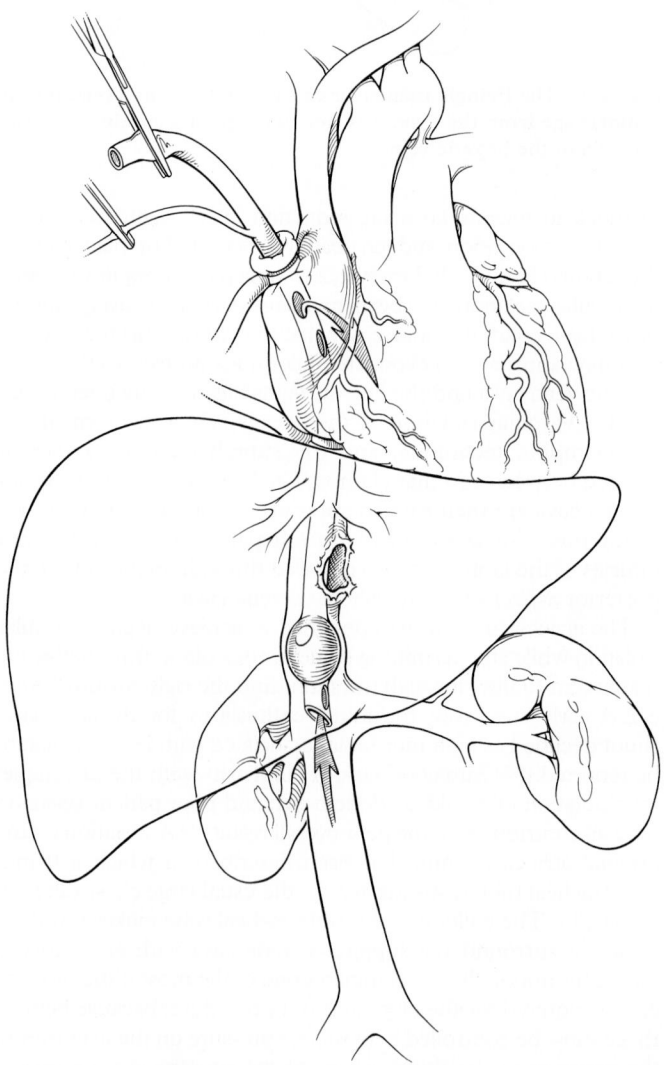

Figure 5 **Shown is a method of achieving hepatic vascular isolation with a 9 mm endotracheal tube.**

Figure 6 Hepatotomy with selective ligation is an important technique for controlling hemorrhage from deep (usually penetrating) lacerations. This technique includes finger fracture to extend the length and depth of the wound (*a*), division of vessels or ducts encountered (*b*), and repair of any injuries to major veins (*c*).

closing the hepatic parenchyma over the bleeding vessels.[13,30] Venous hemorrhage caused by penetrating wounds traversing the central portion of the liver may be managed by closing the entrance and exit wounds with interrupted horizontal mattress sutures. Although this measure may lead to the formation of intrahepatic hematomas that may then become infected, the risk is reasonable compared with the risks posed by an intracaval shunt or a deep hepatotomy. Still, suturing of the hepatic parenchyma is not always successful in controlling hemorrhage, particularly hemorrhage from the larger branches of the hepatic artery. If it fails, one must acknowledge the failure promptly and remove the sutures so that the wound can be explored.

Hepatotomy with selective ligation of bleeding vessels is an important technique that is usually reserved for deep or transhepatic penetrating wounds. Most authorities prefer it to parenchymal suturing[3,4,10,31,32]; some even favor it over placement of an atriocaval shunt for exposure and repair of juxtahepatic venous injuries.[20] The finger-fracture technique is used to extend the length and depth of a laceration or a missile tract until the bleeding vessels can be identified and controlled [*see Figure 6*]. It should be remembered that considerable blood loss may be incurred with the division of viable hepatic tissue in the pursuit of bleeding from deep penetrating wounds.

An adjunct to parenchymal suturing or hepatotomy is the use of the omentum to fill large defects in the liver and to buttress hepatic sutures. The rationale for this use of the omentum is that it provides an excellent source for macrophages and fills a potential dead space with viable tissue.[33] In addition, the omentum can provide a little extra support for parenchymal sutures, often enough to prevent them from cutting through Glisson's capsule.

Hepatic arterial ligation may be appropriate for patients with arterial hemorrhage from deep within the liver[34]; however, it plays only a limited role in the overall treatment of hepatic injuries, because it does not stop hemorrhage from the portal and hepatic venous systems.[35] Its primary role is in the management of deep lobar injuries when application of the Pringle

maneuver results in the cessation of arterial hemorrhage. If the bleeding from the wound stops once the left or right hepatic artery is isolated and clamped, hepatic arterial ligation is a reasonable alternative to deep hepatotomy. Generally, ligation of the right or left hepatic artery is well tolerated; however, ligation of the proper hepatic artery (distal to the origin of the gastroduodenal artery) may produce hepatic necrosis.[36]

An alternative to suturing the entrance and exit wounds of a transhepatic penetrating injury or to performing an extensive hepatotomy is the use of an intrahepatic balloon.[37] These devices are hand-crafted by the surgeon in the OR. One method of fashioning such a device is to tie a 2.5 cm Penrose drain to a hollow catheter [*see Figure 7*]. The balloon is then inserted into the bleeding wound and inflated with a soluble contrast agent. If the hemorrhage is controlled, a stopcock or clamp is used to occlude the catheter and maintain the inflation. (It should be noted that the balloon catheter may not be able to generate sufficient intraparenchymal pressure to tamponade major arterial hemorrhage.) The balloon is left in the abdomen and removed at a subsequent operation after 24 to 48 hours. The hemorrhage may recur when the balloon is deflated.

Resectional debridement is indicated for peripheral portions of nonviable hepatic parenchyma. Except in rare circumstances, the amount of tissue removed should not exceed 25% of the liver. Resectional debridement is performed by means of the finger-fracture technique and is appropriate for selected patients with grade III to grade V lacerations. Because additional blood loss occurs during removal of nonviable tissue, this procedure should be reserved for patients who are in sound physiologic condition and can tolerate additional blood loss.

Perihepatic packing is the most significant advance in the treatment of hepatic injuries to occur in the past 20 years. The practice of packing hepatic injuries is not a new one, but the concepts and techniques associated with it have changed. In the past, liver lacerations were packed with yards of gauze, and one end of the gauze strip was brought out of the abdomen through a separate stab wound[38]; the remainder of the gauze was then teased out of the wound over a period of days. Unfortunately, this approach often led to abdominal infection and failed to control the hemorrhage, and as a result, it eventually fell from favor. The current approach is not to place packing material in the laceration itself but rather to place it over and around the injury to compress the wound by compressing the liver between the anterior chest wall, the diaphragm, and the retroperitoneum.[5-9] The abdomen is closed, and the patient is taken to the SICU for resuscitation and correction of metabolic derangements. Within 24 hours, the patient is returned to the OR for removal of the packs. Perihepatic packing is indicated for grade IV and V lacerations and for less severe injuries in patients who have a coagulopathy caused by associated injuries.

A technique that may be attempted if packing fails is to wrap the injured portion of the liver with a fine porous material (e.g., polyglycolic acid mesh) after the injured lobe has been mobilized.[39,40] Using a continuous suture or a linear stapler, the surgeon constructs a tight-fitting stocking that encloses the injured lobe. Blood clots beneath the mesh, which results in tamponade of the hepatic injury. Although this technique is intuitively attractive, to date it has achieved only limited success.

The final alternative for patients with extensive unilobar injuries is anatomic hepatic resection. In elective circumstances, anatomic lobectomies can be performed with excellent results; however, in the setting of trauma, the mortality associated with this procedure exceeds 50% in most series.[28,29,31,41-43] Consequently, hepatic resection is rarely performed in trauma patients, having been largely replaced by perihepatic packing, resectional debridement, and hepatotomy with selective ligation. Nonetheless, there are two circumstances in which anatomic resection may still be a reasonable choice. The first is prompt resection in patients with extensive injuries of the lateral segment of the left lobe; because hemorrhage from the left lobe is easily controlled with bimanual compression, the risk of uncontrolled blood loss is not as high as with left or right anatomic lobectomies. The second is delayed anatomic lobectomy in patients whose hemorrhage has been controlled but whose left or right lobe is nonviable as a result of ligation or thrombosis of essential blood vessels. Because of the large mass of necrotic liver tissue, there is a high risk of subsequent infection or persistent hyperinflammation, setting the stage for the multiple organ dysfunction syndrome (MODS). The necrotic lobe should be removed as soon as the patient's condition permits.

Hepatic transplantation has been successful in several trauma patients with devastating hepatic injuries who required total hepatectomy.[44-47] In each of these five patients, the mean anhepatic period was approximately 24 hours. All five survived the transplantation, though two died of disseminated viral infections within two months of the procedure. Two others were alive and well 16 and 17 months after the procedure; no follow-up was reported for the fifth patient. Hepatic transplantation represents the ultimate expression of aggressive trauma care. All other injuries must be well delineated (particularly injuries to the CNS), and the patient must have an excellent chance of survival aside from the hepatic injury. High cost and limited availability

of donors restrict the performance of hepatic transplantation for trauma, but it seems probable that this procedure will continue to be performed in extraordinary circumstances.

Subcapsular Hematoma

An uncommon but troublesome hepatic injury is subcapsular hematoma, which arises when the parenchyma of the liver is disrupted by blunt trauma but Glisson's capsule remains intact. Subcapsular hematomas range in severity from minor blisters on the surface of the liver to ruptured central hematomas accompanied by severe hemorrhage [see Table 1]. They may be recognized either at the time of the operation or in the course of CT scanning.

Regardless of how the lesion is diagnosed, subsequent decision making is often difficult. If a grade I or II subcapsular hematoma—that is, a hematoma involving less than 50% of the surface of the liver that is not expanding and is not ruptured—is discovered during an exploratory laparotomy, it should be left alone. If the hematoma is explored, hepatotomy with selective ligation may be required to control bleeding vessels. Even if hepatotomy with ligation is effective, one must still contend with diffuse hemorrhage from the large denuded surface, and packing may also be required. A hematoma that is expanding during operation (grade III) may have to be explored. Such lesions are often the result of uncontrolled arterial hemorrhage, and packing alone may not be successful. An alternative strategy is to pack the liver to control venous hemorrhage, close the abdomen, and transport the patient to the interventional radiology suite for hepatic arteriography and embolization of the bleeding vessels. Ruptured grades III and IV hematomas are treated with exploration and selective ligation, with or without packing.

Perihepatic Drainage

For years, all hepatic injuries were drained via Penrose drains brought out laterally or through the bed of the resected 12th rib;

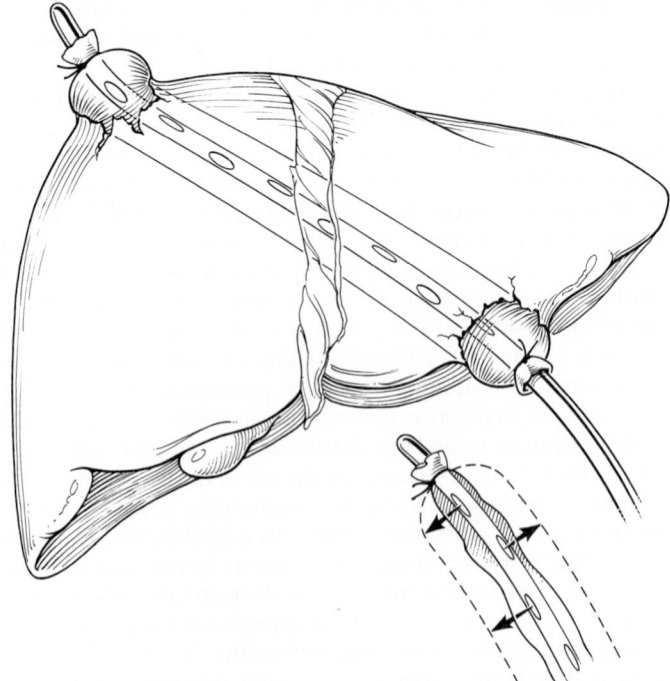

Figure 7 **A hand-made balloon from a Robinson catheter and a Penrose drain may effectively control hemorrhage from a transhepatic penetrating wound.**

recently, the use of large sump drains and closed suction drains has become increasingly popular. Several prospective and retrospective studies have demonstrated that the use of either Penrose or sump drains carries a higher risk of intra-abdominal infection than the use of either closed suction drains or no drains at all.[48-51] It is clear that if drains are to be used, closed suction devices are preferred. What is not clear, however, is whether closed suction drains are better or worse than no drains, particularly in view of the advent of percutaneous catheter drainage. Patients who are initially treated with perihepatic packing may also require drainage; however, drainage is not indicated at the initial procedure, given that the patient will be returned to the OR within the next 48 hours.

MORTALITY AND COMPLICATIONS

Overall mortality for patients with hepatic injuries is approximately 10%. The most common cause of death is exsanguination, followed by MODS and intracranial injury. Three generalizations may be made regarding the risk of death and complications: (1) both increase in proportion to the injury grade and to the complexity of repair; (2) hepatic injuries caused by blunt trauma carry a higher mortality than those caused by penetrating trauma; and (3) infectious complications occur more often with penetrating trauma.

Postoperative hemorrhage occurs in a small percentage of patients with hepatic injuries. The source may be either a coagulopathy or a missed vascular injury (usually to an artery). In most instances of persistent postoperative hemorrhage, the patient is best served by being returned to the OR. Arteriography with embolization may be considered in selected patients. If coagulation studies indicate that a coagulopathy is the likely cause of postoperative hemorrhage, there is little to be gained by reoperation until the coagulopathy is corrected.

Perihepatic infections occur in fewer than 5% of patients with significant hepatic injuries. They develop more often in patients with penetrating injuries than in patients with blunt injuries, presumably because of the greater frequency of enteric contamination. An elevated temperature and a higher than normal white blood cell count after postoperative day 3 or 4 should prompt a search for intra-abdominal infection. In the absence of pneumonia, an infected line, or urinary tract infection, an abdominal CT scan with intravenous and upper gastrointestinal contrast should be obtained. Many perihepatic infections can be treated with CT-guided drainage; however, infected hematomas and infected necrotic liver tissue cannot be expected to respond to percutaneous drainage. Right 12th rib resection remains an excellent approach for posterior infections and provides superior drainage in refractory cases.

Bilomas are loculated collections of bile that may or may not be infected. If a biloma is infected, it is essentially an abscess and should be treated as such; if it is sterile, it will eventually be resorbed. Biliary ascites is caused by disruption of a major bile duct. Reoperation after the establishment of appropriate drainage is the prudent course. Even if the source of the leaking bile can be identified, primary repair of the injured duct is unlikely to be successful. It is best to wait until a firm fistulous communication is established with adequate drainage.

Biliary fistulas occur in approximately 3% of patients with major hepatic injuries.[42] They are usually of little consequence and generally close without specific treatment. In rare instances, a fistulous communication with intrathoracic structures forms in patients with associated diaphragmatic injuries, resulting in a bronchobiliary or pleurobiliary fistula. Because of the pressure differential between the biliary tract and the thoracic cavity, most of these fistulas must be closed operatively; however, we know of one pleurobiliary fistula that closed spontaneously after endoscopic sphincterotomy and stent placement.

Hemorrhage from hepatic injuries is often treated without identifying and controlling each bleeding vessel individually, and arterial pseudoaneurysms may develop as a consequence. As the pseudoaneurysm enlarges, it may rupture into the parenchyma of the liver, into a bile duct, or into an adjacent branch of the portal vein. Rupture into a bile duct results in hemobilia, which is characterized by intermittent episodes of right upper quadrant pain, upper gastrointestinal hemorrhage, and jaundice; rupture into a portal vein may result in portal vein hypertension with bleeding varices. Both of these complications are exceedingly rare and are best managed with hepatic arteriography and embolization.

Injuries to the Bile Ducts and Gallbladder

Injuries to the extrahepatic bile ducts [see Table 1] can be caused by either penetrating or blunt trauma; however, they are rare in either case.[52-55] The diagnosis is usually made by noting the accumulation of bile in the upper quadrant during laparotomy for treatment of associated injuries. Treatment of common bile duct (CBD) injuries after external trauma is complicated by the small size and thin wall of the normal duct, which render primary repair almost impossible except when the laceration is small and there is no tissue loss. When there is tissue loss or the laceration is larger than 25% to 50% of the diameter of the duct, the best treatment option is a Roux-en-Y choledochojejunostomy [see V:11 Biliary Tract Procedures].[56,57] Treatment of injuries to the left or right hepatic duct is even more difficult—so much so that we question whether repair should even be attempted under emergency conditions. If only one hepatic duct is injured, a reasonable approach is to ligate it and deal with any infections or atrophy of the lobe rather than to attempt repair.[58] If both ducts are injured, each should be intubated with a small catheter brought through the abdominal wall. Once the patient has recovered sufficiently, delayed repair is performed under elective conditions. Injuries to the intrapancreatic portion of the CBD are treated by dividing the duct at the superior border of the pancreas, ligating the distal portion, and performing a Roux-en-Y choledochojejunostomy.

The Roux-en-Y choledochojejunostomy is done in a single layer with interrupted 5-0 absorbable monofilament sutures. To prevent ischemia and possible stricture, no circumferential dissection of the duct is performed. A round patch of approximately the same diameter as the CBD is removed from the seromuscular layer of the small bowel, but the mucosa and submucosa are only perforated, not resected. The posterior row of sutures is placed first, with full-thickness bites taken through both the duct and the small bowel. The anterior row is then completed. Finally, three or four 3-0 polypropylene sutures are placed to secure the small bowel around the anastomosis to the connective tissue of the porta hepatis. The only purpose for these sutures is to spare the fragile anastomosis any potential tension. No T tubes or stents are employed. Closed suction drainage is added in the case of injuries to the intrapancreatic portion of the duct or at the surgeon's discretion.

Injuries to the gallbladder [see Table 1] are treated by means of either lateral repair with absorbable sutures or cholecystectomy; the decision between the two approaches depends on which is easier in a given situation. Cholecystostomy is rarely, if ever, indicated.

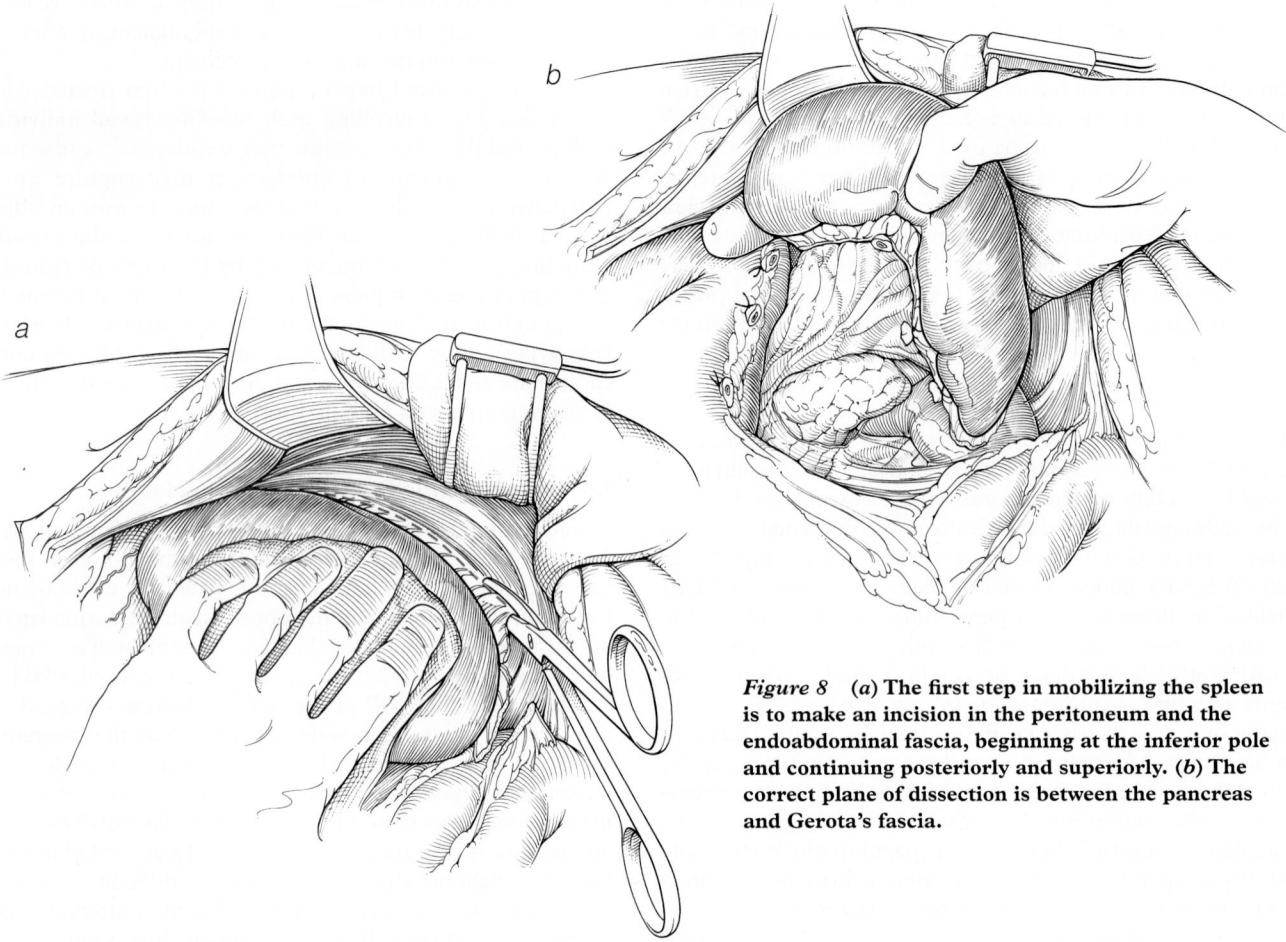

Figure 8 (*a*) **The first step in mobilizing the spleen is to make an incision in the peritoneum and the endoabdominal fascia, beginning at the inferior pole and continuing posteriorly and superiorly. (*b*) The correct plane of dissection is between the pancreas and Gerota's fascia.**

Injuries to the Spleen

Splenic injuries [*see Table 1*] are treated operatively by means of splenic repair (splenorrhaphy), partial splenectomy, or resection, depending on the extent of the injury and the condition of the patient.[59-63] Currently, there is considerable enthusiasm for splenic salvage as a consequence of the evolving trend toward nonoperative management of solid organ injuries and the growing concern about the rare but often fatal complication known as overwhelming postsplenectomy infection (OPSI). OPSI is caused by encapsulated bacteria (e.g., *Streptococcus pneumoniae, Haemophilus influenzae,* and *Neisseria meningitidis*) and is very resistant to treatment: mortality may exceed 50%.[59] OPSI occurs most often in young children and immunocompromised adults and is uncommon in otherwise healthy adults. For this reason, splenic salvage is attempted more vigorously in pediatric patients than in adult ones.

To ensure safe removal or repair, the spleen should be mobilized to the point where it can be brought to the surface of the abdominal wall without tension. To this end, the soft tissue attachments between the spleen and the splenic flexure of the colon must be divided. Next, an incision is made in the peritoneum and the endoabdominal fascia, beginning at the inferior pole, 1 to 2 cm lateral to the posterior peritoneal reflection of the spleen, and continuing posteriorly and superiorly until the esophagus is encountered [*see Figure 8a*]. Care must be taken not to pull on the spleen, so that it will not tear at the posterior peritoneal reflection, causing significant hemorrhage. Instead, the spleen should be rotated counterclockwise, with posterior pressure applied to expose the peritoneal reflection. It is often helpful to rotate the operating table 20° to the patient's right so that the weight of the abdominal viscera facilitates their retraction. A plane is thus established between the spleen and pancreas and Gerota's fascia that can be extended to the aorta [*see Figure 8b*]. With this step, mobilization is complete, and the spleen can be repaired or removed without any need to struggle to achieve adequate exposure.

Splenectomy is the usual treatment for hilar injuries or a pulverized splenic parenchyma. It is also indicated for lesser splenic injuries in patients who have multiple abdominal injuries and a coagulopathy, and it is frequently necessary in patients in whom splenic salvage attempts have failed. Partial splenectomy is suitable for patients in whom only a portion of the spleen (usually the superior or inferior half) has been destroyed. Once the damaged portion has been removed, the same methods used to control hemorrhage from hepatic parenchyma can be used to control hemorrhage from splenic parenchyma [*see Figure 9*]. When horizontal mattress sutures are placed across a raw edge, gentle compression of the parenchyma by an assistant facilitates hemostasis; when the sutures are tied and compression is released, the spleen will expand slightly and tighten the sutures further. Drains are never used after completion of the repair or resection.

If splenectomy is performed, vaccines effective against the encapsulated bacteria are administered. The pneumococcal vaccine is routinely given, and vaccines effective against *H. influenzae* and *N. meningitidis* should also be given if available.

Injuries to the Diaphragm

In cases of blunt trauma to the diaphragm, the injury is on the left side 75% of the time, presumably because the liver diffuses some of the energy on the right side. With both blunt and penetrating injuries [*see Table 1*], the diagnosis is suggested by an abnormality of the diaphragmatic shadow on chest x-ray. Many of these abnormalities are subtle, particularly with penetrating injuries, and further diagnostic evaluation may be warranted. The typical injury from blunt trauma is a tear in the central tendon; often, the tear is quite large. Regardless of the cause, acute injuries are repaired through an abdominal incision. Because of the concave shape of the diaphragm and the overlying anterior ribs, anterior diaphragmatic injuries may be difficult to suture. Repair is greatly facilitated by using a long Allis clamp to grasp part of the injury and evert the diaphragm. Lacerations are repaired with continuous No. 1 monofilament nonabsorbable sutures. Occasionally, with large avulsions or gunshot wounds accompanied by extensive tissue loss, polypropylene mesh is required to bridge the defect.

The explosive growth of laparoscopic procedures has led to the application of this technology for both diagnostic and therapeutic purposes in trauma patients. In a number of patients with low anterior thoracic stab wounds who otherwise were not candidates for a laparotomy, small diaphragmatic lacerations have been identified and repaired with laparoscopy and stapling.

Discussion

Nonoperative Treatment of Blunt Hepatic and Splenic Injury

Only a few years ago, blunt and penetrating hepatic and splenic injuries were managed in a similar fashion on the basis of a positive diagnostic peritoneal lavage or the probability of peritoneal penetration: a laparotomy was performed, and the injured organs were identified and treated. Currently, although penetrating abdominal injuries are still treated in the same way, nearly all children and 50% to 80% of adults with blunt hepatic and splenic injuries are treated without laparotomy.[64-76] This remarkable change was made possible by the development of the high-speed helical CT scanner, the replacement of diagnostic peritoneal lavage by ultrasonography, and the growth of interventional radiology.

The diagnosis of blunt abdominal trauma is suspected on the basis of the mechanism of injury and the presence of associated injuries (e.g., right or left lower rib fractures). In contemporary urban trauma centers, ultrasonographic examination of the abdomen may reveal a fluid stripe in Morrison's pouch, the left upper quadrant, or the pelvis, which suggests a hemoperitoneum. This observation prompts a CT scan of the abdomen, which delineates injuries of the liver or spleen. CT scanning is a less than optimal means of grading hepatic and splenic injuries; however, patients may be observed either in the SICU or on the ward, depending on the apparent severity of the parenchymal injury on the CT scan and the presence and extent of any associated injuries.[77,78]

The primary requirement for nonoperative therapy is hemodynamic stability.[63-72] To confirm stability, frequent assessment of vital signs and monitoring of the hematocrit are necessary. Continued hemorrhage occurs in 1% to 4% of patients.[65,66,68-73] Hypotension may develop, usually within the first 24 hours after hepatic injury but sometimes several days later, especially when splenic injury is present.[79,80] It is often an indication that operative intervention is necessary. A persistently falling hematocrit should be treated with packed red blood cell (PRBC) transfusions. If the hematocrit continues to fall after two or three units of PRBCs, embolization in the interventional radiology suite should be considered.[74] Overall, nonoperative treatment obviates laparotomy in more than 95% of cases.[65,66,68-73]

Out of concern over the risk of delayed hemorrhage or other complications, follow-up CT scans have often been recommended; unfortunately, there is no consensus as to when or even whether they should be obtained. Given that patients with grade I or II hepatic or splenic injuries rarely show progression of the lesion or other complications on routine follow-up CT scans, it is reasonable to omit such scans if patients' hematocrits remain stable and they are otherwise well. Patients with more extensive injuries often have a less predictable course, and CT scanning may be necessary to evaluate possible complications. Routine scanning before discharge, however, is unwarranted. On the other hand, patients who participate in vigorous or contact sports should have CT documentation of virtually complete healing before resuming those activities.

A more convenient and less expensive alternative to follow-up CT scanning is to monitor lesions ultrasonographically. Ultrasonographic monitoring is particularly useful for following up splenic injuries; however, it may not be useful for following up hepatic injuries, because the technology currently available is incapable of reliably imaging the entire liver.

Other complications of nonoperative therapy for blunt hepatic and splenic injuries occur in 2% to 5% of patients; these include missed abdominal injuries, parenchymal infarction,

Figure 9 Methods for controlling hemorrhage from the splenic parenchyma are similar to those for controlling hemorrhage from the hepatic parenchyma. Shown are interrupted mattress sutures across a raw edge of the spleen.

infection, and bile leakage (a complication associated solely with hepatic injuries).[65,68-71] Aseptic infarcts, infected hematomas, and bile collections are suspected on the basis of a clinical picture suggestive of infection and confirmed by CT-guided aspiration. Aseptic infarction usually does not necessitate operative intervention. Fluid collections are drained, with the method depending on the viscosity of the fluid: CT-guided drainage may be effective in treating thin collections, but operative intervention is required for thicker collections, those with solid components, and those for which percutaneous drainage was attempted without success. Extrahepatic bile collections should be drained percutaneously under CT guidance. Most biliary fistulas close spontaneously; endoscopic stent placement may hasten closure in recalcitrant cases.[81] Intrahepatic collections of blood and bile are managed expectantly. Complete absorption of large intrahepatic collections may take several months. If a collection becomes infected, CT-guided aspiration is performed and drainage obtained as described above.

Missed enteric and retroperitoneal injuries are another cause of failed nonoperative treatment. Such injuries are present in 1% to 4% of patients in whom nonoperative treatment is attempted.[65,68-71] High-quality images and expert interpretation minimize the number of missed injuries on CT scans but cannot eliminate them entirely. Therefore, patients must be watched carefully for the development of peritoneal irritation and other signs of intra-abdominal pathology.

References

1. Moore EE, Cogbill TH, Jurkovich GJ, et al: Organ injury scaling: spleen and liver (1994 revision). J Trauma 38:323, 1995

2. Hepatic trauma revisited. Feliciano DV, Pachter HL, Eds. Curr Probl Surg 26, 1986

3. Moore EE: Critical decisions in the management of hepatic trauma. Am J Surg 148:712, 1984

4. Feliciano DV, Mattox KL, Jordan GL, et al: Management of 1000 consecutive cases of hepatic trauma (1979–1984). Ann Surg 204:438, 1986

5. Feliciano DV, Mattox KL, Burch JM, et al: Packing for control of hepatic hemorrhage. J Trauma 26:738, 1986

6. Ivantury RR, Nallathambi M, Gunduz Y, et al: Liver packing for uncontrolled hemorrhage: a reappraisal. J Trauma 26:744, 1986

7. Carmona RH, Peck DZ, Lim RC: The role of packing and planned reoperation in severe hepatic trauma. J Trauma 24:779, 1984

8. Cue JI, Cryer HG, Miller FB, et al: Packing and planned reexploration for hepatic and retroperitoneal hemorrhage: critical refinements of a useful technique. J Trauma 30:1007, 1990

9. Beal SL: Fatal hepatic hemorrhage: an unresolved problem in the management of complex liver injuries. J Trauma 30:163, 1990

10. Pachter HL, Spencer FC, Hofstetter SR, et al: Significant trends in the treatment of hepatic trauma: experience with 411 injuries. Ann Surg 215:492, 1992

11. Murray DH Jr, Borge JD, Pouteau GG: Tourniquet control of liver bleeding. J Trauma 18:771, 1978

12. Heaney JP, Stanton WR, Halbert DS, et al: An improved technic for vascular isolation of the liver. Ann Surg 163:237, 1966

13. Burch JM, Feliciano DV, Mattox KL: The atriocaval shunt: facts and fiction. Ann Surg 207:555, 1988

14. Buechter KJ, Gomez GA, Zeppa R: A new technique for exposure of injuries at the confluence of the retrohepatic veins and the retrohepatic vena cava. J Trauma 30:328, 1990

15. Schrock T, Blaisdell FW, Matthewson C Jr: Management of blunt trauma to the liver and hepatic veins. Arch Surg 96:698, 1968

16. Bricker DL, Morton JR, Okies JE, et al: Surgical management of injuries to the vena cava: changing patterns of injury and newer techniques of repair. J Trauma 11:725, 1971

17. Yellin AE, Chaffee CB, Donovan AJ: Vascular isolation in treatment of juxtahepatic venous injuries. Arch Surg 102:566, 1971

18. Walt AJ: The mythology of hepatic trauma: or Babel revisited. Am J Surg 125:12, 1978

19. Millikan JS, Moore EE, Cogbill TH, et al: Inferior vena cava injuries: a continuing challenge. J Trauma 23:207, 1983

20. Pachter HL, Spencer FC, Hofstetter SR, et al: The management of juxtahepatic venous injuries without an atriocaval shunt. Surgery 99:569, 1986

21. Rovito PF: Atrial caval shunting in blunt hepatic vascular injury. Ann Surg 205:318, 1987

22. Pilcher DB, Harman PK, Moore EE: Retrohepatic vena cava balloon shunt introduced via the sapheno-femoral junction. J Trauma 17:837, 1977

23. Kram HB, Reuben BI, Flemming AW: Use of fibrin glue in hepatic trauma. J Trauma 28:1195, 1988

24. Kram HB, Nathan RC, Stafford FJ, et al: Fibrin glue achieves hemostasis in patients with coagulation disorders. Arch Surg 124:385, 1989

25. Berguer R, Staerkel RL, Moore EE, et al: Warning: fatal reaction to the use of fibrin glue in deep hepatic wounds: case reports. J Trauma 31:408, 1991

26. Ochsner MG, Maniscalco-Theberge ME, Champion HR: Fibrin glue as a hemostatic agent in hepatic and splenic trauma. J Trauma 30:884, 1990

27. Feliciano DV: Continuing evolution in the approach to severe liver trauma (editorial). Ann Surg 216:521, 1992

28. Trunkey DD, Shires GT, McClelland R: Management of liver trauma in 811 consecutive patients. Ann Surg 179:722, 1974

29. Levin A, Gover P, Nance FC: Surgical restraint in the management of hepatic injury: a review of Charity Hospital experience. J Trauma 18:399, 1978

30. Lucas CE, Ledgerwood AM: Prospective evaluation of hemostatic techniques for liver injuries. J Trauma 16:442, 1976

31. Camona RH, Lim RC Jr, Clark GC: Morbidity and mortality in hepatic trauma: a 5 year study. Am J Surg 144:88, 1982

32. Moore FA, Moore EE, Seagrave A: Nonresectional management of major hepatic trauma: an evolving concept. Am J Surg 150:725, 1985

33. Stone HH, Lamb JM: Use of pedicled omentum as an autogenous pack for control of hemorrhage in major injuries of the liver. Surg Gynecol Obstet 141:92, 1975

34. Mays ET: Lobar dearterialization for exsanguinating wounds of the liver. J Trauma 12:397, 1972

35. Flint LM, Polk HC: Selective hepatic artery ligation: limitations and failures. J Trauma 19:319, 1979

36. Lucas CE: Discussion of: Flint LM, Polk HC. Selective hepatic artery ligation: limitations and failures. J Trauma 19:319, 1979

37. Poggetti RS, Moore EE, Moore FA, et al: Balloon tamponade for bilobar transfixing hepatic gunshot wounds. J Trauma 33:694, 1992

38. Madding GF, Lawrence KB, Kennedy PA: War wounds of the liver. Tex State J Med 42:267, 1946

39. Reed RL, Merrell RC, Meyers WC, et al: Continuing evolution in the approach to severe liver trauma. Ann Surg 216:524, 1992

40. Jacobson LE, Kirton OC, Gomez GA: The use of an absorbable mesh wrap in the management of major liver injuries. Surgery 111:455, 1992

41. Lim RC Jr, Knudson J, Steele M: Liver trauma: current method of management. Arch Surg 104:544, 1972

42. Donovan AJ, Michaelian MJ, Yellin AE: Anatomical hepatic lobectomy in trauma to the liver. Surgery 73:833, 1973

43. Defore WW, Mattox KL, Jordan GL, et al: Management of 1590 consecutive cases of liver trauma. Arch Surg 111:493, 1976

44. Esquivel CO, Bernardos A, Makowka L, et al: Liver replacement after massive hepatic trauma. J Trauma 27:800, 1987

45. Angstadt J, Jarrell B, Moritz M, et al: Surgical management of severe liver trauma: a role for liver transplantation. J Trauma 29:606, 1989

46. Ringe B, Pichlmayr R, Ziegler H, et al: Management of severe hepatic trauma by two-stage total hepatectomy and subsequent liver transplantation. Surgery 109:792, 1991

47. Jeng LB, Hsu C, Wang C, et al: Emergent liver transplantation to salvage a hepatic avulsion injury with a disrupted suprahepatic vena cava. Arch Surg 128:1075, 1993

48. Fischer RP, O'Farrell KA, Perry JF Jr: The value of peritoneal drains in the treatment of liver injuries. J Trauma 18:393, 1978

49. Gillmore D, McSwain NE, Browder IW: Hepatic trauma: to drain or not to drain? J Trauma 27:989, 1987

50. Noyes LD, Doyle DJ, McSwain NE: Septic complications associated with the use of peritoneal drains in liver trauma. J Trauma 28:337, 1988

51. Fabian TC, Croce MA, Stanford GG, et al: Factors affecting morbidity after hepatic trauma. Ann Surg 213:540, 1991

52. Posner MC, Moore EE: Extrahepatic biliary tract injury: operative management plan. J Trauma 25:833, 1985

53. Ivatury RR, Rohman M, Nallathami M, et al: The

morbidity of injuries of the extra-hepatic biliary system. J Trauma 25:967, 1985

54. Sheldon GF, Lim RC, Yee ES, et al: Management of injuries to the porta hepatis. Ann Surg 202:539, 1985

55. Feliciano DV, Bitondo CG, Burch JM, et al: Management of traumatic injuries to the extra-hepatic biliary ducts. Am J Surg 150:705, 1985

56. Bade PG, Thomson SR, Hirshberg A, et al: Surgical options in traumatic injury to the extra-hepatic biliary tract. Br J Surg 76:256, 1989

57. Csendes A, Diaz JC, Burdiles P, et al: Late results of immediate primary end to end repair in accidental section of the common bile duct. Surg Gynecol Obstet 168:125, 1989

58. Howdieshell TR, Hawkins ML, Osler TM, et al: Management of blunt hepatic duct transection by ligation. South Med J 83:579, 1990

59. Sherman R: Perspective in management of trauma to the spleen: 1979 presidential address, American Association for the Surgery of Trauma. J Trauma 20:1, 1980

60. Barrett J, Sheaff C, Abuabara S, et al: Splenic preservation in adults after blunt and penetrating trauma. Am J Surg 145:313, 1983

61. Delany HM, Rudavsky AZ, Lan S: Preliminary clinical experience with the use of absorbable mesh splenorrhaphy. J Trauma 25:909, 1985

62. Beal SL, Spisso JM: The risk of splenorrhaphy. Arch Surg 123:1158, 1988

63. Feliciano DV, Spjut-Patrinely V, Burch JM, et al: Splenorrhaphy: the alternative. Ann Surg 211:569 1990

64. Schiffman MA: Nonoperative management of blunt abdominal trauma in pediatrics. Emerg Med Clin North Am 7:519, 1989

65. Cogbill TH, Moore EE, Jurkovich JJ, et al: Nonoperative management of blunt septic trauma: a multicenter experience. J Trauma 29:1312, 1989

66. Meredith JW, Young JS, Bowling J, et al: Nonoperative management of blunt hepatic trauma: the exception or the rule? J Trauma 36:529, 1994

67. Morrell DG, Chang FC, Helmer SD: Changing trends in the management of splenic injury. Am J Surg 170:686, 1995

68. Pachter HL, Hofstetter ST: The current status of nonoperative management of adult blunt hepatic injuries. Am J Surg 169:442, 1995

69. Croce MA, Fabian TC, Menke PG, et al: Nonoperative management of blunt hepatic trauma is the treatment of choice for hemodynamically stable patients. Ann Surg 221:744, 1995

70. Boone DC, Federle M, Billiar TR, et al: Evolution of management of major hepatic trauma: identification of patterns of injury. J Trauma 39:344, 1995

71. Pachter HL, Knudson MM, Esrig B, et al: Status of nonoperative management of blunt hepatic injuries in 1995: a multicenter experience with 404 patients. J Trauma 40:31, 1996

72. Smith JS, Cooney RN, Mucha P: Nonoperative management of the ruptured spleen: a revalidation of criteria. Surgery 120:745, 1996

73. Powell M, Courcoulas A, Gardner M, et al: Management of blunt splenic trauma: significant differences between adults and children. Surgery 122:654, 1997

74. Sclafani SJA, Shaftan GW, Scalea TM, et al: Nonoperative salvage of computed tomography–diagnosed splenic injuries: utilization of angiography for triage and embolization for hemostasis. J Trauma 39:818, 1995

75. Malhotra AK, Fabian TC, Crou MA, et al: Blunt hepatic injury: a paradigm shift from operative to nonoperative management in the 1990's. Ann Surg 231:804, 2000

76. Richardson JD, Franklin GA, Lukan JK, et al: Evolution in the management of hepatic trauma: a 25-year perspective. Ann Surg 232:324, 2000

77. Sutyak JP, Chiu WC, D'Amelio LF, et al: Computed tomography is inaccurate in estimating the severity of adult splenic injury. J Trauma 39:514, 1995

78. Croce MA, Fabian TC, Kudsk KA, et al: AAST organ injury scale: correlation of CT-graded liver injuries and operative findings. J Trauma 31:806, 1991

79. Gates JD: Delayed hemorrhage with free rupture complicating the nonsurgical management of blunt hepatic trauma: a case report and review of the literature. J Trauma 36:572, 1994

80. MacGillivray DC, Valentine RJ: Nonoperative management of blunt pediatric liver injury—late complications: case report. J Trauma 29:251, 1989

81. Sugimoto K, Asari Y, Sakaguchi T, et al: Endoscopic retrograde cholangiography in the nonsurgical management of blunt liver injury. J Trauma 35:192, 1993

Acknowledgments

Figure 1   Marcia Kammerer.
Figures 2 through 9   Susan Brust, C.M.I.

8 INJURIES TO THE STOMACH, DUODENUM, PANCREAS, SMALL BOWEL, COLON, AND RECTUM

Charles E. Lucas, M.D., and Anna M. Ledgerwood, M.D.

Injuries to the stomach, duodenum, pancreas, small bowel, colon, and rectum present a broad spectrum of challenges necessitating widely different solutions. The first priorities are recognizing injury and making the decision to operate.

Initial evaluation of injured patients is addressed more fully elsewhere [see III:1 *Emergency Department Evaluation of the Patient with Multiple Injuries*]. In what follows, we assume that the patient has been stabilized and that injuries to one or more of the organs just mentioned have been recognized. The need for operation varies according to whether the patient has sustained a stab wound, a gunshot wound, or a blunt injury.

Determination of Need for Operation

STAB WOUNDS

It is universally agreed that patients with symptomatic stab wounds (as evidenced by hypotension, peritonitis, or both) should undergo operation immediately.[1] Likewise, most surgeons agree that mentally competent patients with asymptomatic stab wounds are best treated by observation, even if the wounding object has penetrated the peritoneal cavity.[1] For patients who fall into neither of these categories, however, as when there are no signs of injury but the patient is in a compromised state (e.g., as a result of alcohol, drugs, or mental retardation), the diagnostic and therapeutic approach may take a number of different directions. Options include (1) observation with reexaminations until the patient is sober, (2) local wound exploration, (3) diagnostic peritoneal lavage (DPL), (4) laparoscopy, (5) abdominal ultrasonography in the form of the FAST (*Focused Assessment for the Sonographic examination of the Trauma patient* [see V:4 *Ultrasonography: Surgical Applications*]), or (6) contrast abdominal computed tomography. Of these, we prefer immediate FAST, which, if yielding positive results, is followed by DPL. A positive DPL result is defined as the presence of more than 20,000 red blood cells (RBCs) or more than 500 white blood cells (WBCs) per high-power field. When a stab wound to the lower thorax causes hemothorax, pneumothorax, or both, any return of blood on DPL suggests perforation of the diaphragm, for which the recommended treatment is laparotomy and repair.[1]

GUNSHOT WOUNDS

Early operation is indicated for symptomatic patients with gunshot wounds to the abdomen. More than 90% of patients with penetrating gunshot wounds have intra-abdominal

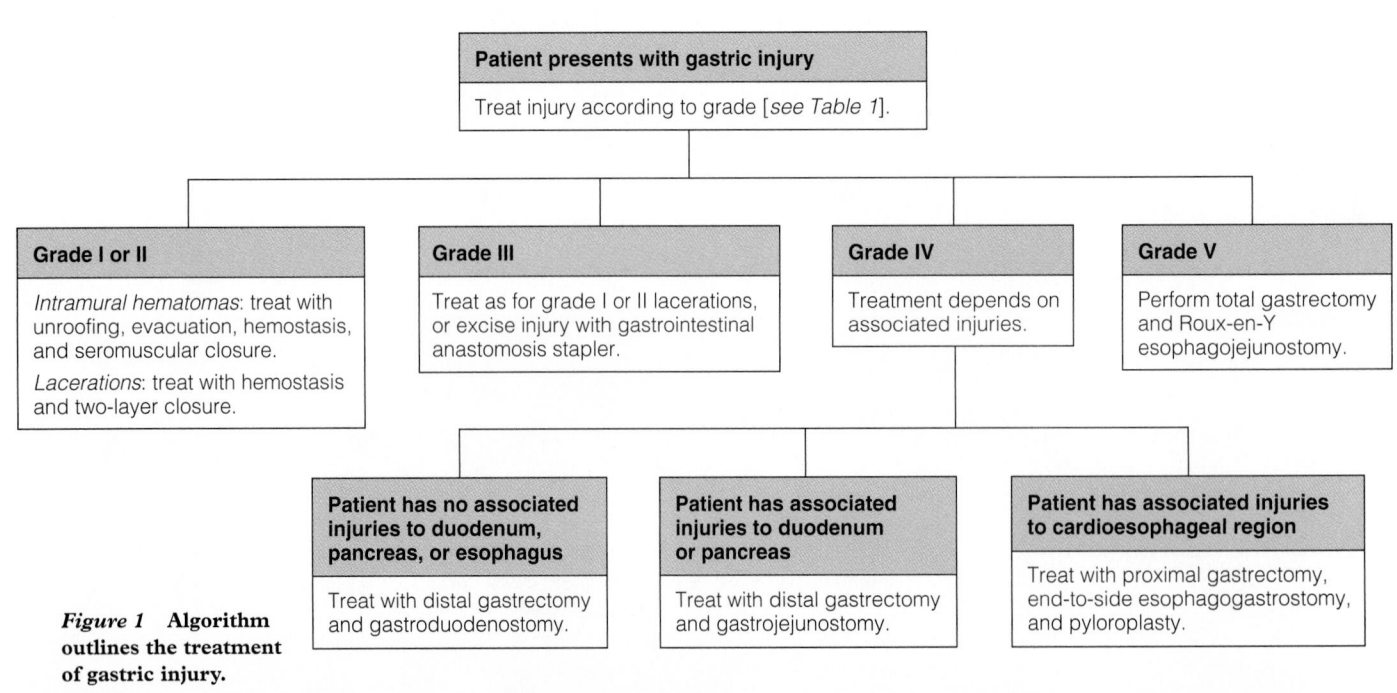

Figure 1 Algorithm outlines the treatment of gastric injury.

Patient presents with gastric injury
Treat injury according to grade [see Table 1].

Grade I or II
Intramural hematomas: treat with unroofing, evacuation, hemostasis, and seromuscular closure.
Lacerations: treat with hemostasis and two-layer closure.

Grade III
Treat as for grade I or II lacerations, or excise injury with gastrointestinal anastomosis stapler.

Grade IV
Treatment depends on associated injuries.

Grade V
Perform total gastrectomy and Roux-en-Y esophagojejunostomy.

Patient has no associated injuries to duodenum, pancreas, or esophagus
Treat with distal gastrectomy and gastroduodenostomy.

Patient has associated injuries to duodenum or pancreas
Treat with distal gastrectomy and gastrojejunostomy.

Patient has associated injuries to cardioesophageal region
Treat with proximal gastrectomy, end-to-side esophagogastrostomy, and pyloroplasty.

Table 1 AAST Organ Injury Scales for GI Tract and Pancreas

Injured Structure	AAST Grade*	Characteristics of Injury	AIS-90 Score
Stomach	I	Intramural hematoma < 3 cm; partial-thickness laceration	2
	II	Intramural hematoma ≥ 3 cm; small (< 3 cm) laceration	2
	III	Large (> 3 cm) laceration	3
	IV	Large laceration involving vessels on greater or lesser curvature	3
	V	Extensive (> 50%) rupture; stomach devascularized	4
Duodenum	I	Single-segment hematoma; partial-thickness laceration	2; 3
	II	Multiple-segment hematoma; small (< 50% of circumference) laceration	2; 4
	III	Large laceration (50%–75% of circumference of segment D2 or 50%–100% of circumference of segment D1, D3, or D4)	4
	IV	Very large (75%–100%) laceration of segment D2; rupture of ampullary or distal bile duct	5
	V	Massive duodenopancreatic injury; devascularization	5
Pancreas	I	Small hematoma without duct injury; superficial laceration without duct injury	2
	II	Large hematoma without duct injury or tissue loss; major laceration without duct injury or tissue loss	2; 3
	III	Distal transection or parenchymal laceration with duct injury	4
	IV	Proximal transection or parenchymal laceration involving ampulla	4
	V	Massive disruption of pancreatic head	5
Small bowel	I	Contusion or hematoma without devascularization; partial-thickness laceration	2
	II	Small (< 50% of circumference) laceration	3
	III	Large (≥ 50% of circumference) laceration without transection	3
	IV	Transection	4
	V	Transection with segmental tissue loss; devascularized segment	4
Colon	I	Contusion or hematoma; partial-thickness laceration	2
	II	Small (< 50% of circumference) laceration	3
	III	Large (≥ 50% of circumference) laceration	3
	IV	Transection	4
	V	Transection with tissue loss; devascularized segment	4
Rectosigmoid and rectum	I	Contusion or hematoma; partial-thickness laceration	2
	II	Small (< 50% of circumference) laceration	3
	III	Large (≥ 50% of circumference) laceration	4
	IV	Full-thickness laceration with perineal extension	5
	V	Devascularized segment	5

*Advance one grade for multiple injuries, up to grade III.
AIS-90—Abbreviated Injury Score, 1990 version   AAST—American Association for the Surgery of Trauma

injuries. If there is any question of possible peritoneal penetration with an anterior or anterolateral wound, diagnostic DPL should be performed; a clear return rules out penetration.[1] Triple-contrast CT helps confirm or rule out penetration in patients with lateral or posterior wounds.

BLUNT TRAUMA

Clinical assessment of stable blunt trauma patients often leads to false positive or false negative conclusions,[1] and the error rate rises in patients whose mental function is compromised. The resultant delay in diagnosis and operative intervention is potentially hazardous. For this reason, FAST and DPL, with or without CT scanning, are essential in mentally compromised patients. When stable patients with no abnormal findings on abdominal examination require operative intervention for nonabdominal injuries, DPL can help identify unsuspected intraperitoneal injuries, and double-contrast CT can help identify unsuspected pancreatic and duodenal injuries.

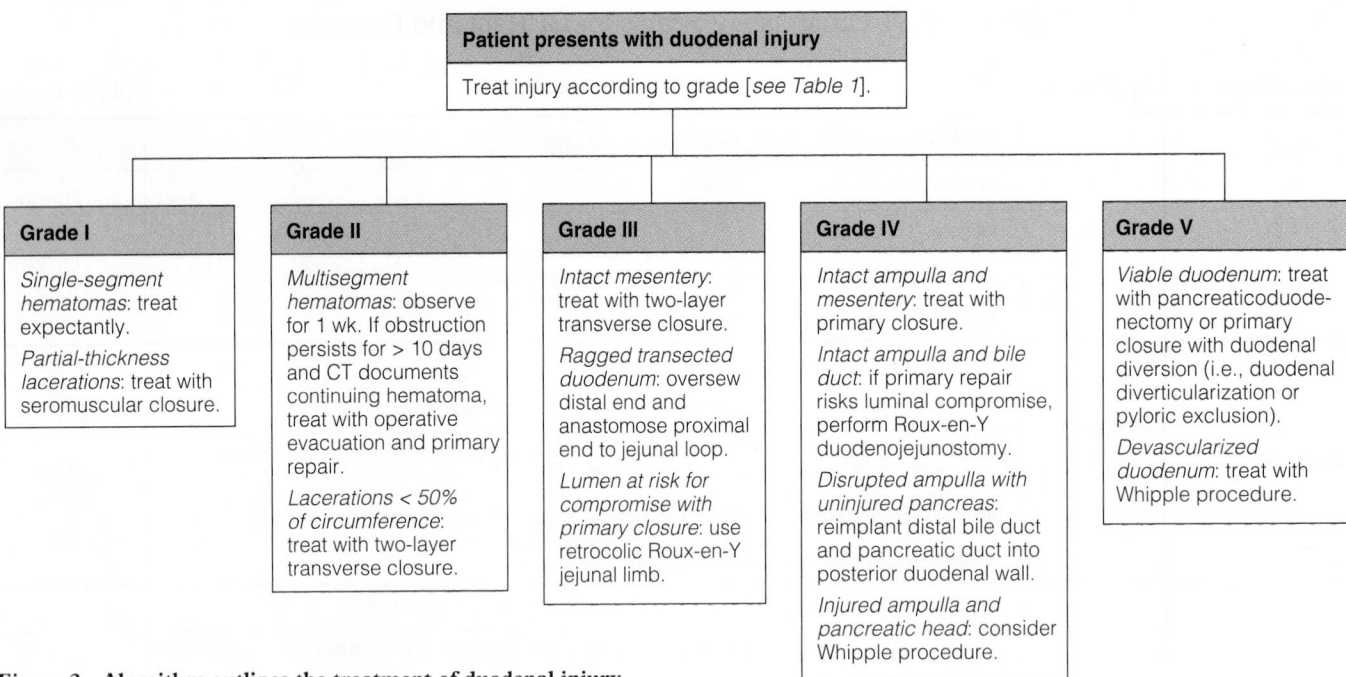

Patient presents with duodenal injury
Treat injury according to grade [*see Table 1*].

Grade I	**Grade II**	**Grade III**	**Grade IV**	**Grade V**
Single-segment hematomas: treat expectantly. *Partial-thickness lacerations*: treat with seromuscular closure.	*Multisegment hematomas*: observe for 1 wk. If obstruction persists for > 10 days and CT documents continuing hematoma, treat with operative evacuation and primary repair. *Lacerations < 50% of circumference*: treat with two-layer transverse closure.	*Intact mesentery*: treat with two-layer transverse closure. *Ragged transected duodenum*: oversew distal end and anastomose proximal end to jejunal loop. *Lumen at risk for compromise with primary closure*: use retrocolic Roux-en-Y jejunal limb.	*Intact ampulla and mesentery*: treat with primary closure. *Intact ampulla and bile duct*: if primary repair risks luminal compromise, perform Roux-en-Y duodenojejunostomy. *Disrupted ampulla with uninjured pancreas*: reimplant distal bile duct and pancreatic duct into posterior duodenal wall. *Injured ampulla and pancreatic head*: consider Whipple procedure.	*Viable duodenum*: treat with pancreaticoduodenectomy or primary closure with duodenal diversion (i.e., duodenal diverticularization or pyloric exclusion). *Devascularized duodenum*: treat with Whipple procedure.

Figure 2 **Algorithm outlines the treatment of duodenal injury.**

Figure 3 **Shown is a grade IV stellate crack to pancreatic head with a grade III (60%) transection of the duodenum (D2). After hemostasis is established, it is possible to perform the so-called duodenal diverticularization, consisting of antrectomy with gastrojejunostomy, tube duodenostomy, vagotomy, and peripancreatic drainage. H₂-receptor blockade precludes the need for vagotomy.**

When DPL is positive for amylase, particulate matter, WBCs, or bowel contents, hollow viscus injury is likely and laparotomy is therefore mandatory.

Injuries to the Stomach

The treatment of gastric injuries varies according to their severity [*see Figure 1 and Table 1*]. Most intramural hematomas (grades I and II) are treated by careful evacuation, hemostasis, and seromuscular closure. Perforations from stabs and bullets are usually small (grade I or II) and can be closed primarily in two layers.[1,2] Because the stomach is quite vascular, even small perforations may bleed profusely, especially along the greater curvature. Consequently, the recommended closure is an inner layer of locked hemostatic sutures followed by an outer inverting layer of sutures.

Large (grade III) injuries near the greater curvature can be closed by the same technique or by excising the injury with a long gastrointestinal anastomosis (GIA) stapler. Careful hemostasis and inversion of the staple line provide extra security when the lumen is not compromised. Extensive (grade IV) injuries may necessitate proximal or distal gastrectomy. The type of resection depends on the presence of associated injuries to the duodenum, the pancreas, or the esophagus. Patients with associated duodenal injuries or pancreatic injuries, or both, are best treated with gastrojejunal reconstruction after distal gastrectomy. In patients who survive extensive injury to the cardioesophageal region, an end-to-side esophagogastrostomy can be performed after proximal gastrectomy; a pyloroplasty is added. When total gastrectomy is performed for grade V injury, Roux-en-Y esophagojejunostomy is advocated [*see V:9 Gastric Procedures*].

Injuries to the Duodenum

The diagnosis of penetrating duodenal injury is usually made during laparotomy performed for hypotension or peritoneal irritation. The decision to explore for isolated blunt duodenal injury is based on the physical examination and roentgeno-

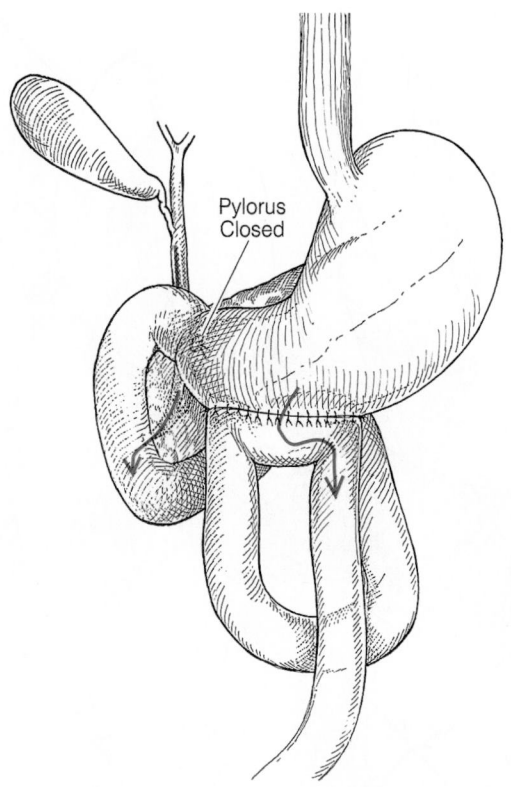

Figure 4 Duodenal exclusion consists of closure of the pylorus from within the stomach, followed by gastrojejunostomy. The procedure eliminates discharge of gastric acid into the duodenum, thus minimizing the stimulation of pancreatic secretion and reducing morbidity if there is breakdown of a repair.

graphic findings. Duodenal injury may be present despite negative findings from DPL, and the symptoms of duodenal injury are often slow to evolve.[3] Roentgenograms made within 2 hours of injury typically show scoliosis and partial obliteration of the right psoas shadow. Retroperitoneal gas along the right psoas margin, over the right pole of the kidney, or in the lower mediastinum is seen within 6 hours in most patients. Contrast CT generally identifies in the site of perforation.

Treatment varies according to the location (segments D1 through D4) and severity of injury [*see Figure 2 and Table 1*].[4,5] Single-segment (grade I) intramural hematoma usually occurs in segment D1 or D2, seldom leads to obstruction, and can be treated expectantly. Partial-thickness (grade I) lacerations are best treated by simple seromuscular closure. Multisegment hematomas (grade II) often require operative evacuation, especially when the obstruction lasts for more than 10 days and there is CT documentation that the hematoma persists. A generous longitudinal serosal incision along the antimesenteric border permits gentle evacuation without accidental injury to the underlying muscular and mucosal layers. The serosa with attached muscle is carefully reapproximated. Drainage is not necessary. Perforations involving less than 50% of the circumference of the duodenum, whether caused by penetrating wounds or blunt injury, are best treated by simple two-layer closure, preferably in a transverse manner.

Larger perforations that involve more than 50% of the circumference (grade III) require careful suture placement along the mesentery border to prevent unintentional vascular compromise.[6] Near D3 and D4 injuries, careful suture placement and gentle duodenal mobilization help prevent iatrogenic injury to the superior mesenteric vessels. If a transected duodenum is ragged, the distal end may be oversewn and the proximal end anastomosed to a jejunal loop.[7] Alternatively, if primary closure would compromise lumen patency, a retrocolic Roux-en-Y jejunal limb can be used to close large defects.

Large D2 injuries (grade IV) can be closed primarily if the adjacent ampulla and mesentery are spared.[8] If the condition of the distal bile duct is unknown, choledochography through the gallbladder or the proximal bile duct will confirm continuity. When the ampulla and the bile duct are intact but primary repair would cause excessive luminal compromise, a Roux-en-Y duodenojejunostomy is preferred. If the ampulla is disrupted but the pancreas is not injured, primary reimplantation of the distal bile duct and the pancreatic duct into the posterior duodenal wall is preferred. When both the ampulla and the pancreatic head are injured, a Whipple procedure may be needed [*see V:13 Pancreatic Procedures*].

Duodenopancreatic crunch (grade V) is associated with high morbidity and mortality. This injury can sometimes be treated by pancreaticoduodenectomy or by primary closure done in

Patient presents with injury to pancreas

Treat injury according to grade [*see Table 1*].

Grade I or II

Treat with unroofing, hemostasis, evacuation, and closed drainage. Control bleeding with either electrocoagulation or suture ligation.

With grade II injuries, take extra care to rule out duct injury and obtain hemostasis.

Grade III

Treat with distal pancreatectomy, with or without splenic salvage. If it is unknown whether duct is injured, simple drainage may be provided instead. When nonresective therapy is given to patients with known ductal injury, reoperation with later resection or Roux-en-Y drainage may be needed.

Grade IV

Diabetic patients with intact duodenal ampullary complex: treat with closure of duodenal rim of pancreas and distal Roux-en-Y pancreaticojejunostomy.

Nondiabetic patients: treat with primary closure of proximal pancreas and distal pancreatectomy.

Grade V

Unstable patients: treat with duodenal diversion and external drainage.

Stable patients: treat with pancreaticoduodenectomy or Roux-en-Y pancreaticojejunostomy.

Figure 5 Algorithm outlines the treatment of pancreatic injury.

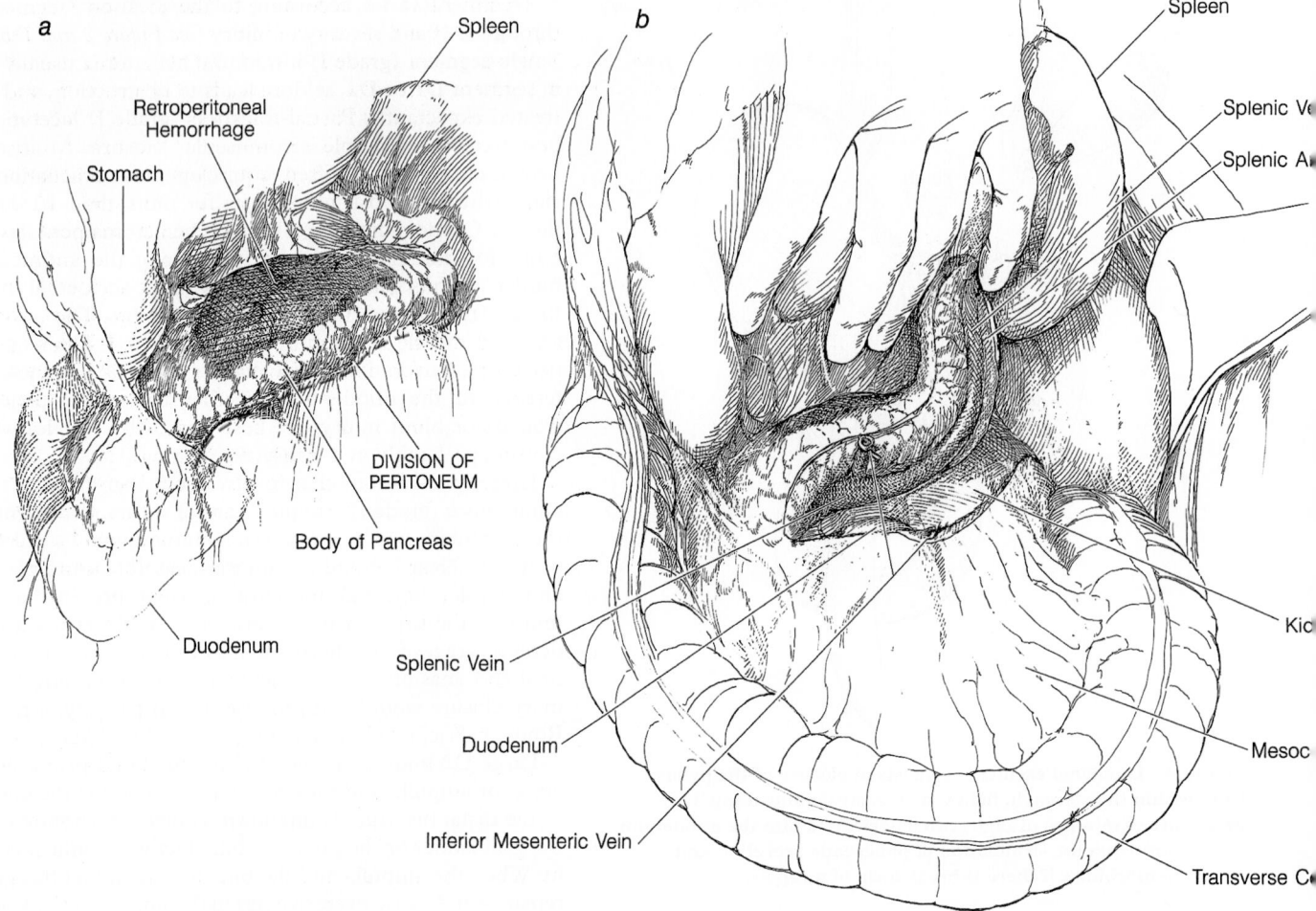

a

Spleen

Retroperitoneal
Hemorrhage

Stomach

DIVISION OF
PERITONEUM

Body of Pancreas

Duodenum

Splenic Vein

Duodenum

Inferior Mesenteric Vein

b

Spleen

Splenic Ve

Splenic A

Kic

Mesoc

Transverse Co

Figure 6 Illustrated is the appearance of a contusion to the body of the pancreas overlying the vertebral column, as seen from the lesser sac (*a*). Such a contusion necessitates mobilization of the pancreas to determine whether a fracture is present and to assess the likelihood of a duct injury. This exposure is best accomplished by dissecting along the inferior border of the gland, dividing the inferior mesenteric vein if necessary, and reflecting the pancreas superiorly (*b*).

conjunction with some type of duodenal diversion. When the injury causes devascularization, resection is mandated. Duodenal bypass is performed by either duodenal diverticularization [*see Figure 3*] or pyloric exclusion [*see Figure 4*]; we prefer the former. Duodenal diverticularization includes antrectomy with gastrojejunostomy, tube duodenostomy, and drainage of the associated pancreatic injury.[6] Tube choledochostomy is added only for overt extrahepatic biliary injury. Duodenal exclusion includes pyloric occlusion by sutures or staples, a side-to-side gastrojejunostomy, and appropriate drainage.[9,10]

Injuries to the Pancreas

The treatment of pancreatic injury depends on its grade and extent [*see Figure 5 and Table 1*].[5] The pancreas is best exposed by dividing the greater omentum just outside the arcades of the gastroepiploic vessels. Assessment of the posterior surface may require mobilization of the inferior border or complete relocation of the spleen and pancreatic tail anteriorly [*see Figure 6*]. A small hematoma (grade I) is best treated by unroofing, hemostasis, evacuation, and drainage. Minor bleed-

ing from unnamed vessels is controlled by either electrocoa ulation or ligature with fine sutures.

Gentle tension-free tying helps avert iatrogenic injury to th soft pancreatic parenchyma. Careful inspection after hemost sis will confirm the presence of a grade I injury, which does n involve a major duct. The site of the unroofed hematoma is le open and drained externally. Closed-suction drainage perm the exit of pancreatic juices. All small pancreatic lesions with out duct injury (grade I) are treated essentially the same wa whether caused by stabs, gunshots, or blunt trauma. If th fluid drained has a high amylase content, skin will not b digested unless the effluent contains enteric juices that activa pancreatic peptidase.[11]

During one 5-year period extending from 1990 throug 1994, the surgical services at Detroit Receiving Hospital trea ed 37 patients with grade I pancreatic injury. All 37 were trea ed with hemostasis, minimal debridement (if tiny fragments loose pancreatic tissue were seen), and external drainage. All the patients survived. Pancreatitis, defined on the basis of elevated serum amylase level lasting more than 5 days, deve oped in two patients, and a pancreaticocutaneous fistula deve oped in two patients whose pancreatic drainage lasted mo than 14 days. All of the complications resolved with nonoperative supportive care, including parenteral nutrition.

Treatment of larger hematomas or lacerations without duct injury (grade II injuries) is similar. Extra care is taken to rule out duct injury and to obtain hemostasis. Once hemostasis has been achieved, the injury is left open and drained. This practice helps prevent the development of a pseudocyst, which may occur if tiny ductules leak pancreatic juices within a closed injury.[12,13]

Although the incidence of postoperative pancreatitis (10%) or persistent pancreatic drainage (20%) seen after grade II injury exceeds that seen after grade I injury, few patients (3%) have refractory drainage lasting more than 30 days. When the external drainage system plugs, percutaneous drainage or reoperation may be needed to reestablish drainage. When reoperation is deemed essential for a peripancreatic abscess, dependent drainage through the bed of the 12th rib helps

avoid the extensive contamination that occurs when laparotomy is performed through the anterior approach.[13]

Grade III lacerations or transections thought to involve the main duct to the left of the superior mesenteric vein are best treated by distal pancreatectomy, with or without splenic salvage [*see Figure 7 and V:13 Pancreatic Procedures*].[11,13] If it is not known whether there is injury to the main pancreatic duct, simple drainage may be provided even though it may result in formation of a pancreaticocutaneous fistula. This approach is more expedient than pancreatic resection in unstable patients, especially those with multiple associated injuries requiring multiple transfusions. Total parenteral nutrition permits such patients to recover from the total insult with minimal morbidity.[11] When nonresective therapy is used for patients known to have a duct injury, reoperation with later resection or Roux-en-Y drainage is often needed.[14]

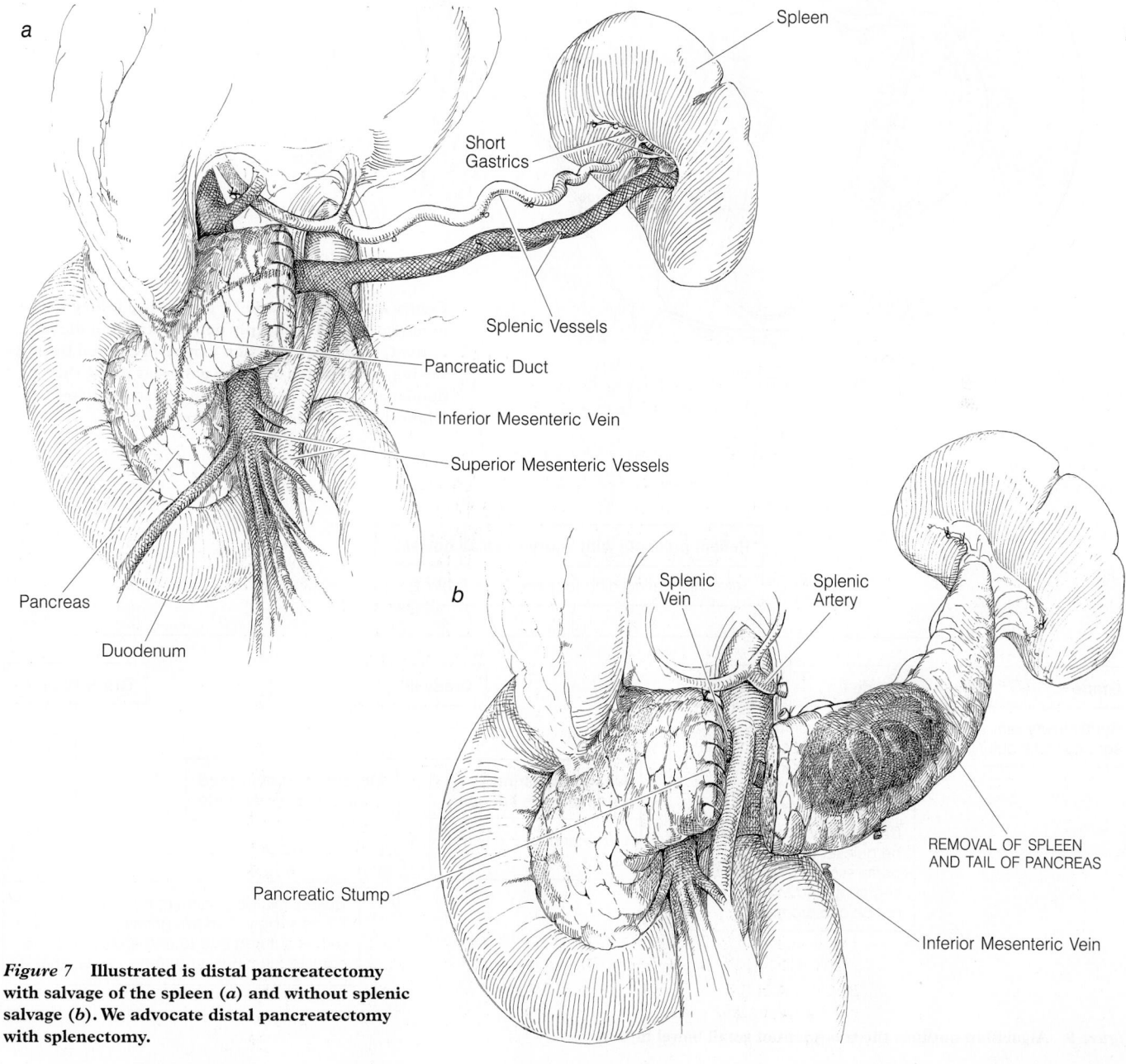

Figure 7 **Illustrated is distal pancreatectomy with salvage of the spleen (*a*) and without splenic salvage (*b*). We advocate distal pancreatectomy with splenectomy.**

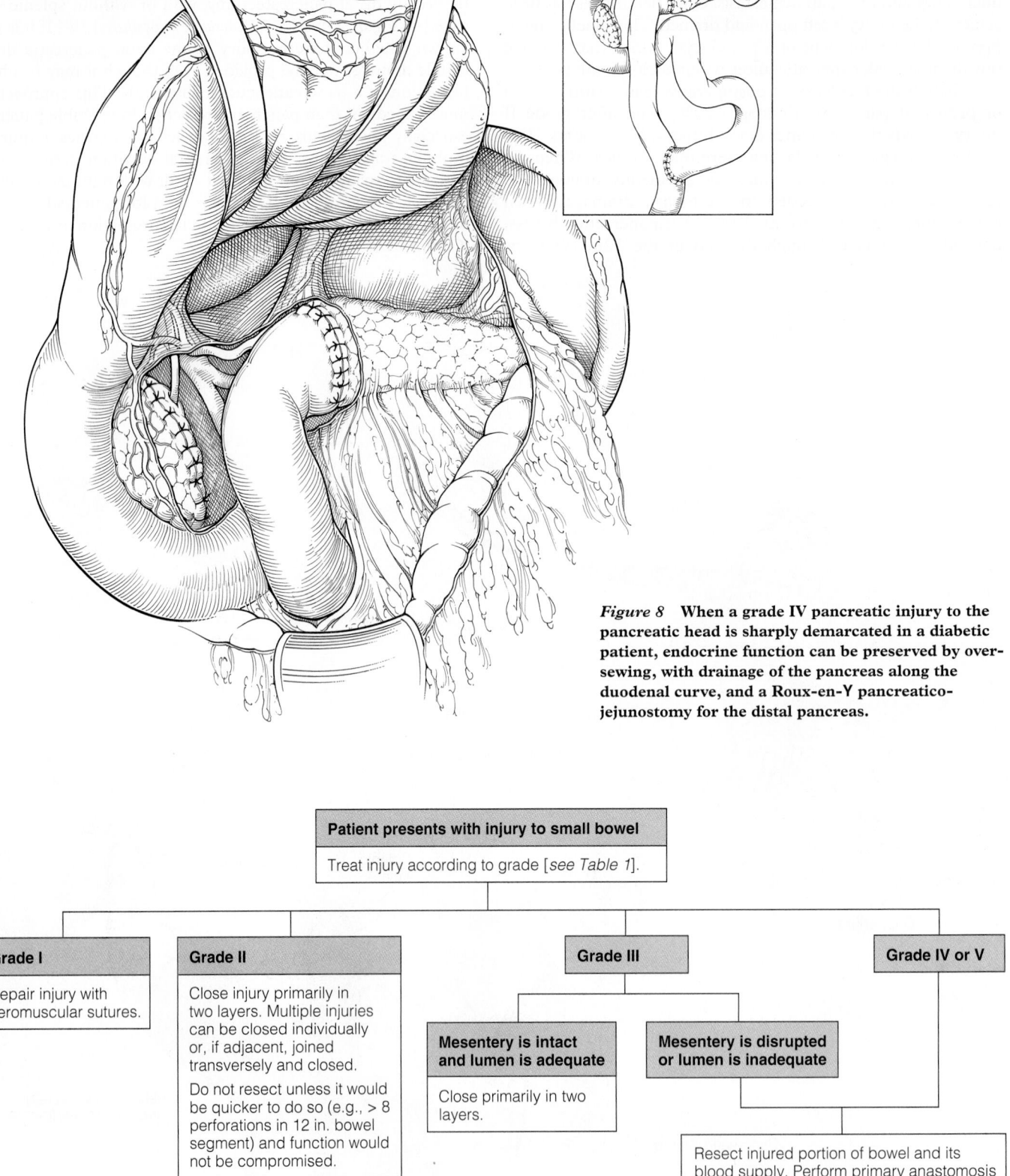

Figure 8 When a grade IV pancreatic injury to the pancreatic head is sharply demarcated in a diabetic patient, endocrine function can be preserved by over-sewing, with drainage of the pancreas along the duodenal curve, and a Roux-en-Y pancreatico-jejunostomy for the distal pancreas.

Patient presents with injury to small bowel

Treat injury according to grade [*see Table 1*].

Grade I

Repair injury with seromuscular sutures.

Grade II

Close injury primarily in two layers. Multiple injuries can be closed individually or, if adjacent, joined transversely and closed.

Do not resect unless it would be quicker to do so (e.g., > 8 perforations in 12 in. bowel segment) and function would not be compromised.

Grade III

Mesentery is intact and lumen is adequate

Close primarily in two layers.

Mesentery is disrupted or lumen is inadequate

Grade IV or V

Resect injured portion of bowel and its blood supply. Perform primary anastomosis (either sutured end-to-end anastomosis or stapled functional end-to-end anastomosis).

Figure 9 Algorithm outlines the treatment of small bowel injury.

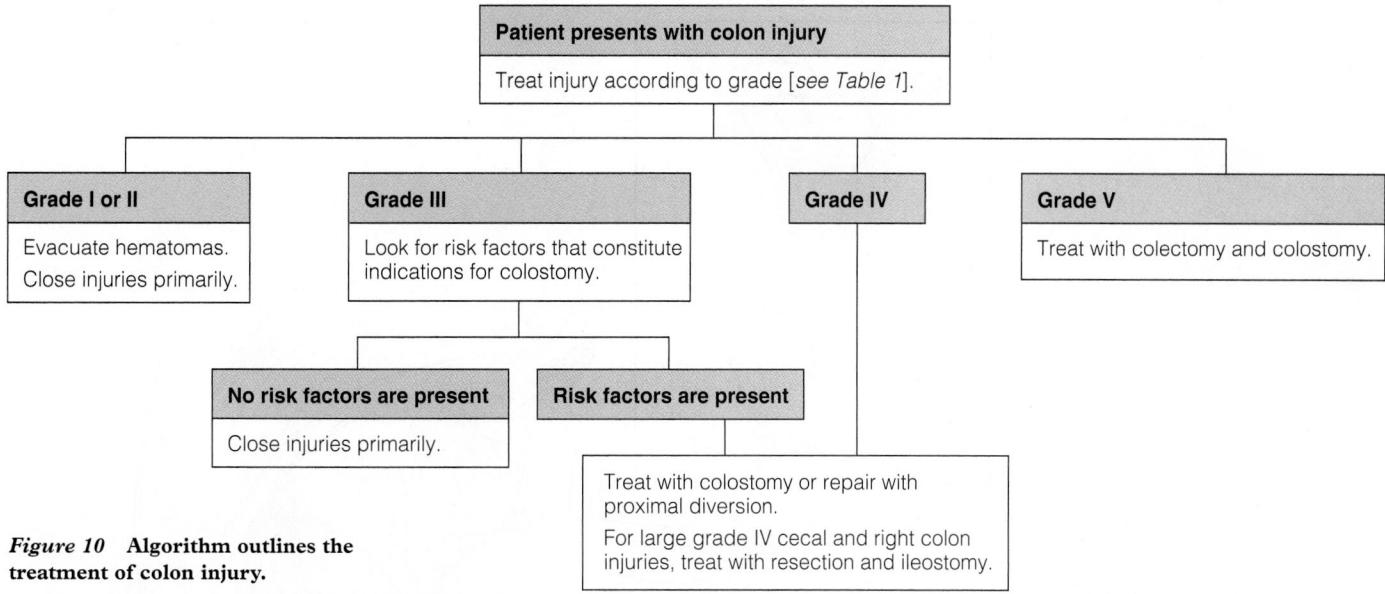

Figure 10 **Algorithm outlines the treatment of colon injury.**

After distal pancreatectomy with primary closure of the pancreatic stump, about 20% of patients have drainage lasting longer than 2 weeks. In most cases, nonoperative supportive therapy leads to resolution. A left upper quadrant abscess may occur, especially in patients with associated colon injury. On rare occasions, a patient with a left upper quadrant abscess experiences bleeding from the pancreatic stump that necessitates reoperation with more proximal ligation of the splenic vessels and better drainage of the left upper quadrant.

A major pancreatic transection or extensive parenchymal disruption near the ampulla (grade IV) presents special challenges. These injuries to the right of the superior mesenteric vein are often lethal when associated with vascular injury. The first priority is hemostasis, which may be accomplished by primary vascular repair or suture ligature of exposed vessels. Gentle retraction helps prevent accidental injury to the supe-

rior mesenteric vein or to unnamed veins draining the uncinate process. When a clean transection is present, a Roux-en-Y pancreaticojejunostomy allows appropriate drainage of the distal pancreas. Simple oversewing of the proximal stump reduces the likelihood that a pancreatic fistula will develop from the transected proximal pancreas [*see Figure 8*]. When the pancreatic head has a stellate laceration that does not extend posteriorly, one should attempt to establish hemostasis and provide for abundant external drainage. Two or more drains are recommended. Although pancreaticoduodenectomy may be used for grade IV injury, the magnitude of this operation in the midst of pancreatic bleeding argues that it should be performed only by the most experienced trauma surgeons.[13,15] Short-term treatment with well-placed drains often permits the patient to recover from the total insult; if a pancreaticocutaneous fistula persists, reoper-

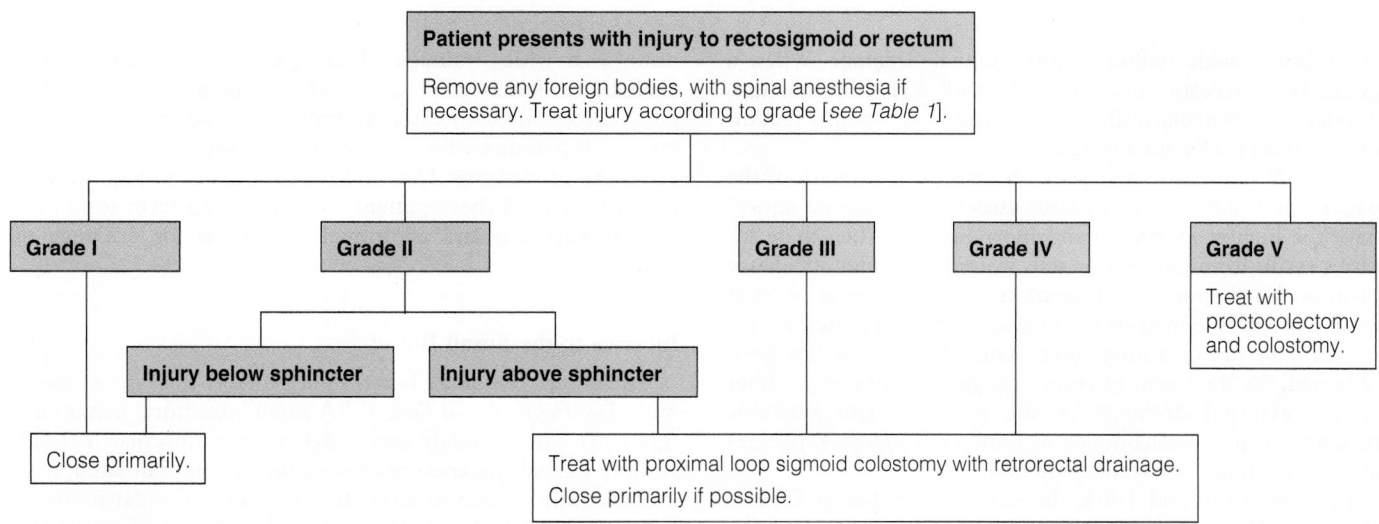

Figure 11 **Algorithm outlines the treatment of rectosigmoid or rectal injury.**

Figure 12 **Presacral drainage is provided through a curved incision midway between the anus and the tip of the coccyx. With blunt dissection, two fingers are inserted between the rectum and the hollow of the sacrum. Penrose drains are inserted and sutured to the skin.**

ation can provide definitive intraluminal drainage. When a grade IV pancreatic injury coexists with a duodenal injury, duodenal diverticularization or duodenal exclusion is recommended; we prefer the former.

Grade V pancreatic injuries with massive disruption of the pancreatic head (with or without associated duodenal injury) have the highest morbidity and mortality.[13,15] When these injuries result from gunshot or stab wounds, the high incidence of injury to the superior mesenteric vein, the superior mesenteric artery, the inferior vena cava, or the aorta often results in death in the operating room. Once hemostasis has been obtained, the treatment of choice for grade V injuries is either simple external drainage of the pancreas (for unstable patients) or pancreaticoduodenectomy or Roux-en-Y pancreaticojejunostomy (for stable patients).

Between 1990 and 1994, the surgical services at Detroit Receiving Hospital treated 18 patients with grade V pancreatic injury. The treatment regimens varied but included duodenal diverticularization, segmental resection of the duode-

num with wide drainage of the pancreatic injury, pyloric exclusion, Roux-en-Y pancreaticojejunostomy, and 95% pancreatectomy with external drainage of the remaining pancreas. All patients who survived the hemorrhagic shock survived the procedures. Hospitalization was prolonged, however, and many of these patients required long-term total parenteral nutrition and additional operations for drainage of abscesses.

Injuries to the Small Bowel

The severity of small bowel injury directs the type of treatment [*see Figure 9 and Table 1*].[5] A small intramural hematoma (grade I) can be safely inverted with seromuscular 4-0 silk sutures. Partial-thickness tears are gently reapproximated, with 4-0 silk sutures used to invert the torn seromuscular tissue. A full-thickness tear (grade II) involving less than 50% of the circumference is treated by primary closure, with a continuous absorbable suture used for the internal layer and interrupted nonabsorbable sutures used for the outer layer.[2] Multiple grade II injuries from penetrating wounds can usually be closed individually in two layers. Adjacent through-and-through wounds are joined transversely and closed in a similar manner.[16,17] Small bowel resection for multiple injuries is not recommended unless (1) resection and anastomosis would take less time than individual closure of the multiple perforations and (2) the amount of tissue sacrificed does not compromise function. If more than eight perforations exist in a 12 in. segment of bowel, resection with primary anastomosis is more expedient than multiple primary closures.

Full-thickness small bowel perforations involving at least 50% of the circumference (grade III) can usually be closed primarily in two layers, provided that adjacent blood vessels are protected and an adequate lumen (greater than 30% of the circumference) is maintained.[18] A transverse closure helps protect lumen patency.

Complete transection (grade IV) is treated by resection of the injured portion and its adjacent blood supply, followed by primary anastomosis.[19,20] This can be accomplished by the hand-sewn end-to-end technique or by fashioning a stapled functional (as opposed to anatomic) end-to-end anastomosis [see V:15 Intestinal Anastomosis]. Stapled small bowel anastomoses may be associated with higher complication rates in injured patients than hand-sewn anastomoses are. A 1999 study[21] found stapled anastomoses to be more prone to leakage, and a 2000 study[22] reported a higher incidence of intra-abdominal abscesses after stapled anastomoses. Neither group of investigators inverted the staple line of the anastomosis. Inversion of all exposed staple lines with 4-0 silk sutures provides added safety.

Extensive destruction of the small bowel or its mesentery (grade V) necessitates resection and reconstruction using the same techniques recommended for grade III and grade IV bowel injuries.[2,17] Treatment of an isolated mesenteric tear without bowel rupture depends on the vascularity of the bowel. If the bowel is necrotic and devascularized, resection is required; if the bowel remains pink and peristalsis is normal, careful closure of the mesenteric tear is sufficient. If vascularity is marginal, simple closure of the mesentery without resection of the bowel may lead to stenosis; thus, resection with primary reconstruction is recommended.

Injuries to the Colon

As with injuries to other organs, the treatment of colon injury depends on its severity [see Figure 10 and Table 1].[5] Because the ascending, descending, and retrosigmoid segments of the colon are located retroperitoneally, they may still have penetrating injuries even when DPL yields negative results.[23] Such injuries may be seen with contrast CT, but the importance of sequential physical examination to an early diagnosis cannot be overemphasized. Blunt injury is uncommon; when present, it is usually located in the cecum or the sigmoid colon.[23,24] Because these injuries seldom cause pneumoperitoneum, early diagnosis depends on careful sequential physical examination.

Most minor injuries (grades I and II) can be treated with primary repair [see Figure 10]. For small hematomas or partial-thickness lacerations, simple closure with inversion is sufficient. Similarly, a partial-thickness contusion should be inverted to preclude subsequent full-thickness necrosis with perforation.[23,25] Grade II hematomas should be evacuated carefully to prevent full-thickness injury and should be closed primarily. Through-and-through injuries with little or no spill and a minimum of associated injuries can be closed primarily throughout the colon.[25,26]

Because the colon has an increased bacterial level, ranging from 10^6 in the cecum to 10^{13} in the rectum, primary closure of colon injuries is associated with a much greater risk of leakage than primary closure of small bowel perforations. Accordingly, many patients are candidates for colostomy; however, primary closure is preferred for most minor injuries. In a prospective, randomized study of primary closure versus colostomy, Stone and Fabian reported that morbidity was much higher in the colostomy patients.[3] On the basis of these and other studies, primary closure appears to be the preferred technique in patients with the following clinical characteristics: (1) injuries with minimal spill; (2) fewer than three associated injuries; (3) no hypotension; (4) minimal blood loss; (5) a short interval between injury and operation; (6) good colonic vascularity; (7) injury involving no more than 50% of the circumference; and (8) an intact abdominal wall.

Figure 13 Irrigation of the distal sigmoid colon and rectum reduces soilage of the retrorectal space through unclosed perforations of the rectum as peristalsis returns. At the completion of the operative procedure, a purse-string suture is placed in the sigmoid colostomy and a large Foley catheter passed into the distal limb. The distal limb is irrigated with saline as the anus is held open. The catheter is then removed, and the colostomy is opened and matured.

ROLE OF COLOSTOMY

Colostomy is preferred in patients with one or more of the following clinical characteristics[3,5,23]: (1) a wound involving more than 50% of the circumference (grade III); (2) extensive free peritoneal fecal spill; (3) associated hypotension; (4) a need for multiple transfusions; (5) three or more associated injuries; (6) colonic devascularization (grade V); (7) a delay of more than 6 hours between injury and operative intervention; (8) an extensive retroperitoneal hematoma from pelvic fractures; (9) an associated abdominal wall defect; and (10) an associated rectal injury.

Specific methods include exteriorization of the segment of injured colon as a loop colostomy; closure of the injured colon, which is then protected by a proximal colostomy; and resection of the injured colon with a proximal end colostomy and a distal mucous fistula (or the Hartmann closure). Simple exteriorization of the injured colon as a loop colostomy is most effective for serious grade III injuries to the right, transverse, left, or sigmoid colon. After the abdomen has been closed, the ostomy is matured primarily to facilitate early fitting with a properly sized appliance. Because exteriorization of the distal sigmoid colon usually is not feasible, such injuries are treated by primary closure with a proximal colostomy (grade III) or by resection of the injury with proximal end colostomy and a distal Hartmann procedure (grades IV and V). For a grade V injury to the distal sigmoid colon with associated devascularization, resection of the injured segment is essential. This type of injury necessitates a proximal end colostomy in conjunction with a Hartmann procedure.

RIGHT COLON INJURY

If the cecum or the first 6 cm of the ascending colon has suffered extensive injury, it may be technically difficult to exteriorize the injured segment as a colostomy.[27] The redundant cecum, including its inferior cul-de-sac, may fill the appliance bag and inconvenience the patient. When large grade IV or V cecal injuries are present, resection with end ileostomy and a distal mucous fistula is safe and effective.

For large cecal and right colon injuries, right hemicolectomy with primary ileotransverse colon anastomosis has been advocated.[23,26] Despite the excellent results reported with right hemicolectomy and primary anastomosis, we recommend that whenever right colon wounds are so extensive that primary closure cannot be done safely, resection with ileostomy should be performed instead. Most patients can tolerate a properly constructed Brooke ileostomy with intraoperative fitting of the appliance [see V:17 Colorectal Procedures].

The so-called closed-loop exteriorization, in which the colon injury is closed primarily and the injured segment then brought out as a temporary exteriorization for 7 to 10 days, is no longer performed. Patients who healed after this procedure probably would have done as well after primary closure. We recommend that whenever there is doubt about the safety of a primary closure, the patient should be treated with a colostomy.

COLOSTOMY CLOSURE

The optimal time for colostomy closure depends on the underlying insult, postoperative morbidity, and the patient's general condition. A patient is ready for a colostomy closure when general health has been restored, appetite has returned, lost weight has been regained, and all wounds have healed. When these criteria are met, mortality associated with colostomy closure should approach zero.[28] Although some colostomies may be closed within days or weeks after injury, those associated with extensive peritonitis and enterocutaneous fistulas are best closed 6 to 12 months after injury.

The safest way of closing loop colostomies involves resection of the exteriorized loop through an oval-shaped incision around the loop, followed by closure with an end-to-end colocolostomy. Sutures are preferred to the staples in this setting because they allow closure of the ostomy through this pericolostomy incision with less mobilization of the proximal and distal ends. When end colostomies are closed, full laparotomy with lysis of all adhesions is required to provide tension-free end-to-end anastomosis and reapproximation of the mesentery. On the whole, we prefer hand-sewn anastomoses for colonic reconstruction.[28]

Injuries to the Rectosigmoid and Rectum

Rectosigmoid and rectal injuries also vary in severity [see Figure 11 and Table 1].[5,29] The agents of injury include knives, bullets, cars, and rectal obturators such as enema tips, thermometers, and sexual toys. The rectosigmoid colon begins near the sacral promontory and extends to the retrovesical fold, where only the anterior bowel wall is covered with peritoneum. Posterior injuries in this 3 to 5 cm zone are retroperitoneal; below this point, the rectum is completely retroperitoneal.

Small, clean, easily accessible rectosigmoid wounds (grades I and II) can be closed primarily if conditions are favorable. Larger wounds require that this segment of bowel be exteriorized or diverted by a proximal colostomy. This can often be accomplished by a proximal sigmoid loop colostomy with primary closure of the rectosigmoid wound.[27,29,30] Massive wounds (grades IV and V) in the rectosigmoid junctional zone require excision, with proximal colostomy and a distal Hartmann procedure.

Penetrating rectal injuries can be diagnosed by means of proctoscopic examination. During laparotomy, the retroperitoneal hematoma associated with rectal injuries often interferes with safe dissection and clear identification of the perforation. Small wounds (grades I and II) can be closed primarily if a proximal colostomy is performed in conjunction with retrorectal drainage. The skin incision for retrorectal drainage is placed between the anus and the coccyx [see Figure 12]. The drain should extend proximal to the perforation. When examination shows that the rectum is filled with stool, the colostomy is opened at the time of operation to facilitate disimpaction and copious distal irrigation with balanced electrolyte solution [see Figure 13]. The anus is kept open only during this irrigation, to facilitate passage of saline and associated stool into an adjacent bucket and to decrease the likelihood that stool will be pushed through the site of injury into retroperitoneal tissues.[28,30] Grade III and grade IV rectal injuries are often more difficult to close primarily; they are usually treated with a proximal colostomy and retrorectal drainage. Massive devascularized grade V rectal injuries are rare; they are treated with resection followed by a proximal end colostomy.

Foreign bodies may produce rectal injuries. Although a thermometer is the most common offending agent in pediatric patients, a larger obturator inserted for pleasure is the usual agent in adults. Such obturators include cans, soft drink bottles, light bulbs, vibrators, and other firm objects. When the offending agent is difficult to remove, spinal anesthesia may be helpful. Once the foreign body has been removed, careful endoscopic examination helps rule out intrinsic injury to the upper rectum or the rectosigmoid. When transanal extraction is impossible, full laparotomy and gentle pushing of the offending agent from above usually permit safe removal. Repair of full-thickness injuries from these obturators follows the guidelines for other types of penetrating injuries.[28]

Extensive grade V rectal injuries associated with close-range shotgun wounds often cause devascularization and intrusion of the bony pelvis. These wounds may require extensive resection of the rectum as well as proximal diversion. Occasionally, these injuries are severe enough to preclude subsequent rectal repair. In rare cases, an industrial accident may result in the same type of extensive injury that is associated with pelvic fractures. For such patients, delayed reconstruction of the rectum may be impossible because of extensive damage to the rectum and the adjacent sacral plexus. Permanent colostomy will be needed in such cases.

References

1. Lucas CE: Splenic trauma: choice of management. Ann Surg 213:98, 1991

2. Wisner DH, Blaisdell FW: Visceral injuries. Arch Surg 127:687, 1992

3. Stone HH, Fabian TC: Management of duodenal wounds. J Trauma 19:334, 1979

4. Kline G, Lucas CE, Ledgerwood AM, et al: Duodenal organ injury severity (OIS) and outcome. Am Surg 60:500, 1994

5. Moore EE, Cogbill TH, Malangoni MA, et al: Organ injury scaling: II. Pancreas, duodenum, small bowel, colon, and rectum. J Trauma 30:1427, 1990

6. Berne CJ, Donovan AJ, White EJ, et al: Duodenal diverticulation for duodenal and pancreatic injury. Am J Surg 127:503, 1974

7. Shorr RM, Greaney GC, Donovan AJ: Injuries of the duodenum. Am J Surg 154:93, 1987

8. Cogbill TH, Moore EE, Feliciano DV, et al: Conservative management of duodenal trauma: a multicenter perspective. J Trauma 30:1469, 1990

9. Degiannis E, Krawczykowski D, Velmahos GC, et al: Pyloric exclusion in severe penetrating injuries of the duodenum. World J Surg 17:751, 1993

10. Vaughan GD 3rd, Frazier OH, Graham DY, et al: The use of pyloric exclusion in the management of severe duodenal injuries. Am J Surg 134:785, 1977

11. Pederzoli P, Bassi C, Falconi M, et al: Conservative treatment of external pancreatic fistulas with parenteral nutrition alone or in combination with continuous intravenous infusion of somatostatin, glucagon, or calcitonin. Surg Gynecol Obstet 163:428, 1986

12. Sugawa C, Lucas CE: The role of endoscopic retrograde cholangiopancreatography in surgery of the pancreas and biliary ducts. Endoscopic Retrograde Cholangiopancreatography. Silvis SE, Rohrmann CA, Ansel HJ, Eds. Igaku-Shoin, New York, 1994, p 3

13. Feliciano DV, Martin TD, Cruse PA, et al: Management of combined pancreatoduodenal injuries. Ann Surg 205:673, 1987

14. Stone A, Sugawa C, Lucas C, et al: The role of endoscopic retrograde pancreatography (ERP) in blunt abdominal trauma. Am Surg 56:715, 1990

15. McKone TK, Bursch LR, Scholten DJ: Pancreaticoduodenectomy for trauma: a life-saving procedure. Am Surg 54:361, 1988

16. Flint LM, Cryer HM, Howard DA, et al: Approaches to the management of shotgun injuries. J Trauma 24:415, 1984

17. Schenk WG 3rd, Lonchyna V, Moylan JA: Perforation of the jejunum from blunt abdominal trauma. J Trauma 23:54, 1983

18. Wisner DH, Chun Y, Blaisdell FW: Blunt intestinal injury: keys to diagnosis and management. Arch Surg 125:1319, 1990

19. Coleman EJ, Dietz PA: Small bowel injuries following blunt abdominal trauma: early recognition and management. NY State J Med 90:446, 1990

20. Sherck J, Shatney C, Sensaki K, et al: The accuracy of computed tomography in the diagnosis of blunt small-bowel perforation. Am J Surg 168:670, 1994

21. Brundage SI, Jurkovich GJ, Grossman DC, et al: Stapled versus sutured gastrointestinal anastomoses in the trauma patient. J Trauma 47:500, 1999

22. Witzke JD, Kraatz JJ, Marken JM, et al: Stapled versus hand-sewn anastomoses in patients with small bowel injury: a changing perspective. J Trauma 49:660, 2000

23. Lucas C, Ledgerwood A: Management of the injured colon. Current Surgery 43:190, 1986

24. Ross SE, Cobean RA, Hoyt DB, et al: Blunt colonic injury—a multicenter review. J Trauma 33:379, 1992

25. George SM Jr, Fabian TC, Voeller GR, et al: Primary repair of colon wounds: a prospective trial in nonselected patients. Ann Surg 209:728, 1989

26. Ivatury RR, Licata J, Gunduz Y, et al: Management options in penetrating rectal injuries. Am Surg 57:50, 1991

27. Strada G, Raad L, Belloni G, et al: Large bowel perforations in war surgery: one-stage treatment in a field hospital. Int J Colorectal Dis 8:213, 1993

28. Ledgerwood AM, Lucas CE: Management of colon injuries. Principles and Practice of Trauma Care. Worth MH, Ed. Williams & Wilkins, Baltimore, 1982, p 117

29. Nelken N, Lewis F: The influence of injury severity on complication rates after primary closure or colostomy for penetrating colon trauma. Ann Surg 209:439, 1989

30. Burch JM, Feliciano DV, Mattox KL: Colostomy and drainage for civilian rectal injuries: is that all? Ann Surg 209:600, 1989

Acknowledgments

Supported by the Interstitial Fluid Fund, Account 4-44966.

Figures 1, 2, 5, 9 through 11   Marcia Kammerer.

Figures 3, 8, 12, 13   Susan Brust, C.M.I.

Figures 4, 6, 7   Carol Donner.

9 INJURIES TO THE GREAT VESSELS OF THE ABDOMEN

David V. Feliciano, M.D.

In patients who have injuries to the great vessels of the abdomen, the findings on physical examination generally depend on whether a contained hematoma or active hemorrhage is present. In the case of contained hematomas around the vascular injury in the retroperitoneum, the base of the mesentery, or the hepatoduodenal ligament, the patient often has only modest hypotension in transit or on arrival at the emergency center; the hypotension can be temporarily reversed by the infusion of fluids and may not recur until the hematoma is opened at the time of laparotomy. This is usually the situation when an abdominal venous injury is present. In the case of active intraperitoneal hemorrhage, the patient typically has significant hypotension and may have a distended abdomen on arrival. Another physical finding that is occasionally noted in association with an injury to the common or external iliac artery is intermittent or complete loss of a pulse in the ipsilateral femoral artery; this finding in a patient with a transpelvic gunshot wound is pathognomonic of an injury to the iliac artery.

Injuries to the great vessels of the abdomen are caused by penetrating wounds in 90% to 95% of cases; accordingly, they are often accompanied by injuries to multiple intra-abdominal organs, including those in the gastrointestinal tract. The general principles governing the sequencing of repairs of injuries to the great vessels and the GI tract are outlined elsewhere [*see III:6 Operative Exposure of Abdominal Injuries and Closure of the Abdomen*].

A hematoma [*see Figures 1 and 2*] or hemorrhage associated with an injury to a great vessel of the abdomen occurs in one of the three zones of the retroperitoneum or in the portal-retrohepatic area of the right upper quadrant [*see III:6 Operative Exposure of Abdominal Injuries and Closure of the Abdomen*]. The magnitude of injury is usually described according to the Abdominal Vascular Organ Injury Scale, devised in 1992 by the American Association for the Surgery of Trauma [*see Table 1*].

Injuries in Zone 1

SUPRAMESOCOLIC

It is helpful to divide midline retroperitoneal hematomas into those that are supramesocolic and those that are inframesocolic. Hematoma or hemorrhage in the midline supramesocolic area of zone 1 is cause to suspect the presence of an injury to the suprarenal aorta, the celiac axis, the proximal superior mesenteric artery, or the proximal renal artery.

When a hematoma is present in the midline supramesocolic area, one usually has time to perform left medial visceral rotation [*see Figure 3 and III:6 Operative Exposure of Abdominal Injuries and Closure of the Abdomen*]. The advantage of this technique is that it allows visualization of the entire abdominal aorta, from the aortic hiatus of the

Figure 1 Algorithm illustrates management of intra-abdominal hematoma found at operation after penetrating trauma.

Figure 2 **Algorithm illustrates management of intra-abdominal hematoma found at operation after blunt trauma.**

diaphragm to the common iliac arteries [*see Figure 4*]. Obvious disadvantages include the 4 to 5 minutes required to complete the maneuver when the surgeon is inexperienced; the risk of damage to the spleen, the left kidney, or the posterior left renal artery as the maneuver is performed; and the anatomic distortion that results when the left kidney and the left renal artery are rotated anteriorly. When the hematoma is near the aortic hiatus of the diaphragm, it may be advisable to leave the left kidney in its fossa, thereby eliminating potential damage to the structure as well as the distortion resulting from rotation. Because of the density of the celiac plexus and the lymphatic vessels surrounding the upper abdominal aorta, this portion of the aorta is difficult to visualize even when left medial visceral rotation has been performed. It is frequently helpful to transect the left crus of the aortic hiatus in the diaphragm at the 2 o'clock

Table 1 AAST Abdominal Vascular Organ Injury Scale

Grade	Characteristics of Injury	OIS Grade	ICD-9	AIS-90
I	Unnamed superior mesenteric artery or superior mesenteric vein branches	I	902.20/902.39	NS
	Unnamed inferior mesenteric artery or inferior mesenteric vein branches	I	902.27/902.32	NS
	Phrenic artery or vein	I	902.89	NS
	Lumbar artery or vein	I	902.89	NS
	Gonadal artery or vein	I	902.89	NS
	Ovarian artery or vein	I	902.81/902.82	NS
	Other unnamed small arterial or venous structures requiring ligation	I	902.90	NS
II	Right, left, or common hepatic artery	II	902.22	3
	Splenic artery or vein	II	902.23/902.34	3
	Right or left gastric arteries	II	902.21	3
	Gastroduodenal artery	II	902.24	3
	Inferior mesenteric artery, trunk, or inferior mesenteric vein, trunk	II	902.27/902.32	3
	Primary named branches of mesenteric artery (e.g., ileocolic artery) or mesenteric vein	II	902.26/902.31	3
	Other named abdominal vessels requiring ligation or repair	II	902.89	3
III*	Superior mesenteric vein, trunk	III	902.31	3
	Renal artery or vein	III	902.41/902.42	3
	Iliac artery or vein	III	902.53/902.54	3
	Hypogastric artery or vein	III	902.51/902.52	3
	Vena cava, infrarenal	III	902.10	3
IV*†	Superior mesenteric artery, trunk	IV	902.25	3
	Celiac axis, proper	IV	902.24	3
	Vena cava, suprarenal and infrahepatic	IV	902.10	3
	Aorta, infrarenal	IV	902.00	4
V†	Portal vein	V	902.33	3
	Extraparenchymal hepatic vein	V	902.11	3 (hepatic vein) 5 (liver + veins)
	Vena cava, retrohepatic or suprahepatic	V	902.19	5
	Aorta, suprarenal and subdiaphragmatic	V	902.00	4

Note: This classification is applicable to extraparenchymal vascular injuries. If the vessel injury is within 2 cm of the parenchyma of a specific organ, one should refer to the injury scale for that organ.

*Increase grade by I if there are multiple injuries involving > 50% of vessel circumference.

†Reduce grade by I if laceration is < 25% of vessel circumference.

AAST—American Association for the Surgery of Trauma   AIS—Abbreviated Injury Scale   ICD—International Classification of Diseases

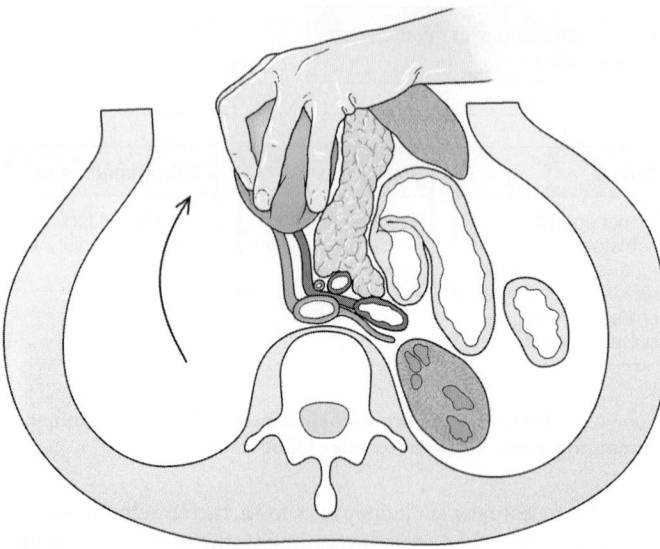

Figure 3 Left medial visceral rotation is performed by means of sharp and blunt dissection with elevation of the left colon, the left kidney, the spleen, the tail of the pancreas, and the gastric fundus.

Figure 4 Shown is an autopsy view of the supraceliac aorta and the celiac axis, the proximal superior mesenteric artery, and the medially rotated left renal artery after removal of lymphatic and nerve tissue.

position to allow exposure of the distal descending thoracic aorta above the hiatus. Visualization of this portion of the vessel is much easier to achieve than visualization of the diaphragmatic or visceral abdominal aorta below, and an aortic cross-clamp can be applied much more quickly at this level.

Active hemorrhage from the midline supramesocolic area is controlled temporarily by packing with laparotomy pads or using an aortic compression device [*see Figure 5*]. The definitive approach is to divide the lesser omentum manually, retract the stomach and esophagus to the left, and manually dissect in the area just below the aortic hiatus to obtain rapid exposure of the supraceliac abdominal aorta; an aortic cross-clamp can then be applied. Distal control of the upper abdominal aorta is difficult to obtain because of the presence of the anteriorly located celiac axis and superior mesen-

teric artery. In young trauma patients who are otherwise healthy, ligation and division of the celiac axis allow easier application of the distal aortic clamp and better exposure of the supraceliac area for subsequent vascular repair.

Small penetrating wounds to the supraceliac abdominal aorta are repaired with a continuous 3-0 or 4-0 polypropylene suture. If two small perforations are adjacent to each other, they can be connected and the defect closed in a transverse fashion. If closure of a perforation would result in significant narrowing of the aorta or if a portion of the aortic wall is missing, patch aortoplasty with polytetrafluoroethylene (PTFE) is indicated. On rare occasions, in patients with extensive injuries to the diaphragmatic or supraceliac aorta, resection of the area of injury and insertion of a vascular conduit are indicated. Even though many of these patients have associated gastric, enteric, or colonic injuries, the most appropriate prosthesis with such a life-threatening injury is a 12 mm or 14 mm Dacron or PTFE graft [*see Figure 6*]. Provided that vigorous intraoperative irrigation is performed after repair of GI tract perforations, that proper graft coverage is ensured, and that perioperative antibiotics are appropriately employed, it is extraordinarily rare for a prosthesis inserted in the healthy aorta of a young trauma patient to become infected.

The aortic prosthesis is sewn in place with a continuous 3-0 or 4-0 polypropylene suture. Both ends of the aorta are flushed before the distal anastomosis is completed, and the distal aortic cross-clamp is removed before the final knot is tied to eliminate air from the system. The proximal aortic cross-clamp is removed very slowly as the

Figure 5 An aortic compression device is used to control hemorrhage from the visceral portion of the abdominal aorta.

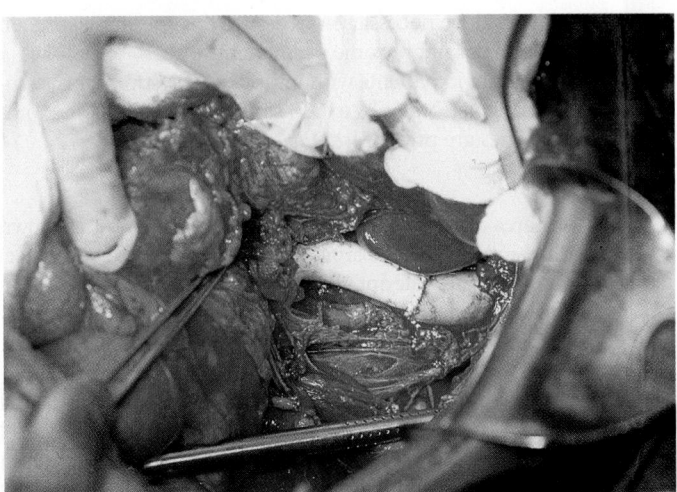

Figure 6 **A 22-year-old man with a gunshot wound to the right upper quadrant had injuries to the prepyloric area of the stomach and to the supraceliac abdominal aorta. The aortic injury was managed by means of segmental resection and replacement with a 16 mm polytetrafluoroethylene (PTFE) graft. The patient went home 46 days after injury.**

anesthesiologist rapidly infuses fluids and intravenous bicarbonate to reverse so-called washout acidosis from the previously ischemic lower extremities. The retroperitoneum is then irrigated with an antibiotic solution and closed over the graft in a watertight fashion with an absorbable suture.

The survival rate in patients with injuries to the suprarenal abdominal aorta had been 30% to 35% but was lower than 10% in one 2001 review.[1]

Injuries to branches of the celiac axis are often difficult to repair because of the amount of dissection required to remove the dense neural and lymphatic tissue in this area. Because most patients have excellent collateral flow in the upper abdomen, major injuries to either the left gastric or the proximal splenic artery generally should be ligated. Because the common hepatic artery may have a larger diameter than either of these two arteries, an injury to this vessel can occasionally be repaired by means of lateral arteriorrhaphy, an end-to-end anastomosis, or the insertion of a saphenous vein graft. One should not worry about ligating the common hepatic artery proximal to the origin of the gastroduodenal artery: there is exten-

sive collateral flow to the liver from the midgut. When the entire celiac axis is injured, it is best to ligate all three vessels and forgo any attempt at repair.

Injuries to the superior mesenteric artery are managed according to the anatomic level of the perforation or thrombosis. On rare occasions, in patients with injuries beneath the neck of the pancreas, one may have to transect the pancreas to obtain proximal control. Another option is to perform left medial visceral rotation (see above) and apply a clamp directly to the origin of the superior mesenteric artery. Injuries to the superior mesenteric artery in this area or just beyond the base of the mesocolon are often associated with injuries to the pancreas. The potential for a postoperative leak from the injured pancreas near the arterial repair has led numerous authors to suggest that any extensive injury to the artery at this location should be ligated [*see Figure 7*].

Because of the intense vasoconstriction of the distal superior mesenteric artery in patients who have sustained exsanguinating hemorrhage from more proximal injuries treated with ligation, the collateral flow from the foregut and hindgut is often inadequate to maintain the viability of the organs in the distal midgut, especially the cecum and the ascending colon. Therefore, it is safest to place a saphenous vein or PTFE graft on the distal infrarenal aorta, away from the pancreatic injury and any other upper abdominal injuries. Such a graft can be tailored to reach the side or the anterior aspect of the superior mesenteric artery, or it can be attached to the transected distal superior mesenteric artery in an end-to-end fashion without significant tension [*see Figure 8*]. Soft tissue must be approximated over the aortic suture line of the graft to prevent the development of an aortoenteric fistula in the postoperative period.

In patients with severe shock from exsanguination caused by a complex injury to the superior mesenteric artery, damage control laparotomy is indicated: the injured area should be resected and a temporary intraluminal Argyle, Javid, or Pruitt-Inahara shunt inserted to maintain flow to the midgut during resuscitation in the surgical intensive care unit. When ligation is indicated for more distal injuries to the superior mesenteric artery, segments of the ileum or even the right colon may have to be resected because of ischemia.

The survival rate in patients with penetrating injuries to the superior mesenteric artery is approximately 50% to 55% overall [*see Table 2*] but only 20% to 25% when any form of repair more complex than lateral arteriorrhaphy is necessary.[1-3]

An injury to the proximal renal artery may also be present under a supramesocolic hematoma or bleeding area. When active hemor-

Table 2 Survival after Injuries to Arteries in the Abdomen

Injured Artery	Asensio et al[2] (2000)		Davis et al[3] (2001)*	Tyburski et al[1] (2001)
	Isolated Injury	With Other Arterial Injury		
Abdominal aorta as a whole	21.7% (10/46)	17.6% (3/17)	39.1% (25/64)	21.1% (15/71)
Pararenal to diaphragm	—	—	—	8.3% (3/36)
Infrarenal	—	—	—	34.2% (12/35)
Superior mesenteric artery	52.4% (11/21)	28.6% (2/7)	53.3% (8/15)	48.8% (20/41)
Renal artery	62.5% (5/8)	33.3% (2/6)	56.2% (9/16)	73.7% (14/19)
Iliac artery				
Common	—	—	55.5% (5/9)	44.7% (17/38)
External	—	—	65.2% (30/46)	62.5% (20/32)

*Excludes patients who exsanguinated before repair or ligation.

Figure 7 An 18-year-old man experienced a gunshot wound to the head of the pancreas and the proximal superior mesenteric artery. A Whipple procedure was performed, and a 6 mm PTFE graft was placed in the artery. The artery-graft suture line dehisced secondary to a pancreatic leak on day 30 after injury, and the patient died on day 42.

rhage is present, control of the supraceliac abdominal aorta in or just below the aortic hiatus must be obtained. When only a hematoma or a known thrombosis of the proximal renal artery is present, proximal vascular control can be obtained by elevating the transverse mesocolon and dissecting the vessel from the lateral aspect of the abdominal aorta. Options for repair of either the proximal or the distal renal artery are described elsewhere [*see* Injuries in Zone 2, *below*].

The superior mesenteric vein is the other great vessel of the abdomen that may be injured in the supramesocolic or retromesocolic area of the midline retroperitoneum. Because of the overlying pancreas, the proximity of the uncinate process, and the close association of this vessel with the superior mesenteric artery, repair of the superior mesenteric vein is quite difficult. As with injuries to the superior mesenteric artery (see above), one may have to transect the neck of the pancreas between noncrushing vascular or intestinal clamps to gain access to a perforation of the superior mesenteric vein. An injury to this vein below the inferior border of the pancreas can be managed by compressing it manually between one's fingers as an assistant places a continuous 5-0 polypropylene suture to complete the repair. When a penetrating injury to the vein has a posterior component, one must ligate multiple collateral vessels entering the vein in this area to achieve proper visualization.

There is now excellent evidence that young trauma patients tolerate ligation of the superior mesenteric vein well when vigorous postoperative fluid resuscitation is performed to reverse the peripheral hypovolemia that results from splanchnic hypervolemia. Typically, ligation is followed almost immediately by swelling of the midgut and discoloration suggestive of impending ischemia. In such cases, temporary coverage of the midgut with a silo, followed by ear-

ly reoperation, may be necessary to reassure the operating surgeon that the ischemia has not become permanent.

The survival rate in patients with injuries to the superior mesenteric vein has ranged from 36% to 71%, depending on whether other vascular injuries are present [*see Table 3*].[1-3]

INFRAMESOCOLIC

The lower area of the midline retroperitoneum in zone 1 is known as the midline inframesocolic area. Injuries to either the infrarenal abdominal aorta or the inferior vena cava occur in this area.

The infrarenal abdominal aorta is exposed by pulling the transverse mesocolon up toward the patient's head, eviscerating the small bowel to the right side of the abdomen, and opening the midline retroperitoneum until the left renal vein is exposed. A proximal aortic cross-clamp is then placed immediately inferior to this vessel [*see Figure 9*]. When there is active hemorrhage from this area, rapid proximal control is obtained in the same fashion or, if necessary, by dividing the lesser omentum and applying the cross-clamp just below the aortic hiatus of the diaphragm. Distal control of the infrarenal abdominal aorta is obtained by dividing the midline retroperitoneum down to the aortic bifurcation, taking care to avoid the left-sided origin of the inferior mesenteric artery.

Injuries to the infrarenal aorta are repaired by means of lateral aortorrhaphy, patch aortoplasty, an end-to-end anastomosis, or insertion of a Dacron or PTFE graft. Much as with injuries to the suprarenal abdominal aorta in young trauma patients, it is rarely possible to place a tube graft larger than 12 or 14 mm. Because the retroperitoneal tissue is often thin at this location in young patients, an appropriate option after the aortic repair is to mobilize the gastrocolic omentum, flip it into the lesser sac superiorly, and then bring it down over the infrarenal aortic graft through a hole in the transverse mesocolon. Another option is to mobilize the gastrocolic omentum away from the right side of the colon and then swing the mobilized tissue into the left lateral gutter just below the ligament of Treitz to cover the graft.

The survival rate in patients with injuries to the infrarenal abdominal aorta had been approximately 45% but was 34% in a 2001 review [*see Table 2*].[1]

Injury to the inferior vena cava below the liver should be suspected when the aorta is found to be intact underneath an inframesocolic hematoma, when such a hematoma appears to be more extensive on the right side of the abdomen than on the left, or when there is active hemorrhage coming through the base of the mesentery of the ascending colon or the hepatic flexure. It is certainly possible to visualize the inferior vena cava through the midline retroperitoneal exposure just described (see above); however, most surgeons are more comfortable with visualizing the vessel by mobilizing the right half of the colon and the C loop of the duodenum [*see III:6 Operative Exposure of Abdominal Injuries and Closure of the Abdomen*]. With this right medial visceral rotation maneuver, the right kidney is left in situ unless there is an associated injury to the posterior aspect of the right renal vein, to the suprarenal vena cava, or to the right kidney itself. Right medial visceral rotation, in conjunction with the Kocher maneuver, permits visualization of the entire vena caval system from the confluence of the iliac veins to the suprarenal vena cava below the liver.

For proper exposure of a hole in a large vein such as the inferior vena cava, the loose retroperitoneal fatty tissue must be dissected away from the wall of the vessel. Active hemorrhage coming from the anterior surface of the inferior vena cava is best controlled by applying a Satinsky vascular clamp. If it is difficult to apply this clamp, one should try grasping the area of the perforation with a pair of vascular forceps or several Judd-Allis clamps; this step may

Figure 8   (*a*) **When complex grafting procedures to the superior mesenteric artery are necessary, it may be dangerous to place the proximal suture line near an associated pancreatic injury. (*b*) The proximal suture line should be on the lower aorta, away from the upper abdominal injuries, and should be covered with retroperitoneal tissue.**

facilitate safe application of the Satinsky clamp. When the perforation in the inferior vena cava is more lateral or posterior, it is often helpful to compress the vessel proximally and distally around the perforation, using gauze sponges placed in straight sponge sticks. On occasion, an extensive injury to the inferior vena cava can be controlled only by completely occluding the entire inferior vena cava with large DeBakey aortic cross-clamps. This maneuver interrupts much of the venous return to the right side of the heart and is poorly tolerated by hypotensive patients unless the infrarenal abdominal aorta is cross-clamped simultaneously.

There are two anatomic areas in which vascular control of an injury to the inferior vena cava below the liver is difficult to obtain: (1) the confluence of the common iliac veins and (2) the junction of the renal veins with the inferior vena cava. One interesting approach to an injury to the inferior vena cava at the confluence of the iliac veins is temporary division of the overlying right common iliac artery, coupled with mobilization of the aortic bifurcation to the patient's left. This approach yields a better view of the common iliac veins and the proximal inferior vena cava and makes repair considerably easier than it would be if the aortic bifurcation were left in place. Once the vein is repaired, the right common iliac artery is reconstituted via an end-to-end anastomosis. The usual approach to injuries to the inferior vena cava at its junction with the renal veins involves clamp or sponge-stick compression of the infrarenal and suprarenal vena cava as well as control of both renal veins with Silastic loops to facilitate the direct application of angled

Table 3   Survival after Injuries to Veins in the Abdomen

Injured Vein	Asensio et al[2] (2000)		Davis et al[3] (2001)*	Tyburski et al[1] (2001)
	Isolated Injury	With Other Venous Injury		
Inferior vena cava as a whole	29.3% (12/41)†	22.2% (8/36)†	56% (47/84)	43% (61/142)
Pararenal to diaphragm	—	—	—	40.3% (31/77)
Infrarenal	—	—	—	46.2% (30/65)
Superior mesenteric vein	47.4% (9/19)	35.7% (5/14)	71.4% (15/21)	56.3% (18/32)
Renal vein	—	44.1% (15/34)	70% (21/30)	68.8% (22/32)
Iliac vein (all)	62.2% (23/37)	33.3% (5/15)	—	—
Common	—	—	81% (17/21)	49% (24/49)
External	—	—	74.5% (41/55)	66.7% (16/24)

*Excludes patients who exsanguinated before repair or ligation.
†Excludes retrohepatic vena cava.

Figure 9 **Shown is a gunshot wound to the infrarenal abdominal aorta viewed through standard inframesocolic exposure.**

vascular clamps. As noted, medial mobilization of the right kidney may permit the application of a partial occlusion clamp across the inferior vena cava at its junction with the right renal vein as an alternative approach to an injury in this area. Another useful technique for controlling hemorrhage from the inferior vena cava at any location is to insert a 5 ml or 30 ml Foley balloon catheter into the caval laceration and then inflate it in the lumen. Once the bleeding is controlled, vascular clamps are positioned around the perforation, and the balloon catheter is removed before repair of the vessel.

Anterior perforations of the inferior vena cava are managed by means of transverse repair with a continuous 4-0 or 5-0 polypropylene suture. Much has been written about visualizing posterior perforations by extending anterior perforations, but in my experience, opportunities to apply this approach have been rare. It is often easier to roll the vena cava to one side to complete a continuous suture repair of a posterior perforation. When both anterior and posterior perforations have been repaired, there is usually a significant degree of narrowing of the inferior vena cava, which may lead to slow postoperative occlusion. If the patient's condition is unstable and a coagulopathy has developed, no further attempt should be made to revise the repair. If the patient is stable, there may be some justification for applying a large PTFE patch to prevent this postoperative occlusion [*see Figure 10*].

Ligation of the infrarenal inferior vena cava is appropriate for young patients who are exsanguinating and in whom a complex repair of the vessel would be necessary. Such patients require vigorous resuscitation with crystalloid solutions in the postoperative period; in addition, both lower extremities should be wrapped with elastic compression wraps and elevated for 5 to 7 days after operation. Patients who have some residual edema during the later stages of hospitalization despite the elastic compression wraps should be fitted with full-length custom-made support hose. Ligation of the suprarenal inferior vena cava is occasionally necessary when the patient has an extensive injury at this location and appears to be in an irreversible shock state during operation. If the patient's condition improves during a brief period of resuscitation in the SICU, reoperation and reconstruction with an externally supported PTFE graft are necessary to prevent renal failure.

The survival rate in patients with injuries to the inferior vena cava depends on the location of the injury; in the past, it ranged from 60% for the suprarenal vena cava to 78% for the infrarenal vena cava but decreased to approximately 33% to 56% if injuries to the retrohepatic vena cava were included. Current studies indicate survival rates of 22% to 56% for inferior vena cava injuries taken as a whole.[2,3] A 2001 review reported survival rates of 46.1% for the infrarenal inferior vena cava and 40.3% for more superior injuries.[1]

Injuries in Zone 2

Hematoma or hemorrhage in zone 2 is cause to suspect the presence of injury to the renal artery, the renal vein, or the kidney.

Figure 10 **Shown is PTFE patch repair of an injury to the infrarenal inferior vena cava.**

Figure 11 **A right perirenal hematoma was not opened at operation, because preoperative abdominal CT documented a reasonably intact kidney.**

Figure 12 **Midline looping of respective renal vessels is performed before entry into any perirenal hematoma.**

In patients who have sustained blunt abdominal trauma but in whom preoperative intravenous pyelography, renal arteriography, or CT of the kidneys yields normal findings, there is no justification for opening a perirenal hematoma if one is found at a subsequent operation [*see Figure 11*].

In highly selected stable patients with penetrating wounds to the flank, there are some data to justify performing preoperative CT. On occasion, documentation of an isolated minor renal injury in the absence of peritoneal findings on physical examination makes it possible to manage such patients nonoperatively. In all other patients with penetrating wounds, when a perirenal hematoma is found dur-

ing initial exploration, the hematoma should be unroofed and the wound tract explored. If the hematoma is not rapidly expanding and there is no active hemorrhage from the perirenal area, one may control the ipsilateral renal artery with a Silastic loop in the midline of the retroperitoneum at the base of the mesocolon [*see Figure 12*]. Control of the left renal vein can be obtained at the same location; however, control of the proximal right renal vein requires mobilization of the C loop of the duodenum and dissection of the vena cava at its junction with this vessel.

If there is active hemorrhage from the kidney through Gerota's fascia or from the retroperitoneum overlying the renal vessels, no central renal vascular control is necessary. In such a situation, the retroperitoneum lateral to the injured kidney should be opened, and the kidney should be manually elevated directly into the abdominal incision. A large vascular clamp should then be applied directly to the hilar vessels of the elevated kidney to control any further bleeding until a decision is reached on repair versus nephrectomy.

Occasionally, a small perforation of the renal artery can be repaired by lateral arteriorrhaphy or resection with an end-to-end anastomosis. Interposition grafting and replacement of the renal artery with either the hepatic artery (on the right) or the splenic artery (on the left) have been used on rare occasions, but such approaches ordinarily are not indicated unless the injured kidney is the only one the patient has. In patients who have sustained multiple intra-abdominal injuries from penetrating wounds or have undergone a long period of ischemia while other injuries were being repaired, nephrectomy is the appropriate choice for a major renovascular injury, provided that intraoperative palpation has confirmed the presence of a normal contralateral kidney.

The role of renal revascularization in patients who have intimal tears in the renal arteries as a result of deceleration-type trauma remains controversial. If a circumferential intimal tear is noted on preoperative arteriography but flow to the kidney is preserved, the decision whether to repair the artery depends on whether laparotomy is necessary for other injuries and whether the opportunity for anticoagulation is available. If there are no other significant injuries and

Figure 13 **With the left renal vein elevated, a hematoma ring may be noted overlying a blunt intimal tear in an occluded left renal artery.**

Figure 14 **In the same patient as in Figure 13, the intimal tear in the left renal artery was resected, an end-to-end anastomosis was performed, and blood flow to the left kidney was restored.**

Figure 15 **A 24-year-old man experienced a gunshot wound to the left external iliac artery and vein. The arterial injury was repaired with segmental resection and insertion of an 8 mm PTFE graft; the venous injury was repaired with segmental resection and an end-to-end anastomosis.**

flow to the kidney is preserved despite the presence of an intimal tear, anticoagulation and a repeat isotope renogram within the first several days may be justified. If occlusion of the proximal renal artery from blunt deceleration-type trauma is documented, the critical factor for renal salvage is the time from occlusion to revascularization. Renal artery occlusion from deceleration-type trauma that is detected within 6 hours of injury is best treated with immediate operation, resection of the area of intimal damage, and an end-to-end anastomosis performed by an experienced vascular trauma team [*see Figures 13 and 14*]. Given proper exposure and medial mobilization of the kidney, this operation is not technically difficult in a young trauma patient whose renal artery is otherwise normal. In a 1998 review,[4] fewer than 20% of kidneys revascularized in this manner regained any significant degree of function. Hypertension develops in 40% to 45% of patients who undergo observation only after thrombosis is detected.

The survival rate in patients with isolated injuries to the renal arteries ranges from 56% to 74% [*see Table 2*].[1,3]

Many patients with penetrating wounds to the renal veins are quite stable as a result of the retroperitoneal tamponade described earlier (see above). Once vascular control is obtained with the direct application of clamps, lateral venorrhaphy is the preferred technique of repair. Nephrectomy should be performed if ligation of the right renal vein is necessary to control hemorrhage, whereas the medial left renal vein may be ligated as long as the left adrenal and gonadal veins are intact. It should be noted, however, that in some series, more postoperative renal complications were noted when this maneuver was used on the left side.

The survival rate in patients with isolated injuries to the renal veins is approximately 70% [*see Table 3*].[1,3]

Injuries in Zone 3

Hematoma or hemorrhage in either lateral pelvic area is suggestive of injury to the iliac artery or the iliac vein.

When lateral pelvic hematoma or hemorrhage is noted after penetrating trauma, compression with a laparotomy pad or the fingers should be maintained as proximal and distal vascular control is obtained. The proximal common iliac arteries are exposed by eviscerating the small bowel to the right and dividing the midline retroperi-

toneum over the aortic bifurcation. In young trauma patients, the common iliac artery usually is not adherent to the common iliac vein, and Silastic loops can be passed rapidly around these vessels to provide proximal vascular control. Distal vascular control is most easily obtained where the external iliac artery and vein come out of the pelvis proximal to the inguinal ligament. Even with proximal and distal control of the common or the external iliac artery and vein, there is often continued back-bleeding from the internal iliac artery. Such bleeding is controlled by elevating the Silastic loops on the proximal and distal iliac artery and then either clamping or looping the internal iliac artery, which is the only major branch vessel that descends into the pelvis.

For transpelvic bilateral iliac vascular injuries resulting from a penetrating wound, a technique of total pelvic vascular isolation has been described. Proximally, the abdominal aorta and the inferior vena cava are cross-clamped just above their bifurcations, and distally, both the external iliac artery and the external iliac vein are cross-clamped, with one clamp on each side of the distal pelvis. Back-bleeding from the internal iliac vessels is minimal with this approach.

Ligation of either the common or the external iliac artery in a hypotensive trauma patient leads to a 40% to 50% amputation rate in the postoperative period; consequently, injuries to these vessels should be repaired if at all possible. The standard options for repair—lateral arteriorrhaphy, completion of a partial transection with an end-to-end anastomosis, and resection of the injured area with insertion of a conduit—are feasible in most situations [*see Figure 15*]. On rare occasions, it may be preferable either to mobilize the ipsilateral internal iliac artery to serve as a replacement for the external iliac artery or to transpose one iliac artery to the side of the contralateral iliac artery. When a patient is in severe shock from exsanguination caused by a complex injury to the common or the external iliac artery, damage control laparotomy [*see* Damage Control Laparotomy, *below*] is indicated. The injured area should be resected and a temporary intraluminal Argyle, Javid, or Pruitt-Inahara shunt inserted to maintain flow to the ipsilateral lower extremity during resuscitation in the SICU.

One unique problem associated with repair of the common or the external iliac artery is the choice of technique when significant enteric or fecal contamination is present in the pelvis. In such cases, there is a substantial risk of postoperative pelvic cellulitis, a pelvic abscess, or both, which may lead to blowout of any type of repair. When extensive contamination is present, it is appropriate to divide the common or external iliac artery above the level of injury, close the injury with a double row of continuous 4-0 or 5-0 polypropylene sutures, and bury the stump underneath uninjured retroperitoneum. If a stable patient has obvious ischemia of the ipsilateral lower extremity at the completion of this proximal ligation, one may perform an extra-anatomic femorofemoral crossover graft to restore arterial flow to the extremity. If the patient is unstable, one should take several minutes to perform an ipsilateral four-compartment below-knee fasciotomy; this step will counteract the ischemic edema that inevitably leads to a compartment syndrome and compromises the early survival of the leg. After adequate resuscitation in the SICU, the patient should be returned to the OR for the femorofemoral graft within 4 to 6 hours.

Injuries to the internal iliac arteries are usually ligated even if they occur bilaterally, because young trauma patients typically have extensive collateral flow through the pelvis.

The survival rate in patients with isolated injuries to the external iliac artery exceeds 80% when tamponade is present. If the injury is large and free bleeding has occurred preoperatively, however, the survival rate is only 45%. Current studies report overall survival rates of approximately 45% to 55% for injuries to the common iliac

Figure 16 Failure to properly dissect out the structures in the porta hepatis after a penetrating wound led to the creation of an iatrogenic hepatic artery–portal vein fistula, which was corrected after the arrival of the attending surgeon.

artery and 62% to 65% for injuries to the external iliac artery [*see Table 2*].[1,3]

Hemorrhage from injuries to the iliac veins can usually be controlled by means of compression with either sponge sticks or the fingers. As noted, division of the right common iliac artery may be necessary for proper visualization of an injury to the right common iliac vein. Similarly, ligation and division of the internal iliac artery on the side of the pelvis yield improved exposure of an injury to an ipsilateral internal iliac vein.

Injuries to the common or the external iliac vein are best treated by means of lateral venorrhaphy with continuous 4-0 or 5-0 polypropylene sutures. Significant narrowing often results, and a number of reports have demonstrated occlusion on postoperative venography. For patients with narrowing or occlusion, as well as for those in whom ligation was necessary to control exsanguinating hemorrhage, the use of elastic compression wraps and elevation for the first 5 to 7 days after operation is mandatory.

The survival rate in patients with injuries to the iliac veins ranges from 33% to 81%, depending on whether associated vascular injuries are present [*see Table 3*].[1-3]

Injuries in the Porta Hepatis or Retrohepatic Area

PORTA HEPATIS

Hematoma or hemorrhage in the area of the portal triad in the right upper quadrant is cause to suspect the presence of injury to the portal vein or the hepatic artery or of vascular injury combined with an injury to the common bile duct.

If a hematoma is present, the proximal hepatoduodenal ligament should be occluded with a vascular clamp (the Pringle maneuver [*see III:7 Injuries to the Liver, Biliary Tract, Spleen, and Diaphragm*]) before the hematoma is entered. If the hematoma is centrally located in the porta, one may also be able to apply an angled vascular clamp to the distal end of the portal structures at their entrance into the liver.

If hemorrhage is occurring, compression of the bleeding vessels with the fingers should suffice until the vascular clamp is in place. Once proximal and distal vascular control is obtained, the three structures in the hepatoduodenal ligament must be dissected out very carefully because of the danger of blindly placing sutures in proximity to the common bile duct [*see Figure 16*].

Injuries to the hepatic artery in this location are occasionally amenable to lateral repair, though ligation without reconstruction is ordinarily well tolerated because of the extensive collateral arterial flow to the liver. If an associated hepatic injury calls for extensive suturing or debridement, ligation of the common hepatic artery will certainly lead to increased postoperative necrosis of the hepatic repair. Moreover, ligation of the common hepatic artery, the right or left hepatic artery supplying the injured lobe, and the portal vein branch to that lobe will lead to necrosis of the lobe and will necessitate hepatectomy. Finally, ligation of the right hepatic artery to control hemorrhage should be followed by cholecystectomy.

Because of the large size of the portal vein and its posterior position in the hepatoduodenal ligament, injuries to this vessel are particularly lethal. Once the Pringle maneuver has been performed, mobilization of the common bile duct to the left and of the cystic duct superiorly, coupled with an extensive Kocher maneuver, allows excellent visualization of any injury to this vein above the superior border of the pancreas. When the perforation extends underneath the neck of the pancreas, it may be necessary to have an assistant compress the superior mesenteric vein below the pancreas and then to divide the pancreas between noncrushing intestinal clamps to obtain exposure of the junction of the superior mesenteric vein and the splenic vein.

The preferred technique for repairing an injury to the portal vein is lateral venorrhaphy with continuous 4-0 or 5-0 polypropylene sutures. Complex repairs that have been successful on rare occasions include end-to-end anastomosis, interposition grafting with externally supported PTFE, transposition of the splenic vein, and a venovenous shunt from the superior mesenteric vein to the distal portal vein or the inferior vena cava. Such vigorous attempts at restoration of blood flow are not justified in patients who are in severe hypovolemic shock, for whom ligation of the portal vein is more appropriate. In addition, if a portosystemic shunt is performed in such a patient, hepatic encephalopathy will result because hepatofugal flow will be present in the rerouted or bypassed portal vein. As with ligation of the superior mesenteric vein, it is necessary to infuse tremendous amounts of crystalloids to reverse the transient peripheral hypovolemia that occurs secondary to the splanchnic hypervolemia resulting from ligation of the portal vein.

Since the early 1980s, the survival rate in patients with injuries to the portal vein has been approximately 50%.

RETROHEPATIC AREA

Retrohepatic hematoma or hemorrhage is cause to suspect the presence of injury to the retrohepatic vena cava, a hepatic vein, or a right renal blood vessel. In addition, hemorrhage in this area may signal injury to the overlying liver [*see III:7 Injuries to the Liver, Biliary Tract, Spleen, and Diaphragm*].

If there is a hematoma that is not expanding or ruptured and clearly has no association with the right perirenal area, a tamponaded injury to the retrohepatic vena cava or a hepatic vein is present. Perihepatic packing around the right lobe of the liver for 24 to 48 hours has been shown to prevent further expansion and should be considered.

If hemorrhage is occurring that does not appear to be coming from the overlying liver, the right lobe of the liver should be compressed posteriorly to tamponade the caval perforation. The Pringle maneuver is then applied, and the surgical and nursing team, the anesthesiologist, and the blood blank are notified. Once the proper instruments and banked blood are in the OR, the overlying injured hepatic lobe is mobilized by dividing the triangular and anterior coronary ligaments and then lifted out of the subdiaphragmatic area. On occasion, an obvious perforation of the retrohepatic or suprahepatic vena cava or an obvious area where a hepatic vein was avulsed from the vena cava may be grasped with a forceps or a Judd-Allis clamp; a Satinsky clamp may then be applied. Because of the copious bleeding that occurs as the liver is lifted and the hole in the vena cava sought, the anesthesiologist should start blood transfusions as the lobe is being mobilized.

If the hemorrhage is not controlled after one or two attempts, another technique must be tried. The most common choice is the insertion of a 36 French chest tube or a 9 mm endotracheal tube as an atriocaval shunt [see III:6 Operative Exposure of Abdominal Injuries and Closure of the Abdomen and III:7 Injuries to the Liver, Biliary Tract, Spleen, and Diaphragm]. The shunt can reduce bleeding by 40% to 60%, but vigorous hemorrhage persists until full control of the perforation is obtained with clamps or sutures. An alternative approach is to isolate the liver and the vena cava by cross-clamping the supraceliac aorta, the porta hepatis, the suprarenal inferior vena cava, and the intrapericardial inferior vena cava. Because profoundly hypovolemic patients usually cannot tolerate cross-clamping of the inferior vena cava, this approach is rarely used.

The retrohepatic vena cava is repaired with continuous 4-0 or 5-0 polypropylene sutures. When the atriocaval shunt is removed from the heart after the vessel has been repaired, the right atrial appendage is ligated with a 2-0 silk tie.

The survival rate in patients undergoing atriocaval shunting and repair of the retrohepatic vena cava who are not in cardiac arrest has ranged from 33% to 50%.

Damage Control Laparotomy

Patients with injuries to the great vessels of the abdomen are ideal candidates for damage control laparotomy: they are uniformly hypothermic, acidotic, and coagulopathic on completion of the vascular repair, and a prolonged operation would lead to their demise. In such patients, packing of minor or moderate injuries to solid organs, packing of the retroperitoneum, stapling and rapid resection of multiple injuries to the GI tract, consideration of diffuse intra-abdominal packing, and towel-clip closure of the skin are all appropriate. If a towel-clip closure cannot be completed because of distention of the midgut (such as may be seen in association with profound shock or after ligation of the superior mesenteric or portal vein), a temporary silo made from a urologic irrigation bag can be used. The silo can be sewn to the skin edges with a continuous 2-0 polypropylene or nylon suture.

The patient is then rapidly moved to the SICU for further resuscitation. Priorities in the SICU include rapid restoration of normal body temperature, reversal of shock, infusion of intravenous bicarbonate to correct a persistent pH lower than 7.2, and administration of fresh frozen plasma, platelets, and cryoprecipitate when indicated. It is usually possible to return the patient to the OR for removal of clot and packs, reconstruction of the GI tract, irrigation, and reapplication of a towel-clip or silo closure within 48 to 72 hours.

When massive distention of the midgut persists after 7 days of intensive care, the safest approach is to convert the patient to an open abdomen (i.e., without closure of the midline incision) and cover the midgut with a double-thickness layer of absorbable mesh. With proper nutritional support and occasional use of Dakin solution to minimize bacterial contamination of the absorbable mesh, most patients are ready for the application of a split-thickness skin graft to the eviscerated midgut within 3 to 4 weeks of the original operation for an injury to a great vessel.

Complications

Besides those already mentioned, major complications associated with repair of injuries to the great vessels in the abdomen include thrombosis, dehiscence of the suture line, and infection. Because of the risk of occlusion of repairs in small vasoconstricted vessels (e.g., the superior mesenteric artery), it may be worthwhile to perform a second-look operation within 12 to 24 hours if the patient's metabolic state suggests that ischemia of the midgut is present. Early correction of an arterial thrombosis in the superior mesenteric artery may permit salvage of the midgut.

As noted [see Injuries in Zone 1, above], dehiscence of an end-to-end anastomosis or a vascular conduit inserted in the proximal superior mesenteric artery when there is an injury to the adjacent pancreas may be prevented by inserting a distal aorta–superior mesenteric artery bypass graft. To prevent adjacent loops of small bowel from adhering to the vascular suture lines, both lines should be covered with soft tissue (retroperitoneal tissue for the aortic suture line and mesenteric tissue for the superior mesenteric arterial suture line). Also as noted [see Injuries in Zone 3, above], when an extensive injury to either the common or the external iliac artery occurs in the presence of significant enteric or fecal contamination in the pelvis, ligation and extra-anatomic bypass may be necessary.

On occasion, vascular-enteric fistulas occur after repair of the anterior aorta or the insertion of grafts in either the abdominal aorta or the superior mesenteric artery. In my experience, such fistulas all occur at suture lines; hence, once again, proper coverage of suture lines with soft tissue should eliminate this complication.

References

1. Tyburski JG, Wilson RF, Dente C, et al: Factors affecting mortality rates in patients with abdominal vascular injuries. J Trauma 50:1020, 2001
2. Asensio JA, Chahwan S, Hanpeter D, et al: Operative management and outcome of 302 abdominal vascular injuries. Am J Surg 180:528, 2000
3. Davis TP, Feliciano DV, Rozycki GS, et al: Results with abdominal vascular trauma in the modern era. Am Surg 67:565, 2001
4. Hass CA, Dinchman KH, Nasrallah PH, et al: Traumatic renal artery occlusion: a 15-year review. J Trauma 45:557, 1998

Recommended Reading

Asensio JA, Britt LD, Borzotta A, et al: Multiinstitutional experience with the management of superior mesenteric artery injuries. J Am Coll Surg 193:354, 2001

Feliciano DV, Burch JM, Graham JM: Abdominal vascular injury. Trauma, 4th ed. Mattox KL, Feliciano DV, Moore EE, Eds. McGraw-Hill, New York, 2000

Wilson RF, Dulchavsky S: Abdominal vascular trauma. Management of Trauma: Pitfalls and Practice. Wilson RF, Walt AJ, Eds. Williams & Wilkins, Baltimore, 1996

Acknowledgments

Figures 1 and 2 Marcia Kammerer.

Figures 3, 5, 8, 12, and 16 Tom Moore.

Figures 4 and 9 From "Abdominal Vascular Injury," by D. V. Feliciano, J. M. Burch, and J. M. Graham, in Trauma, 3rd ed., edited by D. V. Feliciano, E. E. Moore, and K. L. Mattox. Appleton & Lange, Stamford, Connecticut, 1996. Reproduced by permission.

10 INJURIES TO THE UROGENITAL TRACT

Hunter Wessells, M.D., and Jack W. McAninch, M.D.

Hematuria is the hallmark of injury to the urogenital system. Location of the injury and identification of its cause help determine which urologic organs are most likely to have been injured by a particular traumatic event. In penetrating trauma to the abdomen, hematuria signals the need to evaluate the kidneys, ureters, and bladder. Urethral and genital injuries are suspected only with wounds to the pelvis, perineum, and buttocks. When hematuria occurs in association with blunt injuries and pelvic fracture, the entire genitourinary system should be evaluated.

This chapter includes a separate algorithm for each of the major urogenital organs. Injury to both the upper and the lower urinary tract is rare, but a high index of suspicion must be maintained for detection of such an injury. Injury to the female reproductive organs requires special expertise in evaluation and management, particularly if the patient is pregnant or the victim of a sexual assault.

Injuries to the Kidneys

INITIAL EVALUATION

The most reliable sign of injury to the kidney is hematuria, whether microscopic or gross. However, the degree of hematuria is not correlated with the severity of injury, and patients with serious injuries may have no blood in their urine.[1] The same staging system is used to classify blunt injuries and penetrating injuries [*see Figure 1 and Table 1*], and the only significant difference in their management is in the initial evaluation [*see Figure 2*]. For patients with blunt trauma, we recommend the following criteria for radiographic evaluation of injuries to the kidney[2]: adults with microscopic hematuria and systolic blood pressure of at least 90 mm Hg do not require imaging unless serious associated injuries suggest a deceleration injury; all pediatric trauma patients, patients with gross hematuria, and patients with microscopic hematuria and systolic BP lower than 90 mm Hg require radiographic evaluation. Computed tomography is the first-line imaging modality for all cases of suspected blunt renal trauma. We recommend performance of a delayed CT scan 10 minutes after initial imaging to detect any urinary extravasation or injury to the collecting system.[3]

All penetrating injuries of the kidney require exploration unless a complete radiographic evaluation demonstrates that an injury can be managed nonoperatively. CT, which is ideal for study of penetrating injuries, should be the first radiographic method used in hemodynamically stable patients.[4]

Intravenous urography is adequate for the evaluation of trauma only if it includes tomography and does not demonstrate poor visualization, an irregular contour, or extravasation, which should prompt further studies or exploration.[5]

All grade I and II renal injuries, regardless of the mechanism of injury, can be managed without operation. The absolute indications for renal exploration include pulsatile and expanding hematomas and hemodynamic instability resulting from renal injury.[6] In stable patients with adequate staging, grade III and nonvascular grade IV injuries (including devitalized fragments and urinary extravasation) can be observed.[7] In patients requiring laparotomy for associated injuries, we perform renal exploration and reconstruction to reduce the likelihood of delayed complications.[8,9] Shattered kidneys (grade V) and vascular injuries (grades IV and V) require immediate renal exploration. An exception is thrombosis of the renal artery or its branches, which may be treated expectantly if revascularization is not performed expediently in a patient with no associated injuries.

A significant number of patients with a penetrating injury and a minority of those with blunt trauma require immediate laparotomy before they can be evaluated radiographically.[10] Hematuria is the key clinical sign, alerting the surgeon to the possibility of renal injury in inadequately staged patients. The presence of a retroperitoneal hematoma should prompt further evaluation. We obtain a single-shot intravenous pyelogram (IVP) 10 minutes after bolus injection of 150 ml of iodinated contrast material, ensuring the presence of a functioning contralateral unit before exploration. If the injured kidney is imaged adequately and found to be normal, exploration may be omitted.[11] In patients with blunt injuries and gross hematuria or with microscopic hematuria in the presence of shock, intraoperative imaging is required, even in the absence of a retroperitoneal hematoma. If the kidney is not adequately imaged, the possibility of renal artery thrombosis should be considered.

OPERATIVE MANAGEMENT

A midline transabdominal incision permits exploration of the kidneys and abdomen. After areas of bleeding have been packed with laparotomy sponges, the first step is isolation of the renal vasculature before opening Gerota's fascia. This technique, which has reduced our nephrectomy rate, allows rapid control of bleeding from serious injuries.[12] In all renal explorations, regardless of the degree of injury, we begin with isolation of the renal vessels, which is best performed by opening the posterior peritoneum overlying the aorta, preventing premature entry of the retroperitoneal hematoma. Even in the presence of large hematomas, the inferior mesenteric vein serves as a landmark for location of the aorta. Working cephalad along the aorta, the surgeon encounters the left renal vein first and subsequently both renal arteries. The best way to find the right renal artery is to dissect between the aorta and the vena cava; dissection lateral to the vena cava may lead to inadvertent isolation of a seg-

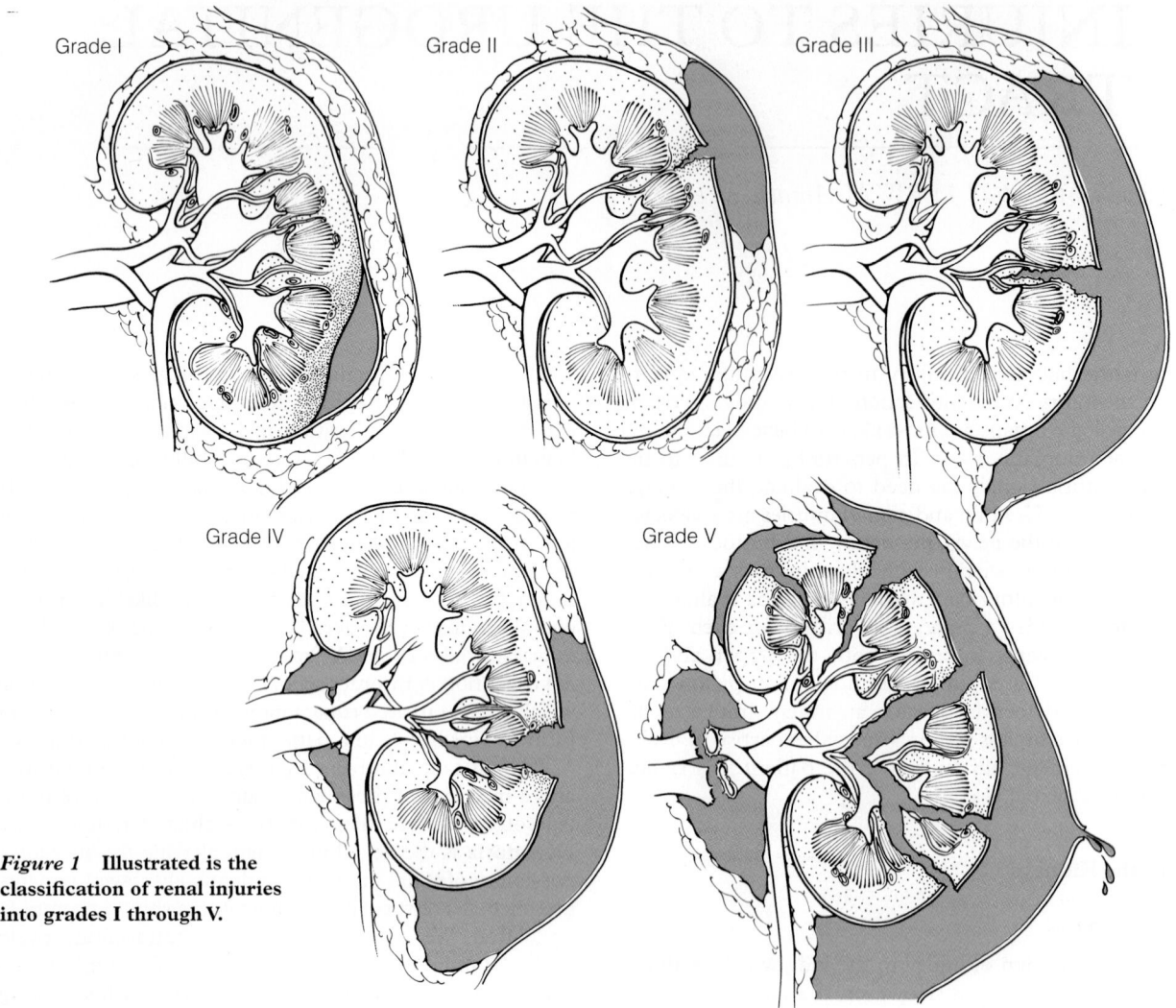

Figure 1 **Illustrated is the classification of renal injuries into grades I through V.**

mental branch of the renal artery. Isolation of the right renal vein may be easier after reflection of the right colon and duodenum. We place vessel loops around the artery and the vein, thus ensuring rapid access to the vessels if significant bleeding occurs. The renal vessels can also be approached laterally if the duodenum or left colon has been mobilized.

Gerota's fascia is opened only after vascular isolation. If release of the tamponade effect causes bleeding, we use Rumel tourniquets or vascular clamps to occlude the renal artery and the renal vein. Clamping of the renal artery alone usually controls bleeding. If it does not, the surgeon should suspect a venous injury and occlude the vein. It is not routine to cool the surface of the kidney after clamping of the renal artery, because patients with trauma are often hypothermic and coagulopathic. Clamp time should be limited to less than 30 minutes, if possible.

Total exposure of the kidney, by means of sharp and blunt dissection, is necessary to rule out injury to the parenchyma, the renal pedicle, and the collecting system. The renal capsule can easily be pulled off the parenchyma if dissection is not meticulous. Once the kidney has been delivered into the field, the extent of injury can be assessed and reconstruction can be planned. Renal reconstruction includes debridement of all devitalized tissue, hemostasis, closure of the collecting system, defect coverage, and drainage [*see Figure 3*]. With these techniques, renal salvage should be possible in close to 90% of kid-

ney explorations.[5] Nephrectomy should be reserved for destroyed kidneys that cannot be reconstructed or for serious renal injury associated with other life-threatening injuries, such as vascular or hepatic trauma.

Debridement of devitalized tissue permits reconstruction with healthy tissue and prevents delayed bleeding and urinary extravasation. If the renal capsule is present at the margins of the wound, it should be peeled back and preserved for subsequent closure. A scalpel is used to remove the devitalized renal parenchyma until bleeding occurs at the margin. Polar injuries can be debrided by guillotine amputation of the parenchyma.

Manual compression usually controls bleeding during the ligation of small vessels. Ligation of individual vessels with absorbable monofilament suture material, such as 4-0 chromic catgut, achieves hemostasis. Temporary release of renal artery occlusion for the assessment of hemostasis is not recommended. Ligation of venous bleeding points generally controls adjacent arterial sources.

Once hemostasis is satisfactory, the collecting system should be scrutinized for evidence of injury. If the extent is unclear, 2 to 3 ml of methylene blue can be injected directly into the renal pelvis, while the ureter is occluded, to identify any openings in the collecting system. Open calyxes or infundibula can be closed with a continuous 4-0 absorbable suture. For injuries to the renal pelvis, interrupted closure is more reliable.

The renal capsule can often be used to cover exposed renal parenchyma. The defect in the parenchyma is filled with folded absorbable gelatin sponges or other hemostatic agents; and with interrupted sutures through the capsule but not the parenchyma, the capsule is closed over the bolsters. If the capsule is not available, options include an omental or perinephric fat flap tacked down over the defect, a patch of Dexon or peritoneum, or an entire sac of Dexon wrapped around the kidney, with the parenchymal edges kept well apposed.[6,13]

At the end of the procedure, the kidney should be returned to its location within Gerota's fascia. Drainage of the renal region is recommended, and either a closed-suction or a Penrose drain is acceptable. If there are significant injuries to the collecting system, a Penrose drain is preferable because it does not exert negative pressure on the repair site. Internalized drains and double J stents generally are not necessary for renal injuries. However, major injuries to the renal pelvis or the ureteropelvic junction (UPJ) should be drained with an internalized stent as well as a retroperitoneal drain.

POSTOPERATIVE CARE

Management of patients after operative or nonoperative intervention for renal trauma depends to a large extent on associated injuries. Bed rest is prescribed until the urine becomes grossly clear, usually within 24 to 48 hours. Ambulation is allowed unless gross hematuria recurs. Drainage of the bladder with a Foley catheter is necessary only until the patient is ambulatory and the urine clear. Nasogastric suction

Table 1   AAST Organ Injury Scales for Urinary Tract

Injured Structure	AAST Grade	Characteristics of Injury	AIS-90 Score
Kidney*	I	Contusion with microscopic or gross hematuria, urologic studies normal; nonexpanding subcapsular hematoma without parenchymal laceration	2; 2
	II	Nonexpanding perirenal hematoma confined to renal retroperitoneum; laceration < 1.0 cm parenchymal depth of renal cortex without urinary extravasation	2; 2
	III	Laceration > 1.0 cm parenchymal depth of renal cortex without collecting system rupture or urinary extravasation	3
	IV	Parenchymal laceration extending through renal cortex, medulla, and collecting system; injury to main renal artery or vein with contained hemorrhage	4; 4
	V	Completely shattered kidney; avulsion of renal hilum that devascularizes kidney	5; 5
Ureter*	I	Contusion or hematoma without devascularization	2
	II	< 50% transection	2
	III	≥ 50% transection	3
	IV	Complete transection with < 2 cm devascularization	3
	V	Avulsion with > 2 cm devascularization	3
Bladder†	I	Contusion, intramural hematoma; partial-thickness laceration	2; 3
	II	Extraperitoneal bladder wall laceration < 2 cm	4
	III	Extraperitoneal bladder wall laceration > 2 cm or intraperitoneal bladder wall laceration < 2 cm	4
	IV	Intraperitoneal bladder wall laceration > 2 cm	4
	V	Intraperitoneal or extraperitoneal bladder wall laceration extending into bladder neck or ureteral orifice (trigone)	4
Urethra*	I	Contusion with blood at urethral meatus and normal urethrography	2
	II	Stretch injury with elongation of urethra but without extravasation of urethrography contrast material	2
	III	Partial disruption with extravasation of urethrography contrast material at injury site with visualization in the bladder	2
	IV	Complete disruption with < 2 cm urethral separation and extravasation of urethrography contrast material at injury site without visualization in the bladder	3
	V	Complete transection with ≥ 2 cm urethral separation or extension into the prostate or vagina	4

*Advance one grade for bilateral injuries, up to grade III.
†Advance one grade for multiple injuries, up to grade III.
AAST—American Association for the Surgery of Trauma AIS-90—Abbreviated Injury Score, 1990 version

should be continued until peristalsis returns. Retroperitoneal drains should be removed within 48 hours unless the output is significant. Often, peritoneal fluid continues to drain. Comparison of the creatinine level in the fluid with the creatinine level in serum can distinguish urinary leakage from serous fluid. If serous fluid is draining, we remove the retroperitoneal drains regardless of output.

Persistent urinary leakage is best evaluated with CT. Evidence of distal ureteral obstruction should be sought and the obstruction alleviated. Many urinomas without concurrent infection resolve without intervention. If the collection is large, the collecting system should be drained with a double J stent or a percutaneously placed nephrostomy tube. With appropriate drainage, uninfected urinomas and extravasation usually resolve.

Infectious complications after renal reconstruction include urinoma formation and perinephric abscesses. Percutaneous drainage of urinomas and abscesses is preferred. Reexploration may force the surgeon to perform a nephrectomy if there is not enough healthy tissue for a trustworthy repair. The renal collecting system should be drained and the collection studied at intervals until the leak has resolved.

Delayed bleeding is a rare but serious complication of renal reconstruction or nonoperative management of major lacerations. Gross hematuria usually, but not invariably, accompanies the bleeding. If there is evidence of significant bleeding (i.e., hypotension or a decreasing hematocrit), the combination of renal angiography and selective embolization is an effective option that should be attempted before reexploration.[14]

Figure 2 **Algorithm illustrates evaluation and treatment of a patient with blunt or penetrating injury to the kidney.**

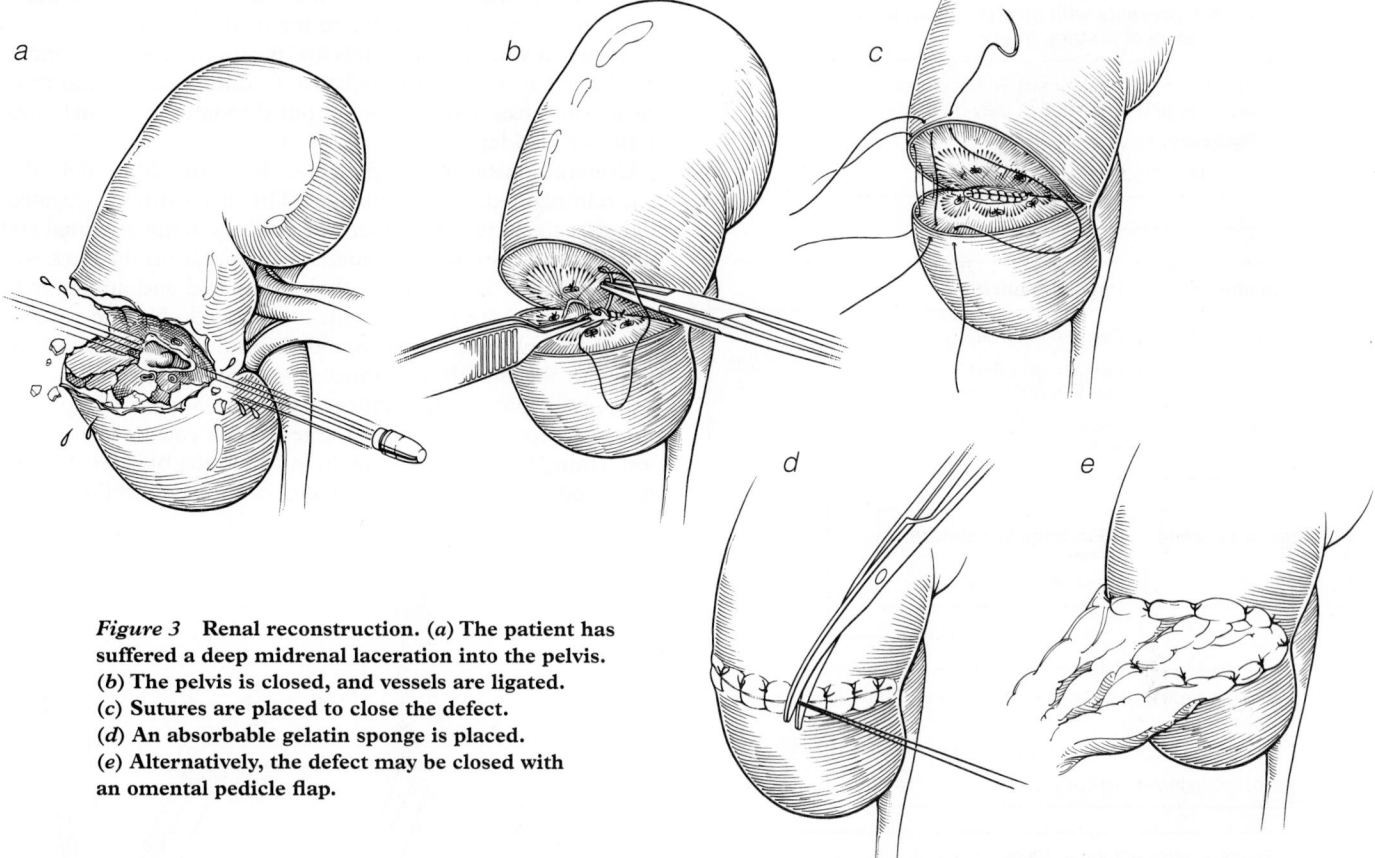

Figure 3 Renal reconstruction. (a) The patient has
suffered a deep midrenal laceration into the pelvis.
(b) The pelvis is closed, and vessels are ligated.
(c) Sutures are placed to close the defect.
(d) An absorbable gelatin sponge is placed.
(e) Alternatively, the defect may be closed with
an omental pedicle flap.

Postoperative imaging is recommended to evaluate renal
function and to rule out the development of hydronephrosis or
stones. The optimal follow-up is intravenous urography or
radionuclide scanning at 3 months and 1 year. If significant
injury to the collecting system was repaired, the imaging study
should be performed before discharge from the hospital.
Hypertension is a rare late complication of renal reconstruction, usually renin-mediated from an ischemic segment of
renal parenchyma. Occasionally, angiography delineates the
ischemic segment of the kidney, and excision of the nonperfused segment or nephrectomy may be required.

Injuries to the Ureters

INITIAL EVALUATION

Ureteral injury [see Table 1] is rare, accounting for fewer than
1% of genitourinary injuries. Although ureteral injury can be
repaired successfully [see Figure 4], it may have serious consequences, including loss of renal function and death,[15] if unrecognized. The absence of physical signs of injury makes diagnosis difficult, and a delayed presentation is not uncommon. Up
to half of all ureteral injuries resulting from blunt trauma are
not recognized immediately, and a high index of suspicion is
necessary to prevent the late complications of urinoma, sepsis,
and nephrectomy.[16]

A penetrating wound is the predominant cause of ureteral
injury, gunshot wounds being the most common cause and
stab wounds the second most common. Deceleration injuries
may result in UPJ disruption, especially in children. The pediatric ureter is prone to injury because hyperextensibility of the

spine can result in avulsion of the ureter at the UPJ.[17] The
patient's history and the physical examination provide little
information about ureteral injuries. Signs and symptoms related to associated injuries predominate. In three series, gross or
microscopic hematuria was present in only 30% to 70% of
ureteral injuries, making vigilance necessary for diagnosis.[15,16,18]

CT with delayed cuts should be performed whenever
ureteral injury is suspected. Intravenous urography is of variable usefulness in the detection of ureteral injuries, but
extravasation of the contrast agent is diagnostic.[19]

Ureteral injury may not be suspected until the time of
laparotomy, when a hematoma is found near the kidney or
ureter. If an on-table IVP is not diagnostic, direct inspection of
the ureter for injury, contusion, and peristalsis is mandatory.
Injection of indigo carmine directly into the collecting system
may identify extravasation. All injuries to the ureter should be
repaired surgically, unless a delay in diagnosis results in an
abscess or a urinoma. For either abscess or urinoma, drainage
by percutaneous nephrostomy and ureteral stenting may allow
the inflamed ureter to heal, whereas an operative approach
may result in nephrectomy.

OPERATIVE MANAGEMENT

Once ureteral injury has been recognized, reconstruction
should proceed. Depending on the type of injury and its location, the reconstructive techniques may include debridement
of devitalized tissue, a spatulated tension-free anastomosis,
watertight mucosal approximation, ureteral stenting, coverage
of the repair with vascularized tissue, and appropriate drainage.[15] Stab wounds generally require less tissue debridement

Figure 4 **Algorithm illustrates evaluation and treatment of a patient with ureteral injury.**

mesocolon to the contralateral side. Anastomosis of the injured ureter to a 1 to 2 cm opening in the medial normal ureter can be achieved without tension. With transureteroureterostomy, a stent (usually a 5 French pediatric feeding tube) should cross the anastomosis and be brought out through the normal lower ureter or bladder.

Ureteral injuries below the pelvic brim should be debrided and reimplanted into the bladder. The distal stump is ligated, and after the anterior bladder wall is opened, the proximal end of the ureter is brought through a new hiatus on the back wall of the bladder. The ureter is then spatulated and approximated to the bladder mucosa with interrupted chromic sutures. One 3-0 anchoring stitch should bring the distal apex of the ureter to the muscle and mucosa; the rest of the sutures are 4-0 only, approximating mucosa. A nonrefluxing reimplantation is acceptable in adults. Large defects can be bridged by performing a vesico-psoas hitch, in which the bladder dome·is mobilized to bridge the ureteral defect and sewn to the central

Figure 5 **Ureteroureterostomy. (*a*) The injured ureter is dissected free. (*b*) The ends are spatulated. (*c*) The ends are approximated over a double J stent. (*d*) The anastomosis is completed with interrupted sutures.**

than gunshot wounds, and partial transections may be closed primarily.

Disruption or transection of the UPJ is repaired by debridement and primary anastomosis of the renal pelvis and ureter. Penetrating low-velocity injuries require minimal or no debridement. Mobilization of the ureter should be limited to avoid compromising the blood supply. Interrupted 5-0 or 6-0 Vicryl sutures are preferred, and a double J ureteral stent or a nephrostomy tube must be inserted before closure of the anastomosis.

Injuries to the abdominal ureter between the UPJ and the pelvic brim are repaired by ureteroureterostomy [*see Figure 5*]. After debridement, the ends are spatulated on opposite sides, and an interrupted approximation is completed over a double J stent. In cases of overlying colonic, duodenal, or pancreatic injury, the anastomosis may be covered with omentum. Large defects in the abdominal ureter may require transureteroureterostomy, in which the injured ureter is passed behind the tendon of the psoas muscle. Three interrupted sutures that enter the detrusor muscle but not the bladder lumen should anchor the dome above the iliac vessels. The dome is mobilized by dividing the obliterated umbilical arteries bilaterally and, if necessary, dividing the contralateral superior vesical artery. Significant bladder or vascular damage may make transureterourerostomy a more attractive option to avoid further dissection in the injured area. A ureteral stent should be used in all ureteral reimplantations. The bladder is closed in two layers with a continuous 2-0 Vicryl suture, and a drain is placed in the Retzius space.

A retroperitoneal drain is essential in all ureteral reconstructions. A large-bore Foley catheter is sufficient for bladder drainage unless there is coexistent bladder injury or prolonged catheterization is expected. In either of these cases, a suprapubic catheter allows better drainage of clots and, in males, has fewer long-term complications.[20]

POSTOPERATIVE CARE

Postoperative care of ureteral trauma relates mainly to the manipulation of drains and management of complications. Retroperitoneal drains may have significant output for several days but are removed once the output is minimal. With severe injuries or persistent output from drains, CT or IVP before discharge from the hospital may help rule out the possibility of extravasation. Bladder catheterization is necessary for 7 days after ureteral reimplantation. In combined bladder and ureteral reconstructions, contrast cystography is indicated before catheter removal. Cystoscopic removal of the double J stent is usually performed with local anesthesia 4 to 6 weeks after operation. Intravenous urography 3 months after removal of the stent rules out the possibility of asymptomatic obstruction.

Fistula formation, usually the result of distal obstruction or necrosis of the ureter, should be managed by antegrade or retrograde drainage of the collecting system using percutaneous or endoscopic techniques. Drainage of periureteral collection may also be necessary. If recognition of an injury or complication is delayed, reconstruction should not be undertaken for at least 3 months, to allow resolution of the inflammatory phase of wound healing. Because hydronephrosis may develop as a result of stricture, retroperitoneal fibrosis, or a urinoma, repeat imaging is appropriate 1 year after injury.

Injuries to the Bladder

INITIAL EVALUATION

Bladder injury [see Table 1] occurs in fewer than 1% of trauma patients.[21] Bladder rupture is most often caused by blunt injuries, including injuries resulting from motor vehicle accidents, falls, and direct blows to the abdomen, and is associated with pelvic fracture in 89% of cases. Overall, 9% of patients with a pelvic fracture have an associated injury to the bladder.[22] Penetrating wounds of the bladder may be caused by gunshot, stabs, or pelvic surgery.

The signs and symptoms of bladder injury are nonspecific [see Figure 6]. Patients may complain of suprapubic pain, dysuria, or an inability to void.[23] Physical examination may reveal tenderness in the suprapubic region, ileus, or an acute abdomen. Bladder rupture is associated with gross hematuria in 95% of cases; in a 1989 report, 3% of patients had no hematuria.[24] Laboratory studies are usually inconclusive unless significant reabsorption of urine causes elevated serum creatinine levels.

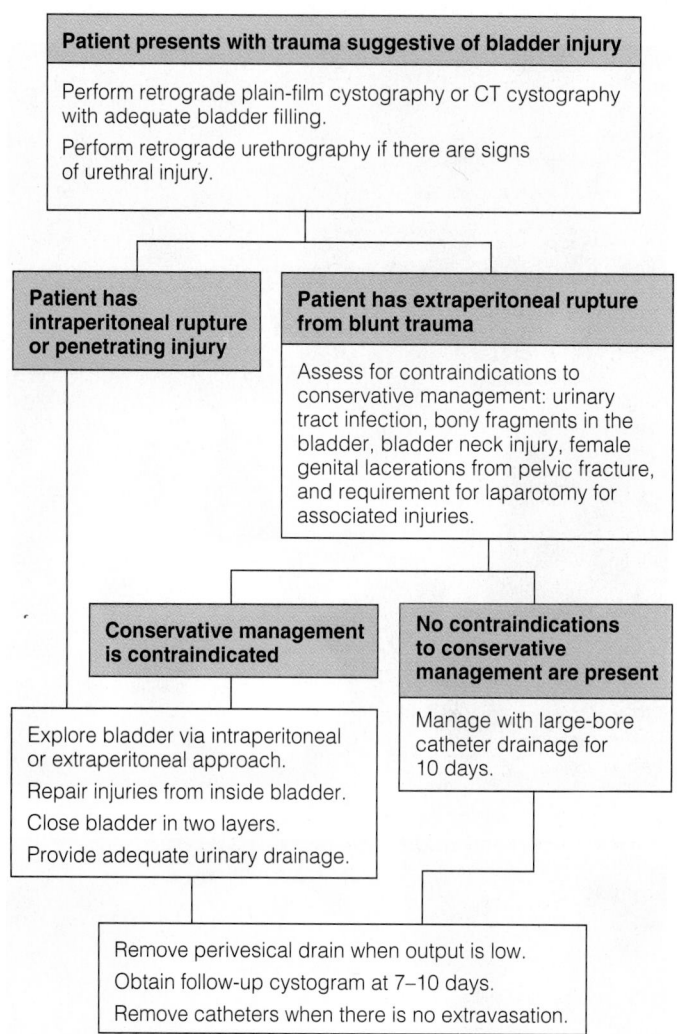

Figure 6   **Algorithm illustrates evaluation and treatment of a patient with bladder injury.**

Bladder rupture can be accurately diagnosed with CT cystography or plain-film cystography. Insufficient instillation of the contrast agent, however, yields false negative results. Standard CT is inadequate for the diagnosis of bladder rupture, because the bladder is not sufficiently distended in most patients. CT cystography involves three sets of images: (1) initial fill images obtained after retrograde instillation of 100 ml of contrast material, (2) complete fill images obtained after instillation of 350 ml, and (3) images obtained after drainage.[25]

A plain-film cystogram is obtained after an initial scout film by instilling 300 to 400 ml of 25% to 30% iodinated contrast through a urethral catheter. An anteroposterior view should be taken with the bladder full and after evacuation. In cases of intraperitoneal bladder injury, extravasation of contrast outlines the bowel loops and may track along the lateral gutters [see Figure 7a]. Extraperitoneal injuries demonstrate flame-shaped extravasation in the pelvis, which may track down into the obturator region, the scrotum, or the thigh [see Figure 7b]. Blunt injuries can cause extraperitoneal, intraperitoneal, or combined rupture. The amount of extravasation has no correlation with the degree of injury and should not influence management.[20]

Figure 7   X-rays show intraperitoneal (*a*) and extraperitoneal (*b*) bladder rupture.

OPERATIVE MANAGEMENT

Extraperitoneal bladder injuries caused by blunt trauma can be managed with catheter drainage for 10 days, unless contraindications exist.[20] After 10 days, plain-film cystography should be used to document healing and allow removal of the catheter. If extravasation persists, cystography should be repeated weekly until healing occurs. Contraindications to nonoperative management include urinary infection; the presence of bony fragments in the bladder; bladder neck injury, which may compromise continence; and female genital lacerations associated with pelvic fracture.

If the patient requires laparotomy for associated injuries and is not critically ill, repair of extraperitoneal bladder injuries is recommended to decrease the possibility of infecting the pelvic hematoma. If the bladder injury is associated with a pelvic fracture in a male patient, the possibility of a urethral injury is

10% to 29% and must be excluded.[24] A successfully placed Foley catheter rules out a complete urethral disruption.

All penetrating injuries and all intraperitoneal ruptures of the bladder are managed by bladder exploration and repair. Bladder exploration can be performed via an intraperitoneal approach. In addition to repair of the bladder, exploration makes it possible to rule out associated injuries, ensure the integrity of the ureters by direct visualization, and, in the case of pelvic fracture, avoid entering the pelvic hematoma. In cases involving early orthopedic reconstruction of the pelvis, we approach the bladder extraperitoneally through the incision used to expose the pubis. Intraperitoneal injuries generally cause a stellate rupture of the dome of the bladder. By enlarging this opening, one can inspect the interior of the bladder to exclude concomitant extraperitoneal injuries, which occur in 8% of cases.[23]

Penetrating injuries and extraperitoneal ruptures are approached by opening the bladder with the electrocautery, vertically at the dome or along the anterior surface, and identifying the sites of rupture intravesically. These lacerations are then debrided (rarely necessary) and closed with interrupted 3-0 chromic catgut or Vicryl sutures, which approximate detrusor muscle and mucosa in one layer and provide hemostasis. In patients with gunshot wounds, entrance and exit sites must be identified. The cystotomy is then closed with two layers of continuous 2-0 or 3-0 Vicryl sutures, the first layer consisting of mucosa and detrusor muscle and the second consisting of detrusor and serosa.

Adequate urinary drainage is essential to successful healing of the repaired bladder. Large-bore (22 French or larger) Foley catheter drainage is sufficient if bladder injuries are not extensive and hemostasis is excellent. Extensive injuries and coagulopathy warrant additional drainage with a suprapubic tube, which allows irrigation of clots and proper decompression of the bladder. If suprapubic cystostomy is chosen, a 24 French Malecot catheter placed through a separate site into the bladder is preferred. In addition, a closed-suction or a Penrose drain near the bladder closure, but not overlying the suture line, is recommended. Like the suprapubic tube, the drain should exit through a separate site in the skin.

POSTOPERATIVE CARE

In the majority of patients with a bladder repair, 7 days of catheter drainage is sufficient to allow healing. Cystography may be indicated in cases of severe bladder injury or persistent output from drains. The perivesical drain can be removed after the output has decreased to an acceptable rate. Because bladder repair is reliable, complications of bladder injury are related to a delay in diagnosis rather than to postoperative morbidity. Azotemia, ascites, and sepsis may result from an intraperitoneal injury that was overlooked. Because an infected pelvic hematoma can have disastrous effects, nonoperative management of extraperitoneal rupture must be undertaken with caution. Bladder neck injury, if unrecognized, may lead to scarring and incompetence of the proximal sphincter mechanism, with resultant incontinence, especially in females.

Injuries to the Urethra

INITIAL EVALUATION

Almost all injuries to the male urethra [*see Table 1*] are caused by blunt trauma. Posterior urethral (prostatic and membranous urethral) injuries in males occur in 5% of pelvic

Figure 8 **Algorithm illustrates evaluation and treatment of a patient with trauma to the urethra.**

fractures, which is the most common cause of posterior urethral injury.[26] Anterior urethral (penile and bulbar urethral) injuries are commonly caused by straddle injury but may be the result of penile fracture or penetrating injuries to the genitalia. Penetrating injury to the posterior urethra often leaves the urethral continuity intact. The female urethra is rarely injured, but when it is, it is invariably associated with bladder injury and pelvic fracture.

Blood at the urethral meatus, the classic sign of injury to the male urethra, indicates that urethrography should be performed immediately. Attempts at catheter placement, which may convert incomplete injuries to complete disruptions,[26] are to be condemned in any case of suspected urethral injury. Because signs of urethral injury are variable, urethrography is the essential diagnostic test.

Retrograde urethrography can document the location and nature of urethral injury. Injection of the contrast agent may be accomplished with a Foley catheter placed in the fossa navicu-

laris, a Brodney clamp, or a catheter tip syringe. The patient is placed in the oblique position, with the penis stretched to delineate the anterior urethra. Extravasation of the contrast agent is evidence of urethral injury. In the absence of extravasation, a Foley catheter may be passed. If a catheter has been placed but its position is unclear, contrast injection will confirm its placement in the bladder. In such cases, the catheter should be left in place until a pericatheter contrast study can document the absence of injury. In cases of pelvic fracture and penetrating posterior urethral injury, bladder injury must be excluded via suprapubic tube cystography or open bladder exploration when the suprapubic tube is placed.

OPERATIVE MANAGEMENT

Management of penetrating injuries to the urethra, which are rare, differs considerably from management of blunt trauma [*see Figure 8*]. Traumatic urethral injuries are usually managed by suprapubic cystostomy, with reconstruction delayed for 3 to 6 months. Straddle injuries to the bulbar urethra should always be managed by urinary diversion and delayed repair because the appearance of the crushed tissue makes it difficult to delineate a healthy margin. The majority of prostatomembranous urethral injuries can be managed with suprapubic cystostomy. Immediate surgical intervention is reserved for the following urethral injuries: selected penetrating anterior urethral injuries without major associated injuries; penetrating posterior urethral injuries; blunt posterior urethral rupture with associated rectal injury, bladder neck injury, or an extremely wide separation of bladder and urethra; and urethral injury associated with penile fracture.[27]

Suprapubic cystostomy allows urinary diversion until all associated injuries and bony fractures have healed. The vast majority of blunt anterior and posterior urethral injuries are managed with this approach. If laparotomy is not indicated for other injuries, the suprapubic tube may be placed percutaneously under fluoroscopic guidance. A cystogram can then be performed via the

suprapubic tube to rule out associated bladder injury. A patient with urethral injury should not be allowed to void (voiding causes urinary extravasation). If open placement of the suprapubic tube is elected, the bladder can be inspected to rule out simultaneous injury, and a cystogram is not necessary.

Use of a lower abdominal incision and an intraperitoneal approach avoids the pelvic hematoma and allows an anterior vertical incision of the bladder. We lead the suprapubic tube (24 French Malecot or Foley catheter) out the superior aspect of the bladder closure and the inferior aspect of the skin wound in the midline, facilitating subsequent tube changes and reconstructive procedures. The bladder is closed in two layers [see Injuries to the Bladder, Operative Management, above]. In 3 to 6 months, a repeat cystogram and a retrograde urethrogram will delineate the residual stricture or rupture defect, which will require repair.

Suprapubic cystostomy should be used for management of penetrating injuries to the anterior urethra if they were caused by high-velocity weapons, leading to extensive tissue loss; if they are associated with serious injuries; or if bony fractures prevent use of the lithotomy position. For stab wounds or isolated low-velocity gunshot wounds, the favored approach is primary repair, which is associated with a lower stricture rate.[28]

Penile urethral injuries are approached by making a circumferential distal penile incision and degloving the penis to expose the urethra. Bulbar injuries are approached through a midline perineal incision. In each case, mobilization of the proximal and distal urethra with debridement of devitalized tissue should allow a spatulated end-to-end anastomosis. We use interrupted 6-0 monofilament absorbable suture over a 16 French Foley catheter. Additional drains are usually not necessary, and the wounds can be closed primarily because of the excellent blood supply of the perineum.

Penetrating injuries to the posterior urethra are rare. The prostate acts as a scaffold, preventing total disruption of the prostatic urethra. If contrast agent used during urethrography reaches the bladder, one can assume an incomplete injury. Endoscopic realignment and placement of a Foley catheter may be sufficient treatment of injury to the posterior urethra. A cystoscope or fluoroscopic guidance is used to place a wire into the bladder, beyond the injury, and a Foley catheter is then advanced over the wire. Positioning is confirmed by contrast instillation. After a month of catheter drainage, a voiding cystourethrogram will document healing.

In cases of prostatomembranous urethral disruption caused by blunt injury, immediate surgical intervention is required in only rare and specific instances. In cases of vascular, rectal, and bladder neck injuries or wide separation of the bladder from the urethra, some authors recommend immediate primary surgical realignment of the urethra.[27] If pelvic exploration is performed for major vascular or orthopedic repair, the urethra can be realigned, and a secondary procedure may not be required.[22] Primary realignment is preferred in such cases because the risk of hardware contamination is considerably lower with a urethral catheter than with a suprapubic cystostomy. Because of the risk of infection to the pelvic hematoma, simultaneous rectal injury should prompt evacuation of the pelvic hematoma, irrigation, placement of drains, and primary realignment of the urethra. Bladder neck injuries, which may compromise the continence mechanism of the proximal sphincter, require reconstruction in patients with posterior urethral rupture (whose external sphincter has been compromised by the injury). At the time of bladder neck repair, primary realignment should be performed. Finally,

---

Patient presents with evidence of gynecologic injury or sexual assault

Examine external genitalia and, by speculum, internal organs.
Notify support services if there is evidence of sexual trauma.

Patient has perineal injury

Look for associated rectal and urinary tract injuries.

Small hematomas: treat conservatively.

Large hematomas: treat with incision, drainage, and ligation of vessels.

Lacerations: treat with irrigation, debridement, and primary closure.

Patient has cervical or vaginal injury

Differentiate between simple and complex injuries.

Patient has pelvic genital organ injury

(Such injury is usually found at laparotomy rather than on examination, and there is a high incidence of associated injuries.)

Close ovarian lacerations primarily; if injury is severe, consider salpingo-oophorectomy.

Repair uterus in two layers.

If bleeding is uncontrolled or uterine artery is avulsed, consider hysterectomy.

Patient has simple vaginal or cervical lacerations

Place antibiotic-soaked vaginal pack and leave for 24 hr.

Give perioperative broad-spectrum antibiotics.

Minor lacerations: close primarily.

Major lacerations: examine via speculum with patient under anesthesia, and repair injury.

Large hematomas: evacuate and drain.

Patient has complex vaginal or perineal lacerations

Evaluate vaginal injuries with patient under anesthesia.

Perform contrast cystography and rigid proctoscopy.

Close vaginal injuries primarily.

Give I.V. antibiotics.

Consider urinary and fecal diversion.

Figure 9 Algorithm illustrates evaluation and treatment of a female patient with trauma to reproductive organs.

when the bladder and prostate are completely avulsed from the urethra and are pushed far up into the abdomen, early intervention makes later reconstruction more successful.

Primary realignment is accomplished through a lower midline abdominal incision. In contrast with suprapubic cystostomy, it is necessary to enter the Retzius space anterior to the bladder, thus disturbing the pelvic hematoma.[29] The bladder is opened along its anterior surface, and catheters are passed from the bladder and the urethral meatus into the pelvic hematoma. The ends of the two catheters are located in the midline anterior to the bladder neck. The two ends are brought up into the wound and attached with a suture, which allows the urethral catheter to be guided into the bladder and reestablishes alignment of the urethra. No traction is necessary, because neither mucosal approximation nor direct anastomosis is the goal. Suprapubic catheter drainage is recommended, and a perivesical drain should be used for 48 hours.[29] Either flexible cystoscopy (from the urethra and via a suprapubic approach)[30] or placement of magnetic urethral catheters[31] may be used for endoscopic realignment of membranous urethral disruption, but not all urologists in the community are familiar with these techniques.

POSTOPERATIVE CARE

The ambulatory patient who has been treated for all injuries may be discharged. In patients with a pelvic fracture, prolonged hospitalization and rehabilitation often postpone definitive care of urethral injuries. Delayed reconstruction of prostatomembranous urethral disruption requires an exaggerated lithotomy position, which may not be possible for months after long-bone or pelvic fractures.

Catheter care is of great importance after urethral reconstruction or suprapubic cystostomy. Urethral catheters should be secured to the abdominal wall in the early postoperative period. After immediate urethral repair or realignment, the Foley catheter should remain in place for 3 to 6 weeks, depending on the nature of the repair. Contrast voiding cystourethrography should be obtained at the time of catheter removal. If extravasation is present, the catheter should be replaced for 1 week and the study repeated. When a suprapubic catheter has been used in addition to a Foley catheter, radiographic studies can be performed via the suprapubic tube.

Patients managed initially with a suprapubic tube alone should have the tube changed after a tract has formed, usually in 4 weeks, and then monthly until reconstruction can be performed. Stricture formation or complete obliteration of the urethra may be the final result after initial management. Subsequent radiographic studies can indicate whether secondary endoscopic or open procedures are needed. Voiding dysfunction may occur after pelvic fracture and sacral nerve root injury.

Injuries to the Vagina, Uterus, and Ovaries

INITIAL EVALUATION

Injuries to the female genitalia [see Table 2] must be regarded as especially morbid because of their association with sexual assault as well as the potential complications of infection and bleeding. Perineal and vaginal injuries, usually the result of blunt trauma, straddle injury, and pelvic fracture, are much more common than cervical and uterine trauma [see Figure 9].[32,33] Enlargement of a reproductive organ predisposes that

organ to injury.[34] Penetrating injuries account for almost all injuries to the fallopian tubes, ovaries, and nongravid uterus.[35]

A history of sexual trauma must be sought and, if elicited, appropriate police and support services notified.[32] In addition, if sexual assault has occurred, informed consent for the rest of the patient assessment must be obtained. This assessment includes a history, physical examination, collection of evidence and laboratory specimens, and treatment, as outlined by the American College of Obstetricians and Gynecologists.[36]

All female patients with evidence of genital injury require examination of the external genitalia as well as a speculum examination of internal organs. The presence of blood implies vaginal laceration. In the presence of pelvic fracture or impalement injury, vaginal laceration warrants complete evaluation (using cystourethrography, proctoscopy, and laparotomy, as indicated) to rule out associated urinary tract and gastrointestinal injuries. Failure to identify vaginal injury associated with pelvic fracture may lead to abscess formation, sepsis, and death.

OPERATIVE MANAGEMENT

Perineal lacerations in the absence of associated urinary tract and rectal injury can be managed in the emergency department. Only large hematomas must be incised and drained, with ligation of vessels. Lacerations of the vulva may be closed primarily after irrigation and debridement. Interrupted absorbable sutures allow any accumulated fluid to drain and eliminate the need for suture removal. Drains are used if there is a large cavity; if hemostasis is suboptimal, the wound may be left open and packed.[32]

Vaginal and cervical lacerations, the result of either blunt or penetrating injury, may bleed extensively if pudendal vessels are injured.[32] If bleeding is not severe, examination and repair under local anesthesia is possible in the ED. If large lacerations are associated with bleeding and hematoma, speculum examination under anesthesia permits more complete assessment and repair of injuries. Vaginal lacerations should be closed with continuous or interrupted absorbable sutures that include mucosal and muscular layers. Antibiotic-soaked vaginal packing should be left in place for 24 hours. Perioperative administration of broad-spectrum antibiotics is sufficient, unless injuries are more complex.

Complex vaginal and perineal lacerations associated with pelvic fracture require much more aggressive management to prevent the morbidity and mortality of open fractures.[32] Evaluation of vaginal injuries under anesthesia, contrast cystography, and rigid proctoscopy are mandatory. The vaginal laceration should be closed with absorbable sutures. Even in the absence of injury to the bladder or rectum, diversion of the urinary and fecal streams should be considered to facilitate care of the wounds.[37] Extraperitoneal bladder rupture associated with vaginal lacerations requires operative repair to prevent infection of pelvic hematoma or the formation of a vesicovaginal fistula. Antibiotic therapy is more prolonged, as appropriate for open fractures.[32] Urologic, gynecologic, and orthopedic consultations are necessary for care of associated injuries.

Injury to the pelvic genital organs is rare in a nongravid patient. Penetrating trauma is the most common cause, and the majority of patients have associated injuries necessitating laparotomy.[34] Blunt injury of the nongravid uterus and pelvic organs occurs in the face of preexisting abnormalities; diagnostic peritoneal lavage demonstrates hemoperitoneum in these instances.[35] The uterus, most commonly injured, is

Table 2 AAST Organ Injury Scales for Female Reproductive Tract

Injured Structure	AAST Grade	Characteristics of Injury	AIS-90 Score
Vagina*	I	Contusion or hematoma	1
	II	Superficial laceration (mucosa only)	1
	III	Deep laceration (into fat or muscle)	2
	IV	Complex laceration (into cervix or peritoneum)	3
	V	Injury to adjacent organs (anus, rectum, urethra, bladder)	3
Vulva*	I	Contusion or hematoma	1
	II	Superficial laceration (skin only)	1
	III	Deep laceration (into fat or muscle)	2
	IV	Avulsion (skin, fat, or muscle)	3
	V	Injury to adjacent organs (anus, rectum, urethra, bladder)	3
Nongravid uterus*	I	Contusion or hematoma	2
	II	Superficial laceration (< 1 cm)	2
	III	Deep laceration (≥ 1 cm)	3
	IV	Laceration involving uterine artery	3
	V	Avulsion or devascularization	3
Fallopian tube†	I	Hematoma or contusion	2
	II	Laceration < 50% of circumference	2
	III	Laceration ≥ 50% of circumference	2
	IV	Transection	2
	V	Vascular injury or devascularized segment	2
Ovary†	I	Contusion or hematoma	1
	II	Superficial laceration (depth < 0.5 cm)	2
	III	Deep laceration (depth ≥ 0.5 cm)	3
	IV	Partial disruption of blood supply	3
	V	Avulsion or complete parenchymal destruction	3
Gravid uterus*	I	Contusion or hematoma (without placental abruption)	2
	II	Superficial laceration (< 1 cm) or partial placental abruption (< 25%)	3
	III	Deep laceration (≥ 1 cm) in second trimester or placental abruption > 25% but < 50%; deep laceration in third trimester	3; 4
	IV	Laceration involving uterine artery; deep laceration (≥ 1 cm) with > 50% placental abruption	4; 4
	V	Uterine rupture in second trimester; uterine rupture in third trimester; complete placental abruption	4; 5; 4–5

*Advance one grade for multiple injuries, up to grade III.
†Advance one grade for bilateral injuries, up to grade III.

repaired with figure-eight sutures or a two-layer closure using Vicryl or chromic catgut sutures.[34] Avulsion of the uterine artery or extensive blast destruction of the uterus may necessitate hysterectomy.[32] When hysterectomy is necessary for trauma, the vaginal cuff may be left open to allow drainage of the operative bed.[38] Lacerations to the ovary or the fallopian tube may be managed by primary closure or salpingo-oophorectomy if contralateral structures are normal.

POSTOPERATIVE CARE

Postoperative care should be dictated by the management of associated injuries. After hysterectomy or repair of vaginal lacerations, a vaginal pack should remain in place for 24 hours. Hemorrhage caused by uterine injury has been treated with oxytocin, which increases uterine tone and controls bleeding.[34] Complex lacerations of the perineum may necessitate bowel rest or colostomy to prevent soilage. Fertility after injury to the

Figure 10   Algorithm illustrates evaluation and treatment of a pregnant female with blunt or penetrating injury to the uterus.

female reproductive organs is not well documented, but patients must be counseled about the possible adverse consequences of uterine and adnexal trauma.

Injuries to the Gravid Uterus

INITIAL EVALUATION

As a result of the increasing incidence of motor vehicle accidents, 6% to 7% of pregnancies are complicated by trauma.[39] Trauma is a leading cause of maternal death, but it more fre-

quently causes death of the fetus.[40-42] Although penetrating injuries are not common, those that do occur are likely to cause uterine injury [see Table 2] and fetal injury because of the size of the uterus.[43] Because of physiologic changes during pregnancy, few signs of injury may be present at initial evaluation, but fetal compromise can easily occur. Conversely, life-threatening hemorrhagic shock may occur with uterine rupture.[38] Maternal survival must remain the first priority, both in initial resuscitation and in the operating room; fetal viability and needs can be managed once the mother's condition has been stabilized.

Table 3 AAST Organ Injury Scales for Male Genitalia

Injured Structure	AAST Grade	Characteristics of Injury	AIS-90 Score
Scrotum	I	Contusion	1
	II	Laceration < 25% of scrotal diameter	1
	III	Laceration ≥ 25% of scrotal diameter	2
	IV	Avulsion < 50%	2
	V	Avulsion ≥ 50%	2
Testis*	I	Contusion or hematoma	1
	II	Subclinical laceration of tunica albuginea	1
	III	Laceration of tunica albuginea with < 50% parenchymal loss	2
	IV	Major laceration of tunica albuginea with ≥ 50% parenchymal loss	2
	V	Total testicular destruction or avulsion	2
Penis†	I	Cutaneous laceration or contusion	1
	II	Laceration of Buck's fascia (cavernosum) without tissue loss	1
	III	Cutaneous avulsion, laceration through glans or meatus, or cavernosal or urethral defect < 2 cm	3
	IV	Partial penectomy or cavernosal or urethral defect ≥ 2 cm	3
	V	Total penectomy	3

*Advance one grade for bilateral injuries, up to grade III.
†Advance one grade for multiple injuries, up to grade III.

All pregnant patients suffering traumatic injury require evaluation [*see Figure 10*]. Ejection from an automobile, presentation in shock, or pelvic fracture increases the likelihood of uterine injury. Estimation of the gestational age is essential for accurate examination of the gravid uterus. Physical signs outlined in the algorithm generally are not useful in determining the status of the fetus. A sterile speculum examination is necessary to evaluate dilation of the cervix and to test for the presence of amniotic fluid.[43] Resuscitation begins by placing the patient in the left lateral decubitus position to minimize obstruction of venous return by the gravid uterus. Once initial evaluation of the mother has been performed, evaluation with external fetal monitoring and real-time ultrasonography provides information on fetal distress, placental abruption, and the general state of the fetus. Most authors agree that real-time ultrasonography gives the most information about the condition of the fetus.[39,44] Kleihauer-Betke testing for fetomaternal hemorrhage has not been predictive of obstetric complications, whereas the maternal Injury Severity Score is correlated with the likelihood of fetal survival.[39,44,45]

Blunt injury and stab wounds to the gravid uterus in a hemodynamically stable female patient should be evaluated by standard methods, with the fetus being shielded as much as possible during radiographic studies but with all available modalities being used, including limited CT if indicated.[43] In the absence of significant injuries, the patient and fetus should be observed and evaluated with external fetal monitoring for at least 4 to 6 hours. In two studies, all complications developed within this time frame.[39,46] Ruptured amniotic membranes, premature labor, or placental abruption should be managed by the obstetric service.

OPERATIVE MANAGEMENT

Pregnant females who experience significant injuries should undergo laparotomy in the following instances: after a gunshot wound to the abdomen; after a defined associated injury necessitating surgery; after a blunt injury or stab wound causes hemodynamic instability; if fetal parts are palpable; and in cases of fetal distress.[43] A midline incision is always selected, and the obstetric consultant should be on hand. Repair of associated injuries can usually be performed by moving the uterus out of the way, permitting subsequent vaginal delivery. Major vascular or rectal injuries may necessitate a cesarean section to provide adequate exposure. Fetal distress or imminent maternal death necessitates an immediate cesarean section. A nonviable fetus, which must be evacuated, is best managed by induced labor at a later date; uterine salvage may be more likely, possibly maintaining reproductive function.[47]

Uterine injuries during pregnancy cause extensive bleeding, but multilayered closure with absorbable sutures should achieve hemostasis. Serious bleeding may be controlled by ligating the hypogastric arteries.[47] In the absence of fetal distress, the abdomen may be closed to allow spontaneous vaginal delivery, even in the perioperative period.[43] If the uterus cannot be salvaged because of bleeding or extensive uterine destruction, a cesarean section and hysterectomy are indicated.

POSTOPERATIVE CARE

External fetal monitoring should be offered when the estimated gestational age is greater than 20 weeks and there is no indication for cesarean section. Monitoring should continue for at least 6 hours after blunt trauma and according to the obstetric recommendations for fetal monitoring after a penetrating injury or laparotomy. $Rh_o(D)$ immune globulin (RhoGAM) should be administered within 72 hours to all Rh-negative mothers, regardless of Kleihauer-Betke test results.[39,40]

Injuries to the Scrotum

INITIAL EVALUATION

Scrotal trauma may result in testicular injury or genital skin loss [see Table 3]. Because blunt injuries to the testicle may be difficult to recognize, high-resolution ultrasonography has become a key element in the evaluation of scrotal trauma [see Figure 11]. When a straddle injury or penetrating mechanism suggests the possibility of urethral injuries, retrograde urethrography is indicated.

Penetrating scrotal injuries commonly involve not only the testis but also the corpora cavernosa, urethra, and spermatic cord. Because of the excellent blood supply of the scrotal skin, most penetrating injuries may be debrided and closed. Exceptions to this general rule include human and animal bites, which are treated with antibiotics and local wound care (or debridement in cases of severe soft tissue infection).[48]

Rupture of the testicle is often immediately painful, with rapid onset of swelling. Falls, straddle injuries, and direct blows are common mechanisms of injury.[49] However, seemingly minor degrees of trauma may be associated with delayed onset of pain, swelling, and ecchymosis; in this scenario, testicular torsion must be included in the differential diagnosis. Physical signs of rupture include scrotal swelling, tenderness, and ecchymosis. Injury to the scrotal wall or tunica vaginalis may cause significant swelling without rupture of the tunica albuginea of the testis; pelvic hematoma caused by fracture may extend down, resulting in massive scrotal swelling. For these reasons, blunt injury to the scrotum should be evaluated by ultrasonography unless findings of the physical examination are normal.

The ultrasonographic characteristics of testicular rupture include loss of normal homogeneity of the testicular parenchyma, loss of continuity of the tunica albuginea, and intraparenchymal hematoma.[50] A discrete break in the tunica is relatively rare. In cases of pelvic fracture with massive scrotal edema, ultrasonography can document the integrity of the testis and allow conservative management of the swelling. If rupture is not documented, conservative treatment with ice packs, analgesics, and elevation allows resolution of swelling.

OPERATIVE MANAGEMENT

Exploration of the scrotum through a vertical incision allows inspection of the scrotal contents and, when spermatic cord injury is discovered, extension of the incision into the groin. The goal is preservation of testicular parenchyma for endocrine and cosmetic purposes; normal sperm production and transport are not expected after repair of rupture. Clots and extruded seminiferous tubules are debrided with scissors to allow closure of the tunica albuginea over the edematous parenchyma. A continuous absorbable suture (3-0 Vicryl) is preferred to prevent palpable knots. When spermatic cord injury is detected, the first priority is determination of the viability of the testis. If this is in doubt, a small incision into the tunica albuginea should cause some bleeding; if the testis is cyanotic and does not bleed when cut, orchiectomy should be performed. If only the vas deferens or spermatic vessels are injured, the testis may

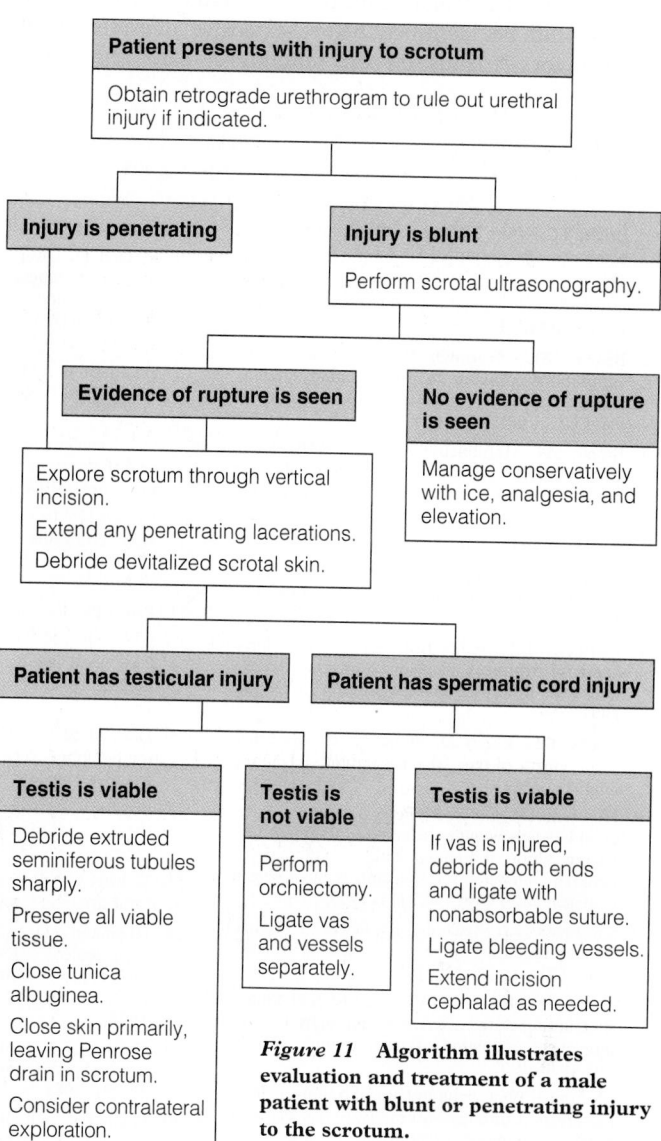

Figure 11 Algorithm illustrates evaluation and treatment of a male patient with blunt or penetrating injury to the scrotum.

remain viable. Ligation of the spermatic vessels is performed in the standard fashion; if vasal ligation is necessary, nonabsorbable suture with long tails is preferable, aiding in later identification for reconstruction if infertility ensues.

Because scrotal skin is well vascularized, it can be closed primarily in almost all instances. Exceptions arise if there is a prolonged delay between injury and definitive care or if grossly contaminated wounds are associated with rectal injuries. Hemostasis should be meticulous because the scrotum will expand massively if bleeding occurs; to prevent such complications, we recommend interrupted suture closure of the tunica dartos and skin in two layers, with a Penrose drain brought out through a separate dependent stab wound. Fluffed gauze should be used for dressing, and a scrotal supporter should be used to keep the scrotum elevated. The Penrose drain is removed on postoperative day 1. There are no major restrictions to activity after scrotal surgery, and patients can be discharged once they have recovered from associated injuries.

Scrotal skin loss caused by burns or electrical or mechanical injury usually spares the testis, which has a separate blood supply. Conservative debridement is possible if there is no infection, but the demarcation between viable and nonviable tissue should be identified before extensive debridement.[51] Management depends on the amount of skin remaining. Options include primary closure, immediate coverage with meshed split-thickness skin grafts, or placement of the testes in subcutaneous pouches in the thigh.

References

1. Bright TC, White K, Peters PC: Significance of hematuria after trauma. J Urol 120:455, 1978

2. Miller KS, McAninch JW: Radiographic assessment of renal trauma: our 15 year experience. J Urol 154:352, 1995

3. Brown SL, Hoffman DM, Spirnak JP: Limitations of routine spiral computerized tomography in the evaluation of blunt renal trauma. J Urol 160:1979, 1998

4. Bretan PN, McAninch JW, Federle MP, et al: Computerized tomographic staging of renal trauma: 85 consecutive cases. J Urol 136:561, 1986

5. Pollack HM: Renal trauma: imaging and intervention. Problems in Urology 8:199, 1994

6. McAninch JW, Carroll PR, Klosterman PW, et al: Renal reconstruction after injury. J Urol 145:932, 1991

7. Matthews LA, Smith EM, Spirnak JP: Nonoperative treatment of major blunt renal lacerations with urinary extravasation. J Urol 157:2056, 1997

8. Cheng DL, Lazan D, Stone N: Conservative management of type III renal trauma. J Trauma 36:491, 1994

9. Husmann DA, Gilling PJ, Perry MO, et al: Major renal lacerations with a devitalized fragment following blunt abdominal trauma: comparison between nonoperative (expectant) versus surgical management. J Urol 150:1774, 1993

10. Sagalowsky AI, McConnel JD, Peters PC: Renal trauma requiring surgery: an analysis of 185 cases. J Trauma 23:128, 1983

11. Morey AF, McAninch JW, Tiller BK, et al: Single shot intraoperative excretory urography for the immediate evaluation of renal trauma. J Urol 161:1088, 1999

12. McAninch JW, Carroll PC: Renal trauma: kidney preservation through improved vascular control, a refined technique. J Trauma 22:285, 1982

13. Corriere JN Jr, McAndrew JD, Benson GS: Intraoperative decision-making in renal trauma. J Trauma 31:1390, 1991

14. Uflacker R, Paolini RM, Lima S: Management of traumatic hematuria by selective renal artery embolization. J Urol 132:662, 1984

15. Presti JC, Carroll PR, McAninch JW: Ureteral and renal pelvic injuries from external trauma: diagnosis and management. J Trauma 29:370, 1989

16. Boone TB, Gilling PJ, Husmann DA: Ureteropelvic junction disruption following blunt abdominal trauma. J Urol 150:33, 1993

17. Corriere JN Jr: Ureteral injuries. Adult and Pediatric Urology, 3rd ed. Gillenwater JY, Grayhack JT, Howards SS, et al, Eds. Mosby–Year Book, St. Louis, 1991

18. Brandes SB, Chelsky MJ, Buckman RF, et al: Ureteral injuries from penetrating trauma. J Trauma 36:766, 1994

19. Medina D, Lavery R, Ross SE, et al: Ureteral trauma: preoperative studies neither predict injury nor prevent missed injuries. J Am Coll Surg 186:641, 1998

20. Corriere JN Jr, Sandler CM: Management of extraperitoneal bladder rupture. Urol Clin North Am 16:275, 1989

21. Fried FA, Rutledge R: A statewide population-based analysis of the frequency and outcome of genitourinary injury in a series of 215,220 trauma patients. J Urol 153:314A, 1995

22. Corriere JN Jr: Trauma to the lower urinary tract. Adult and Pediatric Urology, 3rd ed. Gillenwater JY, Grayhack JT, Howards SS, et al, Eds. Mosby–Year Book, St. Louis, 1991

23. Peters PC: Intraperitoneal rupture of the bladder. Urol Clin North Am 16:279, 1989

24. Cass AS: Diagnostic studies in bladder rupture: indications and techniques. Urol Clin North Am 16:267, 1989

25. Deck AJ, Shaves S, Talner L, et al: Computerized tomography cystography for the diagnosis of traumatic bladder rupture. J Urol 164:43, 2000

26. Sandler CM, Corriere JN Jr: Urethrography in the diagnosis of acute urethral injuries. Urol Clin North Am 16:283, 1989

27. Webster GD: Perineal repair of membranous urethral stricture. Urol Clin North Am 16:303, 1989

28. Husmann DA, Boone TB, Wilson WT: Management of low velocity gunshot wounds to the anterior urethra: the role of primary repair versus urinary diversion alone. J Urol 150:70, 1993

29. Devine CJ Jr, Jordan GH, Devine PC: Primary urethral realignment. Urol Clin North Am 16:291, 1989

30. Guille F, Cipolla B, Leveque S, et al: Early endoscopic realignment of complete traumatic rupture of the posterior urethra. Br J Urol 68:178, 1991

31. Porter JR, Takayama TK, Defalco AJ: Traumatic posterior urethral injury and early realignment using magnetic urethral catheters. J Urol 158:425, 1997

32. Knudson MM, Crombleholme WR: Female genital trauma and sexual assault. Abdominal Trauma. Blaisdell FW, Trunkey DD, Eds. Thieme Medical Publishers, New York, 1993, p 311

33. Mandell J, Cromie WJ, Caldamone AA: Sports-related genitourinary injuries in children. Clin Sports Med 1:483, 1982

34. Quast DC, Jordan GL: Traumatic wounds of the female reproductive organs. J Trauma 4:839, 1964

35. Maull KI, Rozycki GS, Pedigo RE: Injury to the female reproductive system. Trauma, 4th ed. Mattox KL, Moore EE, Feliciano DV, Eds. Appleton-Lange, San Mateo, California, 2000

36. ACOG educational bulletin. Sexual assault. Number 242, November 1997 (replaces No. 172, September 1992). American College of Obstetricians and Gynecologists. Int J Gynaecol Obstet 60:297, 1998

37. Niemi TA, Norton LW: Vaginal injuries in patients with pelvic fracture. J Trauma 25:547, 1985

38. Shires GT: Trauma. Principles of Surgery, 4th ed. Schwartz SI, Shires GT, Spencer FC, et al, Eds. McGraw-Hill, New York, 1984, p 199

39. Towery R, English TP, Wisner D: Evaluation of pregnant women after blunt injury. J Trauma 35:731, 1993

40. Pearlman MD, Tintinalli JE, Lorenz RP: Blunt trauma during pregnancy. N Engl J Med 323:1609, 1990

41. Fildes J, Reed L, Jones N, et al: Trauma: the leading cause of maternal death. J Trauma 32:643, 1992

42. Esposito TJ, Gens DR, Smith LG, et al: Trauma during pregnancy: a review of 79 cases. Arch Surg 126:1073, 1991

43. ACOG educational bulletin. Obstetric aspects of trauma management. Number 251, September 1998 (replaces Number 151, January 1991, and Number 161, November 1991). American College of Obstetricians and Gynecologists. Int J Gynaecol Obstet 64:87, 1999

44. Drost TF, Rosemurgy AS, Sherman HF, et al: Major trauma in pregnant women: maternal/fetal outcome. J Trauma 30:574, 1990

45. Kissinger DP, Rozycki GS, Morris JA, et al: Trauma in pregnancy: predicting pregnancy outcome. Arch Surg 126:1079, 1991

46. Pearlman MD, Tintinalli JE, Lorenz RP: A prospective controlled study of outcome after trauma during pregnancy. Am J Obstet Gynecol 162:1502, 1990

47. Baker DP: Trauma in the pregnant patient. Surg Clin North Am 62:275, 1982

48. Wolf JS, Gomez R, McAninch JW: Human bites to the penis. J Urol 147:1265, 1992

49. Gomez R: Genital injuries. Problems in Urology 8:279, 1994

50. Fournier GR, Laing FC, McAninch JW: Scrotal ultrasonography and the management of testicular trauma. Urol Clin North Am 16:377, 1989

51. McAninch JW: Management of genital skin loss. Urol Clin North Am 16:387, 1989

Acknowledgments

Figures 1, 3, 5 Susan Brust, C.M.I. Adapted from originals by P. Stempen.

Figures 2, 4, 6, 8 through 11 Marcia Kammerer.

11 INJURIES TO THE EXTREMITIES

John T. Owings, M.D., James P. Kennedy, M.D., and F. William Blaisdell, M.D.

Assessment and Management of Extremity Injuries

Trauma to the extremities falls into two basic categories, penetrating and blunt. After penetrating trauma, the primary problem is vascular or neurologic injury. After blunt traumatic injury, the most common problem is fractures and the soft tissue injuries that accompany them. Nonetheless, high-velocity missile injuries can cause complex bone and soft tissue injuries, and blunt trauma can also cause neurologic and vascular injuries.

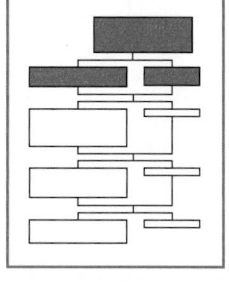

Unless active bleeding is present, injuries to the extremities are less urgent than injuries to the trunk, the head, or the neck: most extremity injuries are not immediately life-threatening and thus can be treated more deliberately. If massive hemorrhage occurs, particularly from a proximal extremity, it can usually be controlled by the application of direct pressure over the bleeding area or, if the conformation of the wound permits, by the introduction of a gloved finger for direct control of the bleeding. In either case, the patient should be directly transferred to the operating room.

Initial Assessment, Temporizing of Fracture-Dislocations, and Secondary Evaluation

Assessment of an injured extremity starts with a history, which can be obtained in parallel with the examination. Failure to elicit the patient's bleeding history at the scene from those transporting the patient may result in failure to recognize the presence of a major vascular injury. The mechanism of injury should also be ascertained.

The initial examination should first be directed toward the circulation. Blood pressure and temperature in both the injured limb and its contralateral counterpart should be determined. Distal pulses should be sought; if they are present and bounding, major vascular injury is unlikely. Injured extremities should be compared with their uninjured counterparts because pulse assessment may be difficult in the face of shock resulting from systemic or torso injuries. If the pulses in one extremity differ significantly from those in the other, vascular injury may be present.

If pulses are absent and a joint dislocation or fracture-dislocation is present, then gentle reduction of the dislocation should be carried out without delay. Frequently, a pulseless extremity with a dislocation regains pulses once the fracture or dislocation is reduced. If pulses return after reduction of the dislocation, assessment may continue on to the next priority. If pulses do not return, vascular injury is assumed, and treatment of such injury becomes the immediate priority.

The circulatory examination should be followed first by a quick neurologic examination aimed at assessing motor function in the hands and feet and ascertaining the presence or absence of sensation and later by a proximal examination of sensory and motor function. Gross deformity is pathognomonic of fracture or dislocation, and appropriate x-rays should be obtained that include portions of the joint above and below the area of suspected injury. Before x-rays are obtained, any gross deformities should be gently reduced to yield a more anatomic alignment of the extremity and splinted to relieve any possible compromise of neural or vascular structures. Finally, soft tissue defects should be noted. If considerable oozing is present, particularly in critical areas such as the hand, proximal application of a tourniquet for a few minutes may facilitate examination, permit definitive control of the bleeding point, and help determine whether significant nerve, muscle, or tendon injury has occurred.

Once the patient's condition has fully stabilized and other injuries have been evaluated, a secondary evaluation of the extremities is appropriate after blunt trauma. The shock, pain, and discomfort associated with more severe truncal injuries may mask the presence of significant extremity injuries. Passive motion of the extremity that results in localized discomfort or crepitation is a signal that x-rays are needed. In the absence of fracture or dislocation, specialized films (e.g., motion or stress studies) may be required if major ligamentous disruption is suspected. Any open wound in the extremity that is associated with a fracture is by definition an open fracture and usually must be explored surgically, ideally within 6 hours of wounding to ensure the removal of any contamination that may have resulted when the bone penetrated the skin.[1] Traumatic penetration of a joint (traumatic arthrotomy) similarly must be expeditiously addressed with prompt irrigation of the joint.

Temporary splinting is in order when definitive treatment of extensive soft tissue injuries, major strains or sprains, or fractures will be delayed. Splints applied in the emergency department must immobilize the injured extremity and prevent movement of the joint above and below the injured area: for example, with a tibial fracture, the leg should be splinted from the toes up to the proximal thigh. Temporary stabilization makes the patient more comfortable and facilitates transfer to the radiology department, the OR, or elsewhere. Immobilization of long bone fractures also helps prevent further soft tissue damage and decrease wound complications. Because most plaster splints obscure radiographic detail, they are best applied after x-rays have been taken. Cardboard splints can be used to stabilize grossly unstable fractures.

Splints vary in width and thickness according to what is appropriate for the extremity. Generally, 15 layers of plaster are applied for arm splints to prevent breakage at the elbow. This thickness is also appropriate for short leg splints; however, 20 to 25 layers may be required for long leg splints. Before being

Assessment and Management of Extremity Injuries

Patient presents with injury to extremity

Management of life-threatening injuries takes priority.

Elicit history (including bleeding history), and ascertain mechanism of injury.

Compare BP, distal pulses, and T° in injured limb and uninjured counterpart.

Check for paralysis or discomfort on motion.

Apply splints or dressing if treatment of fractures or soft tissue injuries must be delayed.

Fracture-dislocation is present, and extremity is pulseless

Reduce fracture-dislocation.

If pulses return, treat as orthopedic injury. If not, assume vascular injury.

No fracture-dislocation is present, and pulses are relatively normal

Major vascular injury is unlikely.

Signs of vascular injury are present

Pulseless extremity from blunt trauma: perform on-table arteriogram.

Pulseless extremity from penetrating trauma: explore or, if location of injury is uncertain, perform on-table arteriogram.

Extremity with pulses but at high risk for vascular injury: perform duplex Doppler evaluation or arteriogram electively.

Repair injuries identified, ideally via primary repair if ≤ 2 cm is resected. If more must be resected, use autogenous vein or a prosthetic graft.

No signs of vascular injury are present

Neurologic injury is present

Penetrating trauma: treat with early debridement and repair unless wound is heavily contaminated or was caused by a gunshot, in which case repair should be delayed.

Blunt trauma: delay repair to allow for possible return of function; these injuries are often contusions rather than lacerations.

No neurologic injuries are present

Orthopedic injuries are present

Open fractures: debride within 6–8 hr of injury, irrigate with saline, and stabilize. Begin antibiotics in ER [*see Figure 3*].

Closed fractures: stabilize.

No orthopedic injuries are present

applied, the splint should be well padded, especially at its edges and at bony prominences, to prevent abrasions, pressure sores, and burns from the exothermic reactions that occur as fiberglass or plaster hardens. Once it has been applied, the splint should be wrapped in such a way as to prevent constriction and held in place with bias-cut stockinette or a similar material.

The ankle should be placed in as close to a neutral position as possible to prevent an equinus deformity. A neutral position can be achieved with a posterior splint bent at 90° or with sugar tong splints applied to the leg medially and laterally. For long leg splints, the knee should be gently flexed. Upper extremity splints should be applied with the limb in the resting position, the wrist extended 20°, and the phalangeal joints gently flexed. An easy way to remember this position is to imagine the hand holding a glass in a drinking position.

The Robert Jones dressing is a very useful all-purpose compressive dressing that immobilizes the injured extremity, helps control swelling, and prevents circulatory compromise. First, a single layer of cast padding is applied to the skin to prevent irritation. Next, one or two layers of thick cotton batting are applied circumferentially or longitudinally and held in place with a roll of cotton bandage. Finally, a splint is applied and kept in place with an elastic bandage or stockinette.

Injuries to Blood Vessels

ARTERIES

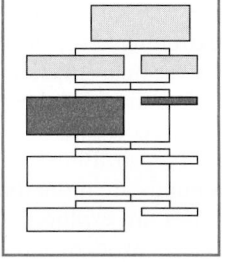

Arterial injuries in an upper extremity are generally a less demanding problem than corresponding injuries in a lower extremity. The main reasons are, first, that upper extremity vessels have much better collateral flow and, second, that even ischemic upper extremities tend to remain viable except when extensive soft tissue damage is present. Moreover, because arteries and veins are smaller in the upper extremities, life-threatening hemorrhages are less common; exceptions are injuries to the subclavian or axillary arteries, which can cause unexpected exsanguination into the chest or present as intrathoracic bleeding.

Blunt and penetrating trauma usually produce different types of injuries. Injuries from blunt trauma usually result in thrombosis of a vessel. Such injuries are primarily stretch injuries rather than transections [see Figure 1]; as the vessel stretches, the tunica intima and the tunica media are disrupted first, leaving the highly thrombogenic tunica externa to maintain temporary vessel continuity. Penetrating injuries that completely divide the vessel may be manifested by thrombosis rather than hemorrhage. If the vessel is only partially divided, however, it contracts and thus will continue to bleed. Accordingly, partial transections are far more dangerous than complete ones.

Bleeding from injured extremity vessels may be ongoing or, if the patient becomes hypotensive, may stop temporarily, only to resume when resuscitation has been initiated. The urgency with which one approaches this type of hemorrhage is governed by whether there is any ongoing limb-threatening ischemia. If limb-threatening ischemia is present, especially in conjunction with anesthesia and paralysis, the extremity is likely to be nonviable: unless vascular repair can be accomplished within 6 hours, normal function is unlikely to return. Moreover, attempts at late repair may be associated with reperfusion injury, the consequences of which also can be life-threatening. If, however, the

Figure 1 Shown is an avulsion injury, in which the artery is stretched, resulting either in partial (*a*) or complete (*b*) intimal disruption or in complete intimal or medial disruption (*c*), with or without pseudoaneurysm formation (*d*) and complete separation of all layers of the vessel wall (*e*).

limb is viable (as indicated by normal or modestly delayed capillary refill, normal sensation, and normal muscle function), then management of other injuries may justifiably assume priority.

Penetrating Trauma

Penetrating vascular injuries generally declare themselves readily. As a rule, the location of a presumed vascular injury can be relatively easily determined by simply noting the path of the penetrating object. If there is evidence of thrombosis or ongoing bleeding, a prompt trip to the OR and an incision placed so as to ensure proximal and distal control are appropriate. If the location of the penetrating injury is obscure or if multiple injuries may exist, angiographic or ultrasonographic evaluation may be appropriate. If the extremity is nonviable, arteriography in the OR is usually preferable to waiting for specific examination in the radiology department. Extremity arteriography in the OR can be performed by injection into the axillary artery (for upper extremity injuries) or the common femoral artery (for lower extremity injuries). Exposure of the x-ray plate immediately after injection of 15 to 20 ml of full-strength contrast material usually results in visualization of the injured area. If it does not, additional films should be obtained; these may be timed according to the progress of the contrast material as estimated from the initial x-ray.

There is considerable controversy regarding whether exploration or angiography is needed when a penetrating injury passes in proximity to a major blood vessel. If the limb appears viable, a duplex Doppler examination may be the best choice: it will identify significant injuries while causing minimal morbidity.[2,3]

Blunt Trauma

Blunt arterial injuries are more difficult to evaluate than penetrating arterial injuries. With blunt trauma, an artery may be completely disrupted, yet pulses may still be present if sufficient collateral blood flow remains. The injured extremity should be compared with its uninjured counterpart; if there are no major differences, it is unlikely that an arterial injury is present. Because the location of an arterial injury is more difficult to discern in cases of blunt trauma, duplex Doppler evaluation or angiography may be indicated when an injury is suspected. If the limb is viable, the definitive diagnostic study can be done electively. If it is not viable, intraoperative angiography should be performed in the OR. Certain injuries, by their very nature, dictate a diagnostic study of the vasculature even in the presence of normal pulses. One example is dislocations of the knee. These injuries usually cause severe stretching of the popliteal artery. Initially, the disruption may constitute only a minor intimal tear, and examination may reveal no evidence of injury [see Figure 2]; however, these internal tears are thrombogenic and result in delayed thrombosis many hours after the initial injury. Because lower extremities are usually splinted to stabilize the extremity, subsequent thrombosis either may not be recognized or may be recognized too late to permit salvage of the limb. Dislocation of the knee with missed popliteal thrombosis is the injury that most often results in subsequent amputation; accordingly, patients with knee dislocations (with a few exceptions) should undergo screening arteriography or duplex Doppler evaluation before any definitive orthopedic treatment of the limb.[4]

VEINS

In the absence of an associated arterial injury, most venous injuries probably go unrecognized. On the whole, the venous system has excellent collateral circulation, and major secondary hemorrhage is rare. Silent venous thrombosis may be responsible for valve damage or may set the stage for subsequent occlusive thrombosis resulting in limb swelling or thromboembolic problems. In the absence of other indications for exploration of the limb, asymptomatic venous injuries need not be repaired; howev-

er, adjusted-dose heparin should be used whenever venous injury is suspected or documented, unless contraindications exist. If there is an associated arterial injury that calls for exposure and operative treatment, the venous injury should be treated simultaneously if the repair is simple. Alternatively, clean ligation may be done; this gives rise to fewer complications than simply ignoring the injury or performing an ill-advised repair of a complex injury. With certain venous injuries, particularly those about the popliteal space or those associated with extensive soft tissue injury, the venous collateral circulation may be inadequate, in which case repair is indicated.

Injuries to Nerves

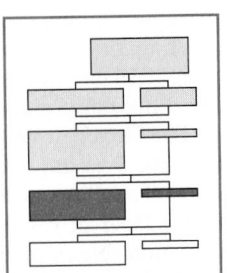

Nerve injury has always been the most challenging aspect of managing trauma to the extremities. It is the principal factor that accounts for limb loss and permanent disability.[5] Some nerve injuries, such as brachial plexus injuries and nerve root injuries, preclude repair.

Because the upper extremities have less muscle and bone mass and more neurologic structures than the lower extremities do, upper extremity injuries are twice as likely to result in nerve damage as lower extremity injuries are. Furthermore, because of the proximity of the upper extremity nerves to arteries, nerve injuries are more common in patients with upper extremity vascular injuries than in patients with lower extremity vascular injuries.

Penetrating injuries from cuts or stab wounds that result in a clean laceration of a nerve are amenable to early intervention and repair. Blunt injuries and penetrating injuries from gunshot wounds are more difficult to assess and manage. When such injuries are explored, one often finds that the nerve is not completely divided, and it is difficult to identify functional injuries—as opposed to anatomic injuries—through visual inspection. Functional loss does not preclude complete recovery without intervention. If exploration reveals complete division of a nerve, it is difficult to determine how much nerve resection may be required to ensure anastomosis of healthy tissue.

CLASSIFICATION

The most practical guide to classification of nerve injuries is that of Sunderland,[6] which comprises five degrees of nerve injury [see Table 1].

First-degree nerve injury results from either concussion or compression of the nerve; electrical conductivity distal to the lesion is preserved. Surgical repair is not necessary. Recovery is spontaneous and rapid, occurring within days or weeks. Because it does not depend on regeneration of any neural element, recovery is usually complete.

Second-degree nerve injury occurs when the anatomic continuity of the nerve and the Schwann sheath is preserved but the axons are interrupted and must recover by means of axonal regeneration. It is characterized by complete motor, sensory, and autonomic paralysis and progressive muscle atrophy. Surgical repair is not necessary. Recovery from secondary injuries is typically complete unless the injury is so proximal that motor end-plate and sensory receptors atrophy before the axon can grow back. The usual rate of axonal regeneration is approximately 1 mm/day or 25 mm/month.

Third-degree nerve injuries involve disruption of endoneural sheaths as well as axons. Thus, when the axons regenerate,

Figure 2 **Knee dislocation is a common mechanism of popliteal artery injury.**

Table 1 Sunderland's Classification of Injuries to Nerves[6]

Degree of Injury	Anatomic Disruption
First	Conduction loss only, without anatomic disruption
Second	Axonal disruption, without loss of the neurilemmal sheath
Third	Loss of axons and nerve sheaths
Fourth	Fascicular disruption
Fifth	Nerve transection

they may enter the nerve sheaths of other axons, resulting in aberrant regeneration. The loss of the sheath leads to increased intraneural fibrosis, which makes it more difficult for the regenerating axons to penetrate the site of injury. The time needed for functional improvement depends on the distance between the injury site and the end organ.

Fourth-degree injuries involve disruption of nerve fasciculi and cause a greater degree of intraneural scarring. To regain function, axons must grow through the scar and reenter the endoneural sheaths. When fourth-degree injuries are minimal, partial resection with meticulous anastomosis of the fasciculi improves outcome.

Fifth-degree nerve injuries involve transection of the entire peripheral nerve. Invariably, there is considerable epineural and perineural hemorrhage and subsequent scarring. Recovery of neural function is impossible without surgical intervention. Fifth-degree injuries may be limited to a very short section of nerve (as with sharp transection) or may affect a very long segment (as with gunshot injury); they may also be associated with stretch injury or compartment syndrome.

How quickly and successfully the nerves regenerate depends on several factors. One such factor is age: the younger the patient, the faster and more complete the recovery. Another is the type of nerve involved: a pure motor or sensory nerve recovers better than a nerve containing both motor and sensory fibers. Thus, the radial and musculocutaneous nerves, which are primarily motor nerves, recover better than the mixed medial nerves, and the tibial division of the sciatic nerve fares better than the peroneal division. A third factor is the level of nerve injury and the duration of denervation. If regenerating axons take more than 12 months to reach denervated muscle, a significant degree of muscle atrophy will have occurred, and the muscle may remain dysfunctional despite some degree of reinnervation. Even when this is the case, it may still be possible to restore some sensation. For example, repair of a divided ulnar nerve near the axilla or the peroneal nerve above midthigh is unlikely to improve motor function; however, median nerve repair near the axilla or tibial nerve at about midthigh may allow the return of at least some protective sensation.

TREATMENT

Whenever an extremity is injured, careful assessment of motor and sensory function is essential. If other life-threatening cranial or truncal injuries are present, evaluation and treatment of nerve injuries may be deferred until these more urgent problems are dealt with. Before any orthopedic manipulation or treatment of vascular injury, an examination must be conducted to assess the integrity of the nerves.

For lacerating nerve injuries, surgical exploration is often indicated. Generally, if the wound is clean or minimally con-

taminated, the feasibility of nerve repair can be considered after the more immediate problems (e.g., vascular injuries) are corrected. If the nerve ends appear to have been sharply divided and there is minimal hemorrhage or contusion, immediate repair is appropriate; identification and approximation of nerve fasciculi are more easily accomplished before extraneural scarring obscures nerve anatomy. If, however, the penetrating object is relatively blunt (e.g., a missile), if the injury is dirty, if there is significant soft tissue damage, if associated fractures are present, or if the vascular repair is particularly tenuous, nerve repair should be delayed. In such circumstances, one should clean and debride the wound, identify the nerve ends if they are divided, and fix them in proximity so that they do not retract; the need for subsequent mobilization at the time of repair will thereby be reduced. After the wound has healed, reexploration is indicated for definitive repair about 3 to 4 weeks after the injury.

A progressing neurologic deficit is another indication for urgent surgical exploration. Such a deficit may result from a false aneurysm associated with vascular injury or from compartment syndrome attributable to hemorrhage and swelling in a fascial compartment. Emergency nerve decompression for a worsening neurologic deficit involves opening any skin, fascia, or muscle constricting the nerve. The decompressed nerve should be covered with some soft tissue, although delayed skin closure may be necessary if the fascia cannot be closed. In cases of compartment syndrome, fascial closure should not be attempted.

In all instances of blunt trauma, delayed repair (usually 2 to 3 months after the injury) is recommended. With neurapraxic lesions, this allows time for recovery, and with axonotmesis lesions, it allows time for possible axonal regrowth through the area of injury. When exploration is delayed, nerve action potential should be recorded intraoperatively to determine whether axonal regeneration has crossed the lesion in continuity. Intraoperative recording of nerve action potentials is much superior to waiting for electromyographic evidence of motor recovery, which requires an average waiting period of 6 months. If no action potentials are recorded crossing the injury, the nerve is resected proximal and distal to the injury until a normal fascicular pattern is obtained. If possible, the nerve is then primarily reapproximated, the epineurium is sutured, or cable nerve grafts are employed.

Open Fractures and Dislocations

The prognosis after an open fracture is very different from that after a closed fracture; treatment of open fractures is much more complex than treatment of simple fractures or traumatic wounds. The existence of an open fracture means that a great deal of energy has been delivered to the bone to produce soft tissue disruption. 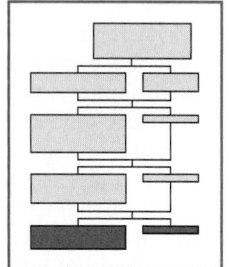 Accordingly, it can be inferred that there has been considerable stripping of muscle, periosteum, and ligament from the bone, resulting in relative devascularization, and that varying degrees of contusion, crushing, and devascularization of the associated soft tissues have occurred. All of these events greatly influence the rate of healing, the incidence of nonunion, and the risk of infection.

The basic principles of management for open fractures are aggressive debridement, open wound treatment, soft tissue and bone stabilization, and systemic administration of antibiotics. These principles have reduced the formerly high mortality associated with open fractures to very acceptable levels.

A simple classification for open fractures exists that is well accepted[7] [see Table 2]. High-velocity gunshot wounds and open fractures must be approached somewhat differently from closed fractures because of the force imparted to the soft tissues. A fracture that looks like a grade I injury because of a small skin wound may behave as a grade III injury because of soft tissue injury. Any open fracture associated with bone loss is treated as a grade III injury, as is any grade I or grade II soft tissue wound that is associated with severe tissue contusion and periosteal stripping. In addition, any fracture associated with gross contamination (e.g., a farmyard injury with vegetable matter or soil within the wound) is treated as a grade III injury because of the risk of clostridial infection and clostridial myonecrosis.

EVALUATION

The injured extremity should undergo orthopedic examination, with particular attention paid to evaluation of neural and vascular status. Compartment syndrome [see Compartment Syndrome, below] should be ruled out in patients at risk; as many as 10% of open tibial fractures are associated with this syndrome as a result of severe soft tissue injury.

The patient's medical condition before the injury, the time elapsed since the injury, the mechanism of injury, and the presence or absence of associated injuries should be noted. If foreign material that is easily removable can be seen, it should be removed promptly, and a quick saline dump (i.e., pouring 1 to 2 L of saline into the wound to help wash out gross contamination and prevent tissue desiccation) is indicated. If the limb is malaligned, gentle gross reduction should be done to relieve any vascular compromise. A sterile dressing moistened with saline or povidone-iodine should then be applied to the wound, and a few minutes should be spent on securing the wound. Ideally, once the wound is assessed and the dressing applied, the dressing should not be removed until the patient is in the OR and preparation for operation is initiated. Once a secure dressing has been applied, a temporary splint should be applied to the limb so that the patient can be transported for x-rays if necessary. Cardboard splints are convenient, inexpensive, and disposable and do not interfere with x-rays.

TREATMENT

When a severe open extremity fracture is accompanied by vascular or neurologic injury, the limb may not be salvageable; such an injury may be essentially a traumatic amputation in which the parts remain connected by a bridge of skin. Although some severely injured limbs can be salvaged, those with both neurologic and vascular injury have a high complication rate and a late amputation rate of 78%. Often, the best treatment in such cases is immediate amputation.

Every open fracture calls for emergency surgical treatment [see Figure 3]. Ideally, treatment should begin within 6 hours of injury: the incidence of infection is directly related to delay in initiating treatment. The factors most helpful in reducing infection (the most severe preventable complication) are antibiotic therapy, timely and aggressive surgical debridement, fracture stabilization, and proper treatment of wounds. Tetanus prophylaxis should be given as needed. Cultures should be obtained in the course of debridement because the results may influence subsequent antibiotic therapy. Patients with grade I or grade II injuries should receive cefazolin in a dosage of 1 g every 4 hours while in the OR and 1 g every 8 hours afterward. Patients with grade III fractures

Table 2 Gradation of Open Fractures[7]

Grade	Wound Size	Extent of Soft Tissue Damage
I	< 1 cm	No or minimal tissue damage
II	> 1 cm	Moderate tissue damage
III	Any size	Major tissue damage; soft tissue loss; bone loss; gross contamination
IIIa		Bone can be covered
IIIb		Bone cannot be covered
IIIc		Vascular injury

or grossly contaminated grade I or II fractures should receive penicillin and gentamicin as well.

WOUND CARE

For all open fractures, irrigation and debridement in the sterile, controlled environment of the OR are required [see Figure 3]. Even apparently minor injures, such as minimal grade I injuries, benefit from thorough examination. The traumatic wound should be extended in such a way as to be compatible with any fracture fixation that may be necessary, and all devitalized or contused soft tissue should be aggressively debrided back to normal, clean, bleeding tissue. It may be a good idea to have a tourniquet in place, but it should be inflated only long enough to control acute hemorrhage; prolonged inflation leads to further tissue ischemia and eliminates muscle contractility, the best indication of muscle viability. If uncontrollable bleeding is encountered, the tourniquet may be inflated for a few minutes until the bleeding point is located and secured. The fracture ends should be delivered into the wound to facilitate inspection and allow adequate irrigation. Any devitalized, stripped, loose bone fragments that are not crucial to reduction or stabilization should be removed, devascularized bone should be debrided, and bleeding fragments should be carefully handled so as to maintain their attachments to the bone and preserve their vascularity.

A pulsatile lavage system should then be used to irrigate the wound and the bone ends with 8 to 10 L of normal saline. At this point, tissue specimens should be obtained and sent for culture. Irrigation is completed by adding another 2 L of fluid containing 100,000 units of bacitracin. Any surgically created wound extensions may then be closed; however, the traumatic wound itself should be left widely open. If the wound is small, a portion of the surgical extension should be left open to allow adequate drainage and to prevent the traumatic wound from sealing off prematurely. Every attempt should be made to cover bone, joint surfaces, implants, and sensitive structures (e.g., tendons, nerves, and blood vessels) with available local soft tissue, but this must be done without tension. Some surgeons are currently investigating wound coverage with primary closure of the primary wound itself. The value of this approach is controversial; however, the need for early and aggressive management of all open fractures is not.[8]

After the initial debridement, the antibiotic regimen is continued for 24 to 48 hours. At this point, if the postdebridement cultures are positive, the regimen is changed to include agents that are appropriate for the infecting organism. If the cultures are negative, the antibiotic regimen may be stopped if the wound appears clean. Any patient who has a grade III fracture or a grade I or II fracture with a positive culture should be returned to the OR every 48 hours for repeat irrigation and debridement until the wound appears healthy and clean. Each

Figure 3 Shown is an algorithm for treatment of grade I, grade II, and grade III open fractures.[7]

time the patient is returned to the OR, new tissue cultures are taken and antibiotics restarted. If the bacterial counts on quantitative culture are higher than 10,000/g tissue, wound infection is probable; lower counts tend to reflect colonization rather than infection. In the case of a grade I or II injury in which the initial culture is negative, the wound may be allowed to close by granulation and secondary intention, or the patient may be returned to the OR in 5 to 7 days for delayed primary closure. For larger wounds, split-thickness skin grafts are often required. For grade III wounds, some type of flap is often required for soft tissue coverage. The flap procedure should be done early, 5 to 10 days after the injury, provided that tissue cultures are negative at this time.

The same protocol used for open fractures is also followed for open dislocations; in addition, the articular surfaces must be kept moist. Cartilage that has been damaged by the force of impact may not be able to tolerate any further insult. Once the

dislocation has been reduced with the patient under anesthesia, the joint should be thoroughly irrigated and debrided as required. The capsule of the reduced joint is closed over a suction drain, and the remaining traumatic wound is left open. In patients who have large grade III injuries associated with soft tissue loss, coverage for the articular surface may not be available, and immediate reconstruction with local or distal flaps may have to be done to keep articular cartilage viable. In these instances, only the joint cartilage should be covered; the remaining portion of the wound must be left open.

FRACTURE STABILIZATION

Operative fixation of open fractures is an extremely complex issue. Many options are open to the orthopedist, and these options change yearly. For open intra-articular fractures, internal fixation is indicated for better healing of cartilage. This is accomplished via anatomic reduction and lag screw fixation, which allow early performance of range-of-motion exercises to minimize permanent loss of range of motion. In addition, any open fractures that are associated with massively traumatized limbs, that occur in patients with multiple injuries to multiple systems, or that are associated with vascular injury should be managed with internal fixation if at all possible.

Generally, it is desirable to stabilize the open fracture during the initial operative procedure. Restoring the anatomy through reduction and stabilization improves circulation; promotes healing of bone and soft tissue; reduces inflammation, bleeding, and dead space; and increases revascularization of devitalized tissue. It also results in earlier mobilization of multiply injured trauma patients and improves their overall status.

Isolated grade I open fractures that are treated promptly can usually be handled with the same techniques as their closed counterparts, with the exception of open tibial fractures. Grade II injuries that occur in ideal circumstances in certain favorable areas (e.g., metaphyseal bone in the forearm and the foot, the humerus, and the femur) can also be treated with the same internal fixation techniques used for closed fractures. Early internal fixation is the optimal method of stabilization for intra-articular fractures.

In other situations, such as those involving open tibial fractures and grade III fractures, the safer approach is conservative treatment with either modified internal fixation techniques or immobilization with external fixators.

Closed Fractures

Of the closed fractures, it is those of the lower extremities with which the trauma surgeon should be most concerned: the prognosis for closed upper extremity fractures is excellent, and these fractures are much less likely to have life-threatening complications than fractures of the lower extremities.

UPPER EXTREMITY FRACTURES

On the whole, fractures of the scapula and the clavicle are relatively benign: they usually heal well, and they typically respond to both conservative and open treatment. Fractures of the neck of the humerus, the shaft, or the condyles (particularly the last) may be associated with vascular complications and may call for immediate fixation. Fractures of the forearm, the wrist, and the hand generally respond to conservative measures and have little or no impact on outcome.

LOWER EXTREMITY FRACTURES

The closed fractures that are of greatest concern for the trauma surgeon and that have the greatest potential effect on outcome are fractures of the femur that involve the acetabulum (with or without hip dislocation), standard hip fractures, and fractures of the shaft of the femur. Other, somewhat less worrisome closed fractures of the lower extremities are fractures that involve the tibial plateau in the knee, fractures that involve the tibia or the fibula, and pilon fractures. Fractures and dislocations of the ankle and the foot, though having the potential to affect long-term morbidity when the ankle joint is involved, generally are not of concern in the immediate overall management of the trauma victim.

Acetabular Fracture and Hip Dislocation

Fractures of the acetabulum and hip dislocations have a common mechanism: they are usually the result of accidents in which a blow is directed down the axis of the femur with the hip and the knee flexed. The telltale sign of soft tissue injury to the knee in an auto accident victim suggests the possibility of hip injury as well. The converse is also true, in that as many as 25% of auto accident victims with posterior hip dislocation also have significant knee injuries. Dislocated hips constitute a pressing orthopedic emergency. Treatment consists of immediate reduction with the patient under general anesthesia to release neurologic compression, restore joint congruency, and reduce any compromise of the femoral head vasculature that may result in aseptic necrosis. This is one situation in which the orthopedist always takes priority over the general surgeon except in the case of impending cardiac arrest. It takes only a few minutes after the induction of anesthesia for the dislocation to be reduced, at which point the case can be turned back over to the general surgeon for definitive treatment of life-threatening emergencies.

Acetabular fractures are of two types. The first type is a fracture associated with hip dislocation; there may be associated cartilage compression with ensuing damage to the joint. The second type results from direct application of force against the pelvis; essentially, it is a pelvic fracture that happens to be intra-articular. The goals of treatment are to obtain anatomic reduction of the articular surfaces and a concentric stable hip joint, to remove intra-articular loose bodies, and to achieve early motion so as to optimize cartilaginous healing. In assessing an acetabular fracture, the most important step is the neurovascular examination, which determines whether any nerve injury has occurred. It is not uncommon to find the nerve entrapped within the sharp edges of a fracture or draped over a displaced fracture under great tension. If a nerve palsy is observed, rapid reduction and stabilization of the fracture are indicated to improve the chances of neurologic recovery. Unless there is an associated hip dislocation, no deformity is noted on examination, but the patient usually complains of deep-seated hip or groin pain. A routine pelvic film usually documents the presence of a fracture; oblique views and computed tomographic scanning permit further localization of the fragments (if necessary) and help determine whether the joint is congruent and the fracture stable.

Although some acetabular fractures (in particular, small chip fractures that have no significant articular component) can be treated with benign neglect, open fixation is usually required if the fracture is displaced or involves the weight-bearing dome of the acetabulum. Fixation may also be necessary for fractures that do not involve the weight-bearing dome if stability is required to prevent recurrent dislocation of the hip. Usually, if an acetabular fracture in a multiply injured patient is displaced severely enough to require internal fixation, intra-articular debris and other indications for open treatment are present. In most situations involving multiple injuries, the best time to fix acetabular injuries is at presentation: at no subsequent point in the early postinjury period will the patient's condition be more favorable and operative fixation easier. If the patient's condition is too unstable to allow immediate fixation, the injury should be treated operatively within 5 to 7 days, before fibrosis and healing begin; once healing has started, mobilization and reduction of the fragments are more difficult. With unstable, displaced fractures, a tibial or femoral traction pin should be inserted if the patient cannot be operated on at presentation or must be stabilized medically before being transferred to a facility that is equipped for operative management of such injuries. In many instances, good reduction can be obtained by using 10 to 15 kg of skeletal traction.

Figure 4 **Shown are five types of hip fractures: (*a*) femoral head fracture, (*b*) subcapital fracture (an intracapsular fracture occurring just below the articular surface at the level of the physeal scar), (*c*) transcervical fracture (also an intracapsular fracture but one that is lower than a subcapital fracture), (*d*) intertrochanteric fracture, and (*e*) subtrochanteric fracture.**

As soon as the patient's level of discomfort has decreased sufficiently, gentle range-of-motion exercise should be started to help mold the cartilage and facilitate its healing. If the patient cannot cooperate with these efforts because of other injuries, continuous passive motion exercise can be started by using a mechanical device with an electric motor.

Hip Fracture

Fracture of the hip is one of the most common conditions seen by orthopedists. A substantial force is required to fracture a hip in a young, healthy accident victim, whereas a minor trauma or fall may be sufficient to do so in an elderly osteoporotic female. Hip fractures may be classified according to their anatomic site: (1) femoral head fractures, (2) intracapsular fractures (including subcapital and transcervical femoral neck fractures), (3) intertrochanteric fractures, and (4) subtrochanteric fractures [*see Figure 4*]. Treatment differs slightly from one type to the next; the primary influence on the choice of treatment is whether the all-important blood supply to the femoral head is preserved or disrupted. With intracapsular fractures, there is a significant risk of disrupting the tenuous blood supply to the joint involved. Such disruption leads to nonunion or avascular necrosis, which can be compounded in the hip by collapse of the femoral head.

Fractures of the femoral head are the most devastating of hip injuries and must be handled as surgical emergencies.[9]

Once a femoral head fracture is recognized, it must be treated operatively within 24 hours of the injury to achieve optimal results. Closed treatment of such injuries yields uniformly poor results. Although operative treatment is usually necessary to provide the best chance of recovery, the initial trauma often is so great as to preclude good results; at best, good results can be obtained in only 50% of cases.[9]

Impaction fractures of the femoral head, however, may be treated in closed fashion with early range-of-motion exercise, particularly if they do not involve a major weight-bearing surface. Internal fixation of these injuries is technically very difficult. Small fracture fragments in the non–weight-bearing inferior portion of the head are probably best excised; large fragments or those involving a significant portion of the weight-bearing dome are best treated with operative fixation. At present, no one form of treatment yields consistently good results. In some patients, particularly physiologically older patients with significant fractures, it may be best to insert a hip prosthesis primarily.

Intracapsular femoral neck fractures carry a high risk of nonunion and avascular necrosis and should be treated on an emergency basis with operative fixation within 12 hours of injury. Even with early optimal surgical treatment, the incidence of avascular necrosis is 20%; if near-anatomic reduction is not obtained, the incidence approaches 50%.[10] The deformity associated with these fractures is not as great as that associated with extracapsular or intertrochanteric fractures. A typical patient with an intracapsular fracture presents with a shortened, externally rotated, and abducted lower extremity. Traction reduces the pain and, more importantly, may allow increased blood flow across the neck by decreasing the external rotation and thus relieving vascular occlusion resulting from compression of a tight, twisted capsule. Treatment consists of early anatomic reduction with fixation to eliminate the risk of displacement and permit rapid mobilization. Closed reduction of displaced fractures should be attempted with the patient under general anesthesia, and it must be gentle to prevent further vascular damage. If closed reduction does not achieve acceptable anatomic results, open reduction is required, with care taken to minimize soft tissue stripping and preserve the blood vessels encountered in the approach. Once anatomic reduction has been accomplished, internal fixation with any of the several types of fixation devices available (e.g., sliding hip screw devices, blade plates, and multiple pins or screws) is indicated. When the patient is physiologically older than 70 years, a primary hip prosthesis is often indicated instead of internal fixation.

Intertrochanteric and subtrochanteric fractures do not threaten the blood supply to the femoral head, because they occur below the extracapsular ring of vessels. As a rule, operative fixation within 24 hours of injury yields optimal results, permitting rapid mobilization and preventing systemic complications as well. A typical patient with an intertrochanteric femoral neck fracture presents with a limb that appears to be markedly shortened and externally rotated. Traction should be used if a delay of more than 12 hours is expected before operation. Almost all patients with these fractures are candidates for internal fixation; the exception is an elderly patient who had significant arthritis of the hip before the fracture, in whom a hip prosthesis may be the best choice. A sliding hip screw

Figure 5 Hip x-ray shows an intertrochanteric fracture stabilized with a sliding hip screw device.

device is most commonly used for fixation [*see Figure 5*]. Operative fixation of subtrochanteric fractures, which are located between the lesser trochanter and a point 5 cm distally, can be more difficult because high bending forces in the region (resulting from the angular shape of the proximal femur) often lead to implant failure before union. Possible management approaches include cross-locking, intramedullary nailing, and the use of plates and screws.

Femoral Shaft Fracture

Fractures of the femoral shaft, like intertrochanteric femoral neck fractures, are associated with significant blood loss. Because of the shape of the thigh, more than 1 L may be lost into this space with little or no external indication. Accordingly, the trauma surgeon must anticipate the blood loss from the fractured femur when formulating the initial management strategy.

The advent of intramedullary nailing has revolutionized the treatment of femoral shaft fractures. With stable femoral shaft fractures that undergo nailing, full weight bearing without crutches is possible within a few days of the operation. Reapproximation of the fracture fragments with nailing also dramatically reduces bleeding into the thigh. Femoral shaft fractures are often associated with injuries to knee ligaments, which are difficult to assess in the presence of the femoral fracture. It is important that, when the patient is under anesthesia for treatment of the fracture, the stability of the knee be assessed as well.

Neurovascular injuries are relatively uncommon with femoral shaft fractures; however, when the fracture is in the distal third of the femur, there is the possibility of injury to either the superficial femoral artery or the popliteal artery as a consequence of the tethering of these vessels against the shaft at the level of the adductor canal [*see Figure 6*]. The most popular method of immobilizing a femoral fracture for transport is the use of a Hare or Thomas splint. These convenient devices consist of a frame buttressed against the ischial tuberosity, along with a nonwound endstrap about the foot for traction. They effectively immobilize the extremity and lessen patient discomfort, and they need not be removed for x-rays to be taken. These splints do, however, exert some pressure on the foot; therefore, the patient should be placed in skeletal traction to maintain the benefits if immediate operation is not feasible. The skeletal traction pin should be placed in the tibia so that the femur is not contaminated by the pin wound. Its placement in the tibia should be distal to the anterior tubercle so that the entire thigh, including the knee joint, can be prepared for operation without the pin site being included.

Very few tenets in orthopedics are held with such absolute conviction as the tenet that femoral fractures are best treated with intramedullary nailing. Nailing lowers the incidence of respiratory distress syndrome, blood loss, and tissue trauma and reduces the patient's need for narcotics. In a multiply injured patient with a fractured femur, nailing should be done immediately to help control hemorrhage to the fracture site and help stabilize the patient hemodynamically. In one study,[11] multiply injured patients with an injury severity score of 18 or higher who underwent nailing more than 48 hours after the injury had a four times greater incidence of pulmonary complications than a similar group of patients who underwent nailing within 24 hours of injury; in addition, they had a longer average stay in the ICU (7.6 days as opposed to 2.8 days). In a patient who does not have multiple injuries, the timing is not crucial, but nailing is easier to perform if it is done within the first 6 to 12 hours, because after this period, hemorrhage and swelling make reduction more difficult. Although virtually all open femoral fractures are best treated with intramedullary nailing, a plate or an external fixator may be indicated as well in isolated instances.

Femoral fractures were once associated with significant morbidity and mortality but now are among the musculoskeletal injuries with the most predictable results after treatment. Most complications are secondary to technical problems at the time of nailing and therefore can be prevented by paying attention to the technical details.

Fracture and Dislocation of the Knee and the Patella

Knee injuries are common in multiply injured patients, partly because of the vulnerability of this joint to dashboard injuries in motor vehicle accidents and to direct trauma in motorcycle accidents.

Intra-articular knee fracture   Fractures about the knee that affect the tibial or femoral condyles are as much an injury to the articular surface of the knee joint as they are a fracture of the periarticular bone. Consequently, even if successful bony union has been achieved, the issues of joint alignment, stability, stiffness, and posttraumatic arthritis must still be taken into account to ensure that the clinical result is not compromised. Knee fractures are characterized by local pain, swelling, and crepitation. A hemarthrosis forms when an intra-articular fracture is present. Such a fracture may be suspected when marrow fat globules are present in the hemarthrosis. With any injury about the knee, ligamentous stressing should not be performed until after x-rays confirm that no fracture is present. If the x-rays show a femoral supracondylar or tibial plateau fracture, x-rays of the entire length of the fractured bone should be obtained to rule out the presence of other fractures.

Unstable intra-articular knee fractures should be treated by means of anatomic reduction, rigid fixation, and early motion. Aspiration of a tense hemarthrosis is sometimes required to decompress the joint and relieve pain. The best results are achieved by means of immediate stabilization through rigid internal fixation; however, if treatment must be delayed for a few days after the injury, acceptable results usually can still be achieved. If delayed fixation is to be done, the extremity should be splinted or placed in balanced traction. Femoral condylar fractures, even when they initially are not displaced, should be treated with rigid fixation to minimize the risk of subsequent displacement from muscle forces or knee motion. Rigid fixation allows early motion to facilitate cartilage healing. Unstable or displaced tibial plateau fractures likewise should be treated with rigid fixation and early motion. Tibial plateau compression fractures are the result of an axial load and are displaced by definition. For active individuals, anatomic reduction and fixation allow early motion and yield the best long-term results. Often, bone grafting is required to maintain elevation of the articular surface.

After rigid stabilization of these fractures, the ligamentous structures about the knee should be evaluated via examination or stress films as warranted: as many as 25% of plateau fractures are associated with ligamentous injuries.[12] Late knee instability may compromise treatment of tibial plateau fractures and is a major cause of unacceptable results.

Patellar fracture   The most common injury to the patella in trauma patients is a stellate comminuted fracture result-

Figure 6   **Vascular injuries resulting from blunt trauma to an extremity are usually associated with fracture. Illustrated here is the mechanism of arterial injury in femoral fracture.**

Adductor Magnus Muscle

Popliteal Artery

ing from a direct blow; the second most common is an avulsion fracture that is a rupture of the extensor mechanism. A patient with a fractured patella exhibits soft tissue swelling about the knee as well as hemarthrosis, which may be tense. Patellar fractures are commonly associated with laceration over the patella; when this is the case, a traumatic arthrotomy must be ruled out. Other injuries, such as cruciate ligament failure and femoral fracture, may be present as well. The most important task in the examination is to make sure that the extensor mechanism is intact. Stellate fractures usually are not associated with extensor ruptures, and the extensor retinaculum keeps many of these fractures from displacing. Avulsion fractures, on the other hand, are associated with tears of the extensor tendon; the patient cannot extend the knee without a lag or perform a straight leg raise against gravity. It may be necessary to infiltrate the joint with local anesthesia so that the patient can attempt the maneuver.

For tensile avulsion fractures, exploration and repair of the fracture are appropriate. Nondisplaced fractures may be treated with a knee immobilizer or a cylindrical cast. Stellate direct blow fractures may be treated initially with simpler immobilization and later with protected motion until the fracture is healed. If the fragments for the joint surface are offset by more than 1 mm, anatomic reduction of the joint surface is necessary to prevent posttraumatic arthritis. Severely comminuted patellar fractures may be irreparable; in such instances, a partial or total patellectomy may be required.

Tibial Fracture, Fibular Fracture, and Pilon Fracture

Tibial fracture   Fractures of the tibia are among the most difficult fractures that orthopedic surgeons are called on to treat. The subcutaneous location of the tibia offers little protection from direct violence, and high-energy fractures are associated with an increased healing time in 50% of cases.[13] Tibial fractures are often fraught with complications, such as compartment syndrome, nonunion, delayed union, malunion, and infection. In their severest manifestations, they often end in amputation.

Tibial shaft fracture is the most common shaft fracture affecting the long bones. Minor fractures take 10 to 16 weeks to heal, with a 2% delayed union rate, and severe fractures take an average of 23 weeks to heal, with a 60% delayed union rate. The reason for the slow healing is that the blood supply to the tibia is notoriously poor; furthermore, because most of the bone is located subcutaneously, a good soft tissue envelope is present only posteriorly and, to a lesser extent, laterally, which means that relatively few areas are available where blood vessels can enter the tibia through muscular attachments. Tibial shaft fractures are easily diagnosed clinically in the emergency room. Whenever such an injury is present, the patient's calf should be palpated for evidence of firmness, which would suggest a possible compartment syndrome. The patient's neurovascular status should then be assessed. If the fracture is grossly angulated or malaligned, gentle restoration of axial alignment helps relieve vascular kinking and compromise. The extremity should be splinted and then x-rayed for full assessment of the fracture. After the x-rays, the tibia should be temporarily stabilized by means of a Robert Jones dressing and a splint or by means of skeletal traction through a calcaneal pin.

For unstable tibial fractures—including long spiral fractures, fractures with butterfly fragments or significant comminution, segmental fractures, and tibial and fibular fractures occurring at the same level—operative fixation is the treatment of choice. For isolated stable tibial fractures in which the fracture line is transverse and there is at least 50% bony apposition, long leg casts with weight bearing may be highly successful. If the patient is comatose or has head injuries, operative fixation should be considered, particularly if the patient is agitated or uncooperative.

The standard treatment for tibial shaft fractures—closed, reamed, intramedullary nailing—has a high success rate and a low complication rate. Although the closed technique helps preserve the extraosseous blood supply, the reaming and nailing lead to loss of the intraosseous vasculature that supplies the inner two thirds of the bone. For rotational or axially unstable fractures, interlocking screws may be required. In those unusual circumstances in which the fracture pattern does not permit insertion of an intramedullary rod, a plate or screws may be used; unfortunately, this form of management is associated with a high rate of nonunion. For open fractures with complex wounds, the standard treatment has been external fixation, which permits stabilization of the fracture, allows access to large open wounds, and facilitates nursing care. Currently, however, nonreamed nailing appears be superior to external fixation in this situation: with proper early treatment and aggressive irrigation and debridement, the infection rates are no higher, the complication rate is lower, and the functional end results are better.

Fibular fracture   Generally, fibular shaft fractures may be ignored; they heal readily, sometimes so readily that they interfere with the union of associated tibial fractures. Isolated midshaft fibular fractures that do not involve the ankle joint may be treated symptomatically, often without a cast. In some instances, plating the fibular fracture stabilizes an unstable tibial shaft fracture; however, rendering the fibula stable may diminish the cyclic compression that occurs with weight bearing at the site of the tibial fracture and may delay healing. For this reason, in most cases of combined tibial and fibular fracture, the fibula is not stabilized.

Fractures at the distal end of the fibula can be a serious problem if the ankle joint is disrupted. In these circumstances, anatomic reduction (usually with internal fixation) is required to prevent chronic pain or late arthritis from altered joint mechanics. The most common problem associated with proximal fibular head injuries is a peroneal nerve palsy, which usually resolves. If the nerve has been lacerated, however, regeneration may take quite a long time.

Pilon fracture   Pilon fracture results from forceful axial compression across the ankle joint, which drives the talus up into the tibial plafond, resulting in a severe intra-articular fracture. It is commonly seen in falls from a height and is usually accompanied by a fracture of the distal fibular diaphysis. Some pilon fractures are so comminuted and severe that reconstruction is technically impossible and primary ankle fusion may be necessary. With severe open fractures, amputation may be required.

Pilon fractures are associated with massive swelling resulting from soft tissue edema and bleeding. Fracture blisters are common. Reconstruction must be done within a few hours of injury; the earlier, the better. If it cannot be done in this period, it must be delayed for 5 to 7 days or longer, until the swelling has decreased. Even with immediate fixation, the swelling can be so great that by the end of the operation, the skin cannot be closed and must be either left open or closed with a skin graft.

The goals of treatment are restoration of ankle joint integrity, congruency and stability, achievement of bony union, and functional painless motion. These are best achieved by means of open reduction and internal fixation, but only if the fracture is amenable to reconstruction. For certain complex fractures, closed treatment may be the only choice.

At best, good surgical technique results in a 50% to 75% return to full function. Accordingly, meticulous attention to detail is essential in performing the procedure. The fibula is usually fixed first through a lateral incision, and the tibia is then fixed via an anterior or medial approach. Dissection should be minimized to prevent further soft tissue injury. Any debris present in the joint should be removed. Plates and screws are necessary for stabilization of the fracture. Bone grafting is often required to fill bony defects and voids. If the tibial fracture is not amenable to reconstruction, the fibula may be plated to help bring the tibia out to length, maintain alignment, and afford some stability. If the fracture cannot be immediately fixed, calcaneal pin traction should be used to bring the limb out to length and permit elevation of the leg to decrease swelling. If posttraumatic arthritic pain is severe, delayed ankle fusion may be required.

Compartment Syndrome

Compartment syndrome is defined as high-pressure swelling within a fascial compartment. The forearm and the lower leg are the classic locations for compartment syndrome—any physician who treats trauma patients will encounter compartment syndromes at these sites—but the syndrome may also occur in the hand or the foot or, less commonly, in the shoulder, the upper arm, the buttock, or the thigh. The reason why compartment syndrome is more common in the forearm and the lower leg than in the less classic sites is that the compartments in these anatomic areas have tighter, better-defined fascial boundaries. Many physicians still believe, incorrectly, that compartment syndrome cannot develop in conjunction with an open fracture because the open nature of the injury provides decompression. This is a dangerous assumption: extensive soft tissue injury is in fact a very common accompaniment to an open fracture, and as many as 10% of open tibial fractures, for example, are associated with compartment syndrome. Alertness to symptoms and physical findings in patients with open fractures is the key to recognizing compartment syndrome.

Compartment syndrome can have any of several causes. The most common cause is hemorrhage and edema in the damaged soft tissue that accompanies a fracture. A dressing or a cast that is too tight can cause external pressure, as can the eschar from a circumferential burn. Massive soft tissue swelling and edema can occur secondary to various toxins found in venomous snakes, spiders, and scorpions. Unintentional infusion of intravenous fluid outside the vascular space can also cause compartment syndrome. A rarer situation is an iatrogenic compartment syndrome induced by the military antishock trousers; several cases have been reported after ill-advised, prolonged occlusion of the extremity with this garment. Disruption of the venous drainage of a limb may also result in edema and high compartment pressures, as may venous thrombosis.

The classic concept of the etiology of compartment syndrome is that as pressure increases within the compartment, it ultimately reaches that of the venous capillary. At this point, complete venous obstruction occurs, which, if arterial flow should continue, would result in continued escalation of compartment pressure. Inevitably, extensive venous obstruction gives rise to reflex spasm of the accompanying arteries, at which point tissues begin to become ischemic. Muscle can tolerate complete ischemia for 3 or 4 hours; after this period, it dies, and limb function is permanently compromised. In advanced ischemia, the microvasculature loses its integrity, with the result that severely ischemic and dead muscle swells and compartment pressure increases. Theoretically, in these circumstances, opening the skin envelope and exposing the dead muscle through fasciotomy would render the tissue vulnerable to infection. With late fasciotomy, when muscle is already necrotic, limb loss occurs primarily as a consequence of loss of skin covering; this consideration should be weighed when fasciotomy is being considered. This issue represents the only significant controversy regarding fasciotomy, which is the treatment of choice for compartment syndrome in all other contexts.

DIAGNOSIS

The key to diagnosis of compartment syndrome is continuous assessment of any extremity injury where there is a chance that the syndrome might develop—for example, fractures of the tibia or the forearm, fractures of the thigh or the upper arm (less likely), and, for that matter, all comminuted fractures associated with severe soft tissue injury. The diagnosis of compartment syndrome is a clinical one: although compartment pressures may be measured, there is no agreement on what constitutes the critical pressure. In fact, it has been shown that there is no specific compartment pressure at which the compartment syndrome occurs. The problem appears to be related more to the difference between the mean arterial pressure and the compartment pres-

sure. As this pressure difference decreases, perfusion of the soft tissues decreases as well, and compartment syndrome occurs. The syndrome is frequently seen when the difference between the mean arterial pressure and the pressure in the involved compartment is less than 40 mm Hg.[14]

The hallmark of the compartment syndrome is the presence of the four Ps: *p*ressure, *p*ain, *p*aresthesia, and intact *p*ulses. On palpation, the compartment will be tense or even boardlike, and this tenseness is usually the critical factor in deciding whether to treat the problem surgically. Pain that is out of proportion to what would be expected for the patient's level of injury and pain that is aggravated by passive stretching of the muscles are also manifestations of compartment syndrome. Muscles are more sensitive to anoxia than nerves are; thus, muscle pain and paralysis occur before paresthesia and anesthesia are noted.

When a patient at risk begins to complain of undue pain, the first step is to remove all circumferential bandages and then split them down to skin to relieve any pressure. If a plaster cast is present, it should be split, spread, or removed; if necessary, maintenance of reduction should be sacrificed. If the clinical picture does not improve after these measures are taken, then a decompressive fasciotomy is indicated.

OPERATIVE TREATMENT

Acute compartment syndrome is treated with wide decompression fasciotomy. To decompress the forearm, two incisions are made, one volar and one dorsal [*see Figure 7*]. A longitudinal dorsal incision provides access to the extensor compartment and the mobile wad. The fascia overlying these compartments must be widely opened. A curvilinear volar incision allows access to

Figure 7 **Shown are incisions for forearm decompression in compartment syndrome.**

Figure 8 **Illustrated is the two-incision technique for lower leg decompression in compartment syndrome. Short transverse incisions are made in the fascia to locate (*a*) the lateral intermuscular membrane dividing the anterior and lateral compartments and (*b*) the posterior membrane dividing the superficial and deep posterior compartments. Fasciotomies are then performed in all four compartments along the dashed lines.**

the flexor compartment from a point proximal to the antecubital fossa to the midpalm. Here, too, it is imperative that fascia be widely opened. In severe cases, the deep intramuscular fascia enveloping the flexor digitorum superficialis, the flexor digitorum profundus, and the flexor pollicis longus may have to be opened as well. The thick transcarpal ligament is divided distally to perform a carpal tunnel release. The proximal end of the incision should release the lacertus fibrosus so as to decompress the median nerve at the elbow.

To decompress the lower leg, again, two incisions are usually made. A lateral incision between the tibial crest and the fibula provides access to the anterior and the lateral compartment. A short transverse incision is then made through the leg fascia to locate the lateral intramuscular membrane. The superficial peroneal nerve lies posterior to this septum in the lateral compartment and must be avoided. The fascia enveloping the two compartments is then widely opened longitudinally with blunt scissors until the muscles are soft and all pressure is dissipated. Next, a medial incision is made 2 cm posterior to the posterior crest of the tibia to provide access to the posterior compartments, with care taken to avoid the saphenous nerve and the saphenous vein. Again, a short

transverse incision is made through the enveloping fascia to identify the septum between the deep compartment and the superficial compartment [*see Figure 8*].

After fasciotomy, both fascia and skin are left widely open. The skin defects may be closed with skin grafts, provided that this is done without tension or pressure. Alternatively, the patient may be returned to the OR after the swelling resolves for delayed closure of the skin (again, with fascia left open) or split-thickness skin grafting, as indicated.

Injuries to Soft Tissue

The main types of soft tissue injuries encountered in patients who have experienced trauma to an extremity are abrasions, contusions, lacerations (including avulsion injuries), hemarthrosis, and sprains and strains. All such injuries should be examined with the goal of determining their nature and severity and ruling out underlying injuries to tendons, arteries, or nerves. Local or systemic analgesia or anesthesia may be required for appropriate examination of injuries. The entire area around the wound should then be prepared with an antiseptic solution and thoroughly inspected, palpated, and, if necessary, probed to ascertain the probable depth and direction of the wound. The position the extremity was in when wounded should be kept in mind; it may be critical for identifying injuries to underlying structures.

When examination reveals that a break in the skin has occurred, tetanus prophylaxis should be given in accordance with the patient's immunization history. For minor, clean lacerations that are not associated with other injuries, prompt debridement and irrigation are indicated. Simple wounds and lacerations that are seen and managed within 6 to 8 hours can usually be closed.

Abrasions are generally minor injuries. Typically, there is some ground-in foreign material, which may give rise to subsequent infection and complicate other injuries. Sometimes, abrasions may be treated in the ED by anesthetizing the injured area and cleaning it with an antiseptic solution and a soft brush to remove any grit and dirt. For abrasions that are more than 10 cm in diameter and are overtly dirty, however, anesthesia and treatment in the OR may be required. Once the abraded area is clean, an occlusive, nonadherent dressing should be applied to ease the pain of dressing changes and promote healing.

Contusion is the result of disruption of and hemorrhage into subcutaneous tissue or muscle as a consequence of blunt trauma. Large contusions that contain expanding hematomas may have to be treated with operative debridement and hemostasis; smaller contusions are usually treated with supportive dressings, with or without counterpressure.

Lacerations range in severity from simple full-thickness skin injuries to complex undermining lacerations and flap avulsions. As noted, simple lacerations can generally be treated in the ED with irrigation, debridement, and closure. Contaminated wounds more than 6 to 8 hours old call for a more conservative approach: once the wound is clean, it should be left open for 3 to 4 days and then closed by secondary intention. The deeper lacerations seen in avulsion injuries usually call for operative exploration, irrigation, and debridement to ensure removal of devitalized tissue and to minimize the risk of retaining foreign material. In some instances, the wound may have to be extended to permit proper inspection of its depth and to ensure adequate cleaning. Copious irrigation with a pulsatile lavage system dilutes the bacterial load and flushes foreign material from the wound. Because muscle takes sutures poorly, no attempt should be made to close muscles unless major tendinous avulsions have occurred. Once the wound has been cleaned and debrided, closure of the overlying fascia results in close approximation of the muscle ends, particularly if closure is accompanied by suction drainage. In the case of avulsion injuries, the likelihood that the flap will slough is high, particularly if the intact portion of the flap is distally based (that is, if the flap derives its blood supply distally). This problem can be dealt with by removing and defatting the skin, converting it to a full-thickness skin graft, and reapplying it to the injured area (provided that the wound is sufficiently clean).

Any laceration in the vicinity of a joint raises the possibility of traumatic arthrotomy. A long knife blade, a shard of glass, or a jagged piece of metal can travel some distance under the skin and can penetrate a joint. Probing the wound often confirms joint penetration, but it does not necessarily rule it out. Air seen in the joint on x-rays confirms penetration. For other wounds in proximity to synovial joints, an arthrogram should be performed. Saline or dilute methylene blue may be injected into the joint; oozing from the wound confirms arthrotomy. Once arthrotomy is confirmed, irrigation of the wound and the joint should be performed on a timely basis in the OR.

An acute joint effusion that occurs within 6 to 8 hours of injury is usually the result of bleeding. The presence of hemarthrosis can be confirmed by joint aspiration, which is also the treatment of choice. After reoperation, hemarthrosis should be treated with bulky, compressive dressings, ice, elevation, and rest until it resolves.

Sprained ligaments and strained muscles of the extremities rarely necessitate urgent surgical treatment. The diagnosis may not even be apparent until the patient has recovered sufficiently from other injuries to note local discomfort when attempting to bear weight on the extremity. Severe sprains and strains in which gross instability of the joint is apparent may be associated with joint dislocation. As a rule, these more extensive injuries need not undergo urgent surgical repair; repair is usually best done later, on an elective basis. Dislocations associated with vascular injury (most commonly, knee dislocations) may necessitate emergency revascularization procedures. In these situations, joint stabilization or reconstruction may be required to protect the vascular repair.

The Mangled Extremity

One of the more difficult decisions for a trauma surgeon is whether to amputate an extremity with multiple severe injuries. A number of scoring systems have been devised to facilitate this decision; however, most are cumbersome and hence too impractical to be used in the very patients most likely to need them—namely, unstable, multiply injured trauma patients. Although the ultimate usefulness of an extremity is related to the presence of intact neurologic function, the decision on when to amputate versus when to attempt complex repair of the mangled extremity is more appropriately based on the patient's overall condition and the vascular supply to the extremity.

In severely injured patients, dead or devitalized tissue can help precipitate the onset of disseminated intravascular coagulation. It is not uncommon for patients with mangled extremities to manifest the systemic inflammatory response syndrome until the extremity is removed, at which point they recover promptly. For this reason, if a mangled extremity is not an acute threat to the patient during the initial resuscitation, it may be best treated with irrigation and debridement (as described with respect to open fractures) and some form of stabilization. If, however, the extremity has no palpable pulses or does not appear viable, then the decision whether to amputate should be based on the functional prognosis of the extremity, which in turn is based on the presence or absence of nerve injury and the orthopedist's judgment of whether long-term bony stabilization is likely to be achievable.

If the decision is made to attempt salvage of the limb, regular rechecking of both the extremity and the patient's overall condition is essential. If the patient's condition deteriorates significantly or the previous prognostic estimate changes for the worse, amputation should be promptly performed within the first 24 hours.[15]

References

1. Allgöwer M, Border JR: Management of open fractures in the multiple trauma patient. World J Surg 7:88, 1983

2. Knudson MM, Lewis FR, Atkinson K, et al: The role of duplex ultrasound arterial imaging in patients with penetrating extremity trauma. Arch Surg 128:1033, 1993

3. Dennis JW, Frykberg ER, Veldenz HC, et al: Validation of nonoperative management of occult vascular injuries and accuracy of physical examination alone in penetrating extremity trauma: 5- to 10-year follow-up. J Trauma 43:196, 1997

4. Wagner WH, Calkins ER, Weaver FA, et al: Blunt popliteal artery trauma: one hundred consecutive injuries. J Vasc Surg 7:736, 1988

5. Visser PA, Hermreck AS, Pierce GE, et al: Prognosis of nerve injuries incurred during acute trauma to peripheral arteries. Am J Surg 140:596, 1980

6. Sunderland S: Nerves and Nerve Injuries. Churchill Livingstone, Edinburgh, 1978, p 127

7. Chapman MW: Operative Orthopaedics. JB Lippincott, Philadelphia, 1988

8. DeLong WG Jr, Born CT, Wei SY, et al: Aggressive treatment of 119 open fracture wounds. J Trauma 46:1049, 1999

9. Epstein HC, Wiss DA, Cozen L: Posterior fracture dislocation of the hip with fractures of the femoral head. Clin Orthop 201:9, 1985

10. Swiontkowski MF, Winquist RA, Hansen ST Jr: Fractures of the femoral neck in patients between the ages of twelve and forty-nine years. J Bone Joint Surg [Am] 66:837, 1984

11. Bone LB, Johnson KD, Weigelt J, et al: Early versus delayed stabilization of femoral fractures: a prospective randomized study. J Bone Joint Surg [Am] 71:336, 1989

12. Delamarter RB, Hohl M, Hopp E Jr: Ligament injuries associated with tibial plateau fractures. Clin Orthop 250:226, 1990

13. Hoaglund FT, States JD: Factors influencing the rate of healing in tibial shaft fractures. Surg Gynecol Obstet 124:71, 1967

14. Heppenstall RB, Sapega AA, Izanty T, et al: Compartment syndrome: a quantitative study of high-energy phosphorus compounds using ^{31}P-magnetic resonance spectroscopy. J Trauma 29:1113, 1989

15. Roessler MS, Wisner DH, Holcroft JW: The mangled extremity: when to amputate? Arch Surg 126:1243, 1991

Acknowledgments

Figures 1, 4, 7, and 8   Tom Moore.

Figures 2 and 6   Carol Donner.

Figure 3   Marcia Kammerer.

12 BURN CARE IN THE EARLY POSTRESUSCITATION PERIOD

Robert H. Demling, M.D.

Approach to the Burn Patient during the Second to Fifth Days after the Burn

Beginning about 36 hours after injury, major physiologic and biochemical changes occur that differ from earlier alterations [*see I:3 Burn Care in the Immediate Resuscitation Period*]. The interval after resuscitation and before the onset of inflammation is generally the most stable period for burn patients. One exception is the patient with a severe inhalation injury, symptoms of which usually become most severe several days after the injury.

Maintenance of Pulmonary Function

ENDOTRACHEAL INTUBATION

Intubation is required for the three Ps:

1. Maintenance of a *patent* airway.
2. *Pulmonary* toilet.
3. *Positive pressure* ventilation.

If edema threatens to compromise airway patency by distortion and compression, intubation is mandatory and should be continued until the upper airway edema begins to resolve, usually between postburn days 2 and 4; elevating the patient's head 30° to 40° allows faster resolution of edema. Oral and facial edema from the burn begins to resolve at this time as well. In the presence of a full-thickness neck burn, tissue edema—including mucosal edema—resolves much more slowly. Positive end-expiratory pressure during this period will help prevent small airway collapse. The injured mucosa is very prone to superinfection because mucosal irritation and increased mucus production persist for several days, whereas clearance is decreased because of the damaged ciliary action of the mucosa. Aggressive mouth care to prevent mucosal infection (particularly with anaerobes) is necessary because aspiration of infected saliva leads to airway infection.

The decision when to extubate is a difficult one because no test of airway patency is foolproof. Laryngoscopy is helpful in that it can determine whether cord edema is present; however, edema of the false cords or the oropharynx, as well as external compression from a neck burn, can impair airway patency even if minimal cord edema is present. As a rule, therefore, extubation should not be performed unless reintubation is technically feasible. If the patient clearly has a severe inhalation injury or a large burn that will necessitate airway protection or ventilatory assistance, a tracheostomy through an unburned or an excised and grafted area of the neck should be done at an early stage (e.g., the first excision and grafting procedure). Percutaneous tracheostomy through unburned skin is an effective approach.

VENTILATION

In the patient without an inhalation injury, lung function during this period is usually surprisingly good if blood volume is not excessively increased. Although massive soft tissue edema is present, lung water measurements are consistently normal or only minimally elevated in both animal and human studies. However, in the presence of inelastic burned tissue and subeschar edema, chest wall compliance may remain significantly decreased. Because the work of breathing is increased, the decreased compliance may result in a diffuse microatelectasis if it is not recognized and aggressively treated.

When initial energy stores are depleted, mechanical ventilatory support may be needed to assist with the increased work load that results from the impaired chest wall function. Although parenchymal pulmonary function may be adequate, it is also important to consider work load and caloric demand before removing ventilatory support. Maintaining the patient in a semierect position improves diaphragmatic function. Oxygen administration to maintain adequate blood oxygen content and tissue oxygen tension is frequently required, for several days at least, after any large burn. Arterial oxygen saturation should be maintained at 90% or greater, preferably with a fraction of inspired oxygen (F_IO_2) of 0.5 or less. In addition, the sequential surgical excisions and wound closure initiated around postburn day 2 or 3 frequently make ventilatory assistance necessary for longer periods because general anesthesia is used every 2 to 3 days and narcotic usage is increased to control postoperative pain, particularly in donor sites. Fluid overload should be carefully avoided to minimize lung dysfunction.

MANAGEMENT OF PULMONARY INJURY

The clearance of soot, mucopurulent exudate, and sloughed mucosa is a major problem during this period, particularly if mucociliary action is impaired by smoke damage. An aggressive surgical approach to the burn wound cannot be undertaken, however, in the absence of good lung function. Airway collapse and atelectasis will result in an increasing shunt and an increasing risk of bronchopneumonia. Bronchodilators, in particular those delivered by aerosol, are very helpful, along with chest physical therapy and frequent repositioning of the patient. Mechanical ventilatory assistance may be necessary in severe cases.

The clinical magnitude of a chemical injury to the smaller airways becomes much more evident during this period. At the very least, mucosal irritation will persist for several days, causing bronchorrhea, increased coughing, and mucus production. Impairment of the ciliary function of the airway lining leads to a high risk of infection, manifested first (in the next 3 to 4 days) by bacterial tracheobronchitis and subsequently by bronchopneumonia. Bacterial colonization is inevitable. When the injury is severe, the damaged mucosa typically becomes necrotic 3 to 4 days after injury and begins to slough. Increased viscous secretions can lead to distal airway obstruction and atelectasis and can place the patient at high risk for rapidly developing bronchopneumonia.

If the chemical burn to the lung occurs in combination with a body burn, the morbidity and mortality of both processes are substantially higher than they would be otherwise.

Diagnosis

In the first several days after injury, soot continues to be present in the airway secretions. Diffuse rhonchi are usually present once inflammation develops. Wheezing often persists as a result of continued bronchospasm and (more frequently) bronchial edema. Continued coughing, as well as the residual airway edema and bronchospasm, increases the work of breathing, which can lead to fatigue and hypoventilation. Secretions then become tenacious and more difficult to clear. In the most severe airway injuries, rales compatible with edema are noted, especially when concomitant volume overload is present. Bacterial tracheobronchitis is common and is followed by bronchopneumonia in a substantial number of patients; the primary pathogen is usually *Staphylococcus aureus.* The symptom complex includes the following: (1) sputum changing from loose to mucopurulent, (2) evidence of necrotic tissue in sputum, (3) increased work of breathing, (4) altered gas exchange, and (5) infiltrates on radiographs (a late finding). The initial presentation is not necessarily an accurate guide to the magnitude of injury: lung function may be deceptively good on day 2, only to deteriorate rapidly on day 3 or 4.

In general, chest radiographs obtained during this period do not reveal the full severity of the lung damage, because the injury usually is initially confined to the airways. Clinical evidence of continued respiratory compromise—dyspnea, tachypnea, diffuse wheezing, and rhonchi—precedes any radiographic changes. The first radiographic indication of lung damage is usually diffuse atelectasis, pulmonary edema, or bronchopneumonia. Parenchymal changes are late findings.

Treatment

Endotracheal intubation may be necessary if clearance of secretions is inadequate. Ventilatory assistance may also be necessary if the patient is fatigued and if gas exchange is deteriorating. Bronchodilators, particularly those delivered by aerosol [*see I:3 Burn Care in the Immediate Resuscitation Period*], are also helpful, as are frequent changes in position to facilitate postural drainage. Continuously rotating beds are ideal for patients with inhalation injury and large body burns, who often find it difficult to move from side to side because of pain and stiffness from tissue edema; the constant postural drainage helps to remove airway plugs.

Infection surveillance is crucial during this early period so that bacterial bronchitis can be detected before pneumonia develops.

Sputum smears should be obtained, and the character of the sputum should be monitored. Systemic antibiotics are not given prophylactically but are administered when a bacterial process becomes evident; it is important not to wait for obvious radiographic evidence of bronchopneumonia, because the process, once well established, is difficult to reverse. Broad-spectrum antibiotics can be used until susceptibility test results become available and a more specific antibiotic regimen can be instituted.

Maintenance of Hemodynamic Stability

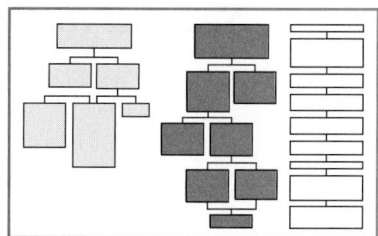

RESTORATION OF BLOOD VOLUME

Although cardiac output may be restored toward normal by fluid resuscitation during the first 24 hours after a burn, blood volume frequently decreases, particularly in the large burn, because of the substantial loss of fluid from the plasma to the interstitial space; edema is maximal at 24 to 36 hours after a burn. Restoration of blood volume is more feasible during the early postresuscitation period. Adequate perfusion pressure must be maintained (i.e., systolic blood pressure greater than 90 mm Hg and urine output 0.5 to 1.0 ml/kg/hr). In the presence of hypovolemia and severe hypoproteinemia (0.5% of normal), plasma protein levels should be restored toward normal to decrease crystalloid needs and to improve gastrointestinal function. Improved gastrointestinal function will be of considerable importance for nutritional support. Protein solutions should be given to replace volume loss [*see I:3 Burn Care in the Immediate Resuscitation Period*]; such solutions should not be administered to patients who are normovolemic or hypervolemic, because volume overload and its complications may result, especially during the fluid mobilization period.

Red blood cells are injured during the burning process and again as a result of the mediator release from burned tissue. Red cell lipid peroxidation is characteristically seen after a burn. The increased fragility leads to a decreased half-life. Red cell hematopoiesis is also markedly impaired. The combination of these processes leads to anemia, beginning during the early postresuscitation period. Red cells should be provided if necessary to maintain a hematocrit of at least 30%, given the increasing oxygen demands in burn patients during this period and the chronic nature of the impaired production.

MAINTENANCE OF FLUID AND ELECTROLYTE BALANCE

A measurable increase in protein permeability in burned tissue vessels persists for days to weeks. The rate of fluid and protein loss into the burned interstitium lessens considerably after the first two postburn days; however, protein loss from the surface of a partial-thickness burn can still be substantial.

After postburn day 2, evaporation from the surface of deep burns becomes a major source of water loss that persists until the wound is closed. Losses are comparable to those expected from an open pan of water with the same surface area. It is possible to calculate a reasonable estimate of water loss from the surface of deep burns [*see Table 1*].

During the early postresuscitation period, however, intravascular fluid is gained from the resorption of edema fluid. Therefore, continued replacement of free water lost from evaporation and of protein lost into burned tissue and from the burned surface must be balanced against these intravascular fluid gains.

Approach to the Burn Patient during the Second to Fifth Days after the Burn

Maintain adequate ventilation

Maintain O_2 sat. > 90%, preferably F_iO_2 < 0.5.

Avoid iatrogenic complications:
- Fluid overload
- Drug-induced hypoventilation

Patient intubated

Maintain ET tube until face, neck, and upper airway edema are adequately resolved.

Assess by laryngoscopy.

Patient not intubated

Continue assessment of airway adequacy for
- Edema
- Secretion clearance
- State of consciousness

No inhalation injury or large chest burn

Extubate when
- Airway edema is resolved
- Patient is alert
- There is no further need for positive airway pressure

Observe closely for pending pulmonary problems:
- Atelectasis
- Fatigue
- Pneumonia

Inhalation injury or large chest burn

Provide positive pressure ventilation as needed.

Remember: Process may worsen during the next 24–48 hr.

Maintain aggressive pulmonary toilet:
- Frequent suctioning
- Position changes
- Bronchodilators

Control infection:
- No prophylactic antibiotics
- Frequent sputum smears and cultures
- Systemic antibiotics with signs of bacterial tracheobronchitis

No inhalation injury or large chest burn

Maintain adequate perfusion

Replace continuing plasma, red blood cell, and evaporative losses.

Maintain
- BP > 90 mm Hg systolic
- Urine output 0.5–1.0 ml/kg/hr
- T° > 37° C

Monitor input and output.

Burns > 20% TBS

Continue I.V. fluid supplementation.

Change fluid to hypotonic salt plus dextrose.

Continue adequate hemodynamic monitoring (BP, pulse, acid-base, urine).

Closely monitor electrolytes, renal function.

Burns < 20% TBS

Can use oral route if patient is extubated, is alert, and has adequate GI function.

Use hemodynamic monitoring as necessary. (The elderly and patients with inhalation injury are at increased risk.)

Patient hemodynamically stable

Watch for ICF to ECF shifts.

Begin nutrition:
- Calories and protein
- Enteral route with peripheral vein supplementation preferred to central line

Patient hemodynamically unstable

Assess for hypervolemia and congestive failure vs. hypovolemia.

Use additional monitoring (e.g., PA catheters) if situation deteriorates.

Hypervolemia or congestive heart failure

Diurese carefully.

Administer inotropes; low-dose dopamine is first choice.

Occasionally, vasodilators are needed; sodium nitroprusside is first choice.

Hypovolemia

Replace blood volume with albumin solution or red blood cells, or both.

Replace evaporative and urine losses with dextrose and hypotonic salt solution.

Consider initiation of nutritional support as soon as feasible

Continue wound management

Control infection

Continue chlorhexidine wash.

Avoid body immersion techniques.

Debride loose eschar.

Use topical antibiotics for deep burns.

Do not give prophylactic systemic antibiotics.

Reassess extent or depth of injury

Look for wound conversion.

Maintain perfusion

Continue elevation of burned extremities.

Consider extending escharotomy if perfusion is impaired.

Avoid excessive heat loss

Maintain warm environment.

Use closed dressings.

Provide adequate pain control

Give premedication, followed by small doses of I.V. narcotics.

Use closed dressings; change twice daily in most areas

Treat infection

Biopsy wound to diagnose infection.

Use systemic antibiotics.

Consider changing topical antibiotic (e.g., to mafenide).

Remove eschar more aggressively.

Close the wound

If burn is not infected, begin wound excision and grafting as soon as patient is hemodynamically stable. Use tangential excision for moderate burns of varying depth; use excision to fascia for large full-thickness burns.

Table 1 Calculation of Evaporative Water Loss and Required Fluid

The patient is a 70 kg male whose burns cover 50% of TBS. His body surface area is 1.7 m².

The patient's output during the previous 24 hours:
Urine: 2,000 ml
Nasogastric tube: pulled

Evaporative water loss (ml/hr) = (25 + % TBS burned) × TBS

In this patient: (25 + 50) × 1.7 = 125 ml/hr
125 ml/hr × 24 hr/day = 3,000 ml/day

Fluid required = evaporative loss + other losses

In this patient: 3,000 ml evaporative loss/day
+ 2,000 ml urine/day

Fluid required = 5,000 ml/day

Give as 5% dextrose in 0.2% normal saline at ~ 200 ml/hr.

The rate of edema absorption depends on the burn depth and subsequent lymphatic damage. It is rapid in superficial burns, beginning at about day 2 or 3 when lymphatics are intact, but much slower after full-thickness injury.

Sodium requirements are usually minimal because of initial sodium loading and because water loss from evaporation is extensive. Therefore, the preferred crystalloid after the resuscitation period is hypotonic salt plus dextrose. Glucose administration is necessary at this point, however, because glycogen stores are totally depleted. Once glucose is administered and tissue utilization improves, large amounts of potassium must be given as well. Potassium administration will be particularly important once nutritional support is initiated because wound healing and new cell formation will increase potassium utilization. Enteral nutrition should begin as soon as the gastric ileus resolves. Nutrition can be supplemented with central or peripheral vein alimentation until the enteral route becomes totally functional [see III:13 Burn Care after the First Postburn Week].

Restoration of blood flow to the burned tissue after resuscitation will result in the resorption of a large load of osmotically active particles made up of solutes from disrupted cells and fragments of denatured proteins. The increased osmotic load is very evident in second-degree burn blisters, which increase dramatically in size and pressure over a period of days. The increased solute load frequently results in an obligate solute diuresis that is manifested by increased output of high–specific gravity urine. It is important that such an increase in urinary output not be mistaken for hypervolemia; therefore, fluids should not be decreased or diuretics initiated. In the diuretic response to hypervolemia, the urine specific gravity is, of course, characteristically low.

TRANSITION FROM HYPOMETABOLISM TO HYPERMETABOLISM

As the hypermetabolic state evolves (beginning at about day 3 or 4), the response of the cardiovascular system changes. Cardiac output begins to increase and exceeds normal values as a hyperdynamic state develops. Mild to modest tachycardia is usually present, partly because of persistently elevated catecholamine levels, which may be even further potentiated by hypothermia, hypoxia, or pain. The tachycardia, however, is usually much less than that seen during the first 24 hours after the burn [see I:3 Burn Care in the Immediate Resuscitation Period]. The early increased systemic vascular resistance (SVR) begins to be replaced by SVR that is lower than normal.

It is important to recognize this transition during the postresuscitation period. The hyperdynamic state is characterized by (1) a 50% to 100% increase in oxygen consumption, (2) a 1° to 2° F rise in body temperature, (3) increased gluconeogenesis, (4) increased secretion of anti-insulin hormones (decreased glucose tolerance), and (5) increased catabolism (increased ureagenesis). The increase in oxygen consumption usually peaks 5 to 10 days after the burn. Body temperature tends to increase further as pyrogen is released from the burn wound. The characteristic rise in body temperature makes it more difficult to diagnose the presence of infection.

The increasing oxygen consumption necessitates increasing oxygen delivery by ensuring adequate blood volume, hematocrit, and oxygen saturation (i.e., lung function and cardiac output must be maintained). Lactic acidosis indicates inadequate oxygen delivery, even if P_aO_2 or oxygen saturation is normal. Oxygen demands are twice normal (100 to 140 ml/min/m² when 50% or more of the total body surface (TBS) has been burned.

Control of Burn Infection

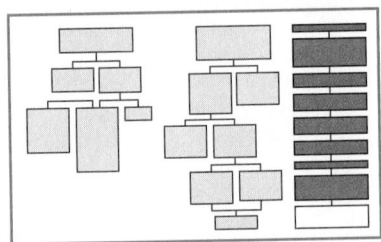

The burn wound is a major site of infection for three reasons: (1) loss of the skin barrier, (2) the presence of dead tissue, and (3) systemic immunosuppression. The stratum corneum is a relatively impermeable barrier to bacterial invasion through the skin. Loss of this barrier as a result of burn injury permits bacteria to populate the underlying tissues. Most of these early colonizing bacteria are endogenous, deriving from heat-injured skin (especially hair follicles, sweat glands, and sebaceous glands), the nares and the oropharynx, the perineum, or stool [see Tables 2 through 4]. The bacteria migrate to the wound by way of wet dressings, immersion in water, hand contact, and, to a lesser extent, aerosolization. The reduced blood flow to the surface of the burn impairs local immune defenses (white blood cells need oxygen to kill bacteria); it also decreases the ability of phagocytes and opsonins to reach the wound. In addition, the wound itself releases a number of immunosuppressive substances that impair both cell-mediated and humoral immunity.

DAILY BURN CARE AND INFECTION CONTROL METHODS

In general, significant bacterial colonization of the burn wound does not occur for several days after injury unless the wound initially is heavily contaminated or inadequately cleaned and treated. The eschar remains intact. Surgical excision of the deep burn is most appropriate during this period because the wound is not yet infected or revascularized [see Wound Closure, below].

Wound conversion is common during this period as injured tissue becomes nonviable. Frequent reassessment of the wound is

Table 2 Organisms Most Commonly Recovered from Burn Wounds in First Week

Organism	% of Patients
Staphylococcus aureus	85
β-Hemolytic streptococcus	5
Pseudomonas aeruginosa	25
Escherichia coli	40
Enterococcus	55
Candida albicans	40

Table 3 Findings Distinguishing Colonization of Burn Wound from Invasive Infection

Findings	Colonization	Invasive Infection
Systemic changes	Variable body temperature	Increased body temperature
	WBC count increased, with mild left shift	WBC count either high or low, with pronounced left shift
	Wound may appear either purulent or benign	Wound may appear purulent, or wound surface may appear dry and pale
Bacterial characteristics	Surface bacterial content ranging from trace to large	Surface bacterial content variable
	Usually < 10^5 bacteria/g tissue on biopsy	Usually > 10^5 bacteria/g tissue on biopsy
	No invasion of normal tissue	Invasion of normal tissue

necessary. In addition, continued edema can still lead to excessive increases in tissue pressure, necessitating additional escharotomies. During this period, burned extremities should remain elevated and active and passive range-of-motion exercises should begin.

Evidence of tissue necrolysis remains absent until neutrophils, bacteria, or both proliferate in the eschar, leading to liberation of proteases and breakdown of tissue. Topical antibiotic therapy rehydrates and softens the eschar more rapidly, thereby allowing inflammatory cells to migrate into the subeschar space. Increased bacterial proliferation is then possible if the amount of topical antibiotic is not sufficient.

The epidemiology of burn wound infection seems to indicate that—in the first week, at least—the primary bacteria present are cutaneous organisms and, to a lesser extent, pulmonary and enteric organisms. This predominance of endogenous bacteria is reflected in the early colonization of the wound by gram-positive bacteria, primarily *S. aureus*, followed in several days by the beginning of gram-negative colonization.

Exogenous bacteria are certainly present in any standard critical care unit; these ordinarily resistant organisms become significant pathogens after the normal flora has been altered by the use of systemic antibiotics. The principal mode of cross-contamination with more resistant strains appears to be direct contact; air is a less significant vehicle. Compulsive hand washing between patient contacts is crucial to minimize this problem. Changes of cap, gown, and mask are also very helpful. Sophisticated isolation techniques (e.g., isolators) are not routinely necessary.

Wound Care

In wounds not amenable to early surgical closure or closure with temporary skin substitutes, daily removal of devitalized tissue, wound exudate, and inactive topical agents is important. A number of approaches are used; the primary objective is to maximize wound cleaning while minimizing patient stress. Hydrotherapy is one approach. Adequate pain control [*see* Stress Control, Analgesia and Sedation, *below*] and adequate safeguards against hypothermia are necessary. It has also become clear that immersion in a hydrotherapy tank can result in significant cross-contamination from perineum to wound or from one burned area to another. Therefore, it is recommended that the patient's head be up on a slanted board or that showers be used so that water runs off the wounds, maximizing mechanical debridement and minimizing stagnation. Another approach, which is very effective, is bedside wound care: each portion of the body is cleaned and rewrapped independently, both to minimize pain and to minimize bacterial cross-contamination. When early excision has been performed, bedside wound care is particularly useful to avoid contamination of clean, grafted wounds and donor sites. In addition, vascular catheters can be protected. A warm environment during burn care, preferably 30° to 35° C (86° to 95° F), is necessary to prevent excessive heat loss when the wound is open. Pyrogen release as a result of wound manipulation can be anticipated. Use of antipyretics before wound care is initiated can significantly attenuate this response.

Topical Antibiotics

Topical antibiotics that are sufficiently water soluble to penetrate the burn eschar will temporarily control bacterial growth in the wound [*see* I:3 Burn Care in the Immediate Resuscitation Period]. Superficial burns do not require topical antibiotics unless they are heavily contaminated—for example, with ground-in dirt. If the burn is extremely deep (i.e., extending into fat or muscle) or clearly infected, mafenide (Sulfamylon) will be more effective in controlling bacterial growth.

Systemic Antibiotics

Systemic antibiotics are used to treat established infection and are not for prophylaxis. Prophylactic antibiotics for small burns

Table 4 Characteristics of Invasive Burn Wound Infection with Specific Etiologic Organisms

Variable	Infecting Organism		
	S. aureus	*P. aeruginosa*	*C. albicans*
Wound appearance	Loss of wound granulation	Surface necrosis; patchy black	Minimal exudate
Clinical course	Slow onset (days)	Rapid onset (hours)	Slow onset (days)
CNS symptoms	Disorientation	Modest changes	Often no change
Temperature	Marked increase	High or low	Modest changes
WBC count	Marked increase	High or low	Modest changes
Blood pressure	Modest decrease	Often severe decrease	Minimal change
Mortality	5%	20% to 30%	30% to 50%

treated on an outpatient basis have also not been shown to be effective in preventing infection. There are only two exceptions. Low-dose penicillin is indicated during the first 24 to 48 hours if the patient is at particular risk for β-hemolytic streptococcus infection; however, this complication is quite uncommon. Systemic antibiotics are also indicated in the 24 to 48 hours before and after burn wound excision to protect against the effects of a transient bacteremia. The agent is selected on the basis of data from the wound culture. The administration of a dose before surgical wound manipulation, followed by continued doses for 24 hours afterward, is common practice.

Systemic antibiotics play no role in treating wound colonization, simply because the agents are incapable of penetrating the nonviable eschar from beneath in sufficient concentration to control bacterial growth. However, if sufficient bacteria ($\geq 10^5$/g eschar) are present in the wound to cause an invasion of underlying viable tissue by breakdown of tissue defense mechanisms, systemic antibiotics are indicated. Values lower than 10^5/g indicate wound colonization that does not require systemic treatment [*see* Table 3]. Diagnosis of infection is difficult to make by wound inspection alone. Full-thickness biopsies of the burn wound with determination of quantitative bacteriology are used to detect infection. However, there is considerable variability in results with this method, particularly if only a superficial biopsy is obtained. Inclusion of viable subeschar tissue is necessary to limit the inaccuracies [*see Sidebar* Technique for Wound Biopsy]. Histologic inspection of the biopsy is a more accurate method for determining tissue invasion.

Wound Closure

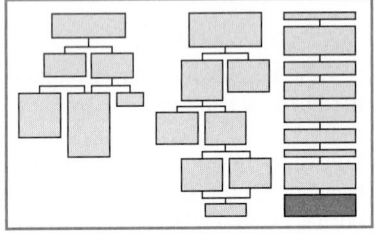

Surgical approaches to the management of large surface burns vary. At one extreme is immediate, complete wound excision to fascia and closure with a combination of autografts and skin substitutes within the first week after the burn. Another method is to initiate sequential excision and graftings, beginning about 2 to 4 days after the burn and continuing every 4 to 5 days until wound closure. The latter appears to be the safer and more common approach.

EARLY EXCISION AND GRAFTING

Risk Assessment

Before the decision is made to proceed with wound excision and grafting, two key judgments must be made:

1. Are the patient's cardiopulmonary status and the operative risk such that the potential benefits of the procedure outweigh the risks?

2. What morbidity may be expected if the wound is not rapidly closed? (This judgment takes into consideration the depth of the wound, the extent of loss of function, and the potential effects of wound inflammation on the host [*see* Table 5].)

General Principles

Four general principles apply to all methods of burn wound excision and grafting.

First, the patient must be hemodynamically stable before excision can be considered. Some degree of pulmonary dysfunction may be expected, but it should not be so severe that the patient cannot be safely moved to the operating room and back.

Second, the potential for significant blood loss must be recognized, and adequate amounts of red cells, plasma, and platelets, if indicated, must be available before treatment is begun. The potential for infection must also be recognized: at this stage, the burn is considered a clean-contaminated wound. Preoperative planning should also include perioperative administration of systemic antibiotics. Given that the initial organisms of concern are gram positive, the drug of choice is usually one of the first-generation cephalosporins.

Third, hypothermia must be avoided. Severe hypothermia is a major hazard in burn patients—particularly if coagulation is crucial, as it is when excision is being done. The operating room temperature should be maintained between 75° and 85° F.

Fourth, the stress induced by anesthesia and the operation must be kept at or below a level that the patient can safely tolerate. Because patients with major burns are potentially highly unstable, the time spent in the operating room should be carefully controlled. A reasonable operating time limit, including anesthesia, is 2 hours—less for elderly or compromised patients. It is better to perform several operations of moderate length at intervals of 1 or 2 days than to perform a single lengthy procedure. Blood loss should be carefully controlled to prevent the development of a coagulopathy: no more than 60% of estimated total blood volume should be lost in the course of any one operation. It is usually possible to stay within this limit, given good timing and careful attention to hemostasis (see below). For large excisions, two operating teams, working simultaneously,

Table 5   Factors Affecting
Burn Wound Morbidity

Infants and the elderly tolerate burn inflammation and infection poorly.

Burns in infants and the elderly are usually deep.

Pulmonary dysfunction from smoke inhalation will be accentuated by burn-induced hypermetabolism, inflammation, and infection.

Burns tend to get deeper over the first several days as a result of necrosis of ischemic areas.

Burns caused by direct contact with flames, hot grease, chemicals, or electricity are invariably deeper than first appearances would suggest.

Burns on the lower back, the scalp, the palms, and the soles usually have sufficient remaining dermis to allow primary healing in 3 to 5 wk.

Small burns—even if they are deep dermal 2° or 3° burns—are not life threatening; therefore, the timing of operation can be much more flexible, depending on the risks to the patient.

Large 3° burns are life threatening until closed.

are required: one is responsible for obtaining the skin grafts and maintaining hemostasis from the donor site, and the other is responsible for excising the wound, maintaining hemostasis, and closing the wound. Any blood lost should be replaced with blood products rather than with crystalloid.

Other issues that must be considered in planning burn wound excision include timing of operation and recovery. Appropriate timing of excision in relation to the changes occurring in the wound itself is crucial for minimizing associated risks. There is a marked increase in blood flow to the burn wound, beginning several days after injury and peaking between days 5 and 14. This increase, which parallels the development of wound inflammation, occurs in the viable tissue beneath the eschar. Excision performed after day 5 or 6 should therefore be expected to cause significantly more blood loss than earlier excision. Any clotting abnormalities present at this stage can thus cause major problems. In addition, the wound undergoes colonization by bacteria during the first week, and manipulation of the wound after this period carries an increased risk of bacteremia.

Types of Surgical Excision

There are two types of surgical procedures for removing eschar: tangential excision and excision to fascia. Each type has advantages and disadvantages [*see Table 6*]. There are also several types of grafts and dressing techniques [*see Grafting, below*].

Tangential (sequential) excision In tangential excision, the wound is excised in thin layers with a blade held at a very acute angle to the skin surface [*see Figure 1*]. The objective is to remove only nonviable tissue while sparing as much viable tissue as possible. This is particularly true with patients who have deep dermal burns, in whom every effort should be made to preserve viable dermis. The dermis is responsible for the elasticity of skin, and it provides an excellent base for grafts. Fat is a less suitable base for skin grafts because of its lesser vascularity and because of the difficulty of determining viable fat on inspection.

Excision is performed with a handheld dermatome to which guards of variable thickness (0.008 to 0.020 in) may be attached. Either a Goulian knife [*see Figure 1*] or a Watson knife is used, depending on the area being excised: the Watson knife, being larger, is used on large, flat surfaces, whereas the Goulian knife is used on curvilinear regions (e.g., bony prominences, fingers, toes, the neck, and, occasionally, the face). Excision over bony surfaces can be facilitated by injecting saline beneath the eschar to flatten the wound and push it away from the bone. For the actual cutting, a back-and-forth motion is used, with very little forward force applied. The depth of the excision is controlled by choosing a guard of the appropriate thickness and by maintaining the blade

at the proper angle to the surface. A sharp blade is needed for this procedure, and frequent blade changes are required.

The end point of excision is brisk punctate bleeding and a completely viable wound base [*see Figure 2*]. Viable dermis is white and shiny; however, one or two large bleeding vessels can make the entire wound look red, which means that careful inspection and considerable experience are needed to assess the adequacy of the wound bed. Nonviable dermis is also white, but punctate bleeding is absent. Nonviable fat is more difficult to recognize because fat often appears to be in better condition than it really is. Healthy fat is light yellow and shiny; any fat that is dark yellow-brown should be removed. It is easy either to underexcise, leaving a poor base for the graft, or to overexcise, thereby removing potentially viable dermis. There is a significant risk of major blood loss, and the procedure must be approached with this risk in mind. Measures must therefore be taken to prepare for the possibility of massive bleeding, and the timing of the procedure must be carefully considered with a view to minimizing this risk [*see General Principles, above*].

Excision to fascia Excision of the burn wound to fascia is appropriate for patients who have very large full-thickness burns or small deep burns that extend well into fat or underlying tissue. This approach is used when the burn is large but only a limited amount of skin is available for grafting. There are three reasons why excision to fascia is suitable for these settings. First, the end point of excision to fascia is well defined, and graft take is always excellent; therefore, less experience is required to define an adequately excised wound surface. Second, wide-mesh grafts can be used because the fascia appears to be less vulnerable to desiccation than fat or dermis is when covered with a skin substitute. Third, when the procedure is performed early, large amounts of most body areas (except for the face and the perineum) can be excised with only modest blood loss. In the case of the small deep wounds, excision to the depth of the fascia or deeper is required because of the extent of the injury itself.

Excision to fascia involves a combination of sharp dissection, constant tension, and electrocauterization; instruments such as those used for tangential excision are not required. The vessels encountered at the fascial plane are less plentiful and larger than those encountered closer to the skin surface and are much easier to control with the electrocautery and ligatures. If the procedure is performed in the first several days after the burn, when the edema fluid separates fascia from overlying subcutaneous tissue, it is actually very easy. Most of the bleeding derives from the wound edge; often, such bleeding can be controlled and exposure of fat on the wound edge minimized if the skin edge is sutured to the fascia. This form of marsupialization may also decrease the total size of the wound as the edges are pulled

Table 6 Advantages and Disadvantages of Tangential Excision and Excision to Fascia

	Advantages	Disadvantages
Tangential excision	Can be performed rapidly Optimal functional and cosmetic results	Substantial blood loss End point of excision difficult to define Greater risk of underexcision or overexcision Greater need for donor skin for coverage
Excision to fascia	Can be performed rapidly, with relatively little loss of blood End point of excision well defined Tourniquets can be used Wide-mesh grafts can be used Excised areas easily covered with skin substitute	Risk of nerve injury Risk of exacerbating distal edema Risk of exposing joints or tendons Potential cosmetic defect

Figure 1 In tangential excision, nonviable tissue is removed in thin layers with a handheld dermatome. Shown at lower right are the components of a Goulian dermatome.

toward the middle. As much as 18% of TBS can be excised with only a 10% to 20% blood loss. Total excision per operation should be limited to 18% to 20% of TBS. Tourniquets may be used when an extremity is being excised to fascia (especially if excision is delayed for several days) because the end point is an anatomic one rather than punctate bleeding (as in tangential excision).

There are a number of disadvantages to this approach that must be carefully weighed against the advantages. The major disadvantage is potential impairment of long-term function of the excised and grafted areas, especially extremities. Removal of superficial veins and lymphatics may result in distal edema; however, in many burn patients, these vessels have already been destroyed by heat. Furthermore, removal of cutaneous nerves leads to impaired sensation in addition to the reduced sensation characteristic of any skin graft in comparison with normal skin, and there is a significant risk of injury to other superficial nerves that have motor function.

The second main disadvantage of fascial excision is cosmetic. A rim of tissue remains at the border between excised and nonexcised tissue and produces a balloonlike effect, especially on the extremities; tapering of the excision at its end points helps minimize this problem. Because fat normally does not regenerate between fascia and skin grafts, the cosmetic defect is persistent, particularly in obese patients. Frequently, fascial excision is combined with tangential excision to maximize the benefits of early wound closure and minimize the complications.

In patients with massive burns, these two disadvantages are outweighed by the excellent graft take and the reliability of the excision end point.

Grafting

Tangential excision Once the wound is excised, the wound bed must be closed. Usually, skin grafts are applied immediately. Meshed skin grafts allow the escape of blood and plasma that would lift a sheet graft off the wound bed. The width of the mesh (e.g., 1.5 to 1 or 3 to 1) depends on the availability of donor skin. Sheet grafts (i.e., nonmeshed grafts) are preferred for the face and

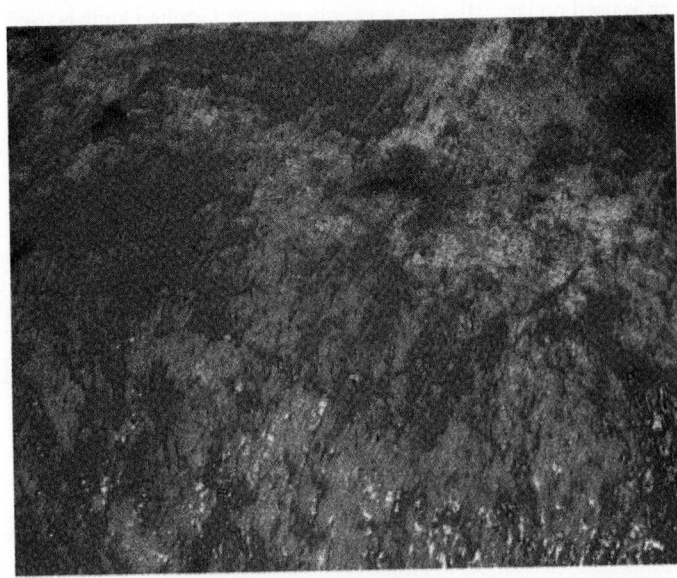

Figure 2 After appropriate tangential excision, brisk punctate bleeding is observed over a completely viable wound base; this is the end point for the procedure.

the hands; however, a 1.5 to 1 mesh opened just slightly for drainage can often be used with excellent cosmetic results. The mesh used for grafting after tangential excision is usually no wider than 1.5 to 1 to prevent excessive exposure of viable tissue (especially fat) so that it does not desiccate and form new eschar [see Figure 3].

Excision to fascia Once excised, the fascial surface must be covered. Given that donor sites are usually limited unless the wound is small, 3 to 1 meshed grafts can be used. Skin substitutes (Biobrane, pigskin, or cadaver skin) are very effective in occluding the fascial wound until the mesh fills in (between days 7 and 10) or until rehealing makes new donor sites available (between days 10 and 14).

Stress Control

The burn itself initiates the stress response to injury, which includes the development of a marked hypermetabolic state. Hypovolemia or tissue hypoxia leads to additional tissue damage, thereby amplifying the host response. Several factors (e.g., pain, anxiety, psychosis, and hypothermia), most of which are largely controllable, further amplify the stress response, exacerbating both physiologic and metabolic abnormalities. All of these factors increase secretion of stress hormones, catecholamines in particular. Psychosis and resulting sleep deprivation also lead to excessive motor activity, further increasing tissue oxygen demand and the risk of oxygen debt.

HEAT LOSS

The loss of the skin barrier increases the rate of heat loss [see I:3 Burn Care in the Immediate Resuscitation Period]. Decreased body temperature is a potent stimulus for catecholamine release. In addition, a core body temperature that falls below what the hypothalamus regards as normal constitutes a strong stimulus for increased heat production (primarily via increased muscle activity).

Heat loss can be controlled by maintaining a warm (30° to 35° C [86° to 95° F]) external environment (e.g., by using radiant overhead heaters), by using occlusive dressings to prevent further convection losses, by minimizing exposure to a wet environment, and by providing adequate oxygen and nutrients. If muscle paralysis proves necessary, the ambient temperature should be further increased, and efforts should be made to achieve additional reduction of heat loss from the wound surface.

HYPERTHERMIA

Severe hyperthermia accentuates the stress response. For every 1° increase in body temperature, oxygen consumption rises by about 5% to 10%. Evaporative water loss increases as well, particularly in patients with large burn wounds. Fluid administration should be stepped up to replace lost water. Nonsteroidal anti-inflammatory drugs may be given; these agents have proved to be very effective in countering hyperthermia in burn patients.

ANALGESIA AND SEDATION

Burn patients experience continuous pain simply from the presence of an open wound. The pain is stimulated by movement and is intensified during dressing changes, debridement, physical therapy, and other burn care–related procedures. Pain increases the stress response and the release of catecholamines, thereby amplifying the hypermetabolic state. The pain-induced increase in sympathetic nervous system activity results in decreased blood flow to skin and soft tissue, which can impair wound healing. Excessive pain also leads to increased release of endogenous

Figure 3 A 1.5 to 1 meshed skin graft has been applied to a tangentially excised wound. Blood and fluid can escape through the interstices of the mesh.

endorphins, which is known to produce both hemodynamic instability and immunosuppression.

Anxiety is also a major problem. Patients suffer from anxiety related to uncertainties about the short- and long-term consequences of their injuries. In addition, many patients experience severe anxiety related to the combination of the stress response and the effects of the ICU environment. There is evidence indicating that the stress response, like pain, leads to increased endorphin release, and it has been well documented that several elements of the ICU environment (e.g., noise, sensory deprivation, and lack of day-to-night cycles) have a major impact on the stress response. Frequent disturbances of sleep patterns may lead to disorientation, greater anxiety, and, eventually, a syndrome loosely described as ICU psychosis. Characteristically, patients with ICU psychosis exhibit a marked increase in muscle activity, which further amplifies the stress response and the hypermetabolic state.

Attempts to control pain and anxiety [see Table 7] are required, as well as increased support during the described maneuvers. Relaxation techniques and hypnosis have advantages over narcotics, which suppress gastrointestinal motility and cause other significant side effects.

For severe burns, I.V. narcotics administered by continuous low-dose infusions or on demand can be quite useful. In addition, sedatives such as diazepam and haloperidol are useful for treating anxiety or psychological aberrations. The addition of sedatives to pain medication or hypnosis, biofeedback, or relaxation techniques is also very useful. For chronic burn pain, give narcotics orally, intramuscularly, or intravenously (either intermittently or via low-dose continuous infusion). In addition, administer sedatives to decrease anxiety.

Table 7 Measures for Controlling Pain and Anxiety in Burn Patients

Patient-controlled analgesia

Continuous regional or intravenous infusion

Early use of benzodiazepines for anxiety and of neuroleptics for ICU psychosis

Avoidance of ICU sensory overload

NUTRITIONAL SUPPORT

Hypermetabolism and nutritional support are discussed in more detail elsewhere [*see III:13 Burn Care after the First Postburn Week and VII:9 Nutritional Support*]. There is, however, one aspect of nutritional management that should be mentioned here— namely, early enteral feeding. Several clinical studies have indicated that initiating enteral feeding soon after the injury (i.e., in the first 48 hours) appears to reduce the degree of subsequent injury-induced hypermetabolism, possibly by preventing early bacterial migration through the gut wall (so-called gut leak). Although the data are not conclusive, it is certainly possible at this point to state that early enteral nutrition is advantageous and that feedings should be started as soon as possible, preferably in the first 48 hours.

GASTRIC pH

Gastrointestinal bleeding from burn stress (i.e., Curling ulcer) was once a major cause of morbidity, but aggressive nutritional support and wound control have decreased this problem. In burn patients as well as in critical care patients in general, maintenance of a gastric pH above 3 has been found to diminish the risk of significant ulceration and bleeding. Scheduled administration of antacids, H_2 receptor blockers, or both can be used to control pH. Continuous tube feeding—or frequent meals, in the absence of a nasogastric tube—is also very effective at decreasing ulceration and maintaining gastric pH at nonulcerogenic levels.

Physical Therapy and Splinting

It is important to maintain as much joint and muscle function as possible during the period of wound closure. If muscle function is not maintained, contraction of the wound by infiltration with myofibroblasts produces permanent impairment of joint motion or a disability requiring extensive reconstructive surgery. Joints must be maintained in the position of function during rest and moved through the limitations of extension, flexion, abduction, and adduction several times a day. Splints are fitted beginning 48 to 72 hours after the burn and refitted as edema resolves.

Recommended Reading

Alexander J: Mechanism of immunologic suppression in burn injury. J Trauma 30:70, 1990

Demling R: Effect of early burn excision and grafting on pulmonary function. J Trauma 24:830, 1984

Desai M, Herdon D, et al: Early burn wound excision significantly reduces blood loss. Ann Surg 211:756, 1990

Dimick P, Heimbach D, Mansen J, et al: Anesthesia assisted procedures in a burn intensive care unit procedure room: benefits and complications. J Burn Care Rehabil 14:446, 1993

Dobke MK, Simoni J, Ninnemann JL, et al: Endotoxemia after burn injury: effect of early excision on circulating endotoxin levels. J Burn Care Rehabil 10:107, 1989

Engrav L, Heimbach D, Reas J, et al: Early excision and grafting vs nonoperative treatment of burns of indeterminate depth. J Trauma 23:1001, 1983

Fuller F, Parrish M, Nance F: A review of dosimetry of silver sulfadiazine cream in burn wound treatment. J Burn Care Rehabil 15:213, 1994

Housinzer T, Lang D, Warden G: A prospective study of blood loss with excisional therapy in pediatric burn patients. J Trauma 34:262, 1993

Hunt J: Is tracheostomy warranted in the burn patient? Indications and complications. J Burn Care Rehabil 7:492, 1986

Lanke K, Liljedahl S: Evaporative water loss from burns, grafts, and donor sites. Scand J Plastic Reconstr Surg 5:17, 1971

Matsumura N, Sugumata A: Aggressive wound closure for elderly patients with burns. J Burn Care Rehabil 15:18, 1994

McDonald W, Deitch E: Immediate enteral feeding in burn patients is safe and effective. Ann Surg 213:177, 1991

Monafo W, Bessey P: Benefits and limitations of burn wound excision. World J Surg 16:37, 1992

Shankowsky H, Callioux L: North American survey of hydrotherapy in modern burn care. J Burn Care Rehabil 15:193, 1994

Acknowledgment

Figure 1   Tom Moore.

13 BURN CARE AFTER THE FIRST POSTBURN WEEK

Robert H. Demling, M.D.

Management of the Burn Patient from 7 Days after the Burn until Complete Wound Closure

Beginning at about postburn day 7, dramatic physiologic and biochemical changes occur, related primarily to the onset of burn wound inflammation. Local and systemic infections also become major factors. The patient with a large burn who was stable during the preceding period frequently becomes unstable again, but the pathophysiologic alterations are much different from those seen during the first postburn week.

Maintenance of Adequate Lung Function

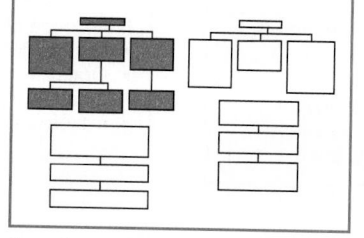

As during the early post-resuscitation period, maintenance of pulmonary function is of major importance. There are two reasons for this: first, oxygen demands and carbon dioxide production are increased, and second, infection risks persist from the immunosuppressed state and from any superimposed smoke damage.

MAINTENANCE OF ADEQUATE ARTERIAL OXYGEN SATURATION

Because oxygen demands nearly double during this period in the patient with a major burn, an arterial oxygen saturation of 95% or greater is preferred, especially if it can be maintained with the fraction of inspired oxygen (F_IO_2) below 0.5, to minimize oxygen toxicity. The shunt fraction therefore must be minimized by maintaining both adequate lung volume and adequate blood volume. Atelectasis from hypoventilation or from secretion-induced obstruction of the small airways must be kept to a minimum.

MAINTENANCE OF ADEQUATE TISSUE OXYGENATION

In burn patients, blood volume, cardiac output, and hemoglobin count must be maintained at levels that optimize oxygen delivery to provide for the increased requirements. Oxygen consumption ($\dot{V}O_2$) increases from the normal value of 125 ml/min/m² to values approaching 300 ml/min/m² in burns exceeding 50% of total body surface (TBS). Pulse rate and cardiac output increase, paralleling the increase in $\dot{V}O_2$. Systemic hypertension is relatively common, as is heart failure, in patients with preexisting cardiac disease, especially the elderly. An obligate urine output of 1 to 2 ml/kg/hr is necessary to remove the increased solute load caused by the hypermetabolic state. Inadequate oxygen delivery is reflected in persistent lactic acidosis or in evidence of early organ failure (in particular, liver dysfunction).

MAINTENANCE OF ADEQUATE MINUTE VENTILATION

The increased carbon dioxide production characteristic of the postburn hypermetabolic state requires a large increase in minute ventilation ($\dot{V}_E$), sometimes twofold or threefold. The increase in $\dot{V}_E$ will depend on how large a portion of the $\dot{V}_E$ is increased dead space ventilation. If excision or grafting is to be performed, the anesthesiologist must be aware that increased ventilation is required to prevent severe hypercapnia.

MECHANICAL VENTILATORY SUPPORT

Frequently, the increased work of breathing necessitates some ventilatory assistance, particularly in the presence of a chest wall burn. Decreased chest wall compliance (in both open and grafted wounds) markedly increases the work necessary to clear the excess carbon dioxide produced. Because oxygen demands are high during this period, mechanical ventilation must be used carefully to allow adequate gas exchange without impeding oxygen delivery. Intermittent mandatory ventilation or, better yet, spontaneous ventilation is preferred to diminish wasted ventilation, provided that adequate energy is available to support the increased work of breathing. In addition, some use of positive end-expiratory pressure (PEEP) may be required to minimize atelectasis. The optimal situation, of course, is adequate spontaneous ventilation, as long as the necessary pulmonary function can be maintained. Any factor that increases carbon dioxide production (e.g., pain, excessive work, or excessive intake of carbohydrate calories) must be controlled.

PULMONARY TOILET

Pneumonia is a major problem during this period, and aggressive maintenance of pulmonary toilet is essential. Among patients in whom the airway mucosal barrier has been injured or actually denuded, pneumonia is particularly frequent and in fact is the major cause of death. The pneumonic process is accentuated by the immunodeficiency state that exists in the presence of the inflamed or infected burn wound.

Careful monitoring of sputum quantity and quality aids in detection of early infection and remains important in preventing the development of a life-threatening pneumonia. In addition, aggressive chest physiotherapy, ambulation, and cough and deep-breathing exercises must be continued until wound closure.

Management of the Burn Patient from 7 Days after the Burn until Complete Wound Closure

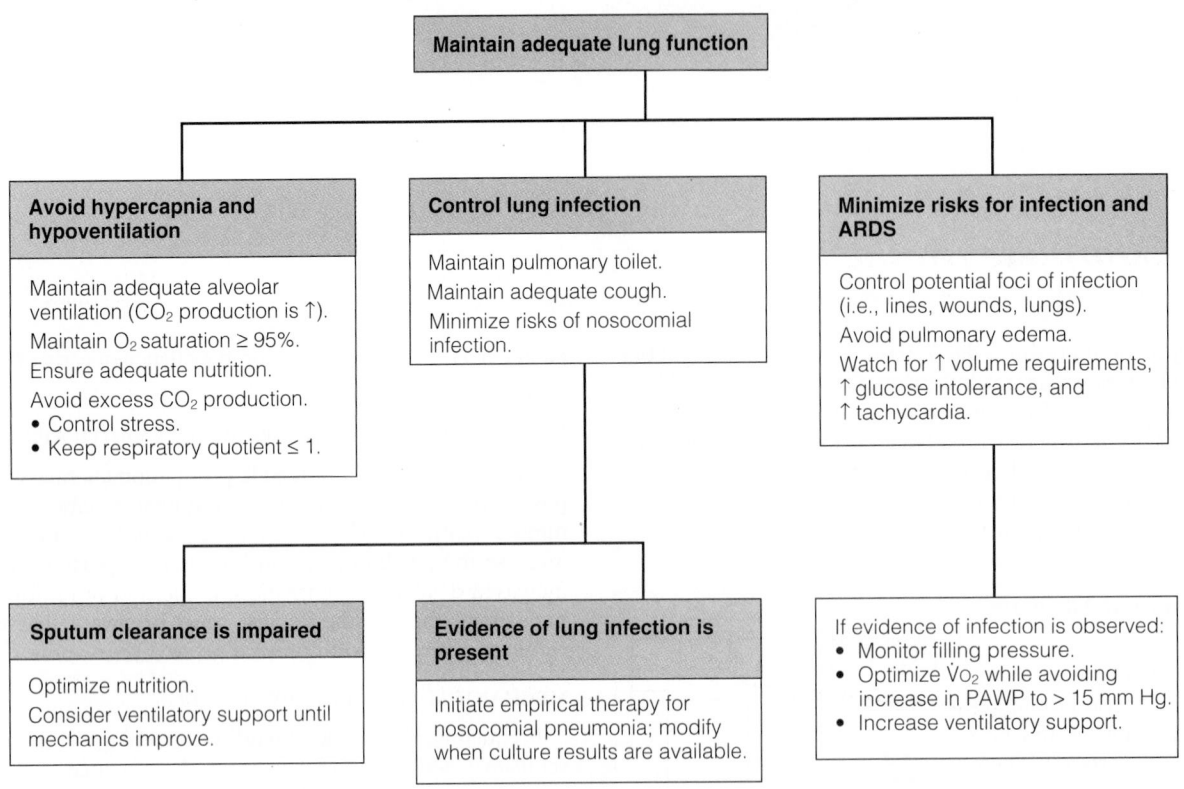

Maintain adequate lung function

Avoid hypercapnia and hypoventilation

Maintain adequate alveolar ventilation (CO_2 production is ↑).
Maintain O_2 saturation ≥ 95%.
Ensure adequate nutrition.
Avoid excess CO_2 production.
• Control stress.
• Keep respiratory quotient ≤ 1.

Control lung infection

Maintain pulmonary toilet.
Maintain adequate cough.
Minimize risks of nosocomial infection.

Minimize risks for infection and ARDS

Control potential foci of infection (i.e., lines, wounds, lungs).
Avoid pulmonary edema.
Watch for ↑ volume requirements, ↑ glucose intolerance, and ↑ tachycardia.

Sputum clearance is impaired

Optimize nutrition.
Consider ventilatory support until mechanics improve.

Evidence of lung infection is present

Initiate empirical therapy for nosocomial pneumonia; modify when culture results are available.

If evidence of infection is observed:
• Monitor filling pressure.
• Optimize $\dot{V}o_2$ while avoiding increase in PAWP to > 15 mm Hg.
• Increase ventilatory support.

Maintain adequate nutritional support

Determine total calories required:
• For burn 20%–40% TBS, 30–35 cal/kg/day.
• For burn ≥ 50% TBS, 35–45 cal/kg/day .
Determine protein requirements:
• Establish calorie-to-nitrogen ratio between 100:1 and 150:1.
Replace lost vitamins and trace elements (e.g., vitamin A, vitamin C, and zinc).

Establish appropriate nutrient mix

Of nonprotein calories, give 70% as carbohydrate.
Of final diet, give 55%–60% as carbohydrate, 20%–25% as fat, 20% as protein.

Select appropriate route

Enteral route is preferred, supplemented by parenteral route as needed.
Consider peripheral vein alimentation with increased water needs.

Maintain hemodynamic stability

Replace lost fluids and electrolytes

Estimate evaporative losses (monitor body weight, urine specific gravity, serum osmolarity, and clinical signs of hydration status).

Replenish evaporative losses: ml/hr = (25 + %TBS burn) × m^2.

Replace lost RBCs and protein.

Monitor electrolyte levels (particularly with nutritional support).

Maintain tissue perfusion

O_2 consumption is 1.5–2 times normal.

Maintain cardiac output at 1.5–2 times normal.

Maintain hematocrit ≥ 30.

Avoid lactic acidosis.

Control stress response

Control the three components of the stress response: (1) systemic inflammation (afferent arc), (2) release of stress hormones (efferent arc), and (3) CNS stimuli such as pain and anxiety (CNS modulation).

Avoid hypothermia:
- Maintain ambient T° ≥ 85° F.
- Minimize heat loss from wound exposure or wet dressings.

Sufficient pain control is essential.

Ensure sufficient sedation to allow for adequate rest.

Burn wound care

Gently debride wound daily.

Graft on clean granulation tissue, if wound is heavily colonized.

Excision should be done cautiously during this period because of increased risks of infection and blood loss.

Control wound infection

Control wound surface bacteria with topical antibiotics.

Treat wound infection with systemic antibiotics.

Monitor plasma levels of antibiotics.

Initiate rehabilitation

Begin and continue joint motion early.

Maintain aggressive muscle-strengthening efforts.

Mobilization should be early and continued.

Apply pressure garments (25 mm Hg) to healed wound.

Use skin moisturizers liberally.

TRACHEOSTOMY

Burn patients are at high risk for lung dysfunction, much of which can be prevented if direct access to excessive secretions can be obtained, the risk of aspirating infected oral secretions can be decreased, and patients can be intermittently rested with partial mechanical support so that the cough reflex can be maintained. A good way of achieving these objectives—given that the time course for correction of a large burn wound or a severe smoke inhalation injury is weeks rather than days—is to perform a tracheostomy. The timing of tracheostomy remains somewhat controversial; however, a tracheostomy through unburned or grafted skin should be considered appropriate if the patient is expected to require an artificial airway for several weeks. Improved pulmonary toilet, enhanced patient comfort, and the elimination of the need for frequent reintubation are all assets. If the high-risk period is short, the burn relatively small, and the patient relatively young, then weaning and extubation are appropriate.

MANAGEMENT OF PULMONARY DYSFUNCTION

Pulmonary problems remain a major cause of morbidity and mortality after the first postburn week. In fact, pulmonary failure and pulmonary infection exceed burn wound infection as causes of death in burn patients. Three major processes occur during this period: (1) nosocomial pneumonia, (2) hypermetabolism-induced respiratory fatigue (power failure), and (3) acute respiratory distress syndrome (ARDS), including low-pressure pulmonary edema. These three processes are closely interrelated. Burn patients are highly vulnerable to infection, particularly after inhalation injury. The hypermetabolic state produces a marked elevation in oxygen requirements and carbon dioxide production; the increased demands placed on the lung as a result may exceed pulmonary functional capacity. ARDS is a severe complication of the septic response; it is very difficult to reverse in burn patients.

Nosocomial Pneumonia

The term nosocomial pneumonia refers to a pneumonia that develops in the hospital in a patient who showed no evidence of lung infection on admission (i.e., to a hospital-acquired pneumonia). Although wound infection, another form of hospital-acquired infection, is more common than nosocomial infection, the latter carries a much higher mortality. Burn patients who have both inhalation injury and a major body burn are at highest risk for nosocomial pneumonia, with the incidence in this population exceeding 50%. This high incidence is attributable to the presence of virulent organisms in the hospital environment and to the immunosuppressed state of burn patients. Once pneumonia is established in a burn patient, it is very difficult to eradicate; consequently, prevention is of primary importance. Preventive measures fall into four main categories: (1) improving systemic host defenses, (2) improving local pulmonary defenses, (3) minimizing oropharyngeal colonization, and (4) minimizing tracheobronchial aspiration [see VI:13 Early Postoperative Pneumonia].

Hypermetabolism-Induced Respiratory Fatigue (Power Failure)

Several processes may impair oxygenation during this period. The severe catabolism initiated by the inflammatory response can lead not only to extremity weakness but also to chest wall muscle weakness. Chronic pain and anxiety can lead to sleep deprivation and fatigue. Heart failure can lead to lung edema, and growing fatigue can lead to hypoventilation-induced atelectasis. As a rule, however, the major problem during this period is not hypoxemia but hypercapnia. Removal of carbon dioxide is directly dependent on alveolar minute ventilation: if carbon dioxide production doubles, alveolar ventilation must also double to maintain normal arterial oxygen tension (P_aO_2). Increased ventilation means increased work of breathing, especially if compliance is decreased or dead space is increased. Large tidal volumes are necessary to maintain adequate alveolar ventilation because small tidal volumes ventilate little more than dead space. Larger tidal volumes call for greater inspiratory force, and the increased work of breathing must be sustained 24 hours a day. Fatigue may then result in impaired clearance of secretions, which can lead to nosocomial pneumonia (see above) as well as hypercapnia.

Serial measurements of tidal volume, vital capacity, and inspiratory force allow one to detect early deterioration of pulmonary function. Measurement of carbon dioxide production allows one to determine whether production exceeds the value predicted on the basis of the burn size alone. Oxygen consumption can also be measured directly by means of either spirometry or the Fick method, and the respiratory quotient can then be calculated directly [see VII:4 Use of the Mechanical Ventilator].

Acute Respiratory Distress Syndrome

ARDS is the name given to the clinical manifestations of a number of indirect lung injury states that are characterized by dyspnea, severe hypoxemia, and decreased lung compliance accompanied by radiographic evidence of diffuse bilateral pulmonary infiltrates. Alveolar consolidation with fluid, protein, and inflammatory cells in the presence of normal pulmonary arterial wedge pressure (PAWP) (i.e., low-pressure pulmonary edema) is also a characteristic finding. Altered permeability results in rapid movement of fluid from plasma to the interstitial space without any increase in PAWP.

ARDS caused by burn inflammation and infection carries an extremely high mortality. The major reason why this is so is that the condition will not resolve until the initiating process is removed. Unfortunately, at this point in the postburn period, burn wounds—especially large ones—cannot be readily excised and closed, because of the increased vascularity of the wound, the presence of colonization or infection, and the further debilitation of the patient. Consequently, efforts must be made to prevent ARDS through early removal of as much of the burn wound (which is a potential source of a systemic inflammatory response) as is feasible [see VII:3 Pulmonary Dysfunction].

Maintenance of Hemodynamic Stability

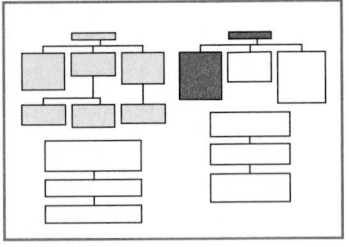

MAINTENANCE OF ADEQUATE HYDRATION

Evaporative loss is greatest from granulation tissue (with its increased blood supply) and least from a third-degree burn (with its thick eschar). Unhealed donor sites must also be considered in the estimation of evaporative loss. In addition, the increased body temperature characteristic of this period increases evaporative loss. Grafted skin restores much of the barrier, but losses may still be greater than evaporation across normal skin until the graft matures. Estimation of these losses depends on close monitoring of body weight, urine specific gravity, serum osmolarity, and clinical signs of hydration status [see III:12 Burn Care in the Early Postresuscitation Period]. Serum sodium is a helpful indicator of the state of hydration. If the value is elevated, more water should be given.

RESTORATION AND MAINTENANCE OF PERFUSION

The Hyperdynamic State

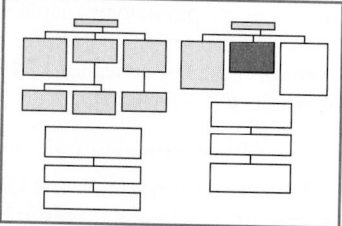

A hyperdynamic state evolves in the postresuscitation period as part of the response to burn injury, peaking about the end of the first postburn week. The degree of hyperdynamism appears to correlate with the degree of initial tissue injury as well as with the degree of initial damage to organs (especially the lungs). The hyperdynamic state is the result of systemic inflammation and the altered hormonal environment: the tissue injury and the secondary inflammatory response it evokes result in increased oxygen demands. Generally, patients remain hemodynamically stable in the postresuscitation period unless volume replenishment is inadequate; however, varying degrees of instability may occur. Physiologic responses range from normal to grossly abnormal or, more specifically, from simple hyperdynamism to the systemic inflammatory response syndrome (SIRS) to septic shock to, finally, the multiple organ dysfunction syndrome (MODS).

It is clear that burn patients who can spontaneously generate a hyperdynamic state in response to injury are capable of supplying enough oxygen to keep up with the increased metabolic demands reflected in increased oxygen consumption. It is also clear that mortality is lower in these patients than in patients who have an oxygen debt. It remains unclear, however, whether patients who cannot spontaneously generate a hyperdynamic response should be artificially maintained in a hyperdynamic state with volume expansion and inotropes, which patients should be so maintained, and what degree of artificial hyperdynamism would be appropriate.

Unfortunately, because of certain direct cellular metabolic changes, lactate concentration is a less sensitive indicator of impaired perfusion in this period than it was in the initial postburn period. Increased quantities of pyruvate are present as a result of the increased glucose utilization. Increased lactate may simply reflect decreased pyruvate utilization. A more reliable indicator of excessive lactate is the lactate-pyruvate ratio. An increase in this ratio would indicate excessive lactate and impaired perfusion. Mixed (or central) venous oxygen saturation may be a less useful monitoring parameter because of inflammation-induced maldistribution of blood flow, which lowers the extraction ratio. Logically, it would appear that maintaining high values for certain physiologic variables might help prevent MODS [see Table 1]; however, this approach has not yet been unequivocally shown to decrease the incidence of MODS during the early stress response.

When bacteria or their by-products are present, a further amplification of the hyperdynamic state occurs, accompanied by increased inflammation; clinical infection may or may not be present. This symptom complex has traditionally been referred to as

sepsis but currently is often referred to as SIRS [see Table 2]. The hyperdynamic state persists, but a degree of hemodynamic instability is now present, necessitating both increased fluid infusion and the administration of inotropes to maintain adequate oxygen delivery and perfusion pressure. Cardiac output remains 1.5 to 2.0 times normal, but vascular pressures decrease gradually as a result of a marked downregulation of both alpha and beta agonists by inflammatory mediators, which leads to hypotension and impaired cardiac function.

A modest lactic acidosis may also be present. If the impairment of blood flow is not corrected, the decreased perfusion leads to damage to vital organs. Neurologic changes (usually increased lethargy or confusion attributable to by-products of the metabolic changes) are also evident. As the hemodynamic changes progress, the hyperdynamic state can actually develop into a hypodynamic state.

Methods for Restoring and Maintaining Perfusion

If the patient is incapable of spontaneously increasing oxygen delivery to meet the increased oxygen demands, one may attempt to improve perfusion using the following approaches.

Volume expansion   Volume expansion is the initial treatment of choice for restoring perfusion in the hypermetabolic burn patient. This primarily involves raising filling pressure to increase cardiac output as well as to reopen underperfused microcirculatory beds. The specific role of colloids in restoring volume remains unclear; however, it seems reasonable to use them to supplement crystalloids. Albumin has a number of important properties in addition to its ability to maintain plasma colloid oncotic pressure, including antioxidant activity and the ability to bind free fatty acids, oxidants, and endotoxin.

Administration of inotropes   Because renal and splanchnic perfusion are often decreased even when overall perfusion appears to be adequate, low-dose dopamine (1 to 3 μg/kg/min) is appropriate for maintaining urine output. Medium-dose dopamine ($\geq$ 4 μg/kg/min) is appropriate for raising the cardiac index when PAWP is normal (14 to 16 mm Hg), and dobutamine

---

Table 1   Physiologic Values to Be Maintained during the Stress Response to Major Burn Injury

Cardiac index > 4 L/min/m²
PAWP 12–16 mm Hg (may have to be as high as 18 mm Hg)
Oxygen delivery 1.5 times normal
Oxygen consumption approximately 1.5 times normal
Normal anion gap (8–12 mEq/L)

Table 2   Unstable Hyperdynamism: Systemic Inflammatory Response Syndrome

Clinical and laboratory findings
   Increased temperature, chills
   Warm, dry skin
   Tachycardia, tachypnea
   Blood pressure: usually decreased
   Mental changes
   Urine changes: variable

Laboratory findings
   White blood cell count: increased
   Metabolic acidosis
   Lactate concentration: 1.5–2.0 mmol/L

Physiologic changes
   Increased O₂ consumption, CO₂ production
   Arterial-venous oxygen difference: normal to low
   PAWP: normal to low
   Cardiac output: increased
   Systemic vascular resistance: decreased
   Local microvascular damage

(usually 5 to 10 μg/kg/min), a nearly pure beta agonist, is used when PAWP is elevated (> 16 mm Hg).

Blood transfusion The ideal hemoglobin concentration for restoring perfusion in the hypermetabolic burn patient remains undefined. It is certain that in previously healthy young patients whose condition is stable, 8 g/dl is adequate. In severely burned patients who have MODS to any degree, on the other hand, a value of 10 g/dl is probably a more appropriate goal, especially in view of the impaired ability of critically ill patients to make new red blood cells.

Patients with Established MODS

In patients with established MODS, it is difficult to improve metabolic function simply by increasing oxygen delivery; inotropes are also often ineffective in these individuals. To date, it has not been documented that maintaining a hyperdynamic state by itself has any beneficial effect on survival once secondary MODS is established; it appears that the stress response–induced metabolic abnormalities must also be minimized for outcome to be improved.

CONTROL OF THE SYSTEMIC STRESS RESPONSE

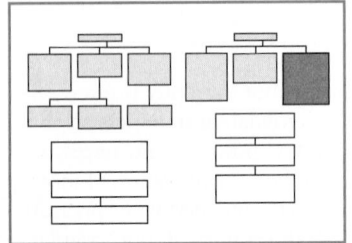

The initial burn insult provokes a reaction on the part of the host. This reaction may be considered a protective mechanism; however, it can in fact produce more injury than the initial insult itself. The components of the stress response are (1) an afferent arc, that is, the inflammatory response; (2) an efferent arc, that is, the release of so-called stress hormones; and (3) a CNS modulation that accentuates the efferent arc, that is, the generation of stimuli such as pain, anxiety, and stress-induced psychosis. The patient's natural response to injury is inflammation, both local and systemic.

Although the physiologic manifestations of the stress response are most evident several days after the injury, cellular biochemical changes caused by activation of this response can be seen very early after injury [*see Figure 1*].

The Afferent Arc: The Inflammatory Response

It has long been known that local inflammation occurs in burn-injured tissue within minutes to hours after injury; it has now also been documented that generalized inflammation also occurs. It is becoming increasingly clear that any severe local tissue trauma can give rise to a massive systemic inflammatory response. Large amounts of cytokines are released soon after major trauma, and inflammatory cells can be found sequestered in the microcirculation in virtually all organs immediately after severe trauma or burn injury. This generalized response appears to be attributable to the systemic activation of a number of inflammatory cascades, including intravascular complement activation. Animal and human studies have found evidence of early tissue oxidant changes, as reflected in elevated levels of circulating lipid peroxides and increased tissue lipid peroxidation.

The inflammatory cell sequestration and adherence to endothelial cells observed initially do not necessarily lead to injury if the inflammatory cells are only primed and not activated. Neutrophils often undergo systemic activation if ischemic or devitalized tissue is not removed or if there is a second insult. Although inflammation begins immediately after injury, physiologic evidence of the systemic response usually is not apparent for several days. The continued presence of devitalized tissue primes the host for a subsequent insult. In addition, the response to any subsequent insult (e.g., endotoxin, vascular catheter bacteremia, or pancreatitis) is amplified, leading to far more tissue damage and hemodynamic instability than would have been expected to result from the same insult in the absence of previous injury or infection.

The observation of this exaggerated response to even modest infection or ischemia on the part of the injured patient has given rise to the so-called two-hit theory of MODS [*see Figure 2*]. The

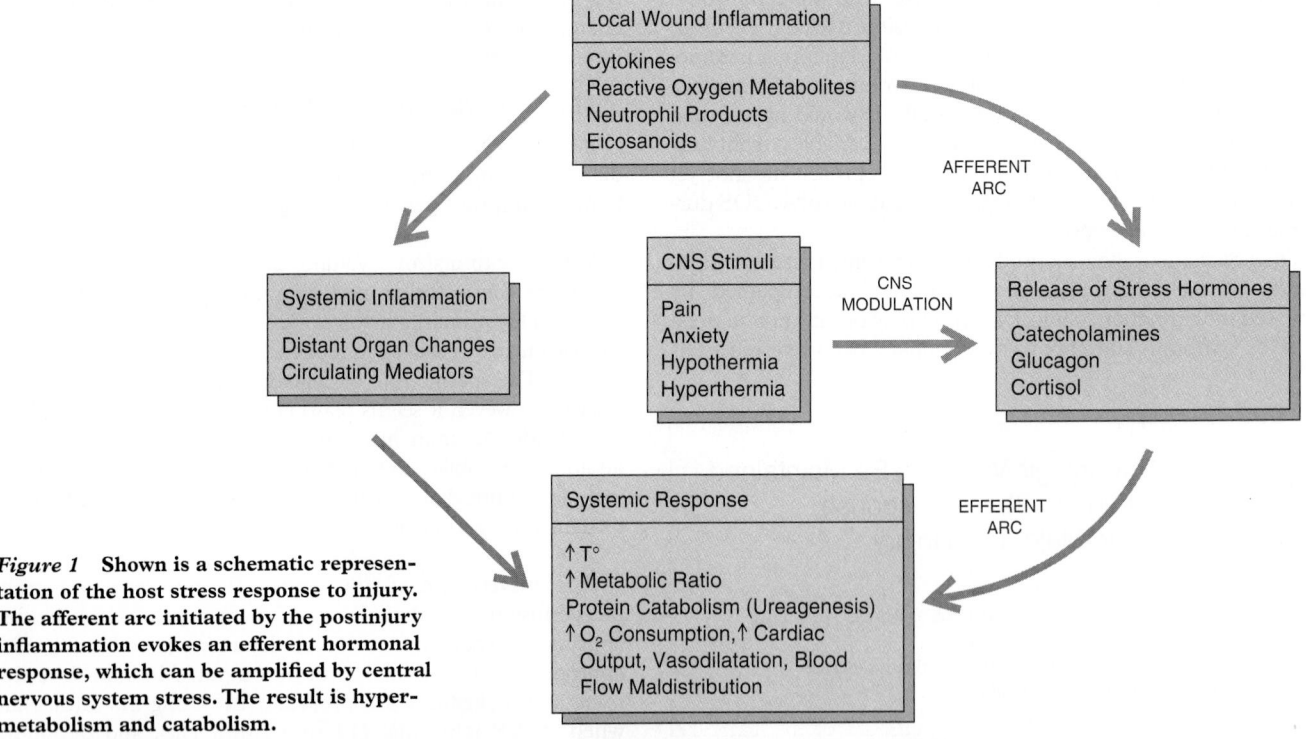

Figure 1 Shown is a schematic representation of the host stress response to injury. The afferent arc initiated by the postinjury inflammation evokes an efferent hormonal response, which can be amplified by central nervous system stress. The result is hypermetabolism and catabolism.

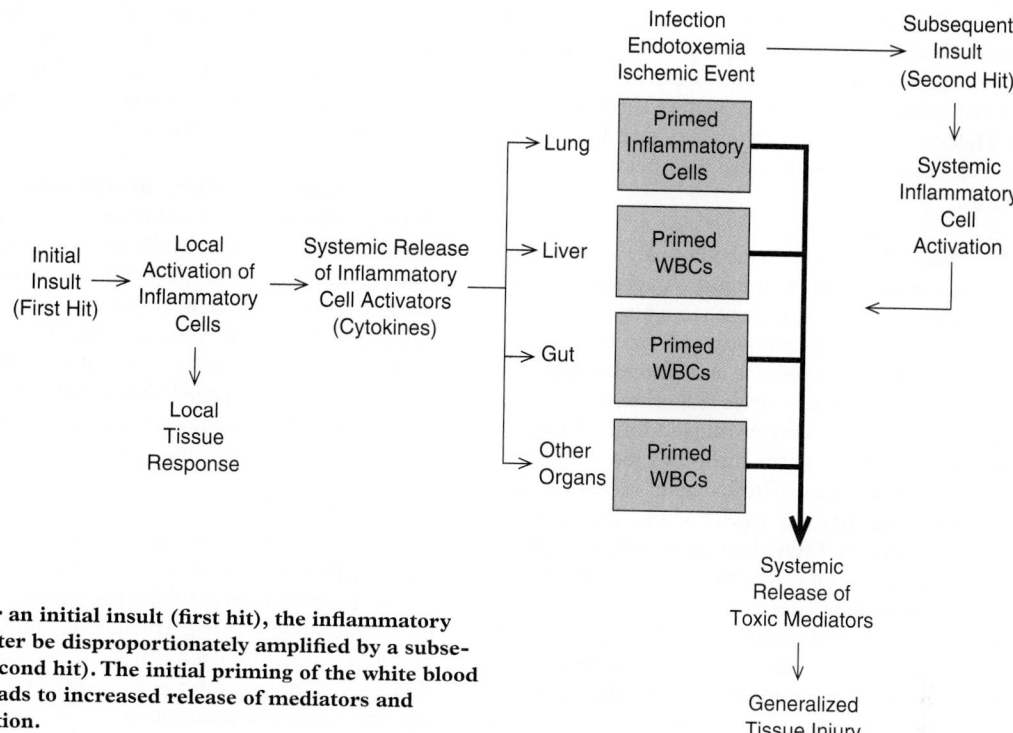

Figure 2 **After an initial insult (first hit), the inflammatory response can later be disproportionately amplified by a subsequent insult (second hit). The initial priming of the white blood cells (WBCs) leads to increased release of mediators and systemic activation.**

initial burn or smoke inhalation injury—the first hit—induces the inflammatory cells to turn on their metabolic machinery; this process usually is not clinically apparent. A subsequent insult—the second hit—causes the mediator factories to synthesize and release larger quantities of toxic compounds than the degree of the second insult would normally call for; these mediators then produce hemodynamic instability and tissue injury. The most prominent mediators of the stress response are the cytokines. These agents activate the inflammatory process and trigger the release of counterregulatory hormones and other potent vasoactive and cytotoxic mediators.

Cytokines are involved in a number of major responses to injury and infection, including hemodynamic changes, tissue inflammation, wound healing, immune defenses, hypermetabolism, and catabolism. Sustained increases in the activity of some of these agents—tumor necrosis factor (TNF) in particular—are thought to be responsible for the organ dysfunction associated with a persistent, progressive inflammatory response. The major cytokines that play a role in the inflammatory response to injury and infection are TNF, interleukin-1 (IL-1), IL-2, IL-6, and interferon gamma.

Endotoxin Endotoxin is a well-known initiator of inflammation and inflammation-induced disease. It activates the release of a number of mediators, including eicosanoids, oxidants, and cytokines (especially TNF). It also leads to generalized immunosuppression, although the mechanism by which it does so remains undefined.

Endotoxemia is considered to play a major role in the postinjury stress response, even when no obvious source of infection is present. In the absence of clinical infection, endotoxin may be absorbed into the circulation from a colonized wound surface or from a leaky GI tract.

Reactive oxygen metabolites Oxygen radicals are unstable metabolites of oxygen that have an unpaired electron in their outer shell and consequently are potent oxidizing agents; two examples are the superoxide anion ($O_2^{\cdot}$) and the hydroxyl

anion ($OH\cdot$). There are other toxic oxygen metabolites that, though not true free radicals, are nonetheless potent oxidants; one example is hydrogen peroxide (H_2O_2). Oxidants are now considered to be involved in several aspects of the response to burn injury and inflammation [*see Table 3*]. Studies have shown that the systemic inflammatory response seen after severe burns is attributable to systemic activation of complement by $OH\cdot$. Toxic oxygen metabolites also cause lipid peroxidation in the lungs, liver, kidneys, and other tissues in the early postburn period. Elevated circulating levels of lipid peroxides have been documented in patients who are injured or infected. This early postinjury lipid peroxidation may not result in immediate organ dysfunction, but it may help amplify the response to a second insult by causing the release of more inflammatory cytokines. Tissues injured by oxidants and proteases are much more vulnerable to further injury by a subsequent insult. The degree of oxidant damage is closely correlated with the adequacy of antioxidant defenses. After the process of inflammation and infection is under way, oxygen metabolites are again involved in tissue injury; during this phase, the primary oxidant source is activated white blood cells, with endotoxin playing a major role in the release of these substances.

Table 3 Effects of Reactive Oxygen Metabolites

Alteration of vascular permeability
Lipid peroxidation, altering function
Initiation and perpetuation of local and systemic inflammation
Disruption of interstitial matrix
Impairment of macrophage phagocytosis
Alteration of cellular DNA
Initiation of arachidonic acid metabolism
Red blood cell hemolysis

At present, a number of antioxidants normally present in tissues (e.g., vitamin C, vitamin E, catalase, superoxide dismutase, and glutathione or its substrate, glutamine) are available for clinical use. Other oxidants (e.g., xanthine oxidase inhibitors, iron chelators, and 21-aminosteroids, a new class of agents with iron chelating and antioxidant properties) are also being developed for use in humans.

Eicosanoids Arachidonic acid metabolites play a role in both the early and the late response to burn injury. Arachidonic acid is released from the cell membrane in response to injury or infection. It is metabolized via two enzymatic pathways: (1) the cyclooxygenase pathway, which yields prostaglandins and thromboxanes, and (2) the lipoxygenase pathway, which yields leukotrienes.

After a burn, both the vasodilator prostaglandin I_2 (PGI_2), or prostacyclin, and the vasoconstrictor thromboxane A_2 (TXA_2) are released in great quantities. Prostacyclin increases local blood flow, thereby accentuating mediator-induced vascular leakage. The local increase in TXA_2 increases platelet aggregation and neutrophil margination in the wound microcirculation, thereby also potentiating tissue ischemia.

CNS production of prostaglandin E is thought to be the cause of the fever associated with the stress response. The characteristic maldistribution of blood flow observed in marked systemic inflammation appears to be related to excessive production of TXA_2 or PGI_2 in various vascular beds.

The Efferent Arc: Release of Stress Hormones

Certain characteristic hormonal alterations take place during the stress response to burn injury. There is an early increase in circulating catecholamine levels, and this increase produces the peripheral vasoconstriction, anxiety, and tachycardia observed in the early postburn period. Catecholamine levels appear to correlate directly with the degree of injury. The sympathetic adrenal response—namely, increased alpha$_1$- and beta$_1$-receptor activity—appears to correlate with the degree of subsequent hypermetabolism and increased oxygen demands. Beta-receptor activity predominates in the hyperdynamic state. The increased sympathetic activity generally persists throughout the period of critical illness.

Cortisol and glucagon levels are also increased during critical illness. Both of these agents are considered anti-insulin hormones because they promote gluconeogenesis and glycogenolysis. Cortisol also promotes catabolism.

Insulin not only increases glycogen production and is essential for glucose utilization at the cell level but also is a potent anabolic hormone that facilitates the incorporation of amino acids into protein. Insulin administration improves both glucose utilization and protein synthesis.

Human growth hormone is the most potent anabolic hormone. It induces marked increases in protein synthesis and gluconeogenesis; in addition, unlike insulin, it causes lipolysis and increased utilization of ketone bodies for fuel, sparing skeletal muscle and decreasing the catabolic response to stress. Growth hormone levels typically are lower than normal in the catabolic phase of severe injury.

Metabolic alterations Significant alterations in normal metabolic activity are observed in patients with SIRS [see Table 4]. In addition to increases in circulating levels of inflammatory mediators (particularly macrophage-derived products), there are large, sustained increases in levels of anti-insulin hormones and catabolic hormones (e.g., catecholamines, cortisol, and glucagon). Although insulin levels are increased as well, insulin activity appears to be outweighed by the anti-insulin

activity of the catabolic hormones. In hypermetabolic patients, calorie requirements are 50% to 100% higher than normal. Because of the altered metabolism, the compensatory mechanisms normally triggered by starvation are absent, and nutrient utilization is substantially affected.

Acute-phase protein production Hepatic protein synthesis is reprioritized. Production of acute-phase proteins is increased, and production of albumin synthetase is decreased. Acute-phase proteins, which have immunoprotective properties, are released from the liver in response to burn injury, severe smoke inhalation injury, or systemic infection; the specific stimulus appears to be the elevated levels of cytokines (IL-6 and IL-1).

Each acute-phase protein has a characteristic function and duration of action. The downregulation of albumin production results in a hypoalbuminemic state that persists throughout the stress response.

CNS Modulation

The CNS significantly affects the efferent response to a burn. Increased CNS stimulation deriving from pain, anxiety, hypothermia, or hyperthermia amplifies the release of catecholamines, thereby accentuating the hypermetabolic state. Occasionally, patients manifest a stress-induced psychosis, which leads to sleep deprivation and excessive motor activity, thereby further increasing oxygen and nutrient consumption.

Methods for Controlling the Stress Response

Removing the inflammatory focus It is critical to remove deep burned tissue as soon as possible. The objective is to remove a potential inflammatory focus before the host stress response takes hold. Once the hyperdynamic state is clinically present, inflammation is already well established. According to current protocols for preventing secondary MODS, devitalized tissue should be removed even if the patient still appears to be stable.

Modulating release of stress hormones It is essential to minimize the likelihood of further stimuli that will amplify the release of stress hormones, especially catecholamines. Infection must of course be controlled, and further ischemic insults must be avoided (see below). Hypothermia usually is readily controlled. To prevent excessive heat loss during care of the burn wounds, the ambient temperature must be maintained at 30° to 35° C (86° to 95° F). Mild hyperthermia generally is not a major problem, but if body temperature exceeds 103° F, deleterious side effects can result.

Pain control helps prevent excessive release of catecholamines in patients at risk for organ dysfunction. Optimum pain control usually cannot be achieved during initial resuscitation, while patients are still hypovolemic; it is possible only when hemodynamic

---

Table 4 **Major Metabolic Abnormalities with Response to Injury**

Sustained increase in body temperature

Marked increase in glucose demand and therefore strong stimulation of liver gluconeogenesis

Rapid skeletal muscle breakdown caused by demand for amino acid substrate for use as a direct energy source, for gluconeogenesis, and for hepatic acute-phase protein production

Stimulation of the liver to produce large quantities of acute-phase proteins

Absence of ketosis, indicating that fat is not the major calorie source

Unresponsiveness of the rate of gluconeogenesis and catabolism to substrate stability is restored. Patients require larger and more frequent doses of pain medication after the first postburn week because during this period, they experience increasing tolerance to analgesic agents as a result of long-term use and the increasing pain of the debriding wound [*see I:3 Burn Care in the Immediate Resuscitation Period and III:12 Burn Care in the Early Postresuscitation Period*]. Self-administration has been found to be quite useful because the patient's perception of the pain is more accurate than that of the care providers. During the postresuscitation period, high-risk patients should receive continuous epidural analgesia or continuous low-dose narcotic infusion to minimize stress.

Anxiety control is crucial. Close attention must be paid to supporting the neuropsychological status of the patient, especially in the presence of organ dysfunction and SIRS. Adequate sleep periods and the avoidance of sensory overload are essential, especially in the ICU. Administration of benzodiazepines, either intermittently or by continuous infusion, can effectively attenuate anxiety-induced stress. The ICU psychosis syndrome [*see III:12 Burn Care in the Early Postresuscitation Period*] usually must be treated by means of a neuroleptic agent, such as chlorpromazine or haloperidol.

Counteracting or augmenting stress hormone activity Excessive production of catecholamines occurs in patients with major burns in the later postresuscitation period. This response increases metabolic demands and is responsible for cardiomyopathy, characterized by focal myofiber necrosis. Rapid pulse rate and hypertension are commonly observed. In moderate doses, beta antagonists can reduce the amount of work the heart must perform and actually decrease metabolic demands, especially in patients with head injuries. Oxygen delivery must not be decreased to the point where it fails to meet oxygen demands.

Recent studies suggest that exogenous administration of human growth hormone may be highly beneficial in patients with massive burns. Human growth hormone, 1 to 2 mg/day, has been shown to improve nitrogen balance in normal elderly men. Levels of endogenous human growth hormone are lower than normal in burn patients. When given to such patients in dosages of 5 to 10 mg/day, human growth hormone markedly improved nitrogen retention and increased the rate of wound healing. Exogenous human growth hormone causes more endogenous fat to be used for fuel and reduces protein catabolism. Its use is associated with some complications, namely, a modest (5% to 10%) increase in oxygen consumption, modest hyperglycemia, and positive salt and water retention, especially during the first several days. Efforts are being made to determine how, when, and to which burn patients human growth hormone should be given.

Preventing a second insult As noted (see above), the addition of a second insult to an already primed system evokes an amplified host stress response. To prevent such an occurrence, extreme vigilance and aggressive institution of preventive measures are required in patients who are at high risk for secondary MODS.

Decreasing leakage from the gut Efforts should be made to minimize bacterial translocation and leakage of endotoxin across the impaired gut barrier. A lack of enteral nutrients rapidly leads to mucosal atrophy, especially during the stress response; early enteral nutrition is considered effective in maintaining the mucosal barrier. Several clinical trials have demonstrated that early enteral nutrition—as compared with early parenteral nutrition or delayed enteral nutrition—decreases secondary MODS in burn patients. Placement of a postpyloric feeding tube is becoming an increasingly common practice.

Table 5 Substances with Antioxidant Effects That May Be Given in Nutritional Solutions

Oxidant scavengers
  Vitamin C: 1–2 g/day
  Vitamin E: 400 mg/day
  β-Carotene: 25,000 IU/day
Antioxidant substrate
  Glutamine: 20–30 g/day (required for glutathione synthesis)
Required cofactors
  Selenium: 40 mg/day (cofactor glutathione peroxidase-reductase)
  Zinc: 20 mg/day parenterally (cofactor superoxide dismutase); alternatively, zinc sulfate, 220 mg t.i.d., p.o.

Administering glutamine The amino acid glutamine is the major fuel for the rapidly dividing enterocytes. Injury is often followed by glutamine deficiency as a result of both increased endogenous utilization and decreased exogenous intake. Glutamine is typically absent from central hyperalimentation solutions and standard tube feedings; however, glutamine-enriched enteral and parenteral solutions are now available. The current recommended daily dose of glutamine for adults is 20 to 30 g or 0.5 g/kg.

Using exogenous inhibitors of inflammation Nonsteroidal anti-inflammatory drugs (NSAIDs), particularly ibuprofen, have been shown to attenuate the response to inflammation and endotoxin in humans. Ibuprofen inhibits cyclooxygenase activity, thereby decreasing eicosanoid production. In addition, NSAIDs have antioxidant, anticytokine, and neutrophil-stabilizing properties. Although it is clear that these agents have significant beneficial potential, it has not been determined whether and to what extent they can actually attenuate the stress response and prevent MODS. The use of NSAIDs during the stress response has not led to an increased incidence of renal complications.

Given the deleterious effects of oxidants, the use of agents that prevent or minimize oxidant activity in some fashion is likely to be beneficial [*see Table 5*]. A host of antioxidants and agents that prevent oxidant release or remove oxidants already released (e.g., vitamin C, vitamin E, and β-carotene) are being used clinically. Optimizing cellular defenses against oxidant activity, particularly by nutritional means, has received considerable attention as a method of preventing inflammation. Marked deficiencies in endogenous antioxidants, resulting from both increased turnover and decreased substrate intake, are known to exacerbate the cellular injury caused by the ongoing inflammatory response. Glutamine, besides being fuel for enterocytes (see above), is also an essential substrate for the endogenous antioxidant glutathione. During critical illness and oxidant stress, tissue glutathione levels decrease.

Nutrition

Adequate nutrition must be provided to meet increased tissue demands by postburn day 7 because early delivery of necessary calories and proteins becomes essential for rapid wound closure and to minimize complications from pulmonary dysfunction and infection. Nutritional support should have begun between postburn days 2 and 5. Increased metabolic activity usually peaks between postburn days 7 and 10, and by then, demands should be completely met.

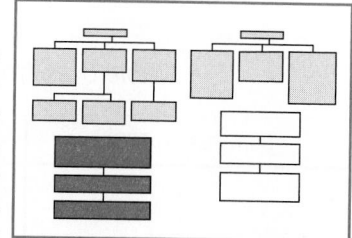

First, energy requirements must be estimated; second, plans for nutrient delivery must be individually tailored according to each patient's requirement for carbohydrate, protein, and fat.

ENERGY REQUIREMENTS

The goal of nutritional support is to provide the necessary calories to meet energy needs. These needs depend on energy expenditure, measurements of which are based on three components: basal metabolic rate (BMR), muscle activity, and stress-induced energy needs.

Basal metabolic rate describes the energy required to maintain cell integrity at the resting state and at thermoneutrality, which for the burn patient is 28° to 30° C ambient (80° to 88° F). Under these environmental conditions, heat loss is minimized and the need to produce additional metabolic heat to maintain body temperature is absent or greatly attenuated. In normal individuals, environmental temperature below thermoneutrality markedly increases sympathetic activity and caloric requirements. The BMR for humans of various ages has been determined and is widely available in chart form. Body size is the principal factor influencing metabolic rate. Other variables include the age and, to a lesser extent, the sex of the patient.

Muscle activity level is a measure of the average amount of energy used by muscles for daily activity. For patients in an ICU, muscle activity is usually quite limited, and the energy cost is usually considered to be no more than 25% above the BMR. The stress of daily exercise, sitting in a chair, and walking all contribute to the additional energy cost. Energy expenditure in bedridden patients can be markedly increased by excessive muscle activity (e.g., in patients who fight the ventilator, who must work excessively hard to breathe, or who are in a combative, disoriented state). Sedation or, if necessary, muscle paralysis will decrease this component of energy expenditure to almost zero. Prolonged muscle paralysis is not desirable, because muscle tone is necessary to maintain strength and positive nitrogen balance; the latter is particularly important for the muscles of respiration.

The third component on which energy requirements are based is stress-induced energy need. A so-called stress factor defines the hypermetabolism that is induced by the burn. The stress factor is a multiple of the basal metabolic rate (normalized to 1.0); its value takes into consideration the size of the burn injury and the average metabolic response that is seen with this size injury [see Table 6].

Oxygen consumption, carbon dioxide production, or both can be measured directly and the metabolic rate calculated. Direct measurement of calorie requirements with an indirect calorimeter (which essentially involves converting oxygen consumption to calorie expenditure) appears to be more accurate than using a formula to estimate calorie requirements; however, formulas can be very useful as guidelines [see Figure 3].

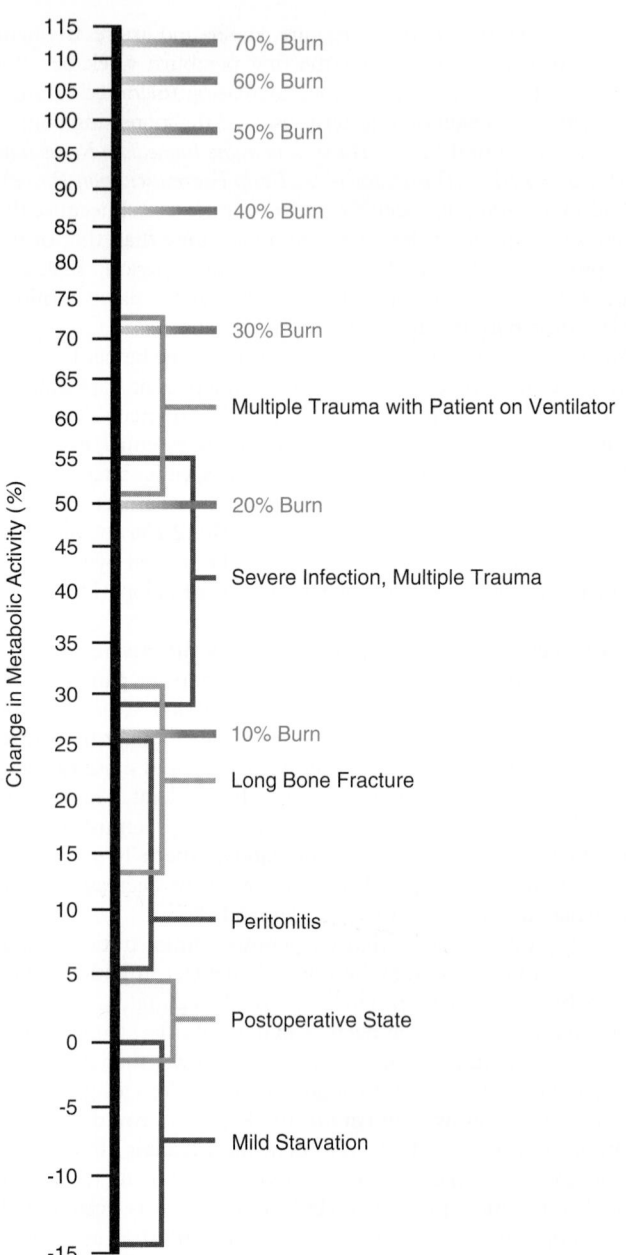

Figure 3 Depicted is the relation between selected injuries and various degrees of change in metabolic activity resulting from these injuries. Major burns cause the largest increases in metabolic rate.

NUTRIENT REQUIREMENTS (CARBOHYDRATE, FAT, AND PROTEIN)

Approximately 70% of estimated nonprotein calorie requirements must be given as glucose to spare nitrogen effectively. If lipid infusions are given, triglyceride levels must be monitored to avoid hypertriglyceridemia. In most burn patients, lipid clearance is not impaired and may in fact be increased. Increasing the proportion of omega-3 fatty acids and decreasing the proportion of omega-6 fatty acids in the infusion may be helpful. Lipids, because of their immunosuppressive effects, should make up no more than 25% of total calories.

When carbohydrates are administered, a large portion is oxidized to carbon dioxide and excreted via the lungs. As the quantity of glucose administered increases, carbon dioxide production

Table 6 Stress Factors

Burn Size (% TBS)	Stress Factor
10	1.25
20	1.50
30	1.70
40	1.85
50	2.00
60–100	2.10

rises and the respiratory quotient shifts from 0.7 (reflecting fat oxidation) toward 1.0 (reflecting carbohydrate oxidation). Excess carbohydrate—that is, more than can be primarily oxidized—is converted to fat. When this conversion occurs, the respiratory quotient exceeds 1.0, and the result may be an increased ventilatory load for the patient.

Protein requirements are also calculated in a number of ways. An estimate of 1.5 to 2.0 g of protein per kilogram of body weight can be used for all major burns. A more specific quantitative estimate can be based on a calorie-nitrogen ratio. (The nitrogen content of protein is determined by dividing the amount of protein by 6.25.) A 150:1 ratio is usually used to calculate protein requirements, but some investigators are now proposing that a 100:1 ratio is preferable. Thus, the final diet provides approximately 20% protein, 55% to 60% carbohydrate, and 20% to 25% fat.

VITAMIN AND TRACE-ELEMENT REQUIREMENTS

The burn patient loses a number of vitamins in increased quantities. Vitamins A and C are of particular concern because they are essential for healing. Vitamin A must usually be replaced in a daily dose of 10,000 to 15,000 units and vitamin C in a daily dose of 1 to 2 g. Zinc, a trace element required for healing, is also lost in increased amounts. Replacement is usually 220 mg of zinc sulfate, given orally three times a day. Administering microminerals in the form of a high-potency vitamin-mineral pill or elixir is necessary to provide trace elements.

ADMINISTRATION OF NUTRITION

Nutritional support is best managed during this period by the enteral route, usually with a combination of balanced tube feeding and voluntary intake. Parenteral supplementation through a peripheral vein may be necessary in the patient with a very large burn (i.e., a burn exceeding 50% of TBS). Central venous feedings are occasionally required if the GI tract is not functioning adequately, as sometimes occurs in patients receiving ventilatory assistance or in patients with SIRS.

For patients with large burns (in whom obligate fluid requirements are high), most of the required calories and protein can be infused through a peripheral vein. Enteral feeding via a nasogastric or postpyloric tube can usually be initiated within 2 to 3 days after a burn. As emphasized elsewhere [see III:12 Burn Care in the Early Postresuscitation Period], the sooner enteral nutrition can be instituted the better [see VII:9 Nutritional Support]. Ideally, it should begin on postburn day 1 or 2, with a small feeding tube placed through the duodenum.

Burn Wound Care

DIAGNOSIS AND TREATMENT OF BURN WOUND INFECTION

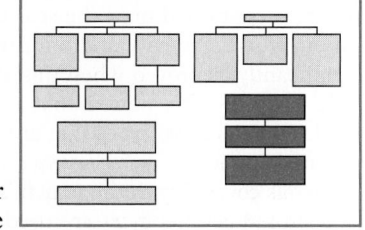

The primary indication for systemic antibiotics in the treatment of the burn wound is (1) evidence of increased bacterial content (i.e., > 10^5 organism/g tissue or histologic evidence of invasion) or (2) cellulitis or other evidence that the wound is increasing in depth or invading adjacent, noninfected tissue. In addition, systemic antibiotics are indicated in the perioperative period (24 to 48 hours) preceding and following debridement and skin grafting [see III:12 Burn Care in the Early Postresuscitation Period]. The initial topical agent is usually silver sulfadiazine. Mafenide, povidone-iodine, gentamicin, and bacitracin are commonly used topical agents when the wound becomes infected or when bacterial overgrowth retards wound healing.

CHANGES IN THE BURN WOUND

By the second postburn week, the burn wound has changed considerably from its state during the first several days. Superficial burns are healing rapidly by this point. Deep second-degree burns are beginning to debride and are becoming much more uncomfortable and prone to infection. Full-thickness burns are now colonized and revascularized, and the eschar is beginning to separate. Deep burns, being now inflamed, hyperemic, and colonized (or infected) with bacteria, must be managed much more gently than in earlier phases. Any vigorous wound manipulation can lead to bacteremia and endotoxemia. Antibiotic-resistant organisms also become more common.

During the first 6 days after the burn, wound inflammation begins and the various components of healing are initiated [see III:12 Burn Care in the Early Postresuscitation Period]. In superficial burns, epidermal regeneration is relatively rapid if the wound environment is optimized; this is achieved by providing sufficient amounts of oxygen, nutrients, and wound-healing factors (e.g., vitamin A and vitamin C), by keeping the wound surface from drying out, and by taking steps to prevent infection. The injured dermal elements are usually covered by new epithelium within 2 weeks. The hyperplasia of dermal fibroblasts then begins to resolve, and healing is complete with only modest amounts of collagen deposited. The wound usually becomes relatively pliable with time, and wound contraction is minimal. Superficial second-degree burns typically result in little or no long-term scarring.

The histology of the wound, however, changes dramatically if it has not been closed by 2 weeks after the burn, as would be the case with nongrafted deep dermal or full-thickness burns. Fibroblasts and macrophages become the predominant cells. Large numbers of myofibroblasts—modified fibroblasts that have some of the contractile properties of smooth muscle—also enter the wound. Microfilament bundles can be seen in their cytoplasm, lined parallel to each other and to the direction of contraction. Cells are linked together via extracellular extensions that allow transmission of the contractile forces. This results in a synchronized contractile process similar to that in smooth muscle. More than 75% of the cells in granulating wounds are myofibroblasts; in hypertrophic scars, the number of myofibroblasts present correlates with the rate of wound contraction. Besides leading to contraction, myofibroblasts continue to deposit large quantities of collagen and glycosaminoglycans.

Closure of the wound by reepithelialization or grafting does not eliminate the stimulus for ongoing scar formation. Angiogenesis continues, as does production of mucopolysaccharides and collagen. A marked increase in the proteoglycan content of chondroitin sulfate A can be seen as well. Chondroitin sulfate A, which is usually found in firm tissues such as cartilage, produces a harder, less pliable wound. As myofibroblasts contract, thereby shortening the scar, the deposition of the mucopolysaccharides and ground substances results in the fusion of the collagen fibers in the contracted site. The process of wound contraction leads to joint contractures.

Collagenase is also released by inflammatory cells. Synthesis of new collagen and lysis of old collagen are ongoing processes: any exaggeration of lysis or retardation of synthesis results in the dissolution of the new tissue.

CHANGES IN WOUND CARE

A marked pyrogen release resulting from manipulation of the wound causes a rise in body temperature, which accentuates the stress response and increases oxygen requirements. Use of antipyretics just before burn care begins attenuates the subsequent pyrogen response; the best agent for this purpose appears to be ibuprofen. Quantitative biopsies of the eschar are useful for diagnosing invasive infection and determining whether systemic antibiotics should be added or the topical antibiotic should be changed. Any pockets of suspected purulence below the eschar should be unroofed. Loose eschar should be removed from the wound to lower the bacterial content and to reduce surface exudation and inflammation, which can injure the new tissue being formed. Sharp dissection should not be continued into viable tissue beneath the eschar; if it is continued, substantial blood loss and bacteremia may result. Hypertrophic granulation tissue continues to be formed until the wound is surgically closed. Wound contraction reduces the surface area of the wound somewhat, but at the cost of mobility and function.

SURGICAL MANAGEMENT

As during the early postresuscitation period, surgical management of the burn wound is complicated by both anesthesia-related and wound-related problems.

Anesthesia

After the first postburn week, patients are highly hypermetabolic, and maintenance of anesthesia can be quite complex. The following are the essential components of anesthesia management in burn patients:

1. Airway maintenance and intubation.
2. Provision for increased ventilatory needs.
3. Choice of anesthetic agent.
4. Monitoring.
5. Maintenance of temperature and hemodynamic stability.

It is well known that the skeletal muscle neuromuscular receptors begin to be more sensitive to depolarizing muscle relaxants about 4 or 5 days after a burn injury and that this change results in the release of large amounts of K^+ and potentially fatal hyperkalemia during muscle fasciculations. Depolarizing agents are therefore contraindicated; a nondepolarizing agent is used when paralysis is indicated.

Adequate cardiopulmonary monitoring is extremely important in patients with major burns, who are potentially highly unstable. The relative lack of sites for invasive monitoring—and even for noninvasive monitoring—in these patients calls for considerable ingenuity on the part of the anesthesiologist. Some of the access problems can be avoided by using needle electrocardiographic electrodes, pulse oximetry, and end-tidal carbon dioxide concentrations (obtained from air expired from the ventilator). Advance knowledge of the patient's ventilatory and hemodynamic status and maintenance of preoperative values are essential.

Accurate assessment of blood loss depends on frequent communication between the surgeon and the anesthesiologist. Any blood lost should be replaced with blood products; crystalloid should be given to replace evaporative losses, not blood losses. Blood and blood products should be present in the room before management of a major case begins. The operating room must be warm (at least 80° F), and heating blankets, warm fluids, and similar adjuvants should be available. The operating time should be limited to two hours in patients who have large burns, especially if any significant cardiopulmonary instability is present.

Surgical Procedures

Surgical procedures done in burn patients during the inflammation period should be performed according to the same guidelines that are applicable in the first postburn week [*see III:12 Burn Care in the Early Postresuscitation Period*]: the duration of the operation must be limited, blood loss must be minimized, and the grafted area must be carefully immobilized. The patient must be hemodynamically stable before the operation. Perioperative antibiotics are indicated. The choice of an agent is governed by the results of the preoperative wound culture: if no specific organism predominates, a first-generation cephalosporin is usually preferred because it provides reasonable coverage of *Staphylococcus aureus* and the more common gram-negative bacteria. *S. aureus* is the most common organism affecting the skin graft and the donor site.

The wound is colonized with bacteria during this period; thus, the potential for producing significant bacteremia also increases. Certainly, endotoxemia develops and inflammatory mediators are released; SIRS results postoperatively. Perioperative antibiotics help combat the bacteremia but do not block the absorption of endotoxins and pyrogens already present in the wound. If the wound infection cannot be controlled by nonoperative management, limited sequential excision can be lifesaving. The primary caution is to avoid large or long procedures that might have been easily tolerated in the first week but that are not as well tolerated during this period.

Wound Remodeling and Scar Formation

HYPERTROPHIC SCARRING

Pressure is the standard means of controlling hypertrophic scarring and accelerating the maturation process. When dressings are still required, pressure is provided by Ace wraps. Form-fitted pressure garments are used later. The pressure is expected to exceed surface vessel capillary pressure and should reach 25 mm Hg or higher. Pressure immediately reduces hyperemia and wound edema, which in turn prevents blister formation. Over a period of several weeks, a decrease in the chrondroitin sulfate content becomes evident, as does a decline in mast cells and myofibroblasts. One theory is that by impeding blood flow to scars, pressure decreases fibroblast and inflammatory cell numbers by means of surface ischemia and thereby decreases overall excess collagen synthesis. In addition, because the water content is decreased, ground substance production is also decreased. The pressure must be continuous to be effective (i.e., about 23 hours every day for up to a year). Therapy with pressure garments is continued until the scar demonstrates complete maturation. Muscle activity and joint motion have been found to be significantly improved when this approach is employed.

It is during this period that permanent skin substitutes are used. There are two types that are commonly used clinically: (1) cultured autologous keratinocytes and (2) bilayer skin with generic dermis covered with the patient's own dermis.

Cultured keratinocytes are used as follows. In the first several days after the burn, the decision is made that cultured keratinocytes will be required to help cover a large burn surface. Full-thickness skin biopsies are then taken for cell preparation, the wound is excised and covered (preferably with cadaver skin), the cells are grown in tissue media for 3 weeks, the skin substitute is removed, the cultured cells are applied, and the area is immobilized. Graft take ranges from 20% to 80%; the best results are obtained with flat surfaces that can be immobilized.

Bilayer skin consists of a dermis, which is absorbed and replaced by the host, and an artificial epidermis in the form of a Silastic sheet, which is eventually replaced by the patient's own epidermis. Bilayer skin, despite its greater potential for providing a dermis and its superior flexibility, is at present less commonly used than cultured keratinocytes, primarily because it is still undergoing developmental changes.

There are a number of experimental skin substitutes in various stages of development. It is likely that before long, skin substitutes will be available that can replace both layers in a predictable fashion.

SKIN LUBRICATION

Because the burn patient's sebaceous glands have been impaired or destroyed, natural skin lubrication is absent; drying, pain, and markedly impaired pliability result. Skin moisturizers will be necessary for months to years to maintain optimal skin function.

Recommended Reading

Alexander W: The role of infections in the burn patient. The Art and Science of Burn Care. Boswick J, Ed. Aspen Publishers, Rockville, Maryland, 1982, p 103

Beeker W: Fungal burn wound infection, a 10 year experience. Arch Surg 126:44, 1991

Bingham H, Gallagher T, Powell R: Early bronchoscopy as a predictor of ventilatory support for burned patients. J Trauma 27:1286, 1987

Bone R, Balk R, Cerra F, et al: Definitions for sepsis and organ failure and guidelines for the use of innovative therapies in sepsis. Chest 101:1644, 1992

Boukoms A: Pain relief in the intensive care unit. J Intens Care Med 3:32, 1988

DeBandt S, Chollet M, Lowry S, et al: Cytokine response to burn injury: relationship with protein metabolism. J Trauma 36:624, 1994

DeBiasse M, Wilmore D: What is optimum nutritional support? New Horizons. Zalaga G, Ed. Society for Critical Care Medicine, Fullerton, California, 1994, p 122

Deitch E: Intestinal permeability is increased in burn patients shortly after injury. Surgery 167:411, 1990

Demling R: Effect of early burn excision and grafting on pulmonary function. J Trauma 24:830, 1984

Demling R: Fluid replacement in burned patients. Surg Clin North Am 67:15, 1987

Demling R, Orgill D: Current concepts and approaches to wound healing. Crit Care Med 16:899, 1988

Demling R, Pomposelli J: Burn wound infection. Surgical Infections: Diagnosis and Treatment. Meakins JL, Ed. Scientific American, Inc, New York, 1994, p 369

Dobke M, Deitch E, Baxter C: Oxidant activity of polymorphonuclear leukocytes after thermal injury. Arch Surg 124:856, 1989

Dong Y, Abdullah K, Yan T, et al: Effect of thermal injury and sepsis on neutrophil function. J Trauma 34:417, 1993

Fong Y, Moldawer L, Shires T, et al: The biologic characteristics of cytokines and their implications in surgical injury. Surg Gynecol Obstet 170:363, 1990

Gatzen C, Scheltinga M, Kimbrough T, et al: Growth hormone attenuates the abnormal distribution of body water in critically ill surgical patients. Surgery 112:181, 1992

Goodwin C, Wilmore D: Surgery and burns. Clinical Nutrition. Paige D, Ed. CV Mosby Co, St Louis, 1988, p 372

Gore D, Honeycutt D, Jahoor F, et al: Effect of exogenous growth hormone on whole body and isolated limb protein kinetics in burned patients. Arch Surg 126:38, 1990

Gottleich M, Warden G: Vitamin supplementation in the patient with burns. J Burn Care Rehabil 11:375, 1990

Hirsch C, Kaemerek R, Stanek K: Work of breathing during CPAP and PSV imposed by the new generation mechanical ventilators. Respir Care 36:815, 1991

Jahoor F, Shangraw RE, Miyoshi H, et al: Role of insulin and glucose oxidation in mediating the protein catabolism of burns and sepsis. Am J Physiol 257:E323, 1989

Jeevandra M, Ramias L, Shamos R, et al: Decreased growth hormone levels in the catabolic phase of severe injury. Surgery 111:495, 1992

Law E, Blecher K, Still J: Enterococcal infections as a cause of mortality and morbidity in patients with burns. J Burn Care Rehabil 15:236, 1994

Machin L, Bendich A: Free radical tissue damage: protective role of antioxidant nutrients. FASEB J 1:441, 1990

Moore E, Jones T: Benefits of immediate jejunostomy feeding after major abdominal trauma: a prospective randomized study. J Trauma 26:874, 1986

Moore F, Haenel J, Moore E, et al: Incommensurate oxygen consumption in response to maximal oxygen availability products post injury multiple organ failure. J Trauma 33:58, 1992

Munster A: Cultured epidermal autograft in the management of burn patients. J Burn Care Rehabil 13:121, 1992

Paxton J, Williamson J: Nutrient substrate: making choices in the 1990s. J Burn Care Rehabil 12:198, 1991

Pinsky M, Matuschak G: A unifying hypothesis of multiple system organ failure: failure of host defense homeostasis. J Crit Care 5:108, 1990

Pruitt B: Infection and the burn patient. Br J Surg 77:1081, 1990

Rodriguez J, Miller C, Till G, et al: Correlation of the local and systemic cytokine response with clinical outcome following thermal injury. J Trauma 34:684, 1993

Servent R, Hansbrough J: Cytotoxicity to human leukocytes by topical antimicrobial agents used for burn care. J Burn Care Rehabil 14:132, 1993

Taddonio T, Thomson P: A survey of wound monitoring and topical antimicrobial therapy practices in the treatment of burn injury. J Burn Care Rehabil 11:423, 1990

Tobin M: Respiratory monitoring. JAMA 264:244, 1990

Wallace B, Caldwell F, Cone J: Ibuprofen lowers body temperature and metabolic rate of humans with burn injury. J Trauma 32:159, 1992

Ward P, Warren J, Johnson K: Oxygen radical inflammation and tissue injury. Free Rad Biol Med 5:403, 1988

Waymack JP, Herndon DN: Nutritional support of the burned patient. World J Surg 16:80, 1992

Wilmore D: Metabolic changes after thermal injury. The Art and Science of Burn Care. Boswick J, Ed. Aspen Publishers, Rockville, Maryland, 1987

Winchurch R, Thupari J, Munster A: Endotoxemia in burn patients, levels of circulating endotoxins are related to burn size. Surgery 102:808, 1987

Woolf P: Hormonal responses to trauma. Crit Care Med 20:216, 1992

Xia Z, Coolbaugh M, He F, et al: The effects of burn injury on the acute phase response. J Trauma 32:245, 1992

Youn Y, Demling R: The role of mediators in the response to thermal injury. World J Surg 16:30, 1992

Acknowledgments

Figures 1 through 3   Talar Agasyan.

Table 1   Adapted from *Metabolic Management of the Critically Ill*, by D. W. Wilmore. Plenum Publishing Corporation, New York, 1977, p 22.

Robert H. Demling, M.D.

Management of Miscellaneous Thermal Injuries

Electrical Injury

Electrical burn injuries account for fewer than 5% of admissions to major burn centers. Compared with skin burns, however, these injuries are much more complex and are associated with higher morbidity and mortality. The mortality is reported to be between 3% and 15%, with about 1,000 deaths a year in the United States attributed to electrical current. More than 90% of injuries occur in males, most of whom are between 20 and 34 years of age. Electrical injuries can be grouped into three categories: high voltage, involving contact with more than 1,000 volts; low voltage, caused by contact with less than 1,000 volts; and those caused by lightning.

HIGH-VOLTAGE INJURY

Diagnosis

The heat generated by arcing (jumping) of a high-voltage current from a high-tension wire toward a human being reaches several thousand degrees and produces a flash skin burn comparable to that caused by any explosion of a volatile substance. The intense heat frequently causes clothes to catch fire, resulting in deep burns of the skin. In the presence of a large skin burn, health care providers may overlook severe injury from an electrical burn. The subsequent soft tissue edema and pain can easily be misinterpreted as the result of thermal injury rather than concomitant damage from the passage of current. Careful history-taking and physical examination are critical to avoiding this error. This type of thermal burn is managed in essentially the same way as any other burn would be [*see Figure 1*], except that a higher urine output will be necessary if myoglobinuria is present [*see Fluid Management, below*].

Physical evidence of an entrance site [*see Figure 2*] and of an exit site [*see Figures 3 and 4*] is pathognomonic of the passage of a significant amount of electrical current through the body. Because the depth of injury and the degree of tissue damage cannot be determined by superficial assessment, victims of electrical injuries must be hospitalized for observation. A history of the event is critical in estimating the extent of injury.

Muscle necrosis Electrical burns more closely resemble crush injuries than thermal burns. Damage below the skin, where the current passes, is usually far greater than the appearance of the overlying skin would indicate [*see Table 1*]. The immediate damage is caused by heat destruction of cells, which is usually patchy in distribution along the course of the current. Other effects are devascularization, caused by injured blood vessels; tissue infection; and compartment syndrome, with pressure necro-

sis especially prominent in nerve tissue and muscle enveloped by nonyielding fascia.

Early necrosis does not follow the anatomic division of muscles but is uneven, reflecting the passage of current through the body. In the first few hours after injury, it is difficult to distinguish between normal muscle and muscle that is irreparably damaged but not immediately coagulated. Progressive necrosis is usually evident over the next 4 to 5 days. It is common to find dead muscle in the presence of excellent local blood supply, indicating that the muscle damage is not totally vascular in origin and that the temperature required to kill muscle cells is less than that required to coagulate blood vessels.

Damage to muscle tissues is evident within minutes to hours of injury, when the still perfused muscles begin to swell. The finite boundaries of the fascial envelope cause a rapid increase in tissue pressure; when the microvascular hydrostatic pressure exceeds 25 mm Hg, there is additional ischemia and compression nerve injury in local tissues. Tissue pressure exceeding 30 mm Hg is clearly abnormal and must be decreased to avoid further damage. Edema increases over the next 24 to 48 hours.

Because of current-induced damage to vessels, vascular thrombosis can occur immediately and over the following 3 to 4 days. The progressive devascularization causes additional loss of muscle tissue. The combination of endothelial cell damage and weakening of vessel walls can lead to local thrombosis and tissue hemorrhage. These processes, the uneven nature of the necrosis, and, in particular, the damage to muscles and nerves closest to bone seriously impair function, resulting in a high rate of amputation (30% to 40%). Muscle atrophy and replacement of injured muscle by fibrous tissue cause subsequent dysfunction.

Monitoring

Cardiopulmonary monitoring and supportive care are clearly necessary, given the high incidence of cardiac arrhythmias and pulmonary dysfunction in patients with electrical injuries [*see Table 2*]. Urinalysis is essential to verify that renal perfusion is adequate and to screen for myoglobinuria, which calls for special management. Measurement of blood gases and the acid-base balance are important for assessment of lung function and peripheral perfusion. Acidosis must be corrected to prevent excess myoglobin in the renal tubules.

Monitoring of peripheral perfusion and palpation of muscle compartments are important for assessment of compartment syndromes caused by muscle edema. Compartment pressure can be monitored by one of the available systems. Indications for fas-

High-voltage injury (≥ 1,000 V)

Evidence of entrance site and exit site is pathognomonic of injury.
Ensure patent airway and assess cardiopulmonary function.
Consider possibility of muscle necrosis or blunt trauma.
Take careful history.
Hospitalize patient for observation.

Monitoring

- ECG
- Arterial and venous pressures (consider pulmonary arterial catheter)
- Urine output, pH, and myoglobin
- Serum electrolytes (especially K^+), myoglobin, and coagulation factors
- Compartment pressures (via wick catheter or solid-state transducer)
- Flow to distal extremity (via Doppler flowmeter)
- Central and peripheral nerve function (for possible compression neuropathy)

Fluid management

Give lactated Ringer's solution, along with colloids and blood as necessary.
Anticipate need for > 4 ml/kg/% TBS burned in first 24 hr.
If myoglobin is present, ensure urine output of ≥ 1 ml/kg/hr:
- Mannitol, 25 g bolus followed by 12 g q. 2–4 hr
- Sodium bicarbonate added to I.V. solution to maintain urine pH > 7 and blood pH ≤ 7.5
- Low-dose dopamine if large amounts of fluid must be given
- Loop diuretics if pigment load persists for > 18 hr

Wound care

Infection control

Debride wound as soon as patient is stable.
Give tetanus prophylaxis.
Do not initiate broad-spectrum antibiotic prophylaxis.
Administer topical antibiotics to burned regions and necrotic areas.

Escharotomy and fasciotomy

Perform escharotomy if there is a circumferential deep burn and distal perfusion is impaired.
Perform fasciotomy if there is electrical injury to underlying tissue or if compartment pressure is increased. Electrocautery may be required.

Aggressive surgical treatment

Remove dead or dying muscle as soon as patient is hemodynamically stable.
Amputate nonviable extremities.

Figure 1 **Shown is an algorithm for treatment of high-voltage electrical injury.**

ciotomy and escharotomy are tissue pressure greater than 40 mm Hg and tissue pressure within 30 mm Hg of diastolic pressure.

The signs of increased compartment pressure include decreased peripheral pulse rate, evidence of nerve compression, paresthesias, decreased sensation or increased pain, and increased muscle turgor. Excessive tissue turgor is the most useful sign of underlying muscle damage and the need for fasciotomy. Motor nerve dysfunction is more difficult to assess because it may be impossible to distinguish nerve damage from muscle damage.

Fluid Management

The principles of fluid management that apply to thermal burns also apply to electrical burns. The primary resuscitation fluid is lactated Ringer's solution (or hypertonic lactated saline), but the unpredictable nature of the tissue damage precludes the use of a standard formula. In general, for a given percentage of total body surface burned, the fluid requirements in patients with electrical burns are 1.5 to 2 times the requirements in patients with skin burns alone, reflecting additional soft tissue injury associated with electrical burns.

The rate of fluid administration is the amount necessary to maintain adequate systemic perfusion. The presence of myoglobin

in the urine, other evidence of early renal impairment, or high levels of creatine kinase in plasma indicate the need for adjustments in fluid administration. If the urine is red or reddish black (evidence of massive myoglobin release from muscle), a urine flow of

Figure 2 **Typical entrance site of high voltage shows desiccation of tissue.**

Figure 3 **Current often exits the body from the foot, through small, round, punctate areas.**

at least 1 ml/kg/hr is needed until the pigment load decreases.

The appropriate treatment regimen is as follows:

1. Mannitol (25 g bolus, followed by 12.5 g every 2 to 4 hours) in addition to fluids until the pigment clears from the urine.
2. Sodium bicarbonate, added to the intravenous solution, to maintain urine pH above 7 without raising blood pH above 7.5.
3. Low-dose dopamine, if excessive amounts of fluid are required to increase renal blood flow and subsequent urine output.
4. Loop diuretics, added to fluid infusion, if the pigment load persists longer than 8 hours.

Infection Control

Infection in areas of tissue necrosis and ischemia begins several days after injury, particularly if a skin burn potentiates cross-contamination from wound to wound. Infection is generally controlled by early wound debridement. Tetanus prophylaxis is required because of the risks of deep tissue necrosis in a relatively anaerobic environment. Prophylactic use of broad-spectrum antibiotics is not indicated, but perioperative antibiotic therapy is, as in the management of thermal burns.

Figure 4 **Severe damage was caused at this ground point, where current left the body.**

Table 1 Common Complications of Electrical Burns	
Ventricular fibrillation and other rhythm abnormalities	Muscle necrosis
Respiratory arrest	Fractures
Seizures	Hemolysis
Coma	Renal failure
Mental changes	Hemorrhage
Hypertension	Limb loss
Retinal detachment	Anemia
Cataract (delayed)	Paresis, complete paralysis, and other neurologic disorders (delayed)

Escharotomy and Fasciotomy

In general, an escharotomy is necessary if there is a circumferential deep burn and any evidence of impaired distal perfusion. Fasciotomy is indicated if there is concomitant electrical injury to underlying tissue and increasing compartment pressure, evident in increased myoglobin levels, rigid muscle compartments, or nerve or vessel compression.

Wound Management

In general, if there are large amounts of necrotic muscle in burns caused by high-voltage contact, treatment must be aggressive, with surgical debridement. These measures minimize subsequent organ dysfunction, infection, and eventual mortality and maximize the salvage of marginal tissue, which is highly susceptible to infection. If gross myoglobinuria is present for several hours, if exit sites are large, if there is mummification of a large entrance wound, or if muscle feels woody, hard, and nonfunctional, a large amount of dead muscle is a virtual certainty.

Early excision of dead muscle is performed as soon as the patient is hemodynamically stable, preferably 1 to 2 days after the injury. The risks of renal failure increase the longer that large amounts of dead and dying muscle remain in the wounds. Muscle of indeterminate viability should be spared, but guillotine amputation should be used on obviously nonsalvageable limbs—a measure that can be lifesaving. After surgery, the wounds should be covered with biologic dressings or moist, dilute antibiotic solutions.

The goal of subsequent surgical procedures is to conserve viable tissue while removing neighboring dead tissue. The uneven nature of injuries makes this approach difficult and time consuming. Small scattered areas of injured muscle will be reabsorbed and replaced by fibrous tissue. A high fever and tachycardia, however, may be physiologic evidence that infected dead tissue remains. The tissue along the bone is often the site of greatest muscle necrosis.

One approach that has shown excellent potential for minimizing long-term disability is early aggressive debridement, followed immediately by reconstruction with rotation flaps and free flaps, if needed, to cover remaining viable tissue, nerves, vessels, and bone.

Managing Entrance and Exit Sites

Entrance and exit sites of electrical current are thermal burns (that is, they are the result of heat generation), but they are more complex than standard skin burns. Heat generated at the skin surface depends on the local resistance to flow. A dry hand in contact with high voltage may generate heat in excess of 1,000° C, leading to mummification at the entrance site. The result is a well-defined charred wound at the site of contact. The skin surface is depressed,

Table 2 Monitoring Patients with Electrical Burns

Evaluation of Systemic Changes	Evaluation of Local Changes
Vital signs Urine output, pH, and myoglobin Serial hematocrits Serum electrolytes (especially K⁺), myoglobin, and clotting factors	Frequent Doppler ultrasound measurement of blood flow in injured extremity Frequent assessment for nerve compression Frequent palpation of muscle compartments
Consider Arterial line Central line Pulmonary arterial catheter (to monitor perfusion in injured CNS, myocardium, and kidneys) Electrocardiography (to monitor arrhythmias)	*Consider* Measurement of compartment pressures

demonstrating the effect of high temperature on the water content of the tissue. Some entrance wounds may resemble deep flame burns, but in such a case, the injury extends well below the dermis.

If there is moderate exposure to current, the appearance at the exit site is similar to small skin ulcerations, with depressed centers and elevated edges. With passage of a large current, multiple exit sites may be seen along the route of the current, suggesting the effects of an explosion. Pieces of cutaneous tissue may be blown out by the immense energy of the exiting current.

In accordance with the principles used for thermal burns, devitalized tissue below the skin at the entrance and exit sites should be debrided. After 3 to 5 days, residual necrotic tissue should be debrided, and the wounds should be closed with skin grafts or flaps. Tissue defects may necessitate soft tissue coverage by a soft tissue flap. Coverage of large wounds with skin grafts may have to be postponed until the patient's condition is more stable.

Other Effects of High-Voltage Injury

Cardiovascular injury Immediate cardiac arrest is the most common cause of death resulting from electrical injury. The current alters rhythm, leading to fibrillation, or depresses respiration, leading to hypoxia. The immediate mortality associated with passage of a high-voltage current from one hand to the other is 60%. The cardiac arrhythmia is often reversible, however, and cardiac resuscitation should be initiated at the scene of the accident. The most common electrocardiographic changes, other than fibrillation, are sinus tachycardia and nonspecific ST-T wave changes.

Major vessel thrombosis occurs, as does delayed rupture of large vessels, with massive hemorrhage; rupture of these vessels in the absence of surrounding tissue damage indicates low resistance to flow within the vessels. Although rare, aneurysms can occur weeks to months after injury; good follow-up measures should be instituted in the light of this possibility.

Renal injury Renal failure is reported in at least 10% of victims of high-voltage electrical burns. Myoglobin and hemoglobin from damaged muscle and red blood cells can precipitate in the renal tubules, producing acute tubular necrosis. The combination of myoglobin, which is colorless in circulating plasma, and hemoglobin produces pink to red urine. Myoglobin precipitation is accentuated by acid urine and decreased by alkaline urine. Muscle necrosis, which can result in distant organ dys-

function, may affect the kidneys; the low-flow state caused by hypovolemia will aggravate the tissue injury. Another cause of renal vascular damage is direct attack by high-voltage current.

Pulmonary injury The pulmonary abnormalities are the result of CNS-induced hypoventilation and chest wall dysfunction. Impaired respiratory center activity and severe CNS damage lead to hypoventilation, often the cause of immediate death.

Neurologic injury Both immediate and delayed neurologic abnormalities are common. Acute CNS dysfunction—with coma, seizures, motor deficits, and, to a lesser extent, sensory deficits—has been well described. Many of these abnormalities are permanent. Delayed injuries include both peripheral neuropathies and cord damage with paralysis. The mechanisms believed to be responsible for the delayed injuries are delayed vascular thrombosis, leading to ischemia, and progressive demyelination following passage of electrical current through the body.

Orthopedic injury Contact with high-tension current causes severe muscle spasm, which can produce long bone fractures and dislocation at major joints. The next most common orthopedic injury in patients who have been in contact with high-tension sources is heat necrosis of local periosteum, with subsequent production of nonviable bone and sequestration formation. Less common is devascularization of bone, caused by the vascular injury affecting other tissues.

Ocular and otic injury Again, both immediate and delayed injuries are noted. Early changes include conjunctival and corneal burns as well as ruptured eardrums. Late changes, occurring up to 1 year after the injury, include cataract formation, tinnitus, and decreased hearing.

LOW-VOLTAGE INJURY

The most common result of low-voltage injury is a cardiac arrhythmia, especially ventricular fibrillation. This cardiac abnormality can be life threatening because only a small proportion of the population has been trained in cardiopulmonary resuscitation. A less common effect of low-voltage injury is suffocation caused by tetany of chest wall muscles. This effect is less common because it takes several minutes to occur, and assistance is often available to move the patient away from the source of injury. Central nervous system abnormalities, if any, are usually the result of hypoxia caused by cardiopulmonary arrest. Because of the possibility of myocardial injury, it is good practice to hospitalize patients for 24 hours and to observe them with cardiac monitors. Fractures may occur as a result of tetany and muscle spasm from alternating current (AC). Treatment is based on the standard approach to the most common injuries, cardiopulmonary arrest and tetany-induced fractures [*see Figure 5*].

Oral Burns

Low-voltage electricity is the leading cause of electrical injury in children, especially those 1 to 2 years of age [*see Figure 6*]. Sucking an extension cord is responsible for more than half of the injuries, and biting an electrical cord accounts for about 30%. The most common mechanism is the production of an electrical arc by the bared wires, conducted by the child's saliva. Intense local heat is generated, destroying tissues in the mouth. The burn may involve the lip, tongue, or oral mucosa and underlying bone, but the most frequent site is the lip, particularly the commissure area between the upper and lower lips [*see Table 3*]. The burn is typically grayish

Low-voltage injury (< 1,000 V)

Diagnosis rests primarily on history.
Ensure patent airway and assess cardiopulmonary function.
Be alert for
- Cardiac arrhythmias (especially ventricular fibrillation)
- Tetany of chest wall muscles
- CNS abnormalities

Monitoring

- ECG (routine)
If ECG is normal, further monitoring is not needed unless there is a history of cardiac events.

Wound care

Infection control

Provide tetanus prophylaxis.
Do not administer systemic prophylactic antibiotics.

Local care

Oral burns

Hospitalize patient.
Wash wound gently, and apply petroleum-based ointment.
Control local bleeding with pressure.
Delay debridement for at least 1 wk.
Place intraoral splint after initial edema resolves. Leave splint in place for 6–12 mo, then, if necessary, perform minor surgery on residual defect.

Burns at other sites

Provide standard outpatient local wound care.

Figure 5 **Shown is an algorithm for treatment of low-voltage electrical injury.**

white and indented at the center because of tissue necrosis. Severe swelling develops as venous thrombosis impedes blood return.

The edema of the lips may be intense, impairing control of saliva. The orbicularis oris muscle is often involved, further impairing control. Edema subsides over the next 5 to 10 days, and local necrotic tissue begins to slough. Bleeding from the labial artery, which occurs in 20% of patients during the period of slough (7 to 21 days), should be anticipated. Granulation tissue then develops, followed by collagen deposition and wound remodeling. Local adhesions and microstomia may develop over a period of 3 to 5 months. Injury to the underlying bone results in dental abnormalities over time.

Hospitalization is recommended to treat the local burn and examine the patient for related injuries. Tetanus prophylaxis is necessary, but systemic antibiotics do not appear to be beneficial. Local wound care consists of gentle washing followed three to four times daily by application of a petroleum-based antibiotic ointment. Feeding by tube, syringe, or a straw is helpful to avoid additional local pressure. Occasionally, vessel ligation is required.

Figure 6 **Typical oral burn, caused by biting an electrical cord, shows tissue necrosis at the corner of the mouth.**

Because the extent of injury cannot be determined for several days, surgical debridement is delayed for at least a week. The present treatment of choice is the placement of a prosthetic intraoral splint after the initial edema resolves, generally 5 to 10 days after the injury. Use of a splint reduces the scarring effect of adhesion formation, thus decreasing the need for cosmetic surgery.

LIGHTNING

Properties and Effects

Lightning is the result of an atmospheric electrical discharge occurring between a positive charge in an upper cloud level and a negative charge at a lower cloud level. A lightning flash occurs when the potential difference between the layers exceeds the insulating properties of air. Air crossed by the lightning is rapidly heated and expands to develop a shock wave, which decays to a sound wave perceived as thunder. The power of a lightning bolt is estimated at 10,000 to 20,000 amperes of current with more than 20 million volts of electromotive force. The four mechanisms of injury are direct strike, flash discharge, ground current, and shock wave.

A direct strike results when a person who is outdoors acts as the grounding site. Mortality is high, with head entry being common. A flash discharge, more common than a direct strike, occurs when the lightning changes direction to hit another object. Injury is still severe, but not as great as in a direct strike.

Ground currents can develop from a strike on the ground. A person standing may generate a sufficient potential difference between legs and ground for current to develop. Overall mortality from lightning injury is about 30%, and approximately two thirds of survivors experience permanent sequelae of the accident.

Table 3 Classification of Electrical Burn of the Lip

Severity	Description
Minor	Injury to less than one third of upper or lower lip, sparing commissure
Moderate	Injury to more than one third of lip, sparing commissure, or injury to commissure alone
Severe	Loss of skin and muscle of more than one third of lip, including commissure

In the phenomenon of flashover, lightning travels along the outside of the conductor—namely, the victim. The current vaporizes skin moisture and destroys clothing but spares the body tissues. The shock wave produced by the heating and expansion of air produces tissue damage comparable to the effects of any large explosion. This form of tissue trauma is often overlooked.

Diagnosis

If the victim is unconscious, if no one witnessed the lightning injury, and if there is no evidence of fire or flames, diagnosis is difficult. Treatment, however, must be based on recognition that the patient was struck by lightning. Understanding of the magnitude of energy involved in the injury minimizes the risk that serious tissue damage, both immediate and delayed, will be overlooked. The general principles of treatment are the same as those for high-voltage electrical burns.

Specific Problems

Cardiovascular injury The direct current of lightning produces myocardial depolarization and arrest. Treatment is supportive.

Central nervous system injury Damage to the CNS is caused by electrical current or by mechanical trauma. At least three fourths of patients with a lightning injury have at least a transient loss of consciousness. More than two thirds experience temporary paralysis of the upper or lower extremities, which resolves over hours to days. Permanent sequelae are common, especially those resulting from anoxia following cardiorespiratory arrest. Treatment is supportive.

Skin injury Injuries to the skin vary from the burns seen after contact with a high-voltage current to a superficial skin abnormality sometimes referred to as feathering or lightning prints. The latter process is characterized by linear fernlike erythematous skin markings that do not blanch. The markings, probably caused by the flashover phenomenon as static electricity is transmitted along the superficial vasculature, fade in several days. Recognition of this skin change in a comatose person can help make the diagnosis of a lightning injury. Treatment of localized deep burns is the same as that of other electrical burns.

Musculoskeletal injury A typical high-tension injury with muscle necrosis is accompanied by compartment syndrome, myoglobinuria, and renal failure. Treatment is the same as that outlined for high-voltage injury.

Ocular and otic injury Lightning may also injure the eyes or the ears. Cataracts are the most common intraocular injury caused by lightning. One type of cataract is traumatic, resulting from the initial concussion; the onset of the second type, which is caused by the current itself, is delayed for several months. Lid lesions from a burn and conjunctivitis are also common. Treatment depends on the injuries produced.

More than 50% of persons struck by lightning have ear injuries, caused by both the concussion (ruptured tympanic membrane) and the current (direct nerve damage). Treatment depends on the specific injuries produced.

Cold Injury

There are three common types of cold injury: tissue-freezing injury (e.g., frostbite), nonfreezing injury (e.g., trench foot and chilblain, or pernio), and hypothermia. Hypothermia is commonly a major complicating factor of cold injury to tissues and is usually the most life-threatening aspect of the injury [*see VII:10 Fever, Hyperpyrexia, and Hypothermia*].

FROSTBITE

Frostbite occurs when tissue freezes, resulting in the formation of intracellular ice crystals and microvascular occlusion. Patients who have frostbite are able to use the frostbitten body part; however, frostbitten tissue is desensitized, so the patient should take care when using the affected body part. In general, rewarming is contraindicated when there is potential for refreezing because refreezing dramatically increases tissue damage.

Risk factors for frostbite are similar to those for hypothermia [*see Table 4*]. However, the effect of windchill can drastically increase the severity of injury.

Treatment

The first steps in treatment of frostbite [*see Figure 7*] are to assess the patient's overall status and to commence total body rewarming. Next, the depth of injury should be determined [*see Table 5*]. The frostbitten area should be rapidly rewarmed by placing the affected part in a warm-water bath (42° C) for approximately 30 minutes. Care should be taken to maintain appropriate water temperature. A direct dry-heat source should never be used for rewarming, because burns may occur.

Rewarming can be extremely painful, often necessitating narcotics. Tetanus toxoid booster should be administered according to a standard protocol. After total body rewarming, wounds should be assessed for possible cleaning and conservative debridement. Clear blisters may be removed. Hemorrhagic blisters indicate deeper tissue involvement and should be temporarily left intact if fluid is infected. The affected area should be elevated to decrease tissue edema. Use of systemic antibiotics is controversial and should generally be limited to patients with suspected or documented infections. Surgical management of frostbite should be of an expectant and conservative nature, quite different from that

---

Table 4 **Risk Factors Associated with Frostbite Injury**

Flow-related
  Peripheral vascular disease
  Cardiac disease

CNS and mental status
  Dementia; history of psychiatric illness
  Injury to brain or spinal cord

Medications
  Same as with hypothermia—ergot alkaloids, theophylline derivatives (e.g., aminophylline and caffeine), and Fiorinal
  Vasoconstrictors

Age
  Elderly
  Very young

Race
  African Americans at greater risk than whites

Other
  Ethanol ingestion
  Previous cold exposure
  Tobacco use
  Malnutrition

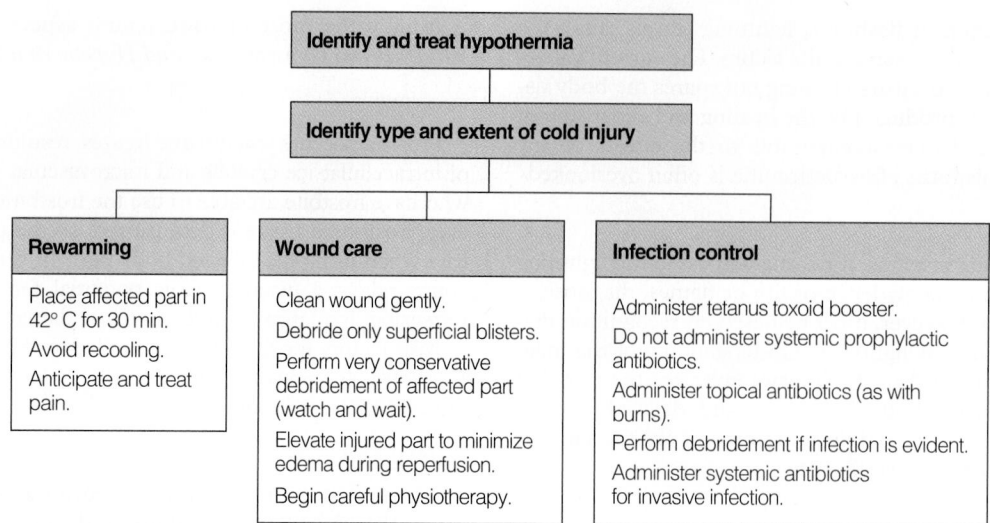

Figure 7 Shown is an algorithm for treatment of cold injury.

of a heat burn. Escharotomy is obviously warranted if vascular compromise occurs. Early debridement or amputation may be necessary if the affected tissue is causing an uncontrollable septic response or disseminated intravascular coagulation. Otherwise, surgical intervention consists of conservative debridement and reconstruction, beginning several weeks after injury. This period allows for adequate tissue demarcation and minimizes any viable tissue loss from an aggressive early debridement.

Concomitant fractures or dislocations should be treated when the patient arrives at the emergency room. As with any trauma patient, open fractures warrant immediate intraoperative management.

Adjuvant Therapy

Many forms of adjuvant therapy have been explored. Thromboxane synthetase inhibitors and ibuprofen, a cyclooxygenase inhibitor, appear to be effective in reducing the postwarming inflammatory response by blocking the formation of prostanoids and leukotrienes. Arterial dilators such as reserpine, tolazoline, and nifedipine have also been used but have not been clearly proved to be effective. Antiplatelet and thrombolytic agents such as dextran, heparin, urokinase, and streptokinase have also shown some clinical efficacy. Use of calmodulin antagonists has shown good results.

Attempts at chemical and surgical sympathectomy and, more recently, electrostimulation of the spinal cord have yielded mixed results. Although sympathectomy may offer benefits in decreasing postfrostbite sequelae, it has not been demonstrated to improve tissue salvage.

Long-Term Complications

Sequelae of frostbite vary in severity. Hyperhidrosis, Raynaud's disease, peripheral neuropathy, hypersensitivity to cold, bony deformity, and atrophy of the nails, hair, and muscle are common problems.

IMMERSION FOOT AND TRENCH FOOT

Immersion foot occurs when a foot exposed to nonfreezing temperatures of 10° C or lower loses heat because it is wet and experiences poor vascular flow because it is constricted and immobile. Symptoms include numbness, tingling, pain, and itching. Skin is initially swollen and red and gradually takes on a gray-blue discoloration. The entire foot may appear black, but deep tissue destruction may not be present. After a few days, a hyperemic state sets in. Between 2 and 6 weeks later, these symptoms gradually subside, but the extremity may still be sensitive to cold. Superficial gangrene may be present.

Management is similar to that of second-degree frostbite. Elevation of the foot and careful wound management are essential. Physical therapy is used to maintain range of motion.

CHILBLAIN (PERNIO)

Chilblain occurs when the skin is exposed to cold for extended periods but the core of the body remains warm. For example, mountain climbers, whose skin is exposed to cold but whose body core is kept warm by exertion, are at risk for chilblain. Exposure to dry air that is just above freezing results in superficial ulceration of the skin similar to that seen in second-degree frostbite. As with frostbite, treatment consists of rewarming and very conservative tissue management.

OPHTHALMIC INJURY

Corneal injury caused by freezing of the eye as a result of exposure to high windchill and reflected ultraviolet radiation at high altitudes can cause keratitis with opacification and corneal pitting. Eyewear that screens out ultraviolet radiation and protects the eyes from wind is recommended to prevent corneal injury. Treatment consists of aggressive ophthalmologic intervention with cycloplegia, mydriasis, and antibiotics.

Toxic Epidermal Necrolysis

Toxic epidermal necrolysis (TEN) is not a thermal injury per se but the name given to a group of dermatologic disorders

Table 5   Classification of Frostbite

Degree of Injury	Features
First degree	Hyperemia and edema, without skin necrosis
Second degree	Vesicle formation along with hyperemia, edema, and partial-thickness skin necrosis
Third degree	Full-thickness skin necrosis
Fourth degree	Full-thickness skin necrosis, including necrosis of underlying muscle and bone, with subsequent gangrene

characterized by inflammation-induced separation of epidermis and dermis followed by epidermal skin sloughing. The denuded areas are comparable to those affected by a second-degree burn. Oral mucosal sloughing is also characteristic of TEN. Complications such as infection, malnutrition, negative nitrogen balance, severe wound pain, and multiple organ dysfunction syndrome are identical to those seen in patients with major burns. Mortality is very high if these complications are not optimally managed. Patients should be treated in a burn center, especially for wound care and control of infectious complications [*see Figure 8*]. The role of the dermatologist is to define the diagnosis and determine the potential etiology.

CLINICAL MANIFESTATIONS

A prodrome of TEN usually consists of signals of upper respiratory tract infection, such as high fever, sore throat, and malaise. Then, 1 to 2 days after these symptoms appear, the skin of the face and extremities usually becomes tender and erythem-

atous. Lesions appear either as large surfaces of red skin or as target lesions that are 2 cm in diameter and consist of concentric rings of erythema.

These lesions soon combine to form large affected areas. In 24 to 96 hours, the involved skin begins to form small blisters or large bullae. Moderate traction of the erythematous skin results in separation of the epidermis from the dermis, a positive Nikolsky's sign. When the bullae rupture, large denuded areas of skin become apparent over the patient's entire body. Fingernails, toenails, and the skin of the palms and soles may also slough.

The most characteristic feature of this disease is severe inflammation of the mouth. Blisters develop on the oral mucosa, leaving a very raw, red surface. The lips may be swollen and crusted with clotted blood. The lesions may be confined to the oral cavity or may extend to the larynx or even to the trachea, the bronchi, and the esophagus. The patient is often unable to eat. The eyelids swell as conjunctival inflammation develops. Conjunctival infection, usually caused by *Staphylococcus aureus*,

Figure 8 Shown is an algorithm for treatment of toxic epidermal necrolysis (TEN).

may lead to scarring and permanent blindness. The nasal and urethral mucosa may also become inflamed, and erosions can develop on the genital and perianal skin.

Systemic signs of the disease include high fever and leukocytosis. In severe cases, gastrointestinal bleeding is common. Renal failure can also occur as a result of hypovolemia, the septic response, or membranous glomerulonephritis. In up to 50% of cases, there are abnormalities in liver enzymes, including modest increases in aspartate aminotransferase (AST) and alanine aminotransferase (ALT). Bilirubin also shows a modest increase. The mechanism of these increases, which appear to be a part of the toxic component of TEN, is unknown.

TREATMENT

There are three main components to treatment of TEN that should be initiated after the skin sloughing has occurred. The first step is restoration and maintenance of cardiopulmonary stability. The second step is aggressive wound management, similar to that of a massive second-degree burn, in which the emphasis is on optimizing healing and controlling infection. The third step is optimizing nutrition and modulating the hypermetabolic response caused by the toxic elements of the underlying disease process and by the lesion itself. Treatment also includes the use of nutritional supplements to attenuate the inflammation-induced disease.

Restoration of Cardiopulmonary Stability

Lung function is often impaired early as a result of aspirated secretions from involved oral mucosa. Reduced clearance of secretions because of oral pain and overall weakness also impairs lung function. Pain control, rest periods, and aggressive pulmonary toilet to assist the patient's cough are the first line of defense. Suctioning can lead to significant bleeding and should be used either sparingly or only after the patient has an endotracheal tube in place. The patient should be intubated if lung function is progressively impaired by a disease process that is expected to last at least 10 to 14 days. Partial ventilatory assistance is often required if the patient is intubated, because chest wall pain, systemic toxicity, and weakness can severely impair spontaneous ventilatory efforts.

Cardiovascular function is initially impaired as a result of hypervolemia caused by fluid loss into the wounds, increased skin losses, and decreased oral intake. As in the treatment of a burn, intravascular volume replacement and evaporative water replacement are required. Controlling the febrile response will also help decrease fluid losses, vasodilatation, and the resulting hyperadrenergic response. Careful use of nonsteroidal anti-inflammatory drugs is often needed to keep the patient's temperature below 102° F (38.9° C). The use of an ibuprofen or acetaminophen elixir along with antacids is usually successful in lowering temperature.

Wound Management and Infection Control

Early in the course of TEN, the wounds evolve into a skin slough at the epidermal-dermal junction. In severe cases, the basal lamina of the dermis is destroyed. If the patient is seen before the wounds progress to superinfection, the blisters can be removed and the surface covered with an antibiotic grease gauze (e.g., Xeroform), a skin substitute, and then a soft outer gauze dressing to soak up secretions. The advantage of this approach is that the wound becomes occluded, which decreases pain, fluid loss, and risk of superinfection and improves healing rate. The outer gauze should be changed as needed to remove the plasma leak (usually twice a day). Leaving the inner dressing in place

optimizes the wound environment for healing and minimizes pain. Cultures of the wound surface and exudate should be performed frequently to monitor for superinfection. If an infection is detected early in the course of TEN (i.e., days 1 to 5), the pathogen is almost always *S. aureus*.

If the wounds are already infected when the patient is first seen, gentle debridement followed by administration of topical antibiotics (e.g., silver sulfadiazine) is required, especially if there is an exudate or eschar on the skin surface. Use of immersion hydrotherapy or showers for these painful superficial wounds may not be feasible, because they may be too painful and because there is a risk that the infection will be spread to clean wounds [see Table 6]. Adequate pain control is essential. Morphine, given as a continuous I.V. infusion or as oral long-acting tablets (e.g., MS Contin), is a good choice.

The role of corticosteroids in the treatment of TEN remains unclear. If started before the skin sloughing occurs, when the disease process is just beginning, corticosteroids can attenuate the process, resulting in less sloughing. However, once vesicles have formed and the separation has occurred, corticosteroids no longer effectively attenuate skin sloughing; in fact, they retard the rate of healing. Aggressive oral care is critical because of the high risk of local mouth infection and consequent wound and lung infection. Early and continued assessment and aggressive management of corneal involvement are required. Administration of ophthalmic antibiotic ointments and gentle breaking of adhesions between conjunctiva and eyelids with a small glass rod are the standard treatment.

Optimizing Nutrition

Nutrition is a major component of care. Total nutrition often cannot be delivered orally because of oral lesions. Delivery of nutrition by a small gastric feeding tube is preferred, if the tube can be accurately placed. If esophagitis is severe, tube placement may be difficult. A nutritional regimen comparable to that prescribed for a person with a large burn is indicated. This regimen includes 30 to 35 calories/kg body weight and a protein content of 1.5 to 2 g/kg body weight. Supplements can be beneficial: additional glutamine (30 g/day) can help heal the gut and skin epithelium and restore cell glutathione levels. In addition, increased daily doses of vitamin C (2 to 4 g), vitamin E (400 units), zinc sulfate (440 mg), selenium (50 mg), and vitamin A (25,000 units) will assist in the wound-healing process and augment tissue antioxidant levels. If adequate nutrition cannot be provided enterally, parenteral supplementation is needed.

Table 6 Wound Management in Toxic Epidermal Necrolysis

Stage and Type of Wound	Treatment
Early, uninfected	Debride blisters Cover wound with Xeroform gauze or skin substitute Cover wound with soft outer gauze dressing; change b.i.d. until drainage decreased Administer antibiotic for *Staphylococcus aureus*, if identified
Late, infected	Debride after initiating systemic antibiotic treatment if infection is invasive Apply topical antibiotics b.i.d.

Discussion

Terminology of Electrical Burns

Familiarity with the appropriate terminology is necessary for an understanding of injuries caused by electrical current [see Table 7].

VOLTAGE AND AMPERAGE

Electrical injuries are classified as low voltage (less than 1,000 volts) and high voltage (usually greater than 1,000 volts). Injuries associated with low voltage are most likely to occur in the home, electrocutions in bathtubs and by electric hair dryers being the most common causes of death associated with low voltage. Injuries caused by high voltage typically occur outdoors, near power sources and lines. Electrical current can arc (jump) 1 in. from a power source or line for every 10,000 volts being carried, so that a person does not have to touch the source to sustain injury.

The severity of injury to tissues depends on the amperage, that is, the amount of current passing through the tissues. Because of the variability of resistance and exposure time, it is impossible to quantify precisely the amperage at the time of an accident, but the amperage can be inferred from the voltage of the source. A low-voltage source is capable of producing serious cardiopulmonary complications and death if a current passing across the chest is strong enough to initiate ventricular fibrillation.

A high-voltage source is usually required to produce tissue necrosis along the path of the current [see Table 8]. The damage is caused by both heat production and direct current. Initial resistance to the flow of current—namely, skin or clothing—is overcome by the heat generated by high voltage. Tissue necrosis occurs with continued contact. Over a short period of time,

a dry hand may have sufficient resistance to avoid the passage of current from a low-voltage source. However, contact with several thousand degrees of heat from a high-tension source causes immediate local coagulation and disruption of the electrical barrier. Because water is an excellent conductor, the current can pass more readily through tissues with a high water content. Tissue damage at the contact site can be seen with low voltage as well, again because of local heat generation. A good example is the oral burn seen in children who have bitten an electrical cord.

Besides heat injury, there is tissue damage from the current itself. The mechanism of tissue damage is not completely understood, but there is clearly injury to the nerves, blood vessels, and muscle from the current itself, damaging the cells. When endothelial cells are injured, there is no protection against local clotting and microvascular thrombosis, resulting in tissue devascularization.

RESISTANCE

The resistance of tissues to the passage of current depends in large part on water content, water being a good conductor. In decreasing order, tissue resistance is highest in bone and lower in fat, tendons, skin, muscles, vessels, and nerves. Skin resistance also depends on its moisture content, a moist hand having 10 to 100 times less resistance to the passage of current than a dry hand. With high voltage, however, the current readily passes through all tissues indiscriminately. Heat produced as the current passes is proportional to tissue resistance (heat = $amp^2 \times R$). High voltage can generate local heat of sufficient degree (more than 1,000° C) to cause bone destruction and total coagulation necrosis of surrounding tissues. Heat produced as the current enters and exits the body also leads to coagulation necrosis of the skin and underlying tissues.

PATHWAY OF CURRENT

The pathway of current can be unpredictable, but current generally passes from a point of entry through the body to a grounded site, that is, a site that has lower resistance to flow than does air, which is a poor conductor. Extremely high voltage sources usually exit in multiple areas in an explosive fashion. When current passes from hand to hand or hand to thorax, there is a higher risk of cardiac fibrillation than when current follows a hand-to-foot path. If current passes through the head, it is likely to cause an initial respiratory arrest and subsequent severe neurologic impairment.

Table 7 Terminology of Electrical Burns

Voltage (electrical or energy potential) is electromotive force generated by the power source.

Amperage (intensity) is the amount of current flowing per unit of time.

Resistance to flow is measured in ohms.

$$Resistance = \frac{Voltage}{Amperage} \qquad Amperage = \frac{Voltage}{Resistance}$$

Household current = 110 to 220 volts
Residential power lines = 5,000 to 10,000 volts
High-tension wire = Up to 100,000 volts

Heat: Electrical current produces heat when it meets a resistance to flow. This process is defined by Joule's law, with the heat production defined in terms of joules (J): $J = I^2RT$, where I = amperage, R = resistance, and T = contact time

Electrical current produces tissue damage in two ways:
  1. Local generation of heat during passage of current
  2. Direct tissue damage by current

The degree of tissue injury depends on the following:
  Voltage of the source
  Amperage of current passing through the tissues
  Resistance of tissues traversed by current
  Duration of contact
  Pathway of current
  Type of current: alternating (AC) or direct (DC)

Table 8 Effect of Current on Severity of Injury

Type of Current	Effect
High-tension source: ≥ 5,000 mA	Destruction of tissue by heat and coagulation Cardiopulmonary failure

Household source:
  60 mA
  30 mA
  5 mA
	
	Cardiac fibrillation
	Respiratory muscle tetany; suffocation
	Pain

mA—milliamperes

TYPE AND DURATION OF CURRENT

Most household current is alternating. Low-voltage AC is more dangerous than direct current (DC) of the same voltage because it produces muscle tetany. The tetany is caused by rapid depolarization and repolarization, impeding attempts at escape from the source of electricity. Injuries caused by high-voltage AC are also more severe than those caused by high-voltage DC, although both have devastating effects. The severity of injury is directly proportional to the duration of current flow, but even brief exposure to high amperage produces massive tissue damage.

Recommended Reading

ELECTRICAL INJURY

Bhatt D, Lee R: Rhabdomyolysis due to pulsed electrical fields. Plast Reconstr Surg 86:1, 1990

Bingham H: Electrical burns. Clin Plast Surg 13:75, 1986

Daniel R, Ballard P, Heroux P, et al: High voltage electrical injury: acute pathophysiology. J Hand Surg 13:44, 1988

Grossman R, Tempereau C: Auditory and neuropsychiatric behavior patterns after electrical injury. J Burn Care Rehabil 14:169, 1993

Grube B, Heimbach P: Acute and delayed neurological sequelae of electrical injury. Electrical Trauma. Lee R, Ed. Cambridge University Press, New York, 1992, p 133

Hiestant D, Colice G: Lightning-strike injury. J Intens Care Med 3:303, 1988

Hunt J, Mason A, Masterson T, et al: The pathophysiology of acute electrical injuries. J Trauma 16:335, 1976

Hunt J, Sato R, Baxter C: Acute electric burns. Arch Surg 115:434, 1980

Lee R, Gaylor D: Role of cell membrane rupture in the pathogenesis of electrical trauma. J Surg Res 44:709, 1988

Lee R, Kolodney M: Electrical injury mechanisms: dynamics of the thermal response. Plast Reconstr Surg 80:663, 1987

Luce E: Electrical injuries. Reconstructive Plastic Surgery. McCarthy, Ed. WB Saunders Co, Philadelphia, 1990, p 110

COLD INJURY

Arregui R, Morandeira JR, Martinez G, et al: Epidural neurostimulation in the treatment of frostbite. PACE Pacing Clin Electrophysiol 12:713, 1989

Beitner R, Chen-Zion M, Sofer-Bassukevitz Y, et al: Treatment of frostbite with the calmodulin antagonists thioridazine and trifluoperazine. Gen Pharmacol 20:641, 1989

Bourne M, Prepcorn M, et al: Analysis of microvascular changes in frostbite injury. J Surg Res 40:26, 1986

Britt LD, Dascombe WH, Rodriguez A: New horizons in management of hypothermia and frostbite injury. Surg Clin North Am 71:345, 1991

Galloway H, Suh JS, Parker S, et al: Radiologic case study: late sequelae of frostbite. Orthopedics 14:191, 1991

Gregory JS, Flancbaum L, Townsend MC, et al: Incidence and timing of hypothermia in trauma patients undergoing operations. J Trauma 31:795, 1991

Heggers J, McCauley R, Robson M: Cold-induced injury: frostbite. Total Burn Care. Herndon D, Ed. WB Saunders Co, Philadelphia, 1996, p 39

Vogel JE, Dellon AL: Frostbite injuries of the hand. Clin Plast Surg 16:565, 1989

TOXIC EPIDERMAL NECROLYSIS

Dajani AS: The scalded-skin syndrome: relation of phage-group II staphylococci. J Infect Dis 125:548, 1972

Keleman J, Cioffi W, McManus W, et al: Burn center care for patients with toxic epidermal necrolysis. J Am Coll Surg 180:273, 1995

Murphy J, Purdue G, Hunt J: Toxic epidermal necrolysis. J Burn Care Rehabil 18:417, 1997

Acknowledgment

Figures 1, 5, 7, and 8   Marcia Kammerer.

IV PREOPERATIVE PREPARATION

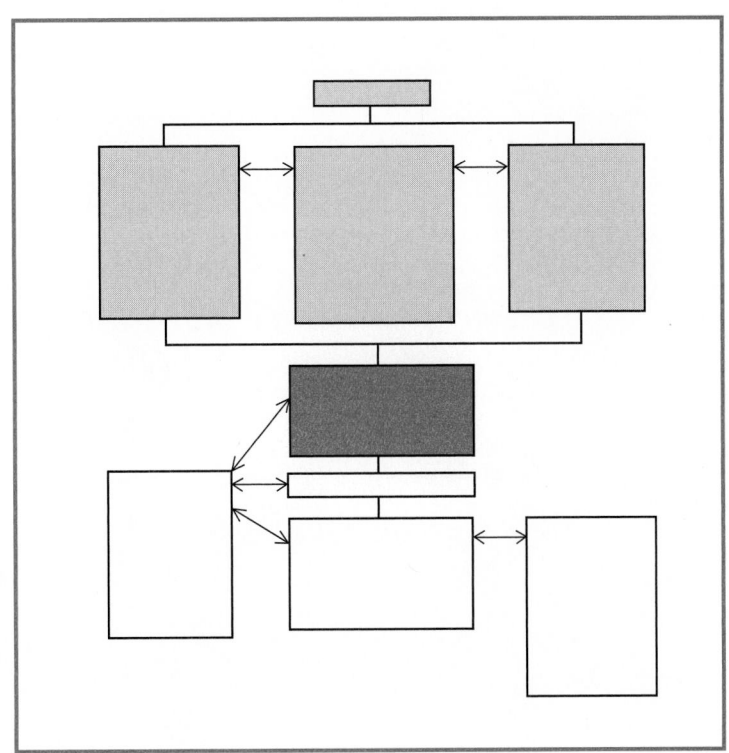

1 ELEMENTS OF COST-EFFECTIVE NONEMERGENCY SURGICAL CARE

Robert S. Rhodes, M.D., and Charles L. Rice, M.D.

The cost and quality of health care concern all industrialized nations, and the responses to these concerns often reflect each nation's particular culture and philosophy. Health care costs in the United States have risen inexorably since 1960 [*see Table 1*].[1] A variety of attempts have been made to control this rise in costs, including price controls (during the Nixon administration) and the introduction of the prospective payment system (during the Reagan administration). Because none of the remedies attempted thus far has been successful, the United States has chosen to address these problems through a number of mechanisms loosely referred to as managed care. In addition to reducing fees paid to providers, managed care focuses on the decision-making aspects of health care: about 75% of the costs of health care result from physician recommendations. As a result, managed care has affected both surgeons' income[2] and their autonomy.

The increased role of managed care in medical decision making has raised concerns that managed care is more about managing cost than about managing care. These concerns are fueled by reports of refusal of care, premature discharges, and termination of care. Growing patient dissatisfaction with such management has produced a backlash.[3]

The issues raised by health care professionals and patients have caused attention to be focused on the cost-effectiveness of medical care. In general terms, cost-effectiveness is defined as cost divided by net benefits. The numerator (cost) is expressed in dollars, and the denominator (net benefits) is expressed as beneficial outcomes minus adverse outcomes. Although the primary goal of cost-effectiveness is to maximize benefits in relation to available resources, cost-effectiveness is also a reflection of health care quality.

In this chapter, we outline the basic principles of cost-effectiveness and address some of the complexities involved. (We do not, however, intend this chapter as a cookbook; modern surgical practice is too dynamic and too diverse for such an approach.) We begin by reviewing the strengths and weaknesses of methods used to assess quality and the relation of quality to cost. We then focus on specific skills and attributes that contribute to cost-effective care. Throughout, we emphasize use of electronic reference sources for access to up-to-date information. An appreciation of the principles, strategies, and tactics of cost-effective surgical care should help surgeons to better serve their patients and their profession as well as help reestablish surgeons' authority in surgical care.

Relation between Quality and Cost

To grasp what cost-effective care is, one must, first, possess an adequate definition of quality and, second, understand the relation between quality and cost. These tasks are more problematic than might at first appear. Traditionally, quality was understood in terms of appropriateness. In the light of this understanding, the relation between cost (expenditure) and quality was viewed exclusively as positive: increased health care expenditure was associated

Table 1   U.S. Health Care Expenditures: Selected Years, 1960–1997[1]

Year	Expenditure for Health Services and Supplies ($ billion)	Total Health Care Expenditure ($ billion)	U.S. Population (million)	Expenditure per Capita ($)	GDP ($ billion)	Expenditure as Percentage of GDP (%)
1960	25.2	26.9	190	141	527	5.1
1970	67.9	73.2	215	341	1,036	7.1
1980	235.6	247.3	235	1,052	2,784	8.9
1990	674.8	699.4	260	2,690	5,744	12.2
1994	917.2	947.7	271	3,500	6,947	13.6
1995	963.1	993.7	273	3,637	7,270	13.7
1996	1,010.6	1,042.5	276	3,781	7,662	13.6
1997	1,057.5	1,092.4	278	3,925	8,111	13.5

GDP—gross domestic product

Table 2 Percentage of GDP Spent on Health Care in Selected Countries: 1960, 1990, and 1997[4]

Year	Expenditure as Percentage of GDP (%)						
	Canada	France	Germany	Japan	United Kingdom	United States	OECD Median for 29 Countries
1960	5.5	4.2	4.8	3.0	3.9	5.2	3.8
1990	9.2	8.9	8.7	6.0	6.0	12.6	7.2
1997	9.0	9.6	10.4	7.3	6.7	13.5	7.5

GDP—gross domestic product   OECD—Organisation for Economic Co-operation and Development

with increased quality and vice versa. However, appropriateness is difficult to define, and even when it is defined, it is difficult to measure. Without accurate definitions or measurements, the relation between cost and quality becomes somewhat theoretical. Thus, with the traditional view of quality, the strongly held positions of providers, purchasers, and patients regarding health care quality (and their subsequent actions) were actually governed more by perceptions than by data.

Several factors eroded this traditional view. One was the realization that even though the United States spends a larger fraction of its gross domestic product (GDP) on health care than does any other industrialized country [*see Table 2*], United States citizens are less healthy—often by wide margins—than citizens of comparable countries [*see Table 3*].[4] Although health status can be significantly influenced by factors outside the health care system (e.g., standard of living, nutrition, sanitation, and safety), the disparity between health care cost and health status in the United States suggested that extravagant health care expenditure did not automatically improve health status.

A second factor, which became apparent before the introduction of managed care, was the growing amount of information on problems with quality in the health care system. For instance, there were data suggesting that one fourth of hospital deaths might be preventable,[5] that one third of hospital procedures might be exposing patients to unnecessary risk, that one third of drugs might not be indicated, and that one third of abnormal laboratory test results might not be followed up by physicians.[6] Reviews of medical records also revealed alarming error rates,[7,8] with as many as half of the adverse events associated with errors in surgical care.

A third factor challenging the traditional relation between quality and cost was the increasing recognition that appropriateness was an insufficient criterion of quality. Without question, some studies of appropriateness had identified valid quality concerns. For instance, researchers at the Rand Corporation, after assessing the appropriateness of carotid endarterectomy, coronary angiography, and upper GI endoscopy, concluded that 32%, 17%, and 17% of these procedures, respectively, were undertaken inappropriately.[9] In another example, an analysis of seven health plans revealed that one in six hysterectomies was inappropriate.[10] Nevertheless, the continued difficulty of measuring appropriateness[11] undermined its value as a standard.[12] For instance, retrospective assessments often judged appropriateness on the basis of outcome alone, without considering processes of care.[13] In addition, appropriateness tended to be judged differently when decisions were made for groups rather than individuals.[14]

A telling blow to the traditional view of the quality-cost relation was the growing awareness of the great disparity in the frequency of surgical procedures within small areas.[15-17] (In addition to these frequency variations, there are also cost variations for seemingly similar services.) The frequency variations proved to be procedure specific. For instance, procedures with highly specific indications (e.g., repair of hip fracture, inguinal herniorrhaphy, and appendectomy) generally exhibited relatively little frequency variation, but carotid endarterectomy, hysterectomy, and coronary angiography exhibited a great deal of variation.[18] The variation also appeared to be related to provider capacity (i.e., number of hospital beds/1,000 persons): one study of the effect of provider capacity on variation noted a close relation between the intensity of local diagnostic testing and invasive cardiac procedures.[19]

Table 3 Health Status and Outcomes in Selected Countries: 1996

	Canada	France	Germany	Japan	United Kingdom	United States	OECD Median for 29 Countries
Percentage of population 65 yr of age or older (%)	12.0	15.4	15.6	14.6	15.6	12.7	14.4
Life expectancy at birth (years)							
Female	81.5	82.0	79.9	83.6	79.3	79.4	80.3
Male	75.4	74.1	73.6	77.0	74.4	72.7	74.0
Infant mortality (per 1,000 live births)	6.0	4.9	5.0	3.8	6.1	7.8	5.8
Potential years of life lost, 1995 (per 100,000 life years)							
Female	3,284	3,092	3,337	2,399	3,616	4,591	3,256
Male	5,451	6,861	6,505	4,443	5,690	8,401	6,281

OECD—Organisation for Economic Co-operation and Development

Several physician factors, such as physician style, a community's so-called practice signature, and physician uncertainty, also appear to be related to variations in the frequency of surgical procedures[20]; this finding lends support to the idea that many medical decisions are based on opinion rather than on evidence.[21] One study even concluded that only about 15% of common medical practices had a documented foundation in any sort of medical research.[22] This conclusion does not necessarily mean that only 15% of care is effective, but it does raise concerns about the lack of hard evidence for most care. In contrast, a subsequent study at a British hospital revealed that 95% of in-hospital surgical patients received treatment based on satisfactory evidence.[23] The different conclusions of these two studies, however, can be accounted for in a number of ways.

Variations in the use of medical services do not correlate with differences in incidence of disease or appropriateness of use.[24] Economic incentives for physicians also appear to have relatively little influence. Thus, there is considerable variation in utilization rates among Veterans Health Administration medical facilities[25] and within countries without fee-for-service reimbursement.

Whether the high utilization rates observed are too high or the low utilization rates are too low is still the subject of debate. The possibility that low frequency of use may reflect restricted access to care is a particular concern, given the association between variation and the ratio of hospital beds to population.[26] Currently, however, the tendency is to believe that the high rates are too high. Moreover, despite the usage variations noted from area to area, providers in each area claim, and often document, equivalent patient health status. This finding led one author to conclude that "marked variability in surgical practices and presumably in surgical judgment and philosophy must be considered to reflect absent or inadequate data by which to evaluate surgical treatment...."[27] The net effect of these developments was to fuel skepticism about the validity of the traditional relation between quality and cost.

The abandonment of the traditional concept of quality as appropriateness was facilitated by the emergence of a new concept of quality,[28] which has three major components: structure (faculties, equipment, and services), process (content of care), and outcomes. This new concept uses many of the industrial quality-control techniques pioneered by W. Edwards Deming and seeks to overcome the shortcomings of the appropriateness criterion. Deming's goal was to minimize quality variations by examining production systems—which, in the case of medicine, are the systems of care. Accordingly, total quality management and continuous quality improvement are increasingly being applied to health care.

This new concept of quality and its relation to cost can be illustrated diagrammatically [see Figure 1].[29] The traditional notion of a positive relation between quality and cost still exists in zones 1 and 2, but the slope of the curve flattens in zone 3 and actually becomes negative in zone 4, where further cost increases are associated with decreased quality. The basis of this effect is that as health care volume increases, the cost-benefit curve flattens but the cost-harm curve does not (i.e., side effects are just as common in patients with mild disease as in those with severe disease).[28] The implication is that reducing use of health care resources in zones 3 and 4 may not detract from quality but actually improve it.

This new concept of quality has intellectual appeal, but like the traditional concept, it remains somewhat theoretical. Because quality itself remains difficult to define, the new construct still oversimplifies the issues. To be more relevant, any definition of the relation of quality to cost should also consider overuse, underuse, and misuse.[30] Despite the shortcomings in definition and measurement, the new three-part concept of quality is widely accepted and has become the template for many profound changes in the United States health care system.

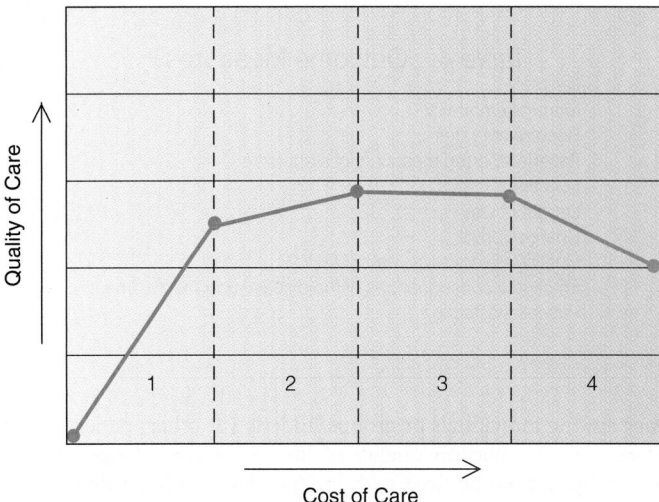

Figure 1 **Illustrated is the new concept of quality and cost.**[29]

The traditional concept of quality as appropriateness persists today and is at least partly responsible for the fears many patients and health care professionals have about the impact of managed care on quality. The lack of clear data on quality has led to a buyer's market, in which health care purchasers use the apparent similarity in quality, despite variations in frequency and cost, as a rationale for contracting for less expensive care. Purchasers assume that even in an atmosphere of decreasing income and increasing constraints, providers will not knowingly or willingly sacrifice quality. Indeed, they believe that competition may spark a drive to exceed patients' expectations. The medical profession, whose authority was once strong enough to forestall system change, now bears the burden of proof. Practitioners and other providers have become primary targets of those calling for assessment and accountability in health care.

Assessment of Outcome

Of the three components of the new concept of quality, outcome assessment has received the most attention.[30] The list of traditional outcome measures [see Table 4][31] is now being superseded by one that is increasingly diverse. Length of stay, costs, and patient satisfaction are increasingly important. The current focus on treatment outcomes also emphasizes long-term health status. Thus, in addition to the immediate morbidity and mortality of a given procedure, there is interest in long-term functional status.

A preferred measure of these long-term outcomes is the health care quality of life or quality-adjusted life years (QALYs),[32,33] a summary measure of the length of time one experiences a given health status. Of the several systems that quantify this health status,[34] some include objective measures (e.g., functional status), whereas others use subjective estimates of well-being. The latter often involve patients' estimates of the meaningfulness of a given functional status. For instance, patient A may not be able to walk as far as patient B, but one cannot conclude that patient A therefore has a poorer quality of life unless that functional status is placed in a context that is meaningful to patient A.[35]

Although health status is thought to be more easily quantified than appropriateness, its measurement still involves considerable subjectivity. For instance, a given individual's estimate of the future value of an outcome measure may vary with time or according to the specific circumstances at assessment. QALYs may also

---

Table 4 Outcome Measures[31]

Morbidity/mortality
Recurrence rates
Patient-reported measures of symptoms
Functional status
Length of stay
Charges/costs
Quality-adjusted life years (QALYs)
Emotional consequences of the disease and the treatment
Patient satisfaction

---

vary among individuals or groups. Elderly (or other) patients may place greater value on quality of life and less on longevity if a longer life cannot be lived with independence.[36] Such differences underscore the impact of ethnicity, religious beliefs, socioeconomic status, and attitudes about health care. Because outcomes have experiential, physiologic, and resource dimensions, patients, providers, and health care purchasers may have entirely different views about which measure is best for judging the outcome of a given intervention. Further complexities may result if there is a discrepancy among measures (e.g., an outcome that is deemed successful by a provider but does not satisfy the patient).

Outcome measures must also take into account health status and severity of illness before treatment,[37] and the necessary adjustments can be difficult. Measuring outcomes may also pose other problems.[38,39] For instance, if outcome measures are valid indices for improving quality of care, the implication is that they must also be intimately related to the processes of care.[30]

Despite concerns that managed care focuses more on cost than on care, managed care organizations are taking significant steps toward assuring quality. At present, the leading organization in this area is the National Committee for Quality Assurance (NCQA) (http://www.ncqa.org). Self-described as a "nonprofit watchdog organization," the NCQA is dominated by the managed care industry it is supposed to evaluate and by large employers. Its two most significant activities are (1) accrediting health care plans and (2) developing and refining the Healthplan Employer Data and Information Set (HEDIS). HEDIS measures focus primarily on utilization and management, but with each revision, more attention is given to the quality of clinical care. Most of the HEDIS measures involve screening, preventive measures (e.g., mammography or smoking cessation), or both.

The Foundation for Accountability (FACCT) (http://www.facct.org) is an independent organization that is establishing standards of care. The National Forum for Health Care Quality Measurement and Reporting (http://www.qualityforum.org) is another important organization. Several recent reports summarize the broader scope of organizational efforts to improve quality in health care.[40-42] Although such efforts will undoubtedly produce some improvements in care, surgeons should recognize that the greatest impact on surgical care is likely to emanate from individual efforts at the grassroots level.

Skills Required for Evidence-Based Decision Making

The most cost-effective care (i.e., the highest-quality care at the lowest cost) will be delivered through evidence-based medical practice. However, such practice requires skills that often are not emphasized during undergraduate and graduate medical education, such as statistical analysis, critical literature analysis, and technology assessment. Acquiring these skills, together with the

computer literacy essential for their application, creates the infrastructure for quality improvement.

STATISTICAL ANALYSIS

Statistical analysis is essential for understanding variations in outcomes, interpreting the medical literature, and evaluating one's own performance. Before the Medicare Prospective Payment System and diagnosis-related groups (DRGs) were implemented, hospital Medicare reimbursement was based on cost. Variations in the use of hospital resources were primarily of academic interest and had relatively few fiscal implications. Under prospective payment, however, hospital reimbursement changed to a system based on national averages rather than actual costs. As a result, the Healthcare Financing Administration transferred the concern over the fiscal implications of these cost variations to the hospitals, and private payers now follow Medicare's lead.

The distribution of variation in medical outcomes tends to have a characteristic shape. Instead of having normal distributions, many outcomes, such as cost and length of hospital stay, tend to have skewed distributions, with the tail toward higher costs or longer stay [*see Figure 2*]. Thus, the mean (or average) value is likely to be greater than the median (or middle) value. However, the overall cluster around the mean or median and the width of the curve vary according to the specific procedure and provider. The longer the tail, the less characteristic of a particular outcome the mean value is. Because the distribution is skewed, the mean is often calculated as the mean of the logarithm of the individual values. This logarithmic average, also known as the geometric mean, is the basis of the length-of-stay calculations of the DRGs.

Currently, the variation in many medical costs and other outcomes is relatively large, often exceeding 200% to 300%. Some of this variation is an expected part of many biologic processes, and some can be accounted for by differences in severity. Consequently, it would probably be difficult to achieve the industry-standard low variation sought by Deming. Still, there is considerable room for improvement [*see* Assessment of Performance, *below*].

Health care purchasers are well aware of cost variations among providers and use low-cost providers as benchmarks toward which other providers are expected to strive. These benchmarks, which occupy the extreme left portion of the curve, are considered to

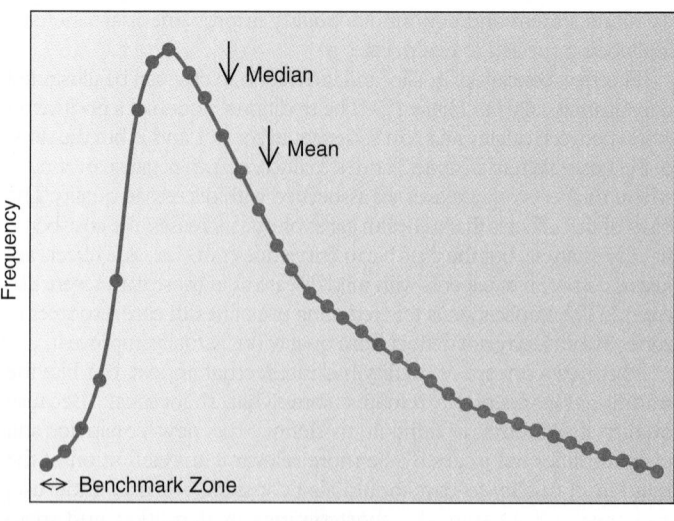

Figure 2 Shown is the skewed distribution curve associated with health care outcomes such as cost or length of stay.

represent best practice and are believed likely to contain lessons for management of similar patients. Such benchmarks, however, often reflect an ideal (i.e., exceptional) patient population rather than a normal one[43]; consequently, applying them to more complicated patients who need more care may increase the risk of adverse outcomes in this setting. Still, understanding the meaning and significance of variation in outcome measures is essential to assessing one's own practice.

Another vital application of statistical analysis to cost-effectiveness is in laboratory and radiologic testing. Such testing accounts for some of the largest increases in health care costs and much of the cost variation. Traditionally, the value of a test was often determined on the basis of its sensitivity (i.e., ability to positively identify patients with a disease) or specificity (i.e., ability to identify patients without a disease).[44] Today, however, these characteristics, by themselves, should no longer be considered sufficient justification for a particular test. The test's value or utility—characteristics that take disease prevalence into account—must also be considered.

For instance, if a test with a 98% sensitivity and a 98% specificity is applied to a group of patients with a disease prevalence of 50% (i.e., a group in which half the patients have the disease being tested for), 245 of every 500 patients tested ($500 \times 0.98 \times 0.5$) will have true positive results and five ($500 \times 0.02 \times 0.5$) will have false positive results. If, however, this same test is applied to 500 members of a population with a disease prevalence of 10%, 49 patients ($500 \times 0.98 \times 0.1$) will have true positive results and nine ($500 \times 0.02 \times 0.9$) will have false positive results. Thus, for a given sensitivity, the ratio of true positives to false positives increases with increasing prevalence of disease in a given patient population, and the opposite holds true as well. Given that most tests are neither as sensitive nor as specific as the one used in this example, the incidence of false positives in the real world is likely to be that much greater. This relation between disease prevalence and the incidence of false positives helps explain why a test with relatively little value as a screening test for a given disease in general practice can be valuable for specialists who see many more patients with that disease.

Increases in diagnostic testing tend to parallel increases in clinically relevant downstream procedures.[45] For instance, there is a known association between the intensity of local diagnostic testing and the frequency of invasive cardiac procedures.[19] Any increase in the number of patients who undergo cardiac catheterization as a result of false positive screening test results increases the number of patients with negative findings who may have complications of catheterization; preoperative evaluation of cardiac function in patients undergoing peripheral vascular surgery provides a specific example. Moreover, the difference in shape between cost-benefit and cost-harm curves demonstrates that besides raising costs, exposing patients to the risks of unnecessary tests may reduce the net benefits of outcomes. The problem of false positives affects both the numerator and the denominator of cost-effectiveness.

Another example of the application of test utility to clinical decision making is found in the functional assessment of incidental adrenal masses.[46] Analysis shows that in the absence of concrete signs and symptoms, measuring specific hormone levels may be of little value. Close inspection of many other routine preoperative tests reveals that they, too, may have little value.[47,48] More selective ordering of tests may be particularly important in capitated systems to minimize the so-called nonfee costs of tests that contribute little or nothing to diagnosis, treatment, or outcome.

Another application of statistical analysis is in clinical decision analysis, in which the effect or impact of each option involved in a medical decision is quantified to yield the probability statistics for that decision. Through the use of a decision tree, the components of deci-

sion making (i.e., the underlying assumptions) become explicit, which then enables one to appreciate or discount the role of factors perhaps not previously considered.[49] Thus, clinical decision analysis is valuable for reducing uncertainty and for estimating cost-effectiveness.[50-52] Although some clinicians may be intimidated by the mathematics involved and others may be bothered by what may seem a cookbook approach to health care, it is clear that sensitivity analyses can yield estimates of the importance of specific facets of care that might be difficult to obtain otherwise. Several reviews of surgery-related decision analyses have been published.[53]

CRITICAL LITERATURE ANALYSIS

Surgeons also need to be better at critical literature analysis, which involves both finding evidence on which to base decisions and being able to judge the quality of that evidence. Access to the Internet is essential because of the high number of useful Web sites and the speed of information retrieval. Three Web sites offer a good sampling of the level of information available. MEDLINE and other databases of the National Library of Medicine (http://www.ncbi.nlm.nih.gov/entrez/query.fcgi?db=PubMed), access to which is free, are particularly useful resources. Another site is the Cochrane Collaboration (http://www.update-software.com/ccweb/cochrane/cdsr.htm), an international network of clinicians and epidemiologists who systematically review the best available evidence on medical care.[54] The Cochrane Collaboration includes sources not always accessible through MEDLINE, but a subscription is required. A third useful resource is the British National Health Services Centre for Evidence-Based Medicine (http://cebm.jr2.ox.ac.uk).

Assessing the evidence is as important as finding it. The randomized, controlled trial is often considered the gold standard for evaluating health care, and the number of such trials is growing rapidly.[30] Many such trials pertain to surgery and are accessible through MEDLINE or the Cochrane Collaboration. Yet these trials also have several shortcomings. One is that the methods for reporting them have not been standardized.[55] Another is that stringent inclusion criteria may limit the applicability of the results to certain defined subgroups. Even when it appears that the findings do apply to a particular patient, it may be difficult to reproduce them in a setting that differs from the carefully controlled conditions under which the original trial was conducted. Thus, a test or treatment that is efficacious under the ideal circumstances of a trial may not be effective under less than ideal circumstances.

Carotid endarterectomy provides an excellent example of the crucial distinction between efficacy and effectiveness. Randomized, controlled trials have shown this procedure to be efficacious when performed by surgeons with low perioperative mortality and stroke rates.[56,57] Yet the effectiveness of the procedure depends on continued performance with a similarly low incidence of complications: as the incidence of stroke and other complications increases, carotid endarterectomy may become less effective or entirely ineffective.[58-60] This example illustrates the strong ethical reasons for being familiar with one's results. If patients are to give truly informed consent, they should have access to information about the outcomes their surgeon has achieved in similar patients.

The extent to which results can be generalized is a concern that applies to all studies, not just to randomized, controlled trials. In a study of the value of computed tomography in the diagnosis of appendicitis, the clinical likelihood of appendicitis in 100 patients was estimated by the referring surgeon and assigned to one of four categories: (1) definitely appendicitis (80% to 100%), (2) probably appendicitis (60% to 79%), (3) equivocally appendicitis (40% to 59%), and (4) possibly appendicitis (20% to 39%).[61] These estimates were then compared with the estimated probability of appendicitis determined via CT; the pathology (or lack thereof) was confirmed by operation or recovery. The CT interpretations had a sensitivity of 98%, a specificity of 98%, a positive predictive value of 98%, a negative predictive value of 98%, and an accuracy of 98% for either diagnosing or ruling out appendicitis. The actual incidences of appendicitis in each of the categories were 78%, 56%, 33%, and 44%, respectively. The difference between the true incidence and the initial clinical estimates indicates that surgeons' estimates of outcomes can differ from the actual data. A second point worth emphasizing in this study concerns the extent of cost savings. The authors calculated a savings of $447 per patient; however, costs (and any savings) are likely to vary in conjunction with a number of factors, including surgeons' estimates of the clinical likelihood of appendicitis, the availability of less expensive alternatives to in-hospital observation, and the use of the ED for triage. In this study, 53% of the patients had appendicitis; in other studies, as few as 30% of patients with an admitting diagnosis of appendicitis eventually underwent appendectomy.[62] Thus, the applicability of study results is likely to vary from institution to institution.

Another aspect of literature analysis concerns the distinction between relative and absolute risk reduction. This issue often arises in reports addressing the effectiveness of cancer therapies. A treatment that reduces recurrence from 5% to 4% and one that reduces it from 50% to 40% can both be said to achieve a 20% relative reduction in risk. Clearly, reporting effectiveness in terms of relative improvement may be misleading if the baseline outcome is ignored.[63] Patients' interest in adjuvant therapy (and their willingness to tolerate side effects) may be affected more by absolute reductions in risk than by relative reductions.

Another pitfall in assessing outcomes arises with tests that allow diagnosis at an earlier stage of disease. Earlier diagnosis does not necessarily mean longer survival: it simply means that a patient with presymptomatic disease identified by screening is aware of the condition for a longer time. The equation of earlier awareness with extended survival is referred to as lead-time bias. In general, advances in diagnostic imaging increase the likelihood of such bias and overestimate disease prevalence.[64]

Additional information on critical analysis of the medical literature can be found in a number of excellent references.[21,65-73]

Finally, critical literature analysis is essential for keeping pace with patients' growing access to medical information. There are now more than 15,000 health-related Web sites [see Table 5],[74] and it is estimated that in 1999, well over 20 million adults found health information online. Because some of this information may be inaccurate, misleading, or unconventional,[75] surgeons must be aware of what their patients may know—or, even more to the point, may believe they know.

TECHNOLOGY ASSESSMENT

Explosive technological growth has increased the need for technology assessment. Inarguably, many technological advances have greatly improved surgical care. Moreover, there is a prevailing societal attitude equating the latest with the best, which places considerable pressure on surgeons and hospitals to acquire the newest equipment and techniques, even when these have not been fully tested. Nevertheless, not every new technology proves successful. For example, laser endarterectomy and the use of gastric freezing machines to control upper GI bleeding represented sizable investments in technology but turned out to be of little value.

Surgeons must recognize how factors affecting decisions about technology acquisition contribute to excess capacity within the health care system. The pressure to acquire technology is often strongest in communities with the greatest competition among health care providers. Out of a compulsion to be first, providers often rush to acquire new technology before its value is proved, with other providers, fearing to be left behind, often following right behind. The result can be double jeopardy: if the new technology is unsuccessful, it has added to cost without increasing benefit; if it is successful, more of it will probably be put in place than the community needs. Competition among health care providers can help restrain the growth in health care costs; however, when driven by the so-called technological imperative, it can also contribute to inflationary increases in these costs.

The American College of Surgeons has developed a series of questions to be answered before a new surgical technology is applied to patient care [see Table 6].[76] Although these questions seem both reasonable and straightforward, the answers may be difficult to find, slow in coming, or contradictory. For example, laparoscopic cholecystectomy became rapidly diffused throughout the surgical community before the answers to these questions were known. Fortunately, in this case, the answers appear to be favorable.

An interesting paradox of new technology is that lower cost per procedure may, as a result of increases in volume, actually increase aggregate costs. Such is the case with laparoscopic cholecystectomy.[77] It also exemplifies how patients and purchasers of health care might reach differing opinions as to the "value" of new technology.

Preventive Approaches and Process Measures

COORDINATION OF CARE AND DISEASE MANAGEMENT

Coordination of care is having a growing impact on the quality of medical care. By preventing duplication of tests and unnecessary delays, coordination of care both improves patient satisfaction and saves money. In one analysis, the most frequent cause of delay was scheduling of tests (31%), followed by unavailability of postdischarge facilities (18%), physician decision making (13%), discharge planning (12%), and scheduling of surgery (12%).[78] Given the current patchwork nature of the health care system, however, preventing delays can be difficult and time-consuming. Increased consolidation of health care purchasers may alleviate some of the delays.

The growing number of patients with a given health problem in a single system is also leading to the use of what is known as disease management. This practice, which represents a step beyond coordination of care, involves an explicit, systematic population-based approach that identifies patients at risk, intervenes with specific programs of care, and measures clinical and other outcomes.[79] Disease management is a distinctly preventive approach.

CRITICAL PATHWAYS

Although outcome assessment is the aspect of the new concept of quality that has received the most attention, the importance of structure and process must not be minimized. Some would even argue that measures of process (i.e., what is done to a patient) are more sensitive indicators of quality of care than measures of outcome (i.e., what happens to a patient) because poor outcomes do not occur every time an incorrect decision is made.[39] The concept of process measurement is embodied in critical pathways, an increasingly common method of standardizing treatments of high-volume diagnoses. The purpose of critical pathways is to minimize variation by displaying optimal goals for both patients and providers. Such pathways have been developed by a number of groups and organizations and are available commercially, through surgical societies,[80] and in focused publications.[81] The Agency for

Table 5   Selected Internet Health Care Sites

Site Name	Web Address (URL)	Topics and Formats
Adam.com	www.adam.com	Men's, women's, and children's health, as well as diet and nutrition, first aid, and mental health
AMA Health Information	www.ama-assn.org/ama/pub/category/ 3457.htm	Easily understood information for consumers, plus the capability to search for physicians, hospitals, and medical subjects
AmericasDoctor.com	www.americasdoctor.com	News, bulletin boards, and shopping, plus the ability to chat one-on-one with a health professional
Centers for Disease Control and Prevention	www.cdc.gov	Statistics, news, consumer fact sheets, and other resources on diseases
drkoop.com	www.drkoop.com	Health news and resources for patients
Drug Infonet	www.druginfonet.com	A broad range of pharmaceutical information
Hardin Meta Directory	www.lib.uiowa.edu/hardin/md/index.html	Medical links grouped by category
Health on Oxygen	www.oxygen.com/health	Magazine-style approach on women's health issues
HealthAnswers.com	www.healthanswers.com	Summaries of health news, a drug database, and "health centers" on specific topics
HealthCentral.com	www.healthcentral.com	General interest health site
Healthfinder	www.healthfinder.gov	Government directory of authoritative health information
HealthAtoZ.com	www.healthatoz.com	Family-oriented site with personalization features
InteliHealth	www.intelihealth.com	Joint venture of Aetna and Johns Hopkins, summarizing news and rounding up the latest tools and references
iVillageHealth.com	www.ivillage.com	Magazine-type health coverage
MayoClinic.com	www.mayoclinic.com	Timely health information from the Mayo Clinic
Med Help International	www.medhelp.org	Resources for patients and families
MedicineNet.com	www.medicinenet.com	Health news and resources
Medscape from WebMD	www.medscape.com	Customized home pages on medical topics for physicians
National Institutes of Health	www.nih.gov/health	Umbrella site for the government's health research institutes, including the National Library of Medicine
WebMD	www.webmd.com	Medical news, personalized health information, and support communities; now includes OnHealth

Healthcare Research and Quality (AHRQ) has also established practice guidelines, which are available online (http://www.ahrq. gov or http://www.guideline.gov) or through evidence-based practice centers. The guideline.gov site is part of the National Guideline Clearinghouse, a comprehensive repository for clinical practice guidelines and related materials.

Their current popularity notwithstanding, critical pathways do have limitations. Perhaps the most significant of these is that they focus on quality and efficiency of care *after* the decision has been made to admit the patient or perform a procedure. Another limitation is that standardization per se is not tantamount to quality improvement. A third is that not all guidelines adhere to established methodological standards.[82-85] Summaries of the process of pathway development, implementation, and troubleshooting are readily available elsewhere.[86,87]

Assessment of Performance

Given the impact physician decision making has on health care costs, those who pay these costs will naturally seek to assess physician performance. Surgical interventions are particularly ripe for scrutiny because the costs are easily identified, surgical illnesses generally are of relatively short duration, and outcomes are readily quantified. In contrast, the starting and end points of nonsurgical interventions are often difficult to define.

Calls for assessing surgeon performance are typically met with varying degrees of disinterest or, in some cases, defensiveness. Such was the case roughly 100 years ago in Boston, when E. A. Codman crusaded for hospitals and surgeons to publicize their results.[88] It is human nature for each surgeon to believe that he or she is among the best, but the data clearly show considerable variation in outcomes from one surgeon to another.[89] Health care purchasers and hospitals, equipped with modern information systems, are well aware of this variation; large health care purchasers, in particular, use claims data to create provider performance profiles characterizing hospital and physician costs and outcomes.

The issue is not whether such assessments will be made but who will use them and for what purposes. It seems paradoxical that the data used by purchasers to create these profiles often are not readily available to the surgeons who generate them. Even if surgeons are not aware of their practice profiles, they should be aware that these profiles are likely to have personal economic consequences. One survey of managed care organizations found that in the initial physician selection process, 39% of the organizations were moderately or largely influenced by the physician's previous patterns of costs or utilization, and nearly 70% profiled their member physicians.[90] As health care purchasers merge and expand, their profile data will become increasingly centralized; the use of these profiles as economic credentials is then likely to become more widespread. At least one HMO recently noted that practices with high scores on service and quality indicators attracted significantly more new enrollees than practices with lower scores.[91] By preemptively becoming familiar with their outcome data and with how these data are interpreted and used, surgeons will be better positioned to initiate self-assessment and to respond appropriately to external review.

At present, the main limitation of practice profiles is that they cannot fully account for disease severity factors that affect outcome. The data used to make adjustments for disease severity are usually derived either from claims or administrative data or from medical record review.[92] Medical record review is capable of identifying many more severity factors, but it is much more cumbersome and costly, and it still leaves much of the cost variation unaccounted for.[93] Health care purchasers usually make severity adjustments from claims or administrative data instead; accordingly, the validity of this severity adjustment is particularly distrusted. Moreover, in many claims/administrative databases, the frequency of miscoding may be 10% or higher.

Another limitation of practice profiles is that many of the factors known to affect variations in cost and length of stay are not under surgeons' direct control.[94,95] Patient-related variation may result from age, gender, and cultural, ethnic, and socioeconomic factors extrinsic to the medical care system.[96] Selection bias may also affect reports of outcomes.[97] High rates of inadequate functional health literacy are known to have an adverse effect on compliance (and hence outcomes).[98]

Despite these shortcomings, attempts have been made, and continue to be made, to use currently available methods of severity adjustment to compare providers. These attempts have been associated with considerable controversy. In an early effort, HCFA calculated mortality data for individual hospitals using a risk-adjustment model based on DRGs. After many years, HCFA acknowledged the flaws in the associated mortality model and stopped releasing these data. Subsequently, both HCFA (using Medicare data) and some states publicly disclosed provider-specific data on outcomes of cardiac surgery. Their intent was to educate the public regarding the choice of health care providers. Although these educational efforts used more criteria than were available through DRGs alone,[99,100] the profiles remained highly controversial because they still did not adequately account for all the differences in case severity. Because current severity adjustment may not reflect differences attributable to patient selection, surgeons operating on truly high-risk patients will, all other factors being equal, have poorer outcomes than surgeons operating on truly low-risk patients. However, all other factors may not be equal. If the latter group of surgeons operated on the former group's patients, the outcomes might even be worse, and if the former group operated on the latter group's patients, the outcomes might even be better. Such patient selection among practices is a well-recognized phenomenon.[101]

In addition to these concerns, public release of such data may have unintended consequences. It has been suggested that publicizing provider profiles creates incentives to avoid treating high-risk patients so as to lower risk-adjusted mortality.[102,103] Although consumer guides containing these data appeared to improve quality of care, they also appeared to have limited credibility among cardiovascular specialists.[103] Surveys also indicated that the data were of limited value to the target audience (i.e., patients undergoing cardiac surgery).

Nevertheless, provider report cards are increasingly being made available to the general public. One Web site (http://www.healthgrades.com) contains hospital specialty data on cardiac, orthopedic, neurologic, pulmonary, and vascular surgery. Data on transplantation outcomes are available from the United Network for Organ Sharing (http://www.unos.org). Information on obstetrics and oncology will soon be available at a site that will draw information from the HCFA MEDPAR database.

Two self-assessment projects now under way are worth a brief mention here. One study, under the auspices of the American College of Surgeons,[89,104] compares surgeon outcomes for laparoscopic cholecystectomy, radical prostatectomy, total hip replacement, and lumbar laminectomy by using disease response, patient satisfaction, resource utilization, and severity of illness as the outcome measures. The other study is from the Northern New England Cardiovascular Disease Study Group, which has developed a multi-institutional regional model for the continuous improvement of surgical care.[105] The group possesses certain important characteristics: there is no ambiguity of purpose, the data are not owned by any member or subgroup of members, members have an established safe place to work, a forum is set up for discussion, and regular feedback is provided. Using a systems approach, this group effected a 24% reduction in hospital mortality for cardiac surgery and reduced variation in outcomes among group members. The decrease in mortality was significantly greater than that reported by HCFA and by state report cards on similar procedures. Despite concerns that release of such findings would produce unfavorable publicity, no such reaction occurred. It is noteworthy that the process did not level personal criticism at anyone or attempt to identify the proverbial bad apple. Three important conclusions can be drawn from this study: (1) physician-initiated interventions seem more effective than external review in improving quality, (2) a systems approach to quality improvement is better than the bad-apple approach, and (3) it is possible to conduct quality improvement among practice groups that might otherwise be viewed as competitors.

Table 6 **American College of Surgeons Criteria for Use of New Technology**

Has the new technology been considered adequately tested for safety and efficacy?

Is the new technology at least as safe and effective as existing, proven techniques?

Is the individual proposing to perform the new procedure fully qualified to do so?

Is the new technology cost-effective?

Although self-assessment of quality and cost-effectiveness may seem somewhat daunting, the most difficult step may be the willingness to initiate the process. One must accept from the outset that self-assessment is an ongoing process: as with peeling an onion, the initial step will almost inevitably lead to a more involved procedure. Simple data charts may reveal changes or patterns in a surgeon's outcomes or resource consumption that might not otherwise be obvious.[106] Sometimes, merely standardizing a process is enough to improve outcomes significantly. With time, strategies for optimal practice emerge.[107,108]

A number of studies have reported that increased surgeon or hospital volume is associated with favorable outcomes.[109-114] Such findings led the National Cancer Policy Board of the Institute of Medicine and the National Research Council to conclude that patients requiring complicated cancer operations or chemotherapy should be treated at facilities that perform a large number of these procedures. There also appears to be an inverse relation between hospital volume and cost[115,116]; thus, high-volume institutions may have advantages in both the numerator and the denominator of cost-effectiveness. Similar arguments have been made with regard to the issue of surgical subspecialty training.[117]

One must remember, however, that the data in these studies represent probabilities, not absolute relationships.[118] Thus, one cannot conclude that low volume is always associated with poorer outcomes and high volume with better outcomes. Because some measures can be convincingly assessed only in large patient populations, outcome comparisons can be highly problematic when one is dealing with unusual or infrequent cases. Moreover, the relative importance of hospital volume and surgeon volume may vary with specific procedures: complex, team-dependent procedures (e.g., coronary artery bypass grafting) may be more dependent on hospital volume, whereas less complicated procedures may be more dependent on surgeon volume. A large study of eight common surgical procedures used medical record data rather than claims data but was still unable to establish any correlation between institutional operative volume and postoperative mortality.[119] It therefore remains unclear whether practice makes perfect or perfect makes practice.

The empirical relation between surgical volume and outcome delineated in these studies has prompted discussion of regionalization of care,[120] which has proved effective in trauma care. Given the potential for adverse or unintended consequences, however, some believe that it is too soon to use these data as final determinants of quality.[121]

Economics of Surgical Care

To increase cost-effectiveness, surgeons must understand the basis of costs as well as the essential distinction between costs and charges. Charges reflect the price structure but are a poor reflection of actual cost; therefore, there are often substantial variations among institutions regarding the relation between charges and costs. Even when costs alone are considered, there is often considerable variation with apparently similar services. Such cost variation arises because there are substantial differences in cost attribution, even for a relatively standardized accounting system such as that required by HCFA.

The complexity of calculating costs is expressed in the statement "cost is a noun that never really stands alone."[122] Costs are often categorized according to a decision maker's specific needs. Four general categories of health-related costs are commonly used [see Table 7]. From a surgeon's perspective, perhaps the two most important of these are the traceability of costs and the behavior of cost in relation to output or activity.

Cost traceability is classified as direct or indirect. Examples of direct costs are salaries, supplies, rents, and utilities; examples of indirect costs are depreciation and employee benefits. However, not all costs classified as indirect may actually be indirect. In some situations, they could be defined as direct costs, and the specific classification may depend on the given cost objective.

Cost behavior is a particularly important classification method. Variable costs, such as supplies, change in a constant proportional manner with changes in output; fixed costs do not change in response to changes in volume. Semivariable costs (e.g., utilities) include elements of both fixed and variable costs: there is a fixed basic cost per unit of time but also a direct, proportional relation between volume and cost. Semifixed, or step, costs may change with changes in output; however, the changes are not proportional but occur in discrete steps. An example of a semifixed cost is the number of full-time equivalents (FTEs) required for a particular output. If one FTE can produce 2,000 widgets, every 2,000-unit change in widget output will be associated with a change in labor cost: for every 2,000-unit increment in output, one more FTE is needed (with a concomitant increase in costs), and for every 2,000-unit decrement, one fewer FTE is needed (with a concomitant decrease in costs). Unless the step threshold is attained, costs do not change. Thus, a semifixed cost might be considered either a variable cost or a fixed cost, depending on the size of the steps relative to the range of output. Articles that re-

Table 7 Categories and Types of Hospital Costs

Category	Type	Example or Definition
Traceability to the object being costed	Direct Indirect	Salaries, supplies, rents, and utilities Depreciation and employee benefits
Behavior of cost in relation to output or activity	Variable Fixed Semivariable Semifixed	Supply Depreciation Utilities Number of full-time equivalents per step in output
Management responsibility for control	—	Often limited to direct, variable costs
Future versus historical	Avoidable costs Sunk costs Incremental costs Opportunity costs	Costs affected by a decision under consideration Costs not affected by a decision under consideration Changes in total costs resulting from alternative courses of action Value forgone by using a resource in a particular way instead of in its next best alternative way

port cost analyses of clinical interventions may not include this information, thereby further complicating comparisons. A standardized protocol may help resolve this problem.[123]

One can use cost traceability in conjunction with cost behavior by creating a matrix of the two. For example, variable costs can be direct or indirect, and direct costs can be variable, semivariable, semifixed, or fixed. The subcategory to which a given cost is assigned, however, often depends on whose point of view is assumed—the purchaser, the provider, or the patient.[124,125]

Given the nature of costs, the claim that physicians' decisions affect roughly 75% of health care costs is deceiving. A large proportion of health care expenditure is indeed related to the decision to provide care. In most cases, however, the prime consideration is not whether to provide care but which options for care should be selected. Thus, the only potential savings lie in the relatively small differences between these options. Moreover, physicians can affect costs directly only to the extent that they can influence variable costs, which typically constitute no more than 15% to 35% of hospital costs.[125,126]

Even if physicians alone have less power to affect costs than is commonly believed, it is nonetheless true that there is still substantial variation in costs and considerable room for reduction. For instance, data collected in 1996[127] indicated that whereas best practice in regard to expense per 100 minutes of OR time was $511, the national median was $938—a 46% variance.

Improvement of OR efficiency is a universal goal, and specific methods of addressing this issue have been developed.[128-130] Slow turnover times, a common complaint, are variously attributed to nurses, anesthesiologists, and surgeons themselves. Large inventories to satisfy the preferences of individual surgeons also contribute to higher costs. The emergence of laparoscopy has added new dimensions to this challenge.[131] The issues include reusable versus disposable equipment, the different costs of specific types of equipment used to accomplish the same task, and just-in-time inventory. Major pieces of equipment are often duplicated to allow simultaneous performance of similar cases even if this means that they lie unused much of the time. More efficient use of such equipment reduces costs, but such efficiency requires cooperation and coordination among surgical staff members—something that, to date, has not been widespread.

Many institutions find it difficult to identify and then rectify OR inefficiency. To improve efficiency, the surgical team must think of the OR less as a workshop and more as a factory. Surgeons often have a hard time relinquishing the concept of the surgeon as "captain of the ship" and embracing in its stead the idea that all members of the surgical team have interdependent quality and financial goals. However, even if a surgeon becomes substantially more cost-effective, this change alone may not have much effect if the individual surgeon's cost-effectiveness is offset by high hospital or facility costs.

Although ambulatory surgery is frequently touted as a cost-saving measure, the actual cost savings achieved are likely to depend on existing OR capacity and specific payer issues.[132] Team efforts to reduce the costs of trauma care have been demonstrated to be effective.[133,134] Efforts to reduce ICU costs have also shown considerable potential; a specific example is the use of protocols to guide ventilator weaning.[135,136]

Determination of Cost-Effectiveness

In simple terms, cost-effectiveness reflects the cost of a health care intervention in relation to outcome. It is distinct both from cost-benefit analysis, which assesses return on investment (with both the numerator and the denominator expressed in dollars), and from efficiency, which measures outputs divided by inputs (i.e., productivity). Determining the cost-effectiveness of health care is not simple, because analyses of cost-effectiveness may vary widely with respect to the costs and health effects they consider and consequently may produce very different cost-effectiveness ratios for the same intervention. An investigator's perspective often affects attribution of cost, and the effects of comorbid conditions on cost and outcome are also difficult to sort out.

A 1996 consensus statement on these issues recommended standards for improving study comparability and quality.[33,137,138] The consensus panel advocated that calculations be based on the perspective of society as a whole rather than on that of patients, providers, or purchasers. It concluded that "costs incurred by patients or others, such as outpatient medication or home care after hospital discharge, may be irrelevant from [the purchaser] perspective. They may also disregard some outcomes. For example, it may matter little to the HMO or government program how soon patients return to work after an illness, although it may matter a great deal to individuals, their employers, or the government agency responsible for disability payments." Most surgeons probably agree with this approach.

Cost-effective analysis, by definition, compares two approaches to a given problem. In some cases, the comparison is between two interventions, whereas in others, an intervention is compared with no treatment. The numerator of the cost-effectiveness ratio is the difference in cost, and the denominator is the difference in outcome. A particularly powerful form of cost-effectiveness analysis combines clinical decision analysis with sensitivity analysis. Such models estimate cost-effectiveness and identify the criteria that affect care decisions. They have, for example, been applied to management of penetrating colon trauma[139] and to use of carotid endarterectomy in asymptomatic patients.[140]

Like any ratio, the cost-effectiveness ratio may be affected by changes in either the numerator (costs) or the denominator (quality). In addition, it must be remembered that QALYs (often used in the denominator) comprise two distinct aspects: quality of life and the duration of that quality. Thus, an intervention can achieve cost-effectiveness either through relatively low cost or through a relatively high impact on quality, with the quality impact reflected in quality per se, duration, or both. The relative influence of the numerator and the denominator has been studied with respect to a number of surgical procedures [see Table 8]. The interval from the intervention to the point of measurement also affects the estimate of cost-effectiveness.[141,142] Patients are likely to take a long-term perspective on value, whereas providers and purchasers may focus on the short term (e.g., the term of a health care contract).

Cost-effectiveness analysis may be well suited to examination of concerns that delays in surgical referrals may adversely affect outcomes (e.g., with appendicitis).[143] One report noted that for each 10% increase in the accuracy with which appendicitis was diagnosed, there was a 14% increase in the perforation rate.[144] In this case, the cost (i.e., increased morbidity from perforation) may be the price paid for the benefit derived (i.e., greater diagnostic accuracy). Any upfront savings may be lost in the long run because of more advanced or complicated illness.

Data are available on the relative cost-effectiveness of some common medical interventions [see Table 9].[145] According to these data, the median medical intervention cost is $19,000 per year of life. Currently, many place the cost-effectiveness threshold at roughly $50,000 per year of life saved, but this figure is only a framework for decisions. Such thresholds remain both arbitrary and relative and are not necessarily indicative of an intervention's

Table 8   Cost-Effectiveness Studies of Selected Surgical Procedures

Procedure	$/QALY	Δ QALY	Comment
Carotid endarterectomy in asymptomatic patients[139]	8,000	+0.25	The initial cost of endarterectomy is offset by the high cost of care after a major stroke; the relative cost of surgical treatment increases substantially with increasing age, increasing perioperative stroke rate, and decreasing stroke rate during medical management
Routine radiation therapy after conservative surgery for early breast cancer[167]	28,000	+0.35	The ratio is heavily influenced by the cost of radiation therapy and the quality-of-life benefit that results from a decreased risk of local recurrence
Total hip arthroplasty for osteoarthritis of the hip: 60-year-old woman[168]	117,000 in cost savings	+6.9	The cost savings result from the high cost of custodial care associated with dependency
Total hip arthroplasty for osteoarthritis of the hip: 85-year-old man[168]	4,600	+2	—
Endoscopic versus open carpal tunnel release[169]	195	+0.235	Cost-effectiveness is very sensitive to a major complication such as median nerve injury
Lumbar diskectomy[170]	29,200	+0.43	Cost-effectiveness results from the moderate costs of lumbar diskectomy and its substantial effect on quality of life

QALY—quality-adjusted life year

societal value. The prioritized list of benefits of the Oregon state health plan are not based on a stratified list of $/QALYs but on broad input from stakeholders. This plan initially provoked strong criticism, but after several years of operation, it appears to be functioning well.[146] It is noteworthy that a physician-legislator spearheaded this plan.

Challenges for Academic Health Centers

Academic medical centers are not immune to the current changes in health care[147]: they, too, face special challenges. Traditionally, hospital charges were 15% to 30% higher at these centers than at community hospitals, partly because they provided certain highly specialized services and partly because they subsidized a great deal of teaching, research, and social outreach—activities that were implicitly, if not explicitly, considered valuable by society. Currently, as academic medical centers compete in the open market, they carry the burden of having to subsidize education and research from clinical incomes that are becoming increasingly restricted. Moreover, because of their involvement in teaching and research, these institutions have more specialists than are needed for clinical care alone.[148] Estimates of the network size needed to sustain current faculty levels and income are often physically, if not politically, impractical. Not surprisingly, despite their higher costs, teaching hospitals have demonstrated better outcomes (e.g., with hip fracture),[149] even for rather low-technology interventions.[150]

Information about the potential impact of the changing health care environment on academia and future academic practice is now emerging.[151] A study of medical schools in the United States demonstrated an inverse relation between growth in National Institutes of Health awards and managed care penetration during the past decade.[152] Two other studies indicated that increased competitiveness of health care markets seemed to hinder the capacity of academic health centers to conduct clinical research and foster the careers of young faculty members.[153,154] Graduate medical education, another integral part of academic medical centers' overall mission, is also facing change. Support for such education has traditionally been financed solely through HCFA, but this support is being reduced and may be eliminated entirely.

The implication of these changes is that academic medical centers may lose the capacity for producing the evidence on which cost-effective practice must be based—an event that could be tantamount to eating the proverbial seed corn.[155] Managed care organizations have been reluctant to address this issue, and they have yet to find common ground with academic medical centers.[156] One suggestion for reversing this worrisome trend is to change from a cost-based research mission to a value-based one.[157]

Ethical and Legal Issues

With managed care, health professionals increasingly face conflicts between the ethic of undivided loyalty to patients and the pressure to use clinical methods and judgment for social purposes and on behalf of third parties. Although resolving these tensions is certain to be difficult,[158] the medical profession is no stranger to such conflicts. The vast majority of physicians have avoided the temptations inherent in fee-for-service care, and at least as many appear to be avoiding incentives to undertreat. Physicians must also balance their responsibilities to individual patients with their responsibilities to society as a whole. Although some believe that evidence-based practices derived from large populations may not be readily applicable to individual patients, the rationale for this belief is not clear.

The high costs of the terminal stages of life, particularly among patients who languish in critical care units, are also being scrutinized. In this arena, tremendous expenditures are often incurred to secure even the slightest chance of survival. To avoid the dilemma inherent in a physician's making life-ending decisions, increasing emphasis is being placed on patient self-determination; still, active efforts to follow the choices of patients or their families in this situation have not led to reduced costs or improved outcomes.[159] Some studies suggest that the actual savings may be small.[160]

Professional liability under managed care is an important but complex topic.[161] There is no evidence that increasing use of clinical pathways has increased surgeon liability. There is also little question that competition among surgeons will increase and that health care purchasers are likely to use such competition to help negotiate lower fees. Any collective actions surgeons take against this tactic may render them vulnerable to antitrust action.

Table 9 Cost-Effectiveness of Common Surgical Interventions[144]

Intervention	Cost-effectiveness ($/QALY)
Mammography and breast exam (versus exam alone) annually for women 40–49 yr of age	95,000
Mammography and breast exam (versus exam alone) annually for women 40–64 yr of age	17,000
Postsurgical chemotherapy for premenopausal women with breast cancer	18,000
Bone marrow transplant and high (versus standard) chemotherapy for breast cancer	130,000
Cervical cancer screening every 3 yr for women older than 65 yr	≤ 0*
Cervical cancer screening annually (versus every 3 yr) for women older than 65 yr	49,000
Cervical cancer screening annually for women beginning at age 20	82,000
One stool guaiac colon cancer screening for persons older than 40 yr	660
Colonoscopy for colorectal cancer screening for persons older than 40 yr	90,000
Left main coronary artery bypass graft surgery (versus medical management)	2,300
Coronary artery bypass surgery for octogenarians[171]	10,424
Exercise stress test for asymptomatic men 60 yr of age	40
Compression stockings to prevent venous thromboembolism	≤ 0*
Preoperative chest x-ray to detect abnormalities in children	360,000

*Saves more resources than it consumes.
QALY—quality-adjusted life year

The Future

Although American health care is being reshaped, what the final shape will be is by no means clear, in part because there is no agreement on the best strategies for dealing with the current problems. Marketplace competition is attractive because these forces are familiar and have been effective in other aspects of our economy by redistributing income, providing consumer choice, ensuring producer autonomy, increasing economic efficiency, and generating equity. However, market forces fail to address other important economic and cultural aspects of health care[162]; for example, they are difficult to reconcile with the view of health care as a right, with the often strong inverse relation between illness and the ability to pay for health care, with the great pressure for risk selection among purchasers and providers, and with the asymmetry of knowledge between provider and consumer. As a result, market forces are unlikely to be the sole long-term solution to the current problems in health care.

For the medically indigent, managed care has exacerbated the problems of access to health care, and every indication is that these problems will worsen in the near future. Physicians involved with managed care plans and those who practice in areas with high managed care penetration tend to provide less charity care.[163] Teaching hospitals provide a disproportionate share of care to the medically indigent and consequently have become the safety nets of our health care system. There is great concern that managed care will jeopardize the fragile social contracts under which the faculty at academic medical centers contribute unreimbursed and underreimbursed time.[164]

The high cost of health care is undoubtedly a multifactorial problem, with some factors being inherent in the current system and others resulting from the medicalization of social problems. A quick fix is unlikely. A more prudent policy for improving overall health status might be to redirect health care expenditures toward alleviating the social problems contributing to poor health. The problems of health care for the indigent and the uninsured are integrally related to the dysfunctional aspects of the entire system.

Physicians undoubtedly have a role in the ongoing discussion and debate on the future of the health care system in the United States. The magnitude of their input in this debate may depend on their ability to address the larger issues of quality. Specifically, they must address variation in outcomes and variation in intervention rates. Medical decision making must increasingly be based on evidence. If wide variations persist, especially for procedures with clearly proven indications (e.g., carotid endarterectomy), health care purchasers may choose to reimburse only for proven indications and for surgeons with suitably low morbidity and mortality. Such was the case with pneumoreductive surgery for end-stage chronic pulmonary obstructive disease. This procedure became increasingly popular, but there were no hard data to support its long-term efficacy. HCFA then announced that it would pay for the procedure only if it was performed as part of a clinical trial to prove its efficacy; other payors quickly followed suit.[165]

It is curious that at present, quality is not the foremost concern among health care purchasers: competition over price seems to be a much more urgent issue than competition over quality.[166] It seems logical, however, that at some point concerns about how much is being paid will give way to questions about why something is being paid. If surgeons cannot practice within proven indications, they may have little chance of regaining lost autonomy.

Physicians must embrace the vision that it is possible to have a cost-effective health care system with an acceptable balance of choice, quality, and access. Managed care has disrupted many aspects of the health care system, but this may be but a phase on the path toward a better one. To ensure choice quality and access, surgeons must participate in the process of reform of the health care system. Although it appears that physicians are losing more and more autonomy, they are the only parties with the knowledge and skills needed to address the challenges of identifying cost-effective care. The path toward resolution of these issues is likely to produce some dilemmas (i.e., true conflicts in established ethical principles) and some hard choices (i.e., conflicts between these ethical principles and self-interest). Yet if physicians wish to retain (or even recover) their status, they must maintain the profession's highest priorities: quality of care and patient advocacy.

References

1. Iglehart JK: The American health care system: expenditures. N Engl J Med 340:70, 1999

2. Simon CJ, Born PH: Physician earnings in the managed care environment. Health Aff (Millwood) 15:124, 1996

3. Bodenheimer T: The HMO backlash—righteous or reactionary? N Engl J Med 335:1601, 1996

4. Anderson GF, Poullier J-P: Health spending, access, and outcomes: trends in industrialized countries. Health Aff (Millwood) 18:178, 1999

5. Dubois RW, Brook RH: Preventable deaths: who, how often, and why? Ann Intern Med 109:582, 1988

6. Brook RH, Kamberg CJ, Mayer-Oakes A, et al: Appropriateness of health care for the elderly: an analysis of the literature. Health Policy 14:225, 1990

7. Leape LL, Brennan TA, Laird N, et al: The nature of adverse events in hospitalized patients: results of the Harvard Medical Practice Study II. N Engl J Med 324:377, 1991

8. Gawande AA, Thomas EJ, Zinner MJ, et al: The incidence and nature of surgical adverse events in Colorado and Utah in 1992. Surgery 126:66, 1999

9. Chassin MR, Kosecoff J, Park RE, et al: Does inappropriate use explain geographic variations in the use of health services? A study of three procedures. JAMA 253:2533, 1987

10. Bernstein SJ, McGlynn EA, Siu AL, et al: The appropriateness of hysterectomy: a comparison of care in seven health plans. JAMA 269:2398, 1993

11. Phelps CE: The methodologic foundations of studies of the appropriateness of medical care. N Engl J Med 329:1241, 1993

12. Kassirer JP: The quality of care and the quality of measuring it. N Engl J Med 329:1263, 1993

13. Caplan RA, Posner KL, Cheney FW: Effect of outcome on physician judgments of appropriateness of care. JAMA 265:1957, 1991

14. Redelmeir DA, Tversky A: Discrepancy between medical decisions for individual patients and for groups. N Engl J Med 322:1162, 1990

15. Wennberg J, Gittelsohn A: Variations in medical care among small areas. Sci Am 246(4):120, 1982

16. Chaissin MR, Brook RH, Park RE, et al: Variations in the use of medical and surgical services by the Medicare population. N Engl J Med 314:285, 1986

17. The Dartmouth Atlas of Health Care. American Hospital Publishing, Chicago, 1998

18. Birkmeyer JD, Sharp SM, Finlayson SR, et al: Variation profiles of common surgical procedures. Surgery 124:917, 1998

19. Wennberg DE, Kellett MA, Dickens JD, et al: The association between local diagnostic intensity and invasive cardiac procedures. JAMA 275:1161, 1996

20. Eddy DM: Variations in physician practice: the role of uncertainty. Health Aff (Millwood) 3:74, 1984

21. Muir Gray JA: Evidence-Based Health Care: How to Make Health Policy and Management Decisions. Churchill Livingstone, New York, 1997

22. Williamson JW, Goldschmidt PG, Jillson IA: Medical practice information demonstration project: final report. Office of the Asst Secretary of Health, US Department of Health, Education, and Welfare, contract #282-77-0068GS. Policy Research Inc, Baltimore, 1979

23. Howes N, Chagla L, Thorpe M, et al: Surgical practice is evidence based. Br J Surg 84:1220, 1997

24. Leape LL, Park RE, Solomon DH, et al: Does inappropriate use explain small-area variations in the use of health care services? JAMA 263:669, 1990

25. Ashton CM, Petersen NJ, Souchek J, et al: Geographic variations in utilization rates in Veterans Affairs hospitals and clinics. N Engl J Med 340:32, 1999

26. Health Services Research Group: Small area variations: what are they and what do they mean? Can Med Assoc J 146:467, 1992

27. Bunker JP: Surgical manpower: a comparison of operations and surgeons in the United States and in England and Wales. N Engl J Med 282:135, 1970

28. Donabedian A: The Definition of Quality and Approaches to Its Assessment. Explorations in Quality Assessment and Monitoring, vol 1. Health Administration Press, Ann Arbor, Michigan, 1980

29. Stoline AM, Weiner JP: The New Medical Marketplace: A Physician's Guide to the Health Care System in the 1990s. Baltimore, Johns Hopkins University Press, 1993, p 138

30. Chassin MR, Galvin RW: The urgent need to improve health care quality: Institute of Medicine National Roundtable on health care quality. JAMA 280:1000, 1998

31. Reemtsma K, Morgan M: Outcomes assessment: a primer. Bull Am Coll Surg 82:34, 1997

32. Testa MA, Simonson DC: Assessment of quality of life outcomes. N Engl J Med 334:835, 1996

33. Russell LB, Gold MR, Siegel JE, et al: The role of cost-effectiveness analysis in medicine. JAMA 276:1172, 1996

34. Velanovitch V: Using quality of life instruments to assess surgical outcomes. Surgery 126:1, 1999

35. Leplege A, Hunt S: The problem of quality of life in medicine. JAMA 278:47, 1997

36. Eiseman B: Surgical decision making and elderly patients. Bull Am Coll Surg 81:8, 1996

37. Kreder HJ, Wright JG, McLeod R: Outcomes studies in surgical research. Surgery 121:223, 1996

38. Garvin DA: Afterword: Reflections on the future. Curing Health Care: New Strategies for Quality Improvement: A Report on the National Demonstration Project on Quality Improvement in Health Care. Berwick DM, Godfrey AB, Roessner J, Eds. Jossey-Bass Publishers, San Francisco, 1990, p 159

39. Brook RH, Kamberg CJ, McGlynn EA: Health system reform and quality. JAMA 276:476, 1996

40. Bodenheimer T: The American health care system: the movement for improved quality in health care. N Engl J Med 340:488, 1999

41. Epstein AE: Rolling down the runway: the challenges ahead for quality report cards. JAMA 279:1691, 1998

42. Campion FX, Rosenblatt MS: Quality assurance and medical outcomes in the era of cost containment. Surg Clin North Am 76:139, 1996

43. Rutledge R: An analysis of 25 Milliman & Robertson guidelines for surgery: data-driven versus consensus-driven clinical practice guidelines. Ann Surg 228:579, 1998

44. Rigelman RK: Studying a Study and Testing a Test: How to Read the Medical Literature. Little, Brown & Co, Boston, 1981

45. Verrilli D, Welch GH: The impact of diagnostic testing on therapeutic interventions. JAMA 275:1189, 1996

46. Ross NS, Aron DC: Hormonal evaluation of the patient with the incidentally discovered adrenal mass. N Engl J Med 323:1401, 1990

47. Velanovich V: Preoperative laboratory test evaluation. J Am Coll Surg 183:79, 1996

48. Marcello PW, Roberts PL: "Routine" preoperative studies: which studies in which patients? Surg Clin North Am 76:11, 1996

49. Richardson WS, Wilson MC, Guyatt GH, et al: Users' guides to the medical literature: XV. How to use an article about disease probability for differential diagnosis. JAMA 281:1214, 1999

50. Sox HC, Blatt MA, Higgins MC, et al: Medical Decision Making. Butterworth-Heinemann, Boston, 1988

51. Birkmeyer JD, Welch HG: A reader's guide to surgical decision analysis. J Am Coll Surg 184:589, 1997

52. Millilli JJ, Philiponis VS, Nusbaum M: Predicting surgical outcome using Bayesian analysis. J Surg Res 77:45, 1998

53. Birkmeyer JD, Birkmeyer NO: Decision analysis in surgery. Surgery 120:7, 1996

54. Taubes G: Looking for evidence in medicine. Science 272:22, 1996

55. Meinert CL: Beyond CONSORT: need for improved reporting standards for clinical trials. JAMA 279:1487, 1998

56. North American Symptomatic Carotid Trial Collaborators: Beneficial effect of carotid endarterectomy in symptomatic patients with high-grade carotid stenosis. N Engl J Med 325:445, 1991

57. Executive Committee for the Asymptomatic Carotid Atherosclerosis Study: Endarterectomy for asymptomatic carotid artery stenosis. JAMA 273:1421, 1995

58. Tu JV, Hannan EL, Anderson GM, et al: The fall and rise of carotid endarterectomy in the United States and Canada. N Engl J Med 339:1441, 1998

59. Wennberg DE, Lucas FL, Birkmeyer JD, et al: Variation in carotid endarterectomy in the Medicare population: trial hospitals, volumes, and patient characteristics. JAMA 279:1278, 1998

60. Chassin MR: Appropriate use of carotid endarterectomy. N Engl J Med 339:1468, 1998

61. Rao PM, Rhea JT, Novelline RA, et al: Effect of computed tomography of the appendix on treatment of patients and use of hospital resources. N Engl J Med 338:141, 1998

62. Gill BD, Jenkins JR: Cost-effective evaluation and management of the acute abdomen. Surg Clin North Am 76:71, 1996

63. Wright JC, Weinstein MC: Gains in life expectancy from medical interventions—standardizing data on outcomes. N Engl J Med 339:380, 1998

64. Black WC, Welch HG: Advances in diagnostic imaging and overestimations of disease prevalence and the benefits of therapy. N Engl J Med 328:1237, 1993

65. Naylor CD, Guyatt GH: Users' guides to the medical literature: X. How to use an article reporting variations in the outcomes of health services. JAMA 275:554, 1996

66. Naylor CD, Guyatt GH: Users' guides to the medical literature: XI. How to use an article about clinical utilization review. JAMA 275:1435, 1996

67. Guyatt GH, Naylor CD, Juniper E, et al: Users' guides to the medical literature: XII. How to use articles about health related quality of life. JAMA 277:1232, 1997

68. Drummond MF, Richardson WS, O'Brien BJ, et al: Users' guides to the medical literature: XIII. How to use an article on economic analysis of clinical practice. A. Are the results of the study valid? JAMA 277:1552, 1997

69. O'Brien BJ, Heyland D, Richardson WS, et al: Users' guides to the medical literature: XIII. How to use an article on economic analysis of clinical practice. B. What are the results and will they help me in caring for my patients? JAMA 277:1802, 1997

70. Dans AL, Dans LF, Guyatt GH, et al: Users' guides to the medical literature: XIV. How to decide on the applicability of clinical trials to your patients. JAMA 279:545, 1998

71. Richardson WS, Detsky AS: Users' guides to the medical literature: VII. How to use a clinical decision analysis. A. Are the results of the study valid? JAMA 273:1292, 1995

72. Barratt AA, Irwig L, Glasziou P, et al: Users' guides to the medical literature: XVII. How to use guidelines and recommendations about screening. JAMA 281:2029, 1999

73. Randolph AG, Haynes RB, Wyatt JC, et al: Users' guides to the medical literature: XVIII. How to use an article evaluating the clinical impact of a computer-based clinical decision support system. JAMA 282:67, 1999

74. Davis R, Miller L: Millions scour the Web to find medical information. USA Today, July 14, 1999

75. Soot LC, Moneta GL, Edwards JM: Vascular surgery and the Internet. J Vasc Surg 30:84, 1999

76. Statement on issues to be considered before new surgical technology is applied to the care of patients. Bull Am Coll Surg 80:46, 1995

77. Legorreta AP, Silber JH, Constantino GN, et al: Increased cholecystectomy rate after the introduction of laparoscopic cholecystectomy. JAMA 270:1429, 1993

78. Selker HP, Beshansky JR, Paulker SG, et al: The epidemiology of delays in teaching hospitals. Med Care 27:112, 1989

79. Epstein RS, Sherwood LM: From outcomes research to disease management: a guide to the perplexed. Ann Intern Med 124:832, 1996

80. Gadacz TR, Adkins RB, O'Leary JP: General surgical clinical pathways: an introduction. Am Surg 63:107, 1997

81. Cost Effectiveness in Surgery. Rossi RL, Cady B, Eds. Surg Clin North Am 76:1, 1996

82. Hayward RSA, Wilson MC, Tunis SR, et al: Users' guides to the medical literature. VIII. How to use clinical practice guidelines. A. Are the recommendations valid? JAMA 274:570, 1995

83. Wilson MC, Hayward RSA, Tunis SR, et al: Users' guides to the medical literature. VIII. How to use clinical practice guidelines. B. What are the recommendations and will they help you in caring for your patients? JAMA 274:1630, 1995

84. Shaneyfelt TM, Mayo-Smith MF, Rothwangl J: Are guidelines following guidelines? The methodological quality of clinical practice guidelines in the peer-reviewed medical literature. JAMA 281:1900, 1999

85. Cook D, Giacomini M: The trials and tribulations of clinical practice guidelines. JAMA 281:1950, 1999

86. Pearson SD, Goulart-Fisher D, Lee TH: Critical pathways as a strategy for improving care: problems and potential. Ann Intern Med 123:941, 1995

87. Hoyt DB: Clinical practice guidelines. Am J Surg 173:32, 1997

88. Passaro E, Organ CH: Ernest A. Codman: the improper Bostonian. Bull Am Coll Surg 84:16, 1999

89. Tunner WS, Christy JP, Whipple TL: System for outcomes-based report card. Bull Am Coll Surg 82:18, 1997

90. Gold MR, Hurley R, Lake T, et al: A national survey of the arrangements managed-care plans make with physicians. N Engl J Med 333:1678, 1995

91. Larkin H: Doctors starting to feel report cards' impact. AMA News 42:1, 1999

92. Risk Adjustment for Measuring Health Care Outcomes. Iezzoni LI, Ed. Health Administration Press, Ann Arbor, Michigan, 1994

93. Horn SD, Sharkey PD, Buckle JM, et al: The relationship between severity of illness and hospital length of stay and mortality. Med Care 29:305, 1991

94. Rhodes RS, Sharkey PD, Horn SD: Effect of patient factors on hospital costs for major bowel surgery: implications for managed health care. Surgery 117:443, 1995

95. Kalman PG, Johnston KW: Sociological factors are major determinants of prolonged hospital stay following abdominal aneurysm repair. Surgery 119:690, 1996

96. Salem-Schatz S, Moore G, Rucker M, et al: The case for case-mix adjustment in practice profiling: when good apples look bad. JAMA 272:871, 1994

97. Melton JL: Selection bias in the referral of patients and the natural history of surgical conditions. Mayo Clin Proc 60:880, 1985

98. Williams MV, Parker RM, Baker DW, et al: Inadequate functional health literacy among patients at two public hospitals. JAMA 274:1677, 1995

99. Hannan EL, Kilburn H, Racz M, et al: Improving the outcomes of coronary artery bypass surgery in New York State. JAMA 271:761, 1994

100. Green J, Winfield N: Report cards on cardiac surgeons: assessing New York State's approach. N Engl J Med 332:1229, 1995

101. Rhodes RS, Krasniak CJ, Jones PK: Factors affecting length of stay for femoropopliteal bypass: implications of the DRGs. N Engl J Med 314:153, 1986

102. Chaissin MR, Hannan EL, DeBunno BA: Benefits and hazards of reporting medical outcomes publicly. N Engl J Med 334:394, 1996

103. Schneider EC, Epstein AM: Influence of cardiac surgery performance report cards on referral practices and access to care. N Engl J Med 335:251, 1996

104. Turner WS: Committee on Socioeconomic Issues. Bull Am Coll Surg 83:40, 1998

105. O'Connor GT, Plume SK, Olmstead EM, et al: A regional intervention to improve the hospital mortality associated with coronary artery bypass graft surgery. JAMA 275:841, 1996

106. Hansen FC: What does your future hold: capitation or decapitation? Bull Am Coll Surg 81:12, 1996

107. Ruffin M: Developing and using a data repository for quality improvement: the genesis of IRIS. Jt Com J Qual Improv 21:512, 1995

108. Clare M, Sargent D, Moxley R, et al: Reducing health care delivery costs using clinical paths: a case study on improving hospital profitability. J Health Care Finance 21:48, 1995

109. Sosa JA, Bowman HM, Tielsch JM, et al: The importance of surgeon experience for clinical and economic outcomes from thyroidectomy. Ann Surg 228:320, 1998

110. Sosa JA, Bowman HM, Gordon TA, et al: Importance of hospital volume in the overall management of pancreatic cancer. Ann Surg 228:429, 1998

111. Birkmeyer JD, Finlayson SRG, Tosteson ANA, et al: Effect of hospital volume on in-hospital mortality with pancreaticoduodenectomy. Surgery 125:250, 1999

112. Begg CB, Cramer LD, Hoskins WJ, et al: Impact of hospital volume on operative mortality for major cancer surgery. JAMA 280:1747, 1998

113. Pearce WH, Parker MA, Feinglass J, et al: The importance of surgeon volume and training in outcomes for vascular surgical procedures. J Vasc Surg 29:768, 1999

114. Harmon JW, Tang DG, Gordon TA, et al: Hospital volume can serve as a surrogate for surgeon volume for achieving excellent outcomes in colorectal resection. Ann Surg 230:404, 1999

115. Trends in the concentration of six surgical procedures under PPS and their implications for patient mortality and medicare cost. Technical report #E-87-08. Project Hope, Chevy Chase, Maryland, 1988

116. Gordon TA, Burleyson GP, Tielsch JM, et al: The effect of regionalization on cost and outcome for one general high-risk surgical procedure. Ann Surg 221:43, 1995

117. Porter GA, Soskolne CL, Yakimets WW, et al: Surgeon-related factors and outcome in rectal cancer. Ann Surg 277:157, 1998

118. Houghton A: Variance in outcome of surgical procedures. Br J Surg 81:653, 1994

119. Khuri SF, Henderson WG, Hur K, et al: The relationship of surgical volume to outcome in eight common operations: results from the VA National Quality Improvement Program. Ann Surg 230:414, 1999

120. Luft HS, Bunker JP, Enthoven AC: Should operations be regionalized? the empiric relation between surgical volume and mortality. N Engl J Med 301:1364, 1979

121. Hannan EL: The relation between volume and outcome in health care. N Engl J Med 340:1677, 1999

122. Cleverly WO: Essentials of Healthcare Finance, 2nd ed. Aspen Publishers Inc, Rockville, Maryland, 1986, p 191

123. Balas EA, Kretschmer RAC, Gnann W, et al: Interpreting cost analyses of clinical interventions. JAMA 279:54, 1998

124. Rhodes RS: How much does it cost? how much can be saved? Surgery 125:102, 1999

125. Roberts RR, Frutos PW, Ciavarella GG, et al: Distribution of variable vs fixed costs of hospital care. JAMA 281:644, 1999

126. Taheri PA, Butz DA, Griffes LC, et al: Physician impact on the total cost of care. Ann Surg (in press)

127. The Rising Tide. Emergence of a New Competition Standard in Health Care. Advisory Board Co, Washington, DC, 1996

128. Kanich DG, Byrd JR: How to increase efficiency in the operating room. Surg Clin North Am 76:161, 1996

129. Clockwork Surgery. Re-engineering the Hospital, Vol I. The Advisory Board Company, Washington, DC, 1992

130. The Surgery Capacity Ceiling. Re-engineering the Hospital, Vol II. The Advisory Board Company, Washington, DC, 1992

131. Newman RM, Traverso LW: Cost-effective minimally invasive surgery: what procedures make sense? World J Surg 23:415, 1999

132. Rhodes RS: Ambulatory surgery and the societal cost of surgery. Surgery 116:938, 1994

133. Taheri PA, Wahl WL, Butz DA, et al: Trauma service cost: the real story. Ann Surg 227:720, 1998

134. Taheri PA, Butz DA, Watts CM, et al: Trauma services: a profit center? J Am Coll Surg 188:349, 1999

135. Horst HM, Mouro D, Hall-Jenssens RA, et al: Decrease in ventilation time with a standardized weaning process. Arch Surg 13:483, 1998

136. Thomsen GE, Pope D, East TD, et al: Clinical performance of a rule-based decision support system for mechanical ventilation of ARDS patients. Proc Annu Symp Comput Appl Med Care 1993, p 339

137. Weinstein MC, Siegel JE, Gold MR, et al: Recommendations of the Panel on Cost-Effectiveness in Health and Medicine. JAMA 276:1253, 1996

138. Siegel JE, Weinstein MC, Russell LB, et al: Recommendations for reporting cost-effectiveness analyses. JAMA 276:1339, 1996

139. Brasel KJ, Borgstrom DC, Weigelt JA: Management of penetrating colon trauma: a cost-utility analysis. Surg 125:471, 1999

140. Cronenwett JL, Birkmeyer JD, Nackman GB, et al: Cost-effectiveness of carotid endarterectomy in asymptomatic patients. J Vasc Surg 25:298, 1997

141. Schermerhorn ML, Birkmeyer J, Gould DA, et al: The impact of operative mortality on cost-effectiveness in the UK small aneurysm trial. J Vasc Surg 31:217, 2000

142. Heudebert GR, Marks R, Wilcox CM, et al: Choice of long-term strategy for the management of patients with severe esophagitis: A cost-utility analysis. Gastroenterology 112:1078, 1997

143. Cacioppo JC, Dietrich NA, Kaplan G, et al: The consequences of current restraints on surgical treatment of appendicitis. Am J Surg 157:276, 1989

144. Wen SW, Naylor CD: Diagnostic accuracy and short-term surgical outcomes in cases of suspected acute appendicitis. CMAJ 153:888, 1995

145. Tengs TO, Adams ME, Pliskin JS, et al: Five-hundred life-saving interventions and their cost-effectiveness. Risk Anal 15:369, 1995

146. Bodenheimer T: The Oregon health plan—lessons for the nation. N Engl J Med 337:651, 720, 1997

147. Iglehart J: Support for academic medical centers: revisiting the 1997 Balanced Budget Act. N Engl J Med 341:299, 1999

148. Billi JE, Wise CG, Bills EA, et al: Potential effects of managed care on specialty practice at a university medical center. N Engl J Med 333:979, 1995

149. Taylor DH, Whelan DJ, Sloan FA: The effects of admission to a teaching hospital on the cost and quality of care for Medicare beneficiaries. N Engl J Med 340:293, 1999

150. Kassirer JP: Hospitals, heal yourselves. N Engl J Med 340:309, 1999

151. Simon SR, Pan RJD, Sullivan AM, et al: Views of managed care: a survey of students, residents, faculty, and deans at medical schools in the United States. N Engl J Med 340:928, 1999

152. Moy E, Mazzaschi AJ, Levin RJ, et al: Relationship between National Institutes of Health research awards to US medical schools and managed care market penetration. JAMA 278:217, 1997

153. Campbell EG, Weissman JS, Blumenthal D: Relationship between market competition and the activities and attitudes of medical school faculty. JAMA 278:222, 1997

154. Weissman JS, Saglam D, Campbell EG, et al: Market forces and unsponsored research in academic health centers. JAMA 281:1093, 1999

155. Thompson JC: Seed corn: impact of managed care on medical education and research. Ann Surg 223:453, 1996

156. LaRosa JC, Whelton P, Litwin MS: Academic medicine and managed care: seeking common ground. Acad Med 74:488, 1999

157. Krauss K, Smith J: Rejecting conventional wisdom: how academic medical centers can regain their leadership positions. Acad Med 72:571, 1997

158. Bloche MG: Clinical loyalties and the social purposes of medicine. JAMA 281:268, 1999

159. The SUPPORT Principal Investigators: A controlled trial to improve care for seriously ill hospitalized patients. JAMA 274:1591, 1995

160. Emanuel EJ, Emanuel LL: The economics of dying—the illusion of cost saving at the end of life. N Engl J Med 330:540, 1994

161. Manuel B: Physician liability under managed care. J Am Coll Surg 183:537, 1996

162. Ginsberg E: A cautionary note on market reforms in health care. JAMA 274:1633, 1995

163. Cunningham PJ, Grossman JM, St Peter RF, et al: Managed care and physicians' provision of charity care. JAMA 281:1087, 1999

164. Shea S, Nickerson KG, Tenebaum J, et al: Compensation to a department and its faculty members for teaching of medical students and house staff. N Engl J Med 334:162, 1996

165. Bodily KC: Surgeons and technology. Am J Surg 177:351, 1999

166. Kassirer JP, Angell M: Quality and the medical marketplace—following elephants. N Engl J Med 335:883, 1996

167. Hayman JA, Hillner BE, Harris JR, et al: Cost-effectiveness of routine radiation therapy following conservative surgery for early-stage breast cancer. J Clin Oncol 16:1022, 1998

168. Chang RW, Pellisier JM, Hazen GB: A cost-effectiveness analysis of total hip arthroplasty for osteoarthritis of the hip. JAMA 275:858, 1996

169. Chung KC, Walters MR, Greenfield ML, et al: Endoscopic versus open carpal tunnel release: a cost-effectiveness analysis. Plast Reconstr Surg 102:1089, 1998

170. Malter AD, Larson EB, Urban N, et al: Cost-effectiveness of lumbar discectomy for the treatment of herniated intervertebral disc. Spine 21:1048, 1996

171. Sollano JA, Rose EA, Williams DL, et al: Cost-effectiveness of coronary artery bypass surgery in octogenarians. Ann Surg 228:297, 1998

2 RISK STRATIFICATION, PREOPERATIVE TESTING, AND OPERATIVE PLANNING

Nicolas V. Christou, M.D., Alden H. Harken, M.D., Douglas W. Wilmore, M.D., and Jyoti Arya, M.D.

The purpose of an operation is to make a patient's subsequent life better than it would have been if the operation had not been performed. Intrinsic to the fulfillment of this purpose is the necessity of carefully considering the risk of complications and taking into account the immediate (and, in some cases, prolonged) disability associated with the operation.

Quantification of Surgical Risk

Ideally, risk should be expressed in terms of the number of occurrences of complications per 100,000 operations performed. In reports of large case series performed in a single institution and retrospectively reviewed, however, both the complication rate and the 30-day mortality are usually expressed in terms of a percentage of the total number of cases. The figures from such reports tend to be low in comparison with those from the surgical community at large because the comparisons often have not been adjusted to take into account comorbid conditions. In addition, single-center studies may not reflect the standards of care prevalent in the broader surgical community. Moreover, it has been argued that 30-day mortality by itself is not a sufficiently precise measure of operative risk and that mortality should also be recorded 6 months after the procedure.[1] The basis for this argument is the gradual deterioration in function that occurs in some individuals during the first 6 months after a major illness.

For accurate calculation of an individual patient's level of operative risk, large databases are needed. Such databases are available for coronary artery bypass surgery,[2] and it is now possible to make accurate risk estimates on the basis of the anatomic location of the obstructive lesion or lesions in the coronary vasculature, the level of cardiac function present (measured according to some index of cardiac output), and the presence or absence of associated comorbid conditions (e.g., diabetes mellitus or pulmonary insufficiency).[2] Unfortunately, it is not yet possible to make such estimates for the wide range of elective general surgical procedures; thus, to inform patients about the risks associated with these operations, surgeons must rely on large case series or on regionally reported mortalities and morbidities and length of hospital stay [see Table 1]. Until more specific quantification of risk can be achieved, patients undergoing operations for which accurate risk estimates are unavailable (i.e., the great majority of elective and semielective procedures) may generally be classified into three categories: (1) low risk, corresponding to a mortality of 2% or lower; (2) moderate risk, corresponding to a mortality higher than 2% but not higher than 6%; or (3) high risk, corresponding to a mortality higher than 6%.

Assessment of Surgical Risk

BASIC RISK STRATIFICATION

A number of guidelines for risk stratification have been proposed, and prospective studies have correlated the categories generated by these systems with postoperative differences in complication rate, mortality, and duration of hospital stay. The most universally used classification system is the one proposed by the American Society of Anesthesiologists (ASA), which is based on the patient's functional status and the comorbid conditions present [see Table 2].[3] The ASA index generally associated poorer overall health with increased postoperative complications, longer hospital stay, and higher mortality.[4] In relation to the general categories already mentioned (see above), ASA classes I and II correspond to low risk, class III to moderate risk, and classes IV and V to high risk.

HISTORY AND PHYSICAL EXAMINATION

The history and the physical examination are the most effective means of identifying risk factors associated with coexisting disease [see Figure 1]. Diagnostically, the history is three times more productive than the physical examination and 11 times more effective than routine laboratory tests; combined with the physical examination, the history is diagnostic in 75% to 90% of patients. Information about the patient's current disease or any other disease processes present helps guide subsequent testing during the initial visit.[5]

The patient's current medications should be listed and any allergies noted. A careful social history should be obtained to uncover risk factors associated with smoking, alcohol ingestion, and drug abuse. If there is a significant history of smoking, further evaluation of cardiac, vascular, and respiratory function may be required. Cessation of smoking for 4 to 6 weeks before operation is usually recommended; cessation for shorter periods may

Table 1 Length of Stay and 30-Day Mortality for Selected Procedures: Health Care Utilization Project[79]

Operation	Length of Stay (days)	Mortality (%)
Gastric, esophageal, or duodenal procedures; age > 17 years	12.3	9.0
Hepatobiliary or pancreatic procedures	13.9	14.7
Rectal resection	4.9	1.9
Major small and large bowel procedures		
With complications	11.4	5.7
Without complications	6.3	—
Mastectomy	2.1–2.8	—
Major thoracic procedures (noncardiac)	9.5	4.5

Table 2 American Society of Anesthesiologists' Physical Status Classification: Nonemergency Surgery[3]

Classification	Description	Examples
Class I	Normal, healthy patient	An inguinal hernia in a fit patient or a fibroid uterus in a healthy woman
Class II	Patient with mild systemic disease—a mild to moderate systemic disorder related to the condition to be treated or to some other, unrelated process	Moderate obesity, extremes of age, diet-controlled diabetes, mild hypertension, chronic obstructive pulmonary disease
Class III	Patient with severe systemic disease that limits activity but is not incapacitating	Morbid obesity, severely limiting heart disease, angina pectoris, healed myocardial infarction, insulin-dependent diabetes, moderate to severe pulmonary insufficiency
Class IV	Patient with incapacitating systemic disease that is life threatening	Organic heart disease with signs of cardiac insufficiency; unstable angina; refractory arrhythmia; advanced pulmonary, renal, hepatic, or endocrine disease
Class V	Moribund patient not expected to survive 24 hr without an operation	Ruptured aortic aneurysm with profound shock, massive pulmonary embolus, major cerebral trauma with increasing intracranial pressure

be associated with a hyperactive inflammatory response in the respiratory system.[6] In a 2002 trial, when preoperative smoking cessation was achieved, the incidence of postoperative complications was reduced from 52% to 18%.[7] Long-term abuse of alcohol is often associated with CNS and hepatic dysfunction as well as with malnutrition. Alcohol abusers, even when they exhibit no overt alcohol-related organ dysfunction, have higher morbidities than nonabusers do and take longer to recover after an operation.[8] In one study of alcohol abusers undergoing colonic surgery, however, patients subjected to an intervention approach that included preoperative alcohol abstinence for 4 weeks exhibited less of the expected increase in postoperative morbidity than did patients who continued their drinking habits.[9] Long-term intravenous drug abuse may be associated with venous thrombosis, hepatitis, AIDS, malnutrition, subacute bacterial endocarditis, or psychiatric disturbances—any of which constitutes an indication for additional preoperative evaluation.

Existing infection—in particular, urinary tract infection and pneumonia—must be identified and treated before operation. This is an especially relevant consideration in patients who are to receive a prosthetic implant (e.g., an artificial heart valve or an aortic graft). Bacteremia resulting from manipulation of an infected urinary tract can predispose to graft infection. Any infection identified preoperatively in these patients should be treated before elective surgery.

Finally, the referring physician may have carried out tests that are pertinent to the patient's current illness, and the results of these tests can be extremely useful in planning the operation. Copies of all laboratory test results and radiologic images should be requested. For example, a patient with cholelithiasis may have undergone preoperative ultrasonography, or a patient referred for hepatic resection may have undergone preoperative angiography. The original angiograms, CT scans, barium enema films, and other images should be personally reviewed with a radiologist. In cases of equivocal diagnosis, slides of pathology specimens obtained by the referring physician must be reviewed.

EVALUATION OF INDIVIDUAL ORGAN SYSTEMS

Cardiovascular System

Cardiovascular risk factors account for by far the greatest portion of postoperative risk [*see Figure 1*]. Significant cardiovascular risk factors include angina pectoris, dyspnea and evidence of

right-sided or left-sided heart failure, arrhythmias or other sinus arrhythmia, more than five ventricular ectopic beats a minute, aortic stenosis with left ventricular hypertrophy, mitral regurgitation, and previous myocardial infarction (MI).

The risk of intraoperative or postoperative MI is much higher in patients who recently had an infarction. In large retrospective reviews, 37% of patients experienced reinfarction when they were operated on within 3 months of an infarction. The incidence of reinfarction decreased to 16% when the operation was performed between 3 and 6 months after infarction and to 4.5% when the operation was performed more than 6 months afterward.[10] The presence of a murmur is an indication for full evaluation of cardiac function and, in certain cases, for antibiotic prophylaxis.

Likewise, the presence of a carotid thrill or bruit may be an indication for further testing to determine whether a carotid endarterectomy should be performed before elective surgery. Hypertension is frequently associated with increased peripheral resistance, cardiac hypertrophy, increased ventricular stroke work, and impaired renal blood flow. The sudden onset of hypertension or a persistent increase in blood pressure in a patient whose BP has been well controlled by antihypertensive medications may warrant postponement of elective surgery. Selective screening of high-risk patients for primary hyperaldosteronism, pheochromocytoma, renal vascular disease, and Cushing syndrome should be undertaken.[11-13] Patients with essential hypertension should not undergo elective surgery until their BP is adequately controlled by pharmacologic means.

To develop a logical strategy for preventing or reducing risk, it is crucial to determine, as far as is possible, which factors contribute most to risk (and are modifiable). A landmark 1977 study by Goldman and colleagues related more than 70 preoperative parameters to perioperative morbidity and mortality in 1,001 patients older than 40 years who underwent noncardiac surgical procedures [*see Table 3*].[14] Not surprisingly, the most significant adverse outcome measures in this study (perioperative MI, congestive heart failure, ventricular tachycardia or fibrillation, and death) were all cardiac problems, and the most robust predictors of these problems were antecedent heart diseases. The implication of these findings is that cardiac risk accounts for by far the largest portion of overall surgical risk and that, for practical purposes, the two are nearly congruent.

The Goldman index of risk is readily correlated with the ASA index: ASA classes I and II correspond with Goldman class I (0

Figure 1 Algorithm depicts recommended approach to cardiac assessment before noncardiac surgery.[14-16,45,47,49,50,53,73-78] (CAD—coronary artery disease; CABG—coronary artery bypass grafting; PTCA—percutaneous transluminal coronary angioplasty)

Table 3 Preoperative Factors Related to Perioperative Morbidity and Mortality[14]

Factor	Description	No. of Points
Ischemic heart disease	MI within 6 mo	10
Congestive heart failure	S_3 gallop or jugular venous distention	11
Cardiac rhythm	Nonsinus rhythm or PACs on last preoperative ECG	7
	> 5 PVCs/min at any point before operation	7
Valvular heart disease	Significant aortic stenosis	3
General medical status	Po_2 < 60 mm Hg or Pco_2 > 50 mm Hg; K$^+$ < 3.0 mmol/L or HCO_3^- < 20 mmol/L; BUN > 50 mg/dl (18 mmol/L) or creatinine > 3.0 mg/dl (260 mmol/L); abnormal AST; signs of chronic liver disease or patient bedridden from noncardiac causes	3
Age	> 70 yr	5
Type of surgery	Intraperitoneal, intrathoracic, or aortic	3
	Emergency	4

AST—aspartate aminotransferase BUN—blood urea nitrogen MI—myocardial infarction PAC—premature atrial contraction Pco_2—partial pressure of carbon dioxide Po_2—partial pressure of oxygen PVC—premature ventricular contraction

to 5 points), ASA class III corresponds to Goldman class II (6 to 12 points), and ASA class IV corresponds to Goldman class III [*see Table 4*]. Goldman and associates remarked, however, that the "subjective" ASA system "could not match" their own system in its ability to isolate 18 "especially high risk patients," in whom 10 of their 19 reported cardiac fatalities occurred.[14]

If it is postulated that a patient with preoperative evidence of heart disease is more likely to suffer perioperative cardiac complications, and if such complications account for the bulk of overall surgical risk, preexisting cardiac disease is probably the most robust predictor of a possible adverse outcome resulting from the stress posed by a noncardiac surgical procedure. This view is supported by the work of Lee and colleagues, who distilled the standard preoperative risk assessment strategies into a prospectively validated index that assigns 1 point to each of the following six clinical factors[15,16]:

1. A high-risk surgical procedure (defined as an intraperitoneal procedure, an intrathoracic procedure, or a suprainguinal vascular procedure).
2. A history of ischemic heart disease.
3. A history of congestive heart failure.
4. A history of cerebrovascular disease.
5. Insulin-dependent diabetes.
6. A serum creatinine level of 2.0 mg/dl or higher.

The resulting score is used to classify risk as mild, intermediate, or high [*see Table 4*]. If diabetes and an elevated creatinine concentration (a frequent cause of renal compromise) are accepted as indicators of vascular disease, five of the six clinical factors can be understood as identifying patients with systemic cardiovascular disease. The logical conclusion to be drawn is that any patient with a history (or cardiovascular test results) suggestive of cardiac problems who is scheduled for a major noncardiac operation (clinical factor 1) is at significantly increased risk from the procedure, and strategies for reducing that risk should be considered.

Respiratory System

Testing of pulmonary function may be indicated on the basis of physical findings (e.g., cough, wheezing, dyspnea on exertion, rales, or rhonchi) or a history of cigarette smoking [*see VI:1 Pulmonary Insufficiency and VII:3 Pulmonary Dysfunction*]. Limited pulmonary reserve may be revealed by observing the patient for dyspnea while he or she is climbing one or two flights of stairs. Forced expiratory volume can be directly measured with a handheld spirometer in all cases where there is a question of possible pulmonary compromise.[17] Once identified, patients with pulmonary compromise may benefit from a preoperative program that includes smoking cessation,[7] use of bronchodilators, physiotherapy, and, if indicated, administration of specific antibiotics.

Nutritional Status

In 1936, Studley demonstrated that weight loss was a basic indicator of operative risk.[18] Loss of more than 15% of body weight during the previous 6 months is associated with an increased incidence of postoperative complications, including delayed wound healing, decreased immunologic competence, and inability to meet the demand for respiratory effort. Peripheral edema and signs of specific vitamin deficiencies are suggestive of severe malnutrition. A global nutritional assessment has been

Table 4 Cardiac Risk Stratification Systems Correlated with ASA Classification

General Risk Category	ASA*			Lee et al[15,16]		Goldman et al[14,73]		
	Class	Description		Points†	Cardiac Morbidity (%)	Risk Class	Points‡	Cardiac Morbidity (%)
Low	I	Normal, healthy patient		0	~0.2	I	0–5	1
	II	Mild disease		1	~1.0			
Moderate	III	Severe but not incapacitating disease		2	~5.0	II	6–12	7
High	IV	Incapacitating disease		≥ 3	~10.0	III	13–25	14
	V	Moribund patient				IV	> 25	78

*See Table 2.
†One point is recorded for each of the following: (1) high-risk operation, (2) ischemic heart disease, (3) congestive heart disease, (4) cerebrovascular disease, (5) insulin-dependent diabetes, and (6) serum creatinine ≥ 2.0 mg/dl.
‡See Table 3.

Table 5 Features of Subjective Global Assessment (SGA)[19]

(Select appropriate category with a checkmark, or enter numerical value where indicated by "#")

A. History

1. Weight change: % weight loss _____

2. Dietary intake change (relative to normal)

_____ No change

_____ Change _____ duration in number of weeks: _____

3. GI symptoms (that persisted for > 2 wk)

_____ None _____ Nausea _____ Vomiting

_____ Diarrhea _____ Anorexia

4. Functional capacity

_____ No dysfunction (e.g., full capacity)

_____ Working suboptimally

_____ Ambulatory

_____ Bedridden

5. Disease and its relation to nutritional requirements

Primary diagnosis (specify)_____

Metabolic demand (stress): _____ No stress _____ Low stress

_____ Moderate stress _____ High stress

B. Physical (for each trait specify: 0 = normal, 1 + = mild, 2 + = moderate, 3 + = severe)

_____ Loss of subcutaneous fat (triceps, chest)

_____ Muscle wasting (quadriceps, deltoids)

_____ Edema

C. Rating (select one)

_____ A = Well-nourished (< 5% weight loss)

_____ B = Moderately nourished (or suspected of being malnourished; 5%–12% weight loss)

_____ C = Severely malnourished (> 12% weight loss)

shown to identify patients who are at increased risk as a result of nutritional deficiencies [*see Table 5*].[19] Individuals with macronutrient deficiencies may benefit from preoperative nutritional supplementation [*see VII:9 Nutritional Support*].

Obese patients frequently require operations for biliary disease, osteoarthritis, hernia, and other common disorders. Preoperative weight loss is encouraged, but the results are usually disappointing. Morbidly obese patients present specific challenges in preoperative management [*see VI:5 Obesity*]; they are at particular risk for cardiovascular and respiratory complications, wound infection, and thromboembolism, and these problems may have to be specifically addressed before the procedure.

Endocrine System

Endocrine-related risk factors are present in patients with hyperthyroidism, hypothyroidism, diabetes mellitus [*see VI:3 Diabetes Mellitus*], pheochromocytoma, or adrenal insufficiency [*see VI:4 Adrenal Insufficiency*] and in those who have received steroid therapy within the preceding 6 months. Certain endocrine conditions should be corrected, or at least stabilized, while the patient awaits admission. Graves disease, for example, calls for a specific preoperative protocol, including administration of thyroid hormone blockers, iodine, and beta blockers. Hypothyroidism is treated with synthetic thyroid hormone. Patients with pheochromocytoma should not undergo operation until adrenergic blockade is adequate.

Hematologic System

Clotting abnormalities are best detected by questioning the patient about familial or personal episodes of unusual bleeding [*see I:5 Bleeding and Transfusion*]. Corroborative findings on physical examination may include petechiae, purpura, or splenomegaly.[20] Risk factors for postoperative phlebothrombosis and, secondarily, pulmonary embolism include hypercoagulability (from antithrombin III deficiency, oral contraceptives, or malignancy), stasis (from obstructed venous outflow, congestive heart failure, or immobility), and vascular endothelial injury (from operation or trauma). Further laboratory evaluation is indicated in patients with any of these conditions.

PREOPERATIVE TESTING

It was once generally agreed that surgical patients should undergo a series of routine screening tests before operation. This approach has not been found to be helpful; it can be confusing, and it is certainly expensive.

It has been observed that the more tests are ordered, the more abnormal values are obtained.[21] On the reasonable assumption that a test performed in a healthy person will yield an abnormal result 5% of the time, when 10 such tests are ordered, there is a 50% probability of an abnormal test result. When an SMA 20 is ordered, the probability of an abnormal test result is quite high. Moreover, although these abnormalities are reported, they rarely alter the physician's behavior or result in cancellation or postponement of the operation [*see Table 6*].[21] Accordingly, current practice is to take a much more selective approach to preoperative laboratory evaluation. Many hospitals now have preoperative testing centers managed by physicians (usually anesthesiologists) who make decisions about which specific preoperative tests are required.

Healthy patients younger than 40 years need not undergo any preoperative laboratory evaluation unless a specific test is indicated by a relevant detail in the history or the physical examination (for example, a finger-stick hematocrit in a young woman with dysmenorrhea). There are, however, certain tests that may be useful in older patients: some authors recommend obtaining

Table 6 Effect of Abnormal Screening Test Results on Physician Behavior[21]

Screening Test	Abnormal Test Results (%)	Resulting Management Change (%)
Hemoglobin level	5 (for < 10 g/dl; < 9 g/dl was rare)	Abnormal result rarely led to change
Total leukocyte count	< 1	Abnormal result rarely led to change
Bleeding time	3.8	Abnormal result rarely led to change
Coagulation time	4.8	
Partial thromboplastin time	15.6	
Chest x-ray	2.5–3.7	2.1
ECG	4.6–31.7	0–2.2
Sodium, potassium	1.4 2.5 5.2	Abnormal result rarely led to change
Urinalysis	1–34.1	0.1–2.8

electrocardiograms, chest x-rays, serum creatinine levels, glucose levels, and hemoglobin concentrations in patients older than 40 years [see Table 7].[22]

Cardiac Tests

Despite the preeminence of cardiac risk as a component of overall surgical risk and despite the comfort to be gained from obtaining so-called cardiology clearance, there is no more justification for routine preoperative cardiac testing than for any other form of routine preoperative testing. To assess surgical risk not only accurately but also cost-effectively, one must take a selective and thoughtful approach to the use of cardiac tests.

The most powerful predictor of cardiac risk comes from the information obtained by communicating with the patient. Talking to the patient is an invaluable first step; frequently, in fact, it is the only essential step. Accordingly, the extent to which the patient is willing or able to communicate can have a pronounced effect on the subsequent course of cardiac evaluation. If the patient reports no exertional angina, fatigue, shortness of breath, or syncope and if a resting ECG (if performed) reveals no evidence of coronary artery disease, the surgeon may proceed with elective surgery without further testing [see Figure 1]. If the patient does not or cannot communicate well or coronary artery disease is a possibility, an exercise ECG should be obtained.

Resting electrocardiogram   Although the heart, like most organs, typically does not exhibit dysfunction until stressed, many physicians, for practical and economic reasons, continue to screen patients with a resting ECG. A previous MI—indicated by the presence of a Q wave 0.04 second or wider in any of the 12 standard ECG leads—is accepted as evidence of coronary artery disease; however, the absence of pathologic Q waves is not necessarily indicative of a healthy heart.[23] Although perioperative risk increases with left ventricular hypertrophy or a nonsinus rhythm (which is easily detected by palpating the patient's pulse) and 3% to 4% of adults exhibit a previously undiagnosed MI, the resting ECG is not a powerful predictor of cardiac complications.

Exercise electrocardiogram   The Seattle Heart Watch collected data on thousands of persons—some of whom had cardiac disease and some of whom did not—to assess the predictive value of exercise ECGs.[24,25] The investigators carefully related exercise level to (1) heart rate, (2) heart rate multiplied by systolic BP (rate-pressure product), and (3) calculated total-body oxygen uptake. Four indicators of ischemic heart disease were observed:

1. ST segment depression (≥ 2 mm).
2. Exercise-induced hypotension (≥ 10 mm Hg fall in systolic BP).
3. Complex ventricular ectopy (three or more consecutive premature ventricular depolarizations).
4. Symptomatic chest pain.

A later study that specifically focused on the assessment of 185 patients undergoing noncardiac surgery found that ST segment depression as small as 1.0 mm was an independent predictor of perioperative cardiac complications.[26]

Relevance of gender.   Traditionally, when measured against coronary angiography, exercise electrocardiography has been considered relatively inaccurate in females: false positive rates as high as 40% have been recorded in women, compared with rates

Table 7   Minimal Preoperative Test Requirements* at the Mayo Clinic[22]

Age (yr)	Tests Required
< 40	None
40–59	Electrocardiography, measurement of creatinine and glucose
≥ 60	Complete blood cell count, electrocardiography, chest roentgenography, measurement of creatinine and glucose

*In addition, the following guidelines apply. (1) A complete blood cell count is indicated in all patients who undergo blood typing and who are crossmatched. (2) Measurement of potassium is indicated in patients taking diuretics or undergoing bowel preparation. (3) Chest roentgenography is indicated in patients with a history of cardiac or pulmonary disease or with recent respiratory symptoms. (4) A history of cigarette smoking in patients older than 40 years who are scheduled for an upper abdominal or thoracic surgical procedure is an indication for spirometry (forced vital capacity).

lower than 10% in men.[27] This discrepancy may be partially attributable to the use of identical ST segment criteria for both males and females.[28] A 2001 study from the Mayo Clinic evaluated the accuracy of exercise ECG testing in 3,213 women and 5,458 men.[29] In relative terms, there was a noticeable gender-related difference between the two groups, in that there was a higher prevalence of false positive ECG tests in the female patients. In absolute terms, however, this difference was not of critical import, in that the false positive rate was not particularly high (< 15%) in either men or women. The investigators concluded that gender should not be used as a justification for selecting expensive stress imaging over standard treadmill testing.

In patients whose anticipated risk of coronary artery disease is low, the sensitivity of an exercise ECG may be as low as 45%.[30] Even so, it is clear that a thoughtful physician can interpret an exercise ECG in concert with a careful history and thereby accomplish a highly precise cardiac risk assessment.[16] Like all other components of preoperative risk evaluation, the exercise ECG should never be considered in a vacuum.

Ambulatory electrocardiogram   Ambulatory monitoring demonstrates that silent (asymptomatic) ischemia occurs in almost all patients with chronic stable angina and in more than 75% of patients with diagnosed coronary artery disease.[23] Unfortunately, a nonischemic ambulatory ECG does not preclude the diagnosis of cardiac muscle damage as identified by perfusion imaging.[31] If myocardial perfusion scanning is taken as the standard, the ambulatory ECG has both low sensitivity and low specificity for the detection of ischemic heart disease.[23] Conversely, cardiac arrhythmias do not invariably indicate coronary artery or cardiac disease.[32]

Stress cardiac imaging   The strength of stress cardiac imaging studies is that they are capable of differentiating healthy from ischemic from scarred myocardium. The surgeon's primary preoperative concern in this regard is to identify those patients with ischemic myocardium that may give rise to a perioperative MI; scarred myocardium is a less immediate concern, in that it represents an old infarction and is relatively stable.

Radionuclide scanning (e.g., with thallium 201) after exercise or pharmacologically induced stress is a useful method of identifying zones of potential ischemia. For patients who cannot exercise, the requisite level of stress can be generated by administering agents such as dobutamine or dipyridamole. Dipyridamole is a potent coronary vasodilator, but it can only dilate normal coronary arteries, which means that a dipyridamole thallium study essentially diverts available coronary blood flow away from the fixed (i.e., nondilatable) atherosclerotic coronary vessels. Thus, exercise and dipyridamole thallium scans should be interpreted as provocative coronary perfusion imaging studies. Such scans can provide a great deal of valuable data and are reported to be as specific as and more sensitive than exercise ECGs.[33,34]

Echocardiographic stress imaging appears to be as successful as radionuclide stress imaging at identifying jeopardized zones of ischemic myocardial tissue.[35] The heart (like all organs) is incapable of storing oxygen; what is more, it has a prodigious metabolic rate. As a result, there is an observable decrease in myocardial contractility within seconds of the time that oxygen demand exceeds supply. If echocardiography detects decreased wall motion in association with stress, the myocardium is considered to be at risk. There are now multiple studies available indicating that both radionuclide and echocardiographic stress imaging provide more diagnostic information than exercise electrocardiography does.[16]

Exercise capacity as a surrogate measure of perioperative risk It would seem intuitively obvious that a patient's cardiovascular resilience in the face of the stress generated by a major surgical procedure ought to correlate well with his or her exercise capacity. Indeed, treadmill exercise testing is an accepted screening measure for cardiovascular disease; however, it can also provide objective quantification of exercise capacity in terms of metabolic equivalents (METs).

In a 2002 study, Myers and colleagues examined the relation between exercise capacity (expressed in METs) and all-cause mortality in more than 6,000 men.[36] Slightly more than half of the patients had abnormal exercise tolerance test results and were designated as having cardiovascular disease; the remainder had normal test results and were designated as healthy. Although advancing age was associated with an increasing risk of death, absolute peak exercise capacity was a more robust predictor of survival than was the percentage of the age-adjusted exercise value achieved. This finding held true for both healthy patients and patients with cardiovascular disease. Indeed, peak exercise capacity was a stronger predictor of survival than were such commonly used variables as a history of hypertension; the presence of chronic obstructive pulmonary disease or diabetes; a history of smoking; a high body mass index; and an elevated total cholesterol level. The survival relationship was highly linear, with each 1 MET improvement in peak treadmill performance conferring a 12% survival advantage. This graded inverse relation between exercise capacity and all-cause mortality has been reported in both men and women[37] as well as in both healthy and unhealthy men.[38]

Strictly speaking, the results of the Myers study are applicable only to men. When women undergo stress testing using default criteria specific to men, the results are predictably imprecise.[39] It would seem logical, however, to assume that the stresses of life and of surgery should be essentially similar in men and women; there is little, if any, reason to believe that such stresses are gender specific.[40]

If the association between peak exercise capacity and survival reported in these studies is accepted, the question then arises of whether it is invariably necessary for surgeons to subject their preoperative patients to the vicissitudes of an exercise tolerance test. Activities of normal living can also be quantified in terms of METs, and the ability to perform such activities may be used as an indicator of peak exercise capacity. For example, the energy expended in sitting comfortably at rest is equivalent to 1 MET or, in hemodynamic terms, an oxygen consumption of 3.5 ml/kg/min. The energy expended in shopping for groceries or doing housework is equivalent to approximately 4 METs. The energy expended in climbing several flights of stairs comfortably is equivalent to 5 to 8 METs. The energy expended in vigorous exercise (e.g., jogging, swimming, and energetic dancing) is equivalent to more than 8 METs. In both the Myers study[36] and the Blair study that included men and women,[37] the risk of death was twice as high in patients capable of less than 5 METs as it was in patients capable of at least 8 METs, even when all the usual comorbid conditions were ignored.

Admittedly, exercise capacity is not a foolproof guide to cardiovascular risk: even fit patients may die as a consequence of surgical treatment. All cardiologic clearance strategies now in use are flawed to some extent, and some of them carry both a degree of inherent risk and a significant physiologic or financial price. In the absence of any perfect preoperative screening algorithm, it can be argued that the Myers[36] and Blair[37,38] studies provide a sufficiently sound epidemiologic foundation for a highly practical preoperative assessment that does not require an exercise tolerance test. From this perspective, if a patient older than 40 years requires an elective surgical procedure and is known to be capable of walking up several flights of stairs (i.e., capable of more than 5 METs), it is reasonable for the surgeon simply to begin administering beta blockers and then proceed with the operation.

Reduction of Perioperative Cardiac Risk

Once patients at significant risk for cardiac complications have been identified, the logical next step is to attempt to reduce the risk to the extent feasible. Ideally, such attempts should be firmly based on scientific data. There are several risk-reduction approaches for which a significant degree of scientific support exists.

For a patient admitted to the hospital with a working diagnosis of MI, the projected 30-day mortality would be approximately 15%.[41] If the same patient had had a prior MI and experienced another MI during a routine sigmoid resection for diverticulitis, the projected 30-day mortality might be as high as 69%.[42] In a medical setting, a patient with an MI is treated with pharmacologic agents such as heparin, nitroglycerin, morphine, thrombolytics, beta blockers, angiotensin-converting enzyme inhibitors, and statins,[41] whereas in the surgical setting, a patient with an MI is faced with the stress imposed by elevated catecholamine levels, hemodynamic compromise, anesthesia, and incisional pain.[42]

At the current state of our knowledge, it is possible to attenuate the cardiac stress associated with noncardiac surgery to a significant degree (though not to eliminate it entirely). One approach to accomplishing this is to maintain intraoperative normothermia. Operating rooms are cold, and the use of general anesthesia impairs the body's normal defense mechanisms against cold exposure. Patients who undergo major procedures lasting more than 2 hours frequently become mildly hypothermic (defined as a 1° to 3° reduction in core temperature), and this hypothermia is associated with an outpouring of catecholamines, cortisol, and other stress hormones. In one randomized trial, use of a patient-warming device to prevent intraoperative mild hypothermia led to a substantially reduced incidence of postoperative morbid cardiac events (1.4% versus 6.3% in the hypothermic control subjects; $P = 0.04$).[43] The incidence of ventricular tachycardia was reduced in this group as well (2.4% versus 7.9%; $P = 0.04$).

Another approach to mitigating the surgical stress response is to employ epidural anesthesia, which blocks afferent nerve traffic to the brain and thus attenuates sympathetic nervous stimulation. A meta-analysis published in 2000 found that the incidence of postoperative MI was about 30% lower in patients who received regional anesthesia than in those who received general anesthesia.[44]

Yet another approach is to maintain scrupulous control of heart rate and BP in the perioperative period in an effort to achieve a lower cardiac event rate and improved surgical survival. A 1983 study retrospectively reviewed 364 patients who underwent noncardiac surgery, all of whom had experienced an MI either 0 to 3 months or 4 to 6 months before the procedure; these patients constituted what was admittedly a high-risk control group.[45] The investigators then prospectively studied 733 similar patients who had recently had an MI and were scheduled for noncardiac surgery. Throughout the perioperative period, this latter group received prompt pharmacologic intervention for any BP or pulse rate deviation of more than 10% from resting preoperative values, whereas the control group did not. In the control group, perioperative reinfarction occurred in 36% of patients whose MIs had occurred 0 to 3 months earlier and in 26% of patients whose MIs had occurred 4 to 6 months earlier. In the group whose heart rates and BPs were meticulously controlled, however, the corresponding perioperative reinfarction rates were only 5.7% and 2.3%, respectively ($P < 0.05$). In the intervention group, there was significantly less use of vasopressors and more use of vasodilators, inotropes, beta blockers, and antiarrhythmic agents.

Still another approach is to administer beta blockers perioperatively. A prospective study from 1996 randomly assigned 200 noncardiac surgical patients to receive either the beta blocker atenolol or placebo.[46] Atenolol was administered intravenously before and immediately after surgery; it was then continued orally until the end of hospitalization, at which point it was stopped. Of the original 200 patients, 194 survived hospitalization, and 192 were followed for 2 years. Mortality, even after hospital discharge and discontinuance of beta blockade, was significantly lower in atenolol-treated patients than in control subjects both at 6 months (0% versus 8%; $P < 0.001$) and at 2 years (10% versus 21%; $P = 0.019$). These findings, though somewhat puzzling, have sparked considerable enthusiasm for perioperative beta blockade[47-51]; however, some clinicians have expressed reservations.[52]

In 1999, a Dutch echocardiographic cardiac risk evaluation study group published a prospective, randomized, multicenter study of perioperative beta blockade in extremely high risk vascular surgical patients.[53] Of the 1,351 patients screened, 846 exhibited cardiac risk factors that would have made them moderate- or high-risk patients according to either Goldman's or Lee's classification system. Of these 846 patients, 173 had positive results on dobutamine stress echocardiography, and 112 of the 173 agreed to undergo randomization. Of these 112 patients, 59 patients were randomly assigned to perioperative beta blockade with bisoprolol, and 53 served as control subjects. Of the patients undergoing beta blockade, 3.4% died of cardiac causes or experienced a nonfatal MI, compared with 34% of the control subjects ($P < 0.001$). Admittedly, this is a study of very high risk patients; nonetheless, the conclusions are striking, and it is tempting to extrapolate them to lower-risk noncardiac surgical patients. In the human heart, alpha$_1$-, beta$_1$-, and beta$_2$-adrenergic receptors promote inotropy, chronotropy, myocyte apoptosis, and direct myocyte toxicity.[47] Expanded use of beta-adrenergic receptor inhibition in the perioperative period has been supported by a number of authors.[54-58]

Prophylactic use of other agents (e.g., aspirin, alpha$_2$-adrenergic agents, nitroglycerin, and calcium channel blockers) has been studied, but at present, the data are insufficient to support routine use of any of them for this purpose.[57,59]

Patient Education

Once appropriate diagnostic information has been obtained, the operative plan should be discussed with the patient and the risks and benefits of the procedure outlined. When the surgeon is satisfied that the patient is fully informed in this regard, a consent form should be signed. The patient should then be told what to expect during the perioperative period.

Education of the patient about the postoperative care plan plays a major role in modifying his or her response to the operative experience. Classic studies demonstrated that well-informed patients require less analgesia in the postoperative period and, at the same time, experience significantly less pain than less well informed patients.[60] Subsequent investigations supported the conclusion that preoperative information facilitates coping, reduces preoperative anxiety, and may also enhance postsurgical recovery.[61,62] Such information can be provided verbally (by the surgeon or a member of his or her staff) or in the form of educational tools (e.g., videotapes and information booklets). In addition, an overly anxious patient often benefits from visiting a satisfied patient who has recently undergone the same operation.

Finally, the patient should receive a checklist of instructions outlining specific actions to be taken in preparation for the procedure (e.g., adjustments of medications or steps to follow in the course of bowel preparation). The time and place at which the patient is to be admitted to the hospital should also be clearly recorded.

Discussion

Epidemiology of Surgical Risk

Various investigators have prospectively studied the outcomes of surgical procedures in efforts to identify variables related to poor results. One such study comes from the Department of Veterans Affairs, which initiated a quality improvement program aimed at prospectively determining factors related to outcome. Initial results were reported from 23,919 patients undergoing one of 11 noncardiac operations performed by surgeons from five specialties (general surgery, urology, orthopedic surgery, vascular surgery, and neurosurgery).[63] The authors demonstrated that prolonged hospital stay could be related to (1) preoperative patient characteristics, (2) intraoperative events, and (3) postoperative occurrences. The specific preoperative patient characteristics associated with prolonged hospitalization included advanced age,

---

Table 8 Factors Associated with Prolonged Hospitalization[63]

Preoperative factors
  Advanced age (> 60 yr)
  Diminished functional status (fully dependent vs fully or partially independent)
  ASA class III or IV
Intraoperative factors
  Transfusion of ≥ 1 unit of blood
  Operating time ≥ 5 hr
Postoperative factors
  Return to OR
  Occurrence of ≥ 2 complications

---

diminished functional status, and higher ASA class [*see Table 8*]. Other preoperative patient characteristics were associated with increased morbidity and mortality [*see Table 9*].[64,65]

A similar approach was taken by investigators in New Zealand, who predicted the risk of surgical morbidity on the basis of operating time, operation category, the hospital status of the patient (inpatient versus outpatient), and the organ system on which the procedure was performed.[66]

Such attempts to predict surgical outcome are laudable, in that they establish standards of care and allow comparisons between institutions, both of which are useful for upgrading underperforming surgical services. It must be pointed out, however, that approaches of this type offer little opportunity for improving outcome for individual patients. Age and disease are reasonably fixed. Skilled surgeons work to minimize operating time and blood loss; a longer than usual procedure or greater than normal blood loss is usually related to the extent of the patient's disease or to the technical difficulty associated with the operation, neither of which is easily modified before or during the operation.

In the hope of actually effecting improvements in individual outcomes, other investigators proposed testing methodologies aimed at identifying specific risks in specific patients and, ideally, facilitating reduction of these risks before operation. For example, Buzby and associates proposed a method of nutrition assessment whose results were related to outcome.[67] In this method, a prognostic index was calculated by determining the serum albumin and transferrin levels and assessing the patient's response to skin testing. Presumably, if this index suggested an unsatisfactory outcome, nutritional intervention could be carried out preoperatively to correct the deficiency, thereby improving outcome. Subsequently, a trial done by a study group of the Department of Veterans Affairs determined that preoperative nutritional intervention was necessary only in the most severely nutritionally depleted patients (> 15% body weight loss), and weight loss became the sole metric used in determining the need for preoperative nutritional support.[68]

Christou and associates used delayed-type hypersensitivity skin test responses to predict septic events in surgical patients[69]; they hoped that immunologic stimulation or nutritional support might improve host resistance in anergic patients. Although, initially, an association was found between skin test reactivity and predicted outcome, over time, surgical care improved and overall mortality fell as a result [*see Table 10*]. The relation between septic events and delayed-type hypersensitivity in elective surgical patients lost its significance, so that intervention of the type the investigators originally envisioned was not possible.[70]

Cost-Effectiveness

A 1999 study assessed the cost-effectiveness of various cardiac diagnostic strategies in terms of cost in relation to each quality-adjusted life year (QALY) saved.[71] Although the question this study was designed to answer was slightly different from the one surgeons typically address before noncardiac surgery, several instructive findings emerged.

1. For a 55-year-old man with typical chest pain, the incremental cost-effectiveness ratio for routine coronary angiography versus exercise echocardiography was $36,400/QALY saved.
2. For a 55-year-old man with atypical chest pain, the incremental cost-effectiveness ratio for exercise electrocardiography versus no testing was $57,700/QALY saved.
3. The incremental cost-effectiveness ratio for exercise echocardiography versus stress electrocardiography was $41,900/QALY saved.

Table 9 Preoperative Predictors of Morbidity and Mortality in General Surgical Patients[64,65]

Rank	Predictor of Morbidity	Predictor of Mortality
1	Albumin concentration	Albumin concentration
2	ASA class	ASA class
3	Complexity of operation	Emergency operation
4	Emergency operation	Disseminated cancer
5	Functional status	Age
6	History of COPD	DNR status
7	BUN > 40 mg/dl	Platelet count < 150,000/mm³
8	Dependency on ventilator	Weight loss > 10%
9	Age	Complexity of operation
10	WBC count > 11,000/mm³	BUN > 40 mg/dl

Table 10 Hospital Mortality in Elective Surgical Patients in a Single Hospital over a 20-Year Period,* Stratified by Admission Skin Test Response[70]

Admission Skin Test Response	Period	N	Alive (%)	Dead (%)
Reactive	1973–1979	896	877 (97.8)	19 (2.1)
	1980–1989	629	611 (97.1)	18 (2.9)
	1990–1994	615	606 (98.5)	9 (1.5)
Relatively anergic	1973–1979	114	106 (93.0)	8 (7.0)
	1980–1989	117	111 (94.9)	6 (5.1)
	1990–1994	163	159 (97.5)	4 (2.5)
Anergic	1973–1979	142	109 (76.8)	33 (23.2)
	1980–1989	199	149 (74.9)	50 (25.1)
	1990–1994	206	193 (93.7)	13 (6.3)

*$\chi^2 = 27.4$; $P < 0.000001$.

Table 11 Effectiveness of Selected Risk Indicators as Predictors of Cardiac Events

Risk Indicator	Study (Year)	Type of Study	Findings	Comments
Age	Mangano et al[73] (1995)	Retrospective: 1,001 patients > 40 yr undergoing general anesthesia	10-fold increase in perioperative death in patients > 70 yr	—
History of congestive heart failure	Kumar et al[80] (2001)	Prospective: 1,121 patients with known or suspected cardiac problems	90% increase in severe or serious complications	Prospective cohort study from urban VA hospital
History of ischemic heart disease or cerebrovascular disease	Lee et al[81] (1999)	Prospective: 4,315 patients undergoing elective major noncardiac surgery	Increased risk of major perioperative cardiac complications	Risk stratification improved by including high-risk surgery, history of CHF, preoperative insulin therapy, and serum creatinine > 2.0 mg/dl
Recent MI	Fleisher[52] (1999)	Retrospective: 587 patients with prior MI who underwent general anesthesia	MI < 3 mo ago: perioperative MI in 27% MI 3–6 mo ago: perioperative MI in 11% MI > 6 mo ago: perioperative MI in 5%	75% of perioperative MIs silent; 69% of MIs fatal Though old, study yields good stratification of risk by antecedent MI timing
Exercise stress testing	Gauss et al[26] (2001)	Prospective: 204 intermediate-risk patients undergoing noncardiac surgery	0.1 mV (1 mm) ST segment depression associated with 420% increase in perioperative cardiac events	Risk stratification improved by combining stress test results with clinical variables
Reduced ejection fraction	Rohde et al[82] (2001)	Prospective: 570 patients undergoing major noncardiac surgery who were assessed with transthoracic echocardiography	140% increase in major cardiac complications	Risk stratification improved by including clinical variables
Echocardiography vs SPECT vs PET	Garber et al[33] (1999)	Meta-analysis: men and women at intermediate risk for coronary artery disease	Echocardiography was most cost-effective; incremental cost-effectiveness ratio was $75,000/QALY for SPECT and $640,000/QALY for PET	—
ASA index vs Goldman index vs Canadian Cardiovascular Society index	Gilbert et al[83] (2000)	Prospective: 2,035 patients seen before elective or urgent noncardiac surgery	All indices performed well and did not differ significantly from each other with respect to assessment of preoperative risk	—

ASA—American Society of Anesthesiologists   PET—positron emission tomography   QALY—quality-adjusted life year   SPECT—single photon emission computed tomography

The literature makes it clear that none of the available diagnostic strategies are more cost-effective than communication with the patient [see Table 11]. Neither routine noninvasive testing nor routine coronary angiography (even when done before vascular surgery) is cost-effective; however, selective screening in advance of vascular surgery is cost-effective and may improve 5-year survival [see Table 11].[72] A simple rule of thumb is that any chest pain or historical evidence of systemic cardiovascular or cerebrovascular disease is a sign that caution should be exercised in subjecting the patient to the stress of noncardiac surgery.

References

1. Shiell AM, Griffiths RD, Short AIK, et al: An evaluation of the costs and outcomes of adult intensive care in two units in the UK. Clin Intens Care 1:256, 1990

2. Ferguson TB Jr, Dziuban SW Jr, Edwards FH, et al: The STS National Database: current changes and challenges for the new millennium. Committee to Establish a National Database in Cardiothoracic Surgery, the Society of Thoracic Surgeons. Ann Thorac Surg 69:680, 2000

3. Dripps RD, Echenhoff JE, Vandom D: Introduction to Anesthesia: The Principles of Safe Practice. WB Saunders Co, Philadelphia, 1988, p 17

4. Cullen DJ, Apolone G, Greenfield S, et al: ASA physical status and age predict morbidity after three surgical procedures. Ann Surg 220:3, 1994

5. Hampson JR, Harrison MAG, Mitchell JAR, et al: Relative contributions of history-taking, physical examination, and laboratory investigation to diagnosis and management of medical outpatients. BMJ 2:486, 1975

6. Jackson CV: Preoperative pulmonary evaluation. Arch Intern Med 148:2120, 1988

7. Møller AM, Villebro N, Pedersen T, et al: Effect of preoperative smoking intervention on postoperative complications: a randomised clinical trial. Lancet 359:114, 2002

8. Tonnesen H, Kehlet H: Preoperative alcoholism and postoperative morbidity. Br J Surg 86:869, 1999

9. Tonnesen H, Rosenberg J, Nielsen HJ, et al: Effect of preoperative abstinence on poor postoperative outcome in alcohol misusers: randomised controlled trial. BMJ 318:1311, 1999

10. Tarhan S, Moffit EA, Taylor WF, et al: Myocardial infarction after general anesthesia. JAMA 220:1451, 1972

11. Gomez-Sanchez CE, Gomez-Sanchez EP, Yamakita N: Endocrine causes of hypertension. Semin Nephrol 15:106, 1995

12. Ross NS: Epidemiology of Cushing's syndrome and subclinical disease. Endocrinol Metab Clin North Am 23:539, 1994

13. Bickler SW, McMahon TJ, Campbell JR, et al: Preoperative diagnostic evaluation of children with Cushing's syndrome. J Pediatr Surg 29:671, 1994

14. Goldman L, Caldera DL, Nussbaum S, et al: Multifactorial index of cardiac risk in noncardiac surgical procedures. N Engl J Med 297:845, 1977

15. Lee TH: Reducing cardiac risk in noncardiac surgery. N Engl J Med 341:1838, 1999

16. Lee TH, Boucher CA: Clinical practice: noninvasive tests in patients with stable coronary artery disease. N Engl J Med 344:1840, 2001

17. Kispert TF, Kazmers A, Roitman L: Preoperative spirometry predicts postoperative pulmonary complications after major vascular surgery. Am Surg 58:419, 1992

18. Studley HO: Percentage of weight loss: basic indicator of surgical risk in patients with chronic peptic ulcer. JAMA 106:458, 1936

19. Detsky AS, McLaughlin JR, Baker JP, et al: What is subjective global status of nutritional state? JPEN J Parenter Enteral Nutr 11:8, 1987

20. Messmore HL Jr, Godwin J: Medical assessment of bleeding in the surgical patient. Med Clin North Am 78:625, 1994

21. MacPherson DS: Preoperative laboratory testing: should any tests be "routine" before surgery? Med Clin North Am 77:289, 1993

22. Narr BJ, Hansen TR, Warner MA: Preoperative laboratory screening in healthy Mayo patients: cost-effective elimination of test and unchanged outcomes. Mayo Clin Proc 66:155, 1991

23. Baszko A, Ochotny R, Blaszyk K, et al: Correlation of ST-segment depression during ambulatory electrocardiographic monitoring with myocardial perfusion and left ventricular function. Am J Cardiol 87:959, 2001

24. Bruce RA: Exercise testing for evaluation of ventricular function. N Engl J Med 296:671, 1977

25. Bruce RA, Hornstein TR: The exercise stress testing in evaluation of patients with ischemic heart disease. Prog Cardiovasc Dis 11:371, 1969

26. Gauss A, Rohm HJ, Schauffelen A, et al: Electrocardiographic exercise stress testing for cardiac risk assessment in patients undergoing noncardiac surgery. Anesthesiology 94:38, 2001

27. Judelson DR: Examining the gender bias in evaluating coronary disease in women. Medscape Womens Health 2:5, 1997

28. Okin PM, Kligfield P: Gender-specific criteria and performance of the exercise electrocardiogram. Circulation 92:1209, 1995

29. Mille TD, Roger VL, Milavetz JJ, et al: Assessment of the exercise electrocardiogram in women versus men using tomographic myocardial perfusion imaging as the reference standard. Am J Cardiol 87:868, 2001

30. Froelicher VF, Lehmann KG, Thomas R, et al: The electrocardiographic exercise test in a population with reduced workup bias: diagnostic performance, computerized interpretation, and multivariable prediction. Ann Intern Med 128:965, 1998

31. Kontos MC, Kurdziel KA, Ornato JP, et al: A nonischemic electrocardiogram does not always predict a small myocardial infarction: results with acute myocardial perfusion imaging. Am Heart J 141:360, 2001

32. Chung KY, Lee SJ: Cardiac arrhythmias in F-16 pilots during aerial combat maneuvers (ACMS): a descriptive study focused on G-level acceleration. Aviat Space Environ Med 72:534, 2001

33. Garber AM, Solomon NA: Cost-effectiveness of alternative test strategies for the diagnosis of coronary artery disease. Ann Intern Med 130:719, 1999

34. Yao SS, Rozanski A: Principal uses of myocardial perfusion scintigraphy in the management of patients with known or suspected coronary artery disease. Prog Cardiovasc Dis 43:281, 2001

35. Pingitore A, Picano E, Varga A, et al: Prognostic value of pharmacological stress echocardiography in patients with known or suspected coronary artery disease: a prospective, large-scale, multicenter, head-to-head comparison between dipyridamole and dobutamine test. J Am Coll Cardiol 34:1769, 1999

36. Myers J, Prakash M, Froelicher V, et al: Exercise capacity and mortality among men referred for exercise testing. N Engl J Med 346:793, 2002

37. Blair SN, Kohl HW III, Paffenbarger RS Jr, et al: Physical fitness and all-cause mortality: a prospective study of healthy men and women. JAMA 262:2395, 1989

38. Blair SN, Kohl HW III, Barlow CE, et al: Changes in physical fitness and all-cause mortality: a prospective study of healthy and unhealthy men. JAMA 273:1093, 1995

39. Shaw LJ, Hachamovitch R, Redberg RF: Current evidence on diagnostic testing in women with suspected coronary artery disease: choosing the appropriate test. Cardiol Rev 8:65, 2000

40. Balady GJ: Survival of the fittest—more evidence. N Engl J Med 346:852, 2002

41. Daneman N, Austin PC, Tu JV: Investigating the determinants of decreasing postmyocardial infarction mortality: an analysis of in-hospital data from 1992 and 1997. Can J Cardiol 17:771, 2001

42. Steen PA, Tinker JH, Tarhan S: Myocardial reinfarction after anesthesia and surgery. JAMA 239:2566, 1978

43. Frank SM, Fleisher LA, Breslow MJ, et al: Perioperative maintenance of normothermia reduces the incidence of morbid cardiac events: a randomized clinical trial. JAMA 277:1127, 1997

44. Rodgers A, Walker N, Schug S, et al: Reduction of postoperative mortality and morbidity with epidural or spinal anaesthesia: results from overview of randomised trials. BMJ 321:1493, 2000

45. Rao TL, Jacobs KH, El-Etr AA: Reinfarction following anesthesia in patients with myocardial infarction. Anesthesiology 59:499, 1983

46. Mangano DT, Layug EL, Wallace A, et al: Effect of atenolol on mortality and cardiovascular morbidity after noncardiac surgery: multicenter study of perioperative ischemia research group. N Engl J Med 335:1713, 1996

47. Selzman CG, Miller SA, Zimmerman MA, et al: The case for beta-adrenergic blockade as prophylaxis against perioperative cardiovascular morbidity and mortality. Arch Surg 136:286, 2001

48. Petros JA: Effect of atenolol on mortality and cardiovascular morbidity after noncardiac surgery. N Engl J Med 336:1452, 1997

49. Leung JM: Beta blockade in non-cardiac surgical patients. Anesthesiology 89:795, 1998

50. Warltier DC: Beta-adrenergic blocking drugs: incredibly useful, incredibly underutilized. Anesthesiology 88:2, 1998

51. Isaacson JH: Should patients with documented or probable coronary artery disease routinely be placed on beta-blockers before noncardiac surgery? Cleve Clin J Med 68:273, 2001

52. Fleisher LA: Con: beta-blockers should not be used in all patients undergoing vascular surgery. J Cardiothorac Vasc Anesth 13:496, 1999

53. Poldermans D, Boersma E, Bax JJ, et al: The effect of bisoprolol on perioperative mortality and myocardial infarction in high-risk patients undergoing vascular surgery. Dutch Echocardiographic Cardiac Risk Evaluation Applying Stress Echocardiography Study Group. N Engl J Med 341:1789, 1999

54. Feldman T, Fusman B, McKinsey JF: Beta-blockade for patients undergoing vascular surgery. N Engl J Med 342:1051, 2000

55. Dickerson LM, Carek PJ: Bisoprolol prevents mortality and myocardial infarction after vascular surgery. J Fam Pract 49:203, 2000

56. Jones KG, Powell JT: Slowing the heart saves lives: advantages of perioperative beta-blockade. Br J Surg 87:689, 2000

57. Fleisher LA, Eagle KA: Lowering cardiac risk in noncardiac surgery. N Engl J Med 345:1677, 2001

58. Auerbach AD, Goldman L: β-Blockers and reduction of cardiac events in noncardiac surgery. JAMA 287:1435, 2002

59. Madi A, Plavec M, Nawaz H, et al: Peri-operative aspirin can prevent post-operative ischemia and thrombosis. Med Hypotheses 55:164, 2000

60. Egbert LD, Bant GE, Welch CE, et al: Reduction of postoperative pain by encouragement and instruction of patients. N Engl J Med 207:824, 1964

61. Daltroy LH, Morlino CI, Eaton HM, et al: Preoperative education for total hip and knee replacement patients. Arthritis Care Res 11:469, 1998

62. Klafta JM, Roizen MF: Current understanding of patients' attitudes toward and preparation for anesthetic: a review. Anesth Analg 83:1314, 1996

63. Collins TC, Daley J, Henderson WH, et al: Risk factors for prolonged length of stay after major elective surgery. Ann Surg 230:251, 1999

64. Khuri SF, Daley J, Henderson W, et al: Risk adjustment of the mortality rate for the comparative assessment of the quality of surgical care: results of the National Veterans Affairs Surgical Risk Study. J Am Coll Surg 185:315, 1997

65. Daley J, Khuri SF, Henderson W, et al: Risk adjustment of postoperative morbidity rate for the comparative assessment of the quality of surgical care: results of the National Veteran's Affairs Surgical Risk Study. J Am Coll Surg 185:328, 1997

66. Pillai SB, van Rij AM, Williams S, et al: Complexity- and risk-adjusted model for measuring surgical outcome. Br J Surg 86:1567, 1999

67. Buzby GP, Mullen JL, Matthews DC, et al: Prognostic nutritional index in gastrointestinal surgery. Am J Surg 139:160, 1980

68. Perioperative total parenteral nutrition in surgical patients. Veteran's Affairs Total Parenteral Nutrition Study Group. N Engl J Med 325:525, 1991

69. Christou NV, Tellado-Rodriques J, Chartrand L, et al: Estimating mortality risk in preoperative patients using immunologic, nutritional and acute phase response variables. Ann Surg 210:69, 1989

70. Christou NV, Meakins JL, Gordon J, et al: The delayed hypersensitivity response and host resistance in surgical patients 20 years later. Ann Surg 222:534, 1995

71. Kuntz KM, Fleischmann KE, Hunink MG, et al: Cost-effectiveness of diagnostic strategies for patients with chest pain. Ann Intern Med 130:709, 1999

72. Glance LG: Selective preoperative cardiac screening improves five-year survival in patients undergoing major vascular surgery: a cost-effectiveness analysis. J Cardiothorac Vasc Anesth 13:265, 1999

73. Mangano DT, Goldman L: Preoperative assessment of patients with known or suspected coronary disease. N Engl J Med 333:1750, 1995

74. Krupski WC, Nehler MR, Whitehill TA, et al: Negative impact of cardiac evaluation before vascular surgery. Vasc Med 5:3, 2000

75. Jones RH, Kesler K, Phillips HR 3rd, et al: Long-term survival benefits of coronary artery bypass grafting and percutaneous transluminal angioplasty in patients with coronary artery disease. J Thorac Cardiovasc Surg 111:1013, 1996

76. Hertzer NR, Young JR, Beven EG, et al: Late results of coronary bypass in patients presenting

with lower extremity ischemia: the Cleveland Clinic Study. Ann Vasc Surg 1:411, 1987

77. Hertzer NR, Young JR, Beven EG, et al: Late results of coronary bypass in patients with peripheral vascular disease. II. Five-year survival according to sex, hypertension, diabetes. Cleve Clin J Med 54:15, 1987

78. Greenbaum BA, Califf RM, Jones RH, et al: Comparison of medicine alone, coronary angioplasty, and left internal mammary artery-coronary artery bypass for one-vessel proximal left anterior descending coronary artery diasese. Am J Cardiol 86:1322, 2000

79. Health Care Utilization Project. Agency for Healthcare Research and Quality, Rockville, Maryland, http://www.ahrq.gov/data/chup/hcupnet.htm

80. Kumar R, McKinney WP, Raj G, et al: Adverse cardiac events after surgery assessing risk in a veteran population. J Gen Intern Med 16:507, 2001

81. Lee TH, Marcantonio ER, Mangione CM, et al: Derivation and prospective validation of a simple index for prediction of cardiac risk of major noncardiac surgery. Circulation 100:1043, 1999

82. Rohde LE, Polanczyk CA, Goldman L, et al: Usefulness of transthoracic echocardiography as a tool for risk stratification of patients undergoing major noncardiac surgery. Am J Cardiol 87:505, 2001

83. Gilbert K, Larocque BJ, Patrick LT: Prospective evaluation of cardiac risk indices for patients undergoing noncardiac surgery. Ann Intern Med 133:356, 2000

Recommended Reading

Fischer SP: Cost-effective preoperative evaluation and testing. Chest 155:96S, 1999

Detsky AS, Abrams HB, McLaughlin JR, et al: Predicting cardiac complications in patients undergoing non-cardiac surgery. J Gen Intern Med 1:211, 1986

Larsen SF, Olesen KH, Jacobsen E, et al: Prediction of cardiac risk in non-cardiac surgery. Eur Heart J 8:179, 1987

3 OUTPATIENT SURGERY

Richard B. Reiling, M.D., and Daniel P. McKellar, M.D.

A safe and cost-effective approach to elective surgery begins with a careful history, a thorough physical examination, well-chosen laboratory tests, and consultation as appropriate and proceeds to selection of the optimal procedure, assessment of patient suitability, and choice of the most appropriate site in which to perform the procedure. In what follows, we address these issues specifically as they pertain to outpatient surgery: from selection of suitable patients and procedures to determination of appropriate outpatient settings in which to perform the procedures, to perioperative management (e.g., premedication, anesthesia, monitoring, and immediate postoperative care), to discharge and postoperative pain control.

Selection of Patients for Inpatient and Outpatient Procedures

Just as inpatient and outpatient procedures must be carefully selected with an eye to difficulty and severity of illness, so too should patients be carefully selected. The following six questions should be asked:

1. Is the facility adequately equipped and appropriate for the intended procedure, and are quality standards maintained?
2. Can the procedure routinely be performed safely without hospital admission?
3. Is the patient at risk for major complications if the operation is performed in the facility?
4. Do concomitant or comorbid conditions present unnecessary risks in the intended setting?
5. Will the patient require any special instructions or emotional counseling before the operation?
6. Do the patient and the family understand their own obligations regarding postoperative care in an outpatient setting?

Surgeons and anesthesiologists have gained an immense amount of experience in outpatient management of many difficult procedures that were once considered best suited for more controlled inpatient environments. Procedures that were regarded as unsafe in an outpatient setting as late as the mid-1990s are now being performed in ambulatory centers, and there is evidence that this shift has not increased patient risk.[1-3] Certain relative contraindications to outpatient surgical procedures have been identified, but these vary depending on the patient, the physician, and the setting [see Table 1]. The pronounced shift toward outpatient surgery has been accompanied by an equally impressive technological revolution, which has led to the development of operative approaches that require less postoperative care (e.g., inguinal herniorrhaphy with mesh plugs and the growing number of laparoscopic abdominal and pelvic operations).

The surgeon is responsible for detecting undiagnosed and unsuspected acute and chronic conditions before operation. The anesthesiologist is also responsible for uncovering potential preoperative problems. In addition, the surgical unit plays a role in determining which types of patients can be treated. Hospital-affiliated units or units in immediate proximity to a full-service hospital that have an agreement for rapid transfer are better able to accept patients with more serious concomitant illnesses than facilities physically separated from the acute care hospital. Surgeons also tend to select certain apparently higher-risk patients for treatment in hospital outpatient or ambulatory surgical units rather than in freestanding day surgical units, as reflected in the higher rate of admission for hospital-based units [see Tables 2 and 3].[4]

Some reimbursement plans, including the Center for Medicare and Medicaid Services (CMS), possess a curious feature by which patients are considered outpatients if they are discharged from the facility within 24 hours. Obviously, an outpatient who stays overnight is effectively an inpatient, even if the length of stay is less than 24 hours. Outpatient facilities exist that are physically separated from an inpatient hospital but that also can accept patients for this 24-hour arrangement. Such freestanding facilities must clearly ensure safety and quality in the unit to the same extent as facilities approved by the Joint Commission on Accreditation of Healthcare Organizations (JCAHO).

Recently, the concept of recovery care was introduced for facilities that provide postoperative care. In this concept, facilities are classified according to the defined length of stay (e.g., extended recovery and 23-hour care).[5] The idea of classifying units according to level of service, in the same way as the American College of Surgeons (ACS) has classified units according to type of surgery performed and level of anesthesia available, is a sensible one that is likely to be more fully developed and more widely applied in the coming years.

If any patient or any responsible relative of the patient does not accept or is extremely critical of nonadmission surgical care and cannot be easily convinced of its advantages, inpatient treatment is indicated regardless of the policy of the third-party payor. Certain complicating factors, such as substantial distance

---

Table 1 Relative Contraindications to Outpatient Surgery

Procedures with an anticipated significant blood loss

Procedures associated with significant postoperative pain

Procedures necessitating extended postoperative I.V. therapy

ASA class IV (or III if the systemic disease is not under control, as with unstable angina, asthma, diabetes mellitus, and morbid obesity)

Known coagulation problems, including the use of anticoagulants

Inadequate abillity or understanding on the part of caretakers with respect to requirements for postoperative care

Table 2 Surgical Categories

Category 1

Generally noninvasive procedures with minimal blood loss and with minimal risk to the patient independent of anesthesia

Anticipated blood loss less than 250 ml

Limited procedure involving skin, subcutaneous, eye, or superficial lymphoid tissue

  Breast biopsy

  Superficial lymph node biopsy

  Removal of minor skin lesions

  Myringotomy tubes

  Circumcision

  Carpal tunnel repair

  Repair of digits without repair to bone

  Retinal surgery

  Cataract extraction

Entry into body without surgical incision

  Cystoscopy

  Hysteroscopy

  Fiberoptic bronchoscopy

Excludes the following:

  Open exposure of internal body organs, repair of vascular or neurologic structures, or placement of prosthetic devices

  Entry into abdomen, thorax, neck, cranium, or extremities other than wrist, hand, or digits

  Placement of prosthetic devices

  Postoperative monitored care setting (ICU, ACU)

Category 2

Procedures limited in their invasive nature, usually with minimal to mild blood loss and only mild associated risk to the patient independent of anesthesia

Anticipated blood loss less than 500 ml

Limited entry into abdomen, thorax, neck, or extremities for diagnostic or minor therapy without removal or major alteration of major organs

  Diagnostic laparoscopy

  Fallopian tubal ligation

  Laparoscopic lysis of adhesions

  Percutaneous lung biopsy, not including mediastinal structures

  Arthroscopy

  Tonsillectomy

  Adenoidectomy

  Rhinoplasty

  Dilatation and curettage

  Inguinal hernia repair

  Umbilical hernia repair

Extensive superficial procedure

Cosmetic surgery to the face or extremities

Excludes the following:

  Open exposure of internal body organs or repair of vascular or neurologic structures

  Placement of prosthetic devices

  Postoperative monitored care setting (ICU, ACU), with no open exposure of abdomen, thorax, neck, cranium, or extremities other than wrist, hand, or digits

Category 3

More invasive procedures and those involving moderate blood loss with moderate risk to the patient independent of anesthesia

Anticipated blood loss 500–1,500 ml

Open exposure of the abdomen

  Hysterectomy

  Myomectomy

  Cholecystectomy

  Resection or reconstructive surgery of the digestive tract

Reconstructive work on hip, shoulder, knees

  Hip replacement

  Laminectomy

Excludes the following:

  Open thoracic or intracranial procedure

  Major vascular repair (e.g., aortofemoral bypass)

  Major orthopedic reconstruction (e.g., spinal fusion)

  Planned postoperative monitored care setting (ICU, ACU)

Category 4

Procedures posing significant risk to the patient independent of anesthesia or in one or more of the following categories:

Procedure for which postoperative intensive care is planned

Procedure with anticipated blood loss greater than 1,500 ml

Cardiothoracic procedure

  Cardiac surgery

  Pneumonectomy or lobectomy

Intracranial procedure

Major procedure on the oropharynx

  Resection of tumors of the head and neck

  Radical neck dissection

Major vascular, skeletal, or neurologic repair

  Aortic aneurysm repair

  Major vessel bypass procedure

  Kyphosis repair

  Scoliosis repair

  Procedure on the spinal cord

---

from the facility, the lack of sufficient support at home, and the presence of significant comorbid diagnoses, also call for inpatient treatment regardless of the payor's policy. It then becomes the responsibility of the surgeon to notify the third-party payor of these contingencies in a simple and nonconfrontational manner as well as to explain to the patient and family why it is necessary to deviate from the more usual outpatient approach for which the payor would more readily provide reimbursement. Efforts to coerce the patient or the family to accept outpatient surgery not only engender bad will between physician and patient but also tend to give rise to more postoperative problems (either real or factitious).

Third-party payors, for their part, must understand and accept that some patients, for whatever reason, will refuse non-admission surgery. It is the responsibility of third-party payors and their customers (i.e., corporations or employers) to provide adequate information to those covered (i.e., employees and families) about the advantages of outpatient surgery. Such education should be provided well before surgical intervention is sought or needed. Too often, the patient and the family are unaware of the payor's guidelines. Finally, patients and their families must also realize the need for cost-effective care and be willing to play their part in achieving it.

SPECIFIC PATIENT RISK FACTORS

It is well attested that careful monitoring and improvement of the patient's physical status before operation reduce mortality and morbidity. Therefore, one should accept a patient with

Table 3 Guidelines for Selection of Outpatient versus Inpatient Surgery

ASA Class	Surgical Category			
	1	2	3	4
I	Outpatient procedure with local anesthesia	Outpatient procedure with general or regional anesthesia	Inpatient procedure	Inpatient procedure
II	Outpatient procedure with local anesthesia*	Outpatient procedure with local, regional, or general anesthesia*	Inpatient procedure	Inpatient procedure
III	Inpatient procedure (unless operation can be done with local anesthesia)*	Inpatient procedure	Inpatient procedure	Inpatient procedure
IV	Inpatient procedure (unless operation can be done with local anesthesia)*	Inpatient procedure	Inpatient procedure	Inpatient procedure

*Patient must be watched carefully.
ASA—American Society of Anesthesiologists

a poor preoperative physical status for outpatient treatment only when it is clear that concomitant disease is well controlled and that there will be adequate postoperative monitoring and treatment in the patient's home.

In evaluating the risk factors for any surgical intervention, the following variables should be considered: (1) the patient's age, (2) the proposed anesthetic approach (type and duration), (3) the extent of the surgical procedure (including the surgical site), (4) the patient's overall physiologic status, (5) the presence or absence of concomitant diseases, (6) baseline medications, and (7) the patient's general mental status. The aim is to return the patient to the preoperative functional level with respect to respiration, cardiovascular stability, and mental status; no deviations should be acceptable. These are the standards used by peer review organizations (PROs) in retroactive evaluation of surgical interventions in Medicare recipients.

Several studies aimed at determining reasons for admission after ambulatory surgical procedures indicate that the major reasons for admission are to an extent related to the patient's preoperative cardiovascular and respiratory status, but the major reason for admission is still uncontrollable nausea and vomiting.[3] Moreover, most complications are related to intraoperative performance and not to the setting of the surgical procedure (outpatient or inpatient). Admission to the hospital after ambulatory surgery because of urinary retention, for example, is related to the use of general anesthesia, the age of the patient, and the administration of more than 1,200 ml of I.V. fluids before, during, and after the operation.[6]

When undergoing relatively short procedures, ASA class III (or even class IV) patients [see *IV:2 Risk Stratification, Preoperative Testing, and Operative Planning*] are appropriate candidates for ambulatory surgery if their systemic diseases are medically stable.

Age

Extremes of age by themselves automatically increase the ASA classification from I to II. Even though age is not correlated with hospital admission after ambulatory surgery, elderly patients often have concomitant conditions that may have gone unrecognized but should be brought to light before the operation. This is the obvious justification for the higher ASA classification—that is, to make the surgical team aware of the potential increased risk. In addition, the family or social support networks available to elderly patients are often of questionable value and may even pose their own risks after the operation.

Young children—especially neonates—present separate problems that must be independently evaluated by the surgeon and the anesthesiologist.

Drug Therapy for Preexisting Disease

Two questions must be answered about a patient taking medication for preexisting disease. First, should the drug or drugs be discontinued or the dosage altered before operation [see *Table 4*]? Second, do the medications necessitate special laboratory evaluations before operation (e.g., a prothrombin time or international normalized ratio [INR] for patients taking anticoagulants)?

Whereas dosages of some medications, such as adrenocorticosteroids, may have to be temporarily increased, certain oral agents may have to be replaced during the immediate perioperative period with agents that can be delivered intravenously. In particular, oral antiarrhythmic drugs (e.g., quinidine sulfate,

Table 4 Disposition of Current Medications before Outpatient Surgery[90]

Continue
    Antihypertensives
    Beta blockers
    Calcium channel blockers
    ACE inhibitors
    Vasodilators
    Bronchodilators
    Antiseizure medications
    Tricyclic antidepressants
    MAO inhibitors (controversial)
    Corticosteroids
    Thyroid preparations
    Anxiolytics
Discontinue or withhold
    Diuretics
    Insulin
    Digitalis
    Anticoagulants (may change to short-acting agent such as heparin)

ACE—angiotensin-converting enzyme   MAO—monoamine oxidase

procainamide, and disopyramide) should be discontinued 8 hours before the operation.[7] Patients taking aspirin should be instructed to stop at least 1 week before elective operation because aspirin's antiplatelet effect lingers for the life of the affected platelets. Patients receiving warfarin require uninterrupted anticoagulation; hence, the drug should be stopped only in the immediate preoperative period. Fresh frozen plasma may be required intraoperatively if excessive bleeding occurs. If warfarin is to be discontinued for a longer period, I.V. or subcutaneous heparin can be given.

In a study of nearly 18,000 ambulatory surgical patients in a major surgical center, almost 2,000 patients had preexisting systemic disease, and more than 900 of them were taking specific drugs for their disease.[8] Nearly half of these patients were taking at least one antihypertensive medication; a significant number were taking one or more heart medications, including cardiac glycosides, beta blockers, diuretics, antiarrhythmics, vasodilators, and anticoagulants. Other drugs that were being used included insulin and asthma medications. However, none of the complications recorded were related to preoperative drug use.

In any case, patients should bring all of their medications—both prescribed and self-administered—on the day of the operation. (Herbals and other over-the-counter medications are often overlooked and underreported by patients. Some of these medications may well influence the procedure and subsequent recovery.)

Hypertension

In general, hypertension should be under control before the operation. It is advisable to discontinue monoamine oxidase (MAO) inhibitors, if possible, 2 weeks before operation because these agents have unpredictable cardiac effects and may lead to hypertension in patients receiving meperidine or vasopressors; however, whether preoperative discontinuance of MAO inhibitors is absolutely necessary remains somewhat controversial. All antihypertensive agents should be continued until the day before the operation; beta blockers can be taken on the day of the operation.

Abrupt withdrawal of clonidine, which is used to treat chronic essential hypertension, is particularly dangerous because it is often associated with an increase in the plasma catecholamine level. Accordingly, clonidine should be continued throughout the perioperative period.

Heart Disease and Congestive Heart Failure

Patients with serious heart disease or congestive heart failure fall into ASA class III or IV and thus should not be considered for outpatient surgery unless the procedure is a minor one necessitating only local or regional anesthesia. Patients with less serious heart disease should take any cardiac glycosides, beta blockers, or antiarrhythmics that have been prescribed with a small amount of water when they awake on the day of the operation.

Bronchopulmonary Disease

Patients with bronchopulmonary disease must be evaluated individually. The degree of impairment is determined by means of a careful history and appropriate testing; a chest x-ray should always be obtained. The history should also reveal factors that initiate attacks of asthma or bronchospasm as well as identify the medications being taken. Many patients with bronchopulmonary disease need corticosteroids and antibiotics preoperatively.

Diabetes Mellitus

Patients whose diabetes is controlled with oral hypoglycemics or controlled low dosages of insulin (i.e., less than 25 U/day) can be adequately managed by withholding the medication on the day of the operation. In general, patients with more severe insulin-dependent diabetes mellitus should not undergo outpatient procedures. Those who do undergo such procedures are best managed by the administration of a fraction of the insulin dose on the day of the operation along with an I.V. dextrose solution (usually 5%), beginning shortly after the patient's arrival at the surgical facility. Ideally, such administration should be scheduled as early in the day as possible. Patient status is monitored by measuring either the blood glucose level or the urine glucose level, both of which can be easily and rapidly determined at the bedside.

Obesity

In general, moderately to severely obese patients should not undergo outpatient surgery. The hazards and risks of surgery in the obese are often unrecognized. Morbid obesity exerts stress on the cardiopulmonary system, and morbidly obese patients easily become, or already are, hypoxemic. In addition, such patients usually have concomitant preexisting conditions, such as diabetes, hypertension, liver disease, or cardiac failure. Moderate obesity increases the ASA classification from I to II; morbid obesity increases it to III. Careful consideration is essential before a morbidly obese patient is released from skilled observation after major anesthesia. Obese children often are not recognized as being at risk. There is some controversy over whether the ability to swallow water in a recovering obese pediatric patient is an acceptable condition for discharge. Minor procedures have ended in tragedy after a seemingly recovered obese patient was discharged.

Adrenocortical Steroid Therapy

Patients taking adrenocortical steroids for 6 to 12 months before operation should usually receive supplemental steroids in the preoperative period. It should be remembered that many patients fail to inform the surgeon of transdermal corticosteroid use. Short-term steroid overdosage has virtually no complications, but inadequate adrenocortical support may have serious repercussions.

Alcohol and Drug Abuse

Alcohol and drug abusers (a category that may also include self-medicated patients and those who are taking a large number of physician-directed medications) are also poor candidates for outpatient surgery. Chronic alcoholism is associated with a number of serious metabolic disorders, and chronic drug abusers often have many medical problems that are related to the habit (e.g., endocarditis, superficial infections, hepatitis, and thrombophlebitis).

Psychotropic Drug Therapy

Except for MAO inhibitors, most psychotropic drugs do not interact with anesthetics. Continuation of anxiolytics probably has a beneficial effect overall.

Psychiatric Illness

Mental instability is a potential problem even in the best of circumstances. A competent adult must be available to provide care for a mentally unstable patient after operation. One benefit of outpatient surgery for such patients, as for very young and very old patients, is that it allows them to return quickly to a familiar environment, which is desirable when safety can be ensured. If safety cannot be ensured, admission is indicated.

Selection of Appropriate Site for Procedure

The following are the four main types of facilities used in the performance of outpatient surgical procedures:

1. Office surgical facilities (OSFs). These include individual surgeons' offices as well as larger group practice units.
2. Free-standing day surgical units. These are often used by managed health care systems and independent contractors.
3. In-hospital day surgical units. These are often associated with inpatient units.
4. In-hospital inpatient units.

At times, these facilities are collectively referred to as ambulatory surgical centers (ASCs); however, the term ASC also has a specific meaning to third-party payors (especially Medicare) for billing purposes.

The primary influences on the choice of setting are the type of procedure to be performed and the condition of the patient. Although there is still disagreement about whether regulations (i.e., legally imposed standards and guidelines) applying specifically to office-based surgical units are advisable or necessary, many states (e.g., New Jersey, California, Pennsylvania, Rhode Island, Texas, Florida, and New York) have already put such regulations in place, and many more are considering doing so.[9]

It is clear that many individually operated units are delivering cost-efficient, safe, and effective care. The imposition of costly regulations and accreditation processes on such units may be fiscally prohibitive. It is equally clear, however, that many such units may well be delivering substandard care, and at present, there is no way of determining quality and safety in these units. Several institutions are currently involved in devising guidelines, standards, and even regulations. Already, some payors, such as Medicare, do not provide reimbursement for care delivered in nonaccredited facilities.

Accordingly, it is wise to have an outpatient surgical facility accredited by JCAHO or another major outpatient surgical accrediting organization. At present, besides JCAHO, only two accrediting organizations are approved by Medicare—the American Association for Accreditation of Ambulatory Surgery Facilities (AAAASF) and the Accreditation Association for Ambulatory Health Care (AAAHC)—and full accreditation by JCAHO, AAAASF, or AAAHC is time-consuming and costly. CMS requires certification by one of these three bodies before a facility can be classified as an ASC for reimbursement purposes. Thus, if reimbursement for Medicare patients is a goal, appropriate certification should be a priority. It is merely a matter of time before the lead taken by those states that already require accreditation of outpatient facilities is followed by most, if not all, of the remaining states.

The ACS has developed guidelines for office-based surgery and continues to reevaluate these guidelines periodically.[10] (The third edition is currently available from the ACS, at http://www.facs.org/commerce/guidelines.html.) However, in contrast with its accrediting activities in cancer and trauma, the ACS does not certify outpatient surgery facilities. The goal of the ACS initiative is simply to present readily acceptable guidelines that meet a minimum standard for surgical care without the necessity of a costly and time-consuming accreditation process. It is the intent of the ACS that these guidelines be acceptable to legislative bodies in lieu of more involved and expensive accreditation approaches. The guidelines are "intended to ensure and maintain superior quality of care for the surgical patient who undergoes an outpatient procedure in an office-based or ambulatory surgical facility."[10]

The concept of governance in an ASC is key to quality. In effect, governance comprises the rules and regulations that determine how the facility does business. The ultimate authority and responsibility reside with the governing body. The processes outlined in the governance manual should include the following[10]:

1. Specifying mission and goals, including the types of services provided.
2. Defining organizational structure.
3. Adopting policies and procedures for the orderly conduct of the ASC.
4. Adopting a quality assurance program.
5. Reviewing and taking appropriate action on all legal affairs of the unit and its staff.
6. Ensuring financial management and accountability.
7. Establishing a policy on patients' rights.
8. Approving all arrangements for ancillary medical care delivered in the ASC, including laboratory, radiologic, pathologic, and anesthesia services.
9. Conducting the operation of the unit without discrimination on any basis (including the presence of disabilities).

There are other regulatory agencies that also must be taken into account in the management of an ASC, especially if laboratory, x-ray, and pharmacy services are being offered. Examples include the Clinical Laboratory Improvement Amendments (CLIA) of 1988 and the Occupational Safety and Health Administration (OSHA) standards on hazard communication (29CFR1910-1200) and blood-borne pathogens (29CFR1910.1030). In addition, compliance with local and state fire and safety regulations and state nuclear regulatory agencies is essential.

An important aspect of the ACS guidelines is that they take into account the differing capabilities of individual facilities. The ACS classifies ambulatory surgical facilities into three categories—classes A, B, and C—on the basis of the level of anesthesia provided, the types of procedures performed, and the degree of sedation employed.[10] The suggested guidelines for each class of unit differ; for example, less resuscitation equipment would be required in a class A facility than in a class C facility. This differentiation makes it easier for a small OSF to demonstrate compliance with reasonable guidelines, in that the relevant requirements are not as extensive as they would be for a more comprehensive center.[10]

Hospital-based ambulatory care units that are extensions of inpatient facilities obviously have many advantages for the surgeon and the patient, but they are often less efficient and convenient than other ambulatory facilities. On the other hand, it is easier to assess the safety and quality of hospital-based units, in that the quality assurance (QA) functions of the hospital must extend to such units. JCAHO is now well established in the voluntary accreditation process for ambulatory health care facilities as well as for inpatient facilities. Even though accreditation is still voluntary, it is clear that a mandate already exists for some sort of QA for ambulatory facilities.

In 1993, the Office of the Inspector General (OIG) reported on the appropriateness of the surgical setting, the medical necessity of the surgical procedure, and the quality of care performed in physicians' offices.[11] The data were obtained from the 1989 Part B Medicare Annual Data and thus are somewhat dated; however, it is likely that the situation has not changed greatly over the past decade. The 1993 report contained disturbing findings: in 20% of the medical records, reasonable quality of care was not documented; in 13%, an indication for surgery was not documented; for a small number of operations, the physician's office was not an appropriate setting; and in 16% of sample cases, procedure codes did not match the operations performed.

Performance of the Operation

PREMEDICATION

Premedication is an important adjunct to local and regional general anesthesia [see Table 5].[12] It can facilitate performance of the procedure by alleviating fear and anxiety, supplementing analgesia, reducing gastric acidity and volume, reducing oral and airway secretions, decreasing histaminic effects in patients with multiple allergies, limiting postoperative nausea and vomiting (PONV), and controlling infection.

On the other hand, premedication, especially with narcotics, can also delay recovery: in fact, patients may actually take longer to recover from premedication and local anesthesia than from general anesthesia. Still, no patient should be denied premedication out of fear that it might delay discharge. Some studies have shown that premedication with agents other than long-acting narcotics does not prolong recovery time [see Table 6].[13] Narcotic premedications are the usual cause of postoperative nausea and vomiting and one of the major reasons for admission of outpatients to the hospital.

The five major categories of agents used for premedication are (1) anticholinergic drugs, (2) narcotics, (3) anxiolytics, (4) antinauseants and antiemetics, and (5) antacids and histamine antagonists.

Anticholinergic Drugs

Atropine and scopolamine are not routinely indicated for outpatient premedication, because newer anesthetics are less irritating than those previously used and because use of anticholinergic agents may increase the incidence of cardiac irregularities. If an anticholinergic is needed, glycopyrrolate, 0.2 to 0.3 mg I.M. or I.V., is a better alternative in that it does not cross the blood-brain barrier and causes less tachycardia than atropine does.

Table 5 Premedications

Class	Drug	Recommended Dose and Route of Administration
Anxiolytics (sedatives)	Midazolam	Titrate in 0.5–1.0 mg aliquots I.V. (total, ~ 2–3 mg)
	Diazepam	4–10 mg (0.05–0.15 mg/kg) I.V. or 5–10 mg p.o.
Narcotics*	Fentanyl	0.5–1.0 µg/kg I.V. or I.M.
	Sufentanil	0.1–0.25 µg/kg

*The use of long-acting narcotics such as meperidine and morphine is usually not recommended for outpatient surgery.

Table 6 Premedication and Recovery Time[12]

Type	Number of Patients	Recovery Time* (min)
No premedication	1,015	179 ± 113
Diazepam	98	168 ± 104
Pentobarbital	25	231 ± 88
Narcotics (meperidine, morphine)	388	208 ± 101
Hydroxyzine	92	192 ± 120

*Values are ± SD.

Narcotics

The primary effect of narcotics is the relief of pain; however, they also have significant side effects that limit their usefulness for outpatient procedures. Fentanyl is appropriate for outpatient surgery because of its short duration of action and its limited side effects; it should be given within 30 minutes of the actual induction of anesthesia. Long-acting narcotics, especially meperidine and morphine, are usually not indicated in the outpatient setting.

As outpatient surgical procedures become more lengthy and complex, larger doses of short-acting narcotics such as fentanyl are being used. As the doses increase, however, the advantages of short-acting drugs over long-acting drugs become less pronounced. Newer short-acting narcotics are now available, but they have side effects of their own.

Anxiolytics

Most barbiturates are long-acting agents and thus are not indicated for outpatient procedures. Very short acting barbiturates, such as thiopental, are occasionally used during anesthesia. Nonbarbiturate tranquilizers, such as midazolam or diazepam, are being used more often, primarily because they act without causing much sleepiness and because they may reduce the amount of anesthetic required. In addition, they are useful in stopping convulsions.

Antinauseants

Administration of antinauseants is often begun in the preoperative setting.[14] Given that PONV is a common cause of prolongation of recovery and subsequent hospital admission, preventive measures aimed at high-risk patients are preferable to treatment.

Antacids and Histamine Antagonists

Antacids and histamine antagonists are sometimes used in an effort to diminish the risk of gastric aspiration and the consequent deleterious effects of acidic gastric contents on the respiratory tract, but they have not been proved to be beneficial in this respect. It is important to remember that most of the commonly used antacid preparations are composed of particulate matter, and thus, aspiration of the antacid can itself be a serious problem. Patients who are assumed to be at high risk for aspiration (e.g., diabetic, obese, or pregnant patients or patients with gastroesophageal reflux disease [GERD], stroke, or swallowing difficulties) should be premedicated with an H_2 receptor antagonist on the evening before and the morning of the operation. Alternatively, these high-risk patients may be premedicated with a nonparticulate (i.e., clear) antacid, such as sodium citrate; a 50 ml dose of sodium citrate 1 hour before the operation raises the pH to a safe level, albeit at the expense of a slightly increased gastric residual volume.[15] Rapid infusions of H_2 inhibitors at the time of surgery are discouraged because of possible bradycardia.

ANESTHESIA

It is beyond the scope of this chapter to address general anesthesia in depth. We merely note that one should be prepared to meet all of the contingencies that can accompany general anesthesia, especially when anesthesia is delivered by someone other than an anesthesiologist and is not immediately supervised by an anesthesiologist. The patient's cardiac activity, blood pressure, temperature, respiration, and neuromuscular activity should be properly monitored.

Local Anesthetics for Local and Regional Anesthesia

As outpatient surgery has become more popular, there has been an increase in the use of local anesthetics for local and regional control of pain [see VIII:2 Postoperative Pain]. Local anesthetics are usually administered by the surgeon. It is crucial that the patient accept and be psychologically suited to this type of anesthesia: obviously, local or regional anesthesia can be very disturbing and disruptive when administered inadequately or when given to an emotionally unstable patient. During the preoperative conference or at the time of the discussion of the operation with the patient, the surgeon, the anesthesiologist, or both should make a point of describing how the anesthetic will be administered and what sensations will ensue.

Local anesthetics can be classified into three groups according to their potency and duration of action: (1) low potency and short duration (e.g., procaine and chloroprocaine), (2) moderate potency and intermediate duration (e.g., lidocaine, mepivacaine, and prilocaine), and (3) high potency and long duration (e.g., tetracaine, bupivacaine, and etidocaine) [see Table 7].

Most local anesthetics are administered by infiltration into the extravascular space or, in the case of epidural administration, by injection into cerebrospinal fluid. In some areas, especially the hands, intravascular (I.V. regional) infiltration has been used with considerable success; however, inadvertent intravascular administration of epidural doses of the high-potency agents can lead to life-threatening complications [see Toxicity and Allergy, below]. Although such complications have not been reported in association with inadvertent intravascular administration during infiltration for local anesthesia, it is advisable to check carefully to be sure that the injecting needle is not located in an intravascular site. Intravascular injection can usually be prevented by constantly aspirating during infiltration and by infiltrating only when the needle is withdrawn.

Mixing local anesthetics is an effective means of obtaining the advantages of more than one drug at once. At the Lichtenstein Hernia Institute in Los Angeles,[16] patients undergoing repair of inguinal hernias receive a 50-50 mixture of 1% lidocaine and 0.5% bupivacaine with epinephrine in a 1:200,000 dilution. The maximum therapeutic dose of lidocaine is 300 mg alone and 500 mg with epinephrine; the maximum therapeutic dose of bupivacaine is 175 mg alone and 225 mg with epinephrine. The addition of 1 mEq/10 ml of sodium bicarbonate to the solution shortens the onset time[17] as well as reduces discomfort by raising the pH. This combination of drugs has several advantages: (1) lidocaine has a rapid onset, whereas bupivacaine prolongs the duration of the effect; (2) the negative chronotropic and inotropic action of lidocaine may well counteract the cardiac excitability of bupivacaine; and (3) use of multiple drugs makes it less likely that the maximum therapeutic dose of any single agent will be exceeded.

Regional anesthesia, usually in the form of a regional nerve block, is generally administered by an anesthesiologist but can be adequately administered by a knowledgeable surgeon.

The use of epinephrine with local anesthetics prolongs the duration of the anesthetic effect without delaying its onset; however, epinephrine should not be used with anesthetics at sites where the vascular supply distal to the site of infusion is marginal (e.g., fingers, toes, the nose, and the external ears). In addition, adrenergic drugs should not be used in unstable cardiac patients unless absolutely necessary.

Administration of long-acting local anesthetics (e.g., 0.25% bupivacaine, injected in the skin edges at the end of the procedure) seems to limit postoperative pain and thus to encourage early activity and ambulation. Often, this technique not only postpones pain but reduces it as well. Bupivacaine is not, however, recommended for patients younger than 12 years.

Adjunctive Use of Local Anesthetics to Prolong Anesthetic Effect

It is clear that even when regional anesthetics, general anesthetics, or both are employed, adjunctive use of local anesthetics at the end of the procedure prolongs the anesthetic effect. In addition, once the patient realizes that ambulation is possible without discomfort, he or she is more likely to leave the hospital sooner and less likely to need additional postoperative analgesia. Several centers are currently experimenting with administering local anesthetics before operation; the hypothesis—still unproven—is that preoperative administration may result in decreased use of postoperative analgesics and a prolonged anes-

Table 7 Local Anesthetics for Infiltration

Drug		Plain Solutions		Epinephrine-Containing Solutions	
		Maximum Adult Dose (mg)	Duration (min)	Maximum Adult Dose (mg)	Duration (min)
Short-acting	Procaine 1%–2%	800	15–30	1,000	30–90
Intermediate-acting	Lidocaine 0.5%–2.0%	300	30–60	500	120–360
	Mepivacaine 1%–2%	300	45–90	500	120–360
Long-acting	Bupivacaine* 0.25%–5.0%	175	180+	225	240+

*Not recommended for children younger than 12 yr.

thetic effect in comparison with administration at the end of the procedure.

Injection of joint capsules with long-acting anesthetics and narcotics (e.g., morphine sulfate) relieves a great deal of postoperative pain. Bathing of wounds with bupivacaine is a safe and effective method of decreasing postoperative pain.[18] The addition of epinephrine can extend the prolongation of analgesia to 12 hours after operation.

Nonsteroidal Anti-inflammatory Drugs

Some centers use nonsteroidal anti-inflammatory drugs (NSAIDs) to reduce inflammation and thus pain [*see VIII:2 Postoperative Pain*]. In addition, it has been shown that NSAIDs significantly reduce the need for opioid analgesics after abdominal procedures. Administration of ketorolac over a short period (i.e., 5 days or less), first at the time of operation (60 mg I.M. in the OR; lower doses for patients weighing less than 50 kg, those older than 65 years, and those with impaired renal function) and then every 6 hours thereafter (10 to 15 mg p.o.), has improved recovery after many operations, especially perianal and inguinal procedures. (Ketorolac is, however, contraindicated as a preoperative prophylactic analgesic.) Other NSAIDs can be given in transdermal patches (which are not recommended for children) or transnasally.

Toxicity and Allergy

Whenever local anesthetics are used, and especially when they are administered regionally for major nerve blockade, the possibility of systemic toxicity should be considered. Such toxicity often results from inadvertent intravascular injection of these agents, leading to a sudden increase in systemic concentration.[13] The rate of injection is inversely related to the patient's tolerance of the drug: the higher the injection rate, the lower the tolerance. In general, arterial infusion is less likely to cause a toxic reaction than venous infusion because of the delay in circulation through the distal capillary network. Other factors that can lead to toxic reactions are a diminished drug detoxification rate, systemic acidosis, and individual sensitivities, which are highly variable.

In the CNS, toxic reactions range from drowsiness to frank convulsions. One study found that the incidence of mild toxic reactions to local and regional anesthetics was 0.38%, and the incidence of convulsions was 0.12%.[19] In the cardiovascular system, toxicity is initially manifested by elevated blood pressure; eventually, depression of systemic resistance and myocardial contractility leads to cardiovascular collapse. The myocardial depression associated with intravascular injection of 0.75% bupivacaine for epidural anesthesia has been reported to be strongly resistant to treatment in pregnant women.[20] Systemic toxicity is also manifested by alterations in the metabolic system, such as derangement of acid-base balance. (Respiratory or metabolic acidosis leads to an increased sensitivity to local anesthetics.) All such reactions are best managed by prevention. Constant vigilance is necessary to ensure that inadvertent intravascular injection does not occur at the time of infiltration. Any serious reactions (e.g., convulsions and cardiovascular collapse) that arise despite precautions are treated with standard measures.

Many patients claim to be allergic to anesthetics (which they often refer to generically as Novocain), but true allergic reactions are rare.[21] A careful history of allergic drug reactions should be taken, including reactions to concomitant medications such as epinephrine. It is important to explain to the patient the nature of any reaction that occurs so that if the reac-

Table 8 Treatment of Allergic Reactions to Local Anesthetics

Agent	Route of Administration	Recommended Dose
Epinephrine	I.M. or subcutaneously	0.3–0.5 ml of 1:1,000 dilution
Diphenhydramine	Systemically	0.5–1.0 mg/kg
Aminophylline	I.V.	3–5 mg/kg
Corticosteroids	I.V.	1 g

tion was not in fact an allergic one, the patient will understand this point and thus will not give a history of allergy to anesthetics in the future.

Allergic reactions are mediated by the release of histamine. Previous exposure to the offending local anesthetic can lead to the production of IgE antibodies, which initiate anaphylaxis on subsequent exposure; however, anesthetics can also initiate complement-mediated release of histamine without previous exposure. Histamine release leads to characteristic symptoms: skin erythema, followed by erythema in various regions of the body and edema of the upper airway. Abdominal cramps and cardiac instability may also be present.

If an allergic reaction occurs, administration of the drug should be stopped immediately. Epinephrine, 0.3 to 0.5 ml of a 1:1,000 dilution I.M. or subcutaneously, should immediately be given either locally or, if the reaction is severe, systemically.[22] Diphenhydramine, 0.5 to 1.0 mg/kg, should also be given systemically. If bronchospasm occurs, aminophylline, 3 to 5 mg/kg I.V., should be administered. Corticosteroids have been used in this setting, but there is little evidence that such therapy is helpful [*see Table 8*].

One common cause of allergic reactions is sensitivity to paraben derivatives, which are preservatives used in local anesthetics. Paraben preservatives resemble para-aminobenzoic acid (PABA), a metabolic breakdown product of ester-type anesthetics (e.g., procaine, benzocaine, and tetracaine). PABA is a member of a class of compounds that are highly allergenic. Patients sensitive to sunscreens containing PABA often show cross-sensitivity to ester-type local anesthetics. Patients who are allergic to a local anesthetic usually can be safely given a preservative-free anesthetic of unrelated structure. An intradermal skin test, in which 0.1 ml of the anesthetic drug is injected intradermally into the volar aspect of the forearm, may be tried. A negative reaction indicates that the drug probably can be used safely; nevertheless, resources for handling major cardiopulmonary irregularities should be available when anesthetics are used in previously sensitized patients.[22]

Control of Nausea and Vomiting

Many predisposing factors play a role in causing PONV. Not all of these factors can be managed. Nevertheless, it behooves the surgeon and the anesthesiologist to identify patients at risk so as to minimize the incidence of this debilitating syndrome, which is responsible for a large number of hospital admissions after outpatient surgical procedures.

Some of the more common causes of nausea are often overlooked. Pain is in itself capable of causing nausea and vomiting. Accordingly, adequate control of pain must be obtained, and the patient must not be deprived of analgesics under the false assumption that the medications are the only cause of the nausea. Changes in body activity, especially assumption of the upright position by a patient with possible hypotension, can also cause nausea, as is experienced before a vasovagal attack. In some patients who are prone to motion sickness, the sensation of motion is aggravated by the surgical procedure, the anesthetics, and pain. A preoperative history of frequent attacks of motion sickness is often a signal that the patient is prone to nausea and vomiting.

The use of narcotics in premedication, as well as in induction and maintenance of anesthesia, is definitely a cause of increased postoperative nausea and vomiting; however, some of the newer opioid analgesics (e.g., fentanyl, sufentanil, and alfentanil), when given judiciously as premedications [see Table 5], appear to reduce anxiety, decrease anesthetic requirements, and relieve pain in the early postoperative period.[23] One should have a thorough understanding of the proper use of these medications before employing them in the ambulatory setting.

Benzquinamide, trimethobenzamide, promethazine, and prochlorperazine have all been used in an effort to control PONV but with only limited success.[24] Droperidol received a so-called black-box warning from the Food and Drug Administration in December 2001; consequently, it is now rarely used.[25] Metoclopramide acts specifically on the upper GI tract and is a useful premedication because it also encourages gastric emptying and prevents aspiration; however, it is a short-acting agent and thus may have to be given again after a long procedure. The usual dose of metoclopramide for the average adult patient is 10 to 20 mg.[26,27]

Given that a history of motion sickness is a good predictor of increased risk for nausea and vomiting, it is not surprising that dimenhydrinate is effective in many cases—in some cases, significantly more effective than droperidol.[28]

Postoperative Care

The cornerstone of postoperative care in outpatient surgery is a well-instructed and well-informed patient. Many postoperative problems can be avoided if patients fully understand the nature of the proposed procedure, the potential side effects of the operation, and the role they must play in their own postoperative care. Facilitating such understanding not only helps prevent potential problems but also increases patients' overall satisfaction with the process of outpatient surgery.

RECOVERY

The process of postoperative recovery may be divided into three phases—I, II, and III—as follows.[29,30]

Phase I

The first phase of recovery—phase I, or early recovery—includes the patient's return to consciousness and recovery of vital reflexes. Generally, phase I takes place in the postanesthesia care unit (PACU). Currently, however, as a result of increasing use of newer anesthetics and conscious sedation, this phase sometimes occurs in the OR, thus eliminating the need for recovery in the PACU. This fast-tracking approach is being adopted more frequently in ambulatory surgery settings, where patients typically undergo shorter, less invasive procedures.[31] It is attractive because if patients can recover in the ASC[1] and avoid the PACU, they can be discharged sooner, and costs can thereby be reduced.

Several significant problems (e.g., PONV, pain, hypotension, and respiratory depression) may arise during phase I. Accordingly, the patient's vital signs, including oxygen saturation, must be closely monitored. Frequent reassessment in the PACU is indicated. A useful way of determining whether the patient is ready for discharge to phase II is to employ a scoring system such as the modified Aldrete system, which assigns scores from 0 to 2 in each of five categories (activity, respiration, circulation, consciousness, and oxygen saturation) [see Table 9].[32,33] A score of 9 signifies that the patient is ready for transfer to phase II of recovery in the ASC.

Phase II

Phase II, or intermediate recovery, is the period between immediate clinical recovery and the time when the patient is ready to be discharged home. This phase usually takes place in the ASC or the stepdown unit. Patients still need periodic monitoring during this period because they often have not yet fully recovered from the effects of the anesthetic and the surgical procedure. As in phase I, patients must be thoroughly assessed according to predetermined criteria to determine whether they are ready to be discharged to the next phase of recovery.[34] Before discharge to phase III, patients should be provided with both verbal and written discharge instructions. A responsible adult must be present to accompany the patient home; often, the absence of such a person serves to delay completion of phase II.

Phase III

Phase III, or late recovery, takes place outside the health care facility, usually at home. Because the anesthetic may still be affecting patients 24 to 48 hours after the procedure (and sometimes considerably longer), they should be cautioned not to drive, operate heavy machinery, or make important decisions during this period. It is in phase III that patients may experience various postoperative problems [see Postoperative Problems, below] that require specific management. Patients should also be informed about warning signs and symptoms and should be carefully instructed as to when to call the health care provider or return to the health care facility.

Table 9 Modified Aldrete Phase I Postanesthetic Recovery Score[32,33]

Patient Sign	Criterion	Score
Activity	Able to move 4 extremities*	2
	Able to move 2 extemities*	1
	Able to move 0 extremities*	0
Respiration	Able to breathe deeply and cough	2
	Dyspnea or limited breathing	1
	Apneic, obstructed airway	0
Circulation	BP +/− 20% of preanesthetic value	2
	BP +/− 20%–49% of preanesthetic value	1
	BP +/− 50% of preanesthetic value	0
Consciousness	Fully awake	2
	Arousable (by name)	1
	Nonresponsive	0
Oxygen saturation	SpO_2 > 92% on room air	2
	Requires supplemental O_2 to maintain SpO_2 > 90%	1
	SpO_2 < 90% even with O_2 supplement	0

*Either spontaneously or on command.
SpO_2—pulse oximetry

Table 10 Issues Addressed in Postoperative Instructions

Activity	Possible complications or side effects (of procedure, anesthesia, or medications)
Medication	Follow-up testing or treatments
Diet	Pain relief
Wound care	

DISCHARGE INSTRUCTIONS

Ideally, ambulatory surgery patients should be given their discharge instructions during the preoperative conference in the office. A variety of patient education tools (e.g., pamphlets, detailed written instructions, and videos) may be used to help educate patients about their operations and subsequent postoperative care.[30] Verbal reinforcement of written instructions by the surgeon is an important component of patient education. Communications from the surgeon should be consistent with the other materials (pamphlets, brochures, preprinted instruction sheets, and the like) provided to the patient. The instructions the patient is given before leaving the ASC must also be consistent with what the patient or family has previously been told, whether orally or in writing, by the surgeon. Providing careful perioperative instructions can yield several significant benefits, including increased patient satisfaction, improved outcomes, decreased patient anxiety, improved compliance, and even reduced costs.[35]

There are several barriers to comprehension of or adherence to instructions that the surgeon must take into account.[36] The most obvious barrier is that patients simply may not understand or remember the instructions given. It has been shown that patients' ability to understand written instructions may be a few grades lower than their actual education level[37]; accordingly, instructions should be written in such a way as to be easily understood by patients. In addition, patients may not be able to remember long, detailed verbal instructions well, even if they understood them on first hearing; thus, supplemental written instructions should be provided.

Another barrier to comprehension and compliance is that patients' perception of when postoperative recovery is complete may be inaccurate. Many patients, mistakenly believing that they are fully recovered, resume driving, working, or other strenuous activities prematurely. Surgeons must therefore stress the necessity of following discharge instructions exactly, even if patients feel that they are completely recovered.

Postoperative instructions should include several specific categories of information [see Table 10], preferably in writing. In addition, a follow-up appointment should be made, and patients should be given clear directions regarding access to postoperative care in the event of an emergency.[29,35,38] As a rule, it is best to present these instructions at the time of the preoperative evaluation, but it is probably advisable to present them again at the time of discharge from the ASC.

Activity instructions should address exercise or activity level, driving or operating machinery, return to work, and showering or bathing. If patients are likely to need someone to assist them in their routine daily activities, they should be informed, so that suitable arrangements can be made preoperatively.

Detailed wound care instructions, including directions for removing or changing dressings, applying ice or heat, and ele-

vating the affected area, are essential. In addition, patients should be told what to do when they see signs of wound problems, such as redness, drainage, or bleeding. Patients should also be taught drain or catheter care, if pertinent, before the operation. If the outputs of these devices must be measured, patients or caretakers should be taught how to do this as well.

It is vital that patients or caretakers be advised regarding resumption of preoperative medications. In addition, patients should be provided with specific information about pain medications, including drug names, dosages, potential side effects, and drug interactions. If patients are taking analgesic preparations that contain acetaminophen, they must be cautioned not to take other acetaminophen-containing medications, because of the potential for hepatotoxicity.

As part of the postoperative instructions, patients or caretakers should be given a list of items that require them to notify the physician [see Table 11].

Access to postoperative care in the event of an emergency is mandatory. Whether such access is available in a given instance often plays a role in determining whether ambulatory surgery is appropriate for that patient. The patient should be given the telephone number of the surgeon and the ASC as well as the location and telephone number of the appropriate emergency care facility.[29] Providing careful and thorough postoperative instructions, however, should help minimize unnecessary telephone calls to the surgeon and inappropriate visits to an emergency facility.[39]

POSTOPERATIVE PROBLEMS

Delayed Discharge or Unexpected Hospital Admission

The overall rate of unanticipated hospital admission after ambulatory surgery ranges from 0.15% to 2.5%[3,40-42]; it may vary considerably depending on what types of procedures are performed at the facility, how patients are selected for outpatient surgery, and whether the facility is hospital-based or independent. Many ASCs use unexpected hospital admission after ambulatory surgery as a quality indicator. Analysis of such admissions may be useful in helping a facility develop appropriate patient and procedure selection criteria.[42] It may also be helpful for developing discharge criteria and identifying patients who will require additional monitoring before discharge.

Factors leading to hospital admission from an ASC may be classified into three general categories: procedure-related factors, anesthetic-related factors, and patient-related factors.

Procedure-related factors Length of operation has been shown to be an independent predictor of increased admission rates after ambulatory surgery.[42,43] Other procedure-related factors associated with increased admission rates include a procedure that is more extensive than planned, inappropriate book-

Table 11 Reasons for Notification of the Surgeon[29]

Persistent nausea and vomiting	Persistent uncontrolled pain
Bleeding	Excessive redness or drainage from incision
Fever (usually > 101° F [38.3° C])	Urinary retention

ing of the case, the need for a subsequent procedure, and intra-operative adverse events (e.g., bleeding or bowel perforation during laparoscopy). Uncontrolled pain related to the procedure is a significant cause of admission from an ASC.[41] Accordingly, measures to prevent and control excessive pain should be taken [see Pain, below].

Anesthetic-related factors   One of the most common of the anesthetic-related factors necessitating hospital admission is PONV [see Nausea and Vomiting, below]. Other adverse reactions to anesthesia that call for admission or observation include delayed emergence from the anesthetic, excessive drowsiness, and delayed resolution of a regional block; more serious reactions include pulmonary aspiration of gastric contents and malignant hyperthermia.

Patient-related factors   Patient-related factors leading to admission after ambulatory surgery may be further divided into three subcategories: medical factors, social factors, and system-related factors.

Many of the medical factors are related to preexisting conditions[44]; for example, it has been shown that patients with preexisting congestive heart failure stay longer in the ASC.[45] Such findings underscore the need for appropriate selection of ambulatory surgery patients and the importance of optimizing treatment of any preexisting medical conditions.

As many as 41% of delays in discharge from the ASC are related to social factors. The most common social reason for delayed discharge is the lack of an adult escort to accompany the patient home.[46,47] To prevent this occurrence, patients should be counseled preoperatively in the office on the need for someone to accompany them home from the ASC, and the availability of the escort should be verified when the patient presents to the ASC before the scheduled procedure.

System-related factors that may delay discharge or increase the postoperative admission rate from the ASC include patient prescriptions that are not ready, nurses who are too busy to instruct and discharge patients, and the unavailability of someone to transport the patient out of the ASC.[47] Because the PACU may close before the patient is fully recovered, some patients need to remain in the ASC until their recovery is complete.[42]

Nausea and Vomiting

PONV is distressing to patients and is a common source of patient dissatisfaction with ambulatory surgery and anesthesia.[38,48-52] In addition, PONV often causes delayed discharge from the ASC or unplanned hospital admission, thereby inconveniencing patients as well as increasing the cost to the ASC.[29,45] Patients who experience PONV report more difficulty in resuming normal activities and may require a longer recovery period.[53] PONV may also precipitate wound problems (e.g., bleeding or dehiscence).

The etiology of PONV is complex and includes procedure-related causes, anesthetic-related causes, and patient-related causes. Certain operations, including ophthalmic procedures, orchiectomy, and middle-ear procedures, are associated with a high incidence of PONV. Certain anesthetics (e.g., narcotics, etomidate, and ketamine) have been shown to carry a greater risk of PONV than other agents do.[48] Use of propofol as an induction agent is known to decrease the incidence of PONV.[54] Other anesthetic-related causes include gastric distention during mask ventilation, hypotension related to regional anesthesia,

and vagal stimulation. Of the patient-related causes, younger age, anxiety, pain, underlying medical conditions such as gastroparesis, and a previous history of PONV are also known to be associated with a higher incidence of PONV.

Prevention of PONV depends on a clear understanding of the etiology and on an accurate assessment of the patient's level of risk for this complication. Given the cost and side effects of the medications required, prophylaxis for all patients undergoing ambulatory surgery is not advisable[48]; however, prophylaxis for patients known to be at high risk for PONV may result in decreased cost to the patient and facility as well as in greater patient satisfaction and fewer associated complications.

PONV prophylaxis should include both pharmacologic and nonpharmacologic interventions. Preoperative sedation to alleviate anxiety may facilitate control of PONV, as may adequate management of postoperative pain [see Pain, below]. Judicious selection of anesthetic agents also helps reduce the incidence of PONV. Limiting patient motion after certain operations (e.g., ophthalmic procedures) may be beneficial. A more flexible approach to postoperative fluid intake may be helpful as well. One study that evaluated the practice of requiring pediatric patients to drink liquids before being discharged from an ASF found that patients required to ingest fluids had a higher incidence of PONV.[55] A similar study of adult patients, however, did not document increased risk of PONV in patients required to drink fluids before discharge, nor did it document decreased risk in patients who were not so required.[56] Given these findings, we believe that patients should be allowed to choose whether they want to drink fluids before discharge; oral fluid intake should not be a mandatory discharge criterion.

Several categories of antiemetic agents are available for prevention and treatment of PONV, the most common of which are the antihistamines, the antidopaminergics, and the anti-serotoninergics.[48]

The antihistamines have long been used to treat motion sickness and other disturbances of the vestibular pathway. They may be more effective than other antiemetics after middle-ear procedures. Common side effects include dry mouth and sedation.

One of the most commonly used antidopaminergic antiemetics is promethazine. This agent possesses both antihistaminic and anticholinergic properties and is therefore useful for treating motion sickness.[48] Droperidol has also been widely used for prevention of PONV. However, because of the December 2001 black-box warning from the FDA—the most serious warning an FDA-approved drug can carry—and because of studies documenting slower recovery from anesthesia with droperidol than with other agents, the current consensus is that the use of droperidol should be limited.[57] Side effects of antidopaminergic agents include anxiety, dizziness, drowsiness, extrapyramidal effects, and hypotension. These effects are dose related and may continue after discharge.[48,57]

The selective serotonin receptor antagonist ondansetron is very effective in preventing and treating PONV.[58] The optimal prophylactic dose for adults is 4 mg.[59] Common side effects seen with antihistamine agents (e.g., blurred vision, dry mouth, and diplopia) are rare with ondansetron.[57,60]

Metoclopramide reduces PONV by increasing lower esophageal sphincter pressure and increasing gastric emptying. This agent may be useful in counteracting the effects of narcotics on gastric motility. Because it does not affect the vestibular system, it is usually employed as an adjunct to other agents in the treatment of PONV.[48] The synthetic glucocorticoid dexamethasone is also a safe and effective agent in preventing PONV.[61-64] The delayed onset of action and prolonged effectiveness of dexamethasone make it ideal for use in conjunction with other agents in patients who are at particularly high risk for PONV.[60] Dexamethasone has few side effects and is more cost-effective than other agents.[65]

Pain

Effective pain management after ambulatory surgery depends on a clear understanding of the mechanisms of pain, a careful assessment of the type and degree of pain, and appropriate selection of pain-control methods so as to optimize patient comfort while minimizing side effects. Incomplete pain control is associated with several significant complications, such as PONV, reduced mobility, and inability to cough and breathe deeply. In addition, pain is associated with delayed discharge from phase II of recovery, more frequent return visits by the patient to a health care facility, and higher rates of unplanned hospital admission.[66-68] Postoperative pain also can be physiologically harmful, causing increased release of catecholamines with resultant elevation of blood pressure and pulse rate. Inadequate postoperative pain control is a significant source of patient dissatisfaction with ambulatory surgery. Moreover, inability to manage pain adequately after certain procedures makes it difficult (or even impossible) for surgeons to perform these procedures in an ambulatory setting.[66]

Assessment of postoperative pain requires careful communication between the surgeon and the patient. Patients have varying sensitivity to pain and respond differently to pain medication. Use of a measurement tool such as the verbal analogue scale can facilitate assessment of postoperative pain. A 1998 study found that 40% of patients reported moderate to severe pain in the first 24 hours after ambulatory surgery and that the best predictor of severe pain at home was inadequate pain control during the first few hours after the operation.[68] It is therefore crucial to assess patients' pain and treat it aggressively before discharging them from the ASC.

A key component of pain control after ambulatory surgery is education of patients regarding the degree of postoperative pain they may experience. It is not uncommon for patients to complain that they were given no information about how much pain to expect and how to manage it. During the preoperative visit, patients should be informed about various nonpharmacologic methods of alleviating pain. Depending on the procedure to be performed, appropriate methods may include application of ice, elevation of an affected extremity, wearing of loose-fitting clothing, sitz baths, or modified sleeping positions.[69] During the same visit, patients should also be informed about the medications they will be given for pain control—specifically, names, dosages, potential side effects, drug interactions, and precautions. Finally, patients should be told how to notify their physician if they continue to experience excessive pain.

The best pharmacologic strategy for controlling postoperative pain is to employ regimens comprising multiple analgesics that work synergistically.[66] So-called balanced analgesia involves giving medications from three different analgesic groups: nonopioids, opioids, and adjuvants.[70]

The nonopioid agents most commonly used after outpatient surgery are the nonsteroidal anti-inflammatory drugs (NSAIDs) and acetaminophen. NSAIDs act peripherally and have anti-inflammatory, analgesic, and antipyretic effects. They are very effective against mild to moderate pain. Side effects include gastric mucosal irritation and inhibition of platelet aggregation;

however, newer NSAIDs that inhibit the cyclooxygenase-2 (COX-2) enzyme exhibit these effects to a much lesser degree.[71] One of the most commonly used NSAIDs in ambulatory surgery patients is ketorolac, which may be administered either I.V. or I.M. Its onset of action occurs approximately 30 minutes after administration, with peak effect coming at about 75 minutes.[70] This agent causes reversible inhibition of platelet aggregation, which resolves 24 to 48 hours after the drug is stopped; it also has an adverse affect on renal function. Accordingly, ketorolac should be used with caution in elderly patients and in patients with altered renal function.[72]

Acetaminophen acts to alleviate pain by a central mechanism. It lacks the antiplatelet effects of NSAIDs and has few side effects. Acetaminophen should not be given to patients with liver disease or chronic alcoholism. The maximum daily dose of acetaminophen in adults is 4,000 mg; thus, as noted [*see* Discharge Instructions, *above*], patients must be cautioned not to take any other acetaminophen-containing medications. This is a matter of particular concern because many of the commonly used oral narcotic pain preparations already include a significant amount of acetaminophen, which patients may not realize.[70]

Overall, opioids are the most commonly used pain medications after ambulatory surgery. They can be delivered via several different routes, including oral, I.V., I.M., transcutaneous, intranasal, oral transmucosal, and subcutaneous.[66] The main concerns with respect to opioid use are the side effects and the potential for abuse. Common side effects include respiratory depression, sedation, reduction of rapid eye movement sleep, impaired GI motility, urinary retention, PONV, and allergic reactions. PONV is a particular problem; however, if other agents (e.g., NSAIDs and adjuvants) are being used as well, the opioid dosage can be reduced and the incidence of PONV thereby lowered.[72]

Adjuvant methods of controlling pain include infiltration of local anesthetics (e.g., bupivacaine) into the surgical site, continuous or patient-controlled regional anesthesia (PCRA) systems, local nerve blocks, and transcutaneous electrical nerve stimulation (TENS). Often, these measures add substantially to control of pain after ambulatory surgery. In particular, PCRA is very effective in certain procedures.[72] In this approach, a catheter is placed in the surgical site or near local peripheral nerves and attached to an elastometric (balloon) pump containing bupivacaine; the patient can then control administration of the local anesthetic.

Infection

The incidence of postoperative infection in ambulatory surgery patients varies depending on the procedure performed and the risk factors for infection present. Overall, however, infection rates after ambulatory surgery tend to be substantially lower than those after inpatient surgery.[73,74] Actual infection rates can be difficult to quantify in ambulatory surgery patients but should nonetheless be measured both as an indicator of quality and as an aid to reducing the incidence of infection.[75] As a rule, infection rates in ambulatory surgery patients are determined on the basis either of surveys sent to surgeons asking them to self-report infections or of telephone interviews with patients.[76-79]

Patients should be given a list of potential signs of infection—redness, drainage, excessive pain around the incision, and fever—and instructed to call the physician if these appear. The presence of any of these signs is an indication for examination by a physician. Most of the postoperative surgical site infections that occur in ambulatory surgery patients can be treated in the office with local wound care.

Many other types of infection may occur in ambulatory surgery patients, of which pneumonia, urinary tract infections, and prosthetic device infections are the most common. Generally, these infections develop several days after the procedure; thus, it is important to schedule a postoperative visit around this time.

Urinary Retention

Postoperative urinary retention occurs in 0.5% to 5% of ambulatory surgery patients.[80,81] Patients at high risk for this complication are those who have previously experienced urinary retention and those who are undergoing particular types of procedures (e.g., herniorrhaphy and anal procedures). Other predisposing factors are advanced age,[81] spinal anesthesia,[80] use of anticholinergics, bladder overdistention, use of analgesics, unrelieved pain, preoperative use of beta blockers,[82] and a history of preoperative catheterization.

Surgeons often require ambulatory surgery patients to void before discharge. This practice unnecessarily delays discharge of low-risk ambulatory surgery patients. A 1999 study showed that low-risk patients could be safely discharged without voiding and did not benefit from being required to void spontaneously before discharge.[80] The incidence of postoperative urinary retention in these patients was 0%. In low-risk patients who were discharged without voiding, the mean time to voiding after discharge was 75 minutes, indicating that discharge had been expedited by at least that length of time. In high-risk patients, however, catheterization before discharge should be considered if they are unable to void. In addition, once discharged, high-risk patients should have ready access to a medical facility and should be instructed to return if they are still unable to void 8 to 12 hours after discharge.

The presence or absence of symptoms is not a reliable indicator of urinary retention: many patients are asymptomatic even with bladder volumes greater than 600 ml.[80,83] Alternative methods of diagnosing urinary retention, such as ultrasonography or catheterization of patients known to be at high risk for urinary retention and unable to void before discharge, are more reliable.

Bladder overdistention is a significant cause of postoperative urinary retention.[6,80] Judicious use of fluids helps minimize postoperative urinary retention in patients at high risk. Those who are at high risk for retention and are receiving substantial amounts of I.V. fluids should be considered for early catheterization to help prevent excessive distention of the bladder with resultant retention and bladder atony.

Patients who require catheterization more than once postoperatively may be safely discharged home after placement of an indwelling catheter. The catheter should be left in place for 24 to 72 hours, after which time it can be removed in the physician's office. In the absence of any complicating circumstances, there is generally no need to admit patients to a hospital simply because of urinary retention.

Other Postoperative Problems

Other common postoperative problems that may develop in ambulatory surgery patients are headache, insomnia, constipation, bleeding, and pharyngitis. Many of these problems can be handled by providing reassurance and carrying out simple interventions; however, some (e.g., headache and bleeding) may necessitate direct physician intervention to ensure that they do not worsen.

Headache occurs in 10% to 38% of patients in the first 24 hours after the operation.[29] It may be related to caffeine withdrawal, in which case it is easily treated with caffeine-containing beverages, often before discharge. Spinal headache, or postdural puncture headache (PDPH), however, may be much more difficult to treat. This condition results from leakage of CSF from a tear in the dura during spinal anesthesia; thanks to advances in spinal needle design, it is now less common than it once was.[84,85] The most common symptom of PDPH is a frontal or occipital headache that worsens with sitting or standing and lessens with recumbency. Photophobia, diplopia, auditory disturbances, and PONV may be noted as well. How PDPH is treated depends on the severity of the symptoms. For mild symptoms, the patient should be instructed to take appropriate amounts of fluids, remain recumbent, decrease environmental stimuli (e.g., lights and noise), and take analgesics; caffeine may be a helpful adjuvant.[29] For severe, persistent symptoms, the patient may have to undergo a blood patch procedure, in which a small amount of his or her blood is injected epidurally to patch the dural leak.[86]

A small amount of incisional bleeding after ambulatory surgery is common. Patients must be carefully taught how to monitor for excessive bleeding and how to perform initial management of incisional bleeding with direct pressure and dressing changes. They must also be instructed to call the physician if bleeding persists.

Discussion

Growth of Outpatient Surgery

The recent evolution of health care in response primarily to socioeconomic factors has been spectacular, and the process is by no means complete. The most striking result to date is the emergence of ambulatory surgery as the predominant mode for the delivery of surgical health care. Just a few years ago, it was estimated that more than 40% of all operative procedures would be performed in the outpatient setting. By 2000, however, 70% of operative procedures were already being performed on an outpatient basis. In 1996, an estimated 31.5 million procedures were performed during 20.8 million ambulatory surgery visits.[87] The majority (84%) of these ambulatory surgical visits, however, still took place in hospitals, with the remainder in freestanding units.[87] Although procedures such as endoscopies and lens extraction and insertion were predominant at this time, there were also many breast biopsies, herniorrhaphies, and orthopedic procedures.

The explosive growth of ambulatory surgery was initiated by economic factors, but it has had some positive effects on patient care, for the following reasons:

1. Development of new technology. Newer techniques, such as laparoscopic surgery, minimize the need for hospitalization

and decrease the pain and suffering that patients must endure. It is not yet clear, however, that such developments will inevitably lead to a reduction in total health care costs. One study reported that the cholecystectomy rate increased from 1.35 per 1,000 enrollees in an HMO in 1988 to 2.15 per 1,000 in 1990 and that the total cost for cholecystectomies rose by 11.4% despite a unit cost savings of 25.1%.[88] The authors suggested that these results might be attributable to changing indications for gallbladder operations; however, it is much more likely that a significant number of patients suffering from gallbladder dysfunction who were reluctant to undergo an open procedure are now willing to accept the lesser discomfort and inconvenience characteristic of a laparoscopic procedure. What the appropriate cholecystectomy rate may be is a question for the future to answer; in the meantime, many patients are living more comfortably, having had the dysfunctional organ removed. The situation is similar in the treatment of GERD. Repairs to the esophagogastric junction can now be done without a long and difficult postoperative course. In addition, there have been major advances in anesthetic techniques and postoperative management of pain and PONV.

2. Cost savings achieved by Medicare and other payors. In 1987, Medicare approved over 200 procedures as suitable for ASCs. Currently, more than 1,200 procedures are so designated, with more procedures being approved every year. The endorsement of cost-efficient delivery systems by employers and the reduction of employee benefits by insurers are encouraging employees (as both consumers and patients) to be more cost-conscious. When patients are involved in the actual cost of medical care, they tend to accept more efficient modes of delivery. This is even more likely to be the case when they are at risk for the cost of care.

3. Physician concern. The emergence of the concept of managed care has exerted a strong influence on physician involvement in ambulatory surgery. Concerns over the safety of major surgical procedures being performed in the outpatient setting have largely been removed, and surgeons are becoming more aggressive. Clearly, surgeons have benefited from the ease and convenience of outpatient surgery, especially with respect to scheduling and protection from cancellations due to emergencies. Equally clearly, however, they will now have to be more vigilant, given that outpatient surgical facilities tend to be less well monitored and supervised.

4. Patient awareness of quality assurance. Today's patients (or consumers) are more medically knowledgeable than ever before and more concerned with actively seeking out institutions that deliver high-quality and cost-efficient care. Consumers are highly sensitive to the issue of quality, but their definitions of this attribute are not always based on the same criteria that surgeons use. To patients, quality is a combination of effectiveness, safety, cost, convenience, and comfort.

Economic benefits aside, the major issue in the movement of surgical activities out of the hospital and into a more convenient and economical environment is how best to ensure that patients continue to receive safe, high-quality care. This consideration must in all circumstances be the primary issue underlying the planning of elective surgery. More and more, third-party payors expect surgical care to be provided to their clients (patients, to us) in a cost-effective environment. On the whole, this is not a bad thing. If, however, they also expect that surgical care can be provided just as cost-effectively to diabetic patients, morbidly obese patients, and patients with serious cardiac or respiratory disease, there is a real danger that patients' welfare could be compromised. Accordingly, it is crucial that all third parties who are not directly involved in the care of the patient permit the surgeon and the anesthesiologist to exercise sound medical judgment in regard to what type of care is needed and where such care can best be delivered. Surgeons must not delegate their responsibility for safeguarding their patients' well-being.

The ACS has issued several statements on ambulatory surgery.[89] In their 1983 statement, the ACS approved "the concept that certain procedures may be performed in an ambulatory surgical facility" but emphasized that "a prime concern about ambulatory surgery is assurance of quality" and that "a discussion between patient and surgeon about performance of the procedure on an ambulatory basis should result in a mutually agreeable decision."[89] Two decades later, this is still the position of the ACS. The College is continually evaluating evolving medical technology, both inpatient and outpatient.

Outpatient surgery would seem to have an obvious advantage over inpatient surgery with respect to cost savings, especially if the main focus of the comparison is the high charges for 1 or more days of inpatient care. Such a comparison may be misleading insofar as it suggests that the entire cost of inpatient care can be saved when the procedure is done on an outpatient basis. The hospital inpatient charge reflects the costs of a number of functions associated with early convalescence in the hospital, including nursing, diet, and housekeeping; some of these costs are also associated with immediate postoperative care in the outpatient recovery area and consequently will be reflected in the outpatient facility's bill as well. The comparison may also be misleading insofar as it ignores the inherent costs of outpatient surgery. In some cases, medical personnel perform functions that do not appear on the bill, such as follow-up care, care by phone, and home visits to evaluate recovery, as well as dressing changes and other services similar to those provided by family members or friends. The costs associated with buying or renting durable medical equipment (e.g., beds and commodes), preparing meals, and various other activities must also be taken into account. Clearly, there are avenues for development in the postoperative setting that might raise expenses for outpatient surgery, but certainly not to the level of an inpatient stay.

It is to be hoped that new Medicare and state regulations mandating evaluation of quality of care in outpatient surgical facilities by PROs will provide definitive statistics for evaluation of actual cost savings. Cost data must be analyzed thoroughly if we are to assess the true contribution of outpatient surgery to cost containment.

References

1. Warner MA, Shields SE, Chute CG: Major morbidity and mortality within 1 month of ambulatory surgery and anesthesia. JAMA 270:1437, 1993

2. Laffafye HA: The impact of an ambulatory surgical service in a community hospital. Arch Surg 124:601, 1989

3. Gold BS, Kitz DS, Lecky JH, et al: Unanticipated admission to the hospital following ambulatory surgery. JAMA 262:3008, 1989

4. Maini BS: Personal communication

5. Recovery Care. Federated Ambulatory Surgery Association http://www.fasa.org/recoverycare.html, September 2001

6. Petros JG, Rimm EB, Robillard RJ, et al: Factors influencing postoperative urinary retention in patients undergoing elective inguinal herniorrhaphy. Am J Surg 161:431, 1991

7. Pennock JL: Perioperative management of drug therapy. Surg Clin North Am 65:1049, 1983

8. Natof HE: Ambulatory surgery: preexisting medical problems. Ill Med J 166:101, 1984

9. Sutton JH: Office-based surgery regulation: improving patient safety and quality care. Bull Am Coll Surg 86:8, 2001

10. Guidelines for Optimal Ambulatory Surgical Care and Office-based Surgery, 3rd ed. American College of Surgeons, Chicago, 2000

11. Physician Office Surgery (abstr). Project No. 5079. Office of Evaluation and Inspection, Washington, DC, 1993

12. Philip BK, Covino BG: Local and regional anesthesia. Anesthesia for Ambulatory Surgery, 2nd ed. Wetchler BV, Ed. JB Lippincott Co, Philadelphia, 1991, p 318

13. Meridy HW: Criteria for selection of ambulatory surgical patients and guidelines for anesthetic management: a retrospective study of 1,553 cases. Anesth Analg 61:921, 1982

14. Abramowitz MD, Oh TH, Epstein BS, et al: The antiemetic effect of droperidol following outpatient strabismus surgery in children. Anesthesiology 59:279, 1983

15. Schmidt JF, Schierup L, Banning AM: The effect of sodium citrate on the pH and the amount of gastric contents before general anaesthesia. Acta Anaesthesiol Scand 28:263, 1984

16. Amid PK, Shulman AG, Lichtenstein IL: Local anesthesia for inguinal hernia repair: step-by-step procedure. Ann Surg 220:735, 1994

17. Arthur GR, Covino BG: What's new in local anesthetics? Anesthesiol Clin North Am 6:357, 1988

18. Bays RA, Barry L, Vasilenko P: The use of bupivacaine in elective inguinal herniorrhaphy as a fast and safe technique for relief of postoperative pain. Surg Gynecol Obstet 173:433, 1991

19. Moore DC: Administer oxygen first in the treatment of local anesthetic-induced convulsions (letter). Anesthesiology 53:346, 1980

20. Covino BG: Pharmacology of local anaesthetic agents. General Anaesthesia, 5th ed. Nunn JF, Utting JE, Brown BR Jr, Eds. Butterworths, London, 1989, p 1036

21. Stoelting RK: Allergic reactions during anesthesia. Anesth Analg 62:341, 1983

22. Aldrete JA, Johnson DA: Evaluation of intracutaneous testing for investigation of allergy to local anesthetic agents. Anesth Analg 49:173, 1970

23. Parnass SM: Controlling postoperative nausea and vomiting. Ambulatory Surgery 1:61, 1993

24. Cohen SE, Woods WA, Wyner J: Antiemetic efficacy of droperidol and metoclopramide. Anesthesiology 60:67, 1984

25. Important drug warning (letter). Akorn Pharmaceuticals www.fda.gov/medwatch/SAFETY/2001/inapsine.htm, December 4, 2001

26. Lacroix G, Lessard MR, Trepanier CA: Treatment of postoperative nausea and vomiting: comparison of propofol, droperidol and metoclopramide. Can J Anaesth 43:115, 1996

27. Steinbrook RA, Freiberger D, Gosnell JL, et al: Prophylactic antiemetics for laparoscopic cholecystectomy: ondansetron versus droperidol plus metoclopramide. Anesth Analg 83:1081, 1996

28. Bidwai AV, Meuleman T, Thatte WB: Prevention of postoperative nausea with dimenhydrinate (Dramamine) and droperidol (Inapsine) (abstract). Anesth Analg 68:S25, 1989

29. Marley RA, Swanson J: Patient care after discharge from the ambulatory surgical center. J Perianesth Nurs 16:399, 2001

30. Marshall SI, Chung F: Discharge criteria and complications after ambulatory surgery. Anesth Analg 88:508, 1999

31. Watkins, et al: Fast-tracking after ambulatory surgery. J Perianesth Nurs 16:399, 2001

32. Aldrete JA, Kroulik D: A postanesthetic recovery score. Anesth Analg 49:924, 1970

33. Aldrete JA: The post anesthesia recovery score revisited (letter). J Clin Anesth 7:89, 1995

34. Theodorou-Michaloliakou C, Chung FF, Chua JG: Does a modified postanaesthetic discharge scoring system determine home-readiness sooner? Can J Anaesth 40:A32, 1993

35. Dunn D: Preoperative assessment criteria and patient teaching for ambulatory surgery patients. J Perianesth Nurs 13:274, 1998

36. Correa R, Menezes RB, Wong J, et al: Compliance with postoperative instructions: a telephone survey of 750 day surgery patients. Anaesthesia 56:447, 2001

37. Wilson FL: Measuring patient's ability to read and comprehend: a first step in patient education. Nursingconnections 8:17, 1995

38. Marley RA, Moline BM: Patient discharge from the ambulatory setting. J Post Anesth Nurs 11:39, 1996

39. Twersky R, Fishman D, Homel P: What happens after discharge? Return hospital visits after ambulatory surgery. Anesth Analg 84:319, 1997

40. Mezei G, Chung F: Return hospital visits and hospital readmissions after ambulatory surgery. Ann Surg 230:721, 1999

41. Greenburg AG, Greenburg JP, Tewel A, et al: Hospital admission following ambulatory surgery. Am J Surg 172:21, 1996

42. Mingus ML, Bodian CA, Bradford CN, et al: Prolonged surgery increases the likelihood of admission of scheduled ambulatory surgery patients. J Clin Anesth 9:446, 1997

43. Lau Hung, Brooks DC: Predictive factors for unanticipated admissions after ambulatory laparoscopic cholecystectomy. Arch Surg 136:1150, 2001

44. Chung F, Mezei G, Tong D: Preexisting medical conditions as predictors of adverse events in day-case surgery. Br J Anaesth 83:262, 1999

45. Chung F, Mezei G: Factors contributing to a prolonged stay after ambulatory surgery. Anesth Analg 89:1352, 1999

46. Pavlin DJ, Rapp SE, Polissar NL: Factors affecting discharge time in adult outpatients. Anesth Analg 87:816, 1998

47. Chung F: Recovery pattern and home readiness after ambulatory surgery. Anesth Analg 80:896, 1995

48. Marley RA: Postoperative nausea and vomiting: the outpatient enigma. J Perianesth Nurs 11:147, 1996

49. Tong D, Chung F, Wong D: Predictive factors in global and anesthesia satisfaction in ambulatory surgical patients. Anesthesiology 87:856, 1997

50. Macario A, Weinger M, Carney S, et al: Which clinical anesthesia outcomes are important to avoid? The perspective of patients. Anesth Analg 89:652, 1999

51. Lee PJ, Pandit SK, Green CR, et al: Postanesthetic side effects in the outpatient: which are the most important? Anesth Analg 80:S271, 1995

52. Orkin FK: What do patients want? Preferences for immediate postoperative recovery. Anesth Analg 74:S225, 1992

53. Carroll NV, Miederhoff P, Cox FM, et al: Postoperative nausea and vomiting after discharge from outpatient surgery centers. Anesth Analg 80:903, 1995

54. Jobalia N, Mathieu A: A meta-analysis of published studies confirms decreased postoperative nausea/vomiting with propofol. Anesthesiology 81:A133, 1994

55. Schreiner MS, Nicholson SC, Martin T, et al: Should children drink before discharge from day surgery? Anesthesiology 76:528, 1992

56. Jin F, Norris A, Chung F, et al: Should adult patients drink fluids before discharge from ambulatory surgery? Anesth Analg 87:306, 1998

57. Grond S, Lynch J, Diefenbach C, et al: Comparison of ondansetron and droperidol in the prevention of nausea and vomiting after inpatient gynecologic surgery. Anesth Analg 81:603, 1995

58. Russel D, Kenny GN: 5-HT$_3$ antagonists in postoperative nausea and vomiting. Br J Anaesth 69:63S, 1992

59. Khalil SN, Kataria B, Pearson K, et al: Ondansetron prevents postoperative nausea and vomiting in women outpatients. Anesth Analg 79:845, 1994

60. Henzi I, Walder B, Tramer MR: Dexamethasone for the prevention of postoperative nausea and vomiting: a quantitative systematic review. Anesth Analg 90:186, 2000

61. Splinter WM: Prevention of vomiting after strabismus surgery in children: dexamethasone alone versus dexamethasone plus low-dose ondansetron. Paediatr Anaesth 11:591, 2001

62. Huang JC, Shieh JP, Tang CS, et al: Low-dose dexamethasone effectively prevents postoperative nausea and vomiting after ambulatory laparoscopic surgery. Can J Anaesth 48:973, 2001

63. Aouad MT, Siddik SS, Rizk LB, et al: The effect of dexamethasone on postoperative vomiting after tonsillectomy. Anesth Analg 92:636, 2001

64. Fujii Y, Uemura A: Dexamethasone for the prevention of nausea and vomiting after dilatation and curettage: a randomized controlled trial. Obstet Gynecol 99:58, 2002

65. Subramaniam B, Madan R, Sadhasivam S, et al: Dexamethasone is a cost-effective alternative to ondansetron in preventing PONV after paediatric strabismus repair. Br J Anaesth 86:84, 2001

66. Tong D, Chung F: Postoperative pain control in ambulatory surgery. Surg Clin North Am 79:401, 1999

67. Chung F, Ritchie E, Su J: Postoperative pain in ambulatory surgery. Anesth Analg 85:808, 1997

68. Beauregard L, Pomp A, Choiniere M: Severity and impact of pain after day-surgery. Can J Anaesth 45:304, 1998

69. Doyle CE: Preoperative strategies for managing postoperative pain at home after day surgery. J Perianesth Nurs 14:373, 1999

70. Moline BM: Pain management in the ambulatory surgical population. J Perianesth Nurs 16:388, 2001

71. Reuben SS, Connelly NR: Postoperative analgesic effects of celecoxib or rofecoxib after spinal fusion surgery. Anesth Analg 91:1221, 2000

72. Rawal N: Postoperative pain management in day surgery. Anaesthesia 53:50, 1998

73. Manian FA, Meyer L: Comprehensive surveillance of surgical wound infections in outpatient and inpatient surgery. Infect Control Hosp Epidemiol 11:515, 1990

74. Zoutman D, Pearce P, McKenzie M, et al: Surgical wound infections occurring in day surgery patients. Am J Infect Control 18:277, 1990

75. Vilar-Compte D, Roldan R, Sandoval S, et al: Surgical site infections in ambulatory surgery: a 5-year experience. Am J Infect Control 29:99, 2001

76. Nafzinger DA, Lundstrom T, Chandra S, et al: Infection control in ambulatory care. Infect Dis Clin North Am 11:279, 1997

77. Zoutman D, Pearce P, McKenzie M, et al: Surgical wound infections occurring in day surgery patients. Am J Infect Control 18:277, 1990

78. Flanders E, Hinnant JR: Ambulatory surgery postoperative sound surveillance. Am J Infect Control 18:336,1990

79. Yozzo JC: Is it feasible to track infections in an ambulatory surgery center? J Post Anesth Nurs 4:255, 1989

80. Pavlin DJ, Pavlin EG, Fitzgibbon DR, et al: Management of bladder function after outpatient surgery. Anesthesiology 91:42, 1999

81. Tammela T: Postoperative urinary retention—why the patient cannot void. Scand J Urol Nephrol 175:75, 1995

82. Boulis NM, Mian FS, Rodriguez D, et al: Urinary retention following routine neurosurgical spine procedures. Surg Neurol 55:23, 2001

83. Stallard S, Prescott S: Postoperative urinary retention in general surgical patients. Br J Surg 75:1141, 1988

84. Lynch J, Kasper SM, Strick K, et al: The use of Quincke and Whitacre 27-gauge needles in orthopedic patients: incidence of failed spinal anesthesia and postdural puncture headache. Anesth Analg 79:124, 1994

85. Jost U, Hirschauer M, Weinig E, et al: Experience with G27 Whitacre needle in in-patient and outpatient settings—incidence of post dural puncture headaches and other side effects. Anasthesiol Intensivmed Notfallmed Schmerzther 35:381, 2000

86. Duffy PJ, Crosby ET: The epidural blood patch: resolving the controversies. Can J Anaesth 46:78, 1999

87. Advance Data Number 300. Centers for Disease Control and Prevention/National Center for Health Sciences, 1998

88. Legorreta AP, Silber JA, Costantino GN, et al: Increased cholecystectomy rate after the introduction of laparoscopic cholecystectomy. JAMA 270:1429, 1993

89. Ambulatory surgery. ACS Reports. American College of Surgeons, Chicago, 1983

90. Green CR, Pandit SK Preoperative preparation. The Ambulatory Anesthesia Handbook. Twersky RS, Ed. CV Mosby, St Louis, 1995, p 180

4 FAST TRACK SURGERY

Henrik Kehlet, M.D., Ph.D., and Douglas W. Wilmore, M.D.

Over the past several decades, surgery has undergone revolutionary changes that are leading to improved treatments (involving lower risk and better outcome) for an increasing number of diseases. These salutory developments are the result of more advanced anesthetic techniques, new methods of reducing the perioperative stress response, wider application of minimally invasive techniques, improved understanding of perioperative pathophysiology, and more sophisticated approaches to the prevention of postoperative organ dysfunction. Currently, many operations that once necessitated hospitalization can readily be performed in the outpatient setting; in addition, many major procedures are now associated with a significantly reduced duration of hospitalization and a shorter convalescence.

Although these anesthetic and surgical developments are the result of basic scientific and clinical research, they have also been influenced by governmental and managed care policies aimed at encouraging more cost-effective treatments. Such extraclinical influences, coupled with new clinical developments, have resulted in novel approaches designed to enhance the cost-effectiveness of health care, such as so-called fast track surgery, critical pathways, and various types of clinical guidelines. To understand the true potential value of such approaches, it is essential to recognize that their aim is not merely to ensure that fewer health care dollars are spent but, more important, to ensure that better and more efficient health care is delivered. Although these novel approaches may reduce cost, their primary purpose is to improve surgical management by reducing complications and providing better outcomes. In what follows, we outline the basic concept, primary components, and current results of fast track surgery, which is a comprehensive approach to the elective surgical patient that is designed to accelerate recovery, reduce morbidity, and shorten convalescence.

Basic Concept

Fast track surgery involves a coordinated effort to combine (1) preoperative patient education; (2) newer anesthetic, analgesic, and surgical techniques whose aim is to reduce surgical stress responses, pain, and discomfort; and (3) aggressive postoperative rehabilitation, including early enteral nutrition and ambulation. It also includes an up-to-date approach to general principles of postoperative care (e.g., use of tubes, drains, and catheters; monitoring; and general rehabilitation) that takes into account the revisions to traditional practice mandated by current scientific findings. It is believed that by these means, fast track surgery can shorten the time required for full recovery, reduce the need for hospitalization and convalescence, and lower the incidence of generalized morbidity related to pulmonary, cardiac, thromboembolic, and infectious complications.[1-3]

For an accelerated recovery program of this type to succeed, proper organization is essential. In general terms, fast track surgery must be based on a process of multidisciplinary collaboration that embraces not only the surgeon, the anesthesiologist, the physiotherapist, and the surgical nurse but also the patient. More specifically, fast track surgery depends on the inclusion and integration of a number of key constituent elements (see below).

Constituent Elements

EDUCATION OF THE PATIENT

To obtain the full advantages of a fast track surgical program, it is essential to provide patients with information about their perioperative care in advance of the procedure. Such educational efforts often serve to reduce patients' level of anxiety and need for pain relief, thereby providing a rational basis for collaboration with health care personnel, a process that is crucial for enhancing postoperative rehabilitation.[1-3] Patients can supplement the information they receive directly from health care providers by accessing reference sources such as www.facs.org/public_info/operation/aboutbroch.html, a collection of electronic brochures on specific clinical procedures that is provided by the American College of Surgeons.

OPTIMIZATION OF ANESTHESIA

The introduction of rapid-onset, short-acting volatile anesthetics (e.g., desflurane and sevoflurane), opioids (e.g., remifentanil), and muscle relaxants has enabled earlier recovery from anesthesia and thereby facilitated ambulatory and fast track surgery.[4] Although use of these newer general anesthetic agents has resulted in quicker recovery of vital organ function after minor surgical procedures, it has not been shown to decrease stress responses or mitigate organ dysfunction after major procedures.

Regional anesthetic techniques (e.g., peripheral nerve blocks and spinal or epidural analgesia), on the other hand, have several advantages in addition to providing anesthesia. Such advantages include improved pulmonary function, decreased cardiovascular demands, reduced ileus, and more effective pain relief. Neural blockade is the most effective technique for providing postoperative pain relief, and it has been shown to reduce endocrine and metabolic responses to surgery [*see VIII:2 Postoperative Pain*]. For a pronounced reduction in perioperative stress after a major operation, continuous epidural analgesia for 24 to 72 hours is necessary.[5] A meta-analysis of randomized trials evaluating regional anesthesia (primarily involving patients undergoing operations on the lower body) found that morbidity was 30% lower with regional anesthesia than with general anesthesia.[6]

Perioperative measures should also be taken to preserve intraoperative normothermia. Hypothermia may lead to an augmented stress response during rewarming, impaired coagulation and leukocyte function, and increased cardiovascular demands. Preservation of intraoperative and early postoperative normothermia has been shown to decrease surgical site infection, intraoperative blood loss, postoperative cardiac morbidity, and overall catabolism.[7]

REDUCTION OF SURGICAL STRESS

The neuroendocrine and inflammatory stress responses to surgery increase demands on various organs, and this increased demand is thought to contribute to the development of postoperative organ system complications. At present, the most important of the techniques used to reduce the surgical stress response are regional anesthesia, minimally invasive surgery, and pharmacologic intervention (e.g., with steroids, beta blockers, or anabolic agents).

Neural blockade with local anesthetics reduces endocrine and metabolic (specifically, catabolic) activation and sympathetic stimulation, thereby decreasing the demands placed on organs and reducing loss of muscle tissue; however, regional anesthetic techniques have no relevant effect on inflammatory responses.[5]

Minimally invasive surgical techniques clearly decrease pain and lessen inflammatory responses,[8-10] but they appear to have relatively little, if any, effect on endocrine and metabolic responses.

Pharmacologic intervention with a single dose of a glucocorticoid (usually dexamethasone, 8 mg) given before a minor procedure has led to reduced nausea, vomiting, and pain as well as to decreased inflammatory responses (IL-6), with no observed side effects.[11,12] This intervention may facilitate recovery from minor (i.e., ambulatory) procedures; however, the data from major procedures are inconclusive. The use of perioperative beta blockade to reduce sympathetic stimulation and thereby attenuate cardiovascular demands has been shown to reduce cardiac morbidity[3] as well as to reduce catabolism in burn patients [see IV:2 Risk Stratification, Preoperative Testing, and Operative Planning].[13] Perioperative beta blockade may therefore become an important component of efforts to facilitate recovery in fast track surgical programs.

For patients whose nutritional status is normal, oral feeding ad libitum is appropriate in the postoperative period. For patients who are elderly or nutritionally depleted, nutritional supplementation, administration of an anabolic agent (e.g., oxandrolone,[14] insulin,[15] or growth hormone [GH][16,17]) to enhance deposition of lean tissue, or both may be beneficial. Most of the studies addressing the use of anabolic agents have focused on critically ill catabolic patients, in whom both indirect effects (e.g., improved nitrogen balance[16]) and direct effects (e.g., improved wound healing and decreased length of stay with GH in burned children[17] and decreased mortality with insulin in critically ill patients[15]) on outcome have been demonstrated. In a study published in 2000, a group of elderly patients undergoing operations for hip fracture received either low-dose GH (20 µg/kg/day) or placebo.[18] Among those patients older than 75 years, a higher percentage were able to return to their prefracture living situation after 24 weeks of GH administration than could do so after a comparable period of receiving placebo (93.8% versus 75%; $P = 0.034$). More investigation is needed in this area.

A 1999 study reported increased mortality when GH was administered to ICU patients,[19] but a 2001 meta-analysis failed to confirm this observation.[20] Adequate control of blood glucose with long-term oral administration of a synthetic anabolic steroid may be an exceedingly cost-effective method of meta-

bolic support.[15] More work is necessary before definitive conclusions can be formed in this regard.

CONTROL OF NAUSEA, VOMITING, AND ILEUS

The ability to resume a normal diet after a surgical procedure (whether minor or major) is essential to the success of fast track surgery. To this end, postoperative nausea, vomiting, and ileus must be controlled. Principles for rational prophylaxis of nausea and vomiting have been developed on the basis of systematic reviews[21,22]: for example, H_2 receptor antagonists, droperidol, and dexamethasone have been shown to be effective in this regard, whereas propofol and metoclopramide have proved less so. There is some reason to think that multimodal antiemetic combinations may be superior to single antiemetic agents; unfortunately, the data currently available on combination regimens are relatively sparse. In addition, analgesic regimens in which opioids are cut back or eliminated have been shown to decrease postoperative nausea and vomiting.

Paralytic ileus remains a significant cause of delayed recovery from surgery and contributes substantially to postoperative discomfort and pain. Of the various techniques available for managing ileus,[23] continuous epidural analgesia with local anesthetics is the most effective, besides providing excellent pain relief.[23] Now that cisapride has been taken off the market, no effective anti-ileus drugs are available. In a 2001 study, however, a new peripherally acting mu opioid receptor antagonist significantly reduced nausea, vomiting, and ileus after abdominal procedures, without reducing analgesia.[24] If further studies confirm these findings, use of peripherally acting opioid antagonists may become a popular and effective way of improving postoperative recovery; this treatment is simple and apparently has no major side effects.

ADEQUATE TREATMENT OF POSTOPERATIVE PAIN

Despite ongoing development and documentation of effective postoperative analgesic regimens—such as continuous epidural analgesia in major operations, patient-controlled analgesia (PCA), and multimodal (balanced) analgesia that includes nonsteroidal anti-inflammatory drugs as well as stronger agents[25] [see VIII:2 Postoperative Pain]—postoperative pain still is too often inadequately treated. Improved pain relief, facilitated by an acute pain service, is a central component of any fast track surgery program and is a prerequisite for optimal mobilization and oral nutrition as well as a valuable aid in reducing surgical stress responses.

APPROPRIATE USE OF TUBES, DRAINS, AND CATHETERS

There is substantial support in the literature for the idea that nasogatric tubes should not be used routinely in patients undergoing elective abdominal surgery.[1,2] Randomized trials indicated that drains offered little benefit after cholecystectomy, joint replacements, colon resection, thyroidectomy, radical hysterectomy, or pancreatic resection[1,3,26] but that they might limit seroma formation after mastectomy.[1,3] Such postmastectomy drainage does not necessarily impede hospital discharge, and the patient generally may be treated on an outpatient basis. Urinary catheterization has been routinely performed after many operations, but scientific documentation of the requirement for this measure is often lacking. In general, catheterization beyond 24 hours is not recommended with colorectal procedures, except with the lowest rectal procedures, for which 3 to 4 days of catheterization may be indicated.[3]

Although tubes, drains, and catheters may lead to morbidity only when used for extended periods, they do tend to hinder mobilization, and they can raise a psychological barrier to the patient's active participation in postoperative rehabilitation. Therefore, such devices should be used not routinely but selectively, in accordance with the available scientific documentation.

NURSING CARE, NUTRITION, AND MOBILIZATION

Postoperative nursing care should include psychological support for early rehabilitation, with a particular focus on encouraging the patient to resume a normal diet and become ambulatory as soon as possible. Early resumption of an oral diet is essential for self-care; furthermore, according to a 2001 meta-analysis of controlled trials, it may reduce infectious complications and shorten hospital stay after abdominal procedures, without increasing the risk of anastomotic dehiscence.[27] In addition, early resumption of enteral feeding may reduce catabolism and may be facilitated by the methods used to reduce postoperative nausea, vomiting, and ileus (see above).

Postoperative bed rest is undesirable because it increases muscle loss, decreases strength, impairs pulmonary function and tissue oxygenation, and predisposes to venous stasis and thromboembolism.[3] Accordingly, every effort should be made to enforce postoperative mobilization; adequate pain relief is a key adjuvant measure in this regard.

Organization is essential for good postoperative nursing care: a prescheduled care map should be drawn up, with goals for rehabilitation listed for each day.

DISCHARGE PLANNING

Given that a primary result of fast track surgery is reduced length of hospitalization, discharge planning must be a major consideration in the preoperative patient information program as well as during hospitalization. Careful, detailed discharge planning is essential for reducing readmissions and increasing patient safety and satisfaction. The discharge plan should include (1) detailed information on the expected time course of recovery, (2) recommendations for convalescence, and (3) encouragement of enteral intake and mobilization. For patients with a significant degree of postoperative disability, various acute care facilities are available after hospital discharge. It should be kept in mind, however, that the integrated care approach fundamental to fast track surgery is specifically intended as a way of limiting or preventing such disability, thereby reducing patients' need for and dependence on postdischarge care facilities.

Reported Results

Ongoing efforts to formulate multimodal strategies aimed at improving postoperative outcome have led to the development of a variety of fast track surgical programs [see Table 1]. Most of the studies published to date have been descriptive ones reporting consecutive patient series from single centers, the findings from which have often been confirmed by other groups using the same or a slightly modified fast track care program. On the whole, the preliminary results from these studies are very positive: fast track surgery is associated with shorter hospital stays, reduced or at least comparable morbidities, and low readmission rates, with no apparent decrease in safety.

Studies of fast track surgery in which organ function was assessed postoperatively and compared with organ function after traditional care found fast track surgery to be associated with earlier ambulation,[28,29] superior postoperative muscle function,[29] improved oral nutritional intake,[30] better preservation of lean body mass,[28,30] reduced postoperative impairment of pulmonary

function,[21] and mitigation of the decrease in exercise capacity and impairment of cardiovascular response to exercise that are usually expected after an operation.[28] The few randomized trials performed to date (mostly involving patients undergoing cholecystectomy or mastectomy) reported that fast track programs increased or at least maintained patient satisfaction while achieving major cost reductions.

Future Developments

The initial promising results from the fast track surgical programs studied suggest that such programs can achieve major care improvements in terms of reducing postoperative stay. At present, however, sufficient scientific documentation is lacking for many commonly performed major operations. Thus, there is a need for additional data—in particular, data on the potential positive effects of fast track surgery on postoperative morbidity. The necessary data would probably be best obtained through multicenter trials using identical protocols; randomized trials within the same unit that allocate some patients to suboptimal care recommendations for pain relief, mobilization, and nutrition would be difficult to perform, if not unethical.

As yet, it has not been conclusively demonstrated that reducing the duration of hospitalization necessarily reduces morbidity,[31] though data from studies addressing colonic and vascular procedures suggest that nonsurgical (i.e., cardiopulmonary and thromboembolic) morbidity may be reduced and overall postoperative recovery (assessed in terms of exercise performance and muscle power) enhanced. More study is required in this area. Future trials should also focus on identifying any factors that might be limiting even more aggressive early recovery efforts, so that more effective fast track programs can be designed. Finally, studies are needed to identify potential high-risk patient groups for whom fast track surgery may not be appropriate or who may need to be hospitalized for slightly longer periods to optimize organ function.

There has been considerable interest in whether the use of critical pathways improves postoperative care. Preliminary studies involving coronary artery bypass grafting, total knee replacement, colectomy, thoracic procedures, and hysterectomy suggested that critical pathways may reduce length of hospital stay, but the reduction is no greater than can be observed in neighboring hospitals that do not use critical pathways.[32] Thus, the initial enthusiasm for critical pathways notwithstanding, conclusive evidence that they have a beneficial effect on postoperative care is still lacking. The continuously decreasing length of stay noted in hospitals without fast track programs may be partly attributable to the intense competition within the health care system, which can lead to changes in care principles even without the formal adoption of critical pathways or similar systems.[32]

All of the studies on the economic implications of fast track surgical programs and critical pathways have documented substantial cost savings. It should, however, be borne in mind that the last portion of a hospital stay is much less expensive than the initial portion; thus, the cost savings in this area may turn out to be smaller than they would at first appear.[33,34] This cavil should not hinder further development and documentation of fast track surgery, because inherent in the concept is the idea that revision and optimization of perioperative care may also reduce morbidity, thereby achieving additional cost savings. As noted, the large-scale data with detailed patient description and stratification that are needed to clarify the improvements achieved by fast track surgery are, unfortunately, lacking at present, but so far, all indications are that postoperative morbidity is comparable or reduced.

Table 1   Results from Selected Fast Track Surgical Programs

Type of Operation	Postoperative Hospital Stay	Comments and Other Findings
Abdominal procedures		
Inguinal hernia repair[39,40]	1.5–6 hr	Large consecutive series using local infiltration anesthesia in > 95%, with one series[40] using unmonitored anesthesia; documented low morbidity, with no urinary retention; patient satisfaction ~90%, cost reduction > $250 with local anesthesia
Cholecystectomy (laparoscopic,[41-46] mini-incision[47])	> 80% discharge on same day	Large consecutive series, with documented safety and patient satisfaction > 80%; cost reduction of $750/patient in randomized study[43]; similar results with mini-incision in consecutive series[47]
Fundoplication[48,49]	> 90% < 23 hr	Large consecutive series with documented safety[49]
Open[50-53] and laparoscopic[54,55] colorectal procedures	2–4 days	Consecutive series including high-risk patients; reduced cardiopulmonary morbidity, readmission rates 0%–15%; no documented advantages of laparoscopy-assisted colonic resection; ileus reduced to < 48 hr in > 90% of patients, with improved muscle and pulmonary function in fast track patients and better preservation of postoperative body composition
Complex pelvic-colorectal procedures[56,57]	3–6 days	Short stay[56] (~4–6 days) even with additional stoma; low readmission rate (7%)
Rectal prolapse[58]	80% < 24 hr	Consecutive series (N = 63) with Altemeier repair; 5% readmission rate (nonserious indications)
Pancreaticoduodenectomy,[59,60] complex biliary tract procedures[61]	—	Hospital stay decreased by implementation of clinical pathway
Mastectomy[62-65]	90% < 1 day	Large cumulative series; documented safety and major cost reduction with high patient satisfaction; no increased morbidity with fast track, but less wound pain and improved arm movement and no increase in risk of psychosocial complications
Vascular procedures		
Carotid endarterectomy[66-69]	90% < 1 day	Surgery done with local anesthesia; specialized nurses and wards
Lower-extremity arterial bypass[70]	2–3 days	Large series (N = 130); documented safety
Abdominal aortic aneurysmectomy[71,72]	~3 days	Preliminary studies (N = 50[71] and N = 77[72]); documented early recovery and safety; one study with epidural analgesia,[72] one without[71]
Urologic procedures		
Radical prostatectomy[73]	~75% 1 day	Large consecutive series (N = 252); documented safety and patient satisfaction
Laparoscopic adrenalectomy[74-76]	< 1 day	Small series; safety and low morbidity suggested
Cystectomy[77]	Not assessed	Improved mobilization, bowel function, and sleep recovery with fast track surgery
Laparoscopic donor nephrectomy[78]	< 1 day	Preliminary study (N = 41); low readmission rate (2%)
Pulmonary procedures[79-83]	~1 day in some series,[79,80] ~4–5 days in others	Shortest stay with fast track protocol including revision of drainage principles[79,80]; safety with very early discharge suggested
Other procedures		
Craniotomy[84]	~40% < 24 hr	Large consecutive series (N = 241) including tumor surgery; local anesthesia used; low readmission rate; safety suggested
Parathyroid procedures[85]	~90% ambulatory	Selected consecutive series (N = 100); regional anesthesia and intraoperative adenoma localization employed; documented safety
Vaginal procedures[86]	~1 day	Consecutive series (N = 108); surgery done with local anesthesia

A commonly expressed concern is that fast track surgery might increase the burden on general practitioners and other parts of the nonhospital care system. The evidence currently available clearly indicates that increased use of ambulatory surgery is safe and is associated with a very low readmission rate.[35,36] After major procedures such as colorectal surgery, however, readmissions are often unpredictable, and the readmission rate is not significantly reduced by keeping patients in the hospital for an additional 2 to 3 days.[37,38] Again, it should be emphasized that the basic concept of fast track surgery implies control of perioperative pathophysiology with the aim of enhancing recovery and thereby reducing the need for postdischarge care. The relatively few published studies to address patient functional status after fast track colonic surgery suggested that muscle function and exercise capacity and body composition are better preserved with this approach than with traditional care, in which surgical stress, insufficient nutrition, and prolonged immobilization typically lead to significant deterioration of organ function.

In summary, the basic concept of fast track surgery, which could be expressed as multimodal control of perioperative pathophysiology, seems to be a highly promising approach to improving surgical outcome. We believe that the principles and techniques embodied in this approach will eventually be integrated into the care of all surgical patients. To this end, resources should be allocated for evaluation and documentation of the effects of fast track surgery and related systems on cost, postoperative morbidity, safety, and overall patient well-being.

References

1. Kehlet H: Multimodal approach to control postoperative pathophysiology and rehabilitation. Br J Anaesth 78:606, 1997

2. Wilmore DW, Kehlet H: Management of patients in fast track surgery. BMJ 322:473, 2001

3. Kehlet H, Wilmore DW: Multi-modal strategies to improve surgical outcome. Am J Surg (in press)

4. White PF: Ambulatory anesthesia—advances into the new millennium. Anesth Analg 98:1234, 2000

5. Kehlet H: Modification of responses to surgery by neural blockade: clinical implications. Neural Blockade in Clinical Anesthesia and Management of Pain. Cousins MJ, Bridenbaugh PO, Eds. JB Lippincott Co, Philadelphia, 1998, p 129

6. Rodgers A, Walker N, Schug S, et al: Reduction of post-operative mortality and morbidity with epidural or spinal anaesthesia: results from an overview of randomized trials. BMJ 32:1, 2000

7. Sessler DI: Mild perioperative hypothermia. N Engl J Med 336:1730, 1997

8. Kehlet H: Surgical stress response: does endoscopic surgery confer an advantage? World J Surg 23:801, 1999

9. Vittimberga FJ Jr, Foley DP, Kehlet H, et al: Laparoscopic surgery and the systemic immune response. Ann Surg 227:326, 1998

10 Gupta A, Watson DI: Effect of laparoscopy on immune function. Br J Surg 88:1296, 2001

11. Henzi I, Walder B, Tramer MR: Dexamethasone for the prevention of postoperative nausea and vomiting: a quantitative systematic review. Anesth Analg 90:186, 2000

12. Holte K, Kehlet H: Perioperative single dose glucocorticoid administration—pathophysiological effects and clinical implications. J Am Coll Surg (submitted for publication)

13. Herndon DN, Hart DW, Wolf SE, et al: Reversal of catabolism by beta-blockade after severe burns. N Engl J Med 345:1223, 2001

14. Demling RH, Orgill DP: The anticatabolic and wound healing effects of the testosterone analog oxandrolone after severe burn injury. J Crit Care 15:12, 2000

15. Van der Berghe G, Wouters P, Weekers F, et al: Intensive insulin therapy in critically ill patients. N Engl J Med 345:1359, 2001

16. Jiang ZM, He GZ, Zhang SY, et al: Low-dose growth hormone and hypocaloric nutrition attenuate the protein-catabolic response of a major operation. Ann Surg 210:513, 1989

17. Ramirez RJ, Wolf SE, Barrow RE, et al: Growth hormone treatment in pediatric burns: a safe therapeutic approach. Ann Surg 228:439, 1998

18. Van der Lely AJ, Lamberts SW, Jauch KW, et al: Use of human GH in elderly patients with accidental hip fracture. Eur J Endocrinol 143:585, 2000

19. Takala J, Ruokonen E, Webster NR, et al: Increased mortality associated with growth hormone treatment in critically ill adults. N Engl J Med 341:785, 1999

20. Raguso CA, Genton L, Pichard C: Growth hormone (rhGH) administration to ICU patients: a literature survey. Clin Nutr 20:16, 2001

21. Tramér MR: A rational approach to control postoperative nausea and vomiting: evidence from systematic reviews. Part 1: efficacy and harm of anti-emetic interventions and methodological issues. Acta Anaesthesiol Scand 45:4, 2001

22. Tramér MR: A rational approach to the control of postoperative nausea and vomiting: evidence from systematic reviews. Part 2: recommendations for prevention and treatment, and research agenda. Acta Anaesthesiol Scand 45:14, 2001

23. Holte K, Kehlet H: Postoperative ileus: a preventable event. Br J Surg 87:1480, 2000

24. Taguchi A, Sharma N, Saleem RM, et al: Selective postoperative inhibition of gastrointestinal opioid receptors. N Engl J Med 345:935, 2001

25. Kehlet H: Acute pain control and accelerated postoperative surgical recovery. Surg Clin North Am 79:431, 1999

26. Conlon KC, Labow D, Leung D, et al: Prospective randomized clinical trial of the value of intraperitoneal drainage after pancreatic resection. Ann Surg 234:487, 2001

27. Lewis SJ, Egger M, Sylvester PA, et al: Early enteral feeding versus "nil by mouth" after gastrointestinal surgery: systematic review and meta-analysis of controlled trials. BMJ 323:1,2001

28. Basse L, Raskov HH, Jacobsen DH, et al: Accelerated postoperative recovery program after colonic resection improves physical performance, pulmonary function and body composition. Br J Surg 89:446, 2002

29. Henriksen MG, Jensen MB, Hansen HV, et al: Enforced mobilization, early oral feeding and balanced analgesia improve convalescence after colorectal surgery. Nutrition 18:147, 2002

30. Henriksen MG, Hansen HV, Hessov I: Early oral nutrition after elective surgery: influence of balanced analgesia and enforced mobilization. Nutrition 18:263, 2002

31. Weingarten S, Riedinger MS, Sandhu M, et al: Can practice guidelines safely reduce hospital length of stay? Results from a multicenter interventional study. Am J Med 105:33, 1998

32. Pearson SD, Kleefield SF, Soukop JR, et al: Critical pathways intervention to reduce length of hospital stay. Am J Med 110:175, 2001

33. Weingarten S: Critical pathways: what do you do when they do not seem to work? Am J Med 110:224, 2001

34. Taheri PA, Butz DA, Greenfield LJ: Length of stay has minimal impact on the cost of hospital admission. J Am Coll Surg 191:124, 2000

35. Barkun JS: Relevance of length of stay reductions. J Am Coll Surg 191:192, 2000

36. Twersky R, Fishman D, Homel P: What happens after discharge? Return hospital visits after ambulatory surgery. Anesth Analg 84:319, 1997

37. Mezei G, Chung F: Return hospital visits and hospital readmissions after ambulatory surgery. Ann Surg 230:721, 1999

38. Azimuddin K, Rosen L, Reed JF, et al: Readmissions after colorectal surgery cannot be predicted. Dis Colon Rectum 7:942, 2001

39. Callesen T, Bech K, Kehlet H: One-thousand consecutive inguinal hernia repairs under unmonitored local anesthesia. Anesth Analg 93:1373, 2001

40. Kark AE, Kurzer NM, Belsham PA: Three thousand one hundred seventy-five primary inguinal hernia repairs: advantages of ambulatory open mesh repair using local anesthesia. J Am Coll Surg 186:447, 1998

41. Mjåland O, Raeder J, Aasboe V, et al: Outpatient laparoscopic cholecystectomy. Br J Surg 84:958, 1997

42. Voitk AJ: Establishing outpatient cholecystectomy as a hospital routine. Can J Surg 40:284, 1997

43. Keulemans Y, Eshuis J, deHaes H, et al: Laparoscopic cholecystectomy: day-care versus clinical observation. Ann Surg 228:734, 1998

44. Calland JF, Tanaka K, Foley E, et al: Outpatient laparoscopic cholecystectomy: patient outcomes after implementation of a clinical pathway. Ann Surg 233:704, 2001

45. Richardson WS, Fuhrman GS, Burch E, et al: Outpatient laparoscopic cholecystectomy. Surg Endosc 15:193, 2001

46. Bringman S, Anderberg B, Heikkinen T, et al: Outpatient laparoscopic cholecystectomy: a prospective study with 100 consecutive patients. Amb Surg 9:83, 2001

47. Seale AK, Ledet WP: Minicholecystectomy: a safe, cost-effective day surgery procedure. Arch Surg 134:308, 1999

48. Trondsen E, Mjåland O, Raeder J, et al: Day-case laparoscopic fundoplication for gastroesophageal reflux disease. Br J Surg 87:1708, 2000

49. Finley CR, McKernan JB: Laparoscopic antireflux surgery at an outpatient surgery center. Surg Endosc 15:823, 2001

50. Basse L, Hjort Jakobsen D, Billesbølle P, et al: A clinical pathway to accelerate recovery after colonic resection. Ann Surg 232:51, 2000

51. Basse L, Hjort Jakobsen D, Billesbølle P, et al: Accelerated rehabilitation after colonic resection. Ugeskr Læger 163:913, 2001

52. Di Fronzo LA, Cymerman J, O'Connell TX: Factors affecting early postoperative feeding following elective open colon resection. Arch Surg 134:941, 1999

53. Smedh K, Strand E, Jansson P, et al: Rapid recovery after colonic resection using Kehlet's multimodal rehabilitation program. Läkartidningen 98:2568, 2001

54. Bardram L, Funch-Jensen P, Kehlet H: Rapid rehabilitation in elderly patients after laparoscopic colonic resection. Br J Surg 87:1540, 2000

55. Senagore AJ, Whalley D, Delaney P, et al: Epidural anesthesia-analgesia shortens length of stay after laparoscopic segmental colectomy for benign pathology. Surgery 129:672, 2001

56. Delaney CP, Fazio VW, Senagore AJ, et al: Fast track postoperative management protocol for

patients with high co-morbidity undergoing complex abdominal pelvic colorectal surgery. Br J Surg 88:1533, 2001

57. Archer SB, Burnett RJ, Flesch LV, et al: Implementation of a clinical pathway decreases length of stay and hospital charges for patients undergoing total colectomy and ileal pouch/anal anastomosis. Surgery 122:699, 1997

58. Kimmins MH, Evetts BK, Isler J, et al: The Altemeier repair: outpatient treatment of rectal prolapse. Dis Colon Rectum 44:565, 2001

59. Brooks AD, Marcus SG, Gradek C, et al: Decreasing length of stay after pancreatoduodenectomy. Arch Surg 135:823, 2000

60. Porter GA, Pisters PTW, Mansyur C, et al: Cost and utilization impact of a clinical pathway for patients undergoing pancreatico-duodenectomy. Ann Surg Oncol 7:484, 2000

61. Pitt HA, Murray KP, Bowman HM, et al: Clinical pathway implementation improves outcomes for complex biliary surgery. Surgery 126:751, 1999

62. Warren JL, Riley GF, Potosky AL: Trends and outcomes of outpatient mastectomy in elderly women. J Natl Cancer Inst 90:833, 1998

63. Ferrante J, Gonzalez E, Pal N, et al: The use and outcomes of outpatient mastectomy in Florida. Am J Surg 179:253, 2000

64. Bundred N, Maguire P, Reynolds J, et al: Randomized controlled trial of effects of early discharge after surgery for breast cancer. BMJ 317:1275, 1998

65. Margolese RG, Jean-Claude M: Ambulatory surgery for breast cancer patients. Ann Surg Oncol 7:181, 2000

66. Collier PE: Are one-day admissions for carotid endarterectomy feasible? Am J Surg 170:140, 1995

67. Bourke BM: Overnight hospital stay for carotid endarterectomy. Med J Aust 168:157, 1998

68. Kaufman JL, Frank D, Rhee SW, et al: Feasibility and safety of 1-day postoperative hospitalization for carotid endarterectomy. Arch Surg 131:751, 1996

69. Littooy FN, Steffen G, Greisler HP, et al: Short stay carotid surgery for veterans: an emerging standard. J Surg Res 95:32, 2001

70. Collier PE: Do clinical pathways for major vascular surgery improve outcomes and reduce cost? J Vasc Surg 26:179, 1997

71. Podore PC, Throop EB: Infrarenal aortic surgery with a 3-day hospital stay: a report on success with a clinical pathway. J Vasc Surg 29:787, 1999

72. Renghi A, Brustia P, Gramaglia L, et al: A clinical program to enhance recovery following abdominal aortic surgery. Ann Surg (submitted for publication)

73. Kirsh EJ, Worwag EM, Sinner M, et al: Using outcome data and patient satisfaction surveys to develop policies regarding minimum length of hospitalization after radical prostatectomy. Urology 56:101, 2000

74. Gill IS, Hobart MG, Schweizer D, et al: Outpatient adrenalectomy. J Urol 163:717, 2000

75. Edwin B, Ræder I, Trondsen E, et al: Outpatient laparoscopic adrenalectomy in patients with Conn's syndrome. Surg Endosc 15:589, 2001

76. Rayan SS, Hodin RA: Short-stay laparoscopic adrenalectomy. Surg Endosc 14:568, 2000

77. Brodner G, Van Aken H, Hertle L, et al: Multimodal perioperative management—combining thoracic epidural analgesia, forced mobilization, and oral nutrition—reduces hormonal and metabolic stress and improves convalescence after major urologic surgery. Anesth Analg 92:1594, 2001

78. Kuo PC, Johnson LB, Sitzmann JV: Laparoscopic donor nephrectomy with a 23-hour stay. Ann Surg 31:772, 2000

79. Tovar EA, Roethe RA, Weissing MD, et al: One-day admission for lung lobectomy: an incidental result of a clinical pathway. Ann Thorac Surg 65:803, 1998

80. Tovar EA: One-day admission for major lung resections in septuagenarians and octogenarians: a comparative study with a younger cohort. Eur J Cardiothorac Surg 20:449, 2001

81. Cerfolio RJ, Pickens A, Bass C, et al: Fast-tracking pulmonary resections. J Thor Cardiovasc Surg 122:318, 2001

82. Zehr KJ, Dawson PB, Yang SC, et al: Standardized clinical care pathways for major thoracic cases reduce hospital costs. Ann Thorac Surg 66:914, 1998

83. Wright CD, Wain JC, Grillo HC, et al: Pulmonary lobectomy patient care pathway: a model to control cost and maintain quality. Ann Thorac Surg 64:299, 1997

84. Blanchard HJ, Chung F, Manninen PH, et al: Awake craniotomy for removal of intracranial tumor: considerations for early discharge. Anesth Analg 92:89, 2001

85. Udelsman R, Donovan PI, Sokoll LJ: One hundred consecutive minimally invasive parathyroid explorations. Ann Surg 232:331, 2000

86. Petros PEP: Development of generic models for ambulatory vaginal surgery—a preliminary report. Int Urogynecol J 9:19, 1998

5 PREVENTION OF POSTOPERATIVE INFECTION

Jonathan L. Meakins, M.D., D.Sc., Byron J. Masterson, M.D., and Ronald Lee Nichols, M.D., M.S.

Epidemiology of Surgical Site Infection

Historically, the control of wound infection depended on antiseptic and aseptic techniques directed at coping with the infecting organism. In the 19th century and the early part of the 20th century, wound infections had devastating consequences and a measurable mortality. Even in the 1960s, before the correct use of antibiotics and the advent of modern preoperative and postoperative care, as much as one quarter of a surgical ward might have been occupied by patients with wound complications. As a result, wound management, in itself, became an important component of ward care and of medical education. It is fortunate that many factors have intervened so that the so-called wound rounds have become a practice of the past. The epidemiology of wound infection has changed as surgeons have learned to control bacteria and the inoculum as well as to focus increasingly on the patient (the host) for measures that will continue to provide improved results.

The following three factors are the determinants of any infectious process:

1. The infecting organism (in surgical patients, usually bacteria).
2. The environment in which the infection takes place (the local response).
3. The host defense mechanisms, which deal systemically with the infectious process.[1]

Wounds are particularly appropriate for analysis of infection with respect to these three determinants. Because many components of the bacterial contribution to wound infection now are clearly understood and measures to control bacteria have been implemented, the host factors become more apparent. In addition, interactions between the three determinants play a critical role, and with limited exceptions (e.g., massive contamination), few infections will be the result of only one factor [*see Figure 1*].

Definition of Surgical Site Infection

Wound infections have traditionally been thought of as infections in a surgical wound occurring between the skin and the deep soft tissues—a view that fails to consider the operative site as a whole. As prevention of these wound infections has become more effective, it has become apparent that definitions of opera-

tion-related infection must take the entire operative field into account; obvious examples include sternal and mediastinal infections, vascular graft infections, and infections associated with implants (if occurring within 1 year of the procedure and apparently related to it). Accordingly, the Centers for Disease Control and Prevention currently prefers to use the term surgical site infection (SSI). SSIs can be classified into three categories: superficial incisional SSIs (involving only skin and subcutaneous tissue), deep incisional SSIs (involving deep soft tissue), and organ/space SSIs (involving anatomic areas other than the incision itself that are opened or manipulated in the course of the procedure)[2,3] [*see Figure 2*].

Standardization in reporting will permit more effective surveillance and improve results as well as offer a painless way of achieving quality assurance. The natural tendency to deny that a surgical site has become infected contributes to the difficulty of defining SSI in a way that is both accurate and acceptable to surgeons. The surgical view of SSI recalls one judge's (probably apocryphal) remark about pornography: "It is hard to define, but I know it when I see it." SSIs are usually easy to identify.

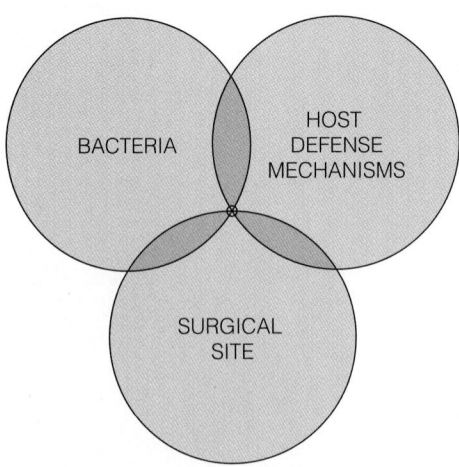

Figure 1 In a homeostatic, normal state, the determinants of any infectious process—bacteria, the surgical site, and host defense mechanisms (represented by three circles)—intersect at a point indicating zero probability of sepsis.

Figure 2 Surgical site infections are classified into three categories, depending on which anatomic areas are affected.[3]

Bacteria

Clearly, without an infecting agent no infection will result. Accordingly, most of what is known about bacteria is put to use in major efforts directed at reducing their numbers by means of asepsis and antisepsis. The principal concept is based on the size of the bacterial inoculum.

Wounds are traditionally classified according to whether the wound inoculum of bacteria is likely to be large enough to overwhelm local and systemic host defense mechanisms and produce an infection [*see Table 1*]. One study showed that the most important factor in the development of a wound infection was the number of bacteria present in the wound at the end of an operative procedure.[4] Another study quantitated this relation and provided insight into how local environmental factors might be integrated into an understanding of the problem [*see Figure 3*].[5] In the years before prophylactic antibiotics as well as during the early phases of their use, there was a very clear relation between the classification of the operation (which is related to the probability of a significant inoculum) and the rate of wound infection.[6,7] This relation has persisted but is now less dominant than it once was; therefore, other factors have come to play a significant role.[8,9]

CONTROL OF SOURCES OF BACTERIA

Endogenous bacteria are a more important cause of SSI than exogenous bacteria are. In clean-contaminated, contaminated, and dirty-infected operations, the source and the amount of bacteria

are functions of the patient's disease and the specific organs being operated on.

Operations classified as infected are those in which infected tissue and pus are removed or drained, providing a guaranteed

inoculum to the surgical site. The inoculum may be as high as 10^{10} bacteria/ml, some of which may already be producing an infection. In addition, some bacteria could be in the growth phase rather than the dormant or the lag phase and thus could be more pathogenic. The heavily contaminated wound is best managed by delayed primary closure. This type of management ensures that the wound is not closed over a bacterial inoculum that is almost certain to cause a wound infection, with attendant early and late consequences.

Patients should not have elective surgery in the presence of remote infection, which is associated with an increased incidence of wound infection.[6] In patients with urinary tract infections, wounds frequently become infected with the same organism. Remote infections should be treated appropriately, and the operation should proceed only under the best conditions possible. If operation cannot be appropriately delayed, the use of prophylactic and therapeutic antibiotics should be considered [*see Sidebar Antibiotic Prophylaxis of Infection and Tables 2, 3, and 4*].

Preoperative techniques of reducing patient flora, especially endogenous bacteria, are of great concern. Bowel preparation, antimicrobial showers or baths, and preoperative skin decontamination have been proposed frequently. These techniques, particularly preoperative skin decontamination [*see Sidebar Preoperative Decontamination of the Operative Site*], may have specific roles in selected patients during epidemics or in units with high infection rates. As a routine for all patients, however, these techniques are unnecessary, time-consuming, and costly in institutions or units where infection rates are low.

The preoperative shave is a technique in need of reassessment. It is now clear that shaving the evening before an operation is associated with an increased wound infection rate. This increase is secondary to the trauma of the shave and the inevitable small areas of inflammation and infection. If hair removal is required,[10,11] clipping is preferable and should be done in the operating room or the preparation room just before the operative procedure. Shaving, if ever performed, should not be done the night before operation.

Bowel preparation [*see Sidebar Bowel Preparation and Tables 5, 6, and 7*] has a clear role in colon and rectal surgery. The suggestion has been made that selective gut decontamination (SGD) may be useful in major elective procedures involving the upper gastrointestinal tract and perhaps in other settings. At present, SGD for prevention of infection cannot be recommended in either the preoperative or the postoperative period.

When infection develops after clean operations, particularly those in which foreign bodies were implanted, endogenous infecting organisms are involved but the skin is the primary source of the infecting bacteria. The air in the operating room and other OR sources occasionally become significant in clean cases; the degree of endogenous contamination can be surpassed by that of exogenous contamination. Thus, both the operating team—surgeon, assistants, nurses, and anesthetists—and OR air have been reported as significant sources of bacteria. In fact, personnel are the most important source of exogenous bacteria.[12-14] In a study by the National Academy of Sciences–National Research Council, ultraviolet light (UVL) was efficacious only in the limited situations of clean and ultraclean cases.[6] There were minimal numbers of endogenous bacteria, and UVL controlled one of the exogenous sources.

Clean air systems have very strong advocates, but they also have equally vociferous critics [*see IV:6 Preparing the Operating Room*]. It is possible to obtain excellent results in clean cases with implants without using these systems. However, clean

Epidemiology of Surgical Site Infection

Wound infection is caused by exogenous or endogenous bacteria; infection is influenced not only by the source of the infecting inoculum but also by the bacterial characteristics.

Ensure that prophylactic antibiotics, if indicated, are present in tissue in adequate concentrations at beginning of operation.

Endogenous factors or sources of bacteria

Bacterial characteristics of importance (virulence and antibiotic resistance)

Exogenous factors or sources of bacteria

Remote sites of infection

Postpone elective operation if possible. Treat remote infection appropriately.

Skin

Bowel

Nature and site of operation

Is the operation
• Clean
• Contaminated
• Clean-contaminated
• Dirty or infected

Size of inoculum required to produce infection

Varies in different clinical situations.

Operating team–related

• Comportment
• Use of impermeable drapes and gowns
• Surgical scrub [*see Sidebar* The Surgical Scrub].

Operating room–related

• Traffic control
• Cleaning
• Air

Surveillance and quality assurance

Preventive measures to control bacteria

• Decontamination of patient's skin [*see Sidebar* Preoperative Decontamination of the Operative Site]
• Bowel preparation [*see Sidebar* Bowel Preparation]
• Additional antibiotics if indicated, depending on likelihood of contamination and on bacterial inoculum and properties [*see Sidebar* Antibiotic Prophylaxis of Infection]

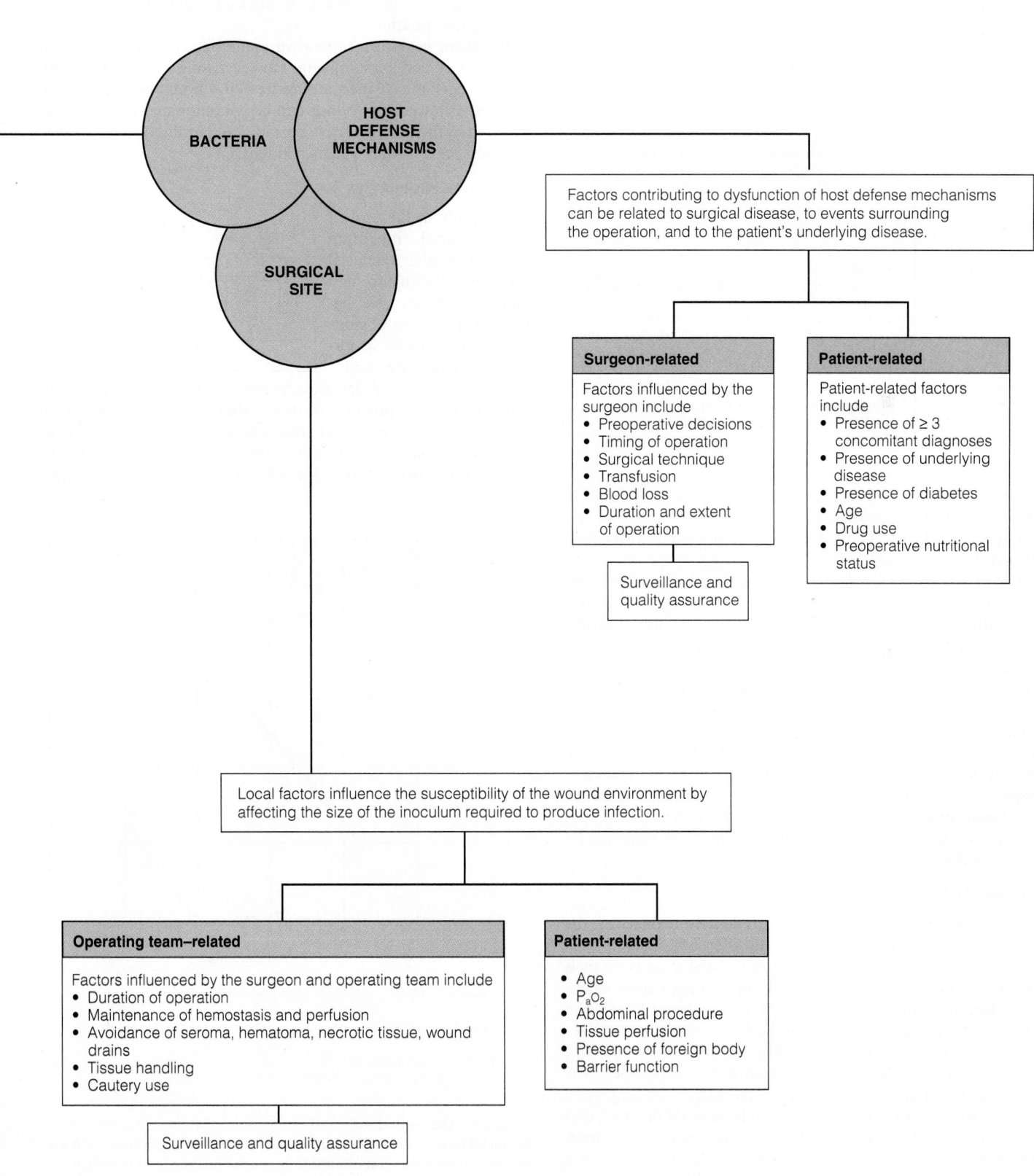

BACTERIA

HOST
DEFENSE
MECHANISMS

SURGICAL
SITE

Factors contributing to dysfunction of host defense mechanisms
can be related to surgical disease, to events surrounding
the operation, and to the patient's underlying disease.

Surgeon-related

Factors influenced by the
surgeon include
- Preoperative decisions
- Timing of operation
- Surgical technique
- Transfusion
- Blood loss
- Duration and extent
  of operation

Surveillance and
quality assurance

Patient-related

Patient-related factors
include
- Presence of ≥ 3
  concomitant diagnoses
- Presence of underlying
  disease
- Presence of diabetes
- Age
- Drug use
- Preoperative nutritional
  status

Local factors influence the susceptibility of the wound environment by
affecting the size of the inoculum required to produce infection.

Operating team–related

Factors influenced by the surgeon and operating team include
- Duration of operation
- Maintenance of hemostasis and perfusion
- Avoidance of seroma, hematoma, necrotic tissue, wound
  drains
- Tissue handling
- Cautery use

Surveillance and quality assurance

Patient-related

- Age
- P_aO_2
- Abdominal procedure
- Tissue perfusion
- Presence of foreign body
- Barrier function

Table 1 National Research Council Classification of Operative Wounds[21]

Clean (class I)	Nontraumatic No inflammation encountered No break in technique Respiratory, alimentary, or genitourinary tract not entered
Clean-contaminated (class II)	Gastrointestinal or respiratory tract entered without significant spillage Appendectomy Oropharynx entered Vagina entered Genitourinary tract entered in absence of infected urine Biliary tract entered in absence of infected bile Minor break in technique
Contaminated (class III)	Major break in technique Gross spillage from gastrointestinal tract Traumatic wound, fresh Entrance of genitourinary or biliary tracts in presence of infected urine or bile
Dirty and infected (class IV)	Acute bacterial inflammation encountered, without pus Transection of "clean" tissue for the purpose of surgical access to a collection of pus Traumatic wound with retained devitalized tissue, foreign bodies, fecal contamination, or delayed treatment, or all of these; or from dirty source

air systems are here to stay. Nevertheless, the presence of a clean air system does not mean that basic principles of asepsis and antisepsis should be abandoned, because endogenous bacteria must still be controlled.

The use of impermeable drapes and gowns has received considerable attention. If bacteria can penetrate gown and drapes, they can gain access to the wound. The use of impermeable drapes may therefore be of clinical importance.[15,16] When wet, drapes of 140-thread-count cotton are permeable to bacteria. It is clear that some operations are wetter than others, but generally, much can be done to make drapes and gowns impermeable to bacteria. For example, drapes of 270-thread-count cotton that have been waterproofed are impermeable, but they can be washed only 75 times. Economics plays a role in the choice of drape fabric because entirely disposable drapes are expensive. Local institutional factors may be significant in the role of a specific type of drape in the prevention of SSI [*see IV:6 Preparing the Operating Room*].

PROBABILITY OF CONTAMINATION

The probability of contamination is largely defined by the nature of the operation [*see Table 1*]. However, other factors contribute to the probability of contamination; the most obvious is the expected duration of the operative procedure, which, whenever examined, has been significant in the wound infection rate.[4,7,8] The longer the procedure lasts, the more bacteria accumulate in a wound; the sources of bacteria include the patient, the operating team (gowns, gloves with holes, wet drapes), the OR, and the equipment. In addition, the patient undergoing a longer operation is likely to be older, to have other diseases, and to have cancer of—or to be undergoing operation on—a structure with possible contamination. A longer duration, even of a clean operation, represents increased time at risk for contamination. These points, in addition to pharmacologic considerations,

suggest that the surgeon should be alert to the need for a second dose of prophylactic antibiotics [*see Sidebar* Antibiotic Prophylaxis of Infection].

Abdominal operation is another risk factor.[8] Significant disease and age play a role in outcome; however, because the major concentrations of endogenous bacteria are located in the abdomen, abdominal operations are more likely to involve bacterial contamination.

In recent years, postoperative contamination of the wound has been considered unlikely. However, one report of SSI in sternal incisions cleaned and redressed 4 hours postoperatively clearly shows that wounds can be contaminated and become infected in the postoperative period.[17] Accordingly, use of a dry dressing for 24 hours seems prudent.

BACTERIAL PROPERTIES

Not only is the size of the bacterial inoculum important; the bacterial properties of virulence and pathogenicity are also significant. The most obvious pathogenic bacteria in surgical patients are gram-positive cocci (e.g., *Staphylococcus aureus* and streptococci). With modern hygienic practice, *S. aureus* should be found mostly in clean cases, with a wound infection incidence of 1% to 2%. Surveillance can be very useful in identifying either wards or surgeons with increased rates. Operative procedures in infected areas

Figure 3 **The wound infection rate is shown here as a function of bacterial inoculum in three different situations: a dry wound with an adequate concentration of antibiotic (cephaloridine > 10 μg/ml), a dry wound with no antibiotic (placebo), and a wet wound with no antibiotic (placebo, wound fluid hematocrit > 8%).[5]**

Antibiotic Prophylaxis of Infection

Selection

Spectrum. The antibiotic chosen should be active against the most likely pathogens. Single-agent therapy is almost always effective, except in colorectal operations, small-bowel procedures with stasis, emergency abdominal operations in the presence of a polymicrobial flora, and penetrating trauma; in such cases, a combination of antibiotics is usually used because anaerobic coverage is required.

Pharmacokinetics. The half-life of the antibiotic selected must be long enough to maintain adequate tissue levels throughout the operation.

Administration

Dosage, route, and timing. A single preoperative dose that is of the same strength as a full therapeutic dose is adequate in most instances. The single dose should be given I.V. immediately before skin incision. Administration by the anesthetist is most effective and efficient.

Duration. A second dose is warranted if the duration of the operation exceeds either 3 hours or twice the half-life of the antibiotic. No additional benefit has been demonstrated in continuing prophylaxis beyond the day of the operation, and mounting data suggest that the preoperative dose is sufficient. When massive hemorrhage has occurred (i.e., blood loss equal to or greater than blood volume), a second dose is warranted. Even in emergency or trauma cases, prolonged courses of antibiotics are not justified unless they are therapeutic.[50,51,55,56,107]

Indications

CLEAN CASES

Prophylactic antibiotics are not indicated in clean operations if the patient has no host risk factors or if the operation does not involve placement of prosthetic materials. Open heart operation and operations involving the aorta or the vessels in the groin require prophylaxis.

Patients in whom host factors suggest the need for prophylaxis include those who have more than three concomitant diagnoses, those whose operations are expected to last longer than 2 hours, and those whose operations are abdominal.[8] A patient who meets any two of these criteria is highly likely to benefit from prophylaxis. When host factors suggest that the probability of a surgical site infection is significant, administration of cefazolin at induction of anesthesia is appropriate prophylaxis. Vancomycin should be substituted in patients who are allergic to cephalosporins or who are susceptible to major immediate hypersensitivity reactions to penicillin.

When certain prostheses (e.g., heart valves, vascular grafts, and orthopedic hardware) are used, prophylaxis is justified when viewed in the light of the cost of a surgical site infection to the patient's health. Prophylaxis with either cefazolin or vancomycin is appropriate for cardiac, vascular, or orthopedic patients who receive prostheses.

Catheters for dialysis or nutrition, pacemakers, and shunts of various sorts are prone to infection mostly for technical reasons, and prophylaxis is not usually required. Meta-analysis indicates, however, that antimicrobial prophylaxis reduces the infection rate in CSF shunts by 50%.[108] Beneficial results may also be achievable for other permanently implanted shunts (e.g., peritoneovenous) and devices (e.g., long-term venous access catheters and pacemakers); however, the studies needed to confirm this possibility will never be done, because the infection rates are low and the sample sizes would have to be prohibitively large. The placement of such foreign bodies is a clean operation, and the use of antibiotics should be based on local experience.

CLEAN-CONTAMINATED CASES

Abdominal procedures. In biliary tract procedures (open or laparoscopic), prophylaxis is required only for patients at high risk: those whose common bile duct is likely to be explored (because of jaundice, bile duct obstruction, stones in the common bile duct, or a reoperative biliary procedure); those with acute cholecystitis; and those older than 70 years. A single dose of cefazolin is adequate. In hepatobiliary and pancreatic procedures, antibiotic prophylaxis is always warranted because these operations are clean-contaminated, because they are long, because they are abdominal, or for all of these reasons. Prophylaxis is also warranted for therapeutic endoscopic retrograde cholangiopancreatography.[7,9] In gastroduodenal procedures, patients whose gastric acidity is normal or high and in whom bleeding, cancer, gastric ulcer, and obstruction are absent are at low risk for infection and require no prophylaxis; all other patients are at high risk and require prophylaxis. Patients undergoing operation for morbid obesity should receive double the usual prophylactic dose[109]; cefazolin is an effective agent.

Operations on the head and neck (including the esophagus). Patients whose operations are of significance (i.e., involve entry into the oral cavity, the pharynx, or the esophagus) require prophylaxis.

Gynecologic procedures. Patients whose operation is either high-risk cesarean section, abortion, or vaginal or abdominal hysterectomy will benefit from cefazolin. Aqueous penicillin G or doxycycline may be preferable for first-trimester abortions in patients with a history of pelvic inflammatory disease. In patients with cephalosporin allergy, doxycycline is effective for those having hysterectomies and metronidazole for those having cesarean sections. Women delivering by cesarean section should be given the antibiotic immediately after cord clamping.

Urologic procedures. In principle, antibiotics are not required in patients with sterile urine. Patients with positive cultures should be treated. If an operative procedure is performed, a single dose of the appropriate antibiotic will suffice.

(continued)

---

have an increased infection rate because of the high inoculum with actively pathogenic bacteria.

The preoperative hospital stay has been found frequently to be an important contributing factor to wound infection rates.[7] The usual explanation is that during this stay either more endogenous bacteria are present or commensal flora is replaced by hospital flora. With respect to bacterial changes, one must recognize that the patient's clinical picture is usually a complex one, often entailing exhaustive workup of more than one organ system, various complications, and a degree of illness that changes radically the host's ability to deal with an inoculum, however small. Therefore, multiple factors combine to transform the hospitalized preoperative patient into a susceptible host.

Bacteria with multiple antibiotic resistance can be associated with significant SSI problems. In particular, staphylococci, with their natural virulence, present an important hazard if inappropriate prophylaxis is used. Many surgeons feel it is inappropriate or unnecessary to obtain good culture and sensitivity data on SSIs and instead simply drain infected wounds, believing that they will heal. However, there have been a number of reports of SSIs caused by unusual organisms[14,17,18]; these findings underscore the usefulness of culturing pus or fluid when an infection is being drained. SSIs caused by antibiotic-resistant organisms or unusual pathogens call for specific prophylaxis, perhaps other infection control efforts, and, if the problem persists, a search for a possible carrier or a common source.[12-14,17,18]

SURGEONS AND BACTERIA

The surgeon's perioperative rituals are designed to reduce or eliminate bacteria from the operative field. Many old habits are obsolete [see *Sidebar* The Surgical Scrub *and* IV:6 *Preparing*

Antibiotic Prophylaxis of Infection (*continued*)

CONTAMINATED CASES

Abdominal procedures. In colorectal procedures, bowel preparation using antibiotics active against both aerobes and anaerobes, along with a parenteral cephalosporin, is recommended. In appendectomy, SSI prophylaxis requires an agent or combination of agents active against both aerobes and anaerobes; a single dose of cefoxitin, 2 g I.V., or, in patients who are allergic to β-lactam antibiotics, metronidazole, 500 mg I.V., is effective. A combination of an aminoglycoside and clindamycin is effective if the appendix is perforated; a therapeutic course of 3 to 5 days is appropriate but does not seem warranted unless the patient is particularly ill. A laparotomy without a precise diagnosis is usually an emergency procedure and demands preoperative prophylaxis. If the preoperative diagnosis is a ruptured viscus (e.g., the colon or the small bowel), both an agent active against aerobes and an agent active against anaerobes are required. Depending on operative findings, prophylaxis may be sufficient or may have to be supplemented with postoperative antibiotic therapy.

Trauma. The proper duration of antibiotic prophylaxis for trauma patients is a confusing issue—24 hours or less of prophylaxis is probably adequate, and more than 48 hours is certainly unwarranted. When laparotomy is performed for nonpenetrating injuries, prophylaxis should be administered. Coverage of both aerobes and anaerobes is mandatory. The duration of prophylaxis should be less than 24 hours. In cases of penetrating abdominal injury, prophylaxis with either cefoxitin or a combination of agents active against anaerobic and aerobic organisms is required. The duration of prophylaxis should be less than 24 hours, and in many cases, perioperative doses will be adequate. For open fractures, management should proceed as if a therapeutic course were required. For grade 1 or 2 injuries, a first-generation cephalosporin will suffice, whereas for grade 3 injuries, combination therapy is warranted; duration may vary. For operative repair of fractures, a single dose of cefazolin may be given preoperatively, with a second dose added if the procedure is long. Patients with major soft tissue injury with a danger of spreading infection will benefit from cefazolin, 1 g I.V. every 8 hours for 1 to 3 days.

DIRTY OR INFECTED CASES

Infected cases require therapeutic courses of antibiotics; prophylax-

is is not appropriate in this context. In dirty cases, particularly those resulting from trauma, contamination and tissue destruction are usually so extensive that the wounds must be left open for delayed primary or secondary closure. Appropriate timing of wound closure is judged at the time of debridement. Antibiotics should be administered as part of resuscitation. Administration of antibiotics for 24 hours is probably adequate if infection is absent at the outset. However, a therapeutic course of antibiotics is warranted if infection is present from the outset or if more than 6 hours elapsed before treatment of the wounds was initiated.

Prophylaxis of Endocarditis

Studies of the incidence of endocarditis associated with dental procedures, endoscopy, or operations that may result in transient bacteremia are lacking. Nevertheless, the consensus is that patients with specific cardiac and vascular conditions are at risk for endocarditis or vascular prosthetic infection when undergoing certain procedures; these patients should receive prophylactic antibiotics.[110-114] A variety of organisms are dangerous, but viridans streptococci are most common after dental or oral procedures, and enterococci are most common if the portal of entry is the GU or GI tract. Oral amoxicillin now replaces penicillin V or ampicillin because of superior absorption and better serum levels. In penicillin-allergic patients, clindamycin is recommended; alternatives include cephalexin, cefadroxil, azithromycin, and clarithromycin. When there is a risk of exposure to bowel flora or enterococci, oral amoxicillin may be given; if an I.V. regimen is indicated, ampicillin may be given, with gentamicin added if the patient is at high risk for endocarditis. In patients allergic to penicillin, vancomycin is appropriate, with gentamicin added in high-risk patients. These parenteral regimens should be reserved for high-risk patients undergoing procedures with a significant probability of bacteremia.[114]

In patients receiving penicillin-based prophylaxis because of a history of rheumatic fever, erythromycin rather than amoxicillin should be used to protect against endocarditis.[110] There is no consensus concerning prophylaxis for orthopedic prostheses and acquired infection after transient bacteremia. In major procedures, where the risk of bacteremia is significant, the above recommendations are pertinent.

---

the Operating Room]. Nonetheless, it is clear that surgeons can influence SSI rates.[9] The refusal to use delayed primary closure or secondary closure is an example. Careful attention to the concepts of asepsis and antisepsis in the preparation and conduct of the operation is important. Although no single step in the ritual of preparing a patient for the operative procedure is indispensable, it is likely that certain critical standards of behavior must be maintained to achieve good results.

The measurement and publication of data about individuals or hospitals with high SSI rates have been associated with a diminution of those rates[7,9,19] [*see Table 8*]. It is uncertain by what process the diffusion of these data relates to the observed improvements. Although surveillance has unpleasant connotations, it provides objective data that individual surgeons are often too busy to acquire but that can contribute to improved patient care.

Environment: Local Factors

Local factors influence the development of an SSI because they affect the size of the bacterial inoculum that is required to produce

an infection: in a susceptible wound, a smaller inoculum produces infection [*see Figure 2*].

THE SURGEON'S INFLUENCE

Most of the local factors that make a surgical site favorable to bacteria are under the control of the surgeon. Although Halsted usually receives, deservedly so, the credit for having established the importance of technical excellence in the OR in preventing infection, individual surgeons in the distant past achieved remarkable results by careful attention to cleanliness and technique.[20] The Halstedian principles dealt with hemostasis, sharp dissection, fine sutures, anatomic dissection, and the gentle handling of tissues. Mass ligatures, large sutures, necrotic tissue, and the creation of hematomas or seromas must be avoided, and foreign materials must be judiciously used because these techniques and materials change the size of the inoculum required to initiate an infectious process. Logarithmically fewer bacteria are required to produce infection in the presence of a foreign body (e.g., suture, graft, metal, or pacemaker) or necrotic tissue (e.g., that caused by gross hemostasis or injudicious use of electrocautery).

The differences in inoculum required to produce wound infections can be seen in a model in which the two variables are wound hematocrit and the presence of antibiotic [*see*

Table 2 Parenteral Antibiotics Recommended
for Prophylaxis of Surgical Site Infection

	Antibiotic	Dose	Route of Administration
For coverage against aerobic gram-positive and gram-negative organisms	Cefazolin	1 g	I.V. or I.M. (I.V. preferred)
If patient is allergic to cephalosporins or if methicillin-resistant organisms are present	Vancomycin	1 g	I.V.
Combination regimens for coverage against gram-negative aerobes and anaerobes	Clindamycin *or*	600 mg	I.V.
	Metronidazole *plus*	500 mg	I.V.
	Tobramycin (or equivalent aminoglycoside)	1.5 mg/kg	I.V. or I.M. (I.V. preferred for first dose)
For single-agent coverage against gram-negative aerobes and anaerobes	Cefoxitin	1–2 g	I.V.
	Cefotetan	1–2 g	I.V.

Figure 3]. Ten bacteria in the absence of an antibiotic and in the presence of wound fluid with a hematocrit of more than 8% yield a wound infection rate of 20%. In a technically good wound with no antibiotic, however, 1,000 bacteria produce a wound infection rate of 20%.[5]

Drains

The use of drains varies widely and is very subjective. All surgeons are certain that they understand when to use a drain. However, certain points are worth noting. It is now recognized that a simple Penrose drain can function not only as a drainage route but also as an access route for pathogens to the patient.[21] It is important that the operative site not be drained through the wound. The use of a closed suction drain further reduces the potential for contamination and infection.

Duration of Operation

In most studies,[4,7,8] contamination certainly increases with time (see above). Wound edges can dry out, become macerated, or in other ways be made more susceptible to infection (i.e., requiring fewer bacteria for development of infection). Speed and poor technique are not suitable approaches; expeditious operation is appropriate.

Electrocautery

The use of electrocautery devices has been clearly associated with an increase in superficial SSI. However, when the unit is properly used to provide pinpoint coagulation (for which the bleeding vessels are best held by fine forceps) or to divide tissues under tension, there is minimal tissue destruction, no charring, and no change in the wound infection rate.[21]

PATIENT FACTORS

Local Blood Flow

Local perfusion can greatly influence the development of infection, as is seen most easily in the tendency of the patient with peripheral vascular disease to acquire infection of an extremity. As a local problem,

inadequate perfusion reduces the number of bacteria required for infection, in part because inadequate perfusion leads to decreased tissue levels of oxygen. Shock, by reducing local perfusion, also greatly enhances susceptibility to infection. Fewer organisms are required to produce infection during or immediately after shock [*see Figure 4*]. To counter these effects, the arterial oxygen tension (P_aO_2) must be translated into an adequate subcutaneous oxygen level (determined by measuring transcutaneous oxygen tension); this, together with adequate perfusion, will provide local protection by increasing the number of bacteria required to produce infection.

Barrier Function

Inadequate perfusion may also affect the function of other organs, and the resulting dysfunction will, in turn, influence the patient's susceptibility to infection. For example, ischemia-reperfusion injury to the intestinal tract is a frequent consequence of hypovolemic shock and septicemia. Inadequate perfusion of the GI tract may also occur during states of fluid and electrolyte imbalance or when cardiac output is marginal. Experimental studies have associated altered blood flow with breakdown of bowel barrier function—that is, inability of the intestinal tract to prevent bacteria, their toxins, or both from moving from the gut lumen into tissue at a rate too fast to permit clearance by the usual protective mechanisms. A variety of experimental approaches aimed at enhancing bowel barrier function have been studied; at present, however, the most clinically applicable method of bowel protection is initiation of enteral feeding (even if the quantity of nutrients provided does not satisfy all the nutrient requirements) and administration of the amino acid glutamine. Glutamine is a specific fuel for enterocytes and colonocytes and has been found to aid recovery of damaged intestinal mucosa and enhance barrier function when administered either enterally or parenterally.

Advanced Age

Aging is associated with structural and functional changes that render the skin and subcutaneous tissues more susceptible to infection. These changes are immutable; however, they must be evaluated in advance and addressed by excellent surgical technique and, on occasion, prophylactic antibiotics [*see Sidebar* Antibiotic Prophylaxis of Infection].

Table 3 Conditions and Procedures
That Require Antibiotic Prophylaxis
against Endocarditis[110,111]

CONDITIONS

Cardiac
Prosthetic cardiac valves (including biosynthetic valves)
Most congenital cardiac malformations
Surgically constructed systemic-pulmonary shunts
Rheumatic and other acquired valvular dysfunction
Idiopathic hypertrophic subaortic stenosis
History of bacterial endocarditis
Mitral valve prolapse causing mitral insufficiency
Surgically repaired intracardiac lesions with residual hemodynamic
    abnormality or < 6 mo after operation

Vascular
Synthetic vascular grafts

PROCEDURES

Dental or oropharyngeal
Procedures that may induce bleeding
Procedures that involve incision of the mucosa

Respiratory
Rigid bronchoscopy

Incision and drainage or debridement of sites of infection

Urologic
Cystoscopy with urethral dilatation
Urinary tract procedures
Catheterization in the presence of infected urine

Gynecologic
Vaginal hysterectomy
Vaginal delivery in the presence of infection

Gastrointestinal
Procedures that involve incision or resection of mucosa
Endoscopy that involves manipulation (e.g., biopsy, dilatation,
    or sclerotherapy) or ERCP

Host Defense Mechanisms

The systemic response is designed to control and eradicate infection. Many factors can inhibit systemic host defense mechanisms; some are related to the surgical disease, others to the patient's underlying disease or diseases and the events surrounding the operation.

SURGEON-RELATED FACTORS

There are a limited number of ways in which the surgeon can improve a patient's systemic responses to surgery. Nevertheless, when appropriate, attempts should be made to modify the host. The surgeon and the operation are both capable of reducing immunologic efficacy; hence, the operative procedure should be carried out in as judicious a manner as possible. Minimal blood loss, avoidance of shock, and maintenance of blood volume, tissue perfusion, and tissue oxygenation all will minimize trauma and will reduce the secondary, unintended immunologic effects of major procedures.

When abnormalities in host defenses are secondary to surgical disease, the timing of the operation is crucial to outcome. With acute and subacute inflammatory processes, early operation helps restore normal immune function. Deferral of definitive therapy frequently compounds problems.

PATIENT FACTORS

Surgeons have always known that the patient is a significant variable in the outcome of operation. Various clinical states are associated with altered resistance to infection. In all patients,

Table 4 Antibiotics for Prevention of Endocarditis[60,110]

Manipulative Procedure	Prophylactic Regimen*	
	Usual	In Patients with Penicillin Allergy
Dental procedures likely to cause gingival bleeding; operations or instrumentation of the upper respiratory tract	*Oral* Amoxicillin, 2.0 g 1 hr before procedure	*Oral* Clindamycin, 600 mg 1 hr before procedure *or* Cephalexin or cefadroxil,† 2.0 g 1 hr before procedure *or* Azithromycin or clarithromycin, 500 mg 1 hr before procedure
	Parenteral Ampicillin, 2.0 g I.M. or I.V. 30 min before procedure	*Parenteral* Clindamycin, 600 mg I.V. within 30 min before procedure *or* Cefazolin, 1.0 g I.M. or I.V. within 30 min before procedure
Gastrointestinal or genitourinary operation; abscess drainage	*Oral* Amoxicillin, 2.0 g 1 hr before procedure *Parenteral* Ampicillin, 2.0 g I.M. or I.V. within 30 min before procedure; if risk of endocarditis is considered high, add gentamicin, 1.5 mg/kg (to maximum of 120 mg) I.M. or I.V. 30 min before procedure‡	Vancomycin, 1.0 g I.V. infused slowly over 1 hr, beginning 1 hr before procedure; if risk of endocarditis is considered high, add gentamicin, 1.5 mg/kg (to maximum of 120 mg) I.M. or I.V. 30 min before procedure‡

*Pediatric dosages are as follows: oral amoxicillin, 50 mg/kg; oral or parenteral clindamycin, 20 mg/kg; oral cephalexin or cefadroxil, 50 mg/kg; oral azithromycin or clarithromycin, 15 mg/kg; parenteral ampicillin, 50 mg/kg; parenteral cefazolin, 25 mg/kg; parenteral gentamicin, 2 mg/kg; parenteral vancomycin, 20 mg/kg. *Total pediatric dose should not exceed total adult dose.*

†Patients with a history of immediate-type sensitivity to penicillin should not receive these agents.

‡High-risk patients should also receive ampicillin, 1.0 g I.M. or I.V., or amoxicillin, 1.0 g p.o., 6 hr after procedure.

Preoperative Decontamination of the Operative Site

Preparation of Skin

The sole reason for preparing the patient's skin before an operation is to reduce the risk of wound infection. A preoperative antiseptic bath is not necessary for most surgical patients, but their personal hygiene must be assessed and preoperative cleanliness established. Multiple preoperative baths may prevent postoperative infection in selected patient groups, such as those who carry Staphylococcus aureus on their skin or who have infectious lesions. Chlorhexidine gluconate is the recommended agent for such baths.[115]

Hair should not be removed from the operative site unless it physically interferes with accurate anatomic approximation of the wound edges.[116] If hair must be removed, it should be clipped in the OR.[10] Shaving hair from the operative site, particularly on the evening before operation or immediately before wound incision in the OR, increases the risk of wound infection. Depilatories are not recommended, because they cause serious irritation and rashes in a significant number of patients, especially when used near the eyes and the genitalia.[117]

In emergency procedures, obvious dirt, grime, and dried blood should be mechanically cleansed from the operative site by using sufficient friction. In one study, cleansing of contaminated wounds by means of ultrasound debridement was compared with high-pressure irrigation and soaking. The experimental wounds were contaminated with a colloidal clay that potentiates infection 1,000-fold. The investigators irrigated wounds at pressures of 8 to 10 psi, a level obtained by using a 30 ml syringe with a 1.5 in. long 19-gauge needle and 300 ml of 0.85% sterile saline solution. High-pressure irrigation removed slightly more particulate matter (59%) than ultrasound debridement (48%), and both of these methods removed more matter than soaking (26%).[118] Both ultrasound debridement and high-pressure irrigation were also effective in reducing the wound infection rate in experimental wounds contaminated with a subinfective dose of S. aureus.

For nonemergency procedures, the necessary reduction in microorganisms can be achieved by using povidone-iodine (10% available povidone-iodine and 1% available iodine) or chlorhexidine gluconate both for mechanical cleansing of the intertriginous folds and the umbilicus and for painting the operative site. The intertriginous folds and the umbilicus often require mechanical scrubbing to generate sufficient friction to remove entrapped microorganisms. In other areas of the skin, simply applying the agent (for example, by painting or spraying[119,120]) is an effective means of disinfection. Before the antiseptic is applied, the patient's history should be assessed for evidence of sensitivity to the antiseptic (particularly if the agent contains iodine) to minimize the risk of an allergic reaction. What some patients report as iodine allergies are actually iodine burns. Iodine in alcohol or in water is associated with an increased risk of skin irritation,[66] particularly at the edges of the operative field, where the iodine concentrates as the alcohol evaporates. Iodine should therefore be removed after sufficient contact time with the skin, especially at the edges. Iodophors do not irritate the skin and thus need not be removed.

Preparation of the Vagina

The purpose of preoperative preparation of the vagina is to reduce the number of bacteria and thereby decrease the risk of postoperative infection. The protocols for vaginal procedures almost always call for prophylactic antibiotics. Apparently, however, no additional benefit is gained from the preoperative use of a vaginal antiseptic.[121] Rather, the quantity of bacteria can be reduced by irrigating the vagina with saline solution.

---

but particularly those at high risk, SSI creates not only wound complications but also significant morbidity (e.g., reoperation, incisional hernia, secondary infection, impaired mobility, increased hospitalization, delayed rehabilitation or permanent disability) and occasional mortality.[13] The Study on the Efficacy of Nosocomial Infection Control (SENIC) has proposed that the risk of wound infection be assessed not only in terms of probability of contamination but also in relation to host factors.[8] According to this study, patients most clearly at risk for wound infection are those with three or more concomitant diagnoses; others clearly at risk are those undergoing a clean-contaminated or contaminated abdominal procedure or any procedure expected to last longer than 2 hours. These past two risk groups are affected by a bacterial component, but all those patients who are undergoing major abdominal procedures or lengthy operations generally have a significant primary pathologic condition and are usually older, with an increased frequency of concomitant conditions.

Shock has an influence on the incidence of wound infection [see Figure 4]. Although this influence is most obvious in cases of trauma, maintenance of blood volume, hemostasis, and oxygen-carrying capacity have significant implications for all patients. The effect of shock on the risk of infection appears to be not only immediate (i.e., its effect on local perfusion) but also late because systemic responses are blunted as local factors return to normal.

Advanced age, transfusion, and the use of steroids and other immunosuppressive drugs, including chemotherapeutic agents, are associated with an increased risk of SSI.[22,23] Often, these factors cannot be altered; however, the proper choice of operation, the appropriate use of prophylaxis, and meticulous surgical technique can reduce the risk of such infection by maintaining patient homeostasis, reducing the size of any infecting microbial inoculum, and creating a wound that is likely to heal primarily.

The basal nutritional state is known to affect immune response; this may be determined either by the patient (motivated

Table 5 Suggested Approach to Preoperative Preparation for Elective Colon Resection

TWO DAYS BEFORE SURGERY (At Home)

Dietary restriction: low residue or liquid diet

Magnesium sulfate, 30 ml of 50% solution (15 g) p.o., at 10:00 A.M., 2:00 P.M., and 6:00 P.M.

Fleet enemas until diarrhea effluent clear in the evening

DAY BEFORE SURGERY (At Home or in Hospital)

Clear liquid diet, I.V. fluids as needed if hospitalized

Magnesium sulfate, in dosage given above, at 10:00 A.M. and 2:00 P.M.

or

Whole gut lavage with GoLYTELY (1 L/hr for 2–4 hr until diarrhea effluent clear) before administration of oral antibiotic, starting at 9:00 A.M.

No enemas

Neomycin and erythromycin base, 1 g each p.o., at 1:00 P.M., 2:00 P.M., and 11:00 P.M.

DAY OF SURGERY

Operation at 8:00 A.M.

Optional: one dose of antibiotic with broad-spectrum activity given I.V. by anesthesia personnel in the operating room just before incision

Bowel Preparation

Elective Colon Operation

The human colon and distal small intestine contain an enormous reservoir of aerobic and anaerobic bacteria that are excluded from the rest of the body by a mucous membrane.[122] If this membrane barrier is disturbed by disease or trauma or if the colon is opened to the peritoneal cavity during operation, bacteria may escape into adjacent tissues and cause serious infection. One technique used to minimize this risk is mechanical cleansing of the colon; however, mechanical cleansing does not kill bacteria but merely removes some bacteria-laden waste material from the colon. To prevent infection, the colonic microflora must be suppressed. A reliable method of sterilization has been a long-standing goal of surgeons. In the past 30 years, results of clinical trials have clearly shown that to reduce infectious complications significantly after elective colon surgery, it is necessary to employ antibiotics that act against both colonic aerobes such as *Escherichia coli* and colonic anaerobes such as *Bacteroides fragilis*. There is still some controversy over what the best antibiotic regimen is and how it should be administered.[123] It is clear, however, that mechanical cleansing coupled with preoperative oral antibiotics or perioperative parenteral antibiotics provides excellent control of SSI. It is hard to imagine that any further studies are required to address SSI in large bowel surgery.

MECHANICAL PREPARATION

Mechanical cleansing of the colonic lumen before elective colon resection is a time-tested procedure that, when done appropriately, reduces total fecal mass, thus facilitating operative manipulation of the colon and enhancing the action of oral antibiotics. Vigorous mechanical cleansing alone, however, whether it includes lavage or follows the classic approach (dietary restriction, enemas, and cathartics), does not significantly reduce the number of microorganisms in residual colonic material.[124]

Today, approaches to mechanical cleansing vary considerably. Modern approaches fall into two general categories: (1) whole gut lavage with an electrolyte solution, 10% mannitol, or polyethylene glycol on the day before operation and (2) standard mechanical cleansing, which utilizes dietary restriction, cathartics, and sometimes enemas for 1 to 2 days.[92,125] The two procedures may also be combined.

Two European studies that investigated the necessity of performing mechanical cleansing before elective colon resection found no differences in the rates of anastomotic dehiscence or of infectious complications between patients who received mechanical cleansing and those who did not.[126,127] The investigators relied on I.V. antibiotics for preoperative intestinal antisepsis and did not employ oral regimens. In North America, some form of mechanical cleansing in addition to antibiotics in preparing for elective colon resection is standard practice.[128] Those surgeons who consider oral antibiotics important to the success of preoperative bowel preparation continue to realize the necessity of effective outpatient mechanical cleansing of short duration (i.e., 24 hours) before operation.[96,97] This combination of mechanical preparation and antibiotic preparation (oral, parenteral, or both) is time-tested and has yielded excellent clinical results.[129]

ANTIBIOTIC PREPARATION

Many surgeons now employ antibiotics as well as mechanical cleansing in preparing patients for elective colon resection. It is generally agreed that the antibiotics used should be able to suppress both aerobes and anaerobes,[81,130] but there is less agreement about which agents are ideal and which route of administration is preferred. Advocates of oral administration of antibiotics typically emphasize the importance of reducing the number of microorganisms in the colonic lumen before opening the colon, whereas advocates of parenteral administration emphasize the importance of adequate tissue levels of antibiotics. That these two approaches yield equivalent results when properly employed suggests that there is no need to be dogmatic.

Oral antibiotics. An effective intestinal antiseptic has three major requirements: (1) rapid, highly bactericidal activity against GI pathogenic organisms, (2) low local and systemic toxicity, and (3) limited ab-

sorption from the intestine. Two oral regimens are now primarily used: (1) an aminoglycoside with an erythromycin base and (2) an aminoglycoside with metronidazole. The regimen most often chosen in the United States is neomycin–erythromycin base, which was introduced in 1972.[128,131] In Europe and Australia, physicians often prefer kanamycin-metronidazole or neomycin-metronidazole.[132,133]

The timing of the administration of these oral agents appears to be critical. It is recommended that 1 g each of neomycin and erythromycin base be given at 1:00 P.M., 2:00 P.M., and 11:00 P.M. on the day before operation (6 g total). The procedure should then be scheduled for about 8:00 A.M. the next day. If the operation must be scheduled for later in the day, the times at which the oral agents are administered should be changed accordingly to preserve the 19 hours of preparation time. Giving more than three doses of oral antibiotics as prophylaxis is unwarranted and may induce the emergence of resistant flora. There appears to be no convincing evidence to suggest that the erythromycin base is superior to metronidazole in this clinical setting, or vice versa. The pharmacokinetics of the oral neomycin–erythromycin base preparation has been studied in healthy volunteers[134] and in patients undergoing elective colon resection.[135] The findings suggest that when adequate mechanical preparation is also carried out, significant intraluminal (local) and serum (systemic) levels of erythromycin and significant local levels of neomycin are present and that both techniques help prevent infection after colon operation. It is likely that significant local and systemic levels of metronidazole can be achieved in this fashion as well.

Parenteral antibiotics. Parenteral agents that are effective in bowel preparation for elective colon resection, either alone or in combination with an aminoglycoside, include cefoxitin,[90,136-139] cefotetan,[82,83] metronidazole,[139-141] and doxycycline.[142,143] One study, reported by the Norwegian Study Group for Colorectal Surgery, advocated mechanical cleansing together with single preoperative I.V. doses of doxycycline for aerobic coverage and tinidazole for anaerobic coverage.[84] Other studies have shown that a single dose of cefotetan is as effective as multiple doses of cefoxitin.[82,83] For elective operations, most investigators recommend restriction of parenteral antibiotic prophylaxis to one to five doses given during a 24-hour period beginning shortly before operation; longer periods of administration have been associated with the development of antibiotic-resistant strains in the colonic lumen.[144] A recent study makes it clear that there are many effective antibiotic combinations.[145] The two keys to antibiotic effectiveness are (1) coverage of both aerobes and anaerobes and (2) adequate levels in the tissues at the time of contamination.

Combination of parenteral and oral antibiotics. Many surgeons now use both oral and parenteral antibiotics along with mechanical cleansing in preoperative preparation for elective colon resection.[146] In a survey of more than 500 surgeons in 1979, only 8% used systemic antibiotics alone, 37% used oral antibiotics alone, and 49% used both oral and systemic antibiotics before colon surgery.[147] In a later survey of 372 board-certified colon and rectal surgeons, 88% used both oral and systemic antibiotics in their preoperative preparation, 3% used oral agents alone, and 8% used parenteral antibiotics alone.[128] The combined oral-parenteral approach has obvious appeal in that it theoretically provides both intraluminal bacterial suppression and high serum and tissue levels of antibiotics; however, it has not been conclusively shown to be superior to the other antibiotic regimens now in use.

Studies using newer systemic agents with both aerobic and anaerobic coverage (e.g., cefoxitin, cefonicid, or ceftizoxime) in addition to oral neomycin–erythromycin base have shown a low incidence of infection.[148-150] Although the evidence is conflicting, it now appears that supplementing mechanical and oral antibiotic preparation with a single parenteral dose of a cephalosporin with aerobic and anaerobic activity (given I.V. within 30 minutes of incision) may be beneficial, particularly in operations expected to last longer than 3 hours. The parenteral antibiotic serves as a fail-safe mechanism when the oral agents have been administered at the wrong times or when the operation has been delayed. *(continued)*

Bowel Preparation (*continued*)

Emergency Colon Operation

Among the clinical conditions that most often necessitate emergency colon operation are acute bleeding, perforated diverticulum or perforated carcinoma, ischemic intestinal disease, obstructing lesions, and trauma involving the colon. Under emergency conditions, the operation must be performed without any bowel preparation because oral antibiotic prophylaxis and mechanical cleansing are either impossible or potentially harmful.

INTRAOPERATIVE LAVAGE

Several techniques for performing intraoperative lavage have been described. In one, 8 to 10 L of saline is introduced into the colon during a period of 20 to 30 minutes through a balloon catheter in the distal ileum; the balloon is inflated to occlude the ileocecal valve. This technique results in uniform cleansing of the unprepared colon; a team approach is necessary to prevent spillage or other mishaps. This method of lavage allowed primary resections and anastomoses in 10 patients who otherwise would have undergone staged procedures (Nichols RL, unpublished data).

PARENTERAL ANTIBIOTICS

Prevention of infectious complications after emergency colon operation depends on proper operative technique, sound judgment, and appropriate choice and administration of parenteral antibiotics.[151] As in elective operation, the antibiotics chosen should be active against both aerobic and anaerobic colonic microflora.[22] They should be given I.V. in appropriate doses, starting shortly before the operation and continuing postoperatively for 1 to 7 days. The duration of administration is governed by the operative findings and by whether the antibiotic regimen is intended to be prophylactic (in which case the antibiotics are given for 1 day) or therapeutic, to manage the intra-abdominal infection for which operation is required (in which case antibiotics are given for 2 days or longer). Many single agents and combinations appear to be equally efficacious and are currently recommended. The choice of an agent or a combination of agents, therefore, depends on local hospital prices, toxicity profiles, and the surgeon's familiarity with the agents. Arguably, potent therapeutic agents such as imipenem have no place in antibiotic prophylaxis before elective colon resection.[152]

TOPICAL ANTIBIOTICS OR ANTISEPTICS

Some surgeons advocate direct application to the wound or irrigation of the wound with either antibiotics or povidone-iodine during colon resection. Solutions containing povidone-iodine should almost never be placed in the peritoneal cavity, because they are likely to be absorbed and subsequently to cause toxic effects.

---

by an interest in self-care, by socioeconomic conditions, or by underlying diseases) or by the surgeon. Of late, considerable attention has been focused on the beneficial effects of daily multivitamin supplements on infectious morbidity in individuals older than 65 years. In addition, there is some evidence that ingestion of certain antioxidants (e.g., beta-carotene, vitamin C, and vitamin E) and trace metals (e.g., selenium and zinc) can enhance host responses to inflammation or infection. A large body of clinical data (particularly in patients with active rheumatoid arthritis) indicates that reducing the quantity of fat in the diet and substituting omega-3 fatty acids (found in high concentrations in fish oil) for omega-6 fatty acids reduces the clinical signs and symptoms of inflammation. Animal studies suggest that similar beneficial effects are observed in the presence of infection; human studies using this approach have yet to be performed. Dietary supplementation with arginine, glutamine, or both also appears to increase resistance to infectious challenge.

Pharmacologic therapy can affect host response as well. Nonsteroidal anti-inflammatory drugs that attenuate the production of certain eicosanoids can greatly alter the adverse effects of infection by modifying fever and cardiovascular effects. Operative procedures involving inhalational anesthetics result in an immediate rise in plasma cortisol concentrations. The steroid response and the associated immunomodulation can be modified by using high epidural anesthesia as the method of choice; pituitary adrenal activation will be greatly attenuated. Some drugs that inhibit steroid elaboration (e.g., etomidate) have also been shown to be capable of modifying perioperative immune responses.

INTEGRATION OF DETERMINANTS

As operative infection rates slowly fall, despite increasingly complex operations in patients at greater risk, it is certain that surgeons are approaching the control of infection with a broader view than simply that of asepsis and antisepsis. It is apparent that this new, broader view must take into account many variables, some of which have no relation to bacteria, but all of which play a role in SSI [*see Table 9*].

To estimate risk, one must integrate the various determinants of infection in such a way that they can be applied to patient care. Much of this exercise is vague. In reality, the day-to-day practice of surgery includes a risk assessment that is essentially a form of logistic regression, and although not recognized as such, each surgeon's assessment of the probability of whether an SSI will occur takes into account the determining variables:

$$\text{Probability of SSI} = x + a\,(\text{bacteria}) + b\,(\text{environment: local factors}) + c\,(\text{host defense mechanisms: systemic factors})$$

Discussion

Antibiotic Prophylaxis of Surgical Site Infection

It is difficult to understand why antibiotics have not always prevented SSI successfully. Certainly, surgeons were quick to appreciate the possibilities of antibiotics; nevertheless, the efficacy of antibiotic prophylaxis was not proved until the late 1960s.[5] Studies before then had major design flaws, principally the administration of the antibiotic some time after the start of the operation—often in the recovery room. The failure of studies to demonstrate efficacy and the occasional finding that prophylactic antibiotics worsened rather than improved outcome led in the late 1950s to profound skepticism about prophylactic antibiotic use in any operation.

The principal reason for the apparent inefficacy was inadequate understanding of the biology of SSIs. Fruitful study of antibiotics and how they should be used began after physiologic groundwork established the importance of local blood flow, maintenance of local immune defenses, adjuvants, and local and systemic perfusion.[24]

Table 6 Oral and Parenteral Antibiotic Regimens in Patients Receiving Mechanical Cleansing: Prospective Studies, 1983 to 1994

Year	Patients (N)	Neomycin and Erythromycin Base Given to All Patients	Antibiotic	Route	Infection Rate (%)
1983[90]	119	No	Neomycin-erythromycin *plus* cefazolin Cefoxitin	Oral Parenteral Parenteral	3 12*
1983[148]	241	Yes	No additional antibiotics Cefoxitin	 Parenteral	18 7†
1983[139]	100	No	Cefoxitin Metronidazole-gentamicin	Parenteral Parenteral	12 12*
1983[85]	1,082	Yes	Placebo Cephalothin	Parenteral Parenteral	8 6*
1984[150]	57	Yes	Cefonicid Cefoxitin	Parenteral Parenteral	6 10*
1984[157]	93	No	Neomycin-erythromycin Metronidazole-gentamicin	Oral Parenteral	9 27†
1985[84]	267	No	Tinidazole-doxycycline Tinidazole	Parenteral Parenteral	3 10†
1986[158]	86	No	Moxalactam Metronidazole-gentamicin	Parenteral Parenteral	12 13*
1986[159]	60	No	Neomycin-erythromycin Metronidazole-ceftriaxone	Oral Parenteral	41 10†
1987[160]	100	Yes	Cefazolin Cefoxitin Cefotaxime	Parenteral Parenteral Parenteral	3* 3* 14
1988[82]	239	Variable	Cefotetan Cefoxitin	Parenteral Parenteral	12 8*
1988[161]	119	No	Neomycin-metronidazole *plus* metronidazole Metronidazole	Oral Parenteral Parenteral	14 28†
1988[162]	102	No	Neomycin-erythromycin *plus* cefazolin Metronidazole	Oral Parenteral Parenteral	11 32†
1988[91]	310	No	Neomycin-erythromycin *plus* cefoxitin Cefoxitin	Oral Parenteral Parenteral	5 18†
1989[83]	403	No	Cefoxitin Cefotetan	Parenteral Parenteral	11 9*
1989[163]	54	No	Neomycin-erythromycin Metronidazole-ceftriaxone	Oral Parenteral	4* 7
1990[164]	146	No	Neomycin-erythromycin Cefoxitin Neomycin-erythromycin *plus* cefoxitin	Oral Parenteral Oral Parenteral	11 12 8
1990[165]	197	Yes	Neomycin-erythromycin Neomycin-erythromycin *plus* cefoxitin	Oral Oral Parenteral	15 5†
1990[166]	943	No	Cefotaxime-metronidazole Cefuroxime-metronidazole	Parenteral Parenteral	7 7
1992[167]	221	No	Amoxicillin-clavulanate Cefotetan	Parenteral Parenteral	11 13
1993[168]	164	No	Amoxicillin-clavulanate Cefotaxime-metronidazole	Parenteral Parenteral	11 9
1994[169]	128	No	Ampicillin-sulbactam Gentamicin-metronidazole	Parenteral Parenteral	10 11
1994[170]	327	No	Piperacillin *plus* ciprofloxacin Piperacillin	Parenteral Oral Parenteral	11 23†

*Not significant. †Significant at $P < 0.05$.

Table 7 Parenteral Antibiotics Commonly Used for Broad-Spectrum Coverage of Colonic Microflora

COMBINATION THERAPY OR PROPHYLAXIS
Aerobic Coverage
(to be combined with a drug having anaerobic activity)

Amikacin	Ciprofloxacin
Aztreonam	Gentamicin
Ceftriaxone	Tobramycin

Anaerobic Coverage
(to be combined with a drug having aerobic activity)

Chloramphenicol	Metronidazole
Clindamycin	

SINGLE-DRUG THERAPY OR PROPHYLAXIS
Aerobic-Anaerobic Coverage

Ampicillin-sulbactam	Imipenem-cilastatin*
Cefotetan	Piperacillin-tazobactam
Cefoxitin	Ticarcillin-clavulanate
Ceftizoxime	

*This agent should be used *only* for therapeutic purposes; it should not be used for prophylaxis.

The Surgical Scrub

The purpose of cleansing the surgeon's hands is to reduce the numbers of resident flora and transient contaminants, thereby decreasing the risk of transmitting infection. Although the proper duration of the hand scrub is still subject to debate, evidence suggests that a 120-second scrub is sufficient, provided that a brush is used to remove the bacteria residing in the skin folds around the nails.[69] The nail folds, the nails, and the fingertips should receive the most attention because most bacteria are located around the nail folds and most glove punctures occur at the fingertips. Friction is required to remove resident microorganisms, which are attached by adhesion or adsorption, whereas transient bacteria are easily removed by simple hand washing.

Solutions containing either chlorhexidine gluconate or one of the iodophors are the most effective surgical scrub preparations and have the fewest problems with stability, contamination, and toxicity.[65,153] According to one review article, chlorhexidine gluconate (4%) in a sudsing base is the preferred agent because of its initial effectiveness, its residual activity, and its limited toxicity.[154] Another study showed that chlorhexidine gluconate achieves significant, immediate reduction of microorganisms and has persistent and residual efficacy.[155,156] In a comparative study of chlorhexidine gluconate, povidone-iodine, parachlorometaxylenol (PCMX or chloroxylenol), and alcohol, only chlorhexidine gluconate achieved significant antimicrobial efficacy in all parameters.

Alcohols applied to the skin are among the safest known antiseptics, and they produce the greatest and most rapid reduction in bacterial counts on clean skin.[66] A vigorous 1-minute scrub with enough alcohol to wet the hands completely has been shown to be the most effective method for hand antisepsis. A 1-minute immersion or scrub with alcohol is as effective as 4 to 7 minutes of skin preparation with other antiseptics, and washing with alcohol for 3 minutes is as effective as scrubbing for 20 minutes.[66] The main disadvantages of the alcohols are (1) their drying effects on the skin and (2) their volatility and flammability, which necessitate extreme caution when electrosurgery or laser procedures are performed. Although the alcohols are less commonly used in the United States, consistent, immediate, and effective reduction of skin flora makes them useful agents for preoperative skin cleansing.

All variables considered, chlorhexidine gluconate followed by an iodophor appears to be the best option.

The key antibiotic study, which was conducted in guinea pigs, unequivocally proved the following about antibiotics:

1. They are most effective when given before inoculation of bacteria.
2. They are ineffective if given 3 hours after inoculation.
3. They are of intermediate effectiveness when given in between these times [*see Figure 5*].[25]

Although efficacy with a complicated regimen was demonstrated in 1964,[26] the correct approach was not defined until 1969.[5] Established by these studies[5,25] are the philosophical and practical bases of the principles of antibiotic prophylaxis of SSI in all surgical arenas: that prophylactic antibiotics must be given preoperatively within 2 hours of the incision, in full dosage, parenterally, and for a very limited period. These principles remain essentially unchanged despite minor modifications from innumerable subsequent studies.[27-30] Prophylaxis for colorectal operations is discussed elsewhere [*see Bowel Preparation for Colonic Surgery, below*].

PRINCIPLES OF PATIENT SELECTION

Patients must be selected for prophylaxis on the basis of either their risk for SSI or the cost to their health if an SSI develops (e.g., after implantation of a cardiac valve or another prosthesis). The most important criterion is the degree of bacterial contamination expected to occur during the operation. The traditional classification of such contamination was defined in 1964 by the historic National Academy of Sciences–National Research Council study.[6] The important features of the classification are its simplicity, ease of understanding, ease of coding, and reliability. Classification is dependent on only one variable—the bacterial inoculum—and the effects of this variable are now controllable by antimicrobial prophylaxis. Advances in operative technique, general care, antibiotic use, anesthesia, and surveillance have reduced SSI rates in all categories that were established by this classification [*see Table 10*].[7-9,26]

In 1960, after years of negative studies, it was said, "Nearly all surgeons now agree that the routine use of prophylaxis in clean operations is unnecessary and undesirable."[31] Since then, much has changed: there are now many clean operations for which no competent surgeon would omit the use of prophylactic antibiotics, particularly as procedures become increasingly complex and prosthetic materials are used in patients who are older, sicker, or immunocompromised.

A separate risk assessment that integrates host and bacterial variables (i.e., whether the operation is dirty or contaminat-

Table 8 Effect of Surveillance and Feedback on Wound Infection Rates in Two Hospitals[19]

		Period 1	Period 2*
Hospital A	Number of wounds	1,500	1,447
	Wound infection rate	8.4%	3.7%
Hospital B	Number of wounds	1,746	1,939
	Wound infection rate	5.7%	3.7%

*Periods 1 and 2 were separated by an interval during which feedback on wound infection rates was analyzed.

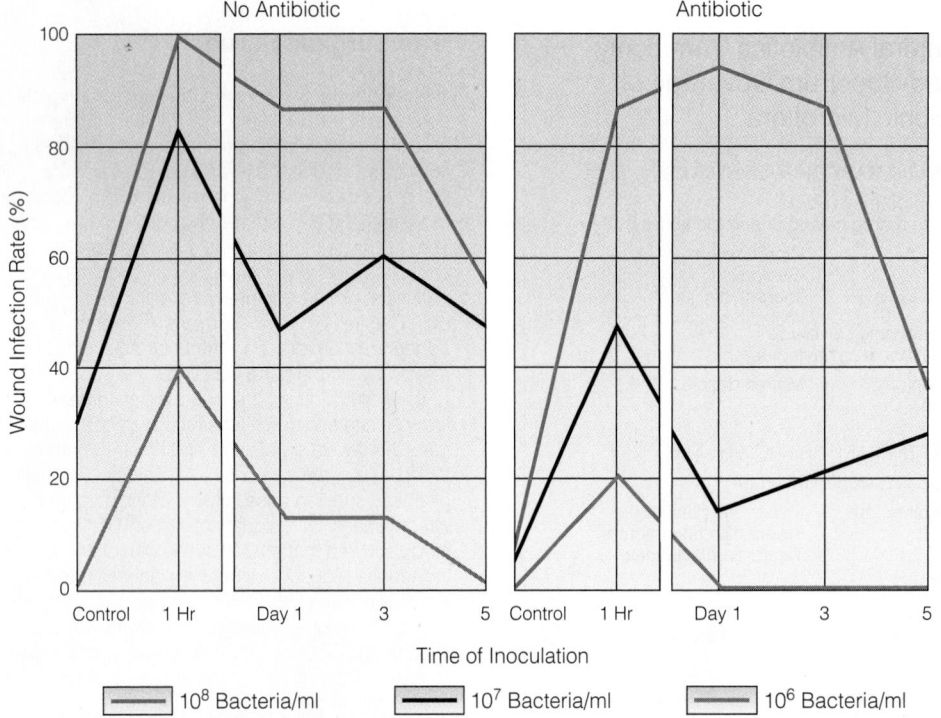

Figure 4 **Animals exposed to hemorrhagic shock followed by resuscitation show an early decreased resistance to wound infection. There is also a persistent influence of shock on the development of wound infection at different times of inoculation after shock. The importance of inoculum size (10^6/ml to 10^8/ml) and the effect of antibiotic on infection rates are evident at all times of inoculation.**[102]

ed, is longer than 2 hours, or is an abdominal procedure and whether the patient has three or more concomitant diagnoses) segregates more effectively those patients who are prone to an increased incidence of SSI [*see* Integration of Determinants of Infection, *below*]. This approach enables the surgeon to identify those patients who are likely to require preventive measures, particularly in clean cases, in which antibiotics would normally not be used.[8]

It has been implied that antibiotic prophylaxis for two types of clean surgery—hernia repair and breast surgery—represents the standard of practice.[32] However, in the study from which these conclusions were drawn, SSI and urinary tract infection rates were higher than many would have predicted, sample sizes were not large, and potential hazards of widespread antibiotic use were not addressed; neither was the evolution to minimal excisions for breast surgery addressed. Without significantly more supportive data, prophylaxis for clean cases cannot be recommended unless specific risk factors are present.[8,33,34]

Data suggest that prophylactic use of antibiotics may contribute to secondary *Clostridium difficile* disease; caution should be exercised when widening the indications for prophylaxis is under consideration.[35] If local results are poor, surgical practice should be reassessed before antibiotics are prescribed.

ANTIBIOTIC SELECTION AND ADMINISTRATION

When antibiotics are given more than 2 hours before operation, the risk of infection is increased.[30,36] I.V. administration in the OR or the preanesthetic room guarantees appropriate

Table 9 Determinants of Infection and Factors That Influence Wound Infection Rates

Variable	Determinant of Infection		
	Bacteria	Wound Environment (Local Factors)	Host Defense Mechanisms (Systemic Factors)
Bacterial numbers in wound[4]	A		
Potential contamination[4,7,8]	A		
Preoperative shave[7]	A		
Presence of 3 or more diagnoses[8]			C
Age[4,7]		B	C
Duration of operation[4,7,8]	A	B	C
Abdominal operation[8]	A	B	C

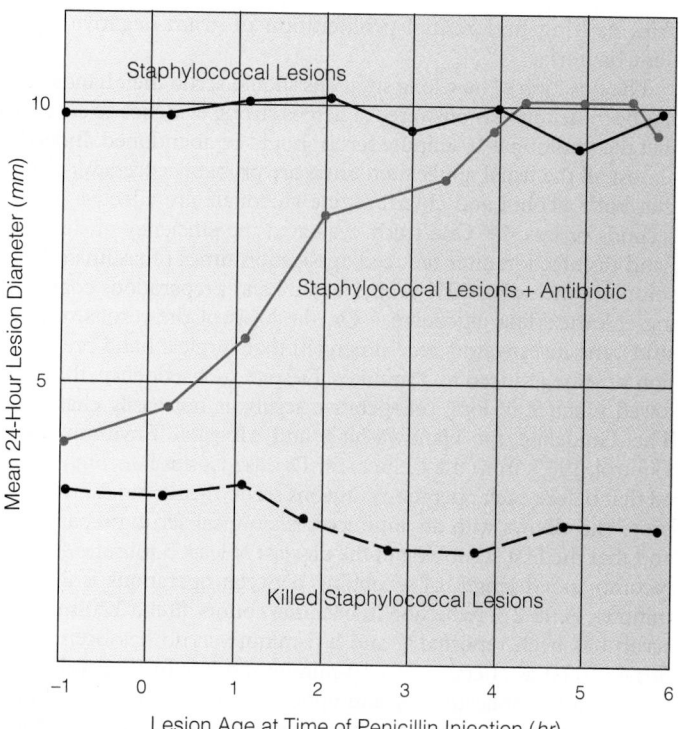

Figure 5 In a pioneer study of antibiotic prophylaxis,[25] the diameter of lesions induced by staphylococcal inoculation 24 hours earlier was observed to be critically affected by the timing of penicillin administration with respect to bacterial inoculation.

levels at the time of incision. The organisms likely to be present dictate the choice of antibiotic for prophylaxis. The cephalosporins are ideally suited to prophylaxis: their features include a broad spectrum of activity, an excellent ratio of therapeutic to toxic dosages, a low rate of allergic responses, ease of administration, and attractive cost advantages. Mild allergic reactions to penicillin are not contraindications for the use of a cephalosporin.[37]

Physicians like new drugs and often tend to prescribe newer, more expensive antibiotics for simple tasks. First-generation cephalosporins (e.g., cefazolin) are ideal agents for prophylaxis. Third-generation cephalosporins are not: they cost more, are not more effective, and promote emergence of resistant strains.[38-40]

The most important first-generation cephalosporin for surgical patients continues to be cefazolin. Administered I.V. in the OR at the time of skin incision, it provides adequate tissue levels throughout most of the operation. A second dose administered in the OR after 3 hours will be beneficial if the proce-

dure lasts longer than that.[36,41] Data on all operative site infections are imprecise, but SSIs can clearly be reduced by this regimen. No data suggest that further doses are required for prophylaxis.

Fortunately, cefazolin is effective against both gram-positive and gram-negative bacteria of importance, unless significant anaerobic organisms are encountered. The significance of anaerobic flora has been disputed,[42] but for elective colorectal operation,[43,44] abdominal trauma,[45,46] appendicitis,[47] or other circumstances in which penicillin-resistant anaerobic bacteria are likely to be encountered, coverage against both aerobic and anaerobic gram-negative organisms is strongly recommended and supported by the data.

Despite several decades of studies, prophylaxis is not always properly implemented. Unfortunately, didactic education is not always the best way to change behavior. Preprinted order forms[48] and a reminder sticker from the pharmacy[49] have proved to be effective methods of ensuring correct utilization.

The commonly heard decision "This case was tough, let's give an antibiotic for 3 to 5 days" has no data to support it and should be abandoned. Differentiation between prophylaxis and therapeusis is important. A therapeutic course for perforated diverticulitis or other types of peritoneal infection is appropriate. Data on casual contamination associated with trauma or with operative procedures suggest that 24 hours of prophylaxis or less is quite adequate.[50-54] Mounting evidence suggests that a single preoperative dose is good care and that additional doses are not required.[55,56]

Trauma Patients

The efficacy of antibiotic administration on arrival in the emergency department as an integral part of resuscitation has been clearly demonstrated.[45] The most common regimens have been (1) a combination of an aminoglycoside and clindamycin and (2) cefoxitin alone. These two regimens or variations thereof have been compared in a number of studies.[22,46,57-59] They appear to be equally effective, and either regimen can be recommended with confidence. For prophylaxis, there appears to be a trend toward using a single drug: cefoxitin[37] or cefotetan.[60] If therapy is required because of either a delay in surgery, terrible injury, or prolonged shock, the combination of an agent that is effective against anaerobes with an aminoglycoside seems to be favored. Because aminoglycosides are nephrotoxic, they must be used with care in the presence of shock.

In all the trauma studies just cited, antibiotic prophylaxis lasted for 48 hours or longer. Subsequent studies, however, indicated that prophylaxis lasting less than 24 hours is appropriate.[52-54,61] Single-dose prophylaxis is appropriate for patients with closed fractures.[62]

Table 10 Historical Rates of Wound Infection

Wound Classification	Infection Rate (%)				
	1960–1962[26] (15,613 patients)	1967–1977[7] (62,937 patients)	1975–1976[8] (59,353 patients)	1977–1981[9] (20,193 patients)	1982–1986[106] (20,703 patients)
Clean	5.1	1.5	2.9	1.8	1.3
Clean-contaminated	10.8	7.7	3.9	2.9	2.5
Contaminated	16.3	15.2	8.5	9.9	7.1
Dirty-infected	28.0	40.0	12.6	—	—
Overall	7.4	4.7	4.1	2.8	2.2

COMPLICATIONS

Complications of antibiotic prophylaxis are few. Although data linking prophylaxis to the development of resistant organisms are meager, resistant microbes have developed in every other situation in which antibiotics have been utilized, and it is reasonable to expect that prophylaxis in any ecosystem will have the same result,[63] particularly if selection of patients is poor, if prophylaxis lasts too long, or if too many late-generation agents are used.

A rare but important complication of antibiotic use is pseudomembranous enterocolitis, which is induced most commonly by clindamycin, the cephalosporins, and ampicillin[35] [see VI:14 Nosocomial Infection]. The common denominator among different cases of pseudomembranous enterocolitis is hard to identify. Diarrhea and fever can develop after administration of single doses of prophylactic antibiotics. The condition is rare, but difficulties occur because of failure to make a rapid diagnosis.

CURRENT ISSUES

The most significant questions concerning prophylaxis of SSIs already have been answered. Important issues that remain are the proper duration of prophylaxis in complicated cases, trauma, and the presence of foreign bodies. No change in the criteria for antibiotic prophylaxis is required in laparoscopic procedures; the risk of infection may actually be lower in such cases.[64] Cost factors are important and may justify the endless succession of studies that compare new drugs in competition for appropriate clinical niches.

Further advances in patient selection may take place but will require analysis of data from large numbers of patients and a distinction between approaches to infection of the wound, which is only a part of the operative field, and approaches to infections directly related to the operative site. These developments will define more clearly the prophylaxis requirements of patients whose operations are clean but whose risk of wound or operative site infection is increased.

Skin Preparation

As the first line of defense against infection, the skin is remarkable in its complexity and efficiency. Surgeons must respect this organ and carefully manage preparation of both their own skin and their patients' skin. None of the topical antibacterial agents now in use are totally harmless; their destructive effect on the skin's natural defense mechanisms must be recognized and taken into account.

Although the importance of skin preparation cannot be denied, in healthy tissue, a wound contaminated with many microorganisms is amazingly resistant to infection. Admittedly, skin preparation has a relatively minor influence on wound infection as compared with surgical technique and host factors; nonetheless, it consumes OR time and the time of health care personnel, both of which are expensive. Therefore, choosing the most effective agent and method for skin preparation is an important economic decision as well as a surgical decision.

CLEANSING THE SURGEON'S HANDS

Scrubbing

Method The dry microenvironment of the hands is inhabited by coagulase-negative staphylococci and coryneform bacteria. Rubber gloves convert this dry microenvironment to wet skin, causing preferential proliferation of gram-negative resident bacteria.

The question of how long surgeons should scrub their hands has not been definitively answered. There is strong evidence to suggest that the traditional 10-minute scrub should be abandoned. Indeed, almost all the usual application times are probably excessive, given that both alcohol and chlorhexidine gluconate are effective in 60 seconds or less.[65,66] One study evaluated the efficiency of surgical hand disinfection after reduced application times of antimicrobial solutions, including 60% propyl alcohol and preparations containing chlorhexidine gluconate.[67] On the basis of the results of this study, the investigators recommended that surgical hand preparation time be reduced to 3 minutes. Despite such evidence, the hallowed practice of long preoperative scrubs is not easily changed. The Guideline for Handwashing and Hospital Environmental Control, 1985, from the Centers for Disease Control, recommended that before each operation surgeons scrub their hands and arms up to the elbows with an antimicrobial surgical scrub preparation and that the first scrubbing of the day last at least 5 minutes.[68] The recommended length of scrubbing between operations is 2 to 5 minutes. A 98.2% reduction in bacterial counts after a 120-second scrub has been reported,[69] and a 5-minute scrub has been confirmed to be as effective as a 10-minute scrub.[70] In England, a 2- to 3-minute application of antiseptic without using a scrubbing brush is recommended.[71] Shorter hand preparation times are further supported by the rarity of infections resulting from the destruction of bacteria by such applications.[71] The weight of the evidence suggests that a preoperative scrub of at least 120 seconds that includes brushing of the nail and fingertip areas adequately disinfects the hands. It must be remembered, however, that successful preparation of the surgeon's hands is impossible when dermatitis is present.

Agent The ideal surgical scrub preparation should be effective and persistent in reducing the numbers of a broad spectrum of microorganisms without irritating intact skin. Although the question of what level of reduction in microorganisms is sufficient to prevent transmission of infection has never been resolved, at least five commonly used agents or classes of agents have a significant antimicrobial effect: the alcohols, the iodophors, chlorhexidine gluconate [see Table 11], hexachlorophene, and benzalkonium. However, hexachlorophene and benzalkonium need not be considered: they have such problems with stability, contamination, and toxicity that they should not be used. Other agents, such as parachlorometaxylenol and triclosan, have also been used, but these agents as well have various properties that make them less attractive.[66,72]

The most commonly used iodophor is povidone-iodine. A formulation containing 7.5% is widely used as a surgical hand scrub; 10% solutions in applicators and various 2% solutions are also available. Use of iodophors sometimes elicits skin reactions, and as yet little is known about their chronic toxicity. A 5-minute scrub with a povidone-iodine preparation results in absorption of more than four times the normal daily intake of iodine through the skin.[73]

Chlorhexidine gluconate is offered in several formulations, of which the most commonly used is 4% chlorhexidine gluconate in a detergent base. Chlorhexidine gluconate is more persistent than the iodophors and slightly less irritating, but both types of agent are acceptable in this regard.[66] An alcohol-based hand rinse containing 0.5% chlorhexidine gluconate is also used; the rapid effect of alcohol and the persistence of chlorhexidine gluconate would seem to be a particularly desirable combination.

Table 11 Characteristics of Three Topical Antimicrobial Agents Effective against Both Gram-Positive and Gram-Negative Bacteria[66]

Agent	Mode of Action	Antifungal Activity	Comments
Chlorhexidine	Cell wall disruption	Fair	Poor activity against tuberculosis-causing organisms; can cause ototoxicity and eye irritation
Iodine/iodophors	Oxidation and substitution by free iodine	Good	Broad antibacterial spectrum; minimal skin residual activity; possible absorption toxicity and skin irritation
Alcohols	Denaturation of protein	Good	Rapid action but little residual activity; flammable

Studies have shown chlorhexidine gluconate to be a more effective surgical scrub than povidone-iodine. In one trial, chlorhexidine gluconate (4%) detergent caused a greater initial reduction of both resident and transient flora than either povidone-iodine (7.5%) surgical scrub or hexachlorophene (3%) emulsion.[74] Repetitive use of each agent produced a further reduction in resident flora. However, chlorhexidine gluconate was the most effective agent and the only one to reduce transient flora further.

In another comparative study, a solution of 4% chlorhexidine digluconate (British Pharmacopoeia) in a detergent base containing 25% poloxamer 237 and 3.7% dimethyl lauryl amine oxide caused a significantly greater initial reduction in skin flora than a povidone-iodine detergent or 0.75% chlorhexidine detergent.[75] Data from this study on the cumulative effect of multiple applications of antiseptic generally favor chlorhexidine gluconate over povidone-iodine as well.

On hands gloved for 3 hours, chlorhexidine gluconate (4%) detergent reduced microorganisms more persistently than povidone-iodine (10%) detergent.[71] Significant regrowth of bacteria on gloved hands disinfected with povidone-iodine has been documented.[74]

When gloves are used in the operating field, it is important to remember that pathologic changes are produced by surgical glove dusting powders. Several investigators have studied both the anatomic and the cellular changes induced by surgical glove powders and the effects of the powders on adhesion formation.[76,77] The protection of the surgeon's skin—particularly during an operation being performed on a woman of reproductive age—should be accomplished with powder-free gloves.

Skin changes resulting from latex sensitivity have become an increasingly important finding, especially among health care workers. In a study by the Association of Operating Room Nurses, 369 (21%) of 1,738 nurses reported reactions to latex.[78] The most commonly reported localized reaction is contact dermatitis, but more severe systemic reactions have also been documented. At present, there is no safe and effective method of diagnosing latex sensitivity in both health care workers and patients at risk for potentially severe reactions.

On the evidence of almost all the considerable literature on the use of topical agents for preparation of the surgeon's hands and the patient's skin, chlorhexidine gluconate is the most effective agent [*see Table 11*]. Povidone-iodine is a relatively poor second. Although 70% isopropyl alcohol is effective and inexpensive, it is not heavily marketed: besides being inflammable, it irritates skin with repetitive use.

Washing

The purpose of washing the hands after surgery is to remove microorganisms that are resident, that flourished in the warm, wet environment created by wearing gloves, or that reached the hands by entering through puncture holes in the gloves. On the ward, even minimal contact with colonized patients has been demonstrated to transfer microorganisms.[79] As many as 1,000 organisms were transferred by simply touching the patient's hand, taking a pulse, or lifting the patient. The organisms survived for 20 to 150 minutes, making their transfer to the next patient clearly possible. Viruses have been shown to survive for 20 to 30 minutes on the hands.[80]

A return to the ancient practice of washing hands between each patient contact is warranted. Nosocomial spread of numerous organisms, including *C. difficile*, antibiotic-resistant bacteria, and viruses (e.g., HIV and hepatitis B virus), is a constant threat. As an example, two million or more North Americans are seropositive for HIV, and most of them are unaware of their seroconversion. This likely is the case as well for most other relevant viruses.

Hand washing on the ward is complicated by the fact that overwashing may actually increase bacterial counts. Dry, damaged skin harbors many more bacteria than healthy skin and is almost impossible to render even close to bacteria free. Although little is known about the physiologic changes in skin that result from frequent washings, the bacterial flora is certainly modified by alterations in the lipid or water content of the skin.

Bowel Preparation for Colon Surgery

The results of the numerous studies of antibiotic bowel preparation that have been done [*see Table 6*] suggest that many different approaches may be equally effective in reducing infection after elective colonic resection. Certain features, however, appear to be common to most of the studies:

1. Oral antibiotic regimens with both aerobic and anaerobic activity (e.g., neomycin–erythromycin base and neomycin-metronidazole) were employed.
2. The oral agents were given in limited doses the day before operation.
3. Addition of systemic antibiotic agents without broad-spectrum coverage to the oral antibiotics generally did not improve the results.
4. Use of broad-spectrum parenteral antibiotic agents alone was associated with a lower infection rate than use of systemic agents with only limited coverage.
5. Addition of a broad-spectrum parenteral antibiotic to the oral antibiotics may further reduce the postoperative infection rate.
6. Parenteral or oral antibiotics should be administered only for short amounts of time during the perioperative period. A single parenteral dose given just before operation may be sufficient.[81-84]

A 5-year cooperative Veterans Administration study of more than 1,000 patients undergoing elective colon operations compared two groups of patients receiving oral neomycin–erythromycin base: one group received only the oral preparation, whereas the other also received parenteral perioperative cephalothin.[85] The infection rates were not significantly different in the two groups and in fact were below 9% in both; however, there was a trend toward lower infection rates in patients receiving both oral and parenteral antibiotics. The authors concluded that if appropriate mechanical cleansing and oral neomycin–erythromycin base therapy are employed, no benefit can be gained from adding parenteral antibiotic prophylaxis. Similar single-hospital studies concluded that the addition of systemic cefazolin to the oral neomycin–erythromycin base preparation did significantly reduce postoperative infections,[86,87] whereas others found no extra benefit from the addition of older systemic antibiotics.[88,89]

Various studies have demonstrated that the duration of colorectal operations affects both the risk of infection and the choice of the optimal preoperative antibiotic preparation. In one study, in operations lasting less than 4 hours, combinations of oral and parenteral antibiotics were not superior to parenteral antibiotics alone; however, in operations lasting longer than 4 hours, combination regimens achieved significantly better results than parenteral agents alone.[90] In another study, combination regimens were found to be superior in operations lasting less than 3 hours and 35 minutes but in which rectal resection was required.[91]

The mechanical cleansing technique employed is a matter of preference. Traditional bowel preparation, if carried out for unnecessarily long periods (3 to 5 days), is associated with less patient compliance and a higher incidence of fatigue and other related symptoms than are other cleansing techniques. Whole gut irrigation as recommended in the past—that is, using large amounts of fluid (10 to 15 L)—should be discouraged. Some authors recommend the use of mannitol in varying concentrations in lavage solutions.[92] Others emphasize that clinical dehydration may develop when 15% mannitol is used or that electrocautery may lead to colonic explosions when mannitol is used without oral antibiotics.[93] Lavage with polyethylene glycol–electrolyte solution appears to be the preferred cleansing method before elective colorectal surgery.[93,94] A study comparing the efficacy of 2-day routine mechanical cleansing with that of lavage performed once on the day before operation demonstrated no difference between the two approaches: 1-day lavage was both safe and economical, and the authors preferred it to 2-day mechanical cleansing.[95] Subsequent studies reported no differences in the adequacy of colon cleansing whether bowel preparation was performed in the inpatient setting or the outpatient setting.[96,97]

Integration of Determinants of Infection

The significant advances in the control of wound infection during the past several decades are linked to a better understanding of the biology of wound infection, and this link has permitted the advance to the concept of SSI.[2] In all tissues at any time, there will be a critical inoculum of bacteria that would cause an infectious process [see Figure 3]. The standard definition of infection in urine and sputum has been 10^5 organisms/ml. In a clean dry wound, 10^5 bacteria produce a wound infection rate of 50% [see Figure 3].[5] Effective use of antibiotics reduces the infection rate to 10% with the same number of bacteria and thereby permits the wound to tolerate a much larger number of bacteria.

All of the clinical activities described are intended either to reduce the inoculum or to permit the host to manage the number of bacteria that would otherwise be pathologic. One study in guinea pigs has shown how manipulation of local blood flow, shock, the local immune response, and foreign material can enhance the development of infection.[98] This study and two others[25,98,99] define an early decisive period of host antimicrobial activity that lasts for 3 to 6 hours after contamination. Bacteria that remain after this period are the infecting inoculum. Processes that interfere with this early response (e.g., shock, altered perfusion, adjuvants, foreign material) or support it (e.g., antibiotics or total care) have a major influence on outcome.

One investigation demonstrated that silk sutures decrease the number of bacteria required for infection.[100] Other investigators used a suture as the key adjuvant in studies of host manipulation,[101] whereas a separate study demonstrated persistent susceptibility to wound infection days after shock.[102] The common variable is the number of bacteria. This relation may be termed the inoculum effect, and it has great relevance in all aspects of infection control. Applying knowledge of this effect in practical terms involves the following three steps:

1. Keeping the bacterial contamination as low as possible via asepsis and antisepsis, preoperative preparation of patient and surgeon, and antibiotic prophylaxis.
2. Maintaining local factors in such a way that they can prevent the lodgment of bacteria and thereby provide a locally unreceptive environment.
3. Maintaining systemic responses at such a level that they can control the bacteria that become established.

These three steps are related to the determinants of infection and their applicability to daily practice. Year-by-year reductions in wound infection rates, when closely followed, indicate that it is possible for surgeons to continue improving results by attention to quality of clinical care and surgical technique, despite increasingly complex operations.[6,9,19-21] In particular, the measures involved in the first step (control of bacteria) have been progressively refined and are now well established.

The integration of determinants has significant effects [see Figures 3 and 4]. When wound closure was effected with a wound hematocrit of 8% or more, the inoculum required to produce a wound infection rate of 40% was 100 bacteria [see Figure 3]. Ten bacteria produced a wound infection rate of 20%. The shift in the number of organisms required to produce clinical infection is significant. It is obvious that this inoculum effect can be changed dramatically by good surgical technique and further altered by use of prophylactic antibiotics. If the inoculum is always slightly smaller than the number of organisms required to produce infection in any given setting, results are excellent. There is clearly a relation between the number of bacteria and the local environment. The local effect can also be seen secondary to systemic physiologic change, specifically shock. One study showed the low local perfusion in shock to be important in the development of an infection.[98,99]

One investigation has shown that shock can alter infection rates immediately after its occurrence [see Figure 4].[102] Furthermore, if the inoculum is large enough, antibiotics will not control bacteria. In addition, there is a late augmentation of infection lasting up to 3 days after restoration of blood volume. These early and late effects indicate that systemic determinants come into play after local effects are resolved. These observations call for further study, but obviously, it is the combined abnormalities that alter outcome.

Table 12   Comparison of Wound Classification Systems[8]

Traditional Wound Classification System	Simplified Risk Index					
	Low Risk	Medium Risk	High Risk			All from Traditional Classification
	0	1	2	3	4	
Clean	1.1	3.9	8.4	15.8		2.9
Clean-contaminated	0.6	2.8	8.4	17.7		3.9
Contaminated		4.5	8.3	11.0	23.9	8.5
Dirty-infected		6.7	10.9	18.8	27.4	12.6
All from SENIC index	1.0	3.6	8.9	17.2	27.0	4.1

SENIC—Study of the Efficacy of Nosocomial Infection Control

Systemic host responses are important for the control of infection. The patient has been clearly implicated as one of the four critical variables in the development of wound infection.[8] In addition, the bacterial inoculum, the location of the procedure and its duration, and the coexistence of three or more diagnoses were found to give a more accurate prediction of the risk of wound infection. The spread of risk is defined better with the SENIC index (1% to 27%) than it is with the traditional classification (2.9% to 12.6%) [see Table 12]. The importance of the number of bacteria is lessened if the other factors are considered in addition to inoculum. The inoculum effect has to be considered with respect to both the number of organisms and the local and systemic host factors that are in play. Certain variables were found to be significantly related to the risk of wound infection in three important prospective studies [see Table 12].[4,7,8] It is apparent that the problem of SSI cannot be examined only with respect to the management of bacteria. Host factors have become much more significant now that the bacterial inoculum can be maintained at low levels by means of asepsis, antisepsis, technique, and prophylactic antibiotics.[103]

Important host variables include the maintenance of normal homeostasis (physiology) and immune response [see 88 Immunomodulation]. Maintenance of normal homeostasis in patients at risk is one of the great advances of surgical critical care.[103] The clearest improvements in this regard have come in maintenance of blood volume, oxygenation, and oxygen delivery.

One group demonstrated the importance of oxygen delivery, tissue perfusion, and P_aO_2 in the development of wound infection.[104] Oxygen can have as powerful a negative influence on the development of SSI as antibiotics can.[105] The influence is very similar to that seen in other investigations. Whereas a P_aO_2 equivalent to a true fractional concentration of oxygen in inspired gas (F_IO_2) of 45% is not feasible, maintenance, when appropriate, of an increased F_IO_2 in the postoperative period may prove an elementary and effective tool in managing the inoculum effect.

Modern surgical practice has reduced the rate of wound infection significantly. Consequently, it is more useful to think in terms of SSI, which is not limited to the incision but may occur anywhere in the operative field; this concept provides a global objective for control of infections associated with a surgical procedure. Surveillance is of great importance for quality assurance. Reports of recognized pathogens (e.g., *S. epidermidis* and group A streptococci) as well as unusual organisms (e.g., *Rhodococcus* [*Gordona*] *bronchialis*, *Mycoplasma hominis*, and *Legionella dumoffii*) in SSIs highlight the importance of infection control and epidemiology for quality assurance in surgical departments.[12-14,17,18] (Although these reports use the term wound infection, they are really addressing what we now call SSI.) The importance of surgeon-specific and service-specific SSI reports should be clear[7,9,106] [see Table 8] and their value in quality assurance evident.

References

1. Meakins JL: Host defence mechanisms: evaluation and roles of acquired defects and immunotherapy. Can J Surg 18:259, 1975

2. Consensus paper on the surveillance of surgical wound infections. The Society for Hospital Epidemiology of America; The Association for Practitioners in Infection Control; The Centers for Disease Control; The Surgical Infection Society. Infect Control Hosp Epidemiol 13:599, 1992

3. Horan TC, Gaynes RP, Martone WJ, et al: CDC definitions of nosocomial surgical site infections, 1992: a modification of CDC definitions of surgical wound infections. Infect Control Hosp Epidemiol 13:606, 1992

4. Davidson AIG, Clark C, Smith G: Postoperative wound infection: a computer analysis. Br J Surg 58:333, 1971

5. Polk HC Jr, Lopez-Mayor JF: Postoperative wound infection: a prospective study of determinant factors and prevention. Surgery 66:97, 1969

6. Report of an Ad Hoc Committee of the Committee on Trauma, Division of Medical Sciences, National Academy of Sciences–National Research Council: Postoperative wound infections: the influence of ultraviolet irradiation of the operating room and of various other factors. Ann Surg 160(suppl):1, 1964

7. Cruse PJE, Foord R: The epidemiology of wound infection: a 10-year prospective study of 62,939 wounds. Surg Clin North Am 60:27, 1980

8. Haley RW, Culver DH, Morgan WM, et al: Identifying patients at high risk of surgical wound infection: a simple multivariate index of patient susceptibility and wound contamination. Am J Epidemiol 121:206, 1985

9. Olson M, O'Connor M, Schwartz ML: Surgical wound infections: a 5-year prospective study of 20,193 wounds at the Minneapolis VA Medical Center. Ann Surg 199:253, 1984

10. Alexander JW, Fischer JE, Boyajian M, et al: The influence of hair-removal methods on wound infections. Arch Surg 118:347, 1983

11. Olson MM, MacCallum J, McQuarrie DG: Preoperative hair removal with clippers does not increase infection rate in clean surgical wounds. Surg Gynecol Obstet 162:181, 1986

12. Boyce JM, Potter-Bynoe G, Opal SM, et al: A common-source outbreak of Staphylococcus epidermidis infections among patients undergoing cardiac surgery. J Infect Dis 161:493, 1990

13. Mastro TD, Farley TA, Elliott JA, et al: An outbreak of surgical-wound infections due to group A

streptococcus carried on the scalp. N Engl J Med 323:968, 1990

14. Richet HM, Craven PC, Brown JM, et al: A cluster of *Rhodococcus (Gordona) bronchialis* sternal-wound infections after coronary-artery bypass surgery. N Engl J Med 324:104, 1991

15. Moylan JA, Kennedy BV: The importance of gown and drape barriers in the prevention of wound infection. Surg Gynecol Obstet 151:465, 1980

16. Garibaldi RA, Maglio S, Lerer T, et al: Comparison of nonwoven and woven gown and drape fabric to prevent intraoperative wound contamination and postoperative infection. Am J Surg 152:505, 1986

17. Lowry PW, Blankenship RJ, Gridley W, et al: A cluster of legionella sternal-wound infections due to postoperative topical exposure to contaminated tap water. N Engl J Med 324:109, 1991

18. Wilson ME, Dietze C: Mycoplasma hominis surgical wound infection: a case report and discussion. Surgery 103:257, 1988

19. Cruse PJE: Surgical wound sepsis. Can Med Assoc J 102:251, 1970

20. Wangensteen OH, Wangensteen SD: The Rise of Surgery: Emergence from Empiric Craft to Scientific Discipline. University of Minnesota Press, Minneapolis, 1978

21. Cruse PJE: Wound infections: epidemiology and clinical characteristics. Surgical Infectious Disease, 2nd ed. Howard RJ, Simmons RL, Eds. Appleton and Lange, Norwalk, Connecticut, 1988

22. Nichols RL, Smith JW, Klein DB, et al: Risk of infection after penetrating abdominal trauma. N Engl J Med 311:1065, 1984

23. Jensen LS, Andersen A, Fristup SC, et al: Comparison of one dose versus three doses of prophylactic antibiotics, and the influence of blood transfusion, on infectious complications in acute and elective colorectal surgery. Br J Surg 77:513, 1990

24. Miles AA, Miles EM, Burke J: The value and duration of defense reactions of the skin to the primary lodgment of bacteria. Br J Exp Pathol 38:79, 1957

25. Burke JF: The effective period of preventive antibiotic action in experimental incisions and dermal lesions. Surgery 50:161, 1961

26. Bernard HR, Cole WR: The prophylaxis of surgical infection: the effect of prophylactic antimicrobial drugs on incidence of infection following potentially contaminated wounds. Surgery 56:151, 1964

27. Chodak GW, Plaut ME: Use of systemic antibiotics for prophylaxis in surgery: a critical review. Arch Surg 112:326, 1977

28. Di Piro JT, Bivens BA, Record KE, et al: The prophylactic use of antimicrobials in surgery. Curr Probl Surg 20:72, 1983

29. Conte JE Jr, Polk HC Jr: Antibiotic Prophylaxis in Surgery: A Comprehensive Review. JB Lippincott Co, Philadelphia, 1984

30. Classen DC, Evans RS, Pestotnik SC, et al: The timing of prophylactic administration of antibiotics and the risk of surgical-wound infection. N Engl J Med 326: 282, 1992

31. Finland M: Antibacterial agents: uses and abuses in treatment and prophylaxis. RI Med J 43:499, 1960

32. Platt R, Zaleznik DF, Hopkins CC, et al: Perioperative antibiotic prophylaxis for herniorrhaphy and breast surgery. N Engl J Med 322:153, 1990

33. Taylor EW, Byrne DJ, Leaper DJ, et al: Antibiotic prophylaxis and open groin hernia repair. World J Surg 21:811, 1997

34. Platt R, Zucker JR, Zaleznik DF, et al: Prophylaxis against wound infection following hernia or breast surgery. J Infect Dis 166:556, 1992

35. Yee J, Dixon CM, McLean APH, et al: Clostridium difficile disease in a department of surgery: the significance of prophylactic antibiotics. Arch Surg 126:241, 1991

36. Galandiuk S, Polk HC Jr, Jagelman DG, et al:

Reemphasis of priorities in surgical antibiotic prophylaxis. Surg Gynecol Obstet 169:219, 1989

37. Kaiser AB: Antibiotic prophylaxis in surgery. N Engl J Med 315:1129, 1986

38. Meijer WS, Schmitz PI, Jeekel J: Meta-analysis of randomized, controlled clinical trials of antibiotic prophylaxis in biliary tract surgery. Br J Surg 77:283, 1990

39. Rotman N, Hay J-M, Lacaine F, et al: Prophylactic antibiotherapy in abdominal surgery: first- vs third-generation cephalosporins. Arch Surg 124:323, 1989

40. Choice of cephalosporins. Med Lett Drugs Ther 32:109, 1990

41. Shapiro M, Muñoz A, Tager IB, et al: Risk factors for infection at the operative site after abdominal or vaginal hysterectomy. N Engl J Med 307:1661, 1982

42. Polk HC Jr: Contributions of alimentary tract surgery to modern infection control. Am J Surg 153:2, 1987

43. Clarke JS, Condon RE, Bartlett JG, et al: Preoperative oral antibiotics reduce septic complications of colon operations: results of prospective, randomized, double-blind clinical study. Ann Surg 186:251, 1977

44. Washington JA III, Dearing WH, Judd ES, et al: Effect of preoperative antibiotic regimen on development of infection after intestinal surgery. Ann Surg 180:567, 1974

45. Fullen WD, Hunt J, Altemeier WA: Prophylactic antibiotics in penetrating wounds of the abdomen. J Trauma 12:282, 1972

46. Gentry LO, Feliciano DV, Lea AS, et al: Perioperative antibiotic therapy for penetrating injuries of the abdomen. Ann Surg 200:561, 1984

47. Heseltine PNR, Yellin AE, Appleman MD, et al: Perforated and gangrenous appendicitis: an analysis of antibiotic failures. J Infect Dis 148:322, 1983

48. Girotti MJ, Fodoruk S, Irvine-Meek J, et al: Antibiotic handbook and pre-printed perioperative order forms for surgical prophylaxis: do they work? Can J Surg 33:385, 1990

49. Larsen RA, Evans RS, Burke JP, et al: Improved perioperative antibiotic use and reduced surgical wound infections through use of computer decision analysis. Infect Control Hosp Epidemiol 10:316, 1989

50. Stone HN, Haney BB, Kolb LD, et al: Prophylactic and preventive antibiotic therapy: timing duration and economics. Ann Surg 189:691, 1978

51. Rowlands BJ, Clark RG, Richards DG: Single-dose intraoperative antibiotic prophylaxis in emergency abdominal surgery. Arch Surg 117:195, 1982

52. Fabian TC, Croce MA, Payne LW, et al: Duration of antibiotic therapy for penetrating abdominal trauma: a prospective trial. Surgery 112:788, 1992

53. Sarmiento JM, Aristizabal G, Rubiano J, et al: Prophylactic antibiotics in abdominal trauma. J Trauma 37:803, 1994

54. Weigelt JA: Role of anaerobic bacteria in antibiotic prophylaxis for trauma. Infect Dis Clin Pract 5(suppl 3):S92, 1996

55. Strachan CJL, Black J, Powis SJA, et al: Prophylactic use of cephazolin against wound sepsis after cholecystectomy. Br Med J 1:1254, 1977

56. Di Piro JT, Cheung RPF, Bowden TA Jr, et al: Single dose systemic antibiotic prophylaxis of surgical wound infections. Am J Surg 152:552, 1986

57. Hofstetter SR, Pachter HL, Bailey AA, et al: A prospective comparison of two regimens of prophylactic antibiotics in abdominal trauma: cefoxitin versus triple drug. J Trauma 24:307, 1984

58. Heseltine PNR, Berne TV, Yellin AE, et al: The efficacy of cefoxitin vs clindamycin/gentamicin in surgically treated stab wounds of the bowel. J Trauma 26:241, 1986

59. Jones RC, Thal ER, Johnson NA, et al: Evaluation of antibiotic therapy following penetrating abdominal trauma. Ann Surg 201:576, 1985

60. Antimicrobial prophylaxis in surgery. Med Lett Drugs Ther 41:75, 1999

61. Dellinger EP: Antibiotic prophylaxis in trauma: penetrating abdominal injuries and open fractures. Rev Infect Dis 13:5847, 1991

62. Boxma H, Broekhuisen T, Patka P, et al: Randomized controlled trial of single-dose antibiotic prophylaxis in surgical treatment of closed fractures: the Dutch Trauma Trial. Lancet 347:1133, 1996

63. Archer GL, Armstrong BC: Alteration of staphylococcal flora in cardiac surgery patients receiving prophylaxis. J Infect Dis 147:642, 1983

64. Illig KA, Schmidt E, Cavanaugh J, et al: Are prophylactic antibiotics required for elective laparoscopic cholecystectomy? J Am Coll Surg 184:353, 1997

65. Casewell MW, Law MM, Desai N: A laboratory model for testing agents for hygienic hand disinfection: handwashing and chlorhexidine for the removal of *Klebsiella*. J Hosp Infect 12:163, 1988

66. Larson E: Guideline for use of topical antimicrobial agents. Am J Infect Control 16:253, 1988

67. Hingst V, Juditzki I, Heeg P, et al: Evaluation of the efficacy of surgical hand disinfection following a reduced application time of 3 instead of 5 min. J Hosp Infect 20:79, 1992

68. Garner JS, Favero MS: CDC guidelines for the prevention and control of nosocomial infections: guideline for handwashing and hospital environmental control, 1985. Am J Infect Control 14:110, 1986

69. Lowbury EJL, Lilly HA, Bull JP: Methods for disinfection of hands and operation sites. Br Med J 2:531, 1964

70. Dineen P: An evaluation of the duration of the surgical scrub. Surg Gynecol Obstet 129:1181, 1969

71. Ayliffe GAJ: Surgical scrub and skin disinfection. Infect Control Hosp Epidemiol 5:23, 1984

72. Sebben JE: Sterile technique and the prevention of wound infection in office surgery: part II. J Dermatol Surg Oncol 15:38, 1989

73. Knolle P, Glöbel B, Glöbel H, et al: Release of iodide from povidone-iodine (PVP-I) in PVP-I preparations: a review of iodide tolerances and a comparative clinical pharmacological study. Proceedings of the International Symposium on Povidone. Digenis GA, Ansell J, Eds. University of Kentucky College of Pharmacy, Lexington, 1983, p 342

74. Peterson AF, Rosenberg A, Alatary SD: Comparative evaluation of surgical scrub preparations. Surg Gynecol Obstet 146:63, 1978

75. Lowbury EJL, Lilly HA: Use of 4% chlorhexidine detergent solution (Hibiscrub) and other methods of skin disinfection. Br Med J 1:510, 1973

76. Ellis H: Pathological changes produced by surgical dusting powders. Ann R Coll Surg Engl 76:5, 1994

77. Tang X-M, Chegini N, Rossi MJ, et al: The effect of surgical glove powder on proliferation of human skin fibroblast and monocyte/macrophage. J Gynecol Surg 10:139, 1994

78. Zaza S, Reeder JM, Luenda EC, et al: Latex sensitivity among perioperative nurses. AORN J 60:806, 1994

79. Casewell M, Phillips I: Hands as route of transmission for Klebsiella species. Br Med J 2:1315, 1977

80. Schürmann W, Eggers HJ: Antiviral activity of an alcoholic hand disinfectant: comparison of the in vitro suspension test with in vivo experiments on hands, and on individual fingertips. Antiviral Res 3:25, 1983

81. Gorbach SL, Condon RE, Conte JE Jr, et al: General guidelines for the evaluation of new anti-infective drugs for prophylaxis of surgical infections. Clin Infect Dis 15(suppl 1):S313, 1992

82. Jagelman DG, Fabian TC, Nichols RL, et al: Single

dose cefotetan versus multiple dose cefoxitin as prophylaxis in colorectal surgery. Am J Surg 155 (suppl 5A):71, 1988

83. Periti P, Mazzei T, Tonelli F, et al: Single dose cefotetan versus multiple dose cefoxitin—antimicrobial prophylaxis in colorectal surgery. Dis Colon Rectum 32:121, 1989

84. Norwegian Study Group for Colorectal Surgery: Should antimicrobial prophylaxis in colorectal surgery include agents effective against both anaerobic and aerobic microorganisms? A double-blind, multicenter study. Surgery 97:402, 1985

85. Condon RE, Bartlett JG, Greenlee H, et al: Efficacy of oral and systemic antibiotic prophylaxis in colorectal operations. Arch Surg 118:496, 1983

86. Stone HH, Hooper CA, Kolb LD, et al: Antibiotic prophylaxis in gastric, biliary and colonic surgery. Ann Surg 184:443, 1976

87. Portnoy J, Kagan E, Gordon PH, et al: Prophylactic antibiotics in elective colorectal surgery. Dis Colon Rectum 26:310, 1983

88. Barber MS, Hirschberg BC, Rice CL, et al: Parenteral antibiotics in elective colon surgery? A prospective, controlled clinical study. Surgery 86:23, 1979

89. Eisenberg HW: The use of new antibiotics in colorectal surgery. Am J Proctol Gastroenterol Colon Rectal Surg 6:9, 1981

90. Kaiser AB, Herrington JL, Jacobs JK, et al: Cefoxitin versus erythromycin, neomycin and cefazolin in colorectal operations: importance of the duration of the surgical procedure. Ann Surg 198:525, 1983

91. Coppa GF, Eng K: Factors involved in antibiotic selection in elective colon and rectal surgery. Surgery 104:853, 1988

92. Jagelman DG, Fazio VW, Lavery IC, et al: A prospective, randomized, double-blind study of 10% mannitol mechanical bowel preparation combined with oral neomycin and short-term, perioperative, intravenous Flagyl as prophylaxis in elective colorectal resections. Surgery 98:861, 1985

93. Beck DE, Harford FJ, DiPalma JA, et al: Bowel cleansing with polyethylene glycol electrolyte lavage solution. South Med J 78:1414, 1985

94. Fleites RA, Marshall JB, Eckhauser ML, et al: The efficacy of polyethylene glycol-electrolyte lavage solution versus traditional mechanical bowel preparation for elective colonic surgery: a randomized prospective, blinded clinical trial. Surgery 98:708, 1985

95. Wolff BG, Beart RW Jr, Dozois RR, et al: A new bowel preparation for elective colon and rectal surgery. Arch Surg 123:895, 1988

96. Frazee RC, Roberts J, Symmonds R, et al: Prospective, randomized trial of inpatient vs. outpatient bowel preparation for elective colorectal surgery. Dis Colon Rectum 35:223, 1992

97. Handelsman JC, Zeiler S, Coleman J, et al: Experience with ambulatory preoperative bowel preparation at The Johns Hopkins Hospital. Arch Surg 128:441, 1993

98. Miles AA, Miles EM, Burke J: The value and duration of defence reactions of the skin to the primary lodgement of bacteria. Br J Exp Pathol 38:79, 1957

99. Miles AA: The inflammatory response in relation to local infections. Surg Clin North Am 60:93, 1980

100. Alexander JW, Alexander WA: Penicillin prophylaxis of experimental staphylococcal wound infections. Surg Gynecol Obstet 120:243, 1965

101. Polk HC Jr: The enhancement of host defenses against infection: search for the holy grail. Surgery 99:1, 1986

102. Livingston DH, Malangoni MA: An experimental study of susceptibility to infection after hemorrhagic shock. Surg Gynecol Obstet 168:138, 1989

103. Meakins JL: Surgeons, surgery and immunomodulation. Arch Surg 126:494, 1991

104. Knighton D, Halliday B, Hunt TK: Oxygen as an

antibiotic: a comparison of the effects of inspired oxygen concentration and antibiotic administration on in vivo bacterial clearance. Arch Surg 121:191, 1986

105. Rabkin J, Heurt TK: Infection and oxygen. Problem Wounds: The Role of Oxygen. Davis JC, Heurt TK (Eds). Elsevier, New York, 1987, p 1

106. Olson MM, Lee JT Jr: Continuous, 10-year wound infection surveillance: results, advantages, and unanswered questions. Arch Surg 125:794, 1990

107. Oreskovich MR, Dellinger EP, Lennard ES, et al: Duration of preventive antibiotic administration for penetrating abdominal trauma. Arch Surg 117:200, 1982

108. Langely JM, Le Blanc JC, Drake J, et al: Efficacy of antimicrobial prophylaxis in placement of cerebrospinal fluid shunts: meta-analysis. Clin Infect Dis 17:98, 1993

109. Forse RA, Karam B, MacLean LD, et al: Antibiotic prophylaxis for surgery in morbidly obese patients. Surgery 106:750, 1989

110. Dajani AS, Taubert KA, Wilson W, et al: Prevention of bacterial endocarditis: recommendations by the American Heart Association. JAMA 277:1794, 1997

111. Durack DT: Prevention of infective endocarditis. N Engl J Med 332:38, 1995

112. Prevention of bacterial endocarditis. Med Lett Drugs Ther 32:112, 1990

113. Kaye D: Prophylaxis for infective endocarditis: an update. Ann Intern Med 104:419, 1986

114. Petersen EA: Prevention of bacterial endocarditis. Arch Intern Med 150:2447, 1990

115. Hayek LJ, Emerson JM, Gardner AMN: A placebo-controlled trial of the effect of two preoperative baths or showers with chlorhexidine detergent on postoperative wound infection rates. J Hosp Infect 10:165, 1987

116. Garner JS: CDC guidelines for the prevention and control of nosocomial infections: guideline for prevention of surgical wound infections, 1985. Am J Infect Control 14:71, 1986

117. Hamilton HW, Hamilton KR, Lone FJ: Preoperative hair removal. Can J Surg 20:269, 1977

118. McDonald WS, Nichter LS: Debridement of bacterial and particulate-contaminated wounds. Ann Plast Surg 33:142, 1994

119. Brown TR, Ehrlich CE, Stehman FB, et al: A clinical evaluation of chlorhexidine gluconate spray as compared with iodophor scrub for preoperative skin preparation. Surg Gynecol Obstet 158:363, 1984

120. Ritter MA, French MLV, Eitzen HE, et al: The antimicrobial effectiveness of operative-site preparative agents: a microbiological and clinical study. J Bone Joint Surg [Am] 62A:826, 1980

121. Amstey MS, Jones AP: Preparation of the vagina for surgery: a comparison of povidone-iodine and saline solution. JAMA 245:839, 1981

122. Nichols RL, Condon RE: Preoperative preparation of the colon. Surg Gynecol Obstet 132:323, 1971

123. Bartlett SP, Burton RC: Effects of prophylactic antibiotics on wound infection after elective colon and rectal surgery 1960–1980. Am J Surg 145:300, 1983

124. Nichols RL, Gorbach SL, Condon RE: Alteration of intestinal microflora following preoperative mechanical preparation of the colon. Dis Colon Rectum 14:123, 1971

125. Bowden TA Jr, DiPiro JT, Michael KA: Polyethylene glycol electrolyte lavage solution (PEG-ELS): a rapid, safe mechanical bowel preparation for colorectal surgery. Am Surg 53:34, 1987

126. Burke P, Mealy K, Gillen P, et al: Requirement for bowel preparation in colorectal surgery. Br J Surg 81:907, 1994

127. Santos JCM Jr, Batista J, Sirimarco MT, et al:

Prospective randomized trial of mechanical bowel preparation in patients undergoing elective colorectal surgery. Br J Surg 81:1673, 1994

128. Solla JA, Rothenberger DA: Preoperative bowel preparation: a survey of colon and rectal surgeons. Dis Colon Rectum 33:154, 1990

129. Nichols RL: Antibiotic prophylaxis in surgery. Curr Opin Infect Dis 7:647, 1994

130. Nichols RL: Update on preparation of the colon for resection. Current Surg 41:75, 1984

131. Nichols RL, Condon RE, Gorbach SL, et al: Efficacy of preoperative antimicrobial preparation of the bowel. Ann Surg 176:227, 1972

132. Goldring J, McNaught W, Scott A, et al: Prophylactic oral antimicrobial agents in elective colon surgery: a controlled trial. Lancet 2:7943, 1975

133. Matheson DM, Arabi Y, Baxter-Smith D, et al: Randomised multicentre trial of oral bowel preparation and antimicrobials for elective colorectal operations. Br J Surg 65:597, 1978

134. Nichols RL, Condon RE, DiSanto AR: Preoperative bowel preparation: erythromycin base serum and fecal levels following oral administration. Arch Surg 112:493, 1977

135. DiPiro JT, Patrias JM, Townsend RJ, et al: Oral neomycin sulfate and erythromycin base before colon surgery: a comparison of serum and tissue concentrations. Pharmacotherapy 5:91, 1985

136. Panichi G, Pantosti A, Giunchi G, et al: Cephalothin, cefoxitin or metronidazole in elective colon surgery? A single blind randomized trial. Dis Colon Rectum 25:783, 1982

137. Slama TG, Carey LC, Fass RJ: Comparative efficacy of prophylactic cephalothin and cefamandole for elective colon surgery: results of a prospective, randomized, double-blind study. Am J Surg 137:593, 1979

138. Hoffmann CEJ, McDonald PJ, Watts JM: Use of perioperative cefoxitin to prevent infection after colonic and rectal surgery. Ann Surg 193:353, 1981

139. McDonald PJ, Karran SJ: A comparison of intravenous cefoxitin and a combination of gentamicin and metronidazole as prophylaxis in colorectal surgery. Dis Colon Rectum 26:661, 1983

140. Eykyn SJ, Jackson BT, Lockhart-Mummery HE, et al: Prophylactic perioperative intravenous metronidazole in elective colorectal surgery. Lancet 2:761, 1979

141. Feathers RS, Lewis AAM, Sagor GR, et al: Prophylactic systemic antibiotics in colorectal surgery. Lancet 2:4, 1977

142. Nygaard K, Hognestad J: Infection prophylaxis with doxycycline in colorectal surgery: a preliminary report. Scand J Gastroenterol 15(suppl):37, 1980

143. Ivarsson L, Darle N, Kewenter JG, et al: Short-term systemic prophylaxis with cefoxitin and doxycycline in colorectal surgery—a prospective, randomized study. Am J Surg 144:257, 1982

144. Kager L, Ljungdahl I, Malmborg AS, et al: Antibiotic prophylaxis with cefoxitin in colorectal surgery—effect on the colon microflora and septic complications—a clinical model for prediction of the benefit and risks in using a new antibiotic in prophylaxis. Ann Surg 193:277, 1981

145. Song J, Glenny AM: Antimicrobial prophylaxis in colorectal surgery: a systematic review of randomized controlled trials. Br J Surg 85:1232, 1998

146. Peck JJ, Fuchs PC, Gustafson ME: Antimicrobial prophylaxis in elective colon surgery—experience of 1,035 operations in a community hospital. Am J Surg 147:633, 1984

147. Condon RE, Bartlett JG, Nichols RL, et al: Preoperative prophylactic cephalothin fails to control septic complications of colorectal operations: results of controlled clinical trial. Veterans Administration cooperative study. Am J Surg 137:68, 1979

148. Coppa GF, Eng K, Gouge TH, et al: Parenteral and

oral antibiotics in elective colon and rectal surgery: a prospective and randomized trial. Am J Surg 145:62, 1983

149. Maki DG, Aughey DR: Comparative study of cefazolin, cefoxitin and ceftizoxime for surgical prophylaxis in colo-rectal surgery. J Antimicrob Chemother 10(suppl C):281, 1982

150. Fabian TC, Mangiante EC, Boldreghini SJ: Prophylactic antibiotics for elective colorectal surgery or operation for obstruction of the small bowel: a comparison of cefonicid and cefoxitin. Rev Infect Dis 6(suppl 4):S896, 1984

151. Nichols RL: Surgical wound infection. Am J Med 91(suppl 3B):54S, 1991

152. Karran SJ, Sutton G, Gartell P, et al: Imipenem prophylaxis in elective colorectal surgery. Br J Surg 80:1196, 1993

153. Aly R, Maibach HI: Comparative antibacterial efficacy of a 2-minute surgical scrub with chlorhexidine gluconate, povidone-iodine, and chloroxylenol sponge-brushes. Am J Infect Control 16:173, 1988

154. Kaul AF, Jewett JF: Agents and techniques for disinfection of the skin. Surg Gynecol Obstet 152:677, 1981

155. Paulson DS: Comparative evaluation of five surgical hand scrub preparations. AORN J 60:246, 1994

156. Proposed recommended practices for surgical hand scrubs. AORN Recommended Practices Committee. AORN J 60:270, 1994

157. Figueras-Felip J, Basilio-Bonet E, Lara-Eisman F, et al: Oral is superior to systemic antibiotic prophylaxis in operations upon the colon and rectum. Surg Gynecol Obstet 158:359, 1984

158. McCulloch PG, Blamey SL, Finlay IG, et al: A prospective comparison of gentamicin and metronidazole and moxalactam in the prevention of septic complications associated with elective operations of the colon and rectum. Surg Gynecol Obstet 162:521, 1986

159. Weaver M, Burdon DW, Youngs DJ, et al: Oral neomycin and erythromycin compared with single-dose systemic metronidazole and ceftriaxone prophylaxis in elective colorectal surgery. Am J Surg 151:437, 1986

160. Jones RN, Wojeski W, Bakke J, et al: Antibiotic prophylaxis of 1,036 patients undergoing elective surgical procedures. Am J Surg 153:341, 1987

161. Playforth MJ, Smith GMR, Evans M, et al: Antimicrobial bowel preparation—oral, parenteral or both? Dis Colon Rectum 31:90, 1988

162. Khubchandani IT, Karamchandani MC, Sheets JA, et al: Metronidazole vs. erythromycin, neomycin and cefazolin in prophylaxis for colon surgery. Dis Colon Rectum 32:17, 1989

163. Kling PA, Dahlgren S: Oral prophylaxis with neomycin and erythromycin in colorectal surgery—more proof for efficacy than failure. Arch Surg 124:705, 1989

164. Stellato TA, Danziger LH, Gordon N, et al: Antibiotics in elective colon surgery: a randomized trial of oral, systemic, and oral/systemic antibiotics for prophylaxis. Am Surg 56:251, 1990

165. Schoetz DJ Jr, Roberts PL, Murray JJ, et al: Addition of parenteral cefoxitin to regimen of oral antibiotics for elective colorectal operations: a randomized prospective study. Ann Surg 212:209, 1990

166. Rowe-Jones DC, Peel ALG, Kingston RD, et al: Single dose cefotaxime plus metronidazole versus three dose cefuroxime plus metronidazole as prophylaxis against wound infection in colorectal surgery: multicentre prospective randomised study. BMJ 300:18, 1990

167. Arnaud JP, Bellissant E, Boissel P, et al: Single-dose amoxycillin–clavulanic acid vs. cefotetan for prophylaxis in elective colorectal surgery: a multicentre, prospective, randomized study. J Hosp Infect 22(suppl A):23, 1992

168. Kwok SPY, Lau WY, Leung KL, et al: Amoxycillin and clavulanic acid versus cefotaxime and metronidazole as antibiotic prophylaxis in elective colorectal resectional surgery. Chemotherapy 39:135, 1993

169. AhChong K, Yip AWC, Lee FCW, et al: Comparison of prophylactic ampicillin/sulbactam with gentamicin and metronidazole in elective colorectal surgery: a randomized clinical study. J Hosp Infect 27:149, 1994

170. Taylor EW, Lindsay G, West of Scotland Surgical Infection Study Group: Selective decontamination of the colon before elective colorectal surgery. World J Surg 18:926, 1994

Acknowledgment

Figures 3 and 4   Albert Miller.

6 PREPARING THE OPERATING ROOM

Ramon Berguer, M.D., Denise Joffe, M.D., Rene Lafreniere, M.D., C.M., James T. Lee, M.D., Ph.D.,
Joseph LoCicero III, M.D., Edward J. Quebbeman, M.D., Ph.D., H. David Reines, M.D.,
Cynthia Spry, R.N., M.S.N., and Karen Stanley Williams, M.D.

The operating room should provide an environment that is safe for the patient and efficient for the personnel who work there. These seemingly simple requirements are achieved only by giving attention to many details, including the physical features of the room, the equipment brought into the room, and the procedures followed by surgeons, nurses, anesthesiologists, and other support personnel. These considerations, in turn, must be evaluated for cost-effectiveness, potential for litigation, and, of course, tradition and personal preference.

Physical Aspects of the Operating Room

DESIGN AND CONSTRUCTION

The exact specifications for new construction and major remodeling of ORs are usually dependent on state and local regulations, which commonly incorporate standards published by the U.S. Department of Health and Human Services.[1] In addition to the primary construction standards document published by this agency, a large number of codes and recommendations generated by specialty associations and regulatory agencies also require consideration.[2]

The minimum size recommended for an OR is generally 20 by 20 ft; however, 24 by 24 ft may be needed for specialized cardiac, orthopedic, or neurosurgical procedures that require additional equipment. Generally, an OR should provide enough space for the following: gowning of the operating team, draping of the patient, movement of other personnel without contaminating sterile areas, and accommodation of large pieces of equipment, if necessary. Smaller rooms may be adequate for such procedures as cystoscopy and eye surgery. To ensure optimal scheduling efficiency, all operating rooms should ideally be large and equipped to accommodate any operative procedure; however, construction and maintenance costs would then increase.

Ceiling height should be at least 10 ft to allow for ceiling mounting of operating lights, microscopes, and other equipment. An additional 1 to 2 ft of ceiling height may be needed if x-ray equipment is to be permanently mounted. Conductive flooring is no longer necessary, but the floor should be seamless, hard, and easily cleaned.

A preoperative staging area should be included to allow preparation of the patient and to reduce the amount of time spent in the OR.[3] The staging area, the operating rooms, and the recovery rooms should be in close proximity to the intensive care unit. Unfortunately, as they are typically designed, the patient holding and transfer areas, personnel locker rooms, and, especially, equipment and supply storage areas are often much too small.

TRAFFIC FLOW

Today, floor plans for basic operating suites incorporate the concept of separating clean traffic from dirty traffic; typically, a peripheral corridor with access to a central sterile supply area is constructed around each OR. Consequently, sterile supplies arrive and are stored separately from contaminated materials. Although this concept is theoretically sound, it has not been shown to lower wound infection rates.[2,4] In one study, for example, investigators measured environmental contamination before and after changing from an old operating suite with a single corridor, which received so-called street traffic, to a new operating suite characterized by strictly controlled surgical traffic.[5] Environmental contamination was decreased in the new suite, but the investigators found that the improvement was "substantially less than anticipated." More important, the wound infection rate was unchanged. Furthermore, the considerable traffic back and forth between ORs (the lowest bacterial reservoir in the hospital) and the ICU (the highest bacterial reservoir) has not been shown to increase the risk of septic complications.

The absence of measurable benefit following separation of surgical traffic from the rest of the hospital traffic may be related to several factors:

1. The primary source of perioperative infection is the patient. The secondary source is the OR team. Neither of these sources is influenced by OR traffic-control schemes.

2. It is very difficult to control environmental contamination of horizontal surfaces such as floors. In one study, multiple cultures were obtained from the floors of an operating suite that had separated traffic patterns. The highest degree of contamination was found in the staff changing rooms, and the lowest was found in the public corridor outside the changing rooms.[6] Bacterial counts in the theoretically clean corridor and the dirty corridor were not different. The OR floors had low bacterial counts, obviously caused by frequent washing with detergent, but counts increased rapidly after the first case of the day.

3. The OR staff may not adhere to the traffic-control scheme. In one study, for example, personnel took the shortest route when walking from one point to another.[2]

4. The rate of redispersal of bacteria from the OR floor into the air caused by personnel moving about is either very low or nil, as reported in two studies.[7,8] These investigations also demonstrated that appropriate ventilation rapidly clears bacteria from the air (see below). If these findings are valid, the degree of floor contamination should not contribute to increased infection rates. However, movement of the personnel within the OR (including movement toward or away from the operative field and into or out of the OR) during a procedure does correlate with deposition of colony-forming units of bacteria on settle plates.[9] Movement may be reduced by determining equipment needs in advance, designing proper storage areas in the OR, and instituting policies limiting unnecessary visitation and observation.

AIR HANDLING

The concentrations of airborne particulate matter and bacteria in most ORs are equivalent to concentrations found in specialized clean rooms used in high-tech industries.[10] These low concentrations are achieved by changing room air 20 to 25 times each hour and passing the inflow air through a high-efficiency particulate air (HEPA) filter, which removes 99.97% of particles larger than 0.3 mm in diameter. Thus, the filter efficiently removes bacteria and fungi but not viruses. Bacteria present in OR air exist in association with particles (e.g., skin flakes, floor dust, lint) and dried droplets (e.g., saliva, nasal secretions). With optimal air-handling practices, particle counts can be kept as low as 1 to 5/cu ft, but most ORs have particle counts of 15 to 20/cu ft. The length of time that particles remain suspended in air varies with their size: large particles (100 μm) will fall 10 ft in 10 seconds; however, 10 μm particles, the size of particles that typically carry bacteria,[11] may remain suspended for 17 minutes, and tiny particles (< 3 μm) may remain suspended indefinitely.

Although the OR and its incoming air may be very clean, the numbers of particles and viable bacteria increase substantially once people enter the room because of shedding of skin scales, lint, and other particles.[10,12-15] These particles are then dispersed by the air turbulence caused by people moving about and by heat sources such as lights. Consequently, some investigators recommend increasing the number of air changes per hour to remove even more bacteria and restricting the number of people in the OR and their movements.[12]

Attempts to reduce infection risk further have led to the development of ultraclean air and laminar airflow technologies. However, these approaches are valid only in operations classified as clean, because in other types of operations, the major sources of infection are within the patient and the operative site. The orthopedic literature frequently reports reduced infection rates, particularly for total hip and knee replacement procedures, in ORs equipped with laminar airflow. In one study, for example, the wound infection rate for total hip or knee replacement procedures performed in a conventional operating room was 2.3%.[16] The rate decreased to 0.7% with use of ultraclean air and to 0.6% with use of prophylactic antibiotics. Another institution, however, achieved an infection rate of 1.9% for total hip replacement without using laminar airflow or even HEPA filtration technology.[17]

Although such findings indicate that improvements in the OR environment can reduce wound infection risk, several alternatives to laminar airflow technology exist, including changing operating garments frequently, limiting access to the OR, decreasing talking, updating old ventilation systems, using better skin preparation, and improving surgical technique.[18]

Bacterial viability in the harsh environment of air is limited to a few types of organisms; these include staphylococci, streptococci, bacterial spores, mycobacteria, and various viruses, yeasts, and fungi. Some of these organisms, especially *Aspergillus* and *Legionella*, have caused human infection after growing in hospital ventilation systems. Staphylococci and streptococci, which are frequent causes of postoperative infection, may be transmitted via OR air but are more likely to be spread either by direct contact with the operating team or from an endogenous source within the patient.

Although viable organisms are certainly present in the air of an occupied OR and bacteria are regularly recovered from surgical wounds,[19] organisms recovered from air are often not those that cause wound infection. Many studies that demonstrated reduced infection rates with improvement in air quality failed to show that the organisms eliminated were the causative agents of the previous infections.[20,21] One study analyzed the epidemiology of wound infection before and after the construction of a modern surgical suite that incorporated 20 air changes per hour and controlled traffic flow in the ORs.[5] The investigators found that the most common source of infection was the patient, followed by the surgical personnel. Only infrequently was the OR air implicated as a possible source of infection. They suggested that major changes in air quality would not significantly alter wound infection rates.

Current recommendations for handling OR air are that the air inflow be diffused over the 10 by 10 ft area of ceiling directly over the operating table and that the exhaust sites be located peripherally at the baseboard level. This pattern of airflow may decrease turbulence at the operating table and prevent entrainment of air from the periphery. The pressure in the operating room should be positive (0.125 to 0.25 cm H_2O) relative to the outside corridor to prevent particles and bacteria from entering the room.[4,22]

TEMPERATURE AND HUMIDITY

The ambient temperature of the OR often represents a compromise between the needs of the patient and those of the staff; the temperature desired by staff is itself a compromise between the needs of personnel who are dressed in surgical gowns and those who are not. In Europe and North America, OR temperatures vary from 18° to 26° C (64.4° to 78.8° F). A higher temperature is necessary during operations on infants and burn patients because conservation of body heat is critical in these patients. Generally, surgeons who are actively working and fully gowned prefer a temperature of 18° C (64.4° F), but anesthesiologists prefer 21.5° C (70.7° F).[23]

Humidity in the OR is generally maintained at between 50% and 60%; humidity greater than 60% may cause condensation on cool surfaces, whereas humidity less than 50% may not suppress static electricity.

LIGHTING

Well-balanced illumination in the OR provides the surgeon with a clear view of the operative field, prevents eye strain, and provides appropriate light levels for nurses and anesthesiologists. Much of our factual knowledge of OR illumination has been gained through the efforts of Dr. William Beck and the Illuminating Engineering Society.[24,25] Both the task (operating) light and the general room lights should be flexible, adjustable, and controllable. The ratio of brightness from the center of the operative site to the periphery of the operative site to the periphery of the OR should be 5:3:1. A general illumination brightness of up to 200 footcandles (ft-c) is desirable in new constructions. The lighting sources should not produce glare or undesirable reflection.

The amount of light required during an operation varies with the surgeon and the operative site. In one study, general surgeons operating on the common bile duct found 300 ft-c sufficient; because the reflectance of this tissue area is 15%, the required incident light level would be 2,000 ft-c. Surgeons performing coronary bypass operations required a level of 3,500 ft-c.[25] Surgeons have also expressed preferences for the color of light emitted. Many prefer a light equivalent to 5,000° K, but individual preferences range from 3,500° to 6,500° K. Whether changes in the color of light can improve discrimination of different tissues is unknown.

Other aspects of OR lighting known to vary with surgeon, specialty, and procedure include depth of focus, directionality of the light fixture, ability to decrease shadowing, size of the operative field, and ability to change position or focus of the light in a sterile manner. Light sources that contain multiple elements will continue to emit some light if one element burns out, which is a desirable feature. Ready availability of replacement elements is also desirable.

Another facet of OR lighting is heat production. Heat may be produced by infrared light emitted either directly by the light source or via energy transformation of the illuminated object. The maximum incident light energy value recommended at the wound level is 25,000 μW/cm².[24] If several light sources are used to illuminate a wound or if fiberoptic sources are utilized, this value may be exceeded. However, most of the infrared light emitted by OR lights can be eliminated by filters or by heat-diverting dichroic reflectors.

Equipment

Modern surgery uses an ever-increasing number of devices in the OR [see Table 1] to support and protect the patient and to assist the work of the surgical team. All OR equipment should be evaluated with respect to three basic concerns: maintenance of patient safety, maximization of surgical team efficiency, and prevention of occupational injuries.

BASIC CONCERNS

Patient Safety

Patient safety, the first order of business in the OR,[26] begins with proper handling of patients and their tissues, which is particularly important where patients are in direct contact with medical devices. It is imperative that physicians, nurses, and technicians protect patients from injuries caused by excessive pressure, heat, abrasion, electrical shock, chemicals, or trauma during their time in the OR. Equipment must be properly used and maintained because equipment malfunction, especially in life-support or monitoring systems, can cause serious harm.

Surgical Team Efficiency

Despite increased financial constraints, the United States health care system expects high-quality surgical care and access to advanced technology.[27] This goal can be achieved only by increasing the efficiency of surgical operations. Thus, proper storage, maintenance, arrangement, and use of OR equipment are paramount considerations. Both small and large devices used during each operation should be spatially arranged to allow unimpeded flow of persons, supplies, and additional equipment before, during, and after operation. Each member of the surgical team should be able to perform his or her function with minimal delay and the least amount of physical and mental effort. Manufacturers should be encouraged to provide standardized devices for the OR environment, and future OR designs should take into account "human factor" issues so that the myriad devices needed for modern surgery can be most efficiently integrated.

Occupational Injuries

Work-related musculoskeletal injuries are a major cause of decreased productivity and increased litigation costs in the United States.[28] In the OR, occupational injuries can be caused by excessive lifting, improper posture, collision with devices, electrical or thermal injury, puncture by sharp instruments, or exposure to bodily tissues and fluids. Temporary musculoskeletal injuries resulting from poor posture (particularly static posture) or excessive straining are less commonly acknowledged by members of the surgical team but occur relatively frequently during some operations.

To reduce injuries from awkward posture and excessive straining, OR devices should be positioned in an ergonomically desirable manner, so that unnecessary bending, reaching, lifting, and twisting are minimized. Visual displays and monitors should be placed where the surgical team can view them comfortably. Devices that require adjustment during operations should be readily accessible. Placement of cables and tubes across the OR workspace should be avoided if possible. The patient and the operating table should be positioned so as to facilitate the surgeons' work while maintaining patient safety. Lifting injuries can be prevented by using proper transfer technique and obtaining adequate assistance when moving patients in the OR. Thermal, electrical, and mechanical injury can occur if surgical devices and instruments are used improperly or if there are faulty equipment connections, inadequate physical protection, or a cluttered work environment.

OR DEVICES

Life-Support, Anesthetic Delivery, and Monitoring Devices

Life-support, anesthetic delivery, and physiologic monitoring devices are the most important equipment in the OR. These devices are typically integrated into a large, semimobile platform controlled by the anesthesiologist.[29] Power, gas, and data connections for this equipment are often provided via ceiling-mounted columns and should be routed to avoid tangles and hazards. Connections to the patient include the respiratory circuit, I.V. catheters, and monitoring devices such as ECG electrodes and pulse oximetry. More advanced monitoring may require additional bulky equipment for transesophageal echocardiography, electroencephalography, or measurement of somatosensory evoked potentials.

Traditionally, a sterile drape connected to two I.V. poles at the head of the bed (a so-called ether screen) has been used to separate the anesthesiologist's territory from the surgeon's. This arrangement is not necessary and can limit access to the area around the patient, especially when devices such as endoscopic imaging systems and alternative surgical power sources are used. A flexible approach to the arrangement of the anesthetic and surgical teams is most efficient, provided that asepsis and patient safety can be maintained.

Table 1 Devices Used in the Operating Room

For support of the patient	Anesthesia delivery devices
	Ventilator
	Physiologic monitoring devices
	Warming devices
	I.V. fluid warmers and infusers
For support of the surgeon	Sources of mechanical, electrical, and thermal power, including power tools and electrocautery, laser, and ultrasound instruments
	Mechanical retractors
	Lights mounted in various locations
	Suction devices and smoke evacuators
	Electromechanical and computerized assistive devices, such as robotic assistants
	Visualization equipment, including microscopes; endoscopic video cameras; and display devices such as video monitors, projection equipment, and head-mounted displays
	Data, sound, and video storage and transmission equipment
	Diagnostic imaging devices (e.g., for fluoroscopy, ultrasound, MRI, and CT)
For support of the OR team	Surgical instruments, usually packaged in case carts before each operation but occasionally stored in nearby fixed or mobile modules
	Tables for display of primary and secondary surgical instruments
	Containers for disposal of single-use equipment, gowns, drapes, etc.
	Workspace for charting and record keeping
	Communication equipment

Heating and Insulating Devices

Maintenance of the patient's normal body temperature during anesthesia and operation is important because it decreases complications[30] (although mild hypothermia may have a protective effect in certain situations where cardiac or central nervous system ischemia is unavoidable). All patients undergoing general anesthesia should be considered at risk for hypothermia due to radiation, conduction, convection, and evaporation heat loss.[23] Preventing hypothermia is especially important for infants, the elderly, and burn patients, all of whom have limitations of thermoregulation.

The safest and most effective manner of protecting the patient from hypothermia is to use forced-air warmers with specialized blankets placed over the upper or lower body; alternatively, one may place a warming water mattress under the patient or drape the patient with an aluminized blanket. Second-line therapy for maintaining normothermia is to warm all I.V. fluids. Irrigation fluids used in surgery should always be warmed at or slightly above body temperature before use. Radiant heating devices placed above the operative field may be especially useful during operations on infants. Use of a warmer on the inhalation side of the anesthetic gas circuit can also help maintain the patient's body temperature during an operation.

Electrosurgical Devices

The electrosurgical device is a 500 W radio-frequency generator that is used to cut and coagulate tissue. Although it is both common and necessary in the modern OR, it is also a constant hazard and therefore requires close attention.[31] When in use, the electrosurgical unit generates an electrical arc that has been associated with explosions. This risk has been lessened because explosive anesthetic agents are no longer used; however, explosion of hydrogen and methane gases in the large bowel is still a real—if rare—threat, especially when an operation is performed on an unprepared bowel.[32] Because the unit and its arc generate a broad band of radio frequencies, electrosurgical units interfere with monitoring devices, most notably the electrocardiographic monitor. Interference with cardiac pacemaker activity also has been reported.[33]

The most frequently reported hazard of the electrosurgical unit is a skin burn. Such burns are not often fatal, but they are painful, occasionally require skin grafts, and provide a potential for litigation. The burn site can be at the dispersive electrode, ECG monitoring leads, esophageal or rectal temperature probes, or areas of body contact with grounded objects. The dispersive electrode should be firmly adhered to a broad area of dry, hairless skin, preferably over a large muscle mass.[32]

Lasers

Lasers generate energy that is potentially detrimental. Lasers have caused injuries to both patients and staff, including skin burns, retinal injuries, injuries from endotracheal tube fires, pneumothorax, and damage to the colon and arteries.[34] Some design changes in the OR are necessary to accommodate lasers. The OR should not have windows, and a sign should be posted that indicates that a laser is in use. The walls and ceiling in the room should be nonreflective. Equipment used in the operative field should be nonreflective and nonflammable. The concentration of O_2 and N_2O in the inhaled gases should be reduced to decrease the possibility of fire. In addition, personnel should wear goggles of an appropriate type to protect the eyes from laser damage. A smoke evacuator should be attached to the laser to improve visualization, reduce objectionable odor, and decrease the potential for papillomavirus infection from the laser smoke plume.[35]

Radiologic Devices

Safety requirements during x-ray use must be understood by the surgical team.[36] Unnecessary exposure to radiation should be avoided. Personnel who participate regularly in procedures involving fluoroscopy should wear a badge dosimeter to measure total exposure. If required to remain in the room during exposures, they should stay at the maximal distance from the machine because radiation exposure decreases in proportion to the square of the distance from the source. If these precautions cannot be followed, it is necessary to use lead shielding in the form of lead aprons, thyroid shields, movable leaded barriers for the OR team members to stand behind, or all three. Whenever possible, devices for holding cassettes should be employed, or shielded gloves should be used in the x-ray field.

Portable fluoroscopy units are best employed when the use of x-ray equipment is infrequent. Portable units are awkward to maneuver in a crowded OR and require additional draping to prevent contamination of the surgical field. Fixed x-ray units are more versatile and produce better output; however, they require specialized fluoroscopy OR tables and occupy a significant part of the OR ceiling space. Rooms with built-in x-ray equipment should have lead-lined walls and doors and a separate shielded control booth.

Ultrasonic Devices

Instruments that allow hemostatic division of tissues via high-frequency vibration have become commonplace. So-called ultrasonic scalpels are particularly useful for rapid hemostatic division of vascular pedicles.[37] Ultrasonic dissectors with attached suction are more commonly used for the precise division of vascular solid organs such as the liver.[38] The main advantage of these devices is that no electrical current passes through the tissues. Instead, the instrument tip vibrates ultrasonically to denature proteins, with the result that tissue is divided hemostatically with no risk of burn or electrical shock to OR personnel or the patient. Another advantage is that these devices generate less lateral thermal damage to surrounding tissues than conventional electrocautery devices. Ultrasonic devices require a power generator and are usually pedal operated. The handpieces and connective tubing can be awkward and often require special assembly and cleaning by the surgical scrub nurse.

Powered Devices

The most common powered device in the OR is the surgical table. Central to every operation, this device must be properly positioned and adjusted to ensure the safety of the patient and the efficient work of the surgical team. Manually adjustable tables are simple, but those with electrical controls are easier to manage. OR table attachments, such as the arm boards and leg stirrups used to position patients, must be properly maintained and secured to prevent injuries to patients or staff. During transfer to and from the OR table, care must be taken to ensure that the patient is not injured and that life-support, monitoring, and I.V. systems are not disconnected. Proper transfer technique, personnel assistance, and the use of devices such as rollers will help prevent musculoskeletal injuries to the OR staff during this maneuver.

Other powered surgical instruments common in the OR include those used to obtain skin grafts, open the sternum, and perform orthopedic procedures. Powered saws and drills can cause substantial aerosolization of body fluids, thereby creating a potential infectious hazard for OR personnel.[39,40]

Viewing and Imaging Devices

OR microscopes are required for microsurgical procedures. Floor-mounted units are the most flexible, whereas built-in microscopes are best employed in rooms dedicated to this type of procedure.[41] Microscopes are bulky and heavy devices that can cause obstructions and collision hazards in the OR.

The development of video-assisted surgery in most of the body cavities has had a major impact on modern OR equipment.[42] Laparoscopy, thoracoscopy, arthroscopy, and other minimally invasive video-assisted procedures require a halogen light source and a video camera connected to the endoscope to provide a magnified color image of the operating field. This image is typically displayed for the surgical team on a conventional CRT monitor. Gas or fluid usually must be injected into the cavity being explored via specialized insufflators or pumps. This collection of devices should be arranged (not necessarily together) on wheeled carts or ceiling-mounted booms to facilitate their use and their sterile connection to the surgical field. In all cases, cables and connections should be placed so that OR traffic can flow freely and the surgical team's movements can be relatively unrestricted. All controls and displays must be properly positioned at or below the user's line of sight to allow comfortable and unobstructed viewing.

Today's less invasive operations require more accurate intraoperative assessment of the relevant surgical anatomy through the use of x-ray, computed tomography, magnetic resonance imaging, and ultrasonography. Intraoperative fluoroscopy and ultrasonography are most commonly used for this purpose. Intraoperative ultrasonography requires a high-quality portable ultrasound unit and specialized probes. Depending on the procedure and the training of the surgeon, the presence of a radiologist and an ultrasound technician may be required. The ultrasound unit must be positioned near the patient, and the surgical team must be able to view the image comfortably. In some cases, the image may be displayed on OR monitors by means of a video mixing device. Intraoperative CT and MRI are used less commonly, mostly in neurosurgical cases. Dedicated open radiologic units are usually installed either in the OR proper or immediately adjacent to the OR to permit intraoperative imaging of the selected body area. As image-guided procedures become more commonplace, OR designers will have to accommodate such devices within the OR workspace in a user-friendly manner.

Additional Devices

The use of sequential compression stockings (SCDs), with or without additional medical anticoagulation, has become the standard of care for the prevention of venous thromboembolism in the majority of operations for which direct access to the lower extremities is not required.[43] This is particularly true in operations lasting more than 4 hours with the patient in the lithotomy position. SCDs come in knee-high and thigh-high lengths and must be connected to a powered pump that inflates and deflates the stockings at a prescribed rate. This pump must often be placed near the patient on the floor or on a nearby cart. The pressure tubing from the stockings to the pump must be routed out of the way of the surgical team to prevent hazards and entanglements, particularly during operations requiring perineal access.

Suction devices are ubiquitous in the OR, assisting the surgeon in the evacuation of blood and other fluids from the operative field. A typical suction apparatus consists of a set of canisters on a wheeled base that receive suction from a wall- or ceiling-mounted source. The surgeon's aspirating cannula is sterilely connected to these canisters. Suction tubing is a common tripping hazard in the OR, and the suction canisters fill rapidly enough to require repeated changing.

Portable OR lights or headlights are often used when the lighting provided by standard ceiling-mounted lights is insufficient or when hard-to-see body cavities prove difficult to illuminate. Headlights are usually preferred because the beam is aimed in the direction the surgeon is looking; however, these devices can be uncomfortable to wear for prolonged periods. The fiberoptic light cord from the headset tethers the surgeon to the light source, which can exacerbate crowding near the surgical team.

Case Carts and Instrument Tables

In the case cart system, prepackaged instruments and linen for each scheduled operation are put together in one or more packs on a single cart and delivered from the central sterile supply to the OR area well before the start of the operation. Advocates of this system claim that it increases efficient use of personnel and thereby reduces costs.[44] However, there are no available data that compare the case cart system with the older, traditional method of packing and sterilizing specific instruments for each operation. Less frequently used instruments are kept in nearby fixed or mobile storage modules for ready access when required.

Traditionally, ORs contain a primary instrument table on which all the instruments specified for the operation are laid out, along with a smaller, secondary stand that can be moved to bring the most needed instruments close to the operating field. The primary table is rectangular or curved, is sterilely covered, and is placed close to the scrub nurse or technician. The secondary stand should be movable and adjustable in height (like, for instance, a Mayo stand). Other tables and stands, also sterilely draped, may be used to provide instruments to a second operating team or to support specific instruments and devices (e.g., drills). The most efficient placement of the instrument tables has been a subject of debate over the years, and each team must choose what works best for them. The goal, regardless of the specific placement, is to provide the surgical team with easy and rapid access to primary and secondary instruments and supplies.

The use of disposable instrumentation and drapes has added to the amount of waste generated by modern surgical procedures. Biohazardous waste must be properly disposed of in labeled red disposal bags. Small wheeled containers (so-called kickbuckets) can be useful for collecting small items near the operating field. Small racks or stands with handy impermeable bags for immediate disposal facilitate counting of used surgical sponges and gauze.

Surgical team members usually must complete some administrative tasks in the OR. Often, paper-based charting is used by the circulating nurse to document the details of the procedure and by the physicians to make perioperative notations. The OR should contain a designated area for such paperwork. A small folding desktop in the corner of the OR will suffice; however, physician dictating and charting rooms are sometimes provided adjacent to the surgical suite.

Communication Equipment

Every operation requires communication with the outside. Telephones should be placed in every OR where the circulating nurse can reach them easily without disturbing the surgical team. Most ORs have a computer terminal or a networked personal computer for routine charting options; this should be placed in a proper compact workstation located inside the OR. Information is being transferred in and out of the modern OR in an increasing variety of forms, including live video images and patient physiologic data. Modern OR design must incorporate facilities for safe and efficient communication of data between the surgical team and the outside.

Housekeeping Procedures

FLOORS AND WALLS

Despite detailed recommendations for cleaning the operating room [see Table 2],[45] the procedures that are optimal to provide a clean environment for the patient and are still cost-effective have not been critically analyzed.

Only a few studies have attempted to correlate surface contamination of the OR with wound infection risk. In one study, for example, ORs were randomly assigned to either a control group or an experi-

Table 2 OR Cleaning Schedules

Areas requiring daily cleaning	Surgical lights and tracks Fixed ceiling-mounted equipment Furniture and mobile equipment, including wheels OR and hall floors Cabinet and push-plate handles Ventilation grills All horizontal surfaces Substerile areas Scrub and utility areas Scrub sinks
Areas requiring routinely scheduled cleaning	Ventilation ducts and filters Recessed tracks Cabinets and shelves Walls and ceilings Sterilizers, warming cabinets, refrigerators, and ice machines

mental group.[46] The control rooms were cleaned with a germicidal agent and wet-vacuumed before the first case of the day and between cases; in the experimental rooms, cleaning consisted only of wiping up grossly visible contamination after clean and clean-contaminated cases. Both rooms had complete floor cleanup after contaminated or septic cases. The investigators found that bacterial colony counts obtained directly from the floors were lower in the control rooms but that counts obtained from other horizontal surfaces did not differ between the two OR groups. In addition, wound infection rates were the same in the control rooms and the experimental rooms and were comparable with rates reported in other series. Another study found that floor disinfectants decreased bacterial concentration on the floor for only 2 hours; colony counts then returned to pretreatment levels as personnel walked on the floor.[47] These investigators recommended discontinuing routine floor disinfection.

Even when an OR floor is contaminated, the rate of redispersal of bacteria into the air is low, and the clearance rate is high. It is unlikely, therefore, that bacteria from the floor contribute to wound infection. Consequently, routine disinfection of the OR floor between clean or clean-contaminated cases appears unnecessary.

According to the guidelines issued by the Centers for Disease Control and Prevention (CDC) for prevention of surgical site infection, when visible soiling of surfaces or equipment occurs during an operation, an Environmental Protection Agency (EPA)–approved hospital disinfectant should be used to decontaminate the affected areas before the next operation.[48] This statement is in keeping with the Occupational Safety and Health Administration (OSHA) requirement that all equipment and environmental surfaces be cleaned and decontaminated after contact with blood or other potentially infectious materials. Disinfection after a contaminated or dirty case and after the last case of the day is probably a reasonable practice, although it is not supported by directly pertinent data. Wet-vacuuming of the floor with an EPA-approved hospital disinfectant should be performed routinely after the last operation of the day or night.

MACHINES FROM "OUTSIDE"

Recording equipment, monitors, and other devices not routinely used in the operating suite occasionally may be brought in to meet a special need. Such "outside" equipment is often viewed as contaminated, and elaborate rituals of washing or wiping with alcohol or other antibacterial agents are sometimes enforced. However, there are no data to support these practices. It seems reasonable to wipe away visible dust and dirt, but elaborate cleaning of visiting outside equipment that will not come into direct contact with the sterile operative field appears to be unnecessary.

DIRTY CASES

Operations are classified or stratified into four groups in relation to the epidemiology of surgical wound infections.[49] Clean operations are those elective cases in which the GI tract or the respiratory tract is not entered and there are no major breaks in technique. The infection rate in this group should be less than 3%. Clean-contaminated operations are those elective cases in which the respiratory or the GI tract is entered or during which a break in aseptic technique has occurred. The infection rate in such cases should be less than 10%. Contaminated operations are those cases in which a fresh traumatic wound is present or gross spillage of GI contents occurs. Dirty operations include those in which bacterial inflammation occurs or in which pus is present. The infection rate may be as high as 40% in a contaminated or dirty operation.

Fear that bacteria from dirty or heavily contaminated cases could be transmitted to subsequent cases has resulted in the development of numerous and costly rituals of OR cleanup. However, there are no prospective studies and no large body of relevant data to support the usefulness of such rituals. In fact, one study[6] found no significant difference in environmental bacterial counts after clean cases and after dirty ones. Numerous authorities have recommended that there be only one standard of cleaning the OR after either clean or dirty cases.[6,45,50] This recommendation is reasonable because any patient may be a source of contamination caused by unrecognized bacterial or viral infection; more important, the other major source of OR contamination is the OR personnel.

Rituals applied to dirty cases include placing a germicide-soaked mat outside the OR door, allowing the OR to stand idle for an arbitrary period after cleanup of a dirty procedure, and using two circulating nurses, one inside and one outside the room. None of these practices has a sound theoretical or factual basis.

Traditionally, dirty cases have been scheduled after all the clean cases of the day. However, this restriction reduces the efficiency with which operations can be scheduled and may unnecessarily delay emergency cases. There are no data to support special cleaning procedures or closing of an operating room after a contaminated or dirty operation has been performed.[51] Tacky mats placed outside the entrance to an operating room or suite have not been shown to reduce the number of organisms on shoes or stretcher wheels, nor do they reduce the risk of surgical site infection.[52]

Protecting the Patient

POSITIONING

Patient positioning is the responsibility of the entire OR staff. The final position must allow adequate surgical exposure without compromising patient safety.

In many cases, one can use the preanesthesia visit to determine whether the patient will be able to tolerate a position by having him or her assume the anticipated posture and verifying that it is not painful. Occasionally, it may be necessary to modify the desired position. The organ systems most affected by changes in position are the cardiopulmonary system, the musculoskeletal system, and the peripheral nervous system.

Effects on Organ Systems

The cardiovascular system is especially vulnerable to changes in position. For any given position, the effect of gravity on the heart and vascular system created by tilting the bed can cause significant hemodynamic changes.[53] The reverse Trendelenburg position causes pooling of blood in the extremities, leading to a decrease in preload. Compressive leg stockings can help reduce venous pooling when the legs are below the level of the heart. The Trendelenburg position causes an increase in venous pressure that not only can affect the heart but also can cause venous pooling and engorgement in the head, resulting in altered cerebral blood flow and swelling of soft tissue.[54]

The vena cava and, less commonly, the aorta are prone to compression, which can cause dramatic changes in preload and perfusion. Inappropriate positioning of bolsters in the prone position can cause caval and abdominal compression,[53] affecting preload as well as giving rise to increased abdominal venous pressure, which is then transmitted to veins in the spinal canal. This increase in spinal pressure can result in excessive bleeding during operations on the spine.

Excessive pressure on the abdomen caused by surgical factors (e.g., retractors) can also compress the vena cava. Uterine compression in the obstetric patient is one of the most common causes of caval compression.[55] Aortic compression can also develop in these patients[56]; hence, it is vital to ensure left uterine displacement so as not to compromise fetal and maternal perfusion.

The pulmonary system is also vulnerable to position changes. Such changes can alter the ventilation-perfusion ratio and exert significant effects on oxygenation. The most dramatic changes occur in lateral positions, in which the height of the chest wall is highest and the effect of gravity on pulmonary blood flow is greatest. The dependent portions of the lung are most affected by the abdominal contents elevating the diaphragm; decreased pulmonary compliance results. Dead space also increases substantially in the lateral position and can affect measurement of the end-tidal CO_2–arterial CO_2 gradient.[57]

The musculoskeletal and peripheral nervous systems are especially vulnerable to injury because they are prone to compression and stretching. This category of injuries generates a multitude of medicolegal complaints against anesthesiologists.[58] The following are the nerves that are most vulnerable.

1. The peroneal nerve, which may be compressed between the head of the fibula and the support bars of stirrups (in the lithotomy position) or the OR table (in the lateral decubitus position).

2. The femoral nerve, which may be compressed by the inguinal ligament when the hip is in flexed position.

3. The saphenous nerve, which may be injured by pressure over the medial femoral condyle.

4. The obturator nerve, which may be stretched when the hip is in flexion.

5. The brachial plexus, which may be stretched when the arm is above the shoulder plane, stretched by exaggerated rotation of the head away from an extended arm, compressed by axillary structures (in the lateral decubitus position), or compressed by shoulder braces.

6. The ulnar nerve, which may be compressed between the medial humeral epicondyle and the olecranon.

7. The radial nerve, which may be compressed by the humerus.

Regardless of the final position, all pressure points must be protected with padding. For long procedures, extra padding between the patient and the bed provides additional protection against decubitus injury. However, the mechanisms of some injuries are not clear. For example, many cases of ulnar injury (one of the most common causes of litigation) have been demonstrated to have causes unrelated to padding and position of the arm.[59] Men at the extremes of body habitus who require prolonged hospitalization are most likely to be

affected despite appropriate supination of the hand and padding of the elbow.

Position may affect other organ systems as well. It is important to ensure that the breasts and genitals are not compressed or pulled. In addition, a soft head support should be used to prevent pressure alopecia.[60] The eyes and ears should be carefully examined. The eyes should be closed, and pressure on the globe should be eliminated. This is especially important in the prone position. Cases of blindness related to pressure on the globe have been reported.[61] Any compression injuries, regardless of the cause, may be exacerbated by hypoperfusion and hypothermia.

Concerns Related to Specific Positions

A number of specific concerns exist regarding specific positions (other than supine), and certain recommendations may be made.

Prone position   Cardiac effects can be minimized by avoiding increases in intra-abdominal pressure and vena caval compression. Pulmonary effects can be minimized by ensuring that the abdomen is not compressed, thereby preventing decreases in lung compliance and lung volume. Musculoskeletal effects can be minimized by ensuring that when the patient's arms are up, the axilla is not tense or stretched; if the patient's arms are at his or her side, they should be supinated.

Lateral position   Cardiac effects can be minimized by keeping the body flat (so that there is no hydrostatic pressure difference); lateral flexion of the legs can compress the cava. Pulmonary effects can be minimized by addressing any abnormalities in oxygenation and arterial CO_2–end-tidal CO_2 gradient (see above). Musculoskeletal effects can be minimized by ensuring that the cervical spine is aligned with the thoracolumbar spine (to prevent injury and jugular venous compression). Peripheral nervous system effects can be minimized by using an axillary roll to relieve compression of the thorax on the brachial plexus. Adequate padding should be placed on decubitus parts and between the legs.

Sitting position   Cardiac effects of note in this position include marked decreases in preload and increases in peripheral and pulmonary vascular resistance and in heart rate (which may be attenuated, depending on the anesthetic). In addition, the risk of air emboli is greatest with the patient in the sitting position.[62] Musculoskeletal effects can be minimized by ensuring that the chin is not forced into the suprasternal notch, which can decrease spinal cord perfusion and venous drainage; cases of tetraplegia and massive swelling of the face and pharynx have resulted.[63,64]

Many other patient positions are commonly used. Most, however, are hybrids of the positions just listed, and their effects on organ systems are a combination of the changes characteristic of the positions from which they derive. It is incumbent on the OR team to ensure that positioning is appropriate: improper positioning can compromise patient care and contribute to multisystem organ dysfunction.

Protecting the Surgeon and Staff

ENVIRONMENTAL HAZARDS

Anesthetic Gases

Anesthetic gases are the most common environmental pollutants in the OR. A study evaluating the distribution of leaked gases in ORs found that anesthesiologists were exposed to the highest levels, although lower levels of gases were detected at the periphery of the room where circulating nurses worked. No OR was completely free of leaks, though exposure could be significantly decreased with proper scavenging.[65]

The major risks of chronic exposure to anesthetic gases are not well known, because many studies of the effects of long-term exposure have yielded inconclusive results. Inhaled agents, such as the halogenated hydrocarbons (e.g., halothane, isoflurane, and enflurane) and nitrous oxide, may be associated with an increased risk of spontaneous abortion among female physicians, nurses, and technicians. Presumably, newer inhaled agents that have not been studied (e.g., desflurane and sevoflurane) have similar effects. Other problems that have been attributed to chronic exposure include an increased incidence of congenital anomalies, liver and kidney disease, and decreased behavioral performance[66-71]; however, the studies supporting the occurrence of these complications are seriously flawed because of their retrospective design, and they induced bias in many participants.[66-71]

Despite the weak scientific evidence for any danger associated with chronic exposure to inhaled anesthetic agents, it is prudent to minimize chronic exposure. The time-weighted exposure limits suggested by the National Institute of Occupational Safety and Health are less than 25 ppm for nitrous oxide, less than 2 ppm for halogenated agents alone, and 0.5 ppm for halogenated agents in combination with nitrous oxide.[72] Scavenging systems can decrease levels by about 90%. If anesthetic vapors are detected by smell, then the levels are at least 33 ppm.[73]

Anesthetic gases may escape into the OR from either anesthetic equipment or the patient. The largest volume of anesthetic gases escapes from the exhalation side of the rebreathing anesthesia circuit via the pop-off valve. Scavenging equipment connects the exhalation side of the rebreathing circuit to a vacuum line, thereby preventing venting of gases into the air. This is a crucial measure used to reduce levels of gases. Although leaks may occur in the anesthetic machine, gas is more likely to come from incomplete isolation of the patient's airway (e.g., from an incompletely sealed ventilation mask, from leaks around endotracheal tubes, or from the patient's mouth after extubation). Meticulous attention to preventing unnecessary leaks from the patient helps decrease the vapor concentration even further.

In many institutions, scavenging is available only in the OR and not in other areas that use anesthetic vapors (i.e., the radiology department). This limited availability should be taken into account in the choice of an anesthetic technique in such areas. Ideally, I.V. anesthesia should be used whenever possible in these situations. Periodically, gas concentrations should be measured in all areas where anesthesia is provided to ensure proper functioning of the anesthesia and scavenging equipment.

Ethylene Oxide

Ethylene oxide (EO), a powerful alkylating agent, is commonly used to sterilize heat- and moisture-sensitive items. EO is a highly penetrating gas with toxic residuals that must be driven from devices that are sterilized. In humans, EO residuals can cause anaphylactic sensitization, contact burns of the skin or the mucous membranes, hemolysis and edema, and other adverse reactions in the respiratory and GI tracts. EO is a known carcinogen.[74]

OSHA has set the permissible exposure limit (PEL) for EO at 1 part EO to 1 million parts of air (1 ppm) as an 8-hour time-weighted average. Sterilization with EO must be followed by lengthy aeration times of 8 to 12 hours or longer in a mechanical aerator to remove toxic residuals. Personnel who operate EO sterilizers must be informed of the associated hazards, and employers are required to provide administrative and engineering controls to protect workers. Annual safety-education programs, badges for monitoring personal

exposure, and alarm systems that activate in the event of an EO leak are three such controls.

Originally, EO gas was combined with a chlorofluorocarbon stabilizing agent in a preparation containing 12% EO and 88% chlorofluorocarbons (referred to as 12/88 EO). The chlorofluorocarbons were phased out in December 1995 under the provisions of the Clean Air Act. (Under that legislation, they were classified as a class 1 substance because of scientific evidence linking them to destruction of the earth's ozone layer.) Some states began to require the use of EO abatement technology to reduce the amount of EO being released into ambient air by 90% to 99.9%.

The EO sterilizer is typically located outside the OR, and OR personnel may not be responsible for operating it. It is important, however, that OR personnel be knowledgeable about EO hazards and aeration times and not request or accept less than complete aeration cycles. No matter how pressing the desire to abort the aeration cycle to retrieve an item, it should not be gratified. The composition of the item to be sterilized and the parameters of the aerator determine the length of required aeration. Mechanical aerators generally have standard aeration cycles with an option to extend the cycle as desired. The aeration times supplied by the manufacturer of the item must be strictly adhered to. Although standard aeration times range from 8 to 12 hours, some items require 24 hours or longer.

If a mechanical aerator is not available, aeration with ambient air will extend aeration times to as much as a week or longer. With items not intended for sterilization that are not made of suitable materials, such as children's toys or instruments created in a home workshop, it may be impossible to reach safe levels of residuals.

Because of the hazards associated with EO and the lengthy cycle times, several new sterilization technologies, including liquid peracetic acid and hydrogen peroxide gas plasma, have been introduced. Both technologies offer cycle times of less than 1 hour, and neither requires aeration of sterilized instruments or devices. Liquid peracetic sterilization is a point-of-use process, and the sterilizer is usually installed adjacent to the OR. At the completion of the cycle, items are wet and should be used immediately. Hydrogen peroxide gas plasma, on the other hand, is a dry process. Sterilized items are wrapped and may be either used immediately or stored for future use. The principal by-products of the process are vaporized water and oxygen; because there are no toxic residuals, no aeration is required. The sterilizer may be located in the central processing department; however, many institutions have placed units within the OR. Because of the short cycle time and the lack of toxic residuals, an increasing number of heat- and moisture-sensitive items are now processed by this means.

INFECTIOUS HAZARDS

Awareness of the emergence of new infectious diseases, the increasing prevalence of antibiotic-resistant strains of bacteria, and the ubiquitous presence of infectious viruses with the potential to cause severe and fatal diseases have encouraged health care workers to practice standard and transmission-based precautions on a routine basis to protect both their patients and themselves.

The most common virus, causing the most work-related deaths in health care workers in the United States (200/year), is the hepatitis B virus (HBV), but the one causing the most concern is HIV. Although the risk of acquiring HIV after an accidental parenteral exposure to blood from a known HIV-infected patient is estimated to be 0.3%,[75] the severe and fatal nature of the resulting disease makes HIV transmission a paramount concern.

Currently, there is concern about the incidence of hepatitis C virus. This pathogen is transmitted by percutaneous inoculation from needle sticks, cuts, and open wounds or breaks in the skin and through contact with infectious fluids and materials. Potentially infectious material includes blood, serum, and any other human bodily fluids, tissues, or organs to which the health care worker may be exposed in the practice setting.

In 1991, OSHA formulated its blood-borne pathogens standard, which mandates the use of universal precautions (to reduce the risk of transmission of blood-borne pathogens) and body substance isolation (to reduce the risk of pathogen transmission from moist body substances). The use of universal precautions requires engineering and work-practice controls, provision of personal protective equipment, an exposure-control plan, exposure documentation, methods of compliance, availability of HBV vaccine, postexposure evaluation, labels and warning signs where appropriate, and employee training.

OR practices associated with universal precautions include but are not limited to the following:

1. Precautions to prevent injuries caused by scalpels and other sharp instruments. A hands-free technique is used to create a neutral zone in which sharps are placed instead of being handed directly to scrubbed personnel. Oral confirmation is provided whenever a scalpel or sharp is passed. A needle holder is used to remove scalpel blades from knife handles.

2. Precautions to prevent exposure. Personnel with open lesions do not scrub. Inexperienced health care workers should not scrub when the patient is known to be HIV positive. Pregnant personnel should not participate in operations on patients with AIDS because of the increased risk of exposure to other infectious agents often carried by AIDS patients, particularly cytomegalovirus and *Toxoplasma gondii*, which may have detrimental effects on the developing fetus. Scrubbed personnel wear gowns that are appropriate for the procedure (e.g., gowns with suitable barrier properties when a large amount of potentially infectious material is anticipated). They also wear two pairs of gloves when the procedure is likely to be lengthy and when loss of glove integrity is a significant possibility. Gloves are regularly checked for integrity during a surgical procedure. Scrubbed personnel wear protective eyewear with a splash shield or goggles with side shields. Attire that becomes contaminated is removed as soon as possible and is placed in an appropriate waste container. Specimens are placed in leakproof containers.

All sites of blood spillage and gross soilage from the operative procedure should be cleaned as soon as possible. Spills should be cleaned with a lint-free cloth saturated with a 1:10 solution of household hypochlorite bleach or with a hospital grade EPA disinfectant or detergent-disinfectant.

Transmission-based precautions should be used in addition to standard precautions for patients who are known or believed to be infected with epidemiologically important and highly transmissible pathogens.[76]

Personnel should wear masks when in the presence of patients known to have an infection caused by an airborne pathogen, such as rubella, varicella, or tuberculosis. Such patients should also wear a mask during transport to prevent generation of airborne particles. Elective procedures on patients with active tuberculosis should be delayed until the patient is no longer infectious. If a procedure cannot be delayed, it should be performed in an operating suite with an anteroom, and only necessary personnel should be allowed to enter the room during the operation. If possible, the operation should take place when there are no other patients in the OR or when traffic is minimal.

Table 3   Criteria for Defining a Surgical Site Infection (SSI)[85]

Superficial incisional SSI

Infection occurs within 30 days after the operation, *and* infection involves only skin or subcutaneous tissue of the incisions, *and* at least *one* of the following:

1. Purulent drainage, with or without laboratory confirmation, from the superficial incision
2. Organisms isolated from an aseptically obtained culture of fluid or tissue from the superficial incision
3. At least one of the following signs or symptoms of infection: pain or tenderness, localized swelling, redness, or heat; *and* superficial incision is deliberately opened by surgeon, *unless* incision is culture negative
4. Diagnosis of superficial incisional SSI by the surgeon or attending physician

Do *not* report the following conditions as SSI:

1. Stitch abscess (minimal inflammation and discharge confined to the points of suture penetration)
2. Infection of an episiotomy or newborn circumcision site
3. Infected burn wound
4. Incisional SSI that extends into the fascial and muscle layers (see deep incisional SSI)

Note: Specific criteria are used for identifying infected episiotomy and circumcision sites and burn wounds

Deep incisional SSI

Infection occurs within 30 days after the operation if no implant* is left in place or within 1 yr if implant is in place and the infection appears to be related to the operation, *and* infection involves deep soft tissues (e.g., fascial and muscle layers) on the incision, *and* at least *one* of the following:

1. Purulent drainage from the deep incision but not from the organ/space component of the surgical site
2. A deep incision spontaneously dehisces or is deliberately opened by a surgeon when the patient has at least one of the following signs or symptoms: fever (> 38° C [100.4° F]), localized pain, or tenderness, unless site is culture negative
3. An abscess or other evidence of infection involving the deep incision is found on direct examination, during reoperation, or by histopathologic or radiologic examination
4. Diagnosis of a deep incisional SSI by a surgeon or attending physician

Notes:

1. Report infection that involves both superficial and deep incision sites as deep incisional SSI
2. Report an organ/space SSI that drains through the incision as a deep incisional SSI

Organ/space SSI

Infection occurs within 30 days after the operation if no implant* is left in place or within 1 yr if implant is in place and the infection appears to be related to the operation, *and* infection involves any part of the anatomy (e.g., organs or spaces), other than the incision, which was opened or manipulated during an operation, *and* at least *one* of the following:

1. Purulent drainage from a drain that is placed through a stab wound† into the organ/space
2. Organisms isolated from an aseptically obtained culture of fluid or tissue in the organ/space
3. An abscess or other evidence of infection involving the organ/space that is found on direct examination, during reoperation, or by histopathologic or radiologic examination
4. Diagnosis of an organ/space SSI by a surgeon or attending physician

*National Nosocomial Infection Surveillance definition: a nonhuman-derived implantable foreign body (e.g., prosthetic heart valve, nonhuman vascular graft, mechanical heart, or hip prosthesis) that is permanently placed in a patient during surgery.

†If the area around a stab wound becomes infected, it is not an SSI. It is considered a skin or soft tissue infection, depending on its depth.

HAZARDS DURING PREGNANCY

Pregnant women working in the OR may place the fetus at risk for several work-related complications. Exposure to anesthetic agents has been implicated in an increased risk of spontaneous abortions and congenital anomalies. Exposure to radiation and infectious agents has also been associated with fetal abnormalities.

The evidence that low levels of anesthetic agents give rise to an increased risk of abortions and congenital anomalies is very weak. The published studies are flawed by their retrospective nature, their reporting bias, and their inadequate control of confounding variables such as work-related stress, noise, sleep deprivation, and numerous lifestyle differences among participants.[66-70] In addition, the high incidence of spontaneous abortions in the general population makes differences hard to demonstrate. Furthermore, even if there is a risk to the fetus associated with chronic exposure to anesthetic agents, newer anesthesia machines and improved scavenging systems may make old data hard to extrapolate to today's ORs. Nevertheless, it is prudent for all personnel to minimize exposure to inhaled gases.

As with anesthetic vapor–induced hazards of pregnancy, it is often hard to show a strong causal relationship between radiation exposure in health care workers and adverse effects because the incidence of spontaneous congenital defects, spontaneous mutations, and spontaneous abortions is so high in the general population.[77] The most sensitive gestational period for teratogenesis is between 8 and 17 weeks.[78] Rare consequences of prenatal radiation exposure include a slight increase in the incidence of childhood leukemia, genetic mutations, and spontaneous abortions.[79-82] In addition, there seems to be a definite increase in the incidence of microcephaly and mental retardation.[78,80] Some of these complications may also occur with radiation exposure before conception.[81]

The level of radiation exposure above which the risk of complications increases significantly is unknown, but it has been suggested that exposure not exceed 0.5 cGy for the 9-month gestation period.[82] No single diagnostic study exceeds this maximum. The use of fluoroscopy exposes personnel to the greatest amount of radiation.[82]

Radiation exposure can be avoided or reduced in several ways: the pregnant woman can (1) be assigned to cases in which radiation will not be used or will at least be minimized, (2) leave the room while the x-ray is being taken, (3) use lead aprons and screens (levels of radiation exposure beneath leaded aprons are comparable to environmental exposure),[82] or (4) stay as far from the source as possible (a distance of at least 3 ft is recommended).[83] If radiation film badges are routinely used, the actual risk for an individual will be known and appropriate precautions can be taken to lower exposure.

The dangers of exposure to infectious agents during pregnancy are more concrete.[83,84] Several viral infections, if acquired during pregnancy, can have devastating consequences on fetal development and even result in fetal death. Some may induce chronic illness in the child. These viruses include rubella, cytomegalovirus, varicella-zoster virus (VZV), HBV, and HIV.

The risk of infection can be decreased by ensuring that employee immunization status is up to date. It is recommended that employees be immunized against VZV (if they are not already immune) and HBV, in addition to the standard childhood vaccines.[83,84] Viral infections are common in immunocompromised patients, and caring for these patients may represent an increased risk for pregnant personnel who are not appropriately immunized. It is generally believed, however, that the use of universal precautions will prevent almost all transmission. The viruses are transmitted by close personal contact or contact with secretions, excretions, or blood. Avoidance of these known modes of transmission should provide adequate protection. Some advocate that pregnant women who have never been infected with VZV or who have not been immunized should not care for high-risk

---

Table 4 Site-Specific Classifications of Organ/Space Surgical Site Infection[85]

Arterial or venous infection
Breast abscess or mastitis
Disk space
Ear, mastoid
Endocarditis
Endometritis
Eye, other than conjunctivitis
Gastrointestinal tract
Intra-abdominal, not specified elsewhere
Intracranial, brain abscess or dura
Joint or bursa
Mediastinitis
Meningitis or ventriculitis
Myocarditis or pericarditis
Oral cavity (mouth, tongue, or gums)
Osteomyelitis
Other infections of the lower respiratory tract (e.g., abscess or empyema)
Other male or female reproductive tract
Sinusitis
Spinal abscess without meningitis
Upper respiratory tract
Vaginal cuff

---

patients because of the highly contagious nature of the virus.[83,84] The OR environment is a safe workplace for pregnant women if appropriate safety precautions are adhered to.

Asepsis

Infections related to surgical procedures (traditionally referred to as surgical wound infections) have been redefined by the CDC as surgical site infections (SSIs). The current definition classifies such infections as either incisional SSIs or organ/space SSIs [*see Table 3*]. Incisional infections are further classified as superficial incisional SSIs or deep incisional SSIs,[85] and organ/space SSIs are classified by site [*see Table 4*]. The classification of surgical wounds as clean, clean-contaminated, contaminated, or dirty helps determine benchmarks for the development of SSIs.[85] SSIs that occur in clean operations are often caused by bacteria introduced by OR personnel or derived from a source in the patient. This is particularly true of operations in which prosthetic devices or materials are implanted.

Numerous aseptic OR procedures and rituals have been developed to protect patients from environmental sources of infection. These procedures came under scrutiny in the 1990s. A task force, the Hospital Infection Control Practices Advisory Committee (HICPAC), was formed in 1991 under the auspices of the CDC and published its findings in 1999[85]; this document supplants earlier guidelines.[86,87] Part II of the 1999 guidelines comprises a set of recommendations for the prevention of SSIs. Each recommendation has been categorized by HICPAC. Category I recommendations include the subcategories IA (strongly recommended and supported by well-designed studies) and IB (strongly recommended for implementation and supported by some studies). Category II recommendations are suggested for implementation and supported by suggestive clinical epidemiologic studies or a theoretical rationale. The final category, labeled as "no recommendation" or "unresolved issue," includes practices for which there is insufficient evidence or no consensus regarding efficacy. There are, however, certain practices required by federal regulation in these areas (see below). The CDC's position is that all category I recommendations should be accepted by health care facilities. In what follows, we place primary emphasis on this category of recommendation.

SKIN PREPARATION

Because the patient is the most common source of bacteria leading to SSIs, attempts should be made to reduce bacterial counts on the patient's skin. Preventive antiseptic showers or baths decrease skin microbial counts; chlorhexidine gluconate is more effective than povidone-iodine and is most effective when repeat applications are used.[87,88] Although showers have not been shown to reduce the incidence of SSIs, a category IB recommendation is that patients be required to shower or bathe with an antiseptic agent the night before the operative day or just before the operation. This recommendation does not address minimally invasive procedures or procedures restricted to the face or the extremities.

Preoperative shaving with a razor is associated with an SSI rate as high as 5.6% versus 0.6% for those not shaved.[89] Depilatory creams or electric clippers lower preoperative SSI rates significantly,[89-91] but it has not been determined which of these methods is safest. Depilatories occasionally cause cuts, skin irritation, or allergic reactions. The CDC IA recommendation is that hair not be removed preoperatively unless it interferes with the operation. If hair removal is indicated, it should be done with electric clippers immediately before the operation.

An antiseptic should be used for skin preparation.[87] Alcohol is effective, fast acting, and inexpensive, although flammable; it is also drying. Although povidone-iodine is widely used, chlorhexidine gluconate achieves greater reduction in skin microflora and has greater residual activity.[92-94] Great care must be taken when these products are used around mucous membranes and the eyes. The incisional area should be free of gross contamination,[95] and the antiseptic should be applied in concentric circles, beginning in the area of the proposed incision (category II recommendation). There is minimal evidence to support the view that antiseptic-impregnated adhesive drapes or scrubbing all wounds affects the incidence of SSIs.

HAND WASHING

The surgical scrub is traditionally performed before sterile gowns and gloves are donned. At present, it remains unclear what the ideal scrubbing agent is and how long it must be applied. Numerous agents are available. Although alcohol is effective, its irritating effect on skin and its flammability limit its use in the United States. Povidone-iodine and chlorhexidine gluconate are currently the agents of choice among surgical teams.[96] No differences in SSI rates have been associated with particular agents, but chlorhexidine gluconate is known to have greater residual microbial activity than other agents.[17]

Scrubbing for at least 2 minutes has been found to be as effective as the traditional 10-minute scrub.[96] The CDC therefore recommends that surgeons scrub for 2 to 5 minutes (category IB recommendation) with an antiseptic solution up to the elbows. Nails should be kept short and clean before the first scrub of the day.

SURGICAL ATTIRE AND DRAPES

Surgical attire includes scrub suits, hair and shoe covers, gloves, gowns, and masks. Perhaps surprisingly, given conventional wisdom and the experimental data showing that live organisms are shed from the hair, skin, and mucous membranes of OR personnel, there are few controlled studies relating the use of surgical attire to the incidence of SSIs.[97,98] It would seem intuitively obvious that a sterile gown can keep body bacteria from falling into a wound, but small amounts of bacteria still escape from exposed areas. In addition, it would seem obviously prudent to use barriers to minimize patients'

exposure to bacteria from OR personnel, but even the use of impermeable plastic gowns and helmets with their own air supply has not been shown to lower the incidence of SSIs significantly.

A two-piece cotton scrub suit composed of pants and a shirt is the standard attire for OR personnel. The use and laundering of scrub suits has not been carefully studied, but the Association of periOperative Registered Nurses (AORN) recommends that scrubs be changed between operations only when visibly soiled, contaminated, or penetrated by blood or possibly infected matter[99] (category IB recommendation). This practice also meets OSHA regulations. How to launder surgical scrubs and whether a coat is needed to cover scrubs when the person is not in the OR are unresolved issues.

The material used in gowns and drapes must be impermeable to liquids and viruses, comfortable, and cost-effective. Thick plastic fits the bill but is intolerably hot and causes increased sweating. More practical fabrics, both disposable and reusable, are now available. The most common disposable materials are spun-lace cloth (a wood pulp–polyester blend manufactured by the hydroentanglement process) in a spun-bond/melt-blown/spun-bond (SMS) laminate of 100% polypropylene. Formerly, the most commonly reusable fabrics were worn woven cotton or a 50%/50% cotton-polyester blend treated with a water-repellent chemical. However, these fabrics are being replaced by very high thread count polyester fabrics and fabrics made of expanded polytetrafluoroethylene (PTFE).

Gowns vary in their ability to prevent blood strike-through. These variations have been measured in the laboratory and in the OR[100,101] and are determined by the kind of material used and the manufacture and design of the gown. No single type of gown can be recommended as the best for all circumstances. In addition to impermeability, comfort, and cost, the conditions to which the gown will be subjected must also be taken into account. If, for instance, no blood comes in contact with the outside of the gown, then any gown is safe because no blood can strike through; however, if large amounts of blood come in contact with the gown, strike-through is almost inevitable (occurring in 93% of cases), and most gowns will eventually fail. The amount of blood on the outside of the gown is one of the most important factors; however, physical stresses on the fabric (such as abrasion, pressure, or stretching) and increasing the duration of exposure through blood will also degrade gown performance and allow blood strike-through.

Additional barriers used to separate sterile and nonsterile areas during the operative procedure include adhesive plastic barrier sheets and plastic ring drapes. Adhesive incise drapes have been evaluated in several studies; whether or not they are impregnated with iodine, they have not proved superior to standard skin preparation and draping procedures in controlling SSI. However, if the adhesive plastic drape becomes separated from the skin during the operation, the infection rate increases.[17,102] Plastic ring drapes are inserted into the wound to cover the wound edges during a procedure. As with the adhesive plastic drape, use of plastic ring drapes has not been shown to decrease SSI rates.[103]

The final CDC recommendation is to use surgical gowns and drapes that resist liquid penetration and remain effective barriers when wet (category IB recommendation).

The rubber sterile drapes worn by all scrubbed members of the surgical team serve two purposes: (1) they protect patients against transmission of microorganisms from the hands of the team, and (2) they protect the team from the patient's contaminated blood and fluids. If a glove is punctured or torn, it should be changed as promptly as is safe. One study found a 13% incidence of punctured gloves at the end of a procedure but could not correlate this with increases in bacterial counts.[104]

The use of double gloving, the length of the procedure, and the type of procedure affect the penetration rate.[104,105] OSHA recommends that all members of the scrubbed surgical team put on sterile gloves after donning a sterile gown (category IB recommendation).

Surgical masks are traditionally worn to prevent potential bacterial contamination of the operative field. Even this belief has come into question.[106] In a series of studies in which no masks were worn for 6 months, the SSI rate compared favorably with the rates reported in the preceding 4 years, when masks were required.[107] Other studies have demonstrated no patient benefit from masks. Masks, can, however, protect the wearer from inadvertent exposure to bodily fluids and blood. OSHA regulations therefore require masks to be used in combination with protective eyewear (e.g., goggles or glasses with shields) whenever spray, splatter, droplets, or potentially infected fluids may be generated and facial contamination can be reasonably anticipated.[108] In addition, a respirator certified with a protection factor of N95 or higher is required for staff members working directly with patients who have suspected or proven infectious tuberculosis. The recommendation is to wear a mask that fully covers the nose and mouth when entering an OR with sterile instruments exposed and to wear this mask throughout the operation (category IB recommendation, OSHA).

Surgical caps or hoods that fully cover head or facial hair can reduce contamination from the hair and scalp. They are required by OSHA and should be worn on entry into a sterile OR (category IB recommendation).

Although shoe covers have never been shown to decrease SSI rates or bacterial counts in the OR floor,[109] they may protect members of the surgical team from exposure to blood and fluids. OSHA regulations require that shoe covers or boots be worn when gross contamination can reasonably be anticipated (e.g., during orthopedic procedures or in cases of penetrating trauma)[110] (category IB recommendation).

The CDC and AORN recommendations, taken together, represent the best current approaches to codifying the traditions and data available for the OR. Unfortunately, in many cases, the data are insufficient either to support the efficacy of a given OR procedure or to permit a rational choice among alternatives. Acquisition of randomized data is inherently difficult and, for many issues, is unlikely to be forthcoming. The most rational approach to the OR environment combines CDC recommendations and OSHA regulations into a logical, cost-effective, and safe approach to the problems of OR asepsis.

SSI Surveillance

SSI prevention attracts the attention of hospital quality-improvement programs because SSIs, though rarely lethal, result in the expenditure of extra health care dollars.[110] SSI prevention is largely the responsibility of surgeons and other members of surgical teams. With careful use of information obtained by SSI surveillance activity, it may be possible to demonstrate that a practice should more closely address specific SSI prevention techniques. Up-to-date standards for SSI prevention are available from the CDC in a comprehensive, detailed clinical-practice guideline.[85,111]

SSI surveillance entails detection and analysis of SSIs within 30 days of an operation; an infection control nurse is usually in charge of this activity. It is essential to report SSI rates and certain facts regarding each patient with an SSI to surgeons.[112] Such case facts must include whether antibiotic prophylaxis was used correctly, the details of skin wound management, and various characteristics of the patient that may be considered risk factors for SSI development. It is also prudent to gather ancillary information, such as laboratory culture results.

Although it is impossible to establish in scientifically rigorous clinical experiments that performance of SSI surveillance favorably influences SSI risk in practice, there is suggestive evidence to support the notion.[85,110] It is recommended that SSI surveillance information be reported regularly to surgical teams, but there is no evidence that a particular reporting interval for SSI case facts and rates is optimal. Many hospitals with surveillance programs make such reports monthly or quarterly.

Finally, it is not necessary that every kind of operation performed be subjected to SSI surveillance. The CDC recommends focusing SSI surveillance on particular segments of a hospital's surgical caseload, as determined by procedure volume or intrinsic SSI risk.[85]

References

1. Requirements of construction and equipment for hospitals and medical facilities. Health and Human Services Publication (HRS-M-HF-84-1), Rockville, Maryland, 1984

2. Symposium on operating room hazard control. Laufman H, Ed. Arch Surg 107:552, 1973

3. Klebanoff G: Operating-room design: an introduction. Bull Am Coll Surg 64(11):6, 1979

4. Laufman H: The control of operating room infection: discipline, defense mechanisms, drugs, design, and devices. Bull NY Acad Med 54:465, 1978

5. Drake CT, Goldman E, Nichols RL, et al: Environmental air and airborne infections. Ann Surg 185:219, 1977

6. Hambraeus A, Bengtsson S, Laurell G: Bacterial contamination in a modern operating suite: II. Effect of a zoning system on contamination of floors and other surfaces. J Hyg [Camb] 80:57, 1978

7. Hambraeus A, Bengtsson S, Laurell G: Bacterial contamination in a modern operating suite: III. Importance of floor contamination as a source of airborne bacteria. J Hyg [Camb] 80:169, 1978

8. Ritter MA, Sieber JM, Carlson SR: Street shoes vs surgical footwear in the operating room. Infect Surg 3:81, 1984

9. Quraishi ZA, Blais FX, Sottile WS, et al: Movement of personnel and wound contamination. AORN J 38:146, 1983

10. Belkin NL: Clean room technology and aseptic practices in the surgical suite. J Environ Sciences 27:30, 1984

11. Noble WC, Lidwell OM, Kingston D: The size distribution of airborne particles carrying microorganisms. J Hyg 61:385, 1963

12. Sukuki A, Yoshimichi N, Matsuura M, et al: Airborne contamination in an operating suite: report of a five-year survey. J Hyg 93:567, 1984

13. Anderson PA, Hambraeus A, Zettersten U, et al: A comparison between tracer gas and tracer particle techniques in evaluating the efficiency of ventilation in operating theatres. J Hyg 91:509, 1983

14. Fitzgerald RH Jr: Microbiologic environment of the conventional operating room. Arch Surg 114:772, 1979

15. Walter CW, Kundsin RB: The airborne component of wound contamination and infection. Arch Surg 107:588, 1973

16. Lidwell OM, Lowbury EJL, Whyte W, et al: Infection and sepsis after operations for total hip or knee-joint replacement: influence of ultraclean air, prophylactic antibiotics and other factors. J Hyg 93:505, 1984

17. Cruse PJ, Foord R: The epidemiology of wound infection: a 10-year prospective study of 62,939 wounds. Surg Clin North Am 60:27, 1980

18. McQuarrie DG, Glover JL: Laminar airflow systems: a 1991 update. Am Coll Surg Bull 76:18, 1991

19. Howe CW: Bacterial flora of clean wounds and its relation to subsequent sepsis. Am J Surg 107:696, 1964

20. Maki DG, Alvarado CJ, Hassemer CA, et al: Relation of the inanimate hospital environment to endemic nosocomial infection. N Engl J Med 307:1562, 1982

21. Howe CW, Marston AT: Qualitative and quantitative bacteriologic studies on hospital air as related to postoperative wound sepsis. J Lab Clin Med 61:808, 1963

22. Beck WC, Frank F: The open door in the operating room. Am J Surg 125:592, 1973

23. Chinyanga HM: Temperature regulation and anesthesia. Pharmacol Ther 26:147, 1984

24. Beck WC: Choosing surgical illumination. Am J Surg 140:327, 1980

25. Beck WC: Operating room illumination: the current state of the art. Bull Am Coll Surg 66(5):10, 1981

26. Kern KA: The National Patient Safety Foundation: what it offers surgeons. Bull Am Coll Surg 83:24, 1998

27. Fuchs VR: Economics, values, and health care reform. Am Econ Rev 86:1, 1996

28. National Academy of Science/National Institute of Medicine/National Research Council: Work-related musculoskeletal disorders: a review of the evidence. National Academy Press, Washington, DC, 1998

29. Weinger MB, Englund CE: Ergonomic and human factors affecting anesthetic vigilance and monitoring performance in the operating room environment. Anesthesiol 73:995, 1990

30. Schmied H, Kurz A, Sessler DI, et al: Mild hypothermia increases blood loss and transfusion requirements during total hip arthroplasty. Lancet 347:289, 1996

31. AORN Recommended Practices Subcommittee: Recommended practices: electrosurgery. AORN J 41:633, 1985

32. Pearce J: Current electrosurgical practice: hazards. J Med Eng Technol 9:107, 1985

33. Bochenko WJ: A review of electrosurgical units in the operating room. J Clin Eng 2:313, 1977

34. Lobraico RV: Laser safety in health care facilities. An overview. Bull Am Coll Surg 76:16, 1991

35. Gloster HM Jr, Roenigk RK: Risk of acquiring human papillomavirus from the plume produced by the carbon dioxide laser in the treatment of warts. J Am Acad Dermatol 32:436, 1995

36. AORN Recommended Practices Subcommittee: Recommended practices: radiation safety in the operating room (including lasers). AORN J 42:920, 1985

37. Cuschieri A, Shimi S, Banting S, et al: Endoscopic ultrasonic dissection for thoracoscopic and laparoscopic surgery. Surg Endosc 7:197, 1993

38. Hurst BS, Awoniyi CA, Stephens JK, et al: Application of the cavitron ultrasonic surgical aspirator (CUSA) for gynecological laparoscopic surgery using the rabbit as an animal model. Fertil Steril 58:444, 1992

39. Wisniewski PM, Warhol MJ, Rando RF, et al: Studies on the transmission of viral disease via the CO_2 laser plume and ejecta. J Reprod Med 35:1117, 1990

40. Jewett DL, Heinsohn P, Bennett C, et al: Blood-containing aerosols generated by surgical techniques: a possible infectious hazard. Am Ind Hyg Assoc J 53:228, 1992

41. Patkin M: Ergonomics and the operating microscope. Adv Ophthalmol 37:53, 1978

42. Alarcon A, Berguer R: A comparison of operating room crowding between open and laparoscopic operations. Surg Endosc 10:916, 1996

43. Walenga JM, Fareed J: Current status on new anticoagulant and antithrombotic drugs and devices. Curr Opin Pulm Med 3:291, 1997

44. Pitts W: Is a case cart system justified? Hosp Mater Manage Q 8:71, 1986

45. Peers JG: Cleanup techniques in the operating room. Arch Surg 107:596, 1973

46. Weber DO, Gooch JJ, Wood WR, et al: Influence of operating room surface contamination on surgical wounds: a prospective study. Arch Surg 111:484, 1976

47. Daschner F: Patient-oriented hospital hygiene. Infection 38(suppl):243, 1980

48. Mangram AJ, Horan TC, Pearson ML, et al: The Hospital Infection Control Practices Advisory Committee. Guideline for prevention of surgical site infection, 1999. Am J Infect Control 27:98, 1999

49. Report of an Ad-Hoc Committee of the Committee on Trauma, Division of Medical Sciences, National Academy of Sciences-National Research Council: Postoperative wound infections: the influence of ultraviolet irradiation of the operating room and of various other factors. Ann Surg 160(suppl):1, 1964

50. McWilliams RM: There should be only one way to clean up between all surgical procedures. J Hosp Infect Contr 3:64, 1976

51. Nichols RL: The operating room. Hospital Infections, 3rd ed. Bennett JV, Brachman PS, Eds. Little, Brown & Co, Boston, 1992, p 461

52. Ayliffe GA: Role of the environment of the operating suite in surgical wound infection. Rev Infect Dis 13(suppl 10):S800, 1991

53. Martin JT: Patient positioning. Clinical Anesthesia, 2nd ed. Barash PG, Cullen BF, Stoelting RK, Eds. JB Lippincott Co, Philadelphia, 1992

54. Shapiro HM: Intracranial hypertension. Anesthesiol 43:445, 1975

55. Kerr MG, Scott DB, Samuel E: Studies of the inferior vena cava in late pregnancy. Br Med J 1:532, 1964

56. Bieniarz J, Yoshida T, Romero-Salinas G, et al: Aortocaval compression by the uterus in late human pregnancy. IV. Circulatory homeostasis by preferential perfusion of the placenta. Am J Obstet Gynecol 103:19, 1968

57. Wahba RW, Tessler MJ: Misleading end-tidal CO_2 tensions. Can J Anaesth 43:862, 1996

58. Cheney FW, Domino KB, Caplan RA, et al: Nerve injury associated with anesthesia: a closed claims analysis. Anesthesiol 90:1062, 1999

59. Warner MA, Warner ME, Martin J: Ulnar neuropathy. Anesthesiol 81:1332, 1994

60. Abel RR, Lewis GM: Postoperative alopecia. Arch Dermatol 81:72, 1960

61. Alexandrakis G, Lam BL: Bilateral posterior ischemic optic neuropathy after spinal surgery. Am J Ophthalmol 127:354, 1999

62. Venous air emboli in sitting and supine patients undergoing vestibular schwannoma resection. Neurosurgery 42:1282, 1998

63. Dominguez J, Rivas JJ, Lobato RD, et al: Irreversible tetraplegia after tracheal resection. Ann Thorac Surg 62:278, 1996

64. Tattersall MP: Massive swelling of the face and tongue: a complication of posterior cranial fossa surgery in the sitting position. Anaesthesia 39:1015, 1984

65. Brown DG, Wetterstroem N, Finch J: Anesthetic gas exposure: protecting the OR environment. AORN J 41:590, 1985

66. Buring JE, Hennekens CH, Mayrent SL, et al: Health experiences of operating room personnel. Anesthesiol 62:325, 1985

67. Spence AA, Cohen EN, Brown BW Jr, et al: Occupational hazards for operating room-based physicians: analysis of data from the United States and the United Kingdom. JAMA 238:955, 1977

68. Spence AA: Environmental pollution by inhalation anaesthetics. Br J Anaesth 59:96, 1987

69. Tannenbaum TN, Goldberg RJ: Exposure to anesthetic gases and reproductive outcome: a review of the epidemiologic literature. J Occup Med 27:659, 1985

70. Vessey MP: Epidemiological studies of the occupational hazards of anaesthesia—a review. Anaesthesia 33:430, 1978

71. Bruce DL, Bach MJ: Effects of trace anaesthetic gases on behavioral performance of volunteers. Br J Anaesth 48:871, 1976

72. National Institute for Occupational Safety and Health: Criteria for a recommended standard: occupational exposure to waste anesthetic gases and vapors. US Department of Health, Education and Welfare (NIOSH) Publication No. 77-140, Washington, DC, 1977

73. Flemming DC, Johnstone RE: Recognition thresholds for diethyl ether and halothane. Anesthesiol 46:68, 1977

74. Working Committee of the International Agency for Research: Cancer, Feb. 1994. Health Indus Manufac Assoc Bull, Washington, DC, 1994

75. Tokars JI, Marcus R, Culver DH, et al: Surveillance of HIV infection and zidovudine among healthcare workers after occupational exposure to HIV infected blood. Ann Intern Med 118:913, 1993

76. Association of Operating Room Nurses: Recommended practices for standard and transmission-based precautions in the perioperative practice setting. AORN J 69:404, 1999

77. Sever LE, Gilbert ES, Hessol NA, et al: A case-control study of congenital malformations and occupational exposure to low-level ionizing radiation. Am J Epidemiol 127:226, 1988

78. Dunn K, Yoshimaru H, Otake M, et al: Prenatal exposure to ionizing radiation and subsequent development of seizures. Am J Epidemiol 131:114, 1990

79. Draper GJ, Little MP, Sorahan T, et al: Cancer in the offspring of radiation workers: a record linkage study. BMJ 8:1181, 1997

80. Swartz HM, Reichling BA: Hazards of radiation exposure for pregnant women. JAMA 239:1907, 1978

81. Goldberg MS, Mayo NE, Levy AR: Adverse reproductive outcomes among women exposed to low levels of ionizing radiation from diagnostic radiography for adolescent idiopathic scoliosis. Epidemiology 9: 271, 1998

82. Krueger KJ, Hoffman BJ: Radiation exposure during gastroenterologic fluoroscopy: risk assessment for pregnant workers. Am J Gastroenterol 87:429, 1992

83. Arnold WP: Environmental safety including chemical dependency. Anesthesia, 3rd ed. Miller RD, Ed. Churchill Livingstone, New York, 1990, p 2409

84. Berry AJ, Katz JD: Hazards of working in the operating room. Clinical Anesthesia, 2nd ed. Barash PG, Ed. JB Lippincott Co, Philadelphia, 1992, p 98

85. Mangram AJ, Horan TC, Pearson ML, et al: The Hospital Infection Control Practices Advisory Committee: guideline for prevention of surgical site infection, 1999. Infect Cont Hosp Epidemiol 20:247, 1999

86. Simmons BP: Guidelines for the prevention of surgical wound infections. Infect Control 3:188, 1982

87. Garibaldi PA: Prevention of intraoperative wound contamination with chlorhexidine shower and scrub. J Hosp Infect 11(suppl B):5, 1988

88. Kaiser AB, Kernodle DJ, Barg NL, et al: Influence of preoperative showers on staphylococcal stain colonization: a comparative trial of antiseptic skin cleansers. Ann Thorac Surg 45:38, 1998

89. Seropian R, Reynolds BM: Wound infections after pre-operative depilatory versus razor preparation. Am J Surg 121:251, 1971

90. Alexander JW, Fischer JE, Boyajian M, et al: The influence of hair removal methods on wound infections. Arch Surg 118:347, 1983

91. Masterson TM, Rodeheaver GT, Morgan RF, et al: Bacteriologic evaluation of electric clippers for surgical hair removal. Am J Surg 148:301, 1984

92. Lowbury EJ, Lilly HA: Use of 4% chlorhexidine detergent solution and other methods of stain disinfection. Br Med J 1:510, 1973

93. Peterson AF, Rosenberg A, Alatary SD: Comparative evaluation of surgical scrub preparations. Surg Gynecol Obstet 146:63, 1978

94. Association of Operating Room Nurses: Recommended practices for skin preparation of patients. AORN J 645:813, 1996

95. Hardin WD, Nichols RL: Handwashing and patient skin preparations. Critical Issues in Operating Room Management. Malangoni MA, Ed. Lippincott-Raven, Philadelphia, 1997, p 133

96. Aly R, Maiboch HI: Comparative antibacterial efficacy of a 2 minute surgical scrub with chorhexidine gluconate, povidone-iodine, and chloroxylenol spongebrushes. Am J Infect Control 16:173, 1998

97. Coop G, Mailhot CB, Zalarm, et al: Cover gowns and the control of operating room contamination. Nurs Rev 35:263, 1986

98. Dineen P: The role of impervious drapes and gowns preventing surgical infection. Clin Orthop 96:210, 1973

99. Best practices for the prevention of surgical site infection. Education Design. Association of Operating Room Nurses, Chicago, 1998

100. Smith JW, Nichols RL: Barrier efficiency of surgical gowns: are we really protected from our patients' pathogens? Arch Surg 126:756, 1991

101. Quebbeman EJ, Telford GL, Hubbard S, et al: In-use evaluation of surgical gowns. Surg Gynecol Obstet 174:369, 1992

102. Lewis DA, Leaper DJ, Speller DCF: Prevention of bacterial colonization of wounds at operation: comparison of iodine-impregnated ('Ioban') drapes with conventional methods. J Hosp Infect 5:431, 1984

103. Nystrom PO, Broome A, Hojer H, et al: A controlled trial of a plastic wound ring drape to prevent contamination and infection in colorectal surgery. Dis Colon Rectum 27:451, 1984

104. McCue SF, Berg EW, Sanders EA: Efficacy of double-gloving as a barrier to microbial contamination during total joint anthroplasty. J Bone Joint Surg 63:811, 1981

105. Dodds RD, Guy PJ, Peacock AM, et al: Surgical glove perforation. Br J Surg 75:966, 1988

106. Tunevall TG, Jorbeck H: Influence of wearing masks on the density of airborne bacteria in the vicinity of the surgical wound. Eur J Surg 158:263, 1992

107. Tunevall TG: Postoperative wound infections and surgical face masks: a controlled study. World J Surg 15:383, 1991

108. US Department of Labor, Occupational Safety and Health Administration: Occupational exposure to bloodborne pathogens: final rule (29 CFR Part 1910.1030). Fed Register 56:64004, 1991

109. Humphreys H, Marshall RJ, Ricketts VE, et al: Theatre over-shoes do not reduce operating theatre floor bacterial counts. J Hosp Infect 17:117, 1991

110. Lee J: Surgical wound infections: surveillance for quality improvement. Surgical Infections. Fry DE, Ed. Little, Brown & Co, Boston, 1995, p 145

111. Horan TC, Gaynes RP, Martone WH, et al: CDC definitions of nosocomial surgical site infections, 1992: a modification of CDC definitions of surgical wound infections. Infect Contr Hosp Epidemiol 13:606, 1992

112. Lee JT, Olson MM: Wound infection surveillance for 85,260 consecutive operations. J Surg Outcomes 2:27, 1999

V OPERATIVE MANAGEMENT

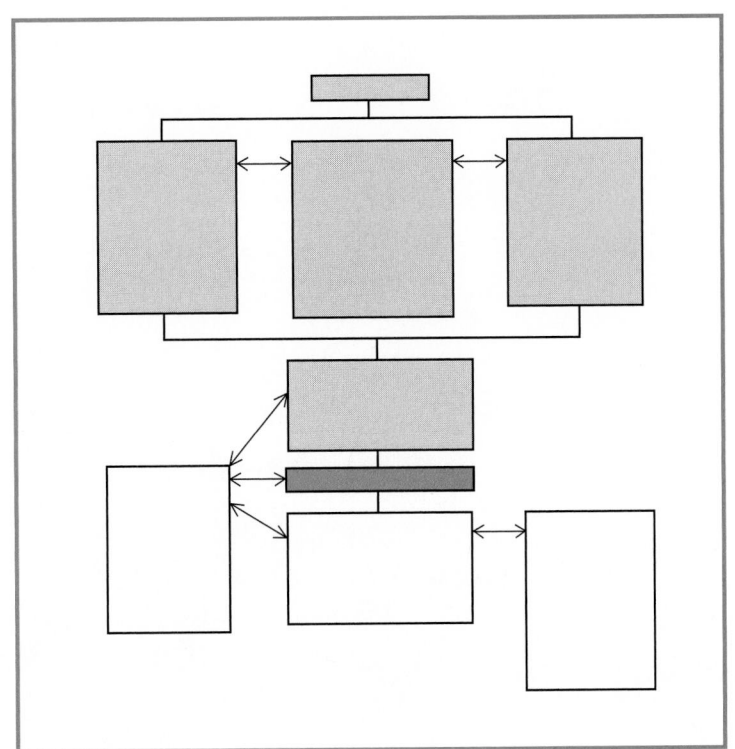

1 THYROID AND PARATHYROID PROCEDURES

Gregg H. Jossart, M.D., and Orlo H. Clark, M.D.

Thyroidectomy

OPERATIVE PLANNING

If the patient has had any hoarseness or has undergone a neck operation before, indirect or direct (ideally, fiberoptic) laryngoscopy is essential to determine whether the vocal cords are functioning normally. All patients scheduled for thyroidectomy should be euthyroid at the time of operation; in all other respects, they should be prepared as they would be for any procedure calling for general anesthesia.

Optimum exposure of the thyroid is obtained by placing a sandbag between the scapula and a foam ring under the occiput; in this way, the neck is extended, and the thyroid can assume a more anterior position. The head must be well supported to prevent postoperative posterior neck pain. The patient is placed in a 20° reverse Trendelenburg position. The skin is prepared with 1% iodine or chlorhexidine.

OPERATIVE TECHNIQUE

General Troubleshooting

Thyroid and parathyroid operations should be performed in a blood-free field so that vital structures can be identified. Operating telescopes (magnification: ×2.5 or ×3.5) are also recommended because they make it easier to identify the normal parathyroid glands and the recurrent laryngeal nerve. If bleeding occurs, pressure should be applied. The vessel should be clamped only if (1) it can be precisely identified or (2) the recurrent laryngeal nerve has been identified and is not in close proximity to the vessel.

As a rule, dissection should always be done first on the side where the suspected tumor is; if there is a problem with the dissection on this side, a less than total thyroidectomy can be performed on the contralateral side to prevent complications. There is, however, one exception to this rule: if the tumor is very extensive, the surgeon will sometimes find it easier to do the dissection on the "easy" side first to facilitate orientation with respect to the trachea and the esophagus.

Step 1: Incision and Mobilization of Skin Layers

A Kocher transverse incision paralleling the normal skin lines of the neck is made 1 cm caudad to the cricoid cartilage [*see Figure 1*]. As a rule, the incision should be about 4 to 6 cm long and should extend from the anterior border of one sternocleidomastoid muscle to the anterior border of the other and through the platysma. Five straight Kelly clamps are placed on the dermis to facilitate dissection, which proceeds first cephalad in a subplatysmal plane anterior to the anterior jugular veins and posterior to the platysma to the level of the thyroid cartilage notch and then caudad to the suprasternal notch. Skin towels and a self-retaining retractor are then applied.

Troubleshooting   Placing the incision 1 cm below the cricoid locates it precisely over the isthmus of the thyroid gland. The course of the incision should conform to the normal skin lines or creases. The length of the incision should be modified as necessary for good exposure. Patients with short, thick necks, low-lying thyroid glands, or large thyroid tumors require longer incisions than those with long, thin necks and small tumors. Patients whose necks do not extend also require longer incisions for adequate exposure. A sterile marking pen should be used to mark the midline of the neck, the level at which the incision should be made (i.e., 1 cm below the cricoid), and the lateral margins of the incision (which should be at equal distances from the midline so that the incision will be symmetrical). A scalpel should never be used to mark the neck: doing so will leave an unsightly scar in some patients. To mark the incision site itself, a 2-0 silk tie should be pressed against the neck [*see Figure 1*].

The upper flap is dissected first by placing five straight Kelly clamps on the dermis and retracting anteriorly and superiorly. Lateral traction with a vein retractor or an Army-Navy retractor

Figure 1   **The initial incision in a thyroidectomy is made 1 cm below the cricoid cartilage and follows normal skin lines. A sterile marking pen is used to mark the midline of the neck, the level of the incision, and the lateral borders of the incision. A 2-0 silk tie is pressed against the neck to mark the incision site itself.[2]**

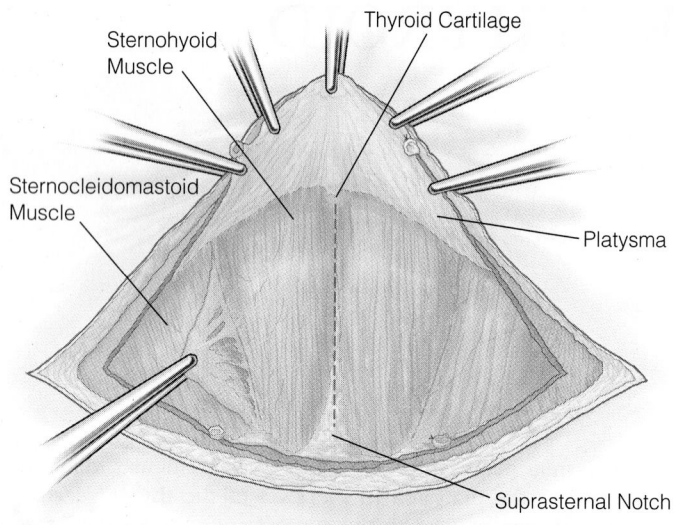

Figure 2 **To expose the thyroid, a midline incision is made through the superficial layer of deep cervical fascia between the strap muscles. The incision is begun at the suprasternal notch and extended to the thyroid cartilage.**[3]

helps identify the semilunar plane for dissection. This blood-free plane is deep to the platysma and superficial to the anterior jugular veins. Cephalad dissection can be done quickly with the electrocautery or a scalpel, and lateral dissection can be done bluntly. The same principles are applied to dissection of the lower flap. In thin patients, the surgeon must be careful not to dissect through the skin from within, especially at the level of the thyroid cartilage.

Step 2: Midline Dissection and Mobilization of Strap Muscles

The thyroid gland is exposed via a midline incision through the superficial layer of deep cervical fascia between the strap muscles. Because the strap muscles are farthest apart just above the suprasternal notch, the incision is begun at the notch and extended to the thyroid cartilage [*see Figure 2*].

On the side where the thyroid nodule or the suspected parathyroid adenoma is located, the more superficial sternohyoid muscle is separated from the underlying sternothyroid muscle by blunt dissection, which is extended laterally until the ansa cervicalis becomes visible on the lateral edge of the sternothyroid muscle and on the medial side of the internal jugular vein. The sternothyroid muscle is then dissected free from the thyroid and the prethyroidal fascia by blunt or sharp dissection until the middle thyroid vein or veins are encountered laterally.

A 2-0 silk suture is placed deeply through the thyroid lobe for retraction to facilitate exposure. This stitch should never be placed through the thyroid nodule: doing so could cause seeding of thyroid cancer cells. The thyroid is retracted anteriorly and medially and the carotid sheath laterally; this retraction places tension on the middle thyroid veins and helps expose the area posterolateral to the thyroid, where the parathyroid glands and the recurrent laryngeal nerves are situated. The middle thyroid veins are divided to give better exposure behind the upper lobe of the thyroid [*see Figure 3*].

Troubleshooting As a rule, it is not necessary to divide the strap muscles; however, if they are adherent to the underlying thyroid tumor, the portion of the muscle that is adhering to the

tumor should be sacrificed and allowed to remain attached to the thyroid. Separation of the sternohyoid muscle from the sternothyroid muscle provides better exposure of the operative field. The middle thyroid veins should be cleaned of adjacent tissues to prevent any injury to the recurrent laryngeal nerve when these veins are ligated and divided. It is always safest to mobilize tissues parallel to the recurrent laryngeal nerve.

Step 3: Division of Isthmus

When a thyroid lobectomy is to be performed, the isthmus of the thyroid gland is usually divided with Dandy or Colodny clamps at an early point in dissection to facilitate the subsequent mobilization of the thyroid gland. The thyroid tissue that is to remain is oversewn with a 2-0 silk ligature. To minimize the chance of invasion into the trachea or to avoid a visible mass in patients with compensatory thyroid hypertrophy, thyroid tissues should not be left anterior to the trachea.

Troubleshooting With larger glands, we divide the isthmus first. This step facilitates the lateral dissection by making the gland more mobile.

Step 4: Mobilization of Thyroid Gland and Identification of Upper Parathyroid Glands

Once the isthmus has been divided, dissection is continued superiorly, laterally, and posteriorly with a small sponge on a peanut clamp. The superior thyroid artery and veins are identified by retracting the thyroid inferiorly and medially. The tissues lateral to the upper lobe of the thyroid and medial to the carotid sheath can be mobilized caudally to the cricothyroid muscle; the recurrent laryngeal nerve enters the cricothyroid muscle at the level of the cricoid cartilage, first passing through Berry's ligament [*see Figure 4*]. The superior pole vessels are individually identified, skeletonized, double- or triple-clamped, ligated, and divided low on the thyroid gland [*see Figure 5*]. To prevent injury to the external laryngeal nerve, the vessels are divided and ligated on the thyroid surface, the thyroid is retracted laterally and caudally, and dissection is carried out on the medial edge of the thyroid gland and lateral to the cricothyroid muscle. The tis-

Figure 3 **The middle thyroid veins are divided to give better exposure behind the upper lobe of the thyroid.**[2]

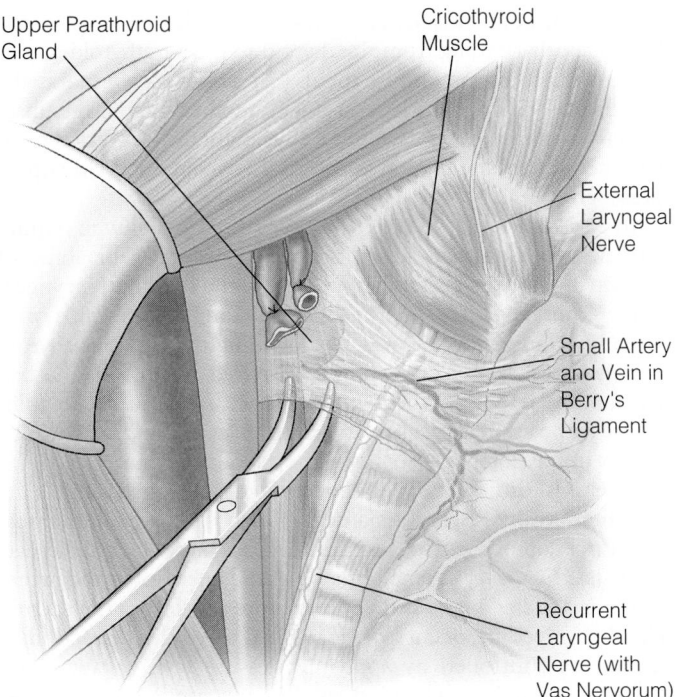

Figure 4 **The recurrent laryngeal nerve enters the cricothyroid muscle at the level of the cricoid cartilage, first passing through Berry's ligament.**[2]

sues posterior and lateral to the superior pole that have not already been mobilized can now be easily swept by blunt dissection away from the thyroid gland medially and anteriorly and away from the carotid sheath laterally. The upper parathyroid gland is often identified at this time at the level of the cricoid cartilage.

Troubleshooting It is essential to keep from injuring the external laryngeal nerve. This nerve is the motor branch of the superior laryngeal nerve and is responsible for tensing the vocal cords; it is also known as the high note nerve or the Amelita Galli-Curci nerve. In about 80% of patients, the external laryngeal nerve runs on the surface of the cricothyroid muscle; in about 10%, it runs with the superior pole vessels; and in the remaining 10%, it runs within the cricothyroid muscle. Given that this nerve is usually about the size of a single strand of a spider web, one should generally try to avoid it rather than to identify it. Injury to the external laryngeal nerve occurs in as many as 10% of patients undergoing thyroidectomy. The best ways of preventing such injury are (1) to provide gentle traction on the thyroid gland in a caudal and lateral direction and (2) to ligate the superior pole vessels directly on the capsule of the upper pole individually and low on the thyroid gland rather than to cross-clamp the entire superior pole pedicle.

The internal laryngeal nerve is the sensory branch of the superior laryngeal nerve; it provides sensory innervation to the posterior pharynx. Injury to this nerve can result in aspiration. Because the internal laryngeal nerve typically is cephalad to the area of dissection during thyroidectomy and runs cephalad to the lateral portion of the thyroid cartilage, it usually is at risk only when the surgeon dissects cephalad to the thyroid cartilage. Such dissection is necessary only when laryngeal mobilization is performed to relieve tension on the tracheal anastomosis after tracheal resection.

Step 5: Identification of Recurrent Laryngeal Nerves and Lower Parathyroid Glands

When the thyroid lobe is further mobilized, the lower parathyroid gland is usually seen; this gland is almost always located anterior to the recurrent laryngeal nerve and is usually located inferior to where the inferior thyroid artery crosses the recurrent laryngeal nerve [*see Figure 6*]. The carotid sheath is retracted laterally, and the thyroid gland is retracted anteriorly and medially. This retraction puts tension on the inferior thyroid artery and consequently on the recurrent laryngeal nerve, thereby facilitating the identification of the nerve. The recurrent laryngeal nerve is situated more medially on the left (running in the tracheoesophageal groove) and more obliquely on the right. Dissection should proceed cephalad along the lateral edge of the thyroid. Fatty and lymphatic tissues immediately adjacent to the thyroid gland are swept from it with a peanut clamp, and small vessels are ligated. No tissue should be transected until one is sure that it is not the recurrent laryngeal nerve.

Troubleshooting The upper parathyroid glands are usually situated on each side of the thyroid gland at the level where the recurrent laryngeal nerve enters the cricothyroid muscle [*see Figure 6*]. Because the recurrent laryngeal nerve enters the cricothyroid muscle at the level of the cricoid cartilage, the area cephalad to the cricoid cartilage is relatively safe.

The right and left recurrent laryngeal nerves must be preserved during every thyroid operation. Although both nerves enter at the posterior medial position of the larynx in the cricothyroid muscle, their courses vary considerably. The right recurrent laryngeal nerve takes a more oblique course than the left recurrent laryngeal nerve and may pass either anterior or posterior to the inferior thyroid artery. In about 0.5% of persons, the right recurrent laryngeal nerve is in fact nonrecurrent and may enter the thyroid from a superior or lateral direction.[1] On rare occasions, both a recurrent and a nonrecurrent laryn-

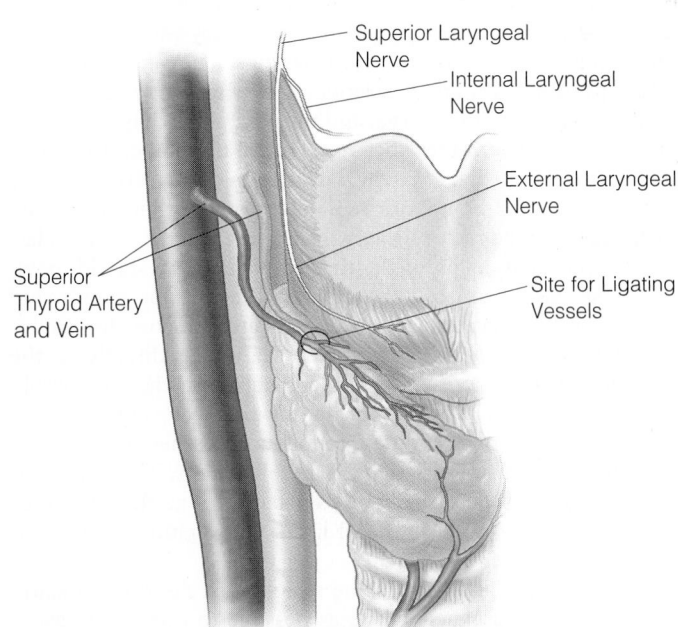

Figure 5 **The superior pole vessels should be individually identified and ligated low on the thyroid gland to minimize the chances of injury to the external laryngeal nerve.**[2]

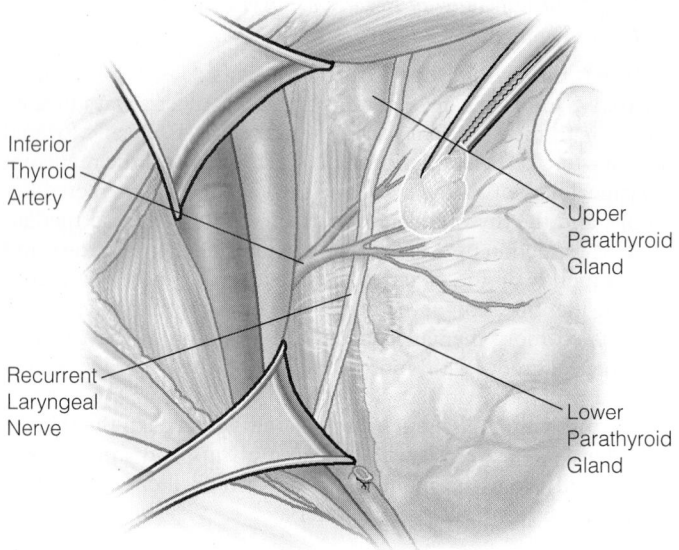

Figure 6 **The upper parathyroid glands are usually situated on either side of the thyroid at the level where the recurrent laryngeal nerve enters the cricothyroid muscle. The lower parathyroid glands are usually anterior to the recurrent laryngeal nerve and inferior to where the inferior thyroid artery crosses this nerve.**[2]

Labels on figure: Inferior Thyroid Artery; Recurrent Laryngeal Nerve; Upper Parathyroid Gland; Lower Parathyroid Gland

geal nerve may be present on the right. The left recurrent laryngeal nerve almost always runs in the tracheoesophageal groove because of its deeper origin within the thorax as it loops around the ductus arteriosus. Either recurrent laryngeal nerve may branch before entering the larynx; the left nerve is more likely to do this. Such branching is important to recognize because all of the motor fibers of the recurrent laryngeal nerve are usually in the most medial branch.

In identifying the recurrent laryngeal nerves, it is helpful to remember that they are supplied by a small vascular plexus and that a tiny vessel runs parallel to and directly on each nerve [*see Figures 4 and 6*]. In young persons, the artery usually is readily distinguished from the recurrent laryngeal nerve; however, in older persons with arteriosclerosis, the white-appearing artery may be mistaken for a nerve, and thus the nerve may be injured as a result of the misidentification. Lateral traction on the carotid sheath and medial and anterior traction on the thyroid gland place tension on the inferior thyroid artery; this maneuver often helps identify the recurrent laryngeal nerve where it courses lateral to the midportion of the thyroid gland. One should, however, be careful not to devascularize the inferior parathyroid glands by dividing the lateral vascular attachments: to remove the thyroid lobe, it is best to divide the vessels directly on the thyroid capsule to preserve the blood supply to the parathyroid glands. It is usually safest to identify the recurrent laryngeal nerve low in the neck and then to follow it to where it enters the cricothyroid muscle through Berry's ligament. The recurrent laryngeal nerves can usually be palpated through the surrounding tissue in the neck; they feel like a taut ligature of approximately 2-0 gauge.

Parathyroid glands should be swept from the thyroid gland on as broad a vascular pedicle as possible to prevent devascularization. When it is unclear whether a parathyroid gland can be saved on its own vascular pedicle, one should biopsy the gland to confirm that it is parathyroid and then autotransplant it in multiple 1 × 1 mm pieces into separate pockets in the ster-

nocleidomastoid muscle. At times, it is preferable to clip the blood vessels running from the thyroid to the parathyroid glands rather than to clamp and tie them. Clipping not only marks the parathyroid gland (which is useful if another operation subsequently becomes necessary) but also enables the gland to remain with minimal manipulation and with its remaining blood supply preserved.

In patients who have extensive thyroid tumors or who require reoperation, extensive scarring is often present. For some of these patients, it is preferable to identify the recurrent laryngeal nerve from a medial approach by dividing the isthmus with Colodny clamps and ligating and dividing the superior thyroid vessels. By carefully dissecting the thyroid away from the trachea, one can identify the recurrent laryngeal nerve at the point where its position is most consistent (i.e., at its entrance into the larynx immediately posterior to the cricothyroid muscle).

The most difficult part of dissection in a thyroidectomy is the part that involves Berry's ligament, which is situated at the posterior portion of the thyroid gland just caudal to the cricoid cartilage [*see Figure 4*]. A small branch of the inferior thyroid artery traverses the ligament, as do one or more veins from the thyroid gland. If bleeding occurs during this part of the dissection, it should be controlled by applying pressure with a gauze pad. Nothing should be clamped in this area until the recurrent laryngeal nerve is identified. In some patients (about 15%), the peduncle of Zuckerkandl, a small protuberance of thyroid tissue on the right, tends to obscure the recurrent laryngeal nerve at the level of Berry's ligament.

Step 6: Mobilization of Pyramidal Lobe

The pyramidal lobe is found in about 80% of patients. It extends in a cephalad direction, often through the notch in the thyroid cartilage to the hyoid bone. One or more lymph nodes are frequently found just cephalad to the isthmus of the thyroid gland over the cricothyroid membrane (so-called Delphian nodes) [*see Figure 7*]. The pyramidal lobe is mobilized by retracting it caudally and by dissecting immediately adjacent to it in a cephalad direction. Small vessels are coagulated or ligated.

Step 7: Thyroid Resection

Once the parathyroid glands have been carefully swept or dissected from the thyroid gland and the recurrent nerve has been identified, the thyroid lobe can be quickly resected. For total thyroidectomy, the same operation is done again on the other side.

Troubleshooting The thyroid lobe or gland should be carefully examined after removal. If a parathyroid gland is identified, a biopsy of it should be performed to confirm that it is parathyroid and then autotransplanted. In a thyroid procedure, every parathyroid gland should be treated as if it is the last one, and at least one parathyroid gland should be definitely identified. As a rule, biopsies should not be performed on normal parathyroid glands during a thyroid procedure.

Step 8: Closure

The sternothyroid muscles are approximated with 4-0 absorbable sutures, and a small opening is left in the midline at the suprasternal notch to make any bleeding that occurs more evident and to allow the blood to exit. The sternohyoid muscles are reapproximated in a similar fashion, as is the platysma. The skin is then closed with butterfly clips, which are hemostatic and inexpensive and permit precise alignment of the skin edges. (In children, the skin is closed with a subcuticular stitch and Steri-

Strips instead.) A sterile pressure dressing is applied.

Special Concerns

Invasion of the trachea or the esophagus On rare occasions, thyroid or parathyroid cancers may invade the trachea or the esophagus. As much as 5 cm of the trachea can be resected safely, without impairment of the patient's voice. If the invasion is not extensive and is confined to the anterior portion of the trachea, a small section of the trachea that contains the tumor should be excised, and a tracheostomy may be placed at the site of resection. If the invasion is more extensive or occurs in the lateral or posterior portion of the trachea, a segment of the trachea measuring several centimeters long is resected, and the remaining segments are reanastomosed. To prevent tension on the anastomosis, the trachea should be mobilized before resection, the recurrent laryngeal nerves should be preserved and mobilized from the trachea, and the mylohyoid fascia and muscles should be divided above the thyroid cartilage to drop the cartilage. Pains must be taken not to injure the internal laryngeal nerves during this dissection, given that these nerves course from lateral to medial just above the lateral aspects of the thyroid cartilage. After resection, the trachea is reapproximated with 3-0 Maxon sutures. One or two Penrose drains should be left near the resection site to allow air to exit. The drains are removed after several days, when there is no more evidence of air leakage.

If the esophagus is invaded by tumor, the muscular wall of the esophagus can be resected along with the tumor, with the inner esophageal layer left in place.

Neck dissection for nodal metastases Lymph nodes in the central neck (medial to the carotid sheath) are frequently involved in patients with papillary, medullary, and Hürthle cell cancer. These nodes should be removed without injury to the parathyroid glands or the recurrent laryngeal nerves. In most patients, it is relatively easy to remove all tissue between the carotid sheath and the trachea. In some patients with extensive lymphadenopathy, it is necessary to remove the parathyroids, perform biopsies on them to confirm that they are in fact parathyroid, and autotransplant them into the sternocleidomastoid muscle.

When lymph nodes are palpable in the lateral neck, a modified neck dissection is performed through a lateral extension of the Kocher collar incision to the anterior margin of the trapezius muscle (a MacFee incision). The jugular vein, the spinal accessory nerve, the phrenic nerve, the vagus nerve, the cervical sympathetic nerves, and the sternocleidomastoid muscle are preserved unless they are directly adherent to or invaded by tumor.

In patients with medullary thyroid cancer, a meticulous and thorough central neck dissection is necessary. When a primary medullary tumor is larger than 1 cm or the central neck nodes are obviously involved, these patients will also benefit from a lateral modified radical neck dissection (with the structures just mentioned preserved). During the dissection, all fibrofatty lymph node tissues should be removed from the level of the clavicle to the level of the hyoid bone. The deep dissection plane is developed anterior to the scalenus anticus muscle, the brachial plexus, and the scalenus medius muscle. The phrenic nerve runs obliquely on the scalenus anticus muscle. The cervical sensory nerves can usually be preserved unless there is extensive tumor involvement.

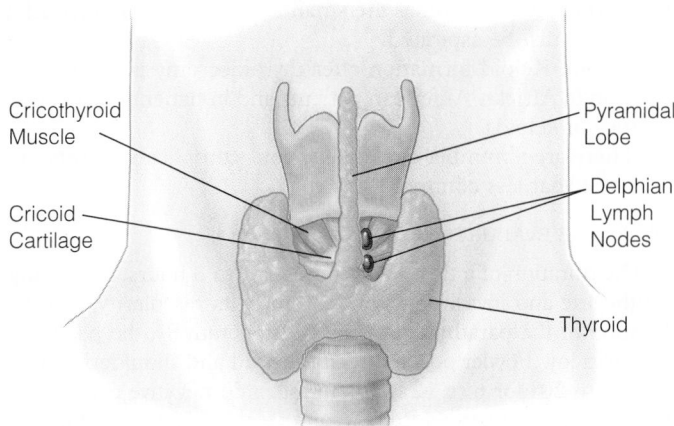

Figure 7 Delphian lymph nodes may be found just cephalad to the isthmus over the cricothyroid membrane.

Median sternotomy A median sternotomy is rarely necessary for removal of the thyroid gland because the blood supply to the thyroid gland, the thymus, and the lower parathyroid glands derives primarily from the inferior thyroid arteries in the neck. Metastatic lymph nodes frequently extend inferiorly in the tracheoesophageal groove into the superior mediastinum; these nodes can almost always be removed through a cervical incision without any need for a sternotomy. On rare occasions, metastatic nodes spread to the aortic pulmonary window and can be identified preoperatively on CT or MRI. If a median sternotomy proves necessary, the sternum should be divided to the level of the third intercostal space and then laterally on one side at the space between the third rib and the fourth. Median sternotomy provides excellent exposure of the upper anterior mediastinum and the lower neck.

COMPLICATIONS

The following are the most significant complications of thyroidectomy.

1. Injury to the recurrent laryngeal nerve. Bilateral injury to the recurrent laryngeal nerve may result in vocal cord paresis and stridor and may have to be treated with a tracheostomy.
2. Hypoparathyroidism. This complication may arise as the result of removal of, injury to, or devascularization of the parathyroid glands. As noted [*see* Operative Technique, *above*], we recommend leaving parathyroid glands on their own vascular pedicle; however, if one is concerned about possible devascularization of a parathyroid, biopsy should be performed on the gland to confirm its identity and then autotransplanted in 1 × 1 mm pieces into separate pockets in the sternocleidomastoid muscle.
3. Bleeding. Postoperative bleeding can be life threatening in that it can compromise the airway. Any postoperative respiratory distress can be thought of as attributable to a neck hematoma until proved otherwise. Most bleeding occurs within four hours of operation, and virtually all occurs within 24 hours.
4. Injury to the external laryngeal nerve [*see* Operative Technique, *above*].
5. Infection. This complication is quite rare after thyroidectomy. Any patient with acute pharyngitis should not undergo this procedure.

6. Seroma. Most seromas are small and resorb spontaneously; some must be aspirated.
7. Keloid. Keloid formation after thyroidectomy is most common in African-American patients and in patients with a history of keloids.
8. There are a number of miscellaneous complications that are somewhat less common.

OUTCOME EVALUATION

The duration of a thyroid operation is 1 to 3 hours, depending on the size and invasiveness of the tumor, its vascularity, and the location of the parathyroid glands. Postoperatively, the patient is kept in a low Fowler position with the head and shoulders elevated 10° to 20° for 6 to 12 hours to maintain negative pressure in the veins. The patient typically resumes eating within 3 to 4 hours, and an antiemetic is ordered as needed (many patients experience postoperative nausea and emesis).

The serum calcium level is measured approximately 5 to 8 hours after operation in patients who have undergone bilateral procedures; no tests are required in those who have undergone unilateral procedures. On the first morning after the thyroidectomy, the serum calcium and serum phosphate levels are measured. If the patient is still hospitalized on postoperative day 2, these tests are repeated on the second morning as well. Oral calcium supplements are given if the serum calcium is below 7.5 mg/dl or if the patient experiences perioral numbness or tingling. A low serum phosphate level (< 2.5 mg/dl) usually is a sign of so-called bone hunger and suggests that there is little reason to be concerned about permanent hypoparathyroidism, whereas a high level (> 4.5 mg/dl) should prompt concern about permanent hypoparathyroidism.

The surgical clips are removed on postoperative day 1, and Steri-Strips are applied to prevent tension on the healing wound. Patients usually are discharged on the first day, are given a prescription for thyroid hormone (L-thyroxine, 0.1 to 0.2 mg/day orally) if the procedure was more extensive than a thyroid lobectomy, and are told to take calcium tablets for any tingling or muscle cramps. Patients with papillary, follicular, or Hürthle cell cancer should receive enough L-thyroxine to keep their serum levels of thyroid-stimulating hormone (TSH) below 0.1 mIU/ml. The Steri-Strips are removed on day 10, the pathology is reviewed, and further management is discussed in the light of the pathologic findings. In patients with thyroid cancer, values for serum calcium, TSH, and thyroglobulin are obtained; in patients with coexisting hyperparathyroidism, values for serum calcium, phosphorus, and parathyroid hormone (PTH) are obtained.

Most patients can return to work or full activity in 1 to 2 weeks. Patients with benign lesions who have undergone hemithyroidectomy may or may not require thyroid hormone; those with multinodular goiter, thyroiditis, or occult papillary cancer typically do, whereas those with follicular adenoma typically do not. Patients who have undergone total or near-total thyroidectomy will require thyroid hormone. Patients with papillary or follicular cancer who have undergone total or near-total thyroidectomy appear to benefit from radioactive iodine scanning and therapy. (It is necessary to discontinue L-thyroxine for 6 to 8 weeks and L-triiodothyronine for 2 weeks before scanning.) Those considered to be at low risk (age < 45 years, tumor confined to the thyroid and not invasive, and tumor diameter < 4 cm) may receive radioactive iodine on an outpatient basis in a dose of approximately 30 mCi. Those who are considered to be at high risk should receive approximately 100 to 150 mCi. Long-term (20-year) mortality is about 4% in low-risk patients and about 40% in high-risk patients. Serum thyroglobulin levels should be determined before and after discontinuance of thyroid hormone; such levels are very sensitive indicators of persistent thyroid disease after total thyroidectomy.

Parathyroidectomy

OPERATIVE PLANNING

The preparation for parathyroidectomy is the same as that for thyroidectomy. Patients who have profound hypercalcemia (serum calcium ≥ 12.5 mg/dl) or mild to moderate renal failure should be vigorously hydrated and given furosemide before operation. On rare occasions, such patients require additional treatment—for example, administration of diphosphonates, mithramycin, or calcitonin. Any electrolyte abnormalities (e.g., hypokalemia) should be corrected.

We recommend bilateral exploration for most patients undergoing initial operations for primary or secondary hyperparathyroidism. For some patients with sporadic primary hyperparathyroidism in whom one abnormal gland has been identified by sestamibi scanning, a focused operation using intraoperative PTH assay is an acceptable alternative approach. Preoperative localization studies (e.g., ultrasonography, MRI, sestamibi scanning, and CT scanning) are generally unnecessary: they provide useful information in about 75% of patients, but they are not considered cost-effective, because an experienced surgeon can treat hyperparathyroidism successfully 95% to 98% of the time. Such studies are, however, essential when reoperation for persistent or recurrent hyperparathyroidism is indicated and when a focused approach with intraoperative PTH assay is to be used. We do not believe that using the gamma probe is any better than preoperative sestamibi scanning. All patients requiring reoperation should undergo direct or indirect laryngoscopy before operation for evaluation of vocal cord function.

OPERATIVE TECHNIQUE

Steps 1 through 4

Steps 1, 2, 3, and 4 of a parathyroidectomy are virtually identical to steps 1, 2, 4, and 5 of a thyroidectomy (see above), and essentially the same troubleshooting considerations apply.

Troubleshooting About 85% of people have four parathyroid glands, and in about 85% of these persons, the parathyroids are situated on the posterior lateral capsule of the thyroid. Normal parathyroid glands measure about $3 \times 3 \times 4$ mm and are light brown in color. The upper parathyroid glands are more posterior (i.e., dorsal) and more constant in position (at the level of the cricoid cartilage) than the lower parathyroid glands, which typically are more anteriorly placed (on the posterior-lateral surface of the thyroid gland). Both the upper and the lower parathyroid glands are supplied by small branches of the inferior and superior thyroid arteries in most patients. About 15% of parathyroid glands are situated within the thymus gland, and about 1% are intrathyroidal. Other abnormal sites for the parathyroid glands are (1) the carotid sheath, (2) the anterior and posterior mediastinum, and (3) anterior to the carotid bulb or along the pharynx (undescended parathyroids).

The upper parathyroid glands are usually lateral to the recurrent laryngeal nerve at the level of Berry's ligament; their position makes them generally easier to preserve during thyroidectomy and easier to find during both parathyroid and thyroid surgery. When the upper parathyroids are not found at this site, they often can be found in the tracheoesophageal groove or in the posterior mediastinum along the esophagus. The lower parathyroid glands are almost always situated anterior to the recurrent laryngeal nerves and caudal to where the recurrent laryngeal nerve crosses the inferior thyroid artery; they may be surrounded by lymph nodes. When the lower parathyroids are not found at this site, they usually can be found in the anterior mediastinum (typically in the thymus or the thymic fat).

Step 5: Parathyroid Resection

Abnormal parathyroid glands are removed. In about 80% of patients with primary hyperparathyroidism, one parathyroid gland is abnormal; in about 15%, all glands are abnormal (diffuse hyperplasia); and in about 5%, two or three glands are abnormal and one or two normal. Parathyroid cancer occurs in about 1% of patients with primary hyperparathyroidism. About 50% of patients with parathyroid cancer have a palpable tumor, and most exhibit profound hypercalcemia (serum calcium ≥ 14.0 mg/dl).

Troubleshooting In some patients, parathyroid tumors and hyperplastic parathyroid glands are difficult to find. If this is the case, the first step is to explore the sites where parathyroids are usually located, near the posterolateral surface of the thyroid gland. (About 80% of parathyroid glands are situated within 1 cm of the point where the inferior thyroid artery crosses the recurrent laryngeal nerve.) When a lower gland is missing from the usual location, it is likely to be found in the thymus; this possibility can be confirmed by mobilizing the thymus from the anterior-superior mediastinum. In all, about 15% of parathyroid glands are found within the thymus. If an upper parathyroid gland cannot be located, one should look not only far behind the thyroid gland superiorly but also in a paraesophageal position down into the posterior mediastinum. A thyroid lobectomy or thyroidotomy should be done on the side where fewer than two parathyroid glands have been located and no abnormal parathyroid tissue has been identified. The carotid sheath and the area posterior to the carotid, as well as the retroesophageal area, should also be explored. In rare cases, there may be an undescended parathyroid tumor anterior to the carotid bulb.

Although we do not recommend routine biopsy of more than one normal-appearing parathyroid gland, we do recommend biopsy (not removal) and marking of all normal parathyroid glands that have been identified when no abnormal parathyroid tissue can be found. When four normal parathyroid glands are found in the neck, the fifth (abnormal) parathyroid gland is usually in the mediastinum. The surgeon's responsibility is to make sure during parathyroidectomy that the elusive parathyroid adenoma is not in or removable through the cervical incision used for the initial operation and to minimize complications. The risk of permanent hypoparathyroidism or injury to the recurrent nerve should be less than 2%.

Step 6: Closure

Closure is essentially the same for parathyroidectomy as for thyroidectomy.

COMPLICATIONS

The complications of parathyroidectomy are similar to those of thyroidectomy but occur less often. Patients with a very high serum alkaline phosphatase level and osteitis fibrosa cystica are prone to profound hypocalcemia after parathyroidectomy. In such patients, both serum calcium and serum phosphorus levels are low. In contrast, patients with hypoparathyroidism exhibit low serum calcium levels but high serum phosphorus levels.

OUTCOME EVALUATION

Outcome considerations are essentially the same as for thyroidectomy. The patient should have a normal voice and be normocalcemic. The overall complication rate should be less than 2%.

References

1. Henry JF, Audiffret J, Denizot A, et al: The nonrecurrent inferior laryngeal nerve: review of 33 cases, including two on the left side. Surgery 104:977, 1988
2. Clark OH: Endocrine Surgery of the Thyroid and Parathyroid Glands. CV Mosby, St Louis, 1985
3. Cady B, Rossi R: Surgery of thyroid gland. Surgery of the Thyroid and Parathyroid Glands. Cady B, Rossi R, Eds. WB Saunders Co, Philadelphia, 1991

Acknowledgment

Figures 1 through 7   Tom Moore.

Recommended Reading

Chen H, Sokol LJ, Udelsman R: Outpatient minimally invasive parathyroidectomy: a combination of sestamibi-spect localization, cervical block anesthesia, and intraoperative parathyroid hormone assay. Surgery 126:1016, 1999

Clark OH: Total thyroidectomy and lymph node dissection for cancer of the thyroid. Mastery of Surgery, 2nd ed. Nyhus LM, Baker RJ, Eds. Little, Brown and Co, Boston, 1992, p 204

Clark OH: Total thyroid lobectomy. Atlas of Surgical Oncology. Daly JM, Cady B, Low DW, Eds. CV Mosby Co, St. Louis, 1993, p 41

Gordon LL, Snyder WH, Wians JR, et al: The validity of quick intraoperative hormone assay: an evaluation of seventy-two patients based on gross morphology criteria. Surgery 126:1030, 1999

Irvin GL, Molinari AS, Figuero C, et al: Improved success rate in reoperative parathyroidectomy with intraoperative PTH assay. Ann Surg 229:874, 1999

Tezelman S, Shen W, Shaver JK, et al: Double parathyroid adenomas: clinical and biochemical characteristics before and after parathyroidectomy. Ann Surg 218:300, 1993

2 BREAST PROCEDURES

Barbara L. Smith, M.D., Ph.D., and Wiley W. Souba, M.D., Sc.D.

Since the 1970s, surgical procedures for cancer of the breast have become progressively less extensive while maintaining excellent control of local recurrence. Updates of multiple prospective, randomized trials continue to demonstrate that survival after lumpectomy, axillary dissection, and radiation therapy does not differ significantly from survival after mastectomy.[1-3] Local recurrence rates after lumpectomy and radiation therapy remain in the 10% range. At present, there are almost no remaining indications for the Halsted radical mastectomy.

The issue of the precise extent of surgical intervention necessary for evaluation and treatment of breast lesions continues to be reexamined. With the increased availability of screening mammography, a higher proportion of cancers are being detected at a nonpalpable stage (as in situ carcinomas or small invasive lesions), for which long-term survival rates range from 90% to 95% or higher. The efficacy of wide local excision without radiation in the treatment of in situ lesions is being investigated, and the need for axillary dissection in the treatment of small invasive cancers and cancers in elderly patients is being reconsidered. Improvements in imaging technology—including more refined mammographic techniques, improved breast ultrasonography, and the development of magnetic resonance imaging of the breast—are yielding enhanced diagnostic sensitivity and specificity. Stereotactic and ultrasound-guided core-needle biopsy of nonpalpable breast lesions has proved to be a less invasive and less costly alternative to open surgical biopsy that is appropriate for many patients. Fine-needle aspiration (FNA) biopsy is increasingly replacing open surgical biopsy in the diagnosis of palpable breast malignancies and is proving useful in the diagnosis of many palpable benign lesions as well.

In what follows, we describe our approach to selected common surgical procedures currently employed in the diagnosis and treatment of breast lesions, taking into account various technical and nontechnical issues raised by the growth of new technologies and the evolution of our understanding of the biology of breast diseases.

Breast Biopsy

OPTIONS FOR PALPABLE MASSES

Tissue diagnosis of a palpable breast mass may be obtained by means of FNA biopsy, core-needle biopsy, or open incisional or excisional biopsy. Needle biopsy techniques are less invasive and less costly than open biopsy but are significantly more likely to yield false negative results. The choice of a biopsy technique must be based on the clinical and radiographic features of the lesion.

Fine-Needle Aspiration Biopsy

FNA biopsy is best performed by an experienced operator. It is an appropriate first step in diagnosing most discrete palpable breast masses encountered in clinical practice. The procedure is less useful in evaluating areas of vague thickening or nodularity: such lesions often contain normal tissue mingled with malignant tissue, and the small samples obtained with FNA biopsy may not include any of the malignant cells. FNA biopsy also is not particularly useful for small masses: the mass must be large enough to permit the biopsy needle to be moved back and forth within the lesion without passing out into surrounding normal tissue and contaminating the specimen with excessive amounts of normal cells. FNA biopsy of lesions less than 1 cm in diameter is associated with an unacceptably high rate of sampling error. FNA biopsy is usually the diagnostic procedure of choice for T3 and T4 primary lesions and for chest wall and axillary recurrences for which systemic therapy or irradiation is indicated as the first treatment modality.

Discrete masses discovered on physical examination may be either cystic or solid. Unless previous ultrasonographic examination has shown the mass to be solid, the needle used should be large enough to permit aspiration of potentially viscous fluid if the lesion proves to be cystic (i.e., 20 or 21 gauge). If the mass is known to be solid, a smaller needle (22 to 25 gauge) is sufficient for obtaining diagnostic tissue and will cause the patient less discomfort. For sufficient suction to be generated, a syringe with a capacity no smaller than 10 ml should be used. A variety of syringe holders are available that facilitate application of suction with a single hand.

Technique The skin of the breast is prepared with alcohol or iodine, and the lesion to be biopsied is held steady between the thumb and the index finger of the nondominant hand. A local anesthetic is usually not necessary; if it is used, it should be injected so as to create only a small skin wheal, so that there will be minimal distortion of the approach to the lesion. To facilitate visualization of the collected sample, 1 to 2 ml of air is introduced into the biopsy syringe before the needle enters the skin. The tip of the needle is advanced into the lesion before any suction is applied to minimize collection of tissue outside the lesion. Once the tip is in place, strong suction is applied, and the needle is moved back and forth within the lesion repeatedly along a 5 to 10 mm long track to loosen and collect cells. (This oscillation of the needle along the same track is the most effective way of obtaining a cellular, diagnostic specimen.) The back-and-forth movement of the needle within the lesion is continued until tissue becomes visible in the hub of the needle. Suction is released while the needle is still within the lesion (again, to prevent collection of contaminating tissue from outside the lesion).

The needle is then withdrawn from the lesion, and its contents are expelled onto prepared glass slides, spread into a thin smear, and fixed according to the preferences of the cytology laboratory. Additional passes through the lesion may be made to ensure that a sufficiently cellular sample has been obtained, and the syringe may be rinsed so that a cell block can be prepared for further analysis. An adhesive bandage is applied to the biopsy site. If the lesion proves to be cystic, all fluid should be aspirated; this should cause the mass to disappear. The fluid need not be sent for analysis unless it is bloody or a palpable mass remains after as much fluid as possible has been aspirated.

The patient is reexamined 4 to 8 weeks after successful aspiration. If the same cyst has recurred, it should be aspirated again and the fluid sent for cytologic analysis.

Interpretation of results Analysis by an experienced cytologist is critical for accurate interpretation of FNA biopsy results. Many cytology laboratories are able to perform immunohistochemical analysis for hormone receptors on FNA specimens if an appropriate fixative has been used. In most cytology labs, the false positive rate for a diagnosis of malignancy in an FNA biopsy of a breast mass is only 1% to 2%. Thus, a diagnosis of malignancy that is based on cytologic analysis of an FNA specimen may generally be believed, and definitive surgery may be planned without further biopsy. It should be remembered, however, that FNA does not distinguish between invasive and in situ breast cancer; intraoperative frozen section should be performed if necessary to determine the need for axillary dissection.

The false negative rate for identifying breast malignancy, however, is high: FNA fails to diagnose as many as 40% of cancers. Any cellular atypia on FNA biopsy is an indication for open biopsy. A diagnosis of normal or fibrocystic breast tissue should also be viewed with suspicion; subsequent open biopsy is usually indicated if the physical examination or a mammogram of the biopsied lesion gives rise to even a minor degree of concern about malignancy. If the cytologic analysis is diagnostic of a specific benign lesion (e.g., a fibroadenoma or a lactating adenoma), it may generally be relied on if it is in keeping with the clinical features of the lesion, and no further workup is necessary. It has been suggested that no further workup is required when the so-called triple negative criteria (a physical examination suggestive of a benign lesion, a normal mammogram, and negative results from FNA biopsy) are present, particularly in younger women.

Core-Needle (Cutting-Needle) Biopsy

As its name suggests, a core-needle biopsy removes a narrow cylinder of tissue from the biopsied lesion. The tissue undergoes standard pathologic rather than cytologic analysis; consequently, this technique is preferable if a skilled cytologist is not available for interpretation of FNA biopsy specimens. Nonetheless, FNA biopsy has supplanted core-needle biopsy in the investigation of most palpable lesions. It should be noted that the false negative rate associated with core-needle biopsy for palpable lesions performed without ultrasonographic or stereotactic guidance is as high as or higher than that of FNA biopsy.[4] The technical difficulty of accurately placing and firing the core needle in small mobile lesions or in lesions surrounded by dense fibrocystic tissue makes FNA biopsy preferable in these set-

tings. Core-needle biopsy is, however, ideal for sampling large lesions or chest wall recurrences in which the larger samples permit more detailed pathologic analysis and easy determination of hormone receptor levels.

Technique If the mass is palpable, the surgeon can perform the core-needle biopsy in the office. A large needle (usually 14 gauge) is placed either by hand or with a biopsy gun device. Injection of a local anesthetic is usually required—again, in a quantity that will create only a small skin wheal. A nick is made in the skin with a No. 11 blade to permit easy entry of the biopsy needle into breast tissue and into the lesion. As with FNA biopsy (see above), the lesion is held steady in the nondominant hand while the biopsy needle is advanced into the lesion and a core sample obtained.

Interpretation of results Atypia on core-needle biopsy is an indication for open biopsy of the sampled lesion. In addition, any core-needle biopsy (especially one done without stereotactic or ultrasonographic guidance) that yields benign or fibrocystic tissue should be viewed with some suspicion because of the risk of technical or sampling error. Open biopsy should be considered if there is any discordance between a benign core-needle biopsy result and the clinical or mammographic features of the lesion.

Open Biopsy

The vast majority of open breast biopsies are now performed with either local anesthesia alone or the use of local anesthesia with intravenous sedation. General anesthesia is reserved for situations in which multiple lesions must be excised and the amount of local anesthetic required would exceed the maximum safe dose.

Technique Open biopsy incisions should generally be curvilinear and should be placed directly over the lesion to minimize tunneling through breast tissue [*see Figure 1*]. Because the possibility of malignancy must always be taken into account, all open biopsy incisions should also be oriented so that they will be included within any subsequent mastectomy incision. Accordingly, if an open biopsy is to be done at an extremely lateral or medial site, it may be best approached via a radial incision placed over the lesion rather than via a more vertical curvilinear incision.

The incision should be long enough to provide adequate exposure and to ensure that the mass can be excised as a single tissue fragment with a small margin of grossly normal tissue. Specimen margins should be inked by the pathologist. Meticulous hemostasis should be achieved before closure. Deep breast tissue should be approximated only if such approximation does not result in significant deformity of breast contour. A cosmetic subcuticular closure is preferred.

OPTIONS FOR NONPALPABLE MASSES

The increasingly widespread use of screening mammography has led to the identification of more and more nonpalpable breast masses for which tissue diagnosis is required. In most series,[5-7] 15% to 30% of such lesions prove to be malignant. Nonpalpable masses may be approached via core-needle biopsy or open biopsy with wire localization.

Image-Guided Core-Needle Biopsy

Needle biopsy techniques are increasingly being used to diagnose nonpalpable breast lesions. In general, FNA biopsy of nonpalpable lesions is inadvisable because of its high false negative rate. Little is lost by attempting an FNA biopsy of a palpable lesion in the office setting, but performing a stereotactic or ultrasound-guided FNA biopsy of a nonpalpable mass carries a significant cost in terms of time, patient discomfort, and expense. The diagnostic accuracy currently achievable with FNA biopsy in this setting does not justify this cost. Consequently, image-guided core-needle biopsy is the preferred approach for needle biopsy of nonpalpable lesions.

In choosing core-needle biopsy, both patient and physician must be comfortable with the fact that the lesion will only be sampled rather than excised, must recognize that the possibility of a sampling error that will cause the examiner to miss the lesion is higher with core-needle biopsy than with open biopsy, and must realize that equivocal findings will necessitate follow-up with open biopsy. The trade-off for these limitations is that core-needle biopsy generally costs less than open biopsy, takes less time, and leaves only a tiny scar. After a core-needle diagnosis of malignancy, the surgeon may proceed directly to wide local excision and will often be able to obtain clean margins with a single open procedure.[8]

Stereotactic versus ultrasound-guided biopsy Whenever feasible, core-needle biopsy is performed with ultrasonographic guidance, which permits real-time documentation of needle position within the lesion. Stereotactic mammography-guided core-needle biopsy is performed if the lesion is not visualized ultrasonographically. Stereotactic biopsy is appropriate for lesions that are favorably located within the breast (i.e., that can be stably positioned in the biopsy window of the machine). Lesions very close to the chest wall or the areola may not be accessible to stereotactic biopsy and are best approached via open biopsy with needle localization (see below).

Clustered microcalcifications may also be approached by stereotactic core-needle biopsy. If the cluster is not large enough for calcifications to remain to guide subsequent wide excision if a malignancy is found, a clip should be placed to mark the biopsy site.

Interpretation of results The introduction of large core-biopsy needles (11- and 14-gauge), coupled with the use of vacuum assistance to draw additional tissue into the needle, has markedly improved the false negative rate for core-needle biopsy. Currently, false negative rates for this procedure fall into the 1% to 2% range,[9,10] results that compare favorably with those reported for wire-localized open surgical biopsy. It is now routine to perform radiography of core-needle biopsy specimens to confirm that targeted calcifications have been removed. When the targeted lesion comprises dense tissue rather than calcifications, care must be taken to confirm that the lesion was adequately sampled and thus ensure that the findings can be interpreted reliably. Immediate postbiopsy radiography may be performed to demonstrate that a hole was made in the lesion. A finding of benign or fibrocystic tissue on such a biopsy should be viewed with some suspicion and interpreted in relation to the lesion sampled. One must decide whether the pathologic findings adequately account for the lesion visualized. If any concern remains, open biopsy is indicated.

Because false positive results are rare, a diagnosis of malignancy may be believed and acted upon without further biopsy. In planning treatment after core-needle biopsy that shows only carcinoma in situ, one should remember that the lesion was only sampled and that invasive tumor may still be found when

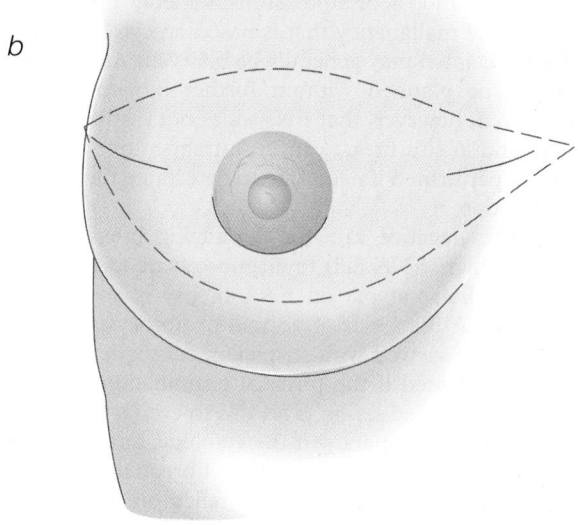

Figure 1 **Open breast biopsy.** (*a*) **In most cases, a curvilinear incision is preferred. If the mass is close to the areola, a periareolar incision may be used.** (*b*) **Extremely lateral or medial incisions may be radial. In any case, incisions should be placed directly over the lesion and should be oriented so that they will be included within a subsequent mastectomy incision if margins prove positive and mastectomy is indicated.**

the lesion is completely excised. The likelihood of finding invasive tumor on surgical excision after a core-needle biopsy indicative of ductal carcinoma may be as high as 20%.[10]

A finding of atypical ductal hyperplasia on core-needle biopsy is an indication for wire-localized open biopsy. Open biopsy after a core-needle biopsy indicative of atypical ductal hyperplasia may reveal ductal carcinoma in situ (DCIS) in as many as 50% of patients; this may be a less frequent finding when a larger (e.g., 11-gauge) needle was used for the core-needle biopsy.[10]

Follow-up Whether short-interval mammographic follow-up is necessary after core-needle biopsy depends on the patho-

a

b

c

Figure 2 **Needle-localized breast biopsy.**[13] (*a*) **The mammographic abnormality is localized immediately before operation. The relation between the wire, the skin entry site, and the lesion is noted by the surgeon. (*b*) The skin incision is placed over the expected location of the mammographic abnormality. The dissection is accomplished with the wire as a guide. (*c*) The tissue around the wire is removed en bloc with the wire and sent for specimen mammography. Tunneling and piecemeal removal are to be avoided.**

logic findings and the mammographic appearance of the lesion. With a well-circumscribed lesion that pathologic evaluation shows to be a fibroadenoma or with calcifications that pathologic evaluation shows to be located in benign fibrocystic tissue, no special follow-up is required, and routine screening at normal intervals may be resumed. In general, if the pathologic findings are equivocal or discordant with the appearance of the lesion, immediate open excision is preferable to a 6-month repeat mammogram. To ensure appropriate follow-up, there should be close communication between the physician ordering the core-needle biopsy, the physician performing the biopsy, and the pathologist analyzing the specimen.

Open Biopsy with Needle (Wire) Localization

As is the case for open biopsy of palpable lesions, the vast majority of needle-localized breast biopsies are now performed with local anesthesia or local anesthesia with intravenous sedation. General anesthesia is reserved for excision of multiple lesions or other special circumstances.

Technique The lesion to be excised is localized by inserting a thin needle and a fine wire under mammographic or ultrasonographic guidance immediately before operation. To facilitate incision placement, images should be sent to the operating room with the wire entry site indicated on them. With superfi-

cial lesions, the wire entry site is usually close to the lesion and thus may be included in the incision. With some deeper lesions, the wire entry site is on the shortest path to the lesion and so may still be included in the incision. The incision is placed as directly as possible over the mass to minimize tunneling through breast tissue. Once the incision is made, a core of tissue is excised around and along the wire in such a way as to include the lesion [*see Figure 2*]. (This process is easier and involves less excision of tissue if the localizing wire has a thickened segment several centimeters in length that is placed adjacent to or within the lesion. One then follows the wire itself into breast tissue until the thick segment is reached and only then extends the excision away from the wire to include the lesion in a fairly small tissue fragment.)

With many lesions, the wire entry site is in a fairly peripheral location relative to the position of the lesion, which means that including the wire entry site in the incision would result in excessive tunneling within breast tissue. In such cases, the incision is placed over the expected position of the lesion [*see Figure 3*], the dissection is extended into breast tissue to identify the wire a few centimeters away from the lesion itself, and the free end of the wire is pulled up into the incision. A generous core of tissue is then excised around the wire. (Again, this process is easier if the thick segment of the localizing wire is placed adjacent to or within the lesion.)

Figure 3 **Needle-localized breast biopsy.**[13] (*a*) **It is sometimes necessary to insert the localizing wire from a peripheral site to localize a deep or central lesion. The incision should be placed directly over the expected location of the lesion, not over the wire entry site.** (*b*) **Once the skin incision is made, the dissection is extended into breast tissue to identify the wire a short distance from the lesion. The free end of the wire is pulled into the wound, and the biopsy is performed as in Figure 2.**

Radiography should immediately be performed on all wire-localized biopsy specimens to confirm that the lesion has been excised. The patient should remain on the operating table with the sterile field preserved until such confirmation has been received. If the mass was missed and the surgeon has some idea of the likely location of the missed lesion, another tissue sample may be excised immediately. If, however, the surgeon suspects that the wire was dislodged before or during the procedure, the incision should be closed. After the patient has healed sufficiently to be able to tolerate repeat mammography, another mammogram is obtained, and repeat localization and biopsy are performed.

Directional Vacuum-Assisted Breast Biopsy (Mammotomy)

Directional vacuum-assisted biopsy (DVAB), or mammotomy, is a special procedure for obtaining specimens from single or multiple breast lesions (e.g., microcalcifications, circumscribed masses, and spiculated masses). DVAB is a diagnostic procedure and is not intended for therapeutic purposes. On the whole, it is safe, and the complication rate is acceptably low.

In comparison with core-needle biopsy, DVAB is more successful at removing microcalcifications, can obtain more specimens in the course of a single procedure, and is more sensitive in detecting ductal carcinoma in situ and atypical duct hyperplasia. DVAB also appears to diagnose nonpalpable breast lesions more effectively than stereotactically guided core-needle biopsy does. It may, in fact, be helpful to perform DVAB after core-needle biopsy when the diagnosis of atypical duct hyperplasia is being considered; this practice may lead to a decrease in the number of open biopsies performed.

Suitable candidates for DVAB include patients with nonpalpable but mammographically visible clusters of suspicious calcifications, those with well-defined masses that are likely to be benign, and those with suspicious masses. Target lesions must be clearly visible on digital images and identifiable on stereo-

tactic projections. DVAB is not recommended for patients with certain lesions located very posteriorly or very anteriorly in the breast, those with very small or very thin breasts, and those who, for one reason or another, cannot be properly positioned for the procedure or cannot cooperate with the surgeon. The procedure is done on an outpatient basis and usually can be completed in 1 hour or less. Patients are restricted from engaging in strenuous activity for 24 hours after DVAB.

The probe employed for the procedure consists of an outer trocar cannula, a sliding inner hollow coaxial cutter, a so-called knockout shaft, a distal sampling notch, and a proximal tissue retrieval chamber; in addition, it has a thumbwheel, which is used for manual advancement, cutting, and retrieval of biopsy specimens. It must be used under the guidance of an imaging modality (e.g., ultrasonography or roentgenography), and it may be either mounted or handheld. The device is connected to a suction machine, which acts first to draw the target tissue into the sampling notch and then to facilitate retrieval of tissue into the proximal collection chamber.

Stereotactic digital imaging is then performed to visualize the target and calculate its location in three dimensions, and a suitable trocar insertion site is identified. The skin is prepared, and a small amount of buffered 1% lidocaine with epinephrine (usually 10 ml or less) is administered. The skin at the insertion site is punctured with a No. 11 blade, the probe is manually advanced to the prefire site, and the position of the probe is confirmed by means of stereotactic imaging. The device is then fired, repeatedly cutting, rotating, and retrieving samples until the desired amount has been removed. If the lesions being removed are calcifications, the sufficiency of the sampling may be confirmed through x-rays of the specimens.

Figure 4 **Terminal duct excision (single duct).**[14] (*a*) **A periareolar incision is made.** (*b*) **The involved duct is identified by means of blunt dissection.** (*c*) **The duct is removed along with a core of breast tissue.**

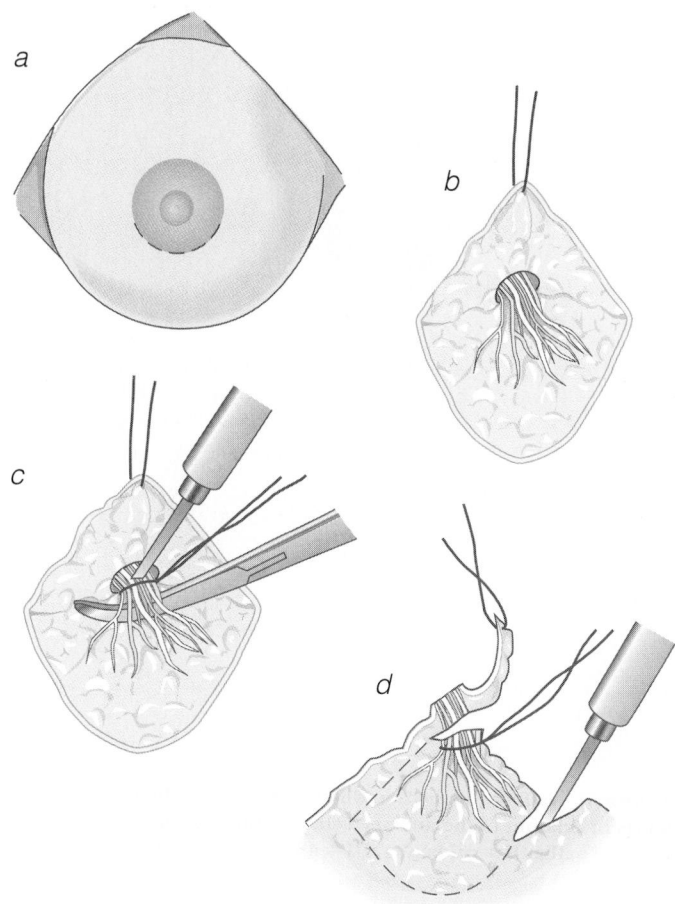

without sedation (as for breast biopsy) is generally sufficient for this procedure. The goal is to excise the duct from which the discharge arises along with as little additional tissue as possible. To this end, the surgeon should carefully note the precise position of the discharging duct at the time of the initial examination. Ductograms generally are not helpful in directing the surgical procedure and need not be performed.

OPERATIVE TECHNIQUE

The patient is instructed not to attempt to express her discharge for several days before operation. The breast skin is prepared, and drapes are placed. The surgeon then attempts to express the discharge so that the offending duct can be precisely identified. If discharge is obtained, the mark for the incision should be made at the areolar border in the same quadrant, extending for about one third of the areola's circumference [see Figure 4a]. A local anesthetic is then administered, the edge of the nipple is grasped with a forceps, and a fine lacrimal duct probe (000 to 0000) is gently inserted into the discharging duct. An incision is then made as marked at the areolar border, the nipple skin flap is raised, and the duct containing the wire is excised with a margin of surrounding tissue from just below the nipple dermis into the deeper breast tissue [see Figure 4b, c].

If it is not possible to pass the lacrimal duct probe into the discharging duct, the skin incision is made and the nipple skin flap raised as described. The surgeon then bluntly dissects among the subareolar ducts to identify the dark, secretion-filled abnormal duct. If the duct is identified, it is excised along its length from the nipple dermis to a depth of 4 to 5 cm within breast tissue. An option at this point is to incise the duct and insert a lacrimal duct probe to facilitate identification of its course. If no single secretion-filled duct is identified, the entire subareolar duct complex must be excised from immediately beneath the nipple dermis to a depth of 4 to 5 cm within breast tissue [see Figure 5].

In all variants of this procedure, the electrocautery should not be used in the superficial portions of the dissection: it could cause devascularization of the nipple-areola complex and result in an electrocautery artifact that could interfere with pathologic analysis. If the patient has a history of periductal infection, the contents of the duct should be sent for culture and the area copiously irrigated with an antibiotic solution before wound closure. Good hemostasis should be obtained at the completion of the procedure. Breast tissue should be reapproximated beneath the nipple before skin closure to prevent retraction of the nipple or indentation of the areola.

Surgical Options for Breast Cancer

There are several surgical options for primary treatment of breast cancer; indications for selecting among them are reviewed elsewhere [see II:3 Breast Complaints]. It should be emphasized that for most patients, wide local excision (lumpectomy) to microscopically clean margins coupled with axillary dissection and radiation therapy yields long-term survival equivalent to that associated with modified radical mastectomy. Currently, indications for mastectomy include patient preference, inability on the part of the surgeon to achieve clean margins without unacceptable deformation of the remaining breast tissue, the presence of multiple primary tumors, previous chest wall irradiation, pregnancy, and the presence of severe collagen vascular disease (e.g., scleroderma). Nonmedical indications for mastectomy include the lack of access to a radiation therapy

Figure 5 Terminal duct excision (entire ductal complex).[14] (a) A periareolar incision is made. (b) The nipple skin flap is raised. (c) The ductal complex is identified by means of blunt dissection and transected. (d) The entire subareolar ductal complex is excised from immediately beneath the nipple dermis to a depth of 4 to 5 cm within breast tissue.

Once the biopsy is complete, an inert metallic clip is deployed into the biopsy site through the trocar so as to mark the lesion for future reference in case it can no longer be visualized after biopsy; deployment and positioning are confirmed by stereotactic imaging. The biopsy device is then removed, the edges of the skin incision are approximated with Steri-Strips, and a compressive bandage is applied. Any bleeding occurring after removal of the biopsy device should be controlled by manual pressure before the final bandage is applied. Typically, 1 g of tissue (equivalent to approximately 10 to 12 samples with an 11-gauge probe) is sufficient for diagnosis of benign disease, atypical duct hyperplasia, or carcinoma.

Complications are uncommon. Brisk bleeding may occur during and immediately after the procedure. Bruising and discoloration may result but generally resolve within days. Less frequently still, hematomas may form, fat necrosis may occur, or the patient may note a palpable lump. Caution is advisable in women who are receiving anticoagulants. Surgical site infection has been reported as well, but it is rare.

Terminal Duct Excision

Terminal duct excision is the procedure of choice in the surgical treatment of nipple discharge. Local anesthesia with or facility and any other patient factors that would prevent completion of a full course of radiation therapy.

Lumpectomy

Lumpectomy—also referred to, more precisely, as wide local excision or partial mastectomy—involves excision of all cancerous tissue to microscopically clean margins. Reexcision or lumpectomy without axillary dissection may be performed with the patient under local anesthesia, but sedation or general anesthesia is usually advisable if a significant amount of tissue is to be excised or if there is tenderness from a previous biopsy. Lumpectomy with axillary dissection usually calls for general anesthesia, but it may be performed with thoracic epidural anesthesia supplemented by local anesthesia as needed.

OPERATIVE TECHNIQUE

Like open breast biopsy incisions [see Breast Biopsy, above], lumpectomy incisions should generally be curvilinear, should be placed directly over the lesion, and should also be oriented so as to be included within a subsequent mastectomy incision if margins prove positive [see Figure 1]. Extremely lateral or medial incisions may be better approached via a radial incision placed over the lesion. Because accurate assessment of margins is of central importance in a lumpectomy, it is critical that the incision be long enough to allow removal of the specimen in one piece rather than several.

Along with the mass itself, it is generally necessary to remove a 1 to 1.5 cm margin of normal-appearing tissue beyond the edge of the palpable tumor or, if excisional biopsy has already been performed, around the biopsy cavity. In the case of nonpalpable lesions diagnosed via needle biopsy, the position of the lesion must be determined by means of wire localization, and 2 to 3 cm of tissue should be excised around the wire to obtain an adequate margin. The specimen should be oriented by the surgeon and the margins inked by the pathologist; this orientation is useful if reexcision is required to achieve clean margins. Reexcision of any close margins may be performed during the same surgical procedure if the specimen margins are assessed immediately by the pathologist.

In the closure of the incision, hemostasis should be meticulous: a hematoma may delay administration of radiation therapy or chemotherapy. Deep breast tissue should be approximated only if such closure does not result in significant deformity of breast contour. A cosmetic subcuticular closure is preferred.

Lymphatic Mapping and Sentinel Lymph Node Biopsy

Lymphatic mapping and sentinel lymph node (SLN) biopsy [see V:3 Lymphatic Mapping and Sentinel Lymph Node Biopsy] is a relatively new procedure that allows the surgeon to confirm or rule out axillary node involvement without performing a standard axillary dissection.[11,12] The technique is based on the theory that the lymphatic channels draining the primary breast tumor initially drain to a single SLN in the regional basin, which can be identified by means of intradermal injection of a vital blue dye, a radiocolloid, or both. A small incision is then made in the regional basin (which is usually the axilla in breast cancer patients), and the stained SLN is identified (either with a handheld gamma probe or by direct visualization), excised, and analyzed histologically.

Because SLN biopsy involves analysis of only one or two nodes, the pathologist can carry out a more detailed examina-

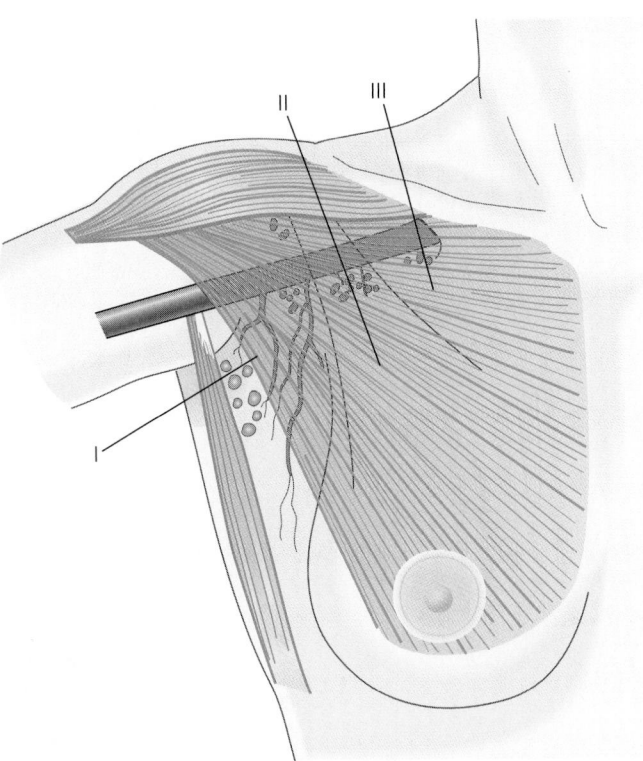

Figure 6 **Axillary dissection. Shown are axillary lymph node levels in relation to the axillary vein and the muscles of the axilla (I = low axilla, II = midaxilla, III = apex of axilla).**[15]

tion than would be possible with a standard axillary lymphadenectomy specimen, which contains multiple nodes. Newer techniques (e.g., immunohistochemical and molecular assays) can also be used to identify micrometastases that light microscopy would fail to detect, but the therapeutic and prognostic significance of tumor cells identified by such means remains unclear.

Although there is a significant learning curve for intraoperative lymphatic mapping, with sufficient experience, the SLN can be identified at least 80% to 90% of the time. Currently, standard axillary dissection is recommended for patients who have a positive SLN; however, prospective, randomized trials are now under way with a view to determining to what extent this step is necessary in node-positive patients. A number of studies have confirmed that the absence of metastases in the SLN reliably predicts the absence of metastases in the remaining axillary nodes.

Contraindications to SLN biopsy include the use of neoadjuvant chemotherapy, the presence of palpable axillary nodes suggestive of metastatic disease, the presence of large or locally advanced breast cancers, prior axillary surgery, and pregnancy or lactation.

Axillary Dissection

Axillary dissection for breast cancer includes resection of level I and level II lymph nodes and the fibrofatty tissue within which these nodes lie [see Figure 6]. The superior border of the dissection is formed by the axillary vein laterally and the upper extent of level II nodes medially; the lateral border of the dissection is formed by the latissimus dorsi muscle from the tail of

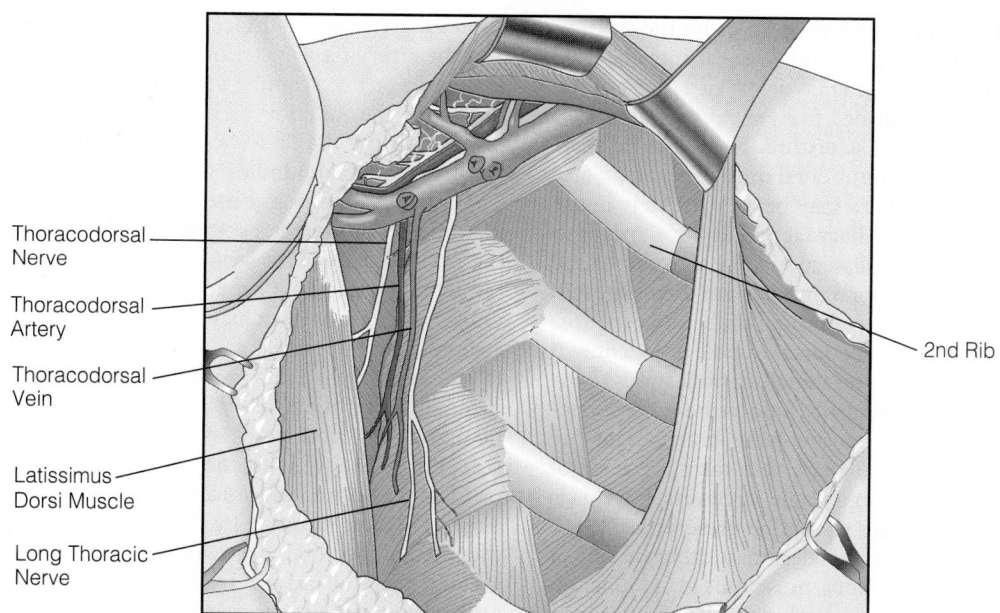

Figure 7 **Axillary dissection. Shown is a view of the structures of the axilla after completion of axillary dissection.**[16]

the breast to the crossing point of the axillary vein; the medial border is formed by the pectoral muscles and the anterior serratus muscle; and the inferior border is formed by the tail of the breast. Level II nodes are easily removed by retracting the greater and smaller pectoral muscles medially; it is not necessary to divide or remove the smaller pectoral muscle. In general, level III nodes are not removed unless palpable disease is present.

Axillary dissection, either alone or in conjunction with lumpectomy or mastectomy, usually calls for general anesthesia, but it may also be performed with thoracic epidural anesthesia supplemented by local anesthesia as needed. To facilitate identification and preservation of motor nerves that pass through the axilla, the anesthesiologist should refrain from using neuromuscular blocking agents. In the absence of neuromuscular blockade, any clamping of a motor nerve or too-close approach to a motor nerve with the electrocautery will be signaled by a visible muscle twitch.

STRUCTURES TO BE PRESERVED

There are a number of vascular structures and nerves passing through the axilla that must be preserved during axillary dissection [*see Figure 7*]. These structures include the axillary vein and artery; the brachial plexus; the long thoracic nerve, which innervates the anterior serratus muscle; the thoracodorsal nerve, artery, and vein, which supply the latissimus dorsi muscle; and the medial pectoral nerve, which innervates the lateral portion of the greater pectoral muscle.

The axillary artery and the brachial plexus should not be exposed during axillary dissection. If they are, the dissection has been carried too far superiorly, and proper orientation at a more inferior position should be established. In some patients, there may be sensory branches of the brachial plexus superficial (and, rarely, inferior) to the axillary vein laterally near the latissimus dorsi muscle; injury to these nerves results in numbness extending to the wrist. To prevent this complication, the axillary vein should initially be identified medially, under the greater pectoral

muscle. Medial to the thoracodorsal nerve and adherent to the chest wall is the long thoracic nerve of Bell. The medial pectoral nerve runs from superior to the axillary vein to the undersurface of the greater pectoral muscle, passing through the axillary fat pad and across the level II nodes; it has an accompanying vein whose blue color may be used to identify the nerve. If a submuscular implant reconstruction [*see Breast Reconstruction after Mastectomy, below*] is planned, preservation of the medial pectoral nerve is especially important to prevent atrophy of the muscle.

The intercostobrachial nerve provides sensation to the posterior portion of the upper arm. Sacrificing this nerve generally leads to numbness over the triceps region. In many women, the intercostobrachial nerve measures 2 mm in diameter and takes a fairly cephalad course near the axillary vein; when this is the case, preservation of the nerve will not interfere with node dissection. Sometimes, however, the nerve is tiny, has multiple branches, and is intermingled with nodal tissue that should be removed; when this is the case, one should not expend a great deal of time on attempting to preserve the nerve. If the intercostobrachial nerve is sacrificed, it should be transected with a knife or scissors rather than with the electrocautery, and the ends should be buried to reduce the likelihood of postoperative causalgia.

OPERATIVE TECHNIQUE

The incision for axillary dissection should be a transverse one made in the lower third of the hair-bearing skin of the axilla. For cosmetic reasons, it should not extend anteriorly onto the greater pectoral muscle; however, it may be extended posteriorly onto the latissimus dorsi muscle as necessary for exposure. Skin flaps are raised to the level of the axillary vein and to a point below the lowest extension of hair-bearing skin, either as an initial maneuver or after the initial identification of key structures.

The key to axillary dissection is obtaining and maintaining proper orientation with respect to the axillary vein, the thoracodorsal bundle, and the long thoracic nerve. After the incision has been made, the dissection is extended down into the true axillary fat pad through the overlying fascial layer. The fat of the axillary fat pad may be distinguished from subcutaneous fat on the basis of its smoother, lipomalike texture. There may be aberrant muscle slips from the latissimus dorsi muscle or the greater pectoral muscle; in addition, there may be an extremely dense fascial encasement around the axillary fat pad. It is important to divide these layers early in the dissection. The borders of the greater pectoral and latissimus dorsi muscles are then exposed, which clears the medial and lateral borders of the dissection.

The axillary vein and the thoracodorsal bundle are identified next. As discussed (see above), the initial identification of the axillary vein should be made medially, under the greater pectoral muscle, to prevent injury to low-lying branches of the brachial plexus. Sometimes, the axillary vein takes the form of several small branches rather than a single large vessel. If this is the case, all of the small branches should be preserved.

The thoracodorsal bundle may be identified either distally at its junction with the latissimus dorsi muscle or at its junction with the axillary vein. The junction with the latissimus dorsi muscle is within the axillary fat pad at a point two thirds of the way down the hair-bearing skin of the axilla, or approximately 4 cm below the inferior border of the axillary vein. Occasionally, the thoracodorsal bundle is bifurcated, with separate superior and inferior branches entering the latissimus dorsi muscle; this is particularly likely if the entry point appears very high. If the bundle is bifurcated, both branches should be preserved. The thoracodorsal bundle may be identified at its junction with the latissimus dorsi muscle by spreading within axillary fat parallel to the border of the muscle and looking for the blue of the thoracodorsal vein. The identification is also facilitated by lateral retraction of the latissimus dorsi muscle. The long thoracic nerve lies just medial to the thoracodorsal bundle on the chest wall at this point and at approximately the same anterior-posterior position. It may be identified by spreading tissue just medial to the thoracodorsal bundle and then running the index finger perpendicular to the course of the long thoracic nerve on the chest wall to identify the cordlike nerve as it moves under the finger. Once the nerve is identified, axillary tissue may be swept anteriorly away from the nerve by blunt dissection along the anterior serratus muscle; there are no significant vessels in this area.

The junction of the thoracodorsal bundle with the axillary vein is 1.5 to 2.0 cm medial to the point at which the axillary vein crosses the latissimus dorsi muscle. The thoracodorsal vein enters the posterior surface of the axillary vein, and the nerve and the artery pass posterior to the axillary vein. There are generally one or two scapular veins that branch off the axillary vein medial to the junction with the thoracodorsal vein. These are divided during the dissection and should not be confused with the thoracodorsal bundle.

The axillary vein and the thoracodorsal bundle having been identified, the greater pectoral muscle is retracted medially at the level of the axillary vein, and the latissimus dorsi muscle is retracted laterally to place tension on the thoracodorsal bundle. Once this exposure is achieved, the axillary fat and the nodes are cleared away superficial and medial to the thoracodorsal bundle to the level of the axillary vein. Superiorly, dissection proceeds medially along the axillary vein to the point where the fat containing level II nodes crosses the axillary vein. To improve exposure, the fascia overlying the level II extension of the axillary fat pad should be incised to release tension and expose the lipomalike level II fat. As noted [see Structures to Be Preserved, above], the medial pectoral nerve passes onto the underside of the greater pectoral muscle in this area and should be preserved. One or more small venous branches may pass inferiorly from the medial pectoral bundle; particular attention should be paid to preserving the nerve when ligating these venous branches.

The next step in the dissection is to reflect the axillary fat pad inferiorly by dividing the medial attachments of the axillary fat pad along the anterior serratus muscle. Care must be taken to preserve the long thoracic nerve. Because there are no significant vessels or structures in the tissue anterior to the long thoracic nerve, this tissue may be divided sharply, with small perforating vessels either tied or cauterized. Finally, the axillary fat is freed from the tail of the breast with the electrocautery or a knife.

There is no need to orient the axillary specimen for the pathologist, because treatment is not affected by the anatomic level of node involvement. A closed suction drain is placed through a separate stab wound. (Some practitioners prefer not to place a drain and simply aspirate postoperative seromas as necessary.) A long-acting local anesthetic may be instilled into the axilla—a particularly helpful practice if the dissection was done as an outpatient procedure.

Mastectomy

The goal of a mastectomy is to remove all breast tissue, including the nipple and the areola, while leaving well-perfused, viable skin flaps for primary closure or reconstruction. This is

Figure 8   **Mastectomy. Shown are common incisions used for mastectomy.[13] Any previous biopsy incisions should have been done in such a way as to be included within the boundaries of the mastectomy incision.**

Figure 9 **Breast reconstruction after mastectomy. Shown is an algorithm outlining the major steps in breast reconstruction.**

the case whether the mastectomy is performed for treatment of breast cancer or for prophylaxis in high-risk patients. Proper skin incisions and good exposure throughout the procedure are the key components of a well-performed mastectomy. The borders of dissection extend superiorly to the clavicle, medially to the sternum, inferiorly to where breast tissue ends (on the costal margin, below the inframammary fold), and laterally to the border of the latissimus dorsi muscle. The fascia of the greater pectoral muscle forms the deep margin of the dissection and should be removed with the specimen.

Mastectomy usually calls for general anesthesia, but it may be performed with thoracic epidural anesthesia supplemented by local anesthesia as needed. When a simple mastectomy is to be performed in a frail patient for whom general anesthesia poses unacceptable risks (particularly if the patient is elderly and has a narrow-based, pendulous breast), local anesthesia with sedation is appropriate.

OPERATIVE TECHNIQUE

Skin-sparing mastectomy performed in conjunction with immediate reconstruction is discussed elsewhere [see Breast Reconstruction after Mastectomy, below]. In a modified radical or simple mastectomy without reconstruction, the goal is to leave a smooth chest wall that permits comfortable wearing of a bra and a prosthesis. It is important to remove a sufficient amount of skin to ensure that no dog-ears or lateral skin folds are left on the anterior chest wall. This undesirable result can be prevented by extending the incision far enough medially and laterally to remove all skin that contributes to the forward projection of the breast skin envelope.

The incision may be either transverse across the chest wall or angled upward toward the axilla as necessary to include the nipple-areola complex and any incisions from previous biopsies, and care should be taken to make the upper and lower skin flaps of similar length so that there is no redundant skin on either flap [see Figure 8]. The boundaries of the incision can be determined in the following five steps: (1) the lateral and medial end points of the incision are marked, (2) the breast is pulled firmly downward, (3) the upper incision is defined by drawing a straight line from one end point to the other across the upper surface of the breast, (4) the breast is pulled firmly upward, and (5) the lower incision is defined by drawing a straight line from one end point to the other across the lower surface of the breast. The outlined incision is then checked to ensure that it can be closed without either undue tension or redundant skin. (The closure should be fairly snug intraoperatively, when the patient's arm is positioned perpendicular to the torso for exposure, because a significant amount of slack is created when the arm is returned to a more normal position at the patient's side.) The medial and lateral end points of the incision may be adjusted upward or downward to include any previous biopsy incisions in the specimen.

Flaps

In most patients, there is a fairly well-defined avascular plane between subcutaneous fat and breast tissue. This plane is identified by pulling the edges of the incision upward with skin hooks and beginning a flap that is 8 to 10 mm thick and extends approximately 1 cm from the skin edge. After this initial release of the skin edge, the desired plane is developed by applying firm tension to pull breast tissue downward and away from the skin at a 45° angle. The fine fibrous attachments between breast tissue and subcutaneous fat (Cooper's ligaments) are then divided with the electrocautery or a blade, and crossing vessels are

Figure 10 **Breast reconstruction after mastectomy. Shown is the recommended placement of incisions for skin-sparing mastectomy. T-shaped incisions extending from the areola to remove previous biopsy incisions may be used if necessary. A separate axillary incision may be necessary when axillary dissection is being done.**

coagulated or ligated as they appear. To protect both arterial supply to and venous drainage from the skin flap, one must refrain from excessive ligation or cauterization of vessels on the flap.

Completed mastectomy flaps are perfused through the network of fine subdermal vessels that remains after dissection. The viability of the flaps is determined by their length, the quality of the vessels they contain, the damage sustained by the vessels during the dissection, and the tension imposed by the final closure. For most women, flap viability is not an issue. It is, however, a serious consideration for diabetics and other patients with diffuse small vessel disease. In such patients, flaps should be carefully planned so that they are no longer than necessary and there is no excess tension, and extra care should be taken to preserve flap vessels. Patients should be warned that even with these additional efforts, there may be some necrosis along the edges of the incision. Such necrosis is best treated with gradual debridement of the dark eschar that forms as epithelialization proceeds from viable tissue.

Borders of Dissection

Flaps are raised superiorly to the clavicle, medially to the sternum, inferiorly to where breast tissue ends on the costal margin (generally below the inframammary fold), and laterally to the border of the latissimus dorsi muscle. The plane between breast tissue and subcutaneous fat is followed down to the greater pectoral muscle and through the pectoral fascia both superiorly and medially. Inferiorly, the fascia of the abdominal muscles is not divided. The greater pectoral muscle, the abdominal muscles, and the anterior serratus muscle form the deep border of the dissection. The pectoral fascia is removed with the breast specimen and may be separated from the muscle with either the electrocautery or a blade.

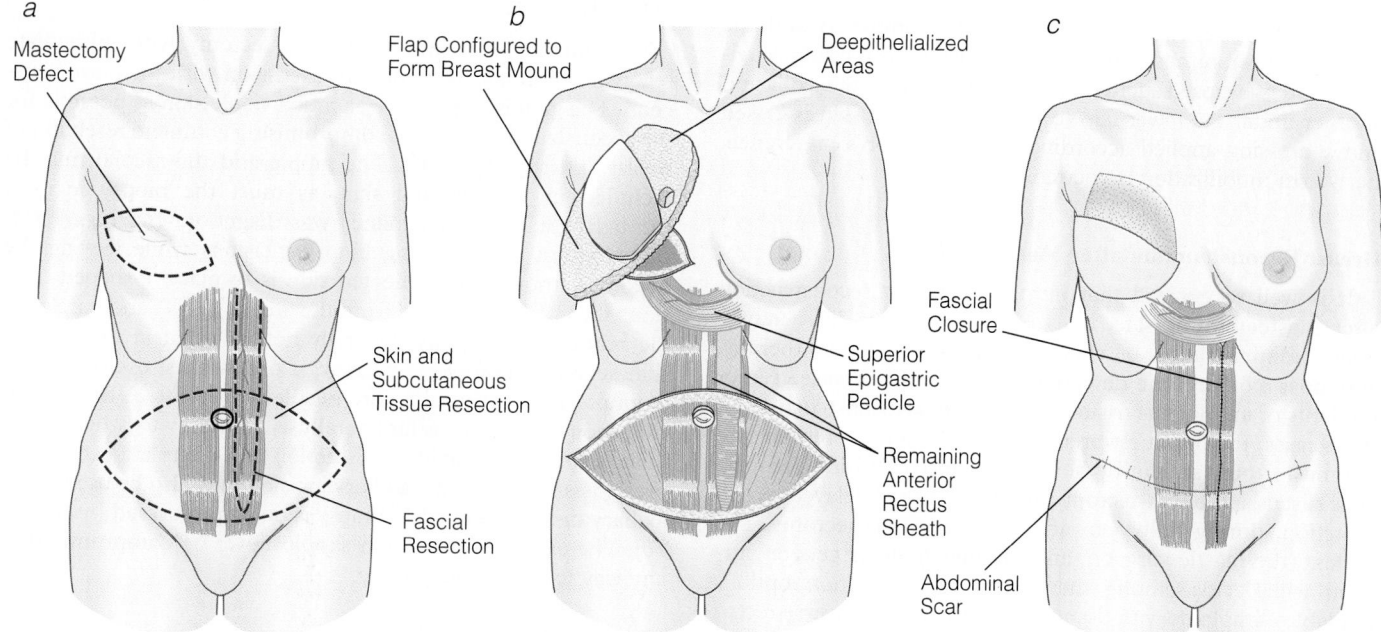

a
Mastectomy Defect

Skin and Subcutaneous Tissue Resection

Fascial Resection

b
Flap Configured to Form Breast Mound

Deepithelialized Areas

Superior Epigastric Pedicle

Remaining Anterior Rectus Sheath

c
Fascial Closure

Abdominal Scar

Figure 11 **Breast reconstruction after mastectomy. Shown is autologous tissue reconstruction with a transverse rectus abdominis myocutaneous (TRAM) flap. The infraumbilical flap is designed (*a*). The TRAM flap is tunneled subcutaneously into the chest wall cavity. Blood supply to the flap is maintained from the superior epigastric vessels of the rectus abdominis muscle. Subcutaneous fat and deepithelialized skin are positioned under the mastectomy flaps as needed to reconstruct the breast mound (*b*). The fascia of the anterior rectus sheath is approximated to achieve a tight closure of the abdominal wall defect and to prevent hernia formation. The umbilicus is sutured into its new position (*c*).**

To maintain the skin tension needed for the development of skin flaps, an assistant holds the flaps taut manually with skin hooks, dull-toothed rakes padded with damp sponges, or Deaver retractors. Care must be taken to obtain adequate tension and exposure so that as much breast tissue as possible can be removed without undue damage to the skin flaps.

Simple versus Modified Radical Mastectomy

Simple mastectomy is performed (1) to treat DCIS, (2) as a prophylactic measure, (3) as a follow-up to lumpectomy and axillary dissection if lumpectomy margins are positive for malignancy, (4) to treat local recurrence of breast cancer after lumpectomy, node dissection, and irradiation, and (5) in elderly patients in whom coexisting medical conditions or other factors constitute contraindications to axillary dissection. Simple mastectomy is also indicated for treatment of sarcomas of the breast: lymphatic spread to axillary nodes is not part of the natural history of this disease.

Modified radical mastectomy is performed to treat invasive breast cancer when (1) there are contraindications to breast preservation or (2) the patient or the physician prefers mastectomy. Simple mastectomy in conjunction with SLN biopsy is an increasingly common alternative to modified radical mastectomy for patients with clinically negative axillary nodes. If the nodes are positive for tumor on pathologic examination, the surgeon may then elect to perform a completion axillary dissection.

Simple mastectomy As described earlier (see above), a skin incision is made, and thin flaps are raised to allow removal of all breast tissue. Laterally, the dissection is extended to the border of the latissimus dorsi muscle, and breast tissue is removed anterior to the long thoracic nerve. The dissection proceeds around the lateral edge of the greater pectoral muscle but stops before entering the axillary fat pad. If one wishes to sample the low axillary nodes (as, for example, in a patient with extensive DCIS of comedo histology), one may remove the lower portion of the axillary fat pad between clamps. (In so doing, one must avoid the long thoracic nerve and the thoracodorsal nerve and keep the dissection low enough to ensure that the intercostobrachial sensory nerve is not damaged.) The breast is then taken off the underlying muscles, and the pectoral fascia is included with the specimen.

A single closed suction drain is placed through a separate stab wound laterally to extend under the lower flap and a short distance upward along the sternal border of the dissection. The skin is closed and a dressing applied according to the surgeon's preference. Early arm mobilization is encouraged.

Modified radical mastectomy The incision is placed and flaps are raised as for simple mastectomy. At the lateral edge of the dissection, the border of the latissimus dorsi muscle is exposed, as is the lateral border of the pectoral muscle. Some surgeons prefer to proceed with axillary dissection first, leaving the breast attached to the chest wall, whereas others prefer to remove the breast from the chest wall first and then use it to provide tension for the axillary dissection. In either case, mechanical or manual retraction of the latissimus dorsi muscle and the greater pectoral muscle generally provides excellent exposure for axillary dissection. The landmarks of the axillary dissection are identified as described earlier [*see* Axillary Dissection, *above*]. The thoracodorsal bundle can often be seen running along the latissimus dorsi muscle as the muscle is retracted laterally.

Once the axillary dissection has been completed and the breast has been removed from the chest wall, the incision is irrigated and two closed suction drains placed, one in the axilla and another under the lower flap to the midline. The skin is closed and a dressing applied according to the surgeon's preference. Early arm mobilization is encouraged.

Breast Reconstruction after Mastectomy

It is well recognized that immediate breast reconstruction after mastectomy is safe, does not significantly delay subsequent administration of chemotherapy or radiation therapy, and does not prevent detection of recurrent disease. Either implants or autologous tissue may be used in reconstruction. In most cases, the option of breast reconstruction is presented to the mastectomy patient by her breast surgeon during preoperative discussion of mastectomy or, in the case of delayed reconstruction, during follow-up after an earlier mastectomy. The patient, the plastic surgeon, and the oncologic or general surgeon will decide among the several reconstruction options available—implants with tissue expansion, the transverse rectus abdominis myocutaneous (TRAM) flap, the latissimus dorsi myocutaneous flap, and various free flaps—on the basis of patient preference and lifestyle, the availability of suitable autologous tissue, and the demands imposed by any additional cancer therapies required [see Figure 9]. Familiarity with the strengths and drawbacks of these reconstruction options facilitates this decision.

OPERATIVE TECHNIQUE

Placement of the incision for mastectomy with immediate reconstruction is determined in discussion with the plastic surgeon. The goal is to preserve as much viable skin as possible for the reconstruction without compromising complete resection of breast and axillary tissue. The nipple and the areola must be included in the resected skin, as must the biopsy incision through which the malignancy was diagnosed [see Figure 10]. (One option for removing biopsy incisions while leaving the maximal amount of unaffected skin is to place T-shaped incisions that extend outward from the areola.) FNA and core-needle biopsy incisions are generally not included in the excised skin segment; however, one may, if one wishes, excise a small amount of skin around a core-needle biopsy site. A linear incision should be made as far laterally as necessary to provide adequate exposure for axillary dissection and complete excision of breast tissue. A separate axillary incision may also be used when axillary dissection or SLN biopsy is being performed [see Figure 10]. The extent of dissection should never be compromised in any way for cosmetic reasons.

Reconstruction Options

Implants Perhaps the simplest method of reconstruction is to place a saline-filled implant beneath the greater pectoral muscle and the anterior serratus muscle to recreate a breast mound. Even after a skin-sparing mastectomy, the greater pectoral muscle is usually so tight that unless the patient is small-breasted, expansion of this muscle and the skin is necessary

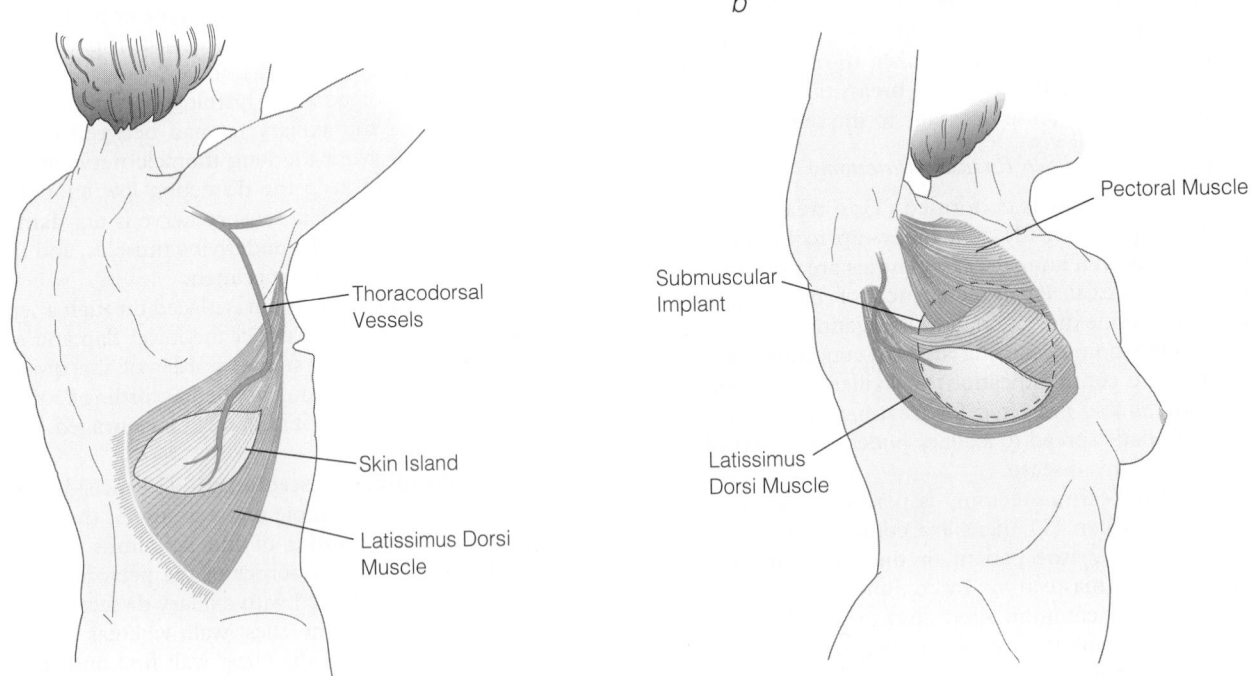

Figure 12 Breast reconstruction after mastectomy. Shown is autologous tissue reconstruction with a latissimus dorsi myocutaneous flap in conjunction with a submuscular implant. (An implant is often required to provide the reconstructed breast with adequate volume and projection.) The myocutaneous flap is elevated; it is important to maintain the blood supply to the flap from the thoracodorsal vessels (*a*). The flap is tunneled subcutaneously to the mastectomy defect (*b*). The latissimus dorsi muscle is sutured to the greater pectoral muscle and the skin of the inframammary fold, so that the implant is completely covered by muscle.

before an implant that matches the opposite breast can be inserted. Serial expansions are performed on an outpatient basis: saline is injected into the expander every 10 to 14 days until an appropriate size has been attained. A second operative procedure is then required to exchange the expander for a permanent implant. A nipple and an areola are constructed at a later date.

The major advantage of implant reconstruction is that there is no need to harvest autologous tissue, and thus the patient is spared the discomfort, scarring, and loss of muscle function that would occur at the donor site. Accordingly, implant reconstructions are commonly performed in patients who require bilateral mastectomies and reconstructions. The initial operative time is significantly shorter for implant reconstruction than for autologous tissue reconstruction, and there is no need for autologous blood donation or transfusion. Hospital stay and recuperation time are also significantly shorter. The main drawbacks are the prolonged time and the multiple office visits required to achieve a symmetrical reconstruction if tissue expansion is required and the necessity of a second surgical procedure to place the permanent implant. In addition, the final cosmetic result often is not as good as what can be achieved with autologous tissue reconstruction, and it may deteriorate over time as a consequence of capsule formation or implant migration. The implant-reconstructed breast is significantly firmer than the contralateral breast. The life expectancy of currently available saline implants has not been established, but it may be less than a decade, which means that many patients who have received or are receiving implants may need replacements at some point. Patients who have previously undergone irradiation of the breast or the chest wall may have tissue that cannot be adequately expanded and thus is unsuitable for implant reconstruction. If the final pathologic evaluation of the mastectomy specimen indicates that radiation therapy is needed for local control, one may consider irradiating the chest wall before expansion with an expander in place; however, this is not an ideal solution.

Autologous tissue   A second approach to reconstruction is to transfer vascularized muscle, skin, and fat from a donor site to the mastectomy defect. The most commonly used myocutaneous flaps are the TRAM flap [see Figure 11] and the latissimus dorsi flap [see Figure 12]. Use of the free TRAM flap is advocated by certain centers; other free-flap options, including the free gluteus flap, are used in special circumstances, when other donor sites are unsuitable.

The major advantage of autologous tissue reconstruction is that it generally yields a superior cosmetic result. Often, the size and shape of the opposite breast can be matched immediately, with no need for subsequent office or operative procedures. The reconstructed breast has a soft texture that is very similar to that of the contralateral breast. In addition, the cosmetic result is stable over time. The main drawbacks are the magnitude of the surgical procedure required for the reconstruction (involving both a prolonged operative time and longer inpatient hospitalization), the potential need for autologous blood donation or transfusion, and the pain, scarring, and loss of muscle function that arise at the donor site. Smokers and patients with significant vascular disease may not be ideal candidates for autologous tissue reconstruction. Partial necrosis of the transferred flap may create firm areas; on rare occasions, complete necrosis and consequent loss of the flap can occur.

A number of factors are considered in choosing between the TRAM flap and the latissimus dorsi flap. In a TRAM flap reconstruction, the contralateral rectus abdominis muscle is transferred along with overlying skin and fat to create a breast mound. This procedure yields a flatter abdominal contour but calls for a long transverse abdominal incision and necessitates repositioning of the umbilicus. A major advantage of the TRAM flap is that it can provide enough tissue to match all but the largest contralateral breasts. Some patients, however (e.g., those who have undergone an abdominal procedure that compromises the TRAM flap's vascular supply) are not ideal candidates for TRAM flap reconstruction. Postoperative discomfort is greater with TRAM flap reconstruction than with other flap reconstructions because of the extent of the abdominal portion of the procedure. In young, healthy, and motivated patients who require bilateral reconstructions, it is often possible to perform two TRAM flap procedures in the same operation.

In a latissimus dorsi myocutaneous flap reconstruction, the ipsilateral latissimus dorsi muscle is transferred along with overlying skin and fat to create a breast mound. Either a horizontal or a vertical donor site incision may be made on the back. The operative technique for the latissimus dorsi flap reconstruction is complex, requiring two intraoperative changes in patient position (from supine to lateral decubitus and from lateral decubitus back to supine for mastectomy, muscle harvest, and final inset of the flap). Patients who have undergone irradiation of the breast, chest wall, or axilla (including irradiation of the thoracodorsal vessels) may not be eligible for this procedure.

A major advantage of the latissimus dorsi flap is that its donor site is associated with less postoperative discomfort than the abdominal donor site of the TRAM flap. In addition, transfer of the latissimus dorsi muscle results in substantially less functional impairment than transfer of the rectus abdominis muscle. A drawback of the latissimus dorsi flap is that in many women, the latissimus dorsi muscle is not bulky enough to provide symmetry with the contralateral breast. In such cases, an implant must be added to the flap to match the size and shape of the opposite breast, which means that the drawback of the implant's limited life span is added to the drawbacks already associated with autologous tissue reconstruction.

Free-flap reconstruction options are utilized primarily when other autologous and implant reconstruction options are not available, do not provide sufficient tissue volume, or have failed. They are more complex procedures, requiring microvascular anastomoses and carrying a higher risk of total flap loss. The two most commonly employed free-flap options are the free TRAM flap and the free gluteus flap.

References

1. Fisher B, Redmond C, Poisson R, et al: Eight-year results of a randomized trial comparing total mastectomy and lumpectomy without irradiation in the treatment of breast cancer. N Engl J Med 320:822, 1989

2. Veronesi U, Luini A, Del Vecchio M, et al: Radiotherapy after breast-preserving surgery in women with localized cancer of the breast. N Engl J Med 328:1587, 1993

3. Sarrazin D, Le M, Rouesse J, et al: Conservative treatment versus mastectomy in breast cancer tumours with mascroscopic diameter of 20 millimetres or less. Cancer 53:1209, 1984

4. Shabot MM, Goldberg IM, Schick P, et al: Aspiration cytology is superior to "Tru-cut" needle biopsy in establishing the diagnosis of clinically suspicious breast masses. Ann Surg 196:122, 1982

5. Gisvold JJ, Martin JK: Prebiopsy localization of non-palpable breast lesions. AJR Am J Roentgenol 143:477, 1984

6. Meyer JE, Kopans DB, Stomper PC, et al: Occult breast abnormalities: percutaneous preoperative needle localization. Radiology 150:355, 1984

7. Rosenberg AL, Schwartz GF, Feig SA, et al: Clinically occult breast lesions: localization and significance. Radiology 162:167, 1987

8. Smith DN, Christian R, Meyer JE: Large-core needle biopsy of nonpalpable breast cancers: the impact on subsequent surgical excisions. Arch Surg 132:256, 1997

9. Parker SH, Lovin JD, Jobe WE, et al: Nonpalpable breast lesions: stereotactic automated large-core biopsies. Radiology 180:403, 1991

10. Meyer JE, Smith DN, Lester SC, et al: Large-core needle biopsy of nonpalpable breast lesions. JAMA 281:1638, 1999

11. Krag D, Weaver D, Ashikaga T, et al: The sentinel node in breast cancer: a multicenter validation study. N Engl J Med 339:941, 1998

12. Giuliano AE, Jones RC, Brennan M, et al: Sentinel lymphadenectomy in breast cancer. J Clin Oncol 15:2345, 1997

13. Souba WW, Bland KI: Indications and techniques for biopsy. The Breast: Comprehensive Management of Benign and Malignant Diseases. Bland KI, Copeland EM III, Eds. WB Saunders Co, Philadelphia, 1991, p 527

14. Morrow M: Management of common breast disorders. Breast Diseases, 2nd ed. Harris JR, Hellman S, Henderson IC, et al, Eds. JB Lippincott Co, Philadelphia, 1987

15. Kinne DW: Primary treatment of breast cancer. Breast Diseases, 2nd ed. Harris JR, Hellman S, Henderson IC, et al, Eds. JB Lippincott Co, Philadelphia, 1987

16. Kinne DW, DeCosse JJ: Modified radical mastectomy for carcinoma of the breast. Am Surg 48:543, 1982

Acknowledgments

The authors wish to thank David Van Hook, M.D., Chief of Mammography, Department of Radiology, Penn State Hershey Medical Center, Hershey, Pennsylvania, for his assistance in preparing the section on directional vacuum-assisted breast biopsy (mammotomy).

Figures 1 through 8, 10   Kerry G. Nicholson.

Figure 9   Marcia Kammerer.

Figures 11 and 12   Tom Moore.

3 LYMPHATIC MAPPING AND SENTINEL LYMPH NODE BIOPSY

Douglas Reintgen, M.D., Rosemary Giuliano, A.R.N.P., Claudia Berman, M.D., Frank Glass, M.D., Jane Messina, M.D., and Charles Cox, M.D.

There is an epidemic of melanoma in the United States: in 2000, 43,000 cases of invasive melanoma and 40,000 cases of melanoma in situ were diagnosed.[1] Moreover, melanoma affects young persons who are in the most productive years of their lives; accordingly, it constitutes a major public health problem. Since the early 1990s, the care of patients with melanoma has changed dramatically with the development of new lymphatic mapping techniques that reduce the cost and morbidity of nodal staging, the emergence of more sensitive assays for occult melanoma metastases, and the identification of interferon alfa-2b as an effective adjuvant therapy for melanoma patients who are at high risk for recurrence. Accurate staging of melanoma patients has become increasingly important in the light of a 1996 report[2] demonstrating improved survival in patients with T4 (tumor thickness > 4.0 mm) or stage III (nodal metastases) melanoma who were treated with adjuvant interferon alfa-2b.

Breast cancer is one of the most common of the malignancies that surgeons encounter in their practices: approximately 186,000 new cases are diagnosed each year in the United States, and the incidence is likely to increase in the next 10 years because the maturation of the baby-boomer population will result in a larger population at risk. It was one of the first tumors for which adjuvant therapy (i.e., treatment of patients who show no evidence of disease but who are at substantial risk for recurrence and death from the disease) was found to be effective. Most authorities believe that axillary nodal staging is an important part of primary breast cancer therapy in that it facilitates identification of patients who are candidates for more aggressive chemotherapy and enhances regional control of disease. Whether axillary node dissection contributes to survival remains controversial, however, and this issue is currently the subject of a national multicenter trial being performed by the American College of Surgeons. That most women with invasive breast cancers will receive either adjuvant chemotherapy or hormone therapy calls into question the necessity of axillary node dissection. Complete axillary node dissection is associated with significant morbidity, and physical problems resulting from the dissection are the complaints women voice most frequently after undergoing breast cancer surgery, once they have dealt with the psychological impact of having an incision on their breast or perhaps even losing the breast.

The development of intraoperative lymphatic mapping and selective lymphadenectomy has made it possible to map the lymphatic flow from a primary tumor and to identify its so-called sentinel lymph node (SLN) in the regional basin. Integration of this technique, in association with detailed pathologic examination of the SLN, into the surgical treatment of melanoma and breast cancer offers the potential for more conservative operations that not only result in lower morbidity but also permit more accurate staging. In what follows, we describe the technical aspects of this new approach, as well as certain related issues.

Lymphatic Mapping and SLN Biopsy for Melanoma

RATIONALE

Many factors are known to predict the risk for metastatic disease in melanoma patients. In evaluating treatments for melanoma, it is crucial to take into account prognostic factors that can accurately categorize patients into different risk groups for metastasis. If this is not done, it is difficult or impossible to determine whether differences between treatment regimens (or the absence thereof) are due to the treatments themselves or merely reflect imbalances of prognostic factors.

The presence or absence of lymph node metastases is the single most powerful predictor of recurrence and survival in melanoma patients: the 5-year survival rate is approximately 40% lower in patients who have lymph node metastases than in those who do not. A great deal of time, effort, and money has been expended on identifying prognostic factors based on primary tumor variables (e.g., Breslow's tumor thickness, ulceration, primary site, and sex); however, multiple regression analyses performed on many collected populations in the literature indicate that once melanoma metastasizes to the regional nodes, such prognostic factors contribute relatively little to the prognostic model compared with the patient's lymph node status. This finding suggests that many melanoma patients might benefit from an accurate nodal staging procedure.

Nodal Staging

Elective lymph node dissection Elective lymph node dissection (ELND) has been the mainstay of the surgeon's armamentarium for nodal staging of melanoma patients. ELND removes clinically negative nodes, as opposed to therapeutic dissection, which removes nodes with gross tumor involvement. Opinions are divided as to whether ELND actually extends survival or whether it is solely a staging procedure. Two prospective, randomized trials failed to demonstrate improved survival in melanoma patients treated with ELND in comparison with patients who underwent wide local excision (WLE) alone as primary surgical therapy.[3,4] Retrospective studies using large databases, however, suggested that there were subpopulations of melanoma patients who did benefit from ELND.[5,6]

The controversy may have been laid to rest by the results of the Intergroup Melanoma Trial, which was the first randomized study to prove enhanced survival after surgical treatment of clinically occult metastatic melanoma. Only patients with intermediate-thickness melanoma (tumor thickness, 1.0 to 4.0 mm) were eligible. In addition, the Intergroup Melanoma Trial was the first prospective study to require preoperative lymphoscintigraphy in all patients to identify and remove all basins at risk for metastasis. Without preoperative lymphoscintigraphy to provide a map for the surgeon, ELND may be misdirected in more than 50% of head and neck dissections and trunk dissections[7]; moreover, so-called in transit nodes (defined as nodes outside the classic anatomic basin between the primary site and the regional nodes), which are equally at risk for metastasis, may be missed in 5% of patients.[8]

In the Intergroup Melanoma Trial, overall survival was not significantly longer in patients who underwent WLE and ELND than in those who underwent WLE of the primary site coupled with observation of the regional basins. There were, however, two well-defined subsets of the ELND group that exhibited a significant increase in overall survival: patients with melanomas 1.1 to 2.0 mm thick and patients younger than 60 years.[9] Stratification by tumor thickness was part of the original design of the trial, but the age-related benefit only became apparent with retrospective subgroup analysis.

A subsequent report from the same group that included 10 years of follow-up indicated that the survival curves of the two groups continued to separate secondary to late recurrences and deaths in the group treated with WLE alone. In addition, the *P* value for survival differences across the entire study decreased from 0.25 to 0.09 over the longer follow-up period, suggesting that surgery in the regional nodal basin, in and of itself, may confer a survival benefit.[10]

Three national prospective, randomized trials—the Eastern Cooperative Oncology Group (ECOG) trials[2,11,12]—have investigated adjuvant interferon alfa-2b; the first of these, ECOG 1684,[2] was the impetus for FDA approval of interferon alfa-2b as the first effective adjuvant therapy for patients at high risk for recurrent melanoma. ECOG 1684 and ECOG 1694 reported significant overall survival benefits, but ECOG 1690 did not (though it did report a significant disease-free survival [DFS] benefit). Statistical analysis of the three ECOG trials shows that given three prospective, randomized trials with a predictive power of 0.8 and a statistical signif-

Choice of Radiocolloid and Vital Blue Dye for Lymphatic Mapping

Choice of Radiocolloid

Little work has been done to determine which radiocolloid is best suited to either preoperative or intraoperative mapping. The ideal radiocolloid for intraoperative SLN mapping would have small particles (< 100 nm) that are uniformly dispersed, would be highly stable, and would have a short half-life that would not complicate the handling of the excised specimen. Technetium (^{99m}Tc)-labeled compounds, being gamma emitters, satisfy most of these requirements. In a direct comparison between filtered (0.1 μm filter) ^{99m}Tc-labeled sulfur colloid (^{99m}Tc-SC) and ^{99m}Tc-labeled antimony trisulfide colloid (^{99m}Tc-ATC), which has a particle size of 3 to 30 nm, filtered ^{99m}Tc-SC was transported more quickly to the nodal basin and emitted less radiation to the liver, the spleen, and the whole body.[90] Unfiltered ^{99m}Tc-SC contains relatively large particles (100 to 1,000 nm), and some investigators have found it to migrate more slowly from the injection site; however, other investigators have found it to be slow to flow through the first SLN to higher secondary nodes, which is actually an advantage.

In comparisons between ^{99m}Tc-labeled human serum albumin (^{99m}Tc-HSA), ^{99m}Tc-labeled stannous phyate, and ^{99m}Tc-ATC with respect to lymphoscintigram quality, the last of these provided the best images for preoperative lymphoscintigraphy.[91] In an animal study comparing ^{99m}Tc-HSA and filtered ^{99m}Tc-SC, ^{99m}Tc-SC was actually concentrated in the SLN over a period of 1 to 2 hours, whereas ^{99m}Tc-HSA passed rapidly through the SLN.[34] As a result, ^{99m}Tc-SC yielded higher activity ratios at intraoperative mapping, improved the success rate of localization, made the technique easier, and thus was a superior reagent for this application.[33,34]

The Sydney Melanoma Unit (SMU) prefers to use ^{99m}Tc-ATC because it seems to have smaller, more uniform particles that rapidly migrate into the lymphatic channels but still are appropriately trapped and retained by the SLN.[92] At SMU, use of this compound allows injection of the radiocolloid and imaging to be performed the day before operation. These investigators find that hot spots in the regional basin are maintained even if 24 hours have elapsed from the time of the injection. The radioactivity in the basin over the hot spot (i.e., the SLN) is decreased because four half-lives of the technetium have been expended and because some of the radiocolloid has passed through, but the ex vivo activity ratio (i.e., SLN:neighboring non-SLN) is not substantially affected. In the United States, ^{99m}Tc-ATC has been removed from the market and is unavailable for clinical use.

Other investigators have obtained very good intraoperative mapping results with unfiltered ^{99m}Tc-SC; however, they have not obtained good planar images for lymphoscintigraphy and have been unable to identify cutaneous lymphatic flow to any basin in 10% of the patients.[21]

At MCC, we use filtered (0.2 μm filter) ^{99m}Tc-SC. This particle size gives good images on lymphoscintigraphy and is trapped and concentrated in the SLN over a significant period, so that the hot spot over the

SLN actually becomes hotter compared with surrounding tissue for 2 to 6 hours after injection, making the SLN easier to find. It also has an advantage over unfiltered ^{99m}Tc-SC in that it results in less shine-through of radioactivity from the primary site.

Choice of Vital Blue Dye

Several vital blue dyes have been investigated with an eye to their potential applicability to cutaneous lymphatic mapping. Among these are methylene blue (American Regent Lab, Shirley, New York); isosulfan blue, 1% in aqueous solution (Lymphazurin; United States Surgical Corporation, Norwalk, Connecticut); patent blue-V (Laboratoire Guerbert, France); Cyalume (American Cyanamid Company, Bound Brook, New Jersey); and fluorescein dye. All substances tested were known to be nontoxic in vivo and were injected intradermally as provided by the supplier. In a feline study,[13] patent blue-V and isosulfan blue were the most accurate in identifying the regional lymphatic drainage pattern. These dyes entered the lymphatics rapidly, with minimal diffusion into the surrounding tissue. Their bright-blue color was readily visible and allowed easy identification of the exposed lymphatics.

Isosulfan blue has worked extremely well for intraoperative SLN mapping. In some patients with thin skin, the afferent lymphatics can be seen through the skin after the injection of isosulfan blue. In addition, when the dye enters the SLN, it stains part of the node a pale blue, thus clearly distinguishing the SLN from the surrounding non-SLNs. The other dyes have largely been abandoned as unsatisfactory because they diffuse too rapidly into surrounding tissue and are not retained by the lymphatic channels in sufficient concentrations to stain the SLN. The fluorescent dyes fluorescein and Cyalume are readily visualized, but a dark room is necessary for optimal visualization; moreover, because of their diffusion into surrounding tissue, the background fluorescence is unacceptably high. Methylene blue is relatively poorly retained by the lymphatic vessels and thus stains the SLN too lightly.

Use of vital blue dyes has not given rise to any significant complications. Although allergic reactions, including anaphylactic reactions, have been reported on rare occasions in the literature, they have not occurred in large study populations.[17,18] Blue dye can be retained at the primary site for more than a year. The color gradually fades with time; however, patients can be left with a permanent tattoo if the injected dye is not removed with wide local excision (WLE) of the primary site or, in the case of breast cancer, with lumpectomy. Fortunately, in the head and neck area, where a permanent tattoo would be unacceptable, the richness of the cutaneous lymphatics allows rapid clearance of the blue dye from the skin and the subcutaneous tissues. A small amount of residual dye may be left behind after WLE, but this typically disappears rapidly and poses no real problem. All patients report the presence of dye in the urine and the stool during the first 24 hours. In some cases, the dye can interfere with transcutaneous oxygen monitoring during anesthesia.

Figure 1 **Lymphatic mapping and SLN biopsy for melanoma. Primary sites for both melanoma and breast cancer may have four to six afferent lymphatics emerging from the tumor location, but as the lymphatics travel to the regional basin, they converge into one or two SLNs. Shown are four afferent lymphatics converging into one SLN.**

icance of 0.95, if two of them report a survival benefit and the third does not, the statistical probability that these results will be obtained with an effective therapy is 0.38. On the other hand, the statistical probability that these results will be obtained with an ineffective therapy is only 0.008. Thus, the evidence that high-dose interferon alfa-2b is an effective adjuvant therapy for patients with stage III melanoma is compelling.

Given the results from the Intergroup Melanoma Trial and the three ECOG trials,[9-12] one can make a strong argument that when the risk of nodal metastasis reaches a certain defined level, a nodal staging procedure should be done. At our institution (H. Lee Moffitt Cancer Center [MCC], Tampa, Florida), the level of primary melanoma thickness at which nodal staging is considered is 0.76 mm or greater. The nodal staging procedure we recommend and perform is lymphatic mapping and SLN biopsy.

Intraoperative lymphatic mapping and selective lymphadenectomy Intraoperative lymphatic mapping and selective lymphadenectomy was developed as a method of assessing regional lymph node status more accurately than ELND could while reducing both morbidity and expense. This technique relies on two concepts: first, that different regions of the skin have specific patterns of lymphatic drainage to the regional lymphatic basin; and second, that for a given skin region, there is a specific lymph node (i.e., an SLN) in the basin to which the cutaneous lymphatic vessels drain first. These concepts were borne out by initial animal studies using either vital blue dye[13] or radiocolloid[14] (which has been shown to map the same lymphatic pathways and label the same nodes as vital blue dye) [see Sidebar Choice of Radiocolloid and Vital Blue Dye for Lymphatic Mapping].

Intraoperative lymphatic mapping and selective lymphadenectomy was initially proposed by Morton and associates,[15,16] who used a vital blue dye method. These investigators showed that the SLN is the first node in the lymphatic basin into which the primary melanoma consistently drains (though not necessarily the closest to the primary). They also hypothesized that the status of the SLN, if it was negative for metastases, would reflect the status of higher nodes (i.e., nodes farther down the lymphatic drainage pathway, also termed second-tier nodes). Subsequent work on intraoperative

mapping and selective lymphadenectomy confirmed that the SLN is the first site of metastatic disease and demonstrated that if the SLN is histologically negative, then the remainder of the lymph nodes in the basin are histologically negative as well.[17,18] These findings suggest that melanoma patients can be accurately staged with procedures that are less extensive than complete dissection.

SLNs can be mapped from different primary site locations, and more than one node in the same basin can be an SLN, depending on the primary site. Fine dermal lymphatic vessels coalesce to form several major lymphatic trunks that eventually drain to the regional lymphatic basin. Because cutaneous lymphatic vessels converge rather than diverge [see Figure 1], one can perform intraoperative mapping from various skin sites and still harvest only one or two SLNs from the basin. The small number of specimens facilitates detailed pathologic examination: the pathologist can readily perform serial sections of the nodes and use immunohistochemical methods to look for micrometastatic disease. More intensive pathologic examination of one or two SLNs appears to identify patients with micrometastatic lymph node metastases more accurately than routine examination of all the regional lymph nodes.

Unusual or ambiguous drainage patterns. Lymphoscintigraphy has been used in live patients to map patterns of lymphatic drainage from various primary skin sites. Early assessments of lymphatic flow patterns, such as those of the 19th century anatomist Sappey,[19] were based on anatomic dissections of cadavers and do not accurately reflect lymphatic flow patterns in living humans. The watershed areas of the body are much larger than originally described by Sappey, and there is no clinically predictable lymphatic flow from a melanoma until it is located 10 cm off the midline or 10 cm off Sappey's line (a line running between the umbilicus and L2) [see Figure 2]. In addition, the entire head and neck region is a watershed area. Cutaneous lymphatic flow frequently cannot be predicted on the basis of anatomic site, and areas of ambiguous or multidirectional flow are

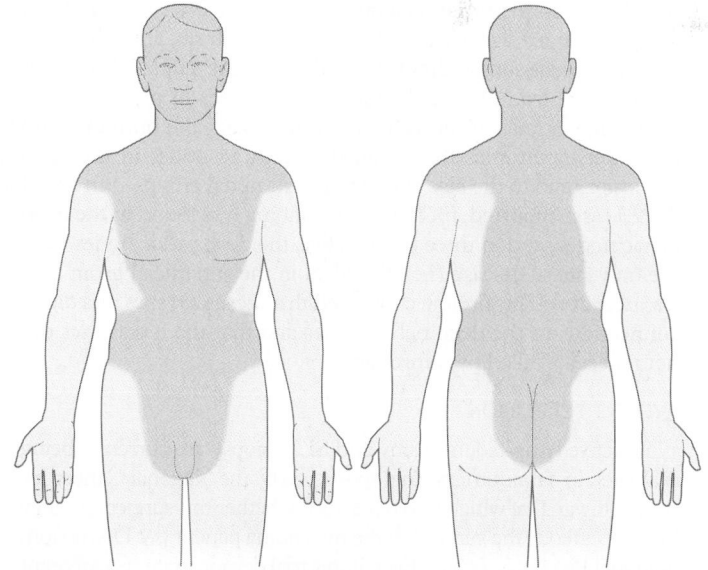

Figure 2 **Lymphatic mapping and SLN biopsy for melanoma. The watershed areas of the body where multidirectional cutaneous lymphatic flow is found are much more extensive than classical descriptions predicted. One does not find unidirectional cutaneous lymphatic flow until lesions are 10 cm off the midline or 10 cm off Sappey's line, which runs between the umbilicus and L2. The entire head and neck area is also unpredictable.**

Figure 3 **Lymphatic mapping and SLN biopsy for melanoma. Shown is an intermediate-thickness melanoma of the left back in a 40-year-old man. Preoperative lymphoscintigraphy identified flow from the primary site into the left axilla and separate flow into an in transit node located at the tip of the left scapula. Vital blue dye was injected into the dermis around the primary site, and a small incision was made over the tattoo marking the location of the in transit node, which could then be visualized and harvested.**

significantly more extensive than classical descriptions predicted.[20]

A number of unusual drainage patterns and pathways have been noted in Australia[20]: 26% of melanomas on the back drained to an in transit node near the scapula in the intermuscular space [*see Figure 3*], 20% of melanomas near the umbilicus drained to an internal mammary node, some posterior scalp melanomas drained to lymph nodes at the base of the neck, and at least one forearm melanoma drained directly to a lymph node in the ipsilateral neck. Krag and coworkers[21,22] have also noted some unusual lymphatic drainage patterns: one melanoma on the right upper back drained directly to a node in the right midclavicular space, almost at the apex of the right lung; another melanoma on the lower back drained to an SLN along the neurovascular bundle under the 12th rib; and two lower extremity melanomas drained to SLNs in the popliteal fossa. A 2001 report from MCC documented 23 cases of primary cutaneous melanomas around the lower abdomen, the buttocks, and the lower extremities that drained directly to nodes in the deep pelvic area and to the iliac and hypogastric nodal groups.[23] In five of the 23 cases reported, metastatic melanoma was found in the deep pelvic nodes, and in three of these five, the deep pelvic nodes were the only site of disease (i.e., the SLN in the superficial groin area was negative). This finding confirmed that these skin sites had direct connections to the deep pelvic nodes and that the metastases did not reflect so-called pass-through.

PATIENT SELECTION

Selective lymphadenectomy and SLN biopsy are currently being evaluated in a randomized trial sponsored by the National Cancer Institute, the goal of which is to determine whether this surgical strategy by itself extends the survival of the melanoma patient [*see* Discussion, National Protocols, *below*]. Even if this trial demonstrates no inherent survival benefit, there are additional considerations that support use of the procedure in certain populations. Data from the interferon alfa-2b trial cited earlier[2] suggest that all patients whose melanoma is more than 1.0 mm thick should undergo a nodal staging procedure so that adjuvant otherapy can be administered in a selective fashion. If T4N0 patients are removed from the analysis of this trial and only patients with lymph node metastases are considered, DFS increas-

es by 82% ($P = 0.0006$) with adjuvant therapy; overall survival increases by 24% as well ($P = 0.006$). Given such a substantial difference in both DFS and overall survival, one would naturally want to offer these patients interferon alfa-2b therapy. Accordingly, one would need to identify patients with nodal metastases who might benefit from such therapy. Lymphatic mapping and SLN biopsy is the least morbid and most cost-effective way of determining which melanoma patients have lymph node metastases.[24]

In female patients with melanomas less than 0.76 mm thick, the risk of nodal metastasis is less than 1%; thus, SLN biopsy is not indicated in this population. In male patients whose primary site is on the trunk, however, the incidence of occult nodal metastases may be as high as 9%, even if the primary lesion is less than 0.76 mm thick; lymphatic mapping may be considered in this population.

In patients whose tumor is 0.76 to 1.0 mm thick, the risk of nodal metastasis is less than 6%; the procedure can be offered as an option in this population. In our experience, these patients usually elect to undergo SLN biopsy despite the low risk of occult nodal metastasis: the morbidity of the procedure is low, and the finding of a positive SLN can radically affect subsequent treatment decisions. Several prognostic factors have been shown to identify patients with thin melanomas who are at higher risk (approximately 10%) for metastatic disease and death at 5 years: tumors at Clark level III or greater, ulcerated primaries, regressed lesions, male gender, and axial melanomas.[25] Patients with four or five of these five prognostic factors should be treated as if they have thicker lesions, and their SLNs should be harvested even if the primary lesions are less than 0.76 mm thick.

Patients whose melanoma is of intermediate thickness (1.0 to 4.0 mm) probably have the most to gain from lymphatic mapping and SLN biopsy. The procedure may be used for staging, so that patients can be offered adjuvant therapy in an appropriately selective fashion, and it may also increase survival, as the long-term follow-up data from the Intergroup Melanoma Trial suggest.[10]

In patients with thick (> 4.0 mm) melanomas, the rate of occult systemic metastasis is 70%, and that of occult nodal metastasis is 60% to 70%. Consequently, in the past, procedures involving the regional nodes (i.e., ELND) were not recommended, because there was no survival benefit. Now that effective adjuvant therapy is available, however, lymphatic mapping and SLN biopsy should be offered to these patients as a staging procedure. Survival is decreased in patients with thick melanomas and documented nodal microscopic disease compared with patients with thick melanomas and no sign of nodal spread[26]; accordingly, some medical oncologists observe T4 patients unless nodal metastasis is documented.

A crucial question to be answered is, what is the standard of surgical care for melanoma patients with tumors thicker than 1.0 mm? Given that the histology of the SLN has been shown to be indicative of the histology of the rest of the nodes in the basin, one can conclude that if the surgeon has adequate support from nuclear medicine and pathology services, there is no need to perform ELND. If such support is unavailable, if intraoperative mapping cannot be done (as, perhaps, when WLE of the primary melanoma has already been performed), or if the results of mapping are equivocal, then the ELND guidelines from the Intergroup Melanoma Surgical Trial[9] should be followed. If this approach is taken, ELND should be guided by preoperative lymphoscintigraphy for identification and dissection of all basins at risk for metastasis.

Finally, previous extensive primary site surgery constitutes a general technical contraindication to lymphatic mapping. Patients who have undergone rotational flap closure or Z-plasty reconstruction are considered ineligible for this procedure.

TECHNIQUE

The technique of intraoperative mapping varies considerably from center to center. We will describe the nuances of the technique as it is performed at MCC, detailing the steps that are important for successful mapping. It cannot be emphasized enough that successful intraoperative SLN mapping requires close collaboration between the surgeon, the nuclear radiologist, and the pathologist, with each member of the team playing a critical role.

An initial caveat regarding the timing of the procedure in relation to WLE is in order. Data from MCC indicate that when lymphatic mapping is done after WLE, the dissection tends to be more extensive than it need have been. More SLNs are removed and more regional basins dissected than when lymphatic mapping is done before WLE; moreover, the rate at which so-called skip metastases are detected appears to be increased. With lymphatic mapping and SLN biopsy becoming the standard of care in the United States for nodal staging to identify melanoma patients who are candidates for adjuvant therapy and a possible survival benefit, it is essential that patient care not be compromised by extensive primary site surgery before lymphatic mapping.

Step 1: Preoperative Lymphoscintigraphy

Patients come to the nuclear medicine suite early on the day of operation and undergo preoperative lymphoscintigraphy with the injection of 450 µCi in 1 ml of filtered technetium-99–labeled sulfur colloid (^{99m}Tc-SC) [*see Sidebar* Choice of Radiocolloid and Vital Blue Dye for Lymphatic Mapping]. Dynamic scans are performed 5 to 10 minutes after injection of the radiocolloid, and the location of the SLN in the basin is marked with an intradermal tattoo. All regional lymphatic basins at risk for metastatic spread, along with in transit nodes and SLNs, are identified and marked for harvesting.

Comment Preoperative lymphoscintigraphy serves as a road map for planning the surgical procedure and is used for four distinct reasons:

1. To identify all nodal basins at risk for metastatic disease.[7] This is especially important with melanomas of the trunk or the head and neck, whose lymphatic drainage patterns cannot be reliably predicted by clinical judgment or classic anatomic guidelines.[27]

2. To identify any in transit nodes that can be tattooed by the nuclear radiologist for later harvesting [*see Figure 4*]. An example is afforded by the case of a forearm lesion with an afferent lymphatic vessel flowing to an epitrochlear in transit node and a separate afferent vessel flowing from that node to the axillary basin [*see Figure 4a*]. The SLNs in both locations were harvested, and only the epitrochlear SLN was histologically positive. In this case, mapping with the blue dye alone would have yielded histologically negative axillary SLNs and understaged the patient. In addition, the tumor containing an epitrochlear in transit node would have been left in place and thus might later have seeded the axillary nodes or distant metastatic sites.

3. To identify the location of the SLN in relation to the rest of the nodes in the basin.[28-30] Because the location of the SLN may vary within a basin, it is important to mark the position of the SLN in reference to other nodes so that harvesting may be done with local anesthesia through a minimal incision. Preoperative lymphoscintigraphy can accomplish this task quite well, especially in the groin and the head and neck area, where the lymph nodes are more superficial. The axilla is the most difficult area to map: here, the best preoperative lymphoscintigraphy can do is to determine

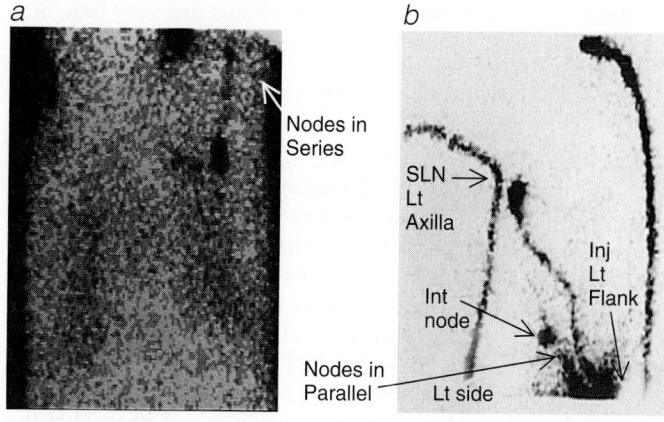

Figure 4 Lymphatic mapping and SLN biopsy for melanoma. In transit nodal areas are identified in 5% of melanoma patients; this is the reason why preoperative lymphoscintigraphy is performed for primary sites on either the upper or the lower extremity. In a patient with a melanoma on the left hand (*a*), the injection site and the left hand are raised above the head, and cutaneous lymphatic flow can be seen into an epitrochlear node. This in transit node then emits a lymphatic vessel flowing to the left axilla. By definition, the SLN is the first node in the chain that receives primary lymphatic flow. The epitrochlear node and any axillary nodes are nodes in series. Hence, the epitrochlear node is the SLN and thus is the only node that must be harvested. In a patient with a primary melanoma on the left flank (*b*), there are two separate afferent lymphatics, one leading to an SLN in the left axilla and the other leading to an in transit node on the left flank. These are nodes in parallel in that they both receive primary lymphatic flow from the skin site. Hence, the two nodes are equally at risk for metastatic disease, and both are considered SLNs and must be harvested.

whether the node is located anteriorly, posteriorly, superiorly, or inferiorly in the basin. Use of hand-held gamma probes during SLN mapping has reduced the need to mark SLN locations during preoperative lymphoscintigraphy; however, intradermal tattooing to mark the location of the SLN can confirm the site and thereby make the surgical procedure more efficient.

4. To estimate the number of SLNs in the regional basin that will have to be harvested.

The timing of the injection of the mapping reagent has an impact on the success of the procedure. Whereas vital blue dyes typically travel to the regional basin within a matter of minutes, most radiocolloids are concentrated in the SLN over a period of hours. Activity ratios (see below) for ^{99m}Tc-SC are highest 2 to 6 hours after injection, which is helpful to the surgeon in three respects. First, the higher ratios make the SLN easier to locate. Second, the radiocolloid can be injected by the nuclear radiologist hours before the actual operation, and the surgeon does not need a special license for radioactivity handling. Third, cases are easier to schedule because there is a 2- to 6-hour window during which the intraoperative mapping can be easily accomplished.

Several groups have shown that lymphatic mapping for melanoma can still be effectively performed as long as 16 to 24 hours after injection of the radiocolloid.[31] Because of the short half-life of technetium (6 hours), the measured radioactivity around the injection site is substantially less when mapping is delayed to this extent. Nevertheless, it is usually possible to recognize the hot spot representing the concentration of radiocolloid in the SLN because once the radiocolloid enters the first node, it tends to be trapped there by the dendritic cells of the node, which means that very little of it passes through to second-tier nodes.

Step 2: Intraoperative Lymphatic Mapping and Identification of SLN

The patient is taken to the OR 2 to 24 hours later, and 1 ml of 1% isosulfan blue dye (Lymphazurin) [see Sidebar Choice of Radiocolloid and Vital Blue Dye for Lymphatic Mapping] per direction of drainage is injected around the primary site. The primary site and the regional basin are prepared and draped, and 10 minutes is allowed for the vital blue dye to travel to the SLN. Attention is then directed initially to the regional basin. The radioactive hot spot in the regional basin is identified with the hand-held gamma probe, and the in vivo activity ratio (see below) is noted. If shine-through from the radioactivity of the radiocolloid injected at the primary site is a problem, WLE of the primary may be performed first. An incision is made over the hot spot, and small flaps are created in all directions to allow identification of the blue-stained afferent lymphatic vessels. Surgical dissection is aided by visualization of the stained afferent lymphatic vessel leading down to the blue-stained node and by the use of the hand-held gamma probe to direct dissection down to the SLN. If, as is sometimes the case, one becomes confused as to what is proximal and what is distal on the afferent lymphatic vessel, the probe can be used to identify the direction of dissection.

Comment Radiocolloid and vital blue dye mapping techniques are complementary, and there is no reason why the two approaches should not be used simultaneously to improve the chances of locating the SLN successfully. Either may be crucial in a given instance, depending on the location of the primary in relation to the regional basin. If the primary site is close to, overlying, or in a direct line to the basin, so that the gamma probe is likely to encounter shine-through, use of vital blue dye may be the only technique that permits successful mapping. Only 1% to 5% of the injected radiocolloid dose is delivered to the regional basin; thus, even if the radioactivity from the primary site is reduced by performing WLE first, enough radioactivity may remain at that site (thanks to diffusion of the injectate) to increase the background level in the basin to the point where mapping with the radiocolloid alone is impossible. On the other hand, when one is mapping a fatty axilla or the head and neck region, it may be impossible to follow a wisp of blue-stained afferent lymphatic vessel to the SLN. Large flaps are especially to be avoided in the head and neck area because of the surrounding vital structures; in this setting, the ability of the gamma probe to locate the hot spot through the skin before the incision is made is a tremendous advantage.

A key issue with intraoperative radiocolloid mapping is how to define an SLN in terms of accumulated radioactivity. To do this, clinicians must use so-called activity (or localization) ratios. Measurement of the absolute level of radioactivity in a node is not sufficient, because in each harvest, there are a number of crucial variables: different radiocolloid doses are injected at the primary site, the injection is sometimes unevenly distributed around the primary site, the time interval between injection and harvest is not constant, the distance between the primary site and the regional basin is not always the same, and varying degrees of shine-through may be present. The effects of these variables can be eliminated by determining the in vivo activity ratio (i.e., the ratio of the radioactivity in the SLN to the background radioactivity). In vivo radioactivity is measured in counts/10 sec with the SLN fully exposed. Background activity is estimated by counting four areas in the basin equidistant from the injection site and away from the SLN. Perhaps more help-

ful is the ex vivo activity ratio (i.e., the ratio of the radioactivity in an excised SLN to that in an excised neighboring non-SLN), which has the virtue of eliminating all shine-through. At MCC, we define an SLN as a node with an activity ratio of 3:1 or higher in vivo or 10:1 or higher ex vivo. In our experience, 98% of SLNs exhibit these ratios.

Occasionally, pass-through of the blue dye or the radiocolloid occurs but rarely, if ever, to the point where it results in mistaken identification of a higher node as an SLN. That is, one typically does not see non-SLNs that are stained blue or that have activity ratios of 3:1 in vivo or 10:1 ex vivo. When the radiocolloid does pass through the SLN, it is distributed to multiple higher nodes, thereby helping to raise the background radiation level; however, it is not concentrated to any large extent in any one higher node.

Step 3: Removal of SLN

Once the SLN is identified, the entire node is removed by means of sharp dissection or the electrocautery. Afferent and efferent lymphatic vessels entering and exiting the SLN, some of which (i.e., the afferent vessels) are stained blue, are controlled with hemostatic clips because the electrocautery will not seal these vessels. This measure decreases the risk of postoperative wound seroma. If the opportunity presents itself without the risk of increased morbidity, a neighboring non-SLN may be removed to provide an internal control, and the ex vivo activity ratio may be calculated.

The radioactivity level in the excised SLN is checked with the hand-held gamma probe to confirm that the node has been correctly identified as the SLN. The residual radioactivity in the basin is then checked with the probe to verify that all SLNs have been removed. If radioactivity has not fallen to the background level, the probe should be used to direct additional dissection aimed at removing any additional SLNs present.

Comment The directed dissection achievable with the help of radio-guided mapping allows the surgeon to perform axillary and head and neck harvests without having to identify the motor nerves running through the basin. A series of 30 head and neck melanoma patients with SLN drainage to the parotid gland showed that the SLNs could be harvested with directed dissection without formal identification of fascial motor nerves.[32] The technique recommended by the authors—which may be adaptable to other basins where dissection passes close to a motor nerve—involved eliminating paralyzing agents with anesthesia, incising the parotid fascia, then, with blunt dissection under gamma-probe guidance, shelling out the SLN in the parotid gland. The success rate of SLN identification in the parotid gland was higher than 90%, and there were no instances of fascial nerve dysfunction. Likewise, in more than 2,000 axillary SLN mappings at MCC, there has been no evidence of prolonged postoperative thoracic or thoracodorsal dysfunction. Dissections in the posterior cervical triangle are performed similarly when in close proximity to the spinal accessory nerve.

A secondary benefit of radiocolloid mapping is its ability to provide immediate verification that all SLNs have been removed from the lymphatic basin: if all of the radiolabeled SLNs have in fact been excised, the radioactivity in the basin must return to its background level. When only vital blue dye is used for mapping, it often proves necessary to perform further dissection (and create more flaps) to locate additional blue-stained lymphatics and verify that all SLNs have been excised.

In addition, as noted [see Step 1: Preoperative Lymphoscintigraphy, above], the radiocolloid has a much longer retention time than the dye and tends to be concentrated in the SLN. When harvest occurs 2 to 24 hours after injection of the radiocolloid, activity ratios are double what they are when mapping is done immediately after injection.[33,34]

Step 4: Pathologic Examination of SLN

Once the SLN has been harvested, it is submitted for detailed pathologic examination. The examination may include serial sectioning, immunohistochemical staining with S-100 and HMB-45 monoclonal antibodies, and perhaps reverse transcriptase–polymerase chain reaction (RT-PCR) analysis.

COMPLICATIONS

Complications of lymphatic mapping are rare. All SLN harvests are performed without any postoperative drainage, and this contributes to the low morbidity of the procedure. A seroma develops in about 10% of patients, but it is easily handled with percutaneous aspiration. Surgical site infections are rare, and wound healing is better than with ELND because large flaps are not needed for the dissection.

In a 2001 report, investigators from the Sun Belt Melanoma Trial compared complication rates for lymphatic mapping in 1,202 patients who underwent SLN dissection alone with complication rates in 277 patients who required complete lymph node dissection (CLND) as part of the trial.[35] The incidences of seroma, lymphedema, and wound problems were 3%, 0.7%, and 1.7%, respectively, in the first group and 7.9%, 9.8%, and 11.9% in the second.

REPORTED RESULTS

In the initial report by Morton and associates,[15] in which mapping was done with vital blue dye alone, SLNs were successfully identified in 194 of 237 lymphatic basins, and 40 (21%) of the 194 specimens contained metastatic melanoma detected either by routine histologic examination with hematoxylin-eosin staining (12%) or by immunohistochemical staining exclusively (9%). Metastases were present in 47 (18%) of 259 SLNs, whereas non-SLNs were the exclusive site of metastasis in only two of 3,079 nodes from 194 dissections, for a false negative rate of 1% (with nodes rather than patients as the unit of analysis).

Given that lymphatic mapping can be evaluated only in patients with metastatic disease—because these are the only patients in whom a skip metastasis (i.e., a metastasis in which the SLN is histologically negative but nodes farther down the drainage pathway are histologically positive) could be documented—the investigators' findings in these patients are of considerable interest. Of 40 patients with histologically positive nodes, SLN mapping identified 38, for a 5% false negative rate. In 72% of basins, a particular primary site drained to a single SLN; in 20%, to two SLNs; and in 8%, to three or more SLNs. Surgeons successfully identified SLNs in 72% to 96% of attempts, depending on where the surgeons were on the learning curve. Overall, groin mappings were the most successful (89% of attempts); axillary mapping was generally successful as well (78% of attempts). The investigators concluded that a learning curve of 60 cases would be necessary, which meant that the procedure would have to be restricted to major medical centers that treat large numbers of melanoma patients. This caveat notwithstanding, the new technique clearly was capable of accurately identifying patients with occult lymph node metastases who might benefit from radical lymphadenectomy.[15,16]

Surgical trials at several other institutions confirmed two essential points.[8,17,18,21,22] First, nodal metastasis from cutaneous primary sites follows an orderly, nonrandom, progressive pattern. Second, SLNs in the lymphatic basins can be individually identified, and their status reflects the presence or absence of melanoma metastases in the remaining nodes in the basins. In an initial study of 42 patients with intermediate-thickness melanomas,[17] SLN harvesting

was followed by complete node dissection to confirm the low incidence of skip metastases in this population. None of the patients in this study had skip metastases: eight had a positive SLN, with the SLN as the only site of disease in seven of the eight, and 34 had a histologically negative SLN, with the rest of the nodes in the basin also histologically negative. Analysis of the results proved that the SLN was the first and favored site of metastatic disease. Preoperative lymphoscintigraphy was performed in this trial to define all basins at risk for metastatic disease, and intraoperative mapping was performed with isosulfan blue dye. The rate of technical failure was 10%.

A trial at the University of Vermont employed radiocolloid for intraoperative mapping after it was determined that in some cases, use of the vital blue dye was difficult if not impossible.[36] The investigators studied 100 patients with melanoma arising at a wide variety of primary sites. All of the patients underwent lymphoscintigraphy 1 to 24 hours before intraoperative mapping and SLN excision. A hand-held gamma probe was used to facilitate accurate identification and removal of the SLNs. Incisions were made directly over the hot spot to minimize dissection; further dissection, if needed, was guided by the probe. The SLNs were successfully located in 98% of the patients, a markedly better result than was obtained in previous reports.

Subsequently, this same melanoma consortium published updated findings.[21] Between February 1993 and October 1994, 121 patients with invasive melanomas and clinically negative nodes were enrolled in a study comparing two different approaches to intraoperative mapping. In one group (64% of patients), mapping involved only injection of a radiocolloid (unfiltered ^{99m}Tc-SC, ^{99m}Tc–human serum albumin [^{99m}Tc-HSA], or Microlite [Dupont, Billerica, Massachusetts]) around the primary site and use of a hand-held gamma probe; the SLN was successfully identified in 97.6% of the patients in this group. In the other group (36% of patients), both vital blue dye and radiocolloid were used. All of the blue-stained SLNs also yielded radioactive hot spots, and in four patients the blue dye was not identified in any of the lymph nodes, which meant that mapping would have been unsuccessful if blue-staining had been the only mapping technique applied. Preoperative lymphoscintigraphy was used in 93% of the patients, with a technical failure rate of 10%. The radiolabeled SLNs could not be successfully imaged in these 12 patients preoperatively, but with the help of the hand-held gamma probe, the SLNs could be identified intraoperatively. This result suggests that a hand-held gamma probe is more sensitive at identifying SLNs than a scintillation camera. The reason may be that the probe accumulates data for scanning the basin in seconds, compared with the 2 to 6 minutes needed for the camera to produce images. This difference probably also explains why multiple nodes are sometimes imaged on preoperative lymphoscintigraphy when 1 to 2 hours have elapsed between radiocolloid injection and imaging. Intraoperative mapping, on the other hand, readily identifies the SLN and does not find multiple nodes to be hot, even when it is done 2 to 24 hours after the lymphoscintigram—provided that ^{99m}Tc-SC is used as the mapping agent.[33] Micrometastatic disease was present in 15 (12.4%) of the 121 patients studied, and the SLN was the only metastatic site in 10 (8.3%). After a minimum follow-up of 220 days, one regional nodal recurrence was observed in an SLN-negative patient.

The addition of intraoperative radiolymphoscintigraphy to vital blue dye lymphatic mapping made SLN localization easier and more widely applicable.[21,33,37] The initial study from MCC on the use of this combined approach included 106 consecutive patients with cutaneous melanoma thicker than 0.75 mm at all primary site locations.[33] A total of 200 SLNs and 142 neighboring non-SLNs were harvested from 129 basins; 70% of the SLNs demonstrated blue staining, and 84% were identified as radioactive hot spots. When the two intraoperative mapping techniques were used in conjunction, the SLN could be identified in 96% of the nodal basins sampled. Routine histology identified SLN micrometastases in 15% of patients, and two patients had micrometastatic disease in nodes that were hot but not blue-stained. These data suggest that radiocolloid localization identifies more SLNs, some of which are clinically important in that they contain micrometastatic disease.[33]

In another study, a combination of vital blue dye and radiocolloid (^{99m}Tc-HSA) mapping was used in a series of 30 patients with melanoma from all primary sites.[37] The SLN stained blue and was the most radioactive site in 27 patients (90%). In five of 13 patients undergoing groin dissection, radiolymphoscintigraphy identified two SLNs in the drainage basin. In each case, the presence of the second inguinal SLN was suggested by the high residual radioactivity after removal of the first node, not by the blue dye; radioactivity decreased to background levels after excision of the second node. The investigators concluded that radiolymphoscintigraphy can be used not only to confirm blue-dye identification of an initial SLN but also to detect additional SLNs that are not easily identified with the dye technique alone.

In a subsequent MCC trial that used isosulfan blue dye and ^{99m}Tc-SC as mapping agents,[29] only patients with a positive SLN underwent complete node dissection. After 3 years of follow-up, two recurrences in regional basins were observed in patients whose previous SLN biopsy was negative. Serial sectioning and immunohistochemical staining of the SLN block found no abnormal cells; however, both patients' SLNs were RT-PCR–positive for messenger RNA (mRNA) for the tyrosinase gene,[38] which suggests the presence of micrometastatic disease that was missed by more conventional tests.

In another study, the Sydney Melanoma Unit reported an 87% success rate in identifying SLNs.[39] There was a pronounced learning curve, in that the success rate for the last 100 patients was 97%. Cutaneous lymphoscintigraphy was performed in 800 melanoma patients and was used to guide subsequent SLN harvesting; 23% of patients were found to have micrometastatic disease. Initially, the SLNs underwent frozen sectioning for occult metastases, but the 9% false negative rate led the investigators to switch to permanent sections, an approach that allowed the pathologist 2 to 5 days to perform a detailed examination. Patients found to have a positive SLN were returned to the OR for complete node dissection. When preoperative lymphoscintigraphy was followed by intraoperative mapping using vital blue-dye staining in conjunction with radiocolloid (^{99m}Tc-ATS) injection and a hand-held gamma probe, a 1.9% false negative rate was reported.

Finally, valuable findings are anticipated from the National Cancer Institute–sponsored prospective trial now under way [see Discussion, National Protocols, below]. Survival data from this trial are unlikely to be available before 2005.

Current data suggest that lymphatic mapping is applicable to all primary sites of the body, including the head and the neck (probably the most technically demanding sites).[31,40] The best results are achieved with a combination mapping approach that employs both vital blue dye and radiocolloid. The procedure is associated with slightly higher false negative rates in patients with head and neck melanoma than in those with extremity and trunk melanoma (10% versus 1% to 2%). Nevertheless, the false negative rates are still low enough to justify offering lymphatic mapping to patients with head and neck melanoma—especially given that the only alternative method of obtaining the nodal staging information is CLND, a more radical procedure that carries a higher morbidity.

Patterns of Failure after Negative SLN Biopsy

Several of the earlier studies found that SLN mapping had a false negative rate—defined as a negative SLN with positive higher nodes—of less than 4%, as determined by concomitant formal lymph node dissection[15-18]; however, they did not clearly establish the long-term risk of failure within the mapped nodal basin after a negative SLN alone. This issue was addressed by a joint study from MCC and the M. D. Anderson Cancer Center (Houston, Texas).[41] In this study, patients with cutaneous melanoma whose tumor was at least 1.0 mm thick or was categorized as Clark level IV or higher were eligible for mapping and SLN biopsy. All patients underwent preoperative lymphoscintigraphy, and only those with a histologically positive SLN underwent complete lymphadenectomy. A total of 618 patients underwent mapping with successful identification of at least one SLN; of these, 518 had histologically negative SLNs. After a minimum follow-up of 3 months and a median follow-up of 18 months, 32 (6%) of the 518 patients had recurrent disease; nine (1.7%) of the 518 had their first recurrence in a basin where the SLN was negative at the previous mapping. Patients with a histologically negative SLN had significantly better DFS ($P < 0.001$) and distant disease–free survival ($P < 0.001$) than those with a histologically positive SLN. When SLNs from the nine patients whose SLNs were determined to be free of metastatic disease on initial review were retrospectively reexamined by serial sectioning or immunohistochemistry, occult nodal metastases were present in seven (77%) of the nine. These data established the durable long-term accuracy of lymphatic mapping and SLN biopsy.

Optimal nodal staging requires not only accurate identification of the SLN but also careful examination of the SLN with special pathologic techniques. It is likely that many false negative SLN biopsies do not actually reflect true skip metastases but are the result of micrometastases missed on routine pathologic examination. In the study cited, it is clear, given the subsequent recurrences, that the missed micrometastases represented clinically relevant disease. The recurrences could have been prevented if the SLNs had undergone detailed histologic examination initially, the micrometastases had been found, and complete node dissection had been performed.

Other explanations of false positive SLN biopsies have been proposed. One is that after a negative SLN biopsy, some regional basins are seeded with metastatic cells from in transit metastases or local recurrences. In transit metastasis occurs in 2% to 3% of patients and could be a source of skip metastases.[8]

Clinical Implications

The information generated by all this experience is being used to change the standards for surgical management of melanoma so that only patients with evidence of nodal metastatic disease are subjected to the morbidity and expense of complete node dissection.[3-6] Initial studies showed the usefulness of lymphatic mapping with either vital blue dye or radiocolloid in obtaining such evidence; however, it is now clear that the success rate of SLN identification increases markedly when the two mapping approaches are combined as described [see Technique, above]. A combined mapping approach identifies SLNs both more accurately and more completely: it removes more SLNs and results in a lower incidence of positive nodes on subsequent CLND.

In 85% to 94% of melanoma patients, the SLN is the only site of metastasis. At MCC, we have seen no patients with melanomas less than 2.8 mm thick in whom nodes other than SLNs harbored metastases. It has been hypothesized that a melanoma must reach a certain thickness before it sheds enough cells to involve higher nodes beyond the SLN, and this hypothesis is supported by data from the M. D. Anderson Cancer Center showing no positive higher nodes after a positive SLN biopsy in patients with melanomas less than 2.5 mm thick. It appears that metastatic cells are concentrated in SLNs in much the same way that vital blue dyes and radiocolloids are. Thus, for many melanoma patients (in particular, those whose tumors have not reached the critical thickness just specified), to locate the SLN is essentially to define the limit of metastatic spread. Accordingly, lymphatic mapping, by identifying SLNs (and thus defining the extent of disease) with a high degree of accuracy, can be extremely useful in helping clinicians make more informed therapeutic decisions—for example, regarding eligibility for adjuvant therapy or the possibility of forgoing CLND.

On the basis of these data, a multicenter regional trial (the Florida Melanoma Trial II) has been initiated that will randomize patients with a microscopic positive SLN into either a group receiving adjuvant therapy alone or a group receiving CLND and adjuvant therapy. This trial will attempt to answer the question of what role CLND plays in the treatment of low-volume metastatic disease in a regional basin. It will also be the first trial to use molecular staging procedures (e.g., RT-PCR analysis) to define SLN-positive disease and to make treatment decisions on the basis of such staging procedures.

The findings of the studies cited demonstrate that intraoperative lymphatic mapping and SLN biopsy yields accurate pathologic staging, does not lower care standards, decreases morbidity (e.g., lymphedema is absent, and early return to work or normal activity is facilitated), makes possible rational yet less aggressive surgical and adjuvant medical approaches, and reduces costs.[24] A 2001 report examining a comprehensive database (including more than 25,000 melanoma patients) assembled from the major melanoma centers throughout the world by the AJCC melanoma staging committee lent support to these findings.[42] In this report, melanoma patients with intermediate-thickness (> 1.0 mm) melanomas who were determined to be node negative through clinical examination had a 5-year survival rate of 65%, and those who were determined to be node negative through ELND had a 5-year survival rate of 75%. In contrast, a similar population of melanoma patients who were determined to be node negative through lymphatic mapping and SLN biopsy had a 5-year survival rate of 90%. These statistically significant differences in survival suggest that lymphatic mapping misses less micrometastatic disease than either clinical examination of the nodal basin or ELND and hence identifies a purer population of truly node-negative patients. Accordingly, lymphatic mapping should be considered the preferred staging method for melanoma patients, particularly in clinical trial settings.

Additional improvements in survival rates can be expected for staged populations when the RT-PCR assay is added to the pathologic examination of the SLN. So-called ultrastaging may yield even further increases in survival for node-negative patients. The process involves serial examination and sampling of other immune compartments of the body besides the SLN, including peripheral blood and bone marrow, followed by analysis of the samples with very sensitive assays of occult metastases (based on RT-PCR technology). The potential value of ultrastaging is that it would allow monitoring of patient status as therapy is administered and might bring clinicians closer to being able to identify patients who have been surgically cured of their disease. That is to say, if both pathologic examination of the SLN and analysis of serial peripheral blood and bone marrow samples with sensitive RT-PCR assays determine that a melanoma patient is free of metastatic disease, that patient has been staged more accurately than would have been possible with ELND and superficial examination of all the nodes in the basin, and he or she is probably closer to being identified as a surgical cure.

The available staging data tend to support this hypothesis. In the literature, when melanoma patients were staged according to the traditional system—that is, by means of either clinical examination of the regional nodal basin or ELND—stage I patients had an 85% 5-year survival rate, stage II patients had a 70% survival rate, and stage III patients had a 47% survival rate. This older staging system yielded a reasonably good separation of the staging groups; however, a significant proportion of stage I and stage II patients (15% and 30%, respectively) experienced recurrences and died of their disease within 5 years of the initial diagnosis. It is instructive to compare these survival rates with those for melanoma patients who are staged by means of lymphatic mapping and RT-PCR assay, which typically approach 100%.

Lymphatic Mapping and SLN Biopsy for Breast Cancer

RATIONALE

For breast cancer, as for most solid tumors, the most powerful prognostic factor is the status of the regional nodes: the presence of regional metastases decreases 5-year survival by approximately 28% to 40%.[43,44] As for melanoma, many prognostic factors for breast cancer have been defined on the basis of primary tumor characteristics, yet regression analyses indicate that such factors add very little to the prognostic model once lymph node status is considered. Hence, the rationale for nodal staging is essentially the same as with melanoma.

Nodal Staging

Currently, surgical management of breast cancer is more conservative than it once was: breast conservation is now considered an acceptable alternative to modified radical mastectomy in as many as two thirds of patients. Management of the axilla in breast cancer patients remains controversial. It is generally accepted that axillary dissection is not indicated for patients with ductal carcinoma in situ (DCIS), because of the low likelihood of axillary node involvement.[45-47] The main point at issue is whether axillary dissection is indicated for patients with small invasive primary lesions. Some authors recommend that patients with T1a lesions be spared a dissection[48]; however, even when an invasive cancer is smaller than 1 cm, a significant percentage (14% to 37%) of patients have axillary nodal metastases.[49,50]

Breast tumors were once thought to have a random nodal metastatic pattern. Accordingly, investigators initially performed sampling procedures of anatomically defined first-station nodal basins in an effort to achieve accurate pathologic staging. These procedures were based on arbitrary assignment of node clusters in the axillary region to various levels (I, II, or III) rather than on intraoperative mapping of the SLN. Unfortunately, this approach led to a high (15%) prevalence of skip metastases (defined in this context as metastases to level II and III axillary nodes without involvement of level I nodes).[51] As a result, investigators abandoned sampling as a nodal staging technique for patients with breast cancer. Subsequent work demonstrated, however, that when lymphatic mapping is performed in patients with upper outer quadrant tumors, about 10% to 15% of them show direct drainage to level II axillary nodes, and skip metastases are not found. In previous studies, these patients would have been classified as having skip metastases; given the available data, it is likely that the earlier investigators simply were using insufficiently accurate staging techniques that were unable to map the SLNs or the levels of the axilla accurately.

More accurate staging involves more than just stage shifting[52]: it can improve survival in the breast cancer population by identifying patients who will gain a survival advantage associated with either the surgical procedure itself (complete axillary dissection)[53] or the accompanying adjuvant therapy.[44] In addition, it keeps a percentage of the population from being exposed to the complications of the more extensive surgical procedure or to the toxicities of the adjuvant therapy. In particular, the ability to limit full axillary lymph node dissection (ALND) to women with documented nodal metastases would be a major advance in the surgical treatment of breast cancer. Now that modern techniques have made breast conservation a viable option for so many women, the main physical complaints patients voice after operation have to do with the side effects of axillary dissection (i.e., lymphedema of the arm, reduced range of motion, and paresthesia). If node-negative patients could be protected from having to experience these side effects, that would be every bit as significant a therapeutic advance as the realization that breast cancer could be treated effectively with lumpectomy and radiation therapy.

PATIENT SELECTION

Any woman with invasive breast cancer is a potential candidate for lymphatic mapping and SLN biopsy. In patients with DCIS, the incidence of nodal metastasis on SLN biopsy with a more detailed examination of the node is 8.4%. In most cases, these apparent metastases are low-volume lesions that are discoverable only with cytokeratin staining of the SLN; there is disagreement as to whether they represent true viable metastases. In patients with invasive tumors more than 5 cm in diameter, the incidence of nodal metastasis on SLN biopsy with detailed examination is 75%. Clinicians must decide for themselves whether these patients should undergo nodal staging; however, at MCC, we routinely offer them the procedure because if nodal metastases are found, the subsequent treatment recommendations will be different.

Contraindications to the procedure are multifocal disease, inflammatory cancer, and extensive previous surgery or radiation therapy (e.g., breast reconstruction with implants above the pectoral muscle).

TECHNIQUE

Step 1: Preoperative Lymphoscintigraphy

Lymphoscintigraphy is performed in much the same way for breast cancer as for melanoma, except that the radiocolloid is injected into the breast parenchyma around the primary tumor. The radioactivity dose is the same as for melanoma (450 µCi), but larger volumes (6 ml) are administered because the breast lymphatics are not as rich as the cutaneous lymphatics. For this reason, the first images are not available until 30 to 40 minutes after injection [*see Figure 5*].

The injection must be diffuse enough around the tumor to allow the radiocolloid to be taken up by the breast lymphatics. If the tumor was detected mammographically, localization wires are placed under either mammographic or ultrasonographic guidance, and the radiocolloid is injected around the wire and the tumor. Injection must not be performed through the localization needle, because the needle will act as a wick, allowing the radiocolloid to flow back out and possibly contaminate the skin. The localization wire is left in place to guide subsequent injection of vital blue dye. If the tumor is palpable, injection is straightforward and is done tightly around the circumference of the tumor. If an excisional biopsy was performed, injection is done under ultrasonographic guidance so that the radiocolloid is placed in the breast parenchyma around the biopsy cavity. If the radiocolloid is placed in the tumor or the biopsy cavity, it will not migrate.

Alternative injection techniques have been described that include injecting the mapping agents either into the subareolar plexus (SAP) (because the breast lymphatics from all quadrants initially migrate to the SAP before traveling to the axilla) or into the skin above the tumor.[54,55] For axillary mapping, these alternative injection techniques seem to work as well as intraparenchymal injection. One potential disadvantage is that the breast lymphatics that drain into the internal mammary chain are located deep in the breast and pass through the pectoralis fascia, and these lymphatic vessels are not visualized with subareolar or intradermal injection. For most surgeons performing lymphatic mapping, successful axillary mapping is the most important aim, and the alternative injection techniques should make axillary mapping easier and its results more reproducible. In so doing, these newer techniques should effectively reduce the steepness of the learning curve.

Comment The timing of radiocolloid injection is not highly critical as long as enough time (2 to 24 hours) is allowed between injection and SLN harvesting for the mapping agent to migrate into the SLN. As the radiocolloid migrates, it is concentrated in the SLN. In most cases, this concentration results in an identifiable radioactive hot spot. When this happens, SLN harvesting becomes easier. Axillary hot spots have been identified up to 24 hours after radiocolloid injection. Harvesting can therefore be done as long as 24 hours after injection, provided that some level of radioactivity remains detectable in the axilla.[56,57]

One may question the need to image the patient after radiocolloid injection, given that the standard of care is to stage the patient according to the status of the axillary nodes alone. Lymphoscintigraphy can be used to identify women whose primary tumors drain bidirectionally to the axilla and to the internal mammary (IM) nodes (about 10% of patients, most of whom have inner-quadrant or central cancers). A 2001 report from MCC clinicians described a series of 30 breast cancer patients in whom lymphoscintigraphy showed bidirectional lymphatic drainage to both axillary and IM SLNs.[58] All axillary and IM SLNs were harvested. In five (16.7%) of the 30 patients, micrometastases were documented in the IM SLN; and in two of those five, the IM SLN was the only site of disease.[58] In two (6.6%) of the 30 patients, IM SLN sampling changed the staging. At MCC, patients whose IM SLN biopsy yields positive results subsequently undergo

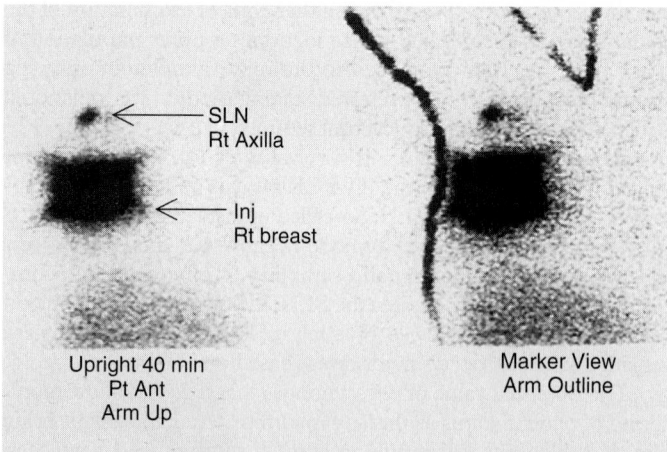

Figure 5 **Lymphatic mapping and SLN biopsy for breast cancer. Whereas flow of the radiocolloid to the SLN takes 5 to 10 minutes for melanoma mapping, it takes 30 to 40 minutes for breast cancer mapping. In addition, the primary site is usually closer to the regional basin in breast cancer than it is in melanoma, and shine-through from the primary site may be a problem. Invariably, the lumpectomy or mastectomy is performed first, followed by axillary SLN harvesting.**

Figure 6 **Lymphatic mapping and SLN biopsy for breast cancer. Isobars of radioactivity are drawn equidistant from the primary site (upper right), and hot spots are identified along each of the isobars. These hot spots represent the location of the afferent lymphatic leading to the SLN in the axilla.**

irradiation of the remainder of the IM chain if they have chosen lumpectomy and radiation therapy to treat their primary breast cancer. Other groups take a broader approach, electing to irradiate the IM chain whenever bidirectional drainage is demonstrated on preoperative lymphoscintigraphy.

The importance of IM SLN harvesting is currently under investigation by a national trial being performed by the National Surgical Adjuvant Breast and Bowel Project (NSABP). Until the results of this trial are available, clinicians should concern themselves primarily with performing accurate mapping of axillary lymph nodes. Given proper training and enough cases to fill out the learning curve, surgeons have demonstrated that they can readily incorporate SLN biopsy into their breast cancer practices in the regional and community hospital setting.[59]

The variations in breast lymphatic drainage revealed by lymphatic mapping (e.g., to level II and III axillary lymph nodes, to subclavian and supraclavicular lymph nodes, and to IM SLNs) will inevitably lead to changes in breast cancer staging, much as has already occurred with melanoma staging. At present, breast cancer patients with micrometastatic disease in the axilla are classified as having stage II disease, those with disease in the IM nodes as having stage III disease, and those with micrometastases in the supraclavicular nodes as having stage IV disease. Lymphatic mapping data, however, suggest that in some patients, all of these scenarios may represent the same biologic phenomenon—that is, regional nodal spread of the breast cancer.

Step 2: Intraoperative Lymphatic Mapping and Identification of SLN

Intraoperative lymphatic mapping and SLN identification follow much the same course in breast cancer patients as in melanoma patients. Patients come to the OR 2 to 24 hours after the injection of the radiocolloid in the nuclear medicine suite. If the tumor is palpable, 5 ml of 1% isosulfan blue dye is injected around the circumference of the primary tumor 10 to 15 minutes before the surgical procedure. If the tumor is nonpalpable, the dye is injected around the localization wire left in place after preoperative lymphoscintigraphy. After injection of the vital blue dye, the breast is massaged for 5 minutes to facilitate migration of the mapping agents.

Given that the newer injection techniques described earlier appear to identify axillary SLNs as reliably as injection into the breast

parenchyma does, a reasonable alternative approach is to split the dose of vital blue dye between intraparenchymal injection around the tumor or the biopsy cavity and injection into the SAP. Injection into the SAP need only cover the 9 to 12 o'clock area in the right breast and the 12 to 3 o'clock area in the left breast because those are the areas where the main SAP lymphatic vessels leading to the axilla branch off.[60] SAP injection is more appealing than intradermal injection above the tumor in that the clinician does not have to know exactly where the tumor is located in the breast. In addition, SAP injection does not involve an injection around an excisional biopsy scar, which is occasionally a complicating factor with intradermal injection.

Before a skin incision is made, a hand-held gamma probe is used to identify the most radioactive area in the axilla. If there is sufficient distance between the primary site and the regional basin, isobar levels of radioactivity [see Figure 6] are drawn emanating from

Figure 7 **Lymphatic mapping and SLN biopsy for breast cancer. The hand-held gamma probe is used to trace the afferent lymphatic through the skin to a hot spot in the regional basin, under which the SLN is located.**

Figure 8 **Lymphatic mapping and SLN biopsy for breast cancer. In the same patient as in Figure 7, a small incision is made in the axilla, and with the gamma probe directing the dissection, a blue-stained afferent lymphatic is seen leading into a blue-stained node. This node is hot as well as blue; it is the SLN and is the first site of metastatic disease.**

the primary site, and hot spots of radioactivity are marked along each of the isobars. If possible, the afferent lymphatic is mapped and followed to a hot spot in the axilla that corresponds to the location of the SLN [*see Figure 7*]. A small (2 to 4 cm) axillary incision is made over the hot spot, dissection is directed through the axillary fat with the probe, and the SLN is identified [*see Figure 8*]. Ideally, the SLN should be both hot and blue. If the hot spot corresponds to a cluster of nodes, the blue staining will help distinguish the SLN from the non-SLNs. The in vivo activity ratio is determined to confirm that the node fulfills the criteria of an SLN. Care must be taken to ensure that the in vivo activity ratio is not being influenced by shine-through from the primary site or from other SLNs in the axilla. For this reason, the ex vivo activity ratio is more helpful in defining an SLN (though not particularly helpful when the surgeon is trying to decide whether to remove the axillary node or leave it in place). Careful dissection is performed to identify the blue-stained afferent lymphatics, which can then be followed to the pale blue–stained SLN or SLNs [*see Figure 8*].

Comment As with melanoma, mapping becomes simpler, more accurate, more complete, and more widely applicable when the vital blue dye method and the radiocolloid method are combined.[61,62] Either method may play a more important role in a given instance, depending on the circumstances. A unique feature of breast lymphatic mapping that makes it more technically demanding than melanoma mapping is that breast cancer primary sites are closer to their regional basins than most melanoma primaries are to theirs. As a result, there may be so much shine-through of radioactivity from the primary site that imaging of the axilla becomes impossible. This may also be the case intraoperatively, when one is trying to identify the axillary SLN, even if lumpectomy is performed first. In such circumstances, vital blue dye mapping takes on a more important role in finding the axillary SLN. On the other hand, radiocolloid mapping takes on a more important role when the blue dye is slow to travel to the regional basin or when the axillary SLN is full of tumor. In such instances, though one typically sees a dilated, blue-stained lymphatic vessel going into the SLN, the node itself may take up relatively little of the blue dye; however, a radioactive hot spot can usually be identified when the very sensitive handheld probe is placed directly at the level of the nodes in the basin.

When newer injection techniques (e.g., more diffuse injection of the radiocolloid around the primary tumor or biopsy cavity, intradermal injection, and subareolar injection) are used in conjunction with breast massage in the nuclear medicine suite, the axillary SLN is successfully imaged in as many as 85% to 90% of breast cancer patients. This is a significant improvement over the results cited in previous reports that examined only intraparenchymal injection, without breast massage. Surgeons may still be able to locate the SLN in the remaining 10% to 15% by using the handheld gamma probe (which is more sensitive than the camera) intraoperatively to find the axillary hot spot and direct dissection toward the SLN.

Activity (localization) ratios are used to eliminate uncontrolled variables that might affect identification of an SLN [*see Lymphatic Mapping and SLN Biopsy for Melanoma, Technique, above*]. The higher the activity ratio, the easier mapping will be and the more likely it is that SLN harvesting will be successful. A major reason for waiting 2 to 24 hours to allow the radiocolloid to migrate and become concentrated in the SLN before intraoperative mapping is that activity ratios are highest at this point. The alternative injection techniques described allow more of the radiocolloid to migrate to the SLN. As a result, SLN harvesting becomes easier, the axillary

SLN identification rate becomes closer to 100%, and the learning curve becomes less steep.[63]

A node is considered to be the SLN if it meets one of three criteria:

1. The node is blue.

2. The node has a blue-stained afferent lymphatic leading to it. Occasionally, a node is full of tumor and has a dilated blue-stained lymphatic vessel leading to it, but it does not take up the dye or the radiocolloid readily. This scenario is easily realized intraoperatively because the node is hard on direct palpation. Despite the lack of uptake of the mapping reagent, such nodes must be considered SLNs.

3. The node has an in vivo activity ratio of 3:1 or an ex vivo activity ratio of 10:1.

Step 3: Removal of SLN

Once the SLN is identified, it is removed. A neighboring non-SLN may also be removed so that the ex vivo activity ratio may be calculated. The blue-stained afferent lymphatics that have been visualized are clipped or tied off. The Bovie electrocautery does not seal lymphatic vessels, and the goal is to perform the dissection without the requirement for postoperative drainage. The central bed is then reexamined for radioactivity. If radioactivity is 150% of the background level or higher, dissection is continued in search of additional SLNs. The mean number of axillary SLNs removed in breast lymphatic mapping is 2.0/patient.

Step 4: Pathologic Examination of SLN

Once SLNs are dissected away from surrounding tissue, they are bivalved intraoperatively and examined for any gross evidence of metastatic disease. All of the excised nodal tissue is submitted for pathologic evaluation. Tissue contents are classified into three categories: SLNs, adjacent non-SLNs, and axillary contents. SLNs 5 mm or less in maximum diameter are bivalved, and those greater than 5 mm in diameter are serially sectioned at 2 to 3 mm intervals to maximize surface area for touch-print cytology and intraoperative immunohistochemistry (IHC). (To prevent loss of tissue in the cryostat, we do not perform frozen sections of the SLNs.) Imprints are made with a single gentle touch on each cut surface of the SLN. The slides are air-dried and stained with Diff-Quick stain, then sent for intraoperative interpretation. Approximately 5 to 8 minutes from the specimen's entry into the pathology laboratory, the intraoperative diagnosis (negative, indeterminate, or positive) is rendered. At MCC, we use an intraoperative IHC cytokeratin stain on the cytologic touch imprints as an adjunct to the Diff-Quick stain; this approach may enhance detection of micrometastases, especially with infiltrating lobular carcinoma or well-differentiated (low-grade) ductal carcinoma. If the diagnosis is positive, one can convert to CLND intraoperatively. Primary diagnoses are made and lumpectomy margins examined with the same touch-print cytology technique[64] [*see Figure 9*]. The utility of this intraoperative technique has been confirmed by the findings from a large series at the University of Arkansas.[65]

Each SLN is placed in a separate formalin container by the nuclear medicine department staff and quarantined in a dedicated refrigerator with the lumpectomy or mastectomy specimen for 48 hours (six half-lives of ^{99m}Tc) to allow decay of the radioisotope. After this period, the SLNs are catalogued, and one or two blocks of tissue per SLN are submitted for permanent histology. Each block is sectioned at one to three levels per slide, depending on the size of the tissue in each block. In addition, any SLNs that appear free of metastasis both grossly and on hematoxylin-eosin staining are stained with IHC using the avidin-biotin complex technique with diaminobenzidine chromogen.

a   *b*

Figure 9 **Lymphatic mapping and SLN biopsy for breast cancer. In touch-print cytology, slides are touched to tissue from a "hot" specimen, and cells on the section or the margin are exfoliated onto the slide for cytologic preparation. Shown are (*a*) permanent histology of an infiltrating ductal carcinoma extending down to an inked margin and (*b*) a touch preparation demonstrating bizarre malignant cells from the sampling of the margin. The advantages of this technique are that the entire margin can be sampled and that tissue is not lost in the cryostat.**

Comment One of the greatest advantages of lymphatic mapping is that the surgeon gives the pathologist only one or two SLNs, which allows more detailed examination with such procedures as serial sectioning, immunohistochemical staining, and perhaps RT-PCR analysis.[66,67] Incorporating a more detailed examination into routine practice enables clinicians to detect lesser degrees of disease and upstage a number of breast cancer patients. It was once believed that micrometastatic disease in a single lymph node was clinically unimportant in breast cancer patients because such patients were thought to have the same survival as node-negative patients. This belief has been challenged by studies demonstrating poorer survival in patients who are upstaged with serial sectioning,[68] immunohistochemical staining,[69-71] or RT-PCR analysis.[66,67] In fact, since 1996, immunohistochemical staining and new molecular biology assays for occult metastases have consistently been reported to upstage patients with melanoma,[38] breast cancer,[72] colon cancer,[73] neuroblastoma,[74] prostate cancer,[75] and stomach cancer,[76] and in most cases, this upstaging has proved clinically relevant.

In a series of 255 breast cancer patients who underwent SLN harvesting with detailed pathologic examination at MCC, intraoperative imprint cytology (IIC) with both Diff-Quick and cytokeratin staining was compared with the gold standard, permanent histology with both hematoxylin-eosin and IHC staining.[77] IIC identified only 50% of the patients with metastatic disease. Another way of stating this result, however, is to say that IIC enabled intraoperative conversion to CLND in 50% of patients with axillary metastatic disease, thereby sparing a substantial number of patients a second trip to the OR. Cytokeratin staining of permanent sections was responsible for the detection of disease in 36.2% of patients with metastases; this disease would have been missed by routine examination of one or two nodal sections and hematoxylin-eosin staining. Detailed examination of SLNs reveals nodal metastases in (i.e., upstages) 9.4% of histologic negative patients[77] [*see Figure 10*].

In another series from MCC, cytokeratin IHC staining was performed on 196 SLNs from 95 patients with comedo DCIS.[78] Eight of the 95 (8.4%) had positive SLNs. Routine histology identified the metastatic disease in only two (25%) of the eight patients, whereas cytokeratin IHC staining identified metastases in six (75%). CLND was performed in seven of the eight patients, and the SLN was the only site of disease in all of them. Previous studies have reported that when CLND is performed in DCIS patients, fewer than 1% turn out to have metastatic disease in the regional basin; accordingly, many clinics have eliminated CLND from primary surgical treatment of these patients. Review of these studies, however, shows that the pathologic examination of the nodes in the CLND specimen was superficial. Lymphatic mapping and SLN biopsy permits a more detailed examination of the one or two nodes most likely to contain disease and, consequently, yields a higher rate of identification of metastases: 2% (2/95) with hematoxylin-eosin staining and 6.2% (6/95) with IHC staining in this study.

A major reason to consider lymphatic mapping and SLN biopsy in patients with DCIS is that as many as 20% of cases of DCIS diagnosed by means of stereotactic breast biopsy are subsequently upstaged to invasive cancer when the formal lumpectomy is performed. In addition, lymphatic mapping and SLN biopsy is not as accurate after excisional biopsy or lumpectomy, particularly for lesions in the upper outer quadrant, where the majority of breast cancers are found. At present, it is probably prudent for surgeons at regional and community hospitals to refrain from performing lymphatic mapping for DCIS patients (except under protocol) until the utility of the technique in this subgroup of patients is established by university centers and national trials.

Currently, the utility of cytokeratin staining of the SLN is being questioned in some quarters. Several breast pathologists (most notably David Page, M.D., of Vanderbilt University) have suggested that in some instances, isolated cytokeratin-positive cells in the SLN may in fact be benign ductal epithelial cells pushed into the afferent lymphatics and lodged in the SLN as a result of trauma to the breast (i.e., the manipulation and massage associated with lymphatic mapping). Nonetheless, at MCC, cytokeratin staining of the SLN is still considered potentially useful for directing the pathologist's search for metastatic disease. It is MCC's policy that before an SLN can be considered positive for metastatic disease, the cytokeratin-positive cells must be confirmed to be malignant through hematoxylin-eosin staining and cytologic evaluation. Only when malignancy has been verified in this way can the patient be classified as having stage II disease.

Figure 10 **Lymphatic mapping and SLN biopsy for breast cancer. Cytokeratin immunohistochemical staining finds metastatic cells in 9.4% of breast cancer patients whose SLNs are histologically negative on routine examination.**

COMPLICATIONS

The complications of the procedure are similar to those of melanoma mapping. Surgical site infections occur in fewer than 1% of cases; a seroma develops in about 10%. In our experience, no patients have complained of paresthesia or lymphedema after lymphatic mapping for breast cancer, in contrast to what is usually noted after CLND. Clearly, the complication rate is significantly lower after SLN biopsy alone than when CLND is required as well.[79] Discomfort, impaired mobility, paresthesias, lymphedema, and lancinating sensations are all less common in patients who undergo only SLN biopsy.

REPORTED RESULTS

MCC's initial experience with lymphatic mapping and SLN biopsy for breast cancer was gained between April 1994 and December 1995. All patients who presented to the Comprehensive Breast Cancer Program at MCC with suspected breast cancer were evaluated for enrollment into the study.[53] Enrollment criteria included invasive breast cancer documented by fine-needle aspiration (FNA) or core-needle biopsy [see V:2 Breast Procedures] rather than excisional biopsy (which meant that the breast lymphatic vessels were unlikely to have been disrupted) and a clinically negative axilla on physical examination. Exclusion criteria included previous incisional or excisional biopsy of the breast cancer [see V:2 Breast Procedures], a tumor that could not be adequately localized by palpation or stereotaxis, and pregnancy. A total of 62 women were enrolled in the study; their mean age was 60 years (range, 32 to 81 years). Axillary mapping was successful in 57. Of these 57 patients, 51 (89%) had a histologic diagnosis of invasive ductal carcinoma, four (7%) had invasive lobular carcinoma, one (2%) had invasive medullary carcinoma, and one (2%) had invasive tubular carcinoma. The mean tumor size was 2.2 cm (range, 0.4 to 8.0 cm).

All 62 patients were scheduled to undergo either lumpectomy and axillary node dissection (63%) or modified radical mastectomy (37%), depending on the clinical presentation and patient preference. Intraoperative lymphatic mapping with isosulfan blue dye and filtered ^{99m}Tc-SC was performed, followed by SLN biopsy and immediate complete axillary node dissection [see V:2 Breast Procedures]. In this way, the skip metastasis rate (and hence the false negative rate) could be calculated. Shine-through from the primary site was handled by making a blind incision in the axilla (usually one fingerbreadth beneath the distal edge of the hair-bearing area of the axilla) and dissecting down to the level of the axillary nodes. The handheld gamma probe could then be positioned directly at the level of the nodes, as close as possible to the location of the SLNs and as far as possible from the primary site. This maneuver facilitated recognition of the SLN while reducing the effects of radioactivity from the primary site on the measurements. Accuracy was further enhanced by setting the energy threshold on the probe high enough to eliminate low-energy radioactivity from the primary site, which otherwise could have been redirected into the probe (the Compton effect).

The SLNs were identified and sent to the pathology laboratory as separate specimens. An average of 15.5 non-SLNs per patient and 2.2 SLNs per patient were obtained from the 57 women in whom lymphatic mapping was successful. Eighteen (32%) of the 57 had metastatic disease to the axilla; the number of nodes involved ranged from one to seven. In all 18, the SLNs were positive; thus, there were no skip metastases (i.e., no false negatives). In 12 of the 18, the SLN was the only metastatic site. The metastatic distribution was significantly in favor of SLN involvement ($P \leq 0.001$): 55% of the SLNs were positive for metastatic disease, compared with only 5% of the non-SLNs. The ex vivo activity ratio averaged 39.2. Addition of the radiocolloid technique to the vital blue dye tech-

nique improved the success rate of mapping from 73% to 92% and increased the average number of SLNs harvested per patient from 1.2 to 2.2. In none of the patients was metastatic disease documented in a hot SLN that was not also stained blue. In 12% of patients (mostly women with upper outer quadrant tumors), lymphatic drainage skipped level I nodes and proceeded directly to level II nodes; no direct drainage to level III nodes was observed in these patients.

In 1997, this experience was updated with a report of 466 women with breast cancer who underwent lymphatic mapping and SLN biopsy at MCC after any type of initial diagnostic procedure, including excisional biopsy.[80] Mapping was successful in 440 of the 466. An average of 1.92 SLNs per patient were harvested. One hundred five (23.8%) of the patients had metastases in the SLN; one patient, who had undergone an excisional biopsy, had a skip metastasis, for a false negative rate of less than 1%. Lymphatic mapping was performed in 87 patients with comedo DCIS, and four patients (4.6%) were found to have positive SLNs. As tumor size increased, the number of patients with a positive SLN also increased.

This series currently includes more than 2,000 patients. The success rate for identifying axillary SLNs remains high (about 98%), and the SLN is positive in 25.3% of patients. No additional skip metastases have been identified. For the last 1,850 patients, however, the false negative rate is being determined on the basis of nodal recurrence in long-term follow-up after a negative SLN; the reason is that these patients are not undergoing CLND when the SLN is negative. After a mean follow-up of 36 months, no axillary nodal recurrences have been observed in this patient group.[81]

If mapping fails in vivo, CLND is performed and an attempt is made to identify an axillary hot spot ex vivo. Occasionally, the SLN can be located when the axillary contents are removed and mapped on the back table to eliminate any shine-through. Although this approach exposes the patient to the morbidity of a CLND, it has an important advantage—namely, that if the SLN can be identified, it can be submitted separately to the pathology laboratory for detailed examination and more accurate staging.

At MCC, when excisional biopsy is done before lymphatic mapping, an average of 2.2 SLNs are removed per patient. In 26% of these cases, three or more SLNs are harvested, and this is the population in which the only skip metastasis has occurred. When lymphatic mapping is done with the tumor intact, an average of 1.8 SLNs are removed per patient. In only 16% of these cases are three or more SLNs excised. Excisional biopsy, whether for palpable tumors or for lesions detected mammographically with needle localization, may well become a thing of the past. In the future, when physical examination or mammography suggests the presence of breast cancer, the diagnosis is likely to be made with minimally invasive techniques, such as FNA or core-needle biopsy. Once the diagnosis is made, lymphatic mapping can be done to minimize unnecessary dissection.

Clinical Implications

It has been suggested that axillary dissection should no longer be performed in women with breast cancer[62,82,83]; however, given the importance of regional node status, it makes sense to continue to perform an axillary staging procedure. The problem is that axillary nodal dissection is associated with significant complications that can lengthen hospital stay, increase cost, and cause the patient considerable discomfort.[84-86] There are numerous reports in the literature suggesting that lymphatic mapping techniques can be used in breast cancer patients to reduce this morbidity.[53,87,88] Initial reports from the John Wayne Cancer Center in Santa Monica,

California,[87] (using blue dye only) and the University of Vermont[88] (using radiocolloid only) documented success rates of 65% and 71%, respectively, for SLN identification; combining the two mapping techniques, as is done at MCC, increases the success rate of SLN localization and makes the technique easier and more widely applicable. Those patients who are SLN negative (approximately 75% of all patients) can be spared having to undergo CLND.

Breast cancer centers across the world have now studied more than 10,000 women with breast cancer who have undergone lymphatic mapping and SLN harvesting. The mapping techniques vary slightly from center to center; however, most have attained similarly high success rates, which argues strongly for the viability of the procedure. Sensitivity and diagnostic accuracy rates for SLN identification have consistently been higher than 95%, and the false negative rate has ranged from 0% to 10%. This combined experience suggests that lymphatic mapping has the potential for changing the standards for surgical management of breast cancer in the same way that it has already changed the standards for surgical management of melanoma in the United States.

Discussion

Training and Credentialing

Credentialing criteria for new operative procedures have traditionally been under the jurisdiction of local hospital credentialing committees. When new technology becomes available, adequate training is essential, both to ensure that surgeons can perform the new procedure with confidence and to minimize any medicolegal problems. The American College of Surgeons has a committee (the Committee on Emerging Surgical Technology and Education) that monitors this activity. With some new techniques (e.g., laparoscopic cholecystectomy and image-guided breast biopsy), hospitals have required surgeons to attend formal training courses and to have their first cases proctored by surgeons experienced in the new technique before they are allowed to perform the procedure on their own.

National organizations continue to struggle with the problem of educating and credentialing surgeons to perform new procedures. This problem takes on increasing urgency as medicolegal issues proliferate, as other specialists begin to move into areas once generally considered to be the domain of surgeons (e.g., radiologists doing breast biopsies), and as new technical developments promise to revolutionize surgical care. In an effort to address this problem as it bears on lymphatic mapping, the American College of Surgeons, in association with MCC, has initiated a program designed to investigate how best to train teams (comprising surgeons, nuclear medicine physicians, radiologists, and pathologists) in the new technology. The formal training course is a 2-day session composed of didactic lectures, live surgery (including extensive surgeon-audience interaction during the procedure), and a hands-on animal laboratory. The program offers mentoring of initial cases as registrants go back to their institutions, maintains national registries on the World Wide Web so that different experiences with the technique can be compared, and, finally, facilitates the participation of other university and community physicians in national protocols [see National Protocols, below]. Further information may be obtained from the Center for Minimally Invasive Surgical Techniques (888-456-2840; www.slnmapping.org). Participation in programs such as this one provides a certain degree of protection against medicolegal risk as new technology and procedures are introduced.

The varied experience reported to date provides some idea of the learning curves associated with lymphatic mapping. For melanoma, the learning curve for mapping with vital blue dye alone is about 60 cases, which is more than many surgeons see in their entire career.[15,16] In contrast, gamma probe–guided resection of radiolabeled lymph nodes is readily mastered: even with minimal experience, the success rate of SLN localization approaches 98%. Combination mapping techniques further increase the success rate and abbreviate the learning curve.

For breast cancer, it has been suggested that the learning curve for lymphatic mapping is about 30 cases. In all of these first 30 patients, SLN harvesting should be followed by CLND; perhaps 10 of the 30 will have metastatic disease. The success rate for finding the axillary SLN should be 85% or higher, with no more than one skip metastasis identified in the first 10 patients with metastatic disease, before one can consider dropping CLND in SLN-negative patients. More than one surgeon can train on the same case, and the final decision as to when an institution is ready to drop full dissection after a negative SLN should be made in conjunction with the medical and radiation oncologists at the institution as well as with the credentialing committee. Clinicians at MCC examined the learning curves of five surgeons who performed more than 700 lymphatic mappings to find axillary SLNs in patients with breast cancer.[89] Learning curves were generated for each surgeon by plotting the failure rate against the number of cases. The failure rate was high (20% to 30%) in the first 20 patients but fell rapidly thereafter. The results of the study indicate that 23 cases and 53 cases are required to achieve success rates of 90% and 95%, respectively. The alternative (subareolar and intradermal) injection techniques mentioned earlier, by making SLNs easier to identify and harvest, should help make the learning curves somewhat less steep.

National Protocols

The first national multicenter study addressing lymphatic mapping for melanoma was the Multicenter Selective Lymphadenectomy Trial (Donald Morton, M.D., principal investigator), which began in 1998 and remains in progress under the sponsorship of the NCI (Grant No. PO1 CA29605-12). This trial focuses on the effect of lymphatic mapping and SLN biopsy on survival. Melanoma patients with intermediate or thick tumors (≥ 1.0 mm) are randomly selected to receive either WLE plus observation of the nodal basins or WLE plus SLN harvesting. The study differs from previous studies of ELND in that only some of the patients (i.e., those with a positive SLN) undergo CLND. If this study demonstrates a survival benefit, then there will be two good reasons to perform SLN: (1) to remove the node at highest risk for metastatic disease, so that CLND may be performed with a view to improving survival, and (2) to identify patients who are candidates for adjuvant therapy.

The second national trial that has been initiated to examine the role of this new procedure in treating melanoma is the industry-sponsored Sunbelt Melanoma Trial, in which 60 institutions across the country, equally divided between university centers and community hospitals, are participating. In this study, melanoma patients whose tumors are at least 1.0 mm thick are undergoing lymphatic mapping and SLN harvesting. SLNs are examined with routine histology, serial sectioning, and immunohistochemical staining. If an SLN is negative on the initial screen, an RT-PCR assay based on a panel of four melanoma-specific markers (at least two of which must be positive for a positive result) is performed. Patients whose SLNs are negative on histology and RT-PCR assay are observed; patients whose SLNs are histologically negative but positive on RT-PCR assay are randomly selected to undergo either observation, CLND, or CLND plus adjuvant interferon alfa-2b. It is conceivable that patients in the second category might have a very small volume of tumor that is confined to the SLN and thus might be cured with SLN harvesting alone, thereby avoiding the side effects attendant on CLND or adjuvant interferon therapy. Another arm of this trial is designed to focus on the role of adjuvant interferon alfa-2b in patients with microscopic nodal disease. In the cooperative group study that found interferon alfa-2b to be effective adjuvant therapy,[2] 85% of the patient population had gross nodal disease. It remains to be determined whether patients with minimal disease in the regional basin (i.e., those with only one positive microscopic SLN) benefit from this adjuvant therapy. This study has now enrolled more than 1,000 patients.

In July 2001, the Florida Melanoma Trial II was initiated (Douglas Reintgen, M.D., principal investigator). This trial involves the random selection of SLN-positive melanoma patients to undergo either observation of the remaining nodes in the basin plus adjuvant therapy or CLND plus adjuvant therapy. The data suggest that the SLN is the only site of disease in 80% to 94% of cases (depending on whether the initial SLN was harvested with a single-agent or a combination mapping technique); thus, the focus of this study would be on defining the role of CLND in patients with microscopic stage III disease documented by SLN biopsy. This trial is also the first national study to use molecular staging (through RT-PCR assay) to determine SLN status.

In fall 1998, the American College of Surgeons Oncology Group initiated a trial (Armando Giuliano, M.D., principal investigator) in which women with invasive breast cancer undergo lymphatic mapping and SLN biopsy. If the SLN is negative, patients are observed and a blinded cytokeratin analysis is performed; bone marrow staging is also investigated in this part of the study. If the SLN is positive, patients undergo either CLND or observation of the regional basin. It is assumed that all of these women will receive appropriate radiation therapy and postoperative adjuvant therapy. The aims of this trial are (1) to define the role of CLND in women with invasive breast cancer and (2) to begin to assess the clinical relevance of upstaging with IHC, not only in the SLN but also in the bone marrow of women with clinical stage I breast cancer.

In the North American Fareston Tamoxifen Adjuvant (NAFTA) trial (Michael Edwards, M.D., principal investigator), perimenopausal or postmenopausal women are staged with the lymphatic mapping technique; if the SLN is negative, no further surgery is performed. Those patients found to have estrogen receptor–positive or progesterone receptor–positive tumors are then eligible to be randomly selected to receive either tamoxifen or the newer antiestrogen toremifene (Fareston).

Finally, the NSABP (David Krag, M.D., principal investigator) will perform lymphatic mapping and SLN biopsy in women with invasive breast cancer who are undergoing breast conservation. Patients will be randomly selected to undergo either SLN biopsy, followed by CLND only if the SLN is positive, or CLND. Radiation therapy to the breast will be provided to all patients. The goal of the study is to determine whether lymphatic mapping coupled with selective use of CLND is as effective as the standard surgical approach to women with invasive breast cancer (i.e., axillary dissection including level I and II nodes).

Radiation Exposure Guidelines and Policies

The amount of radioactivity injected in the course of lymphatic mapping is minimal: about 450 µCi, on average. By comparison, the amount of radioactivity injected in the course of a typical bone scan is 20 mCi—44 times the lymphatic mapping dose. For the first 100 mappings done at MCC, surgeons and pathologists wore radiation detection badges and rings throughout the procedure, and nuclear medicine technicians swiped the relevant areas in the OR and the pathology laboratory after each case. No significant radiation exposure could be documented. Currently, MCC nuclear medicine technicians routinely come into the OR to calibrate and run the gamma probes, and once the specimen has been removed and processed by the surgeon, they handle the specimen and monitor the radioactivity in each one as it is transported from the OR into the pathology laboratory. A separate room is designated for intraoperative handling of specimens; this is particularly important with breast cancer specimens, for which diagnosis, lumpectomy margin, and SLN status may all be determined intraoperatively. In addition, fresh tissue specimens are removed and snap-frozen for RT-PCR assays and estrogen and progesterone receptor assays. As noted [see Lymphatic Mapping and SLN Biopsy for Breast Cancer, Technique, above], specimens are then placed in formalin for 48 hours, stored in a dedicated refrigerator, and later removed for routine processing.

Our experience in handling specimens at MCC notwithstanding, as investigators begin to create lymphatic mapping programs at their own institutions, state regulatory policies must be consulted and procedures put into place to meet each individual state's requirements. Clinicians may have to reinvent the wheel, in a sense, to convince their hospitals and their colleagues that lymphatic mapping and SLN biopsy can be performed safely and results in no significant radiation exposure or health risk.

Cost Considerations

A cost analysis was performed at MCC in an effort to ascertain the impact of lymphatic mapping on both cost and quality of care for patients with malignant melanoma.[24] A series of 98 consecutive patients registered at the Cutaneous Oncology Clinic from July 1993 to August 1994 were entered into the study and separated into four treatment groups, depending on their primary surgical therapy. Group 1 patients (29%) had thin melanomas (< 1.0 mm thick) and underwent 1.0 cm WLE under local anesthesia as outpatients in the clinic. Group 2 patients (13%) underwent WLE and nodal staging by ELND. Group 3 patients (47%) underwent WLE and nodal staging by lymphatic mapping and SLN biopsy under general anesthesia in the OR. As surgeons became comfortable with lymphatic mapping, it became evident that the procedure could be performed with straight local anesthesia, particularly for groin dissections. Group 4 patients (11%) underwent WLE and lymphatic mapping under local anesthesia. CLND was performed in SLN-positive group 3 and group 4 patients, and the costs of the additional surgery were entered into the analysis. The WLEs of the primary sites were closed primarily in all patients. Patients were discharged immediately after the procedure.

Significant cost savings were achieved in group 4 patients compared with group 3 patients ($t = 5.56$; $P = 0.001$); however, no significant cost savings were achieved in group 3 patients compared with group 2 patients ($t = 0.847$; $P = 0.40$). Morbidity was significantly lower in groups 3 and 4, with an earlier projected return to work or normal activity. The study findings suggest that, given an incidence of approximately 43,000 new cases of invasive melanoma in the United States each year, use of lymphatic mapping to stage the regional nodal basin could, by itself, save the health care system close to $120 million annually. This study illustrates that clinicians can maintain quality of care, reduce complications, and lower costs by incorporating this new technique into the care of melanoma patients. These benefits can be achieved without compromising the essential nodal staging data that are the criteria for entry into adjuvant therapy programs—a crucial point, in that adjuvant therapy is offered only to patients whom it has been proved to benefit.

For breast cancer, lymphatic mapping may yield more dramatic cost savings. It is conceivable that the combination of a number of emerging technologies and techniques (e.g., touch-print cytology for making the diagnosis and examining lumpectomy margins and lymphatic mapping and SLN harvesting for nodal staging) could lead to a scenario in which women with mammographic abnormalities can come to the clinic, have their breast lesion diagnosed, and receive at least surgical treatment (lumpectomy for clear margins and SLN biopsy) within a 3- to 4-hour period. With such "one-stop shopping," the patient need not be admitted to a hospital, enter a formal OR, be subjected to general anesthesia, or undergo axillary drainage after CLND.

References

1. Greenlee RT, Murray T, Bolden S, et al: Cancer statistics, 2000. CA Cancer J Clin 50:7, 2000

2. Kirkwood JM, Strawderman MH, Ernstoff MS, et al: Adjuvant therapy of high-risk resected cutaneous melanoma: the Eastern Cooperative Oncology Group Trial EST 1684. J Clin Oncol 14:7, 1996

3. Veronesi U, Adamus J, Bandiera DC, et al: Inefficacy of immediate node dissection in stage I melanoma of the limbs. N Engl J Med 297:627, 1977

4. Sim FH, Taylor WF, Pritchard DJ, et al: Lymphadenectomy in the management of stage I malignant melanoma: a prospective randomized study. Mayo Clin Proc 61:697, 1986

5. Balch CM, Soong SJ, Milton GW, et al: A comparison of prognostic factors and surgical results in 1,786 patients with localized (stage I) melanoma treated in Alabama, USA, and New South Wales, Australia. Ann Surg 196:677, 1982

6. Reintgen DS, Cox EB, McCarthy KS, et al: Efficacy of elective lymph node dissection in patients with intermediate thickness primary melanoma. Ann Surg 198:379, 1983

7. Norman J, Cruse CW, Wells K, et al: A redefinition of skin lymphatic drainage by lymphoscintigraphy for malignant melanoma. Am J Surg 162:432, 1991

8. Reintgen DS, Albertini J, Berman C, et al: Accurate nodal staging of malignant melanoma. Cancer Control: Journal of the Moffitt Cancer Center 2:405, 1995

9. Balch CM, Soong SJ, Bartolucci AA, et al: Efficacy of an elective regional lymph node dissection of 1 to 4 mm thick melanomas for patients 60 years of age and younger. Ann Surg 224:255, 1996

10. Balch CM, Soong SJ, Ross MI, et. al: Long-term results of a multi-institutional trial comparing prognostic factors and surgical results for intermediate thickness melanomas (1.0 to 4.0 mm). Intergroup Melanoma Surgical Trial. Ann Surg Oncol 7:87, 2000

11. Kirkwood J, Ibrahim JG, Sondak V, et al: High- and low-dose interferon alfa 2-b in high-risk melanoma: first analysis of intergroup trial E1690/S9111/C9190. J Clin Oncol 18:2444, 2000

12. Kirkwood J, Ibrahim JG, Sosmon JA, et al: High-dose interferon alfa-2b significantly prolongs relapse-free and overall survival compared with the GM2-KLH/QS-21 vaccine in patients with resected stage IIB-III melanoma: results of intergroup trial E1694/S9512/C509801. J Clin Oncol 19:2370, 2001

13. Wong JH, Cagle LA, Morton D: Lymphatic drainage of skin to a sentinel lymph node in a feline model. Ann Surg 214:637, 1991

14. Alex JC, Krag DN: Gamma-probe-guided localization of lymph nodes. Surg Oncol 2:137, 1993

15. Morton DL, Wen DR, Wong JH, et al: Technical details of intraoperative lymphatic mapping for early stage melanoma. Arch Surg 127:392, 1992

16. Morton DL, Wen DR, Cochran AJ: Management of early-stage melanoma by intraoperative lymphatic mapping and selective lymphadenectomy or "watch and wait." Surg Oncol Clin North Am 1:247, 1992

17. Reintgen DS, Cruse CW, Berman C, et al: An orderly progression of melanoma nodal metastases. Ann Surg 220:759, 1994

18. Ross M, Reintgen DS, Balch C: Selective lymphadenectomy: emerging role of lymphatic mapping and sentinel node biopsy in the management of early stage melanoma. Semin Surg Oncol 9:219, 1993

19. Sappey MPC: Injection, preparation et conservation des vaisseaux lymphatiques. Thèse pour le doctorat en médecine, No. 241. Paris, Rignoux Imprimeur de la Faculté de Médecine, 1843

20. Uren RF, Hoffman-Giles RB, Shaw HM, et al: Lymphoscintigraphy in high-risk melanoma of the trunk: predicting draining node groups, defining lymphatic channels and locating the sentinel node. J Nucl Med 34:1435, 1993

21. Krag DN, Meijer SJ, Weaver DL, et al: Minimal-access surgery for staging of melanoma. Arch Surg 130:654, 1995

22. Krag D, Meijer S, Weaver D, et al: Minimal access surgery for staging regional nodes in malignant melanoma (abstr). Presented at the 48th Cancer Symposium, Society of Surgical Oncology, Boston, 1995

23. Puleo C, Cruse CW, Lowe J, et al: Re-definition of pelvic cutaneous lymphatic drainage based on lymphatic mapping principles (abstr). Presented at the 54th Annual Cancer Symposium, Society of Surgical Oncology, Washington, DC, March 15–18, 2001

24. Reintgen DS, Einstein A: The role of research in cost containment. Cancer Control: Journal of the Moffitt Cancer Center 2:429, 1995

25. Slingluff C, Vollmer R, Reintgen D, et al: Lethal thin malignant melanoma. Ann Surg 208:150, 1988

26. Heaton KM, Sussman JJ, Gershenwald JE, et al: Surgical margins and prognostic factors in patients with thick (> 4 mm) primary melanoma. Ann Surg Oncol 5:322, 1998

27. Meyer CM, Lecklitner ML, Logie JR, et al: Technetium-99m sulfur-colloid cutaneous lymphoscintigraphy in the management of truncal melanoma. Radiology 131:205, 1979

28. Godellas CV, Berman C, Lyman G, et al: The identification and mapping of melanoma regional nodal metastases: minimally invasive surgery for the diagnosis of nodal metastases. Am J Surg 61:97, 1995

29. Norman J, Wells K, Kearney R, et al: Identification of lymphatic basins in patients with cutaneous melanoma. Semin Surg Oncol 9:224, 1993

30. McCarthy WH, Thompson JF, Uren RF: Minimal access surgery for staging of malignant melanoma (invited commentary). Arch Surg 130:659, 1995

31. Byrd D, Nason K, Eary J, et al: Utility of sentinel lymph node dissection in patients with head and neck melanoma (abstr). Presented at the 54th Annual Cancer Symposium, Society of Surgical Oncology, Washington, DC, March 15–18, 2001

32. Wells K, Reintgen DS, Cruse CW, et al: Parotid gland sentinel lymphadenectomy in malignant melanoma (abstr). Presented at the International Congress on Melanoma, Sydney, Australia, 1997

33. Albertini J, Cruse CW, Rapaport D, et al: Intraoperative radiolymphoscintigraphy improves sentinel lymph node identification in melanoma patients. Ann Surg 223:217, 1996

34. Nathanson SD, Anaya P, Karvelis KC, et al: Sentinel lymph node uptake of two different technetium-labeled radiocolloids. Ann Surg Oncol 4:104, 1997

35. Wrightson WR, Reintgen DS, Edwards M, et al: Morbidity of sentinel lymph node biopsy (abstr). Presented at the 54th Annual Cancer Symposium, Society of Surgical Oncology, Washington, DC, March 15–18, 2001

36. Alex JC, Weaver DL, Fairbank JT, et al: Gamma-probe-guided lymph node localization in malignant melanoma. Surg Oncol 2:303, 1993

37. Essner R, Foshag L, Morton D: Intraoperative radiolymphoscintigraphy: a useful adjunct to intraoperative lymphatic mapping and selective lymphadenectomy in patients with clinical stage 1 melanoma (abstr). Presented at the 47th Cancer Symposium, Society of Surgical Oncology, Houston, Texas, 1994

38. Wang X, Heller R, VanVoorhis N, et al: Detection of submicroscopic metastases with polymerase chain reaction in patients with malignant melanoma. Ann Surg 220:768, 1994

39. Thompson JF, McCarthy WH, Robinson E, et al: Sentinel lymph node biopsy in 102 patients with clinical stage 1 melanoma undergoing elective lymph node dissection (abstr). Presented at the 47th Cancer Symposium, Society of Surgical Oncology, Houston, Texas, 1994

40. Medina-Franco H, Beenken S, Heslin M, et al: Sentinel lymph node biopsy for cutaneous melanoma of the head and neck (abstr). Presented at the 54th Annual Cancer Symposium, Society of Surgical Oncology, Washington, DC, March 15–18, 2001

41. Gershenwald J, Thompson W, Mansfield P, et al: Patterns of failure in melanoma patients after successful lymphatic mapping and negative sentinel node biopsy (abstr). Presented at the 49th Cancer Symposium, Society of Surgical Oncology, Atlanta, Georgia, 1996

42. Dessureault S, Soong S, Ross M, et al: Improved survival for node-negative patients with intermediate-to-thick melanomas (>1.0 mm) staged with sentinel lymph node (SLN) biopsy (abstr). Presented at the 54th Annual Cancer Symposium, Society of Surgical Oncology, Washington, DC, March 15–18, 2001

43. Haagensen CD: Treatment of curable carcinoma of the breast. Int J Radiat Oncol Biol Phys 2:975, 1977

44. Bonadonna G: Conceptual and practical advances in the management of breast cancer: Karnofsky Memorial Lecture. J Clin Oncol 7:1380, 1989

45. Balch CM, Singletary ES, Bland KI: Clinical decision-making in early breast cancer. Ann Surg 217:207, 1993

46. Frazier TG, Copeland EM, Gallaher HS, et al: Prognosis and treatment in minimal breast cancer. Am J Surg 133:697, 1977

47. Silverstein MJ, Rosser RJ, Gierson ED, et al: Axillary lymph node dissection for intraductal carcinoma: is it indicated? Cancer 59:1819, 1987

48. Silverstein MJ, Gierson ED, Waisman JR, et al: Axillary lymph node dissection for T1a breast carcinoma: is it indicated? Cancer 73:664, 1994

49. Baker LH: Breast Cancer Detection Demonstration Project: five-year summary report. CA 32:194, 1982

50. Dewar JA, Sarazin D, Benhamou E, et al: Management of the axilla in conservatively treated breast cancer: 592 patients treated at Institut Gustave-Roussy. Int J Radiat Oncol Biol Phys 13:475, 1987

51. Veronesi U, Rilke F, Luini A, et al: Distribution of axillary nodal metastases by level. Cancer 59:682, 1987

52. Feinstein AR, Sosin DM, Wells CK: The Will Rogers phenomenon: stage migration and new diagnostic techniques as a source of misleading statistics for survival in cancer. N Engl J Med 312:1604, 1985

53. Albertini J, Lyman G, Cantor A, et al: Lymphatic mapping and sentinel node biopsy in the breast cancer patient. JAMA 276:1818, 1996

54. Povoski SP, Dauway E, Ducatman BS: Sentinel lymph node mapping and biopsy for breast cancer at a rural-based university hospital: initial experience with intradermal and intraparenchymal injection routes (abstr). Presented at the 54th Annual Cancer Symposium, Society of Surgical Oncology, Washington, DC, March 15–18, 2001

55. Bauer TW, Bedrosian I, Spitz F, et al: Subareolar injection simplifies sentinel lymph node mapping for breast cancer (abstr). Presented at the 54th Annual Cancer Symposium, Society of Surgical Oncology, Washington, DC, March 15–18, 2001

56. McCarter M, Yeung H, Yeh S, et al: Radioisotope localization of the sentinel lymph node in breast cancer: identical results with same day vs day-before injection protocols (abstr). Presented at the 54th Annual Cancer Symposium, Society of Surgical Oncology, Washington, DC, March 15–18, 2001

57. Winchester DJ, Sener SF, Winchester DP, et al: Sentinel lymphadenectomy for breast cancer: experience with 180 consecutive patients: efficacy of filtered technetium 99m sulphur colloid with overnight migration time. J Am Coll Surg 188:597, 1999

58. Cox C, Dupont E, Peltz E, et al: Pre-operative detection of internal mammary lymph nodes using lymphoscintigraphy and intraoperative lymphatic mapping for breast cancer encourages excision (abstr). Presented at the 54th Annual Cancer Symposium, Society of Surgical Oncology, Washington, DC, March 15–18, 2001

59. Reintgen DS, Cox C, Shivers S, et al: Final results of the DoD multi-center breast lymphatic mapping trial (abstr). Presented at the 54th Annual Cancer Symposium, Society of Surgical Oncology, Washington, DC, March 15–18, 2001

60. Kern KA: Sentinel lymph node mapping in breast cancer using subareolar injection of blue dye. J Am Coll Surg 189:539, 1999

61. Nathanson SD, Nelson L, Karvelis KC: Rates of flow of technetium 99m-labeled human serum albumin from peripheral injection sites to sentinel nodes. Ann Surg Oncol 3:329, 1996

62. Cady B: The need to reexamine axillary lymph node dissection in invasive breast cancer. Cancer 73:505, 1994

63. Faddis D, Martin D, Recabaren J: The myth of the learning curve in breast sentinel node biopsy (abstr). Presented at the 54th Annual Cancer Symposium, Society of Surgical Oncology, Washington, DC, March 15–18, 2001

64. Cox C, Nicosia S, Ku NN, et al: Touch preparation cytology of breast lumpectomy margins. Arch Surg 126:490, 1991

65. Henry-Tillman R, Johnson A, Massoll N, et al: Intraoperative Touch Prep for Sentinel Lymph Node Biopsy (abstr). Presented at the 54th Annual Cancer Symposium, Society of Surgical Oncology, Washington, DC, March 15–18, 2001

66. Noguchi S, Aihara T, Motomura K, et al: Detection of breast cancer micrometastases in axillary lymph nodes by means of reverse transcriptase-polymerase chain reaction. Am J Pathol 148:649, 1996

67. Schoenfeld A, Lugmani Y, Smith D, et al: Detection of breast cancer micrometastases in axillary lymph nodes by using polymerase chain reaction. Cancer Res 54:2986, 1994

68. International Ludwig Breast Cancer Study: Prognostic importance of occult axillary lymph node micrometastases from breast cancers. Lancet 335:1565, 1990

69. Trojani M, de Mascarel I, Bonichon F, et al: Micrometastases to axillary lymph nodes from carcinoma of the breast: detection by immunohistochemistry and prognostic significance. Br J Cancer 55:303, 1987

70. Springall SJ, Rytina ERC, Millis RR: Incidence and significance of micrometastases in axillary lymph nodes detected by immunohistochemical techniques. J Pathol 160:174, 1990

71. Hainsworth PJ, Tjandra JJ, Stillwell RG, et al: Detection and significance of occult metastases in node negative breast cancer. Br J Surg 80:459, 1993

72. Fields K, Moscinski L, Trudeu W, et al: The use of polymerase chain reaction (PCR) for amplification of cytokeratin 19 (K19) to detect bone marrow micrometastases in breast cancer (abstr). Presented at the annual meeting of the American Society of Clinical Oncology, 1994

73. Greeson JK, Isenhart CE, Rice R, et al: Identification of occult micrometastases in pericolic lymph nodes of Duke's B colorectal cancer patients using monoclonal antibodies against cytokeratin and CC49: correlation with long-term survival. Cancer 73:563, 1994

74. Moss TJ, Reynolds CP, Sather HN, et al: Prognostic value of immunocytologic detection of bone marrow metastases in neuroblastoma. N Engl J Med 324:219, 1991

75. Moreno JG, Crose CM, Fisher R, et al: Detection of hematogenous micrometastases in patients with prostate cancer. Cancer Res 52:6110, 1992

76. Maehara Y, Oshiro T, Endo K, et al: Clinical significance of occult micrometastases in lymph nodes from patients with early gastric cancer who died of recurrence. Surgery 119:397, 1996

77. Ku NN: Pathologic examination of sentinel lymph nodes in breast cancer. Surg Oncol Clin North Am 8:469, 1999

78. Pendas S, Dauway E, Giuliano R, et al: Upstaging DCIS breast cancer patients using cytokeratin staining of the sentinel lymph nodes (abstr). Presented at the annual meeting of the American Society of Clinical Oncology, 1998

79. Temple LKF, Baron R, Fey J, et al: Postoperative symptoms in breast cancer patients are significantly fewer and less severe with SLN biopsy than with axillary lymph node dissection (ALND): baseline and 3-month results from a prospective study (abstr). Presented at the 54th Annual Cancer Symposium, Society of Surgical Oncology, Washington, DC, March 15–18, 2001

80. Cox C, Pendas S, Cox J, et al: Guidelines for sentinel node biopsy and lymphatic mapping of patients with breast cancer. Ann Surg 227:645, 1998

81. Dessureault S, Dupont E, Shons A, et al: Breast cancer patients with a negative sentinel lymph node (SLN) do not need a complete axillary lymph node dissection (CALND) for local control (abstr). Presented at the San Antonio Breast Cancer Conference, San Antonio, Texas, December 2000

82. Morrow M: Role of axillary dissection in breast cancer management. Ann Surg Oncol 3:233, 1996

83. Baxter N, McCready D, Chapman JA, et al: Clinical behavior of untreated axillary nodes after local treatment for primary cancer. Ann Surg Oncol 3:235, 1996

84. Lin PP, Allison DC, Wainstock J, et al: Impact of axillary node dissection on the therapy of breast cancer patients. J Clin Oncol 11:1536, 1993

85. Ivens D, Hoe AL, Podd TJ, et al: Assessment of morbidity from complete axillary dissection. Br J Cancer 66:136, 1992

86. Recht A, Houlihan MJ: Axillary lymph nodes and breast cancer: a review. Cancer 76:1491, 1995

87. Giuliano AE, Kirgan DM, Guenther MD, et al: Lymphatic mapping and sentinel lymphadenectomy for breast cancer. Ann Surg 220:391, 1994

88. Krag DN, Weaver DL, Alex JC, et al: Surgical resection and radio localization of the sentinel lymph node in breast cancer using a gamma probe. Ann Surg Oncol 6:553, 1999

89. Cox CE, Bass SS, Boulware D, et al: Implementation of a new surgical technology: outcome measures for lymphatic mapping of breast carcinoma. Ann Surg Oncol 6:553, 1999

90. Tanabe KK: Lymphatic mapping and epitrochlear node dissection for melanoma. Surgery 121:102, 1997

91. Hung JC, Wiseman GA, Wahner HW, et al: Filtered technetium-99m-sulfur colloid evaluated for lymphoscintigraphy. J Nucl Med 36:1895, 1995

92. Uren RF, Nowman RB, Thompson JF, et al: Lymphoscintigraphy in melanoma patients (abstr). Presented at the Sixth World Congress on Cancers of the Skin, Buenos Aires, Argentina, 1995

Acknowledgment

Figure 2   Tom Moore.

4 ULTRASONOGRAPHY: SURGICAL APPLICATIONS

Grace S. Rozycki, M.D.

Although the scientific principles underlying ultrasonography first began to be elucidated in the 19th century [*see Sidebar* Ultrasonography in Surgery: Historical Perspectives], it was not until the second half of the 20th century that this technology could be effectively applied to medicine. In particular, surgeons in the United States have now embraced ultrasonography as a key diagnostic tool in many areas of clinical practice. Because ultrasonography is noninvasive, portable, rapid, and easily repeatable, it is especially well suited to surgical practice. In addition, computer-enhanced high-resolution imaging and multifrequency specialized transducers have made ultrasonography increasingly user friendly, enhancing its applicability to a variety of surgical settings.

Physics and Instrumentation

Before the application of ultrasound devices to patient evaluation is addressed, it is worthwhile to briefly review certain basic physical principles and terminology associated with ultrasonography [*see Tables 1 through 3*].[1-5] Nowhere in diagnostic imaging is the understanding of wave physics more important than in ultrasound diagnostic imaging, because ultrasonography is highly operator dependent. To perform an ultrasound examination correctly, a surgeon must be able to interpret echo patterns, determine artifacts, and adjust the machine appropriately so as to obtain the best images.

In diagnostic ultrasonography, the transducer or probe interconverts electrical and acoustic energy [*see Figure 1*].[6] To accomplish

Ultrasonography in Surgery: Historical Perspectives

Ultrasonography has become an important diagnostic modality. Although its potential for medical diagnostic imaging was first recognized in the 1930s and 1940s, when attempts were made to use ultrasound to diagnose brain tumors, it was not until the 1970s that the early pioneering work on ultrasound truly came to fruition. With technological advances, ultrasound machines evolved from large, cumbersome devices that produced suboptimal images to portable, user-friendly, sophisticated instruments that produced detailed and useful images. This evolution required years of research and the marriage of physics with physiology, medicine, engineering, and government.

Milestones in Sound Research

One line of sound research that had a direct bearing on the development of ultrasonography was the invention of SONAR (*SO*und *N*avigation *A*nd *R*anging). The way was paved for this invention by 19th-century inquiries into the measurement of the speed of sound in water. The earliest precursors of SONAR date back to 1838, when Bonnycastle attempted to map the ocean floor by echo-sounding, an operation necessary for the placement of telegraph lines and the safe navigation of large ships. Later, the Swiss physicist Jean-Daniel Colladon[97] determined the speed of sound in water to help confirm his data about the compressibility of liquids. Colladon's experiment, considered the birth of modern underwater acoustics, consisted of striking an underwater bell in Lake Geneva and simultaneously igniting gunpowder. Colladon observed the flash from the gunpowder from 10 miles away, and he also heard the sound of the bell with an underwater trumpet. By measuring the time interval between these two events, he calculated the speed of the sound in Lake Geneva to be 1,435 m/sec, a value that differs from current calculations by only 3 m/sec.[98]

Later, in 1877, John William Strutt published *The Theory of Sound*, which became the foundation for the science of ultrasound. His contributions were deemed so significant that he was appointed to Great Britain's Board of Invention and Research, the body that supervised the development of SONAR during World War I.[99] After the sinking of the *Titanic* and of German U-boats, increased effort was applied to the development of SONAR in the hope that it would help detect underwater objects. It was not until April 1914, however, that iceberg detection was accomplished with the help of Reginald Aubry Fessenden's electromagnetic moving-coil arrangement.[98] Although this technology was well accepted, it was primarily used for underwater signaling and navigation of World War I submarines. In 1915, Constantin Chilowsky, in conjunction with the eminent French physicist Paul Langevin, developed a working hydrophone.[100] This pioneering work considerably enhanced scientists' knowledge of how ultrasound waves were generated and received—an important part of the pulse-echo principle of SONAR. Research and development focusing on underwater acoustics and transducers thrived during this period, and important discoveries were made that advanced the progress of ultrasound technology.

By 1928, with the help of Langevin's contributions, the French ocean liner *Ile de France* had a fully operational device for monitoring the ocean floor and an underwater transmitter for intership communication.[101] The Canadian scientist Donald Sproule led the research efforts that developed the first echo-sounder with a range display for the Canadian navy. Sproule unexpectedly discovered that the echo-sounder not only could display the depth of ocean bedrock but also was capable of detecting schools of fish.[102] This discovery proved to be key for later medical uses of ultrasound.

Another important milestone in sound research was the discovery of piezoelectricity. In 1880, Pierre and Jacques Curie observed that when pressure was applied to crystals of quartz or Rochelle salt, an electric charge was generated that was directly proportional to the force applied to the crystals. The Curies called this phenomenon piezoelectricity, from the Greek word *piezein*, meaning "to press."[97] In addition, they demonstrated the reverse piezoelectric effect that occurred when a rapidly changing electric potential was applied to the crystal and caused it to vibrate. The ultrasound transducers currently in use contain piezoelectric crystals that expand and contract to interconvert electric and mechanical energy; this action is the essence of the ultrasound transducer.

In the post–World War II era, the industrial work of Tom Brown and Ian Donald played a vital role in the development of the first handheld contact ultrasound machine. Donald and colleagues also investigated many of the earliest clinical applications of ultrasound.

Pioneers of Medical Ultrasound

Karl Theodor Dussik, a psychiatrist and neurologist, along with his brother Friederich, a physicist, began studying the clinical uses of ultrasonography in the late 1930s. In 1937, the Dussik brothers used a 1.5
(continued)

this interconversion, the transducer contains the following essential components:

1. An active element. Electrical energy is applied to the piezoelectric crystals within the transducer, and an ultrasound pulse is thereby generated via the piezoelectric effect. The pulse distorts the crystals, and an electrical signal is produced. This signal causes an ultrasound image to form on the screen via the reverse piezoelectric effect.

2. Damping or backing material. An epoxy resin absorbs the vibrations and reduces the number of cycles in a pulse, thereby improving the resolution of the ultrasound image.

3. A matching layer. This substance reduces the reflection that occurs at the transducer-tissue interface. The great difference in density (i.e., the impedance mismatch) between the soft tissue and the transducer results in reflection of the ultrasound waves. The matching material decreases this reflection and facilitates the transit of the ultrasound waves through the body and into the target organ.

Transducers are classified according to (1) the arrangement of the active elements (array) contained within the transducer and (2) the frequency of the ultrasound wave produced. Transducer arrays contain closely packed piezoelectric elements, each with its own electrical connection to the ultrasound instrument.[7] These elements can be excited individually or in groups to produce the ultrasound beam. There are four main transducer arrays: (1) the rectangular linear array, which yields a rectangular image, (2) the curved array, which yields a trapezoidal image, (3) the phased array, a small transducer in which the sound pulses are generated by activating all of the elements in the array, and (4) the annular array, in which the elements are arranged in a circular fashion. The advantage of transducer arrays is that the ultrasound beam can be electronically steered without any moving mechanical parts (except for the annular array) and focused.[7,8] In the clinical setting, this arrangement allows the operator to adjust the focal zone so that he or she can accurately image a large organ (e.g., the liver) while still being able to obtain fine details of a lesion.

The frequency of the transducer is determined by the thickness of the piezoelectric elements within the transducer: the thinner the piezoelectric elements, the higher the frequency.[7,8] Although diagnostic ultrasonography makes use of transducer frequencies ranging from 1 MHz to 20 MHz, the most commonly used frequencies for medical diagnostic imaging are those between 2.5 and 10 MHz [see Table 4]. Ultrasound beams of different frequencies have different characteristics: higher frequencies penetrate tissue poorly but yield excellent resolution, whereas lower frequencies penetrate well but at the cost of compromised resolution. Accordingly, transducers are generally chosen on the basis of the depth of the structure to be imaged.[9] For example, a 7.5 MHz transducer is a suitable choice for imaging a superficial organ such as the thyroid, but a 3.5 MHz transducer would be preferable for imaging a deep structure such as the abdominal aorta.

Ultrasound machines vary in complexity, but each has the following essential components:

Ultrasonography in Surgery: Historical Perspectives *(continued)*

MHz transmitter to record variations in the amplitude of the energy detected in scanning the human brain.[102] Their experiments were deemed to be faulty, however, and research funding for medical uses of ultrasound in the United States was greatly curtailed for the next decade.[102-104]

G. D. Ludwig and F. W. Struthers, working at the Naval Medical Research Institute in Bethesda, Maryland, were among the first investigators to study the use of the pulse-echo technique in biologic tissue; unfortunately, because Ludwig was employed by the military, many of his findings were considered to be restricted information and consequently were not published in medical journals. These studies investigated the transmission velocity of ultrasound waves in slabs of beef and human extremities and determined that the mean propagation speed of ultrasound in soft tissue was 1,540 m/sec. This important achievement had far-reaching consequences that affect how ultrasound software is constructed to this day.

In 1950, the English-trained surgeon John Julian Wild published his preliminary findings on ultrasound-determined bowel wall thickness and the properties of a specimen of gastric cancer.[105] Wild, Donald Neal, and, subsequently, J. M. Reid noted that malignant tissue seemed to be more echogenic than benign tissue.[105,106] Intellectual and financial support for Wild's research was minimal because of his unconventional research methods and his personality differences with his scientific contemporaries. Wild wanted to find immediate clinical applications for ultrasound technology rather than design experiments based on theories. His various difficulties notwithstanding, Wild managed to develop a scanning device that was used to screen patients for breast cancer; he also developed transrectal and transvaginal transducers. With this instrument, he was able to image a brain tumor in a pathology specimen and to localize a brain tumor in a patient after a craniotomy.

Another pioneer from the 1940s, Douglass Howry, played an important role in the development of ultrasound and ultrasonic devices. Working with W. Roderic Bliss, an electrical engineer, Howry began building the first B-mode scanner in 1949. Unlike Wild, Howry was as interested in the behavior of ultrasound waves in tissue as he was in the construction of a functional ultrasound machine. In the early 1960s, W. Wright and E. Meyers joined Howry's research team. The result of this team effort was the production of a direct contact scanner. In 1961, Meyers and Wright incorporated to form Physionics Engineering, and within a year,

they produced the prototype for the first handheld contact scanner in the United States.[107] This scanner had an articulated arm with positioning mechanisms at each joint to integrate information obtained from the transducer.

Ian Donald and another gynecologist, John McVicar, along with Tom Brown, an engineer from Kelvin & Hughes Scientific Instrument Company, developed the first contact compound scanner. Donald's contributions were well accepted in the field of medicine: they essentially solidified the concept that ultrasound would have a major role in medical diagnostic imaging.

In 1955, Bernard Jaffe discovered the piezoelectric properties of polarized solid solutions of lead zirconate titanate. This important finding eventually led to smaller and better ultrasound transducers. Inge Edler of Sweden and Carl Hellmuth Hertz were the principal pioneers in the field of echocardiography.

Christian Doppler and the Doppler Effect

Special mention should be made of the Austrian mathematician and physicist Christian Johann Doppler. In 1841, Doppler gave a speech entitled "On the Colored Light of the Double Stars and Certain Other Stars of the Heavens" to an audience consisting of five people and a transcriber.[108] Doppler's treatise proposed that the observed color of a star was caused by a spectral shift of white light that occurred because of the relative motion of the star to the earth. To provide a basis for his theory, Doppler used analogies based on the transmission of light and sound. Although his theory on light was in error, Doppler's theory on the frequency changes in sound waves was correct. The Doppler effect, as the sonic phenomenon he described came to be known, is defined as "the observed changes in frequency of transmitted waves when relative motion exists between the source of the wave and an observer."[108] This theory has been applied to many aspects of science, including astronomy and medicine.

The first application of the Doppler effect in medicine involved the measurement of differences in the transit time between two transducers of ultrasonic waves traveling "upstream" and "downstream" through flowing blood. Since then, research into the clinical use of the Doppler principle has been carried out simultaneously at numerous centers throughout the global scientific community.

Table 1 Ultrasound Physics Terminology Relevant to Ultrasonographic Imaging[4-6]

Term	Definition	Significance
Ultrasound	High-frequency (> 20 kHz) mechanical radiant energy transmitted through a medium	
Frequency	Number of cycles/sec (10^6 cycles/sec = 1 MHz) Diagnostic ultrasound: 1–20 MHz	Increasing frequency improves resolution
Wavelength	Distance traveled by wave per cycle: as frequency becomes higher, wavelength becomes smaller	Wavelength is related to spatial resolution of object: shorter wavelengths yield better resolution but poorer penetration
Amplitude	Strength or height of wave	Amplitude and intensity are reduced (attenuated) as waves travel through tissue; time-gain compensation circuit compensates for this attenuation
Attenuation	Decrease in amplitude and intensity of wave as it travels through a medium; attenuation is affected by absorption, scattering, and reflection	
Absorption	Conversion of sound energy into heat	
Scattering	Redirection of wave as it strikes a rough or small boundary	
Reflection	Return of wave toward transducer	
Propagation speed	Speed with which wave travels through soft tissue (1,540 m/sec)	Propagation speed (determined by density and stiffness of medium) is greater in solids than in liquids and greater in liquids than in gases

1. A monitor (for displaying the ultrasound image).
2. A keyboard (for labeling the image and making adjustments to produce a quality image).
3. A transducer (for interconverting electrical and acoustic energy).
4. An image recorder (for producing copies of the ultrasound images).

Finally, there are three scanning modes, A, B, and M; these modes evolved over several years.[10] A mode (amplitude modulation), the most basic form of diagnostic ultrasonography, yields a one-dimensional image that displays the amplitude or strength of the wave along the vertical axis and the time along the horizontal axis. Therefore, the greater the signal returning to the transducer, the higher the "spike." B mode (brightness modulation), the mode most commonly used today, relates the brightness of the image to the amplitude of the ultrasound wave. Thus, denser structures appear brighter (i.e., whiter, more echogenic) on the image because they reflect the ultrasound waves better. M mode relates the amplitude of the ultrasound wave to the imaging of moving structures, such as cardiac muscle. Before real-time imaging became available, M-mode scanning formed the basis for echocardiography.[10,11]

Clinical Applications of Ultrasonography in Surgical Practice

As an extension of the physical examination, ultrasonography is a valuable adjunct to surgical practice in the office, the emergency de-

partment, the operating room, and the surgical intensive care unit. Once surgeons have learned the essential principles of ultrasonography, they can readily build on this experience and extend the use of this technology to various specific aspects of surgery. In what follows, I list and briefly describe several clinical areas in which surgeon-performed ultrasonography has proved to be an effective diagnostic and interventional tool.

BREAST

Ultrasound-directed biopsy of breast lesions is now a common office procedure for general surgeons. The increase in the number of screening mammograms performed since the late 1970s has led to the detection of more nonpalpable breast lesions. The traditional choice for further evaluation of such masses has been open surgical excision, but the yield of malignancies with this approach has been only about 20%.[12-14] Advances in ultrasound technology, including automated biopsy needles and high-resolution transducers,[15] have prompted a surge of interest in fine-needle and core biopsy tissue sampling as an alternative to open biopsy. Such procedures are appealing because they are minimally invasive, are about as accurate as open biopsy,[16] and can be performed by the surgeon in the office setting.

Current indications for breast ultrasonography include (1) evaluation of a nonpalpable, new, or growing mass detected on mammog-

Table 2 Essential Principles of Ultrasound

Principle	Explanation
Piezoelectric effect	Piezoelectric crystals expand and contract to interconvert electrical and mechanical energy
Pulse-echo principle	When ultrasound wave contacts tissue, some of signal is reflected while some is transmitted into tissue; these waves are then reflected to crystals within transducer, generating electrical impulse comparable to strength of returning wave
Acoustic impedance	Acoustic impedance = density of tissue × speed of sound in tissue Strength of returning echo depends on difference in density between two structures imaged: structures of different acoustic impedance (e.g., bile and gallstone) are relatively easy to distinguish from one another, whereas those of similar acoustic impedance (e.g., spleen and kidney) are more difficult to distinguish

Table 3 Terminology Used in Assessment of Ultrasonograms[3,109]

Term	Definition
Echogenicity	Degree to which tissue echoes ultrasonic waves (generally reflected in ultrasound image as degree of brightness)
Anechoic	Showing no internal echoes, appearing dark or black
Isoechoic	Having appearance similar to that of surrounding tissue
Hypoechoic	Less echoic or darker than surrounding tissue
Hyperechoic	More echoic or whiter than surrounding tissue
Resolution	Ability to distinguish between two different structures; spatial resolution improves as frequency increases
Lateral	Resolution transverse to ultrasound wave; relates to width of structure
Axial	Resolution parallel to ultrasound wave; relates to depth of structure

Figure 1 **Shown are the basic components of an ultrasound transducer.**

raphy, (2) evaluation of duct size in the presence of nipple discharge, (3) assessment of a dense breast or a vaguely palpable mass, (4) differentiation between a solid palpable mass and a cystic one, and (5) guidance of percutaneous drainage of an abscess.[17-21]

GASTROINTESTINAL TRACT

Endoscopic and endorectal ultrasonography have added a new dimension to the preoperative assessment and treatment of many GI lesions. Endoscopic ultrasonography (EUS) involves the visualization of the GI tract via a high-frequency (12 to 20 MHz) ultrasound transducer placed through an endoscope. With the transducer near the target organ, images of the gut wall and the surrounding parenchymal organs can be obtained that are detailed enough to define the depth of tumor penetration with precision and to detect the presence of involved lymph nodes as small as 2 mm. When done preoperatively, EUS is 80% to 90% accurate at predicting the stage of the tumor; if an endoscopically directed biopsy attachment is used, the diagnostic potential is even higher.[22]

Indications for EUS include (1) preoperative staging of GI malignancies, (2) preoperative localization of pancreatic endocrine tumors, particularly insulinomas, (3) evaluation of submucosal lesions of the GI tract, and (4) guidance of imaging during interventional procedures (e.g., tissue sampling and drainage of a pancreatic pseudocyst).[23-25]

Endorectal ultrasonography is used in the evaluation of patients with benign and malignant rectal conditions.[26-34] It is commonly performed with an axial 7.0 or 10.0 MHz rotating transducer that produces a 360° horizontal cross-sectional view of the rectal wall. This special transducer is 24 cm long and is covered with a water-filled latex balloon. After the transducer is advanced above the rectal lesion, the balloon that surrounds the transducer is filled with degassed water to create an acoustic window for ultrasound imaging. The transducer is gradually withdrawn while the examiner views the layers of the rectal wall [see Figure 2] by means of real-time imaging.[35,36] These layers are important landmarks in ultrasonographic staging, just as they are in postoperative pathologic staging. For example, if the middle white line (i.e., the submucosa) is intact, a be-

Table 4 Clinical Applications of Selected Transducer Frequencies

Frequency	Applications
2.5–3.5 MHz	Renal Aortic General abdominal
5.0 MHz	Transvaginal Pediatric abdominal Testicular
7.5 MHz	Vascular Foreign body in soft tissue Thyroid

nign lesion may be removed via a submucosal resection. A classification of preoperative tumor staging called uTNM has been proposed that is analogous to the TNM classification for tumor staging.[37] This classification is based on ultrasonographic determination of the infiltrative tumor depth (the prefix *u* stands for ultrasonography).

The sensitivity of ultrasonography in determining the depth of tumor invasion is about 85% to 90%; however, it can sometimes overestimate the extent of invasion in the presence of tissue inflammation and edema.[28] Further research is needed to assess the accuracy of ultrasonography in detecting recurrent cancer after surgery.[38] Errors in staging are likely to occur with tumors that invade the lamina muscularis mucosae or are associated with inflammation of the lamina propria mucosae.[39] In addition, lesions characterized by ultramicroscopic invasion of the submucosa may be misstaged because the technology currently available cannot provide the fine resolution necessary to assess such invasion.[28,40]

Endoanal ultrasonography is an important part of the evaluation of anal incontinence because it is capable of detecting defects in the internal and external sphincters.[41-45] It is done in much the same way as endorectal ultrasonography, except that the 10 MHz transducer is covered with a sonolucent hard plastic cone instead of a water-filled balloon. Although endoanal ultrasonography does not measure sphincter function, ultrasound-detected sphincter disruption correlates well with pressure measurements[46,47] and operative findings.[45,48] Additional indications for endoanal ultrasonography include evaluation of patients with an exophytic distal rectal tumor (e.g., a villous adenoma) and assessment of patients who have a perianal abscess, fistula in ano, a presacral cyst, or a rectal ulcer.

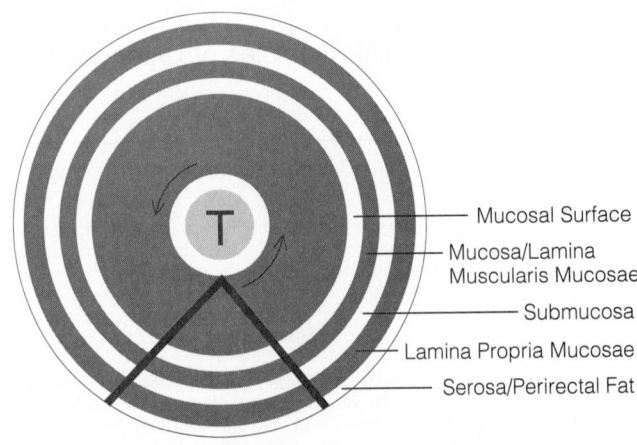

Figure 2 **Depicted is the five-layer model of rectal wall anatomy as delineated by endorectal ultrasonography.**[110]

ACUTE CONDITIONS

Traumatic

The FAST (*F*ocused *A*ssessment for the *S*onographic examination of the *T*rauma patient) is a rapid diagnostic test developed for the evaluation of patients with potential truncal injuries. Historically, its development is rooted in several fundamental studies that demonstrated the high sensitivity of ultrasonography in detecting small degrees of ascites,[49] splenic injury,[50] and hemoperitoneum in the hepatorenal space and the pelvis.[51] The FAST determines the presence or absence of blood in the pericardial sac and three dependent abdominal regions, including Morison's pouch, the splenorenal recess, and the pelvis.

Nontraumatic

In the acute nontraumatic setting, surgeons are currently using ultrasonography for the following purposes:

1. Assessment for multiple loculations and drainage of a soft tissue abscess.[52,53]
2. Early diagnosis of wound dehiscence through visualization of the fascial defect [*see Figure 3*].
3. Detection of a foreign body in soft tissue.[54-56]
4. Evaluation of a patient with abdominal pain (e.g., from gallstones).[52,53,57,58]
5. Confirmation of the reduction of an incarcerated hernia through identification of the fascial defect and observation of the reduction occurring with real-time imaging [*see Figure 4*].[59]
6. Identification of an abdominal aortic aneurysm in a patient who presents with back pain and hypotension. Intramural calcification and intraluminal thrombus are common findings [*see Figure 5*]. If the aortic aneurysm ruptures into the peritoneal cavity, the FAST can detect the presence of hemoperitoneum.

LAPAROSCOPY AND INTRAOPERATIVE USE

Examination with intraoperative or laparoscopic ultrasonography is an integral part of many hepatic, biliary, and pancreatic surgical procedures. With this tool, surgeons can detect previously undiagnosed lesions or bile duct stones,[60] avoid unnecessary dissection of vessels or ducts, clarify tumor margins, and perform biopsy and cryoablation procedures.[61] Compared with preoperative imaging modalities, intraoperative ultrasonography is much more sensitive in detecting malignant or benign lesions.[62] The precision with which intraoperative ultrasonography can delineate small lesions (5 mm) and define their relationship to other structures facilitates resection, reduces operative time, and frequently alters the surgeon's operative strategy.[62-65]

Intraoperative ultrasonography makes use of both contact scanning and so-called standoff scanning for imaging.[66] In contact scanning, the transducer is directly applied to the organ so that the deepest part of the organ is accurately depicted. This technique is most often used for imaging large organs (e.g., the liver). In standoff scanning, the transducer is placed about 1 to 2 cm away from the structure in a pool of sterile saline solution that permits the transmission of ultrasound waves. This technique is often used to image blood vessels, bile ducts, or the spinal cord; it allows good visualization of the structure without compression by the transducer. The size, shape, and type of ultrasound transducer used for intraoperative scanning depend on the anatomic structure to be examined. For example, a pencillike 7.5 MHz transducer is used for scanning the common bile duct, whereas a side-viewing T-shaped 5 MHz transducer is preferable for imaging a cirrhotic liver. Intraoperative ultrasound examinations are conducted systematically to ensure that no subtle pathology is missed and that the examination is reproducible. For example, the liver is imaged sequentially according to a system based on Couinaud's anatomic segments.[67]

Figure 3 **Ultrasound image shows midline abdominal wound dehiscence. Transducer orientation is sagittal with respect to long axis of wound. Interruption in horizontal white line (arrows) represents separation of fascia.**

Figure 4 **Sagittal ultrasound image shows ventral hernia with fascial defect (arrow).**

Similar principles apply to laparoscopic ultrasonography, except that the transducers are made to adapt to the laparoscopic equipment.[68,69] Indications for this modality include detection of common bile duct stones, staging of pancreatic cancer to prevent unnecessary celiotomy, and resection or cryoablation of hepatic metastases.[69]

VASCULAR SYSTEM

Color flow duplex imaging and endoluminal ultrasonography have significantly expanded the diagnostic and therapeutic aspects of vascular imaging. Vascular diagnostic imaging is commonly used for diagnosing arterial disease or deep vein thrombosis (DVT); however, it is also helpful for diagnosing other disorders, such as Raynaud's disease and thoracic outlet syndrome. In the office setting, surgeons use ultrasonography to screen for abdominal aortic aneurysm or to follow patients with a diagnosed aneurysm, because it is capable of detecting change in aortic diameter as small as a few millimeters.[70] In patients who have

Figure 5 **Transverse ultrasound image shows abdominal aortic aneurysm with intraluminal thrombus.**

undergone repair of an abdominal aortic aneurysm, color flow duplex imaging is highly specific for the diagnosis of anastomotic false aneurysms. In one study, this modality was compared with B-mode ultrasonography, CT, digital subtraction arteriography, and magnetic resonance imaging and emerged as the diagnostic test of choice when the accuracy, cost, safety, and availability of each method were assessed.[71]

Color flow duplex scanning is also used to examine the patency and size of the portal vein and the hepatic artery in patients who have undergone liver transplantation, to assess the resectability of pancreatic tumors, to diagnose superior mesenteric artery occlusion, and to diagnose a pseudoaneurysm or an arteriovenous fistula after percutaneous arterial catheterization.[72,73] In the acute setting, several investigators have found color flow duplex imaging to be a reliable, time-saving, noninvasive alternative to arteriography for the detection of arterial injury.[74-78]

Duplex imaging of the lower extremity is used to assess the patency of the deep venous system and is capable of detecting DVT reliably.[79] The addition of color flow imaging facilitates the examination by making the artery and its associated vein easier to identify. By per-

Figure 6 **Sagittal ultrasound image demonstrates pleural effusion.**

forming serial duplex venous ultrasound imaging to detect DVT, one group of investigators was able to identify a subgroup of injured patients who were at highest risk for pulmonary embolism; they suggested that these patients be given DVT prophylaxis and undergo close surveillance with duplex imaging.[79]

Intraoperative duplex imaging can be used to detect technical errors in vascular anastomoses as well as abnormalities in flow.[80] Arteriography assesses the patency of an anastomosis and measures distal arterial runoff, but it is invasive. Intraoperative duplex imaging, on the other hand, permits rapid visualization of the anatomic and hemodynamic aspects of a vascular reconstruction, and it is noninvasive, easily repeatable, and less time-consuming than arteriography.

SURGICAL INTENSIVE CARE UNIT

Indications for surgeon-performed ultrasonography in the SICU include localization of a central vein or an artery for hemodynamic monitoring[81] and detection of a pleural effusion [*see Figure 6*]. Not only are fewer lateral decubitus x-rays ordered when ultrasonography is done in the SICU, but the safety of thoracentesis is also enhanced when it is performed under ultrasound guidance.[82,83]

General Considerations for Diagnostic Ultrasound Examinations

INSTRUMENTATION

Before an ultrasound examination is performed, the following three steps should be observed:

1. The correct ultrasound machine and transducer should be chosen for the specific type of examination to be done. For example, if a vascular study is to be performed, the machine should have Doppler capability and, ideally, color flow capability as well.
2. The transducer should be chosen according to the structure or organ to be imaged. It must provide both sufficient depth of penetration to image the entire organ and sufficient resolution to allow the examiner to distinguish the details of lesions.
3. Although many machines have preset controls for power and gain, a standard image should be obtained to confirm that the settings are correct for the specific examination being done. For example, the FAST begins with an image of the heart so that blood can be identified and the gain controls adjusted (if necessary) to permit accurate detection of hemoperitoneum.

PATIENT POSITIONING

The patient should be positioned so that all of the images required for a particular examination can be readily obtained. The surgeon should take time to review the scanning planes [*see Figure 7*] and understand the orientation of the patient on the monitor screen in relation to the transducer. It is also important to follow conventional scanning protocols so that when the images are reviewed, a lesion can be accurately located and the scan can be reproduced even by another ultrasonographer. An example of such a protocol is the radial-scanning technique recommended for examination of the breast [*see Technique for Selected Surgical Applications of Ultrasonography, Breast Examination, below*].

DOCUMENTATION

The machine's annotation keys are used to record the patient's name and identification number, the area of interest, and the scanning plane. Most machines have function keys that automate the recording of these data. Furthermore, the internal clock automatically labels each image with the date and time (accurate to 0.01 second).

Figure 7 **Depicted are scanning planes used in ultrasonography.**

Transverse Plane

Coronal Plane

Sagittal Plane

TECHNICAL TIPS

The following generic technical tips should prove useful in a wide range of ultrasonographic applications:

1. The ultrasound machine should be inspected according to the guidelines of the institution's department of biomedical engineering to ensure that it is functioning properly.

2. The patient's orientation on the monitor or screen relative to the position of the transducer should be checked by applying gel to the transducer's footprint (i.e., the part of the transducer that is in contact with the patient's skin) and then rubbing the footprint with a finger near the indicator line of the transducer. Motion on the left side of the screen indicates that the transducer is properly oriented.

3. Liberal amounts of gel should be applied to the area being examined. The gel acts as an acoustic coupler, helping to transmit the ultrasound waves and reduce their reflection. If not enough gel has been applied, the waves will not be transmitted properly, and a dark area will appear on the ultrasound image.

4. The transducer should be manipulated with small movements (not wide sweeps), and gentle pressure should be applied initially. This second point is especially important in imaging the breast or the thyroid: the tissues are superficial, and too much pressure can easily compress them and distort the ultrasound image.

5. The gain and time-gain compensation settings should be rechecked for each new examination. For example, after completing a breast examination, the sonographer should not begin an examination of the carotid vessels without confirming that these settings are correct.

Any hard copies of the ultrasound images that may be required should be printed, saved, and reviewed. Ideally, the ultrasound images should be videotaped, because the dynamic real-time image provides more information than still images, thereby increasing the confidence level associated with each observation.

CONTINUOUS PERFORMANCE IMPROVEMENT

As part of the performance improvement process, ultrasound images should be routinely reviewed, with special attention paid to false positive or false negative examinations. The goal of this process is to help identify any correctable factors associated with such examinations and thereby minimize or prevent their recurrence. Some studies have noted the presence of a pronounced learning curve, as a result of which the sensitivity and specificity initially achieved by new surgeon-ultrasonographers have been relatively low[57,84-86]; however, there is evidence that surgeons' performance may be improved with the help of an ultrasound training course that focuses on those pitfalls of imaging that were found to be problems in the clinical setting. For example, in one study, surgeons learned both to perform examinations correctly and to interpret positive results accurately in patients with minimal as well as pronounced ascites; as a result, they were better able to distinguish relatively subtle differences within the spectrum of positive FAST results.[86] Other suggestions for improving performance are (1) to perform the ultrasound examination initially on normal tissue (as in evaluation of a breast mass) and (2) to perform the examinations on patients with known disease (e.g., a palpable breast mass, ascites, gallstones, or benign pericardial effusion). The rationale for the latter suggestion is that it should help the surgeon learn more rapidly how to recognize lesions with varying degrees of pathology.

Figure 8 **FAST. Shown are four transducer positions used in FAST: (1) pericardial area, (2) right upper quadrant, (3) left upper quadrant, and (4) pelvis.**[84]

a

b

Figure 9 FAST. (*a*) Sagittal ultrasound image of heart shows pericardium as single echogenic (white) line; normal findings. (*b*) Sagittal ultrasound image of heart shows separation of pericardial layers by blood.

6. Normal tissue should be examined ultrasonographically before the sonographer turns to the area of interest. For example, if the goal is to assess an abscess or DVT in one extremity, the first step should be to inspect the other extremity to see what the corresponding normal tissue looks like. This helps to sensitize the examiner to subtle pathologic changes in the abnormal tissue.

7. The patient should be asked to take a deep breath so that the motion of the diaphragm and the organs can be observed. If the motion of these structures is impaired, inflammation or an abscess may be present.

8. If the left upper quadrant is difficult to examine (as is sometimes the case in the FAST), a nasogastric tube should be in-

serted to decompress the stomach and minimize the presence of air so that it does not interfere with the transmission of the ultrasound waves.

9. Although B-mode ultrasound is usually sufficient to identify blood vessels, it sometimes is unable to distinguish the artery from the vein because of pulsations transmitted from the artery. In such cases, use of the Doppler mode, compression of the vessel (veins compress very easily), or having the patient perform the Valsalva maneuver can help differentiate arterial from venous anatomy. In addition, the vena cava is more readily identified as the patient completes inspiration.

10. A full bladder is needed for pelvic ultrasound examinations: it acts as an acoustic window, facilitating visualization of the pelvic

a

b

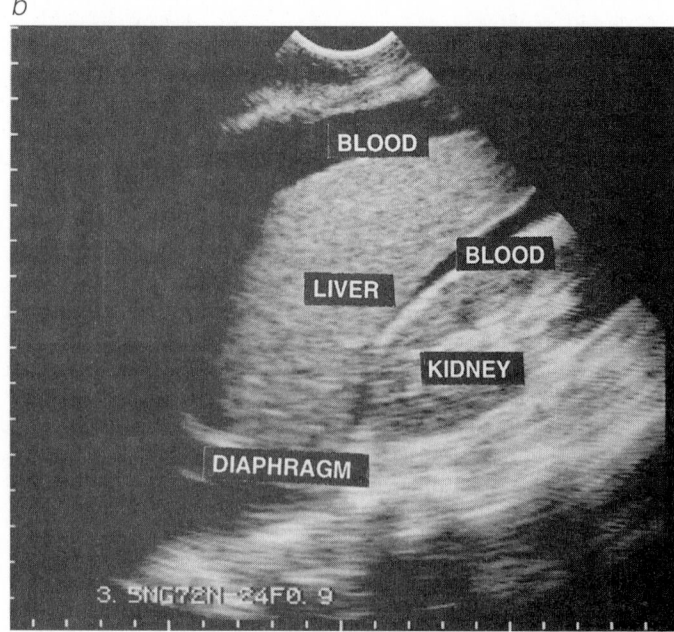

Figure 10 FAST. (*a*) Sagittal ultrasound image of liver, kidney, and diaphragm yields normal findings. (*b*) Sagittal ultrasound image of right upper quadrant shows blood between liver and kidney and between liver and diaphragm.

a

b

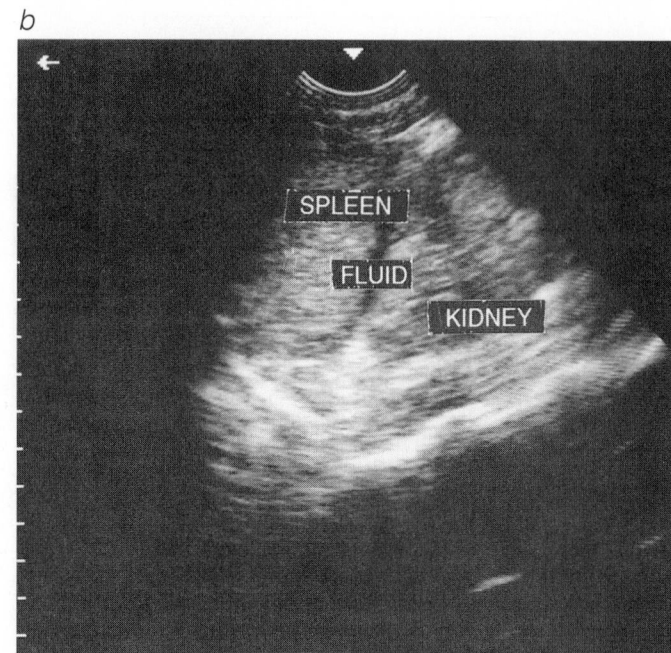

Figure 11 **FAST. (*a*) Sagittal ultrasound image of spleen and kidney yields normal findings. (*b*) Sagittal ultrasound image of left upper quadrant shows blood between spleen and kidney.**

a

b

Figure 12 **FAST. (*a*) Coronal ultrasound image of pelvis shows full bladder; normal findings. (*b*) Coronal ultrasound image of pelvis shows full bladder surrounded by blood.**

structures. It should not, however, be so full that it is overdistended. If the bladder is not full enough, the urinary catheter can be clamped to allow it to fill; if it is too full, the catheter can be unclamped to allow it to drain. In this way, hematomas in the pelvis can be more easily detected.

Technique for Selected Surgical Applications of Ultrasonography

FOCUSED ASSESSMENT FOR THE SONOGRAPHIC EXAMINATION OF THE TRAUMA PATIENT

The FAST is performed during the Advanced Trauma Life Support secondary survey while the patient is in the supine position

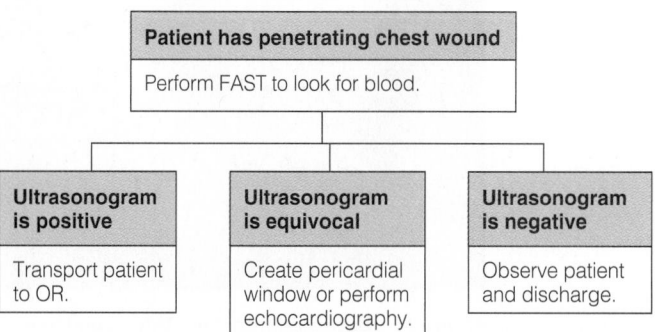

Figure 13 **FAST. Shown is an algorithm for use of ultrasonography in evaluation of patients with penetrating precordial wounds.[111]**

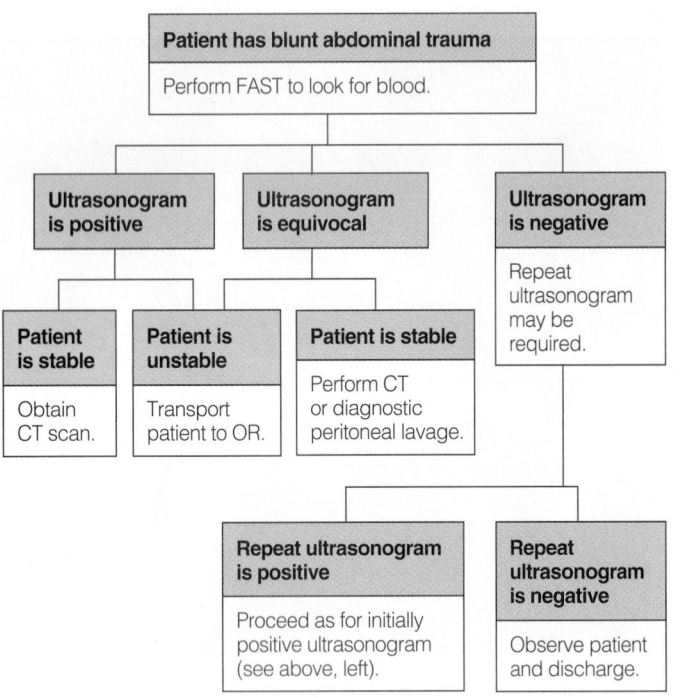

| Patient has blunt abdominal trauma |
| Perform FAST to look for blood. |

Ultrasonogram is positive

Ultrasonogram is equivocal

Ultrasonogram is negative
Repeat ultrasonogram may be required.

Patient is stable
Obtain CT scan.

Patient is unstable
Transport patient to OR.

Patient is stable
Perform CT or diagnostic peritoneal lavage.

Repeat ultrasonogram is positive
Proceed as for initially positive ultrasonogram (see above, left).

Repeat ultrasonogram is negative
Observe patient and discharge.

Figure 14 **FAST. Shown is an algorithm for use of ultrasonography in evaluation of patients with blunt abdominal trauma.**[111]

[*see I:2 Trauma Resuscitation*]. With the thoracoabdominal area exposed, warmed hypoallergenic, water-soluble ultrasound transmission gel is applied to the abdomen in four specific areas. A focused, limited examination for the detection of blood in these four regions is conducted in sequence as follows: (1) the pericardial area, (2) the right upper abdominal quadrant, (3) the left upper abdominal quadrant, and (4) the pouch of Douglas [*see Figure 8*].

The transducer is oriented for sagittal sections and placed in the subxiphoid region. The heart is then identified, with the density of blood used as a standard. The subxiphoid approach through the longitudinal axis is taken to enable the examiner to identify the heart and to look for blood in the pericardial region [*see Figure 9*].

The transducer is then placed in the right midaxillary line region between the 11th and 12th ribs to enable the examiner to identify the liver, the kidney, and the diaphragm and to look for blood in Morison's pouch [*see Figure 10*].

Next, the transducer is positioned on the left posterior axillary line between the 10th and 11th ribs to enable the examiner to visualize the spleen and the kidney and to look for blood in the space between these organs and posterior to the spleen [*see Figure 11*].

The transducer is then oriented for transverse sections and placed in the midline approximately 4 cm superior to the symphysis pubis to determine whether there is blood around the full bladder [*see Figure 12*].

An analysis of 1,540 injured patients undergoing FAST examinations performed by surgeon-ultrasonographers reached the following conclusions[86]:

1. Ultrasonography should be the initial diagnostic adjunct for the evaluation of patients with precordial wounds and blunt truncal injuries because it is rapid and accurate and augments the surgeon's diagnostic capabilities.

2. Surgeon-performed FAST is most accurate when used for the evaluation of patients with precordial or transthoracic wounds and a possible hemopericardium and for the evaluation of hypotensive patients with blunt torso trauma.

3. Because of the high sensitivity and specificity of ultrasonography when it is used for the evaluation of patients with precordial or transthoracic wounds and hypotensive patients with blunt torso trauma, immediate operative intervention is justified in these patients when the ultrasound examination is positive [*see Figures 13 and 14*].

Although the FAST accurately detects the presence or absence of hemoperitoneum in patients with blunt trauma, it does not readily identify intraparenchymal or retroperitoneal injuries. Therefore, a computed tomographic scan of the abdomen may be needed

Figure 15 **Breast examination. Ultrasound image shows simple cyst (arrow) of breast characterized by sharp, smooth margins and homogeneous, anechoic interior.**

Figure 16 **Breast examination. Ultrasound image shows malignant breast lesion (arrow) with indistinct, jagged margins, few internal echoes, and slight posterior shadowing.**

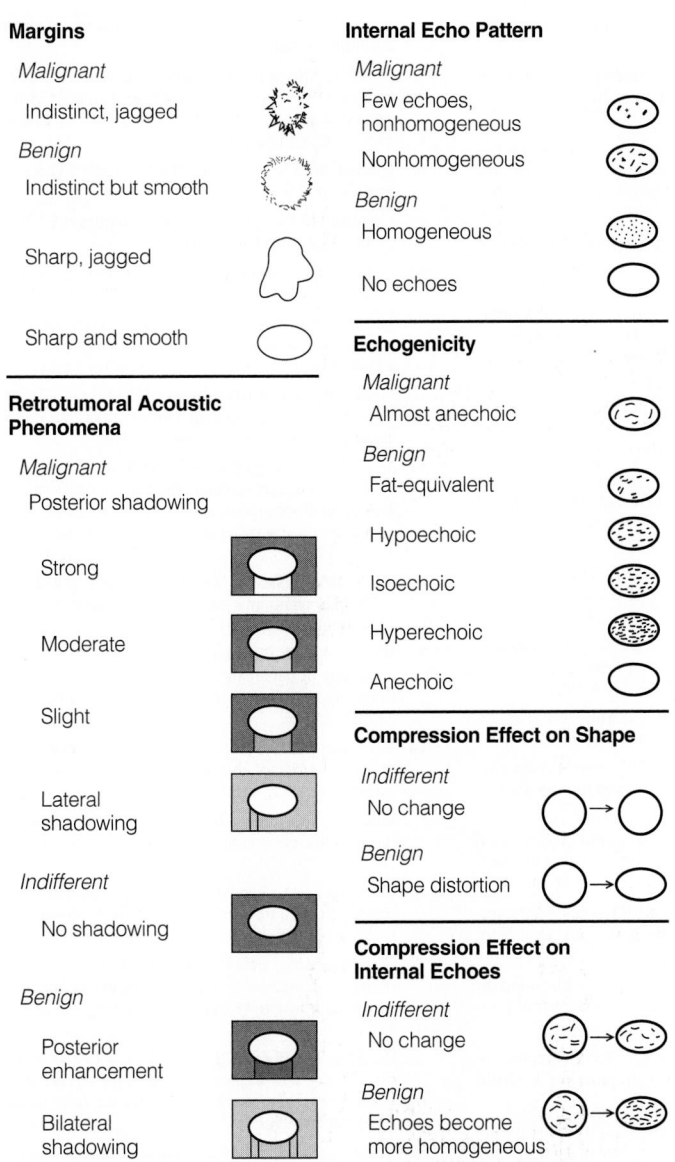

Margins

Malignant

Indistinct, jagged

Benign

Indistinct but smooth

Sharp, jagged

Sharp and smooth

Retrotumoral Acoustic Phenomena

Malignant

Posterior shadowing

Strong

Moderate

Slight

Lateral shadowing

Indifferent

No shadowing

Benign

Posterior enhancement

Bilateral shadowing

Internal Echo Pattern

Malignant

Few echoes, nonhomogeneous

Nonhomogeneous

Benign

Homogeneous

No echoes

Echogenicity

Malignant

Almost anechoic

Benign

Fat-equivalent

Hypoechoic

Isoechoic

Hyperechoic

Anechoic

Compression Effect on Shape

Indifferent

No change

Benign

Shape distortion

Compression Effect on Internal Echoes

Indifferent

No change

Benign

Echoes become more homogeneous

Figure 17 **Breast examination. Shown is a schematic representation of analytic criteria for the interpretation of breast sonograms.**[91]

The increase in surgeon-performed ultrasound examinations has led to decreased performance of diagnostic peritoneal lavage and CT scanning in the trauma setting. It has become apparent that the FAST can replace central venous pressure monitoring in the diagnosis of hemopericardium and can replace diagnostic peritoneal lavage in the detection of hemoperitoneum in many injured patients. Although CT scanning remains a valuable diagnostic test, the indications for its use in the evaluation of injured patients are now narrower than they once were.

BREAST EXAMINATION

The surgeon must be thoroughly familiar with the ultrasonographic anatomy of normal breast tissue to be able to recognize a mass, discern its ultrasonographic characteristics, and determine whether it is likely to be benign [*see Figure 15*] or malignant [*see Figure 16*].[91,92] Analytic criteria for the interpretation of focal lesions detected on breast ultrasound examinations have been well described and depicted elsewhere [*see Figure 17*].[91]

As noted, breast examination should be done according to a specific scanning protocol. The recommended approach is the radial-scanning technique reported by Teboul.[93] A 7.5 MHz linear-array transducer is used, and the patient is placed in the supine position with the ipsilateral arm behind the head. The transducer is placed at the 6 o'clock position; the breast tissue is scanned, and the transducer is then advanced toward the periphery beyond the breast tissue. Next, the 5 o'clock region is evaluated in the same manner. Each sector (or "hour") of the breast is then scanned in a sequential counterclockwise fashion until the process is completed. Some experts recommend that the nipple be used as a visual pivot point during scanning, remaining in the upper left corner of the monitor throughout the ultrasound examination.[94]

To image the nipple-areola complex, the transducer is placed next to the nipple and angled toward the retroareolar area. Several transverse scans are performed to assess the uniformity of the ligamentous structures and to detect any small tumor that may be present between these structures. Finally, the axilla is scanned with transverse and longitudinal sweeps of the transducer to inspect for lymph nodes.[94]

An important principle in the performance of breast ultrasonography is that the examination must be performed in a consistent and methodical manner so that findings can be accurately described and reproduced. If this principle is followed, a trained examiner can probably identify 80% to 90% of mammographically detected nonpalpable breast masses.[95] One important drawback to remember, however, is that ultrasonography generally will not reveal lesions less than 5 mm in diameter or lesions with an isoechoic appearance.[96]

to complement the FAST and reduce the incidence of missed injuries.[84,86-89] There is some evidence that false negative results are more common in patients with pelvic ring fractures, which suggests that CT of the abdomen is routinely indicated in such patients.[90]

References

1. Maggio M, Sanders RC: Basic physics. Clinical Sonography: A Practical Guide. Sanders RC, Ed. Little, Brown and Co, Boston, 1991, p 4

2. Hedrick WR, Hykes L, Starchman DE: Ultrasound Physics and Instrumentation. Mosby, St. Louis, 1995, chap 1, p 23

3. Miner NS: Basic principles. Clinical Sonography: A Practical Guide. Sanders RC, Ed. Little, Brown and Co, Boston, 1991, p 33

4. Kremkau F: Diagnostic Ultrasound: Principles, Instrumentation and Exercises. WB Saunders Co, Philadelphia, 1984, chap 2, p 6

5. Hedrick WR, Hykes L, Starchman DE: Ultrasound Physics and Instrumentation. Mosby, St. Louis, 1995, chap 1, p 8

6. Dubinsky T, Horii S, Odwin CS: Ultrasonic physics and instrumentation. Appleton & Lange's Review for the Ultrasonography Examination. Odwin CS, Dubinsky T, Fleischer AC, Eds. Appleton & Lange, Norwalk, Connecticut, 1993, p 8

7. Zagzebski JA: Physics of diagnostic ultrasound. Essentials of Ultrasound Physics. Zagzebski JA, Ed. Mosby, St. Louis, 1996, p 20

8. Hedrick WR, Hykes L, Starchman DE: Ultrasound Physics and Instrumentation. Mosby, St. Louis, 1995, chap 4, p 96

9. Hedrick WR, Hykes L, Starchman DE: Ultrasound Physics and Instrumentation. Mosby, St. Louis, 1995, chap 2, p 55

10. Sanders RC, Miner NS: Introduction. Clinical Sonography: A Practical Guide. Sanders RC, Ed. Little, Brown and Co, Boston, 1991, p 10

11. Kremkau F: Doppler ultrasound: principles and instruments. Ultrasound: Principles, Instrumentation

and Exercises. WB Saunders Co, Philadelphia, 1995, chap 7, p 123

12. Sailors DM, Crabtree JD, Land RL, et al: Needle localization for nonpalpable breast lesions. Am Surg 60:186, 1984

13. Wilhelm NC, DeParedes ES, Pope T: The changing mammogram: a primary indication for needle localization biopsy. Arch Surg 121:1311, 1986

14. Miller RS, Adelman RW, Espinosa MH: The early detection of non-palpable breast carcinoma with needle localization: experience with 500 patients in a community hospital. Am Surg 58:193, 1992

15. Schlecht L, Hadijuana J, Hosten N, et al: Ultrasonography of the female breast: comparison 7.5 MHz versus 13 MHz. Akt Radiol 6:69, 1996

16. Saarela AO, Kiviniemi HO, Rissanen TJ, et al: Nonpalpable breast lesions: pathologic correlation of ultra-

sonographically guided fine-needle aspiration biopsy. J Ultrasound Med 15:549, 1996

17. Jackson VP: The role of ultrasound in breast imaging. Radiology 177:305, 1990

18. Muttarak M: Abscess in the non-lactating breast: radiodiagnostic aspects. Australas Radiol 40:223, 1996

19. Dempsey PJ: Breast sonography: historical perspective, clinical application, and image interpretation. Ultrasound Q 6:69, 1988

20. Guyer PB, Dewbury KC: Ultrasound of the breast in the symptomatic and x-ray dense breast. Clin Radiol 36:69, 1985

21. Jackson VP, Hendrick RE, Feit SA, et al: Imaging of the radiographically dense breast. Radiology 188:297, 1993

22. Vilmann P, Jacobsen GK, Henriksen FW, et al: Endoscopic ultrasonography with guided fine needle aspiration biopsy in pancreatic disease. Gastrointest Endosc 38:172, 1992

23. Rosch T, Lightdale CJ, Botet JF: Localization of pancreatic endocrine tumors by endoscopic ultrasonography. N Engl J Med 326:1721, 1992

24. Scheiman JM: Endosonography: is it sound for the masses? J Clin Gastroenterol 19:2, 1994

25. Wiersema MJ, Kochman ML, Cramer HM, et al: Real-time endoscopic ultrasound-guided fine-needle aspiration of a mediastinal lymph node. Gastrointest Endosc 39:429, 1993

26. de Lange EE: Staging rectal carcinoma with endorectal imaging: how much detail do we really need? Radiology 190:633, 1994

27. Waizer A, Powsner E, Russo I: Prospective comparative study of magnetic resonance imaging versus transrectal ultrasound for preoperative staging and follow-up of rectal cancer: preliminary report. Dis Colon Rectum 34:1068, 1991

28. Herzog U, von Flue M, Tondelli P, et al: How accurate is endorectal ultrasound in the preoperative staging of rectal cancer? Dis Colon Rectum 36:127, 1993

29. Glaser F, Friedl P, Schlag P, et al: Influence of endorectal ultrasound on surgical treatment of rectal cancer. Eur J Oncol 16:304, 1990

30. Solomon MJ, McLeod RS, Cohen EK: Reliability and validity studies of endoluminal ultrasonography for anorectal disorders. Dis Colon Rectum 37:546, 1994

31. Kusunoki M, Yanagi H, Gondoh N, et al: Use of transrectal ultrasonography to select type of surgery for villous tumors in the lower two thirds of the rectum. Arch Surg 131:714, 1996

32. Beynon J: An evaluation of the role of rectal endosonography in rectal cancer. Ann R Coll Surg Engl 71:131, 1989

33. Milsom JW, Lavery I, Stolfi V, et al: The expanding utility of endoluminal ultrasonography in the management of rectal cancer. Surgery 112:832, 1992

34. Anderson B, Hann L, Enker W, et al: Transrectal ultrasonography and operative selection for early carcinoma of the rectum. J Am Coll Surg 179:513, 1994

35. Saclarides TJ: Endorectal ultrasonography for malignant disease. Ultrasound for the Surgeon. Staren ED, Arregui ME, Eds. Lippincott-Raven, Philadelphia, 1997, p 75

36. Beynon J, Foy DM, Temple LN, et al: The endosonic appearances of normal colon and rectum. Dis Colon Rectum 29:810, 1986

37. Hildebrandt U, Feifel G: Preoperative staging of rectal cancer by intrarectal ultrasound. Dis Colon Rectum 28:42, 1985

38. Romano G, Escercizio L, Santangelo M, et al: Impact of computed tomography vs. intrarectal ultrasound on the diagnosis, resectability, and prognosis of locally recurrent rectal cancer. Dis Colon Rectum 36:261, 1993

39. Hulsmans F, Tio TL, Fockens P, et al: Assessment of tumor infiltration depth in rectal cancer with transrectal sonography: caution is necessary. Radiology 190:715, 1994

40. Sentovitch SM, Blatchford GJ, Falk PM, et al: Transrectal ultrasound of rectal tumors. Am J Surg 166:638, 1993

41. Burnett S, Bartram C: Endosonographic variations in the normal internal anal sphincter. Int J Colorect Dis 6:2, 1991

42. Gantke B, Schafer A, Enck P, et al: Sonographic, manometric and myographic evaluation of the anal sphincter's morphology and function. Dis Colon Rectum 36:1037, 1993

43. Law PJ, Kamm MA, Bartram CI: Anal endosonography in the investigation of faecal incontinence. Br J Surg 78:312, 1991

44. Burnett S, Speakman CT, Kamm MA, et al: Confirmation of endosonographic detection of external anal sphincter defects by simultaneous electromyographic mapping. Br J Surg 78:448, 1991

45. Deen KI, Kumar D, Williams JG: Anal sphincter defects: correlation between endoanal ultrasound and surgery. Ann Surg 218:201, 1993

46. Felt-Bersma RJ, Cuesta MA, Koorevaar M: Anal endosonography: relationship with anal manometry and neurophysiologic tests. Dis Colon Rectum 37:468, 1992

47. Falk PM, Blatchford GJ, Cali RL: Transanal ultrasound and manometry in the evaluation of fecal incontinence. Dis Colon Rectum 37:468, 1994

48. Sultan AH, Kamm MA, Talbot IC: Anal endosonography for identifying external sphincter defects confirmed histologically. Br J Surg 81:463, 1994

49. Goldberg BB, Goodman GA, Clearfield HR: Evaluation of ascites by ultrasound. Radiology 96:15, 1970

50. Asher WM, Parvin S, Virgillo RW, et al: Echographic evaluation of splenic injury after blunt trauma. Radiology 118:411, 1976

51. Chambers JA, Pilbrow WJ: Ultrasound in abdominal trauma: an alternative to peritoneal lavage. Arch Emerg Med 5:26, 1988

52. Parys BT, Barr H, Chantarasak ND, et al: Use of ultrasound scan as a bedside diagnostic aid. Br J Surg 74:611, 1987

53. Peiper HJ, Schmid A, Steffens H, et al: Ultrasound diagnosis in acute abdomen and blunt abdominal trauma. Chirurg 58:189, 1987

54. Blyme PJH, Lind T, Schantz K: Ultrasonographic detection of foreign bodies in soft tissue. Arch Ortho Trauma Surg 110:24, 1990

55. Schlager D, Sanders A, Wiggins D: Ultrasound for the detection of foreign bodies. Ann Emerg Med 20:189, 1991

56. Manthey DE, Storrow AB, Milbourn JM, et al: Ultrasound versus radiography in the detection of soft-tissue foreign bodies. Ann Emerg Med 28:7, 1996

57. Williams RJ, Windsor AC, Rosin RD, et al: Ultrasound scanning of the acute abdomen by surgeons in training. Ann R Coll Surg Engl 76:228, 1994

58. Imhof M, Raunest J, Rauen U, et al: Acute acalculous cholecystitis in severely traumatized patients: a prospective sonographic study. Surg Endosc 6:68, 1992

59. Yokoyama T, Munakata Y, Ogiwara M, et al: Preoperative diagnosis of strangulated obturator hernia using ultrasonography. Am J Surg 174:76, 1997

60. Barteau JA, Castro D, Arregui ME, et al: A comparison of intraoperative ultrasound versus cholangiography in the evaluation of the common bile duct during laparoscopic cholecystectomy. Surg Endosc 9:490, 1995

61. Ravikumar TS, Kane R, Cady B: Hepatic cryosurgery with intraoperative ultrasound monitoring for metastatic colon carcinoma. Arch Surg 102:403, 1987

62. Rafaelsen SR, Kronborg O, Larsen C, et al: Intraoperative ultrasonography in detection of hepatic metastases from colorectal cancer. Dis Colon Rectum 38:355, 1995

63. Machi J, Isomoto H, Kurohiji T, et al: Detection of unrecognized liver metastases from colorectal cancers by routine use of operative ultrasonography. Dis Colon Rectum 29:405, 1986

64. Castaing D, Emond J, Kunstlinger F, et al: Utility of operative ultrasound in the surgical management of liver tumors. Ann Surg 204:600, 1986

65. Kern KA, Shawker TH, Doppman JL, et al: The use of high-resolution ultrasound to locate parathyroid tumors during reoperations for primary hyperparathyroidism. World J Surg 11:579, 1987

66. Machi J, Sigel B: Operative ultrasonography in general surgery. Am J Surg 172:15, 1996

67. Couinaud C: Le Foie, Etudes Anatomiques et Chirurgicales. Masson et Cie, Paris, 1957

68. Schirmer B: Laparoscopic ultrasonography: enhancing minimally invasive surgery. Ann Surg 220:709, 1994

69. John TG: Superior staging of liver tumors with laparoscopy and laparoscopic ultrasound. Ann Surg 220:711, 1994

70. Cook TA, Galland RB: A prospective study to define the optimum rescreening interval for small abdominal aneurysm. Cardiovasc Surg 4:441, 1996

71. Bastounis E, Georgopoulos S, Maltezos C, et al: The validity of current vascular imaging methods in the evaluation of aortic anastomotic aneurysms developing after abdominal aortic aneurysm repair. Ann Vasc Surg 10:537, 1996

72. Turetschek K, Nasel C, Wunderbaldinger P, et al: Power Doppler versus imaging in renal allograft evaluation. J Ultrasound Med 15:517, 1996

73. Wren SM, Ralls PW, Stain SC, et al: Assessment of resectability of pancreatic head and periampullary tumors by color flow Doppler sonography. Arch Surg 131:812, 1996

74. Klyachkin ML, Rohmiller M, Charash WE, et al: Penetrating injuries of the neck: selective management evolving. Am Surg 63:189, 1997

75. Ginzburg E, Montalvo B, LeBlang S, et al: The use of duplex ultrasonography in penetrating neck trauma. Arch Surg 131:691, 1996

76. Demetriades D, Theodorou D, Cornwell E, et al: Evaluation of penetrating injuries of the neck: prospective study of 223 patients. World J Surg 21:41, 1997

77. Knudson MM, Lewis FR, Atkinson K, et al: The role of duplex ultrasound arterial imaging in patients with penetrating extremity trauma. Arch Surg 128:1033, 1993

78. Bergstein JM, Blair JF, Edwards J, et al: Pitfalls in the use of color-flow duplex ultrasound for screening of suspected arterial injuries in penetrating extremities. J Trauma 33:395, 1992

79. Knudson MM, Collins JA, Goodman SB, et al: Thromboembolism following multiple trauma. J Trauma 32:2, 1992

80. Bandyk DF, Mills JL, Gahtan V, et al: Intraoperative duplex scanning of arterial reconstructions: fate of repaired and unrepaired defects. J Vasc Surg 20:426, 1994

81. Gualtieri E, Deppe SA, Sipperly ME, et al: Subclavian venous catheterization: greater success rate for less experienced operators using ultrasound guidance. Crit Care Med 23:692, 1995

82. Sisley AC, Rozycki GS, Ballard RB, et al: Rapid detection of traumatic effusion using surgeon-performed ultrasound. J Trauma 44:291, 1998

83. Kohan JM, Poe RH, Israel RH: Value of chest ultrasonography versus decubitus roentgenography for thoracentesis. Am Rev Respir Dis 133:1124, 1986

84. Rozycki GS, Ochsner MG, Jaffin JH, et al: Prospective evaluation of surgeons' use of ultrasound in the evaluation of trauma patients. J Trauma 34:516, 1993

85. Tso P, Rodriguez A, Cooper C, et al: Sonography in blunt abdominal trauma: a preliminary progress report. J Trauma 33:39, 1992

86. Rozycki GS, Ballard RB, Feliciano DV, et al: Surgeon-performed ultrasound for the assessment of truncal injuries: lessons learned from 1,540 patients. Ann Surg 228:557, 1998

87. Rozycki GS, Ochsner MG, Schmidt JA, et al: A prospective study of surgeon-performed ultrasound as the primary adjuvant modality for injured patient assessment. J Trauma 39:492, 1995

88. Boulanger BR, Brenneman FD, McLellan BA, et al: A prospective study of emergent abdominal sonography after blunt trauma. J Trauma 39:325, 1995

89. Chiu WC, Cushing BM, Rodriguez A, et al: Abdominal injuries without hemoperitoneum: a potential limitation of focused abdominal sonography for trauma (FAST). J Trauma 42:617, 1997

90. Ballard RB, Rozycki GS, Newman PG, et al: An algorithm to reduce the incidence of false-negative FAST examination in patients at high risk for occult injury. J Am Coll Surg 189:145, 1999

91. Leucht W: Analytic criteria for the interpretation of focal sonographic lesions. Teaching Atlas of Breast Ultrasound. Leucht D, Madjar H, Eds. Thieme, New York, 1996, p 23

92. Staren ED: Physics and principles of breast ultrasound. Am Surg 62:103, 1996

93. Teboul M: A new concept in breast investigation: echo-histological acino-ductal 13-analysis or analytic echography. Biomed Pharmacother 42:289, 1988

94. Khattar S, Staren ED: Diagnostic breast ultrasound. Ultrasound for the Surgeon. Staren ED, Arregui ME, Eds. Philadelphia, Lippincott-Raven, 1997, p 85

95. Staren ED: Surgical office-based ultrasound of the breast. Am Surg 61:619, 1995

96. Staren ED, Fine R: Breast ultrasound for surgeons. Am Surg 62:108, 1996

97. Hendee WR: Cross sectional medical imaging: a history. RadioGraphics 9:1155, 1989

98. White DN: Neurosonology pioneers. Ultrasound Med Biol 14:541, 1988

99. Hackmann W: Seek and Strike. Crown, United Kingdom, 1984, p xxiv

100. Hackmann W: Seek and Strike. Crown, United Kingdom, 1984, p 1

101. Hackmann W: Seek and Strike. Crown, United Kingdom, 1984, p 11

102. Hackmann W: Seek and Strike. Crown, United Kingdom, 1984, p 73

103. Meire HB: Basic Ultrasound. John Wiley & Sons, New York, 1995, p 1

104. Wells PNT: Developments in medical ultrasonics. World Med Electron 4:272, 1966

105. Wild JJ: The use of ultrasonic pulses for the measurement of biologic tissues and the detection of tissue density changes. Surgery 27:183, 1950

106. Wild JJ, Reid JM: Diagnostic use of ultrasound. British Journal of Physical Medicine 248, 1956

107. Goldberg BB, Gramiak R, Freimanis AK: Early history of diagnostic ultrasound: the role of American radiologists. AJR Am J Roentgenol 160:189, 1993

108. Maulik D: Doppler Ultrasound in Obstetrics and Gynecology. Springer, New York, 1997

109. Sanders RC, Topper IW: Equipment care and quality control. Clinical Sonography: A Practical Guide. Sanders RC, Ed. Little, Brown and Co, Boston, 1991, p 475

110. Wong WK: Endorectal ultrasonography for benign disease. Ultrasound for the Surgeon. Staren ED, Arregui ME, Eds. Lippincott-Raven, Philadelphia, 1997, p 66

111. Rozycki GS, Shackford SR: Ultrasound: what every trauma surgeon should know. J Trauma 40:1, 1996

Acknowledgments

Figures 1 and 7   Dimitry Schidlovsky.

Figures 2, 13, 14, and 17   Marcia Kammerer.

Figure 8   Tom Moore.

5 VIDEO-ASSISTED THORACIC SURGERY

Raja M. Flores, M.D., and Valerie W. Rusch, M.D.

The technique of thoracoscopy was first described in 1910 by Jacobeus, a Swedish physician who used a cystoscope to examine the pleural space.[1] Although thoracoscopy was initially performed for diagnostic purposes, it later evolved into a therapeutic procedure. During the 1930s and 1940s, it was used to lyse intrapleural adhesions after collapse therapy for tuberculosis. During the 1950s, when effective antituberculous chemotherapy became available, thoracoscopy fell into disuse in the United States[2]; however, it remained popular in Europe, where it was employed in diagnosing and treating problems such as pleural effusion, empyema, traumatic hemothorax, persistent air leak after pulmonary resection, and spontaneous pneumothorax.[3-5] During the 1970s and 1980s, a few North American surgeons revived the practice of thoracoscopy, both to manage pleural disease and to perform small peripheral lung biopsies in patients with diffuse pneumonitis.

In the first stages of its revival, thoracoscopy was often performed with open endoscopes that were originally designed for other procedures (e.g., mediastinoscopes).[6,7] As optics and lighting systems improved, smaller-caliber endoscopes were created specifically for thoracoscopic applications[8]; however, these instruments were limited in that only one person could visualize the operative field at a given time. In 1991, the application of video technology to thoracoscopy revolutionized the procedure because it allowed several persons to see the operative field simultaneously and to operate together as they would during an open procedure. In addition, the development of endoscopic instruments, particularly endoscopic staplers, enabled surgeons to perform major operations using minimally invasive techniques. The impact of this new technology was so profound that within a 2-year period, traditional thoracoscopic techniques were abandoned in favor of video-assisted thoracic surgery (VATS).[9,10] In what follows, therefore, we focus on current VATS procedures rather than traditional thoracoscopic techniques. There are numerous accepted diagnostic and therapeutic indications for VATS [*see Table 1*]. Accordingly, there are numerous operations that can be performed by VATS; we describe the most important of these, with the exception of esophageal myotomy and fundoplication, which are covered elsewhere [*see V:8 Minimally Invasive Esophageal Procedures*].

A major force driving surgeons to perform VATS procedures has been patient demand. Unfortunately, the application of VATS has not always been accompanied by careful evaluation of outcomes. Feasibility has sometimes been confused with success. Although VATS appears to have beneficial effects in terms of cosmesis and postoperative pain in the short term, it has not yet been proved to have beneficial effects on pulmonary function and return to normal activity in the long term.[11,12]

Questions remain about the oncologic soundness of some VATS procedures. It appears that levels of cytokines and other acute-phase reactants are lower with minimally invasive proce-

dures than with the corresponding open procedures[13,14]; however, it remains to be determined whether this decrease will ultimately result in decreased tumor growth or reduced recurrence rates. Rigorous evaluation in the setting of well-designed clinical trials is needed to determine how VATS may be most appropriately and safely employed, especially in cancer patients.

Table 1 Indications and Contraindications for VATS Procedures

Diagnostic indications
  Undiagnosed pleural effusion
  Indeterminate pulmonary nodule
  Undiagnosed interstitial lung disease
  Pulmonary infection in the immunosuppressed patient
  To define cell type in known thoracic malignancy
  To define extent of a primary thoracic tumor
  Nodal staging of a primary thoracic tumor
  Diagnosis of intrathoracic pathology to stage a primary extrathoracic tumor
  Evaluation of intrapleural infection

Therapeutic indications
  Lung
    Spontaneous pneumothorax
    Bullous disease
    Lung volume reduction
    Persistent parenchymal air leak
    Benign pulmonary nodule
    Resection of pulmonary metastases (in highly selected cases)
    Resection of primary lung tumor (in highly selected cases)
  Mediastinum
    Drainage of pericardial effusion
    Excision of bronchogenic or pericardial cyst
    Resection of selected primary mediastinal tumors
    Esophageal myotomy
    Facilitation of transhiatal esophagectomy
    ? Resection of primary esophageal tumors
    ? Thymic resection
    Ligation of thoracic duct
  Pleura
    Drainage of a multiloculated effusion
    Drainage of an early empyema
    Pleurodesis

Contraindications
  Extensive intrapleural adhesions
  Inability to sustain single-lung ventilation
  Extensive involvement of hilar structures
  Preoperative induction chemotherapy or chemoradiotherapy
  Severe coagulopathy

Operative Planning

PATIENT PREPARATION AND INTRAOPERATIVE CARE

Patient preparation and positioning are much the same for most VATS procedures. As a rule, the lateral decubitus position offers the best exposure, and it permits easy conversion to a thoracotomy if necessary. There are occasional exceptions to this rule, however, and in such cases the choice of position is dictated by the procedure planned. For instance, if a cervical mediastinoscopy or a Chamberlain procedure is being performed for lung cancer staging and the pleura must be examined to rule out the presence of metastases, the patient can be left in the supine position and the videothoracoscope introduced through the parasternal incision or a separate inferior incision.[15]

Port placement, the use of so-called access incisions (utility thoracotomies), and instrumentation vary from one procedure to the next. In approximately 20% of patients undergoing VATS, intraoperative conversion to a standard thoracotomy will be necessary for any of several reasons, including extensive pleural adhesions and pulmonary lesions that cannot be located thoracoscopically or require a more extensive resection than can be accomplished endosurgically. With experience, one can learn to predict the likelihood of such conversion in a given case. It is important to discuss this possibility with the patient before operation and to obtain informed consent to conversion. Any patient who is likely to require conversion to a thoracotomy or who may be undergoing lobectomy or pneumonectomy should receive the cardiopulmonary evaluation that is usual for such procedures before VATS is performed.

VATS procedures are performed with the patient under general anesthesia. Very limited operations (e.g., pleural biopsies) can be done with a single-lumen endotracheal tube in place, but most procedures should be performed with single-lung ventilation using a double-lumen endotracheal tube or a bronchial blocker. The degree of intraoperative monitoring needed depends on the extent of the planned procedure and on the patient's general medical condition. Standard monitoring techniques, including pulse oximetry, are always used, but arterial lines are placed selectively. A central venous catheter or a Swan-Ganz catheter is inserted only when the patient's baseline cardiac status demands precise hemodynamic monitoring. A Foley catheter is inserted at the beginning of all VATS procedures to monitor urine output because it is not always possible to predict how long the operation will take or whether conversion to thoracotomy will prove necessary.

INSTRUMENTATION

Instrumentation for VATS comprises (1) video equipment, (2) endoscopes and thoracoports, (3) staplers, (4) thoracic instruments (e.g., lung clamps and retractors) modified for endoscopic use, and (5) various devices for tissue cauterization, including lasers. Because immediate conversion to thoracotomy is occasionally necessary, a basic set of thoracotomy instruments should be an integral part of a VATS instrument tray.[16]

Video Equipment

Several companies manufacture excellent video equipment for thoracoscopy. Minor variations in lighting and optics aside, the basic components of all of these systems are similar: a large-screen (21 in.) video monitor, a xenon light source, a video recorder, and a printer for still photography, mounted together on a cart. A second video monitor, also mounted on a cart, is connected by cable to the main monitor and is placed across from it at the head of the operating table. By using two monitors placed in this manner, both the surgeon and the first assistant can look directly at a video display without having to turn away from the surgical field. Alternatively, a single monitor can be placed at the head of the operating table. The only additional item of equipment necessary for laparoscopy is an insufflator. To maximize cost-efficiency, therefore, hospitals acquiring video monitors and endoscopes should coordinate the choice of this expensive equipment among the specialties using it, including thoracic surgery, general surgery, gynecology, and urology. Hospitals performing many endoscopic procedures may find it advisable to dedicate one or more rooms to video endoscopic surgery and to mount video equipment on the ceilings or walls.

Endoscopes and Thoracoports

Most procedures are performed with a forward-viewing (0°) rigid scope; 30°-angled scopes are useful for visualizing the sulci and the superior and posterior mediastinum. In addition to the standard 10 mm thoracoscopes, there are now 5 mm thoracoscopes, whose resolution is nearly as good. The scope is attached to the light source by a light cable and is coupled to the video-monitor system by a camera cable [see Figure 1]. Although camera cables can be sterilized, it is best to cover the camera head and cable with a clear plastic bag so that the camera cable can remain in the OR at all times. Newer videoscopes are now available in which the camera chip is located at the tip of the scope rather than in the connecting camera cable; these will eventually replace the older endoscopes because they provide a sharper image. Flexible thoracoscopes are also available; these look like a short, heavy version of a flexible bronchoscope but have a more rigid distal end. Some surgeons feel that flexible thoracoscopes enhance their ability to visualize the entire pleural space, but these devices are very expensive and thus continue to be premium purchases for most hospitals.

0° Rigid Scope

Detachable Camera Cable

Figure 1 **Shown is a forward-viewing (0°) rigid scope that can be used for either laparoscopy or thoracoscopy. A detachable camera cable is clipped on to the eyepiece of the scope for video endoscopy. The camera cable can be sterilized or enclosed within a plastic sheath if it is used frequently.**

a

10.5mm

Thoracoscopic Port

b

Endoscopic Gastrointestinal
Anastomosis Stapler

c

Endoscopic Lung Clamp

d

Curved Sponge Stick

Figure 2 **Shown are instruments commonly used during VATS. Modified trocar cannulas, called thoracoports (*a*), facilitate access to the pleural space. They are shorter than the cannulas used in laparoscopy and
have a corkscrew configuration on the outside that maintains their position on the chest wall. The trocar is
a blunt-tipped plastic obturator that facilitates passage of the cannula through the chest wall. A thin plastic diaphragm stabilizes the position of the instruments or can be removed to facilitate access to the pleural space. Endoscopic GIA staplers that make incisions between two triple rows of staples (*b*) can be inserted through these ports. Like staplers designed for open procedures, endoscopic GIA staplers are disposable multifire instruments that hold three replacements of the staple cartridge. Another instrument that
can be inserted through these ports is the nondisposable endoscopic lung clamp (*c*), which is available in
various shapes with serrations at the end or along the full length of the clamp. Finally, the port allows
insertion of curved sponge sticks (*d*), which have been modified for endoscopic use as lung clamps or
lymph node holders.**

Originally, thoracoscopy made use of trocar cannulas designed
for laparoscopy to access the pleural space. These devices are too
long and have sharp ends that can injure the lung. Because patients
undergoing thoracoscopy are under general anesthesia and have a
double-lumen endotracheal tube in place, the cannulas need not
maintain an airtight seal, as they do in laparoscopy. Accordingly,
modified trocar cannulas called thoracoports, which are shorter
than laparoscopy cannulas and have a corkscrew configuration on
the outside that stabilizes them within the chest wall, are now routinely used. The trocar is simply a blunt-tip obturator that facilitates
passage of the cannula through the chest wall [*see Figure 2a*].
Thoracoports are available in several sizes (5, 10.5, 12.0, and 15
mm in diameter) to accommodate various instruments.

Staplers

Endoscopic staplers that cut between two simultaneously
applied triple rows of staples (gastrointestinal anastomosis [GIA]
staplers) are available in lengths of 30 and 60 mm and in staple
depths of 2.5, 3.5, and 4.8 mm [*see Figure 2b*]. Like their counterparts designed for open procedures, they are disposable mul-
ticartridge instruments. The endoscopic GIA stapler with 2.5
mm staples is designed for division of pulmonary vessels. Some
surgeons are reluctant to use it on hilar vessels because if the stapler fails mechanically (e.g., cuts without applying both staple
lines properly), life-threatening hemorrhage can ensue. Endoscopic
staplers that do not cut (transverse anastomosis [TA] staplers)
are also available. Endoscopic GIA staplers have revolutionized
surgeons' ability to perform minimally invasive pulmonary resections. These devices are highly reliable, and because they apply triple

rows of staples instead of double rows, they provide excellent
hemostasis and closure of air leaks. There are also stapler cartridges that buttress the staple line with Gore-Tex (W. L. Gore,
Boulder, Colorado) to reduce postoperative air leakage in patients with emphysematous lung tissue.

Standard stapling instruments are also used during some
VATS procedures. They are unnecessary for most pulmonary
wedge resections but may be helpful for more complex procedures, such as lobectomies. Standard GIA and roticulator TA
staplers are the most practical devices for VATS because they can
be inserted and positioned through an access incision.

Instruments

Various types of Pennington and Duval clamps are available
[*see Figure 2c*]. Sponge sticks modified by the introduction of various curves and a line of DeBakey-type teeth on the end can also
be used as lung clamps or lymph node holders [*see Figure 2d*].

Several retractors have been developed for endoscopic
surgery. One such device is a modified Finochietto retractor with
long, narrow blades, which is particularly helpful for retracting
the chest wall soft tissues in an access incision. Others are the
disposable vein retractor [*see Figure 3a*], the tip of which can be
withdrawn into the straight instrument shaft, and the fan retractor, which can be opened and closed like a fan by turning a knob
on the end of the retractor [*see Figure 3b*]. Of these, the fan
retractor is the most useful general retractor for thoracoscopic
procedures. Vein retractors are best suited for gentle retraction of
hilar or mediastinal structures (e.g., vessels, bronchi, esophagus,
or lymph nodes).

a

Disposable Vein Retractor

b

Disposable Fan Retractor

Figure 3 Shown are retractors used for VATS. Vein retractors are best suited for the gentle retraction of hilar or mediastinal structures, such as the vessels, bronchi, esophagus, and lymph nodes. The tip of the disposable vein retractor (*a*) can be extended from or withdrawn into the shaft to allow insertion of the retractor through a 12 mm port. The most useful retractor for general purposes is the fan retractor (*b*). A knob on the end of the handle opens and closes the fan, so that the retractor can be inserted through a port and opened for retraction in the pleural space.

Although biopsy forceps have been specifically created for laparoscopy and thoracoscopy, those used for mediastinoscopy are, in fact, well suited for thoracoscopy. Because laparoscopy instruments were developed before thoracoscopy instruments, many types of grasping forceps are available; however, most are too traumatizing for thoracic surgery. DeBakey forceps, modified for endoscopic use, are the gentlest type available. Various curved and right-angle dissecting clamps, needle holders, and scissors [*see Figure 4*] have been developed. In addition, standard thoracotomy instruments can be inserted through a minithoracotomy incision and used just as they would be in an open procedure.

Devices for Tissue Cauterization

Most scissors have an electrocautery attachment that permits simultaneous cutting and cauterizing. The neodymium:yttrium-aluminum-garnet (Nd:YAG) laser is sometimes applied to VATS resection of pulmonary lesions. This is done by inserting the YAG laser-fiber through angled or straight handpieces [*see Figure 5*]. Laser-assisted pulmonary resection is helpful in removing lesions on the flat surface of the lung, where a stapler cannot be easily applied.[17]

The argon beam electrocoagulator (ABC) (Birtcher Corporation, Englewood, Colorado) is a noncontact form of electrocautery that provides superb hemostasis on raw surfaces, such as denuded pulmonary parenchyma or the chest wall after pleurectomy, and helps seal air leaks from the surface of the lung.[18] The standard disposable ABC handpiece used for open procedures is narrow enough to pass through a thoracoport and thus may be used for VATS. Both the YAG laser and the ABC can be used to cauterize the pleural surface for pleurodesis and to ablate bullous disease, though neither has proved as effective as endoscopic stapling for lung volume reduction surgery (LVRS).

Instrumentation for videothoracoscopy continues to evolve, especially as minimally invasive cardiac surgical procedures become commonplace. Nevertheless, to put together the best set of instruments, it still is necessary to combine disposable and nondisposable instruments from different manufacturers and to borrow instruments originally designed for other procedures, such as mediastinoscopy and thoracotomy. Rather than create separate instrument trays for different VATS procedures, it is best to maintain a single standard tray that includes the basic instruments required for most operations and to add instruments as needed. Again, this tray should also include the instruments needed for conversion to thoracotomy.

Basic Operative Technique

VATS procedures include both true videothoracoscopies and video-assisted procedures that are really a cross between videothoracoscopies and standard thoracotomies. Because VATS procedures are still evolving, there is no firm consensus among surgeons with respect to the number, size, and location of incisions.

The basic videothoracoscopy techniques have been well described.[19] The primary strategy is to place the instruments and the thoracoscope so that all are oriented in the same direction, facing the target disease within a 180° arc [*see Figure 6*]; this posi-

a

Angled Dissecting Clamp

b

Curved Dissecting Clamp

c

Scissors

Figure 4 Various right-angle (*a*) and curved (*b*) dissecting clamps are available. On the angled model shown (*a*), the knob close to the handle rotates the shaft of the clamp 360°. Finally, many types of endoscopic scissors (*c*) are available. Some scissors incorporate an attachment for electrocautery so that the surgeon can cut and cauterize simultaneously.

YAG Laser Fiber

Angled Hand Piece

Figure 5 Shown is an angled handpiece through which an yttrium-aluminum-garnet (YAG) laser can be placed during VATS. The handpiece is narrow enough to be used during thoracoscopy as well as during open procedures.

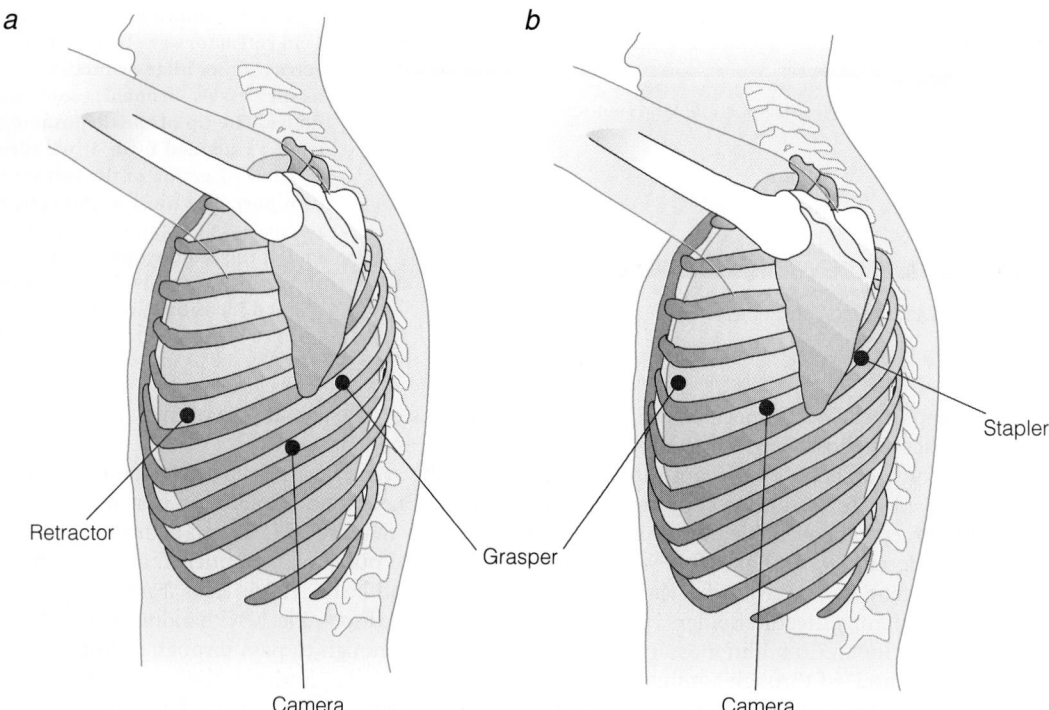

Figure 6 **Basic operative technique. Shown is the typical positioning of instruments and the video camera for patients undergoing VATS for a lesion in the superior segment of the left lower lobe of the lung. Instruments are introduced through two port incisions made anteriorly at approximately the fifth intercostal space in the anterior axillary line and posteriorly parallel to and 2 to 3 cm away from the border of the scapula (*a*). For patients undergoing thoracoscopy for apical bullous disease in the left upper lobe of the lung, the camera port can be placed at the fifth or sixth intercostal space, and one instrument port can be inserted in the axilla and the other port inserted higher on the posterior chest wall at approximately the third intercostal space (*b*).**

tioning prevents mirror imaging. The incisions should also be placed widely distant from each other so that the instruments do not crowd one another.

For most procedures [*see Figure 6a*], the videothoracoscope is inserted through a thoracoport placed in the midaxillary line at the seventh or eighth intercostal space. Instruments are introduced through two thoracoports, one placed at approximately the fifth intercostal space in the anterior axillary line, and the other placed at the fifth space, parallel to and about 2 to 3 cm away from the posterior border of the scapula. If the procedure is converted to a thoracotomy, the two upper incisions can be incorporated into the thoracotomy incision, and the lower incision can be used as a chest tube site. When a patient is being operated upon for an apical lesion (e.g., bullae causing a spontaneous pneumothorax) [*see Figure 6b*], the camera port can be placed at the fifth or sixth intercostal space, and the instrument ports are also moved higher: one in the axilla and the other higher on the posterior chest wall at approximately the third intercostal space. Depending on the location of the lesion being removed, a fourth port incision may be helpful to permit the introduction of additional instruments.

When the lung has to be palpated so that a small or deep-seated lesion can be located or when complex video-assisted procedures are being performed, a small (about 5 cm) intercostal incision is added to the three port incisions. This utility thoracotomy, or access incision, is usually placed in the midaxillary line or in the auscultatory triangle. An infant Finochietto retractor or a

Weitlaner retractor is used to retract the soft tissues without actually spreading the ribs [*see Figure 7*].

These basic concepts regarding incision placement are modified as necessary to accommodate the procedure being performed and the location of the lesion being removed (see below).

VATS Procedures for Pleural Disease

OPERATIVE TECHNIQUE

A double-lumen endotracheal tube is inserted, and the patient is placed in the lateral decubitus position. Two 1.5 cm incisions are made, one for the videothoracoscope and one for the instruments. The videothoracoscope is inserted through a 10.5 mm thoracoport at the seventh or eighth intercostal space in the midaxillary line; the instruments are inserted through a port placed a couple of interspaces higher in the anterior axillary line. If a talc poudrage is performed, both incisions are reused for placement of chest tubes, with a right-angle tube inserted on the diaphragm through the lower incision and a straight tube up to the apex of the pleural space through the upper incision. The addition of a diaphragmatic chest tube helps prevent loculated basilar fluid collections after a talc pleurodesis. If a thoracotomy is subsequently performed, the upper port site is incorporated into the anterior aspect of the incision, and the lower site can be reused as a chest tube site. Proper placement of port incisions is especially important in patients with suspected malignant

Figure 7 **Basic operative technique. Shown are the incisions used for common VATS procedures. The thoracoscope is inserted through the bottom incision. Anterior and posterior incisions are used for the introduction of instruments. Only one additional low anterior incision (arrow) is needed for thoracoscopic pleural procedures. A so-called utility thoracotomy (dotted line) can be added at the fifth intercostal space, if necessary. The tip of the scapula is outlined. These incisions can be incorporated into a standard thoracotomy incision if the VATS procedure is converted to an open procedure.**

mesothelioma because of the propensity of this tumor to implant in incisions and needle tracks.[8,20,21]

Once the videothoracoscope has been inserted, pleural biopsies are obtained under direct vision by introducing a biopsy forceps through a port placed in the upper incision. The mediastinoscopy biopsy forceps is well suited to this task. Pleural fluid is evacuated with a Yankauer or pool-tip suction device. Fibrinous debris can be removed by irrigating the pleural space with a pulsating water jet lavage device (e.g., Water-Pik, Orthotec, Stryker, Kalamazoo, Michigan) designed for debridement of orthopedic wounds. This technique is particularly useful for the debridement and drainage of loculated fibrinopurulent empyemas.[22] At the end of the procedure, intercostal blocks are performed by using a mediastinoscopy aspiration needle, and talc can be insufflated for pleurodesis, if indicated. All of these instruments are introduced sequentially through the upper incision.[23]

An alternative approach is to make a single incision in the midaxillary line at the sixth or seventh intercostal space and to use an operating thoracoscope that incorporates a biopsy forceps. This approach has the advantage of requiring only one incision; however, it does not allow as much latitude in draining or debriding the pleural space. Moreover, the biopsy forceps in an operating thoracoscope is of a smaller caliber than a mediastinoscopy biopsy forceps and thus cannot obtain as large a biopsy specimen.

TROUBLESHOOTING

In patients with loculated effusion, thoracoport placement sometimes must be modified. The preoperative chest computed tomographic scan and chest x-ray should help ensure that the ports are placed in areas when the lung is not adherent to the chest wall.

In some cases, the pleural space is obliterated by adhesions or tumor. This event occurs most frequently in patients who have had severe inflammatory disease (e.g., pneumonia, empyema, or tuberculosis) or extensive pleural malignancy (e.g., locally advanced malignant mesothelioma). In these circumstances, the anterior thoracoport incision can be extended to a length of 5 to 6 cm, the underlying rib section can be resected, and the parietal pleura can be biopsied directly; a full thoracotomy is not required. If thoracotomy is subsequently warranted for therapeutic reasons (e.g, for pleurectomy, decortication, or extrapleural pneumonectomy for mesothelioma), this small incision can be incorporated into the thoracotomy incision.

VATS Pulmonary Wedge Resection

VATS pulmonary wedge resection has become a standard approach to diagnosing small indeterminate pulmonary nodules, especially those not technically amenable to transthoracic needle biopsy.[24,25] It is also an accepted method of diagnosing pulmonary infiltrates of uncertain origin, particularly in immunocompromised patients in whom transbronchial biopsy is either unsafe or inappropriate.[26,27]

The role of VATS wedge resection is less well defined in the management of primary lung cancers. It is an appropriate compromise operation for primary lung cancers in patients whose cardiac or pulmonary function status rules out lobectomy. However, it remains a highly controversial approach to the treatment of pulmonary metastases.[28] In an often-quoted 1993 study,[29] patients with CT-documented pulmonary metastases underwent first thoracoscopic resection and then thoracotomy in the same setting. Many additional lesions, both benign and malignant, were found at thoracotomy that were missed by VATS. The study was terminated early because of the failure of thoracoscopy to identify these lesions. One criticism of the study is that the preoperative CT scans were not comparable to the spiral, or helical, CT scans currently available and therefore probably missed many pulmonary nodules that modern scanning methods would have caught.

A 2000 multicenter study of patients undergoing VATS metastasectomy for colon cancer suggested that minimal residual disease not identified by helical CT and not resected by VATS may not affect survival significantly[30]; however, this conclusion is completely at odds with all of the previously published surgical literature on pulmonary metastasectomy. Improved survival in patients with pulmonary metastases appears to be directly linked to the ability to remove all gross tumor, and VATS does not allow the careful bimanual palpation that is critical to detecting pulmonary metastases that are too small or too deep to be visible endoscopically.[29,31,32] Accordingly, most centers reserve VATS for the diagnosis rather than the treatment of pulmonary metastases. Until a well-designed prospective, randomized trial is conducted with survival as an end point, the standard of care remains thoracotomy and metastasectomy.

Anecdotal reports of port-site recurrence have also raised concerns about VATS as a treatment method in patients with malignancies; however, a 2001 study of 410 patients from a prospective VATS database at the Memorial Sloan-Kettering Cancer

Center (MSKCC) found only one case of port-site recurrence.[33] The authors concluded that the incidence of such recurrences can be kept low if surgical oncologic principles are respected. At MSKCC, these principles include (1) reserving VATS for lesions that can be widely excised, (2) conversion to an open thoracotomy for definitive or extensive operations, and (3) meticulous technique for extraction of specimens from the pleural space, with small specimens removed directly through a thoracoport and larger specimens through specimen bags.

OPERATIVE TECHNIQUE

Once general anesthesia has been induced and a double-lumen endotracheal tube inserted, the patient is placed in the full lateral decubitus position. It is important to stop ventilation to the lung being operated on as soon as the patient is rotated into the lateral decubitus position, so that the lung will be thoroughly collapsed by the time the videothoracoscope is inserted into the pleural space. Small subpleural pulmonary nodules are most easily identified in a fully atelectatic lung because they protrude

Figure 8 **VATS pulmonary wedge resection. A double-lumen endotracheal tube is used to render the lung partially atelectatic. The pulmonary nodule is lifted upward with a lung clamp, and the endoscopic GIA stapler is applied to the lung underneath (top). During the wedge resection, the lung clamp and the endoscopic GIA stapler are alternately inserted through opposite ports to obtain the correct angle for performance of the wedge resection (bottom).**

from the surrounding collapsed pulmonary parenchyma, which is softer.[19,20] Most pulmonary wedge resections are performed as true videothoracoscopic procedures using just three port incisions placed in the triangulated manner already described [*see* Basic Operative Technique, *above*]. The pulmonary nodules to be removed are grasped with an endoscopic lung clamp (Pennington or Duval) inserted through one instrument port, and wedge resection is done with repeated applications of an endoscopic stapler inserted through the opposite port.[24,34] As the resection is performed, it is often helpful to introduce the stapler through each of two instrument ports to obtain the correct angle for application to the lung [*see Figure 8*]. To prevent tumor implantation in the chest wall, small specimens (usually those resected with three or fewer stapler applications) are removed via the thoracoport. Larger specimens are placed in a disposable plastic specimen retrieval bag, which is then brought out through a very slightly enlarged anterior thoracoport incision.

When the wedge resections have been completed, intercostal blocks are performed under direct vision via the mediastinoscopy aspiration needle, and a single chest tube is inserted through the inferior port after the videothoracoscope is withdrawn.[35] The videothoracoscope can be placed through the anterior incision to check the position of the chest tube and confirm reinflation of the lung after the double-lumen endotracheal tube is unclamped. The remaining incisions are then closed with sutures.

TROUBLESHOOTING

Four techniques can be used to locate pulmonary nodules that are either too deep or too small to be easily visible on simple inspection of the lung. All of these should be used in conjunction with a high-quality preoperative chest CT scan to identify the lung segment in which the nodule is located. First, an endoscopic lung clamp can be gently run across the surface of the lung as an extension of digital palpation.[20,36] With some patience and experience, one can achieve considerable success with this technique. Second, ultrasonographic examination of the collapsed lung can also locate deep pulmonary nodules; at present, however, experience with this approach remains very limited.[37] Third, CT-guided needle localization can be used preoperatively if a nodule is likely to be difficult to locate. Localization is accomplished by injecting methylene blue or by inserting a barbed mammography localization needle, which is then cut off at the skin exit site and later retrieved thoracoscopically.[38] Needle localization techniques are effective, but they are also costly and time-consuming and hence not used by most surgeons. Finally, if careful endoscopic examination of the lung does not reveal the location of a nodule, an access incision is added to the videothoracoscopy.[24,39] Each lobe of the lung is sequentially rotated up to this non–rib-spreading utility thoracotomy for direct digital palpation. This technique almost always allows identification of a nodule when other techniques fail. As the endoscopist gains experience with these techniques, conversion to thoracotomy just for the purpose of locating a pulmonary nodule is rarely necessary.[40]

Pulmonary nodules located on the broad surface of the lung may not be amenable to a wedge resection with an endoscopic stapler. Such nodules can be removed by means of electrocauterization, just as in an open thoracotomy. An extension is placed on the handle of the electrocautery, which is then introduced into the pleural space through either a port or an access incision. Another approach is to resect the pulmonary nodule with a laser in either a contact or a noncontact mode. The potassium-titanyl-phosphate

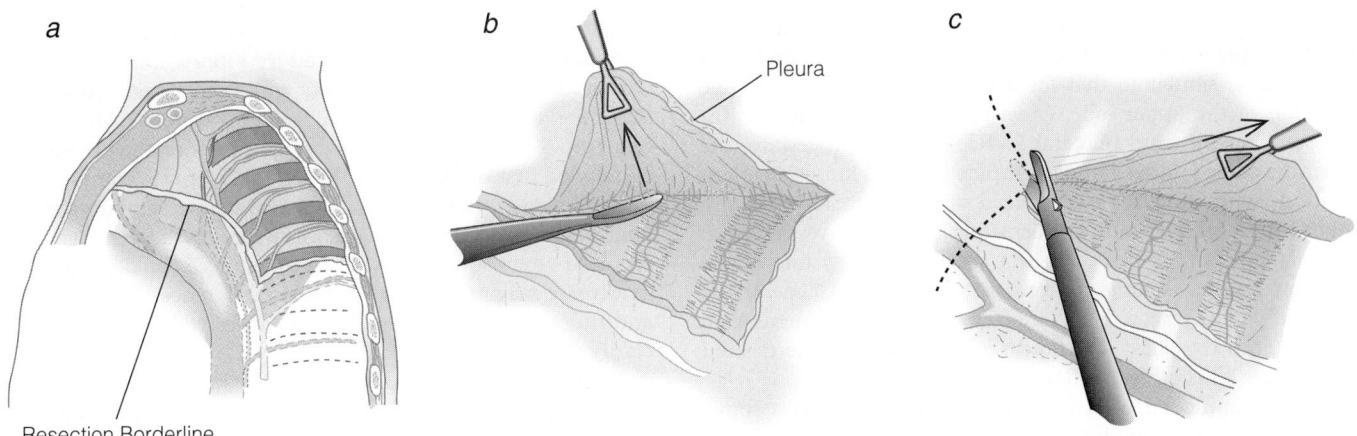

a

Resection Borderline

b

Pleura

c

Figure 9 VATS procedures for spontaneous pneumothorax and bullous disease. Limited apical pleurectomy is a useful alternative to chemical pleurodesis in young patients with spontaneous pneumothorax because these patients may need to undergo thoracotomy later in life. Shown is an outline of the pleural resection (*a*) performed in this procedure. The pleura is grasped at the inferior border with forceps and lifted in the avascular layer in a cranial or ventral direction (*b*). A T-shaped incision is made in the pleura at the level of the subclavian artery or the truncus brachiocephalicus. The dissection of the pleural flap thus created is extended in either the ventral or the parasternal direction and in either the apical or the mediastinal direction (*c*).

(KTP)/YAG laser is particularly suited to this task because it is capable of both cutting and coagulation. To minimize bleeding and air leakage, raw pulmonary surfaces can be cauterized with either the Nd:YAG laser or the ABC.[17] Numerous types of absorbable sealant patches or materials are also available to control air leaks from areas of raw pulmonary parenchyma.

Occasionally, after a wedge resection, it is necessary to suture together the pleural edges over an area of raw pulmonary parenchyma. The suturing can be done directly through a non–rib-spreading minithoracotomy incision or through port sites. In the latter case, the ports are removed, and a 3-0 Prolene suture is passed through the anterior port site with a standard needle holder. A second needle holder is introduced via the posterior port site and used in place of a forceps to pick up and reposition the needle as it is passed through the lung. The surgeon and the first assistant work together to oversew the lung, in contrast with the normal practice for an open procedure, in which the surgeon uses a needle holder and a forceps to place the sutures.

VATS Procedures for Spontaneous Pneumothorax and Bullous Disease

OPERATIVE TECHNIQUE

VATS is now frequently performed for the management of recurrent spontaneous pneumothorax and for bullous disease.[41,42] The approach is similar to that followed in a wedge resection. Three or four port sites are used. The videothoracoscope is inserted at the fifth intercostal space in the midaxillary line. Two other port sites are added at the fourth intercostal space in the anterior and posterior axillary lines.

In patients with spontaneous pneumothorax, the responsible bulla (which is usually apical in location) is identified, and wedge resection is done with an endoscopic stapler.[43,44] Bullae can be excised by applying the stapler across the base of the area of bullous disease. They can also be ablated with the ABC or the Nd:YAG laser, then suture-plicated if necessary; however, this approach may not be as successful over the long term.[45,46]

Some surgeons, noting the lower rate of recurrence, the short-

er hospital stay, and the relative cost-effectiveness, advocate performing VATS for the first episode of spontaneous pneumothorax.[47,48] To justify this approach in patients with primary spontaneous pneumothorax, however, well-designed clinical trials rather than retrospective reviews will be required.

TROUBLESHOOTING

The placement of port incisions should be determined by the location of the bullae. Because bullous disease is generally apical, port sites are correspondingly higher than for the average wedge resection (i.e., at the fourth and sixth intercostal spaces rather than at the fifth or sixth and eighth spaces). The precise placement should, however, be determined by pinpointing the disease site or sites on the preoperative chest x-ray and CT scans.

The main problem after resection for bullous disease is prolonged leakage of air from the staple line. This problem can be minimized by applying commercially available sleeves made of bovine pericardium or Gore-Tex over the arms of the stapler to reinforce the staple line and by performing some form of pleurodesis. Mechanical pleurodesis is done with a small gauze sponge passed through a port site. Some surgeons scarify the pleura by cauterizing it with the ABC or the Nd:YAG laser, but this is not as successful as a mechanical pleurodesis. Chemical pleurodesis by talc poudrage is an appropriate option for older patients with emphysema and bullous disease but is unwise in young patients with spontaneous pneumothorax, who might require a thoracotomy later in life.[49] Another option in younger patients is a limited apical pleurectomy [*see Figure 9*]. Special angulated instruments and blunt dissectors have been designed for this procedure; however, a parietal pleurectomy is also easily performed with combinations of standard blunt and sharp instruments.[50]

VATS Lung Volume Reduction Surgery

OPERATIVE TECHNIQUE

VATS may also be applied to the performance of LVRS. Many candidates for LVRS are receiving steroids and thus are at risk for sternal wound infection; the thoracoscopic approach reduces this risk substantially. If unilateral LVRS is planned, the patient is placed in the lateral decubitus position, and port placement is similar to that for a patient undergoing a wedge resection of the upper lobe. Most patients undergoing LVRS, however, benefit from bilateral LVRS. For this procedure, the patient is placed in the standard supine bilateral lung transplant position, with shoulder rolls placed vertically in an I fashion behind the back and with the arms positioned above the head. The camera port is placed in the anterior axillary line at the sixth interspace. A lung compression clamp is placed on the area that will be resected. A Gore-Tex–reinforced stapler is then inserted into the chest and fired sequentially until the desired area is excised [see Figure 10a].

Another approach used to help buttress the tenuous staple line in emphysematous lung tissue is lung plication [see Figure 10b].[51] In this method, the defunctionalized, bullous lung tissue is stapled to itself to form a plicated autologous buttress [see Figure 11]. Because the diseased bullous lung is not cut, the risk of postoperative air leakage is minimized.

TROUBLESHOOTING

A major cause of morbidity and mortality with this procedure is the occurrence of air leaks, which sometimes are large enough to compromise ventilation significantly. Thus, once LVRS has been done on one side, the lung is reexpanded and any air leaks carefully assessed. If the leak is small, the other side is operated on in the same setting; if the leak is large, the contralateral procedure is put off to a later date. The use of fibrin glue or another commercially available pneumostatic sealant along the staple line should be considered to minimize postoperative air leakage.

VATS Lobectomy and Pneumonectomy

Although VATS lobectomy is much less frequently performed than VATS pulmonary wedge resection, standard techniques have been developed for it.[52] VATS pneumonectomy, on the other hand, is less well accepted. Both operations are done as video-assisted procedures using a utility thoracotomy, which facilitates the insertion of standard thoracotomy instruments, the extraction of the resected specimen from the pleural space, and the performance of the technically complex aspects of the procedure, including dissection of the hilar vessels and of the mediastinal lymph nodes.

A 1998 retrospective study addressing the adequacy of VATS lobectomy as an oncologic procedure reported on 298 patients who underwent VATS lobectomy with mediastinal lymph node dissection for primary non–small cell lung cancer.[53] On the basis of a 70% 4-year survival rate for stage I tumors, the investigators concluded that outcome after VATS lobectomy is comparable to that after open thoracotomy. At 5 years, however, survival rates after VATS are inferior, stage for stage, to the rates generally reported after thoracotomy. Such differences could reflect either inaccurate staging or true oncologic differences between VATS and thoracotomy; additional prospective studies are needed to clarify these issues.

Although VATS lobectomy has not been proved to be an oncologically sound procedure in the long term, there is good evidence that it is safe in acute settings.[54] Therefore, it should certainly be performed to treat benign diseases (e.g., bronchiectasis).[55] As with all minimally invasive procedures, conversion to open thoracotomy is indicated if technical issues require it. Some authors advocate VATS lobectomy for low-grade malignancies (e.g., carcinoids) as well.[56] It must be recognized, however, that although carcinoids have a lower malignant potential than non–small cell lung cancer, they are still malignancies and must be treated appropriately for optimal long-term outcome.

Two approaches to lobectomy have been developed. One involves sequential anatomic ligation of the hilar structures, much as in a standard lobectomy,[57,58] and the other involves mass ligation of the pulmonary vessels and the bronchus. Both approaches require at least two port incisions in addition to the utility thoracotomy. The sequential anatomic ligation approach has been well described.[57]

OPERATIVE TECHNIQUE

Lobectomy

Right-side resections The specific operative approach taken in performing a VATS lobectomy may vary depending on the patient's body habitus and the intraoperative pathology. In our view, however, it is generally the safest strategy to leave the bronchial resection until last, regardless of which lobe is to be resected. When the bronchus is transected first, it may be difficult to gauge the amount of traction placed on the hilum, and accidental traction injury to the pulmonary artery may result in significant hemorrhage.

a

b

Figure 10 **VATS lung volume reduction surgery. Thoracoscopic lung volume reduction can be accomplished through either (*a*) resection or (*b*) plication without cutting.**

Figure 11 VATS lung volume reduction surgery. Shown are the key steps in the plication method of LVRS. (*a*) The apex of the lung area selected for plication is drawn to one side over a lung plication clamp, and the retractable guidebar of the clamp is extended into position. (*b*) The clamp is rotated 180° to fold the lung over itself. (*c*) The guidebar is retracted, a stapler is positioned with its jaws around the folded lung (but not yet closed), and the plication clamp is removed. (*d*) Shown is a cross-section of the folded lung after the stapler has been positioned but before the clamp has been removed. The stapler is then fired to complete the plication.

The first step is to place a camera port at the sixth or seventh interspace between the anterior axillary line and the midaxillary line. Once the camera is inserted and the lung and the pleura have been thoroughly examined for metastatic disease, the access incision is placed under thoracoscopic guidance directly over the interspace that gives the best exposure to the pulmonary hilum; usually the best location is at the fifth interspace in the anterior axillary line. A second thoracoport is placed at the same interspace as the camera port, usually several inches posteriorly but in some cases (depending on patient anatomy) anteriorly. The inferior pulmonary ligament is then divided. A finger is placed through the utility thoracotomy, and an empty sponge stick is placed through the lower thoracoport, thereby allowing digital palpation of the entire lung.

If no other lesions have been identified, the posterior mediastinal pleura is opened to expose the subcarinal (level 7) lymph nodes and the bifurcation of the mainstem bronchus. This maneuver facilitates subsequent division of the major fissure.

The right pulmonary artery is then identified within the fissure by meticulous dissection through the utility thoracotomy. Even when the fissure is incomplete, careful use of the electrocautery can keep bleeding to a minimum. The technique used for dissection of the pulmonary artery in VATS is exactly the same as that in a thoracotomy. The key structures to identify within the fissure are the right pulmonary artery trunk, the right middle lobe artery, the apical posterior segmental artery to the right upper lobe (the recurrent artery), and the artery to the superior segment of the lower lobe. Once these structures have been identified, the various lobes are resected as follows.

Right upper lobe. The superior pulmonary vein is dissected via the access incision in the same manner as in an open lobectomy. The vein is then encircled with a silk tie, and a No. 10 red rubber catheter is placed behind it, with its open end at the inferior portion of the vein. An endovascular stapler is placed via one of the lower thoracoports; to provide the optimal angle for directing the stapler behind the vein, the camera may have to be switched to the posterior port. Once the stapler is inside the chest, it is positioned via the utility thoracotomy so that its open jaw is in the opening of the red rubber catheter. The catheter is then pulled to lead the stapler safely behind the pulmonary vein. Once the stapler is behind the vein, the catheter is removed via the access incision with a DeBakey forceps and the stapler is fired, thereby transecting the superior pulmonary vein.

Once the pulmonary vein has been divided, the pulmonary artery behind the divided vein is dissected, with the middle lobe retracted laterally and posteriorly until the right middle lobe artery is visualized. A tape is then placed around the fissure, just above the right middle lobe artery, and pulled through one of the lower thoracoports. The middle lobe is pulled up to the lateral chest wall with a lung clamp. With the middle lobe vein used as a guide, the minor fissure is completed with an endoscopic GIA stapler. The middle lobe is then moved anteriorly and the lower lobe retracted inferiorly so that a Harken clamp can be placed between the superior segmental artery to the right lower lobe and the recurrent branch to the right upper lobe; the clamp should be aimed toward the area at the bifurcation of the right upper lobe and the bronchus intermedius posteriorly. It may be useful to retract the entire lung anteriorly and dissect this area posteriorly with a peanut sponge to allow better visualization of the bronchial bifurcation. A tape is then passed around the fissure, and an endoscopic GIA stapler is used to complete the fissure.

Once the entire fissure is complete, the recurrent branch is further dissected and stapled with an endovascular stapler passed through the lower anterior port. If it is difficult to place the stapler behind the artery, a red rubber catheter may be used to guide the stapler behind it. The right upper lobe is retracted laterally, and the endovascular stapler is placed via the inferior anterior port and used to divide the truncus anterior. At this point, the only structure remaining to be addressed is the right upper lobe bronchus. This structure is freed of all peribronchial nodal tissue by means of sharp and blunt dissection via the access incision and transected with an endoscopic stapler inserted through the lower anterior port. The specimen is placed in a specimen bag and removed via the access incision, and level 4 and level 7 nodes are either sampled or dissected.

Right lower lobe. Once the right middle lobe artery has been identified, the right lower lobe is retracted posteriorly and laterally to expose the superior aspect of the inferior pulmonary vein. Blunt dissection with a peanut sponge is used to clear the perivascular tissue by pushing up on the lung just superior to the inferior pulmonary vein. A Harken clamp is then placed through the utility thoracotomy, starting at the inferior border of the right middle lobe artery and extending to the area just above the lower lobe vein. The fissure is encircled with a tape and divided with an endoscopic GIA stapler. The lower lobe is retracted via the utility thoracotomy, and an endovascular stapler placed via the lower anterior port is used to transect the vein; the artery is then divided through the same port. Sometimes, the basilar segmental pulmonary artery and the superior segmental artery must be taken separately. The posterior aspect of the major fissure is then completed, and the lower lobe bronchus is transected last.

Right middle lobe. The fissures are completed essentially as already described (see above), with several modifications. The anterior aspect of the major fissure is completed first, as in a lower lobectomy. Next, the middle lobe vein is transected with an endovascular stapler inserted through the inferior thoracoport. The right middle artery is transected from below as well. A peanut sponge is then used to free the superior portion of the right middle lobe bronchus. With the superior pulmonary vein as a guide, the minor fissure is completed, separating the upper and middle lobes. Finally, the bronchus is divided.

Left-side resections   The left side is approached somewhat differently. The initial placement of the camera port should be in the midaxillary line because the apex of the heart prevents good visualization if the camera is inserted in the anterior axillary line. The pulmonary artery is usually easier to identify on the left side than on the right. The lung is retracted anteriorly, and the posterior mediastinal pleura is opened to expose the left main pulmonary artery, the subcarinal space, and the inferior pulmonary vein. The left pulmonary artery, the superior segmental artery to the left lower lobe, and the lingular artery should be clearly identified. The lung is retracted posteriorly, and the bronchial bifurcation between the superior and inferior pulmonary veins is clearly identified by means of sharp and blunt dissection. Once this identification has been made, the fissure between the lingula and the lower lobe is divided with an endoscopic GIA stapler.

Left upper lobe. The fissure having been completed, the superior pulmonary vein is transected. The lingular branches are then transected, usually via the inferior midaxillary port, and the apicoposterior branches of the pulmonary artery are transected via the posterior port, with the camera placed through the utility thoracotomy. The anterior segmental branch of the pulmonary artery may be transected either via the utility thoracotomy or via an extra posterior port placed in the line of the thoracotomy. The bronchus is divided last.

Left lower lobe. The fissure having been completed, the inferior pulmonary vein is transected via either the utility thoracotomy or the most posterior port incision. The lower lobe pulmonary artery is transected via the utility thoracotomy, with the end of the stapler visualized via a lower thoracoport. The bronchus is divided last. Again, a No. 10 red rubber catheter can facilitate passage of endovascular staplers around the vessels.

Mass ligation   The mass ligation approach, or so-called SIS (simultaneous individual stapling) lobectomy, has its advocates as well.[59] Four incisions are made: an incision for the camera port at the seventh intercostal space, a 2 cm incision in the midaxillary line at the sixth intercostal space for the insertion of staplers, and two 3 cm incisions at the fourth intercostal space in the anterior and posterior axillary lines for the insertion of additional instruments. In the initial report of this technique, the bronchus and the pulmonary vessels were ligated separately, but the vessels were stapled en masse.[60] Subsequently, the technique was refined so that the bronchus and the vessels were stapled simultaneously by applying the stapler twice, the first time loosely to obtain closure of the bronchus and the second time more tightly to obtain hemostatic closure of the vessels. Although the early results were satisfactory,[61] concern about the long-term risks of bronchovascular or arteriovenous fistula formation resulting from mass ligation of the hilar structures has prevented universal acceptance of this approach.

Pneumonectomy

A similar approach has been used for VATS pneumonectomy. The thoracoscope is inserted at the seventh intercostal space in the midaxillary line, and a utility thoracotomy is performed at the fourth intercostal space in the same line. Two port sites are then created at the sixth intercostal space in the anterior and posterior axillary lines. The hilar vessels are sequentially isolated, ligated, and divided with endoscopic or standard staplers. The inferior pulmonary vein is done first, followed by the superior pulmonary vein and the pulmonary artery. The bronchus is stapled and divided last.[62,63]

TROUBLESHOOTING

The endoscopic GIA stapler should never be used to divide the hilar vessels: if it fails to fire staples properly, the vessels retract into the pericardium, causing exsanguinating hemorrhage. The hilar vessels can be ligated proximally with a TA stapler, then ligated and divided distally with an endoscopic GIA stapler; alternatively, they can be divided with the scissors after two TA staple rows have been applied. Another option is to doubly ligate or suture-ligate the vessels via the utility thoracotomy, just as is traditionally done during an open procedure.

Most of the reported VATS lobectomies have been performed in patients with stage I lung cancer. If the tumor is invading the chest wall or the mediastinum or if the resection is being performed after induction chemotherapy or chemoradiotherapy,

VATS is inappropriate because it does not provide adequate exposure for complex resections, particularly when significant perihilar fibrosis is present. Since a randomized trial comparing VATS lobectomy to lobectomy performed through a standard muscle-sparing thoracotomy incision failed to show any significant difference between the two with respect to hospital stay or perioperative morbidity, enthusiasm for VATS lobectomy has diminished.[64-66] It is never wise to compromise the quality of a cancer resection for the perceived benefits of a shorter hospital stay or less pain.

Proper specimen extraction is critical. Tumor implantation in the chest wall is now a recognized complication of VATS procedures. Steps should be taken to prevent intrapleural fragmentation of the tumor, and all specimens should be carefully placed in a plastic bag before being withdrawn through the utility thoracotomy incision or a port site.[67,68]

VATS Mediastinal Lymph Node Dissection

OPERATIVE TECHNIQUE

VATS mediastinal lymph node dissection (MLND) can be performed as an alternative to a Chamberlain procedure for biopsy of the aortopulmonary window nodes or anterior mediastinal masses and is thought by some surgeons to provide better exposure and a superior cosmetic result.[69] The thoracoscope is inserted at the fifth or sixth intercostal space in the posterior axillary line. Instruments for retracting the lung inferiorly are introduced via a port at the seventh intercostal space in the midaxillary line. Instruments for dissecting nodes are introduced through ports placed at the fourth intercostal space in the anterior axillary line and in the auscultatory triangle. The lymph nodes are dissected free with graspers, scissors, the electrocautery, and endoscopic hemostatic clips. Curved sponge sticks are ideal lymph node graspers. A similar approach can be used for biopsy of other mediastinal nodes, including the paratracheal and periesophageal nodes. This method has become an accepted approach to the surgical staging of esophageal cancer.[70,71] It is harder to do a complete en bloc subcarinal lymph node dissection, though nodal sampling of this region by VATS is certainly feasible, especially when an access incision is used.

TROUBLESHOOTING

Care should be taken not to injure the phrenic nerve as it courses along the superior vena cava on the right and across the anterior aspect of the aortopulmonary window on the left. The vagus nerve should be visualized, and the origin of the recurrent laryngeal nerve should be avoided during dissection. The recurrent laryngeal nerve is easily injured on the left side, where it passes around the ligamentum arteriosium before traveling under the aortic arch; however, it can also be injured on the right side if MLND is carried too high superiorly along the origin of the innominate artery.

It is unwise to perform a VATS MLND after induction chemotherapy or chemoradiotherapy because the lymph nodes are often densely adherent to surrounding structures. This is especially true on the right side, where the superior mediastinal lymph nodes are usually densely adherent to the superior vena cava, the azygos vein, and the right main pulmonary artery. A thoracotomy, with extensive exposure and sharp dissection, is usually required for a safe and complete MLND.

All lymphatic branches should be ligated during node biopsy or dissection to prevent leakage of chyle. Often, there are large lymphatic branches in the distal right paratracheal area. The thoracic duct can be injured if periesophageal or posterior mediastinal lymph nodes are being removed.

VATS Esophagectomy

OPERATIVE TECHNIQUE

To date, surgeons' experience with thoracoscopic esophageal resection has been limited. VATS esophagectomy can take either a transhiatal or a transthoracic approach.

Transhiatal Approach

The technique for VATS transhiatal esophagectomy[72] is a modification of the open technique advocated by Orringer[73] [see V:7 Open Esophageal Procedures] and allows the esophagectomy to be performed completely under direct vision with the help of a specially designed operating mediastinoscope. This instrument has a partially concave olive tip that distracts the mediastinal tissues away from the mediastinoscope and cradles the esophagus in a stable position during the dissection. The mediastinoscope incorporates an optical system, an irrigation canal, and an operating channel for insertion of scissors, suction devices, and monopolar and bipolar cautery forceps.

The mediastinoscope is introduced through the neck incision used to expose the cervical esophagus after the stomach and the distal esophagus have been mobilized via a laparotomy. The thoracic esophagus is circumferentially freed from the surrounding mediastinal structures, beginning at the thoracic inlet and moving inferiorly to the hiatus, primarily by means of blunt dissection with the suction device. Vessels are cauterized or clipped. Dissection is performed first along the posterior wall of the esophagus, then along both lateral walls, and finally on the anterior surface of the esophagus. At the level of the primary tumor, periesophageal soft tissues are resected en bloc to ensure complete removal of the cancer.

When the esophagus has been fully mobilized down to the diaphragmatic hiatus, a plastic tube is passed into the hiatus, where it is grasped by the mediastinoscope. Both the mediastinoscope and the plastic tube are then withdrawn to the cervical incision. The cervical esophagus is transected at the sternal notch with the GIA stapler, and the plastic tube is sutured to the distal end of the divided esophagus. The tube is then gently pulled back down to the diaphragmatic hiatus, and in the process, the thoracic esophagus is folded onto itself. The mediastinoscope is reintroduced and used to follow the esophagus as it is removed from the mediastinum. Any undivided vessels or lymphatics are easily visualized and are either ligated or cauterized. After the esophagus is extracted, the stomach is passed up to the neck via the posterior mediastinum, and the esophagogastric anastomosis is performed in the standard manner for a transhiatal esophagectomy [see Figure 12].

Transthoracic Approach

The transthoracic thoracoscopic technique for esophagectomy has been described by several authors.[74-76] One group has refined a clinical VATS technique that is based on results from animal studies.[77] A double-lumen endotracheal tube is inserted, the patient is placed in the left lateral decubitus position, and six thoracoports are placed [see Figure 13]. The soft tissue is dissected with endoscopic instruments, including a 10 mm scissors, 5 mm grasping forceps, and a cherry dissector. The mediastinal pleura is opened widely, and the anterior edge is retracted with two stay

a

Mediastinoscope

Optic

Rinsing Canal

Esophagus

Distal Dilating Olive

Dissecting Scissors

b

c

d

Figure 12　VATS esophagectomy. In the transhiatal approach, a specially designed operating mediastinoscope with an olive-shaped tip (*a*) is used. This tip mechanically distracts the mediastinal tissues away from the mediastinoscope and keeps the esophagus in a stable position during dissection. The scope is shown cradling the esophagus with the dissecting scissors inserted. During periesophageal dissection, the distal dilating olive of the mediastinoscope is placed behind the esophagus (*b*). The olive creates and maintains space by careful probing of the periesophageal areolar tissue. When the esophagus has been fully mobilized down to the diaphragmatic hiatus, a plastic tube is passed into the hiatus, where it is grasped by the mediastinoscope. Both the mediastinoscope and the plastic tube are pulled up from the hiatus (*c*). After esophageal resection with an endoscopic GIA stapler, the esophagus is folded over by using endoscopic control (*d*). Structures still attached to the esophagus are placed in traction, coagulated, and divided.

sutures. The azygos vein is divided with an endoscopic stapler. The inferior half of the thoracic esophagus is mobilized away from the aorta and pericardium. The subcarinal lymph nodes are removed en bloc. The upper third of the thoracic esophagus is mobilized away from the trachea, and the right paratracheal lymph nodes are removed, with care taken not to injure the recurrent laryngeal nerve. Once the esophagus has been fully mobilized, the pleural traction sutures are removed, two chest tubes inserted through port sites, and the other port incisions closed. The patient is then moved to the supine position. The stomach is mobilized through a laparotomy and brought up to the neck, where a cervical anastomosis is performed.

TROUBLESHOOTING

The technical problems associated with VATS esophagectomy are similar to those associated with open thoracic esophagectomy, including thoracic duct injury, recurrent nerve palsy, bleeding from the intercostal vessels, and anastomotic leakage [*see V:7 Open Esophageal Procedures*]. These problems are best prevented

by obtaining good visualization of the superior and posterior mediastinum, which can be achieved by using a 30° angled thoracoscope. The most common reason for conversion to thoracotomy is the presence of a locally advanced tumor that necessitates extensive dissection for safe mobilization away from adjacent mediastinal structures.

To date, comparison of the results of VATS esophagectomy with those of open esophagectomy has not shown VATS to yield a significant decrease in major complications, especially postoperative respiratory insufficiency and cardiac arrhythmias. These findings may be attributable in part to the number of port sites required to accomplish a complicated resection and to the necessity of combining VATS with an upper midline laparotomy for mobilization of the stomach.[78,79] As a result, most centers still prefer the standard open transhiatal or transthoracic approaches to esophagectomy.

VATS also plays a useful role in the management of postoperative chylothorax.[80] The thoracic duct can be ligated thoracoscopically, though it is sometimes difficult to identify and ligate

Figure 13 **VATS esophagectomy. Shown are trocar sites for the transthoracic approach.**[77]

the primary site of a postoperative lymphatic leak without reopening the thoracotomy.

VATS Pericardial Window

OPERATIVE TECHNIQUE

Some surgeons create a pericardial window by means of VATS as an alternative to taking the subxiphoid approach or the left anterior thoracotomy approach.[81,82] A double-lumen endotracheal tube is inserted with the patient under general anesthesia, and the patient is rotated into the right lateral decubitus position. Three access sites are used, with the thoracoscope inserted at the seventh intercostal space in the posterior axillary line and instruments introduced through two ports, one at the tip of the scapula and the other at the sixth intercostal space in the axillary line [*see Figure 14a*]. The pericardium is retracted with a grasper forceps, and scissors are used to resect 8 to 10 cm² areas of pericardium both anterior and posterior to the phrenic nerve. If indicated, talc pleurodesis can be performed to control an associated pleural effusion. One or two chest tubes are then inserted through the port-site incisions.

TROUBLESHOOTING

When a pericardial effusion causes cardiac tamponade, a subxiphoid approach is preferable to VATS for creating a pericardial window because it is safer to perform in a hemodynamically unstable patient. A VATS pericardial window is also inadvisable in patients with constrictive physiology or with intrapericardial adhesions discovered at the time of operation. Conversion to an open procedure with formal pericardiectomy is advisable under these circumstances.

VATS Procedures for Mediastinal Masses

A 1998 multicenter trial aimed at defining the role of VATS in the management of mediastinal tumors suggested that VATS can

be used safely to diagnose and resect most middle and posterior mediastinal masses, especially in view of the typically benign nature of these tumors.[83]

VATS thymectomy has been employed to treat myasthenia gravis and thymoma.[84] To date, only anecdotal experience is available, and no studies examining long-term outcome have been published. Although a VATS approach to myasthenia gravis may appear attractive at first, it is not the least invasive approach to the thymus. Transcervical thymectomy is a minimally invasive approach to the thymus that does not require a chest incision, does not violate the pleural space, and allows most patients to be discharged home the next day.[85] There is still a degree of controversy as to whether complete thymic resection, including all ectopic thymic tissue, is necessary to obtain clinical remission in patients with myasthenia gravis.[86] For patients with a thymic mass, we prefer a transsternal approach. For patients with myasthenia gravis who do not have a thymoma, however, we believe that there is a need for prospective studies comparing VATS with other surgical approaches to thymectomy.

OPERATIVE TECHNIQUE

VATS has been used to resect masses in all of the mediastinal compartments. VATS resection is an ideal approach to posterior neurogenic tumors that do not extend into the neural canal.[87,88] With the patient in the lateral decubitus position, the operating table is rotated anteriorly so that the lung falls away from the paravertebral region. The port sites are placed anteriorly; the thoracoscope is inserted at the fifth intercostal space in the midaxillary line, a lung retractor is inserted at the sixth intercostal space in the anterior axillary line, and dissecting instruments are inserted at the second and fourth intercostal spaces in the anterior axillary line [*see Figure 14b*]. The mass is manipulated with a grasper to expose the posteriorly located pedicle, which is then dissected, ligated, and divided with the scissors, clip appliers, and the electrocautery.[89,90]

For removal of anterior mediastinal masses, the port sites are placed in more posterior locations. The thoracoscope is introduced at the fifth intercostal space in the midaxillary or posterior axillary line, and instruments are inserted through two ports, one at the second intercostal space at the midaxillary line and the other at the fifth or sixth intercostal space in the anterior axillary line [*see Figure 14c*]. The mass is retracted with a grasper and dissected free with a combination of sharp and blunt dissection, clip appliers, and the electrocautery.[91,92]

A similar technique is used to resect middle mediastinal masses, most of which are pericardial or bronchogenic cysts.[93,94] The access sites should be chosen according to the location of the mass on the preoperative CT scan. Generally, however, the triangulated site placement used for pulmonary wedge resections provides more suitable exposure than the site placement used for anterior or posterior mediastinal masses.

TROUBLESHOOTING

The placement of the thoracoports and the positioning of the operative team for the resection of posterior mediastinal tumors or for thoracic diskectomy differ significantly from the usual practice in most other VATS procedures. In place of the standard arrangement of trocars in an inverted triangle, the viewing port is placed in the posterior axillary line and the operating ports in the anterior axillary line. The thoracic surgeon and the neurosurgeon both stand on the anterior side of the patient, each viewing a monitor on the opposite side. In addition, a 30° scope is essential for visualizing the intervertebral disk space.[88,90]

Removal of dumbbell neurogenic tumors can be accomplished thoracoscopically if immediately preceded by posterior surgical removal of the spinal component of the tumor via laminectomy and intervertebral foraminotomy. Preoperative MRI scanning is crucial for defining the extent of tumor within the spinal canal.[89] Resection of posterior mediastinal tumors is sometimes associated with significant bleeding from intercostal or spinal arteries; should such bleeding occur, there should be no hesitation in converting to a thoracotomy.

Ideally, anterior mediastinal cysts should be resected in toto to avoid recurrence; however, if the cysts are firmly adherent to vital mediastinal structures, partial excision with cauterization of the endothelial lining may be safer.

VATS Management of Thoracic Trauma

The major contraindication to thoracoscopy in thoracic trauma is hemodynamic instability. For major life-threatening injuries involving the great vessels and the mediastinum, thoracotomy is required to obtain expeditious control of injured structures. However, hemodynamically stable patients with certain thoracic problems—such as diaphragmatic injury, slow continued intrathoracic bleeding, persistent air leakage, and empyema—can be diagnosed and often treated by means of VATS.[95,96]

In the assessment of a trauma patient with a potential diaphragmatic injury, it is important not to ignore the high incidence of associated intra-abdominal injury. If intra-abdominal injury has been ruled out and there is concern about the presence of a diaphragmatic tear, thoracoscopic assessment of the diaphragm is justified. Such assessment allows a more thorough evaluation of the entire diaphragm than the laparoscopic approach, which is limited by the liver on the right side. In the largest series published to date, 60 of 171 patients who underwent thoracoscopy for penetrating chest injuries had diaphragmatic injuries that necessitated repair.[97] For hemodynamically stable patients with suspected diaphragmatic injuries, the VATS approach appears reasonable.

When a patient has an ongoing intrathoracic problem such as persistent bleeding or a large air leak 24 to 48 hours after a traumatic injury, VATS should be considered before a thoracotomy is done because most problems encountered at this time (e.g., chest wall bleeding and laceration of the lung parenchyma) can be managed endoscopically, without the need for a thoracotomy.

TROUBLESHOOTING

The main pitfall in thoracoscopic evaluation of the diaphragm is failure to assess the abdomen appropriately and consequent failure to recognize an occult intra-abdominal injury. When laparoscopy is performed in a patient with a diaphragmatic injury, CO_2 insufflation can cause a tension pneumothorax to develop on the side of the diaphragmatic injury; accordingly, whenever diaphragmatic injury is a possibility, the chest should be included in the operative field to allow chest tube insertion if required. Because thoracoscopy does not require CO_2 insufflation, it is safer in such situations.

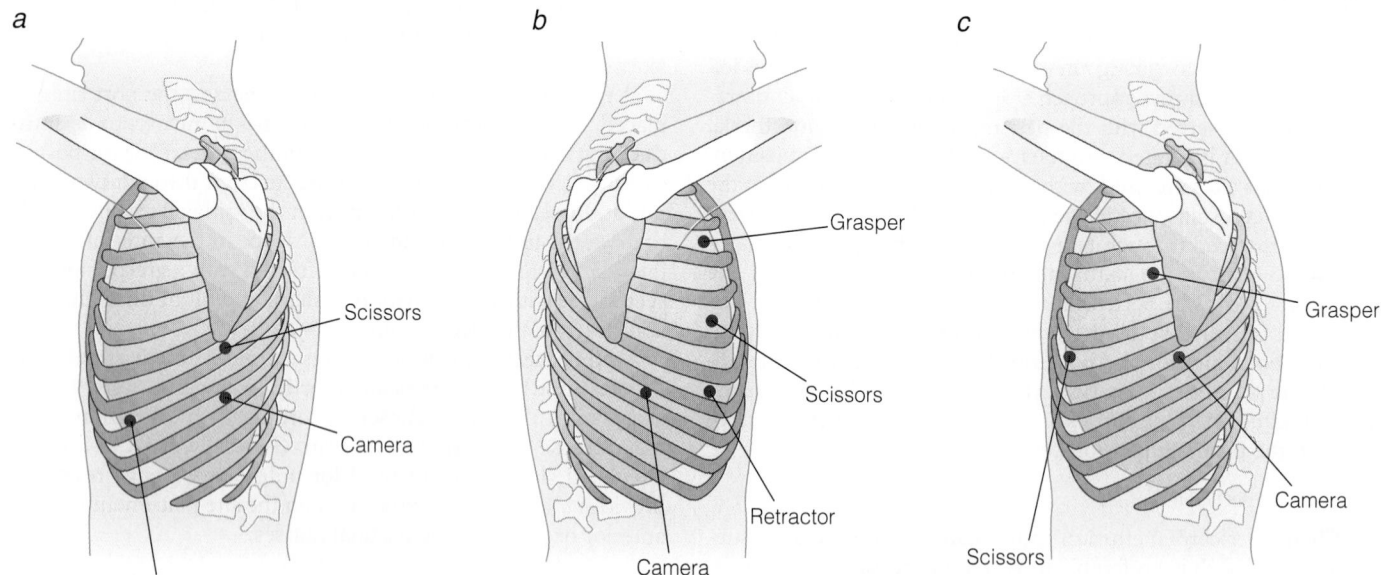

Figure 14 (*a*) **VATS pericardial window. Three access sites are used. The thoracoscope is inserted in the posterior axillary line at the seventh intercostal space, the endoscopic scissors are inserted through one port at the tip of the scapula, and the grasper forceps is inserted through another port in the anterior axillary line at the sixth intercostal space. (*b, c*) VATS procedures for mediastinal masses. For posterior masses, the port sites are placed anteriorly (*b*), and the thoracoscope is inserted at the fifth intercostal space in the midaxillary line. A lung retractor is inserted at the sixth intercostal space in the anterior axillary line, and dissecting instruments are inserted at the second and fourth intercostal spaces in the anterior axillary line. For anterior mediastinal masses and thymectomy, the port sites are placed in more posterior locations (*c*). The thoracoscope is introduced at the fifth intercostal space in the midaxillary or the posterior axillary line, and instruments are inserted through one port at the second intercostal space in the midaxillary line and another at the fifth or sixth intercostal space in the anterior axillary line.**

Figure 15 **VATS splanchnicectomy. Splanchnicectomy may be accomplished by either (*a*) dividing the roots of the splanchnic nerves or (*b*) dividing the splanchnic nerve itself.**

VATS Sympathectomy and Splanchnicectomy

Thoracic sympathectomy is known to be the most effective treatment for upper limb hyperhidrosis, and VATS is now an accepted approach to this operation.

The main indication for splanchnicectomy is intractable abdominal pain from unresectable malignancies (e.g., pancreatic or gastric carcinoma) and chronic pancreatitis. The effects of celiac ganglion blocks are transient, and surgical manipulation of this area is usually very difficult because of the primary disease process, previous operations, or both. In the past, thoracotomy was generally considered too invasive an approach to splanchnic denervation in these patients. Currently, however, because of the less invasive nature of thoracoscopy and the quicker recovery time associated with it, thoracoscopic splanchnicectomy is an attractive therapeutic option.[98]

OPERATIVE TECHNIQUE

Sympathectomy

VATS sympathectomy is performed with the patient under general anesthesia and a double-lumen tube in place. Three port sites are used: one for the thoracoscope at the third intercostal space in the midaxillary line, one at the third intercostal space in the anterior axillary line, and one at the tip of the scapula. The pleura is incised and divided from T2 to T5, and the sympathetic chain is dissected free with scissors. For complete control of upper limb hyperhidrosis, VATS must be done bilaterally.[99,100]

Splanchnicectomy

The technical aspects of VATS splanchnicectomy are quite simple: a sound knowledge of the splanchnic anatomy and a basic set of thoracoscopic instruments are all that is needed. Single-lung ventilation is required. Three thoracoports are placed. A silk stitch is placed in the central tendon of the diaphragm and pulled through the most anterior and inferior port to allow better visualization of the splanchnic nerves. The camera is also placed though this port. An endoscopic grasper and an endoscopic scissors with an electrocautery attachment are used to remove the nerve segment from T5 to T9. The greater

and lesser splanchnic nerves are resected [*see Figure 15*]. The least splanchnic nerve is rarely visualized.

TROUBLESHOOTING

Care should be taken to identify the first and second ribs. Division of the sympathetic trunk at the level of the first rib causes Horner syndrome and does not reduce palmar hyperhidrosis.

Division of the rami communicantes rather than the main sympathetic trunk reduces the incidence of undesirable side effects, especially compensatory hyperhidrosis of the trunk, but its overall success rate in controlling upper limb hyperhidrosis is lower.[99] Abolition of only the T2 and T3 ganglia may control palmar hyperhidrosis without being as likely to result in unacceptable compensatory truncal sweating. Target areas for axillary sweating also include T4 and T5. In addition, an accessory sympathetic nerve fiber that runs lateral to the sympathetic chain (known as the nerve of Kuntz) should be sought and, if identified, divided. Compensatory hyperhidrosis of the inner thighs is a not uncommon complication.

Neuralgia is frequent after VATS sympathectomy. Some authors advocate a 2-day postoperative course of dexamethasone to reduce the incidence of this problem.[100]

Miscellaneous VATS Procedures

Several other procedures have been performed by VATS, including ligation of the thoracic duct[101] and resection of the adrenal gland.[102] For adrenal resection, three incisions are placed at the 9th or 10th intercostal space, extending from the anterior axillary line to the posterior axillary line. A fan retractor is inserted through a radial incision in the diaphragm and used to retract the perirenal fat. The adrenal gland is dissected free and removed, and the associated vessels are clipped or cauterized.[102]

Clinical Considerations

Minimally invasive surgery is currently in high demand, largely as a result of patient preferences. This growing popularity, however, must not be allowed to override clinical concerns. In particular, extreme care must be taken in the treatment of malignant disease because the consequences of cancer surgery are far greater than the consequences of surgery for benign disease. Whether a VATS procedure has good or acceptable long-term results is at least as important as whether it is technically feasible. It is our responsibility as thoracic surgeons to perform these procedures selectively rather than indiscriminately, either in settings where the effectiveness of VATS is clearly proved or, where the role of VATS has not been fully established, within the context of well-designed clinical trials.

Cost Considerations

It is hard to estimate the cost-effectiveness of VATS procedures because the instrumentation, the types of procedures performed, and the surgical expertise with these operations are all still evolving. Initially, VATS procedures proved expensive, for several reasons (e.g., the cost of purchasing video and endoscopic equipment, the cost of disposable instrumentation, and the need for long operating times as surgeons and nursing staff gained experience performing these procedures). Soon after VATS was introduced, a study from the Mayo Clinic compared the cost of performing VATS pulmonary wedge resections with that of the same operation done by thoracotomy.[103] The VATS approach was associated with substantially shorter hospital stays but also with increased OR costs; hence, the use of VATS did not result in any significant overall savings. Since that study, however, as some VATS procedures (e.g., pulmonary wedge resection) have become standard operations and more reusable instrumentation has become available, the cost of VATS has undoubtedly decreased. Whether other, more complex VATS procedures (e.g., thoracoscopic esophagectomy) are cost-effective remains to be determined.

Training and Certification in VATS

Thoracoscopy is most frequently performed by thoracic surgeons.[2] In some centers, however, particularly in Europe, pulmonologists became highly experienced in the application of traditional thoracoscopic techniques for the diagnosis of pleural disease. The experience of Boutin epitomizes the involvement of physicians who do not have specific surgical training.[4,8] The development of small-caliber endoscopes that could be used with local anesthesia outside the OR made it easy for nonsurgeons to perform thoracoscopy.

After the 1950s, thoracoscopy was largely forgotten by surgeons and pulmonologists in the United States until the advent of VATS. The dramatic initial popularity of this technique generated considerable debate about whether nonsurgeons should perform VATS in the same way as they perform other invasive endoscopic procedures.[104-106] During this same period, laparoscopic cholecystectomy became widely practiced, often by persons who lacked adequate training, and reports of serious complications emerged.

Within this context, the Society of Thoracic Surgeons (STS) and the American Association for Thoracic Surgery (AATS) formed a joint committee to establish standards and guidelines for training and certification in VATS [see Sidebar Statement of AATS/STS Joint Committee on Thoracoscopy and Video Assisted Thoracic Surgery].[107] As a result of the educational efforts of this committee, many surgeons were trained within a short time, and VATS was quickly incorporated into thoracic surgical practice and residency training.

The important considerations with respect to the training and practice of VATS have been well articulated.[106,107] VATS is not a minor procedure: it is minimally invasive, complex intrathoracic surgery that should be performed only by persons who are familiar with intrathoracic anatomy and pathology and are fully competent to manage complications and make intraoperative decisions in such a way as to ensure safe outcomes for thoracic surgical patients. The complications encountered during thoracoscopic operations are potentially immediately life-threatening, whereas those encountered during other endoscopic procedures usually are not. For that reason, VATS procedures should not be performed by anyone—surgeon or nonsurgeon—who lacks the training and experience to perform immediate thoracotomy and repair of intrathoracic injuries.

VATS is now an integral part of the practice of thoracic surgery.[108] The direct involvement of the major thoracic societies in the dispersion of this technology has discouraged the casual and unsafe application of VATS and has promoted an ongoing critical appraisal of VATS procedures.

Statement of AATS/STS Joint Committee on Thoracoscopy and Video Assisted Thoracic Surgery[107]

The Councils of the American Association for Thoracic Surgery and the Society of Thoracic Surgeons have formed a Joint Committee on Thoracoscopy and Video Assisted Thoracic Surgery. The purpose of this Committee is to facilitate the education of thoracic surgeons in this new technology and to provide guidelines for appropriate training in and performance of thoracoscopy and video assisted, minimally invasive thoracic surgery.

The following guidelines are recommended by the Joint Committee:

1. In order to ensure optimal quality patient care, thoracoscopy and video assisted thoracic surgery (TVATS) should be performed only by thoracic surgeons who are qualified, through documented training and experience, to perform open thoracic surgical procedures and manage their potential complications. The surgeon must have the judgment, training, and capability to proceed immediately to a standard open thoracic procedure if necessary.

   The preoperative and postoperative care of patients treated by TVATS should be the responsibility of the operating surgeon.

2. It is recommended that TVATS techniques be learned through appropriate instruction:

   a. As part of a formal approved thoracic surgical residency or fellowship program which includes structured and documented experience in these procedures.

   b. For the practicing thoracic surgeon, completion of a course that follows the guidelines approved by the Joint Committee, with hands-on laboratory experience, plus observation of these techniques performed by thoracic surgeons experienced in such procedures.

3. The granting of privileges to perform TVATS remains the responsibility of the credentialing body of individual hospitals.

For the AATS/STS Joint Committee on Thoracoscopy and Video Assisted Thoracic Surgery: Martin F. McKneally, M.D., and Ralph J. Lewis, M.D., co-chairmen; Richard P. Anderson, M.D., Richard G. Fosburg, M.D., William A. Gay, Jr., M.D., Robert H. Jones, M.D., and Mark B. Orringer, M.D.

References

1. Jacobeus HC: The practical importance of thoracoscopy in surgery of the chest. Surg Gynecol Obstet 34:289, 1922

2. Bloomberg AE: Thoracoscopy in perspective. Surg Gynecol Obstet 147:433, 1978

3. Weissberg D, Kaufman M: Diagnostic and therapeutic pleuroscopy: experience with 127 patients. Chest 78:732, 1980

4. Boutin C, Viallat JR, Cargnino P, et al: Thoracoscopy in malignant pleural effusions. Am Rev Respir Dis 124:588, 1981

5. Wihlm JM, Roeslin N, Morand G, et al: Résultats comparés de la ponction, de la biopsie à l'aiguille, de la pleuroscopie et de la thoracotomie dans le diagnostic des pleurésies chroniques. Poumon Coeur 37:57, 1981

6. Rodgers BM, Ryckman FC, Moazam F, et al: Thoracoscopy for intrathoracic tumors. Ann Thorac Surg 31:414, 1981

7. Rusch VW, Mountain C: Thoracoscopy under regional anesthesia for the diagnosis and management of pleural disease. Am J Surg 154:274, 1987

8. Boutin C, Viallat JR, Aelony Y: Practical Thoracoscopy. Berlin, Springer-Verlag, 1991

9. Hazelrigg SR, Nunchuck SK, LoCicero JI: Video Assisted Thoracic Surgery Study Group data. Ann Thorac Surg 56:1039, 1993

10. Krasna MJ, Deshmukh S, McLaughlin JS: Complications of thoracoscopy. Ann Thorac Surg 61:1066, 1996

11. Nakata M, Saeki H, Yokoyama N, et al: Pulmonary function after lobectomy: video-assisted thoracic surgery versus thoracotomy. Ann Thorac Surg 70:938, 2000

12. Kaseda S, Aoki T, Hangai N, et al: Better pulmonary function and prognosis with video-assisted thoracic surgery than with thoracotomy. Ann Thorac Surg 70:1644, 2000

13. Craig SR, Leaver HA, Yap PL, et al: Acute phase responses following minimal access and conventional thoracic surgery. Eur J Cardiothorac Surg 20:455, 2001

14. Yim AP, Wan S, Lee TW, et al: VATS lobectomy reduces cytokine responses compared with conventional surgery. Ann Thorac Surg 70:243, 2000

15. Deslauriers J, Beaulieu M, Dufour C, et al: Mediastinopleuroscopy: a new approach to the diagnosis of intrathoracic diseases. Ann Thorac Surg 22:265, 1976

16. Rusch VW: Instrumentation for video-assisted thoracic surgery. Chest Surg Clin North Am 3:215, 1993

17. Landreneau RJ, Herlan DB, Johnson JA, et al: Thoracoscopic neodymium:yttrium-aluminum garnet laser-assisted pulmonary resection. Ann Thorac Surg 52:1176, 1991

18. Rusch VW, Schmidt R, Shoji Y, et al: Use of the argon beam electrocoagulator for performing pulmonary wedge resections. Ann Thorac Surg 49:287, 1990

19. Landreneau RJ, Mack MJ, Hazelrigg SR, et al: Video-assisted thoracic surgery: basic technical concepts and intercostal approach strategies. Ann Thorac Surg 54:800, 1992

20. Rusch VW, Bains MS, Burt ME, et al: Contribution of videothoracoscopy to the management of the cancer patient. Ann Surg Oncol 1:94, 1994

21. Ohri SK, Oswal SK, Townsend ER, et al: Early and late outcome after diagnostic thoracoscopy and talc pleurodesis. Ann Thorac Surg 53:1038, 1992

22. Angelillo Mackinlay TA, Lyons GA, Chimondeguy DJ, et al: VATS debridement versus thoracotomy in the treatment of loculated postpneumonia empyema. Ann Thorac Surg 61:1626, 1996

23. Hartman DL, Gaither JM, Kesler KA, et al: Comparison of insufflated talc under thoracoscopic guidance with standard tetracycline and bleomycin pleurodesis for control of malignant pleural effusions. J Thorac Cardiovasc Surg 105:743, 1993

24. Landreneau RJ, Hazelrigg SR, Ferson PF, et al: Thoracoscopic resection of 85 pulmonary lesions. Ann Thorac Surg 54:415, 1992

25. Jimenez MF, The Spanish Video-Assisted Thoracic Surgery Group: Prospective study on video-assisted thoracoscopic surgery in the resection of pulmonary nodules: 209 cases from the Spanish Video-Assisted Thoracic Surgery Group. Eur J Cardiothorac Surg 19:562, 2001

26. Ferson PF, Landreneau RJ, Dowling RD, et al: Comparison of open versus thoracoscopic lung biopsy for diffuse infiltrative pulmonary disease. J Thorac Cardiovasc Surg 106:194, 1993

27. Miller JD, Urschel JD, Cox G, et al: A randomized, controlled trial comparing thoracoscopy and limited thoracotomy for lung biopsy in interstitial lung disease. Ann Thorac Surg 70:1647, 2000

28. Dowling RD, Keenan RJ, Ferson PF, et al: Video-assisted thoracoscopic resection of pulmonary metastases. Ann Thorac Surg 56:772, 1993

29. Landreneau RJ, De Giacomo T, Mack MJ, et al: Therapeutic video-assisted thoracoscopic surgical resection of colorectal pulmonary metastases. Eur J Cardiothorac Surg 18:671, 2000

30. McCormack PM, Ginsberg KB, Bains MS, et al: Accuracy of lung imaging in metastases with implications for the role of thoracoscopy. Ann Thorac Surg 56:863, 1993

31. Dowling RD, Ferson PF, Landreneau RJ: Thoracoscopic resection of pulmonary metastases. Chest 102:1450, 1992

32. McCormack PM, Bains MS, Begg CB, et al: Role of video-assisted thoracic surgery in the treatment of pulmonary metastases: Results of a prospective trial. Ann Thorac Surg 62:213, 1996

33. Parekh K, Rusch V, Bains M, et al: VATS port site recurrence: a technique dependent problem. Ann Surg Oncol 8:175, 2001

34. Miller DL, Allen MS, Trastek VF, et al: Videothoracoscopic wedge excision of the lung. Ann Thorac Surg 54:410, 1992

35. Bolotin G, Lazarovici H, Uretzky G, et al: The efficacy of intraoperative internal intercostal nerve block during video-assisted thoracic surgery on postoperative pain. Ann Thorac Surg 70:1872, 2000

36. Normori H, Horio H: Endofinger for tactile localization of pulmonary nodules during thoracoscopic resection. Thorac Cardiovasc Surg 44:50, 1996

37. Shennib H, Bret P: Intraoperative transthoracic ultrasonographic localization of occult lung lesions. Ann Thorac Surg 55:767, 1993

38. Plunkett MB, Peterson MS, Landreneau RJ, et al: Peripheral pulmonary nodules: preoperative percutaneous needle localization with CT guidance. Radiology 185:274, 1992

39. Lewis RJ, Caccavale RJ, Sisler GE, et al: One hundred consecutive patients undergoing video-assisted thoracic operations. Ann Thorac Surg 54:421, 1992

40. Demmy TL, Nielson D, Curtis JJ: Improved method for deep thoracoscopic lung nodule excision. Missouri Med 93:86, 1996

41. Mouroux J, Elkaïm D, Padovani B, et al: Video-assisted thoracoscopic treatment of spontaneous pneumothorax: technique and results of one hundred cases. J Thorac Cardiovasc Surg 112:385, 1996

42. Schrmael FMNH, Sutedja TG, Braber JCE, et al: Cost-effectiveness of video-assisted thoracoscopic surgery versus conservative treatment for first time or recurrent spontaneous pneumothorax. Eur Respir J 9:1821, 1996

43. Hazelrigg SR, Landreneau RJ, Mack M, et al: Thoracoscopic stapled resection for spontaneous pneumothorax. J Thorac Cardiovasc Surg 105:389, 1993

44. Cole FH, Jr, Cole FH, Khandekar A, et al: Video-assisted thoracic surgery: primary therapy for spontaneous pneumothorax? Ann Thorac Surg 60:931, 1995

45. Wakabayashi A: Expanded applications of diagnostic and therapeutic thoracoscopy. J Thorac Cardiovasc Surg 102:721, 1991

46. Wakabayashi A: Thoracoscopic laser pneumoplasty in the treatment of diffuse bullous emphysema. Ann Thorac Surg 60:936, 1995

47. Torresini G, Vaccarili M, Divisi D, et al: Is video-assisted thoracic surgery justified at first spontaneous pneumothorax? Eur J Cardiothorac Surg 20:42, 2001

48. Yim AP: Video-assisted thoracoscopic management of primary spontaneous pneumothorax. Ann Acad Med Singapore 25:668, 1996

49. Colt HG, Russack V, Chiu Y, et al: A comparison of thoracoscopic talc insufflation, slurry, and mechanical abrasion pleurodesis. Chest 111:442, 1997

50. Inderbitzi RGC, Furrer M, Striffeler H, et al: Thoracoscopic pleurectomy for treatment of complicated spontaneous pneumothorax. J Thorac Cardiovasc Surg 105:84, 1993

51. Swanson SJ, Mentzer SJ, DeCamp MM, et al: No-cut thoracoscopic lung plication: a new technique for lung volume reduction surgery. J Am Coll Surg 185:25, 1997

52. Yim APC, Ko K-M, Ma C-C, et al: Thoracoscopic lobectomy for benign diseases. Chest 109:554, 1996

53. McKenna RJ Jr, Wolf RK, Brenner M, et al: Is lobectomy by video-assisted thoracic surgery an adequate cancer operation? Ann Thorac Surg 66:1903, 1998

54. Demmy TL, Curtis JJ: Minimally invasive lobectomy directed toward frail and high-risk patients: a case-control study. Ann Thorac Surg 68:194, 1999

55. Weber A, Stammberger U, Inci I, et al: Thoracoscopic lobectomy for benign disease—a single centre study on 64 cases. Eur J Cardiothorac Surg 20:443, 2001

56. Solaini L, Prusciano F, Bagioni P, et al: Video-assisted thoracic surgery major pulmonary resections: present experience. Eur J Cardiothorac Surg 20:437, 2001

57. Kirby TJ, Mack MJ, Landreneau RJ, et al: Initial experience with video-assisted thoracoscopic lobectomy. Ann Thorac Surg 56:1248, 1993

58. Kohno T, Murakami T, Wakabayashi A: Anatomic lobectomy of the lung by means of thoracoscopy: an experimental study. J Thorac Cardiovasc Surg 105:729, 1993

59. Lewis RJ: Simultaneously stapled lobectomy: a safe technique for video-assisted thoracic surgery. J Thorac Cardiovasc Surg 109:619, 1995

60. Lewis RJ, Sisler GE, Caccavale RJ: Imaged thoracic lobectomy: should it be done? Ann Thorac Surg 54:80, 1992

61. Lewis RJ: Personal communication, 1993

62. Roviaro GC, Rebuffat C, Varoli F, et al: Video-endoscopic thoracic surgery. Int Surg 78:4, 1993

63. Roviaro GC, Varoli F, Rebuffat C, et al: Video-thoracoscopic staging and treatment of lung cancer. Ann Thorac Surg 59:971, 1995

64. Landreneau RJ, Hazelrigg SR, Mack MJ, et al: Postoperative pain-related morbidity: video-assisted thoracic surgery versus thoracotomy. Ann Thorac Surg 56:1285, 1993

65. Kirby TJ, Mack MJ, Landreneau RJ, et al: Lobectomy—video-assisted thoracic surgery versus muscle-sparing thoracotomy: a randomized trial. J Thorac Cardiovasc Surg 109:997, 1995

66. Landreneau RJ, Mack MJ, Hazelrigg SR, et al: Prevalence of chronic pain after pulmonary resection by thoracotomy or video-assisted thoracic surgery. J Thorac Cardiovasc Surg 107:1079, 1994

67. Downey RJ, McCormack P, LoCicero JI, et al: Dissemination of malignant tumors after video-assisted thoracic surgery: a report of twenty-one cases. J Thorac Cardiovasc Surg 111:954, 1996

68. Johnstone PAS, Rohde DC, Swartz SE, et al: Port site recurrences after laparoscopic and thoracoscopic procedures in malignancy. J Clin Oncol 14:1950, 1996

69. Landreneau RJ, Hazelrigg SR, Mack MJ, et al: Thoracoscopic mediastinal lymph node sampling: useful for mediastinal lymph node stations inaccessible by cervical mediastinoscopy. J Thorac Cardiovasc Surg 106:554, 1993

70. Krasna MJ: Minimally invasive staging for esophageal cancer. Chest 112:191S, 1997

71. Krasna MJ, Flowers JL, Attar S, et al: Combined thoracoscopic/laparoscopic staging of esophageal cancer. J Thorac Cardiovasc Surg 111:800, 1996

72. Buess G, Becker HD, Lenz G: Perivisceral endoscopic oesophagectomy. Operative Manual of Endoscopic Surgery. Cuschieri A, Ed. Springer-Verlag, Berlin, 1992, p 149

73. Orringer MB: Transhiatal esophagectomy without thoracotomy for carcinoma of the thoracic esophagus. Ann Surg 200:282, 1984

74. Law S, Fok M, Chu KM, et al: Thoracoscopic esophagectomy for esophageal cancer. Surgery 122:8, 1997

75. Collard J-M, Lengele B, Otte J-B, et al: En bloc and standard esophagectomies by thoracoscopy. Ann Thorac Surg 56:675, 1993

76. Gossot D, Fourquier P, Celerier M: Thoracoscopic oesophagectomy. Ann Chir Gyn Fenniae 83:162, 1994

77. Akaishi T, Kaneda I, Higuchi N, et al: Thoracoscopic en bloc total esophagectomy with radical mediastinal lymphadenectomy. J Thorac Cardiovasc Surg 112:1533, 1996

78. Collard J-M: En bloc and standard esophagectomies by thoracoscopy: update. Ann Thorac Surg 61:769, 1996

79. Peracchia A, Rosati R, Fumagalli U, et al: Thoracoscopic esophagectomy: are there benefits? Sem Surg Onc 13:259, 1997

80. Fahimi H, Casselman FP, Mariani MA, et al: Current management of postoperative chylothorax. Ann Thorac Surg 71:448, 2001

81. Mack MJ, Landreneau RJ, Hazelrigg SR, et al: Video thoracoscopic management of benign and malignant pericardial effusions. Chest 103:390S, 1993

82. Flores RM, Jaklitsch MT, DeCamp MM Jr, et al: Video-assisted thoracic surgery pericardial resection for effusive disease. Chest Surg Clin North Am 8:835, 1998

83. Demmy TL, Krasna MJ, Detterbeck FC, et al: Multicenter VATS experience with mediastinal tumors. Ann Thorac Surg 66:187, 1998

84. Mack MJ, Landreneau RJ, Yim AP, et al: Results of video-assisted thymectomy in patients with myasthenia gravis. J Thorac Cardiovasc Surg 112:1352, 1996

85. Cooper JD, Al-Jilaihawi AN, Pearson FG, et al: An improved technique to facilitate transcervical thymectomy for myasthenia gravis. Ann Thorac Surg 45:242, 1988

86. Jaretzki A, III, Wolff M: "Maximal" thymectomy for myasthenia gravis: surgical anatomy and operative technique. J Thorac Cardiovasc Surg 96:711, 1988

87. Riquet M, Mouroux J, Pons F, et al: Videothoracoscopic excision of thoracic neurogenic tumors. Ann Thorac Surg 60:943, 1995

88. Bousamra M, II, Haasler GB, Patterson GA, et al: A comparative study of thoracoscopic vs open removal of benign neurogenic mediastinal tumors. Chest 109:1461, 1996

89. Vallières E, Findlay JM, Fraser RE: Combined microneurosurgical and thoracoscopic removal of neurogenic dumbbell tumors. Ann Thorac Surg 59:469, 1995

90. Mack MJ, Regan JJ, McAfee PC, et al: Video-assisted thoracic surgery for the anterior approach to the thoracic spine. Ann Thorac Surg 59:1100, 1995

91. Yim APC, Kay RLC, Ho JKS: Video-assisted thoracoscopic thymectomy for myasthenia gravis. Chest 108:1440, 1995

92. Knight R, Ratzer ER, Fenoglio ME, et al: Thoracoscopic excision of mediastinal parathyroid adenomas: a report of two cases and review of the literature. J Am Coll Surg 185:481, 1997

93. Hazelrigg SR, Landreneau RJ, Mack MJ, et al: Thoracoscopic resection of mediastinal cysts. Ann Thorac Surg 56:659, 1993

94. Lewis RJ, Caccavale RJ, Sisler GE: Imaged thoracoscopic surgery: a new thoracic technique for resection of mediastinal cysts. Ann Thorac Surg 53:318, 1992

95. Lang-Lazdunski L, Mouroux J, Pons F, et al: Role of videothoracoscopy in chest trauma. Ann Thorac Surg 63:327, 1997

96. Spann JC, Nwariaku FE, Wait M: Evaluation of video-assisted thoracoscopic surgery in the diagnosis of diaphragmatic injuries. Am J Surg 170:628, 1995

97. Freeman RK, Al-Dossari G, Hutcheson KA, et al: Indications for using video-assisted thoracoscopic surgery to diagnose diaphragmatic injuries after penetrating chest trauma. Ann Thorac Surg 72:342, 2001

98. Le Pimpec-Barthes F, Chapuis O, Riquet M, et al: Thoracoscopic splanchnicectomy for control of intractable pain in pancreatic cancer. Ann Thorac Surg 65:810, 1998

99. Gossot D, Toledo L, Fritsch S, et al: Thoracoscopic sympathectomy for upper limb hyperhidrosis: looking for the right operation. Ann Thorac Surg 64:975, 1997

100. Wong C-W: Transthoracic video endoscopic electrocautery of sympathetic ganglia for hyperhidrosis palmaris: special reference to localization of the first and second ribs. Surg Neurol 47:224, 1997

101. Shirai T, Amano J, Takabe K: Thoracoscopic diagnosis and treatment of chylothorax after pneumonectomy. Ann Thorac Surg 52:306, 1991

102. Mack MJ, Aronoff RJ, Acuff TE, et al: Thoracoscopic transdiaphragmatic approach for adrenal biopsy. Ann Thorac Surg 55:772, 1993

103. Allen MS, Deschamps C, Lee RE, et al: Video-assisted thoracoscopic stapled wedge excision for indeterminate pulmonary nodules. J Thorac Cardiovasc Surg 106:1048, 1993

104. Mathur P, Martin WJ Jr: Clinical utility of thoracoscopy. Chest 102:2, 1992

105. Forum: Who should perform thoracoscopy? Chest 102:1553, 1992

106. Thoracoscopy forum, continuing dialogue. Chest 102:1915, 1992

107. McKneally MF, Lewis RJ, Anderson RP, et al: Statement of the AATS/STS Joint Committee on Thoracoscopy and Video Assisted Thoracic Surgery. J Thorac Cardiovasc Surg 104:1, 1992

108. Mack MJ, Scruggs GR, Kelly KM, et al: Video-assisted thoracic surgery: has technology found its place? Ann Thorac Surg 64:211, 1997

6 GASTROINTESTINAL ENDOSCOPY

Alicia Fanning, M.D., and Jeffrey L. Ponsky, M.D.

Since the beginning of the 1970s, flexible endoscopy of the gastrointestinal tract has been the dominant modality for the diagnosis of gastrointestinal disease. Over the same period, developments in technology and methodology have made possible the use of endoscopy to treat a host of conditions that once were considered to be manageable only by means of open surgical procedures. The integration of flexible endoscopic techniques into the armamentarium of the GI surgeon permits a more multidimensional approach to the treatment of digestive disease. The modern GI surgeon should be conversant in and adept at many of these procedures.

Diagnostic Esophagogastroduodenoscopy

Diagnostic esophagogastroduodenoscopy (EGD) is indicated when a patient has abnormal findings on traditional GI x-ray series, dysphagia, odynophagia, epigastric pain that does not respond to medical therapy, persistent heartburn, or upper GI bleeding; it is also indicated for surveillance of patients at high risk for malignancy and for sampling of GI tissue or fluid. One prepares for the examination by ensuring the patient's hemodynamic stability, having the patient fast for 6 to 8 hours beforehand, and performing conscious sedation, which generally involves applying a topical anesthetic to the posterior pharynx and administering a narcotic and a benzodiazepine intravenously. Monitoring of arterial blood pressure and oxygen saturation throughout the procedure is now standard practice.

TECHNIQUE

With the patient in the left lateral decubitus position, a topical anesthetic is applied to the posterior pharynx and an intravenous sedative administered. The forward-viewing panendoscope—a small-caliber instrument that is long enough to permit examination of the foregut from the mouth to the third portion of the duodenum—is employed.

The endoscope may be introduced either blindly, via finger-guided palpation of the pharynx, or under direct vision. The latter approach is preferable. In this approach, the instrument is advanced slowly until the epiglottis and vocal cords are visualized [*see Figure 1*]; it is then angled posteriorly to the esophageal introitus and gently advanced as the patient is asked to swallow. Insufflation of air is begun to distend the esophagus, which appears as a long, round tube. Frequent peristaltic waves are seen; these are normal. Mucosal surfaces must be closely inspected for signs of ulceration, stricture, tumor, or Barrett's (columnar) epithelium, which manifests itself as orange patches in otherwise pale salmon-pink esophageal (squamous) mucosa. When abnormalities are noted, biopsy, brushing for cytologic evaluation, or both should be performed. Staining of the esophagus with methylene blue may be useful in the search for Barrett's mucosa: the blue dye is avidly absorbed by the intestinal absorptive cells of the columnar epithelium. Darkly stained areas may be biopsied for confirmation.

As the endoscope is advanced, insufflation is continued, and the curve of the lumen is followed to the left as the esophagus traverses the diaphragm to enter the stomach. There is a pinched area where the diaphragm compresses the esophagus; the pinching is exaggerated when the patient is asked to sniff. If gastric folds are seen above this pinched area, a hiatal hernia is present. When the stomach is entered, the tip of the endoscope is elevated so as to center it within the gastric lumen. It should be noted that with the patient lying in the left lateral decubitus position, the stomach is also on its side, with the greater curvature at 6 o'clock, the lesser curvature at 12 o'clock, the posterior wall at 3 o'clock, and the anterior wall at 9 o'clock. Air should be insufflated to distend the stomach fully and permit careful inspection of the mucosal surfaces.

As the instrument is advanced toward the gastric antrum, its tip should be slightly elevated because the stomach has a J shape and the prepyloric region curves upward. The pylorus is normally round and may be seen to open and close with gastric peristalsis. With the tip of the endoscope positioned at the proximal gastric antrum, just under the incisura angularis, a retroflex view of the cardia and the fundus is obtained by elevating the tip of the scope and rotating the shaft to the left. This maneuver provides visual and therapeutic access to the proximal stomach.

After the stomach has been viewed, the instrument is advanced under direct vision through the pylorus and into the duodenal bulb. Insufflation of air should continue as the scope is

Figure 1 **Diagnostic esophagogastroduodenoscopy. As the endoscope is introduced under direct vision, the vocal cords are clearly noted. The esophageal opening is posterior to the cords.**

pressed against the pylorus to facilitate passage of the instrument. The scope tends to pop into the duodenal bulb rather than slide smoothly; it should be pulled back slightly to allow one to observe the mucosal surfaces of the bulb before moving ahead. Unlike the rest of the small bowel, the duodenal bulb has no semicircular folds. The tip of the scope must be rotated slightly to permit examination of the walls of the bulb. It is advisable to pull the instrument back into the stomach while observing the walls of the bulb and the pyloric channel for lesions; several such withdrawals may be required for full assessment of this area.

Once the duodenal bulb has been examined, the endoscope is advanced just past the bulb to the point where the first duodenal folds are observed. Here, the duodenum turns sharply to the rear and downward as it becomes retroperitoneal. Advancement of the scope into the second portion of the duodenum is one of the few endoscopic maneuvers that cannot be accomplished under direct vision. Because of the sharp angle of the turn, one will experience a moment of so-called red out as the tip of the endoscope touches the mucosa during the turn. To ensure that the turn is accomplished safely, the instrument is advanced as far through the bulb as is possible under direct vision. The control handle of the scope is then rotated approximately 90° to the right as the tip of the scope is turned to the right and angled first upward, then downward. As the second portion of the duodenum appears, the scope is rotated back to its neutral position. When done correctly, the turn is actually quite easy. It should never be forced: if the instrument does not proceed easily into the descending duodenum, the scope should be pulled back and the attempt repeated. Pushing against resistance may result in perforation.

Entering the descending duodenum causes the scope to form a large loop in the stomach. Therefore, once the second portion of the duodenum is successfully entered, the shaft of the instrument is pulled back. Paradoxically, as this movement straightens the gastric loop, it also advances the tip of the instrument deeper into the duodenum. Further advancement of the instrument under direct vision often permits entry into the third or even the fourth portion of the duodenum. Once the distal limit of intubation is reached, the scope is withdrawn and the luminal surfaces are carefully examined. Rotating the scope with small right-left movements of the controls and side-to-side movements of the control handle itself will help demonstrate the more subtle details of duodenal anatomy. Often, the upper GI tract is inspected more completely while the instrument is being withdrawn than while it is being advanced.

Mucosal abnormalities should be biopsied; liberal use of brush cytology in combination with biopsy enhances the yield.

COMPLICATIONS

EGD is an extremely safe procedure. Perhaps the most common problems associated with the technique arise from the preparatory sedation and analgesia. Respiratory depression and aspiration may occur during the procedure. Careful attention must be paid to the patient's state of consciousness and airway during the endoscopic procedure, appropriate drugs must be available to reverse sedative effects, and a suction apparatus must be ready for use at all times. Blind advancement of the endoscope by force may lead to perforation of the esophagus; this problem may be avoided by taking care never to advance the instrument against resistance.

Therapeutic Esophagogastroduodenoscopy

CONTROL OF VARICEAL HEMORRHAGE

In patients with massive upper GI hemorrhage, the first priori-

a

b

Figure 2 **Therapeutic esophagogastroduodenoscopy: control of variceal hemorrhage. (*a*) A plastic tip on the endoscope is used to create a chamber. (*b*) An esophageal varix is suctioned into the chamber, and a rubber band is released around it.**

ties are to establish a secure airway and to ensure hemodynamic stability. These priorities must be addressed before endoscopy is attempted. If the bleeding is thought to be coming from esophageal varices, it is frequently useful to perform endotracheal intubation for control of the airway before the endoscopic intervention.

Technique

A rapid but complete diagnostic upper GI endoscopic procedure is performed to determine whether varices are present and to identify the exact site of hemorrhage. Endoscopic therapy for variceal disease is then delivered by means of either sclerotherapy or rubber band ligation.

Sclerotherapy is commenced in the distal esophagus at the site of active or suspected bleeding: 2 to 3 ml of a sclerosant solution (e.g., sodium tetradecyl sulfate) is injected directly into the lumen of the varix. Additional varices can be treated in the same fashion. After the bleeding has stopped, further therapy is usually delivered at weekly intervals until total variceal obliteration is achieved.

Rubber band ligation of varices has become extremely popular in recent years and has been shown to possess some clear advantages over sclerotherapy [*see Figure 2*]. Originally, multiple passages of the endoscope were required to allow for reloading of the bands; however, newer ligating devices permit ligation of as many as 10 varices with a single passage of the endoscope. As with sclerotherapy, the site of active or suspected bleeding is attacked first; it is most often near the esophagogastric junction. The offending varix is centered in the field of view, and suction is applied to pull it into the ligator cup, which sits on the end of the endoscope. When the varix is deep within the cup, the trigger string on the ligator is pulled, and a rubber band is released around the varix. Suction is then released, and the ligated varix is visualized. Additional ligations may be performed at the initial session; follow-up sessions are usually held at weekly intervals until total variceal obliteration is achieved.

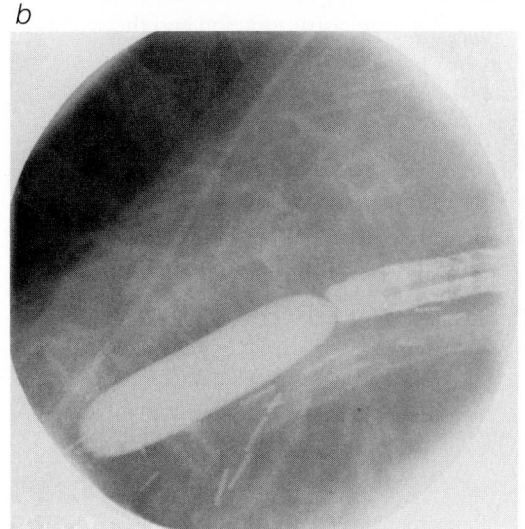

a   *b*

Figure 3   **Therapeutic esophagogastroduodenoscopy: dilation of esophageal strictures. (*a*) A hydrostatic dilating balloon filled with a contrast agent is inflated within the stricture under fluoroscopic guidance. Initially, a "waist" appears at the stricture site. (*b*) Inflation of the balloon is continued until the waist is ablated, which indicates complete dilation of the stricture.**

Complications

Because aspiration of blood and gastric contents may occur during endoscopic control of variceal hemorrhage, endotracheal intubation must be considered when bleeding is massive. In many cases, general anesthesia will permit adequate airway control and a quiet operating field. Violent patient motion when the injection needle is in a varix may result in perforation of the esophagus. This is a rare complication, however; tearing of the varix, with resultant hemorrhage, is more frequent. Injection of excessive amounts of sclerosant may lead to significant ulceration and necrosis of esophageal tissue. Fever, severe infection, pleural effusion, and subsequent esophageal stricture occasionally occur after sclerotherapy. Ulceration and necrosis of tissue, with subsequent stricture, occur after rubber band ligation as well, but severe infection is less common in this setting.

CONTROL OF NONVARICEAL HEMORRHAGE

Bleeding from peptic ulcer disease, gastritis, or vascular malformations is a common indication for EGD. Once the patient has been adequately resuscitated, endoscopy should be performed, and the entire esophagus, stomach, and duodenum should be examined thoroughly. Before the procedure is begun, the stomach should be vigorously irrigated through a large-bore tube so that as much clotted blood as possible can be evacuated. If a pool of blood is noted in the stomach, the position of the patient should be changed so as to move the pool and permit complete examination of the stomach.

The therapeutic modalities available for control of nonvariceal bleeding include (1) the injection of hypertonic saline, epinephrine (in a 1:10,000 solution), or 98% alcohol, (2) bipolar electrocoagulation, (3) the use of heater probes, (4) argon beam coagulation, (5) the application of acrylic glue, (6) the application of hemostatic clips, and (7) the use of the neodynium:yttrium-aluminum-garnet (Nd:YAG) laser.

Technique

The most popular therapeutic modalities are injection therapy, bipolar coagulation, and the use of the heater probe. Injection therapy is performed around the bleeding lesion to create edema and vasospasm in the area. The bipolar coagulator or the heater probe is applied directly to the bleeding lesion in an attempt to coapt the bleeding vessel as heat is delivered. Frequently, injection therapy is employed in conjunction with coagulation; this combination is very effective.

If there is a clot covering the ulcer base, it must be removed with suction or a snare before coagulation is attempted. If a rapidly bleeding lesion is present, the best approach often is injection therapy in adjacent areas to slow or stop the bleeding, followed by coagulation by direct coaptation. Vascular lesions are often multiple or diffuse, as in so-called watermelon stomach. Such lesions are most effectively treated by means of modalities that can be applied in a spraying fashion, such as the Nd:YAG laser or the argon beam coagulator.

Complications

Nonvariceal hemorrhage is successfully controlled by endoscopic means in more than 90% of cases. At times, however, attempts at endoscopic control may exacerbate the bleeding. Several therapeutic modalities should always be available: one may succeed when another fails. Excessive injection therapy or persistent attempts at coagulation may lead to tissue necrosis and subsequent perforation. Although the argon beam coagulator can injure tissue only to a depth of several millimeters, excessive application may result in massive distention of the bowel if care is not taken to aspirate the constantly infused argon gas frequently. The Nd:YAG laser has the potential to cause full-thickness injury to the gastric wall.

DILATION OF ESOPHAGEAL STRICTURES

When patients complain of dysphagia or odynophagia, prompt endoscopic investigation is warranted. Strictures may be secondary to reflux disease, secondary to caustic burns, or of neoplastic origin.

Technique

Endoscopy is performed in the usual fashion. It is imperative that the endoscope be advanced only under direct vision. When a stricture is encountered, its location, morphology, and length should be determined. Biopsy and cytology specimens should be gathered from the circumference of the stricture. When a stricture is present at the esophagogastric junction and the scope can easily be passed by the stricture, it is helpful to view the area from below with the tip of the scope retroflexed.

Stricture dilation can be accomplished in several different ways and with several different kinds of dilators. One commonly employed method is to use the endoscope to guide the passage of a soft-tipped guide wire through the stricture; the scope is then removed, leaving the wire in place. Subsequently, dilators are passed over the guide wire, usually under fluoroscopic control. Another method for endoscopic dilation of strictures is the use of through-the-scope (TTS) hydrostatic dilating balloons. A balloon of the appropriate inflated diameter (usually no larger than 18 mm or 54 French) is selected, passed through the biopsy channel of the endoscope, and advanced under direct vision until its middle portion passes through the stricture. At the stricture site, the balloon is compressed, giving the appearance of a waist. The balloon is then inflated until the waist is fully expanded [*see Figure 3*]. Full expansion is verified by fluoroscopic surveillance and the use of contrast to inflate the balloon. This second method is extremely useful for initial dilation of tight strictures in preparation for the use of other, nonendoscopic dilators or the placement of an esophageal stent.

Complications

Dilation of esophageal strictures may result in bleeding (usually minor) or perforation of the esophagus. When a patient experiences severe pain after dilation, a chest x-ray is imperative. The finding of mediastinal or subcutaneous air should prompt the immediate performance of a contrast study with a water-soluble agent to determine whether a perforation is present. Some small perforations can be managed with intravenous antibiotics and observation, but most must be managed surgically. The incidence of perforation can be minimized by avoiding excessive or forceful dilation.

STENTING OF ESOPHAGEAL TUMORS

Under optimal circumstances, esophageal tumors should be treated by means of extirpative surgery. When surgical cure or palliation seems to have little to offer, placement of an esophageal prosthesis by endoscopic means is a reasonable approach.

Technique

Modern esophageal prostheses are placed under fluoroscopic guidance, frequently after endoscopic balloon dilation of the tumor. During the endoscopic examination, it is useful to inject a small amount of water-soluble contrast material into the muscular wall of the esophagus just above and below the tumor; this enables one to measure the length of the tumor and select the correct stent. Once the tumor has been dilated and marked endoscopically, the scope is removed, and the expandable stent is passed into the esophagus and positioned between the endoscopic injection markings seen on fluoroscopy. The stent is then deployed and allowed to expand [*see Figure 4*]. The endoscope may then be reintroduced to ensure that the prosthesis is patent and is correctly placed.

Complications

Incorrect positioning of the prosthesis is a frequent problem. Attention to the details of endoscopic marking is very important. Also crucial is correct selection of a stent: stents shorten from both ends as they are deployed, and this must be taken into account in selecting the correct stent length. On occasion, the stent may migrate as a result of tumor-related necrosis or incorrect placement. If it migrates into the stomach, it can usually be captured in a snare and retrieved.

RETRIEVAL OF FOREIGN BODIES

Many ingested foreign bodies pass through the GI tract uneventfully, but a good number must be removed by endoscopic means—in particular, foreign bodies in the esophagus, sharp objects that are likely to perforate the bowel, and objects that do not progress from the stomach.

If the ingested object is of an unfamiliar type, it is an extremely good idea to practice with a similar object outside the patient before attempting endoscopic retrieval. This preparatory step allows one to select the most appropriate accessory and technique for removing the object.

Technique

Objects with sharp edges should be removed with the sharp end trailing to prevent perforation. In some cases, this means that the object must be pushed into the stomach and turned

Figure 4 **Therapeutic esophagogastroduodenoscopy: stenting of esophageal tumors. (*a*) An esophageal tumor is dilated. (*b, c*) A compressed expandable metal stent is positioned within the tumor and deployed. (*d*) The expanded stent yields a large enough lumen to permit the patient to continue oral alimentation.**

around before being removed. If multiple foreign bodies are present or if it is highly likely that the foreign body will injure the esophagus if removed in the standard manner, an overtube should be placed over the scope before insertion. The overtube enables one to pass the instrument several times and retrieve any sharp objects without injuring the esophagus; it also helps ensure that the object is not aspirated into the airway. If the patient is a child, general anesthesia may be advisable.

Perhaps the best method of removing foreign bodies is to surround them with a simple polypectomy snare and secure them in the endoscope's grasp. Meat boluses that form in the esophagus or proximal to a gastric band may be extremely difficult to dislodge; the use of a variceal ligator cap to produce a suction chamber can be helpful in such situations.

Complications

Endoscopic removal of foreign bodies is extremely safe and effective. Care must be taken to ensure that the esophagus is not injured during removal of the object. If the object is deeply embedded or refractory to removal, a surgical approach is preferred.

PERCUTANEOUS ENDOSCOPIC GASTROSTOMY

Since 1980, endoscopically guided placement of a tube gastrostomy has been widely employed to provide access to the GI tract for feeding or decompression. Indications for percutaneous endoscopic gastrostomy (PEG) include various disease processes that interfere with swallowing, such as severe neurologic impairment, oropharyngeal tumors, and facial trauma. PEG has also been employed to establish a route for recycling bile in patients with malignant biliary obstruction, to provide supplemental feeding in selected patients with inflammatory bowel disease, and to accomplish gastric decompression in patients with conditions such as carcinomatosis, radiation enteritis, and diabetic gastropathy.

Technique

The patient fasts for 8 hours beforehand, and a single prophylactic dose of an antibiotic is administered just before the procedure is begun. The patient is placed in the supine position, a topical anesthetic is applied to the posterior pharynx, and intravenous sedation is begun. A forward-viewing endoscope is passed into the esophagus and advanced into the stomach. The abdomen is prepared in a sterile fashion and draped. The stomach and the duodenum are then inspected.

The room lights are dimmed, and the light of the endoscope is used to transilluminate the abdominal wall so as to indicate a point where the gastric wall and the abdominal wall are in close proximity. Finger pressure is applied to various areas of the abdomen until a spot is identified at which such pressure produces clear indentation of the gastric wall. An endoscopic snare is deployed through the biopsy channel of the endoscope to cover this spot, and a local anesthetic is infiltrated into the overlying skin [see Figure 5]. A 1 cm skin incision is made at the chosen spot, and a needle is passed through the incision and into the gastric lumen. The endoscopic snare is tightened around the needle, and a wire is passed through the needle and into the gastric lumen. The snare is moved so as to surround the wire, which is then pulled out of the patient's mouth. The gastrostomy tube is fastened to the wire and pulled in a retrograde manner down the esophagus and into the stomach. The gastroscope is subsequently reinserted to ensure that the head of the catheter is correctly positioned against the gastric mucosa [see Figure 6].

An outer crossbar is put in place to prevent inward migration of the tube and to hold the stomach in approximation to the

Figure 5 Therapeutic esophagogastroduodenoscopy: percutaneous endoscopic gastrostomy. The first steps in the procedure involve selecting a proper site in the stomach and using a snare to surround a needle that has been passed through the abdominal and gastric walls.

Figure 6 Therapeutic esophagogastroduodenoscopy: percutaneous endoscopic gastrostomy. After the suture is retrieved from the stomach, it is affixed to the gastrostomy tube and used to pull the tube back into the stomach and out the abdominal wall. The gastroscope is reinserted to follow the process and ensure that the final position of the tube is correct.

abdominal wall. The crossbar should remain several millimeters from the skin to prevent excessive tension, which would cause ischemic necrosis of the underlying tissue.

Complications

Local wound infections are the most common complications of PEG. They can be minimized by administering preoperative antibiotics and ensuring that excessive tension is not applied to the crossbar at the end of the procedure. When such infections do occur, they can usually be treated via simple drainage and local wound care; sacrifice of the gastrostomy is rarely necessary. Several other complications, such as early extrusion of the tube, progressive enlargement of the tract, and separation of the gastric and abdominal walls with leakage of feedings into the abdominal cavity, are also most often attributable to excessive crossbar tension and subsequent ischemia. Gastrocolic fistula can occur after PEG. This problem may not be obvious for months afterward, but severe diarrhea after feedings is grounds for suspicion. Once the PEG tract is mature, gastrocolic fistulas usually close quickly after simple removal of the gastrostomy tube.

Diagnostic Endoscopic Retrograde Cholangiopancreatography

Endoscopic retrograde cholangiopancreatography (ERCP) is an advanced procedure that is technically more challenging than standard upper GI endoscopy; however, it can be mastered by most endoscopists who are willing to dedicate sufficient time to learning the method. ERCP yields a radiologic image of the pancreatic and biliary trees, and in many cases, it provides access for therapy. Indications for ERCP include suspected benign or malignant maladies of the common bile duct (CBD), the ampulla of Vater, or the pancreas. Cholelithiasis per se is not an indication for ERCP unless choledocholithiasis is suspected.

TECHNIQUE

As with standard upper GI endoscopy, the patient fasts for 6 to 8 hours beforehand. Intravenous sedation is administered, and prophylactic antibiotics are given when biliary obstruction is suspected. The patient is initially placed in the left lateral decubitus position but is later rotated to the prone position after the scope is in place in the second portion of the duodenum. A side-viewing endoscope is employed because it allows the best visualization of the ampulla of Vater. The instrument is passed into the esophagus and maneuvered through the stomach, across the pylorus, and into the duodenum. Manipulation of a side-viewing instrument is a bit awkward for the novice but is easily learned.

Once the endoscope is in the second portion of the duodenum, it is pulled back so that the gastric loop is straightened and the tip of the scope occupies a better position with regard to the papilla. This so-called short scope position is generally best for work in the CBD [see Figure 7]. The papilla of Vater (also known as the major duodenal papilla) appears as a small longitudinal nubbin crossing the horizontal semicircular folds of the duodenum, generally in the 12 to 1 o'clock position. At its tip, a small, soft, reticulated area may be noted; this is the papillary orifice. Often, a small mucosal protuberance is seen just proximal and to the right of the papilla of Vater; this is the minor duodenal papilla.

A small plastic cannula is passed through the channel of the endoscope and introduced into the ampullary orifice, and contrast material is injected under fluoroscopic control to provide visualization of the CBD and the pancreatic duct. The two may share a single orifice within the ampulla or may have separate orifices. The CBD exits the papilla in a cephalad direction, tangential to the duodenal wall. The bulge of the ampulla within the duodenum represents the intramural segment of the duct. The orifice of the CBD is typically found at the 11 o'clock position in the ampulla. The pancreatic duct leaves the papilla in a perpendicular fashion. Its orifice is usually in the 1 o'clock area of the papilla [see Figure 8].

COMPLICATIONS

When contrast material is being injected into the pancreatic ductal system, care must be taken to avoid overfilling, which can lead to acinarization, or rupture of the small ductules, with extravasation of contrast material into the pancreatic parenchyma; pancreatitis is a frequent consequence of acinarization. Cholangitis may result when contrast is injected proximal to an obstruction of the biliary tree. When obstruction is demonstrated, drainage of the system by means of stone extraction, stenting, or nasobiliary intubation is important to prevent cholangitis.

Therapeutic Endoscopic Retrograde Cholangiopancreatography

Therapeutic interventions that may be accomplished at the time of ERCP include sphincterotomy for ductal access or ampullary stenosis, removal of CBD stones, dilation of benign and malignant biliary strictures, and insertion of stents to maintain ductal patency. Pancreatic duct interventions include removal of stones, bridging of ductal disruptions, and drainage of pseudocysts.

TECHNIQUE

All therapeutic applications of ERCP must begin with selective cannulation of the duct being treated. Frequently, a guide wire is then introduced deep into the duct to provide a means of obtaining access to the duct on an ongoing basis and to ensure correct

a

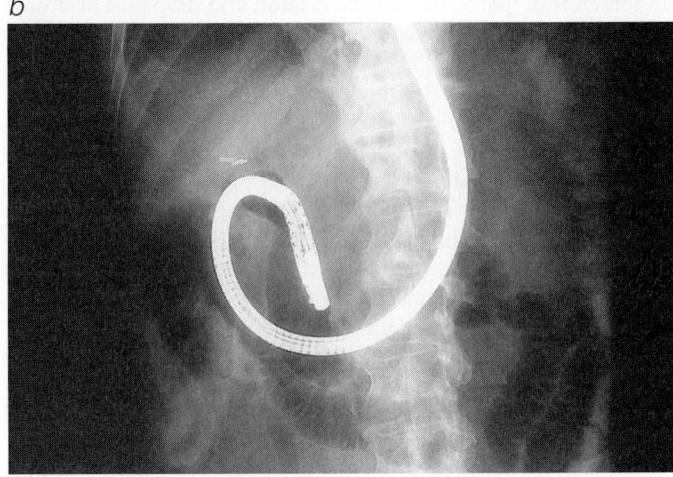

b

Figure 7 **Diagnostic endoscopic retrograde cholangiopancreatography. (*a*) The so-called short scope position, along the lesser curve of the stomach, is usually the most effective in biliary interventions. (*b*) The so-called long scope position may be necessary at times.**

Figure 8 Diagnostic endoscopic retrograde cholangiopancreatography. The so-called long scope position, along the greater curve of the stomach, may be useful in some pancreatic interventions; shown is the pancreatic duct orifice.

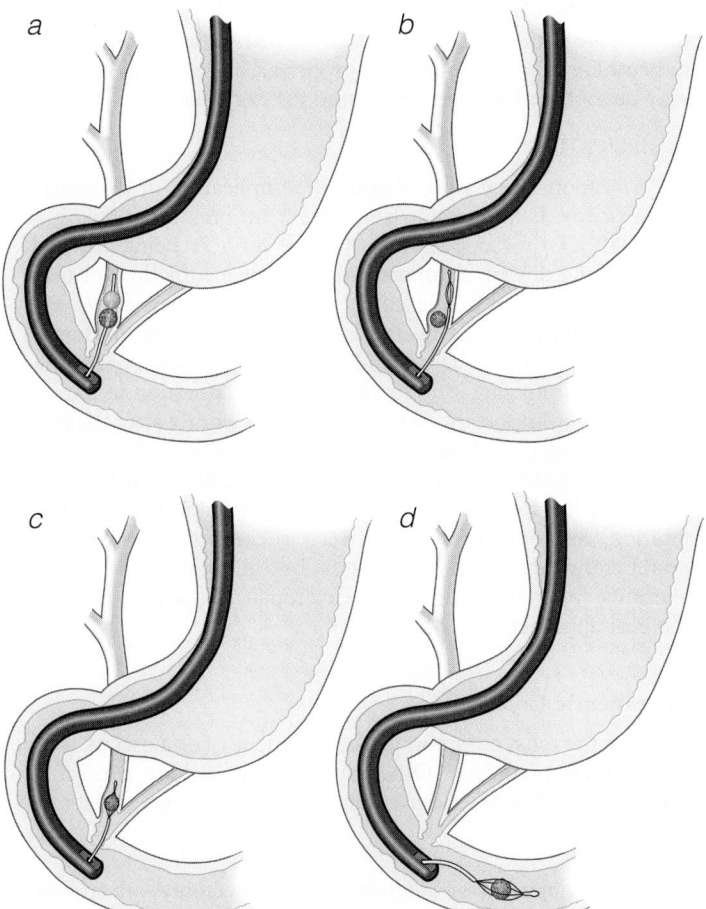

Figure 9 Therapeutic endoscopic retrograde cholangiopancreatography. After endoscopic sphincterotomy, CBD stones may be retrieved with balloons (*a*) or baskets (*b, c, d*).

positioning for intraductal manipulations. After electrosurgical division of the papilla, biliary stones are retrieved with balloon or baskets [*see Figure 9*]. Often, large stones can be captured within the duct in mechanical lithotripsy baskets and crushed before removal.

Strictures should be brushed for cytologic evaluation once they have been traversed by a wire. They may then be dilated with hydrostatic balloons under fluoroscopic guidance and stented [*see Figure 10*]. Plastic stents are used for most benign and many malignant strictures; however, self-expanding metal stents are now being used more frequently for malignant strictures because they remain patent longer [*see Figure 11*].

COMPLICATIONS

Perforation can occur during endoscopic sphincterotomy as a result of extension or tearing of the papilla beyond the junction of the CBD with the duodenal wall. Retroperitoneal or free intraperitoneal air may be seen. In many cases, intravenous antibiotics, hydration, and avoidance of oral intake are sufficient to manage such complications. If the patient's condition deteriorates, surgical exploration is indicated.

Bleeding may also occur with sphincterotomy. It is usually controllable with injection of epinephrine solution (1:10,000), electrocoagulation, or balloon tamponade. Arteriographic embolization of the gastroduodenal artery may be helpful in some cases. As with diagnostic ERCP, pancreatitis may occur; it usually responds to conservative measures.

Diagnostic Colonoscopy

Colonoscopy has become one of the most frequently performed endoscopic examinations. It has revolutionized the diagnosis and treatment of colonic disease and offers the promise of reducing the occurrence of colon cancer. Indications for colonoscopy include iron deficiency anemia, frank or occult rectal bleeding, a history of colonic cancer in the patient or in first-degree family members, a history or suspicion of colonic polyps, inflammatory bowel disease, and a persistent change in bowel habits. Preparation involves purging the bowel mechanically by placing the patient on a clear liquid diet for several days, then giving cathartics and enemas; alternatively, one may use osmotic lavage, in which 1 gal of lavage fluid is administered orally over a period of 4 hours. It is often helpful to administer 10 mg of metoclopramide to enhance gastric motility as preparation begins.

TECHNIQUE

Sedation is accomplished as for upper GI endoscopy, and the patient fasts for 6 to 8 hours before the procedure. With the patient in the left lateral decubitus position, a rectal examination is performed. This step helps relax the anal sphincter in preparation for insertion of the scope and ensures that low-lying rectal lesions are not overlooked.

The colonoscope is introduced into the rectal vault, and insufflation of air is commenced. The instrument is advanced only when the lumen is clearly apparent. At times, only a portion of the lumen may be visible, but this is usually enough to guide advancement of the scope. Frequently, when the lumen itself is not visible, light reflected onto the colonic folds can guide one to the lumen, with the concavity of the fold indicating the direction of the lumen. In contrast with upper GI endoscopy, in which torsion on the shaft of the endoscope is rarely necessary, such torsion is the rule in colonoscopy. The shaft of the instrument is rotated with the right hand to facilitate

Figure 10 **Therapeutic endoscopic retrograde cholangiopancreatography. CBD strictures (*a*), whether benign or malignant, may be dilated effectively with hydrostatic balloons under fluoroscopic guidance (*b*).**

straightening and intubation of the colon. By applying torsion to the shaft frequently and pulling back the scope as necessary, one can pleat the colon on the instrument as it is advanced. Pulling back is one of the most useful techniques for advancing the colonoscope through the colon.

The colon exhibits a number of characteristic anatomic features that are readily observed during colonoscopy. The sigmoid colon, because of its frequent turns, yields elliptical views of the lumen. The descending colon appears as a long, round tunnel with little haustration. The transverse colon has well-defined triangular folds, and the hepatic flexure may exhibit a blue hue resulting from the proximity of the liver. The cecum is recognized on the basis of the appearance of the ileocecal valve on the lateral wall, the convergence of the colonic taenia to form the cecal strap (the so-called Mercedes sign), and the presence of the appendiceal orifice.

Insertion of the colonoscope as far as the hepatic flexure is rarely difficult. Occasionally, the sigmoid colon presents a chal-

lenge, in which case placement of the patient on the back or the abdomen to change the orientation may be helpful. Once again, pulling back and straightening the scope is a highly useful maneuver. Once the scope is in the hepatic flexure looking down the right colon, pulling back, counterclockwise torsion, and the application of suction may all assist in advancing the instrument into the cecum. Changing the patient's position or applying pressure to various points in the abdomen may also be helpful. Once the cecum is reached, the instrument is slowly withdrawn while the colonic parietes are carefully examined. Biopsy and cytologic brushing may be done as appropriate, and colonic contents may be aspirated into a suction trap for examination.

COMPLICATIONS

Perforation is the most common complication of diagnostic colonoscopy. It may result from direct tip pressure, bowing of the shaft of the scope while a large loop is being formed, blowout of a diverticulum secondary to air insufflation, or tearing of an adhesion of the colon to an adjacent structure. The risk of perforation can be minimized by observing the lumen directly as the scope is advanced, avoiding excessive insufflation, and minimizing loop formation. Close attention to patient discomfort is important. If the patient feels poorly after the procedure, an upright chest x-ray, an upright abdominal x-ray, or a lateral decubitus abdominal x-ray should be obtained to determine whether there is any free air, which would indicate a perforation. Such situations have been successfully managed by nonoperative means in some cases, but in most cases, prompt operative intervention with primary repair of the perforation is the best approach.

Therapeutic Colonoscopy

By far the most common use of therapeutic colonoscopy is for the excision of polyps. Other applications include control of bleeding, dilation of strictures, and placement of enteral stents.

TECHNIQUE

The development of colonoscopic polypectomy—electrosurgical excision of the polyp with a wire snare—has rendered operative colotomy unnecessary in the management of colonic polyps. Pedunculated polyps are approached by placing the snare over the polyp's head and tightening the loop around the

Figure 11 **Therapeutic endoscopic retrograde cholangiopancreatography. Self-expanding metal stents may provide effective long-term palliation of malignant biliary obstruction.**

Figure 12 Therapeutic colonoscopy. Shown is removal of a pedunculated colonic polyp by means of snare excision at the stalk.

Figure 13 Therapeutic colonoscopy. Illustrated is piecemeal excision of a sessile colonic polyp.

stalk near the junction of the head and the stalk [*see Figure 12*]. Because the stalk is an extension of normal mucosa, it is unnecessary—and often unwise—to excise the stalk close to the colonic wall; excision near the head of the polyp is usually sufficient. Short bursts of coagulating current are applied to transect the stalk. During excision, the polyps must be moved around to prevent conduction burns to the opposing colonic wall. Once transection is complete, if the polyp is small, it may be suctioned into a trap; if it is large, it may be suctioned onto the tip of the scope and retrieved or captured in a snare or basket. Sessile polyps are more challenging and risky to excise. Accordingly, it is often preferable to excise such polyps in a piecemeal fashion [*see Figure 13*]. The snare is applied several times to successive portions of the polyp until it is excised down to the colonic wall. The excised fragments are then retrieved. Difficult or large sessile polyps may be elevated before excision by injecting epinephrine solution or saline submucosally into the polyp or the surrounding tissue. This maneuver makes transmural injury less likely (see below).

Although the use of colonoscopy to define the site of colonic bleeding is commonplace, its use to treat such bleeding is not.

Figure 14 Therapeutic colonoscopy. Shown is an angiodysplasia of the right colon, a frequent cause of lower GI hemorrhage.

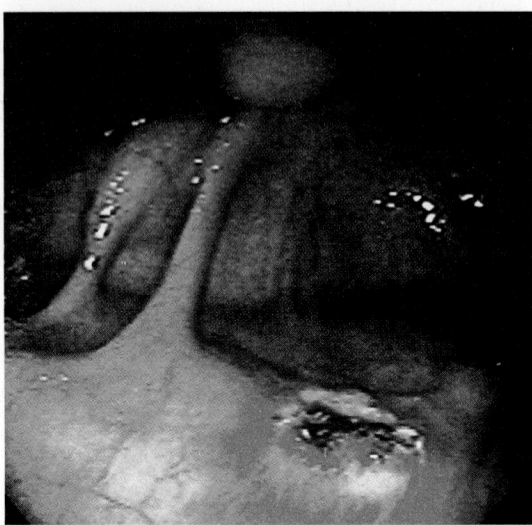

Figure 15 **Therapeutic colonoscopy. Shown is a right colonic angiodysplasia after treatment with bipolar electrocoagulation.**

Diverticular bleeding often stops when colonoscopy is done, and only in rare instances is the actual bleeding diverticulum seen. In such cases, injection of epinephrine solution around the mouth of the offending diverticulum is often effective. Angiodysplasias are frequently found in the right colon, though they are rarely identified while they are bleeding [*see Figure 14*]. They may be treated with a variety of modalities, including bipolar electrocoagulation, injection of a sclerosant solution, and laser therapy [*see Figure 15*]. Currently, the argon plasma coagulator is often employed for obliteration of these lesions. This device has the advantage of being able to obliterate angiodysplasias with minimal wall penetration, thereby increasing the safety of this intervention in the thin-walled right colon.

Strictures may occur in the colon, as in the rest of the GI tract. Colonic strictures usually develop at an anastomosis, though they may also be the result of ischemia. Hydrostatic balloon dilation is very effective in treating such strictures. The balloon is introduced through the lumen of the endoscope, and dilation is carried out under direct vision, often in conjunction with fluoroscopic observation to confirm that dilation is complete. In patients with fully or almost fully obstructing tumors of the colon, self-expanding metal stents may be placed to provide decompression and at least temporary relief of obstruction. This step may avert emergency surgery or, if the tumor is inoperable, provide palliation.

COMPLICATIONS

Perforation may occur as a result of transmural thermal injury during polypectomy. Some perforations are immediately apparent, but others may not be noticed for several days. When perforation is documented, surgical exploration is indicated. Occasionally, a patient may present with fever and abdominal tenderness several days after polypectomy but show no free air on abdominal films. Such a patient may have a thermal injury to the bowel wall or so-called postpolypectomy syndrome and can usually be treated with intravenous fluids, antibiotics, and observation. Bleeding from the stalk of a pedunculated polyp may occur after excision; it may present immediately or may be delayed until the coagulum on the stalk separates 3 to 5 days after polypectomy. Such bleeding is a rare occurrence. When it does occur, it can be treated by injecting epinephrine solution (1:10,000) into the stalk.

Chromoendoscopy

The development of extirpative endoscopy has allowed physicians to treat several conditions that previously required open or laparoscopic surgical procedures. However, it is not always possible to see the difference between diseased and healthy tissue on endoscopy, and this limitation has precluded one-stage procedures. Identification of tissue types required biopsy, and lesion margins were impossible to determine at the time of the procedure.

Chromoendoscopy can help to identify diseased tissue and define lesion borders. This process is essentially an in vivo staining technique in which a variety of specialized stains are applied to tissues to improve their characterization. This differs from carbon-dye injection (tattooing), a technique that is used for later surgical identification, in that the stains used for chromoendoscopy are specific to the anatomic area being examined. Several chromoendoscopic dyes are commercially available in the United States [*see Table 1*]. Selection of a particular agent is based on the type of tissue being studied, the disease state, and physician familiarity.

One of the first agents used for chromoendoscopy was methylene blue. It was initially used in Japan in the 1970s to detect intestinal metaplasia in the stomach. Subsequent studies in the United States, Japan, and Europe independently demonstrated that methylene blue will selectively stain metaplasia in Barrett's esophagus (see above). On routine screening endoscopy in patients with Barrett's esophagus, methylene blue chromoendoscopy offers improved detection of dysplasia and early malignancy compared with four-quadrant random biopsy studies. Other reported applications include esophageal carcinoma, gastric metaplasia, oropharyngeal cancer, mucosal lesions, and heterotopic gastric mucosa.

Endoscopic Mucosal Resection

Endoscopic polypectomy marked the beginning of extirpative procedures. Subsequently, endoscopic resection techniques have continued to advance, as a result of improvements in imaging and instrumentation, along with the development of chromoendoscopy and specific techniques designed as adjuncts to tissue removal. One such technique is endoscopic mucosal resection (EMR).

EMR has its basis in the anatomy of the GI tract. Histologically, the GI tract has three layers: a superficial mucosal, a middle submucosal, and an outer muscular layer. EMR is designed to help the endoscopist remove superficial mucosal tissue while leaving the deeper submucosal and muscular layers intact. These layers can be relatively easily separated from each other by injecting a liquid that spreads within the plane of injection. This step elevates the layers superficial to the injection, thus facilitating the resection of those layers. Advantages over other resection techniques include the preservation of histologic architecture (in contrast to electrocautery or laser ablation), which allows improved pathologic assessment; the ease with which EMR can be combined with endoscopic ultrasonography; and its safety and minimal invasiveness.

EMR was first described in 1955, when submucosal saline injections through a rigid sigmoidoscope were used in the resection of rectal and sigmoid polyps. In 1973, a submucosal saline injection was employed to assist with the removal of sessile polyps throughout the colon. Additional development was accomplished in Japan in 1983, when mucosal resection was used in the treatment of early gastric carcinoma in a technique termed strip-off biopsy. The technique has been refined and is now routinely used for lesions in the esophagus, stomach, duodenum, colon, and rectum. It is widely incorporated into aggressive screening programs designed to detect early GI cancers.

EMR can be used to treat dysplastic and other premalignant lesions, as well as superficial cancers of the GI tract. One must be careful to comply with all standard principles of cancer resection, including knowledge of the depth of the lesion, its radial extent, and staging. Consequently, several criteria must be fulfilled before EMR can be viewed as a curative intervention. Classification of lesions on the basis of their endoscopic appearance can be combined with information obtained through the use of chromoendoscopy and EUS to determine the potential for EMR.

Lesion location within the GI tract is important with respect to long-term outcomes. For example, EMR can be used to treat circumferential colonic lesions but is inappropriate for esophageal lesions that extend beyond one third of the circumference, because of the risk of a late stricture.

Although specific methods differ among practitioners, several generalizations about the technical aspects can be made. First, a liquid must be injected deep to the mucosal layer, allowing separation of the wall components. Although the ideal solution for injection has not been determined, the liquid chosen must be biodegradable, biocompatible, noninflammatory, and have viscoelastic properties allowing the development of an adequate bleb. Saline, hypertonic saline, epinephrine, hyaluronic acid, and glycerol solutions are all in current use. The elevated tissue is then held in place with a grasper or suction mechanism, and snares, needle knives, or lasers are used to cut the tissue at its base. Optimal results are obtained on nonulcerated lesions that are less than 2 cm after elevation; other lesions have a high probability of submucosal lymphatic and vascular invasion.

Although complications can occur, with proper patient selection and procedural refinement they are relatively rare. Perforation has been noted, particularly when submucosal bleb formation is suboptimal. Inadequate blebs may result from insufficient liquid being injected, improper needle depth, or severe scarring of the local tissues. Bleeding has been reported to occur in 1.6% of EMR cases. This complication is relatively easily handled with a combination of electrocautery and epinephrine injection. Infection in the absence of perforation is uncommon.

Overall, EMR provides a minimally invasive means to treat early cancers in favorable locations. Patients must understand that additional resection may be required if histopathologic assessment does not show curative margins. Future development of endoscopic instruments and injection liquids will likely broaden the applicability of the procedure.

Endoscopic Ultrasonography

The 1980s saw the introduction of EUS. Extracavitary ultrasonographic methods have been hampered by the presence of air within the GI tract, which precludes high-resolution imaging. Consequently, they had been relegated to gross estimates of disease and detection of displacement of other tissues or fluid accumulation proximal to stenoses, such as ductal dilation in patients with common bile duct stones.

Three advances have proven invaluable in allowing EUS to carve out a niche in the field of GI diagnosis. First is the improvement in endoscopes that allows transducer and receiver channels to traverse a tortuous path. Second is the development of multiple frequency options in conjunction with circumferential visualization. Higher frequencies provide higher resolutions, allowing useful differentiation of the various layers of the intestinal tract. Third is the evolution of treatment protocols keyed to the accu-

Table 1 Special Stains Used in Endoscopy

Stain	Site of Use	Comment
Lugol solution (2% iodine)	Esophagus	Normal mucosa stains green-brown (as a result of intracellular glycogen); dysplastic cells do not stain
Indigo carmine (0.4% solution)	Stomach, colon	Enhances contour of mucosa, giving tissue a three-dimensional appearance
Toluidine blue	Oropharynx, esophagus	Absorbed by the nucleic acid component of malignant epithelial cells
Congo red	Acid-secreting areas of gastric mucosa	Turns a blue-black color when pH < 3
Methylene blue (0.5% solution)	Intestinal metaplasia, Barrett's esophagus	Absorbed only by dysplastic tissue; however, absorption decreases as severe dysplasia develops

rate staging of tumors—information that is sometimes unobtainable from other imaging techniques.

This technology has now been firmly established as an accurate way to identify carcinoma. More recent developments are allowing EUS to expand from the field of diagnosis into the realm of intervention. Examples of EUS-guided procedures include fine-needle aspiration, lymph node sampling, and drainage of pancreatic pseudocysts.

EUS devices come in both linear and radial transducers. Radial transducers have the advantage of providing circumferential visualization that parallels the standard modes of perceiving the GI tract. Linear images allow EUS-directed biopsies and have the potential to provide color and pulsed Doppler imaging. Probes can be mounted on the top of an oblique viewing fiberoptic scope, or come in an over-the-wire format for use in the pancreaticobiliary tree. A series of frequencies is available, with the higher frequencies providing greater resolution but less tissue depth penetration. Lower-frequency probes allow deeper tissue assessment and a broader view, but at the price of reduced resolution. Nevertheless, any form of EUS will provide better resolution than transcutaneous ultrasonography, allowing markedly improved two-point discrimination and hence more accurate tissue diagnosis.

The benefits of accurate staging of GI tumors paved the way for EUS development. Tissue sampling techniques are further benefited by this technology. The sensitivity of EUS makes it one of the best modalities for the evaluation and detection of pancreatic tumors. Its sensitivity, which is in excess of 95%, contrasts favorably with those of other modalities, including ultrasonography (75%), computed tomography (80%), and angiography (89%). The accuracy of T staging by EUS in esophageal cancer (80% to 90%) is greater than that of staging determined by CT scanning (50% to 60%). This finding has led to the development of several staging schemes that are based solely on EUS findings. EUS has established a role in the identification of early pancreatitis; the detection of common bile duct stones and mediastinal masses; and the assessment of anastomotic strictures, thickened gastric folds, and the integrity of the anal sphincter. It has also proved a useful adjunct in the determination of whether a tumor is amenable to EMR techniques or is better served by adjuvant therapies or surgical interventions.

The sensitivity of EUS is rooted in its ability to delineate the various layers of the alimentary canal. Experienced endoscopists can easily evaluate the submucosa and differentiate intramural from extrinsic masses. Characteristic patterns are readily learned and rapidly recognized, obviating tissue diagnoses in straightforward cases. Criteria have also been established to aid in the differentiation of benign and malignant lesions. With the continued use of this technique, additional algorithms will be established in conjunction with more innovative interventional adjuncts. However, two limitations have caused many practitioners to remain skeptical: cost and training issues. Other imaging modalities, such as CT and magnetic resonance imaging, have also made tremendous strides in the recent past. Although these various modalities are often considered competitors—a view arising from the perceived need for a single imaging modality—the issue of which is superior to the others pales in comparison to the benefits that can be gained from combining imaging techniques in appropriate circumstances.

Endoscopic Suturing

The ability to suture through an endoscope would open up an entire arena of new possibilities, including antireflux procedures, morbid obesity surgery, and advances in the control of acute hemorrhage, as well as improved ability to manage complications of other endoscopic techniques. Despite the development and commercial availability of numerous devices, however, design problems have relegated most applications to investigational status. For such devices to enter clinical practice, they must encompass fundamental surgical techniques: the ability to cut, suture, tie knots, and staple. These are critical for maintaining hemostasis and constructing durable anastomoses. Although these techniques are plausible with modern devices, continued innovation and experience in conjunction with a new paradigm of disease management will direct the future of endoscopic interventions.

Recommended Reading

Abi-Hanna D, Williams SJ: Advances in gastrointestinal endoscopy. Med J Aust 170:131, 1999

Acosta MM, Boyce HW Jr: Chromoendoscopy—where is it useful? J Clin Gastroenterol 27:13, 1998

Brugge WR: Endoscopic ultrasonography: the current status. Gastroenterology 115:1577, 1998

Canto M: Methylene blue chromoendoscopy for Barrett's esophagus: coming soon to your GI unit? Gastrointest Endosc 54:403, 2001

Cotton PB, Williams CB: Practical Gastrointestinal Endoscopy, 3rd ed. Blackwell Scientific, Oxford, 1990

Hawes RH: Endoscopic ultrasound. Gastrointest Endosc Clin N Am 10:161, 2000

Hawes RH: Perspectives in endoscopic mucosal resection. Gastrointest Endosc Clin N Am 11:549, 2001

Inoue H: Endoscopic mucosal resection for the entire gastrointestinal mucosal lesions. Gastrointest Endosc Clin N Am 11:459, 2001

Matsuda K: Introduction to endoscopic mucosal resection. Gastrointest Endosc Clin N Am 11:439, 2001

Ponchon T: Endoscopic mucosal resection. J Clin Gastroenterol 32:6, 2001

Ponsky JL: Atlas of Surgical Endoscopy. Mosby–Year Book, St. Louis, 1992

Ponsky JL, King JF: Endoscopic marking of colonic lesions. Gastrointest Endosc 22:42, 1975

Rosch T, Lightdale CJ, Botel JF, et al: Localization of pancreatic endocrine tumors by endoscopic ultrasound. N Engl J Med 326:1721, 1992

Rosen M, Ponsky JL: Endoscopic therapy for gastroesophageal reflux disease. Semin Laparosc Surg 8:207, 2001

Schrock T: Colon and rectum: diagnostic techniques. Shackelford's Surgery of the Alimentary Tract. Vol 4: Colon and Anorectum, 3rd ed. Condon R, Ed. Philadelphia, WB Saunders Co, 1991, p 22

Schuman BM, Sugawa C: Diagnostic endoscopy of upper gastrointestinal bleeding. Gastrointestinal Bleeding. Sugawa C, Schuman BM, Lucas CE, Eds. Igaku Shoin, New York, 1992, p 222

Soetikno R, Inoue H, Chang KJ: Endoscopic muscosal resection: current concepts. Gastrointest Endosc Clin N Am 10:595, 2000

Swain CP: Endoscopic sewing and stapling machines. Endoscopy 29:205, 1997

Venu RP, Geenen JE: Overview of endoscopic sphincterotomy for common bile duct stone. Endoscopic Approach to Biliary Stones. Kozarek RA, Ed. Gastrointest Endosc Clin N Am 1:3, 1991

Acknowledgment

Figures 2, 4a, 4b, 4c, 5, 6, 9 12, 13   Tom Moore.

7 OPEN ESOPHAGEAL PROCEDURES

John Yee, M.D., and Richard J. Finley, M.D.

The remarkable advances in diagnosis, imaging, and surgical treatment of esophageal diseases over the past decade have resulted in markedly better patient outcomes. Ciné barium swallow remains the most cost-effective method of defining abnormal esophageal anatomy; however, high-quality endoscopic ultrasonography and computed tomography are now widely used to obtain information regarding mass lesions not only in the esophageal wall but also in the surrounding tissues. High-resolution endoscopy combined with photodynamic imaging or vital staining allows accurate diagnosis of dysplastic or malignant esophageal lesions in their earliest stages. Positron emission tomography (PET) and high-resolution CT scanning greatly facilitate identification of metastatic esophageal cancer. Refinements in the use of esophageal manometry, 24-hour esophageal pH tests, and esophageal and gastric nuclear transit studies, combined with improvements in endoscopic and ciné barium swallow techniques, permit more accurate diagnosis and more effective treatment of gastroesophageal reflux disease (GERD) and of functional abnormalities of the esophagus.

In particular, operative techniques for treating esophageal disease have advanced considerably in recent years, as a result of our improved understanding of esophageal anatomy and physiology and the successful introduction of minimally invasive approaches to the esophagus [*see V:8 Minimally Invasive Esophageal Procedures*]. For a number of diseases (e.g., achalasia), minimally invasive procedures have proved to be as effective as their open counterparts while causing less postoperative morbidity. Nevertheless, the growing stature of minimally invasive approaches does not diminish the importance of the equivalent open approaches. In what follows, we describe common open operations performed to excise Zenker's diverticulum, to manage complex GERD, and to resect esophageal and proximal gastric tumors.

General Preoperative Considerations

Patients with obstructing esophageal diseases are often elderly, debilitated, and malnourished. Although months of insufficient nutrition cannot be corrected in the space of a few hours, anemia, dehydration, and electrolyte abnormalities can be mitigated by means of intravenous support and appropriate laboratory monitoring. If esophageal obstruction prevents oral intake, endoscopic dilatation of the stricture accompanied by either nasogastric intubation or percutaneous endoscopic gastrostomy (PEG) [*see V:6 Gastrointestinal Endoscopy*] is indicated. Enteral nutrition, comprising at least 2,000 kcal/day of a high-protein liquid diet, should be administered for at least 10 days before the operation. Cardiovascular, renal, hepatic, and respiratory function should be documented and optimized. If the patient is aspirating, the esophagus should be evacuated and the patient should be given nothing by mouth until after the operation. Aspiration pneumonia should always be corrected preoperatively.

Cricopharyngeal Myotomy and Excision of Zenker's Diverticulum

PREOPERATIVE EVALUATION

Patients who are candidates for cricopharyngeal myotomy usually present with difficulty initiating swallowing, dysphagia or odynophagia, and symptoms of pulmonary aspiration. These symptoms of cricopharyngeal dysfunction may or may not be associated with a Zenker's diverticulum. Ciné barium swallow studies may reveal poor pharyngeal contractility, pulmonary or nasal aspiration, abnormalities of the upper esophageal sphincter, pharyngeal pouches, or structural abnormalities. Zenker's diverticulum is a pulsion diverticulum that arises within the inferior pharyngeal constrictor, between the oblique fibers of the posterior pharyngeal constrictors and the cricopharyngeus muscle. This mucosal outpouching results from a transient incomplete opening of the upper esophageal sphincter: the diverticulum enlarges, drapes over the cricopharyngeus, and dissects behind the esophagus into the prevertebral space. The pouch usually deviates to one side or the other; accordingly, the side on which the deviation occurs must be determined by means of a barium swallow so that the appropriate operative approach can be selected. Esophageal motility studies may show either incomplete upper esophageal relaxation on swallowing or discoordination of the upper esophageal relaxation phase with pharyngeal contractions. Upper GI endoscopy is performed preoperatively to exclude the presence of a pharyngeal or esophageal carcinoma and to assess upper GI anatomy. If there is evidence of GERD, proton pump inhibitors are given.

In symptomatic patients (e.g., those with dysphagia, nocturnal cough, or recurrent pneumonia from aspiration), surgical therapy is indicated regardless of whether a pouch is present or how large it may be. Such treatment involves correcting the underlying cricopharyngeal muscle dysfunction with a cricopharyngeal myotomy. If there is a diverticulum larger than 2 cm, it should be excised in addition to the cricopharyngeal myotomy. Alternatively, the diverticulum can be managed via endoscopic obliteration of the common wall between the pharyngeal pouch and the esophagus with either a stapler or a laser. Cricopharyngeal discoordination may be temporarily relieved by injecting botulinum toxin into the cricopharyngeus muscle.

OPERATIVE PLANNING

The patient is placed on a clear fluid diet for 2 days before the operation. With the patient under general anesthesia, the trachea is intubated with a single-lumen endotracheal tube. A soft roll is placed behind the shoulders to extend the neck. The patient is placed in a 20° reverse Trendelenburg position, and the legs are wrapped with pneumatic calf compressors to prevent deep vein thrombosis (DVT). With the endotracheal tube placed to the left side of the mouth, a preliminary flexible esophagogastroscopy is performed to empty the diverticulum of food and to examine the esophagus and the stomach. The scope is then brought back up

Figure 1 **Cricopharyngeal myotomy and excision of Zenker's diverticulum. A soft roll is placed behind the shoulders to extend the neck. The head is turned to the side opposite the incision. The cricoid cartilage is palpated and marked. The skin is incised obliquely along the sternocleidomastoid muscle, as shown, or transversely in a skin crease at the level of the cricoid.**

into the oropharynx and moved into the pouch. The location of the diverticulum (left or right side) is confirmed by turning the room lights off and noting the light coming from the gastroscope.

OPERATIVE TECHNIQUE

Step 1: Incision and Dissection of Pharyngeal Pouch

The patient lies with the head turned away from the side on which the incision is made. The cricoid cartilage is palpated and marked. A 5 cm skin incision is made, either obliquely along the sternocleidomastoid muscle [*see Figure 1*] or transversely in a skin crease at the level of the cricoid. The platysma is divided in the same line. Self-retaining retractors are inserted. The anterior border of the sternocleidomastoid muscle is incised throughout its length. The omohyoid muscle and the sternohyoid and sternothyroid muscles are retracted [*see Figure 2*]. The sternocleidomastoid muscle is retracted laterally to expose the carotid sheath and the internal jugular vein. The middle thyroid vein is ligated and divided, and the thyroid gland and the trachea are retracted medially by the assistant's finger to minimize the risk of injury to the underlying recurrent laryngeal nerve. The deep cervical fascia is divided. The inferior thyroid artery is divided as laterally as possible. The carotid sheath is retracted laterally, and dissection is carried down to the prevertebral fascia [*see Figure 2*]. The endoscope placed in the diverticulum is palpated, and the pouch is dissected away from the cervical esophagus up as far as the pharyngoesophageal junction. The flexible endoscope is then removed from the pouch and

advanced into the thoracic esophagus so that it can be used as a stent for the cricopharyngeal myotomy. Dissection of the pharyngeal pouch is then completed.

Step 2: Myotomy

The esophageal myotomy is started approximately 3 cm below the cricopharyngeus muscle on the posterolateral esophageal wall [*see Figure 3a*]. The esophageal muscle is divided down to the mucosa, which is recognizable from its bluish coloration with the submucosal plexus overlying it. The esophageal muscle is dissected away from the mucosa with a right-angle dissector and divided with a low-intensity diathermy unit. The myotomy is then continued proximally through the cricopharyngeus muscle and up into the muscular wall of the hypopharynx for 2 cm if there is no diverticulum present. The hypopharynx is distinguished by a pronounced submucosal venous plexus. The muscle is then swept off the mucosa for 120°.

Step 3: Freeing or Excision of Diverticulum

If there is a diverticulum less than 2 cm in diameter, the cricopharyngeus is transected and the muscularis around the diverticulum is freed. The myotomy is extended onto the hypopharynx for 2 cm. The diverticulum may be suspended to the back wall of the pharynx. It should not be sutured to the prevertebral fascia, because the passage of sutures through the diverticulum can contaminate the fascia, leading to an increased risk of fascial infection.

If the diverticulum is more than 2 cm in diameter, it is excised with a linear stapler, which is placed at the base of the sac and pressed firmly against the esophagoscope [*see Figure 3b*]. Particular care must be taken at this point so as not to injure the recurrent laryngeal nerve. The stapler is fired, and the divertic-

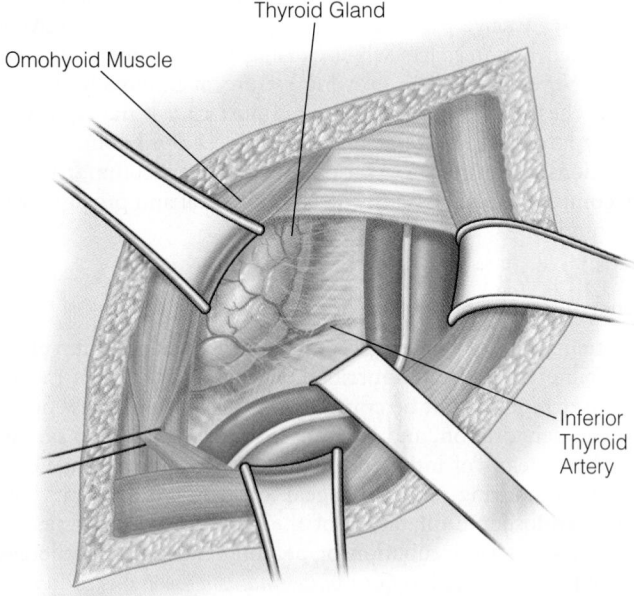

Figure 2 **Cricopharyngeal myotomy and excision of Zenker's diverticulum. The sternocleidomastoid is incised along the anterior border so as to expose the omohyoid muscle and the sternohyoid and sternothyroid muscles, which are retracted. The thyroid gland and the trachea are retracted medially by the assistant's finger, and the inferior thyroid artery is ligated and divided laterally to avoid injury to the recurrent laryngeal nerve.**

Figure 3 **Cricopharyngeal myotomy and excision of Zenker's diverticulum. (*a*) The diverticulum is dissected away from the esophagus, and an esophageal myotomy is started approximately 3 cm below the cricopharyngeus muscle. The myotomy is continued proximally through the cricopharyngeus, and the muscle around the diverticulum is freed. (*b*) A linear stapler is placed at the base of the sac and pressed firmly against the esophagoscope. The stapler is fired, and the diverticulum is excised.**

ulum is excised. The staple line is cleaned with an antiseptic solution, and the incision is filled with saline. The esophagus is insufflated with air to determine whether mucosal leakage has occurred, and the esophagoscope is removed; any mucosal leaks found are closed with fine absorbable sutures. In the absence of a stapler, the best way of excising the sac is to make a series of short incisions through the neck of the sac with scissors, suturing the edges after each cut with absorbable monofilament sutures (the so-called cut-and-sew technique). The esophagoscope ensures that the esophageal lumen is not narrowed.

Step 4: Drainage and Closure

Once hemostasis has been achieved, a short vacuum drain is placed through the skin into the retroesophageal space. The platysma is repaired with absorbable sutures, and the skin is closed with a subcuticular absorbable suture. Nasogastric intubation is unnecessary. Prokinetic agents and proton pump inhibitors are administered to prevent gastroesophageal reflux. A water-soluble contrast study is done on the day of the operation. If the results are normal, the patient is started on a liquid diet, and the drain is removed on postoperative day 1, when the patient is discharged.

COMPLICATIONS

The main complications associated with cricopharyngeal myotomy are recurrent laryngeal nerve trauma (0.5%), hematoma formation, infection (2%), aspiration, and recurrence (4%). Hematomas and infections must be drained promptly. Fistulas usually close once the prevertebral space is drained and the associated infection controlled. Aspiration is the most serious complication after cricopharyngeal myotomy. Gastroesophageal reflux may contribute to oropharnygeal dysphagia. Division of the upper esophageal sphincter in a patient with an incompetent esophagogastric junction may lead to massive tracheobronchial aspiration. Therefore, documented gastroesophageal reflux, gastroesophageal regurgitation, and severe distal esophagitis may be relative contraindications to cricopharyngeal myotomy until the lower esophageal sphincter defect has been remedied with an antireflux operation.

OUTCOME EVALUATION

Of patients with a Zenker's diverticulum, at least 90% experience excellent results from surgical treatment. Of patients without a Zenker's diverticulum, one third experience excellent results, another third show moderate improvement, and the remaining third show no improvement.[1] Patients with poor pharyngeal contractility in conjunction with normal upper esophageal sphincter function show little improvement with cricopharyngeal myotomy. Patients with oropharyngeal dysphagia secondary to neurologic involvement who have intact voluntary deglutination, adequate pulsion of the tongue, and normal phonation may show improvement with cricopharyngeal myotomy. Appropriate selection of patients for cricopharyngeal myotomy leads to better surgical outcomes.

Transthoracic Hiatal Hernia Repair

Unlike most operations on the esophagus, which are extirpative procedures, hiatal hernia repair with fundoplication is a reconstructive procedure. Currently, this repair is often accomplished via minimally invasive approaches; however, such approaches may be hampered by significant perceptual and motor limitations, such as loss of stereosis, reduced tactile feedback, and decreased range of motion for the instruments. In certain patients, laparoscopic reconstruction of a competent gastroesophageal high-pressure zone may be very difficult and may demand a degree of tactile sensitivity that is not yet achievable via videoendoscopy.

The long-term success of antireflux surgery, whether done transthoracically or laparoscopically, depends on three factors: (1) a tension-free repair that maintains a 4 cm long segment of esophagus in the intra-abdominal position, (2) durable approximation of the diaphragmatic crura, and (3) correct matching of the fundoplication technique chosen to the peristaltic function of the esophagus. The transthoracic approach should be considered whenever the standard abdominal approaches carry an increased risk of failure or complication—for instance, in patients who have a foreshortened esophagus, peptic strictures of the esophagus, an associated esophageal motility disorder, or a massive hiatal hernia with the stomach elevated into the chest; those who are morbidly obese; and those who have undergone multiple previous abdominal operations or in whom earlier antireflux procedures have failed.

PREOPERATIVE EVALUATION

Symptomatic Evaluation

All patients being considered for fundoplication to treat GERD must undergo a comprehensive evaluation to determine whether there is indeed an anatomic substrate for their symptoms and what the most appropriate form of repair is. Specifically, a history of heartburn and effortless regurgitation should be sought. Dysphagia and odynophagia are not typical and may reflect the presence of a stricture or a neoplasm. Atypical pain from cholelithiasis, peptic ulcer, or coronary artery disease may also confound the diagnosis.

Imaging

Radiographic investigation should begin with a ciné barium swallow, which may yield valuable information regarding the length of the esophagus, its peristaltic function, and the integrity of the mucosal surface. The gastric views can be used for qualitative assessment of emptying. Next, esophagogastroscopy should be performed to examine the mucosa for the presence of esophagitis, Barrett's mucosa, stricture, or malignancy. The locations of any lesions observed, along with the position of the squamocolumnar junction, should be carefully documented in terms of distance from the incisors. All strictures must undergo brush biopsy to rule out an occult malignancy. The presence of severe esophagitis raises the possibility of acquired shortening of the esophagus secondary to transmural inflammation and contraction scarring. Every effort should be made to measure the length of the esophagus accurately.

Dilatation

If a stricture is found during esophagoscopy, a decision must be made about whether to attempt esophageal dilatation. This procedure carries substantial risk and should only be done after careful consideration. If the stricture is diagnosed at the time of the initial endoscopic examination, it is advisable to perform only the brush biopsy at this point, deferring dilatation to a subsequent visit. Delaying dilatation gives the surgeon time to reassess the anatomy depicted on the barium swallow, to decide whether wire-guided or blind dilatation is indicated, to obtain informed consent, to assemble the requisite equipment, and to plan sedation for what is often an uncomfortable procedure.

The standard adult esophagoscope is approximately 32 French in caliber. In advancing the scope into the stricture, only very gentle pressure should be necessary. The weight of the dilator alone should be sufficient to effect its passage, with little or no forward force applied. As a rule, a mild stricture that is not associated with steep angulation of the esophagus will readily accept passage of the endoscope and will be amenable to subsequent blind dilation with Hurst-Maloney bougies. After successful passage, the scope is removed, and sequential insertion of progressively larger dilators (starting at 32 French) into the stricture is attempted. Although the patient will be able to swallow comfortably only after satisfactory passage of a dilator at least 48 French in caliber, it is essential never to try to force passage. To this end, the surgeon must take careful note of the subtle signs of increasing resistance transmitted through the dilator. Sequential dilation should be stopped whenever significant resistance is encountered or blood streaks appear on the dilator. Sudden pain during dilatation is an ominous sign that calls for immediate investigation with a water-soluble contrast swallow study. Perforation must be definitively ruled out before the patient can be discharged.

Highly stenotic strictures that do not allow the passage of a standard adult endoscope may be associated with a distorted and a steeply angulated esophagus. In such cases, the use of a pediatric endoscope may permit directed placement of a guide wire through the stricture; fluoroscopy is a useful adjunct for this purpose. A series of progressively larger Savary-Gillard dilators may then be passed over the guide wire to enlarge the lumen and allow subsequent endoscopic biopsy. The caveats that apply to blind dilation also apply to wire-guided dilation.

Patients whose esophagus can be dilated to 48 French and who are candidates for antireflux surgery may undergo subsequent intraoperative dilation to 54 to 60 French. Patients who cannot be dilated to 48 French and fail to achieve comfortable swallowing should be classified as having a nondilatable stricture and should be considered for transhiatal esophagectomy [see Resection of Esophagus and Proximal Stomach, below].

Functional Evaluation

Esophageal manometry permits quantitative assessment of peristalsis, a capability that is critically important for determining which type of fundoplication is most suitable for reconstructing a nonoccluding high-pressure zone at the esophagogastric junction. Stationary pH tests measure the capacity of the esophagus to clear acid, its sensitivity to instilled acid, the relationship of reflux episodes to body position, and the correlation between changes in esophageal pH and the subjective symptoms of heartburn. Ambulatory 24-hour pH testing allows further quantification of reflux episodes with respect to duration, frequency, and association with patient symptoms.

OPERATIVE PLANNING

Either a partial fundoplication (as in the 240° Belsey Mark IV procedure) or a complete fundoplication (as in the 360° Nissen procedure) may be performed. The extent of the wrap aside, the two procedures are essentially identical. Acquired shortening of the esophagus may necessitate lengthening of the esophagus by means of a Collis gastroplasty, in which the portion of the gastric cardia along the lesser curvature and directly contiguous to the distal esophagus is fashioned into a tube [see Operative Technique, Step 6a, below].

A thoracic epidural catheter is placed for regional analgesia. General anesthesia is administered, and flexible esophagoscopy is performed by the operating team. Insufflation should be done with the minimum amount of air practical, particularly in the case of large paraesophageal hernias. The extent of the pathologic condition is documented and the absence of malignancy verified. The stomach is decompressed and the endoscope removed. Tracheal intubation is then performed with either a standard single-lumen endotracheal tube or a double-lumen tube. The former requires that the ventilated left lung be retracted cephalad with moist packs during the procedure; the latter allows lung isolation and is preferred by some surgeons. A Foley catheter is placed; central venous access and arterial lines are generally not required. Subcutaneous heparin is administered for prophylaxis against deep vein thrombosis (DVT), and pneumatic calf compression devices are applied. Antibiotic prophylaxis is provided [see IV:5 Prevention of Postoperative Infection].

The patient is positioned for a left thoracotomy. The table is flexed to distract the ribs. An axillary roll is placed to protect the right brachial plexus. The right leg is bent at hip and knee while the left leg is kept straight. Pillows are placed between the legs, and all pressure points are padded. The arms are positioned so that the humeri are at right angles to the chest and the elbows bent 90°.

OPERATIVE TECHNIQUE

Step 1: Incision and Entry into Chest

A standard left posterolateral thoracotomy is performed. The latissimus dorsi muscle is divided. The serratus fascia is incised, but the muscle itself can generally be preserved. The paraspinal muscles are elevated away from the posterior aspect of the ribs, and a 1 cm segment of the seventh rib is resected to facilitate exposure. The chest is entered through the sixth interspace, and the lung and the pleural space are thoroughly inspected. The leaves of the retractor are spread slowly over a period of several minutes so as not to cause iatrogenic rib fractures.

Step 2: Exposure and Mobilization of Esophagus and Vagi

The inferior pulmonary ligament is divided with the electrocautery to the level of the inferior pulmonary vein [see Figure 4]. The mediastinal pleura overlying the esophagus is incised to expose the esophagus from the level of the carina to the diaphragm. Particular care is taken to avoid injury to the vagi. Vessels supplying the esophagus and arising from the adjacent aorta are ligated and divided. The esophagus is encircled just below the inferior pulmonary vein with a Penrose drain [see Figure 4]. The two vagi are mobilized and carried with the esophagus. (The right vagus is located along the right anterior border of the descending aorta and can easily be missed.)

The esophagus is then elevated, and mobilization is circumferentially completed in the direction of the diaphragm. The right pleura is closely approximated to the esophagus for 2 to 5 cm above the diaphragm; in the presence of a substantial hiatal hernia and its sac, it may be difficult to identify. The right pleura should be dissected away from the esophagus without entry into the right chest. If a tear occurs, it should be closed with absorbable suture material to prevent accumulation of blood and fluid on the right side during the operation. Dissection is continued to expose the right and left crura.

Step 3: Division of Phrenoesophageal Membrane and Gastrohepatic Ligament

The esophagus is retracted anteriorly to expose the posteriorly located phrenoesophageal membrane, which is then divided to yield entry into the peritoneum and exposure of the lesser sac. The remainder of the phrenoesophageal membrane is elevated with a right-angle clamp as it courses anteriorly, yielding a view of the spleen below. The esophagus is then mobilized from the left crus. The esophageal branch of the left phrenic artery, visible near the left vagus, is divided near the crus. Dissection proceeds

Figure 4 Transthoracic hiatal hernia repair. The lung is retracted, and the inferior pulmonary ligament is divided to the level of the inferior pulmonary vein. The mediastinal pleura overlying the esophagus is incised to expose the esophagus from the level of the carina to the diaphragm. The esophagus and both vagi are encircled just below the inferior pulmonary vein with a Penrose drain. Vessels supplying the esophagus and arising from the adjacent aorta are ligated and divided.

anteriorly until the distal end of the right crus is encountered at the apex of the hiatus; the right crus is then exposed posteriorly.

The uppermost portion of the gastrohepatic ligament is divided with the electrocautery. Belsey's artery, a communicating branch between the left gastric artery and the inferior phrenic artery, lies in this area and generally must be directly ligated. It is vital to divide the gastrohepatic ligament down to the level of the left gastric artery. The caudate lobe of the liver must be clearly visible. This opening is essential for subsequent passage of the fundoplication wrap behind the esophagus.

Step 4: Completion of Hiatal Dissection, Excision of Hernia Sac, and Ligation of Short Gastric Vessels

Dissection of the hiatus is completed along the right crus to the apex of the hiatus, thus joining the line of incision. Any hernia sac found is then excised. The highest short gastric arteries are ligated between ties to permit mobilization of the fundus. Excessive traction must be avoided to prevent splenic injury. Three or four vessels are usually divided. The esophagogastric junction is then elevated into the chest.

Step 5: Closure of Crura

Because the right crus is often quite attenuated, it is crucial to incorporate an adequate amount of tissue into the repair. An Allis clamp is placed at the apex of the hiatus and into the central tendon so that the crura can be placed under tension. The esophagus is retracted anteriorly, and a No. 1 silk suture is passed through the most posterior aspect of the right crus, with care taken to avoid the adjacent inferior vena cava [see Figure 5]. A notched spoon retractor is placed through the hiatus and into

Figure 5 Transthoracic hiatal hernia repair. The esophagogastric junction is mobilized by dividing the phrenoesophageal ligament and some short gastric vessels. No. 1 silk sutures are passed through the exterior aspect of the right crus (with care taken to avoid the adjacent inferior vena cava) and through the left crus (with care taken to avoid the spleen).

Figure 6 Transthoracic hiatal hernia repair. The anterior fat pad is removed from the esophagus with sharp dissection, with care taken to avoid injury to the vagi.

the abdomen behind the left crus. The spleen is thus protected while the suture is brought through the left crus. Three or four crural repair stitches are then placed at 1 cm intervals, from posterior to anterior. The sutures are held together with hemostats but left untied for the time being. Placement of traction on the last suture should close the defect while still allowing easy passage of one finger along the esophagus. The final decision on whether to tie this last suture or cut it out is made later, after construction of the fundoplication.

Step 6: Assessment of Esophageal Length and Removal of Anterior Fat Pad

After placement of the crural stitches, an assessment of the esophageal length is made. Ideally, the stomach can easily be reduced into the abdomen without placing tension on the thoracic esophagus. When esophageal foreshortening is found, a Collis gastroplasty is performed [*see* Step 6a, *below*].

If an esophageal stricture is present, the assistant performs dilatation by passing a tapered bougie per os while the surgeon supports the esophagus. The anterior fat pad is removed via sharp dissection so as not to injure the vagi located on either side [*see Figure 6*].

Figure 7 Transthoracic hiatal hernia repair. (*a*) If esophageal foreshortening is present, a Collis gastroplasty is performed. A 54 French Maloney bougie is inserted through the esophagogastric junction. A 4 to 5 cm neoesophagus is formed with a 60 mm GIA stapler loaded with 3.5 mm staples. (*b*) Both the fundal staple line and the lesser curvature staple line are oversewn with nonabsorbable monofilament suture.

Step 6a: Collis Gastroplasty

In a Collis gastroplasty for a short esophagus, a stapler is used to form a 4 to 5 cm neoesophagus out of the proximal stomach, thereby effectively lengthening the esophagus and transposing the esophagogastric junction more distally. A large-caliber Maloney bougie (54 French for women, 56 French for men) is placed in the esophagus to prevent narrowing of the lumen. The bougie is advanced well into the stomach, so that its widest portion rests at the esophagogastric junction. The bougie is held against the lesser curvature, and the fundus is retracted away at a right angle to the esophagus. A 60 mm gastrointestinal anastomosis (GIA) stapler loaded with 3.5 mm staples is applied immediately alongside the bougie on the greater curvature side [*see Figure 7a*] and fired, simultaneously cutting and stapling the cardia. The staple line is oversewn with nonabsorbable monofilament suture material on both sides [*see Figure 7b*]. Two metal clips are placed to mark the distal extent of the gastroplasty tube, denoting the new esophagogastric junction.

Step 7: Fundoplication and Reduction of Wrap into Abdomen

The fundus is passed posteriorly behind the esophagus and brought up against the anterior stomach, with care taken to avoid torsion of the fundal wrap. The fundus is then wrapped either over the lower 2 cm of the esophagus, if no gastroplasty was done, or over 2 cm of the length of the gastroplasty tube while the bougie is in place. The seromuscular layer of the fundus is approximated to that of the esophagus or the gastroplasty tube and that of the adjacent anterior stomach with interrupted 2-0 silk sutures [*see Figure 8*]. When tied, the wrap should still be loose enough to accommodate a finger alongside the esophagus. The fundoplication sutures are again oversewn with a continuous seromuscular nonabsorbable monofilament suture. Two clips are placed at the superior aspect of the wrap. These, along with the previously placed clips, will help confirm both the length and the location of the wrap on chest x-ray.

Once the fundoplication is complete, the wrap is reduced into the abdomen. Two mattress sutures of 2-0 silk are placed to secure the top of the fundoplication to the underside of the diaphragm. The crural sutures are then sequentially tied, from the most posterior one to the most anterior. When the final suture is tied, one finger should still be able to pass through the hiatus alongside the esophagus. The dilator is then removed and the mattress sutures tied.

Step 8: Drainage and Closure

A nasogastric tube is passed into the stomach and secured. Hemostasis is verified, and a single thoracostomy tube is placed. The wound is closed in layers. A chest x-ray is performed to verify the position of the tubes and the location of the clips marking the wrap. The patient is then extubated in the OR and transported to the recovery area.

POSTOPERATIVE CARE

Patients typically remain in the hospital for 5 days. The nasogastric tube is left on low suction and removed on postoperative day 3. Patients then begin liquid oral intake, advancing to a full fluid diet as tolerated. Early ambulation is encouraged to prevent respiratory complications. Judicious use of analgesics and antiemetics minimizes nausea and vomiting. The thoracostomy tube is removed as drainage subsides. A barium swallow is performed on postoperative day 5 to verify the position of the wrap, to ensure that no significant obstruction has developed, and to provide a qualitative impression of gastric emptying.

Once patients can tolerate a soft solid diet, they are generally discharged home with instructions about the gradual resumption of a normal diet at home. Large meals and carbonated beverages must be avoided in the early postoperative period.

COMPLICATIONS

The root causes of the complications arising after transthoracic hiatal hernia repair are often technical; thus, the best prevention, in most cases, is meticulous surgical technique. Mobilization of the stomach with ligation of short gastric vessels may result in injury to the spleen. Injury to the vagi predisposes to gastric dysfunction, early satiety, and so-called gas-bloat syndrome. Poor crural approximation increases the chances that the repair will fail. Dehiscence allows upward migration of the wrap into the chest or the development of a paraesophageal hernia. The gastroplasty may leak at the staple line. Overzealous dissection along the lesser curvature can devascularize the cardia and cause ischemic stenosis of the gastroplasty tube. Torsion of the fundus results in perforation and sepsis. Excessive distraction of the ribs can lead to pain, atelectasis, or pneumonia. Inadequate mobilization of the fundus may place excessive tension on the wrap and promote later disruption and recurrent reflux. A so-called slipped Nissen—in which the wrap is inadequately fixed to the esophagus or the gastroplasty tube, and the stomach telescopes through the intact fundoplication and assumes an hourglass configuration—results in heartburn, regurgitation, and dysphagia to varying degrees. A wrap that is too tight or too long results in persistent dysphagia.

Recurrent heartburn and regurgitation call for evaluation with contrast studies and esophagoscopy. If there is an anatomic condition that is responsible for disruption of the fundoplication or failure of the crural repair, reoperation is usually necessary; in such cases, maximal medical treatment for symptoms of reflux has invariably failed already. Dysphagia that is not related to recurrent reflux or ulceration usually responds to dilatation and does not necessitate reoperation.

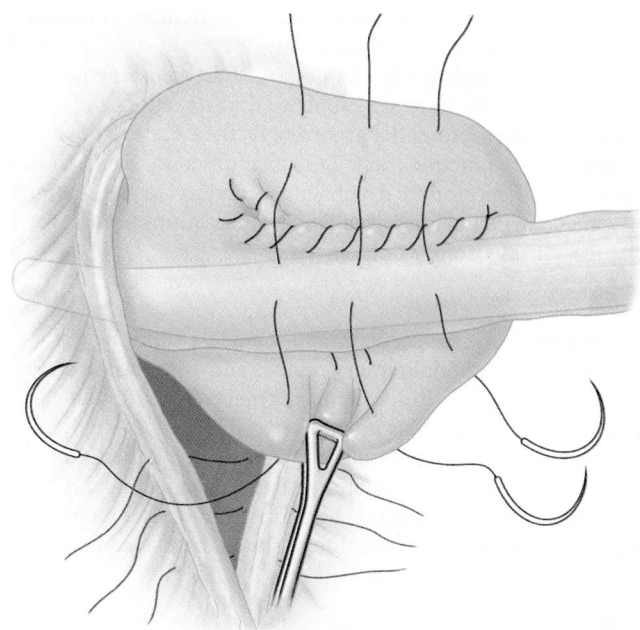

Figure 8 **Transthoracic hiatal hernia repair. The fundus is passed behind the esophagus and sewn to the neoesophagus and the anterior stomach over a 2 cm length with interrupted 2.0 silk sutures.**

OUTCOME EVALUATION

Transthoracic hiatal hernia repair yields good to excellent results in more than 85% of patients undergoing a primary repair. Approximately 75% of patients who have previously undergone hiatal hernia repair experience symptomatic improvement.[2]

Resection of Esophagus and Proximal Stomach

In the remainder of the chapter, we describe the standard open techniques for resection of the esophagus and the esophagogastric junction. Transhiatal esophagectomy is commonly performed to treat end-stage benign esophageal disease and carcinomas of the cardia and the lower esophagus. Esophageal resection through a combined laparotomy–right thoracotomy approach is ideal for cancers of the middle and upper esophagus. The gastric conduit may be anastomosed to the cervical esophagus either high in the right chest (as in an Ivor-Lewis esophagectomy) or in the neck (as in a transhiatal esophagectomy). The left thoracoabdominal approach is indicated for resection of the distal esophagus and the proximal stomach when removal of the stomach necessitates the use of an intestinal substitute to restore swallowing.

PREOPERATIVE EVALUATION

Thorough preoperative preparation is essential for good postoperative outcome. Smoking cessation and a graded regimen of home exercise will help minimize postoperative complications and encourage early mobilization. Schematic diagrams have proved useful for educating patients and shaping their expectations about quality of life and ability to swallow after esophagectomy. Illustrations, by emphasizing the anatomic relations, greatly facilitate discussion of potential complications (e.g., hoarseness from recurrent laryngeal nerve injury, pneumothorax, anastomotic leakage, mediastinal bleeding, and splenic injury). Potential postoperative problems (e.g., reflux, regurgitation, early satiety, dumping, and dysphagia) must be discussed before operation. Such discussion is particularly relevant for patients undergoing esophagectomy for early-stage malignant tumors or for high-grade dysplasia in Barrett's mucosa. These patients generally have no esophageal obstruction and may be completely asymptomatic; accordingly, their expectations about postoperative function may be quite different from those of patients with profound dysphagia secondary to near-complete esophageal occlusion. Realistic expectations improve the chances of satisfactory outcome.

Evaluation of Operative Risk

Preoperative assessment should include a thorough review of the patient's cardiopulmonary reserve and an estimate of operative risk [see IV:2 Risk Stratification, Preoperative Testing, and Operative Planning]. Spirometry, arterial blood gas analysis, and exercise stress testing should be considered. Patients must be able to tolerate a thoracotomy and a laparotomy. Thoracic epidural analgesia should be administered for pain control, and a double-lumen endotracheal tube should be placed for separate lung ventilation.

Imaging

Contrast esophagography, esophagoscopy with biopsy, and contrast-enhanced CT of the chest and the upper abdomen are required before esophagectomy. The esophagogram identifies the location of the tumor and may indicate whether it extends into the proximal stomach. Esophagoscopy allows direct assessment of the mucosa, precise localization of the tumor, and collection of tissue for histologic study. Retroflexion views of the stomach, after distention with air, are particularly important if proximal gastric invasion is suspected, in which case esophagogastrectomy with reconstruction of alimentary continuity by means of intestinal interposition may be required. Thoracic and abdominal CT scans yield information on the extent of any celiac or mediastinal adenopathy, the degree of esophageal thickening, and the possibility of invasion of the adjacent aorta or tracheobronchial tree. The lung parenchyma is assessed for metastatic nodules, as are the liver and the adrenal glands. Suspicious areas may be further assessed by means of either PET scanning or needle biopsy. Invasion of mediastinal structures and distant metastases are contraindications to transhiatal esophagectomy.

Endoscopic ultrasonography, though quite sensitive for detection of paraesophageal adenopathy, is currently incapable of differentiating reactive lymph nodes from nodes invaded by malignancy.

Chemoradiation Therapy

Patients with esophageal cancer who are candidates for resection may benefit from neoadjuvant chemotherapy and concurrent radiation therapy. In particular, patients with good performance status and bulky disease should be considered for such therapy. There are, as yet, no randomized trials that conclusively demonstrate a survival benefit with this approach, but several series have documented a 20% to 30% rate of complete response with no viable tumor found at the time of resection. After chemoradiation, patients are restaged with a barium swallow and CT. If no contraindications to surgical treatment are noted, resection is scheduled 2 weeks later. Previous chemoradiation does not make transhiatal esophagectomy significantly more difficult or complicated. In centers with experience in this approach, the rates of bleeding and anastomotic leakage remain low.

OPERATIVE PLANNING

Transhiatal Esophagectomy

In transhiatal esophagectomy, the stomach is mobilized through a short upper midline laparotomy, the esophagus is mobilized from adjacent mediastinal structures via dissection through the hiatus without the use of a thoracotomy, and the stomach is transposed through the posterior mediastinum and anastomosed to the cervical esophagus at the level of the clavicles. The main advantages of this approach are (1) a proximal surgical margin that is well away from the tumor site, (2) an extrathoracic esophagogastric anastomosis that is easily accessible in the event of complications, and (3) reduced overall operative trauma. Single-center studies throughout the world have shown transhiatal esophagectomy to be safe and well tolerated, even in patients who may have significantly reduced cardiopulmonary reserve. Long-term survival is equivalent to that reported after transthoracic esophagectomy.

Although transhiatal esophagectomy has been used for resection of tumors at any location in the esophagus, it is best suited for resection of tumors in the lower esophagus and at the esophagogastric junction. It should also be considered the operation of choice for certain advanced nonmalignant conditions of the esophagus. Nondilatable strictures of the esophagus may occur as an end-stage complication of gastroesophageal reflux.

Intractable reflux after failed hiatal hernia repair may not be amenable to further attempts at reconstruction of the esophagogastric junction and thus may call for esophagectomy. Because of the high cervical anastomosis, a transhiatal esophagectomy is less likely to predispose to postoperative reflux and recurrent stricture formation than a transthoracic esophagectomy would be. Achalasia may result in megaesophagus and dysphagia that cannot be managed without removal of the esophagus. Transhiatal esophagectomy permits complete removal of the thoracic esophagus and, in the majority of patients, restoration of comfortable swallowing without the need for a thoracotomy.

Generally, patients are admitted to the hospital on the day of the operation. Thoracic epidural analgesia is administered, both intraoperatively and postoperatively, and appropriate antibiotic prophylaxis is provided [see IV:5 Prevention of Postoperative Infection]. Heparin, 5,000 U subcutaneously, is given before induction, and pneumatic calf compression devices are applied. A radial artery catheter is placed to permit continuous monitoring of blood pressure. Central venous access is rarely required. General anesthesia is administered via an uncut single-lumen endotracheal tube. Flexible esophagoscopy is performed by the surgical team. A nasogastric tube is placed before final positioning and draping.

The patient is placed in the supine position with a small rolled sheet between the shoulders. The arms are secured to the sides, and the head is rotated to the right with the neck extended. The neck, the chest, and the abdomen are prepared as a single sterile field. The drapes are placed so as to expose the patient from the left ear to the pubis. The operative field is extended laterally to the anterior axillary lines to permit placement of thoracostomy tubes as needed. A self-retaining table-mounted retractor is used to facilitate upward and lateral traction along the costal margin.

Ivor-Lewis Esophagectomy

At many institutions, Ivor-Lewis esophagectomy is preferred because of the excellent direct exposure it affords for dissection of the intrathoracic esophagus. This procedure should be considered when there is concern regarding the extent of esophageal fixation within the mediastinum. An extensive local lymphadenectomy is easily performed through a right thoracotomy. Whether any regional lymph node dissection is necessary is highly controversial; no significant survival advantage has yet been demonstrated. Long-term survival after Ivor-Lewis resection is equivalent to that after transhiatal esophagectomy.[3]

The main disadvantages of the Ivor-Lewis procedure are (1) the physiologic impact of the two major access incisions employed (a right thoracotomy and a midline laparotomy) and (2) the location of the anastomosis (in the chest, at the level of the azygos vein). Incision-related pain may hinder deep breathing and the clearing of bronchial secretions, resulting in atelectasis and pneumonia. Complications of the intrathoracic anastomosis may be hard to manage. If the anastomosis leaks, drainage will be difficult, empyema may result, and reoperation may prove necessary.

Left Thoracoabdominal Esophagogastrectomy

The left thoracoabdominal approach is indicated for resection of the distal esophagus and the proximal stomach when removal of the stomach necessitates the use of an intestinal substitute to restore swallowing. If the proximal stomach must be resected for adequate resection margins to be obtained, then the distal stomach may be anastomosed to the esophagus in the chest. This operation is frequently associated with significant esophagitis

from bile reflux. Consequently, many surgeons prefer to resect the entire stomach and the distal esophagus and then to restore swallowing with a Roux-en-Y jejunal interposition anastomosed to the residual thoracic esophagus.

OPERATIVE TECHNIQUE

Transhiatal Esophagectomy

Transhiatal esophagectomy is best understood as consisting of three components: abdominal, mediastinal, and cervical. The abdominal portion involves mobilization of the stomach, pyloromyotomy, and a temporary feeding jejunostomy.

Step 1: incision and entry into peritoneum A midline laparotomy is performed from the tip of the xiphoid to the umbilicus. The peritoneum is opened to the left of the midline so that the falciform and the preperitoneal fat may be retracted en bloc to the right. Body wall retractors are placed at 45° angles from the midline to elevate and distract both costal margins. The abdomen is then inspected for metastases.

Step 2: division of gastrohepatic ligament and mobilization of distal esophagus The left lobe of the liver is mobilized by dividing the triangular ligament, then folded to the right and held in this position with a moist laparotomy pad and a deep-bladed self-retaining retractor. Next, the gastrohepatic ligament is divided. Occasionally, there is an aberrant left hepatic artery arising from the left gastric artery [see Figure 9]. The peritoneum over the right crus is incised, and the hiatus is palpated; the extent and mobility of any tumor may then be assessed. The esophagus is encircled with a Penrose drain, and gentle traction is applied to draw the esophagogastric junction upward and to the right.

Step 3: mobilization of duodenum and pyloromyotomy The duodenum is mobilized with a Kocher maneuver. Careful attention to the superior extent of this dissection is critical. Adhesions to either the porta hepatis or the gallbladder must be divided to ensure that the pylorus is sufficiently freed for later migration to the diaphragmatic hiatus.

Gastric drainage is provided by a pyloromyotomy. Two figure-eight traction sutures of 2-0 cardiovascular silk are placed deeply through both the superior and the inferior border of the pylorus; traction is then placed on these sutures to provide both exposure and some degree of hemostasis. The pyloromyotomy is begun 2 to 3 cm on the gastric side of the pylorus. The serosa and the muscle are divided with a needle-tipped electrocautery to expose the submucosa; generally, these layers of the stomach are robust, making the proper plane easy to find. Dissection is extended toward the duodenum with the aid of a fine-tipped right-angle clamp. The duodenal submucosa, recognizable by its fatty deposits and yellow coloration, is exposed for approximately 0.5 cm. The duodenal submucosa is usually much more superficial than expected, and accidental entry into the duodenum often occurs just past the left edge of the circular muscle of the pylorus. Releasing the tension on the traction sutures helps the surgeon visualize the proper depth of dissection. Should entry into the lumen occur, a simple repair using interrupted fine monofilament sutures to close the mucosa is performed. Small metal clips are applied to the knots of the traction sutures before removal of the ends; these clips serve to indicate the level of the pyloromyotomy on subsequent radiographic studies.

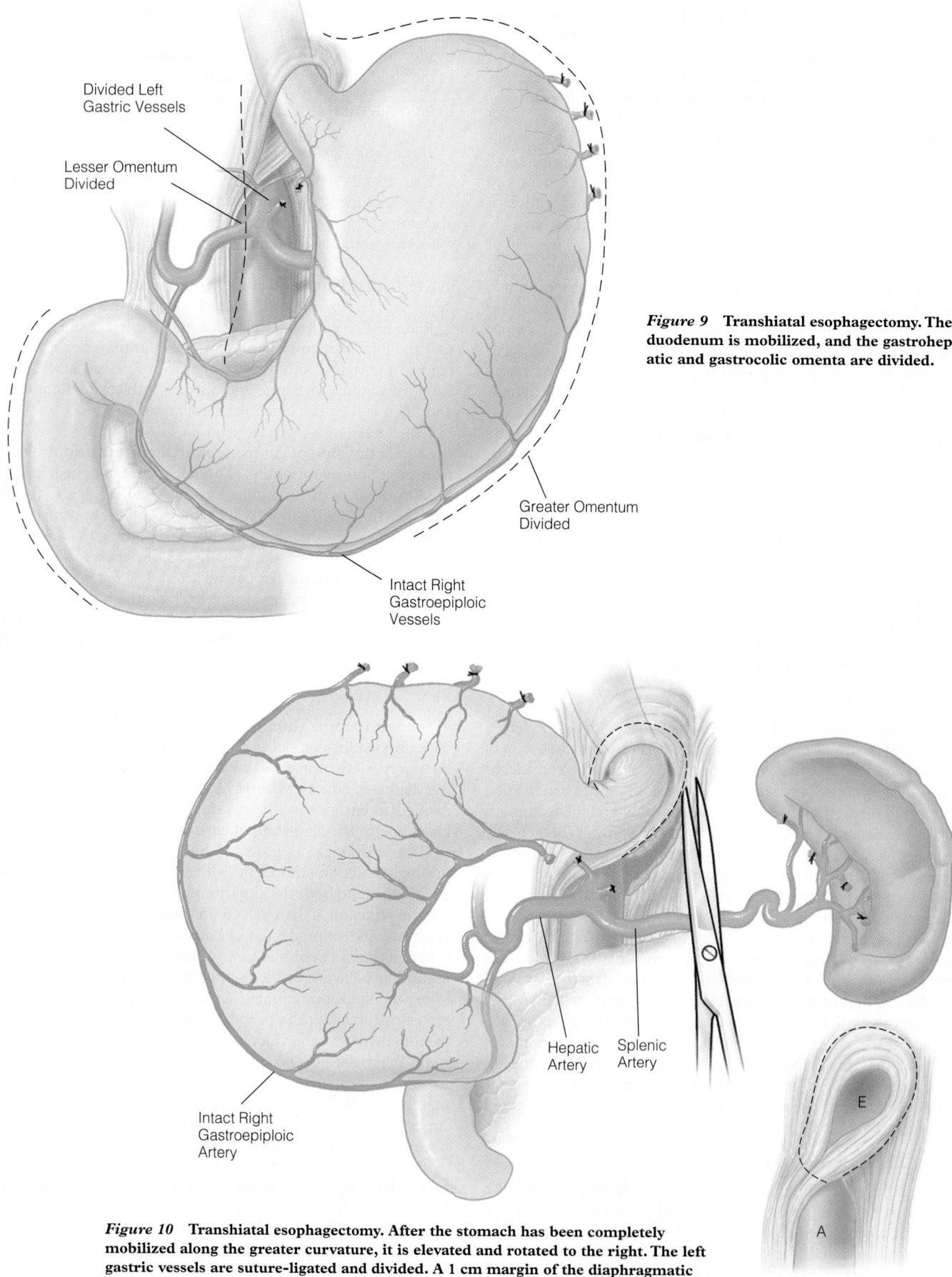

Divided Left
Gastric Vessels

Lesser Omentum
Divided

Figure 9 **Transhiatal esophagectomy. The
duodenum is mobilized, and the gastrohepatic and gastrocolic omenta are divided.**

Greater Omentum
Divided

Intact Right
Gastroepiploic
Vessels

Hepatic
Artery

Splenic
Artery

Intact Right
Gastroepiploic
Artery

E

A

Figure 10 **Transhiatal esophagectomy. After the stomach has been completely
mobilized along the greater curvature, it is elevated and rotated to the right. The left
gastric vessels are suture-ligated and divided. A 1 cm margin of the diaphragmatic
crura is taken in continuity with the esophagogastric junction, providing ample
clearance of the tumor and improved exposure of the lower mediastinum.**

Step 4: mobilization of stomach The greater curvature of the stomach is inspected and the right gastroepiploic artery palpated. The lesser sac is generally entered near the midpoint of the greater curvature. The transition zone between the right gastroepiploic arcade and the short gastric arteries is usually devoid of blood vessels.

Dissection then proceeds along the greater curvature toward the pylorus. The omentum is mobilized from the right gastroepiploic artery. Vessels are ligated between 2-0 silk ties, and great care is exercised to avoid placing excessive traction on the arterial arcade. A 1 cm margin is always maintained between the line of dissection and the right gastroepiploic artery. Venous injuries, in particular, can occur with injudicious handling of tissue. The ultrasonic scalpel is particularly efficient and effective for mobilization of the stomach; again, this instrument must be applied well away from the gastroepiploic arcade. Dissection is continued rightward to the level of the pylorus. It should be noted that the location of the gastroepiploic artery in this area may vary; often, it is at some unexpected distance from the stomach wall. Posterior adhesions between the stomach and the pancreas are lysed so that the lesser sac can be completely opened.

The assistant's left hand is then placed into the lesser sac to retract the stomach gently to the right and place the short gastric vessels on tension. Dissection along the greater curvature proceeds cephalad. The vessels are divided well away from the wall of the stomach to prevent injury to the fundus. Clamps should never be placed on the stomach. A high short gastric artery is typically encountered just adjacent to the left crus. Precise technique is required to prevent injury to the spleen. The previously placed Penrose drain [see Step 2, above] is exposed as the peritoneum is opened over the left crus.

Once the stomach has been completely mobilized along the greater curvature, it is elevated and rotated to the right [see Figure 10]; the left gastric artery and associated nodal tissues can then be visualized via the lesser sac. The superior edge of the pancreas is visible, and the remaining posterior attachments of the stomach are divided along the hiatus and the left crus.

If the operation is being done for malignant disease, a final determination of resectability can be made at this point. Tumor fixation to the aorta or the retroperitoneum can be assessed. Celiac and paraaortic lymph nodes can be palpated and, if necessary, sent for biopsy. The left gastric artery and vein are then ligated proximally. All nodal tissue is dissected free in anticipation of subsequent removal en bloc with the specimen.

Step 5: feeding jejunostomy A standard Weitzel jejunostomy completes the abdominal portion of the transhiatal esophagectomy.

Step 6: exposure and encirclement of cervical esophagus The cervical esophagus is exposed through a 6 cm incision along the anterior edge of the left sternocleidomastoid muscle [see Figure 1] that is centered over the level of the cricoid cartilage. The platysma is divided to expose the omohyoid, which is divided at its tendon. The strap muscles are divided low in the neck. The esophagus and its indwelling nasogastric tube can be palpated.

The carotid sheath is retracted laterally, and blunt dissection is employed to reach the prevertebral fascia. The inferior thyroid artery is ligated laterally; the recurrent laryngeal nerve is visible just deep and medial to this vessel. No retractor other than the surgeon's finger should be applied medially: traction injury to

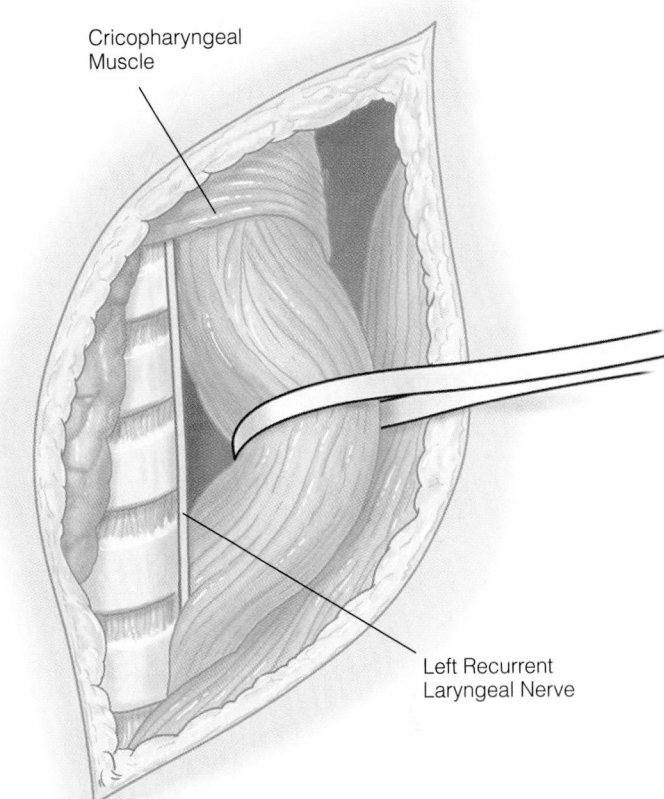

Cricopharyngeal Muscle

Left Recurrent Laryngeal Nerve

Figure 11 **Transhiatal esophagectomy. Once the cervical esophagus is exposed through an incision along the left sternocleidomastoid muscle, strap muscles are divided and retracted, and the cervical esophagus is dissected away from the left and right recurrent laryngeal nerves.**

the recurrent laryngeal nerve will result in both vocal cord palsy and uncoordinated swallowing with aspiration. The tracheoesophageal groove is incised close to the esophageal wall while gentle finger traction is applied cephalad to elevate the thyroid cartilage toward the right. This measure usually suffices to define the location of the nerve.

The esophagus is then encircled by passing a right-angle clamp posteriorly from left to right while the surgeon's finger remains in the tracheoesophageal groove. The tip of the clamp is brought into the pulp of the fingertip. The medially located recurrent laryngeal nerve and the membranous trachea are thereby protected from injury. The clamp is brought around, and a narrow Penrose drain is passed around the esophagus [see Figure 11]. Blunt finger dissection is employed to develop the anterior and posterior planes around the esophagus at the level of the thoracic inlet.

Step 7: mediastinal dissection Three specific maneuvers are now carried out. First, the plane posterior to the esophagus is developed [see Figure 12]. The surgeon's right hand is advanced palm upward into the hiatus, with the fingers closely applied to the esophagus. The volar aspects of the fingers run along the prevertebral fascia, elevating the esophagus off the spine. A moist sponge stick is placed through the cervical incision, also posterior to the esophagus. The sponge is advanced toward the right hand, which is positioned within the mediastinum. As the sponge is advanced into the right palm, the posterior plane is completed. A 28 French mediastinal sump is then passed from the cervical incision into the abdomen along the

Figure 12 Transhiatal esophagectomy. The plane posterior to the esophagus is developed by placing the surgeon's right hand into the hiatus along the prevertebral fascia. A moist sponge-stick is placed through the cervical incision posterior to the esophagus, and the posterior plane is completed.

posterior esophageal wall and attached to suction. Any blood loss from the mediastinum is collected and monitored.

Second, the anterior plane is developed [*see Figure 13*]. This is often much more difficult than developing the posterior plane because the left mainstem bronchus may be quite close to the esophagus. Again, the surgeon's right hand is placed through the hiatus, but it is now palm down and anterior to the esophagus. The fingertips enter the space between the esophagus and the left mainstem bronchus. The hand is gently advanced, and the airway is displaced anteriorly. A blunt curved suction handle is employed from above as a substitute finger. It is advanced along the anterior aspect of the esophagus through the cervical incision. The right hand guides the tip of the suction handle beneath the bronchus. Lateral displacement of the handle allows further mobilization of the bronchus away from the esophagus. Completion of the anterior and posterior planes usually results in a highly mobile esophagus.

Third, the lateral attachments of the esophagus are divided. Upward traction is applied with the previously placed encircling Penrose drain, allowing further dissection at the level of the thoracic inlet. Lateral attachments are pushed caudally into the mediastinum, and traction applied to the esophagus from below allows these attachments to be visualized through the hiatus, then isolated with long right-angle clamps and divided with the electrocautery. Caution must be exercised so as not to injure the

azygos vein. Dissection on the right side must therefore be kept close to the esophagus. Once the last lateral attachment is divided, the esophagus is completely free and can be advanced into the cervical wound.

Step 8: proximal transection of esophagus and delivery into abdomen   The nasogastric tube is retracted to the level of the cricopharyngeus muscle, and the esophagus is divided with a cutting stapler 5 to 6 cm distal to the muscle. The esophagus is then removed via the abdomen [*see Figure 14*]. Narrow curved Harrington retractors are placed into the hiatus and used to elevate the pericardium. Caudal traction is placed on the esophagus, allowing excellent visualization of the hiatus and the distal esophagus. Paraesophageal lymph nodes are removed either en bloc or as separate specimens. Dissection is continued cephalad with the electrocautery and a long-handled right-angle clamp. The two vagi are divided, the remaining periesophageal adhesions are lysed, and the esophagus is delivered into the abdomen.

Close monitoring of arterial blood pressure is maintained throughout. Transient hypotension may occur as a result of mediastinal compression and temporary impairment of cardiac venous return. Vasopressors are never required for management: simple repositioning of the retractors or removal of the dissecting hand usually results in prompt restoration of normal BP.

Figure 13 Transhiatal esophagectomy. The anterior plane is developed by placing the surgeon's right hand through the hiatus anterior to the esophagus. The fingertips enter the space between the esophagus and the left mainstem bronchus, to be met by a blunt suction handle passed downward through the cervical incision. The lateral attachments of the esophagus are divided from above downward as far as the aortic arch.

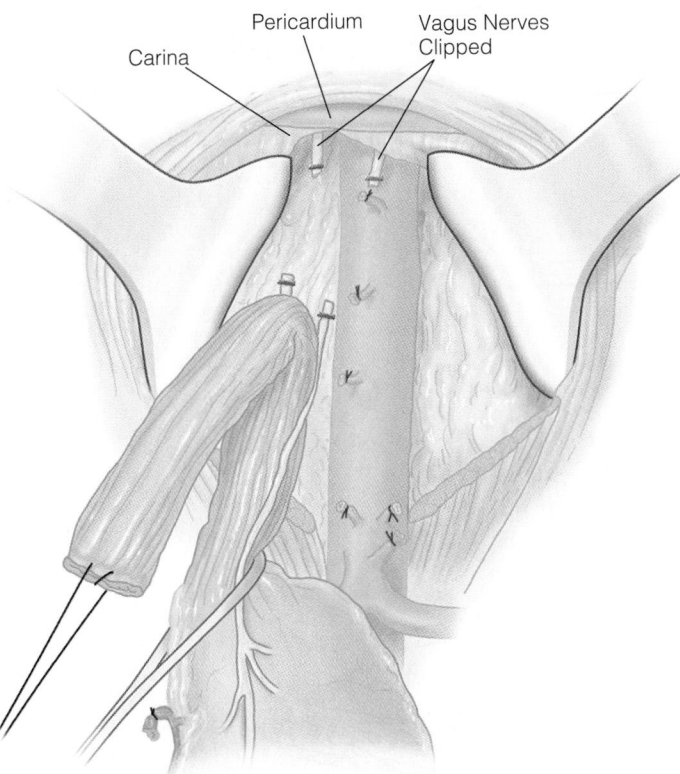

Carina Pericardium Vagus Nerves Clipped

Figure 14 **Transhiatal esophagectomy. The esophagus is divided in the neck and delivered into the abdomen. Retractors are placed in the hiatus, and any vessels entering into the esophagus are clipped and divided. The vagi are also clipped and divided.**

Figure 15 **Transhiatal esophagectomy. A gastric tube is formed by stapling along the lesser curvature of the stomach from the junction of the right and left gastric vessels to the top of the fundus. This staple line is oversewn with a continuous 3-0 suture, with care taken not to foreshorten the gastric tube.**

Placement of the patient in a slight Trendelenburg position is often helpful. Retractors are placed in the hiatus, and the mediastinum is inspected for hemostasis. The sump is removed. Both pleurae are inspected. The lungs are inflated so that it can be determined which pleural space requires thoracostomy drainage. The mediastinum is packed with dry laparotomy pads from below. A narrow pack is placed into the thoracic inlet from above. Chest tubes are then placed as required along the inframammary crease in the anterior axillary line.

Step 9: excision of specimen and formation of gastric tube The gastric fundus is grasped, and gentle tension is applied along the length of the stomach. The esophagus is held at right angles to the body of the stomach, and the fat in the gastrohepatic ligament is elevated off the lesser curvature; all lymph nodes are thus mobilized. A point approximately midway along the lesser curvature is selected. The blood vessels traversing this area from the right gastric artery are ligated to expose the lesser curvature. The distal resection margin is then determined; it should be 4 to 6 cm from the esophagogastric junction, extending from the selected point on the lesser curvature to a point medial to the fundus. A 60 mm GIA stapler loaded with 3.5 mm staples is then used to transect the proximal stomach, proceeding from the lesser curvature toward the fundus [*see Figure 15*]. Resection of the cardia along with the adjacent portion of the lesser curvature effectively converts a J-shaped stomach into a straight tube.

For maximizing the length of the gastric tube, there are several technical points that are critical. Tension must be maintained on the stomach as the stapler is serially applied cephalad. The stapler should be simply placed on the stomach and fired: no attempt should be made to telescope tissue into the jaws, because to do so would effectively reconstitute the curve of the stomach and diminish its upward reach. Multiple staple loads will be required.

The specimen is removed, and frozen section examination is done on the distal margin. The completed staple line is then oversewn with a continuous Lembert suture of 4-0 polypropylene. Once again, tension is maintained along the stomach to prevent any foreshortening of the lesser curvature. The use of two separate sutures, each reinforcing half of the staple line, is helpful in this regard.

Step 10: advancement of stomach into chest or neck The mediastinal packs are removed, and hemostasis is verified in the chest. The stomach is inspected as well. The ends of any short gastric vessels that were divided with the ultrasonic scalpel are now tied so that subsequent manipulation does not precipitate bleeding. The stomach is oriented so that the greater curvature is to the patient's left. There must be no torsion. The stomach can usually be advanced through the posterior mediastinum without any traction sutures or clamps. The surgeon's hand is placed palm down on the anterior surface of the stomach, with the fingertips about 5 cm proximal to the tip of the fundus. The hand is then gently advanced through the chest, pushing the stomach ahead of itself. The tip of the fundus is gently grasped with a Babcock clamp as it appears in the neck. To prevent trauma at this most distant aspect of the gastric tube, the clamp should not be ratcheted closed.

No attempt should be made to pull the stomach up into the neck: the position of the fundus is simply maintained as the surgeon's hand is removed from the mediastinum. Further length in the neck can usually be gained by gently readvancing the hand along the anterior aspect of the stomach. This measure uniformly distributes tension along the tube and ensures proper torsion-free orientation in the chest. The stomach is pushed up into the neck rather than drawn up by the clamp.

A useful alternate approach for positioning the gastric tube involves passing a large-bore Foley catheter through the mediastinum from the neck incision. The balloon is inflated, and a 50 cm section of a narrow plastic laparoscopic camera bag is tied onto the catheter just above the balloon. The gastric tube is positioned within the bag, and suction is applied through the catheter, creating an atraumatic seal between the stomach and the surrounding plastic bag. As the bag is drawn upward through the neck with gentle traction on the Foley catheter, the stomach advances through the mediastinum. A small dry pack is placed in the neck behind the fundus to prevent retraction into the chest. The stomach is not secured to the prevertebral fascia in any way. The viability of the fundus is checked periodically as the feeding jejunostomy is brought out through the abdomen and the laparotomy incision is closed.

Step 11: esophagogastrostomy The construction of the esophagogastric anastomosis is the most important part of the entire operation: any anastomotic complication will greatly compromise the patient's ability to swallow comfortably. Accordingly, meticulous technique is essential.

A seromuscular traction suture of 4-0 Vicryl is placed through the anterior stomach at the level of the clavicle and drawn upward, thus elevating the fundus into the neck wound and greatly facilitating the anastomosis. The pack behind the fundus is then removed.

The site of the anterior gastrotomy is then carefully selected: it should be midway between the oversewn lesser curvature staple line and the greater curvature of the fundus (marked by the ligated ends of the short gastric vessels). The staple line on the cervical esophagus is removed, and the anterior aspect of the esophagus is grasped with a fine-toothed forceps at the level of the planned gastrotomy. A straight DeBakey forceps is then applied across the full width of the esophagus to act as a guide for division. The esophagus is cut with a scalpel at a 45° angle so that the anterior wall is slightly longer than the posterior wall; the anterior wall then forms the hood of the anastomosis. The fine-toothed forceps is used to maintain orientation of the esophagus throughout. Two full-thickness stay sutures of 4-0 Vicryl are placed, one at the midpoint of the anterior cut edge of the esophagus and one at the corresponding location posteriorly. The posterior stitch is placed from inside the lumen, and the needle is left on the suture for later use.

A 2 cm gastrotomy is then performed with a needle-tipped electrocautery using cutting current. The incision is obliquely oriented, with the cephalad extent proceeding medially. The needle from the stay suture previously placed on the posterior wall of the esophagus is then passed the full thickness of the cephalad aspect of the gastrotomy [*see Figure 16a*]. Traction on this untied suture brings the esophagus toward the stomach. An endoscopic stapler loaded with 3.5 mm staples is used to form the back wall of the anastomosis. The thicker portion of the device (the cartridge) is advanced cephalad into the stomach, with the narrower portion (the anvil) in the esophageal lumen [*see Figure 16b*]. The tip of the stapler should be aimed toward the patient's right ear. Tension is applied to the stay suture holding the esophagus and stomach together so as to bring tissue into the jaws of the device. The portion of the fundus extending beyond the stapler is then rotated medially to ensure that the

Figure 16 Transhiatal esophagectomy. (*a*) After the proximal end of the stomach tube is delivered into the neck, the esophagus is cut at a 45% angle so that the anterior wall is longer than the posterior wall. A gastrotomy is placed between the oversewn lesser curvature staple line and the greater curvature of the fundus. A full-thickness suture is placed through all layers of the esophagus and all layers of the gastrotomy. (*b*) An endoscopic GIA stapler is used to form the back wall of the anastomosis. The thicker (cartridge) portion of the device is placed into the stomach, while the narrow (anvil) portion is placed into the esophageal lumen. The tip of the stapler should be aimed toward the patient's right ear. The staple line must be well away from the lesser curvature staple line. Two suspension sutures are placed on either side of the closed stapler, one toward the tip and the other near the heel of the jaws. (*c*) The stapler is fired to complete the posterior portion of the anastomosis.

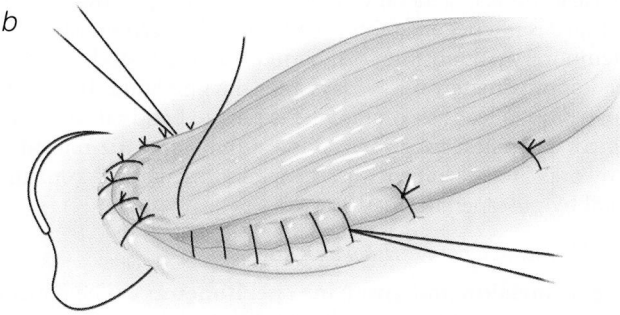

Figure 17 Transhiatal esophagectomy. The anterior portion of the anastomosis is completed with (*a*) an inner layer consisting of a continuous 4.0 PDS suture and (*b*) an outer layer consisting of interrupted sutures.

new staple line is well away from the one previously placed along the lesser curvature. This is a crucial point: crossing of the two staple lines may create an ischemic area that can give rise to a large leak in the postoperative period.

The stapler is then closed, holding the esophagus and stomach together, but not yet fired. Two suspension sutures are placed on either side of the closed stapler, one toward the tip and the other near the heel of the jaws. These sutures alleviate any potential tension on the staple line by approximating the muscular layer of the esophagus to the seromuscular layer of the stomach. The suspension sutures are tied, and the stapler is fired, thereby completing the posterior portion of the anastomosis [*see Figure 16c*].

The anterior portion of the anastomosis is closed in two layers. The inner layer consists of a continuous 4-0 polydioxane (PDS) suture placed as full-thickness inverting stitches, and the second layer consists of interrupted seromuscular Lembert sutures [*see Figure 17*]. The lateral and medial corners of the anastomosis, where the staple line meets the hand-sewn portion, merit extra attention. These corners are quite fragile, and excessive traction may result in dehiscence progressing cephalad along the staple line in a zipperlike fashion. The inner layer should therefore be started at each corner. Once several stitches have been placed from the two corners, the nasogastric tube can be passed through the anastomosis. The inner layer is then completed as the two sutures are tied at the midpoint.

Step 12: drainage, closure, and completion x-ray A small Penrose drain is placed in the thoracic inlet below the anastomosis and brought out through the inferior end of the neck incision. The drain is secured, and the incision is irrigated. The strap muscles are not reapproximated but are merely attached loosely to the underside of the sternocleidomastoid muscle with two interrupted 4-0 Vicryl sutures. The platysma is reconstituted with interrupted 4-0 Vicryl sutures. The nasogastric tube is secured. A chest x-ray is obtained in the OR to verify the position of the drains and the absence of any abnormal collections in the chest. Patients are extubated in the OR and transported to the anesthetic recovery area. Once they are awake and alert, which is usually 3 to 4 hours after the operation, they are taken to the general ward.

In certain patients, a stapled anastomosis may be impractical. In patients with a bull-neck habitus, for example, a partial sternal split may be required for adequate exposure of the cervical esophagus, and a hand-sewn true end-to-end anastomosis may be necessary. In addition, patients who have previously undergone antireflux surgery may have a relatively short gastric tube that will necessitate an end-to-end reconstruction.

Ivor-Lewis Esophagectomy

Steps 1 through 5 Esophagoscopy is performed to confirm the location of the tumor. Steps 1, 2, 3, 4, and 5 of an Ivor-Lewis esophagectomy are virtually identical to the first five steps (i.e., the abdominal portion) of a transhiatal esophagectomy. Once complete mobilization of the stomach is verified, the pylorus is manually advanced to the level of the diaphragm to ensure that it is not being tethered by the duodenum or the greater omentum. The stomach is then placed back into the anatomic position, and the laparotomy is closed.

Step 6: exposure and mobilization of esophagus The patient is shifted to the left lateral decubitus position and redraped. Single-lung ventilation is instituted, and the chest is entered through a right fifth or sixth interspace thoracotomy. The inferior pulmonary ligament is divided, and the lung is retracted cephalad. The esophagus is mobilized from the level of the diaphragm to a point above the azygos vein [*see Figure 18*], which is typically divided with a vascular stapler. The pleura overlying the esophagus is divided to the level of the thoracic inlet, superior to the azygos vein. The esophagus is encircled with a Penrose drain in the retrotracheal region. The pleura is then divided to the level of the diaphragm, with care taken to stay close to the right bronchus and the pericardium and avoid injury to the thoracic duct. The soft tissue between the esophagus and the aorta posteriorly and between the esophagus and the trachea or the pericardium anteriorly is dissected free and maintained en bloc with the esophagus. Periesophageal and subcarinal nodes are thereby mobilized.

Step 7: excision and removal of specimen The hiatus is incised and the abdomen entered. The stomach is drawn up into the chest, with care taken not to place excessive traction on the gastroepiploic pedicle. The esophagus is divided with a stapler proximally at least 5 cm away from any grossly evident tumor. A margin is sent for frozen section examination. The distal resection margin is completed in a similar manner, and the esophageal specimen is removed from the operative field [*see Figure 19*]. The gastric staple line is oversewn, and the stomach is positioned in the posterior mediastinum.

Step 8: esophagogastrostomy The site of the esophagogastric anastomosis should be about 2 cm above the divided azygos vein. Several interrupted sutures are used to secure the transposed stomach to the adjacent pleura. The staple line on the esophagus is removed, and a gastrotomy is performed in

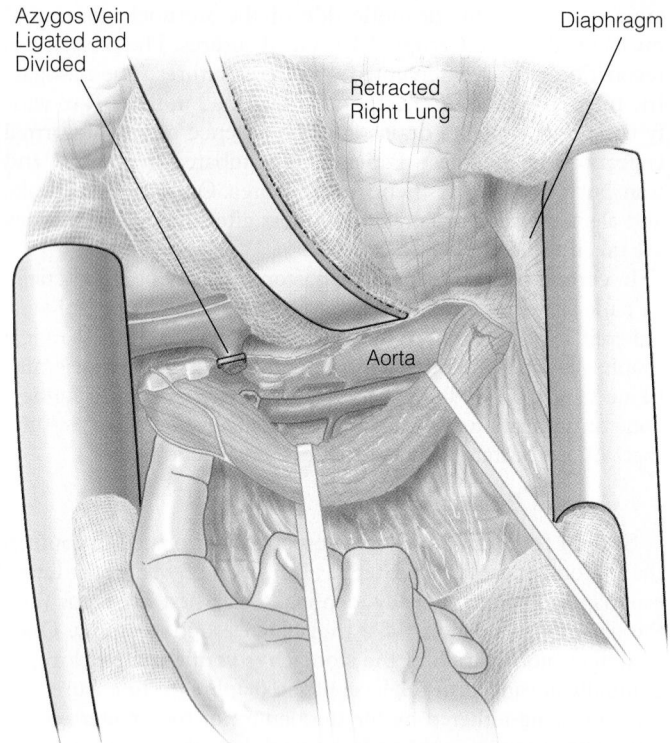

Figure 18 Ivor-Lewis esophagectomy. The lung is retracted, and the azygos vein is stapled and divided. The esophagus and the vagi are mobilized from the level of the diaphragm to the thoracic inlet.

preparation for a side-to-side functional end-to-end anastomosis [*see Figure 20*]. With the aid of full-thickness traction sutures, the esophagus is positioned along the surface of the stomach and well away from the oversewn staple line defining the gastric resection margin. The posterior aspect of the anastomosis is completed with an endoscopic GIA stapler as described earlier [*see* Transhiatal Esophagectomy, Step 11, *above, and Figures 16 and 17*]. A nasogastric tube is passed, and the anterior wall is completed in two layers. The first layer consists of a full-thickness continuous 3-0 PDS suture; the second consists of interrupted absorbable sutures approximating the seromuscular layer of the stomach to the muscular layer of the esophagus.

Two alternative methods of anastomosis are sometimes used: (1) a totally hand-sewn end-to-side anastomosis and (2) a totally stapled end-to-end anastomosis. The latter technique involves opening the previously placed gastric staple line and advancing the handle of an end-to-end anastomosis (EEA) stapler through the stomach. The proximal esophagus is dilated sufficiently to accommodate at least a 25 mm head. The anvil is placed into the distal esophagus and secured with a purse-string suture. The tip of the stapler is brought out through the apical wall of the stomach and attached to the anvil. The stapler is then fired to create the end-to-end anastomosis, and the gastrotomy is closed. The advantages of this technique are its relative simplicity and the theoretical security of a completely stapled anastomosis; the main potential disadvantage is the risk of postoperative dysphagia resulting from an overly narrow anastomotic ring.

After completion of the anastomosis, the stomach is inspected for any potential redundancy or torsion in the chest. To prevent torsion, the stomach is anchored to the pericardium with nonabsorbable sutures. The diaphragmatic hiatus is then inspected:

it should allow easy passage of two fingers into the abdomen alongside the transposed stomach. Interrupted sutures may be used to approximate the edge of the crura to the adjacent stomach wall, thereby preventing any later herniation of abdominal contents into the pleural space.

Step 9: drainage and closure Two chest tubes are placed through separate stab incisions. The tip of the posterior drain is positioned alongside the stomach at the level of the anastomosis. Fine gut sutures secured to the adjacent parietal pleura will help maintain the position of the tube. The thoracotomy is then closed in the standard fashion.

Patients should begin walking on postoperative day 1. The nasogastric tube is generally removed on postoperative day 3. Oral intake is not begun at this point; feeding is accomplished via the temporary jejunostomy. A barium contrast study is performed approximately 5 to 7 days after the operation. If there is no anastomotic leakage, oral intake is initiated and advanced as tolerated. The chest tubes are removed only after the reinstitution of oral intake. Patients are generally discharged from the hospital by postoperative day 8 to 10.

Left Thoracoabdominal Esophagogastrectomy

Step 1: incision and entry into peritoneum The patient is placed in the right lateral position, with the hips rotated backward about 30°. An exploratory laparotomy is performed through an oblique incision extending from the tip of the sixth costal cartilage to a point about halfway between the sternum and the umbilicus. The peritoneal cavity is carefully examined to rule out peritoneal and hepatic metastases. The region of the cardia is palpated and the mobility of the tumor assessed. If there is minor involvement of the crura or the tail of the pancreas, resection may still be possible; however, if the tumor is firmly fixed or there are peritoneal or hepatic metastases, resection should be

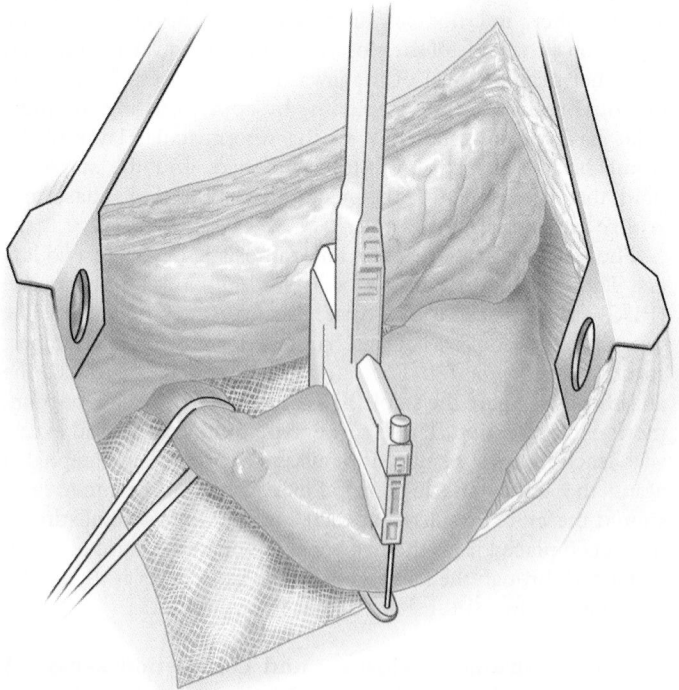

Figure 19 Ivor-Lewis esophagectomy. The esophagus and the proximal stomach are divided and stapled at least 5 cm away from the gross tumor.

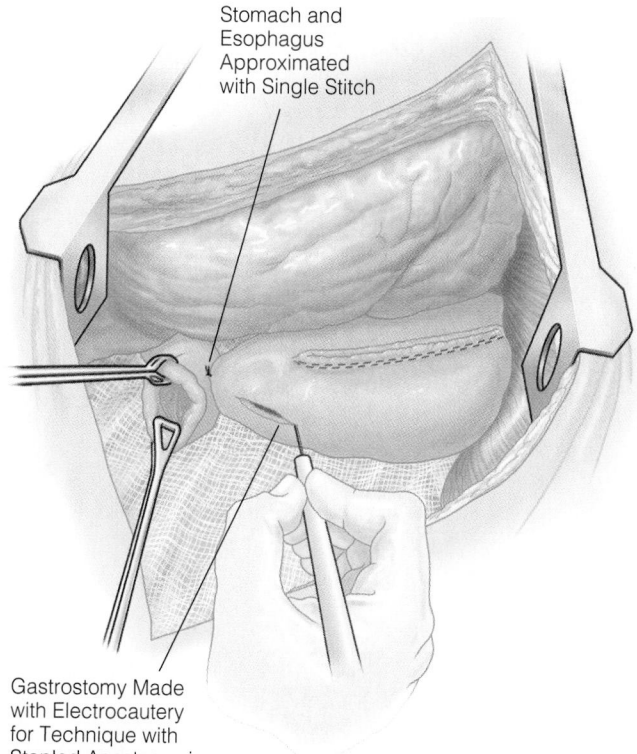

Stomach and
Esophagus
Approximated
with Single Stitch

Gastrostomy Made
with Electrocautery
for Technique with
Stapled Anastomosis

Figure 20 **Ivor-Lewis esophagectomy. The transposed stomach is sutured to the adjacent pericardium, and a gastrotomy is carried out halfway between the lesser curvature staple line and the greater curvature. The anastomosis is completed as in a transhiatal esophagectomy [*see Figures 16 and 17*].**

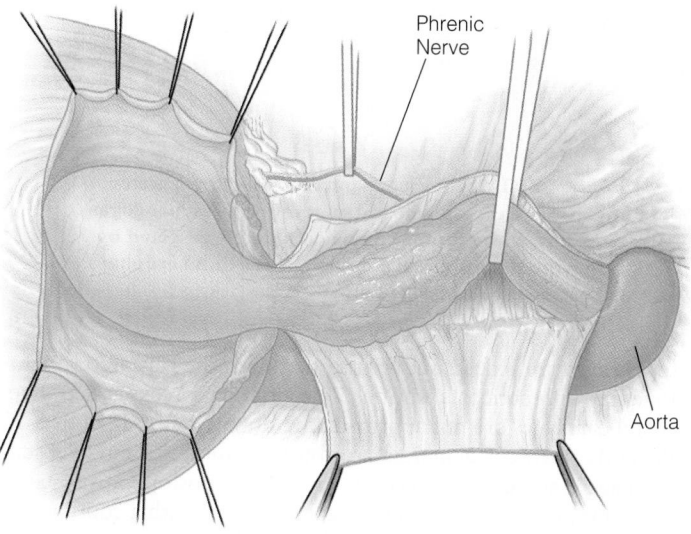

Phrenic
Nerve

Aorta

Diaphragm Sutures

Figure 21 **Left thoracoabdominal esophagogastrectomy. The diaphragm is incised radially. The branches of the pericardial phrenic artery are suture-ligated, and the sutures are left long to be used as diaphragmatic retractors. The pulmonary ligament is divided, and the esophagus is mobilized above the tumor and retracted with a Penrose drain. The esophageal vessels are ligated and divided. The tumor and the esophagus are mobilized off the aorta down to the hiatus; 1 cm of the diaphragmatic crura is taken in continuity with the tumor to provide local clearance. The stomach is then mobilized in much the same way as in a transhiatal esophagectomy [*see Figure 9*].**

abandoned. A feeding jejunostomy, an esophageal stent, or both may be inserted to improve swallowing and allow nutrition.

Step 2: assessment of gastric involvement and incision of diaphragm The extent to which the tumor involves the stomach determines whether a total gastrectomy or a proximal gastrectomy is indicated along with the distal esophagectomy. If no metastases are found, the incision is extended and the chest is opened with a left posterolateral incision through the sixth interspace. If the thoracic component of the tumor appears to be resectable, the costal margin is divided. It is advisable to remove a 1 to 2 cm segment of the costal margin to facilitate repair of the diaphragm at the end of the operation and reduce postoperative costal margin pain. The diaphragm is incised radially [*see Figure 21*]. Branches of the pericardiophrenic artery are suture-ligated, and the sutures are left long so that they can be used as diaphragmatic retractors. Alternatively, a circumferential incision may be made about 2 cm from the costal margin to reduce the risk of postoperative diaphragmatic paralysis.

Step 3: division of pulmonary ligament and mobilization of esophagus and stomach The pulmonary ligament is divided, and the mediastinal pleura is incised over the esophagus as far as the aortic arch. The esophagus is mobilized above the tumor and is retracted by a Penrose drain [*see Figure 21*]. The esophageal vessels are carefully dissected, ligated, and divided. The tumor is then mobilized; the plane of the dissection is kept close to the aorta on the left, and if necessary, the right parietal pleura is taken in continuity with the lesion. About 1 cm of the crura is taken in continuity with the tumor to provide good local clearance. The stomach is then mobilized in much the same way as in a transhiatal esophagectomy [*see Figure 9*].

Step 4: assessment of pancreatic involvement and hepatic viability The lesser sac is opened through the greater omentum so that it can be determined whether the primary tumor involves the distal pancreas. If so, it is reasonable to resect the distal pancreas, the spleen, or both in continuity with the stomach; if not, the short gastric vessels are ligated and divided, with the spleen preserved. The lesser omentum is detached from the right side of the esophagus and the hilum of the liver, then divided down to the area of the pylorus, with the right gastric artery and vein preserved. There is often a hepatic branch from the left gastric artery running through the gastrohepatic omentum. If this hepatic branch is of significant size, a soft vascular clamp should be placed on the artery for 20 minutes so that the viability of the liver can be assessed. If the liver is viable, the artery is suture-ligated and divided.

Step 5: division of greater omentum and short gastric vessels The greater omentum is divided, with care taken to preserve the right gastroepiploic artery and vein. These two vessels are suture-ligated and divided well away from the stomach. Ligation and division of the short gastric vessels allow complete mobilization of the greater curvature of the stomach. Dissection is extended downward as far as the pylorus. The stomach is turned upward, and the left gastric vessels are exposed through the lesser sac [*see Figure 10*]. The lymph nodes along the celiac axis and the left gastric artery are swept up into the specimen, and the gastric vessels are either suture-ligated or stapled.

Step 6: choice of partial or total gastrectomy At this time, the surgeon determines whether the whole stomach must be resected to remove the gastric part of the cancer or whether a partial (i.e., proximal) gastrectomy will suffice.

Proximal esophagogastrectomy with esophagogastrostomy. If the surgeon decides that resection of the proximal stomach will remove all of the tumor while leaving at least 5 cm of tumor-free stomach, a proximal esophagogastrectomy is performed [*see Figure 22*]. A gastric tube is fashioned with a linear stapler [*see* Transhiatal Esophagectomy, Step 9, *above, and Figure 15*]. The staple line is oversewn with inverting 3-0 sutures. Because the vagus nerves are divided and gastric stasis may result, a pyloromyotomy is performed, much as in a transhiatal esophagectomy.

The proximal gastric resection margin is covered with a sponge and turned upward over the costal margin. The stomach tube is then brought up through the hiatus and into the thorax behind the proximal esophageal resection margin. The margin should be at least 10 cm from the proximal end of the esophagogastric cancer. If the esophageal resection margin is not adequate, the stomach tube is mobilized and brought to the left neck, then anastomosed to the cervical esophagus through a left neck incision; alternatively, the left colon is interposed between the gastric stump and the cervical esophagus. If the resection margin is adequate, the tip of the stomach tube is sewn to the posterior wall of the esophagus [*see Figure 23*].

The anastomosis is then performed with the stapling technique previously described for transhiatal esophagectomy [*see Figures 16 and 17*]. A nasogastric tube is passed down into the gastric remnant. The tube is sewn to the pericardium and the endothoracic fascia to prevent anastomotic dehiscence.

Total gastrectomy with Roux-en-Y esophagojejunostomy. If the surgeon decides that a total gastrectomy is necessary, the right gastroepiploic and right gastric vessels are suture-ligated and divided distal to the pylorus. The duodenum is divided just distal to the pylorus with a linear stapler. The staple line is inverted with interrupted 3-0 nonabsorbable sutures and covered with omentum to prevent duodenal stump blowout.

The esophagus is then mobilized up to the level of the inferior pulmonary vein. Two retaining sutures are placed in the esophageal wall. A monofilament nylon purse-string suture is placed around the circumferance of the proximal esophagus in preparation for stapling. A No. 24 Foley catheter with a 20 ml balloon is advanced into the esophagus and gently inflated to distend the esophageal lumen. The resected specimen is sent to the pathologist for examination of the margins.

A jejunal interposition is then fashioned by using the Roux-en-Y technique. One or two jejunal arteriovenous arcades are divided to mobilize enough jejunum to allow anastomosis to the thoracic esophagus [*see Figure 24*]. After removal of the Foley catheter, a 25 or 28 mm EEA stapler is passed through the jejunum into the esophagus, fired, and removed. The jejunum is anchored to the pericardium and the proximal esophagus. The duodenal loop is anastomosed to the jejunum at least 45 to 50 cm distal to the esophageal jejunal anastomosis to minimize bile reflux [*see Figure 24*]. The blind end of the jejunal loop is then stapled closed.

After careful irrigation of the chest, the first step in the closure is to repair the diaphragm around the hiatus. The gastric or jejunal interposition is sewn to the crura with interrupted nonabsorbable sutures. The remainder of the diaphragm is closed with interrupted nonabsorbable 0 mattress sutures. A chest tube is placed into the pleural space close to but not touching the anastomosis. The final sutures in the peripheral part of the

Figure 22 **Left thoracoabdominal esophagogastrectomy: proximal esophagogastrectomy with esophagogastrostomy. If the tumor can be completely resected by removing the proximal stomach, a proximal esophagogastrectomy is carried out.**

diaphragm are placed but are not tied until the ribs are brought together with pericostal sutures. The left lung is reexpanded. The costal cartilages are not approximated but are left to float free. If the ends of the costal margin are abutting, another 2 cm of costal cartilage should be removed to reduce postoperative pain. Thoracic and abdominal skin layers are closed with a continuous absorbable suture. The skin and the subcutaneous tissue are closed in the usual fashion.

POSTOPERATIVE CARE

As a rule, patients are not routinely admitted to the ICU after esophagectomy; however, individual practices depend on the distribution of skilled nursing and physiotherapy personnel. Early ambulation is the mainstay of postoperative care. As a rule, patients are able to walk slowly, with assistance, on postoperative day 1. Patient-controlled epidural analgesia is particularly useful in facilitating good pulmonary toilet and minimizing the risk of atelectasis or pneumonia.

Figure 23 **Left thoracoabdominal esophagogastrectomy: proximal esophagogastrectomy with esophagogastrostomy. The esophagus is sewn to the tip of the stomach tube, halfway between the lesser curvature suture line and the greater curvature. An anastomosis is then fashioned with the stapling technique used in transhiatal esophagectomy [*see Figures 16 and 17*].**

The nasogastric tube is removed on postoperative day 3; jejunostomy tube feedings are gradually started at the same time. Once bowel function normalizes, patients are allowed small sips of liquids. Chest tubes are removed as pleural drainage subsides. By postoperative day 6, most patients have progressed to a soft solid diet. Dietary education is provided, focusing primarily on eating smaller and more frequent meals, avoiding bulky foods (e.g., meat and bread) in the early postoperative period, and taking measures to minimize postprandial dumping. Patients are also taught how to care for their temporary feeding jejunostomy. Consumption of caffeine and carbonated beverages is usually limited during the first few weeks after discharge.

A barium swallow is performed on postoperative day 7 to verify the integrity of the anastomosis and the patency of the pyloromyotomy. Patients are usually discharged on postoperative day 7 or 8. The feeding jejunostomy is left in place until the first postoperative evaluation, which usually takes place 2 to 3 weeks after the operation. The feeding tube is removed during that visit if oral intake and weight are stable.

COMPLICATIONS OF ESOPHAGECTOMY

Pulmonary Impairment

Atelectasis and pneumonia should be considered preventable complications of esophagectomy. Patients with recognized pre-

operative impairment of pulmonary reserve should be considered for transhiatal esophagectomy. Existing pulmonary function can be optimized through incentive spirometry, use of bronchodilators, and physical rehabilitation. Chronic nocturnal aspiration from esophageal obstruction should be watched for in the preoperative patient. Effective pain control is essential to prevent postoperative atelectasis. Routine use of patient-controlled thoracic epidural analgesia should be considered. Deep breathing, early ambulation, and chest physiotherapy encourage the clearing of bronchial secretions. Certain patients will require nasotracheal aspiration or bronchoscopy for pulmonary toilet.

Tracheobronchial Injury

Laceration of the membranous trachea or the left mainstem bronchus may occur during esophagectomy. When such injuries occur during transthoracic resection, management is relatively simple, thanks to the already excellent operative exposure. Direct suture repair and tissue reinforcement with adjacent pleura or a

Figure 24 **Left thoracoabdominal esophagogastrectomy: total gastrectomy with Roux-en-Y esophagojejunostomy. A jejunal interposition is fashioned with the Roux-en-Y technique. One or two jejunal arteriovenous arcades are divided to mobilize enough jejunum for anastomosis to the thoracic esophagus. A 25 or 28 mm EEA stapler is passed through the jejunum into the esophagus. The jejunum is anchored to the pericardium and the proximal esophagus. The duodenal loop is anastomosed to the jejunum at least 45 to 50 cm distal to the esophageal-jejunal anastomosis. The blind end of the jejunal loop is then stapled closed.**

pedicle of intercostal muscle provide safe closure in almost all cases. When tracheobronchial injuries occur during transhiatal esophagectomy, they are less obvious but no less urgent. This rare complication arises during mediastinal dissection. Typically, the anesthetic team notes a loss of ventilatory volume, and the surgeon may detect the smell of inhalational agents in the operative field. Bronchoscopy should be promptly performed to identify the site of the injury. The uncut endotracheal tube is then advanced past the site of the laceration to restore proper ventilation. High tracheal injuries can usually be repaired by extending the cervical incision and adding a partial sternotomy. Injury to the carina or the left mainstem bronchus must be repaired via a right thoracotomy.

Bleeding

Hemorrhage should be rare during esophagectomy. The blood supply to the esophagus consists of small branches coming from the aorta, which are easily controlled and generally constrict if left untied. Splenic injuries sometimes occur during mobilization of the stomach. The resultant hemorrhage can be immediate or delayed; blood loss may be significant, and splenectomy is usually required. Precise dissection around the left gastric artery is vital: the bleeding vessels may retract, and attempts at control may result in injury to the celiac artery or its hepatic branches.

Bleeding that arises during the mediastinal stage of the transhiatal esophagectomy generally subsides with packing if it derives from periesophageal arterial branches. Brisk loss of dark blood usually signifies injury to the azygos vein. The first step in addressing such injuries is to pack the mediastinum quickly so as to allow the anesthetic team to stabilize the patient and infuse fluid. Chest tubes are immediately placed to allow detection of any free hemorrhage into the pleural space. Precise localization of the bleeding site may then follow. Injury to the azygos vein may be addressed via an upper sternal split; however, when the exposure is poor, the surgeon should not hesitate to proceed to a full sternotomy. Bleeding from the subcarinal area is usually bright red and may involve bronchial arteries or small periesophageal vessels arising from the aorta, both of which can usually be controlled through the hiatus.

Laryngeal Nerve Injury

Injury to the recurrent laryngeal nerve is a major potential complication of transhiatal esophagectomy. Traction neuropraxia may be temporary and require no specific treatment. Permanent injury will lead to hoarseness and impaired protection of the airway during deglutition. Meticulous protection of the nerve during the cervical stage should minimize the incidence of this complication.

Of particular concern is the risk of bilateral nerve injury after a transthoracic esophagectomy with a cervical esophagogastric anastomosis (i.e., a so-called three-hole esophagectomy). Any dissection of the upper esophagus performed through the right chest should be done as close to the esophagus as possible to avoid placing traction on the right recurrent laryngeal nerve; the subsequent left cervical dissection may put the left recurrent laryngeal nerve at risk for damage. Bilateral paralysis of the vocal cords is very poorly tolerated and has a devastating impact on quality of life.

Chylothorax

Thoracic duct injuries typically present by postoperative day 3 or 4. Dyspnea and pleural effusion may be noted if thoracostomy tubes are not in place. Thoracocentesis yields an opaque, milky fluid. In patients who already have a chest drain in place, there is typically a high volume of serous drainage in the first 2 postoperative days. As enteral nutrition is established and dietary fat reintroduced, the fluid assumes a characteristic milky appearance. In most cases, the gross appearance is diagnostic, and there is rarely a need to confirm the diagnosis by measuring the triglyceride level. A thoracostomy drain is placed to monitor the volume of the chyle leak. Chest x-rays should be obtained to verify complete drainage of the pleural space and full expansion of the lung.

Patients with chylothorax should be converted to fat-free enteral nutrition. Persistent drainage exceeding 500 ml/8 hr is an indication for early operation and ligation of the thoracic duct; high-volume chyle leaks are unlikely to close spontaneously. Prolonged loss of chyle causes significant electrolyte, nutritional, and immunologic derangements that may prove fatal if allowed to progress. Accordingly, patients with persistent chyle leakage should undergo operation within 1 week of diagnosis. A Dobbhoff feeding tube is placed in the duodenum before operation if a jejunostomy tube is not already in place. Jejunal feeding with 35% cream at a rate of 60 ml/hr is maintained for at least 4 hours before operation. Feeding is continued even during the procedure: the enteral fat stimulates a brisk flow of chyle and greatly facilitates visualization of any thoracic duct injury.

Right-side chyle leaks are approached via either a thoracotomy or video-assisted thoracoscopy. The magnification and excellent illumination associated with thoracoscopy are partially counterbalanced by the constraints imposed by port placement and limited tissue retraction. The inferior pulmonary ligament is divided, and the posterior mediastinum is inspected for extravasation of milky fluid. Any visible sources of chyle leakage can be controlled with clips or suture ligatures. In some cases, mass ligation of the thoracic duct at the level of the diaphragm, incorporating all the soft tissue between the aorta and the azygos vein, may be required.

Left-side leaks can be difficult to manage. The subcarinal area is typically involved; this is the level at which the thoracic duct crosses over from the right. Exploration should begin on the left side. If the leak cannot be visualized, a right-side approach may be necessary to control the thoracic duct as it first enters the chest.

Anastomotic Leakage

The consequences of anastomotic complications after esophagectomy vary considerably in severity, depending on their location and their cause. The cervical anastomotic leaks that may develop after transhiatal esophagectomy are generally simple to treat. Leaks in the early postoperative period are usually related to technical factors, such as excessive tension across the anastomosis. Any possibility of ischemia in the transposed stomach must be addressed promptly, given that a nonviable stomach may not give rise to obvious signs. Tachycardia, confusion, leukocytosis, cervical wound drainage, and neck tenderness may or may not be present.

The morbidity of an open cervical wound is not great—certainly less than that of an untreated leak. Accordingly, any clinical suspicion of a leak should prompt a diagnostic contrast swallow study using dilute barium. Large leaks are manifested as persistent collections of contrast material outside the esophagus. Although such leaks rarely extend into the pleural space, any fluid in the chest must be drained so that its nature can be determined. The neck wound is opened by removing the sutures and performing gentle digital exploration of the prevertebral space behind the esophagus as the finger is advanced into the mediastinum; this is usually done at the bedside and requires little, if any, patient sedation.

Saline-moistened gauze packing is changed three or four times a day. Prolonged or copious cervical drainage may call for supplemental deep wound aspiration with a Yankauer suction handle. Administering water per os during aspiration facilitates removal of any necrotic debris. A fetid, malodorous breath associated with sanguineous discharge from the nasogastric tube and purulent fluid in the opened neck incision are ominous signs that should prompt early esophagoscopy. Diffuse mucosal ischemia may indicate the presence of a nonviable stomach; reoperation with completion gastrectomy and proximal esophagostomy is required to treat this catastrophic complication.

Generally, leaks that occur more than 7 days after operation are small and are related to some degree of late ischemic disruption along the anastomosis. They can usually be managed by opening the cervical wound at the bedside and packing the site with gauze. Oral diet is advanced as tolerated. It may be noted that the volume of the leak is markedly greater or less depending on the position of the head during swallowing. Accordingly, before discharge, patients are taught how to temporarily adjust their swallowing as well as how to manage their dressing changes. Applying gentle pressure to the neck wound and turning the head to the left may help the patient ingest liquids with minimal soiling of the open neck incision. Dysphagia, even with an opened neck incision, should be treated by passing tapered esophageal dilators per os between 2 and 4 weeks after surgery. When a bougie at least 48 French in caliber can be passed through the anastomosis, the patient can usually swallow comfortably. The size of the leak often decreases after dilatation as food is allowed to proceed preferentially into the stomach.

When a routine predischarge barium swallow after transhiatal esophagectomy raises the possibility of an anastomotic leak in an asymptomatic patient, the question arises of whether the wound should be opened at all. For small, contained leaks associated with preferential flow of contrast material into the stomach, observation alone may suffice in selected cases. Patients must be closely watched for fever or other signs of major infection. Given that cervical wound exploration carries quite a low morbidity, the surgeon should not hesitate to drain the neck should the patient's condition change.

The incidence of anastomotic leakage is low after Ivor-Lewis resection, but the consequences are significant. Leaks presenting early in the postoperative period are usually related to technical problems and are difficult to manage; those presenting later are generally related to some degree of ischemic tissue loss. Patients who have received radiation therapy or are nutritionally depleted may be especially vulnerable to problems with anastomotic healing. A contrast swallow with dilute barium is the best method of evaluating the anastomosis. Leaks may be manifested either as a free flow of contrast into the pleural space or as a contained fluid collection.

Small leaks that drain immediately into properly placed thoracostomy tubes can usually be managed by giving antibiotics and withholding oral intake. Local control of infection generally results in spontaneous healing. Anastomotic disruptions that are large or are associated with a major pleural collection typically necessitate open drainage with decortication; percutaneous drainage may be considered as a preliminary approach in selected patients. Persistent soiling of the mediastinum and the pleural space is fatal if untreated.

Early esophagoscopy is strongly advised to evaluate the viability of the gastric remnant. Ischemic necrosis of the stomach necessitates reexploration, decortication, takedown of the anastomosis, gastric debridement, return of any viable stomach into the abdomen, closure of the hiatus, and proximal diversion with a cervical esophagostomy. Repair or revision of the anastomosis in an infected field is certain to fail and should never be considered. In certain cases, diversion via a cervical esophagostomy and a completion gastrectomy may be required.

Late Complications

At every postoperative visit, symptoms of reflux, regurgitation, dumping, poor gastric emptying, and dysphagia must be specifically sought: these are the major quality-of-life issues for postesophagectomy patients.[4] Reflux and regurgitation may complicate any form of alimentary reconstruction after esophagectomy, though cervical anastomoses are less likely to be associated with symptomatic reflux than intrathoracic anastomoses are. Reflux symptoms generally respond to dietary modifications, such as smaller and more frequent meals. Regurgitation is usually related to the supine position and thus tends to be worse at night; elevating the bed and avoiding late meals may suffice for symptom control. Dumping is exacerbated by foods with high fat or sugar content. Dysphagia may be related to narrowing at the anastomosis or, rarely, to poor emptying of the transposed stomach. Anastomotic strictures are most commonly encountered as a sequel to postoperative leakage, resulting either from anatomic distortion of the transposed stomach or from simple atony. Specific tests for gastric atony include nuclear medicine gastric emptying studies using radiolabeled food.

Any form of anastomotic leak will increase the incidence of late stricture. Dysphagia may be treated by means of progressive dilatation with Maloney bougies. This procedure is performed in the outpatient clinic and does not require sedation or any other special patient preparation. Complications are rare if due care is exercised during the procedure. As noted elsewhere [*see* Transthoracic Hiatal Hernia Repair, Preoperative Evaluation, Dilatation, *above*], it is essential that the caliber of the dilators be increased gradually and that little or no force be applied in advancing them. The appearance of blood on a withdrawn dilator signals a breach of the mucosa; further dilatation should be done cautiously lest a transmural injury result. Comfortable swallowing is usually achieved after the successful passage of a 48 French bougie. For late strictures that are particularly difficult to dilate, endoscopic examination and histologic evaluation may be required to rule out a recurrent tumor. CT of the chest should also be performed whenever there is unexplained weight loss late after esophagectomy.

The Savary system of wire-guided dilators has been particularly helpful in the management of tight or eccentric strictures. Patients are generally treated in the endoscopy suite. Temporary sedation with I.V. fentanyl and midazolam is required. Fluoroscopy is used to confirm proper placement of a flexible-tip wire across the stricture. Serial wire-guided dilation can then be performed with confidence and increased patient safety.

OUTCOME EVALUATION

Transhiatal Esophagectomy

A 1999 study from the University of Michigan presented data on 1,085 patients who underwent transhiatal esophagectomy without thoracotomy, of whom 74% had carcinoma and 26% had nonmalignant disease.[5] Transhiatal esophagectomy was completed in 98.6% of the patients; the remaining 1.4% were converted to a transthoracic esophagectomy as a result of either thoracic esophageal fixation or bleeding. Previous chemotherapy or radiation therapy did not preclude performance of a transhiatal esophagectomy. Nine patients experienced inordinate intraoperative blood loss; three died as a result. The overall hospital mortality was 4%. The overall 5-year survival rate for patients undergoing transhiatal esophagectomy is approximately 20% for adenocarcinoma of the cardia and the esophagus and 30% for squamous cell carcinoma of the esophagus.

The stapled anastomosis described earlier [see Operative Technique, Transhiatal Esophagectomy, Step 8, above] reflects numerous refinements introduced at the University of Michigan. The endoscopic GIA stapler has a low-profile head that is ideally suited to the tight confines of the neck, enabling the surgeon to fashion a widely patent side-to-side functional end-to-end anastomosis with three rows of staples along the back wall. The rate of anastomotic stricture is markedly lower with this anastomosis than with a totally hand-sewn anastomosis. As regards postoperative function, stomach interposition through the posterior mediastinum after transhiatal esophagectomy is associated with low rates of aspiration and regurgitation. Esophageal reflux and esophagitis—commonly seen with intrathoracic esophagogastric anastomoses—are usually not clinically significant problems with this approach. Patients are advised to elevate the head of their bed and to continue taking proton pump inhibitors for about 3 months after the operation. Approximately one third will require esophageal dilatation for dysphagia after the operation. Some 7% to 10% experience postvagotomy dumping symptoms, which in most cases can be controlled by simply avoiding high-carbohydrate foods and dairy products.

Ivor-Lewis Esophagectomy

Ivor-Lewis esophagectomy is associated with anastomotic leakage rates and operative mortalities of less than 3%.[3,6] Approximately 5% of patients will require anastomotic dilatation. Again, patients are advised to elevate the head of the bed and to continue taking proton pump inhibitors. In some patients, the gastric interposition rotates into the right posterolateral thoracic gutter, resulting in postprandial gastric tension and rendering them more susceptible to aspiration. The 3-year survival rate is approximately 18% to 25%.

Left Thoracoabdominal Esophagectomy

Left thoracoabdominal esophagogastrectomy is also associated with anastomotic leakage rates and operative mortalities of less than 3%.[7] Approximately 5% of patients will require esophageal dilatation. Reconstructions involving anastomosis of the distal stomach to the esophagus are associated with a high incidence of delayed gastric emptying and bile gastritis and esophagitis. Of all the operations we have described, this one results in the lowest postoperative quality of life. Accordingly, most surgeons prefer to carry out a total gastrectomy. Swallowing is restored with a Roux-en-Y jejunal interposition.

References

1. Lahey FH, Warren K: Esophageal diverticula. Surg Gynecol Obstet 98:1, 1954

2. Stirling MC, Orringer MB: Continued assessment of the combined Collis-Nissen operation. Ann Thorac Surg 47:224, 1989

3. Mathiesen DJ, Grillo HC, Wilkens EW Jr: Transthoracic esophagectomy: a safe approach to carcinoma of the esophagus. Ann Thorac Surg 45:137, 1988

4. Finley RJ, Lamy A, Clifton J, et al: Gastrointestinal function following esophagectomy for malignancy. Am J Surg 169:471, 1995

5. Orringer MB, Marshall B, Iannettoni MD: Transhiatal esophagectomy: clinical experience and refinements. Ann Surg 230:392, 1999

6. King RM, Pairolero PC, Trastek VF, et al: Ivor Lewis esophagogastrectomy for carcinoma of the esophagus: early and long-term results. Ann Thorac Surg 44:119, 1987

7. Akiyama H, Miyazono H, Tsurumaru M, et al: Thoracoabdominal approach for carcinoma of the cardia of the stomach. Am J Surg 137:345, 1979

Acknowledgment

Figures 1 through 24   Tom Moore.

8 MINIMALLY INVASIVE ESOPHAGEAL PROCEDURES

Marco G. Patti, M.D., and Piero M. Fisichella, M.D.

During the 1970s and the 1980s, operations for benign esophageal disorders were often withheld or delayed in favor of less effective forms of treatment in an effort to prevent the postoperative discomfort, the long hospital stay, and the recovery time associated with open surgical procedures. For instance, pneumatic dilatation became the first line of treatment for achalasia, even though studies had shown that surgical management was clearly superior.[1]

Since the beginning of the 1990s, thanks to the advent of minimally invasive techniques, there has been a revolution in the field of general surgery and, in particular, in the management of benign esophageal disorders. In the first part of the 1990s, it became clear that treatment of these conditions with minimally invasive procedures yielded results comparable to those of treatment with traditional operations while causing minimal postoperative discomfort, reducing the duration of hospitalization, shortening recovery time, and permitting earlier return to work.[2,3] Consequently, minimally invasive surgery was increasingly considered as first-line treatment for achalasia, and laparoscopic fundoplication was considered more readily and at an earlier stage in the management of gastroesophageal reflux disease (GERD).

In the latter part of the 1990s and the first few years of the 21st century, minimally invasive esophageal procedures continued to evolve, thanks to better instrumentation and improved surgical expertise. In addition, as experience with these procedures accumulates and the follow-up period lengthens, it becomes possible to analyze techniques and their results more rigorously. For instance, whereas 7 years ago a left thoracoscopic Heller myotomy was considered the procedure of choice for achalasia, the current procedure of choice is a laparoscopic Heller myotomy with partial fundoplication, which is now known to be better at relieving dysphagia and controlling postoperative reflux.[4-7] Similarly, whereas total fundoplication and partial fundoplication were initially considered equally effective in treating GERD,[8] long-term follow-up indicates that total fundoplication is clearly superior in controlling reflux and should be used whenever feasible.[9]

In what follows, we do not address the standard open esophageal operations, which are described elsewhere [*see V:7 Open Esophageal Procedures*]. Instead, we focus on minimally invasive techniques for the treatment of abnormal gastroesophageal reflux and motility disorders of the esophagus.

Laparoscopic Nissen Fundoplication

PREOPERATIVE EVALUATION

All patients who are candidates for a laparoscopic fundoplication should undergo a preoperative evaluation that includes the following: (1) symptomatic evaluation, (2) an upper GI series,

(3) endoscopy, (4) esophageal manometry, and (5) ambulatory pH monitoring.

Symptomatic Evaluation

The presence of both typical symptoms (heartburn, regurgitation, and dysphagia) and atypical symptoms of GERD (cough, wheezing, chest pain, and hoarseness) should be investigated, and symptoms should be graded with respect to their intensity both before and after operation. Nonetheless, a diagnosis of GERD should never be based solely on symptomatic evaluation. Many authorities assert that the diagnosis of GERD can be made reliably from the clinical history,[10] so that a complaint of heartburn should lead to the presumption that acid reflux is present; however, testing of this diagnostic strategy demonstrates that symptoms are far less sensitive and specific than is usually believed.[11] For instance, our group found that of 822 consecutive patients referred for esophageal function tests with a clinical diagnosis of GERD (based on symptoms and endoscopic findings), only 70% had abnormal reflux on pH monitoring.[12] Heartburn and regurgitation were no more frequent in patients who had genuine reflux than in those who did not; thus, symptomatic evaluation, by itself, could not distinguish between the two groups.

The response to proton pump inhibitors is a better predictor of abnormal reflux. For example, in our study, 75% of patients with GERD reported a good or excellent response to these agents, compared with only 26% of patients without GERD.[12] Similarly, a 1999 multivariate analysis of factors predicting outcome after laparoscopic fundoplication concluded that a clinical response to acid suppression therapy was one of three factors predictive of a successful outcome, the other two being an abnormal 24-hour pH score and the presence of a typical primary symptom (e.g., heartburn).[13]

Upper Gastrointestinal Series

An upper GI series is useful for diagnosing and characterizing an existing hiatal hernia. The size of the hiatal hernia helps predict how difficult it will be to reduce the esophagogastric junction below the diaphragm. In addition, large hiatal hernias are associated with more severe disturbances of esophageal peristalsis and esophageal acid clearance.[14] Esophagograms are also useful for determining the location, shape, and size of a stricture and detecting a short esophagus.

Endoscopy

Endoscopy is typically the first test performed to confirm a symptom-based diagnosis of GERD. This approach has two pitfalls, however. First, even though the goal of endoscopy is to assess the mucosal damage caused by reflux, mucosal changes are absent in about 50% of GERD patients.[12] Second, major interobserver variations have been reported with esophageal

Leg Holder

Bean Bag

Figure 1 **Laparoscopic Nissen fundoplication. Shown is the operating table used for laparoscopic fundoplication.**

endoscopy, particularly for low-grade esophagitis.[15] For instance, our group found that of 247 patients with negative results on pH monitoring, 60 (24%) had been diagnosed as having grade I or II esophagitis.[12] Accordingly, we believe that endoscopy is most valuable for excluding gastric and duodenal pathology and for detecting the presence of Barrett's esophagus.

Esophageal Manometry

Esophageal manometry provides useful information about the motor function of the esophagus by determining the length and resting pressure of the lower esophageal sphincter (LES) and assessing the quality (i.e., the amplitude and propagation) of esophageal peristalsis. In addition, it allows proper placement of the pH probe for ambulatory pH monitoring (5 cm above the upper border of the LES).

Ambulatory pH Monitoring

Ambulatory pH monitoring is the most reliable test for the diagnosis of GERD, with a sensitivity and specificity of about 92%.[16] It is of key importance in the workup for the following four reasons:

1. It determines whether abnormal reflux is present. In our study, pH monitoring yielded normal results in 30% of patients with a clinical diagnosis of GERD,[12] thereby obviating the continuation of inappropriate and expensive drugs (e.g., proton pump inhibitors) or the performance of a fundoplication. In addition, pH monitoring prompted further investigation that in a number of cases pointed to other diseases, such as cholelithiasis and irritable bowel syndrome.

2. It establishes a temporal correlation between symptoms and episodes of reflux. Such a correlation is particularly important when atypical symptoms (e.g., cough and wheezing) are present because 50% of these patients experience no heartburn and 50% do not have esophagitis on endoscopy.[17]

3. It allows staging of patients according to disease severity. Specifically, pH monitoring identifies a subgroup of patients characterized by worse esophageal motor function (manifest-

ed by a defective LES or by abnormal esophageal peristalsis), more acid reflux in the distal and proximal esophagus, and slower acid clearance. These patients more frequently experience stricture formation and Barrett metaplasia and thus might benefit from early antireflux surgery.[18]

4. It provides baseline data that may prove very useful postoperatively if symptoms do not respond to the procedure.

OPERATIVE PLANNING

The patient is placed under general anesthesia and intubated with a single-lumen endotracheal tube. Abdominal wall relaxation is ensured by the administration of a nondepolarizing muscle relaxant, the action of which is rapidly reversed at the end of the operation. Adequate muscle relaxation is essential because increased abdominal wall compliance allows increased pneumoperitoneum, which yields better exposure. An orogastric tube is inserted at the beginning of the operation to keep the stomach decompressed; it is removed at the end of the procedure.

The patient is placed in a steep reverse Trendelenburg position, with the legs extended on stirrups. The surgeon stands between the patient's legs. To keep the patient from sliding as a result of the steep position used during the operation, a bean bag is inflated under the patient [*see Figure 1*], and the knees are flexed only 20° to 30°. A Foley catheter is inserted at the beginning of the procedure and usually is removed in the postoperative period. Because increased abdominal pressure from pneumoperitoneum and the steep reverse Trendelenburg position decrease venous return, pneumatic compression stockings are always used as prophylaxis against deep vein thrombosis.

The equipment required for a laparoscopic Nissen fundoplication includes five 10 mm trocars, a 30° laparoscope, a hook cautery, and various other instruments [*see Table 1*]. In addition, we use a three-chip camera system that is separate from the laparoscope.

OPERATIVE TECHNIQUE

In all patients except those with very poor esophageal motility—for whom partial fundoplication [*see* Laparoscopic Partial

(Guarner) Fundoplication, *below*] is preferable—we advocate performing a 360° wrap of the gastric fundus around the lower esophagus as described by Nissen, but we always take down the short gastric vessels to achieve what is called a floppy fundoplication. This type of wrap is very effective in controlling gastroesophageal reflux.[1] The operation can be divided into nine key steps as follows.

Step 1: Insertion of Trocars

Five 10 mm trocars are used for the operation [*see Figure 2*]. Port A is placed about 14 cm below the xiphoid process; it can also be placed slightly (2 to 3 cm) to the left of the midline to be in line with the hiatus. This port is used for insertion of the scope. Port B is placed at the same level as port A, but in the left midclavicular line. It is used for insertion of the Babcock clamp; insertion of a grasper to hold the Penrose drain once it is in place surrounding the esophagus; or insertion of the clip applier, the ultrasonic coagulating shears (LaparoSonic Coagulating Shears [LCS], Ethicon Endo-Surgery, Inc.), or both to take down the short gastric vessels. Port C is placed at the same level as the previous two ports but in the right midclavicular line. It is used for insertion of the fan retractor, the purpose of which is to lift the lateral segment of the left lobe of the liver and expose the esophagogastric junction. We do not divide the left triangular ligament. The fan retractor can be held in place by a self-retaining system fixed to the operating table. Ports D and E are placed as high as possible under the costal margin and about 5 to 6 cm to the right and the left of the midline, so that they are about 15 cm from the esophageal hiatus; in addition, they should be placed in such a way that their axes form an angle of 60° to 120°. These ports are used for insertion of the graspers, the electrocautery, and the suturing instruments.

Troubleshooting   A common mistake is to place the ports too low in the abdomen, thereby making the operation more difficult. If port C is too low, the fan retractor will not retract the lateral segment of the left lobe of the liver well, and the esophagogastric junction will not be exposed. If port B is too low, the Babcock clamp will not reach the esophagogastric junction, and when the LCS or the clip applier is placed through the same

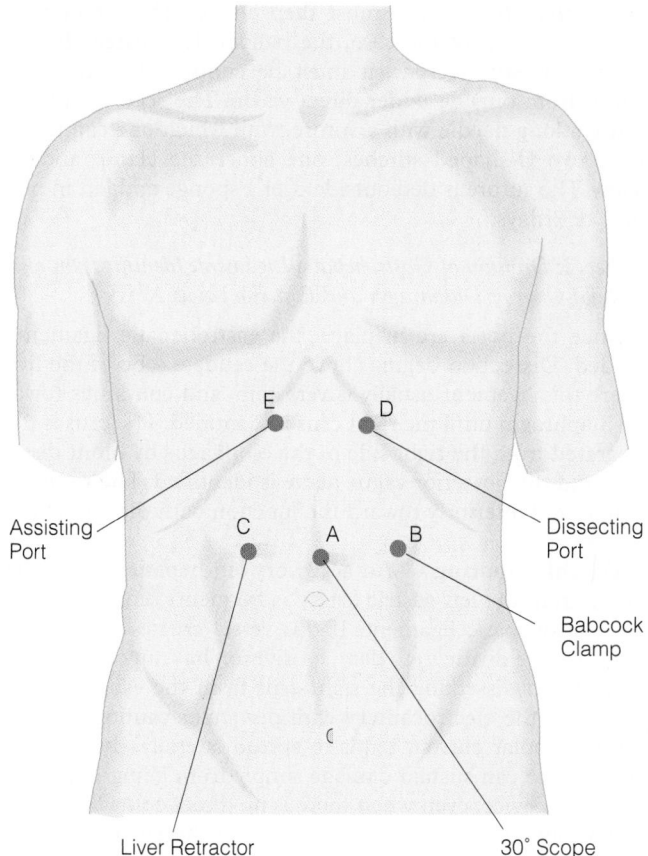

Figure 2 **Laparoscopic Nissen fundoplication. Illustrated is the recommended placement of the trocars.**

port, it will not reach the upper short gastric vessels. If ports D and E are too low, the dissection at the beginning of the case and the suturing at the end are problematic.

Other mistakes of positioning must be avoided as well. It is important not to place port C too medially, because the fan retractor may clash with the left-hand instrument; the gallbladder fossa is a good landmark for positioning this port. Port A must be placed with extreme caution in the supraumbilical area: its insertion site is just above the aorta, before its bifurcation. Accordingly, we recommend initially inflating the abdomen to a pressure of 18 mm Hg just for placement of port A; increasing the distance between the abdominal wall and the aorta reduces the risk of aortic injury. We also recommend directing the port toward the coccyx. A Hasson cannula can be used in this location, particularly if the patient has already had one or more midline incisions. Maintaining the proper angle (60° to 120°) between the axes of the two suturing instruments inserted through ports D and E is also important: if the angle is smaller, the instruments will cover part of the operating field, whereas if it is larger, depth perception may be impaired. Finally, if a trocar is not in the ideal position, it is better to insert another one than to operate through an inconveniently placed port.

If the surgeon spears the epigastric vessels with a trocar, bleeding will occur, in which case there are two options. The first option is to pull the port out, insert a 24 French Foley catheter with a 30 ml balloon through the site, inflate the balloon, and apply traction with a clamp. The advantage of this maneuver is that the vessel need not be sutured; the disadvan-

---

Table 1 **Instrumentation for Laparoscopic Nissen Fundoplication**

Five 10 mm trocars

30° scope

Graspers

Babcock clamp

L-shaped hook cautery with suction-irrigation capacity

Scissors

Laparoscopic clip applier

Ultrasonic coagulating shears

Fan retractor

Needle holder

Penrose drain

2-0 silk sutures

56 French esophageal bougie

tage is that the surgeon must then choose another insertion site. At the end of the case, the balloon is deflated. If some bleeding is still present, it must be controlled with sutures placed from outside under direct vision. The second option is to use a long needle with a suture, with which one can rapidly place two U-shaped stitches, one above the clamp and one below. The suture is tied outside over a sponge and left in place for 2 or 3 days.

Step 2: Division of Gastrohepatic Ligament; Identification of Right Crus of Diaphragm and Posterior Vagus Nerve

Once the ports are in place, the gastrohepatic ligament is divided. Dissection begins above the caudate lobe of the liver, where this ligament usually is very thin, and continues toward the diaphragm until the right crus is identified. The crus is then separated from the right side of the esophagus by blunt dissection, and the posterior vagus nerve is identified. The right crus is dissected inferiorly toward the junction with the left crus.

Troubleshooting An accessory left hepatic artery originating from the left gastric artery is frequently encountered in the gastrohepatic ligament. If this vessel creates problems of exposure, we divide it; to date, its division has not caused problems. When dissecting the right crus from the esophagus, we try to use the electrocautery with particular caution. Because the monopolar current tends to spread laterally, the posterior vagus nerve can sustain damage simply from being in proximity to the device, even when there is no direct contact. The risk of neuropraxia can be reduced by using the cut mode rather than the coagulation mode when the electrocautery is close to the nerve. The cut mode has problems of its own, however, and is not recommended in most laparoscopic procedures. A better alternative is to use bipolar scissors.

Step 3: Division of Peritoneum and Phrenoesophageal Membrane above Esophagus; Identification of Left Crus of Diaphragm and Anterior Vagus Nerve

The peritoneum and the phrenicoesophageal membrane above the esophagus are divided with the electrocautery, and the anterior vagus nerve is identified. The left crus of the diaphragm is dissected downward toward the junction with the right crus.

Troubleshooting During this part of the dissection, pains should be taken not to damage the anterior vagus nerve or the esophageal wall. To this end, the nerve should be left attached to the esophageal wall, and the peritoneum and the phrenicoesophageal membrane should be lifted from the wall by blunt dissection before they are divided.

Step 4: Creation of Window between Gastric Fundus, Esophagus, and Diaphragmatic Crura; Placement of Penrose Drain around Esophagus

The esophagus is retracted upward by means of a Babcock clamp applied at the level of the esophagogastric junction. Via blunt and sharp dissection, a window is created under the esophagus between the gastric fundus, the esophagus, and the diaphragmatic crura. The window is enlarged with the cautery. Sometimes, one or two short gastric vessels can be divided via this exposure. A Penrose drain is then passed around the esophagus. This drain is used for traction instead of the Babcock clamp from this point on to decrease the chances of damage to the gastric wall.

Troubleshooting There are two main problems to watch for during this part of the procedure: (1) creation of a left pneumothorax and (2) perforation of the gastric fundus.

A left pneumothorax is usually caused by dissection done above the left crus in the mediastinum rather than between the crus and the gastric fundus. This problem can be avoided by properly dissecting and identifying the left crus; the use of curved instruments is also helpful.

Perforation of the gastric fundus is usually caused by pushing a blunt instrument under the esophagus and below the left crus without having done enough dissection. Care must be exercised in taking down small vessels from the gastric fundus when the area behind the esophagus is approached from the right: the anatomy is not as clear from this viewpoint, and perforation can easily occur. Sometimes, perforation is caused by the use of a monopolar electrocautery for dissection. An electrocautery burn can go unrecognized during dissection and manifest itself in the form of a leak during the first 48 hours after operation.

Step 5: Division of Short Gastric Vessels

The clip applier or the LCS is introduced through port B. A grasper is introduced by the surgeon through port D, and an assistant applies traction on the greater curvature of the stomach through port E. Dissection begins at the level of the middle portion of the gastric body and continues upward until the most proximal short gastric vessel is divided and the Penrose drain is reached.

Troubleshooting Again, there are two main problems to watch for during this part of the procedure: (1) bleeding, either from the gastric vessels or from the spleen, and (2) damage to the gastric wall.

Bleeding from the gastric vessels is usually caused by excessive traction or by division of a vessel when the clips are not completely occluding the vessel on both sides. Vessels up to 5 mm in diameter can be taken down with the LCS; this process requires about half of the amount of time needed when only clips are used. The lower blade has a sharp, oscillating inferior edge that must always be kept in view to prevent damage to other structures (e.g., the pancreas, the splenic artery and vein, and the spleen).

Damage to the gastric wall can be caused by a burn from the electrocautery used to dissect between vessels or by traction applied via the graspers or the Babcock clamp.

Step 6: Closure of Crura

The diaphragmatic crura are closed with interrupted 2-0 silk sutures on a curved needle; the sutures are tied intracorporeally. Exposure during this phase is provided by retracting the esophagus upward and toward the patient's left with the Penrose drain. The lens of the 30° laparoscope is angled slightly to the left by moving the light cable of the scope to the patient's right. The first stitch should be placed just above the junction of the two crura. Additional stitches are placed 1 cm apart, and a space of about 1 cm is left between the uppermost stitch and the esophagus.

Troubleshooting Pains must be taken not to spear the posterior wall of the esophagus with either the tip or the back of the needle. We do not place the bougie inside the esophagus during this part of the procedure; to do so would limit the space available for suturing.

Step 7: Insertion of Bougie into Esophagus and through Esophagogastric Junction

The esophageal stethoscope and the orogastric tube are removed, and a 56 French bougie is inserted by the anesthesiologist. The bougie is passed through the esophagogastric junction under the view provided by the laparoscope. The crura must be snug around the esophagus but not too tight: a closed grasper should be able to slide easily between the esophagus and the crura.

Troubleshooting The most worrisome complication during this step is perforation of the esophagus. This can be prevented by lubricating the bougie and instructing the anesthesiologist to advance the bougie slowly and to stop if any resistance is encountered. In addition, it is essential to remove any instruments from the esophagogastric junction and to open the Penrose drain; these measures prevent the creation of an angle between the stomach and the esophagus, which can increase the likelihood of perforation. The position of the bougie can be confirmed by pressing with a grasper over the esophagus, which will feel full when the bougie is in place.

Step 8: Wrapping of Gastric Fundus around Lower Esophagus

The gastric fundus is gently pulled under the esophagus with the graspers. The left and right sides of the fundus are wrapped above the fat pad (which lies above the esophagogastric junction) and held together in place with a Babcock clamp introduced through port B. (The Penrose drain should be removed at this point because it is in the way.) Usually, three 2-0 silk sutures are used to secure the two ends of the wrap to each other. The first stitch does not include the esophagus and is used for traction; the second and the third include a bite of the esophageal muscle. Two coronal stitches are then placed between the top of the wrap and the esophagus, one on the right and one on the left. Finally, two additional sutures are placed between the right side of the wrap and the closed crura. It is important to pass the bougie into the stomach after the first stitch is placed to gauge the size of the wrap. If the wrap seems at all tight, the stitch is removed and repositioned more laterally.

To avoid the risk of injuring the inferior vena cava at the beginning of the dissection, some surgeons use a different method—the so-called left crus approach.[19] In this approach, the operation begins with identification of the left crus of the diaphragm and division of the peritoneum and the phrenicoesophageal membrane overlying it. The next step is division of the short gastric vessels, starting midway along the greater curvature of the stomach and continuing upward to join the area of the previous dissection. When the fundus has been thoroughly mobilized, the peritoneum is divided from the left to the right crus, and the right crus is dissected downward to expose the junction of the right and left crura. With this technique, the vena cava is never at risk. In addition, the branches of the anterior vagus nerve and the left gastric artery are less exposed to danger. We feel that this technique is very useful, particularly for management of very large paraesophageal hernias and for second antireflux operations [see Reoperation for GERD, *below*].

Troubleshooting To determine whether the wrap is going to be floppy, the surgeon must deliver the fundus of the stomach under the esophagus, making sure that the origins of the short gastric vessels that have been transected are seen.

Essentially, the posterior wall of the fundus is being used for the wrap. If the wrap remains to the right of the esophagus without retracting back to the left, then it is floppy, and suturing can proceed. If not, the surgeon must make sure that the upper short gastric vessels have been transected. If tension is still present after these maneuvers, it is probably best to perform a partial wrap [see Laparoscopic Partial (Guarner) Fundoplication, *below*].

Damage to the gastric wall may occur during the delivery of the fundus. Atraumatic graspers must be used, and the gastric fundus must be pulled gently and passed from one grasper to the other. Sometimes, it is helpful to push the gastric fundus under the esophagus from the left. The wrap should measure no more than 2 to 2.5 cm in length and, as noted, should be done with no more than three sutures. The first stitch is usually the lowest one; it must be placed just above the fat pad where the esophagogastric junction is thought to be.

If the anesthesiologist observes that peak airway pressure has increased (because of a pneumothorax) or that neck emphysema is present (because of pneumomediastinum), the pneumoperitoneum should be reduced from 15 mm Hg to 7 to 8 mm Hg until the end of the procedure. Pneumomediastinum tends to resolve without intervention within a few hours of the end of the procedure. Small pneumothoraces (usually on the left side) tend to reabsorb spontaneously, and thus, the insertion of a chest tube is unnecessary. Larger pneumothoraces (> 20%) call for the insertion of a small chest tube (18 to 20 French).

Step 9: Final Inspection and Removal of Instruments and Ports from Abdomen

After hemostasis is obtained, the instruments and the ports are removed from the abdomen under direct vision.

Troubleshooting If any areas of oozing were observed during the procedure, they should be irrigated and dried with sponges rolled into a cigarettelike shape before the ports are removed. In addition, if some grounds for concern remain, the oozing areas should be examined after the pneumoperitoneum is decreased to an intra-abdominal pressure of 7 to 8 mm Hg to abolish the tamponading effect exerted by the high intra-abdominal pressure.

All the ports should be removed from the abdomen under direct vision so that any bleeding from the abdominal wall can be readily detected. Such bleeding is easily controlled, either from inside or from outside.

COMPLICATIONS

A feared complication of laparoscopic Nissen fundoplication is esophageal or gastric perforation. As noted, this complication is caused by traction applied with the Babcock clamp or a grasper to the esophagus or the stomach (particularly when the stomach is pulled under the esophagus) or by inadvertent electrocautery burns during any part of the dissection. A leak will manifest itself during the first 48 hours. Peritoneal signs will be noted if the spillage is limited to the abdomen; shortness of breath and a pleural effusion will be noted if spillage also occurs in the chest. The site of the leak should always be confirmed by a contrast study with barium or a water-soluble contrast agent. Perforation is best handled by means of laparotomy and direct repair. If a perforation is detected intraoperatively, it may be closed laparoscopically.

About 50% of patients experience mild dysphagia postoperatively. This problem usually resolves after 4 to 6 weeks, during which period patients receive pain medications in an elixir form and are advised to avoid eating meat and bread. If, however, dysphagia persists beyond this period, one or more of the following causes is responsible.

1. A wrap that is too tight or too long. The wrap should be performed without tension over a 56 French bougie. The total length of the wrap should not exceed 2.5 cm.
2. Lateral torsion with corkscrew effect. If the wrap rotates toward the right (either because of tension from intact short gastric vessels or because the fundus is small), a corkscrew effect is created.
3. A wrap made with the body of the stomach rather than the fundus. The relaxation of the LES and the gastric fundus is controlled by vasoactive intestinal polypeptide and nitric oxide[20,21]; after fundoplication, the two structures relax simultaneously with swallowing. If part of the body of the stomach rather than the fundus is used for the wrap, it will not relax as the LES does on arrival of the food bolus.
4. Choice of the wrong procedure. In patients who have severely abnormal esophageal peristalsis (as in end-stage connective tissue disorders), a partial wrap should be performed. A 360° wrap will control reflux, but it may cause postoperative dysphagia and gas bloat syndrome.

If the wrap slips into the chest, the patient becomes unable to eat and prone to vomiting. A chest radiograph shows a gastric bubble above the diaphragm, and the diagnosis is confirmed by means of a barium swallow. This problem can be prevented by using coronal sutures and by ensuring that the crura are closed securely.

Paraesophageal hernia may occur if the crura have not been closed or if the closure is too loose. In our view, closure of the crura not only is essential for preventing paraesophageal hernia but also is important from a physiologic point of view, in that it acts synergistically with the LES against stress reflux. Sometimes, it is possible to reduce the stomach and close the crura laparoscopically. More often, however, because the crural opening is very tight and the gastric wall is edematous, laparoscopic repair is impossible and laparotomy is preferable.

OUTCOME EVALUATION

Outcome evaluation of laparoscopic Nissen fundoplication is discussed elsewhere in conjunction with outcome evaluation of partial fundoplication [see Laparoscopic Partial (Guarner) Fundoplication, Outcome Evaluation, below].

Laparoscopic Partial (Guarner) Fundoplication

PREOPERATIVE EVALUATION AND OPERATIVE PLANNING

Preoperative evaluation and operative planning are essentially the same for partial (Guarner) fundoplication as for Nissen fundoplication. This operation should be performed only in patients with the most severe abnormalities of esophageal peristalsis: it has been shown to be less effective than a 360° wrap for long-term control of reflux.[9] In addition, laparoscopic partial fundoplication may be performed after laparoscopic Heller myotomy for achalasia.[22]

OPERATIVE TECHNIQUE

The first seven steps in a Guarner fundoplication are identical to the first seven in a Nissen fundoplication. The wrap, however, differs in that it extends around only 240° to 280° of the esophageal circumference. Once the gastric fundus is delivered under the esophagus, the two sides are not approximated over the esophagus. Instead, 80° to 120° of the anterior esophagus is left uncovered, and each of the two sides of the wrap (right and left) is separately affixed to the esophagus with three 2-0 silk sutures, with each stitch including the muscle layer of the esophageal wall. The remaining stitches (i.e., the coronal stitches and those between the right side of the wrap and the closed crura) are identical to those placed in a Nissen fundoplication.

OUTCOME EVALUATION

Initially, our average OR time for a laparoscopic fundoplication was about 3 hours. As we gained more experience and began using the LCS to take down the short gastric vessels, the average operating time decreased: it is now some 60 minutes shorter. We start patients on a soft mechanical diet on the morning of postoperative day 1 and usually discharge them after 23 to 48 hours. The recovery time for the operation is about 7 to 10 days. Long-term follow-up indicates that whereas total fundoplication controls reflux symptoms in about 90% of patients, partial fundoplication has a success rate of about 60% to 70%.

Laparoscopic Heller Myotomy with Partial Fundoplication

It has been demonstrated that minimally invasive surgical procedures for primary esophageal motility disorders (achalasia, diffuse esophageal spasm, and nutcracker esophagus) yield results that are comparable to those of open procedures but are associated with less postoperative pain and with a shorter recovery time.[23] Today, laparoscopic Heller myotomy with partial fundoplication is considered the procedure of choice for esophageal achalasia, replacing the left thoracoscopic approach that was initially favored.[4-7] Long-term studies demonstrated that even though left thoracoscopic myotomy led to resolution of dysphagia in about 85% to 90% of patients, it had the following four drawbacks:

1. Gastroesophageal reflux developed postoperatively in about 60% of patients because no fundoplication was performed in conjunction with the myotomy.[4] With the laparoscopic approach, in contrast, a partial fundoplication can easily be performed, and this prevents reflux in the majority of patients[4,5] as well as corrects many instances of preexisting reflux arising from pneumatic dilatation.[4]
2. The extension of the myotomy onto the gastric wall (clearly the most critical and challenging part of the operation) proved difficult because of poor exposure, with the consequent risk of a short myotomy and persistent dysphagia. With the laparoscopic approach, in contrast, excellent exposure of the esophagogastric junction is easily achieved, and the myotomy can be extended onto the gastric wall for about 2 cm.[4]
3. Double-lumen endotracheal intubation and single-lung ventilation were required, with the patient in the right lateral decubitus position. In contrast, the setting for a laparoscopic myotomy, being the same as that for a laparoscopic fundoplication, is much easier for the patient, the anesthesiologist, and the OR personnel. In addition, most surgeons have by now acquired substantial experience with laparoscopic antireflux procedures and thus are more familiar and comfortable with laparoscopic exposure of the distal esophagus and the esophagogastric junction.

4. After a thoracoscopic myotomy, patients remained in the hospital for about 3 days because of the chest tube left in place at the time of the operation and the discomfort arising from the thoracic incisions. After a laparoscopic Heller myotomy, the hospital stay is only 1 or 2 days; there is no need for a chest tube, and patients are more comfortable.

Because of these drawbacks, left thoracoscopic myotomy is now largely reserved for patients with achalasia who have undergone multiple abdominal operations (which may rule out a laparoscopic approach) and for patients with diffuse esophageal spasm or nutcracker esophagus involving the lower half of the esophagus.

PREOPERATIVE EVALUATION

All candidates for a laparoscopic Heller myotomy should undergo a thorough and careful evaluation to establish the diagnosis and characterize the disease.[24]

An upper GI series is a useful diagnostic test. A characteristic so-called bird beak is usually seen in patients with achalasia. A dilated, sigmoid esophagus may be present in patients with long-standing achalasia. A corkscrew esophagus is often seen in patients with diffuse esophageal spasm.

Endoscopy is performed to rule out a tumor of the esophagogastric junction and gastroduodenal pathology.

Esophageal manometry is the key test for establishing the diagnosis of esophageal achalasia. The classic manometric findings are (1) absence of esophageal peristalsis and (2) a hypertensive LES that fails to relax appropriately in response to swallowing.

Ambulatory pH monitoring should always be done in patients who have undergone pneumatic dilatation to rule out abnormal gastroesophageal reflux. In addition, pH monitoring should be performed postoperatively to detect abnormal reflux, which, if present, should be treated with acid-reducing medications.[24]

In patients older than 60 years who have experienced the recent onset of dysphagia and excessive weight loss, secondary achalasia or pseudoachalasia from cancer of the esophagogastric junction should be ruled out. Endoscopic ultrasonography or computed tomography can help establish the diagnosis.[25]

OPERATIVE PLANNING

Patient preparation (i.e., anesthesia, positioning, and instrumentation) is identical to that for laparoscopic fundoplication.

OPERATIVE TECHNIQUE

Many of the steps in a laparoscopic Heller myotomy are the same as the corresponding steps in a laparoscopic fundoplication. In the ensuing description, we focus on those steps that differ significantly.

To prevent the development of gastroesophageal reflux, a Dor or Guarner fundoplication [see Laparoscopic Partial (Guarner) Fundoplication, *above*] is often performed in conjunction with a Heller myotomy. The Dor fundoplication is an anterior 180° wrap. Its advantages are that (1) it does not require posterior dissection and the creation of a window between the esophagus, the stomach, and the left pillar of the crus; (2) it covers the exposed esophageal mucosa after completion of the myotomy; and (3) it is effective even in patients with GERD.[26] Its main disadvantage is that achieving the proper geometry can be difficult, and a wrong configuration

can lead to dysphagia even after a properly performed myotomy.[27] The advantages of the Guarner fundoplication are that (1) it is easier to perform; (2) it keeps the edges of the myotomy well separated; and (3) it might be more effective than a Dor procedure in preventing reflux. Its main disadvantages are that (1) it requires more dissection for the creation of a posterior window and (2) it leaves the esophageal mucosa exposed.

Steps 1 through 6

Steps 1, 2, 3, 4, 5, and 6 of a laparoscopic Heller myotomy are essentially identical to the first six steps of a laparoscopic fundoplication. Steps 4 and 6, however, are necessary only if a posterior partial fundoplication is to be performed. Care must be taken not to narrow the esophageal hiatus too much and push the esophagus anteriorly.

Step 7: Intraoperative Endoscopy

The esophageal stethoscope and the orogastric tube are removed, and an endoscope is inserted. The endoscopic view allows easy identification of the squamocolumnar junction, so that the myotomy can be extended downward onto the gastric wall for about 2 cm distal to this point. In addition, if possible mucosal perforation is a concern, the esophagus can be covered with water from outside while air is insufflated from inside; bubbling will be observed over the site of any perforation present.

At the beginning of a surgeon's experience with laparoscopic Heller myotomy, intraoperative endoscopy is a very important and helpful step; however, once the surgeon has gained adequate experience with this procedure and has become familiar with the landmarks between esophageal and gastric musculature from a laparoscopic perspective, it can be omitted.

Troubleshooting   The most worrisome complication during this step is perforation of the esophagus. This complication can be prevented by having an experienced endoscopist who is familiar with achalasia perform the procedure intraoperatively.

Step 8: Initiation of Myotomy and Entry into Submucosal Plane at Single Point

The fat pad is removed with the LCS to provide clear exposure of the esophagogastric junction. A Babcock clamp is then applied over the junction, and the esophagus is pulled downward and to the left; this maneuver exposes the right side of the esophagus. The myotomy is performed at the 11 o'clock position. It is helpful to mark the surface of the esophagus along the line through which the myotomy will be carried out [see Figure 3]. The myotomy is started about 3 cm above the esophagogastric junction. Before it is extended upward and downward, the proper submucosal plane should be reached at a single point; in this way, the likelihood of subsequent mucosal perforation can be reduced.

Troubleshooting   The myotomy should not be started close to the esophagogastric junction, because at this level the layers often are poorly defined, particularly if multiple dilatations or injections of botulinum toxin have been performed. It is easier to start about 3 cm above the esophagogastric junction, where the esophageal wall is usually normal. As a rule, we do not open the entire longitudinal layer first and then the circular layer; we find it easier and safer to try to reach the submucosal plane at one point and then move upward and down-

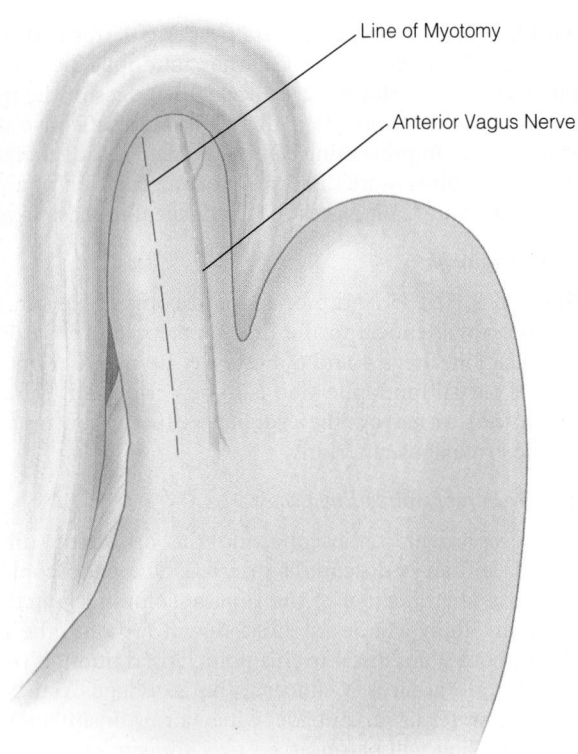

Figure 3 **Laparoscopic Heller myotomy with partial fundoplication. The proposed myotomy line is marked on the surface of the esophagus.**

Figure 4 **Laparoscopic Heller myotomy with partial fundoplication. The myotomy is extended proximally and distally.**

ward from there. In the course of the myotomy, there is always some bleeding from the cut muscle fibers, particularly if the esophagus is dilated and the wall is very thick. After the source of the bleeding is identified by irrigation, the electrocautery must be used with caution. The most troublesome bleeding comes from the submucosal veins (which are usually large) encountered at the esophagogastric junction. In most instances, gentle compression is preferable to electrocautery. A sponge introduced through one of the ports facilitates the application of direct pressure.

Step 9: Proximal and Distal Extension of Myotomy

Once the mucosa has been exposed, the myotomy can safely be extended proximally and distally [*see Figure 4*]. Distally, we extend the myotomy for about 2 cm onto the gastric wall. Proximally, we extend it for about 6 cm above the esophagogastric junction. Thus, the total length of the myotomy is typically about 8 cm [*see Figure 5*].

Troubleshooting It is vital to identify the course of the anterior vagus nerve before the myotomy is started. If this nerve crosses the line of the myotomy, it must be lifted away from the esophageal wall, and the muscle layers must then be cut under it. In addition, care must be taken not to injure the anterior vagus nerve while removing the fat pad. Treatment with botulinum toxin occasionally results in fibrosis with scarring and loss of the normal anatomic planes; this occurs more frequently at the level of the esophagogastric junction.

If a perforation seems possible or likely, it should be sought as described earlier [*see* Step 7, *above*]. Any perforation found should be repaired with 5-0 absorbable suture material, with interrupted sutures employed for a small perforation and a

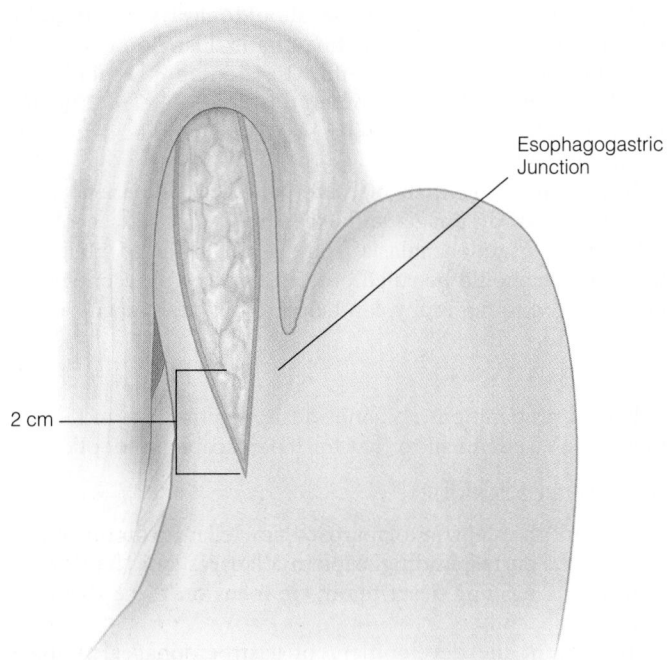

Figure 5 **Laparoscopic Heller myotomy with partial fundoplication. The myotomy is approximately 8 cm long, extending distally for about 2 cm onto the gastric wall and proximally for about 6 cm above the esophagogastric junction.**

continuous suture for a larger one. When a perforation has occurred, an anterior fundoplication is usually chosen in preference to a posterior one because the stomach will offer further protection against a leak.

Step 10 (Dor Procedure): Anterior Partial Fundoplication

Two rows of sutures are placed. The first row (on the left side) comprises three stitches: the uppermost stitch incorporates the gastric fundus, the esophageal wall, and the left pillar of the crus [*see Figure 6*], and the other two incorporate only the gastric fundus and the left side of the esophageal wall [*see Figure 7*]. The gastric fundus is then folded over the myotomy, and the second row (also comprising three stitches) is placed

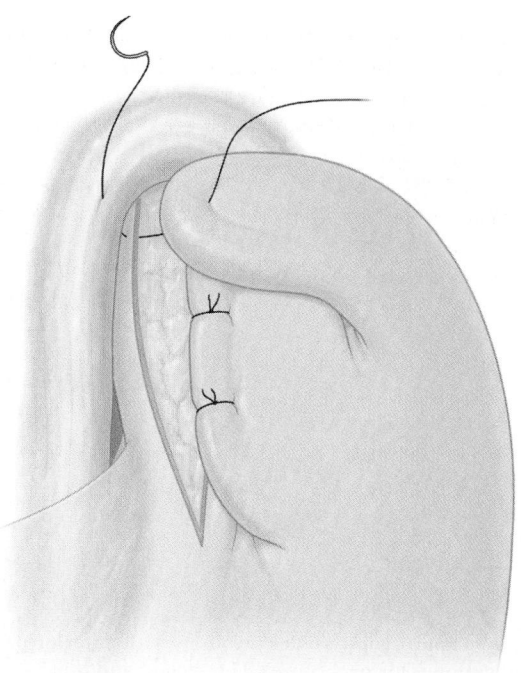

Figure 8 **Laparoscopic Heller myotomy with anterior partial fundoplication (Dor procedure). The uppermost stitch in the second row incorporates the fundus, the esophageal wall, and the right crus.**

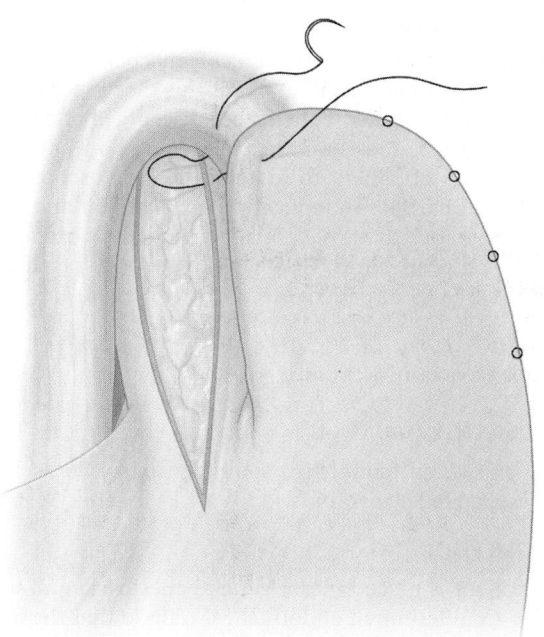

Figure 6 **Laparoscopic Heller myotomy with anterior partial fundoplication (Dor procedure). The uppermost stitch in the first row incorporates the fundus, the esophageal wall, and the left pillar of the crus.**

on the right side between the fundus and the right side of the esophageal wall, with only the uppermost stitch incorporating the right crus [*see Figures 8 and 9*]. Finally, two additional stitches are placed between the anterior rim of the hiatus and the superior aspect of the fundoplication [*see Figure 10*].

Troubleshooting Efforts must be made to ensure that the fundoplication does not become a cause of postoperative dysphagia. To this end, we always take down the short gastric vessels, even though some authorities suggest that this step can be omitted.[5,26] In addition, the gastric fundus rather than the body of the stomach should be used for the wrap, and only the uppermost stitch of the right row of sutures should incorporate the right pillar of the crus.[27]

Step 10 (Guarner Procedure): Posterior Partial Fundoplication

Alternatively, a posterior 220° fundoplication may be performed. The gastric fundus is delivered under the esophagus, and each side of the wrap (right and left) is attached to the esophageal wall, lateral to the myotomy, with three sutures [*see Figure 11*].

Step 11: Final Inspection and Removal of Instruments and Ports from Abdomen

Step 11 of a laparoscopic Heller myotomy is identical to step 9 of a laparoscopic Nissen fundoplication.

POSTOPERATIVE COMPLICATIONS

Delayed esophageal leakage, which is most often the result of an electrocautery burn to the esophageal mucosa, may occur during the first 24 to 36 hours after operation. The characteristic signals are chest pain, fever, and a pleural effusion on the chest x-ray. The diagnosis is confirmed by an esophagogram. Treatment options depend on the time of diagnosis and on the

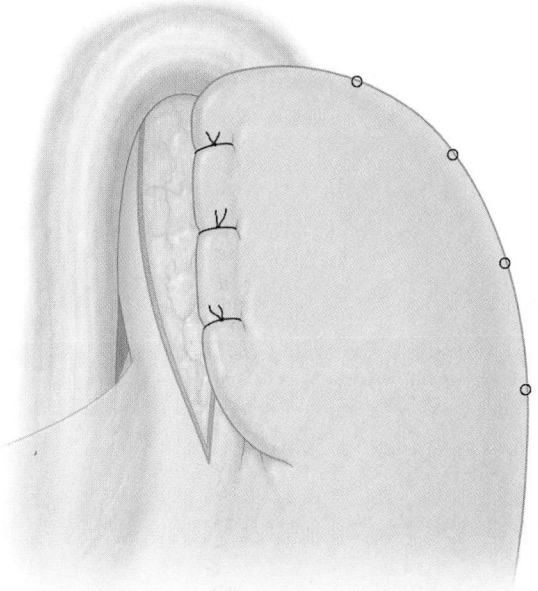

Figure 7 **Laparoscopic Heller myotomy with anterior partial fundoplication (Dor procedure). The second and third stitches in the first row incorporate only the fundus and the left side of the esophageal wall.**

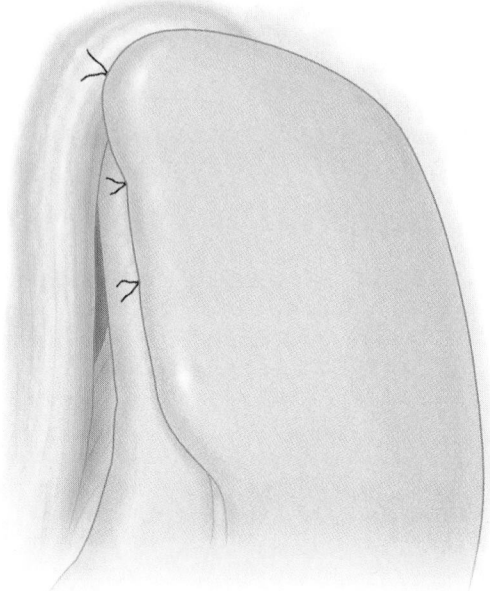

Figure 9 **Laparoscopic Heller myotomy with anterior partial fundoplication (Dor procedure). The second and third stitches in the second row incorporate only the fundus and the right side of the esophageal wall.**

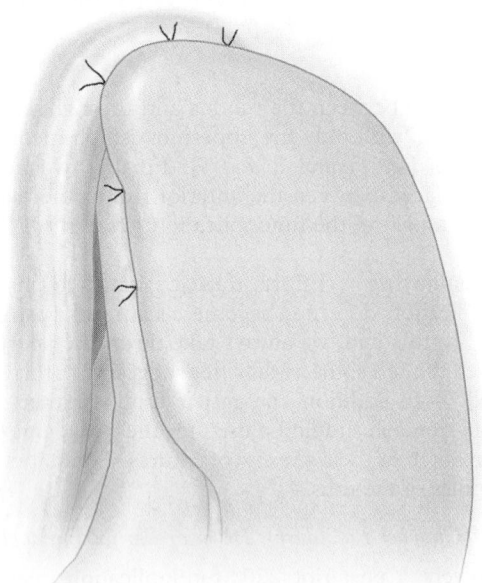

Figure 10 **Laparoscopic Heller myotomy with anterior partial fundoplication (Dor procedure). Two final stitches are placed between the superior portion of the wrap and the anterior rim of the hiatus.**

size and location of the leak. Early, small leaks can be repaired directly. If the site of the leak is high in the chest, a thoracotomy provides the best approach for the repair; if the site is at the level of the esophagogastric junction, a laparotomy provides the best approach, and the stomach can be used to reinforce the repair. If the damage to the esophagus is too extensive to permit repair, a transhiatal esophagectomy [see V:7 *Open Esophageal Procedures*] is indicated.

Dysphagia may either persist after the operation or recur after a symptom-free interval. In either case, a complete

workup is necessary, and treatment is individualized on the basis of the specific cause of dysphagia. Reoperation may be indicated [see Reoperation for Esophageal Achalasia, *below*].

Abnormal gastroesophageal reflux occurs in 7% to 20% of patients after operation.[4,5] Because most patients are asymptomatic, it is essential to try to evaluate all patients postoperatively with manometry and prolonged pH monitoring. Reflux should be treated with acid-reducing medications.

OUTCOME EVALUATION

We do not routinely obtain an esophagogram before initiating feeding. We start patients on a soft mechanical diet on the morning of postoperative day 1, and this diet is continued for the rest of the first week. Patients are discharged after 24 to 48 hours and are able to resume regular activities in 7 to 14 days.

The results obtained to date with laparoscopic Heller myotomy and partial fundoplication are excellent and are generally comparable to those obtained with the corresponding open surgical procedures: dysphagia is reduced or eliminated in more than 90% of patients.[4-7]

Left Thoracoscopic Myotomy

PREOPERATIVE EVALUATION

Preoperative evaluation is essentially the same as that for laparoscopic Heller myotomy.

OPERATIVE PLANNING

The patient is placed under general anesthesia and intubated with a double-lumen endotracheal tube so that the left lung can be deflated during the procedure.

The patient is placed in the right lateral decubitus position over an inflated bean bag, as for a left thoracotomy.

The instrumentation for this procedure is similar to that for a laparoscopic Nissen or Guarner fundoplication. Instead of

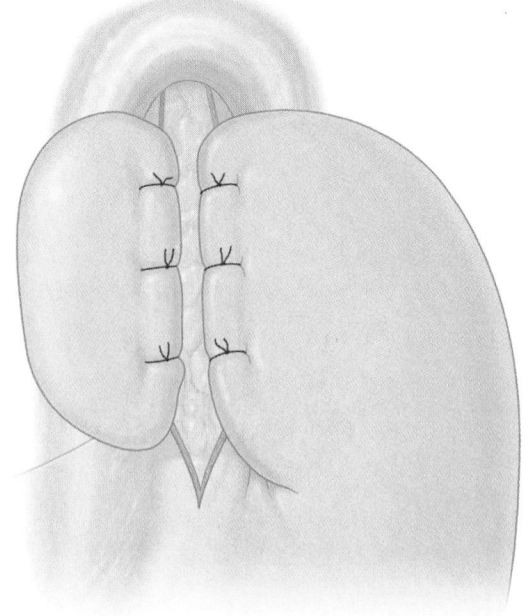

Figure 11 **Laparoscopic Heller myotomy with posterior partial fundoplication (Guarner procedure). Each side of the posterior 220° wrap is attached to the esophageal wall with three sutures.**

conventional trocars, we use four or five thoracoports with blunt obturators because insufflation of the thoracic cavity is not required. The myotomy can be performed with a monopolar hook cautery, bipolar scissors, or an ultrasonic scalpel (e.g., the Harmonic Scalpel, Ethicon Endo-Surgery, Inc.). A 30° scope and a 45° scope are essential instruments for the performance of thoracoscopic procedures. In addition, an endoscope is used for intraoperative endoscopy.

OPERATIVE TECHNIQUE

Step 1: Insertion of Thoracoports

Five ports are usually placed [*see Figure 12*]. Port A is inserted in the sixth intercostal space about 3.5 to 5 cm behind the posterior axillary line. This port is used for the 30° scope. Port B is placed in the third intercostal space about 1.25 to 2.5 cm anterior to the posterior axillary line. This port is used for the lung retractor. Port C is placed in the sixth intercostal space in the anterior axillary line. It is used for insertion of a grasper. Port D is placed in the seventh intercostal space in the midaxillary line. It is used for insertion of the instrument used for the myotomy. Port E is placed in the eighth intercostal space between the anterior axillary line and the midaxillary line. This port is optional: it is needed in about 30% of cases to allow the surgeon to obtain further exposure of the esophagogastric junction through retraction of the diaphragm.

Troubleshooting   A common mistake is to insert port A too anteriorly. This port must be placed well beyond the posterior axillary line to provide the best angle for the 30° scope. Often, the other ports are placed one or two intercostal spaces too high. This mistake hampers the performance of the most delicate portion of the operation, the myotomy of the distal portion of the esophagus and the stomach.

Sometimes, bleeding occurs from the chest wall as a result of the insertion of the ports. The dripping blood will obscure the operating field, and consequently, it is essential to stop the bleeding before the intrathoracic portion of the procedure is begun. Bleeding can be stopped either by using the cautery from the inside or by applying a stitch from the outside if an intercostal vessel has been damaged.

Step 2: Retraction of Left Lung and Division of Inferior Pulmonary Ligament

Once the ports are in place, the deflated left lung is retracted cephalad with a fan retractor introduced through port B. This maneuver places tension on the inferior pulmonary ligament, which is then divided. After the ligament is divided, the fan retractor can be held in place by a self-retaining system fixed to the operating table.

Troubleshooting   Before the inferior pulmonary ligament is divided, the inferior pulmonary vein must be identified to prevent a life-threatening injury to this vessel. If oxygen saturation decreases, particularly in patients with lung disease, the retractor should be removed and the lung inflated intermittently.

Step 3: Division of Mediastinal Pleura and Dissection of Periesophageal Tissues

The mediastinal pleura is divided, and the tissues overlying the esophageal wall are dissected until the wall of the esophagus is visible. This maneuver varies in difficulty depending on

Figure 12   **Left thoracoscopic myotomy. Illustrated is the recommended placement of the thoracoports.**

the width of the space between the aorta and the pericardium (which sometimes is very small) and on the size and shape of the esophagus. Large (sigmoid) esophagi tend to curve to the right, which makes identification of the wall difficult. If the esophagus is not immediately apparent, it can be easily identified in the groove between the heart and the aorta by means of transillumination provided by an endoscope [*see Figure 13*].

Troubleshooting   The endoscope placed inside the esophagus at the beginning of the procedure plays an important role. In the early stages of the procedure, it allows identification of the esophagus via transillumination. When the light intensity of the 30° scope is turned down, the esophagus appears as a bright structure. In addition, tilting the tip of the endoscope brings the esophagus into view as it is lifted from the groove between the aorta and the heart.

Step 4: Initiation of Myotomy and Entry into Submucosal Plane at Single Point

As in a laparoscopic Heller myotomy, it is helpful to mark the surface of the esophagus along the line through which the myotomy will be carried out. The myotomy is started halfway between the diaphragm and the inferior pulmonary vein. Again, the proper submucosal plane should be reached at a single point before the myotomy is extended upward and downward.

Troubleshooting   Troubleshooting for this step is essentially the same as that for step 8 of a laparoscopic Heller myotomy, with the exception that here the myotomy is started 4 to 5 cm (rather than 3 cm) above the esophagogastric junction.

Step 5: Proximal and Distal Extension of Myotomy

Once the mucosa has been exposed, the myotomy can safely be extended proximally and distally [*see Figure 14*]. We usually extend the myotomy for about 5 mm onto the gastric wall, without adding an antireflux procedure.[3,4] Typically, the total length of the myotomy is about 6 cm for patients with achalasia.

Troubleshooting   Proximally, we extend the myotomy all the way to the inferior pulmonary vein only in cases of vigorous

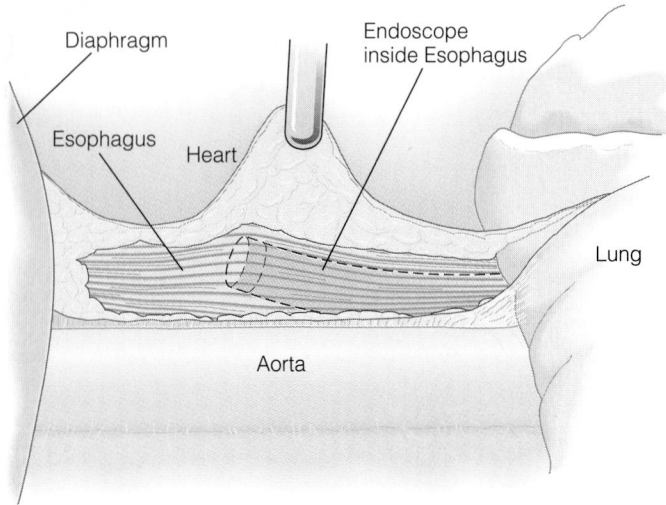

Figure 13 **Left thoracoscopic myotomy. The esophagus may be identified by means of transillumination from the endoscope.**

achalasia (high-amplitude simultaneous contractions associated with chest pain in addition to dysphagia) or diffuse esophageal spasm; otherwise, we limit the myotomy to the distal 5 to 6 cm of the esophagus. If a longer myotomy is needed, the lung is displaced anteriorly and the myotomy extended to the aortic arch.

Distally, we continue the myotomy for 5 mm past the esophagogastric junction. We use the endoluminal view provided by the endoscope to assess the location of the esophagogastric junction. Often, the stomach is distended by the air insufflated by the endoscope and pushes the diaphragm upward, thereby limiting the view of the esophagogastric junction. If sucking air out of the stomach does not resolve this problem, an additional port (i.e., port E) may be placed in the eighth intercostal space, and a fan retractor may be introduced through this port to push the diaphragm down.

Because the myotomy of the gastric wall is the most challenging part of the operation, good exposure is essential. It is at

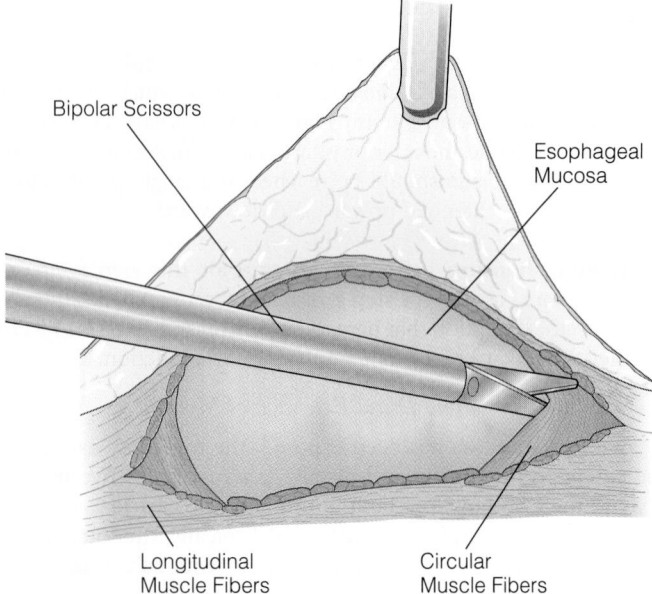

Figure 14 **Left thoracoscopic myotomy. Shown are the distal and proximal extensions of the myotomy.**

this level that an esophageal perforation is most likely to occur. The risk is particularly high in patients who have undergone pneumatic dilatation or injection of botulinum toxin, both of which may lead to the replacement of muscle layers by scar tissue and the consequent loss of the regular planes. Perforations recognized in the OR can be repaired by thoracoscopic intracorporeal suturing or, if this fails, by thoracotomy and open repair. The gastric fundus can be used to buttress the repair. If it is unclear whether a perforation has occurred, the esophagus should be covered with water and air insufflated through the endoscope as described earlier [*see* Laparoscopic Heller Myotomy with Partial Fundoplication, Operative Technique, Step 7, *above*].

Step 6: Insertion of Chest Tube and Removal of Thoracoports

A 24 French angled chest tube is inserted under direct vision through port D or port E. The ports are removed under direct vision, and the thoracic wall is inspected for bleeding.

POSTOPERATIVE COMPLICATIONS

As with laparoscopic Heller myotomy, delayed esophageal leakage is a common postoperative complication, and treatment options are similar.

If the myotomy is not extended far enough onto the gastric wall, residual dysphagia occurs. To prevent this problem, the distal extent of the myotomy should be assessed by the endoscopist, who will confirm that the myotomy includes 5 mm of the gastric wall. Patients with residual dysphagia must be evaluated by means of esophageal manometry, which will document the extent of and the pressure in the residual high-pressure zone. The myotomy can be easily extended by a laparoscopic approach, and a Dor fundoplication can be added.

If, on the other hand, the myotomy is extended too far onto the gastric wall, abnormal gastroesophageal reflux occurs. Some patients present with heartburn; others are asymptomatic. It is essential to evaluate patients postoperatively with manometry and prolonged pH monitoring. Mild reflux can be treated with acid-reducing medications, particularly in elderly patients. In younger patients, abnormal reflux should be corrected by means of a laparoscopic partial fundoplication (e.g., Dor fundoplication).

OUTCOME EVALUATION

We start patients on a liquid diet the morning of postoperative day 1; on postoperative day 2, we start them on a soft mechanical diet, which is continued for the rest of the first week. We do not routinely obtain an esophagogram before starting feedings. The chest tube is removed after 24 hours if the lung is fully expanded and there is no air leak. Patients are discharged after 48 to 72 hours and are able to resume regular activities in 7 to 10 days.

The results obtained with thoracoscopic esophageal myotomy are generally comparable to those obtained with open surgical procedures. Of the first 30 patients with achalasia whom we treated in this fashion, 26 (87%) experienced good or excellent results [*see Table 2*].[4]

Right Thoracoscopic Myotomy

A long myotomy from the diaphragm to the thoracic inlet, performed via a right thoracoscopic approach, is the preferred procedure for patients who have nutcracker esophagus or dif-

Table 2 Results of Thoracoscopic Myotomy in 30 Patients with Achalasia

Results	Patients (% of Total)
Excellent (no dysphagia)	21 (70)
Good (dysphagia < once/wk)	5 (17)
Fair (dysphagia > once/wk)	3 (10)
Poor (persistent dysphagia)	1 (3)

fuse esophageal spasm involving the entire length of the esophagus but who have normal LES function. On the whole, this procedure is technically simpler than a left thoracoscopic myotomy: because there is no need to go through the esophagogastric junction, perforation, postoperative dysphagia, and abnormal gastroesophageal reflux are largely prevented.

PREOPERATIVE EVALUATION

Preoperative evaluation of patients being considered for right thoracoscopic myotomy is essentially the same as that of patients being considered for left thoracoscopic myotomy.

OPERATIVE PLANNING

Operative planning is similar to that for a left thoracoscopic myotomy. The double-lumen tube is used to deflate the right lung rather than the left.

The patient is placed in the left lateral decubitus position over an inflated bean bag, as for a right thoracotomy.

The instrumentation is identical except for the endovascular 30 mm stapler used to transect the azygos vein. It is essential to have a thoracotomy tray ready in case an emergency thoracotomy is necessary to control bleeding.

OPERATIVE TECHNIQUE

Step 1: Insertion of Thoracoports

Only port B is inserted where it would be for a left thoracoscopic myotomy. All the other ports are inserted one intercostal space higher because the myotomy need not be extended all the way to the stomach but must be extended to the thoracic inlet. Usually, only four ports are used; however, an additional port can be placed in the fourth intercostal space in the anterior axillary line to facilitate the proximal extension of the myotomy.

Step 2: Dissection of Periesophageal Tissues and Division of Azygos Vein

The periesophageal tissues above and below the azygos vein are dissected away from the esophagus. A tunnel is created between the azygos vein and the esophagus with a dissector, a right-angle clamp, or both. The azygos vein is then transected with an endovascular 30 mm stapler. (Alternatively, the azygos vein can be spared and simply lifted off the esophagus with umbilical tape.)

Troubleshooting Dissection of the azygos vein is the most critical part of this procedure. We have found that it is easier to transect the azygos vein than to keep the vein lifted away from the esophagus and perform the myotomy under it.

Steps 3, 4, and 5

Steps 3, 4, and 5 of a right thoracoscopic myotomy are virtually identical to steps 4, 5, and 6 of a left thoracoscopic myotomy, with a few minor exceptions. Once the submucosal plane is reached, the myotomy is extended distally to the diaphragm and proximally to the thoracic inlet. The endoscope plays a less critical role in this procedure than in a left thoracoscopic myotomy because the esophagus is easily identified and because the myotomy is not extended through the esophagogastric junction. Instead, we place a 52 to 56 French bougie inside the esophagus. This facilitates the division of the circular fibers and separates the edges of the myotomy nicely.

COMPLICATIONS

A delayed esophageal leak is the most common postoperative complication. It should be handled as described earlier [see Laparoscopic Heller Myotomy with Partial Fundoplication, Postoperative Complications, above].

OUTCOME EVALUATION

The postoperative course of patients who have undergone this procedure is usually identical to that of patients operated on for achalasia. Complete relief of chest pain is obtained in about 75% to 80% of patients.[23]

Reoperation for GERD

Over the past 10 years, we have seen an increasing number of patients being referred to the UCSF Swallowing Center for evaluation and treatment of foregut symptoms after laparoscopic antireflux surgery. In what follows, we describe our approach to this highly challenging group of patients.

PREOPERATIVE EVALUATION

Some degree of dysphagia, bloating, and abdominal discomfort is common during the first 6 to 8 weeks after a fundoplication. If these symptoms persist or heartburn and regurgitation occur, a thorough evaluation (with barium swallow, endoscopy, esophageal manometry, and pH monitoring) is carried out with the aim of answering the following three questions:

1. Are the symptoms attributable to persistent gastroesophageal reflux?
2. Are the symptoms attributable to the fundoplication itself?
3. Can the cause of the failure of the first operation be identified and corrected by a second operation?

Many patients report heartburn after a fundoplication. It is often assumed that this symptom must be the result of a failed operation and that acid-reducing medications should be restarted. In the majority of patients, however, this assumption is mistaken: postoperative pH monitoring yields abnormal results in only about 20% of patients.[28] The value of manometry lies in its ability to document the changes caused by the operation at the level of the LES and the esophageal body. The pH monitoring assesses the reflux status and determines whether there is a correlation between symptoms experienced by the patient and actual episodes of reflux. If abnormal reflux is in fact present, the therapeutic choice is between medical therapy and a second operation.

Other patients complain of dysphagia arising de novo after the operation. This symptom is usually attributable to the operation itself, and it can occur in the absence of abnormal reflux. In addition to manometry and pH monitoring, a barium swallow is essential to define the anatomy of the esophagogastric junction. As shown by investigators from the University of Washington,[29] the anatomic configurations observed can generally be divided into three main types: (1) type I hernia, in which the esophagogastric junction is above the diaphragm (further subdivided into type IA, in which both the esophagogastric junction and the wrap are above the diaphragm, and type IB, in which only the esophagogastric junction is above the diaphragm); (2) type II hernia, a paraesophageal configuration; and (3) type III hernia, in which the esophagogastric junction is below the diaphragm and there is no evidence of hernia but in which the body of the stomach rather than the gastric fundus is used to perform the wrap. In 10% of patients, however, the investigators could not identify the cause of the failure preoperatively.[29]

Some patients present with a mix of postprandial bloating, nausea, and diarrhea. These symptoms may be the result of damage to the vagus nerves. Radionuclide evaluation of gastric emptying of solids and liquids often helps quantify the problem.

OPERATIVE PLANNING

Patient preparation (i.e., anesthesia, positioning, and instrumentation) for operations for reflux is identical to that for the initial laparoscopic fundoplication.

OPERATIVE TECHNIQUE

We routinely attempt a second antireflux operation laparoscopically; however, if the dissection does not proceed smoothly, a laparotomy is performed. To provide a stepwise technical description that would be suitable for all reoperations for reflux is impossible because the optimal procedure depends on the original approach (open versus laparoscopic), the severity of the adhesions, and the specific technique used for the first operation (total or partial fundoplication). The key goals of reoperation for reflux are as follows:

1. To dissect the wrap and the esophagus away from the crura. This is the most difficult part of the operation. The major complications seen during this part of the procedure are damage to the vagus nerves and perforation of the esophagus and the gastric fundus.
2. To take down the previous repair. The earlier repair must be completely undone and the gastric fundus returned to its natural position. If the short gastric vessels were not taken down during the first procedure, they must be taken down during the second.
3. To dissect the esophagus in the posterior mediastinum so as to have enough esophageal length below the diaphragm and avoid placing tension on the repair.
4. To reconstruct the cardia. We follow the same steps described for a first time repair. If, after extensive esophageal mobilization, the esophagogastric junction remains above the diaphragm (short esophagus), esophageal lengthening can be accomplished by adding a thoracoscopic Collis gastroplasty to the fundoplication. In our entire laparoscopic experience to date, however, we have not yet found this step to be necessary.

POSTOPERATIVE COMPLICATIONS

The risk of gastric or esophageal perforation or of damage to the vagus nerves is much higher during a second antireflux operation. Accordingly, the surgeon must stand ready to convert to a laparotomy if the dissection proves too cumbersome or the structures are not properly identified. Most perforations are recognized and repaired intraoperatively. A leak will manifest itself during the first 48 hours. Peritoneal signs will be noted if the spillage is limited to the abdomen; shortness of breath and a pleural effusion will be noted if spillage also occurs in the chest. The site of the leak should always be confirmed by means of a contrast study with barium or a water-soluble contrast agent. Perforation is best handled through laparotomy and direct repair.

OUTCOME EVALUATION

Whereas the success rate is around 90% for a first antireflux operation, it falls to 75% to 80% for a second such operation. In our opinion, a second operation should be attempted by an expert team only if medical management fails to control heartburn or pneumatic dilatation has not relieved dysphagia.

Reoperation for Esophageal Achalasia

Laparoscopic Heller myotomy improves swallowing in more than 90% of patients. What causes the relatively few failures reported is still incompletely understood. Typically, a failed Heller myotomy is signaled either by persistent dysphagia or by recurrent dysphagia that develops after a variable symptom-free interval following the original operation.

A complete workup (routinely including barium swallow, endoscopy, manometry, and pH monitoring) is required before treatment is planned. In addition, it is our practice to review the video of the first operation to search for technical errors that might have been responsible for the poor outcome. Such errors typically fall into one of the following three categories.

1. A too-short myotomy. The myotomy can be too short either distally or proximally. If the myotomy is too short distally, a barium swallow shows persistent distal esophageal narrowing and manometry shows a residual high-pressure zone. If the myotomy is too short proximally, it will be apparent from the barium swallow.
2. A constricting Dor fundoplication. Often, manometry and pH monitoring yield normal results, but a barium swallow shows slow passage of contrast media from the esophagus into the stomach. In our own experience,[27] problems with Dor fundoplications occurred in four (4%) of 102 patients. Analysis of the video records of the first operations showed that in three of the four patients, all the stitches in the right suture row had incorporated the esophagus, the right pillar of the crus, and the stomach, thereby constricting the myotomy. In one patient, the short gastric vessels had not been taken down, and the body of the stomach rather than the gastric fundus had been used for the fundoplication.
3. Transmural scarring caused by previous treatment. In patients treated with intrasphincteric injection of botulinum toxin, transmural fibrosis can sometimes be found at the level of the esophagogastric junction. This unwelcome finding makes the myotomy more difficult and the results less reliable.

There are two treatment options for persistent or recurrent dysphagia after Heller myotomy: (1) pneumatic dilatation and (2) a second operation tailored to the results of preoperative evaluation. In a 2002 study,[30] pneumatic dilatation was successfully used to treat seven of 10 patients who experienced dysphagia postoperatively; of the remaining three patients, two required a second operation and one refused any treatment.

Our own experience has been different: we found pneumatic dilatation to be effective in only one (short distal myotomy) of the eight patients in whom it was tried.[27] The only one of our patients who was helped by dilatation was the one with a short distal myotomy; none of the four patients with dysphagia resulting from a poorly constructed Dor fundoplication derived any benefit. In two patients who had a short proximal myotomy, we successfully extended the myotomy to the inferior pulmonary vein through a left thoracoscopic approach. Of the four patients with a constricting Dor fundoplication, two underwent a second operation during which the Dor was taken down, and one of these two had a second myotomy. Both patients are free of dysphagia; however, they experience abnormal reflux and are currently being treated with acid-reducing medications.

Reoperation for achalasia is a technically challenging procedure. It is of paramount importance to avoid perforating the exposed esophageal mucosa during the dissection. A small hole can be repaired, but a larger laceration might necessitate an esophagectomy. This option should always be discussed with the patient before the operation.

Overall, about 10% of patients have some degree of dysphagia after a Heller myotomy. Pneumatic dilatation, a second operation, or both should always be tried before a radical procedure such as esophagectomy is decided on.

References

1. Csendes A, Braghetto I, Henriquez A, et al: Late results of a prospective randomized study comparing forceful dilatation and oesophagomyotomy in patients with achalasia. Gut 30:299, 1989

2. Hinder RA, Filipi CJ, Wetscher G, et al: Laparoscopic Nissen fundoplication is an effective treatment for gastroesophageal reflux disease. Ann Surg 220:472, 1994

3. Pellegrini CA, Wetter LA, Patti MG, et al: Thoracoscopic esophagomyotomy: initial experience with a new approach for the treatment of achalasia. Ann Surg 216:291, 1992

4. Patti MG, Pellegrini CA, Horgan S, et al: Minimally invasive surgery for achalasia. An 8 year experience with 168 patients. Ann Surg 587:230, 1999

5. Zaninotto G, Costantini M, Molena D, et al: Treatment of esophageal achalasia with laparoscopic Heller myotomy and Dor partial anterior fundoplication: prospective evaluation of 100 consecutive patients. J Gastrointest Surg 282:4, 2000

6. Ackroyd R, Watson DI, Devitt PG, et al: Laparoscopic cardiomyotomy and anterior partial fundoplication for achalasia. Surg Endosc 683:15, 2001

7. Finley RJ, Clifton JC, Stewart KC, et al: Laparoscopic Heller myotomy improves esophageal emptying and the symptoms of achalasia. Arch Surg 892:136, 2001

8. Patti MG, Arcerito M, Feo CV, et al: An analysis of operations for gastroesophageal reflux disease: identifying the important technical elements. Arch Surg 600:133, 2001

9. Horvath KD, Jobe BA, Herron DM, et al: Laparoscopic Toupet fundoplication is an inadequate procedure for patients with severe reflux disease. J Gastrointest Surg 583:3, 1999

10. Sonnenberg A, Delco F, El-Serag HB: Empirical therapy versus diagnostic tests in gastroesophageal reflux disease: a medical decision analysis. Dig Dis Sci 1001:43, 1998

11. Johnsson F, Joelsson B, Gudmundsson K, et al: Symptoms and endoscopic findings in the diagnosis of gastroesophageal reflux disease. Scan J Gastroenterol 714:22, 1987

12. Patti MG, Diener U, Tamburini A, et al: Role of esophageal function tests in the diagnosis of gastroesophageal reflux disease. Dig Dis Sci 597:46, 2001

13. Campos GM, Peters JH, DeMeester TR, et al: Multivariate analysis of factors predicting outcome after laparoscopic Nissen fundoplication. J Gastrointest Surg 292:3, 1999

14. Patti MG, Goldberg HI, Arcerito M, et al: Hiatal hernia size affects the lower esophageal sphincter function, esophageal acid exposure, and the degree of mucosal injury. Am J Surg 182:171, 1996

15. Bytzer P, Havelund T, Moller Hansen J: Interobserver variation in the endoscopic diagnosis of reflux esophagitis. Scan J Gastroenterol 119:28, 1993

16. Fuchs KH, DeMeester TR, Albertucci M: Specificity and sensitivity of objective diagnosis of gastroesophageal reflux disease. Surgery 575:102, 1987

17. Patti MG, Arcerito M, Tamburini A, et al: Effect of laparoscopic fundoplication on GERD-induced respiratory symptoms. J Gastrointest Surg 143:4, 2000

18. Diener U, Patti MG, Molena D, et al: Esophageal dysmotility and gastroesophageal reflux disease. J Gastrointest Surg 260:5, 2001

19. Horgan S, Pellegrini CA: Surgical treatment of gastroesophageal reflux disease. Surg Clin North Am 1063:77, 1997

20. Guelrud M, Rossiter A, Souney PF, et al: The effect of vasoactive intestinal polypeptide on the lower esophageal sphincter in achalasia. Gastroenterology 103:377, 1992

21. Tottrup A, Svane D, Forman A: Nitric oxide mediating NANC inhibition in opossum lower esophageal sphincter. Am J Physiol 260:385, 1991

22. Champion JK, Delisle N, Hunt T: Laparoscopic esophagomyotomy with posterior partial fundoplication for primary esophageal motility disorders. Surg Endosc 746:14, 2000

23. Patti MG, Pellegrini CA, Arcerito M, et al: Comparison of medical and minimally invasive surgical therapy for primary esophageal motility disorders. Arch Surg 130:609, 1995

24. Patti MG, Diener U, Molena D: Esophageal achalasia: preoperative assessment and postoperative follow-up. J Gastrointest Surg 11:5, 2001

25. Moonka R, Patti MG, Feo CV, et al: Clinical presentation and evaluation of malignant pseudoachalasia. J Gastrointest Surg 456:3, 1999

26. Watson DI, Liu JF, Devitt PG, et al: Outcome of laparoscopic anterior 180-degree partial fundoplication for gastroesophageal reflux disease. J Gastrointest Surg 486:4, 2000

27. Patti MG, Molena D, Fisichella PM, et al: Laparoscopic Heller myotomy and Dor fundoplication for achalasia: analysis of successes and failures. Arch Surg 870:136, 2001

28. Lord RVN, Kaminski A, Oberg S, et al: Absence of gastroesophageal reflux disease in a majority of patients taking acid suppression medications after Nissen fundoplication. J Gastrointest Surg 6:3, 2002.

29. Horgan S, Pohl D, Bogetti D, et al: Failed antireflux surgery: what have we learned from reoperations? Arch Surg 809:13, 1999

30. Zaninotto G, Costantini M, Portale G, et al: Etiology, diagnosis and treatment of failures after laparoscopic Heller myotomy for achalasia. Ann Surg 186:235, 2002.

Acknowledgment

Figures 1 through 14   Tom Moore.

9 GASTRIC PROCEDURES

John L. Sawyers, M.D.

In most patients who will undergo gastric procedures, a definitive diagnosis will already have been made by means of esophagogastroduodenoscopy, upper GI tract x-rays, or both. Major gastric procedures are done with the patient under general anesthesia and lying supine on the operating room table.

Initial Incision

The abdomen is opened through an upper midline incision from the left of the xiphoid to the umbilicus. It is not necessary to excise the xiphoid process. Adjacent to the cephalad end of the xiphoid is a small artery that may cause troublesome bleeding; such bleeding can be readily controlled with electrocoagulation. The incision in the linea alba is made with the cutting current of the electrocautery. If further exposure is needed, the incision may be extended around the umbilicus on either side. The wound edges are protected by the application of moist laparotomy pads or a plastic wound protector. A Balfour retractor is then inserted. An upper hand retractor lifts the costal margins to facilitate exposure of the upper abdomen. Some surgeons prefer to use a Buckwalter retractor.

Vagotomy

Since the 1940s, when Dragstedt reintroduced vagotomy as surgical therapy for duodenal ulcer,[1] parasympathetic denervation of the parietal cell mass in the stomach has been the basis for the operative treatment of this disease. Three types of vagotomy—truncal vagotomy, selective vagotomy, and highly selective vagotomy (also known as proximal gastric vagotomy or parietal cell vagotomy)—have been described, all of which result in reduced acid secretion. Of these, selective gastric vagotomy, which denervates the entire stomach but none of the other intra-abdominal organs, is the one that has been least frequently used.

TRUNCAL VAGOTOMY

After entering the abdomen, the surgeon may divide the left triangular ligament of the liver to permit retraction of the left lobe of the liver to the patient's right side. This is not always necessary; often, the left lobe is retracted cephalad. The Weinberg retractor (Joe's hoe) is useful for elevating the left lateral hepatic segment.

The stomach is retracted downward, and the peritoneum overlying the abdominal esophagus is incised transversely. A previously placed nasogastric tube facilitates identification of the esophagus. The esophagus is mobilized circumferentially by a combination of blunt and sharp dissection and encircled with a Penrose drain [*see Figure 1a*]. The drain is passed behind the esophagus either by using a gooseneck clamp or by inserting two fingers posterior to the esophagus and pulling the drain through this opening.

The anterior vagal trunk usually lies on the anterior wall of the esophagus. It can be identified by palpation with a finger as the stomach is retracted caudally with the Penrose drain; it feels like a guitar string. The anterior trunk is mobilized from the esophagus up into the lower mediastinum. Any branches that pass downward toward the esophagogastric junction are divided. A 2 in. segment of the anterior trunk is resected [*see Figure 1b*], and the severed ends are secured with ligating clips or fine (3-0) silk ties.

The posterior vagal trunk is usually larger than the anterior vagal trunk. Its location is variable. Sometimes, it lies directly behind the esophagus and thus is held by the Penrose drain; more often, however, it lies medially and may be found adjacent to the abdominal aorta or in the areolar tissue just medial to the right crus of the diaphragm. Applying traction caudad to the stomach or the Penrose drain will put tension on the posterior vagal trunk, thereby making it easier to identify. As with the anterior trunk, a 2 in. segment is resected [*see Figure 1c*], and the severed ends are secured with ligating clips or silk ties; clips are quicker and easier to use.

Any additional vagal fibers that may arise cephalad to the severed vagal trunks are located and divided. A careful search around the circumference of the esophagus is done to ensure that the vagotomy is complete [*see Figure 1d*].

The esophagus is retracted to the patient's left with the Penrose drain, and the diaphragmatic crura are approximated posterior to the esophagus with one or more heavy (0) silk sutures in such a way that the hiatus is tightened around the esophagus with the indwelling nasogastric tube to a snugness of one finger's breadth.

Because truncal vagotomy denervates the entire stomach (including the gastric antral pyloric pump mechanism), emptying of liquids and solid food is decreased. Gastric stasis may occur; consequently, a drainage procedure (pyloroplasty or gastrojejunostomy) or distal gastric resection (antrectomy) is required.

Transthoracic (Supradiaphragmatic) Vagotomy

Transthoracic truncal vagotomy is usually reserved for cases in which reoperation is necessary because an incomplete previous vagotomy resulted in a recurrent ulcer. The patient is placed on his or her right side, and a left posterior lateral thoracotomy is done in the seventh interspace. The inferior lobe of the left lung is retracted, and the inferior pulmonary ligament is exposed and then divided with the electrocautery. The left lung is either deflated (with a double-lumen endotracheal tube) or retracted upward,

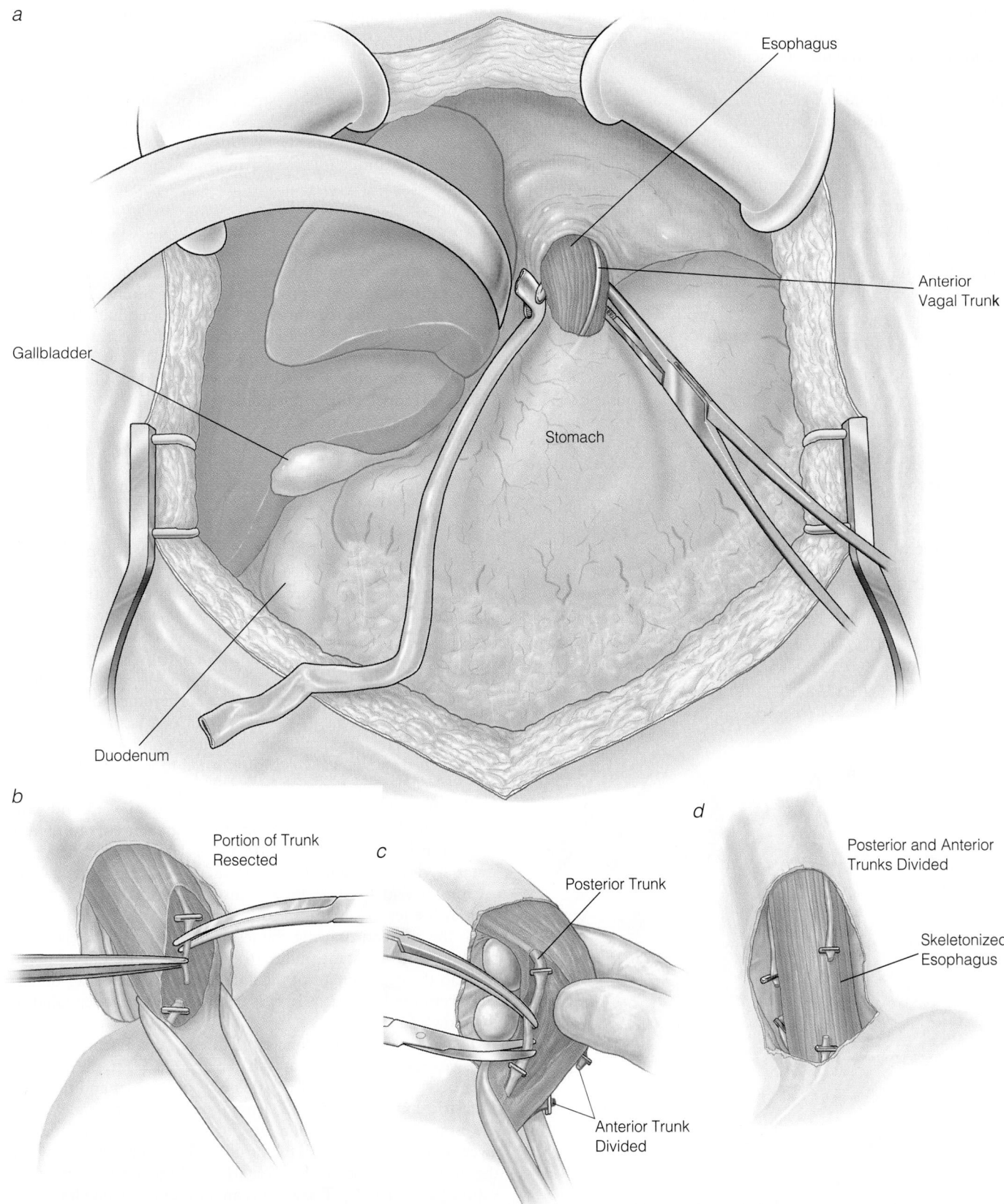

a

Esophagus

Anterior
Vagal Trunk

Gallbladder

Stomach

Duodenum

b

Portion of Trunk
Resected

c

Posterior Trunk

Anterior Trunk
Divided

d

Posterior and Anterior
Trunks Divided

Skeletonized
Esophagus

Figure 1   **Truncal vagotomy. (*a*) The esophagus is mobilized by blunt and sharp dissection and encircled with a Penrose drain. (*b*) The anterior vagal trunk is identified and mobilized, and a 2 in. segment of the trunk is resected. (*c*) The posterior vagal trunk is identified and mobilized, and a 2 in. segment of this trunk is resected. (*d*) Any additional small vagal fibers are divided, and a careful search is made around the esophagus to confirm that the vagotomy is complete.[23]**

and the pleura over the distal esophagus is incised longitudinally. The esophagus is identified by palpating the nasogastric tube previously inserted into the stomach. It is mobilized by blunt dissection until a finger can be passed beneath it. The vagus nerves can then be seen and palpated on each side of the esophageal wall. Because of the patient's rotated position on the table, the left vagus is found on the upper surface of the esophagus, and the right vagus is found beneath the esophagus.

Next, the vagi are freed from the esophagus. At this level, the vagi usually form a single trunk; however, each may consist of two or more fibers. Hence, to be certain of dividing all the fibers, it is advisable to clean all of the adventitia away from the esophagus around its circumference for a length of 5 cm. The vagi are isolated and divided between silk ligatures or ligating clips just above the diaphragm [see Figure 2]. Removal of a segment of nerve is permissible but not necessary. The pleura is then closed over the esophagus.

With the increased use of endoscopic surgical procedures, instruments have been developed that allow transthoracic vagotomy to be performed through a thoracoscope. If no adhesions from a previous thoracotomy are present, the thoracoscopic approach is an easy method of dividing the thoracic vagal nerves. After thoracoscopic vagal nerve resection, the patient may go home the same day or the next day and is spared the discomfort of a thoracotomy incision. This is now my method of choice for transthoracic vagotomy.

HIGHLY SELECTIVE (PROXIMAL GASTRIC) VAGOTOMY

After the anterior and posterior vagal trunks enter the abdomen, the anterior trunk gives off the hepatic vagal branch (or branches) and continues as the anterior gastric nerve of Latarjet, which courses medial to the lesser curvature of the stomach in the anterior leaf of the lesser (or gastrohepatic) omentum. The posterior vagal nerve gives off the celiac branch and continues as the posterior gastric nerve of Latarjet, which parallels the course of the anterior gastric nerve but lies in the posterior leaf of the lesser omentum. These two gastric nerves terminate in fanlike branches that together make up what is called the crow's foot. The crow's foot is located approximately 7 cm proximal to the pylorus along the lesser curvature of the stomach [see Figure 3a]. It is an important anatomic landmark because it coincides with the antral–parietal cell junction.

Adequate exposure of the upper abdominal cavity is essential to the performance of a proximal gastric vagotomy. Such exposure may be obtained through an upper midline abdominal incision, as noted [see Initial Incision, above]. An upper hand retractor with two blades is used to lift up the costal margins. The operating table is tilted to place the patient in a head-up (reverse Trendelenburg) position.

The lateral segment of the left lobe of the liver is retracted upward. Some surgeons prefer to incise the left triangular ligament and to retract the lateral segment medially during the dissection of the vagi. The left lobe is returned to its normal location before the abdomen is closed.

The anterior vagal trunk is identified and encircled with a vessel loop; any ancillary anterior nerve trunks should also be identified at this time. The esophagus is then dissected from its bed. An empty sponge forceps is placed parallel to the esophagus and the diaphragmatic crura and used to free the lateral esophagus attachments. The posterior wall of the esophagus is freed by gentle finger dissection, and a narrow Penrose drain is passed around the esophagus. The posterior vagal trunk is then identified; it is usually anterior to the aorta rather than directly behind the esophagus. A second vessel loop is passed around this trunk. Both vagal trunks are kept intact and retracted to the right of the esophagus, which is returned to its normal position with the encircling Penrose drain still in place.

The stomach is then retracted to the patient's left and caudally by applying Babcock clamps to the greater curvature over a previously placed nasogastric tube. The anterior nerve of Latarjet, descending in the lesser omentum to reach the gastric antrum, is visualized. A finger is inserted through the avascular area in the lesser omentum to place tension on the omentum. With the surgeon drawing the lesser omentum to the patient's right and the assistant pulling the greater gastric curvature to the left, the detachment of the anterior leaf of the lesser omentum from the lesser gastric curvature is begun just cephalad to the crow's foot.

The lesser omentum consists of three layers. Each layer contains vessels and nerves that must be divided. First, the anterior layer between the anterior gastric nerve of Latarjet and the lesser gastric curvature is divided from the crow's foot distally up to the esophagogastric junction [see Figure 3a]; second, the middle layer is divided; and third, the posterior layer is divided between the posterior gastric nerve of Latarjet and the lesser gastric curvature [see Figure 3b]. These steps are best done by dividing each individual neurovascular bundle between two hemostats (e.g., Crile clamps) and tying each neurovascular pedicle with fine silk. The temptation to hurry this part of the dissection by incorporating large amounts of tissue in the clamps must be resisted. Hemostatic clips and diathermy coagulation should not be used:

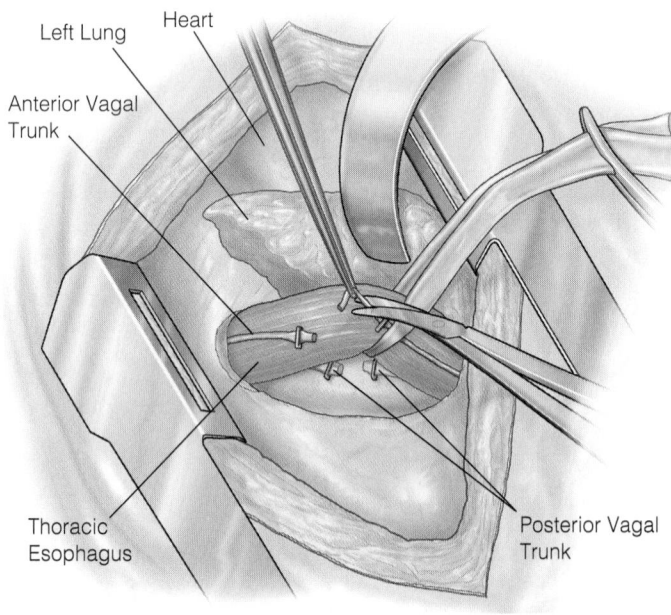

Left Lung

Heart

Anterior Vagal
Trunk

Thoracic
Esophagus

Posterior Vagal
Trunk

Figure 2 **Transthoracic (supradiaphragmatic) vagotomy. Through a left posterior lateral thoracotomy, the vagus nerves are identified, freed from the esophagus, isolated, and divided just above the diaphragm; the pleura is then closed over the esophagus. The procedure may also be performed through a thoracoscope; this is in fact my current method of choice.**

a

7 cm

b

c

Figure 3 **Highly selective (proximal gastric) vagotomy. After the anterior and posterior vagal trunks enter the abdomen, they give off branches and continue as the anterior and posterior gastric nerves of Latarjet. These gastric nerves terminate in fanlike branches that make up a structure known as the crow's foot. This structure, which is about 7 cm proximal to the pylorus along the lesser gastric curvature, coincides with the antral–parietal cell junction. (*a*) The lesser omentum is detached from the lesser gastric curvature. First, the anterior layer of the lesser omentum is divided from the crow's foot distally to the esophagogastric junction; second (not shown), the middle layer is divided. (*b*) Third, the posterior layer is divided between the posterior gastric nerve of Latarjet and the lesser gastric curvature. (*c*) The esophagus is elevated from its bed, and the dissection is extended 7 cm above the esophagogastric junction, with pains taken to detect and divide the so-called criminal nerve. The bare area of the lesser curvature is then closed.**

they may result in bleeding, which leads to hematomas in the lesser omentum that obscure visualization of the gastric nerves.

After the lesser gastric curvature is freed from the anterior and posterior gastric nerves of Latarjet up to the esophagogastric junction, the esophagus is elevated from its bed by traction on the Penrose drain. The dissection is extended 7 cm above the esophagogastric junction to sever any vagal fibers supplying the gastric fundus [*see Figure 3c*]. There is usually a constant vagal branch arising from the posterior vagal trunk that courses along

the left lateral wall of the esophagus to enter the gastric fundus. This branch—aptly termed the criminal nerve because it so often escapes untouched[2]—must be divided.

Finally, the bare area of the lesser gastric curvature is closed by plicating the anterior and posterior leaves of the lesser omentum with interrupted silk sutures from the esophagogastric junction down to the crow's foot [*see Figure 3c*]. This maneuver is thought to reduce the risk of both lesser curvature necrosis (see below) and vagal sprouting.

I generally do not test the completeness of the vagotomy either by performing pH metering with an intragastric electrode or by observing the color changes on the Congo red test. These tests are tedious, lengthen the operation, and are of questionable value. Intraoperative testing appears to offer no significant advantages.[3]

Rosati and coworkers have recommended resecting about 3 cm of the right gastroepiploic neurovascular bundle along the greater gastric curvature opposite the crow's foot or the upper limit of the pyloric antrum.[4] A vagal branch coming off the pyloric nerve may extend proximally up to the parietal cell mass on the greater curvature. I do not routinely divide the neurovascular bundle at this site.

Complications

Proximal gastric vagotomy has the lowest reported mortality of any operation used to treat duodenal ulcer disease. In one series of 5,000 patients, mortality was 0.26 percent.[5] In 500 patients operated on at Vanderbilt University, mortality was only 0.2 percent; the sole postoperative death was the result of a pulmonary embolus.

An early postoperative complication uniquely associated with proximal gastric vagotomy is lesser curvature necrosis, which occurs during the first week after operation. It may be caused by ligation or electrocoagulation performed too close to the lesser gastric curvature. The area of necrosis is located on the lesser gastric curvature between the antral–parietal cell border and the esophagogastric junction. The incidence of this complication is low, typically less than one percent; it may be further reduced by reperitonealizing the lesser curvature. Early recognition of lesser curvature necrosis can be confirmed by meglumine diatrizoate contrast studies of the stomach. Although reoperation to close the site of perforation is usually successful, there are two reported instances in which gastric resection was necessary in a patient with extensive lesser curvature necrosis.[6]

Dysphagia has been reported as an early complication of proximal gastric vagotomy in 10 to 30 percent of patients.[7] The cause is thought to be the intensive lower esophageal dissection necessary to ensure complete vagal denervation of the parietal cell mass. Postvagotomy dysphagia usually subsides spontaneously in two to three months; in rare instances, esophageal dilation with a Hurst or Maloney bougie may be necessary.

Tears of the splenic capsule occur in about four percent of operations but can usually be controlled with hemostatic agents.

In rare cases, perforation of the esophagus may occur as the surgeon attempts to free the esophagus from the posterior mediastinum by passing the Penrose drain behind the esophagus. If this happens, immediate repair of the perforation with interrupted silk sutures should prevent any esophageal leak. The repair may then be reinforced with fundoplication overlying it.

Because the emptying of solid foods remains normal, the incidence of postgastrectomy sequelae (e.g., dumping, diarrhea, and reflux gastritis) after proximal gastric vagotomy is less than that after gastric operations that destroy the integrity of the pyloric sphincter. No dietary restrictions are required after the operation. Dumping generally is not a problem, nor is postvagotomy diarrhea or alkaline reflux gastritis.

Concern has been expressed about the recurrence rate after highly selective vagotomy. Studies have been published that cover more than 15 years of follow-up. In these studies, ulcer recurrence rates have ranged from two to 23 percent[8]; however, when highly selective vagotomy is done by a surgeon who has

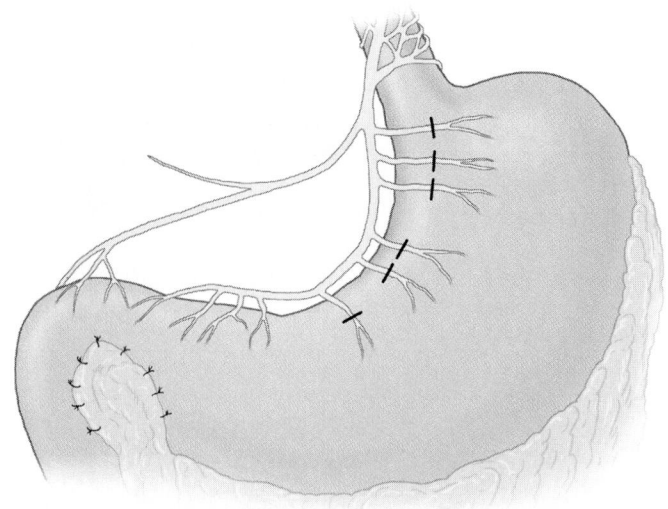

Figure 4 **Patch closure with highly selective vagotomy for perforated duodenal ulcer. An omental patch is placed over the perforation and secured with interrupted 3-0 silk sutures. The peritoneal cavity is thoroughly irrigated, and highly selective vagotomy is performed.[8]**

extensive experience with the procedure, recurrence rates generally range from five to 10 percent.[9] Proximal gastric vagotomy should not be used to treat pyloric or prepyloric ulcers, because patients with these conditions tend to have higher recurrence rates than those with duodenal ulcers. Recurrent ulcers after proximal gastric vagotomy are likely to respond to medical treatment with H_2-receptor antagonists. If a recurrent ulcer makes reoperation necessary, antrectomy with truncal vagotomy is the procedure of choice.

Patch Closure with Highly Selective Vagotomy for Perforated Duodenal Ulcer

Highly selective vagotomy may be added to patch closure for perforated duodenal ulcer.[10] Highly selective vagotomy prevents undesirable postgastrectomy complications and controls the ulcer diathesis. Omentum is placed over the perforation as a patch and secured with interrupted 3-0 silk sutures [*see Figure 4*]; closure of the hole with sutures is unnecessary and may narrow the duodenal lumen. After the patch is secured, highly selective vagotomy is performed as described earlier (see above).

LAPAROSCOPIC VAGOTOMY

Techniques have been developed to perform proximal gastric vagotomy through a laparoscope by means of an approach similar to that described earlier [*see* Highly Selective (Proximal Gastric) Vagotomy, *above*]. Some laparoscopic surgeons prefer to do a posterior truncal vagotomy combined with highly selective vagotomy of the anterior vagal trunk or an anterior seromyotomy.

Laparoscopic highly selective vagotomy is usually done with the patient under general anesthesia and in the reverse Trendelenburg position. Some surgeons prefer the lithotomy position, with the surgeon between the patient's legs. Five trocars are inserted. A 30° telescope is placed through the supraumbilical port; the stomach is grasped and retracted to the left through the left ports; the left lobe of the liver is retracted cephalad through the superior right port; and dissection is performed through the inferior right port. The peritoneum over the esophagus is incised, and the esophagus is retracted to the left. The posterior vagal trunk is divided and the ends clipped; the anterior vagal trunk is not divided but is retracted to the right. Each neurovascular bundle between the anterior nerve of Latarjet and the lesser curvature is clipped and divided, from the crow's foot cephalad to the esophagogastric junction. The vagal fibers running from the anterior trunk to the proximal stomach are divided with the electrocautery.

An alternative method of laparoscopic vagotomy is to perform an anterior gastric seromyotomy with posterior truncal vagotomy.[11] Performing a seromyotomy is quicker and technically easier than dividing each neurovascular bundle in the anterior leaf of the lesser omentum. The immediate results have been good.

Distal Subtotal Gastric Resection (Antrectomy) for Benign Disease

Distal subtotal gastric resection for benign duodenal ulcer usually consists of antral resection in conjunction with truncal vagotomy. The initial abdominal incision is made as previously

Figure 5 **Distal subtotal gastric resection (antrectomy) for benign disease. This procedure usually consists of antral resection combined with truncal vagotomy. After truncal vagotomy, the distal 40 percent of the stomach is excised. The division point on the lesser curvature is more proximal than that on the greater curvature because the antrum extends further cephalad on the lesser curvature.[24]**

described [*see* Initial Incision, *above*]. After truncal vagotomy is performed, the distal 40 percent of the stomach is excised. Because the antrum extends further cephalad on the lesser curvature, the lesser curvature is divided at a point closer to the esophagogastric junction than to the pylorus, whereas the greater curvature is divided halfway between the pylorus and the fundus [*see Figure 5*].

Babcock forceps are placed on the greater gastric curvature, and the organ is lifted up and forward. The arcade of vessels along the middle portion of the greater curvature is divided and ligated with silk. The lesser peritoneal cavity, thus widely opened, is explored, and all fibrous attachments between the posterior gastric wall and the pancreatic pseudocapsule are divided. At this point, an excellent view of the pancreas is obtained, and the organ is carefully inspected for possible adenoma or other pathological findings. The greater curvature is mobilized from the pylorus to a point midway to the fundus. The dissection is extended several centimeters above the incisura angularis on the lesser curvature, and the vessels along the lesser curvature are likewise secured. The descending branch of the left gastric artery is divided and transfixed with silk.

With traction applied to the greater curvature by means of the Babcock forceps, the mobilized stomach is fanned out, and a point along the greater curvature that is approximately midway between the pylorus and the fundus is selected for division; this point is usually just to the right of the first of the vasa brevia. A second point along the lesser curvature that is just proximal to the midway point between the pylorus and the esophagogastric junction is similarly selected for division; this point is usually 3 to 4 cm above the crow's foot.

The stomach is divided between two straight Kocher or Allen clamps placed at right angles to the long axis of the stomach at the selected division point along the greater curvature. The proximal clamp defines the size of the gastroenteric stoma that is to be constructed. A gastrointestinal anastomosis (GIA) stapling device may also be used for this purpose, but I prefer to use the clamps. Next, a TA-60 gastric stapler is placed obliquely along the lesser curvature up to the point previously selected for division. A maneuver that aids in clearing the lesser curvature is to use the left index finger and thumb to place traction medially on the gastrohepatic ligament and to insert a curved hemostat adjacent to the gastric wall, thereby opening a space through which the assistant can place two Kelly clamps across the gastrohepatic ligament in preparation for its division. This piece of tissue, which contains the descending branch of the left gastric artery, is a rather large one and thus is ligated with 2-0 silk. This maneuver quickly clears the lesser curvature and facilitates placement of the linear gastric stapler or GIA stapler. The stomach is then transected at the selected point. The staple line may be inverted with interrupted 3-0 silk sutures.

The resulting gastric remnant assumes a tubular shape. The distal transected stomach is then reflected to the right. At this point, the entire pancreas can again be fully visualized and examined. If traction is applied to the distal transected stomach, the stomach can serve as a handle, and dissection of the pylorus and the duodenal bulb is thereby greatly facilitated. In my experience, this method is much easier and more efficacious than other methods in which the duodenum is mobilized before the stomach is divided. The division is extended distally onto the duodenum far enough to ensure that all antral tissue is removed.

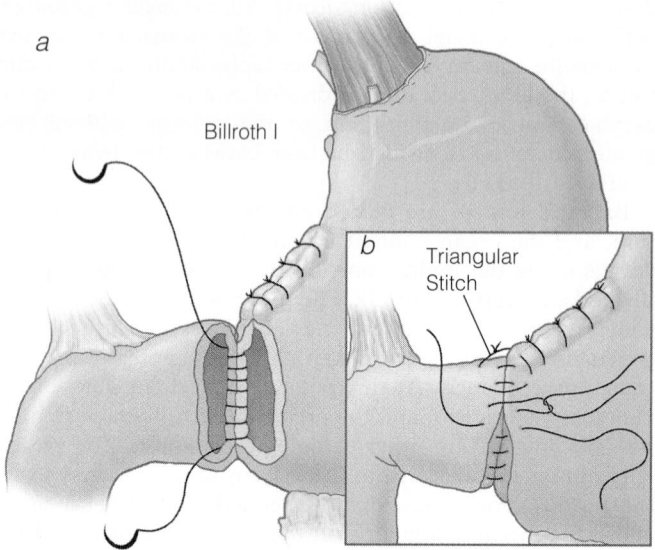

Figure 6 Billroth I gastroduodenostomy. (*a*) **The opposing poste-**
rior gastric and duodenal walls are approximated with a continu-
ous fine chromic catgut suture that commences in the midline with
two separate needles. The suture is continued anteriorly, the oppos-
ing anterior walls are inverted with an over-and-over suture (or,
alternatively, a Connell inverting suture), and the suture ends are
tied in the midline. (*b*) An outer layer of interrupted 4-0 silk sutures
is placed, and the angle of sorrow—the potential weak spot—is closed
with a triangular stitch.[25]

BILLROTH I RECONSTRUCTION

For establishing gastrointestinal continuity, a Billroth I gastroduodenostomy is the preferred procedure; I have used it in
90 percent of my patients. Gastroduodenostomy offers certain
physiologic advantages over gastrojejunostomy: many nutritional studies have indicated that maintaining the duodenum in alimentary continuity causes less loss of fecal fat and nitrogen,
enhances iron absorption, and reduces the incidence of reflux
gastritis.

A duodenal lumen of normal width, without constriction at
or distal to the ulcer, is essential to the performance of an end-
to-end gastroduodenostomy. If a satisfactory lumen is not already present, it must be produced surgically; a Horsley longitudinal incision of the anterior duodenal wall is one way of
accomplishing this.

The ulcer need not be removed if there is no evidence of cicatricial stenosis at or distal to the site of ulceration in the duodenum. In fact, it is better to leave a difficult penetrating ulcer in situ
than to be too aggressive in attempting to remove it: unwarranted aggressive attempts to remove the ulcer may increase mortality and morbidity related to anastomotic leaks, infection, or pancreatitis. When a large penetrating ulcer of the posterior wall is
encountered and scarring extends around the entire circumference of the duodenum—particularly if the patient is obese—I
often elect to close the duodenal stump with a long anterior wall
cuff of duodenum. This long cuff is buttressed to the bed of the
ulcer with two inverting layers of catgut sutures, and the pseudocapsule of the pancreas is approximated to the duodenal serosa
with interrupted silk sutures. A retrocolic Hofmeister reconstruction using a short afferent loop is then done.

As a rule, the duodenum need not be kocherized except in
unusual circumstances: routine use of the Kocher maneuver is
neither necessary nor preferred. After the distal stomach is
mobilized beyond the pylorus, the gastric pouch is placed in
direct apposition to the posterior duodenum. The two structures to be anastomosed must be approximated without the
slightest amount of tension. With the distal stomach still attached to the freed duodenum, a row of interrupted seromuscular silk sutures is placed between the posterior gastric wall
and the posterior duodenal wall distal to the ulcer site. The so-
called rule of nine (according to which the two end sutures are
placed first, followed by the middle suture) may be helpful in
spacing the sutures. These sutures are rendered taut, and the
first assistant approximates the gastric pouch to the posterior
duodenal wall by applying gentle traction to the structures. The
surgeon then ties the sutures and removes the specimen with
the electric cutting current.

A continuous 3-0 chromic catgut suture is placed with two
needles through the entire thickness of the posterior gastric and
duodenal walls; this placement also serves to approximate the
opposing mucosal surfaces [*see Figure 6a*]. The interrupted seromuscular silk sutures placed earlier are held elevated by an assistant as the continuous suture is being placed posteriorly; this
maneuver allows improved visualization of the opposing gastric
and duodenal mucosae. The continuous catgut suture is started
in the middle of the posterior wall, and the posterior row is locked
to prevent purse-stringing of the lumen. As the continuous suture
is advanced, the interrupted silk sutures are cut close to the knots.
The continuous suture is then continued anteriorly, and the opposing gastric and duodenal walls are inverted with an over-and-
over suture (or, as some surgeons prefer, a Connell inverting
suture). An outer layer of interrupted 4-0 silk completes the anastomosis, and the ends of the suture are tied in the midline. It is
essential to close the potential weak spot of the anastomosis—the
so-called angle of sorrow—by placing a triangular silk suture at
the lesser curve of the anastomosis in such a way as to include
both the anterior gastric wall and the posterior gastric wall as well
as the lesser curve of the duodenum [*see Figure 6b*]. If there is any
appreciable discrepancy between the opposing structures to be
anastomosed, the antimesenteric border of the duodenum may
be divided for 1 to 2 cm before the anterior row of sutures is completed (Horsley's maneuver). The resulting gastroduodenal stoma
is usually just wide enough to admit the surgeon's thumb; it
should not be larger.

The nasogastric tube is then irrigated by a member of the OR
staff before the abdomen is closed to ensure that all blood clots
have been removed from the gastric pouch. I prefer to remove
the nasogastric tube after the first 24 hours, provided that the
operation has progressed smoothly. At present, I extubate approximately 75 percent of my patients early. If the operation was
done on an emergency basis, particularly for an acute ulcer perforation in which there was extensive peritoneal soiling, the tube
should be left in place for approximately 72 hours or until the
patient expels flatus. In addition, when massive bleeding occurs
to the point where the GI tract is filled with blood, adynamic
ileus may be anticipated postoperatively, and a few days of nasogastric suction is appropriate.

During the first 72 hours after operation, the patient is
given nothing but parenteral fluids. Small amounts of tap
water are allowed on postoperative day 4, and a liquid diet
usually is begun on day 5. A postgastrectomy diet is begun on

day 6 or 7. The patient can get out of bed and walk on postoperative day 1.

BILLROTH II RECONSTRUCTION

A Billroth II gastrojejunostomy may be indicated when technical reasons rule out a Billroth I gastroduodenostomy. The usual indication for a Billroth II procedure is a high gastric resection involving two thirds to three fourths of the stomach.

After the distal end of the stomach is mobilized, the duodenum is divided with a GIA stapler. The duodenal stump may be oversewn with interrupted 3-0 silk sutures. The lesser curve of the gastric reservoir is closed with a stapler (TA-60 or GIA) and oversewn with interrupted 3-0 silk sutures.

A short-loop retrocolic gastrojejunostomy is done by identifying the ligament of Treitz, bringing the proximal jejunum through an avascular space in the transverse mesocolon, and performing a two-layer anastomosis to the clamped greater gastric curvature. The posterior row consists of interrupted 3-0 silk Lembert sutures. The inner layer is sutured with a continuous double-ended 3-0 chromic catgut suture that is begun in the middle of the posterior row, extended around to close the anterior layer with an over-and-over stitch, and locked. If preferred, a Connell inverting suture may be used on the anterior surface. The anastomosis is reinforced with an anterior row of interrupted 3-0 silk sutures. The lesser curvature–jejunum junction is reinforced with a triangular silk suture that passes through the anterior wall of the stomach, then through the jejunum, and finally back through the posterior wall of the stomach. The mesocolon is sutured to the stomach to keep it from sliding down the jejunal limb and causing obstruction [see Figure 7a].

An antecolic gastrojejunostomy can be performed in the same manner by bringing a short afferent loop of jejunum anterior to the omentum and the transverse colon [see Figure 7b].

A Billroth II anastomosis may also be performed with a GIA stapler. An antecolic jejunal loop is placed 2 to 3 cm above the stapled end of the gastric reservoir on the posterior wall. The GIA instrument is inserted through 1 cm stab wounds in the jejunum and the stomach. Firing the stapler creates an anastomosis between the jejunum and the stomach. The stab wounds are closed with silk sutures.

The Difficult Duodenal Stump

Two methods are available for dealing with duodenal stumps that cannot be closed with either staples or sutures. The time-honored method is to insert a 16 French red rubber duodenostomy catheter through the open end of the duodenum. The duodenum is inverted around the catheter with two purse-string sutures and reinforced with omentum. If the duodenal stump has been sutured but there is concern about the closure, a 16 French catheter is inserted through the lateral margin of the

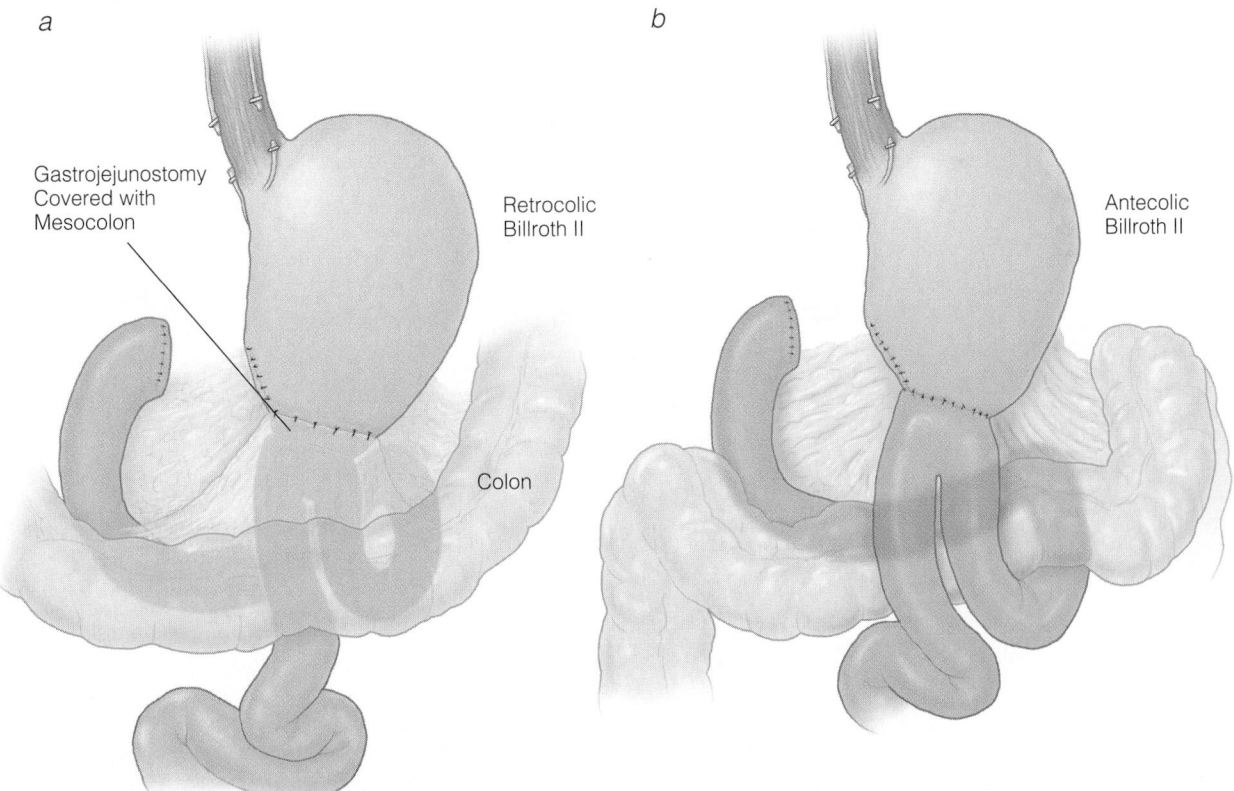

Figure 7 **Billroth II gastrojejunostomy. (a) A retrocolic Billroth II procedure is done by bringing the proximal jejunum through an avascular space in the transverse mesocolon and anastomosing the jejunum to the greater gastric curvature. The anastomosis is reinforced with an anterior row of interrupted 3-0 silk sutures. As in the Billroth I procedure, the potential weak spot of the anastomosis is closed with a triangular stitch. The mesocolon is then sutured to the gastric wall. (b) The antecolic version of the procedure is similar, except that the jejunal loop is brought up anterior to the omentum and the transverse colon.**

duodenum by using two inverting sutures, much as in a Stamm gastrostomy [*see* Stamm Gastrostomy, *below*]. A closed wound suction (Jackson-Pratt) drain is placed alongside the duodenal stump and brought out through a stab wound.

The other major method of dealing with difficult duodenal stumps is to perform a Roux-en-Y reconstruction.[12] This reconstruction is particularly useful when giant duodenal ulcers, large perforations, or dense inflammatory adhesions involving the duodenal area are present. The isolated Roux limb may be used either as a serosal patch to cover the duodenal defect or as an open end-to-side anastomosis [*see Figures 8a and 8b*]. Roux-en-Y reconstruction reroutes fluid and gastric contents from the afferent limb, thus reducing intraluminal afferent limb pressure and reducing the tension being applied to the closed duodenal stump. The afferent limb is kept short to prevent obstruction, and anastomotic traps are carefully closed.

Fashioning a Roux-en-Y jejunal limb The ligament of Treitz is identified. The jejunum is divided close to this ligament, but pains must be taken to preserve an arterial arcade to each side of the jejunum. Usually, the jejunum is divided between the first and the second arcade with a GIA stapler. The stapler should be perpendicular to the jejunum rather than at an angle to avoid compromising the vascularity of the ends. It is possible to obtain a longer Roux limb by dividing the mesentery, but again, one arcade must be preserved on each side of

the divided jejunum. A Roux limb should be at least 45 cm (18 in.) long to prevent reflux of bile and other alkaline secretions; however, it should not be longer than 60 cm, to prevent delayed transit through the limb (Roux syndrome). Lengths between 45 and 60 cm have been used with considerable success.

Anastomosis of the stomach or the esophagus to the Roux limb is best done to the side of the jejunum, not to the end of the divided jejunum; either stapling or hand suturing in two layers is acceptable. The afferent limb is then stapled with a GIA stapler or sutured in two layers to the Roux limb at least 45 cm from the proximal anastomosis.

A Roux jejunal limb may be a useful method for restoring gastrointestinal continuity after resection of a high-lying gastric ulcer or tumor near the esophagogastric junction on the lesser curvature in cases in which closure of the lesser curvature might compromise the lumen of the esophagus. A Roux-en-Y jejunal limb may be brought up antecolically and anastomosed to the entire open end of the gastric pouch and distal esophagus. This maneuver is called a Csendes gastrojejunostomy.

Total Gastrectomy for Cancer

Total gastrectomy is generally performed through an upper midline incision,[13] although some surgeons prefer a bilateral subcostal incision. Exposure is obtained as outlined earlier [*see* Initial Incision, *above*]. The suspensory ligament of the lateral

Figure 8 **Closure of a difficult duodenal stump with a jejunal limb. (*a*) An isolated Roux jejunal limb may be used either as a serosal patch to cover the duodenal defects or as an end-to-side anastomosis. (*b*) Truncal vagotomy–antrectomy is completed with a Billroth II anastomosis in the Roux duodenojejunostomy. The afferent limb is stapled or sutured to create a Roux limb at least 45 cm long.[12]**

Figure 9 Total gastrectomy for cancer. (*a*) Resection should be extensive enough to include at least N1 and N2 lymph nodes (a so-called R2 resection).[26] (*b*) The esophagojejunal anastomosis is done in an end-to-side fashion with an end-to-end anastomosis (EEA) stapler.[13] (*c*) Shown is a completed Roux-en-Y esophagojejunostomy; the isoperistaltic jejunal limb should be 45 to 60 cm long.[13]

segment of the left lobe of the liver is divided so that the lobe may be retracted to the patient's right.

Once abdominal exposure is obtained, the abdominal contents are explored, with the emphasis on the detection of metastatic disease. The greater omentum is detached from the transverse colon with the electrocautery, and the lesser omentum is incised at the liver and reflected downward. Dissection of the peritoneum is continued upward to expose the abdominal esophagus and then around to the spleen to join the dissection of the greater omentum at the splenic flexure. Lymph node dissection begins at the hilum of the liver and is continued until all lymph nodes, lymphatic vessels, and fatty areolar tissue are stripped from the common bile duct, the portal vein, and the hepatic artery. Further dissection exposes the common hepatic artery and the celiac axis. The preaortic area is cleared of all lymph nodes

and areolar tissue. This process skeletonizes the structures in the hepatoduodenal ligament and is termed an N2 node dissection. (The N1 nodes are located in the perigastric area along the greater and lesser curvatures; the N2 nodes are located around the blood vessels arising from the celiac axis that supply the stomach, including the common hepatic, splenic, and left gastric arteries; the N3 nodes are located in the hepatoduodenal ligament, the retropancreatic area, and the celiac plexus, as well as near the superior mesenteric artery; and the N4 nodes are in the para-aortic area.)

The left gastric artery is then ligated, transfixed, and divided. The duodenum is transected 3 cm distal to the pylorus with a GIA stapler and oversewn with interrupted 3-0 silk sutures. The stomach is retracted upward to the left; the resulting excellent exposure of the pancreas permits dissection from the anterior capsule of the pancreas and clearance of the lymph nodes along the splenic artery. The splenic vessels are divided near the caudal end of the pancreas, and the spleen is freed from its ligaments. The abdominal esophagus is then divided about 6 cm above the esophagogastric junction, and the gastrectomy specimen is sent to the surgical pathology laboratory for frozen section examination of the resected margins. This resection includes N1 and N2 nodes and is known as an R2 gastric resection in Japan [see Figure 9a]. (An R0 resection is gastrectomy with incomplete removal of N1 nodes; an R1 resection includes omentectomy along with removal of all N1 nodes; an R3 resection includes removal of all N1, N2, and N3 nodes; and an R4 resection includes removal of all four node groups.)

Alimentary reconstruction takes the form of a Roux-en-Y esophagojejunostomy. The isoperistaltic jejunal limb should be 45 to 60 cm long to prevent alkaline reflux into the esophagus. End-to-end anastomosis should be avoided because the incidence of leakage is unacceptably high, about 16 percent. With end-to-side anastomosis, the incidence of leakage rate is only about two percent, thanks to the superior blood supply.[14] To make an end-to-side esophagojejunal anastomosis, an end-to-end anastomosis (EEA) stapler is inserted through the end of the jejunal segment. The anvil of the stapler is placed in the open end of the esophagus and held in place with a purse-string suture [see Figure 9b]. After the anastomosis is done, the excess portion of the jejunal limb is stapled with a linear stapling device and excised. The proximal jejunum is then anastomosed to the isoperistaltic jejunal limb in an end-to-side fashion with sutures or a GIA stapler [see Figure 9c].

The esophageal connection to the jejunum may be accomplished by creating a jejunal pouch.[15-17] A 1989 review of a century's worth of literature on the pathophysiological and nutritional effects of various types of gastric replacement pouches after total gastrectomy concluded that Roux-en-Y esophagojejunostomy was adequate for reconstructing the alimentary tract and that complicated pouches are not needed.[18] The author did, however, advocate further study of the use of distal jejunojejuneal pouches at Roux-en-Y sites.

Fat and protein malabsorption caused by failure of adequate food intake is often seen after total gastrectomy. This condition abates with time. Initially, patients with end-to-side Roux-en-Y esophagojejunostomies must eat a number of small meals in the course of the day, but after a few months, they can usually resume eating three regular meals a day. With a Roux-en-Y esophagojejunostomy, the transit of food through the small intestine is slower than normal. The proximal jejunum limb does not act as a reservoir, but because it empties rapidly during eating, patients are able to eat a normal-sized meal. The only nutrient that must be replaced on a continuing basis after total gastrectomy is vitamin B$_{12}$, which is given to prevent megaloblastic anemia.

Subtotal Gastrectomy for Cancer

Cancers in the gastric antrum or the distal third of the stomach are becoming less frequent but still account for about one third of all gastric adenocarcinomas.[19] Because these tumors tend to cause obstruction, they are generally diagnosed earlier than proximal gastric carcinomas (which, in contrast, are increasing in frequency).

Radical distal subtotal gastrectomy that includes regional lymph node removal is the operation of choice for distal gastric

carcinoma [see Figure 10]. Resection of 75 to 80 percent of the stomach, including the lesser curvature, leaves enough of a gastric reservoir to minimize postgastrectomy sequelae. My preference is to perform this procedure through an upper abdominal incision [see Initial Incision, above]. The duodenum is divided 3 cm distal to the pylorus with a GIA stapler. The duodenal stump may be oversewn. The stomach is divided at least 6 cm proximal to gross tumor. Frozen-section histologic examination is performed to evaluate the surgical margins before alimentary reconstruction. The greater and lesser omenta are removed. The lymph nodes in the pyloric area, along the common hepatic artery, and in the celiac axis are excised with the stomach. The left gastric artery is divided at its origin. The spleen and the tail of the pancreas are not removed. Gastrointestinal continuity is established via the Schoemaker modification of the Billroth II anastomosis; some surgeons, however, prefer to perform a Billroth I anastomosis or a Roux-en-Y gastrojejunostomy in this setting.

Stamm Gastrostomy

Gastrostomy may be indicated either for gastric decompression or for gastric tube feeding. At present, most tube gastrostomies are performed percutaneously with the aid of an endoscope; however, if stricture or tumor prevents passage of an endoscope into the stomach or previous abdominal operations make percutaneous tube placement hazardous, then an open abdominal procedure may be done to insert a gastrostomy tube with the Stamm technique.

A 7 to 8 cm upper midline abdominal incision is made, and the stomach is grasped with two Babcock clamps. Two concentric

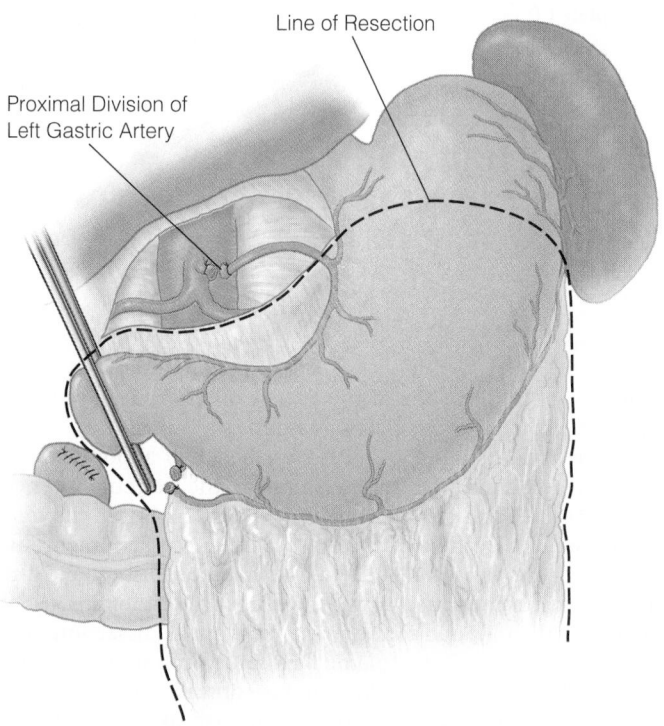

Line of Resection

Proximal Division of
Left Gastric Artery

Figure 10 **Radical distal subtotal gastrectomy for cancer. From 75 to 80 percent of the stomach is resected, including the lesser gastric curvature, and regional lymph nodes are removed.**[26]

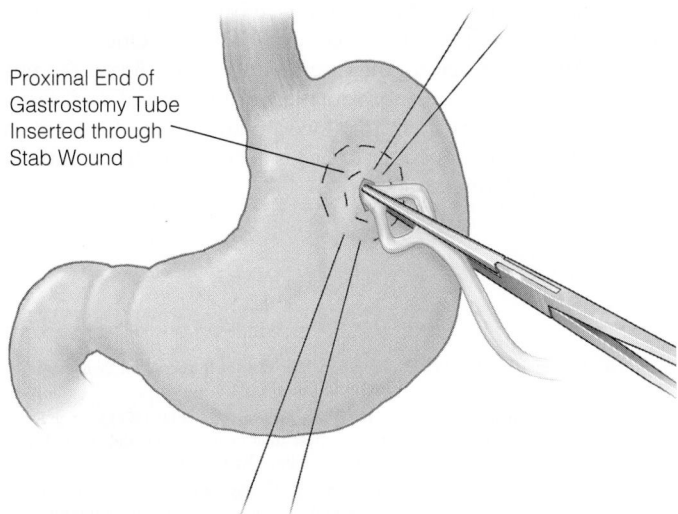

Figure 11 **Stamm gastrostomy. Two concentric purse-string sutures are placed on the anterior gastric wall, about 2.5 cm apart. A Malecot or mushroom catheter is inserted into the stomach through an opening made in the center of the inner suture. A stab wound in the left upper abdominal quadrant serves as the exit site for the tube.**[27]

purse-string sutures of 2-0 silk are placed on the anterior gastric wall, about 2.5 cm apart. An opening into the stomach is made with the electrocautery in the center of the inner purse-string suture. A Malecot or mushroom catheter (about 24 French) is inserted into the gastric opening [*see Figure 11*]. The inner purse-string suture is tied, then the outer purse-string suture. A stab wound is made with the electrocautery in the left upper abdominal quadrant. A Kelly clamp is passed through this opening and used to grasp the end of the gastrostomy tube, which is pulled through the abdominal wall. The skin exit site should be at least 2 cm from the costal margin and not too far laterally, so that the stomach is not distorted; a useful guideline is to place the stab wound at a point about one third of the way from the left midclavicular line at the costal margin to the umbilicus.

The anterior gastric wall around the gastric opening is affixed to the abdominal wall near the exit site with four interrupted 2-0 silk sutures, one suture to each quadrant surrounding the tube. The gastrostomy tube is then used to pull the stomach up to approximate the abdominal wall, and the sutures are tied. One or two 3-0 nylon sutures are placed in the skin, tied loosely at the skin level, wrapped spirally around the tube, and tied snugly. Because these sutures may be left in place for several weeks, nylon is preferred to silk, which is more likely to cause skin irritation.

Some surgeons like to suture omentum around the gastrostomy site to protect against leaks, but I find this practice troublesome and unnecessary. In addition, some surgeons prefer to use a Foley catheter for the gastrostomy tube. A Foley catheter would be first inserted through the abdominal wall stab wound and then placed into the stomach through the concentric purse-string sutures.

The gastrostomy tube is connected to straight drainage. If the tube is to be used for nutritional purposes, feedings are initiated when normal gastric emptying resumes, which is usually within 24 hours.

Pyloroplasty

Pyloroplasty is performed after truncal vagotomy for duodenal ulcer disease or after esophagectomy. It is appropriate only if the anterior surface of the pylorus is minimally involved and the duodenum is mobile enough to make the operation technically feasible.

WEINBERG PYLOROPLASTY

Heineke in 1886 and Mikulicz[20] in 1888 independently described a pyloroplasty in which a longitudinal incision was made through the pylorus, extending from the distal antrum to the proximal duodenum, and the incision was closed transversely in two layers, which resulted in ablation of the continuity of the pyloric sphincter and an increase in the diameter of the outlet of the pylorus. Weinberg[21] modified the closure so that it consisted of only one layer of nonabsorbable sutures; this resulted in a larger opening through the pyloric channel.

My approach to this procedure is as follows. The pylorus is identified, and the duodenum is mobilized by Kocher's maneuver. If the location of the pylorus is difficult to determine, a small incision should be made in the area of the pylorus; once entrance into the stomach or the duodenum is achieved, the pyloric ring can usually be located by palpation from the inside. Two traction sutures are placed about 1 cm apart on the anterior surface of the pylorus. A longitudinal incision is made between the two traction sutures, extending 2.5 to 3.5 cm proximally onto the antrum and a similar distance distally onto the duodenum. Any bleeding that occurs is controlled with electrocoagulation. To ensure adequate closure and a good outlet, the longitudinal incision must be made very carefully. Some surgeons extend the incision slightly further on the gastric side than on the duodenal side; this practice may yield better alignment when the incision is closed transversely. The total length of the incision should be at least 5 cm to ensure that the outlet is adequate after transverse closure. Generally, however, the incision should not be longer than 7 cm, or the surgeon may find it difficult to close the incision transversely without applying excessive tension.

Figure 12 **Closure of a Weinberg pyloroplasty. A pyloroplasty may be closed with the Gambee stitch, as shown. Once all of the sutures have been placed, they are tied.**[28]

I prefer to close a pyloroplasty with the Gambee stitch[22] [see Figure 12]. The suture is started from the serosa of the stomach and passed through all layers, including the mucosa. It is then passed back through the mucosa to the junction of the submucosa and the muscularis on the gastric wall. Mucosal approximation between the stomach and the duodenum is obtained by next passing the suture on the duodenal side from the junction of the submucosa and the muscularis through the mucosa, then back through all layers of the duodenal wall from the mucosa to the serosa. Once all of the sutures have been placed, they are tied; this helps invert the mucosa and improves the approximation of the serosal surfaces. A simple full-thickness stitch that incorporates more of the serosal surface than of the mucosal surface is also an effective technique for closing a pyloroplasty.

References

1. Dragstedt KR, Owens FM Jr: Supra-diaphragmatic section of the vagus nerves in treatment of duodenal ulcer. Proc Soc Exp Biol Med 53:152, 1943

2. Grassi G, Orecchia C: A comparison of intraoperative tests of completeness of vagal section. Surgery 75:155, 1974

3. Amdrup E, Anderson D, Jenson HE: Parietal cell (highly selective or proximal gastric) vagotomy for peptic ulcer disease. World J Surg 1:19, 1977

4. Rosati I, Serantoni C, Cianni PA: Extended selective proximal vagotomy: observations on a variant in technique. Chir Gastroenterol 10:33, 1976

5. Johnston D: Operative mortality and post-operative morbidity of highly selective vagotomy. Br Med J 5:545, 1975

6. Kennedy T, Magill P, Johnston GW, et al: Proximal gastric vagotomy, fundoplication and lesser curve necrosis. Br Med J 1:1455, 1979

7. Guelrud M, Zambrand-Ricones V, Simon C, et al: Dysphagia and lower esophageal sphincter abnormalities after proximal gastric vagotomy. Am J Surg 149:232, 1985

8. Sawyers JL, Goligher JC: Proximal gastric vagotomy. Surgery of the Stomach, Duodenum and Small Intestine, 2nd ed. Scott HW Jr, Sawyers JL, Eds. Blackwell Scientific Publications, Boston, 1992, p 510

9. Jordan PH, Thornby J: Should it be parietal cell vagotomy or selective vagotomy-antrectomy for treatment of duodenal ulcer: a progress report. Ann Surg 205:572, 1987

10. Sawyers JL, Herrington JL Jr: Perforated duodenal ulcer managed by proximal gastric vagotomy and suture plication. Ann Surg 185:656, 1977

11. Taylor TV, Gunn AR, MacLeod DAD, et al: Anterior lesser curve seromyotomy and posterior truncal vagotomy in the treatment of chronic duodenal ulcer. Lancet 2:846, 1982

12. Herrington JL Jr, Bluett MK: The surgical management of recurrent ulceration. Contemporary Surgery 28(2):15, 1986

13. Sawyers JL: Gastric carcinoma. Curr Probl Surg, Feb 1995, p 153

14. Inberg MV, Linna MI, Scheinin TM, et al: Anastomotic leakage after excision of esophageal and high gastric carcinoma. Am J Surg 122:540, 1971

15. Hunt CJ: Construction of food pouch from segment of jejunum as substitute for stomach in total gastrectomy. Arch Surg 64:601, 1952

16. Lawrence W: Reservoir construction after total gastrectomy: an instructive case. Ann Surg 155:191, 1962

17. Paulino F, Roselli A: Carcinoma of the stomach: with special reference to total gastrectomy. Curr Probl Surg, Dec 1973, p 1

18. Nadrowski L: Is a gastric replacement reservoir essential with total gastrectomy? Pathophysiologic update. Current Surgery 46:276, 1989

19. Cady B, Rossi R, Silverman ML, et al: Gastric adenocarcinoma: a disease in transition. Arch Surg 124:303, 1989

20. Mikulicz J, 1886: Cited in Mikulicz J: Zur operativen Behandlung des stenosier enden Magengeschwures. Arch Klin Chir 37:79, 1888

21. Weinberg JA, Stempien SJ, Movius JJ, et al: Vagotomy and pyloroplasty in treatment of duodenal ulcer. Am J Surg 92:202, 1956

22. Gambee LP: A single layer open intestinal anastomosis applicable to the small as well as the large intestine. West J Surg 59:1, 1951

23. Cameron JA: Atlas of Surgery, Vol 2. Mosby–Year Book, St. Louis, 1994

24. Scott HW Jr, Sawyers JL, Gobbel WG Jr, et al: Definitive surgical treatment in duodenal ulcer disease. Curr Probl Surg, Oct 1968, p 11

25. Herrington JL Jr: Vagotomy and antrectomy. Surgery of the Stomach, Duodenum and Small Intestine, 2nd ed. Scott HW Jr, Sawyers, JL, Eds. Blackwell Scientific Publications, Boston, 1992, p 533

26. Scott HW Jr, Longmire WP, Gray GF: Carcinoma of the stomach. Surgery of the Stomach, Duodenum and Small Intestine, 2nd ed. Scott HW Jr, Sawyers, JL, Eds. Blackwell Scientific Publications, Boston, 1993, p 333

27. Sabiston DC Jr: Atlas of General Surgery. WB Saunders Co, Philadelphia, 1994, p 231

28. Sawyers JL: Selective vagotomy and pyloroplasty. Mastery of Surgery. Nyhas LM, Baker RS, Eds. Little, Brown, Boston, 1984, p 525

Reviews

Atlas of General Surgery. Sabiston DC Jr, Ed. WB Saunders Co, Philadelphia, 1994

Atlas of Surgery, Volume 2. Cameron JL, Ed. Mosby–Year Book, St Louis, 1994

Acknowledgment

Figures 1 through 12   Tom Moore.

10 GASTRIC PROCEDURES FOR MORBID OBESITY

Eric J. DeMaria, M.D., and Harvey J. Sugerman, M.D.

It is clear that severe obesity is associated with a significant increase in morbidity[1] and a decreased life expectancy.[2] Morbid obesity has been shown to have a significant genetic basis.[3,4] To date, attempts to manage morbid obesity with medical weight reduction programs have met with an unacceptably high incidence of recidivism.[5] The approach that has had the greatest and longest-lasting success in achieving weight loss is bariatric surgery.

Choice between Gastric Bypass and Gastric Restriction

The gastric operations performed for morbid obesity include gastric bypass (GBP) procedures and gastric restrictive procedures (i.e., gastroplasty). Randomized, prospective trials have conclusively shown that GBP is as effective for weight control as jejunoileal (JI) bypass and results in significantly fewer complications.[6,7] JI bypass is associated with a substantial incidence of both early complications (e.g., acute cirrhosis, electrolyte imbalance, and fulminant diarrhea)[8] and late complications (e.g., cirrhosis, interstitial nephritis, arthritis, enteritis, nephrocalcinosis, and recurrent oxalate renal stones).[9] If evidence of cirrhosis, renal failure secondary to interstitial nephritis, or other complications mandates reversal of a JI bypass, the patient, if not extremely ill, should be converted to a GBP; otherwise, all the lost weight is sure to be regained, and the obesity-related comorbidity will return. Admittedly, however, many patients have done well after JI bypass and do not need to have the operation reversed.

Several randomized, prospective trials have found that horizontal gastroplasty yields poorer results than GBP.[10-12] Failure of horizontal gastroplasty has generally been attributed to technical causes, such as enlargement of the proximal pouch or the stoma or disruption of the staple line. Vertical banded gastroplasty (VBG) was developed by Mason in the hope that it would solve these technical problems and yield weight loss comparable to that seen after GBP without incurring the significant risk of iron, calcium, and vitamin B_{12} deficiencies associated with GBP. Although VBG appears to be an excellent procedure from a technical point of view,[13] one randomized, prospective trial found it to be significantly less effective than standard GBP.[14] In this trial, patients addicted to sweets lost much more weight after GBP than after VBG because they experienced symptoms of dumping syndrome when ingesting sweets. The failure rate was high after VBG because these patients experienced no difficulties when eating candy or drinking nondietetic sodas.

Two subsequent randomized, prospective trials confirmed the superiority of GBP.[15,16] Furthermore, weight loss after GBP appears to continue for as long as 10 years after operation: in the average patient, weight loss amounts to about two thirds of excess weight at 1 to 3 years after operation, three fifths at 5 years, and more than half in years 5 through 10.[17,18] It has been suggested that standard, or proximal, GBP will fail in 10% to 15% of patients because these patients will frequently nibble on high-fat snacks (e.g., corn chips, potato chips, and buttered popcorn). Such patients may have to be converted to a combined restrictive and malabsorptive procedure, such as partial biliopancreatic bypass (BPB).[19]

The original BPB involves hemigastrectomy and anastomosis of the distal 250 cm of intestine to the stomach; the bypassed small intestine is reanastomosed to the ileum 50 cm from the ileocecal valve. However, BPB has been associated with a high incidence of deficiencies of fat-soluble vitamins, hypocalcemia-induced osteoporosis, and protein-calorie malnutrition.[20] These nutritional deficiencies may be more common in the United States, where fat intake is high, than in many other countries. In Italy, for example, starch intake (as in pasta) probably outstrips fat intake; still, a number of Italian patients have had to be readmitted for parenteral nutrition and extension of the common absorptive intestinal tract because of refractory malnutrition. In some patients, it might be possible to convert a failed proximal GBP into a modified BPB with a 150 cm absorptive ileal limb; however, these patients also must be monitored carefully for deficiencies of fat-soluble vitamins, osteoporosis, and malnutrition.

Superobese patients, defined as those whose weight is 225% of ideal body weight or greater or whose body mass index (BMI) is 50 kg/m² or higher, will lose, on average, only about half of their excess weight, rather than two thirds, after standard GBP. In these patients, a 150 cm proximal Roux-en-Y procedure (so-called long-limb GBP [*see* Proximal Gastric Bypass, Operative Technique, *below*]) has been found to increase weight loss to two thirds of excess weight without causing an increase in nutritional complications.[21]

Preparation for Operation

Many surgeons, fearing increased perioperative morbidity and mortality, hesitate to operate on morbidly obese patients. It is true that such patients are at greater risk for complications and adverse results. Nevertheless, severely obese patients can undergo major abdominal surgery for weight loss with a remarkably low complication rate and a low mortality. These results, however, can only be achieved if a comprehensive program for preoperative and postoperative surgical care is rigorously planned and followed. The key elements of preparation for operation in the morbidly obese patient are discussed in greater detail elsewhere [*see VI:5 Obesity*].

Vertical Banded Gastroplasty

OPERATIVE TECHNIQUE

The first step in VBG is to make a circular stapled opening in the stomach 5 cm from the esophagogastric junction. A 90 mm bariatric stapler with four parallel rows of staples is then applied once between this opening and the angle of His. (At this point, ac-

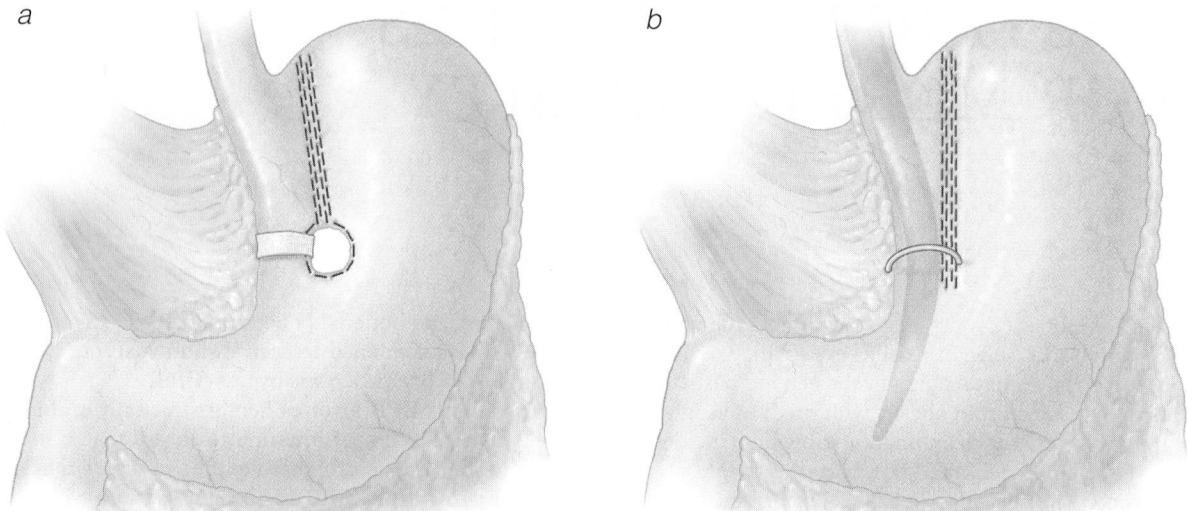

Figure 1 Vertical banded gastroplasty. Depicted are (*a*) standard VBG and (*b*) Silastic ring gastroplasty, a variant of VBG in which the stoma is reinforced with a Silastic tube.

cording to Mason, the originator of the procedure, the volume of the pouch should be measured by means of an Ewald tube placed by the anesthetist; ideally, pouch volume should be 15 ml.) Next, a strip of polypropylene mesh is wrapped around the gastrogastric outlet on the lesser curvature and sutured to itself—but not to the stomach—in such a way as to create an outlet with a circumference of 5 cm for the small upper gastric pouch [*see Figure 1a*]. Some surgeons have used a stomal outlet 4.5 cm in circumference, but this smaller outlet has not led to better weight loss; in fact, many patients with the 4.5 cm outlet exhibit maladaptive eating behavior, drinking high-calorie liquids because meat tends to get caught in the small stoma.

Silastic ring gastroplasty [*see Figure 1b*] is a variant of VBG that uses a vertical staple line and a stoma reinforced with Silastic tubing.

COMPLICATIONS

Complications of VBG include erosion of the polypropylene mesh used to restrict the gastroplasty stoma into the gastric lumen, enlargement of the pouch, stomal stenosis, reflux esophagitis, and mild vitamin deficiencies.[22] To date, mesh erosion has been infrequently observed after VBG. Pouch enlargement is fairly common with horizontal gastroplasty but is much less likely to occur with VBG, in which the vertical staple line is placed in the thicker, more muscular part of the stomach. In addition, stomal diameter remains fixed with the mesh band. If mesh erosion, pouch enlargement, stomal stenosis, disabling GI reflux, or recurrent vomiting occurs, it is probably best to convert the patient to GBP. In particular, patients with a Silastic ring VBG may exhibit intractable vomiting of solid foods with no evidence of mechanical obstruction. In our experience, conversion of these patients to GBP yields good results and eliminates the vomiting problem. Finally, vitamin deficiencies may be prevented by having VBG patients take a multivitamin daily for life.

Laparoscopic Adjustable Gastric Banding

Gastric banding is another form of gastroplasty, in which a polypropylene or Silastic band is placed around the stomach just below the esophagogastric junction. In several series, gastric

banding has had markedly variable results with respect to achievement of weight loss. Furthermore, it has been associated with slipping or kinking of the banded stoma, obstruction at the band, and intractable vomiting.

In the past few years, laparoscopic approaches to gastric banding have been developed and brought into use at a number of centers around the world. Laparoscopic adjustable gastric banding is potentially a significant advance over open gastric banding procedures, primarily because of the adjustability of the band. Open gastric banding procedures have used a variety of materials to constrict the gastric lumen and carry a recognized risk of postoperative nausea and vomiting that do not respond to any treatment short of reoperation. The adjustable gastric band (BioEnterics, Carpinteria, California) used in the laparoscopic procedure [*see Figure 2*] is a silicone device with an inflatable reservoir that can be inflated or deflated postoperatively through a subcutaneous port placed deep in the abdominal wall for percutaneous access. Saline is injected into or withdrawn from the reservoir through the port to adjust gastric luminal diameter, as measured by barium contrast evaluations. Thus, if intractable vomiting develops, saline can easily be removed from the band to alleviate the problem; similarly, if the patient fails to lose weight after operation, additional saline may be injected into the band to narrow the gastric lumen further.

Figure 2 Laparoscopic adjustable gastric banding. Shown is the adjustable gastric banding device used in the procedure.

Figure 3 **Laparoscopic adjustable gastric banding. Once in the correct position on the proximal stomach, the adjustable band is locked into place.**

As of July 2000, use of the laparoscopically placed adjustable gastric band has not been approved by the Food and Drug Administration (FDA). The FDA has, however, authorized a prospective trial involving 300 patients at seven centers in the United States. Enrollment in this initial trial is now complete; after a mandatory 3-year follow-up period, currently under way, the FDA plans to consider approval of this implantable device. No outcome data have been reported yet.

OPERATIVE TECHNIQUE

Laparoscopic adjustable gastric banding is performed by using a six-port technique. Initial abdominal access is obtained via a supraumbilical trocar, and the remaining five ports are placed sequentially along the right and left costal margins. The liver is retracted via the right lateral port, and the proximal stomach is visualized via a laparoscope inserted through the subxiphoid port. A 20 ml balloon catheter is placed perorally into the proximal stomach to define an appropriately small pouch size. Dissection is then begun at the equator of the balloon with a hook electrocautery placed immediately alongside the gastric wall. The retrogastric tunnel should be above the posterior peritoneal reflection so that the free space of the lesser sac posterior to the stomach is not entered. Additional dissection is carried out laterally at the angle of His to open the peritoneum and start clearing a plane behind the proximal stomach. Once the plane is completely cleared from the lesser curve to the angle of His, a specially designed implement is inserted behind the stomach and used to grasp the tubing of the banding device and pull it around the stomach. The banding device is then locked into place at a spot overlying a pressure-sensitive location on the specially designed balloon catheter; this step allows one to confirm that the band is properly closed in the correct position and that the lumen is sufficiently tightened [*see Figure 3*]. The band tubing is then brought through the left midclavicular trocar port, which is placed via the left midclavicular line subcostal trocar incision and fixed to the abdominal wall fascia with sutures. The tubing is connected to the reservoir, which is filled with saline.

TROUBLESHOOTING

It is essential to place the band properly during the initial procedure. Early results suggest that the proximal pouch must be very small to optimize weight loss. In addition, proper placement minimizes—though it does not eliminate—the risk of band slippage and the complications thereof.

It remains controversial whether posterior fixation of the band is necessary to prevent band slippage. Anterior fixation is routinely performed, with interrupted sutures of nonabsorbable

a

b

Figure 4 **Laparoscopic adjustable gastric banding. Contrast studies illustrate (*a*) a normally positioned laparoscopic adjustable gastric band and (*b*) a slipped band.**

material placed between the distal and the proximal stomach to allow tissue to be apposed over the band and held in place. Several techniques have been suggested for posterior fixation of the band, but they are more difficult than anterior fixation techniques. If, as recommended (see above), the band is tunneled above the peritoneal reflection posteriorly, posterior fixation may not be necessary.

Although laparoscopic adjustable gastric banding appears easier than many of the procedures done to treat obesity, there is a definite learning curve. A number of surgical misadventures have been reported, including gastric perforation, splenic injury, and malposition of the band.

COMPLICATIONS

Band slippage (usually posterior rather than anterior) may occur even after proper placement, resulting in intolerance of oral intake and vomiting. Such complaints are an indication for an upper GI series, which usually reveals dilatation of the proximal pouch and rotation of the band [see Figure 4]. Initial treatment consists of evacuating all saline from the band. Frequently, however, the proximal pouch does not return to its normal size, and symptoms recur or fail to resolve. Laparoscopic or open revision of the banding procedure is then required; if the patient also has not lost a sufficient amount of weight, conversion to GBP may be recommended. It is noteworthy that band erosion into the stomach, a not infrequent complication of the use of mesh in VBG or in the Angelchik prosthesis for gastroesophageal reflux treatment, has not been frequently reported to date. Longer follow-up will be necessary to evaluate the true extent of this risk.

As after any form of gastroplasty, the patient may fail to lose weight or may regain lost weight. Inappropriate eating behaviors (e.g., intake of high-calorie sweets) are the most likely cause. If obesity-related comorbid conditions persist, conversion to proximal GBP is appropriate.

OUTCOME EVALUATION

How successful laparoscopic adjustable gastric banding is at achieving weight loss over the long term remains unclear. The adjustability and reversibility of the operation, as well as the decreased disability that results, make it attractive to both patients and physicians. The procedure appears to avoid some of the major postoperative complications associated with open gastric bypass procedures (e.g., incisional hernia, marginal ulcer, and stomal stenosis. Band slippage remains a major postoperative concern, however, though the incidence of slippage does appear to decrease as one's experience with the procedure increases. More significant, there appears to be a high frequency of failed weight loss—as high as 15% to 20% of all patients undergoing the procedure and possibly even higher. European and Australian data confirm that there is a significant failure rate but also suggest that the remaining patients achieve a degree of weight loss approaching that seen with proximal GBP. Whether these reports will withstand the scrutiny of long-term follow-up remains to be seen.

Laparoscopic adjustable gastric banding may come to play an important role in the management of some morbidly obese patients in the United States. If it receives the authorization of the FDA, it may quickly become a frequently performed surgical procedure. On the basis of our participation in the clinical trial, we believe that at present, it is premature to authorize general use of this implantable banding device. It is undeniable, however, that in the United States, the prevalence of severe obesity is increasing at an alarming rate. This worrisome increase, coupled with the disappointingly poor results of medical therapy, the observation that more than 30,000 of these

Figure 5 **Proximal gastric bypass. Depicted is the completed procedure.**

banding devices have already been implanted in patients worldwide, and the potential political consequences of failure to allow use of a potentially helpful device, may spur the FDA to approve laparoscopic adjustable gastric banding prematurely.

Proximal Gastric Bypass

Proximal GBP results in greater weight loss than the gastric restrictive procedures (see above) and carries a lower incidence of weight regain; consequently we consider it the superior procedure. Our focus since the beginning of the 1990s has been on developing techniques for minimizing complications after proximal GBP. In our view, any surgeon currently performing this procedure ought to be able to achieve a gastrojejunal anastomotic leakage rate lower than 5%; many groups, in fact, report rates lower than 3%. In addition, we believe that other postoperative complications (e.g., acute dilatation of the excluded portion of the stomach) are usually preventable if strict attention is paid to mastering the technical aspects of the operation.

Compared with the version of GBP we perform at our institution, the original GBP created a much larger proximal gastric pouch and a much wider anastomotic opening, and it was often associated with inadequate weight loss. In our version of GBP, three superimposed 55 or 90 mm staple lines are placed across the proximal stomach in such a way as to create a gastric pouch no larger than 30 ml with a 45 cm Roux limb and a stoma no larger than 1 cm [see Figure 5].

OPERATIVE TECHNIQUE

Step 1: Initial Incision and Abdominal Exploration

Once the patient is anesthetized, the abdomen receives a thorough, careful cleansing with Betadine and is draped in a sterile fashion. An upper midline incision is made and extended through the fascia alongside the xiphoid process to facilitate cephalad exposure. We routinely carry the incision down to the supraumbilical area. The deep layer of subcutaneous fat can often be separated bluntly with aggressive lateral traction applied by the surgeon and the assistant, and the midline usually can then be identified for fascial incision. We use the electrocautery to enter the abdominal cavity and often encounter a thick layer of subfascial preperitoneal fat before entry into the peritoneal cavity. Abdominal exploration is undertaken in every patient, including examination of the liver for possible signs of liver disease. Other incidental findings may become apparent as well.

Troubleshooting On a number of occasions, we have discovered unexpected significant liver disease at the time of operation. If the patient has cirrhosis without portal hypertension, one should perhaps proceed with bypass if the patient's comorbid conditions make it mandatory; liver transplantation carries increased risk in morbidly obese patients. The gallbladder should be palpated for gallstones, which, if found, we consider an indication for cholecystectomy at the time of the bypass procedure. If there are no visual or palpable gallbladder abnormalities, we use intraoperative ultrasonography to examine the gallbladder and perform cholecystectomy if small stones, sludge, or polyps are identified.

It is not unusual to discover previously unrecognized conditions during GBP, primarily because symptoms may not be obvious in morbidly obese patients and because their large size tends to make radiologic imaging difficult or even impossible. For example, intraoperative discovery of pelvic cysts and tumors is not uncommon in obese female patients. Such lesions may be excised during GBP; on occasion, if they appear benign and their location prevents safe excision, they may be managed with careful follow-up.

Step 2: Mobilization of the Esophagus

The bypass procedure itself is begun by mobilizing the distal esophagus and encircling it with a soft rubber drain 0.5 in. in diameter. The gastrohepatic omentum is bluntly entered at a point overlying the caudate lobe, with care taken to look for and avoid injury to an aberrant left hepatic artery. The phrenoesophageal ligament overlying the anterior and lateral distal esophagus is sharply incised to facilitate subsequent blunt mobilization of the distal esophagus. To prevent esophageal injury, the nasogastric tube is carefully palpated within the lumen of the esophagus during mobilization, and blunt dissection proceeds widely around this important landmark. Laterally, dissection must be at the level of the esophagus or higher.

Troubleshooting If dissection is too low laterally, it may result in blunt injury to the short gastric vessels, bleeding, and the need for urgent splenectomy, which is no easy task in a morbidly obese patient. In addition, it may lead to creation of an inappropriately large pouch by keeping the surgeon from recognizing that some of the stomach is above the level at which the encircling rubber drain is placed.

Step 3: Division of the Mesentery and Dissection around the Stomach

Once the esophagus is mobilized, the assistant's left hand is placed through the gastrohepatic omental opening behind the stomach wall on the lesser curvature. The space between the first and second branches of the left gastric artery is then identified as a landmark for location of the gastric staple line, both to ensure that the pouch created is no larger than 30 ml and to prevent

Figure 6 **Proximal gastric bypass. After dissection of the avascular tissue on the posterior gastric wall, a red rubber catheter is passed through the resulting space to encircle the stomach.**

injury to the left gastric artery, which usually runs cephalad to this location. With the surgeon's posterior finger pressing anteriorly to place tension on the tissue, a fine-tip right-angle clamp and the electrocautery pencil are used to divide the mesentery carefully at this level immediately alongside the stomach wall so as to create a mesenteric opening that will admit a large right-angle clamp. The avascular tissue on the posterior wall of the stomach is then bluntly dissected between the opening in the gastrohepatic omentum and the lateral angle of His, which is identified by the encircling rubber drain. The blunt tip of a large 28 French red rubber tube is placed behind the stomach in a medial-to-lateral direction along this dissected path to encircle the stomach [*see Figure 6*]. The open end of the red rubber tube is subsequently brought through the previously created mesenteric opening with a large right-angle clamp. The stomach is now ready for stapling, and the red rubber tube serves as a guide for introduction of the stapler. At this point, all intraluminal tubes and devices (e.g., the nasogastric tube and the esophageal stethoscope) are removed from the esophagus by the anesthetist.

Troubleshooting When a tube is inadvertently stapled within the stomach, excising it from the staple line can become a technical nightmare. To remove the stapled tube, it is usually necessary to transect the stomach, thereby creating the potential for significant injury to the gastric tissue and possibly compromising the eventual anastomosis.

Step 4: Creation and Mobilization of the Roux Limb and Jejunojejunostomy

The ligament of Treitz is identified, and the jejunum is measured to a point 45 cm beyond the ligament, where the jejunum is divided with a stapler. An 8 to 12 cm segment of jejunum is resected at this point to create a larger mesenteric defect, which we believe facilitates mobilization of the limb to the proximal stomach. Mesenteric dissection is carried posteriorly in fat with the sequential application of clamps until further dissection appears either unnecessary for mobilization or unwise (i.e., likely to cause mesenteric vascular injury).

A side-to-side jejunojejunostomy is then created with a 60 mm linear stapler either 45 cm beyond the initial point of jejunal division, for standard proximal GBP, or 150 cm downstream, for the long-limb modification of the procedure used in superobese patients [*see* Choice between Gastric Bypass and Gastric Restriction, *above*]. It is important not to narrow the efferent lumen at the jejunojejunostomy site, particularly with the long-limb modification, in which the lumen at the distal end of the Roux limb may be quite small. The enterotomies made to allow placement of the stapler can usually be closed with a 55 mm stapler loaded with 3.5 mm staples; however, if stapling would cause undue narrowing of the lumen, the closures should be handsewn instead.

Troubleshooting We generally proceed to mobilization of the Roux limb before committing to stapling the stomach so that we can determine whether the limb can be extended to reach the proximal stomach without tension being placed on it. In those rare cases in which the mesentery is too foreshortened to permit the limb to reach the proximal stomach, we advocate changing the procedure to VBG rather than creating a gastrojejunal anastomosis under tension and incurring the increased risk of leakage.

Step 5: Gastric Stapling and Gastrojejunostomy

The Roux limb is brought through the mesentery of the transverse colon with blunt dissection and then brought up to the proximal stomach. The 55 or 90 mm stapler, loaded with 4.8 mm staples, is guided behind the stomach by inserting its open-mouthed end into the lumen of the previously positioned red rubber tube. Once it is determined that the staple line will reach completely across the stomach and that the stomach is not folded on itself, the stomach is stapled three times in such a way that the three staple lines are superimposed [*see Figure 7*].

A 1 cm anastomosis is created between the proximal stomach pouch and the Roux limb, with an outer layer composed of interrupted 3-0 silk sutures and an inner layer composed of a continuous absorbable 2-0 polyglycolic acid (Dexon) suture. When the posterior aspect of the anastomosis is complete, a 30 French dilator is placed with the patient under anesthesia and is guided

through the anastomosis by the surgeon to ensure that the stoma has the appropriate diameter [*see Figure 8*]. The anterior aspect of the anastomosis is then completed.

Troubleshooting A significant concern for many bariatric surgeons has been a high incidence of staple line disruption causing failed weight loss or weight regain; in one series, the incidence of such disruption was 35%. To minimize this risk, some surgeons advocate transecting the stomach. This is done by inserting two parallel TA-90 staplers and cutting between them with a scalpel after the staplers are fired. Other surgeons, however, prefer to oversew the staple line. By using the technique of three superimposed staple lines, we have decreased the incidence of staple line disruption to less than 2%; consequently, we believe that gastric transection is unnecessary on a routine basis (though occasionally useful in selected cases) and may increase the risk of the procedure. Another advantage of gastric transection besides reduction of staple line disruption is that it allows the Roux limb to be brought up to the gastric pouch via a retrocolic and retrogastric tract, which is significantly shorter and places less tension on the limb. This approach is particularly helpful in severely obese patients with a fatty and foreshortened mesentery, in whom it is difficult to free the Roux limb sufficiently to reach the proximal stomach without tension. The possibility that gastric transection may prove helpful in a specific patient is another reason why it is advisable to delay stapling the stomach until the Roux limb is mobilized.

Step 6: Assessment of the Anastomosis

When the entire anastomosis is complete, the dilator is removed and the tip of an 18 French nasogastric tube is advanced by the anesthetist and carefully guided through the anastomosis by the surgeon. The Roux limb is occluded with the assistant's left hand or with an atraumatic intestinal clamp, and the anesthetist injects a series of 10 ml aliquots of methylene blue dye through the nasogastric tube to determine whether the anastomosis is leaking. A total of 30 to 60 ml of methylene blue must usually be injected; lesser amounts will not stress the suture line enough to constitute an adequate test.

Figure 7 Proximal gastric bypass. The stomach is stapled to create the small proximal pouch. The stapler is fired three times to create three superimposed staple lines, thereby decreasing the risk of staple line disruption.

Figure 8 Proximal gastric bypass. When the posterior aspect of the gastrojejunal anastomosis has been completed, a 30 French dilator is placed through the stoma to confirm that the opening is correctly sized.

Troubleshooting When an intraoperative leak is identified, we oversew the area of leakage with silk sutures until injection of additional methylene blue dye via the nasogastric tube yields no further leakage. The most difficult area to repair is the posterior suture line, which is quite close to the gastric staple line. Posterior leaks are usually repaired by reinforcing the posterior suture line with additional sutures between the excluded stomach and the jejunal limb; often, we oversew the entire posterior suture line. In addition, a viable pedicle of omentum may be mobilized and placed around the anastomosis for additional reinforcement. Closed suction drains may also be placed in this area, both to detect possible postoperative leakage and to control a postoperative fistula.

Finally, a gastrostomy tube is placed in the excluded portion of the stomach. This measure provides postoperative decompression, which should prevent the development of undue tension on the Roux limb as a result of gastric distention, and establishes a route for enteral feeding if a fistula develops. Fortunately, such fistulas are rare. When they do occur, they often heal if (1) they are well drained, (2) there is no distal obstruction or local abscess, and (3) the patient is receiving nutritional support with no oral intake. A gastrostomy tube should also be placed in the distal gastric pouch when extensive adhesions from a previous procedure or a difficult gastric reoperation prevents postoperative dilatation of the pouch.

Step 7: Closure

When the absence of leakage is confirmed or when any leaks identified have been controlled, the tip of the nasogastric tube can be positioned further down in the Roux limb and left to continuous suction overnight. All mesenteric defects—at the jejunojejunostomy, at the mesocolon, and behind the Roux limb—are then closed to prevent a Petersen hernia. The abdominal fascia is reapproximated with a continuous No. 2 nonabsorbable suture, subcutaneous tissues are irrigated with a crystalloid solution containing 1% neomycin, and the skin is closed with skin staples. No subcutaneous sutures or drains are used in routine cases.

COMPLICATIONS

Proximal GBP is associated with a significant incidence of stomal stenosis and with marginal ulcer.[23] The former responds to endoscopic stomal dilatation, and the latter usually responds to H_2 receptor blocker or proton pump inhibitor therapy.

Iron, vitamin B_{12}, and folic acid deficiencies may occur but can usually be corrected with oral supplements[22]; accordingly, GBP patients, like VBG patients, should be advised to take a multivitamin daily for life. Compared with VBG, GBP results in significantly lower serum hemoglobin and iron concentrations. This is primarily a problem in menstruating women. All menstruating women who have undergone GBP should be treated prophylactically with supplemental oral ferrous sulfate, 325 mg/day. As many as six iron tablets a day may be required if menstrual bleeding is heavy. On occasion, intramuscular iron injections or, rarely, hysterectomy may be necessary. The risk of vitamin B_{12} deficiency is higher after GBP than after VBG, but this condition can be prevented with supplemental oral vitamin B_{12}, 500 mg/day. A few patients may require (or prefer) monthly B_{12} injections, which they can learn to administer themselves.

Concerns have been expressed that GBP can lead to other divalent cation deficiencies. We have not encountered zinc deficiencies 5 to 9 years after GBP. We have, however, observed calcium deficiencies leading to osteoporosis, which may take many years to become manifest and may not be biochemically evident because of normal serum calcium levels. We therefore recommend that all our GBP patients take oral calcium supplements. Magnesium deficiencies should be treated with $MgSO_4$ supplementation.

Nutritional deficiencies do not appear to be a greater problem with long-limb GBP than with standard proximal GBP. We do monitor patients for possible malabsorption of the fat-soluble vitamins A, D, and E after long-limb GBP.

BPB may be associated with all of the complications seen after GBP. In addition, patients who undergo BPB may experience diarrhea, severe protein malnutrition (manifested as hypoalbuminemia), and deficiencies of vitamins A (manifested as severe night blindness), D (manifested as severe osteoporosis), and E.[20] Hypoalbuminemia may respond to oral pancreatic enzymes but often must be treated with total parenteral nutrition. In some patients, it may prove necessary to lengthen the absorptive intestinal tract from 50 cm to 200 cm.

OUTCOME EVALUATION

In our series of 672 open proximal GBP procedures,[17] we reported a 1.2% incidence of anastomotic leak with peritonitis, a 4.4% incidence of severe wound infection (defined as infection serious enough to delay hospital discharge), an 11.4% incidence of minor wound infections and seromas (which were easily treated at home), a less than 1% incidence of gastric staple line disruption with the use of three superimposed applications of a 90 mm linear stapler, a 15% incidence of stomal stenosis, a 13% incidence of marginal ulcer, a 16.9% incidence of incisional hernia, and a 10% incidence of cholecystitis necessitating cholecystectomy. Gallstones developed in 32% of the GBP patients who had a normal intraoperative gallbladder ultrasonogram within 6 months of surgery, and sludge was observed in another 10%. In a multicenter randomized prospective trial,[24] we and others were able to reduce the incidence of gallstones within 6 months of GBP from 32% to 2% by giving patients ursodeoxycholic acid, 300 mg twice daily. Gallstone formation is very rare beyond 6 months. The operative mortality in our series was less than 1%. Patients with respiratory insufficiency of obesity had a 2.2% operative mortality, whereas those without pulmonary dysfunction had a 0.4% mortality.

Neither the data from our randomized, prospective trial nor the data from selective studies support the contention that VBG is safer than GBP. Although GBP includes one more anastomosis than VBG, complications such as leaks and peritonitis occur with both operations. A common criticism of GBP is that it is difficult to evaluate the distal gastric pouch and duodenum after the operation. Such evaluation, however, can be done in 75% of patients by means of retrograde passage of an endoscope into the duodenum and the stomach and in others by means of percutaneous distal distention gastrography (DeMaria EJ, Sugerman HJ, unpublished data, 2000). To our knowledge, bleeding from either the distal gastric pouch or a duodenal ulcer has occurred in only one of our more than 1,200 GBP patients. In one patient, a perforation of the proximal gastric pouch developed after administration of high-dose nonsteroidal anti-inflammatory medication. Gastric mucosal metaplasia of the bypassed portion of the stomach was noted in 5% of patients after retrograde endoscopy, a finding that has raised concerns regarding the risk of carcinoma arising at that location. However, tens of thousands of these procedures have been performed since 1967, and only one case of cancer in the bypassed stomach has been reported to date. We have also had one such case but have not published it.

Laparoscopic Gastric Bypass

Laparoscopic gastric bypass is a relatively new alternative to standard open GBP. One would anticipate that laparoscopic GBP would yield much the same weight loss results as open

GBP but with less pain, reduced disability, and a shorter hospitalization period. In addition, one would anticipate a decrease in major wound infections as well as fewer incisional hernias. On the face of it, it seems likely that the laparoscopic procedure, though more expensive, would be cost-effective, but proving it is so will probably require an analysis of long-term follow-up that documents decreased subsequent hospitalizations for wound infections, hernia repairs, and complications of intra-abdominal adhesions (e.g., bowel obstruction), given that early results cannot demonstrate a dramatic reduction in the length of hospitalization after the procedure. If the additional benefit of reduced disability-related absence from work is realized, this would help reduce overall costs as well.

TOTAL INTRACORPOREAL LAPAROSCOPIC GASTRIC BYPASS

Laparoscopic GBP poses significant technical challenges, even for surgeons with advanced laparoscopic skills. Most of the variations seen at different institutions are related to creation of the gastrojejunal anastomosis, with most groups favoring the use of a circular rather than a linear stapler. The anvil of the circular stapler may be placed within the proximal gastric pouch either by means of flexible upper GI endoscopy, through an approach similar to the snare-and-wire technique used for placement of a percutaneous endoscopic gastrostomy (PEG) tube, or by means of a gastrotomy of the pouch for intra-abdominal anvil placement followed by staple closure of the gastrotomy. Peroral placement of the stapler's anvil can be problematic: even the small 21 French anvil is hard to pass through the proximal esophagus in some patients. Nevertheless, we will describe this approach in some detail because it seems to be favored by most surgeons at present and it is easier to perform.

Figure 10 **Laparoscopic gastric bypass: total intracorporeal approach. Much as in open GBP, a linear endoscopic GIA stapler is fired three times to transect the stomach and create the gastric pouch.**

Operative Technique

Step 1: initial access and trocar placement Initial access to the abdomen is obtained through a left subcostal incision with either a Veress needle or a commercially available device that allows direct vision through the scope while a 12 mm trocar is inserted. Gas is then insufflated into the abdomen to a pressure of 15 mm Hg; on occasion, a pressure of 18 mm Hg may be necessary. Additional trocars are placed in specific locations [*see Figure 9*]. To retract the liver, we employ a metal Nathanson liver retraction device anchored to the bed, which is inserted after a 5 mm sharp trocar is used to enter the abdominal cavity and peritoneum and removed. If the left lateral segment of the liver is very large (as in patients with steatosis), additional liver retraction may be necessary.

The falciform ligament is then dissected from the anterior abdominal wall with an ultrasonic scalpel. This dissection allows the trocar incision to be placed quite high in the epigastrium, which facilitates proximal gastric exposure. A 12 mm port placed in the right paramedian position near the costal margin serves as the surgeon's primary operative port; two lateral subcostal 5 mm ports allow both surgeon and assistant to employ two-handed techniques for the entire procedure.

Step 2: dissection around the stomach and creation of the gastric pouch Dissection is performed along the lesser curvature of the stomach between the neurovascular bundle and the gastric wall; the ultrasonic scalpel is the best instrument for this purpose. Dissection posterior to the stomach is performed in the avascular free plane of the lesser sac. Additional dissection along the lesser curvature is not recommended, because it may increase the devascularization of the pouch. Further dissection is done with the ultrasonic scalpel at the angle of His to create a connection with the posterior gastric space. A linear endoscopic gastrointestinal anastomosis (GIA) stapler loaded with 3.5 mm staples in 60 mm cartridges is then used to transect the stomach and create the proximal gastric pouch; three firings are usually necessary [*see Figure 10*].

Step 3 (circular stapling): placement of the stapler in the gastric pouch As noted (see above), surgeons use several different techniques to complete the gastrojejunal anastomosis.

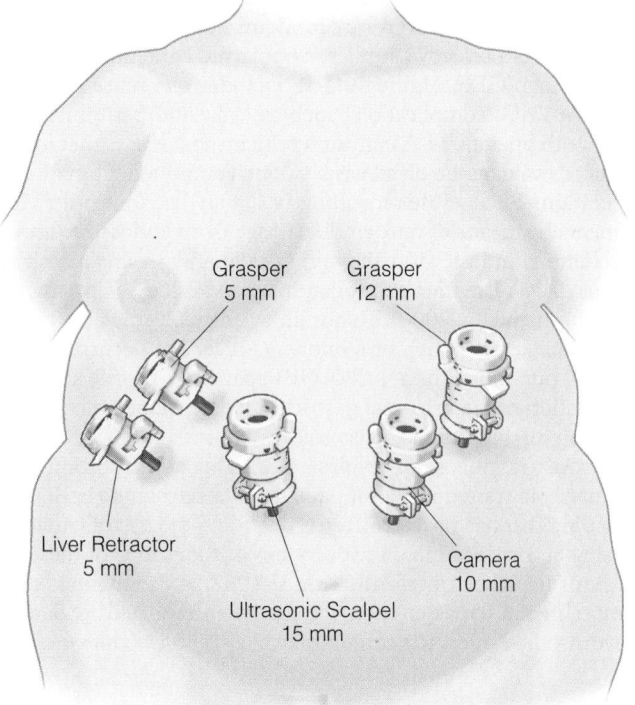

Figure 9 **Laparoscopic gastric bypass: total intracorporeal approach. Shown are the trocar incision sites for laparoscopic GBP.**

Initially, we employed the technique reported in Wittgrove's original description of the procedure,[25] which involved passing the anvil of a circular stapler down the patient's esophagus in a manner resembling placement of a PEG tube. With this approach, the next step in the procedure is to have an assistant perform flexible upper GI endoscopy of the gastric pouch. The pouch wall is transilluminated by the endoscope light, and a site is chosen for the gastrojejunostomy. The endoscopist then places an endoscopic snare, which can be seen pressing against the tissue of the pouch wall. A small opening is made in the pouch with the electrocautery scissors so that the snare can be pushed through the gastric wall at this location. The snare is then used to grasp a wire placed through a needle across the abdominal wall in the left abdomen, and snare and wire are withdrawn through the mouth along with the scope.

The anvil of the stapler is attached to the end of the wire that was drawn through the mouth, and the surgeon pulls on the other end of the wire to deliver the anvil through the mouth, down the esophagus, and into the gastric pouch, where it can be visualized. The electrocautery attached to the scissors is used to enlarge the opening in the gastric wall slightly, and the stem of the stapler is then brought through the gastrotomy. To prevent anastomotic leakage after stapling, the gastrotomy should be no larger than the diameter of the stem; if it is too large, it can be closed around the stem by placing one or two simple sutures.

Troubleshooting. Difficulty in passing the anvil perorally may arise at the level where the trachea separates from the esophagus in the deep pharynx. This difficulty can usually be overcome either by having the endoscopist perform a jaw-thrust maneuver or by placing a large laryngoscope blade deep in the pharynx to make the anvil visible in the proximal esophagus and then nudging the anvil forward with either the tip of the blade or a McGill forceps. Deflating the endotracheal tube balloon may also help. Occasionally, we use the large esophageal dilator to place pressure on the tip of the anvil. Given the potential for esophageal injury if the anvil will not advance, it is important not to apply excessive force. We have seen a case in which the anvil became lodged in the proximal esophagus beyond the laryngoscopic view and the long suture holding it broke; retrograde passage of an esophageal dilator was required to dislodge the anvil. Other surgeons who use wire to draw the anvil down the esophagus have identified nontransmural esophageal injuries on postoperative contrast studies or have seen subcutaneous emphysema in the neck after operation.

Step 3 (linear stapling)   Currently, we prefer a technique in which a linear stapler, rather than a circular one, is used to create the gastrojejunal anastomosis. In this approach, therefore, we proceed directly from creation of the gastric pouch to creation of the Roux limb for subsequent anastomosis to the pouch.

Step 4: creation and mobilization of the Roux limb and jejunojejunostomy   In most reports of laparoscopic GBP, regardless of how the gastrojejunostomy is done, the approach to creating the Roux limb is essentially the same. The patient is placed in a supine position, and graspers are used to bring the omentum upward into the upper abdomen so that the transverse colon and the underlying mesocolon are exposed. Graspers are then placed on the transverse mesocolon and used to elevate it anteriorly so that the ligament of Treitz is exposed. The position of the ligament of Treitz is confirmed by careful manipulation and verification that the bowel is attached to the retroperitoneum at

this location; this may be a more difficult task in patients who have previously undergone abdominal procedures.

With the help of a measuring instrument inserted into the abdomen, the small bowel is measured to a point 30 to 40 cm from the ligament of Treitz, where it is transected with the endoscopic GIA stapler, loaded with 2.5 mm staples. A 0.5 in. Penrose rubber drain is sutured to the cut end of the Roux limb so that it is not confused with the other cut end of the bowel. The Roux limb is then measured to a length of 45 to 60 cm. (As in open GBP, the Roux limb may have to be significantly longer—up to 150 cm—if the long-limb modification is being performed.) The afferent side of the previously transected small bowel is then attached with a simple absorbable suture to the proposed jejunojejunostomy site on the Roux limb. Intracorporeal suturing is facilitated by using an automatic suturing device. Positioning is important: the afferent limb should be kept to the patient's left, with the Roux limb more medial.

A small enterotomy is then made in preparation for passage of the linear stapler, loaded with 2.5 mm staples in a 60 mm cartridge, into the bowel. Two sutures are placed, one anterior to the enterotomy and the other posterior, to help manipulate the bowel onto the stapler. The stapler is then fired, creating a 60 mm side-to-side anastomosis. A third suture is placed at the midpoint of the enterotomy, and all three sutures are grasped to facilitate closure of the enterotomy with another application of the linear stapler. Once completed, the anastomosis is inspected both for integrity and for possible narrowing. At this point, anterior traction is applied to the three sutures to facilitate placement of interrupted or continuous sutures to close the mesenteric defect.

Next, a retrocolic, retrogastric tunnel (which we consider clearly superior to an antecolic approach) is created so that the Roux limb can be advanced to the proximal stomach for anastomosis. The ligament of Treitz is once again identified by lifting the transverse mesocolon anteriorly, and a spot 1 to 2 cm anterior and to the left of the ligament is chosen as the starting point for dissection with the ultrasonic scalpel. The middle colic artery should be visualized medial to this point of entry into the mesocolon. The goal of the dissection is to identify the posterior wall of the stomach, which may be difficult in patients who are extremely obese, have a fatty, foreshortened mesocolon, or have previously undergone abdominal surgery. Once the stomach is visible, it is grasped and elevated through the mesocolic window, and the end of the Penrose drain is grasped and brought through the mesocolic defect into the lesser sac. When the Penrose is in place in the lesser sac, the omentum is pulled down from the epigastrium to allow visualization of the drain, now posterior to the divided distal stomach. The Penrose drain is grasped, and the patient is placed back into a steep reverse Trendelenburg position. Traction is applied to the Penrose drain to deliver the cut end of the Roux limb up into the lesser sac for anastomosis.

Troubleshooting. Some surgeons place the Roux limb in the antecolic position and divide the fatty omentum with the ultrasonic scalpel to decrease the tension on the limb. This technique appears to be inferior to the retrocolic approach, in that it does not decrease the tension on the limb and the anastomosis sufficiently and it necessitates more aggressive transection of the small bowel mesentery to achieve adequate mobilization. For these very reasons, many bariatric surgeons do not favor the antecolic approach during open GBP; thus, to use this approach during laparoscopic GBP violates a basic principle of modern surgery, according to which the application of minimally invasive techniques to an operation must not compromise the quality of the procedure. There are also some surgeons who prefer to create a loop gastrojejunostomy, thus avoiding the technical challenges of creating a Roux limb laparoscopically. This approach was abandoned years ago in open GBP because of postoperative bile reflux and an increased severity of complications resulting from high output of digestive juices when a leak occurs at the gastrojejunal anastomosis; it should be abandoned in laparoscopic GBP as well. We firmly believe that the practice of using such suboptimal methods for the purpose of performing this complex operation more expeditiously is poorly conceived and is to be condemned.

Step 5 (circular stapling): gastrojejunostomy In the circular stapling technique, the stapled end of the Roux limb is open to permit introduction of the stapler. The 12 mm trocar site in the left upper quadrant is dilated so that the circular stapler can be inserted through the abdominal wall without the need for a trocar; lubrication is helpful for this step. The stapler then cannulates the Roux limb. This step is facilitated by holding the open mouth of the limb in three locations, with one of the three holds involving traction on the Penrose drain previously sutured to the bowel. The stapler is advanced 3 to 4 cm down the limb, and the spike on the stapler is brought through the antimesenteric portion of the bowel by unscrewing the stapler under direct vision. Once the stapler has been opened completely, it is laparoscopically joined to the anvil and the gastric pouch, then closed and fired.

Once fired, the stapler is removed from the abdominal wall, and a balloon trocar device is used to close the dilated abdominal wall opening. A single firing of the endoscopic GIA stapler, loaded with 2.5 mm staples, is often all that is required to reclose the cut end of the small bowel. Interrupted or continuous absorbable sutures are then placed around the stapled anastomosis for added security.

Figure 11 **Laparoscopic gastric bypass: total intracorporeal approach. A 30 French dilator is placed into the proximal gastric pouch before closure of the gastrojejunal anastomosis with the endoscopic GIA stapler.**

Step 5 (linear stapling): gastrojejunostomy For the linear stapling technique that we currently prefer, it is not necessary to dilate a trocar site, which appears to increase postoperative pain. Two holding sutures are placed to secure the antimesenteric Roux limb to the posterior gastric pouch toward the lesser curvature. Between the two sutures, an enterotomy and a gastrotomy are performed that are large enough to admit the jaws of the endoscopic GIA stapler, which is loaded with 3.5 mm staples in a 30 mm cartridge for a side-to-side anastomosis [*see Figure 11*]. Applying traction to the sutures facilitates placement of the stapler into the lumen of the bowel and the stomach by means of the same techniques employed in creation of the jejunojejunostomy. A 30 French dilator is then passed into the pouch by the anesthetist and guided through the anastomosis by the surgeon under direct vision to maintain the appropriate stomal diameter (10 to 12 mm) during closure of the open end. Placement of a third suture between the first two holding sutures allows anterior traction and facilitates amputation of the tissue to close the openings. The stapler, loaded with 3.5 mm staples in a 60 mm cartridge, should be placed so as to amputate a significant amount of tissue during this closure; the esophageal dilator preserves the stomal diameter.

We have found that using the linear GIA stapler simplifies the procedure, decreases operative time, and eliminates the concerns about injury to the body of the esophagus that arise with passage of the circular stapler.

Step 6: assessment of the anastomosis In every case, regardless of which stapling technique is employed, flexible upper GI endoscopy is performed to assess the anastomosis. The Roux limb is occluded with an intestinal clamp to prevent excessive bowel and distal gastric dilatation. The patient is placed in the supine position, and the area around the anastomosis is irrigated with saline; the presence of air bubbles, easily detectable in the irrigant, indicates that the anastomosis is leaking. In most cases, we are able to distend the pouch and the Roux limb tightly, and we reinforce even tiny air leaks with additional sutures. The anastomosis and the staple lines are visualized, and the endoscope is navigated through the anastomosis into the Roux limb whenever possible. After adequate visualization and testing, the gas is suctioned from the intestine, the Roux limb is unclamped, and the endoscope is removed.

Step 7: closure Finally, a 10 mm closed suction drainage tube is placed adjacent to the anastomosis to permit monitoring for postoperative leaks. This drain is removed after the patient begins oral intake if an upper GI series reveals no postoperative leakage [*see Figure 12*]. The liver retractor is removed under direct vision to ensure that no bleeding occurs. Trocar sites 10 mm in diameter or larger are closed by using a needle suture passer to place 0 absorbable sutures under direct endoscopic visualization. Skin wounds are closed with skin staples or absorbable subcutaneous sutures.

HAND-ASSISTED LAPAROSCOPIC GASTRIC BYPASS

Because total intracorporeal laparoscopic GBP is such a challenging technical adventure, we initially developed a technique for a hand-assisted version of the procedure based on work done by others.[26] We viewed this technique as a bridge to the total intracorporeal approach, in that it enabled us to learn the technical aspects of a difficult, highly advanced laparoscopic procedure while enjoying the security provided by the presence of an intra-abdominal hand for palpation and manipulation during the procedure. This added security is the major advantage of the hand-

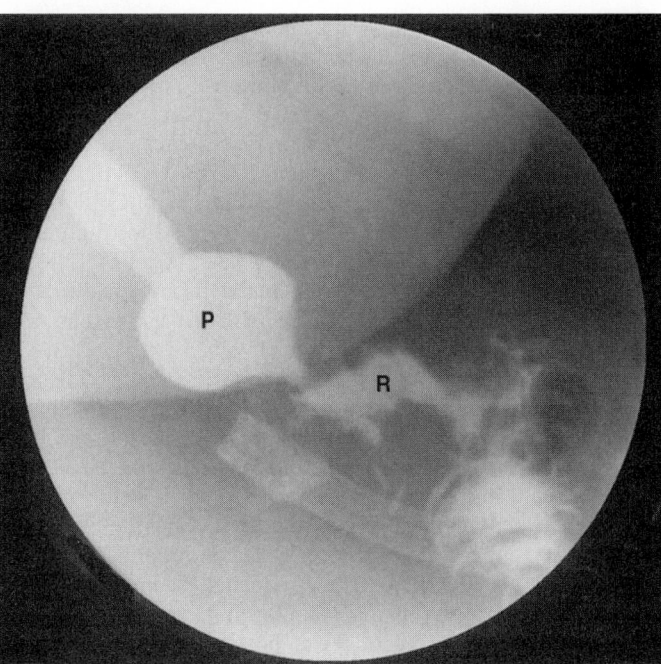

Figure 12 **Laparoscopic gastric bypass: total intracorporeal approach. Flexible upper GI endoscopy is performed to assess the completed anastomosis.**

assisted approach. The major disadvantage is the potential for complications at the incision used for manual access. The complications seen at this site are reminiscent of those seen after open GBP, including major wound infection, dehiscence, and hernia formation. In our series of hand-assisted laparoscopic GBP procedures, we have seen one major wound infection in the hand incision and one instance of postoperative fascial dehiscence.

Operative Technique

Step 1: initial access and placement of the hand-assisted device A left subcostal incision is made, a Veress needle is inserted, and gas is insufflated into the abdomen to a pressure of 15 mm Hg. A periumbilical location for a midline incision is then identified. This incision will allow insertion of the hand at a later point in the procedure; thus, its length in centimeters should roughly correspond to the surgeon's glove size. To provide the assisting hand with access to the abdomen, we use a device called the Pneumo Sleeve (Dexterity Surgical, Inc., Roswell, Georgia). This device includes a ring system at one end. Once pneumoperitoneum is obtained, the ring is glued to the skin of the abdominal wall in such a way that the proposed line of incision is in the middle of the ring.

Step 2: creation and mobilization of the Roux limb, jejunojejunostomy, and creation of the gastric pouch With the ring of the Pneumo Sleeve secured to the skin, the small midline incision is opened and extended directly through the midline fascia. The pneumoperitoneum is released as this incision is opened, and the ligament of Treitz is identified by palpation. Retractors are placed into the incision, and the Roux limb is constructed with an open surgical technique. The small bowel is mobilized into the wound to the extent possible and is transected 20 to 30 cm from the ligament of Treitz. A side-to-side stapled jejunojejunostomy is then constructed with an open technique. In our experience, using an endoscopic GIA stapler rather than a

traditional surgical stapler for this step is both technically superior and more cost-efficient.

Once the anastomosis is created and the enterotomy is closed, the mesenteric defect is sutured in the usual fashion with an open technique. A Penrose drain is sutured to the cut end of the Roux limb. The surgeon, standing on the patient's left side, attaches the Pneumo Sleeve to the nondominant hand and places this into the abdominal cavity. Pneumoperitoneum is reestablished. The ligament of Treitz can then be manually identified, and a blunt mesocolic dissection into the retrogastric space can be performed. This manipulation can be visualized through a laparoscope with the placement of additional trocars, including two in the right subcostal area (as in total intracorporeal laparoscopic GBP); we usually place the laparoscope through a left subcostal trocar site. The Penrose drain is then grasped with the surgeon's fingers and advanced through the mesocolic tunnel into the retrogastric space. The hand is then brought anterior to the stomach, and the patient is placed in a steep reverse Trendelenburg position.

The Nathanson liver retractor is inserted through a subxiphoid puncture as described earlier [*see* Total Intracorporeal Laparoscopic Gastric Bypass, *above*] and positioned to allow visualization of the esophagogastric junction and proximal stomach. The gastrohepatic ligament is bluntly opened, and the surgeon's hand is extended behind the stomach into the lesser sac to retrieve the Penrose drain. The hand is then used to facilitate the mesenteric dissection on the lesser curvature of the stomach 2 to 3 cm from the esophagogastric junction. An endoscopic GIA stapler loaded with 3.5 mm staples in 60 mm cartridges is fired three times to create the gastric pouch (as in total intracorporeal laparoscopic GBP).

Step 3: gastrojejunostomy Again, the gastrojejunal anastomosis can be created with either a circular stapler or a linear stapler [*see* Total Intracorporeal Laparoscopic Gastric Bypass, *above*]. The Roux limb is manipulated into view with the surgeon's hand. In the circular stapling technique, the stapler is placed into the Roux limb with the help of the intra-abdominal hand so that it can be opened, penetrating the antimesenteric portion of the bowel, and joined to the anvil in the gastric pouch. The hand also facilitates removal of the circular stapler, which is occasionally difficult.

Step 4: assessment of the anastomosis The open end of the Roux limb is then stapled closed, and flexible upper GI endoscopy is performed as in total intracorporeal laparoscopic GBP, with the hand (rather than an intestinal clamp) occluding the limb to allow insufflation and testing of the anastomosis. Additional absorbable sutures can be placed around the anastomosis for added security; we use an automatic suturing device such as the Endostitch (United States Surgical, Norwalk, Connecticut) for this purpose. If the sutures are left long, the surgeon can actually tie knots intra-abdominally, using the sleeved hand in a one-handed technique.

Step 5: closure Except for the hand incision, closure is accomplished in the same way as for total laparoscopic GBP. Although the hand incision is small, it may be difficult to close in severely obese patients who have a thick layer of subcutaneous fat. We use a continuous fascial closure with a heavy No. 1 or 2 nonabsorbable suture.

POSTOPERATIVE CARE

The basic principles of care after bariatric surgery [*see* Postoperative Management, *below*] generally apply to laparoscopic cases as well, but with some differences. Unlike patients who have undergone open GBP, those who have undergone laparoscopic GBP do not have a nasogastric tube left in place. In addition, a contrast study of both the pouch and the anastomosis is ordered on postoperative day 1. A water-soluble contrast agent is initially used for this study, followed by barium if no leak or abnormality is identified. The patient may then begin to drink small amounts of liquids and may advance to a pureed diet with no sugar or concentrated sweets as soon as he or she can tolerate it. Discharge usually takes place 2 or 3 days after operation.

COMPLICATIONS

The complications observed to date after laparoscopic GBP include the usual problems that occur in some patients after open GBP, including marginal ulcer and stenosis at the gastrojejunal anastomosis necessitating dilatation. We have seen one gastrogastric fistula leading to a treatment-resistant marginal ulcer. The major advantage of laparoscopic GBP over open GBP is likely to be reduced wound complications (e.g., major wound infection and incisional hernia). We have seen several relatively minor trocar site infections but none carrying the long wound care disability characteristic of a major wound infection after open GBP. In our experience to date, weight loss with laparoscopic GBP is identical to that with open GBP.

Postoperative Management

For optimal results after bariatric surgery, postoperative management must be as well planned as preoperative preparation. The basic principles of postoperative care, including intubation, ambulation, feeding, and monitoring for complications (e.g., anastomotic leakage, abdominal catastrophe, acute gastric distention, and internal hernia), are discussed more fully elsewhere [*see VI:5 Obesity*].

FAILED WEIGHT LOSS AND WEIGHT REGAIN

A postoperative problem that deserves special mention is the risk of failed weight loss or weight regain. This is one of the greatest problems associated with bariatric surgery and may arise after any gastric procedure for morbid obesity. Approximately 20% of

VBG patients have difficulty with solid foods and come to exhibit a maladaptive eating behavior involving frequent ingestion of high-calorie liquid carbohydrates; in about 10% of VBG patients, the procedure fails for this reason. We have converted 53 VBG patients to GBP.[27] After VBG, the average loss of excess weight was 31 ± 5%; 2 years after conversion to GBP, it was 67 ± 2%, a value virtually identical to that in our primary GBP group. Thirteen patients became sweets eaters and had lost only 15 ± 5% of their excess weight more than 1 year after VBG, though there were no radiographically demonstrated problems with the procedure; 1 year after conversion to GBP, they had lost an average of 78 ± 11% of their excess weight.

Inadequate weight loss is also seen in GBP patients. In some, stomal dilatation eventually develops after the procedure; however, no correlation between stomal size and weight loss has been demonstrated for GBP patients, and reoperation to make the pouch or the stoma smaller has not yielded any benefit when the initial procedure has failed. In our experience, failure of GBP is generally due either to the loss or absence of dumping syndrome symptoms in a small percentage of patients, leading to resumption of high-calorie sweets ingestion, or, more often, to frequent ingestion of high-fat junk foods (e.g., potato or corn chips, microwave popcorn, or peanut butter crackers) that crumble easily and empty quickly from the pouch, thereby keeping the patient from feeling full. Repeated dietary counseling over a period of years is required to educate patients to eat low-calorie, high-fiber foods (e.g., raw carrots, broccoli, cauliflower, apples, and oranges) that will stay in the small gastric pouch longer and provide a sensation of early satiety.

Our philosophy is to make clear to patients, well in advance of the operation, that bariatric surgery is designed to help them help themselves. Obesity is easily beaten by surgical treatment, but to maintain the victory, patients must continue to make good food choices and exercise appropriately for the rest of their lives. In our experience, patients who begin to eat more than 1,100 kcal/day will begin to gain weight; even if weight gain is only 0.5 lb/month, this amounts to 6 lb/year, or 60 lb in 10 years. We strongly believe, therefore, that bariatric surgical patients need lifelong nutritional counseling to optimize the results of surgical management of morbid obesity.

References

1. Van Itallie TB: Obesity: adverse effects on health and longevity. Am J Clin Nutr 32:2723, 1979
2. Drenick EJ, Bale GS, Seltzer F, et al: Excessive mortality and causes of death in morbidly obese men. JAMA 243:443, 1980
3. Stunkard AJ, Foch TT, Hrubec Z: A twin study of human obesity. JAMA 256:51, 1986
4. Stunkard AJ, Sorensen TIA, Hanis C, et al: An adoption study of human obesity. N Engl J Med 314:193, 1986
5. Johnson D, Drenick EJ: Therapeutic fasting in morbid obesity: long-term follow-up. Arch Intern Med 137:1381, 1977
6. Griffen WO, Young VL, Stevenson CC: A prospective comparison of gastric and jejunoileal bypass procedures for morbid obesity. Ann Surg 186:500, 1977
7. Buckwalter JA: A prospective comparison of the jejunoileal and gastric bypass operations for morbid obesity. World J Surg 1:757, 1977
8. Halverson JD, Wise L, Wazna MF, et al: Jejunoileal bypass for morbid obesity: a critical appraisal. Am J Med 64:461, 1978
9. Hocking MP, Duerson MC, O'Leary PJ, et al: Jejunoileal bypass for morbid obesity: late follow-up in 100 cases. N Engl J Med 308:995, 1983
10. Pories WJ, Flicinger EG, Meelheim D, et al: The effectiveness of gastric bypass over gastric partition in morbid obesity: consequences of distal gastric and duodenal exclusion. Ann Surg 196:389, 1982
11. Lechner GW, Elliott DW: Comparison of weight loss after gastric exclusion and partitioning. Arch Surg 118:685, 1983
12. Linner JH: Comparative effectiveness of gastric bypass and gastroplasty: a clinical study. Arch Surg 117:695, 1982
13. Mason EE: Vertical banded gastroplasty for obesity. Arch Surg 117:701, 1982
14. Sugerman HJ, Starkey JV, Birkenhauer R: A randomized prospective trial of gastric bypass versus vertical banded gastroplasty for morbid obesity and their effects on sweets versus non-sweets eaters. Ann Surg 205:613, 1987
15. Hall JC, Watts JM, O'Brien PE, et al: Gastric surgery for morbid obesity: the Adelaide Study. Ann Surg 211:419, 1990
16. MacLean LD, Rhode BM, Sampalis J, et al: Results of the surgical treatment of obesity. Am J Surg 165:155, 1993
17. Sugerman HJ, Kellum JM, Engle KM, et al: Gastric bypass for treating severe obesity. Am J Clin Nutr 55(suppl 2):560S, 1992
18. Pories WJ, MacDonald KG Jr, Morgan EJ, et al: Surgical treatment of obesity and its effect on diabetes: 10-year follow-up. Am J Clin Nutr 55(suppl 2):582S, 1992
19. Scopinaro N, Bachi V: Evoluzione del bypass biliopancreatico parziale per l'obesita. Minerva Chir 39:1299, 1984
20. Liszka TG, Sugerman HJ, Kellum JM, et al: Risk/benefit considerations of distal gastric bypass. Int J

Obes 12(suppl A):604, 1988

21. Brolin RE, Kenler HA, Gorman JH, et al: Long-limb gastric bypass in the superobese: a prospective randomized study. Ann Surg 215:387, 1992

22. MacLean LD, Rhode BM, Shizgal HM: Nutrition following gastric operations for morbid obesity. Ann Surg 198:347, 1983

23. Sanyal AJ, Sugerman HJ, Kellum JM, et al: Stomal complications of gastric bypass: incidence and outcome of therapy. Am J Gastroenterol 87:1165, 1992

24. Sugerman HJ, Brewer WH, Shiffman ML, et al. A multi-center, placebo-controlled, randomized, double-blind, prospective trial of prophylactic ursodiol for the prevention of gallstone formation following gastric bypass-induced rapid weight loss. Am J Surg 169:91, 1995

25. Wittgrove AC, Clark GW, Schubert KR: Laparoscopic gastric bypass: Roux-en-Y technique and results in 75 patients with 3-30 month follow-up. Obes Surg 6:500, 1996

26. Naihoth T, Gagner M: Laparoscopically assisted gastric bypass surgery using Dexterity Pneumo Sleeve. Surg Endosc 11:830, 1997

27. Sugerman HJ, Kellum JM, DeMaria EJ, et al: Conversion of failed or complicated vertical banded gastroplasty to gastric bypass in morbid obesity. Am J Surg 171:263, 1996

Acknowledgment

Figures 1, 2, 3, 5, and 9   Tom Moore.

Bryce R. Taylor, M.D., and Bernard Langer, M.D.

Over the past few decades, remarkable advances in imaging technology have been made that allow more accurate diagnosis of biliary tract diseases and better planning of surgical procedures and other interventions aimed at managing these conditions. Operative techniques have also improved as a result of a better understanding of biliary and hepatic anatomy and physiology. In what follows, we describe common operations performed to treat diseases of the biliary tract, emphasizing details of operative planning and intraoperative technique and suggesting specific strategies for preventing common problems. It should be remembered that complex biliary tract procedures are best done in specialized units where surgeons, anesthetists, intensivists, and nursing staff all are accustomed to handling the special problems and requirements of patients undergoing such procedures.

Preoperative Evaluation

IMAGING STUDIES

It is essential to define the pathologic anatomy accurately before embarking on any operation on the biliary tract. Extensive familiarity with the numerous variations of ductal and vascular anatomy in this region is crucial. High-quality ultrasonography and computed tomography are noninvasive and usually provide excellent information regarding mass lesions, the presence or absence of ductal dilatation, the extent and level of duct obstruction, and the extent of vessel involvement. Cholangiography—percutaneous transhepatic cholangiography (PTC), endoscopic retrograde cholangiopancreatography (ERCP), or magnetic resonance cholangiopancreatography (MRCP) [see II:6 Jaundice]—can supply more detailed information about ductal anatomy and is used when CT and ultrasonography yield insufficient information. Angiography is rarely required to determine resectability. Magnetic resonance imaging and MRCP, which are noninvasive, are preferred where available. As newer MRCP technology becomes available, further improvements in definition of biliary anatomy appear to be obtainable. In the near future, it may prove possible to avoid the complications associated with ERCP (a more invasive alternative), at least for diagnostic indications.

MANAGEMENT OF BILIARY OBSTRUCTION

Although jaundice by itself does not increase operative risk, biliary obstruction has secondary effects that may increase operative mortality and the incidence of complications. There is little evidence to support the practice of routine preoperative biliary drainage in all jaundiced patients, but there are some elective situations in which preoperative drainage is required.

Infection

Patients with clinical cholangitis, whether spontaneous or induced by duct intubation (via PTC or ERCP), should be treated with biliary drainage and appropriate antibiotics until they are infection free; the recommended duration of treatment is at least 3 weeks. In addition, perioperative antibiotic prophylaxis with cefazolin or another agent with a comparable spectrum of activity should be employed routinely before any intervention or operation involving the biliary tract. For certain patients with biliary tract infection (e.g., associated with choledocholithiasis), urgent surgical decompression may be necessary, especially if antibiotics and endoscopic or transhepatic drainage are not immediately effective.

Renal Dysfunction

The combination of a high bilirubin level and hypovolemia is a significant risk factor for acute renal failure, which can occur in the presence of a number of additional factors, such as acute infection, hypotension, and the infusion of contrast material. Patients with biliary obstruction should therefore be well hydrated before receiving I.V. contrast agents or undergoing operative procedures. In patients with acute renal dysfunction secondary to biliary obstruction, decompression of the bile duct until renal function returns to normal is advisable before any major elective procedure for malignant disease.

Impaired Immunologic Function or Malnutrition

Patients with long-standing biliary obstruction have impaired immune function and may become malnourished. Decompression of the bile duct until immune function and nutritional status are restored to normal is indicated before any major elective procedure is undertaken; this may take as long as 4 to 6 weeks.

Coagulation Dysfunction

Prolonged bile duct obstruction may lead to significant deficits in clotting factors. These deficits should be corrected with fresh frozen plasma and vitamin K before an operative procedure is begun. Even if there is no measurable coagulation dysfunction, vitamin K should be given to all patients with obstructive jaundice at least 24 hours before operation to replenish their depleted vitamin K stores.

Projected Major Liver Resection

If resection of an obstructing bile duct tumor is likely to necessitate major liver resection (e.g., a right trisegmentectomy), it may be advisable to decompress the liver segments that are to be retained for approximately 4 to 6 weeks.

Operative Planning

PATIENT POSITIONING

The patient is placed in the supine position on an operating table that can be rotated and elevated. An x-ray cassette and machine should be available during major resections. Slight elevation of the right portion of the chest with an I.V. bag facilitates exposure of the liver and the biliary structures. A choledochoscope and equipment for intraoperative ultrasonography should also be available. Access to a pathology department that can perform cytologic or frozen section examination of tissue is essential in operations intended as treatment of malignant disease.

GENERAL TECHNICAL CONSIDERATIONS

Exposure of Subhepatic Field

A right subcostal incision provides excellent exposure for most open procedures on the gallbladder and biliary tract. For more extensive resections or reconstructions, the right subcostal incision can be extended laterally below the costal margin and across the midline to the left as a chevron incision. In patients with very narrow costal margins, a vertical midline incision may be more suitable for limited operations on the gallbladder and biliary tract, and a combination of a unilateral or bilateral subcostal incision and a midline vertical extension to the xiphoid may be required for more extensive operations. In any case, the incision must be long enough to allow sufficient visualization for safe performance of the procedure.

Adequate exposure and lighting are essential. The best retractors are those that can be fixed to the table while remaining flexible in terms of placement and angles of retraction. Modern high-intensity lights with focusing capabilities and headlamps are especially useful when the surgeon wears magnifying glasses.

Good access to the hepatoduodenal ligament and the structures in the porta hepatis is critical. In patients who have never undergone an abdominal procedure, identification of these structures is straightforward. In patients who have undergone previous operations or have a local inflammatory process, however, there may be considerable obliteration of planes. If this is the case, the following techniques may be useful in defining the anatomy.

1. *Using the falciform ligament as a landmark.* In reoperative surgery, the key to opening up the upper abdomen is the falciform ligament. This structure should be found immediately after the opening of the abdominal wall and retracted superiorly. The omentum, the colon, and the stomach are then dissected inferiorly, and a plane that leads to the hepatoduodenal ligament and the porta hepatis is thereby opened.

2. *Taking the right posterolateral approach.* When the colon and the duodenum are adherent to the undersurface of the right lobe of the liver, separation may be difficult. In most patients, an open space remains that can be approached by sliding the left hand posteriorly to the right of these adhesions and into the (usually open) subhepatic space in front of the kidney and behind the adhesions. Anterior retraction allows identification of the adherent structures by palpation and permits dissection of the adhesions in a lateral-to-medial direction. The undersurface of the liver is thus cleared, and the hepatoduodenal ligament can be approached.

3. *Taking the lesser sac approach.* Ordinarily, the foramen of Winslow is open, and the left index finger can be passed through it from the right subhepatic space. When the foramen of Winslow is obliterated, however, one should approach it from the left, dividing the lesser omentum and passing an index finger from the lesser sac behind the hepatoduodenal ligament to reopen the foramen of Winslow by blunt dissection.

4. *Using the round ligament to find the true porta hepatis.* Patients who have already undergone one or more operations on the

bile duct often have adhesions between the hepatoduodenal ligament and segment 4 of the liver. If one dissects this area via the anterior approach, one may think that the actual porta hepatis has been reached but notice that the hepatoduodenal ligament looks unusually short. In most cases, one can find the true porta more easily by tracing the round ligament to the point where it joins the left portal pedicle (including the ascending branch of the left portal vein) and then following that to the right along the true porta. The adhesions between the hepatoduodenal ligament and segment 4 can then be more easily divided from the left than from the front.

5. *Using aids to dissection.* Usually, structures in the hepatoduodenal ligament can be identified by inspection and palpation, especially if there is a biliary stent in place. In cases in which such identification is not easily accomplished, an intraoperative Doppler flow detector may be useful in identifying the hepatic artery and the portal vein, intraoperative ultrasonography may be helpful in identifying the bile duct as well as vessels, and needle aspiration may also be used before the duct is incised if there is any doubt about its location. Either blunt or sharp dissection is effective in this area. Our preference is to use a long right-angle clamp (Mixter) to obtain exposure in a layer-by-layer fashion; we then electrocoagulate or ligate and divide the exposed tissue.

Guidelines for Biliary Anastomosis

As a rule, biliary anastomoses, whether of duct to bowel or of duct to duct, heal very well provided that the principles of preservation of adequate blood supply, avoidance of tension, and accurate placement of sutures are followed. In preparing the bile duct for anastomosis, it is essential to define adequate margins while avoiding excessive dissection that might compromise the blood supply to the duct. In repairs that follow acute injuries, it is important to resect crushed or devascularized tissue; however, in late repairs, it is not necessary to resect all scar tissue as long as an adequate opening can be made in the proximal obstructed duct through normal healthy tissue and as long as mucosa, rather than granulation tissue, is present at the duct margin. The length of the corresponding opening in the jejunal loop should be significantly smaller than the bile duct opening because the bowel opening tends to enlarge during the procedure.

Mucosa-to-mucosa apposition is essential for good healing and the prevention of late stricture. Sutures should be of a monofilament synthetic material (preferably absorbable) and should be as fine as is practical (e.g., 5-0 for a normal duct and 4-0 for a thickened duct). Because the bile duct wall has only one layer, biliary anastomoses should all be single layer. Sutures should pass through all layers of the bowel, taking sizable bites of the seromuscular layer and much smaller bites of the mucosa, and should take moderate-sized (1 to 3 mm, depending on duct diameter) bites in the bile duct. Interrupted sutures are used when access is difficult or the duct is small; continuous sutures, when access is easy and the duct is larger. Sutures should be securely placed but should not be so tight as to injure the tissues. It is sometimes wise to vary the spacing of the stitches: placing many stitches close together may cause ischemia of the suture line in a postage-stamp pattern. Magnification with loupes is particularly useful in anastomosing small ducts. Stents are not routinely required for biliary anastomoses, and drainage of the operative field is seldom necessary.

There are several principles of suture placement that can be applied to most biliary anastomoses, whether end to side or side to side. When the bile duct opening has a vertical configuration (as in side-to-side choledochoduodenostomy or choledochojejunostomy), stay sutures are placed inferiorly and superiorly in the duct and at corresponding points in the intestine. Traction is placed on these sutures to line up the adjacent walls. The right side of the anastomosis is done first; the bowel is then rotated 180°, and the other side is completed [see Figure 1]. This maneuver may be facilitated by retracting the first interrupted posterior stitch leftward to serve as a pivotal stitch. It is advisable to sew about two thirds of the right wall and two thirds of the left wall, leaving the anterior third of the circumference (the easiest part) to be closed last. This technique can also be used for end-to-side choledochojejunostomy and allows all the knots to be tied outside the lumen. When the bile duct opening lies transversely, as in bifurcation reconstruction, lateral stay sutures are placed first, and the posterior wall stitches are placed from inside the lumen. If interrupted sutures are used, they are all placed individually before any of them are tied, with the untied tails carefully arranged in order. When the posterior wall sutures have been tied, the anterior wall can then be sutured with either continuous or interrupted sutures [see Figure 2].

When the intended anastomosis is intrahepatic and access is particularly difficult because of some combination of an unfavorable position, a previous scar, or, perhaps, a stiff liver that is difficult to retract, another technique may be useful. All of the anterior wall stitches are placed into the duct, grouped together on a single retracting forceps with the needles left attached, and retracted superiorly to promote better exposure of the posterior duct wall [see Figure 2c]. The posterior stitches are placed into the duct and the bowel as described, tied in order, and cut; the anterior wall stitches are then completed by being placed into the bowel and tied.

When the duct is small, there are three techniques that may be useful for increasing the size of the lumen.

1. An anterior longitudinal incision can be made in a small common bile duct (CBD), and the sharp corners can be trimmed to enlarge the opening [see Figure 3a].
2. If the cystic duct is present alongside a divided CBD, an incision can be made in the shared wall to create a single larger lumen [see Figure 3b].
3. If the bifurcation has been resected, two small ducts can be brought together and sutures placed into their adjoining walls to form a single larger lumen [see Figure 3c].

Construction of Roux Loop

When the jejunum is used for long-term biliary drainage, a Roux loop is used to prevent reflux of small bowel content into the biliary system. In the creation of the loop, it is important to select a segment of jejunum with a well-defined vascular arcade that will be long enough to support a tension-free anastomosis. If access to the biliary system will be required in the future (e.g., in an operation for recurrent intrahepatic stones), the loop

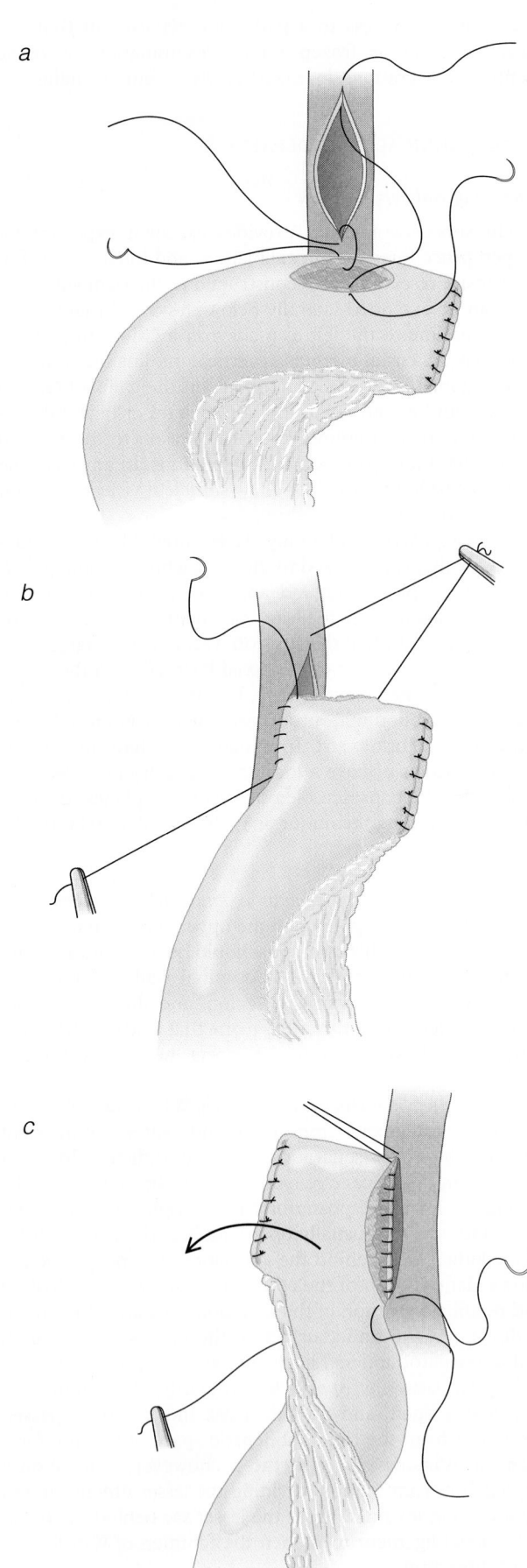

a

b

c

Figure 1 Technical issues in biliary anastomosis. Shown is a side-to-side choledochojejunostomy using a vertical incision in the bile duct. The same technique can be used for choledochoduodenostomy or end-to-side choledochojejunostomy. (*a*) Inferior and superior corner continuous sutures are placed. (*b*) The right side of the anastomosis is sewn. (*c*) The bowel is rotated 180° so that the left side is exposed. The left side of the anastomosis is then sewn.

Figure 2 **Technical issues in biliary anastomosis. Shown is an end-to-side choledochojejunostomy using a transverse opening in the bile duct. This technique can be used at any level. (*a*) Corner sutures and posterior wall sutures are all placed before being tied. (*b*) The posterior wall is completed, and the anterior wall is sewn. (*c*) In difficult cases, the anterior wall sutures may be placed first, then retracted superiorly.**

should be long enough to allow one to place a tube jejunostomy, fixing the loop to the abdominal wall with nonabsorbable sutures. The site of attachment should be marked with metallic clips to facilitate future percutaneous puncture and cannulation and removal of recurrent or persistent stones. The tube can be removed after postoperative imaging studies confirm that the biliary tree is free of stones.

Open Cholecystectomy

Most of the cholecystectomies done for gallstone disease are performed laparoscopically [*see V:12 Laparoscopic Cholecystectomy*]. The decision between the laparoscopic approach and the open approach is based largely on operator experience and the technology available. The open method is more likely to be used in pregnant patients and patients with acute cholecystitis or multiple adhesions; sometimes, it is used as part of a major open procedure (e.g., resection of the stomach or the colon or major hepatic lobectomy). It is also used when the presence of a gallbladder tumor is suspected, when a cholecystostomy has already been done, or when there is a recognized cholecystenteric fistula. Surgeons should not be reluctant to choose the open approach whenever they feel, for any reason, that it is safer in a given situation than the laparoscopic approach; conversion of a laparoscopic procedure to the open method for any reason should not be regarded as a complication.

OPERATIVE TECHNIQUE

Step 1: Identification of Anatomic Structures

The important anatomic structures must be identified and the common anatomic variations kept in mind. The cystic duct and the cystic artery are identified by retracting the duodenum to the left and retracting Hartmann's pouch downward and to the right [*see Figure 4*]. The cystic node is the landmark for the position of the cystic artery. The window in Calot's triangle can then be opened between the cystic artery and the liver bed, and the fatty and areolar tissue can be cleared away from the cystic duct and the cystic artery via sharp and blunt dissection. Verification of the identity of the cystic duct is more safely accomplished by dissecting proximally to the duct's junction with the gallbladder neck than by dissecting distally to its junction with the CBD.

Step 2: Cholangiography

Cystic duct cholangiography is ordered routinely by some surgeons and selectively by others. It is mandatory if there is any question about local anatomy or if CBD exploration is contemplated (e.g., for possible choledocholithiasis). Visualization of the CBD on cholangiography is facilitated by elevating the patient's left side on an I.V. fluid bag to prevent superimposition of the bile duct image on the lumbar spine.

Step 3: Excision of Gallbladder

The gallbladder can be removed in either a prograde or a retrograde fashion. The dissection must stay close to the gallbladder wall to minimize the risk of injury to the right hepatic artery (which may be coursing close to Hartmann's pouch) and prevent entry into the subcapsular plane of the liver (which results in bleeding, especially in cirrhotic patients). The cystic artery and the cystic duct must be cleared around their entire circumference before being divided. Once divided, they can be either ligated or occluded with a carefully applied clip. Postoperative drainage is not routinely used.

TROUBLESHOOTING

In the face of chronic inflammation, the planes may be obscured, rendering dissection difficult. The cystic duct may be shortened and the relationship to the CBD poorly defined. In this situation, manual palpation of the cystic duct may allow identification of the relevant structures, especially after one has rolled the tissues between finger and thumb to squeeze out the liquefied fat and edema fluid [*see Figure 5*]. This technique is

Figure 3 Technical issues in biliary anastomosis. Shown are three methods of enlarging a small duct. (*a*) An anterior longitudinal incision can be made in the duct wall. (*b*) A wall shared by the CBD and the cystic duct can be divided. (*c*) Adjoining walls of two small ducts can be sutured together to make a single opening for anastomosis.

especially useful in the presence of acute cholecystitis. When chronic fibrosis is present and the structures cannot be readily identified either visually or with palpation, it may be better to open the gallbladder, remove the stones, and then identify the cystic duct by using a sound in the gallbladder. In the face of extensive scarring or inflammation of the gallbladder neck, removal of the gallstones accompanied by cholecystostomy may be safer than continued dissection without landmarks.

On occasion, it may not be possible to cannulate the cystic duct. In this situation, the cystic duct can be dissected distally, with care taken to ensure that there are no cystic duct stones, and the incision in the duct can be enlarged and dilated gently with sounds. If cannulation is not possible and cholangiography is mandatory, needle cholangiography directly into the CBD should be considered.

Chronic scarring or severe inflammation may make identification of the correct plane between the gallbladder and the liver

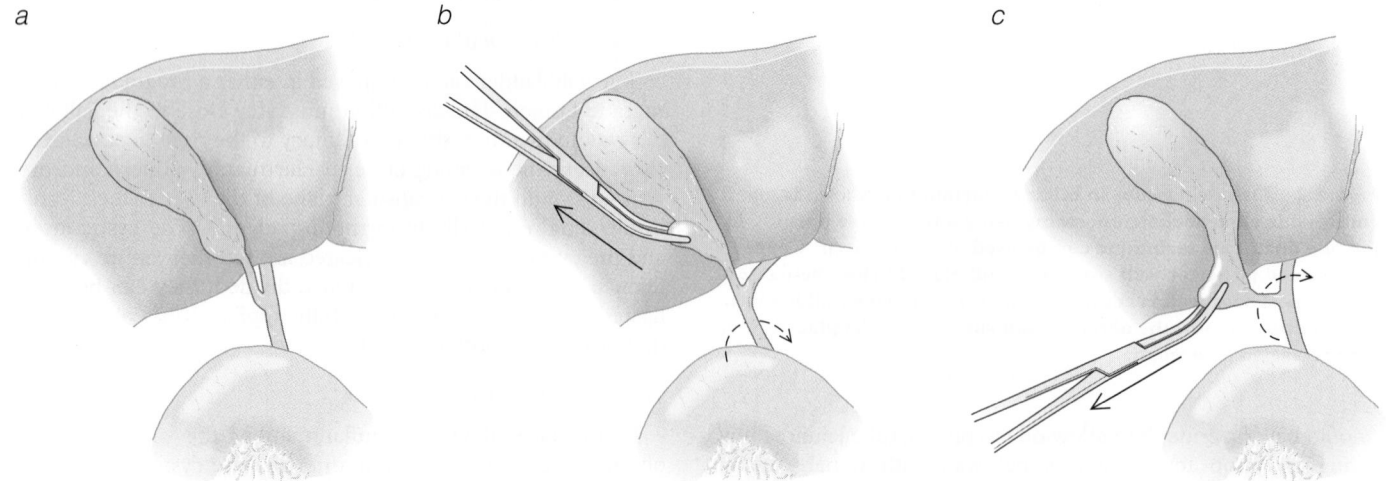

Figure 4 Open cholecystectomy. (*a*) Shown are the resting positions of the cystic duct and the CBD (with Calot's triangle closed). (*b*) Improper upward retraction of Hartmann's pouch lines up the CBD and the cystic duct so that one can easily encircle the CBD or clamp the cystic duct and the CBD. (*c*) Correct downward and rightward retraction opens Calot's triangle; dissection proceeds lateral to the CBD.

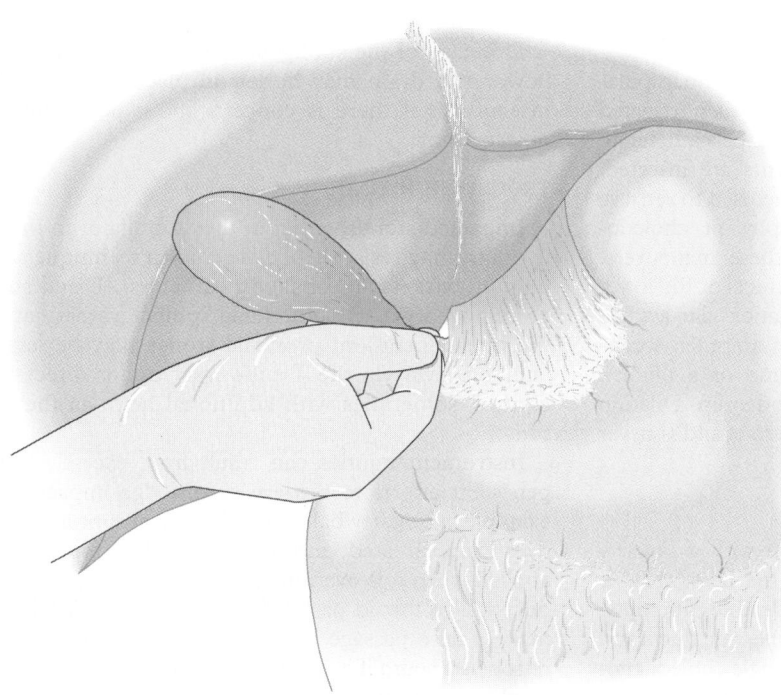

Figure 5 **Open cholecystectomy. Shown is the right finger-thumb technique for identifying the cystic duct and the cystic artery.**

impossible. In this situation, the gallbladder may be opened and the stones removed. Then, with the surgeon's finger in the gallbladder lumen, the gallbladder wall is dissected away from the liver, with the finger used for control. Alternatively, the free portion of the gallbladder wall may be resected, with the part adjacent to the liver left in situ, or the gallbladder may be left in place and a cholecystostomy performed if the cystic duct and the cystic artery are still patent.

As noted, dissection in the subcapsular liver plane may lead to bleeding from the gallbladder bed, especially in cirrhotic patients. This problem can be largely prevented by proper operative technique (see above). If bleeding does occur, however, it usually can be managed without great difficulty. If the bleeding is venous and comes from the liver parenchyma, local pressure should be applied, along with Surgicel or Avitene packing. Surface cauterization is appropriate for smaller vessels, and sutures may be required in cirrhotic patients. If the bleeding is arterial, one should not use the electrocautery or clamps indiscriminately until the source of the bleeding has been accurately identified. A Pringle maneuver should be performed, initially with the fingers and then with a noncrushing clamp, to identify the exact source of the arterial bleeding. The bleeding is then controlled with a hemostat, a small clip, or fine sutures, as appropriate.

COMPLICATIONS

Postoperative infection and bleeding are uncommon complications unless problems were encountered in the course of the operation. Injury to the biliary tract is also an uncommon complication; it can almost always be prevented if the anatomic landmarks are carefully identified before any structures are clamped or divided. Ligation of the CBD will result in obstructive jaundice within a few days. In the case of a transected but not occluded CBD, abdominal symptoms may be mild and nonspecific, and the development of jaundice may be delayed as bile accumulates in the peritoneal cavity. The most useful initial test in a patient with suspected CBD injury is a radiolabeled biliary scan. If a CBD injury is diagnosed, ERCP (with or without PTC) should be performed to define the nature and extent of the injury

before any corrective intervention is initiated. As MRCP continues to evolve, it may prove useful in this setting as well.

Common Bile Duct Exploration (Open)

Most CBD explorations are performed in patients known or believed to have common duct stones; a minority are done in patients with undiagnosed distal bile duct obstruction. Whenever possible, the nature of the pathologic process should be confirmed via cholangiography before exploration is begun.

OPERATIVE TECHNIQUE

Step 1: Identification of Anatomic Structures and Evaluation of CBD

All of the important anatomic structures, including the CBD, the hepatic artery, and the duodenum, must be clearly seen. In a patient undergoing CBD exploration for the first time, the duct usually is easily identified by its slightly greenish-blue color, which is visible through the peritoneum, especially if the patient is thin. In a reoperative situation, exposure of the CBD may be somewhat more involved [*see* Operative Planning, General Technical Considerations, Exposure of Subhepatic Field, *above*]. A limited Kocher maneuver allows the surgeon, standing on the patient's left and using the left hand, to palpate the distal CBD between the fingers behind the pancreatic head and the thumb in front of it. Preoperative evaluation of the duct is desirable; if it is not possible, preexploration cholangiography is advisable, especially in the case of stone disease.

Step 2: Entry into CBD

The CBD is opened by making a vertical incision on its anterior surface to avoid the main arterial blood supply, which runs vertically at the 3 o'clock and 9 o'clock positions. The incision may be facilitated by placing two stay sutures in the duct wall. The opening is then enlarged with scissors to accommodate the largest palpable stone and any exploring instruments required. If the duct is small, care must be taken to avoid the back wall.

Step 3: Extraction of Stones

Many stones can be removed with gentle manual manipulation of the duct. This is done first, and the duct is then irrigated proximally and distally through a 12 or 14 French catheter to wash out mobile stones before any instruments are inserted. Stone forceps, baskets, and balloon catheters are used to retrieve stones identified via palpation, cholangiography, or choledochoscopy. Care must always be taken with these maneuvers: smaller sounds can perforate thin intrahepatic ducts or the lower end of the CBD, and vigorous proximal irrigation can lead to impaction of small stones. The patency of the ampulla is confirmed by gentle passage of a 3 French sound or a filiform catheter through the ampulla and into the duodenum. Dilation of the ampulla with sounds is potentially dangerous and is never indicated.

Step 4: Choledochoscopy

Choledochoscopy facilitates stone extraction with a Fogarty balloon catheter or a Dormia basket and is the most reliable method of verifying complete removal. A flexible fiberoptic choledochoscope yields a good view of the intrahepatic ducts and the distal CBD; in most patients, a rigid right-angle choledochoscope or nephroscope also provides adequate visualization.

Step 5: Closure and Postoperative Care

The incision in the CBD is usually closed over a T tube so that immediate cholangiography can be done to confirm that the duct is clear. If there is concern that some stones might have been left behind, a 14 French T tube should be left in place to allow extraction of stones through the tube tract at a later date. The T tube should take a slightly curved route from the CBD to the abdominal wall—that is, curved enough to prevent dislodgment from the duct by abdominal wall movement but not so curved as to make subsequent percutaneous stone removal difficult [see Figure 6].

The T tube is left to free drainage until GI function has resumed. The follow-up cholangiogram is obtained on postoperative day 4 or 5, and if there is free passage of contrast material into the duodenum with gravity flow only, the tube can be clamped. The T tube may be removed after 14 days (4 weeks if the patient is receiving steroids or immunosuppressive agents), provided that the follow-up cholangiogram is normal. If retained stones are discovered on follow-up cholangiography, the T tube should be left in place for a total of 4 weeks, and the stones should then be removed through the T tube tract or, if this approach fails, via ERCP.

Drainage of the subhepatic space is not routinely required; however, a drain may be left in place if the CBD closure is insecure or if there is concern about persistent distal CBD obstruction.

TROUBLESHOOTING

Impacted stones, either at the ampulla or in the intrahepatic ducts, may resist the usual removal techniques (i.e., manipulation, baskets, and balloon catheters). Distal stones should be removed via transduodenal sphincterotomy at the time of the open operation; proximal stones may be left behind for later retrieval via the T tube tract under direct fluoroscopic control, sometimes with additional help via the transhepatic route.

Instrument injuries can result from excessively vigorous or persistent efforts to retrieve or dislodge impacted stones. For example, a Fogarty balloon catheter can rupture an intrahepatic duct if overinflated, and it can strip duct mucosa if traction is applied when it is overinflated. A Dormia basket can perforate a duct wall if forced past an impacted stone. A CBD sound can make a false passage into the duodenum, the pancreas, or the retroperitoneum if it is forced past an impacted stone or through a tight ampulla of Vater. The primary solution to these problems is simple prevention. All instrument manipulations in the CBD must be done gently. The maxim "If it doesn't go easily, you're in the wrong place" is appropriate here.

The T tube may migrate out of the CBD if there is not enough slack in the tube between the anchoring stitches in the CBD and the abdominal wall as a result of patient movement or abdominal distention. Accordingly, it is important, as noted [see Operative Technique, above], to ensure that the course the tube follows is slightly curved (but not too much so) [see Figure 6].

Choledochoduodenostomy

Choledochoduodenostomy is a relatively straightforward side-to-side biliary-enteric bypass procedure that is effective in certain restricted circumstances and has the advantage of being simpler and safer than transduodenal sphincteroplasty. It is most commonly used in patients with multiple bile duct stones when there is concern about leaving residual stones at the time of CBD exploration as well as in patients with recurrent bile duct stones when endoscopic papillotomy either cannot be done or has been unsuccessful. It is also used in patients with benign distal biliary obstruction (e.g., from chronic pancreatitis) and occasionally in patients with malignant distal CBD obstruction

Figure 6   **CBD exploration (open). Proper placement of a T tube is shown. The route the tube takes should be neither straight (*a*) nor very curved (*b*) but only slightly curved (*c*).**

a

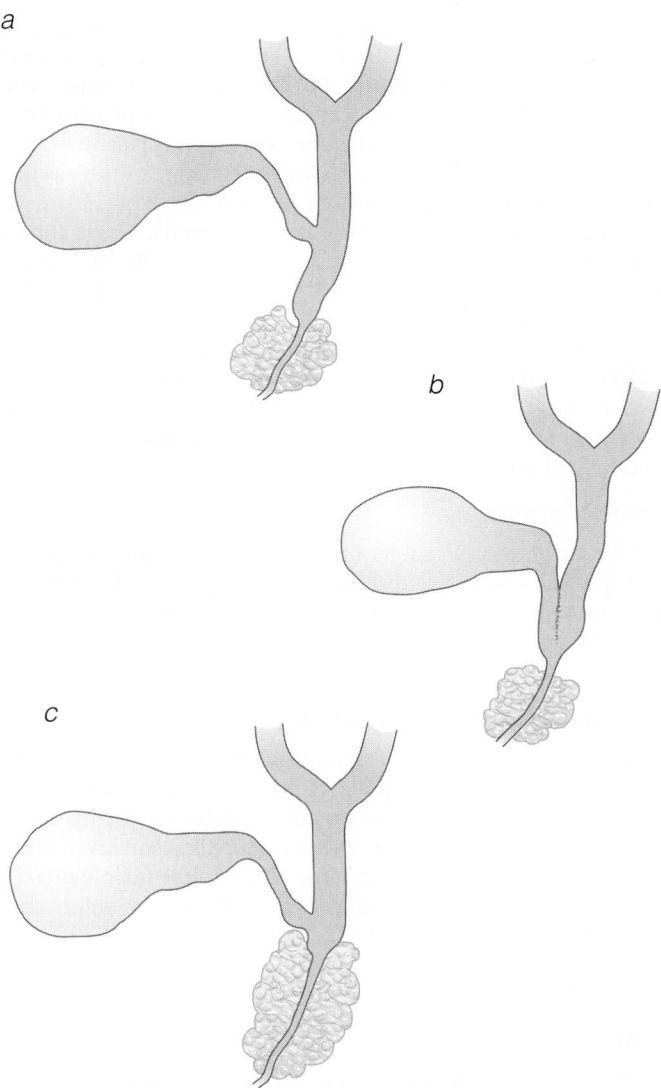

Figure 7 **Cholecystojejunostomy. Cholangiography is essential for determining whether the anatomy is suitable (*a*) or unsuitable (*b, c*) for the procedure.**

whose life expectancy is short. Choledochoduodenostomy works best if the CBD is at least 1 cm in diameter; it should not be used in patients with actual or potential duodenal obstruction.

OPERATIVE TECHNIQUE

The duodenum is mobilized to allow approximation to the CBD without tension. Ordinarily, the first part of the duodenum can easily be rolled up against the CBD; however, in patients who have chronic pancreatitis or have previously undergone an abdominal procedure, extensive kocherization may be required. If satisfactory approximation is not achieved with this maneuver, a choledochojejunostomy should be performed.

The CBD is exposed as described earlier [see Operative Planning, General Technical Considerations, Exposure of Subhepatic Field, *above*]. Longitudinal incisions are made in both the duodenum and the duct [see *Figure 1*], and the anastomosis is carried out as described previously [see Operative Planning, General Technical Considerations, Guidelines for Biliary Anastomosis, *above*].

COMPLICATIONS

Late closure or stricture of the anastomosis may occur if the CBD is small or malignant disease is present. Alternative methods of biliary decompression should be considered in these situations.

Cholangitis related to the presence of food in the CBD distal to the anastomosis (so-called sump syndrome) is an uncommon occurrence. The larger the anastomosis, the smaller the likelihood that this complication will occur.

Cholecystojejunostomy

Cholecystojejunostomy may be performed to treat malignant biliary obstruction in selected patients who are found to be unresectable at operation and whose life expectancy is expected to be short. Occasionally, it is indicated for patients in whom endoscopic or percutaneous stenting has been unsuccessful. This operation is not the preferred procedure for long-term decompression.

Laparoscopic cholecystojejunostomies and choledochojejunostomies have been performed; however, these procedures are still evolving and should be attempted only by surgeons with a high level of laparoscopic expertise.

OPERATIVE TECHNIQUE

Step 1: Verification of Feasibility of Procedure

The cystic duct must be patent. Its junction with the CBD must be at least 1 cm above the tumor obstruction [see *Figure 7*]. The suitability of the anatomy for cholecystojejunostomy may have been verified by cholangiography preoperatively; if not, intraoperative cholangiography via the gallbladder or the CBD is mandatory. If one still cannot be certain that the operation is feasible, the CBD should be opened and a choledochoenterostomy performed. The finding of a bile-filled gallbladder is not sufficient evidence that the patient is a suitable candidate for a cholecystojejunostomy. The gallbladder should be normal: there should be no evidence of cholecystitis or stones. Normal status is verified by inspection, palpation, and, if necessary, needle cholecystography. Finally, for the anastomosis to be feasible, one should be able to approximate the jejunum to the gallbladder easily.

Step 2: Preparation for Anastomosis

A site near the fundus is selected for the anastomosis, and an appropriate segment of proximal jejunum is anchored to the gallbladder with two fine stay sutures in anticipation of a transverse incision in the gallbladder and a longitudinal incision in the antimesenteric border of the bowel.

Step 3: Anastomosis

A 2 cm opening is made in the gallbladder and the adjacent segment of the jejunum, and a single-layer anastomosis is constructed with a continuous monofilament absorbable suture or a stapler.

Step 4: Optional Additional Procedures

A Roux loop, rather than a simple jejunal loop, may be used in the construction of the choledochojejunostomy, and a gastrojejunostomy [see V:9 Gastric Procedures] may be added in patients with pancreatic head cancer in whom duodenal obstruction is either present or anticipated in the near future.

COMPLICATIONS

Bile leakage may occur if there is excessive tension on the anastomosis. In addition, jaundice may persist if there is unrecognized cystic duct obstruction resulting from inflammation or an unnoticed stone in the cystic duct or the gallbladder. Recurrent jaundice is usually the result of extension from an obstructing tumor that has involved the cystic duct–CBD junction.

Choledochojejunostomy

Choledochojejunostomy, one of the most commonly performed biliary tract procedures, is done to provide biliary drainage after CBD resection, repair of ductal injury, or relief of benign or malignant stricture. To reduce the likelihood of reflux of intestinal contents into the biliary tract, a Roux-en-Y jejunal loop is usually used for the anastomosis [see Operative Planning, General Technical Considerations, Construction of Roux Loop, above]. If long-term access to the biliary tract is required (e.g., in patients with recurrent intrahepatic strictures or stones), the Roux limb may be anchored to the abdominal wall rather than left free in the abdominal cavity.

When the operation is performed after CBD resection, an end-to-side choledochojejunostomy using the proximal transected duct is made. When the operation is performed for bile duct obstruction resulting from tumor or stricture and no resection has been performed, a side-to-side anastomosis is constructed. If a stent has already been placed endoscopically or percutaneously, the bile duct is often thickened.

OPERATIVE TECHNIQUE

Step 1: Preparation for Anastomosis

Preparation for an end-to-side anastomosis includes resection of any crushed or devitalized tissue. The CBD should be trimmed back to healthy, viable, bleeding duct wall. If the lumen of the duct is small, a short incision on the anterior wall will effectively increase its circumference to facilitate the anastomosis [see Figure 3a]. If the CBD has been transected at the level of the cystic duct, the lumina of the CBD and the cystic duct may be combined by incising and oversewing their common wall [see Figure 3b].

If a side-to-side anastomosis is being performed for stricture or tumor, the proximal duct is almost always dilated and has thicker walls, and thus a vertical incision is made on the anterior surface. When the procedure is being done for malignant disease, the incision should be made as high as possible above the malignancy to delay the eventual obstruction of the anastomosis by tumor growth.

Step 2: Anastomosis

When the duct is large, a secure, tension-free anastomosis can be constructed by means of the techniques previously illustrated [see Figures 1 and 2]. When the duct is small, extra effort must be made to place sutures carefully to prevent narrowing of the lumen.

TROUBLESHOOTING

It is essential to preserve the blood supply to the CBD. Adequate debridement of injured ducts is mandatory even if this means extending the resection of the duct to the bifurcation. Incisions should not be made in the medial or lateral portions of the CBD, where the major longitudinal blood supply is found. Finally, extensive mobilization of the duct from the surrounding tissues should be avoided so as to preserve the ductal blood supply.

Meticulous surgical technique is critical for ensuring good healing and preventing stricture. The finest suture material that will do the job should be employed, and magnifying devices should be used to facilitate the accurate placement of sutures. In very small ducts, the temporary placement of a small T tube at the anastomosis will allow most of the circumference to be completed without the risk of either picking up the opposite wall or placing sutures incorrectly. The T tube is then removed and the anastomosis completed. Routine use of postoperative stents is unnecessary but may be helpful in those rare cases in which mucosal apposition cannot be accomplished. In these situations, sutures may have to be placed in surrounding liver or scar tissue in much the same way as in a Kasai procedure. In difficult cases of proximal stricture, the surgeon may incise the liver plate and seek out viable duct above the bifurcation.

COMPLICATIONS

The main complications of choledochojejunostomy are bile leakage, late stricture, and recurrent jaundice as a result of tumor extension [see Cholecystojejunostomy and Choledochoduodenostomy, above].

Transduodenal Sphincteroplasty

Transduodenal sphincteroplasty is often indicated when an impacted stone at the ampulla of Vater cannot be removed via choledochotomy. It is also sometimes useful for clarifying the nature of an obstructive process at the ampulla, definitively treating ampullary stenosis, and gaining access to the main pancreatic duct if ERCP has been unsuccessful. Pancreatic sphincteroplasty may be added in selected cases.

OPERATIVE TECHNIQUE

Step 1: Exposure of Ampulla

Mobilization of the duodenum and the pancreatic head is necessary for obtaining exposure of the lateral portion of the second part of the duodenum. The ampulla is located by palpation, which may be facilitated by passage of a sound down the CBD, out the ampulla, and into the duodenum. A longitudinal incision is made on the lateral surface of the duodenum; it should be at least 3 cm long to ensure good exposure. The duodenal edges are retracted gently. Crushing forceps should not be used; they may cause hematomas.

Step 2: Cannulation

If the bile duct has been opened, cannulation of the CBD is done from above. A metal sound may be used; alternatively, a filiform catheter with a flexible follower may be inserted, and the ampulla can then be gently cannulated and elevated into the field [see Figure 8]. This step facilitates accurate placement of an incision in the ampulla. If the duct has not been opened, cannulation is accomplished from below with a sound. Use of a grooved director may simplify the sphincterotomy.

Step 3: Sphincteroplasty

To prevent injury to the pancreatic duct, the incision in the ampulla is placed at the 11 o'clock position with either scissors or a scalpel rather than the electrocautery. A so-called cut-and-sew approach, using interrupted 5-0 monofilament absorbable sutures placed 2 mm apart, is followed. The incision is started at the papillary orifice and extended above the ampullary sphinc-

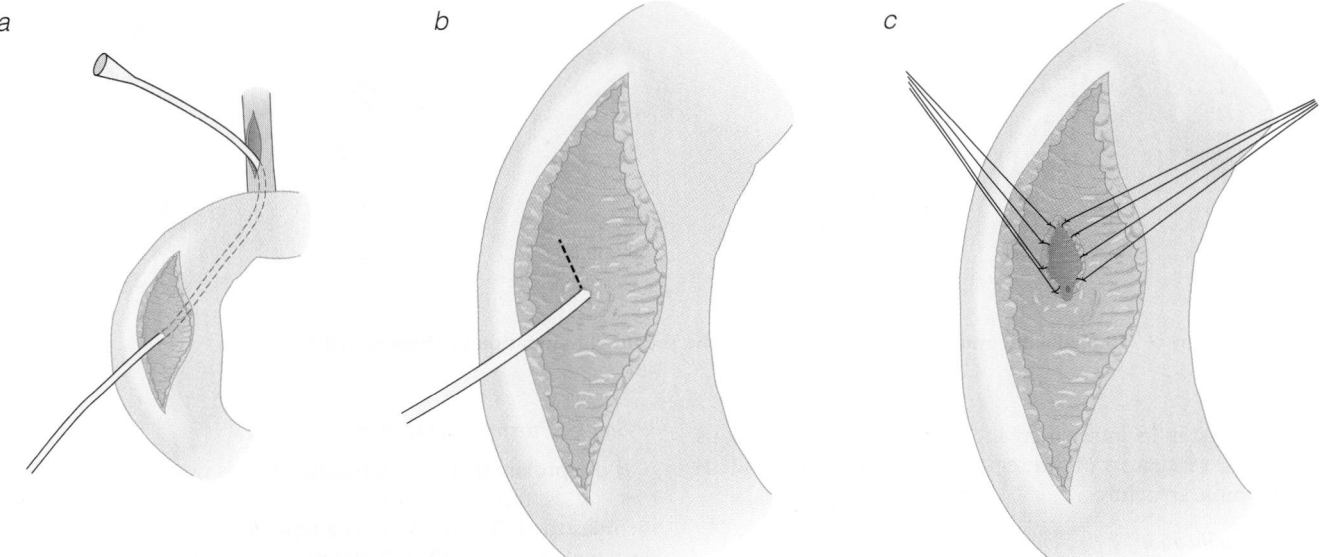

a   *b*   *c*

Figure 8 **Transduodenal sphincteroplasty. (*a*) A longitudinal incision is made in the duodenum, and a fili-form catheter and a follower are used to find and elevate the ampulla. (*b*) An incision is made at the 11 o'clock position with scissors or a scalpel. (*c*) Interrupted sutures are placed through the bile duct wall and the duodenal wall. Lateral traction is applied.**

ter. The sutures should include both the bile duct and the duodenal wall. Once the sutures have been placed, lateral traction is applied to provide exposure of the bile duct lumen and to make each subsequent step in the cut-and-sew procedure easier. The pancreatic duct opening (usually found at the 4 o'clock position) must be identified and protected from being incorporated in the sutures.

Step 4: Exploration of CBD

Exploration of the bile duct should be completed from below with sounds and choledochoscopy to ensure that all stones are removed. If the presence of a tumor is suspected, biopsies of any suspicious areas should be performed.

Step 5: Closure and Postoperative Care

The duodenum is then closed in the direction in which the incision was made. This can be done in either one or two layers, provided that care is taken to prevent inversion and preserve the luminal diameter. Routine drainage is not necessary unless there is concern about the duodenotomy closure or the choledochotomy closure. If a T tube has been left in place, a cholangiogram should be obtained before it is removed.

TROUBLESHOOTING

There may be an impacted stone at the distal end of the CBD that prevents cannulation from either above or below. Such a stone can usually be felt through the duodenal wall, in which case a vertical incision can be made in the medial duodenal wall directly onto the stone. Once the stone has been extracted, the incision can be extended down through the ampulla with a sound used as a guide.

Occasionally (e.g., in some patients with chronic pancreatitis), a long stricture of the CBD may extend above the ampulla. In such cases, the sphincteroplasty may have to be extended proximally to the point where it communicates with the retroperitoneal space. This will not be a problem as long as the duodenum-to-CBD repair is carefully executed. If the obstruction cannot be managed with an extended sphincteroplasty, a differ-

ent decompressive procedure, such as choledochojejunostomy or choledochoduodenostomy, must be chosen.

Postoperative pancreatitis may develop if there was excessive manipulation of the ampulla, if the electrocautery was used at the ampulla, or if the pancreatic duct orifice is occluded by one of the sphincteroplasty sutures.

Choledochal Cyst Resection

Choledochal cysts are generally categorized according to the Todani classification [*see Figure 9*]. More than 80% are type I cysts that involve the CBD in its accessible portion. The following discussion addresses the resection of type I cysts and those type IV cysts that include the proximal right or left hepatic ducts.

Most choledochal cysts are related to an abnormal junction of the pancreatic duct and the distal CBD. Preoperative cholangiography to clarify the anatomy is important for preventing injury to the pancreatic duct, especially when an intrapancreatic resection may be required. Occasionally, intraoperative cholangiography is required to clarify abnormal anatomy. Patients may be symptomatic as a result of stones within the cyst, infection, or malignancy, any of which is an indication for operation. Because of the high incidence of such conditions and the extremely high mortality associated with carcinoma in this setting, prophylactic cyst resection seems justified even in asymptomatic patients.

The objectives of treatment are (1) to remove the cyst completely, along with the gallbladder and any stones that remain in the bile ducts proximal to the cyst, and (2) to achieve free biliary drainage. Resection of a choledochal cyst may be made more difficult by several factors, such as previous operations, recurrent bouts of infection and inflammation in the cyst, and portal hypertension, which may develop as a result of long-standing cholangitis or portal vein thrombosis.

OPERATIVE TECHNIQUE

Resection of a choledochal cyst may be difficult and bloody, especially if inflammation is present. In addition, dissection of a

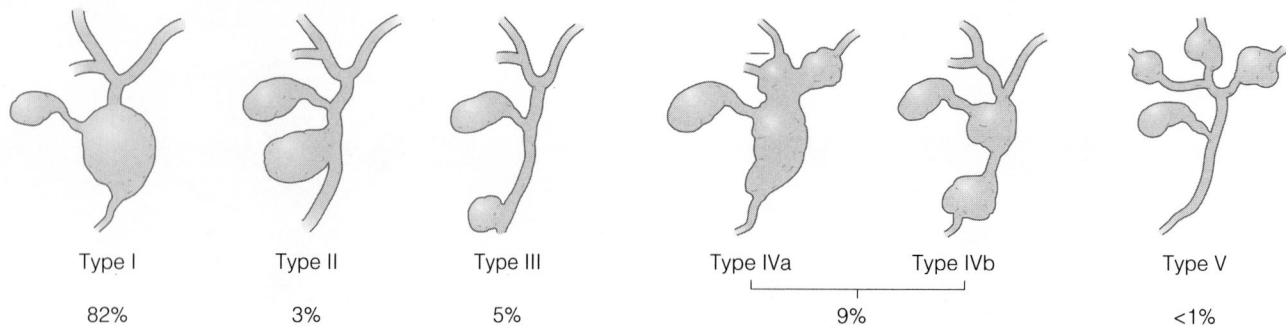

Type I	Type II	Type III	Type IVa	Type IVb	Type V
82%	3%	5%		9%	<1%

Figure 9 **Choledochal cyst resection. Illustrated is the Todani classification of choledochal cysts.**

choledochal cyst in its intrapancreatic portion may be hazardous because of the vascularity of this region and the difficulty of identifying anatomic structures.

Step 1: Clarification of Anatomy

The proximal and distal extent of the cyst and the presence or absence of stones or tumor may be determined preoperatively, as noted, but in many cases, intraoperative verification of the findings is necessary. Intraoperative cholangiography can be carried out by inserting a catheter through the gallbladder, by directly needling the cyst, or both. If cholangiography does not yield an accurate definition of the anatomy of the cyst, the cyst may then be opened and digital exploration and choledochoscopy used to clarify the anatomy.

Step 2: Initial Dissection

If the gallbladder is still in place, it is dissected free of the liver and left attached to the cyst via the cystic duct, then retracted to the right. If the patient has already undergone a cystoenteric anastomosis, this should be taken down at the beginning of the procedure, and the opening in the bowel should be carefully closed.

Step 3: Mobilization of Cyst

As noted, the vascularity of the region and the presence of inflammation may render dissection difficult. Rather than cleaning off the hepatic artery and the portal vein and dissecting them off the cyst, the surgeon should find a plane immediately adjacent to the wall of the cyst and remain close to it [*see Figure 10*]. This approach differs significantly from the corresponding approach in resection of a bile duct malignancy [*see* Resection of Middle-Third and Proximal Bile Duct Tumors, Operative Technique, *below*]. If necessary, the cyst may be opened and the dissection continued with a finger inside the cyst to yield a more accurate definition of its boundaries. The cyst should be cleared circumferentially in the middle third of the CBD so that a tape can be passed around it and traction applied to separate the cyst from the hepatic artery, the portal vein, and any remaining soft tissue in the hepatoduodenal ligament.

Step 4: Distal Dissection

Dissection then proceeds distally along the wall of the cyst until the junction of the cyst with the normal portion of the CBD is reached. If the intrapancreatic portion of the CBD is involved, the cyst must be separated from pancreatic tissue. There are a number of small vessels that must be individually identified and ligated to minimize the risk of early or delayed bleeding. If the cyst is close to the pancreatic duct junction, considerable care must be exercised not to injure the pancreatic duct.

Step 5: Proximal Dissection

If the proximal common hepatic duct is normal (as in a type I cyst), it is transected above the cyst. If the cystic dilatation includes the bifurcation (as in a type IVa cyst), a small button of proximal cyst is usually left attached to the intrahepatic ducts [*see Figure 11*].

Step 6: Reconstruction

Reconstruction is accomplished via an end-to-side anastomosis to a Roux jejunal loop to minimize the likelihood of reflux of enteric contents into the biliary tract.

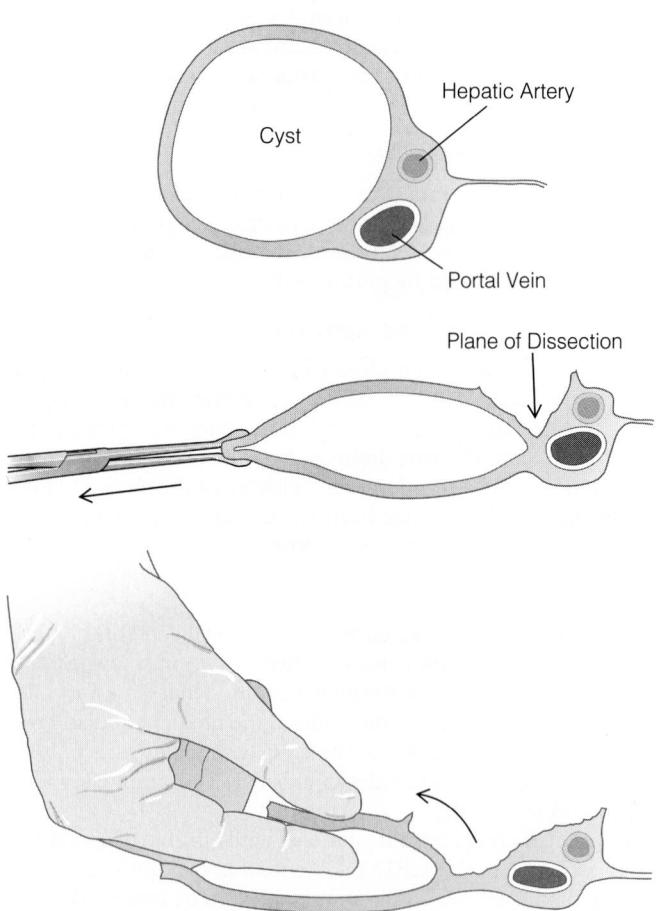

Figure 10 **Choledochal cyst resection. Illustrated is the proper plane of dissection in removal of a choledochal cyst. If necessary, dissection can be done with a finger inside the cyst.**

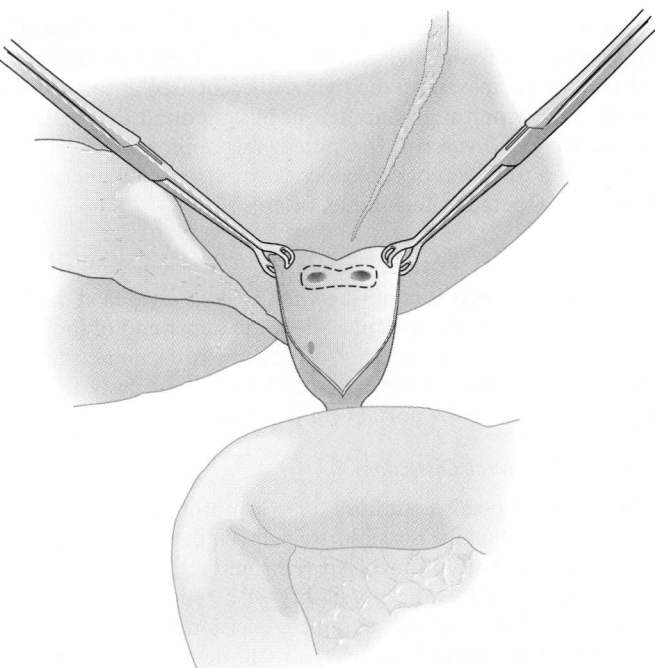

Figure 11   **Choledochal cyst resection. If a cyst extends proximally past the bifurcation (e.g., a type IVa cyst), it may be necessary to open the cyst widely to identify the hepatic duct orifices. A small button of cyst wall is left attached to the hepatic ducts.**

Step 7: Closure

The abdomen is closed in the standard fashion. Stenting is not required, but the area should be drained with closed suction drains if an intrapancreatic resection has been done.

TROUBLESHOOTING

If dissection of the cyst is carried distally into the pancreas, care must be taken to keep from injuring the pancreatic duct. The cyst should be transected as distally as possible, and the end should be carefully oversewn with absorbable sutures. Somatostatin, 100 µg subcutaneously during the operation and every 8 hours for 5 days afterward, should be given to reduce the likelihood of pancreatitis and pancreatic fistula. Occasionally, intraoperative cholangiography is useful to confirm the relationship of the cyst and the CBD to the pancreatic duct.

If the cystic process extends to include the bifurcation (type IVa), the hepatic ducts should be identified from within the cyst and their orifices preserved by leaving a small button of cyst wall in situ; this is preferable to performing an intrahepatic dissection to remove the entire cyst. The presence of this button simplifies and facilitates the anastomosis to the Roux loop.

COMPLICATIONS

Bleeding and pancreatitis are the main early complications of cystectomy. These can be largely prevented by meticulous dissection and ligation of all fine bleeding vessels as well as tissue adjacent to an intrapancreatic cyst. Late stricture of the anastomosis is an uncommon complication but may occur, especially if a small button of proximal cyst is left in place for the anastomosis; this particular complication is considered an acceptable hazard in a difficult situation.

OUTCOME EVALUATION

The immediate expected outcome is the relief of pain, jaundice, and cholangitis and the return of liver function to normal. The long-term expected outcome is the absence of any recurrence of symptoms of stone disease, cholangitis, or malignancy. Because of the rarity of this condition, no good data on the recurrence rate of problems are available.

Resection of Middle-Third and Proximal Bile Duct Tumors

The most common bile duct tumor is adenocarcinoma. Because this tumor responds poorly to irradiation and chemotherapy, surgical resection offers the best opportunity for cure. The appropriate operative approach depends on the location and extent of the tumor [*see Figure 12*]. Tumors in the distal third of the CBD (the pancreatic portion) are treated by means of a Whipple procedure that includes bile duct and periductal tissues right up to the bifurcation [*see V:13 Pancreatic Procedures*]. Those in the middle third or the proximal third are treated by means of bile duct resection, with or without liver resection (see below).

There are certain basic principles underlying bile duct resection for tumor that must be followed. First, the proximal extent of the tumor must be identified so that the correct procedure can be planned. Preoperative PTC is usually not required for staging if high-quality ultrasonography and MRCP are available. Some authorities advocate bilateral percutaneous drainage to facilitate intraoperative dissection. We do not routinely use preoperative drainage tubes, because of the risk of cholangitis.

Second, given that bile duct tumors spread by local extension to lymphatics, along perineural spaces, and along the bile radicles themselves directly into the liver, wide local excision beyond the visible edges of the tumor is required in the performance of curative resections. In proximal tumors, such excision necessitates resection of the adjacent segments of the liver. The principles of en bloc resection beyond tumor margins must be closely adhered to: dissection into or even close to the tumor must be avoided.

Third, intraoperative biopsy of the tumor should not be done, because of the difficulty of making a firm pathologic diagnosis on the basis of frozen section examination and because of the risk of tumor dissemination.

Finally, given that liver resection is required in most cases, one must be careful to preserve enough healthy liver tissue to allow regeneration of the remnant. If there has been long-standing obstruction, biliary drainage on the side to be preserved is important for recovery of function in that portion of the liver. Some authors advocate preoperative portal vein embolization on the contralateral side to stimulate hepatic regeneration in the segments to be preserved, especially if the future remnant is marginal in size.

In recent years, we have generally become more aggressive in treating proximal tumors, for two main reasons: (1) the accompanying liver resection can now be done with greater safety, and (2) this more radical approach has been shown to yield improved long-term results. For middle-third or type I proximal tumors, we favor resection of the bifurcation in conjunction with intrahepatic cholangiojejunostomy. For types II, IIIa, and IV, we recommend additional liver resection: a right trisegmentectomy (segments 5, 6, 7, 8, 4A, 4B, and 1) for types II, IIIb, and IV and a formal left hepatic lobectomy (segments 1, 2, 3, 4A, and 4B) for type IIIb.

OPERATIVE TECHNIQUE

Step 1: Assessment of Resectability

Before any dissection of the tumor or the CBD is done, a careful search for peritoneal metastases is undertaken. Spread within the liver is evaluated via palpation and intraoperative ultrasonography. Lymph nodes are assessed in the immediate and secondary drainage areas. Biopsies of any suspicious areas outside the planned resection margins are carried out. If tumor is found, stenting or a bypass procedure is indicated.

During dissection, determination of resectability is often difficult, especially with respect to assessment of tumor extension into the liver and the degree of vessel involvement. Therefore, any firm commitment to resection (e.g., dividing the blood supply) should be deferred until resectability is confirmed.

The gallbladder is mobilized from the liver bed by entering the usual plane superficial to the liver capsule without dissecting or dividing the cystic artery and the cystic duct. Exposure is improved by mobilizing the gallbladder and, if necessary, emptying the gallbladder of bile. The gallbladder can also be used as a retractor on the bile duct.

Dissection is then begun from below. The common hepatic artery and the portal vein are identified just above the neck of the pancreas and circumferentially cleared of all tissue. Dissection then proceeds proximally, with the hepatic artery retracted to the left and the portal vein to the right. Adjacent areolar tissue, nerve trunks, and lymph nodes are left in place around the CBD and the tumor [see Figure 13]. As noted, this approach differs from that used in resection of choledochal cysts [see Choledochal Cyst Resection, Operative Technique, above].

Step 2: Division of CBD

Once resectability is confirmed, the CBD is divided at the level of the pancreas. A clamp is placed on the upper end of the divided duct, which is then used as a retractor to facilitate the most proximal dissection of the CBD and the tumor away from the hepatic artery and the portal vein [see Figure 14].

Step 3: Proximal Dissection

With middle-third tumors or Bismuth type I proximal tumors, it is usually possible to palpate the proximal tumor margin and identify uninvolved right and left hepatic ducts. If this is not the case, the possibility of a type II or III tumor should be considered, and complete excision of the bifurcation, with or without part of the liver, should be planned.

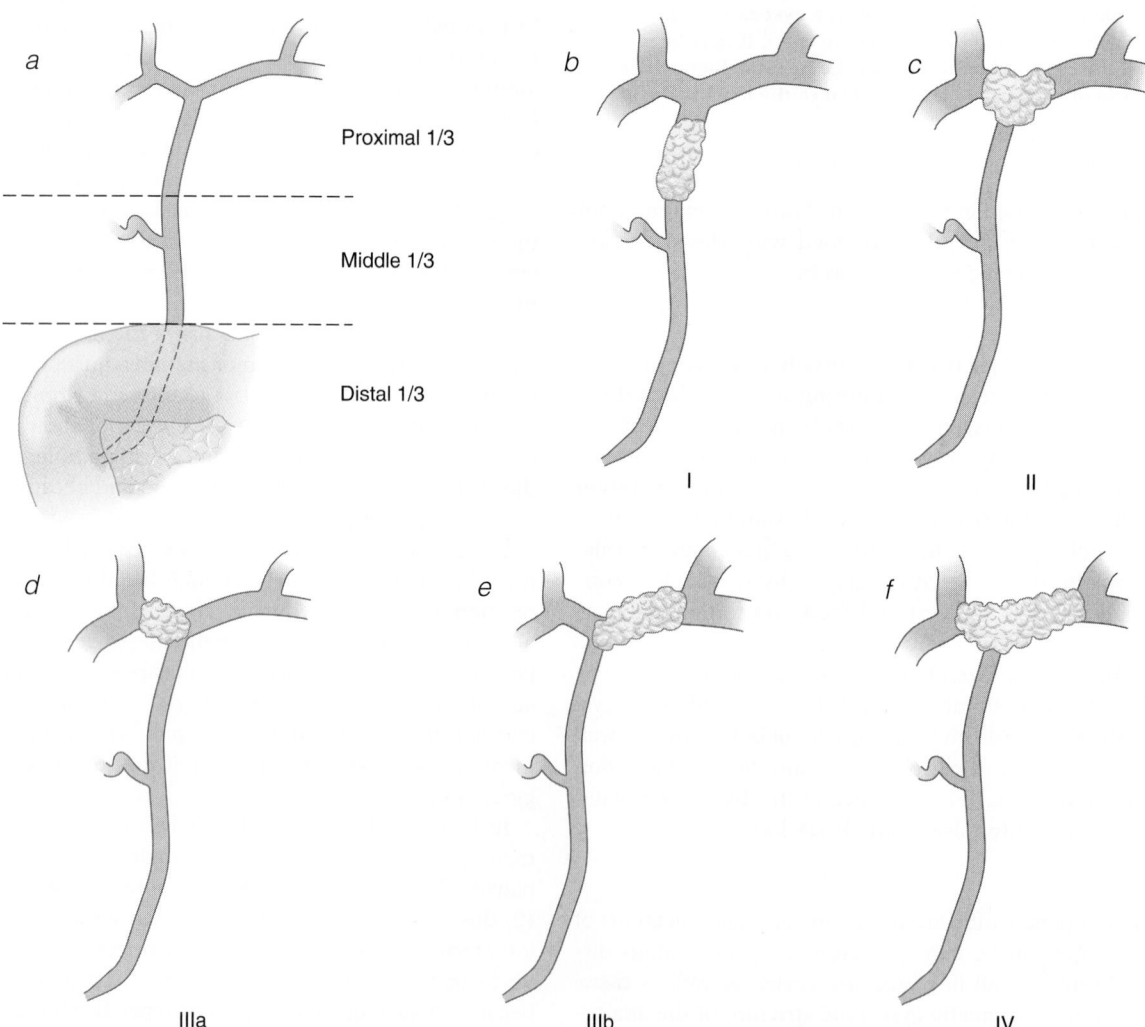

Figure 12 **Resection of middle-third and proximal bile duct tumors. The appropriate operation depends on the location and extent of the tumor. (*a*) Broadly, tumors may be localized to the proximal third, the middle third, or the distal third of the biliary tract. (*b through f*) Proximal tumors may be further categorized according to the Bismuth classification.**

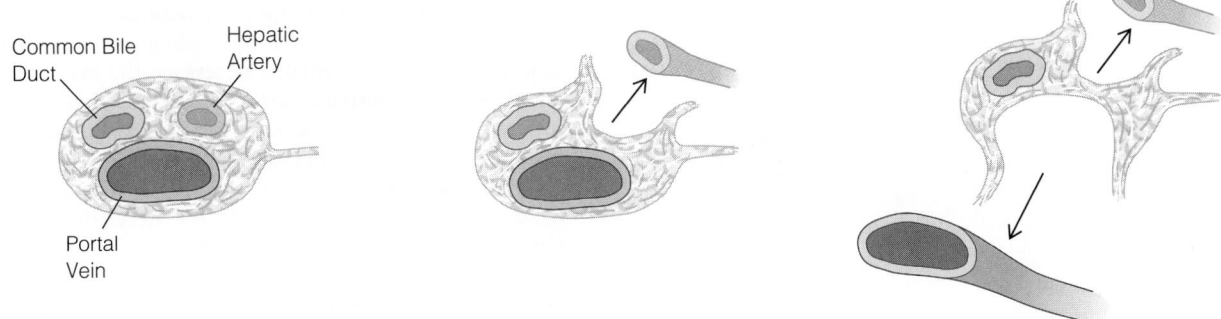

Figure 13 **Resection of middle-third and proximal bile duct tumors. Shown is the proper plane of dissection in the removal of a bile duct cancer. Except for the hepatic artery and the portal vein, all tissue stays with the CBD to be resected.**

The hepatic artery is dissected by retracting the vessel anteriorly and to the left, dividing and ligating the cystic artery where it originates from the right hepatic artery, and clearing all tissue off the right and left branches at least 1 cm proximal to the proximal margin of the tumor. Involvement of the right or left hepatic artery by tumor is almost always a sign of extensive spread on the corresponding side and an indication for resection of that half of the liver.

The portal vein is dissected by retracting the bile duct and the tumor anteriorly and the hepatic artery to the left. All tissue is then cleanly dissected away from the portal vein to expose the bifurcation and the region proximal to it [*see Figure 14*]. At this point, the duct may be found to be tethered down to the caudate lobe by several small branches. If these branches are clearly proximal to the tumor, they are divided and carefully ligated, and the caudate lobe is preserved. If there is tumor in this area, the caudate lobe is resected along with the bifurcation tumor.

The level at which the proximal bile ducts are transected depends on the proximal extent of the tumor. For all middle-third or proximal tumors that are at least 1 cm beyond the bifurcation, proximal resection should usually be above the level of the bifurcation. For type I or type II proximal tumors, proximal resection should always include all of the bifurcation along with the proximal right and left bile ducts out as far as the first major branch [*see Figure 15*]. With type III or IV proximal tumors, the proximal extent of the tumor cannot be determined in both right and left ducts unless the main pedicles are dissected out of the liver. Because these tumors tend to infiltrate locally, such dissection is not advisable. A decision on whether liver resection is indicated should be made at an early stage so that the chances of a cure are not compromised. Intraoperative ultrasonography may help verify the extent of tumor at this point in the operation. Any major liver resection for type III or IV bile duct cancer should include the caudate lobe [*see Figure 16*].

Once the decision to resect part of the liver has been made, the operation consists of dissecting the hepatic artery and the portal vein branch to the part of the liver to be saved away from the tumor area. The hepatic artery and the portal vein branch to the side to be resected are then divided; this allows the tumor to be retracted further and provides better exposure of the duct to the side to be preserved [*see Figures 17 and 18*]. In selected cases, resection of an involved portal vein bifurcation may be carried out at this point [*see Figure 19*]; an end-to-end anastomosis is then fashioned.

The point at which the hepatic parenchyma will be divided is marked, and the parenchymal transection is performed. Division of the hepatic duct (or ducts) to the part of the liver being preserved is done as far from the tumor as possible.

Step 4: Reconstruction

After resection of the bifurcation or intrahepatic bile ducts, an intrahepatic cholangiojejunostomy is performed [*see* Intrahepatic Cholangiojejunostomy, *below*]. The duct tissue is usually healthy enough and the duct lumen large enough to allow mucosa-to-

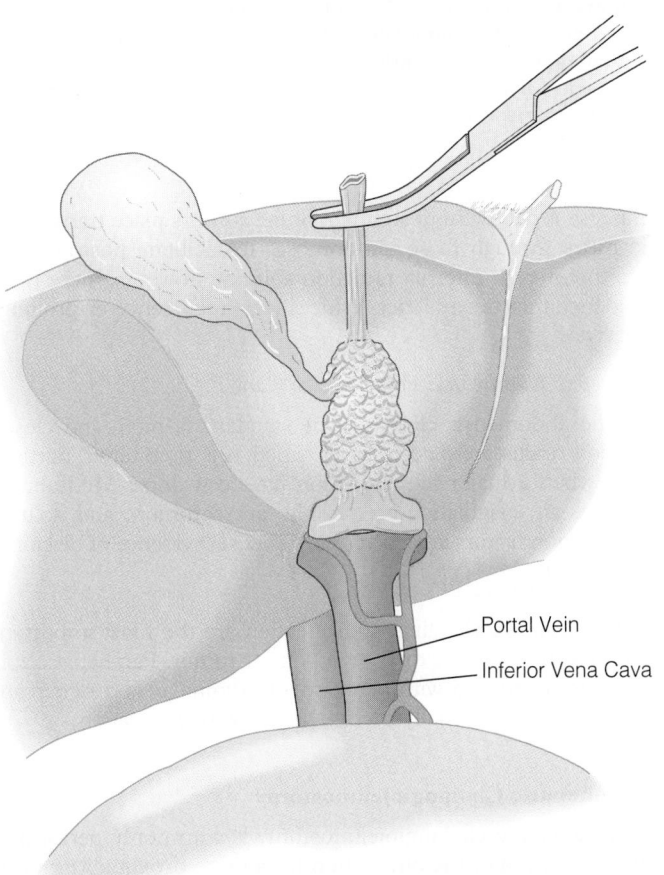

Figure 14 **Resection of middle-third and proximal bile duct tumors. When resectability is confirmed, the CBD is transected at the duodenum. The proximal portion of the divided duct is retracted anteriorly, and the CBD is cleaned off the portal vein up to a point above the bifurcation.**

Figure 15 **Resection of middle-third and proximal bile duct tumors. Illustrated is the level of resection for middle-third and type I proximal tumors. The CBD is resected from the pancreas to a point above the bifurcation. Reconstruction is accomplished via Roux-en-Y hepaticojejunostomy (involving either one or two separate anastomoses).**

mucosa repair without stenting. Some authors place transhepatic tubes through these anastomoses to facilitate postoperative treatment with internal radiation sources; however, there is no evidence that this practice reduces local recurrence or prolongs survival.

Step 5: Closure and Postoperative Care

The abdomen is closed in the standard fashion, and closed suction drains are placed. Liver function is monitored, particularly when a major liver resection has been done. Mild abnormalities in coagulation test results are common, and soluble coagulation factors are given only if there is evidence of bleeding.

COMPLICATIONS

Bile leakage, bleeding, and infection are the most important complications of bile duct resection for tumor. Parahepatic collections are treated with percutaneous drainage, and significant early bleeding is usually best managed by reexploration.

Intrahepatic Cholangiojejunostomy

Intrahepatic cholangiojejunostomy is commonly performed after resection of the bifurcation for a more proximal tumor; it is also performed to manage injury or stricture at the level of the bifurcation and to bypass an unresectable bifurcation tumor.

Because the ducts are smaller, have thinner walls, and are more adherent to the areolar tissue of the pedicles than either the portal vein branches or the hepatic artery branches, dissec-

tion of the ducts must be more meticulous. Magnification is an important aid, particularly in dealing with undilated ducts. Good exposure is essential; if necessary, the liver may be split to allow adequate visualization, access, and lighting. Anatomic mucosal suturing can be achieved in most situations. In rare instances, excessive inflammation, scarring, or tumor makes such suturing impossible, in which case periductal sutures are used and a stent is placed. As described [*see* General Considerations, Technical Issues in Biliary Anastomosis, *above*], separate ducts that are close together can be first sutured together at their adjacent walls to create a single larger proximal duct lumen so that a safer anastomosis can be created [*see Figure 3c*].

OPERATIVE TECHNIQUE

Step 1: Definition of Tissues for Anastomosis

In the case of injury, crushed, cauterized, or devitalized tissue must be debrided back to normal healthy tissue before reconstruction is begun. In the case of bile duct resection for tumor, there should be no attempt to clear a length of duct from surrounding areolar or liver tissue; the suturing should take place in situ, with the stitches passed through the duct wall and the areolar tissue of the portal pedicles. In the case of bypass for unresectable cancer, the duct being used should be opened as far from the tumor as possible. The left main hepatic duct can be approached between the bifurcation and the umbilical fis-

a Types II, IIIa, IV

b Type IIIb

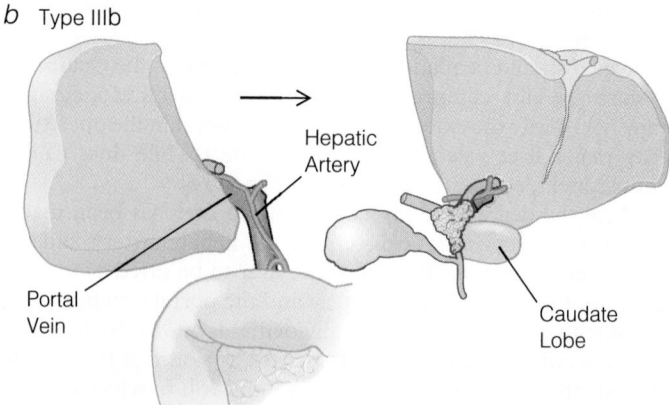

Figure 16 **Resection of middle-third and proximal bile duct tumors. Illustrated are (*a*) a right trisegmentectomy for types II, IIIa, and IV tumors and (*b*) a left hepatic lobectomy (including the caudate lobe) for type IIIb tumors.**

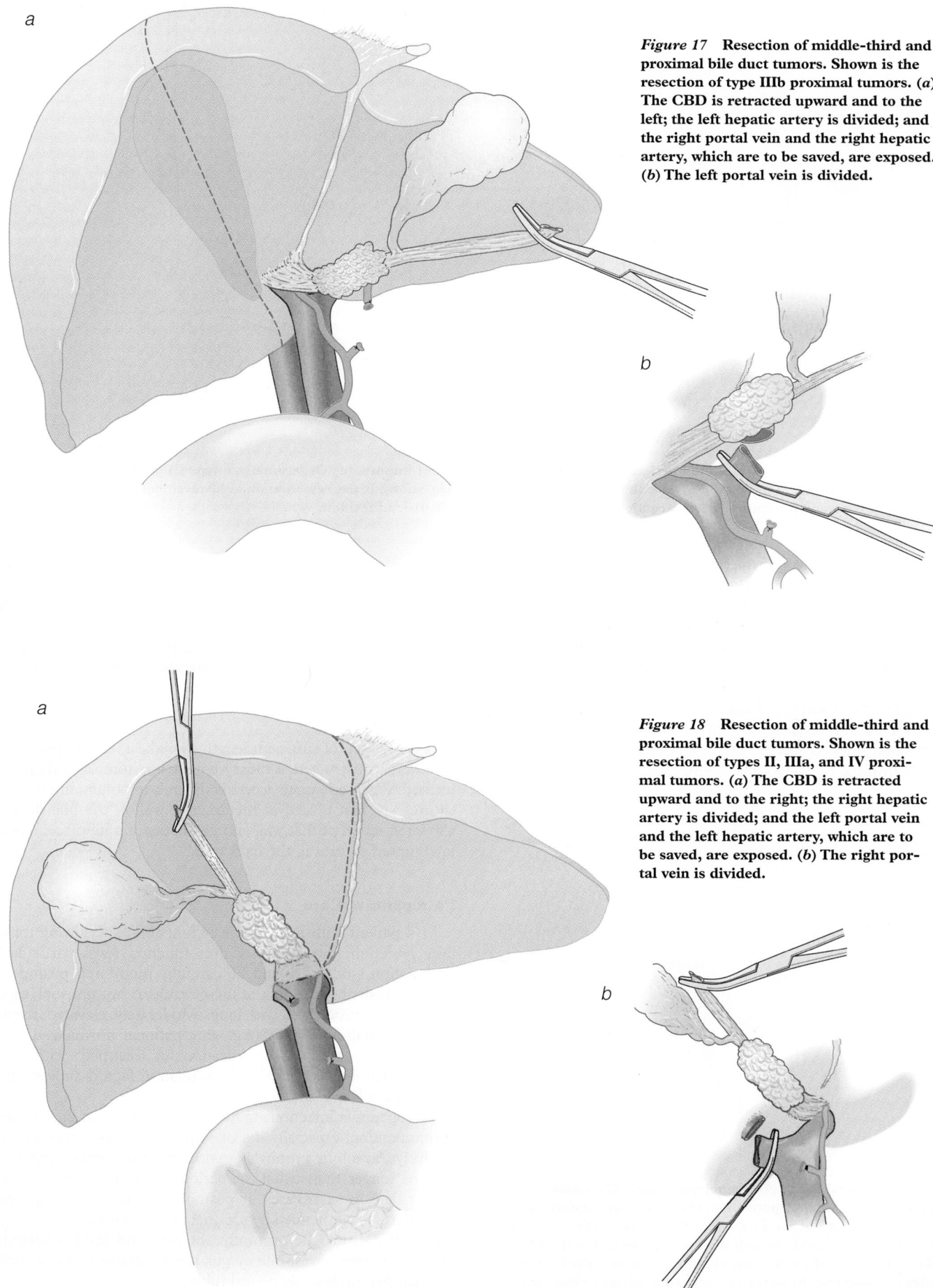

Figure 17 Resection of middle-third and proximal bile duct tumors. Shown is the resection of type IIIb proximal tumors. (*a*) The CBD is retracted upward and to the left; the left hepatic artery is divided; and the right portal vein and the right hepatic artery, which are to be saved, are exposed. (*b*) The left portal vein is divided.

Figure 18 Resection of middle-third and proximal bile duct tumors. Shown is the resection of types II, IIIa, and IV proximal tumors. (*a*) The CBD is retracted upward and to the right; the right hepatic artery is divided; and the left portal vein and the left hepatic artery, which are to be saved, are exposed. (*b*) The right portal vein is divided.

a   *b*

Figure 19 **Resection of middle-third and proximal bile duct tumors. (*a*) Occasionally, a type III or IV proximal tumor will involve the portal vein bifurcation. (*b*) Shown is the resection of an involved portal vein bifurcation. Reconstruction is accomplished in an end-to-end fashion.**

sure. If the tumor involves the left main hepatic duct, the branch to segment 3 of the liver can be used instead; it can be approached in the umbilical fissure, above the round ligament. Occasionally, incision into the liver or excision of a wedge of liver tissue is necessary to provide adequate exposure [*see Figure 20*]. If an intrahepatic anastomosis is required for a bifurcation stricture, resection of the stricture is not necessary; however, it is important to identify a normal duct above the level of the bifurcation. If there is no communication from right to left, a horizontal incision can be made in the left duct and carried across into the right duct just above or through the bifurcation

Figure 20 **Intrahepatic cholangiojejunostomy. If a tumor involves the left main hepatic duct, the branch of the duct that supplies segment 3 of the liver may be used instead for anastomosis to the jejunum. This branch may be approached in the umbilical fissure, above the round ligament. Incision into the liver or wedge excision may be necessary to ensure adequate exposure.**

stricture, so that a single anastomosis can be made that incorporates both ducts. Duct openings can be enlarged by making a small longitudinal incision in the most accessible portion of the duct. This is easier to accomplish in the left hepatic duct (because of its extrahepatic transverse position) than in the right hepatic duct (which tends to run laterally and posteriorly directly in the liver substance).

Step 2: Anastomosis

A Roux loop of sufficient length to make a tension-free anastomosis is constructed. A biliary-enteric anastomosis is then performed. When adequate access is difficult to obtain, interrupted sutures are first placed in the anterior wall of the bile duct to allow retraction of that wall and facilitate accurate placement of interrupted sutures in the back wall.

Postoperative Care

In a patient with impaired liver function or following major liver resection, the results of liver function tests, particularly coagulation studies, should be carefully monitored postoperatively. Transient worsening of these results is not unusual, especially if the procedure was long. Moderately elevated results from coagulation studies (e.g., international normalized ratio [INR] < 2.0) are not an indication for treatment with fresh frozen plasma or concentrated coagulation factors unless clinical bleeding is evident.

Postoperative infections may occur as a result of biliary tract contamination, especially if a bile duct stent was placed preoperatively. Antibiotic prophylaxis with broad-spectrum agents for periods longer than usual for perioperative treatment may be appropriate in such cases. If postoperative fever occurs, especially if it is accompanied by unusual pain and tenderness, imaging studies should be promptly obtained and fluid collections sought. In most cases, bile or pus can be drained satisfactorily through percutaneously placed tubes.

Recommended Reading

Bismuth H, Nakache R, Diamond T: Management strategies in resection for hilar cholangiocarcinoma. Ann Surg 215:31, 1992

Bornman PC, Terblanche J: Subtotal cholecystectomy: for the difficult gallbladder in portal hypertension and cholecystitis. Surgery 98:1, 1985

Braasch JW, Rossi RL: Reconstruction of the biliary tract. Surg Clin North Am 65:273, 1985

Fry DE: Surgical techniques in the management of distal biliary tract obstruction. American Surgeon 49:138, 1983

Gallinger S, Gluckman D, Langer B: Proximal bile duct cancer. Advances in Surgery, vol 23. Cameron JL, Ed. Year Book Medical Publishers, St. Louis, 1990, p 89

Lillemoe KD, Pitt HA, Cameron JL: Current management of benign bile duct strictures. Advances in Surgery, vol 25. Cameron JL, Ed. Year Book Medical Publishers, St. Louis, 1992, p 119

Russell E, Hutson DG, Guerra JJ Jr: Dilatation of biliary strictures through a stomatized jejunal limb. Acta Radiologica: Diagnosis 26:283, 1985

Smadja C, Blumgart LH: The biliary tract and the anatomy of biliary exposure. Surgery of the Liver and Biliary Tract. Blumgart LH, Ed. Churchill Livingstone, New York, 1988, p 11

Stain SC, Guthrie CR, Yellin AE, et al: Choledochal cyst in the adult. Ann Surg 222:128, 1995

Strom PR, Stone HH: A technique for transduodenal sphincteroplasty. Surgery 92:546, 1982

Acknowledgment

Figures 1 through 20   Tom Moore.

12 LAPAROSCOPIC CHOLECYSTECTOMY

Gerald M. Fried, M.D., Liane S. Feldman, M.D., and Dennis R. Klassen, M.D.

Cholecystectomy is the treatment of choice for symptomatic gallstones because it removes the organ that contributes to both the formation of gallstones and the complications ensuing from them. The morbidity associated with cholecystectomy is attributable to injury to the abdominal wall in the process of gaining access to the gallbladder (i.e., the incision in the abdominal wall and its closure) or to inadvertent injury to surrounding structures during dissection of the gallbladder. Efforts to diminish the morbidity of open cholecystectomy have led to the development of laparoscopic cholecystectomy, made possible by modern optics and video technology.

Erich Mühe performed the first laparoscopic cholecystectomy in Germany in 1985; by 1992, 90% of cholecystectomies in the United States were being performed laparoscopically. Compared with open cholecystectomy, the laparoscopic approach has dramatically reduced hospital stay, postoperative pain, and convalescent time. However, rapid adoption of laparoscopic cholecystectomy as the so-called gold standard for treatment of symptomatic gallstone disease was associated with complications, including an increased incidence of major bile duct injuries.

Since the early 1990s, considerable advances have been made in instrumentation and equipment, and a great deal of experience with laparoscopic cholecystectomy has been amassed worldwide. Of particular significance is the miniaturization of optics and instruments, the aim of which is to reduce the morbidity of the procedure by making possible ever smaller incisions. With proper patient selection and preparation, laparoscopic cholecystectomy is being safely performed on an outpatient basis in many centers.

The primary goal of laparoscopic cholecystectomy is removal of the gallbladder with minimal risk of injury to the bile ducts and surrounding structures. Our approach is designed to maximize the safety of both routine and complicated laparoscopic cholecystectomies. In what follows, we describe our approach and discuss current indications and techniques for imaging and exploring the common bile duct (CBD).

Preoperative Evaluation

To plan the surgical procedure, assess the likelihood of conversion to open cholecystectomy, and determine which patients are at high risk for CBD stones, the surgeon must obtain certain data preoperatively. Useful information can be obtained from the patient's history, from imaging studies, and from laboratory tests.

PREOPERATIVE DATA

History and Physical Examination

A good medical history provides information about associated medical problems that may affect the patient's tolerance of pneumoperitoneum. Patients with cardiorespiratory disease may have difficulty with the effects of CO_2 pneumoperitoneum on cardiac output, lung inflation pressure, acid-base balance, and the ability of the lungs to eliminate CO_2. Most bleeding disorders can also be identified through the history. A disease-specific history is important in identifying patients in whom previous episodes of acute cholecystitis may make laparoscopic cholecystectomy more difficult, as well as those at increased risk for choledocholithiasis (e.g., those who have had jaundice, pancreatitis, or cholangitis).

Physical examination identifies patients whose body habitus is likely to make laparoscopic cholecystectomy difficult and is helpful for determining optimal trocar placement. Abdominal examination also reveals any scars, stomas, or hernias that are likely to necessitate the use of special techniques for trocar insertion.

Imaging Studies

Ultrasonography is highly operator dependent, but in capable hands, it can provide useful information. It is the best test for diagnosing cholelithiasis, and it can usually determine the size and number of stones. Large stones indicate that a larger incision in the skin and the fascia will be necessary to retrieve the gallbladder. Multiple small stones suggest that the patient is more likely to require operative cholangiography (if a policy of selective cholangiography is practiced) [*see* Operative Technique, Step 5, *below*]. A shrunken gallbladder, a thickened gallbladder wall, and pericholecystic fluid on ultrasonographic examination are significant predictors of conversion to open cholecystectomy. The presence of a dilated CBD or CBD stones preoperatively is predictive of choledocholithiasis. Other intra-abdominal pathologic conditions, either related to or separate from the hepatic-biliary-pancreatic system, may influence operative planning.

Preoperative imaging studies of the CBD may allow the surgeon to identify patients with CBD stones before operation. Such imaging may involve endoscopic retrograde cholangiopancreatography (ERCP) [*see V:6 Gastrointestinal Endoscopy*], magnetic resonance cholangiopancreatography (MRCP) [*see Figure 1*], or endoscopic ultrasonography (EUS). These imaging modalities also provide an anatomic map of the extrahepatic biliary tree, identifying unusual anatomy preoperatively and helping the surgeon plan a safe operation. Endoscopic sphincterotomy (ES) is performed during ERCP if stones are identified in the CBD. MRCP has an advantage over ERCP and EUS in that it is noninvasive and does not make use of injected iodinated contrast solutions. Most surgeons would probably recommend that preoperative cholangiography be performed selectively in patients with clinical or biochemical features associated with a high risk of choledocholithiasis. The specific modality used in such a case varies with the technology and expertise available locally.

Figure 1 **Laparoscopic cholecystectomy. Preoperative MRCP alerts the surgeon to abnormal anatomy and the presence of stones in the distal CBD. (GB—gallbladder, containing stones; RHD—right hepatic duct; LHD—left hepatic duct; CHD—common hepatic duct; Acc—accessory duct entering common hepatic duct near neck of gallbladder; PD—pancreatic duct; Duo—duodenum)**

Laboratory Tests

Preoperative blood tests are important for evaluation of liver function and for detection of unsuspected abnormalities of renal function, electrolyte balance, or coagulation. Abnormal liver function test results may reflect choledocholithiasis or primary hepatic dysfunction.

SELECTION OF PATIENTS

Patients Eligible for Outpatient Cholecystectomy

Patients in good general health who have a reasonable amount of support from family or friends and who do not live too far away from adequate medical facilities are eligible for outpatient cholecystectomy, especially if they are at low risk for conversion to laparotomy [*see* Special Problems, Conversion to Laparotomy, *below*]. These patients can generally be discharged home from the recovery room 6 to 12 hours after surgery, provided that the operation went smoothly, their vital signs are stable, they are able to void, they can manage at least a liquid diet without vomiting, and their pain can be controlled with oral analgesics.

Technically Challenging Patients

Before performing laparoscopic cholecystectomy, the surgeon can predict which patients are likely to be technically challenging. These include patients who have a particularly unsuitable body habitus, those who are at high risk for multiple and dense peritoneal adhesions, and those who are likely to have distorted anatomy in the region of the gallbladder.

Morbidly obese patients present specific difficulties [*see* Operative Technique, Step 1, Special Considerations in Obese Patients, *below*]. Small, muscular patients have a noncompliant abdominal wall, resulting in a small working space in the abdomen and necessitating high inflation pressures to obtain reasonable exposure.

Patients with a history of multiple abdominal operations, especially in the upper abdomen, and those who have a history of peritonitis are likely to pose difficulties because of peritoneal adhesions. These adhesions make access to the abdomen more risky and exposure of the gallbladder more difficult.

Patients who have undergone gastroduodenal surgery, those who have any history of acute cholecystitis, those who have a long history of recurrent gallbladder attacks, and those who have recently had severe pancreatitis are particularly difficult candidates for laparoscopic cholecystectomy. These patients may have dense adhesions in the region of the gallbladder, the anatomy may be distorted, the cystic duct may be foreshortened, and the CBD may be very closely and densely adherent to the gallbladder. Such patients are a challenge to the most experienced laparoscopic surgeon. When such problems are encountered, conversion to open cholecystectomy should be considered early in the operation.

Predictors of Choledocholithiasis

CBD stones may be discovered preoperatively, intraoperatively, or postoperatively. The surgeon's goal is to clear the ducts but to use the smallest number of procedures with the lowest risk of morbidity. Thus, before elective laparoscopic cholecystectomy, it is desirable to classify patients into one of three groups: high risk (those who have clinical jaundice or cholangitis, visible choledocholithiasis, or a dilated CBD on ultrasonography), moderate risk (those who have hyperbilirubinemia, elevated alkaline phosphatase levels, pancreatitis, or multiple small gallstones), and low risk.

In our institution, where MRCP and EUS are available and reliable and where ERCP achieves stone clearance rates higher than 90%, we recommend the following approach: (1) preoperative ERCP and sphincterotomy (if required) for high-risk patients and (2) MRCP, EUS, or intraoperative fluoroscopic cholangiography for moderate-risk patients. Patients at low risk for CBD stones do not routinely undergo cholangiography [*see Figure 2*]. Laparoscopic CBD exploration and postoperative ERCP appear to be equally effective in clearing stones from the CBD.

Ultimately, surgeons and institutions must establish a reasonable approach to choledocholithiasis that takes into account the expertise and equipment locally available.

Contraindications

There are few absolute contraindications to laparoscopic cholecystectomy. Certainly, no patient who poses an unacceptable risk for open cholecystectomy should be considered for laparoscopic cholecystectomy, because it is always possible that conversion will become necessary. Of the relative contraindications, surgical inexperience is the most important.

Neither ascites nor hernia is a contraindication to laparoscopic cholecystectomy. Ascites can be drained and the gallbladder visualized. Large hernias may present a problem, however, because with insufflation, the gas preferentially fills the hernia. Patients with large inguinal hernias may require an external support to minimize this problem and the discomfort related to pneumoscrotum. Patients with umbilical hernias can have their hernias repaired while they are undergoing laparoscopic cholecystectomy. For such patients, the initial trocar should be placed by open insertion according to the Hasson technique [see Operative Technique, Step 1, below], with care taken to avoid injury to the contents of the hernia. The sutures required to close the hernia defect can be placed before insertion of the initial trocar. A similar technique can be applied to patients with incisional hernias, although for large incisional hernias, laparoscopic cholecystectomy may have no advantages over open cholecystectomy if a large incision and dissection of adhesions are required. Patients with stomas may also undergo laparoscopic cholecystectomy, provided that the appropriate steps are taken to prevent injury to the bowel during placement of trocars and division of adhesions.

Patients with cirrhosis or portal hypertension are at high risk for morbidity and mortality with open cholecystectomy. If absolutely necessary, laparoscopic cholecystectomy may be attempted by an experienced surgeon. The risk of bleeding can be minimized by rigorous preoperative preparation, meticulous dissection with the help of magnification available through the laparoscope, and use of the electrocautery.

Patients with bleeding diatheses, such as hemophilia, von Willebrand disease, and thrombocytopenia, may undergo laparoscopic cholecystectomy. They require appropriate preoperative and postoperative care and monitoring, and a hematologist should be consulted.

Questions have been raised about whether laparoscopic cholecystectomy should be performed in pregnant patients; it has been argued that the increased intra-abdominal pressure may pose a risk to the fetus. Because of the enlarged uterus, open insertion of the initial trocar is mandatory, and the positioning of other trocars may have to be modified according to the position of the uterus. Inflation pressures should be kept as low as possible, and prophylaxis of deep vein thrombosis (DVT) is recommended. Despite these potential problems, safe performance of laparoscopic cholecystectomy and other laparoscopic procedures in pregnant patients is increasingly being described in the literature. If cholecystectomy is necessary before delivery, the second trimester is the best time for it.

Patients in whom preoperative imaging gives rise to a strong suspicion of gallbladder cancer should probably undergo open surgical management.

Operative Planning

ANTIBIOTIC PROPHYLAXIS

Some surgeons recommend routine preoperative administration of antibiotics to all patients undergoing laparoscopic cholecystectomy, on the grounds that inadvertent entry into the gallbladder is not uncommon and can lead to spillage of bile or stones into the peritoneal cavity. Other surgeons, however, recommend using the same guidelines for antibiotic prophylaxis in patients undergoing laparoscopic cholecystectomy as in those undergoing open cholecystectomy. Resolution of this controversy awaits proper prospective trials. We recommend selective use

Figure 2 **Laparoscopic cholecystectomy. Shown is an algorithm outlining the use of preoperative cholangiography in patients at moderate or high risk for CBD stones.**

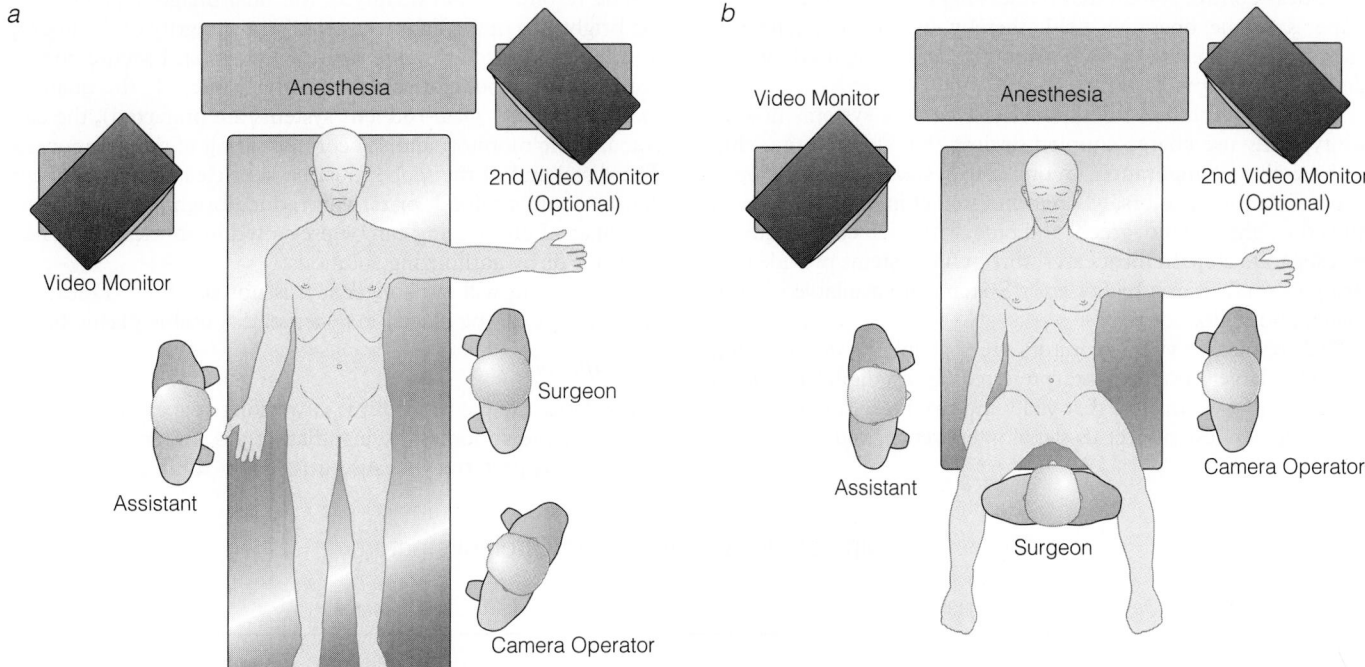

Figure 3 **Laparoscopic cholecystectomy. A patient undergoing laparoscopic cholecystectomy should be positioned so as to allow easy access to the gallbladder and a clear view of the monitors. Shown are the positions of the surgeon, the camera operator, and the assistant in the OR according to (*a*) North American positioning and (*b*) European positioning.**

of antibiotic prophylaxis for patients at highest risk for bacteria in the bile (including those with acute cholecystitis or CBD stones, those who have previously undergone instrumentation of the biliary tree, and those older than 70 years) and for patients with prosthetic heart valves and joint prostheses.

PROPHYLAXIS OF DVT

The reverse Trendelenburg position used during laparoscopic cholecystectomy, coupled with the positive intra-abdominal pressure generated by CO_2 pneumoperitoneum and the vasodilatation induced by general anesthesia, leads to venous pooling in the lower extremities. This consequence may be minimized by using antiembolic stockings or by wrapping the legs with elastic bandages. Subcutaneous heparin and pneumatic compression devices may be employed for patients at increased risk for DVT [*see VI:2 Thromboembolic Problems*]. As yet, however, there is no convincing evidence that the incidence of DVT is higher with laparoscopy than with open surgery.

PATIENT POSITIONING

The patient should be positioned so as to optimize exposure of the gallbladder and to give the surgeon, the camera operator, and the assistant easy access to the patient and a clear view of the video monitor or monitors. There should be a direct line from the surgeon to the laparoscope to the gallbladder. This can be accomplished with the patient in the supine position and the surgeon on the patient's left (North American positioning) [*see Figure 3a*] or with the patient in low stirrups and the surgeon on the patient's left or between the patient's legs (European positioning) [*see Figure 3b*].

With North American positioning, in which the patient is supine, the camera operator usually stands on the patient's left to the left of the surgeon, while the assistant stands on the patient's right. The video monitor is positioned on the patient's right above

the level of the costal margin. If a second monitor is available, it should be positioned on the patient's left to the right of the surgeon, where the assistant can have an unobstructed and comfortable view. Exposure can be improved by tilting the patient in the reverse Trendelenburg position and rotating the table with the patient's right side up. Gravity pulls the duodenum, the colon, and the omentum away from the gallbladder, thereby increasing the working space available in the upper abdomen.

The OR table should allow easy access for a fluoroscopic C arm, to facilitate intraoperative cholangiography. The table cover should be radiolucent.

EQUIPMENT

The equipment required for laparoscopic cholecystectomy [*see Table 1*] includes an optical system, an electronic insufflator, trocars (cannulas), surgical instruments, and hemostatic devices.

Optical System

The optical system consists of a laparoscope, a high-intensity light source, a miniature video camera and camera box, and a high-resolution video monitor. A videotape recording system is desirable but not essential. A video printing system and a digital-image capturing system are also valuable for documenting operative findings.

The laparoscope can provide either a straight, end-on (0°) view or an angled (30° or 45°) view. Scopes that provide an end-on view are easier to learn to use, but angled scopes are more versatile. Scopes with a 30° angle cause less disorientation than those with a 45° angle and are ideal for laparoscopic cholecystectomy. Excellent 30° scopes are currently available in diameters of 10 mm, 5 mm, and 3.5 mm.

Illumination in the abdomen is provided by a separate high-intensity light source (usually xenon or metal halide) that generates 150 to 300 watts. Most light sources have an automatic brightness-control system that reduces light output the closer the scope is to the operative field, thereby diminishing reflective glare. Some cameras also have a control that can be used for regulating light output.

The high-resolution miniature video camera systems now in use typically use charge-coupled devices (CCDs) in a one-chip or three-chip configuration. In one-chip systems, a single chip is responsible for all colors, whereas in three-chip systems, a prism splits the light into red, green, and blue, with each color acquired by a separate chip. In most cases, three-chip systems provide better images, albeit at a higher cost. Systems are available in both analog and digital formats.

High-resolution video monitors are available in various sizes; generally, larger monitors are preferred. Fully digital flat-panel displays are now available that yield improved resolution, take up less space, are less subject to signal interference, and require less power.

The resolution and quality of the final image depend on (1) the brightness of the light source; (2) the integrity of the fiberoptic cord used to convey the light; (3) clean and secure connections between the light source and the scope; (4) the quality of the laparoscope (glass-rod lens systems are preferred), the camera, and the monitor; and (5) correct wiring of the components. The distal end of the scope must be kept clean and free of condensation: bile, blood, or fat will reduce brightness and distort the image. Lens fogging can be prevented by immersion in heated water or by antifogging solutions.

The camera will last longer if it is not sterilized. During the operation, it can be placed in a sterile, disposable plastic bag.

Insufflator

For laparoscopic procedures, a working space must be created within the abdomen by insufflating gas under positive pressure. CO_2 is preferred because it is highly soluble in water and

Table 1 Equipment for Laparoscopic Cholecystectomy

Instrument/Device	Number	Size	Comments

Laparoscopic cart
  High-intensity halogen light source
    (150–300 watts)
  High-flow electronic insufflator (minimum
    flow rate of 6 L/min)
  Laparoscopic camera box
  Videocassette recorder (optional)
  Digital still image capture system (optional)			

Laparoscope	1	3.5–10 mm	Available in 0° and angled views; we prefer to use a 30° 5 mm diameter laparoscope
Atraumatic grasping forceps	2–4	2–10 mm	Selection of graspers should allow surgeon choice appropriate to thickness and consistency of gallbladder wall; insulation is unnecessary
Large-tooth grasping forceps	1	10 mm	Used to extract gallbladder at end of procedure
Curved dissector	1	2–5 mm	Should have a rotatable shaft; insulation is required
Scissors	2–3	2–5 mm	One curved and one straight scissors with rotating shaft and insulation; additional microscissors may be helpful for incising cystic duct
Clip appliers	1–2	5–10 mm	Either disposable multiple clip applier or 2 manually loaded reusable single clip appliers for small and medium-to-large clips
Dissecting electrocautery hook or spatula	1	5 mm	Available in various shapes according to surgeon's preference; instrument should have channel for suction and irrigation controlled by trumpet valve(s); insulation required
High-frequency electrical cord	1		Cord should be designed with appropriate connectors for electrosurgical unit and instruments being used
Suction-irrigation probe	1	5–10 mm	Probe should have trumpet valve controls for suction and irrigation; may be used with pump for hydrodissection
10-to-5 mm reducers	2		Allow use of 5 mm instruments in 10 mm trocar without loss of pneumoperitoneum; these are often unnecessary with newer disposable trocars and may be built into some reusable trocars
5-to-3 mm reducer	1		Allows use of 2–3 mm instruments and ligating loops in 5 mm trocars
Ligating loops			
Endoscopic needle holders	1–2	5 mm	
Cholangiogram clamp with catheter	1	5 mm	Allows passage of catheter and clamping of catheter in cystic duct
Veress needle	1		Used if initial trocar is inserted by percutaneous technique
Allis or Babcock forceps	1–2	5 mm	Allow atraumatic grasping of bowel or gallbladder
Long spinal needle	1	14-gauge	Useful for aspirating gallbladder percutaneously in cases of acute cholecystitis or hydrops
Retrieval bag	1		Useful for preventing spillage of bile or stones in removal of inflamed or friable gallbladder; facilitates retrieval of spilled stones

because it does not support combustion when the electrocautery is used. The CO_2 should be insufflated with an electronic pump capable of a flow rate of at least 6 L/min; most current systems have a maximum flow rate of 20 L/min or higher. The insufflator is connected to one of the trocars by means of a flexible tube and a stopcock.

When intra-abdominal pressure drops below a preset value (usually 12 to 15 mm Hg), gas flow begins at the preset rate. The insufflator should provide digital readouts of the actual gas flow rate, the actual intra-abdominal pressure, and the total amount of CO_2 used during the procedure. It should also have a control for adjusting maximum flow rate and a control for setting the pressure above which gas flow is automatically shut off. An audible alarm should sound when the measured pressure exceeds a certain preset value.

Whenever multiple trocars are used, there is a certain unavoidable loss of gas around and through the trocars. The insufflator rapidly replaces this gas. Because the rate of gas flow is influenced by the diameter of the port through which the gas is infused, insufflators capable of flow rates higher than 6 L/min are rarely used to their full potential. Insufflators that can provide heated gas minimize heat loss and fogging and may offer hemodynamic benefits.

Trocars

The trocars through which access to the abdominal cavity is gained are available in a variety of sizes; selection depends on the external diameter of the instruments to be placed through them.

For cholecystectomy, at least one trocar site must be large enough to allow passage of the gallbladder and any stones removed. Most surgeons prefer to use a 10/12 mm trocar at the umbilicus for this purpose. The other trocars can range from 2 to 12 mm, depending on the size of the laparoscope, the grasping forceps, and the clip appliers being used. The conventional approach is to use 10/12 mm trocars at the umbilicus and the operating port site and 5 mm trocars for the other instruments; however, if a 5 mm laparoscope and a 5 mm clip applier are used, the operating port size can be reduced to 5 mm.

Currently, 2 mm instrumentation is growing in popularity. It must be remembered, however, that as a rule, the smaller the working port, the less versatile the instruments. In our experience, the combination of a 10 mm umbilical trocar, a 5 mm operating port, and 2 mm ports for grasping forceps is a good one: optical quality is maintained, little flexibility is lost with respect to selecting operating instruments, trocar size is minimized, and the cosmetic result is excellent.

Surgical Instruments

The choice of surgical instruments from the large array now available is clearly a personal one. Many instruments are available in both disposable and reusable forms. Reusable instruments tend to be sturdier and better designed, but their design may rapidly become obsolete, and like reusable trocars, they must be checked periodically. Disposables are more current in design, are consistently sharp, and are excellent to have as backups in case nondisposables break down. Instruments are also available in both insulated versions (to allow use of the electrocautery) or noninsulated versions (to reduce maintenance costs).

A minimal set of instruments for laparoscopic cholecystectomy would include graspers, dissectors, clip appliers, scissors, a dissecting electrocautery hook or spatula (or both), probes, reducers, ligating loops, a Veress needle, needle holders, and a cholangiography catheter system [see Table 1]; other instruments may be considered as options.

For clip appliers, curved scissors, and curved dissectors, a rotatable shaft can afford the surgeon more comfortable and convenient working angles. The shaft should be easily locked once it is at the appropriate angle so that it does not rotate during use.

Suction and irrigation probes are available with either trumpet valves or stopcock attachments. Reusable instruments must be checked periodically to ensure that the valves do not stick or leak. Irrigation can be provided under pressure by means of a commercial pump system, a system that uses high-pressure gas, or a pressure bag like those used for infusion of blood products. If a pressure bag is used, it should be pressurized to approximately 300 mm Hg, and either normal saline or lactated Ringer solution can be used as an irrigant.

A retrieval bag system is also useful. When the gallbladder has been perforated, it and any spilled stones should be placed into a bag before removal. This measure minimizes further bile spillage and stone loss and greatly simplifies removal. Although special self-opening retrieval bags are available, many surgeons take a less expensive approach and simply use sterilized food storage bags.

Hemostatic Devices

Hemostasis can be achieved with monopolar or bipolar electrocauterization. Electrocautery units are widely available, safe, inexpensive, and familiar to all surgeons, and they provide excellent hemostasis. A monopolar electrocautery can be connected to most available instruments; however, it is likely that bipolar electrocauterization will eventually prove safer. With a monopolar electrocautery, depth of burn is less predictable, current can be conducted through noninsulated instruments and trocars, and any area of the instrument that is stripped of insulation may conduct current and result in a burn. Caution is essential when the electrocautery is used near hemostatic clips because delayed sloughing may occur.

Electrocauterization should be avoided near the CBD because delayed bile duct injuries and leaks may occur as a result of sloughing from a burned area and devascularization of the duct. Care must be exercised when a cautery is employed near the bowel and when intra-abdominal adhesions are being taken down. The electrocautery can be used with a forceps, scissors, hooks (L or J shaped), a spatula, and other instruments. Some cautery probes incorporate nonsticking surfaces to prevent buildup of eschar. The use of hand-activated cautery probes and the presence of a channel that allows suction and irrigation through the cautery probes are especially convenient.

More advanced energy sources and instruments are also available. Bipolar devices designed to weld tissues have proved capable of achieving superb hemostasis. Ultrasonic dissecting shears can also be used to dissect and coagulate tissues effectively and precisely. For laparoscopic cholecystectomy, however, such advanced—and costly—devices are rarely needed.

Operative Technique

STEP 1: PLACEMENT OF TROCARS AND ACCESSORY PORTS

Placement of Initial Trocar

The first step in laparoscopic cholecystectomy is the creation of pneumoperitoneum and the insertion of an initial trocar through which the laparoscope can be passed. This step is critical because complications resulting from improper placement may cause serious morbidity and death. The surgeon may use either a percuta-

a

b

c

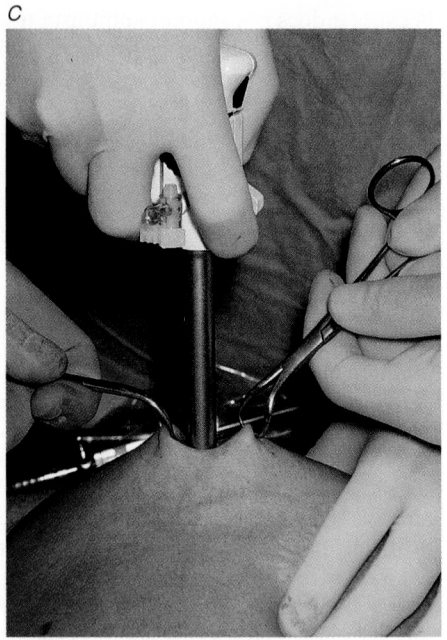

Figure 4 **Laparoscopic cholecystectomy. Illustrated is percutaneous placement of the initial trocar. (*a*) A Veress needle is used for percutaneous entry into the peritoneal cavity. It is angled toward the sacral hollow (where the distance from the anterior to the posterior abdominal wall is greatest) and toward an area below the bifurcation of the aorta. This space can be enlarged by tilting the patient in the Trendelenburg position, allowing the free intestinal loops to fall cephalad. (*b*) With the stopcock on the Veress needle in the closed position, a drop of saline is placed into the hub of the needle. The stopcock is then opened and the abdominal wall elevated. Lifting the abdominal wall creates negative pressure in the peritoneal cavity. Thus, if the tip of the needle is properly positioned within the cavity, the drop of saline should be drawn into the abdomen. (*c*) The abdominal wall is elevated, and a sharp 10/12 mm trocar is inserted into the peritoneal cavity along the same path as the Veress needle. Disposable trocars with a retracting plastic sheath provide further protection against perforation of viscera or vessels.**

neous technique or an open technique. We prefer the open technique, which eliminates the risks inherent in the blind puncture.

Percutaneous technique   For percutaneous trocar insertion, a small curvilinear incision is made in the area of the umbilicus and extended downward through the subcutaneous fat. A Veress needle is then inserted through the fascia and the peritoneum into the abdominal cavity [*see Figure 4a*]. This is best accomplished by elevating the abdominal wall and slightly angling the needle toward the pelvis, with the patient in the Trendelenburg position. The tip of the needle should be directed toward the hollow of the sacrum. Entry of the needle into the peritoneal cavity can usually be confirmed by a popping sensation as the resistance of the peritoneum is overcome. A 10 ml syringe is then attached to the needle and aspiration attempted. If the aspirate contains any blood or bowel contents, the needle is clearly in an inappropriate position.

If the aspirate is clear, the next step is to confirm proper positioning by means of the saline drop test [*see Figure 4b*]. The surgeon then attaches the insufflator to the needle and begins inflating the abdomen at a rate of approximately 1 L/min. The intra-abdominal pressure should be very low when insufflation is started, usually about 2 to 5 mm Hg; high pressure suggests improper needle placement. As the abdomen is distended with CO_2, the surgeon percusses the abdomen to ensure even distribution of the gas. When a pressure of approximately 15 mm Hg is reached (which requires about 5 L of gas in an average-sized patient), the Veress needle is withdrawn, and a sharp 10/12 mm trocar is percutaneously inserted through the same incision into the abdominal cavity, following the same route as the needle.

Because this procedure is done blindly, it may be advisable to enhance its safety by using disposable trocars with a spring-loaded protective plastic mechanism [*see Figure 4c*]. Once the initial trocar is inserted, proper positioning is confirmed by placing the laparoscope. Insufflation of CO_2 through the trocar then resumes, maintaining pneumoperitoneum.

Open insertion technique   The advantage of the open technique is that the trocar is inserted into the peritoneal cavity under direct vision; no Veress needle is required. Although it is certainly possible to injure the bowel inadvertently when placing the trocar, the injury almost always can be identified immediately and usually can be repaired easily through the same incision. Injury to the blood vessels or the bladder should virtually never occur with the open technique.

The umbilical skin is elevated with a sharp towel clip, and a 1 cm incision is made just inferior to the umbilicus [*see Figure 5a*]. Dissection is carried down through the subcutaneous tissue. The skin flap is raised, and a raphe can be seen connecting its undersurface to the midline fascia of the abdominal wall. The raphe is followed down to the fascia, which is then elevated between vertically placed forceps and incised [*see Figure 5b*]. The peritoneum is grasped next and pulled up into the wound, where it is incised. Entry into the abdominal cavity is easily confirmed by inserting a finger or a blunt instrument into the peritoneum [*see Figure 5c*]. Stay sutures are then placed on either side of the fascial incision, and a blunt olive-tipped 10/12 mm trocar, designed to occlude the fascial defect around it, is placed into the abdomen under direct vision. These sutures are then used to fasten the trocar to the wound and to prevent any leakage of gas. Because proper

a *b* *c*

Figure 5 **Laparoscopic cholecystectomy. With the open insertion technique, the initial trocar is placed under direct vision. (*a*) The umbilical skin is elevated with a sharp towel clip. A curvilinear incision is made in the inferior umbilical fold. The skin flap is elevated, and the raphe leading from the dermis to the fascia is thereby exposed. (*b*) The fascia is grasped in the midline between forceps and elevated. The fascia and the underlying peritoneum are incised under direct vision. (*c*) A blunt instrument is placed into the peritoneum to ensure that the undersurface of the peritoneum is free of adhesions. The opening can be enlarged sufficiently to allow placement of a blunt 10/11 mm trocar.**

positioning of the trocar is obvious and needs no further confirmation, pneumoperitoneum can be created rapidly. The additional time expended on the dissection needed for insertion of the trocar is more than outweighed by the increased speed with which pneumoperitoneum is created and facilitates removal of the gallbladder at the end of the procedure. The stay sutures can also be used at the end of the procedure to close the fascial defect.

Scars

Patients who have previously undergone abdominal surgery are at risk for adhesions, both to the undersurface of the abdominal wall and intra-abdominally. Adhesions to the undersurface of the abdominal wall make access to the abdominal cavity potentially hazardous, particularly when the percutaneous method is used for placement of the initial trocar. Scars from previous operations may affect insertion of the initial trocar, depending on its orientation and location. If a patient has a scar in the lower abdomen (e.g., from a Pfannenstiel incision or an incision in the right lower quadrant for an appendectomy), the position of the initial trocar need not be changed. If the scar is in the upper abdomen, the initial trocar may be inserted below the umbilicus in the midline. If there is a long midline scar that is impossible to avoid, careful dissection of the peritoneum through a somewhat longer vertical incision than usual affords safe access to the peritoneum in most cases.

An alternative is to insert the initial trocar high in the epigastrium or in the right anterior axillary line, where bowel adhesions are less common. The laparoscope is inserted through this trocar and used to examine the undersurface of the old scar for a clear site near the umbilicus where a 10 mm trocar can be placed. Previous laparoscopy, which rarely creates significant intra-abdominal adhesions, rarely necessitates modification of trocar insertion.

The surgeon should also consider the reason for the previous surgery. For example, a patient who underwent an appendectomy for perforating appendicitis may have had diffuse peritonitis and may have adhesions well away from the old scar.

Placement of Accessory Ports

In most cases, four ports are necessary. The first port is for the laparoscope; the remaining ports are for grasping forceps, dissectors, and clip appliers. The precise position of the accessory ports depends on the surgeon's preference, the patient's body habitus, and the presence or absence of previous scars or intra-abdominal adhesions. A rigid approach to port placement is inappropriate: trocar placement determines operative exposure, and improper placement will haunt the surgeon throughout the procedure. In some cases, a fifth trocar is required to elevate a floppy liver or to depress or retract the omentum or a bulky hepatic flexure of the colon. In trocar placement, as in patient positioning, European practice tends to differ from North American practice [*see Figure 6*].

Most surgeons elect to place one of the grasping forceps on the fundus of the gallbladder through an accessory port placed approximately in the anterior axillary line below the level of the gallbladder. Because the level of the gallbladder varies from patient to patient, the placement of this accessory port should not be decided on until the gallbladder is visualized. If the gallbladder is low lying and the trocar is placed too high, it is difficult for the surgeon to achieve the appropriate angle of retraction. As a general rule, positioning the trocar in the anterior axillary line approximately halfway between the costal margin and the anterosuperior iliac spine provides the appropriate exposure. A 2 to 5 mm port usually suffices at this site because its only likely function is to allow retraction of the gallbladder. In some cases of acute cholecystitis, however, a larger port may be preferable, so that a larger grasper can be inserted and used to hold the gallbladder without tearing it.

A second accessory port (also 2 to 5 mm) allows the surgeon to grasp the gallbladder in the area of Hartmann's pouch for retraction. This port is usually positioned just beneath the right costal margin. Some surgeons prefer it to be approximately at the midclavicular line; others prefer it to be higher and more medial, just to the right of the falciform ligament.

The main operating port should be 5 or 10 mm in diameter, so that clip appliers can be readily placed through it and the laparoscope can be moved to this port at the end of the procedure. The positioning of this port is determined by the surgeon's preference and, in particular, by the patient's body habitus. The optimum placement is at about the same horizontal level as the gallbladder or slightly higher, so that during the operation, the laparoscope and the operating instrument form an angle of about 90°. Some surgeons prefer to place the operative port in the midline, to the right of the falciform ligament; others prefer to place it to the left of the falciform, passing the trocar underneath the ligament and elevating it with the trocar.

Surgeons should be encouraged to use both hands when performing laparoscopic cholecystectomy. One hand should control the grasping forceps holding Hartmann's pouch, so that the gallbladder can be moved to provide the best possible exposure. The other hand should control the dissecting instruments placed through the operating port.

Special Considerations in Obese Patients

Obese patients pose specific problems that affect port placement. The problems may be related to the thick abdominal wall, the large amount of intra-abdominal fat, or both. A thick abdominal wall makes it more difficult to rotate the trocar around the normal fulcrum point in the abdominal wall. Consequently, it is essential to place the trocar at the angle most likely to be used during the procedure. When a trocar is tunneled through the abdominal wall, more of the cannula is within the abdominal wall than if the trocar had been placed perpendicularly; accordingly, the trocar is less mobile. If the trocars are not easily rotated, the instruments placed through them will be difficult to manipulate smoothly. Thus, in the patient with a very thick pannus, a standard-length trocar may be too short. Displacement of

trocars can lead to insufflation into the abdominal wall and consequently to subcutaneous emphysema, which further thickens the abdominal wall and hinders exposure.

To prevent such problems, special extra-length trocars designed for morbidly obese patients have been developed. It may also be necessary to place the trocars closer to the area of the gallbladder to ensure that the operating instruments can reach the gallbladder. For example, the initial port may have to be placed above the umbilicus.

In obese patients, the bulky falciform ligament and the large omentum may adversely affect exposure. A 30° laparoscope may help the surgeon see over the omentum and the high-lying hepatic flexure of the colon. In some cases, it is useful to place a fifth port so that the surgeon can retract the hepatic flexure downward. Fat may envelop the cystic duct and artery and the portal structures, obscuring normal anatomic landmarks. When the electrocautery is used, the heat melts the fat and causes it to sizzle and spray onto the lens of the laparoscope, resulting in a blurry image. To prevent this, the camera operator should pull the scope slightly away from the operative field during electrocauterization, then advance the scope during dissection. This should also be done when an ultrasonic dissector is being used.

Given that obese patients are more difficult candidates for open cholecystectomy and have a higher complication rate with laparotomy, the advantages of laparoscopic cholecystectomy in these individuals justify the effort needed to overcome the technical problems.

STEP 2: EXPOSURE OF GALLBLADDER AND CALOT'S TRIANGLE

Dissection of Adhesions

Adhesions must be dissected to provide an unimpeded view of the gallbladder through the laparoscope. Not all intra-abdominal

Figure 6 **Laparoscopic cholecystectomy. Illustrated are the differences between typical North American practice (*a*) and typical European practice (*b*) with respect to the placement of the trocars and the instruments inserted through each port.**

adhesions must be taken down, just enough to allow entry of accessory trocars under direct vision and thus permit access to the gallbladder. This process is facilitated by pneumoperitoneum, which provides traction on adhesions to the abdominal wall, and by the magnification provided by the optical system, which allows identification of the avascular plane of attachment.

The most difficult problem is positioning the dissecting instruments so that they can reach the undersurface of the anterior abdominal wall. A rigid trocar inserted through the anterior abdominal wall cannot be rotated enough to allow scissors passed through this port to cut adhesions to the anterior abdominal wall. In such cases, one or two trocars should be placed laterally, near the anterior axillary or midaxillary line. Instruments passed through these ports can easily be angled parallel to the anterior abdominal wall, and the adhesions can then be dissected without difficulty.

Bowel adhesions should be taken down with endoscopic scissors at their insertion to the abdominal wall, where they are least vascular. Electrocauterization, generally unnecessary, should be avoided because of the risk of thermal injury to the bowel. Interloop adhesions, which rarely interfere with exposure of the gallbladder, need not be dissected. Frequently, adhesions to the gallbladder occur as a reaction to inflammatory attacks [see Figure 7]. They are usually relatively avascular. Dissection of these adhesions should begin at the fundus of the gallbladder and should then proceed down toward the neck of the gallbladder. The best way to take them down is to grasp the gallbladder with one grasping forceps at the site where the adhesions attach, gradually placing traction on the adhesions with the other hand. Usually, the adhesions peel down in an avascular plane. Dissection should continue until all adhesions to the inferolateral aspect of the gallbladder have been taken down. It is not necessary to divide adhesions between the superior surface of the liver and the undersurface of the diaphragm unless they impede superior retraction of the liver.

Exposing Calot's Triangle

Obtaining adequate exposure of Calot's triangle is a key step. First, the patient is placed in a reverse Trendelenburg position,

Figure 7 Laparoscopic cholecystectomy. Adhesions of duodenum and omentum to gallbladder wall obscure view of structures of Calot's triangle.

Figure 8 Laparoscopic cholecystectomy. Initial view of gallbladder and related structures is facilitated by appropriate tilting of the operating table. Hartmann's pouch (HP), the cystic duct (CD), and the common bile duct (CBD) can be readily identified before any dissection.

with the table rotated toward the left side. Next, the fundus of the gallbladder and the right lobe of the liver are elevated toward the patient's right shoulder. One grasping forceps, inserted through the most lateral right-side port and held by an assistant, is placed on the fundus of the gallbladder [see Figure 8], and the gallbladder is retracted superiorly and laterally above the right hepatic lobe. This maneuver straightens out folds in the body of the gallbladder and permits initial visualization of the area of Calot's triangle. If Calot's triangle is still obscured, the patient can be placed in a steeper reverse Trendelenburg position, the stomach can be emptied of air via an orogastric tube inserted by the anesthetist, or, if necessary, a fifth trocar can be inserted on the patient's right side to push down the duodenum.

In some patients, such as those with acute cholecystitis and hydrops of the gallbladder, the gallbladder is tense and distended, making it difficult to grasp and easy to tear. In these patients, retraction of the fundus is difficult, and exposure of Calot's triangle is unsatisfactory. This problem is best managed by aspirating the contents of the gallbladder either percutaneously with a 14- or 16-gauge needle inserted into the fundus of the gallbladder under laparoscopic vision or by using the 5 mm trocar in the right upper abdomen to puncture the fundus and then aspirate with the suction irrigator. After the needle is withdrawn, a large atraumatic grasping forceps can be used to hold the gallbladder and occlude the hole; a 10 mm forceps may be preferred if the wall is markedly thickened. An alternative is to place a stitch or a ligating loop around the fundus of the collapsed gallbladder; the tail of the suture can then be grasped with a forceps to achieve a secure grip and also prevent further leakage of gallbladder contents from the needle hole.

Once the fundus of the gallbladder is retracted superiorly by the assistant, the surgeon places a grasping forceps in the area of Hartmann's pouch. Using both hands, the surgeon controls the grasper on Hartmann's pouch as well as the operating instrument. The surgeon maneuvers Hartmann's pouch to provide various angles for safe dissection of Calot's triangle. Initially, lateral and inferior traction are placed on Hartmann's pouch, opening up the angle between the cystic duct and the common ducts [see Figure 9], avoiding their alignment [see Figure 10].

A large stone impacted in the gallbladder neck may impede the surgeon's ability to place the forceps on Hartmann's pouch. This problem can usually be managed by dislodging the stone early in the operation, as follows: the gallbladder is grasped as low as possible with one grasping forceps; a widely opening dissecting instrument, such as a right-angle dissector, a Babcock forceps, or a curved dissector, is used to dislodge the stone and milk it up toward the fundus; with the same forceps or another large grasper, the stone is held up and away from the neck of the gallbladder, and appropriate retraction is provided.

If the stone cannot be disimpacted, an instrument can be used to elevate the infundibulum of the gallbladder superiorly, allowing exposure of Calot's triangle. Alternatively, one can attempt to crush the stone, but small pieces of the stone may fall into the cystic duct. A third option is to place a stitch in Hartmann's pouch and grasp the end of the stitch to provide exposure.

Figure 11 **Laparoscopic cholecystectomy. The gallbladder-cystic duct (GB-CD) junction can be identified as lateral traction is applied to the area of Hartmann's pouch.**

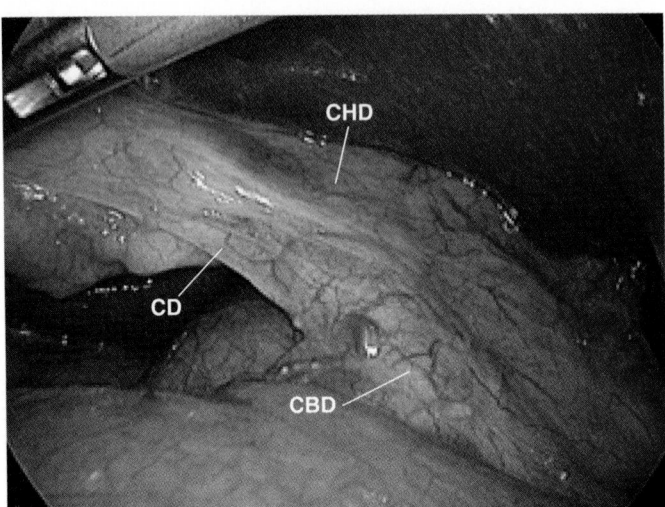

Figure 9 **Laparoscopic cholecystectomy. The area of Hartmann's pouch is retracted laterally. The cystic duct (CD) is seen at an angle to the common hepatic duct (CHD) and the common bile duct (CBD).**

Figure 10 **Laparoscopic cholecystectomy. In this case, the gallbladder is retracted cephalad. The cystic duct (CD) can be seen running in the same direction as the common bile duct (CBD). The CBD may be misinterpreted as being the cystic duct and consequently is at risk for injury.**

Figure 12 **Laparoscopic cholecystectomy. A view from below with a 30° laparoscope demonstrates the point for beginning dissection (arrow), where the gallbladder funnels down to its junction with the cystic duct. Just below this point can be seen a cleft in the liver known as Rouvier's sulcus. This cleft, present in 70% to 80% of livers, reliably indicates the plane of the CBD.**

STEP 3: STRIPPING OF PERITONEUM

The key to avoiding injury to the major ducts during laparoscopic cholecystectomy is accurate identification of the junction between the gallbladder and the cystic duct [*see Figure 11*]. Unless the gallbladder–cystic duct junction is immediately obvious upon examination of Calot's triangle anteriorly, our approach is to begin dissection of Calot's triangle posteriorly [*see Figure 12*]. From this approach, the insertion of the gallbladder neck into the cystic duct is usually more clearly identified, especially with the aid of a 30° laparoscope. Exposure is obtained by retracting Hartmann's pouch superomedially and is facilitated by looking from below with a 30° scope.

Figure 13 **Laparoscopic cholecystectomy. The peritoneum is dissected from the gallbladder–cystic duct junction (arrow), as seen from below through a 30° angled laparoscope.**

Figure 14 **Laparoscopic cholecystectomy. Arterial bleeding can be seen (arrow) from a branch of the cystic artery injured during dissection from the posterior approach.**

Dissection should always start high on the gallbladder and hug the gallbladder closely until the anatomy is identified clearly. Using a curved dissector, the surgeon gently teases away peritoneum attaching the neck of gallbladder to the liver posterolaterally to visualize the funneling of the neck of the gallbladder into the cystic duct [*see Figure 13*]. Only the posterior layer of peritoneum is dissected; care must be taken not to dissect deeply in this area because of the risk of injury to the cystic artery [*see Figure 14*].

In some problem cases, edema, fibrosis, and adhesions make identification of the gallbladder–cystic duct junction very difficult. An anatomic landmark on the liver known as Rouvier's sulcus may be helpful in such circumstances [*see Figure 12*]. This sulcus, or the remnant of it, is present in 70% to 80% of livers and usually contains the right portal triad or its branches. Its location is consistently to the right of the hepatic hilum and anterior to the caudate process (Couinaud segment 1). This landmark reliably indicates the plane of the CBD. Therefore, dissection dorsal to it should be done with caution.

Once the funneling of the gallbladder into the cystic duct has been identified, the area of Hartmann's pouch should be again pulled laterally and inferiorly so that the anterior peritoneum can be dissected, while the 30° scope is angled to view the area. The two-handed technique facilitates the surgeon's movement between the posterior and anterior aspects of Calot's triangle, providing complete visualization. Dissection should always take place at the gallbladder–cystic duct junction, staying close to the gallbladder to avoid inadvertent injury to the CBD. A curved dissecting forceps is used to strip the fibroareolar tissue just superior to the cystic duct. The superior border of the cystic duct can then be identified and the cystic duct gently and gradually dissected [*see Figure 15*]. The cystic duct lymph node is a useful landmark at this location and may facilitate identification of the gallbladder–cystic duct junction.

When traction is placed as described, the cystic artery tends to run parallel and somewhat cephalad to the cystic duct. This artery can often be identified by noting its close relation to the cystic duct lymph node. Complete dissection of the area between the cystic duct and the artery develops a window through which the liver should be visible. The cystic duct is then encircled with a curved dissecting instrument or an L-shaped hook. Downward traction should be applied to the cystic duct to open this window and ensure that there is no ductal structure running through this space in Calot's triangle to join the cystic duct (i.e., the right hepatic duct).

Dissection of Calot's triangle should be completed before the cystic duct is clipped or divided. This is best accomplished by dissecting the neck of the gallbladder from the liver bed. Unequivocal identification of the gallbladder–cystic duct junction is imperative. The cystic duct should be dissected for a length sufficient to permit secure placement of two clips; it is not necessary, and indeed may be hazardous, to attempt to dissect the cystic duct–CBD junction.

The cystic artery is exposed next [*see Figure 16*]. A small vein can usually be identified in the space between the cystic duct and the cystic artery; it can usually be pulled up anteriorly and cauterized. Because dissection is done near the gallbladder, it is not unusual to encounter more than one branch of the cystic artery. Each of these branches should be dissected free of the fibroareolar tissue. Care should also be taken to ensure that the right hepatic artery is not inadvertently injured as a result of being mistaken for the cystic artery.

STEP 4: CONTROL AND DIVISION OF CYSTIC DUCT AND CYSTIC ARTERY

At this point, the cystic duct is clipped on the gallbladder side, and a cholangiogram is obtained if desired [*see Step 5, below*]. If a cholangiogram is not desired, three or four clips should be placed on the cystic duct and the cystic duct divided between them. Two or three hemostatic clips are placed on the cystic artery, and the vessel is divided. It is prudent to incise the artery partially before transecting it completely to ensure that the clips are secure and that there is no pulsatile bleeding. Once the artery is completely divided, the proximal end will retract medially, making it more difficult to expose and control the artery safely if bleeding occurs. Electrocauterization should be avoided near the cystic duct and all metallic clips. Electrical current will be conducted through metallic clips and may result in delayed sloughing of the duct or a clip. Delayed injuries to the CBD may be caused by a direct burn to the duct or by sparking from noninsulated instruments or clips during dissection. As an alternative, locking polymer clips that fit through 5 mm ports, clip across a greater width of tissue, and do not conduct electricity may be used.

Control of Short or Wide Cystic Duct

Edema and acute inflammation may lead to thickening and foreshortening of the cystic duct, with subsequent difficulties in dissection and ligation. If the duct is edematous, clips may cut through it; if the duct is too wide, the clip may not occlude it completely. A modified clipping technique can be employed, with placement of an initial clip to occlude as much of the duct as possible. The occluded portion of the duct is then incised, and

Figure 15 Laparoscopic cholecystectomy. The superior border of the cystic duct has been dissected. Funneling of the gallbladder into the cystic duct is clearly seen (arrow).

Figure 16 Laparoscopic cholecystectomy. Dissection of Calot's triangle further exposes the cystic duct (CD) and the cystic artery (CA) near their entry into the gallbladder (GB) in preparation for clipping and division.

a second clip is placed flush with the first so as to occlude the rest of the duct. Alternatively, wider polymer clips may be used.

Because this technique is not always possible, the surgeon should be familiar with techniques for ligating the duct with either intracorporeal or extracorporeal ties. It is extremely helpful to know how to tie extracorporeal ties so that the cystic duct can be ligated in continuity before it is divided. In some cases, the duct can be divided, held with a forceps, and controlled with a ligating loop. If there is concern about secure closure of the cystic duct, a closed suction drain may be placed. If inflammation, as in cholecystitis, has caused the duct to be shorter than usual, dissection must be kept close to the gallbladder to avoid inadvertent injury to the CBD. A short cystic duct is often associated with acute cholecystitis. Patient blunt dissection with the suction-irrigation device may be the safest technique.

Cystic Duct Stones

Stones in the cystic duct may be visualized or felt during laparoscopic cholecystectomy. Every effort should be made to milk them into the gallbladder before applying clips. Placing a clip across a stone may push a fragment of the stone into the CBD and will increase the risk that the clip will become displaced, leading to a bile leak. If the stone cannot be milked into the gallbladder, a small incision can be made in the cystic duct (as is done for cholangiography), and the stone can usually be expressed and retrieved. Given that cystic duct stones are predictive of CBD stones, cholangiography or intraoperative ultrasonography is indicated.

STEP 5: INTRAOPERATIVE CHOLANGIOGRAPHY

Whether intraoperative cholangiography should be performed routinely is still controversial. Advocates believe that this technique enhances understanding of the biliary anatomy, thus reducing the risk of bile duct injury; at present, however, there are no objective data to confirm this impression. Cholangiography is not a substitute for meticulous dissection, and injuries to the CBD can occur before cystic duct dissection reaches the point at which cholangiography can be performed. Catheter-induced injuries and perforations of the biliary tree have been reported, and cholangiograms have been misinterpreted. On the other hand, one of the main advantages of cholangiography is that injuries can be recognized during the operation and promptly repaired. Another advantage of routine cholangiography is that it helps develop the skills required for more complex biliary tract procedures, such as transcystic CBD exploration.

The two methods of laparoscopic cholangiography differ in their technique for introducing the cholangiogram catheter into the cystic duct. In both approaches, a clip is placed at the gallbladder–cystic duct junction and a small incision made in the anterior wall of the cystic duct. In the first technique, a specially designed 5 mm cholangiogram clamp (the Olsen clamp) with a 5 French catheter is inserted via a subcostal trocar. For easy guidance of the catheter into the incision in the cystic duct, the catheter should be parallel, rather than perpendicular, to the cystic duct. This angle is facilitated by placing the subcostal port directly below the costal margin, near the anterior axillary line. A fifth trocar may occasionally be needed if exposure is lost when one of the grasping forceps is removed to allow passage of the cholangiogram clamp. The clamp and the catheter are then brought to the cystic duct under direct vision, and the catheter is steered into the duct [*see Figure 17*]. The clamp is then closed, holding the catheter in position and sealing the duct to avoid extravasation of dye.

Figure 17 **Laparoscopic cholecystectomy. The cystic duct has been clipped, a small incision has been made for placement of the cholangiogram catheter, and the catheter has been advanced through the specialized cholangiogram clamp into the cystic duct.**

In the second method, the cholangiogram catheter is introduced percutaneously through a 12- to 14-gauge catheter, inserted subcostally as described (see above). The surgeon then grasps the cholangiogram catheter and directs it into the cystic duct. A hemostatic clip is applied to secure the catheter in place. If passage of the catheter into the cystic duct is prevented by Heister's valve, a guide wire can be passed initially.

If the cystic duct is tiny and it is anticipated that cannulation will be difficult or impossible, the gallbladder can be punctured, bile aspirated, and contrast material injected through the gallbladder until the biliary tree is filled.

The cannulas and operating instruments should be positioned so as not to obstruct the view of the biliary tree. If the cannulas cannot be positioned outside the x-ray window, radiolucent cannulas should be used, or the cannulas should be removed and replaced after the cholangiogram. A cholangiogram that does not visualize the biliary tree from the liver to the duodenum is inadequate.

Fluoroscopic cholangiography [*see Figure 18*] may be performed either with hard-copy film or with digital imaging and storage. After the C arm is positioned, with the operating staff protected behind a lead screen, full-strength contrast is slowly injected under fluoroscopic control. The goal is to visualize the biliary tree in its entirety, including the right and left hepatic ductal systems as well as the distal duct. Once the cholangiogram is obtained, the catheter is removed, and the cystic duct is double-clipped and transected.

Laparoscopic Ultrasonography

An emerging alternative for evaluation of the biliary tree is intraoperative laparoscopic ultrasonography, which appears to be as accurate as intraoperative fluorocholangiography in identifying biliary stones. This modality has several advantages over conventional cholangiography: it does not expose patients and staff to radiation; contrast agents are unnecessary; there is no need to cannulate the cystic duct; significantly less time is required; the capital cost of most ultrasound units is less than that of fluoroscopic equipment; and disposable cholangiogram catheters are not needed.

Most of the laparoscopic ultrasound devices in use at present are 7.5 MHz linear-array rigid probes 10 mm in diameter. Flexible probes capable of multiple frequencies are also currently available, and it is likely that future probes will be increasingly versatile. The probe is inserted through a 10/12 mm port (usually a periumbilical or epigastric port) and placed directly on the porta hepatis, perpendicular to the structures of the hepatoduodenal ligament. The probe is then moved to the cystic duct–CBD junction. The transverse image obtained should show the three tubular structures of the hepatoduodenal ligament in the so-called Mickey Mouse head configuration: the CBD, the portal vein, and the hepatic artery [*see Figure 19*]. As the probe is moved distally, it is rotated clockwise to allow identification of the distal CBD and the pancreatic duct where they unite at the papilla. Instillation of saline into the right upper quadrant can enhance acoustic coupling and improve visualization.

Because of its many advantages, intraoperative laparoscopic ultrasonography may eventually replace fluorocholangiography in this setting, particularly for surgeons who practice routine intraoperative evaluation of the CBD. Although the learning curve for effective performance of laparoscopic ultrasound examination is not long, surgeons should receive expert mentoring and formal instruction in ultrasonography before attempting it. During the first few attempts, it may be instructive to perform intraoperative laparoscopic ultrasonography in conjunction with fluorocholangiography.

It should be emphasized that intraoperative laparoscopic ultrasonography is not a replacement for intraoperative cholangiography if the purpose of the examination is to define an anomalous anatomy or to evaluate a suspected injury or leak.

Figure 18 **Laparoscopic cholecystectomy. Shown is a normal intraoperative cholangiogram.**

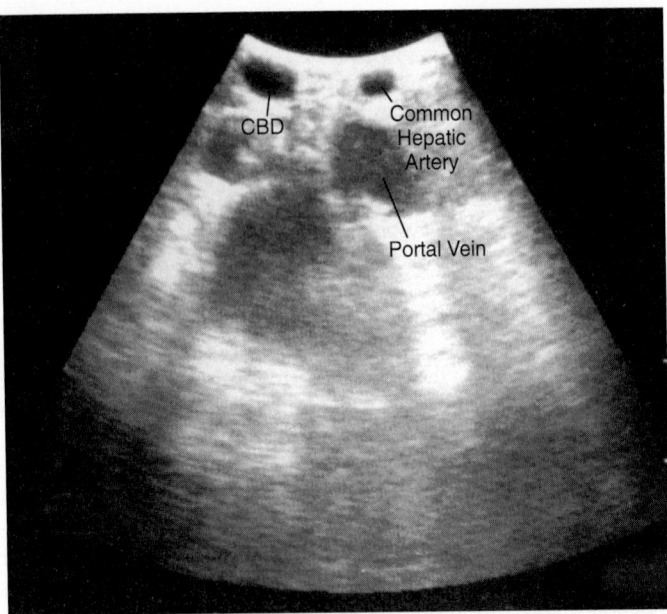

Figure 19 **Laparoscopic cholecystectomy. A transverse intraoperative ultrasound scan of the hepatoduodenal ligament reveals a typical "Mickey Mouse head" appearance. Visible are the CBD, the common hepatic artery, and the portal vein.**

STEP 6: DISSECTION OF GALLBLADDER FROM LIVER BED

The gallbladder is grasped near the cystic duct insertion and pulled down toward the right anterosuperior iliac spine, placing the areolar tissue between the gallbladder and liver anteriorly under tension. The areolar tissue is cauterized with an L-shaped hook dissector or spatula, and dissection is carried upward as far as possible for as long as there is sufficient exposure. When exposure begins to diminish, the cystic duct end of the gallbladder should be pulled up toward or over the left lobe of the liver to expose the posteroinferior attachments of the gallbladder. A two-handed approach by the surgeon facilitates this dissection. It is sometimes helpful to apply downward and lateral traction on the forceps grasping the fundus. Bleeding during this stage generally indicates that the surgeon has entered the wrong plane and dissection has entered the liver. Bleeding can usually be readily controlled with the electrocautery. In some difficult cases (e.g., an intrahepatic gallbladder), it may be prudent to leave some of the posterior wall of the gallbladder in situ and cauterize it rather than persist with an excessively bloody dissection.

Dissection continues until the gallbladder is attached only by a small piece of peritoneum at the fundus. Before the last attachment to the gallbladder is completely divided, the vital clips are reinspected to ensure that they have not slipped off, and the operative field is checked for hemostasis and the presence of any bile leakage. The final attachment to the gallbladder is then divided. The gallbladder is placed over the right lobe of the liver and laterally so that it can be found again to be retrieved. The grasping forceps on the gallbladder should not be removed.

Perforation of Gallbladder

The gallbladder may be accidentally breached at some point in the operation, with the result that bile and stones are spilled into the peritoneal cavity. Efforts should be made to suction the spilled bile, which accumulates in the suprahepatic space, the right subhepatic space, and the lower abdomen because of the

patient's position. Each of these areas should be irrigated and the effluent aspirated until it is clear.

Stones should be located and removed whenever possible. An effective way of removing small stones is to irrigate the subhepatic space copiously. Cholesterol stones usually float on the irrigation fluid and can then be suctioned through a 10 mm suction probe or through a 32 French chest tube passed through the 10 mm operating port. Unfortunately, small stones may be lost in the omentum or between bowel loops. In such cases, it is probably appropriate to leave the stones within the peritoneum rather than perform a laparotomy to attempt to retrieve them. However, there have been reports of serious morbidity, including intra-abdominal abscess, fistula, empyema, and bowel obstruction, resulting from lost stones.

If the gallbladder is perforated and it seems likely that multiple stones will be spilled, the surgeon should introduce a sterile bag into the peritoneal cavity, placing it close to the perforation. Spilled stones can then be transferred immediately into the bag. After the gallbladder is removed from the liver bed, it too is placed in the bag, affording some protection to the wound when it is removed from the abdominal cavity.

STEP 7: EXTRACTION OF GALLBLADDER

The laparoscope is moved to the epigastric port, and a large-tooth grasping forceps is inserted through the umbilical port to grasp the gallbladder at the area of the cystic duct. Under direct vision, the gallbladder is then retrieved and pulled out as far as possible through the umbilical port. If the gallbladder is small enough, it can be drawn right into the trocar sleeve, and it and the trocar can then be removed together. It is sometimes necessary to stretch the fascial opening with a Kelly clamp or to aspirate bile from the gallbladder. It is far preferable to enlarge the incision than to have stones or bile spill into the abdominal cavity from a ripped gallbladder. Enlargement of this incision is easier if initial access was obtained via the Hasson technique. All of the other ports are then removed from the abdominal wall under direct vision to ensure that there is no bleeding. All residual CO_2 should be removed to prevent postoperative shoulder pain. The fascial opening at the umbilicus should be sutured closed to prevent subsequent herniation, and all skin incisions should be closed.

Need for Drainage

The decision to place a drain after laparoscopic cholecystectomy should be governed by the same principles applied to patients undergoing open cholecystectomy. There are two main indications for drainage: (1) the cystic duct was not closed securely, and (2) the CBD was explored by either a direct or a transcystic approach.

Drain placement is easily accomplished. A closed suction drain is inserted intra-abdominally through the 10 mm operative port. A grasping forceps placed through the right lateral port is used to pull one end of the drain out through the abdominal wall. The other end is then positioned according to the surgeon's preference, usually in the subhepatic space.

Complications

INTRAOPERATIVE

Veress Needle Injury

A syringe must always be attached to the Veress needle, and fluid must be aspirated before insufflation is initiated: failure to do so may lead to insufflation into a vessel and consequently to massive gas embolism. If the aspirate from the syringe attached to the Veress needle contains copious amounts of blood, a major vascular injury may have occurred, and immediate laparotomy is indicated. Because the problem at this point is a needle injury, it can usually be repaired easily and without serious sequelae.

Puncture of the bowel by a Veress needle is usually signaled by aspiration of bowel contents through the needle. If this occurs, the needle should be withdrawn and the approximate course and direction of the puncture remembered. The initial trocar should then be inserted by means of the open technique, under direct vision, to ensure that the undersurface of the abdominal wall is free of adherent bowel. Once pneumoperitoneum is created, careful examination of the abdomen through the laparoscope is undertaken. In most cases, either further leakage of bowel contents, staining of the serosal surface with bowel contents, or an ecchymosis on the serosal surface of the bowel helps the surgeon locate the site of the bowel injury. If ecchymosis is present without spillage of bowel contents, the bowel loop should be marked with a suture and reinspected at the end of the procedure. If ongoing leakage of bowel contents is noted, the injured loop of bowel can be either repaired by means of laparoscopic suturing or grasped with an atraumatic forceps and gently withdrawn through an enlarged umbilical incision for suture repair. The bowel is returned to the peritoneal cavity and the laparoscopic cholecystectomy completed.

Improper placement of the Veress needle into the omentum, the retroperitoneum, or the preperitoneal space may be signaled by high inflation pressures, uneven distribution of the gas on percussion, or marked subcutaneous emphysema. If such misplacement goes unrecognized, creation of a safe intraperitoneal space is impossible, and subsequent blind insertion of the trocar may result in injury to an intraperitoneal structure.

Trocar Injury

Trocar injury to blood vessels or bowel is much more dangerous than Veress needle injury to the same structures. Major vascular injuries virtually never occur when trocars are placed under direct vision; however, they remain a potentially lethal—though rare—complication of percutaneous trocar insertion. If active bleeding follows removal of the trocar from the cannula, prompt laparotomy is mandatory; if bleeding passes unnoticed and insufflation begins, massive air embolism will result. At the time of laparotomy, both the anterior and the posterior wall of the vessel must be examined after proximal and distal control of the vessel have been obtained.

Bowel injuries can result from either percutaneous or open insertion of the initial trocar. With open insertion, the bowel injury should be immediately obvious and can be repaired after the injured bowel is pulled through an enlarged umbilical incision; laparoscopic cholecystectomy can then proceed. Bowel injuries caused by percutaneous insertion may occur even in the absence of abdominal wall adhesions and can be managed in the same way as those caused by open insertion. The one caveat is that it is possible to spear the bowel in a through-and-through fashion so that when the laparoscope is inserted through the trocar, the view is normal and the injury is not recognized. This type of injury can be diagnosed only if the laparoscope is repositioned to the operating port at some time during the procedure and the undersurface of the umbilical site is carefully examined. This step is mandatory during the course of the operation, preferably early.

Bleeding

Abdominal wall Bleeding from the abdominal wall can usually be prevented by careful trocar placement. The abdominal wall should be transilluminated before percutaneous trocar insertion and the larger vessels avoided. If a vessel is speared, the cannula usually tamponades the bleeding reasonably effectively during the procedure.

Once the procedure is completed, each trocar is removed under direct vision. If bleeding follows the removal of a trocar, the puncture hole can be occluded with digital pressure to maintain pneumoperitoneum and the bleeding controlled by cauterization or suture repair. Alternatively, the surgeon may place a Foley catheter through the trocar site with a stylet, inflate the balloon, and place traction on the catheter for 4 to 6 hours; however, tissue ischemia can make this technique quite painful.

Omental or mesenteric adhesions Generally, omental adhesions can be bluntly teased from their attachments to the gallbladder, with the plane of dissection kept close to the gallbladder, where the adhesions are less vascular. Adhesions to the liver should be taken down with the electrocautery to prevent capsular tears. Persistent bleeding from omental adhesions is unusual but can be managed by means of electrocauterization (with care taken to avoid damage to the duodenum or colon) or the application of hemostatic clips or a pretied ligating loop.

Cystic artery branch Arterial bleeding encountered during dissection in Calot's triangle is usually due to loss of control of the cystic artery or one of its branches. Biliary surgeons must be aware of the many anatomic variations in the vasculature of the gallbladder and the liver. Because the main cystic artery frequently branches, it is common to find more than one artery if dissection is maintained close to the gallbladder. If what seems to be the main cystic artery is small, a posterior cystic artery may be present and may have to be clipped during the dissection.

Prevention of arterial bleeding begins by dissecting the artery carefully and completely before clipping and by inspecting of the clips to ensure that they are placed completely across the artery without incorporating additional tissue (e.g., a posterior cystic artery or right hepatic artery). When arterial bleeding is encountered, it is essential to maintain adequate exposure and to avoid blind application of hemostatic clips or cauterization. The laparoscope should be withdrawn slightly so that the lens is not spattered with blood. The surgeon should then pass an atraumatic grasping forceps through a port other than the operating port and attempt to grasp the bleeding vessel. An additional trocar may have to be inserted for simultaneous suction-irrigation. Once proximal control is obtained, the operative field should be suctioned and irrigated to improve exposure. Hemostatic clips are then applied under direct vision; in addition, a sponge may be introduced to apply pressure to the bleeding vessel. Conversion to open cholecystectomy is indicated whenever bleeding cannot be promptly controlled laparoscopically.

Liver bed Bleeding from the liver bed may be encountered when the wrong plane is developed during dissection of the gallbladder. Patients who have portal hypertension, cirrhosis, or coagulation disorders are at particularly high risk. Control of bleeding requires good exposure, accomplished via lateral and superior retraction of the gallbladder; hence, all bleeding should be controlled before the gallbladder is detached from the liver bed. Most liver bed bleeding can be controlled with the electrocautery, and

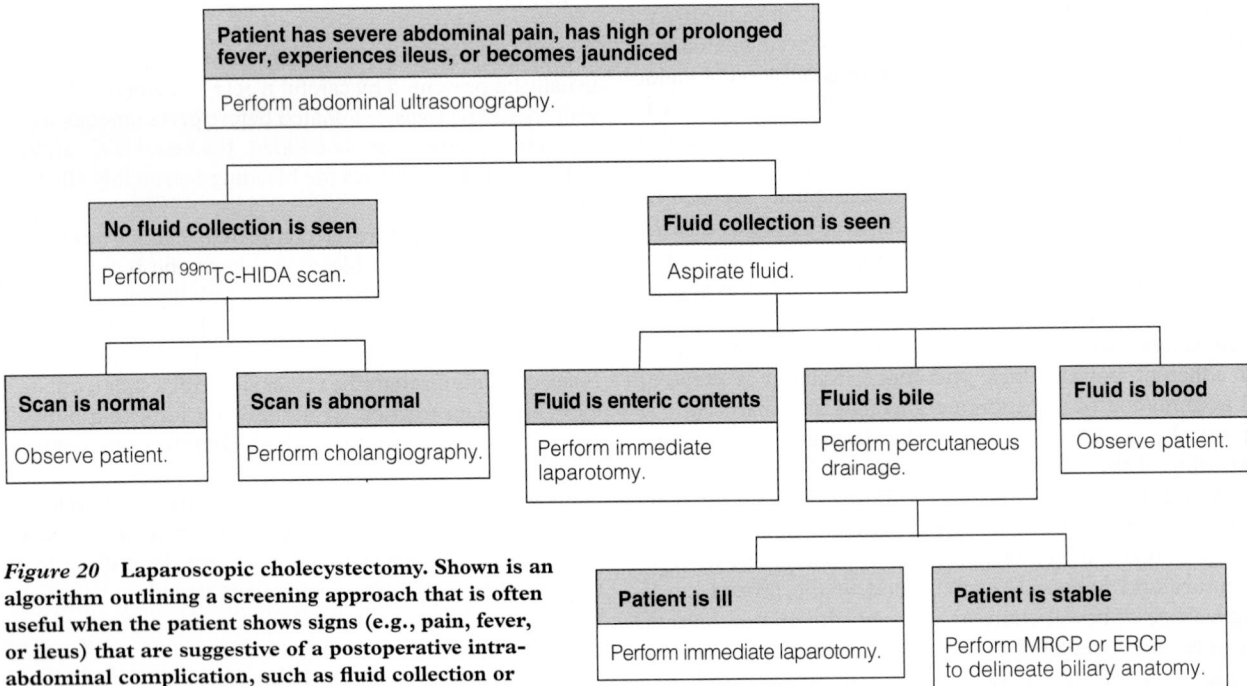

Figure 20 **Laparoscopic cholecystectomy. Shown is an algorithm outlining a screening approach that is often useful when the patient shows signs (e.g., pain, fever, or ileus) that are suggestive of a postoperative intra-abdominal complication, such as fluid collection or bile leakage.**

it should be controlled as it is encountered to allow exposure of the specific bleeding site. Either a hook-shaped or a spatula-shaped coagulation electrode is effective. If oozing continues, oxidized cellulose can be placed as a pack through the operative port and pressure applied on the raw surface of the liver. If needed, fibrin glue can be applied to the bleeding raw surface.

POSTOPERATIVE

If a patient (1) complains of a great deal of abdominal pain necessitating systemic narcotics, (2) has a high or prolonged fever, (3) experiences ileus, or (4) becomes jaundiced, an intra-abdominal complication may have occurred. Blood should be drawn so that the white blood cell count, the hemoglobin concentration, liver function, and the serum amylase level can be assessed. Abdominal ultrasonography may help diagnose dilated intrahepatic ducts and subhepatic fluid collections [*see Figure 20*].

Fluid Collection or Bile Leakage

When a significant fluid collection is seen, it should be aspirated percutaneously under ultrasonographic guidance. If the fluid is blood and the patient is hemodynamically stable and requires no transfusion, observation of the patient and culture of the fluid are usually sufficient. If the fluid is enteric contents, immediate laparotomy is indicated. If the fluid is bile and the patient is ill, immediate laparotomy should be considered; if the patient is stable and the appropriate facilities are available, MRCP or ERCP may be performed to identify the site of bile leakage, determine whether obstruction is also present, and assess the integrity of the extrahepatic biliary tree. If the bile ducts are in continuity and the bile is coming from the cystic duct stump or a small lateral tear in the bile duct, ES, with or without stenting, usually controls the leak. Percutaneous placement of a drain under ultrasonographic guidance allows control of the bile leakage and measurement of the quantity of fluid present.

Fever

Postoperative fever is a common complication of laparoscopic cholecystectomy. As noted, it may be indicative of a postopera-

tive complication such as a bile collection or bile leakage. Other common reasons for postoperative fever (e.g., atelectasis) should also be considered.

Abnormal Liver Function

When postoperative blood tests indicate significantly abnormal liver function, possible causes include injury to the biliary tree and retained CBD stones [*see Figure 21*]. Cholangiography is required, even if it was performed intraoperatively. If MRCP or ERCP yields normal results, observation is sufficient; the abnormalities may be attributable to a passed stone or drug-related cholestasis. If stones are present, ES can usually solve the problem. If ERCP demonstrates extravasation of bile, it is important to establish whether the CBD is in continuity. If the duct is interrupted, early reoperation, ideally at a specialized center, is the best option. If the duct is in continuity, endoscopic and radiologic techniques may successfully resolve the problem without substantial morbidity. Percutaneous drainage is instituted to control the fistula, and sphincterotomy or stenting is useful to overcome any resistance at the sphincter of Oddi. Any retained stones causing distal obstruction should also be removed.

Major ductal injuries usually call for operative repair. When such an injury is identified at operation, the surgeon must decide whether to attempt repair immediately or not; this decision should be based on the surgeon's experience with reconstructive biliary surgery and on the local expertise available. At a minimum, adequate drainage must be established. Most major ductal injuries are not in fact identified intraoperatively. When such an injury is identified postoperatively, adequate drainage must be established and the anatomy of the injury clarified as well as possible before repair. MRCP or transhepatic cholangiography may be required to delineate the anatomy of the proximal biliary tree when ERCP does not opacify the biliary tract above the injury. If surgical repair is indicated, it should be performed by a surgeon experienced in complex biliary tract procedures. Often, referral to a specialized center is the most appropriate decision, especially in the case of more proximal biliary injuries.

Postoperative liver function tests yield abnormal results

Perform ERCP to detect biliary tree injury or retained CBD stones.

ERCP yields normal results

Observe patient.

ERCP reveals presence of CBD stones

Perform ES.

ERCP reveals leakage of bile

Determine whether CBD is in continuity.

Duct is completely interrupted or lacks continuity

Reoperate at an early stage.

Duct is in continuity

Perform percutaneous drainage in conjunction with ES or endoscopic stenting.

Remove any retained stones.

Figure 21 **Laparoscopic cholecystectomy. Shown is an algorithm outlining an approach to abnormal liver function test results after laparoscopic cholecystectomy.**

Special Problems

CONVERSION TO LAPAROTOMY

Conversion from laparoscopy to laparotomy may be required in any laparoscopic cholecystectomy, in accordance with the judgment of the surgeon. The most common reason for such conversion is the inability to identify important anatomic structures in the region of the gallbladder. Distorted anatomy may be the result of previous operations, inflammation, or anatomic variations. Conversion may also be required because of an intraoperative complication [*see* Complications, Postoperative, *above*]. Ideally, the surgeon would wish to convert before any complication occurs. It must be emphasized that conversion to open surgery should not be considered a failure or a complication. Rather, it should be considered a prudent maneuver for achieving the desired objective—namely, safe removal of the gallbladder. Accordingly, every patient consent obtained for a laparoscopic cholecystectomy must explicitly allow for the possibility of conversion to an open procedure.

Attempts have been made to predict the probability of conversion on the basis of preoperative information. It is clearly useful to stratify patients according to likelihood of conversion. This information is helpful in selecting patients for laparoscopic cholecystectomy in an outpatient versus hospital setting, in determining the resources required in the OR, and in assisting patients in planning their work and family needs around the time of surgery.

Factors found to be predictive of an increased probability of conversion include acute cholecystitis, either at the time of surgery or at any point in the past; age greater than 65 years; male sex; and thickening of the gallbladder wall to more than 3 mm as measured by ultrasonography. Other factors more variably associated with an increased likelihood of conversion are obesity, previous upper abdominal operations (especially gastroduodenal), multiple gallbladder attacks over a long period, and severe pancreatitis. Factors not associated with an increased likelihood of conversion are jaundice, previous ES, previous lower abdominal procedures, stomas, mild pancreatitis, and diabetes.

On the basis of our data, a 45-year-old woman with no history of acute cholecystitis and no gallbladder wall thickening has a probability of conversion lower than 1%; such a patient is a good candidate for laparoscopic cholecystectomy in an outpatient setting. Conversely, a 70-year-old man with acute cholecystitis and ultrasonographic evidence of gallbladder wall thickening has a probability of conversion of about 30%; such a patient would be better managed in a traditional hospital environment.

ACUTE CHOLECYSTITIS

Laparoscopic cholecystectomy has been shown to be safe and effective for treating acute cholecystitis. There are, however, several technical problems in this setting that must be addressed if the procedure is to be performed with minimal risk. It should also be recognized that the probability of conversion to laparotomy is greatly increased in these circumstances. There appears to be no advantage to delaying surgery in patients with acute cholecystitis, even if rapid improvement is noted with nonoperative management. Many patients return within a short time with recurrent attacks, and delaying surgery does not reduce the probability of conversion.

Technical difficulties associated with cholecystectomy for acute cholecystitis include dense adhesions, the increased vascularity of tissues, difficulty in grasping the gallbladder, an impacted stone in the gallbladder neck or the cystic duct, shortening and thickening of the cystic duct, and close approximation of the CBD to the gallbladder wall.

The surgeon should not hesitate to insert additional ports (e.g., for a suction-irrigation apparatus) if necessary. Because the tense, distended gallbladder is difficult to grasp reliably, it should be aspirated through the fundus early in the procedure, as previously described. If the graspers fail to grasp the wall or cause it to tear, exposure of Calot's triangle can be achieved by propping up or levering the neck of the gallbladder and the right liver with a blunt instrument. A sponge can be used for this purpose, thereby reducing the potential trauma of the retraction. This maneuver is also useful when an impacted stone in the neck of the gallbladder prevents the surgeon from grasping the gallbladder in the area of Hartmann's pouch. Dense adhesions that may be present between the gallbladder and the omentum, duodenum, or colon should be dissected bluntly (e.g., with a suction tip). Because the tissues are friable and vascular, oozing may be encountered. Electrocauterization should be only sparingly employed until the vital structures in Calot's triangle are identified. Instead, the surgeon should move to another area of dissection, allowing most of the oozing to coagulate on its own. Liberal use of suction and irrigation will keep the operative field free of blood.

In the identification of anatomic structures, it is important to keep dissection close to the gallbladder wall, working down from the gallbladder toward Calot's triangle. Dissection of the lower part of the gallbladder from the liver bed early in the operation may aid in identification of the gallbladder neck–cystic duct junction (analogous to an open, retrograde dissection). The surgeon should be aware that edema and acute inflammation may cause foreshortening of the cystic duct. If the anatomy cannot be identified, preliminary cholangiography through the emptied gallbladder may indicate the position of the cystic duct and the CBD.

Often, the obstructing stone responsible for the acute attack is in the neck of the gallbladder; thus, the cystic duct will be normal and easily secured with clips. If the stone is in the cystic duct, it must be removed before the duct is clipped or ligated. A thickened, edematous cystic duct is better controlled by ligation with an extracorporeal tie or a ligating loop than by clipping. If closure of the cystic duct is tenuous, closed suction drainage is advisable. Obviously, conversion to open cholecystectomy is indicated if the anatomy remains obscure. Conversion should also be considered if no progress is made after a predesignated period (e.g., 15 minutes) because at this point, the surgeon is unlikely to make any headway.

CBD STONES

Identification of Patients at Risk

About 10% of all patients undergoing cholecystectomy for gallstones will also have choledocholithiasis. To select from the various diagnostic and therapeutic options for managing choledocholithiasis, it is helpful to know preoperatively whether the patient is at high, moderate, or low risk for stones. Patients with obvious clinical jaundice or cholangitis, a dilated CBD, or stones visualized in the CBD on preoperative ultrasonography are likely to have choledocholithiasis (risk > 50%). Patients who have a history of jaundice or pancreatitis, elevated preoperative levels of alkaline phosphatase or bilirubin, or ultrasonographic evidence of multiple small gallstones are somewhat less likely to have choledocholithiasis (risk, 10% to 50%). Patients with large gallstones, no history of jaundice or pancreatitis, and normal liver function are unlikely to have choledocholithiasis (risk < 5%).

Diagnostic and Therapeutic Options

One argument for routine intraoperative cholangiography is that it is a good way of identifying unsuspected CBD stones. However, more selective approaches to diagnosing choledocholithiasis make use of preoperative cholangiography via MRCP, EUS, or, more invasively, ERCP [see V:6 Gastrointestinal Endoscopy]. Preoperative identification of choledocholithiasis allows the surgeon to attempt preoperative clearance of the CBD by means of ES or intraoperative clearance during laparoscopy, depending on his or her expertise. Preoperative cholangiography is suggested when the patient's history and the results of laboratory and diagnostic tests suggest that there is a moderate or high risk of CBD stones. It is our practice to have patients at high risk for CBD stones undergo ERCP and ES if warranted. For patients at moderate risk, MRCP or EUS is done first, followed by therapeutic ERCP if CBD stones are identified. Intraoperative cholangiography can also be used to identify choledocholithiasis. ERCP with ES may result in pancreatitis, perforation, or bleeding and carries a mortality of approximately 0.2%.

When stones are detected during the operation, the options include laparoscopic transcystic duct exploration, laparoscopic choledochotomy and CBD exploration, open CBD exploration, and postoperative ERCP/ES. If a single small (2 mm) stone is visualized, it can probably be flushed into the duodenum by flushing the CBD via the cholangiogram catheter and administering glucagons 1 to 2 mg I.V., to relax the sphincter of Oddi. Even if a stone of this size does not pass intraoperatively, it will usually pass on its own postoperatively.

Laparoscopic Transcystic CBD Exploration

Access to biliary tree   The cholangiogram is reviewed; the size of the cystic duct, the site where the cystic duct inserts into the CBD, and the size and location of the CBD stones all contribute to the success or failure of transcystic CBD exploration. For example, transcystic exploration is extremely challenging in a patient who has a long, spiraling cystic duct with a medial insertion. The size of the stones to be removed dictates the approach to the CBD: stones smaller than 4 mm can usually be retrieved in fluoroscopically directed baskets and generally do not necessitate cystic duct dilatation; larger stones (4 to 8 mm) are retrieved under direct vision with the choledochoscope.

A hydrophilic guide wire is inserted through the cholangiogram catheter into the CBD under fluoroscopic guidance. The cholangiogram catheter is then removed. If the largest stone is larger than the cystic duct, dilatation of the duct is necessary, not only for passage of the stone but also to allow passage of the choledochoscope, which may be 3 to 5 mm in diameter.

Dilatation is accomplished with either a balloon dilator or sequential plastic dilators. Because plastic dilators may cause the cystic duct to split, balloon dilatation is recommended. A balloon 3 to 5 cm in length is passed over the guide wire and positioned with its distal end just inside the CBD and its proximal end just outside the incision in the cystic duct. The balloon is then inflated to the pressure recommended by the manufacturer and observed closely for evidence of shearing of the cystic duct. The cystic duct should not be dilated to a diameter greater than 8 mm. Larger stones in the CBD may be either fragmented with electrohydraulic or mechanical lithotripsy, if available, or removed via choledochotomy.

Once dilatation is complete, the guide wire may be removed or left in place to guide passage of a choledochoscope or baskets. When the choledochoscope is used, a second incision in the cystic duct, close to the CBD, avoids Heister's valve and allows removal of the guide wire. If baskets are used, a 6 French plastic introducer sheath may be inserted through the trocar used for cholangiography into the cystic duct. This sheath is especially useful if multiple stones must be removed.

Fluoroscopic wire basket transcystic CBD exploration
Stones smaller than 2 to 4 mm that do not pass with irrigation through the cholangiocatheter after injection of glucagon can usually be retrieved by using a 4 French or 5 French helical stone basket passed into the CBD over a guide wire under fluoroscopic guidance. The baskets can be passed alongside the cholangiocatheter or inserted via a plastic sheath replacing the cholangiocatheter. The basket is opened in the ampulla of Vater, pulled back into the CBD, and rotated clockwise until the stone is entrapped. The stone and basket are then removed together. A Fogarty catheter should not be used, because the stones are likely to be pulled up into the hepatic ducts, where they are much more difficult to remove.

Endoscopic transcystic CBD exploration   When stones are 4 to 8 mm in diameter, the helical stone basket wires are generally too close together to permit retrieval. Hence, choledochoscopic basketing is utilized. A 7 to 10 French choledochoscope with a working channel is either passed over the guide wire or inserted directly into the cystic duct. Because the usual grasping forceps may damage the choledochoscope, forceps with rubber-covered jaws should be used. A separate camera should be inserted onto the choledochoscope, and the image it produces can be displayed on the monitor by means of an audiovisual mixer (i.e., a picture within a picture) or displayed on a separate monitor.

Once the choledochoscope enters the cystic duct, warm saline irrigation is begun under low pressure to distend the CBD and provide a working space. The choledochoscope usually enters the CBD rather than the common hepatic duct. When a stone is seen, a 2.4 French straight four-wire basket is inserted through the operating port. The stones closest to the cystic duct are removed first, by advancing the closed basket beyond each stone, opening the basket, and pulling the basket back, thereby trapping the stone. The basket is then closed and pulled up against the choledochoscope so that they can be withdrawn as a unit. Multiple passes may be required until the duct is clear. A completion cholangiogram is done to ensure that the duct is clear and to rule out proximal stones. The dilated, traumatized cystic duct is ligated with a ligating loop rather than a hemostatic clip. If drainage is required, a red rubber catheter can be inserted into the CBD via the cystic duct.

Because of the angle created by the cephalad and superior retraction of the gallbladder, it may be difficult to pass the choledochoscope into the proximal ducts. If a common hepatic duct stone is seen on the cholangiogram, the patient is placed in a steep reverse Trendelenburg position. In this position, any nonimpacted stones may fall into the distal duct for retrieval. It may be possible to pass the choledochoscope into the proximal ducts by applying caudal traction to the cystic duct so as to align it with the common hepatic duct. An additional access port in the right upper quadrant may be needed. If the cystic duct is long or spiraling or inserts medially, this measure may not be feasible, in which case access must be obtained by means of choledochotomy.

Laparoscopic CBD Exploration

Large stones (> 1 cm), as well as most stones in the common hepatic ducts, are not retrievable with the techniques described above. Ductal clearance can be achieved via choledochotomy if the duct is dilated and the surgeon is sufficiently experienced.

The anterior wall of the CBD is bluntly dissected for a distance of 1 to 2 cm. When small vessels are encountered, it is preferable to apply pressure and wait for hemostasis rather than use the electrocautery in this area. Two stay sutures are placed in the CBD. An additional 5 mm trocar is placed in the right lower quadrant for insertion of an additional needle driver. A small longitudinal choledochotomy (a few millimeters longer than the circumference of the largest stone) is made with curved microscissors on the anterior aspect of the duct while the stay sutures are elevated. A choledochoscope is then inserted and warm saline irrigation initiated. In most cases, baskets should suffice for stone retrieval; however, lithotriptor probes and lasers are available for use through the working channel of the choledochoscope. The choice of approach depends on availability and individual surgical experience.

Subsequently, a 12 or 14 French latex T tube is fashioned with short limbs, placed entirely intraperitoneally to prevent CO_2 from escaping, and positioned in the CBD. The choledochotomy is then closed with fine interrupted absorbable sutures. The first suture is placed right next to the T tube, securing it distally, and the second is placed at the most proximal end of the choledochotomy; lifting these two sutures facilitates placement of additional sutures. Intracorporeal knots are preferred to avoid sawing of the delicate tissues. The end of the T tube is then pulled out through a trocar, and cholangiography is performed after completion of the procedure.

Bibliography

GENERAL REFERENCES

Asbun HJ, Rossi RL: Techniques of laparoscopic cholecystectomy: the difficult operation. Surg Clin North Am 74:755, 1994

Barkun JS, Barkun AN, Sampalis JS, et al: Randomised controlled trial of laparoscopic versus mini cholecystectomy. The McGill Gallstone Treatment Group. Lancet 340:1116, 1992

Bass EB, Pitt HA, Lillemoe KD: Cost-effectiveness of laparoscopic cholecystectomy versus open cholecystectomy. Am J Surg 165:466, 1993

Crist DW, Gadacz TR: Laparoscopic anatomy of the biliary tree. Surg Clin North Am 73:785, 1993

Deziel D: Complications of cholecystectomy: incidence, clinical manifestations and diagnosis. Surg Clin North Am 74:809, 1994

Kane RL, Lurie N, Borbas C, et al: The outcomes of elective laparoscopic and open cholecystectomies. J Am Coll Surg 180:136, 1995

Lam D, Miranda R, Hom SJ: Laparoscopic cholecystectomy as an outpatient procedure. J Am Coll Surg 185:152, 1997

Management of the complicated gallbladder. Semin Laparosc Surg Vol 5 No 2. Cuschieri A, MacFadyen BV Jr, Eds, 1998

Mühe E: Die erste: cholecystecktomie durch das laparoskop. Langenbecks Arch Klin Chir 369:804, 1986

National Institutes of Health Consensus Development Conference Statement on Gallstones and Laparoscopic Cholecystectomy. Am J Surg 165:390, 1993

Society of American Gastrointestinal Endoscopic Surgeons: Guidelines for the clinical application of laparoscopic biliary tract surgery. Surg Endosc 8:1457, 1994

Traverso LW, Hargrave K: A prospective cost analysis of laparoscopic cholecystectomy. Am J Surg 169:503, 1995

Wherry DC, Rob CG, Marohn MR, et al: An external audit of laparoscopic cholecystectomy performed in medical treatment facilities of the Department of Defense. Ann Surg 220:626, 1994

PATIENT SELECTION

Amos JD, Schorr SJ, Norman PF, et al: Laparoscopic surgery during pregnancy. Am J Surg 171:435, 1996

Angrisani L, Lorenzo M, De Palma G, et al: Laparoscopic cholecystectomy in obese patients compared with nonobese patients. Surg Laparosc Endosc 5:197, 1995

Curet MJ: Special problems in laparoscopic surgery: previous abdominal surgery, obesity, and pregnancy. Surg Clin North Am 80:1093, 2000

Curet MJ, Allen D, Josloff RK, et al: Laparoscopy during pregnancy. Arch Surg 131:546, 1996

Fried GM, Clas D, Meakins JL: Minimally invasive surgery in the elderly patient. Surg Clin North Am 74:375, 1994

Lacy AM, Balaguer C, Andrade E, et al: Laparoscopic cholecystectomy in cirrhotic patients: indication or contraindication? Surg Endosc 9:407, 1995

SAGES Committee on Standards of Practice. SAGES Guidelines for Laparoscopic Surgery During Pregnancy. SAGES Publication #0023. Society of American Gastrointestinal Endoscopic Surgeons (SAGES), Santa Monica, California, 2000

Steinbrook RA, Brooks DC, Datta S: Laparoscopic cholecystectomy during pregnancy: review of anesthetic management, surgical considerations. Surg Endosc 10:511, 1996

Tanner AG, Hartley JE, Darzi A, et al: Laparoscopic surgery in patients with human immunodeficiency virus. Br J Surg 81:1647, 1994

ESTABLISHMENT OF PNEUMOPERITONEUM

Bhoyrul S, Vierra MA, Nezhat CR, et al: Trocar injuries in laparoscopic surgery. J Am Coll Surg 192:677, 2001

Sigman HH, Fried GM, Garzon J, et al: Risks of blind versus open approach to celiotomy for laparoscopic surgery. Surg Laparosc Endosc 3:296, 1993

CHOLANGIOGRAPHY AND THE MANAGEMENT OF COMMON BILE DUCT STONES

Abboud PC, Malet PF, Berlin JA, et al: Predictors of common bile duct stones prior to cholecystectomy: a meta-analysis. Gastrointest Endosc 44:450, 1996

Barkun AN, Barkun JS, Fried GM, et al: Useful predictors of bile duct stones in patients undergoing laparoscopic cholecystectomy. McGill Gallstone Treatment Group. Ann Surg 220:32, 1994

Barkun JS, Fried GM, Barkun AN, et al: Cholecystectomy without operative cholangiography: implications for common bile duct injury and retained common bile duct stones. Ann Surg 218:371, 1993

Clair DG, Brooks DC: Laparoscopic cholangiography: the case for a selective approach. Surg Clin North Am 74:961, 1994

Cotton PB: Endoscopic retrograde cholangiopancreatography and laparoscopic cholecystectomy. Am J Surg 165:474, 1993

Crawford DL, Phillips EH: Laparoscopic common duct exploration. World J Surg 23:343, 1999

Cuschieri A, Lezoche E, Morino M, et al: E.A.E.S. multicenter prospective randomised trial comparing two-stage vs single-stage management of patients with gallstone disease and ductal calculi. Surg Endosc 13:952, 1999

Freeman ML, Nelson DB, Sherman S, et al: Complications of endoscopic biliary sphincterotomy. N Engl J Med 335:909, 1996

Guibaud L, Bret PM, Reinhold C, et al: Bile duct obstruction and choledocholithiasis: diagnosis with MR cholangiography. Radiology 197:109, 1995

Halpin VJ, Dunnegan D, Soper NJ: Laproscopic intracorporeal ultrasound vs fluoroscopic intraoperative cholangiography. Surg Endosc 16:336, 2002

Hunter JG, Trus T: Laparoscopic cholecystectomy,

intraoperative cholangiography, and common bile duct exploration. Mastery of Surgery, 3rd ed, Nyhus LM, Baker RJ, Fischer JE, Eds. Little, Brown & Co, New York, 1997

Hunter JG: Laparoscopic transcystic common bile duct exploration. Am J Surg 163:53, 1992

Hunter JG, Soper NJ: Laparoscopic management of bile duct stones. Surg Clin North Am 72:1077, 1992

Jones DB, Soper NJ: Common duct stones. Current Surgical Therapy, 5th ed, Cameron JL, Ed. Mosby-Year Book, St. Louis, 1995

Korman J, Cosgrove J, Furman M, et al: The role of endoscopic retrograde cholangiopancreatography and cholangiography in the laparoscopic era. Ann Surg 223:212, 1996

Liberman MA, Phillips EH, Carroll BJ, et al: Cost-effective management of complicated choledocholithiasis: laparoscopic transcystic duct exploration or endoscopic sphincterotomy. J Am Coll Surg 182:488, 1996

Mahmud S, Hamza Y, Nassar AHM: The significance of cystic duct stones encountered during laparoscopic cholecystectomy. Surg Endosc 15:460, 2001

Menack MJ, Arregui ME: Laparoscopic sonography of the biliary tree and pancreas. Surg Clin North Am 80:1151, 2000

Musella M, Barbalace G, Capparelli G, et al: Magnetic resonance imaging in evaluation of the common bile duct. Br J Surg 85:16, 1998

National Institute of Health State-Of-The-Science Conference statement. Endoscopic retrograde cholangiopancreatography (ERCP) for diagnosis and therapy. Draft statement, January 14–16, 2002

Ohtani T, Kawai C, Shirai Y, et al: Intraoperative ultrasonography versus cholangiography during laparoscopic cholecystectomy: a prospective comparative study. J Am Coll Surg 185:274, 1997

Park AE, Mastrangelo MJ: Endoscopic retrograde cholangiopancreatography in the management of choledocholitiasis. Surg Endosc 14:219, 2000

Paul A, Millat B, Holthhausen U, et al: Diagnosis and treatment of common bile duct stones (CBDS): results of a consensus development conference. Surg Endosc 12:856, 1998

Petelin JB: Laparoscopic approach to common duct pathology. Am J Surg 165:487, 1993

Phillips EH: Choledochotomy in laparoscopy. Operative Laparoscopy and Thoracoscopy. MacFadyen BV, Ponsky JL, Eds. Lippincott-Raven Publishers, Philadelphia, 1996

Phillips EH: Laparoscopic transcystic duct common bile duct exploration-outcome and costs. Surg Endosc 9:1240, 1995

Phillips EH: Controversies in the management of common duct calculi. Surg Clin North Am 74:931, 1994

Phillips EH, Carroll BJ, Pearlstein AR, et al: Laparoscopic choledochoscopy and extraction of common bile duct stones. World J Surg 17:22, 1993

Rhodes M, Sussman L, Cohen L, et al: Randomized trial of laparoscopic exploration of common bile duct versus postoperative endoscopic retrograde cholan-giography for common bile duct stones. Lancet 351:159, 1998

Soper NJ, Brunt LM: The case for routine operative cholangiography during laparoscopic cholecystectomy. Surg Clin North Am 74:953, 1994

Voyles CR, Sanders DL, Hogan R: Common bile duct evaluation in the era of laparoscopic cholecystectomy: 1050 cases later. Ann Surg 219:744, 1994

Wu JS, Dunnegan DL, Soper NJ: The utility of intra-corporeal ultrasonography for screening of the bile duct during laparoscopic cholecystectomy. J Gastrointest Surg 2:50, 1998

Zucker KA, Josloff RK: Transcystic common bile duct exploration. Operative Laparoscopy and Thoracoscopy. MacFadyen BV, Ponsky JL, Eds. Lippincott-Raven Publishers, Philadelphia, 1996

CONVERSION TO OPEN CHOLECYSTECTOMY

Fried GM, Barkun JS, Sigman HH, et al: Factors determining conversion to laparotomy in patients undergoing laparoscopic cholecystectomy. Am J Surg 167:35, 1994

Sanabria JR, Gallinger S, Croxford R, et al: Risk factors in elective laparoscopic cholecystectomy for conversion to open cholecystectomy. J Am Coll Surg 179:696, 1994

Schrenk P, Woisetschlager R, Wayand WU: Laparoscopic cholecystectomy: cause of conversions in 1300 patients and analysis of risk factors. Surg Endosc 9:25, 1995

COMPLICATIONS OF LAPAROSCOPIC CHOLECYSTECTOMY

Bernard HR, Hartman TW: Complications after laparoscopic cholecystectomy. Am J Surg 165:533, 1993

Branum G, Schmitt C, Baillie J, et al: Management of major biliary complications after laparoscopic cholecystectomy. Ann Surg 217:532, 1993

Deziel DJ: Complications of cholecystectomy: incidence, clinical manifestations, and diagnosis. Surg Clin North Am 74:809, 1994

Deziel DJ, Millikan KW, Economou SG, et al: Complications of laparoscopic cholecystectomy: a national survey of 4,292 hospitals and an analysis of 77,604 cases. Am J Surg 165:9, 1993

Fletcher DR, Hobbs MST, Tan P, et al: Complications of cholecystectomy: risks of the laparoscopic approach and protective effects of operative cholangiography. Ann Surg 229:449, 1999

Halevy A, Gold-Deutch R, Negri M, et al: Are elevated liver enzymes and bilirubin levels significant after laparoscopic cholecystectomy in the absence of bile duct injury? Ann Surg 219:362, 1994

Hunter JG: Avoidance of bile duct injury during laparoscopic cholecystectomy. Am J Surg 162:71, 1991

Jatzko GR, Lisborg PH, Pertl AM, et al: Multivariate comparison of complications after laparoscopic cholecystectomy and open cholecystectomy. Ann Surg 221:381, 1995

Lillemoe KD, Martin SA, Cameron JL, et al: Major bile duct injuries during laparoscopic cholecystectomy: follow-up after combined surgical and radiologic management. Ann Surg 225:459, 1997

MacFadyen BV, Vecchio R, Ricardo AE, et al: Bile duct injury after laparoscopic cholecystectomy: the United States experience. Surg Endosc 12:315, 1998

Martin RF, Rossi RL: Bile duct injuries: spectrum, mechanisms of injury, and their prevention. Surg Clin North Am 74:781, 1994

McGahan JP, Stein M: Complications of laparoscopic cholecystectomy: imaging and intervention. AJR Am J Roentgenol 165:1089, 1995

Millitz K, Moote DJ, Sparrow RK, et al: Pneumoperitoneum after laparoscopic cholecystectomy: frequency and duration as seen on upright chest radiographs. AJR Am J Roentgenol 163:837, 1994

Olsen D: Bile duct injuries during laparoscopic cholecystectomy. Surg Endosc 11:133, 1997

Ponsky JL: Endoscopic approaches to common bile duct injuries. Surg Clin North Am 76:505, 1996

Ress AM, Sarr MG, Nagorney DM, et al: Spectrum and management of major complications of laparoscopic cholecystectomy. Am J Surg 165:655, 1993

Soper NJ, Flye MW, Brunt LM, et al: Diagnosis and management of biliary complications of laparoscopic cholecystectomy. Am J Surg 165:663, 1993

Strasberg SM, Hertl M, Soper NJ: An analysis of the problem of biliary injury during laparoscopic cholecystectomy. J Am Coll Surg 180:101, 1995

Woods MS, Traverso LW, Kozarek RA, et al: Characteristics of biliary tract complications during laparoscopic cholecystectomy: a multi-institutional study. Am J Surg 167:27, 1994

ACUTE CHOLECYSTITIS

Koo KP, Thirlby RC: Laparoscopic cholecystectomy in acute cholecystitis: what is the optimal timing for operation? Arch Surg 131:540, 1996

Lo CM, Liu CL, Lai EC, et al: Early versus delayed laparoscopic cholecystectomy for treatment of acute cholecystitis. Ann Surg 223:37, 1996

Rattner DW, Ferguson C, Warshaw AL: Factors associated with successful laparoscopic cholecystectomy for acute cholecystitis. Ann Surg 217:233, 1993

Zucker KA, Flowers JL, Bailey RW, et al: Laparoscopic management of acute cholecystitis. Am J Surg 165:508, 1993

Acknowledgments

Figures 2, 3, 6   Tom Moore.
Figure 19   Courtesy of Nathaniel J. Soper, M.D., Washington University School of Medicine, St. Louis.

13 PANCREATIC PROCEDURES

Keith D. Lillemoe, M.D., and John L. Cameron, M.D.

Pylorus-Preserving Pancreaticoduodenectomy (Whipple Procedure)

Surgical resection of a periampullary carcinoma can be accomplished by means of either a pylorus-preserving pancreaticoduodenectomy or the classic resection (including an antrectomy). The decision is usually made on the basis of individual surgeon preference (unless there is obvious tumor encroachment on the first portion of the duodenum). Neither approach appears to have a proven advantage in terms of either relative ease of performance or short- or long-term outcome (including survival). In the ensuing technical description, we focus primarily on the pylorus-preserving modification but also refer to certain important components of the classic Whipple resection.

The peritoneal cavity is entered through either an upper midline or a bilateral subcostal incision, and the abdomen is thoroughly explored. The head of the pancreas and the duodenum are extensively mobilized out of the retroperitoneum via the Kocher maneuver. (This extensive kocherization allows one to palpate the superior mesenteric artery to confirm that the tumor has not extended from the uncinate process to involve the vessel. It is distinctly unusual for the tumor to extend directly posteriorly into the aorta or the inferior vena cava.) If there is no evidence of local or regional spread to serosal surfaces or the liver, the gallbladder is mobilized out of the liver bed. The common hepatic duct is identified, circumferentially dissected, and then divided [*see Figure 1*]. A complete rim of the duct is sent for frozen section examination.

Once the common hepatic duct has been divided, the anterior surface of the portal vein is easily and quickly identified. The lymph node tissue lateral to the hepatic duct and the portal vein should be dissected off the structures to be included in the surgical specimen. A replaced right hepatic artery is a commonly found anatomic variant in this location; if present, it must be recognized and preserved. If one finds the appropriate plane directly on the anterior surface of the portal vein, one can use a combination of sharp and blunt dissection to develop a plane between the vein and the first portion of the duodenum and the neck of the pancreas; usually, there are no veins joining the anterior surface of the portal vein, and the maneuver can be carried out with no resistance. If this maneuver is difficult, the gastroduodenal artery should be identified where it comes off the common hepatic artery. This artery should first be clamped with a nonoccluding vascular clamp to ensure that the pulse in the hepatic artery is preserved. (Loss of a hepatic artery pulse may suggest misidentification of the vessel or an aberrant blood flow pattern attributable to a congenital variant or to acquired celiac stenosis.) If the hepatic artery pulse is preserved, the gastroduodenal artery is divided between 2-0 silk ties, with a Prolene suture placed on the proximal stump. This step, by providing improved access, often facilitates dissection of the portal vein from the undersurface of the pancreas.

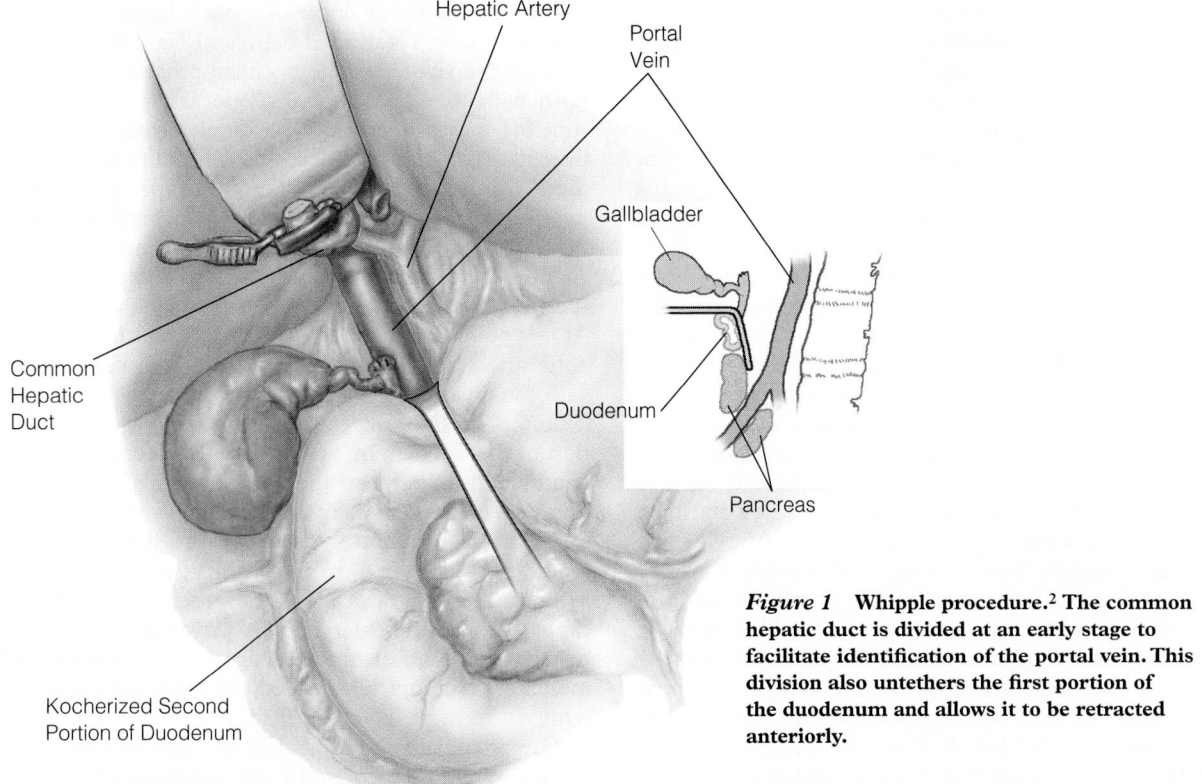

Figure 1 Whipple procedure.[2] The common hepatic duct is divided at an early stage to facilitate identification of the portal vein. This division also untethers the first portion of the duodenum and allows it to be retracted anteriorly.

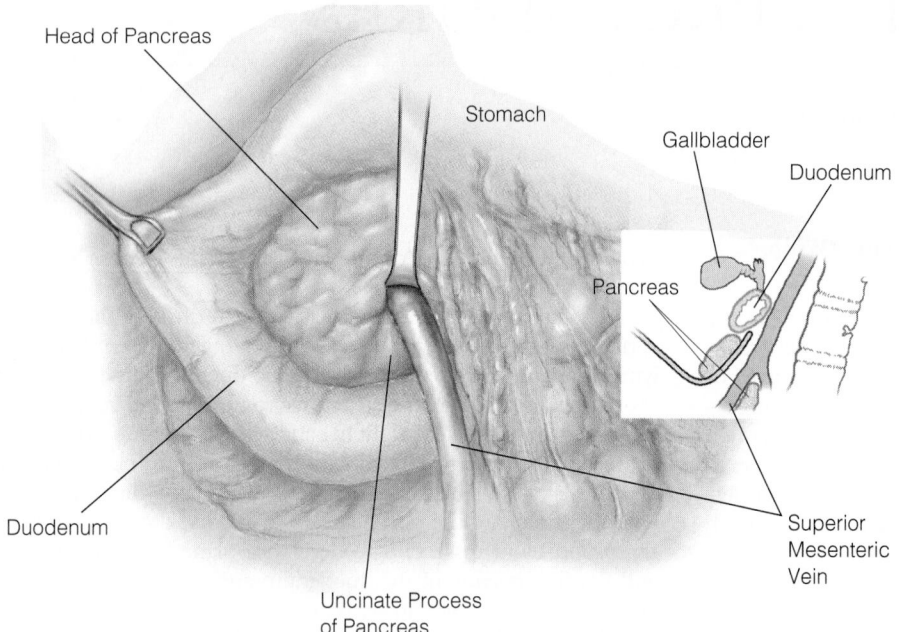

Head of Pancreas

Stomach

Gallbladder

Duodenum

Pancreas

Duodenum

Superior
Mesenteric
Vein

Uncinate Process
of Pancreas

Figure 2 **Whipple procedure.**[2]
Kocherization of the duodenum is continued along the third portion until the superior mesenteric vein is reached. This vein can then be easily cleaned up to its connection with the portal vein.

The third portion of the duodenum is then further kocherized until the superior mesenteric vein is identified [*see Figure 2*]. The superior mesenteric vein is cleaned along its anterior surface under the neck of the pancreas up to its connection with the portal vein. (Identification of the superior mesenteric vein is far easier by this anterior approach than by the traditional route through the lesser sac and is associated with virtually no blood loss.) Once this anterior plane is fully developed, the right lateral surface of the vein should be assessed for tumor involvement. This step, in conjunction with preoperative spiral CT assessment of arterial and venous involvement, helps confirm that the tumor can be resected with negative margins.

The first portion of the duodenum is mobilized from the neck of the pancreas and divided with a gastrointestinal anastomosis (GIA) stapler approximately 2 cm distal to the pylorus. If the surgeon chooses to carry out a classic pancreaticoduodenectomy, an antrectomy is performed. The right gastroepiploic arcade and the right gastric vessels are divided to permit mobilization of the antrum. The stomach is then divided with a GIA stapler, usually at the level of the incisura. A Babcock clamp is then placed on the proximal first portion of the duodenum, which is reflected medially. The posterior surface of the proximal first portion of the duodenum is dissected until the lesser sac is entered. At this point, the soft tissue attachments from the inferior border of the duodenum to the inferior border of the pancreas are divided; the right gastroepiploic vessels, which can be sizable, are clamped, divided, and ligated with 2-0 silk. In a similar fashion, the soft tissue areolar attachments found superiorly are divided with the electrocautery or else clamped, divided, and ligated with 2-0 silk. (Care must be taken to identify and preserve the right gastric artery, which comes off the common hepatic artery and actually joins the foregut along the proximal part of the first portion of the duodenum.) If the gastroduodenal artery was not divided earlier, it is now identified and divided as described earlier (see above).

The neck of the pancreas is divided with the electrocautery. A rush of pancreatic juice is the signal that the enlarged pancreatic duct has been divided. A 1 mm thick complete cross section of the pancreas is taken at this time and sent for frozen

section examination. (Margins should be sent for frozen section as they become available so that one is not delayed in proceeding with the reconstruction while the pathologist takes the margin off the pancreaticoduodenectomy specimen at the end of the formal resection.)

The portal vein and the superior mesenteric vein are mobilized from the uncinate process of the pancreas. It is often necessary to place vessel loops around one or both of these veins so that one can retract them far enough medially to remove them completely from the uncinate process. (There are amazingly few veins that must be ligated and divided in this region.) Dissection should proceed until the superior mesenteric artery, clearly palpable with the index finger of the left hand, is visualized. The uncinate process is divided between Reinhoff clamps and ligated with 2-0 silk ties. The uncinate process should be divided flush with the superior mesenteric artery [*see Figure 3*]. The superior mesenteric artery is completely exposed during this dissection, which proceeds from cephalad to caudad. Generally, there are two large veins joining the superior mesenteric vein inferiorly (the superior and inferior pancreaticoduodenal veins) that one must dissect free, doubly ligate, and divide.

After the uncinate process has been completely divided, the specimen is attached only by the third portion of the duodenum. At this point, the upper abdomen is copiously irrigated with an antibiotic solution and packed. The transverse colon, along with the greater omentum, is reflected cephalad. The proximal jejunum and the ligament of Treitz, along with the fourth portion of the duodenum, are dissected free, and the dissection is continued until it meets the right-side upper abdominal dissection. At a convenient point where there is a wide vascular arcade, the proximal jejunum is divided with a GIA stapler approximately 10 to 12 cm from the ligament of Treitz. The proximal jejunum is then grasped with a Babcock clamp and retracted cephalad. The mesentery to the proximal jejunum is divided between Reinhoff clamps and ligated with 2-0 silk. When the mesentery is completely divided, the specimen is free and can be removed from the operative field.

The proximal jejunum is then brought up through a rent in the transverse mesocolon. In our technique of choice, end-to-

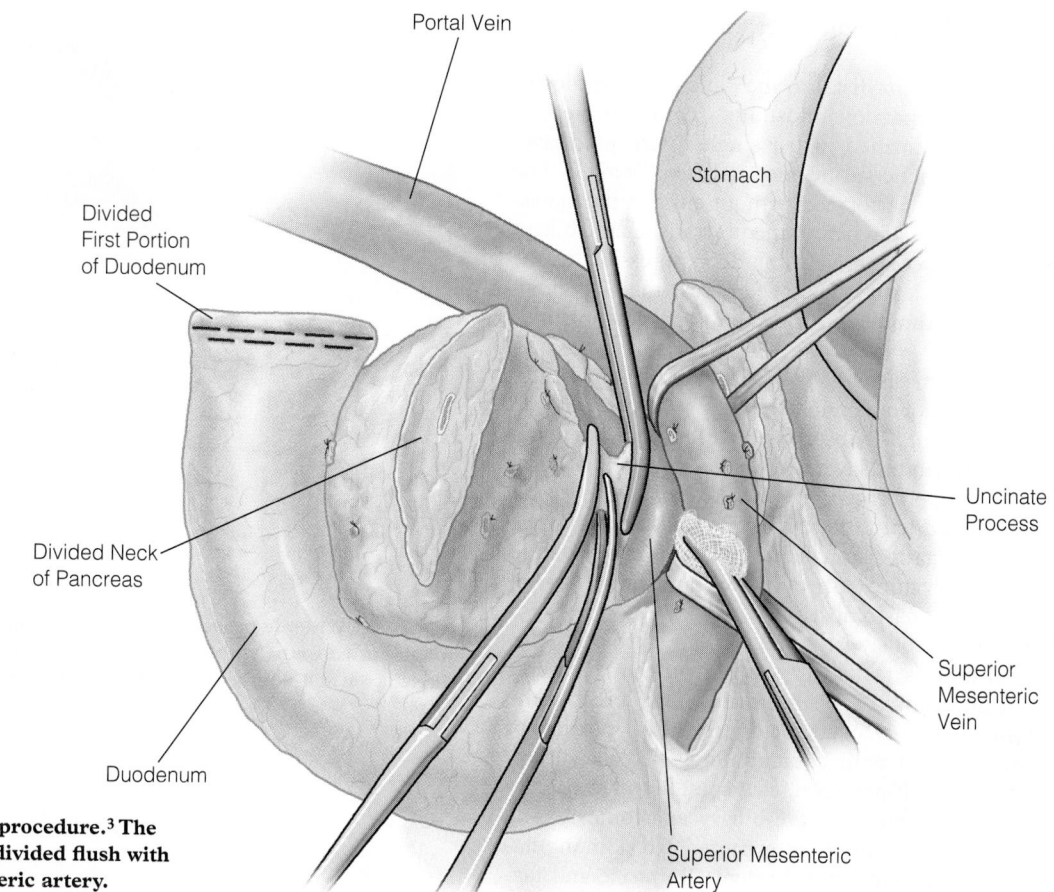

Figure 3 **Whipple procedure.[3] The uncinate process is divided flush with the superior mesenteric artery.**

end or end-to-side pancreaticojejunostomy is performed. In our technique of choice, the end of the pancreas is invaginated into the jejunum for approximately 2 cm. This anastomosis is performed with an outer interrupted layer of 3-0 silk and an inner continuous layer of 3-0 absorbable synthetic suture material [*see Figure 4a*]. The inner layer incorporates the dilated pancreatic duct with several throws, both posteriorly and anteriorly. This invagination technique may be performed in either an end-to-end or an end-to-side manner. As an alternative, an end-to-side mucosa-to-mucosa anastomosis may be performed [*see Figure 4b*]. An outer layer of interrupted 3-0 silk sutures is placed between the capsule of the gland and the seromuscular layer of the bowel. An inner layer of interrupted 4-0 absorbable synthetic sutures is then placed between the pancreatic duct and a

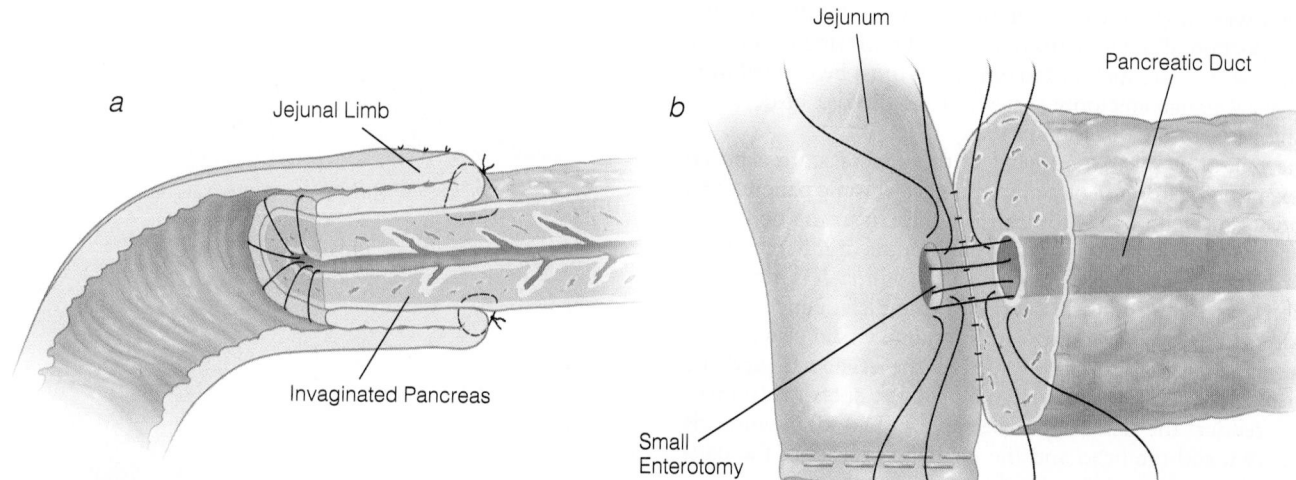

Figure 4 **Whipple procedure.[3] (*a*) In the authors' preferred approach to pancreaticojejunostomy, the end of the pancreas is invaginated into the end of the jejunum for approximately 2 cm. The anastomosis is done with an outer interrupted layer of 3-0 silk and an inner continuous layer of 3-0 absorbable synthetic suture material. (*b*) In an alternative approach, an end-to-end mucosa-to-mucosa pancreaticojejunostomy is again done in two layers with an outer layer of interrupted 3-0 silk sutures and an inner layer of interrupted 4-0 absorbable synthetic sutures.**

small enterotomy in the jejunum, either with or without a pancreatic duct stent.

Approximately 4 to 6 cm distal to the pancreaticojejunostomy, an end-to-side hepaticojejunostomy (common hepatic duct to jejunum) is performed with a single interrupted layer of 4-0 absorbable synthetic suture material [see Figure 5]. The anastomosis is generally performed without either a transanastomotic stent or a T tube. If a percutaneous transhepatic biliary catheter was placed preoperatively for decompression of the obstructed biliary tree, it may be placed across the anastomosis and left to gravity drainage during the early postoperative period.

Approximately 20 cm distal to the biliary-enteric anastomosis, an end-to-side duodenojejunostomy is performed with an inner continuous layer of 3-0 absorbable synthetic suture material and an outer interrupted layer of 3-0 silk [see Figure 6]. If an antrectomy has been performed, the medial half of the gastric staple line is reinforced with interrupted 3-0 silk seromuscular Lembert sutures. The gastrojejunal anastomosis is completed to the lateral (greater curvature) aspect of the staple line as a two-layer Hofmeister-style anastomosis.

The abdomen is copiously irrigated with an antibiotic solution. The jejunal loop is tacked to the rent in the transverse mesocolon with interrupted 3-0 silk sutures. The defect in the retroperitoneum previously occupied by the third portion of the duodenum is closed with a continuous 3-0 silk suture. Closed suction Silastic drains (two, as a rule) are placed adjacent to both the pancreatic and the biliary anastomosis. The abdomen is closed with multiple interrupted No. 1 monofilament sutures placed through and through all muscle and fascial layers. The subcutaneous tissues are irrigated with an antibiotic solution and closed with a continuous 3-0 absorbable synthetic suture. The subcuticular layer is closed with a continuous 4-0 absorbable synthetic suture. Steri-Strips are applied.

Distal Pancreatectomy for Chronic Pancreatitis

The peritoneal cavity is entered through an upper midline incision, and the abdomen is thoroughly explored. The omentum is taken off the transverse colon, and the lesser sac is exposed widely. (One can enter the lesser sac by dividing the middle portion of the omentum instead of removing it from the colon; however, so much of the omentum must be divided during a distal pancreatectomy that one runs the risk of devascularizing some of the distal omentum.)

The tail, body, neck, and head of the pancreas are exposed and examined. (In some patients who have chronic pancreatitis, the posterior wall of the stomach is adherent to the body and tail of the pancreas because of repeated bouts of inflammation. If this is the case, the posterior wall of the stomach is mobilized via both sharp and blunt dissection. If the distal pancreatectomy were being done to remove a tumor, one would also have to be certain that vital structures such as the celiac axis and the superior mesenteric vessels were not involved; such involvement might render the lesion unresectable.) The duodenum is kocherized, and the head and the uncinate process of the pancreas are palpated and visualized.

The splenic artery is identified as it comes off the celiac axis, and a vessel loop is placed around it. This step gives one control of the splenic artery and allows one to ligate it early in the procedure if bleeding should occur. Occasionally, patients with chronic pancreatitis have a thrombosed splenic vein and left-

Common Hepatic Duct

Jejunum

Figure 5 Whipple procedure.[3] The common hepatic duct is anastomosed to the jejunum in an end-to-side fashion with a single layer of 4-0 interrupted absorbable synthetic sutures.

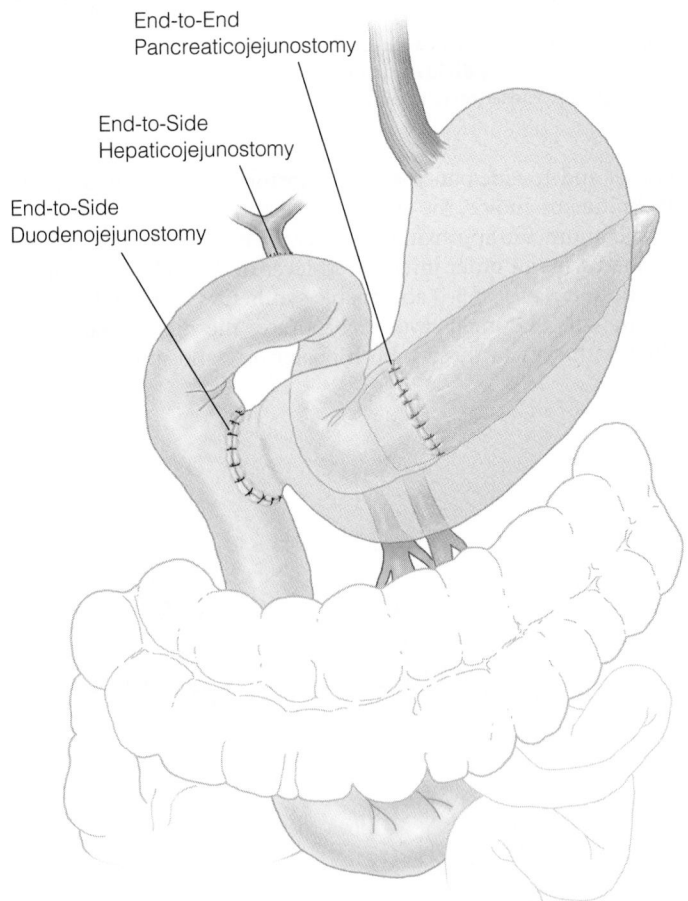

End-to-End
Pancreaticojejunostomy

End-to-Side
Hepaticojejunostomy

End-to-Side
Duodenojejunostomy

Figure 6 Whipple procedure.[3] After the end-to-end pancreaticojejunostomy and the end-to-side hepaticojejunostomy, the duodenum is anastomosed to the jejunum in an end-to-side fashion with an inner continuous layer of 3-0 absorbable suture material and an outer interrupted layer of 3-0 silk.

side portal hypertension. If this is the case, there are usually multiple collateral vessels leading from the spleen to the stomach via the vasa brevia and involving the omentum. In such circumstances, it is usually preferable to ligate and divide the splenic artery early in the procedure.

The spleen is mobilized out of the retroperitoneum. This task is made easier if a splenic pack has been placed beneath the left flank of the patient to elevate the left retroperitoneum before preparation and draping. The spleen is retracted toward the midline with the left hand; it should be compressed medially toward the spine rather than retracted anteriorly. As one opens up the retroperitoneum with the electrocautery, the assistant, standing to the left of the patient, grasps the retroperitoneal serosa. Once the serosa has been divided, the retroperitoneum usually consists of loose areolar tissue that is easily mobilized. One must be careful not to dissect too deeply and injure the kidney or its vessels.

The tail of the pancreas is mobilized out of the retroperitoneum via both sharp and blunt dissection. The omental attachments anterior to the hilum of the spleen are divided between Kelly clamps and ligated with 2-0 silk. (The line of division is easily determined if the omentum has previously been completely taken off the transverse colon. As the division extends up toward and then along the greater curvature of the stomach, the vasa brevia are encountered and are doubly clamped, divided, and ligated.) The splenic flexure of the colon is carefully dissected away from the inferior pole of the spleen, and the peritoneal attachments that make up the splenocolic ligament are divided.

The tail and body of the pancreas are further mobilized out of the retroperitoneum by retracting the spleen and the tail of the pancreas medially. (In the course of this mobilization, one must be careful not to injure the left adrenal gland, which often occupies a fairly superficial position in the retroperitoneum, anterior and medial to the superior pole of the left kidney.) The splenic vein is easily identified in the middle portion of the posterior aspect of the pancreas. The inferior mesenteric vein, which joins the splenic vein at the middle of the body of the pancreas, is identified in the retroperitoneum just lateral to the ligament of Treitz. (Although the inferior mesenteric vein can be divided and ligated with impunity, one should try to preserve it.)

Further mobilization of the pancreas to the midline exposes the point where the splenic artery comes off the celiac axis. (Whereas the splenic vein invariably resides in a groove in the middle portion of the posterior surface of the gland, the splenic artery usually runs along the superior aspect of the gland and is easily identified by palpation where it arises from the celiac axis.) The splenic artery is clamped and divided with 2-0 silk ties and a 3-0 Prolene suture ligature on the proximal stump of the vessel.

The junction of the inferior mesenteric vein and the splenic vein is identified, and the splenic vein is mobilized just distal to this junction. (Because the splenic vein resides in a groove or trough on the posterior aspect of the pancreas, one must be careful when mobilizing the splenic vein out of the pancreatic parenchyma. There are several small venous branches that can be injured if the mobilization is not done fastidiously.) The splenic vein is triply clamped and divided just distal to its junction with the inferior mesenteric vein. The splenic vein is then mobilized from the posterior surface of the pancreas from this point onward to its junction with the superior mesenteric vein and the portal vein [see Figure 7]. If there is a pancreatic tumor arising from the proximal body of the gland, the splenic vein may be ligated flush with the superior mesenteric vein. At this location, it is best to

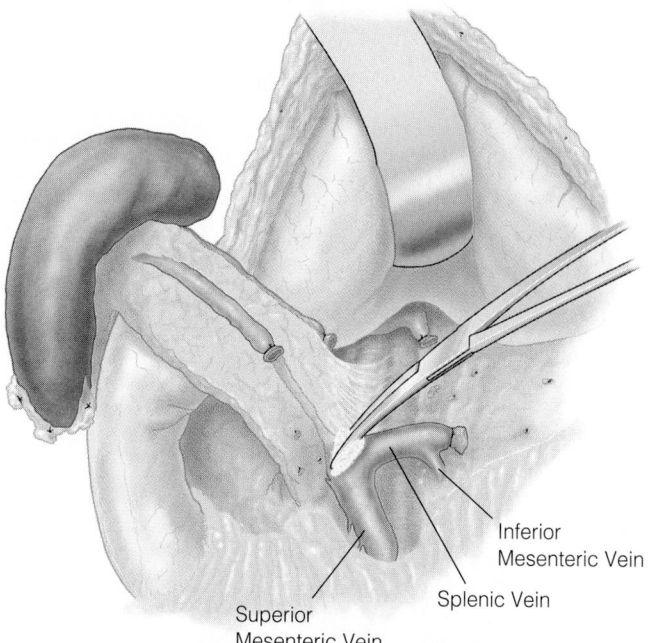

Figure 7 Distal pancreatectomy.[3] The splenic vein is divided just distal to its junction with the inferior mesenteric vein and then dissected away from the posterior surface of the pancreas from this point up to where it joins the superior mesenteric vein to form the portal vein.

Labels in figure:
Inferior Mesenteric Vein
Splenic Vein
Superior Mesenteric Vein

oversew the vein with a continuous 3-0 Prolene suture so as not to compromise the superior mesenteric vein–portal vein complex.

The portal vein and the superior mesenteric vein are carefully dissected away from the undersurface of the neck of the pancreas. (At the neck, the pancreas is often very thinned out and narrow before expanding into the substantially thicker head and uncinate process.) A row of overlapping horizontal mattress sutures of 3-0 absorbable synthetic material is placed in the neck of the pancreas just proximal to the point where it is to be divided. (Using large needles that have been straightened makes this task simple even if the head-neck junction through which the needles are passed is thickened.) The neck of the pancreas is then divided with the electrocautery. A row of figure-eight sutures of 3-0 absorbable synthetic suture material is placed over the end of the pancreas [see Figure 8]. If the pancreatic duct can be identified, it should be separately oversewn with a figure-eight or mattress suture (again, of 3-0 absorbable synthetic suture material).

The abdomen is copiously irrigated with an antibiotic solution. The pancreatic remnant is drained with a closed suction Silastic drain brought out through a stab wound in the left upper quadrant. There is no need to drain the splenic bed. The abdominal wall is closed with a single layer of interrupted No. 1 nonabsorbable synthetic monofilament sutures placed through and through all muscle and fascial layers. The subcutaneous tissues are irrigated with an antibiotic solution and closed with a continuous 3-0 absorbable synthetic suture. The subcuticular layer is closed with a continuous 4-0 absorbable synthetic suture. Steri-Strips are applied.

Longitudinal Pancreaticojejunostomy (Puestow Procedure)

The abdomen is entered through an upper midline incision. The lesser sac is entered by removing the greater omentum

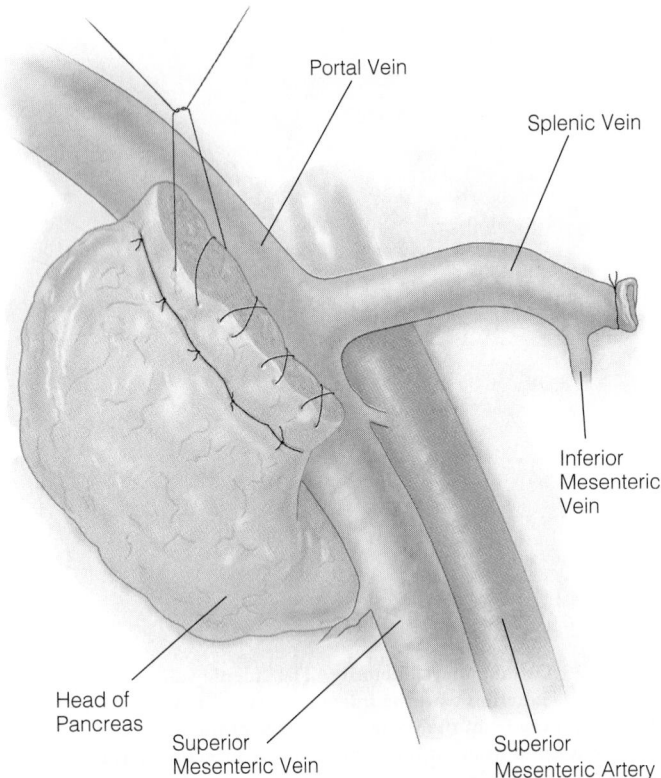

Figure 8 **Distal pancreatectomy.**[3] **A row of overlapping horizontal mattress sutures is placed in the neck of the pancreas just proximal to where it is to be divided, the neck is divided with the electrocautery, and a row of figure-eight sutures of 3-0 absorbable synthetic suture material is placed over the end of the pancreas.**

from the transverse colon along virtually its entire length, thereby exposing the entire tail, body, neck, and head of the pancreas. The pancreas often appears markedly fibrotic and scarred. The posterior wall of the stomach may be adherent to a portion of the body of the pancreas as a result of multiple episodes of inflammation; if it is adherent, it is easily dissected free. The duodenum is kocherized, and the head and the uncinate process of the pancreas are palpated from both an anterior and a posterior direction. In many cases, the pancreatic duct is markedly dilated and can actually be palpated through the anterior surface in the middle portion of the body of the pancreas. The rest of the abdomen is explored to check for the presence of other pathologic conditions. To confirm the position of the dilated pancreatic duct, a 20-gauge needle on a 10 ml syringe is used to aspirate the duct. Once pancreatic juice is obtained, the syringe is removed from the needle hub, with the needle left in place.

The pancreatic duct is entered by dividing the pancreatic parenchyma with the electrocautery on either side of the needle. A large right-angle clamp is then inserted, and the duct is filleted open with the electrocautery both proximally and distally [*see Figure 9*]. Small pancreatic ductal concretions are carefully removed. (Experience has demonstrated that at least 6 cm of the duct must be opened to yield a good chance of long-term success. Ideally, if the duct is dilated all the way out to the tail, it can be filleted open virtually to the tip of the pancreas. In the proximal direction, the duct can easily be opened as far as the neck of the pancreas. Beyond this point, however, the duct passes posteriorly and inferiorly into the head of the pancreas;

because the head can be very thick, opening up the duct any further can be difficult.)

A Bakes dilator is carefully passed proximally through the open pancreatic duct, down through the pancreatic duct in the unopened head, through the ampulla of Vater, and into the duodenum. (If a Bakes dilator cannot be passed into the duodenum, some surgeons elect to open the duodenum and perform a sphincteroplasty, so that by working both from within the duodenum and from within the open pancreatic duct, they can ensure the patency of the entire pancreatic duct.)

A Roux-en-Y jejunal loop approximately 60 cm long is constructed. The most proximal loop of jejunum in which there is a good vascular arcade is selected. A 2 cm segment of this loop is cleaned and divided with a GIA stapler. The small bowel mesentery is divided between clamps down through the arcade vessel and is ligated with 3-0 silk. The end of the distal jejunum is oversewn with a layer of 3-0 silk Lembert sutures. A 60 cm length is then measured. Alimentary tract continuity is reestablished by means of an end-to-side jejunojejunostomy, in which the most proximal portion of the divided jejunum is anastomosed to the side of the Roux-en-Y jejunal loop 60 cm distally with an inner continuous layer of 3-0 absorbable synthetic suture material and an outer interrupted layer of 3-0 silk. The defect in the small bowel mesentery is closed with a continuous 4-0 silk suture.

The Roux-en-Y jejunal loop is brought up into the lesser sac in a retrocolic position through a small rent in the transverse mesocolon. A side-to-side pancreaticojejunostomy is performed in two layers. Before the Roux loop is opened, an outer interrupted layer of 3-0 silk is placed between the jejunal loop and the pancreatotomy, passing through the capsule of the pancreas and out through the opened pancreatic parenchyma along the inferior border of the pancreas. When this layer is complete, an enterotomy approximately 2 mm from the jejunal suture line is

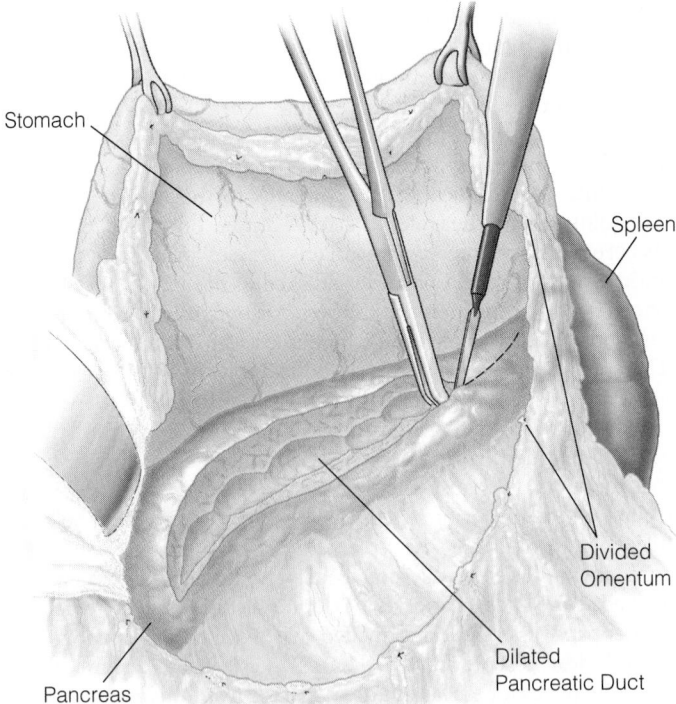

Figure 9 **Puestow procedure.**[3] **The dilated pancreatic duct is filleted open with the electrocautery both proximally and distally. At least 6 cm of the duct should be opened.**

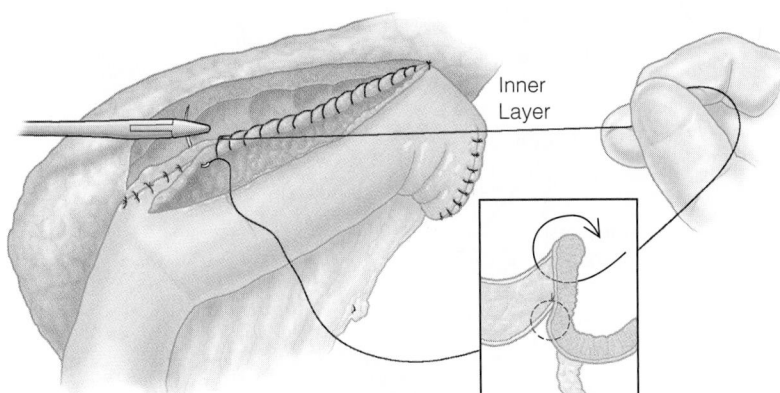

Inner Layer

Figure 10 **Puestow procedure.[3] When the diameter of the dilated pancreatic duct is 1 cm or wider, a side-to-side pancreaticojejunostomy should be done in two layers. Once an outer layer of interrupted 3-0 silk sutures is placed between the jejunal loop and the pancreatotomy, an enterotomy is made along the entire length of the jejunal suture line, and an inner layer consisting of a continuous 3-0 absorbable synthetic suture is placed.**

made along the entire length of this line. Starting at the distal pancreatic tail, an inner continuous layer of 3-0 absorbable synthetic suture material is placed in an over-and-over locking fashion through the entire wall of the jejunum and the entire divided surface of the pancreas and into the duct [*see Figure 10*]. The inner layer of the superior suture line is placed in an over-and-over fashion without locking, again with a continuous 3-0 absorbable synthetic suture. The outer layer of the superior suture line consists of interrupted 3-0 silk sutures placed in a Lembert fashion. (When the pancreatic duct is dilated to a diameter of 1 cm or greater, a two-layer anastomosis is possible and is in fact preferred. However, when the diameter of the duct is between 5 mm and 1 cm, a two-layer anastomosis is generally difficult, and a one-layer anastomosis is preferred. A single layer of interrupted 3-0 silk sutures is placed so that the knots are tied on the outside. This is easily accomplished with the superior suture line. With the inferior suture line, which is placed first, the suture passes from outside inward on the pancreas and then from inside outward on the jejunum. In a single-layer side-to-side pancreaticojejunostomy, the jejunotomy must be performed before any sutures are placed.) The Roux-en-Y jejunal loop is then tacked to the rent in the transverse mesocolon with interrupted 3-0 silk sutures.

The longitudinal pancreaticojejunostomy anastomosis is drained with closed suction Silastic drains that are placed on either side of the anastomosis and brought out through separate stab wounds in the left upper quadrant. The abdomen is copiously irrigated with an antibiotic solution. The midline incision is closed with a single interrupted layer of No. 1 nonabsorbable synthetic monofilament sutures passed through and through all muscle and fascial layers. The subcutaneous tissues are irrigated with an antibiotic solution and closed with a continuous 3-0 absorbable synthetic suture. The subcuticular layer is closed with a continuous 4-0 absorbable synthetic suture. Steri-Strips are applied.

Drainage of Pancreatic Pseudocyst into a Roux-en-Y Jejunal Loop

The peritoneal cavity is entered through a midline incision, and the abdomen is explored. Typically, a substantial mass that is cystic and easily ballotable is palpable posterior to the stomach. The duodenum and the head of the pancreas are kocherized so that the head may be palpated both anteriorly and posteriorly. The physical characteristics of chronic pancreatitis are usually present. The body and the tail of the pancreas are palpated as well; the pancreas is usually fibrotic, firm, and somewhat enlarged. The rest of the abdomen is explored to check for the presence of other pathologic conditions. (At this point, the size

and configuration of the cyst are compared with the size and configuration on the preoperative CT scan. If the CT scan shows a unilocular solitary cyst and if, at the time of laparotomy, there appears to be a mass that coincides exactly with what is seen on the CT scan, there is no need to enter the lesser sac. The lesion can be drained into a Roux-en-Y jejunal loop through the transverse mesocolon, and the lesser sac need not be explored. Most pseudocysts are formed by anterior disruptions of the main pancreatic duct. When pancreatic secretions leak out into the lesser sac, the body walls off the leak through its inflammatory response. The transverse mesocolon becomes adherent to the posterior wall of the stomach, which in turn becomes adherent to other adjacent structures in and around the retroperitoneum, and the leak is sealed off. Thus, the transverse mesocolon is usually the inferior and most dependent portion of the pseudocyst, and this site is the ideal location for drainage [*see Figure 11*].)

The transverse colon is retracted cephalad, and the cyst is easily visualized and palpated through the transverse mesocolon. The location of the cyst is confirmed by aspirating pancreatic juice through the transverse mesocolon with a 10 ml syringe and a 20-gauge needle. (One must be careful to identify and avoid the middle colic vessels.) A 60 cm long Roux-en-Y jejunal loop is constructed. The proximal jejunum is divided with a GIA stapler at the first convenient arcade. The small bowel mesentery is divided down through the arcade. The distal end of the jejunum is inverted with an interrupted layer of 3-0 silk Lembert sutures.

Alimentary tract continuity is reestablished by means of an end-to-side jejunojejunostomy, in which the proximal jejunum is anastomosed to the side of the Roux-en-Y jejunal loop 60 cm from the inverted end. This anastomosis is performed with an inner continuous layer of 3-0 absorbable synthetic suture material and an outer interrupted layer of 3-0 silk. The rent in the small bowel mesentery is closed with a continuous 3-0 silk suture.

A side-to-side cystojejunostomy is performed with an outer interrupted layer of 3-0 silk and an inner continuous layer of 3-0 absorbable synthetic suture material. The posterior outer layer of the anastomosis consists of a series of 3-0 silk sutures passed through and through the jejunal loop and through and through the transverse mesocolon (which is the inferior wall of the pseudocyst) [*see Figure 12*]. The suture line should be approximately 2.5 to 5 cm long. After the posterior layer has been secured, a cystotomy is performed with the electrocautery. An ellipse of cyst wall is removed and sent for frozen section examination. (No matter how convinced one is that one is dealing with a pseudocyst, a specimen from the cyst wall should always be sent for frozen section examination. Some cystic

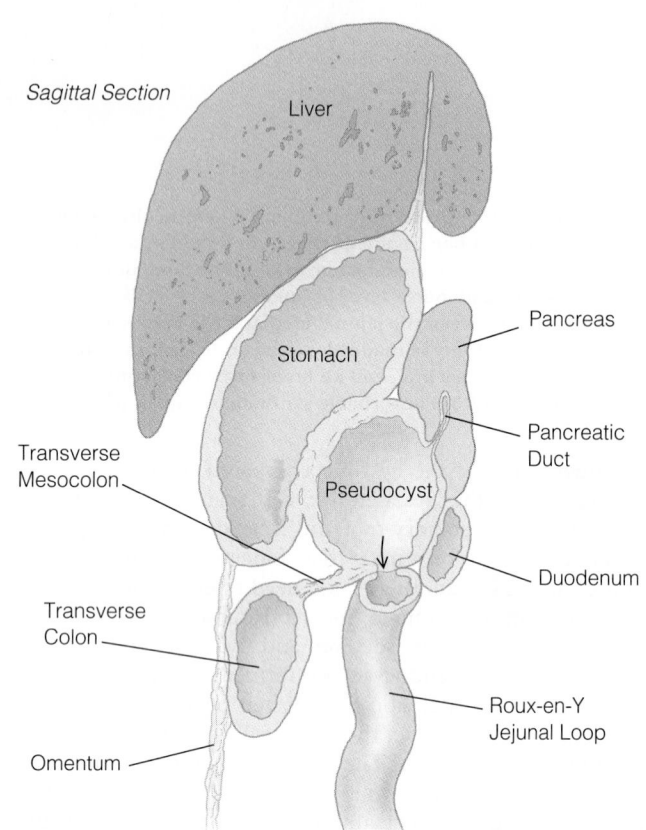

Figure 11   **Drainage of pancreatic pseudocyst into Roux-en-Y jejunal loop.**[3] **The transverse mesocolon is usually the most inferior and dependent part of a pancreatic pseudocyst; thus, drainage through the transverse mesocolon into a Roux loop is usually the ideal approach.**

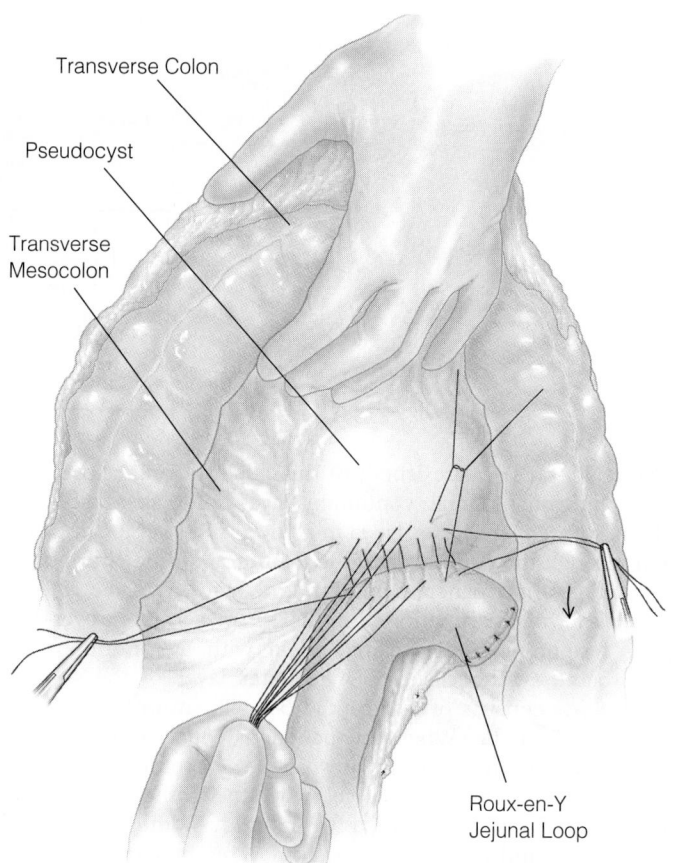

Figure 12   **Drainage of pancreatic pseudocyst into Roux-en-Y jejunal loop.**[3] **The outer posterior layer of the side-to-side cystojejunostomy comprises a series of 3-0 silk sutures placed through and through the jejunal loop and the transverse mesocolon.**

lesions of the pancreas are cystic neoplasms, which must be resected rather than drained. If no epithelial lining is found on frozen section examination, one can assume that the lesion is not a cystic neoplasm but a pancreatic pseudocyst and may proceed accordingly.) A parallel enterotomy is made in the jejunum. An inner continuous layer of 3-0 absorbable synthetic suture material is placed inferiorly in a locking fashion and then brought around superiorly in a Connell stitch. An outer interrupted layer of 3-0 silk is placed superiorly. With the cyst decompressed, one should easily be able to palpate a sizable lumen in the anastomosis between the cyst and the jejunal loop.

A closed suction Silastic drain is left near the anastomosis and brought out through a stab wound in the left upper quadrant. The abdomen is copiously irrigated with an antibiotic solution. The wound is closed with multiple interrupted No. 1 nonabsorbable synthetic monofilament sutures placed through and through all muscle and fascial layers. The subcutaneous tissues are irrigated with an antibiotic solution and closed with a continuous 3-0 absorbable synthetic suture. The subcuticular layer is closed with a continuous 4-0 absorbable synthetic suture. Steri-Strips are applied.

Drainage of Pancreatic Pseudocyst into the Stomach

The peritoneal cavity is entered through an upper midline incision, and the abdomen is explored. Typically, a pseudocyst that is not amenable to drainage through the transverse mesocolon presents as a mass that is cystic and is palpable through the anterior wall of the stomach and the lesser omentum in the upper abdomen; the mass generally is not palpable through the root of the transverse mesocolon with the transverse mesocolon reflected cephalad and thus is not easily drained into a Roux-en-Y jejunal loop. The duodenum and the head of the pancreas are kocherized and the head of the pancreas is palpated. Signs of chronic pancreatitis are invariably present. The body and tail of the pancreas are palpated through the transverse mesocolon and show changes characteristic of chronic inflammation. The rest of the abdomen is explored to check for the presence of other pathologic conditions. (A cyst that is situated high in the abdomen and presents more through the lesser omentum is not accessible to dependent drainage with a Roux-en-Y loop through the transverse mesocolon. Because bringing a Roux-en-Y loop anterior to the stomach to drain the cyst through the lesser omentum is unsatisfactory, such cysts are best drained into the stomach.)

Stay sutures of 3-0 silk are placed in the body of the stomach. A transverse gastrotomy is made with the electrocautery. The cyst wall is easily palpable through the posterior wall of the stomach. The location of the cyst is confirmed by aspirating pancreatic juice through the back wall of the stomach with a 10 ml syringe and a 20-gauge needle [*see Figure 13*]. (The mass palpated at the time of operation is compared with the cyst as it appears on the preoperative CT scan. If the CT scan shows a solitary unilocular cyst that corresponds to the palpable mass identified at the time of laparotomy, one can be certain that the cyst is solitary and can be drained effectively into the stomach.)

A transverse incision is made with the electrocautery through the posterior wall of the stomach, through the cyst wall, and into the pseudocyst. It is often desirable to leave the 20-gauge needle in place and to perform the posterior wall gastrotomy on either side of the needle. An ellipse of cyst wall is sent for frozen section examination. (Again, no matter how obvious it seems that one is dealing with an inflammatory cyst, a portion of the cyst wall should always be sent for frozen section examination to rule out a neoplasm.) A continuous locking suture of 3-0 absorbable synthetic material is placed through and through the posterior wall of the stomach and the anterior wall of the cyst [see Figure 14]. (This step may or may not actually be important for achieving long-term patency of the opening between the cyst and the posterior wall of the stomach, but it does ensure good hemostasis.) The anterior gastrotomy is closed with an inner continuous layer of 3-0 absorbable synthetic suture material in a Connell stitch and an outer interrupted layer of 3-0 silk.

The abdomen is copiously irrigated with an antibiotic solution. The wound is closed with a single layer of interrupted No. 1 nonabsorbable synthetic monofilament sutures. The subcutaneous tissues are irrigated with an antibiotic solution and closed with a continuous 3-0 absorbable synthetic suture. The subcuticular layer is closed with a continuous 4-0 absorbable synthetic suture. Steri-Strips are applied.

Palliative Bypass for Unresectable Pancreatic Cancer

The peritoneal cavity is entered through an upper midline incision. The head of the pancreas (containing a mass) and the duodenum are mobilized out of the retroperitoneum via the Kocher maneuver. The rest of the abdomen is examined for evidence of liver metastases or serosal spread. (Such evidence may

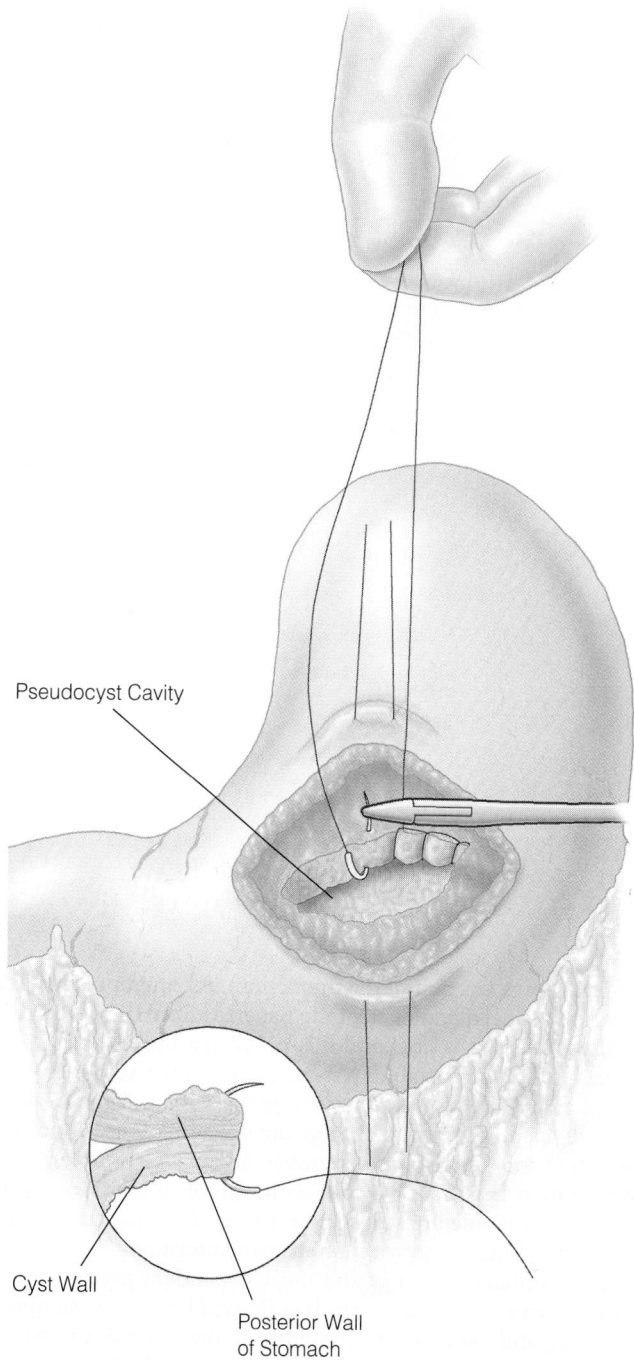

Figure 14 **Drainage of pancreatic pseudocyst into stomach.[3] Once an incision has been made through the posterior wall of the stomach, through the cyst wall, and into the pseudocyst, a continuous locking 3-0 absorbable synthetic suture is placed through and through the posterior wall of the stomach and the cyst wall.**

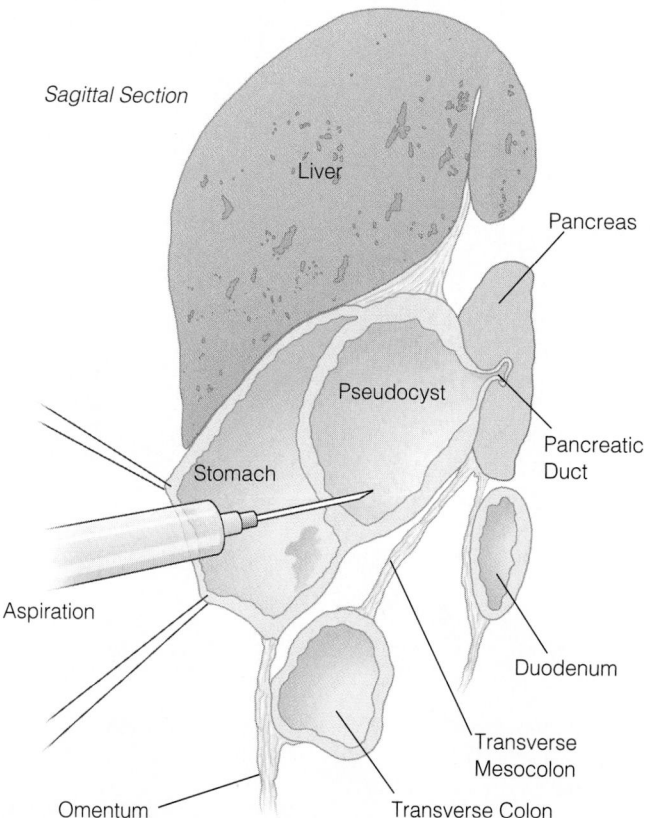

Figure 13 **Drainage of pancreatic pseudocyst into stomach.[3] The location of the pseudocyst is confirmed by aspirating pancreatic juice through the back wall of the stomach.**

be absent; thus, at this stage, the lesion may appear to be resectable.) The gallbladder is mobilized out of the liver bed. The common hepatic duct is circumferentially mobilized and divided. (Dividing the common hepatic duct early often facilitates identification and dissection of the portal vein. Even if the lesion proves to be unresectable, the gallbladder would not be used for the biliary bypass, given that we consider a hepaticojejunostomy preferable to a cholecystojejunostomy.)

Once the common hepatic duct is divided, the portal vein is easily identified. The anterior surface of the vein is cleaned

Gastrotomy and
Enterotomy

Stomach

Duodenum

Opening in
Greater Omentum

Opening in
Transverse Mesocolon

Proximal
Jejunum

Figure 15 **Palliative double bypass for
unresectable pancreatic cancer.**[3] **The
duodenum is bypassed with a retrocolic
gastrojejunostomy.**

under the first portion of the duodenum. An attempt is made to
separate the head and neck of the pancreas from the portal vein.
In many cases, it is not until this point that the lesion is ascertained to be unresectable. (As an example, the tumor may be
found to be directly invading the portal vein, but the invasion
was not apparent from the preoperative staging tests.) Once it is
clear that the tumor is unresectable, a palliative double bypass
procedure is begun, in which the duodenum is bypassed with a
retrocolic gastrojejunostomy [*see Figure 15*] and the distally
obstructed biliary tree with a hepaticojejunostomy.

Approximately 4 cm of the most dependent portion of the
greater curvature of the stomach is cleaned by doubly clamping,
dividing, and ligating attachments of the greater omentum.
Once this is accomplished, a small rent is made in the transverse
mesocolon, and a proximal loop of jejunum is brought up
through this rent and anastomosed to the greater curvature of
the stomach in a side-to-side fashion. The anastomosis is performed with an outer interrupted layer of 3-0 silk and an inner
continuous layer of 3-0 absorbable synthetic suture material.
(In the past, palliative duodenal bypasses for pancreatic cancer
were performed by carrying out an anterior antecolic gastrojejunostomy. Unfortunately, delayed gastric emptying is frequent
after an anterior gastrojejunostomy. A posterior retrocolic
gastroenterostomy virtually eliminates this complication.
Historically, surgeons have been reluctant to perform retrocolic

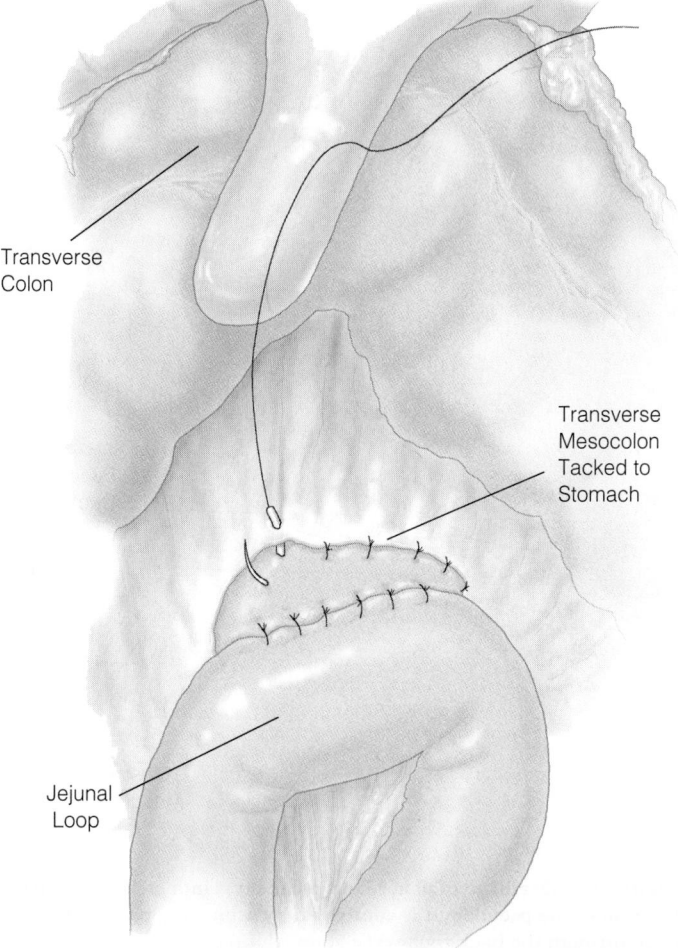

Transverse
Colon

Transverse
Mesocolon
Tacked to
Stomach

Jejunal
Loop

Figure 16 **Palliative double bypass for unresectable pancreatic
cancer.**[3] **Once the retrocolic gastrojejunostomy is complete, the
anastomosis is tacked to the rent in the transverse mesocolon on
the gastric side with interrupted 3-0 silk sutures.**

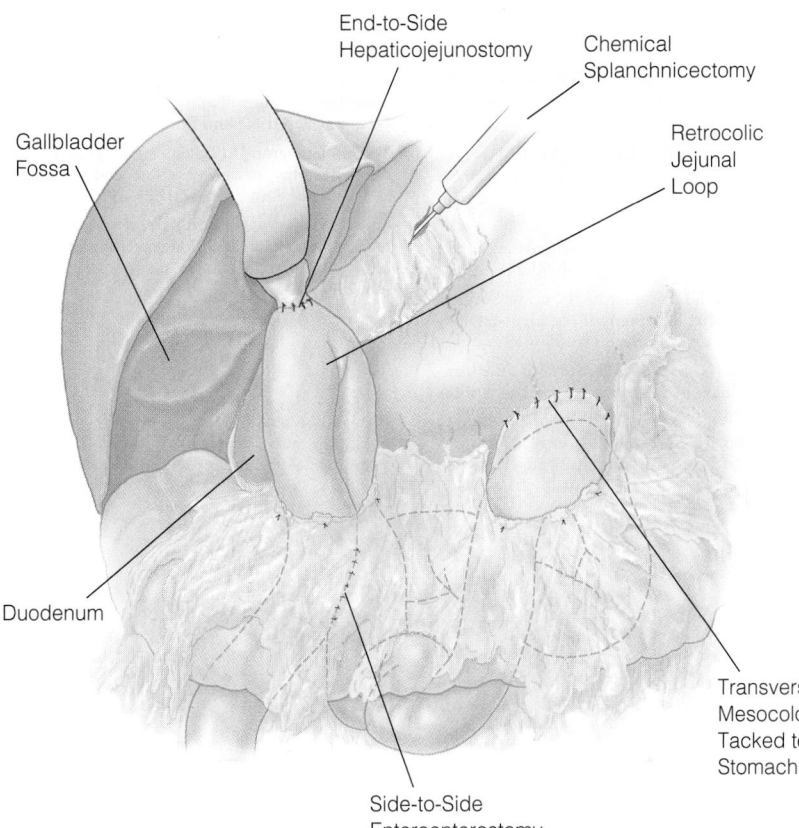

Gallbladder Fossa

End-to-Side Hepaticojejunostomy

Chemical Splanchnicectomy

Retrocolic Jejunal Loop

Duodenum

Transverse Mesocolon Tacked to Stomach

Side-to-Side Enteroenterostomy

Figure 17 **Palliative double bypass for unresectable pancreatic cancer.[3] An end-to-side hepaticojejunostomy is performed, followed by a side-to-side jejunojejunostomy between the afferent loop leading to the biliary anastomosis and the efferent loop leading from it. An opening is made in the lesser omentum, and a chemical splanchnicectomy is performed by injecting alcohol into the celiac plexus.**

gastroenterostomies for pancreatic cancer, fearing that tumor growth would occlude the anastomosis; however, at our institution, we have performed well over 200 such posterior retrocolic gastroenterostomies in this setting and have yet to demonstrate any tumor ingrowth into the anastomosis.) Once the posterior gastroenterostomy is complete, the anastomosis is tacked to the rent in the transverse mesocolon on the gastric side with multiple interrupted 3-0 silk sutures [*see Figure 16*]. (The purpose of this step is to prevent the afferent and efferent jejunal limbs from herniating up through the rent in the transverse mesocolon and becoming obstructed.)

The gallbladder is removed, and the distal biliary segment is oversewn with interrupted 3-0 silk sutures. (The distal biliary segment is routinely oversewn because there is a possibility that if a common channel is present, pancreatic secretions might reflux up the distal biliary tree and out into the peritoneal cavity.)

Approximately 30 cm distal to the gastrojejunostomy, a loop of jejunum is brought up into the right upper quadrant through a second rent in the transverse mesocolon. An end-to-side hepaticojejunostomy is performed with one layer of interrupted 4-0 absorbable synthetic sutures [*see Figure 17*].

A side-to-side anastomosis is performed between the afferent jejunal loop leading to the biliary anastomosis and the efferent jejunal loop leading from it [*see Figure 17*]. This short side-to-side anastomosis is placed below the rent in the transverse mesocolon. It is performed with an inner continuous layer of 3-0 absorbable synthetic suture material and an outer interrupted layer of 3-0 silk. The two limbs are tacked to the rent in the transverse mesocolon to prevent herniation. Alternatively, a Roux limb may be used to provide a conduit for biliary drainage.

The lesser omentum is divided, and a chemical splanchnicectomy is performed by injecting 20 ml of 50% alcohol into the celiac plexus on either side of the aorta at the level of the celiac axis [*see Figure 17*]. The level of the celiac axis is easily determined by palpating the thrill that is invariably present in the common hepatic artery as it comes off the celiac axis. (A prospective, randomized, double-blind study performed at our institution[1] demonstrated that chemical splanchnicectomies performed in this fashion in patients with unresectable pancreatic cancer were, in most cases, markedly effective in decreasing or eliminating pain for the remaining months of life. In addition, this procedure decreased or eliminated patients' narcotic requirements. Moreover, patients who underwent chemical splanchnicectomy actually survived significantly longer than those who did not. The improved survival was attributed to better nutritional intake in the pain-free patients.)

A closed suction Silastic drain is left posterior to the area of the hepaticojejunostomy and brought out through a stab wound in the right upper quadrant. If tissue confirmation of the presence of adenocarcinoma of the head of the pancreas was not obtained preoperatively, it should be obtained during operation. As a rule, this is most easily accomplished by performing a needle biopsy with a Tru-Cut needle transduodenally. The abdomen is irrigated with an antibiotic solution and then closed with multiple interrupted No. 1 nonabsorbable synthetic sutures placed through and through all muscle and fascial layers. The subcutaneous tissues are irrigated with an antibiotic-containing saline solution and closed with a continuous 3-0 absorbable synthetic suture. The subcuticular layer is closed with a continuous 4-0 absorbable synthetic suture. Steri-Strips are applied.

References

1. Lillemoe KD, Cameron JL, Kaufman HS, et al: Chemical splanchnicectomy in patients with unresectable pancreatic cancer: a prospective randomized trial. Ann Surg 217:447, 1993
2. Cameron JL: Rapid exposure of the portal and superior mesenteric veins. Surg Gynecol Obstet 176:395, 1995
3. Cameron JL: Atlas of Surgery. Mosby-Year Book, Inc., St. Louis, 1994

Selected Readings

Cameron JL, Pitt HA, Yeo CJ, et al: One hundred and forty-five consecutive pancreaticoduodenectomies without mortality. Ann Surg 217:430, 1993

Fernandez-del Castillo C, Rattner DW, Warshaw AL: Standards for pancreatic resection in the 1990s. Arch Surg 130:295, 1995

Lillemoe KD, Cameron JL, Hardacre JM, et al: Is prophylactic gastrojejunostomy indicated for unresectable periampullary cancer? a prospective randomized trial. Ann Surg 230:322, 1999

Lillemoe KD, Yeo CJ, Cameron JL: Pancreatic cancer: state-of-the-art care. CA Cancer J Clin 50:241, 2000

Sohn TA, Lillemoe KD, Cameron JL, et al: Surgical palliation of unresectable periampullary adenocarcinoma in the 1990s. J Am Coll Surg 188:658, 1999

Trede M, Schwall G, Saeger HD: Survival after pancreatoduodenectomy: 118 consecutive resections without an operative mortality. Ann Surg 211:447, 1990

Yeo CJ, Cameron JL, Lillemoe KD, et al: Does prophylactic octreotide decrease the rates of pancreatic fistula and other complications after pancreaticoduodenectomy? results of a prospective randomized placebo-controlled trial. Ann Surg 232:419, 2000

Yeo CJ, Cameron JL, Lillemoe KD, et al: Pancreaticoduodenectomy for cancer of the head of the pancreas: 201 patients. Ann Surg 221:721, 1995

Yeo CJ, Cameron JL, Sohn TA, et al: Six hundred fifty consecutive pancreaticoduodenectomies in the 1990s: pathology, complications, and outcomes. Ann Surg 226:248, 1997

Acknowledgments

Figures 1, 2, and 4   Tom Moore.
Figures 3 and 5 through 17   Tom Moore. Adapted from original illustrations by Corinne Sandone.

14 LAPAROSCOPIC SPLENECTOMY

Eric C. Poulin, M.D., M.Sc., Christopher M. Schlachta, M.D., and Joseph Mamazza, M.D.

Medicine is not an exact science, and nowhere is this observation more appropriate than in the operating room when a spleen is being removed.[1]

The first reported splenectomy in the western world was performed by Zacarello in 1549, though the veracity of his operative description has been questioned. Between this initial report and the 1800s, very few cases were recorded. The first reported splenectomy in North America was performed by O'Brien in 1816. The patient was in the act of committing a rape when his victim plunged a large knife into his left side. As in this case, most early splenectomies were done in patients who had undergone penetrating trauma; often, the spleen was protruding from the wound and the surgeon proceeded with en masse ligation. The first elective splenectomy was performed by Quittenbaum in 1826 for sequelae of portal hypertension, and soon afterward, Wells performed one of the first splenectomies using general anesthesia; both patients died. In 1866, Bryant was the first to attempt splenectomy in a patient with leukemia. Over the following 15 years, 14 splenectomies were attempted as therapy for leukemia; none of the patients survived. In a 1908 review of 49 similar cases, Johnston reported a mortality of 87.7%.[2] These dismal results led to the abandonment of splenectomy for leukemia. In 1916, Kaznelson, of Prague, was the first to report good results from splenectomy in patients with thrombocytopenic purpura.

As the 20th century progressed, splenectomy became more common in direct proportion to the increase in the use of the automobile. The eventual recognition of the syndrome known as overwhelming postsplenectomy sepsis (OPSS) made splenic conservation an important consideration. Partial splenectomy had initially been described by the French surgeon Péan in the 19th century. This procedure received little further study until almost 100 years later, when the Brazilian surgeon Campos Cristo reevaluated Péan's technique in his report of eight trauma patients treated with partial splenectomy.[3] Simpson's report on 16 children admitted for splenic trauma to the Hospital for Sick Children in Toronto between 1948 and 1955 was instrumental in establishing the validity of nonoperative treatment of splenic trauma[4] [*see III:7 Injuries to the Liver, Biliary Tract, Spleen, and Diaphragm*].

In late 1991 and early 1992, four groups working independently—Delaître in Paris, Carroll in Los Angeles, Cushieri in the United Kingdom, and our group in Canada—published the first reports of laparoscopic splenectomy in patients with hematologic disorders.[5-7] Since then, the development of operative techniques for partial laparoscopic splenectomy has tested the limits of minimally invasive surgery and encouraged clinical research regarding methods of simplifying the execution of the operation.[8,9] With the benefit of years of experience with laparoscopic splenectomy, it is possible to articulate a rational approach to this procedure that takes into account the technical lessons learned so far.

Preoperative Evaluation

Currently, we consider all patients evaluated for elective splenectomy to be potential candidates for laparoscopic splenectomy. Contraindications to a laparoscopic approach include severe portal hypertension, uncorrectable coagulopathy, severe ascites, and most traumatic injuries to the spleen. Extreme splenomegaly remains a relative contraindication as well. Because most patients scheduled for laparoscopic splenectomy have hematologic disorders, they undergo the same hematologic preparation that patients scheduled for open surgery do—namely, steroids and γ-globulins (when required). Ultrasonography is performed to determine the size of the spleen. Spleen size is expressed in terms of the maximum interpole length (i.e., the length of the line joining the two organ poles) and is generally classified into three categories: (1) normal spleen size (< 11 cm), (2) moderate splenomegaly (11 to 20 cm), and (3) severe splenomegaly (> 20 cm).[10] Because extremely large spleens present special technical problems that test the current limits of laparoscopic surgery, we make use of a fourth category for spleens longer than 30 cm, which we call megaspleens [*see Table 1*]. The ultrasonographer is also asked to try to identify any accessory spleens that may be present. The results of the ultrasound examination often determine whether the surgeon employs the anterior or the lateral approach to the procedure. Computed tomography is done when there is doubt about the exactness of the ultrasonographic measurement; such measurement is sometimes inaccurate at the upper pole and with spleens longer than 16 cm.

Patients receive thorough counseling about the consequences of the asplenic state. Polyvalent pneumococcal vaccine is administered at least 2 weeks before operation in all cases; preoperative *Haemophilus influenzae* vaccination is also advisable. Heparin prophylaxis for thrombophlebitis is administered according to standard guidelines, provided that there is no hematologic contraindication [*see VI:2 Thromboembolic Problems*]. Nonsteroidal anti-inflammatory drugs (NSAIDs) are often given in suppository form before operation to minimize postoperative pain; however, on empirical grounds, NSAIDs are not used when heparin prophylaxis is employed. Platelets are rarely, if ever, required when laparoscopic splenectomy is performed for idiopathic (immune) thrombocytopenic purpura (ITP).

Operative Planning

Laparoscopic splenectomy presents special problems, such as the necessity of dealing with a fragile and richly vascularized organ that is situated close to the stomach, the colon, and the pancreas and the difficulty of devising an extraction strategy that is compatible with

Table 1 Classification of Spleens According to Spleen Length*

Spleen Class	Spleen Length
Normal-size spleen	7–11 cm
Moderate splenomegaly	12–20 cm
Massive splenomegaly	21–30 cm
Megaspleen	> 30 cm

*Spleen length is defined as interpole length, measured along a straight line connecting the two poles.

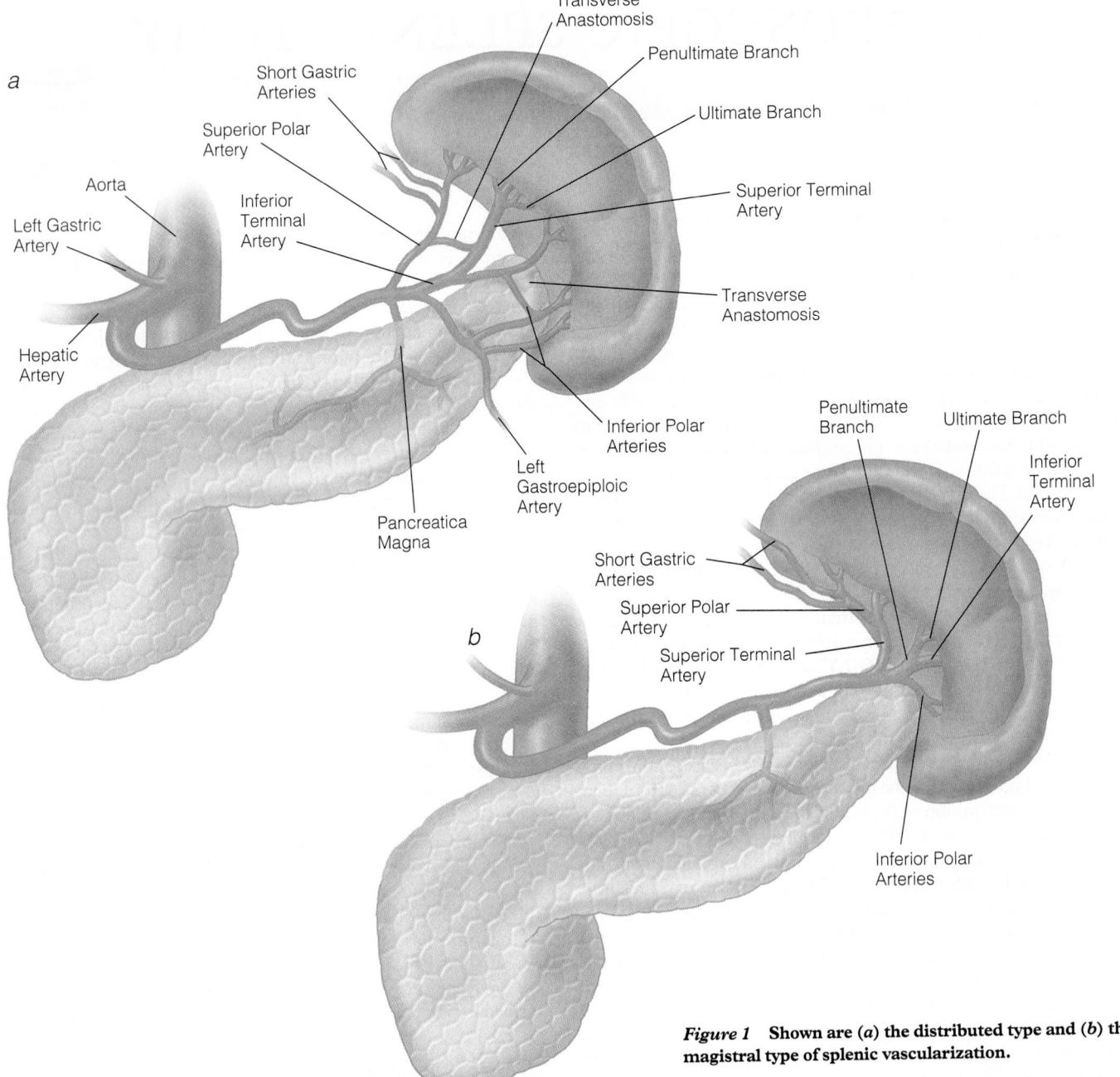

a

Transverse Anastomosis

Penultimate Branch

Ultimate Branch

Short Gastric Arteries

Superior Polar Artery

Aorta

Left Gastric Artery

Inferior Terminal Artery

Hepatic Artery

Superior Terminal Artery

Transverse Anastomosis

Inferior Polar Arteries

Left Gastroepiploic Artery

Pancreatica Magna

b

Penultimate Branch

Ultimate Branch

Inferior Terminal Artery

Short Gastric Arteries

Superior Polar Artery

Superior Terminal Artery

Inferior Polar Arteries

Figure 1 Shown are (*a*) the distributed type and (*b*) the magistral type of splenic vascularization.

proper histologic confirmation of the pathologic process while maintaining the advantages of minimal access surgery. For successful performance of laparoscopic splenectomy, a detailed knowledge of both splenic anatomy and potential complications is essential. It is the anatomic features—which may vary considerably from patient to patient (see below)—that largely determine the operative strategy.[11]

ANATOMIC CONSIDERATIONS

Most anatomy texts suggest that the splenic artery is constant in its course and branches; however, as the classic essay by Michels made clear, each spleen has its own peculiar pattern of terminal artery branches.[12]

Splenic Artery

The celiac axis is the largest but shortest branch of the abdominal aorta: it is only 15 to 20 mm long. The celiac axis arises above the body of the pancreas and, in 82% of specimens, divides into three

primary branches: the left gastric artery, which is the first branch, and the hepatic and splenic arteries, which derive from a common stem. In rare instances, the splenic artery originates directly from the aorta; even less often, a second splenic artery arises from the celiac axis. There are numerous other possible variations, in which the splenic artery may originate from the aorta, the superior mesenteric artery, the middle colic artery, the left gastric artery, the left hepatic artery, or the accessory right hepatic artery. As a rule, however, the splenic artery arises from the celiac axis to the right of the midline, which means that the aorta must be crossed to reach the spleen and that selective angiography is likely to be difficult at times. The splenic artery can take a very tortuous course, particularly in patients who are elderly patients or who have a longer artery.

In his study of 100 cadaver spleens,[12] Michels divided splenic arterial geography into two types, distributed and magistral [*see Figure 1*]. In the distributed type, found in 70% of dissections, the splenic trunk is short, and six to 12 long branches enter the spleen over approximately 75% of its medial surface. The branches originate between 3 and 13 cm from the hilum [see Figure 1a]. In the magistral type, found in the remaining 30% of dissections, there is a long main splenic artery that divides near the hilum into three or four large, short terminal branches that enter the spleen over only 25% to 35% of its medial surface. These short splenic branches originate, on average, 3.5 cm from the spleen, and they reach the center of the organ as a compact bundle [see Figure 1b]. Early identification of the type of splenic blood supply present can help the surgeon estimate how difficult a particular splenectomy is likely to be. Operation on a spleen with a distributed vascular anatomy usually involves dissection of more blood vessels; however, the vessels, being spread over a wider area of the splenic hilum, are relatively easy to deal with. Operation on a spleen with a magistral-type blood supply typically involves dissection of fewer vessels; however, because the hilum is narrower and more compact, dissection and separation of the vessels are more difficult.

Branches of Splenic Artery

The splenic branches vary so markedly in length, size, and origin that no two spleens have the same anatomy. Outside the spleen, the arteries also frequently form transverse anastomoses with each other that, like most collaterals, arise at a 90° angle to the vessels involved [see Figure 1].[13] As a consequence, attempts to occlude a branch of the splenic artery by means of clips or embolization, if carried out proximal to such an anastomosis, may fail to devascularize the corresponding splenic segment. Before the splenic trunk divides, it usually gives off a few slender branches to the tail of the pancreas. The most important of these is called the pancreatica magna (a vessel familiar to vascular radiologists); occlusion of this branch with embolic materiel has been reported to result in pancreatitis. Next, the splenic artery divides into two to six first and second terminal branches, and these branches undergo two further levels of division into two to 12 penultimate and ultimate branches. Segmental and subsegmental division can occur either outside or inside the spleen. The number of arteries entering the spleen ranges from six to 36. The size of the spleen does not determine the number of arteries entering it; however, the presence of notches and tubercles usually correlates well with a higher number of entering arteries.

A reasonable general scheme of splenic artery branches might include as many as seven principal branches at various division levels and in various anatomic arrangements: (1) the superior terminal artery, (2) the inferior terminal artery, (3) the medial terminal artery, (4) the short gastric arteries, (5) the left gastroepiploic artery, (6) the inferior polar artery, and (7) the superior polar artery [see Figure 2]. Veins are usually located behind the corresponding arteries, except at the ultimate level of division, where they may be either anterior or posterior.

First terminal division branches   A classic study from 1917 found that 72% of specimens had three terminal branches (superior polar, superior terminal, and inferior terminal) and 28% had two[14]; the medial terminal artery was observed in only 20% of cases. When the superior terminal artery is excessively large, the inferior terminal is rudimentary, with an added blood supply often coming from the left gastroepiploic and polar vessels.

Second terminal division branches   *Superior polar artery.* The superior polar artery is present in 65% of patients. It usually arises from the main splenic trunk (75% of cases) or the superior terminal artery (20% of cases), but on occasion, it may originate from the inferior terminal artery or separately from the celiac axis (thus providing the spleen with a double splenic artery). In most instances, the superior polar artery gives rise to one or two short gastric branches; rarely, it gives rise to the left inferior phrenic and pancreatic rami. The presence and size of this artery appear to be correlated with tubercle formation, in that it is more prominent in spleens with large tubercles. The superior polar artery is frequently very long and slender and thus easily torn during splenectomy; accordingly, it was suggested in 1928 that ligation of splenic branches be started from the inferior pole of the spleen.[15]

Inferior polar artery. The inferior polar artery is present in 82% of cases. As many as five collateral branches may arise from the

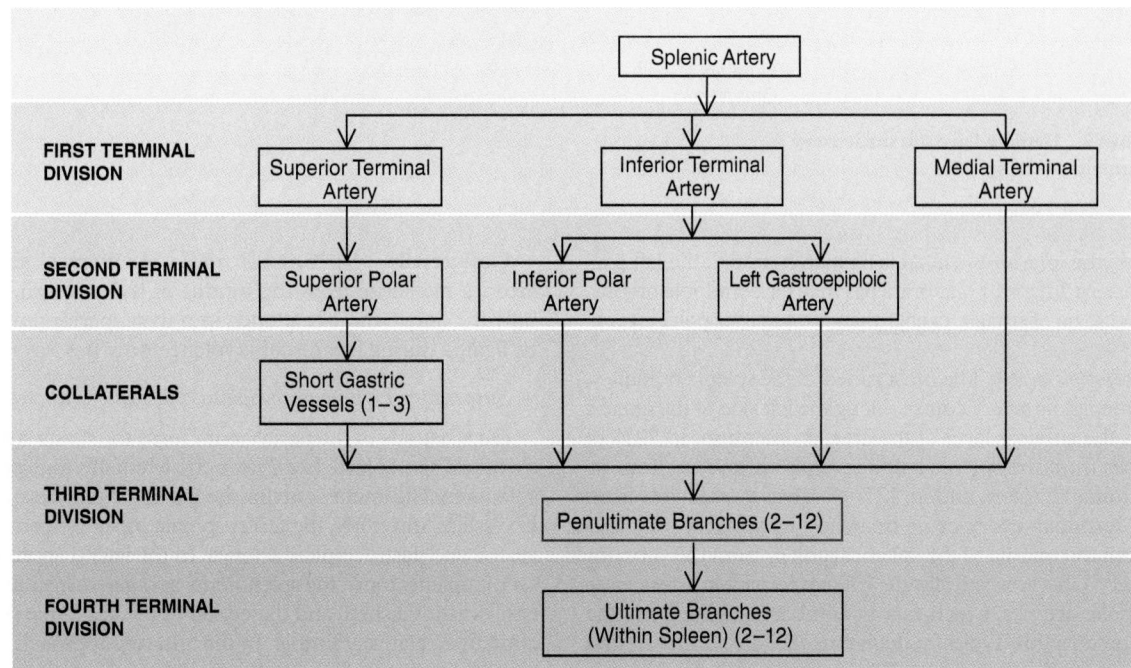

Figure 2   **Outlined is a general scheme of the levels of division of the splenic artery branches.**

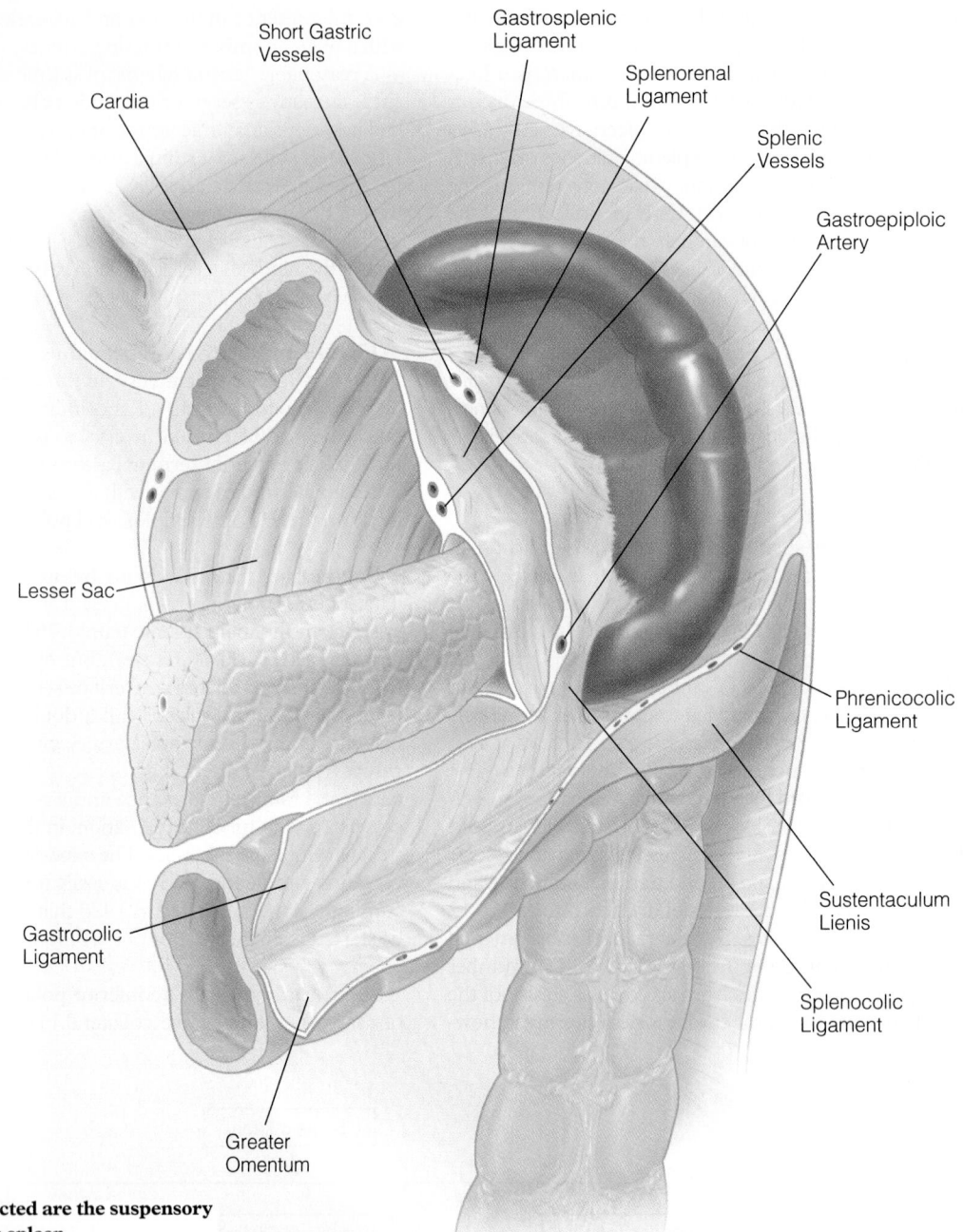

Figure 3 Depicted are the suspensory ligaments of the spleen.

splenic trunk, the inferior terminal artery, or, as noted, the left gastroepiploic artery. Inferior polar branches may have multiple origins, and they tend to be of smaller caliber than the superior polar artery.

Left gastroepiploic artery. The most varied of the splenic branches, the left gastroepiploic artery courses along the left side of the greater curvature in the anterior layer of the greater omentum. In 72% of cases, it arises from the splenic trunk several centimeters from its primary terminal division, and in 22% of cases, it originates from the inferior terminal artery or its branches; however, it may also originate from the middle of the splenic trunk or from the superior terminal artery. Characteristically, the left gastroepiploic artery gives off inferior polar arteries, which vary in number (ranging from one to five), size, and length. Typically, these branches are addressed first during laparoscopic splenectomy. When they are small, they can usually be controlled with the electrocautery.

Collaterals *Short gastric arteries.* As many as six short gastric arteries may arise from the fundus of the stomach, but as a rule, only the one to three that open into the superior polar artery must be ligated during laparoscopic splenectomy [*see Figure 1*].

Suspensory Ligaments of Spleen and Tail of Pancreas

Duplications of the peritoneum form the many suspensory ligaments of the spleen [*see Figure 3*]. Medially and posteriorly, the splenorenal ligament contains the tail of the pancreas and the splenic vessels. Anteriorly, the gastrosplenic ligament contains the short gastric and gastroepiploic arteries. In the lateral approach to laparoscopic splenectomy, the splenorenal and gastrosplenic ligaments are easily distinguished, and dissection of the anatomic structures they contain is relatively simple. In the anterior approach, these two ligaments lie on top of each other, and to separate them correctly and safely requires considerable experience with splenic anatomy.

The phrenicocolic ligament courses laterally from the diaphragm to the splenic flexure of the colon; its upper portion is called the phrenicosplenic ligament. The attachment of the lower pole on the internal side is called the splenocolic ligament. Between these two, a horizontal shelf of areolar tissue, known as the sustentaculum lienis, is formed on which the inferior pole of the spleen rests. The sustentaculum lienis is often molded into a sac that opens cephalad and acts as a support for the lower pole. This structure, often overlooked during open procedures, is readily visible through the laparoscope. The phrenicocolic ligament, the splenocolic ligament, and the sustentaculum lienis are usually avascular, except in patients who have portal hypertension or myeloid metaplasia.

A 1937 study found that the tail of the pancreas was in direct contact with the spleen in 30% of cadavers.[16] A subsequent report confirmed this finding and added that in 73% of patients, the distance between the two structures was no more than 1 cm.[17] Care must be exercised to avoid damage with the electrocautery during dissection as well as damage with the linear stapler in the course of en masse ligation of the splenic hilum (a maneuver more easily performed via the lateral approach to laparoscopic splenectomy).

Operative Technique

LATERAL APPROACH

This approach was first described in connection with laparoscopic adrenalectomy and is currently used for most laparoscopic splenectomies.[18] At present, the only indication for the anterior approach to laparoscopic splenectomy is the presence of massive splenomegaly or a megaspleen. Typically, this alternative approach is taken when a spleen reaches or exceeds 23 cm in length or 3 kg in weight.

Step 1: Placement of Trocars

The patient is placed in the right lateral decubitus position, much as he or she would be for a left-side posterolateral thoracotomy. The operating table is flexed and the kidney bolster raised to increase the distance between the lower rib and the iliac crest. Usually, four 12 mm trocars are used around the costal margin so that the camera, the clip applier, and the linear stapler can be interchanged with maximum flexibility [*see Figure 4*]. The trocars must be far enough apart to permit good working angles. Some advantage may be gained from tilting the patient slightly backward; this step gives the operating team more freedom in moving the instruments placed along the left costal margins, especially during lifting movements, when it is easy for instrument handles to touch the operating table. For the same reason, it is also advisable to place the anterior or abdominal side of the patient closer to the edge of the operating table.

A local anesthetic is infiltrated into the skin at the midpoint of the anterior costal margin, and a 12 mm incision is made. The first trocar is inserted under direct vision, and a symmetrical 15 mm Hg pneumoperitoneum is created. The locations of the remaining trocars are determined by considering the anatomic configuration in relation to the size of the spleen to be excised. In most cases, the fourth posterior trocar cannot be inserted until the splenic flexure of the colon has been mobilized. Accordingly, the procedure is usually started with three trocars in place.

Troubleshooting *Open insertion of first trocar.* After years of using the Veress needle, we now prefer the open method of inserting the first trocar. It is true that use of the Veress needle is for the most part safe; however, the small number of catastrophic complications that occur with blind methods of first trocar insertion are more and more difficult to justify. Admittedly, these complications are infrequent, and thus, it is unlikely that even a large randomized trial would be able to show any significant differences between various methods of first trocar insertion. Nevertheless, even though complications occur with the open method of first trocar insertion as well, they are very uncommon and tend to be limited to trauma to the intestine or the omental blood vessels; they do not have the same serious consequences as the major vessel injury that may arise from blind trocar insertion.

Figure 4 **Laparoscopic splenectomy: lateral approach. Shown is standard trocar placement. Four trocars are used. In most cases, the procedure is begun without the posterior trocar in place.**

Alternative trocar placement. More experienced surgeons (or those simply wishing to make the procedure easier) may choose to replace one or two 12 mm trocars with 5 mm trocars [*see Figure 5a*]. The procedure can also be performed with only three trocars. In leaner patients, one of the trocars can be inserted into the umbilicus to gain a cosmetic advantage. The advent of needlescopic techniques has made it possible to replace some of the 5 and 12 mm trocars with 3 mm trocars. The ultimate (i.e., least invasive) technique, usually reserved for lean patients with ITP and normal-size spleens, involves one 12 mm trocar placed in the umbilicus and two 3 mm trocars placed subcostally [*see Figure 5b*]. This approach requires two different camera-laparoscope setups, so that a 3 mm laparoscope can be interchanged with a 10 mm laparoscope as necessary to permit application of clips or staplers through the umbilical incision once the dissection is completed. The specimen is then retrieved through the umbilicus. Because the use of 3 mm laparoscopes is accompanied by a decrease in available intra-abdominal light and focal width, a meticulously bloodless field and sophisticated surgical judgment are critical for successful performance of needlescopic splenectomy.

Step 2: Search for and Retrieval of Accessory Spleens

The camera is inserted, and the stomach is retracted medially to expose the spleen. Then a fairly standard sequence is followed. A thorough search is then made for accessory spleens. To maximize retrieval, all known locations of accessory spleens should be carefully explored [*see Figure 6*]. Any accessory spleens found should be removed immediately; they are considerably harder to locate once the spleen is removed.

Troubleshooting It is especially important to retrieve accessory spleens from patients with ITP, in whom the presence of overlooked accessory spleens has been associated with recurrence of the disease. Remedial operation for excision of missed accessory spleens has been reported to bring remission of recurrent disease; such operation can be performed laparoscopically. The overall retrieval rate for accessory spleens should fall between 15% and 30%.

Splenic activity has been demonstrated after open and laparoscopic splenectomy for trauma and hematologic disorders[19,20]; accordingly, it is advisable to wash out and recover all splenic fragments resulting from intraoperative trauma at the end of the procedure. This step is particularly important for patients with ITP, in whom intraoperative trauma to the spleen is thought to contribute to postoperative scan-detectable splenic activity. As of this writing, we have recovered accessory spleens in 33% of ITP cases treated laparoscopically.

Step 3: Control of Vessels at Lower Pole, Demonstration of "Splenic Tent," and Incision of Phrenicocolic Ligament

The splenic flexure is partially mobilized by incising the splenocolic ligament, the lower part of the phrenicocolic ligament, and the sustentaculum lienis. The incision is carried slightly into the left side of the gastrocolic ligament. This step affords access to the gastrosplenic ligament, which can then be readily separated from the splenorenal ligament to create what looks like a tent. This maneuver cannot be accomplished in all cases, but when it can be done, it simplifies the procedure considerably. The walls of this so-called splenic tent are made of the gastrosplenic ligament on the left and the splenorenal ligament on the right, and the floor is made up of the stomach. In fact, this maneuver opens the lesser sac in its lateral portion (a point that is better demonstrated with gentle upward retraction of the splenic tip) [*see Figure 7*].

The branches of the left gastroepiploic artery are controlled with the electrocautery or with clips, depending on the size of the branches. The avascular portion of the gastrosplenic ligament, situated between the gastroepiploic artery and the short gastric vessels, is then incised sufficiently to expose the hilar structures in the splenorenal ligament. To accomplish this, the lower pole is gently elevated; in this position, the spleen almost retracts itself as it naturally falls toward the left lobe of the liver. At this point, the surgeon can usually assess the geography of the hilum and determine the degree of difficulty of the operation. The fourth trocar, if needed, is then placed posteriorly under direct vision, with care taken to avoid the left kidney. Caution must also be exercised in placing the trocars situated immediately anterior and posterior to the iliac crest. The iliac crest can impede movement and hinder upward mobilization of structures if the trocars are placed over it rather than in front of or behind it [*see Figure 8*].

Finally, the phrenicocolic ligament is incised all the way to the left crus of the diaphragm, either with a monopolar electrocautery with an L hook or with scissors. A small portion of the ligament is left to keep the spleen suspended and facilitate subsequent bagging. The

a

b

Figure 5 **Laparoscopic splenectomy: lateral approach. Shown are alternative trocar placements. (a) In some patients (e.g., thin patients with normal-size spleens), a 12 mm trocar may be placed in the umbilicus to gain a cosmetic advantage, and most of the other trocars may be downsized to 5 mm. (b) In the needlescopic approach, only three trocars are placed: a 12 mm trocar in the umbilicus and two 3 mm subcostal trocars. Two camera-laparoscope setups (3 mm and 10 mm) are required.**

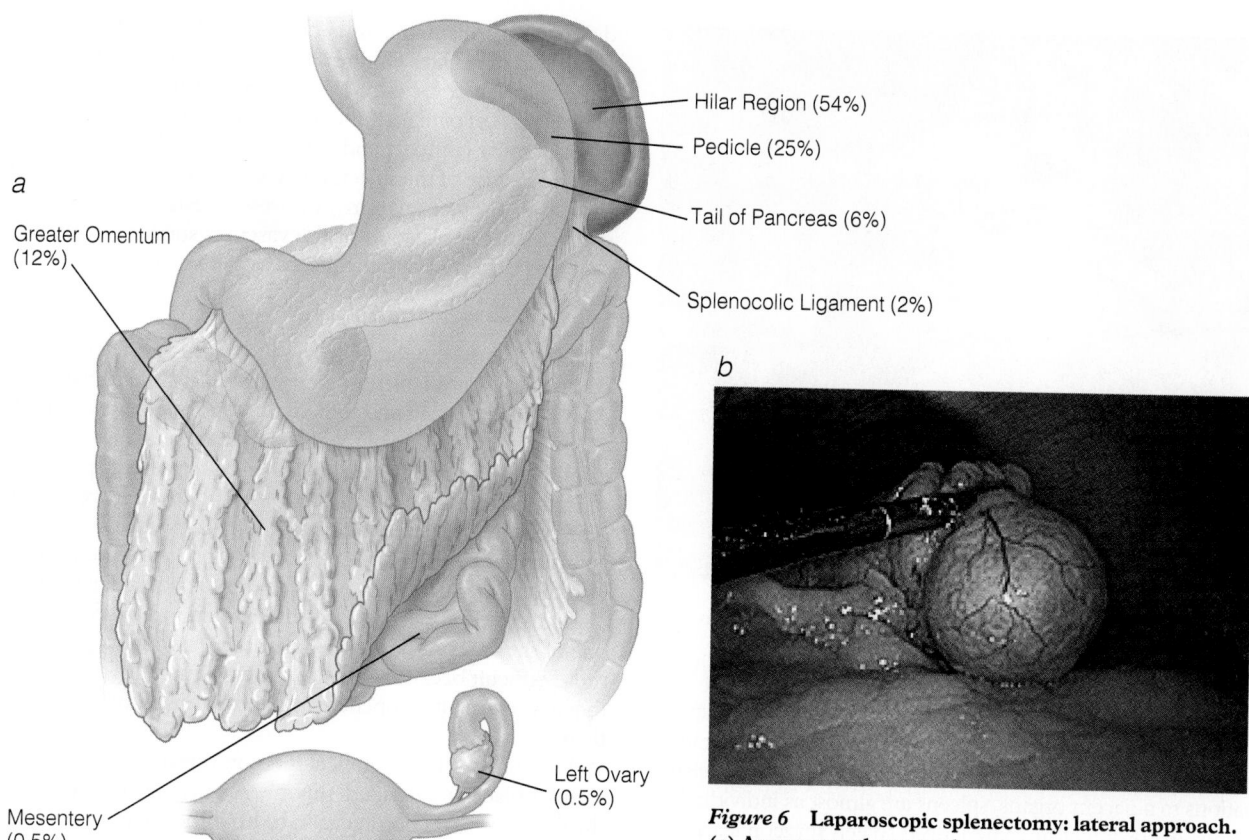

a

Greater Omentum (12%)

Hilar Region (54%)

Pedicle (25%)

Tail of Pancreas (6%)

Splenocolic Ligament (2%)

Mesentery (0.5%)

Left Ovary (0.5%)

b

Figure 6 **Laparoscopic splenectomy: lateral approach. (a) Accessory spleens are known to occur at specific sites. (b) Shown is an accessory spleen.**

phrenicocolic ligament is avascular except in patients with portal hypertension or myeloproliferative disorders (e.g., myeloid metaplasia). Leaving 1 to 2 cm of ligament all along the spleen side facilitates retraction and handling of the spleen with instruments.

Troubleshooting Remarkably few instruments are needed for laparoscopic splenectomy [*see Figure 9*]: most of the operation is done with three reusable instruments. A dolphin-nose 5 mm atraumatic grasper is used to elevate and hold the spleen. It is also used to separate tissue planes and vessels with blunt dissection because its atraumatic tip is easily insinuated between tissue planes. A gently curved 5 mm fine-tip dissector (Crile or Maryland) and a 10 mm 90° right-angle dissector are the only other tools required for cost-efficient dissection.

When a powered instrument is called for, we use a monopolar electrocautery with an L hook or a gently curved scissors [*see Figure 9*]. An ultrasonic dissector can also be used.

Step 4: Dealing with Splenic Hilum and Tailoring Operative Strategy to Anatomy

It is advisable to base one's operative strategy on the specific splenic anatomy. If a distributed anatomy is present, the splenic branches are usually dissected and clipped. This is not only the least costly approach but also the simplest, in that the vessels are spread over a wider area of the splenic hilum and are easier to dissect and separate [*see Figure 10*].

A magistral anatomy lends itself more to a single use of the linear stapler, provided that the tail of the pancreas is identified and dissected away when required. When possible, a window is created above the hilar pedicle in the splenorenal ligament so that all structures can

be included within the markings of the linear stapler under direct vision [*see Figure 11*]. The angles provided by the various trocars make this maneuver much easier via the lateral approach than via the anterior approach. Dissection continues with individual dissection and clipping of the short gastric vessels; occasionally, these vessels can also be taken en masse with the linear stapler. So far, we have not used sutures in this setting, except once to control a short gastric vessel that was too short to be clipped safely. This portion of the operation is performed while the spleen is hanging from the upper portion of the phrenicocolic ligament, which has not yet been entirely cut.

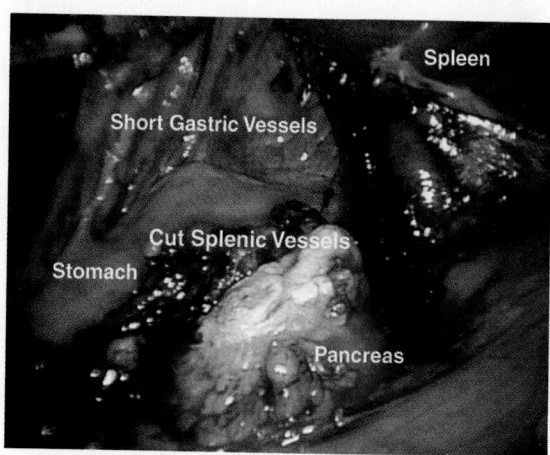

Spleen

Short Gastric Vessels

Cut Splenic Vessels

Stomach

Pancreas

Figure 7 **Laparoscopic splenectomy: lateral approach. The so-called splenic tent is formed by the gastrosplenic and splenorenal ligaments laterally and the stomach below.**

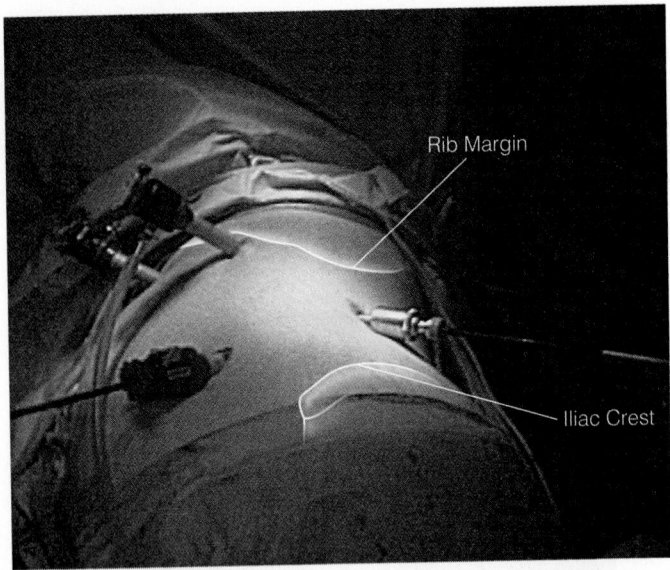

Figure 8 **Laparoscopic splenectomy: lateral approach. Shown is the recommended trocar placement around the iliac crest.**

Troubleshooting It is at this point in the procedure that experience in designing the operative strategy pays off in reduced operating time. Because of the many variations in size, shape, vascular patterns, and relations to adjacent organs, spleens are almost as individual as fingerprints. Accordingly, an experienced spleen surgeon learns to keep an open mind with regard to operative strategy and must be able to call on a wide range of skills to facilitate the procedure.

The surgeon should start by looking at the internal surface of the spleen. If the splenic vessels cover more than 75% of the internal surface (as is the case in 70% of patients), a distributed anatomy is present, which means that the spleen can be expected to have more vessels spread out over a wider area. The number of splenic branches is also related to the presence of notches on the spleen surface. With a distributed vascular anatomy, the vessels tend to be easier to

Figure 9 **Laparoscopic splenectomy: lateral approach. Laparoscopic splenectomy can be done with a few basic instruments: (*a*) a 5 mm laparoscopic grasper, (*b*) a 5 mm laparoscopic dissector, (*c*) a 10 mm right-angle dissector, (*d*) a curved laparoscopic scissors, and (*e*) a monopolar electrocautery with an L hook.**

dissect and isolate and thus can be readily (and cost-effectively) controlled with clips. On the other hand, if the splenic vessels entering the spleen cover only 25% to 35% of the inner surface of the hilum (30% of patients), the pattern is magistral. In such cases, the hilum is more compact and fewer vessels can be expected, especially if the surface of the spleen is smooth and without notches. With a magistral vascular anatomy, the vessels can usually be controlled with a single application of the vascular stapler across the hilum, provided that the tail of the pancreas can be protected.

Step 5: Extraction of Spleen

A medium-size or large heavy-duty plastic freezer bag, of the sort commercially available in grocery stores, is used to bag the spleen. This bag is sterilized and folded, then introduced into the abdominal cavity through one of the 12 mm trocars [*see Figure 12*]. The bag is unfolded and the spleen slipped inside to prevent splenosis during the subsequent manipulations. Grasping forceps are used to hold the two rigid edges of the bag and to effect partial closure. Bagging is facilitated by preserving the upper portion of the phrenicocolic ligament. After final section of the phrenicocolic ligament and any diaphragmatic adhesions present, extraction is performed through one of the anterior port sites. Extraction through a posterior site is more difficult because of the thickness of the muscle mass; usually, the incision must be opened, and more muscle must be fulgurated than is desirable.

The subcostal or umbilical incision through which extraction is to take place is extended slightly. A grasping forceps is inserted through the extraction incision to hold the edges of the bag inside the abdomen. Gentle traction on the bag from outside brings the spleen close to the peritoneal surface of the umbilical incision and then out of the wound [*see Figure 13*]. Specimen retrieval bags have been developed that can accommodate a normal-size spleen and thus make bagging much easier, but they are costly.

A biopsy specimen of a size suitable for pathologic identification is obtained by incising the splenic tip. The spleen is then fragmented with finger fracture, and the resulting blood is suctioned. The remaining stromal tissue of the spleen is then extracted through the small incision, hemostasis is again verified, and all trocars are removed. No drains are used. The incisions are closed with absorbable sutures and paper strips. After verification of hemostasis, the trocar sites are closed with absorbable sutures and paper strips.

Troubleshooting The freezer bags can be more easily introduced into the abdomen if they are pulled in rather than pushed in [*see Figure 12*]. This may be accomplished by bringing out a 5 mm toothed grasper through the introduction trocar from another properly angled trocar, grasping the specimen bag, and pulling the bag back down through the trocar.

Slipping the spleen into a freezer bag is also an acquired skill that takes some time to master. It is an important skill that is useful in many other instances where specimen retrieval is needed (e.g., in procedures involving the gallbladder, the appendix, the adrenal glands, or the colon). In addition, it is highly cost-effective, in that these commercially available bags cost only a few cents each. Admittedly, laparoscopic retrieval bags are easier to use, but their substantially higher cost can become a factor in a busy minimally invasive surgery unit. We recently started to use a powerful suction machine (–70 mm Hg) and a custom-made sharp beveled 10 mm cannula to suction splenic tissue from the plastic retrieval bag [*see Figure 14*].

ANTERIOR APPROACH

The anterior approach is seldom used nowadays; however, it remains the preferable approach in some patients with massive spleno-

a *b*

Figure 10 **Laparoscopic splenectomy: lateral approach. (*a, b*) Clipping is well suited to controlling short gastric or gastroepiploic vessels. It is also appropriate for distributed-type splenic vasculatures, in which more splenic vessels are spread over a wider area of the hilum.**

megaly (21 to 30 cm long) and all patients with megaspleens (> 30 cm or > 3 kg). Very large spleens are extremely heavy and difficult to manipulate with laparoscopic instruments, and it is complicated to lift them so as to gain access to the phrenicocolic ligament posteriorly. The anterior approach can also be considered if another procedure (e.g., cholecystectomy) is being contemplated; alternatively, in this situation, the lateral approach can be used, and the patient can be repositioned for the secondary procedure.

Step 1: Placement of Trocars

Under general anesthesia, the patient is placed in a modified lithotomy position to allow the surgeon to operate between the patient's legs and to allow the assistants to stand on each side of the patient. The procedure is performed through five trocars in the upper abdomen [*see Figure 15*], with the patient in a steep Fowler position with left-side elevation. A 12 mm trocar is introduced through an umbilical incision, and a 10 mm laparoscope (0° or 30°) is connected to a video system. A 12 mm trocar is placed in each upper quadrant, and two 5 mm trocars are inserted close to the rib margin on the left and right sides of the abdomen. Alternatively, trocars can be deployed in a semicircle away from the left upper quadrant. Trocar sites are carefully selected to optimize working angles. The 12 mm ports are used to allow introduction of clip appliers, staplers, or the laparoscope from a variety of angles as needed.

Troubleshooting With increasing experience, we find that we prefer to do as many laparoscopic splenectomies as possible via the lateral approach because it is so much easier, even with spleens that are longer than 20 cm and are readily palpable. The decision is arbitrarily made on the basis of estimated available working space. If the spleen comes too close to the iliac crest or the midline, the anterior approach should be taken instead.

Step 2: Isolation of Lower Pole and Control of Blood Supply

The left hepatic lobe is retracted, and the stomach is retracted medially to expose the spleen. Accessory spleens are searched for, and the phrenicocolic ligament, the splenocolic ligament, and the sustentaculum lienis are incised near the lower pole with an electrocautery and a hook probe or with scissors. Vascular adhesions—frequently found on the medial side of the spleen—are cauterized. The gastrocolic ligament is carefully dissected close to the spleen, and the left gastroepiploic vessels are ligated one by one with metallic clips or, if small, simply cauterized. The upper and lower poles of the

spleen are gently lifted with one or both palpators (placed through the 5 mm ports) to expose the splenic hilum and the tail of the pancreas within the splenorenal ligament, thereby facilitating individual dissection and clipping of all the branches of the splenic artery and vein close to the spleen. The short gastric vessels are then identified and ligated with clips or, occasionally, with staples. No sutures are used. Alternatively, the splenic artery itself can be isolated and clipped within the lesser sac before extensive dissection of the lower pole and suspensory ligaments.

When preoperative splenic artery embolization is employed [*see Preoperative Splenic Artery Embolization, below*], the dissection plane is situated between the sites of distal embolization of splenic artery branches and the site of proximal embolization of the splenic artery itself. Because of the segmental and terminal distribution of splenic arteries, it is easy to determine the devascularized portions of the spleen: these segments exhibit a characteristic grayish color, whereas the vascularized segments retain a pinkish hue. When the organ is completely isolated, it is left in its natural cavity, and hemostasis is verified.

Troubleshooting If one elects first to clip the splenic artery within the lesser sac, there are a few precautions that must be taken. First, the clipping must be done distal to the pancreatica magna artery to prevent pancreatic injury. Second, one must make sure that the splenic artery proper is clipped, not one of its branches (e.g., the superior terminal branch). This is an easy mistake to commit with the distributed type of splenic vasculature [*see Figure 1*] because the splenic artery itself is short and the branches can take off very early. Third, one must always keep in mind the possibility of an anastomotic branch between the major splenic branches, as described by Testut.[13] Should a major terminal branch be clipped rather than the splenic artery proper, there will be no spleen ischemia if such an anastomosis is present [*see Figure 1*].

Yet another challenge posed by the anterior approach is that if bleeding occurs, the blood tends to pool in the area of the hilum and obscure vision even more, whereas in the lateral approach, the blood tends to flow away from the operative field. One quickly learns that there is a steep price to pay for cutting corners during the dissection. The dissection must be meticulous, especially behind branches of the splenic vein.

Step 3: Extraction of Spleen

Given that the anterior approach is now used only in cases of

a

b

c

Figure 11 **Laparoscopic splenectomy: lateral approach. (*a through c*) Stapling is particularly well suited to the compact hilum found in the magistral-type distribution of splenic vessels. As shown, all of the vascular structures are within the stapler markers, and the tail of the pancreas is well protected.**

massive splenomegaly or megaspleen, bagging can be problematic. The largest commercially available freezer bag we have seen measures 27 by 28 cm, and the largest spleen we have been able to bag in one of them was 24 cm long. Furthermore, an accessory extraction incision is often required; a Pfannenstiel incision gives better cosmetic results, but a left lower quadrant incision can also be used. A plastic sleeve designed to maintain pneumoperitoneum is also a useful adjunct for vessel dissection and extraction in patients with very large spleens.

Figure 12 **Laparoscopic splenectomy: lateral approach. Illustrated is the introduction of a sterile freezer bag for specimen extraction via the pull method. A toothed grasper is passed across the abdomen between two trocars and brought out through the 12 mm umbilical trocar site. This grasper is used to pull the extraction bag back into the abdomen.**

If the spleen cannot be bagged, it may be fragmented in the pelvis before extraction, provided that the abdomen is copiously washed and cleaned of any residual spleen fragments before closure to prevent splenosis. Most patients with large spleens have hematologic malignancies; thus, residual splenic activity is not as crucial an issue in these patients as it would be in others.

Troubleshooting Many surgeons advocate the use of pneumatic sleeves as an adjunct to laparoscopic splenectomy. Most such sleeves require at least a 7.5 cm incision for introduction. In our view, use of these sleeves tends to work against the ultimate goal of minimally invasive surgery, which is to produce good surgical outcomes with as little trauma as possible; however, it can be a very helpful aid while one is learning laparoscopic splenectomy as well as in certain special circumstances (e.g., laparoscopic splenectomy for large spleens).

The incision for the pneumatic sleeve may be placed either transversely in the right upper quadrant or vertically in the upper midline. Alternatively, a Pfannenstiel incision may be employed: it has

Figure 13 **Laparoscopic splenectomy: lateral approach. Shown is the position of the specimen bag position before finger fragmentation or pulp suction.**

Figure 14 **Laparoscopic splenectomy: lateral approach. A beveled 10 mm suction cannula is used for subcapsular volume reduction in patients with megaspleens. This custom-made suction cannula can also be used to aspirate splenic pulp from the plastic retrieval bag during laparoscopic splenectomy in patients with normal-size or moderately enlarged spleens.**

cosmetic advantages over upper abdominal incisions and may result in fewer pulmonary complications. Use of the pneumatic sleeve may facilitate hilar dissection by improving retraction (especially in the upper pole) and by guiding placement of linear staples or clips. It may also facilitate retraction of enlarged spleens to improve access to all of the suspensory ligaments.

LAPAROSCOPIC PARTIAL SPLENECTOMY

Concern regarding the risk of OPSS has encouraged the practice of preserving splenic tissue and function whenever possible. For this reason, partial splenectomy has occasionally been indicated for treatment of benign tumors of the spleen and for excision of cystic lesions.[21] Its use has been described in connection with the management of type I Gaucher disease, cholesteryl ester storage disease, chronic myelogenous leukemia, and thalassemia major as well as the staging of Hodgkin disease.[22,23] Partial splenectomy has also been an option in the management of splenic trauma when the pa-

tient's condition is stable enough to permit the meticulous dissection required for the operation.[24,25]

Operative Technique

Like standard laparoscopic splenectomy, laparoscopic partial splenectomy is performed with the patient in the right lateral decubitus position. Trocar placement is similar as well. The splenocolic ligament and the lower part of the phrenicocolic ligament are incised to permit mobilization of the lower pole of the spleen. If the lower portion of the spleen is to be excised, branches of the gastroepiploic vessels supplying the lower pole are dissected and clipped close to the parenchyma. An appropriate number of penultimate branches of the inferior polar artery are then taken in such a way as to create a clear line of demarcation between normal spleen and devascularized spleen. This process is continued until the desired number of splenic segments are devascularized. Next, a standard monopolar electrocautery is used to score the splenic capsule circumferentially, with care taken to ensure that a 5 mm rim of devascularized splenic tissue remains in situ; this is the most important technical point for this procedure [*see Figure 16*]. The incision is then carried into the splenic pulp. Atraumatic intestinal graspers are also used to fracture the splenic pulp in a bloodless fashion. The laparoscopic L hook and scissors provide excellent hemostatic control.

Once the spleen has been allowed to demarcate, resection is remarkably bloodless, provided that the 5 mm rim of ischemic tissue is left in place. Complete control of the splenic artery is not required before splenic separation, because division occurs in an ischemic segment of spleen.[9] The feasibility of leaving portions of ischemic spleen in situ has been demonstrated in a large prospective, randomized trial involving partial splenic embolization as primary treatment of hematologic disorders.[26]

If the superior pole is to be removed, the phrenicocolic ligament must be incised almost entirely so that the spleen can be easily mobilized and the proper exposure achieved. The short gastric branch-

Figure 15 **Laparoscopic splenectomy: anterior approach. Shown is standard trocar placement. The umbilical site is used for the camera. The remaining trocars are placed in the left and right upper quadrants, the epigastrium, and the right subcostal region. Depending on the size of the spleen, the trocars can also be disposed in a semicircle away from the left upper quadrant.**

Figure 16 **Laparoscopic splenectomy: partial splenectomy. (*a, b*) The splenic capsule is scored with the monopolar cautery, and a 5 mm margin of devitalized tissue is left. (*c*) The splenic pulp is fractured with an atraumatic grasper. The electrocautery with the L hook is also used to control parenchymal bleeding. (*d*) Shown is the cut surface of the spleen after transection. The operative field remains remarkably dry.**

es are taken first, along with the desired number of superior polar artery branches.

Laparoscopic partial splenectomy can be performed either with or without the aid of selective preoperative arterial embolization. Radiologists are capable of cannulating the desired segmental splenic arterial branch and embolizing the segment that is to be resected. We have removed the superior pole in a patient with a class IV isolated splenic injury sustained while skiing[8]; partial laparoscopic splenectomy was made possible largely by the accuracy of selective arterial embolization, which permitted control of the bleeding and allowed laparoscopy to be performed in unhurried conditions.[27]

PREOPERATIVE SPLENIC ARTERY EMBOLIZATION

Preoperative splenic artery embolization is used as an adjuvant in a few patients to make laparoscopic splenectomy possible and to reduce blood loss. Although it is now infrequently used, it remains a useful tool in the armamentarium of spleen surgeons.

Preoperative splenic artery embolization is usually performed on the morning of operation to reduce the duration of the pain caused by the procedure. Approximately 45% of patients undergoing embolization experience some degree of pain, which is easily controlled by administering narcotics or instituting patient-controlled analgesia. In some patients, thrombosis extends to the venous side of the splenic blood supply when embolization is done on the day before operation. Whether this occurrence translates into any measurable advantage remains to be determined.

Generally speaking, the technique involves embolization of the spleen with coils placed proximally in the splenic artery and absorbable gelatin sponges and small coils placed distally in each splenic arterial branch (the double embolization technique), with care taken to spare vessels supplying the tail of the pancreas [*see Figure 17*]. More specifically, splenic artery embolization is performed through a 5 French catheter (typically a cobra catheter, though sidewinder and various other types are also used) inserted into the right groin with the patient under local anesthesia. The catheter tip is placed in the splenic artery and advanced to the splenic hilum proximal to the left gastroepiploic artery (or the great pancreatic artery) so that distal pancreatic branches of the splenic artery can be observed. At this level, either iohexol 65% or iothalamate 60% is forcefully injected and a digital substraction angiogram done to verify the pattern of the splenic blood supply.

If no pancreatic branches are opacified, there are several techniques that may be used. In particular, 3 to 5 mm microcoils are placed in the hilar branches of the splenic artery; alternatively, absorbable gelatin sponges are used. The catheter is then pulled back 2 to 4 cm, and one or two 5 to 8 mm microcoils are launched into the main trunk of the splenic artery distal to the great pancreatic artery to prevent pancreatitis or pancreatic necrosis. The surgical plane of dissection is therefore situated between the proximal and distal embolization sites.

The procedure is ended when it is estimated radiologically that 80% or more of the splenic tissue has been successfully embolized.

In most cases, successful embolization is achieved with both proximal and distal emboli; in a minority of cases, it is achieved with proximal emboli alone or with distal emboli alone.[28]

Troubleshooting Preoperative splenic artery embolization is safe, provided that two main principles are adhered to. First, embolization must be done distal to the great pancreatic artery to minimize pancreatic damage. Second, neither microspheres nor absorbable gelatin powder should be used, because particles of this small size may migrate to unintended target organ capillaries and cause tissue necrosis; only coils and absorbable gelatin sponge fragments should be used. If these precautions are taken, embolization is safe and remains a useful tool for difficult cases.

Postoperative Care

Postoperative care for patients who have undergone laparoscopic splenectomy is usually simple. The nasogastric tube inserted after induction of general anesthesia is removed either in the recovery room, once stomach emptying has been verified, or the next morning, depending on the duration and the degree of technical difficulty of the procedure. The urinary catheter is usually removed before the patient leaves the recovery room. The patient is allowed to drink clear fluids on the morning after the operation; when clear fluids are well tolerated, the patient is allowed to proceed to a diet of his or her choice.

If the patient has no history of ulcer or dyspepsia, a 100 mg indomethacin suppository is inserted before induction of anesthesia and again every 12 hours for a total of three to five doses. Postoperative pain medication is given on an individualized basis with a view to ensuring complete patient comfort. Meperidine injections (1 mg/kg) are administered during the first night, followed by oral acetaminophen (1 g every 6 hours). If pain is not well controlled, coanalgesia with an NSAID is added; this combination produces the best results. Because of its side effects (i.e., nausea, vomiting, abdominal fullness, and constipation), codeine is currently avoided if at all possible. When indomethacin is used, prophylactic doses of subcutaneous heparin are avoided on empirical grounds, especially if the platelet count is low or platelet function is abnormal.

Patients receiving I.V. cortisone are given oral steroids on postoperative day 1 after an overlap I.V. injection; thereafter, steroids are gradually tapered. Patients are allowed to shower 48 hours after

surgery and are advised to keep the paper strips covering the trocar incisions in place for 7 to 10 days. No drains are used. No limitations are imposed on physical activity, and patients are allowed to tailor their activities to their degree of asthenia or discomfort.

Complications

Postoperative complications directly related to splenectomy include intraoperative and postoperative hemorrhage; left lower lobe atelectasis and pneumonia; left pleural effusion; subphrenic collection; iatrogenic pancreatic, gastric, and colonic injury; and venous thrombosis.[24-31]

Successful laparoscopic splenectomy depends to a large extent on proper preparation. Recognition of anatomic elements and their arrangement is paramount. As with other laparoscopic procedures, the keys are avoiding complications and minimizing technical misadventures. Vascular structures should be cleanly isolated and dissected from surrounding fat; they then can usually be controlled with two clips proximally and distally. Staplers should be used with care and should not be applied blindly. The stapler tip should be clearly seen to be free of tissue before it is closed; otherwise, hemorrhage from partial section of a major splenic branch might occur after the instrument is released. Blind application of the stapler may also result in damage to the tail of the pancreas, which often lies in close proximity to the inner surface of the spleen. If both clips and a linear stapler are used, it is vital to prevent interposition of clips in the staple line, which will cause the stapler to misfire and possibly to jam.

Improper use of the electrocautery during the procedure can cause iatrogenic injury to the stomach, the colon, or the pancreas. In a smoke-filled environment, where controlling vessels is difficult and time consuming, blind fulguration of fat in the hilum can lead to bleeding. Structures close to the lower pole in the gastrocolic ligament can be approached more aggressively, but not those in the hilum. To prevent arcing and spot necrosis, which may result in delayed perforation and sepsis, the instrument should be activated only in proximity to the target organ.

The assistants also play an important role in preventing complications. All instruments, including those handled by assistants, should be moved under direct vision. Especially in the anterior approach, retraction of the liver and stomach and elevation of the spleen require constant concentration if lacerations and subsequent hemorrhage or perforation are to be avoided.

Special Considerations

EXTRACTION OF SPECIMENS

Spleens removed via the anterior approach are extracted through the umbilical trocar site after finger fragmentation in a plastic bag. It is rarely necessary to enlarge the umbilical incision to more than 2 or 3 cm. When the lateral approach is used, extraction is more easily performed through one of the ports situated anteriorly. This extraction site also requires little or no enlargement. On occasion, for a spleen longer than 20 cm, a 7.5 to 10 cm Pfannenstiel incision is made, and the operator's forearm is introduced into the abdomen to deliver the spleen into the pelvis for extraction in large fragments under direct vision. Pneumatic sleeves may also be used to facilitate hand-assisted surgery. The abdomen is copiously irrigated before closure.

Special mention should be made of laparoscopic splenectomy in patients with malignant disease. If lymphoma or Hodgkin disease is suspected, neither preoperative splenic artery embolization nor finger fragmentation in a plastic bag should be performed, for fear of

Figure 17 **Laparoscopic splenectomy: splenic artery embolization. Shown are splenic angiograms of a patient with thrombotic thrombocytopenic purpura before (left) and after (right) splenic artery embolization with 3 cm, 5 cm, and 7 cm coils and absorbable gelatin sponge fragments.**

making the histologic diagnosis difficult. Extraction of intact spleens through a small left subcostal or median incision has also been employed when preservation of tissue architecture is required. The various techniques of fragmentation and extraction of splenic tissue during laparoscopic splenectomy should be discussed and agreed on with the pathologist ahead of time to ensure that proper pathologic diagnoses are not compromised by either necrotic tissue (in the case of preoperative splenic artery embolization) or altered tissue architecture (in the case of finger fragmentation), especially if malignancy is suspected but not proven. In practice, however, we have found that the diagnosis is made preoperatively in more than 90% of patients with benign and malignant hematologic disease; hence, the issue rarely arises.

MASSIVE SPLENOMEGALY AND MEGASPLEENS

Massive splenomegaly is defined as the presence of a spleen with an interpole length exceeding 20 cm on ultrasonography or a weight exceeding 1,000 g. Laparoscopic removal of spleens of this size is fraught with problems, mostly related to the size of the organ and its components. Large spleens, besides being heavy and hard to manipulate, carry a high risk of serious hemorrhage. Consequently, preoperative splenic artery embolization is sometimes done beforehand because it helps control arterial flow preoperatively. If embolization is performed long enough before operation, it may even be possible to control the venous side of the blood supply through retrograde thrombosis; that blood clots are occasionally expelled from sections of splenic veins during laparoscopic splenectomy attests to the occurrence of this phenomenon. Finding a sensible way to retrieve the specimen also presents an important challenge.

When a spleen longer than 20 cm is to be removed, some modifications must be made to the technique of laparoscopic splenectomy. Once sectioning of the vessels and the suspensory ligaments is complete, a 7.5 to 10 cm Pfannenstiel incision is made at the pubic hairline. Through this incision, hand revision of the operative site under laparoscopic control can be accomplished, and if necessary, any remaining vessels or ligamentous attachments can be sectioned under video control. Adequate pneumoperitoneum can be maintained with the forearm placed through the lower abdominal incision. Whenever possible, the spleen is placed in a plastic bag; however, to date, we have not been able to bag a spleen longer than 24 cm.

That extraction of a very large specimen requires fragmentation of the spleen in the pelvis and extraction through a Pfannenstiel incision raises the possibility of postoperative splenosis. To minimize this problem, after reconstitution of the pneumoperitoneum, the abdomen is copiously irrigated and reviewed for fragments of spleen and accessory spleens, which can be done very thoroughly with laparoscopy.[32]

For a long time, we had no success with laparoscopic splenectomy for spleens longer than 30 cm (i.e., megaspleens): our conversion rate was 100%. Currently, we use preoperative embolization for these spleens. We also take the anterior approach, using five trocars, and are experimenting with a technique for subcapsular volume reduction with a sharp beveled 10 mm suction cannula connected to a powerful –70 mm Hg aspirator. Megaspleens are next to impossible to move with laparoscopic instruments, and the space constraints make our usual laparoscopic approaches futile. We therefore insert the –70 mm Hg aspirating cannula into the spleen and proceed to reduce the splenic volume so that the spleen can be sectioned into more manageable pieces that can be bagged and extracted in the usual fashion. At present, it is too early to tell whether laparoscopic splenectomy will have a place in the management of megaspleens.

Outcome Evaluation

No randomized, prospective trials comparing open splenectomy with laparoscopic splenectomy have yet been conducted. At present, such trials are unlikely to be held, for a variety of reasons. For one thing, randomization is difficult with procedures that are still in evolution. At one end of the spectrum, laparoscopic splenectomy is done for patients with ITP, who usually are relatively healthy and have normal-size spleens. In many of these patients, needlescopic instruments (< 3 mm) can be used in conjunction with a single 12 mm port site in the umbilicus. This approach permits hospital discharge within 24 hours of operation in a significant number of cases. At the other end of the spectrum, laparoscopic splenectomy is done for patients with myeloid metaplasia and spleens longer than 30 cm. In this setting, a laparoscopic approach poses formidable challenges, and the optimal technique and its justification remain to be determined. The window of opportunity for randomized comparative trials may have been lost.

Large case series and nonrandomized comparative trials, however, have consistently reported better outcomes from laparoscopic splenectomy than from open splenectomy.[33-40] For example, in one set of 528 patients [see Table 2],[35-38] the rate of postoperative pneumonia was 1.1% (6/528), and no subphrenic abscesses occurred as postoperative complications. Many surgeons who have completed the learning curve associated with the procedure feel that there is still room for improvement regarding complication rates and length of stay for pa-

Table 2   Clinical Results of Laparoscopic Splenectomy

Authors	N	ITP/Non-ITP	Conversion Rate (%)	OR Time (min)	Morbidity (%)	Mortality (%)	Length of Stay (days)	Accessory Spleen Present (%)
All diagnoses								
Katkhouda et al (1998)[37]	103	67/36	3.9	161	6	0	2.5	16.5
Targarona et al (2000)[35]	122	54/68	7.4	153	18	0	4.0	12
Park et al (2000)[36]	203	129/74	3.0	145	9	0.5	2.7	12.3
Poulin et al (2001)[38]	100	50/50	8.0	180	15	4	3.0	25
ITP								
Trias et al (2000)[39]	48	—	4.2	142	12	N/A	4.0	11
Poulin et al (2001)[38]	51	—	3.9	160	5.9	0	2.0	32
Malignancy								
Schlachta et al (1999)[40]	14	—	21	239	18	9	3.0	—
Trias et al (2000)[39]	28	—	14*	171	28	N/A	5.5	—

*71% required accessory incision because of spleen size.

tients with ITP and other relatively benign conditions necessitating laparoscopic splenectomy. The more serious conditions and the mortality seen in conjunction with the procedure tend to occur in patients with advanced hematologic malignancies or mega-spleens. In such cases, most of the adverse results are related to the disease state rather than to the operation, and it remains to be seen whether laparoscopic splenectomy will have a positive effect on outcome.

One of the great attractions of minimally invasive surgery has been the prospect of significant cost reductions. At this early point in the development of laparoscopic splenectomy, however, we are reluctant to place too much trust in premature cost analyses that do not take into account the "work in progress" nature of minimally invasive surgery. Most surgeons can now perform most cases of laparoscopic splenectomy with simplified trays of reusable instruments. Our

basic laparoscopic tray contains a few instruments and two sizes of reusable clip appliers with inexpensive clips. As noted [see Operative Technique, above], clips are used for distributed-type spleens, single-use linear staplers mostly for magistral-type spleens. To reduce costs, ultrasonic dissectors are rarely used. In addition, the use of commercially available freezer bags instead of laparoscopic retrieval bags further reduces the cost of specimen extraction. Finally, even if intraoperative costs are higher with laparoscopic splenectomy, our experience is that the increase is offset by reductions in postoperative stay.

We, like most authorities, believe that as a surgeon gains experience with laparoscopic splenectomy, operating time tends to fall until it approaches that of open splenectomy. We also concur with many authors who have suggested that once laparoscopic splenectomy is mastered, use of blood products tends to decrease substantially.

References

1. Cole F: Is splenectomy harmless? Surg Gynecol Obstet 133:98, 1971
2. Johnston GB: Splenectomy. Ann Surg 48:50, 1908
3. Campos Cristo M: Segmental resections of the spleen: report on the first eight cases operated on. O Hosp (Rio) 62:205, 1962
4. Upadhyaya P, Simpson JS: Splenic trauma in children. Surg Gynecol Obstet 126:781, 1968
5. Delaitre B, Maignien B: Splénectomie par voie laparoscopique, 1 observation. Presse Médicale 20:2263, 1991
6. Carroll BJ, Phillips EH, Semel CJ, et al: Laparoscopic splenectomy. Surg Endosc 6:183, 1992
7. Thibault C, Mamazza J, Létourneau R, et al: Laparoscopic splenectomy: operative technique and preliminary report. Surg Laparosc Endosc 2:248, 1992
8. Poulin EC, Thibault C, DesCôteaux JG, et al: Partial laparoscopic splenectomy for trauma: technique and case report. Surg Laparosc Endosc 5:306, 1995
9. Seshadri PA, Poulin EC, Mamazza J, et al: Technique for laparoscopic partial splenectomy. Surg Laparosc Endosc 10:106, 2000
10. Goerg C, Schwerk WB, Goerg K, et al: Sonographic patterns of the affected spleen in malignant lymphoma. J Clin Ultrasound 18:569, 1990
11. Poulin EC, Thibault C: The anatomical basis for laparoscopic splenectomy. Can J Surg 36:485, 1993
12. Michels NA: The variational anatomy of the spleen and splenic artery. Am J Anat 70:21, 1942
13. Testut L: Traité d'anatomie humaine, 7th ed. Librairie Octave Doin, Paris, 1923, p 942
14. Lipshutz B: A composite study of the coeliac axis artery. Ann Surg 65:159, 1917
15. Henschen C: Die chirurgische Anatomie der Milzgefässe. Schweiz Med Wochenschr 58:164, 1928
16. Ssoson-Jaroschewitsch A: Zür chirurgischen Anatomie des Milzhilus. Zeitsch f. d. ges. Anat I Abt 84:218, 1937
17. Baronofsky ID, Walton W, Noble JF: Occult injury to the pancreas following splenectomy. Surgery 29:852, 1951
18. Gagner M, Lacroix A, Bolte E, et al: Laparoscopic adrenalectomy: the importance of a flank approach in the lateral decubitus position. Surg Endosc 8:135, 1994
19. Gigot JF, Jamar F, Ferrant A, et al: Inadequate detection of accessory spleens and splenosis with laparoscopic splenectomy: a shortcoming of the laparoscopic approach in hematologic diseases. Surg Endosc 12:101, 1998
20. Nielsen JL, Ellegard J, Marqversen J, et al: Detection of splenosis and ectopic spleens with 99mTc-labeled heat damaged autologous erythrocytes in 90 splenectomized patients. Scand J Haematol 27:51, 1981
21. Pachter HL, Hofstetter SR, Elkowitz A, et al: Traumatic cysts of the spleen: the role of cystectomy and splenic preservation: experience with seven consecutive patients. J Trauma 35:430, 1993
22. Guzetta PC, Ruley EJ, Merrick HFW, et al: Elective subtotal splenectomy: indications and results in 33 patients. Ann Surg 211:34, 1990
23. Hoeckstra HJ, Tamminga RY, Timens W: Partial instead of complete splenectomy in children for the pathological staging of Hodgkin's disease. Ned Tijdschr Geneeskd 137:2491, 1993
24. Sheldon GF, Croom RD, Meyer AA: The spleen. Textbook of Surgery, 14th ed. Sabiston DC, Ed. WB Saunders Co, Philadelphia, 1991, p 1108
25. Jalovec LM, Boe BS, Wyffels PL: The advantages of early operation with splenorrhaphy versus nonoperative management for the blunt splenic trauma patient. Am Surg 59:698, 1993
26. Mozes MF, Spigos DG, Pollak R, et al: Partial splenic embolization, an alternative to splenectomy: results of a prospective randomized study. Surgery 96:694, 1984
27. Poulin E, Thibault C, Mamazza J, et al: Laparoscopic splenectomy: clinical experience and the role of preoperative splenic artery embolization. Surg Laparosc Endosc 3:445, 1993
28. Poulin EC, Mamazza J, Schlachta CM: Splenic artery embolization before laparoscopic splenectomy: an update. Surg Endosc 12:870, 1998
29. Hoeffer RA, Scullin DC, Silver LF, et al: Splenectomy for hematologic disorders: a 20 year experience. J Ky Med Assoc 89:446, 1991
30. Ly B, Albrechtson D: Therapeutic splenectomy in hematologic disorders. Effects and complications in 221 adult patients Acta Med Scand 209:21, 1981
31. Macrae HM, Yakimets WW, Reynolds T: Perioperative complications of splenectomy for hematologic disease. Can J Surg 35:432, 1992
32. Poulin EC, Thibault C: Laparoscopic splenectomy for massive splenomegaly: operative technique and case report. Can J Surg 38:69, 1995
33. Poulin EC, Mamazza J: Laparoscopic splenectomy: lessons from the learning curve. Can J Surg 41:28, 1998
34. Cathode N, Hurwitz MB, Rivera RT, et al: Laparoscopic splenectomy: outcome and efficacy in 103 consecutive patients. Ann Surg 228:568, 1998
35. Targarona EM, Espert JJ, Bombuy E, et al: Complications of laparoscopic splenectomy. Arch Surg 135:1137, 2000
36. Park AE, Birgisson G, Mastrangelo MJ, et al: Laparoscopic splenectomy: outcomes and lessons learned from over 200 cases. Surgery 128:660, 2000
37. Katkhouda N, Hurwitz MB, Rivera RT, et al: Laparoscopic splenectomy: outcome and efficacy in 103 consecutive patients. Ann Surg 228:568, 1998
38. Poulin EC, Schlachta CM, Mamazza J: Unpublished data, February 2001
39. Trias M, Targarona EM, Espert JJ, et al: Impact of hematological diagnosis on early and late outcome after laparoscopic splenectomy: an analysis of 111 cases. Surg Endosc 14:556, 2000
40. Schlachta CM, Poulin EC, Mamazza J: Laparoscopic splenectomy for hematologic malignancies. Surg Endosc 13:865, 1999

Acknowledgment

Figures 1, 3, 4, 6a, and 15   Tom Moore.

15 INTESTINAL ANASTOMOSIS

Zane Cohen, M.D., and Barry Sullivan, M.D.

Intestinal anastomosis is one of the most commonly performed intra-abdominal procedures [*see Sidebar* Intestinal Anastomosis: Historical Perspective]. It is required to reestablish gastrointestinal continuity after surgical resection, traumatic disruption, or bypass procedures. There are several principles that are crucial for obtaining successful results [*see Table 1*]. Of these, surgical technique is widely regarded as the most important for maintaining anastomotic integrity, given that intersurgeon rates of anastomotic breakdown vary by as much as a factor of 60.[1] Anastomotic leakage greatly increases the morbidity and mortality associated with surgical procedures. It has been shown to double the length of hospital stay and increase the chance of dying threefold to 10-fold.[2] Dehiscence, when it occurs, has been associated with one fifth to one third of all postoperative deaths in patients who underwent intestinal anastomosis.[3] Reported leakage rates range from 1.5 percent[4] to 2.2 percent,[5] depending on the type of anastomosis performed and the clinical scenario (i.e., elective or emergency).

Unfortunately, anastomotic dehiscence can occur even in ideal circumstances. This unwelcome fact has stimulated a great deal of debate regarding the reliability of various methods and approaches. In what follows, we address certain fundamental technical issues in the performance of an intestinal anastomosis and attempt to summarize what is known about how these issues relate to the reliability of various anastomotic techniques. We also describe our own approach to performing certain of these procedures [*see* Operative Technique for Selected Anastomoses, *below*].

Intestinal Anastomotic Healing

The process of intestinal anastomotic healing mimics that of wound healing elsewhere in the body in that it can be arbitrarily divided into an acute inflammatory (lag) phase, a proliferative phase, and, finally, a remodeling or maturation phase. As Halsted[6] demonstrated, most of the bowel wall's strength is provided by the collagenous connective tissue layer in the submucosa [*see Figure 1*]. Collagen is thus the single most important molecule for determining intestinal strength, which makes its metabolism of particular interest for understanding anastomotic healing.

Collagen is secreted from fibroblasts in a monomeric form called tropocollagen; this is a large stiff molecule that can be visualized by electron microscopy. Collagen itself can be divided into subtypes on the basis of differences in composition (i.e., different combinations of α_1 and α_2 chains). Type I predominates in mature organisms; type II is found primarily in cartilage; and type III is associated with type I in remodeling tissue and in elastic tissues such as the aorta, the esophagus, and the uterus. Synthesis of collagen is an intracellular process that occurs on polysomes. A critical stage in collagen formation is the hydroxylation of proline to produce hydroxyproline; this process is believed to be important for maintaining the three-dimensional triple-helix conformation of mature collagen, which gives the molecule its structural strength. The amount of collagen found in a tissue is indirectly determined by measuring the amount of hydroxyproline, although no significant statistical correlation between hydroxyproline content and objective measurements of anastomotic strength has ever been demonstrated.[7] Vitamin C deficiency results in impaired hydroxylation of proline and the accumulation of proline-rich, hydroxyproline-poor molecules in intracellular vacuoles.

The degree of fiber and fibril cross-linking relates to the maturity of the collagen and is probably important in determining the overall strength of the scar tissue. Of equal importance is the orientation of the fibers and their weave. The bursting pressure of anastomoses has often been used to gauge the strength of the healing process. This pressure has been found to increase rapidly in the early postoperative period, reaching 60 percent of the strength of the surrounding bowel by three to four days and 100 percent by one week.[8,9]

Collagen synthesis is a dynamic process that is dependent on the balance between synthesis and collagenolysis. Degradation of mature collagen begins in the first 24 hours and predominates for the first four days. By one week, collagen synthesis is the dominant force, particularly proximal to the anastomosis. After five to six weeks, there is no significant increase in the amount of collagen in a healing wound or anastomosis, though turnover and thus synthesis are extensive. The strength of the scar continues to increase for many months after injury. Local infection increases collagenase activity and reduces levels of circulating collagenase inhibitors.[10,11]

Collagen synthetic capacity is relatively uniform throughout the large bowel but less so in the small intestine: synthesis is significantly higher in the proximal and distal small intestine than in the midjejunum. Overall collagen synthetic capacity is somewhat less in the small intestine. Although no significant difference has been found between the strength of ileal anastomoses and that of colonic anastomoses at four days, colonic collagen formation is much greater in the first 48 hours.[12] It is noteworthy that the synthetic response is not restricted to the anastomotic site but appears to be generalized to a significant extent.[13]

Factors Influencing Incidence of Anastomotic Breakdown

ASSOCIATED DISEASES AND SYSTEMIC FACTORS

Resections for Crohn's disease appear to carry a significant risk of anastomotic dehiscence (12 percent in one prospective study[5]) even when macroscopically normal margins are obtained. Strictureplasty has therefore become an attractive alternative to resectional management of Crohn's disease even in the presence of moderately long strictures, diseased tissue, or sites of previous anastomoses.

The glucocorticoid response to injury may attenuate physio-

Intestinal Anastomosis: Historical Perspective

Intestinal anastomosis has a long history. Hippocrates is known to have referred to intestinal suturing as early as 460 B.C., and Celsus is reported to have written about using the glover's stitch to suture colonic perforations and close intestinal fistulas between 30 B.C. and 30 A.D.[73] In the second century, Galen, probably the most influential physician of the time, took a different view, opposing intestinal anastomosis because of the significant risks of stricture and subsequent obstruction. Unfortunately, this view prevailed throughout most of Europe during the Dark Ages. Toward the end of the first millennium, Abulkasim of the Muslim school was experimenting with the so-called ant closure, in which the pincers of ants were allowed to grasp the two intestinal edges to be joined and bring the edges together; the bodies of the ants were then pinched off, and the subsequent spasm of the pincers kept the edges apposed. This closure is considered by many to be the forerunner of the Michel clip, which was developed later in France. Abulkasim also experimented with the glover's stitch for closing enterotomies, using sheep-gut filaments as sutures.

In the 11th century, the School of Salerne was founded by the so-called Four Masters. These physicians reviewed the principles of Hippocrates and Celsus regarding closure of intestinal injuries, maintenance of aseptic technique, and wound closure. They devised a method of closure that made use of a variety of stents to prevent the stricture so feared by Galen. These stents were made of a number of different materials, including elder wood and goose trachea. The Four Masters were also the first to use interrupted sutures as opposed to the glover's stitch. This new practice reduced the incidence of stricture further and, coupled with the use of stents, caused less narrowing of the intestinal lumen. The sutures themselves were not tied; in fact, they were brought out through the skin to be removed once healing had been achieved.

The Four Masters greatly influenced a contemporary group of Benedictine monks, who used dried animal intestine as the stent of choice along with removable sutures. The Four Monks closure, as it became known, was practiced throughout many parts of Europe for nearly a century. In the 12th century, however, Papal ordinances forbade members of the clergy to perform surgical procedures on the grounds that doing so distracted them from ministering to the souls of their

flocks. As a result, the somewhat less well educated barbers became the practitioners of surgery. This development was accompanied by a return to Galenic principles, including the use of the running glover's stitch. The high incidence of leakage and obstruction that resulted soon led the barbers to abandon intestinal procedures, except for repair of partial transverse or colonic wounds. Attempts were made to close bowel injuries and to approximate the repaired area to the abdominal wall or to other organs with the goal of imitating natural adhesion formation. In the 1700s, Palfyn and Peyronie brought the closed intestinal injury out into the wound so that if primary healing failed to occur, an enterocutaneous fistula would develop; this was the first description of a rudimentary stoma. Verduc and von de Wyl carried this principle to its logical conclusion and developed the so-called artificial anus for use in cases of complete transection. In 1730, Ramdohr intussuscepted one segment of bowel into another, fixing it in place with a single transfixing suture. The resultant mucosa-to-serosa coaptation healed poorly and exhibited a high leakage rate.

Stoma formation and stenting with removable sutures followed by approximation to the abdominal wound remained the standards of care until as recently as the 19th century, when Larrey first described his attempts at a two-layer anastomosis. These attempts were followed closely by Travers's description in 1812 of an agglutination substance that was necessary to approximate the wounded intestinal edges. Meanwhile, Bell was experimenting with the baseball stitch and a tallow plug stent that was ultimately melted by body heat, and Lembert at the Charité de Paris was describing the use of interrupted inverting sutures to obtain serosa-to-serosa apposition. Lembert used fine-caliber silk sutures that incorporated all layers except the mucosa and were left in situ. An interesting historical note is that another French surgeon, Jobert, had actually described a full-thickness interrupted inverting stitch for intestinal anastomoses two years earlier, but he was not nearly as vocal a proponent of his approach as Lembert was of his. Many other surgeons were experimenting with different methods of closure throughout the 19th century. For example, Henroz described a self-securing system of metallic rings that was the precursor of the modern Murphy's button or Valtrac system, and Wolfer described a secure two-layer interrupted method of anastomosis.

logic responses to other mediators whose combined effects could be deleterious to the organism.[14] In animal experiments, wound healing, as measured by bursting pressure of an ileal anastomosis one week after operation, was strongly influenced by the maintenance level of corticosterone.[15] Optimal healing occurred at a plasma corticosterone level that maintained maximal nitrogen balance and corresponded to the mean corticosterone level of normal animals. Both supranormal and subnormal cortisol levels resulted in significantly impaired wound healing, probably through different mechanisms. It is believed that slow protein turnover is responsible for delayed anastomotic healing in

adrenalectomized animals,[16] whereas negative nitrogen metabolic balance is responsible for increased protein breakdown and delayed healing in animals with excess glucocorticoid activity.[15] Nonsteroidal anti-inflammatory drugs (NSAIDs) may help increase anastomotic bursting pressure by decreasing perianastomotic inflammation,[17,18] but this effect has not been well studied.

Systemic factors such as diabetes mellitus, anemia, vitamin deficiencies, malnutrition (hypoalbuminemia), exposure to ionizing radiation, and systemic chemotherapy all may influence the rate of anastomotic healing.

PATIENT PREPARATION

Patients must be fit and stable to maximize the chances that the intestinal anastomosis will heal uneventfully. Ideally, patients should be well nourished, should have a minimum of active intercurrent illness, and should receive adequate preoperative antibiotic prophylaxis, steroid coverage as required, and bowel preparation.

At least two studies have suggested that mechanical bowel preparation may not be essential for successful healing.[19,20] In one of these, a series of 72 patients underwent elective colonic anastomosis without any mechanical bowel preparation and a single preoperative dose of intravenous antibiotics.[19] No anastomotic dehiscence was observed, nor were any differences in wound infection rates (8.3 percent) or overall mortality (2.7 per-

Table 1 Principles of Successful Intestinal Anastomosis

Well-nourished patient with no systemic illness

No fecal contamination, either within the gut or in the surrounding peritoneal cavity

Adequate exposure and access

Well-vascularized tissues

Absence of tension at the anastomosis

Meticulous technique

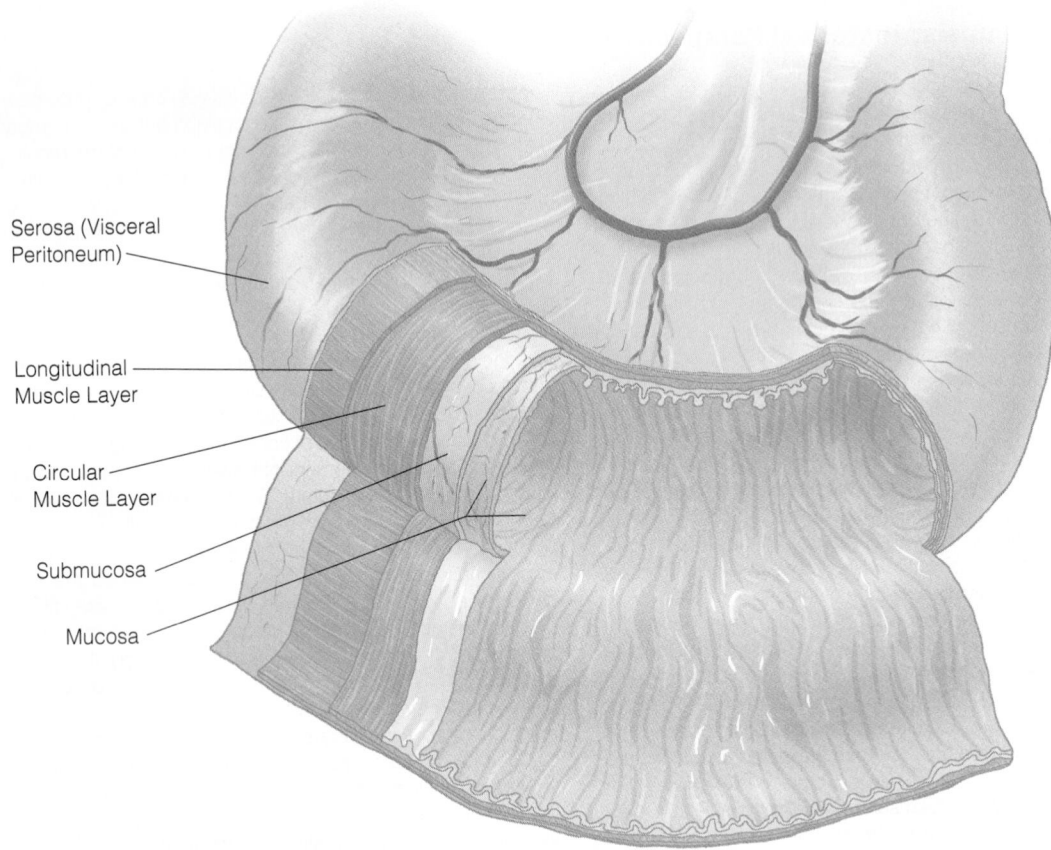

Serosa (Visceral Peritoneum)

Longitudinal Muscle Layer

Circular Muscle Layer

Submucosa

Mucosa

Figure 1   Shown are the tissue layers of the jejunum. Most of the bowel wall's strength is provided by the submucosa.

cent) noted in comparison with published reports of series of patients who underwent full bowel preparation.

On the other hand, a 1989 study reported significantly increased anastomotic bursting pressure and reduced anastomotic dehiscence rates in dogs that underwent mechanical bowel cleansing before low anterior resection.[21] This observation was further supported by a study showing that increasing fecal loading impaired colonic anastomotic healing in rats and by one showing that adding oral erythromycin and kanamycin to bowel preparation led to significantly increased bursting pressure at seven days after operation.[22] In addition, a number of clinical series have been published in which inadequate bowel preparation clearly increased the incidence of anastomotic complications.[23,24]

At our institution, two bottles of Fleet enema are given at 9:00 A.M. and 7:00 P.M. on the day before operation. Patients receive only clear fluids for 24 hours before operation, remain on NPO status after midnight, and then receive tap water enemas on the morning of surgery (for colon and rectal procedures). Neomycin, 500 mg orally, and metronidazole, 500 mg orally, are given at 1:00 P.M., 2:00 P.M., and 10:00 P.M. on the day before operation, and routine I.V. antibiotic prophylaxis is provided on an on-call basis to the OR. Perioperative steroid coverage is important in those patients who may have adrenal suppression as a result of long-term or high-dose steroid therapy. Heparin is administered subcutaneously two hours before operation to all patients scheduled to undergo intestinal anastomosis.

TYPE AND LOCATION OF ANASTOMOSIS

As a rule, for any given technique, the location of the anastomosis seems not to influence the overall leakage rate. The one

exception is low anterior anastomoses, which are associated with leakage rates ranging from 4.5 percent to an incredible 70 percent.[21,23]

Animal studies have demonstrated improved transmission of the intestinal migrating myoelectric complex (MMC) across hand-sewn end-to-end anastomoses in comparison with stapled or sewn side-to-side or end-to-side anastomoses or stapled functional end-to-end anastomoses.[25] This may be of importance to patients with diseases affecting small bowel motility.

Hand-Sewn versus Stapled Anastomoses

Stapled anastomoses are said to heal by primary intention, whereas sutured anastomoses are said to heal by secondary intention, though further experimentation is needed to confirm this distinction.[26] Titanium staples are ideal for tissue apposition at anastomotic sites because they provoke only a minimal inflammatory response and provide immediate strength to the cut surfaces during the weakest phase of healing. Initially, tissue eversion at the stapled anastomosis was a major concern, given that everted hand-sewn anastomoses had previously been shown to be inferior to inverted ones; however, the greater support and improved blood supply to the healing tissues associated with stapling tend to counteract the negative effects of eversion. In fact, one study found that bursting strength for canine colonic end-to-end anastomoses was six times greater when the procedure was performed with an end-to-end anastomosis (EEA) stapler than when it was done with hand-sewn interrupted Dacron sutures.[27] Another study demonstrated a significantly reduced radiographic anastomotic leakage rate with staples applied by an EEA stapler as opposed to a double layer of hand-sewn sutures.[28]

Various prospective randomized trials have demonstrated no differences in clinical and subclinical leakage rates, length of hospital stay, or overall morbidity.[29-31] Even when the anastomosis had to heal under adverse conditions (e.g., carcinomatosis, malnutrition, previous chemotherapy or radiation therapy, bowel obstruction, anemia, or leukopenia), no significant differences were apparent between stapled anastomoses and hand-sewn ones. Stapling did, however, shorten the time required to perform the procedure, especially for low pelvic anastomoses.

Cancer recurrence rates at the site of the anastomosis have been reported to be higher or lower depending on the technique used. Certainly, suture materials engender a more pronounced cellular proliferative response than titanium staples do, particularly with full-thickness sutures as opposed to seromuscular ones,[32] and malignant cells have been shown to adhere to suture materials.[33] One clinical report suggested that stapling anastomoses after resection for cancer can reduce anastomotic recurrence by 40 percent and cancer-specific mortality by 50 percent.[34] This finding has not yet been supported by other work.

At present, it remains unclear whether stapling or suturing is safer from an oncologic perspective. The exception is a very low rectal anastomosis, in which a better margin can sometimes be obtained through double-stapling.

Unusual Techniques

In 1892, Murphy[35] introduced a two-part metal stud that was designed to hold wound edges in apposition without suturing until adhesion had occurred. Thereafter, the stud was voided via the rectum. Several modifications of this technique have been described since then, primarily focusing on the composition of the rings or stents. In 1968, Hopcroft[36] described a casein prosthesis that ultimately dissolved under the influence of intestinal proteolytic enzymes. In 1977, Sognen and associates[37] described a mixture of gelatin and barium sulfate that was molded into a tubular stent for use in veterinary surgery. This structure was meant to provide a firm base for suturing and to shorten the time required for anastomosis; the purpose of the barium was to facilitate radiographic localization of the stent in the postoperative period. More recently, dissolvable polyglycolic acid systems have been developed. These so-called biofragmentable anastomotic rings leave a gap of 1.5, 2.0, or 2.5 mm between the bowel ends to prevent ischemia of the anastomotic line.

The use of adhesive agents such as methyl-2-cyanoacrylate to approximate the divided ends of intestinal segments has been studied.[38] There was only a moderate inflammatory response at the wound, which persisted for two to three weeks. Leakage rates were high, however, and many technical problems remained (e.g., how to stabilize the bowel edges while they underwent adhesion).

CONTROVERSIAL AREAS

The question of the importance of inversion (as described by Lembert in the early 1800s) versus eversion of the anastomotic line has been a controversial one. It has been argued that the traditional inverting methods ignore the basic principle of accurately opposing clean-cut tissues. Halsted,[6] in 1887, was the first to clearly demonstrate the importance of the submucosa as the strength layer of intestinal anastomoses. He initially proposed an interrupted extramucosal technique, which has since been assessed in retrospective[1] and prospective[5] reviews and found to have a low leakage rate (1.3 to 6.0 percent) in a wide variety of circumstances. A 1969 study reported greater anastomotic strength, less luminal narrowing, and less edema and inflammation in everted small intestinal anastomoses in dogs.[39] Subsequent laboratory and clinical studies have not been able to

confirm these findings and, in fact, have often yielded quite the opposite results: lower bursting pressure,[40] slower healing,[41] and more severe inflammation[42] have all been associated with an everted suture line.

The advisability of routine nasogastric decompression in patients undergoing a procedure involving an intestinal anastomosis has remained somewhat controversial over the years. In retrospective[43] and prospective[44] randomized controlled trials, routine use of a nasogastric tube conferred no significant advantage. There was, in fact, a trend toward an increased incidence of respiratory tract infections in patients who underwent routine gastric decompression.[45] Nonetheless, one study found that nearly 20 percent of patients required insertion of a gastric tube in the early postoperative period.[44] We no longer place nasogastric tubes routinely; however, it is still important to be alert to the potential for gastric dilatation in these patients.

There has been a great deal of controversy regarding the ability of abdominal drainage to "protect" the anastomosis. Even before World War I, the old dictum "when in doubt, drain" was called into question by Yates,[46] who wrote that the peritoneal cavity could not be effectively drained because of adhesions and rapid sealing of the drain tract. Six decades later, one study showed a dramatic increase in the incidence of anastomotic dehiscence (from 15 percent to 55 percent) after the placement of perianastomotic drains in dogs.[47] This increase was associated with a significant increase in mortality. Yet another study reported the severe inflammatory reaction caused by drains at anastomoses.[48]

At our institution, intra-abdominal drains are occasionally used when it appears that there is a specific area (e.g., the pelvis) where there is a higher than usual risk that a fluid collection will develop (e.g., after a very low anterior resection or a coloanal anastomosis without diversion). Rectal tubes are commonly employed after subtotal colectomy for acute colitis and after two-stage pelvic pouch procedures.

Hand-Sewn Sutures: Technical Issues

CHOICE OF SUTURE MATERIAL

Sutures act as foreign bodies in the anastomosis and thus produce an inflammatory reaction.[7] One study that examined the relative efficiency of absorbable and nonabsorbable material concluded that the strength of the anastomosis, expressed as a percentage of normal tissue strength, was essentially the same regardless of the type of suture used. Other studies that examined the amount of inflammation induced at the anastomosis by various types of sutures found that polypropylene (Prolene), catgut, and polyglycolic acid (Dexon) were equivalent in this regard.[49,50] Silk, however, produced a significantly greater cellular reaction at the anastomosis, and the reaction persisted for as long as six weeks.[50] A 1975 study reported on a series of 41 patients who underwent low anterior resection involving a primary side-to-end colorectal anastomosis with 5-0 stainless steel wire.[51] The investigators believed that this material was ideal because of its strength and relative inertness within the tissues and supported their claims with a relatively low clinical leakage rate (7.3 percent).

The ideal suture material—one that causes minimal inflammation and tissue reaction while providing maximum strength during the lag phase of wound healing—has not yet been discovered. Clearly, however, monofilament and coated braided sutures represent an advance over silk and other multifilament materials.

CONTINUOUS SUTURES VERSUS INTERRUPTED SUTURES

Both continuous and interrupted sutures are commonly used in fashioning intestinal anastomoses [see Figure 2]. No randomized trials have addressed the question of whether interrupted sutures have a significant advantage over continuous sutures in a single-layer anastomosis; however, retrospective reviews have not revealed any such advantage.[52-54] Animal studies, on the other hand, have found that perianastomotic tissue oxygen tension was significantly less with continuous sutures than with interrupted sutures.[55] This finding was correlated with an increased anastomotic complication rate and impaired collagen synthesis and healing in a rat model.[56]

SINGLE-LAYER ANASTOMOSES VERSUS DOUBLE-LAYER ANASTOMOSES

Double-layer anastomoses were described in the literature before single-layer ones. They are fairly uniform and consist of an inner layer of continuous or interrupted absorbable sutures and an outer layer of interrupted absorbable or nonabsorbable sutures [see Figure 3]. Traditionally, double-layer anastomoses have been considered more secure; however, for some time, single-layer anastomoses have been performed in difficult locations (e.g., low in the pelvis or high in the chest) or in difficult circumstances (e.g., in a patient who is unstable or has multiple intraabdominal injuries) with good results. Moreover, work from the 1980s suggests that the single-layer technique has significant inherent advantages.[56-59]

Double-layer anastomoses were long believed to be essential for safe healing of the wound; however, subsequent pathological analysis of these anastomoses revealed microscopic areas of necrosis and sloughing of the tissues incorporated in the inner layer as a result of strangulation.[60] Animal studies have confirmed that single-layer anastomoses take less time to create,[61] cause less narrowing of the intestinal lumen,[57-62] foster more rapid vascularization[56] and mucosal healing, and increase the strength of the anastomosis (as measured by the bursting pressure) in the first few postoperative days.[61] Nonetheless, although clinical studies have fairly consistently demonstrated that single-layer anastomoses are associated with improved postoperative return to normal bowel function (as measured by bowel sounds, passage of flatus, and return to oral intake),[42,63] nonrandomized studies of anastomotic leakage rates have not shown any differences between single- and double-layer anastomoses in this regard.[64-66]

Some authors still favor double-layer anastomoses when the tissues are very edematous or friable, are under minimal tension, or lie in highly vascular areas (e.g., the stomach). There are no data to indicate that this practice yields superior results.

Staples: Technical Issues

CHOICE OF STAPLER

Surgical stapling devices were first introduced in 1908 by Hültl. Besides the EEA stapler already mentioned, the types most commonly used are the gastrointestinal anastomosis (GIA) stapler and the transverse anastomosis (TA) stapler. Most stapling devices place two double staggered rows of B-shaped staples and can simultaneously cut between the rows. Staplers may be used to create functional (GIA plus TA) or true anatomic (EEA) end-to-end anastomoses as well as side-to-side anastomoses.

In a functional end-to-end anastomosis, two cut ends of bowel (either open or stapled closed) are placed side by side with their blind ends beside each other. A cutting linear stapler (GIA) is then used to fuse the two bowel walls into a single septum with

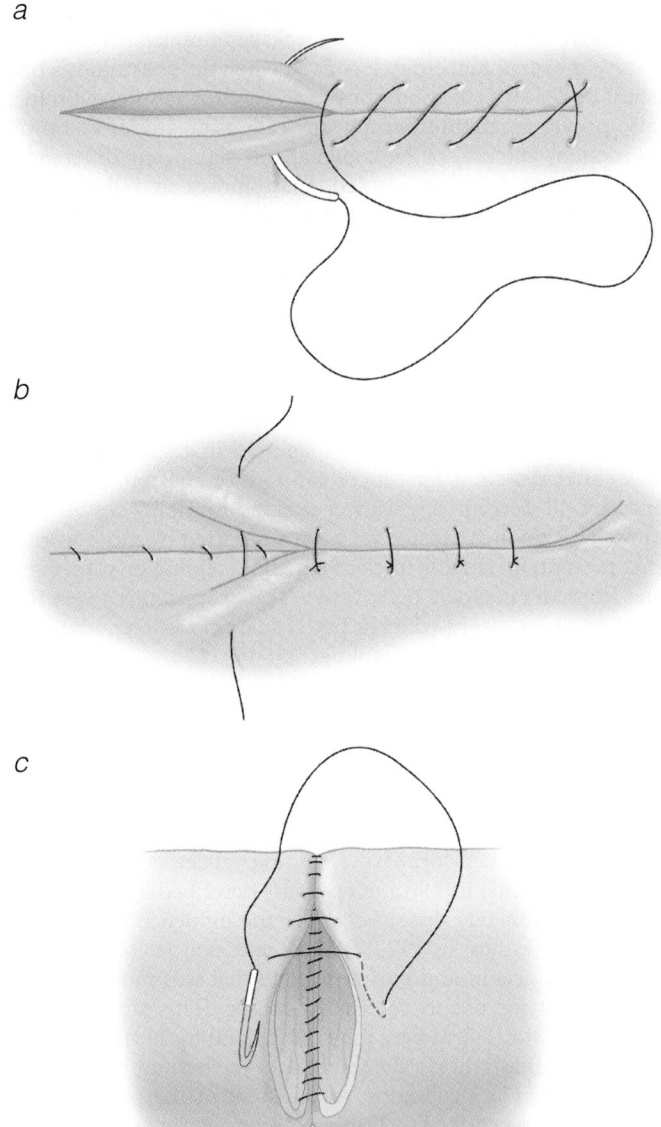

a

b

c

Figure 2 Shown are stitches commonly used in fashioning intestinal anastomoses: (*a*) the continuous over-and-over suture, (*b*) the interrupted Lembert suture, and (*c*) the Connell suture.

two double staggered rows of staples and to create a lumen between the two bowel segments by dividing this septum between the rows. A noncutting linear stapler (TA) is then used to close the defect at the apex of the anastomosis. The cut and stapled edges of the bowel should be inspected for adequacy of hemostasis before the apex is closed. Some authors suggest cauterizing these edges to ensure hemostasis.[67] However, given that electrical current may be conducted along the metallic staple line to the rest of the bowel, it is probably easier and safer simply to underpin bleeding vessels with a fine absorbable suture. It is also important to offset the two inverted staple lines before closing the apex.[68]

True anatomic end-to-end stapled anastomoses may be fashioned with a linear stapler by triangulating the two cut ends, then firing the stapler three times in intersecting vectors to achieve complete closure [see Figure 4]. The creation of end-to-end anastomoses has been considerably facilitated by the development of the EEA stapler. This device places two double circular rows of staples from the inside of the intestinal lumen and cuts between them to create a directly apposed, inverted, stapled end-to-end anastomosis.

STAPLE HEIGHT

A 1987 comparison of anastomotic techniques that used blood flow to the divided tissues as a measure of outcome found that the best blood flow to the healing site was provided by stapled anastomoses in which the height of the staples was adjusted to the thickness of the bowel wall, followed by double-layer stapled and sutured anastomoses, double-layer sutured anastomoses, and tightly stapled anastomoses, in that order.[69] With most modern stapling devices, there is a range within which the stapler can be incompletely closed but the staples placed still function effectively (often indicated by a green or gray shaded region on the closing mechanism of the stapler). Thus, the stapler need not be closed to its maximum if full closure would cause the intervening tissues to be crushed excessively.

SINGLE-STAPLED ANASTOMOSES VERSUS DOUBLE-STAPLED ANASTOMOSES

To accomplish many of these anastomoses, intersecting staple lines are created. Initially, some concern was expressed about the security of these areas and about the ability of the blade in the cutting instruments to divide a double staggered row of staples.

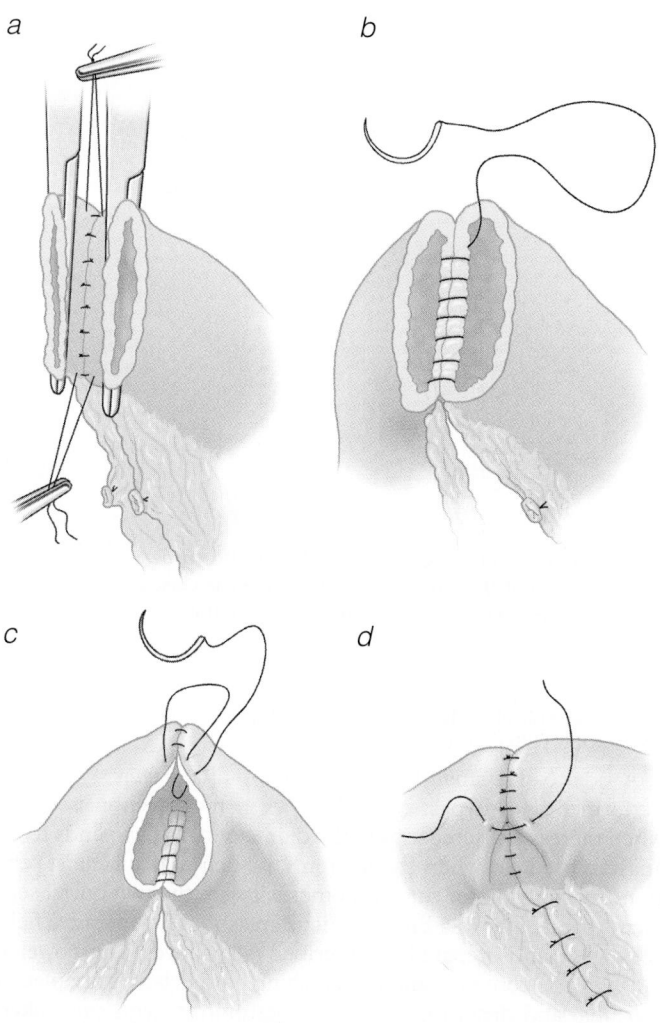

Figure 3 **Double-layer end-to-end anastomosis. (*a*) Interrupted Lembert stitches are used to form the posterior outer layer. (*b*) A full-thickness continuous over-and-over stitch is used to form the posterior inner layer. (*c*) A Connell stitch is used to form the anterior inner layer. (*d*) Interrupted Lembert stitches are used to form the anterior outer layer.**

Subsequent animal studies, however, demonstrated that even though nearly all (> 90 percent) of the staple lines that were subsequently transected by a second staple line contained bent or cut staples, the integrity of the anastomosis was not compromised in any way, nor was its healing adversely affected.[29,70]

Operative Technique for Selected Anastomoses

In what follows, we describe our approach to several operative procedures involving intestinal anastomosis. These procedures are intended not as an exhaustive list but as a representative selection that illustrates the principles already discussed.

A general note about the cosmetic aspect of these procedures is appropriate here. After any of these operations, a close visual inspection of the entire circumference of the anastomosis should be performed. As a general principle, if the divided ends appear well opposed, then the anastomosis is probably sound.

INCISION AND EXPOSURE

Currently, most laparotomies are performed through a standard midline incision with the patient supine and level. Adequate exposure is obtained by ensuring that the skin incision is long enough and using retractors such as a Buchwalter or a Gibson/Balfour type. In procedures involving the small intestine, only the segment of bowel being worked on should be brought out of the abdomen into the operative field; the remainder should be kept warm and tension free inside the abdominal cavity. In colonic procedures, the small intestine may be packed into the left upper quadrant or the right flank region with a damp pack.

The small intestine is quite mobile, and it is rarely difficult to expose a given loop unless adhesions or other disease processes are tethering the bowel. Adequate mobility of the colon is obtained by incising the peritoneal reflection along the white line of Toldt, preferably with a coagulating electrocautery to maintain a bloodless field, and reflecting the retroperitoneal structures posteriorly. For a tension-free primary colonic anastomosis, the splenic and hepatic flexures often must be mobilized.

For rectal procedures, the patient should be placed in Allen stirrups in the lithotomy position. Care must be taken to position the legs and feet properly and secure them so as to prevent pressure points that could lead to ulcers, thrombosis, or neurapraxia. The legs should not be spread too widely or flexed excessively; however, if an EEA stapler is to be used, sufficient maneuvering room must be left between the stirrups. Placing the patient in a 30° Trendelenburg's position and packing the small bowel superiorly also help keep the operative field in the pelvis clear.

BOWEL RESECTION

The technique of bowel resection will not be reviewed in great detail here; a brief summary should suffice. (Colonic resection is covered extensively elsewhere [*see V:17 Colorectal Procedures*].) Appropriate resection margins must be obtained to provide adequate clearance of the lesion or diseased segment. The most important consideration in this regard is the blood supply to the region in question; this is clearly more of an issue in colonic resections than in small bowel resections, given the ample vascular supply of the small bowel. The segment may be removed by first clearing away all mesenteric and serosal attachments with a coagulating electrocautery, then dividing the bowel proximally and distally with either a cutting linear stapler, a combination of a noncutting linear stapler and a crushing bowel clamp, or two

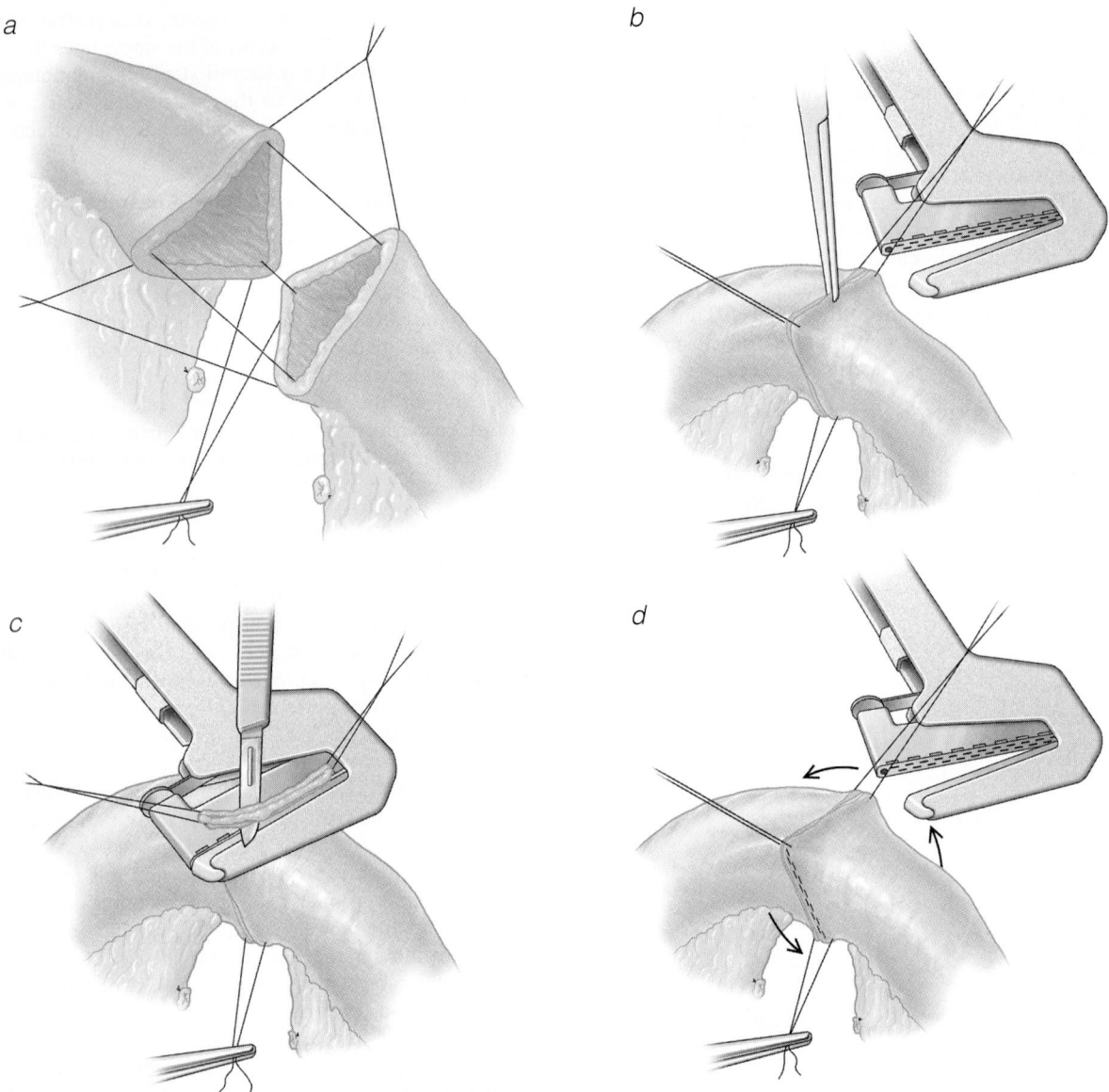

a

b

c

d

Figure 4 **End-to-end anastomosis with linear noncutting stapler. (*a*) The bowel ends are triangulated with three traction sutures. (*b*) A noncutting linear stapler (TA) is placed between two of the sutures. (*c*) The stapler is closed and the excess tissue excised. (*d*) The bowel is rotated, and steps *b* and *c* are repeated twice more to close the remaining two sides of the triangle.**

crushing bowel clamps and a knife or scissors. The tissue to be used for the anastomosis must be well vascularized, viable, and free of its fatty attachments. The pinch-burn technique is particularly useful in clearing the mesenteric attachments close to the bowel wall itself; ties often bunch tissues excessively, resulting in angulation or distortion of the free edge of the intestine. In the pelvis, an angulated noncutting linear stapler is often used to obtain as much length as possible distal to the lesion. The proximal rectum is clamped with a crushing bowel clamp, and a long knife is used to transect the rectum.

Special mention should be made of the technique of strictureplasty, which is used for a number of benign small bowel strictures (especially those resulting from Crohn's disease) as a means of avoiding small bowel resection and anastomoses. In this procedure, the bowel is opened longitudinally and closed transversely with a single layer of 2-0 polyglycolic acid sutures in a Connell stitch. Excellent functional results have been achieved with this technique.

SINGLE-LAYER SUTURED EXTRAMUCOSAL SIDE-TO-SIDE ENTEROENTEROSTOMY

A side-to-side small bowel anastomosis [*see Figure 5*] may be performed as a bypass procedure when no resection is done, when there is a discrepancy in the diameter of the two ends to be anastomosed, or when the anatomy is such that the most tension-free position for the anastomosis is with the two bowel segments parallel (as in a Finney strictureplasty). The operative field is exposed and prepared as described (see above). The bowel is milked of its contents, and noncrushing bowel clamps are placed proximal and distal to the site of anastomosis, with care taken not to impinge on the mesentery. The two loops in question must lie comfortably within the abdomen, without tension, and must be exposed in such a manner as to minimize or at least contain spillage of intestinal content if it occurs. The field is walled off with clean sponges or packs, and the loops are laid side by side.

Two stay sutures of 3-0 polyglycolic acid are placed approximately 3 in. apart on the inner aspect of the antimesenteric border. A 2 in. enterotomy is made on each loop with an electro-cautery or a blade on the inner aspect of the antimesenteric border. If an electrocautery is used, care must be taken not to injure the mucosa of the posterior wall during this maneuver; placement of a hemostat into the enterotomy to lift the anterior wall will usually prevent this problem. Hemostasis of the cut edges is ensured, and the remaining enteric contents are gently suctioned out. A Betadine-soaked Harris gauze pad may be used at this point to cleanse the lumen of the bowel in the perianastomotic region.

A full-length seromuscular and submucosal stitch of 4-0 polyglycolic acid is placed and tied on the inside approximately 0.25 to 0.5 in. from the far end of the enterotomies. The stitch is not passed through the mucosa: to do so would add no strength to the anastomosis and would hinder epithelialization by rendering the tissue ischemic. A hemostat is placed on the short end of the tied suture, and the assistant applies continuous gentle tension to the long end of the suture. An over-and-over stitch is started in the direction of the surgeon; small bites are taken, and proper inversion of the suture line is ensured with each pass through tissue. When the proximal ends of the enterostomies are reached, this so-called baseball stitch is continued almost completely around to the anterior wall of the anastomosis. A single Connell stitch may be used to invert this anterior layer. Another full-length seromuscular and submucosal suture of 4-0 polyglycolic acid is then inserted and tied at the same location in the posterior wall as the first. If the two sutures are placed close enough together, the short ends need not be tied together and may simply be cut off. The remainder of the posterior wall is sewn away from the surgeon in the same manner as the portion already sewn, and the corners are approximated with the baseball stitch. The anterior wall is then completed with this second suture, either in the Connell stitch or in an over-and-over stitch with the assistant inverting the edges before applying tension to the previous stitch.

When the defect is completely closed, the two sutures are tied across the anastomotic line. The stay sutures are removed, and the anastomosis is carefully inspected. Often, there is no mesenteric defect to close in a side-to-side anastomosis, but if there is one, it should be approximated at this point with continuous or interrupted absorbable sutures, with care taken not to injure the vascular supply to the anastomosis.

DOUBLE-LAYER SUTURED END-TO-SIDE ENTEROCOLOSTOMY

The patient is positioned and control of the operative field obtained as described (see above). The bowel loops are isolated with clean sponges, and noncrushing bowel clamps are used as needed to prevent excessive spillage of intestinal contents. This procedure is often performed when there is a significant discrepancy in luminal diameter between the two segments to be joined, as in ileocolic anastomoses. The distal bowel or colon is divided with a cutting stapler so that a blind end is left. Some surgeons underpin or bury this staple line, although this practice is probably unnecessary. The proximal cut end of the intestine is similarly closed either with staples after division with a cutting linear stapler or with a crushing bowel clamp. This proximal end is brought into apposition with the side of the distal bowel segment at a point no further than 1 to 2 in. from the blind end of the distal segment; this proximity to the cut end is important for prevention of the blind loop syndrome [see Figure 6].

Stay sutures of 3-0 polyglycolic acid are placed between the serosa of the proximal limb about 0.5 to 0.75 in. from the clamp and the serosa of the distal limb. Interrupted seromuscular sutures of 3-0 polyglycolic acid are then placed between these

Figure 5 **Single-layer sutured extramucosal side-to-side enteroenterostomy. A full-length suture is started in the back wall and run through the seromuscular and submucosal layers in the direction of the surgeon; the corners of the enterotomy are approximated with a baseball stitch, and a single Connell stitch is used to invert the anterior layer. A second suture is started at the same spot on the posterior wall and run in the opposite direction, again through all layers except the mucosa; the corners of the enterotomies are approximated with a baseball stitch, and the suture is continued in either the Connell stitch or the over-and-over stitch to complete the anterior wall of the anastomosis.**

stay sutures, spaced about eight to 16 to the inch. These stitches may be tied sequentially or snapped and tied once they are all in place. It is crucial not to apply excessive tension, which could cut the seromuscular layer or render it ischemic. Suction is then readied. The staple line or crushed tissue on the proximal limb is cut off with a coagulating electrocautery or a knife; this maneuver opens the lumen of the proximal limb. All residual intestinal content is gently suctioned.

An enterotomy or colotomy is created on the distal limb opposite the open lumen of the proximal bowel. A full-thickness suture of 3-0 polyglycolic acid is inserted in the posterior wall at a point close to the far end of the enterotomy and run in an over-and-over stitch back toward the surgeon. The corner is rounded with the baseball stitch, and when the anterior wall is reached, the Connell stitch is used. A second full-length 3-0 suture is started at the same point on the posterior wall as the first, and the short ends of the two sutures are tied together and cut. This second suture is then run away from the surgeon to complete the posterior wall, and the anterior wall is completed with the Connell stitch. The two sutures are then tied across the anastomotic line.

A second series of interrupted seromuscular stitches is then placed anteriorly in the same fashion as the seromuscular stitches placed in the posterior wall. It is important not to narrow either lumen excessively by imbricating too much of the bowel wall into this second layer. The lumen of the anastomosis is palpated to confirm patency, and the mesenteric defect is closed if possible with either continuous or interrupted absorbable sutures.

DOUBLE-STAPLED END-TO-END COLOANAL ANASTOMOSIS

Preoperative mechanical and antibiotic bowel preparation is performed, and the patient is optimized medically. The patient is placed in stirrups in the lithotomy position and prepared as described (see above). Laparotomy is performed and colonic and rectal mobilization carried out as described (see above). The patient is then placed in Trendelenburg's position, with the small intestine packed into the upper abdomen and a Gibson retractor placed to provide adequate exposure.

The proximal resection margin is determined and cleared of its mesenteric attachments and its appendices epiploicae with the electrocautery. The operative field is prepared, and the colon is divided between crushing bowel clamps. An angled linear noncutting stapler is fired across the distal resection margin, and another bowel clamp is placed proximal to it. The rectum is divided with a long-handled knife, with care taken to avoid plunging the blade into the pelvic sidewall, which could cause significant neurovascular damage. The specimen is removed and the stapler withdrawn. Adequate pelvic hemostasis is ensured.

Once sufficient mobilization has been achieved, a noncrushing bowel clamp is placed on the colon 10 to 15 cm proximal to the margin, and the crushing clamp is removed. (At this stage, some thought should be given to creating an 8 to 10 cm colonic J pouch, which may improve functional outcome after low anastomoses, especially in the early postoperative period in older patients.) A whip-stitch (or purse-string suture) of 2-0 polypropylene is placed around the colotomy, and the anvil from the appropriately sized curved EEA (C-EEA) stapler is inserted into the open end and secured in place by tying the suture [see Figure 7]. The proximal bowel clamp is removed. A digital rectal examination is performed by the assistant, who may also, if desired,

gently wash out the rectal stump with a dilute Betadine solution. The stapler, with its trocar attachment in place, is then inserted into the anus under the careful guidance of the surgeon. The pointed shaft is brought out through or adjacent to the linear staple line, and the sharp point is removed. The peg from the anvil in the proximal colon is snapped into the protruding shaft of the stapler, and the two edges are slowly brought together. The colonic mesentery must not be twisted, and the ends must come together without any tension whatsoever. The stapler is fired, and a distinctive crunching sound is heard. The anvil is then loosened the appropriate amount, and the entire mechanism is withdrawn through the anus. Finally, the proximal and distal rings of tissue are carefully inspected to confirm circumferential closure of the staple line.

The pelvis is then filled with body-temperature saline, and a Toomey syringe is used to insufflate the neorectum with air. The surgeon watches for bubbling in the pelvis as a sign of leakage from the anastomosis. A rectal tube may then be inserted by the assistant or may be placed at the end of the case.

When the anastomosis is very low or there is some concern about healing, a drain may be placed in the pelvis behind the staple line; however, as noted [see Controversial Areas, above], this practice has not been shown to be beneficial and may in fact impair healing. Some surgeons prefer to protect the anastomosis with a temporary covering loop ileostomy, though recent data suggest that this may not be necessary.[71,72]

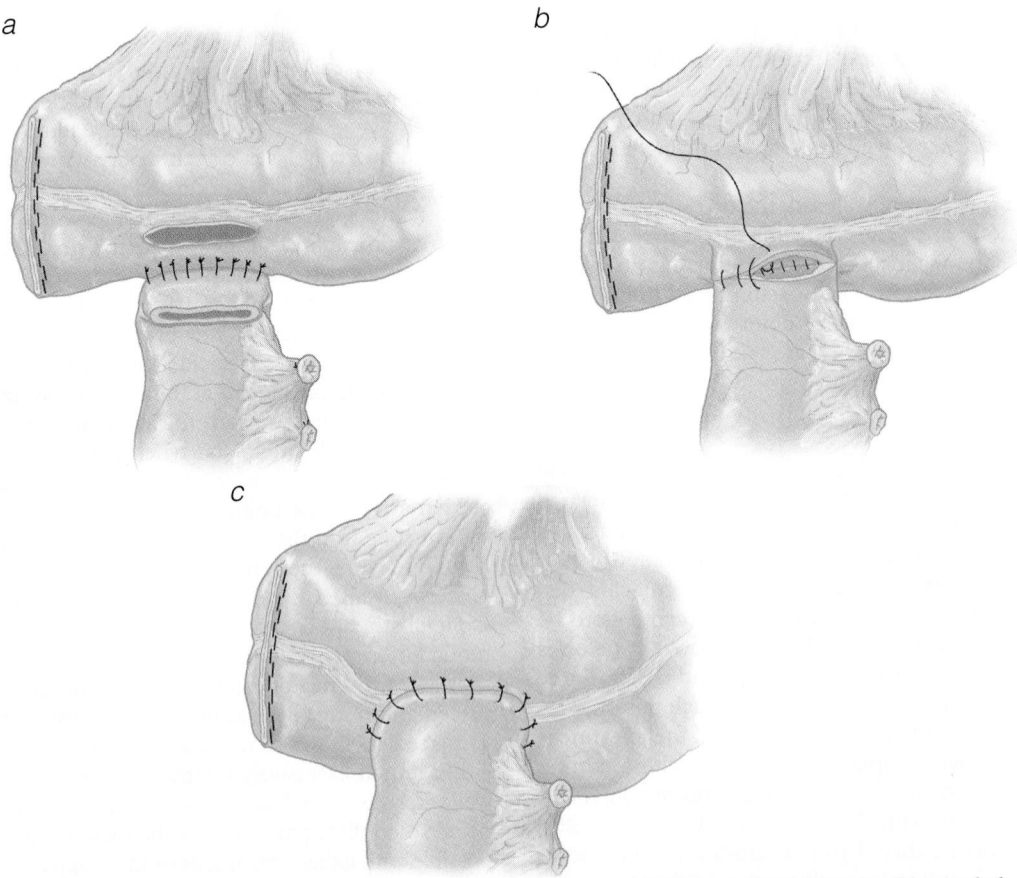

Figure 6 **Double-layer sutured end-to-side enterocolostomy. (*a*) The proximal bowel end is stapled, interrupted Lembert stitches are used to form the posterior outer layer, and a colotomy is made. (*b*) Two continuous sutures are used to form the inner layer of the anastomosis; the posterior portion is done with the over-and-over stitch, the anterior with the Connell stitch. (*c*) Interrupted Lembert stitches are used to form the anterior outer layer.**

Figure 7 **Double-stapled end-to-end coloanal anstomosis. (*a*) The C-EEA stapler comes with both a standard anvil (left) and a trocar attachment (right). (*b*) The rectal stump is closed with an angled linear noncutting stapler. A purse-string suture is placed around the colotomy, and the anvil of the stapler is placed in the open end and secured. (*c*) The stapler, with the sharp trocar attachment in place, is inserted into the anus, and the trocar is made to pierce the rectal stump at or near the staple line, after which the trocar is removed. (*d*) The anvil in the proximal colon is joined with the stapler in the rectal stump, and the two edges are slowly brought together. (*e*) The stapler is fired and then gently withdrawn.**

Conclusion

As far back as 190 years ago, the accepted surgical standards dictated that (1) small bowel transections could not be sutured primarily without a fatal outcome because of dehiscence or stricture formation and obstruction; (2) colonic transections could be sutured over a stent made of autogenous or foreign tissues; and (3) intestinal wounds had to be closed in close approximation to the abdominal wall. Since then, our understanding of the healing of surgical anastomoses and of the optimal technical approaches to performing them clearly has grown considerably. This growth is reflected in lower anastomotic leakage and dehiscence rates, lower operative morbidity, and lower mortality.

Some would argue that much of the improved outcome is attributable to improved anesthesia, more potent antibiotics, and better postoperative monitoring and care. No doubt there is a good deal of truth to this argument. Still, however, we believe it is important to emphasize that one of the most significant determinants of outcome after procedures that include intestinal anastomosis is surgical technique. For this reason, it is essential to continue research into such issues as the best suture material or stapler to be used, the most suitable and best-tolerated type of bowel preparation, the mechanisms and variables involved in wound healing and collagen deposition, and the importance of local and systemic factors in determining overall outcome.

References

1. Smith SRG, Connolly JC, Crane PW: The effect of surgical drainage materials on colonic healing. Br J Surg 69:153, 1982

2. Debas HT, Thompson FB: A critical review of colectomy with anastomosis. Surg Gynecol Obstet 135:747, 1973

3. Schrock TR, Deveney CW, Dunphy JE: Factors contributing to leakage of colonic anastomoses. Ann Surg 177:513, 1973

4. Matheson NA, McIntosh CA, Krukowski ZH: Continuing experience with single layer appositional anastomosis in the large bowel. Br J Surg 72(suppl):S104, 1985

5. Carty NJ, Keating J, Campbell J, et al: Prospective audit of an extramucosal technique for intestinal anastomosis. Br J Surg 78:1439, 1991

6. Halsted W: Circular suture of the intestine—an experimental study. Am J Med Sci 94:436, 1887

7. Hastings JC, Van Winkle W, Barker E, et al: Effects of suture materials on healing of wounds of the stomach and colon. Surg Gynecol Obstet 140:701, 1975

8. Wise L, McAlister W, Stein T, et al: Studies on the healing of anastomoses of small and large intestines. Surg Gynecol Obstet 141:190, 1975

9. Hesp F, Hendriks T, Lubbers E-J, et al: Wound healing in the intestinal wall: a comparison between experimental ileal and colonic anastomoses. Dis Colon Rectum 24:99, 1984

10. Hawley PJ, Hunt TK, Dunphy JE: Aetiology of colonic anastomotic leaks. Proc R Soc Med 63:28, 1970

11. Hawley PJ, Faulk WP: A circulating collagenase inhibitor. Br J Surg 57:900, 1970

12. Martens M, Hendriks T: Postoperative changes in collagen synthesis in intestinal anastomoses of the rat: differences between small and large bowel. Gut 32:1482, 1991

13. Martens M, deMan B, Hendriks T, et al: Collagen synthetic capacity throughout the uninjured and anastomosed intestinal wall. Am J Surg 164:354, 1992

14. Munck A, Guyre M, Holbrook N: Physiological functions of glucocorticoids in stress and their relation to pharmacological actions. Endocrinol Rev 5:25, 1984

15. Matsusue S, Walser M: Healing of intestinal anastomoses in adrenalectomized rats given corticosterone. Am J Physiol 263:R164, 1992

16. Quan Z, Walser M: The effect of corticosterone administration at varying levels on leucine oxidation and whole body protein synthesis and breakdown in adrenalectomized rats. Metabolism 40:1263, 1991

17. Letwin E, Williams HTG: Healing of intestinal anastomosis. Can J Surg 10:109, 1967

18. Gadacz T, Menguy RB: Effects of anti-inflammatory drug oxyphenbutazone on the rate of wound healing and the biochemical composition of wound tissue. Surgery Forum 18:58, 1967

19. Irving AD, Scrimgeour D: Mechanical bowel preparation for colonic resection and anastomosis. Br J Surg 74:580, 1987

20. Hughes ESR: Asepsis in large bowel surgery. Ann R Coll Surg Engl 51:347, 1972

21. O'Dwyer PJ, Conway W, McDermott EWM, et al: Effect of mechanical bowel preparation on anastomotic integrity following low anterior resection in dogs. Br J Surg 76:756, 1989

22. Leveen HH, Wapnicks S, Falk D: Effects of prophylactic antibiotics on colonic healing. Am J Surg 131:47, 1976

23. Goligher JC, Graham NG, DeDombal FT: Anastomotic dehiscence after anterior resection of the rectum and sigmoid. Br J Surg 57:109, 1970

24. Irvin T, Goligher J, Johnston D: A randomized prospective clinical trial of single-layer and two layer inverting intestinal anastomoses. Br J Surg 60:457, 1973

25. Hocking M, Carlson R, Courington K, et al: Altered motility and bacterial flora after functional end-to-end anastomosis. Surgery 108:384, 1990

26. O'Donnell AF, O'Connell PR, Royston D, et al: Suture technique affects perianastomotic colonic crypt cell production and tumour formation. Br J Surg 78:671, 1991

27. Greenstein A, Rogers P, Moss G: Doubled fourth-day colorectal anastomotic strength with complete retention of intestinal mature wound collagen and accelerated deposition following full enteral nutrition. Surgery Forum 29:78, 1978

28. Bubrick MP: Effects of technique on anastomotic dehiscence. Dis Colon Rectum 24:232, 1981

29. Brennan SS, Pickford IR, Evans M, et al: Staples or sutures for colonic anastomosis—a controlled clinical trial. Br J Surg 69:722, 1982

30. Lafrenier R, Ketcham AS: A single layer open anastomosis for all intestinal structures. Am J Surg 149:797, 1985

31. Beart RW, Kelly KA: Randomised prospective evaluation of the EEA stapler for colorectal anastomoses. Am J Surg 141:143, 1981

32. Akyol AM, McGregor JR, Galloway DJ, et al: Recurrence of colorectal cancer after sutured and stapled large bowel anastomoses. Br J Surg 78:1297, 1991

33. O'Dwyer P, Ravikumar TS, Steele G: Serum dependent variability in the adherence to tumour cells to surgical sutures. Br J Surg 72:466, 1985

34. Everett WG, Friend PJ, Forty J: Comparison of stapling and hand-suture for left-sided large bowel anastomosis. Br J Surg 73:345, 1986

35. Murphy JB: A contribution to abdominal surgery, ideal approximation of abdominal viscera without suture. North American Practitioner 4:481, 1892

36. Hopcroft SC: An absorbable intestinal prosthesis for rapid intestinal anastomosis. Expl Med Surg 26:9, 1968

37. Sognen E, Birkeland R, Sohlberg S: A gelatine prosthetic aid for intestinal anastomosis. Journal of Small Animal Practice 18:529, 1977

38. Ballantyne GH: The experimental basis of intestinal suturing: effect of surgical technique, inflammation and infection on enteric wound healing. Dis Colon Rectum 27:61, 1984

39. Getzen L: Intestinal anastomoses. Curr Probl Surg, August 1969, p 3

40. Kratzer GL, Onsanit T: Single layer steel wire anastomosis of the intestine. Surg Gynecol Obstet 139:93, 1974

41. Ravitch MM, Steichen FM: Techniques of staple suturing in the gastrointestinal tract. Ann Surg 175:815, 1972

42. Brunius U, Zederfeldt B: Efffects of antiinflammatory treatment on wound healing. Acta Chir Scand 129:462, 1965

43. Burg R, Geigle C, Faso J, et al: Omission of routine gastric decompression. Dis Colon Rectum 21:98, 1978

44. Reasbeck P, Rice M, Herbison G: Nasogastric intubation after intestinal resection. Surg Gynecol Obstet 158:354, 1984

45. Argov S, Goldstein I, Barzilai A: Is routine use of a nasogastric tube justified in upper abdominal surgery? Am J Surg 139:849, 1980

46. Yates JL: An experimental study of the local effects of peritoneal drainage. Surg Gynecol Obstet 1:473, 1905

47. Berliner SD, Burson LC, Lear PE: Use and abuse of intraperitoneal drains in colon surgery. Arch Surg 89:686, 1964

48. Manz CW, LaTendresse C, Sako Y: The detrimental effects of drains on colonic anastomoses. Dis Colon Rectum 13:17, 1970

49. Koruda MJ, Rolandelli RH: Experimental studies on the healing of colonic anastomoses. J Surg Res 48:504, 1990

50. Munday C, McGinn FP: A comparison of poly-glycolic acid and catgut sutures in rat colonic anastomoses. Br J Surg 63:870, 1976

51. Khubchandani IT: Low end-to-side rectoenteric anastomosis with single-layer wire. Dis Colon Rectum 18:308, 1975

52. Irvin T, Goligher J: Aetiology of disruption of intestinal anastomoses. Br J Surg 60:461, 1973

53. Olsen GB, Letwin E, Williams HTG: Clinical experience with the use of a single-layer intestinal anastomosis. Can J Surg 56:771, 1969

54. Sarin S, Lightwood RG: Continuous single-layer gastrointestinal anastomosis: a prospective audit. Br J Surg 76:493, 1989

55. Shandall A, Lowndes R, Young HL: Colonic anastomotic healing and oxygen tension. Br J Surg 72:606, 1985

56. Jiborn H, Ahonen J, Zederfeldt B: Healing of experimental colonic anastomoses: the effect of suture technique on collagen metabolism in the colonic wall. Am J Surg 139:406, 1980

57. Khoury GA, Waxman BP: Large bowel anastomosis: I. The healing process and sutured anastomoses: a review. Br J Surg 70:61, 1983

58. Abramowitz H: Everting and inverting anastomoses: an experimental study of comparative safety. Rev Surg 28:142, 1971

59. Polglase AL, Hughes ESR, McDermott FT, et al: A comparison of end-to-end staple and suture colorectal anastomosis in the dog. Surg Gynecol Obstet 152:792, 1981

60. O'Neil P, Healey JEJ, Clark RI, et al: Nonsuture intestinal anastomosis. Am J Surg 104:761, 1962

61. Orr NWM: A single layer intestinal anastomosis. Br J Surg 56:77, 1969

62. Templeton JL, McKelvey STD: Low colorectal anastomoses: an experimental assessment of two sutured and two stapled techniques. Dis Colon Rectum 28:38, 1985

63. Goligher J, Morris C, McAdam W: A controlled trial of inverting versus everting intestinal suture in clinical large-bowel surgery. Br J Surg 57:817, 1970

64. Fielding LP, Stewart Brown S, Blesowsky L, et al: Anastomotic integrity after operations for large bowel cancer: a multicentre study. Br Med J 282:411, 1980

65. Leob MJ: Comparative strength of inverted, everted and endon intestinal anastomoses. Surg Gynecol Obstet 125:301, 1967

66. Undre AR: Enteroplasty: a new concept in the management of benign strictures of the intestine. Int Surg 68:73, 1983

67. Chassin JL, Rifkind KM, Turner JW: Errors and pitfalls in stapled gastrointestinal tract surgery. Surg Clin North Am 64:441, 1984

68. Ravitch MM: Intersecting staple lines in intestinal anastomosis. Surgery 97:8, 1985

69. Chung RS: Blood flow in colonic anastomoses: effect of stapling and suturing. Ann Surg 206:335, 1987

70. Julian TB, Ravitch MM: Evaluations of the safety of end-to-end stapling anastomoses across linear stapled closure. Surg Clin North Am 64:567, 1984

71. Gorfine SR, Gelernt IM, Bauer JJ, et al: Restorative proctocolectomy without diverting ileostomy. Dis Colon Rectum 38:188, 1995

72. Grobler SP, Hosie KB, Keighley MR: Randomised trial of loop ileostomy in restorative proctocolectomy. Br J Surg 79:903, 1992

73. Semm N: Enterorophy: its history, technic and present status. JAMA 21:215, 1893

Acknowledgment

Figures 1 through 7   Tom Moore.

16 APPENDECTOMY

Hung S. Ho, M.D.

The vermiform appendix was first depicted in anatomic drawings in 1492 by Leonardo da Vinci and was first described as an anatomic structure in 1521 by Jacopo Berengari da Carpi, a professor of human anatomy at Bologna. Appendicitis became recognized as a surgical disease when the Harvard University pathologist Reginald Heber Fitz reported his analysis of 257 cases of perforating inflammation of the appendix and 209 cases of typhlitis or perityphlitis at the 1886 meeting of the Association of American Physicians. In this landmark paper, Fitz correctly pointed out that the frequent abscesses in the right iliac fossa were often due to perforation of the vermiform appendix, and he referred to the condition as appendicitis.[1] Among his classic observations of the disease was his emphasis on the "vital importance of early recognition" and its "eventual treatment by laparotomy." It was not until 1894 that Charles McBurney first described the surgical incision that bears his name and the technique of appendectomy that was to become the gold standard for appendectomy throughout the 20th century and into the 21st.[2]

Although appendectomy has traditionally been done—and largely continues to be done—as an open procedure, there has been increasing interest in laparoscopic appendectomy since the beginning of the 1990s. In what follows, I describe both approaches to the operation and briefly discuss factors affecting the choice between them.

Open Appendectomy

With the patient in the supine position, general anesthesia is induced and the abdomen is prepared and draped in a sterile fashion so as to expose the right lower quadrant. The skin incision is made in an oblique direction, crossing a line drawn between the anterior superior iliac spine and the umbilicus at nearly a right angle at a point about 2 to 3 cm from the iliac spine. This point, McBurney's point, is approximately one third of the way from the iliac spine to the umbilicus [see Figure 1]. The subcutaneous fat and fascia are incised to expose the external oblique aponeurosis. A slightly shorter incision is made in this aponeurosis; first, a scalpel is used, and then, the incision is extended with scissors in the direction of the fibers of the muscle and its tendon in such a way that the fibers are separated but not cut. The fibers of the internal oblique and transversalis muscles are separated with a blunt instrument at nearly a right angle to the incision on the external oblique aponeurosis. The parietal peritoneum is lifted up, with care taken not to include the underlying viscera, and is opened in a transverse fashion with a scalpel. This incision is then enlarged transversely with scissors. When greater exposure is required, the lateral edge of the rectus sheath is incised and the rectus abdominis muscle retracted medially without being divided [see Figure 2].

A foul smell or the presence of pus on entry into the peritoneum is an indication of advanced appendicitis. The free peritoneal fluid is collected for bacteriologic analysis. The appendix is located by following the cecal taeniae distally. The inflamed appendix usually feels firm and turgid. The appendix, together with the cecum, is delivered into the surgical incision and held with a Babcock tissue forceps. If this step proves difficult, the

appendix can sometimes be swept into the field with the surgeon's right index finger as gentle traction is maintained on the cecum with a small, moist gauze pad held in the left hand [see Figure 3]. Care should be taken at this point not to avulse the friable and possibly necrotic appendix. To deliver a retrocecal appendix, it may be necessary to mobilize the ascending colon partially by dividing the peritoneum on its lateral side, starting from the terminal ileum and proceeding toward the hepatic flexure.

The mesoappendix, containing the appendicular artery, is divided between clamps and ligated with 3-0 absorbable sutures [see Figure 4]. The appendix is held up with a Babcock tissue forceps, and its base is crushed with a straight mosquito arterial forceps. The mosquito forceps is then opened, moved up the appendix, and closed again. The base of the appendix is doubly ligated with 2-0 absorbable sutures at the point where it was crushed, so that a cuff of about 3 mm is left between the forceps and the tie. The appendix is divided by running a scalpel along the underside of the forceps. The mucosa of the appendiceal stump is fulgurated with the electrocautery. The stump is not routinely invaginated into the cecum. In those rare cases in which the viability of the appendiceal base is in question, a 2-0 absorbable purse-string suture is placed in the cecum, and the stump is invaginated as the suture is tied; if this is done, palpation for a patent ileocecal valve is indicated. The operative field is then checked for hemostasis. In cases of perforated appendicitis, the right paracolic gutter and pelvis are irrigated and thoroughly aspirated to ensure that any collected pus or particulate material is removed.

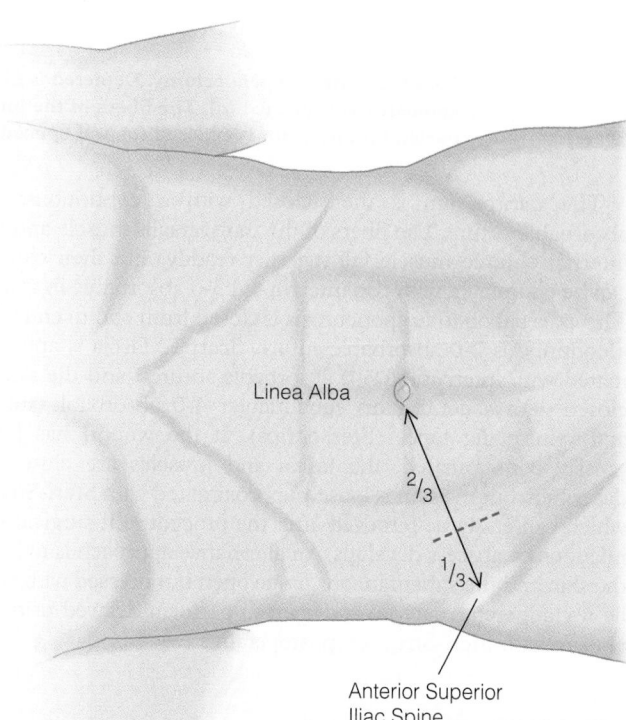

Figure 1 Open appendectomy. Shown are McBurney's point and McBurney's incision.

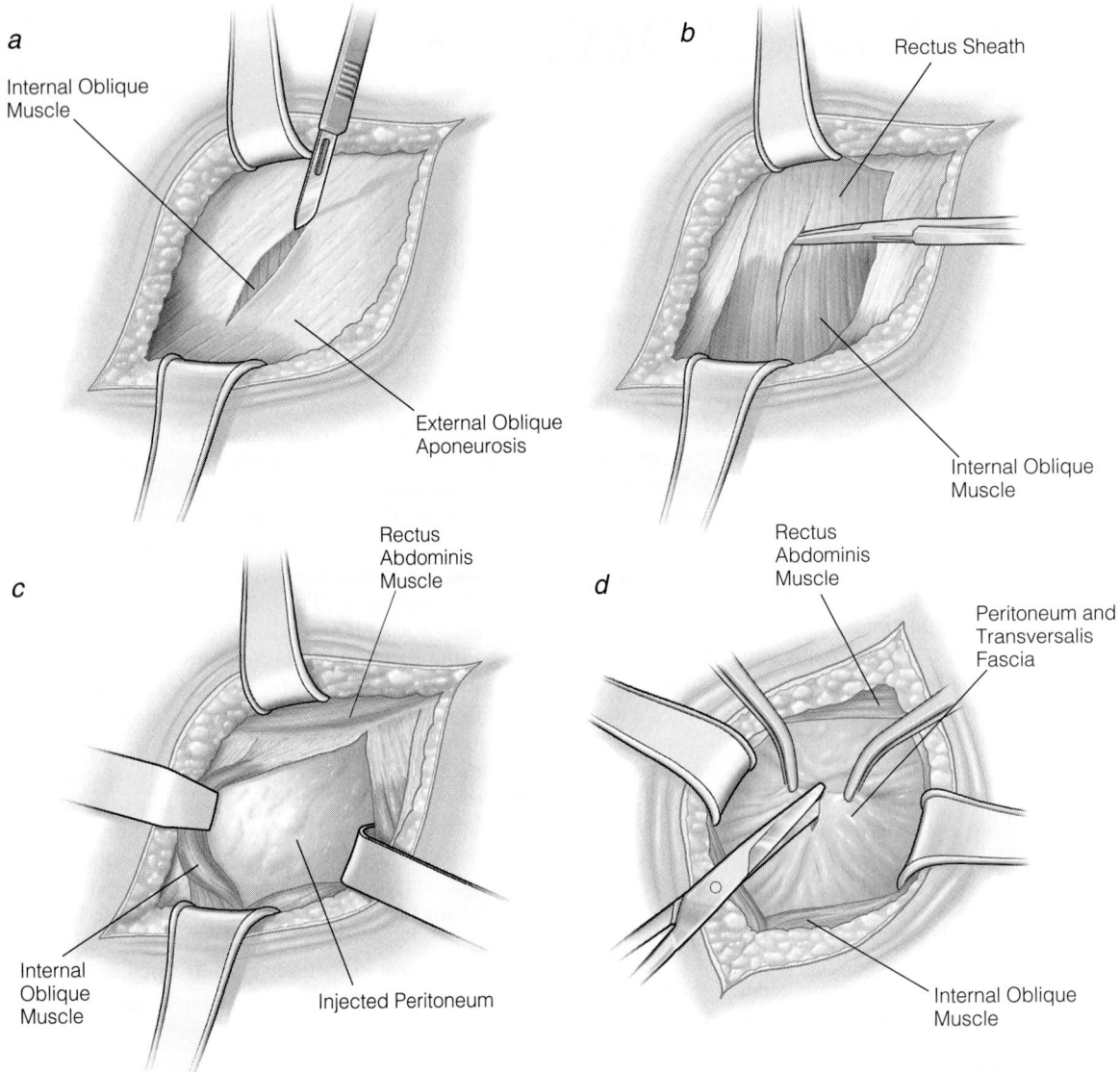

a

Internal Oblique
Muscle

External Oblique
Aponeurosis

b

Rectus Sheath

Internal Oblique
Muscle

c

Rectus
Abdominis
Muscle

Internal
Oblique
Muscle

Injected Peritoneum

d

Rectus
Abdominis
Muscle

Peritoneum and
Transversalis
Fascia

Internal Oblique
Muscle

Figure 2 Open appendectomy. Depicted is exposure of the abdominal cavity. The external oblique aponeurosis is opened (*a*). The fibers of the internal oblique muscle are separated bluntly (*b*). The parietal peritoneum is exposed (*c*) and opened transversely (*d*).

The peritoneum is then closed with a continuous 3-0 absorbable suture. The fibers of the transversalis muscle and the internal oblique muscle fall together readily, and their closure can be completed with two interrupted 3-0 absorbable ligatures. The external oblique aponeurosis is closed from end to end with a continuous 2-0 absorbable suture. Scarpa's fascia is approximated with interrupted 3-0 absorbable sutures, and the skin is closed with a continuous subcuticular 4-0 absorbable suture and reinforcing tapes (Steri-Strips). If the wound has been grossly contaminated, the fascia and muscles are closed as described, but the skin is loosely approximated with Steri-Strips, which can easily be removed after the procedure if surgical site infection or abscess develops. An alternative approach is to leave the skin and the subcutaneous tissue open but dressed with sterile nonadherent material and then to perform delayed primary closure with Steri-Strips on postoperative day 4 or 5.

Laparoscopic Appendectomy

The patient is placed in the supine position, with both arms tucked along the sides, and general anesthesia is induced.

Decompression with a temporary nasal or orogastric tube should be routine, as should placement of a Foley catheter and use of lower-extremity sequential compression devices. The surgeon should stand on the patient's left side, with the assistant (who operates the camera) near the patient's left shoulder [*see Figure 5*]. The monitors are placed on the opposite side of the operating table, so that both the surgeon and the assistant can view the procedure at all times.

The abdomen is prepared and draped in a sterile fashion so as to expose the entire abdomen. A three-port approach is routinely used [*see Figure 5*]. All skin incisions along the midline are made vertically to allow a more cosmetically acceptable conversion to laparotomy, should this become necessary. The suprapubic port must be large enough to accommodate the laparoscopic stapler (usually 12 mm); the other two ports can be smaller (e.g., 5 or 10 mm). The ports are placed as far away from the operative field as possible to permit the application of a two-handed dissection technique. The use of a 25° or 30° angled scope facilitates operative viewing and dissection. With the patient pharmacologically relaxed and in the Trendelenburg position, a Veress needle is inserted into the peritoneal cavity at

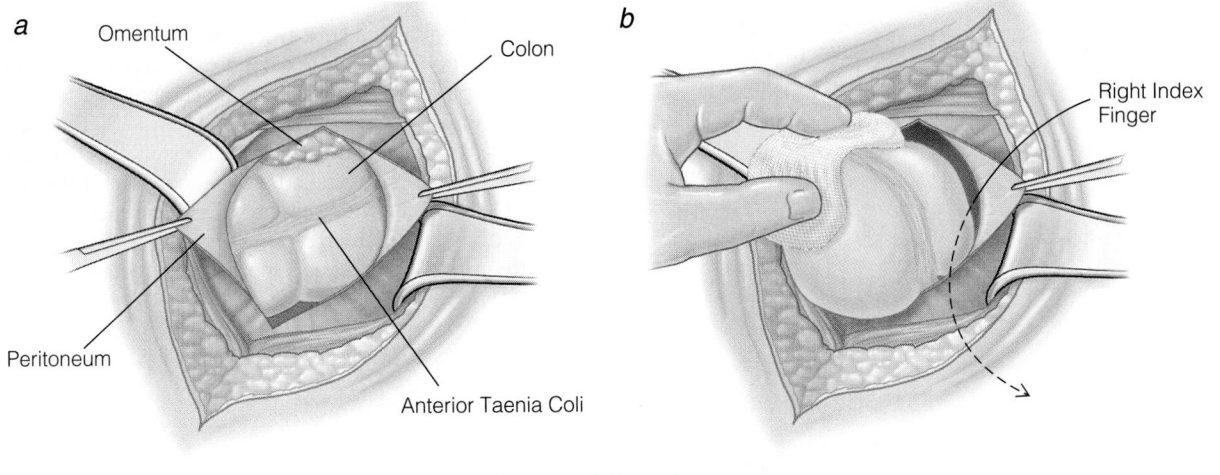

Figure 3 Open appendectomy. Depicted is the mobilization of the appendix. The ascending colon is identified (*a*). The inflamed appendix and the cecum are delivered into the surgical incision; if this is difficult, the appendix can be swept into the field with the right index finger as traction is maintained on the cecum with a gauze pad (*b*). The appendix may be seen to occupy any of a number of potential locations (*c*).

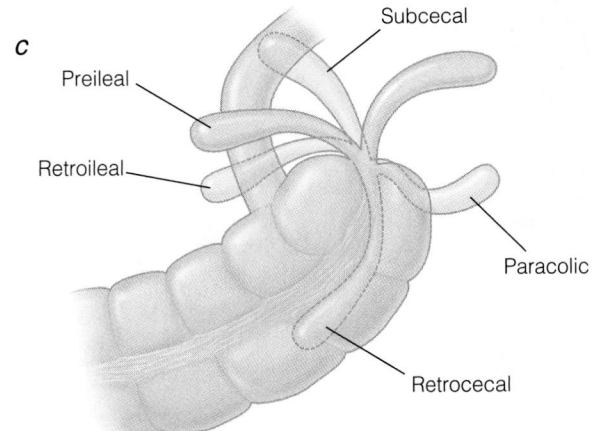

Figure 4 Open appendectomy. The appendicular artery is isolated and controlled (*a*). The mesoappendix is divided and ligated (*b*). The appendix is held up in preparation for its ligation and division (*c*).

Figure 5 Laparoscopic appendectomy. Shown are the positioning and placement of the operative ports, as well as the recommended positions for the surgeon, the camera operator, and the video monitor.

the base of the umbilical ligament. Aspiration and the saline-drop test are performed to ensure that the tip of the needle is correctly positioned. Pneumoperitoneum is established by insufflating CO_2 to an intra-abdominal pressure of 14 mm Hg. The first port is placed at the infraumbilical skin incision, the laparoscope is inserted, and a complete diagnostic laparoscopy is performed. Once the diagnosis of acute appendicitis is confirmed by inspection, the two remaining ports are placed under direct vision. In many cases, however, the diagnosis cannot be confirmed without first placing the second and third ports and exposing the appendix.

The appendix is exposed and traced to its base on the cecum by using an atraumatic retracting forceps. In cases of retrocecal appendix or severe appendiceal inflammation, it is best first to mobilize the cecum completely by taking the lateral reflection of the peritoneum around the terminal ileum and up the ascending colon with an ultrasonic scalpel (e.g., the Harmonic Scalpel, Ethicon Endo-Surgery, Inc.). Surrounding structures, such as the iliac and gonadal vessels and the ureter, should be clearly identified to avoid injury. Dissection of the appendix can then begin. The tip of the appendix is grasped and retracted anteriorly toward the anterior abdominal wall and slightly toward the pelvis; the mesoappendix is thus exposed in a triangular fashion. A window between the base of the appendix and the blood supply is created with a curved dissecting forceps. The mesoappendix is divided either with hemostatic clips and scissors or with a laparoscopic gastrointestinal anastomosis (GIA) stapler loaded with a vascular cartridge [see Figure 6]. If a window on the mesoappendix cannot be safely created because of intense inflammation, antegrade dissection of the blood supply is necessary. The ultrasonic scalpel is a handy (albeit expensive) instrument for this purpose. Endoscopic hemostatic clips usually suffice to control the small branches of the appendicular artery during the course of this dissection.

The base of the appendix is then cleared circumferentially of any adipose or connective tissue and is divided with a laparoscopic GIA stapler loaded with an intestinal cartridge [see Figure

7]. To ensure an adequate closure away from the inflamed appendiceal wall, a small portion of the cecum may have to be included within the stapler. To ensure proper placement of the stapler and to prevent injury to the right ureter or the adjacent small bowel, the tips of the stapler must be clearly visualized before the instrument is closed. The angled scope and the roticulator laparoscopic GIA stapler will facilitate this maneuver. A noninflamed or minimally inflamed appendix can be ligated with sutures, as described earlier [see Open Appendectomy, *above*].

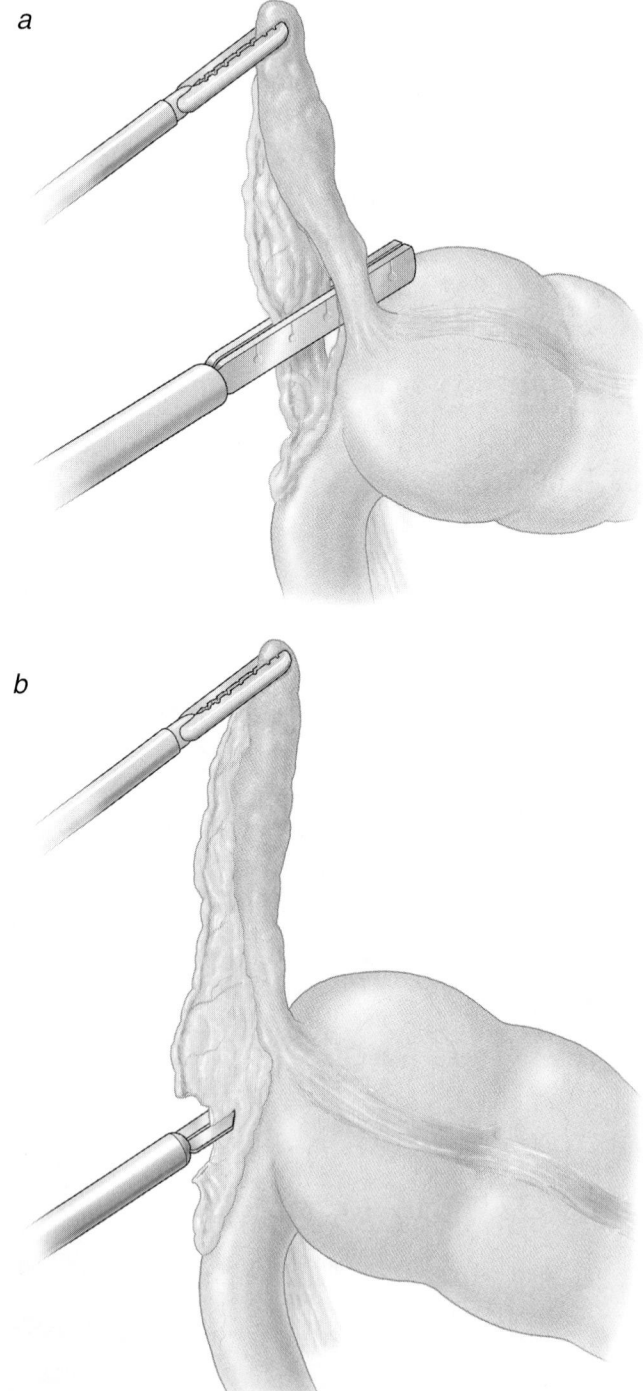

Figure 6 Laparoscopic appendectomy. The mesoappendix is divided either with a laparoscopic GIA stapler (*a*) or with hemostatic clips and scissors (*b*).

Figure 7 **Laparoscopic appendectomy. The mesoappendix having been divided (*a*), the base of the appendix is cleared circumferentially and divided with a GIA stapler (*b*).**

The appendix is removed from the abdominal cavity, with care taken to avoid direct contact with the abdominal wall. A mildly inflamed appendix can be delivered through one of the larger ports; a severely inflamed appendix is often too big and hence should be delivered in a specimen retrieval bag [*see Figure 8*].

The operative field is irrigated and aspirated dry. Hemostasis is confirmed, and the cecum is inspected to ensure proper closure of the appendiceal stump. The ports are removed under direct vision, the absence of back-bleeding from the port sites is confirmed, and the abdomen is completely decompressed. All fascial defects larger than 5 mm are closed with 0 absorbable sutures. The skin incisions are reapproximated with a subcuticular 4-0 absorbable suture and reinforcing Steri-Strips.

Choice between Open and Laparoscopic Appendectomy

To date, 27 reports of randomized, controlled trials comparing laparoscopic appendectomy with open appendectomy have been published as full manuscripts in English [*see Table 1*]. These reports involved a total of 3,755 patients, of whom 1,905 underwent laparoscopic appendectomy and 1,850 underwent open appendectomy.[3-29] Similar incidences of histologically normal appendix were found in the two groups (15.9% with laparoscopic appendectomy versus 16.5% with open appendectomy). The conversion rate from laparoscopic appendectomy to open appendectomy was 11% (range, 0% to 23%). Laparoscopic appendectomy was associated with a lower incidence of postoperative wound infection than open appendectomy was (3.4% versus 7%), but it was also associated with a higher incidence of postoperative intra-abdominal abscess (2.4% versus 1%). The length of stay was slightly shorter after laparoscopic appendectomy (1 to 4.9 days; average, 2.7 days) than after open appendectomy (1.2 to 5.3 days; average, 3.2 days). In men with suspected acute appendicitis, laparoscopic appendectomy has no major advan-

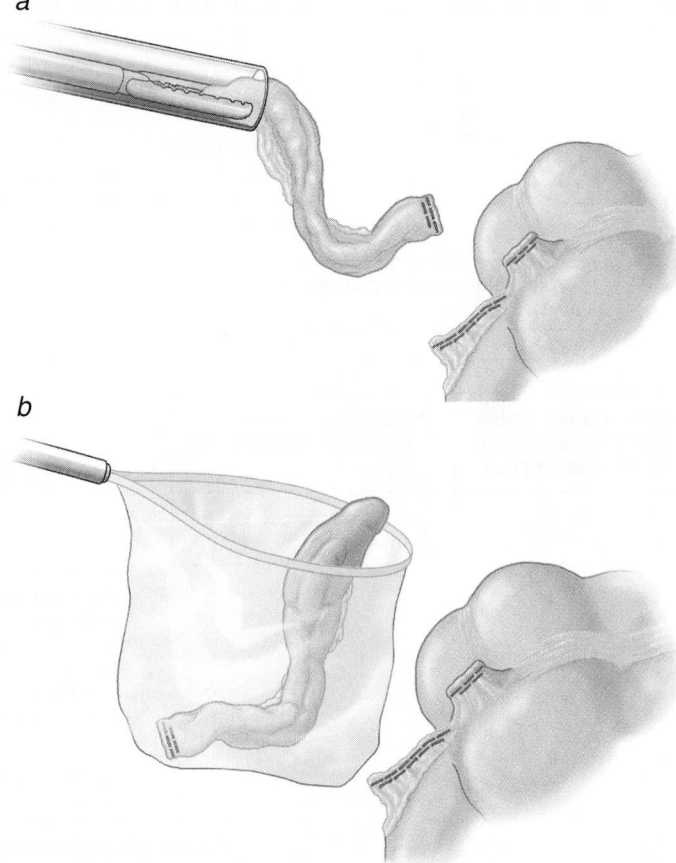

Figure 8 **Laparoscopic appendectomy. The specimen is delivered either through one of the larger ports (*a*) or in a specimen retrieval bag (*b*).**

Table 1   Results of 27 Prospective, Randomized
Trials Comparing Laparoscopic Appendectomy with
Open Appendectomy

Variable	Laparoscopic Appendectomy (N=1,905)		Open Appendectomy (N=1,850)	
	No.	Range	No.	Range
Negative appendix	302 (15.9%)	7.7%–36.0%	305 (16.5%)	0%–35.5%
Conversion to open procedure	205 (10.8%)	0%–23.9%	NA	NA
Surgical site infection	64 (3.4%)	0%–18.3%	129 (7%)	0%–17.3%
Intra-abdominal abscess	45 (2.4%)	0%–7.4%	19 (1%)	0%–4.6%
Days in hospital	2.7	1–4.9	3.2	1.2–5.3

tage over open appendectomy.[10,11] In women of childbearing age and in equivocal cases, laparoscopy may be valuable as a diagnostic tool, but the practice of not removing a normal-looking appendix during exploration for right lower quadrant pain is controversial. Laparoscopic appendectomy appears to offer the potential benefit of less postoperative adhesion formation, but the evidence is inconclusive in the light of the short follow-up times reported in these trials, and the higher incidence of intra-abdominal abscess formation remains cause for concern.

At the beginning of the 21st century, as throughout the 20th, the gold standard for surgical treatment of acute appendicitis remains open appendectomy as described by McBurney in 1894. Meta-analyses of prospective, randomized trials showed that although laparoscopic appendectomy is at least as safe as the corresponding open procedure, it is more time-consuming and more costly. Moreover, it remains questionable whether the benefits of laparoscopic appendectomy—reduced postoperative pain, earlier resumption of oral feeding, shortened hospital stay, quicker return to normal preoperative activities, and lower incidence of surgical site infection—outweigh the doubled incidence of postoperative intra-abdominal abscess formation. Further randomized clinical studies focusing on the efficacy of laparoscopic appendectomy as a diagnostic tool and on the incidence of postoperative intra-abdominal abscess and adhesion formation are needed, as are additional cost analyses. At present, the only patients for whom laparoscopic appendectomy appears to offer significant advan-

Figure 9 **Shown is an algorithm for choosing between treatment options for patients with suspected acute appendicitis.**

tages are female patients of childbearing age, obese patients, and patients with an unclear diagnosis [see Figure 9].

Special Considerations

THE HISTOLOGICALLY NORMAL APPENDIX

Acute appendicitis is the most common cause of acute surgical abdomen in the United States, and it remains one of the most challenging diagnoses to make in the emergency department. Although the use of advanced diagnostic imaging modalities (e.g., ultrasonography and computed tomography) has led to more accurate diagnosis of acute appendicitis in research settings, it has not been shown to reduce the rate of misdiagnosis of acute appendicitis in the general population.[30]

The incidence of histologically normal appendix in patients with clinical signs and symptoms of acute appendicitis ranges from 8% to 41%.[31-40] Nonetheless, appendectomy relieves symptoms in the vast majority of these patients. When extensive sectioning is done on histologically normal specimens, it often happens that a focus of inflammation is found in only a few serial sections. This condition is known as focal appendicitis—so called because the polymorphonuclear infiltration is confined to a single focus, while the remaining appendix is devoid of any polymorphonuclear cells.[41] It is not clear that all cases of acute appendicitis arise from this focal inflammation; however, such inflammatory foci may be the earliest recognizable manifestations of appendicitis in some so-called negative appendectomies. Furthermore, a substantial proportion of histologically normal appendices removed from patients with clinical signs and symptoms of acute appendicitis exhibit significantly increased expression of tumor necrosis factor–α and interleukin-2 messenger RNA (a sensitive marker of inflammation in appendicitis) in germinal centers, the submucosa, and the lamina propria.[42] Therefore, appendectomy is recommended in patients with clinically suspected acute appendicitis even when the appendix does not appear inflamed during exploration.[43]

As noted [see Choice between Open and Laparoscopic Appendectomy, above], the results of numerous randomized, controlled trials indicate that laparoscopic appendectomy does not reduce the incidence of negative exploration in patients with clinically suspected acute appendicitis.[3-29] In these 27 English-language reports, the incidence ranged from 7.7% to 36% (average, 15.9%) with laparoscopic appendectomy and from 0% to 35.5% (average, 16.5%) with open appendectomy [see Table 1].

APPENDICEAL NEOPLASM

Neoplastic lesions of the appendix are found in as many as 5% of specimens obtained with routine appendectomy for acute appendicitis.[44-47] Most are benign. Preoperative detection of such conditions is rare, and intraoperative diagnosis is made in fewer than 50% of cases. Appendectomy alone may be curative for appendiceal mucocele, localized pseudomyxoma peritonei, most appendiceal carcinoids, and other benign tumors. Definitive management of an appendiceal mass unexpectedly encountered during exploration for clinically suspected acute appendicitis depends on whether the tumor is carcinoid, its size and location, the presence or absence of metastatic disease, and histologic and immunohistochemical findings [see Figure 10].

Benign neoplasms of the appendix include mucosal hyperplasia or metaplasia, leiomyomas, neuromas, lipomas, angiomas, and other rare lesions. Appendiceal adenomas tend to be diffuse and to have a predominant villous character. Mucus-producing

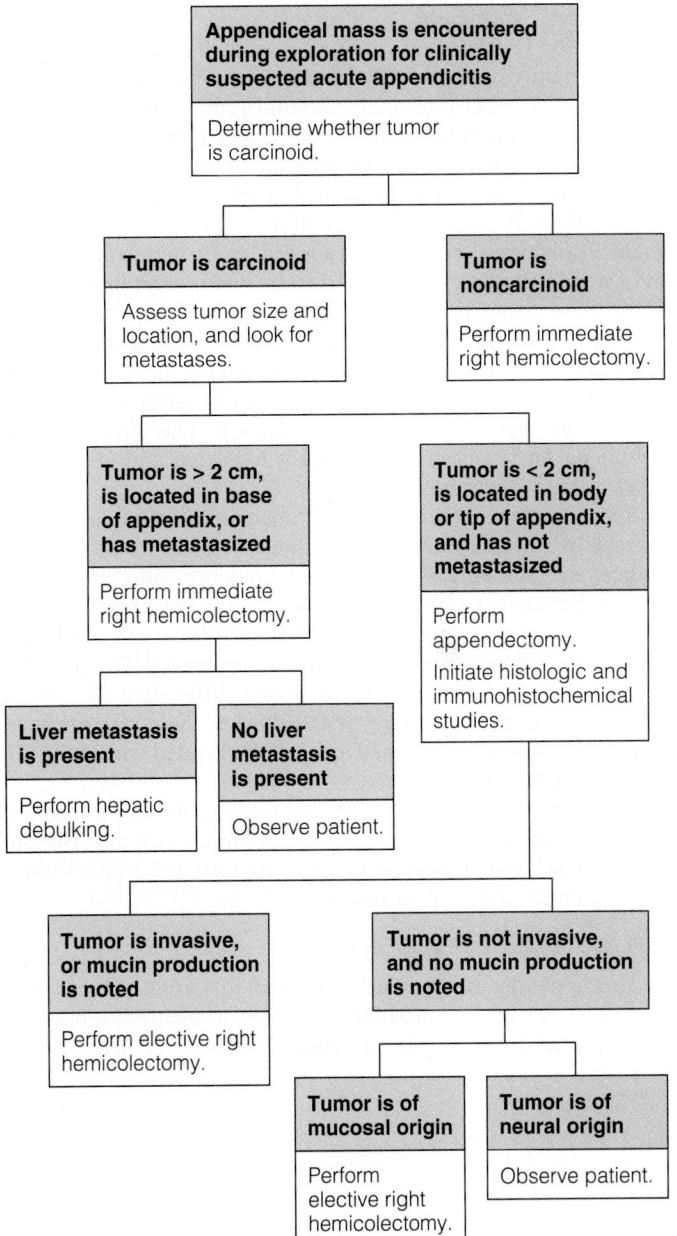

Figure 10 Shown is an algorithm for the management of an appendiceal mass encountered during exploration for clinically suspected acute appendicitis.

cystadenomas predispose to appendiceal mucocele, sometimes accompanied by localized pseudomyxoma peritonei. These lesions are rarely symptomatic and are often encountered incidentally during operation; however, they may also be clinically manifested as acute appendicitis, torsion, intussusception, ureteral obstruction, or another acute condition. If the base of the appendix is free of disease, appendectomy alone is sufficient treatment.

Malignant tumors of the appendix primarily consist of carcinoids and adenocarcinomas; altogether, they account for 0.5% of all GI malignancies.[48] The incidence of malignancy in the appendix is 1.35%.[44] Metastasis to the appendix is rare. Carcinoids are substantially more common than adenocarcinomas in the appendix: as many as 80% of all appendiceal masses are carcinoid tumors. Overall, carcinoid tumors are found in 0.5% of all appendiceal specimens, and appendiceal carcinoid tumors account for 18.9% of all carcinoid lesions.[49] These tumors are predominantly of neural cellular origin and have a better prognosis than all other intestinal carcinoid tumors, which typically are of mucosal cellular origin. If the tumor is less than 2 cm in diameter, is located within the body or the tip of the appendix, and has not metastasized, appendectomy is the treatment of choice. If the lesion is at the base of the appendix, is larger than 2 cm in diameter, or has metastasized, right hemicolectomy is indicated. In addition, secondary right hemicolectomy is indicated if the tumor is invasive, if mucin production is noted, or if the tumor is found to be of mucosal cellular origin at final pathologic examination.[50,51] Patients with metastatic appendiceal carcinoid tumors appear to have a far better prognosis than those with other types of metastatic cancers.[50] Therefore, hepatic debulking for symptomatic control is indicated and justified in cases of liver metastasis.

Primary adenocarcinoma of the appendix is rare, and as yet there is no firm consensus regarding prognosis, treatment of choice, and outcome.[52] Currently, the recommended treatment is right hemicolectomy: a 1993 study found that this approach resulted in an overall 5-year survival rate of 68%, compared with 20% when appendectomy alone was performed.[51] The prognosis is determined by the degree of tumor differentiation and by the histologic stage. As many as one third of these patients have a second primary neoplasm, which will be located within the GI tract about half the time.

Finally, nonepithelial appendiceal tumors, though extremely rare, occur as well. Such lesions include malignant and Burkitt lymphomas, smooth muscle tumors, granular cell tumors, ganglioneuromas, and Kaposi sarcoma.

INFLAMMATORY BOWEL DISEASE

The appendix is frequently involved in Crohn disease and ulcerative colitis (25% and 50% of cases, respectively), but isolated Crohn disease of the appendix is rare.[53-56] When a histologically normal appendix is encountered in a patient with active Crohn disease, appendectomy should be performed because of the high risk of recurrent right lower quadrant pain, fever, and tenderness. Although isolated Crohn disease of the appendix may present as acute appendicitis, it is not clear that this condition will necessarily develop into a more extensive form of Crohn disease. Appendectomy is safe in such cases because fistulas almost never develop after appendectomy in patients with isolated involvement of the appendix.

GYNECOLOGIC CONDITIONS

It is clear that the presentation of right lower quadrant pain in a female patient remains a challenge to the treating physician. Frequently, the causes can be identified by means of proper blood work or ultrasonography, but often they can be revealed only through surgical exploration. In such cases, diagnostic laparoscopy provides an excellent view of the pelvic organs, and it offers the potential for easy continuation on to laparoscopic treatment. Ovarian cysts found in premenopausal women include unilocular clear fluid cysts (e.g., follicular cysts and corpus luteum cysts), dermoid cysts, and endometrial cysts. They can be removed by making an incision on the ovary and separating the cyst from the ovarian cortex. Dermoid cysts should be removed in toto to prevent chemical peritonitis. Endometrial cysts are best evaporated with the laser: complete removal is very difficult and sometimes impossible. Torsion of the fallopian tube or the ovary can be reversed by gentle detorsion of the organ with atraumatic forceps. If there is no evidence of ischemia, no further therapy is indicated. If there is gangrene with no indication of recovery, resection is indicated. If the organ shows partial recovery within 10 minutes after the pedicle is untwisted, a second-look laparoscopy is indicated in 24 hours. Pelvic inflammatory disease should be treated on an individualized basis in accordance with the degree of inflammation, the patient's age and desire to have children, and the microbiologic findings.

References

1. Fitz RH: Perforating inflammation of the vermiform appendix with special reference to its early diagnosis and treatment. Trans Assoc Am Physicians 1:107, 1886

2. McBurney C: The incision made in the abdominal wall in cases of appendicitis, with a description of a new method of operating. Ann Surg 20:38, 1894

3. Attwood SEA, Hill ADK, Murphy PG, et al: A prospective randomized trial of laparoscopic versus open appendectomy. Surgery 112:497, 1992

4. Tate JJT, Dawson JW, Chung SCS, et al: Laparoscopic versus open appendectomy: prospective randomised trial. Lancet 342:633, 1993

5. Kum CK, Ngoi SS, Goh PMY, et al: Randomized controlled trial comparing laparoscopic and open appendicectomy. Br J Surg 80:1599, 1993

6. Frazee RC, Roberts JW, Symmonds RE, et al: A prospective randomized trial comparing open versus laparoscopic appendectomy. Ann Surg 219:725, 1994

7. Ortega AE, Hunter JG, Peters JH, et al: A prospective, randomized comparison of laparoscopic appendectomy with open appendectomy. Am J Surg 169:208, 1995

8. Martin LC, Puente I, Sosa JL, et al: Open versus laparoscopic appendectomy: a prospective randomized comparison. Ann Surg 222:256, 1995

9. Hansen JB, Smithers BM, Schache D, et al: Laparoscopic versus open appendectomy: prospective randomized trial. World J Surg 20:17, 1996

10. Mutter D, Vix M, Bui A, et al: Laparoscopy not recommended for routine appendectomy in men: results of a prospective randomized study. Surgery 120:71, 1996

11. Cox MR, McCall JL, Toouli J, et al: Prospective randomized comparison of open versus laparoscopic appendectomy in men. World J Surg 20:263, 1996

12. Lejus C, Dellie L, Plattner V, et al: Randomized, single-blinded trial of laparoscopic versus open appendectomy in children. Anesthesiology 84:801, 1996

13. Williams MD, Collins JN, Wright TF, et al: Laparoscopic versus open appendectomy. South Med J 89:668, 1996

14. Hart R, Rajgopal C, Plewes A, et al: Laparoscopic versus open appendectomy: a prospective randomized trial of 81 patients. Can J Surg 39:457, 1996

15. Reiertsen O, Larsen S, Trondsen E, et al: Randomized controlled trial with sequential design of laparoscopic versus conventional appendicectomy. Br J Surg 84:842, 1997

16. Laine S, Rantala A, Gullichsen R, et al: Laparoscopic appendectomy—is it worthwhile? a prospective, randomized study in young women. Surg Endosc 11:95, 1997

17. Macarulla E, Vallet J, Abad JM, et al: Laparoscopic versus open appendectomy: a prospective randomized trial. Surg Laparosc Endosc 7:335, 1997

18. Kazemier G, de Zeeuw GR, Lange JF, et al: Laparoscopic versus open appendectomy: a randomized clinical trial. Surg Endosc 11:336, 1997

19. Minne L, Varner D, Burnell A, et al: Laparosopic versus open appendectomy: prospective randomized study of outcomes. Arch Surg 132:708, 1997

20. Hay SA: Laparoscopic versus conventional appendectomy in children. Pediatr Surg Int 13:21, 1998

21. Klinger A, Henle KP, Beller S, et al: Laparoscopic appendectomy does not change the incidence of postoperative infectious complications. Am J Surg 175:232, 1998

22. Hiekkinen TJ, Haukipuro K, Hulkko A: Cost-effective appendectomy: open or laparoscopic? a prospective randomized study. Surg Endosc 12:1204, 1998

23. Hellberg A, Rudberg C, Kullman E, et al: Prospective randomized multicentre study of laparoscopic versus open appendicectomy. Br J Surg 86:48, 1999

24. Ozmen MM, Zulfikaroglu B, Tanik A, et al: Laparoscopic versus open appendectomy: prospective randomized trial. Surg Laparosc Endosc Percutan Tech 9:187, 1999

25. Pedersen AG, Petersen OB, Wara P, et al: Randomized clinical trial of laparoscopic versus open appendicectomy. Br J Surg 88:200, 2001

26. Lavonius MI, Liesjarvi S, Ovaska J, et al: Laparoscopic versus open appendectomy in children: a prospective randomised study. Eur J Pediat Surg 11:235, 2001

27. Long KH, Bannon MP, Zietlow SP, et al: A prospective randomized comparison of laparoscopic appendectomy with open appedectomy: Clinical and economic analyses. Surgery 129:390, 2001

28. Lintula H, Kokki H, Vanamo K: Single-blind randomized clinical trial of laparoscopic versus appendicectomy in children. Br J Surg 88:510, 2001

29. Huang MT, Wei PL, Wu CC, et al: Needlescopic, laparoscopic, and open appendectomy: a comparative study. Surg Laparosc Endosc Percutan Tech 11:306, 2001

30. Flum DR, Morris A, Koepsell T, et al: Has misdiagnosis of appendicitis decreased over time? a population-based analysis. JAMA 286:1748, 2001

31. Chang AR: An analysis of the pathology of 3,003 appendices. Aust NZ J Surg 51:169, 1981

32. Knight PJ, Vassy LE: Specific diseases mimicking appendicitis in childhood. Arch Surg 116:744, 1981

33. Pieper R, Kager L, Nasman P: Acute appendicitis: a clinical study of 1,018 cases of emergency appendectomy. Acta Chir Scand 148:51, 1982

34. Arnbjornsson E, Asp NG, Westin SI: Decreasing incidence of acute appendicitis, with special reference to the consumption of dietary fiber. Acta Chir Scand 148:461, 1982

35. Blind PJ, Dahlgren ST: The continuing challenge of the negative appendix. Acta Chir Scand 152:623, 1986

36. Lau WY: Correlation between gross appeareance of the appendix and histological examination. Ann R Coll Surg Edinb 70:336, 1988

37. Budd JS, Armstrong CP: The correlation between gross appearance at appendix and histological examination. Ann R Coll Surg Edinb 70:395, 1988

38. Blair PM, Bugis PS, Turner LJ, et al: Review of the pathologic diagnosis of 2,216 appendectomy specimens. Am J Surg 165:618, 1993

39. Dahlstom JE, MacArthur EB: *Enterobius vermicularis:* a possible cause of symptoms resembling appendicitis. Aust NZ J Surg 64:692, 1994

40. Pearl RH, Hale DA, Molloy M, et al: Pediatric appendectomy. J Pediatr Surg 30:173, 1995

41. Truji M, Puri P, Reen DJ: Characterization of the local inflammatory response in appendicitis. J Pediatr Gastroenterol Nutr 16:43, 1993

42. Wang Y, Reen DJ, Puri P: Is a histologically normal appendix following emergency appendicectomy always normal? Lancet 347:1076, 1996

43. Grunewald B, Keating J: Should the 'normal' appendix be removed at operation for appendicitis? J R Coll Surg Edinb 38:158, 1993

44. Collins DC: 71,000 human appendix specimens: a final report, summarizing 40 years' study. Am J Proctol 14:265, 1963

45. Chan W, Fu KH: Value of routine histopathological examination of appendices in Hong Kong. J Clin Pathol 40:429, 1987

46. Lenriot JP, Hugier M: Adenocarcinoma of the appendix. Am J Surg 155:470, 1988

47. Gupta SC, Gupta AK, Keswani NK, et al: Pathology of tropical appendicitis. J Clin Pathol 42:1169, 1989

48. Thomas RM, Sobin LH: Gastrointestinal cancer. Cancer 75:154, 1995

49. Modlin IM, Sandor A: An analysis of 8305 cases of carcinoid tumors. Cancer 79:813, 1997

50. Moertel CG, Weiland LH, Nagorney DM, et al: Carcinoid tumor of the appendix: treatment and prognosis. N Engl J Med 317:1699, 1987

51. Gouzi JL, Laigneau P, Delalande JP, et al: Indications for right hemicolectomy in carcinoid tumors of the appendix. Surg Gynecol Obstet 176:543, 1993

52. Nitecki SS, Wolff BG, Schlinkert R, et al: The natural history of surgically treated primary adenocarcinoma of the appendix. Ann Surg 219:51, 1994

53. Yang SS, Gibson P, McCaughey RS, et al: Primary Crohn's disease of the appendix. Ann Surg 189:334, 1979

54. Jahadi MR, Shaw ML: The pathology of the appendix in ulcerative colitis. Dis Colon Rectum 19:345, 1976

55. Ruiz V, Unger SW, Morgan J, et al: Crohn's disease of the appendix. Surgery 107:113, 1990

56. Goldblum JR, Appelman HD: Appendiceal involvement in ulcerative colitis. Mod Pathol 5:607, 1992

Acknowledgments

Figures 1 through 8   Tom Moore.
Figures 9 and 10   Marcia Kammerer.

17 COLORECTAL PROCEDURES

Theodore R. Schrock, M.D.

Total Colectomy with Ileorectal Anastomosis

OPERATIVE PLANNING

Total colectomy involves resection of the entire colon with oversewing of the rectum or construction of an ileorectal anastomosis. Candidates for this operation include certain patients with inflammatory bowel disease, familial adenomatous polyposis, hereditary nonpolyposis colorectal cancer syndromes, chronic constipation, or severe lower gastrointestinal hemorrhage [*see II:9 Lower Gastrointestinal Bleeding*].[1-5] The operation is performed in two stages in patients with fulminant colitis, severe inflammation of the rectum, pelvic abscess, or severe associated disease. Some surgeons perform total colectomy with ileorectal anastomosis via a laparoscopic or laparoscopic-assisted approach[6] [*see V:18 Laparoscopic Colectomy*]; however, in what follows, I address only conventional open techniques.

OPERATIVE TECHNIQUE

Step 1: Positioning and Incision

The lithotomy position, with the lower extremities in Lloyd-Davies leg rests or Allen universal stirrups, has the advantage of providing good access to the anus. The rectum can be examined and irrigated with saline before preparation and draping, and intraoperative colonoscopy, stapling maneuvers, and inspection of the anastomosis for integrity can be performed.

The positioning of the surgical team depends on the experience and the anticipated role of the assistants. If the first assistant is able to dissect under the surgeon's guidance, the surgeon should stand on the patient's left side, a position that gives the surgeon control of retraction and exposure of the right colon and the transverse colon. (I assume this arrangement in the description of the procedure.) When working on the left colon, the assistant retracts with one hand and dissects with the other, while the surgeon displays the tissues to be incised laterally. In the teaching environment, positions sometimes shift around the table.

A midline incision is standard, but a transverse incision below the umbilicus is feasible in slender patients and in patients with long-standing inflammatory bowel disease, which often shortens the colon and the mesocolon.

Step 2: Mobilization and Removal of the Colon

The sigmoid colon is occluded with an encircling ligature of heavy material (e.g., umbilical tape) to prevent perineal soilage from distal passage of colonic contents.

Mobilization of the colon usually begins on the right side. The surgeon pinches the peritoneal surfaces together lateral to the cecum to protect the bowel from injury, and the peritoneum is incised very close to the cecal wall. The surgeon inserts the left index finger into the defect, retracting the cecum and the ascending colon medially while the lateral peritoneum is incised [*see Figure 1*]. The white line of Toldt is ignored on the right side, and the peritoneum is incised as close to the colon as possible. (Incising the peritoneum close to the wall of the right colon makes it unlikely that the surgeon will incise Gerota's fascia and dissect into perinephric fat.) The cecum is pulled laterally, and the medial layer of peritoneum of the distal ileal mesentery is incised proximally as far as necessary. The right ureter is identified.

As the hepatic flexure is approached, the duodenum appears, and the mesocolon is detached from it by dividing filmy tissue containing tiny vessels. In patients with benign disease, separation of the mesocolon from the duodenum up to the pancreas is unnecessary, but it does facilitate division of the mesocolon. In patients with cancer, full mobilization is necessary to ensure that vessels are ligated close to their origin. Hepatic flexure attachments contain vessels of varying size, some of which are large enough to necessitate ligation.

At this point, the surgeon must decide whether to preserve the greater omentum or to remove it. If the omentum is to be preserved, it is detached from the transverse colon; if it is to be removed, the gastrocolic ligament is serially divided and ligated. (I prefer to excise the greater omentum with the colonic specimen because the omentum causes obstruction of the small bowel after total colectomy much more frequently than it does after segmental colectomy.)

The lesser sac is entered to the left of the midline. (One should do this before the hepatic flexure is taken down completely and then work back to the right.) In the lesser sac, adhesions of the stomach to the transverse mesocolon are lysed, the gastrocolic ligament is serially divided and ligated outside the gastroepiploic vessels [*see Figure 2*], and the hepatic flexure is approached from the left. The mesocolon is left intact until it is fully separated from the gastrocolic, duodenal, and pancreatic attachments. The ileocolic, right colic (if present), and middle colic vessels are then divided at a level determined by the pathologic problem being treated [*see Figure 3*]. (Some surgeons preserve the ileocolic vessels in case a pelvic pouch is possible later; however, because I deliberately divide the ileocolic vessels when constructing an ileoanal pouch, I do not preserve them when fashioning an ileorectal anastomosis.) The ileum is divided at the ileocecal valve with a linear cutting stapler or between intestinal clamps.

Once the dissection has reached the distal transverse colon, the sigmoid colon is mobilized so that the splenic flexure can be approached from the left and below. The sigmoid colon and the mesocolon are retracted to the right by the assistant, who remains on the patient's right side. Adhesions of the appendices epiploicae, the colon, and the mesocolon to the parietal peritoneal attachments of the descending colon are incised a little at a time. (If the colonic attachments are divided all the way to the splenic flexure first, one can stray too far laterally and even end up within Gerota's fascia. The surgeon can insert one or two fingers into the space behind the peritoneum to display the next

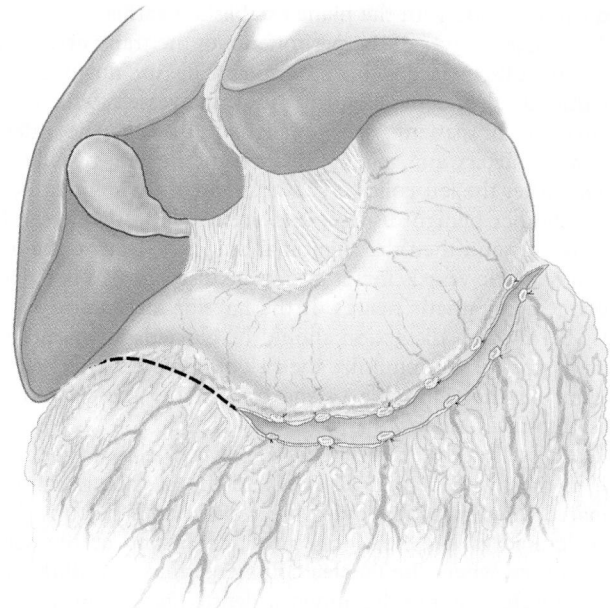

Figure 2 Total colectomy with ileorectal anastomosis. The gastrocolic ligament is serially divided and ligated outside the gastroepiploic vessels, and the hepatic flexure is approached from the left.[33]

Figure 1 Total colectomy with ileorectal anastomosis. The surgeon inserts the left index finger into the peritoneal defect, retracting the cecum and the ascending colon medially while the lateral peritoneum is incised as close to the colon as possible.[33]

toneum are divided. (This must be done in a bloodless plane. No fat should be cut in mobilizing the sigmoid colon. There is no fat in the proper plane; if one is cutting through fat, one is in the wrong plane.)

The sigmoid colon is then pulled farther to the right, and the mesosigmoid is incised at its base. (The incision should be made on the left side, medial to the left ureter. If the ureter is not seen through the intact posterior parietal peritoneum, it should be visible after this incision is made.) The peritoneal incision is extended longitudinally, parallel to the course of the ureter, and the ureter is swept laterally. (Care should be taken to avoid the sympathetic nerves on the surface of the aorta, about 1 cm posterior to the superior hemorrhoidal vessels; injury to these nerves can cause ejaculatory impairment. In men with benign disease, there is no need to risk such impairment. Accordingly, dissection in the vicinity should be minimized once the ureter is seen and protected.)

The splenic flexure is taken down by approaching it from the left, from below, and from behind. The colon and the mesocolon are separated from Gerota's fascia, and the lateral peri-

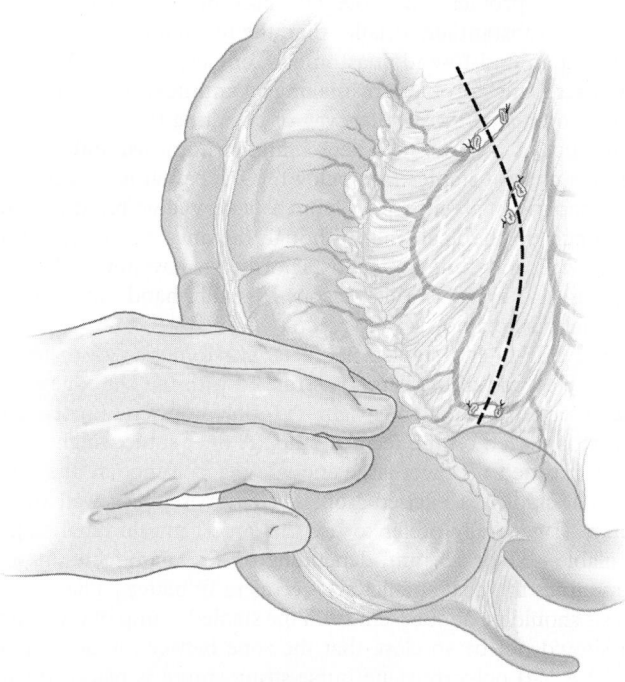

Figure 3 Total colectomy with ileorectal anastomosis. The ileocolic, right colic, and middle colic vessels are ligated and divided at a level called for by the pathologic problem being treated.[33]

portion for incision [*see Figure 4*]. It is important that the path of dissection remain within a few millimeters of the colon as the flexure is taken down. In this way, one follows the plane of attachment of the omentum, which is relatively avascular.) These maneuvers separate the omentum from the colon. If the omentum is to be removed, the remaining portion of the gastrocolic ligament must be divided and ligated so that a connection can be made with the plane established earlier.

The anterior layer of the peritoneum of the transverse mesocolon must be incised to take the splenic flexure down. Behind this thin layer, of course, lie the mesocolic vessels, which must be ligated. In patients with malignant disease, the inferior mesenteric artery and vein are divided and ligated (usually separately) after the left colic vessels are divided. In men with colitis or another benign disease, it is preferable to divide the left colic vessels and then the sigmoidal branches, leaving the inferior mesenteric vessels intact to obviate dissection in the vicinity of the sympathetic nerves. If the inferior mesenteric vessels must be divided, dissection should be carried out as close to them as possible to minimize the risk of nerve injury. The peritoneum on the right side of the base of the mesosigmoid is incised to facilitate vascular division.

The vessels at the rectosigmoid are divided close to the rectal wall in men with benign disease, and the proximal rectum is prepared for transection by division of the mesorectum. (The rectosigmoid is a 4 cm long transitional zone at the sacral promontory, where the taeniae coli merge into a confluent circular muscle coat and the lumen widens.) The rectum is divided between clamps.

Step 3: Ileorectal Anastomosis

Whether an ileorectal anastomosis should be done by hand suturing or by stapling and whether it should be end-to-end or side-to-end are matters of personal preference. My own predilection is for a side-to-end stapled anastomosis, as described here.

A basic problem in ileorectal anastomosis is that the ileal lumen is substantially smaller than the rectal lumen. When performing an end-to-end anastomosis, one can obviate the luminal discrepancy problem by making an antimesenteric slit in the ileum to enlarge it. Another way of obviating the problem is to construct a side-to-end ileorectal anastomosis, either with sutures or with staples (see below). (One caveat is that side-to-end stapling of a very small ileum to a very large rectum seems to bunch up the ileal wall. Although the anastomosis generally heals well and functions satisfactorily, it may not look quite right to the eye. For this reason, I usually hand suture if the luminal discrepancy is very great.)

In a side-to-end stapled ileorectal anastomosis [*see Figure 5*], the stapled end of the ileum is arranged with the cut edge of the mesentery to the patient's right. A 0 polypropylene purse-string suture is placed on the rectal stump. (A finer suture might break when it is tied.) A divot large enough to accommodate the intraluminal stapler is excised from the antimesenteric wall of the ileum. (I generally prefer to use the largest intraluminal stapler available—31 or 33 mm, depending on the manufacturer—but sometimes the next smaller size seems to fit better.) The anastomosis should be about 1 cm from the stapled stump of the ileum. (It should not be so close that the zone between is devascularized.) A 2-0 polypropylene purse-string suture is placed on the ileal defect. The stapler is inserted through the anus and opened, and the distal purse-string suture is tied. (The stapler should have a flat anvil: if the anvil has a protruding knob, it will bump into the opposite wall.) The shaft is separated, and the anvil is secured

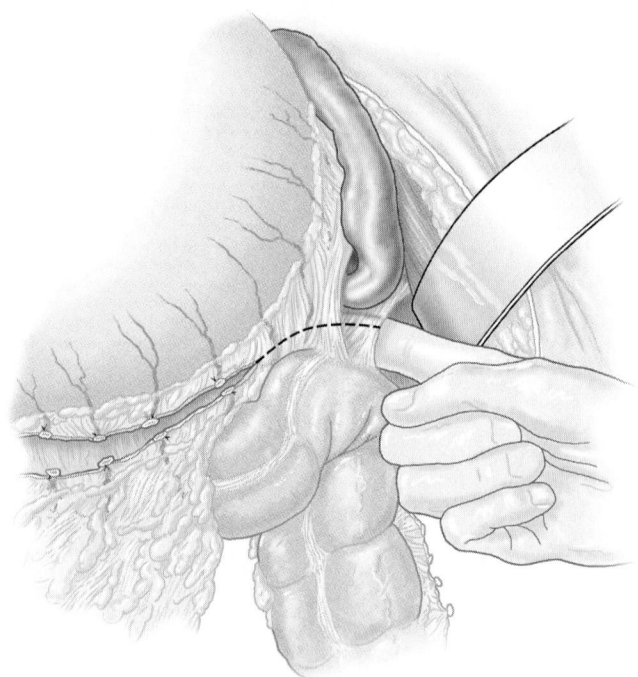

Figure 4 **Total colectomy with ileorectal anastomosis. The surgeon can insert one or two fingers into the space behind the peritoneum to display the next portion for incision.**[33] **The avascular plane is within a few millimeters of the colon as the flexure is taken down.**

in the ileum by tying the proximal purse-string suture. The stapler is then reassembled and fired. Two intact rings of tissue ("doughnuts") should be obtained. The anastomosis is checked for integrity by inserting a rigid sigmoidoscope through the anus and insufflating air with the pelvis filled with saline.

Step 4: Completion

The edge of the ileal mesentery is sutured to the retroperitoneal surface to eliminate the potential hernial defect. Drains are not required. A diverting loop ileostomy is rarely necessary with this procedure.

COMPLICATIONS

Ileus can be prolonged after total colectomy [*see II:7 Intestinal Obstruction*]. Obstruction of the small bowel after total colectomy can be minimized by excising the omentum and closing the mesenteric defect. Anastomotic leakage after ileorectal anastomosis is more common in patients with inflammatory bowel disease than in patients with other conditions; in any case, the incidence of this complication should be lower than 4%.[7] Large leaks necessitate reoperation, takedown of the anastomosis, closure of the rectal stump, and end ileostomy until conditions are right for reconnection of the bowel. Small leaks may be managed nonoperatively.

OUTCOME

Return of function depends on the indication for the operation, the presence or absence of rectal disease, the patient's age, and the presence or absence of comorbid factors.[1,2,4,8,9] Once stools begin, diarrhea is the rule, sometimes accompanied by urgency and even minor incontinence. Loperamide is effective against diarrhea. Generally, otherwise healthy persons who undergo total colectomy with ileorectal anastomosis will have from three to five stools a day for the remainder of their lives. This stool pattern does not interfere with physical activities or daily routine. Incontinence should not be a lingering problem once stools slow and thicken, provided that the preoperative assessment of sphincter adequacy was correct.

Total Proctocolectomy with Conventional Ileostomy

OPERATIVE PLANNING

Proctocolectomy with a permanent ileostomy is appropriate for patients with Crohn colitis and for some patients with familial adenomatous polyposis or ulcerative colitis who are not candidates for restorative proctocolectomy because of obesity, advanced age, or the presence of cancer in the distal rectum.[10-13]

Preoperative education of the patient regarding the ileostomy is essential. Either an enterostomal therapist or the surgeon should, if possible, select the site for the stoma with the patient

a

b

Figure 5 **Total colectomy with ileorectal anastomosis.[33] (*a*) In a side-to-end stapled ileorectal anastomosis, a 0 polypropylene purse-string suture is placed on the rectal stump. A divot is excised from the antimesenteric wall of the ileum, and a 2-0 polypropylene purse-string suture is placed on the ileal defect. (*b*) An end-to-end or intraluminal stapler is inserted through the anus and opened, and the distal purse-string suture is tied. The proximal purse-string suture is tied to secure the anvil in the ileum. The stapler is then reassembled and fired.**

supine, standing, and sitting [*see VIII:3 Stomal Care*]. The ileostomy must pass through the rectus sheath and must be located away from depressions and elevations. The ideal site is nearly always in the right lower quadrant.

OPERATIVE TECHNIQUE

Step 1: Positioning

If the operation is to be performed by two teams, the lithotomy position obviously is necessary. If the entire operation is to be performed by a single surgeon, the patient can be repositioned after the abdomen is closed. The anus is closed with a heavy purse-string suture.

Step 2: Creation of Ileostomy Aperture

The first step in creating the ileostomy aperture is to excise a circle of skin about 2.5 cm in diameter.[14] (This aperture should be made before the abdominal incision so as to maintain normal alignment of the layers of the abdominal wall.) My preferred technique is to grasp the skin with a Kocher clamp and elevate it strongly, then to excise a disk of skin with a heavy curved scissors oriented in the longitudinal direction; stress along Langer's lines converts an elliptical aperture on the vertical axis to a circular opening. Dermis that was crushed but not excised is removed with the electrocautery. (Admittedly, this method looks crude, but it nearly always results in a perfect circle.)

The fat is spread with a clamp, not excised. Dead space is not desirable at an ileostomy site. The anterior rectus sheath is incised longitudinally, the rectus is separated with a clamp, and the posterior rectus sheath is exposed. A moist sponge is stuffed into this space, and the aperture is completed after the main abdominal incision is made. (Care should be taken not to injure the inferior epigastric vessels.)

Step 3: Colectomy and Preparation of Ileal Mesentery

Colectomy is carried out as described earlier [*see* Total Colectomy with Ileorectal Anastomosis, *above*]. (It is important to prepare the ileal mesentery in such a way that the bowel projects straight ahead and is not curved by tension on the mesentery. The ileal mesentery is divided in an L fashion so that the blood supply is preserved but the tissue that is to be brought through the abdominal wall is thinned [*see Figure 6*].)

Step 4: Pelvic Dissection

Dissection proceeds close to the rectal wall until well below the sacral promontory. (In this way, one can usually keep from injuring the sympathetic nerves of the superior hypogastric plexus—that is, the presacral nerves. These nerves lie at the level of the aortic bifurcation and divide into the left and right hypogastric nerves, which extend into the pelvis.)

In the classical method of posterior dissection, the presacral connective tissue was incised for a short distance, the surgeon's hand was inserted, and the mesorectum was separated from the endopelvic fascia by blunt dissection; the separation created a characteristic sucking sound. (This technique crudely tears the soft tissues in what the surgeon can only hope is the proper plane, sometimes injuring the presacral veins, the pelvic nerves, or both. Consequently, it should be abandoned except in the most difficult situations, such as in obese men in whom there is limited visibility of the posterior pelvis.) In the method I use, the rectum is pulled forward with a deep pelvic retractor, and the loose areolar tissue between the intact mesorectum and the intact endopelvic fascia is cut with the electrocautery or

Figure 6 **Total proctocolectomy with conventional ileostomy. The ileal mesentery is divided in an L fashion to thin the tissue that will be brought through the abdominal wall.[14] After the ileocolic vessels are divided and ligated, the mesentery is incised toward the bowel about 1 cm away from the vessels to be preserved; this plane is crossed by no important vessels. The mesenteric incision is then extended at a right angle toward the ileocecal area. Transillumination shows the vessels that must be divided so that the edge of the ileum at the cecum can be reached; there are usually two of these.**

with sharp instruments under direct vision. (This dissection is bloodless or nearly so, and it rarely results in injury to the presacral veins.) Posterior dissection is carried down to the surface of the levator muscles. The pelvic peritoneum is incised bilaterally 1 cm or more medial to the ureters, and the two incisions are connected anteriorly. In men, the rectum is separated from the anterior structures posterior to Denonvilliers' fascia; the seminal vesicles and the prostate are separated from the rectum by blunt dissection or electrocauterization. In women, the rec-

tum is separated from the vagina. If no cancer is present, the lateral dissection should be close to the wall of the rectum. The surgeon's left hand retracts the rectum strongly to the left as the right hand dissects the right side of the pelvis, and the assistant provides the same exposure on the left side. The lateral ligaments are divided completely down to the levators. Either electrocauterization or serial ligation is appropriate.

Step 5: Proctectomy (Perineal Phase)

In patients with benign disease, an intersphincteric proctectomy is performed to minimize the risk of autonomic neurologic sequelae [*see Figure 7*]. In some patients with extensive fistulas, this method is not advantageous or even possible, and an extrasphincteric proctectomy must be done.

For an intersphincteric proctectomy, an elliptical incision is made around the anus over the intersphincteric groove, an easily palpable landmark just at the anal verge. Pennington clamps on the skin edges facilitate retraction. The incision is deepened with the electrocautery or with scissors to display the white fibers of the internal sphincter muscle running circumferentially. (The plane between the internal and external sphincters is fairly obvious laterally and posteriorly because the external sphincter is skeletal muscle and therefore reddish.) Circumferential dissection continues proximally as the longitudinal muscle fibers are cut. Posteriorly, the external sphincter and the puborectalis sling are retracted until the pelvic space is entered by incision through Waldeyer's fascia. The specimen is delivered posteriorly, and the remaining anterior attachments are severed.

Step 6: Closure of Perineal Wound

Sump drains are placed into the pelvic space through the buttocks rather than through the perineal wound itself. The levator muscles are approximated with absorbable sutures, and the soft tissues are closed in layers. The skin is closed with a subcuticular suture. (Primary closure should not be attempted in the presence of anorectal abscesses or complex fistulas.) Closure of the pelvic peritoneum is unnecessary if the perineal wound is sutured primarily.

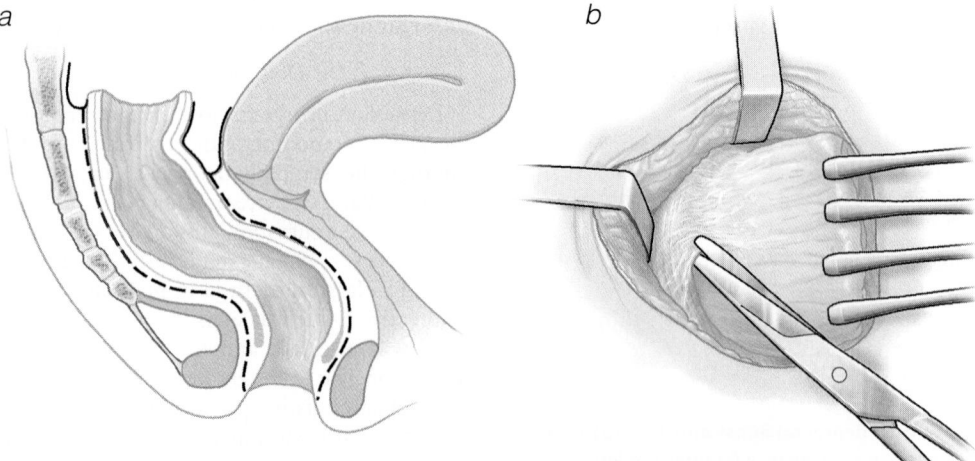

Figure 7 **Total proctocolectomy with conventional ileostomy. The perineal phase usually involves the performance of an intersphincteric proctectomy.[34] (*a*) The pelvic dissection is accomplished from the abdomen, and the perineal dissection preserves the external sphincters and the levators. (*b*) The internal and external sphincters are separated circumferentially by dividing the longitudinal muscle fibers of the gut, which lie in this plane. The specimen is delivered posteriorly (not shown), and the remaining anterior attachments are severed.**

Step 7: Fashioning of Ileostomy

The ileal stump is brought through the aperture so that it projects straight ahead about 5 to 6 cm above the skin.[14] The lateral gutter should be closed to prevent herniation of small bowel around the stoma [*see Figure 8*]. It is unnecessary to suture the bowel to fascia.

A Brooke-type everting ileostomy is fashioned by placing interrupted 4-0 absorbable sutures between the full thickness of the ileal wall and the subcuticular tissue [*see Figure 9*]. One suture in each quadrant also grasps a seromuscular bite of ileum at the skin level. (This facilitates eversion.) The completed stoma should project about 2.5 cm above the skin level. An appliance is placed immediately.

COMPLICATIONS

Early postoperative complications from ileostomy construction include ischemia, paraileostomy abscess, and intestinal obstruction from herniation of small bowel through the gutter.

Perineal wounds may become infected or fail to heal for other reasons. Persistent perineal sinus is a difficult problem that may occur in as many as 50% of patients with Crohn colitis, especially if complex abscesses and fistulas were present at the time of operation.

Postoperative bladder dysfunction is common but is usually transient.

OUTCOME

Operative mortality for proctocolectomy with ileostomy is less than 1% in elective settings; it is higher when the procedure is done on an emergency basis.[8,13] Long-term sequelae include a variety of ileostomy complications, such as retraction, stenosis, prolapse, and paraileostomy hernia. Approximately 90% of patients with a permanent ileostomy are reasonably content, but much depends on the availability of alternatives when the initial operative decision was discussed.[12]

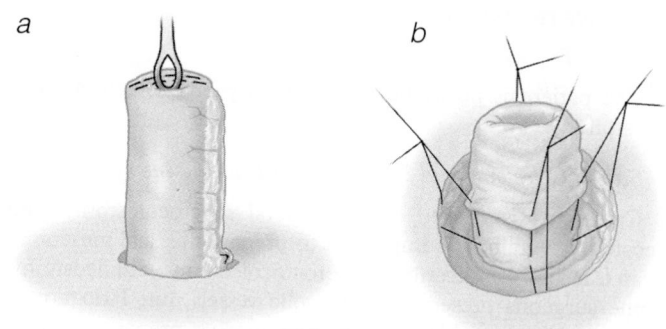

Figure 9 **Total proctocolectomy with conventional ileostomy. A Brooke-type everting ileostomy is fashioned.[14] (*a*) The ileum should project straight ahead for a distance of 5 to 6 cm above the skin. (*b*) One interrupted 4-0 absorbable suture in each quadrant also grasps a seromuscular bite of ileum at the skin level to facilitate eversion. Two additional interrupted sutures (not shown) are placed in each quadrant between the full thickness of the ileal wall and the subcuticular tissue.**

As many as 15% of men who undergo proctocolectomy for benign disease exhibit some postoperative change in sexual function; only about 1% become totally impotent. Some women experience dyspareunia as a result of pelvic fibrosis; others experience sexual dysfunction as a result of altered body image.[15]

Restorative Proctocolectomy with Ileal Pouch–Anal Anastomosis

OPERATIVE PLANNING

Restorative proctocolectomy with ileal pouch–anal anastomosis—complete resection of the colon and rectum and anastomosis of an ileal pouch to the anal canal—is the operation of choice for most patients with ulcerative colitis or familial adenomatous polyposis.[12,15-18] Good anal sphincter function is a requisite. Crohn disease is a contraindication. The operation is difficult but usually possible in obese patients. There is no absolute upper age limit for candidacy for this procedure; however, many elderly, infirm persons may have a better quality of life with an ileostomy. In patients who are acutely ill or malnourished, are receiving huge doses of steroids, or have a significant complication (e.g., perforation), the procedure should be staged.

Whether to perform rectal mucosectomy as part of the procedure is controversial.[19-21] The approach described here involves excising all of the columnar epithelium down to the transitional zone and restoring continuity with a double-stapling technique that renders mucosectomy unnecessary in most patients. The main advantage of this approach is that it minimizes the risk of minor functional impairment resulting from the direct trauma to the sphincters associated with mucosectomy and from the anal dilatation necessary to obtain exposure for mucosectomy. (Insertion of a self-retaining retractor that can be cranked open to improve exposure is risky. Although such devices yield a good view, they can damage the sphincters, often permanently.) The disadvantage of not performing mucosectomy is that one may leave behind some diseased columnar epithelium, which could remain inflamed in patients with ulcerative colitis or become malignant in patients with colitis or polyposis.[21]

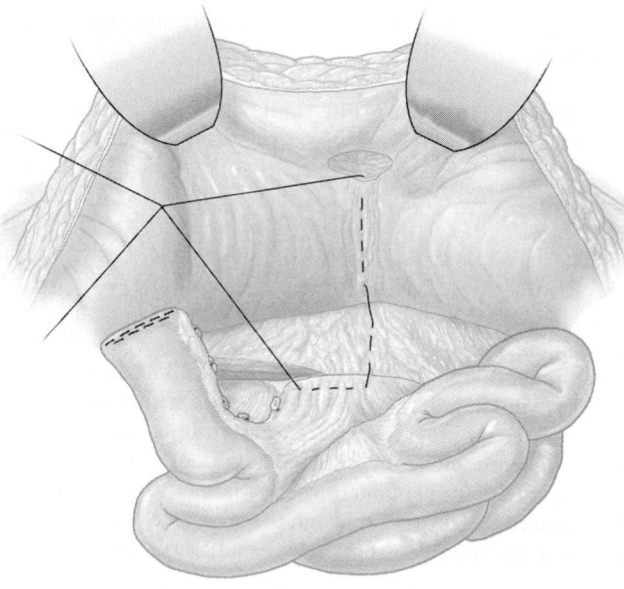

Figure 8 **Total proctocolectomy with conventional ileostomy. One method of closing the gutter uses a purse-string suture passing laterally from the ileostomy aperture to the parietal peritoneum, the retroperitoneal tissue (with care taken to avoid the ureter), and the edge of the mesentery to a point about 8 cm from the ileal stump.[14] The suture is tied and then continued cephalad to the duodenum.**

OPERATIVE TECHNIQUE

Step 1: Positioning

The patient is positioned as for total proctocolectomy with ileostomy.

Step 2: Colectomy and Preparation of Ileal Mesentery

Colectomy is carried out as in total proctocolectomy with ileostomy. (Again, it is important to prepare the ileal mesentery in an L fashion as described for proctocolectomy with ileostomy. Some surgeons preserve the ileocolic vessels, but I do not: if these vessels are divided and the mesentery is prepared properly, the pouch will reach the anus in nearly every instance. It is also important to mobilize the base of the mesocolon and the small bowel mesentery in the hepatic flexure area all the way to the pancreas. Attachments to the duodenum are lysed thoroughly. The peritoneum should be incised on the medial side of the small bowel mesentery all the way up as well.) The ileum is divided with a linear cutting stapler flush with the ileocecal valve.

The ability of the proposed pouch to reach the anus is tested by grasping the ileum about 15 cm proximal to the stapled stump and pulling it to the pubis. If it reaches or extends beyond the lower edge of the pubic bone, there will be no problem; if it does not extend to the lower edge of the pubis, it probably will still reach the anus, but there may be some tension. If additional length is needed, it can be obtained via relaxing incisions through the peritoneum of the mesentery on both sides. (Some surgeons divide mesenteric vessels to gain length, but I have never found this step necessary.) Construction of the pouch is deferred until the colectomy is completed.

Step 3: Proctectomy

The abdominal and pelvic portions of the operation are carried out as described for total proctocolectomy with ileostomy. The rectum is mobilized to the levator muscles circumferentially, but one does not stop at this point: the bowel is dissected from the enveloping puborectal muscles posteriorly and laterally and from urogenital structures anteriorly. (This portion of the large bowel is actually the anal canal. It is lined by columnar epithelium in the upper 1 cm and by transitional epithelium in the lower 1 cm down to the dentate line, though there is anatomic variation in this regard. The pelvic staple line should be in the anal canal rather than the rectum so that diseased mucosa will not be left behind. The surgeon can judge the adequacy of distal mobilization by inserting a finger into the anus from the perineum with the other hand in the pelvis. It is possible to mobilize all the way to the dentate line in most persons, but the intent is to staple across the anal canal 1.0 to 1.5 cm proximal to the dentate line. The end-to-end stapler removes another 1 cm. An assistant can apply pressure to the perineum with a fist, but this is seldom necessary.)

The anal canal is closed off with a right-angle stapler. (I use a 30 mm stapler. If a 30 mm device is too small to close the anal canal across its entire width, one may be certain that mobilization has not been carried far enough distally. The stapler must be aligned so that the distance above the anal verge is uniform.) A crushing intestinal clamp is applied above the stapler, and the bowel is divided and removed. When the stapler is detached, the stump of the anal canal slips within the puborectal muscle.

Step 4: Construction of Ileal Pouch

A J pouch is constructed by approximating two 15 cm limbs measured proximally from the closed end of the ileum [see Figure 10]. (The J pouch and the W pouch are favored over other types that once were more popular.[17,19,20,22,23] Of the two, I prefer the J pouch because it functions as well as the W pouch and is simpler to construct.) Three or four sutures are placed to align the limbs for side-to-side stapling. A divot is excised from the apex of the J with scissors, and an 80 mm linear cutting stapler is inserted with the anvil in one limb and the cartridge in the other. The stapler is fired and reloaded, and the bowel is bunched up in an accordionlike manner for the second firing. Two applications of the stapler are sufficient to construct a pouch 15 cm long.

A 2-0 polypropylene purse-string suture is placed on the cut edge of the apex of the J pouch, and the anvil of an end-to-end stapler is inserted and secured as the purse-string suture is tied. (I prefer to use the largest stapler available—31 or 33 mm—in the hope that all of the staple line on the anal canal stump will thereby be excised to minimize the possibility of leaving an ischemic corner.)

Step 5: Ileoanal Anastomosis

The end-to-end stapler is inserted into the anus with the spike withdrawn into the cartridge. (It is helpful to insert a sequence of progressively larger stapler sizers into the anus to ensure that the anus can accommodate the stapler and also to show the anal canal stump from the pelvic side. At this point, one must be certain that there is adequate separation from surrounding structures, especially the vagina. I find it essential to insert the stapler into the anus with both hands and then to manipulate it into place with the left hand while palpating the anal canal stump with the right hand in the pelvis. The contamination from this maneuver is a small price to pay for the assurance that the stapler is resting firmly against the stump of the anal canal circumferentially. The entire head of the stapler does not slip into the anal canal above the sphincters, as is normally the case in colorectal anastomoses; instead, the stapler rests within the anal sphincters because the anastomosis is so low. If the stapler is not properly positioned, staples may be fired through empty space rather than through tissue.)

The stapler is opened, and the spike is allowed to penetrate the anal stump adjacent to the staple line. The cut edge of the small bowel mesentery is placed toward the patient's right, and a quick check is done to make sure that the pouch has not been rotated 360°. The stapler is then closed and fired. (Before the stapler is closed, one should be sure that the vagina is adequately cleared away and thus will not be caught in the anastomosis. As the stapler is closed, there is inevitably some rotation of the pouch and its mesentery, but this does not seem to cause any problem.)

Two intact doughnuts should be obtained. The anastomosis is tested by palpation and by direct inspection with a rigid sigmoidoscope inserted into the anus. A noncrushing clamp is placed across the ileum above the pouch, and a pool of saline is placed in the pelvis. Air is insufflated to test for leaks. Leaks can usually be repaired by suturing through the anus (see below). In some patients, a diverting ileostomy may be advisable (see below).

Step 6: Optional Steps

Placement of transanal purse-string suture If, for some reason, one cannot use the stapler or if there has been a mishap in the course of the operation (e.g., entry into the lumen), the procedure can be salvaged by transanal placement of a purse-string suture. (This step can be difficult for surgeons who lack experience with the technique. Exposure is limited, and bleeding can obscure the view. A headlight is essential. Separate instruments should be available for the perineal operator.)

Two Gelpi retractors are placed to evert the anus, and a Hill-Ferguson retractor is inserted to expose the anoderm and the epithelium of the anal canal above the dentate line. The full thickness of the wall of the anal canal is incised with a curved scissors in the posterior midline about 1 cm above the dentate line. This incision should provide entry into the pelvic dissection space if the earlier dissection was extended low enough. The entire circumference of the anal canal is divided, and the purse-string suture is placed through the full thickness of the bowel. (I prefer to start this suture in the posterior midline so that it will be easier to tie with the stapler in place. A curved

Figure 10 **Restorative proctocolectomy with ileoanal pouch. Shown is the construction of a J pouch. Two 15 cm limbs, measured proximally from the closed end of the ileum, are aligned; sutures (not shown) may help hold the alignment for stapling. A divot is excised from the apex of the J with scissors. An 80 mm linear cutting stapler is inserted through the resulting opening with the anvil in one limb and the cartridge in the other. Two applications of the stapler are sufficient to construct a 15 cm pouch.**

needle holder is helpful.) The Hill-Ferguson retractor is moved to bring successive portions of the circumference into view. The stapler is inserted and opened, and the shaft is reattached. The distal purse-string suture is tied. The stapler is then closed and fired. (This method is more likely to yield incomplete distal doughnuts.)

Construction of diverting ileostomy If there is concern about anastomotic integrity or the patient's healing capacity, a diverting ileostomy should be constructed. (Diverting loop ileostomy was once routine for all restorative proctocolectomy patients, but I no longer do it in low-risk patients whose anastomosis looks satisfactory and does not leak on testing.[24]) If an ileostomy is constructed, it can be taken down in about 2 months.

Step 7: Completion

Drains are inserted into the pelvis from the abdominal side. The edge of the small bowel mesentery is sutured to the retroperitoneum down to the pelvic brim; it is usually impossible to complete this closure.

COMPLICATIONS

The main complications of this procedure are abscess, anastomotic leakage, and so-called pouchitis. Most abscesses are related to minor anastomotic leaks that are contained in a small area; they tend to be small and easily drained. Large anastomotic or pelvic abscesses or fistulas are uncommon; they may result in failure of the procedure if corrective steps cannot salvage the pouch. So-called cuff abscesses are a complication of mucosectomy in which infected fluid accumulates in the space between the denuded rectal muscle tube and the ileal pouch.

Anastomotic leaks are usually masked by the presence of a diverting ileostomy. They may be revealed by imaging studies before the ileostomy is taken down, or they may remain undetected until the fecal stream is reestablished. If a diverting ileostomy is not performed, leaks become clinically evident in the first few postoperative days. If leakage is significant, laparotomy with ileostomy is the only recourse; however, leakage of this severity is uncommon.[24]

Pouchitis is a late postoperative complication that presumably is related to bacterial overgrowth in the stagnant pouch contents. It is rare in patients with familial adenomatous polyposis and consequently is believed to be related in some way to inflammatory bowel disease.[25] Perhaps 25% of patients with an ileoanal pouch experience pouchitis at some point. The typical manifestations are cramps and diarrhea (sometimes bloody); occasionally, there are systemic symptoms (e.g., fever or arthralgia). The pouch appears inflamed on endoscopy, but this finding is deceptive because some asymptomatic pouches appear red and friable also. Treatment with antibiotics (e.g., metronidazole or a cephalosporin) is usually successful. In a few patients, medical management fails and the pouch must be excised.

OUTCOME

The average patient has about five stools a day after restorative proctocolectomy, but stool frequency may range from two to 10 a day without complications.[15,17-19,22,23] Minor seepage is common in the first weeks after operation, but significant fecal incontinence is uncommon. With the techniques currently in use, infection, pouchitis, incontinence, and other problems lead to failure in about 5% of patients.[20,24]

Low Anterior Resection with Coloproctostomy

OPERATIVE PLANNING

Tumor Assessment

Anterior resection is the procedure of choice for most cancers in or above the midrectum. The goal is to excise the portion of the rectum that contains the tumor and to remove the entire mesorectum as well as pararectal tissue containing lymphatic vessels and lymph nodes. Good technique is critical for minimizing the likelihood of recurrence in the pelvis.[26]

Tumor Assessment

Resection and anastomosis are anatomically impossible when the distal edge of the cancer is lower than about 4 cm above the anal verge (2 cm above the dentate line). In practice, many midrectal cancers that are large, deeply invasive, or poorly differentiated cannot be dealt with by anterior resection either. If the tumor can be moved at all before dissection is begun, it can usually be excised; however, fixity on digital palpation is not a reliable sign that the tumor is unresectable. Computed tomography, magnetic resonance imaging, and endorectal ultrasonography may be helpful. The patient's body habitus and preferences should be taken into account. Sometimes, the final decision regarding sphincter preservation can be made only during the operation. Occasionally, the potential for anastomosis cannot be assessed until the rectum has been mobilized. Extension into the urogenital structures may be apparent, and it should be possible to determine whether the anterior structures (the uterus or the vagina in particular) must be resected en bloc to effect cure.

Excision of the primary tumor is the most effective way of palliating rectal adenocarcinoma. Prevention or relief of tenesmus is a goal worth pursuing, even in patients with distant metastases. Tenesmus is not relieved by fecal diversion, nor is it reliably eliminated by radiation therapy or other forms of local treatment.

OPERATIVE TECHNIQUE

Step 1: Positioning

The patient should be placed in the lithotomy position in Lloyd-Davies leg rests or Allen universal stirrups. Rectal examination is performed to confirm the preoperative assessment of the tumor, and the rectum is irrigated with saline to eliminate any residual stool.

Step 2: Mobilization of Sigmoid and Mesosigmoid

The distal sigmoid is occluded with an encircling umbilical tape to prevent movement of luminal contents from the proximal colon into the rectum and intraluminal migration of malignant cells from the primary rectal cancer into the portion of colon to be retained.

The sigmoid colon and the mesocolon are dissected away from peritoneal attachments, and the left base of the mesosigmoid is incised medial to the ureter as described for total colectomy with ileoanal anastomosis. The splenic flexure is taken down partially or completely, with the redundancy of the sigmoid and the level of the tumor kept in mind. The peritoneum at the base of the mesosigmoid on the right is incised, and the incision is continued cephalad toward the duodenum for a variable distance, depending on the planned level of vessel ligation. (Care should be taken not to injure the preaortic sympathetic nerves during this step. In addition, it is vital that the colon be mobilized in such a way that the proximal end of the bowel will reach the rectal stump with no tension. There must be no compromise on this point.)

Step 3: Ligation of Vessels

There is some controversy regarding the level at which vessels should be ligated during curative resection of rectal cancer. Some surgeons ligate just below the origin of the left colic artery; others ligate at the origin of the inferior mesenteric artery to remove the few nodes that remain with ligation more distally. The data consistently indicate, however, that the level of ligation does not influence survival rates. Today, most surgeons ligate the inferior mesenteric vessels just distal to the origin of the left colic artery.[27]

The mesocolon is divided radially to the point at which the surgeon plans to transect the colon. The colon may be transected either at this time or after the pelvic dissection has been completed.

Step 4: Pelvic Dissection

Dissection is carried out under direct vision.[26] In men, the anterior plane of dissection is anterior to Denonvilliers' fascia if the cancer is nearby; if the lesion is more proximal, dissection can be posterior to Denonvilliers' fascia. In women, the rectum is separated from the vagina, but if there is an anterior lesion invading the vagina, the posterior vaginal wall must be excised. It may be possible to restore colorectal continuity in this situation; however, adjacent suture lines should be avoided, and abdominoperineal resection (see below) may be safer.

The aim of lateral dissection is to leave the pelvis devoid of lateral soft tissue. (To this end, one should remove all of the node-bearing tissue all the way to the pelvic sidewall but not external to the parietal pelvic fascia. One can ligate the middle hemorrhoidal vessels close to the pelvic sidewall and still achieve complete extirpation of soft tissues if this maneuver is conducted under direct vision.) The lateral ligaments are completely divided down to the levator muscles, with the bilobed so-called lipoma of the mesorectum left intact.

Step 5: Removal of Mesorectum

If the tumor is in the midrectum (especially if it is in the distal portion), one should excise the entire mesorectum rather than dissect through it to reach the rectal wall. This approach is referred to as total mesorectal excision.[28] (Residual tumor in the mesorectum is an important cause of local recurrence.) At the levator muscles, the rectal lumen is small, no more than 2.5 to 3.0 cm in diameter; above that point, the rectal lumen enlarges substantially.

Step 6: Anastomosis

Colorectal anastomosis The anastomosis may be done either by hand suturing or by stapling. (Because hand suturing a low anastomosis is tedious, I prefer either the double-staple technique or an open stapled approach.)

In a double-stapled coloproctostomy, the lumen above the planned line of transection is occluded with a right-angled crushing bowel clamp. The distal anorectum is irrigated transanally with dilute povidone-iodine to destroy malignant cells. A 30 mm right-angle stapler (or a device of comparable size) is positioned and fired. (If dissection of the mesorectum is incomplete or if all of the pararectal tissue has not been divided, the 30 mm stapler will not close off the entire rectal stump. One can usually tell when this problem is likely to arise, because the tissue grasped by the stapler will feel unusually bulky. The solution is to remove the stapler without firing it and then to dissect more completely.) The rectum is divided sharply between the stapler and the crushing clamp. A purse-string suture is applied to the colonic stump proximally, and an intraluminal or end-to-end stapler is inserted through the anus. (With a large stapler—31 or 33 mm—one can usually excise the entire original rectal staple line.)

Alternatively, a purse-string suture can be placed distally by hand. (If the rectum is transected deeply in the pelvis, currently available mechanical purse-string appliers do not work well.) The rectum is occluded with a clamp proximal to the proposed site of transection, and the distal portion is irrigated as described for double stapling. The proximal clamp is placed immediately above the planned site of transection so that the bowel can be divided on the distal side flush with the clamp. A beaver blade scalpel with a long handle is used to incise into the rectal lumen in the center, and placement of the purse-string suture is begun with only a portion of the lumen open. (If the rectum is completely divided before the suture is begun, the stump will retract and the mucosa will pout, making the task of suturing unnecessarily difficult.) The rectal transection is completed gradually as the suture is continued.

The anastomosis is tested by digital rectal examination and inspection through a rigid sigmoidoscope as described for ileoanal anastomosis. Drains are placed through a stab wound in the left lower quadrant.

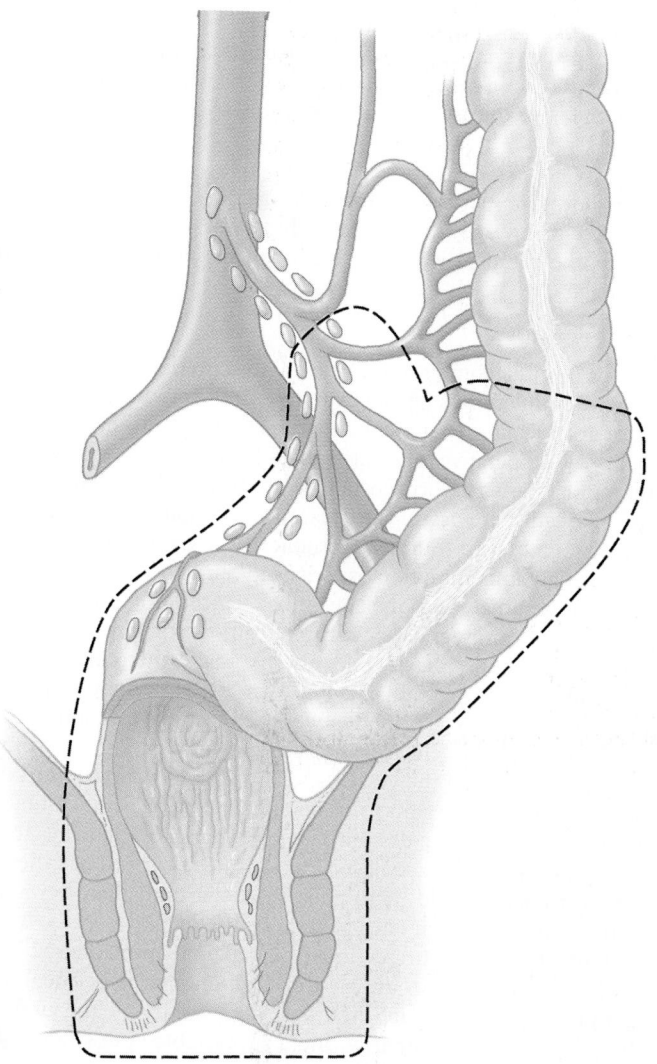

Figure 11 **Abdominoperineal resection. The extent of the resection is outlined.**[35]

Coloanal anastomosis   When a tumor lies in the distal portion of the midrectum but is still high enough for a margin to be obtainable, one may avoid abdominoperineal resection (APR) by performing a coloanal anastomosis. (Coloanal anastomosis is contraindicated in patients with impaired sphincters and persons with infirmities that prevent ready access to bathroom facilities.[29]) Usually, the final decision is made during the operation. This procedure can be performed by means of the double-staple technique or by placing a purse-string suture transanally. Dissection within the levator muscles and the stapling procedure itself are performed as described for restorative proctocolectomy. Postoperative function may be improved by constructing a colonic J pouch and anastomosing the pouch to the anal canal.[30]

COMPLICATIONS

The incidence of clinically significant anastomotic leakage is about 4%.[27] This complication is more common after colorectal anastomoses than after colonic anastomoses, in part because the rectum is devoid of serosa. Tension on the anastomosis is an important—and avoidable—precipitating factor. Infected pelvic fluid can erupt into the lumen and create a leak.

Anastomotic stricture is usually the consequence of a leak, but membranous stenosis can develop in stapled anastomoses. This is rarely a significant problem if large-caliber staplers are used. Digital or sigmoidoscopic stretching of a membranous stenosis usually solves the problem permanently.

OUTCOME

Long-term survival of cancer patients after low anterior resection depends on the tumor stage; it should be no different from survival after APR if patients are selected properly.[31]

The results of very low colorectal or coloanal anastomoses are sometimes functionally unsatisfactory. Mucous leakage is not uncommon. Bowel habits are unpredictable, and patients may experience irregularity and urgency.

Abdominoperineal Resection

OPERATIVE PLANNING

Abdominoperineal resection is the standard procedure for cancers of the distal rectum that are too low to permit preservation of the sphincter [*see Figure 11*].[31,32] Whether APR is appropriate in a given setting depends on the characteristics of the tumor and the general condition of the patient. The tumor is assessed as described for low anterior resection. Ascites is a strong contraindication to APR because ascitic leak through the perineal wound may be troublesome or even fatal if it leads to peritonitis. Palliative APR is worthwhile in many instances.

A colostomy site is selected, and the educational process is begun preoperatively.

OPERATIVE TECHNIQUE

Step 1: Positioning

How the patient is positioned depends on whether APR is to be done in separate stages by a single team or synchronously by two teams. (The synchronous technique is more efficient, but a second experienced surgeon is needed to perform the perineal dissection.) If the two-stage approach is selected, the patient is supine for the abdominal phase and in the lithotomy position or the left lateral decubitus position for the perineal phase. The lateral decubitus position is more cumbersome because the patient must be turned, but it provides superb exposure of the anterior structures. In a difficult patient with an extensive tumor on the anterior wall, the lateral decubitus position is recommended. If the synchronous approach is selected, the patient is in the lithotomy position. If it is certain that APR will be done, the anus is closed with a purse-string suture of heavy material; two sutures should be placed, one within the other. (If there is no doubt about the need for a colostomy, the colostomy aperture is made before the main abdominal incision, as described for total proctocolectomy with ileostomy.)

Step 2: Pelvic Dissection

It is unnecessary to take down the splenic flexure. In men, the anterior pelvic dissection plane is anterior to Denonvilliers' fascia. In women with anterior rectal cancer, the posterior vaginal wall is included with the specimen [see Figure 12]. Hysterectomy is usually advisable in this situation.

Step 3: Management of Pelvic Peritoneal Floor

If the operation is done in separate phases, the sigmoid is divided at this point, and the distal stump is covered with a rubber glove secured with an umbilical tape. The specimen is placed in the pelvis, and the pelvic peritoneum is closed. (If the entire specimen does not fit into the pelvic space, the bowel must be divided again, but this must not be done too close to the tumor.) If the synchronous approach is used, the specimen is passed through the posterior aspect of the perineal wound to the perineal operator. (Some surgeons do not close the pelvic peritoneum routinely; in a few patients, it is impossible to close this layer because of previous pelvic surgery or irradiation. With the pelvic peritoneal floor open, the small bowel falls into the pelvis, but this occurrence probably does not increase the incidence of intestinal obstruction. If postoperative radiation therapy is likely, the pelvic peritoneal floor should be closed, and if there is insufficient peritoneum for this purpose, either omentum or polyglycolate mesh can be used to create a floor.)

Step 4: Colostomy

A conventional sigmoid colostomy is made by bringing the colon straight through the rectus muscle. Once this is done, a space is left lateral to the colon through which small bowel can herniate and become obstructed; this space should be closed. Alternatively, the colostomy can be placed extraperitoneally; however, few surgeons favor this approach, because the advantages of extraperitoneal colostomy do not seem to justify the additional time and effort.

Although protrusion above the skin level is essential for an ileostomy, it is not necessary with a colostomy.

Step 5: Perineal Dissection (Perineal Phase)

An elliptical incision encompassing the anus is made with a scalpel or the electrocautery. The incision is extended through the ischiorectal fat in such a way that much—but not all—of this tissue is included with the specimen. Large rake retractors are used to expose the levator muscles.

The anococcygeal raphe is incised just anterior to the coccyx. (Amputation of the coccyx is unnecessary in routine cases.) With the anus retracted forward, the white Waldeyer's fascia is exposed and incised transversely. The pelvic dissection space is thus entered. The surgeon can insert one or two fingers to locate the levator muscles for division with the electrocautery. (Inadequate levator excision seldom leads to local or regional recurrence; unless the tumor is deeply invasive at this level, a

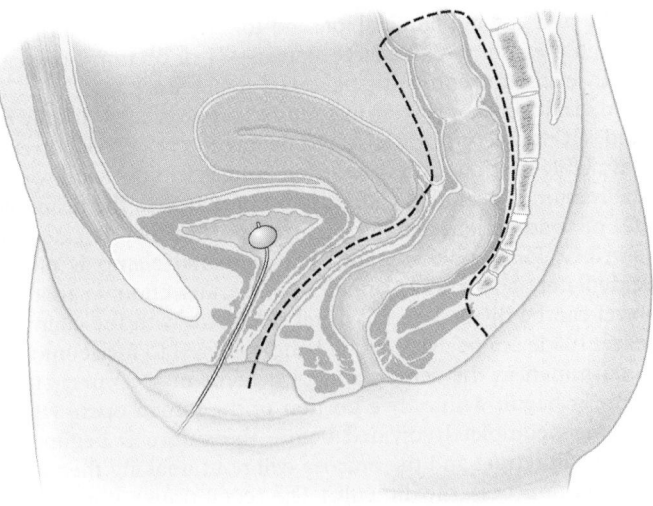

Figure 12 Abdominoperineal resection. In women with anterior rectal cancer, the posterior vaginal wall is included with the specimen.[35] Hysterectomy (not shown) is often done as well.

margin of iliococcygeal muscle can be left laterally to facilitate closure of the perineal wound.)

When the levator muscles have been divided, the specimen is delivered through the posterior part of the perineal wound, with only the anterior attachments left to be severed.

Step 6: Closure of Perineal Wound

If the pelvic peritoneal floor is closed, the perineal wound is sutured in layers with drainage. If bacterial contamination is heavy, the perineal wound is left open or partially closed with drainage.

COMPLICATIONS

The overall complication rate in this predominantly elderly patient population is 35%, but most of the complications—such as atelectasis and postoperative urinary retention—are relatively minor.[31,32] Operative mortality ranges from 0% to 7%; most contemporary series report mortalities of 2% to 3%.[31,32] The majority of deaths are from cardiovascular complications and pulmonary embolism. Surgical complications leading to death are increasingly uncommon in experienced hands.

Intraoperative hemorrhage most commonly arises from injury to the presacral veins. Bulky tumors, previous radiation therapy, a narrow pelvis, and obesity make this complication more likely. If presacral veins are torn, bleeding may stop with pressure. If pressure is ineffective, the bleeding can sometimes be controlled by electrocauterization or ligation with fine sutures; however, if the vessel is torn where it emerges from the bone, these measures may not be effective. (Special metal tacks are manufactured for the purpose of controlling bleeding from these vessels, but I have never found it necessary to use them.) The last resort would be to pack the pelvis and then to return to the operating room later to remove the pack.

Injury to the left ureter must be repaired immediately. The urethra is vulnerable to injury during the anterior perineal dissection; fortunately, such injury is rare. Injury to the urethra should be repaired primarily, and a suprapubic cystostomy tube should be placed.

The rectum can be torn during the posterior pelvic dissection or during the perineal phase. The greatest concern is contamination of the field by malignant cells; bacterial contamination is also problematic but is less worrisome. In the event of entry into the rectal lumen, the field should be irrigated thoroughly with water, a tumoricidal agent (e.g., dilute povidone-iodine), or both.

Colostomy complications include necrosis, retraction, and paracolostomy abscess.

Perineal wound complications occur in about 15% of patients who undergo APR for rectal cancer; the most common such complication is persistent perineal sinus.[23] Perineal hernia is uncommon after APR but is more likely to occur if the levator muscles are excised widely.

OUTCOME

Late colostomy complications are mainly limited to paracolostomy hernia. Prolapse is an uncommon complication of a sigmoid colostomy.

Sexual dysfunction in men after APR is usually neurogenic, but advanced age and psychological factors may play a role as well. Total impotence occurs in 5% to 40% of men after APR.[32] Sexual dysfunction in women may result from psychological problems related to altered body image. Dyspareunia, presumably arising from pelvic fibrosis, is reported by as many as 50% of women after APR.

References

1. Andriesse GI, Gooszen HG, Schipper ME, et al: Functional results and visceral perception after ileo neo-rectal anastomosis in patients: a pilot study. Gut 48:683, 2001

2. Eu KW, Lim SL, Seow-Choen F, et al: Clinical outcome and bowel function following total abdominal colectomy and ileorectal anastomosis in the Oriental population. Dis Colon Rectum 41:215, 1998

3. Mollen RM, Kuijpers HC, Claassen AT: Colectomy for slow-transit constipation: preoperative functional evaluation is important but not a guarantee for a successful outcome. Dis Colon Rectum 44:577, 2001

4. Pastore RL, Wolff BG, Hodge D: Total abdominal colectomy and ileorectal anastomosis for inflammatory bowel disease. Dis Colon Rectum 40:1455, 1997

5. van Duijvendijk P, Slors JFM, Taat CW, et al: Functional outcome after colectomy and ileorectal anastomosis compared with proctocolectomy and ileal pouch-anal anastomosis in familial adenomatous polyposis. Ann Surg 230:648, 1999

6. Milsom JW, Ludwig KA, Church JM, et al: Laparoscopic total abdominal colectomy with ileorectal anastomosis for familial adenomatous polyposis. Dis Colon Rectum 40:675, 1997

7. Nakamura T, Pikarsky AJ, Potenti FM, et al: Are complications of subtotal colectomy with ileorectal anastomosis related to the original disease? Am Surg 67:417, 2001

8. Ko CY, Rusing LC, Schoetz DJ, et al: Does better functional result equate with better quality of life? Implications for surgical treatment in familial adenomatous polyposis. Dis Colon Rectum 43:829, 2000

9. Soravia C, Klein L, Berk T, et al: Comparison of ileal pouch-anal anastomosis and ileorectal anastomosis in patients with familial adenomatous polyposis. Dis Colon Rectum 42:1028, 1999

10. Bernell O, Lapidus A, Hellers G: Recurrence after colectomy in Crohn's colitis. Dis Colon Rectum 44:647, 2001

11. Hulten L: Proctocolectomy and ileostomy to pouch surgery for ulcerative colitis. World J Surg 22:335, 1998

12. Vasen HF, van Duijvendijk P, Buskens E, et al: Decision analysis in the surgical treatment of patients with familial adenomatous polyposis: a Dutch-Scandinavian collaborative study including 659 patients. Gut 49:231, 2001

13. Yamamoto T, Keighley MR: Proctocolectomy is associated with a higher complication rate but carries a lower recurrence rate than total colectomy and ileorectal anastomosis in Crohn colitis. Scand J Gastroenterol 34:1212, 1999

14. Schrock TR: Ileostomy and colostomy. Gastrointestinal Surgery. Fromm D, Ed. Churchill Livingstone, New York, 1985

15. McLeod RS, Baxter NN: Quality of life of patients with inflammatory bowel disease after surgery. World J Surg 22:375, 1998

16. Gorfine SR, Bauer JJ, Harris MT, et al: Dysplasia complicating chronic ulcerative colitis: is immediate colectomy warranted? Dis Colon Rectum 43:1575, 2000

17. Parc YR, Moslein G, Dozois RR, et al: Familial adenomatous polyposis: results after ileal pouch-anal anastomosis in teenagers. Dis Colon Rectum 43:893, 2000

18. Takao Y, Gilliland R, Nogueras JJ, et al: Is age relevant to functional outcome after restorative proctocolectomy for ulcerative colitis? Prospective assessment of 122 cases. Ann Surg 227:187, 1998

19. Karlbom U, Raab Y, Ejerblad S, et al: Factors influencing the functional outcome of restorative proctocolectomy in ulcerative colitis. Br J Surg 87:1401, 2000

20. Regimbeau JM, Panis Y, Pocard M, et al: Handsewn ileal pouch-anal anastomosis on the dentate line after total proctectomy: technique to avoid incomplete mucosectomy and the need for long-term follow-up of the anal transition zone. Dis Colon Rectum 44:43, 2001

21. O'Riordain MG, Fazio VW, Lavery IC, et al: Incidence and natural history of dysplasia of the anal transitional zone after ileal pouch-anal anastomosis: results of a five-year to ten-year follow-up. Dis Colon Rectum 43:1660, 2000

22. Farouk R, Pemberton JH, Wolff BG, et al: Functional outcomes after ileal pouch-anal anastomosis for chronic ulcerative colitis. Ann Surg 231:919, 2000

23. O'Bichere A, Wilkinson K, Rumbles S, et al: Functional outcome after restorative panproctocolectomy for ulcerative colitis decreases an otherwise enhanced quality of life. Br J Surg 87:802, 2000

24. Sugerman HJ, Sugerman EL, Meador JG, et al: Ileal pouch anal anastomosis without ileal diversion. Ann Surg 232:530, 2000

25. Simchuk EJ, Thirlby RC: Risk factors and true incidence of pouchitis in patients after ileal pouch-anal anastomosis. World J Surg 24:851, 2000

26. Polglase AL, McMurrick PJ, Tremayne AB, et al: Local recurrence after curative anterior resection with principally blunt dissection for carcinoma of the rectum and rectosigmoid. Dis Colon Rectum 44:947, 2001

27. Enker WE, Merchant N, Cohen AM, et al: Safety and efficacy of low anterior resection for rectal cancer: consecutive cases from a specialty service. Ann Surg 230:544, 1999

28. Kapiteijn E, Kranenbarg EK, Steup WH, et al: Total mesorectal excision (TME) with or without preoperative radiotherapy in the treatment of primary rectal cancer: prospective randomised trial with standard operative and histopathologic techniques. Dutch ColoRectal Cancer Group. Eur J Surg 165:410, 1999

29. Di Matteo G, Mascagni D, Keri KP, et al: Evaluation of anal function after surgery for rectal cancer. J Surg Oncol 74:11, 2000

30. Lazorthes F, Chiotasso P, Gamagami RA, et al: Late clinical outcome in a randomized prospective comparison of colonic J pouch and straight coloanal anastomosis. Br J Surg 84:1449, 1997

31. Ferulano GP, Dilillo S, La Manna S, et al: Influence of the surgical treatment on local recurrence of rectal cancer: a prospective study (1980–1992). J Surg Oncol 74:153, 2000

32. Enker WE, Havenga K, Polyak T, et al: Abdominoperineal resection via total mesorectal excision and autonomic nerve preservation for low rectal cancer. World J Surg 21:715, 1997

33. Schrock TR: Total colectomy and ileoanal anastomosis. Mastery of Surgery, 3rd ed. Nyhus LM, Baker RJ, Fischer JE, Eds. Little, Brown & Co, Boston, 1997

34. Schrock TR: Inflammatory disease of the colon and rectum. Gastrointestinal Surgery. Fromm D, Ed. Churchill Livingstone, New York, 1985

35. Schrock TR: Abdominoperineal resection—technique and complications. Cancer of the Colon, Rectum, and Anus. Cohen AM, Winawer SJ, Eds. McGraw-Hill, New York, 1995, p 595

Acknowledgment

Figures 1 through 12   Tom Moore.

18 LAPAROSCOPIC COLECTOMY

Babak N. Rad, M.D., and Robert W. Beart, Jr., M.D.

The growing emphasis on minimally invasive approaches in modern surgery has forced surgeons to reevaluate traditional approaches to proven procedures. Laparoscopic cholecystectomy, laparoscopic appendectomy, and laparoscopic inguinal and incisional herniorrhaphy all have proved to be viable alternatives to their open counterparts.[1] Their success has led to the application of laparoscopy to bowel surgery in an effort to reduce the morbidity associated with conventional open colon resections. There is now considerable published evidence indicating that laparoscopic colectomy is both safe and effective and has certain advantages over open techniques—namely, decreased operative morbidity, decreased pain, shorter length of stay, more rapid return to work, and improved cosmesis.[1-3]

Laparoscopic bowel surgery does require that surgeons acquire a new set of skills. Thus, it should not be surprising that the natural human tendency to resist change has, to date, limited its utilization. If, however, encouraging recent study findings are confirmed by trials now under way, it is likely that laparoscopic colectomy will become the treatment of choice in the future.

Indications

Accepted indications for laparoscopic colectomy include most of the benign colonic diseases (e.g., colorectal polyps, rectal prolapse, diverticular disease, inflammatory bowel disease, intestinal stomas for diversion, cecal or sigmoid volvulus, and symptomatic colonic lipomas).[2] The role of laparoscopic bowel resection in the management of malignant colonic disease, however, remains controversial. Specifically, there are questions about the incidence of port-site recurrence and about long-term survival rates that have not yet been answered.[3-6] These questions have provided the impetus for a number of prospective, randomized studies in several countries. Currently, at least seven such trials are under way, most of which are being conducted at multiple centers. Results from these studies should be forthcoming in the next few years.

Operative Planning

No patient should undergo laparoscopic bowel surgery without a defined diagnosis. Colonoscopy, barium enemas, and computed tomography are all potentially useful in determining the diagnosis before operation; the choice of diagnostic modality should be governed by the patient's initial presenting signs and symptoms. The distance from the tumor to the anal verge is readily measured in the course of colonoscopy, but such measurement does not always result in accurate identification of the corresponding segment of diseased bowel intraoperatively. Furthermore, with the exception of the ileocecal valve (which remains a constant and easily identifiable landmark), the general shape and curves of the colon are indistinct. Therefore, it is recommended that India ink tattooing be used to mark lesions located in segments of the bowel outside the area of the ileocecal valve, thereby facilitating intraoperative localization of the tumor.

Patients who have a history of severe cardiopulmonary disease, hepatic disease, coagulopathy, significant respiratory compromise, or a complex colonic disorder (e.g., obstruction, contained perforation, or colovesical fistula) should not be considered for laparoscopic colectomy, nor should patients who are known to have extensive intra-abdominal adhesions. Patients who have tumors larger than 8 to 10 cm in diameter are also unsuitable candidates for laparoscopic colectomy. Larger specimens inevitably require larger incisions for removal; accordingly, patients with large tumors would benefit from having an appropriately sized incision in place from the beginning of the operation.

Before operation, the surgeon must recognize that the laparoscopic colectomy may have to be converted to an open procedure, and he or she must discuss this possibility with the patient. Standard bowel preparation is provided. An epidural catheter is placed to facilitate postoperative pain control, which is an important consideration for the first 2 days after laparoscopic bowel surgery.

Operative Technique

RIGHT HEMICOLECTOMY

Step 1: Positioning of Patient and Operative Team

The patient is initially placed supine on the operating table. Because the position of the patient is changed several times during the operation, some form of restraining device should be employed to minimize the possibility of a fall; we favor the use of a beanbag that is secured to the table. Pneumatic compression stockings are placed on the patient to minimize the risk of deep vein thrombosis. After induction of general anesthesia, a nasogastric tube and a Foley catheter are placed to decompress the bladder and the stomach so that these organs will not be perforated when the trocars are inserted. The abdomen is then prepared and draped in the usual fashion.

The surgeon and the camera operator stand to the left of the patient, the assistant surgeon and the nurse to the right. The monitors are placed on either side of the patient, adjacent to the shoulders. With this configuration, all members of the operative team can easily view the operative field [*see Figure 1*].

Step 2: Placement of Trocars

We use a standardized trocar placement for all colectomies [*see Figure 2*]. A 12 mm Hasson trocar is inserted through the rectus muscle and into the abdominal cavity via a small left upper quadrant incision placed 3 to 4 cm below the costal margin. The trocar is secured with sutures, and the abdomen is insufflated with CO_2 to achieve pneumoperitoneum. We use a pressure of 10 to 12 mm Hg to minimize the risk of pneumatosis, which can involve the entire body (presumably as a result of dissection through the extraperitoneal tissue planes, which are opened during the operation). After a complete survey of the peritoneal cavity, including the liver, three

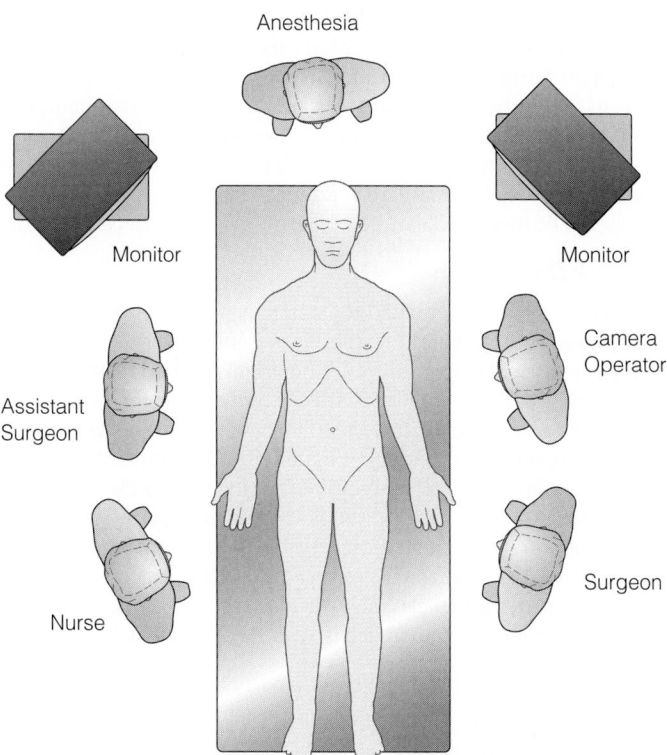

Figure 1 **Laparoscopic colectomy: right hemicolectomy. Shown is the recommended positioning of the operating team.**

additional ports are inserted under direct vision. A 10/12 mm port is placed at the suprapubic location. (Here and at the first site, we recommend the use of 10/12 mm ports to minimize the risk of postoperative port-site herniation.) Two 5 mm ports are placed at sites where stomas could be placed in a conventional procedure. We tend to use a 0° scope for viewing the pelvis, but many surgeons prefer a 30° angled scope. Attempts should be made to close all 10/12 mm ports at the end of the operation.

Step 3: Mobilization of Ascending Colon

The patient is placed in the Trendelenburg position, maximally rotated to the left. This positioning causes the small bowel to fall away from the right colon and allows visualization of the colonic mesentery. Dissecting scissors are inserted through the suprapubic port, and a grasper is inserted through the 5 mm port in the left lower quadrant. The surgeon, standing on the patient's left, operates these two instruments using a two-handed technique. The assistant uses a grasper to retract the peritoneum, taking care not to grasp the bowel but instead to grasp the mesentery or the peritoneum to place the tissues on traction.

The surgeon begins the dissection by incising the peritoneum along the cecum [*see Figure 3*]. The appendiceal and terminal ileal attachments are easily visualized and similarly divided. The bowel is then bluntly reflected from the retroperitoneum. At this point, the ureter can usually be identified in the retroperitoneum. The bowel is further mobilized medially by means of blunt dissection. The dissection is extended upward to the hepatic flexure, and the transverse colon is mobilized as necessary for the diseased bowel segment to be resected. For complete dissection of the transverse colon, it may be necessary to put the patient in the reverse Trendelenburg position. Additional dissection of the colon can also be done under direct vision during the removal of the specimen. The duodenum can usually be visualized during this mobilization.

Step 4: Dissection

The bowel is returned to its normal position, the mesentery is grasped, and the medial aspect of the colon and the ileocolic vessels are placed on traction. With traction placed on the mesentery, the ileocolic vessels are easily visualized. The key technical point here is that on each side of the mesenteric vessels, there exists a clear avascular space, which can be rapidly and readily dissected back into the previously dissected retroperitoneum to create a window [*see Figure 4*]. Once this window is complete, the vessels are isolated and can be controlled with minimal difficulty. The artery and the vein can usually be identified at their origin, separated, and individually clipped. The right colic vessels are then similarly exposed and clipped.

With the dissection of the bowel complete, attention is turned to mobilization and division of the ileocolic and right colic vessels. Once this is accomplished, the bowel is completely mobile and can be retrieved through the abdominal wall. To facilitate creation of the anastomosis, the attachments of the terminal ileum must be completely divided; if this is not done, the surgeon will find it difficult to bring the bowel through the abdominal wall.

Step 5: Anastomosis and Closure

A 5 cm incision is made at the right lower quadrant port site and extended downward through the muscle. Hemostatic techniques must be used: no bleeding should be allowed to occur through this incision. The bowel can then be grasped and brought through the wound with relative ease. Once the bowel is outside the abdomen, any additional mesenteric dissection and ligation that may be needed can be completed under direct vision. Before creating the anastomosis, the surgeon must ensure that the bowel has not been rotated; this can be accomplished by maintaining the orientation of the bowel as it is brought out through the abdominal wall.

The bowel is then divided and reanastomosed either with staples or with sutures. It is not necessary to close the mesenteric defect. The bowel is returned to the peritoneal cavity, and the abdominal wound is closed in layers. The peritoneal cavity is reinsufflated, laparoscopically inspected for hemostasis, and irrigated. The cannulas are removed under direct vision, and the 10/12 mm port sites are closed. Finally, the skin is closed with a subcuticular absorbable suture and Steri-Strips.

Figure 2 **Laparoscopic colectomy: right hemicolectomy. Standard port placement.**

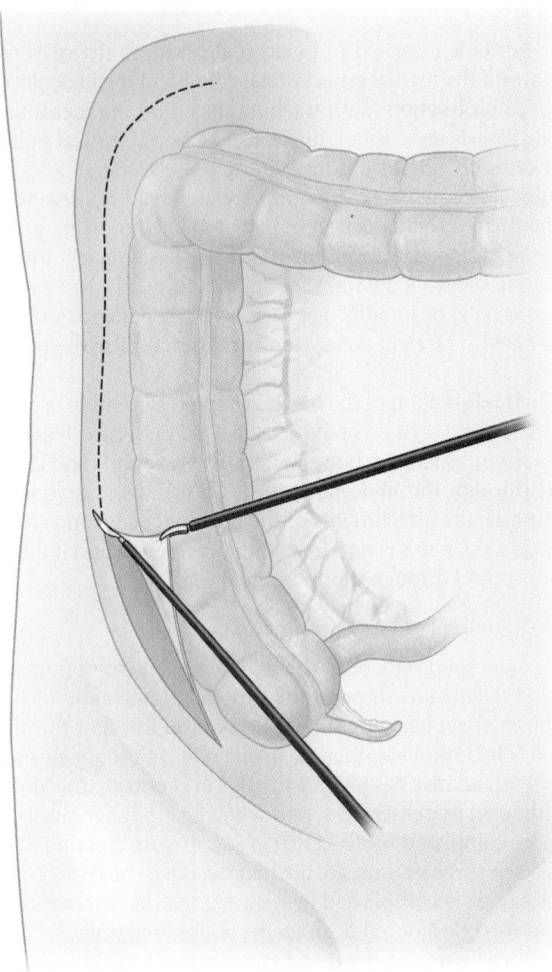

Figure 3 **Laparoscopic colectomy: right hemicolectomy. Right colon mobilization.**

LEFT HEMICOLECTOMY AND SIGMOID RESECTION

Step 1: Positioning of Patient and Operative Team

Initial positioning and preparation of the patient are essentially the same as for a right hemicolectomy (see above). The position of the operative team differs somewhat, in that the surgeon and the nurse stand to the right of the patient, and the camera operator and the assistant stand to the left [*see Figure 5*]. The monitors are placed in the same locations as for a right hemicolectomy.

Step 2: Placement of Trocars

As in a right hemicolectomy, a Hasson trocar is placed in the left upper quadrant via a small incision over the rectus muscle 3 to 4 cm below the costal margin. After pneumoperitoneum is established through this trocar, three additional ports are inserted under direct vision in the same locations used for a right hemicolectomy.

Step 3: Mobilization of Descending Colon

The patient is placed in a steep Trendelenburg position, maximally rotated to the right. For the initial dissection, the laparoscope (either 0° or 30°) is placed in the left upper quadrant port. As the assistant retracts the peritoneal attachments laterally to the left, the surgeon, using the electrified scissors in the suprapubic port and the grasper in the right lower quadrant port, retracts the descending colon cephalad and to the right. The dissection commences along the peritoneal reflection of the sigmoid and descending colon, with

the peritoneum incised along the white line of Toldt. Once the peritoneum has been incised, the colon can be mobilized by blunt reflection off the retroperitoneum.

As in a right hemicolectomy, the ureter must be identified. As a rule, the gonadal vessels appear first, then the ureter. After the ureter is carefully identified and dissected away from the mesentery, the bowel is again laid laterally. To ensure adequate length, the splenic flexure should be mobilized in much the same way as the hepatic flexure.

Step 4: Dissection

After the bowel is returned to its normal anatomic location, the mesentery is grasped and the inferior mesenteric vessels identified. Using the avascular space around the origin of the vessels, the surgeon creates a window that extends laterally to the previously dissected plane. Once the pedicle is isolated, the fat around the vessels can be stripped, and the artery and the vein can be individually controlled and clipped. We use large clips, placing two on the aortic side of the vessels and one on the distal side. In dividing large arteries, it is best to cut partway through the artery and then remove tension from the vessel to make sure that the clips are correctly applied [*see Figure 6*]; alternatively, the pedicle can be divided with a vascular endoscopic stapler. The choice of approach is a matter of individual preference.

Step 5: Anastomosis and Closure

Once the inferior mesenteric artery is ligated, the left colic artery may be divided, depending on which bowel segment is to be removed. A 5 cm incision is then made at the port site in the left lower quadrant. The bowel is grasped and brought up through the incision. The entire bowel can usually be seen, and any additional mesentery can be divided. The bowel is then divided and reanastomosed by means of standard anastomotic techniques. When the anastomosis is complete, the bowel is returned to the abdominal cavity. The fascia is closed in two layers with continuous absorbable sutures, and the skin is closed with a subcuticular absorbable suture.

Figure 4 **Laparoscopic colectomy: right hemicolectomy. Right colon mesenteric dissection.**

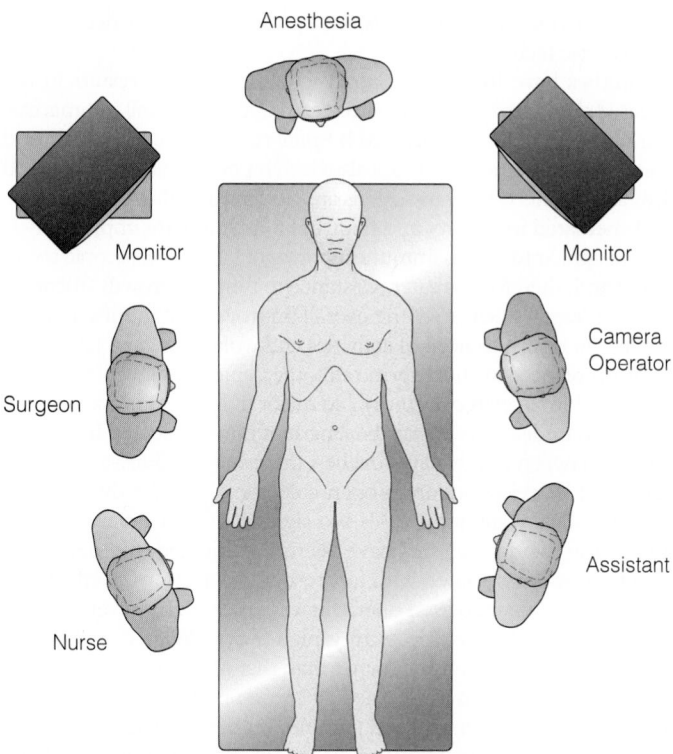

Figure 5 **Laparoscopic colectomy: left hemicolectomy and sigmoid resection. Shown is the recommended positioning of the operating team.**

Postoperative Care

Postoperative care of patients who have undergone laparoscopic colectomy should be similar to that of patients who have undergone open colectomy; however, a shorter recovery period is to be expected with the less invasive procedure. As a rule, patients are started on clear liquids in the evening of the day of surgery and maintained on epidural analgesia until oral intake is adequate. Subsequently, enteral feeding is advanced until patients are on a regular diet, at which point they can be discharged from the hospital. Oral medications are generally adequate for controlling any postoperative pain, and patients are encouraged to pursue desired activities to the extent tolerated. On the whole, it is our impression that patients who have undergone laparoscopic colectomy experience less respiratory and immune dysfunction and can tolerate food more rapidly than those who have undergone open colectomy. They can usually be discharged between postoperative days 3 and 4.

Troubleshooting

A major troubleshooting issue is that of conversion of a laparoscopic bowel resection to an open procedure. Such conversion should not be construed as a failure but rather as the application of sound surgical judgment.

Several findings or conditions may lead to conversion to an open procedure. Inability to identify critical structures (e.g., the ureter or major blood vessels) or concern about appropriate anatomic orientation should encourage the surgeon to open the abdomen. Early in the case, the presence of dense adhesions, which may prolong the procedure excessively, should encourage early conversion to an open procedure. Care and prudence must be exercised during extensive adhesiolysis. In addition, lack of adequate exposure, poor hemostasis, disorientation, inadequate resection or reconstruction,

and the presence of an enterotomy, structure, abscess, or fistula may all prompt early conversion. In particular, we have found it difficult to recognize serosal abrasions and enterotomies, particularly when dissecting over the pelvic brim. Dissecting the small bowel out of the pelvis is difficult. This finding is a common reason for conversion to an open laparotomy.

A key point is that the operation should not be unduly prolonged by troublesome intra-abdominal findings. The decision whether the case can be completed laparoscopically or should be converted to an open laparotomy usually can and should be made rapidly.

Another issue concerns trocar placement. When placing the trocars, we favor a Hasson technique, in which the initial 12 mm port is placed through the left upper quadrant rectus muscle under direct vision. The reason we have come to prefer this location is that in the right upper quadrant, the falciform ligament frequently complicates access to the abdominal cavity. The second, third, and fourth ports are then placed under direct vision. Initial studies reported injuries to major intra-abdominal vessels in the course of port placement, but we have not encountered this problem with our technique.[7] In addition, we favor minimizing the number of 10/12 mm ports used because the larger incisions can be difficult to repair accurately and may be associated with bowel herniation. Bowel herniation has not been reported at 5 mm port sites. The port sizes and instrument sizes necessary for colonic dissection are predictable; thus, a standardized approach, as outlined [*see* Operative Technique, *above*], can be established with little difficulty.

Finally, management of the primary feeding vessels can be an irksome problem. On each side of the ileocolic and inferior mesenteric

Figure 6 **Laparoscopic colectomy: left hemicolectomy and sigmoid resection. Sigmoid mesentery and pelvic dissection.**

vessels, there is a large avascular window. We take advantage of this predictable anatomic finding and aggressively dissect and isolate these vessels. Our usual practice is to separate the vein from the artery with a right-angle dissecting clamp and clip them separately. Occasionally, a fibrotic sheath prevents this separation, in which case we use an endovascular stapler to occlude and divide the vessels.

Complications

Complications associated with laparoscopic colectomy include major vessel injuries and enterotomies (both recognized and unrecognized). These can generally be minimized and managed through careful troubleshooting (see above).

A potential complication that has given rise to considerable concern is recurrence at port sites after laparoscopic colectomy for cancer. Anecdotal reports of wound and port-site recurrences after laparoscopic colon cancer resection were widely published in the early 1990s. A growing body of experience suggests that such recurrences are rare: the average incidence appears to be about 1%, which is comparable to the recurrence rates reported after open procedures.[3-6] Nevertheless, the anecdotal reports of port-site recurrence after laparoscopic colon resection led to a resurgence of the theory that tumoricidal agents may prevent such recurrence. Jacobi and associates found that taurolidine combined with heparin decreased tumor cell growth in a rat model.[8] Basha and coworkers showed that 5% pyrrolidone iodine mixed with 0.5% chloramine killed almost all tumor cells in vitro and prevented their growth in vivo.[9] We demonstrated that povidone decreased tumor cell growth in laparoscopic ports in a murine model.[10] If these results can be confirmed by other studies, placement of a tumoricidal agent in the incisions or on the trocars to prevent port-site recurrence may well become the standard of care.

The best way of putting the issue of port-site recurrence to rest is to perform a prospective, randomized study comparing laparoscopic colectomy with open colectomy in patients with colon cancer. In 1995, the National Cancer Institute initiated a multicenter study designed to address this issue and others having to do with safety, staging, and 5-year survival rates. The results of this study should be available in 2003. The general consensus in the United States is that until the results are in hand, laparoscopic colectomies for cancer should be performed at those centers involved in the study.

Outcome Evaluation

To date, laparoscopic approaches have been most successful for right hemicolectomy, sigmoid resection, and stoma formation. Abdominoperineal resection is also easily and safely performed with laparoscopic techniques.

Studies have found that laparoscopic colectomy results in decreased short-term morbidity, decreased abdominal wall trauma, earlier tolerance of food, shortened hospital stays, and reduced pain and narcotic requirements.[11] It has also been reported that surgical blood loss and the need for transfusions are reduced and that postoperative cell-mediated immunity and neutrophil function are improved.[12,13] There appear to be less immunosuppression after laparoscopic colectomy and, therefore, greater resistance to tumor regrowth (theoretically, at least). Because of the overall improvement in function, patients can return to normal activities and work more quickly.

With respect to short-term outcome, laparoscopic colectomy is comparable to open colectomy. No major differences in the number of lymph nodes resected or the length of bowel resected have been found between the two approaches; there is a trend toward greater length of bowel resection in open colectomy, but the difference is not statistically significant.[14,15] No significant cost differences between the two procedures have been documented: the decreased length of stay associated with laparoscopic colectomy is effectively balanced by the increased operating expenses. If, however, the rate of conversion to open colectomy is high (i.e., > 20%), the cost of laparoscopic surgery may be higher than that of open surgery.

At present, there is a great deal of interest in the use of laparoscopy to resect colon cancers and to minimize the short-term morbidity associated with treatment of malignant diseases. There has been sufficient research into and experience with laparoscopic treatment of colorectal cancer to show that it is a feasible modality offering the same advantages as laparoscopic treatment of benign colonic disease. The heart of the current debate surrounding the application of laparoscopy to malignant colonic disease is the question of how a laparoscopic approach might affect long-term patterns of recurrence and survival.[3,5,6]

Concerns regarding the efficacy of laparoscopic colectomy for cancer have centered on the completeness of the bowel and lymph node resections. As noted, multiple studies have shown no differences between laparoscopic colectomy and open colectomy with respect to proximal and distal margins of resection or the adequacy of lymph node dissection. Most of the concerns regarding the incidence and pattern of recurrence after laparoscopic treatment were generated early in surgeons' experience with laparoscopic colectomy, and subsequent studies tended not to find substantial differences. However, further studies that include long-term follow-up to determine the adequacy of resection and the comparability of cure rates are needed to assess any changes in the long-term staging and survival patterns after laparoscopic colectomy.

References

1. Beart RW Jr: Laparoscopic colectomy: status of the art. Dis Colon Rectum 37(suppl):S47, 1994

2. Monson JRT, Hill ADK, Darzi A: Laparoscopic colonic surgery. Br J Surg 82:150, 1995

3. Ramos JM, Gupta S, Anthone GJ, et al: Laparoscopy and colon cancer: is the port site at risk? a preliminary report. Arch Surg 129:897, 1994

4. Paik PS: Abdominal incision tumor implantation following pneumoperitoneum laparoscopic procedure vs. standard open incision in a syngeneic rat model. Dis Colon Rectum 41:419, 1998

5. Wexner SD, Cohen SM: Port site metastases after laparoscopic colorectal surgery for cure of malignancy. Br J Surg 82:295, 1995

6. Lacy AM, Garcia-Valdecasas JC, Pique JM, et al: Short-term outcome analysis of a randomized study comparing laparoscopic vs open colectomy for colon cancer. Surg Endosc 9:1101, 1995

7. Nordestgaard AG, Bodily KC, Osborne RW Jr, et al: Major vascular injuries during laparoscopic procedures. Am J Surg 169:543, 1995

8. Jacobi C, Ordemann J, Bohm B, et al: Inhibition of peritoneal tumor cell growth and implantation in laparoscopic surgery in a rat model. Am J Surg 174:359, 1997

9. Basha G, Penninckx F, Geboes K, et al: Tumoricidal activity of antiseptics with assessment of cell viability in mice with severe combined immunodeficiency. Tumour Biol 18:213, 1997

10. Hoffstetter W, Ortega A, Chiang M, et al: The effects of topical tumoricidals on port site recurrence of colon cancer. J Soc Laparoendosc Surg (in press)

11. Chen HH, Wexner SD, Iroatulam AJN, et al: Laparoscopic colectomy compares favorably with colectomy by laparotomy for reduction of postoperative ileus. Dis Colon Rectum 43:61, 2000

12. Harmon GD, Senganore AJ, Kilbride MJ, et al: Interleukin-6 response to laparoscopic and open colectomy. Dis Colon Rectum 37:754, 1994

13. Kloosterman T, Von Blomberg ME, Borgstein P, et al: Unimpaired immune function after laparoscopic cholecystectomy. Surgery 113:424, 1994

14. Kockerling F: Prospective multicenter study of the

quality of oncologic resections in patients undergoing laparoscopic colorectal surgery for cancer. Dis Colon Rectum 41:963, 1998

15. Hida J, Yasutomi M, Maruyama T, et al: The extent of lymph node dissection for colon carcinoma: the potential impact on laparoscopic surgery. Cancer 80: 188, 1997

Recommended Reading

Beart RW Jr: Increased tumor establishment and growth after laparotomy vs laparoscopy in a murine model (invited commentary). Arch Surg 130:653, 1995

Dorrance HR, Oien K, O'Dwyer PJ: Effects of laparoscopy on intraperitoneal tumor growth and distant metastases in an animal model. Surgery 126:35, 1999

Fleshman JW, Wexner SD, Anvari M, et al: Laparoscopic *vs.* open abdominoperineal resection for cancer. Dis Colon Rectum 42:930, 1999

Hewitt PM: Laparoscopic-assisted vs. open surgery for colorectal cancer. Dis Colon Rectum 41:901, 1998

Huguet EL, Earnshaw JJ, Heather BP: Major vascular injury during laparoscopy. Br J Surg 84:1479, 1997

Liberman MA, Phillips EH, Carroll BJ, et al: Laparoscopic colectomy vs traditional colectomy for diverticulitis: outcome and costs. Surg Endosc 10:15, 1996

Schwandner O, Schiedeck THK, Bruch HP: Advanced age—indication or contraindication for laparoscopic colorectal surgery? Dis Colon Rectum 42:356, 1999

Solomon MJ, Egan M, Roberts RA, et al: Incidence of free colorectal cancer cells on the peritoneal surface. Dis Colon Rectum 40:1294, 1997

Wolf JS Jr, Stoller ML: The physiology of laparoscopy: basic principles, complications and other considerations. J Urol 152:294, 1994

Acknowledgment

Figures 1 through 6   Tom Moore.

Ira J. Kodner, M.D.

Operative Management of Hemorrhoids

In recent years, the frequency of hemorrhoid surgery has diminished significantly. More patients seem to be achieving adequate symptomatic relief by means of bowel control medications and improved diet (e.g., increased intake of fiber, fruit, vegetables, and grain). It is probable that both for these reasons and because more and better patient information is available, fewer patients today have hemorrhoids that progress to a stage advanced enough to necessitate operative treatment for relief of symptoms.

OPERATIVE PLANNING

It is important to distinguish between internal and external hemorrhoids [*see Figure 1*]. Internal hemorrhoids are treated to relieve specific symptoms, including prolapse and bleeding, not simply because hemorrhoidal tissue was seen on routine examinations. Prolapsing tissue occasionally results in maceration of the perianal skin that may not be clearly evident at the time of examination, especially if the patient is in the prone position. External hemorrhoids are treated because they thrombose and cause pain. There are no other symptoms of the anorectum that should be attributed to the presence of hemorrhoids [*see Table 1*]; in particular, difficulties with bowel movements (e.g., straining, the need for digital evacuation of the rectum, and cramping abdominal pain) must not be ascribed to hemorrhoids.

Accordingly, the ability to recognize and diagnose the spectrum of pelvic floor abnormalities (of which rectal prolapse is the most florid manifestation), especially obstructed defecation, is critical to the decision whether to correct hemorrhoids surgically. Attempting to alleviate nonhemorrhoidal symptoms by means of hemorrhoid surgery is likely to yield unsatisfactory results for both patient and surgeon. It is not uncommon for anal fissure/ulcer disease to coexist with hemorrhoids, in which case the chances of a good operative result can be increased by performing a posterior lateral internal sphincterotomy at the time of hemorrhoid surgery.

Before embarking on the surgical treatment of hemorrhoids, one must always rule out neoplastic disease, compromise of the immune system, and defective clotting mechanisms. Patients with a personal or family history of colorectal cancer and those 50 years of age or older should undergo colonoscopy to eliminate the possibility of polyps or cancer before surgical treatment of hemorrhoids is initiated. The patient's general health status and ability to tolerate pain and an operative procedure should also be taken into account. The postoperative response to anorectal surgery varies enormously among patients. For example, young men tend to strain to have bowel movements after anorectal procedures, and this tendency can lead to bleeding and disruption of postoperative healing. These patients often benefit from the administration of parenteral pain medication for the first 12 to 24 hours after operation, which usually requires hospitalization. Elderly patients, on the other hand, prefer not to be in the hospital. For these patients, single elastic ligation of individual clusters of internal hemorrhoids is performed in the outpatient office.

The next step is to determine the appropriate procedure for the patient. The options include (1) elastic ligation of internal hemorrhoids, (2) excision of thrombosed external hemorrhoids, (3) complete excisional hemorrhoidectomy, and (4) elastic ligation of internal hemorrhoids combined with excision of external hemorrhoids. One should always consider whether complete sigmoidoscopy, rigid or flexible, will be necessary at the time of

INTERNAL HEMORRHOID

Origin above
Dentate Line
(Internal Plexus)

External
Sphincter
Muscle

Intersphincteric
Plane

Internal
Sphincter
Muscle

External Hemorrhoidal Plexus

EXTERNAL HEMORRHOID

Origin below
Dentate Line
(External Plexus)

Internal
Hemorrhoidal
Plexus

Figure 1 **Operative management of hemorrhoids. A key issue is the differentiation of internal hemorrhoids from external hemorrhoids. Internal hemorrhoids (left) originate from the internal hemorrhoidal plexus, above the dentate line. External hemorrhoids (right) originate from the external hemorrhoidal plexus, below the dentate line.**

Table 1 Anal Symptoms Mistakenly Attributed to Hemorrhoids

Symptoms	Cause
Pain and bleeding after bowel movement	Ulcer/fissure disease
Forceful straining to have bowel movement	Pelvic floor abnormality (paradoxical contraction of anal sphincter)
Blood mixed with stool	Neoplasm
Drainage of pus during or after bowel movement	Abscess/fistula, inflammatory bowel disease
Constant moisture	Condyloma acuminatum
Mucous drainage and incontinence	Rectal prolapse
Anal pain with no physical findings	*Caution:* possible psychiatric disorder

the procedure and whether anal sphincterotomy will be indicated, especially in young men with a history of straining. This second consideration is important because many patients are treated for hemorrhoids when in fact their primary disease is anal ulcer/fissure disease, the symptoms of which are pain and some bleeding at defecation. These are not symptoms that can be attributed to hemorrhoids. If a patient undergoes hemorrhoid surgery when the primary disease is anal fissure, proper healing will be impeded.

Finally, one should explain the procedure and its attendant risks to the patient in the outpatient office because in most cases, given the restrictions imposed by health care insurers and managed care administrators, one will not see the patient again until the operating room on the day of operation. Specific complications to be discussed preoperatively include urinary retention, bleeding, and infection. In the event that several symptomatic hemorrhoids are present, surgeon and patient should jointly decide between multiple small procedures done in the office and a single larger procedure done in the OR. Individual economic concerns, as well as employment and lifestyle, should be considered.

Special Situations

Acute thrombosed external hemorrhoids This condition is signaled by acute pain and a swelling blood clot within the skin-covered external hemorrhoid. Often, the clot is eroding through the skin, causing bleeding that may be frightening to the patient but is typically insignificant. If I encounter this problem days after its onset, I generally treat it with bowel control and topical medications as the process resolves. If the hemorrhoid is acutely painful or the clot is eroding, the best therapy is surgical excision of the external hemorrhoid, with the anoderm left intact; this is best done with the patient under adequate local anesthesia. Mere evacuation of the clot is rarely appropriate.

Postpartum hemorrhoids The postpartum rosette of acute thrombosed external (and, often, prolapsed internal) hemorrhoidal tissue is appropriately treated with hemorrhoidectomy (see below), carried out as soon after delivery as is convenient. The risk of infection is minimal, and I know of

no good reason to send a new mother home with hemorrhoids in addition to a new baby and a healing episiotomy.

OPERATIVE TECHNIQUE

Step 1: Positioning

Operative treatment of hemorrhoids, like the vast majority of anorectal procedures, should be done with the patient in the prone-flexed position [see Figure 2]. The transporting stretcher should be kept in the room. The patient will be given I.V. narcotics to allow painless injection of local anesthetics, and if any respiratory compromise results because of the prone-flexed position, the patient can quickly be returned to the supine position on the stretcher until respiration resumes without difficulty.

Step 2: Intravenous Sedation and Local Anesthesia

Before administering a local anesthetic, I usually give the following drugs for sedation: midazolam, 2 to 5 mg, given in the holding area for sedation and amnesia; alfentanil, 0.5 to 1 mg, or fentanyl, 50 to 100 mg, for analgesia to help alleviate the discomfort of the local anesthetic injection; and propofol, 20 to 50 mg, or methohexital, 20 to 50 mg, to achieve patient cooperation with the injection. Sedation is followed by the injection into perianal tissue of 40 ml of bupivacaine (0.5%) along with a buffer that is added immediately before injection (0.5 ml of 8.4% sodium bicarbonate [1 mEq/ml] added to 50 ml of local anesthetic). If resection is anticipated, epinephrine (1:200,000) is usually included with the local anesthetic. To achieve adequate local anesthesia, 5 ml of bupivacaine is injected into the subcutaneous tissue in each quadrant of the tissue immediately surrounding the anus [see Figure 3a]. Next, 10 ml of local anesthetic is injected deep into the sphincter mechanism on each side of the anal canal [see Figure 3b].

Step 3: Anoscopy or Sigmoidoscopy

Anoscopy, sigmoidoscopy, or both should be performed at this point if neither procedure was done before the operation.

Step 4: Sphincterotomy

As noted, sphincterotomy should always be considered, especially if a hypertrophic band of the lower third of the internal

Figure 2 **Operative management of hemorrhoids. The patient is positioned on the operating table in the prone-flexed position, with a soft roll under the hips.**

Figure 3 Operative management of hemorrhoids. (*a*) Five milliliters of bupivacaine is injected into subcutaneous tissue. (*b*) Ten milliliters of local anesthetic is injected deep into the sphincter muscle on each side of the anal canal.

sphincter muscle persists after the local anesthetic has been injected and an anoscope has been inserted. It is always best to obtain permission to do this beforehand on the operative consent form.

Step 5: Treatment of Hemorrhoids

Elastic ligation of internal hemorrhoids This is a very safe operation because by the nature of the banding procedure [*see Figure 4*], bridges of normal mucosa are maintained between treated clusters of hemorrhoids. Any clusters of tissue with squamous metaplasia and obviously friable internal hemorrhoids can be treated in this manner. I find that these tissue clusters are not always confined to the three classic positions

identified for hemorrhoids and that in many cases it is necessary to band three or four clusters. If the bands do not stay on, then the tissue probably need not be treated and no further action need be taken.

I use two rubber bands on each cluster. If one of them breaks, bleeding is unlikely to occur, because the tissue rapidly becomes edematous and necrotic. It is important that the placement of the rubber band be proximal to the mucocutaneous junction; if it is not, the procedure will be too painful, given the extensive innervation of the skin. On the other hand, the band should not be placed so proximally as to incorporate the full thickness of the rectal wall; to do so can be risky for patients in whom difficulties with bowel movements indicate the presence of intus-

Figure 4 Operative management of hemorrhoids. Shown is the elastic ligation technique for internal hemorrhoids. (*a*) The hemorrhoidal tissue is identified. (*b*) The hemorrhoid is grasped and pulled through the drum. (*c*) The elastic band is applied to the base of the hemorrhoid.

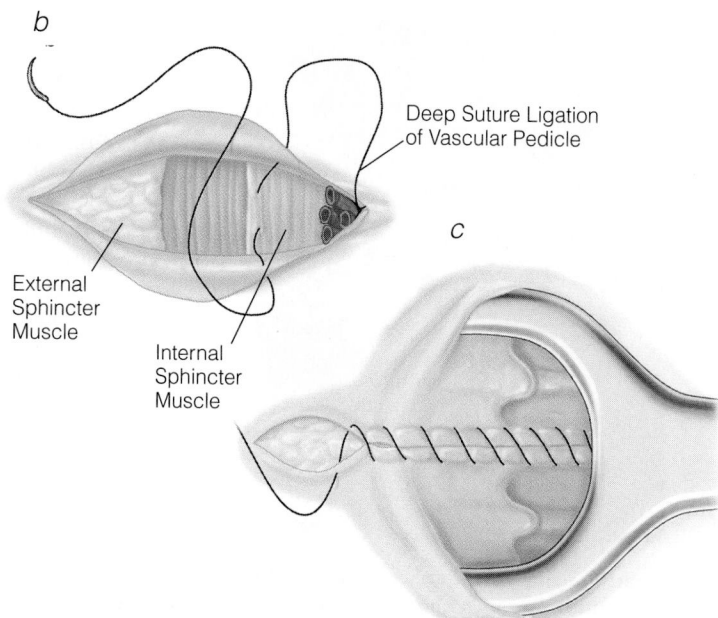

Figure 5 **Operative management of hemorrhoids. Shown is an excisional hemorrhoidectomy. (*a*) An elliptical incision is made in the perianal skin. (*b*) A continuous suture is used in a three-point placement in such a way as to incorporate skin edges and muscle. (*c*) The elliptical defect is closed and the dead space obliterated.**

susception or some other pelvic floor abnormality. Occasionally, the friable tissue gives rise to a suspicion of cancer. If this is the case, rubber bands may be placed at the base, and the tip may be excised for biopsy.

Excision of residual external hemorrhoids Residual external hemorrhoids are rarely treated as a primary problem: true symptoms are few, and the main indication for treatment is maintenance of hygiene. In addition, I find that much of the external tissue is pulled in when the internal hemorrhoids are ligated. Accordingly, I do the internal ligation first and then excise any residual symptomatic external tissue. An elliptical incision is made in the perianal skin, with care taken to protect the underlying sphincter muscle and avoid the previously placed elastic band [*see Figure 5a*]. Although the perianal skin is very forgiving, it is essential to protect the anoderm; this is achieved through careful placement of the rubber band. The elliptical defect is then closed with a continuous absorbable suture in a three-point placement to obliterate the underlying dead space [*see Figures 5b and 5c*]. The suture is tied loosely to allow for swelling. There is no need for separate ligation or coagulation of the small bleeding vessels; this problem is obviated by the continuous suture. It is important not to use slowly absorbable suture material, because it may give rise to infection in this highly susceptible tissue. I prefer to use 3-0 chromic catgut on an exaggeratedly curved needle.

Complete excisional hemorrhoidectomy This procedure is indicated in patients who have large combined internal and external hemorrhoids, patients who are receiving anticoagulants, and patients who have massive edema and thrombosis, as seen in the postpartum rosette of tissue [*see Figure 6*]. I find that even massive edema generally resolves after the local anesthetic is injected and the muscle is allowed to relax. Resolution of edema then permits identification of the specific clusters of hemorrhoids, which can be isolated with a forceps and excised via an elliptical incision. Care must be taken to preserve the underlying muscle, especially in the anterior region in women.

I use 3-0 chromic catgut with a deep stitch at the apex and a continuous three-point suture that is extended on the perianal skin [*see Figure 5b*]. It is important to preserve a bridge of anoderm between the areas of excision. I know of no indications for a radical circumferential procedure (the so-called Whitehead procedure); in fact, I see numerous patients who are seeking a remedy for the stenosis and ectropion that frequently occur after this radical operation [*see Figure 7*].

Currently, a new technique, in which a circumferential band of anorectal mucosa is excised with a special circular stapler, is

Figure 6 **Operative management of hemorrhoids. Massive edema and thrombosis, as seen in the postpartum rosette of tissue, can be reduced after a local anesthetic is injected and the muscle is allowed to relax.**

Figure 7 **Operative management of hemorrhoids. Stenosis and ectropion often result from radical circumferential (Whitehead) procedures.**

under investigation. This technique is intended for patients who have profound prolapsing internal hemorrhoids without much of an external component. Its proponents claim that it results in minimum postoperative discomfort; however, special training with the instrument is required. European centers report excellent success rates, and trials are currently under way in the United States.

Step 6: Postoperative Care

Immediately after the procedure—in fact, after any anorectal procedure—antibiotic ointment and a gauze pad are applied. Pressure dressings are unnecessary. Only a very small amount of adhesive tape should be used, so as to prevent traction avulsion of the perianal skin, an event for which we surgeons too often avoid responsibility by ascribing it to a "tape allergy" on the part of the patient.

TROUBLESHOOTING

The most fundamental way of preventing problems is to make an accurate diagnosis. Surgical treatment of hemorrhoids in a patient whose main disease process is Crohn's disease, a pelvic floor abnormality, or ulcer/fissure disease inevitably yields inferior results. It is especially important to recognize the anal pain and spasm of ulcer/fissure disease because in patients with this condition, excision of hemorrhoidal tissue without sphincterotomy leads to increased postoperative pain and poor wound healing.

I prefer to operate with the patient in the prone-flexed position, using local anesthesia supplemented by I.V. medication. I have found over the years that with this approach, patients retain no unpleasant memories of the OR experience, and good pain control is achieved in the immediate postoperative period.

In the postoperative period, efforts must be made to minimize straining on the part of the patient. To accomplish this, pain must be kept at a low level. I prefer to give only parenteral pain medication, in relatively high doses, on the first night. The patient and the nursing staff must be cautioned that the first sensation of pain, especially after elastic ligation of hemorrhoids, is the urge to defecate. This urge is an indication that pain medication should be given. The patient must not sit on

the toilet and strain; to do so is likely to result in extrusion of the recently ligated tissue.

At least 20% of patients experience some degree of urinary retention. If this occurs, an indwelling catheter should be placed. In-and-out straight catheterization is contraindicated. No bladder stimulants should be given: such agents encourage straining and increase the risk of complications.

Bulk-forming agents and stool softeners are started in the immediate postoperative period. I encourage patients to take warm soaks, either in a bathtub or in a shower, rather than try to squeeze into the disposable sitz-bath mechanisms provided by the hospitals, which are often too small. I also encourage patients to sit on soft cushions rather than the rubber rings marketed for postoperative care; the rings seem to cause more dependent edema and pain.

COMPLICATIONS

Bleeding

Either immediate or delayed bleeding may occur after hemorrhoid surgery. Bleeding within the first 12 to 24 hours after the operation represents a technical error. The only management is to return the patient to the OR, with good anesthesia and adequate visualization, so that the bleeding site can be suture ligated. Frequently, spinal or epidural anesthesia is necessary because the patient is too uncomfortable, and the tissue perhaps too edematous, to allow local anesthesia. Bleeding within 5 to 10 days after the operation usually results from sloughing of the eschar created by suturing or elastic ligation. This delayed bleeding is usually minimal, and the patient is encouraged to rest and to take stool softeners. If the bleeding is significant, examination with adequate anesthesia is indicated to allow cauterization or suture ligation of the bleeding site.

It is important to discourage patients from taking aspirin-containing compounds in the postoperative period, and it is especially important to follow patients taking systemic anticoagulants closely. I prefer to treat these patients with excisional hemorrhoidectomy so that sutures can be placed; in this way, I avoid the risk that the elastic-ligated tissue will slough after 5 to 10 days.

Infection

Infection is unusual after hemorrhoidectomy because perianal tissue is normally well vascularized and extremely resistant to infection despite constant bombardment by bacteria. When it does occur, it is most likely to be in an immunocompromised patient—that is, one who has a blood dyscrasia, diabetes, or AIDS or has recently undergone chemotherapy. In my view, it is imperative to obtain at least a complete blood count and a chemistry profile before embarking on anorectal procedures; if the results are abnormal, elective hemorrhoid surgery is contraindicated.

Any local focus of infection noted in the postoperative period must be drained. I have seen this complication only when slowly absorbable suture material was used, which is the reason why I have returned to using 3-0 chromic catgut. Postoperative perianal infection can be severe and life-threatening, and it is therefore critically important to be familiar with its symptoms and to treat it intensively. Frequently, such infection is initially manifested by pain that is greater than anticipated, urinary retention, and fever. These symptoms have occasionally been reported after elastic ligation of hemorrhoids. In this event, it is critical that the patient be seen on an emergency basis, the elastic bands removed, the patient hospitalized, and parenteral administration of antibiotics begun. In retrospect, I find that all such patients whom I have

Disease Processes That Cause Anorectal Abscess and Fistula in Ano

Cryptoglandular Abscess and Fistula

This condition results from obstruction of the duct of a gland, the body of which resides in the intersphincteric plane. The orifice of the gland is at the base of the crypt. The disease process has both an acute aspect and a chronic aspect.

Abscess is the acute process of the disease. The anatomy is complex because of the tissue planes in the anorectal-perineal area.[2] Surgical drainage, or at least surgical evaluation, is always necessary. Attempts to manage this condition medically can result in progressive tissue destruction and life-threatening infection. It is also essential always to be alert to the possibility of an immunocompromised state. Normally, the anoperineum is quite resistant to microbial invasion; however, in immunocompromised patients, infection can be life-threatening.

Fistula is the chronic process of the disease. Persistent inflammation results in the formation of tracts from the anal duct to the anoperineal skin or to the inside of the anorectum. These tracts can take extremely complex courses. For this reason and because of the complicated tissue planes of dissection, surgical treatment must be carefully planned: the status of the sphincter mechanism may be jeopardized if inappropriate surgical incisions are employed to open a fistula tract.

Crohn's Disease

Anal and perineal infection is a major factor in the clinical course of one third of all patients who have Crohn's disease. The main pathologic process is full-thickness penetration of Crohn's ulcers, occurring at any location in the anal canal (as opposed to uncomplicated cryptoglandular abscess or fistula, which is usually found posteriorly or anteriorly in the midline). The infection associated with Crohn's disease can be massive but is surprisingly well tolerated by the patient. The infectious process can be progressively destructive to the sphincter and to the surrounding tissue. Patients are at lifelong risk for severe diarrhea and loss of rectal distensibility; accordingly, meticulous preservation of the sphincter mechanism is crucial.

The incisional surgical procedures usually employed for infectious foci in the anal canal may be too hazardous, and excisional procedures are never indicated. Given that Crohn's disease tends to persist and recur, long-term drainage may be necessary. Medical management is useful and efficacious, but it should be provided in combination with surgical consultation and drainage of abscesses. Because patients with anal Crohn's disease usually exhibit some degree of intestinal involvement as well, it is important to evaluate the remainder of the GI tract, especially the rectum, before embarking on any surgical treatment of the anus.

Hidradenitis Suppurativa

This condition is caused by blockage and disruption of the apocrine sweat glands in the perianal and perineal tissue. It gives rise to destructive infected sinus tracts in the perineal tissue. Although the destruction can be profound, there is no connection with the intestinal tract (either the rectum or the anus). No specific pathologic diagnosis can be made, because all that is left is the destructive fibrotic reaction to the content of the ruptured gland. Hidradenitis suppurativa occurs in persons with seborrheic skin and in those who perspire profusely; it often involves the axillary, suprapubic, and inguinal areas as well as the perineum.

Because the lesions are actually sinus tracts in the skin, therapy involves simply incising the tracts; biopsy is appropriate at some point during the course of management.

Sepsis Resulting from the Immunocompromised State

Anoperineal infection in an immunocompromised patient is a very serious and possibly life-threatening situation. Because this part of the body is so highly contaminated, failure of immune barriers can be disastrous. This condition is seen in patients who have diabetes mellitus, HIV infection, or other forms of blood dyscrasias; in patients undergoing chemotherapy; and in transplant patients requiring long-term immunosuppression. It is diagnosed on the basis of its symptoms: the clinical findings may be obscured by the absence of pus resulting from leukopenia.

Treatment involves aggressive antibiotic therapy, careful examination with the patient under anesthesia, extremely conservative drainage procedures, and biopsy of the tissue (leukemic infiltrates are occasionally found). The potential consequences of failing to recognize and treat this condition are serious enough to warrant evaluation of all patients with perineal infection for an immunocompromised state before any treatment is undertaken or before these patients are discharged from the surgeon's supervision.

---

seen had preoperative symptoms of a pelvic floor abnormality with difficulty in defecation—not clear symptoms of hemorrhoids.

Urinary Retention

Urinary retention is apparently caused by reflex spasm of the pelvic musculature, which may not become evident until the local anesthesia wears off. Often, a patient still under the influence of local anesthesia seems to be doing exceedingly well for the first few hours after operation, only to go into urinary retention later that night. It may be helpful to reduce the fluid load in the perioperative period. When a patient has trouble urinating, an indwelling urinary catheter should be placed and left in place for at least 12 hours. This, in my view, is one of the major reasons for in-hospital observation after treatment of more than one cluster of hemorrhoids. Placement of the indwelling catheter is of particular importance for the patient's well-being, even if it is not looked on with favor by managed care administrators. Urinary retention is a frightening experience for the patient to undergo at home. What is more, if placement of an indwelling catheter is postponed for 12 to 24 hours, recovery may be delayed. Again, it is important to remember that urinary retention may be an early sign of pelvic infection.

Stricture

Stricture, with or without ectropion, results from circumferential excision of hemorrhoids. I mention this point only to discourage the performance of this procedure.

OUTCOME EVALUATION

Because hemorrhoids are treated only when symptoms—bleeding, prolapse, pain, and difficulty with hygiene—are present, success is determined simply by the extent to which the symptoms are alleviated. If other symptoms were present before operation and persist after the procedure, the primary diagnosis should be called into question. Many elderly patients with a single prolapsing hemorrhoid that causes bleeding or maceration of the perianal skin are well served by outpatient ligation; occasionally, there is a second cluster that requires treatment some months later.

The basic point is that any patient treated surgically for hemorrhoids should experience symptomatic relief. With newer surgical techniques and improved methods of postoperative management, there is no reason for the patient to experience the severe pain described by those who have undergone extensive excisional procedures.

Operative Management of Abscess and Fistula

The conditions that cause suppurative processes in the anoperineum are cryptoglandular abscess and fistula, Crohn's disease, and hidradenitis suppurativa [see Sidebar Disease Processes That Cause Anorectal Abscess and Fistula in Ano]. Accurate diagnosis is essential for proper surgical management. Although these conditions may appear similar at times, each one is managed somewhat differently.

OPERATIVE PLANNING

The most important initial step is to determine the activity and severity of the disease process and the immune status of the patient. For example, a large, fluctuant abscess surrounded by erythema, induration, and superficial necrosis of the skin in an insulin-dependent diabetic is a surgical emergency. On the other hand, a chronic abscess or fistula that drains periodically over a matter of months is not nearly as urgent a problem. Multiple fistula tracts to the perineum in a patient with Crohn's disease require that one perform an adequate study of the intestinal tract and the sphincter mechanism before attempting definitive surgical treatment. It is important to determine the etiology of the process whenever possible. Unfortunately, the determination cannot always be made without examination under anesthesia, during which treatment as well as diagnosis could be accomplished, and this complicates the obtaining of informed consent and the choice of anesthesia.

It is also important to gain as accurate a picture as possible of the complexity of the disease process; this facilitates the planning of the procedure, the choice of anesthesia, and the selection of the information given to patient and family before treatment. For example, in the absence of other significant health problems, a small, well-localized, low intersphincteric abscess often can be easily drained with the patient under local anesthesia if an internal opening can be seen preoperatively on anoscopy, although on occasion even this procedure calls for spinal or epidural anesthesia. (It should be remembered that use of the prone-flexed position [*see Figure 2*], which is my preference, makes general anesthesia more difficult.) Multiple infected tracts associated with undrained infectious foci in a case of rectal Crohn's disease necessitate examination with the patient under spinal or epidural anesthesia. The treating surgeon should perform careful anoscopy and sigmoidoscopy and conservative temporary drainage procedures until consultation with a specialist can be arranged. Severe destruction and suspected deep tissue necrosis, especially in immunocompromised patients, may necessitate extensive resection of tissue and perhaps a completely diverting colostomy.

Bowel preparation should include mechanical cleansing and antibiotics but may not be possible when the situation is urgent (as is most often the case). Appropriate antibiotic coverage (i.e., agents effective against gram-negative organisms and anaerobes) is indicated for all but the simplest cases, with special consideration given to patients who require prophylaxis because of cardiac disease or the presence of prosthetic material.[1] Usually, a urinary catheter should be inserted before operation, especially if the infectious process is located in the anterior region in a man, where the urethra is at risk for injury.

OPERATIVE TECHNIQUE

Many technical elements are common to all operations for conditions that cause suppurative processes in the perineum. The patient should be in the prone-flexed position, with the buttocks taped apart. Conduction anesthesia (spinal, caudal, or epidural) is usually required. The perineum should be examined carefully with an eye to areas of abscess or external drainage sites. Endoscopic examination of the anus, the rectum, and the vagina should be undertaken to search for primary inflammatory bowel disease, internal openings of the fistula, or vaginal openings of the fistula.

Cryptoglandular Abscess and Fistula

The abscess must be located and characterized because drainage will depend on the location of the abscess, the course of the fistula tract, and any related infectious processes [*see Figure 8*]. It is important not to create a fistula through the levator plate of the pelvic floor. This means that an abscess with a low origin must be drained low, with care taken to avoid iatrogenic perforation of the rectum, and an abscess with a high origin (e.g., a high intersphincteric abscess) must be drained high by incising the mucosa and the longitudinal (internal sphincter) muscle of the rectal wall (not a procedure for the occasional rectal surgeon). The internal opening—that is, the crypt where the abscess originated—must be sought; this is best done by means of anoscopy, very careful probing, and sigmoidoscopy to rule out a high source (e.g., Crohn's disease). If the internal opening is found,

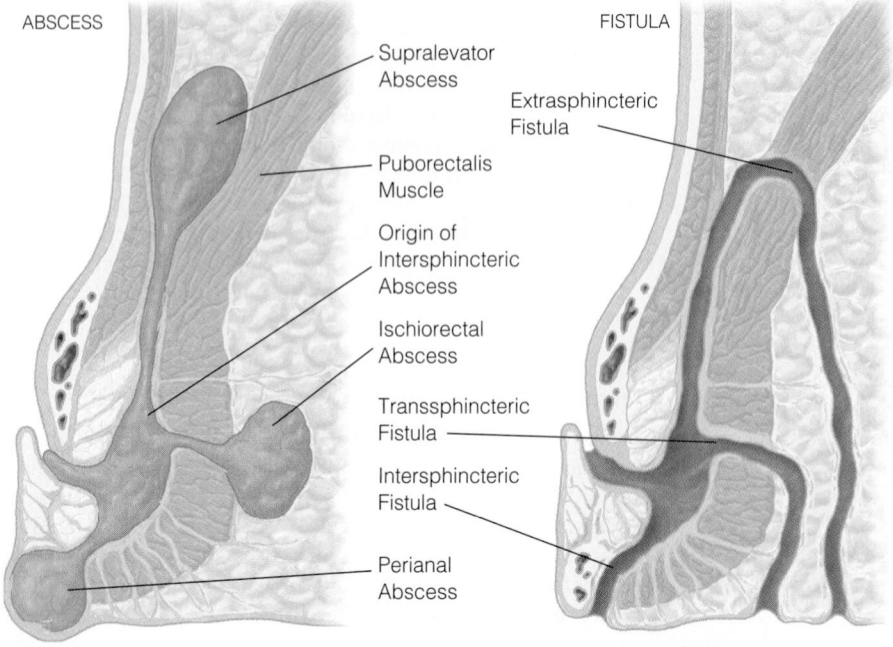

Figure 8 **Abscess and fistula are, respectively, the acute aspect and the chronic aspect of a single disease process. Acute inflammation can lead to different types of abscesses (left), depending on the direction in which the inflammation extends. Chronic inflammation leads to communication of the abscess sites with the surface—that is, fistula tracts (right).**

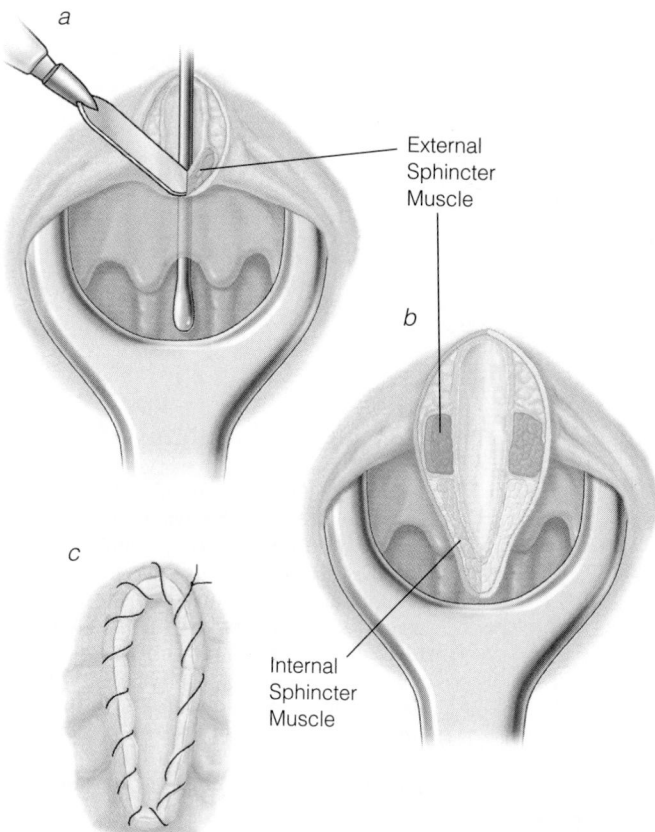

Figure 9 Operative management of abscess and fistula. Shown is a fistulotomy in a patient with cryptoglandular abscess/fistula. (*a*) The fistula tract is carefully probed, a decision is made about which muscle and how much muscle to cut, and the tract is incised. (*b*) Once the tract is open, the involved crypt is excised. (*c*) The defect is marsupialized by sewing skin to the tract.

Figure 10 Operative management of abscess and fistula. Shown is drainage of an ischiorectal abscess. Such abscesses may be palpated above the anorectal ring, even though their location is more inferior. (*a*) The abscess is incised. (*b*) A mushroom-tipped catheter is placed.

the abscess can be drained or a fistulotomy can be performed [*see Figure 9*]. With a fistulotomy, determination of safety is a paramount concern. Careful consideration must be given to which muscle—and how much of the muscle—is to be cut. The anterior location in a woman is especially precarious. If the fistula involves a significant amount of muscle, or any muscle in the anterior region in a woman, either a seton should be placed or a drain should be placed without disruption of the muscle, in preparation for advancement flap closure of the internal opening.

If the internal opening is not found, one should not make one by probing. The abscess should be drained with a mushroom-tipped catheter [*see Figure 10*]; this is preferable to unroofing and eliminates painful packing. The catheter can be left in place for an extended period, and it permits subsequent injection of dye or contrast material. Once the mushroom catheter is in place in the OR, the surgeon can inject diluted methylene blue to search again for internal openings, which, if found, allow one to consider fistulotomy. The drain is usually sutured in place. The patient should be seen a few days after the operation to confirm that the abscess is adequately drained.

After 2 weeks, the patient is seen in the office, and povidone-iodine is injected through the drain while the inside of the anal canal is inspected via an anoscope. If an internal opening is seen, then fistulotomy is planned. If no internal opening is seen (as is the case in about 50% of patients), the drain should be removed 1 week later. This allows any irritant effect of the povidone-iodine to resolve and prevents the abscess from recurring.

If the fistula tract is known to have an external opening and fistulotomy is planned, the following approach should be considered. First of all, fistulectomy is never indicated. Fistulotomy is performed rarely and with great caution in the face of Crohn's disease. To perform the fistulotomy, one must first find the internal opening. In this regard, Goodsall's rule is often helpful: external fistula openings anterior to the midanal line are usually connected to internal openings via short, straight tracts, whereas external openings posterior to this line usually follow a curved course to internal openings in the posterior midline. Dilute methylene blue is injected through the external opening, often via a plastic I.V. catheter.

Careful probing, perhaps with a lacrimal duct probe, is then carried out. If the internal opening still cannot be found, a drain is placed so that the surgeon can return at another time to search for the internal opening. If the internal opening is found, a probe is passed and an effort is made to determine how much muscle and which muscle must be transected to accomplish the fistulotomy and how much muscle will remain to maintain continence [*see Figure 11*].

If the surgeon is not sure of the extent of muscle involvement or of how safe a fistulotomy would be, the infectious process should be drained, and either the patient should be referred to a specialist, or plans should be made for an advancement flap procedure to close the internal opening. If a fistulotomy is done, a biopsy specimen should be obtained from the infected tract, and the tract should be marsupialized to prevent premature healing of the superficial aspect.

It is important to keep in mind that the sphincter mechanism is innervated by a branch of the pudendal nerve that enters the sphincter from the posterolateral aspect. Accordingly, extreme caution must be exercised when a deep fistulotomy is required in the posterolateral perianal quadrants.

There is a growing body of evidence suggesting that injection of commercially available fibrin glue is effective for treatment of fistulas in perianal tissue. Longer tracts appear to respond bet-

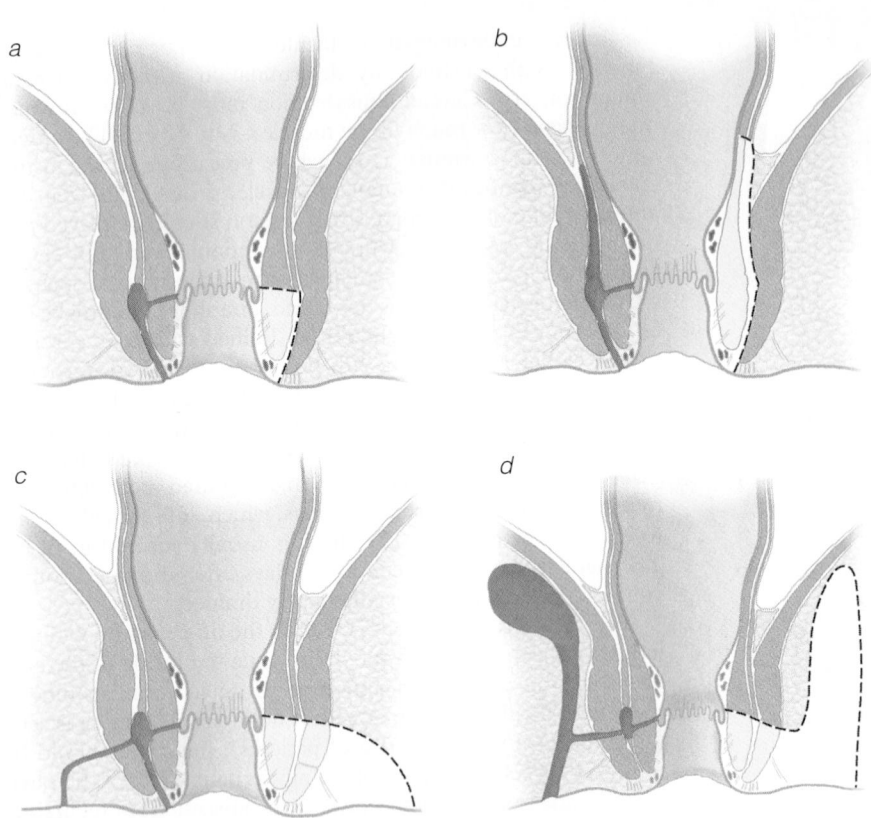

Figure 11 Operative management of abscess and fistula. Shown are examples of the different types of fistulotomies indicated for some of the many types of fistulas: intersphincteric fistula with a simple low tract (*a*), intersphincteric fistula with a high blind tract (*b*), uncomplicated transsphincteric fistula (*c*), and transsphincteric fistula with a high blind tract (*d*). In each image, the left half of the drawing shows the disease process, and the right half illustrates the recommended operation.

ter to this modality than shorter tracts do. The long-term efficacy of this approach remains to be proved.

Special problems   A cryptoglandular abscess that extends into the posterior anal and posterior rectal spaces is often missed as a source of infection. Diagnosis of such abscesses typically involves bidigital examination, often with the patient under anesthesia; needle aspiration may be required as well. Fistulotomy in this area often necessitates opening large amounts of tissue, including partial transection of the sphincter muscle; the tract

may also have to be marsupialized. If one is unsure of the anatomy or has never done the procedure before, the abscess should be drained as simply as possible and the patient referred to a specialist.

The so-called horseshoe abscess [*see Figure 12*] results from an undiagnosed posterior-space abscess that has dissected laterally and may have been drained several times through the lateral extension into one or both ischiorectal fossae. This condition is cured by opening the posterior space and placing a long-term lateral drain, after which healing proceeds by secondary intention (the so-called Hanley procedure). The drain should not be

Figure 12 Operative management of abscess and fistula. Shown is the surgical treatment of a horseshoe fistula. (*a*) The main posterior tract of the fistula is identified by probing. (*b*) The posterior tract is opened, and drains are placed laterally. (*c*) The posterior tract is marsupialized.

removed until there is solid healing in the posterior midline; this may take weeks or even months.

Abscess and Fistula Associated with Crohn's Disease

The goals of treatment are to drain and control the focus of infection, to preserve sphincter function, to plan and implement a staged approach to preservation of anorectal function, and to make the correct diagnosis. To these ends, careful identification of the location and course of the abscess and any associated fistulas is essential; this is accomplished via endoscopic dye injection, probing, and vaginoscopy.

The safest approach, in my view, is to place mushroom catheters in abscesses and complicated fistula tracts or, in some cases, to use setons to allow drainage of the fistulas (not to cut through the tissue, which is often the intended result of seton placement) [see Figure 13]. For optimal resolution of inflammation at the site of the internal opening in anticipation of a possible advancement flap procedure, perirectal mushroom catheters are preferable to setons placed through the internal opening. Superficial fistula tracts may occasionally be managed with fistulotomy if the Crohn's disease is otherwise inactive. Sphincterotomy is never indicated in a patient with Crohn's disease if severe infection is present or the disease is active. When a patient is known or believed to have Crohn's disease, biopsy of the edematous external skin tags that are often present can be a good way of finding granulomatous tissue to confirm the diagnosis.

The newer forms of medical treatment of Crohn's disease, in which a monoclonal antibody to tumor necrosis factor (infliximab) is given either by itself or in combination with immunosuppressive agents, seem to display some of their most beneficial results in patients with complicated anoperineal fistulas. In my view, a good way of managing abscess and fistula associated with Crohn's disease is for the surgeon to drain and control the suppurative process and for the gastroenterologist then to employ the latest medical regimen to force the disease into remission.

Hidradenitis Suppurativa

Patients with infected fistula tracts or abscesses secondary to hidradenitis suppurativa must be positioned in such a way as to allow visualization of and access to all tracts. This is crucial because some of the tracts may extend into the scrotum, the labia, the inguinal areas, or the suprapubic area. Conduction anesthesia is important in that it covers broad areas of the perineum; adequate local anesthesia is impossible unless one is dealing with very small, isolated tracts.

The definitive therapeutic surgical procedure is incision (rather than excision) of these often extensive inflammatory tracts [see Figure 14]. The surgeon should do as much as possible at one time, with the understanding that it is not unusual to leave a few tracts undrained or to return later to address new areas of dissection. Because the primary disease process does not involve the sphincter, intestinal diversion is rarely indicated. Biopsy is indicated because on rare occasions, these long infected tracts exhibit malignant changes or result from an anal malignancy. The perineal skin can tolerate the extensive incisions necessary to cure the process. Special precautions must be taken not only to preserve the sphincter itself but also to avoid damaging the neurovascular bundle that enters the anus from the posterolateral aspect. In male patients, efforts must be made to avoid the urethra during incision in the anterior midline; to this end, a Foley catheter should always be placed before the surgical procedure is begun. Because so many incised skin edges remain after treatment of extensive hidradenitis, it is imperative to achieve adequate hemostasis. The disposable suction cautery units currently available can be especially helpful for this purpose. The wounds may be either left open or loosely packed until good granulation tissue forms.

Bathing the perineum, especially after a bowel movement, is helpful. Often, showers are better for this purpose than the portable minuscule sitz baths commonly used. For patients who have undergone extensive procedures, twice-daily trips to a whirlpool bath (often located in the physical therapy department) are helpful. Despite the multiple lengthy incisions, there is usually little pain, and most of the postoperative care can be done at home. Adequate follow-up is necessary to treat residual or new areas of disease before the dissection becomes extensive again. Care must be taken, especially in the OR, to search for the infected tracts, which may contain little pus

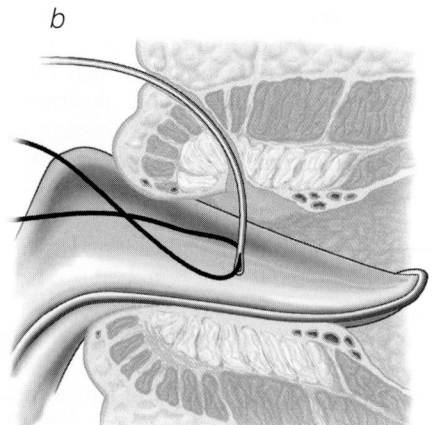

a   b

Figure 13 **Operative management of abscess and fistula. Shown are alternatives for treating abscess or fistula associated with Crohn's disease. In Crohn's disease, multiple perianal and perineal fistulas and abscesses may be seen, often in atypical locations. (*a*) Abscesses may be drained by placing a small mushroom-tipped catheter as close to the anus as possible. A Malecot catheter should not be used. (*b*) In some settings, it is appropriate to place a seton between internal and external openings. This seton may then be left in situ for a time for drainage and for prevention of further disease progression.**

Figure 14 **Operative management of abscess and fistula. In this patient, the causative condition is hidradenitis suppurativa. (*a*) Multiple openings of sinus tracts can be seen and extensive indurated tracts palpated. (*b*) Abscesses are unroofed. (*c*) Indurated tracts are probed. (*d*) All tracts are identified and incised.**

and may be apparent only as indurated cords within the perineal skin.

TROUBLESHOOTING

Most of the important steps for avoiding problems have already been described in the course of addressing preoperative planning and operative technique (see above). The goals in the treatment of all of the processes associated with anorectal abscess and fistula in ano are to preserve sphincter function, to control acute infection, and to eliminate the source of the infection. If it is likely that sphincter function will be compromised at all, a baseline level of sphincter function (including the status of muscles and nerves) must be determined before any surgical procedure is initiated. One should never hesitate to perform an examination with the patient under anesthesia and to inject dilute methylene blue to delineate the extent and location of the infectious process.

Anyone embarking on surgical management of such processes must keep in mind the option of performing an advancement flap procedure to close the internal opening, especially in the anterior region and most particularly in women. If such a procedure is planned, initial drainage should be done external to the rectum with a mushroom catheter rather than through the internal opening with a seton. Simple 3-0 chromic catgut should be used to marsupialize fistula tracts because employing the newer, less quickly absorbable materials may lead to a chronic nidus that gives rise to ongoing infection. Patients should be watched closely in the immediate postoperative period to ensure that all infection is controlled. Not uncommonly, a superficial collection is drained, but a deeper abscess remains that must be sought more aggressively.

One should always take into account the risk of anoperineal infection in immunocompromised patients. Given that the anatomy of the anal tissue planes is complex and can be rendered even more so by multiple surgical procedures, one should not venture beyond one's level of expertise. One should never hesitate to drain an infectious focus with a simple mushroom-tipped catheter and, if appropriate, refer the patient to a colon and rectal surgical specialist who is trained to manage complex anoperineal suppurative processes safely and definitively.

COMPLICATIONS

Complications occur if one or more of the goals just mentioned (see above) have not been achieved. Persistent or recurrent infection is seen with some frequency. In patients with cryptoglandular abscess or fistula, infection usually results from failure to locate the internal opening or to discover a deep posterior midline abscess; such failure is often seen in patients with a horseshoe abscess, in whom repeated lateral drainage procedures may have been undertaken without the primary cavity in the posterior anal or posterior rectal space being discovered and dealt with.

In patients with Crohn's disease, infection can persist if a deeper pocket or extension has gone undiscovered or if the disease has recurred, leading to further penetration and infection in the anoperineum or the perirectal tissue. Extensive examination with the patient under anesthesia, including transrectal ultrasonography or CT scanning, may be required to determine the source and extent of the infection. It is always possible that the infection derives from a superlevator abscess secondary to intestinal disease; consequently, a detailed evaluation of the intestinal tract is indicated in patients with Crohn's disease.

In patients with hidradenitis suppurativa, the most common problems are residual undrained tracts and recurrent disease. Again, examination with the patient under anesthesia and repeated drainage are called for. Because this disease process does not originate in the rectum, care must be taken not to enter the rectum or to cut any of the nerves entering the anus from the posterolateral aspect. It has been reported anecdotally that very chronic or persistent fistula tracts may eventually exhibit malignant changes (squamous cell carcinoma); for this reason, such tracts should be biopsied.

OUTCOME EVALUATION

No sophisticated surveillance is necessary: if drainage persists or some degree of incontinence develops, the patient usually will volunteer the information freely. Either of these complaints could be an indication for a detailed examination, including a sophisticated evaluation of sphincter function.

Figure 15 **Operative management of ulcer/fissure disease. Anal fissure (left) and anal ulcer (right) are, respectively, the acute aspect and the chronic aspect of a single disease process.**

Operative Management of Ulcer/Fissure Disease

Ulcer and fissure are two aspects of a single anorectal disease process with an unclearly defined pathophysiology [*see Figure 15*]. Accurate diagnosis is crucial [*see Sidebar* Ulcer/Fissure Disease: Diagnosis and Treatment]. Not uncommonly, patients are treated for hemorrhoids when the true primary condition is ulcer/fissure disease.

OPERATIVE PLANNING

Fundamental concerns in planning the operation—besides confirming the diagnosis—are to verify that there are no other conditions that could threaten complete healing of an incision in the anal tissue and to make sure that there is no significant incontinence before the sphincterotomy.

For example, a history of diarrhea compatible with the presence of inflammatory bowel disease indicates the need for further evaluation to eliminate the possibility of Crohn's disease; if Crohn's disease is present, the risk of poor healing is greater, and it will be necessary to preserve all of the available sphincter function of the anus for a long period. As another example, a woman who has borne children by vaginal delivery and has any degree of incontinence should undergo manometry, ultrasonography, and perhaps electromyography to confirm that the sphincter is not compromised by a mechanical or neurologic deficiency. Yet another example is a patient with irritable bowel syndrome or a pelvic floor abnormality who experiences a multitude of difficulties with bowel movements. It is important to recognize such conditions and to advise the patient of the need for special attention to maintain adequate bowel function in the postoperative period.

It is essential to clearly explain the nature of the operative procedure (i.e., the incision of a portion of the internal sphincter mechanism) to the patient and to warn him or her that minor incontinence of flatus may persist for as long as a few months postoperatively. To be fair, significant incontinence is highly unusual: in fact, most patients experience very rapid relief of their often distressing symptoms. One should also advise the patient that any other anal procedures that may be indicated (e.g., elastic ligation of internal hemorrhoids or excision of symptomatic external hemorrhoids) can and should be accomplished at the time of sphincterotomy, with or without excision of the anal ulcer, and that he or she should take 3 to 5 days off from work. The risk of urinary

---

Ulcer/Fissure Disease: Diagnosis and Treatment

This condition is a very common one; however, the pathophysiology remains unclearly defined. Like abscess and fistula, ulcer/fissure disease has an acute phase and a chronic phase.

A fissure (the acute phase) results from a tear in the tissue at the mucocutaneous junction of the anal canal. The cause is usually a hard bowel movement that stretches the anal opening and tears the tissue. In fact, fissures are also seen in patients with persistent diarrhea. The anal canal has an extremely rich blood supply, and most fissures heal with bowel control (i.e., bulk-forming agents and stool softeners), warm soaks, and mild analgesics. Patients must be assured that although the condition is extremely painful and is associated with some degree of bleeding, it is not a significant health threat.

For reasons that are not clear, perhaps as many as 50% of fissures do not heal spontaneously. As the opening persists, the surrounding tissue becomes hypertrophied and the process extends into the underlying internal sphincter muscle as an ulcer (the chronic phase) with a sentinel hemorrhoidal tag and a hypertrophied anal papilla (the triad of findings typical of an anal ulcer). Spasm and hypertrophy of the lower third of the internal sphincter muscle of the anal canal are always associated with this condition. Many believe, as I do, that spasm of this involuntary muscle results in diminishment of the blood supply to the anal canal and subsequent poor healing of the acute tear. It seems that as the process persists, the ulcer burrows deeper. The condition then becomes more painful, and the muscular spasm evolves into actual hypertrophy. At present, optimal therapy is based on the principle of incising the hypertrophied band of muscle, releasing the spasm, and improving the relative ischemia, thus allowing the injury to heal.

Ulcer/fissure disease can usually be diagnosed on the basis of the typical history of sudden onset of anal pain (often with a tearing sensation) and bleeding. Symptoms are usually exacerbated during bowel movements and may go on for weeks to months with intermit-

tent healing and recrudescence of the process as the ischemia prevents solid, definitive healing. Diagnosis is complicated in that digital rectal examination can be extremely painful, and most physicians do not have the equipment and skills to perform an adequate anoscopic examination. If examination is too painful, local anesthesia may be necessary. Diagnosis can be facilitated by passage of a lubricated cotton swab to look for the typical streak of blood from the ulcer.

Medical treatment is often begun before the specific diagnosis can be verified. I usually try 2 weeks of medical therapy, often including topical antibiotics and anti-inflammatory suppositories or foam preparations. Once the diagnosis is confirmed, it becomes the patient's choice whether or when to undergo surgical treatment. I explain that the reason for the operation is to relieve discomfort, not to cure a life-threatening condition; however, I also point out that once significant spasm and hypertrophy of the sphincter are identified, definitive cure is unlikely unless a sphincterotomy is performed.

Recently, there has been some enthusiasm for alleviating the muscle spasm and hypertrophy and the subsequent ischemia by using medical rather than surgical measures. The most popular medical approaches are (1) topical application of a low-concentration nitroglycerin paste (a much less concentrated preparation than that used to treat cardiac conditions) and (2) local injection of botulinum toxin. The initial enthusiasm for these modalities notwithstanding, it remains to be seen whether they provide any long-term benefit in comparison with anal sphincterotomy. In addition, some reports have described the use of oral diltiazem to reduce sphincter spasm and ischemia. Again, it remains to be seen whether this approach consistently leads to long-term resolution of the pathologic process.

In my own experience, when a fissure is present, resolution can be achieved with any of a number of nonsurgical maneuvers; however, when an ulcer with muscle hypertrophy is present, surgical management ultimately proves necessary for resolution.

retention, pain, and bleeding must also be discussed. In planning the operative procedure and immediate postoperative care, one must take into account the patient's specific needs, idiosyncrasies, and home environment. Some patients are comfortable undergoing the procedure completely on an outpatient basis, whereas others clearly need to be admitted for short-term observation and parenteral administration of pain medication.

When possible, I keep patients on a liquid diet for 24 hours before operation and use small, self-administered enemas to empty the rectum immediately before the procedure. I advise patients to discontinue any aspirin-containing products and any other anticoagulants, if possible, at least 10 days beforehand.

OPERATIVE TECHNIQUE

Operative treatment of ulcer/fissure disease consists of a posterior lateral internal anal sphincterotomy, in which the internal sphincter is divided but the external sphincter, the anoderm, and the longitudinal muscle remain intact. I generally prefer to place the patient in the prone-flexed position with the buttocks taped apart and adequate local anesthesia in place. The operation can then be performed in one of three ways: (1) as a closed procedure involving the use of a No. 11 blade and digital palpation of the muscle [see Figure 16], (2) as an open procedure without direct visualization of the muscle, or (3) as an open procedure with clear identification of the muscle before its transection. The third option is the one I prefer.

An open procedure with visualization of the muscle is done as follows [see Figure 17]. The first step is anoscopy, preferably with a medium Hill-Ferguson instrument. The hypertrophied band of the lower third of the internal sphincter muscle is clearly identified. If this band is not a distinctly identifiable entity, sphincterotomy should not be performed. The ulcer or fissure itself need not be present, because the disease may be in a relatively inactive state at the time of surgery.

Rigid or flexible sigmoidoscopy should then be performed if it was not done in the immediate preoperative period. The primary purpose of this step is to make sure that no features of Crohn's disease are visible in the rectum. When the endoscopic examination is complete, I usually repeat the preparation of the anal opening.

A 1 cm incision is made in the posterior lateral aspect of the perianal skin, hemostasis is obtained, and a delicate dissection is done with a curved hemostat in the intersphincteric plane. The posterior midline is avoided because healing in this position may result in scar tissue that interferes with perfect continence (the so-called keyhole deformity). The white hypertrophied band of muscle is then elevated into the wound with a curved hemostat. If a rent is made in the anal mucosa, it must be repaired with 3-0 chromic catgut. The band of muscle is then incised with the electrocautery, and pressure is maintained for a few minutes to ensure hemostasis. Digital examination confirms adequate transection of the band. The skin is left open.

Attention is then directed to the ulcer, which may be excised sharply in an elliptical fashion so as to incorporate the entire triad of the ulcer (i.e., the ulcer itself, the sentinel hemorrhoidal tag, and the hypertrophied anal papilla) while avoiding additional transection of the underlying muscle. If I excise the ulcer complex, I usually close the wound with a continuous three-point suture of 3-0 chromic catgut to obliterate any dead space and thus to lower the risk of postoperative infection.

Any additional anal surgery required is then completed, the surgical site is covered with antibiotic ointment, and a very light gauze bandage is applied with a minimum of tape and traction on the perianal skin.

Figure 16 **Operative management of ulcer/fissure disease. Shown is the closed approach to posterior lateral internal sphincterotomy. A No. 11 blade is inserted in the intersphincteric groove and moved upward to the level of the dentate line. Medial movement of the blade divides a portion of the internal sphincter muscle. The anoderm and the other anal muscles are not divided.**

TROUBLESHOOTING

To perform this simple procedure well, one must have a clear understanding of the surgical anatomy of the anal canal and must be able to clearly identify the internal sphincter, the intersphincteric groove, and the external sphincter muscle. The hypertrophied band of muscle must be accurately identified and cleanly transected. No attempt should be made to extend or amplify the procedure by stretching the anal canal and thus bursting the muscle.

Although the procedure and anatomy are simple, the best way of learning the operation is to watch an experienced surgeon perform it. I do not believe this procedure can be learned through reading alone.

COMPLICATIONS

Because the internal sphincter muscle is responsible for resting, involuntary continence, injury to this structure can lead to nocturnal incontinence. Again, special caution is advised with respect to the anterior aspect of the anoperineum in women. On the other hand, incising the posterior midline can also lead to the keyhole deformity, which may cause prolonged anal seepage because of the configuration of the scar tissue; a good analogy is a bent rim on a tubeless tire. It is tempting to close the tiny skin incision at the site of sphincterotomy, but I think it should be left open to reduce the already low risk of infection.

There should be very little postoperative pain. If the patient does complain of significant pain, especially in the presence of fever or urinary hesitancy, one must assume that infection is present in the anoperineum, a structure that is normally highly

a   *b*   *c*

Figure 17   **Operative management of ulcer/fissure disease. Shown is the open approach to posterior lateral internal sphincterotomy. (*a*) The triad of the ulcer complex is visualized. (*b*) Once the hypertrophied band of internal sphincter muscle is identified, a 1 cm incision is made in the posterolateral aspect of the perianal skin. (*c*) The hypertrophied band is elevated into the wound and divided with the electrocautery.**

resistant to microbial invasion. Urgent evaluation, removal of sutures, antibiotic therapy, bowel rest, placement of a urinary catheter, and very close observation in the hospital are indicated.

The major causes of complications are incorrect diagnosis of the disease process (especially overlooking the presence of Crohn's disease) and failure to fully understand the anatomy of the continence mechanism of the anal canal. If too much of the internal sphincter muscle is cut, if this muscle is already compromised, or if the external sphincter muscle is transected by mistake, the patient will be rendered incontinent. On the other hand, if not enough of the internal muscle is transected, the ulcer will not heal and the symptoms will persist.

Overall, the single most common cause of complications that I have observed is the failure even to suspect, much less diagnose, ulcer/fissure disease as the source of a patient's symptoms. I frequently see patients who seem to have failed to heal months after a hemorrhoidectomy. When their symptoms are reviewed and a thorough examination performed, it becomes apparent that the underlying disease process was always ulcer/fissure dis-

ease rather than hemorrhoids and that the hemorrhoidectomy only intensified the anal pain and bleeding. These patients are finally cured when an adequate sphincterotomy is performed.

In very rare instances, drainage continues at the site of the sphincterotomy. If drainage persists for weeks, the patient should be examined under appropriate anesthesia, and the focus of infection should be opened. This is essentially equivalent to a very superficial fistulotomy.

OUTCOME EVALUATION

Again, no sophisticated surveillance is necessary: when the patient returns 2 weeks after the procedure, free of pain and bleeding and able to have bowel movements without difficulty, one may be sure that an acceptable outcome has been achieved. Digital rectal examination should confirm good healing and normal sphincter tone (both while resting and while contracting). For additional confirmation, I have patients continue to take bulk-forming agents and stool softeners and then examine them 1 month later to verify that healing is complete.

References

1. Practice parameters for antibiotic prophylaxis to prevent infective endocarditis or infected prosthesis during colon and rectal endoscopy. Standards Practice Task Force, American Society of Colon and Rectal Surgeons. Dis Colon Rectum 35:277, 1992

2. Kodner IJ, Fry RD, Fleshman JW, et al: Colon, rectum and anus. Principles of Surgery, 6th ed. Schwartz SI, Ed. McGraw-Hill, New York, 1994

Recommended Reading

Corman ML: Colon and Rectal Surgery, 3rd ed. JB Lippincott Co, Philadelphia, 1993

Fry RD, Kodner IJ: Anorectal disorders. Clin Symp 37:6, 1985

Gordon PH, Nivatvongs S: Principles and Practice of Surgery for the Colon, Rectum and Anus. Quality Medical Publishers, St. Louis, 1992

Keighley MRB, Williams NS: Surgery of the Anus, Rectum and Colon, Vols 1 and 2. WB Saunders, London, 1993

Kodner IJ: Differential diagnosis and management of benign anorectal diseases. Gastrointestinal Diseases Today 5:8, 1996

Standards Practice Task Force, American Society of Colon and Rectal Surgeons: Practice parameters for treatment of fistula-in-ano. Dis Colon Rectum 39:1361, 1996

Acknowledgment

Figures 1, 5b, 5c, 8 through 13, 15, 16   Tom Moore. Adapted from original illustrations by John Craig.

20 OPEN REPAIR OF HERNIAS OF THE ABDOMINAL WALL

George E. Wantz, M.D.

Hernias of the abdominal wall are a major recurrent surgical problem. New techniques, modifications of established methods, and even the introduction of synthetic prosthetic screens have not perfected the repair of this type of hernia. Another factor affecting the outcome of a hernia, as in all operations, is the skill and experience of the surgeon.

Classification of Hernias of the Groin

Traditionally, hernias of the groin have been described and classified on the basis of the anterior clinical presentation of the hernial sac (i.e., indirect inguinal, direct inguinal, and femoral). From the posterior, however, this classification is irrelevant because only the neck of the hernial sac and the parietal defect can be seen [*see Figure 1*].

Many attempts to classify hernias and to stage the degree of parietal deterioration have been devised.[1-5] Unfortunately, although the intent of such categorization is to promote a common surgical understanding, the classifications are incomplete and lack unanimity. Until accord is reached, hernias should be described on the basis of the volume of the sac and the location, size, and type of the parietal defect (e.g., a large indirect inguinal hernia with a 3 cm parietal defect).

Fruchaud[6] introduced a concept that unified the various hernias of the groin and simplified our understanding of them. Rather than defining hernias by their clinical presentation, he defined them by their origin and emphasized that all hernias of the groin, no matter the type, begin in a single weak area he called the myopectineal orifice (MPO). Until recently, this concept of groin hernias was little appreciated by surgeons in English-speaking countries.[6,7]

The MPO, a bony muscular framework, is bridged and bisected by the inguinal ligament, traversed by the femoral vessels and the spermatic cord, and sealed on its inner surface by the transverse fascia (endopelvic fascia). The integrity of the MPO depends on the strength of the transverse fascia. A hernia occurs when a peritoneal sac protrudes through the MPO; failure of the transverse fascia to retain the peritoneum is the fundamental cause of all hernias of the groin.

The inguinal ligament along with its recurved lacunar-shaped insertion on the pecten, although only loosely attached to the underlying structures, strongly braces the MPO, serves as the dividing line separating inguinal from femoral hernias, and defines the medial border of the orifice of the femoral canal.

A persistent processus vaginalis peritonei predisposes men and women to indirect inguinal herniation. The descent of the testicle through the abdominal wall predisposes men to direct inguinal herniation. This passage weakens the superior portion of the MPO and changes the function of the inferior portion of the internal oblique abdominal muscle from that of a protective muscle that embraces the floor of the inguinal canal to that of a suspensory muscle of the testicle (cremaster muscle) that embraces the spermatic cord. In women, the increased diameter of the true pelvis compared with that in men proportionately widens the femoral canal and probably predisposes them to femoral herniation.

Essentials of Groin Hernioplasty

Restoring the integrity of the MPO prevents peritoneal protrusion and repairs the hernia. This task may be accomplished in two fundamentally different ways: (1) repairing the parietal defect and (2) replacing the deficient transverse fascia with a synthetic prosthesis.

Access to the MPO may be anterior, through a groin incision, or posterior, through an abdominal incision [*see Figure 2*]. Exposure of the bony and musculoaponeurotic borders of the MPO by the anterior approach requires dissection of the inguinal canal, spermatic cord, and sensory nerves of the groin; by the posterior approach, only reflection of the peritoneum is necessary.

Tension on the suture line is the enemy of successful hernia surgery and must be diligently avoided. Suture tension causes tissue necrosis and, hence, parietal defects and recurrences. It also increases postoperative pain. Sutures must never be drawn up so tightly as to indent tissues.

Permanent synthetic prostheses, usually in the form of a mesh, are now widely employed in the management of hernias of the abdominal wall. At first, there was concern that synthetic prostheses would act like foreign bodies and would easily become infected, but they have not proved to be the bugbear surgeons previously thought they might be.

Finally, recurrence rates may not be a proper measure of the success of classic and prosthetic hernioplasties, because too many variables are involved in hernia recurrence. The outcome of hernia repair depends on the quality of the surgery, the integrity of the tissues, and the amount of suture tension, not on the chosen technique.

Figure 1 Anterior view (top) and posterior view (bottom) of the aponeurosis of the transverse abdominal muscle and the transverse fascia are shown.[53]

Classic Hernioplasties

The classic hernioplasties remain popular and produce excellent results (overall recurrence rates of one to three percent) when expertly performed in appropriate patients.[8-10] Knowledge of the classic hernioplasties is important because they embody the surgical principles and techniques applicable to prosthetic repair.

Only three classic hernioplasties are still in use: the Marcy repair, also known as the simple ring closure; the Bassini repair, either in its original form or in the form developed at the Shouldice Hospital in Toronto; and the Cooper's ligament repair, also known as the McVay-Lotheissen hernioplasty. The three hernioplasties preserve the shutter mechanism of the deep inguinal ring and the obliquity of the inguinal canal; they differ only in the extent to which the MPO is repaired.

OPERATIVE TECHNIQUE

The classic hernioplasties have three stages, namely, dissection, repair, and closure. All use an anterior groin incision.

Dissection

The object of the dissection is to eliminate the hernial sac and to expose the parietal defect in the innermost aponeuroticofascial layer of the abdominal wall. The dissection is performed in several steps. First, the inguinal canal is opened; the ilioinguinal

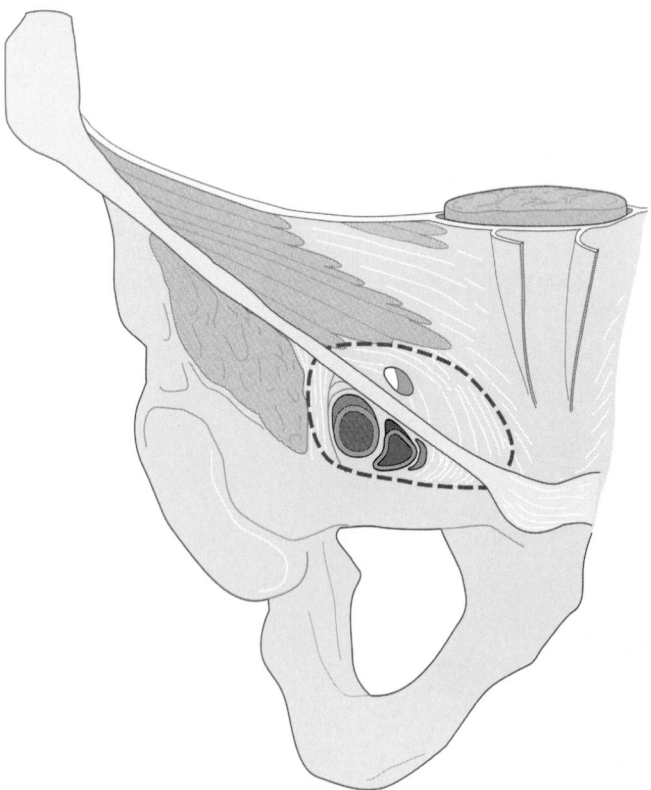

Figure 2 Shown is the anterior view of the myopectineal orifice of Fruchaud. This bony muscular framework is bounded by the iliopsoas muscle, the oblique abdominal muscles, the rectus abdominis muscle, and the pecten of the pubis. It is traversed by the femoral vessels and spermatic cord, bridged by the inguinal ligament, and sealed on the inside by the transverse fascia. Failure of the transverse fascia to retain the peritoneum is the fundamental cause of all hernias of the groin.[53]

Figure 3 Shown is complete anterior dissection of the groin. The spermatic cord has been mobilized and held aside with a Penrose drain. The cremaster muscle and cremaster neurovascular bundle have been divided to enhance the view of the innermost aponeuroticofascial layer of the abdomen. The posterior wall of the inguinal canal has been divided from the deep inguinal ring medially toward the pubic tubercle to a point at which healthy muscle is reached. This division destroys the deep inguinal ring. The transverse aponeurotic arch is an important structure in the repair of hernias and cannot be seen unless the medial flap of the posterior wall is reflected. If a McVay-Lotheissen repair is anticipated, it is also necessary to excise the outlined portion of the iliopubic tract for full exposure of Cooper's ligament and the medial edge of the femoral sheath [*see Figure 4e*].

The aponeurosis of the external oblique muscle is retracted medially to reveal the aponeurosis of the internal oblique muscle. Relaxing incisions are made by vertically incising the aponeurosis of the internal oblique muscle over the belly of the rectus abdominis muscle.

A simple indirect hernial sac is merely divided near the deep inguinal ring, and the distal portion is allowed to remain in situ undissected from the spermatic cord. The proximal portion is dissected from the cord and adjacent structures, ligated or not, and allowed to retract. The spermatic cord should never be dissected beyond the pubic tubercle for fear of damaging the delicate veins of the pampiniform plexus and causing testicular atrophy. The exception to this would be a sliding indirect inguinal hernia when an abdominal viscus is actually a part of the wall of the indirect hernial sac. Sliding indirect hernial sacs and all direct inguinal hernial sacs are simply inverted. Femoral hernial sacs are usually ligated below the inguinal ligament because they are vascular and often contain a lymph node.

a

b

c

Figure 4 (*a*) The Marcy hernioplasty. The deep inguinal ring is tightened and returned to normal size by one or two permanent synthetic monofilament sutures (often called Marcy sutures) placed medially in the transverse aponeurotic arch and laterally in the iliopubic tract or femoral sheath. (*b*) The Bassini hernioplasty. Bassini divided the floor of the inguinal canal as illustrated in Figure 3. Many surgeons omit this step. The three-layer repair consists of approximating with interrupted sutures the internal oblique abdominal muscle, the transverse abdominal muscle, and the transverse fascia to the inguinal ligament and iliopubic tract. (*c*) The Shouldice-Bassini hernioplasty. The floor of the inguinal canal is repaired by imbrication of the innermost aponeurotico-fascial layer of the abdominal wall. The iliopubic tract is fastened to the undersurface of the transverse aponeurotic arch, and the free edge of the transverse aponeurotic arch is attached to the shelving edge of the inguinal ligament with a single continuous to-and-fro monofilament suture. Suturing begins near the pubic tubercle, continues to the deep inguinal ring, and then returns to the starting point. (*d*) The surgeons at the Shouldice Hospital also place a to-and-fro continuous suture affixing the internal oblique abdominal muscle to the inguinal ligament. Most enthusiasts of the technique consider the second suture to be superfluous and therefore leave it out. Sutures should not grasp the periosteum of the pubic tubercle, because this may cause residual postoperative pain. (*e*) The McVay-Lotheissen hernioplasty. This repair consists of attaching the transverse aponeurotic arch to Cooper's ligament, the medial side of the femoral sheath, and the anterior femoral sheath with interrupted sutures. The suture affixing the transverse aponeurotic arch to the medial edge of the femoral sheath is called the transition suture. Relaxing incisions are mandatory[53] [*Figure continued on page 868*].

d

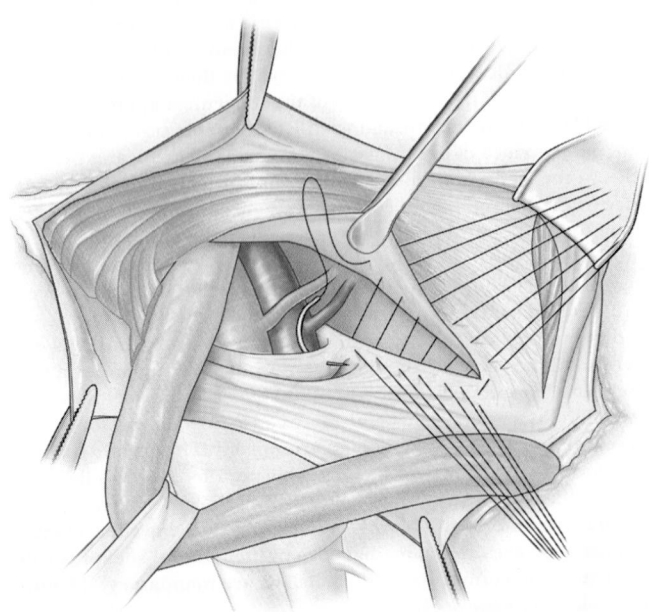

e

nerve is preserved, if possible; the cremaster muscle and neurovascular bundle are divided to expose the deep inguinal ring; and the spermatic cord is mobilized. Then, the posterior wall of the inguinal canal is divided and excised to the extent that it is weak, and the transverse aponeurosis is assessed. Finally, the peritoneal sac is eliminated, cord lipomata are removed, and a relaxing incision is made [see Figure 3].

Division of the cremaster muscle and division of the posterior wall of the inguinal canal are very important steps that many surgeons omit even today, although Bassini routinely performed them and surgeons at the forefront of inguinal hernia repair have repeatedly emphasized their importance.[11] Also important are relaxing incisions, which are required in the Cooper's ligament hernioplasty and are strongly recommended in the Bassini and Shouldice-Bassini hernioplasties. They are not needed in the Marcy repair.

Hernial sacs need not be excised: direct hernial sacs are merely inverted, and indirect hernial sacs are divided near their neck. The proximal sac is dissected from adjacent tissues and may or may not be ligated. The sac is then allowed to retract. The distal sac remains undissected and in situ but should be slit along the avascular border to prevent fluid accumulation. Sliding indirect hernias must be dissected from the spermatic cord and then inverted.

Repair

Common to the repair of all inguinal hernias in men is reconstruction of the deep inguinal ring. The ring cannot be made so tight that it strangles the spermatic cord, because the lateral border of the ring is elastic, muscular, indistinct, undefinable, and nonpalpable. What the surgeon apparently palpates as the deep inguinal ring is actually the inguinal canal, the diameter of which is always reduced when the inguinal ligament is used in the repair. Failure to reconstruct the medial border of the ring adequately is the chief cause of recurrences of indirect hernias. In women, the round ligament should be divided and the deep inguinal ring completely closed.

Marcy hernioplasty The Marcy repair is indicated in men and women with minimally damaged inguinal floors [see Figure 4a].[12,13]

Bassini and Shouldice-Bassini hernioplasties The Bassini and Shouldice-Bassini hernioplasties repair the area of the MPO that is superior to the inguinal ligament, that is, the deep inguinal ring and Hesselbach's triangle. Currently, the Shouldice-Bassini hernioplasty is very popular, produces exceptional results, and is used to manage most indirect and direct inguinal hernias in men. (The Marcy repair remains the most popular procedure in women.)

In the Bassini repair, the triple layer that consists of the internal oblique abdominal muscle, the transverse abdominal muscle, and the transverse fascia is approximated to the iliopubic tract and the shelving edge of the inguinal ligament with interrupted permanent sutures [see Figure 4b]. This differs markedly from the Bassini operation traditionally performed by North American surgeons, in which the posterior wall is plicated beneath sutures approximating the internal oblique muscle and conjoint tendon to Poupart's ligament. In the Shouldice-Bassini repair, the same myoaponeurotic layers are approximated, not edge to edge with interrupted sutures but by precise layered imbrication with continuous sutures [*see Figure 4c and d*].[8,14-16]

The Bassini repair and the Shouldice-Bassini repair are considered nonanatomic because the transverse aponeurosis is sutured to the inguinal ligament. This criticism is academic because the repairs work. Those who object to using the inguinal ligament to repair the MPO favor instead edge-to-edge approximation of the transverse aponeurotic arch and the iliopubic tract. The technique is called the iliopubic tract repair to distinguish it from the Bassini and Shouldice-Bassini repairs, which are inguinal ligament repairs.[17,18]

Cooper's ligament hernioplasty The Cooper's ligament hernioplasty (McVay-Lotheissen repair) addresses the three areas that are most vulnerable for herniation in the MPO, namely, the deep inguinal ring, Hesselbach's triangle, and the femoral canal. Therefore, the Cooper's ligament repair is used to manage femoral hernias and large indirect and direct inguinal hernias.[19-22]

The repair is accomplished by suturing the transverse aponeurotic arch to Cooper's ligament medially and to the femoral sheath laterally [*see Figure 4e*]. To expose Cooper's ligament and the medial border of the femoral sheath, the medial portion of the iliopubic tract must be excised [*see Figure 3*]. This extra step in the dissection is important because it allows the accurate placement of sutures. Relaxing incisions are mandatory in this repair.[23]

Although many enthusiasts employ this repair routinely, McVay himself used it in only about half of the hernioplasties he performed; in patients with smaller defects, he essentially used the Marcy repair.[9] The popularity of the McVay repair has declined in recent years because the operation is more difficult to perform and is associated with more postoperative pain than other repairs. Nevertheless, it is a neat and anatomic procedure.

Closure

The classic hernioplasties are completed by approximating the aponeurosis of the external oblique abdominal muscle. This process closes the inguinal canal and reassembles the superficial inguinal ring. The suture should include the distal stump of the divided cremaster muscle so that the testicle is pulled up.

SPECIAL CONSIDERATIONS

Bilateral inguinal hernias are usually repaired simultaneously because repairing them separately does not improve recurrence rates. Direct hernias are usually bilateral and inherently have a higher recurrence rate than indirect hernias do. This fact has led to the false conclusion that the simultaneous performance of bilateral hernioplasties is associated with increased suture line tension and, therefore, increased recurrence rates. If a hernial sac other than a small indirect one must be removed from the spermatic cord, simultaneous contralateral inguinal hernia repair should not be performed, because bilateral testicular atrophy may occur [*see* Dissection, *above, and* Complications of Groin Hernioplasty, *below*]. Obesity per se is not a contraindication for elective inguinal hernioplasty or a cause of recurrence. However, inguinal hernioplasty is more difficult in obese patients, and general or regional anesthesia is usually required.

In women, femoral hernias with small parietal defects are repaired subinguinally through an anterior groin incision by a few simple sutures (Bassini technique) [*see Figure 5*] or are corked with

Figure 5 Femoral hernias in women can be managed by simple closure of the parietal defect. The lacunar ligament and the femoral canal are incised (top) to enlarge the canal and make it easier to reduce the hernia. The defect is closed (middle) with a running to-and-fro absorbable suture. A flap of fascia from the pectineal muscle can be turned over the suture line to reinforce the repair. Alternatively, a cylindrical plug (bottom) constructed from a 2.0 to 2.5 cm strip of polypropylene mesh can be sutured in the parietal defect. This type of repair, by itself, is not indicated in men because of the high risk of an associated inguinal hernia.[53]

a cylindrical polypropylene prosthetic plug [see Lichtenstein's Tension-Free Hernioplasty, below]. The Cooper's ligament hernioplasty or a properitoneal prosthetic repair [see Figure 5] should be used to repair large femoral hernias in women and all femoral hernias in men, because the latter are usually associated with inguinal hernias. Strangulated femoral hernias should be corrected with a properitoneal repair because this approach provides direct access to the constricting femoral orifices, easy release of the entrapped bowel by incision of the iliopubic and lacunar ligaments, and ample room for bowel resection.[24,25]

In indirect hernias in infants, children, and some young adults, the MPO is not damaged, and a classic repair is unnecessary; simply eliminating the sac repairs the hernia. The operation known as high ligation of the sac consists of opening the inguinal canal and, without mobilizing the spermatic cord, identifying and tracing the sac proximal to the deep inguinal ring and ligating and dividing it there.

CRITIQUE OF THE CLASSIC REPAIRS

The classic hernioplasties have several disadvantages:

1. Considerable experience and skill are required to obtain a recurrence rate of one to two percent.
2. The classic repairs are inadequate for the repair of recurrent hernias.
3. Some unwanted tension will always be present.
4. The problem of continued tissue deterioration is not addressed.
5. There will always be some patients with very poor tissues and some with connective tissue diseases.

These disadvantages have caused many surgeons to use synthetic soft tissue prostheses.

Prosthetic Hernioplasty

Prosthetic hernioplasties are beginning to replace the classic hernioplasties, and a wide variety of permanent synthetic prostheses are readily available. In prosthetic hernioplasty, biomaterials are used to patch or plug the parietal defects, to reinforce the classic repairs, and to replace the transverse fascia (endoabdominal fascia). Enthusiasm for the prosthetic repairs has been stimulated by reports of good results, aggressive promotion by the manufacturers of the prostheses, and recognition in the surgical community that prosthetic infection is not as large a problem as surgeons once thought it was.

SPECIAL CONSIDERATIONS

Synthetic Prostheses for Abdominal Hernioplasty

The permanent synthetic soft tissue prostheses commonly used in hernia surgery are composed of one of the following materials: polypropylene, the polyester Dacron, and expanded polytetrafluoroethylene (Teflon). These materials have replaced the inconvenient biologic grafts, such as fascia lata, and are generally well tolerated.

Marlex mesh, Prolene mesh, and Trelex Natural mesh are composed of loosely knitted monofilament strands of polypropylene. They are semirigid, slightly elastic, and relatively heavy materials that buckle when bent in two directions at once. They have granular surfaces that grip tissue and prevent prosthesis

wandering before incorporation occurs. The three meshes resemble one another and may be used interchangeably.

Surgipro mesh is an open knitted mesh composed of braided strands of polypropylene. Its physical properties resemble those of the knitted monofilament polypropylene meshes, for which it may be substituted.

Mersilene and Lars meshes are open knitted meshes composed of braided strands of Dacron. In contrast to the polypropylene meshes, Dacron meshes are soft, supple, flexible, highly compliant and conforming, elastic in one direction only, and very light. They also have grainy surfaces that grip tissues and prevent the prostheses from wandering when they are not sutured in place.

Gore-Tex is not a mesh but an impervious and pliable material made from Teflon. A patented process expands the material at microscopic intervals so that extremely tiny and complex channels are created that pass completely through the material. Fibroblasts and collagen fibers grasp the material by penetrating these crevices. Gore-Tex is soft, supple, slightly elastic, and smooth.

Absorbable synthetic prostheses are occasionally needed in hernia surgery. The most commonly used materials are Vicryl and Dexon mesh, both of which may be knitted or woven. Vicryl is made from polyglactin 910 acid, Dexon from polyglycolic acid.

Tissue Response

The prostheses made of polypropylene and polyester desirably incite fibroplasia with only minimal inflammation. Therefore, they become quickly integrated into soft tissues. However, the ability to incite fibroplasia can be detrimental if these prostheses are placed intraperitoneally. Troublesome and tightly binding abdominal adhesions may form that are difficult to divide and can cause intestinal obstruction and fistulization.

Binding intra-abdominal adhesions can be prevented by interposing the omentum between an intraperitoneal permanent prosthesis and the abdominal viscera. An absorbable prosthesis made of tightly woven or knitted Vicryl or Dexon may be substituted for the omentum or for peritoneum and posterior rectus abdominis sheath when these structures cannot be approximated. The absorbable prostheses (e.g., those made from Vicryl or Dexon) also cause adhesions. However, they may prevent the viscera from becoming dangerously grafted to the permanent prosthesis because integration of the permanent prosthesis in the mesothelial tissues occurs before the absorbable prosthesis disappears.

Gore-Tex is inert and does not incite fibroplasia or inflammation. Consequently, integration is delayed and may take at least 40 days. This property plus the constant peristaltic intestinal motion usually prevents the formation of adhesions between Gore-Tex and the intestine when the material is placed intraperitoneally.

Infection of a Permanent Prosthesis

All the nonabsorbable synthetic materials can become sequestered, act like a foreign body, and aggravate and prolong infections. Theoretically, mesh made of braided fibers should tolerate infection less well than that made of single strands. Braided yarn contains microscopic interstices 1 to 2 μm in diameter that should conceal bacteria and cellular debris from macrophages, which are 10 mm in diameter, and from tissue fluids that contain antibiotics. In clinical practice, however, this phenomenon happens infrequently. Braided, knitted polyester mesh, such as Mersilene, tolerates infection as well as a nonbraided, solid-fiber, polypropylene mesh, such as Marlex. If either mesh is infected, incorporation rather than rejection usually can be expected, provided that treatment is timely; the wound does not also contain silk, cotton, or coated, heavy-braided Dacron sutures; and the prosthesis is not floating free in the wound but is in firm contact with healthy tissues.

The Dacron yarn in Mersilene and Lars mesh is very fine and pure and is unlike the Dacron sutures, which are heavier and have a reputation for being readily rejected and behaving like foreign bodies. Sutures made from Dacron are typically not pure and are coated with another substance to ensure that they do not drag during their passage through the tissues.

Gore-Tex, although inert, is virtually intolerant of infection because of the delay in integration that occurs when this material is used. When infection occurs in a space that contains Gore-Tex, the material must be removed because the material will not become incorporated in the tissues before bacteria have contaminated the material and occupied microscopic crevices too small for phagocytes to enter.

Management of infection The management of infected wounds that contain a synthetic prosthesis is relatively easy and requires simple application of sound surgical principles. Superficial infection in a wound containing a prosthesis that is positioned deep to the subcutaneous tissues usually can be expected to heal without incident.

Infections involving a prosthesis require vigorous and aggressive treatment. The prosthesis must be exposed without delay; failure to do so leads to chronic sinus formation. Local treatment consists of irrigating away purulent material; lysing cellular, fibrous, and fibrinous debris; and destroying the infectious agent. Interventions such as irrigation with saline or Dakin's solution and application of honey or granulated sugar and topical antimicrobial substances are all useful. Complete incorporation can usually be expected with polypropylene or polyester meshes within three to four weeks of the time when the infection is first recognized. Administration of systemic antibiotics is, of course, also essential.

Delayed infections involving nonabsorbable prostheses may occur months or even years after prosthesis implantation. The cause of delayed infections usually cannot be determined. In delayed infections, reintegration of the prosthesis, regardless of the type, infrequently occurs, and excision of sequestered portions is necessary. Only the sequestered mesh need be removed. Chronically draining sinus tracts involving nonabsorbable prostheses are managed similarly.

Prophylaxis of infection Prophylaxis of infection is essential. Rigid sterile conditions, precise and meticulous surgical technique, and avoidance of seromas and hematomas with the use of closed suction drains are important. When large pieces of mesh are used, broad-spectrum antibiotics should be administered intravenously shortly before the operation begins and should be continued after the operation until the closed suction drains are removed. Topical antibiotics and antimicrobial agents are also commonly used intraoperatively. However, antibiotic prophylaxis is not commonly used in hernia repairs in which small prostheses are used.

Inflammatory granulomas are occasionally encountered during prosthetic hernioplasties for recurrent inguinal and incisional hernias. Gram's staining at the time of operation is not always reliable; consequently, if a granuloma is encountered, a synthetic prosthesis should not be implanted.[26]

Patients with completely integrated soft tissue prostheses are not customarily given preoperative prophylactic antibiotics. They are not at increased risk for infection, as are patients with prostheses that are not integrated into the soft tissues, such as artificial hips and heart valves.

OPERATIVE TECHNIQUE

Anterior Prosthetic Hernioplasty

The anterior groin incision is well known to all surgeons; consequently, it is not surprising that this incision is also the one most commonly used to implant a prosthesis. Usually, the prosthesis is placed on top of the posterior wall of the inguinal canal, although behind it would seem to be the proper site [*see* Posterior (Properitoneal) Prosthetic Hernioplasty, *below*]. Variations and combinations of the following techniques are common.

Lichtenstein's tension-free hernioplasty Synthetic soft tissue patch prostheses have been used for years to buttress the classic repairs, but they have not significantly improved the results. However, when the prosthesis is implanted without a formal repair, thereby obviating tension, results improve dramatically [*see Figure 6*].[27] Lichtenstein credited this original idea to R. Newman of Rahway, New Jersey, but it was Lichtenstein and his associates who championed the tension-free patch hernioplasty and who first reported very favorable results with this technique in a large number of patients.

Lichtenstein, who recognized the importance of tension, was already promoting a tension-free prosthetic plug repair for femoral hernias and for recurrent direct and indirect inguinal hernias. He advocated the use of this technique in situations in which the parietal defect was fibrous, circumscribed, and not too large [*see Figure 7*].[28] Lichtenstein borrowed the idea of the plug hernioplasty from Cheatle, who in 1921 plugged the parietal defect of a femoral hernia with a coil of saphenous vein.[24]

The semirigid knitted polypropylene meshes are the preferred prostheses for Lichtenstein's tension-free patch hernioplasties because they handle well, are easily tailored to the patient, and become integrated quickly. Some surgeons like the feel and the texture of Gore-Tex and prefer it to polypropylene, even though integration is slow with the former.

Originally, Lichtenstein used a 10×5 cm swatch of mesh in his repairs. However, because of recurrences, Lichtenstein's associates now advise using a larger prosthesis (12×6 to 8 cm) and circumcising the cremaster muscle for a snugger fit at the deep inguinal ring. Some proponents of the tension-free patch hernioplasty are concerned about the possibility of indirect hernia recurrences and place a polypropylene cone or an umbrella plug in the deep inguinal ring to ensure against this possibility [*see* Gilbert's Sutureless Hernioplasty, *below*].

The plug employed by Lichtenstein for plug hernioplasty is cylindrical and is made from a 2.0 to 2.5 cm tightly wound strip (or strips) of polypropylene mesh. The plug must occlude the aponeurotic defect completely and must be fixed flush to the defect with four or more permanent synthetic sutures. Polyester and Gore-Tex are not suitable materials for the plugs: polyester meshes are too soft, and coiled Gore-Tex plugs will not be completely integrated. Incompletely integrated prostheses have an increased chance of becoming secondarily infected.

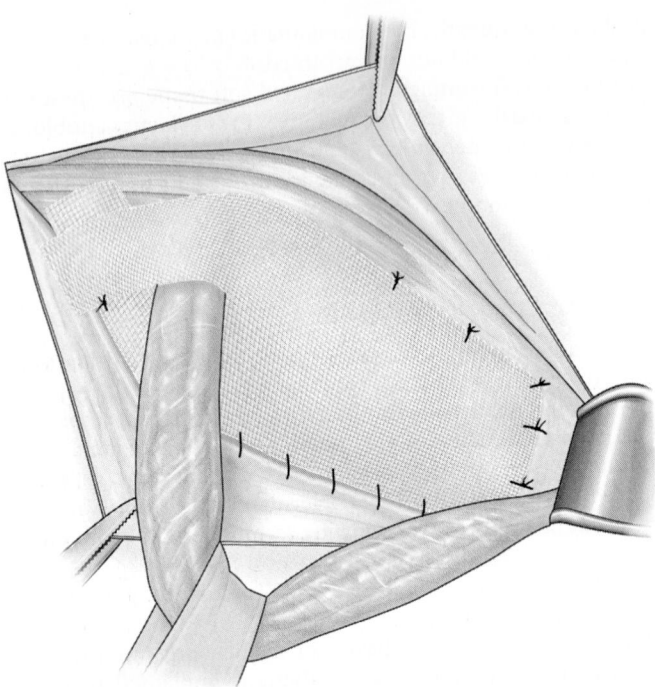

Figure 6 Lichtenstein's tension-free repair for primary hernia. The repair consists of a polypropylene patch laid over the posterior wall of the inguinal canal. The patch is tailored to the patient from a 12 × 8 cm swatch and has a slit to accommodate the spermatic cord. The prosthesis should extend 1.5 to 2.0 cm medial to the pubic tubercle and well lateral to the deep inguinal ring. The patch is sutured to the rectus abdominis sheath and the inguinal ligament. To ensure a snug fit at the deep inguinal ring, Lichtenstein's associates recommend circumcising the cremaster muscle at the level of the ring and crossing the legs of the mesh. The overlapped mesh is fixed with a single suture that grasps the lower edge of both mesh legs and the shelving edge of the inguinal ligament. In lieu of circumcision of the cremaster muscle, a cone plug of polypropylene mesh (like that used by Gilbert) may be placed in the deep inguinal ring [*see Figure 8*]. In a direct hernia, the hernial sac is inverted without tension and secured with a synthetic absorbable suture to ensure a smooth surface on which to place the mesh patch. Once placed, the mesh patch is secured by synthetic absorbable sutures.[53]

Tension-free patch hernioplasties are usually not recommended for recurrent hernias, because remobilization of the spermatic cord greatly increases the chance of testicular atrophy. However, the plug technique does not require remobilization of the spermatic cord, and only a small anterior groin incision directly over the parietal defect is necessary. Local anesthesia is helpful in hernioplasties for recurrent hernias in which plugs have been used, because the hernia can be revealed to the surgeon when the patient coughs. Plug repair for fibrous, small, well-circumscribed indirect and direct defects is very effective. However, recurrent hernias with large or multiple parietal defects are preferably managed by a posterior properitoneal prosthetic repair.

There has been widespread acceptance of the Lichtenstein tension-free patch hernioplasty because postoperative pain is minimal and because the procedure is easy to perform with the patient under local anesthesia. Detractors point out that the technique is not foolproof and that long-term results are not yet

known. Furthermore, even the recommended larger patch does not cover all of the MPO, it contains a slit for potential peritoneal protrusion, it is on the external side of the parietal defect, and it frequently does not fit, because the space is too small or is occupied by a traversing sensory nerve.

Gilbert's sutureless hernioplasty Gilbert placed a 6 × 6 cm cone-shaped swatch of polypropylene mesh through the deep inguinal ring of a patient with a minimally dilated ring and a small indirect hernial sac. Quite astonishingly, the patient could not expel the prosthesis or the hernial sac by coughing and straining. Recognizing the therapeutic possibilities of this observation, Gilbert added to the cone in the deep inguinal ring an unsutured flat patch of polypropylene mesh placed on the floor of the inguinal canal and thereby created the so-called sutureless hernioplasty [*see Figure 8*].[29,30] A slit in the lateral edge of the patch is made to accommodate the spermatic cord.

Gilbert surmised that the gathered mesh unfolded in the properitoneal space and blocked the entrance to the deep inguinal ring. He therefore called the prosthesis an umbrella plug. However, the cone-shaped plug need not unfold in the properitoneal space to be effective, because the textured polypropylene mesh adheres to adjacent tissues and obliterates the entrance of the deep inguinal ring even before integration occurs. Cone-shaped occlusive plugs should always be supplemented with an onlay patch because by themselves, the plugs may deform, collapse, and cease to contain the peritoneal sac.

Gilbert minimizes the dissection of the groin in his technique. The cremaster muscle and vessels are not divided, and the lipomata of the cord and the small, indirect hernial sacs are merely returned to the properitoneal space. The sutureless hernioplasty is used chiefly for indirect hernias with only minimal enlargement of the deep inguinal ring. However, indirect hernias with dilated deep inguinal rings may be managed with this technique if the ring is tightened with one or two Marcy sutures. The repair is simple and produces excellent results.

Rutkow and Robbins adapted Gilbert's sutureless technique to the repair of all types of groin hernias.[31,32] For indirect hernias with patulous deep inguinal rings, a large polypropylene mesh cone plug is implanted in the ring and fixed at the perimeter with interrupted absorbable synthetic sutures. Direct inguinal hernias are similarly managed. Direct hernias are incised at the circumference of the neck to expose properitoneal fat before the cone is implanted and sutured to the fringe of the defect. Combined indirect and direct inguinal hernias are treated with two cone plugs. Plugs are also used in the treatment of femoral and recurrent hernias.

The repairs are completed with a flat piece of polypropylene mesh laid over the inguinal floor. The mesh has a slit at the lateral end that is closed with a suture after it accommodates the spermatic cord. In this procedure, as in Gilbert's original procedure, the dissection of the groin is kept to a minimum. The repairs are easily performed with unassisted local anesthesia, and recovery is fast.

These new and clever repairs are finding favor because they are simple to perform and produce minimal postoperative pain. They are criticized because the onlayed patch is not sutured in place, may not cover the MPO sufficiently, and contains a slit. Furthermore, the cones in the direct and indirect spaces can become deformed by the contracture of the enveloping scar tissue; as they lose their shape, they may fail to occlude the parietal defects. This

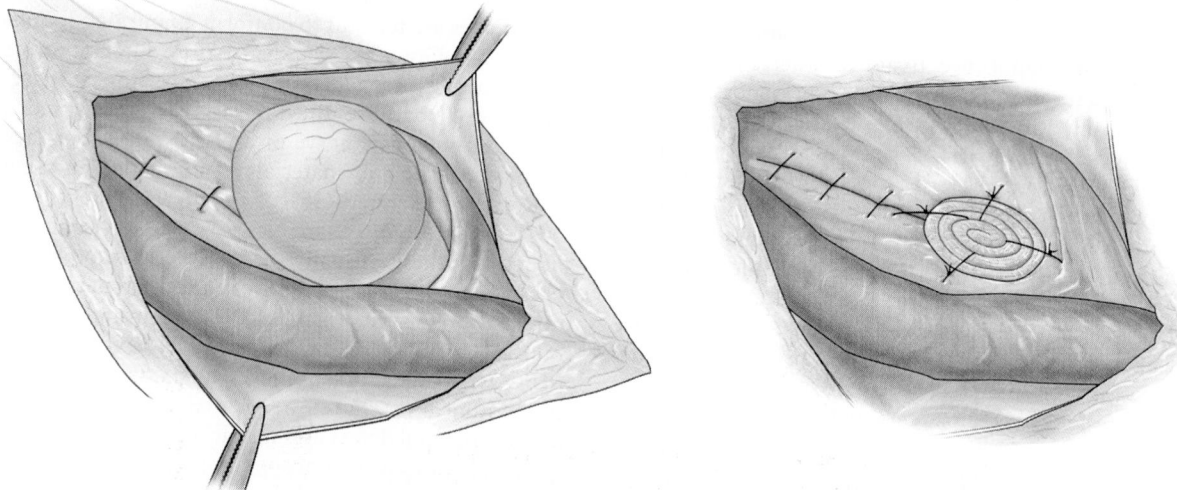

Figure 7 Lichtenstein's recurrent hernia repair. The hernial sac (left), which will be in the subcutaneous tissues under the external oblique aponeurosis, is exposed and returned to the properitoneal space. The plug (right) is made of a strip (or strips) of polypropylene mesh that is 2.0 to 2.5 cm wide and is tightly wound to a diameter that fits snugly in the defect. The plug is fixed in place by four or more interrupted nonabsorbable sutures. Hollow cone-shaped plugs can deform and are not a suitable substitute for the solid cylindrical plugs.[53]

phenomenon has been observed with Lichtenstein's cylindrical plugs that were not tightly rolled and fitted.

Posterior (Properitoneal) Prosthetic Hernioplasty

The properitoneal space is the logical site in which to implant a prosthesis. The prosthesis is held in place by intra-abdominal pressure. It is remote from the relatively avascular subcutaneous tissues and is therefore relatively immune to superficial infection. The myopectineal orifice can be patched or plugged and hernioplasties buttressed with a prosthesis implanted from the posterior approach in the same way as from the anterior approach [*see Figure 9*].[33,34] Although the properitoneal space can be reached through an anterior groin incision, an abdominal incision is preferable because it enables dissection of the inguinal canal to be completely bypassed.

Stoppa's giant prosthetic reinforcement of the visceral sac Stoppa proposed treating hernias of the groin through the use of a large, permanent prosthesis that essentially replaced the transverse fascia.[35-37] The prosthesis adheres to the visceral sac and renders the peritoneum inextensible, so that peritoneum cannot protrude through the MPO or adjacent areas of weakness; repair of the defect in the abdominal wall is then unnecessary. The repair is tension free and sutureless. The operation is technically known by the descriptive phrase "giant prosthetic reinforcement of the visceral sac" (GPRVS), but it is commonly called the Stoppa procedure. Stoppa's innovative and revolutionary properitoneal prosthetic technique was unique: for the first time, hernia repair was focused on retaining the peritoneum rather than on closing the aponeurotic defect.

GPRVS is performed bilaterally or unilaterally. Bilateral GPRVS entails the insertion of a single large prosthesis into the properitoneal space of both groins through a midline or Pfannenstiel's incision [*see Figure 10*].[35,37] The procedure requires general or regional anesthesia and, sometimes, an overnight stay in the hospital. The procedure is ideal for patients with

Figure 8 Gilbert's sutureless hernioplasty. A swatch of polypropylene mesh (6 × 6 cm) is folded into a cone-shaped plug and placed through the deep inguinal ring. The gathered mesh unfolds in the properitoneal space and occludes the deep inguinal ring. Cone-shaped plugs do not have to pass through the deep inguinal ring and into the properitoneal space to be an effective barrier, provided they are sutured in place. Another swatch of mesh slit to accommodate the spermatic cord is tailored to cover the floor of the inguinal canal. Some surgeons use a single suture to fix the distal end of the swatch to the rectus abdominis sheath.

bilateral recurrent hernias, bilateral direct primary hernias, hernias associated with connective tissue disorders, and hernias resulting from fractures of the pelvis. It is quick and exceptionally easy to perform, even in obese patients, for whom it may be the preferred hernioplasty when bilateral hernias are present.

Unilateral GPRVS was developed for use in day surgical centers.[38] The preferred entry route is through a transverse lower quadrant abdominal incision, but an anterior groin incision can be used instead [see Figure 11].[39] Because the abdominal incision circumvents the dissection of the inguinal canal, it is the method of choice for recurrent inguinal hernia in men who have undergone classic and prosthetic anterior repairs. Local anesthesia is suitable for most patients undergoing anterior unilateral GPRVS but only for selected patients undergoing the posterior unilateral procedure.

Ordinarily, a large prosthesis in the properitoneal space requires a slit to accommodate the spermatic cord at the deep inguinal ring [see Figure 9]. The slit, which is sutured closed around the elements of the cord, partially holds the prosthesis in place, but it is also a potential site for peritoneal protrusion. However, a slit in the mesh becomes unnecessary if the elements of the spermatic cord—the vas deferens and the testicular vessels—are dissected from the peritoneum, to which they are attached by a lamina of transverse fascia. Then, the elements of the cord can lie against the wall of the pelvis, and the properitoneal prosthesis will cover them, the deep inguinal ring, and the MPO completely. This technique, called parietalization of structures of the spermatic cord, was devised by Stoppa and facilitates properitoneal prosthetic implantation [see Figure 11].[35,37,39]

Mersilene is the prosthesis of choice for GPRVS because it is supple and elastic, it stays in place without sutures, it conforms to the complex curvature of the pelvis, and it induces prompt fibroblastic integration. In GPRVS, the prosthesis is placed with long abdominal clamps. The prosthesis may be attached with sutures to the anterior abdominal wall, but it is otherwise not fixed.

If prostheses made from materials other than Mersilene are used, peripheral fixation is usually necessary. The polypropylene meshes are too stiff to conform by intra-abdominal pressure alone, and Gore-Tex wanders before integration occurs. The use of sutures and staples in the retroperitoneal space is not recommended, because they may inadvertently include a vital structure, such as a nerve or a blood vessel. For these reasons, Mersilene is the only material recommended for use in GPRVS.

Recurrences after GPRVS occur as a result of technical mishaps—most often an incorrectly sized, shaped, and positioned prosthesis (usually the prosthesis is too small). Another pitfall is an insufficiently cleaved properitoneal space that does not admit the large prosthesis. In these instances, the prosthesis buckles, crimps, and fails to smoothly extend far beyond the MPO when the implantation clamps are withdrawn. Surplus properitoneal fat should be excised because it can pass in and out of a parietal defect and mimic a peritoneal protrusion exactly. Usually, the dissection of the properitoneal space is bloodless, but if it is not or if there is a large retained hernial sac, closed suction drainage is necessary. Hematomas and seromas delay integration, are a good medium for the growth of bacteria, and can also dislodge the unsutured mesh.

Recurrences after GPRVS are usually approached anteriorly and are managed by adding a prosthetic extension to the existing prosthesis. Alternatively, another permanent prosthesis can be implanted transabdominally.

GPRVS is an efficient, anatomic, sutureless, and tension-free repair. It may be the ultimate hernioplasty; when it is correctly performed, all hernias of the groin are cured, even the prevascular femoral hernias. Recovery is very fast and discomfort minimal. GPRVS is the technique I prefer to use for recurrent hernias and for all primary hernias in men when regional or general anesthesia is used.

Complications of Groin Hernioplasty

Testicular atrophy[40-43] and residual neuralgia[44,45] are the important and dreaded complications unique to inguinal hernioplasty. They are more common after anterior hernia repairs than after posterior repairs and are very likely to initiate malpractice suits.

TESTICULAR ATROPHY

Testicular atrophy is a sequela of ischemic orchitis. The clinical manifestations of ischemic orchitis develop insidiously, do not become apparent for two to five days after the hernioplasty, and are frequently misinterpreted at presentation. The testicle and spermatic cord become swollen, hard, tender, painful, and retracted. The process lasts six to 12 weeks and may resolve completely or may end in testicular atrophy. The return of the testicle to normal size and shape does not mean that the process is complete. On occasion, atrophy of the testicle does not become apparent for as long as a year. Gangrene is unusual, and orchiectomy is rarely necessary.

Ischemic orchitis is caused by thrombosis of the spermatic cord, and the testicular pathology is intense venous congestion. The thrombosis is induced by surgical trauma to the cord, especially that associated with the dissection performed to completely remove a large indirect hernial sac. The spermatic cord must always be handled gently, and surgical trauma to the cord must be kept to a minimum. The cord should not be dissected beyond the pubic tubercle, and scrotal pathology should not be dealt with at the time of hernia repair. Trauma to the spermatic

Figure 9 Posterior patch prosthetic hernioplasty. The prosthesis is fixed with synthetic permanent sutures to Cooper's iliopectineal ligament inferiorly and to the abdominal wall superiorly. A slit in the mesh accommodates the spermatic cord.[53]

a

Figure 10 **Bilateral giant prosthetic reinforcement of the visceral sac. (*a*) A large prosthesis is implanted via a midline or a Pfannenstiel incision. The mesh envelops the visceral sac of both groins and extends far beyond the borders of the myopectineal orifice (dotted line). The prosthesis is chevron-shaped and arranged so that the stretch is transverse. The width equals the distance between the anterior superior iliac spines minus 2 cm in a normal patient but can be larger in an obese patient. The vertical dimension equals the distance between the umbilicus and the symphysis. The tails of the chevron are exaggerated to ensure a firm grip of the visceral sac.[53] (*b*) Wide cleavage of the properitoneal space is necessary and easy. The pedicle of an indirect hernial sac is encircled, the sac divided, and the visceral sac closed.[53] (*c*) The vas deferens and the testicular vessels are dissected from the parietal peritoneum. When freed, they will lie against the parietal wall of the pelvis (parietalization), and the prosthesis will cover the entire MPO without a slit having to be made for the cord.[53] (*d*) The prosthesis is implanted by long (30 cm) Wiley or Rochester-Pean clamps, so that it smoothly envelops the visceral sac. The large dead space may require drainage. The prosthesis is fixed with a single suture to the umbilical fascia only[35]** [*Figure continued on page 876*].

cord, especially to the delicate veins of the pampiniform plexus, is the paramount cause of testicular atrophy after inguinal hernioplasty.[40,41] Dissection of an indirect hernial sac in the scrotum damages the delicate veins of the pampiniform plexus, initiates the thrombosis, and coincidentally disrupts the collateral circulation [*see Dissection, above*].

No known successful preventive treatment exists for testicular atrophy. Antibiotics, anti-inflammatory drugs, and massive doses of steroids are often given. Fortunately, the incidence of testicular atrophy can be minimized by reducing surgical trauma to the spermatic cord through such measures as avoiding excision of the distal part of an indirect hernial sac; avoiding

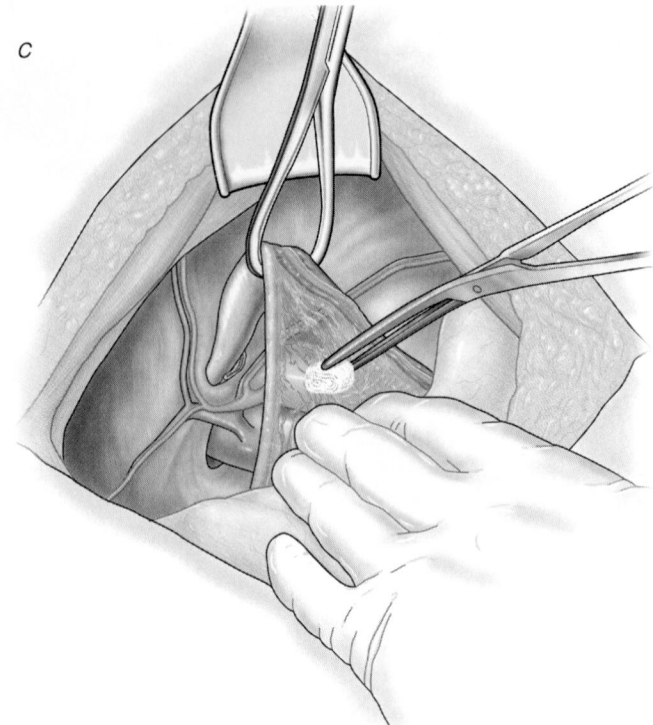

dissection beyond the pubic tubercle; and avoiding redissection of an inguinal canal and spermatic cord in patients who are predisposed to the complication by a previous anterior hernioplasty, vasectomy, hydrocelectomy, or other inguinal or scrotal surgery. In these situations, posterior properitoneal prosthetic hernioplasty is the preferred alternative.

NEURALGIA

Chronic residual neuralgia may result from surgical handling of the sensory nerves in the groin during hernioplasty or from constricting scar tissue or adjacent inflammatory granulomas after hernioplasty. The intraoperative trauma to the nerve, whether caused by division, stretching, contusion, or suture entrapment, is usually not appreciated at the time it occurs. The pain may be localized, diffuse, projected along the course of a nerve, or referred to a nearby site. It may develop early or as late as weeks to months after the operation. In most cases, the pain is accompanied by changes in mood and behavior; depression, disturbed interpersonal relationships, and inability to resume work are common. Management of the neuralgia is frustrating and complicated and benefits from a multidisciplinary approach.

A well-known cause of nociceptive (somatic) residual neuralgia is a neuroma. A neuroma results from a proliferation of nerve fibers outside the neurilemma of a partially or completely divided nerve. The pain from a neuroma varies in intensity, may be induced by changes in position, and is without spontaneous paroxysmal exacerbations. Hyperesthesia is detectable in the area of the lesion, and tapping the site may produce a severe shooting pain.

Deafferentation (central) chronic pain differs from the pain of a neuroma. It is burning and permanent, with intermittent paroxysmal exacerbations. The area of involvement is anesthetic at first but becomes hyperesthetic. Typically, the onset of deafferentation pain is delayed for about a week after the injury, and tapping the site does not produce exquisite pain.

The management of residual neuralgia is often difficult. Neurolysis of the involved nerve may afford relief, especially if it is instituted early. The involved nerve may be identified by local anesthetic nerve blocks. The iliohypogastric and ilioinguinal

nerves can be blocked and divided in the groin. However, a foolproof method of blocking the genitofemoral nerve in the groin does not exist; neuralgia from this nerve is identified by blocking L1 and L2 paravertebrally. Division of the genitofemoral nerve is performed through a flank incision. Other adjunctive therapy includes administration of analgesics, antidepressants, anticonvulsants, and anxiolytic drugs and transcutaneous electrical stimulation. Injections of steroids in the involved area are sometimes helpful.

The prevention of nerve injury is important because the treatment of neuralgic complications is often unsuccessful. Fortunately, such complications are rare. The sensory nerves should be preserved if possible; however, this is not always possible, and some small, not readily visible nerves are invariably divided. Occasionally, major branches of the sensory nerves or the nerve trunks themselves must be divided to accomplish the hernioplasty. Division (usually with ligation) of the genital branch of

Figure 11   **Unilateral giant prosthetic reinforcement of the visceral sac. The prosthesis is shaped somewhat like a diamond and is arranged so that it stretches transversely. It is important that the inferior edge be wider than the superior edge (by 2 to 4 cm) and that the lateral side be longer than the medial side. The long lateral inferior corner ensures a solid prosthetic grip on the lateral visceral sac. The width of the prosthesis at the superior edge equals the distance from the midline to the anterior superior iliac spine minus 1 cm, and the vertical length is approximately 14 cm. The prosthesis is drawn into place (top) under the rectus abdominis muscle and the abdominal wall by three absorbable sutures that affix the prosthesis to the midline, the semilunar line, and the oblique muscles near the anterior superior iliac spine. The abdominal wall is retracted (bottom, left) to expose the properitoneal space. The superior portion of the prosthesis is implanted deep into the muscles of the properitoneal space. Clamps are ready to implant the prosthesis inferiorly. The distal prosthesis is implanted (bottom, right) with long (30 cm) Wiley or Rochester-Pean clamps and positioned so that the prosthesis envelops the peritoneum.**

the genitofemoral nerve is routine in most anterior groin hernio-plasties. This process virtually never produces genital nerve neuralgia, which suggests that complete division of the nerve may be less likely to cause residual neuralgia than other types of nerve trauma. Most nerves require ligation to control bleeding. Fortuitously, the ligature may also confine neuroma formation to within the neurilemma.

Noninguinal Abdominal Wall Hernias

UMBILICAL AND EPIGASTRIC HERNIAS

Umbilical hernias are common in infants and close spontaneously without special treatment if the diameter of the aponeurotic defect is 1.5 cm or less. However, repair is indicated in infants with hernial defects greater than 2.0 cm in diameter and in all children whose umbilical hernia is still present at three to four years of age.

Umbilical hernias in adults are acquired and require repair. They have no relation to umbilical hernias in children. Strangulation of the colon and omentum is fairly common, and rupture occurs in chronic ascitic cirrhosis, in which case an emergency portal decompression is necessary.

Small umbilical hernias are merely closed with a to-and-fro continuous nonabsorbable suture or a small polypropylene plug. Large umbilical hernias should be managed with a prosthetic repair that resembles the prosthetic repair for incisional hernia. The classic repair for umbilical hernias is the Mayo hernioplasty. In this operation, a vest-over-pants imbrication of the superior and inferior aponeurotic segments is performed. However, the Mayo hernioplasty is infrequently used because the results are not as satisfactory as those achieved with the prosthetic repairs.

Epigastric hernias occur between the decussating fibers of the linea alba above the umbilicus. They are managed in the same way as umbilical hernias.

SPIGELIAN HERNIAS

Spigelian hernias are ventral hernias that occur along the subumbilical portion of Spieghel's semilunar line and through Spieghel's fascia.[46] Spigelian hernias are rare, and unless they are large, these hernias are difficult to diagnose because they are

Figure 12 **Rives-Stoppa incisional hernia repair. Parasagittal views showing the site of implantation of the prosthesis (broken line) and suture fixation in (*a*) supraumbilical midline incisional hernias, (*b*) subumbilical midline incisional hernias, and (*c*) subcostal incisional hernias. Cross sections of the abdominal wall anatomy show the implantation of the prosthesis (broken line), the lateral extent of the prosthesis, and suture fixation in the (*d*) epigastric region, (*e*) hypogastric region, and (*f*) right lower quadrant (appendectomy).**

Figure 13 **Mesh placement for repair of incisional hernia. The retromuscular space has been dissected (left), exposing the intercostal vessels and nerves. A Reverdin suture needle (right) facilitates the placement of the sutures for prosthetic fixation.**

interparietal and are contained by the aponeurosis of the external oblique muscle. Sonography and computed tomography often reveal symptomatic spigelian hernias too small to detect clinically. Large spigelian hernias may be mistaken for sarcomas of the abdominal wall, and entrapped anterior cutaneous nerves of T10–T12 produce discomfort resembling spigelian herniation.

Spieghel's fascia is actually aponeurotic and consists of the fused aponeuroses of the internal oblique and transverse abdominal muscles between the belly of these muscles laterally and the rectus abdominis muscle medially. Above the umbilicus, the aponeurotic fibers of these muscles crisscross and form a fairly strong barrier. Below the umbilicus, the fibers are more or less parallel and may split, permitting the peritoneum and properitoneal fat to protrude through a slitlike defect but to be retained by the overlying aponeurosis of the external oblique abdominal muscle. Although spigelian hernias occur anywhere along the semilunar line, they are most common in areas where Spieghel's fascia is widest (between the umbilicus and the line connecting the anterior superior iliac spines) and weakest (just beneath the arcuate line and above the inferior epigastric vessels). Spigelian hernias that occur inferior to the epigastric vessels are a variant of a direct inguinal hernia.

The neck of a spigelian hernia enlarges laterally by spreading apart the broad muscles of the abdomen. The rectus abdominis muscle and sheath inhibit medial enlargement. Small spigelian hernias are simply closed, but large spigelian hernias that are in muscle require a prosthesis.

LUMBAR HERNIAS

Congenital, spontaneous, and traumatic herniations occur through Grynfeltt's superior and Petit's inferior lumbar triangles. They are very rare and are impossible to repair successfully without a prosthesis or a myoaponeurotic flap. Petit's triangle is upright and is bounded by the latissimus dorsi, the external oblique abdominal muscle, and the iliac crest. It is covered by the superficial fascia only. Grynfeltt's triangle is inverted and is

bounded by the 12th rib, the internal oblique abdominal muscle, and the sacrospinal muscle. It is covered by the latissimus dorsi.

The large, diffuse lumbar hernias that occur after kidney excision result in part from muscular paralysis; as a rule, no aponeurotic defects can be identified. These hernias are managed in much the same way as incisional hernias.

PELVIC HERNIAS

Pelvic hernias occur in the obturator fossa, the greater and lesser sciatic foramen, and the perineum. All are very rare and occur mainly in cachectic elderly patients, especially women. Of the hernias in the pelvis, the obturator hernia is the most common. Obturator hernias are almost always strangulated. In about half the patients with obturator hernias, pressure on the obturator nerve causes pain (Howship-Romberg sign) in the region of the hip, the knee, and the inner aspect of the thigh. A palpable mass in the pelvis or the rectum or in the upper medial part of the thigh is occasionally noted. A prosthesis implanted in the properitoneal space over and far beyond the parietal defect in the obturator canal cures the hernia. This method is preferred to suturing of the defect unless septic conditions are present.

Perineal hernias occur through the pelvic diaphragm and may be anterior or posterior to the superficial transverse perineal muscle. The anterior perineal hernia is seen only in women and passes into the labia majora, whereas the posterior perineal hernia enters the ischiorectal fossa in men and passes close to the vagina in women.

PARASTOMAL HERNIAS

Parastomal hernias interfere with colostomy irrigations and the adhesion of stomal appliances. Paracolostomy hernias are more common than paraileostomy hernias, and both are likelier to occur when the stoma emerges through the semilunar line rather than through the rectus abdominis sheath. Parastomal hernias, therefore, are usually lateral to the ostomy.

Moving the stoma to a new location is often the easiest method of management of parastomal hernias. A prosthesis should be used in the repair; otherwise, the operation is likely to fail because the belt muscles lateral to the ostomy lack sufficient aponeurosis. The prosthesis may be implanted extramuscularly on the aponeurotic abdominal wall in the subcutaneous space, retromuscularly or intraperitoneally [see Major Incisional Hernias, below].

Leslie's technique for parastomal hernia repair is easy and effective.[47] In this operation, an incision is made well away from the stoma and the stoma appliance. The skin and subcutaneous tissue are dissected from the abdominal wall and reflected to expose the bowel and the parietal defect. The defect is then closed with sutures. A 12 × 15 cm Mersilene prosthesis is partially slit to accommodate and embrace the bowel. The mesh positioned around the bowel in the subcutaneous tissues is spread out over the repair and the anterior abdominal wall, where it is fixed with staples or sutures. Closed suction drainage is essential until prosthetic integration is assured.

Sugarbaker's parastomal hernioplasty repairs the hernia from within the abdomen without disturbing the stoma.[48] A polypropylene mesh sandwiched between two layers of an absorbable mesh (or, alternatively, a swatch of Gore-Tex) is shaped and sutured to the perimeter of the parietal defect intraperitoneally. The prosthesis creates a flap valve that ensures against recurrence. Success is wholly dependent on the integrity of the sutures unless the prosthesis significantly overlaps the edges of the defect. Sugarbaker's repair should not be used for parastomal hernias involving an ileal conduit, because the method may cause dysfunction by kinking the bowel or ureters.

MAJOR INCISIONAL HERNIAS

Major incisional hernias are serious surgical problems. They have an inordinate tendency to enlarge, are frequently formidable to repair, and are usually accompanied by serious conditions. Patients with incisional hernias are usually obese. In fact, obesity and infection are the two principal causes of this condition. The weight of the panniculus adiposus literally pulls apart the surgical incision, and subsequent wound healing is hampered by infection. Hypertension, cardiac and renal disorders, diabetes, and purulent intertrigo commonly accompany obesity and increase the morbidity associated with the repair.

Pathophysiology

The loss of integrity of the abdominal wall reduces intraabdominal pressure and causes serious pathophysiological disturbances, which Rives appropriately termed eventration disease.[49] The salient abnormality resulting from abdominal weakness is respiratory dysfunction. A large incisional hernia produces paradoxical respiratory abdominal motion similar to that seen in a flail chest. Diaphragmatic function becomes inefficient: the diaphragm no longer contracts against the abdominal viscera but forces them into the hernial sac instead. Appraisal of respiratory function and blood gases is essential.

The detachment of the tendinous insertion of the broad belt muscles of the abdomen aggravates midline incisional hernias. The muscles retract, pull apart the parietal defect, and cause the normally horizontal rectus abdominis muscle to assume a vertical position. Contraction of the rectus abdominis muscle then causes the abdominal viscera to be expelled rather than retained. Ultimately, atrophy, fatty degeneration, and fibrosis of the lateral muscles ensue and make tendinous reinsertion of the belt muscle by the midline approximation of the linea alba difficult. In some midline hernias, actual loss of the abdominal wall may occur as a result of infections, trauma, and repeated laparotomies. However, in most cases, the loss of substance is more apparent than real.

In long-standing large incisional hernias, the viscera are displaced from their normal positions in the abdomen and cannot be restored to them. In such cases, reduction of the viscera at operation can cause death by compression of the inferior vena cava and by respiratory failure caused by forced elevation and immobilization of the diaphragm. The introduction of pneumoperitoneum by Goni Moreno in 1947 made these formerly inoperable hernias reparable.[50]

Reduced intra-abdominal pressure from the hernia also causes edema of the mesentery and stasis in the splanchnic venous system and the inferior vena cava. Distention and atony of the hollow viscera occur and, in conjunction with decreased ability to increase intra-abdominal pressure, produce difficulties with micturition and bowel movements. Back pain is a common complaint and results from lordosis that is caused by retraction of the belt muscles and decreased efficiency of the rectus abdominis muscle.

The skin and subcutaneous tissues overlying large incisional hernias are stretched and damaged, and the skin becomes atrophic, hypoxic, and devoid of subcutaneous fat. Spontaneous ulcerations develop that are typically solitary and occur at the apex of the hernia. These ulcerations are often misdiagnosed as pressure sores. They resist healing, and intensive local and systemic antimicrobial therapy must be administered to prevent infectious complications at the time of hernioplasty.

Obese patients with large incisional hernias are especially at risk for postoperative infectious complications, respiratory dysfunction, and pulmonary emboli.[26] Preoperative and postoperative prophylaxis for these problems is essential.

Progressive pneumoperitoneum is a useful technique to prepare patients for incisional hernioplasty.[51] It overcomes some of the problems associated with eventration disease and enables some patients with massive irreducible incisional hernias to undergo the operation. Pneumoperitoneum stretches the abdominal wall and intra-abdominal adhesions, facilitates the return of the viscera to the abdomen, and improves diaphragmatic function.

The technique of pneumoperitoneum is simple. Air is injected into the peritoneal cavity through a pneumoperitoneum needle that is inserted with the aid of local anesthesia. Insufflation continues until the patient experiences shortness of breath or shoulder pain. At first, the patient may tolerate only small amounts of air; sometimes, as much as 2 to 4 L may be insufflated initially. Thereafter, air is added at one- to three-day intervals as needed. The pneumoperitoneum is maintained for 10 to 20 days. The patient is ready for operation when palpation reveals flabbiness in the flanks. Inability of the patient to tolerate pneumoperitoneum is a contraindication for incisional hernioplasty.

Incisional Hernioplasty

The object of incisional hernioplasty is anatomic reconstruction of the abdominal wall. This process includes closure of the parietal defect, restoration of normal intra-abdominal pressure, and, in midline hernias, tendinous reinsertion of the lateral abdominal muscles.

Most small incisional hernias are managed by simple closure of the aponeurotic defect. However, large incisional hernias with aponeurotic defects greater than 10 cm in diameter have a strong tendency to recur. Repairs performed by edge-to-edge approximation of aponeurosis or by imbrication frequently fail: recurrence rates have been estimated to be as high as 50 percent. Consequently, most incisional hernias and all recurrent incisional hernias call for the insertion of a prosthesis. The Rives-Stoppa procedure is the preferred method for accomplishing the objectives of incisional hernioplasty.[36,49,52] It is applicable to all types of abdominal incisional hernias, including postnephrectomy lumbar hernias.

The Rives-Stoppa incisional hernioplasty consists of implanting a very large Mersilene prosthesis deep to the muscles of the abdominal wall on top of the posterior rectus abdominis sheath or peritoneum [see Figure 12]. The prosthesis extends far beyond the borders of the myoaponeurotic defects and initially is firmly held in place by intra-abdominal pressure (Pascal's principle) and later by fibrous ingrowth. The prosthesis prevents peritoneal eventration in two ways: by rendering the visceral sac indistensible and by solidly uniting and consolidating the abdominal wall. The technique therefore employs the same concept and principles as Stoppa's properitoneal inguinal hernioplasty and likewise is referred to as GPRVS.

The knitted elastic Mersilene prosthesis is arranged so that it expands vertically and is inextensible horizontally. The mesh must extend beyond the lateral borders of the aponeurotic defect by 8 to 10 cm. The distance inferiorly and superiorly is less critical and requires only 4 to 5 cm. Above the umbilicus, the linea alba interferes with the midline placement of the prosthesis, and a slit in the middle of the superior edge of the prosthesis is necessary to allow the prosthesis to protrude upward within the rectus abdominis sheath on either side of the linea alba.

Peripheral fixation by sutures or staples is usually advisable. The preferred technique for fixation is that developed by Rives, in which the mesh is attached to the abdominal wall with traction-fixation sutures every 5 to 6 cm with the aid of the Reverdin suture needle [see Figure 13]. The lateral traction sutures also advantageously stretch the retracted belt muscles, retain the peritoneum, and facilitate midline approximation. Fixation sutures are not needed when the prosthesis extends deep into the space of Retzius or far into the iliac fossa. When the retromuscular space is undissectable, the prosthesis must be implanted intraperitoneally. The intraperitoneal prosthesis must be prevented from touching the viscera either by the omentum or by an absorbable synthetic prosthesis. Likewise, an absorbable prosthesis is used to substitute for the posterior rectus abdominis sheath when the sheath cannot be approximated.

Aponeurotic closure of the parietal defect is important. The midline closure can withstand greater tension because the prosthesis, not the suture line, ultimately unites the abdomen. However, when necessary, tension can be reduced by the use of 1 cm vertical relaxing incisions arranged quincuncially in the rectus abdominis sheath. Each row of overlapping relaxing incisions expands the sheath 1 cm. Long relaxing incisions above the umbilicus are not recommended and should never be made below the umbilicus. Aponeurotic approximation is usually achievable. When it is not, a second absorbable or nonabsorbable prosthesis inlaid in the aponeurotic defect ensures stability of the abdominal wall during the healing process; usually, this inability to achieve approximation occurs in the region of the xiphoid or the symphysis. Dead space created by large prostheses always calls for closed suction drainage to prevent seroma and hematoma formation and to allow quick fibrous incorporation of the prosthesis in the abdominal wall.

References

1. Gilbert AI: An anatomic and functional classification for the diagnosis and treatment of inguinal hernia. Am J Surg 157:331, 1989

2. Nyhus LM, Klein MS, Rogers F: Inguinal hernia. Curr Probl Surg 73:407, 1991

3. Nyhus LM: Clinical update: individualization of hernia repair: a new era. Surgery 114:1, 1993

4. Bendavid R: The TSD classification: a nomenclature for groin hernias. GREPA 15:9, 1993

5. Schumpelick V, Treutner KH, Arlt G: Inguinal hernia repair in adults. Lancet 344:375, 1994

6. Fruchaud H: Le Traitement Chirurgical des Hernies de L'Aine Chez L'Adulte. G Doin, Paris, 1956

7. Fruchaud H: Anatomie Chirurgicale des Hernies de L'Aine. G Doin, Paris, 1956

8. Glassow F: Inguinal hernia repair using local anaesthesia. Ann R Coll Surg Engl 66:382, 1984

9. Halverson K, McVay CB: Inguinal and femoral hernioplasty: a 22-year study of the authors' methods. Arch Surg 101:127, 1970

10. Wantz GE: The Canadian repair: personal observations. World J Surg 13:516, 1989

11. Wantz GE: The operation of Bassini as described by Attilio Catterina. Surg Gynecol Obstet 168:67, 1989

12. Griffith CA: The Marcy repair of indirect inguinal hernia. Surg Clin North Am 51:1309, 1971

13. Griffith CA: The Marcy repair revisited. Surg Clin North Am 64:215, 1984

14. Glassow F: The surgical repair of inguinal and femoral hernias. Can Med Assoc J 108:308, 1973

15. Shearburn EW, Myers RN: Shouldice repair for inguinal hernia. Surgery 66:450, 1969

16. Wantz GE: The Canadian repair of inguinal hernia. Hernia, 3rd ed. Nyhus LM, Condon RE, Eds. JB Lippincott Co, Philadelphia, 1989, p 236

17. Madden JL, Hakim S, Agorogiannis AB: The anatomy and repair of inguinal hernias. Surg Clin North Am 51:1269, 1971

18. Condon RE: The anatomy of the inguinal region and its relation to groin hernia. Hernia, 3rd ed. Nyhus LM, Condon RE, Eds. JB Lippincott Co, Philadelphia, 1989, p 18

19. McVay CB: A fundamental error in current methods of inguinal herniorrhaphy. Surg Gynecol Obstet 74:746, 1942

20. McVay CB: Inguinal hernioplasty: common mistakes and pitfalls. Surg Clin North Am 46:1089, 1966

21. McVay CB: The anatomic basis for inguinal and femoral hernioplasty. Surg Gynecol Obstet 139:931, 1974

22. Rutledge RH: Cooper's ligament repairs: a 25-year experience with a single technique for all groin hernias in adults. Surgery 103:1, 1988

23. McVay CB: The anatomy of the relaxing incision in inguinal hernioplasty. Quarterly Bulletin of the Northwestern University Medical School 36:245, 1962

24. Cheatle GT: An operation for inguinal hernia. BMJ 2:1025, 1921

25. Henry AK: Operation for femoral hernia by a midline, extraperitoneal approach with a preliminary note on the use of this route for reducible inguinal hernia. Lancet 1:531, 1936

26. Houck JP, Rypins EB, Sarfeh IJ, et al: Repair of incisional hernia. Surg Gynecol Obstet 169:397, 1989

27. Lichtenstein IL, Shulman AG, Amid PK, et al: The tension-free hernioplasty. Am J Surg 157:188, 1989

28. Lichtenstein IL, Shore JM: Simplified repair of femoral and recurrent inguinal hernias by a "plug" technic. Am J Surg 128:439, 1974

29. Gilbert AI: Sutureless repair of inguinal hernia. Am J Surg 163:331, 1992

30. Gilbert AI: Inguinal hernia repair: biomaterials and sutureless repair. Perspect Gen Surg 2:113, 1991

31. Rutkow IM, Robbins AW: "Tension-free" inguinal herniorrhaphy: a preliminary report on the "mesh plug" technique. Surgery 114:3, 1993

32. Robbins AW, Rutkow IM: The mesh-plug hernioplasty. Surg Clin North Am 73:501, 1993

33. Read RC: Bilaterality and the prosthetic repair of large recurrent inguinal hernias. Am J Surg 138:788, 1979

34. Nyhus LM, Pollak R, Bombeck TC, et al: The preperitoneal approach and prosthetic buttress repair for recurrent hernia. Ann Surg 208:733, 1988

35. Stoppa RE, Rives JL, Warlaumont CR, et al: The use of Dacron in the repair of hernias of the groin. Surg Clin North Am 64:269, 1984

36. Stoppa RE: The treatment of complicated groin and incisional hernias. World J Surg 13:545, 1989

37. Stoppa RE, Warlaumont CR: The preperitoneal approach and prosthetic repair of groin hernia. Hernia, 3rd ed. Nyhus LM, Condon RE, Eds. JB Lippincott Co, Philadelphia, 1989, p 199

38. Wantz GE: Giant prosthetic reinforcement of the visceral sac. Surg Gynecol Obstet 169:408, 1989

39. Wantz GE: The technique of giant prosthetic reinforcement of the visceral sac performed through an anterior groin incision. Surg Gynecol Obstet 176:497, 1993

40. Fong Y, Wantz GE: Prevention of ischemic orchitis during inguinal hernioplasty with 6454 hernioplasties in male patients. Surg Gynecol Obstet 174:399, 1992

41. Wantz GE: Testicular atrophy and chronic residual neuralgia as risks of inguinal hernioplasty. Surg Clin North Am 73:571, 1993

42. Wantz GE: Testicular atrophy as a risk of inguinal hernioplasty. Surg Gynecol Obstet 154:570, 1982

43. Wantz GE: Ambulatory surgical treatment of groin hernia: prevention and management of complications. Curr Probl Surg 3:311, 1986

44. Chevrel JP, Gatt MT: The treatment of neuralgias following herniorrhaphy: a report of 47 cases. Postgrad Gen Surg 4:142, 1992

45. Starling JR, Harms BA: Diagnosis and treatment of genitofemoral and ilioinguinal neuralgia. World J Surg 13:586, 1989

46. Spangen L: Spigelian hernia. World J Surg 13:573, 1989

47. Leslie D: The parastomal hernia. Surg Clin North Am 64:407, 1984

48. Sugarbaker PH: Prosthetic mesh repair of large hernias at the site of colonic stomas. Surg Gynecol Obstet 150:577, 1980

49. Rives J: Major incisional hernias. Surgery of the Abdominal Wall. Chevrel JP, Ed. Springer-Verlag, New York, 1986, p 116

50. Goni Moreno I: Chronic eventrations and large hernias. Surgery 22:945, 1947

51. Raynor RW, DelGuercio LRM: The place for pneumoperitoneum in the repair of massive hernia. World J Surg 13:581, 1989

52. Wantz GE: Incisional hernioplasty with Mersilene. Surg Gynecol Obstet 172:129, 1991

53. Wantz GE: Atlas of Hernia Surgery. Raven Press, New York, 1991

54. Wantz GE: Abdominal wall surgery. Principles of Surgery, 6th ed. Schwartz SI, Shires GT, Spencer FC, eds. McGraw-Hill, New York, 1994, p 1517

Reviews

Chevrel JP: Surgery of the Abdominal Wall. Springer-Verlag, New York, 1986

Devlin HB: Management of Abdominal Hernias. Butterworth, London, 1988

Lichtenstein IL: Hernia Repair Without Disability, 2nd ed. Ishiyaku Euroamerica, St. Louis, 1986

Nyhus LM, Condon RE: Hernia, 3rd ed. JB Lippincott Co, Philadelphia, 1989

Schumpelick V, Zinner M: Atlas of Hernia Surgery. BC Decker, Philadelphia, 1990

Skandalakis JE, Gray SW, Mansberger AR, et al: Hernia: Surgical Anatomy and Technique. McGraw-Hill, New York, 1989

Wantz GE: Atlas of Hernia Surgery. Raven Press, New York, 1991

Acknowledgment

Figures 1 through 13   Tom Moore.

21 LAPAROSCOPIC HERNIA REPAIR

Liane S. Feldman, M.D., and Marvin J. Wexler, M.D.

The introduction of video-assisted minimal access surgery has dramatically altered patient care over the past decade. Certain laparoscopic procedures, including cholecystectomy and antireflux procedures, have shown obvious benefits (e.g., more rapid and less painful recovery) and have been readily and universally adopted. Others, particularly laparoscopic inguinal hernia repair (first described by Ger in 1990[1]), remain controversial. Laparoscopic inguinal herniorrhaphy has shown a great deal of promise; however, concurrently with its development, open anterior herniorrhaphy has evolved into a tension-free, often sutureless mesh repair that is easily performed with the patient under local anesthesia and that is also associated with rapid recovery and low recurrence rates.[2] Thus, to gain acceptance, laparoscopic inguinal hernia repair must be shown to provide a significant advantage over the tension-free open repair now in use.

The two most common techniques for laparoscopic inguinal hernia repair both involve the insertion of mesh into the preperitoneal space; one makes use of a transabdominal preperitoneal (TAPP) approach, the other a totally extraperitoneal (TEP) approach. Both approaches would appear to offer potential advantages, such as reduced postoperative pain, shortened convalescence, quicker and more accurate assessment and repair of bilateral groin hernias simultaneously, and, in the case of recurrent hernia, avoidance of previously dissected and technically difficult scarred areas. In practice, however, these advantages are not invariably realized: a laparoscopic approach is not always minimally invasive, and various disadvantages accrue from the current requirement for general anesthesia, the need to traverse the abdominal cavity in the TAPP technique, and the increase in operating room time and costs.[3]

Meticulous attention to surgical technique is essential. Because surgeons may be unfamiliar with inguinal anatomy as viewed from inside the abdomen and because the potential for complications necessitating laparotomy is increased with the laparoscopic approach, surgeons must be proficient in laparoscopic techniques and must have a precise knowledge of anatomic relations in the region of the groin as seen from the peritoneal surface.

Since the late 1990s, laparoscopic video techniques have also been increasingly applied to the repair of incisional hernias.[4-8] Laparoscopic repair of large incisional hernias resembles open repair in that mesh is inserted to cover the defect in the abdominal wall fascia. A laparoscopic approach is theoretically attractive because an open approach usually necessitates a large incision as well as extensive and tedious wide dissection to expose the abdominal wall defect, resulting in considerable postoperative pain and a risk of wound complications—problems that a laparoscopic approach to the defect from within might minimize.

It may be many more years before we can determine the true safety and efficacy of laparoscopic herniorrhaphy and establish the correct indications for its use. In the meantime, every repair performed should be subjected to careful classification, documentation, and quality-of-life assessment. Surgeons should not perform laparoscopic herniorrhaphy simply because it is novel or potentially economical: they should perform this procedure only when convinced that it is anatomically and physiologically correct and logical.

In what follows, we discuss laparoscopic repair of both inguinal and incisional hernias. In addition to describing current operative techniques, we address inguinal surgical anatomy, preoperative planning, and complications. Finally, we review selected trials measuring the results of laparoscopic repair against those of open repair and comparing the outcomes of TAPP repair with those of TEP repair.

Laparoscopic Inguinal Hernia Repair

LAPAROSCOPIC INGUINAL ANATOMY

To most surgeons, inguinal anatomy as viewed through the laparoscope appears unfamiliar. The surgical perspective on the pelvic anatomy from the intraperitoneal view has been best described by Skandalakis and coworkers[9] and has been elegantly demonstrated in cadaver dissections by Spaw and colleagues,[10] whose work forms the basis of the descriptions we present in this chapter. Excellent descriptions of the preperitoneal space by Wantz[11] and Condon[12] are also worthy of review.

During laparoscopic herniorrhaphy, a number of structures that are usually visible during open herniorrhaphy (e.g., the inguinal ligament, the pubic tubercle, the lacunar ligament, and the ilioinguinal and iliohypogastric nerves) are not seen initially. Conversely, a number of structures that are visible only after significant dissection in the open approach are easily viewed through the laparoscope [*see Figure 1*]. Identification of the iliopubic tract, Cooper's ligament, and the transverse abdominal arch is mandatory to ensure proper coverage and securing of prosthetic material margins. The obliterated umbilical artery, a structure not encountered in the anterior approach to open herniorrhaphy, must be divided or retracted medially to afford visualization and dissection of the pubic tubercle, Cooper's ligament, and often the entire Hesselbach's triangle.

Peritoneum Intact

Four important landmarks should be seen at initial laparoscopic inspection of the inguinal region [*see Figure 2*]: the spermatic vessels, the obliterated umbilical artery (also referred to as the medial umbilical ligament or bladder ligament by various authors), the inferior epigastric vessels (also referred to as the lateral umbilical ligament), and the external iliac vessels.

Spermatic vessels The testicular artery and vein descend from the retroperitoneum, travel directly over and slightly lateral to the external iliac artery, and enter the internal spermatic ring posteriorly. These vessels are covered only by the peritoneum and are usually well visualized as flat structures in the abdominal cavity that assume a cordlike appearance when joined by the vas def-

a

Internal Oblique Muscle   External Oblique Muscle

Transversus
Abdominis Muscle
and Aponeurosis

Transverse
Fascia

Reflected
External
Oblique
Aponeurosis

Inferior
Epigastric Vessels

Spermatic Cord

Superficial
Inguinal
Ring

b

Transversus Abdominis
Aponeurosis Arch

Semicircular Line

Transverse
Fascia Sling

Spermatic
Cord

Henle's Ligament

Cooper's Ligament

Iliopubic Tract

External Iliac Vessels

Figure 1 Laparoscopic inguinal hernia repair. Shown are (*a*) the anatomy of the left groin region as seen from the traditional anterior approach to herniorrhaphy and (*b*) the anatomy of the right groin from the posterior, or peritoneal, approach. The inguinal canal floor is covered by transverse fascia alone, and a large space separates the transversus abdominis aponeurosis from the inguinal ligament (*a*). A preperitoneal view of the groin region shows the distance between the transversus abdominis tendon and Cooper's ligament, the iliopubic tract, and the inguinal ligament (*b*).

erens immediately before entering the internal spermatic ring. If no hernia is present, a mere dimple will be seen [*see Figure 2*]. An indirect hernia, if present, will be immediately apparent with an obvious opening [*see Figure 3*]. The vas deferens is best identified where it joins the spermatic vessels. From there, the vas can be traced back medially as it courses over the pelvic brim and falls into the pelvis and behind the bladder. There is a small artery that runs with the vas deferens and is not well seen or known. It is white and cordlike in appearance and can usually be seen just beneath the peritoneum.

Obliterated umbilical artery The obliterated umbilical artery is an unfamiliar but sometimes prominent structure that courses along the anterior abdominal wall toward the umbilicus, often with an apparent mesentery. It is most prominent in the region of the medial inguinal space. This ligament is most readily identified when the umbilical laparoscope is directed toward the pelvic midline, where the ligament's bilateral structure can be best seen directed toward the umbilicus. Medial retraction of this structure is usually necessary for full exposure of the medial aspect of the inguinal canal.

Inferior epigastric vessels The inferior epigastric artery and vein lie in the medial aspect of the internal inguinal ring and ascend the rectus abdominis muscle anteriorly. They are frequently difficult to visualize, particularly in obese patients, and are best identified by locating the internal inguinal ring at the junction of

the vas deferens and the testicular artery and vein. At this location, they exit the medial margin of the internal ring. However, the vessels can quickly fade from view as they travel superiorly and medially along the anterior abdominal wall.

Figure 2 Laparoscopic inguinal hernia repair. Shown is a laparoscopic view of the anatomy of the left groin with the peritoneum intact in a patient without a hernia. (IEV—inferior epigastric vessels; IR—internal ring; MUL—medial umbilical ligament; TV—testicular vessels; VD—vas deferens)

Figure 3 Laparoscopic inguinal hernia repair. Shown is a right indirect inguinal hernia. The vas deferens can be seen below the hernia defect. Omentum is in the hernial sac.

Internal inguinal ring The internal inguinal ring is normally identified by a slight indentation of the peritoneum at the junction of the vas deferens and the spermatic vessels. When an indirect hernia is present, however, a true ring or opening is easily identified, and by rotating a 30° laparoscope, one can look directly into the hernial sac or insert the laparoscope into the sac, which often allows the external inguinal ring to be identified more medially. An indirect hernial sac lies anterior and lateral to the spermatic cord at this level, as opposed to the familiar medial cord position seen in the classic exterior groin approach to open herniorrhaphy. The medial border of the internal inguinal ring is formed by the transverse fascia and the inferior epigastric vessels. The inferior border is identified by the iliopubic tract, a distinct structure that is the internal counterpart of the inguinal ligament. Anteriorly, the internal inguinal ring is bordered by the transversus abdominis arch (conjoined tendon), which extends medially to insert into the pubic ramus near the pubic tubercle. As the transversus abdominis arch passes laterally over the internal ring, it forms a very well defined visible edge. The layers of the abdominal wall constituting the lateral border of the internal inguinal ring appear the same as when viewed from the exterior approach, and like all margins of the internal inguinal ring, this border is visible only when an indirect hernia is present.

External iliac vessels The lateral spermatic vessels and the medial vas deferens merge at the internal inguinal ring and enter the inguinal canal, where they form the apex of the so-called triangle of doom. Beneath this triangle lie the external iliac artery and the external iliac vein. More laterally, the femoral nerve can be found. The external iliac vessels are often difficult to visualize, though in an elderly patient, a calcified pulsating artery may be prominent. Extreme care must be taken not to dissect within the triangle of doom because such dissection can result in serious bleeding.

Peritoneum Removed

Removal of the peritoneal covering allows access to and visualization of the preperitoneal space and anatomic landmarks critical for repair [*see Figure 4*].

Iliopubic tract The iliopubic tract originates laterally from the anterior superior spine of the ilium and courses medially, forming the inferior margin of the internal inguinal ring and the roof of the femoral canal before inserting medially into the superior pubic ramus. This tract is formed by the condensation of the transverse fascia with the most inferior portion of the transversus abdominis muscle and aponeurosis, and the tract is usually sturdy along its entire course. All inguinal hernial defects lie above the iliopubic tract, either anterior or superior to it. Conversely, femoral hernias occur below the tract, either posterior or inferior to it. Fibers of the iliopubic tract extend into Cooper's ligament medially, where they become the medial margin of the femoral canal. The iliopubic tract is frequently confused with the inguinal ligament, which, though nearby, is part of the superficial muscu-

Figure 4 Laparoscopic inguinal hernia repair. Shown is the left inguinal region with the peritoneum removed, as seen during laparoscopic herniorrhaphy.

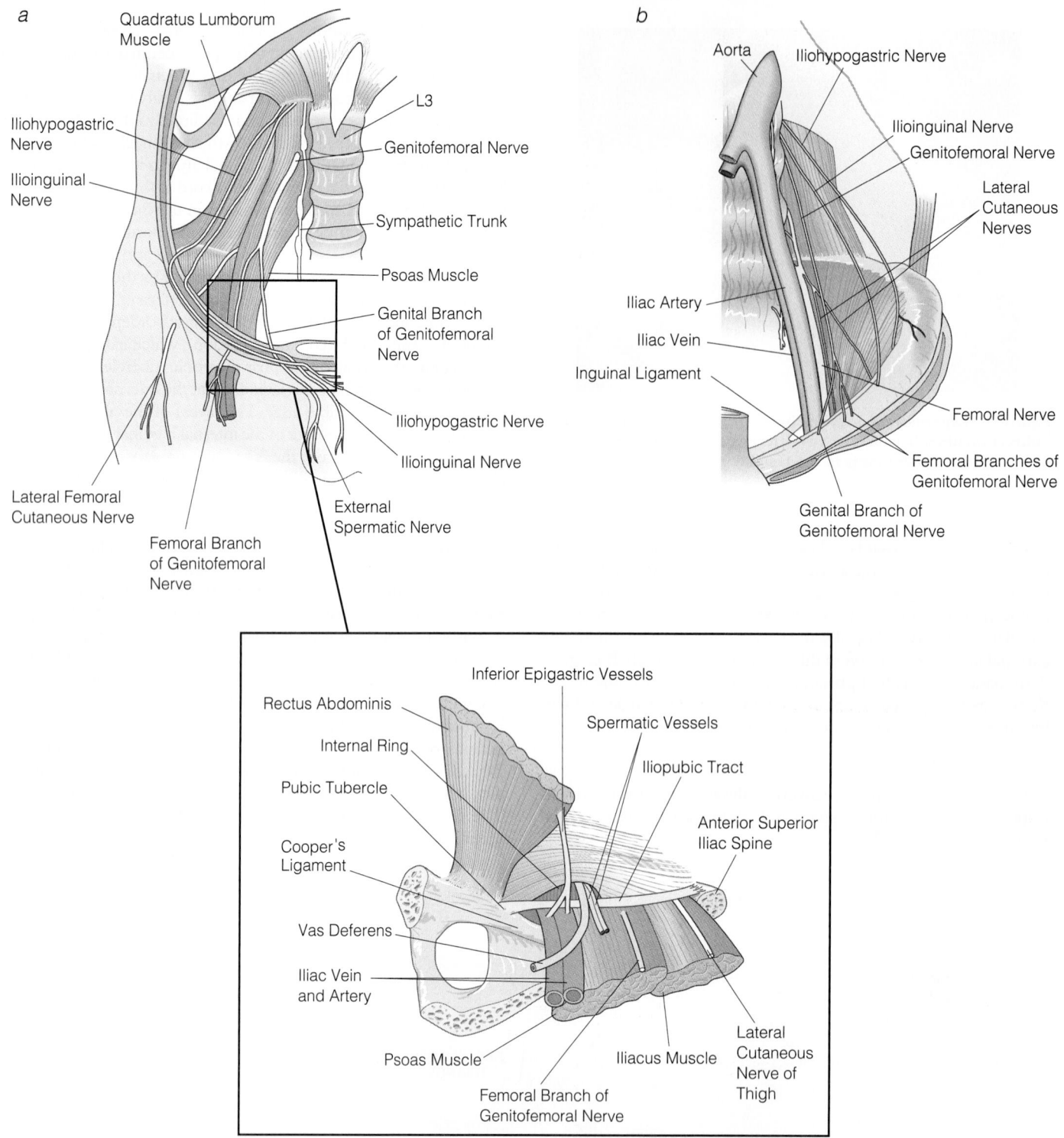

a

Quadratus Lumborum Muscle

Iliohypogastric Nerve

Ilioinguinal Nerve

L3

Genitofemoral Nerve

Sympathetic Trunk

Psoas Muscle

Genital Branch of Genitofemoral Nerve

Iliohypogastric Nerve

Ilioinguinal Nerve

Lateral Femoral Cutaneous Nerve

Femoral Branch of Genitofemoral Nerve

External Spermatic Nerve

b

Aorta

Iliohypogastric Nerve

Ilioinguinal Nerve

Genitofemoral Nerve

Lateral Cutaneous Nerves

Iliac Artery

Iliac Vein

Inguinal Ligament

Femoral Nerve

Femoral Branches of Genitofemoral Nerve

Genital Branch of Genitofemoral Nerve

Inferior Epigastric Vessels

Rectus Abdominis

Internal Ring

Pubic Tubercle

Cooper's Ligament

Vas Deferens

Iliac Vein and Artery

Spermatic Vessels

Iliopubic Tract

Anterior Superior Iliac Spine

Psoas Muscle

Femoral Branch of Genitofemoral Nerve

Iliacus Muscle

Lateral Cutaneous Nerve of Thigh

Figure 5 **Laparoscopic inguinal hernia repair. Shown are the courses of the genitofemoral and ilioinguinal nerves of the right groin (*a*) and of the left groin (*b*). Inset shows the preperitoneal anatomy of the right groin, as seen by the laparoscopic surgeon.**

loaponeurotic layer, which is not seen laparoscopically. The iliopubic tract is part of the deep layer.

Cooper's ligament   Cooper's ligament is a condensation of the transverse fascia and the periosteum of the superior pubic ramus lateral to the pubic tubercle. It can be seen only from within the abdominal cavity once the peritoneum is opened and deflected inferiorly, but a considerable amount of preperitoneal

fat must often be cleaned off the ligament before it can be seen. Initially, it is often easier to palpate the ligament than to see it, but once the ligament has been identified and cleaned, its glistening white fibers are apparent. Care must be taken during dissection to avoid the tiny branches of the obturator vein that often run along the ligament's surface. The iliopubic tract inserts into the superior ramus of the pubis just lateral to Cooper's ligament, blending into it.

Femoral canal   The femoral canal is seen only in the presence of a femoral hernia in the most medial aspect of the femoral triangle. The anterior and medial borders are bounded by the iliopubic tract, the posterior border is formed by the pectineal fascia, and the lateral border is formed by the femoral sheath and vein.

Trapezoid of disaster. Another area worthy of careful attention is the so-called trapezoid of disaster, containing the genitofemoral, ilioinguinal, iliohypogastric, and lateral cutaneous nerves of the thigh, which innervate the spermatic cord, testicle, scrotum, and upper and lateral thigh, respectively. A detailed knowledge of their anatomic course and careful avoidance of the nerves are essential [*see Figure 5*].

Genitofemoral nerve. The genitofemoral nerve arises from the first and second lumbar nerves; pierces the psoas muscle and fascia at its medial border opposite L3 or L4; descends under the peritoneum, on the psoas major muscle; and divides into a medial genital and a lateral femoral branch. The femoral branch descends lateral to the external iliac artery and the spermatic cord, passing posteroinferior to the iliopubic tract and into the femoral sheath to supply the skin over the femoral triangle. The genital branch crosses the lower end of the external iliac artery and enters the inguinal canal through the internal inguinal ring with the testicular vessels. This branch supplies the coverings of the spermatic cord down to the skin of the scrotum. The genitofemoral nerve is the most visible of the cutaneous nerves and is sometimes confused with the testicular vessels if the latter are not well appreciated in their more medial position.

Ilioinguinal and iliohypogastric nerves. When dissected from the anterior position, the ilioinguinal and iliohypogastric nerves lie between the external oblique and the internal oblique muscles above the internal inguinal ring and descend the spermatic cord. In the abdomen, the ilioinguinal and iliohypogastric nerves arise from the 12th thoracic and first lumbar nerve roots, are more laterally located, and run subperitoneally, emerging from the lateral psoas border to pierce the transversus abdominis muscle near the iliac crest and then pierce and course between the internal oblique and the external oblique muscles close to the internal inguinal ring. Aberrant branches sometimes descend with the genital nerve. The ilioinguinal nerve supplies a small cutaneous area near the external genitals.

Lateral cutaneous nerve of the thigh. Supplying the front and lateral aspect of the thigh, the lateral cutaneous nerve of the thigh arises from the second and third lumbar nerves and emerges at the lateral border of the psoas. There, it descends deep to the peritoneum on the iliac muscle and only comes to lie in a superficial position 3 cm below the anterosuperior iliac spine.

PREOPERATIVE EVALUATION

History and Physical Examination

Preoperative assessment is necessary to determine whether a patient is a suitable candidate for laparoscopic herniorrhaphy. A careful surgical history, including both previous hernia repairs and other procedures (particularly those involving the lower abdomen), should be elicited. A cardiovascular history should also be obtained and risk factors for general anesthesia determined.

Physical examination should confirm the presence of an inguinal hernia. If the patient reports a history of a bulge but no hernia is felt on physical examination, an occult hernia may be presumed. If doubt exists, herniography is indicated. Ultrasonography may be helpful for distinguishing an incarcerated groin hernia from other causes of inguinal swelling (e.g., lymphadenopathy).

Selection of Patients

Indications   With the evolution of the open anterior approach to tension-free prosthetic mesh repair, determining which patients will benefit significantly from laparoscopic herniorrhaphy becomes increasingly important. One may choose either (1) to offer laparoscopic repair to all hernia patients in the belief that it is an inherently superior procedure or (2) to reserve laparoscopic repair for specific indications. We prefer the latter choice, believing that these patients are best served when the surgeon has several approaches at his or her command that can be applied to and, if necessary, modified for individual circumstances.

In our opinion, primary unilateral hernias are best treated with an open anterior tension-free repair, preferably with the patient under local or regional anesthesia; possible exceptions include manual laborers and athletes who desire a rapid return to vigorous physical activity and who may benefit from the absence of a sizable incision. We generally reserve laparoscopic inguinal herniorrhaphy for the following clinical situations:

1. Recurrent hernias after previous anterior repair. In such cases, a laparoscopic approach allows one to avoid the scar tissue and distorted anatomy present in the anterior abdominal wall by performing the repair through unviolated tissue, thereby reducing the risk of damage to the vas deferens or the testicular vessels.
2. Bilateral hernias or a unilateral hernia when the presence of a contralateral hernia is strongly suspected. In such cases, a laparoscopic approach allows one to repair both hernias simultaneously and perhaps more rapidly without having to make additional incisions.
3. Repair of an inguinal hernia concurrent with another laparoscopic procedure, provided that there is no contamination of the peritoneal cavity.

Contraindications   We do not treat incarcerated hernias laparoscopically. In patients to whom general anesthesia may pose an increased risk, we prefer open anterior repair using local or regional anesthesia. In infants and young children with indirect hernias, for whom repair of the posterior canal wall is unnecessary, we recommend high ligation of the sac via the anterior approach.

Previous lower abdominal surgery, though not an absolute contraindication, may make laparoscopic dissection difficult. In particular, with respect to TEP repair, previous abdominal wall incisions may make it impossible to safely separate the peritoneum from the abdominal parietes for entry into the extraperitoneal plane. Previous surgery in the retropubic space of Retzius, as in prostatic surgery, is a relative contraindication that is associated with an increased risk of bladder injury[13] and other complications.[14]

OPERATIVE PLANNING

Preparation

General anesthesia administered by inhalation is routinely used. Prophylactic antibiotics are unnecessary. The patient is instructed to void before surgery, which means that preoperative bladder catheterization is unnecessary.

Patient Positioning

The patient is placed in the supine position with both arms tucked against the sides. The anesthesia screen is placed as far toward the

Figure 6 **Laparoscopic inguinal hernia repair. Shown is one of several possible OR setups. The surgeon stands on the side contralateral to the defect, with a nurse on the ipsilateral side. The assistant surgeon stands opposite the surgeon. This positioning may vary, depending on the surgeon's preference and handedness, the visibility of the defect, and the type of defect present, as well as on the prominence of the medial umbilical ligament and the need for its retraction.**

head of the table as possible to allow the surgeon a wide range of mobility with the laparoscope. The skin must be prepared and draped so as to allow exposure of the entire lower abdomen, the genital region, and the upper thighs because manipulation of the hernial sac and the scrotum is frequently necessary. After the laparoscope has been introduced, the patient is placed in a deep Trendelenburg position so that the viscera will fall away from the inguinal areas. Further bowel manipulation is rarely necessary, except to reduce hernial contents. Rotation of the table to elevate the side of the hernia can provide additional exposure, if necessary. A single video monitor is placed at the foot of the bed, directly facing the patient's head.

The surgeon usually begins the repair while standing on the side contralateral to the defect; the assistant surgeon stands opposite the surgeon, and the nurse stands on the ipsilateral side [*see Figure 6*]. Once the key anatomic landmarks and the hernial defect are located and defined, the surgeon should be able to move to either side of the patient, and the surgeon or the assistant should be able to move the camera and the instruments to the ports of preference, the choice of which depends on optimum exposure, angle, right- or left-

handedness, and the designated role of the assistant surgeon as either camera operator or surgical assistant. A two-handed technique provides a distinct technical advantage and also eliminates the need for an additional surgical assistant.

Equipment

Because inguinal hernias occur in the anterior abdominal wall, visualization through the umbilicus requires angling the laparoscope close to the horizontal plane. The view is paralleled anteriorly by the surface of the lower abdominal wall, which may make visualization with a 0° laparoscope difficult. In addition, an indirect hernia is a three-dimensional tubular defect that can be well visualized in its entirety only with an angled lens. For these reasons, we recommend routine use of an oblique, forward-viewing 30° laparoscope. Excellent 30° laparoscopes are currently available in 10 mm, 5 mm, and 3 mm sizes.

A basic set of instruments for laparoscopic hernia repair should include graspers, dissectors, curved scissors, a suction-irrigation device, a hook cautery, and needle drivers. In addition, we use a multifire stapler to fix the mesh and close the peritoneum (though it is certainly possible to use sutures instead). Either a circular tacker or a linear stapler can be employed; both are available in 10 mm and 5 mm sizes. We prefer the linear stapler.

In a TEP repair, besides the equipment needed for a TAPP repair, a blunt trocar is required for gaining access to the preperitoneal space. An operative laparoscope is needed as well. Alternatively, special preperitoneal distention balloon (PDB) systems [*see* Operative Technique, Totally Extraperitoneal Repair, *below*] are also frequently used to develop the preperitoneal space.

OPERATIVE TECHNIQUE

As noted (see above), there are two principal techniques of laparoscopic inguinal hernia repair. The TAPP repair involves insufflating the peritoneal cavity, penetrating the abdomen with trocars, incising the peritoneum overlying the defect, and closing the peritoneum after the repair with a piece of mesh placed in the preperitoneal space. The TEP repair, on the other hand, involves gaining access to the preperitoneal space via trocars placed in a space created between the fascia and the peritoneum, insufflating that space, and placing a piece of mesh between the underside of the anterior abdominal wall and the peritoneum.

We will not describe the intraperitoneal onlay mesh (IPOM) technique, in which polypropylene mesh is fixed directly onto the peritoneum intra-abdominally. This approach has been abandoned by most surgeons out of fear of complications related to adhesions and possible erosion of the mesh into bowel.[3,15]

Transabdominal Preperitoneal Repair

Step 1: placement of trocars Pneumoperitoneum is established through a small vertical infraumbilical incision. Either a closed approach, using a Veress needle, or an open (Hasson) approach, using a 10/12 mm trocar, may be employed. We prefer the open technique, in which the first trocar is inserted into the peritoneal cavity under direct vision. This approach usually prevents injuries to the major blood vessels; although it does not completely prevent bowel injuries, it does facilitate discovery and repair of such injuries.

CO_2 is then insufflated into the abdomen to a pressure of 15 mm Hg. The angled laparoscope is introduced, and both inguinal areas are inspected. Two 10/12 mm accessory ports are then placed at the lateral border of each rectus abdominis muscle at the level of the umbilicus to allow placement of the camera and the instruments [*see Figure 7*]. The 10/12 mm lateral ports can be

Figure 7 **Laparoscopic inguinal hernia repair: TAPP approach. Shown is standard trocar placement for TAPP repair. Usually, three trocar sites are used. The laparoscope is inserted through the umbilical trocar, and two additional trocars are placed in the right and the left midabdomen. To ensure that the first trocar is not placed too close to the surgical field, the first trocar should be placed either in the umbilicus or immediately above it. The two lateral trocars should be placed lateral to the rectus sheath to prevent bleeding and postoperative muscle spasms. At least one trocar must be 10/12 mm to allow insertion of the mesh.**

replaced with 5 mm ports if 5 mm instruments and a 5 mm laparoscope are available. To facilitate port placement, the abdominal wall is transilluminated with the laparoscope so as to delineate the border of the rectus abdominis muscle, which can be difficult to define in muscular or obese males. Additional care is taken to keep from puncturing the large subcutaneous veins that are frequently present in this region. Failure to transilluminate the abdominal wall can result in placement of the trocar through the rectus muscle, which can cause troublesome bleeding.

Step 2: identification of anatomic landmarks The four key anatomic landmarks mentioned earlier [*see* Laparoscopic In-

guinal Anatomy, Peritoneum Intact, *above*]—the spermatic vessels, the obliterated umbilical artery (medial umbilical ligament), the inferior epigastric vessels (lateral umbilical ligament), and the external iliac vessels—are identified on each side. In the presence of an indirect hernia, the internal inguinal ring is easily identified by the presence of a discrete hole at the junction of the vas deferens and the testicular vessels. Identification of a direct hernia can be more difficult [*see Figure 8*]. A direct hernia sometimes appears as a complete circle or hole and sometimes as a cleft, and at other times it is completely hidden by preperitoneal fat and the bladder and umbilical ligament. Visualization can be particularly difficult in obese patients, who may have considerable lipomatous tissue between the peritoneum and the transversalis fascia, or in patients whose hernia consists of a weakness and bulging of the entire inguinal floor rather than a distinct sac. For adequate definition of this type of hernia and deeper anatomic structures, the peritoneum must be opened, a peritoneal flap developed, and the underlying fatty layer dissected.[16] Direct hernial defects are often situated medial to the ipsilateral umbilical ligament, and retraction or even division of this structure is sometimes necessary. Traction on the ipsilateral testicle can demonstrate the vas deferens when visualization is obscured by overlying fat or pressure from the pneumoperitoneum.

Step 3: creation of peritoneal flap The curved cautery scissors or the hook cautery is used to create a peritoneal flap by making a transverse incision along the peritoneum, beginning just above the upper border of the internal inguinal ring and extending medially above the pubic tubercle and laterally 2 cm beyond the internal inguinal ring [*see Figure 9*]. Extreme care must be taken to avoid the inferior epigastric vessels. Bleeding from the epigastrics can usually be controlled by cauterization, but application of hemostatic clips may be necessary on occasion. Another solution is to pass percutaneously placed sutures above and below the bleeding point while applying pressure to the bleeding vessel so as not to obscure the field of vision.

If the monopolar cautery is used to create the peritoneal flap, the entire uninsulated portion of the instrument must be visible at all times. Unlike laparoscopic cholecystectomy, in which the liver acts as a safe backdrop for scatter and dissection is anterosuperior to the colon, laparoscopic herniorrhaphy may bring bowel loops in contact with instruments, an occurrence that can be particularly dangerous if current is applied to a long-nosed forceps or grasper and a backdrop is lacking. The medial umbilical ligament must be retracted for me-

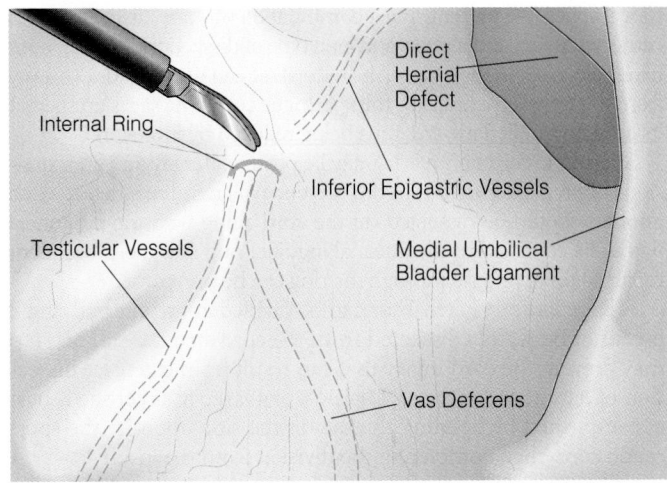

Figure 8 **Laparoscopic inguinal hernia repair: TAPP approach. Shown is a left direct inguinal hernia with the peritoneum intact. The dissector indicates the intact internal ring.**

Figure 9 **Laparoscopic inguinal hernia repair: TAPP approach. Shown is dissection of a left direct inguinal hernia. The hernial sac is inverted and the peritoneum incised superior to the sac.**

Figure 10 **Laparoscopic inguinal hernia repair: TAPP approach. A flap of peritoneum is dissected downward, revealing a hernial defect and the inferior epigastric vessels (arrow) on the left side.**

dial dissection and may have to be divided. Division of this structure does not have any negative sequelae; however, one should be aware that the obliterated umbilical artery may still be patent and should use the cautery or clips.

The incised peritoneum is grasped along with the attached preperitoneal fat and the peritoneal sac and is dissected caudad with blunt and sharp dissection to create a lower peritoneal flap [*see Figure 10*]. Dissection must stay close to the abdominal wall. A significant amount of preperitoneal fat may be encountered, and this should remain with the peritoneal flap so that the abdominal wall is cleared. When the correct preperitoneal plane is entered, dissection is almost bloodless and easily carried out. A smaller superior peritoneal flap is then created, exposing the posterior rectus muscle and the transversus abdominis arch. Scissors, if used, should always have cautery capability so that bleeding from the multiple small vessels beneath the peritoneum can be prevented.

Step 4: dissection of hernial sac The hernial sac, if present, is removed from Hesselbach's triangle or the spermatic cord and surrounding muscle through inward traction, countertraction, and blunt dissection with progressive inversion of the sac until the musculofascial boundary of the internal inguinal ring and the key deep anatomic structures are identified. An endoscopic Kitner dissector or a 2 × 2 in. piece of gauze on a grasper facilitates blunt dissection of the preperitoneal space. We prefer using a combination of sharp dissection with cautery scissors and a push-and-pull type of dissection in which both hands are used. In most cases, the hernial sac can be slowly drawn away from the transverse fascia or the spermatic cord. The sac is grasped at its apex and pulled inward, thus being reduced by inversion.

Spermatic cord lipomas usually lie posterolaterally and are extensions of preperitoneal fat. In the presence of an indirect defect, such lipomas should be dissected off the cord along with the peritoneal flap to lie cephalad to the internal inguinal ring and the subsequent repair so that prolapse through the ring can be prevented.

A large indirect hernial sac can be divided at the internal ring if it cannot be readily dissected from the cord structures. This step may prevent the cord injury that can result from extensive dissection of a large indirect sac. Division of a large indirect sac is best accomplished by opening the sac on the side opposite the spermatic cord, then completing the division from the inside.[13]

Step 5: reidentification and exposure of landmarks Once the peritoneal flap has been created, the key anatomic landmarks

mentioned earlier [*see* Laparoscopic Inguinal Anatomy, Peritoneum Removed, *above*] must be identified and exposed so that neurovascular structures can be protected from injury and the tissues required for reliable mesh fixation can be located. The pubic tubercle is often more easily felt than seen. Cooper's ligament is initially felt and subsequently seen along the pectineal prominence of the superior pubic ramus as dissection continues laterally and fatty tissue is swept off to expose the glistening white structure. Care must be taken to avoid the numerous small veins that often run on the surface of the ligament as well as to avoid the occasional aberrant obturator artery. The iliopubic tract is initially identified at the inferior margin of the internal inguinal ring, with the spermatic cord above, and is then followed in both a medial and a lateral direction. Minimal dissection is carried out inferior to the iliopubic tract so as not to injure the genitofemoral nerve, the femoral nerve, and the lateral cutaneous nerve of the thigh [*see Figure 11*].

Step 6: placement of mesh A 10 × 6 cm sheet of polypropylene mesh is tapered at its medial end, rolled into a cigarette shape and introduced into the abdomen through the 10/12 mm umbilical trocar. Prolene mesh is preferable to Marlex mesh because it is less dense, conforms more easily to the posterior inguinal wall, and has larger pores, which facilitate visualization and subsequent securing with staples. The inherent elasticity and resiliency of Prolene mesh allow it to unroll easily while maintaining its form. The mesh is used to cover the direct space (Hesselbach's triangle), the indirect space, and the femoral ring areas (i.e., the entire inguinal floor). We do not routinely make a slit in the mesh for the cord, because recurrences through the slits have been noted. An alternative is the double-buttress technique, in which a piece of mesh with a slit and a central opening is placed first and a second, uncut piece is then placed on top of the first for added security and reinforcement.[17]

Although not all surgeons consider fixation of the mesh necessary, it is our practice to staple the mesh to prevent any migration. We use an endoscopic multifire hernia stapler to secure the mesh, beginning at the pubic tubercle and proceeding laterally. The upper margin is tacked first to the rectus muscle and the transversus abdominis fascia and arch, with care taken to stay 1 to 2 cm above the level of the internal inguinal ring and avoid the inferior epigastric vessels, up to a point several centimeters lateral to the internal inguinal ring or the indirect hernial defect. Extending mesh fixation to the anterior iliac spine is neither necessary nor desirable. A

Figure 11 **Laparoscopic inguinal hernia repair: TAPP approach. Dissection of the preperitoneal space on the left side allows identification of the anatomic landmarks. The dissector points to the iliopubic tract inferior to the direct hernial defect.**

two-handed technique is recommended for staple placement: one hand is on the stapler, and the other is on the abdominal wall, applying external pressure to place the wall against the stapler. The stapler itself is frequently pushed against the tissues and used as a spreader and palpator; however, it must not be forced too deeply into the abdominal wall superolateral to the spermatic cord so as not to entrap the sensory nerves inadvertently. The stapler can be moved from the left port to the right port, depending on which position more readily allows placement of the staples perpendicular to the mesh and the abdominal wall.

Once the superior margin is fixed, any excess mesh can be trimmed with scissors; however, this step is rarely necessary with a 10 × 6 cm swatch. Fixation of the inferior margin is then easily accomplished, beginning at the pubic tubercle and moving laterally along Cooper's ligament. The mesh is lifted frequently to ensure adequate visualization of the spermatic cord. Care is taken to avoid the adjacent external iliac vessels, which lie inferiorly. Lateral to the cord structures, all staples are placed superior to the iliopubic tract to prevent subsequent neuralgias involving the lateral cutaneous nerve of the thigh or the branches of the genitofemoral nerve. If the surgeon can palpate the stapler through the abdominal wall with the nondominant hand, the stapler is above the iliopubic tract. When an indirect hernia is present, staples are placed circumferentially to the entire musculoaponeurotic ring of the hernia, which can usually be

visualized through the pores of the polypropylene mesh. The mesh should lie flat at the end of the procedure [*see Figure 12*].

For bilateral repairs, we prefer to make two peritoneal incisions and use two pieces of mesh rather than the single large piece advocated by some authorities; we find that this approach makes the mesh easier to manipulate.

Step 7: closure of peritoneum The peritoneal flap, including the redundant inverted hernial sac, is placed over the mesh, and the peritoneum is reapproximated with the tacker by precocking and partially closing the stapler, then hooking the peritoneum on one side and drawing it to the other side [*see Figure 13*]. Reduction of intra-abdominal pressure and external abdominal wall pressure facilitates a tension-free reapproximation. Alternatively, the peritoneum can be sutured over the mesh, but in most surgeons' hands, this closure takes longer.

Step 8: closure of fascia and skin The peritoneal repair is inspected to ensure that there are no major gaps that might result in exposure of the mesh and subsequent formation of adhesions. The trocars are then removed under direct vision, and the pneumoperitoneum is released. The fascia at the 10/12 mm port sites is closed with 2-0 Prolene sutures to prevent incisional hernias. The skin is closed with 4-0 absorbable subcuticular sutures.

Totally Extraperitoneal Repair

The extra-abdominal preperitoneal approach to laparoscopic hernia repair, developed by McKernan,[18] attempts to duplicate the open preperitoneal repair described by Stoppa[19-21] and Wantz.[11,22] In a TEP repair, the trocars are placed preperitoneally in a space created between the fascia and the peritoneum. An operating laparoscope provides access to the preperitoneal space of the groin, where the mesh repair is effected. Ideally, none of the preliminary exploratory trocars penetrates the peritoneum, and the dissection remains in the extra-abdominal plane at all times.

Patient preparation and positioning are much the same as in a TAPP repair. The surgeon stands on the side opposite the hernia.

Step 1: creation of preperitoneal space With the patient in the Trendelenburg position, the fascia is opened through a 1 cm infraumbilical transverse incision placed slightly toward the side of the hernia, which helps one avoid inadvertently opening the peritoneum. An index finger is inserted on the medial aspect of the exposed rectus muscle and slid over the posterior rectus sheath. A

Figure 12 **Laparoscopic inguinal hernia repair: TAPP approach. The mesh is stapled in place.**

Figure 13 **Laparoscopic inguinal hernia repair: TAPP approach. The peritoneum is stapled over the mesh.**

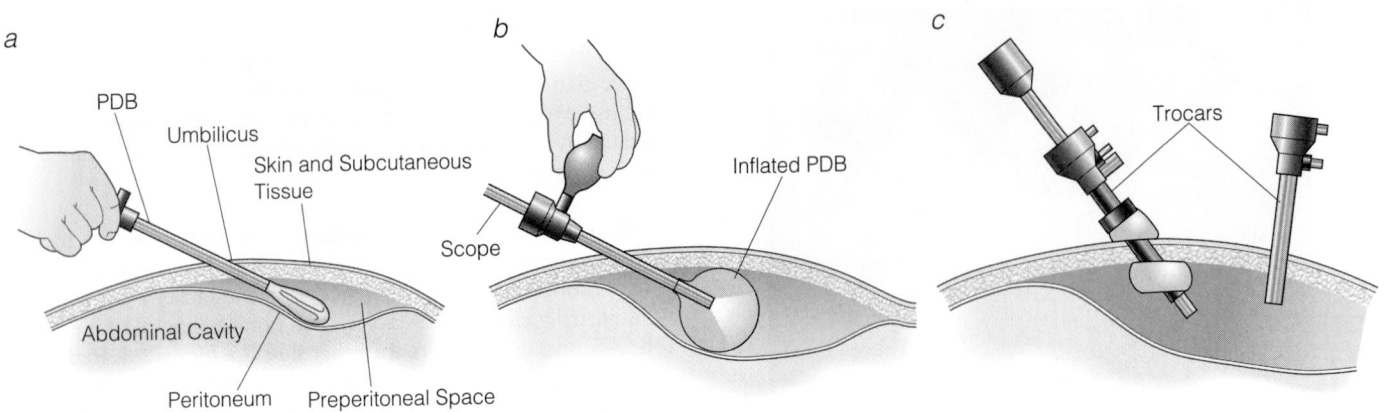

Figure 14 Laparoscopic inguinal hernia repair: TEP approach. Shown is the preperitoneal distention balloon (PDB) system. The PDB is introduced into the preperitoneal space (*a*). As it is tunneled inferiorly toward the pubis, the PDB is inflated under laparoscopic vision (*b*). Once the preperitoneal space is created, the PDB is removed and replaced with a blunt-tip trocar. The preperitoneal space is insufflated under low pressure, additional trocars are placed, and the repair is completed (*c*).

preperitoneal tunnel between the rectus abdominis muscles and the peritoneum is created in the midline with blunt finger dissection. A blunt 10/12 mm trocar is then secured in the preperitoneal space with fascial stay sutures.

An operating laparoscope is inserted through the trocar with a blunt 5 mm probe in the operating channel. Insufflation of the preperitoneal space is begun while the probe depresses the peritoneum and develops the preperitoneal space down to the pubis under direct vision, with the rectus muscles seen anteriorly and the peritoneum posteriorly. Maximum inflation pressure is 8 to 10 mm Hg to prevent disruption of the peritoneum or development of extensive subcutaneous emphysema.

TEP repair can be facilitated by using a preperitoneal distention balloon (PDB) system (Origin Medsystems, Inc., Menlo Park, California). This system consists of a trocar with an inflatable balloon at its tip, which is used to develop the preperitoneal space by atraumatically separating the peritoneum from the abdominal wall. The PDB is inserted into the preperitoneal space below the umbilicus by means of an open Hasson technique and is tunneled inferiorly toward the internal inguinal ring. The preperitoneal working space is developed by gradual inflation of the balloon to a volume of 1 L; the transparency of the balloon permits constant visualization throughout the distention process. Once the working space is created, the PDB is removed and replaced with a blunt sealing trocar. The preperitoneal space is then reinsufflated to a pressure of 8 to 10 mm Hg [*see Figure 14*].

After the peritoneum is dissected away from the rectus muscle, a midline 5 mm trocar is inserted just above the pubis under direct vision, and a 10/12 mm trocar is placed halfway between the pubis and the umbilicus [*see Figure 15*], with care taken not to penetrate the peritoneum. The risk of intraperitoneal entry can be minimized by blunt dissection down to the fascia with a hemostat after the skin incision. If the peritoneum is penetrated, the resulting pneumoperitoneum can reduce the already limited working space. One can try to repair the rent with a suture, but if such repair is unsuccessful, the loss of working space may necessitate conversion to a TAPP approach.

Step 2: dissection of hernial sac The operating laparoscope is replaced by a 45° laparoscope, which facilitates exposure and visualization of this region. Wide dissection of the preperitoneal space is then undertaken with blunt graspers in a two-hand-

ed technique, with the grasper in the left hand depressing the peritoneum. The pubis, Cooper's ligament, and the inferior epigastric vessels are located. If a direct hernia is present, the sac and the preperitoneal contents are carefully dissected away from the fascial defect, with care taken not to enter the peritoneal cavity. The peritoneum is then further dissected cephalad to expose the internal ring and any indirect hernial sac. A small indirect hernial sac is dissected off the spermatic cord and reduced or amputated with an endoscopic ligating loop after reduction of its contents has been ensured. A large indirect hernial sac is transected and closed, with the distal sac left in place and not ligated.

For hernias that are not readily reduced, McKernan[23] suggests making an incision in the groin above the pubis down to the external oblique aponeurosis and severing the adhesions between the sac and the external ring. If this measure does not work, the sac

Figure 15 Laparoscopic inguinal hernia repair: TEP approach. Shown is standard trocar placement for TEP repair. As in TAPP repair, three trocar sites are used. One trocar is placed in the umbilicus; the second is placed in the midline, midway between the umbilicus and the pubis; and the third is placed above the pubic arch. The trocars should not penetrate the peritoneum.

2

2

can be opened through the incision and the adhesions within the sac lysed. If the hernia still cannot be reduced, the TEP repair is abandoned in favor of an anterior approach.

Step 3: placement of mesh A 10×15 cm piece of Prolene mesh is incised vertically, and a 1 cm hole is created centrally for the spermatic cord. The mesh is then folded in half horizontally, with sutures at each corner to maintain the fold, then inserted through the umbilical trocar and drawn behind the cord structures. Once the mesh is well positioned, with the spermatic cord seated in the central hole, the corner sutures are divided, and the mesh is unfolded against the anterior abdominal wall. As in a TAPP repair, the mesh is tacked to key structures, including the pubic tubercle, Cooper's ligament, and the iliopubic tract inferiorly and anteriorly to the posterior aspect of the rectus abdominis muscle. The opening in the mesh is then closed with staples, with great care taken not to compromise cord structures. The mesh must lie flat. No staples are placed inferior to the iliopubic tract lateral to the internal ring. For bilateral hernias, two identical repairs are done, and the two mesh patches are tacked together at the pubis. An additional piece of mesh may be placed cephalad to the pubis for reinforcement.

A major advantage of the TEP approach is avoidance of entry into the peritoneal cavity and thus of the potential risk of adhesions and bowel obstruction. In practice, however, breaches in the peritoneum are common, resulting in decreased operating space and a compromised view of the anatomic structures as pneumoperitoneum ensues. In addition, even when intraperitoneal entry is avoided, the small amount of working space inherent in the nature of the technique can cause the surgeon great difficulty and confusion. For these reasons, considerable experience is required and caution advised before TEP repair is attempted.

Step 4: closure The operative site is inspected for hemostasis. The trocars are removed under direct vision with release of the insufflated CO_2. The fascia at trocar sites larger than 10 mm is closed with 2-0 Prolene sutures, and the skin is closed with subcuticular sutures.

POSTOPERATIVE CARE

Patients are observed in the recovery room until they are able to ambulate unassisted and to void; if they are unable to void at the time of discharge, in-and-out catheterization is performed. Patients are advised to resume their usual activities as they see fit; driving a car is permitted the next day. Outpatient prescriptions for acetaminophen and codeine are given, and follow-up visits in the surgical clinic are scheduled for day 7 after operation. Patients who live alone, who have had an intraoperative complication, who have significant nausea or vomiting, or have unexplained or inordinate pain are admitted overnight.

DISADVANTAGES AND COMPLICATIONS

Disadvantages

Need for general anesthesia The need for pneumoperitoneum and thus for general anesthesia in laparoscopic herniorrhaphy is sometimes considered a major disadvantage. Nausea, dizziness, and headache are more common in the recovery room after TAPP repair than after Lichtenstein repair.[24] It is not necessarily true, however, that local or regional anesthesia is safer than general anesthesia.[25] Anesthesiologic studies critically appraising anesthetic techniques for hernia surgery have shown the choice of general anesthesia over local or regional anesthesia to be safe and, in many cases, advantageous, particularly in patients who are in

poor health. Furthermore, TEP repair has been successfully done with patients under epidural[26] and local[27] anesthesia.

Lower cost-effectiveness The costs of laparoscopic repair exceed those of open repair.[24,28-33] For the most part, the differences are accounted for by longer operative time and the use of disposable equipment. Operative time decreases with experience, and disposable trocars and scissors can be replaced with reusable instruments. Suturing the mesh and peritoneum saves the cost of the stapler but requires more operative time.

The higher operative costs of laparoscopic repair notwithstanding, economic impact studies to date have not shown either approach to be clearly more cost-effective. In terms of effectiveness, the laparoscopic approach fares better on most patient-based outcome measures, including pain and convalescence; however, it remains to be seen whether these savings in disability offset the higher operative costs. One randomized study suggested that the total costs of laparoscopic repair were actually lower than those of the Lichtenstein repair when lost workdays were taken into account.[34]

Complications

Most randomized trials comparing laparoscopic repair with open mesh repair have found comparable numbers of total complications in the two groups [*see Table 1*]. Four studies reported fewer overall complications after laparoscopic repair.[24,32,35,36] In general, although intraoperative complications are more common and potentially more serious in the laparoscopic approach, particularly when a TAPP repair is chosen, postoperative complications tend to be less common.

Complications of access to peritoneal cavity A TAPP hernia repair exposes the patient to several potentially serious risks related to the choice of the transabdominal route. Trocar injuries to the bowel, the bladder, and vascular structures can occur during the creation of the initial pneumoperitoneum or the subsequent insertion of the trocars. Use of an open insertion technique to create the pneumoperitoneum should eliminate major vascular injuries as well as make identification and repair of bowel injuries simpler than they would be with the closed technique. Another complication related to trocar sites is incisional hernia, which can lead to postoperative bowel obstruction.[37]

The use of the transabdominal route also exposes the patient to the risk of adhesions and the potential for late bowel obstruction. Fortunately, evidence from study of herniorrhaphy in pigs[38] and from extensive gynecologic application of laparoscopy in humans over many years suggests that adhesions form significantly less often after laparoscopic procedures than after open procedures.

Complications of dissection Injuries occurring during dissection are often linked to inexperience with laparoscopic inguinal anatomy. If serious enough, they can necessitate laparotomy. Conversion of a laparoscopic procedure to an open one, however, is regarded more seriously in herniorrhaphy patients than in cholecystectomy patients. In laparoscopic cholecystectomy, conversion to laparotomy is acceptable and expected in 4% to 5% of cases, and common bile duct injury is a recognized complication of both open and laparoscopic cholecystectomy. In contrast, some of the complications encountered in laparoscopic herniorrhaphy never occur in classic open anterior herniorrhaphy, and conversion to laparotomy to correct a complication arising during laparoscopic herniorrhaphy is not acceptable. Fortunately, such conversion is rare: in more than 800 laparoscopic herniorrhaphies reported by 19 institutions in a multicenter phase II study, only one bladder injury and one bowel perforation requiring laparotomy for repair were documented.[15]

Table 1 Selected English-Language Randomized Controlled Trials
Comparing Laparoscopic with Open Mesh Repairs

Study Authors	Technique Employed	N	OR Time Needed for Unilateral Repairs (min)	Less Early Pain after Laparoscopic Repair?	Complications*	Recovery† (days)	Recurrences (No.)	Cost
Payne et al (1994)	TAPP	48	68	NA	12%	8.9	0	$3,093
	Lichtenstein	52	56		18%	17‡	0	$2,494‡
Wright et al (1996)	TEP	60	58	Yes‡	15	NA	NA	NA
	Lichtenstein	60	45‡		43			
Champault et al (1997)	TEP	51	NA	Yes‡	4%	17	3	NA
	Stoppa	49			30%‡	35‡	1	
Paganini et al (1997)	TAPP	52	67	No	27%	15	2	$1,249
	Lichtenstein	56	48‡		27%	14	0	$306‡
Wellwood et al (1998)	TAPP	200	45	Yes‡	316	5	0	£747
	Lichtenstein	200	45		452‡	8‡	0	£412‡
Zieren et al (1998)	TAPP	80	61	No	19%	3	0	$1,211
	PP	80	36‡		15%	4	0	$124‡
Khoury (1998)	TEP	150	32	Yes‡	13%	8	4	
	PP	142	31		23%‡	15‡	4	
Johansson et al (1999)	TAPP	205	65	Yes‡	66	18	4	5,988 SEK
	Stoppa	204	38		49	24‡	11	350 SEK
MRC (1999)	TAPP/TEP	468	58	NA	30%	10	7	LH £314
	Mixed open§	460	43‡		44%‡	14‡	0‡	more

*Complications are expressed as percentage of patients affected or total number of complications, as reported in the individual studies.
†Definition of recovery varies from study to study..
‡$P < 0.05$.
§Lichtenstein in 94%.
LH—laparoscopic herniorrhaphy   NA—not available   PP—plug-and-patch   TAPP—transabdominal preperitoneal   TEP—totally extraperitoneal

The most common vascular injuries in laparoscopic herniorrhaphy are those involving the inferior epigastric vessels and the spermatic vessels. The external iliac, circumflex iliac, profunda, and obturator vessels are also at risk. A previous lower abdominal operation is a risk factor.[13] The source of any abnormal bleeding during the procedure must be quickly identified. All vessels in the groin can be ligated except the external iliac vessels, which must be repaired.[13]

Injuries to the urinary tract can also occur. Four bladder injuries requiring repair were documented in a collected series of 762 laparoscopic repairs by different surgical groups.[39] Bladder injuries are most likely to occur when the space of Retzius has been previously dissected (e.g., in a prostatectomy). Renal and ureteral injuries can result from poorly placed trocars. Any urinary tract injuries identified intraoperatively should be repaired immediately. Often, however, these injuries are not apparent until the postoperative period, when they present as lower abdominal pain, renal failure, ascites, dysuria, or hematuria—all of which should be investigated promptly. Although indwelling catheter drainage may constitute sufficient treatment of a missed retroperitoneal bladder injury, intraperitoneal injuries are best treated by direct repair via either laparoscopy or laparotomy.

Complications related to mesh Complications related to the use of mesh include infection, migration, adhesion formation, and erosion into intraperitoneal organs. Such complications usually become apparent weeks to years after the initial repair, presenting as abscess, fistula, or small bowel obstruction.

Mesh infection is very rare. Phillips and colleagues collected information on 2,559 North American patients and found only one patient who required removal of an infected mesh after an IPOM repair.[40] Estour and Mouret reviewed 7,340 patients from 22 European groups and found only seven patients with reported mesh infections.[41] Mesh infection usually responds to conservative treatment with antibiotics and drainage. On rare occasions, the mesh must be removed; this may be accomplished via an external approach. It is noteworthy that removal of the mesh does not always lead to recurrence of the hernia, a finding that may be attributable to the resulting fibrosis.[42]

Mesh migration may lead to hernia recurrence. In a TAPP repair, appropriate stapling of the mesh should reduce this possibility. In a TEP repair, stapling does not appear to be necessary to prevent migration.[43,44]

The risk that adhesions to the mesh will form is substantially augmented if the mesh is left fully exposed to the bowel, as in the case with the IPOM technique. Even with the TAPP approach, the long-term durability and effectiveness of the sometimes flimsy peritoneal coverage have been questioned. Over the past 25 years, however, extensive intraperitoneal use of polypropylene mesh in abdominal wall reconstruction has rarely led to adhesions causing bowel obstruction. Nonetheless, either small bowel[40] or omentum[33] can be incarcerated at a defect in the peritoneal closure site, and reoperation may be required.

Urinary complications Injuries to the urinary tract aside [see Complications of Dissection, *above*], urinary retention, urinary tract infection, and hematuria are the most common complications. Avoidance of bladder catheterization reduces the incidence of these complications, but urinary retention still occurs in 1.5% to 2.0% of patients. General anesthesia and the administration of large volumes of I.V. fluids may also predispose to retention.

Vas deferens and testicular complications Wantz[45] believes that the most common cause of postoperative testicular swelling, orchitis, and ischemic atrophy is surgical trauma to the testicular veins (i.e., venous congestion and subsequent thrombosis). Because spermatic cord dissection is minimized with the laparoscopic approach, the risk of groin and testicular complications resulting from injury to cord structures and adjacent nerves should be reduced. When the hernial sac is left undisturbed, there is less trauma to the cord, its vessels, and adjacent nerves.

Most testicular complications, such as swelling, pain, and epididymitis, are self-limited. Testicular pain occurs in about 1% of patients after laparoscopic repair,[34] an incidence comparable to that seen after open repair.[46] A similar number of patients experience testicular atrophy,[32] for which there is no specific treatment.

The risk of injury to the vas deferens appears to be much the same in laparoscopic repair as in open repair.[13] If fertility is an issue, the cut ends should be reapproximated if the injury is recognized intraoperatively.

Postoperative groin and thigh pain Unlike patients who undergo open anterior herniorrhaphy, in whom discomfort or numbness is usually localized to the operative area, patients who undergo laparoscopic repair occasionally describe unusual but specific symptoms of deep discomfort that are usually positional and are often of a transient, shooting nature suggestive of nerve irritation. The pain is frequently incited by stooping, twisting, or movements causing extension of the hip and can be shocklike. Although these symptoms can frequently be elicited in the early postoperative period, they are usually transient. If a neuralgia is present in the recovery room, however, prompt reexploration is the best approach.[13]

Persistent pain and burning sensations in the inguinal region, the upper medial thigh, or the spermatic cord and scrotal skin region occur when the genitofemoral nerve or the ilioinguinal nerve is stimulated, entrapped, or unintentionally injured. When these symptoms persist, they may result in severe morbidity.[47] A more worrisome symptom is lateral or central upper medial thigh numbness, which is reported in 1% to 2% of patients and often lasts several months or longer. Whether this numbness is related to staple entrapment, fibrous adhesions, cicatricial neuroma, or mesh irritation is unknown. Numbness and paresthesia of the lateral thigh are less frequent and are related to the involvement of fibers of the lateral cutaneous nerve. These problems can be prevented by paying careful attention to anatomic detail and technique.[48] After performing 50 cadaveric dissections to determine the relation of the nerves to the internal ring, Rosen and coworkers concluded that both the genitofemoral nerve and the lateral cutaneous nerve of the thigh will be protected in all cases if no staples are placed further than 1.5 cm lateral to the edge of the internal ring.[49]

A great deal of attention has rightly been focused on the risk of nerve injury with laparoscopic hernia repair as well as on ways of preventing it. At the same time, it is important to note that pain and numbness, including thigh numbness, can also occur after open repair and may in fact be more common in that setting than was previously realized. In one study, groin pain lasting longer than 1 month was present in 8% of patients after Lichtenstein repair but in no pa-

tients after TAPP.[33] A randomized study of 928 patients found that 1 year after operation, the laparoscopic group had a lower rate of persistent groin pain than the open mesh group (30% versus 37%) and a similar incidence of thigh numbness (14% versus 11%).[32]

Miscellaneous complications Early postoperative examination of patients who have undergone laparoscopic hernia repair frequently reveals groin bogginess, a cough impulse, and deep tenderness over the internal inguinal ring, particularly when the hernia was indirect and when the hernial sac was left in situ.[50] True hydroceles are rare. Well-defined, confined masses 1 to 3 cm in diameter are often palpated at the external inguinal ring or near the pubic tubercle. These typically represent hematomas,[50] which are more common when the sac has been dissected in a TAPP repair. Unlike the diffuse hematomas seen with open repair, these hematomas are very well defined and usually asymptomatic; however, they are very slow to disappear. These findings often mimic those of recurrent hernia and call for careful follow-up. Lipomas of the spermatic cord, if left unreduced in patients with indirect hernias, may produce a persistent groin mass and a cough impulse that mimic recurrence, especially to an uninitiated examiner. These lipomas are always asymptomatic.

OUTCOME EVALUATION

Although there is a large body of literature on laparoscopic inguinal hernia repair—including a variety of randomized controlled trials—the benefits of the laparoscopic approach have not yet been clearly defined or widely accepted. One reason may be that the literature can be difficult to summarize and understand. For example, studies have reported conflicting results: several randomized, controlled trials suggested that the laparoscopic technique offered little benefit,[28,29,34,51,52] but many trials reached the opposite conclusion.[24,30-33,35,36,43,53-57] Furthermore, different trials have compared different operations: TAPP repair, TEP repair, or a mixture of the two, on one hand, against open mesh repair, open sutured repair, or a mixture of the two, on the other hand.

Given the low morbidity and relatively short convalescence already associated with the conventional operation, demonstration of any significant improvements that might be associated with the laparoscopic operation would probably require large study samples. Thus, combining existing studies may be illuminating. In a meta-analysis that included studies performed up to March 1997, Chung and Rowland grouped 18 trials according to the operations compared.[58] In group 1, laparoscopic repair (TAPP, in most cases) was compared with open tension-free repair. In group 2, laparoscopic repair was compared with open sutured repair. In group 3, laparoscopic repair was compared with a mixture of open operations ("at the discretion of the surgeon"). In all comparisons, the laparoscopic operation took longer to perform. Compared with sutured repair, laparoscopic operation yielded significantly less postoperative pain and a significantly shorter recovery. Compared with tension-free repair, however, laparoscopic repair showed no significant advantage with respect to pain but resulted in a slightly shorter recovery (though the reduction was of marginal statistical significance). The results of the meta-analysis suggest that the postoperative course of open tension-free repair is different from that of open sutured repair, with the former clearly resulting in less postoperative pain and a shorter recovery. In that open tension-free repair uses mesh, it resembles laparoscopic repair more closely than open sutured repair does and thus is probably a more relevant comparison procedure. Accordingly, we will briefly review the findings of a number of recent studies that compare laparoscopic inguinal herniorrhaphy with open mesh repair.

Laparoscopic Repair versus Open Mesh Repair

At least 12 prospective, randomized trials comparing laparoscopic repair with open tension-free mesh repair were published in English between 1994 and 1999,[24,28-36,46,59] nine of which are summarized elsewhere [*see Table 1*]. The heterogeneity of the studies' designs (particularly with respect to the different types of repairs done and the different outcome measures assessed) makes direct comparisons difficult. For example, the laparoscopic methods used included TAPP repair alone (eight studies[24,28-31,33,34,59]), TEP repair alone (three studies[35,36,46]), and a combination of TAPP and TEP repair (one study[32]). The open methods used included Lichtenstein repair with local anesthesia (four studies[24,28,33,34]), Lichtenstein repair with general anesthesia (four studies[30,32,46,59]), open Stoppa preperitoneal repair with general anesthesia (two studies[31,35]), plug-and-patch repair with local anesthesia (one study[29]), and plug-and-patch repair with general anesthesia (one study[36]). Most of the studies included bilateral along with unilateral hernias.[24,28,32,33,35,36,46] The considerable differences between these 12 studies notwithstanding, several suggestive patterns do emerge.

Convalescence time The most significant short-term outcome measure after hernia repair is convalescence time, defined as the time required for the patient to return to normal activities. One of the most frequently cited benefits of laparoscopic herniorrhaphy is the patient's rapid return to unrestricted activity, including work. Most of the randomized studies comparing laparoscopic with open mesh repair, including the four largest, report a significantly shorter convalescence time after laparoscopic repair.[24,30-33,35,36] For example, in a study of 400 patients specifically designed to detect differences in convalescence at various defined levels, Wellwood and coworkers found that the self-reported time to return to normal household and social activities was significantly shorter after TAPP repair than after Lichtenstein repair with local anesthesia.[24] In a large multicenter cooperative trial of 928 patients in which TAPP or TEP was compared mainly with tension-free mesh repair, the laparoscopic group returned to normal social activities significantly faster than the open group (10 days versus 14 days).[32]

Convalescence time, particularly time off work, is a complex outcome measure that varies as much with patient expectation, motivation, and disability coverage as it does with surgical morbidity.[33,60] Moreover, measurement of convalescence is subject to bias if the assessor is not blinded to the treatment arm. Finally, the operating surgeon may not assess outcome in the same way as other unbiased observers[61] or the patients themselves would.

Postoperative pain After laparoscopic repair, most patients experience minimal immediate postoperative pain and have little or no need for analgesics after postoperative day 1. In addition, patients are generally able to perform some exercises better after laparoscopic repair than after Lichtenstein repair.[33] That patients experience less postoperative pain after laparoscopic repair than after open mesh repair has been reported in several randomized studies.[24,30,31,35,36,46] A meta-analysis of more than 500 patients in five trials, however, found that postoperative pain, measured on the basis either of analgesic administration or of ratings on a visual analog scale (VAS), was not significantly less after TAPP repair than after open tension-free repair.[58] Zieren and colleagues found no difference in postoperative pain assessed by VAS between 80 patients undergoing TAPP repair and 80 patients undergoing open plug-and-patch repair; however, both groups had significantly lower VAS scores than did 80 patients undergoing Shouldice repair[29]—a finding consistent with almost all of the reports comparing laparoscopic repair with open sutured repair.[43]

Quality of life The studies that have assessed quality of life immediately after hernia repair have tended to favor the laparoscopic approach, albeit marginally. Using the SF-36 (a widely accepted general health–related quality-of-life questionnaire), Wellwood and coworkers found that at 1 month, greater improvements from baseline were apparent in the laparoscopic group in every dimension except general health; however, by 3 months, the differences between the two groups were no longer significant.[24] The MRC group also found no differences in any SF-36 domains at 3 months after operation.[32] Filipi and associates, using the Sickness Impact Profile, found some benefit to the laparoscopic approach.[59]

Bilateral hernias Laparoscopy allows simultaneous exploration of the abdominal cavity and diagnosis and treatment of bilateral groin hernias as well as of coexisting femoral hernias (which are often unrecognized preoperatively), without added risk or disability. Many surgeons avoid performing simultaneous bilateral repair during an open procedure because of the resulting increase in swelling, pain, disability, operative time, and the risk of infection and recurrence. One retrospective study found that simultaneous repair of bilateral hernias via the laparoscopic approach resulted in a shorter convalescence time and a quicker return to work than a modified Shouldice repair.[62] In a prospective, randomized study, Paganini and colleagues found in subgroup analysis that the mean operative time did not differ significantly between bilateral laparoscopic repair and bilateral open mesh repair (85.7 ± 32.2 minutes for TAPP repair versus 75.9 ± 43.3 minutes for open repair).[28] Further prospective, randomized trials designed to compare simultaneous bilateral open tension-free repair with bilateral laparoscopic repair should be undertaken.

Hernia recurrence Open mesh repair has been associated with long-term recurrence rates of 1% or less, even when not performed by hernia specialists.[63,64] If the laparoscopic approach is to be a viable alternative to open repair, it should have comparable results.

In fact, the short-term experience with laparoscopic hernia repair is encouraging. Case series of TAPP and TEP repairs demonstrate recurrence rates ranging from 0% to 2%, with especially low recurrence rates reported after TEP repair.[65] Of the 12 randomized studies of laparoscopic repair versus open mesh repair mentioned earlier (see above), only one found a significant difference in recurrence rates, reporting seven recurrences in 468 laparoscopic patients and no recurrences in 460 open repairs.[32] All seven recurrences occurred in patients who underwent TAPP repair, even though TAPP accounted for only 21% of the laparoscopic repairs.

Most reported recurrences after laparoscopic herniorrhaphy come at an early stage in the surgeon's experience with this procedure and soon after operation.[15] The majority can be attributed to (1) the surgeon's imperfect understanding of the preperitoneal anatomy and the anatomic landmarks for mesh fixation, which leads to inadequate preperitoneal dissection; (2) use of an inadequately sized patch, which fails to provide support for the entire inguinal area, including direct, indirect, and femoral spaces; or (3) staple failure. Secure fascial fixation of the prosthesis is a paramount concern, particularly with TAPP repair; accurate stapling technique, with careful placement of each staple, is vital to prevention of recurrence.

Once a hernia recurs after an initial open repair, laparoscopic repair may be a particularly suitable treatment approach.[66] Normal anatomic and cord structures are not distorted by scar tissue in the preperitoneal space, dissection planes are unmarred, and the risk of causing testicular damage is reduced. The recurrence is usually very well seen and better defined from the peritoneal aspect, and the entire myopectineal inguinal floor can be reinforced and repaired without tension and without the need to use scarred or weakened tissue, which predisposes to further recurrence. Unfortunately, there are few controlled studies that have examined recurrent hernias exclusively. In one randomized study of 79 patients in which TAPP repair of recurrent hernias was compared with open preperitoneal repair, patients experienced less pain and had a shorter convalescence after TAPP repair; however, there were seven recurrences after TAPP repair and only one after open repair.[67]

Transabdominal Preperitoneal Repair versus Totally Extraperitoneal Repair

The TAPP approach is easier to learn and perform than the TEP approach, and even experienced laparoscopic hernia surgeons report more technical difficulties with the latter.[68] Nonetheless, there is a growing body of literature to suggest that TEP repair, by avoiding entry into the peritoneal cavity, provides significant advantages over TAPP repair.[3] In particular, the TEP approach should eliminate trocar site hernias, small bowel injury and obstruction, and intraperitoneal adhesions to the mesh. Kald and colleagues consecutively performed TAPP repairs in 339 patients and TEP repairs in 87 patients, then followed the patients for a mean of 23 and 7 months, respectively.[69] Time off work was shorter after TEP. In the 426 patients studied, 15 major complications were noted, including one death, two bowel obstructions, one severe neuralgia, three trocar site hernias, one epigastric artery hemorrhage, and seven recurrences; all except the epigastric artery hemorrhage occurred in the TAPP group. It is possible, however, that these results can be partly explained by the learning curve, in that the TAPP repairs were all done before the TEP repairs. That six TAPP recurrences occurred in the first 31 cases, whereas only one occurred in the subsequent 395 patients, lends support to this possibility.

In a study comparing 733 TAPP repairs with 382 TEP repairs, 11 major complications occurred in the TAPP group (two recurrences, six trocar hernias, one small bowel obstruction, and two small bowel injuries), whereas only one recurrence and no intraperitoneal complications occurred in the TEP group.[70] Seven TEP procedures were converted to TAPP procedures. Time off work was equal in the two groups but was prolonged in patients receiving compensation. As in the Kald study, the TAPP patients were followed longer than the TEP patients, and the TAPP cases occupied the first part of the learning curve. To avoid this type of selection bias would require a randomized study.

Not all surgeons are convinced that TEP repair is the laparoscopic procedure of choice. Cohen and coworkers compared 108 TAPP repairs with 100 TEP repairs.[68] Although the TEP repairs were done only by surgeons who were already familiar with TAPP repair, many of the surgeons still encountered technical difficulties and problems with landmark identification. Overall, complications did not occur significantly more frequently in either group, but they seemed more severe in the TAPP group: four trocar site hernias, one bladder injury, and six seromas were noted in the TAPP group, compared with one cellulitis and six seromas in the TEP group. The authors concluded that because TAPP repair is easier and does not increase complications significantly, it is an "adequate" procedure. The sample size may have been too small to permit detection of small differences in complication rates.

Laparoscopic Incisional Hernia Repair

Incisional hernias develop in approximately 2% to 11% of patients undergoing laparotomy.[71,72] It has been estimated that 90,000 ventral hernia repairs are carried out in the United States every year.[4] Open incisional hernia repair can be a difficult procedure and may carry a high morbidity. Without prosthetic mesh, repair of large incisional hernias is associated with recurrence rates as high as 50%; in addition, it can be associated with significant complications and a substantial hospital stay.

Laparoscopic repair of incisional hernia was initially described in 1992,[8] and it remains an emerging procedure. Taking a laparoscopic approach allows the surgeon to minimize the abdominal wall incisions, avoid extensive flap dissection and muscle mobilization, and eliminate the need for drains in proximity to the mesh, thereby potentially achieving decreases in pain, recovery time, and duration of hospitalization as well as lower rates of surgical site infections. In addition, the improved visualization of the abdominal wall associated with the laparoscopic view may result in better definition of the defect, the discovery of unrecognized hernia sites, and improved adhesiolysis. If this improved visualization permits more precise and accurate placement and tailoring of the mesh, recurrence rates may also be decreased.

Laparoscopic incisional hernia repair is best suited for repairing large incisional hernias, which may be defined as any incisional hernia in which the smallest diameter is greater than 3 cm. With these large defects, prosthetic material must be used to ensure tension-free repair of the hernia, which reduces the risk of recurrence. Smaller hernias can usually be repaired without mesh, often on an outpatient basis; there is little to be gained by adopting a laparoscopic approach to these defects. Both upper abdominal and lower abdominal incisions are amenable to a laparoscopic approach. The so-called Swiss cheese hernia, which comprises multiple small defects, is particularly well suited to this approach: open repair would necessitate a large incision for access to the multiple fascial defects. Incarcerated hernias can also be approached laparoscopically; however, the suspected presence of compromised bowel is an absolute contraindication. An abdomen that has undergone multiple operations and contains dense adhesions presents a challenge in terms of both access to the abdominal cavity and access to the hernia site. If the surgeon cannot obtain safe access to the peritoneal cavity for insufflation, a laparoscopic approach is contraindicated.

To date, very few comparative trials focusing on laparoscopic incisional herniorrhaphy have been reported. We will therefore concentrate on the technique we currently employ for the repair.

OPERATIVE PLANNING

Preparation

Formal mechanical and antibiotic bowel preparation is administered if it is suspected that there is incarcerated bowel in the hernia. With the patient straining, the edges of the hernia defect are marked on the skin whenever possible. If the defect is in the lower abdomen, a Foley catheter is placed in the bladder. Prophylactic antibiotics are not routinely administered. The procedure is performed with the patient under general anesthesia.

Positioning

The patient is placed in the supine position with the arms extended. If the hernia is in the midline, the surgeon can stand on either side of the patient, with the monitor directly opposite. Initially, the assistant stands on the same side as the surgeon; however, he or she may later have to move to the opposite side to help with dissection and stapling. A second monitor on the opposite side of the table is useful. If the defect is subcostal, the surgeon may prefer to operate from between the patient's legs, with a monitor at the head of the bed.

Equipment

Because laparoscopic incisional hernia repair leaves the mesh exposed to the intraperitoneal cavity, some concern has arisen about the risk of adhesion formation and fistulization if polypropylene mesh is used. A polytetrafluoroethylene (PTFE) prosthesis would have a reduced propensity for adhesion formation and could be more safely placed in an intraperitoneal position, but PTFE is much harder to manipulate laparoscopically than polypropylene and is a less effective scaffold for ingrowth of collagen. We currently use Composix mesh (Bard, Davol Inc., Cranston, Rhode Island), which consists of PTFE on the side facing the peritoneal cavity and two layers of polypropylene mesh on the side facing the abdominal wall. This mesh marries the strength of Marlex with the safety of PTFE.

Additional special equipment used for incisional hernia repair includes 2-0 nonabsorbable sutures, a Keith needle, a 2 mm suture passer, a sterile marking pen, and a stapler (typically, a 12 mm 65° device that uses 4.8 mm staples). Atraumatic bowel instruments are required to reduce incarcerated intestines without injuring them. An ultrasonic scalpel is useful if extensive adhesiolysis is required: it helps expedite the procedure while improving hemostasis.

OPERATIVE TECHNIQUE

In essence, the repair consists of the intraperitoneal placement of a large piece of mesh so that it overlaps the defect in the fascia and the abdominal wall. The defect is not closed. The mesh is anchored with a minimum of four subcutaneously tied transfascial sutures placed at the four corners and is further secured between the sutures with intraperitoneally placed staples.

Step 1: Placement of Trocars

Because of the probability of extensive intra-abdominal adhesions, we begin with open insertion of a blunt 12 mm trocar. This trocar is inserted laterally, at the level of the middle of the hernia, rather than in the midline, even though doing so necessitates dissecting through several layers of muscle.

A 30° scope is then inserted. As in inguinal repair, an angled scope is essential because dissection and repair are done on the undersurface of the anterior abdominal wall, which cannot be adequately visualized with a 0° scope. Laparoscopy is performed and the hernial defect identified. Two additional 5 mm ports are then placed on the same side as the surgeon. These ports are placed superior and inferior to the initial trocar and should be lo-

cated as far laterally as possible, with care taken to ensure that the downward movement of the instruments is not limited by the iliac crest or the thigh. Lateral placement is necessary to optimize exposure of the abdominal wall.

Once all adhesions to the abdominal wall have been dissected sufficiently (see below), a fourth port can be placed on the opposite side to facilitate adhesiolysis and mesh fixation. As noted, some of the ports can be 5 mm, depending on the caliber of the instruments available. Ultimately, port placement depends on the hernia's location, the patient's body habitus, and the surgeon's preference.

Step 2: Exposure of Hernial Defect

The edges of the hernial defect are exposed by reducing the contents of the hernia into the abdominal cavity. All adhesions from bowel or omentum to the abdominal wall in the vicinity of the defect must be transected. This dissection may be performed with cautery scissors or a hook cautery. An ultrasonic scalpel may be useful for optimizing hemostasis if extensive vascularized adhesions are encountered. It is not necessary to excise or reduce the hernial sac itself [*see Figure 16*].

Step 3: Tailoring of Mesh

The contours of the hernia defect are marked as accurately as possible on the exterior abdominal wall; the edges may be delineated with a combination of palpation and visualization. A rough pictorial representation of the swatch of mesh that will be required is then drawn on the skin around the hernial defect, with care taken to overlap the edges of the defect by at least 2 cm on all sides [*see Figure 17*]. This template is measured, and the mesh swatch is cut to its dimensions. The four corners of the swatch and those of its representation on the abdominal wall are numbered clockwise from 1 to 4 for later orientation. A mark is made on the inner side of the mesh so that the surgeon can easily determine which side is to face the peritoneum once the mesh is inserted into the peritoneal cavity. A 2-0 Prolene suture is tied in each corner of the mesh swatch, and both ends are left about 15 cm long. Thicker suture material is not easily passed through the abdominal wall.

The mesh swatch is rolled as tightly as possible around a grasping forceps, then introduced into the peritoneal cavity. Small swatches can be inserted through a 12 mm trocar[4]; for larger pieces, we remove a large trocar, enlarge the incision, and insert the mesh directly into the abdomen. The trocar is then repositioned.

a

b

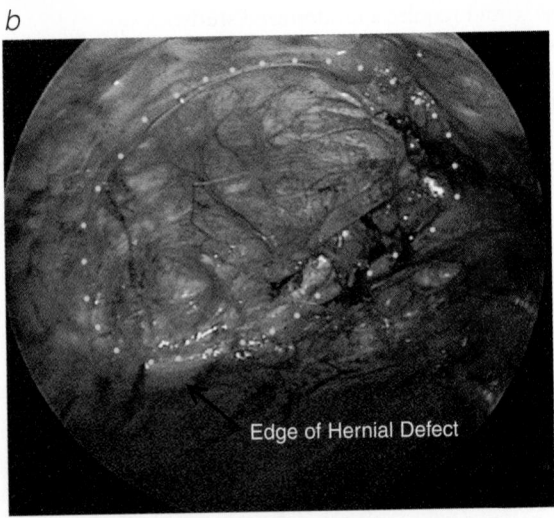

Edge of Hernial Defect

Figure 16 **Laparoscopic incisional hernia repair. (*a*) Shown is dissection of incarcerated small bowel and omentum from an incisional hernia. (*b*) After adhesiolysis, the edges of the defect can be seen.**

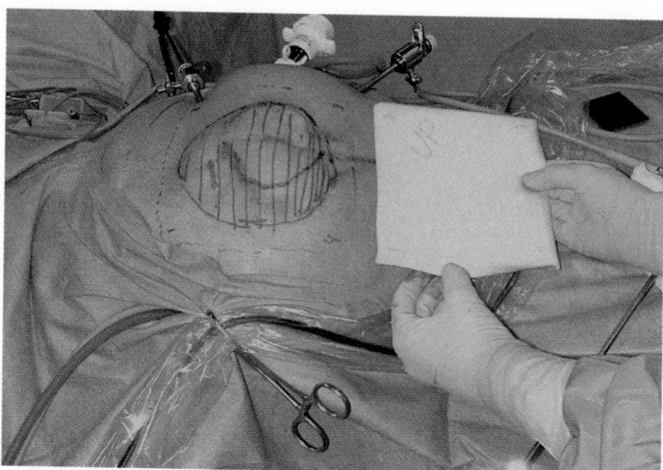

Figure 17 **Laparoscopic incisional hernia repair. An outline of the hernial defect is drawn on the abdominal wall, with a 2 cm margin marked around the defect to serve as a template for tailoring the mesh. The four corners of the mesh swatch and of the template are numbered to facilitate orientation of the mesh once it is inside the peritoneal cavity. Patient's head is to the left.**

Step 4: Fixation of Mesh

Once the mesh swatch has been introduced into the abdomen, it is unfurled and spread out, with the previously placed corner sutures facing the fascia and oriented so that the four numbered corners are aligned with the numbers marked on the abdominal wall. Small skin incisions are then made in two lateral corners. Through each of these incisions, a suture passer is inserted to grasp one tail of the previously placed 2-0 Prolene suture and pull it out through the abdominal wall, then reintroduced through the incision to pull out the second tail. Each suture is then tied and buried in the subcutaneous tissue so as to anchor the mesh to the fascia and maintain its proper orientation. Once two corners are secured, the mesh is spread out tautly and the other two corners secured in a similar fashion. A stapler is then used to tack the mesh circumferentially at 1 cm intervals [*see Figure 18*].

If multiple defects are present over a large area, we overlap multiple swatches of mesh rather than use a single large swatch, which is cumbersome to manipulate laparoscopically.

Step 5: Closure

The pneumoperitoneum is released. The fascia at any trocar site larger than 10 mm is closed. The skin is then closed with subcuticular sutures.

POSTOPERATIVE CARE

The Foley catheter is removed at the end of the procedure. Patients are admitted to the hospital. Oral intake is begun when bowel sounds are present and there is no abdominal distention; when this state is reached varies according to the extent of adhesiolysis and bowel manipulation required to liberate the contents of the hernial sac. Patients are discharged when a full diet is tolerated. Patients are warned that fluid may accumulate at the hernia site. Any fever or redness should be reported.

OUTCOME EVALUATION

Several series of laparoscopic incisional hernia repairs have been reported. In preparation for a randomized trial, Toy and colleagues described 144 patients at multiple centers who were operated on with a standardized technique and followed prospectively.[4] The mean operating time was about 2 hours. Two enterotomies were made intraoperatively. The most common postoperative complication was wound seroma, which occurred in 23 patients (16%). Surgical site infection occurred in five patients (3%). Two patients required removal of the mesh. One experienced bowel obstruction. Recurrences were observed in eight cases (6%) after a mean follow-up of 222 days. In a study of 122 laparoscopic incisional hernia repairs reported by Franklin and associates, there was one recurrence after a mean follow-up of 30.1 months.[6]

Park and colleagues compared 56 prospective laparoscopic incisional hernia repairs with 49 open incisional hernia repairs assessed through retrospective chart review.[7] The groups were comparable in terms of patient characteristics and hernia size. Although the mean operating time was longer in the laparoscopic group (95.4 minutes versus 78.5 minutes), the postoperative length of stay was significantly shorter after laparoscopic repair than after open repair (3.4 days versus 6.5 days). Overall, there were significantly fewer complications after laparoscopic repair. There were fewer recurrences after laparoscopic repair than after open repair (six versus 17); the mean follow-up time was 24.1 months, but follow-up was significantly longer after open repair, for which the data were collected retrospectively.

Carbajo and colleagues compared 30 laparoscopic incisional hernia repairs with 30 open repairs in a randomized trial.[5] There were no intraoperative complications in the laparoscopic group and two enterotomies in the open group. The mean operating time was significantly shorter in the laparoscopic group (87 minutes versus 111.5 minutes), as was the postoperative length of stay (2.23 days versus 9.06 days). One patient in each group required reoperation for bowel obstruction; in the laparoscopic group, this complication was attributable to incarceration of the bowel between the mesh and the abdominal wall. There were fewer wound complications in the laparoscopic group. After a minimum follow-up of 18 months, no recurrences were noted in the laparoscopic group and two in the open group.

Although the results of other large randomized trials are not available yet, preliminary work suggests that the laparoscopic approach to the repair of large incisional hernias is highly promising. The laparoscopic approach seems to confer the well-known benefits of other video-assisted procedures (e.g., quicker recovery) while comparing favorably to the open operation in terms of complication and recurrence rates.

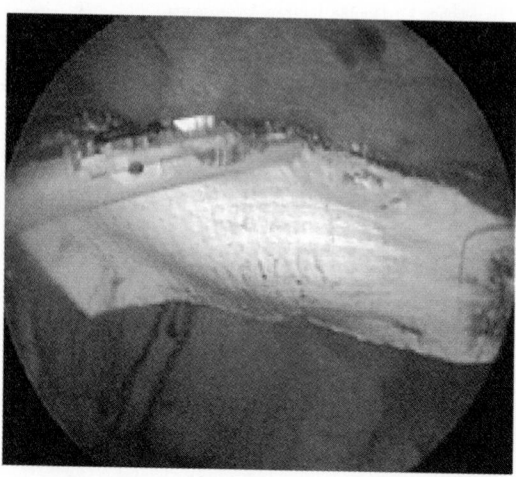

Figure 18 **Laparoscopic incisional hernia repair. The mesh is secured to the peritoneum with sutures and staples.**

References

1. Ger R, Monroe K, Duvivier R, et al: Management of indirect hernias by laparoscopic closure of the neck of the sac. Am J Surg 159:370, 1990

2. Robbins AW, Rutkow IM: Mesh plug repair and groin hernia surgery. Surg Clin North Am 78:1007, 1998

3. Crawford DL, Phillips EH: Laparoscopic repair and groin hernia surgery. Surg Clin North Am 78:1047, 1998

4. Toy FK, Bailey RW, Carey S, et al: Prospective, multi-center study of laparoscopic ventral hernioplasty: preliminary results. Surg Endosc 12:955, 1998

5. Carbajo MA, Martin del Olmo JC, Blanco JI, et al: Laparoscopic treatment vs open surgery in the solution of major incisional and abdominal wall hernias with mesh. Surg Endosc 13:250, 1999

6. Franklin ME, Dorman JP, Glass JL, et al: Laparoscopic ventral hernia repair. Surg Laparosc Endosc 8:294, 1998

7. Park A, Birch DW, Lovrics P: Laparoscopic and open incisional hernia repair: a comparison study. Surgery 124:816, 1998

8. LeBlanc KA, Booth WV: Laparoscopic repair of incisional abdominal hernias using expanded polytetrafluorethylene: preliminary findings. Surg Laparosc Endosc 3:39, 1992

9. Skandalakis JE, Gray SW, Skandalakis LJ, et al: Surgical anatomy of the inguinal area. World J Surg 13:490, 1989

10. Spaw AT, Ennis BW, Spaw LP: Laparoscopic hernia repair: the anatomic basis. J Laparoendosc Surg 1:269, 1991

11. Wantz GE: Atlas of Hernia Surgery. Raven Press, New York, 1991

12. Condon RE: The anatomy of the inguinal region and its relation to groin hernia. Hernia, 3rd ed. Nyhus LM, Condon RE, Eds. JB Lippincott Co, Philadelphia, 1989, p 18

13. Memon MA, Fitzgibbons RJ: Laparoscopic inguinal hernia repair: transabdominal (TAPP) and totally extraperitoneal (TEP). The SAGES Manual. Scott-Connor CEH, Ed. Springer, New York, 1999

14. Ramshaw BJ, Tucker JG, Conner T, et al: A comparison of the approaches to laparoscopic herniorrhaphy. Surg Endosc 10:29, 1996

15. Fitzgibbons RJ Jr, Camps J, Cornet DA, et al: Laparoscopic inguinal herniorrhaphy: results of a multicenter trial. Ann Surg 221:3, 1995

16. Arregui ME. Transabdominal retroperitoneal inguinal herniorrhaphy. Operative Laparoscopy and Thoracoscopy. MacFayden BV, Ponsky JL, Eds. Lippincott-Raven, Philadelphia, 1996

17. Felix H, Michas C: Double buttress laparoscopic herniorrhaphy. J Laparoendosc Surg 3:1, 1993

18. McKernan JB, Laws HL: Laparoscopic repair of inguinal hernias using a totally extraperitoneal prosthetic approach. Surg Endosc 7:26, 1993

19. Stoppa R, Warlaumont C, Verhaeghe P, et al: Dacron mesh and surgical therapy of inguinal hernia. Chir Patol Sper 34:15, 1986

20. Stoppa R, Warlaumont CR: The preperitoneal approach and prosthetic repair of groin hernias. Hernia, 3rd ed. Nyhus LM, Condon RE, Eds. JB Lippincott Co, Philadelphia, 1989

21. Stoppa R: The treatment of complicated groin and incisional hernias. World J Surg 13:545, 1989

22. Wantz GE: Giant prosthetic reinforcement of the visceral sac. Surg Gynecol Obstet 169:408, 1989

23. McKernan JB: Extraperitoneal inguinal herniorrhaphy. Operative Laparoscopy and Thoracoscopy. MacFayden BV, Ponsky JL, Eds. Lippincott-Raven, Philadelphia, 1996

24. Wellwood J, Sculpher MJ, Stoker D, et al: Randomized clinical trial of laparoscopic versus open mesh repair for inguinal hernia: outcome and cost. BMJ 317:103, 1998

25. Amado WJ: Anesthesia for hernia surgery. Surg Clin North Am 73:427, 1993

26. Ferzli G, Sayad P, Hallak A, et al: Endoscopic extraperitoneal hernia repair: a 5-year experience. Surg Endosc 12:1311, 1998

27. Ferzli G, Sayad P, Vasisht B: The feasibility of laparoscopic extraperitoneal hernia repair under local anesthesia. Surg Endosc 13:588, 1999

28. Paganini AM, Lezoche E, Carle F, et al: A randomized controlled clinical study of laparoscopic vs. open tension-free inguinal hernia repair. Surg Endosc 12:979, 1998

29. Zieren J, Zieren H, Jacobi CA, et al: Prospective randomized study comparing laparoscopic and open tension-free inguinal hernia repair with Shouldice's operation. Am J Surg 175:330, 1998

30. Heikkinen T, Haukipuro K, Leppälä J, et al: Total costs of laparoscopic and Lichtenstein inguinal hernia repairs: a prospective study. Surg Lap Endosc 7:1, 1997

31. Johansson B, Hallerbäck B, Glise H, et al: Laparoscopic mesh versus open preperitoneal mesh versus conventional technique for inguinal hernia repair. A randomized multicenter trial (SCUR Hernia Repair Study). Ann Surg 230:225, 1999

32. The MRC Laparoscopic Groin Hernia Trial Group: Laparoscopic versus open repair of groin hernia: a randomised comparison. Lancet 354:185, 1999

33. Payne JH, Grininger LM, Isawa MT, et al: Laparoscopic or open inguinal herniorrhaphy? a randomized prospective trial. Arch Surg 129:973, 1994

34. Heikkinen TJ, Haukipuro K, Hulkko A: A cost and outcome comparison between laparoscopic and Lichtenstein hernia operations in a day-case unit: a randomized prospective study. Surg Endosc 12:1199, 1998

35. Champault GG, Rizk N, Catheline J-M, et al: Inguinal hernia repair. Totally preperitoneal laparoscopic approach versus Stoppa operation: randomized trial of 100 cases. Surg Lap Endosc 7:445, 1997

36. Khoury N: A randomized prospective controlled trial of laparoscopic extraperitoneal hernia repair and mesh-plug hernioplasty: a study of 315 cases. J Laparoendosc Surg 8:367, 1998

37. Phillips EH, Arregui ME, Carroll BJ, et al: Incidence of complications following laparoscopic hernioplasty. Surg Endosc 9:16, 1995

38. Salerno GM, Fitzgibbons RJ Jr, Filipi CJ: Laparoscopic inguinal hernia repair. Surgical Laparoscopy. Zucker KA, Ed. Quality Medical Publishing, St Louis, 1991

39. MacFayden BV Jr, Arregui M, Corbitt J, et al: Complications of laparoscopic herniorrhaphy. Surg Endosc 7:155, 1993

40. Phillips EH, Arregui M, Carroll BJ, et al: Incidence of complications following laparoscopic hernioplasty. Surg Endosc 9:16, 1995

41. Estour E, Mouret PH: Cure laparoscopique des hernies de l'aine. J Coelio Chir 16:15, 1995

42. Avtan L, Avci C, Bulut T, et al: Mesh infections after laparoscopic inguinal hernia repair. Surg Laparosc Endosc 7:192, 1997

43. Leim NSL, Van der Graaf Y, van Steensel CJ, et al: Comparison of conventional anterior surgery and laparoscopic surgery for inguinal hernia repair. N Engl J Med 336:1541, 1997

44. Ferzli GS, Frezza EE, Pecorato AM Jr, et al: Prospective randomized study of stapled versus unstapled mesh in a laparoscopic preperitoneal inguinal hernia repair. J Am Coll Surg 188:461, 1999

45. Wantz GE: Ambulatory surgical treatment of groin hernia: prevention and management of complications. Problems in General Surgery 3:311, 1986

46. Wright DM, Kennedy A, Baxter JN, et al: Early outcome after open versus extraperitoneal endoscopic tension-free hernioplasty: a randomized clinical trial. Surgery 119:552, 1996

47. Starling JR, Harms BA: Diagnosis and treatment of genitofemoral and ilioinguinal neuralgia. World J Surg 13:586, 1989

48. Kraus MA: Nerve injury during laparoscopic inguinal hernia repair. Surg Laparosc Endosc 3:342, 1993

49. Rosen A, Halevy A: Anatomical basis for nerve injury during laparoscopic hernia repair. Surg Laparosc Endosc 7:469, 1997

50. Wexler MJ, Meakins JL, Garzon J: Laparoscopic groin hernia repair: preliminary results from a prospective clinical trial. Can J Surg 36:384, 1993

51. Lawrence K, McWhinnie O, Goodwin, et al: Randomized controlled trial of laparoscopic vs. open repair of inguinal hernia: early results. Br J Surg 311:981, 1995

52. Bassell JR, Baxter P, Riddell F, et al: A randomized controlled trial of laparoscopic extraperitoneal hernia repair as a day surgical procedure. Surg Endosc 10:495, 1996

53. Kald A, Anderberg B, Carlsson P, et al: Surgical outcome and cost-minimization analyses of laparoscopic and open hernia repair: a randomised prospective trial with one-year follow up. Eur J Surg 163:505, 1997

54. Kozol R, Lange PN, Kosir N, et al: A prospective randomized study of open vs. laparoscopic inguinal hernia repair. Arch Surg 132:292, 1997

55. Stoker DL, Spiegelhalter DJ, Singh R, et al: Laparoscopic versus open inguinal hernia repair: randomised prospective trial. Lancet 343:1243, 1994

56. Schrenk P, Woisetschlager R, Reiger R, et al: Prospective randomized trial comparing postoperative pain and return to physical activity after transabdominal preperitoneal, total preperitoneal, or Shouldice technique for inguinal hernia repair. Br J Surg 83:1563, 1996

57. Vogt DM, Curet MJ, Pitcher DE, et al: Preliminary results of a prospective randomized trial of laparoscopic onlay versus conventional inguinal herniorrhaphy. Am J Surg 169:84, 1995

58. Chung RS, Rowland DY: Meta-analysis of randomized controlled trials of laparoscopic vs conventional inguinal hernia repairs. Surg Endosc 13:689, 1999

59. Filipi CJ, Gaston-Johansson F, McBride PJ, et al: An assessment of pain and return to normal activity: laparoscopic herniorrhaphy vs open tension-free Lichtenstein repair. Surg Endosc 10:983, 1996

60. Barkun JS, Keyser EJ, Wexler MJ, et al: Short-term outcomes in open vs. laparoscopic herniorrhaphy: confounding impact of worker's compensation on convalescence. J Gastrointest Surg 3:575, 1999

61. Barkun JS, Barkun AN, Sampalis JS, et al: Randomized controlled trial of laparoscopic versus mini cholecystectomy. Lancet 340:1116, 1992

62. Krähenbühl L, Schäfer M, Schilling M, et al: Simultaneous repair of bilateral groin hernias: open or lap-

aroscopic approach? Surg Laparosc Endosc 8:313, 1998

63. Lichtenstein IL, Shulman AG, Amid PK: The cause, prevention, and treatment of recurrent groin hernia. Surg Clin North Am 73:529, 1993

64. Robbins AW, Rutkow IM: Mesh plug repair and groin hernia surgery. Surg Clin North Am 78:1007, 1998

65. Lowham AS, Filipi CJ, Fitzgibbons RJ, et al: Mechanisms of hernia recurrence after preperitoneal mesh repair: traditional and laparoscopic. Ann Surg 225:422, 1997

66. Memon MA, Rice D, Donohue JH: Laparoscop-

ic herniorrhaphy. J Am Coll Surg 184:325, 1997

67. Beets GL, Dirksen CD, Go PM, et al: Open or laparoscopic preperitoneal mesh repair for recurrent inguinal hernia? A randomized controlled trial. Surg Endosc 13:323, 1999

68. Cohen RV, Alvarez G, Roll S, et al: Transabdominal or totally extraperitoneal laparoscopic hernia repair? Surg Laparosc Endosc 8:264, 1998

69. Kald A, Anderberg B, Smedh K, et al: Transperitoneal or totally extraperitoneal approach in laparoscopic hernia repair: results of 491 consecutive herniorrhaphies. Surg Laparosc Endosc 7:86, 1997

70. Felix EL, Michas CA, Gonzalez MH Jr: Laparoscopic hernioplasty: TAPP vs TEP. Surg Endosc 9:984, 1995

71. Hesselink VJ, Luijendik RW, de Wilt JHW, et al: An evaluation of risk factors in incisional hernia recurrence. Surg Gynecol Obstet 176:228, 1993

72. Santora TA, Roslyn JJ: Incisional hernia. Surg Clin North Am 73:557, 1993

Acknowledgment

Figures 1, 4 through 7, 8 (right), 14, and 15   Tom Moore.

22 VASCULAR AND PERITONEAL ACCESS

Bernard Montreuil, M.D., Laurie Morrison, M.D., Lawrence Rosenberg, M.D., Ph.D., and Carl Nohr, M.D., Ph.D.

Vascular Access via Arteriovenous Fistulas

The number of patients with end-stage renal disease (ESRD) in the United States increased steadily through the 1990s, reaching 300,000 by the end of 1997.[1] Extracorporeal dialysis of blood was introduced in 1943 by Kolff and associates[2]; however, application of this approach was hindered by the requirement for repeated and routine access to the circulation. The full potential of hemodialysis for patient salvage was realized only after the introduction of the external arteriovenous (AV) shunt by Quinton and colleagues in 1960[3] and of the endogenous AV fistula (AVF) by Brescia and coworkers in 1966.[4] The subsequent introduction of synthetic vascular prostheses has permitted continued access in patients who have exhausted peripheral venous sites[5]; however, the long-term performance of such prostheses remains inferior to that of autogenous fistulas. The creation and maintenance of functioning vascular access, along with the associated complications, constitute the most common cause of morbidity, hospitalization, and cost in patients with end-stage renal disease.

The ideal vascular access route permits a flow rate that is adequate for the dialysis prescription (≥ 300 ml/min), can be used for extended periods, and has a low complication rate. The native AVF remains the gold standard. In 1997, the National Kidney Foundation Dialysis Outcome and Quality Initiative (NKF-DOQI)[6] organized multidisciplinary work groups that evaluated all available data on vascular access and concluded that quality of life and overall outcome could be improved significantly for hemodialysis patients if two primary goals were achieved:

1. Increased placement of native AVFs: a minimum of 50% of new dialysis patients should have primary AVFs.
2. Detection of dysfunctional access before thrombosis of the access route occurs.

OPERATIVE PLANNING

At least 4 to 6 weeks—preferably 3 to 4 months—is required for a native AVF to heal and mature before it can be used. Therefore, access planning should be done early in the course of progressive renal failure. Patients should be referred for surgical treatment when creatinine clearance approaches 25 ml/min, the serum creatinine level reaches 4 mg/dl, or dialysis is likely to be necessary within 1 year. Every effort should be made not to puncture forearm veins, particularly the cephalic veins of the nondominant arm; the dorsal hand veins may be used for venipuncture. Subclavian vein catheterization should also be avoided because of the risk of central vein stenosis, which may preclude the use of any part of the ipsilateral arm for vascular access.

Assessment of Venous System

A history of subclavian vein cannulation or transvenous pacemaker placement is associated with a 10% to 40% rate of central vein stenosis or thrombosis.[7] Previous injuries or operative procedures involving the arm, the neck, or the chest, including previous vascular access, also may give rise to significant venous abnormalities. Physical signs of venous outflow obstruction include extremity edema, differences in arm size, and development of collateral veins. All of these historical and physical findings call for investigation by means of phlebography or color flow duplex scanning.[8] Central vein stenosis greater than 50% is a contraindication to creation of an ipsilateral distal AVF: it is a predictor of venous hypertension and edema in the arm and of poor function in the fistula.

Selection of the ideal vein for access is facilitated by distending the veins with a tourniquet around the upper arm. In particular, the cephalic vein is palpated from the region of the anatomic snuffbox to the area above the elbow. Percussion of the vein is performed to confirm that it is patent and to rule out stenosis from previous venipuncture. The fingertips of one hand are positioned over the vein at the elbow, and the vein is gently tapped distally with the other hand. If the vein is patent and of substantial diameter, a fluid wave is felt over the proximal vein.

Assessment of Arterial System

A history of arterial trauma or catheterization, diabetes mellitus, or peripheral arterial disease may be associated with chronic damage to the arterial system. Physical examination involves palpation of the pulses (including both brachial and axillary pulses) and comparison of blood pressure in the arms. A difference of more than 20 mm Hg between the two sides suggests proximal arterial occlusive disease, which may cause the AVF to fail as a result of inadequate inflow. An Allen test is also performed to confirm that the palmar arch is patent, to determine which artery is the dominant vascular supply to the hand, and to ensure that the ulnar artery can support the hand if the radial artery must be divided. Any abnormality on physical examination should be further investigated by means of arterial studies in the vascular laboratory; in select cases, angiography may be indicated.

Noninvasive Preoperative Assessment

Systematic use of noninvasive evaluation in the vascular laboratory permits objective assessment of arterial and venous conduits. If necessary, venous conduits other than the cephalic and basilic veins may be identified,[9] and both arterial and venous segments may be mapped with skin marks to facilitate the operative procedure. The aims are to increase the use of autogenous fistulas and to raise the early and late patency rates by decreasing the use of suboptimal veins and arteries.

Complete noninvasive assessment includes segmental pressure measurements of the upper extremity, arterial waveform recording, and arterial and venous duplex studies. A tourniquet should be placed on the arm, and tapping and stroking maneuvers should be used to distend the vein maximally. Established criteria [see Table 1] are then applied to determine whether venous outflow and arterial inflow are likely to be satisfactory.

Choice of Type of AVF

Multiple varieties of AV fistulas have been used in hemodialysis patients. According to the NKF-DOQI report,[6] the order of preference for AV fistulas in patients requiring long-term hemodialysis is as follows:

1. Wrist (radiocephalic) primary AV fistula.
2. Elbow (brachiocephalic) primary AV fistula.

If neither of these can be constructed, access may be achieved via either of the following:

3. AV graft of synthetic material.
4. Transposed brachiobasilic AV fistula.

All of these fistulas should be established in the nondominant arm, if possible.

The distal radiocephalic AVF remains the gold standard in terms of ease of creation and long-term results. Its advantages considerably outweigh its disadvantages—namely, a higher primary failure rate (10% to 15%) and a long maturation time (1 to 4 months). Radiocephalic AVFs may be constructed either in the anatomic snuff-box or just above the wrist crease. Although the radial artery is smaller in the snuff-box than it is at the classical Brescia-Cimino fistula site, the long-term results at the two sites are comparable if only arteries of adequate diameter are used.[10]

An alternative method of creating an AVF in the forearm that was not mentioned in the NKF-DOQI report is vein transposition.[11] Preoperative duplex ultrasonography often identifies veins that, except for their deep subcutaneous location, are suitable for AVF formation. In addition, the basilic vein in the forearm is often spared and is frequently suitable for AVF formation; however, use of this vein in situ for needle cannulation and hemodialysis may necessitate placing the forearm in an uncomfortable position. In the great majority of cases, such veins can be successfully transposed to a superficial tunnel in the midportion of the volar aspect of the forearm, and the resulting fistula theoretically has the same advantages as a radiocephalic fistula in terms of long-term patency and complication rates. This aggressive approach to autogenous forearm fistula formation also has the advantage of preserving more proximal vessels for future access placement.

If duplex ultrasonography does not identify an adequate forearm vein conduit, a brachiocephalic primary AVF is the next choice. It is easy to create and has the advantage of providing higher blood flow than the wrist fistula. The cephalic vein in the upper arm, because of its position and superficial location, is easy to cannulate and easily covered (a potential cosmetic benefit). The elbow AVF has a theoretical advantage in diabetic patients, in whom medial calcification of the distal radial artery commonly prevents the gradual arterial dilatation required for full maturation of a radiocephalic fistula. In fact, some authors[12] consider an upper-arm autogenous AVF (either a brachiocephalic or a transposed basilic vein fistula) the preferred approach in this particular subgroup of patients. Disadvantages of

brachiocephalic fistulas include higher frequencies of arm swelling and steal syndrome than are seen with forearm fistulas.

If the cephalic vein in the upper arm is unsuitable, the remaining options include a prosthetic graft and transposed basilic vein. An AVF using transposed basilic vein has all the attributes of an autogenous fistula and consequently is preferred to a graft despite being more difficult to create. Its protected, deep subfascial position and large caliber make it a high-quality conduit for hemodialysis access. Its advantages over a prosthetic graft include the avoidance of the distal venous anastomosis (which causes the majority of stenoses in synthetic graft fistulas) and higher primary and secondary patency rates.[13,14] Flow rates are high in basilic vein fistulas because of the large size of the vein, and the infection rate is relatively low. Furthermore, thrombosis of a brachiobasilic fistula does not compromise the integrity of the axillary vein and thus does not preclude subsequent use of a prosthetic conduit at the same site.

If no veins in either upper extremity are suitable for a native AVF, then the use of prosthetic material should be considered. Two options are available. First, if a segment of vein at least 15 cm long is available but is too far from the artery to be used in the creation of a fully native fistula, a jump graft can be constructed between the artery and the vein, and the arterialized vein can be used as the needle conduit for dialysis. Second, the graft itself can be used as the needle conduit for dialysis. The data currently available suggest that extruded polytetrafluoroethylene (ePTFE) is preferable to other biologic and synthetic materials: ePTFE grafts are less likely to disintegrate with infection, they are more widely available, they remain patent longer, and they are easily handled by surgeons. Grafts may be placed in straight, looped, or curved configurations on either the forearm or the upper arm.

OPERATIVE TECHNIQUE

Autogenous AVFs

Radiocephalic fistula The arm is placed on an arm board in 90° of abduction. A tourniquet is applied to the upper arm to distend the cephalic vein, and the vein's course is marked on the skin. The tourniquet is then released.

Local anesthesia using 0.5% or 1% lidocaine without epinephrine is usually adequate for construction of an autogenous AVF at the wrist or the antecubital fossa. General anesthesia may depress cardiac output and thus may, by reducing fistula flow, exert a negative impact on the success of the fistula. Conversely, brachial or supraclavicular regional anesthesia may cause peripheral vasodilatation and thus increase arterial blood flow.

Table 1 Noninvasive Criteria for Selection of Upper-Extremity Arteries and Veins for Dialysis Access Procedures[9]

Venous examination
Venous luminal diameter ≥ 2.5 mm for autogenous AVFs, ≥ 4.0 mm for bridge AV grafts
Absence of segmental stenoses or occluded segments
Continuity with the deep venous system in the upper arm
Absence of ipsilateral central vein stenosis or occlusion

Arterial examination
Arterial luminal diameter ≥ 2.0 mm
Absence of pressure differential ≥ 20 mm Hg between arms
Patent palmar arch

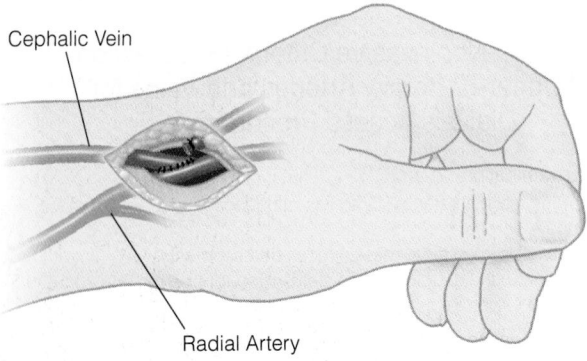

Figure 1 **Vascular access via AVFs: radiocephalic fistula. Shown is the anatomic snuff-box fistula, with the end of the cephalic vein anastomosed to the side of the radial artery.**

Figure 2 **Vascular access via AVFs: radiocephalic fistula. Shown is the Brescia-Cimino fistula. An incision is made midway between the radial artery and the cephalic vein, and the end of the vein is anastomosed to the side of the artery.**

A longitudinal incision is placed either in the anatomic snuff-box, between the tendons of the extensor pollicis longus and the extensor pollicis brevis [*see Figure 1*], or midway between the cephalic vein and the radial artery, proximal to the wrist skinfold [*see Figure 2*]. In the anatomic snuff-box, the cephalic vein overlies the radial artery, so that minimal mobilization is required to approximate the two vessels. Slightly more mobilization is required to approximate the cephalic vein to the radial artery above the wrist without kinking or twisting. A comparable length of radial artery, found under the deep fascia, is also isolated. Care is taken to preserve the superficial branch of the radial nerve, which lies lateral to the radial artery and is separated from it by the brachioradialis muscle.

Four types of anastomoses can be constructed: side to side, end of vein to side of artery, end to end, and end of artery to side of vein. The side-to-side anastomosis [*see Figure 3a*] yields the highest flow through the fistula but may be associated with venous congestion of the hand. Over time, arterial pressure may render the valves of the distal vein incompetent, resulting in retrograde flow toward the hand and venous hypertension. The end of artery–side of vein anastomosis [*see Figure 3b*] also presents a risk of venous hypertension. This configuration reduces the risk of distal steal by preventing retrograde flow into the fistula, but at the price of lower flow through the fistula. Of the four options, the end of artery–end of vein variation [*see Figure 3c*] produces the least distal arterial steal and venous hypertension but yields the lowest flow.

The preferred configuration of the anastomosis is end of vein to side of artery [*see Figure 3d*]. Dividing the vein reduces the risk of venous congestion in the hand; moreover, by allowing retrograde flow from the distal radial artery and the ulnar artery into the vein, which contributes approximately 30% of the total flow of the fistula, this approach yields maximal blood flow through the fistula. There is a risk of steal syndrome with such fistulas, but this problem is easily corrected by ligating the radial artery distal to the fistula, thereby converting the anastomosis to an end-to-end configuration.

Vascular control is obtained with small vessel loops or Heifets clamps. Heparinization is not needed unless the artery is an end artery. A 1 cm arteriotomy is performed, and the vein is ligated and divided distally and tailored to match the arteriotomy. Coronary dilators are then inserted gently to verify patency and to ensure that the vessel lumina are large enough: the artery should easily admit a 2 mm dilator; the vein, a 3 mm dilator. The vessels are then anastomosed in the desired configuration with a fine continuous monofilament suture (6-0 or 7-0 polypropylene) placed by means of standard techniques. The vessels can be probed with the coronary dilators before the anastomosis is completed, to confirm that the vein is not twisted or to overcome any arterial spasm. Once vascular control is released, a thrill should be easily felt over the fistula and for a moderate distance along the venous conduit. The skin is closed with an absorbable suture.

Vein transposition in the forearm The artery and the vein selected for the primary AVF are identified and mapped preoperatively by means of duplex ultrasonography. Positioning and anesthetic considerations are essentially the same as for a radiocephalic fistula.

A longitudinal incision is made directly over the mapped vein, beginning at its distal end and extending toward the antecubital fossa for a distance of at least 15 cm [*see Figure 4a*]. The vein is gently skeletonized and mobilized by ligating and dividing all side branches. The targeted artery (either the radial or the ulnar) is identified and dissected through a separate incision. A superficial subcutaneous tunnel is made between the two incisions with a blunt tunneling instrument, and the vein is passed through the tunnel [*see Figure 4b*]. The vein should be marked along its length with a marking pen before tunneling; this step provides a usual visual check that allows the surgeon to confirm that the vein is not twisted as it passes through the tunnel. A 1 cm anastomosis is then carried out in the same fashion as for a radiocephalic fistula (see above).

Brachiocephalic fistula After adequate local anesthesia, a transverse incision is made 1.5 cm distal to the antecubital crease[15] to expose the superficial antecubital venous system [*see Figure 5a*]. If the median cubital vein is patent, sufficiently wide, and in continuity with the cephalic vein, it is dissected so that the perforating branch of the antecubital venous system (vena mediana cubiti profunda) can be located. The bicipital aponeurosis is divided, and the perforating branch is followed down to the deep system. In the process, the brachial artery is also exposed, as are the origins of the radial and ulnar arteries.

Once the patient is fully heparinized, the confluence of the brachial vein and the perforating vein is identified, and part of the brachial vein is excised so as to form a venous patch. The perforating vein is gently dilated, so that any valves are rendered incompetent, and the proximal median cubital vein is ligated to prevent diversion of blood flow into the basilic vein. The perforating vein is then anastomosed to the brachial artery in an end-to-side fashion [*see Figure 5b*].[16] To prevent subsequent steal syndrome, the arteriotomy should be no larger than 5 to 6 mm.

Figure 3 Vascular access via AVFs: radiocephalic fistula. Four anastomotic configurations are possible for an autologenous radiocephalic fistula: (*a*) side of artery to side of vein, (*b*) end of artery to side of vein, (*c*) end of artery to end of vein, and (*d*) end of vein to side of artery (the preferred configuration).

Other techniques may be used if the perforating vein is very large or very small. If the perforating vein is 5 mm or more in diameter, it may be anastomosed directly to the artery without a patch. If the vein is less than 2.5 mm in diameter, it should not be used; instead, the median cubital vein should be ligated and divided and the cephalic end of the vein anastomosed directly to the brachial artery in an end-to-side fashion [*see Figure 5c*]. If the median cubital vein is too small, the incision is extended laterally and proximally to allow mobilization of the cephalic vein. The length of this incision depends on the extent to which the cephalic vein must be mobi-

a

b

Radial Artery

Figure 4 Vascular access via AVFs: vein transposition in the forearm. (*a*) The selected vein, identified by duplex ultrasonography, is completely mobilized. (*b*) The vein is transposed through a superficial tunnel in the midportion of the volar aspect of the forearm and anastomosed to the radial artery in an end-to-side fashion.

lized to ensure a tension-free end-to-side anastomosis. The accessory cephalic vein, though located far laterally, may also be used.

Repeated venipunctures in the antecubital fossa frequently render the antecubital venous system unsuitable for AVF construction. In such cases, two options are available if the patient has at least 15 cm of good-quality cephalic vein in the upper arm. The first option is to mobilize a sufficient length of the cephalic vein in the distal upper arm through a longitudinal incision, to transpose it medially through a superficial tunnel, and then to anastomose it in an end-to-side fashion to the brachial artery, which has been exposed above the elbow through a separate incision. The second, which avoids extensive dissection of the cephalic vein, is to place two short longitudinal incisions over the brachial artery and the cephalic vein a few centimeters above the elbow crease, to tunnel a short segment of 6 mm ePTFE graft between the two incisions, and to anastomose the ePTFE graft to both the brachial artery and the cephalic vein in an end-to-side fashion [*see Figure 6*].[17] The cephalic vein is used as the needle conduit for this type of bridge AV graft.

Brachiobasilic fistula The technique for constructing a brachiobasilic fistula was described first by Dagher and associates in 1976[18] and then by Logerfo and colleagues in 1978.[19] Local anesthesia can be used, but an axillary block eases the procedure considerably.

An oblique incision overlying the median basilic vein is made in the antecubital fossa, and the vein is mobilized. The brachial artery is exposed as usual by dividing the bicipital aponeurosis. The incision is extended along the medial aspect of the upper arm (the so-called hockey-stick incision), and the basilic vein is mobilized from beneath the fascia, with care taken to preserve the medial cutaneous nerve of the forearm [*see Figure 7a*]. The basilic vein usually pierces the brachial fascia just below the middle of the upper arm, then parallels the course of the brachial artery and vein while remaining superficial to them. At the axillary level, the basilic vein joins the brachial vein to form the axillary vein; this junction constitutes the proximal limit of the dissection.

The distal end of the conduit vein may consist of either the basilic vein or a section of the median cubital vein, which is already exposed. All venous tributaries are ligated and divided. Once this is done, the vein is divided distally, and its anterior surface is

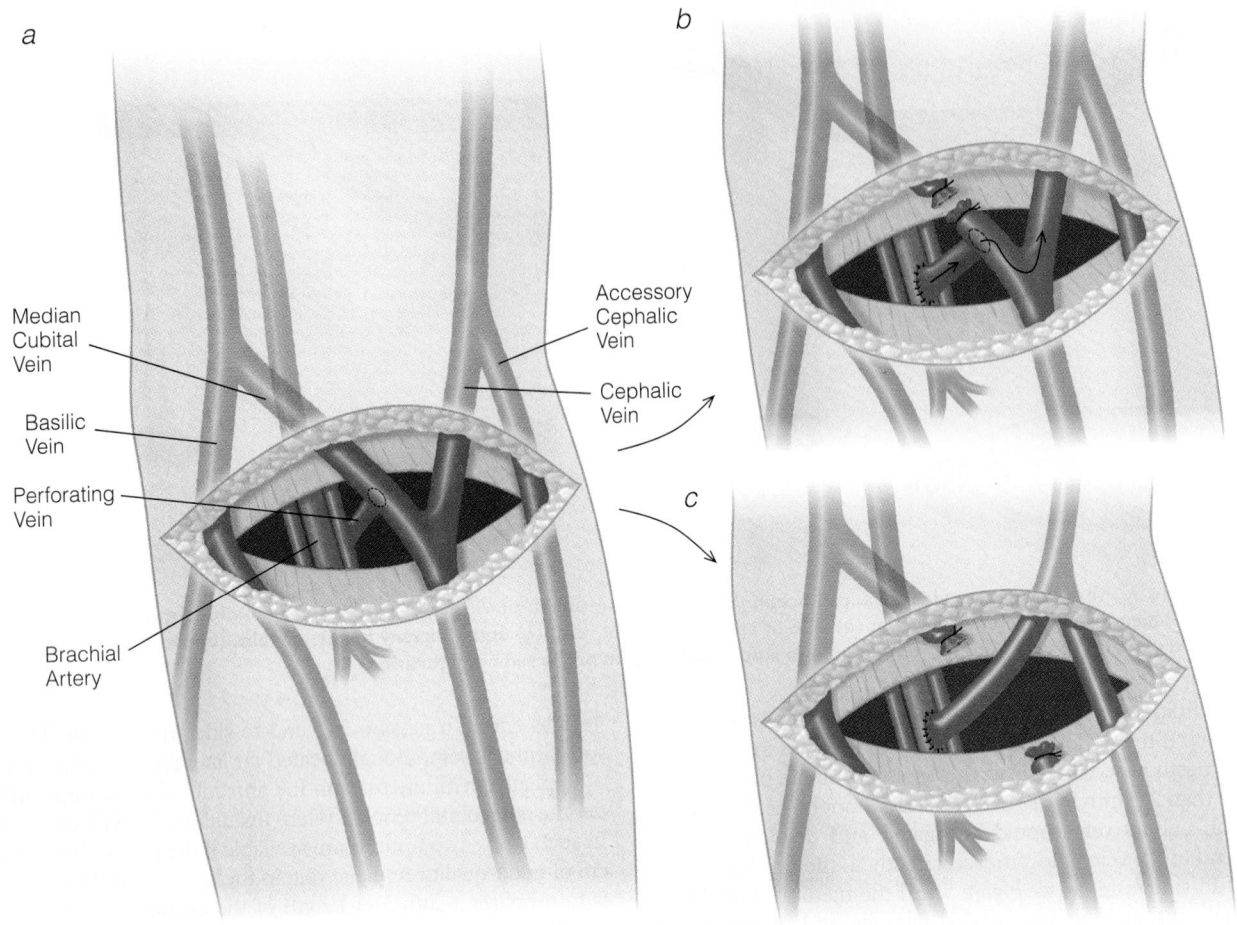

Figure 5 Vascular access via AVFs: brachiocephalic fistula. (*a*) A transverse incision exposes the antecubital venous system (including the perforating branch) and the brachial artery under the bicipital aponeurosis. (*b*) An end-to-side anastomosis is made between the perforating vein and the brachial artery. (*c*) If the perforating vein is too small, the cephalic vein is mobilized and anastomosed to the brachial artery in an end-to-side fashion.

marked to help the surgeon avoid axial rotation during transposition. The vein is then passed through a subcutaneous tunnel on the anterior surface of the arm and anastomosed in an end-to-side fashion to the brachial artery in the antecubital fossa with 6-0 or 7-0 polypropylene [*see Figure 7b*]. This transposition places the vein in a more superficial location and positions it anterolaterally on the arm, thereby facilitating cannulation during hemodialysis sessions. Closure involves approximating the fascia and the subcutaneous tissue in two separate layers.

A modification of the procedure just described is the so-called elevated basilic vein arteriovenous fistula.[20] In this variant, the vein is left in situ rather than transposed anterolaterally, but it is elevated by closing the deep fascia and the subcutaneous tissue beneath the vein. The brachial artery anastomosis is created, and the overlying skin is reapproximated with clips or interrupted sutures. Although the vein remains in its medial location, its new superficial position facilitates cannulation for dialysis.

Bridge AV Grafts

Bridge AV graft procedures involve placing an interposition graft between an artery and a vein and using that graft as the needle conduit for dialysis. In the forearm, the most common configurations are loop grafts between the brachial artery and an antecubital vein (including the brachial veins)[21] and straight bridge AV grafts from the radial artery to an antecubital vein. Most studies report superior patency rates with a loop configuration.[22] Adequate results may be obtained with a straight graft in the forearm if the radial artery is at least 2.5 to 3.0 mm in diameter.

Secondary options for bridge AV graft construction include a variety of unusual configurations, including reverse grafts between the axillary artery and the brachial or the antecubital vein and axilloaxillary grafts, which may be looped in the upper arm or may cross the sternum. It is also possible to construct a looped graft between the proximal superficial femoral artery and the proximal saphenous vein or a straight, reversed graft between the distal superficial femoral or popliteal artery and the proximal saphenous or femoral vein [*see Figure 8*]. Such lower-limb AV grafts are associated with an increased risk of potentially life- or limb-threatening infection and thus are used only as a last resort.

Either local anesthesia or axillary block is usually appropriate for upper-extremity bridge AV grafts. A single dose of a cephalosporin should be given before the procedure. Separate longitudinal incisions are placed to expose the artery and the vein—except when the procedure involves the brachial artery and the antecubital venous system, which are better exposed through a single transverse incision. A 6 mm or a tapered 4 to 7 mm ePTFE graft is then passed through a superficial tunnel between the two incisions. Both anastomoses are constructed in an end-to side fashion, beginning with the venous side. Systemic heparinization is used if an end artery is occluded for the arterial anastomosis.

TROUBLESHOOTING

Autogenous AVFs

Although the quality of the AV conduit is assessed preoperatively by means of physical examination and noninvasive studies, it should also be confirmed intraoperatively for optimal results.

Arterial inflow   Normally, a strong pulse is felt over the targeted artery; however, dissection may cause spasm, which can render intra-operative assessment difficult. The following three measures will help minimize this problem:

1. Elimination of epinephrine from the anesthetic solution.
2. Gentle dissection and avoidance of direct manipulation of the arterial wall. It may be preferable to use a proximal tourniquet for inflow occlusion so that there is no need to place clamps on small arteries.
3. Local application of a papaverine solution, which relaxes vascular smooth muscle.

If spasm occurs, gentle probing of the artery with coronary dilators may help relieve the spasm and restore full flow.

Stiff, calcified arteries can sometimes be successfully used in the creation of fistulas, but it is difficult to assess flow in such vessels. Quantitative and qualitative analyses of the arterial waveform and the intraluminal diameter by means of duplex scanning can help confirm the adequacy of the vessel. Arteries smaller than 1.5 mm are less likely to provide sufficient flow for a fistula. It is particularly important not to place clamps on calcified arteries; a tourniquet is always preferred in this situation.

Venous outflow   A venous diameter of at least 2.5 to 3.0 mm is required for successful maturation of an autogenous fistula. The diameter of the target vein should be known preoperatively from the duplex examination and should be confirmed intraop-

Figure 6   **Vascular access via AVFs: brachiocephalic fistula. If the antecubital venous system is unsuitable for AVF construction, one option is to place an ePTFE interposition graft between the brachial artery and the cephalic vein.**

Figure 7   **Vascular access via AVFs: brachiobasilic fistula. (*a*) The basilic vein is completely mobilized from underneath the fascia in continuity with a section of the median cubital vein in the antecubital fossa. (*b*) The vein is transposed in a subcutaneous tunnel on the anterior surface of the arm and anastomosed to the brachial artery in an end-to-side fashion.**

eratively by calibration with coronary dilators. No attempt should be made to dilate the vein, however, because endothelial injury may result.

Webs, thickened valve leaflets, and areas of sclerosis from previous phlebitis or punctures are common in upper-extremity veins and may be the cause of poor venous outflow and fistula failure. Passage of the coronary dilator helps to localize such obstructive lesions, which should be corrected when found. The patency of the proximal vein can be demonstrated by free flow of injected heparinized saline or by successful passage of a Fogarty catheter. The evoked thrill is also a useful maneuver: intermittent, pulsatile injection of saline into the vein, mimicking arterial flow, should produce a palpable thrill over the proximal vein.[23] The absence of an evoked thrill suggests the presence of stenosis or areas of thickened, nondistensible vein wall proximally. Intraoperative phlebography is indicated in any doubtful situation.

AV anastomosis   Both the artery and the vein should be mobilized sufficiently to ensure that the anastomosis is tension-free once completed. As noted (see above), marking the most superficial aspect of the vein with a sterile pen before mobilization helps ensure that the vein is not rotated when it is approximated to the artery. The ideal anastomosis is constructed by transecting the vein just distal to a bifurcation and using the branch vessel as

Figure 8 **Vascular access via AVFs: bridge AV grafts. Options for bridge graft construction include (*a*) straight forearm AV graft, (*b*) loop forearm AV graft, (*c*) brachioaxillary AV graft, (*d*) loop axilloaxillary AV graft, (*e*) axillary artery–contralateral axillary vein AV graft, (*f*) axillary artery–iliac vein AV graft, (*g*) distal superficial femoral or popliteal artery–saphenous vein AV graft, and (*h*) proximal superficial femoral artery–saphenous vein loop AV graft.**

a patch. Such a spatulated venous conduit facilitates the anastomosis and minimizes the risk of anastomotic stenosis.

For a distal AVF, the anastomosis should be about 10 mm long to ensure that a gradual increase in flow through the fistula can occur. An anastomosis that is too small may impair the normal dilation of the artery and the vein. For AVFs in the antecubital space and the upper arm, in contrast, the arteriotomy should be limited to 5 to 6 mm to prevent excessive shunting.

The anastomosis can be performed with standard vascular techniques. However, construction of the anastomosis with a single continuous suture may have a purse-string effect; accordingly, the use of two separate running sutures may be preferable for small vessels. Interrupted stitches are preferable for very small vessels. Loupes and microvascular instruments are helpful in this setting.

When the anastomosis is completed, vascular control should be released from the proximal vein and the distal artery first; the resultant back-bleeding will confirm the patency of the palmar arch and reveal any major anastomotic defects. Gentle compression is usually sufficient to obtain hemostasis. Any additional sutures deemed necessary should be placed with great caution because of the risk that they may narrow the anastomosis.

The presence of a pulse rather than a thrill in the arterialized vein indicates inadequate outflow, whereas the absence of either a

thrill or a pulse indicates poor inflow. The draining vein should be examined for kinking, twisting, or compression by a fibrous band. If the vein appears to be satisfactory, the anastomosis and the distal vein are inspected and probed with dilators through a venous side branch or a transverse phlebotomy. If no abnormality is identified, the fistula is examined with I.V. contrast studies and fluoroscopy. Focal lesions may be corrected by placement of a vein patch or a short interposition graft or by resection and primary reanastomosis. Alternatively, a short segment of the vein may be excised and the anastomosis repositioned more proximally.

AV Grafts

Skin incisions Incisions should be placed so that neither the graft nor the anastomoses lie directly beneath them. Proper placement reduces the risk of skin erosion, minimizes the risk that the graft will become infected if a surgical site infection occurs, and maximizes the length of conduit available for needle insertion. The subcutaneous tissue and skin should be closed in separate layers to minimize the risk of graft infection in the event of skin dehiscence.

Tunneling The tunnel should be made atraumatically with a Kelly-Wick bidirectional tunneler. It should be superficial to the muscle fascia but no more than 5 mm beneath the skin surface. To decrease the risk of hematoma, there should be a close fit between the diameter of the graft and that of the tunnel, and the graft should be placed before systemic heparinization is initiated.

For a loop configuration, a counterincision at the apex of the tunnel permits the tunnel to be created in two passes of the Kelly-Wick tunneler. This approach gives the tunnel a smooth curve and limits kinking of the graft. In the forearm, this transverse counterincision is usually made 3 to 4 cm proximal to the wrist skinfold [*see Figure 9*]. Careful observation of the stripe on the graft as it is passed through the tunnel helps prevent twisting.

Venous anastomosis   To minimize arterial occlusion time, the venous anastomosis is usually performed first. The vein must be at least 4 mm in diameter; venous diameter and patency are verified by passing coronary dilators or a Fogarty catheter through the vessel and irrigating it with heparinized saline. Before the anastomosis is performed, the vein and all distal branches are ligated to prevent venous hypertension and arm edema.

If no veins of adequate diameter are available, either two adjacent veins or a portion of a transverse communicating vein can be used to construct a venoplasty that will increase the net diameter of the venous outflow tract. Alternatively, the deep brachial or axillary veins can be used for outflow. The latter option is often required when the superficial veins have been exhausted in a patient who has previously had AVFs.

Arterial anastomosis   Systemic heparin is given only if an end artery is occluded for anastomosis. The artery should have a lumen of at least 3 mm, and the arteriotomy should be no more than 6 mm long to prevent distal ischemia. ePTFE sutures are useful for arterial anastomoses: because they have the same diameter as the attached needles, needle-hole bleeding is minimized.

Before the arterial anastomosis is completed, the graft is unclamped and allowed to fill with venous blood; this step prevents air embolism when arterial control is released. When the anastomosis is complete, a thrill should be palpable over the venous outflow tract rather than directly over the graft.

Graft type   The choice between a tapered 4 to 7 mm ePTFE graft and a 6 mm straight graft is a matter of personal preference. The tapered graft was introduced to reduce the incidence of steal syndrome by increasing the resistance to flow through the prosthesis; however, it has not been shown to provide consistent protection from ischemic complications. Both types of graft are also available in either a standard or a thin-wall configuration; the only randomized study published to date reported superior results with the standard configuration.[24] Stretch ePTFE appears to yield better results than the older, nonstretch grafts.[25]

FOLLOW-UP

Upon discharge, the patient is instructed to elevate the arm so as to reduce edema. Regular hand and arm exercise, though not of proven benefit, is nonetheless recommended until the fistula matures.

Physical examination of the fistula, including inspection and palpation for pulse and thrill, should be done on a weekly basis. The patient should also be advised to seek prompt medical attention if the quality of the thrill changes. Normally, a thrill is palpable throughout the cardiac cycle, though it is more intense during systole. Disappearance of the diastolic component of the thrill is generally a consequence of outflow obstruction. Such obstruction (usually from venous or anastomotic stenosis) may also cause intensification of the thrill or bruit. In addition, diminished flow or outflow stenosis may cause the thrill to be converted to a pulse. Any of these abnormal findings is an indication for a diagnostic procedure: salvage attempts are much more likely to succeed if carried out before thrombosis has occurred.

ePTFE AV grafts should not be used until at least 14 days have passed since placement or until the swelling has subsided enough to allow palpation of the graft. This waiting period allows adhesions to form between the subcutaneous tunnel and the graft, thereby decreasing the risk of hematoma in the graft tunnel, which may ruin the access site. A minimum of 1 month is required before a primary AVF may be cannulated. It is preferable, however, to wait until the fistula matures fully, which may take 3 to 4 months.

COMPLICATIONS

Venous Stenosis

Venous stenosis, either at the anastomosis (particularly with ePTFE grafts) or in the body of the vein, is a common complication of AVF construction. Prophylactic intervention for venous stenoses reduces the rate of thrombosis and graft loss, and stenoses detected before thrombosis occurs are more responsive to therapy than those detected afterward. Intervention is indicated when stenosis of 50% or greater (documented by duplex ultrasonography or fistulography) is accompanied by a hemodynamic, functional, or clinical abnormality (e.g., decreased access blood flow, elevated static or dynamic venous pressure, increased recirculation, reduced delivered dialysis dose, or arm edema). Prophylactic intervention for anatomic stenosis is not warranted when such findings are absent.[26]

Although the question of whether angioplasty or surgical revision is the preferable method of intervention remains controversial, experience to date suggests that surgical revision tends to provide better long-term results. This difference may derive from the elasticity of intimal hyperplastic lesions, whose rapid recoil may limit the efficacy of angioplasty. As a rule, if angioplasty is required more than twice within 3 months, the patient should be referred for surgical revision. Treatment options include patch angioplasty for localized or anastomotic stenoses, bypass for longer stenoses, relocation of the venous anastomosis to a new vein, and resection of the stenotic segment with interposition grafting.

Central venous stenosis   Stenotic or occlusive lesions of the central veins develop in as many as 40% of patients who have previously undergone subclavian hemodialysis catheter placement for temporary vascular access.[7] When a vascular access graft or fistula is placed distal to these lesions, they may become symptomatic,

Figure 9 **Vascular access via AVFs: bridge AV grafts. With a loop forearm graft, tunneling of the graft is facilitated by making an incision 1.5 cm distal to the elbow crease to expose the brachial artery and the antecubital venous system, followed by a counterincision at the apex of the tunnel 3 to 4 cm proximal to the wrist skinfold.**

resulting in venous hypertension, arm edema, low access flow, or thrombosis. Percutaneous intervention with transluminal angioplasty is the preferred treatment; the tendency for central venous stenosis to recur soon after treatment[27] may be circumvented by the addition of a stent. Stents are particularly helpful for treating rigid or kinked stenoses, for sealing dissections or circumscribed perforations, and for reestablishing the patency of chronically occluded veins. Surgical repair of central venous obstruction is a major undertaking and is reserved for those occasional cases in which percutaneous procedures have failed in a patient with no alternative access site.

Arterial Stenosis

Arterial stenosis is relatively uncommon. It should be corrected if it is associated with diminished access flow and elevated arterial prepump pressure. Arterial stenosis may be suspected even before dialysis is initiated if a patent vein does not enlarge significantly within several weeks of fistula creation. Angiography provides a definitive diagnosis. Stenosis of the distal artery, the anastomosis, or the distal vein is best treated with reanastomosis proximal to the stenotic area. More proximal stenosis may have to be treated with conventional arterial reconstruction.

Early Thrombosis

Early thrombosis is defined as thrombosis occurring within 3 months of access construction. It is usually the result of technical factors or of inadequate assessment of the arterial or venous conduit. The following are the most common causes of early thrombosis:

1. Inadequate arterial inflow caused by proximal arterial disease.
2. Narrowing of the anastomosis during construction.
3. Kinking or twisting of the vein proximal to the anastomosis or in a subcutaneous tunnel.
4. Undetected occlusion of venous outflow.
5. Compression of the fistula by a hematoma resulting from either inadequate hemostasis during the procedure or early puncture of the fistula with subsequent extravasation of blood.

If early thrombosis is thought to be caused by technical complications and not by the use of marginal vessels, reexploration is worthwhile. Reexploration usually involves takedown of the anastomosis, thrombectomy of the conduit, reevaluation of both arterial inflow and venous outflow, corrective measures as needed, and reanastomosis. Both autogenous AVFs and AV grafts may be profitably reexplored. With an autogenous AVF, reexploration should be done within 24 hours of thrombosis to minimize ischemic endothelial injury.

Late Thrombosis

Autogenous AVFs Little information is available on success rates for treatment of thrombosis in autogenous AVFs; however, it seems that neither percutaneous nor surgical techniques offer good results. Thrombosis of an autogenous AVF most commonly results from an aneurysm of the fistula, hyperplastic stenosis at the anastomosis or in the vein just distal to the anastomosis, fibrosis at an area of repeated needle punctures, or kidney transplantation.

The surgical approach should include exposure of the vein just distal to a clinically apparent or suspected venous stenosis. The vein is opened longitudinally and the thrombus evacuated. Adequacy of venous outflow is assessed with a Fogarty catheter or coronary dilators. If a segment less than 4 mm in diameter is encountered, the problem is corrected with patch angioplasty, vein bypass, or resection and primary anastomosis. (The last of these three approaches is often easy to perform because the tortuosity of the vein allows easy mobilization and length extension.) Central vein stenosis is corrected with intraoperative balloon angioplasty.

When the venous side of the AVF is in satisfactory condition, the thrombus is removed from the arterial limb. Any suspected anastomotic or proximal arterial stenosis should be corrected [see AV Grafts, below]. If the thrombosis resulted from a fistula aneurysm containing adherent thrombus, the aneurysm should be repaired to prevent its recurrence.

AV grafts About 85% of AV graft thromboses are caused by stenosis of the venous anastomosis or of the draining vein (as a result of intimal hyperplasia), and most instances of graft loss are attributable to such stenosis. Treatment of a thrombosed graft has only a 10% chance of success if the underlying venous stenosis is not addressed. Although arterial stenoses are less common causes of late thrombosis, they should be sought out and corrected as well. Before treatment is initiated, information about recent graft performance should be obtained. Signs of venous or outflow stenosis include increasing venous resistance and prolonged bleeding from puncture sites. Inadequate flow rates and increased negative pressures during dialysis are associated with stenosis of the arterial inflow. Hypotension or excessive graft compression can explain spontaneous thrombosis in a previously well-functioning graft.

Graft thrombosis may be corrected either with surgical thrombectomy or with pharmacomechanical or mechanical thrombolysis. On the whole, technical success and long-term patency rates are similar for the two approaches, though there is some evidence for a trend toward longer primary patency with surgical management.[28] The choice between these two approaches continues to be controversial, and the decision should generally be based on local expertise. To date, neither surgical treatment nor endovascular management has produced unassisted patency rates higher than 50% at 6 months. If graft thrombosis occurs repeatedly in a given patient, plans for a new access site should be considered.

If surgical treatment is chosen, it should be carried out in an operating suite with the capacity for intraoperative fluoroscopy. Unless preoperative findings indicate that an arterial lesion is present, the incision is made at the venous anastomosis, and an adequate length of graft and outflow vein is mobilized. A transverse graftotomy is made within 1 or 2 mm of the suture line, any clot found on the venous side is removed with suction and a forceps, and the anastomosis is inspected. The anastomosis is calibrated but not dilated: if a 5 mm dilator passes easily through the venous anastomosis, then thrombectomy alone is often sufficient treatment. A 4 French Fogarty catheter is passed proximally into the right atrium and pulled back slowly with the balloon inflated to check for proximal venous stenosis and to evacuate clot. Any abnormality encountered is an indication for operative phlebography. The presence of a venous abnormality does not rule out the possibility of a coexisting arterial defect; both should be corrected if found.

After the venous anastomosis is examined, a 4 French Fogarty catheter is used to evacuate any clot in the graft itself. Thrombectomy at the arterial anastomosis is delayed until any structural problems in the body of the graft are corrected; this delay permits the structural corrections to be carried out in a bloodless field. Narrowing in the body of the graft is usually caused by fibrous material adherent to the wall, which can be removed with the aid of a curette, an endarterectomy instrument, or suction. Once the body of the graft is clear, any thrombus present at the arterial anastomosis is removed. Free passage of the Fogarty balloon catheter suggests that there is no arterial anastomotic stenosis. The arterial anastomosis may be examined under direct vision if necessary to

Figure 10 **Vascular access via AVFs. Shown are digital photoplethysmographic waveforms on an arm with steal syndrome before and during fistula compression.**

ensure complete removal of the compacted thrombus at the arterial end of the graft.

The graft is filled with heparinized saline before the arterial or the venous anastomosis is repaired. When the arterial side of the graft is involved, a new arterial anastomosis usually suffices to solve the problem. A new arterial site proximal to the old one is selected, and either the graft is moved to the new site or a new free segment is added.

More commonly, the defect is at the venous anastomosis. In this case, the graftotomy is extended longitudinally through the anastomosis. If the stenosis is short, smooth, and hyperplastic, a small patch angioplasty is adequate for repair. If the stenosis is long or if the vein is sclerotic, revision to a new venous outflow site is preferred. The graft can be reanastomosed to another nearby vein, or the stenosis can be bypassed by anastomosing an ePTFE graft of appropriate size to a more proximal segment of the original vein. Joints may be crossed if necessary, in which case an externally supported prosthesis is used.

Steal Syndrome

The incidence of symptomatic steal syndrome has been reported to be approximately 2% for autogenous AVFs and as high as 4% for AV grafts. Ischemic complications result from preferential diversion of arterial flow into the low-pressure venous outflow of the fistula. When collateral arterial flow is inadequate or when proximal or distal occlusive arterial disease is present, distal ischemia occurs. In some cases, the flow into the venous side of the fistula is sufficient to induce reversal of the flow in a portion of the artery distal to the fistula, a phenomenon referred to as steal. Unfortunately, there is no reliable method of predicting the development of symptomatic steal after the construction of an autogenous AVF or AV graft.

The ischemia is usually mild and is characterized by coldness, numbness, and pain during dialysis. In most cases, the problem resolves without treament within a few weeks. If the patient experiences constant pain, severe numbness, a nonhealing ischemic fissure, digital cyanosis or gangrene, or finger contracture, the ischemia should be corrected. The differential diagnosis of vascular steal syndrome includes the neuropathies of uremia and diabetes as well as secondary hyperparathyroidism. Carpal tunnel syndrome—an uncommon but distinct condition occurring in hemodialysis patients—presents with symptoms similar to those of vascular steal but can be differentiated from steal on the basis of the characteristic electromyographic findings.

A classic indicator of clinically significant steal is that digital pulse waves are absent or markedly diminished on digital photoplethysmography (PPG) or pulse volume recordings (PVR) but rise to normal amplitude and contour when the fistula is compressed [*see Figure 10*]. Digital pressures lower than 50 mm Hg and a digital-brachial index lower than 0.47 are also indicative of clinically significant distal ischemia.[29] A significant difference in segmental or digital pressure between the two arms with the fistula compressed may be indicative of superimposed arterial disease proximal or distal to the fistula, in which case arteriography is indicated before surgical correction. Identification of reversed flow distal to the fistula on duplex studies is not, in itself, sufficient reason to conclude that clinically significant steal is present: steal is a common phenomenon and is a physiologic consequence of the rheology of the fistula in 73% of autogenous AVFs and 92% of AV grafts.[30]

The goal of treatment is to reduce steal to a level where there is both adequate residual flow volume for dialysis and adequate perfusion to the hand to eliminate ischemic symptoms. Treatment options include the following:

1. Elimination of the fistula. This is the simplest form of treatment and invariably corrects ischemia; however, it raises the vexing problem of reestablishing access in another extremity.
2. Reducing the flow but maintaining patency. Usually, this option involves narrowing a portion of the access to reduce flow. One technique for accomplishing this narrowing is to excise an elliptical portion of the graft or vein just distal to the anastomosis and reapproximate the edges or to plicate the graft or outflow vein with mattress or continuous sutures[31] [*see Figure 11a through c*]. Another technique is to band the fistula or graft with a crossed ePTFE band.[32] The tails of the band are secured with hemostatic clips, and once the appropriate degree of narrowing has been achieved, the clips are held in place with a figure-eight suture of 5-0 polypropylene [*see Figure 11d*]. Both techniques should narrow the outflow over a fairly long distance ($\geq$ 1 cm). A third technique involves interposing a small-diameter (4 mm) ePTFE graft between the artery and the vein or graft[33] [*see Figure 11e*]; however, this technique does not allow progressive calibration of the narrowing to achieve the desired hemodynamic result.
3. Ligation of the source of steal, with distal revascularization when necessary. When steal occurs in a patient who has a radiocephalic fistula at the wrist with flow reversal in the radial artery distal to the fistula (documented by duplex scans) and whose ulnar artery and palmar arch are patent and competent to perfuse the hand, it is easily treated by ligating the radial artery distal to the fistula.[34] The effect of this treatment is easily demonstrated by compressing the radial artery distal to the fistula, which should relieve the ischemia. With a more proximal fistula, in which ligation of a terminal artery would inevitably result in severe distal ischemia, the distal artery is ligated and an arterial bypass established from a point 5 cm proximal to the fistula to a point just distal to the ligation [*see Figure 12*]. This so-called distal revascularization–interval ligation (DRIL) procedure, originally reported by Schanzer and coworkers,[35] is an elegant way of both preserving adequate flow through the fistula and reversing the ischemia. The pathway of steal is eliminated, and antegrade flow into the extremity is restored through the bypass. This technique is particularly helpful when concomitant arterial stenosis proximal or distal to the fistula contributes to the distal ischemic process, because the bypass can be positioned so as to bypass the arterial stenosis as well.

With any of these techniques, intraoperative assessment is required to ensure adequate residual flow volume in the fistula (assessed by intraoperative duplex scanning) and adequate distal perfusion (assessed by evaluation of digital PPG or PVR waveforms). The goal is to achieve a digital pressure of at least 60 mm Hg, a digital-brachial index of 0.6 or greater, and a residual flow of at least 300 ml/min in the fistula (a level of flow that is adequate both for hemodialysis and for maintenance of patency).[36]

Figure 11 **Vascular access via AVFs. One option for treating steal is to decrease blood flow in the access conduit. Methods that may be used include (a) excision of a portion of the vein or graft, (b) plication with mattress sutures, (c) plication with continuous sutures, (d) placement of a crossed ePTFE band with application of hemostatic clips, and (e) interposition of a 4 mm ePTFE graft.**

Inadequate Maturation of the Vein

Failure of a fistula to mature may result from either inadequate inflow or venous abnormality. Physical examination combined with Doppler ultrasonography or fistulography should identify the underlying cause. If stenosis is not identified in a nonmaturing radiocephalic fistula, venous side branches may be draining critical flow from the primary vessel; ligation of these branches sometimes leads to successful maturation. Median cubital vein ligation may be attempted, as may temporary banding of the main venous channel in the antecubital fossa. Banding is accomplished by narrowing the vein with a 3-0 Vicryl tie over a 4 mm probe. The Vicryl resorbs in 3 to 4 weeks, during which period it is hoped that the increased resistance to flow will cause dilatation of the vein.[37] If none of these measures succeed, another access site should be sought.

True Aneurysm (Autogenous AVFs)

Aneurysmal dilatation of the vein develops in 5% to 8% of autogenous AVFs as a result of high pressure applied to a vein wall weakened by repeated punctures. Usually, the course of such aneurysms is benign and does not preclude use of the fistula; however, large aneurysms containing mural thrombus have been reported to cause late thrombosis and embolization. On rare occasions, progressive enlargement can compromise circulation to the skin above the aneurysmal vein, leading to incomplete hemostasis when the needle is withdrawn and ultimately to graft rupture. Skin compromise and progressive enlargement are therefore indications for surgical correction. Surgical revision is also recommended if the aneurysm involves the arterial anastomosis or is associated with stenosis of the venous outflow.

Options for revision include total excision of the aneurysm with primary reanastomosis, exclusion of the aneurysm with vein bypass grafting, and partial excision in which part of the vein wall is kept as the arterial conduit. The last option frequently results in early recurrence as the vein wall continues to weaken and dilate with time.

Pseudoaneurysm (AV Grafts)

Pseudoaneurysms occur in prosthetic AV grafts and are usually small and asymptomatic. They can be prevented by allowing sufficient time after graft placement to ensure firm fibrous encapsulation of the graft and by avoiding repeated needle insertion at the same site. On occasion, however, pseudoaneurysms are precipitated by underlying venous stenosis, which should be documented and corrected whenever present. Urgent surgical repair is indicated if the pseudoaneurysm is expanding rapidly or is causing ischemia of the overlying skin. Elective repair is indicated if the diameter of the false aneurysm is more than twice that of the graft.

Infection

Infection is the second most common cause of loss of AV access, occurring in 0% to 3% of autogenous AVFs and 6% to 25% of AV grafts. Infection may be acquired during surgery or cannulation of the conduit and is most often caused by *Staphylococcus aureus*.

Autogenous AVFs Infection of an autogenous AVF should be treated aggressively with 6 weeks of antibiotic therapy, much as subacute bacterial endocarditis would be. Local measures, such as

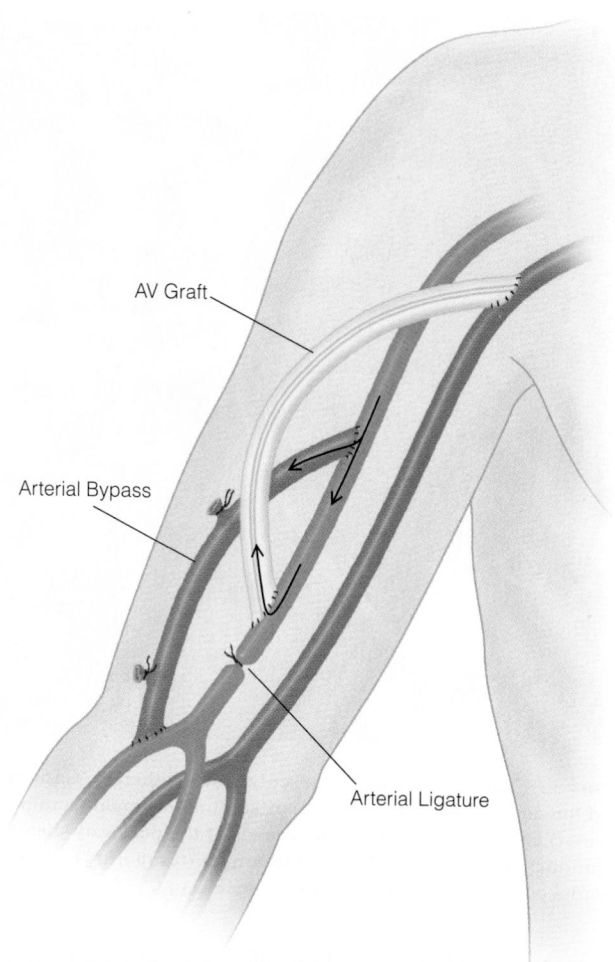

Figure 12 **Vascular access via AVFs. Another option for treating steal is to ligate the source. Shown is the so-called DRIL procedure, which involves arterial ligation distal to the takeoff of the AV graft or the autogenous AVF and arterial bypass from a point 5 cm proximal to the fistula to a point just distal to the ligation.**

drainage of a perifistular abscess, may be necessary. In rare instances, infection-induced anastomotic pseudoaneurysm or septic emboli necessitate takedown of the fistula.

AV grafts Generally, both antibiotic therapy and surgical treatment are necessary for cure. An antibiotic regimen that covers gram-negative organisms, staphylococci, and streptococci should be given until culture results are available. In most cases, complete excision of the prosthetic graft is required,[38] along with vein patch reconstruction of the artery. If the anastomosis is not grossly involved, a small cuff of ePTFE may be left on the arterial side and used to close the arterial defect; this does not seem to alter the prognosis.

In selected cases of well-localized infection, it is possible to resect only the infected portion of the graft and to restore the continuity of the fistula by placing a new conduit in a clean subcutaneous tunnel away from the infected area. A useful approach to managing an infected forearm loop graft is to resect the graft and reconstruct the fistula with an immediate anastomosis between the artery and the arterialized vein remaining after graft excision. Superficial surgical wound infections occurring in the postoperative period can sometimes be treated successfully with aggressive local debridement in combination with systemic administration of antibiotics. Deeper wound infections occurring in the postoperative period must be assumed to involve the entire graft, given that the graft is not yet well incorporated.

OUTCOME EVALUATION

Thrombotic events are the leading cause of access loss. For the most part, they result from venous outflow stenosis that can be detected before thrombosis occurs. An organized monitoring approach that includes regular assessment of the clinical parameters of the access and of the adequacy of the dialysis should be implemented in every dialysis center.[6] Such a proactive approach can be expected to reduce the incidence of thrombosis and increase patency.

Physical examination of the AV graft or autogenous AVF should be performed weekly and should include not only inspection and palpation for changes in the physical characteristics of the pulse or thrill but also a search for indirect signs of graft dysfunction (e.g., arm swelling, prolonged bleeding after needle withdrawal, and aneurysm or pseudoaneurysm). In addition to physical examination, the NKF-DOQI committee recommended routine access monitoring at least monthly with one or more of the following techniques:

1. Intra-access flow assessment using Doppler flow, magnetic resonance imaging, or ultrasound dilution online during dialysis. A trend toward decreasing flow or a flow rate lower than 600 ml/min for an AV graft and lower than 200 to 300 ml/min for an autogenous AVF is predictive of a high likelihood of access stenosis and eventual thrombosis.
2. Static or dynamic venous pressure measurement. Progressively increasing pressures or pressures that exceed the threshold value determined by each center's own protocol are predictive of significant venous outlet stenosis.
3. Urea and nonurea recirculation measurement. Recirculation is defined as the percentage of flow that is recirculated from the venous line into the dialyser inflow by retrograde blood flow through the fistula. A recirculation value exceeding 10% to 20% is significant and usually indicates low arterial blood flow or venous stenosis.
4. Delivered dialysis dose. A decrease is associated with venous outflow stenosis.
5. Arterial prepump pressure. An elevated negative pressure is a sign of inflow insufficiency.

Vascular Access via Percutaneous Catheters

Percutaneous venous catheterization is a useful method of gaining immediate access to the circulation; however, it is associated with significant risks, and the use-life of this type of access is shorter than that of AVFs. Percutaneous catheterization should be reserved for patients with acute renal failure who have an immediate need for dialysis and for patients with chronic renal failure in whom a permanent vascular or peritoneal access route either cannot be established or has not yet matured.

OPERATIVE PLANNING

Patient Assessment

A history is taken, a physical examination is performed, laboratory data are reviewed, and radiologic studies are ordered as for AVFs [*see* Vascular Access via Arteriovenous Fistulas, *above*]. Any finding that might affect the integrity of the central venous system should be noted.

A history or physical signs of previous central venous catheterization, a history of major injury or operation in the area where the catheter is to be inserted, a body mass index greater than 30 or less than 20, and an increasing number of insertion attempts are all known risk factors for perioperative complications from the insertion of venous access devices.[1] If there is any question about the patency of the central venous system, duplex scanning[39] or phlebography is indicated.

On physical examination, the surgeon should note the patient's body type, assess the flexibility of the patient's neck and shoulders, and evaluate the patient's ability to tolerate Trendelenburg's position without dyspnea or discomfort. Chest x-rays are reviewed to verify the patient's pleuropulmonary status and to identify any bony deformities.

The only laboratory study absolutely necessary is a complete blood count (including the platelet count and the differential count); prothrombin and partial thromboplastin times are required if the patient is receiving anticoagulant therapy. The effects of warfarin or heparin should be reversed before the procedure; patients with platelet counts lower than 50,000/mm³ should undergo platelet transfusion immediately before and during catheter placement.[40]

Choice of Type of Catheter

The catheters best suited for hemodialysis are high-flow, large-diameter (12 French or larger) devices with external ports. Silicone catheters are more flexible, are less likely to give rise to injury or thrombosis, and remain patent longer than polyethylene, polyvinyl chloride, and polytetrafluoroethylene catheters. Silicone catheters are available in both noncuffed (temporary) and cuffed (semipermanent) double-lumen configurations through which flow rates of 250 ml/min or higher can be achieved [*see Figure 13*]. The venous and arterial orifices are separated by 1 to 2 cm; recirculation is thereby limited to 5%.

Noncuffed (temporary) catheters Noncuffed catheters can be percutaneously inserted into the internal jugular, subclavian, or femoral vein without the need for fluoroscopic guidance. They are suitable for immediate use and provide acceptable flow rates (250 ml/min). Their main disadvantages are their high rates of infection, thrombosis, and venous stenosis and their short use-life (2 to 3 weeks). For these reasons, noncuffed catheters should be reserved for patients in whom access is expected to be needed for less than 3 weeks, and they should be inserted no earlier than required.

Cuffed (semipermanent) catheters Cuffed catheters are placed in a subcutaneous tunnel under fluoroscopic guidance. They are free of some of the shortcomings of noncuffed catheters; in particular, they are associated with lower infection rates and permit higher flow rates. Cuffed catheters are preferred when temporary access is required for longer than 3 weeks, particularly for patients in whom a primary AV fistula is maturing but who require immediate hemodialysis. Semipermanent catheters have been used for as long as 4 years, but long-term follow-up data on large numbers of patients is lacking.[41] Most patients readily accept this approach to dialysis: cuffed catheters allow so-called no-needle dialysis with high flow rates, they eliminate the problem of vascular steal, and they have no effect on cardiac function. In addition, patients appreciate that the access site is hidden from view, does not limit physical activity, and does not require particular care between treatments.

Choice of Insertion Site

The subclavian veins have given way to the right internal jugular (IJ) vein as the preferred site of primary central access. This site

Figure 13 **Vascular access via percutaneous catheters. Catheters used for hemodialysis include (*a*) cuffed double-lumen (semipermanent) catheters, introduced by means of the peelaway sheath technique, and (*b*) noncuffed double-lumen (temporary) catheters, introduced by means of the Seldinger technique.**

has four main advantages: (1) it offers a consistent, predictable anatomic location with palpable landmarks, (2) it provides a short, straight course to the superior vena cava, (3) success rates are high, and (4) the risk of complications is diminished in comparison with other catheter insertion sites.[42] Of particular importance is that the risk of subclavian vein stenosis is decreased; this complication is a major concern for dialysis patients, who may require subsequent construction of an AVF in the ipsilateral arm. The right IJ vein is preferable to the left IJ vein as an access site because the latter calls for longer catheters, which increase the risk of kinking and diminish flow rates. The left IJ approach is also associated with a high rate of stenosis or thrombosis of the left brachiocephalic vein and may hinder subsequent use of the left arm for an AVF. Placement of the catheter in a subclavian vein either via the percutaneous approach or via cutdown on the cephalic vein should be reserved for cases in which neither jugular vein can be used.[6]

The right IJ vein can be catheterized percutaneously, or it can be surgically exposed and catheterized via direct needle puncture or phlebotomy (venous cutdown). The cutdown approach on the internal jugular vein or the external jugular vein allows greater control over the vessel than the percutaneous approach does and is preferred in patients who have a bleeding diathesis, patients whose body habitus or venous anatomy limits percutaneous access, and patients in whom a percutaneous attempt at placement has failed.

A less commonly used approach is femoral vein catheterization. It is technically easy and has few immediate complications, but it necessitates hospitalization (because the patient cannot ambulate) and is associated with high infection rates that limit use of the catheter to 5 days. Alternatively, access to the inferior vena cava can be gained by cannulating the greater saphenous, inferior epigastric, right gonadal, and lumbar veins. It is also possible to cannulate the azygos vein and the right atrium directly via thoracotomy.

OPERATIVE TECHNIQUE

Right Internal Jugular Vein Approach

Step 1: patient preparation Noncuffed catheters may be inserted at the bedside; cuffed catheters should be inserted in a standard OR with facilities for fluoroscopy.

The anatomy is surveyed before preparation and draping. Important anatomic landmarks include the sternal notch, the clavicle, and the sternocleidomastoid (SCM) muscle. The carotid artery should be palpated lateral to the trachea, under the medial (sternal) head of the SCM. The IJ vein lies lateral and slightly anterior to the carotid artery, between the sternal head and the clavicular head of the SCM muscle.

The patient is placed supine in Trendelenburg's position so that the neck veins are distended and the risk of air embolism is minimized. The head is extended and turned slightly to the left to expose the right side of the neck and keep the chin from interfering with the procedure. The neck should not be overextended or overrotated, however, because either of these actions flattens out the vein, making it more difficult to cannulate, and may increase the risk of arterial puncture by causing the internal jugular vein to overlie the carotid artery.

Step 2: cannulation of right IJ vein The jugular vein is located with a 22-gauge finder needle. This needle is left in place and used to guide the subsequent placement of an 18-gauge needle, through which the guide wire is passed. Use of the smaller needle minimizes the consequences of arterial or pleural puncture occurring during blind attempts at venous puncture.

After local anesthesia is administered, the fingers of the left hand are gently positioned on the carotid pulse to provide an anatomic landmark. The right hand locates the IJ vein by applying negative pressure to the 22-gauge finder needle mounted on a 5 ml syringe [*see Figure 14*]. The needle is inserted at the apex of the triangle formed by the two heads of the SCM muscle and directed toward the ipsilateral nipple at an angle of 30° from the plane of the skin. Alternatively, the needle may be inserted under the medial border of the SCM muscle and directed toward the thoracic inlet while the carotid artery is dislocated medially, or it may be inserted under the lateral border of the SCM muscle and directed toward the contralateral nipple.

Once the vein is located, the syringe is disconnected from the finder needle, which is left in place. The vein is then repunctured with an 18-gauge needle oriented parallel to the finder needle. When venous backflow is obtained, the 18-gauge needle is reoriented at a more acute angle to the skin and is advanced 2 to 3 mm. The syringe is disconnected and the needle hub occluded to prevent air embolism. A 0.035-in. guide wire with either a J tip or a flexible straight tip is then inserted through the needle, and the needle is withdrawn over the wire.

Troubleshooting. Because of the predictable anatomic location of the right IJ vein, the first attempt at cannulation is successful in the majority of cases. If the first attempt fails, the finder needle should be withdrawn and its tip reoriented slightly laterally; however, the needle should not be entirely withdrawn from the skin puncture site. An orderly, systematic search performed in this manner often identifies the vein while posing little risk of carotid artery injury as long as the carotid artery remains palpable medially. To avoid lacerating deep structures, the needle orientation should be changed only when the needle is inserted very superficially. If the vein cannot be located after several passes of the needle, the finder needle is withdrawn completely and the anatomy reassessed. Alternative puncture sites can be attempted. In difficult cases, cannulation may be carried out under ultrasound guidance, or a cutdown can be performed on the external or IJ vein through a small transverse incision.

Figure 14 **Vascular access via percutaneous catheters. The equipment used in percutaneous catheter insertion includes** (*a*) **a 5 ml syringe,** (*b*) **a 22-gauge finder needle,** (*c*) **an 18-gauge needle,** (*d*) **a guide wire,** (*e*) **a dilator,** (*f*) **a peelaway sheath, and** (*g*) **a plastic subcutaneous tunneler.**

When the 18-gauge needle is advanced, the lumen of the jugular vein is often compressed, with the result being that the needle may transfix both front and back walls almost simultaneously. The needle tip should be advanced only slightly beyond the expected depth, then slowly withdrawn, with gentle aspiration maintained on the syringe. Entry into the vein is confirmed by the sudden and easy return of venous blood.

Pulsatile back-bleeding of bright-red blood from the needle usually indicates arterial puncture. If any doubt exists, the aspirated blood can be compared with a simultaneously obtained arterial sample, or the 18-gauge needle can be connected to a pressure transducer. Whenever there is any possibility of arterial puncture, it is preferable to withdraw the needle rather than take the risk of creating a large hole in the artery with a dilator.

The guide wire should be inserted with caution because any forceful movement can result in perforation of the vein wall. The risk is minimized by using a soft-tipped or J-tipped wire. The wire should advance easily into the vein without resistance; if it does not, the guide wire and the needle should be withdrawn together to ensure that the tip of the guide wire is not sheared off and does not embolize.

Step 3 (Seldinger technique): insertion of noncuffed catheter A small nick is made at the point where the guide wire enters the skin [*see Figure 15*]. The dilator is passed over the wire only far enough to enter the vein; it is then removed, and the catheter is inserted over the wire. The catheter tip should be placed in the superior vena cava, above the right atrial junction. This position is typically 15 to 18 cm from the puncture site if the catheter is placed in the right IJ vein; an additional 3 to 5 cm is required for the left IJ approach. The guide wire is then retrieved, venous blood is aspirated from both ports, and each lumen is flushed with heparinized saline. The catheter is anchored to the skin.

Troubleshooting. Dilators are relatively inflexible, and their stiffness increases with size. Consequently, they can easily perforate the vein wall if inserted deeper than the point of entry into the vein. Catheters may also cause perforation, though less commonly. The risk of catheter-related perforation is increased with the left IJ approach and the subclavian approach because catheters inserted from the left side must traverse the innominate vein and enter the superior vena cava at an acute angle, and this course increases the possibility that the tip of the catheter will perforate the right lateral wall of the superior vena cava. No resistance should be felt when the catheter is inserted. In addition, the guide wire should move freely within the catheter during insertion; such free movement suggests that the catheter is not compressing the wire against the wall of the vein.

Manual control of the guide wire must be maintained at all times; without such control, pushing a catheter or dilator over the wire can cause the wire to be completely advanced into the vein.

Inadvertent placement of a dilator or catheter into the carotid artery makes a large hole in the vessel wall, thereby creating the potential for substantial bleeding when the device is removed. In such cases, the catheter should be left in the artery, and a vascular surgeon should be consulted.

Step 3 (peelaway sheath technique): insertion of cuffed catheter A small transverse incision is made at the point where the guide wire enters the skin. Once adequate local anesthesia is achieved, a subcutaneous tunnel is created between the guide-wire entry point and a site on the chest wall at least 10 cm away [*see Figure 16*]. The position of the catheter is estimated by laying the catheter out along its intended tract; the course forms an

Figure 15 Vascular access via percutaneous catheters: Seldinger technique. Shown is a noncuffed (temporary) catheter inserted in the right IJ vein.

inverted U, with the apex at the entry point of the guide wire and the tip of the catheter 5 cm caudad to the angle of Louis (at the second or third intercostal space). The position of the Dacron cuff is noted, and a stab wound is made in such a way that the cuff will be positioned in the subcutaneous tunnel, 2 cm from the wound. This placement simplifies removal of the catheter, prevents the cuff from eroding through the skin, and reduces the incidence of inadvertent catheter dislodgment. The exit wound should be at least 3 to 4 cm from the nipple-areola complex to allow space for the dressing.

A plastic subcutaneous tunneler is attached to the catheter and used to pull the catheter through the tunnel so that the tip emerges adjacent to the guide wire. The venous dilator is then inserted over the wire to effect entry into the vein. Once entry is effected, the dilator is removed and inserted into the peelaway sheath, and sheath and dilator are introduced together into the vein over the guide wire. The guide wire and the dilator are removed, and the open end of the peelaway sheath is occluded with the fingers to prevent air embolism and bleeding. The flushed catheter is then inserted into the peelaway sheath and its position confirmed via fluoroscopy. When the catheter is well positioned, the peelaway sheath is cracked, peeled apart, and removed. Both lumina are tested for easy aspiration of blood and irrigated with heparinized saline. The two incisions are closed with absorbable sutures, and an adequate dressing is applied.

Troubleshooting. Because the procedure is performed under fluoroscopic guidance, fluoroscopy should be used to confirm that the position of the guide wire is satisfactory before the catheter is inserted. If the guide wire is not satisfactorily positioned, a 14-gauge plastic I.V. catheter is placed over the wire into the vein, and the wire is removed and repositioned through the catheter.

The peelaway sheath must be inserted to its full length, which means that the dilator must be inserted to its full length as well. Bending the dilator and the sheath into a gentle curve that matches the curve of the vein minimizes the risk of venous wall perforation, particularly if the left IJ approach or the subclavian vein approach is used.

If resistance is encountered when the catheter is inserted through the sheath, the usual cause is a kink in the sheath. In most instances, partial withdrawal of the sheath resolves the problem. If this step is taken and the catheter still cannot be advanced, the guide wire and the dilator can be reinserted through the sheath, which is then replaced.

Step 4: evaluation The location of the catheter tip should be documented with a chest x-ray after the procedure. To reduce the risk of complications (e.g., central vein thrombosis or perforation of the right atrium), the tip should be located at the junction of the right atrium and the superior vena cava.[43]

Subclavian Vein Approach

The patient is positioned and prepared in much the same way as for the right IJ approach. The arms should be at the sides, and a small roll should be placed between the shoulder blades to allow full exposure of the infraclavicular area. An insertion site is selected 2 to 3 cm caudad to the midpoint of the clavicle, far enough from its inferior edge to allow the needle to remain parallel to the clavicle as it passes beneath its inferior border. A slightly lateral position is preferred to prevent kinking of the peelaway sheath or compression of the soft silicone catheter between the clavicle and the first rib.

Local anesthesia should include the clavicular periosteum. The 18-gauge needle should be advanced into the space between the clavicle and the first rib in the direction of a finger placed in the suprasternal notch. The needle is oriented as horizontally as possible, and the bevel of the needle is oriented downward to decrease the risk that the guide wire will pass upward into the ipsilateral IJ vein.

Careful technique helps prevent pneumothorax and puncture of the subclavian vein. For example, "walking" the tip of the needle down the clavicle, so that it passes as closely underneath the clavicle as possible, reduces the risk of deep puncture and thus of pneumothorax. The rate of complications is directly related to the number of puncture attempts made; consequently, if the subclavian vein is not punctured on the second or third attempt, one should resist the temptation to make additional needle thrusts.

Once the vein is cannulated, the catheter may be inserted by means of either the Seldinger technique or the peelaway sheath technique as previously described [*see* Right Internal Jugular Vein Approach, *above*].

A chest x-ray will confirm the positioning of the tip of the catheter and the presence or absence of kinking. It will also rule out so-called pinch-off, which is a narrowing or notching of the catheter as it pass-

Figure 16 **Vascular access via percutaneous catheters: peelaway sheath technique. Shown is a cuffed (semipermanent) catheter inserted in the right IJ vein and placed in a subcutaneous tunnel.**

es through the tight space between the clavicle and the first rib that may result in transection and embolization of the catheter tip.

Femoral Vein Approach

Femoral venipuncture is performed below the inguinal ligament just medial to the palpated femoral arterial pulse. The catheter is inserted by means of the Seldinger technique. The catheter should be at least 19 cm long to reach the inferior vena cava, thereby minimizing recirculation.

COMPLICATIONS

Early Complications

In more than 5% of catheter insertions, the catheter is improperly positioned. Such malpositioning may cause central venous perforation, venous thrombosis, or device malfunction. The most common positioning error is entry of a subclavian catheter into the ipsilateral IJ vein; less commonly, the catheter tip may inadvertently be placed in an axillary, internal mammary, azygos, or hepatic vein. Placement of the tip within the more cephalad portion of the superior vena cava at an obtuse angle to the venous wall or directly in the heart increases the risk of perforation. Catheter malpositioning is diagnosed by means of fluoroscopy or chest x-ray; management involves immediate repositioning of the catheter with the help of guide wires and fluoroscopy.

Guide-wire embolism can be prevented by being careful not to withdraw the wire through the 18-gauge needle, which can shear off the tip of the wire. Catheter embolism, though rare, may occur when a subclavian venous catheter is inserted too medially and as a consequence is compressed between the costoclavicular ligament, the clavicle, and the first rib. Such compression may lead to biomaterial fatigue, fracture of the catheter, or embolization. Embolized portions of a guide wire or catheter should be removed by means of interventional radiologic techniques to prevent thrombotic complications.

Air embolism occurs when air is inadvertently aspirated into the patient's venous system while the catheter is being inserted, removed, or used. It is easily prevented by using a fingertip to cover all potential communication sites between the venous lumen and the outside air, including the needle hub before guide-wire insertion, the open end of the peelaway sheath just before catheter insertion, and the disconnected external ports of catheters. Patients whose pulmonary status is compromised or who have aspirated large volumes of air may experience respiratory distress. Cardiovascular collapse, caused by obstruction of right ventricular outflow by gas bubbles, can also result. Auscultation may reveal a characteristic millwheel precordial murmur. The patient should be placed in the left lateral decubitus position with the foot of the table elevated so as to trap the air pocket away from the right ventricular outflow tract, and immediate ventilatory support for hypoxemia should be instituted.

Internal hemorrhage may occur at any site, usually as a result of perforation of a central venous or arterial structure during needle puncture or insertion of a guide wire, a dilator, or a catheter. Mediastinal hemorrhage, manifested by mediastinal widening on chest x-ray, occurs in fewer than 1% of all insertions.[44] It is usually self-limited in that the bleeding generally tamponades before hemodynamic compromise occurs.

If both a vascular structure and the parietal pleura are lacerated, hemothorax may result. The chest x-ray will suggest the diagnosis. Treatment includes placement of a thoracostomy tube and early consultation with a thoracic surgeon. Fortunately, the bleeding ceases spontaneously in most cases.

Pericardial tamponade, the most lethal complication of central venous catheterization, may arise as a consequence of perforation into the pericardial space, either through the wall of the vein or through the heart. It can occur immediately, or it can appear hours to days later as a result of delayed perforation by the catheter tip. Proper positioning of the catheter tip is the key to preventing pericardial tamponade. Treatment involves pericardiocentesis, creation of a pericardial window, or median sternotomy, depending on the patient's clinical status.

Cardiac arrhythmias are frequent during catheter insertion: atrial and ventricular arrhythmias occur in as many as 41% and 11% of patients, respectively.[45] These arrhythmias are usually benign; fewer than 1% call for cardioversion.

Pneumothorax occurs in 1% to 4% of attempts at percutaneous catheter placement. The incidence varies according to the experience of the operator and the site selected; in particular, it is higher with the subclavian approach. The presence of pneumothorax may be suggested by air in the syringe during attempts at vein cannulation and may be confirmed by chest x-ray. If the pneumothorax is asymptomatic, with less than 25% lung collapse, it can be treated conservatively; if it is large, symptomatic, or increasing in size, placement of a thoracostomy tube is indicated. Tension pneumothorax is an unusual but important complication that calls for immediate chest tube decompression.

Inadvertent puncture of a lymphatic duct may occur during left subclavian vein or left IJ vein catheterization in patients with hepatic portal hypertension or superior vena caval obstruction. The diagnosis is usually made when clear or milky fluid is aspirated in the syringe during vein cannulation; however, if the duct is punctured at the junction with the vein, the appearance of blood mixed in with the lymphatic fluid may mask the complication. Once lymphatic duct puncture is recognized, the procedure should be abandoned, and pressure should be applied to the site until lymphorrhagia abates. If the complication is recognized late on the basis of spontaneous leakage of lymph around the catheter, either the catheter can be removed or the leak can be stopped with a purse-string suture around the catheter. If persistent fluid drainage, subcutaneous edema, mediastinal enlargement, or chylothorax is noted, the leak is ongoing, and the catheter should be removed.

Late Complications

Central venous thrombosis Catheter-associated central venous thrombosis is more common than was once believed. It is often asymptomatic because of the rich venous collateral circulation in the area. Central venous thrombosis has been estimated to occur in 13% to 35% of catheter insertions[46] and to carry less than a 10% risk of pulmonary embolism and a 19% risk of postphlebitic syndrome. The incidence of catheter-associated thrombosis is correlated with the following factors:

1. Placement site. The incidence of thrombosis or stenosis is as high as 38% with subclavian vein catheters but less than 10% with IJ vein catheters.
2. Site of catheter entry. Surgical cutdown causes less endothelial injury than percutaneous puncture and dilation of the vein and may therefore be less likely to cause thrombosis.
3. Catheter tip position. Catheters placed high in the superior vena cava, near the brachiocephalic vein, are more likely to cause thrombosis.
4. Catheter size. Larger, stiffer catheters are more likely to traumatize the endothelium and to obstruct flow.
5. Catheter material. Silicone is less thrombogenic than other materials.
6. Duration of catheter placement. The incidence of thrombosis increases with the duration of catheter placement.
7. Underlying hypercoagulable state.
8. Associated catheter infection.

The diagnosis is easily made by means of duplex scanning or phlebography. Treatment involves removal of the catheter and administration of anticoagulant therapy. Asymptomatic patients who have no alternative sites for venous access should undergo anticoagulation without removal of the catheter. Thrombolytic therapy through the catheter, though never evaluated in a prospective randomized study, may be useful if the thrombosis is new or symptomatic, is progressing in the face of standard therapy, or is associated with catheter occlusion in a patient with no alternate site of venous access.

Catheter malfunction Catheter malfunction is the most common noninfectious complication of central venous catheterization. Malfunction is defined as either (1) failure to achieve a blood flow rate of at least 300 ml/min on two consecutive occasions or (2) failure to achieve a blood flow rate of 200 ml/min on a single occasion. In addition, partial or complete so-called withdrawal occlusion, in which solutions can be infused but blood cannot be withdrawn, may occur, as may complete occlusion.

Early catheter malfunction is usually caused by improper positioning of the catheter tip proximal to the distal superior vena cava, positioning of the tip against the venous wall, or subcutaneous kinking of the catheter. The precise cause can be determined via chest x-ray and contrast study. Malpositioning of the catheter tip can be corrected by using a tip deflector wire inserted through the lumen of the catheter, by snaring the catheter via the femoral approach and repositioning it, or by replacing the catheter.

Late catheter malfunction is usually caused by intraluminal thrombi; less commonly, it may be caused by extraluminal thrombi (e.g., fibrin tails or sheaths enveloping the distal portion of the catheter) or central venous thrombosis. Most late catheter dysfunction can be successfully managed with thrombolytic therapy. Thrombolysis with urokinase should be attempted first because of its high success rate (up to 90%) and its ease of administration.[47] Multiple protocols have been described. Typically, 5,000 units of urokinase, in a volume sufficient to fill the catheter lumen (usually 1.2 ml), is injected in each port and left in place for 20 to 30 minutes. The urokinase is then withdrawn, and another attempt is made to flush the line. The procedure can be repeated if necessary; the dose and the incubation time may be increased if desired because the urokinase is unlikely to reach the circulation. If catheter function fails to improve, imaging of the catheter with infused contrast material will allow identification and correction of other problems. Residual thrombus in the catheter lumen can be treated by means of intracatheter urokinase infusion (20,000 U/lumen/hr for 6 hours), catheter embolectomy, or catheter exchange over a guide wire. Fibrin sheaths around the catheter can be treated by means of urokinase infusion, fibrin sheath stripping with a snare,[48] or catheter exchange.

Catheter infection Infection is the most common complication of venous catheterization for vascular access, occurring in as many as 30% to 40% of patients. It is also one of the leading causes of catheter removal and morbidity in dialysis patients. Gram-positive bacteria, principally *S. aureus* and *S. epidermidis*, are the most commonly isolated organisms, though gram-negative bacteria and fungi may also be involved.

The clinical spectrum of catheter infection includes exit-site infection, tunnel infection, systemic line sepsis, and suppurative thrombophlebitis.

Exit-site infection. The characteristic signals are localized erythema, induration, tenderness, and exudate at the catheter exit site. Systemic symptoms are absent, and blood cultures are negative.

Treatment involves local wound care and application of topical antibiotics. The catheter need not be removed.

Tunnel infection. If the inflammatory process extends along the entire course of the subcutaneous tunnel, a more extensive cellulitic process, with or without purulent discharge, results. Initially, tunnel infection can be treated with parenteral antibiotics and local measures; however, it usually does not respond to this regimen, and removal of the catheter is often required. If a new catheter is called for, it should use a different tunnel and exit site.

Systemic line sepsis. This condition is manifested by systemic symptoms and signs of bacteremia in a patient who has a central venous catheter in place but exhibits no local evidence of catheter or tunnel infection and has no other identifiable source of infection. It is defined on the basis of the following two criteria: (1) in comparison with peripheral blood, a 10-fold increase in colony-forming units (CFU)/ml blood drawn from the catheter, or (2) in the absence of a positive peripheral blood culture, more than 1,000 CFU from blood drawn through the device. Empirical I.V. antibiotic treatment (including coverage for penicillin-resistant staphylococci) should be administered through the catheter. This measure will eliminate the clinical sepsis syndrome in 70% of patients. Once the antibiotics are discontinued, however, there is a 40% risk of reinfection; for this reason, catheter exchange over a guide wire, using the same tunnel and exit site, is recommended once bactericidal levels have been obtained[49] and the sepsis syndrome has resolved. I.V. antibiotics should be continued for 3 weeks thereafter. If the patient is unstable or still symptomatic after 24 to 36 hours of antibiotic therapy, removal of the catheter is mandatory. The catheter should also be removed if fungemia is suspected or confirmed.

Suppurative thrombophlebitis. When arm edema occurs in addition to systemic sepsis, suppurative thrombophlebitis of a great vein should be suspected. The diagnosis may be confirmed by means of duplex scanning or contrast phlebography. Treatment involves catheter removal, systemic I.V. antibiotic therapy, and heparin anticoagulation and is successful in more than 50% of patients. Vein excision is associated with significant morbidity and consequently is not indicated. Patients who do not respond to treatment can be treated with vena caval filter placement and central vein thrombectomy.

OUTCOME EVALUATION

To improve dialysis outcomes and to maintain or improve quality of care for dialysis patients, percutaneous catheterization should be performed only in selected cases. Given that percutaneous catheterization is associated with higher complication rates, morbidity, and mortality than AV fistulization, the goal should be to use percutaneous catheters in fewer than 10% of hemodialysis patients requiring long-term vascular access. In those cases in which central catheter placement is the best available option, the use of a consistent technique by skilled operators should, according to the NFK-DOQI, reduce the risk of serious complications necessitating intervention to 2% or lower.

Peritoneal Access

OPERATIVE PLANNING

Patient Assessment

For short-term peritoneal access, little formal patient assessment is required. The insertion site should be away from any areas of soft tissue infection and as far from any abdominal scars as is practical.

For long-term peritoneal access, more thorough patient assessment is required. Peritoneal dialysis is absolutely contraindicated in patients who have lost more than 50% of their peritoneal surface area. This degree of loss occurs in some patients who have previously undergone extensive intra-abdominal surgery or have had peritonitis or inflammatory bowel disease. Nonetheless, many patients who have undergone operation have a peritoneal cavity that either is usable for dialysis as is or could be made usable by lysis of adhesions. Patients who have previously undergone intra-abdominal vascular procedures are not candidates for peritoneal dialysis unless the graft is not accessible to the dialysate, so that episodes of peritonitis will not result in graft infection. In addition, adhesions are to be expected in such patients, and preparations to deal with them should be made when catheter insertion is being planned. If active local or distant bacterial infection is present, a permanent catheter should not be inserted until the infection has completely resolved. Advanced age is not a contraindication to peritoneal dialysis, but if the procedure is to be performed in an ambulatory setting, the patient must have sufficient motivation, dexterity, and mental capacity. A prolapsed rectum or uterus is considered a contraindication. Relative contraindications include very large polycystic kidneys, cutaneous stomas, and abdominal hernias. In patients with umbilical or groin hernias, herniorrhaphy may be done either before or at the time of catheter insertion. After herniorrhaphy, it is probably best not to use the catheter for several weeks; a small volume of heparin should be infused every other day while the site of the repair heals.

Choice of Type of Catheter

The catheters used for short-term access to the peritoneal cavity, as in diagnostic peritoneal lavage or short-term peritoneal dialysis, are constructed of rigid plastic and have no Dacron cuff. They may be inserted either percutaneously or under direct vision through small cutdown incisions; the preferred location is the midline.

To obtain long-term access to the peritoneal cavity for chemotherapeutic purposes, the surgeon may elect to place a subcutaneous reservoir to which a catheter is attached in such a way that the unattached end enters the peritoneal cavity. (The same devices are also sometimes used to obtain long-term nondialysis venous access.) The reservoir is accessed with special Huber-point needles; between uses, it is filled with heparinized saline. Alternatively, the surgeon may insert a Dacron-cuffed Silastic catheter [*see* Operative Technique, Step 1: Insertion of Catheter, *below*].

For long-term peritoneal dialysis, transcutaneous catheters made of silicone and equipped with one or two Dacron cuffs are used. These devices are available in a variety of configurations: the intra-abdominal portion may be straight or curved or may have plastic disks attached to it, and the subcutaneous portion may be straight or bent [*see Figure 17*]. The preferred configuration is a pigtail catheter with a preformed bend in the subcutaneous portion.

OPERATIVE TECHNIQUE

General Principles

Long-term peritoneal dialysis catheters may be inserted by means of percutaneous, laparoscopic, or cutdown techniques. Certain general principles apply to all these approaches. The double-cuffed catheter should be placed so that the catheter tip is in the pelvis, the inner cuff is in the rectus abdominis muscle (or adjacent to the linea alba), and the outer cuff is in the subcutaneous tissues. The exit site chosen should permit the patient to see the site to provide local care and should cause minimal interference with clothing. The catheter should exit the skin pointing in a caudal direction;

use of special curved or bent catheter configurations facilitates this. Nearly all patients need only local anesthesia; however, patients who have undergone abdominal operation should be prepared for general anesthesia in case extensive lysis of adhesions is required for satisfactory catheter placement.

What follows is a description of the most commonly used approach to insertion of a long-term peritoneal dialysis catheter, namely, use of a cutdown technique with the patient under local anesthesia [see Figure 18].

Step 1: Insertion of Catheter

Catheter insertion and exit sites are chosen so as to avoid old scars, belt lines, and possible future transplantation incisions. Full sterile precautions are taken. A local anesthetic is infiltrated at the catheter insertion site, and an incision is made down to the anterior rectus sheath. This incision is opened longitudinally, the rectus abdominis muscle is split, and the posterior rectus sheath is exposed. A purse-string suture of 2-0 absorbable material is placed in the posterior rectus sheath, and a small incision is made in the peritoneum.

The catheter is inserted into the peritoneal cavity and directed into the pelvis; if a curled catheter is used, it is directed by means of a lubricated straight metal rod. The inner cuff is positioned just outside the posterior rectus sheath, and the purse-string suture is tied. With the ends of the purse-string suture providing traction, the posterior sheath is held up, and a free tie of absorbable material is placed around the tented-up peritoneum and catheter to keep the insertion site watertight. The barrel of a 50 ml syringe full of saline is then attached to the catheter. When the syringe barrel is held above the abdomen, the fluid should flow freely into the abdomen by gravity alone. Conversely, when the syringe barrel is placed in a dependent position, the fluid should flow rapidly and freely out of the peritoneal cavity and back into the barrel. This test confirms that catheter position is satisfactory.

Troubleshooting   The possibilities for error during placement are numerous: the catheter may be misdirected into the upper abdomen, it may be placed in a pocket of adhesions and blocked from reaching the greater peritoneal cavity, or it may be kinked in the abdomen, in muscle, or in the subcutaneous fascia. Plain radiographs sometimes facilitate recognition of incorrect placement. Surgical management—involving reexploration of the catheter insertion site, laparoscopy, or simple removal of the catheter and replacement at another site—is usually necessary if catheter malpositioning is not recognized at the time of the initial insertion.

Step 2: Tunneling of Catheter

The catheter is then tunneled to the exit site. It should emerge from the skin pointing in a caudal direction; this is more easily achieved with a catheter that has a preformed bend. The anterior sheath is closed snugly around the catheter, with the inner felt cuff left in the rectus abdominis muscle. The skin is closed with subcuticular sutures. If the catheter is to be used immediately, dialysis tubing is connected and a dressing is applied. If the catheter is not to be used immediately, 50 ml of saline containing 5,000 units of heparin is placed in the peritoneal cavity and the catheter is capped; this procedure is repeated every other day until dialysis begins.

Figure 17   Peritoneal access. Four types of peritoneal access catheters are shown: (*a*) a rigid catheter without a cuff, designed for temporary use, (*b*) a pigtail silicone catheter with a straight subcutaneous portion, (*c*) a pigtail silicone catheter with a curved subcutaneous portion, and (*d*) a pigtail silicone catheter with a preformed bend in the subcutaneous portion, which is currently the preferred configuration.

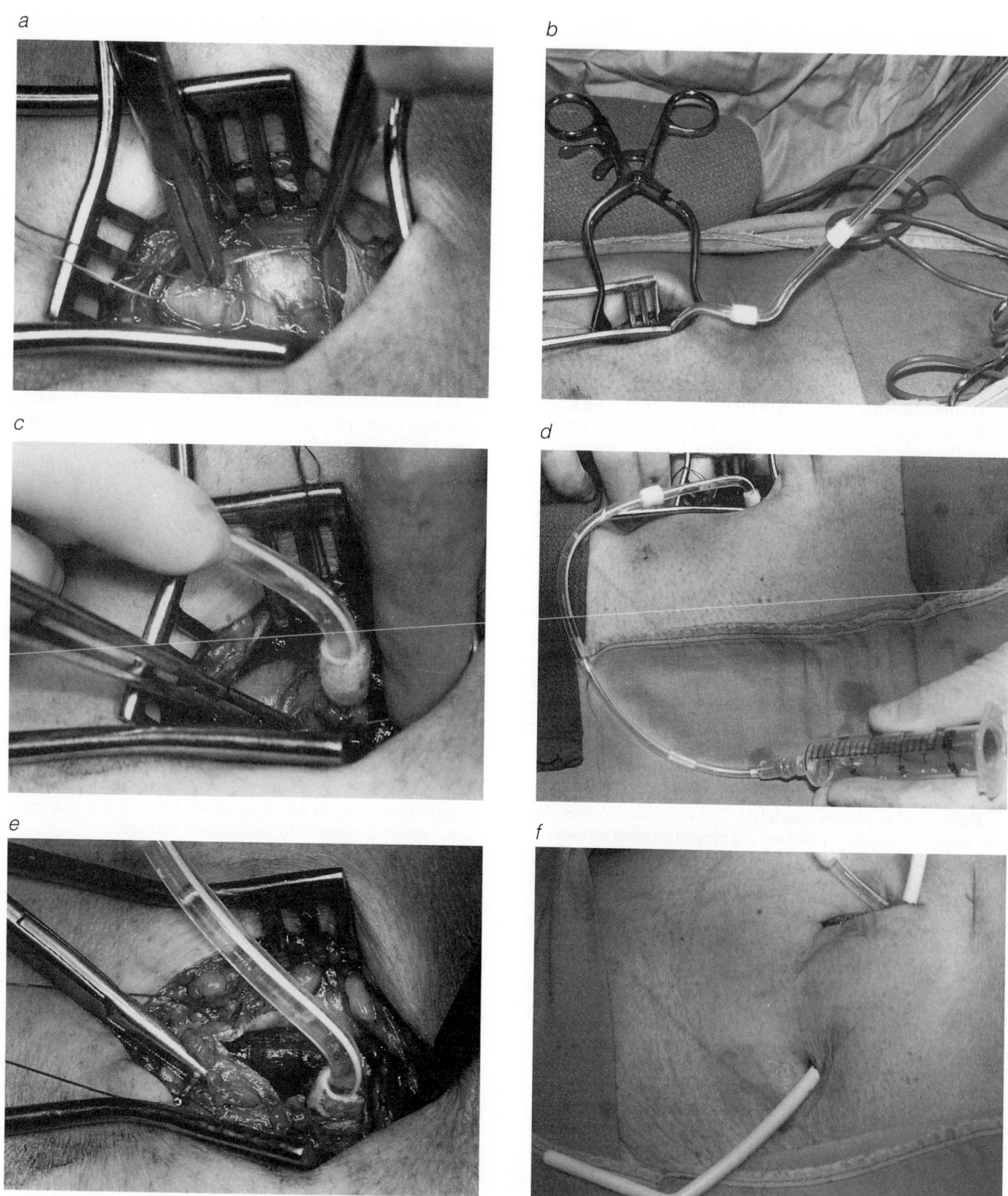

Figure 18 Peritoneal access. Illustrated is the procedure for inserting a peritoneal dialysis catheter by cutdown with the patient under local anesthesia. (*a*) A local anesthetic is infiltrated, the anterior rectus sheath is opened, the rectus abdominis muscle is split, and a purse-string suture is placed in the posterior rectus sheath. (*b*) With the stylet in place, the catheter is inserted in the direction of the pelvis (left). (*c*) With the inner cuff at the level of the rectus abdominis, the purse-string suture is tied and reinforced with an additional circumferential free tie around the peritoneum, if possible. (*d*) A flow test is performed to confirm satisfactory catheter position. (*e*) The anterior rectus sheath is closed over the inner cuff. (*f*) The catheter is tunneled to the exit site so that it emerges pointing inferiorly (left), with the outer cuff in the subcutis.

Step 3: Maintenance of Catheter

Maintenance of the catheter involves use of sterile dressings until the skin sites are healed, after which time a routine of skin cleansing and dressing is maintained. Whenever the catheter is disconnected, sterile precautions are taken to limit the possibility of contamination.

Step 4: Removal of Catheter

A Tenckhoff catheter is removed as follows. First, a local anesthetic is infiltrated into the original insertion site, and the inner Dacron cuff is dissected out of the rectus abdominis muscle (or the linea alba) with the electrocautery. Next, the catheter is divided and the abdominal portion removed. The rectus sheath (or the linea alba) is repaired with sutures, and the incision is closed. The subcutaneous cuff is then dissected out from the outside, and the outer portion of the catheter is removed. Finally, the insertion site is debrided, and the small skin opening is left to heal by second intention.

Troubleshooting Infection of the catheter tunnel or the Dacron cuffs necessitates some modification of this technique. If both the inner Dacron cuff and the outer are infected, salvage is impossible and the entire catheter must be removed. Areas of gross infection are treated with drainage and debridement and left open to heal by second intention. If alternative temporary peritoneal access for dialysis is available, a new catheter is not placed until the skin has healed completely. If no alternative temporary access is available, it may be necessary to insert a new catheter simultaneously at another site that is distant from the original infected location.

If only the outer cuff is infected and no other sites are available for subsequent catheter replacement, salvage may be attempted as follows: the outer cuff is dissected out of the subcutaneous tissue, the Dacron is shaved off, and this portion of the catheter is left outside the skin. This approach may allow resolution of the infection; however, it makes the inner cuff the sole barrier to deep infection and thus should not be used when alternative access is possible.

Special Considerations

Peritoneal access in children The technical considerations for peritoneal access in children are much the same as those for peritoneal access in adults. There are, however, some significant differences. If a Tenckhoff catheter is to be used in a child weighing less than 20 kg (44 lb), it should have only one Dacron cuff, which should be placed in the rectus abdominis muscle. The appropriate length for the catheter must be determined; this is done by measuring the size of the child from the point of insertion to the pelvic basin. Leaks should be prevented by ligating the peritoneum underneath the purse-string suture in the posterior rectus sheath [see Step 1: Insertion of Catheter, above]. General anesthesia is usually required. Postoperative dialysis volumes are selected according to patient size.

Alternative technology Laparoscopic techniques have also been developed for placement of peritoneal catheters. These techniques employ the standard 5 to 10 mm diameter trocars commonly used for laparoscopic procedures.[50] The catheter is inserted into the abdomen through a large cannula. One problem with this technique is that it is difficult to confirm that the deep cuff is placed within the musculature until after the cannula is removed. Moreover, despite the excellent visualization of the peritoneal cavity achieved with catheters placed in this manner, there is a high incidence of pericatheter leakage. Alternatively, one may resort to new techniques using specially designed equipment, such as the Y-Tec 2.2 mm–diameter Peritoneoscope, which always positions the deep cuff tight-

ly within the musculature.[51] In fact, randomized, controlled studies have indicated that catheters placed via peritoneoscopy survive approximately twice as long as catheters placed via traditional surgical dissection.[52] Furthermore, such procedures can always be performed at the bedside with local anesthesia or in an outpatient setting.

COMPLICATIONS

The following are the most significant early complications of peritoneal access procedures:

1. Injury to intra-abdominal organs, most commonly the small bowel, the colon, the bladder, and the fallopian tubes. Immediate exploration is necessary.
2. Leakage of peritoneal dialysate soon after catheter placement. This complication is caused by inadequate closure of the peritoneum around the catheter.
3. Incorrect catheter placement, usually manifested by relatively good inflow but poor outflow.
4. Intra-abdominal bleeding, signaled by a bloody dialysate. Although most episodes of intra-abdominal bleeding are minor and self-limited and consequently do not call for transfusion or specific intervention, investigation to determine the underlying cause is warranted.

The following are the most significant late complications of procedures for peritoneal access:

1. Intra-abdominal bleeding. The most common causes of such bleeding are related to menstruation and ovulation.
2. Erosion of the outer cuff of the catheter through the skin. This complication can be treated by dissecting the remaining cuff completely out of the subcutaneous tissues and shaving off the Dacron [see Operative Technique, Step 4: Removal of Catheter, above]. Because this approach, as noted, leaves only the inner cuff as a barrier to infection, it is usually advisable to treat outer-cuff erosion by removing the catheter completely and replacing it at another site.
3. Catheter breakage. If more than 2 cm remains outside the skin, special repair kits may be used to splice a new external catheter piece onto the original catheter.
4. Tunnel infections. Such infections are typically associated with contamination and infection of the outer cuff. The most common causative organisms are *Staphylococcus* species and *Pseudomonas* species.[53] Nasal carriage of *Staphylococcus* is a risk factor for tunnel infections, and pretreatment with rifampin may help decrease the risk.[54] Although many tunnel infections can be controlled with several weeks of antibiotic therapy and some can even be cured, most eventually necessitate removal of the catheter, especially if there is concomitant peritonitis.[55]
5. Catheter malfunction. Late catheter malfunction is uncommon. Complete obstruction of both inflow and outflow is generally attributable to fibrin plugs and can be corrected by infusing streptokinase. Good inflow coupled with poor outflow frequently signals wrapping of the catheter by omentum. This problem can be corrected by performing an omentectomy either laparoscopically or in an open fashion via a low midline incision.

OUTCOME EVALUATION

When peritoneal dialysis catheter function is poor shortly after operative placement, possible causes to be suspected include misdirection into the upper abdomen, kinking, previous abdominal adhesions, and omental obstruction of the catheter. Most of these complications present with satisfactory inflow but poor drainage.

Plain radiographs of the abdomen (or contrast studies if the catheter is not radiopaque) may reveal the problem. Sometimes, the complications respond to enemas (which may alter the location of the catheter) and to persistent attempts to achieve satisfactory exchange. Frequently, however, abdominal exploration via a lower midline incision is required, followed by omentectomy, redirection of the catheter, or catheter replacement. If omental wrap-ping of the catheter is the problem, the entire omentum should be removed to prevent a recurrence. General anesthesia is often necessary, though in some cases, certain of these procedures can be done with the patient under local anesthesia with sedation or under regional anesthesia. Laparoscopy has also been used to diagnose and treat peritoneal dialysis catheter dysfunction; general anesthesia is usually required.

References

1. US Renal Data System: USRDS 1999 Annual Data Report. The National Institute of Health, National Institute of Diabetes and Digestive and Kidney Disease. Am J Kidney Dis 34(suppl 1):540, 1999

2. Kolff WJ, Berk HT, ter Welle M, et al: The artificial kidney: a dialyzer with a great area. 1944. J Am Soc Nephrol. 8:1959, 1997

3. Quinton WE, Dillard DH, Scribner BH: Cannulation of blood vessels for prolonged hemodialysis. Trans Am Soc Artif Intern Organs 6:104, 1960

4. Brescia MJ, Cimino JE, Appell K, et al: Chronic hemodialysis using venipuncture and surgically created arteriovenous fistula. 1966. J Am Soc Nephrol 10:193, 1999

5. Baker LD, Johnson JM, Goldfarb D: Expanded polytetrafluoroethylene (PTFE) subcutaneous arteriovenous conduit: an improved vascular access for chronic hemodialysis. Trans Am Soc Artif Intern Organs 22:382, 1976

6. National Kidney Foundation DOQI: Clinical Practice Guidelines for Hemodialysis Vascular Access. Am J Kidney Dis 30(suppl 3):S150, 1997

7. Schwab SJ, Quarles LD, Middleton JP, et al: Hemodialysis-associated subclavian vein stenosis. Kidney Int 33:1156, 1988

8. Passman MA, Criado E, Farber MA, et al: Efficacy of color duplex imaging for proximal upper extremity venous outflow obstruction in hemodialysis patients. J Vasc Surg 28:869, 1998

9. Silva MB, Hobson RW, Pappas PJ, et al: A strategy for increasing use of autogenous hemodialysis access procedures: impact of preoperative noninvasive evaluation. J Vasc Surg 27:302, 1998

10. Marx AB, Landmann J, Harder FH: Surgery for vascular access. Curr Probl Surg 28(1):15, 1990

11. Silva MB, Hobson RW, Pappas PJ, et al: Vein transposition in the forearm for autogenous hemodialysis access. J Vasc Surg 26:981, 1997

12. Hakaim AG, Nalbandian M, Scott T: Superior maturation and patency of primary brachiocephalic and transposed basilic vein arteriovenous fistulae in patients with diabetes. J Vasc Surg 27:154, 1998

13. Matsuura JH, Rosenthal D, Clark M, et al: Transposed basilic vein versus polytetrafluoroethylene for brachial-axillary arteriovenous fistulas. Am J Surg 176:219, 1998

14. Coburn MC, Carney WI: Comparison of basilic vein and polytetrafluoroethylene for brachial arteriovenous fistula. J Vasc Surg 20:896, 1994

15. Gracz KC, Ing TS, Soung L, et al: Proximal forearm fistula for maintenance hemodialysis. Kidney Int 11:71, 1977

16. Bender MHM, Bruyninckx CMA, Gerlag PGG: The brachiocephalic elbow fistula: a useful alternative angioaccess for permanent hemodialysis. J Vasc Surg 20:808, 1994

17. Polo JR, Vazquez R, Polo J, et al: Brachiocephalic jump graft fistula: an alternative for dialysis use of elbow crease veins. Am J Kidney Dis 33:904, 1999

18. Dagher FJ, Gelber R, Ramos E, et al: The use of basilic vein and brachial artery as an A-V fistula for long term hemodialysis. J Surg Res 20:373, 1976

19. LoGerfo FW, Menzoian JO, Kumaki DJ, et al: Transposed basilic vein-brachial arteriovenous fistula: a reliable secondary-access procedure. Arch Surg 113:1008, 1978

20. Humphries AL, Colborn GL, Wynn JJ: Elevated basilic vein arteriovenous fistula. Am J Surg 177:489, 1999

21. Benedetti E, Del Pino A, Cintron J, et al: A new method of creating an arteriovenous graft access. Am J Surg 171:369, 1996

22. Santoro TD, Cambria RA: PTFE shunts for hemodialysis access: progressive choice of configuration. Semin Vasc Surg 10:166, 1997

23. Lazarides MK, Staramos DN, Tzilalis VD, et al: Evoked thrill: a simple intraoperative maneuver predicts early patency of arteriovenous fistulas. J Vasc Surg 27:750, 1998

24. Lenz BJ, Veldenz HC, Dennis JW, et al: A three-year follow-up on standard versus thin wall ePTFE grafts for hemodialysis. J Vasc Surg 28:464, 1998

25. Tordoir JH, Hofstra L, Bergmans DC, et al: Stretch versus standard expanded PTFE grafts for hemodialysis access. Vascular Access for Hemodialysis IV. Henry ML, Ferguson RM, Eds. WL Gore & Associates and Precept Press, Chicago, 1995, p 277

26. Lumsden AB, MacDonald MJ, Kikeri D, et al: Prophylactic balloon angioplasty fails to prolong the patency of expanded polytetrafluoroethylene arteriovenous grafts: results of a prospective randomized study. J Vasc Surg 26:382, 1997

27. Shoenfeld R, Hermans H, Novick A, et al: Stenting of proximal venous obstruction to maintain hemodialysis access. J Vasc Surg 19:532, 1994

28. Marston WA, Criado E, Jacques PF, et al: Prospective randomized comparison of surgical versus endovascular management of thrombosed dialysis access grafts. J Vasc Surg 26:373, 1997

29. DeMasi RJ, Gregory RT, Sorrell KA, et al: Intraoperative noninvasive evaluation of arteriovenous fistulae and grafts: "the steal study." J Vasc Tech 18:192, 1994

30. Kwun KB, Schanzer H, Finkler N, et al: Hemodynamic evaluation of angioaccess procedures for hemodialysis. Vasc Surg 13:170, 1979

31. Odland MD, Kelly PH, Ney AL, et al: Management of dialysis-associated steal syndrome complicating upper extremity arteriovenous fistulas: Use of intraoperative digital photoplethysmography. Surgery 110:664, 1991

32. Mattson WJ: Recognition and treatment of vascular steal secondary to hemodialysis prostheses. Am J Surg 154:198, 1987

33. West JC, Evans RD, Kelley SE, et al: Arterial insufficiency in hemodialysis access procedures: reconstruction by an interposition polytetrafluoroethylene graft conduit. Am J Surg 153:300, 1987

34. Bussel JA, Abbott JA, Lim RC: A radial steal syndrome with arteriovenous fistula for hemodialysis. Ann Intern Med 75:1657, 1971

35. Schanzer H, Schwartz M, Harrington E, et al: Treatment of ischemia due to "steal" by arteriovenous fistula with distal artery ligation and revascularization. J Vasc Surg 7:770, 1988

36. Shemesh D, Mabjeesh NJ, Abramowitz HB: Management of dialysis access-associated steal syndrome: use of intraoperative duplex ultrasound scanning for optimal flow reduction. J Vasc Surg 30:193, 1999

37. Beathard GA, Settle SM, Shields MW: Salvage of the nonfunctioning arteriovenous fistula. Am J Kidney Dis 33:910, 1999

38. Zibari GB, Rohr MS, Landreneau MD, et al: Complications from permanent hemodialysis vascular access. Surgery 104:681, 1988

39. Haire WD, Lynch TG, Lieberman RP, et al: Duplex scans before subclavian vein catheterization predict unsuccessful catheter placement. Arch Surg 127:229, 1992

40. Whitman ED: Complications associated with the use of central venous access devices. Curr Probl Surg 33:324, 1996

41. Dunea G, Domenico L, Gunnerson P, et al: A survey of permanent double-lumen catheters in hemodialysis patients. ASAIO Trans 37:M276, 1991

42. Chimochowski GE, Worley E, Rutherford WE, et al: Superiority of the internal jugular over the subclavian access for temporary hemodialysis. Nephron 54:154, 1990

43. The Food and Drug Administration Task Force: Precautions necessary with central venous catheters. FDA Drug Bulletin 15:6, 1989

44. Mansfield PF, Hohn DC, Fornage BD, et al: Complications and failures of subclavian-vein catheterization. N Engl J Med 331:1735, 1994

45. Stuart RK, Shikora SA, Akerman P, et al: Incidence of arrhythmia with central venous catheter insertion and exchange. J Parenter Enteral Nutr 14:152, 1990

46. Horattas MC, Wright DJ, Fenton AH, et al: Changing concepts of deep venous thrombosis of the upper extremity: report of a series and review of the literature. Surgery 104:561, 1988

47. Suchoki P, Conlon P, Knelson M, et al: Silastic cuffed catheters for hemodialysis vascular access: thrombolytic and mechanical correction of HD catheter malfunction. Am J Kidney Dis 28:279, 1996

48. Crain MR, Mewissen MW, Ostrowski GJ, et al: Fibrin sleeve stripping for salvage of failing hemodialysis catheters: techniques and initial results. Radiology 198:41, 1996

49. Schaffer D: Catheter-related sepsis complicating long-term, tunnelled central venous dialysis catheters: management by guidewire exchange. Am J Kidney Dis 25:593, 1995

50. Douglas AF, Deardon DA, Barclay CA, et al: Laparoscopic insertion of CAPD catheters. Proceedings of the 3rd International Congress on Access for Dialysis. Maastricht, 1997

51. Ash SR: Bedside peritoneoscopic peritoneal catheter placement of Tenckoff and newer peritoneal catheters. Adv Peritoneal Dialysis 14:1, 1998

52. Gadallah MF, Pervez A, El-Shahawy M, et al: Peritoneoscopic versus surgical placement of Tenckhoff catheters: a prospective study on outcome. J Am Soc Nephrol 7:A0904, 1996

53. Prevention of peritonitis in CAPD (editorial). Lancet 337:22, 1991

54. Piraino B: A review of *Staphylococcus aureus* exit-site and tunnel infections in peritoneal dialysis patients. Am J Kidney Dis 16:89, 1990

55. Holley JL, Bernardini J, Piraino B: Risk factors for tunnel infections in continuous peritoneal dialysis. Am J Kidney Dis 18:344, 19

Acknowledgments

Figures 1 through 9, 11, 12, 15, and 16 Jean Montreuil, B.Ing, M.Sc. Digitized and adapted by Tom Moore.

23 CAROTID ARTERIAL PROCEDURES

Wesley S. Moore, M.D.

The rationale for operating on patients with carotid artery disease is to prevent stroke. It has been estimated that in 50% to 80% of patients who experience an ischemic stroke, the underlying cause is a lesion in the distribution of the carotid artery, usually in the vicinity of the carotid bifurcation. It would follow, then, that appropriate identification and surgical intervention could significantly reduce the incidence of ischemic stroke.

Carotid endarterectomy for both symptomatic and asymptomatic carotid artery stenosis has been extensively evaluated in prospective, randomized trials. Symptomatic patients have been studied in the North American Symptomatic Carotid Endarterectomy Trial (NASCET),[1] the European Carotid Stenosis Trial (ECST),[2] and the symptomatic carotid stenosis trial from the Veterans Affairs (VA) Cooperative Studies Program.[3] The results of all three trials conclusively demonstrate that symptomatic patients with greater than 50% stenosis on arteriography are at substantially lower risk for stroke after carotid endarterectomy than control subjects receiving medical management alone. Asymptomatic patients with hemodynamically significant stenosis also benefit from surgical treatment: the Asymptomatic Carotid Atherosclerosis Study (ACAS)[4] and the asymptomatic carotid stenosis trial from the VA Cooperative Studies Program[5] show that the risk of both transient ischemic attacks (TIAs) and stroke is markedly lower in patients treated with carotid endarterectomy and best medical management than in control subjects treated with best medical management alone.

Surgical reconstruction of the carotid artery yields the greatest benefits when done by surgeons who can keep complication rates to an absolute minimum. The majority of complications associated with carotid arterial procedures are either technical or judgmental; accordingly, in what follows, I emphasize the procedural details that I consider particularly important for deriving the best short- and long-term results from surgical intervention.

Preoperative Evaluation

PATIENT SELECTION

Indications for carotid artery surgery can be divided into two major categories: (1) asymptomatic critical stenosis and (2) symptomatic hemodynamically significant stenosis.[6]

Asymptomatic Critical Stenosis

ACAS and the VA asymptomatic carotid stenosis study both found that in patients with diameter-reducing stenosis of 60% or greater on angiography, carotid endarterectomy resulted in fewer fatal and nonfatal strokes over a 5-year period than nonoperative treatment with best medical management alone. It is important to keep in mind that there are several different ways of measuring stenosis [*see II:2 Asymptomatic Carotid Bruit*]. The 60% figure cited by ACAS and the VA study was determined according to the North American method rather than the European method. Moreover, it was determined by means of contrast angiography rather than duplex ultrasonography (DUS) or magnetic resonance imaging. If the decision for carotid endarterectomy is to be based on DUS, some conversion of values is required. A patient who has an 80% to 99% stenosis on DUS can generally be assumed to have a diameter-reducing stenosis of at least 60% on angiography; a stenosis that is less than 80% on DUS may fall short of a 60% diameter-reducing stenosis on angiography.

Symptomatic Hemodynamically Significant Carotid Stenosis

Transient ischemic attacks Both NASCET and ECST found that symptomatic patients with hemodynamically significant stenoses experienced fewer fatal and nonfatal strokes after carotid endarterectomy combined with best medical management than after best medical management alone, provided that the perioperative morbidity and mortality from stroke was 6.0% or less. Thus, patients with monocular or hemispheric TIAs are good candidates for carotid endarterectomy. Global ischemic attacks have also been used as an indication for carotid endarterectomy. This practice has not been evalutated in clinical trials; it is usually justified on the basis of the ACAS data alone.

Prior stroke Patients who have previously experienced a hemispheric stroke but who are not disabled and have made a reasonable recovery are also good candidates for carotid endarterectomy if they have a hemodynamically significant stenosis.

IMAGING

Indications for Carotid Duplex Scanning

Identification of a carotid lesion that can be treated with endarterectomy usually begins with a carotid duplex scan. Indications for carotid duplex scanning fall into three main categories: symptoms, signs, and risk factors. Symptoms include classic TIAs and strokes that give rise to clinical suspicion of carotid bifurcation disease. The primary sign is the presence of a carotid bruit on auscultation. Risk factors include cigarette smoking, hypertension, diabetes mellitus, hypercholesterolemia, peripheral vascular disease, and coronary artery disease. As the number of risk factors present increases, the likelihood of associated carotid bifurcation disease increases exponentially.

Other Considerations in Symptomatic Patients

Patients who present with focal ischemic symptoms are likely to have associated carotid bifurcation disease; however, other pathologic conditions (e.g., emboli of cardiac origin, aortic arch disease, intracranial vascular disease, coagulopathy, and brain tumors) can also be responsible for focal symptoms. Accordingly, a complete workup of a symptomatic patient should include cardiac evaluation as well as intracranial imaging.

Additional Arterial Imaging

The accuracy of carotid duplex scanning is highly dependent on the technician performing it and on the laboratory where it is done. A carefully performed carotid duplex scan is often the most accurate indicator of carotid bifurcation disease; however, a hastily or carelessly performed scan can result in overestimation of the extent of the carotid bifurcation disease. For this reason, additional imaging studies (e.g., MRI, computed tomographic angiography, and, when there is serious doubt, contrast angiography) may be indicated.

Operative Planning

Before operation is scheduled, the general health of the patient must be assessed, with particular attention paid to cardiac and pulmonary status. Given that many patients with carotid artery disease are hypertensive or diabetic, good preoperative control of diabetes mellitus and blood pressure is mandatory. Finally, to reduce the risk of thromboembolic complications, patients should receive antiplatelet drugs (e.g., aspirin) up to and on the day of operation.

ANESTHESIA

Surgery on the cervical portion of the carotid artery may be performed with the patient under either general or cervical block anesthesia. Both techniques have their advocates, their advantages, and their disadvantages.

The advantages of general anesthesia include a quiet operative field, maximal patient comfort, good airway control, and convenient blood gas management. In addition, general anesthesia may lead to improved cerebral blood flow and give better protection against reduced blood flow during carotid clamping. The disadvantages of general anesthesia include blood pressure swings during induction and the inability to monitor the patient's conscious response to carotid clamping. Some reports also suggest that the incidence of cardiac complications is higher during general anesthesia than during cervical block anesthesia.

The main advantage of cervical block anesthesia is the ability to monitor cerebral function during carotid clamping: an awake patient can be engaged in conversation and can be asked to carry out motor activities of the extremities. The disadvantages of cervical block anesthesia include possible patient discomfort, restlessness, and intolerance of the longer operations that are sometimes necessary for technical reasons. Another disadvantage is that on occasion, a patient cannot tolerate carotid clamping and demonstrates an immediate neurologic deficit with clamp application. Such an occurrence heightens the anxiety level of the surgical team, thereby increasing the risk that they will commit technical errors in the rush to place an internal shunt.

Besides considering the inherent advantages and disadvantages of these two anesthetic techniques with respect to the patient, it is important to consider their advantages and disadvantages with respect to individual surgical practice. A given surgeon may well work better and achieve better results with one technique or the other.

Whichever anesthetic approach is used, all patients should have a radial arterial line in place to allow continuous blood pressure monitoring as well as provide access for determining blood gas levels. As a rule, there is no need to place a central venous line or a right heart catheter, except in patients with marginal cardiac function.

Figure 1 **Carotid arterial procedures. Shown is the recommended patient positioning.**

PATIENT POSITIONING

Proper positioning of the patient is necessary to provide optimal exposure of the neck from the clavicle up to the mastoid process on the side of the proposed operation [*see Figure 1*]. The patient is placed in the supine position with a folded sheet under the shoulders to induce a mild degree of neck extension. Excessive neck extension should be avoided, however, because it places tension on the artery and actually hinders rather than facilitates exposure. This potential problem can be addressed by placing one or more towels under the head to adjust the neck to the optimal degree of extension. The patient's head is then turned away from the side of the operation to improve cervical exposure further. Finally, the table top may be rotated slightly away from the side of the operation so as to provide a flat surgical field. The head of the table may be elevated slightly if the patient's blood pressure is adequate; this step helps

Figure 2 **Carotid arterial procedures. The incision most commonly used to expose the cervical carotid artery is a vertical one placed along the anterior margin of the sternocleidomastoid muscle and centered over the presumed location of the carotid bifurcation. It may be extended proximally or distally, depending on where the carotid bifurcation turns out to be.**

Figure 3 **Carotid arterial procedures. An alternative incision to the vertical incision is a transverse incision along a skin crease in the vicinity of the carotid bifurcation.**

lower venous pressure and reduce venous bleeding during the operation [*see Figure 1*].

Operative Technique

STEP 1: INITIAL INCISION

Either of two incisions may be used for exposure of the cervical carotid artery. The more common choice is a vertical incision placed along an imaginary line that extends from the sternoclavicular junction to the mastoid process, paralleling the anterior margin of the sternocleidomastoid muscle as well as the course of the carotid artery and the contents of the carotid sheath [*see Figure 2*]. The incision is centered over the presumed location of the carotid bifurcation. The advantage of this incision is that it provides optimal exposure of the cervical carotid artery and can readily be extended either proximally or distally along the aforementioned imaginary line to give additional exposure when needed (e.g., when the carotid bifurcation is unusually high). The disadvantage of this incision is that it runs against Langer's lines; thus, if a keloid occurs, it is likely to be in an unsightly position. In most patients, the incision heals to a fine line, and it usually is not noticeable once healing is complete.

The alternative to the vertical incision is a transverse incision that is placed in a skin crease on the anterior portion of the neck and then curved toward the mastoid process posteriorly [*see Figure 3*]. Skin flaps are raised in a subplatysmal layer, and the incision is deepened along the anterior border of the sternocleidomastoid muscle. The advantage of this alternative incision is that it may be more cosmetically acceptable; however, its inferior portion frequently crosses the neck anteriorly, which may make it more visible than an incision confined to the line of the sternocleidomastoid muscle would be. The disadvantage of this incision is that it requires the raising of skin flaps, which takes additional time and may limit the extent of any proximal exposure that may be required.

STEP 2: EXPOSURE OF CAROTID ARTERY

Once the incision through the platysmal layer has been completed, an avascular areolar plane is developed along the anterior border of the sternocleidomastoid muscle for the full length of the incision so as to expose the carotid sheath. The internal jugular vein is usual-

ly the most visible vessel, and the carotid sheath is opened along this vessel's anterior border. The common facial vein, which drains into the internal jugular vein, is a relatively constant landmark. Because the common facial vein is the venous analogue of the external carotid artery, it can generally be used as a guide to the position of the carotid bifurcation [*see Figure 4*]. On occasion, a patient has several accessory facial veins instead of a single common facial vein. The common facial vein or the accessory facial veins are then divided between ligatures so that the jugular vein can be retracted laterally. The common carotid artery and the carotid bifurcation lie immediately beneath the divided facial veins.

At this point, care must be taken to look for the vagus nerve. This nerve is usually located posterior to the common carotid artery, but it is sometimes rotated into a more superficial position. Another important neurologic structure in this area is the ansa cervicalis, which is formed by the junction of fibers from the hypoglossal (12th cranial) nerve and fibers from the first cervical nerve and which continues inferiorly as a single trunk, providing innervation to the strap muscles. This nerve should be spared if possible, but it can be divided without significant sequelae if it interferes with optimal exposure of the carotid bifurcation. One convenient method of separating the nerve from the artery is to divide the fibers running from the first cervical nerve to the ansa cervicalis; when this is done, the nerve is readily mobilized and retracted anteriorly away from the carotid artery.

The perivascular plane of the common carotid artery is then entered, and the common carotid artery is circumferentially mobilized. The common carotid artery is palpated against a right-angle clamp to determine the proximal extent of the atherosclerotic plaque. If possible, the common carotid artery should be mobilized proximal to the plaque until a circumferentially soft portion of that vessel is

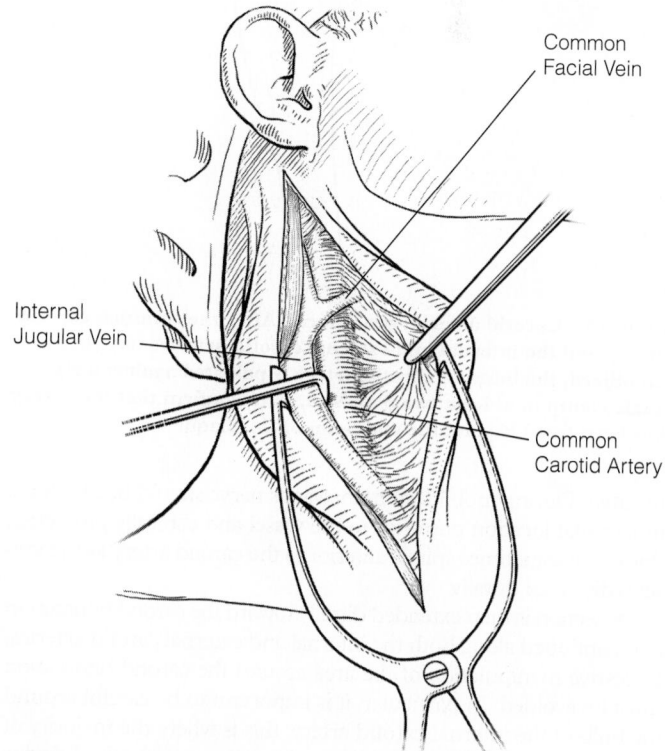

Figure 4 **Carotid arterial procedures. After the sternocleidomastoid muscle is mobilized off the carotid sheath, the jugular vein is identified. The perivascular plane along the jugular vein is opened until the common facial vein is exposed.**

Dissection should then continue distally beyond the bulb of the internal carotid artery to a point where the internal carotid artery is normal. At this point, the relevant portion of the vessel is circumferentially mobilized and palpated against a right-angle clamp in at least two planes to confirm that the atheromatous plaque does not reach up to the level of the proposed clamping [see Figure 5]. Once this is accomplished, the external carotid artery is mobilized beyond the end point of plaque extension in a similar manner.

If the patient has a high carotid bifurcation or if the plaque in the internal carotid artery extends further distally than usual, a more extensive exposure of the carotid bifurcation, the internal carotid artery, or both is required. To provide such exposure, the skin incision is extended all the way to the mastoid process. The sternocleido-mastoid muscle is fully mobilized up to the mastoid process, with

Figure 5 **Carotid arterial procedures. After the common carotid artery and the internal and external carotid arteries have been mobilized, the internal carotid artery is palpated against a right-angle clamp in at least two planes (*a, b*) to confirm that the artery has been freed beyond the end point of the plaque.**

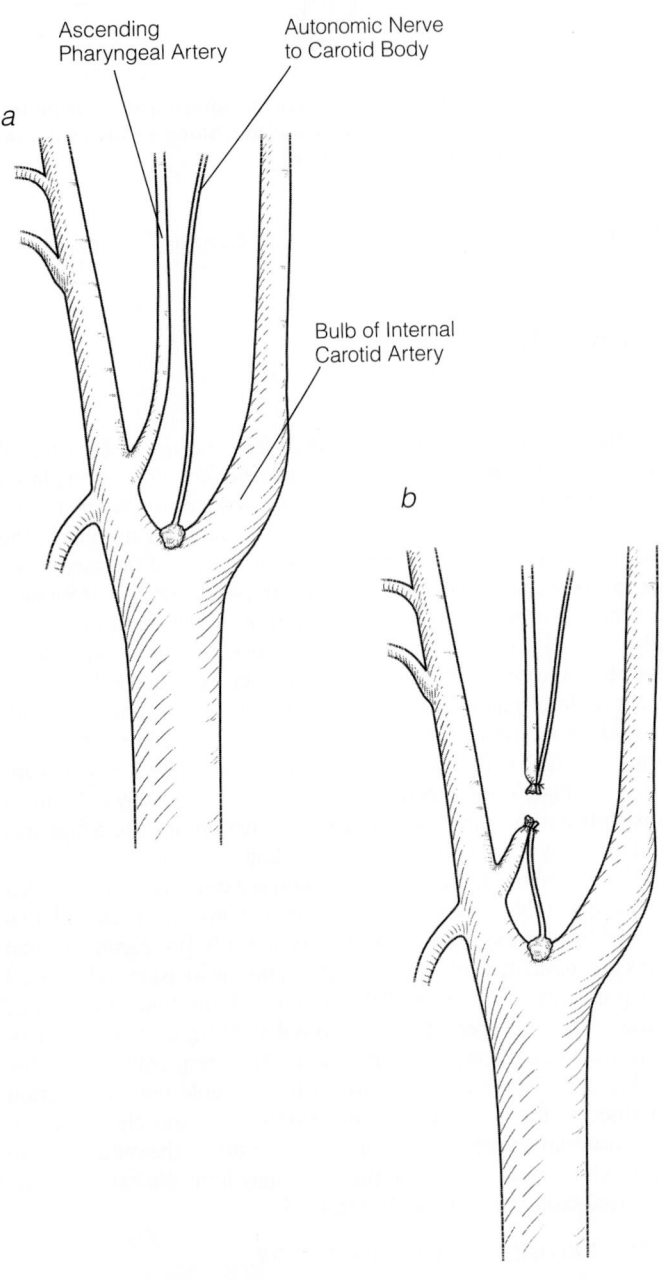

Figure 6 **Carotid arterial procedures. Once the common, internal, and external carotid arteries are fully mobilized, the structures between the internal and external carotid arteries (*a*) are divided (*b*) to allow the carotid bifurcation to drop down.**

reached. During mobilization, the vagus nerve should be identified in its usual location posterior to the vessel and carefully protected; this nerve sometimes spirals anterior to the carotid artery as the vessel is dissected distally.

Dissection is then extended distally toward the carotid bifurcation and continued along both the internal and external carotid arteries. Excessive manipulation of the area around the carotid bifurcation must be avoided. In particular, it is important to be careful around the bulb of the internal carotid artery: this is where the majority of the plaque will be located, and manipulation can easily dislodge plaque or thromboembolic material. With exposure of the carotid bifurcation, the hypoglossal nerve may come into view. Care should be taken not to injure this nerve, though it may have to be mobilized to permit sufficient distal exposure of the internal carotid artery.

Middle Meningeal Artery

Point of Division of Styloid Process

Point of Division of Posterior Belly of Digastric Muscle

Interior Carotid Artery

Exterior Carotid Artery

Inferior Alveolar Artery

Submental Artery

Omohyoid Muscle

Common Carotid Artery

Sternocleidomastoid Muscle

Sternocleidomastoid Muscle

Above Digastric
1. Superficial Temporal Artery
2. Internal Maxillary Artery
3. Posterior Auricular Artery
   Digastric Muscle

Below Digastric
1. Occipital Artery
2. Ascending Pharyngeal Artery
3. Facial Artery
4. Lingual Artery
5. Superior Thyroid Artery

Vertebral Artery

First Rib

Figure 7 **Carotid arterial procedures. Division of the posterior belly of the digastric muscle yields additional exposure of the internal carotid artery. If the internal carotid artery must be mobilized all the way to the base of the skull, further distal exposure is obtained by separating the attachments of the ligaments to the styloid process and dividing the styloid process.**

care taken to look for the spinal portion of the accessory (11th cranial) nerve as it enters the sternocleidomastoid muscle on the medial surface. With the sternocleidomastoid muscle fully mobilized and retractors in place, the internal carotid artery can then be further exposed.

The jugular vein is mobilized up toward the base of the skull, with care taken to look for additional accessory facial branches, which must be divided between ligatures so that the jugular vein can be fully mobilized and moved posteriorly. The perivascular plane of the internal carotid artery is carefully defined, and the artery is gently mobilized with a sharp-tipped clamp applied in a spreading motion; in this way, the more distal portion of the inter-

nal carotid artery can be mobilized downward. If the vessel is still insufficiently mobile, then the nerve to the carotid body and the ascending pharyngeal artery within the crotch between the internal and external carotid arteries are mobilized and divided between ligatures. These two structures often serve as a de facto suspensory ligament for the carotid bulb; dividing them allows the carotid bifurcation to drop down and permits further downward traction of the internal carotid artery as the vessel is gently mobilized distally [*see Figure 6*].

Once the internal carotid artery is further exposed distally and the hypoglossal nerve is mobilized along its vertical portion and moved anteriorly, the posterior belly of the digastric muscle is encountered.

An areolar plane is developed posteriorly and superiorly along the inferior margin of the posterior belly of the digastric muscle, allowing the muscle to be mobilized anteriorly to yield additional exposure of the internal carotid artery. If the resulting exposure is not sufficient, the muscle may be carefully encircled with a right-angle clamp and divided [see Figure 7]. In those relatively uncommon cases in which even further distal exposure is required, the styloid process is palpated and the muscular and ligamentous attachments to the styloid process divided, so that the styloid process can be exposed with a periosteal elevator. Once the styloid process has been completely freed of its muscular and ligamentous attachments and the cranial nerves in the vicinity have been identified and carefully protected, the styloid process is cut close to the base of the skull [see Figure 7].

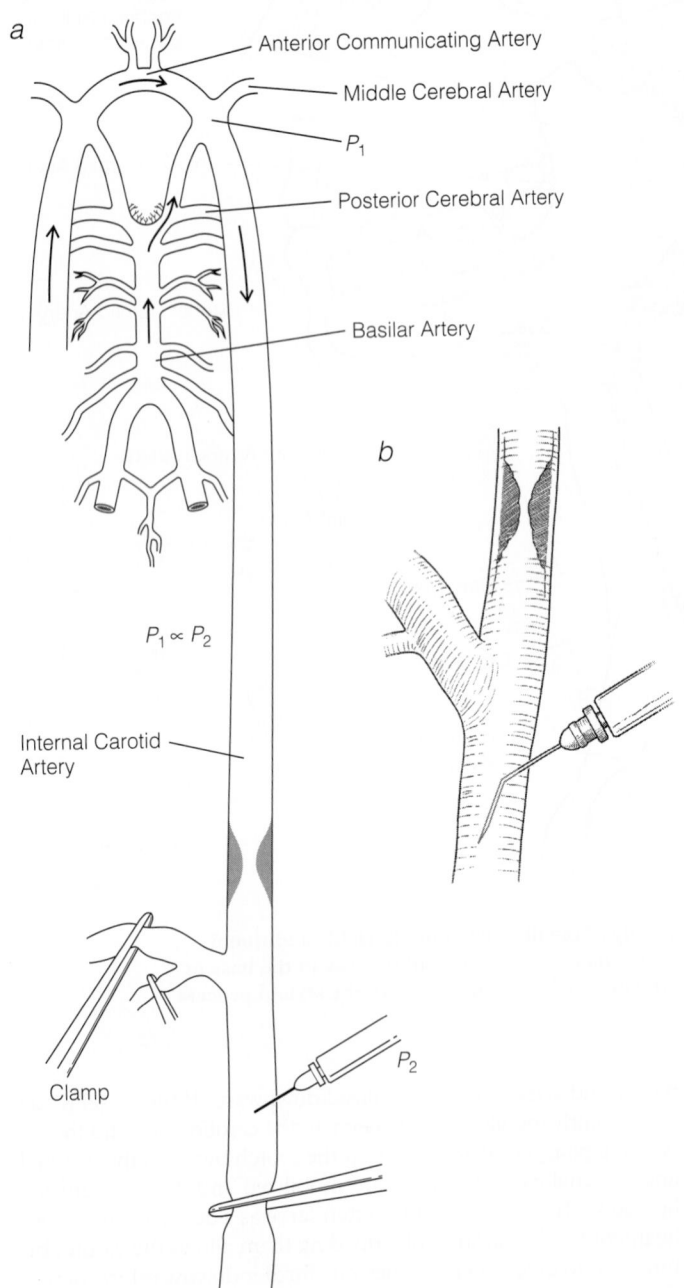

This step yields optimal exposure of the internal carotid artery all the way to the base of the skull.

Additional adjunctive measures for more extensive exposure of the internal carotid artery have been described. These include subluxation or dislocation of the mandible,[7] wiring of the mandible into a subluxed position, and division of the ramus of the mandible with rotation of the mandible away from the base of the skull. In my view, these measures are unnecessary, provided that the sternocleidomastoid muscle and the jugular vein have been adequately mobilized, the plane around the internal carotid artery has been developed, and the carotid bifurcation has been released.

A significant risk associated with extended exposure of the internal carotid artery is possible injury to the vagus nerve, the accessory nerve, or the hypoglossal nerve. Retraction of the vagus nerve may produce either temporary or permanent vocal cord palsy, and extensive retraction of or injury to the hypoglossal nerve causes denervation of the ipsilateral side of the tongue, manifested by tongue deviation to the ipsilateral side on protrusion or difficulty with mastication or swallowing. In addition, posterior exposure of a high carotid bifurcation may result in injury to branches of the glossopharyngeal (ninth cranial) nerve.

A common error in carotid artery mobilization is failure to recognize that the plaque in the internal carotid artery extends beyond the upper limit of the arterial exposure. It is far better to anticipate this problem before clamping and opening the artery than to discover it afterward and be forced to mobilize the vessel after it has been clamped. Once the common carotid and internal carotid arteries have been mobilized sufficiently, they are encircled with umbilical tapes; Rumel tourniquets are used if an internal shunt is required or desired.

STEP 3: CEREBRAL CIRCULATORY SUPPORT

Clamping of the carotid artery necessarily results in interruption of blood flow through the vessel. Patients who have good collateral circulation via the contralateral carotid artery or the vertebral arteries generally (though not always) tolerate the temporary interruption of flow through the clamped artery well.[8] Patients who have inadequate collateral blood flow require cerebral circulatory support, usually in the form of placement of an internal shunt. There are three basic approaches to shunt use: (1) routine use of an internal shunt, (2) selective use of an internal shunt, and (3) routine avoidance of shunting in an attempt to minimize clamp time.

Shunting Options

Routine shunting In approximately 10% of patients undergoing carotid artery surgery, collateral blood flow is inadequate and temporary use of an indwelling shunt is necessary to prevent brain damage; in the remaining 90%, collateral blood flow is adequate and clamping generally well tolerated, and shunting is therefore unnecessary. Clearly, routine use of an internal shunt takes care of the 10% of patients who require shunts. Its disadvantage is that it is an additional procedure that carries its own complications, to which not only the 10% of patients who require shunting but also the 90% who do not are subjected. The potential complications associated with placement of a shunt include intimal injury (including the raising of an intimal flap), atheroma embolization (if atheromatous material is scooped up during shunt placement), and air embolization (if air bubbles are trapped within the shunt and not recognized).

Selective shunting Selective placement of a shunt has an advantage over routine placement in that the procedure and its potential complications are limited to the 10% of patients who actually re-

Figure 8 **Carotid arterial procedures.** (*a*) **Shown is a graphic representation of the measurement of internal carotid artery back-pressure.** (*b*) **The needle is bent at a 45° angle before being inserted into the common carotid artery.**

Figure 9 **Carotid arterial procedures. When a thromboembolic fragment occludes a cortical arterial branch, a central infarct zone develops, surrounded by an ischemic zone that derives some residual blood supply from collateral vessels. In this zone, known as the ischemic penumbra, the residual blood supply is sufficient to maintain viability.**

quire a shunt. Its main disadvantage is that the methods used to identify patients who require shunting may not be entirely reliable.

Selective identification of patients who require shunting can be accomplished in several ways. The most direct—and perhaps safest—method is to employ local or cervical block anesthesia so that the effect of temporary carotid clamping can be assessed in a conscious patient; if clamping leads to a neurologic deficit, then the patient clearly requires an internal shunt. Other methods of identifying patients who require a shunt make use of techniques such as continuous electroencephalographic monitoring, measurement of somatosensory evoked potential, and monitoring of middle cerebral blood flow with transcranial Doppler ultrasonography.

A useful method of determining the adequacy of collateral cerebral blood flow is measurement of back-pressure in the internal carotid artery.[9] Back-pressure has been shown to be a good index of the adequacy of collateral blood flow, and it correlates well with the safety of temporary clamping and thus with the necessity of placing an internal shunt. Back-pressure is measured by placing into the common carotid artery a needle that is connected to pressure tubing and a pressure transducer. The tip of the needle is bent at a 45° angle. Systemic blood pressure is measured, and clamps are placed on the common carotid artery proximal to the needle and on the external carotid artery. The residual pressure in the common carotid artery, which is in continuity with the internal carotid artery, is then allowed to equilibrate; the resulting pressure reading represents internal carotid artery back-pressure [*see Figure 8*]. It has been determined that patients with back-pressures higher than 25 mm Hg can tolerate temporary clamping without incurring brain damage.

Selective shunting is also appropriate for patients who have previously had strokes, regardless of the degree of neurologic recovery. In these patients, a central area of cerebral infarction is surrounded by a zone of relatively ischemic tissue—the so-called ischemic penumbra. The ischemic penumbra is made up of live and potentially functional brain tissue, but its viability is highly dependent on maximization

of cerebral perfusion pressure through collateral channels. Accordingly, any interruption of carotid circulation, regardless of the degree of collateral circulation present, may threaten the ischemic penumbra and extend the infarct [*see Figure 9*]. In my opinion, all carotid endarterectomy patients with prior strokes should receive shunts on a routine basis.

Routine avoidance of shunting The advantage of routinely avoiding the use of shunts is that the technical issues and potential complications associated with the additional procedure are avoided entirely. The disadvantage is that unshunted patients with poor collateral blood flow may sustain ischemic brain damage, particularly if the clamp time turns out to be longer than was anticipated.

Technique of Shunt Placement

Internal shunts must be placed with great care if shunt-associated complications are to be avoided. Of the various shunts currently available, I prefer the Javid shunt, which is tapered, has smooth leading edges, and possesses external bulbous circumferential extensions that permit it to be held in place with a circumferential Rumel tourniquet, thereby minimizing the chances of inadvertent dislodgment. Optimal placement of an internal shunt may be achieved by means of the following steps [*see Figure 10*].

After the patient has been adequately heparinized and the artery clamped and opened, the distal portion of the internal shunt is placed into the internal carotid artery. A clamp is placed on the shunt and briefly opened to allow back-bleeding; good back-bleeding confirms that the shunt is lying free in the lumen of the internal carotid artery. The shunt is then secured by tightening a Rumel tourniquet, and the bulbous portion of the shunt is engaged to prevent dislodgment.

Next, the proximal portion of the shunt is placed into the common carotid artery. As this is done, the clamp is removed from the shunt so that backflow from the shunt will dislodge any loose material and air within the common carotid artery. The shunt is then re-

Figure 10   **Carotid arterial procedures. Shown is the technique of shunt placement, first distally** (*a*) **and then proximally** (*b*).

clamped, and the clamp is removed from the common carotid artery as the proximal portion of the shunt is passed into that vessel.

When the proximal portion of the shunt is in the proper position in the common carotid artery, it is secured by tightening a Rumel tourniquet on the vessel. The clamp on the shunt is then slowly opened so that the surgeon can observe flow through the translucent device and thus verify that no solid particles or air bubbles are passing through it. Because the shunt is relatively long, the surgeon has a reasonable amount of time in which to observe flow. If any particles or air bubbles are identified, the shunt can be quickly clamped, removed from the common carotid artery, and back-bled, and the procedure can then be repeated.

Once the shunt is secured in place and open, its length and redundancy allow it to be easily manipulated medially and laterally; endarterectomy can then be performed without the encumbrance of an inlying shunt.

STEP 4: RECONSTRUCTION OPTIONS

There are four principal reconstructions involving the common carotid artery and the carotid bifurcation: (1) conventional open carotid endarterectomy with either patch angioplasty or primary closure, (2) eversion endarterectomy, (3) reconstruction for proximal lesions of the common carotid artery, and (4) reconstruction for recurrent stenosis with resection of the carotid bifurcation and grafting.

Open Carotid Endarterectomy

Once the carotid bifurcation has been fully mobilized both proximal and distal to the lesion, systemic anticoagulation with heparin is initiated. I generally give 5,000 units, an amount that is sufficient to produce adequate anticoagulation for the duration of carotid clamping but is not large enough to necessitate heparin reversal on completion of the operation. If internal carotid artery back-pressure is to be used to determine whether the patient requires an internal shunt, then it is measured at this time. If cerebral electrical activity is to be the determinant, then the internal, external, and common carotid arteries are clamped and electrical activity is monitored (e.g., via EEG) with the clamps in place. If electrical changes are noted with clamping, an internal shunt is required.

Arteriotomy   The common carotid artery and the carotid bifurcation are rotated so as to be positioned for an arteriotomy that begins on the common carotid artery and extends through the bulb of the internal carotid artery to a point 180° opposite the flow divider [*see Figure 11*]. This incision effectively bivalves the carotid bulb, thus making possible a more accurate primary or patch closure. The arteriotomy continues through the plaque and extends well up into the internal carotid artery, beyond the visible end point of the atherosclerotic plaque.

Plaque removal   A dissection plane separating the atherosclerotic intima from the media and the adventitia is then developed with a sharp-bladed dissector. As a rule, it is easiest to begin the endarterectomy at the point where the plaque is bulkiest. At this point, the medial fibers are usually gone, but as the dissection continues both proximally and distally, more normal medial tissue may be seen. It is important to develop the dissection plane between the intima and the media if possible because doing so permits the creation of a feathered end point distally as dissection proceeds into a relatively normal portion of the internal carotid artery [see Figure 12]. If the dissection plane is between the media and the adventitia, a feathered end point is much harder to achieve. Failure to achieve a feathered end point often results in a sharp shelf at the internal carotid artery level, which increases the risk of subsequent intimal dissection when blood flow is restored.

Once the dissection plane is complete on one side of the arteriotomy at the level of the common carotid artery, a right-angle clamp is gently inserted into the plane and advanced through it to the opposite side of the arteriotomy, thereby separating the plaque from the arterial wall around the entire circumference of the vessel. The clamp is then gently spread and brought downward to complete the circumferential dissection of the plaque proximally. The proximal end point of plaque dissection is obtained by cutting the intima with a No. 15 blade.

With the same depth of dissection now existing on both sides of the open common carotid artery, dissection then continues distally up to the carotid bifurcation. At this point, the plaque within the external carotid artery is carefully separated in a circumferential fash-

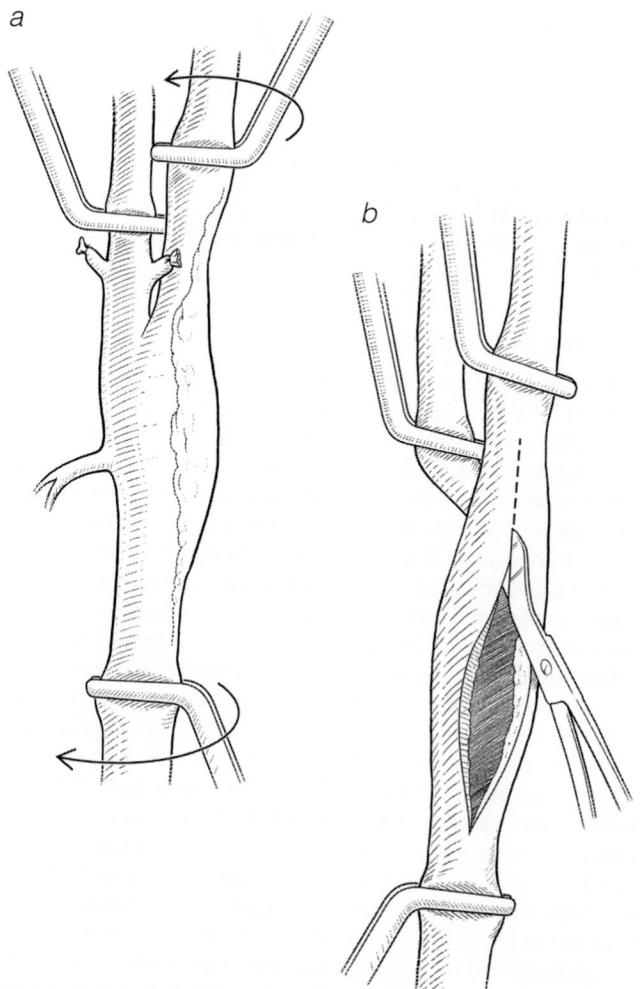

Figure 11 **Carotid arterial procedures: open endarterectomy. Clamps are applied to the common, internal, and external carotid arteries, and the structures are rotated (*a*) so that an arteriotomy can be made in the common carotid artery 180° opposite the flow divider (*b*).**

ion. This is usually done by using a sharp mosquito clamp until all of the plaque has been separated from the vessel wall and dissection has reached normal intima. The freed plaque is gently grasped with the opened mosquito clamp, traction is applied, and the distal end point of plaque dissection in the external carotid artery is obtained.

Dissection then continues up the internal carotid artery, with care taken to leave normal intima behind. Often, the plaque becomes a relatively narrow tongue of atheroma on the posterior wall of the internal carotid artery. If the edge of the atheromatous plaque is followed to its end, a tapered, feathered end point can be achieved.

Irrigation and clearing of debris After removal of the specimen, the intimectomized surface is vigorously irrigated with heparinized saline. Any medial debris present is carefully removed. The distal end point is irrigated to determine whether there is a residual flap that might lead to subsequent intimal dissection; if there is a flap, it is carefully removed. If there is a sharp shelf at the distal end point, it is usually an indication that the endarterectomy has not been carried far enough distally. When this is the case, the arteriotomy should be lengthened so that the endarterectomy can be extended to a point where the intima is completely normal. If the patient has a very high carotid bifurcation, very distal plaque, or both and further dissection is impeded by the base of the skull, it may be necessary to secure the distal end point with tacking sutures. Tacking sutures should be used only in exceptional circumstances because their use may lead to healing abnormalities or to the presence of platelet aggregate material that can cause thromboembolic or occlusive complications.

Once the intimectomized surface is completely clear of debris, the lumen of the external carotid artery should be visually inspected to confirm that all overlying dissected intima has been cleared. Any residual dissected intima can be gently teased out with a mosquito clamp. Once the vessel is completely clear, preparation is made for closure of the arteriotomy.

Closure of arteriotomy If the arteriotomy is relatively short and extends only up to the central portion of the bulb of the internal carotid artery, it can usually be closed primarily with a continuous 6-0 polypropylene suture. Placing very small stitches close together in the internal carotid artery should minimize the risk of vessel narrowing.

If the vessel is relatively small or the arteriotomy was extended well up on the internal carotid artery to ensure a complete endarterectomy, the arteriotomy should be closed with a patch angioplasty. Of the several patch options available, the basic choice is between a prosthetic patch and an autogenous patch composed of a segment of saphenous vein obtained from an extremity. The relative merits of autogenous and prosthetic patches have been extensively debated in the literature, but no definitive conclusions have been reached. One of the disadvantages of an autogenous patch is that surgeons tend to use the entire open portion of the saphenous vein, which then dilates further under arterial pressure, leading to an artery of aneurysmal proportions. Another disadvantage is the potential for patch blowout, which, though rare, has been reported in several series. The main disadvantage of a prosthetic patch is the risk of infection, but this is extremely low.

At present, it would appear that a prosthetic patch is at least as acceptable as an autogenous patch, and the prosthetic patch has an additional advantage in that there is no need to remove a normal saphenous vein segment from an extremity. Prosthetic patches can be composed of either fabric or polytetrafluoroethylene (PTFE). Fabric patches now come impregnated with either collagen or gelatin to make them leakproof; PTFE patches do not leak on the surface, but they are prone to leakage at suture needle puncture sites.

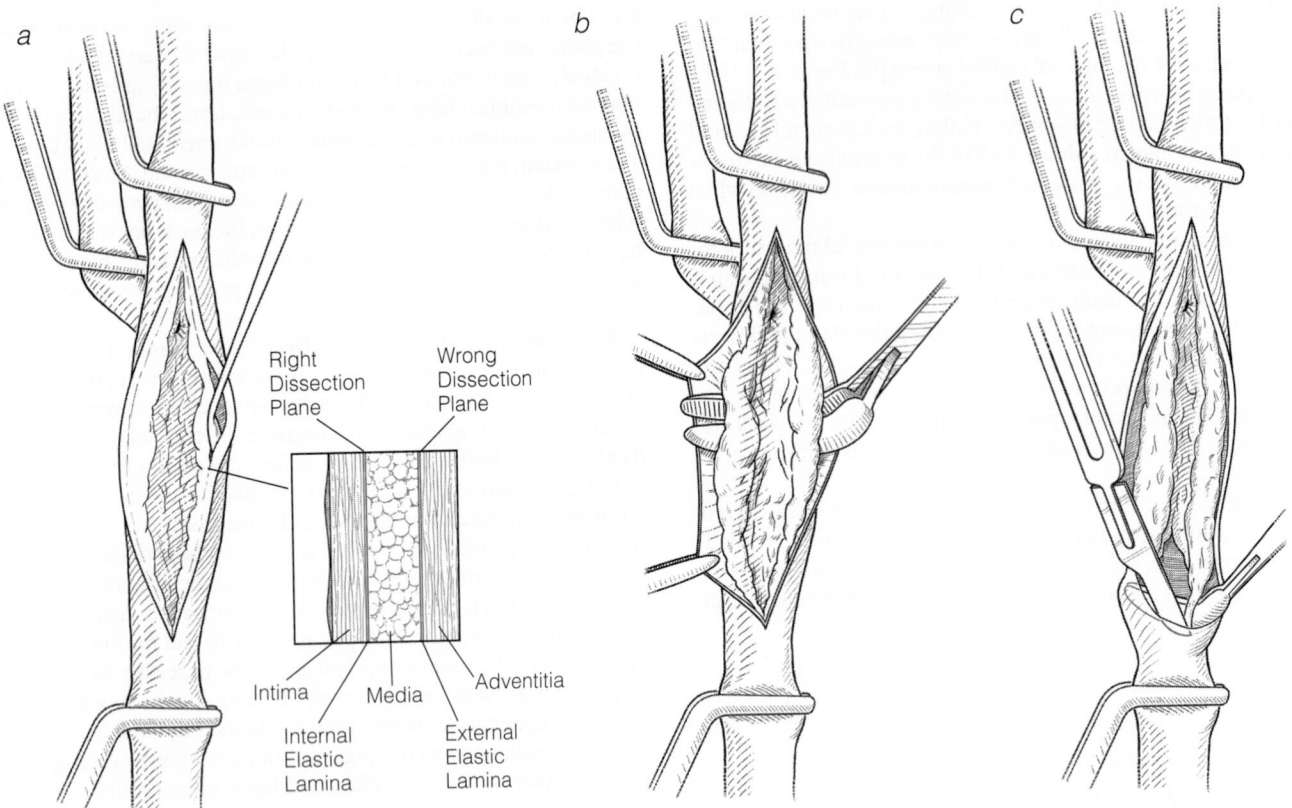

Figure 12 **Carotid arterial procedures: open endarterectomy. (*a*) The endarterectomy plane is started at the point where plaque is thickest and ideally is developed between the diseased intima and the media. Dissection proceeds both proximally and distally along one side of the arteriotomy. (*b*) Once dissection is complete on one side, a right-angle clamp is used to establish the same plane on the opposite side. (*c*) The end point of proximal dissection is established by sharp division of the plague against the clamp.**

Patch size is a crucial consideration: it is important that the patch be neither too wide nor too narrow. If the patch is too narrow, it will not provide the additional material needed to restore the carotid bifurcation to a normal diameter. If the patch is too wide, it will provide too much additional material and create what virtually amounts to a carotid aneurysm; this would represent a significant disadvantage to the patient in terms of flow dynamics and the risk of producing laminated thrombus in the most dilated portion of the carotid bulb. My preference is to use a 6.0 mm wide collagen-impregnated fabric patch for patch angioplasty.

Whichever patch is selected is cut to length, beveled at each end, and sewn in place with a continuous 6-0 polypropylene suture.

Before completion of the closure, the internal carotid artery and the external carotid artery are back-bled, and the common carotid artery is flushed. The arteriotomy is then completely closed. Removing the clamp on the internal carotid artery allows blood flow to fill the carotid bulb and permits one last internal flush. The origin of the internal carotid artery is then occluded with a vascular forceps, and the clamps are removed first from the external carotid artery and then from the common carotid artery to allow resumption of blood flow. After several heartbeats, the forceps on the origin of the internal carotid artery is removed, and blood flow through the internal carotid artery is restored. There may be some leakage of blood along the suture line, which can usually be controlled with the placement of thrombin-soaked absorbable gelatin sponge. If any obvious defect is noted between sutures, an additional stitch should be placed.

Eversion Endarterectomy

Eversion endarterectomy was designed and developed to eliminate the need for a suture line on the internal carotid artery, in the hope that doing so would reduce the incidence of myointimal hyperplasia and consequent restenosis. There is evidence to suggest that the use of eversion endarterectomy has led to some reduction in the incidence of myointimal hyperplasia, but the data are controversial and certainly are not conclusive. Nonetheless, the technique may well have merit, and it should be a part of the vascular surgeon's armamentarium.

Besides the avoidance of a suture line on the internal artery, the advantages of eversion endarterectomy include the simple end-to-side anastomotic closure and the possibility of managing a redundant internal carotid artery by moving it down the common carotid artery. One disadvantage is the potential difficulty of achieving an end point in cases in which the bifurcation is high or plaque extends well up the internal carotid artery toward the base of the skull. Another disadvantage arises with patients who require an internal shunt, in that it is not possible to keep an internal shunt in place for the entire duration of an eversion endarterectomy. Yet another disadvantage is that the distal end point cannot be viewed as clearly as it can in open endarterectomy. A fourth disadvantage is that eversion endarterectomy is poorly suited to cases in which the internal carotid artery is relatively small and contracted and thus better treated with patch angioplasty.

Eversion and plaque dissection After the carotid bifurcation is fully mobilized, the internal, external, and common carotid arteries are clamped. A circumferential incision is placed in an oblique fashion at the junction of the common carotid artery and the bulb of the internal carotid artery to permit division of the bulbous portion of the internal carotid artery from the common carotid [*see Figure 13*]. The edges of the adventitia of the bulb of the internal carotid artery are grasped, and the outer layers of the vessel wall are gradually everted away from the plaque within the artery. Eversion continues cephalad until it reaches the distal end point of the atherosclerotic lesion, which is marked by the presence of a thin, filmy intima that clearly separates with the specimen, leaving normal vessel behind. The plaque in the common carotid artery and the external carotid artery is then removed in the traditional manner; the opening in the common carotid artery may be extended proximally to facilitate this portion of the endarterectomy.

Reversion and reanastomosis   The internal carotid artery is then reverted to its normal anatomic position, and an anastomosis between the end of the divided bulb of the internal carotid artery and the common carotid artery is fashioned with a continuous 6-0 polypropylene suture. If the internal carotid artery is redundant [*see Special Considerations, below*], the arteriotomy on the common carotid artery is extended proximally and the arteriotomy on the medial aspect of the bulb of the internal carotid artery is extended distally so that the carotid bifurcation may be advanced between the internal and common carotid arteries to eliminate the redundancy.

Reconstruction for Proximal Lesions of Common Carotid Artery

Lesions at the origin of the common carotid artery, either at the level of the aortic arch (in the case of the left common carotid artery) or at the innominate bifurcation (in the case of the right common carotid artery), are relatively rare but do occur. Such lesions may arise either in isolation or in combination with carotid bifurcation disease. They can be managed by dividing the common carotid artery and transposing it to the adjacent subclavian artery, provided that there is no occlusive disease in the ipsilateral subclavian artery.

Exposure and mobilization   If the lesion at the origin of the common carotid artery is the only one being treated, both the common carotid artery and the subclavian artery should be exposed through a supraclavicular incision that parallels the clavicle. If a carotid bifurcation lesion is present in conjunction with the lesion at the origin of the common carotid artery, the supraclavicular incision is supplemented with a vertical incision along the sternocleidomastoid muscle to permit exposure of the carotid bifurcation. Exposure of the bifurcation has already been addressed (see above); accordingly, I focus here on exposure of the subclavian artery and the proximal common carotid artery.

A supraclavicular incision is placed approximately 1.5 fingerbreadths above the clavicle and centered over the lateral head of the sternocleidomastoid muscle. The lateral head of the sternocleidomastoid muscle is divided, and the scalene triangle is defined. The scalene fat pad is mobilized off the anterior scalene muscle. The phrenic nerve is identified, mobilized off the scalene muscle, and gently retracted. A plane is developed with gentle dissection between the posterior portion of the anterior scalene muscle and the underlying subclavian artery, and the anterior scalene muscle is divided. Division of the muscle exposes the underlying subclavian artery, a sufficient length of which can then be mobilized in the perivascular plane to permit an anastomosis.

The jugular vein is identified at the medial aspect of the incision and mobilized anteriorly and medially to expose the common carot-

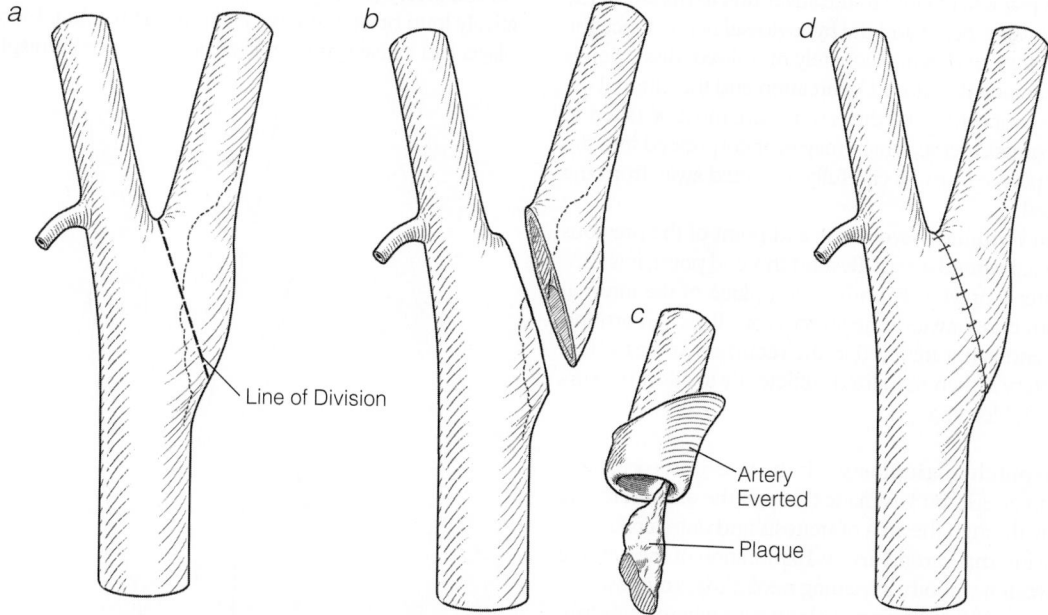

Figure 13 Carotid arterial procedures: eversion endarterectomy. (*a, b*) The internal carotid artery is divided from the common carotid artery in an oblique line. (*c*) The divided internal carotid artery is everted on itself so that it can be separated from the underlying plaque. Eversion proceeds distally until the plaque end point is encountered, and the plaque is removed from the internal carotid artery. Proximal endarterectomy of the common carotid artery and endarterectomy of the external carotid artery are then carried out. (*d*) Once all of the plaque has been removed, the internal carotid artery is reverted and an end-to-side anastomosis is fashioned between the common carotid artery opening and the internal carotid artery.

id artery. The vagus nerve is identified and carefully protected. The common carotid artery is then mobilized both proximally and distally; proximal mobilization should extend as far behind the sternoclavicular junction as the surgeon can comfortably manage.

Transection and anastomosis   The common carotid artery is clamped proximally and distally, then divided; the proximal portion of the vessel is oversewn. The transected common carotid artery is brought posterior to the jugular vein in the vicinity of the subclavian artery. The subclavian artery is clamped proximally and distally, a longitudinal arteriotomy is made, and a small ellipse of subclavian arterial tissue is removed. The end of the common carotid artery is then sewn to the side of the subclavian artery with a continuous 6-0 polypropylene suture.

Before completion, the vessels are back-bled and flushed. Once the anastomosis is complete, blood flow is restored, first to the distal subclavian artery and then to the common carotid artery.

Reconstruction for Recurrent Carotid Stenosis

For an initial recurrence of carotid stenosis that primarily results from myointimal hyperplasia, conversion to a patch angioplasty is generally the best treatment. For second or third recurrences or for recurrences that develop in spite of patch angioplasty, resection of the carotid bifurcation with interposition grafting between the common carotid artery and the normal distal internal carotid artery is the best treatment.

Exposure and mobilization   Exposure of a carotid bifurcation for treatment of recurrent carotid stenosis can be challenging. The initial skin incision is reopened, and dissection is carried down through the scar tissue to the common carotid artery. The common carotid artery is sharply dissected from the surrounding scar tissue, with the dissection plane kept close to the adventitia to minimize the risk of injury to the vagus nerve and the hypoglossal nerve. Once the common carotid artery has been adequately mobilized, dissection is carried distally to include the carotid bifurcation and the internal carotid artery. In the course of distal dissection, care must be taken to watch for the hypoglossal nerve, which may be incorporated into the scar tissue; this structure must be carefully dissected away from the artery and protected.

Distal dissection continues beyond the end point of the previous closure of the internal carotid artery. Beyond this end point, it is usually possible to enter a previously undissected plane of the internal carotid artery; from here onward, the artery typically is soft around its circumference and is not involved in the recurrent stenosis. The external carotid artery is then mobilized sufficiently to allow the surgeon to control back-bleeding.

Conversion to patch angioplasty   If the artery was originally closed primarily, an arteriotomy is made through the old suture line and carried distally through the area of stenosis and onto a relatively normal area of the internal carotid artery. Exploration of the luminal surface usually reveals a smooth, glistening neointima, and observation of the cut section of the artery reveals an area where a whitish, firm thickening of the intimal wall has occurred as a result of myointimal hyperplasia. No attempt should be made to reendarterectomize the stenotic area, because the intimal lesion is not, in fact, plaque but scar tissue. If the intima is removed, the cascade of events that led to the myointimal hyperplasia will simply be reinitiated. Accordingly, the healed intimal surface should be carefully protected. A patch angioplasty across the stenotic area, extending from the common carotid artery proximally to a relatively normal portion of the internal carotid artery distally, is usually sufficient to treat the lesion.

Resection of carotid bifurcation with interposition grafting
If the stenosis is recurring for the second or third time or the artery was originally closed with a patch, the surgeon should proceed with resection and interposition grafting. In most cases, it is necessary to sacrifice the external carotid artery and oversew its origin. The internal carotid artery is divided distal to the intimal hyperplastic lesion, the common carotid artery is divided proximally, and the diseased specimen is removed.

I prefer to use 6.0 mm thin-walled PTFE for the interposition graft. The internal carotid artery distally and the common carotid artery proximally are spatulated by making vertical incisions approximately 6.0 mm in length. The PTFE graft is appropriately beveled both proximally and distally, and beveled or spatulated end-to-end anastomoses are performed, first to the internal carotid artery and then to the common carotid artery.

Before completion, the vessels are back-bled and flushed; once the anastomoses are complete, blood flow is reestablished.

Some surgeons may be tempted to use autogenous saphenous vein for the interposition graft. To use such grafts would appear, on the face of it, to be a good idea; in fact, it is a mistake. For reasons not clearly understood, the use of autogenous saphenous vein in the neck has an extremely poor track record, yielding unacceptably high rates of recurrent stenosis and occlusion in comparison with the use of prosthetic grafts.

Special Considerations

Fibromuscular dysplasia of internal carotid artery   Fibromuscular dysplasia of the internal carotid artery is a congenital or acquired lesion that has been subdivided into four pathologic varieties, of which the most common is medial fibroplasia. On contrast angiography, medial fibroplasia has a characteristic appearance, resembling a string of beads in the extracranial portion of the internal carotid artery [*see Figure 14*]. A common initial manifestation is a relatively loud bruit in the neck of a young woman. Fibromuscular dysplasia can cause symptoms of monocular or hemispheric TIAs, or it

Figure 14   **Carotid arterial procedures: repair of fibromuscular dysplasia. Depicted is the so-called string of beads deformity of the cervical portion of the internal carotid artery, which is characteristic of medial fibroplasia.**

Figure 15 Carotid arterial procedures: repair of fibromuscular dysplasia. (*a*) The proximal portion of the internal carotid bulb is clamped, a transverse arteriotomy is made, and a coronary dilator is passed into the internal carotid artery and advanced up the vessel to the base of the skull. (*b*) The small septa in the internal carotid artery are disrupted by the advancing probe.

may go on to cause a stroke, usually as a consequence of a dissection resulting in thrombotic occlusion. If symptoms develop, they can generally be controlled by means of antiplatelet drugs. Currently, the only indication for surgical intervention is the persistence of symptoms despite antiplatelet therapy.

Treatment of fibromuscular dysplasia has evolved in recent years. The first attempts at surgical repair involved a total resection of the internal carotid artery coupled with interposition of a graft (usually composed of saphenous vein). This technique is now largely abandoned because of the extensive surgical dissection required and the substantial risk of cranial nerve injury; its only remaining application is in cases where there is associated aneurysmal dilatation in the dysplastic segment that calls for resection and graft interposition. At present, the two most popular modes of therapy both involve intraluminal dilatation with disruption of the small septa within the artery. One mode achieves intraluminal dilatation via an open approach, and the other achieves the same end via a percutaneous approach that includes balloon angioplasty. Dilatation and fracturing of the intraluminal septa often result in the release of particles of septal tissue, which in turn can lead to cerebral embolization and infarction. Consequently, open methods, which enable the surgeon to flush out the disrupted segments, are usually favored.

In symptomatic patients with fibromuscular dysplasia, the carotid bifurcation may be exposed in the usual manner. If there is significant redundancy of the internal carotid artery, as documented by preoperative imaging, the artery should be mobilized relatively extensively so that it can be straightened by downward traction before intraluminal dilatation is begun. If, on the other hand, the artery is relatively straight, only minimal mobilization is required. It should be kept in mind that approximately 25% of patients with fibromuscular dysplasia have associated atheromatous disease of the carotid bifurcation that must be dealt with at the time of operation. In addi-

tion, about the same number of patients have associated intracranial aneurysms that should be checked for by means of intracranial imaging studies.

Once the carotid bifurcation has been suitably mobilized and it has been established that no associated atheromatous plaque is present, a small transverse incision is made on the bulb of the internal carotid artery, with flow being maintained between the common and external carotid arteries. Serial intraluminal dilatations are then performed with coronary artery dilators of progressively increasing diameter [see Figure 15]. The first dilator (usually 2.5 mm in diameter) is passed up the carotid artery to the base of the skull under digital control. The dilator is then withdrawn, and the artery is back-bled to flush out any fractured segments. The next larger dilator (3.0 mm in diameter) is passed in a similar fashion. Dilatation is repeated with progressively larger dilators (3.5, 4.0, and possibly 4.5 mm in diameter) to complete the procedure.

The transverse arteriotomy is closed with 6-0 polypropylene suture material and flow is reestablished. A completion angiogram verifies that the dysplastic segment is fully restored.

Coiling or kinking of internal carotid artery Redundancy of the internal carotid artery, often resulting in a 360° coil of the high cervical portion of the internal carotid artery, is usually thought to be developmental in origin [see Figure 16a]. Elongation of the internal carotid artery, which often results in kinking of the vessel, is believed to be related to the degenerative changes that occur with aging and atherosclerosis [see Figure 16b]. Both of these phenomena, in and of themselves, are usually asymptomatic; exceptions occur when an atheromatous plaque develops at the apex of the coil or when kinking of the internal carotid artery is accentuated with changes in head position in a patient who depends on relatively normal blood flow through that vessel. Redundancy of the internal carotid artery often becomes a technical consideration during standard surgical treatment of a carotid bifurcation atheroma. When redundancy occurs, it must be appropriately dealt with to prevent postoperative complications.

Figure 16 Carotid arterial procedures: repair of coiling or kinking of the internal carotid artery. (*a, b*) Redundancy of the internal carotid artery can result in one or more 360° coils in the vessel. (*c*) Degenerative atheromatous changes of the internal carotid artery can cause elongation with associated kinking or buckling.

Anticipated redundancy of the internal carotid artery at the time of carotid bifurcation endarterectomy can usually be managed with a patch angioplasty. Provided that the arteriotomy extends beyond the apex of the kink, the patch should smooth out the curvature of the redundant vessel and eliminate the kink. If it appears that internal carotid artery redundancy is greater than can be corrected by an elongated patch, then detachment of the internal carotid artery followed by eversion endarterectomy and reimplantation is indicated.

If the arteriotomy has already been closed when it becomes apparent that a kink is present, the problem may be dealt with by mobilizing the external carotid artery sufficiently and then resecting a segment of the common carotid artery and pulling down on the carotid bifurcation with a new end-to-end anastomosis to straighten the redundant internal carotid artery [see Figure 17]. Segmental resection of the internal carotid artery itself combined with end-to-end repair has also been described; this approach is less desirable, being more technically demanding and hence more subject to technical error.

Patients with coiling of the internal carotid artery may present a more difficult problem. If the atheromatous plaque involves only the first portion of the internal carotid artery and the vessel beyond that first portion is relatively normal up to the point where coiling begins, the surgeon can simply avoid the problem by leaving the smooth coil in place and not carrying out an extensive distal dissection. If, on the other hand, it appears that there may be plaque in the coil, then the entire coil must be dissected free, and the patient is left with a very redundant internal carotid artery that must be dealt with. Once again, the best method of managing the problem is to resect the redundant segment of the internal carotid artery, with or without eversion endarterectomy, and to reimplant the internal carotid artery onto the distal common carotid artery at the point of transection.

Upon completion of the reconstruction, a completion angiogram should be obtained to verify that the coiling or kinking has been adequately treated.

STEP 5: COMPLETION IMAGING

Given that the majority of neurologic complications after carotid artery surgery are attributable to technical error, it is imperative that the technical accuracy of the reconstruction be confirmed before the incision is closed and the patient is sent to the recovery room. There are two principal methods of determining the technical quality of the reconstruction: on-table angiography and direct-contact duplex scanning of the carotid artery. To perform either of these techniques routinely in all patients adds relatively little time to the surgical procedure and offers significant advantages to both the patient and the surgeon.[10,11]

My preferred method of confirming the quality of the reconstruction is completion angiography using a C-arm with digital imaging. For this reason, the operation is done on a table that has angiographic capability, and the radiology technician and the equipment are called for at the beginning of the arteriotomy closure. A 10 ml syringe is connected to flexible tubing, and a 20-gauge needle is attached to the end of the tubing and bent at a 45° angle. Air bubbles are carefully evacuated from the tubing and the needle. Placing the needle into the artery or, in the case of a patched artery, into the midportion of the patch in a retrograde fashion will provide good stability for the needle, which lies in the lumen of the artery in an axial position. Once the C-arm is in place and the fluoroscopy unit turned on, the contrast material is injected by hand. The resulting image of the carotid bifurcation can be continuously replayed until maximal radiographic opacity of the carotid bifurcation and the intracranial circulation has been attained. The image is then carefully inspected for defects at the end points in the internal and external carotid arteries.

Intimal defects in the internal carotid artery are unusual, though

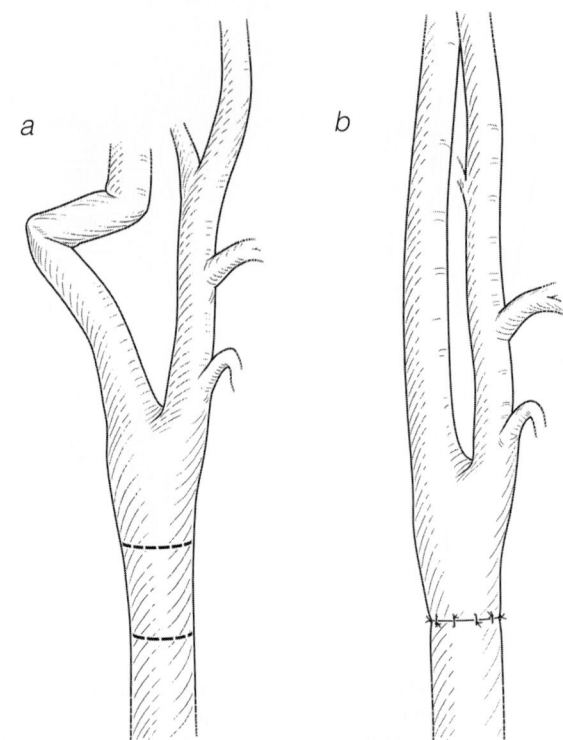

Figure 17 **Carotid arterial procedures: repair of coiling or kinking of the internal carotid artery. Kinking or redundancy of the internal carotid artery can be managed by mobilizing the external carotid artery, then resecting a segment of the common carotid artery (*a*). The surgeon can then draw down the carotid bifurcation for a new primary anastomosis (*b*).**

not unknown. Defects in the external carotid artery are more common because the endarterectomy is essentially done in a blind or closed manner. Defects in the external carotid artery are matters of concern because they may lead to thrombus formation in the external carotid artery; if the thrombus propagates proximally, it may embolize up the internal carotid artery and cause a stroke.[12] For this reason, if a defect is found in the external carotid artery, it is repaired at the time of the operation. To accomplish the repair, clamps are placed on the external carotid artery proximally at its origin and distally beyond the intimal flap. A transverse arteriotomy is made in the external carotid artery to permit identification and removal of the intimal flap. Once the flap has been carefully removed, the transverse arteriotomy is closed with two or three interrupted 6-0 polypropylene sutures and flow is restored.

Completion angiography also has the advantage of permitting the surgeon to image the intracranial circulation. Now that many operations are being performed on the basis of preoperative carotid duplex scanning, intracranial imaging is typically unavailable beforehand, which means that the status of the intracranial circulation with respect to atherosclerotic lesions in the area of the siphon or the middle cerebral artery or with respect to intracranial aneurysms is usually unknown at the start of the procedure. A completion angiogram gives the surgeon the opportunity to rule out these lesions by looking not only at the area around the reconstruction but also at the intracranial circulation.

An alternative to completion angiography is DUS. DUS can be a highly satisfactory way of examining the area of reconstruction, provided that the operating room has duplex scanning capability and that a technologist is available to operate the equipment. Standard B-mode imaging, in conjunction with Doppler ultrasonography, can accurately identify patent or compromised internal and external carotid arteries.

Once the surgeon has confirmed that a good technical reconstruction has been achieved, preparations can be made for closure.

STEP 6: CLOSURE

The dissected area around the reconstructed carotid artery is carefully irrigated with an antibiotic solution, and the wound is meticulously inspected for hemostasis. Even when good hemostasis has been achieved, it is my practice to place a drain overnight—specifically, a 7.0 mm Jackson-Pratt drain brought out through a small separate stab wound. The platysmal layer is closed with a continuous 3-0 absorbable suture, and the skin is closed with a continuous 4-0 subcuticular absorbable suture. A clear adhesive plastic dressing is applied to the skin, and the patient is sent to the recovery room.

Postoperative Management

The main patient variables to be evaluated in the postoperative period are neurologic status, blood pressure, and wound stability.

On awakening from anesthesia, the patient is carefully observed with a view to determining gross cerebral function on the basis of response to commands and movement of extremities. When the patient is fully awake, vagus nerve and hypoglossal nerve function can be tested.

Blood pressure monitoring is of critical importance after carotid endarterectomy. It is essential first to decide on an acceptable blood pressure range for the patient and then to ensure that this pressure is maintained: neither hypertension nor hypotension is acceptable. Patients with severe carotid bifurcation disease who have undergone carotid endarterectomy temporarily lose autoregulation on the side of the operation; therefore, hypertension can result in reperfusion injury to that side of the brain, ranging all the way from simple headache to fatal intracerebral hemorrhage.

The surgical site should be carefully observed for possible wound expansion resulting from hematoma formation. Even when good hemostasis is achieved and a drain is in place, there is still the possibility of delayed bleeding leading to hematoma and airway compromise. If an expanding hematoma is noted, the safest response is to return the patient to the OR so that the hematoma can be evacuated and a bleeding site sought. The earlier this is done, the better.

If the patient is neurologically intact, blood pressure is well controlled, and there is no evidence of an expanding hematoma, then the remaining postoperative care can be provided in a regular hospital room. It is seldom necessary to observe the patient in the intensive care unit, as was once standard practice.

Follow-up

Periodic follow-up examination is essential. There are two major areas of concern: (1) the possibility of recurrent stenosis on the operated side and (2) the possibility of disease developing or progressing in the contralateral carotid artery. It is my practice to see the patient approximately 3 weeks after carotid endarterectomy. In that visit, the patient is examined for quality of wound healing and the presence or absence of carotid bruit on both the operated side and the contralateral side, and a carotid duplex scan is performed. If at this time there are no grounds for concern about the contralateral side, scanning is done only on the side of the operation. The scan serves to establish the new baseline and confirms that the carotid reconstruction is satisfactory. The new baseline is then used as the basis for assessing patient status during subsequent follow-up.

The next patient visit takes place 6 months after operation, at which time a bilateral carotid duplex scan is performed. If the operated side continues to be normal and there are no major problems on the contralateral side, the patient is seen again at the 1-year anniversary of the procedure. If examinations yield satisfactory results at this time, the patient may thereafter be seen at 1-year intervals, with bilateral carotid duplex scanning done at each visit.

Alternatives to Direct Carotid Reconstruction

Stented balloon angioplasty of the carotid bifurcation and the common carotid artery is currently under investigation as an alternative to direct carotid reconstruction. Several phase I studies have been published. Some report unacceptably high incidences of perioperative stroke, but others report complication rates comparable to those of carotid endarterectomy. It appears that a state of clinical equipoise exists. A prospective, randomized trial comparing carotid endarterectomy with stented balloon angioplasty in symptomatic patients is under way. It is anticipated that the trial will be completed by 2006.

References

1. Beneficial effect of carotid endarterectomy in symptomatic patients with high-grade carotid stenosis. North American Symptomatic Carotid Endarterectomy Trial Collaborators. N Engl J Med 325:445, 1991
2. MRC European Carotid Surgery Trial: interim results for symptomatic patients with severe (70-99%) or with mild (0-29%) carotid stenosis. European Carotid Trialists' Collaborative Group. Lancet 337:1235, 1991
3. Mayberg MR, Wilson SE, Yatsu F, et al: Carotid endarterectomy and prevention of cerebral ischemia in symptomatic carotid stenosis. Veterans Affairs Cooperative Studies Program 309 Trialist Group. JAMA 266:3332, 1991
4. Endarterectomy for asymptomatic carotid artery stenosis. Executive Committee for the Asymptomatic Carotid Atherosclerosis Study. JAMA 273:1421, 1995
5. Hobson RW II, Weiss DG, Fields WS, et al: Efficacy of carotid endarterectomy for asymptomatic carotid stenosis. The Veterans Affairs Asymptomatic Cooperative Study Group. N Engl J Med 328:221, 1993
6. Moore WS, Barnett HJM, Beebe HG, et al: Guidelines for carotid endarterectomy—a multidisciplinary consensus statement from the Ad Hoc Committee, American Heart Association. Circulation 91:566, 1995
7. Fisher DF Jr, Clagett GP, Parker JI, et al: Mandibular subluxation for high carotid exposure. J Vasc Surg 1:727, 1984
8. Moore WS, Yee JM, Hall AD: Collateral cerebral blood pressure—an index of tolerance to temporary carotid occlusion. Arch Surg 106:520, 1973
9. Moore WS, Hall AD. Carotid artery back pressure—a test of cerebral tolerance to temporary carotid occlusion. Arch Surg 99:702, 1969
10. Blaisdell FW, Lim R Jr, Hall AD: Technical results of carotid endarterectomy: arteriographic assessment. Am J Surg 114:239, 1967
11. Schwartz RA, Peterson GJ, Noland KA, et al: Intraoperative duplex scanning after carotid reconstruction: a valuable tool. J Vasc Surg 7:260, 1988
12. Moore WS, Martello JY, Quiñones-Baldrich WJ, et al: Etiologic importance of the intimal flap of the external carotid artery in the development of post-carotid endarterectomy stroke. Stroke 21:1497, 1990

Recommended Reading

Eastcott HHG, Pickering GW, Robb C: Reconstruction of internal carotid artery in a patient with intermittent attacks of hemiplegia. Lancet 2:994, 1954

Matsumoto GH, Cossman D, Callow AD: Hazards and safeguards during carotid endarterectomy: technical considerations. Am J Surg 133:485, 1977

Mock CN, Michael PL, McRae RG, et al: Selection of the approach to the distal internal carotid artery from the second cervical vertebra to the base of the skull. J Vasc Surg 13:846, 1991

Moore WS: Surgery for Cerebrovascular Disease, 2nd ed. WB Saunders Co, Philadelphia, 1996

Sundt TM, Sharbrough FW, Anderson E, et al: Cerebral blood flow measurements and electroencephalogram during carotid endarterectomy. J Neurosurg 41:310, 1974

Acknowledgment

Figures 1 through 17 Tom Moore.

24 REPAIR OF INFRARENAL ABDOMINAL AORTIC ANEURYSMS

Frank R. Arko, M.D., and Christopher K. Zarins, M.D.

An arterial aneurysm is defined as a permanent localized enlargement of an artery to a diameter more than 1.5 times its expected diameter. Aneurysms are classified according to morphology, etiology, and anatomic site. The most common morphology is a fusiform, symmetrical, circumferential enlargement that involves all layers of the arterial wall. A saccular morphology is also seen, in which aneurysmal degeneration affects only part of the arterial circumference.

The most common cause of an arterial aneurysm is atherosclerotic degeneration of the arterial wall. The pathogenesis is a multifactorial process involving genetic predisposition, aging, atherosclerosis, inflammation, and localized activation of proteolytic enzymes. Most aneurysms occur in elderly persons, and the prevalence rises with increasing age. Aneurysms also occur in genetically susceptible individuals with Ehlers-Danlos syndrome or Marfan syndrome. Other causes include tertiary syphilis and localized infection resulting in a mycotic aneurysm.

Aneurysms of the infrarenal aorta are by far the most common arterial aneurysms encountered in clinical practice today: they are three to seven times more common than thoracic aneurysms and affect four times as many men as women.[1] Abdominal aortic aneurysms (AAAs) have a tendency to enlarge and rupture, causing death. In the United States, AAAs result in approximately 15,000 deaths each year and are thus the 13th leading cause of death in the United States.[2,3] The only way to reduce the death rate is to identify and treat aortic aneurysms before they rupture.

Preoperative Evaluation

IDENTIFICATION OF RISK FACTORS

For successful surgical reconstruction of AAAs, any significant comorbidities that would increase the risk of operative repair must be identified and managed at an early stage. Patients undergoing the procedure usually are elderly and often have coexisting cardiac, pulmonary, cerebrovascular, renal, or peripheral vascular disease. The major anesthetic risk factors for elective resection of AAAs are similar to those for other major intra-abdominal operations; in particular, they include inadequate cardiopulmonary and renal function. Patients with unstable angina or angina at rest, a cardiac ejection fraction of less than 25%, a serum creatinine concentration higher than 3 mg/dl, or pulmonary disease (manifested by oxygen tension < 50 mm Hg, elevated carbon dioxide tension, or both on room air) are considered to be at high risk.[4,5]

Myocardial ischemia is the most common cause of perioperative morbidity and mortality after arterial reconstruction of the aorta. Optimization of preoperative medical management, perioperative invasive monitoring, and long-term risk factor modification are all facilitated by an accurate preoperative cardiac evaluation. Such evaluation may include transthoracic echocardiography, exercise stress testing, myocardial scintigraphy, stress echocardiography, and coronary angiography; each test has its own merits and limitations with regard to clinical risk assessment. To reduce the mortality associated with resection of AAAs, it is necessary not only to identify high-risk groups but also to institute appropriate preoperative, intraoperative, and postoperative alterations in patient care. Patients who have severe coronary disease (manifested by unstable angina, ischemic congestive heart failure, or recent myocardial infarction [MI]) benefit from invasive cardiac evaluation and possibly from preliminary coronary intervention.

With intensive perioperative monitoring and support in place, resection of AAAs has been successfully performed even in high-risk patients, with operative mortalities of less than 6%.[6-8]

CONFIRMATION OF DIAGNOSIS AND DETERMINATION OF ANEURYSM SIZE

Physical examination suffices for detection of most large aneurysms. To determine the exact size of the aneurysm as well as to identify smaller aneurysms, however, more objective methods are available and should be used. Determination of the size of the aneurysm is extremely important because size is the most important determinant of the likelihood of rupture and plays a crucial role in subsequent management decisions. Imaging modalities commonly employed to diagnose and measure aneurysms include duplex ultrasonography (DUS), aortography, computed tomography, and magnetic resonance imaging.

The main advantages of DUS are its ready availability in both inpatient and outpatient settings, its low cost, its safety, and its good performance; many studies have documented the ability of DUS to establish the diagnosis and accurately determine the size of AAAs [see Figure 1].[9-11] The primary limitations of DUS are that imaging of the thoracic and suprarenal aorta is poor, that the quality of the images is considerably lower in the presence of obesity or large amounts of intestinal gas, and that it must be performed by a skilled imaging technician.

Aortography yields excellent images of the contours of the aortic lumen, but it is not a reliable method for determining the diameter of an aneurysm or even for establishing its presence, because the mural thrombus within the aneurysm tends to reduce the lumen to near-normal size. Nonetheless, aortography can be helpful in determining the extent of an aneurysm, especially when there is iliac or suprarenal involvement, defining associated arterial lesions involving the renal and visceral arteries, and detecting lower-extremity occlusive disease. There are risks associated with aortography that place some restrictions on its use. Among these risks are the potential renal toxicity resulting from the use of contrast agents. In addition, manipulation of catheters through the laminated mural thrombus increases the risk of distal embolization. Finally, local arterial complications may arise at the arterial puncture site.

CT provides reliable information about the size of the entire aorta, thereby allowing accurate determination of both the size and the extent of the AAA [see Figure 2]. Spiral CT scanning permits identification of the visceral and renal arteries and their relationship to the aneurysm. With the administration of I.V. contrast material, the aor-

Figure 1 **Duplex ultrasonography may be used as a screening test as well as to determine the actual size of the aneurysm.**

tic lumen, the amount and location of mural thrombus, and the presence or absence of retroperitoneal hematoma can all be assessed [*see Figure 3*]. Overall, spiral CT scanning is currently the most useful imaging method for evaluation of the abdominal aorta.

MRI is also useful in preoperative evaluation of aortic aneurysms.[12,13] It employs radiofrequency energy and a magnetic field to produce images in longitudinal, transverse, and coronal planes. The advantages of MRI over CT are that no ionizing radiation is administered, multiplane images can be obtained, and no nephrotoxic contrast agents are used.

CLASSIFICATION OF PATIENTS FOR ELECTIVE OR URGENT REPAIR

Patients may usefully be classified into three categories according to how they present for repair: (1) elective patients, (2) symptomatic patients, and (3) patients with ruptured aneurysms.

Elective aneurysm repair is recommended for asymptomatic patients who have aneurysms 5.0 cm in diameter or larger, who have an acceptable level of operative risk, and who have a life expectancy of 1 year or more. Furthermore, elective operation should be considered for patients with aneurysms smaller than 5.0 cm who are not at high operative risk if they are hypertensive or live in a remote area where proper medical care is not readily available. Repair is also appropriate for aneurysms that are between 4.0 and 5.0 cm in diameter and have shown growth of more than 0.5 cm on serial images in less than 6 to 12 months. Peripheral embolization originating from the aneurysm is an indication for repair, regardless of the size of the aneurysm.

Urgent operation is indicated for patients with symptomatic aneurysms, regardless of the size of the aneurysm. Such patients typically present with abdominal or back pain. Sometimes, the back pain radiates to the groin, much as in ureteral colic; this pain may be elicited by palpating the aneurysm. In most cases, DUS, CT, and MRI will reliably detect the presence of periaortic blood; however, the absence of this finding should not delay operation, because actual rupture of the aneurysm can occur at any time.

Emergency operation is indicated for almost all patients with known or suspected rupture of an aneurysm.

Operative Planning

Preoperative planning is essential for a successful outcome after repair of an infrarenal AAA. Like the choice between elective and urgent or emergency repair, operative planning is governed by the presentation of the patient. In patients with ruptured aneurysms, diagnosis is immediately followed by operative repair. In patients with symptomatic aneurysms, the amount of preoperative imaging done is balanced against the risk of impending rupture. In patients presenting for elective repair, it is generally possible to perform extensive imaging to determine whether the repair is best done via an endovascular approach or a standard open approach. Current preoperative imaging methods utilizing CT angiography obviate several common pitfalls. The recent introduction of endovascular techniques for excluding an aneurysm should not alter the patient selection criteria for aneurysm repair. Endovascular grafting does introduce certain morphologic criteria into the process of patient selection, in that stent grafting is appropriate only for patients in whom the infrarenal neck and the iliac arteries are suitable.

Given that the long-term outcome of endovascular grafting is currently unknown, younger patients who are at low operative risk and are expected to survive into the long term are typically better served with open surgical repair. In addition, patients who require additional abdominal or pelvic revascularization procedures, who have small or diseased access vessels, or who have short (< 10 mm) or tortuous infrarenal necks are not candidates for endovascular grafting and should undergo open surgical repair instead.

Preoperative preparation to optimize cardiopulmonary function, administration of preoperative antibiotics, and intraoperative hemodynamic monitoring with appropriate fluid management can significantly reduce the risks associated with AAA repair. Before aortic cross-clamping, appropriate volume loading, combined with vasodilatation, is carried out to help prevent declamping hypotension.

Figure 2 **Shown is a CT angiogram providing a three-dimensional reconstruction of an infrarenal AAA after endovascular repair. Of particular interest is the relation of the graft to the renal arteries and the hypogastric arteries distally.**

Figure 3   CT scanning assesses the size of the aneurysm, the amount of mural thrombus present, and the relation of other intra-abdominal structures to the aneurysm.

Operative Technique

OPEN REPAIR

Step 1: Initial Incision and Choice of Approach

Open surgical repair of infrarenal AAAs is performed through a transperitoneal or retroperitoneal exposure of the aorta with the patient under general endotracheal anesthesia. The aneurysm may be exposed through either a long midline incision (for the transperitoneal approach) or an oblique flank incision (for the retroperitoneal approach) [*see Figure 4a*]. An upper abdominal transverse incision may also be used for either retroperitoneal or transperitoneal exposure. The results with the two exposures are equivalent. The transperitoneal approach is preferred when exposure of the right renal artery is required and when access to the distal right iliac system or to intra-abdominal organs is necessary. The retroperitoneal exposure offers advantages when extensive peritoneal adhesions, an intestinal stoma, or severe pulmonary disease is present and when there is a need for suprarenal exposure. Use of the retroperitoneal approach has been associated with a shorter duration of postoperative ileus, a lower incidence of pulmonary complications, and a reduction in length of stay in the ICU.

Step 2 (Transperitoneal Approach): Exposure and Control of Aorta and Iliac Arteries

When the transperitoneal approach is used, the small bowel (including the duodenum) is retracted to the right, and the retroperitoneum overlying the aneurysm is divided to the left of the midline [*see Figure 4b*]. The duodenum is completely mobilized, and the left renal vein is identified and exposed. The normal infrarenal neck, which is just below the left renal vein, is then exposed and encircled for proximal control. Both common iliac arteries are then mobilized and controlled, with care taken to avoid the underlying iliac veins and ureters that cross over at the iliac bifurcation [*see Figure 5*]. If the common iliac arteries are aneurysmal, then both the internal and the external iliac arteries are controlled. The inferior mesenteric artery is then dissected out and controlled for possible reimplantation into the graft after the aneurysm has been repaired.

Step 2 (Retroperitoneal Approach): Exposure and Control of Aorta and Iliac Arteries

When the retroperitoneal approach is taken, a transverse left abdominal or flank incision is made, and the peritoneum is reflected anteriorly. The left kidney usually is left in place but may be mobilized anteriorly to expose the posterolateral aorta. Exposure of the right iliac system can be achieved by dividing the inferior mesenteric artery early in the course of dissection. The aorta and the iliac arteries are controlled in essentially the same fashion regardless of the type of incision used.

Step 3: Opening of Aneurysm and Creation of Proximal Anastomosis

Systemic anticoagulation with I.V. heparin is then performed. After sufficient time (3 to 5 minutes) has elapsed to permit adequate circulation, the infrarenal neck and the iliac arteries are clamped. To prevent distal embolization, the distal clamps should be applied before the proximal aortic clamp. The aneurysm is then opened longitudinally, the mural thrombus is removed, and back-bleeding lumbar arteries are oversewn. Depending on its degree of backflow and on the patency of the hypogastric arteries, the inferior mesenteric artery may be either ligated or clamped and left with a rim of aortic wall for subsequent reimplantation [*see* Troubleshooting, *below*].

The aortic neck is then partially or completely transected, and an appropriately sized tubular or bifurcated graft is sutured to the aorta with a continuous nonabsorbable monofilament suture [*see Figure 6*]. When the proximal aortic neck is very short, suprarenal aortic clamping may be required for performance of the proximal anastomosis. If suprarenal clamping is necessary, the security of the proximal anastomosis should be verified, and the clamp should then be moved onto the graft below the renal arteries as soon as possible to minimize renal ischemia. If the aorta is especially weak or friable, the anastomosis may be supported with Teflon-felt pledgets.

Step 4: Creation of Distal Anastomosis

When the aneurysm is confined to the aorta, the distal anastomosis is performed by suturing a straight tube graft to the aortic bi-

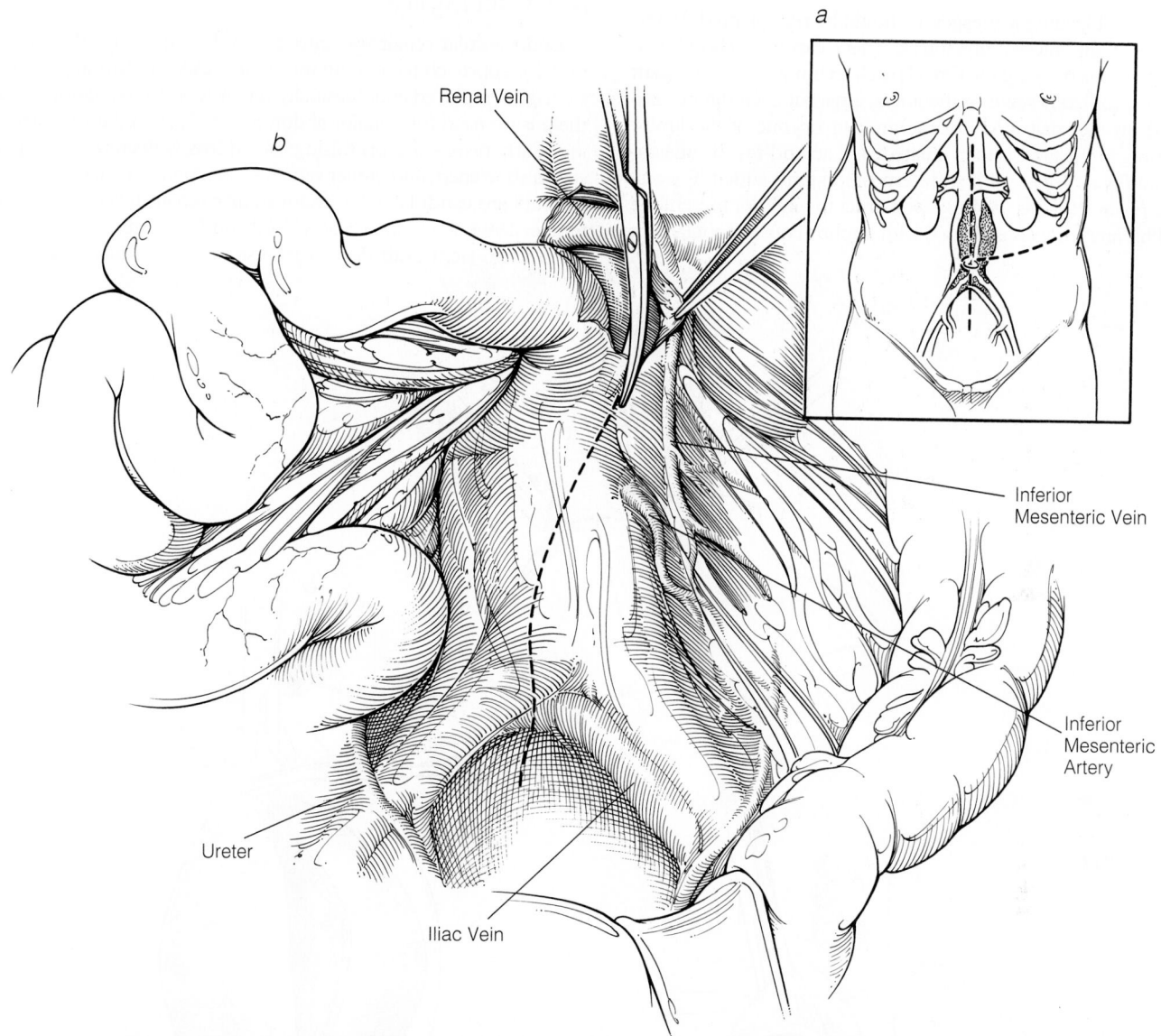

Figure 4 **Open repair of infrarenal AAAs. (a) For the transabdominal approach to the abdominal aorta, a midline or transverse incision is appropriate. For the retroperitoneal approach, an oblique flank incision may be used. (b) The small intestine (including the duodenum) is retracted laterally after the ligament of Treitz is mobilized, and the retroperitoneum is incised in the midline. The left renal vein is the landmark for the infrarenal neck.**

furcation [*see Figure 7*]; straight tube graft reconstructions are used about 30% of the time. Distally, the dissection should avoid the fibroareolar tissue overlying the left common iliac artery because this tissue contains branches of the inferior mesenteric artery and the autonomic nerves that control sexual function in men.

When the aneurysm extends into the common iliac arteries, the distal anastomosis is accomplished by suturing a bifurcated graft to the distal common iliac arteries or, in the case of significant occlusive disease, to the common femoral arteries. In these situations, control of the iliac arteries is best achieved by mobilizing the external and internal arteries and clamping them individually [*see Figure 8*]. It is sometimes easier to control iliac artery back-bleeding by using intraluminal balloon catheters and oversewing the common iliac arteries from within the opened aortic or iliac aneurysms. Care must be taken not to injure the accompanying venous structures or the ureters, which cross anterior to the iliac bifurcation. Every effort should be made to ensure perfusion of at least one hypogastric artery to help minimize the risk of postoperative left colon ischemia.

Declamping hypotension may occur after reperfusion of the lower extremities. It is essential to maintain communication with the anesthesiologist so that blood and fluid replacement can be adjusted in anticipation of lower-extremity reperfusion. Even though the graft and vessels are flushed and back-bled before distal flow is reestablished, it is preferable first to establish flow into one of the hypogastric arteries so as to minimize the chances of distal embolization to the legs.

Before the abdomen is closed, adequate perfusion of the lower extremities and the left colon should be ensured via either direct inspection or noninvasive monitoring. The open aneurysm sac is then sutured closed over the aortic graft to separate the graft from the duodenum and the viscera [*see Figure 9*]. This step reduces the risk of aortoenteric fistula.

Troubleshooting

If the inferior mesenteric artery is small and back-bleeding is adequate, it may be ligated [*see Figure 10a*]; however, if the vessel is large or back-bleeding is meager, it should be reimplanted. Reim- plantation of the inferior mesenteric artery can be accomplished with relative ease by using the Carrel patch technique. After the graft has been completely sewn to the aorta, a partial occluding clamp is placed on the main body of the graft or on one of the limbs. An opening in the graft is then created, and an end-to-side anasto- mosis [*see Figure 10b*]—with an interposition graft added if neces- sary [*see Figure 10c*]—is used to reconstruct the inferior mesenteric artery. This anastomosis is created with a continuous monofilament suture.

ENDOVASCULAR REPAIR

Endovascular repair was introduced during the 1990s as a less invasive approach to treating infrarenal AAAs. In this approach, a stent-graft is placed endoluminally via bilateral groin incisions; thus, there is no need for a major abdominal incision and aortic clamp- ing. Early results are promising: blood loss is decreased, hospital stay is shortened, and earlier return to function is achieved. Not all patients are candidates for endovascular repair, however. In Sep- tember 1999, the United States Food and Drug Administration ap- proved two stent-graft devices for use in surgical management of

Figure 5 **Open repair of infrarenal AAAs. (*a*) Once the aneurysm is exposed, proximal control is obtained by encir- cling the proximal neck with an umbilical tape or heavy Silastic. The inferior mesenteric artery is identified and then either clamped or ligated for possible reimplantation at the end of the procedure. (*b*) The iliac arteries are dissected free, systemic heparin anticoagulation is instituted, and distal control is obtained, followed by proximal control to prevent distal embolization. The aneurysm sac is then opened longitudinally. (*c*) All mural thrombus is removed, and the proximal and distal necks of the aorta are incised.**

Figure 6 **Open repair of infrarenal AAAs. (*a*) Back-bleeding lumbar arteries are over-sewn with figure-eight sutures to control bleeding. (*b, c, d*) The proximal anastomosis is sewn to the back wall of the aorta with a continuous nonabsorbable monofilament suture. (*e*) If the aorta is weak or friable, Teflon-felt pledgets may be used for additional support.**

AAAs: the Ancure device (Guidant, Indianapolis, Indiana), which is a balloon-expandable one-piece bifurcated stent-graft, and the AneuRx device (Medtronic AVE, Santa Rosa, California), which is a self-expanding bifurcated modular device that is fully supported externally by a nitinol stent.

Procedure-Specific Preoperative Preparation

Precise preoperative evaluation that yields accurate measurements will result in proper planning and effective prevention of problems. Both CT angiography and contrast biplane angiography are used for this purpose. Of the two, spiral CT angiography is currently preferred. This imaging modality is capable of obtaining high-quality images of the vascular anatomy and reconfiguring them into detailed three-dimensional images. For optimal evaluation, images should be obtained at 3 mm intervals from the celiac artery to the femoral arteries. Spiral CT angiography accurately defines the proximal and distal characteristics of the AAA as well as detects any sig-

nificant renal, visceral, or iliac occlusive disease. It is particularly helpful in defining the infrarenal neck between the renal arteries and the proximal portion of the aneurysm.

Angiography is employed as a complement to spiral CT angiography in this setting. An arteriogram is useful in that it helps define renal, mesenteric, and distal arterial anatomy; helps characterize tortuosity, calcification, and stenoses in access arteries; and helps determine the angles between the aorta, the proximal neck, and the aneurysm.

Proper patient selection is mandatory for successful outcome. The common femoral arteries must be large enough to accept a 22 French sheath. The proximal infrarenal aortic neck must be suitable for device implantation—that is, its diameter must be between 16 and 25 mm, and it must be longer than 10 mm. The common iliac artery implantation should be at least 10 mm above the hypogastric artery, and the iliac artery diameter must be between 8 and 15 mm. In patients with iliac artery aneurysms, it is possible to land the end

Figure 7 **Open repair of infrarenal AAAs. When the aneurysm does not extend into the iliac arteries, a straight tube graft is used. The distal anastomosis is completed with a continuous suture. Before completion of the anastomosis, the graft is flushed by back-bleeding the iliac arteries and flushing the proximal anastomosis.**

of the stent in the external iliac artery and thereby exclude one internal iliac artery; however, exclusion of both internal iliac arteries should be avoided so as to prevent ischemic sequelae.

Technique for Device Implantation

The methods and technical principles we briefly describe here derive from the personal experience one of us (C.K.Z.) has accumulated with more than 150 modular implants. The ensuing technical description is not intended to be exhaustive, nor is it meant as a substitute for the instructions provided by the manufacturer.

The patient is placed under epidural or general anesthesia. Bilateral femoral artery cutdowns are performed through transverse groin incisions to allow exposure of the common femoral artery from the inguinal ligament to the femoral bifurcation. Proximal control of the femoral arteries is obtained with umbilical tapes. Systemic anticoagulation with I.V. heparin is instituted to prolong the activated clotting time (ACT) to greater than 250 seconds. The ACT is monitored and maintained at this level throughout the procedure, and additional heparin is given as needed.

The femoral arteries are cannulated with an 18-gauge needle, and 0.035-in. guide wires are placed bilaterally under fluoroscopic guidance; 10 French sheaths are then placed over the two guide wires and advanced into the aneurysm under fluoroscopic guidance. A superstiff 0.035-in. guide wire 260 cm in length is inserted into the thoracic aorta, usually from the right limb. In the contralateral iliac artery, a pigtail catheter is placed just above the level of the renal arteries, and an initial roadmapping aortogram is obtained. The 10 French sheath in the right femoral artery is exchanged for a 22 French sheath, which is placed over the superstiff guide wire and carefully advanced into the proximal infrarenal aorta under fluoroscopic guidance. The main stent-graft module, which is chosen on

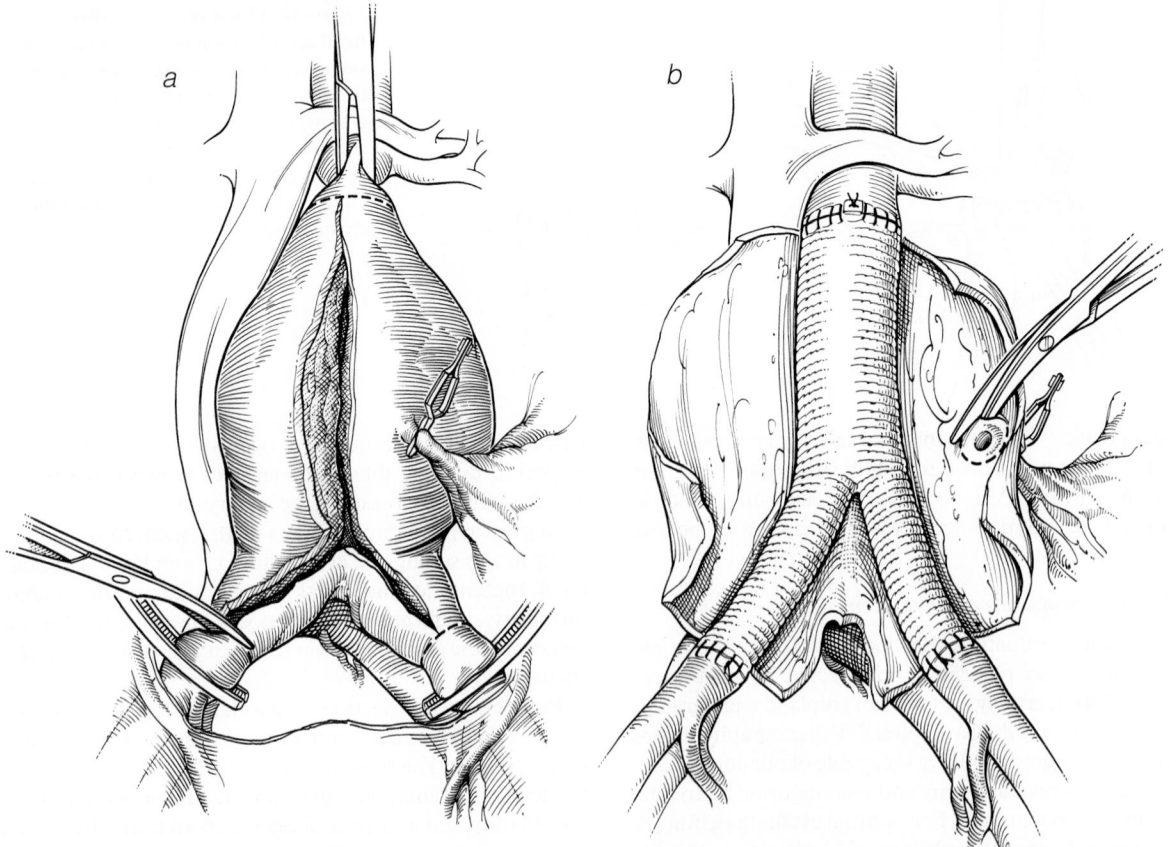

Figure 8 **Open repair of infrarenal AAAs. When the common iliac arteries are aneurysmal, both the internal and the external iliac arteries must be clamped individually (*a*), and a bifurcated graft is sewn to the iliac arteries bilaterally (*b*).**

the basis of preoperative measurements, is then advanced over the guide wire and through the delivery sheath into the perirenal aorta [see Figure 11a]. A second aortogram is performed to verify the position of the renal arteries. Under fluoroscopic guidance, the stent-graft is then gradually deployed by retracting the outer sheath and allowing the graft to expand, and it is positioned directly below the level of the renal arteries [see Figure 11b].

Once the main bifurcation module has been deployed, the 10 French sheath in the contralateral iliac artery is pulled back, and a 0.035-in. angled hydrophilic wire and a guide catheter are inserted into the contralateral limb of the bifurcation module. The hydrophilic wire is then exchanged for a superstiff guide wire, over which a 16 French sheath is advanced into the contralateral limb under fluoroscopic guidance. The contralateral limb is then advanced through the sheath into the contralateral limb and deployed [see Figure 11c]. A final aortogram is then performed to confirm that a satisfactory technical result has been achieved [see Figure 11d]. Proximal and distal extender cuffs may be placed if necessary. The femoral arteriotomies are repaired, and lower-extremity perfusion is reestablished.

Special Considerations

CONCURRENT DISEASE PROCESSES

At times, a concurrent disease process complicates repair of an AAA. The most common problems encountered are hepatobiliary, pancreatic, gastrointestinal, gynecologic, and genitourinary disorders. Careful evaluation of the situation is necessary to determine whether to treat the two disease entities concurrently. As a rule, the more life-threatening disorder is treated first.

There are three key points that should be remembered in the management of patients with AAAs and concurrent diseases. First, a careful preoperative diagnostic workup usually detects any concomitant disease processes. Second, in emergency situations such as ruptured or symptomatic aneurysms, the aneurysm always takes priority unless the other condition is life-threatening and the aneurysm is clearly not the cause of the critical symptoms. Finally, many concomitant intra-abdominal problems can be avoided by taking an endovascular approach.

ANATOMIC VARIANTS

Several anatomic variants may be encountered during repair of AAAs, including horseshoe kidney, accessory renal arteries, and venous anomalies.

Horseshoe Kidney

The incidence of horseshoe kidney in the general population is less than 3%. Most patients with horseshoe kidneys have between three and five renal arteries.[14] To preserve renal function, renal arteries arising from the aneurysm should be reimplanted. In patients with horseshoe kidneys who have more than five renal arteries, there often are multiple small accessory arteries, some of which originate from the aneurysm, the iliac arteries, or both.

The presence of a horseshoe kidney may complicate—but does not preclude—an anterior approach to repair of an infrarenal AAA.[15] In such cases, the left retroperitoneal approach provides excellent exposure of the infrarenal aorta. This approach requires that the surgeon dissect the space between the aneurysm and the left portion and isthmus of the kidney; the kidney can then be reflected to the right and the aneurysm fully exposed. The left ureter crosses the iliac arteries from the right in this position, and duplication of ureters may be noted.

Figure 9 Open repair of infrarenal AAAs. Once the anastomoses have been completed and adequate flow to the lower extremities and the left colon has been confirmed, the open aneurysm sac is sutured closed over the aortic graft.

Venous Anomalies

A number of different venous anomalies may be observed in the course of AAA repair; however, the overall incidence is quite low. Left renal vein variants, such as retroaortic left renal veins and circumaortic venous rings, are the most commonly seen venous anomalies.[16] Azygous continuation of the inferior vena cava and bilateral inferior vena cava have also been noted. Unnecessary bleeding can be prevented by means of careful dissection and meticulous technique.

INFLAMMATORY ANEURYSM

Approximately 5% of infrarenal AAAs are inflammatory.[17] These AAAs have a dense fibroinflammatory rind that typically adheres to the fourth portion of the duodenum; they may also involve the inferior vena cava, the left renal vein, or the ureters. Patients with inflammatory AAAs typically experience abdominal or flank pain and may present with weight loss. The erythrocyte sedimentation rate is usually elevated as well. Inflammatory aneurysms rarely rupture, because most are symptomatic and consequently are treated before rupture can occur. Repair of inflammatory aneurysms poses technical problems because of the involvement of adjacent structures. A retroperitoneal approach is usually advocated for these aneurysms.

RUPTURED ANEURYSM

Infrarenal AAAs can rupture freely into the peritoneal cavity or into the retroperitoneum. Free rupture into the peritoneal cavity is usually anterior and is typically accompanied by immediate hemodynamic collapse and a very high mortality. Retroperitoneal ruptures are usually posterior and may be contained by the psoas muscle and adjacent periaortic and perivertebral tissue. This type of rupture may occur without significant blood loss initially, and the patient may be hemodynamically stable.

When an aortic aneurysm ruptures, immediate surgical repair is indicated. If the patient is unstable and either an abdominal aortic aneurysm was previously diagnosed or a palpable abdominal mass is present, no further evaluation is necessary and the patient should be taken directly to the OR. If the patient is stable and the diagnosis is questionable, CT scanning may be performed to confirm the presence of an aneurysm and determine its extent, the site of the rupture, and the degree of iliac involvement. Bedside ultrasonography may also be used for quick confirmation of the presence of an AAA.

Surgical repair of ruptured aneurysms is performed via a transperitoneal approach. In cases of contained rupture, supraceliac control should be achieved before infrarenal dissection; once the neck of the aneurysm has been dissected free, the aortic clamp may be moved to the infrarenal level. In cases of free rupture, efforts to obtain vascular control may include compression of the aorta at the hiatus and infrarenal control with a clamp or an intraluminal balloon. Once proximal and distal control have been achieved, the operation is conducted in much the same way as an elective repair.

Outcome Evaluation

The mortality associated with repair of AAAs has been greatly re-duced by improvements in preoperative evaluation and perioperative care: leading centers currently report death rates ranging from 0% to 5%.[18] Mortality after repair of inflammatory aneurysms and after emergency repair of symptomatic nonruptured aneurysms continues to be somewhat higher (5% to 10%), primarily as a consequence of less thorough preoperative evaluation. The mortality associated with endovascular repair of AAAs is 1% to 3%—that is, essentially equivalent to that associated with open repair in selected patients.

Overall morbidity after elective aneurysm repair ranges from 10% to 30%. The most common complication is myocardial ischemia, and MI is the most common cause of postoperative death. Mild renal insufficiency is the second most frequent complication, occurring after 6% of elective aneurysm repairs; however, severe renal failure necessitating dialysis is rare in this setting. The third most common complication is pulmonary disease; the incidence of postoperative pneumonia is approximately 5%.

Postoperative bleeding may occur as well. Common sources of such bleeding include the anastomotic suture lines, inadequately recognized venous injuries, and coagulopathies resulting from intraoperative hypothermia or excessive blood loss. Any evidence of ongoing bleeding is an indication for early exploration.

Lower-extremity ischemia may occur as a result of either emboli or thrombosis of the graft and may necessitate reoperation and thrombectomy. So-called trash foot may also develop when diffuse microemboli are carried into the distal circulation.

Figure 10 **Open repair of infrarenal AAAs. (*a*) A small, adequately back-bleeding inferior mesenteric artery may be ligated. (*b*) A large or meagerly back-bleeding inferior mesenteric artery should be reimplanted. A side-biting clamp is applied to the graft, and an end-to-side anastomosis is created with a fine monofilament suture. (*c*) If the inferior mesenteric artery is not long enough for a direct anastomosis, an interposition graft—either a segment of a vein or a prosthetic graft—may be used for added length.**

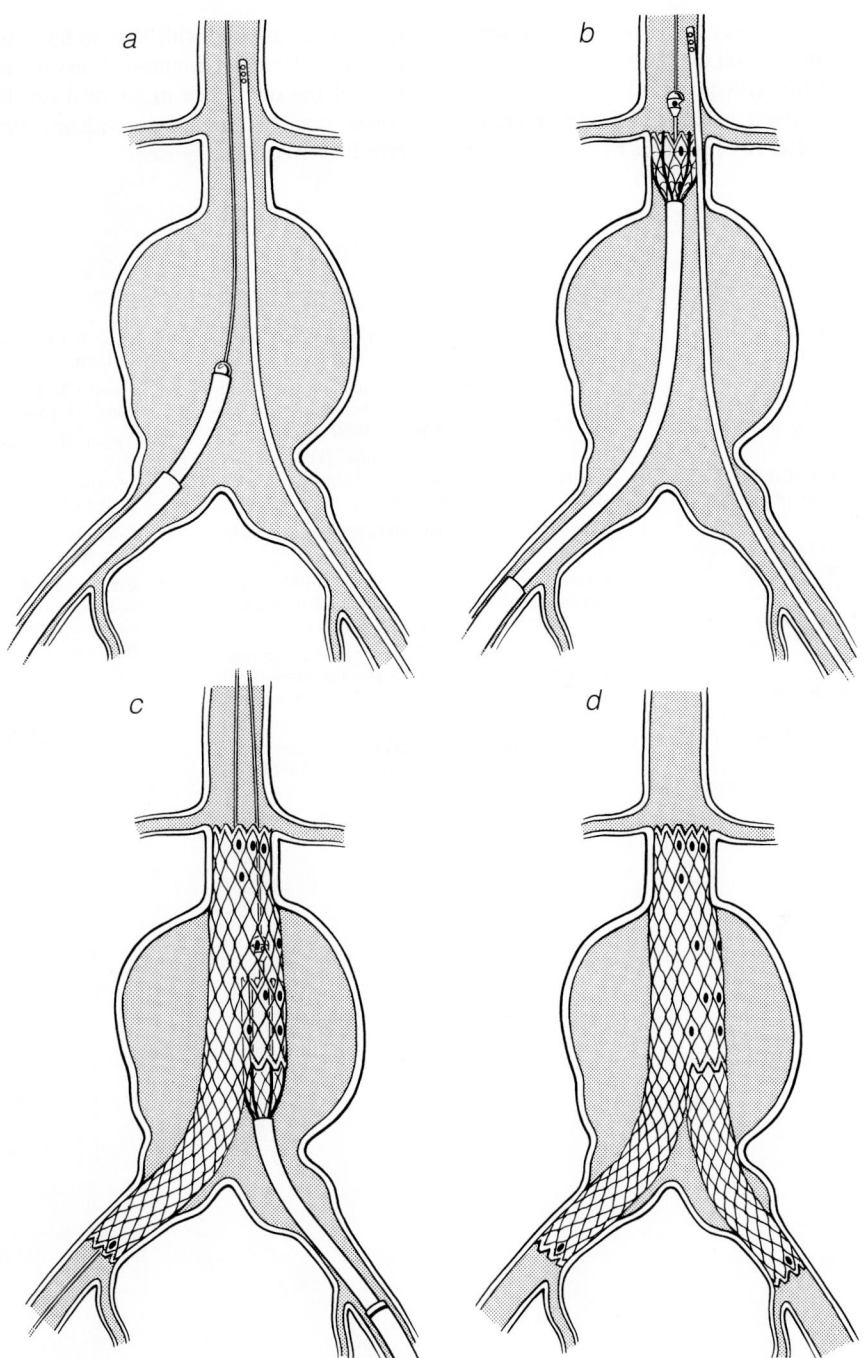

Figure 11 **Endovascular repair of infrarenal AAAs. (*a*) The main bifurcated stent-graft is advanced through the aortoiliac system under fluoroscopic guidance. (*b*) The sheath over the stent-graft is retracted under fluoroscopic guidance. Controlled deployment allows the graft to be gradually positioned directly below the renal arteries. (*c*) With the main body of the stent-graft deployed, the contralateral limb is cannulated. Once this is done, the contralateral limb is positioned within the junction gate and the common iliac artery. (*d*) Shown is proper deployment of the stent-graft within the aortoiliac system, with good proximal and distal fixation of the stent to the arterial wall.**

Colon ischemia develops after 1% of elective aneurysm repairs. Patients usually present with bloody diarrhea, abdominal pain, a distended abdomen, and leukocytosis. Diagnosis is confirmed by sigmoidoscopy, which reveals mucosal sloughing. In cases of transmural colonic necrosis, colon resection and exteriorization of stomas are warranted.

Paraplegia is rare after repair of infrarenal AAAs: the incidence is only 0.2%. Most instances of paraplegia occur after repair of a ruptured aneurysm or when the pelvis has been devascularized. The majority of patients recover at least some degree of neurologic function.

Late complications—such as pseudoaneurysms at the suture lines, graft or graft limb thrombosis, and graft infection—may occur but are extremely rare. Graft infection may be associated with graft-enteric fistula and is notoriously difficult to diagnose and treat.

Long-term survival in patients who have undergone successful AAA repair is reduced in comparison with that in the general population. The 5-year survival rate after AAA repair is 67% (range, 49% to 84%), compared with 80% to 85% in age-matched control subjects, and the mean duration of survival after AAA repair is 7.4 years. Part of the difference in survival can be attributed to associated coronary disease in patients with aneurysms. Late deaths result primarily from cardiac causes.

References

1. Taylor LM, Porter JM: Basic data related to clinical decision-making in abdominal aortic aneurysms. Ann Vasc Surg 1:502, 1980

2. Bickerstaff LK, Hollier LH, Van Peenen HJ, et al: Abdominal aortic aneurysm: the changing natural history. J Vasc Surg 1:6, 1984

3. Melton L, Bickerstaff L, Hollier LH, et al: Changing incidence of abdominal aortic aneurysms: a population based study. Am J Epidemiol 120:379, 1984

4. Darling RC, Messina CR, Brewster DC, et al: Autopsy study of unoperated aortic aneurysms. Circulation 56(suppl 2):161, 1977

5. Thurmond AS, Semler JH: Abdominal aortic aneurysm. Incidence in a population at risk. J Cardiovasc Surg 27:457, 1986

6. Whittemore AD, Clowes AW, Hechtman HB, et al: Aortic aneurysm repair reduced operative mortality associated with maintenance of optimal cardiac performance. Ann Surg 120:414, 1980

7. Pairolero PC: Repair of abdominal aortic aneurysms in high-risk patients. Surg Clin North Am 69:755, 1989

8. Stokes J, Butcher HR: Abdominal aortic aneurysms: factors influencing operative mortality and criteria of operability. Arch Surg 107:297, 1973

9. Quill DS, Colgan MP, Summer DS: Ultrasonic screening for the detection of abdominal aortic aneurysms. Surg Clin North Am 69:713, 1989

10. Bluth EI: Ultrasound of the abdominal aorta. Arch Intern Med 144:377, 1994

11. Gomes MN, Choyke PL: Preoperative evaluation of abdominal aortic aneurysms: ultrasound or computed tomography? J Cardiovasc Surg 28:159, 1987

12. Amparo EG, Hoddick WK, Hricak H, et al: Comparison of magnetic resonance imaging and ultrasonography in the evaluation of abdominal aortic aneurysms. Radiology 154:451, 1985

13. Lee JKT, Ling D, Heiken JP, et al: Magnetic resonance imaging of abdominal aneurysms. Am J Roentgenol 143:1197, 1984

14. Papin E: Chirurgie du rein. Anomalies du rein. Paris, G. Doin, 1928, p 205

15. Zarins CK, Gewertz BL: Atlas of Vascular Surgery. New York, Churchill Livingstone, 1988, p 56

16. Trigaux JP, Vandroogenbroek S, De Wispelaere JF, et al: Congenital anomalies of the inferior vena cava and left renal vein: evaluation with spiral CT. J Vasc Interv Radiol 9:339, 1998

17. Crawford JL, Stowe CL, Safi HJ, et al: Inflammatory aneurysms of the aorta. J Vasc Surg 2:133, 1985

18. Crawford ES, Saleh SA, Babb JW 3d, et al: Infrarenal abdominal aortic aneurysm: factors influencing survival after operation performed over a 25-year period. Ann Surg 193:699, 1981

Acknowledgment

Figures 4 through 11   Susan Brust, C.M.I.

25 INFRAINGUINAL ARTERIAL PROCEDURES

William D. Suggs, M.D., and Frank J. Veith, M.D.

Since the early 1980s, there have been enormous advances in the treatment of lower-extremity ischemia secondary to infrainguinal arteriosclerosis. Effective interventional management strategies have been developed for virtually all patterns of arteriosclerosis underlying limb-threatening ischemia.[1,2] Bypasses to the infrainguinal arteries using segments of autologous vein have become routine for limb salvage. As this technique has evolved, the distal limits of revascularization have been extended. Bypasses to arteries near the ankle or in the foot can now be offered to patients who have no patent arteries suitable for more proximal bypasses. In addition, bypasses to distal tibial or tarsal vessels may be performed in some patients whose popliteal arteries are patent but who have three-vessel distal occlusive disease and forefoot gangrene.[3,4] Frequently, patients who require very distal bypasses have already undergone vascular reconstruction; these patients may be candidates for alternative approaches, such as a popliteal-distal bypass or a tibiotibial bypass.[5-7]

Patients with limbs threatened by distal tibial occlusive disease present an ongoing challenge to the vascular surgeon. Provided that careful attention is paid to obtaining high-quality preoperative angiograms and that the surgeon is willing to consider alternative approaches, it is generally possible to achieve good results from limb salvage procedures.

It should be kept in mind that only patients with threatened limbs—manifested by rest pain, frank gangrene, or nonhealing ulcers—should be considered candidates for infrainguinal bypass. Patients who have gangrene that extends into the deeper tarsal region of the foot, who have a severe organic mental syndrome, or who are nonambulatory are not candidates for limb salvage surgery and should be treated with primary amputation instead.[1,2]

Preoperative Evaluation

HISTORY AND PHYSICAL EXAMINATION

A careful history and a thorough physical examination are crucial for accurate assessment of the extent of the patient's atherosclerotic disease. In the course of the history, the examiner should pay particular attention to distinguishing true rest pain from other causes of pain (e.g., arthritis and neuritis). Significant ischemic pain is usually associated not only with decreased pulses but also with other manifestations of ischemia (e.g., atrophy, decreased skin temperature, marked rubor, and pain that is relieved when the foot is dangled). In the course of the physical examination, the examiner should look for and assess the extent of any underlying infection and should closely examine any surgical scars for clues to the nature and extent of any previous vascular operations involving the use of the saphenous vein. In addition, a careful pulse examination should be performed to assess the patient's baseline arterial status; these baseline measure-

ments provide a basis for comparison if the disease subsequently progresses and may help determine the approach to be used to salvage the threatened limb.

NONINVASIVE TESTING

Noninvasive tests are helpful in that they provide semiquantitative assessment of the circulation and help confirm the diagnosis made on the basis of the history and the physical examination. Such test measurements include the ankle-brachial index (ABI) and pulse volume recordings (PVRs).

The ABI is determined by dividing the ankle pressure in each lower limb by the higher of the two brachial pressures. Normal circulation typically yields an ABI of 1.0 to 1.2; claudication, an ABI of 0.40 to 0.95; and limb-threatening ischemia, an ABI of 0 to 0.5. It is vital to remember, however, that lower-extremity pressure measurements are less reliable in patients with heavily calcified vessels (e.g., diabetics and patients with end-stage renal disease). In these patients, ABIs are falsely elevated as a result of the higher cuff pressures required to occlude calcified vessels, which in some cases are not occluded even with pressures higher than 300 mm Hg.

PVRs are obtained by means of calibrated air-cuff plethysmography. Standard blood pressure cuffs are placed at different levels of the lower extremity, and the increases in pressure within the cuffs resulting from the volume increase during systole are recorded as pulse waves. Tracings exhibiting a brisk rise during systole and a dicrotic notch are characterized as normal, those exhibiting loss of the notch and a more prolonged downslope are characterized as moderately abnormal, and those exhibiting a flattened wave are characterized as severely abnormal. Absolute amplitudes on PVRs are not directly comparable between patients; however, serial PVRs from a single patient are highly reproducible and thus are quite useful for following the course of severe peripheral vascular disease in individual cases.[4] One disadvantage of PVRs is that they cannot differentiate proximal femoral disease from iliac occlusive disease.[8]

IMAGING

Duplex Scanning

Duplex scanning is a useful noninvasive method of assessing the aortoiliac and infrainguinal arterial systems. Several studies have evaluated the ability of duplex scanning to predict iliac artery stenosis. A 1987 trial found that duplex scanning was highly sensitive (89%) and specific (90%) in predicting iliac stenosis of 50% or greater.[9] Three subsequent trials corroborated these findings, reporting sensitivities ranging from 81% to 89% and specificities ranging from 88% to 99%.[10-12] This noninvasive modality may be especially useful for improving evaluation of diabetic patients before invasive procedures (e.g., angiography and angioplasty).[10]

Duplex scanning has also been used to allow infrapopliteal bypasses to be performed without preoperative angiography. In one study, a limb salvage rate of 86% was achieved with this approach, and completion arteriography matched the runoff status predicted by duplex scanning in 96% of cases.[13] In a study from our own institution, we were able to perform femoropopliteal bypasses without preoperative arteriography and were able to perform distal bypasses with confirmatory arteriograms at the time of operation.[14]

Magnetic Resonance Angiography

Magnetic resonance angiography (MRA), a noninvasive modality that does not require contrast agents, often yields good arterial images and may, in fact, be more sensitive than angiography in imaging distal lower-extremity runoff vessels.[15,16] More recently, developments such as gadolinium enhancement, multistation examination, and the floating table technique have further improved the resolution of MRA,[17-19] to the point where many institutions that use current forms of MRA no longer routinely obtain preoperative angiograms. MRA, in combination with arterial duplex scanning, has the potential to replace contrast arteriography in the assessment of patients with distal arterial occlusive disease.

Arteriography

Until MRA and duplex scanning become more widely available, contrast angiography will remain the gold standard for the evaluation of patients with distal arterial occlusive disease. A complete evaluation of the existing arterial disease from the aorta to the pedal vessels is necessary for diabetic patients, who frequently have multilevel occlusive disease. Obtaining intra-arterial pressure measurements at the time of angiography significantly improves detection of clinically significant stenosis. The systolic pressure gradient across the lesion should also be measured: gradients greater than 15 mm Hg are considered hemodynamically significant.[20]

In the general population, arteriography has a complication rate of only 1.7% to 3.3%.[21] Elderly patients with severe aortoiliac or infrainguinal disease must be carefully evaluated before the procedure because they are more likely to experience local and systemic complications than patients in the general population are. For the majority of patients, the transfemoral approach is the safest; however, for patients with weak or nonpalpable femoral pulses, other approaches (e.g., translumbar, transbrachial, or transaxillary) may be preferable. These alternative approaches are associated with higher rates of local complications, including hematomas, pseudoaneurysms, dissections, thrombosis, and embolization.

Renal insufficiency is an important complication of angiography: 6.5% to 8.2% of patients who undergo arteriography experience some degree of impairment associated with contrast agents.[22,23] Patients who have preexisting azotemia and whose baseline creatinine concentrations exceed 2.0 mg/dl are at highest risk for renal complications after angiography. Elderly patients typically have lower creatinine clearances for a given serum creatinine level and thus should always be considered at higher risk for nephrotoxicity. All possible precautions should be taken to limit the renal insult. There is some evidence to suggest that the use of low-osmolar contrast agents can decrease the incidence of renal impairment,[24,25] but the data are not unanimous on this point.[26] Adequate hydration before arteriography is highly effective in diminishing the risk of contrast nephropathy.

Administration of mannitol, which has an osmotic diuretic effect, helps prevent contrast toxicity as well. These measures, coupled with judicious use of contrast agents, should minimize renal impairment associated with arteriography.

Femoropopliteal Bypass

Patients whose limbs are clearly threatened and who have undergone arteriographic examination should undergo femoropopliteal bypass when the superficial femoral artery or the popliteal artery is occluded and when arteriography indicates that a patent popliteal artery segment distal to the occlusion has luminal continuity with any of its three terminal branches (even if one or more of these branches ends in an occlusion anywhere in the leg). Even if the popliteal artery segment into which the graft is to be inserted is occluded distally, femoropopliteal bypass to this isolated segment can still be considered.[27,28] If the isolated popliteal segment is shorter than 7 cm or if there is extensive gangrene or infection in the foot, a femorodistal artery bypass or a sequential bypass is sometimes performed in one or two stages.

OPERATIVE TECHNIQUE

Femoropopliteal bypass may be carried out either above or below the knee.

Above-the-Knee Bypass

For above-the-knee bypass, the patient is placed in the supine position with the thigh externally rotated and the knee flexed approximately 30°. This position affords easy exposure of the femoral and popliteal arteries as well as of the saphenous vein.

Harvesting of saphenous vein The greater saphenous vein is harvested through intermittent skip incisions starting in the groin and proceeding distally toward the knee [see Figure 1]. Multiple short skin incisions heal better than a single long one and are less likely to result in skin necrosis.

Dissection of the saphenous vein begins at the groin. This proximal incision is also used for exposure of the femoral artery. The saphenofemoral junction is carefully mobilized, and the tributaries are ligated with fine silk close to where they enter the main trunk, with care taken not to impinge on the wall of the trunk. As dissection continues distally, the main trunk of the saphenous vein is progressively elevated, and all tributaries are identified and ligated. The vein is then removed from its bed and

Figure 1 **Femoropopliteal bypass: above knee. Shown is the appropriate position of the leg. Interrupted skin incisions are made in the thigh and upper leg to permit harvesting of the saphenous vein.**

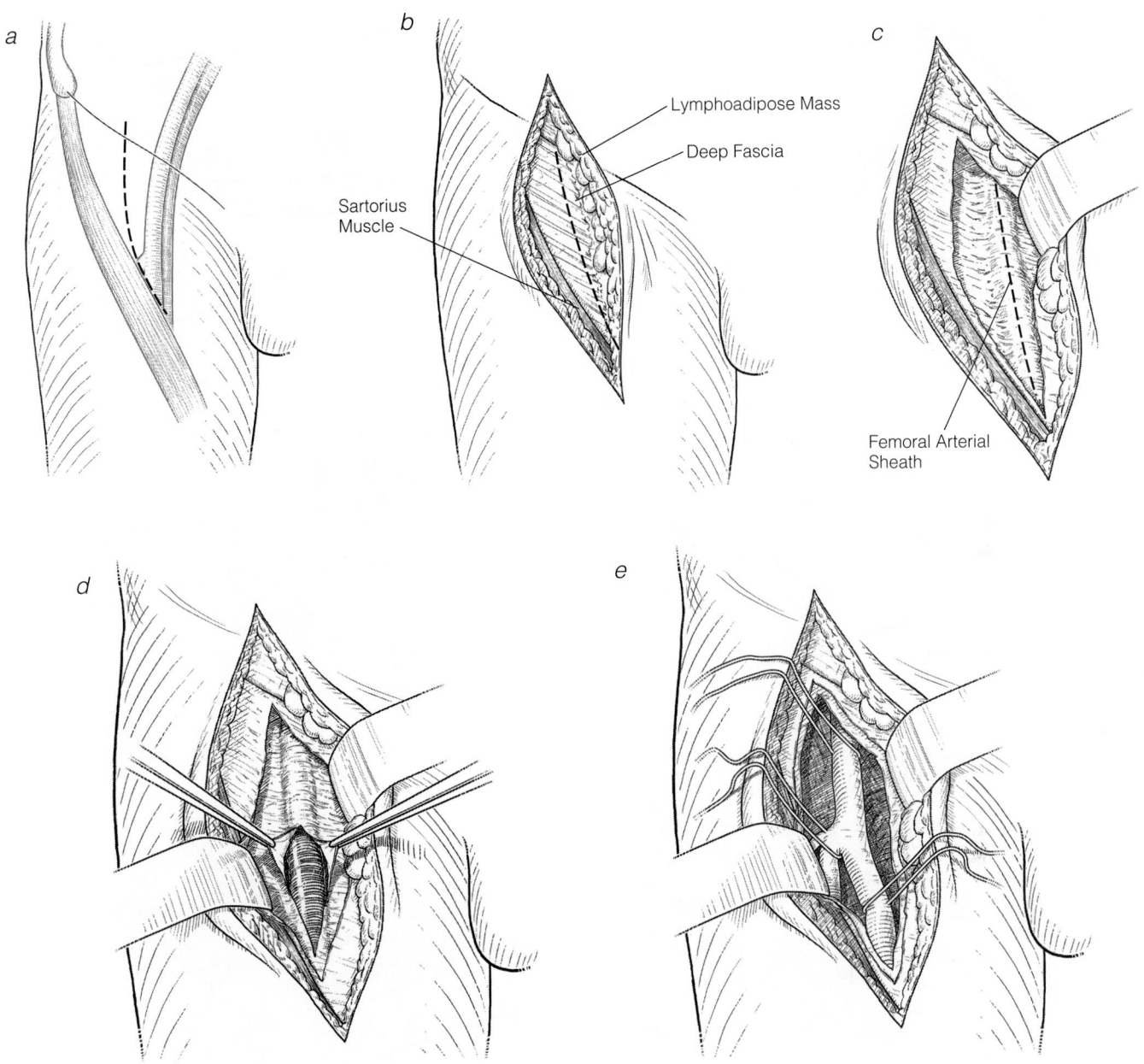

Figure 2 **Femoropopliteal bypass: above knee. Depicted is exposure of the femoral artery. (*a*) A curved 4 to 5 in. skin incision is made slightly lateral to the pulsation of the femoral artery. (*b*) Lymphoadipose tissue is retracted to expose the deep fascia overlying the course of the femoral artery. (*c*) The deep fascia is incised, exposing the femoral arterial sheath, which is then opened along its axis (*d*). (*e*) The common and superficial femoral arteries are mobilized and encircled with Silastic vessel loops.**

immediately placed into a basin containing heparinized saline (or heparinized whole blood) at a temperature of 4° C or cold Hanks solution. A small cannula is passed through the distal end of the divided vein, and the vessel is irrigated with cold Hanks solution to expel any liquid blood or clot and to locate any leaks. If a leak is found, it is repaired with 6-0 Prolene.

Step 1: exposure of femoral artery A slightly curved skin incision, with the concavity facing the medial aspect, is made starting at a point slightly above the inguinal crease and extending distally for 10 to 12.5 cm [*see Figure 2a*]. The incision should be slightly lateral to the pulsation of the femoral artery so as to avoid the lymphatics as much as possible. Any minor bleeding or

divided lymphatic vessels should be controlled with electrocoagulation or fine ligatures. Self-retaining retractors are placed both proximally and distally in the wound, and the lymphoadipose tissue is gently retracted medially [*see Figure 2b*].

The deep fascia is opened along the femoral artery [*see Figure 2c*], and the sheath of the artery is opened along its axis [*see Figure 2d*]. The common and superficial femoral arteries are mobilized, and Silastic loops are placed around them [*see Figure 2e*]. These vessels are then elevated slightly, and the origin of the deep femoral artery comes into view lateral and posterior to the common femoral artery and just proximal to the superficial femoral artery. Dissection of the origin of the deep femoral artery must be done carefully so as not to injure the collateral

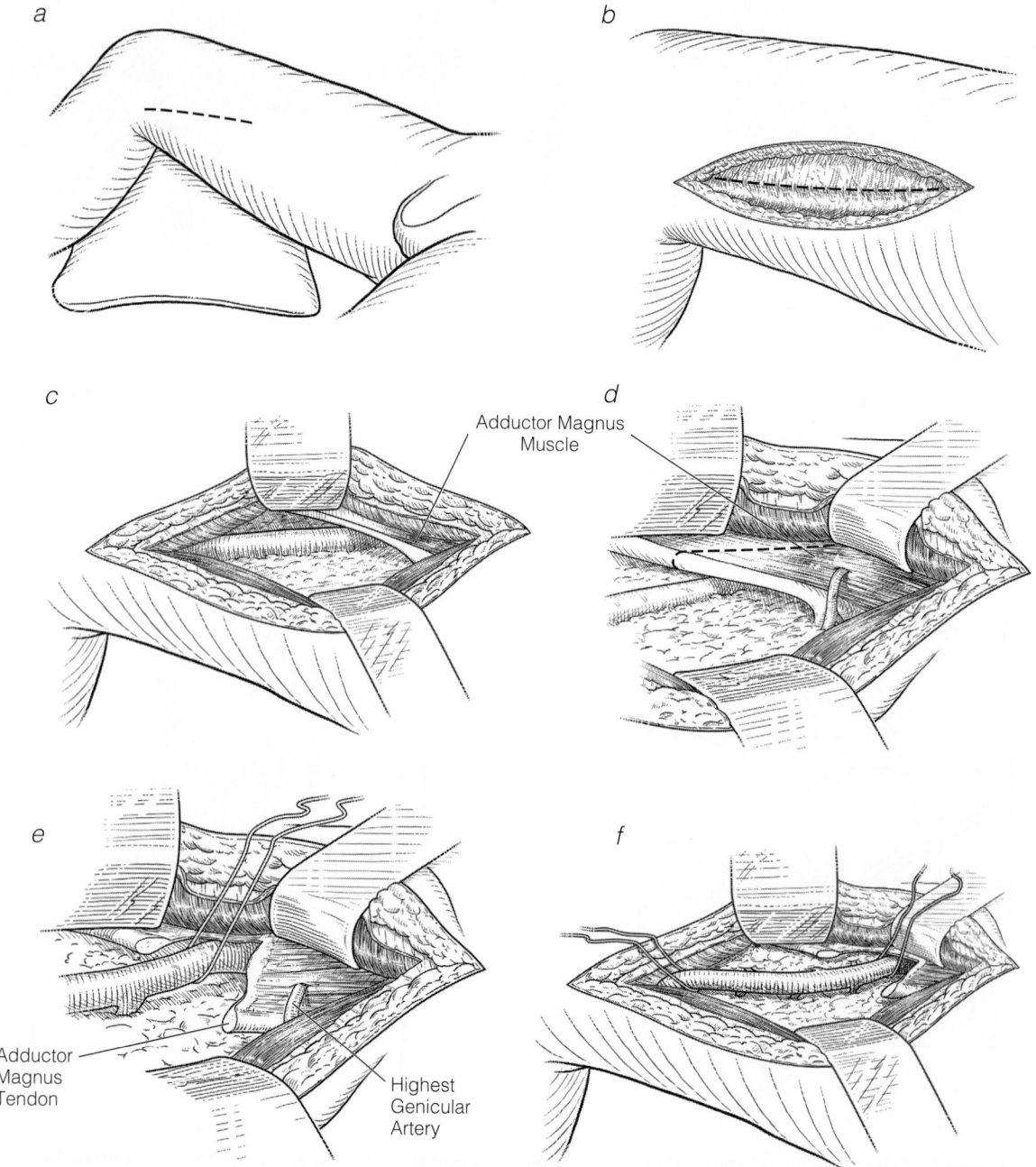

Figure 3 Femoropopliteal bypass: above knee. Depicted is medial exposure of the proximal popliteal artery. (*a*) An incision is made in the lower third of the thigh, anterior to the sartorius muscle. (*b*) The deep fascia is incised, and the sartorius muscle is retracted posteriorly, allowing the popliteal artery to be readily palpated. (*c*) The popliteal arterial sheath is opened, exposing the svessel and its surrounding venules. The adductor magnus tendon may be seen covering the proximal end of the artery (*d*), and it may have to be divided (*e*) to provide better exposure of the artery. (*f*) The popliteal artery, freed of the venous plexus, is mobilized between two vessel loops.

vessels coming off the artery at that level and the one or two branches of the satellite veins that cross the anterior portion of its initial segment. If mobilization of the deep femoral artery proves difficult, the satellite vein branches can be divided and ligated.

Step 2: exposure of proximal popliteal artery For the approach to the popliteal artery, the surgeon moves to the opposite side of the table. An incision is made in the lower third of the thigh anterior to the sartorius muscle and is extended close to the medial aspect of the knee [*see Figure 3a*]. The deep fascia anterior to the sartorius muscle is opened, and the sartorius

muscle is detached from the vastus medialis muscle and retracted posteriorly. The popliteal artery is identified by palpation; it is the most superficial structure palpable through this exposure [*see Figure 3b*]. The overlying fascia is incised, and the adipose tissue usually present at this level is dissected until the vascular bundle is reached.

The sheath of the artery is opened [*see Figure 3c*]. At this level, there is almost always a network of venules surrounding the artery, which must be carefully dissected away from the arterial wall. Division of the adductor magnus tendon may be required to yield adequate exposure of the proximal portion of the popliteal artery [*see Figures 3d and 3e*]. The venous network is separated from the arterial adventitia, and the various branches are divided and ligated. The popliteal vein is then separated from the artery—a process that, because of the intimate connection between the two vessels, is sometimes quite difficult. In separating the vein from the artery, care must be taken not to injure any of the genicular branches of the artery. The popliteal artery is freed for a length of approximately 1.5 to 2 in., and vessel loops are placed around it [*see Figure 3f*].

If the proximal popliteal artery appears markedly sclerotic and unsuitable for anastomosis to the graft, the exposure must be extended to the middle portion of the artery. To achieve this extended exposure, the hamstring muscles and their tendons are mobilized and retracted posteriorly, and the medial head of the gastrocnemius muscle is divided close to the medial condyle of the femur.

Next, the sheath of the popliteal artery is opened farther distally, and the tributaries of the veins surrounding the artery are further dissected away from it. Dissection of the middle portion of the popliteal artery may be facilitated by flexing the knee; this measure relaxes the artery, thereby allowing it to be readily drawn closer to the superficial level of the exposure.

Step 3: creation of tunnel Implantation of the graft may be started in either the popliteal artery or the femoral artery; the former is our usual preference. Before the anastomoses are constructed, a tunnel is created under the sartorius muscle by means of either a tunneler or an aortic clamp with a red rubber catheter attached to it to mark the tunnel.

Step 4: construction of distal anastomosis to popliteal artery Heparin is routinely administered before the vascular clamps are applied. A longitudinal arteriotomy is made in the anterior wall of the artery with a sharp No. 15 knife blade. This arteriotomy is then enlarged with a scalpel or a Potts angled scissors. The length of the opening in the artery should be approximately twice the diameter of the vessel. If the edges of the arteriotomy are calcified and the atheromatous intima overlaps the cut edge, the diseased intima should be excised with arteriotomy scissors.

The saphenous vein segment is then brought into the field. It is reversed so that its proximal end becomes the distal end for the anastomosis. This distal end is then enlarged with a longitudinal incision in its posterior wall, and the right-angle tips of the two sides of the divided posterior wall are cut away. Double-armed sutures are placed through the proximal angle (or heel) of the graft, with the needles going from the outside of the arteriotomy to the inside and then from the inside to the outside. Next, a similar double-armed suture is passed through the distal angle (or toe) of the graft from the outside to the inside and then from the inside to the outside through the end of the arteriotomy.

The edge of the vein is then approximated to that of the arteriotomy with a continuous suture starting at the toe of the graft and proceeding toward the heel [*see Figure 4*]. When half of the anastomosis has been completed, the edge of the vein graft is separated from the edge of the opposite side of the arteriotomy to permit inspection of the arterial lumen and the completed suture. The other half of the anastomosis is then completed by placing a second continuous suture, starting at the heel and proceeding toward the toe. Finally, the two sutures are tied together midway between the heel and the toe to complete the popliteal anastomosis.

Figure 4 **Femoropopliteal bypass: above knee. Shown are details of the anastomotic suturing, which is begun at the distal end and continued to the middle portion of each side of the anastomosis of the artery and the saphenous vein graft. Equal bites of all layers of each vessel are included in each stitch, all of which are placed under direct vision.**

Step 5: placement of graft in tunnel The graft is distended by injecting heparinized saline solution into it to test for leaks either from the vein segment itself or from the anastomotic site. The graft is then marked to ensure that it does not become twisted when brought through the tunnel. The graft is brought through the tunnel either by using an aortic clamp or by attaching it to the previously placed red rubber catheter.

Step 6: construction of proximal anastomosis to femoral artery Before the proximal anastomosis is begun, the proper length of the graft should be determined to ensure that there is no redundancy. The proximal end of the graft is split and enlarged in the same fashion as the distal end, and the resulting right-angle corners are similarly trimmed. The graft is then anastomosed to the arteriotomy made in the femoral artery (which, like the popliteal arteriotomy, should be at least twice as long as the vessel is wide). The graft is attached by double-armed needles at its proximal angle and then in a similar fashion at its distal angle. The anastomosis is then completed from each end toward the center, just as the popliteal anastomosis was.

Below-the-Knee Bypass

When occlusion or marked stenosis renders the proximal and middle portions of the popliteal artery unsuitable for graft implantation, the lower portion of the vessel, which is often relatively free of atherosclerosis, may be used for the distal anastomosis instead.

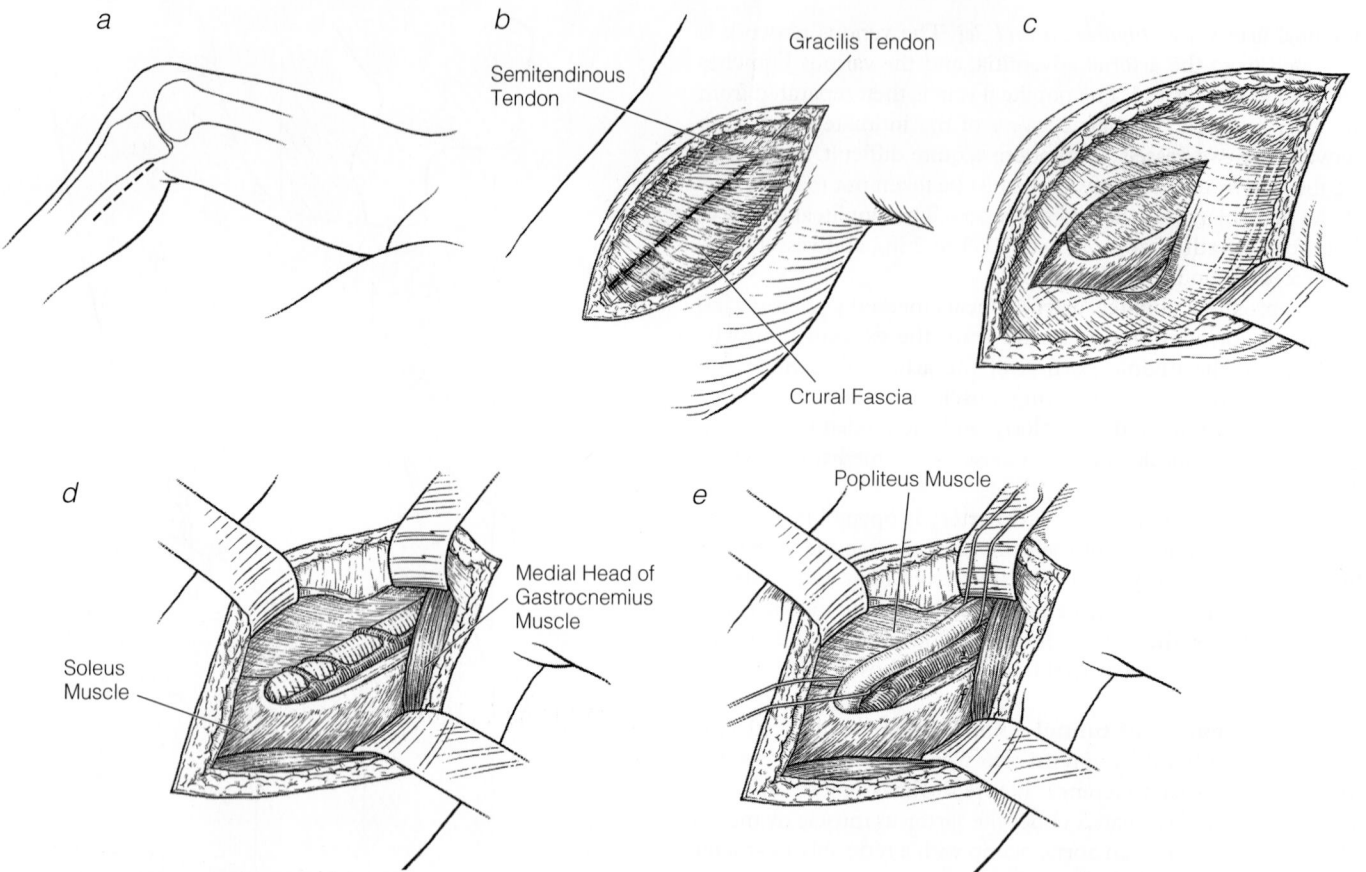

Figure 5 Femoropopliteal bypass: below knee. Depicted is medial exposure of the distal popliteal artery. (*a*) An incision is made just behind the posteromedial surface of the tibia [*see Figure 5a*]. (*b*) The crural fascia is exposed. (*c*) The fascia is incised, exposing the vascular bundle. (*d*) The medial head of the gastrocnemius muscle is retracted posteriorly, exposing the distal popliteal vessels and the arcade of the soleus muscle. (*e*) The distal popliteal artery is freed and mobilized between vessel loops.

Step 1: exposure of popliteal artery With the knee moderately flexed and supported by a rolled sheet placed under it, a vertical skin incision is made just behind the posteromedial surface of the tibia [*see Figure 5a*], exposing the crural fascia [*see Figure 5b*]. Care must be taken to avoid injury to the greater saphenous vein during the skin incision. When a saphenous vein graft is to be used, the same incision can serve both for harvesting of the vein and for exposure of the artery.

The crural fascia is opened along its fibers [*see Figure 5c*], its distal attachments are separated from the semitendinosus and gracilis tendons, and the two tendons are mobilized proximally and, if necessary, divided. The medial head of the gastrocnemius muscle is retracted posteriorly [*see Figure 5d*] to expose the popliteal artery and vein and the posterior tibial nerve as these structures cross the popliteus muscle posteriorly [*see Figure 5e*].

It should be noted that (1) the distal popliteal artery has few branches below the inferior geniculate arteries, (2) atheromatous plaques are rarely present at this level, and (3) the arterial wall is often more suitable for graft implantation in this portion of the popliteal wall than it is above the knee.

Step 2: exposure of femoral artery This exposure is accomplished in essentially the same way as it would be in an above-the-knee bypass.

Step 3: creation of tunnel Tunneling for a below-the-knee femoropopliteal bypass is carried out through Hunter's canal,

through the upper popliteal space, and finally through the region behind the popliteus muscle.

Steps 4 through 6 Steps 4, 5, and 6 of a below-the-knee femoropopliteal bypass—the distal anastomosis of the vein graft to the distal popliteal artery, the placement of the graft in the tunnel, and the proximal anastomosis to the femoral artery—are carried out in much the same way as the corresponding steps in an above-the-knee bypass. A completion angiogram should be obtained to confirm the adequacy of the distal anastomosis and verify the position of the graft in the tunnel [*see Figure 6*].

OUTCOME EVALUATION

Femoropopliteal bypasses performed with segments of the greater saphenous vein are associated with 4-year primary patency rates ranging from 68% to 80% and limb salvage rates ranging from 75% to 80%.[29] Femoropopliteal bypasses performed with polytetrafluoroethylene (PTFE) grafts yield comparable patency and limb salvage rates above the knee but are significantly less successful below the knee.[30]

Newer vein harvesting techniques may help improve outcome further. The use of endoscopic vein harvesting methods has been shown to reduce the incidence of wound complications associated with femoropopliteal bypass.[31] This approach allows above-the-knee bypasses to be performed through two incisions.

Infrapopliteal Bypass

Bypasses to the small arteries beyond the popliteal artery are performed only when femoropopliteal bypass is contraindicated according to accepted criteria [see Femoropopliteal Bypass, above]. Infrapopliteal bypasses are performed to the posterior tibial artery, the anterior tibial artery, or the peroneal artery, in that order of preference. As a rule, a tibial artery is used only if its lumen runs without obstruction into the foot, though bypasses to isolated tibial artery segments and other disadvantaged outflow tracts have been performed and have remained patent for more than 4 years.[2,3] Generally, the peroneal artery is used only if it is continuous with one or two of its terminal branches, which communicate with foot arteries [see Figure 7]. Neither the absence of a plantar arch nor vascular calcification is considered a contraindication to a reconstruction.[2,7] With both femoropopliteal and infrapopliteal bypasses, stenosis of less than 50% of the diameter of the vessel is acceptable at or distal to the site chosen for the distal anastomosis.

OPERATIVE TECHNIQUE

Bypasses to tibial arteries should be performed with autogenous vein grafts, and either the reversed technique (as previously described [see Femoropopliteal Bypass, above]) or the in situ technique [see In Situ Bypass, below] may be used. Placement of a tourniquet above the knee allows the distal anastomosis to be performed without extensive dissection of the tibial vessels or the application of clamps.[32] Exposure of the inflow vessel (i.e., the femoral artery or the popliteal artery) is achieved in the same way as in femoropopliteal bypass. Accordingly, bypasses to tibial and

Figure 7 **Infrapopliteal bypass. An arteriogram from a 65-year-old female with rest pain in the right foot who underwent in situ bypass to the middle portion of the peroneal artery shows communication of the peroneal artery with foot arteries and reconstitution of the dorsalis pedis artery.**

Figure 6 **Femoropopliteal bypass: below knee. A completion arteriogram from a patient who underwent below-the-knee femoropopliteal bypass for a nonhealing toe amputation site shows runoff through all three tibial vessels.**

peroneal arteries are best described in terms of the approaches required for exposure of these vessels and the tunnels required for routing the bypass conduits.

Exposure of Posterior Tibial Artery

The very proximal portion of the posterior tibial artery is aproached via a below-the-knee popliteal incision. The deep fascia is incised, and the popliteal space is entered. The gastrocnemius muscle is retracted posteriorly, and the soleus muscle is separated from the posterior surface of the tibia. The distal portion of the posterior tibial artery is approached via a medial incision along the posterior edge of the tibia [see Figure 8]; deepening this incision along the posterior tibialis muscle and the posterior surface of the tibia allows exposure of the posterior tibial artery. The tunnel from the popliteal fossa to the distal posterior tibial artery is made just below the muscle fascia, ideally with a long, gently curved clamp.

Exposure of Anterior Tibial Artery

To expose the proximal portion of the anterior tibial artery, an anterolateral incision is made in the leg midway between the tibia and the fibula over the appropriate segment of patent artery [see

Figure 8 Infrapopliteal bypass: posterior tibial artery. Shown are incisions for bypasses to the distal regions of the leg.

Figure 9a]. Additional small medial incisions are also required for tunneling. The anterior incision is carried through the deep fascia, and the fibers of the anterior tibial muscle and the extensor digitorum longus muscle are separated to reveal the neurovascular bundle. The accompanying veins are mobilized and their branches divided to allow visualization of the anterior tibial artery, which can then be carefully mobilized [*see Figure 9b*]. With the artery mobilized, further posterior dissection can be performed, and the interosseous membrane can then be visualized and incised in a cruciate fashion.

Careful blunt finger dissection via the anterior incision and from the popliteal fossa via the medial incision facilitates creation of a tunnel without injury to the numerous veins in the area [*see*

Figure 9c]. Alternatively, the tunnel for the bypass may be placed lateral to the knee in a subcutaneous plane.

The distal anterior tibial artery is approached via an anterior incision placed midway between the tibia and the fibula [*see Figure 8*]. A tunnel is made from the distal popliteal fossa across the interosseous membrane (like the tunnel to the peroneal artery) and beneath the deep fascia to a point 5 to 7 cm above the lateral malleolus. Once the distal anastomosis is complete and the graft has been drawn through the tunnel, any tendons that may be distorting or compressing the graft in its course around the tibia are divided; this measure proves necessary in most low anterior tibial bypasses.

Exposure of Peroneal Artery

The peroneal artery is usually approached via the same incision as the posterior tibial artery [*see* Exposure of the Posterior Tibial Artery, *above*]. The artery is located and isolated just medial to the medial edge of the fibula. In its distal third, however, and in patients with stout calves and ankles, the peroneal artery should be approached via a lateral incision [*see Figure 8*], followed by excision of the fibula.

For lateral exposure of the peroneal artery, a long segment of fibula is freed from its muscle attachments with a combination of blunt and sharp dissection; particular care should be taken in dissecting along the medial edge of the bone because the peroneal vessels run just below this edge and are easily injured by instruments. Next, a finger is passed around the fibula [*see Figure 10a*]; once this is done, the free edge of bone is further developed by

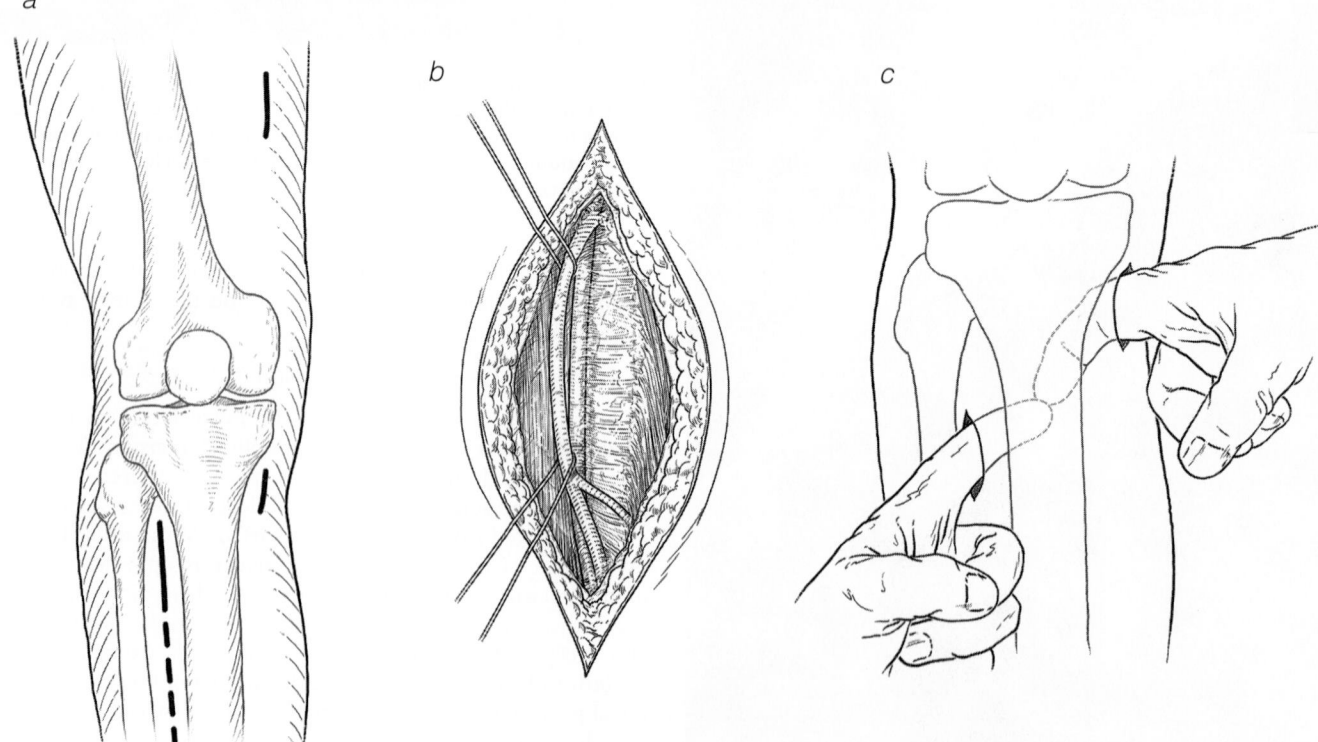

Figure 9 Infrapopliteal bypass: anterior tibial artery. (*a*) An anterolateral incision is made midway between the tibia and the fibula over the artery; small medial incisions are also made for tunneling. (*b*) The anterior incision is carried through the deep fascia, the anterior tibial and extensor digitorum longus muscles are separated, the accompanying veins are mobilized and divided, and the anterior tibial artery is mobilized. (*c*) A tunnel is created with careful blunt finger dissection.

Figure 10 **Infrapopliteal bypass: lateral exposure of peroneal artery. Lateral exposure of the peroneal artery typically requires excision of part of the fibula; this is done by (*a*) passing a finger behind the fibula, developing the free bone edge further with a right-angle clamp, (*b*) passing a right-angle retractor behind the fibula, and dividing the bone with a power saw.**

forcefully pushing a right-angle clamp inferiorly and superiorly [*see Figure 10b*]. A right-angle retractor is passed behind the bone, and the fibula is divided with a power saw. The peroneal artery can then be dissected free from surrounding veins and used in the construction of the distal anastomosis.

Gentle blunt finger dissection is required to develop a tunnel from this lateral wound to the distal popliteal fossa, and great care should be taken to avoid injury to the numerous veins in the area. Because the peroneal artery is the least accessible of the three leg arteries used for infrapopliteal bypasses and normally has the poorest connections with the arteries of the foot, we recommend that it be used as a distal implantation site only when the anterior and posterior tibial arteries are not suitable.

Exposure of Dorsalis Pedis Artery

When no more proximal procedure is possible, a bypass to the ankle region or the foot may be performed. The dorsalis pedis artery is easily approached via a lateral incision on the dorsum of the foot [*see Figure 11a*]. The incision is curved slightly and a flap raised so that the incision will not be directly over the anastomosis [*see Figure 11b*]. If the artery must be approached at the ankle, the extensor retinaculum must be divided. Otherwise, the operation is performed in much the same fashion as a distal anterior tibial bypass [*see Figure 12*]. The posterior tibial artery can be

approached down to a point several centimeters below the medial malleolus.

In Situ Bypass

In situ bypass is an acceptable alternative to reversed vein bypass. Minimally invasive techniques have been developed to reduce the wound complications encountered when in situ bypass is performed with long incisions.

With the help of a side-branch coil occlusion system, in situ bypass can be performed through the two arterial access incisions. The angioscopic coil device is passed through the proximal greater saphenous vein, and the coils are placed into the side branches under angioscopic guidance [*see Figure 13*]. As the device is advanced more distally through the vein, the valves are lysed with a flexible valvulotome.

Another approach to side-branch occlusion involves the use of an endoscopic vein harvesting system. Three skin incisions are made: two incisions for arterial access and one 2 cm incision above the knee for insertion of an endoscopic device to locate and clip the side branches of the saphenous vein. Once the proximal anastomosis is complete, the valves are lysed with a flexible valvulotome passed through the distal end of the vein. Completion cineangiography is then performed to confirm side-branch occlusion and to assess the entire reconstruction.[33]

OUTCOME EVALUATION

Infrapopliteal bypasses should have 5-year primary patency rates ranging from 60% to 67% and limb salvage rates ranging from 70% to 75% whether they are done with the reversed-vein technique or with the in situ technique.[34,35] For all such grafts, close patient follow-up and graft surveillance improve secondary

Figure 11 **Infrapopliteal bypass: dorsalis pedis artery. (*a*) The dorsalis pedis artery is approached via an incision on the dorsum of the foot. (*b*) The incision is curved and a flap raised so that the incision is not directly over the anastomosis.**

patency rates. Reduced complications and decreased length of stay have been reported for patients undergoing distal in situ bypasses using either the endoscopic or the coil occulsion approach.[36,37]

Plantar Bypass

Extension of the standard approaches to limb salvage has led to the performance of bypasses to vessels below the ankle joint [see Figures 14 and 15]. Such bypasses are indicated when the more proximal tibial vessels are occluded, which frequently occurs secondary to failure of a more proximal bypass. The technique required for performing bypasses to secondary branches in the foot is essentially the same as that required for performing bypasses to major infrapopliteal vessels.

Optimal illumination by means of head lamps is important for achieving technical success with plantar bypass, and loupe magnification is helpful when the vessel is less than 1.5 mm in diameter. In addition, visualization of perimalleolar and inframalleolar arteries requires excellent preoperative imaging studies.

Figure 13 **Infrapopliteal bypass: in situ technique. A completion arteriogram from a patient who underwent an in situ bypass with coil occlusion of the side branches shows the two coils (arrows), which have successfully occluded the side-branch veins.**

Posterior Tibial Artery
Peroneal Artery
Anterior Tibial Artery
Lateral Tarsal Artery
Dorsalis Pedis
Arcuate Artery
Deep Plantar Artery
Lateral Plantar Artery
Medial Plantar Artery

Figure 12 **Infrapopliteal bypass: dorsalis pedis artery. Shown is an arteriogram from a 72-year-old diabetic patient who underwent a popliteal artery–dorsalis pedis artery bypass with a reversed saphenous vein graft for a nonhealing great toe amputation.**

Figure 14 **Plantar bypass. Shown are the major arteries of the foot, including the two major branches of the posterior tibial artery.[3] The lateral plantar artery is usually the larger and ends in the deep plantar arch.**

Figure 15 Plantar bypass. A completion arteriogram from a 62-year-old diabetic with nonhealing toe ulcers who underwent a popliteal artery–medial plantar artery bypass with a reversed saphenous vein graft shows the distal anastomosis, with flow visible through a small but patent medial plantar artery.

These very distal bypasses offer a viable alternative to a major amputation. Like infrapopliteal bypasses, they are best described in terms of the anatomic approaches to the distal branch vessels. In what follows, we outline exposure of the plantar and tarsal arteries; exposure of the dorsalis pedis artery is outlined elsewhere [see Infrapopliteal Bypass, *above*].

OPERATIVE TECHNIQUE

Exposure of Lateral and Medial Plantar Arteries

The lateral and medial plantar branches are the continuation of the posterior tibial artery in the foot [see Figure 16]. The lat-

eral plantar artery forms the deep plantar arch and is larger than the medial plantar artery. If the lateral branch is occluded, the medial branch may enlarge and feed the plantar arch through collateral vessels.

The initial incision is made over the termination of the posterior tibial artery below the malleolus. The artery is isolated, and the incision is extended inferiorly and laterally onto the sole. A direct approach to the individual branches is difficult, for several reasons. First, because the skin of the sole is not easily retracted, adequate exposure of the lateral and medial plantar arteries is hard to obtain if the incision does not follow their course exactly. Second, because these arteries are small in diameter and lie deep within the foot, they can be quite difficult to locate. Third, it is sometimes hard to distinguish the lateral plantar artery from the medial plantar artery. Dissection of the termination of the posterior tibial artery can help the surgeon make this distinction. The lateral branch is usually located inferiorly when the foot is externally rotated on the operating table.

Exposure of the proximal 2 to 3 cm of the plantar branches is accomplished by incising the flexor retinaculum and the adductor muscle of the great toe. More distal exposure of these branches can be obtained by dividing the medial border of the plantar aponeurosis and the extensor digitorum brevis muscle.

Exposure of Deep Plantar Artery and Lateral Tarsal Artery

The deep plantar artery and the lateral tarsal artery are branches of the dorsalis pedis artery. The deep plantar artery originates at the metatarsal level, where it descends into a foramen bounded proximally by the dorsal metatarsal ligament, distally by the dorsal interosseous muscle ring, and medially and laterally by the bases of the first and second metatarsal bones. As the deep plantar artery exits from this tunnel, it connects with the lateral plantar artery to form the deep plantar arch [see Figure 17].

A slightly curved longitudinal 3 to 4 cm incision is made over the dorsum of the middle portion of the foot, and the dorsalis pedis artery is dissected distally down to its bifurcation into deep plantar and first dorsal metatarsal branches. The extensor hallucis brevis muscle is retracted laterally—or, if necessary,

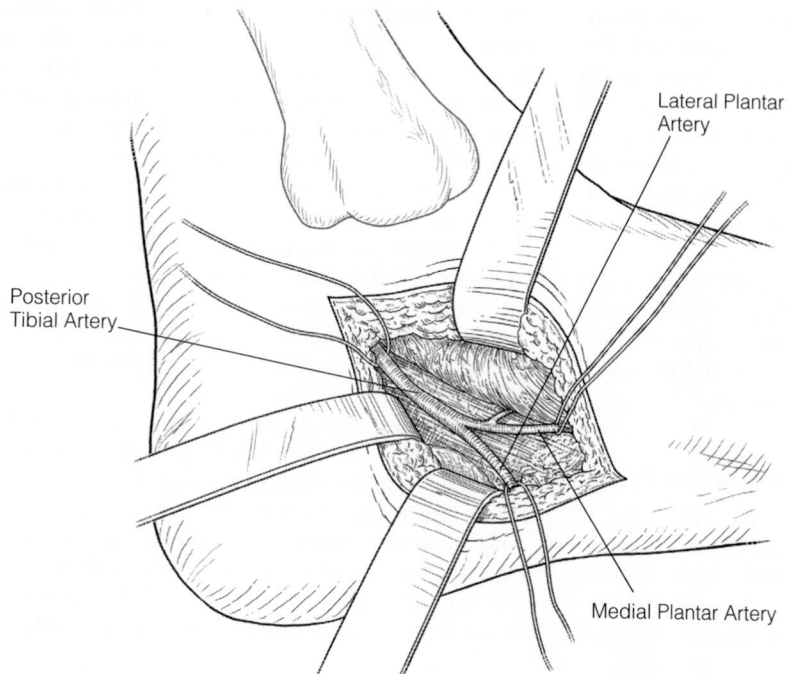

Figure 16 Plantar bypass. Depicted is exposure of the distal portion of the posterior tibial artery. The lateral and medial plantar arteries branch from this vessel and lie beneath the flexor retinaculum and the abductor hallucis muscle, which can be incised.

Lateral Plantar Artery

Posterior Tibial Artery

Medial Plantar Artery

Dorsalis Pedis Artery

Lateral Tarsal Artery

Arcuate Artery

Deep Plantar Artery

Figure 17 **Plantar bypass. Shown is a dorsal view of the arteries of the foot. Exposure of the distal dorsalis pedis artery (insert) highlights the origin of the deep plantar artery and its downward course between the first and second metatarsal bones. This exposure is facilitated by lateral retraction of the extensor hallucis brevis muscle.**

transected—and the dorsal interosseous muscle ring is split to allow better exposure of the proximal portion of the deep plantar artery. The periosteum of the proximal portion of the second metatarsal bone is then incised and elevated. A fine-tipped rongeur is used to excise enough of the metatarsal shaft to permit ample exposure of the deep plantar artery.

OUTCOME EVALUATION

Bypasses to the dorsalis pedis artery and its branches have yielded results comparable to those of bypasses to more proximal tibial vessels, with 3-year primary patency rates ranging from 58% to 60% and limb salvage rates ranging from 75% to 95%.[38-40] In one review, patency rates were higher in patients who had an intact plantar arch than in those who did not; however, failure to visualize the plantar arch on preoperative arteriograms does not preclude the performance of these bypasses for limb salvage. With careful follow-up, the assisted primary patency rates for these grafts have been substantially improved.[41] The available reports emphasize the need to repair failing grafts because their secondary patency was much better than that of failed grafts. In one study, patients who required shorter bypasses or had lower preoperative C-reactive protein levels experienced significantly better outcomes.[42] In some patients, occlusion of the distal tibial vessel necessitates performance of a tibiotibial bypass to achieve wound healing.[7]

Bypasses to plantar or tarsal vessels performed with vein grafts yield 2-year patency rates ranging from 65% to 75% and limb salvage rates higher than 80%.[4,5] In one report, the primary patency rate for these grafts was 74% at 1 year and 67% at 2 years, and the limb salvage rate was 78% at 2 years.[3]

Alternative Bypasses Using More Distal Inflow Vessels

Traditionally, the femoral artery has been the inflow site of choice for infrainguinal bypasses. Since the early 1980s, the superficial femoral, deep femoral, popliteal, and tibial arteries have all been used as inflow sources when these vessels were relatively disease free or when the amount of autologous vein available was lim-

ited. Currently, the superficial femoral artery and the popliteal artery are preferentially used for primary bypasses when they are free of disease.

The strategy of utilizing more distal inflow sources is particularly applicable to inframalleolar bypasses, in which very long vein segments would be required to reach the dorsalis pedis or other pedal arteries from the usual more proximal inflow sites. Two studies from the latter half of the 1980s reported that the patency rates in bypasses originating from the superficial femoral and popliteal arteries were comparable to those in bypasses originating from the common femoral artery.[43,44] In a review of our own experience with popliteal-distal vein graft bypasses,[5] we reported a patency rate of 65% at 4 years—a figure comparable to rates reported for femorodistal bypasses with reversed or in situ vein grafts (67% and 69%, respectively).[34] Given these results, surgeons should not hesitate to employ either the popliteal artery or the superficial femoral artery as an inflow source. Use of these more distal inflow sites results in shorter grafts and allows portions of saphenous vein to be preserved for other purposes.

An increasing number of limb salvage procedures are secondary interventions. These secondary procedures are generally more difficult to perform because the access routes to the arteries have been previously dissected and because there frequently is little good autologous vein left. In some cases, patients present with gangrene developing below a functioning bypass or after a previous failed bypass. Some of these patients need nothing more than a short distal extension of their functioning bypass; others have only enough vein left to make up a short graft. For such patients, a tibiotibial bypass may be an effective alternative revascularization approach.

In 1994, our group reported our 11-year experience with tibiotibial bypasses, comprising 42 procedures in 41 patients.[7] Ten of these bypasses were performed because previous bypasses failed; the remainder were performed because the amount of autologous vein available was limited. Approximately 50% of the bypasses were to pedal or tarsal vessels. At 5 years, the patency rate for these grafts was 65%, and the limb salvage rate was 73%.[7] A subsequent study reported comparable results.[45]

References

1. Veith FJ, Gupta SK, Wengerter KR, et al: Changing arteriosclerotic disease patterns and management strategies in lower-limb–threatening ischemia. Ann Surg 212:402, 1990

2. Veith FJ, Gupta SK, Samson RH, et al: Progress in limb salvage by reconstructive arterial surgery combined with new or improved adjunctive procedures. Ann Surg 194:386, 1981

3. Ascer E, Veith FJV, Gupta SK: Bypasses to plantar arteries and other tibial branches: an extended approach to limb salvage. J Vasc Surg 8:434, 1988

4. Andros G: Bypass grafts to the ankle and foot: a personal perspective. Surg Clin North Am 75:715, 1995

5. Wengerter KR, Yang PM, Veith FJ, et al: A twelve-year experience with the popliteal-to-distal artery bypass: the significance and management of proximal disease. J Vasc Surg 15:143, 1992

6. Veith FJ, Gupta SK, Samson RH, et al: Superficial femoral and popliteal arteries as inflow site for distal bypasses. Surgery 90:980, 1981

7. Lyon RT, Veith FJ, Marsan BU, et al: Eleven-year experience with tibiotibal bypass: an unusual but effective solution to distal tibial artery occlusive disease and limited autologous vein. J Vasc Surg 17:1128, 1994

8. Baker JD, Dix D: Variability of Doppler ankle pressures with arterial occlusive disease: an evaluation of ankle index and brachial-ankle pressure gradient. Surgery 79:134, 1976

9. Kohler TR, Nance DR, Cramer MM, et al: Duplex scanning for diagnosis of aortoiliac and femoropopliteal disease—a prospective study. Circulation 76:1074, 1987

10. Langsfeld M, Nupute J, Hershey FB, et al: The use of deep duplex scanning to predict hemodynamically significant aortoiliac stenosis. J Vasc Surg 7:395, 1988

11. Moneta GL, Yeager RA, Antonovic R, et al: Accuracy of lower extremity arterial duplex mapping. J Vasc Surg 15:275, 1992

12. Legemate DA, Teeuwen C, Hoenveld H, et al: Value of duplex scanning compared with angiography and pressure measurement in the assessment of aortoiliac lesions. Br J Surg 78:1003, 1991

13. Aser E, Mazzariol F, Hingorani A, et al: The use of duplex ultrasound arterial mapping as an alternative to conventional arteriography for primary and secondary infrapopliteal bypasses. Am J Surg 178:162, 1999

14. Wain RA, Berdejo GL, Delvalle WN, et al: Can duplex scan arterial mapping replace contrast arteriography as the test of choice before infrainguinal revascularization? J Vasc Surg 29:100, 1999

15. Owens RS, Carpenter JP, Baum RA, et al: Magnetic resonance imaging of angiographically occult runoff vessels in peripheral arterial occlusive disease. N Engl J Med 326:1577, 1992

16. Carpenter JP, Owen RS, Baum RA, et al: Magnetic resonance angiography of peripheral runoff vessels. J Vasc Surg 16:807, 1992

17. Earls JP, Patel NH, Smith PA, et al: Gadolinium-enhanced three-dimensional MR angiography of the aorta and peripheral arteries: evaluation of a multistation examination using two gadopentetate dimeglumine infusions. AJR Am J Roentgenol 171:599, 1998

18. Fellner F, Janka R, Fellner C, et al: Post occlusion visualization of peripheral arteries with "floating table" MR angiography. Magn Reson Imaging 17:1235, 1999

19. Fenlon HM, Yucel EK: Advances in abdominal, aortic, and peripheral contrast-enhanced MR angiography. Magn Reson Imaging Clin North Am 7:319, 1999

20. Brewster DC, Waltman AC, O'Hara PJ, et al: Femoral artery pressure measurement during aortography. Circulation 60:120, 1979

21. Hessel SJ, Adams DF, Abrams HL: Complications of angiography. Radiology 138:273, 1981

22. Gomes AS, Baker JD, Martin-Paredero V, et al: Acute renal dysfunction after major arteriography. AJR Am J Roentgenol 145:1249, 1985

23. Martin-Paredero V, Dixon SM, Baker JD, et al: Risk of renal failure after major angiography. Arch Surg 118:1417, 1983

24. Nikonoff T, Skau T, Berglund J, et al: Effects of femoral arteriography and low osmolar contrast agents on renal function. Acta Radiol 34:88, 1993

25. Katholi RE, Taylor GJ, Woods WT, et al: Nephrotoxicity of nonionic low-osmolality versus ionic high osmolality contrast media: a prospective double-blind randomized comparison in human beings. Radiology 186:183, 1993

26. Lautin EM, Freeman NJ, Schoenfeld AH, et al: Radiocontrast-associated renal dysfunction: a comparison of lower-osmolality and conventional high-osmolality contrast media. AJR Am J Roentgenol 157:59, 1991

27. Kram HB, Gupta SK, Veith FJ, et al: Late results of two hundred seventeen femoropopliteal bypasses to isolated popliteal artery segments. J Vasc Surg 14:386, 1991

28. Veith FJ, Gupta SK, Daly V: Femoropopliteal bypass to the isolated popliteal segment: is polytetrafluoroethylene graft acceptable? Surgery 89:296, 1981

29. Taylor LM, Edwards JM, Porter JM: Present status of reversed vein bypass grafting: five-year results of a modern series. J Vasc Surg 11:193, 1990

30. Veith FJ, Gupta SK, Ascer E, et al: Six year prospective multicenter randomized comparison of autologous saphenous vein and expanded polytetrafluoroethylene grafts in infrainguinal arterial reconstructions. J Vasc Surg 3:104, 1986

31. Jordan WD, Voellinger DC, Schroeder PT, et al: Video-assisted saphenous vein harvest: the evaluation of a new technique. J Vasc Surg 26:405, 1997

32. Wagner WH, Treiman RL, Cossman DV, et al: Tourniquet occlusion technique for tibial artery reconstruction. J Vasc Surg 18:637, 1993

33. Suggs WD, Sanchez LA, Woo D, et al: Endoscopically assisted in situ lower extremity bypass: a preliminary report of a new minimally invasive technique. J Vasc Surg 34:668, 2001

34. Bergamini TM, Towne JB, Bandyk DF, et al: Experience with in situ saphenous vein bypasses during 1981 to 1989: determinant factors of long-term patency. J Vasc Surg 13:137, 1991

35. Wengerter KR, Veith FJ, Gupta SK, et al: Prospective randomized multi center comparison of in situ and reversed vein infrapopliteal bypasses. J Vasc Surg 13:189, 1991

36. Rosenthal D, Arous EJ, Friedman SG, et al: Endovascular-assisted versus conventional in situ saphenous vein bypass grafting: cumulative patency, limb salvage, and cost results in a 39-month multi center study. J Vasc Surg 21:60, 2000

37. Piano G, Schwartz LB, Foster L, et al: Assessing outcomes, costs, and benefits of emerging technology for minimally invasive saphenous vein in situ distal arterial bypasses. Arch Surg 133:613, 1998

38. Schneider JR, Walsh DB, McDaniel MD, et al: Pedal bypass versus tibial bypass with autogenous vein: a comparison of outcome and hemodynamic results. J Vasc Surg 17:1029, 1993

39. Harrington EB, Harrington ME, Schanzer H, et al: The dorsalis pedis bypass: moderate success in difficult situations. J Vasc Surg 15:409, 1992

40. Panayiotopoulos YP, Tyrrell MR, Arnold FJ, et al: Results and cost analysis of distal [crural/pedal] arterial revascularization for limb salvage in diabetic and nondiabetic patients. Diabet Med 14:214, 1997

41. Rhodes JM, Gloviczki P, Bower TC, et al: The benefits of secondary interventions in patients with failing or failed pedal bypass grafts. Am J Surg 178:151, 1999

42. Biancari F, Alback A, Kantonen I, et al: Predictive factors for adverse outcome of pedal bypasses. Eur J Vasc Endovasc Surg 18:138, 1999

43. Cantelmo NL, Snow JR, Menzoian JO, et al: Successful vein bypass in patients with an ischemic limb and a palpable popliteal pulse. Arch Surg 121:217, 1986

44. Rosenbloom JS, Walsh JJ, Schuler JJ, et al: Long-term results of infragenicular bypasses with autogenous vein originating from the distal superficial femoral and popliteal arteries. J Vasc Surg 7:691, 1988

45. Plecha EJ, Lee C, Hye RJ: Factors influencing the outcome of paramalleolar bypass grafts. Ann Vasc Surg 10:356, 1996

Acknowledgment

Figures 1 through 17   Tom Moore.

26 LOWER-EXTREMITY AMPUTATION FOR ISCHEMIA

William C. Pevec, M.D.

Patients with infected, painful, or necrotic lower extremities can be restored to a better functional level by means of a properly selected and performed amputation. This procedure should be considered reconstructive and restorative. In what follows, I address amputations across the toe, the forefoot, the leg, and the thigh. Because Symes' amputations and hip disarticulations are seldom appropriate on ischemic limbs, I omit discussion of these procedures.

General Preoperative Planning

Selecting the appropriate level of amputation is of primary importance for healing and preservation of function. For an ambulatory patient who has either a palpable pulse over the dorsal pedal or posterior tibial arteries or a functioning infrainguinal arterial bypass graft, amputation on the foot (either toe amputation or transmetatarsal amputation) is appropriate. For an ambulatory patient who has a palpable femoral pulse and a patent profunda femoral artery, whose skin is warm at least to the level of the ankle, and who has no skin lesions on the proposed amputation flaps, amputation below the knee is appropriate. For a nonambulatory patient who has ischemic rest pain, ulceration, or gangrene, amputation above the knee is appropriate. Arterial reconstruction is not indicated if the extremity is nonfunctional. Below-the-knee amputation does not offer nonambulatory patients any functional advantage; moreover, it is less likely to heal and often results in a flexion contracture at the knee that leads to pressure ulceration of the stump. Above-the-knee amputation depends on pulsatile flow into the ipsilateral internal iliac artery for successful healing. Above-the-knee amputation is also necessary for a patient whose skin is cool at or above the midcalf or who has skin lesions at or proximal to the midcalf.

Several adjunctive measurements (e.g., transcutaneous oxygen tension and segmental arterial pressure) have been used to select the level of amputation but have not proved particularly helpful. Generally, these adjuncts can reliably determine a level of amputation at which healing is virtually assured, but they cannot reliably determine the level at which an amputation will not heal. Consequently, reliance on such measures to select the level of amputation will result in an unnecessarily high percentage of more proximal amputations.

In most cases, definitive amputation can be accomplished in a single stage. Local cellulitis can usually be controlled beforehand with bed rest and systemic administration of antibiotics. Undrained pus or recalcitrant cellulitis, however, must be treated with debridement and drainage in advance of definitive amputation. This can be accomplished with local soft tissue debridement, single-toe amputation, or guillotine amputation across the ankle.

Careful preoperative medical assessment is essential. Lower-extremity amputation for ischemia is associated with a mortality of 4.5% to 16%,[1-5] owing to the poor overall condition of the patient population. Accordingly, optimization of cardiac and pulmonary function and control of systemic infection are mandatory.

Finally, the timing of elective amputation is crucial. Because the loss of a limb is a difficult and frightening thing for a patient to accept, there is a natural tendency to delay amputation for as long as possible. This tendency is understandable but must be weighed against the potential problems associated with delay, such as poor preoperative pain control, which leads to an increased incidence of postamputation phantom limb pain, and extended preoperative immobility, which leads to physical deconditioning and makes prosthetic limb rehabilitation more difficult. A preoperative consultation with a physiatrist can allay some of the patient's anxiety by addressing the expected postoperative course of rehabilitation and thereby removing some of the fear of the unknown.

Toe Amputation

Amputation of the toe can be done either across a phalanx or across a metatarsal bone; the latter procedure is commonly referred

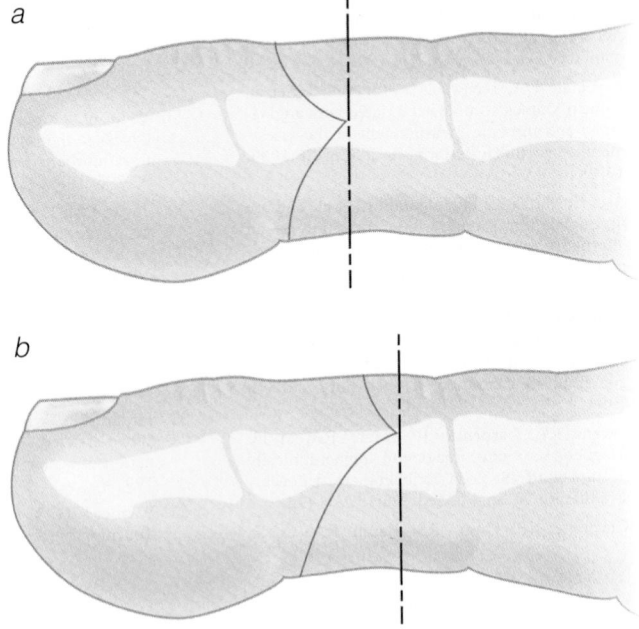

a

b

Figure 1 Toe amputation: transphalangeal amputation. Transphalangeal amputation can be performed either with dorsal and plantar flaps of equal length (*a*) or with a plantar flap that is longer than the dorsal flap (*b*). The phalanx is transected at the level of the apex of the skin flaps (dashed line). The bone is transected through the shaft of the phalanx, never across the joint.

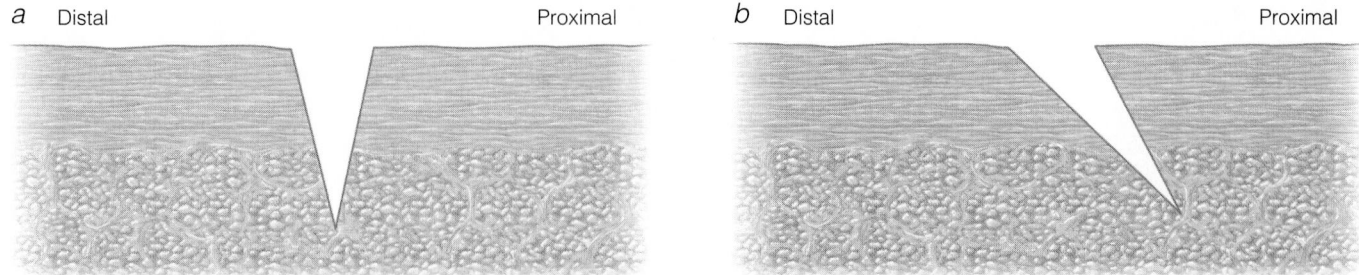

a Distal   Proximal   *b* Distal   Proximal

Figure 2 In a lower-extremity amputation, the skin is always incised perpendicular to its surface (*a*). Given the varying contours encountered during extremity amputation, it can be difficult to maintain the perpendicular orientation of the scalpel; however, an incision that undermines the proximal skin flap (*b*) will devascularize the epidermis and lead to necrosis of the suture line.

to as a ray amputation. Many of the perioperative issues are essentially similar for the two approaches; however, indications and operative details differ somewhat and thus will be described separately.

OPERATIVE PLANNING

As noted (see above), for a toe amputation to heal properly, there must be either a palpable pulse over the dorsal pedal or posterior tibial artery or a functioning bypass graft to an infrapopliteal artery. If tissue necrosis or infection is confined to the distal or middle phalanx, transphalangeal amputation is appropriate; if tissue loss or necrosis involves the proximal phalanx, ray amputation is indicated. If tissue necrosis or infection extends over the metatarsophalangeal joint, either transmetatarsal amputation of the entire forefoot or below-the-knee amputation is usually necessary (see below).

Multiple transphalangeal amputations are functionally well tolerated. If, however, ray amputation of the great toe or of more than one smaller toe is called for, it is preferable to perform a transmetatarsal amputation of the forefoot. Adequate skin coverage is usually difficult to achieve with a great-toe or multiple-toe ray amputation. In addition, ray amputation of more than one of the middle toes often causes central deviation of the remaining outside toes, which can lead to ulcerations secondary to abnormal pressure points. Finally, loss of the first metatarsal head or of several of the other metatarsal heads results in abnormal weight-bearing on the remaining metatarsal heads, which may give rise to late ulceration.

OPERATIVE TECHNIQUE

Transphalangeal Amputation

Digital block anesthesia is ideal for transphalangeal amputation. A 25-gauge needle is inserted into the skin over the medial aspect of the dorsum of the proximal phalanx and advanced until the bone is encountered. The needle is then withdrawn slightly, and a small amount of fluid is aspirated to confirm that the tip of the needle is not in a blood vessel. Next, 0.5 to 1.0 ml of lidocaine, 0.5% or 1.0% without epinephrine, is slowly injected. The needle is then carefully advanced medial to the bone until the tip can be felt pressing against (but not puncturing) the plantar skin. Again, the needle is withdrawn slightly, fluid is aspirated, and 0.5 to 1.0 ml of lidocaine is injected. The same technique is repeated on the lateral aspect of the proximal phalanx. In this way, all four digital nerve branches are blocked. If multiple toe amputations are required, an ankle block, epidural anesthesia, spinal anesthesia, or general anesthesia can be used.

An incision is made to create dorsal and plantar skin flaps. Typically, these flaps are equal in length [*see Figure 1a*]; however, depending on the location of the skin lesion, either the dorsal flap or the plantar flap can be left longer [*see Figure 1b*]. Care must be tak-

en not to create excessively long flaps, which may lack sufficient perfusion for healing, or to create undermined bevels with the scalpel [*see Figure 2*], which will lead to epidermolysis of the suture line.

The incision is extended down to the phalanx, and the soft tissues are gently separated from the bone with a small periosteal elevator. All tendons and tendon sheaths are debrided because the poor vascularity of these tissues may compromise the healing of the toe. The phalanx is transected at the level of the apices of the skin incisions [*see Figure 1*]. Care must be taken not to leave the remaining bone segment too long: this places undue tension on the skin flaps and is a primary cause of poor healing. The best way of transecting the phalanx is to use a pneumatic oscillating saw. Manual bone cutters can splinter the bone, and manual saws can cause extensive damage to the soft tissues. The bone is always transected across the shaft: because of the poor vascularity of the articular cartilage, disarticulation across a joint typically leads to poor healing.

Hemostasis is achieved with absorbable sutures and limited use of the electrocautery. Excessive tissue manipulation and electrocauterization should be avoided. The skin edges are carefully approximated with simple interrupted nonabsorbable monofilament sutures; perfect apposition is necessary to maximize the potential for primary healing. The sutures must not be placed too close to the skin edges, because the heavily keratinized skin of the foot is easily lacerated. The final step is the application of a soft dressing.

Ray Amputation

For ray amputation, spinal, epidural, or general anesthesia can be employed. A so-called tennis racket incision is made—that is, a straight incision along the dorsal surface of the affected metatarsal bone coupled with a circumferential incision around the base of the toe [*see Figure 3a*]. The goal is to save all available viable skin on the toe; this skin is used to ensure a tension-free closure, and any excess skin can be debrided later, at the time of closure. Again, undermined bevels are avoided. The incision is taken down to the bone, and the soft tissues are separated from the distal metatarsal bone with a periosteal elevator. Dissection must be kept close to the affected metatarsal head to prevent injury to the adjacent metatarsophalangeal joint, which can lead to necrosis of the adjacent toe. The metatarsal bone is transected across the shaft with a pneumatic oscillating saw [*see Figure 3b*]. The tendons and the tendon sheaths are debrided.

Meticulous hemostasis is achieved with absorbable sutures and limited use of the electrocautery. The skin is approximated with simple interrupted nonabsorbable monofilament sutures. If sufficient viable skin was preserved, a flap of plantar skin is rotated dorsally, and the incision is closed in the shape of a Y [*see Figure 4a*]. Alternatively, the medial and lateral edges are shifted, one proximally and the other distally, the corners are trimmed, and the incision is

Figure 3   Toe amputation: ray amputation. (*a*) A longitudinal incision is made along the dorsum of the shaft of the metatarsal bone of the affected toe. A circumferential incision is then made around the phalanx. The circumferential incision should be placed as distal on the toe as there is viable skin so that as much skin as possible is retained for closure of the wound. (*b*) The metatarsal bone is transected across its shaft, proximal to the metatarsal head; the joint is never disarticulated.

closed in a linear fashion [*see Figure 4b*]. A soft supportive dressing is applied.

COMPLICATIONS

Complications of toe amputation include bleeding, infection, and failure to heal. Because even a small amount of bleeding under the skin flaps can prevent proper healing, meticulous hemostasis is mandatory. In most cases, infection and failure to heal are attributable to poor patient selection and poor surgical technique; the usual result is a more proximal amputation.

OUTCOME

For optimal healing, there must be an extended period (2 to 3 weeks) during which no weight is borne by the foot that underwent toe amputation. Once healing is complete, the patient should be able to walk normally, with no need for orthotic or assist devices. Beginning ambulation too early can disrupt healing flaps and necessitate more proximal amputation, which lengthens the hospital stay and increases long-term disability. For these reasons, toe amputation in patients with arterial occlusive disease is not an outpatient procedure. Patients are kept on bed rest and instructed in techniques (e.g., use of a wheelchair, a walker, or crutches) that allow them to function without stepping on the foot that was operated on. Hospital discharge is delayed until such techniques are mastered.

Transmetatarsal Amputation

OPERATIVE PLANNING

As noted (see above), transmetatarsal amputation is indicated if there is tissue loss in the forefoot involving the first metatarsal head, two or more of the other metatarsal heads, or the dorsal forefoot. It is contraindicated if there is extensive skin loss on the plantar sur-

face of the foot or on the dorsum proximal to the midshaft of the metatarsal bones. The peroneus longus and peroneus brevis muscles insert on the proximal portions of the fourth and fifth metatarsal bones; if these insertions are sacrificed, inversion of the foot results, eventually leading to chronic skin breakdown from the side of the foot repeatedly striking the ground during ambulation. Transmetatarsal amputation is also contraindicated if there is a preexisting footdrop (peroneal palsy).

OPERATIVE TECHNIQUE

Spinal, epidural, or general anesthesia may be employed. Placement of a tourniquet on the calf is a useful adjunctive measure. This step greatly reduces intraoperative blood loss. More important, the bloodless operative field that results allows more accurate assessment of tissue viability and hence more precise selection of the level of amputation; in a field stained with extravasated blood, it is easy to leave behind nonviable tissue that will doom the amputation. Use of a tourniquet is, however, contraindicated in patients who have a functioning infrapopliteal artery bypass graft.

After sterile preparation and draping, the leg is elevated to help drain the venous blood, and a sterile pneumatic tourniquet is placed around the calf, with care taken to pad the skin under the tourniquet and to position the tourniquet over the calf muscles, where it will not apply pressure over the fibular head (and the common peroneal nerve) or other osseous prominences. The tourniquet is then inflated to a pressure higher than the systolic blood pressure. In patients who do not have diabetes mellitus, a tourniquet inflation pressure of 250 mm Hg is typically employed; in patients who have diabetes mellitus and calcified arteries, a pressure of 350 to 400 mm Hg is preferred.

An incision is made across the dorsum of the foot at the level of the middle of the shafts of the metatarsal bones, extending medially and laterally to the level of the center of the first and fifth metatarsal bones, respectively [*see Figure 5*]. The dorsal incision is curved prox-

Figure 4 Toe amputation: ray amputation. (*a*) **If adequate skin is available, a plantar flap can be rotated dorsally and the skin closed in a Y configuration. This closure is technically easy to perform; however, there is a risk of skin necrosis at corners A and B. (*b*) Alternatively, the skin can be closed in a linear fashion. Corners A and B are gently trimmed. Corner B is shifted distally toward point D as corner A is shifted proximally. A slight dog-ear will result at point E; however, it will diminish with time.**

imally at the medial and lateral edges to ensure that no dog-ears remain at the time of closure. The dorsal incision is continued perpendicularly through the soft tissues on the dorsum down to the metatarsal bones. The plantar incision is extended distally to a point just proximal to the toe crease. Care is taken not to bevel the skin incisions.

A plantar flap is created by making an incision with the scalpel adjacent to the metatarsophalangeal joints; the incision is then carried more deeply to the level of the midshafts of the metatarsal bones on their plantar surfaces. The periosteum of the first metatar-

sal bone is scored circumferentially with the scalpel, and the soft tissue is dissected away from the first metatarsal bone with a periosteal elevator to a point about 1 cm proximal to the dorsal skin incision. The first metatarsal bone is then transected perpendicular to its shaft at the level of the dorsal skin incision with a pneumatic oscillating saw. This process is repeated for each individual metatarsal bone, with care taken to follow the normal contour of the forefoot by cutting the lateral ametatarsal bones at a level slightly proximal to the level at which the more medial bones are transected. All visible digital arteries are clamped and tied with absorbable ligatures. If a

Figure 5 Transmetatarsal amputation. The skin incisions are shown from various angles. The metatarsal shafts are divided in their midportions (dashed line). The metatarsal bone transection is at the level of the apices of the skin incision, and the lateral metatarsal bones are cut slightly more proximally than the medial metatarsal bones, in a pattern reflecting the normal contour of the forefoot.

tourniquet was used, it is deflated at this time. All tendons and tendon sheaths are debrided from the wound.

Meticulous hemostasis is achieved with absorbable sutures and limited use of the electrocautery. Any sharp edges on the metatarsal bones are smoothed with a rongeur or a rasp. The wound is irrigated to flush out devitalized tissue and thrombus. The plantar flap is trimmed as needed. The dermis is approximated with simple interrupted absorbable sutures, and the knots are buried. Because the edge of the plantar flap is generally longer than the edge of the dorsal flap, the sutures must be placed slightly farther apart on the plantar flap than on the dorsal flap if perfect alignment is to be obtained. It is imperative to achieve the correct skin alignment with the dermal suture layer. Once this is accomplished, the skin edges are gently and perfectly apposed with interrupted vertical mattress sutures of nonabsorbable monofilament material. Finally, a soft supportive dressing with good padding of the heel is applied; casts and splints are avoided because of the risk of ulceration of the heel or over the malleoli.

COMPLICATIONS

If a tourniquet is not used, intraoperative blood loss can be substantial; the blood pools in the sponges and drapes, often out of the anesthesiologist's field of view. Consequently, good communication between the surgeon and the anesthesiologist is crucial for preventing ischemic complications secondary to hemorrhage.

Postoperative complications include bleeding, infection, and failure to heal, all of which are likely to result in more proximal amputation. They can best be prevented by means of careful patient selection and meticulous surgical technique.

OUTCOME

For proper healing, postoperative edema must be avoided and the plantar flap protected against shear forces. To prevent swelling, the patient is kept on bed rest with the foot elevated for the first 3 to 5 days. This step is particularly important if the transmetatarsal amputation was performed simultaneously with arterial reconstruction, which carries a high risk of reperfusion edema of the foot. Af-

ter 3 to 5 days, the patient is instructed in techniques for moving in and out of the wheelchair without stepping on the foot. The foot that was operated on should not bear any weight at all for at least 3 weeks; early weight-bearing may disrupt the healing of the plantar flap and necessitate more proximal amputation.

Once healed, patients should be able to walk independently with standard shoes. There is, however, a risk that they may trip over the unsupported toe of the shoe. In addition, the pushoff normally provided by the toes is lost after transmetatarsal amputation, and this change results in a halting, flat-footed gait. These problems can be obviated by using an orthotic shoe with a steel shank (to keep the toe of the shoe from bending and causing tripping) and a rocker bottom (to provide a smooth heel-to-toe motion).

Guillotine Ankle Amputation

OPERATIVE PLANNING

Guillotine amputation across the ankle is indicated when a patient presents with extensive wet gangrene that precludes salvage of a functional foot (e.g., wet gangrene that destroys the heel, the plantar skin of the forefoot, or the dorsal skin of the proximal foot). In such patients, initial guillotine amputation through the ankle is safer than extensive debridement: the operation is shorter, less blood is lost, the risk of bacteremia is reduced, and better control of infection is possible. Guillotine amputation is also indicated in patients with foot infections who have cellulitis extending into the leg. Transection at the ankle, perpendicular to the muscle compartments, tendon sheaths, and lymphatic vessels, allows effective drainage and usually brings about rapid resolution of the cellulitis of the leg, thus permitting salvage of the knee in many cases in which the knee might otherwise be unsalvageable.

OPERATIVE TECHNIQUE

General anesthesia is preferred; regional anesthesia is relatively contraindicated for critically ill patients who are in a septic state. Anesthesia is required for no more than 15 to 20 minutes.

Figure 6 **Guillotine ankle amputation. The skin incision is made circumferentially at the narrowest portion of the ankle. The bones are then transected at the same level (dashed line).**

A circumferential incision is made at the narrowest part of the ankle (i.e., at the proximal malleoli) regardless of the level of the cellulitis [see Figure 6]. This placement takes the line of incision across the tendons, thereby preventing bleeding from transected muscle bellies. The incision is then carried through the skin and soft tissues to the bone. If the arteries are patent, the assistant applies circumferential pressure to the distal calf. The distal tibia and fibula are then divided with a Gigli saw. Hemostasis is achieved with suture ligation and electrocauterization. A moist dressing is applied.

OUTCOME

After the procedure, the patient is kept on bed rest and given systemic antibiotics. Formal below-the-knee amputation can be performed when the cellulitis resolves, usually within 3 to 5 days. Routine dressing changes are unnecessary—first, because they are painful, and second, because the decision to proceed with formal below-the-knee amputation is based on the extent of the cellulitis in the calf, not on the appearance of the transected ankle.

Below-the-Knee Amputation

OPERATIVE PLANNING

Below-the-knee amputation is indicated when the lower extremity is functional but the foot cannot be salvaged by arterial reconstruction or by amputation of one or more of the toes or the forefoot. Healing can be expected if there is a palpable femoral pulse with at least a patent deep femoral artery, provided that the skin is warm and free of lesions at the distal calf. Before formal below-the-knee amputation, infection should be controlled with antibiotic therapy, debridement, and, if indicated, guillotine amputation. It is advisable to obtain consent to possible above-the-knee amputation beforehand in case unexpected muscle necrosis is encountered below the knee.

As with any amputation, the surgeon's preoperative interaction with the patient should be as positive as possible. A constructive perspective to convey is that the amputation, though regrettably neces-

sary, is in fact the first step toward rehabilitation. A well-motivated patient whose cardiopulmonary status is not too greatly compromised can generally be expected to walk again, albeit at an increased energy cost. In this regard, a preoperative discussion with a physiatrist can be very helpful, as can a meeting with an amputee who is doing well with a prosthesis. By inculcating a positive attitude in the patient before the procedure, the surgeon can greatly improve the patient's chances of achieving full rehabilitation as well as decrease the time needed for rehabilitation.

OPERATIVE TECHNIQUE

Epidural, spinal, or general anesthesia is appropriate.

The lines of incision should be marked on the skin. The primary level of amputation is determined by measuring a distance of 10 cm from the tibial tuberosity [see Figure 7]. The circumference of the leg at this level is then measured by passing a heavy ligature around the leg and cutting the ligature to a length equal to the circumference. The ligature is folded into thirds and cut once more at one of the folds, so that two segments of unequal length remain. The longer segment of the ligature, which is equal in length to two thirds of the leg's circumference 10 cm below the tibial tuberosity, is used to measure the anterior transverse incision; this incision is centered not on the tibial crest but on the gastrocnemius-soleus muscle complex. The shorter segment, which is one third of the leg's circumference at this level, is used to measure the posterior flap; the line of the posterior incision runs parallel with the gastrocnemius-soleus complex. To prevent dog-ears, the medial and lateral ends of the anterior transverse incision are curved cephalad before meeting the posterior incision, and the distal corners of the posterior incision are curved as well [see Figure 7].

10 cm

Figure 7 **Below-the-knee amputation. The transverse incision (A) is made 10 cm distal to the tibial tuberosity. Its length is equal to two thirds of the circumference of the leg at that level. The posterior incision (B) is made parallel with the gastrocnemius-soleus muscle complex. The length of the posterior flap is equal to one third of the measured circumference of the leg. The corners of the incisions are curved to avoid dog-ears.**

Posterior   Anterior

Figure 8 **Below-the-knee amputation. In this lateral view of the right leg, the tibia is beveled anteriorly, and the anterior portion is smoothed with a rasp. The fibula is transected at least 1 cm proximal to the level of transection of the tibia.**

Blood loss can be reduced by using a sterile pneumatic tourniquet. A gauze roll is passed around the distal thigh. The leg is elevated to drain the venous blood, and the tourniquet is applied over the gauze roll. The tourniquet is inflated to a pressure of 250 mm Hg (350 to 400 mm Hg if the patient has heavily calcified arteries). The assistant elevates the leg, and the incision on the posterior flap is made first, followed by the anterior transverse incision; this sequence helps prevent blood from obscuring the field while the incisions are being made. The incisions are carried fully through the dermis, and the skin edges are allowed to separate and expose the subcutaneous fat. Care is taken to keep the scalpel perpendicular to the skin so as not to bevel the incision, which can lead to necrosis of the epidermal edges [see Figure 2].

The anterior muscles are transected with the scalpel in a direction parallel to the transverse skin incision. The tibia is scored circumferentially, and a periosteal elevator is used to dissect the soft tissues away from the tibia for a distance of approximately 3 to 4 cm. The tibia is then transected just proximal to the transverse skin incision. Dividing the tibia more than 1 cm proximal to the anterior skin incision will cause the thin skin of the anterior leg to be pulled taut over the cut end of the tibia by the weight of the posterior flap, thereby leading to skin ulceration. The tibia is transected perpendicularly, with a cephalad bevel of the anterior 1 cm to keep from creating a sharp point at the tibial crest [see Figure 8]. The tibia can be transected with either a Gigli saw or an oscillating saw; because of the unpleasant sound of the power saw, the Gigli saw is preferred if the patient is under regional anesthesia. Sedation should be augmented in awake patients before division of the tibia. Benzodiazepines provide good sedation and amnesia.

The lateral muscles are divided, and the fibula is scored circumfer-

entially. A periosteal elevator is used to dissect the soft tissues away from the fibula to a point 2 to 3 cm cephalad to the level at which the tibia was transected. The fibula is then transected with a bone cutter at least 1 cm cephalad to the tibial transection level. The distal end of the tibia is lifted with a bone hook, and division of the posterior muscles is completed with an amputation knife. The specimen is then handed off the field.

The anterior tibial, posterior tibial, and peroneal arteries and veins are clamped, and the tourniquet is released. Clamps are placed on all other bleeding vessels. The posterior tibial and sural nerves are placed on gentle traction and clamped proximally. The distal nerves are transected, and the proximal nerves are allowed to retract into the soft tissues so as to prevent painful neuromas at the end of the stump. All clamped structures are then ligated with absorbable ligatures. The nerves are ligated because their nutrient vessels can bleed significantly. The distal anterior tip of the tibia is smoothed with a rasp to decrease the risk of skin ulceration over this osseous prominence. The stump is gently irrigated to remove all thrombus and devitalized tissue and to reveal any bleeding sites that may have been missed. Electrocauterization is rarely necessary.

The deep muscle fascia—not the Achilles tendon—is approximated with simple interrupted absorbable sutures, with care taken to align the posterior flap with the anterior incision. The dermis is approximated as a separate layer with simple interrupted absorbable sutures; if correctly placed, the dermal sutures should take all tension off the skin. The skin edges are then accurately apposed with interrupted vertical mattress sutures composed of monofilament nonabsorbable material. A carefully padded posterior splint or cast is applied to prevent flexion contracture.

COMPLICATIONS

The most common complications after below-the-knee amputation are bleeding, infection, and failure to heal, all of which are likely to result in a more proximal amputation, frequently accompanied by loss of the knee. Prevention of these complications depends on careful patient selection, preoperative control of infection, and meticulous surgical technique.

To walk with a prosthetic leg, the patient must be able to fully extend and lock the knee; thus, flexion contracture at the knee is a major complication. Such contractures are usually attributable either to poor pain control or to noncompliance with knee extension exercises. Good perioperative analgesia is of vital importance because knee flexion is the position of comfort and the patient will be unwilling to extend the knee if doing so proves too painful. To maintain knee extension, the patient should be placed in either a cast or a splint in the early postoperative period. Once postoperative pain has abated, the splint or cast can be removed. At this point, the patient must be taught extension exercises, in which the quadriceps muscles are contracted to maintain the length of the hamstring muscles. If a patient spends all of his or her time in a sitting position with the knee flexed, a flexion contracture will quickly develop. Once this happens, the patient may find it very difficult to regain full knee extension, and without full knee extension, prosthetic limb rehabilitation is impossible.

Phantom sensation is a common complication after below-the-knee amputation but is rarely of any consequence. Phantom pain, on the other hand, can be devastating. Sometimes, phantom pain develops as a consequence of unintentional suggestions made to the patient by medical personnel who fail to distinguish between the two entities. For example, a patient remarks to a medical attendant that he or she can still feel the amputated foot and toes, and the attendant suggests in response that the patient has phantom pain; the patient then focuses on the sensation and exaggerates the severity of

Figure 9 **Above-the-knee amputation. Broadly based anterior and posterior flaps are created. The femur is transected along the dashed line, at the apices of the skin flaps. The skin flaps and the level of transection of the femur can be placed more proximally if clinically indicated.**

the foot and toe discomfort, setting up a cycle of ever-worsening pain. This scenario is even more likely if the patient has had prolonged ischemic rest pain before the amputation. Phantom pain can be prevented by (1) encouraging early amputation in a patient with a hopelessly ischemic foot (while taking into account the patient's need to come to grips with the prospect of amputation), (2) providing good pain control in the early postoperative period, and (3) assuring the patient that phantom sensation after a below-the-knee amputation is common and that any discomfort in the foot immediately after the operation period will vanish once he or she begins walking again with a prosthetic leg.

Ulceration of the skin over the transected anterior portion of the tibia is another serious complication that may preclude successful prosthetic limb fitting. This complication is also best managed through prevention, which depends on meticulous surgical technique. As noted (see above), the anterior tibial crest must be carefully beveled and smoothed at the level of transection, and the tibia must not be transected more than 1 cm proximal to the anterior skin incision.

OUTCOME

Shortly after the amputation, the patient should be encouraged to start working on strengthening the upper body; upper-body strength is critical for making transfers and for using parallel bars, crutches, or a walker. In patients who have preoperative intractable ischemic rest pain, postoperative administration of epidural analgesia can break

the cycle of pain. Once postoperative pain is adequately controlled, patients are taught to transfer in and out of a wheelchair. A compression garment is used on the stump once the sutures have been removed and the stump is fully healed.

Prosthetic rehabilitation begins when the stump achieves a conical shape. Unfortunately, a number of patients who have undergone amputation for ischemia are unable to walk with a prosthetic limb because of comorbid medical conditions and general debility. In many cases, however, even if full ambulation is impossible, patients can maintain relative independence if the knee is salvaged by using a combination of a prosthetic leg and a walker for transfers and movement around the house.

Above-the-Knee Amputation

OPERATIVE PLANNING

Above-the-knee amputation is indicated if the lower extremity is unsalvageable and there is no femoral pulse. The presence of pulsatile flow into a well-developed ipsilateral internal iliac artery usually ensures healing, but even when there is more severe arterial occlusive disease in the pelvis, healing can sometimes be achieved. Above-the-knee amputation is also indicated if there is tissue necrosis or uncontrollable infection extending cephalad to the midleg. Above-the-knee amputation is the procedure of choice in the case of gangrene or ulceration of a completely nonfunctional lower extremity.

OPERATIVE TECHNIQUE

Epidural, spinal, or general anesthesia may be used.

For the best functional results, it is desirable to keep the femur as long as possible. A longer stump improves the prognosis for prosthetic limb rehabilitation and provides better balance for sitting and transfers. Healing potential, however, is lower with a longer stump; therefore, if the pelvic circulation is severely compromised, a shorter stump should be fashioned.

Anterior and posterior flaps of equal length are marked on the skin. The flaps should be wide and long [*see Figure 9*], and their apices should be centered on the line dividing the anterior and posterior muscle compartments. The posterior incision is made first to minimize the presence of blood in the operative field. The anterior incision is made second and carried through the anterior muscles in a plane parallel to the skin incision. The skin incisions are carried through the dermis, and the skin edges are allowed to separate and expose the subcutaneous fat; as in other amputations, they should be perpendicular to the skin surface so as not to undermine the skin.

If the superficial femoral artery is patent, the artery and vein are isolated and clamped after the sartorius muscle is divided but before the remainder of the anterior muscles are divided. The femur is scored circumferentially. The soft tissues are dissected away from the femur to the level of the apices of the flaps, and the femur is divided with an oscillating saw at this level. If the end of the resected femur extends beyond the apices of the flaps, the wound cannot be closed without tension. The posterior flap is completed with an amputation knife, and the specimen is handed off the field.

All bleeding points are clamped and tied with absorbable sutures. The sciatic nerve is placed on gentle traction, clamped, divided, and ligated, and the transected nerve is allowed to retract into the muscles. The deep fascia is approximated with interrupted absorbable sutures, with adjustments made for any discrepancy in length between the two flaps. The dermis is approximated with interrupted absorbable sutures; the dermal sutures should take all tension off

Figure 10 Above-the-knee amputation. (*a*) After an aerosol tincture of benzoin is applied to the thigh, the hip, and the lower abdomen, a 4 in. wide stockinette is rolled over the amputation stump. The cuff of the stockinette is cut medially at the groin. (*b*) The remainder of the stockinette is then rolled laterally up over the hip, and the cuff is cut on the lateral midline. (*c*) The two resulting strips of cloth are passed around the waist, one anteriorly and one posteriorly, and these strips are tied on the anterior midline to complete the dressing.

the skin. The skin edges are then carefully apposed with interrupted vertical mattress sutures.

A nonadherent dressing is placed on the suture line and covered with dry, fluffed gauze bandages. An aerosol tincture of benzoin is sprayed on the thigh, the hip, and the lower abdomen. When the benzoin is dry, a cloth stockinette with a diameter of 4 in. is stretched over the stump [*see Figure 10*]. The cuff of the stockinette is cut medially at the groin, and the stockinette is rolled laterally above the hip, where the cuff is then cut on the midaxillary line. This process yields two strips of cloth, one anterior and one posterior, which are passed around the patient's waist and tied on the anterior midline.

If the patient is a candidate for prosthetic limb rehabilitation, a traction rope is passed through a hole cut in the distal end of the stockinette and tied. The traction rope is hung over the end of the bed and tied to a 5 lb weight; this step helps prevent flexion contracture at the hip.

The stockinette need not be removed for the wound to be inspected. A window is cut in the distal end of the stockinette, and the gauze is removed. Once the incision has been inspected, fresh gauze is applied, and the window in the stockinette is closed with safety pins.

COMPLICATIONS

Postoperative complications include bleeding, infection, and failure to heal, all of which are likely to result in the need for surgical revision of the amputation stump. Control of preoperative infection and meticulous surgical technique and hemostasis are necessary to prevent these complications.

Flexion contracture of the hip is a major complication of above-the-knee amputation. Such contractures preclude successful prosthetic limb rehabilitation. In dealing with this complication, prevention is far more effective than treatment: once a flexion contracture at the hip becomes fixed, it is very difficult to reverse. If a patient is a candidate for prosthetic limb rehabilitation, the traction weight mentioned earlier (see above) can be very helpful. As soon as postoperative pain is controlled, the patient should be taught to spend three periods daily in a prone position to help extend the hip. He or she should then be taught exercises for maintaining range of motion in the hip before prosthetic limb rehabilitation is initiated. Flexion contracture of the hip is less of a problem in nonambulatory patients; however, it can still lead to wound breakdown and chronic skin ulceration.

OUTCOME

Once postoperative pain has abated, patients are mobilized to wheelchair transfers. The prognosis for successful prosthetic limb ambulation in patients undergoing above-the-knee amputation for ischemia is very poor.

References

1. Reichle FA, Rankin KP, Tyson RR, et al: Long-term results of 474 arterial reconstructions for severely ischemic limbs: a fourteen year follow-up. Surgery 85:93, 1979

2. Maini BS, Mannick JA: Effect of arterial reconstruction on limb salvage. Arch Surg 113:1297, 1978

3. Ellitsgaard N, Andersson AP, Fabrin J, et al: Outcome in 282 lower extremity amputations: knee salvage and survival. Acta Orthop Scand 61:140, 1990

4. Stewart CPU, Jain AS, Ogston SA: Lower limb amputee survival. Prosthet Orthot Int 16:11, 1992

5. Inderbitzi R, Buttiker M, Pfluger D, et al: The fate of bilateral lower limb amputees in end-stage vascular disease. Eur Vasc Surg 6:321, 1992

Acknowledgment

Figures 1 through 10   Tom Moore.

27 LAPAROSCOPIC ADRENALECTOMY

Theresa M. Quinn, M.D., Francesco Rubino, M.D., Michel Gagner, M.D.

Since the introduction of laparoscopic adrenalectomy in 1992, the minimally invasive approach to the adrenal gland has become the preferred option in a number of settings.[1-18] In particular, the small size of the glands, the superior retroperitoneal location, the benign nature of most adrenal tumors, and the lower morbidity associated with smaller incisions have made laparoscopy a valuable tool in endocrine surgery. Several published series[9,16,19,20] have documented the advantages of laparoscopic adrenalectomy over open adrenalectomy, including decreased operative blood loss, reduced narcotic requirements, and shorter hospital stay and recovery time.

Like its open counterpart, laparoscopic adrenalectomy may be performed via an anterior, a lateral, or a posterior approach. Successful laparoscopic adrenalectomy requires advanced laparoscopic skills, a solid understanding of adrenal anatomy, meticulous hemostasis, and delicate tissue handling. A thorough preoperative evaluation that includes clinical examination, biochemical assessment, diagnostic imaging (computed tomography or magnetic resonance imaging) for localization of the adrenal pathology, and, if necessary, venous sampling or fine-needle aspiration (FNA) cytology is essential.

Indications

Laparoscopic adrenalectomy is now the gold standard for adrenalectomy for selected patients with a variety of conditions [see Table 1], including both functional masses and nonfunctioning tumors. There are also several established contraindications [see Table 1], the most prominent of which is a surgeon's lack of experience with the technique. In addition, patients who are believed to have adrenal carcinoma on the basis of radiographic evaluation or who have a lesion greater than 10 cm in diameter should undergo open adrenalectomy to ensure complete excision of the lesion along with en bloc resection of surrounding organs as necessary. Coagulopathy and portal hypertension, conditions that place the patient at undue risk for perioperative bleeding and limit the exactitude of the laparoscopic procedure, are also contraindications to a minimally invasive approach.

Anatomic Considerations

The two adrenal glands are located in the lateral retroperitoneal area, in front of the 12th rib on the right and in front of the 11th and 12th ribs on the left, and are surrounded by perirenal fascia. They weigh approximately 6 g each, measure $5.0 \times 3.0 \times 0.6$ cm, and are placed like caps on the superomedial poles of the two kidneys. The right adrenal and the left adrenal have very similar relationships to the adjoining anatomy dorsally and laterally but substantially different relationships ventrally and medially. There are also significant right-left differences in adrenal blood supply that have important implications for surgical technique.

DORSAL AND LATERAL RELATIONSHIPS

Because the two adrenal glands have virtually identical dorsal and lateral anatomic relationships, there are no significant differences between posterior and lateral approaches to the right adrenal and posterior and lateral approaches to the left adrenal. Through the pararenal fat and the perirenal fascia, the posterolateral aspect of each adrenal is in contact with the superior part of the posterior abdominal wall. Each gland lies in close proximity to the diaphragmatic crus and to the lateral arcuate ligament. The crus and the arcuate ligament separate the adrenals from the reflection of the pleura, from the 11th and 12th ribs, and from the subcostal, sacrospinalis, and latissimus dorsi muscles.

VENTRAL RELATIONSHIPS

Right Adrenal

The main ventrolateral anatomic relationship of the right adrenal is with the peritoneum between the liver and the kidney. Exposure of the gland is achieved by opening the peritoneum after the right lobe of the liver is mobilized cephalad and medially. The main ventromedial anatomic relationship of the right adrenal is with the inferior vena cava. The right adrenal vein emerges from this aspect of the gland before emptying directly into the inferior vena cava.

Left Adrenal

The main ventrolateral relationships of the left adrenal are with the attachments of the kidney and, occasionally, the splenic flexure of the colon. Mobilization of the splenic flexure and incision of the peritoneal layer overlying Gerota's fascia expose the lateral aspect of the left adrenal. The main ventro-

Table 1 Indications for and Contraindications to Laparoscopic Adrenalectomy

Indications	Functional masses
	  Cortisol-secreting adenoma (Cushing syndrome)
	  Aldosterone-secreting adenoma (Conn syndrome)
	  Adrenocortical hyperplasia (Cushing disease) or
	    other hypercortisolism syndrome
	  Pheochromocytoma
	  Virilizing/feminizing syndromes
	Nonfunctional tumors
	  Incidentaloma (> 3 cm or growing)
	  Isolated adrenal metastases
	  Symptomatic angiomyolipoma
	  Symptomatic adrenal cyst

Contraindications	Surgeon inexperience Adrenal carcinoma Adrenal mass > 10 cm Coagulopathy (uncorrected) Portal hypertension

medial relationships of the left adrenal are with the spleen, the pancreas, and the gastric fundus. The splenorenal ligament is divided along the lateral aspect of the spleen to allow medial displacement of the spleen, the tail of the pancreas, and the gastric fundus. The splenic vein can be seen coursing along the posterior margin of the pancreas and the splenic artery along the superior border.

The body of the pancreas separates the adrenal gland from the lesser sac and from the stomach. A second approach to the left adrenal is direct access through the lesser sac after division of the gastrocolic ligament. The adrenal gland can be exposed by means of a peritoneal incision along the inferior or superior border of the pancreatic body. A third approach entails dissection of the transverse mesocolon to provide direct access to the posterior side of the pancreas and the adrenal gland.

BLOOD SUPPLY, LYMPHATIC DRAINAGE, AND INNERVATION

The adrenal glands receive their arterial blood from three sources: a superior adrenal artery arising from the inferior phrenic artery, a middle adrenal artery arising from the abdominal aorta, and an inferior adrenal artery arising from the renal artery.

The arrangement of the adrenal veins is much simpler than that of the adrenal arteries. There is one dominant vein and several smaller accessory veins that follow the arteries. During adrenalectomy for the treatment of a tumor producing excessive amounts of a hormone (especially a pheochromocytoma), the flow of the main adrenal vein is controlled at the beginning of the adrenal dissection.

On the left side, vascular control of the adrenal vein is relatively straightforward because the vein is long (about 30 mm) and empties into either the left inferior phrenic vein or the left renal vein; however, exposure of the left adrenal vein requires more time and more extensive dissection than exposure of the right. Once the inferior pole of the left adrenal has been identified, dissection for 1 to 2 cm along the medial margin of the gland reveals the left adrenal vein. On the right side, vascular control of the adrenal vein is more precarious because the right adrenal vein is much shorter than the left (about 6 mm) and empties directly into the posterior part of the inferior vena cava, an anatomic arrangement that increases the risk of major venous injury. On both sides, numerous accessory adrenal veins follow the arteries and empty into the inferior phrenic vein, the renal vein, or anastomotic branches joining with the azygos system and the posterior gastric veins. These collateral vessels may become significantly enlarged in patients with large adrenal tumors.

Nerves and vessels are ligated simultaneously during adrenalectomy. The nerves are numerous and arise from the sympathetic nervous system. The visceral afferent fibers arise from the celiac ganglia, which is derived from the posterior vagus nerve and the greater and lesser splanchnic nerves. The visceral fibers traverse the cortex to effect direct secretory or indirect vasomotor innervation and finish in the medulla as sympathetic preganglionic fibers.

Preoperative Evaluation

CLINICAL EXAMINATION

The clinical examination should be performed with particular attention to signs and symptoms of aldosterone, catecholamine, or cortisol excess. Nearly all patients with hyperaldosteronism and 60% of patients with pheochromocytoma

have a history of hypertension.[21] About 90% of patients with pheochromocytoma experience nonspecific symptoms, such as headache, diaphoresis, palpitations, abdominal pain, nervousness, nausea, vomiting, chest pain, and weakness. A history of type 2A or 2B multiple endocrine neoplasia can be helpful in diagnosing pheochromocytoma, given that this endocrine tumor ultimately develops in 40% of pheochromocytoma patients. Glucocorticoid-producing adenomas are extremely rare in the absence of the characteristic signs of hypercortisolism (i.e., easy bruising, striae, and myopathy). A functioning adrenocortical carcinoma may be signaled by the abrupt onset of Cushing syndrome or a virilization syndrome, pyrexia, and abdominal pain. Most adrenocortical carcinomas are large (mean diameter, 12.4 cm) and are symptomatic on presentation; only 10% are small and present asymptomatically as incidentalomas.[22]

BIOCHEMICAL ASSESSMENT

Between 0.3% and 5.0% of all abdominal CT scans performed for other reasons reveal incidental adrenal lesions.[23] Determination of hormone levels is important in all such cases because excision of all functioning lesions is recommended. Biochemical evaluation should include measurement of serum potassium concentrations and 24-hour urine collection for determination of metanephrine, vanillylmandelic acid (VMA), 17-hydroxycorticosteroid, and free cortisol levels. A patient with a nonfunctioning adrenal tumor should undergo repeat CT scanning within 6 months so that the evolution of the lesion can be monitored; if the tumor is larger than 4 cm or is found to be growing at the follow-up evaluation, it should be resected.

Hypokalemia in a hypertensive patient suggests primary hyperaldosteronism; an elevated plasma aldosterone level is seen in conjunction with decreased plasma renin activity. Cushing syndrome is caused by excess glucocorticoid secretion; if a glucocorticoid-producing adenoma, an adrenal carcinoma, or macronodular adrenal hyperplasia is noted, resection is indicated. A patient who has a pituitary adenoma or exhibits ectopic production of adrenocorticotropic hormone (ACTH) should undergo bilateral adrenalectomy if pituitary surgery or primary tumor resection fails to control cortisol hypersecretion. Patients with Cushing disease or Cushing syndrome typically have elevated levels of free cortisol and 17-hydroxycorticosteroids. A normal or slightly elevated ACTH level suggests pituitary disease, whereas a markedly elevated level suggests an ectopic source of ACTH. A depressed ACTH level suggests adrenal production of glucocorticosteroids. CT scanning can sometimes differentiate adrenal tumors from macronodular adrenal hyperplasia. Adrenocortical carcinoma is a rare condition but should nonetheless be suspected in patients with large (> 6 cm) adrenal masses, elevated 17-ketosteroid levels, or evidence of local invasion or distant metastasis.

Patients with pheochromocytoma may be normotensive or may have episodic or chronic hypertension. Urinary measurements of metanephrine, VMA, and plasma catecholamine levels allow biochemical confirmation of the diagnosis. CT or MRI is used to localize the tumor. Scintigraphy with 131-metaiodobenzylguanidine may exclude multiple or bilateral tumors or metastasis.[24]

In patients with virilizing syndromes, 24-hour urine collection for 17-ketosteroid, plasma testosterone, and dehydroepiandrosterone levels must be done to confirm the presence of an androgen-producing adrenal tumor.

DIAGNOSTIC IMAGING

Patients with adrenalomas first diagnosed by means of ultrasonography or CT scanning should undergo further evaluation with either helical CT scanning or MRI. In most cases, a thin-cut (3 mm) helical CT scan is capable of localizing the adrenal tumor and determining its size and its relationships with contiguous structures. MRI has the additional advantage of providing T$_2$-weighted images, which can distinguish various adrenal lesions on the basis of differences in adrenaloma-to-liver signal ratios. For instance, on T$_2$-weighted images, pheochromocytomas are markedly brighter in relation to the liver than other tumors are.

ADRENAL VENOUS SAMPLING

In selected patients with suspected aldosterone-producing tumors, venous sampling can be used to differentiate an incidentaloma from a cortical adenoma that produces aldosterone.

FNA CYTOLOGY

At present, FNA cytology plays only a limited role in the assessment of adrenal lesions owing to its inability to distinguish an adenoma from a well-differentiated carcinoma. Moreover, a needle biopsy in a patient with a pheochromocytoma can lead to a fatal hypertensive crisis. Consequently, FNA cytology is generally not recommended in this setting.[25]

Operative Planning

PREPARATION FOR OPERATION

Routine bowel preparation and antibiotic prophylaxis are unnecessary. Intermittent pneumatic compression stockings or subcutaneous heparin should be used to prevent thromboembolism.

Preoperative administration of alpha and beta blockers is recommended for patients with pheochromocytoma, who may experience severe hypertension intraoperatively with mild tumor manipulation or hypotension after tumor removal as a consequence of inadequate volume resuscitation before operation.[21] Of the several options available, we prefer phenoxybenzamine, given for at least 1 week preoperatively. The selective alpha-antagonist prazosin is a reasonable alternative. Success has also been reported with the use of either I.V. phentolamine and esmolol[26] or calcium channel blockers starting the day before the procedure.[27] Beta blockers may be given to control intraoperative arrhythmias but should not be started until after alpha blockade has been achieved. In patients with aldosteronomas, potassium deficits should be corrected before operation. Preoperative administration of spironolactone can counteract the aldosterone-producing activity of the tumor.

PATIENT POSITIONING

After placement of intermittent compression stockings and insertion of a Foley catheter, the patient is placed in the lateral decubitus position on a bean bag with the side of the adrenal pathology facing up [see Figure 1a]. An axillary roll (two rolled towels or a 1 L I.V. bag covered with a towel) is used to protect the brachial plexus and a rolled blanket under the flank to facilitate the opposite flank exposure. The flank must be positioned over the table break [see Figure 1b], so that the table can be flexed at this joint to maximize the distance between the costal margin and the iliac crest. Hyperextension of the table is continued until the flank musculature begins to feel taut. The arms are extended over boards and secured, and pressure sites

are padded. The torso and the legs are secured with 2 in. cloth tape. The table is then tested to verify its capability for the reverse Trendelenburg position and for airplaning (i.e., lateral rotation), both of which will be used to facilitate exposure during the operation.

The surgeon and the assistant stand facing the patient's abdomen. To maximize the degree of freedom with which the instruments can be used, the patient's abdomen is moved close to the edge of the table. The area from the umbilicus to the vertebral column and from the nipple to the middle of the iliac crest is prepared and draped. Video monitors are placed on either side of the head of the table.

EQUIPMENT

For adequate vision of the operative field, a 30° laparoscope is recommended. A fan-type liver retractor is useful for liver retraction in a laparoscopic right adrenalectomy.

The surgeon's nondominant hand typically holds an atraumatic bowel grasper. The flat surface of this instrument is used to grasp and retract the tissue adjacent to the adrenal. The surgeon's dominant hand holds an electrocautery scissors, an electrocautery hook, or an ultrasonic scalpel. Because all of these devices can generate thermal energy, care must be taken not to rest their active areas against tissue that is not to be divided. A 5 mm curved ultrasonic endoscopic shears is particularly valuable for dissection around the adrenal. The adrenal vein can be dissected with a right-angle dissector and clipped with either medium or large titanium clips. Arteries can be either ligated with clips and divided with the endoscopic shears or divided directly with the ultrasonic scalpel.

Laparoscopic ultrasonography using a 5 to 7 MHz probe can be useful for localizing the left adrenal gland when large amounts of perirenal and retroperitoneal fat are present.[28] Intraoperative ultrasonography is particularly useful in patients with small tumors when the tumor is not directly visible, the adrenal appears normal, and a paraganglioma is present; it is also helpful in evaluating the venous anatomy and searching for evidence of invasion or metastasis.

A laparoscopic biopsy forceps should be available for biopsy of the adrenal. An impermeable nylon laparoscopic bag is necessary for gland retrieval to prevent seeding of the abdomen or the trocar sites with tumor cells.

Operative Technique

CHOICE OF APPROACH

Two approaches to laparoscopic adrenalectomy—transperitoneal and retroperitoneal—have been described in the literature. We advocate the transperitoneal approach because the anatomy is more familiar to most surgeons, enlarged glands are more easily approached, and the liver can be assessed for metastases. The retroperitoneal approach, much like the open posterior approach, involves creation of a retroperitoneal space. It has often been recommended for patients who have previously undergone abdominal surgery.[19,29,30] Our experience, however, suggests that this approach may not always be superior in this population: more than half of our transperitoneal laparoscopic adrenalectomies have been performed in patients with prior abdominal operations.

The transperitoneal approach may be either anterior or lateral. The anterior transperitoneal approach was the first to be

Figure 1 **Laparoscopic adrenalectomy. (a) Depicted is the recommended placement of the operating room monitor, the surgeon, the assistant, and the nurse. The patient is placed in the lateral decubitus position, with the side to be operated on facing up; positioning shown is appropriate for a left adrenalectomy. (b) An axillary roll is used to protect the brachial plexus, and a bean bag is used under the flank to facilitate exposure. The flank is positioned over the flex point of the table.**

used but was eventually discarded owing to difficulties in exposing the gland, attributable to the supine positioning of the patient. Currently, the lateral transperitoneal approach is the one most commonly used for laparoscopic adrenalectomy. With the patient in the lateral decubitus position, gravity helps to retract anatomic structures, thereby simplifying exposure of the adrenal glands.

We advocate the lateral transperitoneal approach for most cases of adrenal pathology. Accordingly, the bulk of the ensuing technical description is devoted to this technique. The retroperitoneal approach, in our view, is appropriate primarily for tumors less than 6 cm in diameter.

LEFT ADRENALECTOMY: LATERAL TRANSPERITONEAL APPROACH

Step 1: Placement of Trocars

The operation may be performed with either three or four trocars [*see Figure 2*]. In the classic approach, four 10 mm trocars are placed along the subcostal margin. If a 5 mm 30° angled laparoscope is available, the ports can all be 5 mm; if not, a 10 mm 30° angled laparoscope is used and either all three remaining ports are 10 mm as well or the camera port is 10 mm and the other two are 5 mm. The port that is optional is the most posterior one, at the costovertebral angle. This fourth port is sometimes required for retraction of the spleen, but it can generally be dispensed with if the spleen is adequately mobilized and the patient is positioned so that gravity helps pull the spleen down and away from the operative field.

Via either a percutaneous or an open technique, the first port site is created medial to the anterior axillary line, 2 cm below and parallel to the costal margin. Particular care must be taken with the percutaneous technique, because the Veress needle can easily puncture the spleen. CO_2 is insufflated to a pressure of 15 mm Hg, and the initial trocar (5 or 10 mm) is inserted. The abdomen is then visually explored. Under laparoscopic vision, two additional trocars are inserted, one inferior and slightly medial to the tip of the 11th rib and the other more anterior, medial to the initial trocar but lateral to the rectus sheath (approximately a handsbreadth from the midline) so as to avoid the epigastric vessels. The trocars must be placed at least 5 cm—optimally, 10 cm—apart to ensure adequate mobility of the instruments. The most anterior trocar is used for the camera, and the two lateral ports are used for the grasping and cutting instruments.

Step 2: Mobilization of Spleen

With a laparoscopic bowel clamp in the surgeon's left hand and an ultrasonic endoscopic shears in the right, the splenic flexure is mobilized inferiorly and medially to uncover the inferior pole of the splenorenal ligament [see Figure 3]. This ligament is divided along the lateral border of the spleen, from the inferior pole to the superior pole, all the way to the diaphragmatic attachments. When the short gastric vessels are identified, dissection is complete. Once the spleen is fully mobilized, it falls medially, and the retroperitoneum comes into full view. The lateral and anterior portions of the adrenal gland become visible in the perinephric fat, superior and medial to the kidney.

Troubleshooting Incomplete division of the splenorenal ligament is the most common reason for inadequate exposure

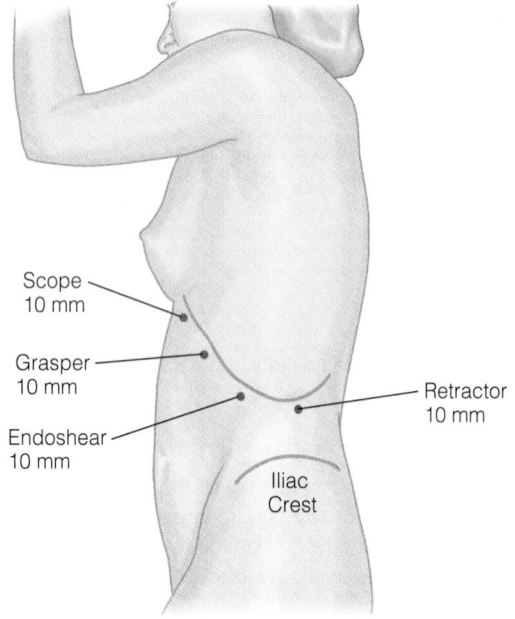

Scope
10 mm

Grasper
10 mm

Endoshear
10 mm

Retractor
10 mm

Iliac
Crest

Figure 2 **Laparoscopic left adrenalectomy: lateral transperitoneal approach. Shown is the recommended trocar placement. The most posterior trocar can often be omitted.**

of the left adrenal. The usual solution involves placement of an additional trocar and prolongation of the operation.

Correct patient positioning is key for exposure of the adrenal. The table is tilted to the reverse Trendelenburg position, thereby displacing the surrounding organs and forcing fluids from irrigation or oozing to collect away from the field of dissection. Airplaning the patient toward the surgeon also helps induce the spleen to fall away from the field.

Step 3: Dissection and Removal of Adrenal Gland

The perinephric fat is grasped, and either the lateral and anterior attachments or the medial and inferior attachments are divided with the electrocautery hook or the ultrasonic scalpel to mobilize the adrenal [see Figure 4]. The superior and posterior attachments are left for last: while in place, they act as an anatomic retractor for the gland, thereby facilitating dissection of the adrenal vein. The initial goal of the dissection is to identify and clip the adrenal vein (with two or three clips placed proximally and two distally). The inferior phrenic vein joins the adrenal vein before junction of the adrenal vein with the renal vein. The adrenal vein is clipped above the junction with the inferior phrenic vein, and any branches from the inferior phrenic vein to the adrenal gland are clipped as dissection continues along the medial superior border of the adrenal. The final portion of the dissection of the adrenal gland is performed in the superior and posterior planes. The shaft of a closed instrument can be used to retract the adrenal or elevate it gently during dissection.

The gland is placed in an impermeable nylon bag and removed through the original trocar site, which is widened by gently spreading the abdominal musculature with a clamp. On occasion, the incision may have to be enlarged to permit removal of the specimen.

Troubleshooting Laparoscopic ultrasonography can be used to identify the adrenal gland or vein in patients who have extensive perinephric fat.[31] If ultrasonography is not available, dissection of the adrenal vein's junction with the renal vein may be necessary to identify the left adrenal.

It is important not to grasp the adrenal gland or the tumor directly. The gland is fragile and prone to tearing. Fracture of the capsule can result in seeding of tumor cells into surrounding tissues, much as sometimes occurs with spleen or parathyroid dissection.

It is not necessary to take the inferior phrenic vein if the adrenal vein is clipped superior to the junction of the two veins and if dissection along the medial superior border of the adrenal stays medial to this vein.

Larger (> 5 cm) adrenal masses may preclude initial access to the adrenal vein. When we encounter a large left adrenal mass, we prefer to dissect laterally and superiorly first, clipping and dividing the inferior phrenic branches to the adrenal. We identify and divide the adrenal vein last.

RIGHT ADRENALECTOMY: LATERAL TRANSPERITONEAL APPROACH

Step 1: Placement of Trocars

In the classic approach to right laparoscopic adrenalectomy, four 10 mm trocars are placed along the subcostal line. If a 5 mm 30° angled laparoscope is available, the ports can all be 5 mm except for the most medial liver retraction port (most liver retractors require a 10 mm trocar). If not, a 10 mm 30° angled laparoscope is used, and either the remaining ports are all 10 mm or the two medial ports (for the camera and the liver retractor) are 10 mm and the remaining one 5 mm.

a

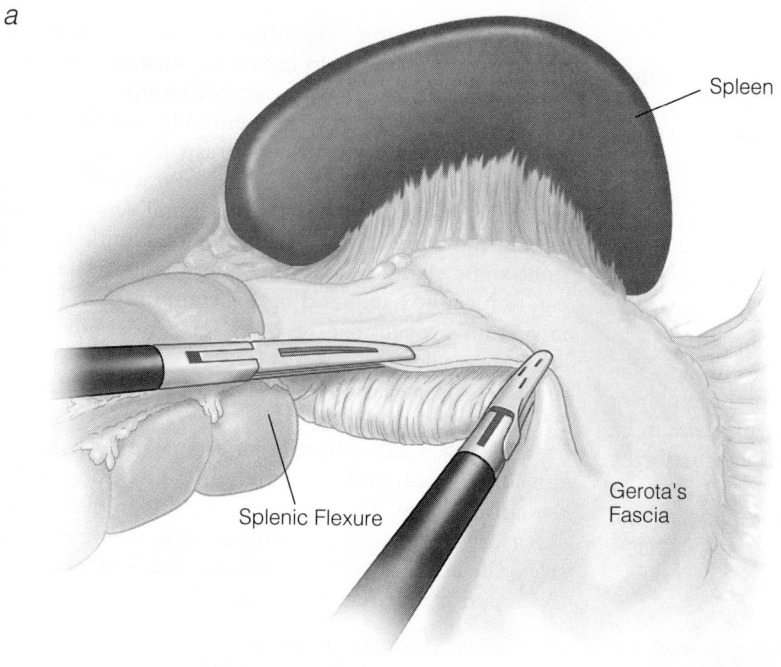

Spleen

Splenic Flexure

Gerota's Fascia

b

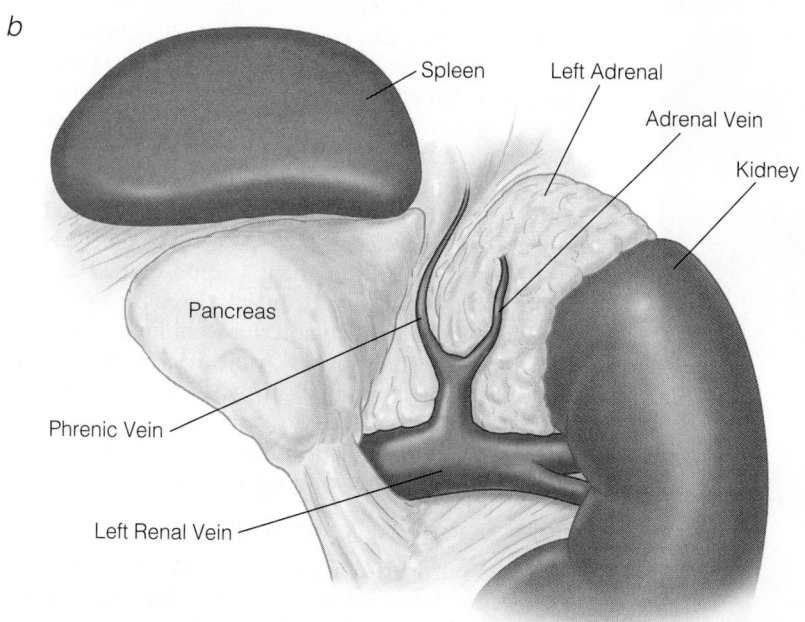

Spleen

Left Adrenal

Adrenal Vein

Kidney

Pancreas

Phrenic Vein

Left Renal Vein

Figure 3 **Laparoscopic left adrenalectomy: lateral transperitoneal approach. Depicted is exposure of the left adrenal. (*a*) The splenorenal ligament is divided and the splenic flexure mobilized, revealing the left adrenal gland. (*b*) After dissection of the lower pole of the adrenal, the adrenal vein and its junctions with the inferior phrenic vein and the left renal vein are revealed.**

Like several other components of a right adrenalectomy, placement of the initial trocar largely mirrors its technical counterpart in a left adrenalectomy (see above), with either percutaneous or open creation of the fascial opening, trocar insertion, insufflation, and visual exploration of the abdomen. The three remaining trocars are then placed under laparoscopic vision at least 5 cm (preferably 10 cm) apart, with one inferior and posterior to the tip of the 11th rib and the other two more anterior and medial. The most medial trocar is placed lateral to the ipsilateral rectus muscle, approximately a handsbreadth from the midline, to avoid the epigastric vessels. The most anterior port is used for the liver retractor, the second port for the camera, and the two lateral ports for the cutting and grasping instruments.

Step 2: Mobilization of Liver

A fan-type liver retractor is inserted through the most anterior port, and the right hepatic lobe is gently reflected medial-ly. The 30° angled laparoscope is inserted into the second trocar, and liver mobilization is begun. With a laparoscopic curved dissector in the surgeon's left hand and an ultrasonic endoscopic shears in the right, the right lateral hepatic attachments and the triangular ligament are divided along the diaphragm [*see Figure 5a*]. The peritoneum between the liver and the vena cava is divided along the upper border of the renal vein up to the triangular ligament. Once this is done, the liver can readily be retracted medially. At this point, the adrenal gland, the perinephric fat, and the vena cava are generally visible.

Troubleshooting Incomplete division of the right hepatic ligament is the most common reason for inadequate exposure of the right adrenal. As with left adrenalectomy (see above), correct patient positioning is key for exposure of the adrenal.

Step 3: Dissection and Removal of Adrenal Gland

The perinephric fat is grasped, and dissection of the adrenal is begun with the electrocautery hook or the ultrasonic endoscopic shears along the lateral inferior margin of the gland. Dissection continues medially and superiorly until the main adrenal vein coming directly off the vena cava is identified. The adrenal vein is then mobilized with a right-angle clamp and clipped [*see Figure 5b*] with medium or large titanium clips (three on the vena cava side and two on the adrenal side). As dissection progresses superiorly, small veins draining the adrenal gland directly into the inferior phrenic vein or the vena cava may be encountered; these must be clipped. The final portion of the dissection is performed in the superior and posterior planes. The shaft of a closed instrument can be used to retract the adrenal gland or to elevate it gently during dissection.

Finally, the adrenal is placed in an impermeable bag and removed exactly as in a left adrenalectomy.

Figure 4 **Laparoscopic left adrenalectomy: lateral transperitoneal approach. Depicted is mobilization of the left adrenal gland. (a) The lower pole of the adrenal is dissected to reveal the clipped adrenal vein. The pancreas is retracted to the left by gravity, with the splenic vein coursing along its posterior margin. The adrenal is retracted to the right with the laparoscopic instrument. The left renal artery (arrow) is visible. (b) The posterior medial attachments of the adrenal are divided with the ultrasonic endoscopic shears. The inferior phrenic vein (arrows) can be seen coursing from the diaphragm along the medial aspect of the adrenal dissection. With sufficient dissection, gravity helps retract the spleen and the gastric fundus from the adrenal.**

Troubleshooting As with a left adrenalectomy, laparoscopic ultrasonography can help define the anatomy; however, it is not needed as often with a right adrenalectomy.

Many problems can be prevented by careful tissue handling. Again, it is important not to grasp the adrenal gland or the tumor directly. In addition, excessive traction during dissection around or clipping of the right adrenal vein can tear the vena cava at the adrenal vein insertion site. Gentle spreading of the right-angle clamp without opening the jaws to their full extent can reduce the likelihood of this complication. The laparoscopic suction tip can also be used for gentle, effective dissection around vessels. If the vein is large, a vascular transverse anastomosis (TA) or gastrointestinal anastomosis (GIA) stapler may be used.

Larger (> 5 cm) adrenal masses may prevent visualization of the adrenal vein and preclude initial dissection and division of the adrenal vein. The solution, again, is to dissect laterally and superiorly first, then continue caudally along the vena cava to reach the adrenal vein. Special care must be taken not to injure the superior pole renal arteries.

BILATERAL ADRENALECTOMY

Most bilateral laparoscopic adrenalectomies are performed to treat Cushing disease or bilateral pheochromocytoma (either benign or malignant). In rare cases, they are performed to treat neoplastic hypercortisolism that cannot be controlled medically or bilateral macronodular hyperplasia associated with Cushing syndrome.

The patient is placed in the lateral decubitus position, with either the left or the right side facing up, depending on which side is to be operated on first. After all wounds have been closed on the first side, the patient is repositioned and redraped to expose the second side. It may be possible to avoid repositioning by making use of an anterior technique, in which trocars are inserted in the anterior subcostal areas on the left and the right, or a posterior technique, in which the patient is prone. Our preference, however, is to start with the left side, with the patient in the lateral decubitus position, then reposition the patient and continue with the right side.

RETROPERITONEAL ADRENALECTOMY

In the retroperitoneal laparoscopic approach to the adrenal gland, first described in 1995,[20,32-35] the patient is placed in the prone position, which enables performance of a bilateral adrenalectomy (if necessary) without repositioning. A retroperitoneal space is created with a balloon dissector. The kidney and the adrenal gland are identified. Dissection is carried out along the inferomedial border of the adrenal, and the renal vein is exposed. The adrenal vein is ligated, and the remainder of the operation proceeds in much the same fashion as with the lateral transperitoneal approach.

The retroperitoneal approach reduces the risk of injury to intra-abdominal organs; however, there are fewer classic anatomic landmarks, the operative field is significantly smaller, and identification of the adrenal glands can be more challenging. In addition, accidental opening of the posterior peritoneal sheath can allow gas to escape into the abdomen, a complication that can further reduce the retroperitoneal space and make dissection even more difficult. A 1997 report that included 111 consecutive retroperitoneal laparoscopic adrenalectomies suggested that this approach is best reserved for management of smaller (< 6 cm) adrenal tumors.[5]

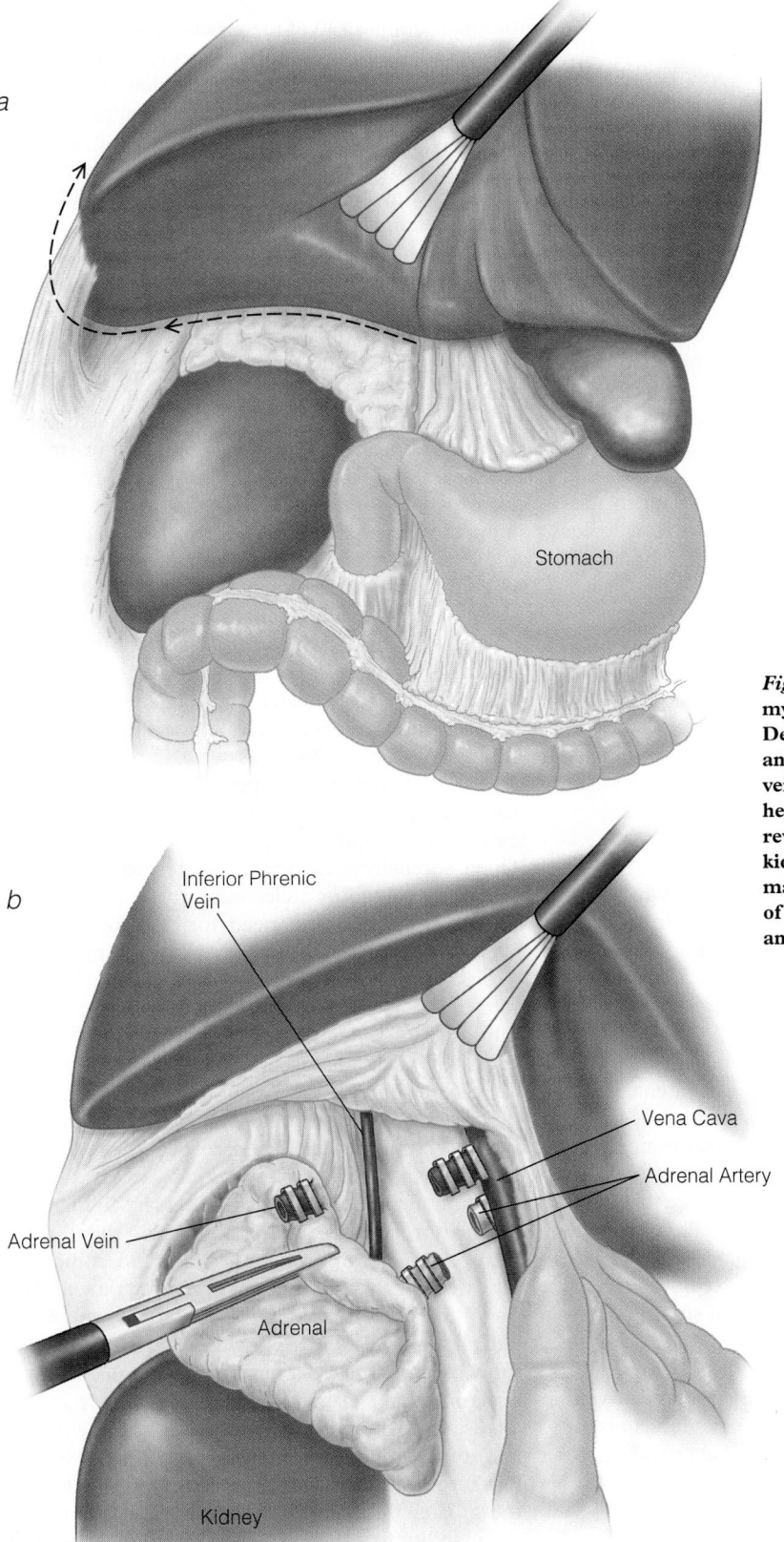

Stomach

Figure 5 **Laparoscopic right adrenalecto-my: lateral transperitoneal approach. Depicted are exposure of the right adrenal and dissection and clipping of the adrenal vein. (*a*) The peritoneal attachments of the hepatic flexure and the liver are divided to reveal the right adrenal gland adjacent to the kidney and the inferior vena cava. (*b*) The main adrenal vein is clipped, along with one of the adrenal arteries arising from the aorta and coursing behind the vena cava.**

Inferior Phrenic Vein

Vena Cava

Adrenal Artery

Adrenal Vein

Adrenal

Kidney

Postoperative Care

Oral fluids are started on the day of the operation. Nasogastric tubes are unnecessary. Most patients need only oral pain medication. The postoperative course is similar to that of laparoscopic cholecystectomy [*see V:12 Laparoscopic Cholecystectomy*], except that some endocrine diseases call for hormonal support. Patients typically are ambulatory on the day of the operation and are discharged on postoperative day 1; however, discharge may be delayed if perioperative administration of stress-dose steroids or adjustment of blood pressure medications is required.

Complications

BLEEDING

Operative bleeding can be prevented by meticulous attention to hemostasis. The retroperitoneal fat can be particularly difficult to dissect in male patients: it is extensive and tends to bleed with even gentle manipulation. In this setting, the ultrasonic scalpel is especially useful.

Careful handling of the adrenal vein is crucial. Opening the jaws of a laparocopic dissector can create significant force that the laparoscopic surgeon may fail to appreciate. Gentle spreading, without opening the jaws to their full extent, helps reduce the chances of tearing the vessel. Use of the laparoscopic suction tip also helps reduce the risk of injury to vessels during dissection.

Double or triple clip application to the distal segment of the adrenal vein reduces the chances of clip dislodgment. The clips should be applied at right angles to the tissue. Twisting the clip applier or applying the clips at acute angles can result in scissoring of the clip and division of the vessel. It is of particular importance not to apply clips indiscriminately or blindly if bleeding occurs; to do so puts the renal vein, the vena cava, and other retroperitoneal structures at risk.

The best way of dealing with bleeding during a laparoscopic adrenalectomy is to apply gentle pressure with an instrument or to place an additional trocar to facilitate pressure or exposure. The assistant holding the camera must stay calm and keep the field in view while being careful not to get blood on the lens. Suction devices should be used only under direct vision in the adrenal bed to prevent removal of the clips by the suction.

DAMAGE TO ADJACENT ORGANS

Damage to the pancreas and the spleen (in a left adrenalectomy), to the liver and the vena cava (in a right adrenalectomy), and to the renal arteries (in a left or a right adrenalectomy) can largely be prevented by a thorough knowledge of the anatomy and close attention to key technical details [see Operative Technique, above].

It is not necessary to identify the adrenal vein–left renal vein junction. Tracing the left adrenal vein back to the adrenal gland suffices to confirm its identity. Adequate mobilization of the spleen renders additional retraction of the spleen or pancreas unnecessary. Damage to the pancreas can present either early (as pancreatitis) or late (as a pancreatic pseudocyst). To reduce the risk of such damage, dissection should be kept close to the adrenal and the top of the kidney after division of the splenorenal ligament. Liver lacerations can be controlled with gentle pressure. Bowel lacerations should be closed by means of intracorporeal suture repair.

DEEP VEIN THROMBOSIS

In our series of 100 patients,[2] the incidence of deep vein thrombosis (DVT) was 3%. We routinely use intermittent compression stockings at the beginning of the operation to minimize the occurrence of this complication.

Outcome Evaluation

To date, more than 1,000 cases of laparoscopic adrenalectomy have been reported in the literature. Although no prospective, randomized trials of this new procedure have been published, there is considerable evidence substantiating its effectiveness and safety. A 2000 review examined all English-language studies published between 1995 and 1999 that consisted of more than 20 cases.[18] A total of 1,052 patients underwent 1,082 adrenalectomies (30 of the procedures were bilateral).[18] Patients ranged in age from 17 to 84 years and were equally distributed between males and females. The lesions ranged in size from 0.5 to 14 cm. The lateral transperitoneal approach was followed in 88% of patients, the posterior retroperitoneal approach in 12%. Rates of conversion to open adrenalectomy ranged from 0% to 18%. The most common indications for adrenalectomy were aldosteronoma (42.7%), Cushing syndrome (18.6%), incidentaloma (16.9%), and pheochromocytoma (14.7%); other, less common indications were angiomyolipoma, metastases, small carcinoma, virilizing adenoma, and macronodular hyperplasia.

The retrospective studies comparing laparoscopic adrenalectomy with open adrenalectomy indicated that the average operating time was shorter with open procedures (149 versus 195 minutes). More recently, however, some authors have reported operating times as short as 109 minutes for laparoscopic operations. One of us (M.G.) has now performed more than 200 laparoscopic adrenalectomies.[18] In the first 100, the mean operating time was 123 minutes, the mean blood loss was 70 ml, and the average length of stay was 2.4 days.[2] Currently, the mean operating time is less than 60 minutes for a benign unilateral lesion, and the median length of stay is 1 day.

These retrospective studies also found that laparoscopic adrenalectomy was associated with reduced blood loss (153 versus 355 ml) and a shorter length of stay (2.6 versus 6.5 days).[18] The overall complication rate was lower in the laparoscopic group (7% versus 24%) as well. Laparoscopic adrenalectomy was associated with postoperative hematoma or need for transfusion in approximately 3% of patients and with wound complications, pulmonary complications, or DVT in fewer than 1%. Open adrenalectomy was associated with respiratory problems (e.g., pneumonia or atelectasis) in 6% of patients, with wound infections in 3%, with need for transfusion in 3%, and with splenic injury (sometimes necessitating splenectomy) in 1.5%. Moreover, the open approach was associated with a 54% overall rate of late complications, namely, chronic pain (14%), flank numbness (10%), and muscle laxity (30%). When performed by an experienced laparoscopic surgeon, laparoscopic adrenalectomy can be completed with no mortality, minimal morbidity, and no recurrence of hormonal excess. In the aforementioned experience with more than 200 cases, conversion to an open procedure was required only for removal of invasive or giant (> 15 cm) tumors; in no case was it necessary to manage bleeding.

The retrospective studies comparing the transperitoneal and retroperitoneal approaches to laparoscopic adrenalectomy reported slight differences in operating time and blood loss but no differences in length of stay.[18] As noted [see Operative Technique, Choice of Approach and Retroperitoneal Adrenalectomy, above], the retroperitoneal approach may have advantages in some settings (e.g., the avoidance of intraperitoneal adhesions from previous operations and the elimination of patient repositioning for bilateral procedures), but it also has certain important disadvantages (e.g., the smaller operative field, the greater difficulty of visualizing the adrenal anatomy, and the inability to survey the liver and the peritoneum for metastases). The choice between the lateral transperitoneal approach to laparoscopic adrenalectomy and the retroperitoneal approach is determined primarily by surgeon preference—except in patients with larger tumors, for whom the lateral transperitoneal approach is clearly superior. In general, the retroperitoneal approach is ideal for a surgeon who is experienced with this approach and who is treating a patient with a benign adrenal tumor less than 6 cm in diameter.

References

1. Gagner M, Lacroix A, Bolte E: Laparoscopic adrenalectomy in Cushing's syndrome and pheochromocytoma (letter). N Engl J Med 327:1033, 1992

2. Gagner M, Pomp A, Heniford B, et al: Laparoscopic adrenalectomy: lessons learned from 100 consecutive procedures. Ann Surg 226:238, 1997

3. Gagner M, Breton G, Pharand D, et al: Is laparoscopic adrenalectomy indicated for pheochromocytoma? Surgery 120:1076, 1996

4. Duh QY, Siperstein AE, Clark OH, et al: Laparoscopic adrenalectomy: comparison of the lateral and posterior approaches. Arch Surg 131:870, 1996

5. Bonjer HJ, Lange JF, Kazemeir G: Comparison of three techniques for adrenalectomy. Br J Surg 84:679, 1997

6. Baba S, Miyajima A, Uchida A, et al: A posterior lumbar approach for retroperitoneoscopic adrenalectomy: assessment of surgical efficacy. Urology 50:19, 1997

7. Gagner M, Lacroix A, Prinz RA, et al: Early experience with laparoscopic approach for adrenalectomy. Surgery 114:1120, 1993

8. Chapuis Y, Maignien B, Abboud B: Adrenalectomy under celioscopy: experience of 25 operations. Presse Med 24:845, 1995

9. Brunt LM, Doherty GM, Norton JA, et al: Laparoscopic adrenalectomy compared to open adrenalectomy for benign adrenal neoplasms. J Am Coll Surg 183:1, 1996

10. Fernandez-Cruz L, Saenz A, Benarroch G, et al: Laparoscopic unilateral and bilateral adrenalectomy for Cushing's syndrome: transperitoneal and retroperitoneal approaches. Ann Surg 224:727, 1996

11. de Canniere L, Michel L, Hamoir E, et al: Multicentric experience of the Belgian Group for Endoscopic Surgery (BGES) with endoscopic adrenalectomy. Surg Endosc 11:1065, 1997

12. Jacobs JK, Goldstein RE, Geer RJ, et al: Laparoscopic adrenalectomy: a new standard of care. Ann Surg 225:495, 1997

13. Filipponi S, Guerrieri M, Arnoldi G, et al: Laparoscopic adrenalectomy: a report on 50 operations. Eur J Endocrinol 138:548, 1998

14. Guazzoni G, Montorsi F, Bocciardi A, et al: Transperitoneal laparoscopic versus open adrenalectomy for benign hyperfunctioning adrenal tumors: a comparative study. J Urol 153:1597, 1995

15. Janetschek G, Finkenstedt G, Gasser R, et al: Laparoscopic surgery for pheochromocytoma: adrenalectomy, partial resection, excision of paragangliomas. J Urol 160:330, 1998

16. Winfield HN, Hamilton BD, Bravo EL, et al: Laparoscopic adrenalectomy: the preferred choice? A comparison to open adrenalectomy. J Urol 160:325, 1998

17. Janetschek G, Altarac S, Finkenstedt G, et al: Technique and results of laparoscopic adrenalectomy. Eur Urol 30:475, 1996

18. Jossart G, Burpee SE, Gagner M: Surgery of the adrenal glands. Endocrinol Metab Clin 29:57, 2000

19. Linos D, Stylopoulos N, Boukis M, et al: Anterior, posterior, or laparoscopic approach for the management of adrenal diseases? Am J Surg 173:120, 1997

20. Thompson GB, Grant CS, van Heerden JA, et al: Laparoscopic versus open posterior adrenalectomy: a case-control study of 100 patients. Surgery 122:1132, 1997

21. Grant C: Pheochromocytoma. Textbook of Endocrine Surgery, 1st ed. Clark OH, Duh Q, Eds. WB Saunders Co, Philadelphia, 1997, p 513

22. Icard P, Louvel A, Chapuis Y: Survival rates and prognostic factors in adrenocortical carcinoma. World J Surg 16:453, 1992

23. Herrera MF, Grant CS, van Heerden JA, et al: Incidentally discovered adrenal tumors: an institutional perspective. Surgery 110:1014, 1991

24. Gross MD, McLeod MK, Sanfield JA, et al: Scintigraphic evaluation of clinically silent adrenal masses. J Nucl Med 35:1145, 1994

25. Silverman SG, Mueller PR, Pinkey LP, et al: Predictive value of image-guided adrenal biopsy: analysis of results of 101 biopsies. Radiology 187:715, 1993

26. Pertsemlidis D: Minimal-access versus open adrenalectomy. Surg Endosc 9:384, 1995

27. Proye C, Thevenin D, Cecat P, et al: Exclusive use of calcium channel blockers in preoperative and intraoperative control of pheochromocytomas: hemodynamics and free catecholamine assays in ten consecutive patients. Surgery 106:1149, 1989

28. Miyake O, Yoshimura K, Yoshioka T, et al: Laparoscopic adrenalectomy: comparison of the transperitoneal and retroperitoneal approach. Eur Urol 33:303, 1998

29. Gasman D, Droupy S, Koutani A, et al: Laparoscopic adrenalectomy: the retroperitoneal approach. J Urol 159:1816, 1998

30. Heintz A, Walgenbach S, Junginger T: Results of endoscopic retroperitoneal adrenalectomy. Surg Endosc 10:633, 1996

31. Heniford BT, Iannitti DA, Hale J, et al: The role of intraoperative ultrasonography during laparoscopic adrenalectomy. Surgery 122:1068, 1997

32. Mercan S, Seven R, Ozarmagan S, et al: Endoscopic retroperitoneal adrenalectomy. Surgery 118:1071, 1995

33. Takeda M, Go H, Watanabe R, et al: Retroperitoneal laparoscopic adrenalectomy for functioning adrenal tumors: comparison with conventional transperitoneal laparoscopic adrenalectomy. J Urol 157:19, 1997

34. Terachi T, Matsuda T, Terai A: Transperitoneal laparoscopic adrenalectomy: experience in 100 patients. J Endourol 11:361, 1997

35. Walz MK, Peitgen K, Saller B, et al: Subtotal adrenalectomy by the posterior retroperitoneoscopic approach. World J Surg 22:621, 1998

Acknowledgment

Figures 1 through 3 and 5   Tom Moore.

28 LAPAROSCOPIC DONOR NEPHRECTOMY

Stephen C. Jacobs, M.D., and Stephen T. Bartlett, M.D.

The number of patients needing renal transplantation far outstrips the number of organs obtainable from cadavers. Expanded application of living renal donor transplantation is currently the only viable option for coping with this gap between demand and supply. Living renal donors have indeed helped bridge the organ supply gap, but historically, the open surgical procurement procedure has proved to be a significant disincentive to donation. Since the latter part of the 1990s, laparoscopic living donor nephrectomy has become established as the surgical approach of choice in most large renal transplant programs.[1-6] It has both enlarged the pool of willing potential renal donors and increased the supply of kidneys for transplantation.[7,8] The spectrum of donors[9] now includes older donors (≤ 72 years),[10] unrelated donors,[11] on-call emergency donors needing concomitant pancreas transplantation,[12] obese donors,[13] consenting incarcerated donors, paired-exchange donors,[14] and Good Samaritan donors.[15] In the United States, paid donors are not knowingly used, but this is not invariably the case outside the United States.[16-18] Neither the use of prisoners as donors against their will nor the use of minors as donors has been reported to date.

Although laparoscopic harvesting is now well developed, there is probably room for further refinement. For instance, systemic vasodilation might improve intraoperative renal blood flow and enhance urine production. The extraction site, however, appears to be optimal as is. Current experience suggests that suprapubic, umbilical, lower quadrant, and dorsal lumbotomy extraction sites are surgically comparable; transvaginal extraction has not yet been performed.

When laparoscopic donor nephrectomy is done by an appropriately experienced surgeon, the recipient typically achieves about the same level of renal function as with an open donor nephrectomy [see Table 1]. Nonetheless, the laparoscopic approach poses risks to both the donor and the allograft recipient. These risks are potentially catastrophic and militate against casual embarkation on a laparoscopic donor nephrectomy program. A good case can be made for restricting laparoscopic donor nephrectomy to a few centers where a large number of cases are done.[19] Few, if any, patients are more easily moved a substantial distance for an operation than a living renal donor.

Contraindications to laparoscopic donor nephrectomy are similar to those to its open counterpart, with the addition of previous intra-abdominal processes that may have caused adhesions. Obesity is not a contraindication to laparoscopic donor nephrectomy, but it does make the procedure more difficult. Obese donors tolerate the procedure as well as lean donors do.[13]

Operative Planning

Donor nephrectomy is a unique operation in that the procedure is performed on a healthy volunteer solely for the benefit of the recipient. The margin for error must be very small.

Kidney donors undergo a standard preoperative evaluation. They should be in reasonably good health and able to tolerate the loss of one kidney without a significant reduction in longevity. Both kidneys are evaluated anatomically by means of computed tomographic angiography; we find that this modality offers superior visualization of the renal parenchyma, the renal venous anatomy, and the remainder of the abdomen while yielding a good view of the renal arterial and ureteral anatomy.[20] Arteries too small to be seen on CT angiography have not proved to be problems intraoperatively.

PREPARATION

Donor nephrectomy is done with the patient under general anesthesia. Although adjuvant epidural anesthesia helps decrease intraoperative and postoperative narcotic requirements in open nephrectomy patients, it has no advantages in laparoscopic nephrectomy patients, because the narcotic requirements are so low.

Table 1   Relative Advantages of Laparoscopic and Open Approaches to Donor Nephrectomy

Areas in Which Laparoscopic Approach Is Equivalent to Open	Advantages of Laparoscopic over Open Approach	Advantages of Open over Laparoscopic Approach
Comparable cost	Less postoperative pain	Shorter warm ischemia time
Similar operative time	Reduced incisional morbidity	Greater number of skilled surgeons available
Equivalent recipient renal function	Enhanced cosmesis	More rapid access to vessels
Similar time to return of bowel function	Shorter hospital stay	Better intraoperative urine output
	Quicker return to normal activity	Lower risk of intraperitoneal organ injury
	Lower risk of pneumothorax	
	Decreased blood loss	
	Greater appeal to recipient	
	Larger overall donor pool	

Figure 1 **Laparoscopic donor nephrectomy. Shown are the recommended positioning of the donor, the trocar sites, and the suprapubic Pfannenstiel extraction site.**

Renal blood flow must be maintained at the highest possible levels until the kidney has been removed. Accordingly, I.V. infusion, at a rate of 1 L/hr, is started as early as possible before operation; a typical laparoscopic kidney donor will receive 4 to 5 L intraoperatively. The flank position tends to decrease renal blood flow. Insufflation of the abdomen with CO_2 markedly lowers urine output, and overhydration is employed as a means of compensating for this reflex oliguria. A brisk diuresis is highly desirable; thus, mannitol, 12.5 g I.V., is given at the onset of abdominal insufflation and again midway through the procedure.

PATIENT POSITIONING

After the induction of general anesthesia, a urethral catheter is placed. With the patient supine, the probable trocar sites are marked with an indelible skin marker. The extraction site is marked as well: for most women, a transverse skin incision 1 to 2 in. above the pubic bone is used for extraction, whereas for most men, a lower midline incision is employed. The midline should also be marked for subsequent use as a reference point to aid in producing a cosmetically appealing scar. Once the patient is placed in the flank position, marking out a symmetrical incision becomes difficult.

The donor is then turned so that the left flank is up and the right iliac crest is just below the kidney rest. This position is the same one used for open flank nephrectomy, except that in the laparoscopic procedure, the patient is moved so that the abdomen is close to the edge of the operating table, whereas in the open procedure, the back is placed at the edge of the table. The kidney rest is elevated and the operating table extended.

Padding of the donor is very important. A right axillary roll is placed under the patient to protect against brachial plexus injury. The neck is then elevated from the table with shock-absorbing material until it is straight. The right ear is positioned inside a gel protector. The right leg is flexed at the hip and the knee for stability, and the left leg is kept straight. Two pillows are placed between the legs to protect against peroneal nerve compression and ankle compression. The Foley catheter is draped ventrally without traction. The right arm is angled fairly high on a table-attached armrest so as to allow room for the camera operator. The elbow and the wrist are cushioned with eggcrate-type soft padding. The upper left arm is positioned either on two pillows between the arms or on a rigid arm support attached to the table. Care must be taken to protect the endotracheal tube from dislodgement, to support the left axilla, and to ensure that no compression occurs at the left elbow.

Given that the operating table may have to be turned from side to side during the procedure to facilitate exposure, the patient must be taped very securely to the table. Two long strips of 4 in. tape are passed from the dorsal sidebar of the table to the ventral sidebar,

crisscrossing over the iliac crest, which is the anchoring location on the patient. The dorsal-side attachment to the table is level with the iliac crest, but the ventral-side attachment angles sharply downward and caudally to provide the necessary exposure of the suprapubic area. A third strip of 4 in. adhesive tape is passed across the chest to anchor it and prevent it from rotating. The adhesive tape should stick firmly to the skin while avoiding the nipple. An electrocautery grounding pad is attached to the left thigh.

Next, the patient is prepared and draped from table to table and from xiphoid to pubis. We employ a Velcro tape holding mechanism to control the multiple cords (i.e., for the electrocautery, the light, the camera, gas, suction-irrigation, and the ultrasonic scalpel) that are now brought onto the table, and we make pockets in the drape ventrally and dorsally to hold all the instruments. The location of the 12th rib and a potential site for an open flank incision are drawn on the skin to facilitate rapid entry should this measure be required.

Before the procedure is begun, it is necessary to confirm (1) that the ice-slush machine is functioning in the donor operating room, (2) that a full open surgical set is open on the scrub table, and (3) that cold intracellular preservation fluid is available in the recipient OR.

EQUIPMENT

In addition to a standard open surgical tray and standard laparoscopic equipment, the following special equipment is necessary:

1. A 15 mm specimen pouch (e.g., Endocatch II; United States Surgical Corp., Norwalk, Connecticut);
2. An 18 French trocar (e.g., Endopath Surgical Transparent Trocar Sleeve with Dilating Obturator 18 French; Ethicon Endo-surgery Inc., Cincinnati, Ohio);
3. A 12 mm endoscopic gastrointestinal anastomosis (GIA) stapler with multiple-fire capability (e.g., Multifire Endo GIA 30-3.5; United States Surgical Corp., Norwalk, Connecticut);
4. A right-angle endoscopic multiple clip applier (e.g., AcuClip; United States Surgical Corp., Norwalk, Connecticut);
5. Papaverine;
6. A cholangiogram catheter; and
7. A cholangiogram catheter grasper.

Operative Technique

STEP 1: PLACEMENT OF TROCARS FOR RENAL DISSECTION

Preemptive analgesia, involving infiltration of 0.5% bupivacaine, is employed before any skin incisions are made. Three trocars are used for the renal dissection phase of the procedure [*see Figure 1*].

The first trocar to be placed (for the surgeon's left hand) is a 5 mm direct-vision type. A skin incision is made 1 in. above the umbilicus at the lateral border of the rectus muscle, the abdomen is insufflated with CO₂ to a pressure of 15 mm Hg via a Veress needle inserted through the skin incision, and the trocar is placed. A 5 mm 30° laparoscope is then used to explore the abdomen, and the other two trocars are placed under direct laparoscopic vision. The second trocar, the uppermost of the three, is 5 mm and is used for the camera. It should be situated as far cephalad as possible and slightly medial to the ribcage (just far enough away from the ribs to prevent levering on the ribcage, which can cause postoperative pain). The third trocar (for the surgeon's right hand) is 12 mm and is placed in the left lower quadrant, midway between the left-hand trocar and the iliac

Figure 2 **Laparoscopic donor nephrectomy. The sustenaculum coli is initially taken down close to the lateral peritoneum. Occasionally, an extensive attachment must be taken down before all ports can be placed under direct vision.**

Figure 3 **Laparoscopic donor nephrectomy. The white line of Toldt is incised with the ultrasonic scalpel. This superficial incision starts centrally and is extended downward all the way to the sigmoid colon and then upward as far as possible.**

crest; placement is aided by transillumination of the abdomen, which helps the surgeon avoid branches of the epigastric vessels. Given that more instrument exchanges are done through this port than through the others, it is more likely to require fixation.

The renal dissection is performed primarily with an ultrasonic scalpel (either 5 mm or 10 mm) in the right hand through the left lower quadrant port and with a grasping instrument in the left hand through the middle port. The camera is connected to the 5 mm 30° scope inserted through the uppermost port.

STEP 2: TAKEDOWN OF COLON

The initial intra-abdominal incision divides the sustenaculum coli, an adhesion of omentum that extends from the splenic flexure to the anterolateral peritoneum [*see Figure 2*]. If done right at the peritoneal surface, the division is bloodless; there are no vessels crossing from the omentum to the peritoneum. The white line of Toldt is then incised all the way from the sigmoid colon to a point above the kidney [*see Figure 3*].

Next, in what is probably the key point for making the renal dissection go easily, the colon and its mesentery are swept medially while Gerota's fascia and its contents are left untouched. The pericolic fat is gently lifted to reveal the fine plane between the colonic mesentery and the anterior surface of Gerota's fascia. This plane is most easily seen inferiorly; hence, separation of mesentery from fascia begins inferiorly and proceeds superiorly. As with the initial intra-abdominal incision, no vessels cross this plane; thus, bleeding indicates violation of either Gerota's fascia or the colonic mesentery. All pulsating arteries go with the colonic mesentery.

As dissection proceeds, the colon, the pancreas, and the spleen fall medially, and the kidney becomes visible within Gerota's fascia [*see Figures 4 and 5*]. Eventually the spleen is retracted medially with the left hand. The peritoneum anchors the spleen laterally and covers structures (such as the pancreas and the splenic vein) that are retroperitoneal but lie outside Gerota's fascia. An incision is made in the peritoneal reflection, initially lateral to and about 1 cm away from the spleen but subsequently curving medially as it is extended above the spleen. If the incision strays from the spleen and comes too close to the diaphragm, the risk of pneumothorax arises. As the spleen is retracted medially, the attachments holding the spleen come under tension and should be divided until the stomach is visible. When the spleen is being retracted, the sharp tip of the left-hand instrument should be advanced past the spleen and its blunt side used to push the organ (so-called pastpointing), because the tip can easily tear the splenic capsule [*see Figure 6*].

The colon is then mobilized medially along with its mesentery up to a point well below the iliac vessels. Any holes made in the colonic mesentery must be closed to eliminate the potential traps that may lead to small bowel herniation. When this portion of the dissection is finished, the spleen, the pancreas, the colon, and the small bowel should have fallen completely medially, and the field should be the entire anterior surface of Gerota's fascia. As Gerota's fascia extends medially, it also angles posteriorly; consequently, the surgeon typically encounters a large amount of periaortic nodal tissue and fat, which must be avoided. When the field is clear, Gerota's fascia is entered fairly medially.

STEP 3: MOBILIZATION OF RENAL VEIN

At this point, the left renal vein can usually be easily seen. Its surface is bluntly dissected very medially (i.e., over the aorta). There are a number of lymphatic vessels and fibers lying just anterior to the renal vein; cutting these with the ultrasonic scalpel markedly facilitates dissection.

Figure 4 **Laparoscopic donor nephrectomy. The kidney lies behind the splenic flexure of the colon and the lower pole of the spleen; these structures will be reflected medially (i.e., toward the floor).**

The superior and inferior surfaces of the vein are bluntly dissected to expose the adrenal vein and the gonadal vein, which are then freed circumferentially at their junctions with the renal vein. Because these two branches are at right angles to the instrument in the right hand, the best tool for freeing them is a 12 mm right-angle dissector; alternatively, the right-angle clip applier itself can be used for this purpose. The adrenal vein and the gonadal vein should each be freed circumferentially for a distance of 1 to 2 cm; these vessels always bifurcate within that distance. Once the vessels have been freed, four clips are applied to each one, and cuts are made with a scissors between the second and third clips [*see Figure 7*].

Before the third major branch of the renal vein—the lumbar vein—can be approached, however, the adrenal gland must be dissected to provide good exposure of all surfaces of the renal vein.

STEP 4: DISSECTION OF ADRENAL GLAND

The adrenal gland is recognizable by its characteristic golden-yellow color. All attachments on the gland's border are cut with the ultrasonic scalpel, first inferiorly and then laterally. Just at the triangular corner pointing toward the renal hilum, there is usually a small venous branch coming out of the renal hilum, which can cause troublesome bleeding if not recognized. The dissection should be kept close to the adrenal gland and away from the renal hilum so as to avoid the various small polar renal vessels coursing nearby. Bleeding vessels in this area should not be controlled with clips or the electrocautery, because damage to major renal branches may result.

With the adrenal attachments severed, the gland itself is peeled back, and the upper-pole renal parenchyma comes into view. The fat behind the adrenal gland and in front of the

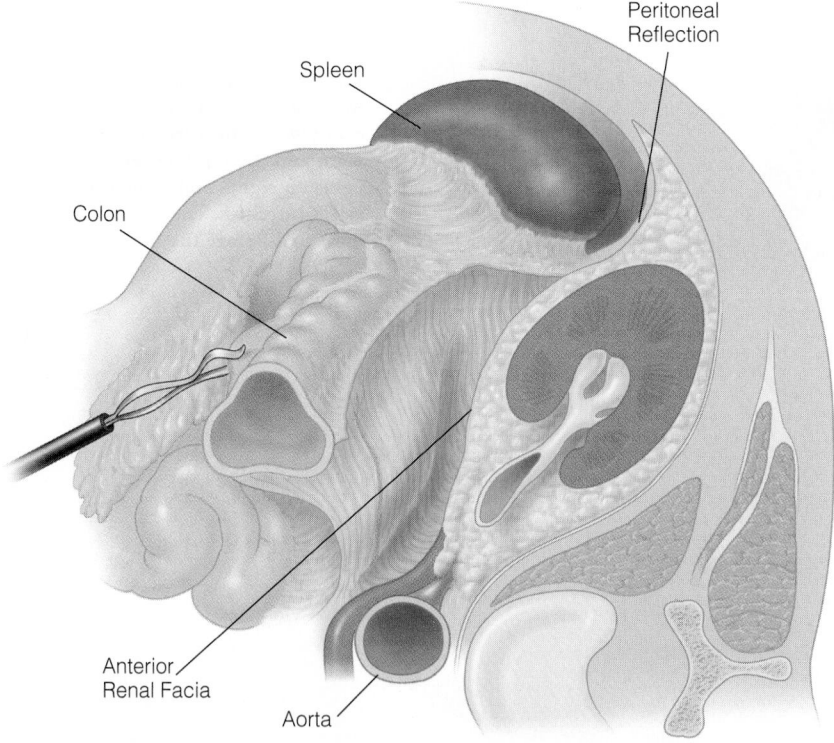

Spleen

Peritoneal Reflection

Colon

Anterior Renal Facia

Aorta

Figure 5 **Laparoscopic donor nephrectomy. Medial visceral rotation of the left colon and the splenic flexure, the spleen, and the pancreas exposes the entire anterior surface of Gerota's fascia. An incision is made in the peritoneal reflection as a continuation of the incision of the white line of Toldt.**

Figure 6 **Laparoscopic donor nephrectomy. The left-hand instrument pastpoints the spleen (left) and retracts it medially to place tension on the peritoneal reflection, which is incised with the ultrasonic scalpel. The contents of Gerota's fascia (right) and the left diaphragm (straight ahead) are visible. To visualize this area for the surgeon, the camera operator must come down and then look back cephalad around the spleen.**

medial upper kidney is then sectioned with the ultrasonic scalpel, and the upper pole thereby gains a modest degree of freedom.

Dissection then continues on the inferior and superior surfaces of the vein until the large lumbar vein, which branches posteriorly from the renal vein, can be readily visualized. As the renal vein is retracted with the left-hand instrument, four clips are applied to the lumbar vein with the right-angle clip applier and the lumbar vein is divided with a scissors. Again, the vein bifurcates before entering the posterior abdominal wall.

STEP 5: MOBILIZATION OF RENAL ARTERY

The course of the renal artery is just superior to that of the lumbar vein; however, the artery can be difficult to locate and dissect because of the multiple lymphatic vessels and nerves covering it. The origin of the renal artery is identified by first exposing the aortic surface just inferior to the renal vein and then carefully sectioning the periaortic lymphatics and nerves. The artery is freed circumferentially at its origin for a distance of about 1.5 cm. To avoid setting off vasospasm, the vessel should not be touched or retracted with any vigor. Topical application of vasodilators helps maintain renal arterial blood flow. A cholangiogram catheter is introduced through the 12 mm port, and 10 ml of papaverine is sprayed into the serosa of the renal artery at several points. The residual papaverine is suctioned out with a suction-irrigator held in the left hand. The vasodilatation also affects the lymphatic network here, leading to copious lymphatic flow into the operative field.

Just cephalad and anterior to the renal artery and cephalad and posterior to the renal vein is a large ganglion that must be cut. This ganglion is tough, and dividing it with the ultrasonic scalpel takes time. Once the ganglion has been divided, the medial kidney becomes a great deal more mobile.

STEP 6: DISSECTION OF URETER

The ureteral dissection takes the form of a wide radical resection. The clipping and cutting described in the preceding steps (see above) cause the caudad gonadal vein to retract somewhat inferiorly. The right-hand and left-hand instruments are placed medial to the clips on the gonadal vein, and the entire contents of Gerota's fascia are gently lifted until the psoas muscle is visualized. The resulting opening is gradually worked in both directions. The lymphatic vessels and neural fibers running behind and parallel to the artery are then cut. Gerota's fascia is incised inferiorly to allow the whole ureteric packet—comprising the gonadal vein, the ureter, and the periureteric fat—to be lifted en bloc off the psoas and the posterior musculature [*see Figure 8*].

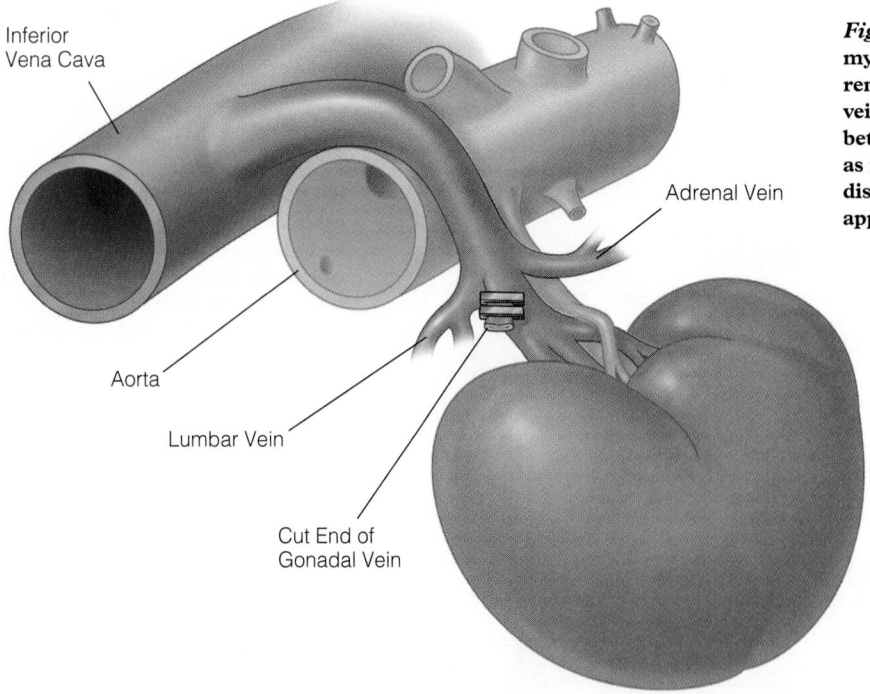

Figure 7 **Laparoscopic donor nephrectomy. Each of the three branches of the renal vein—the adrenal vein, the gonadal vein, and the lumbar vein—is taken between right-angle endoscopic clips just as it bifurcates. The adrenal gland must be dissected before the lumbar vein can be approached.**

Inferior Vena Cava

Adrenal Vein

Aorta

Lumbar Vein

Cut End of Gonadal Vein

Figure 8 **Laparoscopic donor nephrectomy. The gonadal vein and the ureter, along with all the surrounding periureteric fat, are lifted up until the psoas muscle and the posterior body wall musculature are visualized.**

It is crucial, however, not to pull up the fine fascia that covers these muscles: the lateral femoral cutaneous nerve lies just beneath this fascia and is easily traumatized.

After the ureter and the periureteric fat have been freed medially all the way to the level of the common iliac artery, a lateral incision is made in Gerota's fascia, extending from about the level of the lower pole of the kidney to the iliac artery. The ureteric packet is then lifted up to allow the surgeon to verify that the two incisions have met and that the ureteric packet has been freed circumferentially. At the level of the common iliac artery, the ureteric packet thins out, containing primarily the gonadal vein and the ureter.

The advantages of performing such a wide ureteral resection are that it minimizes the chances of trauma to the fine vasculature and diminishes the risks of ureteral necrosis in the transplant recipient.[21]

STEP 7: RETRORENAL DISSECTION

Up to this point in the procedure, the kidney has been held up by the lateral attachments of Gerota's fascia; otherwise, the organ would have moved freely. The lower pole of the kidney is now pulled ventrally with the grasper in the left hand so as to place the fascial attachments under tension. These attachments are then cut with the ultrasonic scalpel in the right hand, starting at the incision above the ureteral packet and continuing all the way to the upper pole. The kidney itself continually falls ventrally. This step in the operation poses a real challenge to the camera operator, who must move the camera from above down around the lower pole and then look back up the posterior surface of the kidney. Once the kidney flops ventrally, the camera operator can move the scope up over the kidney and look down as the many attachments are divided. This part of the dissection is quite avascular. Eventually, the renal artery becomes visible from the posterior side. At this point, both instruments are used to grasp Gerota's fascia and push the kidney back into its natural fossa.

Once the posterior attachments have been taken, a new risk arises: torsion. The still intact ureter is of some help in keeping the kidney oriented, but care must be taken not to twist the kidney and cause ischemia. The two working instruments are placed cephalad and caudad to the renal vessels, and the kidney is lifted up. At this point, it is crucial to make sure that the only structures tethering the kidney to the patient are the renal artery, the renal vein, and the ureter.

STEP 8: CREATION OF EXTRACTION SITE AND PLACEMENT OF 18 FRENCH TROCAR

A Pfannenstiel incision is used for the extraction site; when making this incision, the surgeon may be more comfortable sitting on a stool. The midline rectus fascia is exposed for a distance of at least 7 cm and incised. The posterior rectus fascial fibers are also carefully incised down to the semilunar line so as both to avoid entering the peritoneal cavity and to confirm that there are no strong fibers that would hinder kidney extraction. An 18 French trocar is placed in the incision and angled cephalad. The incision is then visualized from the inside via the laparoscopic camera, and the blunt trocar tip is pushed through the peritoneum. CO_2 leaks can be sealed temporarily with laparotomy pads.

Heparin, 5000 U I.V., is administered by the anesthesiologist. A large bowl of ice-slush solution is prepared. The recipient OR is notified to hang the I.V. bag containing the preservation fluid.

STEP 9: DIVISION OF URETER

A stapler loaded with an endovascular cartridge is used to divide the ureteral packet. The stapler can be introduced either through the 12 French port in the left lower quadrant or through the 18 French suprapubic trocar (with the help of an 18 French–12 French reducer). The jaws of the stapler are opened, placed across the ureteral packet near the iliac vessels, and levered caudad as far as possible to yield the greatest possible ureteral length. This maneuver is facilitated by applying cephalad traction to the ureter with the left-hand instrument.

STEP 10: "PREBAGGING" OF KIDNEY

The kidney is bagged before the renal vessels are divided for two reasons: (1) to make sure that the organ is not too big to fit into the extraction bag and (2) to provide better visualization of the renal vessels during their division [see Figure 9].

Figure 9 **Laparoscopic donor nephrectomy. The kidney is "prebagged" before the renal vessels are divided.**

The specimen pouch is inserted through the 18 French suprapubic trocar under laparoscopic vision. The bag is then deployed out behind the kidney; deployment must be complete (in the case of the Endocatch II, all the way out to the white hub at the base of the bag) to ensure that the bag does not separate prematurely. The direction of the bag must be positioned with its upside to the right (in the case of the Endocatch II, with the green drawstring ring on the handle down). The kidney is then scooped up with the specimen pouch in a clockwise rotational motion. Both poles of the kidney, along with the ureter, are laid inside the bag. Gentle downward pressure is applied to the handle of the bag, lifting the kidney up and exposing its last two attachments, the renal artery and the renal vein. An assistant then holds the specimen pouch in position, freeing the surgeon to return to two-handed surgery.

STEP 11: DIVISION OF RENAL VESSELS

At this point, it is crucial to confirm (1) that vascular cartridges are available for the stapler, (2) that the scrub nurse knows how to change cartridges rapidly, and (3) that extra endoscopic GIA staplers and extra specimen pouches are immediately available in case of equipment failure.

Figure 10 **Laparoscopic donor nephrectomy. The renal artery is divided with the stapler. Care must be taken not to include any of the aorta in the stapler's jaws.**

The stapler (which may be either a straight or an articulating model) is tested to verify that it can go across each vessel smoothly. No earlier than 3 minutes after administration of heparin, the stapler is placed across the entire width of the renal artery and very gently levered downward toward the aorta so as to yield as much arterial length as possible [*see Figure 10*]; however, the device should not be moved down so far that it grasps any of the aortic wall. If, in the attempt to avoid trauma to the aorta, one renal artery is converted into two by stapling, this result (unlike aortic bleeding) can be repaired by the recipient surgeon.[22] The stapler is fired, and the circulating nurse records the start of warm ischemia time. Protamine, 50 mg I.V., is given by the anesthesiologist as soon as the renal artery has been cut.

The stapler is withdrawn, and a new cartridge is loaded. If an articulating stapler was employed, it must be straightened before it can be removed through the trocar. Further upward traction is employed to facilitate exposure of the renal vein, which is then divided with the reinserted vascular stapler [*see Figure 11*]. It is important to ensure that the stapler divides the renal vein below the three sets of endoscopic clips on the vein's branches: trying to staple through the clips will result in a misfire or a locked, irremovable stapler. The stapler is then removed, and the surgeon takes the handle of the retrieval bag from the assistant.

STEP 12: EXTRACTION OF KIDNEY

Once the renal vessels are divided, the camera operator must immediately change the view from the vasculature to the contents of the retrieval bag. Further clockwise rotation of the bag, in conjunction with upward traction and shaking, allows the kidney to fall well inside; pushing with the left-hand instrument is also helpful. The green ring of the drawstring is pushed down and out of its holder and then pulled while the separation of the bag from the metal hoop ring and the closing of the bag are visualized. Next, the handle and the attached hoop ring are removed under direct vision: this must be done carefully, because the metal hoop ring is capable of cutting tissue and vessels and of trapping loops of small bowel.

The 18 French trocar is also removed along with the handle and the hoop ring. The surgeon's two index fingers are inserted into the peritoneal cavity at the point from which the trocar was just removed and are pulled strongly apart to create a peritoneal opening at least 8 cm wide. By pulling on the drawstring, the specimen pouch is drawn out through the extraction site. If the contents of the pouch are too bulky to fit smoothly through the

Figure 11 **Laparoscopic donor nephrectomy. The stapler is reloaded and used to divide the renal vein. To prevent misfiring or locking of the stapler, division must be done below the clips previously placed on the vein's three branches.**

opening, a gentle rocking motion can be used to pull the kidney out. This must be done gently: excessive force will result in a compression injury to the renal parenchyma. Occasionally, the fascial incision is too small to permit smooth extraction and must be enlarged.

STEP 13: IMMERSION AND PERFUSION OF EXTRACTED KIDNEY

The plastic bag containing the kidney is cut open with a scissors, and the kidney is immediately immersed in the ice slush; this action marks the end of warm ischemia time. The kidney is then taken to the recipient OR and perfused. The arterial and venous staple lines are excised, and the renal artery is perfused with preservation solution until the venous effluent is clear. The renal vein branches are tied at their origins and the endoscopic clips removed. The ureteral staple line is excised. The perinephric fat is removed, but a generous amount of periureteral tissue is left with the ureter.

STEP 14: CLOSURE

A continuous 0 suture is placed to close the midline rectus fascia. The abdomen is then reinsufflated, and a careful examination is performed. Bleeding vessels are either fulgurated or clipped. The renal fossa is copiously irrigated with the suction-irrigator. The areas where bleeding is particularly apt to arise are the renal artery and renal vein staple lines, the adrenal gland, the spleen, and the ureteral vein and gonadal vein stumps. The left lower quadrant trocar site is closed with a 0 suture on a Carter-Thomason needle under direct laparoscopic control. The trocars are removed, and CO_2 is expressed from the abdomen. The remaining skin incisions are closed with 4-0 subcuticular absorbable sutures, and dressings are applied.

Postoperative Care

A chest x-ray and a complete blood count (CBC) are obtained in the recovery room. The patient is monitored for signs of bleeding, and a follow-up CBC and creatinine level are obtained on postoperative day 2. Venous compression devices are used until the patient becomes ambulatory. Pain is managed by patient-controlled analgesia with morphine. The postoperative diet begins with clear liquids and progresses as tolerated: typically, the donor takes liquid on postoperative day 1 and solids on postoperative day 2. As with any nephrectomy, slow return of bowel function is to be expected and is typically the major deterrent to very early discharge. In fact, donors may report sluggish bowel function for as long as 7 to 10 days. A 48-hour hospital stay is the goal, but 65 hours is actually the average length of stay. The urethral catheter is removed early on postoperative day 1, and early ambulation is aggressively encouraged.

Troubleshooting

USE OF AUXILIARY 5 MM PORT

Augmenting the initial three ports with an additional 5 mm port can make it much easier for an assistant to move the specimen to provide exposure. This auxiliary port is placed under direct laparoscopic vision midway between the ribcage and the iliac crest in the midaxillary line. The assistant stands on the opposite side of the table from the surgeon and, for the most part, operates in a mirror-image fashion. A grasper is inserted through the auxiliary port and employed to grip Gerota's fascia and move the kidney. During retrorenal dissection, this grasper can be used to help shift the kidney ventrally as well as to bring it back dorsally when the organ is obscuring the surgeon's ports.

TECHNIQUES FOR OPERATING BEHIND STRUCTURES

The dissection of the neural and lymphatic attachments paralleling the renal artery can be difficult to visualize. Great care must be taken in this area because accessory vessels or branches may not be appreciated on the angiogram.

Small bites should be taken with the ultrasonic scalpel, with the active blade kept away from the renal artery. The camera can usually come around from below and show the renal artery quite well; this area is close to the right-hand port and thus is easily reached with the ultrasonic scalpel. The upper side of the renal artery, however, is more difficult to reach. The 30° lens allows the camera to look down at the artery, but it does not clearly show the surgeon how to get to the vessel's upper surface. By switching hands, the surgeon can reach this area with a 5 mm ultrasonic scalpel inserted through the left-hand port. Alternatively, the surgeon can pass the 10 mm ultrasonic scalpel through the right-hand port and behind the renal artery under direct vision, then move the camera and visualize the tip of the scalpel from above. The scalpel tip can then be used for gentle sectioning under direct vision, but it will not be possible to see all of the instrument shaft at one time.

HIBACHI MANEUVER

Before initiating extraction, the surgeon must verify that all attachments except the renal artery, the renal vein, and the ureter have been resected [*see Figure 12*]. This may be accomplished by means of the so-called hibachi maneuver. The left-hand instrument is passed under the specimen just cephalad to the renal vessels and advanced all the way through to the posterior body wall. The right-hand instrument is similarly passed just caudad to the renal vessels and advanced all the way through to the posterior body wall. The two instruments are then lifted simultaneously, allowing the surgeon to view the specimen from above and below and thus to determine whether all extraneous attachments have been cut.

ALTERNATIVE EXTRACTION APPROACHES FOR SPECIMENS THAT CANNOT BE BAGGED

Patients with a high body mass index (stocky male patients, in particular) sometimes have a great deal of perinephric fat. Typically, excessive fat is readily apparent on the preoperative CT scan. Besides being present in supranormal quantity, the fat may also exhibit textural differences: some male patients have extremely thick and sticky fat, with poorly defined planes. As a result, the specimen may be too large to fit into the retrieval bag. With experience, the surgeon can predict which cases are likely to be difficult in this regard and can take appropriate measures. For instance, staying close to the upper pole of the kidney during the initial dissection leaves significant fat with the diaphragm. Sacrificing some of the width of the ureteral resection leaves fat with the posterior body wall and reduces the specimen size. If the specimen still cannot be reduced to the point where it fits into the retrieval bag, either the kidney should be removed manually or an alternative extraction site should be considered.

For manual extraction, the previously created Pfannenstiel incision must be enlarged sufficiently to allow withdrawal of the specimen and the surgeon's hand together. This manual removal can be done under direct vision: insufflation will be maintained because the extraction site still fits tightly around the surgeon's arm. We do not recommend devices such as the Pneumo Sleeve (Dexterity Surgical, Inc., Roswell, Georgia) for this application, because they are expensive and take time to install at a Pfannenstiel site. Such devices are, however, excellent for planned hand-assisted nephrectomies from high sites.

For specimens that cannot be retrieved through the suprapubic extraction incision, whether laparoscopically or manually, the preferred alternative extraction site is a 7 cm incision placed through the left lower quadrant trocar incision; all of the bowel has fallen far away from this site. This alternative extraction incision, though more painful postoperatively than a midline incision would be, is still less painful than a full flank incision would be.

BOWEL RETRACTION VIA PFANNENSTIEL SITE

In obese donors, even after the left colon and the spleen are taken down, the bowel may still hinder visualization. The surgeon should first check to make sure that anesthesia with nitrous oxide, which causes bowel distention, is not being used. The problem can usually be resolved by placing a laparoscopic port through the Pfannenstiel incision and then employing a fan retractor to push the left colon and the small bowel medially.

Complications

NEUROLOGIC

There are two neurologic complications that have an incidence of at least 1% in laparoscopic kidney donors: injury to the left sympathetic chain and injury to the left lateral femoral cutaneous nerve [see Figure 13]. To date, left sympathetic chain injury has not been recognized intraoperatively, but postoperatively, some donors report that their right foot is cool. Recognition of this injury is typically delayed, occurring as long as 1 year after the procedure. Lateral femoral cutaneous nerve injury generally is demonstrable immediately after operation, when donors report diminished sensation over the left lateral thigh. The symptoms (including tingling, numbness, or both) are not disabling and may resolve in 1 to 50 weeks. The lateral femoral cutaneous nerve runs just under the psoas fascia and may be injured in the course of wide resection of the ureter; however, some surgeons believe that it is the flank position itself that leads to this injury, in that the problem may also be seen with open flank nephrectomy.

VASCULAR

Minor bleeding may occur as a result of small incidental lacerations of the spleen, the adrenal gland, or the colonic mesentery. Such bleeding can be controlled with oxidized regenerated cellulose (Surgicel) and pressure. There is a small accessory adrenal vein that derives from the renal hilum and enters the adrenal gland inferolaterally; bleeding from this vessel can be controlled with oxidized regenerated cellulose. The use of endoscopic clips sometimes results in injury to upper pole renal arterial branches. Anticoagulation may lead to resumed bleeding

Fat

Ureter

Figure 12 Laparoscopic donor nephrectomy. The so-called hibachi maneuver is employed to confirm that all attachments to the kidney except the renal artery, the renal vein, and the ureter have been severed.

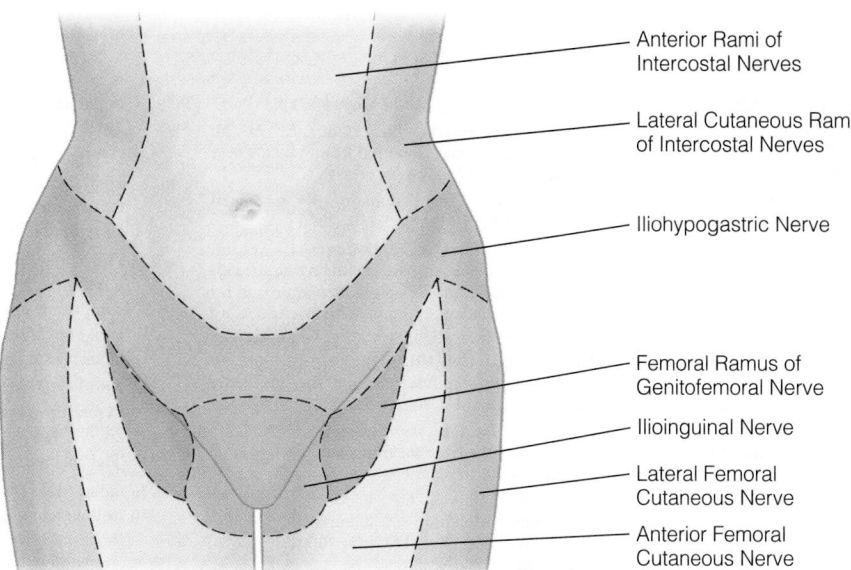

- Anterior Rami of Intercostal Nerves
- Lateral Cutaneous Rami of Intercostal Nerves
- Iliohypogastric Nerve
- Femoral Ramus of Genitofemoral Nerve
- Ilioinguinal Nerve
- Lateral Femoral Cutaneous Nerve
- Anterior Femoral Cutaneous Nerve

Figure 13 **Laparoscopic donor nephrectomy. Shown is the cutaneous nerve distribution in the lower abdomen and the groin. Laparoscopic kidney donors may experience injuries to either the left sympathetic chain or the left lateral femoral cutaneous nerve.**

from previously controlled vessels. Before the trocars are removed at the close of the procedure, all actual and potential bleeding sites should be reexamined.

Injuries to the renal vein can usually be controlled with pressure, endoscopic clips, and, occasionally, suturing; however, any clips used must be safely away from any future endovascular stapler lines. Injuries to the renal artery or the aorta are best handled by immediate conversion to open nephrectomy. As noted earlier [*see* Operative Technique, Step 11: Division of Renal Vessels, *above*], in the placement of the vascular stapler, it is crucial not to take any part of the aortic wall with the device: shorter-than-ideal arterial length and accidental conversion of one renal artery into two can be repaired by the recipient surgeon,[22] whereas aortic bleeding cannot.

Misfiring of the endovascular stapler is rare but not unknown.[23] Venous misfires are usually attributable to locking of the stapler after it hits a clip, whereas arterial misfires are usually attributable to failure to occlude the artery with the three patient-side rows of staples. Arterial misfires have dramatic results: immediate conversion to open nephrectomy, using the open surgical set, is required to prevent exsanguination.

PNEUMOTHORAX

In thin patients, dissection of the upper pole may lead to a pneumothorax, manifested by a fluttering of the diaphragm downward, which obstructs the surgeon's vision. If the hole can be seen, the suction-irrigator is inserted through it, and a figure-eight suture is placed around the device. The CO_2 is evacuated from the chest, and the suture is tied in one quick motion.

Most of the time, once the gas has been evacuated from the abdomen, there is little if any pneumothorax. A small CO_2 pneumothorax is inconsequential. However, if a fluttering diaphragm is obscuring the surgeon's vision intraoperatively, then placement of a small percutaneous thoracic catheter connected to suction in the axillary line allows the pleural space to remain evacuated during the procedure.

MESENTERIC

During takedown of the colon and the colonic mesentery, it is important both to avoid entering Gerota's fascia and to avoid going back through the colonic mesentery and reentering the peritoneum. All mesenteric rents are potentially dangerous and should be repaired if possible. Any such rent can easily lead to internal herniation, with small bowel passing into the now empty renal fossa. All kidney donors with mesenteric openings must be carefully observed for postoperative bowel obstruction.

Outcome Evaluation

At present, it appears that when laparoscopic donor nephrectomy is done by experienced surgeons, it can yield recipient renal function results equivalent to those of open nephrectomy.[2-6] This was not the case early in the laparoscopic experience, when recipient renal function was noticeably worse with laparoscopic grafts than with open grafts 1 week after transplantation[3]; it is unknown whether this early mild impairment will translate into any long-term detriment. Later in the laparoscopic experience, however, graft function with laparoscopic nephrectomy came to equal that with open nephrectomy at intervals ranging from 1 week to 3 years.[5,6] It may be anticipated, then, that whenever a center starts a laparoscopic donor nephrectomy program, there is likely to be some decrease in initial recipient renal function until sufficient experience is amassed.

References

1. Schulam PG, Kavoussi LR, Cheriff AD, et al: Laparoscopic live donor nephrectomy: the initial 3 cases. J Urol 155:1857, 1996
2. Ratner LE, Kavoussi LR, Schulam PG, et al: Comparison of laparoscopic live donor nephrectomy versus the standard open approach. Transplant Proc 29:138, 1997
3. Flowers JL, Jacobs SC, Cho E, et al: Comparison of open and laparoscopic live donor nephrectomy. Ann Surg 226:483, 1997
4. Jacobs SC, Cho E, Dunkin BJ: Laparoscopic donor nephrectomy: current role in allograft procurement. Urology 55:807, 2000
5. Jacobs SC, Cho E, Dunkin BJ, et al: Laparoscopic live donor nephrectomy: the University of Maryland 3 year experience. J Urol 164:1494, 2000
6. Ratner LE, Montgomery RA, Kavoussi LR: Laparoscopic donor nephrectomy: the four year Johns Hopkins University experience. Nephrol Dial Transplant 14:2090, 1999
7. Schweitzer EJ, Wilson J, Jacobs S, et al: Increased rates of donation with laparoscopic donor nephrectomy. Ann Surg 232:392, 2000
8. Ratner LE, Hiller J, Sroka M, et al: Laparoscopic live donor nephrectomy removes disincentives to live donation. Transplant Proc 29:3402, 1997
9. Gridelli B, Remuzzi G: Current concepts: strategies for making more organs available for transplantation. N Engl J Med 343:404, 2000
10. Ramey JR, Swartz DE, Cho E, et al: Laparoscopic kidney donation from patients over the age of fifty. Urology (in press)
11. Levinsky NG: Organ donation by unrelated donors. N Engl J Med 343:430, 2000
12. Farney AC, Cho E, Schweitzer EJ, et al: Simultaneous cadaver pancreas-living donor kidney transplantation (SPLK): a new approach for the type 1 diabetic uremic patient. Ann Surg 232:696, 2000
13. Jacobs SC, Cho E, Dunkin BJ, et al: Laparoscopic nephrectomy in the markedly obese renal donor. Urology 56:926,2000
14. Gridelli B, Remuzzi G: Strategies for making more organs available for transplantation. N Engl J Med 343:404, 2000
15. Matas AL, Garvey CA, Jacobs CL, et al: Nondirected donation of kidneys from living donors. N Engl J Med 343:433, 2000
16. Zargooshi J: Iranian kidney donors: motivations and relations with recipients. J Urol 165:386, 2001
17. Finkel M: This little kidney went to market. New York Times Magazine, May 27, 2001, p 26
18. Radcliffe-Richards J, Daar AS, Guttmann RD: The case for allowing kidney sales. Lancet 351:1950, 1998
19. Hannan EL: The relation between volume and outcome in health care. N Engl J Med 340:1677, 1999
20. Del Pizzo JJ, Sklar GN, Wong You-Cheong J, et al: Helical computerized tomography arteriography for evaluation of live renal donors undergoing laparoscopic nephrectomy. J Urol 162:31, 1999
21. Philosophe B, Kuo PC, Schweitzer EJ, et al: Laparoscopic versus open donor nephrectomy: comparing ureteral complications in the recipients and improving the laparoscopic technique. Transplantation 68:497, 1999
22. Kuo PC, Bartlett ST, Schweitzer EJ, et al: A technique for management of multiple renal arteries after laparoscopic donor nephrectomy. Transplantation 64:779, 1997
23. Chan D, Bischoff JT, Ratner LR, et al: Endovascular gastrointestinal stapler device malfunction during laparoscopic nephrectomy: early recognition and management. J Urol 164:319, 2000

Acknowledgment

Figures 1, 4, 5, 7 through 9, 12, 13   Tom Moore.

29 ORGAN PROCUREMENT

Charles M. Miller, M.D., Felix T. Rapaport, M.D., and Thomas E. Starzl, M.D., Ph.D.

Approach to the Potential Organ Donor

Preliminary Steps

When a patient presents with severe neurologic insult, initial efforts should be directed at saving the injured patient by minimizing cerebral swelling and possible brain herniation [*see III:2 Injuries to the Central Nervous System*]. Often, this is best accomplished by strict fluid restriction and the administration of diuretics and mannitol. However, one of the key advances in clinical 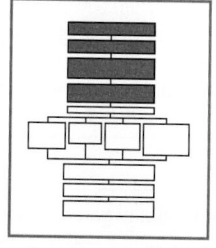 organ transplantation has been improved identification and early referral of potential organ donors. Any patient who has suffered severe brain damage should be considered for organ donation. Causes of such damage include external trauma, motor vehicle accidents, falls, assaults, spontaneous intracerebral hemorrhages, drownings, hangings, primary brain tumors, drug overdoses, and sudden infant death syndrome.

A neurologist, a neurosurgeon, or both should be consulted early in the evaluation of a patient with a severe neurologic insult. Such consultation will be important in an eventual diagnosis of brain death, which can be made on clinical criteria alone[1] but is often confirmed by means of electroencephalography,[2] occasionally by means of a cerebral blood flow scan,[3] and sometimes by means of both. Clinical criteria of brain death include deep coma, lack of spontaneous movement, a positive apnea test, and no response to painful stimuli. In addition, cranial nerve reflexes, such as the oculocephalic reflex (tested with the doll's-eyes maneuver) and the oculovestibular reflex (tested with the caloric test), should be absent. Brain-dead patients have fixed, dilated pupils and do not have protective corneal reflexes. Spinal reflexes may still be present because they do not involve the higher centers of the brain or the brain stem.[4,5] If the patient has stable cardiovascular function, the clinical criteria of brain death usually are documented twice within an interval of six to 12 hours before a final declaration of death is made [*see I:9 Coma, Seizures, Cognitive Impairment, and Brain Death*].

As soon as the possibility of donation is established, the local organ procurement agency should be contacted. (The telephone numbers of these agencies are available in most intensive care units.) The procurement coordinator then evaluates the patient's potential for organ donation, assists in the administrative details necessary for declaration of death, and acts as intermediary between the hospital and the donor's family.

When brain death is confirmed, the attending physician or neurologist should make a pronouncement in the patient's chart and complete the death certificate. The physician, procurement coordi- nator, or both may then formally request consent to donation from the family, making sure that the family members have complete and separate understandings of each of the two distinct issues involved—namely, the diagnosis of brain death and the process of organ procurement.

Donor Evaluation and Management

With the declaration of brain death, efforts must be redirected toward protecting the organs to be transplanted rather than the now dead brain. Usually, primary therapy entails aggressive rehydration. In addition, the procurement coordinator must clearly establish the adequacy of each organ to be used, according to well-recognized sets of standard criteria (see below). A 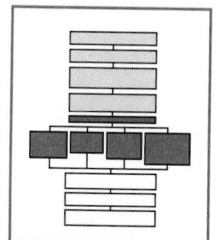 detailed medical history must be obtained that includes the cause of the brain damage as well as the donor's age, height, weight, and blood type. Assessment of acute physiologic status can be made by measuring blood pressure, central venous pressure (CVP), urine output, and arterial blood gases. Serologic analysis must be done for syphilis (Venereal Disease Research Laboratory [VDRL]), hepatitis B surface antigen (HB_sAg), hepatitis B core antibody (HB_cAb), hepatitis C virus (HCV), and cytomegalovirus,[6] as well as for human immunodeficiency virus (HIV)[7] and human T cell lymphotropic virus type I (HTLV-I); otherwise, recipients may be infected with these organisms.

A kidney donor can be between six months and 75 years of age. Levels of serum creatinine and blood urea nitrogen (BUN) should be normal, although elevations may be caused by dehydration or other adverse but reversible acute states. If dehydration is responsible, BUN and creatinine levels should fall after adequate fluid replacement.

Kidneys can be preserved after nephrectomy for up to 72 hours. Thus, there may be time for tissue typing and matching before kidneys are sent to recipients in distant cities. However, the chances that a kidney will function immediately in the recipient diminish greatly with storage for more than 24 hours.

The pancreas may be safely preserved for as long as 20 hours.

With newer preservation solutions, the liver may now be safely preserved for up to 20 hours. Time constraints are more rigid for the thoracic organs, however, and they should be transplanted within six hours after removal from the donor.

There is no consensus on the upper age limit for donors of extrarenal organs. Although an arbitrary limit of 40 to 45 years

Approach to the Potential Organ Donor

Patient has severe neurologic insult

Perform complete neurologic exam. Treat for cerebral edema, if present.

Patient has no signs of cerebral or brain stem function

Consult neurologist or neurosurgeon. Contact local procurement agency.

Neurologist or neurosurgeon confirms and makes formal pronouncement of brain death

Death certificate should be completed.
Request for donation is made by physician, local procurement coordinator, or both.

Consent obtained; patient becomes potential organ donor

Redirect therapy to donor organs. If donor is unstable, resuscitate with appropriate rehydration. Evaluate medical history and physiologic status. Screen for HB_sAg, HB_cAb, HCV, VDRL, HIV, HTLV-I, and CMV.

Evaluate each potential organ

Kidney donors

Kidneys can be preserved after nephrectomy for up to 72 hr. Criteria for donors are flexible:
- Age > 6 mo but < 75 yr.
- Normal or correctable levels of BUN and serum creatinine.

Pancreas donors

Pancreas can be preserved up to 20 hr. Donors can be as young as 10 yr or as old as 45 yr.

Liver donors

Livers can be preserved for up to 18 hr. Donors may be as old as 85 yr. Near-normal or normalizing levels of AST, ALT, and bilirubin should be documented.

Heart and heart-lung donors

Thoracic organs can be preserved for 4 to 6 hr. Donors may be as old as 60 yr. Criteria include the following: no history of cardiac disease; near-normal chest x-ray; no significant abnormality of ECG, echocardiography, or isoenzyme levels; negative Gram's stain and cultures of sputum.

Consult regional and national lists for renal and extrarenal organ placement

Contact the Organ Center of the United Network for Organ Sharing: 1-800-292-9537. Organize and coordinate donor operation.

Move donor to operating room

Include anesthetic team in management of donor. Carry out multiorgan harvesting.

Successful procurement

Store kidneys to await crossmatch. Transport extrarenal organs to transplant centers for back-table preparation and transplantation.

of age had been used to exclude donors, many recent reports have shown that livers have been safely and successfully used from donors as old as 85 years,[8] and hearts can be successfully transplanted from donors as old as 60 years.[9]

If the liver is under consideration for donation, normal or near-normal serum aspartate aminotransferase (AST), serum alanine aminotransferase (ALT), and bilirubin levels must be documented. A history of hepatitis or alcoholism is a warning sign but not necessarily a contraindication to liver transplantation. Very obese donors can be problematic for liver recovery: there is a high likelihood of macrovesicular steatosis that may preclude safe transplantation.

Heart and heart-lung donors must have no history of cardiac disease and should have a normal chest x-ray, electrocardiogram, and physical examination. The arterial oxygen tension (P_aO_2) of heart-lung donors should be 350 mm Hg during ventilation with a fraction of inspired oxygen (F_IO_2) of 1. Sputum cultures and Gram's stains should be negative. In trauma cases, tests of cardiac isoenzymes should also yield negative results.

ABO blood group and organ size are important factors in placing extrarenal organs. Ideally, a liver donor should be slightly smaller than the proposed recipient, but large variations on this generalization may occur, according to the size of the recipient liver that is to be removed. Size is a special concern in pediatric liver transplantation. Because small baby donor organs are scarce, most pediatric centers reduce the size of adult organs by performing right hepatic lobectomies or right hepatic trisegmentectomies and implanting the left lobe itself or the left lateral segment.[10-12] In addition, to maximize the donor potential, partition of the liver into the right lobe and the left lateral segment with subsequent implantation into two separate recipients is becoming more popular. These practices address both the restrictions of size and the scarcity of both pediatric and adult organ donors.

In heart transplantation, the organ of the donor usually should be slightly larger than that of the recipient because cardiomegaly is a common finding in the recipient. The height, weight, and chest circumference of the heart-lung recipient must closely match those of the donor. The donor team is responsible for accumulating the information on which wise recipient selection can be based.

During the evaluation, the donor must be maintained in a stable physiologic state.[13] Basic monitoring should include an arterial line for blood pressure monitoring and blood gas surveillance, a central venous pressure monitor, and an indwelling urinary catheter to measure urine output. Because the basic physiologic situation rarely, if ever, improves in brain-dead patients, the interval between pronouncement of death and procurement surgery should be kept as short as possible. If a donor is unstable, aggressive therapy must be directed at maintaining adequate circulation, ventilation, and diuresis. If the donor is dehydrated from earlier efforts to prevent cerebral edema, rapid repletion is required with crystalloid solutions, colloid solutions, or both.

One relatively simple guide to fluid therapy is to maintain the central venous pressure between 6 and 8 mm Hg if a normal systemic blood pressure can be achieved. However, brain death is sometimes associated with severe neurogenic shock and peripheral vasodilatation. In such cases, the peripheral vascular resistance will not support a normal systemic blood pressure, no matter how well the heart is loaded. In these patients, vasopres-sors, such as dopamine, should be added to restore normal blood pressure. Norepinephrine bitartrate (Levophed) should be used judiciously and metaraminol bitartrate (Aramine) should be avoided because they produce severe visceral and renal vasoconstriction and may injure the organs to be transplanted.

Respiratory care of the potential donor is the same as that of any ventilator-dependent patient in an intensive care setting. Chest x-rays should be obtained at least once a day. Frequent endotracheal suctioning must be done, good pulmonary toilet must be maintained at all times, and arterial blood gases must be monitored frequently. Oxygen saturation should be maintained at no less than 95 percent by adjusting the F_IO_2 settings on the ventilator [see VII:4 Use of the Mechanical Ventilator]. Levels of positive end-expiratory pressure (PEEP) greater than 5 cm H_2O are not recommended, because the higher levels increase intrathoracic and right atrial pressures, which in turn may cause hepatic parenchymal congestion and preclude the use of the liver.

A stable brain-dead donor should produce urine at a rate of at least 1 ml/kg/hr. The most common cause of oliguria is hypovolemia. If the CVP is low, further fluid resuscitation is in order. In some instances, however, oliguria may be the result of acute heart failure that is secondary to excessive fluid resuscitation, and osmotic and loop diuretics, such as mannitol and furosemide, will be needed.

When trauma to the brain is severe, pituitary function often fails. The resulting absence of antidiuretic hormone causes diabetes insipidus, and a large volume diuresis ensues, which can lead to severe volume depletion and donor instability. Most cases of diabetes insipidus can be handled simply by replacing the urine output intravenously with half-normal saline. Serum electrolytes must be monitored frequently during such treatment because hypernatremia can easily be produced. If fluid replacement cannot keep up with the diuresis, intravenous vasopressin may be given, but only with great caution, because the resulting vasoconstriction can cause severe end-organ ischemia.

Coordination of Donor and Recipient Activities

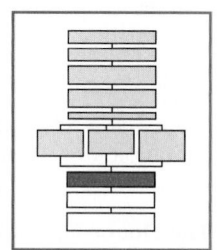

After the donor has been identified, studied, and stabilized, the procurement team contacts regional transplant programs about their needs for renal and extrarenal organs and inquires about needs in other parts of the country. A national computer registry of potential recipients of renal and extrarenal organs is maintained by the Organ Center at the United Network for Organ Sharing (UNOS). (The 24-hour UNOS number is 1-800-292-9537.)

Potential recipients of extrarenal organs are categorized according to ABO blood group, weight, acceptable weight range of the donor, distance the recipient team is willing to travel for procurement, length of time the patient has been on the transplant list, and medical urgency status. Sharing of all organs is based on the principle that organs should be allocated first within the local area, then within a specific geographic region, and finally nationally if no suitable recipients can be found locally or within the region. An exception to this rule exists for renal graft allocation. For kidneys, when there is a six-antigen match (i.e., a perfect histocompatibility match between a donor and a recipient on all six HLA-A, HLA-B, and HLA-DR antigens) or when there is at least phenotypic identity between a donor and a prospective recipient, the kidney must be offered to the matched recipient regardless of geographic location.

Within each of these geographic distributions, whether it is local, regional, or national, organs are shared according to computerized point systems, which are based on a variety of parameters that are slightly different for each organ concerned. A potential kidney recipient may accumulate points for time on the waiting list, the degree of histocompatibility match between donor and recipient, and the degree of previous antibody sensitization. There is no allocation of points for medical urgency in kidney recipients. The variables in the point system for liver recipients include blood type compatibility, time on the waiting list, and medical urgency on a scale of 1 to 4, with 4 being the least urgent and 1 being the most urgent. Finally, distribution of thoracic organs is based on principles similar to those governing distribution of livers. However, there are only two categories of medical urgency in heart and heart-lung recipients. A status 1 recipient is a critically ill patient in the intensive care unit receiving either pressor or mechanical heart support. Status 2 includes all other patients who are waiting either at home or in the hospital but outside of an ICU.

Once recipients for extrarenal organs have been identified, the local procurement team must coordinate the arrival of the participating recovery teams, schedule the operating room for donor surgery, and maintain the stability of the donor. With the recent proliferation of experienced extrarenal transplant centers throughout the United States, it is becoming more common for donor operations for extrarenal organs, especially the liver, to be performed by expert local procurement teams.[14] In the past, the recipient institution was required to send a donor team to retrieve the liver. This change has improved the coordination of the retrieval process, reduced the transportation costs associated with long-distance procurements, and helped ease the burden on the recipient team.

With cooperation from all participants, including promptness, the different procurement teams will arrive as the donor is transported to the operating room. Before actual operation, the renal and extrarenal procurement teams should coordinate their techniques and preferences to avoid unseemly conflicts during a multiple-organ harvest.

The Donor Operation

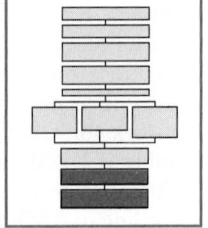

When the donor is brought to the operating room, the anesthetic team begins to participate in donor management. If spinal reflexes persist in the donor, a muscle relaxant such as pancuronium bromide should be administered.

The operation for multiple-organ procurement must proceed in such a way that the kidneys, the pancreas, the liver, the heart, the heart and the lung, or various combinations of these or other organs can be removed without any of them being jeopardized. The basic principle of the procedure is to carry out preliminary dissection of the great vessels of the abdomen and chest. The aorta is isolated at preplanned levels to allow cross-clamping, so that the organs to be removed can be core-cooled

in situ with cold intra-aortic and intraportal infusions (see below).[15] Thus, warm ischemia will be avoided in the donor organs. This technique has been adopted as an international standard. The most refined version of this procedure,[16] commonly known as the rapid-flush technique, can be completed in less than an hour, from beginning to end.

To start, a complete midline incision is made from the suprasternal notch to the pubis [see Figure 1]. If a heart team is on hand for cardiectomy, the pericardium is opened and the heart is inspected. Very minimal dissection is required to prepare the heart for removal. The superior vena cava and the aorta are encircled with tapes to allow eventual occlusion of the inflow and outflow tracts. The heart team can complete its preliminary work in 10 to 15 minutes.

The abdominal team, which consists of hepatic and renal surgeons, then proceeds. The left triangular ligament of the liver is incised, the esophagus is held to the left with a finger, and a longitudinal incision is made in the diaphragmatic crura, between the retrohepatic inferior vena cava and the esophagus [see Figure 2]. The aorta is encircled with a tape at this level.

At this point, the abdominal team's decision on how to proceed is based on the physiologic status of the donor. If the donor

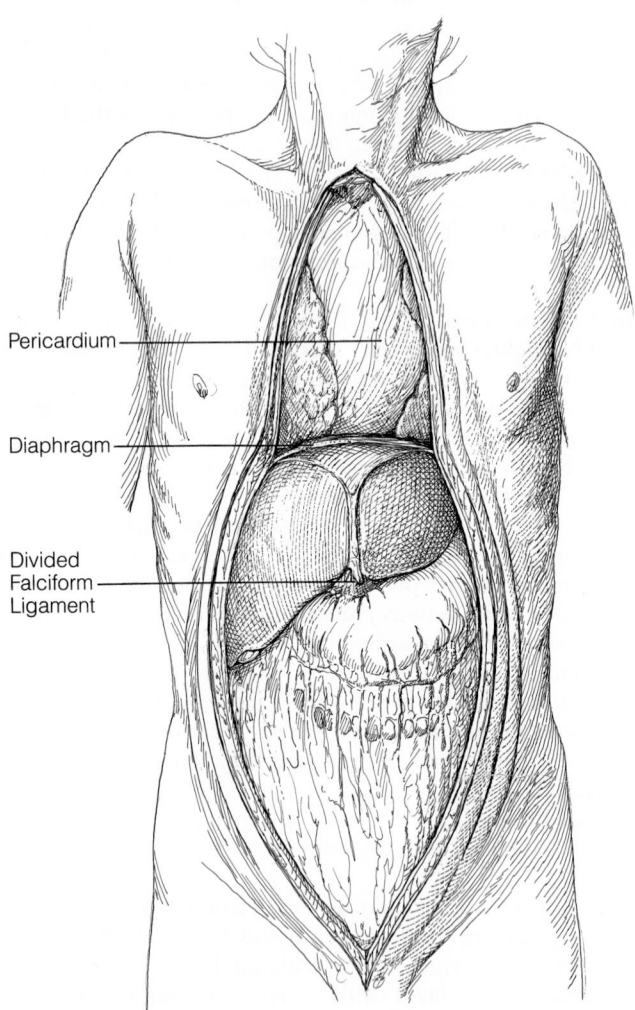

Figure 1 **The incision used for multiple-organ procurement is made from the suprasternal notch to the pubis, as illustrated here.**

cedure, the splenic vein is isolated and ligated and a cannula is advanced to the bifurcation of the splenic and portal veins. Finally, after systemic heparinization, the distal aorta is ligated and the aortic perfusion cannula is inserted [*see Figure 3*].

With the abdominal and cardiac teams coordinated, effective circulation is terminated by cross-clamping the aorta at the predetermined levels [*see Figure 4*]. The cardiac team then proceeds with removal of the heart or heart-lung as expeditiously as possible. The heart is core-cooled with a potassium-rich cardioplegic solution infused via a cannula inserted into the ascending aorta. Blanching of the heart and cardiac arrest from the cardioplegic infusion occur within a few seconds. At the same time, the systemic venous inflow is discontinued by bleeding the inferior vena cava into the pericardium. However, if the cardiac surgeons insist on cross-clamping the inferior vena cava

Figure 2 The crura are divided between the esophagus and the vena cava to facilitate exposure and encirclement of aorta at the diaphragm.

is hemodynamically unstable and efforts at stabilization have failed, the rapid-flush technique should be used: all dissection is accomplished after circulatory arrest and in situ core cooling of the organs. In hemodynamically stable donors, however, many teams, depending on their experience, prefer to perform varying amounts of dissection of the hepatic hilar structures (including the hepatic arterial supply, the common bile duct, and the portal vein) before in situ flushing, especially when use of the pancreas is being considered. In addition, renal surgeons commonly free up the ureters from the bladder to the ureteropelvic junction and perform variable dissections of the renal veins and arteries. During lengthy preliminary dissections, however, undetected periods of ischemia may occur as individual vessels of the kidneys, pancreas, or liver are occluded during skeletonization. Lengthy dissection can be most dangerous in unstable donors. Periods of ischemia produced during these long dissections probably cause a higher incidence of liver graft failure in liver-pancreas procurements.

When the dissection is completed, the abdominal team turns its attention to the more distal aorta, ligating and dividing the inferior mesenteric artery and encircling the aorta at this level [*see Figure 3*]. If the rapid-flush technique is used, the inferior mesenteric vein (IMV) is isolated and ligated. A cannula is inserted into the IMV and advanced superiorly for approximately 5 cm in adults and for lesser distances in children so that the tip is in or just entering the portal vein. In the classic pro-

Figure 3 The inferior mesenteric artery is ligated and divided. Catheters are inserted into the inferior mesenteric vein and into the distal aorta.

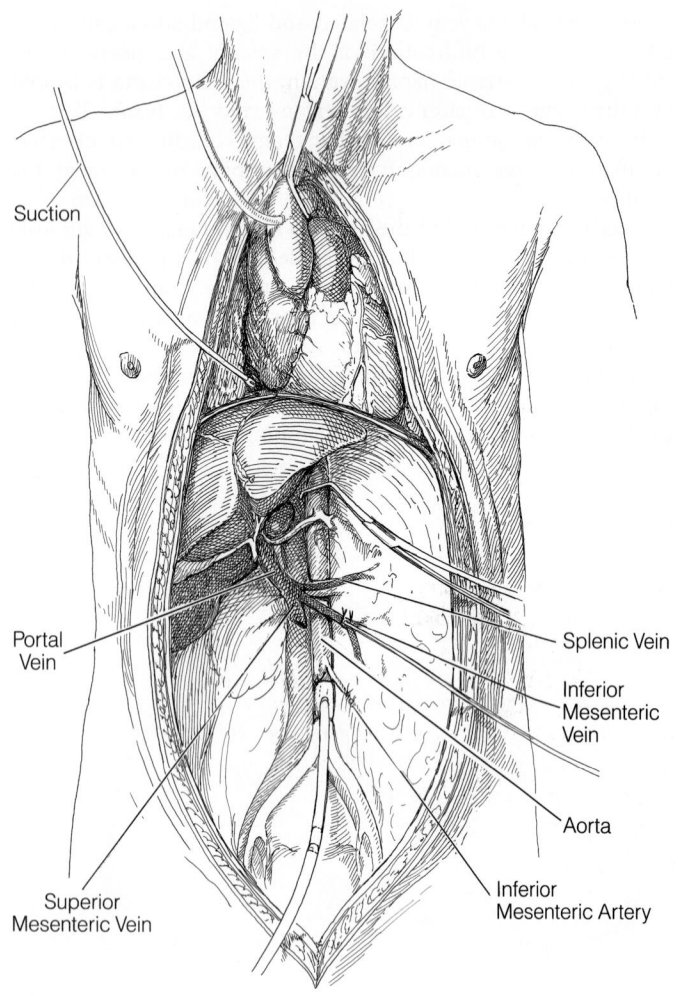

Figure 4 **The aorta is cross-clamped at the diaphragmatic level at the time of rapid infusion.**

within the pericardium, the vena cava must be vented into the lower abdomen to prevent venous hypertension.

Most cardiac teams require five to 10 minutes from the onset of the cardioplegic infusion to remove the heart. However, as soon as the heart team has discontinued effective circulation by occluding vena caval inflow or by cross-clamping the ascending aorta, the previously encircled aorta is cross-clamped at the diaphragmatic level [*see Figure 4*]. Infusion with cold fluid is begun through both the inferior mesenteric (portal) cannula and the terminal aortic cannula. Thus, the liver is blanching and cooling while the cardiac team is completing removal of the heart. The liver is not dissected further until it becomes palpably cold and free of blood. The kidneys participate in the perfusion and cooling process.

After the liver is cold and the heart has been removed, the liver is removed in a bloodless field while the cold infusion is continued. Above the liver, a patch of diaphragm is removed around the lumen of the suprahepatic inferior vena cava [*see Figure 5*]. The surgeon must now complete the hepatic hilar dissection by cutting or ligating the remaining branches of the celiac axis as far as possible from the parent trunk [*see Figure 5*]. By doing so and, especially, by dividing the gastroduodenal artery, the surgeon uncovers the portal vein. The portal vein is followed inferiorly to the junction of the superior mesenteric and splenic veins, which are cut [*see Figure 6*]. The area posterior to the portal vein must be inspected carefully because it is here that an aberrant right hepatic artery originating from the superior mesenteric artery is most commonly found [*see Figure 6*]. The originating vessel (or vessels, in the case of an aberrant right hepatic artery) is traced to its aortic origin and removed with a Carrel patch [*see Figure 7*]. The liver is excised and placed in a sterile, empty sack immersed in a basin of ice-slush solution. Through a small infusion cannula placed in either the superior mesenteric or the splenic vein, the liver is then perfused with approximately 1.0 to

b

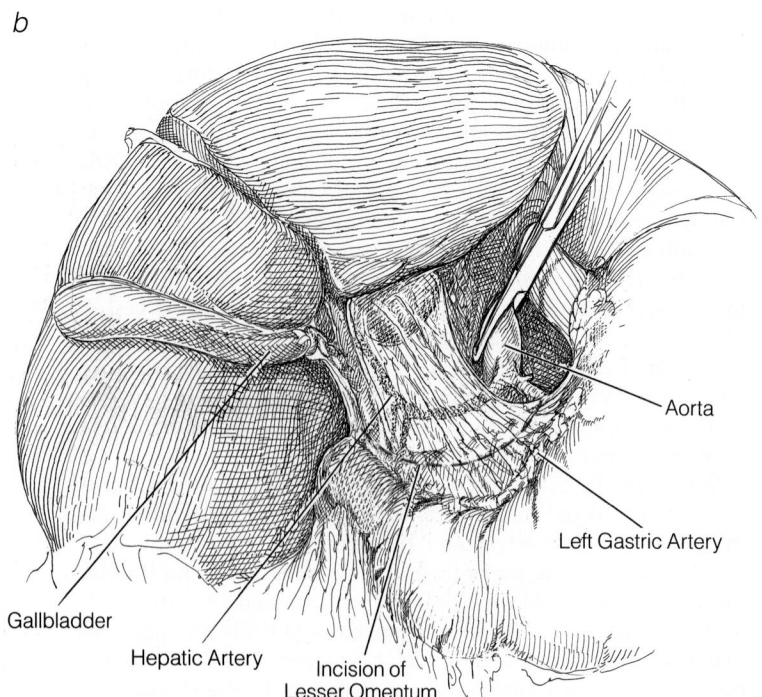

Figure 5 **A patch of diaphragm surrounding the suprahepatic inferior vena cava is removed with the liver (*a*). The approach to the hepatic hilar structures is made in a bloodless field (*b*).**

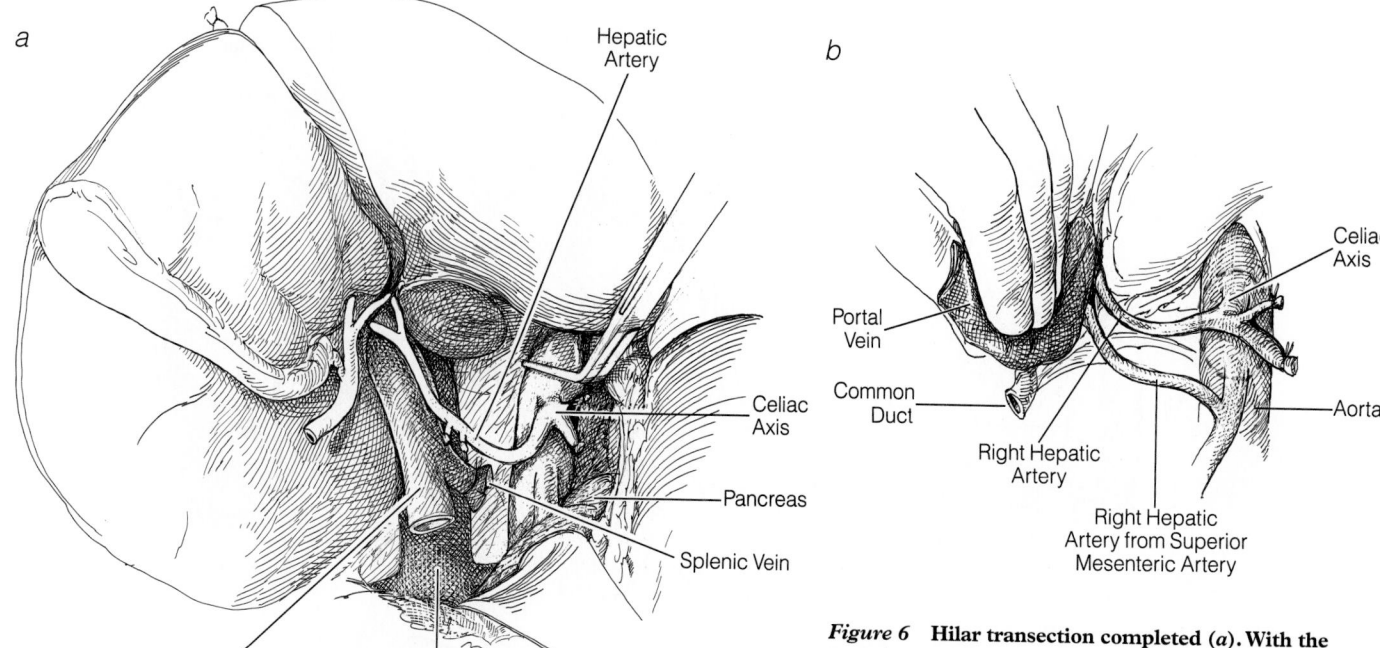

a

Hepatic
Artery

Celiac
Axis

Pancreas

Splenic Vein

Superior
Mesenteric Vein

Vena Cava

b

Portal
Vein

Common
Duct

Right Hepatic
Artery

Right Hepatic
Artery from Superior
Mesenteric Artery

Celiac
Axis

Aorta

Figure 6   **Hilar transection completed (*a*). With the superior mesenteric vein and the splenic vein cut, the portal vein may be folded superiorly with a finger so that an anomalous right hepatic artery may be found posterior to the portal vein (*b*).**

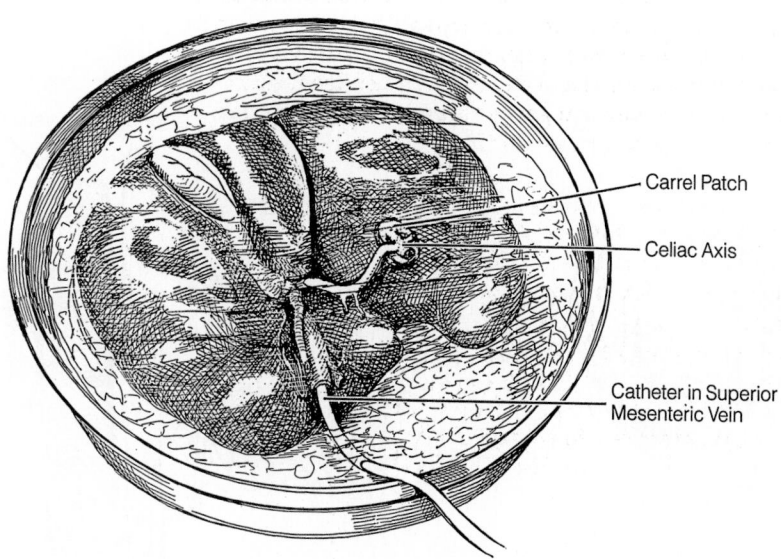

Carrel Patch

Celiac Axis

Catheter in Superior
Mesenteric Vein

Figure 7   **The aortic Carrel patch and the portal cannula used to infuse chilled preservation solution are shown in this illustration of an excised liver in an ice basin.**

1.5 L of University of Wisconsin (UW) preservation solution.[17] The organ is subsequently packed in the effluent that remains in the sack and kept refrigerated in a standard ice chest.

The organ is transported to the recipient hospital, where it is cleaned and prepared for transplantation in a formal back-table procedure that takes approximately 30 minutes.

Removal of the cold and bloodless liver requires 15 to 30 minutes, but during most of this time, effective cold perfusion of the kidneys in situ continues through the aortic cannula. With the liver out of the field, the two kidneys can be removed en bloc; this process takes an additional five to 10 minutes. Removal is best accomplished from below upward [see *Figure 8*].

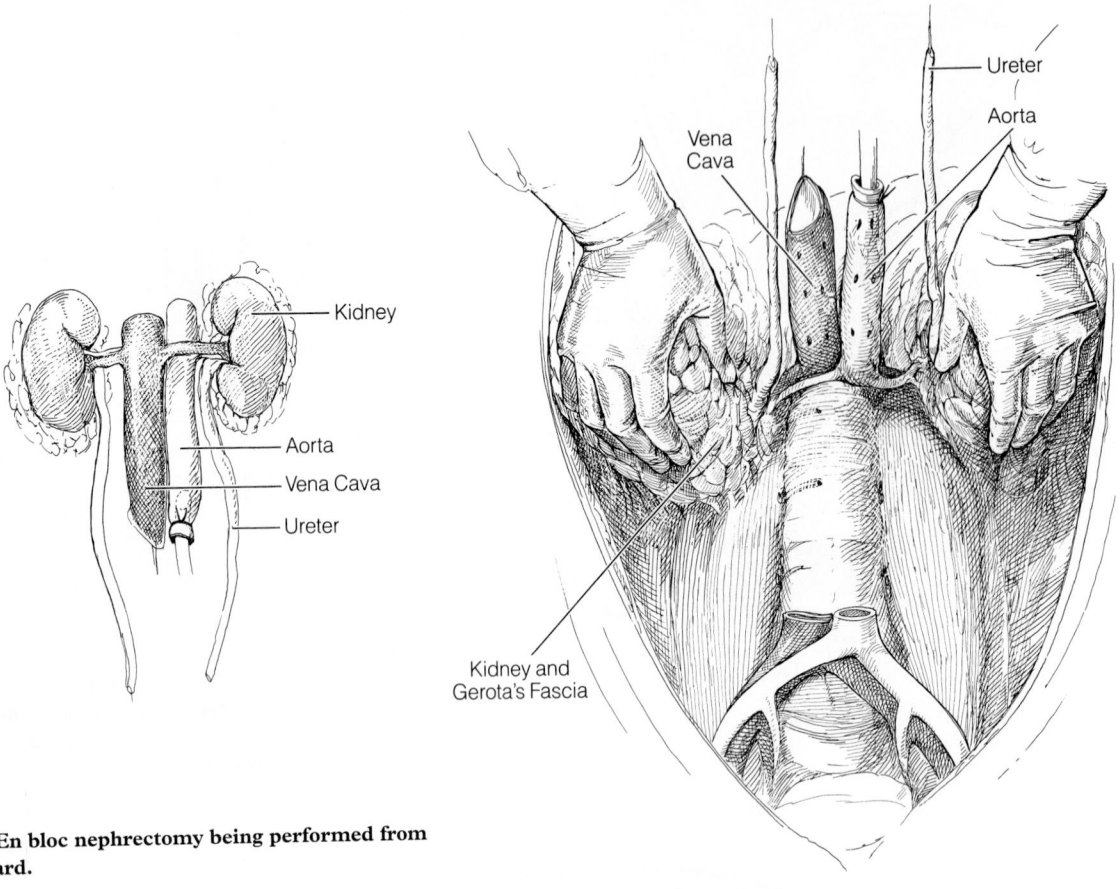

Figure 8 En bloc nephrectomy being performed from below upward.

Figure 9 Kidneys are placed in the ice basin in the anatomic position (*a*). In the posterior orientation (*b*), the left renal vein can be seen transected at its origin from the vena cava.

After the kidneys are removed, they are immersed in an ice bath and reperfused with preservation solution either individually or through the aorta. If the kidneys are to be separated, the left renal vein is transected flush at the point where it enters the inferior vena cava [*see Figure 9*]. The kidneys are then turned over so that the posterior wall of the aorta is accessible. Inserting one blade of a scissors into the aortic lumen, the sur-geon incises the posterior wall of the aorta at the midline. A per-fect guide to the line of aortic incision is the row of lumbar arteries. Then, having an internal view of the renal arterial branches passing laterally, the surgeon incises the anterior wall of the aorta longitudinally from the inside. If continuous perfu-sion is planned for later preservation of the organs, aortic flaps can be fashioned during separation of the kidneys and used for

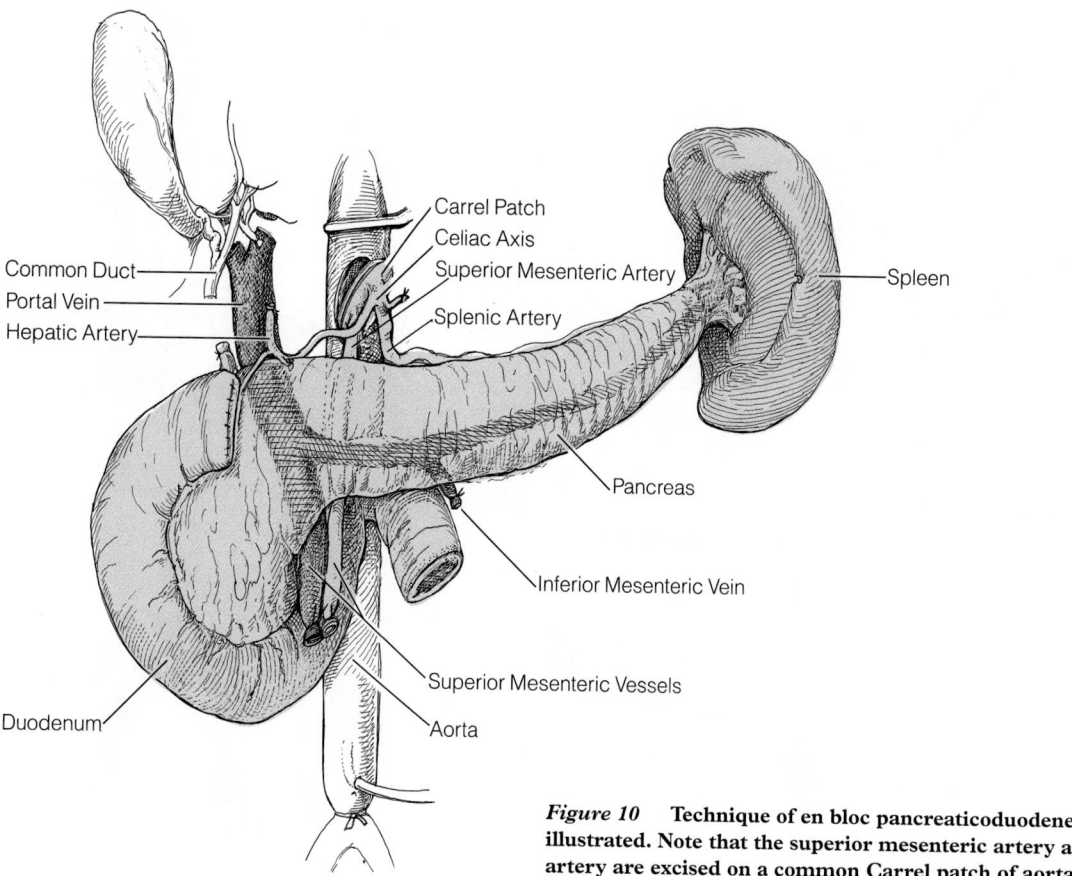

Common Duct
Portal Vein
Hepatic Artery
Carrel Patch
Celiac Axis
Superior Mesenteric Artery
Splenic Artery
Spleen
Pancreas
Inferior Mesenteric Vein
Superior Mesenteric Vessels
Duodenum
Aorta

Figure 10 **Technique of en bloc pancreaticoduodenectomy is illustrated. Note that the superior mesenteric artery and celiac artery are excised on a common Carrel patch of aorta.**

closure so that cannulas need not be placed directly into the renal arteries. Final dissection of the kidneys is performed on a back table at the recipient hospital.

Total or segmental pancreatectomy can be part of the multiple-organ procurement procedure [*see Figure 10*]. The technique differs in details but not in principle from that of the procedures described (see above). The dissection is almost always accomplished before in situ flushing and may require between one and a half and three and a half hours to complete. If the whole pancreas is to be transplanted, a Carrel patch, including the celiac axis and the superior mesenteric artery, can be taken from the abdominal aorta [*see Figure 10*]. This procedure ensures better vascularization of the pancreas graft, and the natural superior-to-inferior pancreaticoduodenal arterial anastomoses are vascularized from both directions.

It was once thought that simultaneous whole organ pancreas and liver recovery could not be done (because both procedures called for retention of the celiac axis and the portal vein), but safe techniques now exist for dividing the vasculature of these organs. The use of free iliac vein and arterial grafts has allowed successful transplantations of liver and pancreas from a single donor.[18] It is now UNOS policy to encourage utilization of both organs from appropriate donors, although many liver teams approach these donors with trepidation because of the lengthy dissection and associated risks of graft nonfunction. For most diabetics, pancreas transplantation is something of a luxury

because of the option of insulin administration, whereas for patients who require liver transplantation, no alternative exists. Therefore, if an anomaly in the donor precludes successful procurement of both the liver and the pancreas, the liver team takes priority.

With the improved technique that makes possible the use of the liver and the whole pancreas, the liver retains almost all of the portal vein, and the short portal vein of the pancreatic specimen is lengthened with an iliac vein graft from the donor [*see Figure 11*]. The donor celiac axis, proximal hepatic artery, and superior mesenteric artery stay with the pancreas. The hepatic artery retained with the liver is lengthened with a free iliac artery graft. Obviously, many variations of this technique are possible with the use of free iliac artery and vein grafts.

The arteries and veins of a multiple-organ donor can be put to many other uses. After all the organs have been removed and packaged, segments of the remaining iliac arteries and veins are routinely removed [*see Figure 12*] and placed in a cold tissue culture solution for refrigeration. The thoracic aorta and pulmonary artery may also be harvested under special circumstances. Vascular grafts can be lifesaving in the event of unexpected technical problems in hepatic recipients, approximately 25 percent of whom require portal vein or hepatic arterial homografts. Vascular grafts are also often employed for reconstruction of renal vessels or for other purposes, including potential pancreas vessel reconstruction.

Figure 11   The addition of an iliac artery graft to the hepatic artery and an iliac vein graft to the portal vein of the pancreas graft allows the use of both organs from a single donor.

Figure 12   After organs have been removed and packaged, segments of iliac arteries, veins, and thoracic aorta are routinely removed, as illustrated here.

Discussion

Principles and Limitations of Current Methods of Organ Preservation

Despite its importance and despite recent advances, organ preservation remains the least developed component of transplantation technology. Preservation techniques begin with the intraoperative infusion of cold fluids; the paramount objective is to avoid warm ischemia. Cooling of organs by intravascular infusions of chilled lactated Ringer's solution at the time of circulatory arrest was first introduced into the laboratory for experimental liver transplantation more than a quarter of a century ago. The procedure was promptly applied clinically to the preservation of kidneys and other organs. Such cooling lengthens the duration of organ viability and allows subsequent application of more sophisticated preservation measures.

Lactated Ringer's solution is low in potassium and nearly isotonic. In 1969, researchers documented that chilled solutions with an electrolyte composition similar to that in cells, such as Collin's solution, extended the permissible time limit of cold renal ischemia beyond that achievable with isotonic solutions.[19] The same effect was demonstrated in livers.[20] Cardiac surgeons

have cooled the heart with various cardioplegic solutions having potassium concentrations of 20 mEq/L or greater.

From 1969 to 1987, these high-potassium preservation solutions were the only means available for inexpensive cold-storage preservation of transplanted organs. In 1987, the University of Wisconsin solution was introduced.[17] This solution immediately extended safe preservation times for the liver and pancreas and provided improved function as well. The allowable cold ischemia time for the liver increased from eight to 18 hours or longer, and pancreas preservation was increased to 20 hours with excellent postoperative function. UW solution is a complex multiconstituent solution, the components of which address a number of theoretical issues in organ preservation. Although the exact function of each constituent in the solution is unknown, it is felt that the parenchymal cells of the liver, pancreas, and kidney are impermeable to the large anion in the solution, lactobionic acid, and that this prevents the cellular swelling that can complicate all forms of hypothermic preservation. UW solution receives its oncotic support from the complex starch hydroxyethyl starch rather than from dextrose or the other complex sugars used in the older solutions. Finally, there are a variety of components, including glutathione, raffinose, and allopurinol, that act as free radical scavengers and help prevent reperfusion injury.[21] UW solution is now internationally accepted as a universal flush and preservation solution, although preference for it over isotonic saline as a flush solution is controversial. Its application to cardiac preservation has been studied extensively in the laboratory, and it has become a popular substitute for potassium-based cardioplegic solutions in cardiac preservation. One of the most profound impacts of UW solution has been felt by liver transplant surgeons, who can temporally separate the complex donor and recipient operations and perform them in an unrushed, meticulous fashion without jeopardizing organ function.

Highly sophisticated and costly techniques for continuous perfusion of these organs exist, but they have been widely used only for kidney grafts. The continuous perfusion technique for kidneys as originally described used an asanguineous and oncotically controlled fluid.[22] The method has proved to be a good one but has not markedly improved the quality of renal preservation in the first 48 hours over that provided by the simpler infusion-and-slush method. In the future, better continuous perfusion techniques may extend preservation time for all organs.

Even with UW solution, it is still essential to appreciate how unpredictable the outcome of a transplantation can be with any of the currently available preservation techniques. The unknown extent to which the donor has suffered organ ischemia caused by the processes of injury and dying contributes to this unpredictability. All experienced transplant surgeons have been dismayed to observe that homografts retrieved from seemingly ideal donors occasionally do not function, whereas organs obtained under seemingly adverse conditions may function perfectly. One study has documented this phenomenon particularly well for liver transplants[23]; no correlation could be found between liver recipient outcome and the use of ideal versus less than ideal donors. What is urgently needed is a simple, discriminating predictive technique for assessing organ viability before the ruthless biologic test of actual transplantation is performed.

Medical, Ethical, and Legal Considerations

THE RETRIEVAL TEAM

Because the stakes are so high in terms of recipient survival, the technical elements of the organ procurement operation must be constantly reassessed. Much attention is now given to the specific training of the donor, or retrieval, surgeon. When kidneys were the only organs transplanted, transplant centers often assigned organ retrieval to local surgeons whose experience was limited to only the occasional case. Frequently, the penalty for this practice was a prolonged period of acute tubular necrosis in the transplanted kidney, with the attendant risks and mortality. The enormously increased sophistication of today's multiple-procurement procedures make this approach undesirable and probably indefensible from the medicolegal standpoint. In addition, it is important to emphasize that surgeons should not delegate to nonphysicians the actual task of excising organs for transplantation from cadaver donors. Today, most transplant centers tend to delegate organ procurement operations to highly trained surgeons with a specific interest and training in transplantation surgery and organ preservation. Only in this way has

it been possible for teams from different institutions to retrieve organs from common donors and to work harmoniously and effectively together. This development reflects the maturation of the field of transplantation.

THE ROLES OF GOVERNMENT AND THE PRIVATE SECTOR

Organ harvesting was once an uncommon, hurried, poorly standardized surgical exercise in which kidneys (or, rarely, other organs) were rapidly excised from a donor whose heart had just stopped beating.[1] The establishment of irreversible neurologic injury, or brain death, as actual death[24] has made it possible for surgeons to procure organs from heart-beating cadavers in a well-organized manner. Legislation sanctioning the concept of brain death has been passed in 44 states, and judicial precedent exists in the other six.[25]

Despite these developments, skepticism, fear, and anxiety regarding the concept of brain death persist.[26] Brain death must be clearly and fully explained to the relatives of a potential donor to allay the common fear that lifesaving measures may be prematurely terminated to gain rapid access to organs for transplantation. This is never the case. The physician in charge of the initial care of the donor is responsible for determining and making the pronouncement of brain death, with the collaboration of experts in the neurosciences. He or she in no way participates in the donation and harvesting procedures. Conversely, the transplant surgeons cannot participate in the determination of death.

The Uniform Anatomical Gifts Act (UAGA), passed by Congress in 1973, has been adopted in some form in all 50 states.[27] This act states that organ donation is a voluntary gift made by either the donor or the family. The UAGA does not include the concept of presumed consent, whereby organs may be removed automatically unless the next of kin objects. Presumed consent has been practiced in many European countries with some success, and strong ethical arguments have been advanced in its favor.[28] The concept of presumed consent has not gained a foothold in transplantation in the United States.

Despite passage of brain-death legislation and of the UAGA, there is still an acute shortage of cadaveric renal and extrarenal organs, which has been aggravated by the burgeoning success of transplantation. Several factors contribute to this shortage. Some physicians do not wish to face the failure implicit in the death of their patients, do not want to burden a grieving family further by requesting donation, are aware of certain religious taboos about organ donation, or have an unrealistic fear of legal recriminations.

The Surgeon General of the United States has made several recommendations for solving these problems, including systematic public education and education of physicians, nurses, and paramedical personnel; recruiting support from the religious community; and sharper delineation of the exact conditions to be met for a pronouncement of brain death.[29] Another strategy for increasing organ donation has been to encourage the signing of donor cards and other forms of living wills.[30]

The organ shortage has prompted a new kind of legislative initiative called required request. Required-request laws have been passed in almost half the states. These laws mandate that each hospital systematically approach the families of all patients who die under circumstances that might make solid-organ donation possible. With such laws, physicians and hospital staff are protected from charges of callousness for asking a grieving family for donation, they are relieved of the fear of legal recrimination, and they can work within an organized administrative channel. Unfortunately, these required-request laws have not been consistently honored and therefore have not helped increase the supply of organs. New initiatives aimed at encouraging voluntary reporting of all deaths by the hospital to the local organ procurement organization, so as not to miss any potential donors, have been tried in pilot programs in a few regions, with promising results.

In 1984, Congress enacted legislation authorizing a task force to study issues in organ procurement and distribution and provided for the creation and funding of an Organ Procurement and Transplant Network (OPTN). In 1986, the federal government awarded the OPTN contract to the United Network for Organ Sharing. Under the terms of the contract, UNOS operates a computer-matching system designed to aid in systematic placement of renal and extrarenal organs and to ensure equitable allocation of organs throughout the country. In addition, UNOS is to keep careful data on all harvested organs to analyze and define patterns of organ procurement in the United States so that resources for future development can be better allocated. In the distribution of extrarenal organs, UNOS acts in an advisory capacity to the organ procurement agency managing a specific donor by supplying a prioritized list of acceptable recipients.

In the first version of this chapter, published in early 1989, we speculated about how this system would change, as more surgeons were trained in extrarenal organ procurement, as regional centers proliferated, as involvement of personnel at the new centers increased, and as additional demands for equitable allocation of organs were made on the distribution network. We predicted that as more powerful immunosuppression and preservation techniques were developed and tissue typing and matching became better understood, smaller organ procurement regions in the country would coalesce into larger, more centralized territories to increase the pool of potential local recipients, improve equity, and ultimately improve transplantation outcomes.

Unfortunately, the system has not evolved as far as we hoped it would have by now. The urgency imposed by current organ preservation techniques is made more pressing by continued reliance on complex tissue typing for renal allocation; these factors place a real strain on any kidney distribution and sharing system covering a large region. Although the restrictive limits of preservation and the logistics of allocation are not as burdensome for the extrarenal organs, influential segments of the transplantation community have resisted any movement to larger regional or national sharing, continuing to rely on the standard renal distribution algorithms despite the clear advantages of larger distribution regions (especially with regard to fairness and justice for patients).

For better or for worse, transplantation of all organs has achieved the level of mass clinical application, even though the field of transplantation has yet to gain full recognition as an established science. Consequently, federal and state governments continue to have a strong interest in regulating transplantation medicine. We agree that the government should collaborate with the transplantation community in developing new health policies; however, we believe that overregulation could stifle the progress of transplantation. The emphasis should be on constructive collaboration, not on domination, but this balance has proved difficult to achieve. Political machinations such as the opposition expressed by the transplantation community to realistic proposals for a true national retrieval and sharing system can have extremely negative repercussions for transplantation medicine and can provoke a demand for greater governmental intervention so as to ensure equity and fairness. The result may be efforts on the part of government to regulate the criteria for patient treatment. Political guidelines must not be allowed a role in judging a candidate's suitability for transplantation. Physicians cannot ethically accept any but strict medical criteria in selecting organ recipients.[31,32]

Since the early 1960s, knowledge in the field of transplantation medicine has grown almost exponentially. The tremendous potential of this field continues to depend on broad research aimed at solving a wide variety of problems in the laboratory and at the bedside as well as on resolution of the issues and controversies that transplantation has generated for the public and the medical community.

References

1. A definition of irreversible coma. Report of the Ad Hoc Committee of the Harvard Medical School to examine the definition of brain death. JAMA 205:337, 1968

2. Silverman D, Saunders MG, Schwab RS, et al: Cerebral death and the electroencephalogram. Report of the Ad Hoc Committee of the American EEG Society on EEG Criteria for Determination of Cerebral Death. JAMA 209:1505, 1968

3. Goodman JM, Heck LL: Confirmation of brain death at bedside by isotope angiography. JAMA 238:966, 1977

4. Ivan LP: Spinal reflexes in cerebral death. Neurology 23:650, 1973

5. Ropper AH: Unusual spontaneous movements in brain-dead patients. Neurology 34:1089, 1984

6. Goldsmith J, Montefusco CM: Nursing care of the potential organ donor. Critical Care Nurse 5:22, 1985

7. Tzakis AG, Cooper MH, Dummer SJ, et al: Transplantation in HIV+ patients. Transplantation 49:354, 1990

8. Emre S, Schwartz ME, Altaca G, et al: Safe use of hepatic allografts from donors older than 70 years. Transplantation 62:62, 1996

9. Teperman L, Podesta L, Mieles L, et al: The successful use of older donors for liver transplantation. JAMA 262:2837, 1989

10. Otte JB, de Ville de Goyet J, Sokal E, et al: Size reduction of the donor liver is a safe way to alleviate the shortage of size-matched organs in pediatric liver transplantation. Ann Surg 211:146, 1990

11. de Hemptinne B, Salizzoni M, Tan KC, et al: The technique of liver size reduction in orthotopic liver transplantation. Transplant Proc 20(suppl 1):508, 1988

12. Broelsch CE, Emond JC, Thistlethwaite JR, et al: Liver transplantation including the concept of reduced size liver transplants in children. Ann Surg 208:410, 1988

13. Montefusco CM, Mollenkopf FP, Kamholz SL, et al: Maintenance protocol for potential organ donors in multiple organ procurement. Hospital Physician 20:9, 1984

14. Miller CM, Teodorescu V, Harrington M, et al: Regional procurement and export of hepatic allografts for transplantation. Mt Sinai J Med 57:93, 1990

15. Starzl TE, Hakala TB, Shaw BW, et al: A flexible procedure for multiple cadaveric organ procurement. Surg Gynecol Obstet 158:223, 1984

16. Starzl TE, Miller C, Broznick B, et al: An improved technique for multiple organ harvesting. Surg Gynecol Obstet 165:343, 1987

17. Kalayoglu M, Sollinger HW, Stratta RJ, et al: Extended preservation of the liver for clinical transplantation. Lancet 1:617, 1988

18. Sollinger HW, Vernon WB, D'Alessandro AM, et al: Combined liver and pancreas procurement with Belzer-UW solution. Surgery 106:685, 1989

19. Collins GM, Bravo-Shugarman M, Terasaki PI: Kidney preservation for transportation. Lancet 2:1219, 1969

20. Benichou J, Halgrimson CG, Weil R III, et al: Canine and human liver preservation for 6–18 hours by cold infusion. Transplantation 24:407, 1977

21. Belzer FO, Southard JH: Principles of solid-organ preservation by cold storage. Transplantation 45:673, 1988

22. Belzer FO, Ashby BS, Dunphy JE: 24-hour and 72-hour preservation of canine kidneys. Lancet 2:536, 1967

23. Makowka L, Gordon RD, Todo S, et al: Analysis of donor criteria for the prediction of outcome in clinical liver transplantation. Trans Proc 19:2378, 1987

24. Guidelines for the Determination of Death: Report of the Medical Consultants on the Diagnosis of Death to the President's Commission for the Study of Ethical Problems in Medicine and Biomedical and Behavioral Research. JAMA 246:2194, 1981

25. Gunby P: Panel ponders organ procurement problem. JAMA 250:455, 1983

26. Lee PP, Kissner P: Organ donation and the uniform anatomical gift act. Surgery 100:867, 1986

27. Sadler AM, Sadler BL, Stason EB, et al: Transplantation—a case for consent. N Engl J Med 280:862, 1969

28. Caplan AL: Sounding board—ethical and policy issues in the procurement of cadaver organs for transplantation. N Engl J Med 311:981, 1984

29. Koop CE: Increasing the supply of solid organs for transplantation. Public Health Rep 98:566, 1983

30. Overcast TD, Evans RW, Bowen LA, et al: Problems in the identification of potential organ donors. JAMA 251:1559, 1984

31. Starzl TE, Hakala T, Tzakis A, et al: A multifactorial system for equitable selection of cadaveric kidney recipients. JAMA 257:3073, 1987

32. Starzl TE, Gordon RD, Tzakis A, et al: Equitable allocation of extrarenal organs: with special reference to the liver. Transplant Proc 20:131, 1988

Acknowledgment

Figures 1 through 12   Carol Donner.

David A. Hidalgo, M.D., and Joseph J. Disa, M.D.

Approach to Surgical Reconstruction

Acute Reconstruction

EVALUATION AND INITIAL TREATMENT OF THE OPEN WOUND

Problem wounds are characterized by one of the following: large size that precludes direct primary closure, gross infection or uncertain bacteriologic status, or threatened loss of critical structures exposed as a result of insufficient soft tissue coverage. Surgically created wounds, which generally pose less of a problem from a bacteriologic standpoint than traumatic wounds, are best managed by an immediate coverage procedure when direct closure is impossible.

Traumatic wounds are more difficult to evaluate than surgical wounds for several reasons. First, in traumatic wounds, the potential for infection is high because of the environment in which the wound is created, the mechanism of injury, and the time that elapses before operative intervention. Second, the mechanism of injury (e.g., crush, avulsion, or gunshot) may extend the zone of injury beyond what is immediately apparent [see Figure 1]. Serious postoperative infection may develop in these cases if definitive wound coverage is provided in the absence of adequate debridement. Third, the long-term functional prospects for the injured part are a key determinant in selecting the method of acute treatment. However, accurate assessment of the chances for recovery of specific structures within the wound is often difficult immediately after injury.

The initial step in the management of problem wounds is to decide whether the wound is suitable for immediate soft tissue coverage. Wounds that are surgically created during the course of an elective procedure are almost always best treated with primary definitive coverage. Traumatic wounds that present within an hour or two of injury and have a minimal crush component are also best treated with a primary definitive coverage procedure after thorough operative debridement.

Injuries with a significant crush component and exposure of critical structures such as nerves, vessels, tendons, or bone are best treated more aggressively. In these cases, thorough debridement requires considerable surgical experience because the tendency is to debride inadequately. The degree of accuracy to which tissue viability can be assessed varies among different types of tissue. For example, skin can be evaluated by its color, the nature of its capillary refill, the quality of its dermal bleeding, or its bleeding response to pinprick. After intravenous fluorescein injection, skin viability can also be assessed qualitatively, by using a Wood's light, or quantitatively, by using a dermofluorometer. Muscle is the most difficult tissue to evaluate. Color, capillary bleeding, and contractile response to stimulation are not always reliable indicators of muscle viability. In severe injuries, they can be misleading. Inadequate debridement may lead to severe consequences resulting from infection. Therefore, serial debridement at 24-hour intervals is essential for accurately establishing the limits of muscle injury. Efforts should be made during debridement to preserve tissues such as major nerves and blood vessels unless they are severely contused. These structures are vital for function and are of small mass compared with other tissues (e.g., skin, fat, and muscle) at risk for necrosis and subsequent infection.

Wound debridement, therefore, should involve careful analysis of the injury from an anatomic point of view; debridement should not consist of indiscriminate excision of blocks of tissue. Between debridement procedures, the wound should be treated with sterile dressings but in an open manner (i.e., without closure by sutures and with wet-to-dry dressings changed three or four times a day). A definitive soft tissue coverage procedure should then be performed as soon after the initial injury as wound conditions permit. When thorough debridement and definitive coverage can be completed within less than a week, the wound will generally heal uneventfully. Inadequate debridement frequently results in the loss of any additional tissue invested to achieve acute soft tissue coverage. The wound becomes grossly infected, and important functional structures within the wound are reexposed.

Infected surgical wounds, neglected wounds, or other complex wounds in which initial wound management fails should be debrided and then treated by open methods. Proper care of these wounds is achieved by a multifaceted approach aimed at converting established gross infection to a much lower level of bacterial contamination, which is then compatible with successful secondary wound closure.

Debridement

Devitalized tissue provides an ideal culture medium for bacteria and isolates them from host defense mechanisms. Surgical debridement must be performed as often as necessary to remove all necrotic tissue.

High-Pressure Irrigation

A useful adjunct to debridement is high-pressure irrigation, which has been shown experimentally to decrease wound infection rates significantly.[1,2] The necessary pressure of 8 psi can be

a
b
c

Figure 1 (*a*) **A so-called bumper injury of the leg is shown after initial debridement and bony stabilization (two days after injury). After the second debridement (*b*), the true extent of devitalization of bone and soft tissue is apparent (four days after injury). (*c*) A latissimus dorsi free flap has been used to reconstruct the soft tissue defect (five days after injury).**

achieved by forceful irrigation through a 35 ml syringe fitted with a 19-gauge needle. Low-pressure irrigation with a bulb-type syringe, for example, has not proved to be beneficial.

Bacterial Counts

The degree of bacterial wound contamination can be accurately quantified. The standard technique of quantitative bacteriology requires several days to complete. In addition to a count, it provides identification and antibiotic sensitivities of the organism. Quantitative bacteriology can also be performed using the rapid slide technique, which provides valuable information about the wound within 20 minutes.[3,4]

The level of bacterial contamination has been shown to be a significant predictor of outcome in wound closure by either skin-graft or flap-coverage techniques. According to the golden-period principle of wound closure, a minimum time interval is necessary for bacteria to proliferate to a certain threshold level. Studies show that contaminated wounds take a mean time of about 5 hours to reach a level of 10^5 bacteria per gram of tissue. Attempts to close wounds that have counts higher than 10^5/g of tissue will fail 75% to 100% of the time, whereas wounds with lower counts are successfully closed more than 90% of the time.[5] β-Hemolytic streptococci are an exception in that much lower concentrations of these organisms consistently result in failure of wound closure. When a β-hemolytic streptococcus is the dominant isolate, the wound should generally be treated openly until cultures become negative.

Systemic Antibiotics

The role of systemic antibiotics in wound management is not clearly defined. Broad-spectrum antibiotics should be given in cases of severe trauma or established, uncontrolled infection. They may also be useful for minor wounds that cannot be closed within 3 hours of injury.

Topical Antibiotics

Certain antibiotics provide broad-spectrum activity when applied topically. Neomycin used at a concentration of 10 mg/ml or a combination of bacitracin, 50 U/ml, and polymyxin B, 0.05 mg/ml, will kill most common wound pathogens. These solutions can be used when wet dressings are indicated.

Topical Antiseptics

A variety of topical antiseptics have been used empirically in wound care. Critical examinations have revealed, however, that these solutions are detrimental to wound healing when used in the concentrations usually recommended. Povidone-iodine (1%), hydrogen peroxide (3%), acetic acid (0.25%), and sodium hypochlorite (0.5%) all have been shown to be lethal to fibroblasts as well as bacteria. More dilute concentrations of povidone-iodine (0.001%) and sodium hypochlorite (0.005%) have been shown to be effective against bacteria while being safe for fibroblasts.[6] A number of these agents also inhibit normal white blood cell function in the wound.

Wet Dressings

Open wounds are treated with wet dressings, generally consisting of gauze soaked in saline or an acceptable topical antiseptic. Wet-to-wet dressings prevent desiccation of exposed vital structures or freshly placed skin grafts. Wet-to-dry dressings are useful for assisting in daily wound debridement. These dressings are allowed to dry on the wound; when they are removed, adherent fibrinous debris is removed with the dressing. Wet dressings of either type should be changed at least three times a day.

Small wounds can be expected to close by contraction and secondary epithelialization after appropriate open management with the techniques described. Large wounds will improve with aggressive open care but will then stabilize into a chronic state of wound colonization of varying degrees. A soft tissue coverage procedure is then necessary to complete closure in these cases.

SELECTION OF THE COVERAGE PROCEDURE

The goals of coverage procedures in the management of acute as well as chronic wounds are to achieve a healed wound and to avoid infection. The treatment of functional problems is generally deferred for secondary reconstruction. The method of coverage depends on whether vital structures, such as vessels, tendons, nerves, and bone, are exposed in the wound. If no vital structures are exposed, skin-graft coverage is indicated. Skin grafts can also be used over tendon if the paratenon is intact, over nerve if the epineurium is intact, and over bone if the periosteum is intact. Skin grafts are the most expendable type of soft tissue available for the coverage of open wounds. They allow the wound to heal completely and set the stage for secondary reconstruction, during which more valuable tissue can be used to achieve other goals at minimal risk.

When vital structures are exposed in the wound, a flap is preferred because it provides more substantial soft tissue coverage of

Acute reconstruction is indicated

Evaluate and treat open wound.

Select coverage procedure to achieve healed wound and avoid infection.

Defer treatment of functional problems for secondary reconstruction.

Wound does not contain exposed bone, cartilage, nerve, or tendon but cannot be closed directly

Apply a skin graft.

Wound is small defect but is in an area where graft contracture is not desirable (e.g., face, hand, or flexion crease)

Apply full-thickness skin graft; donor sites include the ear, upper eyelid, neck, and groin.

Wound has a large surface area or is a small wound in a noncritical area

Apply split-thickness skin graft.

Wound is known to be significantly contaminated

Apply meshed split-thickness skin graft or consider delayed skin graft replacement and open treatment of wound until bacteriologic status is clear.

Secondary reconstruction of chronic defect is indicated

Defect is a small localized scar or a focal scar contracture

Revise with Z-plasty or other local tissue rearrangement procedure.

There is a shortage of skin and subcutaneous tissue only, but skin graft coverage is not desirable

Use tissue expanders (except on hand or foot).

One or more of the following conditions is present:
- Composite defect
- Functional defect of muscle or bone
- Contour deformity
- Unstable soft tissue coverage of vital structure
- Inadequate soft tissue coverage for bone or nerve grafting

Repair with free or local flap.

Approach to Surgical Reconstruction

Bone, cartilage, nerve, or tendon is exposed and cannot be covered by direct wound closure

Perform flap coverage procedure.

Local donor site meets needs and is not involved in the primary process

Use local flap.

- *Small or clean wound:* use local skin flap if possible.
- *Large or contaminated wound:* use regional myocutaneous flap.

Local flap is not possible or would not provide appropriate tissue

Use free flap.

- If wound is clean and thin flap is desired, apply skin or fascial free flap.
- If wound is large or contaminated, apply muscle or myocutaneous free flap.

Muscle flaps require coverage with a meshed split-thickness skin graft.

Head or neck defect

- *Small facial defect with no facial features involved:* use Z-plasty, Limberg flap, or other advancement flap of cheek or forehead.
- *Large defect of neck or lower head:* use regional myocutaneous flap of trapezius, latissimus dorsi, or pectoralis major muscle.

Chest or back defect

In most cases, use regional myocutaneous flap (e.g., pectoralis major, rectus abdominis, latissimus dorsi, or trapezius muscle).

Arm defect

Cover large wounds above the elbow with latissimus dorsi muscle transposed as a pedicled flap.

Hand defect

Free flaps are preferred, but pedicled distant skin flaps from the chest or abdomen are also acceptable. Defects of the digits can be covered with cross-finger flaps or, for tip injuries, with thenar flaps.

Abdominal defect

Use regional flap (e.g., tensor fasciae latae, rectus femoris, or rectus abdominis muscle).

Gluteal or perineal defect

Use regional myocutaneous flap (e.g., gluteus maximus, gracilis, tensor fasciae latae, or biceps femoris).

Thigh, knee, or leg defect

- *Thigh defect:* use regional muscle flap (e.g., tensor fasciae latae, rectus femoris, vastus lateralis, or vastus medialis muscle).
- *Defect of knee or proximal leg:* use gastrocnemius muscle flap.
- *Proximal or midleg defect:* use soleus muscle flap.

Foot defect

- *Plantar:* close defect of weight-bearing heel or midsole with medially based skin rotation flap raised superficial to plantar fascia or with other myocutaneous or fasciocutaneous plantar flap. Cover limited defect of distal plantar surface with toe flap.
- *Posterior heel, Achilles tendon, malleoli:* use either extensor digitorum brevis muscle as pedicled flap or lateral calcaneal artery flap.

Head or neck defect

- *Large defect of scalp or upper face:* cover with latissimus dorsi, scapular, or rectus abdominis free flap.
- *Floor of the mouth:* replace with forearm free flap.
- *Mandible:* reconstruct with various composite free flaps of bone and skin.
- *Oropharynx or cervical esophagus:* use jejunum free flap or forearm flap.

Forearm defect

Cover large forearm wound with free flap of rectus abdominis, scapular, or latissimus dorsi muscle.

Hand defect

- *Exposed tendons on the dorsum:* cover with temporalis fascia free flap.
- *Defect of the web space:* correct with lateral arm free flap.

Knee or leg defect

- *Major wound of the popliteal fossa:* use free flap if the blood supply to the gastrocnemius muscle is compromised.
- *Defect of the lower third of the leg:* use latissimus dorsi, rectus abdominis, scapular, or gracilis free flap.

Foot defect

- *Plantar:* repair very large defect with muscle free flap covered with a skin graft.
- *Dorsum:* use fascial free flap and overlying skin graft, or use thin skin free flap.

the structure. The choice of flap depends on the location of the wound and on its overall size, depth, and topographic configuration (see below).

Skin Grafts

Skin grafts may be either partial thickness (i.e., split thickness) or full thickness. Split-thickness grafts are preferred for wounds with a large surface area. Full-thickness grafts are suitable only for small defects because their donor sites must be closed primarily; the most common donor sites for full-thickness grafts are the ears, upper eyelids, neck, and groin. Full-thickness grafts contract less with time than split-thickness grafts and are therefore particularly suitable for wounds of the hands, extremity flexion creases, nose, eyelids, and other areas of the face.

Successful healing of skin grafts requires immobilization of the recipient site to prevent shearing in the plane between the graft and the wound bed [*see Postoperative Care, below*]. However, although complete immobilization is desirable, the required dressings may preclude observation of a wound that is known to be significantly contaminated. In such cases, a meshed split-thickness graft is indicated, and the wound should be treated in an open fashion. A meshed graft can be placed directly over the muscle of a flap and secured over its irregular contour with staples [*see Figure 2*]. Because the graft is meshed, serum can escape between the interstices and there is little risk of separation from the underlying tissue. A meshed graft is also less vulnerable to disruption by shear forces. An additional advantage of a meshed graft is that it permits the wound to be treated with wet dressings if there is still risk for infection. A mesh expansion ratio of 1.5 : 1.0 is generally preferred, except when the surface area of the wound is very large and the availability of donor sites is limited.

Flap-Coverage Procedures

Flaps consist of tissues that have a self-contained vascular system. They permit a more substantial transfer of tissue bulk than do skin grafts and may consist of either skin and subcutaneous tissue, fascia, muscle, bone, or a combination of several of these tissue types. Local flaps consist of tissue that is mostly detached from surrounding tissue but retains enough connection to preserve an adequate blood supply to the entire flap. Local flaps are either transposed, rotated, or advanced into adjacent defects for purposes of reconstruction. Free flaps are totally detached and have their blood supply reconnected at the recipient site by surgically performed microvascular anastomoses between recipient-site blood vessels and the major vessels that supply the flap.

Local Flaps versus Free Flaps

The choice between a local flap and a free flap is determined by the amount and the type of tissue needed, as well as by the availability of flaps in the immediate area of the wound [*see Figure 3*]. Availability of local flaps, in turn, is determined by the nature of the regional blood supply. The vascular anatomy of a particular area determines the availability of arterialized skin flaps, fasciocutaneous flaps, myocutaneous flaps, and other forms of composite

Figure 2 **A meshed (1.5 : 1.0 ratio) skin graft has been secured to the irregular contour of a muscle free flap with staples. No additional immobilization of the graft is needed. The interstices of the graft allow free drainage of serous exudate from the muscle.**

flaps. Local flaps can be grouped regionally by the types of tissue that they provide [*see Table 1*].

A local flap is generally preferred over a free flap if the two provide similar tissue, primarily because of the additional effort required to move a free flap. A free-flap procedure commonly takes twice as long as a local-flap procedure. The preference for local flaps does not result from fear of performing microvascular anastomoses—experienced surgeons accomplish free tissue transfer with success rates higher than 95%.

Free flaps are indicated in areas where local flaps are unavailable, such as in the distal third of the leg, or when an extremely large flap is needed but is unavailable locally. When regional donor sites are affected by the primary process, free tissue transfer

LOCAL FLAPS   MYOCUTANEOUS FLAPS   FREE FLAPS

Figure 3 **Regional alternatives in flap selection are illustrated. Defects in the central portion of the body are treated with myocutaneous flaps primarily; defects of the peripheral areas are treated with either local flaps or free flaps. In some areas, several options exist, and the choice is influenced by the size of the defect and the specific tissue requirements.**

Table 1 Selection of Local Flaps by Region and Tissue Type

Site	Skin Flaps	Muscle and Myocutaneous Flaps	Fascial and Fasciocutaneous Flaps
Head and neck	Scalp; forehead; nasolabial; cervico-facial; Mustardé; eyelid; lip	Trapezius; latissimus dorsi; pectoralis major	Superficial and deep temporal fascia
Chest and back	Lateral thoracic; deltopectoral	Trapezius; pectoralis major; latissimus dorsi; rectus abdominis (superiorly based)	Scapular
Arm	Medial arm (Tagliacozzi)	Latissimus dorsi; pectoralis major	Lateral arm; forearm
Hand	Cross-finger; thenar; neurovascular island; fingertip advancement	—	Forearm
Abdomen and perineum	Groin	Rectus abdominis (inferiorly based); tensor fasciae latae; rectus femoris; gracilis	Medial thigh
Gluteal area	Sacral; thoracolumbar	Gluteus maximus; gracilis; tensor fasciae latae; biceps femoris	Gluteal thigh
Thigh	—	Tensor fasciae latae; rectus femoris; vastus lateralis; vastus medialis; gracilis; biceps femoris; rectus abdominis	Anterior thigh; anteromedial thigh; posterior thigh
Knee and proximal leg	—	Gastrocnemius	Saphenous artery; posterior calf
Midleg	—	Soleus; tibialis anterior	Anterior leg; lateral leg; posterior leg
Distal leg	—	—	—
Foot	Dorsalis pedis; plantar rotation; lateral calcaneal artery; plantar V-Y	Flexor digitorum brevis; abductor hallucis; abductor digiti minimi; extensor digitorum brevis	—

allows healthy, well-vascularized tissue to be brought into the compromised area. Moreover, if free tissue is transferred, the size of the wound is not extended, because the donor site is not contiguous but instead is located at a distance from the wound.

If expertise in microvascular surgery is available, free flaps are frequently a first-line choice. Free flaps allow selection of the appropriate type of tissue in the most suitable size and configuration for the specific reconstructive problem. Compared with free flaps, local flaps are inefficient ways of moving tissue because only a small portion of a local flap actually reaches the defect itself. The choice of donor site is greater with free flaps because the limitations imposed by local availability are avoided.

Free flaps used in acute reconstruction can be grouped into three major types [see Table 2]. The soft tissue coverage requirements of most wounds can be met by so-called workhorse free flaps. These flaps typically have the advantages of large size, ease of dissection, and a vascular pedicle that is long and of large diameter. The disadvantages, such as awkward patient positioning for flap harvest, are minor. Most workhorse flaps consist of muscle with an optional skin component; they are the flaps of choice for contaminated wounds [see Figure 4]. A second group of free flaps is useful for acute reconstruction of unusually large wounds. These flaps con-

Table 2 Free Flap Selection for Soft Tissue Coverage*

Requirement	Specific Flap	Advantages	Disadvantages
Reliable workhorse flaps	Latissimus dorsi	Ideal pedicle[†]; ease of dissection	Awkward patient positioning
	Rectus abdominis	Ideal pedicle; supine position; ease of dissection	No major disadvantages
	Scapular	Ideal pedicle; skin flap only	Awkward patient positioning
Flaps of very large surface area	Combined latissimus dorsi and scapular	Independent component inset[‡]; primary donor-site closure possible; ideal pedicle	Awkward patient positioning
	Extended tensor fasciae latae and partial quadriceps	Supine position; large skin flap component	Donor-site healing[§]; pedicle configuration[∥]
Small flaps	Gracilis	Small muscle	Small vessels
	Lateral arm	Thin, sensate; convenient for hand trauma	Small vessels; donor-site scar
	Forearm	Thin skin flap; ideal pedicle	Minor hand morbidity; poor donor-site appearance
	Temporalis fascia	Thinnest flap; ideal coverage for exposed tendons[¶]; can transfer hair-bearing scalp	Variable donor-site scar alopecia

*Includes only the more commonly used free flaps for purposes of comparison.
[†]Characterized by large-diameter vessels and long pedicle length.
[‡]Each part can be arranged and sewn into the wound separately.
[§]Donor-site closure requires a skin graft, which may result in delayed healing.
[∥]Pedicle enters middle of undersurface of flap.
[¶]Permits tendon gliding underneath if used on dorsum of the hand or of the foot.

Figure 4 (*a*) A facial tumor has recurred following previous orbital exenteration. (*b*) The defect has been resected. Local flaps and regional myocutaneous flaps are not available for this defect. (*c*) The design for a rectus abdominis myocutaneous free flap is shown. This flap can be designed in other sizes and configurations depending on specific needs. The vascular pedicle is long and of large diameter, and the flap is easily accessible in the supine patient. (*d*) Soft tissue coverage with a reasonable restoration of facial contour has been achieved.

sist of combined vascular territories supplied by a single vascular pedicle. A third category consists of smaller free flaps that provide tissue that is superior in either amount or type to the local flaps that are otherwise available. An additional advantage of these flaps is that they tend not to be bulky. They are frequently used in areas such as the head, hands, distal third of the leg, and feet [*see Figure 5*].

Regional Alternatives in Flap Selection

Head, neck Facial defects of small to moderate size are best treated with local skin flaps. A variety of flaps are available for reconstruction of limited defects

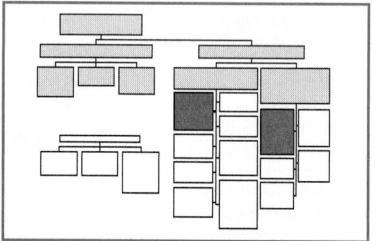

of the eyelids, cheeks, nose, and mouth.[7-9] Small facial defects that do not directly involve the facial features can often be closed with several types of flaps that rearrange the existing tissue in the area—for example, Z-plasty [*see Secondary Reconstruction, Small Localized Scar, below*] or a Limberg flap. Tissues that are difficult to match, such as those of the eyelids or lips, can often be reconstructed with flaps that borrow tissue from their opposite, intact counterparts; the Abbe lip flap is such a flap [*see Figure 6*].

For coverage of some large defects in the head and neck region, the trapezius, latissimus dorsi, and pectoralis major muscles can be used. Each muscle can be raised with an optional skin island. These flaps are generally too bulky to be used on the face, and their reach is limited when used as pedicled flaps: none of them can cover major portions of the scalp or comfortably reach the upper face.

Latissimus dorsi, scapular, and rectus abdominis free flaps are useful for very large defects of the scalp or upper face. Smaller defects of the scalp are best treated with local scalp flaps.

Other free flaps of a specialized nature are superior for reconstruction of the floor of the mouth and mandible, even though local myocutaneous flaps will reach this area. For example, the forearm free flap based on the radial artery is quite thin and pliable and therefore provides an ideal replacement for the floor of the mouth. Composite free flaps that contain both bone and skin, such as those taken from the scapula, ilium, radius, and fibula, provide tissue of the appropriate type and proper configuration for defects of the lower face in which the mandible must be reconstructed along with the intraoral lining, the external skin, or both.

Chest, back Most defects of the chest and back are amenable to treatment with local myocutaneous flaps because of the wide arc of rotation of muscles located in these areas.[10] Midline sternal wounds can be cov-

ered with either pectoralis major or rectus abdominis muscle flaps; lateral chest defects with latissimus dorsi or pectoralis major muscle flaps; and midline back defects with latissimus dorsi or trapezius muscle flaps. Both the pectoralis and latissimus muscles can be divided from their primary vascular supply while retaining their intercostal supply and folded over as local flaps to cover midline defects anteriorly and posteriorly, respectively.

Arm, forearm Large wounds above the elbow can be covered with a latissimus dorsi myocutaneous flap transposed as a pedicled flap, provided that the vascular pedicle of the muscle has not been affect-

ed by the injury. Forearm wounds that require flap closure are best treated with free flaps. A rectus abdominis, scapular, or latissimus dorsi muscle flap can be used for large defects of the arm or forearm. Although soft tissue coverage with simultaneous functional forearm muscle replacement can be achieved with a single flap such as the gracilis muscle, this procedure is not generally recommended; rather, a skin flap such as a scapular free flap is preferred as a first stage of reconstruction to achieve wound healing.

Figure 5 (*a*) A soft tissue sarcoma has recurred in the scar of a previous excision. Reexcision of the defect (*b*) has exposed bone and tendons. No regional flaps are available for satisfactory coverage of this defect. The forearm (*c*) is a source of small, thin free flaps. (*d*) Flap transfer has been completed. The radial artery and venae comitantes have been anastomosed to their dorsalis pedis counterparts.

Hand   Both free flaps and pedicled skin flaps are useful for soft tissue coverage of hand wounds. The temporalis fascia free flap is particularly thin and is ideal for coverage of exposed tendons on the dorsum of the hand. The lateral arm free flap is ideal for reconstruction of a large defect of the first web space; it has sensory potential because it contains a large sensory nerve. Both of these free flaps are small. Pedicled distant skin flaps from the chest or abdomen are available as an alternative form of coverage of sizable hand defects. However, pedicled skin flaps have major disadvantages: wound care is difficult, edema persists because elevation and movement of the hand are seldom possible while it is attached to the trunk, and a second procedure is needed to divide these flaps.

Digital injuries with exposed tendons can be closed with a variety of cross-finger flaps of skin and subcutaneous tissue raised from either the volar or extensor aspect of an adjacent digit. Because these flaps do not contain a great deal of subcutaneous tissue, they are preferred for coverage of digits proximally, where a thick subcutaneous pad is not essential. The thenar flap is useful for fingertip injuries in which the soft tissue pad of the fingertip is lost and bone is exposed. This flap provides an ideal pulp replacement as well as better sensory recovery than skin grafts. Fingertip injuries can also be closed with several types of V-Y advancement flaps

that can be raised from either the volar or lateral surfaces of the end of the finger.

Abdomen   Defects of the abdominal wall that require flap closure are best treated with local muscle flaps such as the tensor fasciae latae and rectus femoris from the thigh. The rectus abdominis also can occa- 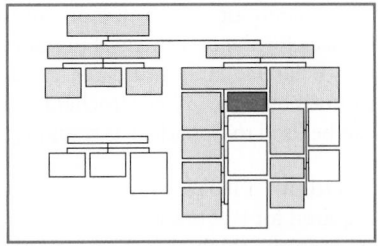 sionally be transposed to cover an abdominal defect. Each of these flaps is harvested along with skin, although a large tensor fasciae latae flap will probably require skin-graft closure of the donor site. The tensor fasciae latae flap has the advantage of including the thickened deep fascia (iliotibial band) of the thigh, which can provide additional strength for abdominal wall closure.

Gluteal area, perineum   Local muscle flaps with or without skin are indicated for defects in this area. They are preferable to large, random-pattern advancement skin flaps from the posterior thigh and thoracolumbar rotation skin

a BILOBED NASAL FLAP

b ABBE LIP FLAP

Figure 6 To close small facial defects, the bilobed nasal flap (*a*) and a variety of local flaps take advantage of skin laxity that exists in certain directions. Specialized tissues such as lip (*b*) and eyelid are frequently reconstructed with the same type of tissue borrowed from the opposite side.

flaps. The gluteus maximus muscle, for example, can be used as a rotation, V-Y advancement, or turnover flap in the treatment of pressure sores. As a turnover flap, it can be proximally or distally based, or it can be split along its longitudinal axis so that only a portion of it is used. Also useful for covering defects in the gluteal area and the perineum is the myofasciocutaneous gluteal-thigh flap, a combination of a gluteus muscle flap and a fasciocutaneous flap from the posterior thigh that is supplied by an extension of the inferior gluteal artery. Because of its size and location, the gracilis muscle is well suited for coverage of defects of the perineum. The gracilis and biceps femoris muscles are generally secondary choices for the treatment of pressure sores over the ischium. The tensor fasciae latae muscle is frequently used for treating open wounds over the greater trochanter. The entire quadriceps muscle can be used to close defects resulting from hemipelvectomy.

Thigh Flaps are rarely required for soft tissue coverage in the thigh area, because critical vital structures are located deep within the thigh and are rarely exposed by injury or by surgical procedures. A number of regional muscle flaps are available, however, including the tensor fasciae latae, rectus femoris, vastus lateralis, and vastus medialis muscles. The gracilis and posterior thigh muscles are rarely used in this area. An anterior defect with exposure of the femoral vessels can be covered with either an ipsilateral or a contralateral rectus abdominis myocutaneous flap. A number of smaller local skin flaps that are supplied with blood from the deep fascia can be raised over portions of the thigh; except for the posterior thigh flap, however, the clinical usefulness of these flaps remains to be demonstrated.

Knee, proximal leg, midleg The two heads of the gastrocnemius muscle can be used either together or independently to cover defects of the knee and proximal leg. The soleus muscle is useful for coverage of defects of the proximal leg and midleg. Local flaps should not be used for major leg wounds if the extent of the injury suggests involvement of the muscle donor site. Instead, a free flap should be used to bring healthy tissue into the area. Therefore, free flaps are a first choice, for example, for coverage of major wounds of the popliteal fossa, knee, and proximal leg that involve the sural artery blood supply to the gastrocnemius muscle.

Skin flaps fed by the fascial blood supply can also be raised over the leg.[11] A number of fasciocutaneous flaps have been described in this area, but they tend to be smaller than muscle flaps and generally less reliable. These flaps are longitudinally oriented over the course of the anterior tibial artery or the peroneal artery. The maximum length at which such fasciocutaneous flaps are safe and their specific applications have not been well established.

Foot The foot is as complex as the hand and the face in that it is composed of separate regions, each of which has a unique set of alternatives for reconstruction. These regions include the plantar surface; the dorsum; and the posterior (non–weight-bearing) heel, Achilles tendon, and malleoli.

Superficial defects that lie completely within the non–weight-bearing portion of the midsole do not need flap coverage. Defects of the weight-bearing heel and midsole area that are less than 6 cm in diameter can be closed with a medially based skin rotation flap that is raised superficial to the plantar fascia.[12] This flap maintains plantar sensation. Limited defects of the distal plantar surface can be treated with local toe flaps that also maintain sensation. Very large plantar defects are best resurfaced with a muscle free flap (e.g., latissimus dorsi or rectus abdominis) covered with a skin graft. Although this type of flap lacks sensation, it appears to provide the most durable form of coverage because it is able to resist shear forces well.[13]

Defects of the dorsum that require flap coverage are best covered either with a fascial free flap (e.g., temporalis fascia) and an overlying skin graft or with a skin free flap that is thin (e.g., from the forearm). The extensor digitorum brevis muscle can be raised from the dorsum as a pedicled flap fed by the dorsalis pedis artery. This flap, which measures approximately 5 × 6 cm, has an arc of rotation that makes it useful for the coverage of defects of the malleolus or the Achilles tendon area. A narrow transposition skin flap fed by the lateral calcaneal artery is useful for coverage of defects approximately 3 cm in diameter that lie over the Achilles tendon or the non–weight-bearing posterior heel.

Secondary Reconstruction

Selection of the proper method for secondary reconstruction requires analysis of the type and extent of tissue deficiency that is present. Superficial defects may require replacement or supplementation of only skin and subcutaneous tissue, whereas more complex defects may require replacement of several types of tissue. Specialized tissue such as vascularized nerve (i.e., a nerve free flap) or intestine may be necessary to provide a functional reconstruction in some cases (see below).

SMALL LOCALIZED SCAR

When small localized scars need reconstruction, soft tissue coverage is generally sufficient and poses no threat of breakdown leading to exposure of important structures. Instead, the reconstructive problem is generally functional in nature. An example is a tight scar band across a flexion crease, commonly seen after a burn injury. A local procedure that rearranges the existing tissue can relieve the tension by making more tissue available in one direction, although the amount of tissue in the area is not actually increased.

The Z-plasty is an example of such tissue rearrangement [see Figure 7]. Two triangular flaps are designed to have a common, or central, limb aligned in the direction that needs to be lengthened. Each of the other two limbs is equal in length to the central limb and diverges from it at an equal angle varying from 30° to 90°. After the flaps are transposed, length is gained in the desired direction, and the original Z is rotated 90° and reversed. An angle of 60°, which is commonly used, will result in a 75% gain in length along the central limb. In theory, the maximum gain in length is achieved by using the greatest angle possible, but practical limitations are imposed by the nature of skin elasticity.

Although Z-plasty is simple in conception, experience is necessary for the surgeon to realize the limitations of the technique and appreciate the subtleties of proper design. Important considerations in the use of Z-plasty include the proper length of the central limb and the proper orientation of the limbs so that the new central limb formed after transposition is parallel to the skin tension lines. Multiple Z-plasties or other procedures, such as W-plasty, may be useful for some localized scars.

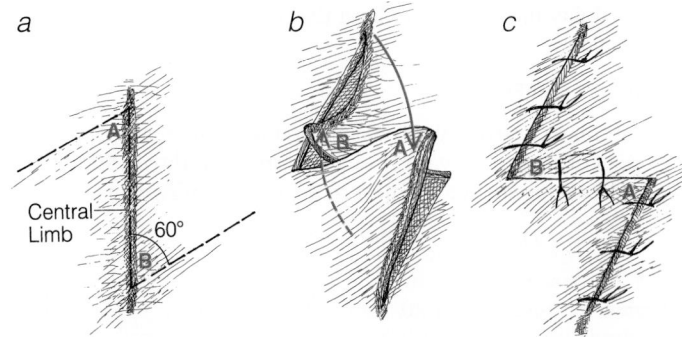

Figure 7 (*a*) **A scar that requires lengthening to eliminate a contracture forms the central limb of a Z-plasty design. Incisions diverging from the scar at a 60° angle will yield an increase of approximately 75% in the direction of the original central limb. (*b*) The flaps are transposed. (*c*) The length from top to bottom has been increased, and the original Z design has been rotated 90° and reversed.**

SHORTAGE OF SKIN AND
SUBCUTANEOUS TISSUE

A shortage of skin and subcutaneous tissue may result from excision of a large scar or of a large congenital defect such as a nevus. Mastectomy commonly leaves a shortage of skin that prevents creation of a breast mound. In these cases, extra tissue can be created locally with the use of tissue expanders. These devices are inflatable plastic reservoirs of various shapes and volumes that are implanted under the skin. The skin over the expander is stretched during a period of several weeks as the expander is gradually filled by percutaneously injecting saline into an incorporated or remote fill port. The expander is then removed as a second procedure, and the expanded area of skin is advanced to cover the defect.

A number of important principles govern the use of tissue expanders. The expanders must be placed in such a way as to allow expansion to occur only in normal skin adjacent to the defect and not in the defect itself. A sufficiently large expander or multiple expanders must be used to ensure adequate expansion. Complications associated with the use of tissue expanders include infection, extrusion, deflation, flipped ports (remote type), and hematoma formation.[14]

Tissue expanders are used in secondary reconstruction only; they do not have a role in acute wound management. They are not indicated for contour defects (see below), because the tissue they provide is of only two dimensions and is deficient in bulk. Nor is expanded tissue adequate for coverage of chronically exposed structures such as bone. Tissue expanders do not provide adequate replacement tissue to establish a suitable bed for nerve or bone grafting. Therefore, they are not a substitute for flaps in general.

The scalp is an ideal location for the use of tissue expanders because no equivalent substitute for this type of hair-bearing tissue exists. Expanders work effectively when implanted over the hard calvarium and are useful in cases of burn alopecia and large nevi involving the scalp. Expanders are also useful for breast reconstruction, for carefully selected large lesions of the face, and for certain scars of the limbs. They are generally not indicated for use in the hands or feet. Although some local flap donor sites, such as the forehead, can be expanded before flap transfer, there is a loss of tissue pliability that appears to limit the usefulness of this particular application.

COMPLEX DEFECTS

Certain reconstructive problems require substantial amounts of tissue of one or more types or of a very specialized type. Either local or free flaps are used to meet these tissue requirements.

Composite Defect

A composite defect may result from resection of an intraoral carcinoma with loss of the mandible and either the lining of the mouth or external skin. Another example is a crush injury of the leg with loss of soft tissue and a segment of weight-bearing bone. These defects require that a composite flap be brought to the area to meet more than one type of tissue deficiency. Local flaps generally do not provide the necessary types of tissue or permit the freedom of design possible with free flaps. The wide variety of free flap donor sites that exists allows tissue in the appropriate quantity and configuration to be selected for a particular defect [*see Figure 8*].

Functional Defect

Functional defects require repair with specialized flaps. Free flaps are frequently used because the specific tissue requirements usually cannot be satisfied by a local flap. A functional defect may result, for example, in the cervical esophagus from tumor resection or in the forearm from Volkmann's contracture. A segment of small intestine can repair the esophageal defect; transfer of a vascularized and innervated muscle such as the gracilis can replace forearm muscle.[15]

a

b

c

d

e

Figure 8 (*a*) **A chronic draining sinus of the ulna with poor overlying soft tissue coverage is shown. Simultaneous replacement of both bone and overlying soft tissue with a composite tissue flap is needed. (*b*) A radiograph shows nonunion of the ulna with orthopedic hardware. A fibular free flap (*c*) provides bone and skin in the appropriate amount and configuration for replacement of the affected tissues in a single stage. (*d*) The segment of ulna and overlying skin has been replaced. A radiograph (*e*) shows the vascularized fibula in place.**

Contour Deformity

Contour defects, such as those that result from mastectomy or from trauma to the lower extremity, can be reconstructed with either local or free flaps. A mastectomy defect, because of its location on the chest, is suitable for reconstruction with one of several myocutaneous flaps from either the back or the abdomen. A free flap from the abdomen or the gluteal area is another alternative. The best reconstructive solution for a particular person is determined by variables such as body habitus and the size and configuration of the contralateral breast.

A contour defect of the lower extremity is best reconstructed with a large myocutaneous free flap that provides tissue of sufficient quantity and flexibility to allow sculpting into the appropriate shape.

Unstable Soft Tissue Coverage

Marginal soft tissue coverage (e.g., skin grafts) may break down after repeated minor trauma. Bones may become exposed and are then at risk for osteomyelitis. This situation can be avoided by elective replacement of the tissue at risk with a more substantial soft tissue covering. As in acute reconstruction, local flaps are the first choice for lesions of the trunk or the proximal extremities, whereas free flaps are often more appropriate for lesions of the distal extremities.

Soft tissue coverage is sometimes inadequate even in a healed wound. For example, certain procedures, such as nerve or bone grafting, require an ideal soft tissue bed to promote adequate graft revascularization. In some cases, it may be necessary first to replace the existing soft tissue coverage as a first-stage procedure before grafting a bone or nerve gap. A skin or muscle flap is most commonly used in these cases. This problem is most common in areas such as the distal extremities, where native soft tissue coverage is not overly abundant and is easily lost from trauma or tumor resection. Free flaps are usually chosen to provide a healthy, well-vascularized soft tissue bed before further functional reconstruction is undertaken.

Postoperative Care

SKIN GRAFTS

The postoperative fate of a skin graft is largely determined by the circumstances of the wound (especially the presence or absence of infection) and the technical execution of the grafting procedure. Successful healing of skin grafts requires immobilization of the recipient site for 5 to 7 days. Immobilization can be accomplished with tie-over bolsters; on extremities, skin grafts can be further immobilized with plaster casts. Proper immobilization is critical for graft survival because it prevents shearing in the plane between the graft and the wound bed. After 5 to 7 days of immobilization, either a gauze dressing such as Xeroform or a lubricating antibiotic ointment should be applied for another 5 to 7 days.

Grafts that are treated by closed methods (i.e., tie-over bolsters) are carefully observed for evidence of infection. Developing erythema or suppuration is an indication for immediate removal of the bolster dressing and inspection of the graft. A graft threatened by infection may be saved by switching to an open method of graft care with wet dressings changed three or four times a day.

Nonmeshed grafts may form a hematoma or seroma that will prevent the graft from taking. Fluid accumulation should be evacuated by puncturing the graft or by rolling cotton-tipped swabs over it until the fluid escapes from under its edges. Survival of the entire graft is possible if fluid is meticulously evacuated within the first few days after graft placement.

Meshed grafts are not subject to the problem of fluid accumulation, nor are they as vulnerable as nonmeshed grafts to the shear forces that can prevent graft survival. For meshed grafts, the postoperative goal is to prevent desiccation, because they are more exposed to the environment. Gauze dressings such as Xeroform should be placed over the graft and changed once a day. After 2 weeks, the dressings can be discontinued, but the graft should be kept well lubricated with either a skin cream or cocoa butter.

Meshed grafts that are placed over wounds at high risk for infection should be aggressively managed postoperatively with wet dressings changed three or four times a day. The dressing changes will not interfere with graft take and will maximize graft survival in the face of heavy bacterial contamination.

Management of Skin-Graft Donor Sites

The donor sites of split-thickness grafts heal by epithelialization. They are best managed by coverage with a gas-permeable polyurethane film dressing such as OpSite. This dressing retains moisture underneath, which favors rapid epithelialization. It is also impermeable to bacteria. It is placed on the donor site after removal of the skin graft, and the area is wrapped with an overlying dressing for 48 hours to prevent formation of a seroma or hematoma under the OpSite. The outer dressing is then removed, and the OpSite is left in place for as long as 2 weeks. This plastic dressing is painless and much better tolerated than more traditional forms of dressing such as Xeroform gauze, which is left to dry out and spontaneously separate.[16]

LOCAL FLAPS

The postoperative care of local flaps is not complex. Flap healing is supported by adequate nutrition and maintenance of a normal hemodynamic state, including normal blood volume. Tension must not be placed on the flap. Tension can develop in flaps on the trunk by changes in patient position or in flaps on the limbs by loss of immobilization. The tip of any local flap is generally not only its most valuable portion but also its most vulnerable area. At the tip, the blood supply is the most precarious, and the detrimental effects of tension are magnified. Unfortunately, no pharmacologic agents are of proven benefit in preventing progressive necrosis of a flap with failing circulation. Any flap necrosis that might develop should be minimized by preventing infection of the necrotic tissue. Necrotic tissue must therefore be debrided after the extent of tissue loss becomes clear. Portions of the flap that are undergoing demarcation but do not appear to be actively infected can be protected by the application of a topical antibiotic such as silver sulfadiazine cream (Silvadene).

FREE FLAPS

Survival of free flaps, unlike that of local flaps, tends to be an all-or-none phenomenon. Careful postoperative monitoring of flap circulation is essential because flap failure is likely to be the result of a problem at the vascular anastomoses. Flaps are usually monitored for 7 days. However, the most critical time for free-flap monitoring is the first 6 to 8 hours because the majority of vascular crises usually occur within this period. Early detection and aggressive investigation of such crises generally allow a flap to be salvaged.

Maintenance of normal blood volume and treatment of hypothermia are important in the early postoperative period to avoid vascular spasm. Spasm causes flaps to appear pale and to exhibit a significant temperature drop.

Free flaps should be monitored on an hourly basis during the early postoperative period. Most free flaps include an exposed skin island, which facilitates evaluation of the flap circulation. The flap is observed for color and for capillary refill. A pale flap generally indicates arterial insufficiency; however, the normal, lighter color of certain donor sites, such as the abdomen, can be misleading. Flaps with venous insufficiency are characteristically blue in color and exhibit rapid capillary refill. Bleeding from the edges of a flap is common in the presence of venous hypertension.

Surface temperature probes are used to monitor free flaps that have a skin island. The advantages of this method are simplicity and reliability. One probe is placed on the flap and another on a nearby area to serve as a control. The flap surface temperature is generally less than the control temperature by 1.0° to 2.5° C. A progressive widening of the temperature difference is ominous and requires critical assessment of the flap circulation. The absolute temperature of the flap probe is also significant: a flap temperature greater than 32° C indicates healthy circulation, whereas a temperature between 30° and 32° C indicates marginal circulation and a temperature less than 30° C usually indicates a vascular problem. In a healthy flap, temperature fluctuations may be caused by a dislodged probe, an exogenous heat source (such as a lamp), cooling of one of the probes from an oxygen mist mask, or cleaning of the flap skin with alcohol (which results in a precipitous drop in skin temperature).

To confirm the presence of an anastomotic problem, flap circulation is assessed directly by a full-thickness puncture of the flap skin with a 19- or 20-gauge needle. If flap circulation is healthy, a drop of bright-red blood should appear at the puncture site within a few seconds, and another drop should appear each time the previous drop is wiped away by an alcohol swab. The failure of blood to appear or the delayed appearance of a clear, serous ooze instead of blood is an indication of arterial insufficiency. Vigorous, dark bleeding confirms a venous problem. Flaps that are pale as a result of vascular spasm are difficult to assess because their bleeding response to needle puncture is poor despite intact anastomoses. Whenever uncertainty exists, however, surgical exploration should be undertaken because the entire flap is in jeopardy.

Free flaps without skin islands are more difficult to monitor accurately. Muscle flaps can be followed in much the same way as skin free flaps by inserting needle temperature probes directly into the muscle belly. A healthy muscle free flap is red in color and typically has a serous ooze between the interstices of the overlying meshed skin graft. A flap with an arterial problem quickly becomes dry and dark in appearance. A muscle flap with a venous problem becomes dark and engorged with blood and exhibits bleeding from

its surface and perimeter. A muscle free flap can be punctured with a needle to assess the quality of the bleeding if its circulatory status is unclear.

Fascial free flaps covered with skin grafts are more difficult to assess. They tend to transmit body core temperature readily because they are quite thin; therefore, needle temperature probes are generally unreliable. It is often possible in these cases either to observe the arterial pulsations in the flap directly or to monitor them with a conventional Doppler device.

Some free flaps are completely buried beneath the skin. Others, such as intraoral skin free flaps, are equally difficult to monitor postoperatively. Specialized transplants, such as jejunum, are particularly vulnerable to short periods of anoxia and are not likely to be salvageable by the time a problem is recognized. Alternative methods of monitoring buried free flaps are being developed, although they are not in wide clinical use. One example is the implantable Doppler monitor. This device is placed in direct contact with the artery distal to the anastomosis to obtain a continuous Doppler signal.

PATIENT POSITIONING

Extremities that are recipient sites for skin grafts or flaps should always be maintained above heart level for a minimum of 1 week postoperatively. Lower extremities with skin grafts or free flaps, particularly below the knee, should remain elevated for a minimum of 10 days to 2 weeks. Patients should be mobilized in a progressive manner, beginning with brief periods of limb dangling. Premature ambulation of patients with lower-extremity skin grafts can result in loss of the skin graft despite an early appearance of complete graft take. Free flaps exhibit venous engorgement when placed in a dependent position up to several weeks postoperatively. Such engorgement is generally not dangerous, although patients with free flaps below the knee should be gradually mobilized in the same fashion as patients with skin grafts in this location.

Free flaps in the head and neck area require that the patient's head motion be restricted somewhat for the first few days. It is important that electrocardiographic leads and tracheostomy tube ties not compress the external jugular vein if it was used as a recipient vessel for anastomosis. If central lines are required postoperatively, they should be placed on the contralateral side of the neck.

Discussion

Wound Healing

The wound healing process consists of several identifiable phases [see I:8 Acute Wound Care]. The first phase is an inflammatory response that includes both vascular and cellular components. The second stage is fibroplasia, during which collagen deposition by fibroblasts increases the tensile strength of the wound. The maturation phase of wound healing begins at about 3 weeks, when the rate of collagen degradation begins to balance the rate of collagen production. The previously random arrangement of collagen fibers becomes more organized, and the type I to type III collagen ratio returns to normal. The wound gradually progresses from a raised, indurated, red scar to a mature form that is flat, soft, lighter in color, and of increased tensile strength. The maturation phase continues for more than a year.

Contraction of open, so-called granulating wounds is caused by myofibroblasts, modified fibroblasts that have smooth muscle characteristics. The number of myofibroblasts within the wound has been found to be proportional to the rate at which the wound

contracts.[17,18] These cells are scattered throughout the wound and pull the edges of the wound toward the center. Skin grafts inhibit wound contraction, apparently by accelerating the life cycle of the myofibroblast.

Skin Grafts

Split-thickness skin grafts include the epidermis and only a portion of the dermis, whereas full-thickness skin grafts include the entire dermis. Skin grafts contract to a degree that is related to their thickness. After their harvest from donor sites, full-thickness grafts will contract to a surface area as small as 40% of their original surface area, whereas split-thickness grafts contract only about half as much. This reduction in area, referred to as primary contraction, is a passive phenomenon caused by elastic tissue within the graft. Secondary contraction occurs as a graft heals at the recipient site. Full-thickness grafts undergo minimal secondary contraction, whereas split-thickness grafts contract to a degree that is inversely proportional to their dermal content. In other words, thick split-thickness grafts contract less than thin split-thickness grafts.

Skin grafts gradually regain sensation by reinnervation from the wound bed. Thick grafts and healthy wound beds contribute to greater sensory recovery. However, the degree of sensation after healing is complete does not equal that of normal skin. Graft thickness also affects recovery of certain other functions of normal skin, such as secretion from sweat glands and sebaceous glands, and of hair growth. These processes will be active only in full-thickness and thick split-thickness grafts. Secretion from sweat glands depends on sympathetic reinnervation of the graft and follows the sweat pattern of the recipient site. Sebaceous glands, on the other hand, secrete independently of graft reinnervation by the recipient bed. Thin split-thickness skin grafts tend to be quite dry because they contain inadequate numbers of functioning sebaceous glands, which are more abundant in thicker grafts.

GRAFT REVASCULARIZATION

A phase of serum imbibition lasts for the first 2 days after placement of a skin graft. During this period, the graft is nourished by passive absorption of nutrients from serum in the recipient bed and not by direct vascular perfusion. The graft gains as much as 40% of extra weight because of fluid absorption. Vessels within the graft gradually dilate and fill with static columns of blood. A fibrin network in the wound bed causes graft adherence during this early phase.

The next phase in revascularization is a period of inosculation, during which anastomoses are formed between vessels in the graft and those in the wound bed. It is not clear, however, whether connections are established between existing vessels in the recipient bed and graft or whether new vessels grow into the graft from the recipient bed. Both processes may occur, and both may be important in graft revascularization. In any case, circulation is sluggish during postoperative days 3 and 4 but gradually increases during postoperative days 5 and 6 to become essentially normal by day 7.[19]

Lymphatic drainage from the graft is established at approximately the same rate as the circulation of blood. Lymphatic flow is present by postoperative day 5 or 6, and the graft starts losing the extra fluid weight it has gained. The graft begins to resume its normal weight by postoperative day 9.

FACTORS AFFECTING GRAFT SURVIVAL

Hematoma formation beneath a skin graft is the most common cause of graft failure. Blood accumulation interferes with graft adherence as well as with both imbibition and inosculation. Early evacuation of blood from beneath a skin graft can result in graft survival. Shear forces that result from inadequate immobilization cause graft failure by preventing or disrupting developing communications between vessels of the graft and the recipient bed. Infection of the recipient bed makes the bed unsuitable for grafting, and such infection is another major cause of graft failure. Proteolytic enzymes produced by microorganisms destroy the fibrin bond between the graft and recipient bed. Bacteria such as β-hemolytic streptococci and *Pseudomonas* are particularly virulent because they produce high levels of plasmin and other proteolytic enzymes. The type of organism present may actually be a more important factor in graft failure than the number of organisms.[20]

HEALING OF DONOR SITES

Donor sites for split-thickness grafts heal by reepithelialization. Epithelial cells from remaining portions of skin appendages, such as hair follicles, sebaceous glands, and sweat glands, migrate across the exposed dermis to establish a new epidermis. Donor sites for thin grafts heal more rapidly and leave less of a scar than those for thick grafts, which take longer to heal and can be associated with significant scarring. The epidermis of a healed donor site is fully differentiated within 3 to 4 weeks. The dermis shows little evidence of regeneration, however. An occlusive dressing such as Op-Site promotes more rapid healing of the donor site than coverage with fine mesh gauze.[16]

Flaps

FLAP NOMENCLATURE

Flaps are described by the types of tissue that they contain, their blood supply, and the method by which they are moved from the donor to the recipient site. Flaps commonly consist of skin and subcutaneous tissue alone. However, they may also consist of skin combined with either muscle, fascia, or bone; in these cases, the flaps would be called myocutaneous, fasciocutaneous, or osteocutaneous, respectively. Flaps of skin and subcutaneous tissue that contain a known major artery are described as axial-pattern, or arterialized, skin flaps. If such a flap is raised at the donor site and remains attached only by the vascular pedicle, it is termed an island flap. The same flap is termed a free flap if the vascular pedicle is severed, the flap is transferred to a distant recipient site, and its circulation is restored by microvascular anastomoses. Local flaps may be called either rotation, advancement, or transposition flaps, depending on how they are moved to reach their recipient sites. The combination of several descriptive terms provides a more complete characterization of flaps. For example, a muscle and skin flap that is rotated to cover an adjacent soft tissue defect is termed a myocutaneous rotation flap, and a skin and bone flap used to reconstruct a distant composite defect is termed an osteocutaneous free flap.

FLAP BLOOD SUPPLY

Plastic surgical reconstruction has evolved with the improved understanding of how blood is supplied to various body tissues. The earliest flaps in common use were skin flaps described as having a so-called random-pattern type of circulation [*see Figures 9 and 10*],[21] because they were supplied by the subdermal capillary plexus rather than by a major, named vessel. The precarious nature of the blood supply of such flaps severely limited flap design and resulted in a preoccupation with maintaining suitable length:width ratios. Greater length:width ratios became possible after the empirical discovery that a more vigorous circulation develops in flaps raised in stages.[22] The reason for this delay phenomenon is accommodation to ischemia, but the precise mechanism is still not well understood.

The next advance in flap technology was the identification of several body sites where a sizable artery coursed directly to a specific cutaneous territory. The groin was the first region where this arrangement was carefully described, and it remains a useful source of flaps for selected applications. Because longer flaps can be made in areas where the blood supply has an axial pattern [*see Figures 9 and 10*], the length:width ratio and delay phenomenon became less important issues in flap design.[23] Identification of a specific vessel as the supply for a certain territory of tissue allows so-called islanding of this tissue from the donor site except for the vascular connection, which is preserved. Such island flaps have greater mobility than do flaps that have a more significant soft tissue attachment to the donor site.

Another major advance in flap technology was an understanding of the important myocutaneous blood supply, a network of vessels that perforate muscles vertically and supply overlying cutane-

RANDOM PATTERN   AXIAL PATTERN   MYOCUTANEOUS

Figure 9   A random–pattern skin flap is supplied by a subdermal plexus of small vessels that do not have an axial orientation. An axial–pattern skin flap is designed parallel to the axis of a known major subcutaneous artery. It can have a greater length : width ratio because its blood supply is more reliable. A myocutaneous flap derives the blood supply of its skin component from vertical perforators from the underlying muscle. The skin can be completely isolated over the muscle as an island.

ous territories. These perforators are not necessarily the exclusive supply to the skin in a specific region, but they are able to support the skin entirely when other sources of blood supply are eliminated [*see Figure 9*]. This arrangement assumed great clinical significance when it was recognized that a skin flap could be designed as an island that is based on a muscle blood supply [*see Figure 10*] and that

such an island could be safely moved anywhere within the arc of rotation of the particular muscle once the muscle was detached from its origin, its insertion, or both.[10]

The revolution in myocutaneous flaps took place in the 1970s. A systematic study of the blood supply to the muscle itself became important in the clinical application of the myocutaneous flap prin-

Figure 10   The blood supply of random–pattern skin flaps is quite limited, and only small flaps, such as thenar flaps (*a*), are consistently reliable. (*b*) An axial–pattern skin flap is shown. The skin and subcutaneous tissue of a myocutaneous flap (*c*) can exist as a complete island because the blood supply is derived from vertical muscular perforators. (*d*) A large free flap of scapular area skin and the entire latissimus dorsi muscle are shown. The subscapular vessels that connect the two will supply both components of the flap after microvascular anastomoses.

TYPE I	TYPE II	TYPE III	TYPE IV	TYPE V

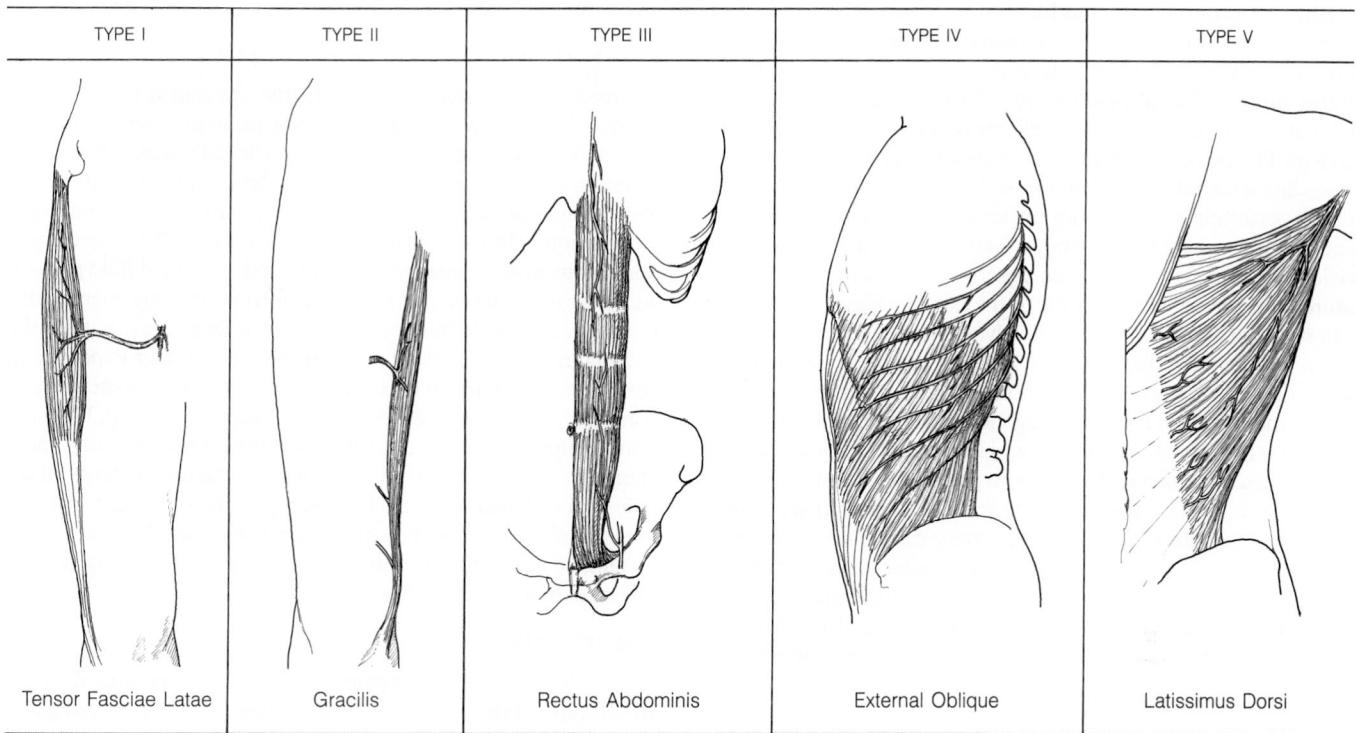

| Tensor Fasciae Latae | Gracilis | Rectus Abdominis | External Oblique | Latissimus Dorsi |

Figure 11 **Schematized are the five basic patterns of blood supply to muscle. Individual muscles are classified on the basis of the dominance, number, and size of the vessels that supply them. Type I is supplied by a single dominant pedicle. Type II is supplied by one dominant vessel and several much smaller vessels. Type III is supplied by two dominant pedicles. Type IV is supplied by multiple vessels of similar size. Type V is supplied by one dominant pedicle and several smaller segmental vascular pedicles.**

ciple. Investigation of the body musculature showed that there were at least five basic patterns of blood supply to muscle, distinguished by the existence of and balance between primary pedicles and secondary sources of supply [*see Figure 11*]. Some muscles can be rotated or transposed as myocutaneous flaps on the basis of either their dominant or secondary blood supply (e.g., pectoralis major and latissimus dorsi). Some muscles have two dominant supplies and can be transposed on either one (e.g., rectus abdominis). Other muscles do not reliably support skin territories supplied by minor pedicles (e.g., gracilis).

TYPE A	TYPE B	TYPE C

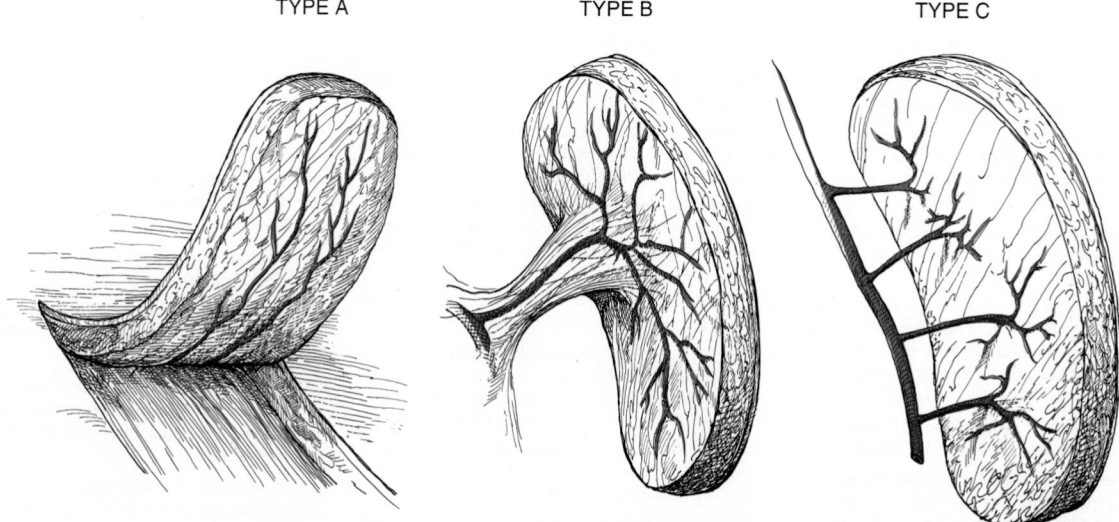

Figure 12 **At least three types of fasciocutaneous flaps exist, categorized by blood supply configuration. Type A is supplied by multiple small, longitudinal vessels that course with the deep fascia. These flaps must retain a base of a certain width and cannot be raised as an island (e.g., longitudinally oriented flaps of skin and fascia on the lower leg). Type B is supplied by a single major vessel within the fascia (e.g., scapular flap). Type C is supplied by multiple perforating segments from a major vessel that courses through intermuscular septa (e.g., forearm flaps).**

Other patterns of cutaneous blood supply were later recognized and quickly assumed clinical importance. The discovery that larger skin flaps can be raised if the deep fascia is included led to more careful study of fascial blood supply. Fasciocutaneous flaps with high length:width ratios can be reliably raised on the trunk, arms, and legs. The blood supply of deep fascia appears to consist of both a deep and a superficial fascial plexus. These fascial vessels connect both to perforating vessels from the underlying muscles and to the subcutaneous tissue vessels above them.[24] At least three types of fasciocutaneous flaps have been described that are based on the nature of the fascial blood supply to the skin [see Figure 12].[25]

In some areas, fascia supplies overlying subcutaneous tissue and skin in a more direct fashion. This arrangement of fasciocutaneous blood supply is most evident in the extremities. There, direct branches from major vessels course through intermuscular septae to reach the deep fascia. The overlying skin and subcutaneous tissue are supplied by these so-called septocutaneous perforators. The forearm has become an important donor site clinically because thin septocutaneous flaps that are fed by the radial artery can be raised either as pedicled or free flaps. Other examples of fasciocutaneous flaps include the lateral arm septocutaneous flap, fed by the profunda brachii artery; the scapular flap, fed by the circumflex scapular artery; and the fibular osteofasciocutaneous flap, fed by the peroneal artery.

FLAP RESISTANCE TO INFECTION

Skin flaps, myocutaneous flaps, and fasciocutaneous flaps have been shown experimentally to vary in their resistance to bacterial infection.[26] Random-pattern skin flaps are not as resistant as myocutaneous flaps. The cutaneous portions of myocutaneous and of fasciocutaneous flaps have similar levels of resistance, but the muscle component of myocutaneous flaps is more resistant than the fascial component of fasciocutaneous flaps in situations where the flap lies over a focus of infection within the wound. Muscle therefore appears to be the type of flap most resistant to infection. Such resistance is of clinical significance in cases of exposed bone with chronic osteomyelitis, for example. This condition can be successfully treated by debridement and immediate coverage with a muscle flap.

FREE FLAPS: THE CONCEPT OF NO-REFLOW

Free tissue transfer is unique in that the flap is completely ischemic for a given period. How long ischemia can be tolerated without resultant flap failure (despite technically satisfactory microvascular anastomoses) is an important clinical question. An increasing duration of ischemia has been associated experimentally with obstruction to blood flow in the microcirculation.[27,28] This obstruction results from cellular edema, increased interstitial fluid pressure, and sludging of blood and thrombus formation. This phenomenon is initially reversible but becomes irreversible as the duration of ischemia increases. After 12 hours of ischemia under experimental conditions, obstruction to blood flow has been demonstrated to be complete, preventing successful reperfusion of the flap. How long uninterrupted ischemia can safely continue is not precisely known clinically, and evidence suggests that the ischemic tolerance of specific types of tissue varies. For example, flaps that are primarily bone are more durable than muscle or bowel flaps. Evidence gained by clinical experience has shown that up to 4 hours of ischemia is safely tolerated by most free flaps.

TISSUE EXPANSION

Histologic changes of expanded skin include thinning of the dermis but not of the epidermis,[29] suggesting a permanent net gain in epidermal tissue only. The mitotic rate in the epidermis has been shown to increase with expansion, but the mechanism for this increase is unclear.[30]

The circulation of expanded skin also changes. An increase in vascularity of expanded tissue is partially explained by the fact that tissue expansion is a form of delay procedure. However, experimental studies suggest that an increased potential for flap survivability is directly attributable to the expansion process and not merely to its delay component.[31-33] The fibrous capsule that forms around the prosthesis during expansion appears to contribute to the increased vascularity of these flaps, and the increased pressure around the expander may stimulate angiogenesis.

References

1. Edlich RF, Jones KC Jr, Buchanan L, et al: A disposable emergency wound treatment kit. J Emerg Med 10:463, 1992

2. Stevenson TR, Thacker JG, Rodeheaver GT, et al: Cleansing the traumatic wound by high pressure syringe irrigation. JACEP 5:17, 1976

3. Hollander JE, Singer AJ, Valentine SM, et al: Risk factors for infection in patients with traumatic lacerations. Acad Emerg Med 8:716, 2001

4. Edlich RF, Rodeheaver GT, Thacker JG: Technical factors in the prevention of wound infection. Surgical Infectious Diseases. Simmons R, Howard R, Eds. Appleton-Century-Croft, East Norwalk, Connecticut, 1981

5. Robson MC, Heggers JP: Delayed wound closures based on bacterial counts. J Surg Oncol 2:379, 1970

6. Teepe RG, Koebrugge EJ, Lowik CW, et al: Cytotoxic effects of topical antimicrobial and antiseptic agents on human keratinocytes in vitro. J Trauma 35:8, 1993

7. Jackson IT: Local Flaps in Head and Neck Reconstruction. CV Mosby, St Louis, 1985

8. Spinelli HM, Forman DL: Current treatment of post-traumatic deformities: residual orbital, adnexal, and soft-tissue abnormalities. Clin Plast Surg 24:519, 1997

9. Luce EA: Reconstruction of the lower lip. Clin Plast Surg 22:109, 1995

10. Mathes SJ, Nahai F: Reconstructive Surgery: Principles, Anatomy, Technique, Vol 1. Churchill Livingstone, New York, 1997, p 37

11. Taylor GI, Giantoutsos MP, Morris SF: The neurovascular territories of the skin and muscles: anatomic study and clinical implications. Plast Reconstr Surg 94:1, 1994

12. Hidalgo DA, Shaw WW: Reconstruction of foot injuries. Clin Plast Surg 13:663, 1986

13. May JW Jr, Halls MJ, Simon SR: Free microvascular muscle flaps with skin graft reconstruction of extensive defects of the foot: a clinical and gait analysis study. Plast Reconstr Surg 75:627, 1985

14. Bennett RG, Hirt M: A history of tissue expansion: concepts, controversies, and complications. J Dermatol Surg Oncol 19:1066, 1993

15. Hidalgo DA, Disa JJ, Cordeiro PG: A review of 716 consecutive free flaps for oncologic surgical defects: refinement in donor site selection and technique. Plast Reconstr Surg 102:722, 1998

16. Smith DJ Jr, Thomson PD, Bolton LL: Microbiology and healing of the occluded skin-graft donor site. Plast Reconstr Surg 91:1094, 1993

17. McGrath MH, Hundahl SA: The spatial and tempo-

ral quantification of myofibroblasts. Plast Reconstr Surg 69:975, 1982

18. Rudolph R: Inhibition of myofibroblasts by skin grafts. Plast Reconstr Surg 63:473, 1979

19. Angel MF, Giesswein P, Hawner P: Skin grafting. Operative Plastic Surgery. Evans GRD, Ed. McGraw-Hill, New York, 2000, p 59

20. Teh BT: Why do skin grafts fail? Plast Reconstr Surg 63:323, 1979

21. Daniel RK, Kerrigan CL: Skin flaps: an anatomical and hemodynamic approach. Clin Plast Surg 6:181, 1979

22. Cederna PS, Chang P, Pittet-Cuenod BM, et al: The effect of the delay phenomenon on the vascularity of rabbit abdominal cutaneous island flaps. Plast Reconstr Surg 99:183, 1997

23. Milton SH: Pedicled skin-flaps: the fallacy of the length:width ratio. Br J Surg 57:502, 1970

24. Lamberty BG, Cormack GC: Fasciocutaneous flaps. Clin Plast Surg 17:713, 1990

25. Cormack GC, Lamberty BG: Arterial Anatomy of Skin Flaps. Churchill Livingstone, Edinburgh, 1987

26. Gosain A, Chang N, Mathes S, et al: A study of the relationship between blood flow and bacterial inoculation in musculocutaneous and fasciocutaneous

flaps. Plast Reconstr Surg 86:1152, 1990

27. Kerrigan CL, Stotland MA: Ischemia reperfusion injury: a review. Microsurgery 14:165, 1993

28. Kirschner RE, Fyfe BS, Hoffman LA, et al: Ischemia-reperfusion injury in myocutaneous flaps: role of leukocytes and leukotrienes. Plast Reconstr Surg 99: 1485, 1997

29. Johnson TM, Lowe L, Brown MD, et al: Histology and physiology of tissue expansion. J Dermatol Surg Oncol 19:1074, 1993

30. Olenius M, Johansson O: Variations in epidermal thickness in expanded human breast skin. Scand J Plast Reconstr Hand Surg 29:15, 1995

31. Babovic S, Angel MF, Im MJ, et al: Effects of tissue expansion on secondary ischemic tolerance in experimental free flaps. Ann Plast Surg 34:593, 1995

32. Matturri L, Azzolini A, Riberti C, et al: Long-term histopathologic evaluation of human expanded skin. Plast Reconstr Surg 90:636, 1992

33. Olenius M, Dalsgaard CJ, Wickman M: Mitotic activity in expanded human skin. Plast Reconstr Surg 91: 213, 1993

Acknowledgment

Figures 3, 6, 7, 9, 11, and 12   Carol Donner.

31 HEPATIC RESECTION

Yuman Fong, M.D., and Leslie H. Blumgart, M.D.

Liver resections were first described centuries ago, but until the latter half of the 20th century, the majority of such resections were performed for management of either injuries or infections. Today, these procedures are performed not only for treatment of acute emergencies (e.g., traumatic injuries or abscesses) but also as potentially curative therapy for a variety of benign and malignant hepatic lesions.

The first planned anatomic resection of a lobe of a liver is credited to Lortat-Jacob, who in 1952 performed a right lobectomy as treatment for metastatic colon cancer.[1] Major hepatectomies, however, did not become commonplace until the 1980s. Since then, the safety of these operations has improved dramatically, and as safety has improved, the indications for hepatic resection have become better refined as well. Currently, resection of as much as 85% of the functional liver parenchyma is being performed at numerous centers with an operative mortality of less than 2%. The duration of hospitalization is typically less than 2 weeks, and almost all individuals regain normal hepatic function.

In what follows, we focus on the technical aspects of hepatic resection, emphasizing efficiency and safety and taking into account recent developments, current controversies, and special operative considerations (e.g., the cirrhotic patient and repeat liver resection). Detailed discussions of the indications for hepatic resection are available elsewhere.[2-4]

Hepatic Anatomy

Familiarity with the surgical anatomy of the liver is essential for safe performance of a partial hepatectomy. The liver can be divided into two lobes (right and left) comprising eight segments [*see Figure 1*]. Each of these segments is a discrete anatomic unit that possesses its own nutrient blood supply and its own venous and biliary drainage. The right lobe consists of segments 5 through 8 and is nourished by the right hepatic artery and the right portal vein; the left lobe consists of segments 1 through 4 and is nourished by the left hepatic artery and the left portal vein. The anatomic division between the right lobe and the left is not at the falciform ligament (the most readily apparent visual landmark on the anterior liver) but follows a line projected through a plane (the principal plane, or Cantlie's line) that runs posterosuperiorly from the medial margin of the gallbladder to the left side of the vena cava.

The venous drainage of the liver consists of multiple small veins draining directly from the back of the right lobe and the caudate lobe to the vena cava, along with three major hepatic veins. These major hepatic veins occupy three planes, known as portal scissurae. The three scissurae divide the liver into four sectors, each of which is supplied by a portal pedicle; further branching of the pedicles subdivides the sectors into the eight segments [*see Figure 1*].[5-7] (Some surgeons refer to these sectors

Figure 1 **The liver is separated into eight anatomic segments, each with an independent nutrient blood supply and venous and biliary drainage. Appreciation of this segmental anatomy is the basis of anatomic resection of the liver.**

Inferior Vena Cava

Right Hepatic Vein

Middle Hepatic Vein

Left Hepatic Vein

Falciform Ligament

Portal Vein

Common Hepatic Artery

Common Bile Duct

Figure 2 (*a*) **The arterial anatomy of the celiac axis is reconstructed from thin-slice CT images. (*b*) The hepatic venous anatomy is similarly reconstructed, with the tumor superimposed on the vascular reconstruction.**

as segments—hence the term trisegmentectomy.) The right hepatic vein passes between the right anterior sector (segments 5 and 8) and the right posterior sector (segments 6 and 7) in the right scissura. This vein empties directly into the vena cava near the atriocaval junction. The middle hepatic vein passes between the right anterior sector and the left medial sector (segment 4) in the central, or principal, scissura, which represents the division between the right lobe and the left. The left hepatic vein runs in the left scissura between segments 2 and 3. In most persons, the left and middle hepatic veins join to form a common trunk before entering the vena cava. Occasionally, a large inferior right hepatic vein is present that may provide adequate drainage of the right lobe after resection of the left even when all three major hepatic veins are ligated.[8]

The portal vein and the hepatic artery divide into left and right branches below the hilus of the liver. Unlike the hepatic veins, which run between segments, the portal venous and hepatic arterial branches, along with the hepatic ducts, typically run centrally within segments [*see Figure 1*]. On the right side, the hepatic artery and the portal vein enter the liver substance almost immediately after branching. The short course of the right-side extrahepatic vessels and the variable anatomy of the biliary tree make these vessels vulnerable to damage during dissection.[9] In contrast, the left branch of the portal vein and the left hepatic duct take a long extrahepatic course after branching beneath segment 4. When these vessels reach the base of the umbilical fissure, they are joined by the left hepatic artery to form a triad, which then enters the left liver substance at this point. It must be emphasized that proximal to the base of the umbilical fissure, the left-side structures are not a triad. A consequence of the long extrahepatic course of the left-side structures is that for tumors that involve the hilus (e.g., Klatskin tumors), when a choice exists between an extended right hepatectomy or an extended left hepatectomy, most surgeons choose the former because the greater ease of dissection on the left side facilitates preservation of the left-side structures. Knowledge of the relative anatomic courses of the portal veins, the hepatic arteries, and the hepatic ducts is the basis of the classical extrahepatic dissection for control of hepatic inflow [*see Operative Technique, Right Lobectomy, Step 6 (Extrahepatic Dissection and Ligation), below*].

The fibrous capsule surrounding the liver substance was described by Glisson in 1654.[10] It was Couinaud,[6] however, who demonstrated that this fibrous capsule extends to envelop the portal triads as they pass into the liver substance. Thus, within the liver, the portal vein, the hepatic artery, and the hepatic duct running to each segment of the liver lie within a substantial sheath. This dense sheath allows rapid control of inflow vessels to specific anatomic units within the liver and permits en masse ligation of these vascular structures in a maneuver known as pedicle ligation [*see Operative Technique, Right Lobectomy, Step 6—Alternative (Intrahepatic Pedicle Ligation), below*].[11]

Preoperative Evaluation

Cross-sectional imaging modalities such as computed tomography, magnetic resonance imaging, and ultrasonography play an important role in enhancing the safety and efficacy of hepatic resection. These modalities, along with biologic scanning techniques such as positron emission tomography (PET), are also invaluable for staging malignancies so as to improve patient selection and thereby optimize long-term surgical outcome.

At a minimum, all candidates for hepatic resection should undergo either CT or MRI. These imaging tests not only identify the number and size of any mass lesions within the liver but also delineate the relations of the lesions to the major vasculature—data that are crucial for deciding whether to operate and which operative approach to follow.

Use of contrast enhancement during CT scanning is vital for accurate definition of the vascular anatomy. In fact, data from thin-slice (1 to 2 mm) images captured by current spiral, or helical, CT scanners can be reconstructed to provide angiographic pictures whose level of detail rivals that of direct angiograms [*see Figure 2*]. Triple-phase scans (including a noncontrast phase, an arterial phase, and a venous phase) are recommended: these yield the best definition and characterization of intrahepatic lesions. For example, some vascular tumors become isodense with liver parenchyma after contrast injection. By first obtaining noncontrast scans and then obtaining contrast scans at two different times after contrast injection, the examiner stands a better chance of visualizing such tumors.

For small tumors, a CT variant known as CT portography is recommended. In this technique, contrast material is injected through the superior mesenteric artery, and images are obtained during the portal venous phase. The normal liver receives the majority of its nutrient blood from the portal vein and is therefore contrast-enhanced in this phase. Tumors, on the other hand, usually derive their nutrient blood from the hepatic artery and therefore appear as exaggerated perfusion defects. CT portography is the most sensitive test available for identifying small hepatic tumors.[12]

MRI may also be valuable for characterizing lesions and defining them vis-à-vis the vasculature. It is particularly helpful in diagnosing benign lesions such as hemangiomas, fibronodular hyperplasia, and adenomas. Whenever any of these benign lesions is suspected, MRI is usually indicated. With regard to surgical planning, MRI angiographic images are useful for identifying the major hepatic veins and clarifying their relations to any tumor masses.[13]

Imaging recommendations may be summed up as follows. A triple-phase CT should be obtained for most patients under consideration for hepatic resection. If diagnostic doubt remains after CT, particularly if the differential diagnosis includes an asymptomatic benign tumor, MRI should be performed. If questions remain after CT as to the extent of hepatic venous or major biliary involvement, MRI or duplex ultrasonography should be considered.[14] If small tumors are encountered, CT portography should be performed. Duplex ultrasonography, by demonstrating the vascular hilar structures, the hepatic veins, and the inferior vena cava, renders angiography unnecessary in many cases.[13,15] Currently, direct hepatic angiography is rarely required, and inferior vena cavography is almost never needed.

Operative Planning

PREPARATION

In general, preparation for hepatic resection is much the same as that for other major abdominal procedures. All patients who are older than 65 years or have a history of cardiopulmonary disease undergo a full cardiopulmonary assessment. It was once commonly believed that patients 70 years of age or older were poor candidates for major liver resection,[16,17] but this notion has been dispelled by more recent data.[18-20] Advanced chronologic age is not a complete contraindication to hepatectomy.

Anemia and coagulopathy, if present, are corrected. All patients are now encouraged to donate two units of autologous blood before a major hepatectomy. Appropriate single-dose antibiotic prophylaxis is administered [see IV:5 Prevention of Postoperative Infection].

ANESTHESIA

Decisions regarding anesthesia should take into account the possibility of baseline hepatic parenchymal dysfunction as well as the postoperative hepatic functional deficits resulting from resection of a major portion of the hepatic parenchyma.

The most important consideration, however, is the possibility of major intraoperative hemorrhage. Suitable monitoring and sufficient vascular access to permit rapid transfusion should be in place. At some centers, fluid resuscitation and blood transfusion are begun early in the course of resection to increase intravascular volume as a buffer against sudden blood loss. At the Memorial Sloan-Kettering Cancer Center (MSKCC), however, we favor the opposite approach, whereby a low central venous pressure is maintained during resection. The rationale for our preference is that generally, most of the blood lost during hepatic resection comes from the major hepatic veins or the vena cava.[21,22] If central venous pressure is kept below 5 mm Hg, there is less bleeding from the hepatic venous radicles during dissection.

Reduction of intrahepatic venous pressure can be facilitated by performing the dissection with the patient in a 15° Trendelenburg position, which increases venous return to the heart and enhances cardiac output. Central venous pressure is maintained at the desired level through a combination of anesthesia and early intraoperative fluid restriction. The minimal acceptable intraoperative urine output is 25 ml/hr.

The need for intraoperative blood transfusion can be minimized by accepting hematocrits lower than the common target figure of 30%: 24% in patients without antecedent cardiac disease and 29% in patients with cardiac disease. If blood loss is estimated to reach or exceed 20% of total volume or the patient becomes hemodynamically unstable, transfusion is indicated.[21]

PATIENT POSITIONING

The patient should be supine: to date, we have not found a lateral position to be necessary even for the largest of tumors. Electrocardiographic leads should be kept clear of the right chest wall and the presternal area in case a thoracoabdominal incision is necessitated by the position of a tumor or by intraoperative hemorrhage. Preparation and draping should therefore also allow for exposure of the lower chest and the entire upper abdomen down past the umbilicus. A crossbar or a similar device that holds self-retaining retractors should be used to elevate the costal margin. Some surgeons prefer ring-based self-retaining retractors. In our experience, although these retractors are adequate for most resections, the rings tend to restrict lateral access, thereby potentially hindering posterior dissection, particularly of the vena cava.

ANATOMIC VERSUS NONANATOMIC RESECTION

The key decision in planning a hepatectomy is whether the resection should be anatomic or nonanatomic. For treatment of malignant disease, anatomic resection is usually favored because the long-term outcome is better. Anatomic resections permit excision of parenchymal areas distal to the index tumors, where there is a high incidence of vascular micrometastases. In addition, they are significantly less likely to have positive margins than nonanatomic resections are. In a large series of hepatectomies for metastatic colorectal cancer, wedge or nonanatomic resections were associated with a 19% rate of positive margins.[23] In a recent examination of our increasing preference for anatomic resections over wedge resections, wedge resections were associated with a 16% rate of positive margins, compared with a 2% rate for anatomic resections.[24]

There are two oncologic settings where nonanatomic resections are favored. In patients with hepatocellular carcinoma, viral hepatitis and cirrhosis are often complicating factors. Cirrhotic patients tolerate resection of more than two segments of functional parenchyma poorly. Accordingly, for these patients, the smallest resection that will achieve complete tumor excision is favored, even if it is a wedge resection. For management of metastatic neuroendocrine tumors, in which resections are merely debulking procedures designed to alleviate symptoms, nonanatomic resections are accepted because cure is highly unlikely.

Hepatic resections for benign hepatic tumors are usually performed for one of three reasons: (1) to relieve symptoms (e.g., pain or early satiety), (2) because the diagnosis is uncertain, or (3) to prevent malignant transformation. A goal of such resections should be to spare as much normal parenchyma as possible. Consequently, lesions such as hemangiomas, adenomas, complex cysts, and fibronodular hyperplasia are often excised by means of enucleation or another nonanatomic resection with limited margins.

Operative Technique

Theoretically, any hepatic segment can be resected in isolation. For practical purposes, however, there are five types of major anatomic resections [*see Figure 3*]. We follow the most commonly used terminology, that of Goldsmith and Woodburne.[25] Some authors prefer other systems of nomenclature, based on the anatomic descriptions of Couinaud[6] or Bismuth.[7]

The essential principles of all anatomic hepatectomies are the same: (1) control of inflow vessels, (2) control of outflow vessels, and (3) parenchymal transection. To illustrate these principles, we begin by outlining the steps in a right lobectomy [*see Figure 3a*] in some detail, describing both extrahepatic vascular dissection and ligation and the alternative approach to inflow control, intrahepatic pedicle ligation. Left lobectomy [*see Figure 3b*] and other common anatomic resections share a number of steps with right lobectomy; accordingly, we discuss them in somewhat less detail. Further detail on these procedures is available in other sources.[26,27]

RIGHT LOBECTOMY

Step 1: Laparoscopic Inspection

Experience from MSKCC[28,29] and other centers[30,31] indicates that laparoscopy allows detection of unresectable disease and prevents the morbidity associated with a nontherapeutic laparotomy. We generally perform laparoscopy immediately before laparotomy during the same period of anesthesia. The laparoscopic port sites are placed in the upper abdomen along the line of the intended incision [*see* Step 2, *below*]. The first two ports are usually 10 mm ports placed in the right subcostal area along the midclavicular line and along the anterior axillary line. These ports allow inspection of the abdomen and of the entire liver, including the dome and segment 7. The port along the right anterior axillary line is particularly suitable for laparoscopic ultrasound devices. If additional ports are necessary, a left subcostal midclavicular port is usually the best choice.

Step 2: Incision

For the majority of hepatic resections, most surgeons use a bilateral subcostal incision extended vertically to the xiphisternum [*see Figure 4*]. Our own preference, however, is to use an upper midline incision extending to a point approximately 2 cm above the umbilicus, with a rightward extension from that point to a point in the midaxillary line halfway between the lowest rib and the iliac crest [*see Figure 4*]. We find that this incision provides superb access for either right- or left-side resection, without the wound complications often encountered with trifurcated incisions (e.g., ascitic leakage and incisional hernia). On rare occasions (e.g., in the resection of large, rigid posterior tumors of the right lobe), a right thoracoabdominal incision may be required. In a recent series of nearly 2,000 resections at MSKCC, however, a thoracoabdominal incision proved necessary in only 3% of patients; the most common indication was repeat liver resection after previous right hepatic lobectomy [*see* Repeat Hepatic Resection, *below*].

Step 3: Abdominal Exploration and Intraoperative Ultrasonography

The liver is palpated bimanually. Intraoperative ultrasonography is systematically performed to identify all possible lesions and their relations to the major vascular structures. This modality is capable of identifying small lesions that preoperative imaging studies and palpation of the liver may miss.[32] The lesser omentum is incised to allow palpation of the caudate lobe and inspection of the celiac region for nodal metastases. A finger is passed from the lesser sac inferior to the caudate lobe through the foramen of Winslow to permit identification of the portal vein and palpation of the portocaval lymph nodes. The hilar lymph nodes are palpated, and any suspicious nodes are removed for frozen section examination. If the operation is being done for cancer, the entire abdomen is inspected for evidence of extrahepatic tumor.

Step 4: Mobilization of Liver

Once the decision is made to proceed with hepatic resection, the liver is fully mobilized by detaching all ligamentous attachments on the side to be resected. (Some surgeons defer completion of mobilization to a later stage in the procedure.) In particular, the suprahepatic inferior vena cava and the hepatic veins above the liver are dissected to facilitate the subsequent approach to the hepatic veins [*see* Step 7, *below*]. Once the liver is mobilized, further palpation is done to detect any small lesions that may have been obscured initially. This additional palpation is particularly important on the right side because before mobilization, the posterior parts of the liver cannot be effectively palpated, and intraoperative ultrasonography may fail to detect small lesions in this area.[32]

If, in the course of mobilization, tumor is found to be attached to the diaphragm, the affected area of the diaphragm may be excised and subsequently repaired.

Step 5: Identification of Arterial Anomalies

Any hepatic arterial anomalies present should be identified before resection is begun. With good preoperative imaging, the arterial anatomy is usually defined with sufficient exactitude before

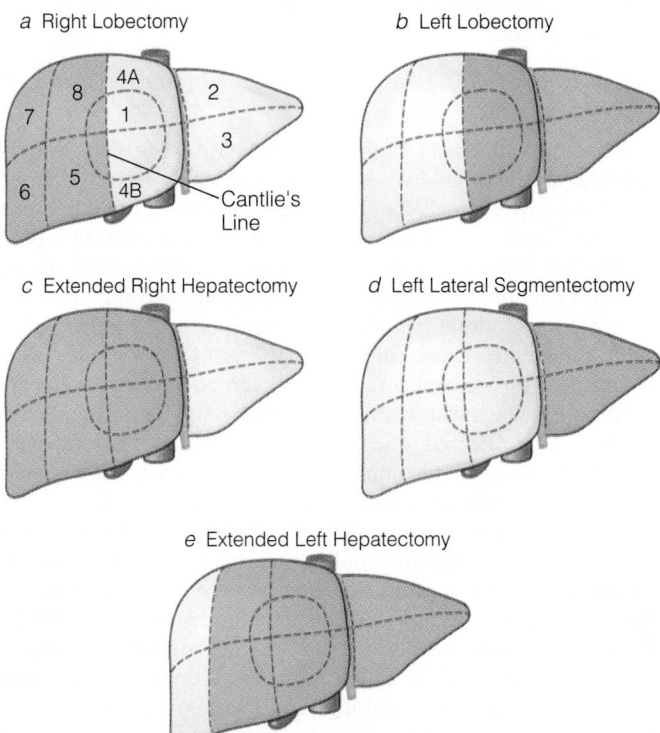

a Right Lobectomy

8 4A 2
7 1
3
6 5 4B
Cantlie's Line

b Left Lobectomy

c Extended Right Hepatectomy

d Left Lateral Segmentectomy

e Extended Left Hepatectomy

Figure 3 **Shown are schematic illustrations of standard hepatic resections, with the shaded areas representing the resected portions: (*a*) right lobectomy, (*b*) left lobectomy, (*c*) extended right hepatectomy (or right trisegmentectomy), (*d*) left lateral segmentectomy, and (*e*) extended left hepatectomy (or left trisegmentectomy).**

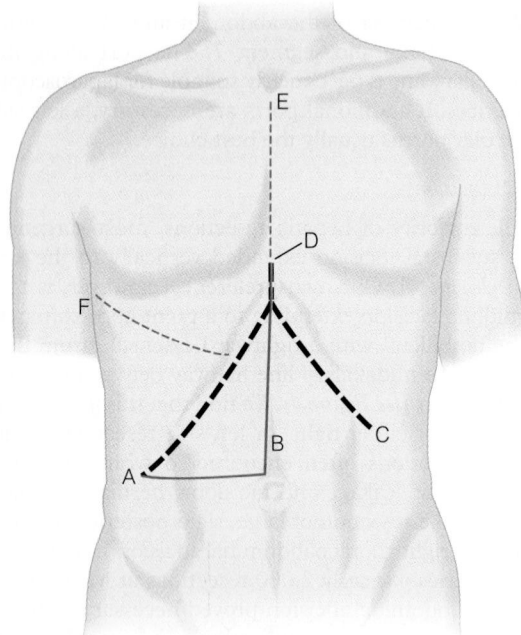

Figure 4 **Right lobectomy. A right subcostal incision (A) with a midline extension to the xiphoid (D) is the most common choice; an extension to the left subcostal area (C) is sometimes added to provide further operative exposure. We prefer a long midline incision from the xiphoid (D) to a point approximately 3 cm above the umbilicus (B) along with a rightward extension (A) because this incision provides superb exposure of both the right side and the left without the wound complications of a trifurcated incision. The chest can be entered through either a median sternotomy (E) or an anterolateral right thoracoabdominal incision (F).**

laparotomy. It is also possible to gain a clear picture of the arterial anatomy intraoperatively by means of simple maneuvers that do not involve major dissection.

The lesser omentum should be examined to determine whether there is a vessel coursing through its middle to the base of the umbilical fissure, and the hepatoduodenal ligament should be palpated with an index finger within the foramen of Winslow to see whether there is an artery in the gastropancreatic fold on its medial aspect. The usual bifurcation of the hepatic arteries occurs low and medially in the hepatoduodenal ligament, and the left hepatic artery normally travels on the medial aspect of the ligament to reach the base of the umbilical fissure. Thus, if an artery is palpable in the medial upper portion of the hepatoduodenal ligament, it is the main left hepatic artery. Any vessel seen in the lesser omentum must therefore be an accessory left artery. If, however, no pulse is found in the medial upper portion of the hepatoduodenal ligament, the vessel in the lesser omentum must be a replaced left hepatic artery. The right hepatic artery usually travels transversely behind the common bile duct (CBD) to reach the base of the cystic plate. A vertically traveling artery on the lateral hepatoduodenal ligament must therefore be either a replaced or an accessory right hepatic artery, probably arising from the superior mesenteric artery.

Step 6 (Extrahepatic Dissection and Ligation): Control of Inflow Vessels

The classic approach to extrahepatic control of the inflow vessels in a right lobectomy involves extrahepatic dissection and ligation [*see Figure 5*]. The cystic duct and the cystic artery are ligated and divided. The gallbladder may be either removed or left attached to the right liver, according to the surgeon's preference. The usual practice is first to ligate the right hepatic duct, then the right hepatic artery, and finally the right portal vein, working from anterior to posterior. Our preference, however, is to work from posterior to anterior, as follows.

The sheath of the porta hepatis is opened laterally. Dissection is then performed in the plane between the CBD and the portal vein. To facilitate this dissection, the CBD is elevated by applying forward traction to the ligated cystic duct. The portal vein is then followed cephalad until its bifurcation into the left and right portal veins is visible. In a small percentage of patients, the left portal vein arises from the right anterior branch of the portal vein. If the main right portal vein is ligated in a patient who exhibits this anatomic variant, the portion of the liver remaining after resection will lack any portal flow. There is usually a small portal branch that passes from the main right portal vein to the caudate process. Ligation of this branch untethers another 1 to 2 cm of the right portal vein, thereby allowing safer dissection and ligation. The right portal vein is usually clamped with vascular clamps, divided, and oversewn with nonabsorbable sutures. Once this is done, the right hepatic artery is visible behind the CBD and can easily be secured and ligated with nonabsorbable sutures. Because of the multitude of biliary anatomic variations, we usually leave the right hepatic duct intact until parenchymal dissection [*see Step 8, below*] is begun, when this structure can be secured higher within the hepatic parenchyma and divided with greater safety.

Staple ligation Vascular staplers may be used for stapling the right or the left portal vein during extrahepatic vascular dissection[33,34]; however, suture ligation of the extrahepatic portal veins is such a straightforward technical exercise that staplers add little except cost.

Step 6—Alternative (Intrahepatic Pedicle Ligation): Control of Inflow Vessels

The observations of Glisson and Couinard (see above) that the nutrient vessels to the liver are contained within a thick connective tissue capsule [*see Figure 6*] were the basis for the initial proposal by Launois and Jamieson[11] that intrahepatic vascular pedicle ligation could serve as an alternative to extrahepatic dissection and ligation for controlling vascular inflow to the liver. This alternative technique has the advantages of being rapid and of being unlikely to cause injury to the vasculature or the biliary drainage of the contralateral liver. Given adequate intrahepatic definition and control of the portal triads supplying the area of the liver to be resected, one can readily isolate the various major pedicles by using simple combinations of hepatotomies at specific sites on the inferior surface of the liver [*see Figure 7*].

The right liver is completely mobilized from the retroperitoneum. The most inferior small hepatic veins are ligated, and the inferior right liver is mobilized off the vena cava. Incisions are then made in the liver capsule at hepatotomy sites A and B [*see Figure 7*]. The first incision is made though the caudate process. The full thickness of the caudate process is divided with a combination of diathermy, crushing, and ligation. The second incision is made almost vertically in the medial part of the gallbladder bed. Both incisions must be fairly substantial and reasonably deep. Care must be taken to avoid the terminal branches of the middle hepatic vein, which are the most common source of significant bleeding. By means of either finger dissection or the passage of a large curved clamp, a tape is then placed around the right main sheath [*see Figure 8*]. This tape can be pulled medial-

Figure 5 **Right lobectomy. For control of the inflow vessels of the right liver, the liver is retracted cephalad to allow exposure of the porta hepatis. (*a*) The gallbladder is resected to allow access to the bile duct and hepatic vessels. (*b*) The right hepatic duct is ligated to allow access to the hepatic artery and the portal vein. (*c*) After the right hepatic artery is divided, the right portal vein is controlled and divided. Alternatively, the vessels may be approached from a posterolateral direction and the portal vein and hepatic artery may be divided first, with the hepatic duct left intact until the parenchymal transection.**

ly to provide better exposure of the intrahepatic right pedicle and to retract the left biliary tree and portal vein away from the area to be clamped and divided. Clamps are then applied, the right pedicle is divided, and the stumps are suture-ligated.

In practice, for right lobectomies, we prefer to isolate the right anterior and posterior pedicles separately [*see Figure 8*] and ligate them individually. This measure ensures that the left-side structures cannot be injured. Any minor bleeding from a hepatotomy

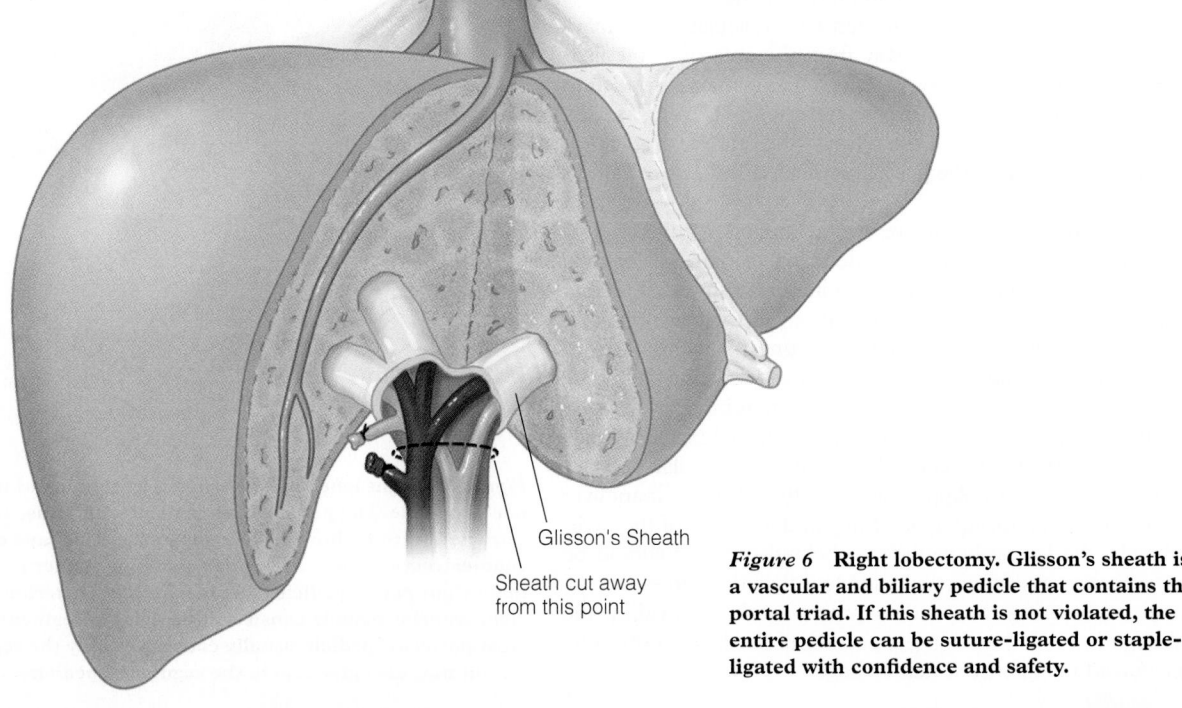

Glisson's Sheath

Sheath cut away from this point

Figure 6 **Right lobectomy. Glisson's sheath is a vascular and biliary pedicle that contains the portal triad. If this sheath is not violated, the entire pedicle can be suture-ligated or staple-ligated with confidence and safety.**

Figure 7 **Right lobectomy. Depicted are sites where hepatotomies can be made to permit isolation of various vascular pedicles. Incisions at sites A and B allow isolation of the right main portal pedicle. Incisions at sites A and D allow isolation of the right posterior portal pedicle. Incisions at sites B and D allow isolation of the right anterior pedicle. Incisions at sites C and E allow isolation of the left main portal pedicle; if the caudate is to be removed, incisions are made at sites C and F.**

usually ceases spontaneously or else stops when Surgicel is placed into the wound.

Staple ligation   The use of staplers is now well established for liver resections,[33-38] and we find that staple ligation greatly increases the speed with which intrahepatic portal pedicle ligations can be performed. To control the intrahepatic portal pedicles for a right lobectomy, incisions are made at hepatotomy sites A and B [*see Figure 7*]. Ultrasonography directed from the inferior aspect of the liver helps determine the depth at which the right pedicle lies, which is usually 1 to 2 cm from the inferior surface. The right main pedicle is then secured either digitally or with a curved blunt clamp (e.g., a renal pedicle clamp), and an umbilical tape is placed around it [*see Figure 9a*]. The hilar plate in the back of segment 4 is lowered via an incision at hepatotomy site C [*see Figure 7*] to ensure that the left-side vascular and biliary structures are mobilized well away from the area of staple ligation. A transverse anastomosis (TA) vascular stapler is applied to the right main pedicle while firm countertraction is being applied to the umbilical tape to pull the hilus to the left [*see Figure 9a*]. The stapler is fired, and the pedicle is divided [*see Figure 9b*].

Troubleshooting   There are several important guiding principles that should be followed in deciding on and performing intrahepatic pedicle ligation. The most important principle is that in patients undergoing operation for cancer, an intrahepatic pedicle approach should not be used when a tumor is within 2 cm of the hepatic hilus. In such cases, extrahepatic dissection should be performed to avoid violation of the tumor margin.

From a technical standpoint, removal of the gallbladder greatly facilitates isolation and control of right-side vascular pedicles in a right lobectomy. Application of the Pringle maneuver decreases bleeding during hepatotomy and isolation of the pedicle. Finally, the lowest hepatic veins behind the liver should be dissected before any attempt is made to isolate the right-side portal pedicles: incising the caudate process without dividing the small hepatic veins draining this portion of the liver to the vena cava can lead to significant hemorrhage.

Step 7: Control of Outflow Vessels

Control of the outflow vasculature begins with division of the hepatic veins passing from the posterior aspect of the right liver directly to the vena cava. After the right lobe is completely mobilized off the retroperitoneum by dividing the right triangular ligament, it is carefully dissected off the vena cava. Dissection proceeds upward from the inferior border of the liver until the right hepatic vein is exposed. Complete mobilization of the right liver

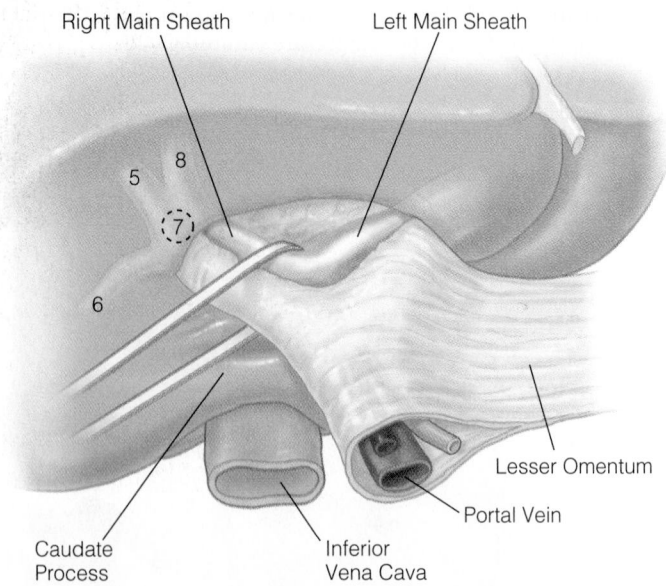

Figure 8   **Right lobectomy. Depicted is isolation of the main right portal pedicle. The pedicle is controlled with a vascular tape and retracted from within the liver substance. This tape can be used for countertraction when a vascular clamp or stapler is applied. The main right portal pedicle has anterior and posterior branches. The right anterior pedicle consists of pedicles to segments 5 and 8. The right posterior pedicle usually consists of only the segment 6 pedicle but may also give rise to the segment 7 pedicle.**

a
b

Figure 9 Right lobectomy. Shown is staple ligation of the right portal pedicle. (*a*) After the liver is incised across the caudate process and along the gallbladder bed, the right main pedicle is isolated and held with an umbilical tape. Countertraction is placed on the umbilical tape while a TA vascular stapler is placed across the pedicle, allowing the left hepatic duct and the left vascular structures to be retracted away from the line of stapling. (*b*) After the stapler is fired, the pedicle is clamped and divided.

is particularly critical for tumors close to the vena cava. The right hepatic vein is then isolated, cross-clamped, divided, and oversewn [*see Figure 10*]. Unless the tumor or lesion involves the middle hepatic vein close to its junction with the vena cava, the middle hepatic vein usually is not controlled extrahepatically for right-side resections and is easily secured during parenchymal transection.

If there is a large tumor residing at the dome of the liver, gaining control of the hepatic veins and the vena cava may prove very difficult. If so, one should not hesitate to extend the incision to the chest by means of a right thoracoabdominal extension. The morbidity of a thoracoabdominal incision is preferable to the potentially catastrophic hemorrhage that is sometimes encountered when the right hepatic vein is torn during mobilization of a rigid right hepatic lobe containing a large tumor.

Staple ligation Staple ligation has proved useful for outflow control during hepatectomy. When the tumor is in proximity to the hepatic vein–vena cava junction, extrahepatic control of the hepatic veins is essential for excision of the tumor with clear margins, and it limits blood loss during parenchymal transection.[39] Ligating the hepatic veins, particularly with a large and rigid tumor in the vicinity, can be a technically demanding and dangerous exercise. Tearing the hepatic vein or the vena cava during this maneuver is the most common cause of major intraoperative hemorrhage.[27] The endoscopic gastrointestinal anastomosis (GIA) stapler is well suited for ligation of the major hepatic veins in that it has a low profile and is capable of simultaneously sealing both the hepatic vein stump on the vena cava side and the one on the specimen side.

For staple ligation of the right hepatic vein, the right liver is mobilized off the vena cava. Any large accessory right hepatic

Vena Cava

Figure 10 Right lobectomy. Once the small perforating vessels to the vena cava have been ligated, further dissection cephalad leads to the right hepatic vein. This vessel is controlled with vascular clamps and divided.

Figure 11 Right lobectomy. As an alternative to clamping and division, the right hepatic vein may be staple-ligated. Once the small perforating tributaries from the right liver to the vena cava have been divided, the right hepatic vein is isolated and ligated with an endoscopic GIA vascular stapler. The safest method for introducing this stapler is to retract the liver cephalad and to the left while advancing the stapler cephalad in the direction of the vena cava.

vein encountered can be staple-ligated, as can the tongue of liver tissue that often passes from the right lobe behind the vena cava to the caudate lobe. The right hepatic vein is then identified and isolated. It is the practice of some authors to introduce the stapler from the top of the liver downward,[34] but we find that in most patients, the liver is sufficiently high in the surgical wound

to render this angle of introduction technically impracticable. Accordingly, we introduce the stapler parallel to the vena cava and direct it from below upward [see Figure 11]. To ensure that the stapler does not misfire, care should be taken to confirm that no vascular clips are near the site where the stapler is applied.

Step 8: Parenchymal Transection

Inflow to the left liver is temporarily interrupted by clamping the hepatoduodenal ligament (the Pringle maneuver) [see III:7 *Injuries to the Liver, Biliary Tract, Spleen, and Diaphragm*]. The safety of temporary occlusion of the vessels supplying the hepatic remnant is well documented. Even in patients with cirrhosis, the warm ischemia produced by continuous application of the Pringle maneuver is well tolerated for as long as 1 hour.[40] Our practice is to apply the Pringle maneuver intermittently for periods of 10 minutes, with 2 to 5 minutes of perfusion between applications to allow decompression of the gut.

Parenchymal division is then begun along the line demarcated by the devascularization of the right liver. The line of transection along the principal plane is marked with the electrocautery and then cut with scissors. Stay sutures of 0 chromic catgut are placed on either side of the plane of transection and used for traction, separation, and elevation as dissection proceeds.

Many special instruments have been proposed for use in parenchymal transection, including electrocauteries, ultrasonic dissectors, and water-jet dissectors. We find that for the majority of hepatic resections, blunt clamp dissection is the most rapid method and is quite safe. In essence, a large Kelly clamp is used to crush the liver parenchyma [see Figure 12]. The relatively soft liver substance dissects away, leaving behind the vascular and biliary structures, which are then ligated. With this technique, the principal plane of the liver can usually be transected in less than 30 minutes.

In cirrhotic patients, the clamp-crushing technique may not work as well because of the firmness of the liver substance: the vessels often tear before the parenchyma does. Accordingly, in

Figure 12 Right lobectomy. The parenchyma can be quickly and safely transected by means of the clamp-crushing technique. Large vessels and biliary radicles are visualized and ligated or clipped. This is usually done in tandem with inflow occlusion (i.e., the Pringle maneuver). Alternatively, the parenchyma can be bluntly dissected away by means of the finger-fracture technique.

cirrhotic patients, ultrasonic dissectors that coagulate while transecting the parenchyma may be a better choice. Water-jet dissectors may be useful in defining the major intrahepatic vascular pedicles or the junction of the hepatic vein and the vena cava, particularly if tumor is in close proximity.

After the specimen is removed, the raw surface of the hepatic remnant is carefully examined for hemostasis and bile leaks. Any oozing from the raw surface may be controlled with the argon beam coagulator. Biliary leaks should be controlled with clipping or suture ligation. The retroperitoneal surfaces should also be examined carefully for hemostasis, and the argon beam coagulator should be used where necessary.

Step 9: Closure and Drainage

The abdominal wall is closed in one or two layers with continuous absorbable monofilament sutures. The skin is closed with staples or with subcuticular sutures. Drains are unnecessary in most routine cases[41]; sometimes, in fact, they may exert harmful effects by leading to ascending infection or fluid management problems if ascites develops. There are four clinical situations in which we will routinely place a drain: (1) clear biliary leakage, (2) an infected operative field, (3) a thoracoabdominal incision, and (4) biliary reconstruction. In the case of the thoracoabdominal incision, a drain is placed to ensure that biliary leakage does not develop into a fistula into the chest.

LEFT LOBECTOMY

Steps 1 through 5

Left lobectomy involves removal of segments 2, 3, 4, and sometimes 1. The first five steps of the procedure are much the same as those of a right lobectomy.

Step 6 (Extrahepatic Dissection and Ligation): Control of Inflow Vessels

Extrahepatic control of vascular inflow vessels can be achieved in essentially the same fashion in a right-side resection. Our preference is to start the dissection at the base of the umbilical fissure. The left hepatic artery is divided first. The left branch of the portal vein is then easily identified at the base of the umbilical fissure. The point at which the left portal vein is to be divided depends on the extent of the planned parenchymal resection [see Figure 13]: if the caudate lobe is to be preserved, the left portal vein is ligated just distal to its caudate branch (line B); if the caudate lobe is to be removed, the left portal vein is ligated proximal to the origins of the portal venous branches to this lobe (line A).

Step 6—Alternative (Intrahepatic Pedicle Ligation): Control of Inflow Vessels

If the hepatectomy is being done to treat benign disease or to remove a malignancy that is remote from the base of the umbilical fissure, we highly recommend performing stapler-assisted pedicle ligation in preference to extrahepatic dissection and ligation.

The left portal pedicle is identified at the base of the umbilical fissure. The hilar plate is lowered through an incision at hepatotomy site C [see Figure 7], and a second incision is made in the back of segment 2 at hepatotomy site E [see Figure 7], thereby allowing isolation of the left portal pedicle with minimal risk of injury to the hilus. If the caudate lobe is to be removed as well, incisions should be made at hepatotomy sites C and F [see Figure 7] to allow isolation of the main left portal pedicle proximal to the vessels nourishing the caudate. The portal pedicle is isolated and secured with an umbilical tape. There is some risk that in the

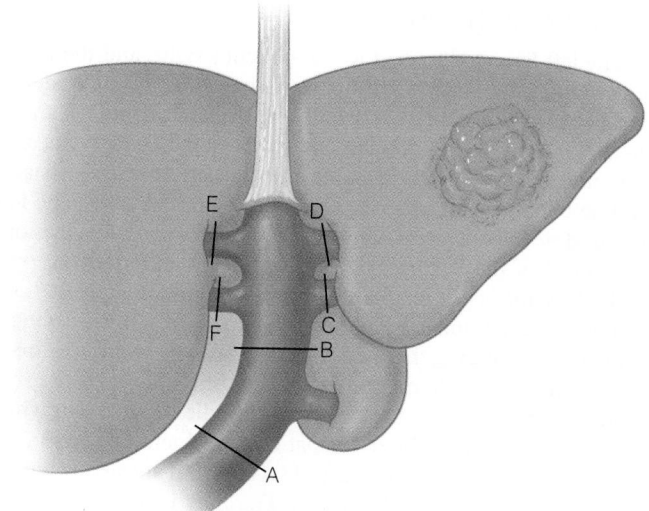

Figure 13 Left lobectomy. Ligation of vascular pedicles at specific sites in the left liver interrupts inflow to specific areas. Ligation at A interrupts inflow to the entire left liver, including the caudate lobe. Ligation at B interrupts blood flow to the left liver while sparing the caudate lobe. Ligation at C devascularizes segment 2, and ligation at D devascularizes segment 3. Ligation at E and F devascularizes segment 4.

course of securing the left portal pedicle, the middle hepatic vein, which lies immediately lateral to the left portal pedicle, may be injured. To minimize this risk, firm downward traction is applied to the umbilical tape, and a TA-30 vascular stapler is placed across the left portal pedicle [see Figure 14]. The pedicle is then stapled and divided.

Figure 14 Left lobectomy. After hepatotomies in segment 4 and in the back of segment 2, the left portal pedicle is isolated, stapled, and divided.

Step 7: Control of Outflow Vessels

The left liver is retracted to the patient's right, and the entire lesser omentum is divided. The ligamentum venosum is identified between the caudate lobe and the back of segment 2 and is then divided near its attachment to the left hepatic vein; this measure facilitates identification and dissection of the left and middle hepatic veins anterior to the inferior vena cava. The left and middle hepatic veins are isolated in preparation for division.

Control of the left hepatic vein is quickly and safely accomplished by means of stapled ligation. In approximately 60% of patients, the left and middle hepatic veins join to form a single trunk before entering the vena cava. In a left lobectomy, the middle hepatic vein is often left intact; accordingly, if this is the surgeon's intent, it is vital to protect the middle hepatic vein while ligating the left. After the left hepatic vein is identified, an endoscopic GIA-30 vascular stapler is directed from above downward [see Figure 15] to ligate this vessel. The liver is retracted to the right to permit visualization of the junction of the left and middle hepatic veins. If ligation of the middle hepatic vein is desired as well, as is the case when there is tumor in proximity to the vessel, this can be accomplished with a stapler directed along the same path used for left hepatic vein ligation.

Steps 8 and 9

Parenchymal transection and closure are accomplished in much the same manner in a left lobectomy as in a right lobectomy (see above).

OTHER ANATOMIC RESECTIONS

In the ensuing discussion of the other major anatomic resections, we focus primarily on the major points in which they differ from right and left lobectomy. More detailed discussions of these operations are available in specialty texts on liver resection.[26,27]

Extended Right Hepatectomy (Right Trisegmentectomy)

An extended right hepatectomy involves removal of the right lobe along with segment 4—that is, all liver tissue to the right of the falciform ligament [see Figure 3c]. The initial steps of this operation are the same as those of a right lobectomy, up through division of the right inflow vessels and the right hepatic vein.

The next step is devascularization of segment 4. The umbilical fissure is dissected to permit identification of the vascular pedicles to segments 2, 3, and 4, which lie within this fissure [see Figure 13]. In most cases, the lower part of the umbilical fissure is concealed by a bridge of liver tissue fusing segments 2 and 3 to segment 4. After this tissue bridge is divided with diathermy, the ligamentum teres is retracted caudally to reveal the vascular pedicles from the umbilical fissure to segment 4 (lines E and F [see Figure 13]). We generally suture-ligate these pedicles before dividing them.

The liver tissue is then transected immediately to the right of the falciform ligament, from the anterior surface back toward the divided right hepatic vein. The middle hepatic vein is generally left intact until it is encountered in the upper part of the dissection, at which point it is controlled and either suture- or staple-ligated.

Left Lateral Segmentectomy

A left lateral segmentectomy involves removal of only segments 2 and 3—that is, all liver tissue to the left of the falciform ligament [see Figure 3d]. These segments are mobilized by dividing the left falciform and triangular ligaments. As this is done, care

Figure 15 Left lobectomy. Staple ligation of the left hepatic vein. After the left lobe is completely mobilized through division of the left triangular ligament and the lesser omentum, the left hepatic vein is isolated and ligated with an endoscopic GIA vascular stapler. The best angle for introducing the stapler is from the xiphoid posteriorly and caudad.

Ligamentum Teres

Caudate Lobe

Vena Cava

must be taken not to injure the left hepatic and phrenic veins, which lie on the medial portion of the left triangular ligament.

The falciform ligament is retracted caudally, and the bridge of liver tissue between segment 4 and segments 2 and 3 is divided with diathermy. Dissection is then performed within the umbilical fissure to the left of the main triad. The vascular pedicles to segments 2 and 3 usually are then readily dissected and controlled (lines C and D [see Figure 13]). Control of these pedicles within the umbilical fissure is particularly important for tumor clearance if tumor is in proximity to the umbilical fissure: if the condition is benign or if tumor is remote from the umbilical fissure, the liver may be split anteroposteriorly just to the left of the ligamentum teres and the falciform ligament, and the vascular pedicles may be identified and ligated as they are encountered in the course of parenchymal transection.

Once the inflow vessels have been ligated, the left hepatic vein is identified and then divided either before parenchymal transection or as the vessel is encountered near the completion of parenchymal transection. If there is tumor near the dome, it is particularly important for tumor clearance that the left hepatic vein be controlled and ligated early and outside the liver.

Extended Left Hepatectomy (Left Trisegmentectomy)

An extended left hepatectomy involves resection of segments 2, 3, 4, 5, 8, and sometimes 1 [see Figure 3e]. In essence, it is a left lobectomy combined with a right anterior sectorectomy; it may or may not include excision of the caudate lobe. This complex resection is usually undertaken to excise large tumors that occupy the left lobe and cross the principal scissura into the right anterior sector.

In this procedure, it is essential to preserve the right hepatic vein, which constitutes the sole venous drainage of the hepatic remnant. Usually, however, parenchymal transection must be performed along the course of this vein; thus, the major potential danger in the operation is injury to the vessel, which could lead to hemorrhage or hepatic failure from venous congestion of the hepatic remnant. In addition, because the blood supply to segment 7 often arises from the right anterior portal pedicle or from the junction of the right anterior and posterior pedicles [see Figure 8], there is a risk that the operation may result in devascularization of a large portion of the hepatic remnant. Finally, because of the great variability of the biliary anatomy and the extensive intrahepatic dissection required in this procedure, there is a significant risk of biliary complications.[42] For all of these reasons, extended left hepatectomies are rarely performed outside major centers.[43]

In the planning of an extended left hepatectomy, particularly close attention must be paid to preoperative imaging investigations so that the right-side intrahepatic vessels and biliary structures can be accurately delineated. Thin-slice CT or MRI images in the form of arterial, portal venous, and hepatic venous reconstructions [see Figure 2] are quite helpful in this regard. For large tumors encroaching on the hepatic hilum or on the junction of the right anterior and posterior pedicles, direct angiography may still be necessary.

The liver is fully mobilized by dividing not only the left triangular ligament but also the ligaments on the right. This step is essential for identifying the correct plane of parenchymal dissection and for ensuring safe dissection along the right hepatic vein.

The initial dissection is the same as for a left lobectomy. The liver is turned to the right side and the portal triad approached. The inflow vessels to the left liver are ligated, and the left hepatic vein and the subdiaphragmatic inferior vena cava are dissected free. The left and middle hepatic veins are controlled and ligated in the extrahepatic portions of their courses.[43] The left liver is thereby freed, and dissection on the right liver is greatly facilitated.

Next, the plane of transection within the right liver is defined. This plane is horizontal and lies lateral to the gallbladder fossa and just anterior to the main right hepatic venous trunk in the right scissura, halfway between the right anterior pedicle and the right posterior pedicle. The plane can be approximated by drawing a line from just anterior to the right hepatic vein at its insertion into the vena cava to a point immediately behind the fissure of Gans. This line can be accurately defined by clamping the portal pedicle to the anterior right sector of the liver.[43] If the tumor is remote from the junction of the right anterior and posterior portal pedicles, the anterior pedicle is controlled as outlined earlier [see Right Lobectomy, Step 6—Alternative (Intrahepatic Pedicle Ligation), above]. A vascular clamp is placed on the pedicle and the line of demarcation on the liver surface inspected before the pedicle is divided. If segment 7 appears to be ischemic as well, further dissection must be done to identify and protect the origins of the vessels supplying segment 7.

Parenchymal dissection is then carried out from below upward, with bleeding controlled by means of low central venous pressure anesthesia and intermittent application of the Pringle maneuver. If the caudate lobe is to be removed as part of the total resection, the veins draining the caudate must be controlled before parenchymal transection.

Segment-Oriented Resection

Each segment of the liver can be resected independently. In addition, resections involving only the right posterior sector (segments 6 and 7) or the right anterior sector (segments 5 and 8) are not uncommon. Extensive and excellent descriptions of so-called segment-oriented hepatic resection are available elsewhere.[44,45]

Postoperative Care

I.V. fluids administered postoperatively should include phosphorus for support of liver regeneration. For large-volume hepatic resections, electrolyte levels, blood count, and prothrombin time (PT) are checked after the operation and then daily for 3 to 4 days. Packed red blood cells are administered if the hemoglobin level falls to 8 mg/dl or lower, and fresh frozen plasma is given if the PT is longer than 17 seconds. Postoperative pain control is best achieved with patient-controlled analgesia (PCA). Because of the decreased clearance of liver-metabolized drugs after a major hepatectomy, selection and dosing of pain medications should be adjusted accordingly. An oral diet can be resumed as early as postoperative day 3 unless a biliary-enteric anastomosis was performed.

Peripheral edema is common after major hepatic resections and may be treated with spironolactone. If an unexplained fever occurs or the bilirubin level rises when other hepatic function parameters are normal, an intra-abdominal bile collection may be present, and a CT scan should be obtained. Percutaneous drain placement usually brings about resolution of such collections after a few days; reoperation is rarely necessary.

Special Considerations

TOTAL VASCULAR ISOLATION FOR CONTROL OF BLEEDING

For control of bleeding during liver parenchymal transection, a technique known as total vascular isolation can be used as an alternative to the Pringle maneuver. In this technique, the liver is isolated by controlling the inferior vena cava (both above and below the liver), the portal vein, and the hepatic artery. This approach is based on techniques developed for liver transplantation and on the observation that the liver is capable of tolerating total normothermic ischemia for as long as 1 hour.[46] Its primary advantage is that while the liver is isolated, little or no bleeding occurs. It does, however, have disadvantages as well. In some patients, temporary occlusion of the inferior vena cava causes hemodynamic instability as a consequence of reduced cardiac output coupled with increased systemic vascular resistance.[47] Cardiac failure with marked hypotension, cardiac arrhythmia, and even cardiac arrest may ensue. In addition, when hepatic perfusion is restored, the sudden return of stagnant potassium-rich blood to the systemic circulation can aggravate the situation. For these reasons and because bleeding is generally well controlled with low central venous pressure anesthesia, we believe that total vascular isolation is useful only in rare cases. The clinical data published to date support this view. A prospective study from 1996 found that total vascular isolation had no major advantages over the approach described earlier [see Operative Technique, Right Lobectomy, Step 8, above] and was actually associated with greater blood loss.[39]

The one setting where we believe that total vascular isolation may have a significant role to play is in the surgical management of hepatic tumors, particularly very large tumors that compromise the vena cava or the hepatic veins. To extend the duration of vascular isolation in this setting, a venovenous bypass that vents the splanchnic blood into the systemic circulation may be used.[48] To further minimize parenchymal injury during vascular isolation, the liver may be perfused with cold organ preservation solutions. For extensive vascular invasion that necessitates major vena caval or hepatic venous reconstruction, some authors have suggested that the liver can be removed during venovenous bypass and resection and reconstruction performed extracorporeally.[49]

Although there are clinical situations that call for venovenous bypass and ex vivo resection, in practice, these techniques are very rarely necessary: short-length vena caval resection and reconstruction can be performed quite safely without resort to them. In fact, involvement of the retrohepatic vena cava at a level below the major hepatic veins can generally be treated with simple excision of the affected segment without replacement,[50] particularly if complete obstruction at this level has already led to established collateral circulation.

THE CIRRHOTIC PATIENT

Cirrhotic patients, by definition, have reduced hepatic functional capacity and reserve. Accordingly, these patients are at higher risk from hepatectomy and require careful assessment of liver function, appropriate selection for surgery and choice of operation, and greater attention to perioperative care.

Operative Planning

Selection of patients Hepatic failure is the major cause of hospital death and long-term morbidity after hepatic resection in cirrhotic patients.[51-55] Consequently, determination of a cirrhotic patient's candidacy for hepatectomy is based on preoperative assessment of baseline liver function.

A variety of tests have been proposed for assessment of hepatic reserve, including measurement of clearance of various dyes and metabolic substrates (e.g., indocyanine green[56,57] and aminopyrine[51]). Measurement of the urea-nitrogen synthesis rate has also been suggested as a way of predicting outcome after resection.[54] Another functional test involves administering lidocaine and measuring levels of monethylglycinexylidide (a metabolite of lidocaine that is generated mostly through the cytochrome P-450 enzyme system in the liver) as a gauge of liver function.[58] Measurement of the hepatic portal venous pressure gradient via invasive radiologic techniques has been found to predict postoperative hepatic failure.[59] Assessment of portal venous hemodynamics by means of noninvasive Doppler ultrasonography has also been found to predict outcome after hepatectomy.[60]

Currently, none of these functional tests are routinely done at most major liver resection centers. In practice, the Child-Pugh score [see II:6 *Jaundice*] is the most commonly employed clinical tool for selection of surgical candidates. A Child-Pugh score higher than 8 is generally accepted as a contraindication to major hepatic resection.[53,55,61-64]

Choice of procedure The appropriate extent of resection for cirrhotic patients may be quite different from that for noncirrhotic patients. In cirrhotic patients, the majority of hepatectomies are performed to eradicate hepatocellular carcinoma. A prime consideration in such resections is the margin needed to ensure tumor clearance. Most clinicians aim for a tumor-free margin of 1 cm. A 1989 study, however, found that in cirrhotic patients with hepatocellular carcinoma, as long as the tumor margin was microscopically clear of cancer, the exact size of the margin was not correlated with the incidence of recurrence.[65] In fact, the acceptance of limited margins, coupled with the acceptance of nonanatomic resections aimed at preserving as much functional parenchyma as possible, is the single change in technical practice that is most responsible for the great improvements in the safety of hepatic resection observed worldwide in cirrhotic patients.

The guiding principle for hepatectomy in cirrhotic patients is that limited resections should be favored, with as much functional parenchyma spared as possible. In general, even for patients with well-compensated Child's grade A cirrhosis, we try to limit resections to less than two segments of functional liver. Patients with large tumors are more likely to tolerate a major resection because little functional parenchyma must be removed along with the tumor. Major hepatic resections involving removal of at least one lobe are now reported to carry an operative mortality of less than 10% in cirrhotic patients.[66,67] Such procedures are usually performed in cirrhotic patients who have large tumors replacing most of one lobe, acceptable liver function, and no atrophy of the uninvolved lobe. Small tumors are often more difficult to manage. For patients with small, deeply placed tumors whose resection would necessitate removal of a large amount of functional parenchyma, an ablative alternative or even transplantation might be more suitable.

In an attempt to preserve as much functional liver as possible, many surgeons resort to more technically challenging operations. Most will perform multiple limited resections in order to avoid performing a full lobectomy.[68,69] Some go so far as to reconstruct the right hepatic vein for the purpose of preserving venous outflow in segments 5 and 6 after resection of segments 7 and 8.

Operative Technique

Hepatic resection in cirrhotic patients is associated with certain specific technical difficulties that substantially increase the complexity of the operation. The liver parenchyma is hard, which makes retraction of the liver difficult. In addition, anatomic landmarks are distorted and difficult to find as a consequence of fibrosis and atrophy-hypertrophy. Finally, portal hypertension and tissue friability contribute to increased blood loss during mobilization and parenchymal transection.

Exposure and mobilization Trifurcated incisions and thoracoabdominal incisions should be avoided in cirrhotic patients because of the potential for ascitic leakage externally or into the chest. The increased firmness of the cirrhotic liver and the consequent difficulty of retraction can lead to significant blood loss from retroperitoneal or phrenic collateral vessels during mobilization. To prevent such bleeding, it may be preferable to use an anterior approach in which the liver parenchyma is split within the principal interlobar plane down to the anterior surface of the vena cava before the right liver is mobilized off the retroperitoneum.[70] The right lobe is then mobilized in a medial-to-lateral direction, and the right hepatic vein is secured during mobilization of the right lobe off the vena cava.

Inflow control At one time, it was widely doubted whether the Pringle maneuver was safe in cirrhotic patients. Subsequently, however, many studies verified that this maneuver can be performed for extended periods in cirrhotic patients without increasing either morbidity or mortality.[71-76] Nevertheless, it is advisable to employ the Pringle maneuver sparingly in this population so as to minimize ischemic stress. Our practice is to clamp the portal triad with a vessel loop tourniquet for 10-minute periods with 5-minute breaks in between. We have not found additional protective maneuvers (e.g., topical cooling[77,78]) to be necessary.

Figure 16 Liver atrophy and hypertrophy occur after right portal vein embolization. Shown are images of the liver (*a*) at baseline and (*b*) 6 weeks after PVE. The right liver is outlined in white.

Parenchymal transection In patients with normal liver parenchyma, most experienced hepatic surgeons use blunt dissection, with either the clamp-crushing technique or the finger-fracture technique, to transect the liver tissue.[79] In patients with cirrhosis, however, the firmness of the parenchyma makes the clamp-crushing technique less than ideal: because the parenchyma is often harder than the underlying vasculature and biliary radicles, blunt dissection is likely to tear these vessels. Accordingly, ultrasonic dissectors that coagulate and seal vessels during dissection are more suitable for parenchymal transection in this population.

Closure and drainage Because of the likelihood of postoperative ascites, the abdominal wall is closed with a heavy continuous absorbable monofilament suture to create a watertight closure. To prevent major fluid and protein losses and ascending infections, abdominal drains generally are not used.[41] Reports specifically examining the role of drainage in cirrhotic patients documented a much lower incidence of postoperative complications and a shorter hospital stay for patients in whom no drains were placed.[80,81]

Postoperative Care

The focus of postoperative care in cirrhotic patients is on management of cirrhosis and portal hypertension. In most such patients who undergo hepatic resection, transient hepatic insufficiency develops postoperatively, with hyperbilirubinemia, ascites formation, hypoalbuminemia, edema, and worsening of the baseline coagulopathy.

In the first 24 hours after the procedure, crystalloid must be administered at a level sufficient to maintain adequate portal perfusion.[82] If patients are stable after the first 24 hours, they are subjected to water and sodium restriction and receive liberal amounts of salt-poor albumin for volume expansion if needed. Spironolactone is started in all patients as soon as oral diet is resumed; furosemide is added as needed. On rare occasions, a peritoneovenous shunt may have to be employed to control postoperative ascites,[83] but this measure is usually unnecessary if patients were properly selected. The PT is checked twice daily

during the immediate postoperative period: a PT longer than 17 seconds is corrected by administering fresh frozen plasma.

Preoperative Portal Vein Embolization

Most liver surgeons would be reluctant to resect more than the equivalent of two segments of functional liver in a patient with documented cirrhosis.[84] Consequently, many cirrhotic patients with technically resectable tumors are relegated to noncurative ablative therapy out of concern over possible postoperative hepatic failure. The situation may be changing, however, with the growing use of preoperative portal vein embolization (PVE), a technique that may extend surgeons' ability to resect tumor in cirrhotic patients.

In PVE, access to the portal vein on the side of the liver to be resected is gained via a percutaneous transhepatic approach. The vein is embolized approximately 1 month before the planned resection so as to produce ipsilateral atrophy along with compensatory hypertrophy of the contralateral future hepatic remnant.[85] The degree of compensatory hypertrophy can be dramatic [*see Figure 16*] and may modulate postoperative hepatic dysfunction. PVE is also employed in patients with normal parenchyma in whom extensive resection may result in a very small hepatic remnant. In patients undergoing extended right hepatectomy, particularly those with congenitally small left lateral sectors, the entire area of the extended hepatectomy, including the main right portal vein and the segmental branches supplying segment 4, can be embolized.[86]

There is substantial evidence that preoperative PVE can be successfully used in patients with cirrhotic livers or impaired liver function and that such use is generally well tolerated.[87-90] This technique can also serve as a test of the regenerative capacity of the hepatic remnant. If no compensatory hypertrophy is seen 4 weeks after PVE, the decision to perform a major hepatectomy should be reconsidered.

Repeat Hepatic Resection

Since 1984, when one of the first reports of repeat hepatic resection was published,[91] a number of reports from around the world have demonstrated that repeat resection can be done safely and with good long-term results even for recurrent malignancies. The morbidity rates and mortalities reported after repeat hepatectomy for metastatic colorectal cancer[92-104] and hepatocellular carcinoma[105-112] are comparable to those reported after initial hepatectomy. Extended survival has been demonstrated, and in some cases, the survival rate is equivalent to or even better than that observed after initial resection.[93,100,107,113] In the following section, we concentrate on the key technical aspects of repeat hepatic resection. Discussions of indications, patient selection, and outcome are available in other sources.[93,100,107,113]

Repeat hepatic resection poses certain technical difficulties that are not commonly encountered during initial resection.[92,114,115] First, adhesions at the previous line of parenchymal transection can make reexposure of the liver difficult. Mobilizing the liver off the vena cava and reexposing the porta hepatis and the hepatic veins can be extremely hazardous if dissection was previously done in these areas. Second, liver regeneration and systemic chemotherapy can induce accumulation of fat within the liver, thereby rendering it more friable[93]; the increased friability further increases the difficulties of reexposure and predisposes to tearing of Glisson's capsule.[114] Third, regeneration alters the normal anatomic configuration of the portal structures [see Figure 17].[116] For example, after a right hepatectomy, the porta hepatis is rotated posteriorly and to the right. The normal relationship among the portal structures is altered, with the bile duct displaced posteriorly and the portal vein displaced anteriorly.

Preoperative imaging is even more important for repeat resections than for primary resections. This is because scarring limits access to the liver for intraoperative assessment via palpation or ultrasonography. Before embarking on a repeat resection, it is essential to know the exact number and locations of the lesions to be treated within the regenerated parenchyma. Preoperative imaging also facilitates operative planning by accurately delineating the vasculature within the regenerated liver.

Figure 17 Repeat hepatic resection. Depicted are the changes in the relations of the portal structures that occur as a result of right liver atrophy or resection and left-side hypertrophy. The structures in the porta hepatis rotate to the right, with the CBD coming to rest laterally rather than anteriorly.

In a repeat resection after a previous major right hepatectomy, it is important to be prepared to convert the incision into a thoracoabdominal incision if necessary. Access through the right chest may be required for mobilization of the liver because of adherence of the previous resection margin to the diaphragm, or it may be required for access to the rotated CBD and portal vasculature at the porta hepatis.

In the dissection of the right upper quadrant after a previous right hepatectomy, three landmarks are particularly helpful in defining the anatomic structures within the regenerated left liver. The first landmark is remnants of the ligamentum teres, which defines the demarcation between the left lateral segment and segment 4; these should be found early on. The ligamentum teres may be followed to the base of the umbilical fissure to define the location of the left hepatic artery. Whether this artery arises from the common hepatic artery or from the left gastric artery, it passes into the liver parenchyma at the base of the umbilical fissure. The second landmark is the caudate lobe. The lesser omentum should be opened early on to reveal this lobe. An index finger should then be passed in front of the caudate toward the obliterated foramen of Winslow to define the porta hepatis and the location of the portal vein. The third landmark is the vena cava. Performing the Kocher maneuver to mobilize the duodenum off the vena cava allows this vessel to be dissected, thus further defining the portocaval plane. Definition of this plane leads to the correct plane for dissection and mobilization of the liver off the vena cava; it also allows isolation of the hepatoduodenal ligament for application of the Pringle maneuver and for extrahepatic dissection of the inflow vessels.

In a repeat resection after a previous left hepatectomy, the main concern with regard to mobilization of the liver is the anterior position of the portal vasculature after right-side hypertrophy. It is therefore prudent to mobilize the right liver, perform a Kocher maneuver, and follow the vena cava caudally to identify the portal vein from the right. The stomach and the colon usually are adherent to the edge of the previous resection and must be carefully dissected free to allow access to the liver. If the middle hepatic vein was preserved in the earlier left hepatectomy, it will lie immediately deep to the plane of the stomach or the colon and thus may be a source of hemorrhage during dissection.

Control of the inflow or outflow vasculature may be compromised by the scarring resulting from the previous operation. If extensive extrahepatic dissection was performed for control of inflow vasculature in the earlier procedure, control of these vessels in the repeat resection is more safely accomplished via intrahepatic pedicle ligation [see Operative Technique, Right Lobectomy, Step 6—Alternative (Intrahepatic Pedicle Ligation), above].

A major concern with repeat hepatectomy is that it is sometimes necessary to perform more limited resections than would otherwise be indicated. Normally, for removal of liver tumors, we avoid wedge excisions because these nonanatomic resections are more often associated with greater blood loss and positive margins than anatomic resections are.[99,117] In a repeat hepatectomy, however, anatomic considerations arising in the regenerated liver may make a wedge resection the best choice.

With appropriate patient selection and careful operative planning, very favorable perioperative and long-term results can be achieved after repeat hepatic resection. It is noteworthy that studies addressing repeat resection have not documented any substantial increases in blood loss, duration of operation, or rate of complications in comparison with the initial resection.[93-97,118]

Figure 18 **Hand-assisted laparoscopic hepatic resection. Introduction of the hand within the abdomen restores tactile sensation to the surgeon and facilitates resection of the liver. The hand is the best liver retractor available and can be used to dissect the parenchyma. The specimen can be extracted through the hand access port.**

Hand-Assisted Laparoscopic Hepatic Resection

In addition to revolutionizing treatment of gallstone disease,[119] laparoscopic techniques are increasingly used for fenestration of benign cysts of the liver[120,121] and for staging of hepatobiliary malignancies to prevent unnecessary laparotomies.[29,122,123] Until recently, however, laparoscopic resection of liver tumors was described only in case reports or small series.[120,124-128] Perhaps the main reason for the strong resistance to laparoscopic hepatic resection has been fear of catastrophic bleeding. If inadvertent damage to a major hepatic vein or the vena cava occurs during an open operation, the bleeding can be controlled with direct manual compression until the vessel is repaired; however, if such damage occurs during a laparoscopic operation, control of the bleeding is considerably more difficult. In addition, damage to a hepatic vein or the vena cava during a laparoscopic procedure can theoretically result in CO_2 embolism. Another concern is that the loss of tactile sensation characteristic of laparoscopic surgery may lead to inadequate tumor clearance. Finally, whereas there are many liver retractors designed to hold the liver in one position, there is no good retractor for repeatedly moving the liver from side to side, as would be necessary during a laparoscopic hepatectomy. The human hand is still the best tool for this purpose.

Laparoscopic hepatic resection has been greatly facilitated by several recent technologic advances, including laparoscopic staplers[129] and ultrasonic dissectors,[130] which can be used for ligation of the hepatic vasculature and transection of liver parenchyma. The most important advance, however, is the hand access port, a small port through which one hand can be introduced into the abdomen for a hand-assisted laparoscopic resection [see Figure 18].[131-133] With this approach, the surgeon not only regains a measure of tactile sensation but also is able to employ the best liver retractor available. Moreover, direct manual compression of any bleeding vessels is once again possible, and the incision made for the hand access port is also used for extraction of the resected specimen.

Patient selection is essential for safe laparoscopic resection of liver tumors. Resection of any two segments along the lower edge of the liver is easily accomplished laparoscopically. At MSKCC, we have laparoscopically resected lesions from all segments.[38]

The procedure starts with the placement of a 10 mm port, usually in the right or left upper quadrant on the side opposite that on which the hand access port will be placed. After staging is performed to ensure that the lesion is resectable, a 5 to 6 cm incision is made for placement of the hand access port. The port site should be chosen so as to allow manual retraction of the part of the liver to be resected, with the falciform and triangular ligaments used to provide countertraction. Once the access port is in place, the abdomen is fully palpated under laparoscopic vision. A laparotomy sponge is placed into the abdomen to facilitate retraction and absorb blood, and a long bulldog clamp is inserted for use in the Pringle maneuver. A long umbilical tape is tied to the bulldog clamp beforehand so that the instrument can be easily located throughout the procedure. Additional ports are then placed as necessary for introduction of the stapler or the ultrasonic scalpel.

The area to be resected is outlined with the electrocautery. The liver is manually retracted, intermittent application of the Pringle maneuver is initiated, and the parenchyma is transected. Liver parenchyma remote from the major portal pedicles and hepatic veins may be transected either with the ultrasonic dissector or by means of finger fracture. Near the major portal pedicles and hepatic veins, an endoscopic GIA vascular stapler may be used. After removal of the specimen, the laparoscopic argon beam coagulator (Conmed Corporation, Utica, New York) and hemostatic agents may be used.

The laparoscopic approach is suitable for minor as well as major hepatic resections. At present, however, it is unclear whether this approach constitutes a significant advance in liver surgery. To clarify this issue, further study of laparoscopic hepatic resection with respect to perioperative outcome, quality of life, and long-term survival is required.

References

1. Lortat-Jacob JL, Robert HG: Hepatectomie droite reglee. Presse Med 60:549, 1952

2. Fong Y: Hepatic colorectal metastasis: current surgical therapy, selection criteria for hepatectomy, and role for adjuvant therapy. Adv Surg 34:351, 2000

3. Jarnagin WR, Fong Y, Blumgart LH: The current management of hilar cholangiocarcinoma. Adv Surg 33:345, 1999

4. Fong Y, Sun RL, Jarnagin W, et al: An analysis of 412 cases of hepatocellular carcinoma at a Western center. Ann Surg 229:790, 1999

5. Couinaud C: Bases anatomiques des hepatectomies gauche et droite reglées. J Chir 70:933, 1954

6. Couinaud C: Le Foie: Etudes Anatomiques et Chirurgicales. Masson, Paris, 1957

7. Bismuth H: Surgical anatomy and anatomic surgery of the liver. World J Surg 6:3, 1982

8. Baer HU, Dennison AR, Maddern GJ, et al: Subtotal hepatectomy: a new procedure based on the inferior right hepatic vein. Br J Surg 78:1221, 1991

9. Smadja C, Blumgart LH: The biliary tract and the anatomy of biliary exposure. Surgery of the Liver and Biliary Tract, 2nd ed. Blumgart LH, Ed. Churchill Livingstone, London, 1994

10. Glisson F: Anatomia Hepatis. O Pullein, London, 1654

11. Launois B, Jamieson GG: The importance of Glisson's capsule and its sheaths in the intrahepatic approach to resection of the liver. Surg Gynecol Obstet 174:7, 1992

12. Soyer P, Levesque M, Elias D, et al: Preoperative assessment of resectability of hepatic metastases from colonic carcinoma: CT portography vs sonography and dynamic CT. AJR Am J Roentgenol 159:741, 1992

13. Hann LE, Schwartz LH, Panicek DM, et al: Tumor involvement in hepatic veins: comparison of MR imaging and US for preoperative assessment. Radiology 206:651, 1998

14. Hann LE, Fong Y, Shriver CD, et al: Malignant hepatic hilar tumors: can ultrasonography be used as an alternative to angiography with CT arterial portography for determination of resectability? J Ultrasound Med 15:37, 1996

15. Gibson RN, Yeung E, Thompson JN, et al: Bile duct obstruction: radiologic evaluation of level, cause and tumor resectability. Radiology 160:43, 1986

16. Fortner JG, Lincer RM: Hepatic resection in the elderly. Ann Surg 211:141, 1990

17. Karl RC, Smith SK, Fabri PJ: Validity of major cancer operations in elderly patients. Ann Surg Oncol 2:107, 1995

18. Fong Y, Blumgart LH, Fortner JG, et al: Pancreatic or liver resection for malignancy is safe and effective for the elderly. Ann Surg 222:426, 1995

19. Hanazaki K, Kajikawa S, Shimozawa N, et al: Hepatic resection for hepatocellular carcinoma in the elderly. J Am Coll Surg 192:38, 2001

20. Fong Y, Brennan MF, Cohen AM, et al: Liver resection in the elderly. Br J Surg 84:1386, 1997

21. Cunningham JD, Fong Y, Shriver C, et al: One hundred consecutive hepatic resections: blood loss, transfusion and operative technique. Arch Surg 129:1050, 1994

22. Melendez J, Ferri E, Zwillman M, et al: Extended hepatic resection: a 6-year retrospective study of risk factors for perioperative mortality. J Am Coll Surg 192:47, 2001

23. Scheele J, Stangl R, Altendorf-Hofmann A, et al: Indicators of prognosis after hepatic resection for colorectal secondaries. Surgery 110:13, 1991

24. Weber SM, Jarnagin WR, DeMatteo RP, et al: Survival after resection of multiple hepatic colorectal metastases. Ann Surg Oncol 7:643, 2000

25. Goldsmith NA, Woodburne RT: The surgical anatomy pertaining to liver resection. Surg Gynecol Obstet 105:310, 1957

26. Blumgart LH, Jarnagin W, Fong Y: Liver resection for benign disease and for liver and biliary tumors. Surgery of the Liver and Biliary Tract, 3rd ed. Blumgart LH, Fong Y, Eds. WB Saunders, London, 2000, p 1639

27. Blumgart LH, Fong Y: Surgical management of colorectal metastases to the liver. Curr Probl Surg 5:333, 1995

28. Jarnagin WR, Conlon K, Bodniewicz J, et al: A clinical scoring system predicts the yield of diagnostic laparoscopy in patients with potentially resectable hepatic colorectal metastases. Cancer 91:1121, 2001

29. Jarnagin WR, Bodniewicz J, Dougherty E, et al: A prospective analysis of staging laparoscopy in patients with primary and secondary hepatobiliary malignancies. J Gastrointest Surg 4:34, 2000

30. Lo CM, Lai EC, Liu CL, et al: Laparoscopy and laparoscopic ultrasonography avoid exploratory laparotomy in patients with hepatocellular carcinoma. Ann Surg 227:527, 1998

31. Callery MP, Strasberg SM, Doherty GM, et al: Staging laparoscopy with laparoscopic ultrasonography: optimizing resectability in hepatobiliary and pancreatic malignancy. J Am Coll Surg 185:33, 1997

32. Castaing D, Kunstlinger F, Habib N: Intraoperative ultrasound study of the liver: methodology and anatomical results. Am J Surg 149:676, 1985

33. McEntee GP, Nagorney DM: Use of hepatic staplers in major hepatic resections. Br J Surg 78:40, 1991

34. Cohen AM: Use of laparoscopic vascular stapler at laparotomy for colorectal cancer. Dis Colon Rectum 35:910, 1992

35. Jurim O, Colonna II JO, Colquhoun SD, et al: A stapling technique for hepatic resection. J Am Coll Surg 178:510, 1994

36. Yanaga K, Nishizaki T, Yamamoto K, et al: Simplified inflow control using stapling devices for major hepatic resection. Arch Surg 131:104, 1996

37. Lefor AT, Flowers JL: Laparoscopic wedge biopsy of the liver. J Am Coll Surg 178:307, 1994

38. Fong Y, Jarnagin W, Conlon KC, et al: Hand-assisted laparoscopic liver resection: lessons from an initial experience. Arch Surg 135:854, 2000

39. Belghiti J, Noun R, Zante E, et al: Portal triad clamping or hepatic vascular exclusion for major liver resection. Ann Surg 224:155, 1996

40. Bothe AJ, Steele G Jr: Is there a role for perioperative nutritional support in liver resection? HPB Surgery 10:177, 1997

41. Fong Y, Brennan MF, Brown K, et al: Drainage is unnecessary after elective liver resection. Am J Surg 171:158, 1996

42. Starzl TE, Iwatsuki S, Shaw BW, et al: Left hepatic trisegmentectomy. Surg Gynecol Obstet 155:21, 1982

43. Blumgart LH, Baer HU, Czerniak A, et al: Extended left hepatectomy: technical aspects of an evolving procedure. Br J Surg 80:903, 1993

44. Scheele J: Segment oriented resection of the liver: rationale and technique in hepato-biliary and pancreatic malignancies. Lygidakis NJ, Tytgat GNJ, Eds. Thieme, Stuttgart, 1989

45. Scheele J, Stangl R: Segment oriented anatomical liver resections. Surgery of the Liver and Biliary Tract. Blumgart LH, Ed. Churchill Livingstone, London, 1994

46. Huguet C, Nordlinger B, Gallopin JJ, et al: Normothermic hepatic vascular occlusion for extensive hepatectomy. Surg Gynecol Obstet 147:689, 1978

47. Pappas G, Palmer WM, Martineau GL, et al: Hemodynamic alterations caused during orthotopic liver transplantation in humans. Surgery 70:872, 1971

48. Shaw BW, Martin DJ, Marquez JM, et al: Venous bypass in clinical liver transplantation. Ann Surg 200:524, 1984

49. Pichlmayr R, Grosse H, Hauss J, et al: Technique and preliminary results of extracorporeal liver surgery (bench procedure) and of surgery on the in situ perfused liver. Br J Surg 77:21, 1990

50. Cunci O, Coste T, Vacher B, et al: Resection de la veine cave inferieure retro-hepatique au cours d'une hepatectomie pour tumeur. Ann Chir 37:197, 1983

51. Lau H, Man K, Fan ST, et al: Evaluation of preoperative hepatic function in patients with hepatocellular carcinoma undergoing hepatectomy. Br J Surg 84:1255, 1997

52. Takenaka K, Kanematsu T, Fukuzawa K, et al: Can hepatic failure after surgery for hepatocellular carcinoma in cirrhotic patients be prevented? World J Surg 14:123, 1990

53. Nagasue N, Yukaya H, Kohno H, et al: Morbidity and mortality after major hepatic resection in cirrhotic patients with hepatocellular carcinoma. HPB Surg 1:45, 1988

54. Paquet KJ, Koussouris P, Mercado MA, et al: Limited hepatic resection for selected cirrhotic patients with hepatocellular or cholangiocellular carcinoma: a prospective study. Br J Surg 78:459, 1991

55. Fan ST, Lai EC, Lo CM, et al: Hospital mortality of major hepatectomy for hepatocellular carcinoma associated with cirrhosis. Arch Surg 130:198, 1995

56. Hasegawa H, Yamazaki S, Makuuchi M, et al: [Hepatectomy for hepatocarcinoma on a cirrhotic liver: decision plans and principles of perioperative resuscitation. Experience with 204 cases.] J Chir (Paris) 124:425, 1987

57. Makuuchi M, Kosuge T, Takayama T, et al: Surgery for small liver cancers. Semin Surg Oncol 9:298, 1993

58. Ercolani G, Grazi GL, Calliva R, et al: The lidocaine (MEGX) test as an index of hepatic function: its clinical usefulness in liver surgery. Surgery 127:464, 2000

59. Bruix J, Castells A, Bosch J, et al: Surgical resection of hepatocellular carcinoma in cirrhotic patients: prognostic value of preoperative portal pressure. Gastroenterology 111:1018, 1996

60. Yin XY, Lu MD, Huang JF, et al: Significance of portal hemodynamic investigation in prediction of hepatic functional reserve in patients with hepatocellular carcinoma undergoing operative treatment. Hepatogastroenterology 48:1701, 2001

61. Franco D, Capussotti L, Smadja C, et al: Resection of hepatocellular carcinomas: results in 72 European patients with cirrhosis. Gastroenterology 98:733, 1990

62. Wu CC, Ho WL, Yeh DC, et al: Hepatic resection of hepatocellular carcinoma in cirrhotic livers: is it unjustified in impaired liver function? Surgery 120:34, 1996

63. Noun R, Jagot P, Farges O, et al: High preoperative serum alanine transferase levels: effect on

the risk of liver resection in Child grade A cirrhotic patients. World J Surg 21:390, 1997

64. Capussotti L, Borgonovo G, Bouzari H, et al: Results of major hepatectomy for large primary liver cancer in patients with cirrhosis. Br J Surg 81:427, 1994

65. Yoshida Y, Kanematsu T, Matsumata T, et al: Surgical margin and recurrence after resection of hepatocellular carcinoma in patients with cirrhosis: further evaluation of limited hepatic resection. Ann Surg 209:297, 1989

66. Vauthey JN, Klimstra D, Franceschi D, et al: Factors affecting long-term outcome after hepatic resection for hepatocellular carcinoma. Am J Surg 169:28, 1995

67. Poon RT, Fan ST, Lo CM, et al: Intrahepatic recurrence after curative resection of hepatocellular carcinoma: long-term results of treatment and prognostic factors. Ann Surg 229:216, 1999

68. Makuuchi M, Hasegawa H, Yamazaki S, et al: Four new hepatectomy procedures for resection of the right hepatic vein and preservation of the inferior right hepatic vein. Surg Gynecol Obstet 164:68, 1987

69. Makuuchi M, Mori T, Gunven P, et al: Safety of hemihepatic vascular occlusion during resection of the liver. Surg Gynecol Obstet 164:155, 1987

70. Lai EC, Fan ST, Lo CM, et al: Anterior approach for difficult major right hepatectomy. World J Surg 20:314, 1996

71. Nagasue N, Uchida M, Kubota H, et al: Cirrhotic livers can tolerate 30 minutes ischaemia at normal environmental temperature. Eur J Surg 161:181, 1995

72. Wu CC, Hwang CR, Liu TJ, et al: Effects and limitations of prolonged intermittent ischaemia for hepatic resection of the cirrhotic liver. Br J Surg 83:121, 1996

73. Kim YI, Kobayashi M, Aramaki M, et al: "Early-stage" cirrhotic liver can withstand 75 minutes of inflow occlusion during resection. Hepatogastroenterology 41:355, 1994

74. Kim YI, Nakashima K, Tada I, et al: Prolonged normothermic ischaemia of human cirrhotic liver during hepatectomy: a preliminary report. Br J Surg 80:1566, 1993

75. Smadja C, Kahwaji F, Berthoux L, et al: [Value of total pedicle clamping in hepatic excision for hepatocellular carcinoma in cirrhotic patients.] Ann Chir 41:639, 1987

76. Elias D, Desruennes E, Lasser P: Prolonged intermittent clamping of the portal triad during hepatectomy. Br J Surg 78:42, 1991

77. Yamanaka N, Furukawa K, Tanaka T, et al: Topical cooling-assisted hepatic segmentectomy for cirrhotic liver with hepatocellular carcinoma. J Am Coll Surg 184:290, 1997

78. Kim YI, Kobayashi M, Nakashima K, et al: In situ and surface liver cooling with prolonged inflow occlusion during hepatectomy in patients with chronic liver disease. Arch Surg 129:620, 1994

79. Lin TY: A simplified technique for hepatic resection: the crush method. Ann Surg 180:285, 1974

80. Smadja C, Berthoux L, Meakins JL, et al: Patterns of improvement in resection of hepatocellular carcinoma in cirrhotic patients: results of a non drainage policy. HPB Surg 1:141, 1989

81. Franco D, Smadja C, Meakins JL, et al: Improved early results of elective hepatic resection for liver tumors: one hundred consecutive hepatectomies in cirrhotic and noncirrhotic patients. Arch Surg 124:1033, 1989

82. Tsuge H, Mimura H, Orita K, et al: Evaluation of preoperative and postoperative sodium and water loading in patients undergoing hepatectomy for liver cirrhosis complicated by hepatocellular carcinoma. Hepatogastroenterology 38(suppl 1):56, 1991

83. Maeda T, Shimada M, Shirabe K, et al: Strategies for intractable ascites after hepatic resection: analysis of two cases. Br J Clin Pract 49:149, 1995

84. Shirabe K, Shimada M, Gion T, et al: Postoperative liver failure after major hepatic resection for hepatocellular carcinoma in the modern era with special reference to remnant liver volume. J Am Coll Surg 188:304, 1999

85. Makuuchi M, Thai BL, Takayasu K, et al: Preoperative portal embolization to increase safety of major hepatectomy for hilar bile duct carcinoma: a preliminary report. Surgery 107:521, 1990

86. Nagino M, Nimura Y, Kamiya J, et al: Right or left trisegmental portal vein embolization before hepatic trisegmentectomy for hilar bile duct carcinoma. Surgery 117:677, 1995

87. Shimamura T, Nakajima Y, Une Y, et al: Efficacy and safety of preoperative percutaneous transhepatic portal embolization with absolute ethanol: a clinical study. Surgery 121:135, 1997

88. Lee KC, Kinoshita H, Hirohashi K, et al: Extension of surgical indications for hepatocellular carcinoma by portal vein embolization. World J Surg 17:109, 1993

89. Wakabayashi H, Okada S, Maeba T, et al: Effect of preoperative portal vein embolization on major hepatectomy for advanced-stage hepatocellular carcinomas in injured livers: a preliminary report. Surg Today 27:403, 1997

90. Azoulay D, Castaing D, Krissat J, et al: Percutaneous portal vein embolization increases the feasibility and safety of major liver resection for hepatocellular carcinoma in injured liver. Ann Surg 232:665, 2000

91. Tomas de la Vega JE, Donahue EJ, Doolas A, et al: A ten year experience with hepatic resection. Surg Gynecol Obstet 159:223, 1984

92. Bismuth H, Adam R, Navarro F: Re-resection for colorectal liver metastasis. Surg Oncol Clin North Am 5:353, 1996

93. Adam R, Bismuth H, Castaing D, et al: Repeat hepatectomy for colorectal liver metastases. Ann Surg 225:51, 1997

94. Fong Y, Blumgart LH, Cohen A, et al: Repeat hepatic resections for metastatic colorectal cancer. Ann Surg 220:657, 1994

95. Petrowsky H, Gonen M, Jarnagin W, et al: Second liver resections are safe and effective treatment for recurrent hepatic metastases from colorectal cancer: a bi-institutional analysis. Ann Surg 235:863, 2002

96. Pinson CW, Wright JK, Chapman WC, et al: Repeat hepatic surgery for colorectal cancer metastases to the liver. Ann Surg 223:765, 1996

97. Tuttle TM, Curley SA, Roh MS: Repeat hepatic resection as effective treatment for recurrent colorectal liver metastases. Ann Surg Oncol 4:125, 1997

98. Nordlinger B, Vaillant JC, Guiguet M, et al: Survival benefit of repeat liver resections for recurrent colorectal metastases: 143 cases. J Clin Oncol 12:1491, 1994

99. Fernandez-Trigo V, Sharmsa F, Sugarbaker PH, et al: Repeat liver resections from colorectal metastasis. Surgery 117:296, 1995

100. Yamamoto J, Kosuge T, Shimada K, et al: Repeat liver resection for recurrent colorectal liver metastases. Am J Surg 178:275, 1999

101. Muratore A, Polastri R, Bouzari H, et al: Repeat hepatectomy for colorectal liver metastases: a worthwhile operation? J Surg Oncol 76:127, 2001

102. Suzuki S, Sakaguchi T, Yokoi Y, et al: Impact of repeat hepatectomy on recurrent colorectal liver metastases. Surgery 129:421, 2001

103. Riesener K-P, Kasperk R, Winkeltau G, et al: Repeat resection of recurrent hepatic metastases: improvement in prognosis? Eur J Surg 162:709, 1996

104. Kin T, Nakajima Y, Kanehiro H, et al: Repeat hepatectomy for recurrent colorectal metastases. World J Surg 22:1087, 1998

105. Farges O, Regimbeau JM, Belghiti J: Aggressive management of recurrence following surgical resection of hepatocellular carcinoma. Hepatogastroenterology 45(suppl 3):1275, 1998

106. Nagasue N, Kohno H, Hayashi T, et al: Repeat hepatectomy for recurrent hepatocellular carcinoma. Br J Surg 83:127, 1996

107. Neeleman N, Andersson R: Repeated liver resection for recurrent liver cancer. Br J Surg 83:893, 1996

108. Lee PH, Lin WJ, Tsang YM, et al: Clinical management of recurrent hepatocellular carcinoma. Ann Surg 222:670, 1995

109. Hu RH, Lee PH, Yu SC, et al: Surgical resection for recurrent hepatocellular carcinoma: prognosis and analysis of risk factors. Surgery 120:23, 1996

110. Shimada M, Takenaka K, Gion T, et al: Prognosis of recurrent hepatocellular carcinoma: a 10-year surgical experience in Japan. Gastroenterology 111:720, 1996

111. Shuto T, Kinoshita H, Hirohashi K, et al: Indications for, and effectiveness of, a second hepatic resection for recurrent hepatocellular carcinoma. Hepatogastroenterology 43:932, 1996

112. Shimada M, Takenaka K, Taguchi K, et al: Prognostic factors after repeat hepatectomy for recurrent hepatocellular carcinoma. Ann Surg 227:80, 1998

113. Sugimachi K, Maehara S, Tanaka S, et al: Repeat hepatectomy is the most useful treatment for recurrent hepatocellular carcinoma. J Hepatobiliary Pancreat Surg 8:410, 2001

114. Elias D, Lasser P, Hoang JM, et al: Repeat hepatectomy for cancer. Br J Surg 80:1557, 1993

115. Hemming AW, Langer B: Repeat resection of recurrent hepatic colorectal metastases. Br J Surg 81:1553, 1994

116. Blumgart LH, Baer HU: Hilar and intrahepatic biliary-enteric anastomosis. Surgery of the Liver and Biliary Tract. Blumgart LH, Ed. Churchill Livingstone, London, 1994, p 1051

117. Polk W, Fong Y, Karpeh M, et al: A technique for the use of cryosurgery to assist hepatectomy. J Am Coll Surg 180:171, 1995

118. Chu QD, Vezeridis MP, Avradopoulos KA, et al: Repeat hepatic resection for recurrent colorectal cancer. World J Surg 21:292, 1997

119. The Southern Surgeons Club: A prospective analysis of 1518 laparoscopic cholecystectomies. N Engl J Med 324:1073, 1991

120. Katkhouda N, Hurwitz M, Gugenheim J, et al: Laparoscopic management of benign solid and cycstic lesions of the liver. Ann Surg 229:460, 1999

121. Jeng KS, Yang FS, Kao CR, et al: Management of symptomatic polycystic liver disease: laparoscopy adjuvant with alcohol sclerotherapy. J Gastroenterol Hepatol 10:359, 1995

122. Cuesta MA, Meijer S, Borgstein PJ, et al: Laparoscopic ultrasonography for hepatobiliary and pancreatic malignancy. Br J Surg 80:1571, 1993

123. Ravikumar TS: Laparoscopic staging and intraoperative ultrasonography for liver tumor management. Surg Oncol Clin North Am 5:271, 1996

124. Asahara T, Dohi K, Nakahara H, et al: Laparoscopy-assisted hepatectomy for a large tumor of the liver. Hiroshima J Med Sci 47:163, 1998

125. Huscher CGS, Lirici MM, Chiodini S: Laparoscopic liver resections. Semin Laparosc Surg 5:204, 1998

126. Kaneko H, Takagi S, Shiba T: Laparoscopic partial hepatectomy and left lateral segmentectomy: technique and results of a clinical series. Surgery 120:468, 1996

127. Rau HG, Meyer G, Cohnert TU, et al: Laparoscopic liver resection with the water-jet dissector. Surg Endosc 9:1009, 1995

128. Yamanaka N, Tanaka T, Tanaka W, et al: Laparoscopic partial hepatectomy. Hepatogastroenterology 45:29, 1998

129. Fong Y, Blumgart LH: Useful stapling techniques in liver surgery. J Am Coll Surg 185:93, 1997

130. Jackman SV, Cadeddu JA, Chen RN, et al: Utility of the harmonic scalpel for laparoscopic partial nephrectomy. J Endourol 12:441, 1998

131. Wolf JSJ, Moon TD, Nakada SY: Hand assisted laparoscopic nephrectomy: comparison to standard laparoscopic nephrectomy. J Urol 160:22, 1998

132. Klingler PJ, Hinder RA, Menke DM, et al: Hand-assisted laparoscopic distal pancreatectomy for pancreatic cystadenoma. Surg Laparosc Endosc 8:180, 1998

133. Nakada SY, Moon TD, Gist M, et al: Use of the pneumo sleeve as an adjunct in laparoscopic nephrectomy. Urology 49:612, 1997

Acknowledgment

Figures 1, 3 through 15, 17, 18   Tom Moore.

VI   SPECIAL PERIOPERATIVE PROBLEMS

1 PULMONARY INSUFFICIENCY

Robert H. Bartlett, M.D.

Approach to Pulmonary Insufficiency

Prevention of Postoperative Pulmonary Insufficiency

Pulmonary insufficiency is the most common complication occurring after operative procedures. It ranges in incidence from five to 50 percent and in severity from minor atelectasis to lethal acute respiratory distress syndrome (ARDS). The lungs are extremely vulnerable in the postoperative period because both ventilation (the anatomy and physiology of breathing) and pulmonary circulation (the anatomy and physiology of the pulmonary endothelium and interstitium) are affected by all the events surrounding tissue injury, anesthesia, and tissue dissection.[1] Abnormal ventilation leads to alveolar collapse, decreased functional residual capacity (FRC), and atelectasis. Abnormal capillary homeostasis leads to lung edema. ARDS comprises a combination of atelectasis and edema, with edema predominating. The term ARDS will be used sparingly in this discussion, to describe the occurrence of pulmonary edema caused by increased capillary permeability.

This discussion will describe the care of patients at risk for pulmonary complications, including the clinical presentation, pathogenesis, prevention, recognition, and treatment of pulmonary insufficiency. Atelectasis and lung edema will be considered as separate events, although it is obvious that the two abnormalities can and do occur simultaneously in the postoperative period. Disorders of the pulmonary parenchyma will be emphasized, as opposed to pulmonary insufficiency secondary to such conditions as cardiac disease, thromboembolism, and central nervous system depression, all of which are covered elsewhere. This discussion is limited to mild pulmonary insufficiency; major insufficiency is discussed elsewhere in this text [*see VII:3 Pulmonary Dysfunction*].

Preoperative Pulmonary Function Testing

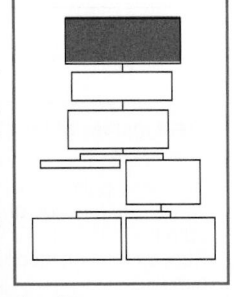

Preoperative assessment of respiratory status is important because identification of high-risk patients can minimize the incidence of pulmonary complications. The history is the most valuable step. Indications for detailed study of pulmonary function include exercise intolerance, dyspnea on exertion, wheezing, cigarette smoking, cough, and sputum production.

Physical examination should include auscultation and percussion of the lung bases during tidal breathing and maximal inspiration to detect hypoventilation in weak or debilitated patients and hyperinflation in patients with chronic airway dis-

ease. The presence of wheezing, rales, or rhonchi should trigger further examination. Any signs of cardiac insufficiency, obesity, clubbing, tobacco stains, or poor oral hygiene are all relative indications for more detailed pulmonary function testing. A chest x-ray should be considered part of the routine physical examination for any patients with an abnormality detected from the history or the physical examination, any patient scheduled to undergo a thoracotomy, and any patient at risk for cardiac or pulmonary disease because of age (i.e., persons older than approximately 60 years).

As part of every physical examination, the patient should be instructed to inhale to the maximum, followed by a vigorous forced expiration (a vital capacity maneuver). Observation of the chest and the sound of the forced expiration can enable the surgeon to estimate the volume of inspiration (in normal adults, at least 1 L/50 kg), forced expiration (in normal adults, at least 2 L/50 kg), and expiratory flow (most of the exhaled volume should come out in the first second without wheezing). The forced expiratory volume (or vital capacity) and the maximum voluntary ventilation (MVV, or maximal breathing capacity) can be directly measured with a handheld turbine spirometer.

Strength and endurance can be estimated by stair climbing.[2] A patient who cannot climb two flights of stairs at a steady pace without dyspnea may have respiratory, cardiac, or joint disease or may be too obese, too weak, too sedentary, or too debilitated to manage mild exercise. Whatever the cause, more detailed evaluation is indicated.

Breathing maneuvers to accomplish maximal inflation must be carefully taught to the patient preoperatively [*see* Postoperative Measures to Prevent Pulmonary Insufficiency, Routine Measures, *below*]. Most patients cannot learn breathing exercises in a painful, narcotized, postoperative state.

Pulmonary function tests (e.g., spirometry) should be performed whenever the history, physical examination, or bedside tests indicate major abnormalities of pulmonary function. The measurements obtained for tidal volume, inspiratory capacity, vital capacity (total and timed intervals), and MVV are compared with tables for normal persons of the same age, sex, and size and the values reported as percentages of the predicted normal. Values of 80 to 120 percent of what was predicted are considered normal. If these tests of lung volume and flow are within the normal range, the risk of pulmonary complications is small—although the tests do not measure endurance. Abnormally high values are not important. Values below 70 percent of predicted indicate one or more of the following: a low expiratory flow rate indicative of small airway or obstructive lung disease, a low vital capacity indicative of loss of lung vol-

Assess pulmonary function preoperatively

Review history; perform physical exam. Evaluate for wheezing, rales, and rhonchi; cough and sputum production; cardiac insufficiency; and obesity. Estimate volume of inspiration, forced expiration, and expiratory flow.

Obtain chest x-ray if abnormality is detected, thoracotomy is planned, or patient is at risk for cardiac or pulmonary disease because of age (e.g., > 60 years).

If pulmonary dysfunction is suspected:

- Measure tidal volume, inspiratory capacity, vital capacity, and maximum voluntary ventilation.
- Obtain baseline blood gas measurements.
- In special circumstances: Measure functional residual capacity. Assess for chronic fibrotic disease. Obtain ventilation-perfusion lung scan if pulmonary resection is contemplated.

Correct abnormalities, and prepare patient before operation

Teach breathing maneuvers, and exercise patient's respiratory muscles.
Reduce risk factors (e.g., smoking).
Assess effects of bronchodilators in patients with bronchospasm.
Provide adequate nutrition.
Augment left ventricular function pharmacologically if signs of LV failure exist.

Follow a pulmonary prophylaxis regimen during and after operation

Inflate all alveoli regularly:

- Use breathing exercise with incentive spirometer. Use intermittent positive pressure breathing (IPPB) if necessary.
- Use mechanical ventilation in high-risk patients.
- Use bronchodilators for bronchospasm.

Maintain normal body fluid volume and composition:

- Give blood and fluids as needed, but not excessively.
- If fluid overload is unavoidable, diurese when stable.

Minimize the risk of venous thrombosis and pulmonary embolism.

Postoperative pulmonary insufficiency does not develop

Postoperative pulmonary insufficiency develops (e.g., dyspnea, tachypnea, tachycardia, confusion, cyanosis, abnormal x-ray)

Rule out mechanical limitation of breathing, bronchospasm, pulmonary embolism, congestive heart failure, and hypovolemia.

Evaluate for atelectasis or pulmonary edema.

General support: Give O_2 during preliminary investigations (10–20 L/min by cannula or mask).

(**Caution:** in patients with preexisting pulmonary disease, supplemental O_2 may result in CO_2 narcosis.)

Approach to Pulmonary Insufficiency

Treat atelectasis

Establish large-volume inflation via deep breathing exercises. If unsuccessful, try IPPB without intubation.

Initiate chest physiotherapy and postural drainage. Administer hydration, nebulized bronchodilators, and mucolytic drugs via airway. Perform bronchoscopy or tracheal suctioning as indicated.

If ventilation is still inadequate: Intubate and initiate mechanical ventilation. Provide nutritional support. Treat coexisting lung edema and lung infection. Maintain fraction of inspired oxygen < 60% and airway pressure < 40 cm H_2O.

Treat increased lung water

Decrease pulmonary hydrostatic pressure by improving left ventricular function pharmacologically. (Monitor changes in cardiac output.)

Reduce total extracellular fluid volume by forced diuresis, dialysis, or hemofiltration.

Increase plasma oncotic pressure by administering colloids during diuresis.

Establish and maintain normal pulmonary microvascular integrity by treating any extrapulmonary site of infection or inflammation.

ume, and localized or generalized muscle weakness. If the expiratory flow is abnormally low, spirometry should be repeated after the administration of aerosolized bronchodilators. Low expiratory flow that improves after bronchodilation indicates bronchospasm, which will require special management during and after operation. An MVV value below 50 percent of predicted correlates most closely with the incidence of postoperative pulmonary complications. The MVV may be abnormally low for many reasons both pulmonary and nonpulmonary.[3]

Arterial blood gas measurements are obtained only if major pulmonary dysfunction is suspected, and they serve primarily as a baseline for postoperative comparison and for decisions regarding postoperative ventilation rather than as a screening test for inadequate pulmonary function. Arterial carbon dioxide tension (P_aCO_2) greater than 45 mm Hg at rest indicates significant alveolar hypoventilation. If the cause is muscular weakness, bronchospasm, or chronic bronchitis, it should be treated before any elective operation. If the arterial oxygen tension (P_aO_2) is less than 70 mm Hg, the patient has one or more of the following: a significant right-to-left shunt, a diffusion block, or ventilation-perfusion mismatch—usually the last. These three causes of hypoxemia can be further identified on the basis of the patient's response to breathing 100 percent oxygen, but this evaluation requires special equipment (a face mask or nasal catheter is not satisfactory), and the effort is generally not worthwhile in preoperative assessment.

More detailed tests of pulmonary function are needed only in special circumstances. The most useful measurement is of functional residual capacity. An FRC greater than 120 percent of predicted indicates air trapping from small airway disease or bronchospasm. These conditions should be treated before any elective operation. An FRC less than 50 percent of predicted indicates loss of lung volume, which may be caused by atelectasis, pneumonia, pleural effusion, or congestive heart failure. Measurement of diffusing capacity by carbon monoxide inhalation is not helpful. When severe fibrotic lung disease is suspected, diffusion can be measured by determination of P_aO_2 while the patient is breathing air and of P_aO_2 while the patient is breathing 100 percent oxygen. Oxygen consumption, CO_2 production, and the respiratory quotient are measurements of systemic metabolism rather than of pulmonary function; therefore, although these measurements may be very helpful in preoperative detection of sepsis or in planning nutritional therapy, they are generally not useful as measurements of pulmonary function. Ventilation-perfusion scan should be added to the regimen of routine preoperative testing in any patient with evidence of compromised pulmonary function in whom pulmonary resection is contemplated.

In summary, history, physical examination, and chest x-ray are sufficient means of preoperative pulmonary assessment in almost all patients. Patients at risk for pulmonary complications, as identified by history or examination, should undergo simple spirometry (pulmonary function testing) to identify abnormalities that can be corrected before elective operations. Arterial blood gases should be measured preoperatively in patients with major respiratory dysfunction to serve as a baseline for postoperative management.

Preoperative Correction of Abnormalities

If the planned operation is totally elective, as much time as is necessary should be spent measuring lung function, correcting the abnormalities and conditions that may predispose to pulmonary complications, and improving physical conditioning, including breathing. This is particularly true in patients with preexisting cardiopulmonary disease. Patients should be advised in the preoperative period to train for a major operation as one would train for an athletic event. The respiratory muscles should be exercised and specific breathing maneuvers learned.

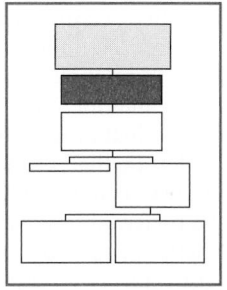

Factors that may decrease the efficiency of ventilation should be corrected, including smoking, gross obesity, and existing bacterial infection, particularly chronic bronchitis. Patients with bronchospasm should become accustomed to bronchodilator treatment preoperatively, and the effect of bronchodilators on pulmonary mechanics should be directly measured, particularly in patients with known bronchospastic disorders, such as asthma.

Preoperative preparation should include adequate nutrition to ensure normal total serum protein concentration and a normal plasma oncotic pressure; inotropic support should be provided if signs of left ventricular failure exist.

The patient with preexisting lung disease requires special consideration. Preparation related to bronchospasm or to chronic bronchitis has been discussed. The patient in whom acute pulmonary insufficiency, increased lung water, or atelectasis is secondary to an acute disorder such as pancreatitis or systemic sepsis will often improve during the operation and with postoperative mechanical ventilation. The condition of the patient with severe chronic obstructive pulmonary disease should be improved as much as possible by means of bronchodilators, therapy for chronic bronchitis, nutritional support, and breathing and coughing training. If the pulmonary disorder is very severe (if P_aO_2 is < 50 mm Hg with the patient breathing room air or if carbon dioxide retention is evident), prolonged postoperative intubation and mechanical ventilation should be anticipated, and the patient should be advised accordingly.

Intraoperative Measures to Prevent Pulmonary Complications

Intraoperatively, several factors may minimize the risk of postoperative pulmonary complications. The operation itself may directly improve pulmonary function (e.g., by repairing an incompetent mitral valve or a large abdominal wall hernia) or may eliminate factors that of themselves are causing pulmonary insufficiency (e.g., empyema, a foreign body, or dead tissue).

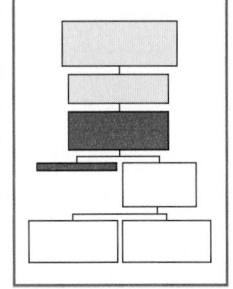

Abdominal incisions should be planned to minimize postoperative pain and to maintain the strength of the abdominal wall for forced inspiration. Transverse incisions should be used whenever possible, particularly in patients with chronic heavy sputum production who will need to cough excessively after the operation. Gastrostomy should be considered to avoid prolonged nasogastric intubation. Bone fragments should be manipulated as gently as possible to avoid marrow embolism. Veins under negative pressure (e.g., in the brain) must be managed carefully to avoid air embolism. If the patient has a history of pulmonary embolism or existing deep vein thrombosis in the legs, prophylactic inferior vena cava plication should be considered when abdominal procedures are performed.

The method of anesthesia may be important in preventing pulmonary complications. Local or spinal anesthesia would seem to be preferred to avoid the respiratory depression of general anesthetic agents. However, general anesthesia gives the anesthesiologist control over the airway with the opportunity to provide optimal inflation and ventilation. In general, the patient who is at high risk for pulmonary complications is best managed with general anesthesia. Epidural anesthesia combined with light general anesthesia intraoperatively and continued for the first few days after operation is ideal for high-risk patients.[4]

During long procedures, alveoli will begin to collapse unless regularly inflated.[5] Sustained inflation to 20 ml/kg or an airway pressure of 30 cm H_2O should be done hourly. Overload with crystalloid fluid should be avoided. Generally, blood or plasma losses that exceed 10 percent of the blood volume should be replaced with blood or plasma. Moderate amounts of saline-type solutions are permissible, but caution should be observed. Saltwater overload does not cause pulmonary insufficiency, but if the pulmonary endothelium is injured, the edematous patient is primed for pulmonary edema.

Mechanical ventilation should be continued postoperatively until the adequacy of spontaneous ventilation has been clearly established. The action of paralytic drugs should be reversed completely and a vital capacity at least twice the tidal volume documented before extubation.

Postoperative Measures to Prevent Pulmonary Insufficiency

ROUTINE MEASURES

In the recovery room, the endotracheal tube should be maintained in place as long as necessary. Patients with preexisting pulmonary dysfunction or those at high risk for pulmonary complications may need to remain intubated and be maintained on mechanical ventilation for hours or days after operation. The well-ventilated alveolus is less susceptible to humoral capillary damage than is the atelectatic alveolus.[6] Elderly, debilitated patients and patients with extensive trauma, multiple fractures, pancreatitis, dead tissue, or severe peritonitis are commonly left intubated and are maintained on mechanical ventilation for at least 12 hours postoperatively. When the patient is fully alert and awake, when perfusion and cardiac status are stable, and when the blood and extracellular fluid volumes are demonstrated to be normal, then the patient is ready for spontaneous ventilation and extubation.

Deep breathing exercises, clearing of sputum and mucus, and avoidance of prolonged periods in the supine position must begin in the recovery room. Profound hypoventilation, ventilation-perfusion imbalance, and the resultant hypoxemia are the rule in the patient awakening from anesthesia. For this reason, moderate amounts (5 to 10 L/min) of supplemental oxygen are commonly administered to all patients in the recovery room. This precaution is wise for the first hour or two after anesthesia, but it is actually prophylactic only against hypoxic arrhythmias and

may actually be slightly detrimental to lung function by suppressing whatever deep breathing may result from moderate degrees of hypoxemia. Consequently, supplemental oxygen should not be administered for more than a few hours after anesthesia unless oximetry indicates significant hypoxemia.

Airway cleaning, suctioning, expectorant drugs, mist inhalation, and mucolytic agents are all useful in patients with preexisting chronic bronchitis or thick, tenacious tracheobronchial secretions. However, these maneuvers and agents may not be necessary in patients who can adequately inflate their lungs by means of inspiratory maneuvers. A compulsion to force patients to cough dominates much of the thinking on postoperative pulmonary care. Coughing may be necessary in patients with chronic bronchitis. In general, however, coughing maneuvers are painful, and they are unnecessary if the lung remains well ventilated.

Breathing maneuvers and devices designed to encourage those maneuvers are important adjuncts to postoperative care.[7] Because shallow breathing, the lack of spontaneous deep breaths, and alveolar collapse are the steps that lead to postoperative pulmonary complications, respiratory maneuvers must emphasize maximal lung inflation. Breathing out (i.e., with coughing, tracheal stimulation, or so-called blow bottles) does nothing to accomplish alveolar inflation, except perhaps for the preparatory inspiration the patient may take before that maneuver. The greater the emphasis placed on the inhaled volume and the inspiratory pressure, the more effective the maneuver will be.

Deep inspiratory maneuvers can be performed spontaneously[8] or with a device that indicates the volume inhaled and rewards the patient's efforts, such as an incentive spirometer. The regular performance of deep breathing exercises using an incentive spirometer has been shown to decrease the incidence of pulmonary complications after laparotomy from about 30 percent to about 10 percent.[7-9]

Another method of preventing postoperative atelectasis is application of continuous positive airway pressure (CPAP) with a tightly fitting face mask.[10] Initial reports of the benefits of this technique show improved alveolar inflation. The potential complications of mask CPAP—gastric distention, vomiting and aspiration, and patient discomfort—did not occur in the initial series but remain a cause for concern. This technique, perhaps combined with intermittent positive pressure breathing (IPPB)—so-called mask IPPB—may prove useful in the management of patients who are extubated but who cannot or will not breathe deeply.

If the patient cannot do deep breathing inspiratory exercise voluntarily, inflation can be achieved with a mechanical ventilator attached to a mouthpiece (IPPB). To be effective, IPPB must be based on volume rather than pressure and should be done frequently (hourly while the patient is awake). In previous studies, infrequent, pressure-limited IPPB did not prevent atelectasis, and this technique was largely abandoned.[11] Properly administered, however, intermittent positive pressure breathing is a very useful method of preventing and treating atelectasis.

Frequent change of position and early ambulation will minimize fluid collection in the dependent portions of the lung. Adequate nutrition should be maintained postoperatively. If the patient must go without enteral feeding for more than four or five days, parenteral nutrition will be required to maintain the strength of the respiratory muscles. Fluids must be managed carefully to avoid overloading the extracellular space and diluting the serum proteins.

Pulmonary thromboembolism from the deep veins of the leg or pelvis is a constant threat in the postoperative period. Obese patients, immobilized patients, and patients with cancer are at particularly high risk. Several methods have been proposed to prevent deep vein thrombosis [see VI:2 Thromboembolic Problems], including administration of anticoagulants or drugs that inhibit platelet function, application of pressure to the legs by means of plastic wraps or stockings, and frequent active or passive exercises for the lower leg. Regular muscle exercise and early ambulation are the easiest of these maneuvers, have the fewest complications, and are advised for all postoperative patients.

Postoperative analgesia should be planned to decrease pain without depressing ventilation. Intramuscular narcotics may suppress deep breathing and contribute to atelectasis. In high-risk patients, therefore, intermittent local or regional blocks, intrathecal narcotics, and catheter epidural analgesia are the preferred methods of pain control[12] [see VIII:2 Postoperative Pain].

PREEXISTING LUNG DISEASE

Patients with chronic disease of the airways or of the pulmonary parenchyma have less pulmonary reserve; consequently, acute respiratory failure may develop after they suffer a minimal insult to the lung. The patient with emphysema or asthma presents an interesting problem. Because of the primary disease, the residual volume and functional residual capacity are abnormally expanded. The patient is protected to a small extent against alveolar collapse secondary to shallow breathing. The affected alveoli are difficult to ventilate, however, even with maximal effort. The dead space is abnormally large, so that the minute ventilation must be higher than normal just to achieve normal carbon dioxide excretion. In addition, carbon dioxide excretion and oxygenation may be decreased because of the presence of alveolar destruction, fibrosis, or bulae. Shallow breathing in such a patient will not produce atelectasis, as would occur in the normal lung, but rather carbon dioxide retention and hypoxemia. Supplemental oxygen may reverse the hypoxemia, but carbon dioxide narcosis may result, particularly if the patient is also sedated with narcotics or anesthetics.

Chronic bronchitis narrows the small airways, increasing susceptibility to inadequate inflation and alveolar collapse. Heavy cigarette smoking has the same effect. For these conditions, treating the airways before elective procedures (with antibiotics or the cessation of smoking, respectively) is advisable. Severe restrictive disease from pulmonary fibrosis, pleural thickening or fibrosis, or chest wall deformities predisposes the patient to atelectasis.

Patients with acute respiratory failure may require operation; in fact, the respiratory failure may be secondary to the indication for operation (e.g., abscess, ischemic tissue, or long-bone fracture). Such patients come to operation with a decreased FRC and increased pulmonary water [see Discussion, Pathogenesis of Postoperative Pulmonary Insufficiency, below]. The respiratory failure may improve with operative resolution of the primary condition, but if improvement in pulmonary function does not occur, these patients cannot afford any worsening of alveolar collapse or pulmonary edema. In these patients, further deterioration of pulmonary function must be prevented by means of prolonged postoperative ventilatory support and by fine-tuning of the hydrostatic pressure and

colloid osmotic pressure in relation to cardiac output and blood volume.

Clinical Presentation of Postoperative Pulmonary Insufficiency

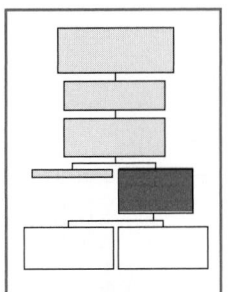

At any time during the first week after a major operation, a patient may manifest the syndrome of pulmonary insufficiency: dyspnea, tachypnea, tachycardia, fever, confusion, and cyanosis. Although the most likely causes of this syndrome are atelectasis and edema, the first step in evaluating the patient is to rule out mechanical limitation of breathing, acute bronchospasm, pulmonary thromboembolism, congestive heart failure, and hypovolemia [see Table 1]. Mechanical limitation of breathing may be caused by gastric or intestinal distention, ascites, pneumothorax, hydrothorax, or splinting of the chest wall because of pain or rib fractures. Mechanical limitation of breathing is diagnosed by physical examination and chest x-ray and treated by removing the limitation.

Bronchospasm occurs in patients with a history of asthma. The diagnosis is made by finding wheezes on physical examination and hyperinflation on x-ray. Treatment consists of the administration of bronchodilators.

Pulmonary embolism is the first consideration when the onset of pulmonary insufficiency is sudden, but it is the least common cause. Small, lobar pulmonary emboli rarely cause symptoms. The patient who is symptomatic from embolism has had a major embolism or a series of minor emboli occluding more than 50 percent of the pulmonary circulation. It is usually easy to differentiate pulmonary embolism from atelectasis by clinical examination and evaluation of blood gases [see Table 1].

Congestive heart failure in the postoperative period may be an exacerbation of a chronic condition or acute cardiac failure secondary to myocardial infarction. In either case, the diagnosis is made by physical and x-ray examination of the chest. The initial management of acutely ill patients with heart failure includes diuresis, administration of supplemental oxygen, review of records of body weight and fluid balance, and transfer to the intensive care unit for more invasive monitoring. In the patient who is fluid overloaded, pulmonary arterial monitoring may be required to differentiate cardiogenic from capillary-injury pulmonary edema.

Hypovolemia is often first manifested by dyspnea, and postoperative shortness of breath should always raise the question of occult bleeding or third-space sequestration. Clinical examination indicates findings of hypovolemia. The chest x-ray is usually clear, and blood gases demonstrate normal oxygenation and carbon dioxide clearance with metabolic acidosis.

In postoperative pulmonary insufficiency caused by atelectasis or edema, physical examination shows diminished breath sounds over one or both lung bases. Rales and rhonchi may be heard in the middle and lower lung fields. Although tidal volume is normal, vital capacity (judged or actually measured) is decreased. Chest x-ray demonstrates incomplete lung inflation, usually with overt collapse or consolidation apparent in the lower lobes. If the pulmonary abnormality is predominantly the result of lung edema, a diffuse increase in lung density is seen, which, when combined with irregular inflation, is often described as

Table 1 Differential Diagnosis of Postoperative Dyspnea

	Atelectasis/ Edema	Pulmonary Embolism	Bronchospasm	Congestive Heart Failure
Lung bases	Not aerated	Clear	Wheezes	Rales
Chest x-ray	Consolidation, general edema	Clear ↑ Diameter of main pulmonary artery	Hyperinflated	Hydrostatic edema ↑ Diameter of main pulmonary artery
Central venous pressure	Normal	Elevated	Normal	Elevated
Pulmonary arterial wedge pressure	Normal	Normal or low	Normal or high	High
Arterial Po_2 (breathing air) (mm Hg)	40–60	40–80	70–90	40–60
Arterial Po_2 (breathing O_2) (mm Hg)	50–100	100–300	200–300	100–300
Arterial Pco_2	Low	Normal or low	High	Normal or high
Lung scan	Regional ischemia	Regional ischemia	± Normal	± Normal
Pulmonary angiogram	Normal	Diagnostic	Normal	Normal

diffuse fluffy infiltrates. This finding can usually be differentiated from radiographic findings of cardiogenic pulmonary edema, which are more apparent in the lower and middle lung fields when the x-ray is taken with the patient sitting or standing. Measurement of arterial blood gases while the patient is breathing air demonstrates hypoxemia, hypocapnia, and respiratory alkalosis.

Supplemental oxygen supplied by nasal catheter or face mask with high-flow oxygen (10 to 20 L/min) supplies approximately 40 percent inspired oxygen (regardless of the settings on the equipment). Supplemental oxygen reverses the hypoxemia caused by ventilation-perfusion mismatch, pulmonary embolism, or cardiogenic pulmonary edema, typically resulting in a P_aO_2 greater than 150 mm Hg. In contrast, supplemental oxygen has a minor effect on hypoxemia caused by atelectasis, with the P_aO_2 typically rising from the 40s to the 80s. Fever and mild leukocytosis often accompany atelectasis, and the differential diagnosis between atelectasis and pneumonia is based primarily on continuing signs of infection without another obvious source, combined with pathogenic organisms on sputum culture. Thickened or copious bronchial secretions may be present in any postoperative patient, particularly if the patient has had endotracheal intubation and general anesthesia during operation. Bronchial secretions are neither the cause nor the result of atelectasis. However, sputum samples should be acquired from every patient with pulmonary complications for Gram's staining and culture.

Treatment of Postoperative Pulmonary Insufficiency Caused by Atelectasis or Edema

GENERAL SUPPORT

Beginning during the preliminary clinical and laboratory examinations, supplemental oxygen should be supplied by nasal cannula or a face mask at 10 to 20 L/min. Special precautions must be taken in patients who have a history of severe pulmonary disease with preoperative hypoxemia and hypercapnia, because supplemental oxygen may correct the hypoxemia but diminish the respiratory drive and result in carbon dioxide narcosis. The patient should be positioned in a way that maximizes diaphragmatic excursion—that is, sitting but not hunched forward; the stomach and abdomen must not be distended.

TREATMENT OF ATELECTASIS

The cornerstone of treatment aimed at alveolar inflation [*see Figure 1*] is to establish large volume inflation by instituting deep breathing exercises [*see* Postoperative Measures to Prevent Pulmonary Insufficiency, *above*]. If adequate volumes cannot be generated by the patient in this manner, then mechanical assistance is necessary, initially with IPPB with a mechanical ventilator, without intubation. Mechanical assistance must be done with direct exhaled-volume measurement and often requires high pressures (30 cm H_2O) with the IPPB device. All of the inflation techniques of mechanical ventilation (positive end-expiratory pressure, sighs, inspiratory hold, CPAP) can be used in patients who have not been intubated [*see VII:4 Use of the Mechanical Ventilator*].

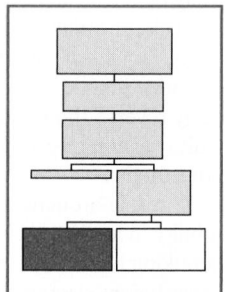

When an area of lung is not ventilated, mucus secreted in the bronchi draining from that segment may become thickened and impacted and hinder efforts at reexpansion. This mucus should be cleared by chest physical therapy (percussion) and postural drainage. Hydration and nebulized bronchodilator and mucolytic drugs may be administered via the airway. Coughing will help expel mucus from airways that have been inflated distally but will not dislodge mucus from airways leading to nonventilated areas of the lung. In this situation, mucus must be removed directly by means of bronchoscopy or tracheal suction.

ALVEOLAR COLLAPSE

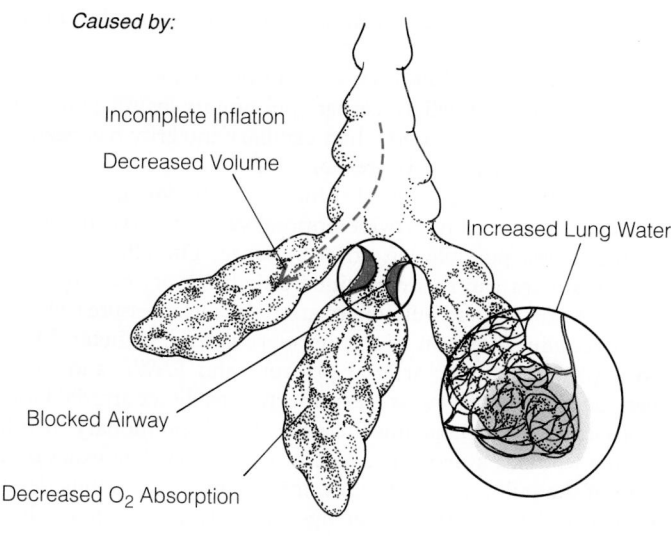

Caused by:

Incomplete Inflation

Decreased Volume

Increased Lung Water

Blocked Airway

Decreased O₂ Absorption

Leads to: Ventilation-Perfusion Imbalance
Hypoxemia
Decreased Functional Residual Capacity
Decreased Compliance
Increased Work

Treatment: Maximum Inflation
Yawn, Mechanical Ventilator, IPPB, CPAP
Maintain Lowest Possible F$_I$O$_2$
Decrease Lung Water
Treat Infection
Optimize Nutrition

Figure 1   **Illustrated are causes and effects of alveolar collapse in postoperative pulmonary insufficiency. (IPPB = intermittent positive pressure breathing; CPAP = continuous positive airway pressure; F$_I$O$_2$ = fraction of inspired oxygen.)**

Tracheal suctioning should be done only if thick mucus cannot be removed with simple methods.[13] The catheter is passed through the nose, verified as passing through the larynx by a change in voice, and connected to oxygen at 5 L/min. Then, 5 ml of saline is injected, and the oxygen is reconnected for several coughing breaths. Suction is applied for no longer than 10 seconds; then, oxygen is resumed. This process is repeated for one to five minutes until the suction return is clear. Electrocardiographic monitoring should be done during and after suctioning. Atropine is given for bradycardia.

In adults, the value of endotracheal suctioning lies primarily in its stimulation of deep breathing associated with the vigorous coughing it produces. Deep breathing can be easily accomplished by other means, however, without the potential vagal complications associated with tracheal suctioning. Routine tracheal suctioning has no rational place in the care of adult patients postoperatively.

Flexible fiberoptic bronchoscopy[14] is preferable to blind tra-

cheal suctioning in the management of atelectasis. Topical anesthesia is administered, and an endotracheal tube is placed without balloon inflation. Bronchoscopy is performed to examine the airways and clear mucus from the atelectatic area. Use of the endotracheal tube facilitates repeated removal and reinsertion of the bronchoscope, which may be necessary if mucus is too thick to be aspirated through the small suction lumen.

If adequate ventilation cannot be established with the methods described earlier, endotracheal intubation and continuous mechanical ventilation are indicated; specific indications are (1) an inspiratory force during a Müller's maneuver of less than 20 cm H$_2$O, (2) a vital capacity less than twice the tidal volume, (3) a respiratory rate consistently greater than 30, or (4) severe hypoxemia (P$_a$O$_2$ < 50 mm Hg, breathing room air). If any one of these indications cannot be reversed, intubation and mechanical ventilation should be considered [*see VII:4 Use of the Mechanical Ventilator*].

If supplemental oxygen has been instituted for the general support of the patient, the amount of oxygen should be kept as low as possible to avoid displacing nitrogen from alveoli and causing absorption atelectasis. Nutritional support should be instituted and a positive nitrogen balance achieved to maintain the strength of respiratory muscles and to optimize host defenses. The amount of nutrition should be based on the measured expenditure of energy to avoid overfeeding, particularly with carbohydrates; carbon dioxide produced in response to excess carbohydrates may add to the pulmonary insufficiency.[15]

TREATMENT OF EDEMA

The amount of lung water can be reduced by decreasing the entire extracellular fluid space, decreasing the hydrostatic pressure in the pulmonary capillary bed, and increasing the plasma oncotic pressure without increasing the oncotic pressure in the interstitial fluid of the lung [*see Figure 2*]. Mechanical positive pressure ventilation is not a means of decreasing lung water. In fact, positive end-

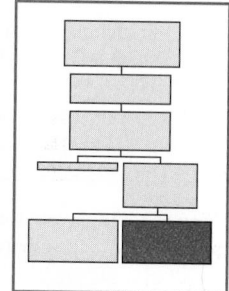

expiratory pressure actually increases lung water slightly, probably by stretching the pulmonary tissue.[16] Mechanical ventilation improves gas exchange in patients with pulmonary edema by overcoming the ventilation-perfusion mismatch associated with bronchodilator or alveolar thickening, but it does not decrease lung water.

If the patient is in renal failure, total extracellular fluid volume must be reduced by forced diuresis, dialysis, or hemofiltration. Diuresis is induced with a potent diuretic such as furosemide or mannitol. The course of diuresis is followed by daily measurement of body weight and hourly measurement of fluid intake and output. Usually, the patient with postoperative pulmonary insufficiency will be found to be 4 to 5 kg overloaded, primarily with extracellular fluid. Diuresis and negative fluid balance greatly improve the chance of survival in patients with pulmonary edema.[17,18]

Adequate treatment of pulmonary edema must include removal of the excess extravascular fluid (i.e., returning the patient to his or her baseline weight). A major decrease in total extracellular fluid volume will be accompanied by a minor decrease in pulmonary extracellular fluid volume, but even this change may be enough to improve pulmonary function greatly.

INCREASED LUNG WATER

Caused by:

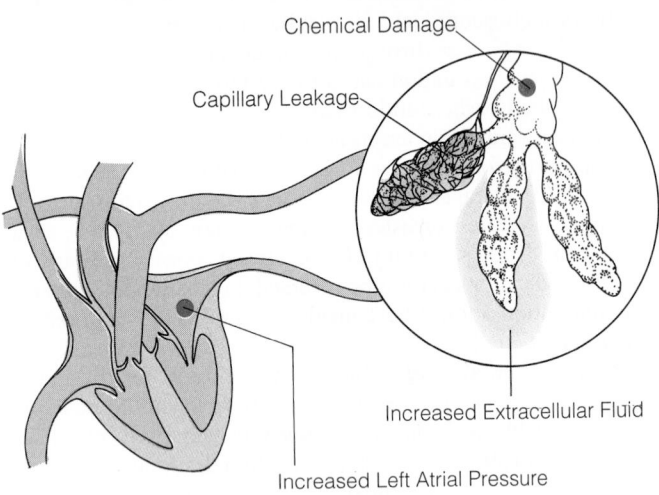

Leads to: Increased Pulmonary Vascular Resistance
Decreased Functional Residual Capacity
Ventilation-Perfusion Imbalance
Infection

Treatment: Decrease Extracellular Fluid
    Diuresis, Decrease Intake
Increase Plasma Oncotic Pressure
Treat Capillaries
Decrease Hydrostatic Pressure

Figure 2 **Illustrated are effects of lung water in postoperative pulmonary insufficiency.**

If the patient becomes hypovolemic because of diuresis, blood volume should be expanded with red blood cells (if the patient is anemic) or colloid solutions; a net loss of sodium and water should be maintained. Diuretic agents will remove water, sodium, and potassium at differing rates, so that all must be monitored carefully and frequently. Usually, water is removed in excess of electrolytes, so that with extreme, forced diuresis a hypernatremic, hyperosmotic state results. Serum sodium concentrations should be monitored closely, and diuresis should be discontinued when the serum sodium level is between 140 and 150 mEq/L.

Diuresis concentrates serum proteins and results in increased plasma oncotic pressure. Diuresis should be combined with colloid loading to further increase plasma oncotic pressure transiently and force the movement of fluid from the extravascular to the intravascular space. The colloids should be administered during the course of diuresis, because most agents used for colloid loading, such as albumin, have a molecular weight between 50,000 and

100,000 and will gradually find their way into the extracellular space within four to 12 hours of infusion. The benefits of colloid loading are gained within the first hour or two of infusion, before the colloid load joins the lymphatic system and is subsequently metabolized.[19]

Administration of albumin without diuresis to a patient who is fluid overloaded will exacerbate pulmonary insufficiency. The technique should be used when capillary integrity has been restored, as determined by response to small initial doses. Diuresis, colloid loading, blood volume adjustment, and inotropic drugs are balanced to provide optimal systemic oxygen delivery at the lowest possible left atrial pressure. The effectiveness of this treatment can be determined only by direct measurement of cardiac output and pulmonary arterial wedge pressure (PAWP). This requires insertion of a pulmonary arterial catheter. Monitoring of pulmonary arterial pressure and PAWP and mixed venous blood sampling are as important as direct arterial blood gas sampling in managing the patient with pulmonary insufficiency who has a major increase in lung water. The exact position of the pulmonary arterial catheter must be carefully determined and the pressure tracings properly interpreted, which requires continuous display on an oscilloscope and careful selection of the end-expiratory point for pressure readings [*see VII:1 Cardiopulmonary Monitoring*].

An effort should be made to establish and maintain normal pulmonary capillary permeability. The most common cause of pulmonary capillary leakage or ARDS is infection or inflammation at a site distant to the lungs.[20] The presence of pulmonary insufficiency in a patient in the postoperative period should always trigger a search for wound infection, deep abscess, pancreatitis, and septic phlebitis. Drugs that inhibit the inflammatory response, block mediators of capillary injury, or prevent fibrosis have been investigated for the prevention or treatment of ARDS. Glucocorticoids definitely diminish the inflammatory response and have been shown to be effective in some disorders, including fat embolism,[21] but the deleterious systemic effects outweigh any advantage.[22] Drugs such as ibuprofen[23] block production of inflammatory mediators more specifically than do steroids. Drugs that inhibit the action of specific mediators (e.g., antihistamines,[24] superoxide dismutase, and catalase[25]) are under investigation in the treatment of lung edema.

Vigorous treatment of alveolar collapse can lead to lung injury and exacerbate lung edema (see below). Specifically, inspired oxygen concentrations greater than 60 percent and airway pressures greater than 40 cm H_2O should be carefully avoided.[26] With these precautions in mind, efforts at maintaining alveolar expansion are an important component of the treatment of interstitial lung edema. The well-ventilated lung appears to be more resistant to capillary injury than the atelectatic lung.

Bacterial infection often complicates atelectasis and edema, and it may occur as a primary event after operation. The progression from atelectasis to pneumonia can be difficult to identify because pulmonary infiltration and consolidation, fever, leukocytosis, and sputum production occur in both conditions. This differential diagnosis is one of the most difficult in postoperative care; decisions must be based on repeated examination of the patient and the sputum [*see VI:13 Early Postoperative Pneumonia*].

Discussion

Pathogenesis of Postoperative Pulmonary Insufficiency

VENTILATION AND PULMONARY MECHANICS

After any major operation, changes occur in lung function. These changes occur in all patients but are not detected on routine examination.[27,28] Aside from shallow tidal ventilation and some decreased breath sounds at the lung bases, most patients show no signs of respiratory abnormality. On direct measurement, lung volumes are decreased (particularly residual volume, expiratory reserve volume, functional residual capacity, and vital capacity). Compliance is decreased because of the decrease in FRC. The work of breathing is increased for the same reason: more pressure is required to inhale a given volume into the decreased lung air space. Further evidence that alveoli are not being ventilated is the presence of absolute or relative arterial hypoxemia, which occurs when the patient is breathing room air or 100 percent oxygen and which indicates transpulmonary shunting (i.e., nonventilated alveoli are being perfused).[29]

These changes in lung function are present immediately after operation, then evolve slowly over one to two days, and return to normal in most patients [see Figure 3]. The extent and duration of abnormality are related to the site of operation, the duration of operation and anesthesia, the quality of postoperative care, and preexisting pulmonary status. The extent and duration are greatest for those operations on the thorax and upper abdomen and progressively decrease for operations situated more distally and more superficially on the body structures. These changes may occur after only one to two hours of general anesthesia if careful attention is not paid to maximal lung inflation during anesthesia. Such changes are superimposed on the patient's preexisting lung status. If, for example, operation is required for complications of pancreatitis two weeks after the onset of disease, the patient may already have pleural effusions, increased pulmonary capillary permeability, and existing transpulmonary shunting and will not tolerate further deterioration of lung function. Likewise, the patient with preexisting chronic obstructive pulmonary disease with high airway resistance, maximal work of breathing, and minimal functional lung tissue may retain carbon dioxide postoperatively if the work of breathing is only slightly increased. Advanced age itself is not a cause of lung dysfunction,[30] but elderly patients may have chronic lung disease or cardiac disease and thus be at greater risk for pulmonary failure. More important, the elderly patient may be weak, and weak respiratory muscles predispose to alveolar collapse.

Several factors contribute to these changes in pulmonary function, but shallow breathing with incomplete alveolar inflation is the common denominator.[31] If spontaneous deep breaths to maximal lung inflation are eliminated from the pattern of breathing, alveolar collapse begins within one hour and progresses rather rapidly to produce significant transpulmonary shunting.[32] Several studies have shown that patterns of spontaneous deep breaths are abnormal in postoperative patients because of severe pain, anesthetics, or narcotics.[28] Supporting this observation is the fact that the postoperative changes in lung function can be returned toward normal by instituting maximal-inflation deep breathing exercises at regular intervals.[33,34] Excessive tracheobronchial secretions, aspiration of oral or gastric contents, and intraoperative fluid over-load can contribute to the postoperative lung abnormalities described earlier.

Within two to four days after operation, it becomes clear whether the pattern of decreased lung volume and shunting is returning to normal or progressing [see Figure 3]. Decreased lung volume is detectable as decreased breath sounds on physical examination, and atelectatic areas may be visible on chest x-ray. Shunt-produced hypoxemia leads to an increased ventilatory rate and the sensation of dyspnea.

Severe hypoxemia may cause cyanosis. Atelectasis causes fever and pooling of mucus in nonventilated areas, leading to an apparent increase in sputum production. Against the background of changes that normally accompany major operations, a more complete picture of pulmonary pathophysiology in the surgical patient can be drawn.

Abnormal ventilation will lead to atelectasis as outlined earlier. The typical postoperative pattern of tidal breathing without spontaneous deep breaths is a good example of this phenomenon. A patient lying on his or her back in bed will preferentially ventilate the superior lobes while the blood will flow preferentially to dependent lobes. This ventilation-perfusion imbalance itself will result in hypoxemia; if it progresses over time, lower lobe alveoli begin to collapse in the pathogenetic pathway. Alveolar collapse will occur in any patient who remains in one position for a prolonged period and in whom the pattern of breathing is that of shallow tidal ventilation. It should be emphasized that normal tidal breaths delivered with a mechanical ventilator will similarly lead to alveolar collapse if regular maximal inflations are not carried out.[4]

EDEMA AND THE PULMONARY INTERSTITIUM

Increased pulmonary hydrostatic pressure, decreased plasma oncotic pressure, and increased capillary permeability may all occur in the surgical patient. All of these states will cause increased pulmonary extravascular water and deterioration of lung function. Edema is the hallmark of ARDS.[35] Edema causes atelectasis in the dependent lung simply by the weight of the fluid.[36,37] This effect can often be reversed by prone positioning of the patient.[38]

Fluid flux is a net function of the hydrostatic pressure that tends to force fluid out of the vascular space, on the one hand, and the oncotic pressure that tends to pull fluid in, on the other hand. High hydrostatic pressure or low plasma oncotic pressure will result in accumulation of fluid in the extravascular space [see Figure 3]. If the pulmonary endothelium is damaged, fluid may leak into the extracellular space at normal hydrostatic or oncotic pressures (the acute respiratory distress syndrome). Pulmonary vascular resistance increases because of periarteriolar cuffing. Ventilation-perfusion imbalance is created by peribronchiolar and alveolar compression. Shunting occurs if the alveoli become completely collapsed or filled with fluid. Finally, boggy atelectatic areas of lung are ideal breeding grounds for bacterial pulmonary infection.

In the normal course of treatment or resuscitation, well-intentioned interventions may result in increased lung water. For example, when blood or plasma is replaced with crystalloid, that fluid must equilibrate into the entire extracellular space, including that in the lung. This effect is compounded by the

Figure 3 **Shaded areas represent normal changes in pulmonary function after an operation. Solid lines represent progression to pulmonary insufficiency. (A-aDo$_2$ = alveolar-arterial difference in oxygen.)**

reduced oncotic pressure that results when protein is lost or replaced with non–colloid-containing fluids. When plasma proteins are diluted in this way, lung interstitial proteins are also diluted; thus, the oncotic gradients stay unchanged,[39] whereas the entire extracellular space expands.

The pulmonary capillary endothelium is the first major vascular bed to be exposed to toxic substances arising from peripheral organ metabolism or perfusion of ischemic or infected tissue. The venous effluent from underperfused tissue arrives directly at the lung, where pulmonary capillary damage occurs. Humoral substances (e.g., lysosomal enzymes) and bacterial endotoxin or particulate materials (e.g., microemboli, platelet aggregates, and fat particles) may lodge in the pulmonary capillary bed.

As these materials are cleared, leaky pulmonary capillaries are left behind, with a resulting accumulation of extravascular fluid despite normal hydrostatic pressure. The pulmonary effects of materials released into the venous blood in shock sets in motion a particularly vicious circle. The increased pulmonary vascular resistance and hypoxia that result from the pulmonary capillary damage lead to a decrease in cardiac output and peripheral oxygen delivery, which adds to the shock state and perpetuates the pulmonary lesion.

Left ventricular failure with increased left atrial pressure will result in pulmonary transcapillary transudation, which may be subtle or grossly obvious, as in congestive heart failure with overt pulmonary edema. Left ventricular pressures may waver at the point of high left atrial pressure for short periods—even minutes—resulting in a transient increase in lung water, and then return to a balanced state. This situation may not lead to severe pulmonary edema in itself, but it probably places the lung in a more vulnerable position when minor capillary damage coexists.

The pulmonary interstitium is particularly vulnerable to the events surrounding an operation. Saltwater infusion usually greatly exceeds losses and increases the extracellular space. Bleeding and venous compression may cause hypotension and necessitate blood transfusion. Mediators from sterile tissue injury or bacterial invasion may injure the pulmonary capillary endothelium. Transient myocardial depression may cause hydrostatic pulmonary edema. With all of these factors, it is remarkable that there is no primary change in lung water volume after uncomplicated operations, even operations including cardiopulmonary bypass.[40] Nonetheless, it should be remembered that the patient usually leaves the operating room overloaded with fluid and primed for the development of lung edema.

Summary

The pathogenesis of pulmonary failure in surgical patients can be characterized as a decrease in functional residual capacity and an increase in interstitial fluid. Decreased FRC is caused by inadequate alveolar inflation; prevention and treatment are aimed at maximal inflation. Pulmonary edema is caused by cardiac failure, fluid overload, and increased capillary permeability; it is prevented and treated by maximizing cardiac function and systemic oxygen delivery, avoiding extracellular space overload, and treating conditions that lead to altered pulmonary capillary permeability. Understanding these aspects of pulmonary pathophysiology and using such understanding to guide prevention and treatment should decrease mortality and morbidity from postoperative pulmonary complications.

References

1. Bartlett RH: Pulmonary pathophysiology in surgical patients. Surg Clin North Am 60:1323, 1980

2. Bolton JWR, Weiman DS, Haynes JL, et al: Stair climbing as an indicator of pulmonary function. Chest 92:783, 1987

3. Tisi GM: Preoperative evaluation of pulmonary function: validity, indications, and benefits. Am Rev Respir Dis 119:293, 1979

4. Cuchieri RJ, Morran CG, Howie JC, et al: Postoperative pain and pulmonary complications: comparison of three analgesic regimens. Br J Surg 72:495, 1985

5. Bendixen HH, Bullwinkel B, Hedley-Whyte J: Atelectasis and shunting during spontaneous ventilation in anesthetized patients. Anesthesiology 25:297, 1964

6. Tilson MD, Bunke MC, Smith JW, et al: Quantitative bacteriology and pathology of the lung in experimental Pseudomonas pneumonia treated with positive end-expiratory pressure (PEEP). Surgery 82:133, 1977

7. Bartlett RH, Gazzaniga AB, Geraghty TR: Respiratory maneuvers to prevent postoperative pulmonary complications: a critical review. JAMA 224:1017, 1973

8. Roukema JA, Carol EJ, Prins JG: The prevention of pulmonary complications after upper abdominal surgery in patients with noncompromised pulmonary status. Arch Surg 123:30, 1988

9. Bartlett RH: Incentive spirometry. Current Respiratory Care. Kacmarek RM, Stoller JK, Eds. BC Decker, Philadelphia, 1988, p 38

10. Greenbaum DM, Millen JE, Eross B, et al: Continuous positive airway pressure without tracheal intubation in spontaneously breathing patients. Chest 69:615, 1976

11. Bartlett RH: Respiratory therapy to prevent postoperative pulmonary complications. Respiratory Intensive Care. Pierson DJ, Ed. Daedalus Enterprises, Dallas, 1986, p 369

12. Bromage PR, Camporesi E, Chestnut D: Epidural narcotics for postoperative analgesia. Anesth Analg 59:473, 1980

13. Demers RR: Complications of endotracheal suctioning procedures. Respir Care 27:453, 1982

14. Ratliff JL: Bronchoscopy in respiratory care. Surg Clin North Am 60:1497, 1980

15. Kemper M, Weissman C, Askanazi J, et al: Metabolic and respiratory changes during weaning from mechanical ventilation. Chest 92:979, 1987

16. Parker JC, Hernandez LA, Peevy KJ: Mechanisms of ventilator-induced lung injury. Crit Care Med 21:131, 1993

17. Simmons RS, Berdine GG, Seidenfeld JJ, et al: Fluid balance and the adult respiratory distress syndrome. Am Rev Respir Dis 135:924, 1987

18. Mitchell JP, Schuller D, Calandrino FS, et al: Improved outcome based on fluid management in critically ill patients requiring pulmonary artery catheterization. Am Rev Respir Dis 145:990, 1992

19. Skillman JJ, Parikh BM, Tanenbaum BJ: Pulmonary arteriovenous admixture: improvement with albumin and diuresis. Am J Surg 119:440, 1970

20. Seidenfeld JJ, Pohl DF, Bell RC, et al: Incidence, site, and outcome of infections in patients with the adult respiratory distress syndrome. Am Rev Respir Dis 134:12, 1986

21. Schonfeld SA, Ploysongsang Y, DiLisio R, et al: Fat embolism prophylaxis with corticosteroids: a prospective study in high-risk patients. Ann Intern Med 99:438, 1983

22. Bernard GR, Luce JM, Sprung CL, et al: High-dose corticosteroids in patients with the adult respiratory distress syndrome. N Engl J Med 317:1565, 1987

23. Johnson A, Malik AB: Pulmonary transvascular fluid and protein exchange after thrombin-induced microembolism: differential effects of cyclooxygenase inhibitors. Am Rev Respir Dis 132:70, 1985

24. Leeman M, Boeynaems JM, Degaute JP, et al: Administration of dazoxiben, a selective thromboxane synthetase inhibitor, in the adult respiratory distress syndrome. Chest 87:726, 1985

25. Flick MR, Hoeffel JM, Staub NC: Superoxide dismutase with heparin prevents increased lung vascular permeability during air emboli in sheep. J Appl Physiol 55:1284, 1983

26. Kolobow T, Moretti MP, Fumagalli R, et al: Severe impairment in lung function induced by high peak airway pressure during mechanical ventilation: an experimental study. Am Rev Respir Dis 135:312, 1987

27. Lee AB, Kinney JM, Turino G, et al: Effects of abdominal operations on ventilation and gas exchange. J Natl Med Assoc 61:164, 1969

28. Okinaka AJ: The pattern of breathing after operation. Surg Gynecol Obstet 125:785, 1967

29. Julien M, Lemoyne B, Denis R, et al: Mortality and morbidity related to severe intrapulmonary shunting in multiple trauma patients. J Trauma 27:970, 1987

30. Bartlett RH: The respiratory system in the elderly. Surgical Care of the Elderly. Meakins JL, McClaran JC, Eds. Year Book Medical Publishers, Chicago, 1988, p 121

31. Zikria BA, Spencer JL, Kinney JM, et al: Alterations in ventilatory function and breathing patterns following surgical trauma. Ann Surg 179:1, 1974

32. Caro CG, Butler J, Dubois AB: Some effects of restriction of chest cage expansion on pulmonary function in man: an experimental study. J Clin Invest 39:573, 1960

33. Bartlett RH, Krop P, Hanson EL, et al: Physiology of yawning and its application to postoperative care. Forum on Fundamental Surgical Problems 21:222, 1970

34. Ward RJ, Danziger F, Bonica JJ, et al: An evaluation of postoperative respiratory maneuvers. Surg Gynecol Obstet 123:51, 1966

35. Bernard GR, Artigas A, Brigham KL, et al: The American-European consensus conference on ARDS: definitions, mechanisms, relevant outcomes and clinical trial coordination. Am J Respir Crit Care Med 149:818, 1994

36. Pelosi P, D'Andrea L, Vitale G, et al: Vertical gradient of regional lung inflation in adult respiratory distress syndrome. Am J Respir Crit Care Med 149:8, 1994

37. Gattinoni L, D'Andrea L, Pelosi P, et al: Regional effects and mechanism of positive end-expiratory pressure in early adult respiratory distress syndrome. JAMA 269:2122, 1993

38. Lamm WJE, Graham MM, Albert RK: Mechanism by which the prone position improves oxygenation in acute lung injury. Am J Respir Crit Care Med 150:184, 1994

39. Demling RH, Manohar M, Will JA, et al: The effect of plasma oncotic pressure on the pulmonary microcirculation after hemorrhagic shock. Surgery 86:323, 1979

40. Shires GT III, Peitzman AB, Albert SA, et al: Response of extravascular lung water to intraoperative fluids. Ann Surg 197:515, 1983

Acknowledgments

Figures 1 and 2   Dana Burns-Pizer.

Figure 3   Albert Miller.

2 THROMBOEMBOLIC PROBLEMS

F. William Blaisdell, M.D., and John T. Owings, M.D.

Approach to Venous Thromboembolism

Superficial Thrombophlebitis

CLINICAL MANIFESTATIONS

Superficial thrombophlebitis has several characteristic clinical manifestations [*see Figure 1*]. Pain is usually present, and slight swelling of the extremity can be seen, with most of the edema occurring over the course of the involved vein. Unless the patient is obese, with a heavy layer of subcutaneous tissue, a palpable, very tender subcutaneous cord is usually found; the presence of this cord is pathognomonic of the disease. There is usually some edema in the adjacent subcutaneous tissue and erythema in the overlying skin. The main conditions to be considered in the differential diagnosis are cellulitis and streptococcal lymphangitis. For both conditions, there should be a proximal source (e.g., an open wound); neither condition will be associated with a palpable cord or with evidence of increased superficial collateral circulation.

If there is overt limb swelling (i.e., one limb is at least several centimeters larger in diameter than the other) in a patient who appears to have superficial phlebitis, associated deep thrombophlebitis should be assumed, and appropriate treatment [*see* Deep Thrombophlebitis, *below*] should be initiated.

Superficial thrombophlebitis, which is largely a benign disease, is often overtreated out of fear that infection may be contributing to the phlebitis. It is therefore important to differentiate between sterile superficial thrombophlebitis and septic superficial thrombophlebitis. The two are often confused because they may have many of the same manifestations (e.g., redness and induration).

STERILE THROMBOPHLEBITIS

Sterile thrombophlebitis can be assumed with minimal risk of misdiagnosis if there has been no invasion in or near the superficial vein involved. The condition is best treated not with immobilization of the patient or the extremity but with administration of aspirin (one tablet daily) or dipyridamole (50 mg four times daily).

If the phlebitis persists or continues to extend and there is significant morbidity, interruption of the vein may be appropriate, particularly when a lower extremity saphenous vein is involved. This is especially true when the phlebitis is affecting a previously varicose vein; because these dilated veins can accommodate a large amount of clot, considerable disability can result. The choice of treatment is between interrupting the vein above the area of palpable thrombosis and stripping and removing the vein. The second alternative carries a higher morbidity than simple interruption, but it can be used effectively when there are associated varicosities and the thrombosis is not responding to treatment. Stripping of the channels above and below

the phlebitic process as well as the phlebitic area itself will remove the risk of extension of the phlebitis and subsequent recurrence.

SEPTIC THROMBOPHLEBITIS

When the vein has been invaded or when there are systemic manifestations of severe infection (e.g., fever and an elevated white blood cell count), septic thrombophlebitis is likely. In addition, the induration, tenderness, and redness over and along the course of the vein are usually more extensive than with sterile thrombophlebitis.

If the phlebitis is associated with an intravenous catheter, the device should be removed, the tip cultured, and the patient's response observed [*see VI:14 Nosocomial Infection*]. If the patient has no overt systemic signs of infection, treatment is similar to that of sterile phlebitis. If the patient has systemic signs, antibiotics should be administered; if a skin organism is the presumed source of infection, antistaphylococcal drugs are appropriate. If the patient is a drug addict or the phlebitis is associated with a contaminated wound, blood samples for culture and a Gram's stain should be obtained by aspirating the vein with a small syringe and needle. Specific antibiotic therapy directed toward the organisms seen on Gram's stain or culture should then be instituted.

If the patient is in a toxic state from presumed septic phlebitis in a subcutaneous vein or is not responding to treatment, it may be appropriate to ligate the vein, to drain it by cutting down on the phlebitic process with the patient under local or general anesthesia and laying the vein open, or to combine ligation with drainage. Moist compresses are then applied, the area is immobilized, and antibiotics are administered. Heparin may occasionally be of value, particularly when the process appears to be extending into the deep venous system (e.g., into the saphenofemoral junction).

Deep Thrombophlebitis

CLINICAL MANIFESTATIONS

Deep thrombophlebitis can involve either obstructive clots, which affect the drainage of venous blood from an extremity, or nonobstructive clots, which are relatively asymptomatic [*see Figure 2*]. Obstructive clots may also occur in association with nonobstructive clots. The latter are more dangerous because they are not circumferentially attached to the vein wall, do not elicit much vein inflammation, and are prone to embolization—the lethal complication of deep thrombophlebitis.

Deep thrombophlebitis may be divided into three main forms: nonocclusive thrombophlebitis, occlusive thrombophlebitis, and phlegmasia cerulea dolens (massive thrombophlebi-

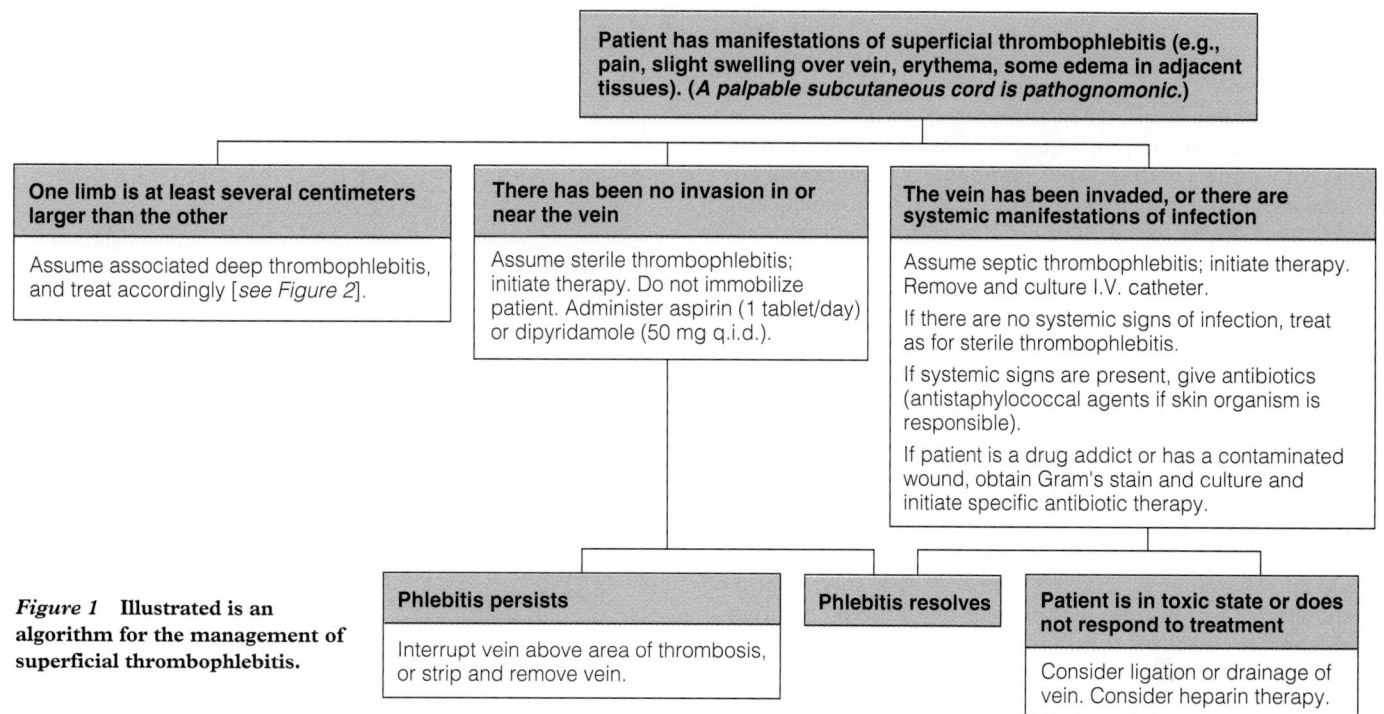

Patient has manifestations of superficial thrombophlebitis (e.g., pain, slight swelling over vein, erythema, some edema in adjacent tissues). (*A palpable subcutaneous cord is pathognomonic.*)

One limb is at least several centimeters larger than the other

Assume associated deep thrombophlebitis, and treat accordingly [*see Figure 2*].

There has been no invasion in or near the vein

Assume sterile thrombophlebitis; initiate therapy. Do not immobilize patient. Administer aspirin (1 tablet/day) or dipyridamole (50 mg q.i.d.).

The vein has been invaded, or there are systemic manifestations of infection

Assume septic thrombophlebitis; initiate therapy. Remove and culture I.V. catheter.

If there are no systemic signs of infection, treat as for sterile thrombophlebitis.

If systemic signs are present, give antibiotics (antistaphylococcal agents if skin organism is responsible).

If patient is a drug addict or has a contaminated wound, obtain Gram's stain and culture and initiate specific antibiotic therapy.

Phlebitis persists

Interrupt vein above area of thrombosis, or strip and remove vein.

Phlebitis resolves

Patient is in toxic state or does not respond to treatment

Consider ligation or drainage of vein. Consider heparin therapy.

Figure 1 **Illustrated is an algorithm for the management of superficial thrombophlebitis.**

tis). Each form gives rise to different clinical problems and therefore is discussed separately.

NONOCCLUSIVE THROMBOPHLEBITIS

Nonocclusive thrombophlebitis, sometimes referred to as phlebothrombosis, is a frequent complication in postoperative surgical patients. Unfortunately, its presence all too often is not suspected until an embolic complication occurs. In many instances, it is the development of pulmonary embolism that precipitates the search for asymptomatic deep vein thrombosis. There may be absolutely no manifestations of clot on clinical examination, or there may be some nonspecific swelling in an extremity; rarely is there sufficient pain or tenderness to suggest the presence of deep thrombophlebitis. Consequently, it is essential to be aware of the major risk factors for this condition [*see Table 1*].

When thrombophlebitis develops or appears likely to develop in an outpatient, every effort should be made to determine the cause because apparent spontaneous onset of this condition is often the manifestation of a congenital clotting tendency that will necessitate lifelong treatment [*see* Approach to Acquired and Congenital Thrombotic Syndromes, *below*]. Conversely, when risk factors for deep thrombophlebitis (e.g., injury, the postoperative state, or systemic infection) are identified in a hospitalized patient, it can be assumed that the etiology is acquired and that the clotting tendency will be reversed when the patient recovers from his or her illness. If there is no contraindication to anticoagulation, moderate- or high-dose heparin therapy can be initiated on an empirical basis. Even if tests reveal no clot at the moment, the patient remains at risk for thrombophlebitis.

Once anticoagulant therapy is begun, the diagnosis, if not already clinically obvious, should be verified. The differential diagnosis includes muscle contusion, plantar muscle rupture, gastrocnemius muscle rupture, ruptured Baker's cyst, popliteal artery aneurysm, arthritis of the knee or the ankle, cellulitis, and myositis. The gold standard for diagnosis of deep thrombophlebitis is phlebography. However, study of the entire lower extremity venous system often involves injection of dye not only at

the foot or ankle level but also at the groin level so that the iliac and femoral veins can be adequately visualized. This approach is uncomfortable for the patient and is associated with morbidity; in critically ill ICU patients, it may not be feasible. For these reasons, noninvasive techniques of evaluating the veins are favored.

The most sensitive noninvasive technique is iodine-125 (^{125}I)–labeled fibrinogen scanning. This test is so efficient at detecting small calf vein thrombi that it frequently detects minor disease that is of little or no clinical significance. Calf vein thrombi, by themselves, are almost always clinically insignificant: although they occur in as many as 30 to 40 percent of hospitalized patients, they usually resolve spontaneously. It is thrombi in the major deep veins of the thigh and the pelvis that place the patient at high risk for morbidity and mortality. Clots in these vessels are not diagnosed well by ^{125}I-labeled fibrinogen scanning. In addition, this technique yields false positives in patients who have had bleeding or inflammation. Consequently, this study, despite its sensitivity, is no longer used in most centers.[1-3]

Various modifications of plethysmographic techniques have been used.[4,5] For instance, impedance plethysmography measures alterations in calf circumference by recording changes in electrical impedance. These techniques are strictly noninvasive and are accurate only when there is at least 50 percent obstruction of the lumen of a deep vein. The presence of large collateral vessels may result in a false negative test result as well.

Doppler ultrasonography can be performed quickly and easily. It measures alterations in venous flow velocity during compression and during respiratory excursion. Interpretation of the results, however, requires considerable experience. Because Doppler ultrasonography is a physiologic method that depends on alterations in flow and the presence of obstruction, it has the same drawbacks as plethysmography.[4]

Real-time B-mode (duplex) ultrasonography, originally developed to visualize extracranial cerebrovascular disease, has recently proved valuable in detecting deep thrombophlebitis.[4,6,7] B-mode ultrasonography can actually visualize the thrombus within a vessel. Inability to obliterate the vein with probe compression is additional evidence of thrombus. Often, experienced users can even differentiate between new and old thrombi: the former are compressible, whereas the latter are not.

B-mode ultrasonography is quite sensitive and specific in patients with suspected deep vein thrombosis; the addition of color flow imaging may further enhance its diagnostic qualities. Its sensitivity is similar to that of impedance plethysmography, and it has in fact become the noninvasive procedure of choice for assessment of clot in the neck and the extremity vessels. Unfortunately, it is less specific above the axilla and the inguinal ligament because in these regions it is difficult to compress the vessels. B-mode ultrasonography is particularly valuable for detecting associated conditions that may confuse the diagnosis (e.g., muscle hematomas or a popliteal cyst).[7]

Ultimately, ascending phlebography is the most accurate method of assessment.[8,9] This approach requires cannulation of a vein of the foot; if the iliac veins are not well visualized or the vena cava is suspect, it may be necessary to inject the contrast agent into the femoral vein [see Figure 3]. If a good contrast study fails to demonstrate the presence of clot, venous thrombophlebitis is effectively ruled out.

Once nonocclusive phlebitis is diagnosed, the treatment of choice is medium-dose heparin anticoagulation. After three or four days, depending on the response, heparin can be replaced with an oral anticoagulant, such as warfarin. If anticoagulation is contraindicated because of the presence of fresh wounds or a bleeding disorder, low-molecular-weight dextran may be of some benefit.

OCCLUSIVE THROMBOPHLEBITIS

Leg Thrombophlebitis

In the lower extremity, deep thrombophlebitis that produces venous obstruction is usually associated with swelling; however, if good collateral circulation or duplicate veins are present, especially in the thigh, only local manifestations of inflammation may be apparent. The typical findings include pain and tenderness over the involved veins as well as swelling in the distal limb (which may be minimal with the patient in the supine position). The differential diagnosis is essentially the same as for nonocclusive thrombophlebitis. Lower leg occlusive thrombophlebitis is characterized by pain, swelling, and tenderness of the limb in the segment below the phlebitic process. In addition, lower extremity thrombophlebitis can be associated with pulmonary embolism: free-floating clot may occur in conjunction with occlusive (inflammatory) clot, although the latter is inevitably firmly adherent to the vein wall.

If the entire leg is swollen, the proximal portion of the clotting process must be in the iliac veins. If both legs are involved, involvement of the cava is likely. If the swelling is limited to the lower leg below the knee, the thrombotic problem is probably in the superficial femoral vein. If the manifestation is simply calf tenderness with only minimal to moderate swelling, then the thrombus is probably limited to the sural vein, the gastrocnemius vein, or both.

If the patient has a history of thrombophlebitis, is hospitalized, and has risk factors for deep thrombophlebitis, it is appropriate to begin treatment with moderate-dose heparin without ordering further diagnostic studies if there is no contraindication to anticoagulation. If the patient is an outpatient, if the patient is hospitalized but has no risk factors for deep thrombophlebitis, or if there appears to be a potential contraindication to anticoagulation, then the diagnosis should be

a

Nonocclusive thrombophlebitis is suspected

Patient may be asymptomatic, or there may be nonspecific extremity swelling. Pulmonary embolism is a common signal. Consider major risk factors, and attempt to determine cause.

Onset is apparently spontaneous

Consider congenital clotting tendency.

Risk factors for thrombophlebitis are identified

Assume acquired clotting tendency. If anticoagulation is not contraindicated, initiate moderate- to high-dose empirical heparin therapy.

Verify diagnosis

Perform noninvasive tests (^{125}I-labeled fibrinogen scan, plethysmography, Doppler or B-mode ultrasonography). If noninvasive tests are inconclusive, perform ascending phlebography.

Initiate definitive therapy for nonocclusive thrombophlebitis

Give moderate-dose heparin. After 3 or 4 days, depending on response, switch to warfarin. If anticoagulation is contraindicated, consider low-molecular-weight dextran.

Figure 2 **Illustrated are algorithms for the management of deep thrombophlebitis. The treatment approach depends on whether the thrombophlebitis is nonocclusive (*a*), occlusive (*b*), or massive (*c*).**

confirmed by means of the same techniques that are recommended for nonocclusive thrombophlebitis. In such patients, the accuracy of noninvasive assessment is excellent because any clot present must be occlusive. Impedance plethysmography, Doppler and B-mode ultrasonography, and phlebography can all be used with confidence. If diagnostic studies yield equivocal results and phlebography is difficult or impossible, treatment should proceed as if the diagnosis had been confirmed.

Table 1 Risk Factors for the Development of Acute Deep Thrombophlebitis

Hypercoagulability
    Congenital hypercoagulability
    Malignancy
    Oral contraceptives
    Polycythemia
    Thrombocytosis
Venous stasis
    Immobility
    Varicose veins
    Advanced age
    Congestive heart failure
    Obesity
Endothelial injury
    Trauma
    Recent surgery
    Severe infection

b

Signs of occlusive thrombophlebitis are present

Patient has signs of leg phlebitis (pain, tenderness over vein, swelling, possible pulmonary embolism)

Patient has signs of arm phlebitis (pain, tenderness over vein, swelling); may be relatively asymptomatic

Patient has history of thrombophlebitis, is hospitalized, and has risk factors

Do not await diagnostic studies. If anticoagulation is not contraindicated, begin empirical treatment with moderate-dose heparin.

Patient is outpatient, patient is hospitalized but has no risk factors, or treatment is contraindicated

Confirm diagnosis via noninvasive tests or phlebography. If these modalities are inconclusive, proceed as if diagnosis had been confirmed.

Patient has no systemic signs of infection

Assume that patient has sterile thrombophlebitis. If diagnosis is in doubt, utilize noninvasive tests or phlebography.

Patient has systemic signs of infection

Assume that patient has septic thrombophlebitis.

Initiate definitive treatment

Immobilize patient in bed and elevate leg (with or without elastic compression). Give moderate-dose heparin, followed by 6 mo of warfarin.

Treat sterile thrombophlebitis

Give moderate-dose heparin immediately. Consider lytic therapy. If arm veins are compressed after lytic therapy or spontaneous recovery from thrombosis, consider first-rib resection.

Treat septic thrombophlebitis

Remove any foreign body, culture tip, and do a Gram's stain of any clot. Give moderate-dose heparin. Give broad-spectrum antibiotics until organism is identified, then initiate specific antibiotic therapy.

Phlebitis resolves

Phlebitis persists

Consider ligation or drainage of vein.

c

Signs of phlegmasia cerulea dolens are present

Limb is massively swollen, bluish, and mottled distally. Gangrene is noted. Acute fluid losses may lead to hypovolemic shock.

Treat phlegmasia cerulea dolens

Replace fluids and elevate limb. Give high-dose heparin.

Phlebitis resolves

Phlebitis persists

Consider thrombectomy.

The treatment of choice is immobilization in bed, elevation of the limb (with or without elastic compression), and moderate-dose heparin, usually followed by three to six months of warfarin therapy. If the episode is mild, recovery is usually prompt. If the pain and swelling do not respond promptly to anticoagulation, either the diagnosis is wrong or the anticoagulation is inadequate [*see* General Principles of Anticoagulation and Lytic Therapy, *below*]. The combination of lytic therapy and heparin anticoagulation may be superior to heparin anticoagulation alone, leading to better clearance of clot from the valves with improved function and less risk of postphlebitic syndrome.[10]

Arm Thrombophlebitis

For all practical purposes, deep thrombophlebitis of the upper extremity involves only the axillary, the subclavian, or the innominate vein (or a combination thereof). Involvement of the superior vena cava is rare; when it does occur, it is usually in chronic conditions, such as malignancy in the medi-

astinum and long-term venous catheterization. Arm thrombophlebitis is characterized by pain and swelling in the involved limb with tenderness over the involved vein. In many instances, however, the condition is relatively asymptomatic: because of the excellent collateral circulation in the arm, particularly about the shoulder, the thrombosis must be extensive to produce marked swelling.

Spontaneous onset of axillary or subclavian vein thrombosis can occur in association with thoracic compression syndromes or as a complication of so-called Saturday night palsy (the result of an alcoholic's sleeping with his or her axilla compressed by the arm of a chair); investigation into the etiology [*see Table 2*], which includes the acquired and congenital clotting disorders [*see* Approach to Acquired and Congenital Thrombotic Syndromes, *below*] in the absence of mechanical factors that might explain the condition, is called for. The onset of swelling, tenderness, or fever in a patient with a central venous catheter is an indication for removal of the foreign body. If the patient is not bacteremic or febrile, if there has been a foreign body in the vein, and if the problem developed spontaneously, the presumption is that he or she has a sterile thrombophlebitis.

Subclinical nonocclusive clot is probably of little significance because documented pulmonary embolism from the upper extremity is quite rare. For this reason, the need for diagnosis of thrombophlebitis is less compelling in the upper extremity than in the lower extremity. Most of the noninvasive tests described earlier [*see* Nonocclusive Thrombophlebitis, *above*] usually yield positive results when the upper extremity is involved.[8] Moreover, catheterization of the distal veins is easy, and phlebography is relatively uncomplicated. These techniques should be used whenever the diagnosis is in doubt.

Figure 3 Shown is a phlebogram of the lower extremities. Injection of dye into the dorsal foot veins demonstrated occlusion of the iliac veins with excellent pelvic collateral circulation.

The morbidity of symptomatic upper extremity venous thrombosis can be quite significant. Thus, if the patient presents with massive swelling of the upper limb, moderate-dose heparin anticoagulation should be initiated immediately, and consideration should be given to lytic therapy (i.e., streptokinase, urokinase, or tissue plasminogen activator [t-PA]) [*see* General Principles of Anticoagulation and Lytic Therapy, *below*].[10] If phlebography shows compression of arm veins at the thoracic inlet after lytic therapy or spontaneous recovery from the thrombotic process, first-rib resection may be indicated, particularly if positional morbidity is present.

Septic deep thrombophlebitis is more common in the upper extremity than in the lower extremity. This is so primarily because the upper extremity veins are more frequently catheterized, as well as because they are the vessels most often used by drug addicts. If the phlebitis occurs in a critical care setting and there is an intravenous catheter in the vein at the time of clinical manifestations of fever and sepsis, the foreign body should be removed immediately, the tip cultured, and a Gram's stain done on any clot present. Broad-spectrum antibiotics (e.g., gentamicin, 80 mg four times daily, or metronidazole, 500 mg four times daily) should be administered until the organism can be identified and more specific antibiotic therapy instituted. Moderate-dose heparin anticoagulation is the primary treatment unless strictly contraindicated.

Ligation and drainage are not as practical for deep veins as they are for superficial veins, but one or the other, or both, may be indicated on rare occasions if the process does not respond to conventional therapy within three or four days and marked swelling and fever persist. Drainage is done on the most accessible portion of the phlebitic process. For ligation, the proximal end of the obstructive process should be identified via surgery or phlebography and the vein then ligated proximally.

PHLEGMASIA CERULEA DOLENS

Phlegmasia cerulea dolens is most apt to occur in dehydrated, cachectic patients and is usually superimposed on another critical illness, such as peritonitis or terminal malignancy. It can involve either the upper or the lower extremity but more commonly affects the latter. The swelling is severe because of massive thrombosis of all the main channels and their collateral vessels. In the lower extremity, there is usually simultaneous thrombosis of the iliac, the femoral, the common femoral, and the superficial femoral vein. The limb is massively swollen, bluish, and mottled in its most distal portion. Eventually, the limb becomes nonviable as arterial flow stops because of intense arterial vascular spasm associated with massive venous outflow obstruction. The clinical problem is compounded by acute massive fluid loss into the limb that can result in hypovolemic shock.

Treatment involves massive fluid replacement, elevation of the limb, and high-dose heparin anticoagulation. If the patient does not respond, thrombectomy may be considered, provided that the associated disease does not carry a fatal prognosis.[11] The procedure is best done via the transfemoral route with a limited incision so that anticoagulation can be continued postoperatively. If anticoagulation cannot be continued after thrombectomy, the thrombophlebitis will immediately recur.

Table 2 Etiology of Upper Extremity Thrombophlebitis
Congenital hypercoagulability
Thoracic outlet syndrome
Axillary vein compression
Stress injury
Central venous catheters
Mediastinal malignancy
Shoulder trauma

Approach to Pulmonary Embolism

All authorities agree that pulmonary embolism is a grossly under-diagnosed disease. In the United States, pulmonary embolism is believed to be associated with approximately 200,000 deaths a year, and it is probable that most episodes of pulmonary embolism (perhaps as many as 90 percent) are unsuspected because they are clinically insignificant or are misdiagnosed as other conditions.[1-3,12] Clinical manifestations include dyspnea, hemoptysis, pleurisy, heart failure, and cardiovascular collapse; however, each of these symptoms or signs is also associated with a number of other conditions [see Table 3]. The risk factors for pulmonary embolism in postoperative patients are similar to those for thrombophlebitis [see Table 4].

It is worthwhile to distinguish pulmonary embolism from pulmonary infarction. Of the approximately 10 percent of all emboli that are recognized clinically, only 10 percent are associated with pulmonary infarction.[13] Because the collateral circulation of the lung is excellent, obstruction of the larger pulmonary arteries rarely leads to death of lung tissue. When pulmonary infarction does occur, the diagnosis is usually obvious; hemoptysis, pleuritic chest pain, and a wedge-shaped density on chest x-ray are the classic manifestations. In most patients with pulmonary embolism (i.e., those who do not have pulmonary infarction), the chest x-ray is relatively normal.

From the standpoint of clinical diagnosis and treatment, pulmonary embolism is best classified as minor (or suspected) pulmonary embolism, moderate pulmonary embolism, or catastrophic pulmonary embolism [see Figure 4].

Minor Pulmonary Embolism

Minor pulmonary embolism undoubtedly occurs frequently in critically ill medical and surgical patients.[12] Manifestations may include transient tachypnea, with perhaps a slight change in blood gas values, and cardiac irritability, with frequent premature beats or tachyarrhythmias.[14-16] These changes may resolve in a few moments, and the patient may then appear perfectly normal. In these circumstances, it is probable that the embolus either is small or is composed of relatively fresh clot that produces only transient obstruction when it enters the pulmonary vascular tree.

If risk factors for pulmonary embolism are present [see Table 4], the differential diagnosis should be considered[15]; this includes acute respiratory distress syndrome, aspiration, atelectasis, heart failure, pneumonia, and systemic infection. If the diagnosis is not obvious but the risk of pulmonary embolism is substantial and there is no contraindication to anticoagulation, moderate-dose heparin therapy should be instituted while the diagnostic tests are being selected and performed. (Alternatively, one can simply assume the diagnosis of pulmonary embolism and continue therapy for as long as the patient is at risk.)

If pulmonary embolism is unlikely, if the risk from anticoagulation is high, or if there are other serious conditions in the differential diagnosis that are likely and cannot be ruled out, then specific studies should be ordered. These consist of laboratory studies for intravascular coagulation and noninvasive peripheral vascular studies to document the presence or absence of clot in leg veins, ventilation-perfusion lung scanning, or venous or pulmonary angiography.

Most patients with pulmonary embolism will have laboratory evidence of intravascular coagulation; however, the coagulation process may also be activated by severe infection, very

recent soft tissue trauma, or devitalization of tissue. The most accurate tests for detection of intravascular clotting are the test for the presence of fibrin degradation products (FDPs) and that for the presence of D-dimer, which is the particle cleaved off cross-linked (clotted) fibrin. The latter test is more specific because the presence of D-dimer signals the fibrinolytic breakdown of cross-linked fibrin, whereas fibrin degradation products can result from fibrinolytic dissolution of fibrinogen as well as fibrin.[16,17] High levels of both FDPs and D-dimer constitute strong indirect evidence of intravascular clotting. Although such a finding does not necessarily establish the diagnosis of pulmonary embolism, it strongly suggests the presence of clot somewhere in the vascular system and the need for anticoagulation, if only to prevent subsequent clotting complications. If both tests yield negative results, the probability of clotting anywhere in the vascular system is low. It must be remembered, however, that with both tests, fibrinolysis must be relatively intact for a positive result to be possible; if fibrinolysis is defective, these tests could, in theory, yield negative results even in the presence of clotting.

Noninvasive assessment (e.g., duplex scanning) aimed at detecting clot in the major leg veins may facilitate diagnosis. When definitive evaluation that includes phlebography is done, as many as 70 percent of patients with pulmonary embolism are found to have clot in the thigh or abdominal veins. This finding

Table 3   Clinical Features of Pulmonary Embolism: Differential Diagnosis

Clinical Feature	Other Conditions Associated with Feature
Dyspnea	Aspiration Atelectasis Pneumonia Pneumothorax Pulmonary edema Systemic infection
Heart failure	Cardiac tamponade Intracardiac injury Myocardial contusion Myocardial infarction
Hemoptysis	Bronchial injury Pulmonary contusion Tracheal erosion Unsuspected neoplasm
Pleurisy	Chest wall injury Pneumonia Pneumothorax Subphrenic inflammation
Cardiovascular collapse	Air embolism Cardiac tamponade Hypovolemia Myocardial infarction Severe hypoxemia Systemic infection Tension pneumothorax

---

Table 4 Risk Factors for Pulmonary Embolism

Major surgery
Surgical complications
Severe trauma
Lower extremity fractures
Obesity
Immobilization
Old age
Previous thrombotic events
Heart failure

---

in itself is usually an indication for treatment, even if pulmonary embolism is not present.

The initial enthusiasm for the use of lung scans to diagnose or screen for pulmonary embolism has receded somewhat.[18,19] It was thought that a negative scan rules out pulmonary embolism; however, in one study,[18] patients with negative or near-negative scans (14 percent of the total) still had a four percent incidence of pulmonary embolism when they were evaluated by means of angiography. A high-probability scan, on the other hand, did establish the presence of pulmonary embolism: the diagnosis was verifiable in 86 percent of cases when pulmonary angiography was done concomitantly.[18] Unfortunately, patients with high-probability scans

accounted for only 13 percent of the total and only 40 percent of those who later proved to have embolism. In the low- to moderate-probability group, which contained 72 percent of the patients with possible pulmonary embolism, 21 percent of the patients in the group proved to have pulmonary embolism on angiography. Although most of the patients with pulmonary embolism had scans ranging from low to moderate probability, so too did most of the patients in whom pulmonary embolism was initially suspected on clinical grounds but later excluded. Overall, therefore, whereas the sensitivity of scanning is high (96 percent), the specificity is low (10 percent). Even if patients with negative or near-negative scans are excluded, most patients will still require pulmonary angiography to confirm the diagnosis.

Because patients who are critically ill tolerate diagnostic testing poorly, pulmonary angiography is a more appropriate initial study in these patients than lung scanning; at present, it is the gold standard for diagnosis[1,3,20] [see Figure 5]. If the pulmonary angiogram is done immediately after the clinical episode, particularly if the patient is still symptomatic, a negative result rules out pulmonary embolism. However, pulmonary emboli frequently lack integrity and break up quickly. Thus, if the patient improves or recovers before the angiogram is done, the implication is that the clot was minimal, that it has disappeared into the microcirculation, or that it has been disposed of by the natural lytic process. Because angiography is not reliable in diagnosing clot in the subsegmental arteries,[21] a negative angiogram in a patient who is no longer symptomatic does not

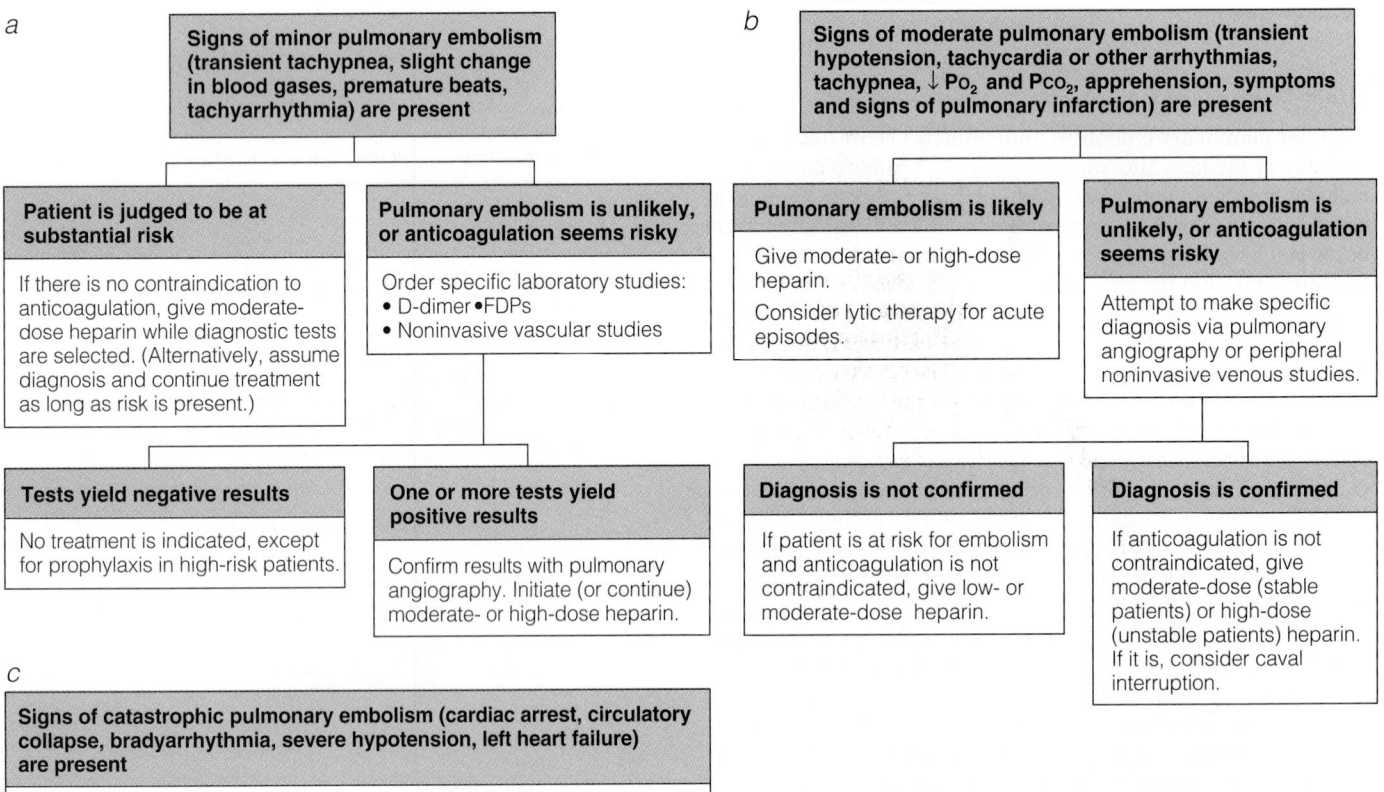

Figure 4 **Illustrated is an algorithm for the management of minor (*a*), moderate (*b*), and catastrophic (*c*) pulmonary embolism.**

rule out a pulmonary embolus, although it can establish the degree of patency of the pulmonary vasculature, which affects the prognosis. Alternative studies using magnification or balloon occlusion techniques may eventually be able to diagnose clot in vessels as small as 2 mm in diameter. Conceivably, studies of this type may show that some perfusion defects documented by scanning actually are related to pulmonary embolism.[21,22]

If all diagnostic tests for pulmonary embolism yield negative results, treatment may not be indicated, except for prophylaxis in patients at risk. If the tests are suggestive or indicative of pulmonary embolus, heparin anticoagulation should be continued at a moderate to high dosage, depending on the clinical significance of the embolic episode.

Moderate Pulmonary Embolism

The manifestations of moderate pulmonary embolism include transient hypotension, tachycardia or other cardiac arrhythmias, tachypnea with a significant fall in arterial oxygen tension and carbon dioxide tension, apprehension, and symptoms or signs of pulmonary infarction.[14,16] There may be signs of right heart failure as documented by increased central venous pressure, right ventricular heave, and an accentuated pulmonic second sound. Electrocardiography is rarely helpful in the differential diagnosis. Although acute right axis deviation, new incomplete right bundle branch block, and changes in S_1, Q_3, or T_3 are thought to characterize this disorder, they are found in only a small percentage of patients with proven pulmonary embolism.

If the diagnosis is probable and there are no likely alternative diagnoses, anticoagulant therapy (moderate- to high-dose heparin, depending on the symptoms) should be initiated. Lytic therapy can be used for acute episodes; however, its mortality has not been significantly lower than that of heparin, and it carries a much higher risk of bleeding.[1,3] Moreover, lytic therapy is often contraindicated because of recent surgery, injury, or vascular punctures.

If there is a relative contraindication to anticoagulation (e.g., an acute surgical wound, a previous bleeding episode, or an allergic reaction to heparin) or alternative diagnoses are likely, specific diagnosis is required. This is best achieved by means of pulmonary angiography. Peripheral noninvasive venous studies may be helpful because if they show significant venous obstruction, the likelihood of pulmonary embolism increases and the need for therapy is documented. As noted earlier, ventilation-perfusion scanning is only valuable if strongly positive.

If the diagnosis is not confirmed but the patient is at risk for embolic complications and there is no contraindication to heparin therapy, either low-dose or moderate-dose heparin anticoagulation should be initiated.[23,24] If the diagnosis is verified, the treatment is moderate-dose to high-dose heparin therapy, depending on the stability of the patient. If the patient is stable, moderate-dose therapy is sufficient; if the patient is unstable, high-dose therapy is indicated.[25-28]

When heparin therapy is contraindicated, caval interruption is appropriate. This approach is also indicated for patients who have documented pulmonary embolism despite what seems to be adequate systemic anticoagulation. Caval interruption can be done percutaneously via either the jugular or the femoral route; however, if it is done by the latter route, phlebography should be performed first to document the absence of clot along the planned route. The use of filters, such as those of Greenfield, is the most popular method.[29-31] If there is an indication for operation or a complication develops that necessitates operative intervention in the abdomen, caval ligation or caval clipping at

Figure 5 **A pulmonary angiogram shows nonequivocal filling defects in multiple arteries.**

the infrarenal level is the most appropriate therapy. Caval ligation at the juxta-infrarenal level is the most certain means of preventing further embolic episodes. This approach does not produce an area of relative stasis above the clip or ligature; clot has been shown to propagate through filters and embolize when there is such an area between the filter and the renal veins.

Catastrophic Pulmonary Embolism

Catastrophic pulmonary embolism is most apt to be superimposed on a critical illness or a major operation. The peak incidence is seven to 10 days after the procedure or the onset of clinical illness. The reason for this delay is that a clot must mature in the vascular system before it has integrity when it embolizes, and this process requires a considerable amount of time. As noted earlier, fresh clot breaks up readily and disappears promptly into the microvasculature, and thus it tends to produce transient problems; mature clot is resistant to lysis and can produce acute pulmonary obstruction and acute right heart failure.[14] Occlusion of large portions of the vasculature is associated with hemodynamic catastrophe.

Typically, the clinical onset of catastrophic pulmonary embolism comes when the patient, having just been mobilized after surgery, has his or her first postoperative bowel movement. If in the course of the bowel movement the patient performs a vigorous Valsalva maneuver, the great abdominal veins distend, and any clot present tends to be stripped loose. If a large clot embolizes, immediate collapse and cardiac arrest may result; in some cases, bradyarrhythmia or severe hypotension precedes the actual arrest. Immediate emergency treatment comprises administration of 100 percent oxygen by endotracheal tube, massive doses of heparin, and, if cardiac arrest occurs, cardiopulmonary resuscitation. A Swan-Ganz catheter should be inserted as soon as possible so that the effects of therapy can be monitored. Cardiotonic agents (e.g., dopamine, 2.0 to 5.0 μg/min, or dobutamine, 2.5 to 10.0 μg/kg/min) should be administered to strengthen myocardial function. If sudden arrest occurs in cir-cumstances that permit emergency thoracotomy, Trendelenburg's procedure can be performed; however, this procedure is rarely indicated and even more rarely successful. If the patient survives the initial emergency treatment and improves, high-dose heparin therapy should be continued and lytic therapy considered.[27,29]

Approach to Arterial Embolism

Arterial embolism has been much less common in recent decades, thanks to a decreased incidence of congenital heart disease, improved prevention of rheumatic heart disease, and better initial treatment of acquired heart disease.[32-34] The manifestations of arterial embolism result from sudden occlusion of a major artery, which characteristically is associated with overt clinical catastrophe (because previously patent arteries generally have very little collateral circulation). Sudden catastrophic arterial thrombosis can also occur, as a consequence of sudden elevation of an arteriosclerotic plaque; however, in most instances, the onset of arterial thrombosis is gradual, the danger is less, and the condition is easily distinguished from arterial embolism [see Table 5]. Spontaneous thrombosis of small arteries can be a complication of congenital clotting syndromes and autoimmune states [see Approach to Acquired and Congenital Thrombotic Syndromes, below]. Because arterial thrombosis is almost invariably superimposed on underlying occlusive disease, it will not be discussed further here.

The most common site for an embolic lodgment is the common femoral bifurcation[32-34] [see Figure 6]. Next in incidence is the aortoiliac region, followed by the popliteal artery and the brachial artery. The carotid bifurcation may be involved 20 to 25 percent of the time, but embolic lodgment at this site may be difficult to distinguish from occlusion secondary to carotid atherosclerosis. The superior mesenteric arterial circulation and the renal arterial circulation are involved five to 10 percent of the time, but as with carotid bifurcation involvement, the source of the occlusion may be hard to ascertain. Diagnosis of superior mesenteric arterial embolism is often delayed until the bowel is irreversibly damaged. The true incidence of renal artery involvement is more difficult to determine. Because of the bilaterality of the kidneys and because an isolated embolus typically has little or no impact on renal function, the diagnosis sometimes is not made.

When arterial embolism is likely or probable, two steps should be taken simultaneously: treatment should be begun, and an attempt should be made to determine the source of the embolus. Treatment involves immediate initiation of anticoagulation with heparin in moderate to high dosages (depending on the severity of the symptoms), followed by specific treatment for the site of lodgment. Discussion of specific diagnosis and treatment will be limited to visceral embolism and extremity embolism because these are the types of arterial embolism most often seen by the surgeon in the emergency setting. Carotid artery embolism is rarely managed surgically in the initial stages.

In most cases, arterial emboli have their origin in the heart; less commonly, they derive from the great vessels [see Figure 7]. If the patient is known to have an underlying cardiac disorder, such as atrial fibrillation, myocardial infarction, valvular heart disease, or thrombus formation on an artificial heart valve, then it can be assumed that the heart is the source. If cardiac evaluation, including ultrasonography, yields negative results, the large blood vessels are the probable source. The most common kind of embolic material is thrombus from aortic aneurysms or debris associated with atherosclerosis (usually involving the abdominal aorta). Ultrasonography can be rapidly performed in most environments; if there is evidence of aneurysm, the patient can be evaluated further with CT scanning. Alternatively, aortography may reveal atherosclerotic irregularities that explain the source of the embolic event.

Visceral Embolism

Early diagnosis of visceral arterial occlusion depends on a high degree of suspicion. When abdominal pain develops suddenly in a patient who is in the arteriosclerotic age group, has underlying heart disease, or is known to be at risk for embolism, the diagnosis should be suspected. Typically, in the first few hours, the pain is out of proportion to the clinical findings; on examination, the abdomen seems relatively normal, and only after several hours have passed is some tenderness apparent [see Figure 8]. If the patient is seen acutely and the diagnosis is suspected, immediate operative intervention is indicated. On rare occasions, arteriographic evaluation of the visceral circulation may be indicated if the index of suspicion is low or if nonocclusive causes (e.g., low cardiac output or shock-induced mesenteric venous thrombosis) are likely.

Mesenteric arterial occlusion is usually diagnosed late. After six to eight hours of ischemia, the diagnosis becomes obvious when abdominal tenderness and rebound develop and the patient becomes hemodynamically unstable. Mucus mixed with blood (currant jelly stool) is the characteristic finding on rectal examination if the colon is ischemic; often, however, gross, dark blood is found.

When the diagnosis of mesenteric arterial occlusion is suspected or documented, urgent laparotomy is indicated. If the diagnosis is made at an early stage and the bowel is still viable, mesenteric embolectomy or autogenous vein aortomesenteric bypass is indicated. If the intestine has been deprived of circulation for many hours, it is usually no longer viable; the only possible treatment may be resection of the dead portion of bowel. More often

Table 5 Differentiation of Arterial Embolism and Arterial Thrombosis

	Arterial Embolism	Arterial Thrombosis
History	Preexisting symptoms of vascular disease uncommon	Preexisting symptoms of vascular disease common
	Sudden onset usual	Sudden onset uncommon
	Symptoms usually severe	Symptoms usually moderate
Examination	Opposite limb usually normal	Usually vascular disease in opposite limb
	Chronic skin changes absent	Chronic skin changes usual
	Ischemia profound (no preexisting collateral)	Ischemia moderate (preexisting collateral)

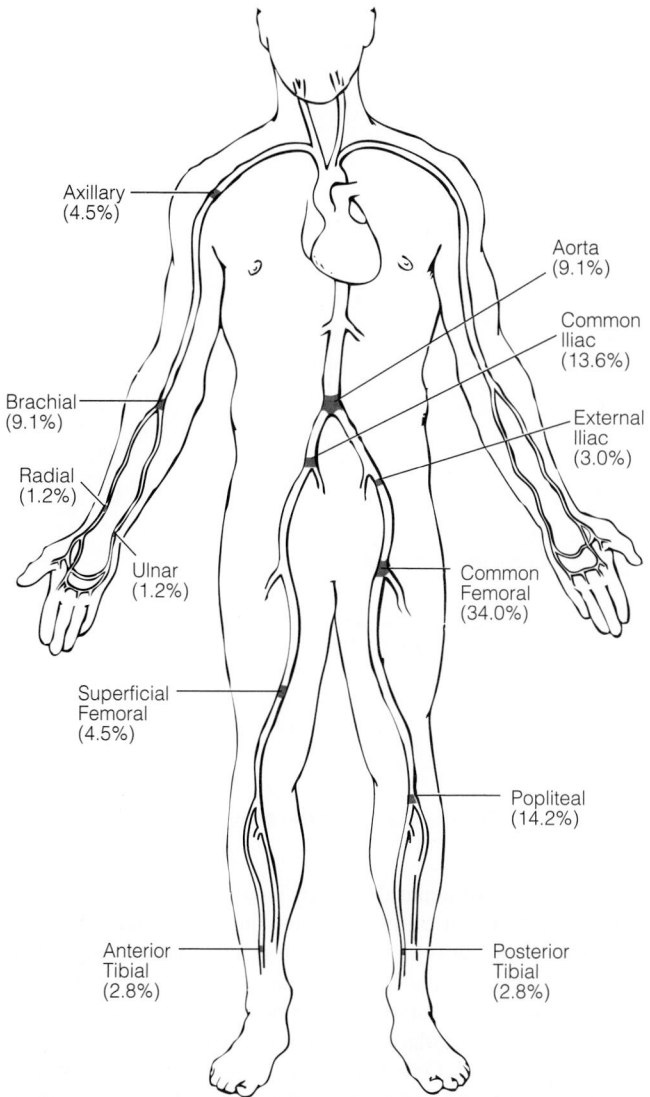

Axillary
(4.5%)

Brachial
(9.1%)

Radial
(1.2%)

Ulnar
(1.2%)

Superficial
Femoral
(4.5%)

Anterior
Tibial
(2.8%)

Aorta
(9.1%)

Common
Iliac
(13.6%)

External
Iliac
(3.0%)

Common
Femoral
(34.0%)

Popliteal
(14.2%)

Posterior
Tibial
(2.8%)

Figure 6 **Arterial embolism occurs with varying frequency in different peripheral arteries. The most common sites of embolic lodgment are shown.**

than not, the entire portion of the bowel supplied by the mesenteric artery is nonviable, and the condition is untreatable. If the bowel appears to be marginally viable, resection should be conservative, the mesenteric artery should be repaired if possible, and a second-look operation should be performed within 24 hours to reassess the viability of the remaining portion of the bowel.

In addition, the attempts to determine the source of the embolus that were begun earlier (see above) should be continued, and the underlying condition should be corrected if possible. Low- or moderate-dose heparin anticoagulation should be initiated (if not contraindicated by operation) 24 to 48 hours

after surgery and continued for two to three days, provided that no bleeding complication develops. Because long-term prophylactic anticoagulation is indicated, the patient should be transferred to warfarin after this initial period of heparin therapy.

Renal arterial embolism is usually manifested by the onset of flank pain, with or without microscopic hematuria, in a patient at risk for embolism. These findings constitute an indication for further diagnostic evaluation with renal scanning, arteriography, or both. Failure to identify blood flow on the renal scan and the demonstration of arterial occlusion on arteriography are indications for treatment. Once the diagnosis is made, the therapeutic choice is between moderate-dose heparin anticoagulation, direct catheter infusion of a thrombolytic agent, and surgery. If the kidney appears viable, surgical treatment involves exploration combined with restoration of circulation by embolectomy or autogenous vein aortorenal bypass; if the kidney is not viable, exploration is combined with nephrectomy.

Extremity Embolism

Arterial embolism to a limb results in acute limb ischemia, manifested by pain, paralysis, or anesthesia in the involved extremity [*see Figure 9*]. The presence of anesthesia, paralysis, or both is an indication of nonviability if allowed to persist. If the patient is seen promptly (within six to eight hours), immediate restoration of the circulation by means of thromboembolectomy is indicated, followed by high-dose heparin and then warfarin. If, however, more than six to eight hours has passed, the muscles are firm, and the skin is blue and mottled, then the process is unlikely to be reversible[35-37]; if it is reversible, it carries a high risk of mortality secondary to the reperfusion syndrome. In such cases, the best treatment is high-dose heparin anticoagulation for two to three days. This regimen allows sharp demarcation of the nonviable region from the rest of the limb, which permits successful amputation at the lowest possible level—ideally, no higher than just below the knee.

Pain and coldness coupled with retained sensation and muscle function indicate that the limb is still viable. When these signs and symptoms are first noted (usually in the emergency room), anticoagulation should be initiated with a large bolus of heparin (10,000–20,000 units) as the limb is evaluated. If the limb is viable when anticoagulation is begun, viability will improve as collateral flow is mobilized.[38] It is important not only to treat the initial ischemia but also to minimize the possibility of recurrent embolism. The heparin dosage, which should be high initially, can gradually be titrated downward over a period of two or three days, after which the patient can be transferred to warfarin.[39]

If the patient has minimal disability in the limb after this treatment, he or she should be followed and anticoagulation continued as clinically appropriate. The source of the embolus should be identified and treated if possible. If the patient has moderate or severe disability in the ischemic limb, elective revascularization can be carried out later.

General Principles of Anticoagulation and Lytic Therapy

Heparin Anticoagulation

LOW-DOSE HEPARIN

Low-dose heparin therapy is usually initiated with a 3,000 to 5,000 unit bolus given intravenously.[40] Next, 1,000 units/hr is

given by continuous intravenous infusion; this method of administration permits more precise control than subcutaneous administration. The activated partial thromboplastin time (PTT) should be elevated to at least five points above the normal value for the laboratory involved and should be maintained at this level for

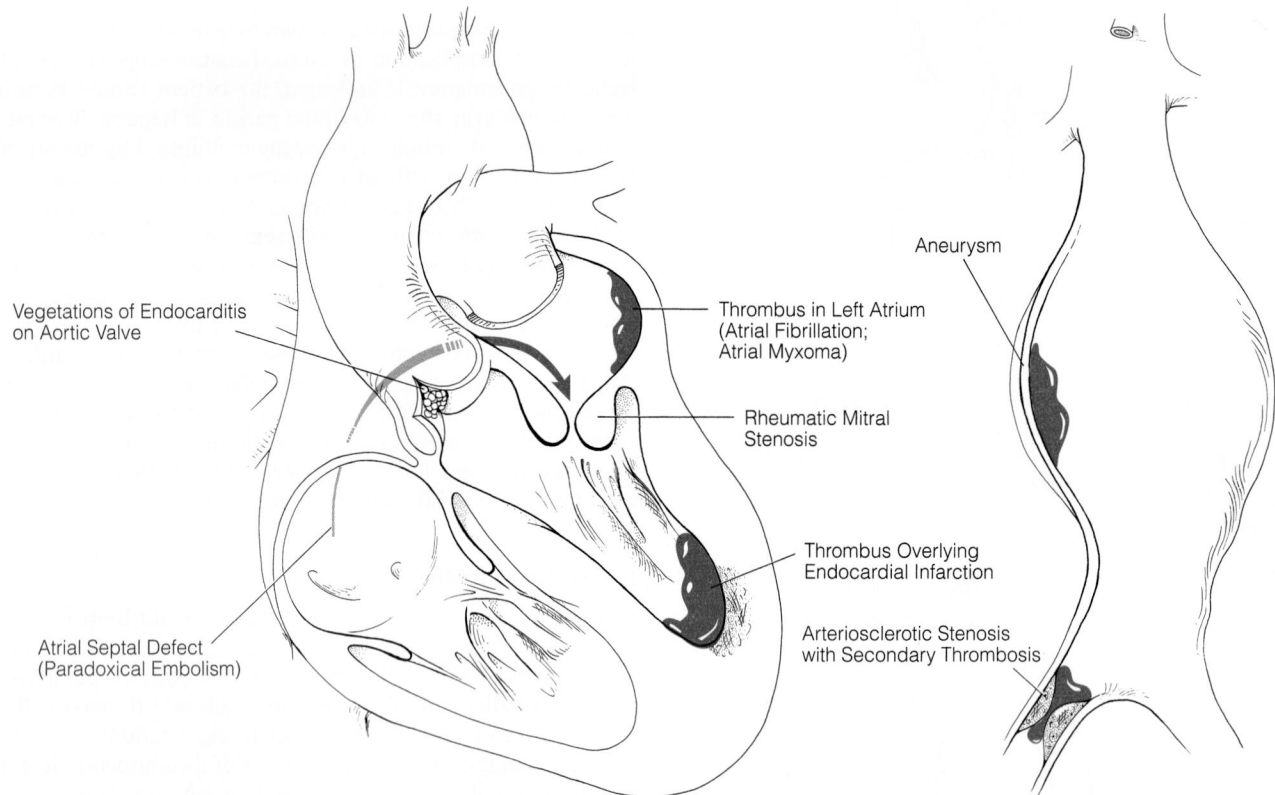

Figure 7 **Most arterial emboli originate in the heart; less commonly, emboli arise in the great vessels.**

the entire period of risk for clotting. If the initial PTT is more than five points above the laboratory's normal value, the heparin dosage should be gradually titrated downward to maintain the PTT at the appropriate level. If the patient is able to take nourishment and if anticoagulation for a week or longer is appropriate, warfarin therapy can be started in parallel with heparin anticoagulation, and heparin can be discontinued when the prothrombin time (PT) reaches a standard international ratio of about 2.0 to 3.0 [*see* Oral Anticoagulation, Dosage, *below*]. When the patient is active and mobile, anticoagulation with heparin or warfarin can be discontinued.

MODERATE-DOSE HEPARIN

Moderate-dose heparin could also be referred to as conventional anticoagulation.[41-43] This regimen may be appropriate for patients with non–life-threatening clotting complications (e.g., pulmonary embolism causing minimal morbidity or deep thrombophlebitis). Before therapy is begun, a clotting battery should be performed, consisting of the PTT, the PT, the platelet count, and levels of fibrinogen, antithrombin III, FDPs, fibrin monomer, and D-dimer. High fibrinogen levels and platelet counts are seen in patients with chronic clotting syndromes,[44] probably representing overcompensation for increased utilization. Elevated levels of fibrin monomer indicate low-grade clotting, and elevated levels of FDPs and D-dimer suggest clotting and activation of fibrinolysis. If these tests all strongly suggest intravascular clotting, high-dose heparin may be more appropriate initially, unless it is contraindicated by imminent or very recent surgery or by the presence of open lesions.

In the average patient, moderate-dose heparin anticoagulation begins with an arbitrary dose, 10,000 units, followed by continuous intravenous administration at a rate sufficient to double the PTT. This rate varies greatly but averages about 2,000 units/hr. When dosages higher than 2,000 units/hr are required, preexisting antithrombin depletion is highly probable.

Tight control of heparin therapy is not as important as monitoring the patient for evidence of bleeding and platelet depletion. Clinical evidence of bleeding does not necessarily contraindicate continuing anticoagulation. Minimal amounts of blood may be lost in the urine or through the GI tract; if the patient has a clear-cut need for anticoagulation, these minor bleeding complications should be accepted. Only when transfusion is indicated to maintain the hematocrit must the risk-benefit ratio of continuing therapy be considered. At that point, if the risks of bleeding seem to outweigh the benefits of anticoagulation, heparin can be discontinued or reduced to the low-dose level. One of the most important aspects of monitoring is watching for falls in hematocrit that indicate significant bleeding. The most common sites for hemorrhagic complications are surgical wounds and the retroperitoneum. The latter is a silent area.

HIGH-DOSE HEPARIN

High-dose heparin therapy consists of the administration of arbitrary large doses of heparin without regard to PTT monitoring. The PTT is used only to ensure that the heparin is having an appropriate effect. The maximum PTT that can be measured by our laboratory is 150 seconds; in high-dose heparin treatment, the PTT should be greater than this value. Given that a fully anticoagulated patient cannot form clot at all, the PTT in this circumstance theoretically should be infinite.

In most patients, high-dose therapy begins with a 20,000 unit I.V. bolus, followed by infusion of 5,000 units/hr I.V. Such high dosages are necessary in most patients with arterial ischemia to produce complete anticoagulation and prevent distal propagation of clot.[38,39,45-47] Clinical evidence of improved collateral circulation in a patient being treated for arterial ischemia or venous thrombosis is a sign that the dosage is adequate. Pulmonary function should improve in patients being treated for pulmonary embolism.

Visceral embolism is suggested by sudden abdominal or flank pain in a patient who is in the arteriosclerotic age group, has underlying heart disease, or is at risk for embolism

Early diagnosis requires high degree of suspicion. Pain is typically out of proportion to the clinical findings.

Patient is hemodynamically unstable, with abdominal tenderness with rebound; rectal exam shows gross, dark blood or mucus mixed with blood

Suspect mesenteric arterial occlusion; perform urgent laparotomy. (Condition is usually diagnosed late, after 6–8 hr of ischemia.)
- *If bowel is viable*: Perform mesenteric embolectomy or autogenous vein aortomesenteric bypass.
- *If bowel is marginally viable:* Resect conservatively, repair mesenteric artery (if possible), and perform second-look procedure within 24 hr.
If possible, identify source of embolus and treat underlying condition.

Provide long-term prophylaxis

Give low- or moderate-dose heparin (if not contraindicated and if no bleeding develops) for 2–3 days, then switch to warfarin.

Patient has flank pain, with or without microscopic hematuria

Suspect renal arterial occlusion. Perform renal scanning, arteriography, or both.

Failure to identify blood flow on renal scan and demonstration of occlusion on arteriography are indications for treatment

Treat via
- Heparin anticoagulation,
- Lytic therapy, or
- Surgical exploration combined with embolectomy or autogenous vein aortorenal bypass (*if kidney is viable)* or with nephrectomy (*if kidney is nonviable*).

Figure 8 **Illustrated is an algorithm for the management of visceral embolism.**

Complete anticoagulation is the essential principle of high-dose heparin therapy. Therefore, there is no need to be concerned about an upper limit for the dosage: if the patient cannot clot, doubling or even tripling the dosage will not, in theory, increase the risk of bleeding. Moreover, because the incidence of bleeding is very low in the first two or three days of therapy, regardless of the heparin dosage,[46,47] high initial dosages will not be associated with an unacceptable risk of bleeding. After the heparin has been observed to have an effect and the prolonged PTT has been documented, the high dosage should continue for at least 24 hours. The dosage can then be decreased by 500 to 1,000 units/hr in the next 24 hours. If the clinical effect is maintained and the patient continues to improve, the dosage can be decreased once again in the following 24 hours by another 500 to 1,000 units/hr. In theory, if all clotting has stopped, levels of natural antithrombins (which are depleted by clotting) should recover, and lower dosages of heparin

will be effective. After three or four days of therapy, it may be appropriate to reduce the dosage still further, to more conventional levels, such as the moderate level described earlier [see Moderate-Dose Heparin, *above*].

If the improvement initially noted is lost, the dosage should be increased to its previous level, and the elevated dosage should be maintained for several days before any attempt is made to reduce it again. Careful monitoring of the platelet count and the hematocrit is appropriate. The hematocrit should be monitored at least four times a day, and heparin should be discontinued or the dosage reduced only when the risks posed by bleeding and transfusion exceed the benefits provided by anticoagulation. In a monitored environment, patients very rarely die of hemorrhage; rather, they die of the consequences of the clotting. The primary hemorrhagic risk is intracranial bleeding. Fortunately, this is a quite rare complication of heparin anticoagulation. The risk of

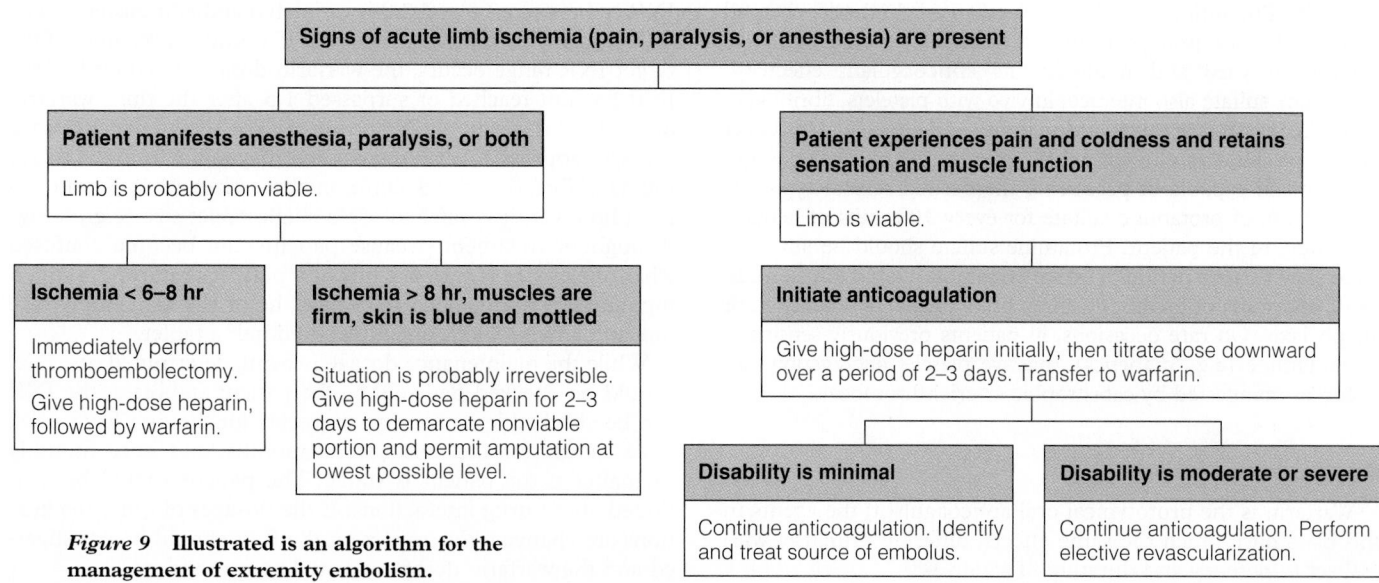

Figure 9 **Illustrated is an algorithm for the management of extremity embolism.**

Signs of acute limb ischemia (pain, paralysis, or anesthesia) are present

Patient manifests anesthesia, paralysis, or both

Limb is probably nonviable.

Ischemia < 6–8 hr

Immediately perform thromboembolectomy.
Give high-dose heparin, followed by warfarin.

Ischemia > 8 hr, muscles are firm, skin is blue and mottled

Situation is probably irreversible. Give high-dose heparin for 2–3 days to demarcate nonviable portion and permit amputation at lowest possible level.

Patient experiences pain and coldness and retains sensation and muscle function

Limb is viable.

Initiate anticoagulation

Give high-dose heparin initially, then titrate dose downward over a period of 2–3 days. Transfer to warfarin.

Disability is minimal

Continue anticoagulation. Identify and treat source of embolus.

Disability is moderate or severe

Continue anticoagulation. Perform elective revascularization.

intracranial bleeding is greatest in elderly patients, particularly women[42]; however, it is small in comparison with the obvious risks posed by the clotting episode. Nevertheless, the existence of the risk makes it appropriate to use high-dose heparin primarily in life-threatening conditions.

COMPLICATIONS

Two forms of acute heparin-induced thrombocytopenia have been reported.[48-51] Mild thrombocytopenia occurs in two to five percent of patients two to 15 days after the initiation of therapy. The platelet count usually remains at about 100,000/mm³, and treatment can be continued without undue risk of bleeding. Severe thrombocytopenia is much less frequent. It usually occurs about seven to 14 days after the initiation of heparin therapy (perhaps depending on the type of heparin being used) and is reversible once the drug is discontinued. This severe form of heparin-induced thrombocytopenia has been associated with thrombotic complications, including arterial thrombosis with platelet fibrin clots, which may cause myocardial infarction or stroke or necessitate amputation of the limb. Thrombocytopenia appears to be less common when porcine rather than bovine heparin is used.

Unlike warfarin, heparin does not cross the placenta and has not been associated with fetal malformations; therefore, it is the drug of choice for thrombotic complications of pregnancy. Heparin can be administered for periods of three to six months by subcutaneous injection in an outpatient setting. Osteoporosis and spontaneous vertebral fractures can occur with long-term administration.[52] Thrombocytopenia excepted, allergic reactions to heparin are rare.

An extremely rare complication of heparin therapy is adrenal hemorrhage, which can result in adrenal insufficiency[42] [see VI:4 Adrenal Insufficiency]. If acute adrenal insufficiency is suspected, anticoagulant therapy should be discontinued, and high-dose steroid therapy, preferably with hydrocortisone, should be initiated. Treatment should not be delayed until laboratory confirmation can be obtained. CT scanning may be useful in diagnosing this condition. Heparin may also suppress aldosterone synthesis, especially with prolonged use.[42]

REVERSAL OF HEPARIN EFFECT

The anticoagulant effect of heparin disappears within hours after the drug is discontinued. If the effect must be reversed quickly, the patient should be given protamine sulfate intravenously. Protamines are low-molecular-weight basic charged proteins that are isolated from fish sperm. They bind tightly to heparin in vitro and neutralize its anticoagulant effect.[42,43] Protamine sulfate also interacts in vivo with platelets, fibrinogen, and other plasma proteins and may have an anticoagulant effect of its own. Therefore, it should be given in the smallest dosages that are still capable of producing the desired result—typically, about 1 mg of protamine sulfate for every 100 units of heparin remaining in the patient. Protamine sulfate should be administered slowly over a period of five to 10 minutes; rapid infusion can cause shortness of breath, flushing, bradycardia, hypotension, or anaphylaxis. On rare occasions, in patients previously sensitized to protamine (e.g., diabetics), massive platelet aggregation can occur, as manifested by catastrophic arterial thrombosis.

Oral Anticoagulation

Warfarin is the prototypical oral anticoagulant; the agents in this class have much the same effects, differing primarily with respect to potency and duration of action.[42,43]

Table 6 Recommendations for Use of Varying Dosages of Warfarin

The dosage of warfarin is regulated by monitoring the INR. A less intense therapeutic range (INR = 2.0 to 3.0, corresponding to a PT 1.3 to 1.5 times normal with a WHO-designated thromboplastin) is appropriate for the following applications:

1. The prevention of venous thromboembolism in high-risk patients.

2. The treatment of venous thrombosis and pulmonary embolism after an initial course of heparin.

3. The prevention of systemic embolism (a) in patients with tissue heart valves, (b) in selected patients with atrial fibrillation, (c) in patients with acute anterior wall myocardial infarction, and (d) in patients with valvular heart disease.

A more intense therapeutic range (INR = 3.0 to 4.5, corresponding to a PT 1.5 to 2.0 times normal with a WHO-designated thromboplastin) is appropriate for patients with mechanical prosthetic valves and patients with recurrent systemic embolism.

INR—international normalized ratio PT—prothrombin time WHO—World Health Organization

---

DOSAGE

Historically, the dosage of warfarin has been regulated by monitoring the PT. A PT that is 1.5 to 2.5 times the normal value (11 or 12 seconds) has generally been considered to represent the optimal therapeutic level. However, wide variation in the PT has been reported because of the different thromboplastins used by different laboratories.[53] The World Health Organization (WHO) has recommended converting the PT ratio into an international normalized ratio (INR) so that all laboratory assessments will be comparable. This involves comparing the various thromboplastins with a single standard, a WHO-designated human brain thromboplastin. An INR of 2.0 to 3.0 corresponds to a PT that is 1.3 to 1.5 times normal and represents a moderate dose; an INR of 3.0 to 4.5 corresponds to a PT that is 1.5 to 2.0 times normal and represents a high dose. When bleeding and recurrence rates were measured in patients with high-dose and moderate-dose INRs, the incidence of bleeding was 20 percent in the first group versus five percent in the second, and the therapeutic benefit was equivalent in the two groups.[53] Consequently, the lower ratios are recommended for all but extremely high-risk patients[53] [see Table 6].

Initially, the daily dose of warfarin required to increase the INR to between 2.0 and 3.0 is estimated and administered. The INR is then checked every morning. If a sudden overshoot of the target INR range occurs, the warfarin dosage is reduced. If the INR has not reached or surpassed 1.5 after the third warfarin dose, the dosage should be increased. The maintenance dosage averages approximately 5 mg/day but may range from 2.5 to 7.5 mg/day. Warfarin tablets come in three sizes (2.5, 5, and 7.5 mg); however, it is safer to use a single tablet size (e.g., 5 mg) throughout treatment because patients can become confused when tablet size is varied. Thus, if a patient requires 7.5 mg, 5 mg, and 2.5 mg on successive days, he or she can simply take one and a half tablets, one tablet, and half a tablet.

While the maintenance dosage is being determined, the INR should be checked daily. Once the patient stabilizes, the INR can be checked less often: twice weekly for the first few weeks, once weekly for the next several months, and once monthly thereafter if the patient is stable. The patient should be cautioned about drug interactions. If the dosages of other medications are changed, the impact on the INR should be investigated and the warfarin dosage adjusted as appropriate.

DRUG INTERACTIONS

The patient's response to warfarin is affected not only by various bodily factors but also by interactions with numerous drugs [see Table 7]. Interactions are most dangerous when the drugs administered in parallel are taken intermittently.[42,43] Increased metabolic clearance of the drug, secondary to activation of hepatic enzymes, can result from administration of barbiturates, rifampin, or phenytoin; chronic use of alcohol; ingestion of large amounts of vitamin K; and rich foods. Elevated levels of coagulation factors during pregnancy also decrease the effectiveness of the drug.

Decreased metabolism or displacement from protein binding sites caused by phenylbutazone, sulfinpyrazone, metronidazole, disulfiram, allopurinol, cimetidine, amiodarone, or acute intake of ethanol can increase the INR and increase the risk of hemorrhage. Relative deficiency of vitamin K, resulting from inadequate diet or the elimination of the intestinal flora by antimicrobial agents, may have similar effects.

There are some serious interactions that increase the risk of bleeding without altering the INR. These include inhibition of platelet function by drugs such as aspirin and gastritis or gastric ulceration induced by anti-inflammatory drugs.

COMPLICATIONS

Bleeding is the major toxic complication of oral anticoagulation. Whereas tight control of heparin therapy is usually not crucial, tight control of warfarin therapy is definitely necessary to minimize bleeding complications. Bleeding is rare when the INR is kept below 3; when bleeding does occur, it suggests a preexisting lesion. If the bleeding is minor, the warfarin dosage should be adjusted, and if it is major, the drug may have to be discontinued. As with heparin, the risk of intracerebral or subdural hematoma is greater in patients older than 50 years. If the patient shows any sign of hemorrhage, the next dose of anticoagulant should be withheld and the PT measured. For continued or serious bleeding, 5 to 10 mg of vitamin K_1 oxide (phytonadione) I.V. is an effective antidote. Several hours may pass before significant improvement in hemostasis becomes apparent, and 24 hours or longer may be needed for maximal effect. If immediate restoration of hemostatic competence is necessary, levels of vitamin K–dependent coagulation factors can be raised by giving fresh frozen plasma, 10 to 20 ml/kg body weight. Vitamin K_1 oxide should be given simultaneously.

Because administration of warfarin during pregnancy can cause birth defects and abortion, it is contraindicated under these circumstances. Warfarin-induced skin necrosis is a rare complication of oral anticoagulant therapy.[50] First noted in 1943, this syndrome is characterized by the appearance of skin lesions shortly after treatment is initiated. It may be the result of depressed protein C and S levels.

Lytic Therapy

Although heparin is used primarily as an anticoagulant, there is evidence that it may also promote lysis of clot. This phenomenon has been observed in vivo, and a sophisticated group of experiments utilizing cultured mesothelial cells has shown that when heparin is added, these cells are also capable of lysing fibrin.[54] However, lytic therapy is generally understood to refer to administration of streptokinase, urokinase, or tissue plasminogen activator.[42,43,55-58] These agents act by different mechanisms on the endogenous fibrinolytic system to convert plasminogen to plasmin [see I:5 Bleeding and Transfusion]. Streptokinase indirectly promotes plasmin formation by combining with plasminogen to form streptokinase-plasminogen complexes that are converted to streptokinase-plasmin complexes. These activator complexes convert residual plasminogen to plasmin.[42,58] Urokinase directly cleaves a peptide bond in the plasminogen molecule to form plasmin. Tissue plasminogen activator binds to fibrin via lysine binding sites at the N-terminal.

The thrombolytic agents are most effective when treatment can be initiated in a matter of hours. Lytic therapy is worth attempting when the clot has been present for less than one week, particularly if it has been present for less than three days. When lytic therapy is begun, heparin therapy usually is temporarily discontinued because of the theoretical possibility of increased bleeding risk; anticoagulation may be resumed immediately upon completion of lytic therapy. If, however, the problem is immediately life threatening (e.g., myocardial infarction or massive pulmonary embolism), anticoagulation should probably be carried out in parallel with lytic therapy to prevent rethrombosis.

INDICATIONS AND CONTRAINDICATIONS

The indications for lytic therapy are being extended.[58] Streptokinase and urokinase are being used for venous thrombotic conditions, such as symptomatic obstruction of major veins in the upper extremities. The morbidity of axillary vein thrombosis can be considerable; clearance of clot may not only help restore patency but also help identify the underlying cause, if it is unknown. In the lower extremities, more thorough clearance of clot should, in theory, help restore valve function and prevent so-called postphlebitic syndrome.[57,59]

Lytic therapy is also of some use in patients with arterial embolism. Although acute arterial ischemia may become irreversible before lytic agents can take effect, the ability of these agents to clear clot from peripheral bypass grafts and arterial venous shunts may not only result in restoration of vascular

Table 7 Factors Influencing
Response to Warfarin

Factors Leading to Increased Response	Factors Leading to Decreased Response
Drugs	Drugs
Allopurinol	Barbiturates
Amiodarone	Cholestyramine
Aspirin	Diuretics
Cephalosporins	Ethanol (chronic use)
Cimetidine	Phenytoin
Clofibrate	Rifampin
Disulfiram	Vitamin K
Ethanol (acute intoxication)	Foods
Heparin	Green leafy vegetables
Metronidazole	Bodily factors
Sulfinpyrazone	Hereditary resistance
Trimethoprim-sulfamethoxazole	Hypometabolic states
Bodily factors	Pregnancy
Age	Uremia
Congestive heart failure	
Dietary inadequacy	
Hypermetabolic states	
Intestinal flora loss	
Liver disease	

function but also permit identification of the lesion that precipitated the embolism. Lytic agents may also clear clot sufficiently to permit correction of underlying anatomic defects by means of balloon angioplasty or local surgical procedures.[58]

There are several contraindications that preclude the use of thrombolytic therapy: surgery in the previous 10 days, serious gastrointestinal bleeding in the previous three months, a history of hypertension, an active bleeding or hemorrhagic disorder, a previous cerebrovascular accident, or an active intracranial process. As with heparin, the risk of intracranial bleeding is increased in older patients. Use of t-PA appears to be associated with a higher risk than use of streptokinase or urokinase.

STREPTOKINASE

Streptokinase is a 47 kd protein produced by β-hemolytic streptococci. Because streptokinase is not an endogenous protein, circulating antibodies to it are often already present in plasma; these antibodies result from previous streptococcal infections. When streptokinase is administered via a traditional intravenous infusion, a loading dose must be given to overcome these antibodies. It is essential to ensure that the desired therapeutic effects are achieved. This is done by documenting a rise in the thrombin time (TT), a fall in the fibrinogen level, or an abrupt rise in the D-dimer level. At times, a large loading dose may be necessary to overcome the inactivating antibodies. Once the antibodies are depleted, the half-life of streptokinase is about 80 minutes.

Because streptokinase may deplete circulating plasminogen after a few hours, the optimal therapeutic approach may be to administer it for six hours by continuous infusion every 24 hours for a period of two or three days and then to administer heparin in the intervals between streptokinase infusion.

UROKINASE

Urokinase is a 34 kd globulin that was originally found in human urine and is now isolated from cultured human cells. It has a half-life of 15 minutes and is metabolized by the liver. For catheter clearance, a solution containing 5,000 units/ml should be infused into the obstructed tubing. Like streptokinase, urokinase lacks fibrin specificity and therefore produces a systemic lytic state. Its primary disadvantage is that it costs far more than streptokinase.

TISSUE PLASMINOGEN ACTIVATOR

Tissue plasminogen activator is an enzymatic glycoprotein composed of 527 amino acids that is produced from a human melanoma cell line by means of recombinant DNA technology. The half-life of t-PA is approximately four minutes; it is metabolized by the liver, and approximately 80 percent of the dose is excreted in the urine within 18 hours. It is not antigenic and does not promote antibody formation. Theoretically, t-PA should be somewhat more specific for fibrin clot than urokinase or streptokinase: t-PA invades clot locally, and the t-PA that reaches the systemic circulation is largely deactivated by circulating t-PA inhibitor. In practice, however, the effects of t-PA have not been clinically distinguishable from those of urokinase. Like urokinase, t-PA is extremely expensive.

TECHNIQUE OF ADMINISTRATION

Several methods of administering thrombolytic therapy are currently in use. The traditional method, venous infusion, has been widely used to treat coronary artery thrombosis[60]; however, it has shown only modest effectiveness against peripheral arterial occlusion and is associated with a high rate of hemorrhagic com-

plications.[61] Over time, administration of thrombolytic agents has evolved to become more focused on the site of occlusion, particularly with the development of intra-arterial infusion techniques. A 1974 study reported success with lower total doses of streptokinase administered directly into the occluded artery.[62] The theoretical advantages of this approach were (1) that it decreased the systemic dose of the thrombolytic drug and the concomitant risk of bleeding and (2) that it improved the local effect, as demonstrated by increased 90-minute patency rates. Since that study, intra-arterial infusions have been provided either via a drip proximal to the thrombosis or via a pulse spray directly into the clot through a specialized catheter.

For patients with acute occlusion of a peripheral artery, direct infusion of urokinase into the affected artery in a dosage of 4,000 IU/min for four hours, then in a dosage of 2,000 IU/min for up to 48 hours, has proved as efficacious as immediate surgery.[63] The survival and amputation rates associated with this method of therapy are not significantly different from those associated with a standard primary surgical approach.

Use of thrombolytic agents as the primary therapy has both advantages and disadvantages. One advantage is that it gives the surgeon time to optimize the patient's condition for the stress of an operative procedure. Another is that once the thrombus has been dissolved, it may be easier to identify the underlying atherosclerotic lesion, which would permit better operative planning. The concurrent disadvantages are that there is a one to two percent rate of bleeding at the skin insertion site for the catheter as well as a similar rate of arterial thrombosis at the site where the catheter enters the arterial tree.

Thrombolytic therapy for acute pulmonary embolism has a number of attractive theoretical benefits; however, clinical trials have not shown that such therapy has any significant practical advantages, except in patients who are hemodynamically unstable as a result of an embolus. In these patients, thrombolysis, compared with heparin alone, achieves greater improvements in intermediate end points, such as right ventricular function, but does not increase survival.[64]

MONITORING

Although monitoring of thrombolytic therapy is less standardized than monitoring of anticoagulant therapy, there are several principles that should be followed. First, the effect should be monitored from both a clinical and a laboratory perspective. Clinical monitoring involves following improvements in the angiographic images. Laboratory monitoring has three components. First, D-dimer levels should be measured; a marked increase should be noted, signaling that cross-linked fibrin is undergoing breakdown. Second, adequate stores of the effector protein plasminogen should be documented; without plasminogen, none of the thrombolytic drugs are effective. Third, fibrinogen levels should be followed to prevent exhaustion of native clotting. Most authorities recommend that thrombolytic therapy be discontinued once fibrinogen levels fall below 50 mg/dl. Previously, the TT had been used for monitoring thrombolysis; however, given the current recommendation for concurrent use of heparin,[60] the TT is of little value in this setting.

COMPLICATIONS

The major toxicity of all three thrombolytic agents is hemorrhage. The incidence of bleeding is many times higher after lytic therapy than after anticoagulant therapy and is dependent on both the dosage and the duration of lytic therapy. With careful administration of thrombolytic agents, the incidence of major hemorrhage is less than five percent and the incidence of intracranial hemorrhage is less than one percent.[58] Hemorrhage is the result of two factors: (1) the lysis of physiologic thrombi occurring at sites of vascular injury (e.g., venipuncture sites) and (2) a systemic lytic state caused by the systemic formation of plasmin, which results in fibrinogenolysis and destruction of other coagulation proteins, especially factors V and VIII.

A potential major complication is distal embolism of partially lysed clot. In theory, this possibility should contraindicate use of these agents to treat thrombus in the heart or in the cerebrovascular system.[58] Surprisingly, dislodgment of intracardiac clot as a result of lytic therapy is rare.

There are several adverse reactions that are caused by streptokinase but not by urokinase or t-PA. When streptokinase was first produced, it was associated with a very high incidence of antigenicity and severe pyrogenic reactions. The current purified formulation is relatively free of pyrogens and has a reduced incidence of allergic side effects. It is still antigenic, however, and its use may cause allergic reactions or, in rare instances, anaphylaxis resulting from the presence of preformed streptococcal antibodies. Streptokinase may also induce the formation of additional antibodies that eliminate the possibility of retreatment. In contrast, patients may be re-treated with urokinase as often as necessary with minimal risk of allergic reactions.

Approach to Acquired and Congenital Thrombotic Syndromes

It is well known that certain patients seem to have a tendency to clot spontaneously. Although it has long been postulated that so-called hypercoagulability states exist, such states have been difficult to document except on clinical grounds. Over the past several decades, however, a clearer picture of the nature of these clotting tendencies has emerged.[65] A major impetus for this development was the recognition of the role of antithrombins in exposing clotting. If an antithrombin deficiency exists and clotting goes unchecked, the activation of a clotting cascade could theoretically progress to clotting throughout the entire vascular system. Another important discovery in the understanding of thrombotic syndromes was the recognition of natural lytic substances in the blood that tends to remove the clot after clotting has occurred. Deficiencies of these lytic substances may also exist and may result in a clinical thrombotic tendency. Both types of deficiency can be either acquired or congenital.

Screening

When the etiology of a clotting episode is unclear, the family history should be reviewed for evidence of a congenital disorder. If the history is negative, the patient should be screened for the acquired disorders; if it is positive or if initial screening for acquired disorders yields negative results, the patient should be screened for the congenital disorders [see Figure 10].

ACQUIRED CLOTTING CONDITIONS

Screening for acquired clotting conditions [see Table 8] is based on the history, physical examination, and laboratory assessment. The history should include medications, diseases, and surgical procedures or other injuries.[66-68] Examination may disclose causes of hypercoagulability.[69] Soft tissue injury, for example, whether from surgery, injury, or vascular damage, is a potent activator of the coagulation system. If the injury is severe enough, as in a mangled extremity, it may by itself be capable of causing a severe acquired coagulopathy. The problem is usually obvious, but on occasion, detailed study may be necessary to identify tissue damage or ischemic injury to bowel or extremities. Hypovolemia—especially hypovolemic shock—markedly reduces the clotting time: blood from a patient in profound shock may clot instantaneously in the syringe as it is being drawn. The breakdown of red cells in a hemolytic transfusion reaction can cause clotting. Severe infection, especially from gram-negative organisms, is a potent activator of coagulation.[70]

Laboratory screening may facilitate the diagnosis. A complete blood count may document the presence of polycythemia or leukemia. Thrombocythemia may be a manifestation of a hypercoagulable disorder, and thrombocytopenia after the administration of heparin raises the possibility of intravascular platelet aggregation. A prolonged PTT is suggestive of lupuslike anticoagulant. The presence of increased levels of D-dimers, FDPs, or fibrin monomers in the plasma may document the presence of low-grade intravascular coagulation.

CONGENITAL CLOTTING CONDITIONS

Congenital clotting tendencies can result from deficiencies in thrombosis inhibitors (antithrombin III, protein C, protein S, and possibly heparin cofactor II), dysfibrinogenemias, or dysfibrinolysis (defects in fibrinolysis) [see Table 9]. Most of the congenital clotting defects are transmitted as an autosomal dominant trait. A negative family history, however, does not preclude inherited thrombophilia, because the defects have a low penetrance and fresh mutations may have occurred.

Initial Laboratory Assessment

If the TT and the euglobulin clot lysis time are used in initial laboratory assessment, the following approach, described by Rodgers and Shuman,[71] can be taken.

If the TT is prolonged, dysfibrinogenemia is likely. Further assessment using the reptilase test and specific functional assays for fibrinogen will confirm the diagnosis (see below).

A prolonged euglobulin clot lysis time is suggestive of dysfibrinolysis. This possibility can be verified by applying a tourniquet. If venous blood specimens are taken before and after 10 to 20 minutes of venous occlusion midway between systolic and diastolic pressure, the second specimen should show a shorter lysis time because the application of the tourniquet activates t-PA. If a fibrinolytic defect is evident, the nature of the defect can be determined by means of specific assays for plasminogen, t-PA, and t-PA inhibitor (see below).

If the TT and the euglobulin clot lysis time are normal, specific tests for the antithrombins (antithrombin III, protein C, protein S, and heparin cofactor II) should be carried out (see below).

Specific Causes of Thrombotic Tendency

Dysfibrinogenemia More than 100 qualitative abnormalities of fibrinogen (dysfibrinogenemias) have been reported.[72] Dysfibrinogenemias are inherited in an autosomal dominant manner, with most patients being heterozygous. Most patients with dysfibrinogenemia have either no clinical symptoms or symptoms of a bleeding disorder; a minority (about 11 percent) have clinical features of a recurrent thromboembolic disorder, either venous or arterial.[73,74] Congenital dysfibrinogenemias associated with thrombosis account for about one percent of cases of unexplained venous thrombosis occurring in young individuals. The most commonly observed functional defect in dysfibrinogenemias associated with thrombosis is abnormal fibrin monomer polymerization combined with resistance to fibrinolysis. In recently described cases, decreased binding of plasminogen and increased resistance to lysis by plasmin have been noted.

In addition to the routine prolongation of the TT, patients who have dysfibrinogenemia associated with thromboembolism may also have a prolonged INR. The diagnosis is confirmed if the reptilase time is also longer than normal. When measured with clotting techniques, fibrinogen levels may be slightly or moderately low; however, when measured immunologically, levels may be normal or even increased.

Dysfibrinolysis The plasma fibrinolytic system can be impaired by inherited deficiencies of plasminogen, defective release of t-PA from the vascular endothelium, and high plasma levels of regulatory proteins such as t-PA inhibitors.[74,75] In addition, a deficiency of factor XII (contact factor) may induce failure of fibrinolysis activation.

Inherited plasminogen deficiency is believed to be only rarely responsible for unexplained deep thrombophlebitis in young patients. The defect is transmitted as an autosomal dominant trait. In heterozygous persons with a thrombotic tendency, plasminogen activity is about one half the normal level (normal, 3.9 to 8.4 μmol/ml. As noted earlier, the euglobulin clot lysis time is prolonged. Functional assays should be carried out, and there should be full transformation of plasminogen into plasmin activators. Several commercial methods are now available.

The important role of t-PA inhibitors in the regulation of fibrinolysis is now well defined.[75,76] Two such inhibitors have been purified, t-PA inhibitor I and t-PA inhibitor II. In normal plasma, t-PA inhibitor I is the primary inhibitor for both t-PA and urokinase. Release of t-PA inhibitor I by platelets results in locally increased concentrations where platelets accumulate. The ensuing

Figure 10 **Illustrated is an algorithm for screening for acquired and congenital thrombotic syndromes. The direction screening should take depends on the family history.**

Table 8 Etiology of Acquired Hypercoagulability

Tissue and cellular damage
  Shock
  Trauma
  Surgery
  Tissue necrosis
  Transfusion necrosis
Drugs
  Estrogens
  Drug reactions and interactions
  Heparin platelet antibody
  Warfarin
Disease
  Blood dyscrasias
  Cancer
  Diabetes
  Homocystinuria
  Hyperlipidemia
  Presence of lupuslike anticoagulant
  Severe infection
Pregnancy

local fibrinolysis inhibition may help stabilize the hemostatic plug. t-PA inhibitor II was first identified in extracts of human placenta and is present in and secreted by monocytes and macrophages.

Factor XII deficiency is a rare cause of impaired fibrinolysis. Initial contact activation of factor XII not only results in activation of the clotting cascade (with generation of thrombin) and of the inflammatory response (with generation of kinins, complement, and thromboxane) but also leads to plasmin generation. This intrinsic activation of fibrinolysis requires factor XII, prekallikrein, and high-molecular-weight kininogen. Studies of 121 patients with factor XII deficiency found that 10 (8.3 percent) experienced thrombotic episodes.[72] Patients with factor XII deficiencies can be identified by a prolonged activated partial thromboplastin time (aPTT) in the absence of clinical bleeding.[65,71]

Resistance to activated protein C The resistance of human clotting factors to inactivation by activated protein C was first reported in 1993 and is now believed to be the most common inherited procoagulant disorder.[77] The prevalence of this disorder has been estimated to range from one percent to five percent in the general population and may be as high as 45 percent in patients with venous thromboembolism.[78]

Activated factor V is normally degraded by activated protein C in the presence of membrane surface as part of the normal regulation of thrombosis. Activated protein C resistance is caused by a single substitution mutation (guanine for adenine) in the factor V gene. This mutation is passed in an autosomal dominant fashion, and the mutant factor V that results has been termed factor V Leiden. Factor V Leiden is resistant to inactivation by activated protein C and thus has a greater ability to activate thrombin and accelerate clotting.

Two techniques are commonly used to diagnose this disorder. The first is a functional assay that compares a standard aPTT to one performed in the presence of exogenous activated protein C. If the latter aPTT does not exhibit significant prolongation, then the patient is probably resistant to activated protein C. The second technique involves analysis of the patient's DNA with a polymerase chain reaction to detect the mutation directly.

Antithrombin deficiency Antithrombin III (now termed simply antithrombin because there is no antithrombin I or II) is a 65 kd protein that decelerates the coagulation system by inactivating activated factors.[79,80] Its principal activity is to inactivate factor Xa and thrombin; it also inactivates activated factors XII, XI, and IX. Antithrombin therefore acts as a scavenger of activated clotting factors. Its activity is enhanced 100-fold by the presence of heparans on the endothelial surface and 1,000-fold by administration of exogenous heparin.

Antithrombin deficiency is one of the more common congenital hypercoagulable states.[79] Its prevalence is approximately 0.01 to 0.05 percent in the general population and two to four percent in patients with venous thrombosis. The trait is passed on as an autosomal dominant trait, with the heterozygous genotype being incompatible with life. Antithrombin-deficient patients are at increased risk for thromboembolism when their antithrombin activity falls below 70 percent of normal.[81]

Patients with congenital antithrombin deficiency frequently present after a stressful event, such as childbirth, surgery, or trauma. These patients usually have deep thrombophlebitis but sometimes have pulmonary embolism. If anticoagulation is not contraindicated, the treatment of choice is heparin at a dosage sufficient to raise the aPTT to the desired level, followed by warfarin. If anticoagulation is contraindicated (as it is during the peripartum period), antithrombin concentrate should be given to raise the antithrombin activity to 80 to 120 percent of normal during the period when anticoagulants cannot be given.

Acquired antithrombin deficiency is now a well-recognized entity. In most patients undergoing severe systemic stress (e.g., major surgical procedures or trauma), antithrombin levels fall below normal.[82] Furthermore, patients with the classic risk factors for venous thromboembolism tend to have the lowest antithrombin levels.

Protein C and protein S deficiency Protein C is a 62 kd glycoprotein with a half-life of six hours. Because it is vitamin K dependent, a deficiency will develop in the absence of vitamin K. Acquired protein C deficiency is seen in liver disease, malignancy, infection, the postoperative state, and disseminated intravascular coagulation (DIC).[11]

Protein C deficiency occurs in approximately four to five percent of patients younger than 40 to 45 years who present with

Table 9 Congenital Clotting Disorders

Deficiencies in thrombosis inhibitors
  Antithrombin III deficiency
  Proteins C and S deficiency
  Activated protein C resistance
Dysfibrinogenemias
Dysfibrinolysis
  Hypoplasminogenemia
  Impaired release of t-PA
  High levels of t-PA inhibitor
  Factor XII deficiency

unexplained venous thrombosis.[83] It is transmitted as an autosomal dominant trait, and the family history is usually positive for a clotting tendency.

Protein C levels range from 70 to 164 percent of normal in patients who do not manifest a clotting tendency; levels below 70 percent of normal are associated with a thrombotic tendency. The most appropriate tests for screening, however, are functional assays, because there are cases of dysfunctional protein C deficiency in which levels of protein C antigen are normal but levels of protein C activity are low, and these would not be detected by the usual immunoassays.

Protein S is a vitamin K–dependent protein that functions as a cofactor for activated protein C by enhancing protein C–induced inactivation of activated factor V. The incidence of protein S deficiency is similar to that of protein C deficiency: about five percent of young patients with unexplained venous thrombosis.[83] Like protein C deficiency, it is transmitted as a dominant trait, and the family history is often positive for a thrombotic tendency.

Treatment

Treatment of a clinical hypercoagulable state involves both prophylaxis [see Discussion, Prophylaxis of Thromboembolism, below] and specific treatment.[84] Prophylaxis in postoperative patients consists primarily of maintaining good hydration, ensuring normal cardiac output, and early mobilization. Administration of low-dose heparin, use of intermittent pneumatic compression, administration of low-molecular-weight dextran, or any combination of these may also be appropriate for a specific patient.

Treatment of thromboembolism associated with dysfibrinogenemia involves moderate-dose heparin anticoagulation followed by long-term warfarin anticoagulation.

Treatment of thromboembolic disorders associated with abnormalities of fibrinolysis is essentially the same as that of dysfibrinogenemia. It is possible that patients with these qualitative plasminogen defects and acute massive thrombotic events might not respond to fibrinolytic treatment with urokinase or streptokinase.

Patients with activated protein C resistance who present with venous thrombosis should be treated with heparin in the standard fashion. They also should receive genetic counseling and refrain from using oral contraceptives.

Treatment of antithrombin deficiency associated with active clotting involves initiating anticoagulation with the appropriate doses of heparin so as to ensure a significant rise in the PTT. Warfarin is the drug of choice for long-term prophylaxis and should be given in a dose sufficient to maintain an INR of 2.0 to 3.0. For patients with a contraindication to anticoagulation, a purified form of antithrombin is available that can be administered directly. Patients with acquired antithrombin deficiency should receive prophylaxis for thromboembolism in the form of heparin in dosages sufficient to raise the aPTT five seconds above the upper limit of the normal laboratory value.

Treatment of the clotting states related to protein C or protein S deficiency involves administering fresh frozen plasma or factor IX concentrate. Low-dose heparin followed by warfarin may be appropriate for long-term treatment.

Discussion

Development of Venous Thrombosis

PATHOPHYSIOLOGY

In 1856, Virchow described a triad of factors that predisposed to venous thrombosis: venous stasis, endothelial damage, and hypercoagulability.[85] Whether all three are required to induce an intravascular thrombotic episode or not, it is certainly true that when all three factors are present, the tendency toward clotting is overwhelming.

Vascular stasis occurs primarily in the great veins of the body, which constitute the blood reservoirs; at any given moment, approximately 70 percent of the total blood supply is contained in the venous system. Muscular activity, with the resultant compression of the great veins, is the pump that promotes return of blood to the heart. When a portion of the body is immobilized, the blood flow slows, and there is a tendency toward stagnation in the veins draining that region. In one experiment, contrast material was administered through the dorsal vein of the foot to patients who had no history of venous disease.[86] The dye tended to be retained in the valve pockets of the thigh and calf veins and in the venous saccules of the calf muscles. Moreover, in supine, completely immobilized patients, the clearance time of the dye was 21 minutes in the thigh and 27 minutes in the lower leg. The retention of dye was substantially reduced by both muscle contractions and elevation of the leg by 15° or more.[87] Patients who suffer from quadriplegia, paraplegia, or hemiplegia have an increased incidence of thrombosis in the paralyzed limbs; in fact, thrombosis is almost universal in this group of patients.[88] Inactivity also results in a relative paralysis of the lytic system, which further encourages propagation of thrombus.[89,90]

Although there is no question that endothelial damage is associated with a thrombotic tendency, it is uncertain whether or how this component of Virchow's triad plays a significant role in the tendency toward venous thrombosis. Certainly, whenever the endothelium of a blood vessel has been directly injured by trauma or by placement of a prosthetic graft or other surgery, blood is exposed to a thrombogenic surface. Exposure of basement membranes to the circulation results in platelet adhesion, platelet release reaction, platelet aggregation, thrombin generation, and clot formation. A 1974 study found no microscopic damage to valve pockets in patients with venous thrombosis.[91] A later study, however, suggested that hypoxic injury to the endothelium plays a role in the formation of deep thrombophlebitis.[92] The endothelium in the venous valve cusp receives little or no oxygen from the adjoining avascular tissue and depends on the oxygen content of the blood. In hypokinetic conditions, oxygen supply to the valve cusp endothelium is reduced. The investigators sampled oxygen tension (P_{O_2}) values in various areas of the valve pocket and in the saphenous vein of humans undergoing operations to remove varicose veins. They found that the P_{O_2} in the deepest part of the valve pocket was lower than that in the saphenous vein and concluded that venous thrombi were initiated as a result of hypoxic endothelial damage. The investigators postulated that freshly oxygenated leukocytes and platelets adhere more readily to hypoxic endothelium and that the damaged endothelium therefore was the initiating site of thrombus formation. One could also speculate that hypoxic damage to endothelium interferes with the release of plasminogen activator, thereby allowing any clotting process that is initiated to progress.

Hypercoagulability, the third factor in the triad, undoubtedly plays a large role in thrombogenesis. Acquired and congenital disorders that promote the hypercoagulable state are present in surgical patients and surgical disease states, particularly trauma and vascular disease. As noted earlier [see Approach to Acquired and Congenital Thrombotic Syndromes, above], this hypercoagulable state could result from depletion of antithrombins, compromise of the lytic system, or the entrance of procoagulants into the bloodstream from injured tissues. Precipitation of clot would tend to occur in areas of stasis or sites of endothelial damage.

Most spontaneous venous clots occur in the deep venous system of the lower half of the body. In immobilized postoperative patients, the initial site of most thrombus formation appears to be the valve pockets, where flow is stagnant and eddies form. Thrombi grow by the progressive deposition of layers of thrombotic material, forming in the direction of blood flow. Initially, the thrombus is attached at the point of origin on the vessel wall, with the tail floating freely in the lumen. Most clots that form in this manner promptly lyse or fragment and break loose. Small fragments that reach the pulmonary vascular system lyse and disappear. If persistent stasis is present, antithrombin activity is reduced, or lytic activity is impaired, the clot will continue to grow. It may elicit an inflammatory response in the vein wall and become circumferentially adherent (and therefore obstructive), or it may remain primarily free floating, except for a localized attachment.

Alternatively, the clot may take a combined form, with some portions adherent and the propagating tail free floating, depending on how much vein wall inflammation the thrombus induces. Obstructive clot may well propagate backward down the vein, aggravating the obstruction by blocking collateral vessels.

Normally, the hydrostatic pressure on the arterial side of the capillary loop is approximately 30 mm Hg, that on the venous side is approximately 12 mm Hg, and that in the surrounding external tissue is approximately 2 to 3 mm Hg. Venous hypertension caused by obstructive clot raises the hydrostatic pressure in the distal venous capillary bed, thereby increasing the transfer of fluid from the vascular compartment into the interstitium. Eventually, the interstitial extravasation of fluid increases tissue tension and counterbalances Starling forces, preventing further accumulation of fluid.

Leg swelling causes passive muscle engorgement and dilation of muscle fibrils. These, in turn, activate pain receptors located in the muscle spindle and account for the muscle discomfort. Stretching the muscle aggravates the discomfort—hence, the positive Homans' sign (pain in the calf on forced dorsiflexion of the foot).

Stable clot does not release inflammatory mediators, but actively proliferating clot releases serotonin, histamine, thromboxane, and other mediators. These activate vein wall afferent receptors and account for most of the pain and the tenderness in the vein containing the thrombus. Inflammatory mediators pass through the vein wall and, in the superficial veins, are associated with redness and swelling of the overlying skin.[3]

INCIDENCE

It is estimated that 2.5 million people a year suffer from deep thrombophlebitis.[93] The incidence of deep thrombophlebitis in surgical patients varies widely depending on the method of study. In a review of eight series in which venography or autopsy was used to verify the diagnosis, the incidence of deep thrombophlebitis ranged from 18 to 90 percent (average, 42 percent).[94]

Estimates of the incidence of pulmonary embolism also vary widely, but reviews suggest that about 700,000 individuals suffer from this complication each year and that about 200,000 die as a result.[1,2] In the absence of prophylaxis, fatal pulmonary embolism has been reported in four to seven percent of hip surgery patients and in 0.1 to 0.8 percent of general surgery patients.[1,95] In about 40 to 60 percent of patients who die of pulmonary embolism, the diagnosis is not made clinically. Pulmonary embolism may be responsible for as many as five percent of postoperative deaths, and it may occur in as many as 25 percent of patients admitted to the hospital.[96,97] Pulmonary infarction occurs in about 10 percent of patients with clinical evidence of pulmonary embolism.[13]

Development of Arterial Embolism

PATHOPHYSIOLOGY

The sequential changes secondary to sudden vascular occlusion can be clearly followed when the site of embolic lodgment is in a major artery. Sudden obstruction of a vessel leads to immediate accretion of platelets and clot on the embolus and the downstream release of inflammatory mediators, including histamine, serotonin, thromboxane, complement, and kinins. These mediators cause reflex spasm in all the vessels distal to the obstruction, and the skin becomes pale, cold, and ischemic. The spasm is actually protective to an extent, in that it prevents propagating thrombus from filling the lumina of the main vessels distal to the obstruction. Most of the small side branches of these main channels essentially close.[39]

A small, thin string of clot may propagate, but if collateral flow subsequently develops, there is room for nutritive blood flow alongside the thrombotic cord. If collateral flow is not sufficient to meet the minimal nutritional needs of the organ or limb, function will be lost in the critical tissues, particularly those most distal to the obstruction. Ischemia of sensory nerves of the extremities will result in numbness and anesthesia. Muscle will become paralyzed and nonfunctional. If collateral flow is subsequently mobilized in response to stimulation by the low pressures distal to the obstruction, this event may be sufficient to ensure viability; the numbness may improve and muscle function may return even if the limb remains pale and cool.

If collateral flow continues to be inadequate, the tissues distal to the obstruction ultimately die. The initial manifestations of irreversibility are loss of tone in smooth muscle that has been in spasm and microvascular dilation, usually occurring after six to eight hours of ischemia. When an extremity is involved, there will be bluish mottling of the overlying skin, which signals that capillaries have reopened and vascular stasis is present[35] [see Figure 11]. Initially, the bluish mottling is patchy and varies in its location; finally, however, it becomes confluent. At this point, major feeding channels thrombose, and muscle goes into rigor, becoming firm, hard, and patchily necrotic.[36,37] In absolute ischemia associated with thigh tourniquet shock, muscle starts to die at approximately three hours, and extensive areas of necrosis are present by six to eight hours.[37] At this point, attempts to open major channels and extract thrombus will be unsuccessful because clotted branches of the main arterial channels feeding dead or markedly ischemic tissue will not accept flow. Moreover, clot will begin to accumulate in the venules and major veins, further compromising capillary flow. Finally, the limb becomes irreversibly ischemic, as indicated by failure of the bluish areas of the skin to blanch with pressure.

It should be remembered that skin can tolerate prolonged periods of ischemia much better than any of the underlying structures (except perhaps bone and tendon) can: irreversible thrombosis of skin capillaries occurs only after 24 hours of ischemia. Theoretically, therefore, late reestablishment of circulation to an ischemic extremity could be associated with death of muscle and irreversible damage to nerves, but the skin could still be viable. In the final analysis, limbs are lost when the skin is lost, not when muscle is lost. This is a crucial point when fasciotomy is under consideration.

Figure 11 **The bluish, mottled appearance of the skin of the left foot and ankle denotes irreversible ischemia.**

OUTCOME CONSIDERATIONS

The act of extracting clot and restoring circulation, especially when done on the lower extremity through a femoral incision with the patient under local anesthesia,[98] seems benign; however, the literature clearly documents a high mortality associated with embolic occlusion in an extremity.[99-103] This average mortality has improved very little in recent years.

Almost all studies of extremity embolic occlusions that are associated with low mortalities document the importance of heparin anticoagulation given preoperatively, intraoperatively, and postoperatively.[39,104] If reperfusion can be reestablished before the organ is irreversibly damaged—preferably while it is still completely viable—then systemic morbidity will be acceptable and the end result optimal.

Both the bowel and skeletal muscle remain viable for six to eight hours after interruption of circulation. After six or eight hours of profound ischemia, attempts to revascularize major segments of bowel or extremities in which there is a large mass of ischemic muscle tissue not only meet with little success in reestablishing flow but also carry a high risk of mortality from the reperfusion insult.[105-109] In advanced ischemia involving the entire lower leg below the knee, reperfusion will result in death for most older patients, and in advanced ischemia of the entire leg, reperfusion will be life threatening for even young patients.

There are two main problems associated with reperfusion. The first is the acute metabolic problem produced by reperfusion of a large mass of ischemic tissue. There is an obligatory diffuse vascular dilation in the ischemic limb, and the dilated vascular bed can temporarily sequester large volumes of blood when flow is initially reestablished. Peripheral resistance is lost, and reperfusion flow can be three times normal or even greater,

creating a demand for increased cardiac output that a patient with poor cardiac reserve may be incapable of meeting.[107] Large quantities of potassium and lactate are washed out of the distal circulation[106]; serum potassium may reach critically high levels when the mass of tissue reperfused is equivalent to an entire leg. These high levels, coupled with systemic acidosis from lactate release, can compromise myocardial function.

Fresh clot that formed in the venous system during stasis is washed out into the systemic circulation and is eventually filtered out by the lung. This clot, along with inflammatory mediators released from devitalized cells in the ischemic limb, induces diffuse systemic inflammation, increased vascular permeability, and third-spacing (transudation of fluid into the extravascular space). Pulmonary function is impaired, and the hypovolemia caused by the third-spacing may result in systemic organ damage.[105,107,108] Systemic release of myoglobin and other tissue procoagulants leads to systemic hypercoagulability and thus to intravascular coagulation. Intravascular coagulation results in further release of inflammatory mediators and, on rare occasions, disseminated intravascular coagulation with diffuse, uncontrollable hemorrhage. Thrombotic renal cortical necrosis may lead to renal shutdown.

The second problem associated with reperfusion of severely ischemic limbs is fascial compartment swelling. When fasciotomy is carried out on these ischemic limbs, dead muscle is usually found. The question that must then be answered is whether the compartmental swelling resulted from permeability alterations in viable muscle or whether the muscle was irreversibly damaged and capillary permeability increased as a direct result of the vascular occlusion. The answer has important implications for treatment. On one hand, if it is only irreversibly ischemic muscle that swells enough to produce high compartmental pressures, opening the skin and the fascia to relieve pressure would expose dead muscle. In theory, this should increase the risk of loss of limb because exposed nonviable muscle inevitably becomes infected. On the other hand, if viable muscle is being compromised by the swelling, early exposure should prevent muscular death and facilitate salvage of extremities. It is of therapeutic interest that in one study, early administration of heparin to animals with ischemic limbs markedly diminished local vascular permeability and muscle swelling.[110]

There is no question that when compartment syndromes involve primary swelling resulting from high venous pressure, direct hemorrhage, or muscle contusion, fasciotomy is beneficial. If, however, the muscle is already dead or irreversibly ischemic secondary to the proximal arterial occlusion, fasciotomy is not beneficial and might even be harmful. We have found that when fasciotomy is required to relieve high compartmental pressures after proximal arterial occlusion, limb loss is extremely high, and significant mortality may be expected. For this reason, our policy—admittedly a controversial one—is not to do fasciotomy routinely after restoration of extremity blood flow. If revascularization is carried out within six to eight hours, severe muscle swelling is rare. Moreover, attempts to enhance reperfusion of severely ischemic or dead muscle by means of fasciotomy may increase mortality. It is better to risk the loss of a limb than the loss of a patient.

INCIDENCE

The incidence of arterial embolism is much lower than it once was[34]; however, reliable figures are not currently available. In most series, the incidence of cerebral embolism is not well documented, because it is often confused with other causes of stroke—in particular, local atherosclerotic obstruction and intracranial hemorrhage.[34]

Prophylaxis of Thromboembolism

The optimal means of treating a thromboembolic event is to prevent its occurrence. This is particularly true for certain groups known to be at high risk for thromboembolic complications.[111,112] Patients older than 60 years should be considered for prophylaxis if they are about to undergo major surgery or are significantly injured. Immobilized patients are at high risk for thromboembolism because prolonged immobilization results in stasis in lower leg veins. Any patient with a major injury (particularly a pelvic fracture) is at risk for thromboembolism as well, perhaps because the trauma may involve stretch injuries to pelvic and iliac veins, which then become the source of thrombus. Finally, any patient with a history of a spontaneous thrombotic event, either after surgery or de novo, is at high risk for subsequent thromboembolism.

There are a number of techniques that can be used to prevent thromboembolic complications. The most effective of these is early ambulation. It is known and universally accepted that surgical patients immobilized for prolonged periods have a very high incidence of thrombotic events.[2,93-95,111] Elastic stockings have been used for decades as prophylaxis for thromboembolism. Unfortunately, most commercial stockings neither fit adequately nor provide adequate compression; thus, they probably offer little or no benefit.[2] Low-molecular-weight dextran, which lowers blood viscosity and inhibits platelet aggregation, is helpful in certain instances but is not completely protective.[112] In theory, it should prevent arterial clots (which are primarily composed of platelets) more effectively than venous clots (which are primarily composed of fibrin). Dextran may provide a fair degree of prophylaxis. A 2 unit priming dose is given in the first 24 hours, followed by 1 unit/day for three or four days in the postoperative period.

A newer modality that seems to have a significant impact on the incidence of thromboembolic complications is intermittent pneumatic compression. The original rationale for this technique was based on the concept that massage of the lower legs would empty the veins and improve venous efflux. This rationale was faulty in that venous efflux cannot possibly be increased unless arterial influx is increased in parallel, which, of course, is not the case. Moreover, the clots that cause fatalities form in the large veins of the upper thigh and the pelvis, and massage of the calf and the lower thigh would do nothing for these veins. Although intermittent pneumatic compression does not have the effect originally predicted, it probably has a more important one: massage of the leg veins is known to activate t-PA and thus the fibrinolytic system,[113] thereby providing not only local but also systemic benefit. Massage of upper extremities decreases clotting in lower extremity veins, and massage of one leg decreases clotting in the other leg. As a result, intermittent pneumatic compression has proved to be a safe, although somewhat uncomfortable, method of preventing clots in patients who are immobilized for prolonged periods. It has found particular favor in critical care units, where other forms of prophylaxis are inapplicable or contraindicated.[111]

Finally, there is prophylactic anticoagulation. A major British study of thromboembolic prophylaxis in patients undergoing surgical therapy for hip fractures found that subcutaneous administration of 5,000 units of heparin two or three times daily before, during, and after the operation was not associated with a significantly increased incidence of bleeding and substantially lowered the incidence of thromboembolic complications.[95] This low-dose protocol has been criticized as being insufficiently individualized for specific high-risk patients. The mode of action of low-dose heparin is to markedly augment the antithrombotic effect of antithrombin[114]; therefore, if antithrombin levels are reduced, low-dose heparin might not be effective, and moderate-dose heparin might be more appropriate in high-risk settings.

Recently, a new form of heparin has appeared on the market: low-molecular-weight heparin. This form of heparin uses the same pentasaccharide chain to potentiate the effects of antithrombin (thereby achieving anticoagulation) as unfractionated (standard) heparin does. Like unfractionated heparin, it is ineffective if antithrombin levels have been depleted. The main advantage of low-molecular-weight heparin is that it has a more dependable half-life and bioavailability than unfractionated heparin. For this reason, it has been given without any monitoring of the drug's effect or the patient's plasma heparin levels.

Several clinical trials in Europe and in the United States have documented the efficacy of low-molecular-weight heparin. The majority of the trials have been in patients undergoing elective hip[115,116] or knee operations; however, a few have addressed other patient populations, such as trauma patients.[117] In these studies, the rates of deep thrombophlebitis for patients receiving unmonitored low-molecular-weight heparin therapy have, for the most part, been compared with those of patients receiving either placebo[115] or so-called minidose heparin therapy[116,117] (5,000 units of unfractionated heparin given subcutaneously twice or three times daily). Several studies from the 1980s have shown the superiority of so-called adjusted-dose heparin therapy to either placebo or the minidose approach.[118,119] (The adjusted-dose approach is identical to the low-dose approach described earlier [see General Principles of Anticoagulation and Lytic Therapy, Heparin Anticoagulation]; we use the latter term to clarify the relation of this approach to the other two regimens that we recommend, moderate dose and high dose.)

From the available information on low-molecular-weight heparin, it appears that it can be recommended for both elective and emergency trauma patients in place of placebo or minidose heparin. Whether it is superior to adjusted-dose therapy with unfractionated heparin remains uncertain. An unmonitored low-molecular-weight heparin regimen is clearly simpler to manage than an adjusted-dose unfractionated heparin regimen. In settings where compliance with monitoring and dose-adjusting protocols is an issue, unmonitored low-molecular-weight heparin therapy may well be preferable because it may lead to improved compliance.

Warfarin may be used instead of heparin in some patients.[112,120] Warfarin anticoagulation must be started three or four days before the surgical procedure, and the patient must be able to continue taking oral medications in the immediate postoperative period. Consequently, this approach is of limited value for abdominal procedures, although it has proved to be a useful alternative to heparin for orthopedic procedures. The INR should be kept below 3.0 to prevent excessive bleeding. Warfarin is not as easy to regulate tightly as heparin, and it is not as easily turned on and off; that is, several days are needed for the therapeutic effect to be achieved and several more days for the effect to wear off. Recently, it has been shown that use of low-dose warfarin (as little as 1 mg/day) may offer prophylactic benefit.[120]

Rationale for Varying Heparin Dosage

For many years after the introduction of heparin therapy into surgery in 1936,[121-123] the dosages used were arbitrary. In 1955, however, a series of experiments in dogs showed that when a ligature was applied to the jugular vein and sufficient heparin administered to increase the clotting time of blood in a test tube to 2.5 times normal (corresponding to a Lee-White clotting time of 20 to 30 minutes), thrombus formation was prevented distal to the ligature.[124] Because the prolonged periods of observation necessary for the Lee-White clotting time are not practical in modern clinical laboratories, other tests, such as the activated PTT and the activated clotting time, have been introduced; these represent practical modifications to the original Lee-White clotting time. An activated PTT of 1.5 to 2.0 times normal and an activated clotting time of 200 seconds are considered to be therapeutically equivalent to a Lee-White clotting time of 30 minutes.

Heparin therapy is still plagued by several misconceptions. One is that the extent of anticoagulation is necessarily correlated with prolongations of the activated PTT or the activated clotting time.[38,45,125] All the experimental studies on which this misconception is based are concerned with anticoagulation in normal animals or normal humans, who have normal levels of antithrombins.

Another misconception is the idea that pathological bleeding correlates directly with the prolongation of the clotting time and that bleeding complications can be prevented by tight control of anticoagulation. In fact, there is no evidence of any correlation between the bleeding risk and the anticoagulatory effect.[46,47,125] In normal patients, anticoagulation for as long as three or four days is rarely associated with bleeding unless a prior sensitivity to heparin has been induced.

Still another misconception is the idea that a relative degree of anticoagulation can be achieved that effectively counteracts the clotting yet is free of the risk of bleeding. The fallacy of this idea is best illustrated by considering the therapeutic problem presented by the ischemic limb. An ischemic limb is, to an extent, isolated from the circulation. This means that a dose of heparin that is sufficient to produce the desired anticoagulation, according to conventional measures, may be relatively ineffective in the ischemic area, distal to the obstruction. For therapeutic purposes, it is the clotting status in the ischemic area that is crucial; therefore, conventional monitoring, which provides information only about the clotting status in a peripheral vein,[38] must be disregarded. To ensure adequate anticoagulation in the involved limb, arbitrary high doses of heparin are required.[39] Similar principles apply to the treatment of major pulmonary embolism. Downstream from the embolus, the inflammatory products released by the proximal clot will result in both vascular and bronchiolar spasm. These inflammatory mediators also impair collateral circulation and potentiate clotting in the region of vascular stasis. Administration of high doses of heparin is necessary to prevent further propagation of clot distal to where the embolism is lodged.[126]

Determination of the optimal heparin dose is further complicated by the fact that the shock state itself markedly augments the clotting tendency. Two hundred years ago, Hewson observed that when he bled patients, "the blood that emerged last clotted first, the blood that emerged first clotted last."[127] Nearly every clinician who works with shock patients has noted that in some instances, the blood of the patient clots in the syringe before it can be placed in the anticoagulant. Presumably, this is a survival mechanism, in that enhanced spontaneous thrombosis would result in prompter cessation of hemorrhage.

Out of frustration at the apparent unreliability of current tests of clotting status, one of us (F.W.B.) and others measured the survival of radioactive-labeled fibrinogen as a means of documenting the effectiveness of anticoagulation under various experimental and clinical conditions.[38,45,68] In patients on cardiopulmonary bypass or extracorporeal membrane oxygenation, the fibrinogen half-life remained abnormal despite what appeared to be adequate anticoagulation according to the activated PTT. Dosages three times as large as the "adequate" dosage were required to normalize the fibrinogen half-life and to anticoagulate the patient fully. In a canine study, the adequacy of anticoagulation after administration of thrombin and thrombin-heparin was assessed according to both the activated PTT and the half-life of fibrinogen.[55] Once again, the fibrinogen half-life remained grossly abnormal despite what appeared to be adequate anticoagulation according to the activated PTT.

In all the experiments, particularly the clinical ones, it was apparent that when full anticoagulation was obtained in a clinical clotting situation, vascular spasm decreased, as manifested by improvement in collateral flow. When adequate anticoagulation was achieved in an ischemic limb, the level of demarcation inevitably dropped, and the pain decreased.[45-47] In venous thrombotic conditions, the findings were even more dramatic: when adequate anticoagulation was achieved, pain inevitably disappeared, and swelling and signs of inflammation improved within hours.[46,47] An interesting corollary of this finding is that in patients with venous thrombosis, conventional doses of anticoagulant controlled in a conventional fashion were associated in most instances with immediate improvement,[45] whereas in patients with arterial ischemia, this was almost never true—much higher doses of anticoagulant were required than the conventional tests suggested.[38,39]

Therefore, to meet the varying needs of patients with thromboembolic complications, we use three degrees of heparin anticoagulation: low dose, moderate dose, and high dose [see General Principles of Anticoagulation and Lytic Therapy, Heparin Anticoagulation, above].

References

1. Hirsh J, Hull RD: Venous Thromboembolism: Natural History, Diagnosis, and Management. CRC Press, Boca Raton, Florida, 1988

2. Bergqvist D: Postoperative Thromboembolism: Frequency, Etiology, Prophylaxis. Springer-Verlag, New York, 1983

3. LeClerk JR: Venous Thromboembolic Disorders. Lea & Febiger, Philadelphia, 1991, pp 54, 176

4. Bergqvist D, Bergentz SE: Diagnosis of deep vein thrombosis. World J Surg 14:679, 1990

5. Hirsh J: Reliability of non-invasive tests for the diagnosis of venous thrombosis (editorial). Thromb Haemost 65:221, 1991

6. Krupski WC, Bass A, Dilley RB, et al: Propagation of deep venous thrombosis identified by duplex ultrasonography. J Vasc Surg 12:467, 1990

7. Lensing AW, Prandoni P, Brandjes D: Detection of deep-vein thrombosis by real-time B-mode ultrasonography. N Engl J Med 320:342, 1989

8. Haire WD, Lynch TG, Lund GB: Limitations of magnetic resonance imaging and ultrasound directed (duplex) scanning in the diagnosis of subclavian vein thrombosis. J Vasc Surg 13:391, 1991

9. Barnes RW, Nix ML, Barnes CL: Perioperative asymptomatic venous thrombosis: role of duplex scanning versus venography. J Vasc Surg 9:25, 1989

10. Hirsh J, Turpie AG: Use of plasminogen activators in venous thrombosis. World J Surg 14:688, 1990

11. Lord RS, Chen FC, DeVine TJ, et al: Surgical treatment of acute deep venous thrombosis. World J Surg 14:694, 1990

12. Smith GT, Dammin GJ, Dexter L: Postmortem arteriographic studies of the human lung in pulmonary embolization. JAMA 188:143, 1964

13. Dalen JE, Haffajee CI, Alpert JS 3rd, et al: Pulmonary embolism, pulmonary hemorrhage and pulmonary infarction. N Engl J Med 296:1431, 1977

14. Moser KM, Hull R, Saltzman HA, et al: Recent advances in diagnosis of pulmonary embolism and deep venous thrombosis. Am Rev Respir Dis 138:1046, 1988

15. Coon WW: Risk factors in pulmonary embolism. Surg Gynecol Obstet 143:385, 1976

16. Boneu B, Bes G, Pelzer H, et al: D-dimers, thrombin antithrombin III complexes and prothrombin fragments 1 + 2 diagnostic value in clinically suspected deep vein thrombosis. Thromb Haemost 65:28, 1991

17. Speiser W, Mallek R, Koppensteiner R: D-dimer and

TAT measurement in patients with deep venous thrombosis: utility in diagnosis and judgment of anticoagulant treatment effectiveness. Thromb Haemost 64:196, 1990

18. PIOPED Investigators: Value of ventilation/perfusion scan in acute pulmonary embolism: results of prospective investigation of pulmonary embolism diagnosis (PIOPED). JAMA 263:2753, 1990

19. Hull RD, Hirsh J, Carter CJ, et al: Diagnostic value of ventilation-perfusion lung scanning in patients with suspected pulmonary embolism. Chest 88:819, 1985

20. Hull RD, Raskob GE, Hirsh J: The diagnosis of clinically suspected pulmonary embolism: practical approaches. Chest 89:417S, 1986

21. Ferris EJ, Holder JC, Lim WN, et al: Angiography of pulmonary emboli: digital studies and balloon-occlusion cineangiography. Am J Roentgenol 142:369, 1984

22. Hull RD, Hirsh J, Carter CJ, et al: Pulmonary angiography, ventilation lung scanning, and venography for clinically suspected pulmonary embolism with abnormal perfusion lung scan. Ann Intern Med 98: 891, 1983

23. Atik M, Broghamer WL Jr: The impact of prophylactic measures on fatal pulmonary embolism. Arch Surg 114:366, 1979

24. Collins R, Scrimgeour A, Yusuf S, et al: Reduction in fatal pulmonary embolism and venous thrombosis by perioperative administration of subcutaneous heparin: overview of results of randomized trials in general, orthopedic, and urologic surgery. N Engl J Med 318:1162, 1988

25. Geerts WH: Pulmonary embolism. Conn's Current Therapy 1992. Rakel RE, Ed. WB Saunders Co, Philadelphia, 1992, p 179

26. Moser KM: State of the art: pulmonary embolism. Am Rev Respir Dis 115:829, 1977

27. Thomas DP: Therapeutic role of heparin in acute pulmonary embolism. Curr Ther Res 18:21, 1975

28. Silver D: Pulmonary embolism: prevention, detection and nonoperative management. Surg Clin North Am 54:1089, 1974

29. Rohrer MJ, Scheidler MG, Wheeler HB, et al: Extended indications for placement of an inferior vena cava filter. J Vasc Surg 10:44, 1989

30. Fink JA, Jones BT: The Greenfield filter as the primary means of therapy in venous thromboembolic disease. Surg Gynecol Obstet 172:253, 1991

31. Wells I: Inferior vena cava filters and when to use them. Clin Radiol 40:11, 1989

32. Zimmerman JJ, Fogarty TJ: Acute arterial occlusion. Textbook of Surgery: The Biological Basis of Modern Surgical Practice, 13th ed. Sabiston DC, Ed. WB Saunders Co, Philadelphia, 1986, p 1904

33. Imparato AM, Riles TS: Peripheral arterial disease. Principles of Surgery, 5th ed. Schwartz SI, Shires GT, Spencer FC, Eds. McGraw-Hill Book Co, New York, 1989, p 933

34. Haimovici H: Peripheral arterial embolism: a study of 330 unselected cases of embolism of the extremities. Angiology 1:20, 1950

35. Stallone RJ, Blaisdell FW: Analysis of morbidity and mortality from arterial embolectomy. Surgery 65: 207, 1969

36. Dunant JH, Edwards WS: Small vessel occlusion in the extremity after various periods of arterial obstruction: an experimental study. Surgery 73:240, 1973

37. Mullick S: The tourniquet in operations upon the extremities. Surg Gynecol Obstet 146:821, 1978

38. Blaisdell FW, Graziano CJ, Effeney DJ: In vivo assessment of anticoagulation. Surgery 82:827, 1977

39. Blaisdell FW, Steele M, Allen RE: Management of acute lower extremity arterial ischemia due to embolism and thrombosis. Surgery 84:822, 1978

40. Leyvraz PF, Richard J, Bachmann F, et al: Adjusted versus fixed dose heparin in the prevention of deep vein thrombosis after hip replacement. N Engl J Med 309:954, 1983

41. Rooke TW: Deep venous thrombosis of the extremities. Conn's Current Therapy 1992. Rakel RE, Ed. WB Saunders Co, Philadelphia, 1992, p 289

42. Majerus PW, Broze GJ Jr, Miletich JP, et al: Anticoagulant, thrombolytic and antiplatelet drugs. Goodman & Gilman's The Pharmacological Basis of Therapeutics. Goodman AG, Rall TW, Nies AS, et al, Eds. Pergamon Press, New York, 1990, p 1311

43. USP DI, Drug Information for the Health Care Professional, Vol IB. The United States Pharmacopeial Convention, Inc, Rockville, Maryland, 1992, pp 1505, 2357, 2658

44. Owen CA Jr, Bowie EJ, et al: Chronic intravascular coagulation syndromes: a summary. Mayo Clin Proc 49:673, 1974

45. Blaisdell FW, Graziano CJ: Assessment of clotting by the determination of fibrinogen catabolism. Am J Surg 135:436, 1978

46. Conti S, Daschbach M, Blaisdell FW: A comparison of high-dose versus conventional-dose heparin therapy for deep vein thrombosis. Surgery 92:972, 1982

47. Kashtan J, Conti S, Blaisdell FW: Heparin therapy for deep venous thrombosis. Am J Surg 140:836, 1980

48. Silver D, Kapsch DN, Tsoi EK: Heparin induced thrombocytopenia, thrombosis and hemorrhage. Ann Surg 198:301, 1983

49. Becker PS, Miller VT: Heparin-induced thrombocytopenia. Stroke 20:1449, 1989

50. Celoria GM, Steingart RH, Banson B, et al: Coumarin skin necrosis in a patient with heparin-induced thrombocytopenia: a case report. Angiology 39:915, 1988

51. Walker AM, Jick H: Predictors of bleeding during heparin therapy. JAMA 244:1209, 1980

52. Ginsberg JS, Kowalchuk G, Hirsh J, et al: Heparin effect on bone density. Thromb Haemost 64:286, 1990

53. Hirsh J, Poller L, Deykin D, et al: Optimal therapeutic range for oral anticoagulants. Chest 95(2 suppl): 5s, 1989

54. Grulich-Henn J, Preissner KT, Müller-Berghaus G: Heparin stimulates fibrinolysis in mesothelial cells by selective induction of tissue plasminogen activator but not plasminogen activator inhibitor-1 synthesis. Thromb Haemost 64:420, 1990

55. Blaisdell FW: Hemostasis and thrombosis. Vascular Surgery: A Comprehensive Review, 2nd ed. Moore WS, Ed. Grune & Stratton, New York, 1986, p 909

56. Meyerovitz MF, Goldhaber SZ, Reagan K, et al: Recombinant tissue-type plasminogen activator versus urokinase in peripheral arterial and graft occlusions: a randomized trial. Radiology 175:75, 1990

57. Turpie AG: Thrombolytic agents in venous thrombosis. J Vasc Surg 12:196, 1990

58. Marder VJ, Sherry S: Thrombolytic therapy: current status. N Engl J Med 318:1585, 1988

59. Goldhaber SZ, Buring JE, Lipnick RJ, et al: Pooled analyses of randomized trials of streptokinase and heparin in phlebographically documented acute deep venous thrombosis. Am J Med 76:393, 1984

60. The effects of tissue plasminogen activator, streptokinase, or both on coronary-artery patency, ventricular function, and survival after acute myocardial infarction. The GUSTO Angiographic Investigators. N Engl J Med 329:1615, 1993

61. Amery A, Deloof W, Vermylen J, et al: Outcome of recent thromboembolic occlusions of limb arteries treated with streptokinase. Br Med J 4:639, 1970

62. Dotter CT, Rosch J, Seaman AJ: Selective clot lysis with low-dose streptokinase. Radiology 111:31, 1974

63. Ouriel K, Veith FJ, Sasahara AA: Thrombolysis or peripheral arterial surgery: phase I results. TOPAS investigators. J Vasc Surg 23:64, 1996

64. Meyer GJ, Sors H, Charbonnier B, et al: Effects of intravenous urokinase versus alteplase on total pulmonary resistance in acute massive pulmonary embolism: a European multicenter double-blind trial. The European Cooperative Study Group for Pulmonary Embolism. J Am Coll Cardiol 19:239, 1992

65. Schafer AI: The hypercoagulable states. Ann Intern Med 102:814, 1985

66. Baehner RL: Alterations in blood coagulation with trauma. Pediatr Clin North Am 22:289, 1975

67. Jansson IG, Hetland O, Rammer LM, et al: Effects of phospholipase C, a tissue thromboplastin inhibitor, on pulmonary microembolism after missile injury of the limb. J Trauma 28:S222, 1988

68. Effeney DJ, McIntyre KS, Blaisdell FW, et al: Fibrinogen kinetics in major human burns. Surg Forum 29:56, 1978

69. Blaisdell FW: Acquired and congenital clotting syndromes. World J Surg 14:664, 1990

70. Hauptman JG, Hassouna HI, Bell TG, et al: Efficacy of antithrombin III in endotoxin induced disseminated intravascular coagulation. Circ Shock 25:111, 1988

71. Rodgers GM, Shuman MA: Congenital thrombotic disorders. Am J Hematol 21:419, 1986

72. Rocha E, Paramo JA, Aranda A, et al: Congenital dysfibrinogenemias: a review. Ric Clin Lab 15:205, 1985

73. Liu Y, Lyons RM, McDonagh J: Plasminogen San Antonio: an abnormal plasminogen with a more cathodic migration, decreased activation and associated thrombosis. Thromb Haemost 59:49, 1988

74. Nilsson IM, Ljungner H, Tengborn L: Two different mechanisms in patients with venous thrombosis and defective fibrinolysis: low concentration of plasminogen activator or increased concentration of plasminogen activator inhibitor. Br Med J 290:1453, 1985

75. Kruithof EK, Gudinchet A, Bachmann F: Plasminogen activator inhibitor 1 and plasminogen activator inhibitor 2 in various disease states. Thromb Haemost 59:7, 1988

76. Juhan-Vague I, Roul C, Alessi MC, et al: Increased plasminogen activator inhibitor activity in non insulin dependent diabetic patients—relationship with plasma insulin. Thromb Haemost 61:370, 1989

77. Dahlbäck B, Carlsson M, Svensson PJ: Familial thrombophilia due to a previously unrecognized mechanism characterized by poor anticoagulant response to activated protein C: prediction of a cofactor to activated protein C. Proc Natl Acad Sci USA 90: 1004, 1993

78. Bertina RM, Reitsma PH, Rosendaal FR, et al: Resistance to activated protein C and factor V Leiden as risk factors for venous thrombosis. Thromb Haemost 74:449, 1995

79. Egeberg O: Inherited antithrombin deficiency causing thrombophilia. Thrombosis et Diathesis Haemorrhagica 13:516, 1965

80. High KA: Antithrombin-III, protein-C, and protein-S: naturally occurring anticoagulant proteins. Arch Pathol Lab Med 112:28, 1988

81. Bauer KA, Goodman TL, Kass BL, et al: Elevated factor Xa activity in the blood of asymptomatic patients with congenital antithrombin deficiency. J Clin Invest 76:826, 1985

82. Owings JT, Bagley M, Gosselin R, et al: Effect of critical injury on plasma antithrombin activity: low antithrombin levels are associated with thromboembolic complications. J Trauma 41:396, 1996

83. Gladson CL, Scharrer I, Hach V, et al: The frequency of type I heterozygous protein-S and protein-C deficiency in 141 unrelated young patients with venous thrombosis. Thromb Haemost 59:18, 1988

84. Blaisdell FW: What's new in clotting and anticoagulation. Progress in Vascular Surgery. Najarian JS, Delaney JP, Eds. Year Book Medical Publishers, Chicago, 1988, p 75

85. Virchow R: Gesammelte Abhandlungen zur wissenschaftlichen Medizin. Von Meidingersohn, Frankfurt am Main, Germany, 1856

86. McLachlin AD, McLachlin JA, Jory TA, et al: Venous stasis in the lower extremities. Ann Surg 152:678, 1960

87. McLachlin J, Paterson JC: Some basic observations

on venous thrombosis and pulmonary embolism. Surg Gynecol Obstet 93:1, 1951

88. Cope C, Reyes TM, Skversky NJ: Phlebographic analysis of the incidence of thrombosis in hemiplegia. Radiology 109:581, 1973

89. Dooijewaard G, deBoer A, Turion PN, et al: Physical exercise induces enhancement of urokinase-type plasminogen activator (u-PA) levels in plasma. Thromb Haemost 65:82, 1991

90. Hansen J-B, Wilsgård L, Olsen JO, et al: Formation and persistence of procoagulant and fibrinolytic activities in circulation after strenuous physical exercise. Thromb Haemost 64:385, 1990

91. Sevitt S: The structure and growth of valve-pocket thrombi in femoral veins. J Clin Pathol 27:517, 1974

92. Hamer JD, Malone PC, Silver IA: The Po_2 in venous valve pockets: its possible bearing on thrombogenesis. Br J Surg 68:166, 1981

93. Dunmire SM: Pulmonary embolism. Emerg Med Clin North Am 7:339, 1989

94. Shackford SR, Moser KM: Deep venous thrombosis and pulmonary embolism in trauma patients. J Intensive Care Med 3:87, 1988

95. Kakkar VV, Stringer MD: Prophylaxis of venous thromboembolism. World J Surg 14:670, 1990

96. Bell WR, Simon TL: Current status of pulmonary thromboembolic disease: pathophysiology, diagnosis, prevention and treatment. Am Heart J 103:239, 1982

97. Sabiston DC Jr: Pathophysiology, diagnosis and management of pulmonary embolism. Am J Surg 138:384, 1979

98. Fogarty TJ, Cranley JJ, Krause RJ, et al: A method for extraction of arterial emboli and thrombi. Surgery 116:241, 1963

99. Gregg RO, Chamberlain BE, Myers JK, et al: Embolectomy or heparin therapy for arterial emboli. Surgery 93:377, 1983

100. Ricotta JJ, Scudder PA, McAndrew JA, et al: Management of acute ischemia of the upper extremity. Am J Surg 145:661, 1983

101. Jivegård L, Holm J, Bergqvist D: Acute lower limb ischemia: failure of anticoagulant treatment to improve one month results of arterial thromboembolectomy: a prospective randomized multi-center study. Surgery 109:610, 1991

102. Kendrick J, Thompson BW, Read RC, et al: Arterial embolectomy in the leg: results in a referral hospital. Am J Surg 142:739, 1981

103. Balas P, Bonatsos G, Xeromeritis N, et al: Early surgical results on acute arterial occlusion of the extremities. J Cardiovasc Surg 26:262, 1985

104. Dale WA: Differential management of acute peripheral arterial ischemia. J Vasc Surg 1:269, 1984

105. Stallone RJ, Lim RC Jr, Blaisdell FW: Pathogenesis of the pulmonary changes following ischemia of the lower extremities. Ann Thorac Surg 7:539, 1969

106. Haimovici H: Proceedings: myopathic-nephrotic-metabolic syndrome associated with massive acute arterial occlusions. J Cardiovasc Surg 14:589, 1973

107. Kontaxis AN, Skalkas G, Sechas M, et al: Proceedings: effect of acute arterial ischemia of the extremities on cardiac and pulmonary functions. J Cardiovasc Surg 14:605, 1973

108. Anner H, Kaufman RP, Valeri CR, et al: Reperfusion of ischemic lower limbs increases pulmonary microvascular permeability. J Trauma 28:607, 1988

109. Jivegård L, Holm J, Schersten T: Acute limb ischemia due to arterial embolism or thrombosis: influence of limb ischemia versus pre-existing cardiac disease on postoperative mortality rate. J Cardiovasc Surg 29:32, 1988

110. Hobson RW 2nd, Neville R, Watanabe B, et al: Role of heparin in reducing skeletal muscle infarction in ischemia-reperfusion. Microcirc Endothelium Lymphatics 5:259, 1989

111. Blaisdell FW: Preventing postoperative thromboembolism. West J Med 151:188, 1989

112. Reilly DT: Prophylactic methods against thromboembolism. Acta Chir Scand Suppl 550(suppl): 115, 1989

113. Skillman JJ, Collins RE, Coe NP, et al: Prevention of deep vein thrombosis in neurosurgical patients: a controlled randomized trial of external pneumatic compression boots. Surgery 83:354, 1978

114. Rosenberg RD: Action and interactions of antithrombin and heparin. N Engl J Med 292:145, 1975

115. Turpie AG, Levine MN, Hirsh J, et al: A randomized controlled trial of a low-molecular-weight heparin (enoxaparin) to prevent deep-vein thrombosis in patients undergoing elective hip surgery. N Engl J Med 315:925, 1986

116. Levine MN, Hirsh J, Gent M, et al: Prevention of deep vein thrombosis after elective hip surgery: a randomized trial comparing low molecular weight heparin with standard unfractionated heparin. Ann Intern Med 114:545, 1991

117. Geerts WH, Jay RM, Code KI, et al: A comparison of low-dose heparin with low-molecular-weight heparin as prophylaxis against venous thromboembolism after major trauma. N Engl J Med 335:701, 1996

118. Leyvraz PF, Richard J, Bachmann F, et al: Adjusted versus fixed-dose subcutaneous heparin in the prevention of deep-vein thrombosis after total hip replacement. N Engl J Med 309:954, 1983

119. Owings JT, Blaisdell FW: Low-dose heparin thromboembolism prophylaxis. Arch Surg 131:1069, 1996

120. MacCallum PK, Thomson JM, Poller L: Effects of fixed minidose warfarin on coagulation and fibrinolysis following major gynaecological surgery. Thromb Haemost 64:511, 1990

121. Crafoord C: Preliminary report on post-operative treatment with heparin as a preventive of thrombosis. Acta Chir Scand 79:407, 1937

122. Murray GDW, Jaques LB, Perrett TS, et al: Heparin and the thrombosis of veins following injury. Surgery 2:163, 1937

123. Murray GDW, Best CH: The use of heparin in thrombosis. Ann Surg 108:163, 1938

124. Wessler S, Morris LE: Studies in intravascular coagulation: IV. The effect of heparin and dicumarol on serum-induced venous thrombosis. Circulation 12:553, 1955

125. Wessler S, Gitel SN: Heparin: new concepts relevant to clinical use. Blood 53:525, 1979

126. Holm HA, Finnanger B, Hartmann A, et al: Heparin treatment of deep venous thrombosis in 280 patients: symptoms related to dosage. Acta Med Scand 215:47, 1984

127. Gulliver G: The Works of William Hewson. Printed for the Sydenham Society, London, 1846, p 5

3 DIABETES MELLITUS

Maha F. Ansara, M.D., Philip E. Cryer, M.D., and David W. Scharp, M.D.

Perioperative Management of the Diabetic Patient

Patients with diabetes have a 50 percent chance of undergoing surgical procedures during their lifetime.[1] In the past, operation in these patients was associated with a mortality of four to 13 percent,[2,3] usually attributed to cardiovascular complications. This statistic suggests the risks of performing operative procedures in diabetic patients. Any improvement in this situation has probably been offset by the increasing age of patients with diabetes and the larger variety of procedures they undergo.

The perioperative management of diabetic patients is complicated by the metabolic abnormalities of the disease and, if present, the effects of atherosclerotic disease, diabetic nephropathy, and autonomic neuropathy. There is also an increased risk of postoperative wound infection.

Nomenclature

The term insulin-dependent diabetes mellitus (IDDM) is applied to all forms of diabetes in which exogenous insulin is required to prevent diabetic ketoacidosis, regardless of the etiology. IDDM is not, however, synonymous with type I diabetes, which is the term applied to diabetes that results from autoimmune destruction of beta cells, regardless of whether the destruction is sufficient to cause ketoacidosis. The term non–insulin-dependent diabetes mellitus (NIDDM) can be applied to any form of diabetes in which endogenous insulin production is sufficient to prevent diabetic ketoacidosis. NIDDM is not synonymous with type II diabetes; the latter term should be restricted to patients with NIDDM who do not have autoimmune destruction of beta cells (type I diabetes), diabetes secondary to pancreatic disease, or other hyperglycemic conditions. Thus, IDDM is distinguished from NIDDM on the basis of the need for exogenous insulin for survival, whereas type I diabetes is distinguished from type II on the basis of the presence of autoimmune beta cell destruction.

Type I diabetes accounts for approximately three percent of all new cases of diabetes diagnosed each year in the United States. Although type I is much less common in the general population than type II, it is by no means rare among children and young adults. The estimated annual incidence of new cases of type I diabetes in children is one per 7,000, making this disorder three to four times more common than chronic childhood diseases such as cystic fibrosis, peptic ulcer, juvenile rheumatoid arthritis, and leukemia and nearly 10 times more common than nephrotic syndrome, muscular dystrophy, or lymphoma.

After 20 years of age, the yearly incidence of type I diabetes decreases to five per 100,000. The incidence is similar in men and women, lower in African Americans than in whites, and still lower in Latinos, Asian Americans, and Native Americans. Two to five percent of the siblings of persons with type I diabetes will acquire the disorder; among identical twins, one of whom has type I diabetes, concordance rates are only 50 percent.

Criteria for Diagnosis

Possible causes of perioperative hyperglycemia [see Table 1] must be carefully evaluated before operation. Diabetes is diagnosed de novo in a significant number of patients admitted for routine procedures. The measurement of blood glucose, glycosylated hemoglobin, or even urine glucose in outpatients could lead to earlier diagnosis, preventing last-minute detection of diabetes. If perioperative hyperglycemia is diagnosed in the hospital, major procedures should be delayed until patients have received proper metabolic and cardiovascular assessment. For patients with mild glycemic disturbances and those undergoing minor procedures, metabolic adjustments can be made quickly.

Fasting plasma glucose levels greater than 140 mg/dl (7.8 mmol/L) or random plasma glucose levels in excess of 200 mg/dl (11.1 mmol/L) are indicative of diabetes. Other signs and symptoms are polyuria, polydipsia, polyphagia, weight loss, and blurred vision. If the fasting plasma glucose levels are below 140 mg/dl (7.8 mmol/L), the diagnosis may be established by the results of an oral glucose tolerance test [see Table 2].

Table 1 Possible Causes of Perioperative Hyperglycemia

Diabetes mellitus
  Insulin-dependent (IDDM)
  Non–insulin-dependent (NIDDM)

Impaired glucose tolerance (secondary diabetes mellitus)
  Pancreatic disease
  Endocrinopathies (e.g., acromegaly, Cushing's syndrome, pheochromocytoma, glucagonoma, and primary aldosteronism)
  Chemical agents (e.g., estrogen, glucocorticoids, catecholamines, certain antihypertensive agents, thiazides, and psychoactive agents)
  Insulin-receptor abnormalities (e.g., acanthosis nigricans)
  Genetic disorders (e.g., hyperlipidemia, Huntington's disease, and muscular dystrophies)
  Miscellaneous conditions (e.g., malnutrition)

Perioperative Management of the Diabetic Patient

Diabetic patient is scheduled to undergo operation

Perform patient evaluation:

History: Look for recent fluctuations in blood glucose levels; consider timing and dosages of current medications; watch for diabetic complications (e.g., neuropathy, nephropathy, peripheral vascular disorders, cardiac disease).

Physical examination: Assess eyes, skin, neurologic system, and cardiovascular system.

Laboratory tests: Measure levels of plasma glucose (after fasting and 2 hr after eating), HbA1c, electrolytes, ketones, serum creatinine; obtain blood gas values; perform ECG with Valsalva maneuver to rule out cardiac autonomic neuropathy.

Before operation

Monitor metabolic status: If glycemic control is not achieved before admission, schedule admission for 12–16 hr before operation to allow time to optimize control of diabetes. Target values for blood glucose are < 125 mg/dl (fasting) and < 180 mg/dl (postprandial). If emergency operation is required in a patient with a severe metabolic derangement, provide 6–8 hr of intensive treatment. Substitute intermediate-acting insulins for long-acting and, in NIDDM, short-acting sulfonylureas for long-acting. Discontinue metformin. Correct any dehydration.

Assess cardiovascular and renal systems: Watch particularly for cardiac autonomic neuropathy. On ECG, ratio of longest RR interval to shortest during Valsalva maneuver is normally ≥ 1.21; 1.11–1.20 is borderline, and ≤ 1.10 is abnormal. Look for hypoglycemia (in patients taking beta blockers) and thrombosis. Measure BUN, serum creatinine, electrolytes, and urine protein. Consider monitoring central venous pressure or pulmonary arterial wedge pressure.

During operation

Administer insulin, glucose, or both.

Elective major procedures

If patient has type I diabetes, takes insulin for type II, or has type II that is not controlled by drugs or diet, give glucose and short-acting insulin. Target value for blood glucose is between 125 and 200 mg/dl.

Minor procedures

If patient fasted, withhold morning dose of insulin or oral hypoglycemic agent, give short-acting insulin every 2–4 hr, and resume normal dosing after procedure. If patient ate breakfast, give normal morning does, give 4 U of short-acting insulin if blood glucose > 250 mg/dl, and resume normal dosing after procedure.

Emergency procedures

If emergency operation precipitates metabolic decompensation, manage patient conservatively at first, emphasizing correction of any underlying metabolic cause. If problem is metabolic, it should resolve or improve in 3–4 hr; if it is surgical, it will remain the same or worsen over the same period.

Prevent renal dysfunction: Use contrast agents with caution, choosing the least invasive procedure that will provide adequate data; give mannitol and furosemide from 1 hr before to 6 hr after the study; give saline in D5W with potassium.

After operation

Administer insulin and glucose: Infusion should be continued until patient can tolerate oral feeding. If patient is receiving TPN, give insulin only.

Assess cardiovascular and renal systems: If patient is older, has long-standing type I diabetes, or has heart disease, perform serial ECGs. Watch for MI and orthostatic hypotension. Monitor BUN and serum creatinine levels, ensure adequate hydration, and correct any electrolyte abnormalities.

Evaluation of the Diabetic Patient

HISTORY

In the preoperative history, attention should be directed to any recent fluctuation in blood glucose as well as to the type of therapy used to control the patient's diabetes. Inquiries should cover the timing and dosage of medication, especially if the patient is using a long-acting insulin or an oral hypoglycemic. The degree of control of diabetes in the perioperative period, which has an impact on the patient's postoperative recovery, could be affected by certain medications, such as antihypertensive agents. The presence of diabetic complications (e.g., neuropathy, peripheral vascular disorders, nephropathy, and cardiac disease) should be documented because they may have serious effects during and after operation.

The incidence of peripheral neuropathy increases with the age of the patient and the duration of diabetes.[4] Diabetic neuropathies, which mimic many syndromes, should be considered in the differential diagnosis of all patients who are candidates for operation. Patients with cardiac autonomic neuropathy, who are at risk for sudden cardiorespiratory arrest, may have orthostatic hypotension that is not associated with tachycardia, evidence of peripheral neuropathy, and manifestations of other autonomic neuropathies such as nocturnal diarrhea and gustatory sweating.[5]

Diabetic nephropathy alters the clearance of numerous drugs and increases the renal threshold for glucose, making it possible for a patient to produce a urine sample that is negative for glucose even though the plasma glucose level is higher than 300 mg/dl. This condition should be suspected if the patient has overt proteinuria, hypertension, or decreasing insulin requirements. Diabetic nephropathy increases the risk of acute renal failure after the administration of iodinated contrast agents. In some patients, contrast-associated renal failure results in permanent impairment of kidney function, necessitating dialysis.

PHYSICAL EXAMINATION

Specific areas for attention on physical examination are the eyes, the skin, and the neurologic and cardiovascular systems.

Diabetic retinopathy is often asymptomatic in its most treatable stages. Unfortunately, only 45 percent of the diabetic population receives adequate ophthalmic care.[6] Retinopathy rarely occurs in patients who have had type I diabetes for less than five years; after 10 years, however, some degree of retinopathy is present in 60 percent. Proliferative diabetic retinopathy (PDR) is unusual before the disorder has been present for 10 years but is present in 26 percent of type I diabetes patients after 15 years. Diabetic retinopathy is present in approximately 20 percent of patients with type II diabetes at the time of diagnosis; after 15 years, the percentage increases to 60 to 85 percent. PDR is present in three to four percent of the patients who have had type II diabetes for less than four years; after 15 years, five to 20 percent of type II diabetes patients have PDR.[6] Cataracts are four to six times more likely to develop at a young age.

The progressive signs of diabetic retinopathy are the formation of microaneurysms, the development of new vessels elsewhere on the retina (with or without periretinal or vitreous hemorrhage), contraction of the vitreous humor, and retinal detachment. Dia-

---

Table 2 Diagnostic Criteria for Diabetes Mellitus, Gestational Diabetes, and Impaired Glucose Tolerance

Diabetes mellitus

In nonpregnant adults, diagnosis should be restricted to those meeting *one* of the following criteria:

- Random plasma glucose level ≥ 200 mg/dl *plus* classic signs and symptoms of diabetes mellitus.
- Fasting plasma glucose level ≥ 140 mg/dl on at least two occasions
- Fasting plasma glucose level < 140 mg/dl *plus* sustained elevated plasma glucose levels during at least two oral glucose tolerance tests. The 2-hr sample and at least one other from the first 2 hr after a 75 g glucose dose should be ≥ 200 mg/dl. Oral glucose tolerance testing is not necessary if the patient has a fasting plasma glucose level ≥ 140 mg/dl.

In children, diagnosis should be restricted to those meeting *one* of the following criteria:

- Random plasma glucose level ≥ 200 mg/dl *plus* classic signs and symptoms of diabetes mellitus.
- Fasting plasma glucose level ≥ 140 mg/dl on at least two occasions *plus* sustained elevated plasma glucose levels during at least two oral glucose tolerance tests. The 2-hr sample and at least one other from the first 2 hr after a glucose dose (1.75 g/kg of ideal body weight, up to 75 g) should be ≥ 200 mg/dl.

Gestational diabetes

The diagnosis can be made if, on two occasions, oral intake of 100 g of glucose results in plasma glucose values that are (1) ≥ 105 mg/dl while the patient is fasting or (2) ≥ 190 mg/dl at 1 hr, ≥ 165 mg/dl at 2 hr, or ≥ 145 mg/dl at 3 hr postprandially.

Impaired glucose tolerance

In nonpregnant adults, the diagnosis should be restricted to those meeting *all* of the following criteria:

- Fasting plasma glucose level < 140 mg/dl.
- 2-hr oral glucose tolerance test result between 140 and 200 mg/dl.
- Intervening oral glucose tolerance test result ≥ 200 mg/dl.

In children, the diagnosis should be restricted to those who have *both* of the following:

- Fasting plasma glucose concentration < 140 mg/dl.
- 2-hr oral glucose tolerance test result > 140 mg/dl.

---

betic macular edema, which occurs at any level of diabetic retinopathy, is best detected by stereoscopic examination of macules with a slit-lamp biomicroscope or a funduscope. Diabetic macular edema may be associated with nonproliferative diabetic retinopathy, which is manifested by formation of retinal microaneurysms, hard exudate, and intraretinal microvascular abnormalities. The nonproliferative form may advance to proliferative diabetic retinopathy, in which new vessels form, with or without preretinal or vitreous hemorrhage. Panretinal photocoagulation has beneficial effects for all eyes threatened by retinopathy.

Diabetic dermopathy is characterized by multiple hyperpigmented macules on the extensor surface of the distal lower extremities. The individual lesions are oval or circular, ranging in size from 0.5 to 2.0 cm, and are sometimes associated with atrophy and scaling. These skin changes, also referred to as shin spots or pigmented pretibial patches, occasionally occur in persons with no evidence of glucose intolerance. Except for its appearance, the dermopathy is generally asymptomatic. No effective treatment has been described.

Necrobiosis lipoidica diabeticorum (NLD) is characterized by red to red-brown to violet plaques that enlarge, often becoming yellow at the center. The overlying skin is usually shiny and transparent because of epidermal atrophy. In 90 percent of patients, this condition is most likely to occur on the shins, but it can also be found on the scalp, face, arms, and trunk. NLD lesions, especially in the distal lower extremities, may ulcerate. There is no well-established treatment for the condition, but some success has been reported with pentoxifylline (400 mg three times daily), dipyridamole (50 to 75 mg three or four times daily) plus low-dose aspirin (325 mg/day), and intralesional corticosteroids (5 mg/ml of triamcinolone acetonide). With triamcinolone acetonide, there may be breakdown of skin lesions.[7]

Lipodystrophy may appear as atrophic or hypertrophic lesions that are thought to be caused by a local response to insulin administration. Use of a less antigenic form of insulin, deeper insulin injections, and frequent changes of injection sites are recommended. When subcutaneous fat has disappeared, improvement has been reported after the injection of purified insulin into the edge of the lipoatrophy.

In tissues affected by vascular insufficiency, minor trauma may lead to infection. Patients with peripheral sensory neuropathy may not be aware of these minor injuries and may fail to treat them. Infections may undermine extensive amounts of tissue, especially in the feet or at pressure points (bedsores). These infections are caused by both aerobic and anaerobic organisms.

The peripheral polyneuropathy of diabetes is distributed in a stocking-glove pattern. The lancinating pain of diabetic radiculopathy is dramatic and can mimic abdominal pain caused by other disorders. Confirmation of the diagnosis of diabetic neuropathy may depend on electromyography and, in rare cases, nerve biopsy.

LABORATORY TESTS

Plasma levels of glucose should be measured while the patient is fasting and two hours after he or she has eaten; long-term diabetic control can be assessed by measurement of glycosylated hemoglobin (HbA_{1c}) concentrations. The potential for metabolic disturbances can be gauged from measurement of electrolyte and ketone levels and arterial blood gas values. Serum creatinine levels can be used to monitor renal function, and an ECG performed in conjunction with the Valsalva maneuver can rule out cardiac autonomic neuropathy.

Preoperative Management

METABOLIC MONITORING

All diabetic patients who are candidates for elective surgical procedures require careful preoperative assessment, including metabolic monitoring [see Table 3]. Ideally, diabetic patients achieve glycemic control before being admitted to the hospital. It may be more realistic, however, to schedule admission for 12 to 16 hours before the operation to allow time to optimize metabolic control in all insulin-dependent patients and in non–insulin-dependent patients who have inadequate metabolic control. In general, preoperative blood glucose targets should be less than

125 mg/dl (6.9 mmol/L) during fasting and less than 180 mg/dl (10.0 mmol/L) postprandially. If emergency operation is required in patients with severe metabolic derangements (diabetic ketoacidosis or hyperosmolar nonketotic states), six to eight hours of intensive treatment usually improves their general condition. This brief period permits clarification of the diagnosis in patients with acute abdominal pain, which may be the consequence of diabetic ketoacidosis rather than the so-called surgical abdomen.

The current practice in preparing diabetic patients for operation is to stop all use of long-acting insulins (Ultralente preparations), replacing them with intermediate-acting insulins (the neutral protamine Hagedorn [NPH] or Lente preparations). In patients with NIDDM, use of long-acting sulfonylureas such as chlorpropamide and glyburide should be stopped because of the risk of hypoglycemia; a short-acting preparation should be substituted. Use of metformin should be stopped because of the risks of lactic acidosis when renal function is impaired, as it may be during any procedure requiring anesthesia. Chronically hyperglycemic patients are frequently dehydrated, and this condition must be corrected before operation.

CARDIOVASCULAR AND RENAL ASSESSMENT

Coronary artery disease and hypertensive vascular disease are common in diabetic patients. Thorough evaluation of a patient's cardiovascular condition should include careful assessment of the autonomic nervous system because of the known risks of cardiorespiratory arrest in patients with auto-

---

Table 3 **Preoperative Assessment and Preparation of the Diabetic Patient**

Assessment
  Cardiovascular
    History (hypertension, angina, infarction)
    Blood pressure
    Full examination, including peripheral pulse rates
    Electrocardiogram
  Neurologic
    Peripheral neuropathy
    Autonomic examination: RR interval
  Renal
    Proteinuria
    Serum creatinine levels
    Urinalysis
  Metabolic
    Home glucose control
    Glycosylated hemoglobin
    Electrolytes (sodium, potassium)

Preparation
  Patients with insulin-dependent diabetes mellitus (IDDM)
    Stop administration of long-acting insulin
    Substitute b.i.d. intermediate-acting insulin (NPH or Lente) combined with t.i.d. regular insulin before meals
  Patients with non–insulin-dependent diabetes mellitus (NIDDM)
    Stop administration of long-acting sulfonylureas (e.g., chlorpropamide), but substitute a short-acting one if necessary
    Stop administration of metformin
    Reinforce dietary advice

nomic neuropathy. Cardiac autonomic neuropathy can usually be diagnosed preoperatively by means of electrocardiography. One method calculates the ratio of the longest RR interval to the shortest RR interval during the Valsalva maneuver. The normal ratio is 1.21 or higher, a borderline ratio is 1.11 to 1.20, and an abnormal ratio is 1.10 or lower.[8] (Occasionally, however, older nondiabetic patients have a ratio lower than 1.03.) The poor prognosis of patients with cardiac autonomic neuropathy, in whom mortality reaches 50 percent within 2.5 years of diagnosis,[9] may influence the decision to perform an elective procedure in this group.

Well-controlled hypertension does not pose special risks during operation, but hypoglycemia may develop without warning in patients receiving beta blockers, who should be monitored accordingly. Patients with type I diabetes (resulting from autoimmune destruction of beta cells) who use beta blockers are also at greater risk for prolonged episodes of insulin-induced hypoglycemia. All diabetic patients are at increased risk for thrombosis. Unless its use is specifically contraindicated, 5,000 units of heparin should be administered subcutaneously every eight to 12 hours to diabetic patients who are confined to bed, whether before or after operation.

Measurement of blood urea nitrogen, serum creatinine, electrolytes, and urine protein should be performed before operation. Azotemic patients may have problems with fluid management, and monitoring of central venous or pulmonary arterial wedge pressure may be necessary. Hyperkalemia, often seen in patients with mild to moderate kidney failure, can precipitate acute cardiac arrhythmia. This metabolic finding usually results from hyporeninemic hypoaldosteronism. Hypokalemia, if present, may be aggravated by use of insulin and glucose therapy.

Intraoperative Management

METABOLIC EFFECTS OF OPERATION AND ANESTHESIA

Surgical procedures and anesthesia have profound metabolic effects that are exacerbated by insulin deficiency or hyposecretion and by insulin insensitivity. The effects of operation are amplified in patients who are in a catabolic state, as are diabetic patients with poor metabolic control.

During anesthesia and operation, endogenous insulin secretion is suppressed but the plasma levels of counterregulatory hormones (glucagon, epinephrine, cortisol, and growth hormone) increase in nondiabetic as well as diabetic patients. The increased secretion of these hormones in the setting of low insulin levels stimulates hepatic glucose production. In nondiabetic persons, major procedures are frequently associated with blood glucose levels of 150 to 200 mg/dl (8.3 to 11.1 mmol/L). In diabetic persons, the metabolic abnormality varies according to the extent and duration of the surgical procedure and the impairment of insulin secretion.

Two studies in patients with stable IDDM have shown blood glucose levels rising from about 180 mg/dl (10.0 mmol/L) to about 270 mg/dl (15.0 mmol/L) postoperatively, with ketone body levels rising to about twice the levels in nondiabetic control subjects.[10,11] The situation is similar metabolically even in patients with NIDDM who undergo minor procedures that generate relatively little stress—blood glucose levels rising to 180 mg/dl (10.0 mmol/L), with higher than normal levels of ketone bodies and free fatty acids.[12]

Autonomic neuropathy can cause severe hypotension during induction of anesthesia. Diabetic nephropathy complicates fluid management, usually resulting in electrolyte abnormalities. All diabetic patients are at higher risk for postoperative myocardial infarction, which is often asymptomatic. Poor nutrition and impaired phagocytosis make diabetic patients more susceptible to infection and slower to heal.

INSULIN AND GLUCOSE ADMINISTRATION

Elective Major Procedures

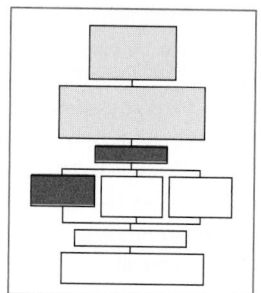

In a patient undergoing general anesthesia, regardless of the duration of the operation, infusion of insulin and glucose is recommended if the patient has type I diabetes, takes insulin for type II diabetes, or uses drugs or diet therapy (or both) but has not achieved satisfactory control of type II diabetes. Several methods of insulin administration have been recommended for use during the perioperative period. Most of the protocols include the intravenous administration of short-acting insulin and five to 10 percent glucose.

In some of the protocols, the glucose and insulin are administered in a single infusion. The advantage of this approach is that if the glucose infusion is accidentally disconnected or obstructed, the insulin infusion is as well, so that the risk of hypoglycemia is eliminated. The disadvantage of this method is that it is impossible to change the delivery rate of one agent without changing the delivery rate of the other. The administration of insulin and glucose in separate bags but through the same vein (that is, piggybacked) allows either infusion rate to be changed without affecting the other. The insulin infusion rate is progressively increased, and the glucose infusion rate is progressively decreased, according to the capillary blood glucose levels, measured hourly [see Table 4]. With this protocol, a blood glucose level in the range of 125 to 200 mg/dl (6.9 to 11.1 mmol/L) is easily maintained during the entire perioperative period. Close observation of blood glucose levels and prompt adjustment of insulin and glucose delivery are mandatory to achieve a stable blood glucose level. Electrolyte supplementation is administered via a separate infusion.

In patients who are fluid restricted or those receiving large amounts of other solutions, 10 percent dextrose in water (D10W) can be substituted for the five percent dextrose (D5W) solution. If D10W is not available, it can be made by adding 100 ml of 50 percent dextrose in water (D50W) to 1 L of D5W. D50W can be administered in the central line in patients with severe congestive heart failure or end-stage renal disease, whose fluid intake is severely restricted. For a person weighing 70 kg, this corresponds to a glucose infusion rate of 2 mg/kg/min. Clinical judgment dictates changes in the infusion protocol as necessary, the glucose infusion rate remaining constant while the insulin infusion rate is modified. The blood glucose level must be monitored hourly. Capillary blood glucose levels can be measured with glucose oxidase strips and a reflectance meter in the operating and recovery rooms. With appropriate adjustments of the insulin-glucose infusion algorithm, blood glucose levels will remain between 125 and 200 mg/dl (6.9 and 11.1 mmol/L).

Table 4 Representative Protocol for Insulin-Glucose Infusion during the Perioperative Period

1. Infuse 5% dextrose in water (D5W) I.V. via pump.

2. Make insulin solution with 0.5 U/ml of short-acting insulin (i.e., 250 U of regular insulin in 500 ml of normal saline). Administer in piggyback fashion via infusion pump into D5W infusion.

3. After initiating glucose-insulin infusion, stop all subcutaneous insulin therapy.

4. Measure capillary blood glucose levels every hour.

5. On the basis of hourly blood glucose levels, adjust each infusion according to the following schedule:

Blood Glucose (mg/dl)	Insulin Infusion		D5W Infusion (ml/hr)
	(ml/hr)	(U/hr)	
< 70*	1.0	0.5	150
71–100	2.0	1.0	125
101–150	3.0	1.5	100
151–200	4.0	2.0	100
201–250	6.0	3.0	100
251–300	8.0	4.0	75
> 300	12.0	6.0	50

*Give 10 ml D5W I.V. and repeat blood glucose measurement 15 min later.

Minor Procedures

Diabetic patients who fast before minor operations (for example, endoscopy or procedures performed with the patient under local anesthesia) should omit the morning dose of insulin or oral hypoglycemic agent. Their capillary blood glucose level should be measured every two to four hours. Supplemental subcutaneous short-acting 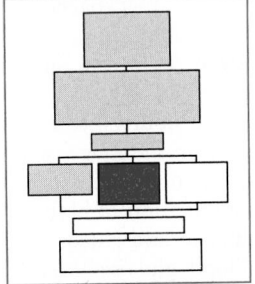 insulin can be administered according to a variable insulin schedule, and the usual insulin or oral agent can be taken after the procedure [see Table 5]. This method of administration, which is associated with unpredictable absorption and variable plasma insulin levels, is restricted to surgical patients undergoing minor procedures and should not be used in patients undergoing major operations.

Emergency Procedures

Diabetic patients may be more likely than nondiabetic patients to undergo emergency operation, which can cause rapid metabolic decompensation with dehydration, hyperglycemia, and ketoacidosis. Uncontrolled diabetes may also be precipitated in patients with no history of diabetes. Management depends, to a large extent, on the patient's metabolic condition. In a patient with a so-called surgical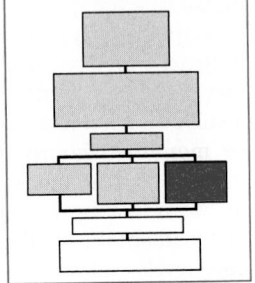

abdomen, it is crucial to ascertain whether there may be a metabolic cause for the condition. The sensible approach is to manage the patient conservatively at first, with an emphasis on metabolic correction. If the problem is metabolic, it should resolve or improve in three to four hours; a surgical problem will remain the same or worsen in three to four hours.

PREVENTION OF RENAL DYSFUNCTION

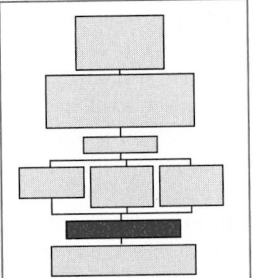

Injudicious use of contrast agents can cause permanent impairment of renal function, necessitating dialysis. In patients with preexisting renal disease, certain measures can prevent contrast-associated renal failure. These include selection of the least invasive procedure that will provide adequate diagnostic information. The following recommendations can be used for patients whose serum creatinine is at or above 2 mg/dl (≥ 176.9 mmol/L) at baseline: one hour before the contrast study, begin infusing 20 ml/hr of a solution of 500 ml of 20 percent mannitol with 200 mg of furosemide added; continue this infusion uninterrupted for six hours after completion of the study; and give 0.5 N saline in D5W with 30 mEq/L of potassium to replace the urine output. Although this regimen has not been validated by controlled studies, it appears to be safe. Many clinicians recommend the use of nonionic low-osmolar contrast agents in diabetic patients with renal insufficiency to reduce the risk of significant renal ischemia, but there is no evidence justifying the considerable cost of the newer agents.[13]

Table 5 Management of Diabetes in Patients Undergoing Minor Surgical Procedures[20]

If patient fasted

1. Withhold morning dose of insulin or oral agent.

2. Measure capillary blood glucose level before procedure and every 2–4 hr thereafter.

3. Give short-acting insulin every 2–4 hr, as follows:

Blood Glucose (mg/dl)	Short-Acting Insulin (U)
< 150	0
151–200	2
201–250	3
251–300	5
> 300	6

4. After procedure, give usual dose of insulin or oral agent.

If patient ate breakfast

1. Give normal morning dose of insulin or oral agent.

2. Measure blood glucose levels before and after procedure.

3. Give supplemental 4 U of short-acting insulin if blood glucose level exceeds 250 mg/dl.

4. After prodecure, give usual afternoon dose of insulin or oral agent.

Postoperative Management

INSULIN AND GLUCOSE ADMINISTRATION

After a minor procedure, a diabetic patient should receive glucose and insulin by infusion until the metabolic condition is stable and oral feeding can be tolerated. To prevent ketosis, the insulin and glucose infusions should be continued for at least one hour after the administration of subcutaneous short-acting insulin. After a major procedure, the patient should receive glucose and insulin infusions until he or she is able to take solid food without difficulty. The regimen of multiple subcutaneous injections of short-acting insulin before meals and intermediate-acting insulin twice daily is recommended during the first 24 to 48 hours after cessation of the insulin and glucose infusions and before resumption of the patient's usual insulin regimen [see Table 6].

Total parenteral nutrition (TPN), often required during the postoperative period, can cause serious metabolic derangements in diabetic patients. A variable insulin infusion schedule [see Table 4], with hourly determinations of blood glucose, is recommended under these circumstances, but additional glucose is not needed, because it is included in the TPN solution. Initially, the insulin should be given as a continuous infusion separate from the TPN solution. Once a stable dose of insulin is reached (usually within 24 to 48 hours), the total amount of insulin required over 24 hours can be added to the TPN bag. This amount may be high—often more than 100 units daily. At this point, capillary blood glucose levels can be measured every two to four hours.

CARDIOVASCULAR AND RENAL ASSESSMENT

Serial postoperative electrocardiograms are recommended for older diabetic patients, those with long-standing type I diabetes, and those with known heart disease. Postoperative myocardial infarction, which may be silent, has a high mortality. When the patient begins to walk, the possibility of orthostatic hypotension must be considered.

Careful monitoring of blood urea nitrogen and serum creatinine levels facilitates the detection of acute kidney failure, which may occur after procedures involving the administration of iodinated contrast material. If a contrast agent is used, the patient should be well hydrated before and after the procedure. Electrolyte abnormalities, such as elevated or decreased levels of potassium, must be treated aggressively.

INFECTION

Wound infection is common in diabetic patients with poor metabolic control. Impaired granulocyte function, resulting from hyperglycemia, may predispose to bacterial infections. If autonomic neuropathy is present, it may lead to difficulty in postoperative voiding, which increases the risk of urinary tract infection. Poor circulation as a result of macroangiopathy or microan-

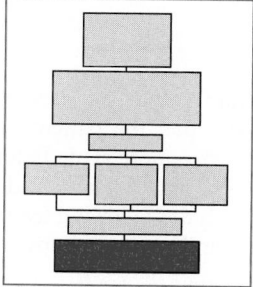

Table 6 Postoperative Management When Diabetic Patient Can Take Solid Food

1. Continue intravenous insulin-glucose infusion for 1 hr after subcutaneous administration of insulin dose.
2. Measure capillary blood glucose before meals, at 10:00 P.M., and at 3:00 A.M. If the patient is hypoglycemic at 3:00 A.M., reduce the insulin dose at 10:00 P.M.
3. Administer preprandial short-acting insulin according to the following variable-dosage schedule:

Blood Glucose (mg/dl)	Short-Acting Insulin (U)			
	Breakfast	Lunch	Dinner	10:00 P.M.
< 70	3	2	2	0
71–100	4	3	3	0
101–150	6	4	4	0
151–200	8	6	6	0
201–250	10	8	8	1
251–300	12	10	10	2
> 300	14	12	12	3

4. Administer 10–20 U of intermediate-acting insulin at 10:00 P.M. (in addition to the dose of short-acting insulin scheduled for this time).
5. Provide three meals and three snacks, for a total of 20 to 30 kcal/kg/day.

giopathy can also contribute to the likelihood of postoperative infection.

Tight metabolic control during the perioperative period can decrease the risk of postoperative infection. If wound infections occur, they are usually caused by mixed flora, including aerobic and anaerobic organisms such as *Escherichia coli*, Enterobacteriaceae, various streptococci, *Staphylococcus aureus*, and *Bacteroides fragilis*. Several organisms produce gas, resulting in crepitation in patients with the so-called diabetic foot. This must be distinguished from the much less common and more acutely devastating clostridial gas gangrene and necrotizing fasciitis.

Surgical debridement and drainage, if needed, should be performed early. Cultures should be obtained during drainage procedures and, ideally, before antibiotic therapy is started. However, it may be preferable to initiate empirical therapy for the most likely organisms until the results of cultures are available. Swarming of *Proteus* organisms may obscure other pathogens on culture plates. Unless the patient is clearly manifesting a septic response, aminoglycosides should not be used because of their nephrotoxicity and the likelihood that diabetic patients may have underlying kidney disease. If severe infections do not respond to antibiotic therapy, the presence of *Candida* or other fungal species [see VI:18 Fungal Infection] should be suspected.

Discussion

Developments in Diabetic Management

PREVENTION OF INSULIN-DEPENDENT DIABETES MELLITUS

Diabetologists' ultimate goal is to find a means of preventing diabetes. It is now known that IDDM is an autoimmune disorder strongly associated with the class II alleles DR3 and DR4, and it is thought that alleles of the HLA-DQ β chain are primarily responsible for susceptibility (and resistance) to autoimmune destruction of beta cells. This theory has generated a series of studies on immunosuppression induced by cyclosporine, azathioprine, or steroids in patients newly diagnosed with IDDM, with the goal of delaying or preventing the autoimmune destruction of beta cells. Cyclosporine has proved to be relatively effective in delaying insulin dependence and inducing prolonged remission, but diagnosis must be made during the prediabetes phase because more than 90 percent of beta cells have been destroyed by the time IDDM is diagnosed.

There are ethical obstacles to using broad-spectrum immunosuppression in patients at risk for IDDM, because conventional insulin therapy has increased the life expectancy of patients with this disorder. The Barts Windsor study[14] has shown that islet cell antibodies develop many years before the onset of clinical diabetes in the nondiabetic siblings of patients with IDDM. A series of studies from New Zealand,[14] largely uncontrolled and unconfirmed, suggest that nicotinamide induces remission in patients with newly diagnosed IDDM and delays the onset of diabetes in antibody-positive nondiabetic children. Additional studies are needed to substantiate these findings.

The prospect of being able to intervene in the prediabetic state is an exciting one, but it must be remembered that these early studies are limited in scope, focusing on first-degree relatives (even though familial cases of diabetes constitute a minority of all cases) and relying on strategies that are not totally harmless. Immunosuppression and administration of nicotinamide, subcutaneous insulin, oral insulin, and glutamic decarboxylase have been proposed as means of intervention. Even subcutaneous insulin is not totally harmless, and nicotinamide, though a natural substance, was used in these studies in doses higher than the recommended daily allowance. Well-designed multicenter studies are needed for the development of acceptable means of preventing IDDM.

INSULIN PUMPS

Results of the Diabetes Control and Complications Trial[15] (DCCT) may prompt many physicians to advocate intensive insulin therapy. The DCCT clearly demonstrated that intensive therapy delays the development and progression of retinopathy, nephropathy, and neuropathy. Hypoglycemic reactions, however, were more frequent in the group receiving intensive therapy than in the conventional-therapy group.

Insulin pump therapy or continuous subcutaneous insulin infusion (CSII) is a highly adjustable method offering type I diabetes patients an alternative to multiple daily injections. Effective use of intensive insulin therapy requires that the health care provider possess a great deal of knowledge about diabetes and that the patient, the family, and the health care team be highly motivated. Before beginning treatment with an insulin pump, the patient and health care provider should be familiar with the following features of intensive insulin therapy in general and pump therapy in particular:

1. The patients most likely to achieve improved glycemic control with insulin pump therapy are those who monitor their capillary blood glucose concentration at least four times daily.

2. Target levels of blood glucose should be selected with care to reduce the risk of hypoglycemia. Pump therapy per se does not increase the frequency of serious hypoglycemia, but attempts to achieve blood glucose values within the normal range substantially increase the risk of serious hypoglycemia—a danger in patients who are unaware of their hypoglycemic states.

3. Care of the skin at infusion sites must be meticulous. Patients with a history of recurrent staphylococcal skin infections and those who are nasal carriers may be at higher risk.

4. Plugging of infusion sets and leaks in infusion-set connections are common. These problems can be identified with self-monitoring of blood glucose and corrected with adjustment of the infusion system, but ketoacidosis may occur if interruption of insulin delivery is not detected. An insulin syringe and vial should be kept for backup.

5. Insulin pump therapy demands more time, effort, and money than treatment with conventional injections. Many people develop a sense of well-being while using a pump, but those with a history of emotional problems or stress may not be able to cope with the increased demands of intensive insulin therapy.

Initiating Pump Therapy in Type I Diabetes Patients

Before using the pump, the patient should practice loading and programming the unit and changing infusion sets. The best sites are usually far from bony prominences and belt lines. The infusion set is secured with an occlusive dressing or paper tape and is generally changed every two to three days to prevent infection.

Pump therapy is often initiated during a two- to three-day hospital stay. In general, blood glucose targets are 80 to 140 mg/dl (4.4 to 7.8 mmol/L) for the average of values taken before each meal and at bedtime. Target averages for pregnant patients are usually somewhat lower, generally not exceeding 100 mg/dl (5.5 mmol/L). Targets for patients who have been unaware of their hypoglycemia or who have a history of recurrent severe hypoglycemia should be higher, at least at the beginning of infusion pump therapy.

If pump therapy is started outside the hospital, a friend or relative should be available to assist in the event of serious hypoglycemia. The patient should be instructed not to undertake unusual activity for several days, until approximate insulin doses have been established.

The initial programming of insulin dosages is based on the total daily prepump dosages, as follows:

1. The basal rate is initially set at 50 percent of the total prepump dosage. Breakfast, lunch, dinner, and bedtime boluses are initially written as 16, 12, 16, and 6 percent, respectively, of the total prepump insulin dosage. Capillary blood glucose concentrations are checked before each meal and at bedtime, and basal and bolus doses are altered by 10 to 20 percent every one to two days to move toward target values.

2. The basal rate is adjusted to achieve the target fasting blood glucose level, with mealtime boluses adjusted to achieve similar values before the next meal. Peak blood glucose elevations between meals can be blunted by giving the premeal bolus 30 to 45 minutes before eating.

3. A prebreakfast increase in blood glucose may require a preprogrammed basal rate step-up in the early morning, but multiple complex changes in basal rate throughout the day are usually not necessary. In general, the proportion of insulin delivered over 24 hours should begin at approximately 50 percent of the total for the basal and bolus modes, allowing for flexibility in delivering bolus doses. Increases in basal rate and bolus doses are usually required if hyperglycemia occurs during intercurrent illness.

Benefits

Approximately 90 percent of patients changing from two conventional injections daily to insulin pump therapy achieve improved glycemic control. Fifty percent of patients using pumps achieve at least temporary normalization of glycosylated hemoglobin concentration, and 15 percent are able to maintain normal yearly averages of glycosylated hemoglobin for at least three years.[16] Most patients appreciate the greater flexibility of intensive insulin therapy, which matches insulin administration to variations in diet and exercise.

Complications

Insulin therapy is not without complications. In approximately 30 percent of patients, infections develop at infusion sites, usually caused by coagulase-positive *S. aureus*. Cellulitis is often responsive to dicloxacillin (250 mg orally four times daily for one week). Abscesses should be incised and drained promptly. Ketoacidosis is the second most common acute complication of pump therapy, occurring in 15 percent of patients using pumps in one large series. Capillary blood glucose levels should be measured four times daily. If the patient's blood glucose level exceeds 240 mg/dl (13.3 mmol/L), the infusion set should be checked. If the blood glucose level remains elevated after one to two hours, the infusion set should be changed. The infusion set should also be changed if the patient becomes ill unexpectedly and the blood glucose level exceeds 240 mg/dl (13.3 mmol/L).[17] Finally, CSII therapy, like any other intensive insulin regimen, may be associated with an increased incidence of hypoglycemic reactions.

Although insulin pumps more closely approximate the physiologic secretion of insulin than other methods of insulin administration do, they have some of the drawbacks of conventional regimens. The appearance of insulin in the circulation is not regulated by the plasma glucose concentration, and absorption from subcutaneous injection sites is variable and unpredictable. These shortcomings limit the efficacy and safety of pump therapy when attempts are made to approach a normal metabolic state.

PANCREAS AND ISLET TRANSPLANTATION

The DCCT sponsored by the National Institutes of Health established that more intensive insulin therapy reduces the risk of multiorgan microvascular and macrovascular complications.[15] This reduced risk is accompanied, however, by a threefold increase in serious hypoglycemic episodes that necessitate the intervention of another person. In addition, the treatment goal of normal glycosylated hemoglobin levels has not been achieved, which suggests that alternatives to intensive insulin therapy would be beneficial if normoglycemia could be achieved without these risks.

Pancreas transplantation clearly achieves normoglycemia and normal glycosylated hemoglobin levels, with a 75 percent rate of one-year graft function (comparable to the success achieved with kidney or liver transplantation).[18] This approach, unfortunately, necessitates lifelong immunosuppression, with engraftment only in patients with end-stage complications. Thus, although pancreas transplantation provides normoglycemia in patients requiring immunosuppression, it is not an option for most diabetic patients.

Islet transplantation has recently advanced from a technique used in laboratory animals to one that has achieved insulin independence in a few patients.[19] Although islet transplantation offers normoglycemia to a few recipients, its use, like that of pancreas transplantation, is limited to immunosuppressed individuals. This cellular transplant, however, has the potential of being protected from the immune system by means of immunoisolation (e.g., encapsulated islets) or the development of tolerance. Additional study will be required before islet transplantation can be offered to more patients with diabetes.

References

1. Root HF: Preoperative medical care of the diabetic patient. Postgrad Med 40:439, 1966

2. Galloway JA, Shuman CR: Diabetes and surgery: a study of 667 cases. Am J Med 34:177, 1963

3. Alberti KGMM, Marshall SM: Diabetes and surgery. Diabetes Annual/4. Alberti KGMM, Krall LP, Eds. Elsevier Science Publishers, Amsterdam, 1988, p 248

4. Clements RS Jr: Diabetic neuropathy—new concepts of its etiology. Diabetes 28:604, 1979

5. Fraser DM, Campbell IW, Ewing DJ, et al: Peripheral and autonomic nerve function in newly diagnosed diabetes mellitus. Diabetes 26:546, 1977

6. Aiello LM, Cavallerano JD: Ocular complications. Therapy for Diabetes Mellitus and Related Disorders. Lebovitz HE, Ed. American Diabetes Association, Alexandria, Virginia, 1991, p 226

7. Bolognia JL, Braverman IM: Skin and subcutaneous tissues. Therapy for Diabetes Mellitus and Related Disorders. Lebovitz HE, Ed. American Diabetes Association, Alexandria, Virginia, 1991, p 204

8. Page MM, Watkins PJ: Cardiorespiratory arrest and diabetic autonomic neuropathy. Lancet 1:14, 1978

9. Ewing DJ, Campbell IW, Clarke BF: Mortality in diabetic autonomic neuropathy. Lancet 1:601, 1976

10. Alberti KG, Thomas DJ: The management of diabetes during surgery. Br J Anaesth 51:693, 1979

11. Walts LF, Miller J, Davidson MB, et al: Perioperative management of diabetes mellitus. Anesthesiology 55:104, 1981

12. Thompson J, Husband DJ, Thai AC, et al: Metabolic changes in the non–insulin-dependent diabetic undergoing minor surgery: effect of glucose-insulin-potassium infusion. Br J Surg 73:301, 1986

13. Bennett WM: Drug-induced renal dysfunction. Therapy for Diabetes Mellitus and Related Disorders. Lebovitz HE, Ed. American Diabetes Association, Alexandria, Virginia, 1991, p 241

14. Alberti KG: Preventing insulin dependent diabetes mellitus (editorial). BMJ 307:1435, 1993

15. The effect of intensive treatment of diabetes on the development and progression of long-term complications in insulin-dependent diabetes mellitus. Diabetes Control and Complications Trial Research Group. N Engl J Med 329:977, 1993

16. Skyler JS: Insulin treatment. Therapy for Diabetes Mellitus and Related Disorders. Lebovitz HE, Ed. American Diabetes Association, Alexandria, Virginia, 1991, p 127

17. Mecklenburg RS, Benson EA, Benson JW Jr, et al: Acute complications associated with insulin infusion pump therapy: report of experience with 161 patients. JAMA 252:3265, 1984

18. Sutherland DER, Gruessner A, Moudry-Munns K: Analysis of United Network for Organ Sharing (UNOS) United States of America (USA) Pancreas Transplant Registry data according to multiple variables. Clinical Transplants 1992. Terasaki PI, Cecka JM, Eds. UCLA Tissue Typing Laboratory, Los Angeles, 1992, p 45

19. Hering BJ, Browatzki CC, Schultz A, et al: Clinical islet transplantation—registry report, accomplishments in the past and future research needs. Cell Transplantation 2:269, 1993

20. Surgery: practical guidelines for diabetes management. Clinics in Diabetes 5:49, 1987

4 ADRENAL INSUFFICIENCY

Valerie J. Halpin, M.D., and Jeffrey A. Norton, M.D.

Recognition and Management of Adrenal Insufficiency

Adrenal glucocorticoid or mineralocorticoid insufficiency is a rare clinical problem. It may be the direct result of a primary adrenal lesion (primary adrenal insufficiency), or it may be secondary to an abnormality in the pituitary or the hypothalamus (secondary adrenal insufficiency) (see below). Either primary or secondary adrenal insufficiency may lead to so-called adrenal crisis (acute adrenal insufficiency) perioperatively if the hypothalamus-pituitary-adrenal (HPA) axis is unable to generate an appropriate stress level of cortisol [*see Discussion, below*]. Adrenal crisis is an uncommon occurrence; however, if adrenal insufficiency is left untreated, the consequences may be severe.[1,2] Accordingly, it is essential that surgeons know how to recognize adrenal insufficiency and how to identify those patients who will benefit from perioperative glucocorticoid coverage.

Recognition and Classification

A fundamental issue is how to determine which patients need perioperative adrenal steroid replacement and which do not. Involved in this issue

is the question of whether the insufficiency is primary or secondary [*see Sidebar* Causes of Primary and Secondary Adrenal Insufficiency]. The initial clues should come from the history and the physical examination. Patients who have been receiving prednisone or another steroid preparation [*see Table 1*] for extended periods after organ transplantation or as treatment for systemic diseases such as systemic lupus erythematosus or rheumatoid arthritis are at risk for secondary adrenal cortical insufficiency. Their serum cortisol levels are unlikely to increase in response to surgical stress. Patients who are receiving small doses of prednisone every other day or who have received a short course of high-dose corticosteroid therapy in the recent past are at lesser risk for secondary insufficiency. They may be able to generate an appropriate stress cortisol response during some procedures.

On physical examination, persons with secondary insufficiency may be identified by various clinical features of Cushing's syndrome or hypercortisolism (e.g., hypertension, diabetes, weight gain, truncal obesity, hirsutism, muscle weakness, osteoporosis, striae, buffalo hump, and easy bruising).

Persons with primary adrenal insufficiency or Addison's disease may be identified by their thin, hyperpigmented appearance and by various characteristic complaints (e.g., fatigue, weakness, nausea, abdominal pain, diarrhea, postural dizziness, myalgias, and arthralgias).

It is essential to be alert for any signs of possible adrenal crisis. Patients in acute adrenal crisis present with a constellation of symptoms that may include unexplained hypotension, fever, nausea, vomiting, abdominal pain, weakness, or dizziness. These symptoms are not unique to acute adrenal insufficiency and may resemble those of severe infection. In fact, the clinical picture of adrenal crisis may mimic that of septic shock. Acute blood loss, severe dehydration, significant infection, or any of a number of other stressful conditions may precipitate an adrenal crisis. Patients at risk for acute hypocortisolism include those who have active tuberculosis, those who are actively bleeding, and those who are receiving maintenance glucocorticoid therapy after a recent adrenalectomy for correction of hypercortisolism.

Management

ADRENAL CRISIS

If the diagnosis of adrenal crisis is suspected, hydrocortisone should immediately be given intravenously, and steps should be taken to correct precipitating factors.

First, blood is drawn and sent for measurement of serum levels of cortisol, glucose, sodium, potassium, blood urea nitrogen (BUN), and creatinine. A complete blood count is obtained. Treatment then proceeds before the laboratory results come in. A 200 mg bolus of hydrocortisone is rapidly administered intravenously, followed by infusion of glucose and saline to correct dehydration and maintain volume. If the patient has acute adrenal insufficiency, there should be a rapid response to I.V. hydrocortisone: blood pressure should return to normal within one to two hours. If there is no response to the hydrocortisone bolus, adrenal crisis is unlikely. Steroid therapy is discontinued, and a search for another cause of the clinical condition is initiated.

If the patient is improving clinically and the results of the

Recognition and Management of Adrenal Insufficiency

History or physical examination is suggestive of adrenal insufficiency

Clues include a history of steroid use; clinical features of Cushing's syndrome or hypercortisolism (hypertension, diabetes, weight gain, truncal obesity, hirsutism, muscle weakness, osteoporosis, striae, buffalo hump, easy bruising); a thin, pigmented appearance; and various characteristic complaints (fatigue, weakness, nausea, abdominal pain, diarrhea, postural dizziness, myalgia, arthralgia).

Be particularly alert for signs or symptoms of acute adrenal insufficiency (adrenal crisis): unexplained hypotension, fever, nausea, vomiting, abdominal pain, weakness, dizziness.

Attempt to determine whether insufficiency is primary (caused by damage to adrenal) or secondary (caused by inadequate adrenal stimulation) [*see Sidebar* Causes of Primary and Secondary Adrenal Insufficiency].

Patient exhibits signs or symptoms of adrenal crisis

Patient has known or suspected adrenal insufficiency

Treat immediately

Draw blood for measurement of serum cortisol, glucose, Na$^+$, K$^+$, BUN, and creatinine. Obtain CBC. *Do not wait for lab results to return.*

Give 200 mg bolus of hydrocortisone I.V., followed by glucose and saline infusion.

Patient has primary adrenal insufficiency or secondary insufficiency from long-term steroid therapy

---

Serum cortisol < 20 μg/dl with < 7 μg/dl increase over baseline

HPA axis function is abnormal. Steroid supplementation is necessary.

Patient does not respond to hydrocortisone

Discontinue steroids.

Search for another cause of clinical condition.

Patient responds to hydrocortisone, and lab results support diagnosis

Continue hydrocortisone, first at 100 mg q. 8 hr for 2 days, then 50 mg q. 8 hr for 2 days, then 25 mg q. 8 hr for 2 days, and finally 15 mg/m^2/day.

If patient has primary insufficiency, give fludrocortisone, 0.1–0.2 mg/day, when hydrocortisone dosage < 50 mg/day.

When patient stabilizes, perform ACTH test to confirm diagnosis.

Determine cause of adrenal crisis.

Determine amount of steroid coverage needed according to magnitude of surgical procedure

---

Major procedure

Give hydrocortisone, 100–150 mg I.V., before operation.

Continue hydrocortisone, first at 50 mg I.V. q. 8 hr for 2 days, then 25 mg I.V. q. 8 hr for 3 days.

If there are no complications, resume usual steroid dosage.

Procedure of moderate magnitude

Give hydrocortisone, 50–75 mg I.V., before operation.

Give an additional 50–75 mg over remainder of operative day.

Give 50–75 mg on postoperative day 1.

Resume usual steroid dosage on postoperative day 2.

Minor procedure

Give hydrocortisone, 25 mg I.V., before operation.

Give usual daily dose on operative day.

Resume usual steroid dosage on postoperative day 1.

Patient once took steroids but no longer does or else is taking low doses every other day

Perform ACTH stimulation test.

Serum cortisol > 20 μg/dl with > 7 μg/dl increase over baseline

HPA axis function is normal. No steroid supplementation is necessary.

Patient is undergoing surgical correction of endogenous hypercortisolism

Glucocorticoid replacement is always necessary. Do *not* give steroids preoperatively.

Give hydrocortisone, 100 mg I.V., intraoperatively once tumor or second adrenal is removed.

Initiate replacement therapy, first at 50 mg I.V. q. 8 hr for 2 days, then 25 mg I.V. q. 8 hr for 3 days, and finally 12–15 mg/m^2/day.

Patient underwent unilateral adrenalectomy

Replacement therapy continues until HPA axis function returns.

Perform ACTH stimulation test 6 mo after procedure and every 3–6 mo thereafter to determine when steroids can be discontinued.

Patient underwent bilateral adrenalectomy

Replacement therapy continues on permanent basis.

When hydrocortisone dosage < 50 mg/day, give fludrocortisone, 0.1 mg/day.

Causes of Primary and Secondary Adrenal Insufficiency

Primary Insufficiency

In primary adrenal insufficiency, the adrenal cortex is incapable of producing sufficient amounts of adrenal hormones, usually because of a disease process that destroys the adrenal gland. Secretion of both glucocorticoids and mineralocorticoids is deficient. Although primary adrenal insufficiency is rare, its etiology is varied. In the industrialized world, autoimmune disease is the most common cause. There are two associated autoimmune polyendocrine syndromes, type 1 and type 2. Type 1 includes adrenal insufficiency, hypoparathyroidism, mucocutaneous candidiasis, and, less commonly, hypogonadism, pernicious anemia, chronic active hepatitis, and alopecia. Type 2 is associated with autoimmune thyroid disease, diabetes mellitus, and adrenal insufficiency.

Worldwide, tuberculosis remains the most prominent cause of hypocortisolism. Other granulomatous diseases, such as sarcoidosis and some fungal infections, may exhibit a similar clinical picture. Primary adrenal insufficiency may occur in association with adrenal hemorrhage; it is usually attributable to anticoagulation or severe infection but may also be seen after trauma or severe hypertension. Adrenal metastases from a primary lesion elsewhere are not unusual, but metastases rarely cause inadequate adrenocortical function. The cancers most often associated with adrenal metastases are breast cancer, lung cancer, stomach cancer, colon cancer, melanoma, and lymphoma.

Other possible causes of primary adrenal insufficiency are congenital disorders, the acquired immunodeficiency syndrome (AIDS), and the demyelinating syndromes, including adrenoleukodystrophy and adrenomyeloneuropathy.

Secondary Insufficiency

In secondary adrenal insufficiency, hypocortisolism is caused by inadequate stimulation of the adrenal gland. Mineralocorticoid production is normal because aldosterone secretion is regulated via the renin-angiotensin system, independently of pituitary adrenocorticotropic hormone (ACTH) secretion. The etiology of secondary adrenal insufficiency has three main components: adrenal suppression after the administration of exogenous glucocorticoid or ACTH, adrenal suppression after the surgical correction of endogenous hypercortisolism, and ACTH insufficiency resulting from abnormalities of the hypothalamus or the pituitary gland.

The most common specific cause of secondary adrenal insufficiency is long-term prescription of exogenous glucocorticoids to treat other diseases. Any patient receiving glucocorticoids on a daily basis just before operation is clearly at risk for adrenal insufficiency. Furthermore, any patient who has taken the equivalent of 20 to 30 mg/day of prednisone [see Table 1] for longer than five consecutive days in the previous 12 months is at risk.[18] It is difficult to know in advance which patients will experience hypothalamus-pituitary-adrenal (HPA) axis suppression: neither the glucocorticoid dosage nor the duration of therapy is predictive of the eventual degree of adrenal suppression.[8] Because patients may not think to mention steroid therapy that started and stopped several months ago, the surgeon must make a point of inquiring about steroid use if the patient has a medical problem that is commonly treated with glucocorticoids (e.g., asthma, rheumatoid arthritis, autoimmune diseases, collagen vascular diseases, or immunosuppression in transplant recipients).

Pituitary failure can also lead to secondary adrenal insufficiency, but it is a much less common cause. In patients who have undergone transsphenoidal surgery, decreased production of ACTH may occur and may result in secondary adrenal insufficiency.

---

initial laboratory evaluation support the diagnosis, glucocorticoid replacement is continued. (Laboratory findings consistent with the diagnosis of acute adrenal crisis include a serum cortisol level lower than 20 µg/dl, hyponatremia, hyperkalemia, hypoglycemia, and azotemia. The complete blood count may show anemia, leukopenia, lymphocytosis, and eosinophilia.) After the initial bolus of hydrocortisone, hydrocortisone is given intravenously at a dosage of 100 mg every eight hours for two days. The hydrocortisone dosage is reduced by half every two days, first to 50 mg I.V. every eight hours and then to 25 mg I.V. every eight hours. Finally, a replacement regimen is initiated at a dosage of 15 mg/m²/day. Patients with primary adrenal insufficiency require mineralocorticoid replacement (fludrocortisone, 0.1 to 0.2 mg/day) when the hydrocortisone dosage is less than 50 mg/day.

Once the patient's condition is stable, the diagnosis of adrenal crisis is confirmed by means of an adrenocorticotropic hormone (ACTH) stimulation test [see Table 2]. Finally, the cause of the adrenal crisis is determined.

KNOWN OR SUSPECTED
ADRENAL INSUFFICIENCY

Patients known to have primary adrenal insufficiency or chronic secondary adrenal insufficiency caused by long-term glucocorticoid treatment for another disease process must receive glucocorticoid

treatment during surgical procedures. On the other hand, patients who had previously been treated with glucocorticoids but are no longer taking them and patients who are currently receiving glucocorticoids in low doses every other day may in fact be able to generate an appropriate stress cortisol response during operation and consequently may not need perioperative

Table 1 Selected Corticosteroid Preparations

Preparation	Equivalent Doses (mg)	Glucocorticoid Activity*	Mineralocorticoid Activity*
Short-acting (8–12 hr)			
Hydrocortisone	20	1	1
Cortisone	25	0.80	0.80
Intermediate-acting (12–36 hr)			
Prednisone	5	4	0.80
Prednisolone	5	4	0.80
Methylprednisolone	4	5	0
Triamcinolone	4	5	0
Long-acting (36–54 hr)			
Betamethasone	0.60	25	0
Dexamethasone	0.75	30	0
Mineralocorticoid			
Fludrocortisone	—	10	125

*Ranked on a scale rating hydrocortisone as 1.

Table 2 ACTH Stimulation Test

1. Measure baseline serum cortisol level
2. Give 250 µg of ACTH by I.V. bolus or I.M. injection
3. Draw blood, and measure serum cortisol level 30 and 60 min after administration of ACTH
4. Interpret results:
   - If serum cortisol level > 20 µg/dl and an increase > 7 µg/dl is noted after ACTH administration, HPA axis function is normal
   - If serum cortisol level < 20 µg/dl and an increase > 7 µg/dl is noted after ACTH administration, HPA axis function is abnormal

ADRENAL INSUFFICIENCY AFTER SURGICAL CORRECTION OF ENDOGENOUS HYPERCORTISOLISM

Cushing's syndrome is a hypercortisolemic state that results either from overproduction of cortisol by an adrenocortical adenoma or carcinoma or from overproduction of ACTH by a pituitary tumor or another ACTH-producing tumor. The hypercortisolemia causes suppression of the HPA axis in much the same way that long-term steroid use does, via suppression of the hypothalamus or the pituitary gland [see Figure 1]. Adrenal insufficiency is manifested after surgical removal of the tumor.

All patients undergoing surgical treatment of endogenous

glucocorticoid replacement. If enough time is available before an elective surgical procedure, an ACTH stimulation test can be performed to ascertain whether the stress response is abnormal and thus whether glucocorticoid replacement is called for. If the ACTH stimulation test yields normal results, then HPA axis function is adequate and there is no need for any perioperative steroid coverage.

If, however, the ACTH test yields abnormal results or the patient is known to have chronic adrenal insufficiency, the amount of cortisol coverage required must be assessed. This assessment is made on the basis of the magnitude of the surgical procedure (i.e., major, moderate, or minor). The stress response to surgery ranges from minimal elevation of the cortisol level after minor procedures to a total cortisol production of 200 mg/day after major procedures.[3-5] Perioperative steroid coverage should approximate the expected stress cortisol response but need not exceed it.[6] If the patient's maintenance glucocorticoid dosage equals or exceeds the expected stress cortisol production, he or she may receive the maintenance dosage equivalent of cortisol preoperatively, with no additional supplementation. Preferably, cortisol should be administered intravenously in an easily hydrolyzable form (e.g., hydrocortisone hemisuccinate or hydrocortisone phosphate).

Coverage for major, moderate, and minor procedures is provided as follows. Patients undergoing major surgical procedures (e.g., the Whipple procedure, esophagogastrectomy, coronary artery bypass grafting, and thoracotomy) should receive 100 to 150 mg of hydrocortisone intravenously before operation. Hydrocortisone coverage is continued at a dosage of 50 mg I.V. every eight hours for two days. The dosage is then reduced to 25 mg I.V. every eight hours for an additional three days. After this period, the usual dosage may be resumed, provided that there are no complications. Patients undergoing surgical procedures of moderate magnitude (e.g., cholecystectomy, appendectomy, joint replacement, colectomy, and hysterectomy) should receive hydrocortisone, 50 to 75 mg I.V., before operation and then an additional 50 to 75 mg I.V. over the remainder of the day of the operation. Another 50 to 75 mg I.V. is given on postoperative day 1, and the usual steroid dosage may be resumed on postoperative day 2. Patients undergoing procedures done under local anesthesia (e.g., herniorrhaphy and dental procedures) should receive hydrocortisone, 25 mg I.V. (or the equivalent), preoperatively on the day of the procedure; the usual dosage may be resumed on postoperative day 1.

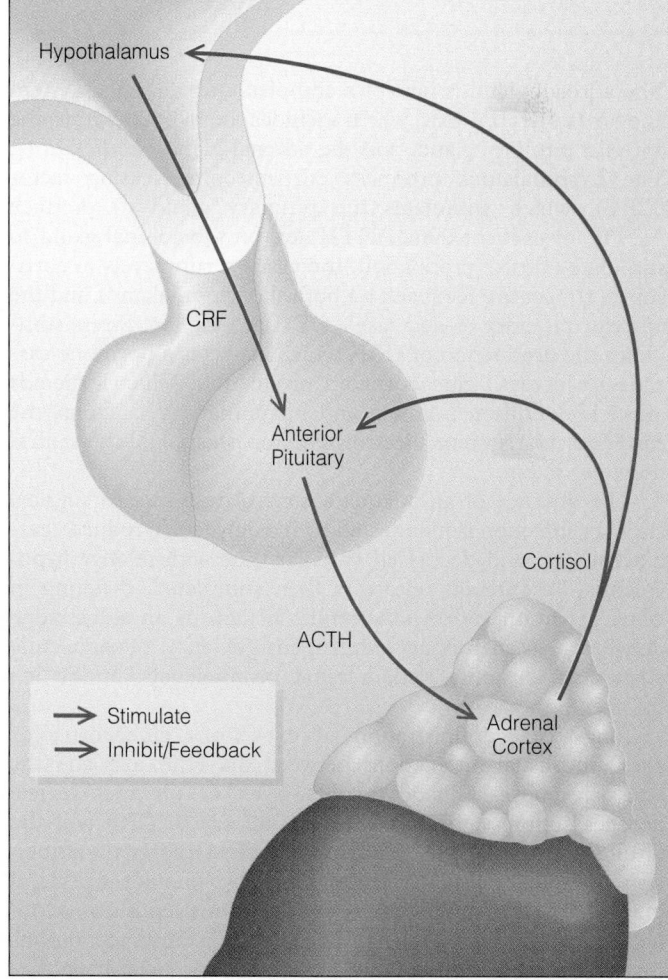

Figure 1 Shown is a schematic representation of the hypothalamus-pituitary-adrenal (HPA) axis. The hypothalamus produces corticotropin-releasing factor (CRF), which stimulates the pituitary to release adrenocorticotropic hormone (ACTH), or corticotropin. ACTH acts on the adrenal, stimulating production of cortisol. When serum levels of cortisol rise, negative feedback prompts the pituitary and the hypothalamus to decrease ACTH production.

hypercortisolism require glucocorticoid replacement. Corticosteroids are not administered preoperatively, because these patients are already hypercortisolemic. Instead, hydrocortisone, 100 mg I.V., is given intraoperatively once the cortisol- or ACTH-producing tumor—or, in patients with primary adrenocortical hyperplasia, the second adrenal gland—has been removed. Administration of hydrocortisone is continued at a dosage of 50 mg I.V. every eight hours for two days and then at a dosage of 25 mg I.V. every eight hours for an additional three days. The final replacement dosage is 12 to 15 mg/m²/day. This dosage may be adjusted as necessary to prevent symptoms and signs of adrenal insufficiency. All patients should be advised to wear a medical identification bracelet notifying health care workers that adrenal insufficiency may result from any condition that evokes the stress response.

In patients who have undergone unilateral adrenalectomy for hypercortisolemia, replacement therapy continues until the hypothalamus-adrenal-pituitary axis recovers. To assess the status of the hypothalamus-adrenal-pituitary axis, an ACTH stimulation test is performed six months after operation and again every three to six months thereafter until the cortisol response returns to normal (> 20 μg/dl and a > 7 μg/dl increment over baseline levels). Once the response is normal, the daily replacement dosage of steroids can be rapidly tapered and eventually discontinued.[7] In patients who have undergone bilateral adrenalectomy, replacement hydrocortisone therapy continues indefinitely. Mineralocorticoid replacement is also required when the hydrocortisone dosage is less than 50 mg/day; the standard starting regimen is fludrocortisone acetate, 0.1 mg/day orally. Normal serum sodium and potassium levels, normal blood pressure, and the absence of postural hypotension indicate that replacement therapy is efficacious. Again, patients should be advised to wear a medical identification bracelet.

Discussion

The adrenal gland is part of a complex interglandular system known as the HPA axis, which includes the hypothalamus, the anterior pituitary gland, and the adrenal gland [see Figure 1]. The hypothalamus produces corticotropin-releasing factor (CRF), which stimulates the pituitary gland to produce ACTH, or corticotropin. ACTH acts on the adrenal gland to stimulate cortisol production. Increased serum levels of cortisol exert negative feedback on both the hypothalamus and the anterior pituitary to decrease ACTH production. Stress stimulates the production of CRF, which activates a hormone cascade to increase glucocorticoid production. Glucocorticoids affect metabolism, immune and inflammatory reactions, the cardiovascular system, electrolyte homeostasis, and the central nervous system.

The absence of an adequate cortisol response to surgical stress or infection is manifested by hypoglycemia, reduced cardiac output, and decreased vascular tone with relative hypovolemia. Vasopressin release is then stimulated, resulting in water retention and hyponatremia. If there is an aldosterone deficiency, as in primary adrenal insufficiency, hyperkalemia ensues. If left untreated, adrenal insufficiency can be life threatening.

Long-term administration of exogenous glucocorticoids alters the usual interactions between the HPA axis and the stress response. Glucocorticoids given at pharmacological dosages suppress the hypothalamic release of CRF and the pituitary release of ACTH. The inadequate adrenal stimulation that results leads to adrenal atrophy. The adrenal gland may be able to maintain adequate daily function but may not be able to produce sufficient glucocorticoids during conditions that evoke a maximal stress response, such as general anesthesia and major surgical procedures. The HPA axis may recover if the glucocorticoid dosage is reduced to maintenance levels or if glucocorticoids are given in low doses every other day; however, neither low dosages, shortened duration of therapy, nor an every-other-day regimen guarantees recovery of the normal glucocorticoid stress response.[8] HPA axis testing, specifically the ACTH stimulation test [see Table 2], must be done unless stress doses of glucocorticoids are administered.

Endogenous hypercortisolism, or Cushing's syndrome, affects the hypothalamus and pituitary in much the same way as long-term administration of exogenous glucocorticoids. The HPA axis is suppressed immediately after operation and in the postoperative period. In patients receiving maintenance glucocorticoid therapy (hydrocortisone, 12 to 15 mg/m²/day), the time to recovery of HPA axis function ranges from nine months to two years.[7] Assessment of the HPA axis by means of ACTH testing should begin six months after operation and should be repeated every three to six months thereafter until normal function has been regained. Once adrenal function has returned to normal, as defined by a normal ACTH stimulation test result, maintenance hydrocortisone therapy can be discontinued. Thus, the ACTH stimulation test can be used as a guide to the optimal duration of postoperative glucocorticoid replacement after the resection of a cortisol-secreting tumor.[7]

There is evidence to suggest that some patients receiving exogenous glucocorticoids may not require perioperative stress-dose glucocorticoid coverage.[9-11] This evidence derives from studies in which patients underwent surgery without any glucocorticoid coverage and experienced no untoward effects; however, because the incidence of adrenal insufficiency is so low, the effect of steroid coverage could not be defined with certainty on the basis of the relatively small numbers of patients included in these studies. In one animal study, subphysiologic levels of cortisol replacement had detrimental effects on clinical outcome (including increased mortality) after cholecystectomy in adrenalectomized primates.[2] Given the impossibility of predicting the degree of HPA suppression and the adequacy of the patient's cortisol response to surgical or anesthetic stress, one cannot assume that the patient will be able to generate the necessary physiologic levels of cortisol. Therefore, either HPA axis function must be assessed via an ACTH stimulation test or steroids must be administered perioperatively in amounts approximately equivalent to the expected stress glucocorticoid response.[12]

Some investigators have suggested that elements of the surgical stress response may actually be detrimental to the patient.[13] The production of neuroendocrine hormones (including cortisol) and the local release of cytokines increase metabolism, heart rate, and coagulability and alter immune function. As a consequence, the stress response may increase cardiac and vascular morbidity and foster postoperative immunosuppression and infection. A few studies have examined the results of modifying the biochemical parameters of the stress response.[14-17] It has been clearly demonstrated that the cortisol response is modified—and, in some cases, completely abolished—by epidural anesthesia. Studies comparing stress response and postoperative morbidity in patients undergoing general anesthesia with those in patients undergoing epidural anesthesia suggest that epidural anesthesia has a beneficial effect.[17] At present, the data are insufficient to establish a clear relation between reduction of the stress response and reduction of cardiac and vascular morbidity. More work is necessary to elucidate which components of the stress response are beneficial and which are not. The results of such work may have a significant bearing on the necessity of perioperative cortisol replacement. Until the effects of the surgical stress response can be further defined, perioperative steroid coverage must be continued. Studies have also shown, however, that the glucocorticoid dosage can be significantly reduced when the surgical procedure is one that evokes a relatively minor stress response.[6]

References

1. Kehlet H: Clinical course and hypothalamic-pituitary-adrenocortical function in glucocorticoid-treated surgical patients. FADL's Forlag, Copenhagen, 1976

2. Udelsman R, Ramp J, Gallucci WT, et al: Adaptation during surgical stress—a reevaluation of the role of glucocorticoids. J Clin Invest 44:539, 1986

3. Udelsman R, Norton J, Jelenich SE, et al: Responses of the hypothalamic-pituitary-adrenal and renin-angiotensin axis and the sympathetic system during controlled surgical and anesthetic stress. J Clin Endocrinol Metab 64:986, 1987

4. Peterson RE: The miscible pool and turnover rate of adrenocortical steroids in man. Recent Prog Hormone Res 15:231, 1959

5. Peterson RE, Nokes G, Chen PS, et al: Estrogens and adrenocortical function in man. J Clin Endocrinol Metab 20:495, 1960

6. Salem M, Tainsh RE Jr, Bromberg J, et al: Perioperative glucocorticoid coverage: a reassessment 42 years after emergence of a problem. Ann Surg 219:416, 1994

7. Doherty G, Nieman LK, Cutler GB Jr, et al: Time to recovery of the hypothalamic-pituitary-adrenal axis after curative resection of adrenal tumors in patients with Cushing's syndrome. Surgery 108:1085, 1990

8. Schlaghecke R, Kornely E, Santen RT, et al: The effect of long-term glucocorticoid therapy on pituitary-adrenal responses to exogenous corticotropin-releasing hormone. N Engl J Med 326:226, 1992

9. Bromberg JS, Alfrey EJ, Barker CF, et al: Adrenal suppression and steroid supplementation in renal transplant recipients. Transplantation 51:385, 1991

10. Roberts C, LaFond J, Fitt CT, et al: New patterns of transplant nephrectomy in the cyclosporine era. J Am Coll Surg 178:59, 1994

11. Friedman RJ, Schiff CF, Bromberg JS: Use of supplemental steroids in patients having orthopaedic operations. J Bone Joint Surg 77A:1801, 1995

12. Kehlet H, Binder C: Value of an ACTH test in assessing hypothalamic-pituitary-adrenocortical function in glucocorticoid-treated patients. Br Med J 2:147, 1973

13. Kehlet H: The surgical stress response: should it be prevented? Can J Surg 34:565, 1991

14. Downing R, Davis I, Black J, et al: Effect of intrathecal morphine on the adrenocortical and hyperglycaemic responses to upper abdominal surgery. Br J Anaesth 58:858, 1986

15. Rittmaster R, Cutler GB Jr, Sobel DO, et al: Morphine inhibits the pituitary-adrenal response to ovine corticotropin-releasing hormone in normal subjects. J Clin Endocrinol Metab 60:891, 1985

16. Enquist A, Brandt MR, Fernandes A, et al: The blocking effect of epidural analgesia on the adrenocortical and hyperglycemic responses to surgery. Acta Anaesth Scand 21:330, 1977

17. Liu S, Carpenter RL, Neal JM: Epidural anesthesia and analgesia, their role in postoperative outcome. Anesthesiology 82:1474, 1995

18. Axelrod L: Glucocorticoid therapy. Medicine (Baltimore) 55:39, 1976

Acknowledgment

Figure 1   Seward Hung.

5 OBESITY

Harvey J. Sugerman, M.D.

Approach to the Morbidly Obese Patient

Many surgeons are afraid to operate on the morbidly obese patient (i.e., a patient whose weight is 100 lb greater than ideal body weight or who has a body mass index [BMI] greater than 35 kg/mg2) because they presuppose a marked increase in perioperative morbidity and mortality. Although the morbidly obese patient is certainly at greater risk, this risk can be markedly reduced by paying careful attention to detail in preoperative and post-

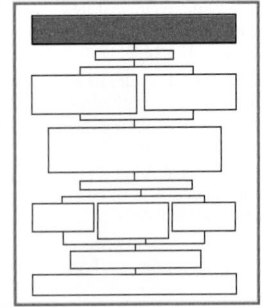

operative care. The increased risks encountered in these patients include wound infection, dehiscence, thrombophlebitis, pulmonary embolism, anesthetic calamities, acute postoperative asphyxia in patients with obstructive sleep apnea syndrome (SAS), acute respiratory failure, right ventricular or biventricular cardiac failure, and missed acute catastrophes of the abdomen, such as an anastomotic leak. In a series of about 2,000 gastric procedures for morbid obesity itself, we have observed the following incidence of complications: wound infection that delayed hospital discharge, 5%, as well as minor infections or seromas in an additional 10%; clinically apparent phlebitis, 0.4%; clinically diagnosed fatal pulmonary embolism, 0.15%; and pneumonia, 0.5%. We reported a 0.4% operative mortality. Although many of these patients had severe preoperative morbidity (respiratory insufficiency, pseudotumor cerebri, or insulin-dependent diabetes), the risks of complication approach the risks associated with major abdominal operation in nonobese patients. In what follows, I focus on issues that the surgeon should carefully consider when operating on an extremely overweight patient.

Cardiac Dysfunction

Morbidly obese patients are at significant risk of coronary artery disease as a result of an increased incidence of systemic hypertension, hypercholesterolemia, and diabetes. Because of this increased risk for cardiac dysfunction, preoperative electrocardiography should be performed on all obese patients 20 years of age or older.

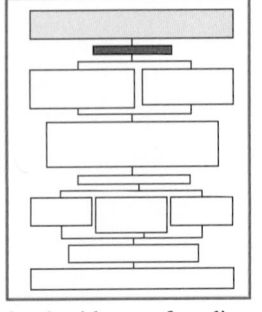

Most morbidly obese patients have minimal evidence of cardiac dysfunction as detected by Swan-Ganz catheterization. Markedly elevated pulmonary arterial pressure (PAP) and pulmonary arterial

wedge pressure (PAWP) values will frequently be noted in patients with the respiratory insufficiency of obesity, especially those with obesity hypoventilation syndrome (OHS) [*see* Respiratory Insufficiency, Obesity Hypoventilation Syndrome, *below*].[1] Intubation and ventilation in these patients will often be followed by a vigorous diuresis, and it is not unusual for a patient to lose 50 lb or more of retained fluid. In a few obese patients, acute respiratory insufficiency will be caused by a greatly expanded central blood volume and heart failure. Abnormal blood gas values in these individuals will be corrected by vigorous diuresis alone. As with most other abnormalities related to morbid obesity, weight loss will also correct cardiac dysfunction.

Respiratory Insufficiency

Morbidly obese patients may suffer from obstructive SAS or OHS. The simultaneous presence of SAS and OHS is known as the pickwickian syndrome [*see* Discussion, Respiratory Insufficiency of Obesity, *below*].[2-4]

SLEEP APNEA SYNDROME

SAS is a potentially fatal complication of morbid obesity. A diagnosis of SAS should be suspected when there is a history of loud snoring, frequent nocturnal awakening with shortness of breath, and daytime somnolence. It is estimated that 2% of middle-aged women and 4% of middle-aged men in the United States workforce have SAS, and the incidence is markedly higher in the severely obese.[5]

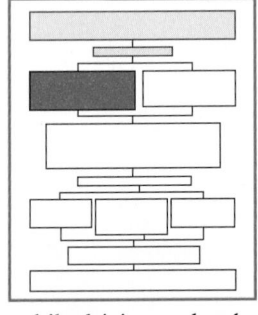

Patients will often admit to falling asleep while driving and waking up with their car on the road's median strip or bumping its guardrail. It is extremely important that trauma surgeons be aware of the relation between obesity and somnolence should a morbidly obese patient be seen in the emergency room after an automobile accident in which he or she fell asleep at the wheel. Elective patients with suspected sleep apnea syndrome should undergo preoperative polysomnography at a sleep center to confirm the diagnosis. Medications are usually ineffective. Stimulants, such as methylphenidate hydrochloride (Ritalin), should not be used. If a patient has more than 25 apneic episodes per hour of sleep or has cardiac arrhythmias in association with apnea, treatment by nocturnal nasal continuous positive airway pressure (nasal CPAP) should be provided. If the patient does not respond with elimina-

Approach to the Morbidly Obese Patient

Patient is morbidly obese (current weight at least 100 lb > ideal body weight, body mass index ≥ 35 kg/m², or both)

Increased risks include
- Missed abdominal catastrophe
- Respiratory failure
- Cardiac failure

- Anesthetic calamities
- Pulmonary embolism
- Internal hernia
- Acute gastric distention

- Wound infection
- Postoperative asphyxia
- Dehiscence
- Thrombophlebitis

↓

Evaluate cardiopulmonary status preoperatively

Patient reports loud snoring, frequent nocturnal awakening, and daytime somnolence, or trauma victim has fallen asleep at the wheel

Suspect sleep apnea syndrome (SAS).

Confirm SAS by polysomnography in elective patients. Provide nocturnal nasal CPAP if apneic episodes are ≥ 25/hr of sleep or are associated with arrhythmias. If patient does not respond to — or does not tolerate — CPAP, perform tracheostomy with extra-long tube.

Patient has heart failure or extreme shortness of breath

Suspect obesity hypoventilation syndrome (OHS).
OHS is confirmed by $P_aO_2 ≤ 55$ mm Hg or $P_aO_2 ≥ 47$ mm Hg
- If PAWP ≥ 18 mm Hg, try I.V. furosemide.
- If PAP ≥ 40 mm Hg, consider insertion of Greenfield vena caval filter.
- If Hb ≥ 16 g/dl, phlebotomize to Hb of 15 g/dl.

Give prophylaxis against thromboembolism, induce anesthesia, and intubate

Administer regular or low-molecular-weight heparin 30 min preoperatively and at appropriate intervals thereafter until the patient is ambulatory.

Use intermittent sequential venous compression boots during anesthesia induction and throughout operation.

Two anesthesia personnel are required for induction and intubation of patients with SAS or OHS (one to hold the mask and one to squeeze the ventilation bag).

Insert oral airway after administration of succinylcholine and sodium pentobarbital. Ventilate with 100% O_2 for several minutes before intubation. If intubation is unsuccessful, reinsert oral airway and ventilate with a mask. Patient should be in reverse Trendelenburg's position.

In the recovery room, keep patient in reverse Trendelenburg's position

Patient does not have respiratory insufficiency of obesity

Extubate in recovery room when patient is fully alert and ventilatory effort is adequate; return patient to room.

Patient has SAS

In the absence of OHS, wean and extubate the day after operation. If patient was on nasal CPAP before operation, reinstitute on second night after operation. Monitor for prolonged apnea or arrhythmia; if either occurs, awaken patient.

Patient has OHS

Continue mechanical ventilation after operation until pain of breathing resolves. Wean to preoperative arterial blood gas levels; several days may be required.

Encourage early postoperative ambulation

Use intermittent sequential venous compression boots until patient is fully ambulatory.

Maintain high index of suspicion for recognition of abdominal catastrophes

Guarding, tenderness, and rigidity may be absent. Signs of infection (fever, tachypnea, tachycardia) may be absent. Acute respiratory failure may be secondary to peritonitis. Radiographic contrast studies and laparotomy may be indicated even when clinical signs are few.

tion of the apneic episodes or cannot tolerate nasal CPAP, a tracheostomy should be performed. An extra-long tracheostomy tube is usually necessary because of the depth of the trachea in the morbidly obese patient.

OBESITY HYPOVENTILATION SYNDROME

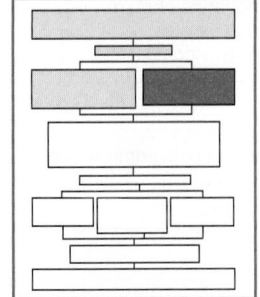

OHS should be suspected in patients who present with heart failure or extreme shortness of breath. Diagnosis is confirmed when the patient's arterial oxygen tension (P_aO_2) is 55 mm Hg or less or the arterial carbon dioxide tension (P_aCO_2) is 47 mm Hg or greater. These patients often have marked elevations in mean PAP, mean PAWP, or both, as well as severe polycythemia. In patients with obesity hypoventilation syndrome, a Swan-Ganz catheter should be inserted as part of the preoperative evaluation. If PAWP is 18 mm Hg or greater, diuresis with intravenous furosemide is indicated. In many of these patients, however, an elevated PAWP is necessary to maintain adequate cardiac output; such patients do not have congestive heart failure, despite a markedly elevated filling pressure [*see* Discussion, *below*]. Little can be done for the pulmonary hypertension that is seen in many of these patients; raising the P_aO_2 above 60 mm Hg usually will not lower PAP acutely.

Polycythemia can significantly increase the incidence of phlebothrombosis. If the hemoglobin (Hb) concentration is 16 g/dl or greater, phlebotomy to a concentration of 15 g/dl should be performed to reduce the postoperative risk of venous thrombosis. If PAP is 40 mm Hg or greater, consideration should be given to prophylactic insertion of a Greenfield vena caval filter because of the high risk of a fatal pulmonary embolism in these patients.[6] Placement of this filter can be a challenge because the appropriate landmarks cannot be identified in the operating room with fluoroscopy. It is necessary before operation to tape a quarter to the patient's back over the second lumbar vertebra with the aid of fixed radiographs and then during operation to aim for the quarter with the insertion catheter, using fluoroscopy. Because these patients are usually too heavy for angiography tables, the Greenfield filter usually cannot be inserted percutaneously in the radiology department.

Embolism

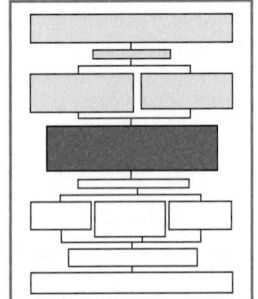

The risk of deep vein thrombosis [*see* *VI:2 Thromboembolic Problems*] increases with a prolonged operation or a postoperative period of immobilization, and it increases even further in the morbidly obese patient. Standard or low-molecular-weight heparin should be administered subcutaneously 30 minutes before operation and at appropriate intervals thereafter (depending on the type of heparin used) for at least 2 days or until the patient is ambulatory. Because respiratory function in the morbidly obese patient is greatly enhanced with the reverse Trendelenburg's position, intermittent sequential venous compression boots should be used to counteract the increased venous stasis and the propensity for clotting. It is important that the intermittent venous compression boots be used before induction of anesthesia and throughout the operative procedure. Compression boots are usually part of a standard preoperative protocol in gastric procedures for weight control; their use should not be unintentionally neglected in preparation for other elective or emergency procedures on morbidly obese patients. As noted (see above), prophylactic insertion of a Greenfield vena caval filter should be considered in OHS patients with a high PAP.

Anesthesia in Patients with Respiratory Insufficiency

Morbidly obese patients can be intimidating to the anesthesiologist because they are at significant risk for complications from anesthesia, especially during induction. The risk is particularly great for obese patients with respiratory insufficiency. An obese patient often has a short, fat neck and a heavy chest wall, which make intubation and ventilation a challenge. If endotracheal intubation proves difficult, however, these patients can usually be well ventilated with a mask. Awake intubation can be performed, with or without fiberoptic aids, but is quite unpleasant and unnecessary.

It is extremely important that at least two anesthesia personnel be present during induction and intubation for patients with respiratory insufficiency of obesity. An oral airway is inserted after muscle paralysis with succinylcholine and sodium pentobarbital induction. One person elevates the jaw, hyperextends the neck, and ensures a tight fit of the mask, using both hands. To ensure adequate oxygen delivery, a second person compresses the ventilation reservoir bag, using two hands because of the resistance to air flow from the poorly compliant, heavy chest wall. After ventilation with 100% oxygen for several minutes, intubation is attempted. If difficulties are encountered within 30 seconds, the steps above should be repeated until the patient has been successfully intubated. A volume ventilator is required during operation. Placing the patient in the reverse Trendelenburg's position expands total lung volume and facilitates ventilation[7]; however, the reverse Trendelenburg's position increases lower extremity venous pressure and therefore mandates the use of intermittent sequential venous compression boots [*see* Embolism, *above*]. It is helpful to monitor blood gases through a radial arterial line or digital pulse oximeter.

Postoperative Management

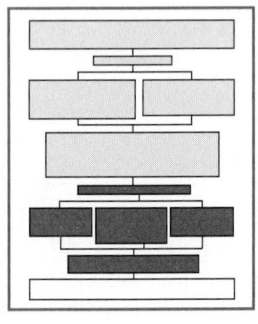

After operation, the obese patient should be kept in the reverse Trendelenburg's position and should not be extubated until he or she is fully alert and showing evidence of adequate ventilatory effort [*see VII:4 Use of the Mechanical Ventilator*]. In the absence of respiratory insufficiency, most obese patients can be extubated in the OR or the recovery room and returned to a standard hospital room.

Patients with SAS, however, should be managed with overnight mechanical ventilation in the ICU. In the absence of concomitant OHS, they can usually be weaned and extubated the day after operation. Patients who were receiving ventilatory support with nasal CPAP before operation should have this treatment reinstituted the second night after operation; monitoring for prolonged apnea should be continued in the ICU or in a stepdown unit with digital oximetry. If apnea occurs, simply waking the patient should correct the problem. Patients who required tracheostomy can also usually be weaned from the ventilator the morning after operation.

Patients with OHS require prolonged mechanical volume ventilation until the pain of breathing resolves. One cannot expect such patients to manifest normal arterial blood gas levels, and they should be weaned to their preoperative values. This weaning process may require several days. It is important that these patients remain in the reverse Trendelenburg's position to maximize diaphragmatic excursion. Positive end-expiratory pressure (PEEP) ventilation may be detrimental in patients with OHS because it can overdistend alveoli, thereby leading to capillary compression, decreased cardiac output, and increased dead space, all of which can exacerbate retention of carbon dioxide.

Swan-Ganz catheters, inserted preoperatively in patients with severe OHS, are useful in monitoring postoperative intravascular volume and oxygen delivery status. Excessive diuresis or restriction of fluids should be avoided [*see* Discussion, *below*].

It is extremely important to encourage early postoperative ambulation for the morbidly obese patient. These patients have surprisingly little pain, and it is not unusual to see them walking in the afternoon or early evening after a major abdominal procedure. If the patients have been advised preoperatively of the merits of early postoperative ambulation and know it is for their own welfare, they are usually willing to cooperate.

Complications of Gastric Surgery for Obesity

Current gastric procedures for obesity include gastric bypass (GBP) and gastroplasty, in which the stomach is stapled so as to create small and large pouches connected via a small stoma. The procedures themselves are described in more detail elsewhere [*see V:10 Gastric Procedures for Morbid Obesity*]; the following are some of the main complications associated with any abdominal operation in a severely obese patient.

ABDOMINAL CATASTROPHE

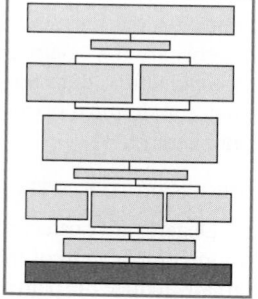

It may be very difficult to recognize an abdominal catastrophe in patients who are very young, very old, or morbidly obese or who are receiving high doses of steroids. The obese patient, for example, may present in the emergency room with a perforated duodenal ulcer or a ruptured diverticulum, complaining of abdominal pain, and yet on abdominal examination have no evidence of peritoneal irritation (no guarding, tenderness, or rigidity). This situation has been well documented in patients in whom an anastomotic or gastric leak has developed after operation for morbid obesity.[8] Symptoms include shoulder pain, pelvic or scrotal pain, back pain, tenesmus, urinary frequency, and, of great importance, marked anxiety. Signs of infection (e.g., fever, tachypnea, and tachycardia) may be absent. Patients with peritonitis often have clinical symptoms and signs suggesting a massive pulmonary embolus: severe tachypnea, tachycardia, and sudden hypotension. Such acute pulmonary failure is probably secondary to sepsis-induced acute respiratory distress syndrome (ARDS). Thus, peritonitis must be suspected in any morbidly obese patient with acute respiratory failure.

Because a high index of suspicion of peritonitis is required to detect the condition in morbidly obese patients, radiographic contrast studies with water-soluble agents such as diatrizoate meglumine (Gastrografin) may be indicated even when there are few clinical signs. If a perforated viscus is suspected, an exploratory laparotomy may be necessary despite normal findings on radiographic contrast study.

INTERNAL HERNIA

GBP places patients at risk for internal hernia with a closed-loop obstruction, leading to bowel strangulation. There are three potential locations for these internal hernias: the Roux-en-Y anastomosis; the opening in the transverse mesocolon through which the retrocolic Roux limb is brought; and the Petersen hernia, which is located behind the retrocolic Roux limb. The primary symptom of an internal hernia is periumbilical pain, usually in the form of cramping consistent with visceral colic. These internal hernias may be very difficult to diagnose. An upper gastrointestinal radiographic series is often normal, providing a false sense of security. The resulting assumption that no problem exists may be devastating for the patient should bowel infarction occur as a consequence of closed-loop obstruction. One should always carefully inspect the plain abdominal radiograph for the abnormal placement or spreading of the Roux-en-Y anastomotic staples. The safest course of action in patients with recurrent attacks of periumbilical pain is abdominal surgical exploration.

ACUTE GASTRIC DISTENTION

After GBP, massive gaseous distention occasionally develops in the distal bypassed stomach; this can lead to a gastric perforation or disruption of the gastrojejunostomy. The primary symptoms of this complication are hiccups and a bloated feeling. Massive gastric dilatation can lead to severe left shoulder pain and shock. The problem is usually secondary to edema at the Roux-en-Y anastomosis but can also be secondary to a mechanical problem. The diagnosis is made by means of an urgent upright abdominal radiograph, which reveals the markedly dilated and air-filled bypassed stomach. Occasionally, the stomach is filled with fluid, and the diagnosis may be more difficult. In those few cases in which the dilatation is primarily caused by air, the problem can be relieved by percutaneous transabdominal skinny-needle decompression with subsequent passage of gas and gastric and biliopancreatic juices through the Roux-en-Y anastomosis. Should the dilatation recur or the patient be in serious difficulty, an emergency laparotomy with insertion of a gastrostomy tube should be performed and the jejunojejunostomy evaluated. If a patient has extensive adhesions from previous abdominal surgery, a gastrostomy tube should be inserted at the time of GBP to prevent gastric dilatation.

Diabetes Mellitus

Type 2 (non–insulin-dependent) diabetes mellitus, a nonketotic form of diabetes that is usually noted after age 40, is markedly exacerbated by obesity. Patients with this type of diabetes often require large amounts of insulin for blood glucose control because of a significant reduction in insulin receptors. It is not unusual, however, to note a complete absence of the requirement for insulin in the immediate postoperative period in morbidly obese patients. Therefore, insulin should be withheld on the morning of operation. There is often a marked reduction in the requirement for insulin throughout the postoperative period and even at discharge in morbidly obese patients who have undergone GBP, probably because of increased release of gastric inhibitory peptide (GIP) from the proximal small bowel. Therefore, regular subcutaneous insulin should be administered to GBP patients according to a sliding scale after operation until insulin requirements can be determined. Before discharge, the patient should be taking an appropriate dose of neutral protamine Hagedorn (NPH) or Lente insulin but must perform frequent finger-stick blood glucose determinations afterward, given that the need for insulin will decrease progressively with weight loss.

In one study of 23 patients with type 1 (insulin-dependent) diabetes mellitus who underwent gastric bariatric operation, the average requirement for insulin decreased from 74 units/day before operation to 8 units/day after operation.[9] Fourteen of the 23 patients were able to discontinue insulin completely, 11 by the time of discharge from the hospital 1 week after operation. These benefits were maintained during long-term follow-up to 39 months and were a result of a major decrease in insulin resistance that was associated with decreased food intake as well as weight loss.

Wound Care

Morbidly obese patients have been reported to have an increased risk of wound infection and dehiscence. However, the incidence of these complications in this group of patients can be very low. In a randomized, prospective trial comparing a running, continuous absorbable No. 2 polyglycolic acid suture with a No. 28 stainless-steel wire in morbidly obese patients who weighed an average of 320 lb, there was no significant difference in complications, including the incidence of incisional hernia, between the types of closure.[10] However, the running absorbable suture closure required significantly less time. Similar results comparing continuous with interrupted sutures have been noted by others.[11] Subcutaneous sutures should not be used, because the subcutaneous fat becomes reapproximated during skin closure, and subcutaneous sutures have been found to increase the risk of wound infection.[12] Obese patients undergoing clean-contaminated intestinal procedures should be given a parenteral antibiotic immediately before the operation and for only 24 hours after the operation[13]; it is important to note that morbidly obese patients should receive a double dose of prophylactic antibiotics because of the increased volume of distribution. If a gastric or gallbladder operation is planned, only aerobic bacterial coverage is necessary; a colon operation will necessitate anaerobic coverage as well.

It has been our experience that the incidence of incisional hernia is much higher in morbidly obese patients than in thin patients with ulcerative colitis who are taking large doses of corticosteroids and who undergo the same fascial wound closure with running No. 2 polyglycolic acid sutures.[14] This increased risk in morbidly obese patients is probably secondary to the increased intra-abdominal pressures (IAP) present in patients with central, or android, obesity.[15]

Obese diabetic patients are at risk for rapidly spreading panniculitis secondary to mixed aerobic and anaerobic organisms.[16] Subcutaneous gas and extensive necrosis, which usually does not involve the underlying muscle, are often present. It is uncommon to culture clostridia from these wounds. Even after extensive and repeated debridement, mortality remains high [*see II:11 Soft Tissue Infection*].

Other Obesity-Related Diseases

GALLSTONES

Approximately one third of morbidly obese patients either have had a cholecystectomy or may have had gallstones noted at the time of another intra-abdominal operative procedure, such as gastric operation for morbid obesity. Preoperative evaluation of the gallbladder may be technically quite difficult in morbidly obese patients because gallstones may be missed with either ultrasonography or oral cholecystography. Intraoperative sonography is probably much more accurate. Should stones be present in a patient undergoing gastric operation for obesity, the gallbladder should be removed. In the past, obese patients with intermittent attacks of biliary colic were told to lose weight before an elective cholecystectomy for fear of significant morbidity and mortality from an elective operation. This attitude is no longer valid, because among the large numbers of obese patients who now undergo major elective abdominal procedures, morbidity is similar to that seen in thin patients if appropriate precautions are taken. Furthermore, obese patients have great difficulty losing large amounts of weight by diet alone and should be allowed to undergo definitive corrective operative procedures before weight reduction.

Rapid weight loss may lead to the development of gallstones in 25% to 40% of patients who undergo GBP. The risk of cholelithiasis in this setting can be reduced to 2% by administering ursodeoxycholic acid, 300 mg orally twice daily.[17]

PSEUDOTUMOR CEREBRI

Pseudotumor cerebri is an unusual complication of morbid obesity that is associated with benign intracranial hypertension, papilledema, blurred vision, headache, and elevated cerebrospinal fluid pressures.[18] It has been our experience that patients with pseudotumor cerebri are not at any additional perioperative risk and that cerebrospinal fluid does not have to be removed before anesthesia and major abdominal operation. Weight reduction will cure pseudotumor cerebri.[19,20]

DEGENERATIVE OSTEOARTHRITIS

Degenerative osteoarthritis of the knees, hips, and back is a common complication of morbid obesity. Weight reduction alone may greatly reduce the pain and immobility that afflict these patients, although the damage may be so extensive that a total joint replacement may be desirable. However, joint replacement in patients who weigh more than 250 lb is associated with an unacceptable incidence of loosening.[21] Weight reduction by means of a gastric bariatric operation may be the most sensible initial approach, to be followed by joint replacement after weight loss if pain and dysfunction persist.

Discussion

Morbidity Associated with Central Fat Deposition

Much has been written about the increased health risks inherent in central, or android, fat deposition as compared with peripheral, or gynoid, fat deposition. It is thought that in the former, the increased metabolic activity of mesenteric fat is associated with increased metabolism of amino acids to sugar, which leads to hyperglycemia and hyperinsulinism. Hyperinsulinism gives rise to increased sodium absorption and hypertension. Furthermore, central obesity has been linked to hypercholesterolemia. Hence, these patients have a significantly higher incidence of diabetes, hypertension, hypercholesterolemia, and gallstones[22]—which explains the higher mortality of the

apple distribution of body fat as compared with the pear distribution. In the past, fat distribution was measured on the basis of the waist-to-hip ratio; however, computed tomography scans have shown that abdominal circumference is a more accurate measurement of central fat distribution.[23] We have found that morbidly obese women have significantly increased IAP and that this is associated with stress and urge overflow urinary incontinence.[24] With weight loss comes a significant decrease in bladder pressure and correction of incontinence. We have found IAP, as reflected in bladder pressure, to be closely correlated with sagittal abdominal diameter but not with waist-to-hip ratio (many morbidly obese patients have both central and peripheral obesity). We have also found that the increased IAP associated with central obesity may cause additional comorbid factors, including venous stasis ulcers, OHS, gastroesophageal reflux, and inguinal and incisional hernias.

Respiratory Insufficiency of Obesity

Obese patients are at risk for respiratory difficulties, which may be present before operation or may be exacerbated by an operation. The term pickwickian syndrome (which derives from *The Posthumous Papers of the Pickwick Club*, by Charles Dickens) was resurrected from the late 1800s to describe a morbidly obese man 52 years of age who fell asleep in a poker game while holding a hand containing a full house.[2] He was taken to the hospital by friends who presumed he was ill. The pickwickian syndrome is now known to comprise two pulmonary syndromes associated with morbid obesity: obstructive SAS and OHS.[3]

Patients with SAS suffer from repeated attacks of upper airway obstruction during sleep. The cause is probably related to a large, fat tongue as well as to excessive fat deposition in the uvula, pharynx, and hypopharynx. The normal genioglossus reflex is depressed, but this depression may be secondary to the excessive weight of the tongue. These patients are notorious snorers. As a result of inadequate stage IV and rapid eye movement (REM) sleep, they are markedly somnolent during the day.

Patients with SAS are at great risk for acute upper airway obstruction and respiratory arrest after operation and general anesthesia. A high index of suspicion is necessary before operation. Patients with severe SAS often have ventricular arrhythmias and sinus arrest during their apneic episodes, thereby placing them at even greater risk. A history of heavy snoring, early morning headaches, frequent awakening at night with shortness of breath, severe daytime somnolence (including falling asleep at the wheel), and frequent headaches should prompt further study. The syndrome is confirmed by sleep polysomnography, which is available at sleep centers in most major cities.

In most instances, severe SAS can be treated with nocturnal nasal CPAP. With this technique, air flowing through a nasal mask against a constant airway resistance enters the nasal pharynx and pushes the tongue forward to prevent recurrent obstruction.[25] The pressure can be adjusted for each patient. Unfortunately, many patients cannot tolerate the device, because it is cumbersome and noisy and tends to dry out the upper airway, although dryness can be prevented with an inexpensive room humidifier. If nasal CPAP cannot be tolerated by the patient, or if it is ineffective and the problem is severe (i.e., causing cardiac arrhythmias or severe hypoxia), tracheostomy is indicated. This procedure can be very difficult and dangerous and therefore should not be relegated to the youngest house officer in a surgical residency program. Because of the extremely deep neck in obese patients, a standard tracheostomy tube is usually inadequate, and a special tube with a deep bend should be used.

OHS is a condition associated with morbid obesity in which an individual suffers from hypoxemia and hypercapnia when breathing room air while awake but resting.[26] Spirometry reveals decreases in forced vital capacity, residual lung volume, expiratory reserve volume, functional residual capacity, and maximum minute volume ventilation, usually without obstruction to airflow [*see Figure 1*]. The most profound decrease is that in expiratory reserve volume; it is probably secondary to increased intra-abdominal pressure and a high-riding diaphragm. Thus, these patients have restrictive rather than obstructive pulmonary disease. The decreased expiratory reserve volume implies that many alveolar units are collapsed at end-expiration, which leads to perfusion of unventilated alveoli, or shunting. Patients with OHS often are heavy smokers or have addi-

tional pulmonary problems, such as asthma, sarcoidosis, idiopathic pulmonary fibrosis, or recurrent pulmonary emboli. One study of patients who underwent operation for morbid obesity showed no statistically significant difference in weight between those who had OHS and those who did not.[3]

As a result of chronic and severe hypoxemia, patients with OHS are often markedly polycythemic. The polycythemia further increases their already significant risk for venous thrombosis and pulmonary embolism. Because we have had several patients who later had a subclavian venous thrombosis and one patient who probably had a transient sagittal sinus thrombosis, patients with OHS should probably undergo phlebotomy to a hemoglobin concentration of 15 g/dl before elective operation.

Chronic hypoxemia also leads to pulmonary arterial vasoconstriction and severe pulmonary hypertension[1,27] and eventually to right-sided heart failure or cor pulmonale with neck vein distention, tricuspid valvular insufficiency, right upper quadrant tenderness secondary to acute hepatic engorgement, and massive peripheral edema. Such patients may also have significantly elevated PAWP, which suggests left ventricular dysfunction.[1] All morbidly obese patients should have preoperative determinations of blood gas values. If an abnormality is detected, spirometry can be performed, although it would probably be of little additional diagnostic value. If arterial blood gas measurement reveals severe hypoxemia (i.e., $P_aO_2 \leq 55$ mm Hg), severe hypercapnia ($P_aCO_2 \geq 47$ mm Hg), or both, the patient should undergo Swan-Ganz catheterization. If PAWP is 18 mm Hg or greater, intravenous furosemide should be administered for diuresis before elective operation. However, some patients may require a high ventricular filling pressure. A low cardiac output and hypotension may follow diuresis, necessitating volume reexpansion. If mean PAP is 40 mm Hg or greater, consideration should be given to the prophylactic insertion of a Greenfield inferior vena caval filter [*see* Thrombophlebitis, Venous Stasis Ulcers, and Pulmonary Embolism in the Morbidly Obese Patient, *below*].

It is highly probable that some of the elevated PAP and PAWP measurements are caused by the increased IAP in the morbidly obese[15,28] [*see Figure 2*]. This leads to an elevated diaphragm, which in turn increases intrapleural pressure and thereby PAP and PAWP; if the pleural pressure is measured with an esophageal transducer, the transmyocardial pressure can be estimated. For this reason, these patients may require a markedly elevated PAWP to maintain an adequate cardiac output, and excessive diuresis may lead to hypotension. The same reasoning may be applied to a patient with a distended abdomen resulting from peritonitis and pancreatitis in whom what seem to be unusually high cardiac filling pressures are

*P < 0.01 Compared with Preoperative Values

Figure 1 **Impaired pulmonary function in the morbidly obese improved significantly after weight loss induced by gastric operation.**[3]

necessary. Therefore, one must rely on relative changes in cardiac output in response to either volume challenge or diuresis to determine the optimal PAWP in morbidly obese patients.

Patients with OHS respond rapidly to supplemental oxygen. However, oxygen administration is occasionally associated with significant CO_2 retention, which necessitates intubation and mechanical ventilation. Because their pulmonary disease is restrictive rather than obstructive, these patients are usually easy to ventilate without high peak airway pressures. Arterial blood gases need not return to normal before extubation; it is only necessary that they return to their preoperative values. These values are achieved, on average, 4 days after major upper abdominal operation, when the patients no longer have abdominal pain.[3]

It is important to emphasize that morbidly obese patients, especially those with respiratory insufficiency, should be placed in the reverse Trendelenburg's position to maximize diaphragmatic excursion and to increase residual lung volume.[7] These patients will often complain of air hunger and respiratory distress when they lie supine. So-called breaking of the bed at the waist may exacerbate the problem by pushing the abdominal contents into the chest, thereby raising the diaphragm and further reducing lung volumes. Placing these patients in the leg-down position may predispose them to venous stasis, phlebitis, and pulmonary embolism, which should be offset with intermittent venous compression boots [see Thrombophlebitis, Venous Stasis Ulcers, and Pulmonary Embolism in the Morbidly Obese Patient, below].[29]

Both SAS and OHS can be completely corrected with weight reduction after gastric operation for morbid obesity: the nocturnal apneas resolve, the P_aO_2 rises, and the P_aCO_2 falls to normal as lung volumes improve.[3]

Cardiac Dysfunction in the Morbidly Obese Patient

Cardiac dysfunction in the morbidly obese patient is usually associated with respiratory insufficiency of obesity, especially OHS.[2] Elevated PAP in these patients may be secondary to hypoxemia-induced pulmonary arterial vasoconstriction, to elevated left atrial pressures secondary to left ventricular dysfunction, or to a combination of these; they may also be secondary to the increased pleural pressures arising from an elevated diaphragm secondary to increased IAP.[1,28,29] It is unusual for morbidly obese patients without respiratory insufficiency to experience significant cardiac dysfunction in the absence of severe coronary artery disease. Morbidly obese patients often have systemic hypertension, which can aggravate left ventricular dysfunction; however, mild left ventricular dysfunction can be documented in many morbidly obese patients in the absence of systemic hypertension.[30,31] Circulating blood volume, plasma volume, and cardiac output increase in proportion to body weight.[31] Massively obese patients may occasionally present with acute heart failure: it is reasonable to assume that the enormous metabolic requirements of such patients can present a greater demand for blood flow than the heart can provide. Vigorous diuresis will often correct such acute heart failure. Significant weight loss will correct pulmonary hypertension [see Figure 3] as well as left ventricular dysfunction associated with respiratory insufficiency.[1,32]

Thrombophlebitis, Venous Stasis Ulcers, and Pulmonary Embolism in the Morbidly Obese Patient

Morbidly obese individuals have difficulty walking; tend to be sedentary; have a large amount of abdominal weight resting on their inferior vena cava; and have increased intrapleural pressure, which impedes venous return.[27,28] All of these conditions increase the ten-

Figure 2 In a porcine model,[28] raising IAP caused cardiac index to fall and PAWP to rise. At an IAP of 25 mm Hg, saline was given to restore intravascular volume; cardiac index returned to baseline levels, but PAWP remained elevated. (IAP—intra-abdominal pressure; PAWP—pulmonary arterial wedge pressure)

dency toward phlebothrombosis. The patient is most at risk when immobilized in the supine position for long periods in the operating room. These patients have also been shown to have low levels of antithrombin III, which may increase their tendency toward venous thrombosis.[33] It has also been suggested that starvation, particularly in the postoperative period, may be associated with high levels of free fatty acids, which may predispose to perioperative thrombotic complications.[34]

Intermittent venous compression boots have been shown in randomized trials to reduce the incidence of deep vein thrombosis.[29] Administration of low-dose subcutaneous heparin must be started immediately before operation. However, because morbidly obese patients show a significant improvement in pulmonary function when placed in the reverse Trendelenburg's position,[7] and because this position further increases venous pressure in the legs and the tendency toward stasis, it is preferable to use this position and intermittent venous compression boots. All patients, but especially the

Figure 3 Mean pulmonary arterial pressure was significantly improved in 18 patients 3 to 9 months after gastric surgery–induced weight loss of 42% ± 19% of excess weight.[1]

morbidly obese, should make every attempt to walk during the evening after operation.

Because pulmonary embolism is quite unusual when the appropriate precautions have been taken, acute air hunger, tachypnea, and hypoxemia should suggest the equal likelihood that sepsis-induced ARDS is present secondary to an intra-abdominal anastomotic leak.

Patients with severe OHS often have noticeably elevated PAP, which can lead to right-sided heart failure and can increase the risk of venous stasis and thrombosis. Investigators have noted that patients with primary idiopathic pulmonary hypertension are at significant risk for fatal pulmonary embolism.[5] For this reason, it has been our policy to place a prophylactic Greenfield vena caval filter in patients with respiratory insufficiency of obesity and a mean PAP of 40 mm Hg or greater. With this approach (in which a vena caval filter was used in 15 patients), we have had one fatal pulmonary embolus in 156 patients with respiratory insufficiency of obesity who have undergone gastric bariatric procedures. The fatality was a patient whose mean PAP was initially 40 mm Hg but fell to 35 mm Hg with diuresis and who was not considered to require a filter.

Venous stasis ulcers can be quite difficult to treat in a thin individual; they are almost impossible to cure in a patient with morbid obesity [see Figure 4]. The most important goal in management of these ulcers is weight loss, which almost invariably leads to healing of the ulcer, probably as a result of decreased IAP.

Pseudotumor Cerebri in the Morbidly Obese Patient

Pseudotumor cerebri (also known as idiopathic intracranial hypertension) associated with obesity is almost certainly secondary to increased IAP. The rise in IAP causes a rise in intrathoracic pressure, which in turn raises central venous pressure and PAWP [see Figure 2], thus decreasing venous drainage from the brain.[28] This sequence of events has been reproduced in a porcine model.[35] The elevated intracranial pressure (ICP) can be prevented by means of median sternotomy and pleuropericardiotomy [see Figure 5].[36] In humans studied 3 years after weight-reduction surgery, surgically induced weight loss was associated with a significant decrease in ICP (from 353 ± 35 mm H₂O to 168 ± 12 mm H₂O; $P < 0.001$) and with relief of headache and pulsatile tinnitus.[19,20]

Conclusion

Although the morbidly obese patient is potentially at risk for significant perioperative morbidity and mortality, attention to detail in preoperative preparation as well as in postoperative management should reduce this risk almost to that of the general population. A high index of suspicion for peritonitis must be maintained after an intra-abdominal procedure or when the patient complains of abdominal pain in the emergency room. Awareness of the problems associated with respiratory insufficiency in obese patients should enable the surgeon to avoid pitfalls when managing the patient with obstructive SAS or OHS. These patients may require preoperative pulmonary arterial catheterization for optimal fluid management before and after operation. The risks of venous thrombosis and pulmonary embolism are high, but the use of intermittent compression boots and early ambulation can minimize the dangers. The obese patient with non–insulin-dependent diabetes has been surprisingly easy to manage after major operation.

Weight reduction by diet is associated with a 95% incidence of recidivism. The average morbidly obese patient can be expected to lose two thirds of the excess weight within 1 year after a standard GBP or, if superobese, after a long-limb gastric bypass. Further-

Figure 4 This chronic venous stasis ulcer was present for several years in a morbidly obese patient. Healing promptly followed weight loss induced by a gastric operation.

more, recent reports note that this weight loss is long-lasting and averages 60% of excess weight at 5 years and more than 50% of excess weight up to 10 years after operation. This weight loss is associated with the correction of insulin-dependent diabetes, obstructive SAS, OHS, pseudotumor cerebri, hypertension, chronic venous stasis ulcers, stress incontinence, gastroesophageal reflux, and female sex hormone abnormalities, which may be related to dysmenorrhea, infertility, hirsutism, and an increased risk of endometrial carcinoma. Weight loss can markedly improve the patient's self-image and employability. Because techniques for operation for morbid obesity continue to change as understanding of pathophysiology improves, it is important for surgeons to keep abreast of the latest developments.

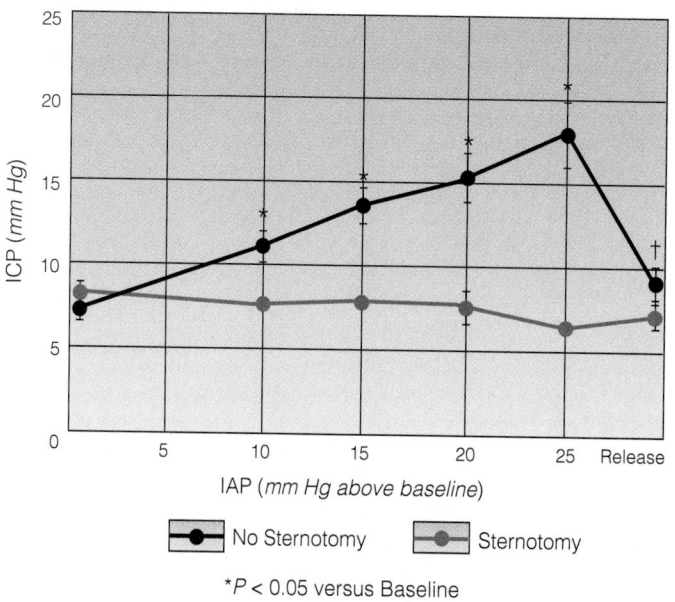

*P < 0.05 versus Baseline
†P < 0.05 versus Maximum IAP

Figure 5 In a porcine model,[36] IAP was increased to 25 mm Hg in 12 animals, of which three underwent median sternotomy and pleuropericardiotomy (red line) and nine did not (black line). Sternotomy and pleuropericardiotomy prevented the expected increase in ICP. (ICP—intracranial pressure)

References

1. Sugerman HJ, Baron PL, Fairman RP, et al: Hemodynamic dysfunction in obesity hypoventilation syndrome and the effects of treatment with surgically induced weight loss. Ann Surg 207:604, 1988

2. Burwell CS, Robin ED, Whaley RD, et al: Extreme obesity associated with alveolar hypoventilation—a pickwickian syndrome. Am J Med 21:811, 1956

3. Sugerman HJ, Fairman RP, Baron PL, et al: Gastric surgery for respiratory insufficiency of obesity. Chest 89:81, 1986

4. Sugerman HJ, Fairman RP, Sood RK, et al: Long-term effects of gastric surgery for treating respiratory insufficiency of obesity. Am J Clin Nutr 55(2 suppl): 597S, 1992

5. Young T, Palta M, Dempsey J, et al: The occurrence of sleep-disordered breathing among middle-aged adults. N Engl J Med 328:1230, 1993

6. Greenfield LJ, Scher LA, Elkins RC: KMA-Greenfield® filter placement for chronic pulmonary hypertension. Ann Surg 189:560, 1979

7. Vaughan RW, Bauer S, Wise L: Effect of position (semirecumbent versus supine) on postoperative oxygenation in markedly obese subjects. Anesth Analg 55:37, 1976

8. Mason EE, Printen KJ, Barron P, et al: Risk reduction in gastric operations for obesity. Ann Surg 190:158, 1979

9. Herbst CA, Hughes TA, Gwynne JT, et al: Gastric bariatric operation in insulin-treated adults. Surgery 95:209, 1984

10. McNeill PM, Sugerman HJ: Continuous absorbable vs interrupted nonabsorbable fascial closure: a prospective, randomized comparison. Arch Surg 121:821, 1986

11. Richards PC, Balch CM, Aldrete JS: Abdominal wound closure: a randomized prospective study of 571 patients comparing continuous vs. interrupted suture techniques. Ann Surg 197:238, 1983

12. De Holl D, Rodeheaver G, Edgerton MT, et al: Potentiation of infection by suture closure of dead space. Am J Surg 127:716, 1974

13. Stone HH, Hooper CA, Kolb LD, et al: Antibiotic prophylaxis in gastric, biliary, and colonic surgery. Ann Surg 184:443, 1976

14. Sugerman HJ, Kellum JM, Reines HD, et al: Incisional hernia: greater risk with morbidly obese than steroid dependent patients; low recurrence rate with prefascial polypropylene mesh repair. Am J Surg 171:80, 1996

15. Sugerman H, Windsor A, Bessos M, et al: Intra-abdominal pressure, sagittal abdominal diameter, and obesity co-morbidity. J Intern Med 241:71, 1997

16. Rouse TM, Malangoni MA, Schulte WJ: Necrotizing fasciitis: a preventable disaster. Surgery 92:765, 1982

17. Sugerman HJ, Brewer WH, Shiffman ML, et al: A multicenter, placebo-controlled, randomized, double-blind, prospective trial of prophylactic ursodiol for the prevention of gallstone formation following gastric-bypass-induced rapid weight loss. Am J Surg 169:91, 1995

18. Corbett JJ, Mehta MP: Cerebrospinal fluid pressure in normal obese subjects and patients with pseudotumor cerebri. Neurology 33:1386, 1983

19. Sugerman HJ, Felton WL, Salvant JB, et al: Effects of surgically induced weight loss on pseudotumor cerebri in morbid obesity. Neurology 45:1655, 1995

20. Sugerman HJ, Felton WL III, Sismanis A, et al: Gastric surgery for pseudotumor cerebri associated with severe obesity. Ann Surg 229:634, 1999

21. Goldin RH, McAdam L, Louie JS, et al: Clinical and radiologic survey of the incidence of osteoarthritis among obese patients. Ann Rheum Dis 35:349, 1976

22. Kissebah AH, Vydelingum N, Murray R, et al: Relation of body fat distribution to metabolic complications of obesity. J Clin Endocrinol Metab 54:254, 1982

23. Kvist H, Chowdhury B, Grangard U, et al: Total and visceral adipose-tissue volumes derived from measurements with computed tomography in adult men and women: predictive equations. Am J Clin Nutr 48:1351, 1988

24. Bump RC, Sugerman HJ, Fantl JA, et al: Obesity and lower urinary tract function in women: effect of surgically induced weight loss. Am J Obstet Gynecol 167: 392, 1992

25. Sullivan CE, Issa FG, Berthon-Jones M, et al: Reversal of obstructive sleep apnoea by continuous positive airway pressure applied through the nares. Lancet 1:862, 1981

26. Rochester DR, Enson Y: Current concepts in the pathogenesis of the obesity hypoventilation syndrome: mechanical and circulatory factors. Am J Med 57: 402, 1974

27. Alexander JK, Amad KH, Cole VW: Observations on some clinical features of extreme obesity, with particular reference to cardiorespiratory effects. Am J Med 32:512, 1962

28. Ridings PC, Bloomfield GL, Blocher CR, et al: Cardiopulmonary effects of raised intra-abdominal pressure before and after volume expansion. J Trauma 39:1168, 1995

29. Coe NP, Collins RE, Klein LA, et al: Prevention of deep vein thrombosis in urological patients: a controlled, randomized trial of low-dose heparin and external pneumatic compression boots. Surgery 83:230, 1978

30. Kaltman AJ, Goldring RM: Role of circulatory congestion in the cardiorespiratory failure of obesity. Am J Med 60:645, 1976

31. De Divitiis O, Fazio S, Petitto M, et al: Obesity and cardiac function. Circulation 64:477, 1981

32. Alpert MA, Terry BE, Kelly DL: Effect of weight loss on cardiac chamber size, wall thickness and left ventricular function in morbid obesity. Am J Cardiol 55: 783, 1985

33. Batist G, Bothe A, Bern M, et al: Low antithrombin III in morbid obesity: return to normal with weight reduction. JPEN 7:447, 1983

34. Printen HJ, Miller EV, Mason EE, et al: Venous thromboembolism in the morbidly obese. Surg Gynecol Obstet 147:63, 1978

35. Bloomfield GL, Ridings PC, Blocher CR, et al: Effects of increased intra-abdominal pressure upon intracranial and cerebral perfusion before and after volume expansion. J Trauma 40:936, 1996

36. Bloomfield GL, Ridings PC, Blocher CR, et al: A proposed relationship between increased intra-abdominal, intrathoracic, and intracranial pressure. Crit Care Med 25:496, 1997

Acknowledgments

Figures 1 and 3   Albert Miller.

Figures 2 and 5   Marcia Kammerer.

6 NON-AIDS IMMUNOSUPPRESSION

Carl Nohr, M.D., Ph.D.

Approach to Patients with Host Defense Defects

Evaluation of Host Defense Mechanisms in Surgical Patients

Immunosuppression is a biologic state characterized by detrimental alterations in aspects of host anatomy and physiology normally dedicated to defense against infections and malignancy. Because of the invasive nature of surgery and because defects in systemic immunity have been observed in most major illnesses, it is reasonable to state that all, or nearly all, surgical patients are immunosuppressed at some point. The nature and degree of immunosuppression in a particular patient is the sum of several disease-related or iatrogenic changes.

An understanding of normal immune mechanisms is important to the recognition of immunodeficiency. Host defense mechanisms may be broadly categorized as either local or systemic. Local host defenses include epithelial coverings, specialized cells, and secretions. Systemic defense mechanisms include phagocytic cells as well as complement, humoral, and cell-mediated immune mechanisms. There are major interactions at many levels between the various local and systemic immune processes. Comprehensive descriptions of actual immune processes appear elsewhere.[1] The following sections of this chapter are limited to the clinical and laboratory evaluation of host defense defects [*see Figure 1*].

Immunodeficiency may be primary or acquired secondary to illness or iatrogenic intervention. In most primary immunodeficiency diseases, defects in systemic host defenses can be clinically detected and have a clear relation to the kinds of infection for which the patient is at risk. In the more common acquired immunodeficiencies, however, the relation of host defense defects to the pathogenesis of infections is generally less clearly defined. Nevertheless, tests of immune function can help define underlying defects in local and systemic host defense mechanisms in patients with an acquired increased susceptibility to local and systemic infection with or without the septic response.

LOCAL HOST DEFENSES

The human body is a complex tube covered by skin and lined with mucosa. Various mechanical, cellular, microbiological, and biochemical properties of these coverings account for local host defense mechanisms.[1] When these coverings are broken or disrupted, the defense mechanisms may be compromised. Evaluation of breaks in local host defenses thus begins with determining the location and number of invasive devices or procedures and the duration of their use. Such interventions include endotracheal tubes, tracheostomies, nasogastric tubes, bladder catheters, and central venous catheters. Intracranial pressure monitors, chest tubes, drains, external fixation devices, and implanted prostheses also produce changes in local host defenses.

The presence and condition of burn wounds, fistulas, decubitus ulcers, and open or closed surgical wounds should be noted.

Mechanical aspects of the urinary, respiratory, and gastrointestinal systems should be evaluated. Obstruction or stasis in any of the lumina of these systems will alter the local microflora and change the efficacy of local secretions and ciliated and phagocytic cells, thus predisposing to invasive infection. The condition of the gastrointestinal system is especially important in this regard because the gut may be the major source of bacterial infection resulting in sepsis and organ failure in critically ill surgical patients.[2,3]

Changes in local microflora are important considerations, especially in hospitalized patients. Prolonged hospitalization results in gram-negative colonization.[4] Changes in gastric pH can allow overgrowth of some bacterial species.[5] Prolonged broad-spectrum antibiotic treatment is associated with fungal superinfection. Although changes in the local microflora can be evaluated by culture of body fluids and mucosal surfaces, the status of many other important aspects of local immunity cannot be determined reliably by clinical means at present. Measurement of cellular and immunoglobulin contents of respiratory, urinary, and gastrointestinal secretions is not clinically feasible. Evaluation of local defenses of the peritoneum, which are very important to the control of the septic response to infection, is also not feasible.[6]

SYSTEMIC HOST DEFENSES

For purposes of study, systemic immunity may be classified as either antigen specific or nonspecific. Humoral immunity and cell-mediated immunity provide antigen-specific immunity, whereas phagocytes and complement provide nonspecific immunity. There are many interactions between these arbitrary divisions. At the present time, little therapy is available for most of the deficiencies discussed (see below), with the exception of some primary immunodeficiencies. Immunomodulation is an active area of research, however, and the biologic description of acquired immunodeficiencies will assume increasing importance as corrective methodologies evolve.

Surgical patient manifests defects in host defense

Assess present state of patient's local and systemic defenses.

Take history, and perform physical examination, radiologic and laboratory studies, and specific tests of immune function.

Significant immunosuppression is present

Treat any correctable immunodeficiency (e.g., by administering immunoglobulin for defects in B cell function or by reducing dosage of immunosuppressive agents in patients receiving such therapy).

Immunity is slightly impaired

Optimize overall medical and surgical care to help restore immune function

Reassess need for invasive devices.

Remove any infected foreign bodies.

Restore blood volume, and optimize tissue perfusion.

Treat any fistulas, decubitus ulcers, or other wounds.

Correct any underlying nutritional deficiency.

Provide surgical intervention as appropriate: e.g., drain abscesses, resect tumors, and excise burns, if present.

Diagnose and treat any local or systemic infections.

Assess need for vaccination.

Use prophylactic antibiotics when indicated.

For patients who are receiving immunosuppressive therapy, institute appropriate prophylaxis to prevent specific complications.

Optimize renal function, using dialysis if necessary.

Correct hyperglycemia in patients with diabetes mellitus.

Institute therapy to optimize cardiac function.

Candidate for transplantation is to be deliberately immunosuppressed

Perform preimmunosuppression workup, including:

- History and physical examination
- Blood work
- Radiologic studies
- Nuclear medicine scans
- Other studies and tests

Workup should address the following:

- Nervous system
- Cardiovascular system
- Respiratory system
- Digestive system
- Genitourinary system
- Musculoskeletal system
- Endocrine system
- Dermal system
- Hematologic system
- Immune system
- Preexisting infection
- Nutritional state
- Psychological, social, and financial assessment

Patient has no invasive infection or malignant disease

Treat any underlying correctable conditions (e.g., local infection around foreign bodies).

Provide appropriate prophylaxis to prevent complications.

Patient has active invasive infection or malignant disease

Do not proceed with immunosuppression.

Proceed with transplantation, and institute immunosuppressive therapy

Approach to Patients with Host Defense Defects

1110

Immunosuppression suspected in patient scheduled for operation

Evaluate patient's immune status.

Take patient's history and perform physical examination

History should cover the following:
- Patient's age
- Underlying disease or other medical conditions
- Weight loss
- Previous infections
- Splenectomy
- Radiation therapy
- Immunosuppressive medications
- Blood transfusions
- Foreign bodies (e.g., prosthetic valve)

Physical examination should focus on the following:
- Preexisting infection
- Signs of organ failure
- Fistulas
- Bowel obstruction
- Open wounds
- Any invasive device (e.g., bladder catheter, endotracheal tube or tracheostomy, central venous catheter, nasogaastric tube, external-fixation device, intracranial pressure monitor)
- Nutritional status

Perform radiographic and laboratory studies

Chest x-ray
Blood count with differential
Urinalysis
Serum albumin
Liver and kidney function tests
Culture of infected sites
Serology for hepatitis B surface antigen, cytomegalovirus, HIV

Perform specific tests to evaluate function of patient's T cells, B cells, polymorphonuclear neutrophils (PMNs), and complement

T cell function:
- Delayed-type hypersensitivity skin testing
- Number of circulating T cells
- T cell phenotypic analysis
- In vitro T cell function
- Thymic hormone assay
- Lymphokine assays

PMN function:
- Absolute neutrophil count
- Adherence
- Chemotaxis
- Cell delivery to a skin window
- Phagocytosis and killing assays
- Assessment of oxidative metabolism
- Leukocyte adhesion molecule assay

B cell function:
- Serum immunoglobulin levels
- Response to natural or common antibodies, including isohemagglutinins
- Antibody response to vaccination
- Circulating B cell numbers
- In vitro B cell function
- Bone marrow and lymph node biopsy

Complement function:
- CH_{50} assay
- C3 and C4 assay

Diagnose nature and extent of immunosuppression on the basis of history, physical, and laboratory findings and results of immunologic studies

Institute therapy if patient has an immunodeficiency that responds to therapeutic intervention.

Figure 1 Illustrated is a diagnostic approach to suspected immunosuppression in a patient scheduled for operation.

Cell-Mediated Immunity

The most useful test of cell-mediated immunity in surgical patients is the delayed-type hypersensitivity (DTH) skin-test reaction.[7] Many disease processes, including malnutrition,[8] cancer,[9] and thermal injury,[10] alter DTH testing. Results of the test provide a global assessment of host defense function that, together with age, sex, and serum albumin, can be used to calculate the probability of infection in a particular patient.[11,12] DTH is assessed by determining the reaction to the intradermal injection of several antigens to which the patient presumably has had previous exposure, including *Candida* antigen, *Trichophyton* antigen, tuberculin, streptokinase-streptodornase, and mumps antigen. The response may be measured at either 24 or 48 hours after injection of the antigens. It may be expressed as the sum of the diameters of induration of all antigens, or it may be defined as a positive response if two or more antigens produce more than 5 mm of induration each.

The next echelon of tests evaluates T cell function. Populations of T cells are measured precisely with the use of monoclonal antibodies. These antibodies bind to cell surface receptors that distinguish between functional subpopulations of lymphocytes. The ratio of helper to suppressor T cells—that is, CD4+ to CD8+—is frequently used as a measure of immune function. The normal ratio is 1.8:2.2.

Testing of in vitro T cell function is largely a laboratory process that measures the capacity of mononuclear cells to proliferate, produce lymphokines, or become killer cells after stimulation in culture. Several stimulating agents are used in this process. Such stimulants include antigen to which the cell donor has been previously exposed and T cell mitogens—for example, phytohemagglutinin, concanavalin A, or HLA-dissimilar cells.

With greater understanding of the interactions between immunologically active cells, it is possible to define more precisely the communication signals between cells. Although not yet clinically routine, the study of the ability of cells to produce normal amounts of cytokines and the study of cytokine gene expression will, in time, assume greater importance in the definition of immunosuppression.

Humoral Immunity

As a first measure of humoral immune function, serum levels of IgG, IgM, and IgA are measured. Levels vary with age; IgA and IgM are absent in neonates unless there has been intrauterine infection. Next, determination of natural or commonly occurring antibodies—for example, isohemagglutinins or antibody to diphtheria, tetanus, or common viruses—will indicate a past humoral immune response. The current status of humoral immune function can best be evaluated by testing antibody response to active vaccination. Tetanus toxoid[13] and pneumococcal vaccine[14] may be used to test antibody responses to protein and polysaccharide antigens, respectively.

In-depth investigation of humoral immunity involves examination of cell surface markers and in vitro B cell function. B cells are characterized by the presence of surface immunoglobulin or other cell surface markers. Bone marrow, lymph node, and blood mononuclear cells may be examined to determine the prevalence of B cells. Spontaneous and mitogen- or drug-induced proliferation of B cells in vitro, as well as their maturation into plasma cells that produce immunoglobulin, may be studied by a variety of research laboratory methods.[8]

Neutrophil Function

Most of the functions of polymorphonuclear neutrophils (PMNs) can be tested. Adherence, a first step in ingress toward sites of inflammation, is tested by measuring the attachment of neutrophils to nylon wool. Chemotaxis, the directed motion toward a stimulus, can be quantitated by several techniques. Cell delivery to skin abrasions is a useful test of phagocyte function. Phagocytosis and killing assays measure the ability of host PMNs to ingest and kill test organisms. Oxidative metabolism of PMNs, important to normal function, can be measured with myeloperoxidase assay, nitroblue tetrazolium reduction, or chemoluminescence studies.[8]

Complement

Overall integrity of the complement cascade is determined by measuring the amount of serum needed to lyse 50 percent of antibody-coated sheep red cells; this measurement is called the CH$_{50}$ test. An abnormal CH$_{50}$ is followed by assay of individual complement components, usually C3 and C4.

Therapeutic Approach to Immunocompromised Surgical Patients

The approach to the care of the immunocompromised surgical patient focuses on ways of promoting wound healing and host resistance to infection. At present, there is little specific anti-immunosuppressive treatment for the broad-based acquired immunodeficiencies seen in surgical patients. Management therefore depends on minimizing immunosuppressive procedures and treatments and ensuring that overall care is as good as possible.

The surgical approach to the care of the immunocompromised patient begins with a complete evaluation of the present state of local and systemic immunity. The possibility of reduced dosages of immunosuppressive medications is considered in cases in which these drugs are the cause of the immunocompromised state. (In transplant recipients, the benefits of decreasing immunosuppressive medications must be balanced against the risk of allograft rejection.) The need for invasive devices is reviewed. Foreign bodies are removed if infected. Physiologic conditions are improved by restoring blood volume and optimizing tissue perfusion. Nutritional deficiencies are corrected. Fistulas, decubitus ulcers, and other wounds are treated. Local and systemic infections are diagnosed and treated. Prophylactic or therapeutic antibiotics are used when indicated. Appropriate measures are instituted to stop ongoing hemorrhage so transfusion requirements can be minimized. Abscesses are drained, malignancies treated, and burns excised where appropriate. The need for any vaccination is assessed. In some patients, evaluation of systemic immunity may indicate a need for specific treatment—for example, immunoglobulin infusions.

The first two goals of immunomodulatory therapy in surgical patients are anatomic and physiologic restoration and assurance of good local microcirculation. Host anatomy and physiology determine the microenvironmental milieu in which wound healing and antimicrobial resistance mechanisms operate. Regional blood flow, concentration of protein and hormones in plasma and interstitial fluid, tissue oxygenation, and other systemic physiologic parameters determine not only the microenvironmental conditions in which defense mechanisms operate but also the ability of the body to produce resistance factors and deliver them to inflammatory sites. All treatments, procedures, and agents designed to restore and maintain normal anatomy and physiology are therefore useful in the care of the immunosuppressed patient.

Restoration of nutritional status by oral or intravenous feeding has been shown to be beneficial for several abnormalities of host defense,[8] including skin-test reactivity; lymphocyte transformation, serum immunoglobulin levels, specific antibody responses, and neutrophil chemotaxis may also be restored in this manner. For patients with a functional intestinal tract, enteral feeding is preferred over parenteral nutrition [see VII:9 Nutritional Support].

Although surgical intervention is generally immunosuppressive, it can help restore immune function by treating disease. For example, the depressed DTH test responses of cancer patients, which are associated with an increased risk of infection and mortality, can be improved by tumor resection.[15,16] Correction of biliary tract disease, bowel obstruction, hypovolemia, and visceral abscesses can also improve responses to DTH tests.[17] Similarly, early burn excision decreases immunosuppression. Care in administering prophylactic antibiotics, handling tissue, and controlling contamination and blood loss will produce the best outcomes.

Two aspects of the host response to bacterial infection—a critical interval termed the decisive period and the so-called inoculum effect—are of special importance to the timing of surgical intervention. After subcutaneous injection of bacteria in guinea pigs, there is a decisive period of only a few hours during which the administration of antibiotics can prevent the development of infection and the septic response.[18] The inoculum effect describes the important observation that a large inoculum (i.e., large numbers of bacteria) is more likely to cause invasive infection than a small inoculum. Incorporating the concepts of a decisive period during the process of infection and an inoculum effect is an important aspect of the philosophy of surgical care. Minimizing the quantity and duration of bacterial contamination through early diagnosis and definitive surgical therapy is important in the care of the immunocompromised patient.

Some preexisting illnesses—for example, renal failure or diabetes mellitus—are also immunosuppressive. Because these abnormalities are regarded as part of an acquired immunodeficiency syndrome caused by illness, optimization of organ system function should also help restore immune function. The restoration of red cell mass, use of dialysis, correction of hyperglycemia, and treatment of heart failure are examples of general care that can improve local and systemic host defense and wound-healing mechanisms.

Vaccination, either active or passive, is an important topic in the care of the immunocompromised patient. Live vaccines, such as those for smallpox, measles, rubella, polio (oral vaccine), mumps, and yellow fever, must not be given to immunosuppressed patients. Vaccination against tetanus, diphtheria, pneumococcus, and meningococcus is permitted, as is subcutaneous vaccination for polio, all with the same indications as in nonimmunosuppressed patients. In immunosuppressed patients, there is one additional indication for vaccination with pneumococcal and meningococcal polysaccharide—namely, patients who have been splenectomized or who are scheduled to undergo splenectomy. In the latter case, the vaccine is preferably administered two weeks before splenectomy.

Passive vaccination against gram-negative organisms may be available soon. Gram-negative bacterial organisms are antigenically complex, but many share a common core glycolipid antigen system. Polyclonal or monoclonal antibodies to this moiety may be useful in the management of bacterial infection in the immunocompromised surgical patient.[17] Vaccination may also be useful in viral infections other than polio. Vaccine against cytomegalovirus (CMV) has undergone clinical trial but is not universally used. Passive vaccination with CMV hyperimmune globulin or prophylactic administration of ganciclovir may be more practical approaches to the prevention of CMV infections in transplant recipients.[19-21] Early treatment with ganciclovir, rather than universal prophylaxis, in patients with positive surveillance cultures for CMV may also be effective in reducing the incidence and severity of symptomatic infection.[22]

The use of drugs and other agents specifically intended to improve host defense mechanisms is at present experimental. In general, such agents act by removing suppressor influences, replenishing supplies of endogenous host defense factors, restoring deficient mechanisms to normal, or hyperstimulating already functioning host defense mechanisms.[17]

Prophylaxis of certain disease processes is a special topic in the care of immunocompromised patients. Several measures are commonly used or are under study for the prevention of complications in such patients [see Table 1].

SPECIAL CONSIDERATIONS

Prevention of infection is preferable to treatment. However, if clinical illness develops, outcome will be determined by the speed with which a specific diagnosis is reached and the correct therapy instituted.

Approach to Suspected Infection

Several factors must be considered in the workup of a possibly infected immunosuppressed patient [see Table 2]. Two aspects of infection in the immunosuppressed patient are especially important. One is the effect of immunosuppression on the presentation of infections and on their natural history and response to treatment. The other is the increased susceptibility of so-called septic patients to infections by opportunistic microorganisms [see Table 3]. When a diagnosis of infection is being considered in febrile allograft recipients, it is important to remember that other causes of fever, such as rejection and malignancy, may also be present.

Signs and symptoms of many infectious processes are altered or absent in immunosuppressed patients. Low-grade fever, confusion, acidosis, tachypnea, unexplained third-space fluid loss, or tachycardia may be the only manifestations of infection and should be worked up and treated vigorously. It is frequently appropriate to treat speculatively with antibiotics early while pursuing aggressive diagnostic procedures. This approach is especially important in neutropenic patients. Failure to respond to therapy indicates the need for more aggressive diagnostic procedures and changes in antibiotic treatment.

All body fluids and tissue specimens must be studied microbiologically and, frequently, histologically for conventional bacteria, viruses, acid-fast bacteria, fungi, and protozoa. DNA hybridization may be useful in the diagnosis of latent infection in cells.

Table 1 Prevention of Complications in Immunosuppressed Patients

Complication	Preventive Measure
Bacteremia	Preimmunosuppressive dental work Prophylaxis for later dental work Low-bacterial-content diet ? Protected environment ? Gut decontamination
Pneumocystis pneumonia	Trimethoprim-sulfamethoxazole
Listeria infection	Trimethoprim-sulfamethoxazole
Nocardia infection	Trimethoprim-sulfamethoxazole
Mycobacterium infection	Isoniazid
Cryptococcus infection	Fluconazole
Urinary tract infections	? Preimmunosuppressive nephrectomy for chronic pyelonephritis (in renal transplant candidates) Trimethoprim-sulfamethoxazole
Hepatitis A	? Postexposure prophylaxis with hyperimmune globulin
Hepatitis B	Vaccination
Cytomegalovirus infection	Avoid seropositive-to-seronegative transplants ? Vaccination ? Hyperimmune globulin ? Prophylactic acyclovir or ganciclovir
Varicella-zoster virus	Hyperimmune globulin
Influenza	Vaccination
Influenza A	? Amantadine prophylaxis
Postsplenectomy infection with septic response	Nonoperative treatment Splenic salvage Pneumococcal polysaccharide vaccine Meningococcal polysaccharide vaccine ? Prophylactic antibiotics
Candidal esophagitis	Nystatin swish and swallow
Peptic ulcer disease	Avoidance of acetylsalicylic acid and anti-inflammatory agents Antacids H_2-receptor antagonists
Acute cholecystitis	Preimmunosuppressive cholecystectomy
Perianal ulceration	Stool softeners Antiseptic lotions
Skin carcinoma	Avoidance of sun exposure Use of sunscreens
Osteopenia	Antiresorptive therapy

Wound infections in transplant recipients are caused by common pathogens such as *Staphylococcus* species and mixed bacterial species. They may present, however, with very few local findings as long as years after operation. Diagnostic aspiration of fluid collections is helpful [*see Table 4*].

Mycobacterial or fungal infection of the skin may cause ulcerated, nodular lesions. Although some fungi produce characteristic skin lesions, biopsy may be necessary to distinguish species of *Candida, Torulopsis, Histoplasma, Cryptococcus, Aspergillus, Blastomyces, Actinomyces,* and *Nocardia*. If such organisms are found, systemic infection should be strongly suspected and probably treated even if unproved. Viral infections of the skin are common. Herpes simplex usually causes characteristic vesicular mucocutaneous lesions, whereas varicella-zoster causes chicken pox or shingles. In the immunocompromised patient, either of these viruses may produce disseminated disease as well. Amebic infections may also present initially as skin infection before progressing to systemic infection. Biopsy is diagnostic.

Headache, seizures, altered mentation, or focal neurologic signs suggest central nervous system infection. Viral encephalitis and viral, bacterial, or fungal meningitis are possible. Computed tomographic scanning, with or without infusion of a contrast agent, can rule out space-occupying lesions such as abscess or lymphoma. Funduscopic examination may show evidence of local or systemic infection. For some viral encephalitides, an electroencephalogram or magnetic resonance imaging is diagnostically useful. The most important test for CNS infection, however, is lumbar puncture. Specimens must be stained with Gram's stain and India ink stain and examined for cell count, protein content, and the presence of cryptococcal and bacterial antigens. Finally, brain biopsy may be necessary. *Cryptococcus, Listeria,* and *Aspergillus* are the most important causes of meningitis.

Infection of the cardiovascular system is suggested by bacteremia, new heart murmurs, worsening of congestive heart failure, mycotic aneurysms, or metastatic infarcts or abscesses. Blood cultures and echocardiography are the mainstays of diagnosis.

Any conventional bacteria or mycobacteria may cause pneumonia in the immunosuppressed patient. The major opportunistic agents are CMV, *Aspergillus, Nocardia, Cryptococcus,* and *Pneumocystis* species. This variety of microorganisms in immunosuppressed patients requires a more aggressive diagnostic approach than in nonimmunosuppressed patients. Patterns of infiltration, consolidation, or cavitation on chest radiographs may suggest specific etiologies but are not diagnostic. Detection of *Aspergillus* on throat and nasopharyngeal cultures may indicate the presence of invasive infection caused by this organism elsewhere. Although chest radiographs, sputum examination and culture, thoracentesis, nuclear scanning, and CT scanning are useful in the diagnosis of pneumonitis and empyema, bronchoscopy is frequently required to provide an accurate and timely diagnosis. Minimal abnormalities on chest radiograph, pulmonary function studies, or blood gas measurement should be taken as indications for bronchoscopy. Bronchoalveolar lavage specimens are examined for *Pneumocystis* species, viral inclusion bodies, and CMV antigen, and they are cultured for bacteria, mycobacteria, viruses, and fungi. Transtracheal aspiration can also be used but may be complicated by bleeding and cervical cellulitis. Transbronchial biopsy, open-lung biopsy, and video thoracoscopic lung biopsy are final steps if the diagnosis has not been made.[23,24]

Table 2 Components of Workup for Infection
in Immunocompromised Patients

Patient Subgroup	Components of Workup
All patients	History Review travel, exposure to illness, animal contact Physical examination Blood count and differential count Serum electrolyte levels Liver profile Serum amylase levels Serum cryptococcal antigen Culture of blood, sputum, nasopharyngeal secretions, and urine for aerobes, anaerobes, viruses, and fungi Serum titers of antibodies to herpes simplex virus, cytomegalovirus, and Epstein-Barr virus Chest x-ray ECG Arterial blood gas concentrations
Patients with cutaneous or systemic symptoms or signs	Skin biopsy Fine-needle aspiration Bone marrow aspiration
Patients with neurologic symptoms or signs	Ophthalmoscopic examination CT scan of head MRI scan of head EEG Examination and culture of CSF: cell count, protein content, glucose level, India ink stain, Gram's stain, cryptococcal antigen, bacterial antigens Brain biopsy
Patients with sinus symptoms or signs	Sinus x-rays CT scan of sinuses Sinus aspiration
Patients with cardiac symptoms or signs	Echocardiogram Myocardial biopsy
Patients with pulmonary symptoms or signs	Lung scan CT scan Pulmonary function tests Transtracheal aspiration Bronchoscopy: viral inclusion bodies; cytomegalovirus antigen; culture for bacteria, fungi, and viruses Thoracocentesis: cell count; protein content; glucose level; LDH level; Gram's stain; cytology; culture for bacteria, fungi, and viruses Pleural biopsy Transbronchial lung biopsy Open or thoracoscopic lung biopsy
Patients with abdominal symptoms or signs	Upper and lower endoscopy: biopsy; culture for bacteria, fungi, and viruses Contrast studies of upper and lower GI tract Ultrasonography of abdomen CT scan of abdomen Paracentesis or aspiration
Patients with urinary tract symptoms or signs	Ultrasonography of native and transplanted kidneys Cystoscopy
Patients with bone or joint symptoms or signs	Joint aspiration: cell count; glucose level; Gram's stain; culture for bacteria, fungi, and viruses

---

Table 3 Common Opportunistic Infectious Agents in Immunosuppressed Patients

Bacteria

Brucella species
Legionella species
Listeria monocytogenes
Mycobacterium avium–intracellulare
Nocardia asteroides
Mycobacterium tuberculosis
Salmonella species
Chlamydia species

Fungi

Aspergillus species
Candida species
Cryptococcus neoformans
Histoplasma capsulatum
Rhizopus species

Protozoa and parasites

Cryptosporidium species
Giardia lamblia
Isospora belli
Pneumocystis carinii
Strongyloides stercoralis
Toxoplasma gondii
Trypanosoma species

Viruses

Cytomegalovirus
Epstein-Barr virus
Herpes simplex
Herpes zoster

Sinusitis may present as fever and headache and can be diagnosed by means of radiographs, CT scanning, and aspiration. There are special problems in the diagnosis of gastrointestinal or abdominal infection in the immunosuppressed patient. Evaluation of the oropharynx and esophagus is performed by physical examination and endoscopy. Inspection of the mucosa and biopsy will usually yield a diagnosis of either candidal or viral (CMV or herpes simplex) esophagitis. Systemic treatment of either viral or fungal esophagitis is frequently necessary.

Inflammatory intra-abdominal conditions may not be revealed by history and physical examination. An absence of free intraperitoneal air is not enough to rule out perforation in immunosuppressed patients with infection. A contrast swallow with a water-soluble agent, followed by barium if initially negative, is a definitive test for upper intestinal perforation. A similar diagnostic approach is used for colon perforation. Ultrasonography or CT scanning is used to rule out fluid collections in the abdomen, which are almost invariably present in patients with acute abdominal diseases. Acalculous cholecystitis can be diagnosed by ultrasonography and treated by percutaneous drainage.[25] Paracentesis or radiologically guided aspiration may be useful in cases in which there is demonstrable intra-abdominal fluid but no clear indication for laparotomy [see Table 4].

Viral infections and hepatotoxic drugs such as azathioprine account for most episodes of hepatitis in immunocompromised patients. Most cases of hepatitis are clinically indolent, but hepatic failure and death from systemic opportunistic infection can occur.[26]

Infections in the genitourinary tract can usually be diagnosed by urinalysis, urine culture, and ultrasonography. In renal transplant recipients, infection can occur in either transplanted or native kidneys. Asymptomatic viral excretion in the urine is common after transplantation. Candiduria is also common, especially in diabetic immunosuppressed patients, but it usually reflects colonization rather than invasive infection [see VI:18 Fungal Infection].

Bone and joint infections are caused by either normal pathogens, mycobacterial organisms, or fungi. Persistent sampling of effusions with appropriate microbiological workup is needed.[27]

Management of Neutropenia

Neutropenic patients are a special challenge.[28] The most common cause of important neutropenia is chemotherapy. The white blood cell nadir usually occurs from 10 to 20 days after the start of chemotherapy. Infections produce few local signs of a septic response because there are not enough granulocytes to produce classic signs of inflammation or pus. Asymptomatic pneumonia may present with only slight abnormalities on x-ray. Similarly, urinary tract infection may produce bacteremia without significant symptoms. Mucocutaneous viral infections or dental caries can provide a portal of entry for gram-negative bacteria. Fungal superinfections are common and usually develop after broad-spectrum antibiotic treatment. Diagnosis of invasive fungal sepsis is sometimes difficult, and a clinical response to systemic antifungal treatment may be the best evidence that such an infection is present. Invasive fungal infection is often detected at autopsy.

Perirectal pain may occur in neutropenic patients and is usually caused by ulceration, fissure, or abscess. Diagnosis of a rectal abscess is difficult and may require observation of the clinical response to antibiotics and local treatment. Aspiration of the abscess, which usually yields watery fluid, or examination under anesthesia may be useful. Fluctuance is an indication for drainage.

Even without evidence of primary infection, bacteremia is common.[29] Most of the organisms implicated in bacteremia are derived from the patient's endogenous flora, some of which is acquired nosocomially. These findings suggest that bacteremia originates in the gut or from colonized body surfaces. The classic signs and symptoms of bacteremia are frequently absent in the leukopenic patient, who may present with only hyperventilation or an altered mental state. Immediate institution of broad-spectrum antibiotic therapy is indicated.

Leukocyte transfusions may be useful in the management of neutropenic patients.[29] Most neutrophil functions are preserved in storage up to 24 hours. Clinical studies of efficacy, however, have been hampered by problems of cell isolation and patient variability.[17] The use of colony-stimulating factors for reducing the duration and severity of neutropenia is more promising.[30]

To prevent neutropenic bacteremia, it may be useful to decontaminate the intestine by administering oral nonabsorbable antibiotics, such as combinations of oral nystatin, an aminoglycoside, and polymyxin, while the patient follows a diet containing foods of low bacterial content.[31] However, the benefit of this approach has not yet been proved. A total protected environment has been tried in the care of the neutropenic patient. Sterilized air is provided to the patient, who is decontaminated with skin antiseptics and nonabsorbable antibiotics. The room is sterilized with disinfectants. Although this approach reduces the number of infections, they still occur. At present, bone marrow transplant recipients are candidates for a protected

Table 4 Therapy for Opportunistic Infectious Agents in Immunosuppressed Patients

Organism	Recommended Agent
Central nervous system	
Cryptococcus neoformans	Amphotericin B plus flucytosine
Herpes simplex	Acyclovir
Listeria monocytogenes	Ampicillin or trimethoprim-sulfamethoxazole
Mycobacteria	Multiple drug combinations
Nocardia species	Sulfonamide
Toxoplasma gondii	Trisulfapyrimidines or sulfadiazine plus pyrimethamine
Varicella-zoster	Acyclovir
Gastrointestinal tract	
Cytomegalovirus	Ganciclovir
Cryptosporidium species	None available
Giardia lamblia	Quinacrine or metronidazole
Isospora belli	Trimethoprim-sulfamethoxazole
Salmonella species	Ciprofloxacin, ceftriaxone, trimethoprim-sulfamethoxazole, or chloramphenicol
Lungs	
Aspergillus species	Amphotericin B
Candida species	Fluconazole or amphotericin B
Cryptococcus neoformans	Amphotericin B plus flucytosine
Cytomegalovirus	Ganciclovir
Gram-negative bacteria	Aminoglycoside plus cephalosporin or aminoglycosides plus penicillin
Herpes simplex	Acyclovir
Histoplasma capsulatum	Amphotericin B
Legionella species	Erythromycin
Mycobacterium avium–intracellulare	Combined treatment with antituberculous and antimicrobial agents
Mycobacterium tuberculosis	Antituberculous agents
Pneumocystis carinii	Trimethoprim-sulfamethoxazole or pentamidine
Varicella-zoster	Acyclovir or vidarabine
Oropharynx and sinuses	
Aspergillus species	Fluconazole or amphotericin B
Candida species (esophagus)	Fluconazole or amphotericin B
Candida species (mouth)	Nystatin suspension, clotrimazole troches, oral ketoconazole, or oral fluconazole
Cytomegalovirus	Ganciclovir
Herpes simplex	Acyclovir
Rhizopus species	Fluconazole or amphotericin B
Strongyloides species	Thiabendazole
Skin	
Papillomavirus	Podophyllin, fluorouracil, or interferon
Varicella-zoster	Acyclovir

environment; indications for use in the care of other immunosuppressed patients have not yet been established.[31]

In the granulocytopenic patient, systemic infections with both gram-negative and gram-positive organisms occur. The early institution of empirical therapy before definitive identification of the infection site or causative organism will reduce the risk of mortality. Several antibiotic regimens have been shown to be effective. Patients who are neutropenic and febrile for more than one week while receiving antibacterial therapy should be considered to have a fungal infection and should be treated with systemic antifungal antibiotics. If no source of infection is found, treatment may be stopped when the neutrophil count has returned to normal. If a discrete focus is found, local treatment should be given and the antibiotic therapy continued.

Special acute abdominal conditions requiring surgical intervention occur in neutropenic patients. Neutropenic enterocolitis is characterized by fever, abdominal pain, and tenderness occurring during periods of neutropenia.[32] It is probably a bacterial infection of the wall of the large or small bowel. It may cause hemorrhage in the bowel wall, ischemia, and perforation, frequently accompanied by bacteremia. The condition is treated initially with bowel rest and antibiotics, but laparotomy should be done at any sign of clinical deterioration, an acute abdomen, or free air. Early recognition by frequent physical examination, abdominal radiography, and ultrasonography or CT scanning, followed by surgical intervention, will produce a better outcome than protracted nonoperative care. As is true for other causes of gastrointestinal perforation in the immunocompromised patient, resection and exteriorization is preferred to anastomosis unless conditions are optimal in terms of the patient's condition, expected course of neutropenia, timing after perforation, spillage, and degree of peritoneal reaction.[33]

Evaluation of Patients before Immunosuppressive Therapy

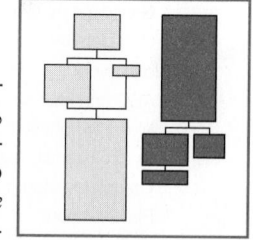

An immunosuppressed state is sometimes deliberately created—for example, to prevent allograft rejection in transplant recipients. Such patients undergo a preimmunosuppression workup [*see Table 5*] that has six objectives: full investigation of the primary disease, optimization of physiologic status, treatment of infections, discovery of occult malignancy, minimization of risk of posttransplant complications, and complete psychological, social, and financial evaluation. Details of the first and last objectives are not considered here. For the other objectives, an organ systems approach is used.

The presence of active invasive infection or active malignant disease is a contraindication to transplantation and immunosuppressive therapy. It is not yet known how much time should elapse between treatment of malignancy and the beginning of immunosuppressive therapy. It seems reasonable to wait until recurrence of malignancy is unlikely, prove that the patient is free of tumor, and proceed after advising the patient that immunosuppressive medication may reactivate malignancy.

Transplantation is also inadvisable when the patient's physiologic state predicts operative mortality, when the anatomic setting is inadequate for technical success, and when the patient has severe psychological, social, or financial problems without evident support or solution.

Table 5 Components of Preimmunosuppression Workup

History
  Review of underlying disease
  Surgical history
    Peptic ulcer surgery
    Cholecystectomy
    Nephrectomy
    Splenectomy
    Cardiac surgery
  Medical history
    Cardiac disease
    Pulmonary disease
    Renal disease
    Parenchymal disease
    Urosepsis
    Gastrointestinal disease
    Cholelithiasis
    Peptic ulcer disease
    Infectious diseases
    Malignancies
    Blood transfusions
    Vaccinations
      Hepatitis B
      Pneumococcal polysaccharide
    Review of current medications
Physical examination
  General examination
  Neurologic examination
  Cardiopulmonary examination
  Abdominal examination
  Breast examination
  Genitourinary examination
  Complete skin examination
Blood work
  ABO and HLA type
  Mixed lymphocyte culture
  Cytotoxic antibody determination
  Complete blood count
  Platelet count
  Prothrombin time and partial thromboplastin time
  Bleeding time
  Electrolytes, urea nitrogen, and creatinine
  Serum calcium and phosphate
  Hepatic enzymes and bilirubin
  Serum albumin, transferrin, and total protein

  Serum protein electrophoresis
  Uric acid, cholesterol, and triglycerides
  Arterial blood gases
  Hepatitis B surface antigen, hepatitis B antibody and core antibody
  Cytomegalovirus, herpes simplex virus, herpes zoster virus, and Epstein-Barr virus titers
  Human immunodeficiency virus test
  VDRL
Radiologic studies
  Chest radiography
  Upper gastrointestinal series
  Gallbladder ultrasonography
  Barium enema
  Voiding cystourethrography
  Doppler examination of abdominal vessels
  Skeletal survey
  Coronary angiography
  Sinus radiography
  CT scan of head, chest, or abdomen
Nuclear medicine scans
  Thallium stress test
  Myocardial kinetic scan
  Liver-spleen scan
  Bone densitometry scan
Other studies and tests
  Electrocardiography
  Treadmill test
  Pulmonary function studies
  Noninvasive vascular laboratory studies
  Urinalysis
  Creatinine clearance
  Quantitative protein excretion
  Hormonal studies
  Occult blood screening
  Upper or lower endoscopy
  Cystometry
  DTH skin testing (includes PPD)
  Pap smear and cervical swab for herpes
  Examination of stool for bacteria, ova, and parasites
  Cultures of urine, stool, and throat for viruses and bacterial pathogens
  Dental consultation
  Ophthalmologic consultation
  Neurologic evaluation
  Psychosocioeconomic consultation

NERVOUS SYSTEM

Examination of the central and peripheral nervous systems should be supplemented by diagnostic tests as indicated to investigate degenerative, vascular, malignant, or infectious processes. The brain and spinal cord can be evaluated by CT and MRI scanning. Cerebrospinal fluid examination may be necessary to rule out demyelinating diseases or infections. Electromyography or the study of visually evoked potentials is necessary in some cases. Ophthalmologic examination should be performed to rule out infectious processes in the eye and to determine the state of the fundus and optic nerve before immunosuppressive therapy is begun. Visual field testing may be useful in the diagnosis of demyelinating diseases and other disease states. Autonomic nervous function is assessed with tests of gastric emptying, the presence or absence of orthostatic hypotension, and heart-rate responses to standing, the Valsalva maneuver, and deep inspiration.

CARDIOVASCULAR SYSTEM

History and physical examination of the heart should focus on determining the presence of intrinsic heart or valvular disease and the functional state of the cardiovascular system. If the cardiac history reveals ischemic heart disease or underlying disease with accelerated atherosclerosis, a treadmill or thallium exercise test should be done. Cardiac performance should also be measured with a gated scan. Because extensive cardiac morbidity occurs after transplantation, preoperative coronary angiography should be considered in patients with a positive cardiac history. At present, however, it is unknown whether the indications for coronary artery dilatation or bypass surgery are different for pretransplant patients than for other patients with ischemic heart disease. The peripheral vascular system is also evaluated. Ischemia in upper and lower extremities should be corrected if possible to diminish the risk of infection in the extremities and a septic response. Carotid arteries should be examined and tested according to usual criteria.

RESPIRATORY SYSTEM

The respiratory system must be able to survive operation and must be free from infection and malignancy. Evaluation should include a chest x-ray, pulmonary function tests, and, if indicated, bronchoscopy, CT scanning of the chest, and lung biopsy. Patients with a history of bronchopulmonary disease must be in the best possible condition before operation. Preoperative chest physiotherapy, bronchodilators, and antibiotics are used to ensure fitness [see VI:1 Pulmonary Insufficiency].

DIGESTIVE SYSTEM

Evaluation of the digestive system begins with dental consultation. Necessary dental work should be performed before immunosuppression. This work frequently involves multiple extractions to minimize the risk of oral infection.

The esophagus may be examined with either contrast radiography or endoscopy. Candidal esophagitis, which is likely to worsen after immunosuppression, should be treated with nystatin, ketoconazole, or, in severe cases, systemic amphotericin B.[34] Disruption of the esophageal mucosal barrier resulting from reflux esophagitis should be decreased with the usual antireflux treatments.

There is no clear solution to the problem of peptic ulcer disease in potential transplant recipients. Available data are from renal transplant studies.[35] The risk of posttransplant ulcer complications is five to 10 percent, but this risk is doubled in patients who have a pretransplant history of peptic ulcer disease.[36] Mortality in those who develop such complications is high.[34] Various protocols have been used for prophylactic gastric surgery. It is not clear, however, that the rate of posttransplant gastroduodenal complications can be decreased by prophylactic surgery.[36] Antacid prophylaxis, however, probably is effective. Although potentially immunostimulatory, cimetidine has also been used effectively for ulcer prevention.[35] Until further data have been accumulated, the following measures are recommended. In asymptomatic patients, routine workup for peptic ulcer disease is optional. Good-risk patients with a definite history of recurrent or complicated ulcer disease should have acid-reducing surgery before immunosuppressive therapy is initiated. Other patients with inactive ulcer disease may be treated with cimetidine before and after transplantation, and all patients should receive antacid prophylaxis.

Prophylactic cholecystectomy has been suggested for patients with asymptomatic gallstones. The justification for this procedure is to eliminate the risk of postoperative cholecystitis and to avoid possible diagnostic confusion in cases in which jaundice or pancreatitis develops after transplantation. In one study, pretransplant cholecystectomy was associated with a lower incidence of morbidity and mortality than surgical treatment for complications of cholelithiasis after transplantation.[37] However, this approach is not universally accepted at present.

Although postoperative pancreatitis is known to occur after transplantation and immunosuppression,[35] there is no predictive or preventive preoperative workup. The functional status of the liver should be evaluated with blood tests and CT scanning if necessary. The presence of infectious or noninfectious hepatitis should be determined by serologic studies, and disease activity should be staged by follow-up blood tests, biopsy, or both.

Infectious or malignant disease of the colon should be ruled out. Screening tests include stool culture, examination for ova and parasites, and tests for occult blood. If test results are positive, barium enema or colonoscopy (or both) is indicated. Digital examination of the rectum is performed to find local pathological lesions, such as fissures, hemorrhoids, or malignant tumors, that may require treatment before the transplantation procedure is undertaken.

GENITOURINARY SYSTEM

Renal function is evaluated by measurement of creatinine clearance, quantitative tests for proteinuria, and renal biopsy if necessary [see VII:5 Renal Failure]. Upper and lower urinary tract infections must be treated. In the case of renal transplantation, pretransplant bilateral nephrectomy may be necessary to eliminate a potential source of infection. Indications for nephrectomy include pyelonephritis and severe ureterovesical reflux, with dilatation of the renal pelvis. Lesser degrees of ureterovesical reflux, polycystic kidney disease, and hypertension are less frequent indications.[38] Bladder infections in anuric patients may be treated with systemic antibiotics with or without antibiotic irrigation.

In women, a gynecologic examination, including a Papanicolaou test and cervical swab for bacterial and viral pathogens, should be performed before immunosuppressive therapy.

MUSCULOSKELETAL SYSTEM AND ENDOCRINE SYSTEM

Steroids occasionally cause avascular necrosis of the hip.[35] Existing skeletal disorders should be studied before transplantation. A suggestive history or physical signs of thyroid or adrenal hyperfunction or hypofunction should be followed by laboratory testing. Thyroid nodules, which are potentially malignant, should be a special focus of physical examination. In some potential recipients, assessment of calcium metabolism with parathyroid hormone assays, skeletal surveys, and bone scans is indicated.

DERMAL SYSTEM

The entire body surface should be examined for malignancies and present or potential sources of infection. All boils and other skin infections should be treated before transplantation. Diffuse skin diseases such as psoriasis should be as fully treated as possible. Anal condylomata, which may contain squamous cell carcinoma, should be removed.[39] Diabetic patients and those with peripheral vascular disease are especially likely to acquire foot infections and should have their feet evaluated. They should be instructed to wear loose-fitting shoes, trim toenails square, and apply lanolin creams frequently.

HEMATOLOGIC SYSTEM

Complete blood count and peripheral smear should be done; abnormal results may call for a bone marrow examination. If the patient has undergone splenectomy or if an underlying disease has resulted in splenic dysfunction, the patient should receive pneumococcal and meningococcal polysaccharide vaccines.

IMMUNE SYSTEM

Unless there is evidence of primary immunodeficiency, little specific treatment is currently available for abnormal immunity. A comprehensive workup before deliberate immunosuppressive therapy is therefore not useful. If desired, however, the acquired immune abnormalities associated with organ failure could be studied [see Table 1].

INFECTIOUS DISEASES

The patient should be examined and treated for bacterial, fungal, viral, and protozoan diseases. Bacterial infections of the CNS, lungs, blood, urinary system, and skin require conventional surgical and antibiotic treatment.

Mycobacterial Infection

Mycobacterial infections are of special concern. Administration of steroids to a patient with latent tuberculosis may precipitate active infection. Patients are screened by history; physical examination of the neck, chest, and abdomen; chest and bone x-rays; urinalysis and urine culture; and skin testing. Active tuberculosis should be treated with conventional therapy: double or triple chemotherapy for 24 months before transplantation, if possible. Patients with positive tuberculin skin tests but no evidence of active infection are given prophylactic isoniazid after immunosuppressive medication is started.

Fungal Infection

Most fungal infections occur in patients who are already seriously immunosuppressed. Candidal esophagitis and cystitis, however, may occur in patients awaiting transplants who are not severely immunosuppressed, especially diabetic patients and patients receiving antibiotics. Oral nystatin may be effective in mild cases of candidal esophagitis, but severe candidal esophagitis should be treated with ketoconazole or with a short course of systemic amphotericin B. Candidal cystitis requires correction of motor abnormalities of the bladder, if possible [see VI:18 Fungal Infection].

Viral Infection

The experience of the recipient's immune system with viral infections can be evaluated serologically. Titers of antibody to CMV, herpes simplex virus (HSV), varicella-zoster virus (VZV), Epstein-Barr virus (EBV), hepatitis B surface antigen (HB_sAg), and human immunodeficiency virus (HIV) are determined. CMV titers may influence the subsequent management of immuno suppression or prophylaxis against CMV. Titers to herpes simplex virus and varicella-zoster virus are mostly useful as baseline measurements for later testing. A positive titer for HB_sAg requires complete evaluation of liver function. It has not been established, however, whether patients with negative tests for HB_sAg should be vaccinated against hepatitis B. A positive test for HIV has a controversial impact. Asymptomatic individuals who are positive for HIV have a life expectancy that may justify transplantation with lifesaving organs such as the heart or liver. As in other patients with similar life expectancy, transplantation may not be justifiable when the organ failure can be treated by other means.

Foreign Bodies

Peritonitis in peritoneal dialysis patients should be treated [see VI:15 Peritonitis and Intra-abdominal Abscesses]; if the infection resolves, transplantation is not contraindicated. If bacterial infections arise around implanted devices, the devices often must be removed before the infection will resolve. In some patients, persistent local infection of hemodialysis shunts, indwelling bladder catheters, and Tenckhoff catheters may be treated by removal of the devices at the time of transplantation and administration of systemic antibiotics.

Local infection around transcutaneous foreign bodies, such as shunts and catheters, can become systemic after immunosuppression or may result in diffuse skin colonization, increasing the risk of wound infection. If possible, all such transcutaneous devices should be removed or local infection controlled before immunosuppression. If only bacterial colonization is present, it is reasonable to remove the device involved at the time of transplantation and to begin antibiotic therapy.

NUTRITIONAL STATE

Malnutrition is frequently present in patients with organ failure and generally worsens the outcome of operation. Despite the lack of clear data, it seems reasonable, when possible, to determine and correct the patient's nutritional state before transplantation. DTH skin testing, anthropometry, measurement of serum proteins, and body composition studies are used to evaluate the patient's nutritional status preoperatively. Treatment may include tube feeding or parenteral nutrition to restore body cell mass before transplantation [see VII:9 Nutritional Support].

PSYCHOLOGICAL, SOCIAL, AND FINANCIAL ASSESSMENT

Potential organ recipients must be psychologically, socially, and financially capable of undergoing transplantation. Discrete criteria depend on the organ being transplanted, local programs for care and support of transplant patients, and availability of financial assistance.

Discussion

Abnormalities of Systemic Immunity in Specific Diseases

PRIMARY IMMUNODEFICIENCY

Primary immunodeficiencies are viewed as defects in cellular differentiation and are classified according to whether the most prominent defect is in neutrophil or T or B cell function. More than 70 such syndromes have been described, but the cumulative prevalence of clinically important cases is approximately one for every 10,000 persons in the population. Approximately half of all primary immunodeficiencies are related to B cell dysfunction, one third to T cell abnormalities, and the remainder to neutrophil or complement deficiencies[40] [*see Table 6*].

Disorders affecting mainly B cell function are characterized by deficiencies in all or some immunoglobulin isotypes with concomitant inability to produce specific antibody responses after vaccination. The clinical presentation is variable, depending on the degree of deficiency and type of immunoglobulin involved. Recurrent pyogenic infections are caused by pneumococci, streptococci, and *Hemophilus* organisms. The most common infections are pneumonia, bronchiectasis, sinusitis, meningitis, and septicemia. Treatment consists of antibiotics and replacement therapy with human immunoglobulin. IgG levels should be raised to between 1 and 3 g/L, which may be done preoperatively.

Cellular immunodeficiency diseases are characterized by an increased incidence of fungal and viral infections, failure to thrive, and an increased incidence of malignancy. Treatment of these conditions yields less satisfactory results than does treatment of B cell defects. There is little experience with surgery in these persons.

ACQUIRED IMMUNODEFICIENCY

The practicing surgeon is unlikely to encounter cases of primary immunodeficiency; most immunosuppression in surgi-

Table 6 Primary Immunodeficiency Diseases

Disorder	Defective Component or Function	Probable Pathogenesis
Predominantly B cell defect		
X-linked agammaglobulinemia	All immunoglobulin classes	Impaired maturation of B cells
Autosomal recessive agammaglobulinemia	All immunoglobulin classes	Impaired maturation of B cells
Immunoglobulin deficiency with increased IgM	IgG	Impaired maturation of B cells
Selective IgA deficiency	IgA	Immature IgA B cells
IgG subclass deficiencies	IgG subclasses	?
IgM deficiency	IgM	?
Common variable agammaglobulinemia	All immunoglobulin classes	Impaired differentiation of plasma cells, presence of autoantibodies, imbalance in regulatory T cells
Predominantly T cell defect		
Severe combined immunodeficiency	Antibodies and T cells	?
Thymic hypoplasia	T cells	Abnormal embryologic development
Cellular immunodeficiency with thymoma	T cells and B cells	?
Wiskott-Aldrich syndrome	Antibodies and T cells	?
Ataxia-telangiectasia	Antibodies and T cells	Impaired maturation of T cells
Chronic mucocutaneous candidiasis	T cells	?
Predominantly neutrophil defect		
Neutrophil dysfunction with high IgE levels	Chemotaxis	?
Actin dysfunction	Phagocyte motility	Actin dysfunction
Glycoprotein deficiency	Phagocyte motility	Glycoprotein deficiency
Chronic granulomatous disease	Microbicidal activity	Enzyme deficiency
Glucose-6-phosphate dehydrogenase deficiency	Miicrobicidal activity	Enzyme deficiency
Myeloperoxidase deficiency	Microbicidal activity	Enzyme deficiency
Chédiak-Higashi syndrome	Microbicidal activity	Lysosomal defect
Leukocyte adhesion deficiency	Cell adhesion molecule deficiency	?
Complement defect		
Deficiency of complement components	Complement function	?
Dysfunction of C1 inhibitor, C3 inactivator, or C5	Complement function	?

Table 7 **Effect of Illness, Injury, or Treatment on Host Defense Mechanisms**

Condition	Local Immunity	T Cell Function	B Cell Function	Phagocytic Function	Complement
Primary immunodeficiencies	↓	↓	↓	↓	↓
Secondary (acquired) immunodeficiencies					
Age	NC	↓	↓	NC	NC
Obesity	↓	?	?	↓	?
Malnutrition	NC	↓	↑ or ↓	↓	↓
Malignancy	NC	↓	↓	NC	NC
Thermal injury	↓	↓	↑ or ↓	↓	↓
Septic response	↓	↓	?	↓	?
Diabetes mellitus	↓	↓	?	↓	?
Renal failure	NC	↓	NC or ↓	↓	?
Liver disease	NC	↓	↓	?	?
Protein-losing diseases	NC	↓	↓	NC	?
Foreign bodies	↓	NC	NC	NC	?
Drugs	NC	↓	↑ or ↓	↓	?
Radiation	↓	?	?	?	?
Trauma or operation	↓	↓	?	↓	?
Anesthesia	NC	↓	?	↓	?
Blood transfusion	NC	↓	?	?	?
Splenectomy	NC	NC	↓	↓	?

NC—no change

cal patients is acquired secondary to disease processes or medical interventions. As mentioned, all or nearly all surgical patients are immunosuppressed to some degree. The nature of the immunodeficiency present in specific conditions or disorders will determine the therapeutic response [see Table 7].

Preexisting Conditions

Age Study of immune alterations in elderly persons is often complicated by the presence of malnutrition. There is a range of age-related changes in the immune system, including changes in both T and B cell function. Lymphopenia is not a feature of old age, but there is a decrease in the number of circulating T cells; in vitro T cell function may be normal or decreased in elderly patients.[41] Serum immunoglobulin levels are normal, and specific antibody responses are decreased.[42] These changes may indicate a tendency to produce more nonspecific immunoglobulin with age because of changes in helper-suppressor T cell function.[43] Chemotaxis and the number of polymorphonuclear neutrophils are normal.[44] The metabolic activity of polymorphonuclear neutrophils is decreased only in persons with evidence of malnutrition.

Obesity Obesity is also associated with abnormalities in host defense. Local wound defense is altered, resulting in the well-known increased risk of wound infections in obese patients [see VI:5 Obesity]. There may also be alterations in systemic immunity, with changes in neutrophil and lymphocyte function.[45]

Medical Conditions

Malnutrition Malnutrition is present in a high percentage of surgical patients. The nature of the immune aberrations in a particular patient depends on the type and extent of malnutrition. Malnutrition predisposes to infection and vice versa. Vitamin and mineral deficiencies that result from malnutrition impair cell-mediated immunity. A lack of protein calories is associated with involution of lymphoid tissue, decreased DTH responses, decreased circulating T cells, abnormal lymphocyte responses in vitro, and changes in cytotoxicity assays and lymphokine production.[8] Thus, defects are found in most tests of T cell function in malnourished patients.

There is, however, no consistent change in B cell function in malnutrition.[8] Circulating numbers of B cells are normal. Serum immunoglobulin levels have been reported in various studies to be normal, elevated, or reduced—a disparity that may be explained by the relation of these levels to intercurrent infection in malnourished patients.

The most important aspect of B cell function—the capacity to produce a specific antibody response to vaccination—has also been studied in malnutrition. Although the capacity to respond to previously encountered antigens may be unimpaired, the response to new antigens is probably reduced. Even short-term acute nutritional deprivation decreases humoral immunity in animal models.[46] Restoring proper nutrition probably restores antibody reactivity quickly.

Although neutropenia is not a feature of malnutrition, defects in polymorphonuclear neutrophil functions, such as chemotaxis and bacterial killing, have been reported.[8] Restoring proper nutrition in malnourished patients can restore killing function. Serum levels of some components of the complement cascade are reduced.[8] Whether this decrease causes a functional defect is unknown.

Malignancy   There are changes in general immunity related to the presence of malignancy as well as complications (e.g., malnutrition) in the host.[9] DTH changes correlate with staging and prognosis. Altered humoral immunity occurs in hematologic and visceral malignancies. Monocyte chemotaxis is reduced, but no major changes in PMN or complement function are known.

Thermal injury   Besides the evident severe disruptions in local host defense, serious systemic changes in immune function occur after thermal injury [*see III:13 Burn Care after the First Postburn Week*]. Changes are more pronounced in cellular than in humoral mechanisms. Circulating T cells are reduced, and ratios of helper to suppressor T cells are changed. DTH responses are reduced, and such changes are clearly correlated with survival. The presence of suppressors of lymphocyte function and monocyte chemotaxis in the serum has been shown. Changes in antibody responses are variable. Data from human burn patients show a functioning humoral immune system, whereas animal studies show decreased or increased responsiveness. There are definite alterations in PMN function: chemotaxis and bacterial killing are reduced. Complement levels decrease, but such declines probably have little significance.

Septic response   In human studies, it is difficult to identify the primary effects of the septic response, with or without infection, on the immune system. It is clear, however, that the surgical resolution of infection can restore some aspects of immune reactivity.[17]

Diabetes mellitus   The local tissue changes caused by neuropathy and angiopathy markedly increase susceptibility to sepsis in diabetic patients. Ischemic areas are susceptible to mixed aerobic and anaerobic infections. Other bacterial and fungal infections are also more common in diabetic patients. Diabetes causes systemic alterations in immunity as well. The ratios of helper to suppressor T cells are altered,[47] and there are defects in monocyte and PMN chemotaxis.[48] Antibody responses are normal.[49]

Renal failure   Both local and systemic derangements contribute to infections in uremic patients. Skin disorders and sensory neuropathy caused by renal failure produce changes in local host defense mechanisms. Lymphoid tissue shrinks, lymphopenia occurs, and DTH reactions are reduced.[50] Impaired in vitro lymphocyte function has been reported in some cases; it may be caused by an inhibitory effect of uremic serum. Humoral immunity is better preserved.[51] Serum immunoglobulin levels are normal. Specific antibody responses are either normal or reduced. Studies of PMN function have shown that adherence and chemotaxis have been reduced but may improve with dialysis.[50] Peritoneal dialysis may be more effective than hemodialysis in reversing some uremia-induced changes in the immune system.[51]

Liver disease   Chronic liver disease is a heterogeneous group of illnesses frequently accompanied by malnutrition. Studies of immunity have shown decreased numbers of lymphocytes and T cells[52] but normal antibody responses.[53]

Protein-losing diseases   Severe protein loss may lead to decreased serum immunoglobulin levels as well as to many of the other immune manifestations of malnutrition.

Medical and Surgical Intervention

Foreign bodies   As mentioned earlier, invasive monitoring devices and permanently implanted foreign bodies impair local host defenses. They may disrupt normally protective surfaces and act as conduits for bacteria from external surfaces. Bacteria can also be protected in a glycocalyx on the surface of implants, and phagocytosis may be limited by increased bacterial adherence to prosthetic surfaces. Even though systemic alterations in immunity are absent, the presence of foreign bodies may produce serious infection and a septic response. Sterile techniques and care in the use of monitoring devices and implanted foreign bodies serve as preventive measures. Technology now in development, such as antibiotic-bonded vascular prostheses, may limit infectious complications even further.

Drugs   Important immunosuppressive medications include chemotherapeutic agents, corticosteroids, cyclosporine, and antilymphocyte antibodies. Chemotherapeutic agents differ in their mechanism of action. Alkylating agents cross-link DNA, thus limiting the division of proliferating cells. Antimetabolites interfere with nucleic acid synthesis, and antibiotics with antitumor activity block RNA synthesis. The tissues at greatest risk for toxicity are those with actively dividing cells—namely, the gastrointestinal epithelium and bone marrow. The most important toxic effect of chemotherapy on host defense is leukopenia. The nadir of white cell counts is variable but usually occurs between 10 and 20 days after initiation of drug treatment. The risk of infection is increased when the absolute neutrophil count is less than 1,500/mm^3 and increases even further when the count is less than 500/mm^3.[54] Toxicity of gastrointestinal epithelium often produces mucositis, which may be a portal of entry for pathogens in some bacteremias. Also, bowel perforation may occur in the treatment of lymphomas that involve the bowel wall.

Corticosteroids are used in the management of conditions such as inflammatory bowel disease, arthritis, and transplantation. Both local and systemic host defenses are affected. Skin is abnormal, and wound healing is delayed.[55]

The most important impact of steroids on systemic immunity is the decrease in leukocyte accumulation at inflammatory sites.[56] The mechanism involved is probably a combination of effects on vascular endothelium and inflammatory cells. Although steroid administration can produce leukocytosis by prolonging the half-life of leukocytes and increasing their release from the marrow, leukocyte adherence is decreased. PMN chemotaxis is preserved, but monocyte chemotaxis is depressed. Consequently, the whole cascade of responses leading to local manifestations of infection is slowed. These effects result in late presentation of serious infections because of diminished clinical signs. Lymphocyte function—especially that of T cells—is also altered by steroid administration.[56] Lymphopenia occurs because of T cell redistribution, with a minor amount of lysis of some groups of T cells. Lymphocyte proliferation is decreased, probably because of diminished interleukin synthesis. Although serum levels of immunoglobulins decline, in vitro immunoglobulin synthesis is either normal or increased by steroids.[57] Antibody responses to vaccination are preserved.

The mechanism of action of corticosteroids is unknown. Likely possibilities include effects on membrane stabilization, prostaglandin metabolism, interleukin synthesis, and free radical mechanisms. Some of these effects may be diminished by administration of prednisone on alternate days instead of daily.

In practice, steroid administration has several important effects.[33] As mentioned, wound healing is slowed, and the ability of parietal cavities to localize infection is reduced. In clinical practice, fascial closures must therefore be secure. Skin stitches should be left in place 50 to 100 percent longer than in normal patients. In the treatment of abdominal infection, peritoneal cleaning should be thorough. For small- and large-bowel perforation, preference should be given to resection and exteriorization rather than to unprotected anastomosis. Duodenal perforation can be managed in the normal manner. It is unclear whether additional ulcer operation should be performed at the same time as closure; assessment should be done on a patient-by-patient basis and should include natural history of the underlying disease, previous treatments, and history of ulcer disease.

Cyclosporine is almost universally used for immunosuppression in transplant recipients. It has little effect on local inflammatory reactions. Lymphocyte accumulation in lymph nodes is decreased, however, and in vitro tests of T and B cell function are abnormal.

Antilymphocyte antibodies are used to prevent or treat allograft rejection in transplant patients. They are either polyclonal heterosera or rodent monoclonal antibodies. Monoclonal antibodies have a uniform antigen specificity. The most commonly used monoclonal antibody at present is OKT3, which is specific for T cell receptors. Polyclonal heterosera manifest various specificities against mononuclear cells. The mechanism of action of antilymphocyte antibodies is probably the elimination of target cells by lysis. As with other immunosuppressive medication, risk of infection increases with cumulative dosage.

Radiation   Local radiation impairs host defenses by affecting tissue vascularity, mucocutaneous barriers, and wound healing. The toxic effect of total-body irradiation on bone marrow is well known. A total-body exposure of approximately 300 rads results in 50 percent mortality.[58] Although leukopenia occurs within days, the highest risk for infection is between two and six weeks after irradiation, during the nadir of white cell counts. There is little information regarding the effect on the systemic immune system of localized therapeutic radiation, but local host defenses can be impaired.

Trauma and operation   Trauma and operation are complex processes whose effects on the immune system are complicated by those of underlying disease, tissue injury, neuroendocrine activation, general anesthesia, and blood transfusion. Sepsis or malnutrition may also supervene.

Total lymphocyte count, total number of T cells, skin-test reactivity, and in vitro T cell tests are all depressed by surgical intervention.[8] Although serum immunoglobulins are decreased, probably by dilution, there are few data on antibody responses. After vaccination with the recall antigen tetanus toxoid, only 17 to 53 percent of surgical patients produced specific antibody; their response depended on their overall clinical condition.[13] The response to pneumococcal polysaccharide antigen was better.[14] These surgical patients, however, may have various underlying medical disorders and hence many possible reasons for altered host defense. The primary effect of injury or surgery on antibody responsiveness is unknown. Neutrophil chemotaxis is depressed soon after trauma, and this change is associated with a suppressive serum factor.[59]

Anesthesia   General anesthetic agents cause a short-term depression of in vitro tests of T cell function.[60] Regional anesthesia has a lesser impact. The difference in impact may be related to differential effects of the two forms of anesthesia on the neuroendocrine system. Studies have shown definite depression of PMN function caused by anesthesia, but there are few data on effects on the humoral immune system.[61] Any depression of antibody responses produced by anesthesia, however, may have very important clinical implications. For example, a depressed antibody response may be significant in cases in which intestinal contents spill into the peritoneal cavity shortly before or during a laparotomy under anesthesia, because this event may be the first antigenic encounter of some patients with potential future pathogens.

Blood transfusion   Although the immunosuppressive effect of blood transfusions has become evident in transplant recipients and cancer patients,[62] it is not clear how susceptibility to infections is affected. Volume of blood transfused relates inversely to outcome in trauma patients, a relation that probably reflects the severity of the injury. Transfusion may exert an independent immunosuppressive effect in these patients as well, however. In principle, blood loss during surgery should be minimized in this already immunosuppressed population.

Splenectomy   The spleen plays two important roles in the immune system.[63] It functions as a filter to remove encapsulated, poorly opsonized bacteria, and it is a site of antibody synthesis. Although it is unclear whether loss of the spleen as an antibody-producing organ is important, splenectomy does cause loss of the phagocytic function, which in turn predisposes to the septic response. The syndrome of overwhelming infection may occur after splenectomy regardless of the reason for the operation, but it is more common when splenectomy is performed to treat a hematologic disorder. The syndrome is characterized by a septic response with shock, disseminated intravascular coagulation, and a high mortality, without evidence of local tissue infection. The usual organisms implicated are pneumococcus, meningococcus, and *Hemophilus*.[64]

Preoperative care of the patient who is undergoing splenectomy focuses on the nature and timing of operation and vaccination, antibiotic prophylaxis, and patient instruction. After traumatic injury, nonoperative treatment or splenic salvage procedures should be performed if possible. Splenic reimplantation has not yet been shown to be effective and is not routinely performed. Vaccination with pneumococcal and meningococcal polysaccharide should be performed before splenectomy if possible. Prophylactic antibiotics may be indicated, especially in patients splenectomized for hematologic diseases, but such prophylaxis is not uniformly practiced. Finally, the patient and family should be instructed to seek medical attention promptly for febrile illnesses, and the patient should carry identification as a postsplenectomy patient.

Malignancy as a Complication of Immunosuppressive Therapy

Immunosuppressive medication, whether given for suppression of allograft rejection or as other medical therapy, is associated with an increase in malignancy.[65,66] Overall, neoplasms develop in approximately six percent of organ transplant recipients. The cause of the increased incidence of malignancy in immunosuppressed patients may be viral transformation of host cells, chronic antigenic stimulation, administration of carcinogenic medications, or impaired immunosurveillance. Lymphoid malignancies are clearly increased, although it does not appear that visceral tumors are increased. Some lymphoid malignancies are associated with evidence of viral infection, which may be a cause.[67] Some organ transplant recipients in whom malignancy develops show lower immune responses than do recipients who are free of cancer.[68,69] The pattern of malignancy may vary with different immunosuppressive regimens.[70] Compared with patients receiving prednisone-azathioprine therapy, those on cyclosporine therapy experience a higher incidence of lymphoma and Kaposi's sarcoma but a lower incidence of gynecologic cancer. The biologic behavior of tumors in immunosuppressed patients may be different from that of tumors in patients who are otherwise well.

Several polyclonal and monoclonal lymphoproliferative diseases have a viral etiology. Most originate in B cells. EBV antigen and nuclear material have been demonstrated in involved tissue.[67] The spectrum of disorders ranges from benign polyclonal hyperplasias to malignant monoclonal lymphomas.[71] Benign polyclonal hyperplasias respond to acyclovir without change in immunosuppression. Malignant monoclonal lymphomas are resistant to acyclovir and respond poorly to any treatment, suggesting that they are independent of viral replication. Diseases that fall between these extremes respond to acyclovir, but their management also requires reduced immunosuppression to prevent progression to a more malignant form.

Anogenital carcinomas are a special problem in transplant recipients,[39] in whom incidence is 100 times normal; the carcinomas occur from one to 15 years after transplantation and range from carcinoma in situ to metastatic disease. Treatment is conventional. A viral etiology is suggested by the association of these lesions with condylomata acuminata. Carcinoma may be an incidental pathological finding in condylomata that are excised after transplantation. Therefore, the location of all such specimens should be marked, and they should be examined by the pathologist.

Table 8 Manifestations of Glucocorticoid Insufficiency

Weakness and easy fatigability
Weight loss, anorexia
Nausea, vomiting, diarrhea
Depression
Fever
Postural or general hypotension
Muscle weakness
Delayed tendon reflexes
Low voltage on ECG
Hyponatremia
Neutropenia
Eosinophilia

The incidence of skin cancer in transplant recipients varies from 10 to 40 percent, depending on degree of pretransplant and posttransplant sun exposure.[72] Prevention involves avoidance of sun exposure and the use of sunscreens, although the latter is not of proven benefit. Treatment is conventional, with excision or irradiation as the mainstay of treatment. In addition, reduction of the dosage of azathioprine has been tried. No good treatment exists for the occasional patient with multiple, recurrent skin cancers.

Perioperative Glucocorticoid Management in Patients Treated with Steroids

Corticosteroids are necessary for normal organ function. They are produced by the adrenal cortex and controlled by the hypothalamic-pituitary-adrenal axis. Adrenal insufficiency is a serious, potentially lethal illness. The circulating corticosteroid level increases in response to stress, including trauma, operation, and anesthesia. The mechanism of action of glucocorticoids in the stress response is not yet fully understood. Knowledge of the interactions between cytokines and glucocorticoids is increasing, however, and it is likely that counterregulatory roles in the stress response will be defined for the adrenal hormone.

The hormonal response to stress includes increases in adrenocorticotropic hormone (ACTH), blood cortisol levels, and

Table 9 Perioperative Glucocorticoid Coverage

Surgical Procedure	Maximal Cortisol Production	Duration of Stress Response	Steroid Coverage (Hydrocortisone or Equivalent) Preoperative (Total, Including Usual Dose)	Postoperative
Minor	25 mg/day	Minimal	25 mg	Usual dose
Moderate	50–75 mg/day	1–2 days	50–75 mg	50–75 mg for 1 day, then usual dose
Major	100–150 mg/day	2–5 days	100–150 mg	50 mg every 8 hr for 1 day, then 25 mg every 8 hr for 1–4 days, then usual dose

urinary cortisol secretion. Although individual variability is substantial, it is possible to describe a spectrum of responses in terms of both the amount of cortisol produced and the duration of stress-induced increases in cortisol levels. The normal daily production of cortisol is 25 to 30 mg a day. Persons who undergo operation of less than one hour's duration under local anesthesia have minimal to no change in glucocorticoid excretion. Maximal amounts produced after major operation are between 100 and 150 mg a day. The increase is measurable one hour postoperatively and reaches maximal levels within the first 24 hours. Levels quickly return to normal, often within 48 hours but in all cases within five days unless complications occur. In surgical stress of a moderate degree, the daily production of cortisol increases to 50 to 75 mg a day and returns to a normal level within 24 hours.[73]

Adrenal insufficiency may be primary or secondary. Primary adrenal insufficiency is a result of adrenocortical failure and therefore includes both glucocorticoid and mineralocorticoid deficiency. The causes of primary insufficiency include autoimmune disease, destruction of the adrenal glands by infection or tumor, bilateral adrenal hemorrhage, and bilateral adrenalectomy. Secondary adrenal insufficiency is a result of pituitary or hypothalamic failure. This is most commonly a consequence of suppression of the hypothalamic-pituitary-adrenal axis from previous glucocorticoid administration.

The clinical manifestations of hypoadrenalism depend on whether the illness is primary or secondary or involves a full adrenal crisis [see Table 8]. Skin pigmentation and electrolyte disturbances are characteristic of primary adrenal insufficiency. Because mineralocorticoid function is generally preserved in secondary adrenocortical failure, electrolyte balance is usually maintained in patients previously treated with exogenous steroids, even if they are experiencing adrenal insufficiency resulting from surgical stress. In an adrenal crisis, patients characteristically present with abdominal pain, nausea, vomiting, fever, and hypovolemic shock.

Surgical patients with any of the following characteristics should be considered at risk for perioperative adrenal insufficiency: (1) those with a previous diagnosis of primary or secondary adrenal insufficiency, (2) those with signs or symptoms of adrenocortical insufficiency [see Table 8], (3) those on exogenous steroid therapy, (4) those who have received exogenous steroid therapy for more than seven days in the preceding 12 months, (5) those with an abnormal ACTH stimulation test (see below), (6) those with a history of lung, breast, or prostate cancer, (7) those who have received ketoconazole treatment, and (8) those who have undergone or will undergo a bilateral adrenalectomy or hypophysectomy. Such patients can be identified by history, physical examination, and laboratory tests. Because the medication history may be inaccurate, it is important to inquire not only about exogenous steroid usage in the past year but also about any illness that may have been treated by steroids.

The clinical and laboratory manifestations of symptomatic adrenal insufficiency are nonspecific (see above). Furthermore, it is impossible to evaluate adrenal reserve by clinical means. Therefore, several provocative tests are used to determine the functional state of the adrenal cortex, particularly its capacity to respond to stress. These tests measure the plasma cortisol response to exogenous corticotropin-releasing hormone, ACTH,

Table 10 Corticosteroid Properties

Corticosteroid	Glucocorticoid Potency*	Mineralocorticoid Potency*	Duration of Action (Hours)
Cortisol	1	1	8
Cortisone	0.8	1	8
Hydrocortisone	0.8	1	8
Prednisone	4	0.8	24
Prednisolone	4	0.8	24
Methylprednisolone	5	0.5	36
Dexamethasone	25	0.0	72

*Values are relative to the potency of the body's natural cortisol.

endogenous pyrogen, insulin-induced hypoglycemia, vasopressin, and metyrapone. If the objective is preoperative assessment of functional adrenal reserve, the best procedure is a short ACTH stimulation test. This is done as follows: 250 μg of synthetic ACTH (cosyntropin) is given intravenously, and blood is drawn 30 minutes later for assay of plasma cortisol. A cortisol level of greater than 500 nmol/L demonstrates a competent adrenal cortex.[74] This test does not demonstrate the etiology of the adrenal insufficiency, only that it is present.

If a patient is identified as having insufficient adrenocortical reserve to produce the additional amount of cortisol normally produced in response to the planned surgical stress, additional glucocorticoid should be administered. The amount and timing of the exogenous steroid coverage should match the physiologic response that would normally occur. It is unnecessary to exceed the expected physiologic response. If the patient is already receiving therapeutic steroid medication in excess of the calculated response to the planned stress, additional coverage is unnecessary. Exceeding the amount of glucocorticoid necessary to compensate for the diminished adrenal reserve would expose the surgical patient to a higher risk of steroid-related complications, particularly in relation to wound healing and immune function. Established protocols are derived from estimates of the average surgical stress for an uncomplicated surgical procedure [see Table 9]. If complications develop, glucocorticoids should be administered continuously, at a dosage that reflects the degree of stress, until improvement occurs. Although tapering is frequently done, there is no rationale for this other than that it mimics the natural stress response.

Several drugs are available [see Table 10]. For most patients, hydrocortisone is sufficient. Patients with liver disease may benefit from prednisolone because hepatic metabolism is unnecessary for biologic action. For patients with lung disease, methylprednisolone may be preferred; the low mineralocorticoid potency will protect the patient from potentially hazardous metabolic alkalosis. Dexamethasone is preferred if the diagnosis of adrenal insufficiency is uncertain because it will not interfere with subsequent testing.

References

1. Howard RJ, Simmons RL: Surgical Infectious Diseases, 2nd ed. Appleton & Lange, East Norwalk, Connecticut, 1988

2. Border JR, Hassett JM: Multiple systems organ failure: history, pathophysiology, prevention, and support. Trauma, Sepsis, and Shock: The Physiological Basis of Therapy. Clowes GHA Jr, Ed. Marcel Dekker, New York, 1988, p 335

3. Marshall JC, Christou NV, Horn R, et al: The microbiology of multiple organ failure: the proximal gastrointestinal tract as an occult reservoir of pathogens. Arch Surg 123:309, 1988

4. Johanson WG Jr, Pierce AK, Sanford JP, et al: Nosocomial respiratory infections with gram-negative bacilli: the significance of colonization of the respiratory tract. Ann Intern Med 77:701, 1972

5. Giannella RA, Broitman SA, Zamcheck N: Influence of gastric acidity on bacterial and parasitic enteric infections. Ann Intern Med 78:271, 1973

6. Hau T: Local host defense in the peritoneal cavity. Surgery and Immunity 2:1, 1989

7. Christou NV: Host-defence mechanisms in surgical patients: a correlative study of the delayed hypersensitivity skin-test response, granulocyte function and sepsis. Can J Surg 28:39, 1985

8. Meakins JL, Nohr CW: Assessment of immunologic responsiveness. Nutrition and Metabolism in the Surgical Patient. Kirkpatrick JR, Ed. Futura Publishing Co, Mt Kisco, New York, 1983, p 107

9. Kirkpatrick JR, Meakins JL, Wilson RF: Gastrointestinal disease: fistulas and malignancy. Nutrition and Metabolism in the Surgical Patient. Kirkpatrick JR, Ed. Futura Publishing Co, Mt Kisco, New York, 1983, p 385

10. Kirkpatrick JR, Meakins JL: The burn patient. Nutrition and Metabolism in the Surgical Patient. Kirkpatrick JR, Ed. Futura Publishing Co, Mt Kisco, New York, 1983, p 425

11. Christou NV: Predicting septic related mortality of the individual surgical patient based on admission host-defence measurements. Can J Surg 29:424, 1986

12. Tellado-Rodriguez J, Christou NV: Clinical assessment of host defense. Surg Clin North Am 68:41, 1988

13. Nohr CW, Christou NV, Rode H, et al: In vivo and in vitro humoral immunity in surgical patients. Ann Surg 200:373, 1984

14. Nohr CW, Latter DA, Meakins JL, et al: In vivo and in vitro humoral immunity in surgical patients: antibody response to pneumococcal polysaccharide. Surgery 100:229, 1986

15. Eilber FR, Morton DL: Impaired immunologic reactivity and recurrence following cancer surgery. Cancer 25:362, 1970

16. Meakins JL, Christou NV, Shizgal HM, et al: Therapeutic approaches to anergy in surgical patients: surgery and levamisole. Ann Surg 190:286, 1979

17. Nohr CW, Meakins JL: Biological response modifiers. Surgical Infection in Critical Care Medicine. Meakins JL, Ed. Churchill Livingstone, New York, 1985, p 309

18. Miles AA, Miles EM, Burke J: The value and duration of defence reaction of the skin to the primary lodgement of bacteria. Br J Exp Pathol 38:79, 1957

19. Snydman DR, Werner BG, Heinze-Lacey B, et al: Use of cytomegalovirus immune globulin to prevent cytomegalovirus disease in renal-transplant recipients. N Engl J Med 317:1049, 1987

20. Suthanthiran M, Strom TB: Renal transplantation. N Engl J Med 331:365, 1994

21. Snydman DR, Rubin RH, Werner BG: New developments in cytomegalovirus prevention and management. Am J Kidney Dis 21:217, 1993

22. Goodrich JM, Mori M, Gleaves CA, et al: Early treatment with ganciclovir to prevent cytomegalovirus disease after allogeneic bone marrow transplantation. N Engl J Med 325:1601, 1991

23. Rubin RH, Greene R: Etiology and management of the compromised patient with fever and pulmonary infiltrates. Clinical Approach to Infection in the Compromised Host. Rubin RH, Young LS, Eds. Plenum Publishing Corp, New York, 1988, p 131

24. Bensard DD, McIntyre RC Jr, Waring BJ, et al: Comparison of video thoracoscopic lung biopsy to open lung biopsy in the diagnosis of interstitial lung disease. Chest 103:765, 1993

25. Klimbert S, Hawkins I, Vogel SB: Percutaneous cholecystostomy for acute cholecystitis in high-risk patients. Am J Surg 153:125, 1987

26. Dienstag JL: Viral hepatitis in the compromised host. Clinical Approach to Infection in the Compromised Host. Rubin RH, Young LS, Eds. Plenum Publishing Corp, New York, 1988, p 325

27. Peterson PK, Simmons RL: Infections in organ transplant recipients. Principles and Practice of Infectious Diseases, 2nd ed. Mandell GL, Douglas RG, Bennett JE, Eds. John Wiley & Sons, New York, 1985, p 1676

28. Joshi JH, Schimpff SC: Infections in special hosts: infections in the compromised host. Principles and Practice of Infectious Diseases, 2nd ed. Mandell GL, Douglas RG, Bennett JE, Eds. John Wiley & Sons, New York, 1985, p 1644

29. Young LS: Gram-negative sepsis. Principles and Practice of Infectious Diseases, 2nd ed. Mandell GL, Douglas RG, Bennett JE, Eds. John Wiley & Sons, New York, 1985, p 452

30. Rusthoven J: The potential role of recombinant hematopoietic colony-stimulating factors in preventing infections in the immunocompromised host. Can J Infect Dis 2:74, 1991

31. Pizzo PA: Empiric therapy and prevention of infection in the immunocompromised host. Principles and Practice of Infectious Diseases, 2nd ed. Mandell GL, Douglas RG, Bennett JE, Eds. John Wiley & Sons, New York, 1985, p 1680

32. Kemeny MM, Brennan MF: The surgical complications of chemotherapy in the cancer patient. Curr Probl Surg 24:609, 1987

33. Cosimi AB: Surgical aspects of infection in the compromised host. Clinical Approach to Infection in the Compromised Host. Rubin RH, Young LS, Eds. Plenum Publishing Corp, New York, 1988, p 649

34. Frick T, Fryd DS, Goodale RL, et al: Incidence and treatment of candida esophagitis in patients undergoing renal transplantation. Am J Surg 155:311, 1988

35. Vincenti F, Parfrey PS, Briggs W: Skeletal, gastrointestinal, hepatic, and hematologic disorders following kidney transplantation. Renal Transplantation. Garovoy MR, Guttman RD, Eds. Churchill Livingstone, New York, 1986, p 233

36. Bansky G, Huynh Do U, Largiadèr F, et al: Gastroduodenal complications after renal transplantation: the role of prophylactic gastric surgery in hyperacid kidney allograft recipients. Clin Transpl 1:209, 1987

37. Graham SM, Flowers JL, Schweitzer E, et al: The utility of prophylactic laparoscopic cholecystectomy in transplant candidates. Am J Surg 169:44, 1995

38. Briggs JD: The recipient of a renal transplant. Kidney Transplantation. Morris PJ, Ed. Grune & Stratton, London, 1984, p 59

39. Penn I: Cancers of the anogenital region in renal transplant recipients: analysis of 65 cases. Cancer 58:611, 1986

40. Rosen FS, Cooper MD, Wedgewood RJP: The primary immunodeficiencies (pts 1 and 2). Medical Progress 311:235, 300, 1984

41. Delafuente JC: Immunosenescence: clinical and pharmacologic considerations. Med Clin North Am 69:475, 1985

42. Kishimoto S, Tomino S, Mitsuya H, et al: Age-related decline in the in vitro and in vivo syntheses of anti-tetanus toxoid antibody in humans. J Immunol 125:2347, 1980

43. Ceuppens JL, Goodwin JS: Regulation of immunoglobulin production in pokeweed mitogen-stimulated cultures of lymphocytes from young and old adults. J Immunol 128:2429, 1982

44. Tsukayama D, Breitenbucher R, Steinberg S, et al: Polymorphonuclear leukocyte, T-lymphocyte, and natural killer cell activities in elderly nursing home residents. Eur J Clin Microbiol 5:468, 1986

45. Chandra RK, Kutty KM: Immunocompetence in obesity. Acta Paediatr Scand 69:25, 1980

46. Nohr CW, Tchervenkov JI, Meakins JL, et al: Malnutrition and humoral immunity: short-term acute nutritional deprivation. Surgery 98:769, 1985

47. Horita M, Suzuki H, Onodera T, et al: Abnormalities of immunoregulatory T cell subsets in patients with insulin-dependent diabetes mellitus. J Immunol 129:1426, 1982

48. Hill HR, Augustine NH, Rallison ML, et al: Defective monocyte chemotactic responses in diabetes mellitus. J Clin Immunol 3:70, 1983

49. Beam TR, Crigler ED, Goldman JK, et al: Antibody response to polyvalent pneumococcal polysaccharide vaccine in diabetes. JAMA 244:2621, 1980

50. Goldblum SE, Reed WP: Host defenses and immunologic alterations associated with chronic hemodialysis. Ann Intern Med 93:597, 1980

51. Glassock RJ: Nutrition, immunology, and renal disease. Kidney Int 24(suppl 16):S194, 1983

52. Fernandez LA, Laltoo M, Fox RA: A study of T cell populations in alcoholic cirrhosis and chronic alcoholism. Clin Invest Med 5:241, 1982

53. Havens WP Jr, Myerson RM, Klatchko J: Production of tetanus antitoxin by patients with hepatic cirrhosis. N Engl J Med 257:637, 1957

54. Bagby GC Jr: Leukopenia. Cecil Textbook of Medicine. Wyngaarden JB, Smith LH, Eds. WB Saunders Co, Philadelphia, 1988, p 961

55. Orgill D, Demling RH: Current concepts and approaches to wound healing. Crit Care Med 16:899, 1988

56. Meuleman J, Katz P: The immunologic effects, kinetics, and use of glucocorticosteroids. Med Clin North Am 69:805, 1985

57. Cupps TH, Edgar LC, Thomas CA, et al: Multiple mechanisms of B cell immunoregulation in man after administration of in vivo corticosteroids. J Immunol 132:170, 1984

58. Hobbs CH, McClellan RO: Radiation and radioactive materials. Casarett and Doull's Toxicology: The Basic Science of Poisons, 2nd ed. Casarett LJ, Doull J, Eds. Macmillan Publishing Co, New York, 1980, p 497

59. Christou NV, McLean APH, Meakins JL: Host defense in blunt trauma: interrelationships of kinetics of anergy and depressed neutrophil function, nutritional status, and sepsis. J Trauma 20:833, 1980

60. Salo M: Effects of anaesthesia and surgery on the immune response. Trauma, Stress and Immunity in Anesthesia and Surgery. Watkins J, Salo M, Eds. Butterworth Publishers, Stoneham, Massachusetts, 1982, p 211

61. Moudgil GC: Update on anaesthesia and the immune response. Can Anaesth Soc J 33:S54, 1986

62. Wu H-S, Little AG: Perioperative blood transfusions and cancer recurrence. J Clin Oncol 6:1348, 1988

63. Bohnsack JF, Brown EJ: The role of the spleen in resistance to infection. Annu Rev Med 37:49, 1986

64. Hau T: Infections of the liver and spleen. Surgical Infectious Diseases, 2nd ed. Howard RJ, Simmons RL. Appleton & Lange, East Norwalk, Connecticut, 1988, p 659

65. Wilson RE: Surgical Problems in Immuno-Depressed Patients. WB Saunders Co, Philadelphia, 1984

66. Sheil AGR: Cancer after transplantation. World J Surg 10:389, 1986

67. Hanto DW, Najarian JS: Advances in the diagnosis and treatment of EBV-associated lymphoproliferative diseases in immunocompromised hosts. J Surg Oncol 30:215, 1985

68. Kelly GE, Sheil AGR, Taylor R: Nonspecific immunological studies in kidney transplant recipients with and without skin cancer. Transplantation 37:368, 1984

69. Birkeland SA: Immune monitoring of tumor development after renal transplantation. Cancer 55:988, 1985

70. Penn I: Cancer in the immunosuppressed organ recipient. Transplant Proc 23:1771, 1991

71. Hanto DW: Polyclonal and monoclonal posttransplant lymphoproliferative diseases (LPD). Clin Transpl 6:227, 1992

72. Harid IR, Strong RW, Hartley LCJ, et al: Skin cancer in Caucasian renal allograft recipients living in a subtropical climate. Surgery 87:177, 1980

73. Napolitano LM, Chernow B: Guidelines for corticosteroid use in anesthetic and surgical stress. Int Anesthesiol Clin 26:226, 1988

74. Salem M, Tainsh RE Jr, Bromberg J, et al: Perioperative glucocorticoid coverage: a reassessment 42 years after emergence of a problem. Ann Surg 219:416, 1994

7 THE ELDERLY SURGICAL PATIENT

James M. Watters, M.D., and Jacqueline C. McClaran, M.D.

Perioperative Management of the Elderly Patient

Principles of Care

Management of surgical illness in geriatric patients is different from that in younger patients and typically more complex. Assessment of surgical problems and physiologic status of the elderly must take into account (1) the marked variability of the changes associated with advancing age, both among individuals and among different organ systems in an individual, (2) changes in the incidence, prevalence, and natural history of certain disease processes, and (3) the increased likelihood of multiple medical diagnoses and polypharmacy.

These factors and others may alter the presentation of surgical illness. Symptoms may be diminished in intensity, nonspecific, indirect, or atypical and therefore may be inappropriately ignored or attributed simply to advanced age. Patients may postpone seeking medical attention, or physicians may fail to recognize the gravity of an acute surgical condition if pain, fever, and acute-phase responses are blunted [see Discussion, Alterations in Clinical Presentation, below]. Furthermore, it may be difficult to obtain the details of the history if the patient is confused or suffers from impaired hearing or memory.

Both the potential benefits and the risks of surgical treatment are more difficult to assess in the elderly. Assumptions about physiologic status and primary treatment goals that are reasonable in younger patients may not be appropriate in older patients. Often, the major concern of elderly patients is whether they will be able to enjoy an independent life after surgery, to at least the extent they did before. Consequently, such patients may find a radical procedure that offers potential cure less desirable than a more conservative procedure (or endoscopic, percutaneous, or nonoperative treatment) that relieves pain or other symptoms, largely restores function, and allows a return to normal surroundings. On the other hand, an early aggressive approach may obviate later procedures and prevent associated morbidity. A thorough knowledge of treatment alternatives and their risks, a close familiarity with the natural history of the disease in relation to life expectancy, and a clear understanding of the patient's goals are paramount in surgical decision making in the elderly.

The risks associated with surgical treatment depend on the nature of the proposed procedure and on the patient's physiologic and medical status [see Risk Assessment, below]. Whereas minor elective procedures done with the patient under local anesthesia can be performed safely regardless of age, emergency thoracotomy and laparotomy are associated with significant mortality in the elderly. Mortality from emergency procedures is markedly higher than mortality from elective procedures. Elective surgery may therefore be indicated when it can be predicted that complications will develop and emergency intervention will be necessary. Cardiovascular and pulmonary complications remain important causes of postoperative mortality in the elderly, much more so than in younger patients.

The elderly population is very heterogeneous. Some elderly persons are wholly independent, have maintained moderate levels of physical activity, have preserved lean body mass and cardiopulmonary function, and have physiologic responses similar to those of younger individuals; in these patients, the risks associated with surgical illness and treatment are relatively low. At the opposite extreme, some elderly persons have multiple illnesses, are capable of only limited activity and independence, and suffer from cardiovascular and pulmonary disease; in these patients, surgery-associated risks are substantial. Physiologic status is a more fundamental determinant of risk than age is. As one surgeon put it as long ago as 1907, "In deciding for or [against] operation we depend upon the condition of the heart, the arteries, the lungs, and kidneys, rather more than the number of years the patient has lived."[1]

Nonetheless, no matter how fit, active, and free of comorbidity the elderly individual appears, there is a gradual loss of physiologic reserve in various organ systems associated with aging [see Table 1]. This is most obvious in the oldest old but occurs to some extent even in younger old patients. In general, maximal physiologic functions decline, with the result that the ability to increase functions as needed is more and more limited. In addition, sensitivity to deviations from physiologic norms is decreased and mechanisms for reestablishing such norms are less efficient, with the result that homeostatic perturbations tend to be exaggerated.[2] These phenomena may have little consequence in healthy daily life but are critical to the elderly patient facing the stress of a major operation or acute illness. The elderly surgical patient is less able to maintain homeostasis and tolerates complications poorly. All aspects of perioperative care must be focused on minimizing the stress of surgery and avoiding the added stresses of complications. The surgical procedure must be carefully chosen and conducted with meticulous technique. Careful attention must be given to drug and fluid and electrolyte therapy. Pain, tubes, and other restraining factors must be kept to a minimum so as to allow prompt resumption of physical activity and minimize the adverse effects of immobility. The potential for impaired cognitive function must also be recognized.

Five factors are critical for obtaining the best outcomes from surgical treatment of elderly patients: (1) careful preoperative preparation of the patient and optimization of medical and physiologic status; (2) minimization of perioperative starvation and inactivity and the stresses of hypothermia, hypoxemia, and pain; (3) meticulous perioperative care, to avoid clinical complications from perturbations of fluid and electrolyte balance, impaired cardiovascular and respiratory function, and inappropriate pharmacotherapy; (4) careful surgical judgment and technique to achieve the desired goals and avoid technical complications; and (5) optimization of physical and cognitive function. Accomplishing such care requires thorough preoper-

Table 1   Physiologic Changes Associated with Aging

	Age-Related Changes	Clinical Consequences	Implications for Care
Respiratory System	Decreased strength and endurance of respiratory muscles Increased stiffness of the chest wall and increased reliance on diaphragm function Decreased vital capacity, FEV_1, maximal inspiratory and expiratory pressures, maximum midexpiratory flow rate, and maximum voluntary ventilation Diminished elastic lung recoil and increased closing volume Increased alveolar-arterial oxygen gradient Decreased arterial oxygen tension Decreased airway sensitivity and efficiency of mucociliary clearance mechanism Decreased compensatory responses to hypoxia or hypercarbia Increased sensitivity to narcotic respiratory depression	Less effective cough Predisposition to aspiration Increased closure of small airways during tidal respiration, especially postoperatively and when supine, leading to increased atelectasis and shunting Predisposition to hypoxemia Tachypnea and increased tidal volume may be less apparent as respiratory failure develops	Encourage early mobilization, assumption of upright rather than supine position Provide effective pain relief to allow mobilization, deep breathing Routinely supply supplemental oxygen in the immediate postoperative period, and then as needed Use nasogastric tubes sparingly Recognize decreased ventilatory responses to hypoxia and hypercarbia
Cardiovascular System	Decreased maximal heart rate, cardiac output, ejection fraction Reliance on increased end-diastolic volume to increase cardiac output Slowed ventricular filling, increased reliance on atrial contribution Decreased inotropic and chronotropic responses to beta-adrenergic stimuli Decreased baroreceptor sensitivity Increased prevalence of coronary artery disease, clinically apparent or occult; may influence cardiac function during acute stress	Greater reliance on ventricular filling and increases in stroke volume (rather than ejection fraction) to achieve increases in cardiac output Intolerance of hypovolemia Intolerance of tachycardia; dysrhythmias, including atrial fibrillation	Employ vigorous fluid resuscitation to achieve optimal ventricular filling Nonvasoconstricting inotropes and afterload reduction may be more effective if pharmacologic support is required Avoid tachycardia; correct significant arrhythmias Recognize potential for preexisting cardiac disease
Renal Function and Fluid-Electrolyte Homeostasis	Decreased sensitivity to fluid and electrolyte perturbations Decreased thirst response Decreased ability to concentrate urine and conserve water and solute Decreased efficiency of solute and water excretion Decreased renal mass, renal blood flow, and glomerular filtration rate Increased renal glucose threshold	Predisposition to hypovolemia Predisposition to extracellular fluid volume expansion, electrolyte disorders (e.g., hyponatremia) Predisposition to hyperglycemia Predisposition to hyperosmolar states	Pay meticulous attention to fluid and electrolyte management Recognize that a "normal" serum creatinine value reflects a decreased creatinine clearance, because muscle mass (i.e., creatinine excretion) is decreased concurrently: estimate creatinine clearance using age-adjusted formulas or measure Select drugs carefully: avoid agents that may be nephrotoxic (e.g., aminoglycosides) or adversely affect renal blood flow (e.g., NSAIDs) Adjust drug dosages as appropriate for altered pharmacokinetics
Body Composition	Significantly decreased muscle mass, accounting for much of the age-related decrease in lean tissue mass Increased fat mass	Erosion of muscle mass during acute illness may result in strength rapidly falling below important clinical threshold (e.g., impaired coughing, decreased mobility, increased risk of venous thrombosis) Altered volumes of drug distribution	Maintain physical function through effective pain relief; avoid tubes, drains, and other "restraints"; encourage early mobilization; and provide assistance with mobilization Minimize fasting, provide early nutritional supplementation or support (both protein-calorie and micronutrient) Adjust drug dosages for volume of distribution
Thermoregulation	Diminished sensitivity to ambient temperature and less efficient mechanisms of heat conservation, production, and dissipation Febrile responses to infection may be blunted in frail or malnourished elderly and those who are extremely old	Predisposition to hypothermia (e.g., decline in body temperature during surgery is more marked unless preventive measures are undertaken) If hypothermic, shivering may result, associated with marked increases in oxygen consumption and cardiopulmonary demands Fever may be absent despite serious infections, especially in frail elderly	Use active measures to maintain normothermia during surgical procedures and to rewarm after trauma: warmed I.V. fluids, humidified gases, warm air Maintaining intraoperative normothermia reduces wound infections, adverse cardiac events, and length of stay

ative assessment and planning and the involvement of a multidisciplinary clinical team knowledgeable about and interested in the elderly surgical patient.[3] With a comprehensive approach, major operations can be completed with low risk, a short hospital stay, and a rapid return to full function.[4]

Goals of Therapy

The goals of an elderly patient with a surgical problem may differ considerably from those of a younger patient. Such goals must be carefully elicited and addressed in the treatment plan. Definitive cure of the presenting problem and maximizing longevity may be very reasonable and achievable goals, regardless of age. As the risks of surgical therapy increase in the very frail and oldest old, however, priorities may shift. The major concern of an elderly patient may be whether he or she will be able to enjoy the same level of function and independence that he or she did before the onset of the problem. Relief of symptoms and maintaining quality of life may be more important than long-term survival. Maintaining reasonable function in the short-term may be of special importance, for example, during the last stages of a spouse's illness or in advance of a landmark event in the family. In some circumstances, the elderly patient may be less willing than a younger patient to accept the risks of major surgical interventions, even if such measures are potentially curative, and more likely to pursue alternatives with less immediate risk and more limited goals. It is, of course, essential to recognize those situations in which timely elective intervention carries little risk and is likely to prevent discomfort, impairment, and the greater risks of emergency intervention in the future.

Clinicians' traditional focus has been on outcomes such as postoperative morbidity and mortality, length of hospital stay, long-term survival, and recurrence rates. Reasonable information about these outcomes in elderly patients is now available for many surgical procedures, though it is important to appreciate the extent to which study design can influence such observations [see Discussion, Studies of Aging and Aged Populations, below]. Unfortunately, however, for most surgical problems and procedures, there is little information about impact on outcomes that may be of particular interest to elderly patients. In addition, it has been suggested that physicians are not especially successful at identifying the aspects of disease and treatment that are most important to individual patients.[5]

Major surgical procedures to maximize longevity may be entirely appropriate in an elderly patient who is fit from physiologic, functional, and cognitive perspectives. Current average expectations for 70-year-old men and women are an additional 12.5 and 15.3 years of life, respectively, and for 85-year-old men and women, an additional 5.3 and 6.3 years, respectively.[6] Thus, the absolute gain in life expectancy from even completely effective interventions declines as the age of the patient increases. Patients and clinicians probably recognize this principle intuitively but may find it difficult to quantify. It is based on an understanding of the effects of competing risks—that is, risks to survival from sources other than the condition of interest—and is reflected in the observation that life expectancy curves for normal individuals and for those with various medical conditions typically grow closer together as age increases [see Figure 1]. Competing risks increase progressively with age, decrease the impact of a new condition on life expectancy, and

decrease the potential life expectancy gain from therapy.[7] For example, cancer-specific survival after resection of a colorectal tumor does not vary with age, whereas overall survival declines progressively as age rises.[8] The implications of competing risks for therapy are (1) that interventions carrying minimal risk are reasonable, regardless of age, and (2) that very elderly patients should select interventions that are clearly effective and are associated with a low complication rate when maximizing longevity is their goal. In the oldest old and those with greater than average competing risks (e.g., major comorbid conditions), net gains in longevity will be very modest indeed.

Discussion of the elderly patient's wishes regarding medical care in the event of serious postoperative complications should be encouraged before a major elective procedure, with family members or other possible substitute decision-makers involved as appropriate, or early after an acute hospital admission. Expectations about convalescence should be discussed and temporary placement after discharge, home care, and other discharge planning arranged as needed [see Planning Convalescence, below]. Patients generally welcome the opportunity to discuss their wishes, and surgeons should not hesitate to raise these issues.

Some elderly patients may be unable to articulate goals and make treatment decisions on their own behalf. In some instances, they have expressed their wishes previously about medical care, perhaps in the form of an advance directive or "living will." (An example of the latter is available from the University of Toronto Joint Centre for Bioethics [http://www.utoronto.ca/jcb].) Discussions that patients may have had with their families, their caregivers, or both may be particularly helpful if they were held recently or were related to the specific situation at hand. When wishes have not been previously expressed, substitute decision-makers must consider what is known about the patient's values and arrive at a judgment about what his or her goals and probable decision would be. Advance directives may provide a context in which to make decisions about limits to treatment, even though they usually apply to conditions that are irreversible or nearly so. In the absence of such information, a decision must be made in the best interests of the patient, taking into account the advantages and disadvantages of the treatment options, likely effects on quality of life,

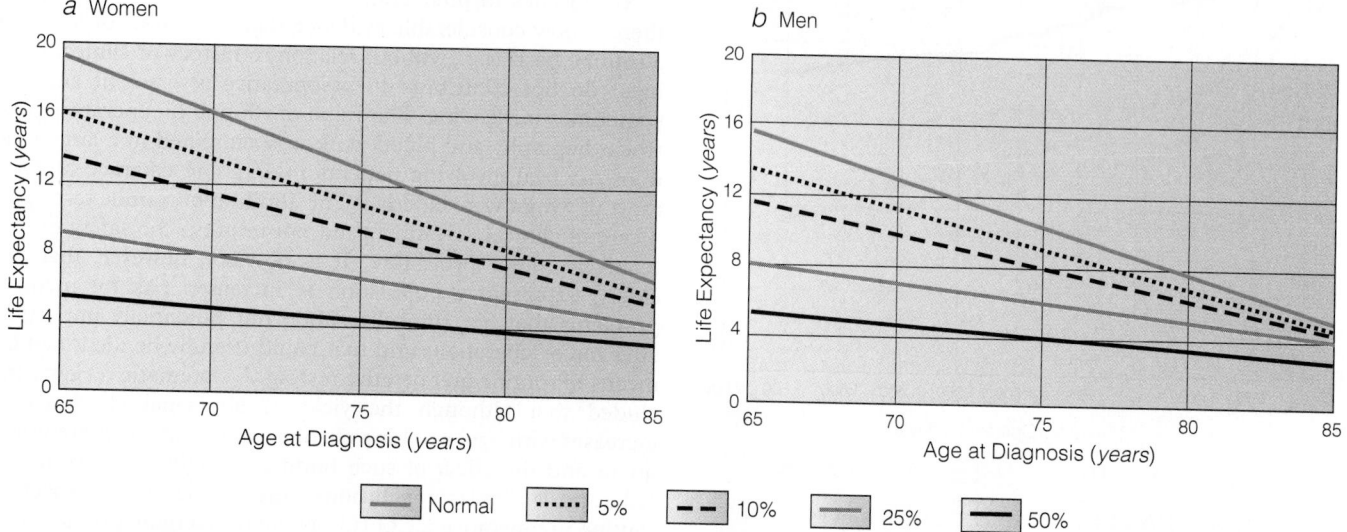

Figure 1 **Illustrated is the effect of disease-related mortality (5%, 10%, 25%, and 50%) on remaining life expectancy for women (*a*) and men (*b*).[7]**

and similar concerns. It should be recognized that individuals may rate their quality of life highly despite significant health impairment and functional problems and that the assessments of physicians and family members may be quite different from those of patients.[5] In general, the literature suggests that significant problems persist in all areas of planning, communicating, and implementing advance care preferences.[9]

Preserving patients' dignity and autonomy and minimizing distress are important health care goals that often are not met in the elderly.[10] Dignity (self-respect and being valued by others) is readily undermined in the health care setting by disrespect for patient privacy and insensitivity to patient needs and desires. Such disrespect and insensitivity may reflect stereotyped, negative attitudes toward the elderly on the part of caregivers. Autonomy is inevitably diminished when sufficient information and opportunity to make informed choices about care are not provided.

Preoperative Management

Preoperative assessment and optimization of cardiovascular, respiratory, nutritional, cognitive, and functional status in the elderly patient will be addressed in some detail (see below). Smoking should be stopped as far in advance of surgery as possible, active respiratory infection resolved, airflow obstruction minimized, and exercise tolerance optimized. Although strategies for preventing cardiovascular complications continue to evolve [see IV:2 Risk Stratification, Preoperative Testing, and Operative Planning], it does appear that beta-adrenergic blockade is well tolerated and should be considered in patients undergoing major elective noncardiac procedures who are at increased risk.[11]

The importance of micronutrients and compounds with antioxidant properties is being increasingly appreciated. Whether or not preexisting deficits are suspected, preoperative multivitamin supplementation should be considered in the elderly. The preoperative period is also the optimal time to address protein-calorie deficiencies, using oral supplements in most malnourished patients, enteral feeding when necessary,

and parenteral feeding when it is the only option. The diminished muscle mass, strength, and functional status that tend to accompany aging [see Nutritional Assessment, below] and the demonstrated effects of physical training in frail elderly nursing home residents raise the possibility that similar programs might minimize the development of muscle weakness and functional impairments after major operations in the elderly.[12] In a recent randomized trial, patients awaiting coronary bypass grafting who underwent supervised exercise training twice weekly and a broadly based educational program had shorter intensive care unit and hospital stays than control subjects did.[13] In an observational study, a home-based strength and aerobic training program was associated with increases in 6-minute walking distance, quality of life, strength, and peak oxygen consumption in patients preparing for lung volume reduction surgery.[14]

RISK ASSESSMENT

Assessment of risk in the elderly must consider patient factors, the surgical problem, and the treatment options. Assessment of the elderly patient is typically more challenging and time-consuming, and it more often involves family members, the primary care physician, anesthetists, and other physicians and health care disciplines. Coexisting medical conditions are common and may markedly increase the risks associated with surgical intervention. The American Society of Anesthesiologists (ASA) physical status scale reflects functional status and comorbidity and is a strong predictor of postoperative and late mortality [see Figure 2].[15]

Although physiologic reserve is diminished and comorbidity common in the elderly, aging is a very heterogeneous process. Great care must be taken in applying generalizations about the elderly population to elderly individuals. Outcomes depend not only on physical or physiologic fitness but also on cognitive and social factors: a careful assessment must go beyond simply establishing a specific diagnosis and include all of these elements.[16] A rational approach to risk assessment should take into account factors that predict important adverse clinical outcomes, allowing risks and treatment goals to be weighed and preparation for surgery and perioperative care to be planned optimally. Decisions about surgical care must rest on criteria that are more specific and strongly predictive than chronologic age is.

Approaches to preoperative testing continue to evolve, but there is now considerable evidence that many tests ordered on a routine basis (i.e., without relation to history or clinical findings) do not contribute to preoperative assessment and are sometimes misleading. The value of routine preoperative electrocardiography and blood work was examined in a large randomized trial involving patients undergoing cataract surgery, most of whom were elderly.[17] The addition of routine testing to a careful clinical assessment did not improve the safety of this relatively minor procedure. It is possible, however, that the elderly represent a population at increased risk for medical problems that are clinically subtle but potentially important after major operations and that could usefully be identified by means of routine preoperative testing. A systematic review concluded that although the yield of abnormal chest x-rays increases with age, resulting changes in management are infrequent and the effect of such findings on clinical outcomes is unknown.[18] Similar conclusions were reached with respect to routine preoperative ECG (in patients undergoing noncardiac surgery), hematology, and biochemistry. A higher incidence of perioperative arrhythmia and a greater need for cardiopul-

Figure 2 Depicted is correlation between ASA grade and postoperative survival.[15]

monary resuscitation are associated with preoperative hypokalemia in patients undergoing elective coronary artery bypass grafting.[19] Additional well-designed studies are needed to evaluate routine testing in populations, such as the elderly, who are at increased risk for postoperative cardiopulmonary and other complications.

RESPIRATORY ASSESSMENT

Respiratory complications are among the most common complications after major surgical procedures and are more frequent in elderly surgical patients.[20-22] Postoperative pulmonary complications are considerably more common than cardiac complications and are equally likely to cause postoperative death after abdominal procedures. In a large prospective study of patients undergoing major noncardiac procedures, predominantly males, the incidence of postoperative pneumonia was 1.5%, compared with 0.7% for cardiac arrest and 0.4% for myocardial infarction.[22] The 30-day mortality was 21% for patients in whom pneumonia developed and 2% for those in whom it did not. The risk of pneumonia was five times greater in patients aged 80 years or older than in those younger than 50 years. In another study, the combination of age 60 years or greater and ASA risk category II or higher identified nearly 90% of patients who experienced respiratory complications after abdominal surgery.[20] Age-related changes in respiratory function [see Table 1] and their interaction with the changes that occur after operation and during acute surgical illness are discussed elsewhere [see Postoperative Management, Respiratory Care, below]. The unadjusted relative risk of postoperative pulmonary complications for patients older than 70 years compared with younger patients ranges from 0.9 to 2.4.[23] In a systematic review of patients undergoing surgical treatment of colorectal cancer, the incidence of respiratory complications was 5% in patients younger than 65 years, 10% in those 65 to 74 years of age, 12% in those 75 to 84 years of age, and 15% in those 85 years of age or older.[8] Much of the unadjusted risk associated with advanced age may be attributable to comorbidities, although some reports have found ASA category and age to be independent, additive risk factors.[24]

Other significant patient-related risk factors for postoperative pulmonary complications are smoking, poor exercise capacity, chronic obstructive pulmonary disease (COPD), active pulmonary infection, and cognitive impairment.[21,23] Smoking should be stopped as far in advance of operation as possible: cessation of smoking 6 to 8 weeks beforehand significantly reduces cardiopulmonary and wound-related as well as overall postoperative complications.[25] Active respiratory infection should be resolved, even if this means delaying the operation. Airflow obstruction should be treated in patients with COPD and asthma. The aim should be to optimize respiratory status, as determined by exercise capacity, physical findings, and perhaps spirometry.[23] Bronchodilators, glucocorticoids, and chest physiotherapy may be helpful.

Procedure-related risk factors are also of some relevance. The site of surgery is the most important procedure-related predictor. The risk of pulmonary complications is greatest after upper abdominal and thoracic procedures and is lower with laparoscopic procedures than with open procedures. On rare occasions, the risk of respiratory complications is considered so great that the choice of surgical procedure is based on the desire to avoid an abdominal (especially an upper abdominal) or thoracic procedure or general anesthesia. Lengthy surgical procedures (> 3 hours) are also accompanied by increased risk.[21]

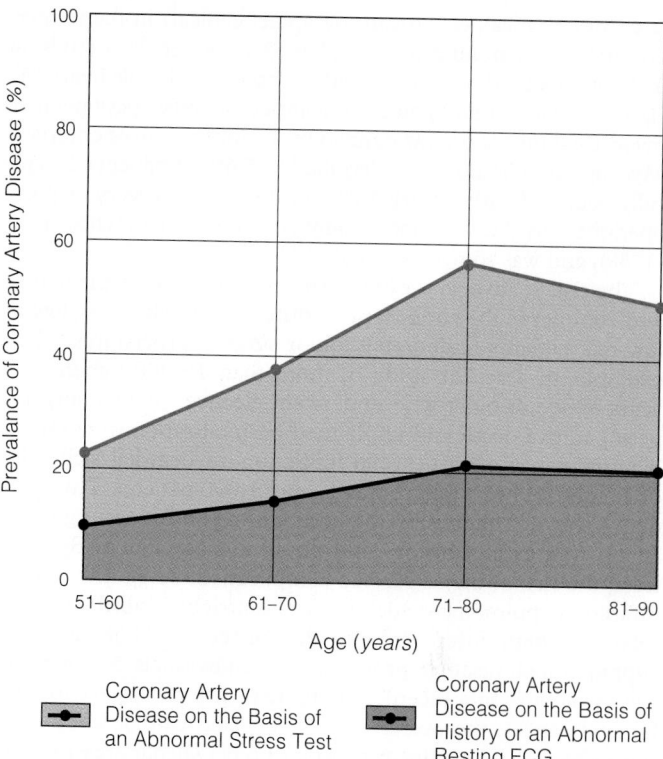

Figure 3 **Shown is an estimate of the prevalence of coronary artery disease in men between 51 and 90 years of age.**[251]

A careful history and a thorough physical examination directed at the risk factors discussed are the most important elements of preoperative assessment and should be completed in elderly patients undergoing abdominal and thoracic procedures. An abnormal chest x-ray is also a risk factor, but whether routine preoperative chest roentgenography is warranted in the healthy elderly patient at low risk for postoperative pulmonary complications is unknown.[18,26] The value of routine preoperative pulmonary function testing (for procedures other than pulmonary resection) in addition to careful clinical assessment is not supported by published reports, many of which have methodologic shortcomings.[23,26,27] Abnormal spirometry results should not be used in isolation to decide against a surgical procedure.[23] Spirometry may be helpful in determining whether the status of a patient with known COPD has been optimized.

CARDIOVASCULAR ASSESSMENT

The presence of coronary artery disease increases with age: significant coronary artery disease is present at autopsy in more than 50% of individuals older than 70 years [see Figure 3]. Perioperative myocardial ischemia and infarction can arise from a number of mechanisms, including increased myocardial oxygen demand, increased shear stresses on atherosclerotic plaques, thrombosis related to changes in coagulability or in vascular tone or endothelial function.[28] In unselected patients older than 40 years, the risk of perioperative myocardial infarction or death has been reported to range from 2.0% to 3.7%, with a pooled average of 2.5%.[29] This rate may be gradually declining.[30] The pooled averages were 4.6% in patients considered to be at high risk (range, 2.7% to 5.8%), and 6.2% in vascular surgical patients (range, 2.2% to 19.0%). Considerable disparity results from the use of inconsistent diagnostic criteria (e.g., biochemical, electrocardiographic, clinical) in the numerous studies examining this problem.[29] However, in a study of 323 patients aged 50 years or older who had ischemic heart disease and were undergoing noncardiac surgery, perioperative myocardial infarction was defined by a combination of criteria.[31] Myocardial infarction was identified in 5.6% of patients; it typically occurred early (nearly 80% on the day of surgery or postoperative day 1), was not usually accompanied by chest pain (17%), and was sometimes fatal (17%).

The risk of adverse cardiac events is influenced by the nature and conduct of the surgical procedure.[32] The risk is very low in low-risk patients undergoing minor surgical procedures.[30] For example, in a recent study of more than 18,000 patients 50 years of age or older who underwent elective cataract surgery, perioperative death and unplanned hospitalization were rare.[17] The incidence of myocardial infarction, myocardial ischemia, or congestive heart failure was 1.2 per 1,000 patients. This incidence was not altered by the addition of routine testing (e.g., ECG) to a careful history and physical examination. By contrast, the risk of major cardiac complications (e.g., myocardial infarction, pulmonary edema, and ventricular fibrillation) is relatively high after abdominal, noncardiac thoracic, and suprainguinal vascular procedures in individuals 50 years of age or older.[33] In a recent systematic review of surgery for colorectal cancer, the overall rate of reported cardiac complications was 2%, with a linear relationship between increasing age and the frequency of such complications.[8]

Assessment of patient-related risk of cardiac complications is based on a careful medical history, physical examination, and ECG. Multifactorial risk indexes may also contribute to the assessment.[33,34] Even major vascular procedures are accompanied by very low risk when cardiac functional status is good, coronary artery disease is absent, and the multifactorial risk index score is low.[35] It is noteworthy that advanced age (70 years or older) did not correlate with cardiac complications in the 1999 revision of a widely cited cardiac risk index.[33] Presumably, this absence of correlation reflects, in part, the inclusion in the index of specific factors (e.g., ischemic heart disease) that are associated with age but are stronger predictors of outcome. It is also noteworthy that cerebrovascular disease, renal insufficiency, and insulin-dependent diabetes are significant predictors of cardiac complications, which suggests that these conditions tend to coexist with coronary artery disease or that disturbances in a variety of organ systems can lead ultimately to cardiac complications.

The concepts pertinent to assessing perioperative and long-term cardiac risk before major elective noncardiac surgery are still evolving [see IV:2 Risk Statification, Preoperative Testing, and Operative Planning], and a number of approaches, guidelines, and algorithms have been published.[33,36-40] According to one algorithm, if functional status is good, coronary disease and risk factors absent, and cardiac risk index score low, then no preoperative cardiovascular testing or nonroutine therapy is warranted. When coronary artery disease or risk factors are present and functional status is equivocal or unclear on routine clinical assessment and ECG, then further testing is warranted. ECG treadmill testing is appropriate for patients able to exercise; dipyridamole thallium scanning, stress echocardiography, and ambulatory ECG monitoring are useful for those who are not. If test results are strongly positive for ischemia, consideration should be given to coronary angiography and angioplasty or coronary revascularization. A conservative approach is appropriate when test results are not strongly pos-

itive, with optimization of cardiac medications and the use of aggressive intraoperative and postoperative monitoring. Aggressive but conservative therapy without further cardiac testing is proposed when functional status is clearly impaired in patients with known coronary artery disease or risk factors. When multiple risk factors for coronary disease are present, then further testing is undertaken if functional status is impaired or indeterminate, but not if it is good. In general, it is reasonable to proceed with elective surgery in patients with coronary artery disease if the patient has had successful coronary revascularization within 5 years, with no recurrent symptoms, or if the patient has recently undergone angiography or stress testing, with favorable or low-risk findings.[37]

COGNITIVE ASSESSMENT

Preexisting impairments of cognitive function are associated with an increased risk of postoperative complications and worse early and 6-month survival.[21,41-43] For example, the risk of postoperative pulmonary complications after abdominal procedures is increased nearly sixfold in patients with preoperative cognitive dysfunction.[21] Patients with end-stage dementia have been reported to have a fourfold higher 6-month mortality (55%) than patients who were cognitively intact (13%).[43] Such patients were fully dependent in activities of daily living (ADL) and unable to remember the names of family members. This poor short-term prognosis, which may even be an overestimate, appeared not to have been generally recognized by caregivers and families and was not reflected in differences in care, palliative measures, or decisions to forgo burdensome interventions or life-sustaining measures. Dementia, delirium, and depression are each associated with increased mortality after hip fracture.[44] The potential for diagnostic delays in cognitively impaired patients, leading to adverse outcomes, has been identified in patients with general surgical problems.[41]

Advanced age is a risk factor for acute confusion or delirium after major surgery.[45-47] Acute postoperative confusion is, in turn, a predictor of prolonged hospital stay and functional decline that persists after hospital discharge.[45,46,48] The incidence of acute postoperative confusion varies with the surgical procedure and may be as high as 15% in general surgical patients and 60% in orthopedic patients.[49] Other risk factors for postoperative confusion are preexisting cognitive impairments, visual impairment, alcohol use, the diagnosis of fracture, and, in hospital, the duration of anesthesia, occurrence of postoperative infection, use of narcotics, and the need for a second operation. Postperative cognitive function has also been studied in the longer term.[47,50,51] Advanced age is a risk factor for cognitive impairment 3 months after major noncardiac surgery, which occurs in approximately 10% of patients but resolves in the majority of patients 1 to 2 years postoperatively. Complaints about changes in cognitive function do not necessarily correlate well with measured performance. Early cognitive dysfunction after cardiac surgery with cardiopulmonary bypass is well recognized, and the likelihood of long-term dysfunction is considerable.[52]

The Mini-Mental State Examination (MMSE) is useful as a preoperative screening instrument for cognitive impairment [see Table 2].[53] The MMSE requires approximately 10 minutes to complete and is suitable for repeated assessments. A modified "telephone" version requires only verbal responses and yields comparable results.[54] A number of alternative instruments are available.[55] An assessment of cognitive function should be completed as a routine in patients older than 75

Table 2 Mini-Mental State Examination for Cognitive Function[53]

Maximum Score	Score	Item
5	( )	*Orientation* "What is the date?" Give 1 point each for year, season, date, day, month.
5	( )	"Where are we?" Give 1 point each for state, county, town, building, floor or room.
3	( )	*Registration* Name three objects. Take 1 second to say each, then ask patient to name all three. Give 1 point for each correct answer. Repeat until patient learns all three (for later testing).
5		*Attention and Calculation* Ask patient to subtract serial sevens, starting at 100. Give 1 point for each correct answer. Stop after five answers. (Alternatively, ask patient to spell "world" backward.)
3	( )	*Recall* Ask patient to name the three objects mentioned previously. Give 1 point for each correct answer.
9	( )	*Language* Point to a pencil and a watch and ask patient to name them. Give 1 point for each correct answer. Ask patient to repeat the following: "No ifs, ands, or buts." Give 1 point if successful. Give patient a three-stage command: "Take a paper in your right hand, fold it in half, and put it on the floor." Give 1 point for each correct action. Ask patient to read and obey the following: "Close your eyes." Give 1 point if patient closes eyes. Ask patient to write a sentence. Give 1 point if sentence has a subject and a verb and makes sense. Ask patient to copy a simple design. Give 1 point if drawing is correct.
30	( )	Total Score*

*A score of 24 or more is considered normal.

years for whom major elective surgery is planned and in patients with existing cognitive impairments or other risk factors for postoperative confusion. A baseline assessment is valuable for assessing risk, implementing preventive strategies, and permitting reliable identification of postoperative deterioration; such deterioration may be the initial manifestation of a serious postoperative complication.

NUTRITIONAL ASSESSMENT

The elderly are at risk for malnutrition for several reasons, even in the absence of acute illness. The dietary range of the elderly may be limited by physical and cognitive disabilities, social isolation, a lack of awareness of the importance of a balanced diet, poverty, poor dentition, and the effects of medication on appetite, taste, nutrient absorption, and metabolism. The prevalence of overt protein-calorie malnutrition among the community-dwelling elderly is modest, but intakes of specific minerals and vitamins may be inadequate, especially to meet the increased demands of acute illness. Micronutrient (vitamin and trace element) supplementation has been shown to improve immune function and lower the incidence of clinical infections in both healthy community-dwelling and institutionalized elderly persons.[56,57] Oral protein-calorie and micronutrient supplements should be prescribed before major elective procedures if there is any question about the adequacy of nutrient intake. Malnutrition is more common in elderly residents of nursing homes and other long-term care facilities. Reported rates vary considerably, ranging from 37% to 85%.[58-60] Malnutrition is quite common in hospitalized elderly patients but is frequently not recognized.[61,62] It is consistently associated with adverse outcomes, which intervention studies suggest can be improved by nutritional therapy.[63,64] Assessment of nutritional status should be routine in elderly patients for whom major elective surgery is planned or who are admitted to hospital with an acute illness.

A large number of anatomic, biochemical, and functional measures of nutritional status have been used, in some instances combining measures by means of multivariate statistical techniques.[65-68] A structured clinical assessment can be completed rapidly, is reliable, and is among the most useful tools for nutritional assessment in the elderly. Subjective Global Assessment (SGA) is one such approach that incorporates relevant features of history and physical examination.[69] The Mini Nutritional Assessment (http://www.mna-elderly.com/index.htm) incorporates brief questions and simple anthropometric measurements in an instrument designed for rapid screening of nutrition status in elderly persons in outpatient, nursing home, and hospital settings.[70]

Decreased muscle mass in older persons is accompanied by decreased strength. Maximal voluntary handgrip strength can be evaluated rapidly and has been reported to be a useful predictor of postoperative complications and length of hospital stay after elective surgery and hip fracture.[71,72]

There is no single accepted standard for assessment of nutritional status, which is unsurprising, given the range of micro- and macronutrients to be considered and the myriad of possible structural and functional consequences of what we perceive as malnutrition. Nonetheless, elderly surgical patients should routinely be screened for malnutrition through thoughtful clinical assessment, at least.

ASSESSMENT OF FUNCTION

Assessment of functional level is important at every stage of care of the elderly surgical patient [see Table 3]. Function assessment assists appropriate surgical decision making, governs perioperative care, and helps set realistic goals for postoperative functional level and quality of life. Tools for function assessment (e.g., the FIM instrument, available from the Uniform Data System for Medical Rehabilitation, http://www.udsmr.org) should address basic activities of daily living, cognition, mood, health-related quality of life, and instrumental ADL [see Table 4]. Functional level is a rich field for surgical outcomes research.[16-22,24]

PROCEDURE-RELATED FACTORS

The site of the operation and the magnitude of tissue injury and physiologic perturbation are risk factors for postoperative complications. The increased risks of cardiac and pulmonary complications associated with major abdominal or thoracic procedures are discussed above. The risk of perioperative complications is very low after relatively minor procedures, such as cataract surgery and hernia repair under local anesthesia.[17,73] Morbidity and mortality are invariably greater for emergency operations than for elective ones, presumably because of the

Table 3 Functional Level Assessment for Elderly Surgical Candidates

Why
  To individualize and adapt therapy
  To assign patients to particular treatment protocols, clinical guidelines, or critical pathways
  To follow individual patients to determine outcome measures
  To follow groups of patients
  To conduct patient and institutional outcome research
  To identify gaps in service

When
  Preoperative planning period
  Preoperative assessment—immediate for baseline measures for elective patients
  By history for nonelective cases
  "Reflective" history for elective patients with functional compromise related to the condition that will receive surgical intervention (e.g., patient waiting for hip replacement—how long has gait been impaired?)

What
  General function level (e.g., FIM)
  Cognition (e.g., Mini-Mental State Examination) [see Table 2]
  Depression (e.g., Geriatric Depression Scale) [see Table 4]
  Quality of life (e.g., SF-36 or SF-12 v2)
  Capacity for self-care (e.g., CSHA–modified OARS)

CSHA—Canadian Study of Health and Aging   FIM—Functional Independence Measure SF-36—Short Form–36 Health Survey SF-12 v2—Short Form–12, version 2 Health Survey   OARS—Older Americans Research Survey

greater physiologic disturbance caused by the condition requiring urgent treatment and the limited opportunity to assess and optimize the patient's general medical condition [see Figure 4].[15,74,75] Mortality for emergency GI procedures, for example, has been reported to be as much as three times higher than that for elective procedures. Elderly surgical patients are less likely than young ones to tolerate the prolonged starvation, pain, immobility, and possible infection that accompany delayed operation and should therefore have a high priority for access to the OR for emergency procedures.[3] Overall operative mortality in the elderly appears to have declined gradually over many years. This may be attributable to better preoperative preparation of patients as well as to improvements in anesthetic and perioperative care and surgical technique.

PSYCHOLOGICAL PREPARATION

Psychological factors are of considerable importance in preparing the elderly patient for elective operation [see Sidebar Establishing Rapport with the Elderly Patient]. Preoperative patient education has been shown to enhance patient confidence and to hasten the resumption of ADL after operation.[76] Acute mental stress has been associated with myocardial ischemia in patients with coronary artery disease. The ischemia was reflected in wall motion abnormalities observed on radionuclide ventriculography, was frequently silent, and was similar in magnitude to that induced by exercise but occurred at a lower heart rate.[77] Preoperative reassurance and education of the patient have been shown to reduce anxiety and the postoperative need for narcotic analgesics. Preoperative teaching probably also improves patient compliance with and the effectiveness of postoperative chest physiotherapy and other respiratory maneuvers.[78] Postoperative psychological adjustment is

enhanced by the physician's caring attitudes, as displayed, for example, in preoperative diagnostic interviews with breast cancer patients, who perceived the actual information given in the interviews as the less important component.[79]

PLANNING CONVALESCENCE

Convalescence should be planned before operation, with full consideration given to both the potential impact of planned surgery on function and the possible duration of functional impairment. During convalescence, the patient has not only medical needs but also personal needs (e.g., clothing to be washed, cooking to be done, and living space to be cleaned). Arrangements must be made to meet these personal needs. A small trial of patients with hip fracture and mild or moderate dementia demonstrated a shorter length of hospital stay and greater likelihood of independent living 3 months later with a program of active geriatric rehabilitation.[80] Systematic reviews of programs of rehabilitative care after hip fracture and of supported discharge home for geriatric patients suggest that there is value to such interventions but that considerable uncertainty remains about the populations most likely to benefit and about optimal program design.[81,82]

In elderly individuals, the lack of any immediate family contributes not only to very long hospital stays but also to the requirement for nursing home placement at discharge. These trends hold true regardless of surgical procedure, surgical service of admission, diagnosis, age, and gender. The adjusted odds ratio for very long hospital stays is 1.85 in patients with no adult child. The adjusted odds ratios for requirement for nursing home placement at discharge are 2.59 in patients with no spouse, 3.27 in patients with no adult child, and 8.47 in patients with neither.[83]

Table 4 Geriatric Depression Scale (Mood Scale) (Short Form)

Patient Name:
Date:

Choose the best answer for how you have felt over the past week:	Give 1 point if answer is:
1. Are you basically satisfied with your life?	No
2. Have you dropped many of your activities and interests?	Yes
3. Do you feel that your life is empty?	Yes
4. Do you often get bored?	Yes
5. Are you in good spirits most of the time?	No
6. Are you afraid that something bad is going to happen to you?	Yes
7. Do you feel happy most of the time?	No
8. Do you often feel helpless?	Yes
9. Do you prefer to stay at home, rather than going out and doing new things?	Yes
10. Do you feel you have more problems with memory than most?	Yes
11. Do you think it is wonderful to be alive now?	No
12. Do you feel pretty worthless the way you are now?	Yes
13. Do you feel full of energy?	No
14. Do you feel that your situation is hopeless?	Yes
15. Do you think that most people are better off than you are?	Yes
Total:	_____

For clinical purposes, a score > 5 points is suggestive of depression and should warrant a follow-up interview. Scores > 10 almost always indicate depression.

The caretaker is typically a daughter 50 to 70 years of age or a frail elderly spouse. The caretaker often has a wide range of concerns in addition to the elderly parent or spouse who is the surgical candidate. Such concerns might include holding down a job, helping her adult children through graduate school, minding her grandchildren, maintaining the traditional homemaker's role, and planning financially for her own retirement. Accordingly, she should plan to do one or more of the following: (1) hire a full-time housekeeper for her parent, (2) miss some work, or (3) arrange for convalescent care for a few weeks after the operation.

If family members are reluctant to participate in planning convalescence or arranging for live-in help or community support, they should be warned that they may eventually need to take as much as 8 weeks off from work to compensate for temporary and minor functional lapses on the part of the patient. For reasons not well understood, the elderly patient may not feel quite like himself or herself postoperatively.

During convalescence, which may go on for weeks after discharge, family members should save their energy for those personal support activities in which they cannot be replaced (e.g., visits and telephone conversations). They should not spend disproportionate amounts of time and effort on activities that another person could be paid to perform, such as washing sheets or delivering provisions. In this way, the family may avoid burnout or family stress, either of which may lead to neglect of the elderly member or to early placement.

The elderly patient should be advised to cultivate healthy habits preoperatively, such as exercising and having regular, balanced meals. Finally, the patient should come to the hospital prepared for an active postoperative period, bringing his or her clothes, jogging suit, shoes, walker or cane, hearing aid, glasses, pictures of loved ones, radio, and calendar.

INFORMED CONSENT AND ASSESSMENT OF COMPETENCE

Inherent in the idea of informed consent is that each patient has both the right to be informed about the therapeutic options available and the right to consent to—or refuse—intervention.

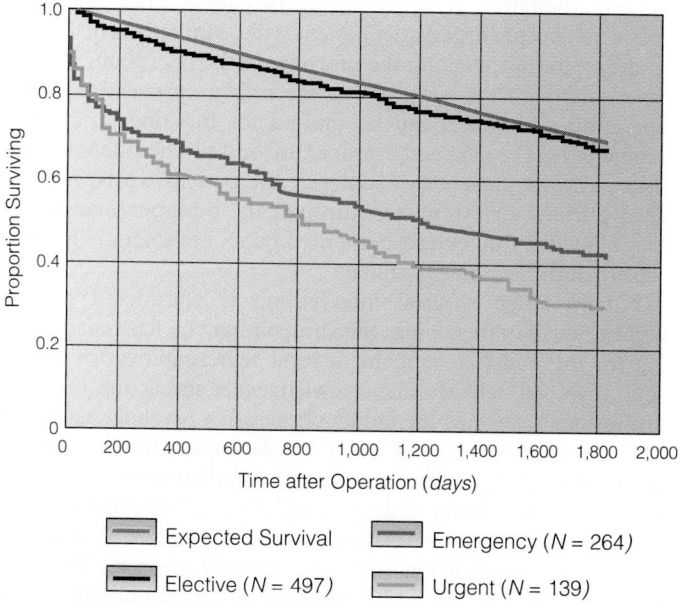

Figure 4 **Depicted is correlation between mode of admission and postoperative survival.**[15]

Establishing Rapport with the Elderly Patient

The surgeon's personal rapport with the patient remains an important element of healing. The patient tends to interpret every aspect of preoperative, intraoperative, and postoperative care—including physiotherapy, nursing, and the ward routine as well as the surgical skills and knowledge displayed—as part of the surgeon's treatment. Older patients are often more in awe of physicians than are younger patients and thus may attribute almost shamanic powers to the surgeon. Such beliefs may be a valuable therapeutic aid.

The elderly generations comprise more disparate styles, cultures, vocabularies, and individual differences than any other generational group. It is therefore especially important that the surgeon attempt to understand and empathize with each patient's attitudes, beliefs, concerns, and modes of communication, some of which have been retained from an earlier time. The result will be a more confident patient, and confident elderly patients have been shown to experience fewer complications. Enhanced feelings of control and autonomy on the part of the patient correlate with a shorter hospital stay. These feelings can be promoted by specific behaviors on the part of the surgeon:

- Never call the patient by his or her first name, even if the patient calls you by yours. Never use "dear," "granny," or any other diminutive or familiar name.
- Address the patient, not the accompanying family member.
- When you speak to the patient, keep your expression calm, smile, bring your face close, and do not turn away. Speak slowly and distinctly, but do not raise your voice.
- Pause from time to time to permit the patient to speak. Do not allow the accompanying family member to fill all the pauses.
- To interrupt or to bring the patient back to the subject you want to discuss, touch him or her slowly on the hand or arm and repeat the question.
- Ask the patient if he or she understands what you have said.
- Ask the patient how he or she feels about what you have said, and address any concerns raised.

It is essential to avoid the appearance of haste or carelessness. If the surgeon is calm and supportive, the patient is likely to be calm and confident. Such nonverbal messages are more important to elderly persons than to younger adults and may be perceived as more valuable than the actual information given.

Confused, demented, or depressed elderly patients are not the only ones who benefit from reassuring nonverbal messages. This style of interaction may be used, for instance, with an active 70-year-old CEO who has sandwiched an appointment with the surgeon between a board meeting and a golf game, even if it seems somewhat exaggerated under the circumstances. Later, when the patient feels confused and cold, cannot see, hear, or smile normally, and has just suffered the indignity of a catheter, he or she will remember the respectful healing behaviors, and the surgeon-patient rapport will be enhanced.

Finally, it should be remembered that aged persons are subject to psychological, physical, and financial abuse. The surgeon should ask the patient directly about these potential problems and should, if necessary, request social and psychiatric assessment and legal intervention.

Obtaining informed consent is more complicated with elderly patients than with younger ones for several reasons: first, older patients may be psychologically or physically dependent on someone else; second, they may be overly deferential to (or suspicious of) the surgeon; third, they may be demented but nonetheless competent to accept or reject a surgical choice. Occasionally, an elderly patient is capable in all the usual areas of function but acts irrationally when asked to accept or forgo a surgical intervention. When told that complications are rare, an older patient may believe the risk to be higher than a younger person would.[84] Older patients may be less interested in obtaining information about complications than younger patients are[85,86]; however, giving detailed information about anesthesia risk does not appear to raise their anxiety level.[87]

The term competence, as we use it here, is defined simply as the capacity to understand the available options and their consequences and the ability to choose freely among these options.[88,89] Competence may refer to either clinical status or legal status. It should be remembered that guidelines allowing a parent or guardian to speak for a child or for a mentally challenged person cannot be generalized to apply to a frail elderly individual whom the surgeon may consider clinically incompetent but who has not yet been determined to be legally incompetent.

To maximize the possibilities for informed consent, the surgeon should arrange to spend some time with the patient, even if the patient seems completely demented. The patient should be asked the following questions:

1. Do you feel comfortable with the idea of surgery?
2. Do you understand what is planned?
3. Do you have any questions for me?

Only after these questions have been answered satisfactorily should the patient be reassured that surgery is in his or her best interests. If the patient is unaccompanied, the surgeon should ask permission to speak with the spouse, a child, or anyone who may be assisting the patient either before or after the surgical procedure. The surgical plan is reviewed with family members and repeated to the patient in the presence of the family. Included in the review should be expectations for the patient's capacity to function in the immediate postoperative period as well as the amount of family support that will be required. Finally, the surgeon should make it very clear to both the patient and the family that although family members can help the patient to understand the available choices, they do not have the right to make the final decision, even if the patient is completely dependent and demented, unless there has been a valid formal delegation of responsibility for health care, including surgery. Definitions and terminology vary among jurisdictions.

When the patient's competence is uncertain, assessment by a psychogeriatrician may be helpful, as may assessments by a geriatrician, a social worker, and the patient's family physician. Some variation of opinion is to be expected because the issue of competence is not a simple one. For example, a patient may be incompetent to manage money but competent to accept operation. Alternatively, a patient may have a borderline status and experience diurnal fluctuations in cognition. A 1994 study of 2,100 internists, surgeons, and psychiatrists concluded that "the common clinical practice of relying on expert medical opinion may introduce bias and produce inaccurate results that undermine patient autonomy."[90] Surgeons performed almost as well as psychiatrists on theoretical issues of competence but surpassed their psychiatric colleagues in the practical application of competence assessment. Practical solutions and common sense must prevail. The patient's values, both cultural and personal, must be taken into account.

When the patient is deemed incompetent, the next step is to establish legal incompetence. Most provinces, states, and hospitals require two psychiatric opinions to declare incompetence and to place the patient under legal guardianship. The efforts of a social worker are usually vital to this process, which can be accomplished immediately in urgent situations, usually through the director of professional services. Once declared incompetent, the patient comes under the protection of the state, which may delegate the role of legal representative to the private sector in the form of family guardianship or the so-called committee of the person. These private-sector guardians are then overseen by the state.

Hospital personnel and family members should be aware that in most North American jurisdictions, power of attorney does not constitute legal guardianship. Power of attorney concerns management of certain delegated acts, such as writing checks and buying and selling certain properties. In fact, as soon as a person becomes incompetent, whether clinically or legally, power of attorney is invalid, because the person is no longer able to decide how these acts should be delegated.

It is vital to consult with, to educate, to reassure, and to work with the family when surgical decisions must be made about a demented elderly patient. Questions to the family should focus on gathering relevant information, such as what the patient's wishes would probably be if he or she could express them and what the patient's functional and biologic status was before the current surgical problem. The family must understand that such questions constitute a request not for permission but rather for information that will help the surgeon in the management of the demented patient.

If the family is the legal representative for health care and refuses operation but the surgeon feels strongly that surgical intervention is in the patient's best interest, legal review should be requested. This request may place the surgeon in a difficult position. In fact, it may relieve some of the burden of decision making carried by the most responsible family member, who may blame himself or herself or be blamed by siblings for everything that goes wrong with the aging parent in the remaining years of life, regardless of whether the problem is related to the surgical intervention.

Rarely, it may happen that even when the patient has been declared legally incompetent, the legal representative for health care has signed the consent form, hospital administrators and the psychogeriatric consultant are supportive of the decision to operate, the family is supportive of the patient, and the patient seems to accept surgery, the patient will adamantly refuse to go to the operating room on the morning of the operation. In such cases, although the surgeon has the right to proceed with the operation and would not be faulted for insisting on it, it is probably best to cancel the procedure and reschedule it for the next day. The presence of someone the patient trusts, such as an old friend or a minister, through the perioperative period may allow the frail elderly demented patient to tolerate the procedure and the surgical milieu.

Finally, when surgical intervention is considered neither urgent nor life threatening, the surgeon may be frustrated waiting for the courts to appoint a legal representative for health care. If so, the help of other knowledgeable and action-oriented professionals, such as the family physician, a psychogeriatrician, or a social worker, may be valuable. New, more flexible mechanisms are being explored in various jurisdictions for management of the well-being of the patient who has lost some autonomy. The newer mechanisms include durable power of attorney, health care proxy, living wills, and judicial advisers. The surgeon's consultants should be able to assist in selecting the most appropriate mechanism, depending on the patient's medical status, prognosis, and family support and on local laws.

Intraoperative Management

POSITIONING

Because elderly patients commonly have diminished range of joint motion, particular attention must be paid to how they are positioned for surgery. The use of regional or general anesthesia may allow positioning that would be uncomfortable and beyond the usual range of motion were the patient not anesthetized. Postoperative back pain is a well-recognized complication of the use of the lithotomy position in the elderly. The remarkable prevalence of osteoporosis and the high incidence of related fractures in the geriatric population emphasize the fragility of these patients and the importance of gentleness and care in turning and positioning them, particularly when discomfort and protective musculoskeletal reflexes have been suppressed by anesthesia. In addition, the skin of elderly individuals is easily injured by tape, adhesive electrodes, cautery pads, and warming blankets. Injury to the skin can occur easily by shearing when elderly patients are lifted and moved or when sheets are pulled from underneath them. Careful padding is necessary to prevent localized pressure, which may result in nerve compression and skin injuries, and to maintain appropriate positioning throughout anesthesia. The head and neck should be kept in a position that is comfortable and limits hyperextension so that cerebral blood flow is not compromised.

MAINTAINING CORE TEMPERATURE

Unless effective preventive measures are taken, a fall in core temperature is common in patients undergoing major surgery, whether general or neuraxial anesthesia is used.[91] The elderly are less well able to maintain normothermia [see Discussion, Thermoregulation, below], and in older studies, the extent and duration of postoperative hypothermia were found to be greater and shivering to be more common in elderly patients.[92] Shivering can result in a severalfold increase in oxygen consumption, which imposes a substantial burden on the cardiac and pulmonary systems in the immediate postoperative period.[93] If the oxygen transport system is unable to meet the increased oxygen demand, myocardial ischemia may result. Maintaining normothermia results in a marked reduction in morbid postoperative cardiac events in patients with cardiac risk factors who have undergone major noncardiac procedures.[94] The incidence of surgical site infection (SSI) is increased by even mild hypothermia, probably in part because of reduced cutaneous blood flow and tissue oxygen delivery.[95] Impaired platelet function and decreased activation of the coagulation cascade are believed to contribute to the increased blood loss and the greater need for blood transfusion associated with hypothermia during elective hip arthroplasty.[96]

Hypothermia should be minimized or prevented in the OR by controlling room temperature, minimizing exposure of body surfaces, warming I.V. fluids and ventilator gases, and using active warming devices (e.g., a warming blanket) as needed. The opportunity to restore an appropriate core temperature without excessive metabolic stress and cardiac work is a reason to consider a brief period of mechanical ventilation when hypothermia was preexisting or is unavoidable (e.g., with major trauma).

PROPHYLAXIS FOR SURGICAL SITE INFECTION AND DEEP VEIN THROMBOSIS

Advanced age is a well-recognized risk factor for the development of postoperative deep vein thrombosis (DVT). Prophylaxis of DVT should be considered in elderly surgical patients [see VI:2 Thromboembolic Problems]. Advanced age has been demonstrated to be associated with an increased incidence of postoperative SSI.[97] In one report, however, the likelihood of SSI (incision or organ/space) after elective resection of the colon and rectum was not influenced by patient age but was influenced by ASA class, male sex, the presence of a stoma, and other factors.[98]

Postoperative Management

RESPIRATORY CARE

For many reasons, elderly patients are predisposed to postoperative respiratory complications, respiratory failure, and inadequate oxygen transport. Such complications remain an important cause of death in this population. Resting arterial oxygen tension and content decrease progressively with advancing age, and the further decrease associated with operation is more marked in the elderly. In addition, the ventilatory responses to both hypoxia and hypercapnia are blunted in older persons. Postoperative hypothermia is more prominent in the elderly, and oxygen demand is markedly increased by postoperative shivering. Abdominal procedures with general anesthesia induce decreases in vital capacity and FEV_1 that last as long as 2 weeks after operation[99]; similar declines in lung volume accompany aging. The combined result is increased closure of small airways, ventilation-perfusion mismatch, and an increased alveolar-arterial oxygen gradient. Impairment of diaphragm function after upper abdominal procedures results in a shift in ventilation away from dependent portions of the lung.[100] Because of stiff chest walls and diminished elastic lung recoil, elderly patients are more reliant on diaphragmatic function than younger patients.[101] Protective airway reflexes are less sensitive in the elderly, mucociliary transport is less efficient, and coughing is less effective because strength, elastic recoil of the lungs, vital capacity, and maximum expiratory flow rate are all diminished. The use of parenteral narcotics for postoperative analgesia has been associated with striking episodic falls in oxygen tension; the increased sensitivity of the elderly to narcotics may further predispose them to such hypoxemia. The presence of coronary artery disease in many older persons underscores the importance of maintaining adequate oxygen delivery and avoiding excessive myocardial oxygen demand in the perioperative period.

Effective analgesia is associated with a partial reversal of postoperative decreases in vital capacity and functional residual capacity and appears to be superior to parenteral narcotic analgesia in this regard.[99] The supine position is accompanied by the closure of small airways in dependent areas of the lung, ventilation-perfusion mismatch, increased alveolar-arterial oxygen gradient, and hypoxemia. Small airway closure occurs at higher lung volumes in older persons, with the result that these adverse effects are more prominent. For this reason, besides adequate analgesia, encouragement and assistance in the early resumption of physical activity must be provided. Simply changing from the supine to the sitting position increases functional residual capacity and improves gas exchange in patients who have undergone abdominal surgery [see Figure 5].[102]

Incentive spirometers, breathing exercises, and intermittent positive-pressure breathing are of some benefit in reducing pulmonary complications after upper abdominal surgery and may help shorten the hospital stay.[103,104] These aids are probably most valuable when used on a regular and frequent basis by patients who are at high risk for pulmonary complications. Supplemental oxygen should be routinely provided to elderly patients who have undergone abdominal or thoracic procedures for a period of several days or until physical mobility is restored—that is, until functional residual capacity is close to preoperative values, ventilation and perfusion are better matched, and oxygen delivery is more reliable. Studies in which patients undergoing elective resection received an inspired oxygen fraction of 80% during surgery and for 2 hours afterward have demonstrated a reduced incidence of both postoperative nausea and vomiting and surgical wound infection compared with those with a 30% inspired oxygen fraction.[105,106]

RENAL FUNCTION AND FLUID AND ELECTROLYTE MANAGEMENT

A 1999 analysis of postoperative deaths in the elderly identified poor fluid and electrolyte management as an important contributor.[3] Inadequate monitoring and documentation were common, and the predisposition of elderly patients to fluid and electrolyte imbalances and their clinical importance was not well recognized. Elderly patients are less able to restore and maintain acid-base, fluid, and electrolyte homeostasis during surgical illness. Compensatory mechanisms that can be relied on in younger patients function less rapidly in older ones. Renal handling of salt and water is less efficient, the physiology of aldosterone and vasopressin is altered, and renal and other mechanisms of acid-base regulation are more limited. As a result, elderly patients are less able to maintain the integrity of the extracellular space and other fluid compartments when challenged. Careful management, based on an understanding of physiologic mechanisms, is necessary if extreme abnormalities of fluid, electrolyte, and acid-base status are to be avoided.

The minimum requirement for water is increased in older patients as a result of increased insensible losses through thinned skin and impairment of the concentrating ability of the kidneys. Thirst is an important response to fluid deprivation, but it is known to be diminished in the elderly.[107] In one study, thirst after a 24-hour period of water deprivation was less in healthy elderly men (67 to 75 years of age) than in younger patients (20 to 31 years of age) despite higher circulating vasopressin levels and higher plasma osmolality; urine osmolality was lower in the first group as well.[108] Hypothalamic responsiveness to osmotic signals appears to increase with age, as manifested by increased release of vasopressin from the posterior pituitary.[109] Unlike the response to osmotic signals, however, the vasopressin response to volume-pressure changes is blunted in the elderly. Renin responses to sodium restriction and postural changes are diminished in older patients, and circulating aldosterone levels are decreased as a result of diminished adrenal sensitivity to both renin-angiotensin and local sodium-potassium signals.[110]

Renal blood flow decreases progressively with advancing age, and the glomerular filtration rate (GFR) falls rapidly after the fifth or sixth decade. The ability of older persons to conserve or excrete water or solute is further reduced by the diminished efficiency of tubular processes, which is a result of decreased osmotic stratification in the medulla and decreased responsiveness to vasopressin.[111] One group of investigators found that healthy young subjects demonstrated a marked decrease in urine flow and a moderate increase in urine osmo-

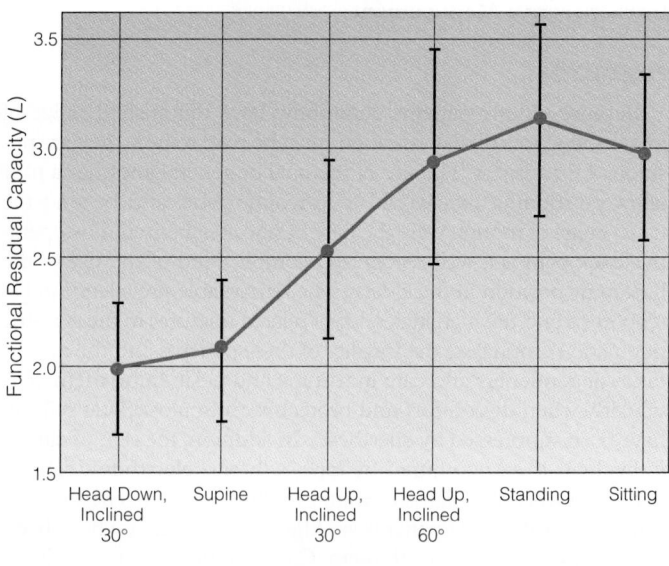

Figure 5 **Shown is functional reserve capacity in selected body positions.**[102]

lality in response to 12 hours of water deprivation, whereas in healthy elderly persons, there was no decrease in urine flow or urine osmolality.[112] Sodium conservation is similarly impaired: the half-time to the achievement of sodium equilibrium in the face of sodium restriction is significantly longer in healthy individuals older than 60 years than in younger individuals.[113] Thus, inefficient renal conservation of salt and water exacerbates hypovolemic states in the elderly patient, and the onset of oliguria may be delayed.

A fall in the GFR also accounts for the decreased ability of the kidneys in the elderly to excrete an acute load of salt or water, predisposing to extracellular fluid volume expansion.[114] Hyponatremia coupled with water intoxication is a serious disorder in the elderly, presenting as anorexia, weakness, lethargy, confusion, and, if severe, seizures or coma. The elderly are prone to excessive secretion of antidiuretic hormone (ADH), particularly during the stress of surgical illness; this excessive ADH secretion is accompanied by extracellular fluid expansion, hyponatremia, and inappropriately concentrated (i.e., less than maximally dilute) urine despite normal renal function.[114]

Although the pH of body fluids is normally only slightly affected by age, the efficiency of acid-base homeostasis is decreased in the elderly.[111] For example, elderly persons (72 to 93 years of age) take twice as long to eliminate an acid load as younger individuals (17 to 35 years of age) do.[115] Maintenance of normal pH depends on chemical buffer systems in body fluids, alterations in ventilation and elimination of carbon dioxide, and renal excretion of excess acid or base. The slight decreases in extracellular volume and in bicarbonate concentration that occur in the elderly may limit the capacity of rapid chemical buffering systems. Similarly, decreased plasma volume and lean body mass and bone demineralization decrease the availability of slower buffers such as plasma and intracellular proteins and hydroxyapatite.[111] Bicarbonate buffering depends on the rapid elimination of carbon dioxide by the lungs. Neither arterial carbon dioxide tension (P_aCO_2) nor minute ventilation changes with age: increased physiologic dead space is compensated for by decreases in metabolic rate and carbon dioxide production. Ventilatory responses to hypercapnia are significantly diminished in healthy elderly persons[116]; however, because ventilation is increased and eucapnia maintained during exercise in the elderly,[117] physiologic pH buffering by respiratory mechanisms probably will not be limited during acute illness except perhaps in the face of a very large acid load.

Renal regulation of acid-base status is based on the variable reabsorption of bicarbonate, the elimination of hydrogen ions in the form of titratable acid, and the regeneration of extracellular bicarbonate accompanying the deamination of glutamine and the synthesis of ammonia.[111] The capacity of each of these mechanisms is presumably limited by the diminished effective renal mass in the elderly.[111] Although the efficiency of bicarbonate reabsorption is maintained and is adequate for handling an acid load, a decreased GFR results in decreased presentation of bicarbonate to the proximal tubule and delayed elimination of bicarbonate in response to an alkaline load. The major buffer used for the generation of titratable acid is phosphate, which is less available in the distal nephron of the aged kidney, primarily as a result of a decreased GFR. The deamination of glutamine in the distal tubule provides ammonia (NH_3), which combines with secreted hydrogen ions to form ammonium (NH_4^+) and is then excreted with chloride and other tubular anions; this process is accompanied by a net increase in bicarbonate in the extracellular fluid. These processes are less effective in the elderly because the capacity of the aged kidney to deaminate glutamine is decreased and lower plasma aldosterone levels limit the exchange of sodium and hydrogen in the distal segment.

The progressive decline in renal function that occurs with advancing age has been well described[118] and appears to be more consistent than changes in other organ systems [see Table 1]. Because of predictable decreases in skeletal muscle mass—and therefore in creatinine production—the serum creatinine concentration is likely to remain within the laboratory normal range despite the substantial concurrent decreases in GFR that occur [see Figure 6]. Increased serum creatinine concentrations reflect a marked impairment of renal function. Creatinine clearance can be estimated from the assumptions that it is 100 ml/min at age 40 years and declines by 1 ml/min each subsequent year. Another approach is based on age, gender, and serum creatinine: for males, creatinine clearance in ml/min = [(140 - age in years) × weight in kg] ÷ (72 × serum creatinine in mg/dl); for females, the result is multiplied by 0.85.[119] Creatinine clearance is most reliably assessed by determining creatinine clearance from 24-hour urine creatinine and serum creatinine concentration.

Nonsteroidal anti-inflammatory drugs (NSAIDs) have a number of potentially detrimental effects on the kidneys of older patients.[120] Inhibition of cyclooxygenase (COX)-catalyzed prostaglandin production by NSAIDs may allow unopposed vasoconstriction and marked decreases in renal blood flow and GFR in hypovolemic states, which may result in acute renal failure. In addition, NSAIDs potentiate hyponatremia and hyperkalemia through their effects on the renin-angiotensin-aldosterone system, and may cause acute interstitial nephritis. Selective inhibition of the COX-2 isoform is associated with the therapeutic effects of NSAIDs. However, COX-2 is present in the kidney, and selective COX-2 inhibition has effects on renal function that are similar to those of nonselective NSAIDs.[121] Both selective and nonselective NSAIDs should be used with caution in the elderly surgical patient, especially with pre-existing renal impairment and during acute illness when multiple factors predisposing to renal injury are frequently present.

CARDIOVASCULAR CARE

Cardiovascular complications are a major cause of postoperative death in elderly patients. The assessment of cardiac risk previously described (see above) should be the basis for preventive and monitoring strategies in the perioperative period. Aggressive reduction of coronary risk factors such as smoking and hypertension should be pursued preoperatively. The effectiveness of perioperative beta-blockers in limiting increases in heart rate and blood pressure and reducing myocardial ischemia and cardiac mortality has been suggested in clinical trials.[11] In practice, however, starting beta-blockers preoperatively is infrequent.[122]

It is in the first 48 to 96 hours after operation that the most significant shifts in fluid between body compartments occur, the onset of congestive heart failure is most frequent, and the hemodynamic abnormalities contributing to myocardial ischemia are most readily identified and treated. When invasive hemodynamic monitoring has been initiated in the OR, consideration should be given to continuing it during this period.

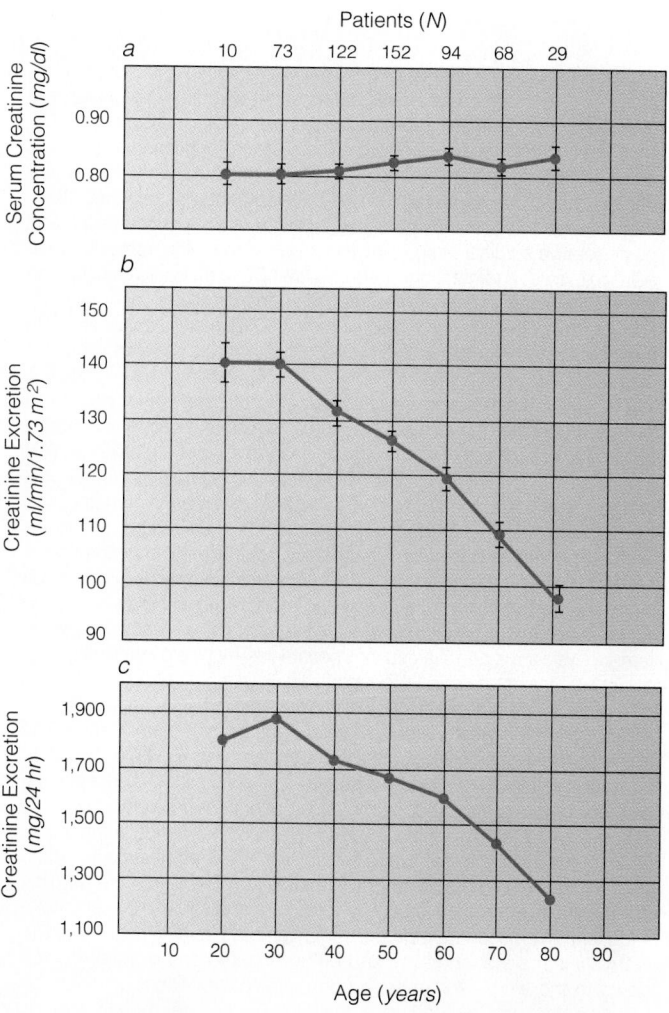

Figure 6 **Illustrated are cross-sectional differences in serum creatinine concentration, creatinine clearance, and creatinine excretion.**[252]

In studies of patients of varying ages, myocardial infarction and reinfarction have tended to occur in the early postoperative period, often painlessly. Continuous ECG monitoring in the postoperative period may be a sensitive method for detecting myocardial ischemia and determining whether intensive therapy is needed. Many studies suggest the need for frequent clinical assessment and continuous ECG monitoring in elderly patients who are at high risk for cardiac complications (considering patient-, diagnosis-, and procedure-related factors) for at least 3 days postoperatively and possibly longer.

PAIN MANAGEMENT

Effective analgesia plays a critical role in allowing early resumption of physical activity, increasing lung volumes, and improving respiratory gas exchange after operation. In addition, postoperative pain is itself a stimulus to the elaboration of stress hormones and stress responses. Activation of the sympathoadrenal axis and other mediators results in increases in overall metabolic demand and in myocardial work. These effects serve no beneficial purpose in the postoperative patient and are detrimental from a physiologic perspective, quite apart from the fundamental clinical goal of preventing or relieving suffering.

Alternatives in the management of postoperative pain are discussed in detail elsewhere [see VIII:2 Postoperative Pain].

Table 5 Stratification of Modified Older Americans Research Survey ADL and IADL in Canadian Study of Health and Aging[256]

Basic Self-Care (Scale 1)	Intermediate Self-Care (Scale 2)	Complex Self-Management (Scale 3)
Toileting (ADL)	Bathing (ADL)	Handling money (IADL)
Dressing (ADL)	Walking (ADL)	Phone use (IADL)
Eating (ADL)	Housework (IADL)	Self-medicating (IADL)
Transferring (ADL)	Meal preparation (IADL)	
Grooming (ADL)	Shopping (IADL)	
	Walking outside (IADL)	

ADL—activities of daily living IADL—instrumental ADL
Each item is scored as follows: 2—task performed without help; 1—task performed with some help; 0—task not performed. Valid for "self-report" and family or proxy report.

Recent developments in anesthetic techniques, minimally invasive surgery, and perioperative care now allow major procedures to be carried out with a very limited postoperative stress response, minimal pain, decreased organ dysfunction and morbidity, very brief periods of starvation and immobility, and early recovery.[123] Continuous blockade of neural signals from

Achievement of Optimal Functional Level

Optimal functional level is the goal of all diagnostics, therapeutics, and management in the elderly patient. According to a 1988 statement by the American College of Physicians, "maintenance of the patient's functional well-being is a fundamental goal of medical practice. Assessment of the impact of illness on physical, mental, and psychosocial functioning is an essential element of clinical diagnosis, a major determinant of therapeutic choices, a measure of their efficacy, and a guide in the planning of long-term care for the dependent elderly."[241]

Functional level assessment is intrinsic to geriatric care and should be practiced throughout the perioperative period to predict rehabilitation potential, to estimate biologic reserve, to follow progress, to signal complications, to identify appropriate social supports at discharge, and to ensure discharge. Functional level assessment is known to improve diagnostic and therapeutic outcomes.[242] Recognition of functional impairment leads to identification of previously undiagnosed conditions that may be treatable preoperatively or managed perioperatively. Another justification for functional level assessment is that disease states do not correlate as well with severity of impairment in elderly patients as they do in younger adults, even when clinical judgment has provided a reliable estimate of degree of aging and all disease states are known.[243,244]

The surgical literature reflects a growing awareness of functional outcomes—both specific outcomes related to pathology and surgery and general outcomes related to the patient's day-to-day activities and quality of life.[245-250]

For assessment of functional level, surgeons need fast, simple tools suitable for all stages of management (preoperative, perioperative, and postoperative) that correlate well with measures of cardiovascular, pulmonary, and renal function and that identify patients who will achieve maximum postoperative function and who need rehabilitation or other community supports at discharge. Unfortunately, no such tool exists; surgeons will probably have to develop one themselves. In the meantime, the ASA scale and other biologic assessments can be complemented with functional assessments borrowed from the medical, psychiatric, and social science literatures.

There are actually hundreds of functional assessment tools, some of which have been validated for use in the geriatric population and some of which were specifically developed for elderly patients. These tools have various goals, ranging from predicting social supports to monitoring deterioration. Most of them address one or more of the following

areas: mobility, falls and balance, continence, cognition, emotional and affective status, nutrition, homeostasis, basic ADL, instrumental ADL, environment, and social supports. The various functional level scales cover items ranging from disability, handicap, and incapacity to independence and ranging from ability to self-development and self-realization.

In selecting functional measures, preoperative, perioperative, and postoperative surgical teams may focus on the following domains: basic ADL (e.g., toilet and nutrition); instrumental ADL (e.g., banking, shopping for and preparing meals, and using public transportation); cognitive function (including memory and language); mood (primarily to validate data available in other domains); and quality of life from the patient's viewpoint [see Table 3].

It is worth remembering that assessments of basic and instrumental ADL and cognition do not explain why a particular function is impaired but simply describe how well a patient is functioning at a given time. Any functional impairment is a signal that further assessment to identify correctable pathologic conditions is indicated. When areas of compromised function have been identified before an elective procedure, it may be wise to request a period of rehabilitation to maximize functional level before admission. For example, continence training may be provided by a community health nurse, and gait and mobility training may be provided by a geriatric physiotherapist. Complementary assessments by the family physician, a psychiatrist, or a geriatrician may help identify ways of achieving maximal function preoperatively.

In general, it is not expected that a preoperative functional impairment will be improved postoperatively unless the surgical intervention was specifically designed to address the impairment. For example, if mobility is compromised by an inguinal hernia, it is reasonable to expect the patient to resume his or her own banking after herniorrhaphy.

The nursing team should be made aware of the patient's functional deficits in the OR, in recovery, and in the ward afterward. To some degree, they may be able to compensate for disability in the surgical environment and may even prevent additional disability. For example, a patient who is encouraged to wear glasses and a hearing aid in recovery is more cooperative and better oriented and is ready to step down to the ward. Nurses who compensate for patient deafness by ensuring that the patient sees their lips when they speak and by speaking slowly and clearly can report patient level of consciousness more reliably.[76]

the operative site for 24 to 48 hours, often with epidural anesthesia, minimizes the stress response to surgery, reducing morbidity substantially and all-cause mortality by one third.[124] When such techniques are not available or applicable, patient-controlled analgesia may be appropriate for the elderly patient who understands and is able to self-administer analgesic medication (usually intravenously).

Of note in elderly patients is the reported CNS stimulation induced by multiple doses of meperidine, which is attributed to accumulation of the metabolite normeperidine; meperidine should therefore be used with caution in these patients. The volume of distribution of morphine is smaller in the elderly patient, plasma and tissue drug levels are greater for a fixed dose, and the drug disappears more slowly from CSF; these differences would account for the more marked respiratory depression and other CNS effects observed in older patients. Plasma morphine concentration and morphine clearance also depend on renal function.

Age-related changes in pharmacokinetics and pharmacodynamics are relevant also to the use of fentanyl, sufentanil, and alfentanil.[125] Elderly patients reportedly obtain greater relief of pain from constant narcotic doses and show more marked CNS depression at given blood levels of benzodiazepines than younger patients do. Parenteral administration of narcotics can be associated with profound arterial oxygen desaturation, particularly in older patients and particularly during sleep, and may not provide optimal relief of pain.[126,127]

NSAIDs have been used in combination with narcotics and other analgesics in the management of postoperative pain. Such agents should be used with caution in elderly surgical patients, as noted above.

MAINTAINING FUNCTION

The goal of postoperative care is maximum function. Achievement of optimal functional level depends on three principal areas—mobility, continence, and cognition—and on how these areas are integrated with the six basic ADL during hospitalization [see Table 5 and Sidebar Achievement of Optimal Functional Level].

Each patient should have a program designed to enhance independence in performing ADL at every stage of recovery. Occasionally, postoperative ADL function may exceed preoperative ADL function, either because the surgery has direct effects on function or because the patient had been unnecessarily limited (by self, family, or caregivers) preoperatively. All stages of step-down care must be individually tailored and modified when medical conditions are present that might inhibit progress.

Physical Function

Mobility and appropriate sensory stimulation should be maximized before and after operation. Even healthy elderly patients have lost a good deal of their muscle strength. The continued loss of strength that accompanies immobility may have marked functional consequences. Elderly patients are at increased risk for atelectasis and other pulmonary complications after operation, and early mobilization helps minimize the incidence of these complications [see Table 6]. Cardiovascular deconditioning occurs regardless of age: the decrease in cardiac output on standing may be considerable after a period of prolonged bed rest and may be accompanied by orthostatic hypotension and tachycardia. Maximum oxygen consumption, cardiac output,

Table 6 Potential Complications of Immobility[257]

Skin	Pressure sores
Musculoskeletal	Muscular deconditioning and atrophy Contractures Bone loss (osteoporosis)
Cardiovascular	Deconditioning Decreased plasma volume Orthostatic hypotension Venous thrombosis, embolism
Pulmonary	Decreased ventilation Atelectasis Aspiration pneumonia
Gastrointestinal	Anorexia Constipation Fecal impaction, incontinence
Genitourinary	Urinary infection Urinary retention Bladder calculi Incontinence
Metabolic	Negative nitrogen balance Impaired glucose tolerance Altered drug pharmacokinetics
Psychological	Sensory deprivation Dementia, delirium Depression

and stroke volume at maximum exercise are all lower after prolonged immobilization. Bed rest results in a significant decrease in tissue sensitivity to insulin, exaggerating age-related glucose intolerance. Bed rest is also associated with an increased incidence of DVT, as is advancing age. Constipation and fecal impaction are frequent in immobilized patients as a result of alterations in gastrointestinal motility (related to inactivity and medications), lack of privacy, and the use of bedpans. Decubitus ulcers are well-recognized complications of immobility to which the elderly are predisposed because of diminished subcutaneous fat and decreased skin elasticity.

Expectations about postoperative mobilization, its importance, and the assistance that will be provided should be communicated preoperatively to patients and their families. Postoperatively, effective pain management is essential. Beginning in the immediate postoperative period, full passive range-of-motion exercises of all joints should be undertaken daily, even after the patient is able to sit up in a chair and walk a short distance in the corridor. These interventions not only conserve the patient's capacity for mobility but also help prevent bedsores. The involvement of a physiotherapist may be required.

Once awake, the patient who requires glasses or a hearing aid should wear them at all times. As soon as the patient is able to sit in a chair, he or she should wear shoes, preferably solid, comfortable jogging shoes with Velcro closures. The patient should wear regular clothes, preferably a jogging suit, as soon as possible. A walker, a cane, or a wheelchair should be kept at the bedside and used as the physiotherapist advises. The patient should be encouraged to walk the full length of the hall each day. Every effort should be made to minimize intravenous lines, drains, catheters, and other forms of physical restraint. Regardless, such devices should not prohibit planned activities but may necessitate accompaniment and assistance. Periods of activity should be systematically alternated with rest periods. The primary nurse is the caregiver best equipped to ensure that this routine is implemented.

These rehabilitation and maintenance efforts must be carried out in the surgical ward. There is no point to sending a frail elderly person down to the physiotherapy/occupational therapy department: the patient will not learn to integrate the new skills into a daily routine. Older persons must work like athletes in the postoperative period. A training effect can be noted in skeletal muscle and in the cardiovascular and pulmonary systems. Accordingly, elderly patients deserve continual congratulations and encouragement.

Aggressive rehabilitation instituted early will certainly lead to better function at discharge. However, a general surgical ward that properly serves elderly patients will also show a higher incidence of hip fracture and minor injuries. These risks must be accepted by staff, patients, and family.

Cognitive Function

In a dark, soundless, weightless chamber without aural, visual, sensory, or vestibular cues, young, fit adults are known to have a high incidence of transitory psychosis, presumably caused by the intense isolation and lack of stimulation. The elderly hospitalized patient who is medicated, deprived of glasses or a hearing aid, and restrained in a dimly lit room may exhibit a similar response, provoked by isolation and lack of cueing. The sensory deprivation characteristic of even brief confinement in a typical hospital setting may be accompanied by changes in affect, impaired cognition and intellectual function, and perceptual distortions in the elderly patient. All staff members who have contact with older patients, including housekeeping personnel and technicians, should continually provide them with orienting cues, such as the weather, the season, the day of the week, the name of the hospital, and their own name and function. Many of the interventions described in the discussions of physical function, continence, and ADL have the added advantage of increasing the amount of appropriate sensory stimulation provided to the patient and thereby contributing to improved cognition.

As discussed [see Risk Assessment and Cognitive Assessment, above], early postoperative confusion is relatively common in elderly patients and is best identified by means of an instrument such as the MMSE [see Table 2], especially if a preoperative baseline assessment is available. The MMSE is a valid, rapid, and reliable assessment tool designed for elderly patients and suitable for repeat assessment. Acute postoperative confusion usually corresponds to delirium characterized by an acute onset of fluctuating inattentiveness, cognitive impairment, and psychomotor changes, which may include agitation, retardation, or both. The diagnosis implies an underlying organic etiology that must be actively sought and corrected. Delirium may be the first manifestation of a postoperative complication such as infection or hypoxemia. Medications must be reviewed, especially sedatives and narcotics. Physical examination should look for potential sources of infection, signs of cardiorespiratory or other organ dysfunction, and focal neurologic deficits. Hematologic tests, blood chemistry, and oxygen saturation or blood gas analysis should be routinely ordered. Chest x-ray, other imaging, ECG, and other investigations should be undertaken as indicated.

Confused patients require close supervision to ensure that they do not harm themselves. Haloperidol or other medication may be necessary to control behavior. Reassurance and reorientation provided by someone familiar, especially family, in a calm, well-lit environment may be very helpful. In a 1999 study of elderly general medical patients, a multicomponent intervention strategy was shown to be effective in reducing the incidence of delirium.[128] The strategy targeted the risk factors of cognitive impairment (orientation), sleep deprivation, immobility, hearing impairment, and dehydration.

Confusion, dementia, and cognitive deficits are not normal consequences of aging. Their presence is an indication for diagnostic and therapeutic intervention.

Continence

Efforts to help the patient achieve and maintain continence should begin preoperatively and should be reestablished postoperatively as soon as possible. Systematic toileting (every 2 hours) should be initiated by the primary nurse, even before the catheter is removed, to maintain bowel function and toileting habits. Catheters should be removed as soon as possible and should not be relied on for monitoring of input and output. Nurses should respond promptly to patient requests for toileting. If urinary incontinence recurs or persists, the toileting interval should be shortened until continence is achieved and then should be lengthened. If urinary continence cannot be established in 48 hours, residual urine should be measured, urinalysis should be performed, and a urine specimen should be sent for culture. Other metabolic causes of urinary incontinence should be sought and urodynamic studies carried out.

Stool incontinence (with or without diarrhea) should be considered the result of impaction, until proved otherwise, even if there is no fecalith palpable on digital examination. Bowel care must be the responsibility of the surgeon and primary nurse. A step-down program for encopresis should be started aggressively with enemas, followed by stool softeners and bulk agents, with suppositories as needed, and toileting 1 hour after each meal as well as in response to urge. A behavioral program should be developed with the patient, who should participate in maintaining the toileting schedule and recording performance. Rewards, even trivial ones such as stick-on stars for clean, dry days and big stars for clean, dry days and nights, can make the program more attractive and enjoyable for the patient and the staff.

It is worth remembering that incontinence is never a normal consequence of aging. In every case, it should be explained by a specific diagnosis, managed, and treated.

Activities of Daily Living

Patients should groom and dress themselves entirely as soon as they able, including putting on aids and prostheses. Self-medication should be introduced gradually, starting as soon as possible after recovery, and should be reviewed twice daily by the nursing staff. Dosette boxes and calendars are useful. Unit dose pharmacy management has no place in geriatric care because it systematically teaches dependence.

The independence of the hospitalized elderly patient is continually undermined. To begin with, insisting on patient independence takes extra nursing time: it is quicker and easier to do things for patients than it is to instruct them. In addition, patients themselves often sabotage nurses' efforts to foster independence, arguing that because they are old and sick they

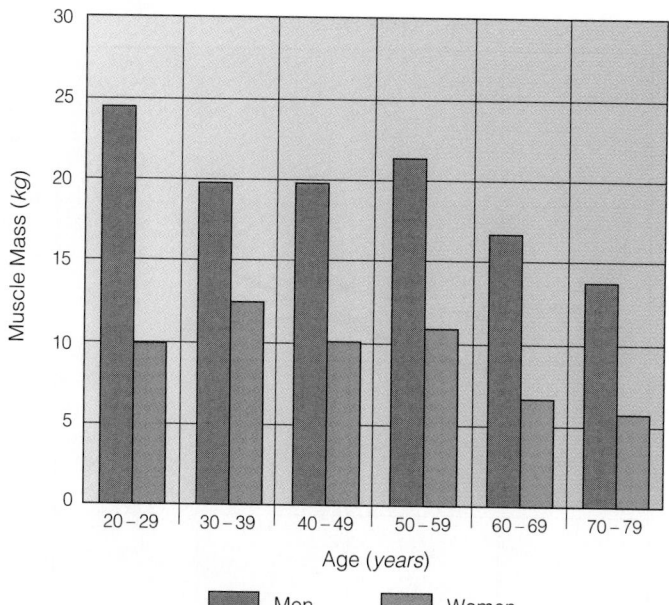

Figure 7   **A substantial portion of the muscle mass present in young adulthood is lost by 70 years of age. Age-related declines in muscle strength have been documented as well.**[149]

should not be expected to do much for themselves. Consequently, nurses who encourage self-care sometimes have patients who feel neglected and who may even become resentful and uncooperative; in some cases, an unhappy family may even complain to the administration.

Families are not naturally helpful in mobilization. Instead, they often insist on doing things for geriatric patients even while scolding them for not doing more for themselves. Families must be taught by nurses and physiotherapists exactly how the elderly persons are to get out of a chair and how far and how often they are to walk.

Persistent stepwise encouragement to regain autonomy is perhaps the most beneficial service nurses can offer elderly surgical patients in the postoperative period. A word from the surgeon to the patient and family may gain the nurse and physiotherapist the patient's willing cooperation. If behavioral problems persist, a behaviorist, a psychiatrist, a geriatrician, or the patient's family physician should be consulted.

Summary

The surgeon should not make the mistake of assuming that paying attention to the patient's functional level in basic ADL is the responsibility solely of the rehabilitation unit or the convalescent unit. Orientation, mobility, and ADL all are significantly and systematically compromised in the traditional surgical ward in just a few days. Once function is lost, even long-term rehabilitation cannot ensure that it will be recaptured. Immobility, inadequate nutrition, and sensory deprivation and other features of the usual acute care hospital environment will contribute to a "cascade to dependency" in vulnerable elderly patients unless actively addressed by a multidisciplinary clinical team.[129]

Other patient skills to be demonstrated before discharge should match the environment to which the patient is going. Occupational and physical therapists should routinely follow geriatric surgical patients and should integrate planning with the nursing staff. Elderly patients are less likely than younger

patients to integrate the skills demonstrated during rehabilitation in a traditional occupational/physical therapy work area or gymnasium into the performance of ADL on the ward and, later, at home. Home visits by the occupational and physical therapists are useful components of assessment and rehabilitation.

NUTRITIONAL CARE

Preexisting malnutrition is relatively common in the elderly (see above) and is exacerbated in hospital by the periods of fasting that are commonplace and by the rapid erosion of skeletal muscle that accompanies the stress of major surgery and acute surgical illness. Such losses of muscle protein may be uniquely detrimental in elderly patients. Lean body mass and body cell mass both decrease considerably with normal aging, largely because of declining muscle mass: a loss of 40% of muscle mass or more is typical between young adulthood and the age of 80 years and is accompanied by a comparable decrease in strength [*see Figure 7*]. For example, the average 80-year-old woman is at the threshold of quadriceps strength necessary to rise from a low, armless chair [*see Figure 8*].[130] Thus, during prolonged or severe illness, the rapid erosion of muscle mass may reduce an elderly patient's muscle strength below that necessary to move about in bed, sit, and cough effectively. Moreover, recovery of strength is impaired in older surgical patients compared with younger patients [*see Figure 9*].[131]

The typical diets followed by older persons may provide adequate vitamins and trace minerals in the absence of stress, though it is worth remembering that there is a general lack of information about specific requirements in the elderly. Stores may be limited, however, and deficiencies may arise during illness. For example, plasma zinc concentration decreases after

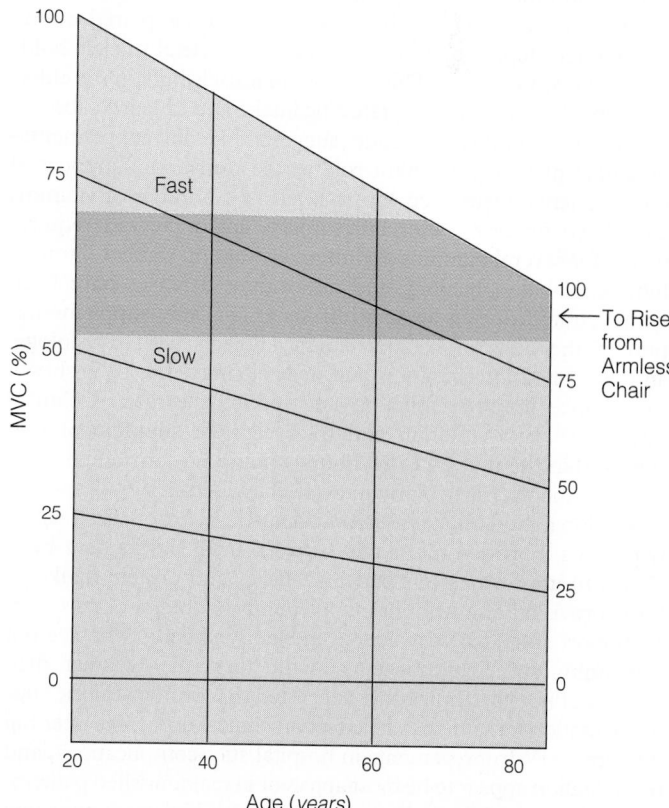

Figure 8   **Depicted is the effect of age on ability to rise from a low, armless chair.**[130] **(MVC—maximal voluntary contraction)**

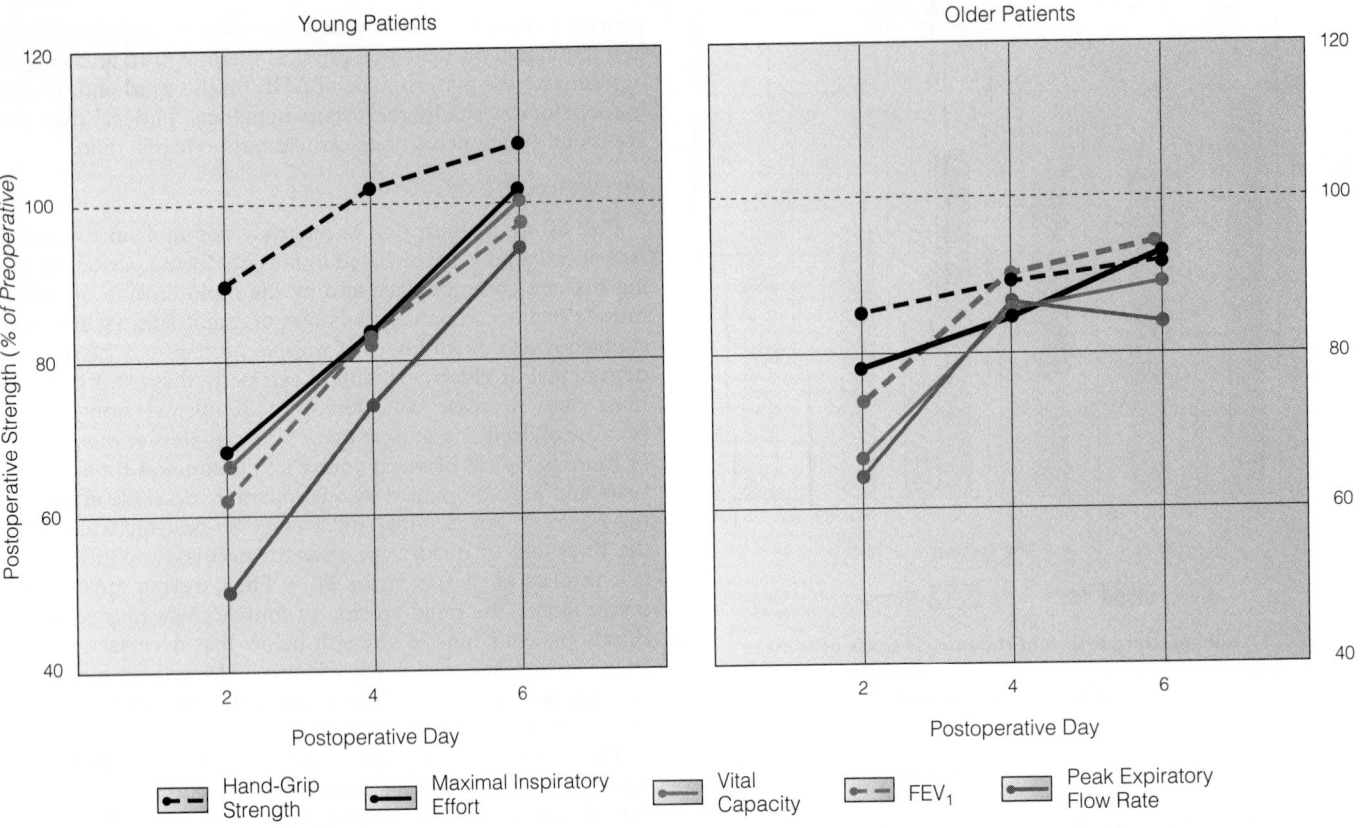

Figure 9 **Illustrated is the recovery of postoperative strength (assessed with respect to five variables) in younger and older patients.**[131]

injury and other stresses, partly as a result of increased urinary losses. Zinc deficiency has been associated with impaired wound healing and depressed immune function. Skeletal muscle holds the largest store of zinc. The decrease in muscle bulk in the elderly, coupled with the inadequate zinc intake and impaired absorption reported in this age group, suggests that zinc supplementation may play an important role in the nutritional support of these patients. Decreased serum levels of a number of vitamins have been observed after burn injury, and increased requirements for several vitamins and minerals that may affect immune function, wound healing, and antioxidant defenses have been demonstrated during acute stress states.[132] Daily supplementation of the diets of healthy elderly subjects with physiologic amounts of various vitamins and trace elements has been shown to enhance immune function and reduce the rate of clinical infection.[56] Early vitamin and trace element supplementation (i.e., within the first 24 to 48 hours) should be considered in all elderly patients, particularly in nonelective settings.

Volitional food intake is often inadequate in hospitalized elderly patients. Fortified meals and between-meal snacks have been shown to improve elderly patients' energy and protein intake.[133] Early provision of nutritional supplements or enteral or parenteral support should be considered in elderly patients who are not consuming sufficient nutrients in the form of a regular diet. Some, but not all, studies have suggested that protein-calorie supplementation has a beneficial effect on clinical outcomes after hip fracture.[134-136] Improvements in hospital stay, complications, and rehabilitation appear to be most apparent in malnourished patients, although methodologic limitations in published trials preclude definitive conclusions. Oral supplements are usually well tolerated and do not necessarily lead to a decrease in volitional intake.

Enteral feeding should be initiated promptly in any elderly patient whose voluntary intake is not adequate. Parenteral feeding can be used alone or as an adjunct when enteral feeding is being established or when prescribed nutrients cannot be fully administered by the enteral route. Energy intake and expenditure in healthy individuals tend to decrease in parallel with advancing age as a result of diminished metabolic body size (i.e., body cell mass) and reduced activity[137] [*see Figure 10*]. The number of calories provided to elderly surgical patients should reflect these changes, although of course the considerable variability among individuals must be taken into account as well. Protein intake should normally be 1 to 2 g/kg/day, depending on the severity of the primary illness and the nature of the associated disease states. Provision of nutritional support via enteral and parenteral routes is discussed in detail elsewhere [*see VII:9 Nutritional Support*].

Whereas the need for nutritional support appears to be greater in elderly patients, such support may be less efficacious and less well tolerated because of the combined influences of aging and acute illness on intermediary metabolism. Glucose tolerance decreases with normal aging, and enteral or parenteral feeding may result in marked hyperglycemia, particularly when coupled with the insulin resistance that accompanies trauma and critical illness.[138] Additionally, insulin responses to glucose loads are markedly diminished in the elderly after injury [*see Figure 11*]. Decreased serum growth hormone and insulinlike growth factor–1 (IGF-1) responses to feeding have also been described in older trauma patients.[139,140] Renal clearance of glucose is normally an important defense against hyperglycemia; however, a reduced GFR and an increased renal threshold for glucose make elderly patients even more prone to hyperglycemia. Uncontrolled hyperglycemia resulting from either an enteral or a parenteral glucose load may give rise to hyperosmolar nonketotic coma, in which serum osmolarity and glucose are markedly elevated in association with a solute diuresis, dehydration, coma, and inappropriately low insulin and ketone levels. This condition is corrected by rehydration and insulin administration. In a trial involving patients admitted to a surgical ICU and given parenteral nutrition, intensive insulin therapy and control of blood glucose levels resulted in less frequent sepsis and organ dysfunction and improved survival.[141]

Hyperglycemia may limit the administration of calories provided in the form of glucose even when insulin is used. Fat emulsion may be used as an alternative energy source in parenteral feeding, but plasma triglyceride levels should be monitored because they tend to increase with age and because lipid clearance may be altered. Because of age-related decreases in GFR, protein loads that might be well tolerated in young

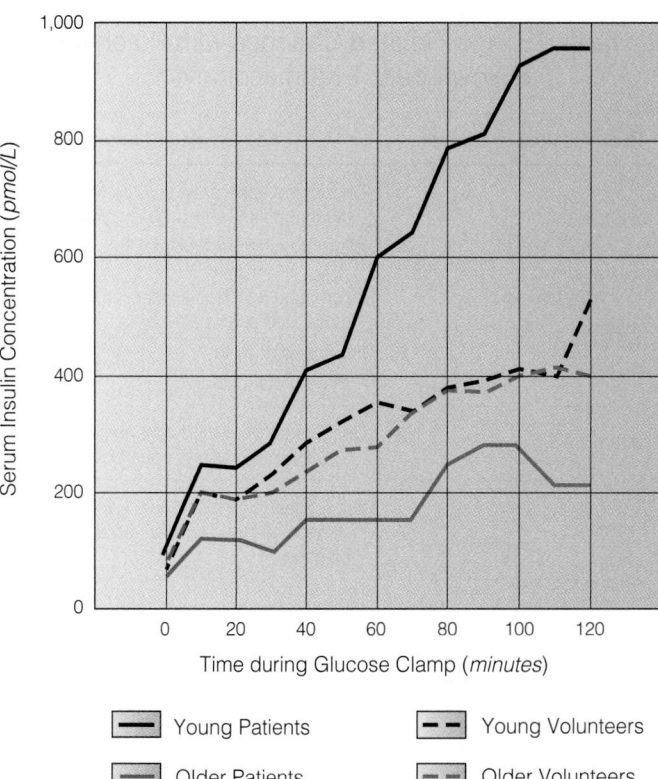

Figure 11 Shown are serum insulin responses to glucose loading (during glucose clamp).[253]

patients can lead to uremia in the elderly. Blood urea values should be monitored.

Nutritional support of the elderly patient should begin early, should take into account age-related changes in body composition, should include appropriate micronutrients, and should anticipate diminished tolerance of substrate and fluid loads.

CLINICAL PHARMACOLOGY

Use of both prescription and nonprescription drugs is heavy in the geriatric population, and a careful history of drug use must be obtained, if necessary by contacting family and pharmacist and examining the drug containers themselves. Noncompliance occurs but is probably no more frequent in elderly patients than in younger ones. Most instances of noncompliance may actually be underadherence, which can be an appropriate response to adverse drug effects. A knowledge of how aging affects clinical pharmacology is important because drugs and doses that would not normally cause toxicity in younger patients can do so in the elderly.[142] Consequently, the incidence of adverse drug reactions increases substantially with age, and drug reactions are an important cause of hospital admission, morbidity, and mortality.[143-145] This increase may reflect the greater use of drugs by older patients (particularly drugs with a low therapeutic index, such as digoxin), polypharmacy and resultant interactions, the presence of multiple and more severe comorbidities in the elderly, and aging-associated alterations in pharmacokinetics and pharmacodynamics [see Table 7].

Pharmacologic considerations include both pharmacokinetics and pharmacodynamics. The term pharmacokinetics refers to the absorption, distribution, protein binding, metabolism, and excretion of drugs and their metabolites (drug disposition), whereas the term pharmacodynamics refers to the interaction of drugs with receptors and the resulting desired or

Figure 10 Depicted are the daily intake and expenditure of calories in normal males of various age groups.[137]

Table 7 Age-Related Changes with Potential Relevance to Pharmacology[258]

Pharmacologic Parameter	Age-Related Changes
Absorption	Decreased absorptive surface, splanchnic blood flow, and gastric acidity Altered gastrointestinal motility
Distribution	Decreased total body water, lean body mass, and serum albumin Increased body fat Altered protein binding
Metabolism	Decreased liver blood flow, enzyme activity, and enzyme inducibility
Excretion	Decreased renal blood flow, glomerular filtration rate, and tubular secretory function
Tissue sensitivity	Altered receptor number, receptor affinity, second-messenger function, and cellular and nuclear responses

undesired physiologic responses (drug response). Alterations in both pharmacokinetics and pharmacodynamics are predictable to a degree and must be taken into account whenever a drug is given to an elderly patient.

Most clinically relevant drugs given orally are absorbed by passive diffusion across the very extensive surface area of the proximal small bowel. Absorption of these drugs is unimpaired in the elderly, although gastric acid secretion may be decreased and the rate of gastric emptying diminished. Changes in body composition—specifically, an increase in the proportion of body fat and a decrease in the proportion of lean tissue [*see* Discussion, Patterns of Change in Body Composition, Organ System Function, and Integrated Responses, *below*]—may influence the distribution of drugs: the volume of distribution of relatively water-soluble drugs tends to decrease, and that of more fat-soluble drugs tends to increase. Altered distribution influences the elimination half-life of drugs, but it does not affect steady-state blood levels with multiple dosing if hepatic and renal drug clearances are unchanged.

Clearance of drugs primarily excreted by the kidneys declines predictably with advancing age and the concomitant decrease in GFR. Creatinine clearance is a much more reliable marker of the GFR than serum creatinine concentration, which depends on muscle mass as well. Drugs for which the dosage may require adjustment according to the patient's level of renal function include aminoglycosides, vancomycin, penicillins, cephalosporins, imipenem-cilastatin, metronidazole, digoxin, and procainamide. Age-related differences in the pharmacokinetics of renally excreted drugs, including the aminoglycosides, are unlikely when the creatinine clearance is greater than 80 ml/min/1.73 m². Drug levels should be monitored, particularly when drugs with a low therapeutic index are used.

Clearance of drugs by the liver depends on the delivery of the drug (i.e., on hepatic blood flow) and on the activity of biotransforming enzymes. Clearance of drugs that are metabolized relatively slowly is dependent on the function of hepatic enzymes; given that hepatic mass decreases with age, clearance of such drugs tends to be reduced.[146] Hepatic blood flow also decreases with age: it is 40% to 45% less in elderly persons than in young adults, and this decrease results in diminished flow-dependent clearance.[146] Age-related reductions in the clearance of diazepam, chlordiazepoxide, theophylline, and propranolol have been suggested on the basis of decreased hepatic biotransformation (whether dependent on blood flow or on enzyme function). Such reductions may be more pronounced in males. Plasma levels of drugs cleared in a flow-dependent fashion may be higher when hepatic blood flow is further decreased, as it is in conditions such as congestive heart failure or chronic liver disease.

The effects of age on the actions of drugs at target sites have not been extensively studied. Reductions in the number of beta-adrenergic receptors may contribute to the diminished effectiveness of sympathetic agonists in the elderly. Synthesis of vitamin K–dependent clotting factors may be more strongly inhibited in older patients at a given plasma warfarin concentration.[147] The elderly also exhibit more marked CNS depression at given blood levels of benzodiazepines.[148]

Discussion

Patterns of Change in Body Composition, Organ System Function, and Integrated Responses

BODY COMPOSITION

Specific changes in body composition are characteristic of advancing age, though they are not inevitable. Whereas weight remains more or less stable, fat mass tends to increase and lean body mass tends to decrease.[149] Lean body mass comprises body cell mass—defined as the "component of body composition containing the oxygen-consuming, potassium-rich, glucose-oxidizing, work-performing tissue"[150]—and extracellular mass. Body cell mass decreases by an average of 23% in men and 25% in women from the third to the eighth decade.[149] Besides decreasing in absolute terms, body cell mass declines as a proportion of lean body mass; this decline is largely accounted for by diminished skeletal muscle mass [*see Figure 7*]. About 40% to 45% of the muscle mass present in young adulthood is lost by the time a person reaches 70 years of age.[149] At the same time, muscle strength and function are lost as well.[151,152] Reductions in FEV_1 and maximal midexpiratory flow rate occur with advancing age; these reductions are partially attributable to a decrease in the strength of the respiratory musculature.[153] Together with decreased physical activity, changes in body composition contribute to decreased resting energy expenditure and therefore to decreased requirements for calories. Food intake decreases with aging in relation to alterations in GI physiology, endocrine function, and cytokine elaboration.[154]

The changes in body composition and muscle function appear to be at least partially determined by the level of habitual physical activity. For example, body weight and proportion of fat were constant in a cross-sectional study of lumberjacks 20 to 70 years of age, in contrast to the gradual increase in weight and body fat seen in men with sedentary occupations.[155]

Another study found that the body composition of male endurance athletes 50 to 75 years of age was very similar to that of younger athletes, whereas both untrained individuals and visually matched lean older individuals had significantly higher levels of body fat.[156] One group of investigators demonstrated increased muscle strength and a modest but significant decrease in body fat in elderly men who underwent 6 weeks of training; significant increases in minute ventilation during exercise and vital capacity were also observed.[157] Another group experienced a 10% increase in lean tissue, a 17% decrease in skinfold thickness, a 4% to 5% increase in body potassium, and an apparent halting of age-related decreases in bone calcium during a 1-year physical-training program in individuals in their seventh decade.[158] Another investigator, who studied age-related muscle fiber atrophy in men 25 to 65 years of age, found that muscle fiber size and strength increased after twice-weekly exercise for 15 weeks, particularly in the older subjects.[159]

ORGAN SYSTEM FUNCTION

Aging is associated with a variety of predictable morphologic, functional, and pathologic changes in major organ systems. Such changes have been best described for cardiovascular, respiratory, and renal systems, which are also the systems most relevant to perioperative care [see Table 1].

INTEGRATED RESPONSES AND FUNCTIONS

Oxygen Transport

The earliest physiologic responses to tissue injury are directed at restoring and maintaining the perfusion of vital organs. These responses rely on rapid activation of the sympathoadrenal axis by signals from the site of injury and from baroreceptors and chemoreceptors. Blood flow to the skin and skeletal muscle is decreased by peripheral vasoconstriction, and cardiac output is redistributed to vital tissues. With advancing age, however, the efficiency of many of these critical responses is diminished, even in healthy individuals. Baroreflex sensitivity is decreased in the elderly, presumably as a result of reduced arterial distensibility.[160] Vasoconstrictor responses are also reduced, probably because of alterations in autonomic neural pathways.[161] In addition, an age-associated decline in the inotropic and chronotropic effects of beta-adrenergic stimulation has been well described.[162] Thus, diminished arterial compliance, impaired vasoconstriction, altered autonomic function and sensitivity to catecholamines, and decreased baroreflex sensitivity all may limit the maintenance of cardiovascular homeostasis.

Delivery of oxygen to the tissues may be impaired in the elderly at every step of the oxygen transport pathway and may be inadequate when oxygen demands are increased.[111,163] Ventilatory responses to both hypoxia and hypercapnia are diminished. The alveolar-arterial oxygen gradient increases, and arterial oxygen tension (P_aO_2) progressively declines. There is substantial variation in most cardiac variables among older individuals, reflecting aging, atherosclerosis and other diseases, and various lifestyle factors that interact and influence cardiovascular function in ways that are often difficult to disentangle.[162] In unselected individuals, cardiac output declines approximately 1% each year, beginning in the fourth decade.[111] Progressive decreases in resting stroke volume and cardiac output with increasing age have been observed in individuals without clinical evidence of cardiovascular disease, both at rest and during exercise[164,165]; in addition, older subjects have had larger arteriovenous oxygen differences and increased arterial lactate concentrations. However, the

older individuals in such studies may well have had clinically occult cardiovascular disease or deconditioning resulting from long-standing limitations of physical activity (e.g., from time spent in nursing homes), and the use of invasive measurement techniques may have influenced observations.

Later studies of nonsedentary individuals who were screened with resting and stress ECG and dipyridamole-thallium scanning have demonstrated that older individuals, assessed noninvasively, maintain resting cardiac output, heart rate, stroke volume, and ejection fraction [see Figure 12].[162] Stiffening of the aorta and of more peripheral vessels tends to be associated with increased peripheral vascular resistance. A normal modest increase in left ventricular wall thickness with aging is exaggerated in persons with hypertension and coronary artery disease. Myocardial relaxation is typically prolonged, and early diastolic filling is slowed and delayed with advancing age.[162,166] Left ventricular end-diastolic volume at rest tends to be increased, with more rapid filling later in diastole; this tendency is associated with left atrial enlargement and an enhanced contribution to filling from atrial contraction.[167] Resting pulmonary arterial pressure and pulmonary vascular resistance increase moderately.[168]

Cardiovascular responses to exercise have been studied in detail and provide insight into the responses associated with acute surgical illness. The maximal heart rate achieved during exercise diminishes consistently with age, whereas changes in stroke volume index are variable (reflecting occult coronary artery disease, fitness level, heart size, and body composition), and maximum cardiac index tends to decline.[162] Older persons who are free of cardiovascular disease rely more on increases in stroke volume to achieve increases in their cardiac index during exercise than younger persons do.[169] Thus, end-diastolic volume index tends to increase in older persons; decreases in end-systolic volume index and increases in ejection fraction are less prominent than in young individuals [see Figure 13].[162,170] In one study of generally healthy persons who were not extensively screened, the likelihood of ventricular wall motion abnormalities during exercise rose consistently with age.[170] In an older study of persons with varying levels of habitual activity, the incidence of ECG abnormalities during and after maximal exercise rose with age and was much higher than the incidence at rest.[164]

The response of healthy older individuals to an increase in afterload differs from that of young persons: significant left ventricular dilatation occurs, and contraction begins from a greater preload than in young persons, presumably as a reflection of a diminished contractile reserve in the older persons.[171] Diminution of the inotropic, chronotropic, and arterial vasodilating effects of beta-adrenergic stimulation with advancing age may contribute to many age-related changes in cardiovascular function.[162] Isoproterenol infusion results in lesser increases in heart rate, left ventricular ejection fraction, and cardiac index in older persons than in younger ones.[172] Dobutamine augments cardiac output and stroke volume to a much lesser extent in elderly patients with decompensated congestive heart failure than in younger patients and provides no additional hemodynamic benefit at infusion rates higher than 5 mg/kg/min.[173]

Thus, older patients are predisposed to hemodynamic compromise related to tachyarrhythmias, atrial fibrillation, increased afterload, and coronary artery disease. Increased end-diastolic volume and stroke volume are compensatory mechanisms that maintain cardiac output in the face of other limitations, and appropriate filling volumes must be achieved. Inotropic drugs may be less beneficial in the elderly, and agents that are nonvasoconstricting (e.g., dobutamine) or have non-

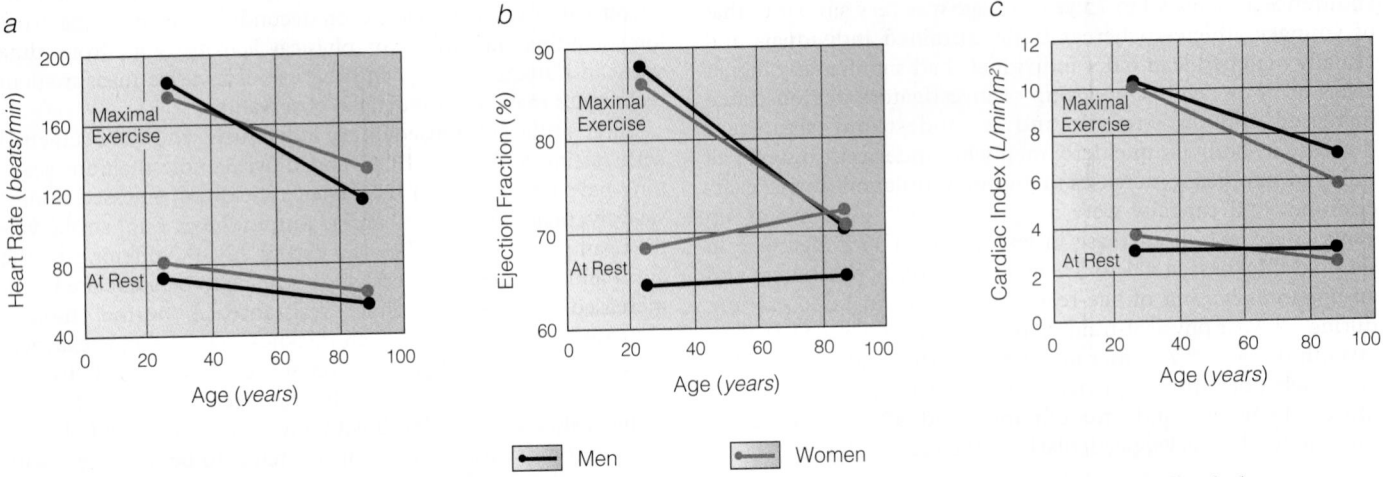

Figure 12 Shown are linear regressions on age of (*a*) heart rate, (*b*) ejection fraction, and (*c*) cardiac index at rest and during maximal cycle ergometry in healthy, sedentary male and female volunteers who had been screened to exclude clinical hypertension and occult coronary artery disease.[254]

adrenergic mechanisms of action (e.g., amrinone) may be useful. Agents that reduce afterload (e.g., angiotensin-converting enzyme inhibitors) may also play a greater role in older patients. Elderly patients are less able to increase oxygen delivery in the face of increased demand and, with a high prevalence of coronary artery disease, are at risk for myocardial ischemia if demands are excessive. Although increases in energy expenditure in hospitalized patients are generally much lower than those in healthy individuals during exercise, maximal oxygen consumption during exercise does decline very substantially with age.[174] It is probably not appropriate to arbitrarily set supranormal goals for cardiac index and oxygen delivery in elderly patients. In addition, every effort must be made to minimize unnecessary stresses that increase metabolic demands, such as hypothermia, shivering, exposure to a cool ambient environment, hypovolemia, acidosis, pain, and inappropriate

weaning from ventilatory support. The principles of physiologic and invasive hemodynamic monitoring are the same in elderly patients as in the young; however, such monitoring is perhaps even more important in the elderly when the direction of therapy is unclear because of the limitations in cardiopulmonary function and homeostatic mechanisms.

Age-associated changes in blood flow to (and, to a lesser extent, oxygen consumption in) specific organs have been investigated. The kidneys receive a diminishing proportion of cardiac output in the elderly; renal plasma flow decreases by about 10% each decade after 40 years of age and decreases in relation to renal mass. Liver volume decreases by more than one third, apparent liver blood flow by one half, and liver perfusion by one fifth from age 24 to age 91.[146] Cerebral blood flow, blood volume, and oxygen consumption decrease by about 0.5% a year in pure gray and white matter regions,

Figure 13 Depicted are relations between end-diastolic volume, end-systolic volume, and cardiac output in young and older patients at rest and during graded upright bicycle exercise.[255]

whereas the oxygen extraction ratio does not change or changes only to a minor degree.[175] Skeletal muscle blood flow at rest appears to be unaffected by age, but maximal blood flow after exercise is diminished in older subjects.[171,176] Average skin blood flow decreases by 30% to 40% from age 20 to age 70.[177]

Thermoregulation

The endogenous temperature set point is typically elevated after operation or injury and during sepsis, and ambient temperature is often kept inappropriately low in hospitals. Alterations in vasomotor activity are normally relied on in the range of temperatures between those that elicit shivering and those that cause sweating. When the core temperature is lower than the thermoregulatory set point and heat conservation is inadequate, shivering is initiated to generate heat. Shivering may be accompanied by a severalfold increase in oxygen consumption, which would constitute a substantial metabolic load. When the core temperature falls below 34° C (93.2° F), thermoregulation becomes impaired, metabolic activity slows, and further decreases in temperature are more rapid. The hypothermic myocardium is prone to intractable arrhythmias that may be triggered by minimal stimulation. Conditions associated with secondary hypothermia, such as hypothyroidism and diabetes mellitus, may be more frequent (or more frequently undiagnosed) in the elderly. The management of hypothermia and hyperthermia is discussed in detail elsewhere [see VII:10 Fever, Hyperpyrexia, and Hypothermia].

The elderly, particularly those older than 80 years, are less sensitive to alterations in environmental temperature and less able to maintain thermal homeostasis.[178] These limitations result in a higher incidence of hypothermia and heatstroke, a lower maximum body temperature during febrile illness, and more marked and prolonged falls in body temperature with surgery.[92,93,178]

Mechanisms of heat conservation, production, and offloading are less efficient in the elderly. Sensitivity to changes in ambient temperature is less precise, and behavioral responses are delayed. Vasoconstrictor responses to a cold stimulus are depressed in some elderly individuals, and shivering is delayed.[179] Moreover, the capacity for metabolic heat production by shivering is limited by the reduced muscle mass characteristic of the aged. With decreased blood flow in the skin, reduced sweat gland density, and delayed and diminished sweating responses, the elderly are less able to offload heat and reduce body temperature than younger individuals are.[111]

Malnutrition may predispose to hypothermia and accidental injury. In a study of 744 elderly women with fractures of the neck of the femur, most of those who were very thin had a core temperature lower than 35°C (95.0°F) on admission, whereas most of those who were well nourished had a temperature higher than 36°C (96.8°F).[180] The increase in the incidence of fractures in cold weather was greatest among the very thin; the finding that most injuries occurred indoors suggested that impaired thermoregulation in the malnourished individuals resulted in hypothermia, lack of coordination, and subsequent injury. In a study of elderly patients exposed to a range of ambient temperatures after femur fracture, vasoconstrictor responses were generally maintained; however, whereas patients who were well nourished could increase metabolic heat production appropriately, those who were undernourished (by anthropometric measurements) could not.[181]

Wound Healing

Advanced age is cited as a risk factor for impaired wound healing, though not consistently. Any association is probably attributable primarily to a higher prevalence of specific risk factors in the elderly, such as malnutrition, malignancy, uremia, diabetes mellitus, and atherosclerosis. Studies of healthy, well-nourished volunteers have shown minor delays in the epithelialization of split-thickness skin wounds in older subjects; collagen synthesis in subcutaneous implants was similar in young subjects and older ones, whereas accumulation of noncollagenous protein was decreased in the latter.[182] In a 2000 study of surgical patients, collagen deposition in subcutaneous implants decreased as a function of age in men but remained unchanged in older women.[183] Anastomotic leak rates after resection of colorectal cancer are not greater in elderly patients.[8] Outcome after abdominal wound dehiscence may be worse in the elderly.[184]

Immune Function

There is abundant evidence that changes in immune function occur with advancing age and that these changes may predispose to infectious, neoplastic, and perhaps vascular disease.[185] However, there is considerable variability among studies in the age definition of elderly, consideration of comorbidity, and the immune functions examined [see Discussion, Studies of Aging and Aged Populations, below]. A 2000 report suggests that many immune functions are relatively well preserved in healthy, independent-living, elderly persons.[186]

The delayed-type hypersensitivity (DTH) response to intradermal challenge with common antigens can be used as a global measure of immune function. For a normal response (i.e., erythema and induration), intact antigen processing and stimulation of lymphocytes, release of soluble mediators, and migration of macrophages to the injection site are necessary. The likelihood of diminished or absent DTH responses to common antigens increases after the eighth decade of life, and the probability of achieving primary sensitization to an antigen to which the individual had not previously been exposed is diminished after 70 years of age.[187,188] Aging-associated changes in cell-mediated and humoral immune responses have been well reviewed elsewhere.[185,186] Overall, responses to foreign antigens are diminished and responses to autologous antigens may be increased. The limited information available on phagocytic responses suggests that polymorphonuclear leukocyte function may decrease with age.

Alterations in Clinical Presentation

The manifestations of surgical illness in the elderly may be considerably different from those in young or middle-aged individuals. Multiple medical disorders are often present, and the symptoms of acute surgical illness may be masked. The CNS is particularly sensitive to the effects of drugs and disease, and the presentation of surgical and medical illness may be nonspecific (e.g., lethargy, confusion, or agitation) or indirect (e.g., an unexplained fall). The clinical presentation will tend to reflect the most vulnerable organ system (often the CNS) in the earliest stages, not necessarily the organ system that is diseased.[142] Relative inactivity may limit the manifestations of important cardiac, pulmonary, or peripheral vascular disease. The patient, the family, or the surgeon may inappropriately attribute relevant symptoms to the supposedly inevitable changes of advancing age. Memory or hearing impairment may make it difficult to obtain a reliable history. To ensure effective communication, the surgeon may have to make an extra effort when taking the history and reviewing the medical records.

Elderly patients may have a higher pain threshold than

younger individuals. Older patients presenting with acute abdominal pain are more likely than younger individuals to require surgical intervention.[189] The localization of abdominal pain in patients with peritonitis may not be as reliable; elderly patients with appendicitis are less likely than younger patients to have pain localized to the right lower quadrant.[190] Abdominal pain is a less frequent presentation of colorectal carcinoma in geriatric patients than in younger patients.[191] These observations suggest that pain is a particularly important symptom in the elderly and that its degree is not necessarily an adequate indication of the gravity of the underlying problem.[192] The perception of pain is complex, however; situational factors and expectations may have a major impact on reactions to injury.

Although febrile responses are generally intact, fever may be less marked in elderly individuals with infectious or inflammatory processes, particularly those older than 80 years. Hypothermia is more common in elderly patients who are seriously ill than in younger patients.

The prevalence and natural history of some pathologic processes, as well as their clinical manifestations, may be altered in the geriatric population. For example, elderly patients presenting with appendicitis are more likely to have gangrenous or perforated appendicitis than younger patients are, and patients with perforated diverticulitis are more likely to have generalized peritonitis.[193] It is not clear whether these observations reflect a change in the onset of symptoms, a difference in the evolution of the pathologic process, or a delay in seeking medical attention. Similarly, elderly patients with symptomatic gallstones are more likely than younger patients to present with perforation, empyema, or gangrene of the gallbladder, acute cholecystitis, or cholangitis and are more likely to require urgent surgery.[194]

Specific Clinical Concerns

Much of the material we have presented to this point is relevant to the care of elderly surgical patients in general and of elderly patients undergoing major elective procedures specifically. In what follows, we discuss specific considerations that arise for elderly patients who have cancer, are seriously injured, are critically ill, or are very frail and have major functional limitations and comorbidities.

TRAUMA

The management of trauma is typically more complex and challenging in elderly patients than in younger ones. The prevalence of preexisting medical conditions increases with age, and such conditions are associated with longer hospital stays and higher mortality after injury.[195,196] Mechanisms of injury change in relative frequency with age, as do the types of injuries that result from a given physical insult and the outcomes that follow a given injury. In the Major Trauma Outcome Study (MTOS), for example, falls were the predominant mechanism of injury in patients 65 years of age or older, but they were relatively infrequent in younger patients.[197]

Motor vehicle crashes are the most common mechanism of injury in younger patients and remain the second most common in older patients. The circumstances and nature of motor vehicle crashes tend to differ in the elderly. Crashes involving older drivers occur mainly in daytime and close to home and more often result from errors of judgment or perception than from high speed, aggressive driving, loss of vehicle control, or the use of alcohol.[198] Older drivers are more likely to be in crashes involving right-of-way conflicts, improper turning or starting, and failure to recognize or obey traffic signals.[199] Older drivers are also more likely to be involved in multivehicle side-impact collisions.[198,200]

The direction of impact influences both the pattern of injuries sustained and mortality.[198] In one study, injuries to the face and the lower extremities were significantly more common in drivers involved in frontal collisions, whereas injuries to the chest, the abdomen, and the pelvis were more frequent in left lateral impacts.[198] Mortality was nearly doubled in left lateral impacts; this increase was independent of both Injury Severity Score and driver age.

The pattern of injuries resulting from a given physical insult also seems to differ to some extent in the elderly: older drivers have a higher incidence of chest injuries, specifically rib and sternal fractures.[201] Greater chest wall stiffness and osteoporotic changes may predispose older persons to rib fractures after relatively minor trauma. Rib fractures or even flail chest may sometimes occur in the elderly without the significant underlying pulmonary contusion that would be anticipated in a younger patient.[202,203] Striking age-related increases in fractures of the vertebrae, the hip, and the distal forearm have been documented, and the pivotal role of osteoporosis in such fractures is well recognized.[204] Patients who have major injuries despite an apparently insignificant mechanism of injury (e.g., a low-level fall) are more likely to be older than 55 years.[205] Burn injuries are more common in the elderly, and these injuries tend to be more severe in terms of both surface area and depth; moreover, inhalation injury is more likely.[206] As a consequence, mortality is higher and hospital stay longer. The increased risk of burn injury in the elderly may be attributable to a diminished sense of smell, impaired hearing or vision, or reduced mobility and reaction time. The tendency to more severe thermal injury may be attributable to age-related changes in skin morphology.

Elderly persons are, in general, less sensitive to deviations from physiologic norms and less able to maintain homeostasis.[207] They are less able to maintain adequate perfusion of vital organs after injury[208] and more likely to arrive in the emergency department hypotensive, cold, and in shock after a given injury than younger patients are. Presumably, reduced homeostatic capacity contributes to the overrepresentation of the elderly with regard to immediate and early trauma deaths as well as late deaths related to infection and multiple organ dysfunction syndrome (MODS). In one study, no elderly patient with a Trauma Score (TS) lower than 7 survived long enough to be admitted to a hospital.[209] Resuscitative measures, though identical in principle to those taken in younger patients, must be carried out with an eye to the physiologic limitations of the elderly, particularly the need for volume loading to achieve increases in cardiac output. Preexisting medical conditions must be identified rapidly via history-taking, physical examination, and investigative studies as needed, and information about previous medication use should be obtained. Because thermoregulatory mechanisms are less efficient in the elderly, measures should be taken to minimize ongoing heat loss from exposure and administration of cool fluids and to prevent the adverse effects of hypothermia.

Unfortunately, even an apparently good physiologic status in the ED (at least as reflected in the TS or the Revised Trauma Score [RTS]) does not guarantee survival for the elderly trauma patient: mortality in elderly patients with high TS or RTS is many times higher than that in younger patients with comparable scores.[197,210,211] MTOS data demonstrate that case-fatality rates are uniformly higher in patients 65 years of age or older than in younger patients for every injury mechanism for which sufficient data were available.[212] Mortality was consistently higher for each range of Injury Severity Scores and for each injury severity–body region combination. Patients 65 years of age or older accounted for 30% of the deaths that were unexpected according to Trauma and Injury Severity Score (TRISS) projections despite representing only 8% of the MTOS study population. Complications (pulmonary, cardiovascular, and infectious) were also more common in the older patients[197,212]; the difference was most striking in patients with mild to moderate injury. Others have noted the high incidence in the elderly of respiratory complications (including pneumonia) as well as cardiac complications that are relatively uncommon in younger patients.[213,214]

Elderly patients are less likely to survive their injuries and be discharged from hospital than younger patients are, but several reports indicate that many older survivors will ultimately return to a satisfactory level of function and independence.[202,213-217] Recent studies should serve as a caveat, however, in that prolonged and profound functional limitations have been identified after major trauma when sophisticated assessments of long-term functional, psychological, and quality-of-life outcomes have been undertaken.[218] Variations in functional recovery and placement status result from a number of factors besides the specific mechanism and nature of the injury. For example, family and social support systems have been shown to be important for achieving discharge-to-home and optimal functional recovery in patients with isolated hip fracture, and some authors have reached similar conclusions with reference to trauma in the elderly in general.[219] Very advanced age, preinjury placement, preinjury functional status, and preexisting medical conditions are also likely to influence postinjury rehabilitation. Injury-causing falls may, in some instances, be a reflection of important underlying problems, such as drop attacks or a poor physical state. The adverse impact of serious head injury on early and delayed mortality has been reported in a number of studies.[211,213,215-217] Admission to an ICU, even if the stay is longer than 2 weeks and even if mechanical ventilation is necessary, does not preclude a very good functional recovery in survivors.[202,213-215]

CANCER

The incidence of most cancers increases with age. One half of new cases of lung and colorectal cancer now occur in persons aged 70 years or older, as do nearly two thirds of new cases of prostate cancer and one third of new cases of breast cancer.[220] The importance of cancer as a cause of surgical illness in the elderly is further indicated by the high proportion of surgical procedures related to malignancy, and its frequency as a cause of death in surgical patients.[221]

The principles of cancer care are similar in the elderly, and surgeons play a central role in determining the application of those principles. There is considerable evidence, however, that the use of diagnostic modalities, the choice of surgical treatment, and other forms of cancer care differ in the elderly.[8,222-226] This difference may be an appropriate response to the increased prevalence of comorbidity or to age-related differences in treatment goals, or it may reflect an inappropriate bias. Older cancer patients may assign greater importance to outcomes other than the traditional ones of survival, response rates, and disease-free intervals than younger patients do.[224,227] They also appear more concerned about the effects of treatment and may be less willing to trade current health-related quality of life for potential survival advantage.[222,228]

Comorbidity in the elderly population may limit potential gains in life expectancy, alter treatment goals, and reduce the ability to tolerate major surgical procedures and other forms of

therapy. Yet adjustments for comorbidity do not fully account for age-related differences in care.[229,230] Moreover, the elderly population is very diverse and includes individuals who are physiologically very fit as well as ones who are very frail. In addition, there is evidence that nondefinitive care is associated with poorer clinical outcomes.[231] Thus, it is inappropriate to generalize cancer care simply on the basis of chronologic age.

The elderly have been underrepresented in clinical studies, with the result that our perceptions of the efficacy and safety of many therapies in the elderly must be based on inference rather than knowledge and may therefore be inaccurate.[232] The development of multidimensional assessment tools for the geriatric cancer patient should allow appropriate enrollment and stratification in clinical trials and permit identification of patients who can expect the most benefit from aggressive therapy.[233,234] There is considerable uncertainty about cancer screening in the elderly, for the reasons discussed. A framework for making decisions about screening has been proposed, incorporating quantitative estimates of risks and benefits in relation to individual preferences and values.[235] When life expectancy is less than 5 years, cancer screening is unlikely to provide any survival benefit.

THE VERY FRAIL PATIENT

Most elderly individuals live independently and function well. Indeed, increases in specialist medical care have been considerably greater for healthy elderly individuals than for those in poor health.[236] Nonetheless, elderly persons in nursing homes or similar facilities are often especially frail, have significant comorbidity and functional limitations, and usually have a limited life expectancy. They experience a range of orthopedic, general surgical, vascular, and other surgical problems that may be relatively advanced and that commonly present as an emergency or in atypical or nonspecific ways.[42] Dementia and other cognitive impairments predict increased mortality [see Cognitive Assessment, above], presumably because of delays in presentation and diagnosis and the comorbidities that are frequently present.

The goals of surgical therapy are usually modest: to correct immediately life-threatening conditions or to address problems related to quality of life. Comfort, function, and dignity—rather than major gains in survival—are more often the primary goals. How well we achieve these goals with current surgical care is uncertain. Precise diagnosis is usually the most satisfactory basis for relieving suffering and achieving the other goals of importance to the frail elderly patient. However, it must be kept in mind that precise diagnosis is just one means to that end and that pathology of various kinds can almost always be identified in such individuals, whether relevant or not.[237]

Advance decisions to limit the use of specific therapies have been made and documented by some elderly individuals. Surgical care should not be denied to patients who have issued a do-not-resuscitate (DNR) order in the event of critical cardiopulmonary deterioration. Outcomes in such patients are not necessarily worse than in other frail patients, and agreement to rescind the DNR order temporarily should be sought because the causes of cardiopulmonary arrest in the immediate perioperative period may be rapidly and readily correctible.

Surgical problems in nursing home patients should be addressed actively, because they can often be managed more easily and safely when elective, rather than when they have evolved into more difficult, high-risk, emergency conditions. The elective setting also provides more opportunity for informed decision-making and treatment planning and the development of consensus among those involved. The care of such very frail patients is especially challenging and should be undertaken by surgeons who are interested in and knowledgeable about the problems that arise, who are prepared to deal with the complexities of comorbidity and cognitive and functional impairment, and who will educate their colleagues, patients, and families about the full range of therapies available for surgical conditions.[42]

Studies of Aging and Aged Populations

Age is an important predictor of many clinical outcomes. Two related concepts must be considered in reviewing studies that are concerned with elderly patients and aged populations or in which age may be a significant variable. First, although age has obvious chronologic meaning, it is a surrogate for a range of biologic, clinical, social and other variables. Some of the variables that we often recognize as changing in association with age are maximal organ system function (physiologic reserve), the prevalence of comorbidity, functional status, patterns of illness (e.g., a preponderance of perforated appendicitis in the elderly), and disease incidence (e.g., cancer). A knowledge of age-related variables in the population being reported on is important in that it can help determine the extent to which findings can be generalized to one's own patients. Age-related variables must be excluded as fully as possible when basic disease mechanisms or causal relationships are being examined.

Second, the method by which elderly research subjects are selected greatly influences the findings of clinical studies. Aging is a highly variable process, both among individual and among different organ systems within an individual. Studies of institutionalized elderly who have multiple comorbidities and functional impairments will give very different results from studies of active, healthy, community-dwelling individuals. Again, such age-associated variables must be addressed to allow proper interpretation of study findings. It must also be remembered that aging is a continuous process. For example, a 65-year-old person and an 85-year-old person, each in good health, could well be very different with respect to physiologic and functional status, even though they would often be grouped together into a single "elderly" category.

Because research subjects cannot be randomized to an age group, prospective clinical studies of aging and of aged populations are necessarily observational in design. As a result, study groups that differ in age, by design, will also unavoidably differ in terms of other variables (covariates), such as those already described. For this reason, although observational studies are very useful for descriptive and prognostic purposes, they are less satisfactory for examining causal relationships. Several strategies for study design and analysis are useful for minimizing or adjusting for imbalances in covariates between groups.[238]

Two basic study designs are employed in clinical studies of the elderly and aged populations: cross-sectional and longitudinal. In cross-sectional studies, subjects of various ages are assembled, and observations are made at one point in time. Such studies are easier and less expensive to conduct than longitudinal studies, but they are subject to bias and confounding variables. For example, elderly patients, when younger, may have been very different from the young patients with whom they are being compared; that is, changes may occur in the population as a whole over time. In addition, elderly individuals (particularly those older than 75 years) make up what may be thought of as a biologically superior group in that they have been selected by the very fact of their survival from a larger group, many of whose members have died. Cross-sectional studies thus may demonstrate differences between current age groups rather than changes that occur with aging. Bias may also arise in relation to referral for surgical care or to particular institutions or from a wide range of other potential sources. A clear description of the source of the data and the basis on which the subjects came to be studied allows others to make judgments about bias and the generalizability of research findings.

In longitudinal studies, a cohort is assembled and followed prospectively, with observations made at planned intervals. Longitudinal studies require a stable, dedicated population observed over a prolonged period and are particularly sensitive to subtle alterations in methods. Among the most comprehensive and widely cited longitudinal studies is the Baltimore Longitudinal Study of Aging, conducted using carefully screened, community-residing, independent adults.[239]

Advanced age has, in the past, been a common exclusion criterion for research studies, with the result that there is a paucity of information pertaining specifically to the elderly in certain important clinical areas.[232] Inferences about age effects on diseases and responses to therapy must then be made, exposing elderly patients to the risks of inaccuracy. In addition, outcomes that are likely to be of particular interest to the elderly (quality of life, for example) may not be well addressed when studies are designed with a focus on younger patients.[240] The unique problems and questions of the elderly must be addressed in surgical research. Concerns about vulnerability and exploitation may sometimes arise, but they do not negate the obligation to conduct research in these individuals; to continue to exclude elderly patients would be to deny the potential benefits of research to a population that has great need of such benefits.

References

1. Smith OC: Advanced age as a contraindication to operation. Med Rec (New York) 72:642, 1907

2. Kenney RA: Physiology of Aging: A Synopsis, 2nd ed. Year Book, Chicago, 1989, p 111

3. Callum K, Gray A, Hoile R, et al: Extremes of Age. The 1999 Report of the National Confidential Enquiry into Perioperative Deaths. National Confidential Enquiry into Perioperative Deaths, London, 1999

4. Bardram L, Funch-Jensen P, Kehlet H: Rapid rehabilitation in elderly patients after laparoscopic colonic resection. Br J Surg 87:1540, 2000

5. Carr AJ, Higginson IJ: Measuring quality of life: are quality of life measures patient centred? BMJ 322:1357, 2001

6. Ventura SJ, Peters KD, Martin JA, et al: Births and deaths: United States, 1996. Mon Vital Stat Rep 46(1 suppl 2):1, 1997

7. Welch HG, Albertsen PC, Nease RF, et al: Estimating treatment benefits for the elderly: the effect of competing risks. Ann Intern Med 124:577, 1996

8. Colorectal Cancer Collaborative Group: Surgery for colorectal cancer in elderly patients: a systematic review. Lancet 356:968, 2000

9. Making Health Care Safer: A Critical Analysis of Patient Safety Practices, Evidence Report/Technology Assessment No. 43. Agency for Healthcare Research and Quality, Rockville, Maryland, 2001 http://www.ahrq.gov/clinic/ptsafety

10. Lothian K, Philp I: Maintaining the dignity and autonomy of older people in the healthcare setting. BMJ 322:668, 2001

11. Auerbach AD, Goldman L: Beta-blockers and reduction of cardiac events in noncardiac surgery: clinical applications. JAMA 287:1445, 2002

12. Fiatarone MA, Oneill EF, Ryan ND, et al: Exercise training and nutritional supplementa-

tion for physical frailty in very elderly people. N Engl J Med 330:1769, 1994

13. Arthur HM, Daniels C, McKelvie R, et al: Effect of a preoperative intervention on preoperative and postoperative outcomes in low-risk patients awaiting elective coronary bypass graft surgery. Ann Intern Med 133:253, 2000

14. Debigare R, Maltais F, Whittom F, et al: Feasibility and efficacy of home exercise training before lung volume reduction. J Cardiopulm Rehabil 19:235, 1999

15. Edwards AE, Seymour DG, McCarthy JM, et al: A 5-year study of general surgical patients aged 65 years and over. Anaesthesia 51:3, 1996

16. Carpenter G, Bernabei R, Hirdes J, et al: Building evidence on chronic disease in old age: standardised assessments and databases offer one way of building the evidence. BMJ 320:528, 2000

17. Schein OD, Katz J, Bass EB, et al, for the Study of Medical Testing for Cataract Surgery: The value of routine preoperative medical testing before cataract surgery. N Engl J Med 342:168, 2000

18. Munro J, Booth A, Nicholl J: Routine preoperative testing: a systematic review of the evidence. Health Technology Assessment 1(12), 1997 http://www.hta.nhsweb.nhs.uk/

19. Wahr JA, Parks R, Boisvert D, et al, for the Multicenter Study of Perioperative Ischemia Research Group: Preoperative serum potassium levels and perioperative outcomes in cardiac surgery patients. JAMA 281:2203, 1999

20. Hall JC, Tarala RA, Hall JL, et al: A multivariate analysis of the risk of pulmonary complications after laparotomy. Chest 99:923, 1991

21. Brooks-Brunn JA: Predictors of postoperative pulmonary complications following abdominal surgery. Chest 111:564, 1997

22. Arozullah AM, Khuri SF, Henderson WG, et al, for the Participants in the National Veterans Affairs Surgical Quality Improvement Program: Development and validation of a multifactorial risk index for predicting postoperative pneumonia after major noncardiac surgery. Ann Intern Med 135:847, 2001

23. Smetana GW: Preoperative pulmonary evaluation. N Engl J Med 340:937, 1999

24. Hall JC, Hall JL: ASA status and age predict adverse events after abdominal surgery. J Qual Clin Pract 16:103, 1996

25. Moller AM, Villebro N, Pedersen T, et al: Effect of preoperative smoking intervention on postoperative complications: a randomised clinical trial. Lancet 359:114, 2002

26. Lawrence VA, Dhanda R, Hilsenbeck SG, et al: Risk of pulmonary complications after elective abdominal surgery. Chest 110:744, 1996

27. De Nino L, Lawrence VA, Averyt EC, et al: Preoperative spirometry and laparotomy: blowing away dollars. Chest 111:1536, 1997

28. Mangano DT: Perioperative cardiac morbidity. Anesthesiology 72:153, 1990

29. Mangano DT: Adverse outcomes after surgery in the year 2001—a continuing odyssey. Anesthesiology 88:561, 1998

30. Mangano DT, Goldman L: Preoperative assessment of patients with known or suspected coronary disease. N Engl J Med 333:1750, 1995

31. Badner NH, Knill RL, Brown JE, et al: Myocardial infarction after noncardiac surgery. Anesthesiology 88:572, 1998

32. Eagle K, Rihal C, Mickel M, et al: Cardiac risk of noncardiac surgery: influence of coronary disease and type of surgery in 3368 operations. CASS Investigators and University of Michigan Heart Care Program. Coronary Artery Surgery Study. Circulation 96:1882, 1997

33. Lee TH, Marcantonio ER, Mangione CM, et al: Derivation and prospective validation of a simple index for prediction of cardiac risk of major noncardiac surgery. Circulation 100:1043, 1999

34. Goldman L, Caldera DL, Nussbaum SR, et al: Multifactorial index of cardiac risk in noncardiac surgical procedures. N Engl J Med 297:845, 1977

35. Golden M, Whittemore A, Donaldson M, et al: Selective evaluation and management of coronary artery disease in patients undergoing repair of abdominal aortic aneurysms: a 16-year experience. Ann Surg 212:415, 1990

36. Eagle K, Brundage B, Chaitman B, et al: Guidelines for perioperative cardiovascular evaluation for noncardiac surgery. Report of the American College of Cardiology/American Heart Association Task Force on Practice Guidelines (Committee on Perioperative Cardiovascular Evaluation for Noncardiac Surgery). J Am Coll Cardiol 27:910, 1996

37. Leppo J, Dahlberg S: The question: to test or not to test in preoperative cardiac risk evaluation. J Nucl Cardiol 5:332, 1998

38. Kelion AD, Banning AP: Is simple clinical assessment adequate for cardiac risk stratification before elective non-cardiac surgery? Lancet 354:1837, 1999

39. Mangano DT: Assessment of the patient with cardiac disease. An anesthesiologist's paradigm. Anesthesiology 91:1521, 1999

40. Romero L, de Virgilio C: Preoperative cardiac risk assessment: an updated approach. Arch Surg 36:1370, 2001

41. Bernstein GM, Offenbartl SK: Adverse surgical outcomes among patients with cognitive impairments. Amer Surgeon 57:682, 1991

42. Zenilman ME, Bender JS, Magnuson TH, et al: General surgical care in the nursing home patient: results of a dedicated geriatric surgery consult service. J Am Coll Surg 183:361, 1996

43. Morrison RS, Siu AL: Survival in end-stage dementia following acute illness. JAMA 284:47, 2000

44. Nightingale S, Holmes J, Mason J, et al: Psychiatric illness and mortality after hip fracture. Lancet 357:1264, 2001

45. Gustafson Y, Brannstrom B, Berggren D, et al: A geriatric-anesthesiologic program to reduce acute confusional states in elderly patients treated for femoral neck fractures. J Am Geriatr Soc 39:655, 1991

46. Marcantonio ER, Goldman L, Mangione CM, et al: A clinical prediction rule for delirium after elective noncardiac surgery. JAMA 271:134, 1994

47. Moller JT, Cluitmans P, Rasmussen LS, et al, for the ISPOCD Investigators: Long-term postoperative cognitive dysfunction in the elderly: ISPOCD1 study. Lancet 351:857, 1998

48. Murray A, Levkoff S, Wetle T, et al: Acute delirium and functional decline in the hospitalized elderly patient. J Gerontol 48:M181, 1993

49. Parikh SS, Chung F: Postoperative delirium in the elderly. Anesth Analg 80:1223, 1995

50. Dijkstra J, Houx P, Jolles J: Cognition after major surgery in the elderly: test performance and complaints. Br J Anaesth 82:867, 1999

51. Abildstrom H, Rasmussen L, Rentowl P, et al: Cognitive dysfunction 1–2 years after non-cardiac surgery in the elderly ISPOCD group. International Study of Post-Operative Cognitive Dysfunction. Acta Anaesthesiol Scand 44:1246, 2000

52. Newman MF, Kirchner JL, Phillips-Bute B, et al, for the Neurological Outcome Research Group and the Cardiothoracic Anesthesiology Research Endeavors Investigators: Longitudinal assessment of neurocognitive function after coronary-artery bypass surgery. N Engl J Med 344:395, 2001

53. Folstein MF, Folstein SE, McHugh PR: "Mini-Mental State": a practical method for grading the cognitive state of patients for the clinician. J Psychiatr Res 12:189, 1975

54. Roccaforte W, Burke W, Bayer B, et al: Validation of a telephone version of the Mini-Mental State examination. J Am Geriatr Soc 40:697, 1992

55. Ritchie K: The screening of cognitive impairment in the elderly: a critical review of current methods. J Clin Epidemiol 41:635, 1988

56. Chandra RK: Effect of vitamin and trace-element supplementation on immune responses and infection in elderly subjects. Lancet 340:1124, 1992

57. Girodon F, Lombard M, Galan P, et al: Effect of micronutrient supplementation on infection in institutionalized elderly subjects: a controlled trial. Ann Nutr Metab 41(2): 98, 1997

58. Shaver HJ, Loper JA, Lutes RA: Nutritional status of nursing home patients. JPEN J Parenter Enteral Nutr 4:367, 1980

59. Pinchcofsky-Devin GD, Kaminski MV: Incidence of protein-calorie malnutrition in the nursing home patient. J Am Coll Nutr 6:109, 1987

60. Rudman D, Feller AG, Nagruj HS, et al: Relation of serum albumin concentration to death rate in nursing home men. JPEN J Parenter Enteral Nutr 11:360, 1987

61. Allison SP: Outcomes from nutritional support in the elderly. Nutrition 14:479, 1988

62. Sullivan DH, Sun S, Walls RC: Protein-energy undernutrition among elderly hospitalized patients: a prospective study. JAMA 281:2013, 1999

63. Bastow MD, Rawlings J, Allison SP: Benefits of supplementary tube feeding after fractured neck of femur: a randomised controlled trial. BMJ 287:1589, 1983

64. Potter J, Langhorne P, Roberts M: Routine protein energy supplementation in adults: systematic review. BMJ 317:495, 1998

65. Klein S, Kinney J, Jeejeebhoy K, et al: Nutrition support in clinical practice: review of published data and recommendations for future research directions. JPEN J Parenter Enteral Nutr 21:133, 1997

66. Omran M, Morley J: Assessment of protein energy malnutrition in older persons, part I: History, examination, body composition, and screening tools. Nutrition 16:50, 2000

67. Apovian CM: Nutritional assessment in the elderly: facing up to the challenges of developing new tools for clinical assessment. Nutrition 17:62, 2001

68. Corish CA: Pre-operative nutritional assessment in the elderly. J Nutr Health Aging 5:49, 2001

69. Detsky AS, McLaughlin JR, Baker JP, et al: What is subjective global assessment of nutritional status? JPEN J Parenter Enteral Nutr 11:8, 1987

70. Vellas B, Guigoz Y, Garry PJ, et al: The Mini Nutritional Assessment (MNA) and its use in grading the nutritional state of elderly patients. Nutrition 15:116, 1999

71. Klidjian AM, Foster KJ, Kammerling RM, et al: Relation of anthropometric and dynamometric variables to serious postoperative complications. BMJ 281:899, 1980

72. Twiston Davies CW, Moody Jones D, Shearer JR: Hand grip—a simple test for morbidity after fracture of the neck of femur. J Royal Soc Med 77:833, 1984

73. Nehme AE: Groin hernias in the elderly: management and prognosis. Am J Surg 146:257, 1983

74. Greenburg AG, Saik RP, Coyle JJ, et al: Mortality and gastrointestinal surgery in the aged: elective versus emergency procedures. Arch Surg 116:788, 1981

75. Seymour DG, Pringle R: A new method of auditing surgical mortality rates: application to a group of elderly general surgical patients. BMJ 284:1539, 1982

76. Gilliss CL, Gortner SR, Hauck WW, et al: A randomized clinical trial of nursing care for recovery from cardiac surgery. Heart & Lung 22:125, 1993

77. Rozanski A, Bairey CN, Krantz DS, et al: Mental stress and the induction of silent myocardial ischemia in patients with coronary artery disease. N Engl J Med 318:1005, 1988

78. Milledge JS, Nunn JF: Criteria of fitness for anaesthesia in patients with chronic obstructive lung disease. Br Med J 3:670, 1975

79. Roberts CS, Cox CE, Reintgen DS, et al: Influence of physician communication on newly diagnosed breast patients' psychological adjustment and decision-making. Cancer 74(1 suppl):336, 1994

80. Huusko TM, Karppi P, Avikainen V, et al: Randomised, clinically controlled trial of intensive geriatric rehabilitation in patients with hip fracture: subgroup analysis of patients with dementia. BMJ 321:1107, 2000

81. Cameron I, Crotty M, Currie C, et al: Geriatric rehabilitation following fractures in older people: a systematic review. Health Technol Assess 4(2), 2000
http://www.hta.nhsweb.nhs.uk

82. Hyde CJ, Robert IE, Sinclair AJ: The effects of supporting discharge from hospital to home in older people. Age Ageing 29:271, 2000

83. McClaran J, Berglas R, Franco E: Long hospital stays and need for alternate level of care at discharge: does family make a difference for elderly patients? Can Fam Physician 42:449, 1996

84. Mazur DJ, Merz JF: How age, outcome severity, and scale influence general medicine clinic patients' interpretations of verbal probability terms. J Gen Intern Med 9:295, 1994

85. Farnill D, Inglis S: Patients' desire for information about anaesthesia: Australian attitudes. Anaesthesia 49:162, 1994

86. Lonsdale M, Hutchison GL: Patients' desire for information about anaesthesia: Scottish and Canadian attitudes. Anaesthesia 46:410, 1991

87. Inglis S, Farnill D: The effect of providing preoperative statistical anaesthetic-risk information. Anaesth Intens Care 21:799, 1993

88. Lella J, Kaye M: Ethics and surgical practice with the elderly. Surgical Care of the Elderly. Meakins JL, McClaran JC, Eds. Year Book Medical Publishers, Chicago, 1988, p 50

89. Langslow A: Nursing and the law: who has the capacity to consent to surgery? Austr Nurs J 2:31, 1995

90. Markson LJ, Kern DC, Annas GJ, et al: Physician assessment of patient competence. J Am Geriatr Soc 42:1074, 1994

91. Sessler DI: Mild perioperative hypothermia. N Engl J Med 336:1730, 1997

92. Vaughan MS, Vaughan RW, Cork RC: Postoperative hypothermia in adults: relationship of age, anesthesia, and shivering to rewarming. Anesth Analg 60:746, 1981

93. Roe CF, Goldberg MJ, Blair CS, et al: The influence of body temperature on early postoperative oxygen consumption. Surgery 60:85, 1966

94. Frank SM, Fleisher LA, Breslow MJ: Perioperative maintenance of normothermia reduces the incidence of morbid cardiac events: a randomized clinical trial. JAMA 227:1127, 1997

95. Kurz A, Sessler DI, Lenhardt R: Perioperative normothermia to reduce the incidence of surgical-wound infection and shorten hospitalization. N Engl J Med 334:1209, 1996

96. Schmied H, Kurz A, Sessler D, et al: Mild hypothermia increases blood loss and transfusion requirements during total hip arthroplasty. Lancet 347:289, 1986

97. Cruse PJE, Foord R: The epidemiology of wound infection: a 10-year prospective study of 62,939 wounds. Surg Clin North Am 60:27, 1980

98. Tang R, Chen H, Wang Y, et al: Risk factors for surgical site infection after elective resection of the colon and rectum: a single-center prospective study of 2,809 consecutive patients. Ann Surg 234:181, 2001

99. Craig DB: Postoperative recovery of pulmonary function. Anesth Analg 60:46, 1981

100. Simonneau G, Vivien A, Sartene R, et al: Diaphragm dysfunction induced by upper abdominal surgery: role of postoperative pain. Am Rev Respir Dis 128:899, 1983

101. Rizzato G, Marrazini L: Thoracoabdominal mechanics in elderly men. J Appl Physiol 28:457, 1970

102. Vaughan RW, Wise L: Postoperative arterial blood gas measurement in obese patients: effect of position on gas exchange. Ann Surg 182:705, 1975

103. Celli BR, Rodriguez KS, Snider GL: A controlled trial of intermittent positive pressure breathing, incentive spirometry, and deep breathing exercises in preventing pulmonary complications after abdominal surgery. Am Rev Respir Dis 130:12, 1984

104. Ford GT, Guenter CA: Toward prevention of postoperative pulmonary complications. Am Rev Respir Dis 130:4, 1984

105. Greif R, Laciny S, Rapf B, et al: Supplemental oxygen reduces the incidence of postoperative nausea and vomiting. Anesthesiology 91:1246, 1999

106. Greif R, Akca O, Horn EP, et al, for the Outcomes Research Group: Supplemental perioperative oxygen to reduce the incidence of surgical-wound infection. N Engl J Med 342:161, 2000

107. Miller PD, Krebs RA, Neal BJ, et al: Hypodipsia in geriatric patients. Am J Med 73:354, 1982

108. Phillips PA, Rolls BJ, Ledingham JG, et al: Reduced thirst after water deprivation in healthy elderly men. N Engl J Med 311:753, 1984

109. Helderman JH, Vestal RE, Rowe JW, et al: The response of arginine vasopressin to intravenous ethanol and hypertonic saline in man: the impact of aging. J Gerontol 33:39, 1978

110. Saruta T, Suzuki A, Hayashi M, et al: Mechanism of age-related changes in renin and adrenocortical steroids. J Am Geriatr Soc 28:210, 1980

111. Kenney RA: Physiology of aging. Clin Geriatr Med 1:37, 1985

112. Rowe JW, Shock NW, DeFronzo RA: The influence of age on the renal response to water deprivation in man. Nephron 17:270, 1976

113. Epstein M, Hollenberg NK: Age as a determinant of renal sodium conservation in normal man. J Lab Clin Med 87:411, 1976

114. Rowe JW: Aging and renal function. Ann Rev Gerontol Geriatr 1:161, 1980

115. Adler S, Lindeman RD, Yiengst MJ, et al: Effect of acute acid loading on urinary acid excretion by the aging human kidney. J Lab Clin Med 72:278, 1968

116. Kronenberg RS, Drage CW: Attenuation of the ventilatory and heart rate responses to hypoxia and hypercapnia with aging in normal men. J Clin Invest 52:1812, 1973

117. Brischetto MJ, Millman RP, Peterson DD, et al: Effect of aging on ventilatory response to exercise and CO_2. J Appl Physiol 56:1143, 1984

118. Rowe JW, Andres R, Tobin JD, et al: The effect of age on creatinine clearance in men: a cross-sectional and longitudinal study. J Gerontol 31:155, 1976

119. Cockcroft DW, Gault MH: Prediction of creatinine clearance from serum creatinine. Nephron 16:31, 1976

120. Garella S, Matarese RA: Renal effects of prostaglandins and clinical adverse effects of nonsteroidal anti-inflammatory agents. Medicine (Baltimore) 63:165, 1984

121. Brater D, Harris C, Redfern J, et al: Renal effects of COX-2-selective inhibitors. Am J Nephrol 21:1, 2001

122. Devereaux P, Ghali W, Gibson N, et al: Physicians' recommendations for patients who undergo noncardiac surgery. Clin Invest Med 23:116, 2000

123. Wilmore DW, Kehlet H: Management of patients in fast-track surgery. BMJ 322:473, 2001

124. Rodgers A, Walker N, Schug S, et al: Reduction of postoperative mortality and morbidity with epidural or spinal anaesthesia: results from overview of randomised trials. BMJ 321:1, 2000

125. Jones AG, Hunter JM: Anaesthesia in the elderly: special considerations. Drugs & Aging 9:319, 1996

126. Catley DM, Thornton C, Jordan C, et al: Pronounced, episodic oxygen desaturation in the postoperative period: its association with ventilatory pattern and analgesic regimen. Anesthesiology 63:20, 1985

127. Wheatley RG, Somerville ID, Sapsford DJ, et al: Postoperative hypoxaemia: comparison of extradural, I.M., and patient-controlled opioid analgesia. Br J Anaesth 64:267, 1990

128. Inouye SK, Bogardius ST, Jr, Charpentier PA, et al: A multi-component intervention to prevent delirium in hospitalized older patients. N Engl J Med 340:669, 1999

129. Creditor MC: Hazards of hospitalization of the elderly. Ann Intern Med 118:219, 1993

130. Young A: Exercise physiology in geriatric practice. Acta Med Scand 711(suppl):227, 1986

131. Watters JM, Clancey SM, Moulton SB, et al: Impaired recovery of strength in older patients after major abdominal surgery. Ann Surg 218:380, 1993

132. DeBiasse MA, Wilmore DW: What is optimal nutritional support? New Horizons 2:122, 1994

133. Gall MJ, Grimble GK, Reeve NJ, et al: Effect of providing fortified meals and between-meal snacks on energy and protein intake of hospital patients. Clin Nutr 17:259, 1999

134. Bastow MD, Rawlings J, Allison SP: Benefits of supplementary tube feeding after fractured neck of femur: a randomised controlled trial. BMJ 287:1589, 1983

135. Delmi M, Rapin C-H, Bengoa J-M, et al: Dietary supplementation in elderly patients with fractured neck of the femur. Lancet 335:1013, 1990

136. Espaulella J, Guyer H, Diaz-Escriu F, et al: Nutritional supplementation of elderly hip fracture patients: a randomized, double-blind, placebo-controlled trial. Age Ageing 29:425, 2000

137. Shock NW: Energy metabolism, caloric intake and physical activity in old age. Symposium on Nutrition in Old Age. 10th Symposium of the Swedish Nutrition Foundation. Carlson LA, Ed. Almqvist and Wiksell, Uppsala, Sweden, 1972, p 12

138. Watters JM, Moulton SB, Clancey SM, et al: Aging exaggerates glucose intolerance following injury. J Trauma 37:786, 1994

139. Jeevanandam M, Holaday NJ, Shamos RF, et al:

Acute IGF-1 deficiency in multiple trauma victims. Clin Nutr 11:352, 1992

140. Jeevanandam M, Ramias L, Shamos RF, et al: Decreased growth hormone levels in the catabolic phase of severe injury. Surgery 111:495, 1992

141. Van den Berghe G, Wouters P, Weekers F, et al: Intensive insulin therapy in critically ill patients. N Engl J Med 345:1359, 2001

142. Resnick NM, Marcantonio ER: How should clinical care of the aged differ? Lancet 350:1157, 1997

143. Lazarou J, Pomeranz B, Corey P: Incidence of adverse drug reactions in hospitalized patients: a meta-analysis of prospective studies. JAMA 279:1200, 1998

144. Pouyanne P, Haramburu F, Imbs J, et al: Admissions to hospital caused by adverse drug reactions: cross sectional incidence study. BMJ 320:1036, 2000

145. Thomas EJ, Brennan TA: Incidence and types of preventable adverse events in elderly patients: population based review of medical records. BMJ 320:741, 2000

146. Wynne HA, Cope LH, Mutch E, et al: The effect of age upon liver volume and apparent liver blood flow in healthy men. Hepatology 9:297, 1989

147. Shepherd AM, Hewick DS, Moreland TA, et al: Age as a determinant of sensitivity to warfarin. Br J Clin Pharmacol 4:315, 1977

148. Reidenberg MM, Levy M, Warner H, et al: Relationship between diazepam dose, plasma level, age, and central nervous system depression. Clin Pharmacol Ther 23:371, 1978

149. Cohn SH, Vartsky D, Yasumura S, et al: Compartmental body composition based on total-body nitrogen, potassium, and calcium. Am J Physiol 239:E524, 1980

150. Moore FD, Olesen KH, McMurrey JD, et al: The Body Cell Mass and Its Supporting Environment: Body Composition in Health and Disease. W B Saunders Co, Philadelphia, 1963

151. Skelton DA, Grieg CA, Davies JM, et al: Strength, power and related functional ability of healthy people aged 65-89 years. Age Ageing 23:371, 1994

152. Metter EJ, Conwit R, Tobin J, et al: Age-associated loss of power and strength in the upper extremities in women and men. J Gerontol Biol Sci 52A:B267, 1997

153. Wahba WM: Influence of aging on lung function: clinical significance of changes from age twenty. Anesth Analg 62:764, 1983

154. Morley J: Anorexia, sarcopenia, and aging. Nutrition 17:660, 2001

155. Skrobak-Kaczynski J, Andersen KL: The effect of a high level of habitual physical activity in the regulation of fatness during aging. Int Arch Occup Environ Health 36:41, 1975

156. Heath GW, Hagberg JM, Ehsani AA, et al: A physiological comparison of young and older endurance athletes. J Appl Physiol 51:634, 1981

157. DeVries HA: Physiological effects of an exercise training regimen upon men aged 52 to 88. J Gerontol 25:325, 1970

158. Sidney KH, Shephard RJ, Harrison JE: Endurance training and body composition of the elderly. Am J Clin Nutr 30:326, 1977

159. Larsson L: Physical training effects on muscle morphology in sedentary males at different ages. Med Sci Sports Exerc 14:203, 1982

160. Gribbin B, Pickering TG, Sleight P, et al: Effect of age and high blood pressure on baroreflex sensitivity in man. Circ Res 29:424, 1971

161. Collins KJ, Exton-Smith AN, James MH, et al: Functional changes in autonomic nervous responses with ageing. Age Ageing 9:17, 1980

162. Lakatta EG: Cardiovascular regulatory mechanisms in advanced age. Physiol Rev 73:413, 1993

163. Davies CT: The oxygen-transporting system in relation to age. Clin Sci 42:1, 1972

164. Strandell T: Circulatory studies on healthy old men: with special reference to the limitation of the maximal physical working capacity. Acta Med Scand 175:1, 1964

165. Brandfonbrener M, Landowne M, Shock NW: Changes in cardiac output with age. Circulation 12:557, 1955

166. Gerstenblith G, Fleg JL, Becker LC, et al: Maximum left ventricular filling rate in healthy individuals measured by gated blood pool scans. Circulation 68(III):101, 1983

167. Miyatake K, Okamoto M, Kinoshita N, et al: Augmentation of atrial contribution to left ventricular inflow with aging as assessed by intracardiac doppler flowmetry. Am J Cardiol 53:586, 1984

168. Davidson WR Jr, Fee EC: Influence of aging on pulmonary hemodynamics in a population free of coronary artery disease. Am J Cardiol 65:1454, 1990

169. Rodeheffer RJ, Gerstenblith G, Becker LC, et al: Exercise cardiac output is maintained with advancing age in healthy human subjects: cardiac dilatation and increased stroke volume compensate for a diminished heart rate. Circulation 69:203, 1984

170. Port S, Cobb FR, Coleman RE, et al: Effect of age on the response of the left ventricular ejection fraction to exercise. N Engl J Med 303:1133, 1980

171. Yin FCP, Raizes GS, Guarnieri T, et al: Age-associated decrease in ventricular response to haemodynamic stress during beta-adrenergic blockade. Br Heart J 40:1349, 1978

172. Stratton JR, Cerqueira MD, Schwartz RS, et al: Differences in cardiovascular responses to isoproterenol in relation to age and exercise training in healthy men. Circulation 86:504, 1992

173. Rich MW, Imburgia M: Inotropic response to dobutamine in elderly patients with decompensated congestive heart failure. Am J Cardiol 65:519, 1990

174. Dehn MM, Bruce RA: Longitudinal variations in maximal oxygen intake with age and activity. J Appl Physiol 33:805, 1972

175. Leenders KL, Perani D, Lammertsma AA, et al: Cerebral blood flow, blood volume, and oxygen utilization. Brain 113:27, 1990

176. Lindbjerg IF: Diagnostic application of the ^{133}xenon method in peripheral arterial disease. Scand J Clin Lab Invest 17:589, 1965

177. Tsuchida Y: Age-related changes in skin blood flow at four anatomic sites of the body in males studied by xenon-133. Plast Reconstr Surg 85:556, 1990

178. Collins KJ, Exton-Smith AN: Thermal homeostasis in old age. 1983 Henderson Award Lecture. J Am Geriatr Soc 31:519, 1983

179. Wagner JA, Robinson S, Marino RP: Age and temperature regulation of humans in neutral and cold environments. J Appl Physiol 37:562, 1974

180. Bastow MD, Rawlings J, Allison SP: Undernutrition, hypothermia, and injury in elderly women with fractured femur: an injury response to altered metabolism? Lancet 1:143, 1983

181. Allison SP: Some metabolic aspects of injury. The Scientific Basis for the Care of the Critically Ill. Little RA, Frayn KN, Eds. Manchester University Press, Manchester, 1986, p 169

182. Holt DR, Kirk SJ, Regan MC, et al: Effect of age on wound healing in healthy human beings. Surgery 112:293, 1992

183. Lenhardt R, Hopf HW, Marker E, et al: Perioperative collagen deposition in elderly and young men and women. Arch Surg 135:71, 2000

184. White H, Cook J, Ward M: Abdominal wound dehiscence. Ann Royal Coll Surg Engl 59:337, 1977

185. Miller RA: Aging and the Immune Response. Handbook of The Biology of Aging, 3rd ed. Schneider EL, Rowe J, Eds. Academic Press, San Diego, 1996, p 355

186. Carson P, Nichol K, O'Brien J, et al: Immune function and vaccine responses in healthy advanced elderly patients. Arch Intern Med 160:2017, 2000

187. Waldorf DS, Willkens RF, Decker JL: Impaired delayed hypersensitivity in an aging population. JAMA 203:831, 1968

188. Pietsch JB, Meakins JL, MacLean LD: The delayed hypersensitivity response: application in clinical surgery. Surgery 82:349, 1977

189. Brewer RJ, Golden GT, Hitch DC, et al: Abdominal pain: an analysis of 1,000 consecutive cases in a university hospital emergency room. Am J Surg 131:219, 1976

190. Albano WA, Zielinski CM, Organ CH: Is appendicitis in the aged really different? Geriatrics 30:81, 1975

191. Rowe JW, Minaker KL: Geriatric medicine. Handbook of the Biology of Aging, 2nd ed. Finch CE, Schneider EL, Eds. Van Nostrand Reinhold, New York, 1985, p 932

192. Fenyö G: Acute abdominal disease in the elderly: experience from two series in Stockholm. Am J Surg 143:751, 1982

193. Watters J, Blakslee J, March R, et al: The influence of age on the severity of peritonitis. Can J Surg 39:142, 1996

194. Irvin TT, Arnstein PM: Management of symptomatic gallstones in the elderly. Br J Surg 75:1163, 1988

195. Sacco WJ, Copes WS, Bain LWJ, et al: Effect of preinjury illness on trauma patient survival outcome. J Trauma 35:538, 1993

196. Morris JA Jr, MacKenzie EJ, Edelstein SL: The effect of preexisting conditions on mortality in trauma patients. JAMA 263:1942, 1990

197. Finelli FC, Jonsson J, Champion HR, et al: A case control study for major trauma in geriatric patients. J Trauma 29:541, 1989

198. Dischinger PC, Cushing BM, Kerns TJ: Injury patterns associated with direction of impact: drivers admitted to trauma centers. J Trauma 35:454, 1993

199. Fatality facts: elderly. Insurance Institute for Highway Safety, Highway Loss Data Institute. Arlington, Virginia, 2002 http://www.hwysafety.org/safety%5Ffacts/fatality%5Ffacts/elderly.htm

200. Viano DC, Culver CC, Evans L, et al: Involvement of older drivers in multivehicle side-impact crashes. Accid Anal & Prev 22:177, 1990

201. McCoy GF, Johnstone RA, Duthie RB: Injury to the elderly in road traffic accidents. J Trauma 29:494, 1989

202. Allen JE, Schwab CW: Blunt chest trauma in the elderly. Am Surgeon 51:697, 1985

203. Richardson JD, Adams L, Flint LM: Selective management of flail chest and pulmonary contusion. Ann Surg 196:481, 1982

204. Riggs BL, Melton LJ: Involutional osteoporosis. N Engl J Med 314:1676, 1986

205. Velmahos GC, Jindal A, Chan LS, et al: "Insignificant" mechanism of injury: not to be taken lightly. J Am Coll Surg 192:147, 2001

206. Linn BS: Age differences in the severity and outcome of burns. J Am Geriatr Soc 28:118, 1980

207. Frankenfield D, Cooney RN, Smith JS, et al: Age-related differences in the metabolic response to injury. J Trauma 48:49, 2000

208. McKinley BA, Marvin RG, Cocanour CS, et al: Blunt trauma resuscitation: the old can respond. Arch Surg 135:688, 2000

209. Osler T, Hales K, Baack B, et al: Trauma in the elderly. Am J Surg 156:537, 1988

210. Pellicane JV, Byrne K, DeMaria EJ: Preventable complications and death from multiple organ failure among geriatric trauma victims. J Trauma 33:440, 1992

211. Knudson MM, Lieberman J, Morris JA, et al: Mortality factors in geriatric blunt trauma patients. Arch Surg 129:448, 1994

212. Champion HR, Copes WS, Buyer D, et al: Major trauma in geriatric patients. Am J Public Health 79:1278, 1989

213. DeMaria EJ, Kenney PR, Merriam MA, et al: Aggressive trauma care benefits the elderly. J Trauma 27:1200, 1987

214. Carrillo EH, Richardson JD, Malias MA, et al: Long term outcome of blunt trauma care in the elderly. Surg Gynecol Obstet 176:559, 1993

215. Day RJ, Vinen J, Hewitt-Falls E: Major trauma outcomes in the elderly. Med J Australia 160:675, 1994

216. van Aalst JA, Morris JA Jr, Yates HK, et al: Severely injured geriatric patients return to independent living: a study of factors influencing function and independence. J Trauma 31:1096, 1991

217. Oreskovich MR, Howard JD, Copass MK, et al: Geriatric trauma: injury patterns and outcome. J Trauma 24:565, 1984

218. Holbrook TL, Anderson JP, Sieber WJ, et al: Outcome after major trauma:12-month and 18-month follow-up from the Trauma Recovery Project. J Trauma 46:765, 1999

219. Koval KJ, Zuckerman JD: Functional recovery after fracture of the hip. J Bone Joint Surg 76A: 751, 1994

220. Canadian cancer statistics. Canadian Cancer Society, Toronto, Ontario, Canada, 2001 http://www.cancer.ca/english/RS_CanCanStats.asp

221. Feldman AR, Kessler L, Myers MH, et al: The prevalence of cancer: estimates based on the Connecticut Tumor Registry. N Engl J Med 315:1394, 1986

222. Newcomb PA, Carbone PP: Cancer treatment and age: patient perspectives. J Natl Cancer Inst 85:1580, 1993

223. Elsaleh H, Joseph D, Grieu F, et al: Association of tumour site and sex with survival benefit from adjuvant chemotherapy in colorectal cancer. Lancet 355:1745, 2000

224. Mahoney T, Kuo Y-H, Topilow A, et al: Stage III colon cancers: why adjuvant chemotherapy is not offered to elderly patients. Arch Surg 135:182, 2000

225. Hodgson DC, Fuchs CS, Ayanian JZ: Impact of patient and provider characteristics on the treatment and outcomes of colorectal cancer. J Nat

Canc Inst 93:501, 2001

226. Yancik R, Wesley MN, Ries LAG, et al: Effect of age and comorbidity in postmenopausal breast cancer patients aged 55 years and older. JAMA 285:885, 2001a

227. Desch CE, Smith TJ: Defining treatment aims and end-points in older patients with cancer. Drugs & Aging 6:351, 1995

228. Yellen SB, Cella DF, Leslie WT. Age and clinical decision making in oncology patients. J Natl Cancer Inst 86:1766, 1994

229. Greenfield S, Blanco DM, Elashoff RM, et al: Patterns of care related to age of breast cancer patients. JAMA 257:2766, 1987

230. Silliman RA: Breast cancer care in old age: where do we go from here? J Natl Cancer Inst 88:701, 1996

231. Goodwin JS, Samet JM, Hunt WC: Determinants of survival in older cancer patients. J Natl Cancer Inst 88:1031, 1996

232. Hutchins LF, Unger JM, Crowley JJ, et al: Underrepresentation of patients 65 years of age or older in cancer-treatment trials. N Engl J Med 341:2061, 1999

233. Bernabei R, Venturiero V, Tarsitani P, et al: The comprehensive geriatric assessment: when, where, and how. Crit Rev Oncol Hematol 33:45, 2000

234. Yancik R, Ganz PA, Varricchio CG, et al: Perspectives on comorbidity and cancer in older patients: approaches to expand the knowledge base. J Clin Oncol 19:1147, 2001

235. Walter LC, Covinsky KE: Cancer screening in elderly patients. A framework for individualized decision making. JAMA 285:2750, 2001

236. Black C, Roos NP, Havens B, et al: Rising use of physician services by the elderly: the contribution of morbidity. Can J Aging 14:225, 1995

237. Goodwin JS: Geriatrics and the limits of modern medicine. N Engl J Med 340:1283, 1999

238. Watters JM, O'Rourke K: Effects of age and gender. Surgical Research. Wilmore DW, Souba WW, Eds. Academic Press, San Diego, 2001

239. Normal Human Aging: The Baltimore Longitudinal Study of Aging. Shock NW, Greulich RC, Andres R, et al, Eds. US Government Printing Office, Washington, DC, NIH Publication No. 84-2450, 1984.

240. MacDonald P, Johnstone D, Rockwood K: Coronary artery bypass surgery for elderly patients: is our practice based on evidence or faith? CMAJ 162:1005, 2000

241. Comprehensive functional assessment for elderly patients. Health and Public Policy Committee, American College of Physicians. Ann Intern Med 109:70, 1988

242. McClaran JC: Preoperative assessment: the geriatrician's viewpoint. Surgical Care of the Elderly. Meakins JL, McClaran JC, Eds. Year Book Medical Publishers, 1988, p 217

243. Katz S: The science of quality of life (editorial). J Chron Dis 40:459, 1987

244. Katz S: Assessing self-maintenance: activities of daily living, mobility, and instrumental activities of daily living. J Am Geriatr Soc 31:721, 1983

245. Haab F, Boccon-Gibod L, Delmas V, et al: Perineal versus retropubic radical prostatectomy for T1, T2 prostate cancer. Br J Urol 74:626, 1994

246. Oxman TE, Freeman DH Jr, Manheimer ED: Lack of social participation or religious strength and comfort as risk factors for death after cardiac surgery in the elderly. Psychosomatic Medicine 57:5, 1995

247. Bombardier C, Melfi CA, Paul J, et al: Comparison of a generic and a disease-specific measure of pain and physical function after knee replacement surgery. Med Care 33(4 Suppl): AS131, 1995

248. Jaeger AA, Hlatky MA, Paul SM, et al: Functional capacity after cardiac surgery in elderly patients. J Am Coll Cardiol 24:104, 1994

249. Weller SJ, Rossitch E Jr: Unilateral posterolateral decompression without stabilization for neurological palliation of symptomatic spinal metastasis in debilitated patients. J Neurosurg 82:739, 1995

250. Munin MC, Kwoh CK, Glynn N, et al: Predicting discharge outcome after elective hip and knee arthroplasty. Am J Phys Med Rehabil 74:294, 1995

251. Lakatta EG: Heart and circulation. Handbook of the Biology of Aging, 2nd ed. Finch CE, Schneider EL, Adelman RC, et al, Eds. Van Nostrand Reinhold Co, New York, 1985, p 413

252. Seely JF: Renal function in the elderly. Surgical Care of the Elderly. Meakins JL, McClaran JC, Eds. Year Book Medical Publishers, Chicago, 1988

253. Watters JM, Moulton SB, Clancey SM, et al: Aging exaggerates glucose intolerance following injury. J Trauma 37:786, 1994

254. Lakatta EG: Cardiovascular reserve capacity in healthy older humans. Aging: Clinical and Experimental Research 6:213, 1994

255. Lakatta EG: Heart and circulation. Handbook of the Biology of Aging, 3rd ed. Schneider EL, Rowe JW, Eds. Academic Press, San Diego, 1990, p 181

256. Thomas VS, Rockwood K, McDowell K: Multidimensionality in instrumental and basic activities of daily living. J Clin Epidemiol 51:315, 1998

257. Kane RL, Ouslander JG, Abrass IB: Essentials of Clinical Geriatrics, 2nd ed. McGraw-Hill Information Services Co, New York, 1989, p 213

258. Kane RL, Ouslander JG, Abrass IB: Essentials of Clinical Geriatrics, 2nd ed. McGraw-Hill Information Services Co, New York, 1989, p 341

Acknowledgments

Figures 2, 4, 8   Marcia Kammerer.

8 THE PEDIATRIC SURGICAL PATIENT

Arnold G. Coran, M.D.

Perioperative care of infants and children presents many management problems that differ significantly from those seen in adults.[1] This chapter is concerned with recognition and management of certain clinical problems that occur frequently in neonates, infants, and children, with special attention paid to seven areas: (1) monitoring, (2) shock, (3) fluid and electrolyte management, (4) infection and antibiotics, (5) ventilatory support, (6) nutritional support, and (7) trauma. More emphasis is placed on the special needs of neonates (i.e., babies younger than 28 days) and infants (i.e., babies 28 days to 1 year of age) because management of these patients diverges more from management of adults than does management of older children. Several special conditions for which pediatric management differs significantly from adult management (e.g., intestinal obstruction, respiratory distress, and abdominal pain) are discussed in more detail [see Sidebars Intestinal Obstruction in the Newborn, Respiratory Distress in the Newborn, Abdominal Pain, Analgesic Dosage Guidelines in Children, and Preparation of the Neonate with Emergency Surgical Problems].

Parameters to Monitor

It is only since the middle to late 1980s that the most advanced techniques for monitoring critically ill patients have been used in neonates, especially in premature and young infants, because of the technical difficulties involved.

TEMPERATURE

Temperature regulation is critical in neonates because in comparison with older children and adults, they have a large body surface area, little subcutaneous fat (and therefore poor thermal insulation), and reduced lean body mass (required for generating and retaining heat). Most of the heat loss from newborns occurs through radiation, convection, and evaporation; very little heat is lost through conduction. Although the role of evaporation in heat loss increases with increasing prematurity, radiation and convection account for the greater part of the heat lost. Incubators are manufactured so as to minimize radiation and convection by decreasing airflow across the skin and by providing a tightly regulated, thermally neutral environment.

Temperature is monitored by measuring both skin temperature and rectal temperature (core temperature); there is normally a 1.5° C difference between the two. Maintaining body temperature in neonates and young infants is critical both in the neonatal intensive care unit and in the operating room. In the neonatal ICU, temperature is regulated by placing the infant in an incubator or on a bed with an overhead radiant heater. In the OR, an overhead radiant heater is also used; however, the most effective way of maintaining body temperature is to keep the extremities of the infant wrapped or covered.

BODY WEIGHT

Measurement of body weight is especially helpful in evaluating neonates and young infants. Most acute changes in body weight result from changes in total body water; serial measurements of body weight are therefore useful guides to fluid replacement [see Fluid and Electrolyte Management, below]. In general, a 1 g loss of body weight is equivalent to a 1 ml loss of total body water. Serial measurements should be made every 8 to 12 hours and possibly more frequently in neonates. It is important to keep in mind that in their first day of life newborns undergo significant diuresis that reduces extracellular fluid (ECF) volume and total body water.

URINE OUTPUT

Urine flow is a very useful guide to fluid management in all age groups [see Fluid and Electrolyte Management, below]. Measurement of urine output requires accurate collections. In critically ill female infants and in all children, a urinary catheter should be inserted for accurate urine collections. I prefer not to catheterize male neonates and infants because of the risk of trauma to the small urethra; in these patients, properly secured collection bags will allow accurate measurement of urine output. An appropriate urine output is 1 to 2 ml/kg/hr with an osmolality of 250 to 300 mOsm/kg. In premature infants, the flow may have to be somewhat higher, and the osmolality may tend to be slightly lower.

CARDIAC FUNCTION

In critically ill patients, even in premature infants, heart rate and rhythm must be monitored by continuous electrocardiography. In addition, continuous measurements of arterial blood pressure are very helpful [see Table 1]. The standard technique of blood pressure measurement with a sphygmomanometer and a stethoscope has significant disadvantages in the pediatric age group, especially in neonates and infants, because it is so dependent on cuff size, which is highly variable among children. Palpation methods are even less reliable. Of all the noninvasive systems, the Doppler ultrasound technique is by far the most accurate. None of the noninvasive techniques can be used for continuous monitoring, however, nor are they as accurate as intra-arterial measurements. In very sick infants and

Table 1 Normal Values for Vital Signs in Children up to 10 Years of Age

Age (yr)	Pulse Rate (beats/min)	Blood Pressure (mm Hg)	Respirations (breaths/min)
0–1	120	80/40	40
1–5	100	100/60	30
5–10	80	120/80	20

1159

children, direct intra-arterial pressure monitoring should be done via a percutaneous or direct cutdown approach to a peripheral artery. The radial artery is most commonly used,[2,3] but the posterior tibial artery and the dorsalis pedis artery can also be utilized if necessary. In neonates, the umbilical artery is easily accessible and can be used for arterial monitoring.

When there are no cardiac abnormalities, central venous pressure correlates roughly with blood volume. The central venous catheter can be inserted percutaneously into the subclavian or internal jugular vein in older children[4,5]; however, cutdown via the external jugular vein is preferred in neonates and infants.[6] If the external jugular vein cannot be used, the internal jugular vein, the facial vein, the basilic vein, and the proximal saphenous vein are acceptable substitutes. Because of the contamination associated with procedures in the groin, the saphenous vein is the least desirable route.

Swan-Ganz catheters are occasionally used in infants and children, even in newborns and premature neonates.[7-9] No. 5 catheters with triple lumens are available, as are No. 4 catheters with double lumens. The No. 4 catheter can be inserted into premature neonates weighing as little as 1,500 g. These catheters allow simultaneous measurement of right atrial pressure, pulmonary arterial pressure, and pulmonary arterial wedge pressure (PAWP). In addition, the No. 5 catheter can be obtained with a thermistor tip for continuous measurement of cardiac output with thermodilution techniques using small volumes of room-temperature standard infusates [see VII:1 Cardiopulmonary Monitoring].

PAWP is a good index of left atrial pressure. If there is no obstruction between the left atrium and the left ventricle, PAWP will reflect left ventricular end-diastolic pressure, which in turn is a measure of left ventricular volume. A low PAWP suggests that blood volume must be expanded for cardiac output to be adequate and for blood flow to improve [see Fluid and Electrolyte Management, below]. A high or normal PAWP in the face of hypotension suggests inadequate myocardial function.

OXYGENATION

Arterial Blood Gases

The umbilical artery can also be used for the collection of specimens for arterial blood gas monitoring. Serial measurement of arterial pH is extremely important in monitoring acid-base status. Metabolic alkalosis is related to electrolyte loss [see Fluid and Electrolyte Management, below], whereas metabolic acidosis is usually the result of poor tissue perfusion. Arterial oxygen tension (P_aO_2) and arterial carbon dioxide tension (P_aCO_2) are excellent measures of the adequacy of oxygenation and ventilation [see Ventilatory Support, below].

Pulse Oximetry

Although the standard and most effective way of monitoring oxygenation in any age group is to measure arterial blood gases, the introduction of pulse oximetry has revolutionized this type of monitoring. Pulse oximetry is based on the comparison of the light absorption properties of oxyhemoglobin with those of reduced hemoglobin. Its advantages are immediate availability of oxygen saturation data, minimal cost, the absence of any need for calibration, and the possibility of leaving the probe in place for several hours.

Shock

The two most common types of shock seen in infants, children, and adults are hypovolemic shock and septic shock; in infants and children, septic shock is the most common.[10] How newborns and infants respond to either type of shock is significantly different from how older children and adults respond. For example, in a neonate affected by profound shock, bradycardia is a common response, rather than tachycardia, which is more common in adults. Moreover, neonates, especially premature neonates, normally have a low blood pressure; consequently, the shock insult often does not evoke a further significant reduction of blood pressure. The hypovolemia caused by the shock results in decreased venous return, which lowers cardiac output; the low cardiac output leads to poor tissue perfusion and the development of lactic acidosis.

Septic shock is usually caused by gram-negative bacteria. Peritonitis resulting from intestinal perforation is a common cause of septic shock in neonates and infants; other causes are urinary tract infections, respiratory tract infections, and contaminated intravascular catheters. Although the pathophysiology of septic shock differs substantially from that of hypovolemic shock, in both states the stasis and pooling of blood in the capillary bed lead to reduction of the circulating blood volume.[11]

TREATMENT

The mainstay of treatment of hypovolemic shock is fluid and blood replacement [see Fluid and Electrolyte Management and Trauma, below]. In neonates, the hematocrit should be maintained at 45% to ensure adequate oxygen delivery. In many infants, hypovolemic shock is caused not by hemorrhage but by dehydration (e.g., from severe gastroenteritis). The subsequent dehydration is usually hypertonic because of the significant loss of hypotonic fluid. As a rule, much more water is lost than electrolytes, which results in serum sodium levels as high as 150 mEq/L. Emergency treatment involves infusion of hypotonic solutions of sodium chloride.

Because septic shock, like hypovolemic shock, is characterized by reduced circulating blood volume, initial therapy involves infusion of large volumes of colloid solutions. Most of the experimental and clinical data suggest that colloid solutions are preferable to crystalloid for treating septic shock, both in children and in adults. In addition, broad-spectrum antibiotics should always be administered. Agents that are effective against anaerobic bacteria, such as clindamycin, metronidazole, and chloramphenicol, must be included as well [see Table 2]. The use of corticosteroids to treat septic shock has been controversial since its introduction in 1964.[12-20] In experimental settings, pharmacologic doses of corticosteroids appear to increase cardiac output and decrease peripheral resistance.[21] Methylprednisolone, administered intravenously in a dosage of about 30 mg/kg every 6 hours, is used in critically ill infants or children in whom other methods of resuscitation have been unsuccessful.

If fluid infusion has achieved its maximal effects, as evidenced by a normal to elevated central venous pressure or PAWP, but hypotension persists, pharmacologic agents must be used to improve myocardial contractility. The agent of choice is dopamine, which is an alpha and beta agonist.[22-28] In low dosages (0.5 to 5.0 µg/kg/min), this agent activates specific dopamine receptors, causing vasodilatation of the renal and mesenteric arteries and, to a lesser extent, of the coronary and cerebral arteries. In higher dosages (5 to 10 µg/kg/ min), it increases myocardial contractility and thus cardiac output. Up to dosages of approximately 10 µg/kg/min, dopamine primarily exerts a beta-adrenergic effect. Above this point, it begins to exert alpha-adrenergic effects—namely, increases in peripheral resistance, which can have a detrimental effect on the course of septic shock. Dobutamine, which has primarily inotropic and vasodilatory effects, can be used instead of dopamine.

Fluid and Electrolyte Management

Fluid and electrolyte management of neonates and infants requires a thorough understanding of the body fluid compartment

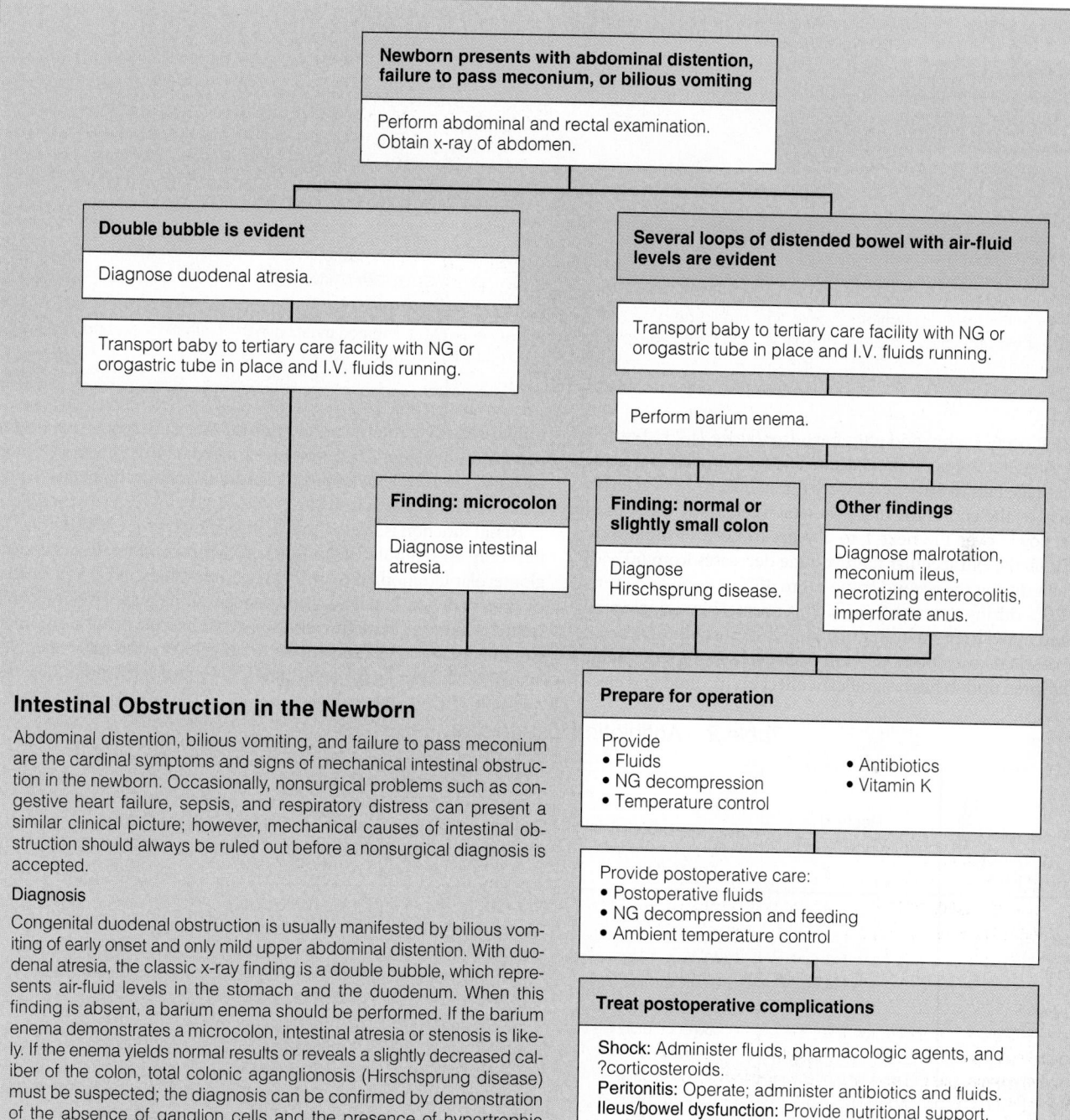

Newborn presents with abdominal distention, failure to pass meconium, or bilious vomiting

Perform abdominal and rectal examination. Obtain x-ray of abdomen.

Double bubble is evident

Diagnose duodenal atresia.

Transport baby to tertiary care facility with NG or orogastric tube in place and I.V. fluids running.

Several loops of distended bowel with air-fluid levels are evident

Transport baby to tertiary care facility with NG or orogastric tube in place and I.V. fluids running.

Perform barium enema.

Finding: microcolon

Diagnose intestinal atresia.

Finding: normal or slightly small colon

Diagnose Hirschsprung disease.

Other findings

Diagnose malrotation, meconium ileus, necrotizing enterocolitis, imperforate anus.

Prepare for operation

Provide
• Fluids
• NG decompression
• Temperature control

• Antibiotics
• Vitamin K

Provide postoperative care:
• Postoperative fluids
• NG decompression and feeding
• Ambient temperature control

Treat postoperative complications

Shock: Administer fluids, pharmacologic agents, and ?corticosteroids.
Peritonitis: Operate; administer antibiotics and fluids.
Ileus/bowel dysfunction: Provide nutritional support.

Intestinal Obstruction in the Newborn

Abdominal distention, bilious vomiting, and failure to pass meconium are the cardinal symptoms and signs of mechanical intestinal obstruction in the newborn. Occasionally, nonsurgical problems such as congestive heart failure, sepsis, and respiratory distress can present a similar clinical picture; however, mechanical causes of intestinal obstruction should always be ruled out before a nonsurgical diagnosis is accepted.

Diagnosis

Congenital duodenal obstruction is usually manifested by bilious vomiting of early onset and only mild upper abdominal distention. With duodenal atresia, the classic x-ray finding is a double bubble, which represents air-fluid levels in the stomach and the duodenum. When this finding is absent, a barium enema should be performed. If the barium enema demonstrates a microcolon, intestinal atresia or stenosis is likely. If the enema yields normal results or reveals a slightly decreased caliber of the colon, total colonic aganglionosis (Hirschsprung disease) must be suspected; the diagnosis can be confirmed by demonstration of the absence of ganglion cells and the presence of hypertrophic nerves on rectal biopsy.

The differential diagnosis of intestinal obstruction in the newborn should also include meconium ileus, meconium plug syndrome, necrotizing enterocolitis, imperforate anus, malrotation and volvulus, and annular pancreas. Of all these conditions, malrotation with midgut volvulus is the one for which prompt diagnosis and treatment are most critical (because of the risk of necrosis of the entire small intestine). The diagnosis of malrotation is best made by means of an upper GI series.

Preoperative Care

All newborns should be given vitamin K I.V. or I.M. before operation because of the normally low levels of prothrombin present in all neonates.

Postoperative Care

Postoperative fluid and electrolyte requirements of infants are easily calculated. One may assume that maintenance fluid requirements are 100 ml/kg/24 hr and that third-space loss into the peritoneal cavity and the intestinal lumen is about half that volume. In general, the maintenance requirements and third-space losses—provided that the third-space losses are relatively small—can be replaced with 5% dextrose in 0.25 normal saline with supplemental potassium chloride at 3 mEq/kg/24 hr. If the third-space losses are large and prolonged, they are best replaced with 5% dextrose in lactated Ringer solution or with plasma. Gastric drainage should be replaced with 5% dextrose in 0.5 normal saline plus 30 mEq/L of potassium chloride.

If total parenteral nutrition (TPN) is required for 2 weeks or less, peripheral TPN is most appropriate; however, if TPN is required for longer than 2 weeks, a central venous Silastic catheter should be inserted.

When an infant on a ventilator becomes clinically stable, weaning should be started by simultaneously reducing the fractional concentration of oxygen in inspired gas (F_IO_2), the backup rate, and the peak inspiratory pressure (because most of the ventilators used on

(continued)

Intestinal Obstruction (*continued*)

infants are pressure controlled). Once the F_iO_2 is down to 21%, the backup rate is further reduced until the baby can be taken off the ventilator.

Postoperative Complications

PERITONITIS

Postoperative peritonitis is often difficult to diagnose in neonates. Tenderness can usually be elicited from the infant but not in every case. Cellulitis of the abdominal wall is a more useful sign. The best way of detecting free air on x-ray examination is with a cross-table lateral view; the free air is usually just under the abdominal wall. If peritonitis is present in the newborn, antibiotic coverage should be broad and should include ampicillin, an aminoglycoside, and metronidazole or clindamycin.

SEPTIC SHOCK

The development of septic shock in newborns can be very subtle and sudden. Because the blood pressure in newborns is normally low, the drop in blood pressure that follows the onset of septic shock may not be very significant. Possibly, a more helpful sign is the development of bradycardia. The initial therapy for septic shock in all age groups, and especially in neonates, is rapid I.V. infusion of colloid after broad-spectrum antibiotics have been administered and the surgical problem has been handled.

ILEUS AND BOWEL DYSFUNCTION

In many newborns, the ileostomy drainage is so high that they cannot tolerate enteral feeding and must have their intestinal tract put at complete rest with parenteral nutrition.

changes that occur before and after birth [*see Figure 1*].[29-34] During the first trimester, total body water accounts for 95% of body weight. This percentage falls to 80% by 32 weeks' gestation, to 78% at term, and to 75% by the end of the first postnatal week. Body water then decreases slowly over the next 1 to 2 years to 60% of total body weight. Similarly, extracellular fluid volume decreases from 60% of body weight during the second trimester to 45% at birth and eventually to 20% during the next 2 years. This normal physiologic process is interrupted in premature neonates, who must diurese excess fetal and postnatal total body water in a relatively short period after birth. This interruption has a significant effect on the fluid and electrolyte requirements of premature infants undergoing major surgery.[35] An expanded ECF volume in a premature infant is a potent stimulus for the release of prostaglandin E_2, which maintains the patency of a ductus arteriosus.[36-38]

Renal function is related to two physiologic processes: glomerular filtration and tubular excretion and reabsorption. In newborns, glomerular filtration rates are 25% of adult values, which are reached by 2 years of age. Likewise, renal concentrating ability is significantly reduced in both premature and full-term infants. A full-term infant can maximally concentrate urine to only 500 to 600 mOsm/kg (versus 1,200 mOsm/kg for an adult)[39,40]; a premature infant has even

Table 2 Antibiotic Dosages for Neonates

Antibiotic	Route of Administration	Dosage (mg/kg/day)			
		Body Weight < 2,000 g		Body Weight > 2,000 g	
		Age 0–7 days	Age > 7 days	Age 0–7 days	Age > 7 days
Amikacin	I.M., I.V.	15 div q. 12 hr	22.5 div q. 8 hr	20 div q. 12 hr	30 div q. 8 hr
Ampicillin	I.V., I.M.	50 div q. 12 hr	75 div q. 8 hr	75 div q. 8 hr	100 div q. 6 hr
Cefazolin	I.V., I.M.	40 div q. 12 hr	40 div q. 12 hr	40 div q. 12 hr	60 div q. 8 hr
Cefotaxime	I.V., I.M.	100 div q. 12 hr	150 div q. 8 hr	100 div q. 12 hr	150 div q. 8 hr
Ceftazidime	I.V., I.M.	100 div q. 12 hr	150 div q. 8 hr	100 div q. 8 hr	150 div q. 8 hr
Ceftriaxone	I.V., I.M.	50 once daily	50 once daily	50 once daily	75 once daily
Cephalothin	I.V.	40 div q. 12 hr	60 div q. 8 hr	60 div q. 8 hr	80 div q. 6 hr
Chloramphenicol	I.V., p.o.	25 once daily	25 once daily	25 once daily	50 div q. 12 hr
Clindamycin	I.V., I.M., p.o.	10 div q. 12 hr	15 div q. 8 hr	15 div q. 8 hr	20 div q. 6 hr
Erythromycin	p.o.	20 div q. 12 hr	30 div q. 8 hr	20 div q. 12 hr	30–40 div q. 8 hr
Gentamicin	I.M., I.V.	5 div q. 12 hr	7.5 div q. 8 hr	5 div q. 12 hr	7.5 div q. 8 hr
Kanamycin	I.M., I.V.	15 div q. 12 hr	22.5 div q. 8 hr	20 div q. 12 hr	30 div q. 8 hr
Methicillin	I.V., I.M.	50 div q. 12 hr	75 div q. 8 hr	75 div q. 8 hr	100 div q. 6 hr
Metronidazole	I.V., p.o.	15 div q. 12 hr	15 div q. 12 hr	15 div q. 12 hr	30 div q. 12 hr
Mezlocillin	I.V., I.M.	150 div q. 12 hr	225 div q. 8 hr	150 div q. 12 hr	225 div q. 8 hr
Oxacillin	I.V., I.M.	50 div q. 12 hr	100 div q. 8 hr	75 div q. 8 hr	150 div q. 6 hr
Nafcillin	I.V.	50 div q. 12 hr	75 div q. 8 hr	50 div q. 8 hr	75 div q. 6 hr
Netilmicin	I.M., I.V.	5 div q. 12 hr	7.5 div q. 8 hr	5 div q. 12 hr	7.5 div q. 8 hr
Penicillin G	I.V.	50,000 U div q. 12 hr	75,000 U div q. 8 hr	50,000 U div q. 8 hr	100,000 U div q. 6 hr
Penicillin G Benzathine	I.M.	50,000 U (one dose)	50,000 U (one dose)	50,000 U (one dose)	50,000 U (one dose)
Procaine		50,000 U once daily	50,000 U once daily	50,000 U once daily	50,000 U once daily
Ticarcillin	I.V., I.M.	150 div q. 12 hr	225 div q. 8 hr	225 div q. 8 hr	300 div q. 6 hr
Tobramycin	I.M., I.V.	4 div q. 12 hr	6 div q. 8 hr	4 div q. 12 hr	6 div q. 8 hr
Vancomycin	I.V.	30 div q. 12 hr	45 div q. 8 hr	30 div q. 12 hr	45 div q. 8 hr

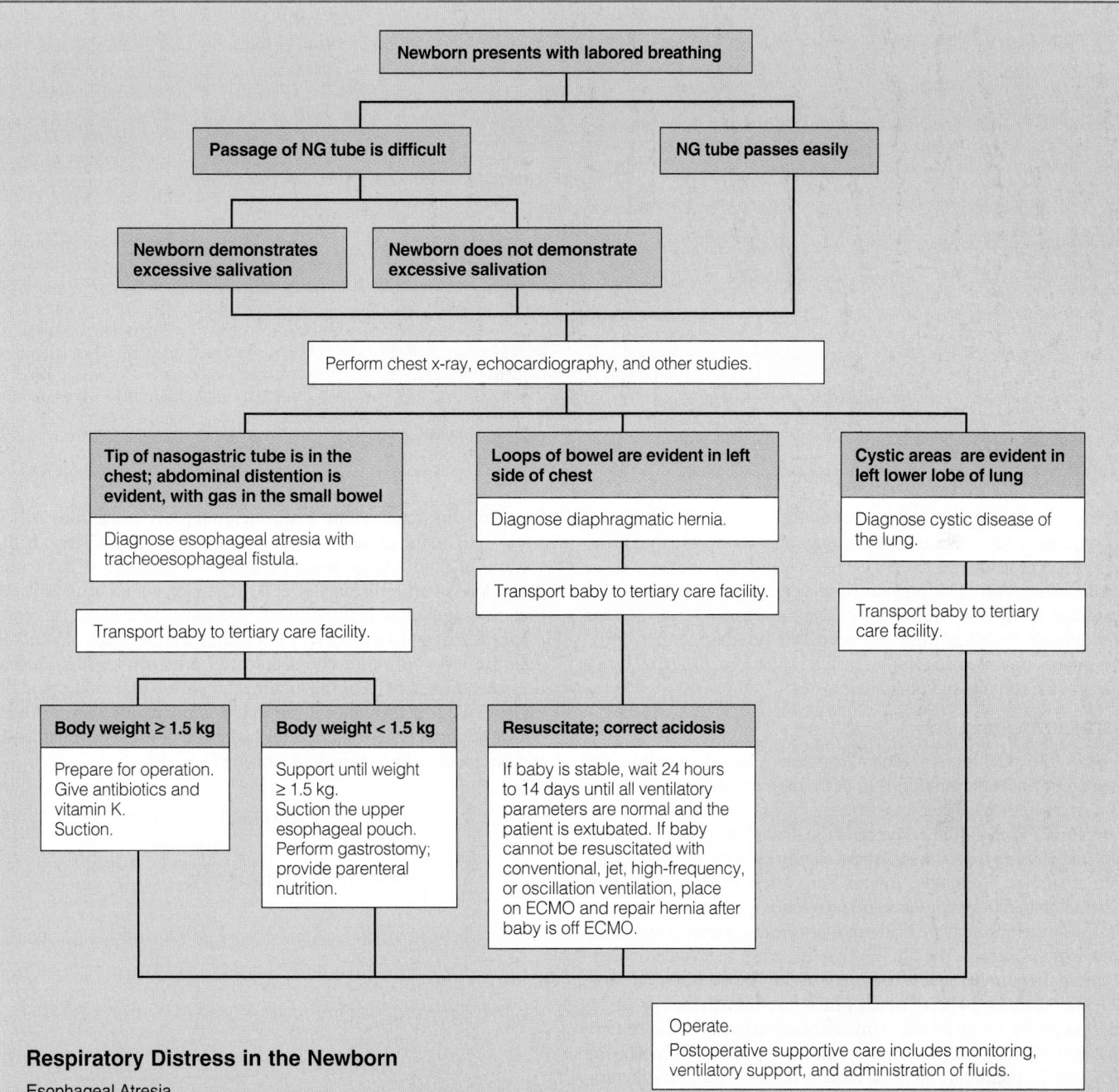

Newborn presents with labored breathing

Passage of NG tube is difficult

NG tube passes easily

Newborn demonstrates excessive salivation

Newborn does not demonstrate excessive salivation

Perform chest x-ray, echocardiography, and other studies.

Tip of nasogastric tube is in the chest; abdominal distention is evident, with gas in the small bowel

Diagnose esophageal atresia with tracheoesophageal fistula.

Transport baby to tertiary care facility.

Loops of bowel are evident in left side of chest

Diagnose diaphragmatic hernia.

Transport baby to tertiary care facility.

Cystic areas are evident in left lower lobe of lung

Diagnose cystic disease of the lung.

Transport baby to tertiary care facility.

Body weight ≥ 1.5 kg

Prepare for operation. Give antibiotics and vitamin K. Suction.

Body weight < 1.5 kg

Support until weight ≥ 1.5 kg. Suction the upper esophageal pouch. Perform gastrostomy; provide parenteral nutrition.

Resuscitate; correct acidosis

If baby is stable, wait 24 hours to 14 days until all ventilatory parameters are normal and the patient is extubated. If baby cannot be resuscitated with conventional, jet, high-frequency, or oscillation ventilation, place on ECMO and repair hernia after baby is off ECMO.

Operate.
Postoperative supportive care includes monitoring, ventilatory support, and administration of fluids.

Respiratory Distress in the Newborn

Esophageal Atresia

In many obstetric units, a nasogastric or orogastric tube is routinely inserted immediately after birth to exclude an esophageal atresia. The most common form of esophageal atresia occurs in combination with a tracheoesophageal fistula; the proximal esophagus ends in a blind upper pouch, and there is a connection between the distal esophagus and the carina of the trachea.[150] Infants with this condition manifest significant respiratory distress within a few hours of birth as a result of salivary aspiration, gastroesophageal reflux of acid into the trachea through the distal fistula, and elevation of the diaphragm as a result of gastric distention with air from the tracheoesophageal fistula.

Diagnosis is confirmed when attempts to pass a nasogastric tube are unsuccessful and chest x-ray reveals the nasogastric tube curled in the esophageal pouch. Aspiration pneumonia should be looked for on the x-ray; its presence suggests that primary repair should be delayed. Echocardiography helps to identify associated cardiac anomalies and also demonstrates the location of the aortic arch. Esophageal anastomosis is most easily accomplished by means of thoracotomy opposite the side of the aortic arch.

PREOPERATIVE CARE

The related pathophysiologic processes must be corrected immediately to stabilize the baby for definitive repair. A sump catheter should be passed into the upper esophageal pouch; constant suction is necessary to prevent pneumonia. A gastrostomy tube (which is only placed if delayed primary repair is contemplated) relieves gastric distention and decreases acid reflux. The infant should be placed in an upright position to prevent gastric reflux.

Once the infant has been stabilized and major associated anomalies have been evaluated, primary repair can be carried out. In a small premature infant (< 1.5 kg) with esophageal atresia, however, it is best merely to perform a gastrostomy within 24 hours of birth and to treat the baby with gastrostomy drainage, sump suction of the upper esophageal pouch, and parenteral nutrition until the infant reaches a weight of 1.5 kg. This approach is better than an early division of the fistula retropleurally and a subsequent primary esophageal anastomosis transpleurally.

(continued)

Respiratory Distress (*continued*)

Diaphragmatic Hernia

Infants with congenital diaphragmatic hernia are usually quite sick at birth. They do not have difficulty swallowing their saliva; however, it may be difficult to pass a nasogastric tube into the stomach because the entire stomach may be in the chest. A plain x-ray will usually confirm the diagnosis of congenital diaphragmatic hernia.

These babies require immediate resuscitation with endotracheal intubation and sodium bicarbonate to correct acidosis. It should be noted that standard sodium bicarbonate solutions are extremely hypertonic and should be diluted before being administered, especially in neonates. Once the baby is relatively stable, it is best to wait 24 hours to as much as 14 days before operating to allow the pulmonary hypertension to decrease or disappear. If the baby cannot be resuscitated with conventional, jet, high-frequency, or oscillation ventilation, then he or she should be placed on extracorporeal membrane oxygenation (ECMO), and the hernia should be repaired after the baby is off ECMO.[151-153] In the OR, the intestines are reduced into the abdominal cavity, and the diaphragmatic defect is repaired. However, this operative procedure usual-ly does not result in significant improvement. Often, the newborn's condition will improve during the first 12 hours postoperatively and then begin to deteriorate. If the baby fails to respond to vasodilators and inotropic agents, ECMO will be required postoperatively. Usually, ECMO permits survival of the infant under circumstances in which the mortality would be close to 100% were ECMO not available.

Cystic Disease of the Lung

Cystic lung disease, especially cystic adenomatoid malformation of the left lower lobe, can mimic diaphragmatic hernia both clinically and radiographically.[154,155] However, in contrast to a newborn with diaphragmatic hernia, a baby with cystic adenomatoid malformation will demonstrate the normal protuberance of a newborn's abdomen. If an infant with cystic adenomatoid malformation of the lungs manifests marked respiratory distress necessitating intubation and mechanical ventilation, it is preferable to perform an emergency lobectomy rather than subject the baby to a period of mechanical ventilation with the attendant risks of barotrauma and oxygen toxicity.

less concentrating ability (up to a maximum of 400 mOsm/kg). As a consequence, newborns tolerate dehydration poorly. Furthermore, the kidneys of newborns cannot excrete a water load as effectively as mature kidneys can. This phenomenon, combined with the low concentrating ability of the newborns' kidneys, makes fluid management very difficult. An initial fluid and electrolyte program for newborns and infants must replace the insensible water loss, the renal water loss, and the sodium and potassium losses.

INSENSIBLE WATER LOSS

Insensible water loss is a result of continuous loss of water from the respiratory tract and the skin.[41] In both full-term and premature infants, transepithelial water loss is the major component of insensible water loss.[42] The stratum corneum is the major barrier to the passive diffusion of water from the superficial capillaries of the skin to the epidermal surface. Premature infants have a less developed stratum corneum than full-term infants and therefore experience a greater diffusion of water through the epidermal surface and a greater insensible water loss through the skin. In full-term neonates, in an environment of thermal neutrality and a humidity of 50%, total insensible water loss is 12 ml/kg/24 hr, of which 7 ml is lost through the skin and 5 ml through the lungs. In full-term infants, overhead radiant heaters and phototherapy may increase insensible water loss from skin by 50%.[43-49] In premature infants, radiant heaters and phototherapy may increase insensible water loss from skin by 50% to 100%.

Full-term babies sweat at birth if body temperature exceeds 37.5° C (99.5° F); however, the amount of water they lose by this mechanism is quite small. Respiratory water loss accounts for about one third of total insensible water loss in full-term infants and is related to the volume of inspired air, respiratory rate, body temperature, and the humidity of the expired air.[50] Premature infants of less than 36 weeks' gestation do not sweat in the first few days of life. In these infants, especially those who are born after less than 32 weeks' gestation, the respiratory water loss is less than it is in full-term infants because the transepithelial water loss is greater.

Insensible water loss from the skin can be minimized by the use of incubators in the neonatal ICU and extremity coverings in the OR. Water loss from the lungs can be decreased by humidifying the inspired gases.

RENAL WATER REQUIREMENTS

The water required for excretion of the products of catabolism is based on the renal solute load, including any exogenous solute load,[51] and on the maximal renal concentrating ability. Therefore, the volume of fluid administered must allow excretion of the entire solute load at an osmolality of 250 mOsm/kg, a level achievable by even the smallest premature infant. The solute load of the newborn is approximately 15 mOsm/kg/24 hr during the first week of life if the infant receives only intravenous fluids; 17.5 mOsm/kg/24 hr during the second week of life if the infant is on partial oral intake; and 30 mOsm/kg/24 hr thereafter if the infant is maintained on formula. The amount of water required for excretion of these osmolar loads can be calculated by using the following formula:

$$H_2O \text{ requirements (ml/kg/24 hr)} = \frac{\text{osmolality of solute load (mOsm/kg)}}{\text{osmolality of urine (mOsm/kg)}} \times 1,000$$

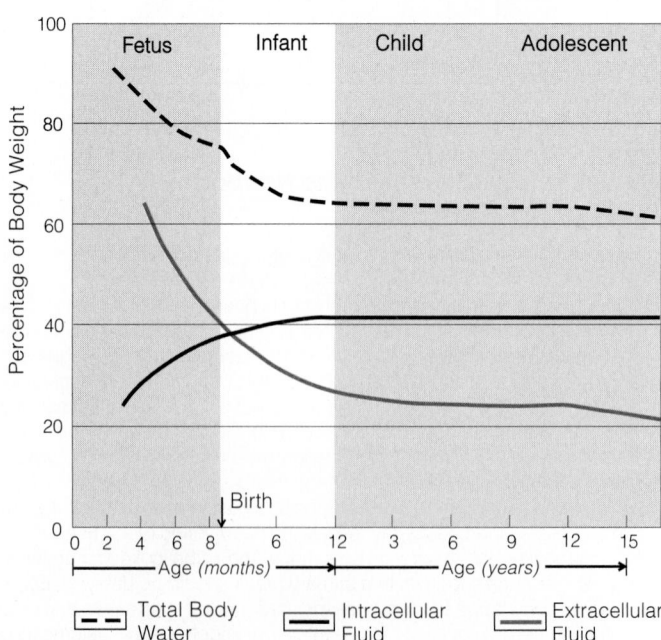

Figure 1 **Total body water (TBW) and extracellular fluid (ECF) decrease between fetal life and adulthood, and intracellular fluid (ICF) increases.**

Abdominal Pain

Abdominal pain in a pubertal female can have many different causes. Acute appendicitis is the most common cause; nevertheless, the differential diagnosis should also include perforated duodenal ulcer, Meckel diverticulum, ulcerative colitis, Crohn disease, ruptured ovarian cyst, pelvic inflammatory disease, pancreatitis, and, in much younger children, intussusception. The diagnosis of appendicitis is based on the presence of localizing physical findings in the right lower quadrant of the abdomen. Even if the history and laboratory data are not typical, the presence of localizing physical findings should allow one to make the diagnosis and to proceed with appropriate operation.

If perforation of the appendix is suspected preoperatively, broad-spectrum antibiotics should be started, and the patient should be given I.V. crystalloid. There is no value in leaving a drain, even if pus is encountered in the peritoneal cavity, because it is impossible to drain the peritoneal cavity adequately. Instead, the cavity should be vigorously irrigated with saline. In most cases of perforated appendicitis, the wound can be closed primarily if irrigation has been adequate. Currently, many pediatric surgeons treat perforated appendicitis nonoperatively with I.V. antibiotics followed by laparoscopic interval appendectomy at 6 weeks.

A pelvic abscess after operation for acute appendicitis typically develops between postoperative days 5 and 7. It is usually manifested by fever and elevation of the white blood cell count and not infrequently by diarrhea. In almost all cases, surgical drainage is not necessary, and treatment with I.V. antibiotics is sufficient.

Very often, a teenager who exhibits the classic signs and symptoms of appendicitis turns out to have Crohn disease of the terminal ileum. This condition will be obvious at operation if the mesenteric fat is seen to be creeping up along the sides of the inflamed ileum. In the past, it was generally agreed that an appendectomy should not be performed under these circumstances because of the theoretical risk that a cecal fistula

---

Patient between the ages of 5 and 14 presents with abdominal pain, fever, and leukocytosis

Establish preoperative diagnosis.

Most likely diagnoses are
- Appendicitis
- Inflammatory bowel disease (ulcerative colitis, Crohn disease)

Less likely diagnoses are
- Perforated ulcer
- Meckel diverticulum
- Pelvic inflammatory disease
- Pancreatitis
- Intussusception
- Ruptured ovarian cyst

Postoperative care includes general support, administration of fluids, and administration of antibiotics.

Avoid complications:
- Wound infection
- Intra-abdominal abscess
- Enterocutaneous fistula
- Malnutrition

---

would develop. In fact, this reservation has not been shown to be well founded, and most surgeons now recommend appendectomy at the time of exploratory laparotomy. When the child has fully recovered from the operation, a definitive workup should be performed to ascertain the extent of the Crohn disease. The workup should include a small-bowel series and a colonoscopy with biopsy. If an enterocutaneous fistula should develop, TPN will be required for a prolonged period.

If the urine osmolality is 250 mOsm/kg, the renal water requirements are 60 ml/kg/24 hr during the first week of life, 72 ml/kg/24 hr during the second week of life, and 84 ml/kg/24 hr thereafter. This rate of fluid infusion will produce a urine output of approximately 2.5 ml/kg/hr. Renal water requirements are modified by a number of factors. An anabolic, growing infant has a lower solute load and therefore a lower water requirement. A certain amount of water is required for active growth, between 10 and 15 ml/kg/24 hr. On the other hand, if the infant has recently undergone an operation or is otherwise stressed, a catabolic state exists, and the solute load will increase. Tissue destruction secondary to trauma or surgery increases the solute load even further.

WATER LOSS FROM THE GASTROINTESTINAL TRACT

In general, water loss from the stool need not be considered in calculating water requirements; such water loss amounts to an expenditure of only 5 to 10 ml/100 kcal. Infants who are receiving nothing through the GI tract will have smaller losses than infants who are being fed orally. Short-bowel syndrome or significant diarrhea increases the stool water loss; phototherapy doubles stool water content. Measurable water and electrolyte losses from the GI tract or other sites should be replaced.

SODIUM REQUIREMENTS

The sodium requirements of full-term infants average 2 mEq/kg/24 hr; preterm infants older than 32 weeks in gestational age require 3 mEq/kg/24 hr; and babies who are of low gestational age or who are critically ill require 4 to 5 mEq/kg/24 hr. Conditions such as intestinal obstruction [see Sidebar Intestinal Obstruction in the Newborn] and peritonitis increase sodium loss and therefore increase the sodium requirements.

Although full-term infants can retain sodium as well as adults do

in the face of a sodium deficit, they are unable to excrete excess sodium as effectively as adults. As a result, excessive infusion of intravenous sodium can rapidly result in hypernatremia. The problem is exaggerated in premature infants. Sodium excretion during the last half of gestation is significant but quickly drops off after birth in full-term infants. Premature neonates excrete large amounts of sodium to complete the normal intrauterine process of sodium excretion, but this ability appears to be fixed; premature infants are unable to respond to an excessive infusion of sodium by increasing sodium excretion, perhaps because of immaturity of the renal tubules or because of unresponsiveness of the renal tubules to aldosterone.

POTASSIUM REQUIREMENTS

Potassium requirements of infants are not well documented. The generally accepted requirements are 2 mEq/kg/24 hr after the first 2 to 3 days of life. The delay in administration has been recommended because of the concern about immature renal function in the first few days of life. In fact, however, potassium requirements are significant in the first few days of life, especially after a major operation, because in the catabolic state, protein breakdown leads to nitrogen loss in the urine and a concomitant potassium loss. Thus, potassium should be administered in the first 1 or 2 days of life after an operation once urine output is established.

Given all the considerations described, the initial fluid used for surgical management of the neonate and infant, both preoperatively and postoperatively, should be 5% or 10% dextrose in 0.2% saline at a dosage of approximately 100 to 150 ml/kg/24 hr [see Table 3].

ACID-BASE STATUS

Metabolic alkalosis caused by electrolyte loss, specifically chloride, may occur with prolonged gastric suction or vomiting and is usually easily corrected by replacement of the appropriate electrolytes (e.g., with potassium chloride). Metabolic acidosis, on the other hand, is usually the result of poor tissue perfusion and lactic acidosis. It is best corrected by treating the underlying cause of the poor perfusion and by temporarily administering buffers, such as sodium bicarbonate, which is usually done when the pH falls below 7.3. Standard sodium bicarbonate solutions are extremely hypertonic and should be diluted before being administered, especially in neonates. The dose can be calculated from the following formula:

$$\text{NaHCO}_3 \text{ dose (mmol)} = \frac{\text{base excess} \times \text{body weight (kg)}}{3}$$

Infection and Antibiotics

INFECTION IN NEONATES

Immediately after birth, bacterial colonization of the newborn begins.[52] This process begins with the skin and shortly thereafter involves the GI tract.[53,54] By 10 days of age, normal newborns have the common aerobic and anaerobic bacteria in their GI tract.[55] Neonates in ICUs undergo delayed colonization with a small number of pathogenic bacteria.[56,57] Normal barriers to invasive infection, especially the skin and GI tract, are underdeveloped in newborns.[58] The normal mucosal barrier to bacterial invasion in the neonatal ileum is defective,[59] which may explain the etiology of neonatal sepsis (see below) and possibly of necrotizing enterocolitis (NEC) as well. Postischemic reperfusion injury may give rise to NEC, in which case serum levels of several cytokines (e.g., tumor necrosis factor, interleukin-1 [IL-1], and IL-6) may rise. Enteral administration of nonabsorbable antibiotics and immunoglobulins may reduce the amount of bacterial translocation that occurs during NEC and may thereby lower the incidence of bacteremia and neonatal sepsis.[60]

Nor are normal host defense mechanisms completely developed at birth: full immunocompetence develops during the first few months of life. In premature infants, antibody levels are not high enough for adequate response to invasive sepsis. Normal full-term infants have adequate levels of IgG antibodies from their mothers, but lack of IgM antibodies, which include many opsonins, makes newborns susceptible to infection with gram-negative bacteria. Secretory IgA antibodies from the intestine do not reach effective levels until 3 weeks of age; they are passively acquired from colostrum in the first few days of life. Phagocytes in breast milk are another source of passive protection for the neonate.[61]

Usually, the first sign of a postoperative infection is fever, except in neonates, who rarely manifest temperature elevation. The usual sites of postoperative infection are the lungs, the surgical wound, the urinary tract, and I.V. catheter sites. The time of onset of postoperative wound infection is usually related to the pathogen involved. For example, wound infection within 48 hours after operation is usually caused by *Clostridium perfringens* or by β-hemolytic streptococcus.

Table 3 Daily Fluid Requirements for Neonates and Infants*

Weight	Volume
Premature < 1.5 kg	150 ml/kg
Neonates and infants 1.5–10 kg	100 ml/kg for first 10 kg
Infants and children 10–20 kg	1,000 ml + 50 ml/kg over 10 kg
Children > 20 kg	1,500 ml + 20 ml/kg over 20 kg

*Maintenance Na+ and K+ requirements range from 2 to 4 mEq/kg; solution can generally be given as 0.2% saline with 5% or 10% dextrose and K+ added.

Analgesic Dosage Guidelines in Children

Drug	Dosage	Comments
Mild Pain		
Acetaminophen	10–15 mg/kg p.o. q. 4 hr 15–20 mg/kg p.r. q. 4 hr	Wide margin of safety
Aspirin	10–15 mg/kg p.o.	For inflammatory disorders
Ibuprofen	3–10 mg/kg p.o. q. 6 hr	For inflammatory disorders
Moderate to Severe Pain*		
Codeine	0.5–1 mg/kg p.o. or I.M. q. 4 hr	
Morphine	0.06 mg/kg/hr continuous I.V. infusion (average effective rate) 0.02 mg/kg/hr (neonates) 0.07–0.1 mg/kg I.V. q. 2 hr 0.1–0.15 mg/kg I.M. q. 3–4 hr 0.2–0.6 mg/kg p.o. q. 4–6 hr	Slow-release preparations can be given two to three times a day
Methadone	0.1 mg/kg I.V. q. 4 hr, first 2 doses only, then 0.05 mg/kg I.V. q. 4–6 hr 0.1–0.2 mg/kg p.o. q. 6–12 hr	Careful titration is required
Fentanyl	0.5–1.5 µg/kg I.V. bolus for short procedures 1–2 µg/kg/hr I.V. continuous infusion	
Hydromorphone	1/5 – 1/4 the comparable morphine dose	
Meperidine	8–10 times the comparable morphine dose	

*Continue acetaminophen, ibuprofen, or other NSAIDs as above if the oral route is available and there is no contraindication.

Staphylococcus aureus wound infection usually occurs between postoperative days 3 and 5. Wound infection from gram-negative bacteria, usually of enteric origin, occurs after postoperative day 5. An infected wound should be opened, packed, and treated with dressing changes until the wound has closed on its own. Intravenous and urinary catheters and endotracheal tubes are common sources of infection in neonates. *S. epidermidis* is the most common cause of infection from indwelling vascular catheters[62]; this type of infection calls for removal of the catheter and treatment with parenteral vancomycin if initial treatment with I.V. vancomycin through the catheter for 7 to 10 days is unsuccessful.[63]

Neonatal Sepsis

Neonatal sepsis is a systemic bacterial infection occurring during the first month of life.[64] Bloodstream invasion is always present. Meningitis develops in about 25% of cases. When overwhelming sepsis intervenes, shock occurs, accompanied by oliguria and coma [see Shock, Treatment, *above*]. Mortality averages about 50%.

Diagnosis of neonatal sepsis is often difficult because the clinical findings are subtle and include such symptoms as lethargy, poor feeding, hypothermia, ileus, hyperglycemia, and respiratory distress. Lab-

Preparation of the Neonate with Emergency Surgical Problems

In many communities, the general surgeon is frequently called to aid in diagnosis and initial care of the neonate with an apparent surgical problem. After preliminary tests to establish a diagnosis along with stabilization of the infant, the baby may be transported to a pediatric center that is specially equipped and staffed to study and treat the specific surgical problem.

The steps in the stabilization of a critically ill neonate before transport are similar to the ABCs of initial care in the adult. By the time the surgeon is consulted, the neonatologist or pediatrician may have accomplished initial stabilization and begun to prepare the baby for transfer. The surgeon may be needed to establish vascular access; in some cases, a peripheral venous cannula may be appropriate, but more often, central catheters are inserted via the umbilical vein or arteries. In the case of babies with omphalocele or gastroschisis, the I.V. line should be placed in the upper extremities or the neck. Appropriate fluids should be provided to prevent dehydration and to restore any fluid and electrolyte deficits. When required, a nasogastric or esophageal pouch suction tube should be placed and decompression initiated. This maneuver is extremely important if transport by air is considered because trapped gases will change with alterations in barometric pressure, and such changes may have particularly deleterious effects on infants with intestinal gas or with pneumothorax or pneumomediastinum.

Vitamin K should be given as the natural K oxide, phytonadione, in a dose of 1 mg I.V. or I.M. (the dose for babies who weigh less than 1,500 g is 0.5 mg). Appropriate antibiotics should also be administered. Finally, the infant should be wrapped and placed in an incubator or radiant warmer to stabilize and maintain normal body temperature.

Sophisticated transport teams with appropriate equipment and supplies frequently participate in moving these babies between hospitals. However, early stabilization and communication with the primary physician and transport team is essential to minimize potential risks and morbidity associated with patient transfer.

Steps in the preparation of the neonate with emergency surgical problems for interhospital transfer are as follows:

Diaphragmatic hernia

Insert NG or OG tube. Ventilation by face mask is contraindicated; if ventilation is required, intubate. Paralyze or anesthetize infant to assist ventilation until operation.

Esophageal atresia

Insert tube to aspirate secretions from pouch (use Replogle tube, if available). If possible, avoid mechanical ventilation; if intubation is required, use high-frequency, low-pressure ventilation to prevent distention and possible perforation of the stomach.

Congenital lobar emphysema

Support normal oxygenation.

Intestinal obstruction

Use nasogastric or orogastric suction. Verify I.V. lines.

Omphalocele/gastroschisis

Use nasogastric or orogastric suction. Cover sac with a nonadherent gauze, and take care not to rupture membrane; cover intestine with saline-soaked gauze. Place I.V. line in upper extremity or neck. Maintain hydration by increasing fluid administration to account for fluid lost from exposed bowel. Support bowel with dressings. Maintain body temperature.

Exstrophy of the bladder

Cover exposed bladder with a nonadherent dressing.

Meningomyelocele

Cover sac with a nonadherent dressing.

---

oratory studies are not very helpful in establishing the diagnosis. In fact, the white cell count is usually normal or low. Very often, the platelet count drops with the onset of sepsis and returns toward normal once the sepsis is under control.[65] When neonatal sepsis is suspected, cultures of blood, cerebrospinal fluid, and urine must be obtained immediately. Broad-spectrum antibiotics, including a penicillin and an aminoglycoside, should be started before the culture results have returned; the antibiotics can be adjusted when culture results become available [see Table 2]. Group B streptococcus and Escherichia coli account for the majority of cases of neonatal sepsis.[66] Anaerobic bacteria rarely cause neonatal sepsis unless the etiology is perforation of the GI tract with peritonitis.

ANTIBIOTICS

In general, the indications for antibiotic use in neonates, infants, and children are the same as those in adults [see VI:12 Antibiotics]. Peritonitis of gastrointestinal origin, for example, is treated with triple antibiotic therapy that includes a penicillin, an aminoglycoside, and clindamycin.[67] Intravenous metronidazole is an appropriate substitute for clindamycin as a potent antianaerobic agent. Some surgeons prefer to administer a third-generation cephalosporin (e.g., moxalactam, cefotaxime, or cefoperazone) instead of triple antibiotic therapy, but patients treated with cephalosporins alone are at risk for sepsis from cephalosporin-resistant Pseudomonas aeruginosa and enterococci.[68,69]

For clean-contaminated elective surgical procedures, such as elective colon operation,[70] the commonly used prophylactic systemic antibiotic regimen in infants and children is either a penicillin with an aminoglycoside or a third-generation cephalosporin; I tend to prefer the latter. The first dose is given just before the operation so that an adequate tissue level is achieved during the procedure. The antibiotics are continued for 24 hours postoperatively.

The side effects of antibiotics in neonates, infants, and children are similar to those seen in adults, with certain important exceptions. Sulfonamide administration is associated with an increased incidence of kernicterus in neonates, and chloramphenicol is associated with the so-called gray syndrome (in which the baby looks gray from drug toxicity); these agents should not be administered to newborns. Tetracyclines cause staining and hypoplasia of the enamel of developing teeth and thus should not be administered to children.

Serum levels of certain antibiotics, especially gentamicin, must be measured to ensure that therapeutic levels are achieved and toxic levels avoided. Patients in a septic state require higher doses of gentamicin to achieve therapeutic levels because they tend to metabolize the agent more rapidly than nonseptic patients. In septic patients, serum levels must be monitored carefully. It is important to remember that the gentamicin dosage schedule in neonates is 7.5 mg/kg/day in two divided doses given every 12 hours, whereas in adults it is 5 mg/kg/ day every 8 hours.

Almost every antibiotic has been implicated in pseudomembranous enterocolitis,[71] which probably develops from the overgrowth of C. difficile after antibiotic suppression of the normal colonic bacteria [see VI:14 Nosocomial Infection].[72] The clinical picture of severe diarrhea is probably secondary to the C. difficile toxin. Treatment consists of oral administration of vancomycin and withdrawal of the antibiotics that caused the syndrome.

Ventilatory Support

Respiratory failure is manifested by either poor oxygenation (hypoxemia) or inadequate ventilation; occasionally, a combination of the two exists. Hypoxemia, or low arterial oxygen tension, is a result either of an alveolar ventilation-perfusion imbalance or of impaired diffusion through the alveolar wall to the pulmonary capillary. Inadequate ventilation results from hypoventilation and leads to elevated arterial CO_2 tension. The hypoventilation may be secondary to depression of the respiratory center; abnormalities of central or peripheral nerves, muscles, or skeleton; ventilation-perfusion mismatch; or excessive CO_2 production. In managing acute respiratory failure, it is important to distinguish between inadequate ventilation and inadequate oxygenation. Mild hypoxemia can usually be treated adequately by increasing the oxygen content of air inspired via nasal cannulas, masks, hoods, and incubators. In general, higher concentrations of oxygen can be produced with cannulas or masks in infants and children than in adults because of the smaller tidal volumes required.[73] Humidification of the gas is important to avoid drying of the nasal and pharyngeal mucosa by otherwise desiccant gases.

If increasing the fraction of inspired oxygen (F_IO_2) is unsuccessful, the transpulmonary distending pressure must be increased, initially with a nasal cannula or prongs. If this measure is unsuccessful, an endotracheal tube should be inserted [see Table 4]. If airway pressure with an endotracheal tube is still inadequate, mechanical ventilation must be started. In critically ill neonates (particularly premature infants), pressure-controlled ventilators are more commonly used than volume-controlled ventilators [see VII:4 Use of the Mechanical Ventilator]. When the ventilator is properly set, tidal volumes average about 8 ml/kg body weight.

The initial approach to mechanical ventilation in the pediatric patient should be intermittent mandatory ventilation (IMV)—that is, unassisted, unrestricted spontaneous respirations supplemented at regular intervals with mechanical breaths. The mechanical minute ventilation should be adjusted so that normal arterial CO_2 tension and pH are achieved. The adequacy of the mechanical ventilation is monitored by intermittent determination of arterial blood gases obtained from an intra-arterial cannula or from arterialized capillary blood. When an infant on a ventilator becomes clinically stable, weaning should be started by decreasing the fixed ventilator breath rate slowly while maintaining a normal arterial CO_2 tension and pH and simultaneously reducing the F_IO_2, the backup rate, and the peak inspiratory pressure. Once the F_IO_2 is down to 21%, the backup rate and the peak inspiratory pressure are further reduced until the baby can be taken off the ventilator.

Other means of elevating airway pressure include continuous positive airway pressure (CPAP), intermittent positive pressure breathing (IPPB), and continuous positive pressure ventilation (CPPV). The principles of mechanical ventilation are much the same in children and adults [see VII:4 Use of the Mechanical Ventilator]. With CPAP, the patient breathes spontaneously through a gas delivery system into which the fresh gas flow exceeds or equals the patient's peak inspiratory flow rate. A valve maintains system pressure by eliminating exiting gas flow when a predetermined threshold is reached during exhalation. An alternative to CPAP is positive end-expiratory pressure (PEEP), in which a reservoir furnishes inspired volume. The reservoir is placed between the patient and the compressed gas source delivering low flow. A valve between the reservoir and the pa-

tient prevents exhaled gases from flowing toward the reservoir and prevents rebreathing.

There are four different techniques for delivering CPPV. The first is controlled ventilation. When a patient is unable to generate any voluntary respiratory effort, because of respiratory center depression, spinal cord respiratory muscle dysfunction, or neuromuscular blockade, for example, the mechanical ventilator must deliver the entire minute ventilation. To avoid atelectasis and to improve gas exchange, PEEP can be added to the system. The second technique is patient-initiated ventilation: a spontaneous respiratory effort by the patient signals the ventilator to initiate a mechanical inspiration. The tidal volume is preset; however, the respiratory rate is determined by the patient's spontaneous efforts. The third technique is supplemental ventilation, in which unrestricted and unassisted spontaneous ventilation is augmented by a mechanical ventilator. The respiratory rate and tidal volume are preset so that a specific minute ventilation is achieved, which will diminish as the spontaneous breathing of the patient improves. The fourth technique is pressure-controlled ventilation, in which a preset expiratory pressure above the patient's own expiratory pressure is maintained during spontaneous respiration.

Because mechanical ventilation decreases venous return, thereby also decreasing cardiac output, and because conventional mechanical ventilation is associated with barotrauma, high-frequency ventilation is often used for neonates and infants.[74] This type of ventilation can be delivered either as positive pressure ventilation through an endotracheal tube or as jet ventilation through a catheter. At present, oscillation ventilation is increasingly being used in neonates to reduce barotrauma.

Mechanical ventilation is associated with a number of other complications as well. Pneumothorax, pneumomediastinum, and subcutaneous emphysema can occur when the inspiratory pressures are high.[75] In addition, the presence of an endotracheal tube in the tracheobronchial tree can result in pulmonary infection.[76] All patients on mechanical ventilators should thus receive antibiotics; the appropriate agent can be determined by culture of tracheal secretions. Moreover, the endotracheal tube can injure the subglottic area, especially in premature infants, and result in subglottic stenosis. Finally, high concentrations of oxygen can result in oxygen toxicity to the lungs and eyes, which can produce bronchopulmonary dysplasia and retrolental fibroplasia in neonates, especially in premature neonates.

Nutritional Support

Whereas the nutritional requirements of children and teenagers do not differ significantly from those of adults [see VII:9 Nutritional Support], the requirements of infants do. Sick infants in need of nutritional support pose therapeutic problems that are different from and frequently more complex than those of their adult counterparts. Not only must the metabolic demands that a major illness or operation imposes on all patients be taken into account, but additionally, special consideration must be given to the unique characteristics of pediatric patients, such as smaller body size, rapid growth, highly variable fluid requirements, and, in newborns, the immaturity of certain organ systems. These characteristics, coupled with low caloric reserves in premature infants and sick children, make adequate nutritional intake particularly important. Consequently, infants whose nutritional needs are not met as a result of a functional or organic disorder of the GI tract can rapidly acquire protein-calorie malnutrition. That a problem indeed exists is clear from one nutritional survey in a pediatric referral center, which demonstrated that one third of hospitalized pediatric patients show evidence of acute malnutrition.[77] Even a relatively short period of inadequate nutrition an lead to decreased host resistance, increased infection, and poor

Table 4 Tracheal Tube Size by Age

Age of Patient	Internal Diameter of Tube (mm)
Premature	2.5
0–3 mo	3.0
3–7 mo	3.5
7–15 mo	4.0
15–24 mo	4.5
2–10 yr	(16 + age) ÷ 4
10–19 yr	6.0–8.0 cuffed

wound healing, which contribute appreciably to morbidity and mortality in infants and children with surgical disease.

NUTRITIONAL REQUIREMENTS

An infant's body contains more water than an adult's body (70% to 75% versus 60% to 65%); therefore, infants require more water per unit of body weight. Healthy infants consume water at a daily rate of 10% to 15% of body weight, in contrast to a rate of only 2% to 4% in adults. They retain only 0.5% to 3% of their fluid intake: about 50% is excreted through the kidneys, 3% to 10% is lost through the GI tract, and 40% to 50% is insensible loss.

Infants also have much higher caloric requirements than older children and adults [see Table 5], and these requirements are further increased by periods of active growth and extreme physical activity.[78-80] Major illness or surgical trauma raises caloric requirements even further: there is a 12% increase for each 1° of fever above 37° C (98.6° F), a 20% to 30% increase with a major operation, a 40% to 50% increase with severe sepsis, and a 50% to 100% increase with long-term growth failure. In general, calories should be provided in the proportions found in a well-balanced diet—that is, 50% carbohydrate, 35% fat, and 15% protein. Carbohydrates contain 3.4 kcal/g, fat contains 9.0 kcal/g, and protein contains 4.0 kcal/g.

Most of an infant's caloric requirements are supplied by carbohydrates. Much less glycogen can be stored in an infant's liver than in an adult's, however; for this reason, fats are the other major nonprotein calorie source in infants. One of the fatty acids, linoleic acid, an 18-carbon chain with two double bonds, cannot be synthesized by the human body. It must be supplied in the diet and is therefore an essential fatty acid. A deficiency of this fatty acid results in a dry, flaky, erythematous skin rash. To prevent this deficiency, a total of 2% to 4% of required kilocalories must be in the form of linoleic acid.

Protein needs of infants are based on the combined requirements for maintenance and growth. Protein constitutes 13% of an infant's body weight, compared with 20% of an adult's. Most of the increase in body protein occurs during the first year of life, which explains why protein requirements are highest in infancy and decrease with age. Of the 20 amino acids that have been identified, eight are essential in adults, but it is thought that nine are essential in infants and 11 are essential in premature infants [see Table 6].

In general, infants require more vitamins and minerals than adults. Increased amounts of calcium and phosphorus are particularly important because of the rapid growth rate of the infant's skeleton.

METABOLIC RESPONSE TO SURGERY

Nutritional management of the surgical patient is complicated by the patient's metabolic response to the stress and trauma of the operation, which in turn affects nutritional requirements and management. This metabolic response to surgery was well described in adults by Francis D. Moore in 1959.[81] Although it was initially thought that infants did not respond to this type of stress in the same way that adults did,[82] later studies confirmed that the response of infants was indeed the same as that of adults.[83-86] Metabolic response to surgery can be divided into four phases: (1) the adrenergic-corticoid phase, (2) the corticoid withdrawal phase, (3) the spontaneous anabolic phase, and (4) the fat gain phase. The length of each phase is directly related to the severity of the trauma: phase 1 usually lasts 2 to 4 days and phase 2 usually lasts 2 to 3 days, whereas the duration of phases 3 and 4 is variable.

During phase 1, which begins on induction of anesthesia, serum and urine levels of glucocorticoids and mineralocorticoids increase. At the same time, there is a significant rise in catecholamine levels and in the secretion of antidiuretic hormone (ADH). The increase in ADH results in early water retention that usually lasts for 36 to 72

Table 5   Kilocalorie and Protein Requirements for Infants and Children

Age (yr)	Kilocalories* (kcal/kg)	Protein (g/kg)
0–1	90–120	2.0–3.5
1–7	75–90	2.0–2.5
7–12	60–75	2.0
12–18	30–60	1.5
18	25–30	1.0

*These numbers represent volume administered when solutions of 1 kcal/ml are used.

hours. The increased secretion of glucocorticoids and mineralocorticoids—especially aldosterone—along with the body's unique response to trauma and surgery leads to increased protein breakdown and elevation of the urinary nitrogen level. The potassium-to-nitrogen ratio in the urine, which is usually 3 mEq of potassium for every gram of nitrogen excreted, increases in the early postoperative period to 6 mEq of potassium per gram of nitrogen excreted.

Phase 2 usually begins on postoperative day 4. In this phase, the adrenal steroid output begins to return to normal, sodium excretion increases, and potassium and nitrogen excretion in the urine decreases. The antidiuretic effect is usually over, and a water diuresis ensues.

In phase 3, protein synthesis begins, and the nitrogen balance changes from negative to positive and thus begins the anabolic phase of recovery. During this time, any weight gain that occurs is usually caused by synthesis of new protein.

In phase 4, most of the increase in body weight is related to accumulation of fat. It is important to remember that infants, because of the rapid growth of their skeletons, have a more severe negative phosphorus balance than adults. A normal adult has a nutritional requirement of 150 nonprotein kcal for every gram of nitrogen administered. Stress and trauma probably increase this requirement, but the precise extent of the increase under these conditions is not known. Infants probably require 230 nonprotein kcal for every gram of nitrogen administered after a major operation.[87] Although the response in neonates is similar to that in adults, the duration of each phase is significantly shorter in neonates (e.g., phase 1 lasts only 48 to 72 hours), and the negative nitrogen balance may be minimal because protein synthesis is diverted away from growth to tissue repair.

NUTRITIONAL ASSESSMENT

In many cases, a sick infant's history and overall appearance provide sufficient grounds for initiating nutritional support. For example, a preterm infant with respiratory distress who is small for his or her gestational age will clearly require parenteral nutrition, as will a newborn with gastroschisis. Physical variables that should be considered in nutritional assessment include weight, length, head circumference, chest circumference, and triceps skin-fold thickness. There are no blood tests sufficiently sensitive to reflect changes in the patient's nu-

Table 6   Essential Amino Acids

Threonine	Lysine	Histidine*
Leucine	Methionine	Tyrosine†
Isoleucine	Phenylalanine	Cystine†
Valine	Tryptophan	

*Essential only in infancy.
†May be essential in premature infants.

tritional status accurately; the serum albumin level is probably the most useful test, and it is both economical and readily obtainable. A serum albumin concentration of 2.8 to 3.5 g/dl indicates moderate malnutrition, and a concentration of less than 2.8 g/dl suggests severe malnutrition (except in newborns, in whom levels are normally low). The serum transferrin level is actually a more sensitive index of nutritional status than the serum albumin level because transferrin has a half-life of only 9 days, whereas albumin has a half-life of 20 days.

ENTERAL FEEDING

The type of nutritional support to be employed depends on the disease affecting the patient and the patient's status. From a physiologic standpoint, enteral feedings are preferable and are the first choice for patients whose GI tract is functioning adequately.[88] Breast milk or a standard infant formula is used for oral or tube feeding of infants younger than 1 year[89] [see Table 7]. A liquid diet of either blenderized food or liquid formula may be used for feeding older children who are unable or unwilling to eat. A number of nutritionally complete liquid formulas are commercially available [see Table 8]. Specialized formulas are available for use in patients who have lactose intolerance or protein sensitivity or who suffer from renal or hepatic failure.

POSTOPERATIVE FEEDING

Infants have more difficulty feeding during the early months of life, especially premature infants, in whom the complex physiology of sucking and swallowing is not yet fully developed. In addition, the work of feeding accounts for most of an infant's caloric expenditure in the early months, and the stressed infant tires easily. For this reason, gavage or gastrostomy tube feedings are generally employed for the early stages of postoperative feeding in infants. Feedings are begun after the resolution of postoperative ileus has been demonstrated by the passage of meconium or stool. Further evidence that the bowel is beginning to function is the disappearance of the bilious green color of the gastric aspirate and the decrease in volume of the aspirate from the nasogastric or gastrostomy tube. The average volume of gastric aspirate in neonates with unobstructed intestines is 50 ml/24 hr. The return of bowel sounds, a helpful sign in older children, is not as sensitive or reliable in determining the resolution of ileus in infants.

Feedings of small volumes of sugar water are given by mouth or by gastrostomy tube. The initial feeding is 10 to 15 ml every 2 to 3 hours, which is increased by 2 to 5 ml increments over the next 12 to 24 hours until the infant is ingesting 30 to 45 ml of sugar water every 3 hours. Administration of half-strength formula is then started, and the infant is fed a similar volume every 3 hours during the next 12 to 24 hours. When the infant is able to tolerate this regimen, the diet is changed to the same amount of full-strength formula. At this point, the nurse or the mother feeds the infant whatever amount the infant will tolerate.

It is almost axiomatic that infants tolerate increases in volume much more readily than increases in osmolarity; it is generally best to use diluted formulas (three-quarters strength, half strength, or quarter strength) and to increase the volume as necessary to supply the calories needed. Inability to tolerate increased osmolarity is usually manifested by diarrhea. Inability to tolerate increased volume is usually evidenced by vomiting or increased residuals in the gastrostomy or nasogastric tube. If a gastrostomy tube is in place in an infant or child, it is usually elevated 8 to 12 in. above the abdominal wall for 12 to 24 hours after bowel function first returns, and the volume and bile content of the gastric reflux are observed; clear color and diminished volume of gastric juice are often the best indications that the patient is ready for oral feeding. The next step is to clamp the tube for 3 hours and then to drain for 1 hour. If there is no significant drainage during the 1-hour period, the infant or child is ready for feeding. If the infant or child has difficulty digesting a standard or lactose-free formula, one of the formulas containing predigested components should be tried. When selecting a predigested formula, one must make sure that the osmolarity of the formulation is not too high.

Elemental or chemically defined diets require a minimum of digestive work and are free of residual bulk [see Table 9]; however, they are unpalatable and thus are usually given by tube. Constant infusion with a pump is the preferred method of administration. Because of the high osmolarity of these diets, bolus feeding induces nausea, cramps, and diarrhea (the dumping syndrome). Accordingly, feedings are started with quarter-strength or half-strength formula and are increased first in volume and then in concentration during a period of 3 to 4 days. Once the patient is able to tolerate formula in sufficiently high concentration and volume to meet nutritional needs, I.V. fluids are no longer required. Patients on elemental diets should be monitored in the same way as those receiving total parenteral nutrition (TPN). When administered by continuous drip through a feeding tube, elemental and chemical diets furnish roughly the same amounts of calories and protein that TPN does, at considerably lower cost.[90] Unfortunately, they are not as well tolerated in infants and neonates as they are in older children and adults and consequently are only infrequently employed in treating these very young patients. Two available forms of the elemental diet, Vivonex and Criticare, are the ones most often used. The ease of gastrointestinal absorption and minimal residue make elemental diets extremely useful as an intermediate step between parenteral nutrition and regular feedings.

TOTAL PARENTERAL NUTRITION

TPN is a well-balanced system of intravenous feeding that was developed to meet the needs of nutritionally compromised patients

Table 7 Composition of Infant Formulas

Formula	Kilocalories		Na (mEq/L)	K (mEq/L)	Ca (mg/L)	P (mg/L)	Fe (mg/L)	Osmolarity (mOsm/L)
	(kcal/oz)	(kcal/ml)						
Breast milk	20	0.67	7	14	340	162	1.5	100
Cow's milk	20	0.67	25	35	1,240	950	1	270
Enfamil	20	0.67	11	19	546	462	trace	285
Nutramigen	20	0.67	14	17	630	473	13	460
Portagen	20	0.67	14	21	630	473	13	210
Pregestimil	20	0.67	14	17	630	473	13	311
ProSobee	20	0.67	18	19	788	525	13	250
Similac 20	20	0.67	11	19	580	430	trace	285
S-M-A	20	0.67	7	15	400	200	12	250

Table 8 Formulas for Routine Infant Feeding

	Mature Human Milk	Enfamil with Iron	Pregestimil	Ross Carbohydrate Free*	Nursoy	Enfamil Premature	Whole Cow Milk†	Peptamen Junior
Protein‡	1.1	1.4	1.9	1.8	2.1	2.0	3.6	3.0
Casein	40%	40%	—	—	—	40%	82%	—
Whey	60%	60%	—	—	—	60%	18%	—
Soy	—	—	—	100%	100%	—	—	100%
Hydrolyzed casein	—	—	100%	—	—	—	—	—
Osmolarity (mOsm/kg H₂O)	300	270	320	70	296	260	290	260
Fat‡	3.9	3.5	2.7	3.7	3.6	3.4	3.7	3.9
Long-chain triglycerides	100%	100%	60%	100%	100%	60%	100%	40%
Medium-chain triglycerides	—	—	40%	—	—	40%	—	60%
Carbohydrate‡	7.2	7.3	9.0	0	6.9	7.4	4.8	13.8
Type	Lactose	Lactose	Partially hydrolyzed starch		Sucrose	Lactose, glucose polymer	Lactose	Maltodextrin, starch
Minerals (selected) (mg/L)								
Sodium§	150	180	315	320	200	260	520	460
Potassium‖	550	720	730	950	700	690	1,480	1,320
Calcium	340	520	630	710	600	400	1,220	1,080
Phosphorus	140	350	415	510	420	550	960	800
Iron	0.5	12	12.5	12	12	12	0.6	14
Energy (kcal/30 ml)	20	20	20		20	20		30
Indication			Malabsorption, hypoallergenic also for short bowel syndrome and biliary atresia	Carbohydrate intolerance (carbohydrate added as tolerated)	Lactose intolerance	For premature, up to full-term birth weight		For child with impaired GI function; 1 to 6 yr of age
Similar formulas		Similac Gerber Carnation	Nutramigen¶ Portagen Alimentum	3232 A	Isomil ProSobee I-Soyalac	Similac Special Care		

*Not a complete formula as provided by the manufacturer and contains no carbohydrates. Carbohydrate can be reintroduced as dextrose, up to 7 g/dl, and slowly changed from dextrose to sucrose.

†For comparison only. Whole cow milk should not be fed to infants until they are at least 6 mo of age and have developed renal maturity.

‡Values stated are percentages of weight per volume.

§To determine mEq/L, divide by 23.

‖To determine mEq/L, divide by 39.1.

¶Lacks medium-chain triglycerides.

who can neither accept nor assimilate foods given enterally. Experience in a large number of institutions confirms the lifesaving potential of TPN in infants and children with inadequate GI tract function. In 1944, Helfrick and Abelson reported the first successful use of TPN in an infant.[91] During the next 20 years, however, efforts to duplicate this achievement met with failure, largely because the peripheral veins were unable to tolerate the infusates. The venous endothelium was damaged by the high osmolality of the glucose solutions, but the high osmolality was necessary to provide sufficient calories for anabolism of the administered amino acids. The alternative, administration of large volumes of a dilute solution of glucose, was equally unsuccessful: it created a different set of complications, mostly related to increased fluid volume (e.g., pulmonary edema, peripheral edema, and congestive heart failure). In an effort to bypass these two alternatives, fat emulsions were administered. At first, this approach also failed, but eventually, after the introduction of Intralipid (soybean oil) in 1962, it proved successful.[92] Fat emulsions have a substantial advantage over glucose solutions in that they have both high caloric density and isotonicity; this advantage allows them to be infused into peripheral veins.[93-95] The most significant breakthrough in TPN, however, occurred in the late 1960s, when Dudrick and associates introduced the concept of TPN based on the infusion of a hypertonic solution of glucose into a central vein.[96,97] In the early years after this group's initial success, this approach to TPN began to be widely used in newborns with GI anomalies.[98,99] Since then, the technique has come to be applied to care of all age groups, with dramatic results [see VII:9 Nutritional Support].

There are essentially two approaches to I.V. nutrition in infants and children[100]: (1) central infusion of hypertonic glucose–amino acid solutions and (2) peripheral infusion of moderately hypertonic solutions of glucose and amino acids, along with a fat emulsion. Each of these techniques induces nitrogen retention and weight gain. In difficult cases, both may be required for an extended period.[101]

Indications

TPN is generally reserved for infants and children threatened by catabolic or nutritional deficits because feeding via the GI tract is either hazardous, inadequate, or impossible. In some instances—for

Table 9 Elemental Diets

	Vivonex High Nitrogen, Vivonex Standard Diet	Criticare HN
Form	Powder	Fluid
Carbohydrate	Glucose and glucose oligosaccharides	Maltodextrin, cornstarch, citrate
Fat	Safflower oil	Safflower oil
Protein	Crystalline amino acids	Casein hydrolysate supplemented by L-amino acids
Essential amino acids (%)	36.25	30.4
Nonessential amino acids (%)	63.75	69.56

example, cases of chronic nonspecific diarrhea—providing TPN and placing the GI tract at rest for a time are sufficient for cure. In others—for example, cases of inflammatory bowel disease—restoration and maintenance of adequate nutrition permit subsequent corrective operative procedures.

Parenteral nutrition is used in the treatment of a wide range of common conditions, including intestinal obstruction caused by congenital disorders; postoperative adhesions; peritonitis; intestinal fistulas; chronic nonspecific diarrhea; necrotizing enterocolitis; short-bowel syndrome; extensive burns; and abdominal neoplasms treated by surgery, chemotherapy, and radiation. Besides being used for nutritional repletion of malnourished children, I.V. nutrition may also be employed as prophylaxis when prolonged starvation is expected, as in cases of gastroschisis. In infants, TPN is indicated if nutrition is inadequate for 4 or 5 days. Older children and adults may tolerate a longer period of inadequate nutrition depending on their nutritional status before operation or at the onset of illness. The benefits of improved nutrition in reducing mortality and morbidity must be weighed against the risks of serious complications secondary to I.V. nutrition (see below), especially sepsis. TPN should not be used when enteral nutrition is possible.

Composition of TPN Solutions

Central vein infusions When administered through a central vein, the basic parenteral nutrition solution contains 25% glucose and 3.5% amino acids [*see Table 10*]. Electrolytes, trace elements, and vitamins are added in the amounts appropriate to the infant's weight. The final solution provides 1 kcal/ml. Infusion of 100 to 120 ml/kg/day of this solution provides the glucose, amino acids, and other nutrients that normal infants need for tissue growth and repair; the volume is lower in older children because their requirements are lower. Iron requirements are met through either blood transfusions or daily addition of 2 mg of iron-dextran to the solution. Linoleic acid, an essential fatty acid, is provided through weekly infusion of a commercial fat emulsion in amounts equivalent to 2% to 4% of the patient's daily caloric requirement. Protein is supplied in amounts not exceeding 3.5 g/day. If fat is used as a nonprotein calorie source in the basic solution, it should account for no more than 50% of the daily calories. Furthermore, no more than 4 g/kg/day of fat should be infused into an infant and no more than 3 g/kg/day into an older child. Fat should be infused in small amounts (1 g/kg/day) initially and gradually raised to maximal levels during a period of 2 to 3 days.

Peripheral vein infusions When the basic parenteral nutrition solution is administered through a peripheral vein, it is made up of equal volumes of 4% amino acids and 20% glucose [*see Table 11*].

The final concentration of this solution is 2% amino acids and 10% glucose, which yields 0.48 kcal/ml. As with the central infusate, electrolytes, trace elements, and vitamins are added to the solution routinely. In neonates, 160 to 200 ml/kg/day is infused, providing 77 to 96 kcal/kg/day; in older children, the volume is reduced according to the caloric need. Unless contraindications are present, it is generally advantageous to use an I.V. fat emulsion as a major calorie source in the peripheral feeding regimen. As much as 4 g/kg/day of fat may be administered to infants and younger children; the nonlipid part of the solution is reduced by a corresponding caloric amount. This formula provides 102 to 121 kcal/kg/day, which is generally adequate for weight gain and growth. In older children, 3 g/kg/day of fat emulsion is given, with the glucose-protein solution supplying the remainder of the caloric needs. If a fat emulsion is not used, the infant's essential fatty acid requirements must be supplied by daily application of sunflower seed oil to the skin of the chest.

Whatever form of parenteral nutrition is used, one of the most important considerations is the ratio of nonprotein calories to grams of nitrogen, which should be somewhere between 150 and 300. This range is necessary to achieve the optimal utilization of the administered amino acids.

Administration

In central parenteral nutrition, hypertonic nutrient solutions are delivered through a central venous catheter to avoid peripheral venous inflammation and thrombosis. In infants, a venous cutdown is performed, and a pediatric silicone rubber (Broviac) catheter is passed through the external or internal jugular vein to the superior vena cava [*see Figure 2*]. This procedure is carried out in an operating room or, if necessary, a neonatal ICU, where adequate exposure, proper instruments, and intraoperative fluoroscopy are available and strict aseptic conditions can be maintained. The venous catheter is tunneled from the point of entry to the vein to a skin exit site 5 to 10

Table 10 Central Parenteral Nutrition in Infants*

Constituent	Amount (per kg/24 hr)
Glucose	15–30 g
Protein	2.0–4.0 g
Sodium	2.4 mEq
Potassium	2.4 mEq
Chloride	3–6 mEq
Magnesium	0.5–1.0 mEq
Calcium	0.5–3.0 mEq
Phosphate	0.5–1.0 mM
Trace elements†	0.1 ml (0.3 ml for neonates)
Multivitamin infusion (MVI)‡	1 vial (diluted to 3 ml)
Heparin	1.0 IU/ml
Glucose-protein volume	60–114 ml
Fat	1–4 g
10% fat emulsion volume	10–40 ml
Total volume	70–154 ml
Total kilocalories	70–154 kcal

*Each 1,000 ml of a standard solution is prepared by mixing 500 ml of 50% dextrose and water with 500 ml of 7% amino acids to give a final concentration of 25% dextrose and 3.5% amino acids. The appropriate amounts of electrolytes, vitamins, and trace elements are added according to the patient's weight.

†Each 0.1 ml of trace element solution (University of Michigan Pharmacy) contains zinc, 100 µg; copper, 20 µg; manganese, 10 µg; chromium, 0.2 µg; and selenium, 1.2 µg. Special neonatal trace element solution contains 300 µg of zinc in 0.3 ml and the same amounts of the other elements.

‡Each vial (diluted to 3 ml) of pediatric MVI (USV Pharmaceutical Corporation) contains vitamin A, 2,300 IU; vitamin D, 400 IU; ascorbic acid, 80 IU; thiamine (vitamin B_1), 1.2 mg; riboflavin (vitamin B_2), 1.4 mg; niacinamide, 17 mg; pyridoxine (vitamin B_6), 1 mg; dexpanthenol, 5 mg; vitamin E, 7 IU; folic acid, 140 µg; cyanocobalamin (vitamin B_{12}), 1 µg; phytonadione (vitamin K_1), 200 µg; and biotin, 20 µg.

Table 11 Peripheral Parenteral Nutrition with Fat in Infants*

Constituent	Amount (per kg/24 hr)
Glucose	15–20 g
Protein	2.0–4.0 g
Sodium	2–4 mEq
Potassium	2–4 mEq
Chloride	3–6 mEq
Magnesium	0.5–1.0 mEq
Calcium	0.5–3.0 mEq
Phosphate	0.5–1.0 mM
Trace elements [see Table 10]†	0.1 ml (0.3 ml for neonates)
Multivitamin infusion (MVI) [see Table 10]‡	1 vial (diluted to 3 ml)
Heparin	1.0 IU/ml
Glucose-protein volume	120–160 ml
Fat	4 g
10% fat emulsion volume	40 ml
Total volume	160–200 ml
Total kilocalories	102–121 kcal

*Each 1,000 ml of a standard solution is prepared by mixing 500 ml of 20% dextrose and water with 500 ml of 4% amino acids to give a final concentration of 10% dextrose and 2% amino acids. The appropriate amounts of electrolytes, vitamins, and trace elements are added according to the patient's weight.
†Each 0.5 ml of trace element solution (University of Michigan Pharmacy) contains zinc, 100 µg; copper, 20 µg; manganese, 10 µg; and chromium, 0.2 µg.
‡Each ml of MVI (USV Pharmaceutical Corporation) contains vitamin A, 2,000 IU; vitamin D, 200 IU; ascorbic acid, 100 IU; thiamine (vitamin B₁), 10 mg; riboflavin (vitamin B₂), 2 mg; niacinamide, 20 mg; pyridoxine (vitamin B₆), 3 mg; dexpanthenol, 5 mg; and vitamin E, 1 IU.

cm away, with the aim of minimizing the likelihood of bloodstream contamination from dressing changes at the skin exit site. The catheter is brought out on the chest wall, where it is easily accessible and not likely to be disrupted by an active patient. When no vein sites are available in the neck, the catheter may be placed in the external iliac vein via a cutdown on the greater saphenous vein and tunneled out on the abdominal wall.[102]

Central venous insertion by percutaneous subclavian vein puncture is often performed in older children and adults; the subclavian percutaneous technique has now been used in infants.[103] Every 48 hours, the dressing is changed aseptically, the skin is cleansed with an antiseptic, and povidone-iodine ointment is applied to the catheter skin junction to protect against bacterial and fungal infection. A millipore filter (0.22 µm) is placed in the line to remove particulate matter, such as calcium salts and microorganisms, that may have contaminated the solution. A calibrated burette is necessary for accurate monitoring of the volume delivered; it is used even when the solution is infused with a volumetric pump. To minimize the risk of infection, an alternate I.V. line should be utilized whenever possible for infusing drugs, measuring central venous pressure, sampling blood, and transfusing blood products. The infusate must be delivered at a uniform rate to ensure proper utilization of the glucose and amino acids. Currently, peripherally inserted central venous catheters (PICC lines) are increasingly being used to provide central venous parenteral nutrition to pediatric patients.

Peripheral parenteral nutrition with fat involves the insertion of a No. 21 or 23 needle into a peripheral vein (in infants, usually a scalp vein). The I.V. tubing from the bottle containing the glucose–amino acid solution is connected to the needle, and the tubing from the fat emulsion bottle is then inserted piggyback into the rubber nipple at the end of the tube from the first bottle. A calibrated burette is placed in each I.V. line, and the two bottles are infused for 24 hours with two separate constant-infusion pumps. Because the fat emulsion will not

pass through a millipore filter, the filter is inserted into the line containing the amino acid solution at a point proximal to that at which the fat solution enters the nipple. The injection site usually must be changed every 2 to 3 days because of infiltration, which is usually bland and nonphlebitic. The same technique is used for peripheral parenteral nutrition without fat; however, the injection sites must be changed more frequently because of the greater tonicity of the infusate.

Monitoring

Infants receiving TPN must be carefully monitored. Essential clinical measurements include body weight (assessed daily), body length (weekly), head circumference (weekly), and intake and output volumes. Urinary glucose and acetone levels are monitored, initially with each voiding and then, after the patient is stable, once each nursing shift. Blood tests must be employed judiciously and sparingly in infants and children because of their small total blood volume. At the start of therapy and once a week thereafter, a complete blood count should be done, blood urea nitrogen should be measured, and

Figure 2 Depicted is the preferred approach for central venous parenteral nutrition in infants.

serum levels of electrolytes, glucose, phosphorus, and albumin should be assessed. Serum levels of liver enzymes, bilirubin, and creatinine should be measured at the start of therapy and every 2 weeks thereafter [see Table 12].

Weight changes during TPN vary according to the patient's overall clinical status. During the first 2 weeks of therapy, significant weight gain is rarely seen in infants and children who are severely malnourished or in a septic state at the start of treatment; pathologic increases in metabolic demands, such as result from sepsis, produce a flatter growth curve. However, weight gains comparable to those seen in normal infants may be expected in patients who are not severely malnourished or in a septic state. The weight gains observed with the two I.V. nutrition techniques are comparable, averaging 15 to 25 g/day in the neonate and 0.5% of total body weight (kg)/day in older children. Greater weight gains may signal excessive fluid administration and fluid retention.

Urine output should be 1 ml/kg/hr or more, with the urine specific gravity falling between 1.005 and 1.015 in the absence of glucosuria. Positive nitrogen balance has been observed in almost all patients studied. Most pediatric patients tolerate the large amounts of I.V. glucose administered in TPN reasonably well and do not need exogenous insulin, which can be dangerous to neonates and infants. Blood glucose generally remains in the high-normal range, and urinary glucose is usually between 0 and 2+. As a rule, hyperglycemia and glucosuria can be counteracted by slowing the infusion rate or lowering the concentration of glucose temporarily, unless the patient is in a septic state. Although TPN usually induces greater excretion of solutes in the urine than oral feeding does, this increased load does not exceed the concentrating ability of normal kidneys. As a result, water balance is usually well maintained.[104,105]

Complications

Most of the complications associated with TPN can be classified into two categories: technical complications and metabolic complications. The technical complications are related to the placement of the central venous catheter and have been greatly reduced by careful attention to technique. Radiologic confirmation of catheter position has substantially lowered the incidence of cardiac arrhythmias caused by catheter irritation. The use of nonreactive silicone catheters in place of polyvinyl catheters has decreased the incidence of foreign-body reactions, vein perforation, and subclavian vein or vena caval thrombosis. Thrombosis of the superior vena cava is still a potential problem, however, especially in critically ill infants with sepsis and inadequate circulation. The thrombosis is usually well tolerated, but the superior vena cava syndrome can occur. Pulmonary embolism has been reported, but it is extremely rare.

The two most common complications related to the central venous catheter itself are thrombosis and infection. The incidence of catheter thrombosis can be decreased by periodic flushing with heparinized saline. If a clot does form, it can often be dislodged by means of vigorous flushing and the instillation of urokinase into the catheter. Catheter infection should initially be treated with I.V. infusion of an antibiotic (usually vancomycin because most such infections are caused by *S. epidermidis*) through the catheter. If this approach is unsuccessful, then the catheter must be removed. If *Candida* is the infecting organism, the first step in management should be removal, followed by 2 to 6 weeks of I.V. amphotericin B.

Almost all the technical complications inherent in central parenteral nutrition can be avoided by switching to peripheral parenteral nutrition, the major complications of which are phlebitis and superficial skin sloughing.

Almost every conceivable metabolic abnormality has been reported to occur during TPN [see Table 13]; the ones most frequently observed

Table 12 Blood Values Monitored Routinely during Total Parenteral Nutrition

Values Monitored at Start of Therapy and Weekly	Values Monitored at Start of Therapy and Every 2 Weeks	Values Monitored as Indicated
Na, K, Cl	AST	Copper
Urea	Lactic dehydrogenase	Zinc
Glucose	Alkaline phosphatase	Iron
Magnesium	Bilirubin (direct/total)	Ammonia
Calcium	Creatinine	Osmolarity
Phosphorus		pH
Albumin		
Hemoglobin		
Hematocrit		
White blood cell count		
Platelet count		

AST—aspartate aminotransferase

are hyperglycemia, hypoglycemia, hypocalcemia, hypercalcemia, hypophosphatemia, and hyperphosphatemia. As a rule, hyperglycemia is best treated by decreasing the I.V. glucose load rather than by administering insulin, especially in infants. Usually, metabolic complications can be prevented by careful attention to the nutrient content of the infusate. Now that trace element solutions are routinely administered at the beginning of therapy, deficiencies of copper and zinc are no longer seen. Likewise, routine administration of fat emulsions has eliminated the syndrome of fatty acid deficiency. Central infusion can lead to osmotic diuresis because of the high concentrations of glucose involved; premature infants, with their underdeveloped renal tubules, are most susceptible to this complication. Fluid overload in the form of pulmonary edema, peripheral edema, or congestive heart failure is rare, provided that patients are properly selected and monitored.[106] In patients with obstructed airways and compromised respiratory function, the large dextrose load provided by TPN can precipitate respiratory failure by increasing production of carbon dioxide, the elimination of which demands increased respiratory effort. If these patients are receiving ventilatory assistance, they may be difficult to wean. This complication may be resolved by decreasing the dextrose load and substituting fat calories for dextrose calories.[107]

Abnormalities in liver function, such as elevations in liver enzyme levels and serum bilirubin (both total and direct), often occur after 1 month of TPN, especially in neonates (premature neonates, in particular). These functional abnormalities result from cholestasis in the small bile ductules of the liver. If TPN is continued, the bilirubin levels, especially the direct fraction, will continue to rise, sometimes reaching 35 mg/dl (half of which is accounted for by the direct fraction). This process can result in cirrhosis and liver failure and ultimately in death. It appears that the cholestasis can be stopped and even reversed by increasing the enteral feedings, even in infants who are unable to tolerate large amounts of food given via the GI tract.[108]

Sepsis continues to be the major complication of central parenteral nutrition in infants and children. Long-term indwelling venous catheters are well-documented sources of bloodstream infection [see VI:14 Nosocomial Infection]. Organisms may enter the bloodstream along the catheter tract, via a contaminated I.V. solution, or may travel from a distant infected site and attach to the catheter, which serves as a foreign-body focus for bacterial growth. Placement of catheters under strict aseptic conditions, together with meticulous care of the catheter site with standardized dressing changes every other day, greatly reduces the incidence of septic complications.

Fever, leukocytosis, unexplained glucosuria, or any combination

Table 13   Potential Metabolic Complications
Resulting from TPN

Electrolyte imbalance	Hyper/hyponatremia Hyper/hypokalemia Hyper/hypochloremia Hyper/hypocalcemia Hyper/hypomagnesemia Hyper/hypophosphatemia
Complications related to carbohydrate administration	Hyper/hypoglycemia Hyperosmolarity and associated osmotic diuresis with dehydration, leading to non-ketotic hyperglycemic coma
Complications related to protein administration	Cholestatic jaundice Azotemia Hyperchloremic metabolic acidosis (with protein hydrolysate)
Complications related to lipid administration	Hyperlipidemia Alteration of pulmonary function Displacement of albumin-bonded bilirubin by plasma free fatty acid Overloading syndrome characterized by hyperlipidemia, fever, lethargy, liver damage, and coagulation disorders—reported in adults but rarely seen in children
Trace element deficiencies	Zinc Copper Chromium
Essential fatty acid deficiency	If lipids not used; manifested by skin rash

of these is often the first indication of catheter sepsis. Infection is confirmed by culturing microorganisms from blood obtained from the central vein through the venous line and from other venous sites. If no other site of sepsis is found, the catheter should be removed. In general, antibiotics should not be administered unless fever persists for longer than 24 hours after removal of the catheter or the patient exhibits a clinical septic response. Peripheral parenteral nutrition has the advantage of being free of most of the septic and technical complications inherent in central parenteral nutrition. In our study of 102 pediatric patients receiving peripheral parenteral nutrition, invasive sepsis was noted in none of the subjects being given fat and in only one of the infants and children not being given fat.

Complications of parenteral nutrition in infants and children are potentially numerous and frequent. Nevertheless, with careful patient selection, proper preparation of the solution, careful monitoring, and meticulous attention to technical details, the benefits of parenteral nutrition far outweigh the risks. Parenteral nutrition has been directly responsible for the survival of many infants and children who in the past would have died of malnutrition.

Special Problems

Infants with short-bowel syndrome pose an extremely difficult management problem. Great skill and patience are demanded of the surgeon, the pediatrician, the nutritionist, and the nurse. A full-term infant is born with approximately 200 cm of small intestine. Although the shortest intestinal length compatible with life has not been clearly defined, most pediatric surgeons agree that survival on oral alimentation is generally impossible when intestinal length is less than 25 to 30 cm with an intact ileocecal valve or less than 50 cm without an intact ileocecal valve. There are a few reports of infants surviving with shorter intestinal lengths, but they represent the exception rather than the rule.

Management of short-bowel syndrome is complex and not well defined. In most cases, treatment rests on a combination of parenteral nutrition, elemental diets, and predigested formulas. Regular feedings are gradually achieved during a period of several weeks to several months. Requirements for growth and development should be kept in mind at all times, and TPN with all of the necessary carbohydrate, fat, and protein calories should be provided continuously while various oral diets are being tried. The infant is gradually weaned from I.V. nutrition as the GI tract adapts to oral feedings. Because babies with short-bowel syndrome have very little tolerance for even moderately hypertonic diets, predigested formulas of high osmolarity must be administered in highly dilute form. The volume is increased gradually during a period of several days to weeks; only after sufficient volume is tolerated is the concentration slowly increased. As the infant grows, the intestine adapts by lengthening and by manifesting villous hypertrophy. It is not unusual for these infants to be hospitalized for several months to a year or even longer. During hospitalization, the infant's condition may improve or deteriorate markedly on several occasions, and it is very easy for parents and medical staff to become discouraged. Such discouragement is understandable, but it must be combated because it invariably results in decreased attention being paid to the critical details and imaginative approaches that are essential for the management of these patients. One of the most important elements of the treatment of infants with short-bowel syndrome is maintenance of high morale among the physicians, nutritionists, and nurses caring for them.

In some patients with short-bowel syndrome or inflammatory bowel disease, complete or partial parenteral nutrition may be required indefinitely. Such patients have benefited from programs designed to deliver parenteral nutrition at home. Although home parenteral nutrition has been used for several years in older children and adults [see VII:9 Nutritional Support], it has only now come to be successfully used in infants. The two main advantages of the program are (1) improved morale for the infant or child and the mother, as a result of placement in the home environment, and (2) significant reduction in cost, as a result of the patient's discharge from the hospital. It should be kept in mind, however, that considerable dedication on the part of the parents is necessary if complications are to be minimized.

Trauma

Whereas accidents are the third most common cause of death in the United States population as a whole, they are the single most common cause of death in children between 1 and 15 years of age.[109,110] Every year, about 20 million injuries occur in children, resulting in approximately 15,000 deaths and 100,000 cases of permanent disability. The consequences of permanent disability in this age group are obvious: these disabled children will place a burden on society for an additional 50 or 60 years after the accident. The first approach to be considered in managing pediatric trauma is clearly prevention; preventive efforts have in fact been gaining momentum, thanks in part to support from federal funds. These efforts have included greater emphasis on the use of pediatric restraint devices in automobiles, the wearing of crash helmets by bicycle and motorcycle riders, improvements in the design of space heaters, the use of fire-retardant material for children's clothes (as dictated by the Flammable Fabrics Act), the proper packing and labeling of poisons and medications, and the installation of proper fencing around swimming pools.

GENERAL PRINCIPLES OF CARE IN CHILDREN

Although the general principles of trauma care are essentially the same for children as for adults, there are several significant differences

Blunt Trauma in Children

Initial resuscitation of children suffering from blunt trauma is no different from that of their adult counterparts. It is important, however, to keep in mind that the vital signs of children are different: blood pressures are lower, and heart rates are higher.

If the child is hemodynamically stable, a nasogastric tube should be inserted early in the course of evaluation because of the high incidence of gastric dilatation after severe trauma in this age group. If severe head injury is present, physical examination of the abdomen is not very reliable. If auscultation of the lungs yields abnormal findings, an immediate portable chest x-ray is helpful for determining whether a pneumothorax is present before more complicated diagnostic studies are initiated. If hypotension is present, the first fluid to be infused should be lactated Ringer solution in a bolus of 20 ml/kg. Cervical spine x-rays should be obtained as well.

Once the child is hemodynamically stable and is receiving ventilatory support through an endotracheal tube, definitive evaluation of the intra-abdominal injuries can be performed. I prefer to assess such injuries with a total-body CT scan because I prefer to manage intra-abdominal solid visceral injuries nonoperatively. Nonoperative management of childhood liver and spleen injuries has been shown to be safe and effective in pediatric trauma centers throughout the world. CT scanning can accurately define injuries to the liver and spleen and precisely estimate the volume of fluid in the peritoneal cavity.

There arises the question of what to do if blood is detected in the peritoneal cavity. Given this finding in adults, most surgeons would proceed to laparotomy. In some cases, the bleeding may have stopped at the time of laparotomy. If the bleeding is restarted in an attempt to determine the extent of the injuries to the spleen, it may not be controllable with suture techniques. If a fractured spleen is discovered at the time of laparotomy, there should be a vigorous attempt to save the spleen with whatever technique is required. Sometimes, however, salvage is not possible, and a splenectomy must be carried out to control the bleeding. If the spleen had not been manipulated at the time of laparotomy, it probably would have

Patient presents with history of blunt trauma

Perform physical examination.

Provide initial care:
- Airway
- Resuscitation

Perform initial tests:
- Chest x-ray
- Cervical spine x-rays
- CT scan

Perform laparotomy

Criteria for operation:
- Hemodynamic instability
- Intestinal perforation

Observe patient (in facility with pediatric ICU)

Criteria for operation:
- Development of hemodynamic instability after stabilization
- Continued unexplained blood loss
- Development of peritonitis

healed on its own postoperatively. The risks of infection after splenectomy, especially in the child, are well known. They may be managed with administration of Pneumovax and the prophylactic use of oral penicillin.

It is not known how long it actually takes a fractured liver or spleen to heal. Usually, a CT scan at 3 months shows complete healing of these two organs. For that reason, I generally recommend abstinence from contact sports for 3 months after an injury.

---

that must be taken into account in the care of pediatric accident victims.[111-116] For example, children do not react to trauma in the same way as adults. They often have difficulty in expressing pain and in articulating their complaints. They are often extremely frightened after an accident, and this fear may cause them to give misleading signals—for instance, by exhibiting signs of an acute abdomen even though no intra-abdominal injury has occurred. Children who experience stress often undergo developmental regression, typically accompanied by severe depression. All these psychological factors must be taken into account in treatment of a pediatric accident victim.

Another key difference between children and adults is that children are still growing. Postoperative metabolic management after any form of stress, whether it is a surgical procedure, trauma, or some other event, must take this difference into account. A small blood loss that is insignificant in an adult can result in marked hemodynamic changes in a small child. Moreover, water and heat loss can be far greater in small children than in older children and adults because of their greater surface area relative to their weight and their relative lack of insulating subcutaneous fat. Hypothermia aggravates acidosis and makes hemodynamic resuscitation much more difficult. Gastric dilatation, which can result in vomiting and pulmonary aspiration, is very common in young children after all forms of trauma. Finally, the nutritional requirements of injured children are greater than those of adults because children, as growing organisms, naturally have a high metabolic rate. Consequently, TPN often must be started earlier in a child than it would be in an adult in a comparable condition.

Not only are there significant physiologic and psychological differences between children and adults after trauma, there are also differences in accident pattern. Most childhood injuries result from blunt

trauma [see Sidebar Blunt Trauma in Children], whereas in adults, blunt trauma is no more common than penetrating trauma.[117] More specifically, head trauma is far more common in children than in adults; in fact, it accounts for most of the morbidity and mortality in the pediatric population. After motor vehicle accidents, which are the major cause of trauma in both children and adults, the next most frequent causes of trauma in children are events that are less important causes in adults: falls, bicycle accidents, drownings, poisonings, and burns from fires. Child abuse and birth trauma are unique and important causes of trauma in children.

Pediatric accident victims must be treated in centers experienced in the care of traumatized children [see Table 14]. Such centers must have an emergency department with a section that is specifically set aside for the care of children and is staffed by nurses and physicians experienced in the management of pediatric trauma. They must have a hospital with a pediatric ICU that is also staffed with experienced medical and paramedical personnel. Finally, they must have a transportation system capable of rapidly transporting critically ill pediatric trauma victims both by air and by land or water.

EMERGENCY MANAGEMENT

As in emergency management of an adult, the first priority in emergency management of an injured child is to ensure and maintain an adequate airway. If the child has several injuries, the neck must be stabilized before assessment of the airway in case the cervical spine has been injured (although this type of injury rarely happens). Stabilization can be accomplished with a collar or with sandbags placed on either side of the neck. The airway must be cleared of regurgitated food, blood, or broken teeth. In some circumstances, it may be appropriate to try an oral airway; in general, however, it is best to proceed immediately to oral tracheal intubation [*see Table 4*]. While the necessary preparations are being made, the airway can be improved by pulling the chin forward, and oxygenation can be improved by administering oxygen through an oral or nasal cannula.

As a rule, uncuffed endotracheal tubes are used. The tube size can be estimated from the size of the child's fifth fingernail or from visual measurements [*see Table 4*]. It is rare that an emergency tracheostomy must be performed in a child in the ED, except when severe facial trauma is present, in which case it is preferable to insert a No. 14 plastic catheter through the cricothyroid membrane and then to proceed to the OR for a tracheostomy under controlled conditions if the patient is otherwise stable.[118] If respiration continues to be labored after an endotracheal tube has been placed, pneumothorax is a strong possibility. Unfortunately, pneumothorax is difficult to diagnose clinically in a young child because breath sounds are so easily transmitted; an immediate portable chest x-ray will help make the diagnosis. The first step in treatment of pneumothorax is the insertion of a plastic cannula into the chest. Later, under more elective conditions, a chest tube can be placed. Hyperventilation is a common response to stress in all age groups, especially in children, and it often results in rapid gastric dilatation, which can be managed easily with the insertion of a nasogastric tube.

Once respiration is under control, I.V. access must be established. Such access is often difficult to achieve when a needle is percutaneously placed into a peripheral vein in a child because the vein is small and becomes markedly vasoconstricted in the presence of hypovolemia. If a needle cannot be rapidly inserted into a peripheral vein, then a cutdown into the greater saphenous vein at the ankle should be performed. An alternative is to insert an interosseous needle into the tibia to begin fluid resuscitation.

Initially, superficial bleeding can be managed by simple pressure on the site of injury or laceration. Large scalp lacerations can lead to significant blood loss; therefore, it is important to place pressure on such lacerations early in the management of the traumatized child.

Almost all cases of shock in traumatized children following an accident are related to hemorrhage. Therefore, shock should be treated initially with relatively rapid infusion of 20 ml/kg of a crystalloid solution such as lactated Ringer solution or normal saline, to which should be added 2 mEq/kg of sodium bicarbonate to correct any acidosis that may be present. If shock continues, a second infusion of crystalloid should be given, followed by uncrossed O negative blood if there is no response. Once hemodynamic stability is established, a Foley catheter should be inserted, and insertion of a central venous line and an arterial catheter should be considered. A stable patient in whom operative intervention is not contemplated should be transferred to a pediatric ICU, where monitoring will be continued. In general, central venous pressure or, if a Swan-Ganz catheter has been inserted, PAWP should be maintained between 5 and 10 mm Hg.

ABDOMINAL TRAUMA

Abdominal trauma in children is usually blunt. Penetrating injuries occur in only about 20% of children who sustain trauma and are managed in essentially the same way in children as in adults [*see III Trauma and Thermal Injury*].

Children who sustain major trauma often suffer intra-abdominal injury. Because gastric dilatation and reflex ileus are far more common in children than in adults after a major injury, the initial clinical evaluation of the child's abdomen may be highly misleading. The early insertion of a nasogastric tube will decompress the stomach and allow more accurate physical examination of the abdomen. In addition, decompression of the stomach with a nasogastric tube will reduce the risk of aspiration pneumonitis. Once the child is stable

Table 14 Pediatric Trauma Score

	Coded Value
Size	
> 20 kg	+2
10–20 kg	+1
< 10 kg	−1
Airway	
Normal	+2
Maintainable	+1
Not maintainable	−1
Systolic Blood Pressure	
> 90 mm Hg	+2
50–90 mm Hg	+1
< 50 mm Hg	−1
In the absence of proper size BP cuff, assess BP by assigning these values:	
Pulse palpable at wrist	+2
Pulse palpable at groin	+1
Pulse not palpable	−1
Central Nervous System Status	
Awake	+2
Partially conscious or unconscious	+1
Comatose or decerebrate	−1
Open Wounds	
None	+2
Minor	+1
Major	−1
Skeletal Injury	
None	+2
Closed fracture	+1
Open/multiple fractures	−1
Score	−6 to +12
Scoring triage criterion for direct transport of the patient to a trauma center	< 9

from a hemodynamic and respiratory point of view, the abdomen should be carefully examined for external evidence of trauma, such as ecchymoses, abrasions, and tire tracks. The abdomen should then be carefully and gently palpated; the examiner should keep in mind that a frightened child will tend to tighten his or her rectus muscles in a way that gives a false impression of intra-abdominal injury. Serial abdominal examinations are essential.

Although peritoneal lavage is an acceptable diagnostic tool for the evaluation of a child with blunt abdominal trauma,[119-121] most pediatric surgeons now prefer to proceed directly to computed tomography of the abdomen, especially when the child has suffered from severe head injuries, which almost always require a CT scan for complete evaluation.[122] The CT scan is extremely accurate in the evaluation of liver and spleen injuries and in the determination of the amount of blood in the peritoneal cavity [*see Figures 3 and 4*]. The CT scan is also useful for detecting pneumoperitoneum resulting from perforation of the intestine.

Because hollow viscus injury is extremely uncommon in children after blunt abdominal trauma, nonoperative treatment is the accepted method of management for most liver and spleen injuries. Although associated fractures of the lower ribs are fairly common in adults with liver and spleen injuries, they are rare in children with such injuries.[123]

The initial plain film of the abdomen will often demonstrate medial and inferior displacement of the gastric bubble caused by an accumulation of blood under the left diaphragm. A CT scan will then accurately confirm the diagnosis of a splenic injury. CT scanning has the additional advantage of allowing postoperative follow-up of the healing of the splenic injury.[124,125] A major reason why nonoperative treatment is recommended for pediatric splenic injuries is that the risk of overwhelming postsplenectomy infection (OPSI) is far higher in children than in adults[126]; the younger the child, the higher the risk of OPSI. OPSI develops in 1.5% of splenectomized patients and carries a mortality of 25% to 50%.

The only type of liver trauma that necessitates surgery is that associated with injury to the hepatic veins or inferior vena cava.[127] Injury to these vascular structures is usually obvious: the patient will hemorrhage extensively into the peritoneal cavity or retroperitoneum and will be hemodynamically highly unstable, even after receiving massive transfusions.

Once a liver or spleen injury has been diagnosed, the child should immediately be transferred to a pediatric ICU staffed with experienced medical and paramedical personnel. The child should remain in the ICU for 2 or 3 days and on bed rest on the hospital ward for the rest of the week; however, some authorities currently advocate earlier discharge for patients with lesser splenic injuries. If hemodynamic instability persists despite significant transfusion of blood, exploratory laparotomy will be necessary.[128] Fortunately, this situation is extremely unusual; in fact, in our institution, we have never had to take a child to the OR for a liver or spleen injury after admission to the ICU.[129] If laparotomy is necessary, the liver and spleen should be repaired. Most liver lacerations can be simply debrided and drained, and most splenic lacerations, even lacerations through the hilum of the spleen, can be repaired with absorbable sutures.

Among the less common injuries to intra-abdominal organs that occur in children are perforation of the stomach when an accident has occurred shortly after eating and the stomach is distended; perforation of the small intestine and large intestine at points of fixation, such as the ligament of Treitz and the cecum; rupture of the left diaphragm; and damage to the duodenum and pancreas. Retroperitoneal perforation of the duodenum can result from blunt abdominal trauma; it is often suggested by the presence of air around the right kidney on a plain abdominal x-ray. Traumatic pancreatitis can be diagnosed by an elevation in serum amylase and lipase levels and by the presence of pancreatic edema on ultrasonography and CT scan. Obviously, perforations of the stomach, the intestine, and the duodenum call for exploratory laparotomy and, in most cases, simple suture repair of the laceration. Traumatic pancreatitis, on the other hand, can usually be managed nonoperatively with nasogastric decompression and I.V. fluids. Fracture of the pancreatic duct is usually secondary to compression of the pancreas against the vertebral column and is quite rare in children.[130] This injury necessitates exploratory laparotomy and distal pancreatectomy with suture closure of the proximal pancreatic duct; however, more recent experience indicates that it can often be successfully treated nonoperatively, though there is a risk that pseudocysts will subsequently develop. Intramural duodenal hematoma is relatively uncommon in children and is usually well managed by nasogastric decompression for about 10 days and institution of TPN.[131]

In the assessment of the child with abdominal trauma, the diagnosis of a pelvic fracture should be seriously considered. Pelvic fractures can result in significant bleeding into the retroperitoneum, in addition to injuries to the bladder and urethra.[132] The diagnosis can be confirmed by x-ray studies of the pelvis. In most cases, the fracture can be treated with bed rest, immobilization, and the replacement of blood loss.

Unless they have sustained head injuries, children with blunt multisystem injuries rarely die if they are alive when brought to an ED.

Figure 3 These three CT scans of children's livers were obtained after blunt abdominal trauma. In *a* and *b*, the areas of radiolucency in the right lobe of the liver (arrows) represent trauma to the liver. In *c*, note the crack at the level of the falciform ligament (arrow), with blood in the porta hepatis.

Figure 4 **This CT scan was obtained after blunt abdominal trauma in a child. Note several large cracks in the spleen (arrow).**

Care of these patients requires aggressive, coordinated efforts on the part of a multispecialty team under the direction of a pediatric surgeon. The evolution of specifically designated pediatric trauma centers around the country was one of the most important developments in the care of children to occur in the 1980s.

CHILD ABUSE

One of the unique varieties of pediatric trauma is child abuse or the battered-child syndrome. Although the exact incidence of child abuse is not known, it is thought that about 50,000 to 100,000 children are abused in the United States every year.[133] In most cases, the children come from a low socioeconomic background and their parents are very young.[112,114,134-136] The children tend to be younger than 2 years, except when sexual abuse is involved, in which case the average age is about 10 years. The abuse can take many different forms, such as physical or mental injury, nutritional or hygienic neglect, delayed or inadequate treatment of disease, sexual abuse, or verbal abuse. Clues to the diagnosis include a marked delay in seeking medical help on the part of the parents, poor hygiene in the child, and marked depression and lack of emotion in the child. The injuries most commonly seen are soft tissue injuries, burns, fractures, and head trauma. X-ray evidence of healing fractures of different ages, a finding described in 1946,[137] is strong evidence of child abuse. Visceral injuries, including liver fractures, splenic fractures, duodenal hematomas, and pancreatic fractures, also occur, although less frequently.

Once a physician suspects child abuse, he or she is both legally and ethically obliged to report the situation to the appropriate team in the hospital dealing with these problems. The typical hospital team usually includes a physician, a social worker, and a nurse. Prompt and full reporting often makes it more likely that the parents will receive positive counseling, which may well reduce their subsequent abuse of the child.

BIRTH TRAUMA

About 0.5% of all births result in trauma to the neonate; in general, larger infants are at greater risk.[138-140] However, routine use of prenatal ultrasonography has reduced the incidence of birth trauma because those infants ascertained to be at risk are now delivered by cesarean section. The injuries typically associated with birth trauma are fractures, nerve injuries, and visceral injuries to the liver, spleen, and adrenal glands.[141-143] Full-term infants are generally at greater risk than premature infants, and infants with preexisting anomalies, such as hydronephrotic kidneys, are at still greater risk.[144]

The fracture most commonly seen is that of the clavicle, usually caused by shoulder dystocia. Treatment is usually expectant because displacement is rare. Fractures in the humerus or the femur are less common and are often epiphyseal.

Peripheral facial nerve paralysis sometimes occurs, generally as a result of direct pressure against the infant's face from the mother's pelvis.[145] Complete recovery is usual by 1 year of age. Erb-Duchenne paralysis, or upper brachial plexus palsy, is usually secondary to shoulder dystocia or breech presentation. This injury results in lack of shoulder motion and winging of the scapula, with no evidence of motor or sensory dysfunction in the hand. The upper arm tends to be abducted, and the forearm cannot be supinated.[146] Klumpke's paralysis, or lower brachial plexus palsy, produces sensory deficits and an ipsilateral Horner's syndrome as a result of damage to the sympathetic fibers of the first thoracic root. In about 5% of cases of Erb-Duchenne paralysis, there is an associated phrenic nerve paralysis resulting in elevation of the ipsilateral diaphragm.

Hemoperitoneum can occur during birth as a result of fracture of the liver, the spleen, or the adrenal gland caused by direct pressure from the birth canal against the newborn's abdomen.[147,148] In these three instances, nonoperative management is appropriate. The baby should be stabilized with blood transfusions and observed. In almost all cases, the bleeding will stop, and no operative intervention will be required. Fracture of the kidneys is extremely rare but has been reported.

Direct birth trauma can disrupt some of the fibers of the sternocleidomastoid muscle, which leads to formation of a hematoma and eventually to a torticollis.[149] Passive and active exercises bring about complete recovery in most infants, although surgical correction is occasionally necessary if recognition of the condition is delayed for any reason.

Pharyngeal or cervical esophageal perforation can occur after a breech delivery, usually because the physician's finger was placed in the baby's mouth. This injury is usually well handled by placing a nasogastric tube, instituting I.V. antibiotics, and giving the baby nothing orally.

References

1. Coran AG: Perioperative care of the pediatric patient (pt 1). Surg Annu 23:31, 1991
2. Adams JM, Rudolph AJ: The use of indwelling radial artery catheters in neonates. Pediatrics 55:261, 1975
3. Barr PA, Sumners J, Wirtschafter D, et al: Percutaneous peripheral arterial cannulation in the neonate. Pediatrics 59(suppl 6):1058, 1977
4. Groff DB, Ahmed N: Subclavian vein catheterization in the infant. J Pediatr Surg 9:171, 1974
5. Hall D, Geefhuysen J: Percutaneous catheterization of the internal jugular vein in infants and children. J Pediatr Surg 12:719, 1977
6. James P: Central venous cannulation. J Pediatr Surg 13:107, 1977
7. Pollock MM, Reed TP, Holbrook PR, et al: Bedside pulmonary artery catheterization in pediatrics. J Pediatr 96:274, 1980
8. Todres ID, Crone RK, Rogers MC, et al: Swan-Ganz catheterization in the critically ill newborn. Crit Care Med 7:330, 1979
9. Wetxel RC, Rogers MC: Pediatric monitoring. Textbook of Critical Care. Shoemaker WC, Thompson WL, Holbrook PR, Eds. WB Saunders Co, Philadelphia, 1984, p 136
10. Wesley JR, Coran AG: Infants and children. Treatment of Shock: Principles and Practice, 2nd ed. Barrett J, Nyhus LM, Eds. Lea & Febiger, Philadelphia, 1986, p 211
11. Holcroft JW, Trunkey DD, Carpenter MA: Extravasation of albumin in tissues of normal and septic baboons and sheep. J Surg Res 26:341, 1979

12. Lillihei RC, Longerbeam JK, Boch JH, et al: The nature of irreversible shock: experimental and clinical observations. Ann Surg 160:682, 1964

13. Spink WW, Weil MH, Melby JC, et al: Clinical experience with corticoids in shock. Corticosteroids in the Treatment of Shock. Schumer W, Nyhus LM, Eds. University of Illinois Press, Urbana, 1970

14. Pierce CH, Briggs BT, Gutelius JR: Methylprednisolone and phenoxybenzamine in experimental cardiovascular dynamics and platelet function. Shock in Low Flow States. Forscher BK, Lillehei RC, Stubbs SS, Eds. Excerpta Medica, Amsterdam, 1972

15. Sambhi MP, Weil MH, Udhoji VN: Acute pharmacodynamic effects of glucocorticoids: cardiac output and related hemodynamic changes in normal subjects and patients in shock. Circulation 31:523, 1965

16. Thomas CS Jr, Brockman SK: The role of adrenal corticosteroid therapy in Escherichia coli endotoxin shock. Surg Gynecol Obstet 126:61, 1968

17. Hinshaw LB, Beller-Todd BK, Archer LT: Current management of the septic shock patient: experimental basis for treatment. Circ Shock 9:543, 1982

18. Schumer W: Steroids in the treatment of clinical septic shock. Ann Surg 184:333, 1976

19. Lucas CE, Ledgerwood AM: The cardiopulmonary response to massive doses of steroids in patients with septic shock. Arch Surg 119:537, 1984

20. Sprung CL, Caralis PV, Marcial EH, et al: The effects of high-dose corticosteroids in patients with septic shock: a prospective controlled study. N Engl J Med 311:1137, 1984

21. Connors RH, Coran AG, Drongowski RA, et al: Combined fluid and corticosteroid therapy in septic shock in puppies. World J Surg 7:661, 1983

22. Chatterjee K: Digitalis versus newer inotropic agents: which to use? Drug Ther 13:77, 1983

23. Goldberg LI: Cardiovascular and renal actions of dopamine: potential clinical applications. Pharmacol Rev 24:1, 1972

24. Goldberg LI: Dopamine—clinical uses of an endogenous catecholamine. N Engl J Med 291:707, 1974

25. Herbert P, Tinker J: Inotropic drugs in acute circulatory failure. Intensive Care Med 6:101, 1980

26. Latts JR, Goldberg LI: Dopamine in the management of shock. Drug Ther 4:25, 1979

27. Loeb HS, Winslow EBJ, Rahimtoola SH, et al: Acute hemodynamic effects of dopamine in patients in shock. Circulation 44:163, 1971

28. Rosenblum R, Tai AR, Lawson D: Dopamine in man: cardiorenal hemodynamics in normotensive patients with heart disease. J Pharmacol Exp Ther 183:256, 1972

29. Friis-Hansen B: The extracellular fluid volume in infants and children. Acta Paediatr 43:444, 1954

30. Friis-Hansen B: Changes in body water compartments during growth. Acta Paediatr [suppl] 207:1, 1957

31. Friis-Hansen B, Holiday M, Stapleton T, et al: Total body water in children. Pediatrics 7:321, 1951

32. Friis-Hansen B: Body water compartments in children: changes during growth and related changes in body composition. Pediatrics 28:169, 1961

33. Friis-Hansen B: Body composition during growth: in vivo measurements and biochemical data correlated to differential anatomical growth. Pediatrics 47:264, 1971

34. Friis-Hansen B: Water distribution in the foetus and newborn infant. Acta Paediatr Scand [Suppl] 305:7, 1983

35. Coran AG, Drongowski RA: Body fluid compartment changes following neonatal surgery. J Pediatr Surg 24:829, 1989

36. Bell EF, Warburton D, Stonestreet BS, et al: High-volume fluid intake predisposes premature infants to necrotising enterocolitis. Lancet 2:90, 1979

37. Stevenson JG: Fluid administration in the association of patent ductus arteriosus complicating respiratory distress syndrome. J Pediatr 90:257, 1977

38. Bell EF, Warburton D, Stonestreet BS, et al: Effect of fluid administration on the development of symptomatic patent ductus arteriosus and congestive heart failure in premature infants. N Engl J Med 302:598, 1980

39. Aperia A, Broberger O, Herin P, et al: Postnatal control of water and electrolyte homeostasis in pre-term and full-term infants. Acta Paediatr Scand [Suppl] 305:61, 1983

40. Aperia A, Broberger O, Thodenius K, et al: Renal control of sodium and fluid balance in newborn infants during intravenous maintenance therapy. Acta Paediatr Scand 64:725, 1975

41. Doyle LW, Sinclair JC: Insensible water loss in newborn infants. Clin Perinatol 9:453, 1982

42. Hammarlund K, Nilsson GE, Oberg PA, et al: Transepidermal water loss in newborn infants: I. Relation to ambient humidity and site of measurement and estimation of total transepidermal water loss. Acta Paediatr Scand 66:553, 1977

43. Baumgart S, Engle WD, Fox WW, et al: Radiant warmer power and body size as determinants of insensible water loss in the critically ill neonate. Pediatr Res 15:1495, 1981

44. Bell EF, Weinstein MR, Oh W: Heat balance in premature infants: comparative effects of convectively heated incubator and radiant warmer with and without plastic heat shield. J Pediatr 96:460, 1980

45. Engle WD, Baumgart S, Fox WW, et al: Effect of increased radiant warmer power output on state of hydration in the critically ill neonate. Crit Care Med 10:673, 1982

46. Oh W, Karecki H: Phototherapy and insensible water loss in the newborn infant. Am J Dis Child 124:230, 1972

47. Tan KI, Jacob E: Effect of phototherapy on neonatal fluid and electrolyte status. Acta Pediatr Hung 22:187, 1981

48. Bell EF, Neidich GA, Cashore WJ, et al: Combined effect of radiant warmer and phototherapy on insensible water loss in low-birth-weight infants. J Pediatr 94:810, 1979

49. Engel WD, Baumgart S, Schwartz JG, et al: Insensible water loss in the critically ill neonate: combined effect of radiant-warmer power and phototherapy. Am J Dis Child 135:516, 1981

50. Sosulski R, Polin RA, Baumgart S: Respiratory water loss and heat balance in intubated infants receiving humidified air. J Pediatr 103:307, 1983

51. Saigal S, Sinclair JC: Urine solute excretion in growing low-birth-weight infants. J Pediatr 90:934, 1977

52. Brook I, Barrett CT, Brinkman CR III, et al: Aerobic and anaerobic bacterial flora of the maternal cervix and newborn gastric fluid and conjunctiva: a prospective study. Pediatrics 63:451, 1979

53. Van Camp J, Drongowski RA, Gorman R, et al: Colonization of intestinal bacteria in the normal neonate: comparison between mouth and rectal swabs and small and large bowel specimens. Surg Forum 44:627, 1993

54. Van Camp J, Drongowski RA, Gorman R, et al: Colonization of intestinal bacteria in the normal neonate: comparison between mouth and rectal swabs and small and large bowel specimens. J Pediatr Surg 29:1366, 1994

55. Long SS, Swenson RM: Development of anaerobic fecal flora in healthy newborn infants. J Pediatr 91:298, 1977

56. Goldman DA, Leclair J, Macone A: Bacterial colonization of neonates admitted to an intensive care environment. J Pediatr 93:288, 1978

57. Lawrence G, Bates J, Gaul A: Pathogenesis of neonatal necrotising enterocolitis. Lancet 1:137, 1982

58. Van Camp J, Tomaselli V, Coran AG: Intestinal bacterial translocation in the newborn. Curr Opin Pediatr 6:327, 1994

59. Walker WA: Gastrointestinal host defense: importance of gut closure in control of macromolecular transport. Ciba Found Symp 70:201, 1979

60. Lelli JL Jr, Drongowski RA, Coran AG, et al: Hypoxia-induced bacterial translocation in the puppy. J Pediatr Surg 27:974, 1992

61. Barlow B, Santulli TV, Heird WC, et al: An experimental study of acute neonatal enterocolitis—the importance of breast milk. J Pediatr Surg 9:587, 1974

62. Noel GJ, Edelson PJ: Staphylococcus epidermidis bacteremia in neonates: further observations and the occurrence of focal infection. Pediatrics 74:832, 1984

63. Scherer LR, West KW, Weber TR, et al: Staphylococcus epidermidis sepsis in pediatric patients: clinical and therapeutic considerations. J Pediatr Surg 19:358, 1984

64. Siegel JD, McCracken GH: Sepsis neonatorum. N Engl J Med 304:642, 1981

65. Rowe MI, Buckner DM, Newmark S: The early diagnosis of gram-negative septicemia in the pediatric surgical patient. Ann Surg 182:280, 1975

66. Freedman RM, Ingram DL, Gross I, et al: A half century of neonatal sepsis at Yale: 1928–1978. Am J Dis Child 135:140, 1981

67. Bell MJ, Ternberg JL, Bower RJ: The microbial flora and antimicrobial therapy of neonatal peritonitis. J Pediatr Surg 15:569, 1980

68. Stone HH, Strom PR, Fabian TC, et al: Third-generation cephalosporins for polymicrobial surgical sepsis. Arch Surg 118:193, 1983

69. Fry DE: Third generation cephalosporin antibiotics in surgical practice. Am J Surg 151:306, 1986

70. Burke JF: The effective period of preventive antibiotic action in experimental incisions and dermal lesions. Surgery 50:161, 1961

71. Rifkin GD, Fekety RF, Silva J Jr, et al: Antibiotic-induced colitis: implication of a toxin neutralised by Clostridium sordellii antitoxin. Lancet 2:1103, 1977

72. Bartlett JG, Chang TW, Gurwith M, et al: Antibiotic-associated pseudomembranous colitis due to toxin-producing clostridia. N Engl J Med 298:531, 1978

73. Shapiro BA, Harrison RA, Trout CA: Clinical Application of Respiratory Care, 2nd ed. Year Book Medical Publishers, Chicago, 1979, p 139

74. Sjostrand U, Borg U, Eriksson I: Minor circulatory interference and improved alveolar gas distribution during continuous positive-pressure ventilation by means of high ventilatory frequency and ventilatory system of negligible compression volume (abstr). Excerpta Medica International Congress Series 452: 516, 1978

75. Kirby RR, Downs JB, Civetta JM, et al: High level positive end expiratory pressure (PEEP) in acute respiratory insufficiency. Chest 67:156, 1975

76. Holzman BH, Scott GB: Control of infection and techniques of isolation in the pediatric intensive care unit. Pediatr Clin North Am 28:703, 1981

77. Merrit RJ, Suskind RM: Nutritional survey of hospitalized pediatric patients. Am J Clin Nutr 32:1320, 1979

78. Dechert R, Wesley J, Schafer L, et al: Comparison of oxygen consumption, carbon dioxide production, and resting energy expenditure in premature and full-term infants. J Pediatr Surg 20:792, 1985

79. Dechert RE, Wesley J, Schafer LE, et al: A water-sealed indirect calorimeter for measurement of oxygen consumption (VO_2), carbon dioxide production (VCO_2), and energy expenditure in infants. JPEN J Parenter Enteral Nutr 12:256, 1988

80. Mendeloff E, Wesley JR, Dechert RE, et al: Comparison of measured resting energy expenditure (REE) versus estimated energy expenditure (EEE) in infants. JPEN J Parenter Enteral Nutr (in press)

81. Moore FD: Metabolic Care of the Surgical Patient. WB Saunders Co, Philadelphia, 1959

82. Rickham PP: The Metabolic Response to Neonatal Surgery. Harvard University Press, Cambridge, Mass, 1957

83. Knutrud O: The water and electrolyte metabolism in the newborn child after major surgery: with special reference to the potassium, phosphorus and magne-

sium metabolism. Norwegian Monographs on Medical Science, Oslo, 1965

84. Schmeling DJ, Coran AG: The hormonal and metabolic response to stress in the neonate. Pediatr Surg Int 5:307, 1990

85. Schmeling DJ, Coran AG: Hormonal and metabolic response to operative stress in the neonate. JPEN J Parenter Enteral Nutr 15:215, 1991

86. Coran AG, Pierro A, Schmeling DJ: Metabolism of the neonate requiring surgery. Principles of Perinatal and Neonatal Metabolism. Cowett RM, Ed. Springer-Verlag, New York, 1996, p 1131

87. Benner JW, Coran AG, Weintraub WH, et al: The importance of different calorie sources in the intravenous nutrition of infants and children. Surgery 86:429, 1979

88. Heymsfield SB, Bethel RA, Ansley JO, et al: Enteral hyperalimentation: an alternative to central venous hyperalimentation. Ann Intern Med 90:63, 1979

89. Johnson LR, Copeland EM, Dudrick SJ, et al: Structural and hormonal alterations in the gastrointestinal tract of parenterally fed rats. Gastroenterology 68:1177, 1975

90. Stephens RV, Randall HT: Use of the concentrated, balanced, liquid elemental diet for nutritional management of catabolic states. Ann Surg 170:642, 1969

91. Helfrick FW, Abelson NM: Intravenous feeding of a complete diet in a child: report of a case. J Pediatr 25:400, 1944

92. Lee HA: Parenteral Nutrition in Acute Metabolic Illness. Academic Press, Inc, San Diego, 1974, p 3

93. Coran AG: The long-term intravenous feeding of infants using peripheral veins. J Pediatr Surg 8:801, 1973

94. Coran AG: Total intravenous feeding of infants and children without the use of a central venous catheter. Ann Surg 179:445, 1974

95. Coran AG: Lipids. Intravenous Feeding of the Neonate. Yu VYH, MacMahon RA, Eds. Edward Arnold, Melbourne, 1992, p 50

96. Dudrick SJ, Wilmore DW, Vars HM, et al: Long-term total parenteral nutrition with growth, development, and positive nitrogen balance. Surgery 64:134, 1968

97. Dudrick SJ, Wilmore DW, Vars HM, et al: Can intravenous feeding as the sole means of nutrition support growth in the child and restore weight loss in an adult: an affirmative answer. Ann Surg 169:974, 1969

98. Filler RM, Eraklis AJ, Rubin VG, et al: Long-term parenteral nutrition in infants. N Engl J Med 281:589, 1969

99. Heird WC, Winters RW: Total parenteral nutrition: the state of the art. J Pediatr 86:2, 1975

100. Wesley JR, Coran AG: Intravenous nutrition for the pediatric patient. Semin Pediatr Surg 1:212, 1992

101. Coran AG, Drongowski RA: Studies on the toxicity and efficacy of a new amino acid solution in pediatric parenteral nutrition. JPEN J Parenter Enteral Nutr 11:368, 1987

102. Fonkalsrud EW, Berquist W, Burke M, et al: Long-term hyperalimentation in children through saphenous central venous catheterization. Am J Surg 143:209, 1982

103. Filston HC, Izant R Jr: The Surgical Neonate: Evaluation and Care. Appleton-Century-Crofts, East Norwalk, Connecticut, 1978, p 56

104. Polley TZ, Benner JW, Rhodin A, et al: Changes in total body water in infants receiving total intravenous nutrition. J Surg Res 26:555, 1979

105. Rhodin AGJ, Coran AG, Weintraub WH, et al: Total body water changes during high volume peripheral hyperalimentation. Surg Gynecol Obstet 148:196, 1979

106. Coran AG, Weintraub WH: Peripheral intravenous nutrition without fat in neonatal surgery. J Pediatr Surg 12:195, 1977

107. Askanazi J, Rosenbaum SH, Hyman AI, et al: Respiratory changes induced by the large glucose loads of total parenteral nutrition. JAMA 243:1444, 1980

108. Drongowski RA, Coran AG: An analysis of factors contributing to the development of total parenteral nutrition-induced cholestasis. JPEN J Parenter Enteral Nutr 13:586, 1989

109. Accident Facts. National Safety Council, Chicago, 1979

110. Accident Facts. National Safety Council, Chicago, 1982

111. Coran AG: Pediatric trauma. Pediatr Surg Int 5:301, 1990

112. Coran AG: Update: pediatric trauma. Compr Ther 17(10):16, 1991

113. Coran AG: Thoracic trauma. Pediatric Emergency Medicine. Reisdorff EJ, Roberts MR, Wiegenstein JG, Eds. WB Saunders Co, Philadelphia, 1992, p 881

114. Coran AG: Abdominal trauma. Pediatric Emergency Medicine. Reisdorff EJ, Roberts MR, Wiegenstein JG, Eds. WB Saunders Co, Philadelphia, 1992, p 886

115. Coran AG, Wesley JR: Shock in pediatric trauma. Pediatric Trauma: Proceedings of the Third National Conference. Coran AG, Harris BH, Eds. JB Lippincott Co, Philadelphia, 1990, p 29

116. Polley TZ Jr, Coran AG: Special problems in management of pediatric trauma. Crit Care Clin 2:775, 1986

117. Mayer T, Walker ML, Johnson DG, et al: Causes of morbidity and mortality in severe pediatric trauma. JAMA 245:719, 1981

118. O'Neill JA: Special pediatric emergencies. Emergency Care. Boswick JA, Ed. WB Saunders Co, Philadelphia, 1981, p 137

119. Drew R, Perry JF Jr, Fischer RP: The expediency of peritoneal lavage for blunt trauma in children. Surg Gynecol Obstet 145:885, 1977

120. DuPriest RW Jr, Rodriguez A, Shatney CH: Peritoneal lavage in children and adolescents with blunt abdominal trauma. Am Surg 48:460, 1982

121. Powell RW, Smith DE, Zarins CK, et al: Peritoneal lavage in children with blunt abdominal trauma. J Pediatr Surg 11:973, 1976

122. Karp MP, Cooney DR, Berger PE, et al: The role of computed tomography in the evaluation of blunt abdominal trauma in children. J Pediatr Surg 16:316, 1981

123. Eichelberger MR, Randolph JG: Thoracic trauma in children. Surg Clin North Am 61:1181, 1981

124. Cooney DR: Splenic and hepatic trauma in children. Surg Clin North Am 61:1165, 1981

125. Adler DD, Blane CE, Coran AG, et al: Splenic trauma in the pediatric patient: the integrated roles of ultrasound and computed tomography. Pediatrics 78:576, 1986

126. Francke EL, Neu HC: Postsplenectomy infection. Surg Clin North Am 61:135, 1981

127. Karp MP, Cooney DR, Pros GA, et al: The nonoperative management of pediatric hepatic trauma. J Pediatr Surg 18:512, 1983

128. Ein SH, Shandling B, Simpson JS, et al: Nonoperative management of traumatized spleen in children: how and why. J Pediatr Surg 13:117, 1978

129. Delius R, Frankel W, Coran AG: A comparison between operative and nonoperative management of blunt injuries to the liver and spleen in adult and pediatric patients. Surgery 106:788, 1989

130. Eichelberger MR, Hoelzer DJ, Koop CE: Acute pancreatitis: the difficulties of diagnosis and therapy. J Pediatr Surg 17:244, 1982

131. Touloukian RJ: Protocol for the nonoperative treatment of obstructing intramural duodenal hematoma during childhood. Am J Surg 145:330, 1983

132. Reichard SA, Helikson MA, Sorter N, et al: Pelvic fractures in children—review of 120 patients with a

new look at general management. J Pediatr Surg 15:727, 1980

133. O'Neill JA, Rowe MI, Grosfeld JL, et al: Pediatric Surgery, 5th ed. CV Mosby, St. Louis, 1996, p 235

134. Holter JC, Friedman SB: Child abuse: early case finding in the emergency department. Pediatrics 42:128, 1968

135. O'Neill JA Jr, Meacham WF, Griffin JP, et al: Patterns of injury in the battered child syndrome. J Trauma 13:332, 1973

136. Rosenberg NM, Myers S, Shackleton N: Prediction of child abuse in an ambulatory setting. Pediatrics 70:879, 1982

137. Caffey J: Multiple fractures in the long bones of infants suffering from chronic subdural hematoma. AJR 56:163, 1946

138. Bauer O, Weidenback A, Thieme R: Die Knochernen Geburtsverletzungen des Neugeborenen. Münchener Medizinische Wochenschrift 109:998, 1967

139. Bianco AJ, Schlein AP, Kruss RL, et al: Birth fractures. Minn Med 55:471, 1972

140. Cohen AW, Otto SR: Obstetric clavicular fractures: a three-year analysis. J Reprod Med 25:119, 1980

141. Gordon M, Rich H, Deutschberger J, et al: The immediate and long-term outcome of obstetric birth trauma. Am J Obstet Gynecol 117:51, 1973

142. Abramson AH: Resuscitation of the Newborn Infant and Related Emergency Procedures in the Perinatal Center Special Care Nursery. CV Mosby Co, St Louis, 1973

143. Schwartz O, Cohn BD: Rupture of the normal spleen in the newborn, with survival. Surgery 59:1124, 1966

144. Tank ES, Davis R, Holt JF, et al: Mechanisms of trauma during breech delivery. Obstet Gynecol 38:761, 1971

145. Garza-Mercado R: Intrauterine depressed skull fractures of the newborn. Neurosurgery 10:694, 1982

146. Valman HB: Birth trauma. Br Med J 2:1566, 1979

147. Goodman JM: Liver trauma in the newborn: a case report. J Trauma 14:427, 1974

148. Monson DO, Raffensperger JG: Intraperitoneal hemorrhage secondary to liver laceration in a newborn. J Pediatr Surg 2:464, 1967

149. Sanerkin NG, Edwards P: Birth injury to the sternomastoid muscle. J Bone Joint Surg [Br] 48B:441, 1966

150. Manning PB, Morgan RA, Coran AG, et al: Fifty years' experience with esophageal atresia and tracheoesophageal fistula: beginning with Cameron Haight's first operation in 1935. Ann Surg 204:446, 1986

151. Bartlett RH, Gazzaniga AB, Toomasian J, et al: Extracorporeal membrane oxygenation (ECMO) in neonatal respiratory failure: 100 cases. Ann Surg 204:236, 1986

152. Stiemle CN, Meric F, Hirschl RB, et al: The effect of extracorporeal life support (ECLS) on survival when applied to all patients with congenital diaphragmatic hernia (CDH). J Pediatr Surg 29:997, 1994

153. Reickert CA, Hirschl RB, Schumacher R, et al: The effect of very delayed repair of congenital diaphragmatic hernia on survival and ECLS use. Surgery 120:766, 1996

154. Wesley JR, Heidelberger KP, DiPietro MA, et al: Diagnosis and management of congenital cystic disease of the lung in children. J Pediatr Surg 21:202, 1988

155. Coran AG: Congenital cystic disease of the tracheobronchial tree in infants and children: experience with 44 consecutive cases. Arch Surg 129:521, 1994

Acknowledgment

Figure 2 Carol Donner.

David C. Brooks, M.D., and Cherie P. Parungo, M.D.

Approach to Abdominal Pain in Pregnant Patients

Since the early 1990s, the number of live births in the United States has ranged from 3.88 to 4.12 million per year.[1] Complications related to nonobstetric surgery are relatively uncommon, occurring in only 1% to 2% of pregnancies.[2] Management of the pregnant patient differs from that of other patients in several ways. First, pregnancy induces a variety of mechanical, hormonal, and chemical alterations that may confuse and mislead even the most experienced surgeon [*see* Discussion, Physiologic Changes in Pregnant Patients, *below*]. Second, a surgeon's natural inclination, when faced with a pregnant patient experiencing abdominal pain, is to temporize. This tendency, which generally arises from the misconception that surgical intervention may injure the fetus, is responsible for delays in diagnosis and ultimately for the unfavorable outcomes often associated with acute abdominal pathology in pregnant patients. Third, pregnant patients require a multidisciplinary approach to care that involves the surgeon, the obstetrician, the radiologist, and the anesthesiologist. Finally, and most important, a surgeon treating a pregnant woman is actually caring for two patients and has the same responsibility to both.

In what follows, we first review urgent surgical problems in the pregnant patient, then discuss the physiologic changes of pregnancy and how these changes help shape general surgical principles in this population. Finally, we address certain nonurgent surgical problems associated with pregnancy.

Initial Management

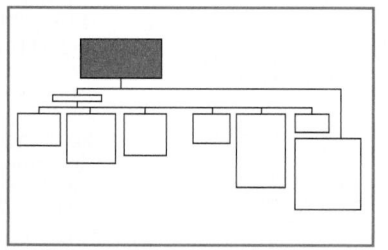

Initial management of any pregnant patient presenting with an acute abdomen or an acute surgical problem should include a thorough history and physical examination [*see II:4 Acute Abdominal Pain*], with particular consideration given to historical aspects of the pregnancy, the expected date of delivery, and the presence of any pregnancy-related complications. Whenever possible, an obstetrician should be consulted and included in the decision-making process. Initial maneuvers should include administration of supplemental oxygen, placement of an I.V. line with the capacity to deliver ample amounts of fluid or blood, insertion of a nasogastric tube if significant vomiting is present, and performance of routine laboratory evaluations, such as a complete blood count, assessment of serum electrolyte levels, and urinalysis. If the pregnancy has passed the 26th week, a fetal monitor should be employed. Radiographic investigations should be kept to a minimum, although abdominal and pelvic ultrasonography may be especially useful not only in assessing the maternal pathology but also in evaluating the fetus.

Acute abdominal surgical problems must be dealt with immediately. Management of less acute problems, however, must take into account the stage of the pregnancy. The risk of spontaneous abortion at operation is highest during the first trimester. The optimal time for elective surgery is during the second trimester because the uterus is smaller at that time than it is in the third trimester and because the fetus can be maintained in a relatively stable condition during the administration of general anesthesia.

Urgent Surgical Problems

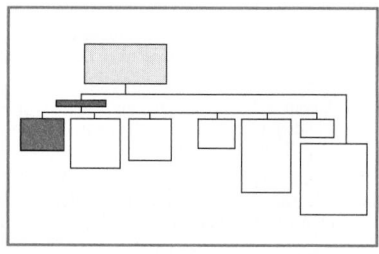

TRAUMA

Trauma is estimated to occur in approximately 6% to 7% of gestations.[3] It remains the leading cause of maternal death, accounting for 46.3% of deaths during pregnancy.[4] Homicide is the most common cause of traumatic maternal death, followed by motor vehicle accidents, accidental injury, and suicide.[5] Motor vehicle accidents account for 55% to 66% of all trauma during pregnancy, falls account for 22%, and domestic abuse and assaults account for 21%. The more severe the injury to the mother, the greater the risk of injury to the fetus. When the mother survives, fetal death is most commonly related to abruptio placentae. Major trauma causes placental abruption in 40% to 66% of cases; minor trauma causes placental abruption in 5% of cases.[6] Fetal death may also result from complications of premature delivery or from direct penetrating injury to the fetus.

Blunt Injury

In the mother, blunt trauma (as in motor vehicle accidents) may cause multiple life-threatening injuries, including head trauma, intra-abdominal hemorrhage, pelvic fracture, and uteroplacental vascular injury. Pelvic fractures are a particular concern: because of the extensive vascular supply in this area, there is a significant risk of substantial hidden blood loss. Uterine blood flow at term is approximately 500 ml/min; thus, pregnant women are at significant risk for massive hemorrhage if the uterus is injured. Uterine expansion displaces the bladder into the abdomen, thereby increasing the risk of traumatic bladder injury. The upper urinary tract is generally spared from injury, however, because the gravid uterus shields the retroperitoneum from direct injury. It should be kept in mind that mild hydroureter is physiologic in pregnancy. Hepatic, splenic, and

12 WEEKS   20 WEEKS   36 WEEKS

Liver

Colon

Stomach

Small
Intestine

Uterus

Figure 1 Enlargement of the uterus to accommodate the developing fetus shifts intra-abdominal contents superiorly and compresses retroperitoneal structures. These effects are particularly important during the second and third trimesters.

uterine injuries are common in high-speed motor vehicle accidents, but injuries to the GI tract, surprisingly, appear to be uncommon, largely because of the protective effects of the gravid uterus.[7] Direct injury to the fetus as a result of blunt trauma is unusual because of the protection afforded by the maternal abdominal wall and the uterus. Blunt trauma may result in fetal skull fractures, fetal intracranial hemorrhage, or abruptio placentae; nevertheless, fetal demise is rare in this setting and usually is secondary to maternal demise.

Many women refrain from using seat belts during pregnancy because of discomfort or out of concern that the seat belt might injure the fetus; however, this practice has no effect on fetal death rates in automobile accidents. When unbelted women are ejected from an automobile, maternal mortality is 33% and fetal mortality is 47%.[8] Three-point restraint is the safest choice for pregnant women in motor vehicles.

Penetrating Injury

Penetrating injury is usually more damaging to the fetus than to the mother. Mortality is actually lower for pregnant women with penetrating injuries than for nonpregnant women with similar injuries, presumably because of the shielding effect of the uterus and the fetus.[9]

Penetrating trauma, however, often results in direct fetal injury. Fetal mortality in this setting ranges from 40% to 70%, whereas maternal mortality ranges from 5% to 10%.[10] In the first trimester, trauma generally poses little direct threat to fetal viability because the uterus is protected within the pelvis. In the second and third trimesters, however, when the uterus is located within the abdomen, penetrating trauma may result in direct fetal injury or rupture of the membranes. With penetrating abdominal trauma, the prognosis depends on which and how many organs are injured.

General principles of trauma management are applied when the need for laparotomy is under consideration. Visceral injury occurs 95% of the time if the peritoneum has been penetrated.[11] For this reason, many authorities advocate exploratory laparotomy for all high-velocity penetrating injury to the abdomen. How best to manage low-velocity penetrating injury remains somewhat controversial. Low-velocity injuries above the fundus of the uterus are almost always associated with visceral injury and thus call for exploratory laparotomy. Injuries below the fundus and anteriorly are seldom associated with visceral injury[7] and thus can generally be managed nonoperatively. Subsequent laparotomy is indicated for worsening maternal symptoms. Subsequent cesarean section is indicated for a viable fetus in distress.

Domestic or partner violence during pregnancy occurs in 7% to 23% of all pregnancies.[12] If the patient is in an abusive relationship, the severity and frequency of assault typically increase during pregnancy.[13] In addition, 20% of abused pregnant women attempt suicide[14] or abuse alcohol or drugs. Abuse has many far-reaching consequences for the mother and the fetus that cannot be accurately measured. Unfortunately, partner violence often goes undiagnosed and hence untreated: as few as 12% of abused women are correctly identified in emergency room settings.[15] Typical presentations of partner abuse include multiple injuries in various states of healing, inconsistent explanations of the injuries, minimization of the injuries, and delay in seeking medical attention.[16] The face and the abdomen are struck more frequently during pregnancy. If a suspicion of partner violence arises, the physician should ask direct questions about threats and should provide appropriate contacts and support. A well-documented evaluation, unedited quotes, and careful drawings or pictures are also necessary in case the patient wishes to take legal action immediately or in the future. In all 50 states, domestic violence is a crime, and in some, failure to report suspected violence is a crime as well.

Management

Trauma is managed in essentially the same way in pregnant patients as in nonpregnant patients [*see I:2 Trauma Resuscitation*

Approach to Abdominal Pain in Pregnant Patients

Pregnant woman presents with acute abdomen

Obtain history, and perform physical examination.

Place I.V. line, and administer fluids as needed.

Insert nasogastric tube if significant vomiting is present.

Perform routine laboratory evaluations (e.g., CBC, serum electrolyte levels, urinalysis). Take into account normal changes in pregnancy.

Use fetal monitor after 26th week.

Use x-rays sparingly (only after first month); avoid radionuclide studies; employ abdominal and pelvic ultrasonography.

Identify conditions that require immediate operation.

Condition requires immediate operation

Trauma

Management: proceed essentially as for nonpregnant patients. *Mother is first priority.* Stabilization of mother improves fetal survival. Determine gestational age, and perform external fetal monitoring as indicated. In the event of acute maternal decompensation, consider cesarean section.

Acute appendicitis

Signs and symptoms: nausea and vomiting (differentiate from morning sickness); pain higher and more lateral in pregnancy; fever not a prominent finding; leukocytosis shifted to left. Pain that lessens when patient is turned to left is most likely of adnexal or ovarian origin. Use graded, real-time ultrasonography.

Management: perform laparotomy; use transverse incision when diagnosis is certain; use low midline incision, right paramedian incision, or exploratory laparoscopy if diagnosis in doubt (to permit examination of peritoneum).

Intestinal obstruction

Signs and symptoms: nausea and vomiting; history of abdominal operation or adhesions. Rule out pseudo-obstruction.

Management: pass nasogastric tube; initiate fluid resuscitation and total parenteral nutrition, if needed. Begin operation as soon as possible. For large-bowel obstruction, perform sigmoidoscopy, resection of threatened bowel, and cecopexy.

Perforated duodenal ulcer

Management: plication of the perforation. Definitive ulcer operation should not be attempted. If patient is close to term, avoid cesarean section because of risk of uterine contamination.

Spontaneous visceral rupture

General signs and symptoms: intra-abdominal hemorrhage, shock, acute abdomen.

- Hepatic rupture: severe right upper quadrant pain; complication of preeclampsia
- Renal rupture: probably secondary to hydronephrosis
- Splenic rupture: occurs in conjunction with splenic artery aneurysm or capsular rupture, usually secondary to hypervolemia and splenomegaly
- Esophageal rupture: may be associated with excessive vomiting during pregnancy (hyperemesis gravidarum)
- Ruptured ectopic pregnancy

Note: in operation for hepatic rupture, cesarean section should be performed simultaneously.

Other conditions requiring urgent operation

Ectopic pregnancy.
Ovarian torsion.

Condition requires operation only if disease does not respond to medical management

Acute cholecystitis: presents with epigastric or upper right quadrant pain, nausea and vomiting, occasional radiation of pain to right scapula; use ultrasonography to visualize. Do not use HIDA scan. Manage nonoperatively during first and third trimesters (fluid resuscitation and antibiotics); during second trimester, perform cholecystectomy. Use intraoperative cholangiography.

Pancreatitis: presents with unremitting visceral pain that may radiate to the back and with raised amylase levels (2,000–3,000 IU). Operative intervention (preferably during second trimester) indicated by evidence of biliary obstruction but no evidence of stone passage or by failure of medical management.

Peptic ulcer disease: treatment is based on symptomatic relief. Prompt operative intervention is indicated in the event of perforated duodenal ulcer.

Inflammatory bowel disease: operative intervention is last resort if medical therapy ineffective. Indications for operation include abscess, fistula, or bowel obstruction (Crohn disease) or toxic megacolon (ulcerative colitis).

and III *Trauma and Thermal Injury*]. The mother is the first priority: stabilization of the mother improves both maternal and fetal survival. Initial measures include efforts to support the airway, breathing, and circulation (the ABCs). The physiologic alterations characteristic of pregnancy affect maternal responses to injury [*see* Discussion, Physiologic Changes in Pregnancy, *below*].

The increased blood volume and enhanced cardiac output mask hypovolemia. Tachycardia and hypotension may not be accurate indicators of hypovolemia: as much as 2 L, or 30% of maternal blood volume, may be lost before hemodynamic instability is detected.[17] The expansion of intravascular fluid volume that occurs in pregnancy affects the amount of replacement fluid needed. In the third trimester, patients should receive 1.5 times the amount of fluid that would ordinarily be given to compensate for this effect. Use of military antishock trousers (MAST) may decrease maternal venous return by compressing the uterus on the inferior vena cava; accordingly, their use is not recommended. Vasoconstrictive agents should never be used for hemodynamic stabilization until hypovolemia has first been treated. Epinephrine and norepinephrine lead to uteroplacental vasoconstriction and fetal compromise; ephedrine and phenylephrine may be used during pregnancy.

An important concern with advancing gestation is the possibility that the expansion of the gravid uterus [*see* Figure 1] can produce aortocaval compression, leading to supine hypotension. Left lateral displacement of the uterus is necessary to improve blood flow to both the mother and the fetus after the 20th week.

There are very few diagnostic procedures for which pregnancy is a contraindication. Radiographic investigation should be performed whenever necessary if the results are expected to affect management. It is usually possible to keep the total absorbed radiation dose below the level that is thought to increase teratogenic risk (i.e., 50 to 100 milliGrays [mGy]) [*see* Table 1].[18] Plain films of the cervical spine provide useful information on head and neck injuries; computed tomographic scanning of the abdomen with contrast may offer the greatest amount of information on injuries to the retroperitoneum, the peritoneum, and the pelvis. Ultrasonography is now being used for acute trauma assessment in both pregnant and nonpregnant patients; the results to date have been good. Peritoneal lavage done in an open fashion through a supraumbilical incision may facilitate rapid assessment of intra-abdominal hemorrhage in cases of blunt trauma.[19] A Kleihauer-Betke test for fetal red blood cells in the maternal circulation will reveal any fetomaternal hemorrhage present. (Fetomaternal hemorrhage is the passage of fetal blood into the maternal vascular system; it occurs more frequently in pregnant women who have suffered traumatic injury than in those who have not, and it can lead to fetal anemia, arrhythmias, and fetal exsanguination.[20]) Rh_o (D) immune globulin and tetanus toxoid should be administered when indicated.

Early determination of gestational age by means of ultrasonography is a critical guide to further management decisions. Ultrasonography can also be used to monitor fetal heart tones, fetal activity, and amniotic volume. After the 20th week of gestation, cardiotocographic monitoring is an important adjunct for determining fetal status after trauma. Such monitoring should also be employed in the event of preterm contractions. As many as 40% of women experience preterm contractions, but only 3% progress to premature delivery.[6] Preterm contractions in a pregnant trauma patient should initiate an evaluation for abruptio placentae, uterine hemorrhage, and intra-abdominal hemorrhage. Given that placental abruption occurs in 66% of cases of major trauma and 5% of cases of minor trauma, the patient should be evaluated for ruptured membranes. Placental abruption usually occurs within 4 hours of injury. Ultrasonography is not sensitive enough to detect this condition[21]; therefore, cardiotocographic monitoring should be continued for 4 to 6 hours after stabilization and longer if any irregularity in the mother or fetus is noted.[22] If the fetus has not yet reached the gestational age of 23 weeks or is not viable, the mother should receive supportive care. In these circumstances, cesarean section is reserved for cases of disseminated intravascular coagulation (DIC). If the fetus is viable and the mother stable, cesarean section can be carried out safely; if the fetus is viable and the mother unstable as a result of trauma, cesarean section should be carried out with the exploratory laparotomy.[6] When the need for concurrent hysterotomy is under consideration, however, each case must be assessed individually. Patients undergoing an emergency cesarean section should receive a broad-spectrum antibiotic preoperatively.

In the event of acute maternal decompensation that does not respond to standard resuscitative measures, a cesarean section may be appropriate. In cases of particularly severe trauma, emergency operative resuscitation should be considered. If the patient is in cardiac arrest, thoracotomy and open chest massage, with concurrent cesarean section if the fetus is viable, have been recommended.[5] Cesarean section may increase maternal circulating volume. Occasionally, cardiopulmonary resuscitation (CPR) is more effective after the gravid uterus is emptied. There is also less risk of supine hypotension after cesarean section, although the associated surgical blood loss may exacerbate maternal instability. Timing is critical: if anoxia is limited to 4 to 6 minutes, the fetus generally will not be harmed. Therefore, any attempt to deliver the fetus should begin within 4 to 6 minutes after maternal cardiac arrest. If the fetus appears to be still viable after this period has passed, cesarean section should be performed; isolated cases of fetal salvage after prolonged maternal anoxia have been reported. Fetal survival after delivery is dependent on its having reached a gestational age greater than 28 weeks. CPR of the mother

Table 1 Radiation Dose Absorbed by Unshielded Gravid Uterus from Radiographic Studies Often Performed in Trauma Patients

Radiographic Study	Unshielded Uterine Dose (mGy)
Cervical spine	No detectable contribution
Chest (AP)	0.003–0.043
Pelvis (AP)	1.42–4.86
Abdomen (AP)	1.33–4.51
IVP	2.02–8.15
Full spine (AP)	1.54–5.27
Femur (AP)	0.016–0.12
Humerus (AP)	< 0.00001
Cystography	1.35–4.41
CT scan	
Head	< 0.5
Thorax	< 10
Upper abdomen	< 30
Cumulative dose (without CT scan)	7.68–27.36
Cumulative dose (with CT scan)	> 7.68–67.86

AP—anteroposterior   IVP—intravenous pyelography

should be continued during and after the delivery because it may improve maternal status and survival.

Two caveats should be kept in mind: (1) cesarean section should not be performed in an unstable patient because of an anticipated cardiac arrest, and (2) if CPR is successful before surgical delivery is attempted, cesarean section should not be performed, because in utero resuscitation is likely.[23]

APPENDICITIS

Appendicitis is the most common surgical problem in pregnancy, occurring in 0.05% to 0.1% of pregnancies, but it occurs no more often in pregnant women than in nonpregnant women.[24,25] The incidence

is approximately the same in all three trimesters. The low maternal mortality—0.5% in 1977 and 0% in recent studies[26]—notwithstanding, of all surgical problems during pregnancy, appendicitis causes the most fetal loss.[27] The particular dangers of appendicitis in pregnancy lie in the varied presentation of symptoms, the higher chance of delayed diagnosis, and the significant risk that surgery presents to the fetus.

The symptoms of appendicitis mimic symptoms of normal pregnancy—namely, anorexia, nausea, vomiting, and abdominal discomfort. The most reliable symptom of appendicitis during pregnancy is periumbilical or diffuse abdominal pain that later localizes to the right lower quadrant.[28] Although as the gravid uterus grows, it pushes the appendix cephalad and posteriorly, right lower quadrant pain remains the most consistent symptom of appendicitis in any trimester.[28]

On physical examination, appendicitis presents with tenderness in the right lower quadrant. It can be differentiated from adnexal or uterine pain with the help of the Adler sign: if the point of maximal tenderness shifts medially with repositioning on the left lateral side, the etiology is generally adnexal or uterine. Abdominal guarding, rebound tenderness, or referred tenderness is present in 60% to 70% of patients with appendicitis; however, these findings are less common during the third trimester because of the laxity of the abdominal wall muscles.[29] Elevated body temperature is not a consistent finding in pregnant patients with appendicitis.[26,28]

Laboratory values can be misleading, in that pregnancy can cause a leukocytosis as high as 15,000 leukocytes/mm³ in the absence of any source of infection.[30] The white cell differential is more useful than the absolute count; increased levels of band cells or immature forms suggest that the leukocytosis may be secondary to an infectious process. A urinalysis is necessary to rule out a urinary tract infection, which occurs in 10% to 20% of pregnant women.

Diagnostic radiology should be employed deliberately and judiciously. Ultrasonography of the lower abdomen or transvaginal ultrasonography can often visualize an inflamed appendix without risk to the fetus. It can also distinguish other causes of abdominal pain, such as an ovarian cyst. The clinical presentation and an ultrasonogram are often sufficient to establish the diagnosis of appendicitis.[31,32]

In very rare cases, a CT study of the pelvis should be done as well to elucidate a complicated presentation. A pelvic CT yields a total radiation dose of 25 mGy, and a directed helical, or spiral, CT study yields a total exposure of 30 mGy. Directed spiral CT has a sensitivity and specificity of 98%.[33] For both

pelvic CT and directed spiral CT, the total radiation doses are well below the threshold of safety established by the International Commission on Radiological Protection (ICRP), which is 100 mGy.[34] With plain films, the chance of obtaining valuable information is seldom worth the risk associated with the radiation. In certain cases, magnetic resonance imaging may be helpful for further delineation of the source of pain without the risk posed by ionizing radiation.

Differential Diagnosis

The condition most often confused with appendicitis is pyelonephritis, which occurs in 1% to 2% of pregnant women. The two diseases may present remarkably similar clinical pictures, especially when pyelonephritis occurs on the right side. Because of the mechanical effects of the gravid uterus on the ureter, pyelonephritis is more common in pregnant women than in nonpregnant ones. Furthermore, urinalysis yields abnormal results—either pyuria or hematuria—in as many as 20% of patients with appendicitis as a result of extraluminal irritation of the ureter by the inflamed appendix.[35] Nephrolithiasis can also be mistaken for appendicitis; it should be seriously considered whenever acute abdominal pain is present on the right side. Management of ureteral stones in pregnant patients presents a substantial challenge to both the surgeon and the urologist. Newer techniques, such as stents[36] and percutaneous nephrostomy tubes,[37] have been successful in obviating surgical intervention.

Right lower quadrant pain during early pregnancy may also be a presentation of ectopic implantation. Typically, a patient misses a period and then experiences some degree of vaginal bleeding or spotting. Abdominal or pelvic pain as well as cervical motion tenderness is present, and a mass is often appreciated on pelvic examination. When ectopic pregnancy is suspected, a serum human chorionic gonadotropin (hCG) assay should be performed along with transvaginal ultrasonography. If the serum hCG level is higher than 2,000 IU/L and an intrauterine gestational sac is not visualized by transvaginal ultrasonography, laparotomy or laparoscopy is indicated.

Torsion of an ovary or an ovarian cyst is also difficult to distinguish from appendicitis.[38] Although rare in pregnant patients, torsion of an ovarian cyst may occur in the early stages of the pregnancy. The physical examination is notable for pain in the right or left adnexa and the occasional presence of a tender mass. Transvaginal ultrasonography will frequently detect the cyst. Treatment requires laparotomy. The differential diagnosis of acute abdominal pain in pregnancy should also include ovarian cysts, mesenteric adenitis, degenerating fibroid tumors, salpingitis, inflammatory bowel disease, cholecystitis, ovarian vein thrombosis, ruptured corpus luteum, rectus hematoma, round ligament pain, abruptio placentae, chorioamnionitis, and adhesions.

Management

When there is evidence of appendicitis and no alternative diagnosis seems likely, operative intervention is warranted no matter what stage the pregnancy has reached.[39] The risk of the procedure to mother and child is minimal in comparison to the risks posed by delayed diagnosis, perforation, and abscess formation. Appendectomy in a pregnant patient does not increase the incidence of congenital malformation or stillbirth.[25] With routine surgical management, maternal mortality is negligible and fetal mortality is 2% to 8%.[26,40] For a ruptured appendix, maternal mortality is 1% and fetal mortality is as high as 35%.[38,41] Negative laparotomy rates of 15% or lower are considered acceptable in the nonpregnant population, but negative laparotomy rates as high as 35% are considered acceptable in pregnant patients in the light of the grave consequences of delayed diagnosis.[41]

For appendectomy in the pregnant patient, a right lower quadrant muscle-splitting approach should be employed over the point of maximal tenderness. With late trimester pregnancies, this point of maximal tenderness may be higher than the traditional McBurney's point [see V:16 Appendectomy]. The patient should also be turned 30° to the left to reduce pressure on the inferior vena cava and to facilitate exposure of the cecum. If there is doubt about the diagnosis, a low midline incision or a right paramedian incision should be made, especially if the patient has diffuse peritonitis. If appendicitis is found at the time of laparotomy, no further investigation for other intra-abdominal processes should be performed; such investigation may disseminate the infectious process and lead to late pelvic or abdominal abscesses. If, however, appendicitis is not found, the surgeon should thoroughly examine the peritoneal contents on the right side of the abdomen, taking care to avoid exerting traction on the uterus, which might lead to preterm labor. Appendectomy is advisable to avoid later confusion. If perforation occurs, the abdomen should be irrigated and drained. Skin closure should be avoided if abscess, advanced perforation, or gangrene is encountered.

Laparoscopic appendectomy, like all laparoscopic procedures, is controversial in the setting of pregnancy [see Discussion, Laparoscopic Surgery in Pregnancy, below]. When the diagnosis of appendicitis is uncertain, a laparoscopic approach can help rule out salpingitis, adnexal mass, or ectopic pregnancy.[29] When diffuse peritonitis is present, however, laparoscopy is associated with higher complication rates than laparotomy is.[29]

For a laparoscopic appendectomy in a pregnant patient, the first trocar (i.e., that for the camera) is placed in the subxiphoid area under direct vision via an open technique; this step allows visualization of all pelvic structures and the appendix. Once the appendix has been visualized, the right upper quadrant and right lower quadrant trocars should be placed under direct vision. If the size and position of the uterus make laparoscopic appendectomy difficult or impractical, the camera can be used to help locate the best available spot for an open incision.[42]

Antibiotics should be given preoperatively. Postoperative wound infection can be minimized if adequate attention is paid to aseptic technique and handling of tissues. If perforation, peritonitis, or abscess formation is noted, I.V. antibiotics should be administered.

The premature delivery rate for pregnant women undergoing appendectomy ranges from 13% to 22%; this increased rate may contribute to the lower birth weights reported after maternal appendectomy.[24,28] The risk of premature delivery is especially high during the first week after appendectomy. Given that tocolytics have never been shown to improve outcome in this setting, beta$_2$ receptor agonists are a better choice[29]; they are indicated when advanced appendicitis is suspected or when active contractions have been documented.

INTESTINAL
OBSTRUCTION

The incidence of bowel obstruction [see II:7 Intestinal Obstruction] in pregnant patients ranges from one in 1,500 to one in 66,000.[43] The most

common cause of small-bowel obstruction during pregnancy is adhesions, which account for 55% of cases; volvulus accounts for 25% of cases, with hernia, cancer, and intussusception accounting for the remainder.[44,45] As the incidence of operative procedures and the average age of the mother at gestation have risen, the likelihood of adhesive obstruction has risen as well. This problem may be further exacerbated by the hypomotility or dysmotility known to occur during pregnancy.[46] The need for laparotomy and lysis of adhesive bands during pregnancy is extremely low; however, when surgical management is necessary, fetal mortality is 26% and maternal mortality 5%. With intestinal obstruction, the main concern is to ensure that diagnosis is not delayed. Accordingly, any pregnant patient presenting with nausea, vomiting, and a history of abdominal surgery should be presumed to have a small-bowel obstruction until it is proved otherwise.

Large-bowel obstruction is less common than small-bowel obstruction but can be seen more often as pregnancy progresses. The most common cause of large-bowel obstruction is cecal or sigmoid volvulus. Volvulus during pregnancy is associated with a 21% to 43% mortality.[47] Colonic pseudo-obstruction, or Ogilvie syndrome, has also been reported late in pregnancy or in the early puerperium.[48] Striking colonic dilatation without anatomic obstruction is apparent, with gas filling the entire length of the colon from cecum to rectum. The danger of cecal perforation is high when the maximum diameter of the cecum exceeds 12 cm.

Management

Any sign of bowel ischemia or perforation in a pregnant patient with intestinal obstruction should prompt immediate operation. For small-bowel obstruction, a nasogastric tube should be inserted, fluid resuscitation should be initiated, a Foley catheter should be placed, and a full battery of blood tests should be performed, including assessment of blood gas levels and electrolyte levels and a complete blood count. Because of the leukocytosis known to occur in pregnancy, close attention should be paid to the differential blood count. Any sign of increasing acute-phase activity may suggest ischemia or perforation. Evaluation of acid-base status may also be useful in assessing bowel viability. A flat-plate and an upright abdominal film can confirm the diagnosis of small-bowel obstruction and rule out free air. The risk of radiation exposure to the fetus must be weighed against the potential morbidity and mortality of a missed diagnosis.

Once ischemia and perforation are ruled out, small-bowel obstruction should be treated with aggressive fluid resuscitation to ensure euvolemia and correction of electrolyte abnormalities. If long-term bowel rest is anticipated, total parenteral nutrition should be considered [see VII:9 Nutritional Support]. If conservative management does not lead to resolution, prompt operative intervention maximizes the chances of an excellent outcome for both fetus and mother.[29] A vertical incision allows the best exposure. The entire bowel must be examined for points of obstruction and assessed for viability. Segments of necrotic bowel should be resected, and an ostomy should be fashioned if necessary.

Large bowel obstruction is usually caused by volvulus. Sigmoid volvulus can usually be reduced by rigid or flexible sigmoidoscopy. If sigmoidoscopy fails, operative intervention with bowel resection and possible colostomy is indicated.[29] Treatment of a recognized cecal volvulus involves prompt operative intervention, resection of any threatened bowel, and cecopexy to prevent recurrence.

Pseudo-obstruction should be managed initially with bowel rest, electrolyte replacement, and the placement of a rectal tube. If these conservative measures fail to reestablish normal peristaltic activity, colonoscopy and intraluminal aspiration of the gas-filled colon should be tried. This approach is effective in as many as 85% of cases; however, it should be undertaken only by a skilled endoscopist because the potential for iatrogenic perforation of the bowel is extremely high. If there is no change in the size of the colon after 72 hours, a cecostomy is indicated.

PERFORATED DUODENAL ULCER

Although rare, perforated duodenal ulcer has been reported. When it occurs, it poses an extremely serious threat to both mother and fetus. There is no place for expectant, nonoperative therapy: prompt operative intervention is crucial. Surgical therapy should be directed at plication of the perforation, and no attempt should be made to perform a definitive ulcer operation. If the woman is close to term, the child should be delivered vaginally rather than by cesarean section because of the prohibitive risk of uterine contamination.

SPONTANEOUS VISCERAL RUPTURE

Spontaneous rupture during pregnancy can involve the liver, the kidney, the spleen, or the esophagus. Spontaneous hepatic rupture during pregnancy is extremely uncommon, occurring no more frequently than one in 50,000 pregnancies and perhaps as infrequently as one in 250,000 pregnancies.[49] It is thought to be an advanced development in preeclampsia or eclampsia. Abdominal trauma and events that increase intra-abdominal pressure (e.g., sudden coughing, sneezing, or unusually strong contractions) have also been implicated as causes of spontaneous rupture. Rupture may occur during the second or third trimester, during delivery, or even in the early postpartum period. Typically, it develops in older, multiparous women in the third trimester.[50] Patients present with several days of severe right upper quadrant or substernal pain radiating to the back. The pain may precede the actual rupture by as much as a few days. Nausea, vomiting, hypertension, coagulopathy, and thrombocytopenia are frequently present. In some cases of rupture, the patient presents with hypovolemic shock. A right upper quadrant ultrasonogram often visualizes the rupture or the preceding subcapsular hematoma.[29]

A limited number of renal ruptures have been described in conjunction with hydronephrotic kidneys; they are thought to be secondary to the physiologic hydronephrosis seen in pregnancy. Ultrasonography is the best imaging technique for diagnosis of renal rupture.[51] Splenic rupture is the most common nonobstetric cause of intra-abdominal hemorrhage during gestation. It usually occurs in conjunction with splenic artery aneurysms or spontaneous capsular rupture. In most cases, it is probably secondary to the increased blood volume and splenic enlargement seen toward the later part of pregnancy.

Esophageal rupture has also been described, generally in association with heavy vomiting. Patients report sudden epigastric pain on vomiting that may radiate to the back and the chest. X-rays may reveal air in the mediastinum. An upper GI series with water-soluble contrast material will demonstrate the site of the rupture. Although esophageal rupture is not more common in pregnancy, it may be associated with the frequent nausea and vomiting seen with hyperemesis gravidarum. Ultrasonography, radionuclide scanning, and, ultimately, angiography may be helpful in diagnosing rupture of the liver, the kidney, or the spleen.

Management

Prompt institution of volume support is essential, followed by emergency surgery and correction of any coagulopathy. Conservative management is reserved for stable patients with nonexpanding subcapsular hematomas. Serial ultrasonography is indicated. If adequate assessment of the hematoma, expanding hematoma, or rupture proves difficult or impossible, the patient should be taken to the OR for surgical treatment.[52]

Operative management of hepatic rupture or expanding hematoma involves debridement of nonviable liver, hemostasis with electrocoagulation or packing, and adequate drainage. Cesarean section should be performed simultaneously, depending on the gestational age and the likelihood of fetal survival. This maneuver, when indicated, is curative. Maternal mortality as high as 50% to 75% has been reported, even with prompt surgical intervention. Fetal mortality can be even higher, reaching nearly 80% in some series.[53] Renal rupture necessitates urgent operative exploration. Every effort should be made to salvage the ruptured kidney. Suspected splenic rupture necessitates immediate laparotomy and splenectomy. Esophageal rupture is treated with immediate repair through the left chest, if the injury is to the lower portion of the esophagus, or through the right chest, if the injury is to the upper portion.

Conditions for Which Medical Management Should Be Attempted

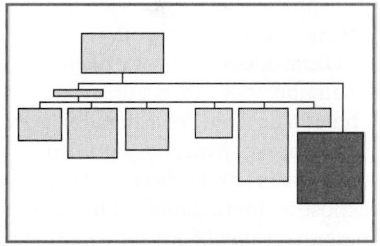

BILIARY TRACT DISEASE

Acute cholecystitis is the second most common nonobstetric emergency in pregnant women. Symptomatic gallstone disease is far more common in women than in men because of the differential effects of the sex steroids on bile lipid composition and cholesterol saturation.[54] The difference in incidence begins at menarche, increases during the childbearing years, and decreases at menopause. By the age of 75 years, at least 35% of women and 20% of men have gallstones.[55]

Gallstone disease is a result of cholesterol supersaturation and biliary stasis, both of which are promoted by pregnancy.[56] The elevated estrogen levels during pregnancy increase cholesterol secretion by the liver. Estrogen increases hepatic cholesterol uptake, increases cholesterol synthesis, and inhibits catabolism of cholesterol to bile acids. High concentrations of cholesterol in the bile overwhelm the solubilizing ability of bile salts, with the result that cholesterol stones form.[57] Elevated progesterone levels lead to bile stasis and decreased gallbladder contraction. Progesterone also causes incomplete emptying of the gallbladder after stimulation by cholecystokinin (CCK).[58] The mechanisms are not understood, but it is thought that progesterone may decrease gallbladder reactivity to CCK.[59] The decrease in small-bowel motility that occurs secondary to progesterone elevation may alter enterohepatic circulation and decrease bile acid return to the liver.[60] The balance of bile salts and cholesterol is further altered in such a way as to favor cholesterol supersaturation and stone formation. Pregnancy also alters the pool of bile acids. The decreased percentage of chenodeoxycholic acid and the increased percentage of cholic acid during pregnancy also promote stone formation.

The incidence of gallstone disease in pregnant women ranges from 3.3% to 12.2%[61] and increases with gestational age; however, only 30% to 40% of patients with gallstones are symptomatic.[62] The relative infrequency of symptomatic biliary disease is a function of the natural history of gallstones and of the time required to precipitate sufficient stones to generate symptoms.[63] Management of biliary colic consists of conservative therapy—namely, hydration, bowel rest if necessary, analgesia, and fetal monitoring. In pregnant patients, elective cholecystectomy for symptomatic gallstone disease should be delayed until after delivery. Fewer than 11% of symptomatic patients progress a more serious complication (e.g., cholecystitis, choledocholithiasis, or pancreatitis). Cholecystectomy during pregnancy is reserved for recurrent biliary colic or the aforementioned complications. It follows that cholecystectomy is rarely necessary in pregnant patients: it is undertaken once in every 10,000 live births.[64]

Gallstone disease causes acute cholecystitis in only 0.05% to 0.08% of births.[64] The clinical symptoms of cholecystitis consist of epigastric or right upper quadrant pain, fever, nausea, vomiting, and occasional radiation of the pain into the right scapula. Physical findings include tenderness in the right upper quadrant and, occasionally, the Murphy sign. Elevated liver function test results indicate that complicated biliary tract disease or choledocholithiasis is likely; however, elevated alkaline phosphatase levels are seen in normal pregnancies and thus are diagnostically unhelpful.

Ultrasonography can diagnose gallstones and biliary ductal dilatation with an accuracy of 97%.[56] It can also detect pericholecystic fluid, reveal gallbladder wall thickening, and elicit a sonographic Murphy sign, all of which are characteristic of cholecystitis.[65] Radionuclide scans introduce the risk of fetal exposure to radiation. This risk almost always outweighs the potential value of any information to be gained from such a scan.

Differential Diagnosis

The differential diagnosis of cholecystitis includes appendicitis (see above), pyelonephritis, nephrolithiasis, acute pancreatitis (see below), myocardial infarction, gastroesophageal reflux disease, peptic ulcer disease (see below), hepatitis, and hepatic liver abscess. Significant hepatic syndromes can occur during pregnancy, such as intrahepatic cholestasis of pregnancy, acute fatty liver of pregnancy, infectious hepatitis, the hemolysis–elevated liver enzymes–low platelet count (HELLP) syndrome, and eclampsia.[66-68] These syndromes should be considered if the clinical signs and symptoms observed in a pregnant patient do not conform to the typical picture of gallstone disease.

Management

Initial management of cholecystitis is conservative, comprising I.V. hydration, bowel rest, administration of meperidine

and antibiotics, fetal monitoring, and, if necessary, nasogastric decompression. This regimen is successful in 84% of patients.[69] Operative intervention is indicated in the presence of any of the following: failure of conservative management, recurrent disease, intractable nausea, maternal weight loss, fetal growth retardation, obstructive jaundice, gallstone pancreatitis, or peritonitis. Thus, serial monitoring of liver function test results and amylase levels is essential during conservative therapy. If cholecystectomy during pregnancy is necessary but not urgent, it is best to perform the operation in the second trimester: fetal mortality from a first-trimester cholecystectomy can be as high as 12%.[70] The rate of fetal loss decreases through gestation; however, beginning in the third trimester, the risk of preterm labor increases. Symptomatic gallstone disease is also a reasonable indication for surgical management.[64,71] Half of patients with symptomatic gallstone disease require repeat hospitalizations; in addition, several investigators have found the incidence of spontaneous abortion, preterm labor, or premature delivery to be higher in patients treated nonoperatively than in those undergoing cholecystectomy.[72] If cholecystectomy is performed in the second or third trimester, fetal mortality is lower than 5%.[73] There remains a degree of controversy regarding the relative merits of conservative management and aggressive surgical intervention for patients with symptomatic gallbladder disease.

Surgical treatment during pregnancy consists of either open cholecystectomy [see V:11 Biliary Tract Procedures] or laparoscopic cholecystectomy [see V:12 Laparoscopic Cholecystectomy]. The advantages of laparoscopic over open cholecystectomy include earlier recovery, earlier mobility, reduced use of narcotics, smaller incisions, and fewer surgical site infections.[72] When carried out with standard precautions, laparoscopic cholecystectomy does not increase the rate of fetal loss (5%) or of spontaneous abortion, nor does it have a greater adverse effect on birth weight, Apgar scores, or the rate of preterm delivery than open cholecystectomy does.[74] Laparoscopic cholecystectomy can be performed safely and effectively throughout pregnancy.[74,75] Routine indications for conversion to open cholecystectomy apply, including uncontrolled bleeding and unclear anatomy. Additionally, conversion during pregnancy is indicated if the gravid uterus has expanded to the point where safe dissection of the gallbladder by laparoscopic means is impossible.[75-79] If the fetus shows signs of distress, deflation of the pneumoperitoneum and conversion to an open cholecystectomy may be necessary. Laparoscopic cholecystectomy is contraindicated in pregnant patients with gallstone pancreatitis.

In patients with choledocholithiasis, intervention should be performed without delay. The common bile duct (CBD) should be explored by means of endoscopic retrograde cholangiopancreatography (ERCP) [see V:6 Gastrointestinal Endoscopy], with fluoroscopy used economically and lead aprons worn to shield the fetus.[29] ERCP with sphincterotomy successfully addresses choledocholithiasis without increasing fetal mortality or the rate of preterm delivery.[80] Surgical management of choledocholithiasis with open or laparoscopic cholecystectomy and CBD exploration should be reserved for patients in whom ERCP fails. Choledocholithiasis with right upper quadrant tenderness, fever, and jaundice (Charcot's triad) suggests cholangitis. The only treatment options for cholangitis when ERCP fails are open cholecystectomy and percutaneous intubation of bile ducts.[81] Intraoperative cholangiography can be used without problems after the second trimester,[82] provided that the fetus is shielded with lead during imaging to limit radiation exposure. Duct imaging should be reserved for patients who have risk factors for CBD stones (e.g., pancreatitis, a history of jaundice, or choledochal dilatation).[29]

PANCREATITIS

Pancreatitis is rare during pregnancy, occurring in every 1,000 to 10,000 pregnancies.[64] Its incidence, like that of gallstone disease, increases with gestational age. Associated gallstone disease is present in 70% to 90% of pregnant women presenting with pancreatitis.[64,80,83] Gallstone pancreatitis is associated with a maternal mortality of less than 37% and a fetal mortality of 10% to 60%.[82] In the nonpregnant population, pancreatitis is associated with biliary tract disease in only 40% of cases, with alcohol-induced pancreatitis accounting for another 40%. In pregnant patients, pancreatitis can be secondary to hypertriglyceridemia[84] as well as to thiazide administration and hyperparathyroidism.[85] At present, there is little evidence to suggest that pregnancy itself is an etiologic mechanism in the development of pancreatitis.[86,87]

The signs and symptoms of pancreatitis in pregnant women are indistinguishable from those seen in the general population. Patients report an unremitting, deep visceral pain that is usually midabdominal but may radiate into the back; nausea, vomiting, and anorexia are also typical symptoms. Findings in severe cases include hypotension, hypovolemia, and a rapid, thready pulse. Jaundice occurs in patients with CBD stones. The hallmark of the condition is diffuse abdominal pain combined with hyperamylasemia[88]; amylase levels may approach 2,000 to 3,000 U/L and may be accompanied by lipase elevations.[89] Albumin, calcium, and bilirubin levels should be measured and liver function tests performed. The results should be interpreted with caution in the light of the alkaline phosphatase elevation known to occur in normal pregnancies. Ultrasonography should be undertaken with the aim of searching for evidence of cholelithiasis and choledocholithiasis. Visualization of the inflamed pancreatic head may be informative; however, this structure is often difficult to locate.

Management

Treatment should be aimed at correction of the hypovolemia that invariably accompanies pancreatitis.[90] Restriction of oral intake is necessary. A nasogastric tube should be placed in cases of intractable nausea. Intramuscular administration of meperidine at a dosage of 50 to 75 mg every 3 to 4 hours provides adequate analgesia. Antibiotics should be reserved for treatment of a specific infectious complication. Calcium levels should be kept within the normal range. Arterial blood gases should be monitored as indicated. Prolonged pancreatitis may necessitate lengthy periods of bowel rest. During extended periods without oral feeding, pregnant women should be maintained on total I.V. hyperalimentation.[91]

In patients with pancreatitis caused by extrahepatic biliary obstruction, endoscopic management has achieved excellent results. ERCP and sphincterotomy [*see V:6 Gastrointestinal Endoscopy*] can both be performed safely during pregnancy. Definitive treatment with cholecystectomy and intraoperative cholangiography can safely be delayed until after delivery. Operative intervention should be reserved for patients with biliary obstruction in whom there is no evidence of stone passage. Efforts aimed at postponing operative intervention have been somewhat successful, though the recurrence rate approaches 50%. Early operative intervention has not been shown to improve fetal survival.[83] During the first trimester, loss of the fetus is common[92]; however, in the second trimester, operative intervention has a good chance of yielding excellent results for both mother and fetus.[93] Although unusual, pseudocyst formation has been reported in pregnant women. It is managed conservatively, without operative intervention. Laparotomy, debridement, drainage, and cholecystectomy are indicated for severe cases with pancreatic necrosis.

PEPTIC ULCER DISEASE

During pregnancy, symptoms of upper abdominal pain, nausea, and vomiting are not uncommon. Peptic ulcer disease usually begins with these same symptoms. Women with peptic ulcer disease usually experience symptomatic improvement during pregnancy. Elevated estrogen levels are believed to decrease gastric acidity during early pregnancy. Maternal gastrin production does not change during pregnancy, but histamine-stimulated acid output is lower. During the third trimester, however, maternal serum gastrin levels rise as a result of placental contribution, and symptomatic peptic ulcer disease may become more likely. During the late third trimester and the early postpartum period, basal and stimulated acid production returns to normal.

The diagnosis is made in much the same way in pregnant patients as in nonpregnant ones, except that physicians treating pregnant women should rely more on clinical information and less on radiologic intervention. Intractable pain that is not relieved by the usual therapeutic interventions should prompt endoscopic evaluation with a tissue biopsy for *Helicobacter pylori* culture.

Management

Safe symptomatic relief can be achieved with direct-acting agents (bismuth salicylate, sucralfate, aluminum hydroxide, and magnesium hydroxide). H_2 blockers and proton pump inhibitors are reserved for symptoms refractory to direct-acting agents. Most gastritis and ulcer disease is caused by infection by *H. pylori*. Treatment with the usual array of antibiotics (clarithromycin, amoxicillin, and metronidazole—but not tetracycline), direct-acting oral agents, and H_2 blockers is also safe in pregnancy.[94] Limitation of intake of nonsteroidal anti-inflammatory drugs (NSAIDs), tobacco, and caffeine also helps mitigate symptoms.

A perforated duodenal ulcer must be treated surgically [*see Urgent Surgical Problems, Perforated Duodenal Ulcer, above*]. Surgery is also indicated if significant hemorrhage—necessitating transfusion of more than six units over a 24-hour period—is observed. In this setting, maternal mortality is 14% after operation; however, it is 44% if surgical treatment is not provided.[95]

INFLAMMATORY BOWEL DISEASE

Pregnancy does not affect either ulcerative colitis or Crohn disease to any great degree, nor do these diseases affect the welfare of the fetus appreciably.[96-98] Active disease flare-ups are most common during the first trimester and during the early postpartum period.[99] In a review of pregnancies in patients with Crohn disease, the outcome of the pregnancy was not adversely affected by the disease. Although patients with active disease generally had poorer outcomes, neither pregnancy nor therapy affected the course of the disease.[100]

In addition to these frank forms of inflammatory bowel disease (IBD), ulcerative or granular proctitis may also occur in pregnancy. This poorly understood disorder is confined entirely to the distal 10 cm of the rectum. Endoscopically, the mucosa manifests multiple diffuse superficial ulcerations and friability. Above the distal 12 to 15 cm of the rectum, the mucosa assumes a normal appearance. Bleeding is observed, ranging from spotting with defecation to measurable loss. The disease is self-limited, almost never progressing to true IBD.

Management

Treatment of ulcerative colitis or Crohn disease involves administration of sulfadiazine, steroids, or both.[101] Treatment with both of these agents is often recommended.[102] Both steroids and sulfadiazine have been reported to cause congenital malformations in animal studies; however, because of the increased risk of fetal and maternal mortality in untreated cases of IBD, it is recommended that steroids and sulfadiazine be administered together as necessary to minimize the active effects of the disease.[103] If the disease does not respond to medical management, operative intervention may be undertaken, but only as a last resort. In patients with ulcerative colitis, the most common indication for operation is toxic megacolon, which, if left untreated, can cause significant infant and maternal mortality. In patients with Crohn disease, the uncommon problems of abscess, fistula formation, and bowel obstruction may force operation; these conditions should be treated in the usual fashion. Greater reliance should be placed on fecal diversion in pregnant patients because of the increased risk of anastomotic dysfunction. Active Crohn disease may necessitate complete bowel rest and maintenance of nutrition by central I.V. feedings.[104,105]

Patients with ulcerative or granular proctitis should not receive systemic treatment with steroids or sulfadiazine because of the potential toxicity to the fetus. Steroid enemas or enemas concocted from an elixir preparation of sulfasalazine may be administered. Low-residue diets may help control particularly bothersome symptoms.

Discussion

Physiologic Changes of Pregnancy

A variety of physiologic alterations occur during pregnancy. These include mechanical, hormonal, chemical, and hematologic changes [see Table 2] that are essential for maintenance of the pregnancy during the 40 weeks of gestation but that may also complicate the evaluation of abdominal problems in the pregnant patient.

RESPIRATORY CHANGES

The respiratory system undergoes several measurable changes as a result of the hormonal and physiologic influences of pregnancy. Elevated progesterone and estrogen levels cause blood volume and cardiac output to increase; as a result, pulmonary blood flow increases. With the added component of decreased blood albumin concentration and thus decreased oncotic pressure, mild lung edema may ensue.[106] Progesterone also acts as a direct respiratory stimulant, increasing the chemosensitivity of the respiratory center to CO_2.

In pregnant patients, both O_2 consumption and CO_2 production increase as gestation progresses. As the progesterone level rises, chemosensitivity to CO_2 and CO_2 production increase, and minute ventilation progressively rises by up to 30%.[107] Progesterone and increased CO_2 production are the main forces behind the condition known as hyperpnea of pregnancy. This condition results in a reduction in P_aCO_2 from 40 mm Hg to 34 mm Hg and an increase in arterial oxygen tension (P_aO_2) from 60 mm Hg to 100 mm Hg. This exaggerated gradient between the mother and the fetus facilitates efficient exchange of gases. With the decreased P_aCO_2, the pregnant patient also experiences respiratory alkalosis in relation to the fetus. The oxyhemoglobin dissociation curve is thus shifted to the right, again facilitating delivery of oxygen to the fetus. To prevent harmful pH increases, the kidneys respond appropriately by excreting bicarbonate.

As pregnancy progresses, tidal volume rises as a result of increases in chest circumference (usually about 5 cm). Although the growing uterus forces the diaphragm upward by as much as 4 cm, tidal volume is maintained, thanks to increased use of accessory muscles. Functional reserve capacity (FRC) decreases by 10% to 25% by week 12 of gestation because of decreased chest wall compliance. Relaxin, the hormone responsible for ligamentous relaxation of the pelvis, may also be responsible for laxity of the chest wall ligaments. As a consequence of this laxity, the subcostal angle increases from 68° to 103°.[108]

As many as 75% of pregnant women are affected by dyspnea. Dyspnea of pregnancy comprises mild pulmonary edema, increased breathing load, increased drive, and greater use of accessory muscles.[106] It can complicate the assessment of any pregnant patient with an underlying surgical issue. In addition,

Table 2 Chemical and Hematologic Alterations in Pregnant Patients[163]

Laboratory Test	Normal Values	
	Nonpregnant	Pregnant
Urinary acetone	Negative	Faint positive
Serum total protein (g/dl)	6.5–8.5	6.8
Serum albumin (g/dl)	3.5–5.0	2.5–4.5
Blood urea nitrogen (mg/dl)	10–25	5–15
Fasting blood glucose (mg/dl)	70–110	65–100
Two-hour postprandial blood glucose (mg/dl)	< 110	< 120 (plasma)
Serum calcium (mEq/L)	4.6–5.5	4.2–5.2
Serum phosphate (mg/dl)	2.5–4.8	2.3–4.6
Alkaline phosphatase (IU/L)	35–48	35–150
Cholesterol (mg/dl)	120–290	177–345
Triglycerides (mg/dl)	33–166	130–400
Serum folic acid (ng/ml)	5–21	4–14
Vitamin B_{12} (pg/ml)	430–1,025	Decreased
Hemoglobin (g/dl)	12	> 11
Hematocrit (%)	36	33
Serum iron (µg/dl)	> 50	> 60
TIBC (µg/dl)	250–400	300–600
% TIBC saturation	30	> 20
Serum zinc (µg/dl)	65–115	55–80
Urinary zinc (µg/dl)	200–450	200–450

TIBC—total iron-binding capacity

pregnant women typically have decreased oxygen reserve and thus are subject to rapid development of hypoxia and hypercapnia with hypoventilation or apnea. This vulnerability becomes especially important when such patients undergo intubation and anesthesia.

CARDIOVASCULAR CHANGES

During pregnancy, cardiac output rises by 30% to 50% [see Table 3]. This rise is attributable to an increased heart rate and, to a lesser extent, an increased stroke volume.[109] The HR increase may begin as early as 6 weeks after conception[110]; by the third trimester, HR is 15 to 20 beats/min faster than the baseline rate. The increase in the plasma volume may be as great as 50%. Despite the increases in cardiac output and blood volume, BP actually decreases because of the overwhelming effect of reduced systemic vascular resistance. BP reaches a nadir in the second trimester and returns to baseline levels by the time of delivery.[111]

The gravid uterus may press on the inferior vena cava, decreasing venous return and causing cardiac output to decrease by as much as 30%. Pregnant women may even experience dizziness or syncope. To optimize cardiac output, the pregnant patient should be placed in the left lateral decubitus position.[107]

Cardiovascular evaluation of the pregnant patient must take into account the altered cardiac output, blood volume, HR, and BP. Hypovolemia may not manifest itself as tachycardia or hypotension, as would normally be predicted; alternatively, tachycardia of pregnancy may be mistaken for hemorrhage. Careful analysis of the data is necessary whenever hypovolemia is under consideration. Additionally, pregnancy-associated signs and symptoms may complicate any evaluation of concurrent heart disease [see Cardiovascular Conditions during Pregnancy, below].[112]

GASTROINTESTINAL CHANGES

Appetite can vary greatly from one pregnant woman to another. The average increase in daily intake is 200 kcal/day during the first trimester. The recommended dietary allowance (RDA) is 300 kcal/day during pregnancy—more if the pregnant patient is an adolescent or especially physically active.[113] As many as 70% of pregnant patients experience nausea and vomiting. Nausea of pregnancy, or morning sickness, frequently occurs between weeks 4 and 16 of gestation. Most patients respond to conservative treatment, including selective eating and avoidance of dehydration. Persistent nausea and vomiting, termed hyperemesis gravidarum, can lead to dehydration, electrolyte imbalance, and organ failure. It is important to exclude other possible causes of nausea before attributing symptoms to nausea of pregnancy. This condition can complicate the diagnosis of appendicitis, gallbladder disease, pancreatitis, or bowel obstruction.

From 40% to 80% of pregnant women experience gastroesophageal reflux disease (GERD).[94] Esophagogastric junction tone decreases as intra-abdominal pressure increases, with reflux the result. In addition, under the influence of estrogen and progesterone, the stomach has decreased motility and an increased emptying time. Transit through the small bowel and the colon is also slowed.

Estrogens and progesterone are thought to influence cholestasis of pregnancy as well. The net effect of the two hormones is to increase the cholesterol concentration in bile. Estrogen also decreases bile flow. Progesterone promotes smooth muscle relaxation and stasis throughout the biliary system.[114] In the evaluation of cholestasis or any liver disease, it is important to remember that placental alkaline phosphatase can increase measured alkaline phosphatase levels by a factor of three or four.

URINARY CHANGES

As cardiac output increases, the glomerular filtration rate increases by 30% to 50%. This increase reaches a peak at the end of the first trimester. Accordingly, creatinine clearance and blood urea nitrogen (BUN) levels fall by 25% over the first trimester. The kidneys themselves increase in size by 1.5 cm as a result of increased vascularity.[115] The ureters become dilated as a consequence of the relaxing effects of progesterone on smooth muscle.[116] Dextrorotation of the uterus causes further dilatation of the right ureter.

HEMATOLOGIC CHANGES

Normal pregnancy causes numerous changes in coagulation and fibrinolysis. Platelets become more reactive, and destruction is enhanced; to compensate, the pregnant patient increases production of platelets. Normal pregnancy increases hepatic and endothelial cell synthesis of many procoagulant factors. Pregnant women have normal anticoagulant factor levels except for a sharp decrease in protein S antigen and activity. In general, fibrinolytic activity is impaired during pregnancy; however, bleeding time and clotting time are unchanged. Overall, pregnancy is a hypercoagulable state.[117] The risk of thromboembolism doubles during pregnancy.[118] Accordingly, compression stockings should be used whenever surgical management is embarked on.

Leukocytosis is normally seen in pregnancy. What the net effect of a decrease in CD4+ cells, an increase in CD8+ cells, and

Table 3 Hemodynamic Values in Healthy Nonpregnant, Pregnant, and Postpartum Subjects[109,164]

Parameter	Nonpregnant	36–38 Weeks' Gestation*	Postpartum
Heart rate (beats/min)	60–100	83 ± 10	71 ± 10
Central venous pressure (mm Hg)	5–10	3.6 ± 2.5	3.7 ± 2.6
Mean pulmonary arterial pressure (mm Hg)	15–20	—	—
Pulmonary arterial wedge pressure (mm Hg)	6–12	7.5 ± 1.8	6.3 ± 2.1
Mean arterial pressure (mm Hg)	90–110	90.3 ± 5.8	86.4 ± 7.5
Cardiac output (L/min)	4.3–6.0	6.2 ± 1.0	4.3 ± 0.9
Stroke volume (ml/beat)	57–71	74.7	60.6
Systemic vascular resistance (dyne · cm · sec^{-5})	900–1,400	1,210 ± 266	1,530 ± 520
Pulmonary vascular resistance (dyne · cm · sec^{-6})	< 250	78 ± 22	119 ± 47

*Values in pregnant patients were determined with patient in left lateral decubitus position.

an unchanged number of B cells may be is the subject of some controversy at present.[119] More important than the higher total number of cells is the altered activity exhibited by all leukocytes, a complicated picture that is still not fully understood.

Although pregnancy may appear to be an anemic state, it is not: blood volume actually increases (see above), and red cell mass rises by 30% [see Table 2].

General Perioperative Considerations in Pregnant Patients

The use of anesthesia in the course of an operation does not pose a teratogenic risk to the fetus.[120] Surgical treatment can be acceptably safe if appropriate attention is given to certain key perioperative considerations—namely, fetal monitoring, radiologic investigation, anesthesia, and the timing of the operation.

FETAL MONITORING

Monitoring consists of measuring uterine contractions with a tocometer, fetal HR with a Doppler transducer, and fetal movement and tone with ultrasonography. Together, these measurements yield a good indication of fetal health. Preoperative ultrasonography can also approximate gestational age when an accurate history cannot be obtained. Gestational age plays a pivotal role in all surgical decision making for a pregnant patient.

The fetal HR is routinely measured both preoperatively and postoperatively.[121] Though the fetal HR can be heard 14 weeks after conception, it serves as an indicator of fetal oxygenation only after week 26. Specific fetal HR abnormalities—absence of variability, late or variable decelerations, and bradycardia—are predictive of impending fetal hypoxia, physical damage, or death. In the absence of these extreme (and hence obvious) fetal HR patterns, interpretation of fetal tracings can be complex.[122] There are no conclusive data to suggest that any single monitoring technique reflects fetal outcome.[121] Optimization of maternal physiologic status is more important than any mode of fetal monitoring.

RADIOLOGIC INVESTIGATION

X-rays and CT scans must be employed judiciously, given the risk that radiation poses to the pregnant patient. Depending on the exposure time and the total dose, radiation may cause failure to implant, malformation, growth retardation, CNS abnormalities, or fetal loss.

The standard units of measure for radiation are the Gray (Gy) and the rad; 1 Gy is equivalent to 100 rad, and 1 rad thus is equivalent to 1 cGy or 10 mGy. The ICRP has stated that radiation doses lower than 100 mGy do not increase the risk of fetal death, malformation, or developmental delay.[34] Doses between 200 to 500 mGy during weeks 8 to 15 of gestation, however, result in measurable IQ reductions, and doses higher than 600 mGy result in growth retardation and CNS damage. Most diagnostic procedures fall within the accepted safe range. The average radiation dose from an abdominal x-ray is 1.4 mGy, that from an abdominal CT scan is 8.0 mGy, that from a pelvic CT scan is 25 mGy, and that from a selective spiral CT scan of the abdomen and the pelvis is 30 mGy.

In many instances, alternate diagnostic modalities that do not employ ionizing radiation, such as ultrasonography and MRI, are sufficient to determine the proper treatment. If, however, diagnostic radiation does prove necessary, the fetus should be shielded, radiation exposure should be minimized,

and radiation doses should be carefully documented.[123] Careful cooperation with the radiologist will help limit radiation exposure. It is of particular importance that the patient be informed of the risks associated with radiation in comparison with the expected benefits of diagnostic radiation in her case.

ANESTHESIA

The physiologic changes associated with pregnancy have implications for anesthetic management. As noted (see above), oxygen reserve decreases with pregnancy. Upon intubation, hypoxia and hypercapnia with hypoventilation or apnea may develop rapidly. In one clinical study of obstetric anesthesia, airway difficulties occurred in 7.9% of intubated patients, compared with 2.5% of nonintubated patients[124]; it is noteworthy that the primary reasons for difficult intubation were airway anatomy and technique, just as would be the case in nonpregnant patients. During intubation, pregnant women are also at increased risk for gastric aspiration owing to the decreased gastroesophageal sphincter tone. Because of this increased risk of aspiration, nasogastric suction should be freely employed. The stomach should be emptied before emergency procedures and continually decompressed throughout the operation and the early postoperative period.

Anesthesia can suppress the normal physiologic compensation for aortocaval compression, in which event hypotension can ensue. Positioning of the patient in a leftward tilt or the left lateral decubitus position can minimize hypotension.[121] Liberal use of indwelling urinary catheters allows gross estimation of the adequacy of blood volume and splanchnic perfusion during general operative procedures. If intra-abdominal operation is necessary after weeks 12 to 16, the bladder must be decompressed to allow adequate exposure in the pelvis and the lower abdomen.

According to retrospective studies, all anesthetic, opioid, sedative-hypnotic, and anxiolytic agents pose some degree of risk to the fetus; none of them appears to be significantly more teratogenic or safer than any other.[121] If vasopressors are necessary, ephedrine is the drug of choice, in that it causes less uterine vasoconstriction than epinephrine or norepinephrine does. Small doses of phenylephrine are also safe for use in pregnant women who are hypotensive [see Table 4].

TIMING OF SURGERY

If a surgical problem arises during pregnancy, the urgency of surgical treatment must be balanced against the risk such treatment poses to the mother and the fetus. Urgent procedures, such as appendectomy, should be carried out in the usual timely fashion [see Urgent Surgical Problems, above]: in such cases, the risks to both mother and fetus outweigh the risks of miscarriage and preterm labor. Semielective procedures are best done during the second trimester.[72] In the first trimester, when organogenesis is ongoing, concerns arise about the teratogenic risks of medications and surgical interventions. During the first trimester, surgical procedures are associated with a miscarriage rate of 12%; during the second trimester, this rate falls to 0% to 5.6%. The incidence of preterm labor with surgical procedures is 5% in the second trimester but rises to 30% to 40% in the third trimester.[125] Elective procedures should be delayed until 6 weeks after delivery.

TOCOLYTICS

Even though surgical procedures have been associated with a higher incidence of preterm labor, especially in the third trimester, routine prophylactic use of tocolytics is not recom-

Table 4 Safety of Various Drugs Used during Pregnancy[165,166]

Drug (FDA Pregnancy Category)	Toxicity	Comments
Analgesics/tranquilizers		
Ibuprofen (B)	Risk of postpartum hemorrhage; premature patent ductus arteriosus closure; no teratogenic effects	Use with caution toward end of pregnancy
Meperidine (B)	Decreased neonatal respiration; CNS depression	Greatest risk near term
Morphine (C)	Small size for gestational age; respiratory depression; fetal death	Greatest risk near term
Codeine (C)	Possible congenital anomalies	Avoid in first trimester
Acetaminophen (B)	None known	Analgesic of choice
Aspirin (C)	Anticoagulation effect; fetal bleeding; possible prolongation of pregnancy; no teratogenesis known	Use with caution, especially toward end of pregnancy; not recommended for routine analgesia
Barbiturates (C)	Fetal addiction; neonatal bleeding; ?teratogenesis	Long-term administration not recommended
Diazepam (D)	?Cleft palate; ?heart defects; hypotonia; hypothermia; withdrawal symptoms	Long-term administration not recommended
Anesthetics		
Bupivacaine (C)	Bradycardia	Use with caution in late pregnancy
Lidocaine (B)	Bradycardia; CNS depression	Use with caution in late pregnancy
Halothane (C)	Uterine relaxation	Can cause abortion in early pregnancy
Nitrous oxide (C)	?Teratogenesis in early pregnancy	Can be used in late pregnancy
Muscle relaxants (C)	Fetal curarization	Relatively safe; incidence of problems extremely low
Antibiotics		
Ampicillin (B)	None known	Safe
Aztreonam (B)	Not teratogenic in rodents	Safety in pregnancy unclear
Cephalosporins (B)	No embryocidal reports	Safe
Clindamycin (B)	None known	Safety in pregnancy unclear
Erythromycin, azithromycin (B)	Risk of cholestatic hepatitis; no reported congenital defects	Avoid in pregnancy
Fluoroquinolones (C)	Irreversible arthropathy in immature animals	Avoid in pregnancy
Gentamicin (C)	Possible 8th nerve toxicity; no reported congenital defects, neonatal ototoxicity, or nephrotoxicity	Avoid in pregnancy
Imipenem (C)	None known	Safety in pregnancy unclear
Metronidazole (B)	Carcinogenic in rodents; possibly teratogenic	Contraindicated in first trimester; use with caution thereafter
Nitrofurantoin (C)	Hemolytic anemia in newborns; no known teratogenic effects	Contraindicated at term
Penicillin G (B)	None known	Safe
Streptomycin (D)	8th cranial nerve abnormality	Contraindicated
Tetracycline (D)	Adverse effects on fetal teeth and bones; maternal hepatotoxicity; congenital defects	Contraindicated
Trimethoprim-sulfamethoxazole (C)	Hemolysis in G6PD-deficient patients; risk of kernicterus	Contraindicated at term
Vancomycin (C)	Potential fetal ototoxicity, nephrotoxicity	Avoid in pregnancy

mended. Tocolytics have a several side effects and have not been shown to improve outcome when used prophylactically. Tocolytics are best employed to treat active uterine irritability. Uterine irritability can also be reduced by controlling maternal pain and anxiety.[126]

Laparoscopic Surgery in Pregnant Patients

The role of laparoscopic surgery in the management of pregnant patients remains to be established. Most current recommendations are based on retrospective and animal studies. Laparoscopy would appear to offer some significant benefits. For example, it leads to rapid postoperative recovery and mobilization and thus reduces the risk of thromboembolism associated with pregnancy. Hospital stays are shorter and hospital costs lower.[127] Often, less narcotic analgesia is required during recovery, and fetal depression from narcotic exposure is thereby minimized. Because laparoscopic surgery makes use of smaller incisions, incisional hernias are less common, and there is less incision-related discomfort as a result of the growing uterus and increasing intra-abdominal pressure.[125] Moreover, laparoscopic surgery involves less manipulation of the uterus and so may be less likely to induce uterine irritability, preterm

labor, premature delivery, or spontaneous abortion.[42] Finally, when the diagnosis is uncertain, the surgeon can often use laparoscopy to identify appendicitis, ovarian masses, ovarian torsion, and ectopic pregnancy.

Pregnancy adds a level of risk to any laparoscopic procedure. Insufflation with CO_2 and increased intra-abdominal pressure lead to decreased uterine blood flow, decreased maternal vena cava return, and decreased maternal functional residual capacity.[75,126] The combination of CO_2 pneumoperitoneum, the reverse Trendelenburg position, general anesthesia, and aortocaval compression by the gravid uterus can decrease maternal cardiac output by 50%.[127] Animal studies suggest that CO_2 pneumoperitoneum may also cause an increase in maternal arterial CO_2 tension (P_aCO_2), resulting in maternal and fetal acidosis[128]; however, there is active controversy as to whether these intraoperative alterations caused by CO_2 pneumoperitoneum actually affect fetal health.[129] Finally, when laparoscopic surgery is performed in a pregnant patient, the uterus is susceptible to direct damage, irritation, or penetration by a Veress needle or trocar.[130]

Certain precautions can be taken to limit the risks associated with laparoscopic surgery during pregnancy.[125] Using the Trendelenburg position (or minimizing use of the reverse

Trendelenburg position) and left uterine displacement enhance venous return. Keeping intra-abdominal pressure below 15 mm Hg can minimize the decreases in uterine blood flow, maternal inferior vena cava return, and maternal functional residual capacity. Limiting the duration of insufflation minimizes the risks associated with CO_2 pneumoperitoneum. During laparoscopy, a transvaginal Doppler transducer should be used for fetal monitoring when possible; any signs of distress can be combated by decreasing intra-abdominal pressure and hyperventilating the mother. Standard noninvasive monitoring methods (e.g., capnography) are sufficient guides to P_aCO_2 values in routine cases.[131] Ventilation should be adjusted in accordance with maternal P_aCO_2 levels. Finally, penetrating injury to the uterus can be minimized by entering the abdomen under direct vision and applying upward countertraction of the abdominal wall while placing a Hasson trocar.[42]

Currently, the general tendency is to limit laparoscopic surgery in pregnant women to the first 28 weeks of gestation. Later in pregnancy, when the uterus is no longer confined within the pelvis and the lower abdomen, laparoscopic surgery becomes substantially more difficult. Although laparoscopic surgery, like laparotomy, increases the likelihood of preterm labor, tocolytics should be administered only in the event of documented or perceived contractions; given the side effects of tocolytics, their prophylactic use is more worrisome than the potential risk of preterm contractions.[74]

When appropriate precautions are employed, laparoscopy poses no more risk to either the mother or the fetus than laparotomy does.[72,130,132] Again, there are no significant differences between the two approaches with respect to preterm delivery rate, birth weight, Apgar score, growth restriction, infant mortality, or risk of fetal malformation.[74,126]

Cardiovascular Conditions during Pregnancy

CARDIAC DISEASE

The incidence of heart disease during pregnancy is 1.5%, with rheumatic heart disease accounting for 60% to 75% of cases.[133] The current trend in the United States, however, is that fewer pregnant women are presenting with rheumatic heart disease and more are presenting with congenital heart disease.[112] Heart disease becomes an active issue during pregnancy because gestation places great stress on the cardiovascular system: cardiac output increases by 30% to 50%, HR by 15 to 20 beats/min, and plasma volume by 50%. Delivery places added stress on the heart as a result of physical exertion, pain, and drastic fluid shifts. There is some blood loss with delivery, but there is also an increase in venous return resulting from the release of the pressure imposed by the gravid uterus on the inferior vena cava. In addition, excess extracellular fluid is drawn into the vasculature after delivery. If the diseased heart has little reserve, pregnancy can push the patient into florid heart failure. Recognition of heart failure may be delayed because normal pregnant patients typically present with peripheral edema, dyspnea, and poor exercise tolerance.

The most common indication for cardiac surgery during pregnancy is native valve disease (36%),[134] of which mitral stenosis is the variety most commonly encountered. Progressive failure from mitral stenosis can cause arrhythmias that exacerbate symptoms. Pregnant women with aortic stenosis or hypertrophic cardiomyopathy may experience angina and syncope in addition to heart failure, and they tolerate arrhythmias

poorly. Aortic disease is the second most common indication for cardiac surgery during pregnancy (31%). Aortic dissection and aneurysm are associated with hypertension, atherosclerosis, and connective tissue disorders (e.g., Marfan syndrome and Ehlers-Danlos syndrome). Approximately 50% of all aortic dissections in women younger than 40 years occur during pregnancy. Other indications for cardiac surgery during pregnancy are prosthetic valve dysfunction (14%), congenital anomalies (e.g., atrial and ventricular septal defects) (7%), pulmonary embolism (6%), cardiac tumors (4%), and coronary artery disease (2%). Overall, cardiac surgery is associated with a maternal mortality of 0% to 3% and a fetal mortality of 12% to 20%.[133,135] The outcome of a cardiovascular operation performed in a pregnant patient is affected by the indication for surgery, the condition of the mother, and the timing of the procedure in relation to the gestational age.[136]

Management

Ideally, women of childbearing age who have heart disease should receive counseling before planned conception. Such counseling should address the risks of pregnancy, the issues related to anticoagulation, and the fetal mortality and morbidity associated with specific clinical situations. Any significant congenital heart condition should be corrected before pregnancy if possible. Vigilance for symptoms of heart failure should be an adjunct to routine prenatal care[137]; if signs of failure develop, the patient should be hospitalized for treatment of volume overload, tachycardia, and possible arrhythmias.[138] If aortic dissection is noted, hypertension should be controlled.

The question of the optimal timing of cardiac surgery during pregnancy introduces a potential maternal-fetal conflict of interest. On one hand, maternal mortality from cardiac surgery is lowest in the first trimester; delaying operative treatment increases maternal mortality substantially.[134] On the other hand, fetal mortality and morbidity from cardiac surgery are highest in the first trimester and decrease as gestation progresses. Hence, the issue of how to time surgical management so as to safeguard both mother and fetus as well as possible is still the subject of some debate. In general, operative intervention should be delayed until the fetus is deliverable, at which time cesarean section can be performed, followed by cardiac surgery or aortic surgery.[133,139] If it is necessary to perform a cardiac operation during the first or second trimester, precautions should be taken to minimize the effects of bypass on the fetus. High-flow, high-pressure bypass is favored by most surgeons, the rationale being that high rates are necessary during pregnancy to ensure perfusion to the fetus, especially in the context of a contracting uterus. Cardiotocographic monitoring should be instituted to measure the level of fetal stress during bypass. Bypass causes uterine contractions through dilution of progesterone, a natural inhibitor of uterine contractions. Patients with documented contractions should receive tocolytics.

Finally, any pregnant woman undergoing cardiac surgery should receive antibiotics as prophylaxis against endocarditis, the most lethal complication of such procedures.[134]

SPLENIC ARTERY ANEURYSMS

Splenic artery aneurysms are rare, with an incidence of less than 1%. They are, however, four times more common in women than in men, and 25% of all splenic artery ruptures in women occur during pregnancy. Several factors contribute to the relatively high incidence of such rupture in pregnant women. Splenic arterial pressure is unusually high during pregnancy as a result of the increased cardiac output, the increased blood volume, and the pressure placed on the abdominal aorta and the iliac arteries by the gravid uterus. Pregnancy is also believed to break down the connective tissue component of the arterial wall. Multiparous women in the third trimester are at highest risk for a ruptured splenic artery aneurysm. In the non-pregnant population, splenic artery rupture is associated with a 25% mortality; however, in pregnant women, it is associated with maternal and fetal mortalities ranging from 75% to 95%,[140] mainly as a consequence of erroneous diagnosis. Upon diagnosis of rupture, immediate operative repair is necessary. If a splenic artery aneurysm larger than 2 cm is found in a woman of childbearing age, elective resection is indicated.[141]

RENAL ARTERY ANEURYSMS

Renal artery aneurysms are uncommon, appearing in 0.09% of the population; most are diagnosed incidentally in the course of CT scanning done for other indications. Renal artery aneurysms not only are associated with brittle hypertension but also carry a high mortality when they rupture. Because of the connective tissue laxity that develops during pregnancy, the risk of rupture is higher in pregnant than in nonpregnant women. When renal artery rupture occurs, immediate operative repair of the aneurysm is necessary. The most important indication for surgery in this situation is hypertension and female gender; the size of the aneurysm is a secondary concern.[142]

Malignancies during Pregnancy

Cancer during pregnancy occurs in 0.07% to 0.1% of births.[143] The types most commonly encountered in this setting are breast cancer (19%), thyroid cancer (17%), cervical cancer (11%), Hodgkin disease (7%), and ovarian cancer (6%).[144] All cancers except for melanoma and hematologic tumors metastasize to the placenta but not to the fetus.[145,146] The major risk factor for malignancy during pregnancy is age greater than 40 years. Pregnant women with malignancies are more likely to experience complicated hospitalizations, as are their babies. Malignancy during pregnancy also increases the chances of low birth weight and premature labor.[144]

The measures commonly employed to treat cancer—surgery, irradiation, and chemotherapy—all pose significant risks to the fetus, especially in the first trimester. The degree of risk associated with operation depends not only on the gestational age but also on the disease, the stage of the cancer, and the nature of the procedure. Chemotherapy during the first trimester can cause fetal malformations, premature delivery, and restricted fetal growth in as many as 25% of cases; however, chemotherapy during the second and third trimester generally has a favorable long-term outcome.[147] Finally, any radiation therapy administered is likely to exceed the safety threshold for fetal radiation exposure.

Thus, treatment of cancer in a pregnant woman should involve close coordination between the oncology team, the obstetrician, and possibly a neonatologist. The patient must be well informed regarding the overall risks of treatment, the specific risks to herself if some components of therapy are delayed, and the specific risks to the fetus associated with each type of therapy.

BREAST CANCER

Pregnancy-associated breast cancer is defined as cancer diagnosed during pregnancy or up to 1 year after delivery.

Pregnancy-associated breast cancer is associated with a worse outcome than other types of breast cancer are. The poorer prognosis may be attributable to aggressive tumor growth in response to hormones of pregnancy. In addition, diagnosis of pregnancy-associated breast cancer is often delayed because of the normal hypertrophic thickening of the breast during pregnancy, the inability of mammography and ultrasonography to differentiate between normal breasts and breasts with malignancies in pregnant women, or the reluctance of surgeons to perform biopsies during pregnancy.[148]

Management

Any suspicious breast mass should be aspirated to rule out the possibility that it is a cyst. If the mass disappears after aspiration, follow-up via physical examination is appropriate; mammography is not advisable, because it may damage the fetus. If the mass does not resolve, a core-needle biopsy or an open biopsy with local anesthesia should be performed [*see V:2 Breast Procedures*], regardless of the stage of pregnancy. Strict attention to hemostasis and to ligature of obvious ductules is necessary to prevent postoperative hematoma or leakage of milk. Another common presentation is nipple discharge [*see II:3 Breast Complaints*], which may signal a papilloma or duct ectasia and thus calls for biopsy. Inflammatory changes in breast skin are generally caused by staphylococcal or streptococcal infections; they occur most frequently in the postpartum period but also are occasionally seen during pregnancy. If inflammation does not resolve rapidly after antibiotics are administered, drainage is indicated and biopsy should be considered.

Management of breast cancer in pregnant patients does not vary greatly from that in nonpregnant patients.[149] Once the diagnosis of breast cancer is made, modified radical mastectomy [*see V:2 Breast Procedures*] should be done expeditiously; it should not be delayed because of the pregnancy.[148] Given the high doses required, radiation therapy is contraindicated during pregnancy. Accordingly, lumpectomy with radiation therapy is an option only if radiation therapy can commence after delivery. As noted, chemotherapy is relatively safe during the second and third trimesters. For patients with stage III or IV breast cancer, termination of pregnancy may be considered to allow unrestricted treatment with chemotherapy and radiation. For all patients, treatment plans should be formulated on an individual basis, taking into account the risks facing both the fetus and the mother.

Burns during Pregnancy

Burns occurring during pregnancy should be evaluated in the same manner as burns occurring in the nonpregnant population [*see III Trauma and Thermal Injury*]. The total body surface (TBS) burned should be measured and documented (ideally with photographs). Adjustments must be made for the increased abdominal surface area seen in the later stages of gestation. Fetal outcome is dependent on the mother's condition: fetal mortality is 89% when the mother has burns over more than 50% of her TBS but falls to 21% when the mother has burns over less than 50% of her TBS.[150]

Management

Generally, burns are treated in much the same way in pregnant patients as in nonpregnant patients; however, special attention should be paid to securing the airway and ensuring adequate breathing. Pregnant patients have a lower FRC and are less able to compensate for hypoxia. Moreover, exposure to burns often puts the mother at risk for carbon monoxide inhalation. The fetus is especially susceptible to carbon monoxide poisoning because fetal hemoglobin has a higher affinity for carbon monoxide than maternal hemoglobin does; thus, carbon monoxide can easily lead to fetal hypoxia.[151] Silver sulfadiazine cream should not be used near term because of its association with kernicterus in the infant. Finally, if the fetus is older than 24 weeks and the mother sustains burns over 50% or more of her TBS, cesarean section is indicated.

Electrical accidents are associated with a fetal mortality of 50%. Any woman who has experienced electric shock should undergo serial ultrasonography until delivery. Maternal mortality with such injuries is minimal.

Minor Surgical Problems of Pregnancy

HEARTBURN

Heartburn is a common complaint of pregnancy that results in part from decreased lower esophageal sphincter pressure and regurgitation of stomach contents.[152] An alkaline reflux gastritis may in part be responsible because gastric acidity is decreased in pregnancy. Toward the later part of the pregnancy, 10% to 15% of pregnant women will also manifest severe reflux that is caused by a frank diaphragmatic hiatus hernia.

Management

Antacids containing aluminum hydroxide or magnesium hydroxide, such as Gelusil and Amphojel, should be taken 30 minutes to 1 hour after meals.[103] Positional changes, such as elevation of the head of the bed and maintenance of an upright posture for several hours after meals, should be encouraged. Chewing gum or sucking on hard candies tends to increase esophageal motility and decrease reflux. In severe cases, sucralfate may be given to soothe and possibly to heal active gastritis and esophagitis. Metoclopramide has also been found to be efficacious in cases of heartburn that is refractory to oral antacids.

CONSTIPATION

Increased levels of sex steroid hormones during pregnancy are thought to produce decreases in smooth muscle motility and subsequent functional decreases in bowel motility. Moreover, the pressure exerted on the bowel by the expanded and displaced uterus is thought to interfere with normal peristaltic activity.

Management

Stressing good bowel care and bowel training is helpful. Nonpharmacologic methods of increasing bowel activity, such as increasing the fiber and roughage in the diet to maximize stool bulk, are also useful. Foods with laxative properties, such as prunes, figs, apples, and citrus fruits, may facilitate stool passage. The patient should take at least eight to 10 extra glasses of fluid a day; water is preferable, but non–caffeine-containing liquids are also acceptable. Increased exercise may help in the passage of stool. A bulk laxative, such as Metamucil, or a stool softener, such as Colace, should be prescribed, regardless of whether the natural roughage foods are effective. Mild laxatives may be given when all other measures are inadequate. Small doses of milk of magnesia and similar osmotic reactive laxatives

are useful. Small amounts of mineral oil may be cautiously administered; prolonged use of mineral oil can cause liver degeneration and interferes with the absorption of fat-soluble vitamins.

HEMORRHOIDS

Nearly 10% of obstetric patients have hemorrhoids at some point during their pregnancy.[153] The development of hemorrhoids during pregnancy results from the decreased motility and the tendency toward constipation that occur in all pregnancies. These changes lead to straining at stool, during which the shearing force generated in the rectal canal can exacerbate and intensify preexisting hemorrhoid disease. Furthermore, the weight and pressure of the uterus itself tends to decrease venous return and increase the amount of pooling in vascular structures in the lower pelvis.[154] Hemorrhoids can present with itching, bleeding, or severe pain if the hemorrhoids thrombose.

Management

The best method of preventing hemorrhoids is to maintain adequate bowel function; when that is not feasible, the following general measures should be taken:

1. Warm sitz baths
2. A local astringent, such as a Tucks pad or witch hazel
3. Supine positioning with the legs elevated whenever that is possible
4. Manual replacement of the hemorrhoids after each bowel movement, regardless of the pain incurred
5. Astringent suppositories or creams, such as Anusol or Anusol HC
6. Minimization of constipation (see above)

Acutely thrombosed hemorrhoids should be incised with the patient under local anesthesia; the clot should be evacuated, astringent ointments applied, and bowel care resumed. Injection with sclerosing agents is not advisable. The potential for submucosal abscess formation and pelvic sepsis, though small, makes the procedure extremely dangerous.

Surgery is seldom indicated. In a study of 12,455 pregnant women, only 25 required surgical excision of the symptomatic tissue, which was done under local anesthesia. There were no maternal or fetal problems as a result of the procedure.[155] On rare occasions, hemorrhoid banding [see V:19 Anal Procedures] may be indicated for excessive bleeding. It should be performed very carefully because of the potential for necrosis and infection.

VARICOSE VEINS

Varicosities become a problem with successive pregnancies. They are generally a minor nuisance in the primipara but become more bothersome the more children a woman has. Thrombophlebitis is not uncommon, but embolism is a rare complication. Varicose veins develop in women who are predisposed to this problem as a result of weakness in the valvular structures in the veins. The increased stasis and venous pressure created by the expansion of the uterus leads to progressive enlargement and engorgement of the veins. Besides cosmetic problems, varicosities can cause muscle aching, swelling, and, in severe cases, ulceration.

Management

Increased exercise that includes regular walking and activity is suggested. Elevation of the legs at rest is advised; prolonged sitting is not. Support stockings and, in poor weather, support panty hose should be used. The stockings should be placed on the legs in the early morning, before substantial pooling has occurred. Injection therapy is contraindicated during pregnancy. Ligation of veins causing ulceration or phlebitis is recommended only in extreme cases. Administration of aspirin or other NSAIDs is also contraindicated. If anticoagulation is necessary, heparin should be given because it does not cause fetal damage and is fairly easily controlled.

DEEP VEIN THROMBOSIS

Pregnant women are more prone to deep vein thrombosis (DVT) [see VI:2 Thromboembolic Problems] during the later stages of pregnancy and the early postpartum period, largely because of alterations in the normal blood coagulation system, such as increased levels of clotting factors and decreased fibrinolytic activity. These intrinsic factors may be exacerbated by the venous stasis and increased blood viscosity that occur during pregnancy. Compression of the iliac veins by the growing uterus also predisposes pregnant women to thrombosis. Although venous thrombosis affects only 4.1% of women during pregnancy,[156] recognition and management of the disorder are important to prevent the potentially life-threatening sequelae of pulmonary embolism.

Leg swelling and prominent superficial veins are common in pregnancy and may delay the diagnosis of DVT. Phlebography is the most accurate, operator-independent study available for confirmation of DVT. Because the iliofemoral system is the most common site of DVT, it is crucial that it be well visualized; however, this may not be possible with the fetus shielded. Serial impedance plethysmography may be effective in diagnosing DVT while eliminating exposure of the fetus to radiation.[157] Doppler ultrasonography is relatively ineffective in predicting isolated pelvic thrombosis but may be attempted. Real-time B-mode ultrasonography is an extremely sensitive examination that is useful in detecting DVT. This technique achieves good visualization of venous thrombi within vessels; however, although it can readily visualize clots in leg veins, it is less specific above the inguinal ligament. Noninvasive screening is not useful during pregnancy because of the high false positive and false negative rates; it is not uncommon for DVT to occur immediately after a screening examination. Any signs or symptoms of DVT or pulmonary embolism are an indication for aggressive testing.[156] Radioactive fibrinogen should not be used near term, because of the potential hazard to the fetal thyroid.

Management

When the diagnosis is made, therapy with a low-molecular-weight heparin (LMWH) should be instituted for the duration of pregnancy, with postpartum antiocoagulation, in the form of an LMWH or warfarin, continued for 6 weeks. LMWH doses should be adjusted according to weight and thus may increase throughout pregnancy and decrease after delivery. Unfractionated heparin can also be used during pregnancy. Current experience with LMWHs suggests that they are as efficacious and safe as unfractionated heparin.[158,159] In addition, LMWHs have certain advantages over unfractionated heparin: once-daily or twice-daily subcutaneous administration, a predictable dose response, reduced passage across the placenta, and lower incidences of heparin-induced thrombocytopenia and heparin-induced osteoporosis. Warfarin should not ordinarily be given for maintenance anticoagulation: it has teratogenic potential during the first trimester and may induce bleeding during the later part of pregnancy.[160]

Prophylaxis of DVT is recommended for subsequent pregnancies. For most women, 4 to 6 weeks of postpartum anticoagulation with an LMWH followed by warfarin is sufficient.[161,162] For patients who are at high risk for DVT because of inherited thrombophilia, DVT outside of pregnancy, multiple episodes of DVT, morbid obesity, or prolonged bed rest, prophylactic anticoagulation may be necessary both ante partum and post partum. When surgery is planned during pregnancy, patients should be fitted with graded compression boots beforehand and should continue to wear them until they are ambulating regularly. Ambulation should commence on the night of the operation whenever possible.

ROUND LIGAMENT PAIN

The general surgeon is occasionally asked to evaluate the pregnant woman in the late stages of her pregnancy with a possible inguinal hernia. Groin hernia in the pregnant patient is extremely uncommon because the expanded uterus acts as a shield against the abdominal wall, preventing incarceration or strangulation of bowel contents. Groin pain is generally caused by excessive traction on the round ligament, usually on the left, during the later part of pregnancy. As the uterus rotates and the patient's position changes, this pain can become quite severe.

Treatment

Local heat and abdominal support are the mainstays of treatment. Positional changes are necessary, and the patient should rest in the supine position.

References

1. National Vital Statistics Report, vol 49, no 1, April 17, 2001

2. Barron WM: The pregnant surgical patient: medical evaluation and management. Ann Intern Med 101:683, 1984

3. Hoff WS, D'Amelio LF, Tinkoff GH, et al: Maternal predictors of fetal demise in trauma during pregnancy. Surg Gynecol Obstet 172:175, 1991

4. Fildes J, Reed L, Jones N, et al: Trauma: the leading cause of maternal death. J Trauma 32:643, 1992

5. Pearlman MD, Tintinalli JE, Lorenz RP: Blunt trauma during pregnancy. N Engl J Med 323:1609, 1990

6. Hanlon D, Duriseti RS: Current concepts in the management of the pregnant trauma patient. Trauma Rep 2:3, 2001

7. Awwad JT, Azar GB, Seoud MA, et al: High-velocity penetrating wounds of the gravid uterus: review of 16 years of civil war. Obstet Gynecol 83:259, 1994

8. Crosby WM, Costiloe JP: Safety of the lap-restraint for pregnant victims of automobile collisions. N Engl J Med 24:78, 1971

9. Kuhlmann RS, Cruikshank DP: Maternal trauma during pregnancy. Clin Obstet Gynecol 37:274, 1994

10. Hill DA, Lense JJ: Abdominal trauma in the pregnant patient. Am Fam Physician 53:1269, 1996

11. Edwards RK, Bennett BB, Ripley DL, et al: Surgery in the pregnant patient. Curr Probl Surg 38:4, 2001

12. Hamberger LK, Ambuel B: Maternity care: spousal abuse in pregnancy. Clin Fam Pract 3:2, 2001

13. Campbell JC: Women's responses to sexual abuse in intimate relationships. Health Care Women Int 10:335, 1989

14. Hilliard PJA: Physical abuse in pregnancy. Obstet Gynecol 66:185, 1985

15. Abbott J: Domestic violence against women: incidence and prevalence in an emergency department population. JAMA 273:1763, 1995

16. Helton AS, Snodgrass FG: Battering during pregnancy: intervention strategies. Birth 14:3, 1987

17. Baker RN: Hemorrhage in obstetrics. Obstet Gynecol Annu 6:295, 1977

18. Drost TF, Rosemurgy AS, Sherman HF, et al: Major trauma in pregnant women: maternal/fetal outcome. J Trauma 30:574, 1990

19. Sorensen VJ, Bivins BA, Obeid FN, et al: Management of general surgical emergencies in pregnancy. Am Surg 56:245, 1990

20. Goodwin TM, Breen MT: Pregnancy outcome and fetomaternal hemorrhage after noncatastrophic trauma. Am J Obstet Gynecol 162:665, 1990

21. Stone IK: Trauma in the obstetric patient. Obstet Gynecol Clin 26:3, 1999

22. Pearlman MD, Tintinalli JE, Lorenz RP: A prospective controlled study of outcome after trauma during pregnancy. Am J Obstet Gynecol 162:1502, 1990

23. Gonik B: Intensive care monitoring of the critically ill pregnant patient. Maternal-Fetal Medicine. Creasy RK, Resnik R, Eds. WB Saunders Co, Philadelphia, 1989, p 867

24. Mazze A, Kalln B: Appendectomy during pregnancy: a Swedish registry study of 778 cases. Obstet Gynecol 77:835, 1991

25. Al-Mulhim AA: Acute appendicitis in pregnan-

cy: a review of 52 cases. Int Surg 81:295, 1996

26. Andersen B, Nielsen T: Appendicitis in pregnancy: diagnosis, management and complications. Acta Obstet Gynecol Scand 78:758, 1999

27. Squires RA: Surgical considerations in pregnancy. Audio Dig Gen Surg 45, 1998

28. Mourad J, Elliot JP, Erickson L, et al: Appendicitis in pregnancy: new information that contradicts long-held clinical beliefs. Am J Obstet Gynecol 182:5, 2000

29. Firstenberg MS, Malangoni MA: Pregnancy and gastrointestinal disorders: gastrointestinal surgery during pregnancy. Gastroenterol Clin 21:1, 1998

30. Lavin JP Jr, Polsky SS: Abdominal trauma during pregnancy. Clin Perinatol 10:423, 1983

31. Adams DH, Fine C, Brooks DC: High-resolution real-time ultrasonography: a new tool in the diagnosis of acute appendicitis. Am J Surg 155:93, 1988

32. Anderson JM, Lee TG, Nagel N: Ultrasound diagnosis of nonobstetric disease during pregnancy. Obstet Gynecol 48:359, 1976

33. Castro MA, Shipp TD, Castro EE, et al: The use of helical computed tomography in pregnancy for the diagnosis of acute appendicitis. Am J Obstet Gynecol 184:5, 2001

34. Pregnancy and medical radiation. Ann ICRP 30:1, 2000

35. Tamir IL, Bongard FS, Klein SR: Acute appendicitis in the pregnant patient. Am J Surg 160:571, 1990

36. Loughlin KR, Bailey RB Jr: Internal ureteral stents for conservative management of ureteral calculi during pregnancy. N Engl J Med 315:1647, 1986

37. Kavoussi LR, Albala DM, Basler JW, et al: Percutaneous management of urolithiasis during pregnancy (pt 2). J Urol 148:1069, 1992

38. Horowitz MD, Gomez GA, Santiesteban R, et al: Acute appendicitis during pregnancy: diagnosis and management. Arch Surg 120:1362, 1985

39. McComb P, Laimon H: Appendicitis complicating pregnancy. Can J Surg 23:92, 1980

40. Hee P, Viktrup L: The diagnosis of appendicitis during pregnancy and maternal and fetal outcome after appendectomy. Int J Gynaecol Obstet 65:129, 1999

41. Masters K, Levine BA, Gaskill HV, et al: Diagnosing appendicitis during pregnancy. Am J Surg 148:768, 1984

42. Curet MJ, Allen D, Josloff RK, et al: Laparoscopy during pregnancy. Arch Surg 131:546, 1996

43. Connolly MM, Unti JA, Nora PF: Bowel obstruction in pregnancy. Surg Clin North Am 75:101, 1995

44. de Paul M, Tew WL, Holiday RL: Perforated peptic ulcer in pregnancy with survival of mother and child: case report and review of the literature. Can J Surg 19:427, 1976

45. Perdue PW, Johnson HW, Stafford PW: Intestinal obstruction complicating pregnancy. Am J Surg 164:384, 1992

46. Milne B, Johnstone MS: Intestinal obstruction in pregnancy. Scott Med J 24:80, 1979

47. Ballantyne GH: Review of surgical volvulus: clinical patterns and pathogenesis. Dis Colon Rectum 25:494, 1985

48. Shaxted EJ, Jukes R: Pseudo-obstruction of the bowel in pregnancy: case reports. Br J Obstet Gynaecol 86:411, 1979

49. Ibrahim N, Payne E, Owen A: Spontaneous rupture of the liver in association with pregnancy. Br

J Obstet Gynaecol 92:539, 1985

50. Hunter SK, Martin M, Benda JA, et al: Liver transplant after massive spontaneous hepatic rupture in pregnancy complicated by preeclampsia. Obstet Gynecol 85:819, 1995

51. Hwang SS, Park YH, Jung YJ: Spontaneous rupture of hydronephrotic kidney during pregnancy: value of serial sonography. J Clin Ultrasound 28:7, 2000

52. Barton JR, Sibai BM: HELLP and the liver diseases of preeclampsia. Clin Liver Dis 3:1, 1999

53. Henny CP, Lim AE, Brummelkamp WH, et al: A review of the importance of acute multidisciplinary treatment following spontaneous rupture of the liver capsule during pregnancy. Surg Gynecol Obstet 156:593, 1983

54. Braverman DZ, Johnson ML, Kern F Jr: Effects of pregnancy and contraceptive steroids on gallbladder function. N Engl J Med 302:362, 1980

55. Wilkinson EJ: Acute pancreatitis in pregnancy: a review of 98 cases and a report of 8 new cases. Obstet Gynecol Surv 28:281, 1973

56. Yates MR, Baron TH: Biliary tract disease in pregnancy. Clin Liver Dis 3:1, 1999

57. Everson GT, McKinley C, Kern F: Mechanisms of gallstone formation in women: effects of exogenous estrogen (Premarin) and dietary cholesterol on hepatic lipid metabolism. J Clin Invest 87:237, 1991

58. Tierney S, Nakeeb A: Progesterone alters biliary flow dynamics. Ann Surg 229:2, 1999

59. Ryan JP: Effect of pregnancy on gallbladder contractility in guinea pig. Gastroenterology 87:674, 1984

60. Kern F Jr, Everson GT, DeMark B, et al: Biliary lipids, bile acids, and gallbladder function in the human female: effects of pregnancy and the ovulatory cycle. J Clin Invest 68:1229, 1981

61. Valdivieso V, Covarrubias C, Siegel F, et al: Pregnancy and cholelithiasis: pathogenesis and natural course of gallstones diagnosed in early puerperium. Hepatology 17:1, 1993

62. Basso L, McCollum PT, Darling MRN, et al: A study of cholelithiasis during pregnancy and its relationship with age, parity, menarche, breastfeeding, dysmenorrhea, oral contraception and a maternal history of cholelithiasis. Surg Gynecol Obstet 175:41, 1992

63. Glenn F, McSherry CK: Gallstones and pregnancy among 300 young women treated by cholecystectomy. Surg Gynecol Obstet 127:1067, 1968

64. Ramin KD, Ramsey PS. Medical complications of pregnancy: disease of the gall bladder and pancreas in preganacy. Obstet Gynecol Clin 28:3, 2001

65. Woodhouse DR, Haylen B: Gall bladder disease complicating pregnancy. Aust NZ J Obstet Gynaecol 25:233, 1985

66. Bynum TE: Hepatic and gastrointestinal disorders in pregnancy. Med Clin North Am 61:129, 1977

67. Cheng YS: Pregnancy in liver cirrhosis and/or portal hypertension. Am J Obstet Gynecol 128:812, 1977

68. Seymour CA, Chadwick VS: Liver and gastrointestinal function in pregnancy. Postgrad Med J 55:343, 1979

69. Landerd D, Carmona R, Cromblehome W: Acute cholecystitis in pregnancy. Obstet Gynecol 69:131, 1987

70. McKellar DP, Anderson CT, Boynton CJ: Cholecystectomy during pregnancy without fetal loss. Surg Obstet Gynecol 174:465, 1992

71. Dixon NP, Faddis DM, Silberman H: Aggressive management of cholecystitis during pregnancy.

Am J Surg 154:292, 1987

72. Curet MJ: Special problems in laparoscopic surgery: previous abdominal surgery, obesity and pregnancy. Surg Clin North Am 80:4, 2000

73. Printen KJ, Ott RA: Cholecystectomy during pregnancy. Am Surg 44:432, 1978

74. Affleck DG, Handrahan DL, Egger MJ, et al: The laparoscopic management of appendicitis and cholelithiasis during pregnancy. Am J Surg 178:6, 1999

75. Gouldman JW, Sticca RP, Rippon MB, et al: Laparoscopic cholecystectomy in pregnancy. Am Surg 64:93, 1998

76. Lanzafame RJ: Laparoscopic cholecystectomy during pregnancy. Surgery 118:627, 1995

77. Morrell DG, Mullins JR, Harrison PB: Laparoscopic cholecystectomy during pregnancy in symptomatic patients. Surgery 112:856, 1992

78. Soper NJ, Hunter JG, Petrie RH: Laparoscopic cholecystectomy during pregnancy. Surg Endosc 6:115, 1992

79. Weber AM, Bloom GP, Allen TR, et al: Laparoscopic cholecystectomy during pregnancy. Obstet Gynecol 78: 958, 1991

80. Baillie J, et al: Endoscopic management of choledocholithiasis during pregnancy. Surg Gynecol Obstet 171:1, 1990

81. Strasberg SM: Laparoscopic biliary surgery. Gastroenterol Clin 28:1, 1999

82. Hunt CM, Sharara AI: Liver disease in pregnancy. Am Fam Phys 59:4, 1999

83. McKay AJ, O'Neill J, Imrie CW: Pancreatitis, pregnancy and gallstones. Br J Obstet Gynaecol 87:47, 1980

84. Glueck CJ, Christopher C, Mishkel MA, et al: Pancreatitis, familial hypertriglyceridemia, and pregnancy. Am J Obstet Gynecol 136:755, 1980

85. Thomason JL, Sampson MB, Farb HF, et al: Pregnancy complicated by concurrent primary hyperparathyroidism and pancreatitis. Obstet Gynecol 57(suppl 6):34S, 1981

86. Young KR: Acute pancreatitis in pregnancy: two case reports. Obstet Gynecol 60:653, 1982

87. Hasselgren PO: Acute pancreatitis in pregnancy: report of two cases. Acta Chir Scand 146:297, 1980

88. Jouppila P, Mokka R, Larmi TK: Acute pancreatitis in pregnancy. Surg Gynecol Obstet 139:879, 1974

89. Strickland DM, Hauth JC, Widish J, et al: Amylase and isoamylase activities in serum of pregnant women. Obstet Gynecol 63:389, 1984

90. Dreiling DA, Bordalo O, Rosenberg V, et al: Pregnancy and pancreatitis. Am J Gastroenterol 64:23, 1975

91. Gineston JL, Capron JP, Delcenserie R, et al: Prolonged total parenteral nutrition in a pregnant woman with acute pancreatitis. J Clin Gastroenterol 6:249, 1984

92. Hiatt JR, Hiatt JC, Williams RA, et al: Biliary disease in pregnancy: strategy for surgical management. Am J Surg 151:263, 1986

93. Vonherzen J, Noe J, Goodlin R: Pancreatitis pseudocyst complicating pregnancy. Obstet Gynecol 45:588, 1975

94. Winbery SL, Blaho KE. Dyspepsia in pregnancy. Obstet Gynecol Clin 28:2, 2001

95. Cappell MS, Garcia A: Gastric and duodenal ulcers during pregnancy. Gastroenterol Clin North Am 27:169, 1998

96. Mogadam M, Korelitz BI, Ahmed SW, et al: The course of inflammatory bowel disease during pregnancy and postpartum. Am J Gastroenterol 75:265, 1981

97. Nielsen OH, Andreasson B, Bondesen S, et al: Pregnancy in Crohn's disease. Scand J Gastroenterol 19:724, 1984

98. Vender RJ, Spiro HM: Inflammatory bowel disease and pregnancy. J Clin Gastroenterol 4:231, 1982

99. Baiocco PJ, Korelitz BI: The influence of inflammatory bowel disease and its treatment on pregnancy and fetal outcome. J Clin Gastroenterol 6:211, 1984

100. Woolfson K, Cohen Z, McLeod RS: Crohn's disease and pregnancy. Dis Colon Rectum 33:869, 1990

101. Warsof SL: Medical and surgical treatment of inflammatory bowel disease in pregnancy. Clin Obstet Gynecol 26:822, 1983

102. Mogadam M, Dobbins WO III, Korelitz BI, et al: Pregnancy in inflammatory bowel disease: effect of sulfasalazine and corticosteroids on fetal outcome. Gastroenterology 80:72, 1981

103. Witter FR, King TM, Blake DA: The effects of chronic gastrointestinal medication on the fetus and neonate. Obstet Gynecol 58(suppl 5):79S, 1981

104. Jacobson LB, Clapp DH: Total parenteral nutrition in pregnancy complicated by Crohn's disease. JPEN J Parent Enteral Nutr 11:93, 1987

105. Rivera-Alsina ME, Saldana LR, Stringer CA: Fetal growth sustained by parenteral nutrition in pregnancy. Obstet Gynecol 64:138, 1984

106. Wise RA, Polito AJ: Asthma and allergy during pregnancy, respiratory physiology changes in pregnancy. Immunol Allergy Clin North Am 20:4, 2000

107. Edwards RK, Bennett BB, Ripley DL, et al: Surgery in the pregnant patient. Curr Probl Surg 38:4, 2001

108. Sherwood OD, Downing SJ, Guico-Lamm ML, et al: The physiological effects of relaxin during pregnancy: studies in rats and pigs. Oxf Rev Reprod Biol 15:143, 1993

109. Clark SL, Cotton DB, Lee W, et al: Central hemodynamic assessment of normal term pregnancy. Am J Obstet Gynecol 161:1439, 1989

110. Stein PK, Hagley MT, Cole PL, et al: Changes in 24-hour heart rate variability during normal pregnancy. Am J Obstet Gynecol 180:4, 1999

111. Katz R, Karliner J, Resnik R: Effects of a natural volume overload state (pregnancy) on left ventricular performance in normal human subjects. Circulation 48:434, 1978

112. Thilen U, Olsson SB: Pregnancy and heart disease: a review. Obstet Gynecol 75:43, 1997

113. Obstetrics: Normal and Problem Pregnancies, 3rd ed. Gabbe SG, Niebyl JR, Simpson JL, Eds. London, Churchill Livingstone, 1996, p 92

114. Fagan EA: Cholestasis: intrahepatic cholestasis of pregnancy. Clin Liver Dis 3:3, 1999

115. Sanders CL, Lucas MJ: Medical complications of pregnancy: renal disease in pregnancy. Obstet Gynecol Clin 28:3, 2001

116. Fried A, Woodring JH, Thompson TJ: Hydronephrosis of pregnancy. J Ultrasound Med 2:225, 1983

117. Deitcher SR, Gardner JF: Pregnancy and liver disease: physiologic changes in coagulation and fibrinolysis during normal pregnancy. Clin Liver Dis 3:1, 1999

118. Martin C, Varner MW: Physiologic changes in pregnancy: surgical implications. Clin Obstet Gynecol 37:241, 1994

119. Heinly TL, Leiberman P: Asthma and allergy during pregnancy: anaphylaxis in pregnancy. Immunol Allergy Clin North Am 20:4, 2000

120. Czeizel AE, Pataki T, Rockenbauer M: Reproductive outcome after exposure to surgery under anesthesia during pregnancy. Arch Gynecol Obstet 261:193, 1998

121. Rosen MA, Weiskopf RB: Management of anes-

thesia for the pregnant surgical patient. Anesthesiology 91:4, 1999

122. Parer JT, King T: Fetal heart rate monitoring: is it salvageable? Am J Obstet Gynecol 182:982, 2000

123. Timins JK: Radiation during pregnancy. NJ Med 98:29, 2001

124. Ezri T, Szmuk P, Evron S, et al: Difficult airway in obstetric anesthesia: a review. Obstet Gynecol Surv 56:631, 2001

125. Fatum M, Rojansky N: Laparoscopic surgery during pregnancy. Obstet Gynecol Surv 56:50, 2001

126. Shay DC, Bhavani-Shankar K, Datta S: Laparoscopic surgery during pregnancy. Anesthesiol Clin North Am 19:57, 2001

127. Steinbrook RA, Brooks DC, Datta S: Laparoscopic cholecystectomy during pregnancy: review of anesthetic management, surgical considerations. Surg Endosc 10:511, 1996

128. Hunter J, Swanstrom L, Thornburgh K: Carbon dioxide pneumoperitoneum induces fetal acidosis in a preganat ewe model. Surg Endosc 9:272, 1995

129. Curet MJ, Vogt DM, Schob O, et al: Effects of CO_2 pneumoperitoneum in pregnant ewes. J Surg Res 63:1, 1996

130. Reedy MB, Galan HL, Richards WE, et al: Laparoscopy during pregnancy: a survey of laparoendoscopic surgeons. J Reprod Med 42:33, 1997

131. Bhavani-Shankar K, Steinbrook RA, Brooks DC, et al: Arterial to end-tidal carbon dioxide pressure difference during laparoscopic surgery in pregnancy. Anesthesiology 93:370, 2000

132. Sharp HT: Gastrointestinal surgical conditions during pregnancy. Clin Obstet Gynecol 37:306, 1994

133. Parry AJ, Westaby S: Cardiopulmonary bypass during pregnancy. Ann Thorac Surg 61:1865, 1996

134. Weiss BM, von Segesser LK, Alon E, et al: Outcome of cardiovascular surgery and pregnancy: a systematic review of the period 1984-1996. Am J Obstet Gynecol 179:6, 1998

135. Pomini F, Mercogliano D, Cavalletti C, et al: Cardiopulmonary bypass in pregnancy. Ann Thorac Surg 61:259, 1996

136. Gei AF, Hankins GDV: Medical complications of pregnancy: cardiac disease and pregnancy. Obstet Gynecol Clin 28:3, 2001

137. Vaska PL: Cardiac surgery in special populations, part 2: women, pregnant patients, and Jehovah's Witnesses. AACN Clinical Issues 8:1, 1997

138. Birincioglu CL, Kucuker SA, Yapar EG, et al: Perinatal mitral valve interventions: a report of 10 cases. Ann Thorac Surg 67:1312, 1999

139. Zeebregts CJ, Schepens MA, Hameeterman TM, et al: Acute aortic dissection complicating pregnancy. 64:1345, 1997

140. Hillemanns P, Knitza R, Muller-Hocker J: Rupture of splenic artery aneurysm in a pregnant patient with portal hypertension. Am J Obstet Gynecol 174:1665, 1996

141. Merbeck M, Horbach T, Putzenlachner C: Ruptured splenic artery aneurysm during pregnancy: a rare case with both maternal and fetal survival. Am J Obstet Gynecol 181:3, 1999

142. Henke PK, Cardneau JD, Welling TH, et al: Renal artery aneurysms. Ann Surg 234:4, 2001

143. Resnik R: Cancer during pregnancy. N Engl J Med 341:120, 1999

144. Smith LH, Dalrymple JL, Leiserowitz GS, et al: Obstetrical deliveries with maternal malignancy in California, 1992 through 1997. Am J Obstet Gynecol 184:7, 2001

145. Catlin EA, Roberts JD Jr, Erana R, et al:

Transplacental transmission of natural-killer-cell lymphoma. N Engl J Med 341:85, 1999

146. Dildy GA III, Moise KJ Jr, Carpenter RJ Jr, et al: Maternal malignancy metastatic to the products of conception: a review. Obstet Gynecol Surv 44:535, 1989

147. Ebert U, Loffler H, Kirch W: Cytotoxic therapy and pregnancy. Pharmacol Ther 74:207, 1997

148. Gemignani ML, Petrek JA, Borgen PI. Breast cancer and pregnancy. Surg Clin North Am 79:5, 1999

149. Barnavon Y, Wallack MK: Management of the pregnancy patient with carcinoma of the breast. Surg Gynecol Obstet 171:347, 1990

150. Rode H, Millar AJ, Cywes S, et al: Thermal injury in pregnancy: the neglected tragedy. S Afr Med J 77:346, 1990

151. Prentice-Bjerkeseth R: Perioperative anesthetic management of trauma in pregnancy. Anesthesiol Clin North Am 17:1, 1999

152. Hey VM, Cowley DJ, Ganguli PC, et al: Gastrooesophageal reflux in late pregnancy. Anaesthesia 32:372, 1977

153. Medich DS, Fazio VW: Hemorrhoids, anal fissure and carcinoma of the colon rectum and anus during pregnancy. Surg Clin North Am 75:77, 1995

154. Hulme-Moir M, Bartolo DC: Hemorrhoids. Gastroenterol Clin 30:1, 2001

155. Saleeby RG Jr, Rosen L, Stasik JJ, et al: Hemorrhoidectomy during pregnancy: risk or relief? Dis Colon Rectum 34:260, 1991

156. Ginsberg JS, Greer I, Hirsh J: Use of antithrombotic agents during pregnancy: sixth ACCP Consensus conference on antithrombotic therapy. Chest 169:122S, 2001

157. Hull RD, Raskob GE, Carter CJ: Serial impedance plethysmography in pregnant patients with clinically suspected deep-vein thrombosis. Ann Intern Med 112:663, 1990

158. Ginsberg JS, Hirsh J, Turner CD, et al: Risks to the fetus of anticoagulant therapy during pregnancy. Thromb Haemost 61:197, 1989

159. Sanson BJ, Lensing AWA, Prins MH, et al: Safety of low-molecular-weight heparin in pregnancy: a systematic review. Thromb Haemost 81:668, 1999

160. Ginsberg JS, Hirsh J: Anticoagulants during pregnancy. Annu Rev Med 40:79, 1989

161. Bolan JC: Thromboembolic complications of pregnancy. Clin Obstet Gynecol 26:913, 1983

162. Brill-Edwards P, Ginsberg JS: Safety of withholding antepartum heparin in women with a previous episode of venous thromboembolism. The Recurrence Of Clot In This Pregnancy (ROCIT) Study Group. N Engl J Med 343:20, 2000

163. MacBurney MM, Wilmore DW: Parenteral nutrition in pregnancy. Parenteral Nutrition. Rombeau JL, Caldwell M, Eds. WB Saunders Co, Philadelphia, 1986

164. Rosenthal MH: Intrapartum intensive care management of the cardiac patient. Clin Obstet Gynecol 24:789, 1981

165. Dashe JS, Gilstrap LC: Antibiotic use in pregnancy. Obstet Gynecol Clin North Am 24:617, 1997

166. Murray L, Seger D: Drug therapy during pregnancy and lactation. Emerg Med Clin North Am 12:129, 1994

Acknowledgment

Figure 1   Carol Donner.

10 CLINICAL AND LABORATORY DIAGNOSIS OF INFECTION

David C. Evans, M.D., and Jonathan L. Meakins, M.D., D.Sc.

Approach to Diagnosis of Surgical Infection

The presence of surgical infectious disease is determined clinically, usually with confirmation and microbiologic diagnosis provided by the laboratory. Identification of an infection is rarely incidental; usually, it is a response to a clinical *signal*. This signal is often fever but may be one of a number of other symptoms and signs or some combination thereof.

Most surgical infections are outpatient conditions that are easily diagnosed and treated. Infections in hospitalized patients, whether related to the primary surgical disease or resulting from surgical therapy, are less easily managed. The greatest challenges in diagnosis and treatment of surgical infections arise in the perioperative and postoperative periods.

Infection versus Sepsis

Before the advent of surgical critical care units, the definitions of a number of key concepts—infection, sepsis, bacteremia, septicemia, septic shock, endotoxemia—were either treated as interchangeable or, if not interchangeable, considered to be of interest primarily to academics with a research orientation. However, as diagnostic possibilities have expanded and our ability to resuscitate and support critically ill patients has improved, classic clinical problems have evolved into new and more complex problems that call for new definitions—especially for the fundamental concepts of infection and sepsis[1] [*see Sidebar* Definitions of Key Concepts]. The crucial point is that infection and sepsis are conceptually distinct: infection is a process, and sepsis is the response to that process. The response provides the clinical signals that lead to diagnosis of the initiating process. As a rule, infection, once diagnosed, is easily treated with antibiotics and drainage. It is the management of sepsis that is difficult [*see VII:7 Multiple Organ Dysfunction Syndrome*].

Normally Responsive versus Compromised or Complex Patients

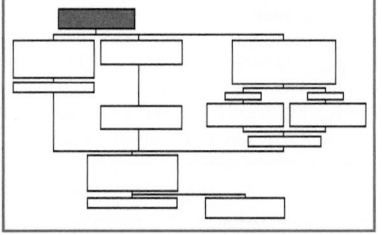

The fact that signs and symptoms of infection in compromised or complex patients differ from those in normally responsive hosts has important diagnostic implications. The normally responsive patient, for whom the physician can obtain a history and perform a physical examination, responds to infection in the classic manner—that is, with fever, elevated white blood cell count, malaise, and other appropriate symptoms. If infection is severe, a normally responsive patient may become compromised. The compromised or complex patient is unable to meet inflammatory or infectious challenges in the normal manner [*see VI:6 Non-AIDS Immunosuppression*]. The clinical response to infection is altered in such a patient: the signals of infection differ from those in the normally responsive patient and often develop at a later stage of infection. A multitude of clinical conditions or physiologic states are represented by compromised or complex patients, who include elderly patients, patients who are immunosuppressed as a result of either disease or medications, patients with thermal injury or major trauma, patients receiving chemotherapy, patients receiving treatment for stable degrees of end-organ failure in intensive care units, and patients with more than one chronic disease. The prevalence of such patients in modern hospital surgical practice is increasing.

The normally responsive patient and the compromised or complex patient are merely extreme points on the clinical spectrum rather than categorically distinct populations.

General Approach to Clinical and Laboratory Diagnosis of Infection

The search for an infection is initiated in response to a clinical signal indicating a problem that requires resolution [*see Table 1*]. The

---

Definitions of Key Concepts

For the purposes of the present discussion, infection, bacteremia, sepsis, severe sepsis, and septic shock will be defined as follows[1]:

- Infection is a microbial phenomenon characterized by an inflammatory response to the presence of microorganisms or the invasion of normally sterile host tissue by these organisms.
- Bacteremia is the presence of viable bacteria in the blood.
- Sepsis is the systemic response to infection. This response is manifested by the occurrence of two or more of the following conditions as a result of infection: (a) temperature higher than 38° C or lower than 36° C, (b) heart rate greater than 90 beats/min, (c) respiratory rate greater than 20 breaths/min or arterial carbon dioxide tension less than 32 mm Hg, and (d) white blood cell count greater than 12,000/ mm^3 or less than 4,000/mm^3, or immature (band) forms accounting for more than 10% of the neutrophils present.
- Severe sepsis is sepsis associated with organ dysfunction, hypoperfusion, or hypotension. Hypoperfusion and perfusion abnormalities may include, but are not limited to, lactic acidosis, oliguria, or acute alteration of mental status.
- Septic shock is sepsis with hypotension, occurring despite adequate fluid resuscitation, along with the presence of perfusion abnormalities that may include, but are not limited to, lactic acidosis, oliguria, or acute alteration of mental status. Patients receiving inotropes or vasopressors may not be hypotensive at the time when perfusion abnormalities are measured.

Approach to Diagnosis of Surgical Infection

Clinical signals of infection in compromised or complex patients differ from those in normally responsive patients

The clinical signal is often fever but may be one of several other symptoms and signs or a combination thereof.

Infection in normally responsive patients usually presents with appropriate signals

Cardinal signs of inflammation are
• Redness • Heat • Pain • Swelling • Loss of function
Other appropriate signals include
• Fever (≥ 38° C) appearing after normal postoperative T° elevation has resolved
• ↑ WBC
• Infectious syndrome (manifested by failure to thrive, unexplained anorexia, and indefinably unsatisfactory clinical course)

Septic shock may be the first signal of infection

Manifestations include tachycardia; tachypnea; hypotension; warm, dry extremities; generalized flushing; other signs of a hyperdynamic, hypermetabolic state.

Diagnosis and therapy should proceed concurrently.

Presence and location of infection (first suggested by clinical findings) are confirmed by directed laboratory assessment

---

Empirical antibiotic therapy is always instituted before diagnosis is completed

Efficacy of empirical antibiotic therapy is assessed on the basis of the patient's clinical course; empirical antibiotic therapy is modified or discontinued accordingly.

General approach to diagnosis of infection

Begin with history and physical examination.

Perform laboratory assessment:
• Obtain Gram's stain and cultures of wound tissue, sputum, urine, and drainage effluent.
• Consider percutaneous aspiration and microbiologic examination of potentially infected fluid.
• Obtain WBC and blood chemistry measurements.
• Obtain chest x-ray; consider ultrasonography or CT scan of operative site.

In normally responsive patients, specific therapy is started on the basis of diagnosis

Infection in compromised or complex patients is often occult

Risk factors include
- Advanced age
- Thermal injury
- Major trauma
- Chemotherapy
- End-organ failure
- Presence of more than one chronic disease

Infection may be clinically manifested by
- Confusion
- Hypotension
- Ileus
- Water retention
- Gastric bleeding
- Delayed wound healing

Fever may or may not be present or related to infection.

Laboratory signs of occult infection include
- Renal, hepatic, or respiratory dysfunction
- Thrombocytopenia
- Hyperglycemia and insulin resistance
- Immune failure

Sepsis is mild to moderate

Empirical antibiotic therapy is sometimes instituted before diagnosis

Efficacy of empirical antibiotic therapy is assessed on the basis of the patient's clinical course; empirical antibiotic therapy is modified accordingly.

Sepsis is severe

Empirical antibiotic therapy is often instituted before diagnosis

Efficacy of empirical antibiotic therapy is assessed on the basis of the patient's clinical course; empirical antibiotic therapy is modified accordingly.

Presence and location of infection must be determined by laboratory tests, with clinical support

---

No infection present

Stop antibiotics. Maintain hemostasis and provide hemodynamic, nutritional, and physiologic support. Search for noninfectious causes of septic response. Support and wait.

Table 1 Fundamental Approach to Diagnosis of Infection

Recognize clinical signal and observe its characteristics:
- Nature
- Intensity
- Rapidity of development

Make best guess as to source and likely pathogen on the basis of
- History of surgical disease
- Physical examination
- Microbiologic examination of stained specimens
- Radiologic findings

Confirm presence of infection by means of
- Laboratory results
- Observation of clinical course
- Invasive procedures (e.g., paracentesis, thoracentesis, interventional radiology, operation)

---

signal represents the response of a patient to an infection and is a function of the patient's ability to react to the liberated stimuli and mediators and to generate a clinical response to the infectious process. All patients may exhibit one or more of these signals. Normally responsive patients tend to show the classic signals, whereas compromised or complex patients tend to show more subtle changes that often are first noted in the course of routine laboratory tests.

Simply stated, the proper approach to diagnosis in a patient with probable infection begins with a thorough history and physical examination followed by directed, specific laboratory tests. The details of the approach must be modified according to patient characteristics and the circumstances of presentation. For example, if a patient has undergone operation or is in the ICU, the list of possibilities to be considered must be modified, and the time allotted to diagnosis must be reduced.

Infection in Normally Responsive Patients

CARDINAL SIGNS OF INFLAMMATION

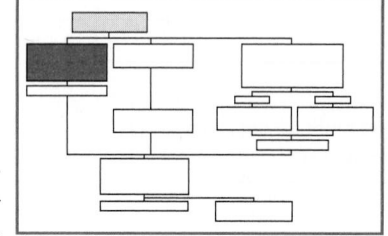

Rubor, calor, dolor, tumor, and functio laesa—that is, redness, heat, pain, swelling, and loss of function—have been considered the cardinal signs of inflammation since the times of Hippocrates and Galen. They remain the primary signals leading to medical consultation for outpatient surgical infections and for many of the infectious complications of operation. They represent the host response to infection and may signal the presence of infection even in cases in which the primary site of infection is a deeply situated organ or tissue. These cardinal signs are clinical manifestations of the infection and its accompanying inflammatory process; they either identify the process or guide the investigation. In the hospital setting, such signs, when present, are important clues to the existence of infection. Often, however, nosocomial infections are signaled in more subtle ways.

FEVER

Fever is the most important and the most common signal that an infectious process is present [see VII:10 Fever, Hyperpyrexia, and Hypothermia]. Postoperative fever is a normal part of the recovery process; understanding the typical febrile course is important in dif-

ferentiating normal from pathologic fever. It is unusual for a sudden, very high fever to be the first signal of an infection. The infection usually begins to manifest itself with a prodrome, recognition of which speeds diagnosis and therapy. Investigation should be started when the patient's temperature reaches 38° C (100.4° F) rather than 40° C (104° F). Although this point may seem obvious, many of the crisis intervention measures required in managing fevers could be avoided if the significance of more modest temperature elevations were recognized more often.

A fever that appears after the normal postoperative temperature elevation has resolved must not be ignored. To simply wait for such a fever to go away is to court disaster. Complete physical examination of the patient and, in the absence of a diagnosis, directed laboratory tests, followed by reexamination as necessary, are required to determine the nature and severity of the problem.

MISCELLANEOUS SIGNALS

A variety of signals reflect a patient status between normal responsiveness and significant compromise. Many of these signals are soft; moreover, they can sometimes be attributed to patient anxiety, neurosis, or a wish to stay longer in the hospital. In the light of current changes in the hospital population (e.g., increased numbers of elderly patients and patients with multiple medical problems or degrees of organ dysfunction), however, these signals should be considered seriously because in compromised patients, each one can be a harbinger of infection.

Altered Heart Rate

A heart rate that is either too high or too low may signal an infection. On rare occasions, changes in rhythm in the elderly (e.g., paroxysmal atrial tachycardia, atrial flutter, or fibrillation) are indicators of an infectious process. An unexplained sustained increase in pulse rate should not be ignored.

Tachypnea

Tachypnea should be recognized as part of either the prodrome or the infectious syndrome itself. Because it may herald other important diagnoses—pulmonary embolus, for example—tachypnea should not be overlooked.

Pain

Pain that persists or is out of proportion to the expected response deserves attention. Infection is only one of the many possible causes of pain. Often, the pain is referred, and the painful area appears normal on examination. Pneumonia that presents with abdominal findings is a classic example, as is a subphrenic abscess that presents with shoulder-tip pain and a normal range of motion.

Confusion

Confusion may be the most common symptom of infection in the elderly; it is also an important signal in patients who had been well and fit. The physician's first response to confusion in an elderly patient in the postoperative period must be to seek a cause, not to order sedation.

Ileus

Ileus has many causes, some of which are not well understood. Prolonged ileus after abdominal operation—as well as almost any ileus after other operations—requires explanation. Infections at remote sites can produce ileus, as if the bowel were a target organ such as the kidney, liver, or lung. Wound infection and pneumonia are common examples of such infections.

THE INFECTIOUS SYNDROME

The normal response to infection includes what might be best described as a flulike syndrome: general malaise, headache, myalgias, fatigue, and loss of appetite. This syndrome is most often seen in outpatients or patients who have not undergone operation.

In hospitalized patients, particularly patients in the postoperative period, the infectious syndrome will be manifest in the form of failure to thrive, unexplained loss of appetite, and an indefinably unsatisfactory clinical course. These symptoms are so-called soft symptoms; that is, they are hard to recognize. In the current health care environment, characterized by adherence to the diagnosis-related group (DRG) system and growing pressure to shorten hospital stays, these symptoms are often not taken seriously.

Infection in Compromised or Complex Patients

The presence of fever remains a common signal of infection in the compromised or complex patient; however, it may be absent, or the patient's temperature may already be elevated as a result of other causes. Cardinal signs of infection, such as decubitus ulcers, may be present. More often, however, the infection is occult, and classic signals are unrelated to the infectious focus. In some very ill immunocompromised patients, findings that usually signal an infection may already be present. Slight changes in clinical status (such as very small temperature elevations, increased fluid requirements, confusion, or ileus) or changes in laboratory findings (such as an elevated white blood cell count, glucosuria, or hyperglycemia) should trigger investigation.

Patients in whom the first signal of an infectious process is organ dysfunction or failure are more ill than patients in whom high fever is the first signal; perhaps more important, however, is that they are a group whose diagnosis and management require more than standard clinical skills. Because the classic septic response may not be present, it is essential to be alert to the signs and symptoms of occult infection (see below). In these patients, the laboratory becomes increasingly important in diagnosing and understanding the evolution of the infection.

CLINICAL SIGNS AND SYMPTOMS OF OCCULT INFECTION

Subtle changes in temperature, mental status, pulse rate, or respiratory rate may signal occult infection, as may the development of pain or ileus.

Intermittent Hypotension and Septic Shock

Septic shock, an important signal of an unrecognized or occult focus of infection, is the original expression of multisystem failure, but it rarely occurs without warning. The prodrome often includes fever and, perhaps, one or two other signals. Intermittent hypotension is the most characteristic signal. It is not catastrophic and responds quickly to fluid resuscitation. Characteristically, it recurs, at which time it may again respond to fluids. Oliguria may accompany the hypotension. If this clinical picture is allowed to progress, the hypotension will lead to renal failure (see below), with a substantial amount of water retention. Septic shock will result if the infection is not identified, treated with antibiotics, and, if necessary, drained.

Both clinical assessment and laboratory studies are necessary to confirm the presence of septic shock, although florid septic shock is easily recognized on clinical examination alone [see I:4 Shock]. Any or all of the following findings may be present in varying degrees in the patient with septic shock: tachycardia; tachypnea; hypotension; warm, dry extremities; generalized flushing; and other signs suggesting a hyperdynamic, hypermetabolic state. Swan-Ganz catheter measurements confirm high cardiac output and low peripheral resistance.

Gastric Hemorrhage

Gastric hemorrhage may be the presenting symptom for serious infection even if prophylactic measures against such hemorrhage have been taken. Gastric acidity and bleeding respond to drainage of an abscess. Hemorrhagic gastritis must be considered a signal of occult infection, which demands prompt diagnosis and treatment.

Delayed Wound Healing

The absence of wound healing can indicate the presence of a significant infection. Typically in such a case, wounds left for delayed primary closure or secondary closure do not exhibit the appropriate granulation tissue and appear pale, dry, and unhealthy. The development of good granulation tissue is a sign that infection is controlled.

LABORATORY SIGNS OF OCCULT INFECTION

Renal Failure

Renal failure is identified by elevations in serum creatinine and blood urea nitrogen (BUN) levels, which can be highly sensitive signals of developing infection. A still more sensitive indicator is an alteration in creatinine clearance, a laboratory test underutilized in the ICU. Such alterations are generally evident before changes in serum levels. Creatinine clearance should be measured at an early stage in high-risk patients. In the presence of shock, renal failure can develop suddenly. Otherwise, loss of renal function is insidious, but it can usually be identified if sought before oliguria or anuria develops. Resolution of infection is associated with return of function.

Hepatic and Respiratory Failure

Hepatic failure, primarily manifested as jaundice, and respiratory failure, initially presenting as a falling arterial oxygen tension and subsequently marked by a need for mechanical ventilation or by a change in the fraction of inspired oxygen (F_IO_2) requirements, can behave in the same way as renal failure (i.e., drainage and control of infection lead to restoration of function).

Thrombocytopenia

Thrombocytopenia may indicate serious infection, although it is not a common signal. If possible, its cause should be identified promptly.

Hyperglycemia and Insulin Resistance

Hyperglycemia and insulin resistance are often reliable signals of the presence of infection in diabetic patients as well as in nondiabetic patients. The degree of insulin resistance can reflect the severity of the infection as well as the effectiveness of infection control.

Immune Failure

Immune failure is discussed in detail elsewhere [see VI:6 Non-AIDS Immunosuppression]. Severe infection is immunosuppressive. The most clinically applicable assessment of immune failure at present is probably wound healing.

Evaluation for Presence of Infection

Essentially the same clinical and laboratory assessments are used to evaluate normally responsive and compromised or complex patients for the presence of infection. There is, however,

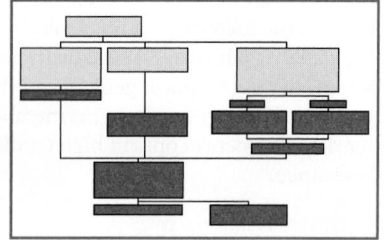

a significant difference in emphasis. In normally responsive patients, the diagnosis of infection is usually made on clinical grounds with laboratory support, whereas in compromised or complex patients, the diagnosis is usually made on the basis of laboratory findings with clinical support.

The ICU patient presents a particular conundrum. Nosocomial infection is identified in an estimated 20% of such patients.[2] Despite the frequency with which it is suspected and reported, it is difficult to prove unequivocally. The perceived prevalence of nosocomial infection has created a strong predisposition toward instituting empirical antibiotic therapy in ICU patients; however, the global value of this action in terms of both patient outcome and the impact on the ecology of the ICU is unconfirmed and requires validation. The enormous inconsistencies in how infections are diagnosed have a tremendous effect on our ability to assess the efficacy of therapy for infection. The current approach to diagnosing infection in surgical patients, particularly those who are critically ill or compromised, is still in great need of clarification and standardization.[3] Until the issues are resolved, the clinician must be familiar with the strengths and limitations of a variety of current diagnostic methodologies and then exercise thoughtfulness and disciplined diligence. The likelihood that a particular patient is infected (i.e., the pretest probability) is as important in the decision to treat as the fulfillment of any particular constellation of diagnostic criteria.

HISTORY AND PHYSICAL EXAMINATION

The history should include all background diseases—such as diabetes, lung disease, cirrhosis, hepatitis, kidney disease necessitating dialysis, and previous important infections—as well as a hospitalization history that covers health status, surgical diagnosis and therapy, additional therapeutic interventions (including interventional radiology, monitoring devices, drains, and drugs), and other related variables.

In the early postoperative period (3 to 6 days after operation), the traditional causes of the signals of infection have their origin in the wound, intravascular lines, the urinary tract, and the lungs. Deep thrombophlebitis, with or without pulmonary embolism, may also give rise to the clinical picture of sepsis. The general physical examination is often unrewarding, but a number of specific examinations should be carefully performed, with emphasis given to (1) all wounds and operative sites, (2) all invasive monitoring or therapeutic devices and surrounding areas, (3) all drainage systems and surrounding tissue, with particular attention paid to the nature of the drainage and whether it has recently changed in character or volume (particularly if it has stopped), (4) the rectal examination (for pelvic or prostatic infection), (5) areas of potential decubitus ulcers, (6) the neck (for central nervous system infection), (7) intravascular lines, surrounding tissue, and proximal vessels, (8) the lungs, and (9) the legs. The physical examination is important as a guide for selecting specimens for microbiologic analysis, particularly when wounds or drainage has recently manifested significant changes. The decision to seek radiologic consultation may depend on the findings on physical examination.

BLOOD TESTS

After physical assessment, laboratory blood tests are routinely relied on to orient the surgeon toward or away from a clinical diagnosis of infection. Leukocytosis, particularly with an increase in band forms, is a usual but not constant marker for infection. The white blood cell (WBC) count is widely used to follow the response of infection to therapy and thus has been adopted as a surrogate indicator of the success or failure of therapy. Surprisingly, however, the documentation supporting this ubiquitous practice is sparse,[4,5] and the daily series of complete blood counts often ordered in conjunction with the initiation of antibiotic therapy usually tells the clinician little about a patient's clinical course that cannot be gleaned at the bedside.

In more complex surgical patients, other biochemical cues are used to varying degrees as means of assessing the likelihood of infection. In addition to thrombocytosis, thrombocytopenia, hyperglycemia, and metabolic acidosis, which commonly reflect the stress of severe infection, changes in the erythrocyte sedimentation rate (ESR) and blood levels of C-reactive protein (CRP), procalcitonin (PCT), interleukin-6 (IL-6), and tumor necrosis factor–α (TNF-α) have a significant association with the presence of clinical infection. Plasma CRP concentration, which has been extensively used in some European countries to monitor the evolution of infection, has been found to be significantly elevated in patients with pulmonary aspiration that has induced bacterial infection rather than sterile pneumonitis.[6] Some investigators have suggested that because CRP concentration appears to be particularly responsive to bacterial infection, it may be useful as a monitor of the efficacy of antibiotic use, thereby guiding discontinuance of treatment.[7] A host of cytokines, cellular adhesion molecules, oxidants, and other biomolecules known to participate in systemic inflammation from numerous causes are being extensively investigated to establish both diagnostic and therapeutic functions. As yet, however, no single mediator of systemic inflammation has been validated as a reliable clinical tool for surveillance of the progression of infection or the response of infection to treatment.

MICROBIOLOGIC STUDIES

As a rule, Gram's stains and cultures of wound tissue, sputum, urine, and drainage effluent are the most useful studies. In some cases, however, a battery of cultures of potential sites of infection may be the only feasible approach. Culture techniques are discussed more thoroughly elsewhere [see VI:11 Blood Cultures and Infection in the Patient with the Septic Response and VI:14 Nosocomial Infection]. The use of polymerase chain reaction technology to detect bacterial DNA is emerging as a potential alternative to microbiologic culture for determining the presence of infection. The accuracy of this methodology remains to be established, but the rapidity with which it yields results makes it highly promising as a potential guide to therapeutic intervention. Future developments are eagerly awaited.

RADIOLOGY

A chest x-ray is mandatory. Ultrasonographic examination of the operative site may be useful. The possibility of acalculous cholecystitis must be kept in mind [see VI:16 Infections in the Upper Abdomen: Biliary Tract, Pancreas, Liver, and Spleen]. Computed tomography of the operative site is often more useful than ultrasonography because the presence of wounds, dressings, and drainage tubes may obscure the findings on ultrasonography. In compromised or complex patients who have not recently undergone an operation, the medical and surgical history combined with the radiologic examination may be the only guide to the potential focus (e.g., ulcer, diverticulitis, cholecystitis or cholangitis, or obstructed ureter). Percutaneous aspiration of potentially infected fluid should be considered; the fluid should be microbiologically examined if possible.

Institution of Therapy

The response to infection must be thought of in terms of a continuum ranging from virtually no clinical expression in the immunosuppressed patient to full-blown septic shock. Sepsis, as defined earlier [see Sidebar Definitions of Key Concepts], represents a mild to moderate response occurring in normally responsive patients as well as in many compromised or complex patients. On the basis of the degree to which other clinical or laboratory signals manifest themselves, the clinician can evaluate the magnitude of the septic response and, therefore, its clinical gravity.

It is the magnitude of the septic response, as well as the nature and condition of the patient, that governs the clinician's use of specific or empirical therapy. The greater the degree of sepsis, the greater the clinical urgency of solving the two fundamental problems involved: resolution of the initiating process (i.e., treatment of the infection) and modulation of the response to that process (i.e., management of sepsis) [see VII:7 Multiple Organ Dysfunction Syndrome]. The therapeutic approach to a given patient is based on the need for speed.

MILD TO MODERATE SEPSIS

The approach to treatment of infection in normally responsive and compromised patients with mild to moderate sepsis includes four steps: (1) if necessary, resuscitation and reestablishment of homeostasis and organ function, (2) diagnosis of the focus of infection by means of microbiologic culture and radiologic examination, (3) treatment with antibiotics, directed as specifically as possible at the presumed cause, and (4) drainage, which often amounts to definitive therapy. In compromised patients, empirical antibiotic therapy is often started before diagnosis and its efficacy gauged by the patient's clinical course [see Discussion, below].

Antibiotic treatment Antibiotic treatment must be directed against a likely cause, as determined by recent history (particularly procedures), past history, and physical examination. Examples of likely causes are (1) urinary manipulation, which indicates coverage against enterococci and gram-negative bacteria with ampicillin and an aminoglycoside, (2) colonic flora, which indicates coverage against anaerobes and aerobes, (3) vascular lines, which indicate coverage against gram-positive organisms, (4) cholangitis, which indicates coverage against aerobic gram-negative bacteria with ceftriaxone or an aminoglycoside, and (5) pneumonia, which indicates coverage against gram-positive and gram-negative aerobes.

Drainage The search for the focus of infection is important because drainage may resolve the entire problem. The clinical state can be changed dramatically by technical or mechanical management of pus behind an obstruction (e.g., in the biliary tree, urinary tract, or tracheobronchial tree) or of pus under pressure (e.g., an abscess), manipulation of a drain, or removal of a foreign body (e.g., an intravascular line or pacemaker). Prompt elimination of all foci of infection that can be drained or are operable is critical. Needle aspiration of peritoneal or pleural fluid may be very helpful. Wounds must be reevaluated constantly and the presence of pressure sores ruled out. Drainage can often be performed percutaneously (e.g., for pyelonephritis in an obstructed ureter or for subphrenic abscess) or endoscopically (e.g., for cholangitis).

SEVERE SEPSIS AND SEPTIC SHOCK

For assessment and management of severe sepsis and septic shock [see Sidebar Definitions of Key Concepts], the four steps in treatment—resuscitation, diagnosis of the infectious focus, antibiotic therapy, and drainage—must be performed concurrently. Specifically, I.V. administration of antibiotics must be initiated immediately, before the diagnostic process is completed, and the potentially drainable focus must be identified via physical examination or radiologic techniques. The choice of antibiotic depends on (1) what the likely source of infection is (e.g., a lung, a perforated viscus, or the biliary tract), (2) whether the infection is hospital acquired (in which case antibiotic resistance must be considered), and (3) whether the patient has previously received antibiotic therapy. No "shotgun" regimen can be universally recommended.

Case Study: Clinical Picture of Sepsis without Infection

Infection is a process; sepsis is the response.

The difficulty of managing the patient who manifests the septic response in the absence of infection is illustrated by the following case:

A 55-year-old insulin-dependent man with peripheral vascular disease presented with evidence of infection in both feet. Hydration and antibiotic therapy did not prevent progression of the infection, and within 18 hours, it was apparent that amputation would be required for source control. In the course of the operation, gas gangrene, more extensive than had been clinically suspected, was discovered. The initial below-the-knee amputations were eventually followed by a hip disarticulation on one side and a high above-the-knee amputation on the other. Over the 36-hour period during which the infectious process was being controlled, classic septic shock, renal failure, coma, and respiratory failure developed. There was no change in the patient's hyperdynamic and hypermetabolic state after the amputations. During the following 3 weeks, he required ventilator support and daily hemodialysis or hemofiltration; became jaundiced and more deeply comatose; received fluids in amounts significantly in excess of output to maintain blood volume; was hyperglycemic despite receiving regular insulin in dosages of 3 to 5 U/hr; and remained in a hyperdynamic state. Shortly after the last operation, an ileus developed, accompanied by gross fluid retention, which further increased the patient's girth.

This state of overt sepsis with hypermetabolism persisted while the wounds healed by primary closure, but no focus of infection could be found.

Antibiotic therapy was stopped 10 days after operation; the patient's clinical status did not change. Frequent searches were made to ensure that no infection had been overlooked. Suggestions—seriously put forward—to explore the patient's abdomen because "there must be something there" were not heeded. At the end of the third week, for no obvious reason, the patient started to urinate, his ileus resolved, and he was gradually weaned from the ventilator. His level of consciousness improved, the massive edema cleared, and the high cardiac output and low peripheral resistance resolved over a period of 72 hours. He was discharged from the surgical ICU 1 day later and from the hospital in 3 weeks. Some noninfectious process that had maintained this patient's persistent septic response had disappeared or had been turned off, and the result was rapid resolution of the septic state and recovery of health.

As noted, initial control of infection, though difficult, was achieved relatively early. Subsequent therapeutic efforts involved providing hemodynamic, metabolic, and physiologic support of the patient's failing organs and organ systems while waiting for the septic response to resolve. The real problem in this case was not the infection but the patient's unremitting septic response, which was initiated by the infection but maintained in its absence.

THE SYSTEMIC INFLAMMATORY RESPONSE IN THE ABSENCE OF INFECTION

In critically ill and traumatized ICU patients, it is not uncommon for clinical signs and symptoms indistinguishable from those of severe sepsis to arise or persist in the absence of any infection [*see Sidebar* Case Study: Clinical Picture of Sepsis without Infection]. Burn injury and pancreatitis are classic examples of conditions that can provoke such a response: both can give rise to a hyperdynamic, hypermetabolic clinical picture identical to that of sepsis or severe sepsis, even when no infection is present. Surgeons have learned, to their cost, not to give antibiotics unless there is evidence of infection. The instinctive reflex to do something must be held in check: "masterful inactivity" is the appropriate response until a specific source that can be controlled is identified.

Discussion

Approaches to Specific Infections in the Complex Surgical Patient

The following infections may occur in all surgical patients. They are, however, much more difficult to identify in complex surgical patients, such as those admitted to intensive care. Because the signals of infection are less specific and extremely difficult to interpret after injury or operation, the approach to diagnosing and treating infection must be cautious and disciplined.

SURGICAL SITE INFECTION

Surgical site infections include all infections occurring within the operative field, from the skin to the actual area of surgery.[8]

The patient history should address previous diseases as well as issues concerning the operation itself, such as classification, duration, difficulty, urgency, use of drains, other details of the procedure, time elapsed since the operation, and whether the patient was immunosuppressed, experienced trauma, or received chemotherapy. Physical examination should focus on the cardinal signs of infection and the absence or presence of a healing ridge.

Deeper infections tend to become apparent later in the postoperative course, often after a period in which the patient appears to be recovering, and are associated with a variety of signals, some of which can appear suddenly. The physical examination is often useless or misleading because of discomfort associated with the operation. Rectal examination is important because it may detect abscess formation or bleeding. Return of ileus after an abdominal operation is a significant clue to the presence of abdominal infection.

Culture is essential because use of the correct antibiotics is particularly vital in treatment of compromised or complex patients. Knowledge of the organism and its sensitivities is the key to identifying epidemic or multiresistant strains.

URINARY TRACT INFECTION

Nearly all patients admitted to the ICU have a urinary catheter in place; of these, it is estimated that about 20% progress to urinary tract infection (UTI).[2] Bacteria adhere to urinary catheter surfaces, where they promote growth of a so-called biofilm composed of microorganisms, bacterial glycocalices, Tamm-Horsfall protein, and urinary salts. Eradication of this infectious nidus is essentially impossible without catheter removal.[9] The standard criterion for the diagnosis of UTI (10^5 bacteria/ml) is difficult to apply in catheterized patients because antibiotic therapy without removal of the catheter and the source of bacteriuria would be ineffective. Furthermore, it is well established that urine cultures demonstrating as few as 10^1 or 10^2 bacteria/ml increase 1,000-fold within 1 to 2 days[10]; therefore, effectively any bacterial growth on a urine culture from a catheterized patient signals heavy colonization, if not infection.

More important than quantifying the degree of bacteriuria is determining whether there is any evidence of tissue invasion by urinary bacteria, which would present as pyelonephritis, cystitis, prostatitis, epididymitis, bacteremia, or systemic sepsis. The patient history should determine whether a Foley catheter was used and for how long; how, when, and why it was inserted; instrumentation (e.g., a so-called in-and-out catheter, cystoscopy, or transurethral resection of the prostate); and whether the patient has had any prior UTIs. The physical examination should ascertain whether there is any costovertebral angle tenderness or evidence of prostatic or epididymal tenderness.

Laboratory tests should include gross and microscopic urinalysis, urine culture, and sensitivity tests. Blood culture is important because it may substantiate the diagnosis, identify the bacteria present, and determine the degree of invasiveness of the infectious process.

VASCULAR CATHETER INFECTION

The most frequent sites of infection postoperatively are intravenous catheters, particularly peripheral ones. Diagnosis of peripheral catheter infection is simple and is made on clinical grounds. Diagnosis of central venous catheter (CVC) infection is more difficult. Because hospitalized patients are increasingly being supported by monitoring or therapeutic modalities that depend on vascular access (e.g., total parenteral nutrition and dialysis), line infections have become more common, with an incidence ranging from two to 30 infections per 1,000 central catheter days.[11] The combined pressures imposed by (1) the need to maintain vascular access in sicker and more complex patients and (2) the increasing predominance of gram-positive CVC infections observed since the late 1970s has led clinicians in many centers to administer empirical therapy without line removal to complex patients as a matter of course; some even advocate 10 to 21 days of vancomycin-based therapy. The problems associated with the latter approach—emerging vancomycin resistance, nephrotoxicity, and rash—are serious and relate specifically to the diagnostic strategy used to manage potential CVC infections. The distinction between contamination, colonization, and true infection is problematic; as a result, a number of diagnostic strategies have been advocated that are predicated more on practicality and cost-effectiveness than on microbiologic reality.

It is believed that CVC infection most commonly arises from invasion by skin microorganisms (*Staphylococcus aureus* or *Staphylococcus epidermidis* in about 80% of cases), which may manifest itself as exit-site purulence with or without local cellulitis, as a tunnel infection that may be clinically difficult to detect, or as catheter-related bloodstream infection (CR-BSI). Of these, CR-BSI, which complicates as many as 5% of line placements, is the most clinically important entity. It is strictly diagnosed by identification of the same microorganism (identical species and antibiogram) grown from both the catheter and a peripheral blood culture. The catheter may be cultured in one of several ways, the most common of which is the roll-plate method [*see VI:14 Nosocomial Infection*]. Because it is theoretically possible that this technique may fail to detect bacteria harbored within the catheter lumen, some authorities advocate the more sensitive sonication method, in which the catheter segment is immersed and agitated in a medium to produce a broth that contains bacteria from both the internal and the external surfaces of the line. This technique is both more costly and more time consuming, in that it requires quantitative cultures that are deemed positive only when more than 10^3 colony-forming units are detected. More often, blood drawn through the CVC or cultured from an exit-site exudate is compared with peripheral cultures, and thus there is no need to remove the line. If quantitative cultures are done, a line-blood culture showing five times more growth than the peripheral sample strongly suggests that the catheter is the source of the bacteremia; on its own, a line-blood culture is not sensitive or specific enough to be diagnostically useful.

PULMONARY INFECTION

Diagnosis and management of nosocomial pneumonia in surgical patients is addressed in detail elsewhere [see VI:13 Early Postoperative Pneumonia]. The central issue is that there is no universal agreement as to how pneumonia—particularly ventilator-associated pneumonia—should be diagnosed. Of the innumerable diagnostic options, none can rely on demonstration of tissue invasion by microorganisms, as would be ideal: all are to some degree nonspecific, and any may be invoked to justify initiation of antibiotic therapy.[12] Randomized trials linking mode of diagnosis to therapeutic strategy and then to outcome are badly needed.[13]

SINUSITIS

All patients undergoing prolonged nasogastric intubation are predisposed to sinus infection. Previous facial trauma and a history of sinusitis are potential contributing factors as well. (Otitis and pharyngitis, which are not often considered, occur in much the same group of patients.) Because maxillary or frontal area tenderness is nonspecific in very ill surgical patients, the diagnosis is usually based on CT demonstration of sinus opacification or air-fluid levels. As a first step, sinus drainage should be reestablished by removal of an unnecessary nasogastric tube. When diagnosis seems urgent, many authorities advocate sinus aspiration for culture before empirical antibiotic therapy is begun.

PAROTITIS

Parotitis is an increasingly common clinical diagnosis in elderly patients. It is usually caused by *S. aureus* and diagnosed on the basis of the presence of the classic local signs of inflammation. Culture of Stensen's duct and blood culture are useful.

PROSTATITIS

Prostatitis (diagnosed by rectal examination) and epididymitis are clinical expressions of Foley catheter–related infection. The aid of prostatic massage is important in obtaining specimens for culture. It should be remembered that a blocked Foley catheter is the most common cause of hospital anuria. This obstruction can lead to devastating purulent cystitis and upper UTI.

PSEUDOMEMBRANOUS ENTEROCOLITIS

Antibiotic-associated pseudomembranous enterocolitis is diagnosed by performing proctosigmoidoscopy and obtaining specimens for serology and culture. *Clostridium difficile* is frequently identified as the causative pathogen. Although pseudomembranous colitis is rarely clinically impressive and is easy to overlook, it can be rapidly fatal. Initial appropriate antibiotic therapy is not always successful; therefore, reevaluation at the end of the treatment course is required.

The Systemic Inflammatory Response Syndrome: Terminology

The human body's physiologic response to systemic infection is well characterized and is often referred to as sepsis. As noted, however [see Infection versus Sepsis, *above*], infection and sepsis are distinct entities that do not always occur concurrently in seriously ill patients. The normal septic response to infection may, in fact, be completely absent in immunosuppressed patients. Most surgeons, for example, have encountered a patient receiving high doses of steroids who has a perforated intra-abdominal viscus and fecal peritonitis but whose leukocyte count, temperature, and blood pressure are all normal. Conversely, the septic response may be present in noninfected patients.[14,15] For example, patients with acute pancreatitis, tissue necrosis, or fractures may manifest physiologic and metabolic changes that are indistinguishable from those associated with bacteremia, even in the absence of infection. Animal studies have confirmed that a sepsislike syndrome can occur without microbial invasion of host tissues.[16]

Accordingly, several clinicians have used the term sepsis syndrome to refer to the group of signs, symptoms, and physiologic changes that result from a variety of sterile inflammatory processes as well as from systemic infection.[15,17] The problem with using the term in this way, however, is that it derives from a Greek word (*sepsis* "decay") that implies infection with microorganisms. The twenty-eighth edition of *Dorland's*[18] defines sepsis as "the presence in the blood or other tissues of pathogenic microorganisms or their toxins; the condition associated with such presence." It is therefore not surprising that application of the term sepsis syndrome to noninfectious settings has led to some confusion.[19,20]

Various attempts have been made to refine the terminology used to describe sepsis and related phenomena. The definitions of infection, bacteremia, sepsis, severe sepsis, and septic shock cited earlier [see Sidebar Definitions of Key Concepts] were derived from an August 1991 consensus conference held by the American College of Chest Physicians and the Society of Critical Care Medicine.[1] In addition to defining these commonly used terms, the conference participants proposed adoption of two new terms, systemic inflammatory response syndrome (SIRS) and multiple organ dysfunction syndrome (MODS), which were defined as follows:

1. SIRS is the systemic inflammatory response to a variety of severe clinical insults (either infectious or noninfectious). The response is manifested by two or more of the following conditions: (a) temperature higher than 38° C (100.4° F) or lower than 36° C (96.8° F), (b) heart rate greater than 90 beats/min, (c) respiratory rate greater than 20 breaths/min or arterial carbon dioxide tension less than 32 mm Hg, and (d) white blood cell count greater than 12,000/mm³ or less than 4,000/mm³, or immature (band) forms accounting for more than 10% of the neutrophils present.
2. MODS is the presence of altered organ function in an acutely ill patient such that homeostasis cannot be maintained without intervention. (This term was recommended as a replacement for multiorgan failure and multiple system organ failure [see VII:7 Multiple Organ Dysfunction Syndrome].)

Clearly, SIRS includes all the signs, symptoms, and physiologic changes characteristic of the sepsis syndrome; however, use of the term SIRS avoids the idea that such manifestations are necessarily the product of infection. Both infectious and noninfectious insults may evoke SIRS. Sepsis may, in fact, be thought of as a special case of SIRS—SIRS associated with infection [see Figure 1]. The term sepsis syndrome, although very useful in guiding clinical thinking,

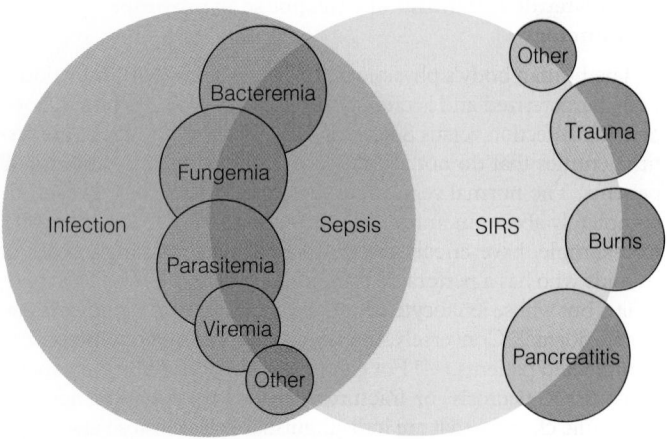

Figure 1 **Depicted are the interrelations among infection, sepsis, and systemic inflammatory response syndrome (SIRS).**

appears to be insufficiently precise for our current needs and probably should no longer be used. The term septicemia probably should not be used either.

The developing views expressed in this evolving terminology have clear therapeutic implications. There are two distinct problems to be faced: the initiating process and the systemic response. Treatment of the initiating process depends on the nature of the process (e.g., infection, trauma, burn, or pancreatitis). Treatment of the response—if indeed desirable—depends on the severity of the response; it should be thought of as independent of the initiating process.

Problems with Empirical Treatment of Infection

The frequent presence of SIRS in complex or critically ill surgical patients usually prompts a reflexive response to "pan culture" the patient if no credible source of infection is apparent. When permissive or loose diagnostic criteria for infection are invoked, the inevitable result is the commencement of empirical antibiotic therapy for suspected infection, which is often, by default, continued for days, if not weeks, pending definitive culture results. This strategy may seem reasonable and is undeniably difficult to resist, but it is potentially deleterious in many ways, and there are many sound objections to its reflexive use.[21] Empirical antibiotic therapy can obfuscate future cultures, predispose to the emergence of resistant organisms (which are associated with increased attributable mortality), promote derepression of homeostasis-maintaining endogenous flora, cause toxic reactions and secondary effects, alter the ecology of the unit in which it is used (as shown by the rising prevalence of methicillin-resistant *S. aureus* and vancomycin-resistant enterococci in both European and North American centers), and raise the cost of patient care. This widely used strategy is largely unvalidated.[4,5] It must be emphasized that the paramount principle of therapy for infection is treatment focused on appropriate microbiologic cultures in the context of strict diagnostic criteria for infection.

Many authorities espouse so-called streamlining of empirically begun broad-spectrum antibiotic therapy in response to microbiologic data once culture results are available; however, it is frequently difficult to discontinue antibiotics once they have been started. When strict diagnostic criteria for infection are not met or, more important, when antibiotic therapy based on nonmicrobiologic evidence of infection yields negligible results, strong consideration should be given to stopping the antibiotics, and an exhaustive effort should be made to identify and control any occult persistent cause of the inflammatory state. Of course, this is easier said than done. Moreover,

positive cultures do not automatically confirm infection, and great discretion must be exercised in determining how the microbiologic information obtained should be used. For example, tracheal aspirates from intubated patients routinely reveal gram-negative flora, but this finding in no way confirms pneumonia. A single blood culture growing *S. epidermidis* is similarly difficult to interpret. Despite ubiquitous use in surgical patients, there is not a great deal of evidence in the clinical literature to substantiate the effectiveness of either empirical or streamlined antibiotic therapy. Further efforts must be made to find such evidence, if it exists, because this practice could theoretically exact a substantial cost from both the patient and the environment in which the patient is cared for. In the meantime, clinicians must approach the development of SIRS or other nonspecific signs of infection in their patients by predicating antimicrobial use on carefully formulated diagnostic criteria for the presence of infection; CDC consensus definitions of infection are a good starting point.

SOURCE CONTROL

In the past, as noted, the term sepsis was loosely used to describe any general systemic inflammatory state. Because such states often arose as a result of infection, it was assumed that antimicrobial therapy was generally appropriate in the management of the "septic" patient. Currently, however, sepsis should be defined exclusively as SIRS in a patient in whom a causative source of infection has been identified; in the absence of proven infection, the term SIRS should be used. This distinction is important because it encourages more discriminating management of this exceedingly common clinical situation.

In the same vein, so-called source control has been developed as a strategy for managing the "septic" patient. Like the term sepsis, the term source control traditionally connotes management of infection rather than, more generally, management of a cause of inflammation. Classically, source control consists of a three-pronged approach employing measures to (1) eradicate a focus of infection, (2) eliminate ongoing microbial contamination, and (3) render the local environment inhospitable to microbial growth and tissue invasion. Diligent source control has long been considered pivotal to successful management of sepsis. Although this traditional approach addresses the infectious causes of local or systemic inflammation very well in a great variety of clinical situations, it must not lead us to become dogmatic about or oversimplify our understanding of which processes are required to overcome infection and inflammation. Challenging convention, a surprising number of investigators have successfully managed many supposedly surgical conditions (e.g., appendicitis[22] and intra-abdominal abscess[23]) without intervention or by using only prolonged antibiotic therapy. Seasoned general surgeons know well that if acute cholecystitis is not operated on urgently, it may certainly harm the patient or cause recurring discomfort, but it may also resolve completely on its own. What actually constitutes adequate source control and how this can be measured are critical questions and are currently the subject of great debate. These questions become particularly problematic with respect to ICU patients, in whom SIRS is highly nonspecific.

It would seem rational to take our current understanding of SIRS as encompassing both infectious and noninfectious pathology and extrapolate it to the concept of source control. Indeed, as regards more complex surgical patients, it may be appropriate to broaden the definition of source control to include control of all causes of SIRS, not merely infectious ones. For example, debriding devitalized injured tissue, removing a rejected allograft, and resolving postoperative atelectasis are all important for successfully abating a systemic inflammatory state that might easily be mistaken for a manifestation of infection. Deemphasizing infection as the predominant cause of SIRS and withholding antibiotic therapy until stricter, more focused diagnostic criteria for infection are met should make treatment paradigms for managing difficult surgical patients, if not altogether more effective, at least more evaluable.

If one assumes that source control is in fact a therapeutic response to the presence of SIRS, one may then think of it as being either assisted or unassisted. This therapeutic response is initiated by the host, with either complete or partial success. Only in the latter instance should one assist the host's efforts at source control by providing antibiotics or taking surgical measures. This is by no means to suggest that one should not search diligently for a correctable cause of infection or inflammation but rather to suggest that when such an effort yields negligible results, one should consider the possibility that SIRS may be not only appropriate but desirable and may represent the patient's own adequate management of the underlying physiologic insult. Thus, in certain situations, source control may be best regarded as an endogenous or unassisted event. For instance, when fever, tachycardia, and leukocytosis are observed in a surgical

patient who is coping well, antibiotics should not necessarily be given automatically. Indeed, such "default therapy" should be actively discouraged. (The reflexive and unnecessary use of antibiotic therapy to manage early acute cholangitis in an otherwise healthy person is a good example.) One should also keep in mind that some forms of injury or insult (e.g., some viral infections) not only are very well managed without intervention but may not even prompt a clinically evident systemic inflammatory response.

The notion that no intervention may be required is understandably difficult for many surgeons to embrace at the bedside. Nonetheless, extensive ongoing research elucidating the complex dynamic of circulating proinflammatory and counterinflammatory mediators (e.g., TNF-α, the interleukins, and a host of other cytokines) suggests that a poorly understood but highly sophisticated biologic apparatus exists for responding to injury and insult. Indeed, it is widely hypothesized (though yet unproved) that this systemic response can be manipulated to restore health in stressed or deteriorating surgical patients. The prospect of untangling the complex biology of systemic inflammation through advances in this field is truly engaging.

References

1. American College of Chest Physicians/Society of Critical Care Medicine Consensus Conference: Definitions for sepsis and organ failure and guidelines for the use of innovative therapies in sepsis. Crit Care Med 20:864, 1992
2. Vincent J, Bihari DJ, Suter PM, et al: The prevalence of nosocomial infection in intensive care units in Europe: results of the European Prevalence of Infection in Intensive Care (EPIC) Study. JAMA 274:639, 1995
3. Casadevall A: Crisis in infectious diseases: time for a new paradigm? Clin Infect Dis 32:790, 1996
4. Lennard ES, Mineshew BH, Dellinger EP, et al: Leukocytosis at termination of antibiotherapy: its importance for intra-abdominal sepsis. Arch Surg 115:918, 1980
5. Stone HH, Bourneuf AA, Stinson LD: Reliability of criteria for predicting recurrent sepsis. Arch Surg 120:17, 1985
6. Adnet F, Borron SW, Vicault E, et al: Value of C-reactive protein in the detection of bacterial contamination at the time of presentation in drug-induced aspiration pneumonia. Chest 112:466, 1997
7. Young B, Gleeson M, Cripps AW: C-reactive protein: a critical review. Pathology 23:118, 1991
8. The Society for Hospital Epidemiology of America, the Association for Practitioners in Infection Control, the Centers for Disease Control, the Surgical Infection Society: Consensus paper on the surveillance of surgical wound infections. Infect Control Hosp Epidemiol 13:599, 1992
9. Stamm WE, Hooton TM: Management of urinary tract infection in adults. N Engl J Med 329:1328, 1993
10. Stark RP, Maki DG: Bacteriuria in the catheterized patient: what quantitative level of bacteriuria is relevant? N Engl J Med 311:560, 1984
11. Bullard KM, Dunn DL: Diagnosis and treatment of bacteremia and intravascular catheter infections. Am J Surg 172(suppl 6A):13S, 1996
12. American Thoracic Society: Hospital-acquired pneumonia in adults: diagnosis, assessment of severity, initial antimicrobial therapy, and preventive strategies: a consensus statement. Am J Respir Crit Care Med 153:1711, 1995
13. Sterling TR, Ho EJ, Brehm WT, et al: Diagnosis and treatment of ventilator-associated pneumonia—impact on survival. Chest 110:1025, 1996
14. Marshall J, Sweeny D: Microbial infection and the septic response in critical surgical illness. Arch Surg 125:17, 1990
15. Meakins JL, Marshall JC: The gut as the motor of multiple system organ failure. Splanchnic Ischemia and Multiple Organ Failure. Marston A, Ed. Edward Arnold, London, 1989, p 339
16. Goris RJA, Boekhorst TAP, Nuytinck JKS, et al: Multiple organ failure: generalized autodestructive inflammation? Arch Surg 120:1109, 1985
17. Bone RC, Fisher CJ Jr, Clemmer TP, et al: Sepsis syndrome: a valid clinical entity. Crit Care Med 17:389, 1989
18. Dorland's Illustrated Medical Dictionary, 28th ed. Philadelphia, WB Saunders Co, 1994, p 1507
19. Bone RC: Let's agree on terminology: definitions of sepsis. Crit Care Med 19:973, 1991
20. Sibbald WJ, Marshall J, Christou N, et al: "Sepsis"—clarity of existing terminology . . . or more confusion? Crit Care Med 19:996, 1991
21. Timsit M, Misset B, Renaud B, et al: Effect of previous antimicrobial therapy on the accuracy of the main procedures used to diagnose nosocomial pneumonia in patients who are using mechanical ventilation. Chest 108:1036, 1997
22. Eriksson S, Granstrom L: Randomised controlled trial of appendectomy versus antibiotic therapy for acute appendicitis. Br J Surg 82:166, 1995
23. Montgomery RS, Wilson SE: Intraabdominal abscess: image-guided diagnosis and therapy. Clin Infect Dis 23:28, 1996

Acknowledgments

The authors wish to thank François Lemaire, Dominique Franco, A.P.H. McLean, and C. Brun-Buisson for their help and Fiorella Delcampe and Maria Betancourt for their secretarial assistance.

11 BLOOD CULTURES AND INFECTION IN THE PATIENT WITH THE SEPTIC RESPONSE

Donald E. Fry, M.D.

Approach to Blood Cultures in Patients with the Septic Response

It has been well established that infection and sepsis are distinct events [see VI:10 Clinical and Laboratory Diagnosis of Infection and Discussion, *below*]. Infection is local activation of the human inflammatory response secondary to local proliferation and invasion of tissue by microorganisms. When infection reaches a critical threshold of severity, the inflammatory response may be activated at a systemic level. Systemic activation of human inflammation is called the systemic inflammatory response syndrome (SIRS). When infection is the putative agent for SIRS, it is called sepsis.[1]

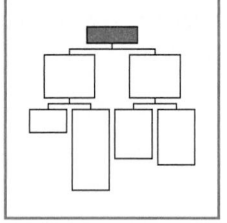

SIRS secondary to infection occurs when (1) whole microorganisms are disseminated from the primary site of infection, usually via the vascular or lymphatic system (e.g., bacteremia); (2) structural components of the cell wall (e.g., gram-negative endotoxin) or secreted exotoxins are systemically disseminated (e.g., toxic shock); or (3) normal autocrine and paracrine signals of inflammation at a local focus reach high systemic concentrations, and these proinflammatory signals (e.g., tumor necrosis factor [TNF]), through their exaggerated endocrine domain of action, activate SIRS.

Although biologic causes other than infection may precipitate SIRS and provoke a syndrome virtually identical to that resulting from invasive infection, infection is the most common cause of SIRS in acutely ill surgical patients. Effective management of infection in these patients requires recognition of the primary site of infection, control of the source of microbial contamination and dissemination (i.e., source control), characterization of the causative microorganism(s), drainage and debridement of inflammatory exudates and necrotic tissue at the primary site, and antibiotic therapy specific for the microbial pathogen.

Positive Blood Culture with Infection

A positive blood culture in a patient with the septic response serves to identify the putative cause of the infection. This identification not only permits institution of appropriate systemic antibiotic therapy [see Figure 1] but also facilitates assessment of potential primary sources of the infection because of the established associations between specific anatomic sites and specific microbial isolates. Although it is not always possible to identify the microorganism or microorganisms responsible for the septic response, organization of

the discussion according to the proven or suspected pathogen that may be recovered in a blood culture is a convenient way of addressing treatment options.

GRAM-POSITIVE COCCI

Staphylococci

The identification of gram-positive organisms from a blood culture immediately arouses suspicion that a *Staphylococcus* species is the likely pathogen. Because staphylococci ordinarily colonize the skin and integument, infection from those sources must be considered responsible for the bacteremia.

In the surgical patient, a positive blood culture for staphylococci must be assumed to arise from an intravascular device until proved otherwise[2] [see Table 1]. Peripheral intravenous catheters, subclavian lines, Swan-Ganz catheters, systemic arterial lines, and even transvenous pacemaker wires are all documented sources for staphylococcal bacteremia [see Table 2]. All lines must be removed and their sites changed. The line and catheter tips should be cultured by semiquantitative methods[3] to document the role of the particular device in question [see VI:14 Nosocomial Infection]. Although this semiquantitative method uses a count of 15 colony-forming units as the threshold for a positive culture of the catheter, devices responsible for bacteremia will usually demonstrate a solid sheet of bacterial growth on the agar [see Figure 2]. Devices causing bacteremia must be removed. Treatment cannot consist of antibiotics alone.

Septic thrombophlebitis may occur at the site of a previously placed device even though the foreign body has been removed.[4,5] Pus within the vein becomes a source of persistent bacteremia until appropriate therapy is employed. Persistent evidence of gram-positive bacteremia after removal of all intravascular lines gives rise to a high index of suspicion for suppurative thrombophlebitis. Previous intravenous sites must be examined for evidence of pus; suspicious sites may even have to be explored with the patient under local anesthesia. When suppurative thrombophlebitis is identified, the entire length of septic vein must be surgically excised. Although many different species of bacteria may be responsible for suppurative thrombophlebitis, *S. aureus* is the most common.

Implantable synthetic prosthetic materials have become a major part of vascular, cardiac, and orthopedic surgery but may become sources of bacteremia secondary to infections resulting from intraoperative contamination. The synthetic implant should be considered the source of blood-borne infection when gram-positive organisms are identified in the blood of patients at risk. As the use of synthetic

Approach to Blood Cultures in Patients with the Septic Response

Patient has septic response

Perform blood culture to identify putative cause of infection.

Blood culture is positive

Common pathogens include
- Gram-positive cocci (staphylococci, streptococci)
- Gram-negative Enterobacteriaceae (*Escherichia coli, Klebsiella, Proteus, Serratia*)
- Anaerobes (*Bacteroides*, clostridia, certain streptococci)
- Fungi (*Candida*)

Attempt to determine whether there is a primary focus of infection.

Blood culture is negative

Attempt to determine whether there is a primary source of infection:
- Perform careful physical examination
- Order appropriate diagnostic studies for each anatomic area
- Aggressively culture suspicious fluids or exudates

Pay particular attention to
- Surgical site
- Insertion sites for monitoring and support devices

Infectious focus is identified

Initiate therapy as appropriate for pathogen identified [*see Figure 1*].

No infectious focus is identified

Presume GI microbial translocation. Likelihood of this diagnosis is increased by presence of "trilogy of translocation" in blood culture:
- Enterococcus
- *Staphylococcus epidermidis*
- *Candida*

Rule out intravascular device infection.
Continue to search for primary infectious focus.
Reinforce gut barrier function via
- Enteral nutritional support
- Patient mobilization
- Addition of glutamine and short-chain fatty acids to nutritional solution
- Possible alteration of antibiotic regimen

Infectious focus is identified

Drain primary focus mechanically.
Initiate empirical antibiotic therapy directed at suspected pathogens while culture and sensitivity data are pending.
Maintain constant vigilance for changing clinical findings, and observe response to empirical therapy carefully.

No infectious focus is identified

Consider noninfectious causes of septic response, such as
- Acute pancreatitis
- Aspiration pneumonitis
- Multiple trauma with extensive soft tissue damage
- Extracorporeal membrane oxygenation

Do not give antibiotics.
Provide supportive care:
- Fluids
- Ventilatory assistance

Positive blood culture identifies putative source of infection

Staphylococcus aureus

Causes soft tissue infection, commonly with a foreign body (e.g., intravascular device or prosthesis). Infected device will have to be removed; may have to excise infected vein.

Antibiotic selection:

If organism is methicillin sensitive, give either nafcillin, 1 g q. 4 hr; oxacillin, 1 g q. 4 hr; or cefazolin, 1–2 g q. 8 hr. If organism is methicillin resistant, give vancomycin, 0.5–1.0 g q. 6 hr.

S. epidermidis

Infection of intravascular device is presumed until proved otherwise; remove infected foreign body. May need to excise infected vein.

Antibiotic selection:

S. epidermidis shows a high frequency of methicillin resistance; vancomycin, 0.5–1.0 g q. 6 hr, will likely be necessary.

Escherichia coli, Klebsiella species

Infection usually arises in peritoneal cavity, biliary tract, or urinary tract. Must ensure adequate drainage and debridement of primary focus of infection.

Antibiotic selection:

Choice of antibiotic is based on sensitivity data. Empirical therapy: gentamicin, 3–5 mg/kg (pharmacokinetically dosed), cefotaxime, 2 g q. 6–8 hr, or ceftizoxime, 2 g q. 8–12 hr.

Enterococcus

Infection of intravascular device (remove device), heart valve, or biliary tract is likely. May occur with *Candida* species as primary bacteremia without anatomic site of infection.

Antibiotic selection:

Give piperacillin, mezlocillin, or ticarcillin at 12–16 g/day; consider ampicillin-sulbactam

Pseudomonas species, Serratia species

Pulmonary sepsis (usually with pulmonary failure), urinary tract sepsis, or infection of intravascular device is likely. Treatment requires aggressive pulmonary toilet, ensurance of unobstructed urinary tract, and removal of potentially infected devices.

Antibiotic selection:

Give gentamicin, 3–5 mg/kg/day, or amikacin, 15 mg/kg/day (depending on sensitivity; pharmacokinetically dosed). The addition of expanded-spectrum penicillin (ticarcillin, mezlocillin, or piperacillin, 12–16 g/day) may be desirable in severe infections.

Bacteroides species, clostridia, anaerobic streptococci

Intra-abdominal sepsis, polymicrobial soft tissue infection, or female genital tract infection is likely. Adequate drainage and debridement of primary site of infection is mandatory.

Antibiotic selection:

Give clindamycin, 900–1,200 mg q. 6–8 hr, or metronidazole, 500 mg q. 6 hr.

Candida species

Primary source of infection is infected central catheters or gastrointestinal translocation. Remove catheters at risk.

Antifungal selection:

Give amphotericin B, 0.5 mg/kg/day (after test dose documents patient tolerance), or fluconazole, 200–800 mg/day.

Figure 1   **Identification of the putative cause of infection permits institution of appropriate antibiotic therapy.**

devices increases, the delayed nature of some infections, particularly when *S. epidermidis* is the pathogen, is now being appreciated. These indolent infections are consequences of intraoperative contamination but may not be clinically evident for months to years after implantation. Because selected species of *S. epidermidis* produce a glycocalix "slime," culturing of the microorganism from the infected prosthesis can be very difficult even after removal of the prosthesis. Recovery of this microorganism from a blood culture is quite uncommon, because presentation of the infection occurs months after the primary operative procedure.[6]

Diagnosis of arterial graft, heart valve, and total-joint arthroplasty infections can be very difficult. Once infection has been established, however, prompt removal of the prosthesis is mandatory. Prosthesis removal is invariably associated with major morbidity because an active infection limits the reconstructive options available. Although antibiotic therapy alone will not eradicate the infection, it may prolong the decision to remove the prosthesis and result in arterial graft failure (e.g., thrombosis, pseudoaneurysm), cardiac valvular insufficiency, or extensive arthroplasty infection (e.g., extrusion, osteomyelitis).

S. epidermidis is being recognized as having a greater role in surgical infection than was previously appreciated.[7] Because *S. epidermidis* normally colonizes skin, it is also a potential contaminant in the blood culture process. The continued emphasis on technique in blood culture is important to minimize this potential artifact in diagnosis. A frequent cause of false positive cultures of this microorganism is use of the arterial line or the central venous catheter, instead of a separate and carefully prepared venipuncture site, for drawing of blood samples. When more than one culture shows *S. epidermidis* or when cultures taken at separate times show the same organism, however, the clinician must assume that the organism is participating in clinical infection.

Staphylococcal bacteremia is a preventable complication of indwelling devices and implants. Aseptic placement of intravascular devices cannot be compromised. Peripheral I.V. catheters should be changed routinely every 48 to 72 hours. Arterial lines that have been present for more than 72 hours are at considerable risk for being foci

Table 1 Pathogens in 159 Cases of Intravascular Device–Associated Bacteremia[119]

Organism	Number of Isolates
Staphylococcus aureus	78
S. epidermidis	33
Serratia marcescens	18
Klebsiella/Enterobacter species	16
Candida species	11
Enterococcus	8
Proteus species	6
Others	6
Total	176*

*The total exceeds 159 because of polymicrobial isolates in several patients.

Figure 2 **Illustrated is a blood agar plate 24 hours after an infected catheter has been cultured by semiquantitative technique. Although colony counts of greater than 15 are associated with a positive culture, the prolific growth noted in this illustration is commonly identified.**

for bacteremia. Catheters devoted to parenteral nutrition must receive ongoing care to prevent septic morbidity [*see VII:9 Nutritional Support*].

The primary therapy for device-related infection is removal of the infected device. Systemic antibiotics cannot overcome the adjuvant effects of the foreign body in supporting bacterial growth. Antimicrobial therapy becomes adjunctive to removal of the primary nidus of infection.

Prevention of infection from prosthetic implants requires that efforts be made to minimize development of a microenvironment in the wound that favors bacterial proliferation. Meticulous technique, appropriate hemostasis, conservative use of the electrocautery, judicious use of suture ligatures, and antibiotics given immediately before operation will reduce infectious morbidity. Cefazolin, 1 g preoperatively, administered either intravenously (by preference) or intramuscularly, is the agent of choice [*see VI:5 Prevention of Postoperative Infection*]. With lengthy operations, repeat doses should be given at 4-hour intervals. Prolonged postoperative administration is of no value.

Before the 1970s, methicillin-resistant staphylococcal infections were rare, and presumptive therapy for bacteremia (including that caused by intravascular devices) could safely employ methicillin, nafcillin, or oxacillin. Methicillin-resistant staphylococci, particularly *S. epidermidis*, are being recognized with increasing frequency; in some series, they account for as many as 40% of clinical isolates. Thus, presumptive antimicrobial therapy for bacteremia arising from an intravascular or implantable device requires vancomycin, 0.5 to 1 g every 6 hours. When culture and sensitivity data are subsequently available, the antimicrobial choice may be modified. When methicillin-resistant species are not a concern, nafcillin, 1 g every 4 hours, is appropriate. Because of the risks of metastatic infectious complications from staphylococcal bacteremia, systemic antibiotics should be continued for a minimum of 7 days.

Table 2 Sites of Intravascular Device–Associated Bacteremia in 159 Patients[119]

Site	Number of Patients
Peripheral I.V. catheter	72
Central venous catheter	49
Arterial line	18
Subclavian dialysis catheter	12
Swan-Ganz catheter	4
Broviac catheter	3
Transvenous pacemaker wire	1

The toxic-shock syndrome, caused by *S. aureus,* gives the clinical impression of being a bacteremic illness.[8] However, blood cultures are infrequently positive in this clinical condition because the SIRS is created by the exotoxin produced by the microorganism, not by bacteremia per se. Initially associated with vaginal tampons, toxic-shock syndrome can be seen in any body cavity or open wound filled with gauze or other packing. Diagnosis of toxic shock requires a high index of suspicion in the septic, hypotensive patient with body packing. Treatment requires removal of the packing, aggressive systemic supportive care of the shock and associated organ-failure complexes, and systemic antibiotics appropriate for staphylococcal infection.

Streptococci

Streptococcal bacteremia occurs less often than staphylococcal blood-borne infection, but some areas of the United States are experiencing an apparent increase in these infections. Invasive group A streptococcal infection with bacteremia is seen in patients with necrotizing soft tissue infections, invasive pharyngeal infections, bone and joint infections, or severe and rapidly advancing pneumonia. About 20% of bacteremias with group A streptococci have no primary source of infection.[9]

Necrotizing soft tissue infection is the setting most likely to result in a positive blood culture of group A streptococci. These fulminant infections are seen after seemingly trivial cutaneous injuries but may also complicate chickenpox in children[10] and may even be seen as complications of elective surgery. The necrotizing infection is characterized by pain, tenderness, and induration around a wound that is out of proportion to the size or mechanism of the injury. The infection dissects along the fascial plane and can evolve from injury to a fatal illness in 24 hours. The diagnosis requires a high index of suspicion in a toxic patient with rapidly advancing cellulitis. The induration of the advancing infection, palpable in thin patients, differentiates this type of infection from clostridial gas gangrene. Although these infections are associated with the toxic-shock–like syndrome, patients with these infections—unlike those with true toxic shock—usually have blood cultures positive for group A streptococci.[8] Unfortunately, the positive blood culture is not available until the patient's fate has already been dictated by earlier clinical decisions.

Therapy requires aggressive debridement of the necrotic tissue, systemic antibiotic therapy, and systemic supportive therapy for the shock and organ-failure syndrome characteristic of severe infections. The antibiotic choice for these serious infections includes both penicillin, 12 to 24 million units/day, and clindamycin, 900 to 1,200 mg every 6 hours, in adult patients. The addition of clindamycin is thought to be important as an inhibitor of protein synthesis, reducing toxin production by the rapidly multiplying bacteria. Clindamycin is also useful because it is thought that large inocula of group A streptococci do not express penicillin-binding proteins.[11]

α-Hemolytic streptococcal bacteremia, well known in patients with endocarditis, is generally associated with this infection when blood cultures are positive for this organism. Echocardiographic confirmation of the diagnosis sets the stage for treatment with penicillin. Therapy is continued until there is conclusive evidence that the infection has been eradicated.

Other groups of streptococci identified by positive blood cultures usually occur in infections secondary to GI contamination. The group B streptococci are identified as bacteremic pathogens in neonates but are now being seen with somewhat greater frequency in adults. In adult bacteremia, the group D (nonenterococcal) streptococci are identified in circumstances similar to those associated with the group B pathogens. Gut-derived streptococcal pathogens are usually quite sensitive to the penicillins.

Enterococci

There continues to be debate concerning the true virulence and pathogenicity of the enterococcus when it is isolated as part of the polymicrobial microflora of a clinical exudate,[12,13] but no one would deny the need for antimicrobial chemotherapy when the organism is isolated in blood cultures. Mortalities in excess of 50% clearly underscore the severity of enterococcal bacteremia.[14]

The primary foci of infection in enterococcal bacteremia include intravascular devices and the biliary and gastrointestinal tracts. Enterococcal bacteremia ordinarily occurs in elderly or chronically ill patients who are being treated with broad-spectrum antibiotics. Cephalosporins in particular have been implicated as favoring enterococcal overgrowth.[15] The enterococcus is usually associated with other bacterial species at the primary site of intra-abdominal or soft tissue infection, and experimental observations suggest that a synergistic relation with other organisms may be part of its pathogenic expression.[16,17]

Therapy for enterococcal bacteremia requires definition of the primary focus of infection. When the enterococcus is a solitary isolate in blood, intravenous devices should be changed and semiquantitatively cultured. Potential biliary sources must be evaluated, with all available clinical data, including those from ultrasound examination of the gallbladder [see VI:16 Infection in the Upper Abdomen: Biliary Tract, Pancreas, Liver, and Spleen], taken into account. Gangrenous, acalculous cholecystitis must be kept in mind because of the type of patient likely to have enterococcal bacteremia.[18] Intra-abdominal abscesses and serious soft tissue infections are customarily associated with polymicrobial isolates, which may include the enterococcus. The urinary tract, however, appears to be an infrequent cause of enterococcal bacteremia in the absence of anatomic obstruction to urine flow.

When the primary focus is identified, removal of the foreign body, drainage and debridement of infected material, and specific antibiotic therapy are indicated. Piperacillin, 12 to 16 g/day, is recommended. Ticarcillin and mezlocillin, 12 to 16 g/day, are alternatives. Although ampicillin appears to have nearly uniform activity against the enterococcus in vitro, the β-lactamase production of synergistic pathogens in the polymicrobial milieu raises serious questions about the effectiveness of this choice. The recent addition of sulbactam to ampicillin has improved enterococcal coverage in mixed infections.

In about 40% of patients with positive blood cultures for the enterococcus, no primary site of infection can be identified.[14] This observation has led to considerable speculation as to whether this organism is a marker of gastrointestinal bacterial translocation [see Positive Blood Culture without Infection, below] or whether the infection arises from a clinically obscure primary focus (e.g., infection at a catheter site).

The emergence of vancomycin-resistant enterococci has created considerable concern.[19] These nosocomial infections, like all enterococcal bacteremias and infections, occur in severely ill hospitalized patients and are associated with intensive care units using large amounts of vancomycin. Specific antibiotic therapy in these infections is highly problematic. Current recommendations are to start with an assessment of the sensitivity of the enterococcal isolate to the aminoglycosides.[20] If the isolate lacks a high level of resistance to aminoglycosides, then the choices for antibiotic treatment include (1) an aminoglycoside plus teicoplanin (if susceptible), (2) an aminoglycoside plus vancomycin (for a low level of resistance), (3) an aminoglycoside plus ampicillin plus vancomycin, and (4) an aminoglycoside plus ciprofloxacin plus rifampin (if susceptible). If the isolate is highly resistant to aminoglycosides, then antibiotic treatment may be (1) teicoplanin (if susceptible), (2) novobiocin plus a quinolone, (3) ampicillin plus a quinolone, or (4) ceftriaxone plus fosfomycin. In vitro susceptibility testing with the combination of quinupristin and dalfopristin has raised the hope that these agents will be of use in the management of vancomycin-resistant enterococcal infections.[21] Because vancomycin resistance is mediated by two separate genes, there is considerable concern in the academic community about transfer of these genes into staphylococci or other gram-positive organisms.

GRAM-NEGATIVE ENTEROBACTERIACEAE

The gram-negative Enterobacteriaceae represent a group of facultative bacteria that are associated with infections of the abdominal cavity, biliary tract, and genitourinary tract. Infections tend to be monomicrobial when the urinary and biliary tracts are involved[22,23] but are nearly always polymicrobial with peritonitis and intra-abdominal abscess.[24] The common gram-negative Enterobacteriaceae include Escherichia coli, Klebsiella species, Enterobacter species, and Proteus species. Because intra-abdominal infection is a polymicrobial process, bacteremia may involve one or more of the Enterobacteriaceae and may likewise occur with several different anaerobic enteric species. Thus, bacteremia with one of these organisms in patients with intra-abdominal infection represents only the tip of the iceberg, with a polymicrobial flora presumed to be present at the focus [see VI:15 Peritonitis and Intra-abdominal Abscesses and VI:16 Infection in the Upper Abdomen: Biliary Tract, Pancreas, Liver, and Spleen].

In the surgical patient, eradication of gram-negative bacteremia requires identification of the primary focus because mechanical therapy is almost always necessary in addition to antibiotic treatment. The intra-abdominal compartment must be the primary consideration. Ultrasound examination of the biliary tract may be useful. Abdominal computed tomography is approximately 90% accurate in the definition of abscess. Urinary cultures may be useful but must be cautiously interpreted because a well-drained urinary tract is an improbable focus for bacteremia. P. vulgaris is a urease-producing organism, and its presence in patients with ileal conduits or staghorn calculi strongly favors a urinary tract source. Gram-negative bacteremia from hospital-acquired pneumonitis is always a possibility but is less common with the Enterobacteriaceae than with Pseudomonas or Serratia species. In general, bacteremia from nosocomial pneumonia is relatively uncommon in the surgical patient. *Klebsiella* and *Enterobacter* species are known pathogens for bacteremia from intravascular devices; appropriate cultures of the primary device are necessary to establish this potential source.

Mechanical treatment is necessary at the primary focus of infection. Defects in the gastrointestinal tract must be managed, pus drained, necrotic tissue debrided, urinary obstruction relieved, and infected catheters removed. Empirical exploration of the abdomen may be necessary in bacteremic patients in whom the likelihood of an intra-abdominal source is great, but CT of the abdominal compartment often eliminates the need for exploratory surgery.

Considerable latitude surrounds appropriate antibiotic therapy for gram-negative bacteremia, particularly when the bacteremia is secondary to intra-abdominal infection. When the infectious process responsible for the bacteremia is community-acquired, an expanded-spectrum β-lactam antibiotic is appropriate[25] [*see Table 3*]. Although anaerobic coverage is a necessary prerequisite in intra-abdominal infection, the expanded-spectrum β-lactam agents appear to have sufficient activity to provide equivalent results when compared with those combinations of drugs that might appear to have preferable anaerobic activity. Furthermore, single-agent treatment with the expanded-spectrum β-lactam antibiotics is less expensive than multiple-drug therapy and eliminates the toxicity and pharmacokinetic dosage complexities of the aminoglycoside alternatives.[26] Newer quinolone antibiotics with both gram-negative and anaerobic activity, as well as long elimination half-lives, may become additional choices for the treatment of bacteremia from intra-abdominal infection sites.[27]

Patients with bacteremia from hospital-acquired infections or infections that represent failures of prior antimicrobial therapy, however, will necessarily require therapy addressed to these more resistant isolates. Single antibiotics that may be chosen to cover hospital-acquired gram-negative bacteria include aminoglycosides, expanded-spectrum penicillins, ceftazidime, aztreonam, quinolones, and the carbapenems. Even though the bacteremic isolate may be sensitive to lesser drugs, a combination of an expanded-spectrum penicillin with an aminoglycoside is commonly chosen to cover potential pathogens [*see Table 4*] because of the synergism between these two types of agents. Culture and sensitivity data from the primary source of infection are par-

Table 4 Expanded-Spectrum Penicillins and Aminoglycosides Used in Combination Regimens in Treatment of Nosocomial Gram-Negative Bacteremia

Drug		Half-life (hr)	Total 24-Hr Dose
Penicillins	Ticarcillin	1.0	16–18 g
	Mezlocillin	1.0	16–18 g
	Piperacillin	1.0	12–18 g
Aminoglycosides*	Gentamicin	2.0	3–5 mg/kg
	Tobramycin	2.0	3–5 mg/kg
	Amikacin	2.0	15–20 mg/kg

*Dosing interval and total dose per day are variable and require pharmacokinetic dosing to avoid toxicity or underdosing.

ticularly important to permit modification of drug therapy. Because the complex patient in the surgical ICU will have an expanded volume of distribution and an altered pattern of excretion of antibiotics,[26] it is essential that aminoglycoside therapy be pharmacokinetically dosed to minimize drug toxicity and ensure adequate therapy. Recently, there has been considerable interest in the use of single daily dosing of aminoglycosides for gram-negative hospital-acquired infections.[28] Because of limited data on the postoperative use of this strategy in surgical patients, it cannot be recommended.

Nosocomial bacteremia with gram-negative organisms is a significant complication in surgical patients [*see VI:14 Nosocomial Infection*]. The principal sites are usually the respiratory and urinary tracts and intravascular devices; the surgical wound is a common site for nosocomial infection but is only infrequently responsible for the septic response or bacteremia.

ANAEROBES

The refinements in anaerobic bacteriology since the early 1970s have resulted in an increased awareness of anaerobic pathogens in surgical infection. Anaerobes of particular significance to surgeons as bacteremic pathogens are principally colonizers of the human GI tract and the female genital tract. Oral or cutaneous anaerobes (e.g., diphtheroids) are rarely identified as bacteremic pathogens, although diphtheroids are commonly recognized skin contaminants of the blood-culturing process. *Bacteroides* species, anaerobic streptococci, and *Clostridium* species tend to be the more commonly identified anaerobic pathogens in blood.

Among all anaerobes, *Bacteroides* species, particularly *B. fragilis*, stand out as the preeminent pathogens. They are customarily identified in infections involving distal ileum or colonic contamination. Intra-abdominal infection must be considered the primary focus of *B. fragilis* bacteremia.[29] Soft tissue infections may also be the source of *Bacteroides* bacteremia, particularly in the presence of a polymicrobial infection or necrotic tissue and particularly in soft tissue infections of the perineum. In one series of patients with *B. fragilis* bacteremia, 80% required operative drainage and debridement as primary treatment.[29]

The selection of antimicrobial therapy for *B. fragilis* must be based on an understanding of the pathogenesis of anaerobic infections. Anaerobic infection in the abdomen and soft tissues is synergistic, wherein anaerobic and aerobic organisms mutually benefit from the polymicrobial environment. The aerobic species decrease the oxidation-reduction potential of the environment, which optimizes conditions for anaerobic proliferation. The anaerobe may then elaborate factors that accelerate the growth cycle of the aerobe, or it may shed a portion of its capsular polysaccharide into the environment and re-

Table 3 Expanded-Spectrum β-Lactam Antibiotics Effective against Enterobacteriaceae

Drug	Half-life (hr)	Dose Interval (hr)	Total 24-Hr Dose (g)
Cephalosporins			
Cefoxitin	0.7–1.0	4–6	12–18
Cefotetan	3.5	12	2–4
Cefotaxime	1.0	6	8–12
Ceftizoxime	1.5	8	6
Ceftazidime	2.0	8	6
Ceftriaxone	6.5–8.0	12–24	2–4
Penicillins			
Ampicillin-sulbactam	1.0	6	12
Ticarcillin-clavulanate	1.0	4	18.6
Piperacillin-tazobactam	1.0	6	13.5
Monobactams			
Aztreonam	2.0	8	6
Carbapenems			
Imipenem-cilastatin	1.0	6	2–4
Meropenem	1.0	6	2–4

tard phagocytosis of all components of the infection.[30] The complexity of this synergistic relation may be further compounded by interactions between the enterococcus and either the gram-negative rod[16] or the anaerobic organism.[17]

Antimicrobial therapy must address both halves of the synergistic pair, with coverage of the aerobic Enterobacteriaceae species being a vitally important component of treatment for the anaerobe. Antibiotic therapy with the expanded-spectrum β-lactam antibiotics appears to provide adequate polymicrobial coverage in intra-abdominal infection. Clindamycin (900 to 1,200 mg every 6 to 8 hours) or metronidazole (500 mg every 6 hours) in combination with an aminoglycoside has been the traditional treatment but poses special problems (as identified earlier in this discussion). *B. fragilis* bacteremia arising from unusual sites (e.g., endocarditis) or bacteremia in the face of β-lactam antibiotic therapy calls for specific clindamycin or metronidazole therapy. It is of utmost importance that treatment of the patient with anaerobic bacteremia include complete drainage and debridement of the primary focus.

Peptostreptococci and, to a lesser degree, peptococci are anaerobic streptococcal species that may cause bacteremia from infection after gastrointestinal contamination. More commonly, their presence should arouse suspicion that bacteremia may be arising from the female genital tract. Puerperal sepsis and pelvic inflammatory disease may have either of these anaerobes as participants, with common gram-negative Enterobacteriaceae or enterococci, or both, being synergistic partners in the infection. *Bacteroides* species may similarly participate in these types of infections.

Bacteremia with anaerobic streptococci secondary to infection in the female genital tract mandates a search for a drainable primary focus. Puerperal sepsis may require dilatation and curettage to eliminate retained products of conception. Pfannenstiel flaps may become potential sources of wound infection that may cause bacteremia and thus necessitate drainage and debridement. Pelvic inflammatory disease may be complicated by tubo-ovarian abscess or extrauterine abscess within the pelvis that will have to be drained.

Appropriate antibiotic therapy for anaerobic streptococcal bacteremia remains unclear. Most anaerobic species likely to cause infection in the female genital tract are sensitive to penicillin, with *Bacteroides* species being a notable exception. Therapy with an anaerobe-specific agent (e.g., clindamycin or metronidazole) in combination with an aminoglycoside, however, appears to offer better clinical results in puerperal infection.[31] The role of the expanded-spectrum β-lactam agents remains poorly defined. Because enterococcus is commonly identified in infections involving the female genital tract, ampicillin is frequently added to the antibiotic regimen, but it is of unproven value.

Clostridium species are gram-positive anaerobic rods that may cause bacteremia in surgical patients. Relatively uncommon in blood cultures, the organism is ordinarily associated with clostridial myonecrosis or cellulitis. Usually, the fulminant nature of the infection is readily identifiable at the primary soft tissue focus, and blood culture is of little assistance in diagnosis. Therapy consists of radical debridement of the primary site of infection and aggressive administration of penicillin [see II:11 Soft Tissue Infection].

Nonhistotoxic clostridial bacteremia has been identified with increased frequency. In a series of 47 patients with such bacteremia, only 25% had a focus of infection[32]; the remaining 75% had no clinically identifiable source. The patients in this latter group either were severely, chronically ill or were alcoholics; thus, the presence of a colonic anaerobe in blood may be evidence of primary bacteremia from the GI tract without a primary focus of infection, and nonhistotoxic clostridial bacteremia may be an expression of failed gastroin-

testinal barrier function rather than infection in the classic sense.

FUNGI

Fungemia in surgical patients has become a major problem since the early 1970s. *Candida* species have been the most common fungal organisms cultured from the blood in these patients. Candidemia is typically seen in a severely ill patient who has had or continues to have bacterial infection and is being treated with a prolonged course (more than 7 days) of broad-spectrum antibiotics.[33,34] Parenteral nutrition and corticosteroid therapy are associated with candidemia. The bacterial microflora becomes suppressed, and colonization by *Candida* organisms of the alimentary tract becomes the reservoir for dissemination.

Candidemia appears to occur principally via two mechanisms. In the first, indwelling catheters (particularly central lines) become colonized. Catheter removal and appropriate culture will document the process and likewise be effective treatment. The alternative mechanism of *Candida* dissemination, however, is gastrointestinal overgrowth with this fungal species, leading to impairment of host barrier function and resultant fungemia.[34] Although peritonitis and intra-abdominal abscess with *Candida* organisms have been identified,[35] translocation of the organisms across the gut barrier is the probable source of contamination.

Prevention of candidemia requires aseptic care of catheters and prompt catheter removal when fungemia is suspected or documented. A reduction in the spectrum and duration of systemic antibiotic therapy is probably the most important way of reducing fungal overgrowth and subsequent risk for dissemination. Oral nystatin, ketoconazole, and fluconazole have been recommended for prophylaxis in patients at risk for candidemia but remain unproven.

In the patient with established candidemia who has had all central lines removed, systemic chemotherapy with amphotericin B is recommended. A dosage of 0.5 to 1.0 mg/kg/day is suggested. The lower dosage (0.5 mg/kg/day) has been reported to be as effective as higher dosages but with reduced toxicity.[35] Fluconazole is a newer antifungal agent that has also been successful in the treatment of candidemia[36]; it is given in a dosage of 200 to as high as 800 mg/day. Because some resistance to fluconazole has been reported,[37] many feel that intravenous amphotericin B is the drug of choice for treatment of severe, life-threatening *Candida* infections. Although cessation of systemic antibiotic therapy has been recommended for the candidemic patient and is certainly desirable, more than 50% of these patients have synchronous bacteremia[33] [see Table 5], which compromises the decision to stop all antibiotics. Diagnosis and treatment of candidemia are discussed in detail elsewhere [see VI:18 Fungal Infection].

Positive Blood Culture without Infection

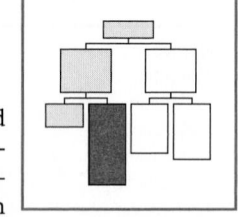

In the late 1950s, Jacob Fine proposed the theory that acute physiologic perturbations (e.g., hemorrhagic shock) could disrupt gastrointestinal barrier function to such a degree that bacteria and their cellular products could escape from the gut reservoir[38-40] and contribute to the patient's clinical illness. In other words, the septic response could be triggered by bacteria or their products (e.g., endotoxin) without infection, in the traditional sense of the term, being present. Although this theory was discredited in the 1960s in germ-free rat experiments,[41,42] it enjoyed a considerable resurgence in the late 1980s, as both experimental[43-47] and clinical[48,49] studies demonstrated that gastrointestinal microbial translocation appears to be a valid biologic event. Consequently, it has been proposed (although not universally accepted[50]) that a co-

Table 5 Bacteria Identified in Blood Culture within 48 Hours of Positive Culture for *Candida* in 83 Patients[33]

Organism	Number of Isolates
Staphylococcus species	25
Enterococcus	25
Klebsiella species	22
Serratia species	20
Pseudomonas species	11
Bacteroides species	9
Enterobacter species	7
Proteus species	6
Escherichia coli	6
Miscellaneous	15
Total	146*

*Only 27 patients in the series did not have associated bacteria in blood culture. In the 56 patients with associated bacteria, the blood-borne infection was truly polymicrobial, with each patient averaging nearly three bacterial isolates in addition to the *Candida* organism.

hort of surgical patients may have the septic response secondary to microorganisms while lacking a primary focus of clinical infection.

MECHANISMS OF GUT BARRIER FUNCTION

For gastrointestinal microbial translocation to be a clinically relevant event, gut barrier function must be impaired. At its most distal site, the lumen of the human GI tract may contain as many as 10^{10} bacteria/g of colon contents. The biologic partition that prevents microbes from escaping from this reservoir is complex and consists of anatomic, physiologic, and immunologic mechanisms.

The physical barrier of the gut is constituted by a contiguous layer of enterocytes and colonocytes. An intercellular matrix exists between the cells. Both types of cell appear to obtain a large part of the nutrients they need directly from the gut lumen. Enterocytes have a specific nutrient requirement for glutamine,[51] and colonocytes require short-chain fatty acids.[52] Deficiencies of these critical nutrients lead to atrophy of the gut lining, which results in a defective physical barrier.

The surface of the gut mucosal cells is covered with the glycoprotein mucin,[53] which is an important component of the gut barrier. The mucin layer has a nonspecific retarding effect on bacterial adherence to mucosal cells. In addition, it has a nonspecific inhibitory effect on bacterial proliferation at the mucosal cell surface, thereby helping prevent invasion by luminal bacteria.

Secretory IgA also prevents the binding of bacteria to mucosal cells.[54] Presumably produced as nonspecific antibody from submucosal gut lymphocytes, IgA does not fix complement and does not have cytotoxic effects on bacteria. Rather, it is thought to bind to bacteria and impede their binding to the mucosal cell lining. The IgA concentration is highest at the mucosal cell surface.

The normal microflora that colonizes the GI lumen appears to make a significant contribution to normal gut barrier function. Anaerobic bacteria play a positive role by virtue of their species-specific adherence to mucosal cell-binding sites and their ability to prevent more noxious aerobic species from adhering to mucosal cells via competitive inhibition.[55,56] This positive role creates a real dilemma for clinicians attempting to formulate antimicrobial regimens for critically ill patients.

Normal gastrointestinal motility is perhaps the most important of the physiologic components of the gut barrier. Movement of luminal contents distally within the gut keeps luminal concentrations of bacteria relatively low in the proximal gut and reduces the risk of adher-

ence and translocation. Conversely, there is considerable evidence to suggest that ileus and intestinal obstruction could be important factors in the so-called gut origin septic response.[57]

FACTORS THAT COMPROMISE BARRIER FUNCTION

In critically ill surgical patients, there are numerous associated clinical factors that compromise the various components of barrier function. Critical illness and injury lead to disordered gastrointestinal motility and ileus. Antibiotic therapy frequently covers the common aerobic and anaerobic members of the normal microflora, which results in overgrowth of the gut with resistant aerobic species. Parenteral nutrient solutions are characteristically deficient in glutamine and short-chain fatty acids, and sustained use of such solutions can cause atrophy of the mucosal barrier. IgA and mucin production may be compromised by the catabolic state typical of severe illness. In essence, all of the components of the gut barrier are potentially vulnerable; microbial translocation (and, subsequently, the systemic septic response) can result from impairment of any or all of them.

RECOGNITION AND MANAGEMENT OF MICROBIAL TRANSLOCATION

The clinical basis for the diagnosis of gastrointestinal microbial translocation is imprecise: there is no distinctive clinical marker of this event. Essentially, the diagnosis is one of exclusion. When all conventional infectious sources for a septic response have been excluded by careful clinical evaluation, microbial translocation is considered to be the cause. This clinical diagnosis is a treacherous one and can only be made presumptively. Even when the clinician is convinced that gastrointestinal microbial translocation is operative, he or she must remain vigilant and continue to search for infectious foci that may be driving the septic response.

Blood cultures that are positive for certain opportunistic microbes imply that gastrointestinal microbial translocation may be present. The so-called trilogy of translocation includes the enterococcus,[14] *S. epidermidis*,[7] and *Candida* species.[33,34,58] These three microbes are common overgrowth organisms after sustained courses of broad-spectrum antibiotic therapy and are commonly identified together in blood culture.[7,14,33] Obviously, when blood cultures are positive for these organisms, infectious sources must be ruled out, particularly bacteremia from intravascular devices.

Fundamental to the prevention and treatment of gastrointestinal microbial translocation is reinforcement of the gut barrier. Enteral rather than parenteral nutritional support is always recommended if the clinical circumstances permit.[59] Intraluminal nutrients are delivered directly to the mucosal cells and promote gastrointestinal motility[60]; moreover, they foster proliferation of a more normal intestinal microflora. Mobilization of the patient from the recumbent position likewise promotes gastrointestinal motility and is considered a critical feature of early fixation of long-bone fractures in multiple-trauma patients.[57,61] Immunonutritional regimens that are enhanced with glutamine, arginine, omega-3 fatty acids, and nucleotides have produced encouraging results in prospective clinical trials.[62]

Given what is known about the critical role of the normal gut microflora in the prevention of microbial translocation, it is important to reevaluate patterns of antibiotic use. Although anaerobes are pathogens that act synergistically with aerobes in intra-abdominal and soft tissue infection, in the gut lumen anaerobes are important components of the gut barrier.[63,64] Because anaerobes are seldom nosocomial pathogens, use of systemic antibiotics that cover anaerobes should be avoided in the ICU-acquired infection unless clearly necessary. Some authors have advocated selective gut decontamination (SGD), in which intraluminal antibiotics are employed to reduce aerobic colonization of the gut while preserving the anaerobic species.[65,66] Although SGD is popular in some areas, its value remains controversial.

Negative Blood Culture with Infection

A positive blood culture is generally accepted as proof that microbial dissemination has occurred and that this process is the stimulus for the septic response (although, as noted [*see* Positive Blood Culture without Infection, *above*], such an assumption is not always warranted). However, most patients who manifest the septic response secondary to severe infection do not have positive blood cultures. Thus, in these patients, it is the septic response, rather than the blood culture itself, that is the most useful clinical indicator of a systemic reaction to infection.

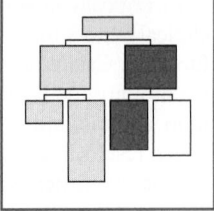

REASONS FOR NEGATIVE CULTURE

Patients with the septic response secondary to infection may have negative blood cultures for any of several reasons. First, the septic response may have been activated by disseminated microorganisms that are sensitive to concurrently administered antibiotic therapy. The patient may actually be bacteremic, but the presence of active antibiotic in the blood prevents bacterial growth in the culture. For certain antibiotics, there are laboratory methods for neutralizing the effects of their concurrent administration (e.g., penicillinase), but for most, this is not the case. Second, it may have been dissemination of bacterial cellular products rather than of whole, viable microorganisms that activated the septic response. Endotoxin is the most notable of the cellular products associated with the septic response. Third, the septic response may have been activated by systemic distribution of cytokine signals from an intense focus of infection (e.g., severe peritonitis), without bacteria or their products being disseminated from the primary site. Fourth, bacteremia is an episodic process, and blood culture a random event; thus, the culture sample may simply have been obtained at a time when the patient was temporarily nonbacteremic. The frequency of positive blood cultures in critically ill surgical patients in the ICU is so low, and the value of the occasional positive culture so minimal, that several authors have recommended discontinuing the practice of drawing blood samples from these patients.[67,68]

EVALUATION AND MANAGEMENT

Nonbacteremic patients who manifest the septic response must still be evaluated just as thoroughly as bacteremic patients would be, with the aim of ascertaining whether there is a primary source of infection. The lungs, the urinary tract, surgical or traumatic wounds, visceral compartments, and intravenous devices must all be sequentially evaluated. Careful physical examination, appropriate diagnostic studies for each anatomic area (e.g., CT scans for the abdomen), and aggressive culturing of suspicious fluids or exudates are indicated. Special emphasis must be placed on the surgical site and on sites where invasive monitoring devices (e.g., a Foley catheter) or support instruments (e.g., an endotracheal tube) have been introduced into the patient; these sites are frequently the source of the patient's problem. Nonbacteremic patients may indeed have the septic response without being infected [*see* Septic Response without Microorganisms, *below*], but this can be determined only after the patient has undergone systematic evaluation for a primary infectious focus.

Once a presumptive source of infection has been identified, the primary focus should be drained mechanically, and empirical antimicrobial therapy directed toward the anticipated pathogens should

Table 6 Common Pathogens Identified in Severely Ill Surgical Patients with Postoperative Pneumonia

Cultured Pathogen	Number of Isolates	
	Rodriguez[69]	Fink[70]
Gram-negative		
Pseudomonas species	38 (22%)	70 (19.5%)
Haemophilus species	16 (9%)	53 (15%)
Enterobacter species	26 (15%)	32 (9%)
Klebsiella species	13 (7.5%)	38 (10.5%)
Escherichia coli	7 (4%)	24 (7%)
Acinetobacter species	12 (7%)	11 (3%)
Proteus species	10 (6%)	11 (3%)
Serratia species	14 (8%)	0
Others	0	46 (13%)
Gram-positive		
Staphylococcus aureus	37 (21%)	48 (13%)
Other	0	26 (7%)
Total	173	359

be initiated while culture and sensitivity data are pending. For intra-abdominal infections, the antibiotic regimen must cover both enteric aerobic and anaerobic bacteria. For postoperative pulmonary infection, it usually must cover the multiresistant gram-negative bacteria of the *Pseudomonas* and *Serratia* species[69,70] [*see* Table 6]. Postoperative urinary tract infections are usually caused by enteric aerobic gram-negative rods [*see* Table 7]. Intravascular device infections are generally attributable to staphylococci but are sometimes caused by gram-negative rods or even fungi.

In many cases, critically ill patients who have undergone operation have already received antibiotic therapy at some time during the course of their management. Culture and sensitivity information must therefore be continuously obtained because the pathogens found in complex ICU patients with the septic response will often be resistant to multiple conventional antibiotics.

Although in many cases the source of the infection and the attendant septic response is readily apparent, in many others the diagnosis

Table 7 Pathogens Cultured in 212 Postoperative Urinary Tract Infections That Occurred in 153 Surgical Patients[22]

Organism	Number of Isolates
Escherichia coli	56
Klebsiella species	38
Pseudomonas species	37
Proteus species	30
Enterobacter species	22
Enterococcus	22
Serratia species	16
Citrobacter species	10
Streptococcus species	9
Staphylococcus epidermidis	8
Providencia species	5
Candida species	3
Total	256*

*The total exceeds 212 because of polymicrobial isolates in a number of patients.

can only be presumptive. Constant vigilance for changing clinical findings and careful observation of the response to empirical therapy are essential. For example, if a postoperative patient with the septic response has a urinary tract culture that is positive for *E. coli* at 10^5 colony-forming units/ml, it does not necessarily follow that the urinary tract is the source of the patient's septic response. In my experience, a well-drained urinary tract is seldom the source of a septic response in a postoperative patient; other sources must be considered even when a positive urinary tract culture has been obtained.

The surgeon without a diagnosis is likely to find it difficult to handle either the infection or the septic response effectively; thus, continued intensive surveillance of these difficult patients is essential. The objective of management is to control, by mechanical and pharmacologic means, the primary infectious source or sources of the disseminated whole microorganisms, microbial cellular products, or inflammatory cytokines that are responsible for the clinical septic response. Unfortunately, this objective is not equally appropriate for all nonbacteremic septic patients: as is now well established, the septic response can be activated by processes other than clinical infection.

Septic Response without Microorganisms

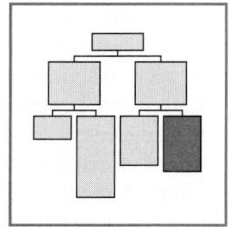

Traditional assumptions notwithstanding, there is no necessary association between the activation of the septic response and the presence of infection. To underscore this point, some authors have advocated use of the term systemic inflammatory response syndrome to the exclusion of the term sepsis.[1] Nevertheless, the term sepsis is commonly used for SIRS that is secondary to infection [*see VI:10 Clinical and Laboratory Diagnosis of Infection*]. Any physiologic event that can trigger a severe local inflammatory response is potentially capable of activating the septic response.[71-73] In much the same way as in severe infection without bacteremia or dissemination of bacterial cellular products, extreme local tissue inflammation without a microbial component can cause the release of inflammatory cytokines into the circulation in sufficient quantities to evoke the septic response.

Several common clinical entities can trigger the systemic septic response. Of these, acute pancreatitis is perhaps the most notable. The clinical course of severe acute pancreatitis managed with aggressive volume resuscitation includes loss of peripheral vascular resistance, elevated cardiac output, elevated white blood cell counts, and fever. Indeed, Ranson's criteria reflect characteristics of systemic inflammation, including end-organ damage to the lungs, the liver, and the kidneys.[74] Patients with severe acute pancreatitis often clearly illustrate the rapid physiologic progression from the initiation of the septic response to multiorgan dysfunction [*see 0VII:7 Multiple Organ Dysfunction Syndrome*]. Other conditions that can activate the septic response are severe aspiration pneumonitis, which initially is a chemical event that evokes an intense inflammatory response, and multiple trauma with extensive soft tissue injury, necrosis at the injury site, and tissue hematoma. Even extracorporeal membrane oxygenation can be associated with acute activation of the complement cascade and a postoperative septic response leading to end-organ failure, without infection or bacteria being involved at all.

When the septic response occurs in a patient with one of these conditions, the clinician often becomes anxious about the possibility of infection and is tempted to initiate antimicrobial therapy, at the very least. The clinical manifestations of the septic response are essentially the same whether it is caused by infection or not. Accordingly, the diagnosis of the septic response secondary to sterile inflammation is one of suspicion and exclusion. The septic response caused by noninfectious inflammatory processes evolves rapidly after the biologic insult and is not associated with clinical evidence of infection at a specific anatomic site; it is this very response, rather than any infection, that is the fundamental problem to be dealt with in these patients. Obviously, then, antibiotic therapy will be ineffective in such cases, and specific treatment must be directed toward the septic response itself.

Effective supportive care is essential to the management of the septic response secondary to sterile inflammation. Volume support to maintain an adequate cardiac output and tissue perfusion is vital. The pulmonary microcirculation is the early target of the septic response; accordingly, support of systemic oxygenation with mechanical ventilation is commonly necessary.

A vexing problem associated with severe pancreatitis or aspiration pneumonia is that a number of separate stimuli capable of activating the septic response will present themselves during the course of protracted management. In a patient with severe pancreatitis, for example, the primary inflammatory focus gives rise to an initial septic response characterized by pulmonary failure. The patient is effectively resuscitated and appears clinically improved by the fourth or fifth day of hospitalization. By this point, however, an infectious focus, in the form of a pancreatic abscess, has often developed, and this focus evokes a second septic response. Multiple operations and prolonged antibiotic therapy then set the stage for gastrointestinal microbial translocation, which results in candidemia and a third septic response.

What is more, not only may a single condition give rise to multiple different stimuli for the elicitation of the septic response, but severely ill surgical patients may also have additional separate inciting causes (either sequentially or simultaneously) during the course of management, each of which may be associated with one or more septic stimuli. Indeed, a major challenge for the future—perhaps the major challenge—is better definition of clinical markers for specific stimuli of the septic response so that treatment can be better directed.

Discussion

Sepsis as Nonspecific Systemic Inflammatory Response

Infection has traditionally been viewed as a local inflammatory response within tissue that is initiated and perpetuated by microorganisms. It is generally agreed that the numerous elements of host defense are designed to both contain and eradicate the microbial provocateurs of this inflammatory process. It is also generally recognized that a threshold exists, the breaching of which results in the dissemination of the infectious process and the elicitation of a systemic inflammatory response. The precise point at which this threshold is passed has not been well defined clinically; however, the clinical expressions of this event are easily recognized [*see VI:10 Clinical and Laboratory Diagnosis of Infection*].

Characteristic systemic manifestations of infection include fever, leukocytosis, hyperglycemia, gastrointestinal ileus, and many other findings, depending on the acuteness and severity of the situation. Blood cultures may be positive (see above), and sophisticated laboratory analysis of peripheral blood may yield evidence of the presence of bacterial cell products, such as gram-negative bacterial endotoxin. In these clinical circumstances, patients are said to be septic, to have sepsis, or to have septicemia because the clinical response has been most closely identified with severe infection.[75]

There is considerable evidence to support the theory that the so-called septic patient has a generalized, systemic activation of the inflammatory cascade. The intricate inflammatory response to injury that is so salutary at the tissue level actually becomes a self-destructive process when activated at the systemic level.[76] Although these septic events have been associated most often with uncontrolled infection, it is now appreciated that the systemic inflammatory response is in fact a nonspecific host response in the same way that soft tissue inflammation is nonspecific. In other words, the septic response, despite its traditional association with severe infection, does not require infection or even the presence of microorganisms to be activated—hence the introduction of the term SIRS.[1]

We can now identify a changing perspective with respect to the stimuli of the septic response in the surgical intensive care unit. Current support technology permits sustained survival of critically ill and severely injured patients to a biologic point never before reached. As a result, the septic response may now be seen as a consequence of (1) microorganisms in the context of infection, (2) microorganisms in the absence of infection, and (3) inflammatory events not associated with either microorganisms or clinical infection.

Elements of the Septic Response

The septic response represents an evolution of multiple physiologic and metabolic changes. These changes do not constitute an either-or phenomenon but instead take place along an ever-changing continuum. Consequently, it is difficult to determine exactly when a patient ceases to manifest an appropriate stress response and begins to manifest a deleterious septic response.

The key physiologic elements of the septic response are (1) reduced peripheral vascular resistance, (2) hyperdynamic cardiac performance, and (3) narrowing of the arteriovenous oxygen content difference. The metabolic features of the septic response are quite complex but can be simplified into five main elements: (1) hypermetabolism, (2) accelerated hepatic gluconeogenesis, (3) accelerated hepatic ureagenesis, (4) increased urinary nitrogen loss, and (5) insulin resistance. These metabolic changes are discussed in greater detail elsewhere [see VII:8 Metabolic Response to Critical Illness].

Reduced peripheral vascular resistance—contrasting dramatically with the increased resistance associated with hypovolemia and cardiac failure—is the sine qua non of the septic response. (It must be emphasized that whereas resistance is reduced for the vascular system as a whole, this may not be the case for each individual tissue bed.) The loss of resistance is particularly interesting in the light of the elevated catecholamine concentrations that are simultaneously identified in these patients. The increases in catecholamine concentration reflect the counterregulatory metabolic milieu of the septic response.[77,78] The alpha-adrenergic effects of the catecholamines are obviously overridden by other peripheral mechanisms.

The systemic vasodilatation has been explained by several mechanisms, but it appears to be principally the result of nitric oxide from endothelial cells in the microcirculation.[79-82] Nitric oxide is a paracrine signal that mediates relaxation of vascular smooth muscle. Its synthesis and release are stimulated by several agonist agents, including endotoxin, bradykinin, and acetylcholine. While other mechanisms include prostacyclin and histamine as potential mediators of vasodilatation, at this time nitric oxide appears to be the principal one.

Hyperdynamic cardiac performance is the obligatory response of the left ventricle when peripheral vascular resistance declines. For cardiac output to increase, however, intravascular volume must be replenished, and the myocardium must possess sufficient physiologic reserve. Thus, elderly patients may not be able to meet the physiologic demands imposed by sepsis-induced afterload reduction, and such inability will result in the hypodynamic septic-shock state. Even in young, healthy patients, the sustained hyperdynamic state will ultimately lead to ventricular failure and low cardiac output.

Narrowing of the arteriovenous oxygen content difference in the hyperdynamic patient is perhaps the most important key to the critical mechanisms responsible for the septic response. Oxygen consumption is inadequate to meet the demands of hypermetabolism,[83,84] and lactate production is the result. When intravascular volume is fully expanded, further increases in cardiac output result in further narrowing of the arteriovenous oxygen content difference. The failure of peripheral oxygen utilization is fundamental to the septic process and underscores that the septic response is not a disease of inadequate myocardial performance until the very late stages in the natural history of the disease.

Natural History of the Septic Response

Studies from the late 1970s[85] provided an important classification system for the natural history of the septic response. This classification identifies exaggeration of the fundamental stress response as the basis for deterioration of the patient from a compensated state (i.e., the stress response) to a decompensated state (i.e., the septic response). The key element to be understood in the natural history of the septic response is the relation between cardiac output and peripheral vascular resistance [see Figure 3].

State A represents the normal adaptive stress response, the first-order response to biologic insults. Cardiac output is modestly elevated, and peripheral vascular resistance is modestly reduced. Systemic oxygen consumption is increased, but lactate concentration is not. This state reflects the postresuscitative physiology of the injured or postoperative patient. The hemodynamic profile progressively returns to normal over the ensuing several days, provided that there is no intercurrent insult (e.g., infection).

State B represents the exaggerated stress response and marks the transition to the beginning of biologic decompensation. Peripheral

Cardiac Output

Systemic Vascular Resistance

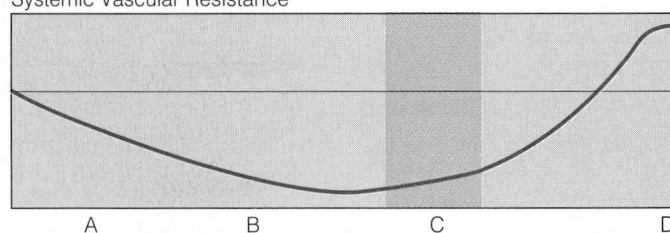

Figure 3 Illustrated is the relation of cardiac output to peripheral vascular resistance during the natural history of the septic response. The area indicated by the box is state C, reflecting the onset of clinical septic shock.

vascular resistance is profoundly reduced. A total peripheral vascular resistance lower than 800 dynes-sec/cm^5 is the commonly recognized threshold for the septic response; resistance may decline to 400 dynes-sec/cm^5 or even lower. The afterload reduction results in dramatic elevation of cardiac output. An acceptable arterial blood pressure can usually be sustained unless intrinsic myocardial disease or hypovolemia is present. The increased capacitance typical of state B necessitates considerable preload support, which often calls for aggressive fluid administration. Measurement of the pulmonary capillary wedge pressure is often necessary to facilitate the expansion of intravascular volume.

State B is also characterized by accumulation of lactate species in the blood before the evolution of frank clinical hypotension. Lactate concentrations in the blood reflect net lactate production in selected tissues minus lactate utilization in other tissues. Because not all tissues are necessarily affected equally by the septic response process, oxidation of lactate by selected well-perfused tissues may compensate for production of lactate by others. Lactic acidemia preceding lactic acidosis is usually seen in patients with sustained state B; compensatory mechanisms prevent acidosis until later in the process. These patients are actually in a state of shock, even though their arterial blood pressure is considered normal, because tissue oxygen utilization is clearly impaired.

State C heralds the beginning of septic shock as it has been traditionally defined—that is, as hypotension in a nonhypovolemic patient that is secondary to severe infection. State C patients fulfill this definition: they have mild to severe hypotension, with systolic arterial blood pressures lower than 80 mm Hg. In this setting, however, septic shock is secondary to the severe and exaggerated loss of peripheral vascular resistance; although cardiac output may be normal or slightly increased (8 to 10 L/min), it is insufficient to compensate for this loss.

State C patients are in so-called hot shock. They are warm to the touch and usually show evidence of diaphoresis. One has the clinical impression that the cutaneous tissues are well perfused, even though the arterial blood pressure is low. The loss of perfusion pressure acts synergistically with the peripheral defect in oxygen utilization to create a severe peripheral oxygen debt that is clearly reflected in the severe lactic acidosis seen in these patients.

State D represents the final phase in the process, in which frank congestive heart failure emerges. Cardiac performance is considerably depressed. Autonomic mechanisms override the vasodilatory influences seen in state C, and peripheral vascular resistance is now increased. In state D, low cardiac output, peripheral vasoconstriction, and peripheral defects in oxygen utilization work simultaneously to produce profound tissue hypoxemia and lactic acidosis. In the absence of dramatic therapeutic and supportive measures, this is the preagonal period before death.

Pathophysiology of the Septic Response

Fundamental to our current understanding of the septic response is the idea that its negative and destructive features are simply the systemic manifestations of what is otherwise a positive and beneficial local inflammatory response to tissue injury. The two types of response involve the same physiologic processes, but their domain and scope are very different. This crucial point can be illustrated by considering the local events that attend soft tissue injury. These events, in essence, are the septic response in microcosm.

LOCAL EVENTS

Soft tissue injury triggers a local inflammatory response that includes disruption of blood vessels, exposure of the collagen matrix, extravasation of red blood cells and plasma proteins, activation of the coagulation cascade, aggregation of platelets, and activation of the complement cascade via the alternative pathway.[86] It is likely that by-products of coagulation and complement activation, among other potential biochemical signals, are the stimuli to mast cells that initiate the first phases of the inflammatory response; the specific cleavage products of complement proteins C3, C4, and C5 (the soluble anaphylatoxins C3a, C4a, and C5a) are known to be the most potent stimuli of mast cell degranulation.[87-89] The production of bradykinin occurs from plasma protein precursors via the stimulation of activated factor XII from the coagulation cascade. Activation of these five initiators of inflammation (coagulation cascade, platelets, complement proteins, mast cells, and bradykinin) produces (1) local vasodilatation, increasing local flow but reducing flow velocity in the area of injury; (2) increased capillary permeability, resulting in extravasation of protein-rich plasma into the injured area, thereby initiating edema; and (3) generation of numerous inflammatory enzyme and protein cleavage products, which serve as chemoattractants.

Diffusion of the chemoattractant signals from the epicenter of injury begins the process of phagocytic infiltration of the injured area. Chemoattractants bind to specific receptor sites on vascular endothelial cells, initiating interaction between endothelial cells and intravascular neutrophils. Neutrophil "rolling" on the endothelial surface, initiated by surface selectin receptors, slows neutrophil transit velocity within the microcirculation and sets the stage for integrin interactions leading to margination of the neutrophil. The gradient of chemoattractant signals from the epicenter of the injury serves as a beacon, directing phagocytic diapedesis toward the site of injury and contamination. The severity of the injury, the extent of necrosis, and the degree of exogenous microbial contamination dictate the intensity of the summed chemoattractant signals that govern the rapidity and the quantity of neutrophil infiltration.

Approximately 24 hours after injury, macrophages infiltrate the area via the same mechanisms for margination and chemotaxis that mobilized the neutrophils. Macrophages orchestrate the severity of the inflammatory response. If necrotic tissue and foreign elements (e.g., bacteria) are minimally present in the area of injury, then the magnitude of the chemoattractant signal will be small, macrophages are minimally activated, and the neutrophils proceed with phagocytosis in an orderly fashion. If, however, bacterial contamination is severe and there is considerable necrotic tissue, then the amplitude of chemoattractant effects will be great, resulting in full activation of macrophages. The fully activated macrophage elaborates multiple proinflammatory cytokines with autocrine, paracrine, and endocrine functions.

One such cytokine, tumor necrosis factor, is itself capable of inducing full macrophage activation.[90] In addition, TNF serves as an activating signal from the macrophages to the neutrophils, causing the neutrophils to enter a state of accelerated and enhanced phagocytic activity and eliciting the extracellular release of reactive oxygen intermediates and lysosomal enzymes. The accelerated phagocytic activity, driven by the TNF and other proinflammatory signals from the macrophages, results in the death of the neutrophils and in the formation of pus. Suppuration at the epicenter of the injury is further enhanced when the TNF signal diffuses into the adjacent microcirculation, where marginated neutrophils, recruited into the inflammatory focus, are fully activated. Activation of these neutrophils, coupled with release of reactive oxygen intermediates and lysosomal enzymes, results in thrombosis of the adjacent microcirculation. This microcirculatory thrombosis is actually beneficial in that it prevents bacteria or their products from gaining systemic access. Indeed, the ultimate function of the inflammatory response is the containment and subsequent eradication of bacterial contaminants.

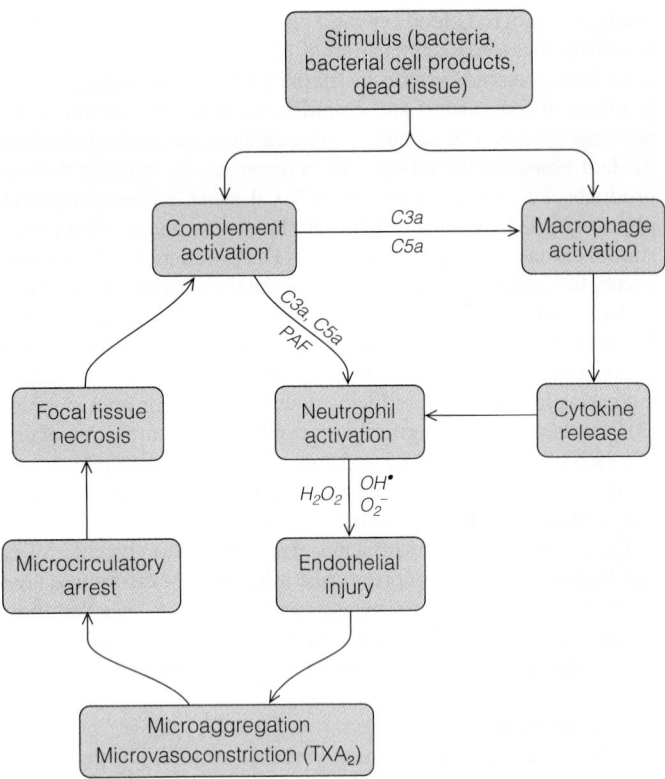

Figure 4 **Shown is the self-energized cycle of tissue-level injury that becomes the end-organ consequences of the septic response. Activation of the inflammatory cascade via several different stimuli results in neutrophil activation, which leads to autodestructive inflammation, tissue ischemia, tissue necrosis, and reactivation of the process.**

SYSTEMIC EVENTS

The systemic septic response comprises the same sequence of events just described, except that the activation of the inflammatory cascade is generalized and lacks the clear directional focus that characterizes the local response. In severe infection, dissemination of bacteria and endotoxins leads to systemic activation of the initiator pathways of human inflammation. Systemic activation of coagulation, platelets, complement proteins, mast cells, and bradykinin results in generalized edema, systemic vasodilatation, and a generalized release of chemoattractant signals. Generalized neutrophil margination occurs. The up-regulation of the generalized inflammatory response results in full activation of marginated neutrophils. From their intravascular and perivascular position, the activated neutrophils subsequently release reactive oxygen intermediates and lysosomal enzymes. The resulting inflammatory injury to the microcirculation leads to aggregation of platelets, damage to the endothelial cells, and release of prostaglandin derivatives that promote vasoconstriction. The consequence of these events is a two-pronged injury comprising the biomechanical blockade caused by the inflammatory aggregate and the vasoconstriction caused by thromboxane A_2.

When an inflammatory focus is sufficiently severe (as, for example, in pancreatitis), it may release so much TNF that macrophages and neutrophils are activated within the circulation. In these circumstances, in situ macrophage cells, such as alveolar macrophages and Kupffer's cells, can be activated, and a generalized inflammatory response is the result. In this scenario, systemic dissemination of the pathogen or its cellular products may not be required for the systemic inflammatory response; instead, only the proinflammatory cytokine signal needs to be disseminated.

This microcirculatory arrest, in turn, leads to the formation of foci of necrotic tissue,[91] which evoke a local inflammatory response that eventually reactivates the septic response. A self-energized and futile cycle is created, in which an initial injury elicits a local response, the local response subsequently expands into a systemic response, and the systemic response finally generates tissue-level injuries that start up the whole process all over again [*see Figure 4*]. The progressive loss of microcirculatory units within the critical organ systems leads to multiorgan failure (now also known as multiple organ dysfunction syndrome) [*see VII:7 Multiple Organ Dysfunction Syndrome*] and ultimately to the death of the host.[92-94]

New Approaches to Management of the Septic Response

A clearer comprehension of the mechanisms involved in the evolution of the septic response and its end-organ effects should facilitate the development of new and better therapeutic regimens. On the basis of what is currently known, numerous new treatments have already been examined in experimental studies, and a few of them have been used on an investigational basis in humans [*see 88 Immunomodulation*]. These newer therapies have had three general areas of focus: (1) neutralization of stimuli that provoke the systemic inflammatory response, (2) inhibition or blockade of the initiator events of inflammation itself, or (3) inhibition or neutralization of effector mechanisms that are the consequence of activation of the systemic inflammatory response.

Efforts to neutralize or inhibit the provocative stimulation of SIRS have focused on bacterial endotoxin as the target. Antiendotoxin antibody has been given to septic patients in an attempt to neutralize the effects of a component of gram-negative bacteria that is a potent activator of the septic response. Although some clinical studies have found that certain groups of septic response patients benefit from administration of polyclonal sera[95-97] or the monoclonal antibody,[98,99] considerable controversy continues to surround this proposed treatment. Favorable reports focusing on beneficial effects in specific subpopulations of patients have not been validated by prospective studies addressed to these cohorts.[100,101] Because endotoxin is only one of numerous stimuli of the septic response, routine use of the very expensive monoclonal antiendotoxin antibody for all septic response patients would be difficult to justify. It appears unlikely that this treatment strategy will be generally deployed in clinical practice.

Numerous experimental studies have explored inhibition of the initiators of inflammation: specifically, inhibition of coagulation,[102] coagulation and platelets,[103-105] bradykinin,[106] mast cell products,[107] and complement proteins.[108,109] Few have been pursued into prospective clinical trials. A prospective multicenter trial of a promising bradykinin antagonist failed to demonstrate any clinical benefit.[110]

A third focus of investigation has been the inhibition or alteration of effector mechanisms or consequences of activation of inflammation. Specific neutralization of TNF[111,112] or receptor blockade of the effects of interleukin-1[113] were initially the most promising prospects. However, clinical trials of both approaches have failed to demonstrate any meaningful benefit.[114-118] Other directions have included antibodies to prevent neutrophil-endothelial interaction; anti–platelet activating factor; neutralization of reactive oxygen intermediates to prevent lipid peroxidation; inhibition of various eicosanoid derivatives; and strategies with dialysis, plasmapheresis, or other means of filtering cytokines or other adverse effector substances. The theme is a constant one, in that experimental data inevitably show promise, but efforts to convert the experimental observations into improved results have consistently failed.

The current explosion in cytokine research has resulted in the identification of numerous new mediators of the inflammatory response. It is likely that still more will be recognized in the near future and that our understanding of the septic response will continue to evolve rapidly. At present, the major problem associated with mediator blockade or neutralization is that there are numerous redundant mechanisms at play in the human inflammatory response. Blockade of a single signal is unlikely to achieve the necessary physiologic effect. Furthermore, these chemical signals play a positive biologic role in the salutary local inflammatory response, which means that neutralization of the inflammatory cascade, while preventing the systemic septic response, could significantly impair host defense.

SIRS represents the same biologic processes that are identified in every wound and in every cutaneous infection. Surgical drainage of a severe soft tissue abscess results in rapid down-regulation of the inflammatory signals. Intrinsic down-regulatory mechanisms for the inflammatory response are obviously operational when inflammation is no longer necessary. A clearer understanding of the natural counterinflammatory mechanisms will likely prove to be the pathway to newer therapies for SIRS and its sequelae.

References

1. American College of Chest Physicians/Society of Critical Care Medicine Consensus Conference: Definitions for sepsis and organ failure and guidelines for the use of innovative therapies in sepsis. Crit Care Med 20:864, 1992

2. Fry DE, Fry RV, Borzotta AP: Nosocomial blood-borne infection secondary to intravascular devices. Am J Surg 167:268, 1994

3. Maki DG, Weise CE, Sarafin HW: A semiquantitative culture method for identifying intravenous-catheter–related infection. N Engl J Med 296:1305, 1977

4. Stein JM, Pruitt BA Jr: Suppurative thrombophlebitis: a lethal iatrogenic disease. N Engl J Med 282:1452, 1970

5. Garrison RN, Richardson JD, Fry DE: Catheter-associated septic thrombophlebitis. South Med J 75:917, 1982

6. Bandyk DF, Bergamini TM, Kinney EV, et al: In situ replacement of vascular prostheses infected by bacterial biofilm. J Vasc Surg 13:575, 1991

7. Burchard KW, Minor LB, Slotman GJ, et al: *Staphylococcus epidermidis* sepsis in surgical patients. Arch Surg 119:96, 1984

8. Stevens DL: The toxic shock syndromes. Infect Dis Clin North Am 10:727, 1996

9. Davies HD, McGeer A, Schwartz B, et al: Invasive group A streptococcal infection in Ontario, Canada: Ontario Group A Streptococcal Study Group. N Engl J Med 335:547, 1996

10. Aebi C, Ahmed A, Ramilo O: Bacterial complications of primary varicella in children. Clin Infect Dis 23:698, 1996

11. Stevens DL, Gibbons AE, Bergstrom R, et al: The eagle effect revisited: efficacy of clindamycin, erythromycin, and penicillin in the treatment of streptococcal myositis. J Infect Dis 158:23, 1988

12. Barie PS, Christou NV, Dellinger EP, et al: Pathogenicity of the enterococcus in surgical infections. Ann Surg 212:155, 1990

13. Nichols RL, Muzik AC: Enterococcal infections in surgical patients: the mystery continues. Clin Infect Dis 15:72, 1992

14. Garrison RN, Fry DE, Berberich S, et al: Enterococcal bacteremia: clinical implications and determinants of death. Ann Surg 196:43, 1982

15. Yu VL: Enterococcal superinfection and colonization after therapy with moxalactam, a new broad-spectrum antibiotic. Ann Intern Med 94:784, 1981

16. Fry DE, Berberich S, Garrison RN: Bacterial synergism between the enterococcus and *Escherichia coli*. J Surg Res 38:475, 1985

17. Onderdonk AB, Bartlett JG, Louie T, et al: Microbial synergy in experimental intra-abdominal abscess. Infect Immun 13:22, 1976

18. Fry DE, Cox RA, Harbrecht PJ: Gangrene of the gallbladder: a complication of acute cholecystitis. South Med J 74:666, 1981

19. Eliopoulos GM: Vancomycin-resistant enterococci: mechanism and clinical relevance. Infect Dis Clin North Am 11:851, 1997

20. Landman D, Quale JM: Management of infection due to resistant enterococci: a review of therapeutic options. J Antimicrob Chemother 40:161, 1997

21. Collins LA, Malanoski GJ, Eliopoulos GM, et al: In vitro activity of RP 59500, an injectable streptogramin antibiotic, against vancomycin-resistant gram positive organisms. Antimicrob Agents Chemother 37:598, 1993

22. Asher EF, Oliver BG, Fry DE: Urinary tract infections in the surgical patient. Am Surg 54:466, 1988

23. Fry DE, Cox RA, Harbrecht PJ: Empyema of the gallbladder: a complication in the natural history of acute cholecystitis. Am J Surg 141:366, 1981

24. Mosdell DM, Morris DM, Voltura A, et al: Antibiotic treatment for surgical peritonitis. Ann Surg 214:543, 1991

25. Fry DE: Third generation cephalosporin antibiotics in surgical practice. Am J Surg 151:306, 1986

26. Niemiec PW Jr, Allo MD, Miller CF: Effect of altered volume of distribution on aminoglycoside levels in patients in surgical intensive care. Arch Surg 122:207, 1987

27. Brighty KE, Gootz TD: The chemistry and biological profile of trovafloxacin. J Antimicrob Chemother 39(suppl B):1, 1997

28. Koo J, Tight R, Rajkumar V, et al: Comparison of once-daily versus pharmacokinetic dosing of aminoglycosides in elderly patients. Am J Med 101:177, 1996

29. Fry DE, Garrison RN, Polk HC Jr: Clinical implications in bacteroides bacteremia. Surg Gynecol Obstet 149:189, 1979

30. Kasper DL, Hayes ME, Reinap BG, et al: Isolation and identification of encapsulated strains of *Bacteroides fragilis*. J Infect Dis 136:75, 1977

31. Ledger WJ, Kriewall TJ, Sweet RL, et al: The use of parenteral clindamycin in the treatment of obstetric-gynecologic patients with severe infections: a comparison of clindamycin-kanamycin with penicillin-kanamycin. Obstet Gynecol 43:490, 1974

32. Fry DE, Klamer TW, Garrison RN, et al: Atypical clostridial bacteremia. Surg Gynecol Obstet 153:28, 1981

33. Dyess DL, Garrison RN, Fry DE: *Candida* sepsis: implications of polymicrobial blood-borne infection. Arch Surg 120:345, 1985

34. Stone HH, Kolb LD, Currie CA, et al: *Candida* sepsis: pathogenesis and principles of treatment. Ann Surg 179:697, 1974

35. Solomkin JS, Flohr AB, Quie PG, et al: The role of *Candida* in intraperitoneal infections. Surgery 88:524, 1980

36. Rex JH, Bennett JE, Sugar AM, et al: A randomized trial comparing fluconazole with amphotericin B for the treatment of candidemia in patients without neutropenia. N Engl J Med 331:1325, 1994

37. Evans TG, Mayer J, Cohen S, et al: Fluconazole failure in treatment of systemic mycoses. J Infect Dis 164:1232, 1991

38. Fine J, Frank ED, Ravin HA, et al: The bacterial factor in traumatic shock. N Engl J Med 260:214, 1959

39. Ravin HA, Fine J: Biological implications of intestinal endotoxins. Fed Proc 21:65, 1962

40. Schweinburg F, Fine J: Evidence for a lethal endotoxemia as the fundamental feature of irreversibility in three types of traumatic shock. J Exp Med 112:793, 1960

41. Zweifach BW: Hemorrhagic shock in germfree rats. Ann NY Acad Sci 78:315, 1959

42. Zweifach BW, Gordon HA, Wagner M, et al: Irreversible hemorrhagic shock in germfree rats. J Exp Med 107:437, 1958

43. Maejima K, Deitch EA, Berg RD: Bacterial translocation from the gastrointestinal tracts of rats receiving thermal injury. Infect Immun 43:6, 1984

44. Baker JW, Deitch EA, Li M, et al: Hemorrhagic shock induces bacterial translocation from the gut. J Trauma 28:896, 1988

45. Deitch EA, Winterton J, Li M, et al: The gut as a portal of entry for bacteremia: role of protein malnutrition. Ann Surg 205:681, 1987

46. Deitch DE, Berg R, Specian R: Endotoxin promotes the translocation of bacteria from the gut. Arch Surg 122:185, 1987

47. Rush BF Jr, Sori AJ, Murphy TF, et al: Endotoxemia and bacteremia during hemorrhagic shock. Ann Surg 207:549, 1988

48. Deitch EA: Simple intestinal obstruction causes bacterial translocation in man. Arch Surg 124:699, 1989

49. Rush BF Jr, Redan JA, Flanagan JJ Jr, et al: Does bacteremia in hemorrhagic shock have clinical significance? A study in germ-free animals. Ann Surg 210:342, 1989

50. Lanser ME: An experimental phenomenon without clinical significance. Multiple System Organ Failure. Fry DE, Ed. Mosby–Year Book, Chicago, 1992, p 382

51. Wilmore DW, Smith RJ, O'Dwyer ST, et al: The gut: a central organ after surgical stress. Surgery 104:917, 1988

52. Roediger WE, Rae DA: Trophic effect of short chain fatty acids on mucosal handling of ions by the dysfunctioned colon. Br J Surg 69:23, 1982

53. McNabb PC, Tomasi TB: Host defense mechanisms at mucosal surfaces. Annu Rev Microbiol 35:477, 1981

54. Tomasi TB Jr, Bienenstock J: Secretory immunoglobulins. Adv Immunol 9:1, 1968

55. Savage DC, Dubos R, Schaedler RW: The gastrointestinal epithelium and its autochthonous bacterial flora. J Exp Med 127:67, 1968

56. Suegara N, Morotomi M, Watanabe T, et al: Behavior of the microflora in the rat stomach: adhesion of lactobacilli to the keratinized epithelial cells of the rat in vitro. Infect Immun 12:173, 1975

57. Border J, Hassett J, LaDuca J, et al: The gut origin septic states in blunt multiple trauma (ISS = 40) in the ICU. Ann Surg 206:427, 1987

58. Alexander JW, Boyce ST, Babcock GF, et al: The process of microbial translocation. Ann Surg 212:496, 1990

59. Moore FA, Moore EE, Jones TN, et al: TEN versus TPN following major abdominal trauma—reduced septic morbidity. J Trauma 29:916, 1989

60. Mochizuki H, Trocki O, Dominioni L, et al: Mechanism of prevention of postburn hypermetabolism and catabolism by early enteral feeding. Ann Surg 200:297, 1984

61. Seibel R, LaDuca J, Hassett JM, et al: Blunt multiple trauma (ISS 36), femur traction, and the pulmonary failure–septic state. Ann Surg 202:283, 1985

62. Kudsk KA, Minard G, Croce MA, et al: A randomized trial of isonitrogenous enteral diets following severe trauma: an immune-enhancing diet (IED) reduces septic complications. Ann Surg 224:531, 1996

63. Berg RD: Promotion of the translocation of enteric bacteria from the gastrointestinal tracts of mice by oral treatment with penicillin, clindamycin, or metronidazole. Infect Immun 33:854, 1981

64. Epstein MD, Tchervenkov JI, Alexander JW, et al: Effect of intraluminal antibiotics on the translocation of *Candida albicans* in burned guinea pigs. Burns 16:105, 1990

65. van der Waaij D: Colonization resistance of the digestive tract: clinical consequences and implications. J Antimicrob Chemother 10:263, 1982

66. Cerra FB, Maddaus MA, Dunn DL, et al: Selective gut decontamination reduces nosocomial infections and length of stay but not mortality or organ failure in surgical intensive care unit patients. Arch Surg 127:163, 1992

67. Theuer CP, Bongard FS, Klein SR: Are blood cultures effective in the evaluation of fever in perioperative patients? Am J Surg 162:615, 1991

68. Henke PK, Polk HC Jr: Efficacy of blood cultures in the critically ill surgical patient. Surgery 120:752, 1996

69. Rodriguez JR, Gibbons KJ, Bitzer LG, et al: Pneumonia: incidence, risk factors, and outcome in injured patients. J Trauma 31:907, 1991

70. Fink MP, Snydman DR, Niederman MS, et al: Treatment of severe pneumonia in hospitalized patients: results of a multicenter, randomized, double-blind trial comparing intravenous ciprofloxacin with imipenem-cilastatin. Antimicrob Agents Chemother 38:547, 1994

71. Goris RJ, Boekholtz WK, van Bebber IP, et al: Multiple-organ failure and sepsis without bacteria: an experimental model. Arch Surg 121:897, 1986

72. Schirmer WJ, Schirmer JM, Naff GB, et al: Systemic complement activation produces hemodynamic changes characteristic of sepsis. Arch Surg 123:316, 1988

73. Schirmer WJ, Schirmer JM, Townsend MC, et al: Femur fracture with associated soft-tissue injury produces hepatic ischemia: possible cause of hepatic dysfunction. Arch Surg 123:412, 1988

74. Ranson JHC, Rifkind KM, Roses DF, et al: Prognostic signs and the role of operative management in acute pancreatitis. Surg Gynecol Obstet 139:69, 1974

75. Bone RC: Sepsis, the sepsis syndrome, multi-organ failure: a plea for comparable definitions (editorial). Ann Intern Med 114:332, 1991

76. Goris RJ, te Boekhorst TP, Nuytinck JK, et al: Multiple organ failure: generalized autodestructive inflammation? Arch Surg 120:1109, 1985

77. Bessey PQ, Watters JM, Aoki TT, et al: Combined hormonal infusion simulates the metabolic response to injury. Ann Surg 200:264, 1984

78. Watters JM, Bessey PQ, Dinarello CA, et al: Both inflammatory and endocrine mediators stimulate host responses to sepsis. Arch Surg 121:179, 1986

79. Moncada S, Palmer RMJ, Higgs EA: The discovery of nitric oxide as the endogenous nitrovasodilator. Hypertension 12:365, 1988

80. Ignarro LJ: Biological actions and properties of endothelium-derived nitric oxide formed and released from artery and vein. Circ Res 65:1, 1989

81. Ignarro LJ: Biosynthesis and metabolism of endothelium-derived nitric oxide. Annu Rev Pharmacol Toxicol 30:535, 1990

82. Vallance P, Collier J, Moncada S: Nitric oxide synthesised from L-arginine mediates endothelium dependent dilatation in human veins in vivo. Cardiovasc Res 23:1053, 1989

83. Siegel JH, Greenspan M, Del Guercio LRM: Abnormal vascular tone, defective oxygen transport and myocardial failure in human septic shock. Ann Surg 165:504, 1967

84. Siegel JH, Farrell EJ, Miller M, et al: Cardiorespiratory interactions as determinants of survival and the need for respiratory support in human shock states. J Trauma 13:602, 1973

85. Siegel JH, Cerra FB, Coleman B, et al: Physiological and metabolic correlations in human sepsis: invited commentary. Surgery 86:163, 1979

86. Pillemer L, Blum L, Lepow IH, et al: The properdin system and immunity: I. Demonstration and isolation of a new serum protein, properdin, and its role in immune phenomena. Science 120:279, 1954

87. Gorski JP, Hugli TE, Muller-Eberhard HJ: Characterization of human C4a anaphylatoxin. J Biol Chem 256:2707, 1981

88. da Silva WD, Eisele JW, Lepow IH: Complement as a mediator of inflammation: III. Purification of the activity with anaphylatoxin properties generated by interaction of the first four components of complement and its identification as a cleavage product of C'3. J Exp Med 126:1027, 1967

89. Shin HS, Snyderman R, Friedman E, et al: Chemotactic and anaphylatoxic fragment cleaved from the fifth component of guinea pig complement. Science 162:361, 1968

90. Beutler B, Cerami A: Cachectin: more than a tumor necrosis factor. N Engl J Med 316:379, 1987

91. Asher EF, Rowe RL, Garrison RN, et al: Experimental bacteremia and hepatic nutrient blood flow. Circ Shock 20:43, 1986

92. Townsend MC, Hampton WW, Haybron DM, et al: Effective organ blood flow and bioenergy status in murine peritonitis. Surgery 100:205, 1986

93. Schirmer WJ, Townsend MC, Schirmer JM, et al: Galactose elimination kinetics in sepsis: correlations of hepatic blood flow with function. Arch Surg 122:349, 1987

94. Haybron DM, Townsend MC, Hampton WW, et al: Alterations in renal perfusion and renal energy charge in murine peritonitis. Arch Surg 122:328, 1987

95. Lachman E, Pitsoe SB, Gaffin SL: Anti-lipopolysaccharide immunotherapy in management of septic shock of obstetric and gynaecological origin. Lancet 1:981, 1984

96. Baumgartner JD, Glauser MP, McCutchan JA, et al: Prevention of gram-negative shock and death in surgical patients by antibody to endotoxin core glycolipid. Lancet 2:59, 1985

97. Ziegler EJ, McCutchan JA, Fierer J, et al: Treatment of gram-negative bacteremia and shock with human antiserum to a mutant *Escherichia coli*. N Engl J Med 307:1225, 1982

98. Ziegler EJ, Fischer CJ, Sprung CL Jr, et al: Treatment of gram-negative bacteremia and septic shock with HA-1A human monoclonal antibody against endotoxin: a randomized, double-blind, placebo-controlled trial. N Engl J Med 324:429, 1991

99. Greenman RL, Schein RMH, Martin MA, et al: A controlled clinical trial of E5 murine monoclonal IgM antibody to endotoxin in the treatment of gram-negative sepsis. JAMA 266:1097, 1991

100. McCloskey RV, Straube RC, Sanders C, et al: Treatment of septic shock with human monoclonal antibody HA-1A: a randomized, double-blind, placebo-controlled trial. CHESS Trial Study Group. Ann Intern Med 121:1, 1994

101. Bone RC, Balk RA, Fein AM, et al: A second large controlled study of E5, a monoclonal antibody to endotoxin: results of a prospective, multicenter, randomized, controlled trial. The E5 Sepsis Study Group. Crit Care Med 23:994, 1995

102. Jansen PM, Pixley RA, Brouwer M, et al: Inhibition of factor XII in septic baboons attenuates the activation of complement and fibrinolytic system and reduces the release of interleukin-6 and neutrophil elastase. Blood 87:2337, 1996

103. Hau T, Simmons RL: Heparin in the treatment of experimental peritonitis. Ann Surg 187:294, 1978

104. O'Leary JP, Malik FS, Donahoe RP, et al: The effects of a minidose of heparin on peritonitis in rats. Surg Gynecol Obstet 148:571, 1979

105. Schirmer WJ, Schirmer JM, Naff GB, et al: Heparin's effect on the natural history of sepsis in the rat (abstr). Circ Shock 21:363, 1987

106. Ridings PC, Blocher CR, Fisher BJ, et al: Beneficial effects of a bradykinin antagonist in a model of gram negative sepsis. J Trauma 39:81, 1995

107. Leeper-Woodford SK, Carey D, Byrne K, et al: Histamine receptor antagonists, cyclooxygenase blockade, and tumor necrosis factor curing acute septic insult. Shock 9:89, 1998

108. Jansen PM, Eisele B, de Jong IW, et al: Effect of C1 inhibition on inflammatory and physiologic response patterns in primates suffering from lethal septic shock. J Immunol 160:475, 1998

109. Mohr M, Hopken U, Opperman M, et al: Effects of anti-C5a monoclonal antibodies on oxygen use in a porcine model of severe sepsis. Eur J Clin Invest 28:227, 1998

110. Fein AM, Bernard GR, Criner GJ, et al: Treatment of severe systemic inflammatory response syndromes and sepsis with a novel bradykinin antagonist, deltibant (CP-0127): results of a randomized, double-blind, placebo-controlled trial. CP-1027 SIRS and Sepsis Study Group. JAMA 277:482, 1997

111. Beutler B, Milsark IW, Cerami AC: Passive immunization against cachectin/tumor necrosis factor protects mice from lethal effect of endotoxin. Science 229:869, 1985

112. Tracey KJ, Fong Y, Hesse DG, et al: Anti-cachectin/TNF monoclonal antibodies prevent septic shock during lethal bacteraemia. Nature 330:662, 1987

113. Wakabayashi G, Gelfand JA, Burke JF, et al: A specific receptor antagonist for interleukin 1 prevents *Escherichia coli*-induced shock in rabbits. FASEB J 5:338, 1991

114. Abraham E, Wunderink R, Silverman H, et al: Efficacy and safety of monoclonal antibody to human tumor necrosis factor alpha in patients with sepsis syndrome: a randomized, controlled, double-blind, multicenter clinical trial. JAMA 273:934, 1995

115. Cohen J, Carlet J: Intersept: an international, multicenter, placebo-controlled trial of monoclonal antibody to human tumor necrosis factor-alpha in patients with sepsis. International Sepsis Trial Study Group. Crit Care Med 24:1431, 1996

116. Reinhart K, Wiegard-Lohnert C, Grimminger F, et al: Assessment of the safety and efficacy of the monoclonal anti-tumor necrosis factor antibody-fragment, MAK 195F, in patients with sepsis and septic shock: a multicenter, randomized, placebo-controlled, dose-ranging study. Crit Care Med 24:733, 1996

117. Fisher CJ Jr, Dhainaut JF, Opal SM, et al: Recombinant human interleukin 1 receptor antagonist in the treatment of patients with sepsis syndrome: results from a randomized, double-blind, placebo-controlled trial. Phase III rhIL-1ra Sepsis Syndrome Study Group. JAMA 271:1836, 1994

118. Opal SM, Fisher CJ Jr, Dhainaut JF, et al: Confirming interleukin-1 receptor antagonist trial in severe sepsis: a phase III, randomized, double-blind, placebo-controlled, multicenter trial. The Interleukin-1 Receptor Antagonist Sepsis Investigation Group. Crit Care Med 25:1115, 1997

119. Fry DE, Fry RV, Borzotta AP: Nosocomial blood-borne infection secondary to intravascular devices. Am J Surg 167:268, 1994

12 ANTIBIOTICS

Nicolas V. Christou, M.D., Ph.D.

Antibiotic Therapy in Surgical Patients

Several important advances in antimicrobial therapy have been made since the early 1980s. Among these advances are (1) improved understanding of the microbiologic spectrum of so-called optimal therapy, (2) better application of pharmacokinetic principles to drug administration, (3) the development of several new classes of anti-biotics, and (4) greater insight into the interplay among host resistance factors, microorganisms, and chemotherapy. Also, the wide range of antibiotics now available has made possible the tailoring of antibiotic therapy to various host factors and various infections.

General Principles of Antimicrobial Therapy

EMPIRICAL THERAPY

Surgeons often treat serious surgical infections without the benefit of microbiologic culture and sensitivity testing of the microbial pathogens. Even with the most rapid bacteriologic tests currently available, it may not be possible to identify a pathogen in less than 24 hours, and antimicrobial sensitivities can rarely be obtained in less than 48 to 72 hours. In seriously ill patients, treatment cannot be delayed for 2 to 3 days until these data become available. If therapy is to be successful, it must be started as soon as a life-threatening infection is diagnosed—or, in some patients, as soon as such an infection is suspected. Which antimicrobial agents are to be used depends on the suspected site of infection and on the organisms that are commonly pathogenic at this site. Therapy is initiated with an agent or combination of agents whose action is broad enough to cover all the suspected microbial pathogens. The application of such broad-spectrum antibiotic therapy in the absence of microbiologic confirmation is termed empirical therapy.

To make a rational decision regarding empirical therapy, the surgeon must be familiar with the organisms that are likely to be encountered when a particular infection (e.g., an intra-abdominal abscess) is suspected. Selection of the agent or agents is based on the history, the physical examination, where the infection was likely to have been acquired, the host defense status, the overall clinical severity of the infection, and the response of the host. Definitive therapy is initiated after the host response to the infection and to the empirical treatment has been monitored and the results from the microbiology laboratory—specifically, identification of the isolated organisms and the minimal inhibitory concentrations (MICs) of various antimicrobial agents—have been assessed. If the surgeon chooses an appropriate antimicrobial therapy, the patient will get well, will experience no adverse reactions, and will leave the hospital in a short time. In addition, the environment will not be harmed, and the cost of therapy will be low.

VARIABLES INFLUENCING TREATMENT

A surgeon planning a course of antimicrobial therapy must take into account a number of variables. One of these is efficacy, which is the ability of an agent to reach the site of the infection and to be active at that site. Therefore, knowledge of the absorption, distribution, and excretion characteristics of the agent is essential for selecting an agent and a method of administration.

Another variable is toxicity, which relates to immediate allergic-type reactions, idiosyncratic reactions that occur subsequently, and dose-dependent end-organ damage. It is vitally important to reduce the risks of treatment to the individual patient as much as possible, but it is also important to consider the broader effects of antimicrobial use. Indiscriminate use of antibiotics may produce microbial resistance that is peculiar to the institution, which increases the risk that other patients will be infected with these resistant organisms.

A third variable is cost, which involves much more than the price of a gram of the agent, the frequency with which doses are given, or the duration of treatment. The most expensive drug may be the most economical and logical choice if it shortens a hospital stay, allows outpatient treatment, or saves a life. Cost must be considered in relation to both efficacy and toxicity.

A fourth variable is dosage. Dosages for antimicrobial agents with a wide margin between therapeutic and toxic blood levels are usually standardized and independent of the adult patient's weight. Dosages for agents with a narrow margin between therapeutic and toxic blood levels (e.g., aminoglycosides), however, are calculated on the basis of body weight.

A fifth variable is route of administration. In patients with severe infections and in all compromised hosts, antimicrobial agents should be given parenterally because this approach is more likely to yield therapeutic blood levels and consequently higher tissue levels. Intravenous administration is also essential in patients who are hypotensive or in shock, because in such conditions, drug absorption from intramuscular sites is poor.

A sixth variable is the duration of antimicrobial treatment, which is dependent on the type and severity of infection, the host response, and the clinical course of the patient. Usually, the antibiotic is continued until the signs and symptoms of the infection resolve, which typically occurs within 5 to 14 days.

A final variable is whether single-agent therapy or multiagent therapy is indicated. In certain situations, administration of multiple agents is essential for optimal antimicrobial therapy.

Many patients who report a history of allergy to antibiotics are not genuinely allergic. Statements about allergic reactions can be neither taken for granted nor disregarded without risk of serious therapeutic consequences, not to mention legal problems. A carefully elicited history may reveal that the symptoms attributed to an allergic reaction are incompatible with such an interpretation. Skin testing with benzylpenicilloyl-polylysine and minor determinant antigens done just before a planned course of therapy with a penicillin, a penicillin derivative, or a cephalosporin may reveal a propensity to an immediate allergic reaction. Because skin testing itself is associated with some risk of reaction, it should be done only when the drug to be tested is clearly superior and is certain to be used if the test result is negative. A good deal of concern remains about possible cross-allergenicity between the penicillins and the cephalosporins. If the reaction is neither immediate nor severe, the patient usually will tolerate the antibiotic. There are numerous other in vivo interactions involving antimicrobials [see Table 1].

A number of antibiotics should be used with caution in pregnant women because they have significant toxic effects on the mother, the fetus, or both [see Table 2].

Laboratory Tests

Many laboratory tests, if used in the proper context, can guide selection of optimal antimicrobial therapy.

In vitro susceptibility tests are indicated when the susceptibility of an organism is not completely predictable or when certain other specific problems arise, such as the necessity of determining whether resistance has developed during the course of therapy. An organism is generally considered susceptible if the concentration of antimicrobial agent necessary to inhibit its growth is lower than that usually attainable in body fluids, particularly blood, cerebrospinal fluid, or urine. The results of these tests may vary from laboratory to laboratory, depending on the preparation of the antimicrobial agent, the size of the inoculum, the duration and temperature of incubation, the definition of inhibitory end points, and the characteristics of the medium used (especially its cation content and pH). For instance, a gentamicin susceptibility test performed at a pH of 7.4 may show considerable activity, but this result may not be clinically valid. The purulent fluid at the infection site may have a much lower pH, and aminoglycoside activity decreases with decreasing pH.

The disk diffusion method has been standardized by the National Committee for Clinical Laboratory Standards (NCCLS)[1] for in vitro susceptibility testing. Commercially available paper disks containing specific amounts of antimicrobial agents are placed on Mueller-Hinton agar plates that contain a standard bacterial inoculum. A zone of inhibition of bacterial growth develops around each active antibiotic after overnight incubation. The size of the zone determines the

organism's susceptibility or resistance; prior studies have correlated zone sizes with MICs obtained through dilution tests. Arbitrary zone-size break points for susceptibility have been established by clinical and laboratory investigators on the basis of such additional factors as achievable serum levels, degree of protein binding, and toxicity. Worldwide, the standardized disk test is probably the most frequently used method for in vitro susceptibility testing, and results should be comparable from laboratory to laboratory. The organism must fall into one of three categories: susceptible, intermediate, or resistant.

The broth dilution method exposes an inoculum of bacteria to various concentrations of an antimicrobial agent during incubation. The MIC of an agent that inhibits growth can be determined, and this value can be correlated with blood, urine, or other body fluid levels of the antimicrobial agent. Moreover, those tubes that show inhibition of growth can be subcultured to an antimicrobial-free medium, and the minimal bactericidal concentration (MBC) can be determined. Unfortunately, this test is not well standardized at present, and its reproducibility is poor when it is subjected to intralaboratory and interlaboratory comparisons.[2]

The agar dilution method works in much the same way as the broth dilution method, except that it employs agar plates that contain various dilutions of antimicrobial agents, and as many as 36 organisms can be efficiently inoculated on each plate by means of a replicator device. The minimal inhibitory concentration is determined by reading inhibition of colony growth on the agar surface. Agar dilution has the advantage of producing MIC data efficiently in a laboratory that performs large numbers of tests daily.

In the serum bactericidal test (SBT), samples of the serum of the treated patient are obtained and incubated with the infecting organism in doubling dilutions with broth to determine the highest dilution that is bactericidal. (Not all antimicrobial agents exhibit bactericidal activity: some exhibit only bacteriostatic activity [see Table 3].) The drawing of serum specimens can be timed to coincide with anticipated peak and trough antimicrobial levels. In effect, this test indirectly assesses both the susceptibility of the organism and the serum concentration of the antimicrobial agent, as well as the interactions between serum and organism and serum and drug. The NCCLS has developed proposed guidelines for the SBT.[3] A comprehensive review of the technical and clinical considerations associated with the SBT has been provided.[4]

Antibiotic Therapy for Infections in Surgical Patients

The antimicrobial agents of choice for various infections (e.g., community-acquired pneumonia[5-8]) in adults are well established [see Table 4], as are their dosages in patients with normal renal function [see Table 5]. No attempt will be made to review all of that material in this discussion. Excellent reviews and practice guidelines have been published.[9,10]

Discussion

Penicillins

Although the original penicillins are still useful against specific bacteria, there are some infections in which both they and the penicillinase-resistant semisynthetic penicillins are ineffective because of the emergence of penicillinase-producing staphylococci and methicillin-resistant staphylococci. The penicillins can be classified

by structure [see Figure 1], β-lactamase susceptibility, and spectrum of action. They have a number of adverse effects [see Table 6].

The action of the penicillins depends on the presence of a bacterial cell wall containing peptidoglycans that are accessible to the agent. In actively growing bacteria, interference with biosynthesis of the peptidoglycan structure—specifically, of

Table 1 In Vivo Drug Interactions Involving Antimicrobials[203,204]

Antimicrobial Agent	Interacting Drug	Adverse Effect	Proposed Mechanism
Aminoglycosides	Amphotericin B	↑ Nephrotoxicity	Synergism
	Ascorbic acid	↓ Antibacterial effect in urinary tract	Urinary acidification
	Bumetanide	↑ Ototoxicity	Additive actions
	Carbenicillin, ticarcillin	↓ Aminoglycoside effect	Inactivation of aminoglycosides by the penicillin at high concentrations
	Cephalosporins	↑ Nephrotoxicity	?
	Cisplatin	↑ Nephrotoxicity	?
	Curarelike drugs	↑ Neuromuscular blockade	Additive actions
	Cyclosporine	↑ Nephrotoxicity	Additive actions (monitoring of levels recommended)
	Digoxin	Probable ↓ digoxin effect with neomycin or gentamicin	↓ Absorption
	Ethacrynic acid	↑ Ototoxicity	Additive actions
	Furosemide	↑ Nephrotoxicity, ↑ ototoxicity	Additive actions
	Magnesium sulfate	Possible ↑ neuromuscular blockade	Additive actions
	Methotrexate	Possible ↑ methotrexate toxicity with kanamycin	?
		↓ Methotrexate effect with oral aminoglycosides	↓ Absorption
	Neuromuscular blocking agents	↑ Apnea, respiratory paralysis	?
	Nonsteroidal anti-inflammatory drugs	↑ Nephrotoxicity	Additive actions
	Polymyxins	↑ Nephrotoxicity, neuromuscular blockade	Additive actions
	Radiographic contrast agents	↑ Nephrotoxicity	Additive actions
Cephalosporins	Alcohol	Disulfiram-like effect with cefamandole, cefoperazone, and moxalactam	Probable inhibition of intermediary metabolism of alcohol
	Aminoglycosides	↑ Nephrotoxicity	?
	Oral anticoagulants	Possible ↑ anticoagulant effect with moxalactam, cefotetan, cefmetazole	?
	Aspirin, heparin	Possible ↑ risk of bleeding with moxalactam, cefotetan, cefmetazole	Additive actions
	Ethacrynic acid	↑ Nephrotoxicity	?
	Furosemide	↑ Nephrotoxicity	?
	Penicillins	Possible ↑ cefotaxime toxicity with azlocillin in azotemic patients	↓ Excretion
Chloramphenicol	Acetaminophen	Possible ↑ chloramphenicol toxicity	↓ Metabolism
	Oral anticoagulants	↑ Anticoagulant effect	Inhibition of microsomal enzymes
	Barbiturates	↑ Barbiturate effect	↓ Metabolism
		↓ Chloramphenicol effect	↑ Metabolism
	Cimetidine	Possible aplastic anemia (single case report)	?
	Etomidate	Prolonged anesthesia	↓ Metabolism
	Oral hypoglycemic agents	↑ Sulfonylurea-induced hypoglycemia	?
	Phenytoin	Possible ↑ chloramphenicol toxicity	?
		↑ Phenytoin toxicity	↓ Metabolism
Clindamycin	Neuromuscular blocking agents	↑ Neuromuscular blockade	Additive actions
	Theophylline	↓ Clindamycin levels, apnea, seizures	?
Erythromycin	Oral anticoagulants	↑ Anticoagulant effect	Possible ↓ metabolism
	Carbamazepine	↑ Carbamazepine toxicity	↓ Metabolism
	Corticosteroids	↑ Methylprednisolone effect and possible toxicity	↓ Excretion
	Cyclosporine	↑ Cyclosporine level	↓ Excretion
	Digoxin	↑ Digoxin effect	↑ Absorption
	Theophyllines	↑ Theophylline effect and toxicity	↓ Metabolism
Imipenem	Cyclosporine	↑ Cyclosporine levels, ↑ CNS effect	?
	Ganciclovir	↑ Seizures	?
Metronidazole	Alcohol	Nausea, cramps, headache, flushing	Possible inhibition of intermediary metabolism of alcohol
	Oral anticoagulants	↑ Anticoagulant effect	Inhibition of microsomal enzymes
	Cimetidine	Possible ↑ metronidazole toxicity	↓ Metabolism
	Ciprofloxacin	↑ Seizures	?
	Disulfiram	Organic brain syndrome	?
	Phenobarbital	↓ Phenobarbital clearance	?

(continued)

Table 1 (continued)

Antimicrobial Agent	Interacting Drug	Adverse Effect	Proposed Mechanism
Penicillins	Beta-adrenergic blockers	Possible ↓ atenolol effect with ampicillin	↓ Absorption
	Allopurinol	↑ Incidence of rashes with ampicillin	?
	Aminoglycosides	↓ Aminoglycoside effect with carbenicillin or ticarcillin at high concentrations	Aminoglycoside inactivation
	Oral anticoagulants	↓ Anticoagulant effect with nafcillin	↑ Metabolism
	Cephalosporins	Possible ↑ cefotaxime toxicity with azlocillin in azotemic patients	↓ Excretion
	Oral contraceptives	↓ Contraceptive effect with ampicillin	↓ Enterohepatic circulation of estrogen
	Lithium	Hypernatremia with ticarcillin	Large sodium load, ↓ renal excretion
	Methotrexate	Possible ↑ methotrexate toxicity	↓ Excretion
Polymyxins	Aminoglycosides	↑ Nephrotoxicity, ↑ neuromuscular blockade	Additive actions
	Neuromuscular blocking agents	↑ Neuromuscular blockade	Additive actions
Quinolones	Antacids	↓ Absorption of quinolones	Binding of aluminum and magnesium antacids to quinolones
	Oral anticoagulants	Possible ↑ anticoagulant effect	Possible alteration of hepatic metabolism; displacement from albumin binding site (warfarin)
	Caffeine	Exaggerated or prolonged effects of caffeine, ↑ half-life	?
	Cimetidine	↑ Quinolone levels	Competitive action
	Cyclosporine	Potentiation of cyclosporine nephrotoxicity	? (monitoring of levels recommended)
	Probenecid	↑ Quinolone levels	↓ Renal excretion
	Sucralfate	↑ Absorption of quinolones	pH changes
	Theophyllines	Possible ↑ theophylline levels, ↑ half-life	Possible alteration of hepatic metabolism
Sulfonamides	Oral anticoagulants	↑ Anticoagulant effect	Displacement from binding sites, decreased metabolism
	Cyclosporine	↓ Cyclosporine levels	?
	Digoxin	Possible ↓ digoxin effect with sulfasalazine	↓ Absorption
	Oral hypoglycemic agents	↑ Sulfonylurea-induced hypoglycemia	?
	Methotrexate	Possible ↑ methotrexate toxicity	Displacement from binding sites, ↓ renal clearance
	Phenytoin	↑ Phenytoin effect (except possibly with sulfisoxazole)	↓ Metabolism
	Monoamine oxidase inhibitors	Possible ↑ phenelzine toxicity	↓ Metabolism
	Pyrimethamine	↑ Hypersensitivity reaction, including fatalities, with sulfadoxine	?
	Thiopental sodium	↑ Thiopental sodium effect	↓ Albumin binding
Tetracyclines	Antacids	↓ Tetracycline effect	↓ Absorption
	Oral anticoagulants	↑ Anticoagulant effect	?
	Barbiturates	↓ Doxycycline effect	Induction of microsomal enzymes
	Bismuth subsalicylate	↓ Tetracycline effect	↓ Absorption
	Carbamazepine	↓ Doxycycline effect	Induction of microsomal enzymes
	Oral contraceptives	↓ Contraceptive effect	Possible ↓ enterohepatic circulation of estrogen
	Digoxin	↑ Digoxin effect	↑ Absorption
	Insulin	↑ Insulin effect	?
	Oral iron salts	↓ Tetracycline and iron effects	↓ Absorption of tetracycline and iron
	Lithium	↑ Lithium toxicity	↓ Renal excretion
	Phenytoin	↓ Doxycycline effect	Induction of microsomal enzymes
	Zinc sulfate	↓ Tetracycline effect	↓ Absorption
Trimethoprim	Amiloride, thiazides	Hyponatremia	Additive actions
	Oral anticoagulants	↑ Anticoagulant effect	↓ Metabolism
	Cyclosporine	↑ Nephrotoxicity	Synergism
	Mercaptopurine	↓ Antileukemic effect	?
	Digoxin	Possible ↑ effect	↓ Renal excretion
Trimethoprim-sulfamethoxazole	Oral anticoagulants	↑ Anticoagulant effect	↓ Metabolism

the cross-linkages between the peptide chains—prevents the bacterium from developing its normal structural firmness, and this lack of firmness leads to lysis. Enzymes located beneath the cell wall (transpeptidases and carboxypeptidases) are involved in synthesis of the cell wall. These penicillin-binding proteins are the sites at which β-lactam drugs bind.[11]

NATURAL PENICILLINS

Aqueous Crystalline Penicillin G

Aqueous crystalline penicillin G is used when a high serum concentration of the agent is required.[12] Its half-life is normally 30 minutes but may be as long as 10 hours in patients with

Table 2 Antibiotics in Pregnancy[203]

Drug	Major Toxic Potential		Pharmacology	
	Maternal	Fetal	Maternal Serum Levels	Excreted in Mother's Milk
Considered safe				
Cephalosporins	Allergies	None known	Decreased	Trace
Erythromycin base	Allergies, GI intolerance	None known	Decreased	Yes
Penicillins	Allergies	None known	Decreased	Trace
Use with caution				
Aminoglycosides	Ototoxicity, nephrotoxicity	Ototoxicity	Decreased	Yes
Clindamycin	Allergies, colitis	None known	Unchanged	Trace
Sulfonamides (contraindicated at term)	Allergies, crystalluria	Kernicterus (at term), hemolysis (G6PD deficiency)	Unchanged	Yes
Avoid if possible				
Metronidazole	Hypersensitivity, alcohol intolerance, neuropathy	None known (teratogenic in animals)	Probably unchanged	Yes
Contraindicated				
Chloramphenicol	Blood dyscrasias	Gray syndrome	Unchanged	Yes
Erythromycin estolate	Hepatotoxicity	None known	Decreased	Yes
Nalidixic acid	GI intolerance	Increased intracranial pressure	?	?
Nitrofurantoin	Allergies, neuropathy, GI intolerance	Hemolysis (G6PD deficiency)	Decreased	Trace
Norfloxacin	GI intolerance	Arthropathies in immature animals	?	?
Tetracyclines	Hepatotoxicity, renal failure	Tooth discoloration and dysplasia, impaired bone growth	Probably unchanged	Yes
Trimethoprim	Hypersensitivity	Teratogenicity	Unchanged	Yes

anuria. Approximately 50% of penicillin G is bound to plasma proteins. Penicillin G sodium contains approximately 2 mEq of sodium in each one million units. Therefore, the potassium salt of penicillin G should be used except in patients with renal insufficiency, who may not be able to tolerate the 1.7 mEq of potassium contained in each one million units. This agent is destroyed by gastric acid when given orally.

Penicillin G Benzathine

Penicillin G benzathine, 1.2 to 2.4 million units I.M., is used in the definitive management of certain infections, such as streptococcal sore throat, and as prophylaxis for several conditions, such as rheumatic fever, in which reinfection by β-hemolytic streptococci is a constant threat.

Penicillin G Procaine

Penicillin G procaine is used intramuscularly when a long-acting preparation is preferred and high blood levels are not required. It is indicated for treatment of pneumococcal pneumonia, uncomplicated cases of which are adequately treated by administration of one or two daily doses of 300,000 units, and for treatment of acute genitourinary gonorrhea, for which a dose of 4.8 million units is divided and injected at two sites and 1 g of probenecid is given orally before the injection.

Penicillin V

Because phenoxymethyl penicillin, or penicillin V, is resistant to gastric acid, it leads to higher serum concentrations when given orally than penicillin G does at similar doses. Penicillin V should not be substituted for parenterally administered penicillin G when such therapy is needed, but it can be given orally to treat mild infections of the throat, the respiratory tract, or soft tissue, in doses of 125 to 500 mg given four to six times daily.

PENICILLINASE-RESISTANT PENICILLINS

The semisynthetic penicillinase-resistant penicillins available for parenteral use are methicillin, oxacillin, and nafcillin; those available for oral use are oxacillin, nafcillin, cloxacillin, and dicloxacillin.

Methicillin

Methicillin is the least protein bound of this group (39%); nafcillin (90%), oxacillin (94%), cloxacillin (95%), and dicloxacillin (98%) all have higher rates of protein binding. Methicillin was the first of the semisynthetic penicillinase-resistant penicillins.[13] It must be administered parenterally and is usually given every 4 to 6 hours in a total daily dose of 100 to 300 mg/kg body weight.

Oxacillin and Nafcillin

Oxacillin seems to be as effective as methicillin against staphylococcal infections, and it causes interstitial nephritis less often. For

Table 3 Bactericidal and Bacteriostatic Agents[203]

Bactericidal Agents	Bacteriostatic Agents
Aminoglycosides*	Chloramphenicol
Aztreonam	Clindamycin
Bacitracin	Erythromycin
Cephalosporins	Sulfonamides
Imipenem	Tetracyclines
Penicillins	Trimethoprim
Polymyxins†	
Quinolones‡	
Vancomycin	

*Including streptomycin, neomycin, kanamycin, gentamicin, tobramycin, amikacin, and netilmicin.
†Including polymyxin B and colistimethate.
‡Including norfloxacin and ciprofloxacin.

parenteral use, oxacillin or nafcillin can be given in dosages of 100 to 300 mg/kg/day for children and up to 4 to 12 g/day for adults.

Cloxacillin and Dicloxacillin

One of the penicillinase-resistant penicillins or cefazolin (a first-generation cephalosporin) should be used as initial therapy for all cases of gram-positive coccal infections before identification and susceptibility testing. If laboratory data indicate that non–penicillinase-producing staphylococci (i.e., staphylococci that are susceptible to penicillin G) are the causative infectious agents, penicillin G is the agent of choice because it is more active against such organisms (i.e., it has a lower MIC), is less toxic, and costs less. If penicillinase-producing organisms are identified or suspected and oral therapy is desired, cloxacillin or dicloxacillin, 1 to 2 g/day, can be given.

AMINOPENICILLINS

Ampicillin

Ampicillin is active against a variety of bacteria, including many strains of *Escherichia coli*, *Proteus mirabilis*, *Salmonella*, *Shigella*, *Listeria*, and *Hemophilus influenzae*. Most strains of *Klebsiella* and all strains of *Pseudomonas aeruginosa* are resistant. The antienterococcal effect of ampicillin may be synergistically enhanced by concurrent administration of an aminoglycoside, which results in bactericidal activity.

Because it is stable in gastric juices, ampicillin is suitable for oral as well as parenteral use. When it is given orally, peak serum levels are reached in about 2 hours, but they seldom exceed 0.3 µg/ml. When it is given intramuscularly, peak serum levels are achieved in 1 hour, and they are both higher and more prolonged than the peak levels achieved after oral administration. About 10% of ampicillin is bound to plasma proteins. The recommended daily dose is 1 to 4 g; parenteral administration of up to 12 g/day is recommended for major systemic infections.

Amoxicillin

Amoxicillin is closely related to ampicillin, both in chemical structure and in spectrum of antibacterial activity.[14] Amoxicillin, however, is more completely absorbed than ampicillin is: approximately 70% of a dose of amoxicillin is absorbed, compared with approximately 50% of a dose of ampicillin. Consequently, the blood levels attainable with a given dose of amoxicillin are usually about twice those attainable with a comparable dose of ampicillin. Amoxicillin is at least as effective as ampicillin in the treatment of respiratory disorders that are caused by susceptible bacteria, including otitis media, sinusitis, and bronchitis.

CARBOXYPENICILLINS

Carbenicillin

Carbenicillin has an antibacterial range similar to that of ampicillin, with the added benefit of activity against certain strains of *P. aeruginosa*,[15] indole-positive *Proteus* species, and *Enterobacter* species.[16] Because carbenicillin is inactivated by penicillinase, penicillinase-producing *Staphylococcus aureus* is resistant to it. *Klebsiella* species are resistant to carbenicillin, as are many *Serratia* organisms. Carbenicillin is bactericidal and is recoverable from blood, urine, lymph, cerebrospinal fluid, and most body tissues. About 50% of the drug is bound to serum proteins.[17] For most gram-negative bacteremias, the MIC for carbenicillin is between 10 and 25 µg/ml; for *P. aeruginosa*, it is between 25 and 100 µg/ml.

Carbenicillin has been used to treat severe infections caused by *P. aeruginosa*, *Proteus* species, and other gram-negative bacteria that are susceptible to it. For systemic and soft tissue infections caused by *P. aeruginosa*, the dosage should be 400 to 500 mg/kg/day by continuous intravenous drip or in divided doses every 4 hours. The dosage should be reduced in patients with renal failure,[18] and close surveillance must be maintained for signs of bleeding. Currently, carbenicillin is used less often than it once was; it has been largely supplanted by ticarcillin and by the ureidopenicillins.

Ticarcillin

The antibacterial spectrum of ticarcillin is similar to that of carbenicillin; however, it is two to four times more active against *P. aeruginosa*. It is frequently preferred to carbenicillin in the treatment of serious gram-negative infections because of its greater potency and the lower incidence of adverse effects.[19] The primary use of ticarcillin is in the treatment of proven or suspected *Pseudomonas* infections. The recommended dosage is 16 to 24 g/day.

UREIDOPENICILLINS

Mezlocillin, Azlocillin, and Piperacillin

Mezlocillin, azlocillin, and piperacillin are semisynthetic penicillins derived from the ampicillin molecule with side-chain adaptations. The side chains of mezlocillin and azlocillin are acyl derivatives of a urea molecule—hence the term ureidopenicillins. The ureidopenicillins are generally bactericidal and act primarily by inhibiting cell wall synthesis in dividing bacteria. Pharmacokinetic studies show them to follow a first-order, two-compartment model. In comparison with the carboxypenicillins carbenicillin and ticarcillin, the ureidopenicillins exhibit less pronounced plasma protein binding, a shorter serum half-life, and a greater volume of distribution.[20-22] They are minimally metabolized (10%) and are primarily excreted in an active form by glomerular filtration and tubular secretion. Unlike carbenicillin and ticarcillin, the ureidopenicillins achieve high concentrations in bile because of increased biliary excretion.

In vitro, the ureidopenicillins are active against streptococci, enterococci, most Enterobacteriaceae, *Pseudomonas*, β-lactamase–negative staphylococci, *Neisseria*, and *Hemophilus*.[23-25] β-Lactamase–producing staphylococci and *H. influenzae* are resistant. The major advantage the ureidopenicillins have over other penicillins in clinical use is their increased activity against *P. aeruginosa* and *Klebsiella*.

The recommended dosages of the ureidopenicillins are 6 to 16 g/day for mild to moderate infections and 18 to 24 g/day for severe to life-threatening infections. Small doses may be given intramuscularly, but large doses must be given intravenously. The dosing interval is usually 4 to 6 hours.

An observed property of the ureidopenicillins that has given rise to some concern is their loss of activity as inoculum size increases; this is known as the inoculum effect. When the bacterial concentration is increased from 10^3 to 10^7 colony-forming units/ml, the MIC and the MBC increase substantially.[26,27] The inoculum effect has been consistently noted not only with *P. aeruginosa* but also with some strains of *E. coli*, *Klebsiella*, *Enterobacter*, and *Morganella*.

Monotherapy with mezlocillin or piperacillin has been efficacious in patients with pneumonia, bacteremia, osteomyelitis,

Table 4   Antimicrobial Drugs of Choice for Various Infections in Adults[203]

	Causative Organism	Drug of Choice	Alternative Drugs

Gram-Positive Cocci	*Staphylococcus aureus*
	   Methicillin-resistant[1]
		Vancomycin,[2] with or without
		   rifampin or gentamicin
			Trimethoprim-sulfamethoxazole (TMP-SMX)[2] with or without rifampin,[2]
			   a fluoroquinolone,[3] minocycline[4]

	Non–penicillinase-producing (uncommon)	Penicillin G[5] or penicillin V	A cephalosporin,[6] vancomycin,[7] clindamycin, imipenem, a fluoroquinolone[3]

	Penicillinase-producing (common)	Penicillinase-resistant penicillin[8]	A cephalosporin,[6] clindamycin, vancomycin,[7] imipenem,[9] ticarcillin-clavulanate,
			   ampicillin-sulbactam, amoxicillin-clavulanate, piperacillin-tazobactam,
			   a fluoroquinolone[3]

	S. epidermidis[10]	Vancomycin,[7] with or without
		   rifampin[2] or gentamicin
			A cephalosporin, a penicillinase-resistant penicillin, imipenem,[9]
			   a fluoroquinolone[3]

	Anaerobic streptococcus (*Peptostreptococcus*)	Penicillin G[5]	Clindamycin, a cephalosporin,[6] vancomycin[7]
	Streptococcus bovis	Penicillin G[5,11]	A cephalosporin,[6] vancomycin[7]

	Enterococcus
	   Endocarditis or other serious
	      infection
		Penicillin or ampicillin, plus
		   gentamicin[12] or streptomycin
			Vancomycin,[7] with gentamicin or streptomycin; ampicillin-sulbactam with
			   gentamicin or streptomycin, teicoplanin,[13] quinupristin/dalfopristin[14]

	Uncomplicated urinary tract infection	Ampicillin (or amoxicillin) or penicillin G	A fluoroquinolone[3] or nitrofurantoin[15]
	Groups A, G, and C streptococci	Penicillin G[5,16] or penicillin V	A cephalosporin,[6] vancomycin,[7] an erythromycin,[17] clindamycin, clarithromycin, azithromycin
	Group B streptococcus	Penicillin G[5,16] or ampicillin	A cephalosporin,[6] vancomycin,[7] an erythromycin
	S. pneumoniae (pneumococcus)	Penicillin G[5,16] or penicillin V	An erythromycin,[16,17] a cephalosporin,[6] chloramphenicol,[7,16] vancomycin[7,16] with or without rifampin, TMP-SMX, azithromycin, clarithromycin
	Viridans streptococcus	Penicillin G,[5,11] with or without gentamicin	A cephalosporin,[6] vancomycin[7]
Gram-Positive Bacilli	*Bacillus cereus, B. subtilis*	Vancomycin	Imipenem,[9] clindamycin
	B. anthracis	Penicillin G	A tetracycline, an erythromycin[2]
	Clostridium difficile	Vancomycin[18] or metronidazole[18]	Bacitracin
	C. perfringens	Penicillin G	Clindamycin, metronidazole, a tetracycline,[4] imipenem,[9] chloramphenicol[7]
	C. tetani	Penicillin G	A tetracycline[4]
	Corynebacterium diphtheriae	An erythromycin	Penicillin G
	Corynebacterium, JK group	Vancomycin	Penicillin G with gentamicin, an erythromycin
	Listeria monocytogenes	Ampicillin with or without gentamicin	TMP-SMX
	Propionibacterium	Penicillin G	Clindamycin, an erythromycin

Gram-Negative Cocci	*Moraxella* (formerly *Branhamella*)
	   catarrhalis
		TMP-SMX	Amoxicillin-clavulanate, an erythromycin, a tetracycline, cefuroxime, third-
			   generation cephalosporins, clarithromycin, azithromycin, a fluoroquinolone[3]

	Neisseria gonorrhoeae[19]	Ceftriaxone[6]	Ampicillin or penicillin, spectinomycin,[20] cefotaxime,[5] a fluoroquinolone[3]
	N. meningitidis Meningitis, bacteremia	Penicillin G	A third-generation cephalosporin,[6] TMP-SMX, chloramphenicol[7]
	Carrier state	Rifampin	Minocycline, ciprofloxacin

Enteric Gram-Negative Bacilli	*Bacteroides*
	   GI tract strains (*B. fragilis*)
		Metronidazole	Clindamycin, cefoxitin, cefotetan, ceftizoxime, or cefmetazole; chloramphenicol[21];
			   imipenem[9]; ticarcillin–clavulanate; ampicillin-sulbactam, piperacillin-tazobactam

	Respiratory tract strains	Penicillin G or clindamycin	Cefoxitin,[6] cefotetan, metronidazole, chloramphenicol[7]
	Campylobacter fetus	Imipenem[9]	Gentamicin
	C. jejuni	A fluoroquinolone,[3] an erythromycin	A tetracycline,[4] gentamicin[7]
	Citrobacter	Gentamicin, a third-generation cephalosporin[6]	A fluoroquinolone,[3] imipenem,[9] tobramycin, chloramphenicol,[7] amikacin

	Enterobacter	Imipenem[9]	A third-generation cephalosporin[6]; for serious infections, use with ciprofloxacin
			   or gentamicin; gentamicin, tobramycin, amikacin, a fluoroquinolone,[3]
			   a carboxypenicillin or acylaminopenicillin,[22] aztreonam,[23] TMP-SMX,
			   chloramphenicol[7]

	Escherichia coli[24]	Ampicillin, a cephalosporin,[6] a fluoroquinolone,[3] TMP-SMX[26]	Gentamicin,[25] tobramycin, amikacin, imipenem,[9] aztreonam,[23] chloramphenicol[7]

	Helicobacter pylori	Tetracycline with metronidazole
		   and bismuth subsalicylate
			Amoxicillin with metronidazole and bismuth subsalicylate; tetracycline with
			   clarithromycin and bismuth subsalicylate; clarithromycin with omeprazole

	Klebsiella[24]	A cephalosporin[6]	Imipenem,[9] gentamicin,[25] tobramycin, amikacin, chloramphenicol,[7] TMP-SMX,[26]
			   a carboxypenicillin or acylaminopenicillin,[22] amoxicillin-clavulanate, ampicillin-
			   sulbactam, ticarcillin-clavulanate, piperacillin-tazobactam, aztreonam,[23]
			   a fluoroquinolone[3]

	Proteus
	   mirabilis[24]
		Ampicillin	A cephalosporin, gentamicin or tobramycin, chloramphenicol,[7]
			   a carboxypenicillin or acylaminopenicillin,[22] imipenem,[9] TMP-SMX,
			   aztreonam,[23] a fluoroquinolone[3]

	non-*mirabilis*,[24] including *P. vulgaris*,
	   Morganella morganii, and
	   Providencia rettgeri
		A second- or third-generation
		   cephalosporin[6]
			Gentamicin, tobramycin, amikacin, a carboxypenicillin or acylaminopenicillin,[22]
			   chloramphenicol,[7] imipenem,[9] aztreonam,[23] ampicillin-sulbactam, ticarcillin-
			   clavulanate, piperacillin-tazobactam, amoxicillin-clavulanate, a fluoroquinolone[3]

Note: all superscript numbers refer to footnotes that follow table.

(continued)

Table 4 (continued)

	Causative Organism	Drug of Choice	Alternative Drugs
Enteric Gram-Negative Bacilli (continued)	*Providencia stuartii*	A second- or third-generation cephalosporin	An aminoglycoside, TMP-SMX,[26] imipenem,[9] aztreonam,[23] a carboxypenicillin or acylaminopenicillin,[22] a fluoroquinolone[3]
	Salmonella typhi	Ceftriaxone or a fluoroquinolone[3]	Chloramphenicol or ampicillin,[27] TMP-SMX
	Other *Salmonella* species	Ceftriaxone or cefotaxime or a fluoroquinolone[3]	Ampicillin or amoxicillin, TMP-SMX, chloramphenicol[7]
	Serratia	A third-generation cephalosporin	Gentamicin or amikacin, a carboxypenicillin or acylaminopenicillin,[22] chloramphenicol,[7] imipenem,[9] aztreonam, a fluoroquinolone[3]
	Shigella	A fluoroquinolone[3]	TMP-SMX, ampicillin, ceftriaxone, cefixime
Other Gram-Negative Bacilli	*Acinetobacter (Herellea)*	Imipenem[9]	Tobramycin, gentamicin, amikacin, doxycycline, minocycline, a carboxypenicillin or acylaminopenicillin,[22] TMP-SMX, a fluoroquinolone,[3] ceftazidime
	Aeromonas hydrophilia	TMP-SMX[2]	A fluoroquinolone,[3] gentamicin, tobramycin, imipenem[9]
	Bartonella henselae		
	(cat-scratch disease)	Ciprofloxacin[3]	TMP-SMX, gentamicin; rifampin
	(bacillary angiomatosis)	An erythromycin	Doxycycline
	Brucella	A tetracycline, with gentamicin or streptomycin	Rifampin[2] with a tetracycline, chloramphenicol[7] with or without streptomycin, TMP-SMX[2] with or without gentamicin, a fluoroquinolone
	Eikenella corrodens	Ampicillin	An erythromycin, a tetracycline,[4] amoxicillin-clavulanate, ampicillin-sulbactam, ceftriaxone
	Francisella tularensis (tularemia)	Streptomycin	Gentamicin, a tetracycline,[4] chloramphenicol[7]
	Fusobacterium	Penicillin	Clindamycin, metronidazole, chloramphenicol,[7] cefoxitin
	Gardnerella (formerly Hemophilus) vaginalis	Metronidazole[2] (oral)	Intravaginal or oral clindamycin
	Hemophilus influenzae		
	Bronchitis, otitis media	TMP-SMX	Ampicillin or amoxicillin; a tetracycline[4]; a sulfonamide with or without erythromycin; amoxicillin-clavulanate, cefuroxime axetil, ceftizoxime, clarithromycin, azithromycin, a fluoroquinolone,[3] cefamandole, cefprozil
	Meningitis, epiglottitis, life-threatening infections	Cefotaxime or ceftriaxone	Chloramphenicol[28]
	Legionella pneumophila (Legionnaires' disease)	Erythromycin	Rifampin,[29] TMP-SMX,[2] clarithromycin, a fluoroquinolone,[3] azithromycin
	L. micdadei	Erythromycin	Rifampin,[2] TMP-SMX[2]
	Pasteurella multocida	Penicillin G	A tetracycline,[4] a cephalosporin,[6] amoxicillin-clavulanate, ampicillin-sulbactam
	Calymmatobacterium granulomatis (granuloma inguinale)	A tetracycline[4]	Streptomycin, TMP-SMX, an erythromycin
	H. ducreyi (chancroid)	Ceftriaxone or erythromycin or azithromycin	A fluoroquinolone
	Pseudomonas aeruginosa		
	Urinary tract infections	A fluoroquinolone[3]	Gentamicin or tobramycin; amikacin; ceftazidime[6] with or without gentamicin or tobramycin; imipenem[9]; aztreonam[23]; a carboxypenicillin or acylaminopenicillin[22]
	Other infections	Gentamicin or tobramycin with or without a carboxypenicillin or acylaminopenicillin,[22] ceftazidime, imipenem,[9] aztreonam[23] with or without gentamicin or tobramycin	Amikacin with or without a carboxypenicillin or acylaminopenicillin,[22] ciprofloxacin[7]
	P. cepacia	TMP-SMX	Chloramphenicol,[7] ceftazidime,[2] imipenem[2,9]
	Streptobacillus moniliformis (rat-bite fever)	Penicillin G	A tetracycline,[4] streptomycin
	Vibrio cholerae	A tetracycline[4]	TMP-SMX, a fluoroquinolone[3]
	V. vulnificus	A tetracycline[4]	Cefotaxime
	Agents of Vincent's stomatitis (trench mouth)	Penicillin G	A tetracycline,[4] an erythromycin
	Xanthomonas (formerly Pseudomonas) maltophilia	TMP-SMX	Minocycline, ceftazidime,[6] a fluoroquinolone[3]
	Yersinia enterocolitica	TMP-SMX[2]	A fluoroquinolone, gentamicin,[2] tobramycin,[2] amikacin, cefotaxime[2,6] or ceftizoxime[2,6]
	Y. pestis (plague)	Streptomycin	A tetracycline,[4] chloramphenicol,[7] gentamicin[2]
Acid-Fast Bacilli	*Mycobacterium avium complex*	Clarithromycin or azithromycin plus one or more of the following: ethambutol, rifabutin, ciprofloxacin, rifampin, clofazimine, amikacin	—
	M. fortuitum	Amikacin,[2] doxycycline,[2] or both	Rifampin,[2] cefoxitin, a sulfonamide
	M. kansasii	Isoniazid with rifampin, with or without ethambutol or streptomycin	Cycloserine, ethionamide, clarithromycin
	M. leprae	Dapsone[7] with rifampin, with or without clofazimine	Minocycline,[4] ofloxacin,[3] clarithromycin
	M. marinum (balnei)[30]	Minocycline	TMP-SMX, rifampin, ethambutol, clarithromycin, doxycycline
	M. tuberculosis[31]	Isoniazid with rifampin, and pyrazinamide with or without ethambutol or streptomycin	Ciprofloxacin or ofloxacin; third-line agent [*see Subsection VIII*]

Note: all superscript numbers refer to footnotes that follow table.

(continued)

Table 4 (*continued*)

	Causative Organism	Drug of Choice	Alternative Drugs
Actinomyces	*Actinomyces israelii*	Penicillin G	A tetracycline,[4] an erythromycin, clindamycin
	Nocardia	TMP-SMX	Minocycline, sulfisoxazole, imipenem,[9] amikacin,[2] cycloserine
Fungi	*Aspergillus*	Amphotericin B[7]	Itraconazole
	Blastomyces dermatitidis	Amphotericin B[7] or itraconazole	Ketoconazole
	Candida	Amphotericin B[7,32] or fluconazole	Ketoconazole, itraconazole, flucytosine,[33] nystatin (oral or topical), miconazole (topical),[34] clotrimazole (topical)
	Coccidioides immitis	Amphotericin B[7] or fluconazole	Ketoconazole, itraconazole
	Cryptococcus neoformans	Amphotericin B[7] with or without flucytosine[35]	Fluconazole, itraconazole
	Histoplasma capsulatum	Amphotericin B or itraconazole	Ketoconazole
	Phycomycetes (e.g., *Mucor*)	Amphotericin B	No dependable alternative
	Sporothrix schenckii (sporotrichosis)	Amphotericin B[7] or itraconazole	Saturated solution of potassium iodide[36]
Chlamydia	*Chlamydia psittaci* (psittacosis)	A tetracycline[4]	Chloramphenicol[7]
	C. trachomatis		
	Inclusion conjunctivitis	An erythromycin (oral or I.V.)	A sulfonamide (topical plus oral)
	Lymphogranuloma venereum	A tetracycline[4]	An erythromycin
	Pneumonia	An erythromycin	A sulfonamide
	Trachoma	Azithromycin	A tetracycline[4] (topical plus oral), a sulfonamide (topical plus oral)
	Urethritis or pelvic inflammatory disease	Doxycycline or azithromycin	Erythromycin, ofloxacin, sulfisoxazole, amoxicillin
	C. pneumoniae	An erythromycin or clarithromycin, a tetracycline	—
Mycoplasma	*Mycoplasma pneumoniae*	An erythromycin[37] or a tetracycline[4]	Clarithromycin, azithromycin
	Ureaplasma urealyticum	An erythromycin	A tetracycline,[4] clarithromycin
Rickettsia	Various rickettsial organisms Rocky Mountain spotted fever, epidemic and endemic (murine) typhus, rickettsial pox, Q fever, scrub typhus	A tetracycline[3]	Chloramphenicol,[7] a fluoroquinolone[3]
Spirochetes	*Borrelia burgdorferi* (Lyme disease)	Doxycycline or amoxicillin or ceftriaxone	Penicillin, an erythromycin, clarithromycin, azithromycin
	B. recurrentis (relapsing fever)	A tetracycline[4]	Penicillin G
	Leptospira	Penicillin G	A tetracycline,[4] an erythromycin
	Treponema pallidum	Penicillin G	A tetracycline,[4] an erythromycin, ceftriaxone
Viruses	Herpes simplex		
	Disseminated	Acyclovir	Vidarabine, foscarnet[2]
	Encephalitis	Acyclovir	Vidarabine
	Genital	Acyclovir	Vidarabine, foscarnet[2]
	Keratitis	Trifluridine (topical)	Idoxuridine (topical), vidarabine (topical)
	Neonatal	Acyclovir	Vidarabine
	HIV[38]	Therapeutic regimens are rapidly evolving	—
	Cytomegalovirus	Ganciclovir or foscarnet[2]	None
	Influenza A	Amantadine or rimantadine	No dependable alternative
	Respiratory syncytial virus	Ribavirin	None
	Varicella-zoster	Acyclovir	Foscarnet
	Hepatitis B or C	Interferon alfa-2b	None

1. Some strains of *S. aureus* and most strains of *S. epidermidis* are resistant to penicillinase-resistant penicillins; these strains are also resistant to cephalosporins.

2. Not approved for this indication by the FDA.

3. For most infections, ciprofloxacin or ofloxacin, either orally or I.V. For urinary tract infection, norfloxacin, lomefloxacin, or enoxacin can be used. None of these drugs is recommended for children.

4. Tetracycline is preferred for most uses. Doxycycline is the safest tetracycline for treatment of extrarenal infections in renal insufficiency. Tetracyclines should be avoided in pregnant women and in children younger than 8 yr.

5. Crystalline penicillin G is administered parenterally in serious infections. For less severe infections caused by pneumococci, group A streptococci, gonococci, or *Treponema pallidum*, procaine penicillin G is administered I.M. once or twice daily. For mild infections caused by streptococci and pneumococci, oral penicillin V is preferable to oral penicillin G. Benzathine penicillin G is given I.M. (once monthly for the prophylaxis of rheumatic fever; a single injection for the treatment of group A streptococcal pharyngitis) when patient compliance for oral medication is questionable and for treatment of syphilis, in one to three doses at weekly intervals, depending on the stage of the disease.

6. Cephalosporins are sometimes used as alternatives to penicillin in patients with suspected penicillin allergy but not in patients with serious hypersensitivity (especially immediate anaphylactic or accelerated urticarial reactions). Patients allergic to penicillin may be hypersensitive to cephalosporins. Only third-generation cephalosporins are effective in bacterial meningitis.

7. In view of the occurrence of adverse reactions, this drug should be used only for serious infections and when less toxic drugs are ineffective.

8. For severe infections, I.V. nafcillin or oxacillin should be used. For mild infections, oral cloxacillin, dicloxacillin, or oxacillin may be employed. One to two percent of *S. aureus* strains are resistant to penicillinase-resistant penicillins (and usually to cephalosporins) but are susceptible to vancomycin. High doses of penicillin G, ampicillin, amoxicillin, carbenicillin, or ticarcillin do not overcome the clinical resistance of penicillinase-producing staphylococci to these drugs.

9. Imipenem is a β-lactam antibiotic that should be used with caution in patients who are allergic to penicillins and cephalosporins. Meropenem is a similar carbapenem.

10. In vitro sensitivity testing with cephalosporins or penicillins may be misleading because of heteroresistance and because these antibiotics may be bacteriostatic only. For serious infections, vancomycin is preferred (see text).

11. The combination of penicillin G with streptomycin for the first two weeks of treatment of endocarditis caused by viridans streptococci is preferred by some.

12. Various aminoglycosides have been used in synergistic combination with penicillin or vancomycin. Because of the appearance of enterococcal strains resistant to the synergistic action with streptomycin (but not gentamicin), gentamicin is preferred for use in the combination.

13. An investigational drug in the United States (Targocid—Hoechst Marion Roussel)

14. An investigational drug in the United States (Synercid—Rhône-Poulenc Rorer)

15. Contraindicated in pregnancy or in the presence of renal insufficiency.

(*continued*)

Table 4 (continued)

16. In patients with major allergy to penicillin, erythromycin is the alternative for respiratory tract infections; chloramphenicol is the preferred alternative for meningitis. Occasional strains of pneumococci have high-level resistance to penicillin and to most other antibiotics except vancomycin.

17. Some strains of pneumococci and group A streptococci are erythromycin resistant.

18. Antibiotics may be administered orally for antibiotic-associated pseudomembranous enterocolitis. Vancomycin has been the drug of choice, but metronidazole appears to be as effective and is much less expensive.

19. Large doses of penicillin G or ampicillin (or amoxicillin) may be required because some strains are resistant to these drugs. Penicillinase-producing gonococci, which are more resistant to penicillin, have appeared in the United States; spectinomycin is the treatment of choice for infections with such strains.

20. Rare strains of gonococci are resistant to spectinomycin; use cefoxitin, cefuroxime, cefotaxime, or TMP-SMX to treat these strains.

21. In CNS infection, metronidazole or chloramphenicol should be used.

22. The carboxypenicillins are carbenicillin and ticarcillin; the acylaminopenicillins are mezlocillin, azlocillin, and piperacillin. When one of these drugs is used for a severe infection, an aminoglycoside is often recommended as well.

23. Aztreonam is a β-lactam antibiotic; cross-sensitivity has not occurred, but use with caution in patients allergic to penicillins, cephalosporins, or imipenem.

24. An oral sulfonamide such as sulfisoxazole is often the initial therapy for an acute uncomplicated urinary tract infection, before the results of culture and susceptibility testing have been obtained. Alternatives include oral ampicillin or amoxicillin. Should the causative agent be a *Klebsiella* organism, an oral cephalosporin can be used; should it be a non-*mirabilis Proteus* organism, carbenicillin indanyl can be employed.

25. In severely ill patients, an aminoglycoside is combined with a cephalosporin.

26. Principally in treatment of uncomplicated urinary tract infections.

27. Ampicillin or amoxicillin may be effective in milder cases.

28. Some encapsulated *H. influenzae* (type b) strains and some unencapsulated strains are resistant to ampicillin, and rare strains are resistant to chloramphenicol. Chloramphenicol plus ampicillin (or chloramphenicol alone) should be used for initial treatment of meningitis or epiglottitis in children until the organism is identified and its susceptibility is determined. In adults with meningitis of unknown etiology and an indeterminate Gram's stain and in whom *H. influenzae* is suspected, chloramphenicol is added to ampicillin (or penicillin G) for the first 24 hours until the results of culture are available. Ampicillin is preferred when the infecting strain of *H. influenzae* is susceptible.

29. Not an FDA-approved use. Evidence for possible efficacy comes only from in vitro susceptibility testing and from treatment of infections in experimental animals. In both cases, *L. pneumophila* is highly susceptible to rifampin.

30. Most infections are self-limited without therapy.

31. Various combination treatments are available [*see Subsection VIII*].

32. I.V. amphotericin B is the drug of choice for systemic candidal infections. If in vitro synergism can be demonstrated with flucytosine, the combination may be indicated in therapy. For GI infections or oral thrush, oral nystatin may be adequate. Topical nystatin, miconazole, or clotrimazole is useful for skin or vaginal infections.

33. Some strains of *Candida* may be resistant to flucytosine, or resistance may develop during treatment. Bone marrow depression may be produced by flucytosine administration in the presence of renal insufficiency.

34. I.V. miconazole appears to have promise in treatment of coccidiodomycosis, particularly when amphotericin B has failed or cannot be tolerated. Its role in treatment of cryptococcal meningitis in patients who cannot tolerate amphotericin B is under study.

35. Combined therapy for cryptococcal meningitis with amphotericin B and flucytosine may provide more rapid sterilization of CSF. Combined therapy may decrease amphotericin B toxicity by allowing some dose reduction without loss in therapeutic effect.

36. For treatment of lymphocutaneous form only.

37. Erythromycin and tetracycline have been equally effective in the treatment of mycoplasmal pneumonia. Because of the initial clinical similarity between mycoplasmal pneumonia and some cases of Legionnaires' disease and because erythromycin is effective in both diseases, it is the drug of choice in patients presumed to have mycoplasmal pneumonia.

38. Guidelines for the treatment of HIV infections are evolving rapidly.

---

soft tissue infections, urinary tract infections, peritonitis, and pelvic infection.[28-31] These agents are usually well tolerated, but bacterial resistance may occur in 10% to 15% of patients. Their use has been limited by concerns about their increased sensitivity to β-lactamase, the inoculum effect, and their reduced bacteriolytic activity. To address the first concern, piperacillin has been given in combination with the β-lactamase inhibitor tazobactam [*see* β-Lactamase Inhibitors, *below*].

Cephalosporins

Cephalosporium acremonium was discovered in 1948. This fungus was found to produce cephalosporin C, from which cephalothin, the first cephalosporin to be introduced, was in turn derived. The basic cephalosporin structure consists of a dihydrothiazine ring fused to a β-lactam ring.

Various side chains have been substituted at the number 3 carbon position of the six-membered ring and at the acyl side chain of this basic cephalosporin nucleus. Changes at position 3 are thought to affect pharmacologic activity primarily. Several cephalosporins, including cefamandole, cefoperazone, moxalactam (not a true cephalosporin but a close relative with very similar characteristics), and ceftazidime, have a methyltetrazolethiol side chain at this position. This substitution results in effects similar to those of disulfiram: alcohol cannot be metabolized, and acetaldehyde accumulates in the blood, causing headache, nausea, flushing, and dizziness. Another side effect associated with this substitution is hypoprothrombinemia, which is usually reversible with pharmacologic doses of vitamin K.

Substitutions at the acyl side chain have led to differences in antibacterial spectrum and β-lactamase stability. The side chains substituted at this position interfere with proper stereotactic binding of the molecule to the β-lactamase active site, thus preventing degradation of the cephalosporin. Some of the side effects involving platelet aggregation that have been observed with the use of moxalactam can be traced to substitutions at this position.

For convenience, cephalosporins are divided into three groups, or generations, according to the nature and extent of their antibacterial spectra. More specifically, the division into generations is based on the number of gram-negative bacterial species against which each cephalosporin demonstrates clinical activity. For example, first-generation cephalosporins are active against three common gram-negative bacteria—*E. coli*, *Klebsiella pneumoniae*, and *P. mirabilis*—but they have a wider range of activity against gram-positive organisms than do second- and third-generation agents. It must be remembered, however, that although the members of each generation are sufficiently similar to be grouped together, they also are different from each other in a number of ways [*see Table 7*].

Three critical variables determine the antimicrobial activity of a cephalosporin: (1) ability to penetrate the outer cell wall of the bacterium, (2) ability to resist β-lactamase activity, and (3) ability to bind and inhibit the penicillin-binding protein enzymes (PBPs) that synthesize the bacterial cell wall. The membrane complexes in the outer cell wall of gram-positive bacteria do not block entry of cephalosporins, whereas those of gram-negative bacteria, especially *P. aeruginosa*, tend to resist cephalosporin penetration. As many as six PBPs can be found in gram-negative bacteria. Each cephalosporin binds best to a different PBP. PBPs 1, 2, and 3 are the most important. Binding to these target proteins results in inhibition of transpeptidation of glycopeptide polymers, the final step in bacterial cell wall synthesis. This action eventually triggers autolytic enzymes in susceptible bacteria, which leads to cell lysis. Because cephalosporins do not bind well to enterococcal PBPs, the MIC of cephalosporins for these bacteria is 64 to 128 times that of penicillin G and ampicillin.

FIRST-GENERATION CEPHALOSPORINS

First-generation cephalosporins have good activity against aerobic gram-positive cocci such as *S. aureus*, group B streptococci, and *Streptococcus pneumoniae*. In addition, they are effective against three aerobic gram-negative bacilli—*E. coli*, *K. pneumoniae*, and *P. mirabilis*—although even among these three, resistance is common, occurring in as many as 30% of cases. First-generation cephalosporins are also active against most anaerobic cocci and bacilli (other than *Bacteroides fragilis*). They have little or no activity against *Enterobacter*, *Serratia*, *Acinetobacter*, *Pseudomonas*, methicillin-resistant *S. aureus*, *S. epidermidis*, and enterococci. They are also inactive against *B. fragilis*, *Citrobacter*, *Listeria monocytogenes*, *Proteus* (except for *P. mirabilis*), and *Providencia*.

First-generation cephalosporins are used for infections caused by gram-positive cocci, such as skin infections and osteomyelitis, although penicillins are the agents of choice for all streptococcal infections and for infections proven by culture to be caused by susceptible staphylococci. First-generation cephalosporins are often combined with aminoglycosides to provide broad-spectrum coverage in patients with hospital-acquired pneumonias; however, this practice is falling out of favor because of the high incidence of resistance to first-generation agents observed in gram-positive organisms. The best use for first-generation cephalosporins is in surgical prophylaxis. For this application, cefazolin sodium is the preferred agent. In fact, cefazolin sodium is the most commonly used first-generation cephalosporin: it is on the drug formulary of more than 90% of United States hospitals.[32]

SECOND-GENERATION CEPHALOSPORINS

Second-generation cephalosporins possess the same spectrum of activity as the first-generation cephalosporins, with the addition of broader coverage of gram-negative organisms, including *H. influenzae*, *Enterobacter aerogenes*, and some *Neisseria* species. Fewer than 5% of *E. coli* and *Proteus* strains are resistant to second-generation cephalosporins. The activity of second-generation agents against *S. pyogenes* and *S. pneumoniae* is equal to that of the first-generation agents, but their activity against staphylococci is variable: the MIC ranges from 0.2 to 25 µg/ml. Of the second-generation agents, the most active against staphylococci is cefamandole, which has an MIC of 0.6 µg/ml for *S. aureus*. Cefotetan and cefoxitin have significant activity against *B. fragilis*. Cefoxitin is less active against *H. influenzae* and *E. aerogenes* than other second-generation cephalosporins are, but it is more active against *Serratia* species. Cefoxitin is resistant to destruction by β-lactamase and is the most potent cephalosporin against *B. fragilis*. For this reason, it is a useful primary agent in mixed infections,[33] which the rest of the second-generation cephalosporins, for the most part, are not. Cefoxitin by itself is effective in patients with community-acquired peritonitis who are unlikely to be infected with *Enterobacter* or *P. aeruginosa*.[34] Cefuroxime and cefamandole have been used with some success in empirical therapy for community-acquired pneumonia.[35] Cefuroxime axetil, an orally administered prodrug formulation of cefuroxime, is active in vitro against many gram-positive organisms and some gram-negative organisms. Its resistance to β-lactamase makes it useful for treating infections caused by β-lactamase–producing strains of *H. influenzae*, *Moraxella* (formerly *Branhamella*) *catarrhalis*, and *S. aureus*. Cefuroxime axetil provides good coverage against the Enterobacteriaceae and moderate coverage against non–*B. fragilis* anaerobes.[36]

Cefotetan, a cephamycin introduced in 1986, has a spectrum of activity very similar to that of cefoxitin.[37] It is as active as cefoxitin against *B. fragilis* but is less active against other strains in the *B. fragilis* group. Unlike cefoxitin, cefotetan is active against *H. influenzae*. Both cefoxitin and cefotetan are active against gonococci and many enteric gram-negative bacilli, but neither is effective against *Enterobacter*, *Pseudomonas*, and *Acinetobacter* species or enterococci. Cefotetan has proved effective and safe in a variety of clinical situations, including gynecologic infections and surgical prophylaxis.[38]

Cefprozil is a new oral agent whose spectrum of activity includes gram-positive and gram-negative pathogens. It has achieved good results in patients with pharyngitis or tonsillitis.[39]

Loracarbef is a new oral agent of the carbacephem class that is active in vitro against the common pathogens associated with skin infections, otitis media, sinusitis, bronchopulmonary infec-

tions, and urinary tract infections.[40] Its in vitro activity against these common outpatient pathogens is similar to that of other oral antimicrobials, such as cefaclor, cefuroxime axetil, cefixime, amoxicillin-clavulanate, and trimethoprim-sulfamethoxazole.

THIRD-GENERATION CEPHALOSPORINS

In the third-generation cephalosporins, activity against gram-positive cocci is replaced by broader gram-negative coverage. This development is illustrated by susceptibility testing done on *S. aureus*: the MIC of first-generation cephalosporins is 1 µg/ml, that of second-generation cephalosporins is 2 µg/ml, and that of third-generation cephalosporins is 3 µg/ml. Third-generation cephalosporins are more active against the enteric gram-negative bacilli covered by first- and second-generation cephalosporins. Their spectrum of activity includes *Serratia* and *Citrobacter*. They are also highly active against *H. influenzae* and *N. gonorrhoeae* and moderately active against *P. aeruginosa* and some anaerobes. At first, the third-generation cephalosporins seemed capable of providing the same spectrum of activity as the aminoglycosides but without their inherent toxicity; however, they have failed to gain wide popularity in the treatment of high-risk patients or patients with extensive infections. The reasons for this failure include their incomplete spectra of activity against the range of organisms likely to be encountered in polymicrobial infections, their unexpected agent-specific toxicity, their suboptimal pharmacokinetic properties, and their high propensity for inducing resistance.

Several new cephalosporins are under development. Cefixime, an orally absorbed iminomethoxyaminothiazolyl cephalosporin, inhibits 90% of *S. pneumoniae*, *H. influenzae*, and *H. parainfluenzae* strains, whether they produce β-lactamase or not, at concentrations of less than 0.25 mg/L. It inhibits 90% of *M. catarrhalis* strains at concentrations of less than 1 mg/L. With respect to in vitro activity, cefixime is generally superior to cefaclor and the other cephalosporins as well as to erythromycin and amoxicillin.[41]

Ceftibuten is an orally active third-generation cephalosporin that possesses increased potency against members of the Enterobacteriaceae.[42] Generally, it is about 16 times more active than cefuroxime, cefaclor, cephalexin, or amoxicillin-clavulanate; its activity is comparable to that of cefixime. Ceftibuten is ineffective against staphylococci and only partially effective against *S. pneumoniae*. *H. influenzae* and *Neisseria* species, however, are highly susceptible to this agent.

Cefepime is a new extended-spectrum parenteral cephalosporin that provides coverage against both gram-positive and gram-negative organisms, including *S. aureus* and *P. aeruginosa*. It has been used to treat patients with pneumonia, with results comparable to those obtained with ceftazidime.[43]

Antimicrobial Spectra of Activity

Enterobacteriaceae such as *E. coli*, *Klebsiella*, *Citrobacter diversus*, *Proteus* species, and *Morganella* are usually highly susceptible to third-generation cephalosporins; in general, *Enterobacter* species, *C. freundii*, *Serratia marcescens*, and *Providencia* species are less susceptible to third-generation cephalosporins, though there is a fair amount of variability among published reports. Frequently, no more than 50% of *P. aeruginosa* isolates are susceptible at cephalosporin levels of 16 µg/ml. For cephalosporins as a group, the MIC is generally 32 to 64 µg/ml for this organism. Cefoperazone tends to be more active against *P. aeruginosa* than are the other third-generation agents: some papers report an MIC of 8 to 16 µg/ml for carbenicillin-susceptible *P. aeruginosa* strains.[44-47] Isolates

Table 5 Antimicrobial Drug Dosages for Treatment of Bacterial Infections in Adults with Normal Renal Function[203]

| Class of Agent | Specific Agent | Trade Names | Modest Infections* | | | |
| | | | Oral | | Intramuscular | |
			Daily Dose	Interval	Daily Dose	Interval
Penicillinase-susceptible penicillins	Penicillin G	—	0.8–3.2 million units	6 hr	1.2 million units	8 hr
	Penicillin G benzathine	Bicillin	—	—	1.2–2.4 million units	See fn. 1
	Penicillin G procaine	Crysticillin, Duracillin, etc.	—	—	0.6–4.8 million units	6–24 hr
	Penicillin V	Pen-Vee K, V-Cillin K, etc.	0.8–3.2 million units (0.5–2.0 g)	6 hr	—	—
Penicillinase-susceptible penicillins with activity against gram-negative bacilli	Amoxicillin	Amoxil, Larotid, etc.	750–1,500 mg	8 hr	—	—
	Ampicillin	Omnipen, Polycillin, etc.	1–4 g	6 hr	1–2 g	6 hr
	Azlocillin	Azlin	—	—	—	—
	Carbenicillin	Pyopen, Geopen	—	—	See fn. 2	See fn. 2
	Carbenicillin indanyl sodium	Geocillin	—	—	—	—
	Mezlocillin	Mezlin	—	—	—	—
	Piperacillin	Pipracil	—	—	See fn. 4	See fn. 4
	Ticarcillin	Ticar	—	—	See fn. 5	See fn.5
Penicillinase-resistant penicillins	Cloxacillin	Tegopen	1–3 g	6 hr	—	—
	Dicloxacillin	Dynapen, Pathocil	1–2 g	6 hr	—	—
	Methicillin	Celbenin, Staphcillin	—	—	4 g	6 hr
	Nafcillin	Nafcil, Unipen	2–4 g[6]	6 hr	2–3 g	4–6 hr
	Oxacillin	Bactocill, Prostaphlin	2–4 g	6 hr	1–2 g	6 hr
Penicillins with clavulanate	Amoxicillin-clavulanate	Augmentin	750–1,500 mg (amoxicillin)	8 hr	—	—
	Ticarcillin-clavulanate	Timentin	—	—	—	—
Cephalosporins	Cefaclor	Ceclor	750 mg–1.5 g	8 hr	—	—
	Cefadroxil	Duricef, Ultracef	500 mg–2g	12–24 hr	—	—
	Cefamandole	Mandol	—	—	2–4 g	6 hr
	Cefazolin	Ancef, Kefzol	—	—	750 mg–1.5 g	8 hr
	Cefonicid	Monocid	—	—	See fn. 8,9	See fn. 8,9
	Cefoperazone	Cefobid	—	—	See fn. 8,9	See fn. 8,9
	Ceforanide	Precef	—	—	See fn. 8,9	See fn. 8,9
	Cefotaxime	Claforan	—	—	See fn. 8,9	See fn. 8,9
	Cefotetan	Cefotan	—	—	See fn. 8,9	See fn. 8,9
	Cefoxitin	Mefoxin	—	—	2–4 g	6 hr
	Ceftazidime	Fortaz, Tazicef, Tazidime	—	—	See fn. 8,9	See fn. 8,9
	Ceftizoxime	Cefizox	—	—	See fn. 8,9	See fn. 8,9
	Ceftriaxone	Rocephin	—	—	See fn. 8,9	See fn. 8,9
	Cefuroxime	Kefurox, Zinacef	—	—	See fn. 8,9	See fn. 8,9
	Cephalexin	Keflex	1–4 g	6 hr	—	—
	Cephalothin	Keflin	—	—	2–3 g	6 hr
	Cephapirin	Cefadyl	—	—	2–3 g	6 hr
	Cephradine	Anspor, Velosef	1–4 g	6 hr	2 g	6 hr
Carbapenems	Imipenem-cilastatin	Primaxin	—	—	—	—
	Meropenem	Merrem	—	—	—	—
Monobactams	Aztreonam	Azactam	—	—	1–2 g	8–12 hr
Aminoglycosides	Amikacin	Amikin	—	—	—	—
	Gentamicin	Garamycin	—	—	3–5 mg/kg[12]	8 hr
	Kanamycin	Kantrex	—	—	—	—
	Neomycin	—	See fn. 16	See fn. 16	—	—
	Netilmicin	Netromycin	—	—	4–6 mg/kg[12,13]	8 hr
	Streptomycin	—	—	—	1–2 g	12 hr
	Tobramycin	Nebcin	—	—	3–5 mg/kg[12]	8 hr
Tetracyclines	Demeclocycline	Declomycin	600 mg	6 hr	—	—
	Doxycycline	Vibramycin, etc.	100–200 mg[18]	12 hr	—	—

Note: all superscript numbers refer to footnotes following table.
*Infections of the upper respiratory tract, soft tissues, etc.

(continued)

Table 5 (*continued*)

Uncomplicated Urinary Tract Infections		Major and Systemic Infections[†]			
Oral		Intramuscular		Intravenous	
Daily Dose	Interval	Daily Dose	Interval	Daily Dose	Interval
—	—	—	—	4–24 million units	2–4 hr
—	—	—	—	—	—
—	—	—	—	—	—
—	—	—	—	—	—
750–1,500 mg	8 hr	—	—	—	—
2–4 g	6 hr	—	—	4-12 g	2–4 hr
—	—	—	—	12–18 g	4 hr
—	—	—	—	30–40 g	3–4 hr
4–8 tablets[3]	6 hr	—	—	—	—
—	—	—	—	12–18 g	4 hr
—	—	See fn. 4	See fn. 4	12–18 g	4 hr
—	—	—	—	16–24 g	3–6 hr
—	—	—	—	—	—
—	—	—	—	—	—
—	—	—	—	6–12 g	4–6 hr
—	—	—	—	4–12 g	4–6 hr
—	—	—	—	4–12 g	4–6 hr
750 mg (amoxicillin)	8 hr	—	—	—	—
—	—	—	—	12–18 g (ticarcillin)	4–6 hr
750 mg–1.5 g	8 hr	—	—	—	—
500 mg–2 g	12–24 hr	—	—	—	—
—	—	—	—	4–12 g	2–4 hr
See fn. 7	See fn. 7	2–3 g	6–8 hr	2–6 g	6–8 hr
—	—	—	—	0.5–2.0 g	12–24 hr
—	—	—	—	2–12 g	6–8 hr
—	—	—	—	1–2 g	12 hr
—	—	—	—	2–12 g	4–6 hr
—	—	—	—	2–6 g	12 hr
—	—	—	—	4–12 g	4 hr
—	—	—	—	2–6 g	8–12 hr
—	—	—	—	2–6 g	8–12 hr
—	—	—	—	1–4 g	12–24 hr
1–4 g	6 hr	—	—	3–6 g	6 hr
—	—	—	—	—	—
—	—	—	—	4–12 g	2–4 hr
2 g	6 hr	—	—	4–12 g	2–4 hr
				3–8 g	4–6 hr
—	—	—	—	1–4 g	6–8 hr
—	—	—	—	3 g	8 hr
—	—	—	—	3–8 g	6–8 hr
—	—	15 mg/kg[10]	8–12 hr	15 mg/kg[11]	8 hr
—	—	3–5 mg/kg	8 hr	3–5 mg/kg[13]	8 hr
—	—	15 mg/kg[14]	8–12 hr	15 mg/kg[15]	8 hr
—	—	—	—	—	—
—	—	4–6 mg/kg	8 hr	4–6 mg/kg[17]	8 hr
—	—	1–2 g	12 hr	—	—
—	—	3–5 mg/kg	8 hr	3–5 mg/kg[17]	8 hr
600 mg	6 hr	—	—	—	—
100–200 mg[18]	12 hr	—	—	100–200 mg[19]	12 hr

[†]Osteomyelitis, peritonitis, bacteremia, meningitis, endocarditis, etc.

(*continued*)

Table 5 *(continued)*

Class of Agent	Specific Agent	Trade Names	Modest Infections*			
			Oral		Intramuscular	
			Daily Dose	Interval	Daily Dose	Interval
Tetracyclines (continued)	Minocycline	Minocin	200 mg[20]	12 hr	—	—
	Oxytetracycline	Terramycin	1–2 g	6 hr	See fn. 22	See fn. 22
	Tetracycline	Achromycin, Panmycin, Sumycin, Tetracyn, etc.	1–2 g	6 hr	See fn. 22	See fn. 22
Erythromycins	Erythromycin	E-Mycin, Erythrocin, Ilotycin	1–2 g	6 hr	See fn. 22	See fn. 22
	Erythromycin estolate[24]	Ilosone	1–2 g	6 hr	—	—
Lincomycins	Clindamycin	Cleocin	600 mg–1.8 g	6 hr	600 mg–1.2 g	6–8 hr
	Lincomycin[25]	Lincocin	1.5–2.0 g	6–8 hr	600 mg–1.2 g	8–12 hr
Polymyxins	Colistimethate	Coly-Mycin M	—	—	—	—
	Polymyxin B	Aerosporin, etc.	—	—	—	—
Sulfonamides	Sulfadiazine	—	2–4 g[27]	6 hr	—	—
	Sulfisoxazole	Gantrisin	2–6 g[27]	6 hr	—	—
	Trimethoprim-sulfamethoxazole	Bactrim, Septra	4 tablets[28]	12 hr	—	—
Miscellaneous antibacterial agents	Chloramphenicol	Chloromycetin	1.5–3.0 g	6 hr	See fn. 29	See fn. 29
	Metronidazole	Flagyl	250 mg	8 hr	—	—
	Spectinomycin	Trobicin	—	—	2 g[31]	Single injection
	Trimethoprim	Proloprim, Trimpex	200 mg	12 hr	—	—
	Vancomycin	Vancocin	2 g[32]	6 hr	—	—
Quinolones	Ciprofloxacin[33]	Cipro	500 mg	12 hr	—	—
	Enoxacin	—	—	—	—	—
	Nalidixic acid	NegGram	—	—	—	—
	Norfloxacin	Noroxin	—	—	—	—
	Ofloxacin	—	—	—	—	—
	Perfloxacin	—	—	—	—	—

Note: all superscript numbers refer to footnotes following table.

*Infections of the upper respiratory tract, soft tissues, etc.

1. Benzathine penicillin G is used primarily in three circumstances. (1) Treatment of streptococcal pharyngitis in cases in which patient compliance is questionable (a single dose of 1.2 million units I.M.). (2) Prophylaxis of rheumatic fever recurrences (1.2–2.4 million units I.M. once monthly). (3) Treatment of syphilis: for primary, secondary, or early (< 1 yr) latent syphilis, a single dose of 2.4 million units I.M.; for late syphilis (late latent, cardiovascular, neurosyphilis, etc.), 2.4 million units I.M. weekly for three doses has been recommended, but many authorities now treat neurosyphilis with high-dose I.V. penicillin.

2. Parenteral carbenicillin is usually used in the treatment of serious infections caused by susceptible *Pseudomonas, Enterobacter,* and non-*mirabilis Proteus* strains and is given in maximal dosage (30–40 g I.V. daily). It is often used in synergistic combination with gentamicin or tobramycin for I.V. treatment of *Pseudomonas* infections. Occasionally, it is given in smaller dosages (1–2 g I.M. or I.V. q. 6 hr) to treat an uncomplicated urinary tract infection caused by the same organisms.

3. Each tablet of carbenicillin indanyl sodium is equivalent to 382 mg of carbenicillin (usual dosage is 1 or 2 tablets p.o., q.i.d.).

4. Piperacillin is most often used in the treatment of serious infections caused by susceptible *Pseudomonas, Klebsiella, Enterobacter,* and non-*mirabilis Proteus* strains; the agent is given in maximal dosage (12–18 g I.V. daily). It is commonly used in synergistic combination with tobramycin or gentamicin for treatment of *Pseudomonas* infections. Occasionally, it is given in smaller dosages (1.0–1.5 g I.M. or I.V. q. 6 hr) to treat an uncomplicated urinary tract infection caused by the same organisms.

5. Ticarcillin, piperacillin, mezlocillin, and azlocillin are usually used in the treatment of serious infections caused by susceptible *Pseudomonas, Enterobacter,* and non-*mirabilis Proteus* strains and are given in maximal dosage (12–24 g I.V. daily). One of these agents is commonly used in synergistic combination with tobramycin or gentamicin for treatment of *Pseudomonas* infections. Occasionally, they are given in smaller dosages (1 g I.M. or I.V. q. 6 hr) to treat an uncomplicated urinary tract infection caused by the same organisms.

6. Nafcillin is not reliably absorbed by the oral route.

7. Cefazolin may be used in the treatment of acute uncomplicated urinary tract infections caused by susceptible gram-negative bacilli (*E. coli, P. mirabilis,* and *Klebsiella*). It is administered I.M. in a dosage of 2 g daily (given as aliquots q. 8 hr).

8. Although the second- and third-generation cephalosporins can be used for milder infections at the lower end of their recommended dosage range, these potent but expensive agents should generally be reserved for treatment of serious infections or for the treatment of resistant organisms when the alternative is a more toxic antimicrobial drug.

9. The I.M. route is acceptable for milder illnesses, but the I.V. route is recommended for serious infections, including bacteremias and meningitis. The range for the I.M. dosage is the same as that for the I.V. dosage.

10. Dosage must be reduced in the presence of renal insufficiency. The daily parenteral dose should not exceed 15 mg/kg, and the total daily amount administered should not exceed 1.5 g, regardless of the patient's weight.

11. The I.V. dose should be infused during a period of 30–60 min q. 8 hr.

12. For urinary tract infections caused by resistant organisms.

13. Dosage must be reduced in the presence of renal insufficiency. The I.V. dose should be administered for a period of 30–60 min q. 8 hr. In patients with meningitis caused by susceptible gram-negative bacilli, intrathecal gentamicin (5 mg for adults, 1–2 mg for infants) is often administered once daily along with parenteral gentamicin until CSF cultures are negative.

14. Dosage must be reduced in the presence of renal insufficiency. The daily parenteral dose should not exceed 15 mg/kg (daily dose should not exceed 1.5 g, regardless of the patient's weight); the total quantity administered in a therapeutic course should not exceed 15 g.

15. The I.V. route should be employed only when I.M. administration is not possible. The I.V. dose should be administered during a period of at least 60 min q. 8 hr.

16. There are no clinical indications for the parenteral administration of neomycin in view of its marked toxicity and the availability of safer alternative drugs. The drug is given p.o. or by nasogastric tube (4–6 g daily in 4 divided doses) to reduce the number of ammonia-forming bacteria in the intestine in the short-term treatment of acute hepatic coma. It is also given in a total daily dose of 2–3 g in long-term therapy for chronic hepatic encephalopathy or episodic hepatic coma. Nephrotoxicity and ototoxicity have followed prolonged high-dose therapy in hepatic coma, particularly in patients with some renal impairment. Neomycin is also used along with vigorous mechanical cleansing of the large bowel as preoperative prophylaxis for bowel surgery. In this situation, it is administered for 1–3 days preoperatively (40 mg/ kg p.o. daily in 6 divided doses).

17. Dosage must be reduced in the presence of renal insufficiency. The I.V. dose should be administered during a period of 30–60 min q. 8 hr.

18. Usually administered as 100 mg p.o. q. 12 hr on the first day of treatment, followed by 50 mg q. 12 hr. For more difficult infections, the dosage may be continued at 100 mg q. 12 hr.

19. Usually administered as 100 mg I.V. q. 12 hr on the first day of treatment. Thereafter, it may be given as 50–100 mg I.V. q. 12 hr. Each I.V. dose should be given during a period of 1–4 hr.

20. Usually administered initially as 200 mg p.o., followed by 100 mg q. 12 hr.

21. Usually given initially as 200 mg I.V., followed by 100 mg q. 12 hr. Maximum dose in any 24-hr period is 400 mg.

22. I.M. administration is generally unsatisfactory because of poor absorption and local irritation.

23. In special circumstances, it may be given in higher doses but not in excess of 500 mg q. 6 hr.

24. Cholestatic hepatitis may develop as a hypersensitivity response to erythromycin estolate

(continued)

Table 5 (continued)

| Uncomplicated Urinary Tract Infections | | Major and Systemic Infections† | | | |
| Oral | | Intramuscular | | Intravenous | |
Daily Dose	Interval	Daily Dose	Interval	Daily Dose	Interval
200 mg[20]	12 hr	—	—	200 mg[21]	12 hr
1–2 g	6 hr	—	—	—	—
1–2 g	6 hr	See fn. 22	See fn. 22	750 mg–1.0 g[23]	6–12 hr
—	—	See fn. 22	See fn. 22	2–4 g	6 hr
—	—	—	—	—	—
—	—	1.2–2.4 g	6–8 hr	1.8–3.0 g	6–8 hr
—	—	1.2–1.8 g	8 hr	1.8–3.0 g	8 hr
—	—	2.5–5.0 mg/kg[26]	6 hr	2.5–5.0 mg/kg	6 hr
—	—	1.5–2.5 mg/kg	6–8 hr	1.5–2.5 mg/kg	6–8 hr
2–4 g[27]	6 hr	—	—	—	—
2–6 g[27]	6 hr	—	—	100 mg/kg[27]	4–6 hr
4 tablets[28]	12 hr	—	—	8–12 mg/kg[28] (trimethoprim)	6 hr[28]
1.5–2.0 g[30]	6 hr	See fn. 29	See fn. 29	2–4 g	6 hr
—	—	—	—	30 mg/kg	6 hr
200 mg	12 hr	—	—	—	—
—	—	—	—	1–2 g	6–12 hr
500 mg–1 g	12 hr	1.5 g p.o.	12 hr	—	—
800 mg	12 hr	800 mg–1.2 g	12 hr	—	—
2–4 mg	6 hr	—	—	—	—
800 mg	12 hr	—	—	—	—
400 mg	24 hr	400–800 mg	24 hr	—	—
400–800 mg	24 hr	800 mg–1.2 g	24 hr	—	—

†Osteomyelitis, peritonitis, bacteremia, meningitis, endocarditis, etc.

but not to the other erythromycin preparations. For this reason, erythromycin base or erythromycin stearate is preferable.

25. Clindamycin has supplanted lincomycin in clinical usage.

26. Dosage usually is 2.5–3.5 mg/kg daily parenterally. Occasionally, the dosage required is as high as 5 mg/kg daily; at this level, paresthesias and more serious neurotoxicity and nephrotoxicity may be manifest in some patients.

27. A loading dose of one half the daily dose is given initially. In severe infections, the dosage of sulfonamide is adjusted to provide a blood level of 10–15 mg/dl. Sulfonamides must be used with caution in patients with renal insufficiency. Sulfisoxazole is the preferred sulfonamide.

28. Each tablet contains 80 mg trimethoprim and 400 mg sulfamethoxazole. Double-strength tablets are also available (usual dosage is 1 tablet q. 12 hr). Pediatric suspensions contain 40 mg trimethoprim and 200 mg sulfamethoxazole/5 ml. Trimethoprim-sulfamethoxazole has also been used in the treatment of typhoid fever in the same dosage as recommended for urinary tract infections. It has been used in a dosage of 4–8 standard tablets daily in the treatment of brucellosis. For pneumonia caused by *Pneumocystis carinii*, the oral dosage is 20 mg/kg trimethoprim and 100 mg/kg sulfamethoxazole/24 hr (equally divided doses q. 6 hr). The I.V. dosage of trimethoprim-sulfamethoxazole ranges from 8 mg/kg trimethoprim and 40 mg/kg sulfamethoxazole/24 hr to 20 mg/kg trimethoprim and 100 mg/kg sulfamethoxazole/24 hr.

The lower dosage range is used in the treatment of urinary tract infections that require parenteral antimicrobial therapy and in the treatment of shigellosis; the larger dosage is employed in the treatment of *P. carinii* pneumonia.

29. Chloramphenicol sodium succinate, the parenteral preparation, should only be used I.V. It is ineffective when administered I.M.

30. Chloramphenicol should not be used in the treatment of a urinary tract infection that could be managed with another, safer, effective antimicrobial.

31. The only approved indication for the use of spectinomycin is in the treatment of anogenital and urethral gonorrhea in a penicillin-allergic patient or when the infecting organism is highly penicillin resistant. In geographic areas where antibiotic-resistant gonococci are prevalent, treatment with 4 g of spectinomycin (2 g in each gluteal region) may be indicated.

32. Vancomycin is not absorbed through the GI tract. Its use orally is for treatment of staphylococcal enterocolitis or antibiotic-associated enterocolitis.

33. Ciprofloxacin has been used with success in a variety of serious systemic infections, including pneumonias and osteomyelitis. The use of oral antibiotics in seriously ill patients must be weighed against the much greater experience with parenteral therapy; in particular, oral therapy may not be effective in those patients who have adynamic ileus and therefore may not reliably absorb drugs from the GI tract.

of *L. monocytogenes*, *Acinetobacter* species, *P. cepacia*, *Xanthomonas maltophilia*, *P. putida*, and *P. fluorescens* are variably sensitive to the third-generation cephalosoporins[48-51]; consequently, these drugs should not be relied on clinically.

Combinations of third-generation cephalosporins with aminoglycosides often exert additive or synergistic effects against gram-negative bacilli in vitro,[52,53] but this phenomenon has been demonstrated only in infections in neutropenic patients; these effects may not be achievable in all patients with intra-abdominal infections.

Despite their resistance to β-lactamase hydrolysis, all third-generation cephalosporins are subject to an inoculum effect; that is, the MIC and MBC are significantly increased when larger bacterial inocula (more than 10^5 organisms/ml) are tested in vitro. This is particularly true with *S. marcescens* and *P. aeruginosa*.[54] The clinical relevance of this effect is not known, but it may explain the failure of certain β-lactam compounds against infections in which large numbers of organisms may be present (e.g., pleural effusion with empyema or large intra-abdominal abscesses).

One piece of information that may help determine which cephalosporin is most active against a known infecting organism is the kill ratio, which is the ratio obtained by dividing the highest achievable blood or tissue level of an antibiotic by its average MIC for the organism. A kill ratio of 2 or greater is considered predictive of the eradication of the organism and thus of clinical cure. The following example illustrates the significance of the kill ratio as well as the importance of understanding the pharmacokinetics of antibacterial agents.

The mean MIC of cephalothin for *S. aureus* is 0.5 µg/ml, and that of cefazolin is 1.0 µg/ml. The obvious conclusion would be that cephalothin is twice as active against *S. aureus* as cefazolin. In fact, the reverse is true if the achievable serum concentrations are considered and kill ratios are constructed. The maximum attainable serum level of cephalothin after a 2 g dose is about 100 µg/ml, and the maximum attainable serum level of cefazolin after a 1 g I.V. dose is about 200 µg/ml. Therefore, the kill ratio is 200 for both cephalothin and cefazolin, but cefazolin achieves this ratio with a 1 g dose, whereas cephalothin does so with a 2 g dose.

A final concern regarding the in vitro activity of third-generation cephalosporins is their ability to induce chromosomally mediated β-lactamases in a variety of gram-negative bacilli.[55] The clinical implications of β-lactamase induction are not entirely clear, but this process is probably responsible for the development of resistance to these agents and others during therapy. Organisms that have become resistant include some *Enterobacter* species, *S. marcescens*, and *P. aeruginosa*.

Pharmacokinetics

After intravenous administration, third-generation cephalosporins conform to an open, two-compartment model, characterized by an initial rapid distribution phase followed by a slower terminal elimination phase. Peak serum concentrations attained after a 2- to 30-minute intravenous infusion of 1 g are highest for cefoperazone and ceftriaxone.[56,57] Because these two agents are very highly bound to serum proteins, they possess small apparent distribution volumes that are roughly equivalent to the volume of the intravascular space. In contrast, the distribution volume of free ceftriaxone is large, approximately 17 L.[58]

The relatively long elimination half-lives of many of the newer β-lactam antibiotics make less frequent dosing possible. Most third-generation cephalosporins are primarily eliminated renally, with two exceptions: cefoperazone and ceftriaxone. Cefoperazone is primarily eliminated unchanged in the bile, and only about 25% of an administered dose is recovered in the urine after 24 hours.[59] Peak biliary concentrations of cefoperazone approach or exceed 2,000 µg/ml after a 2 g I.V. dose.[60] Because cefoperazone's elimination half-life is essentially unaltered in patients with renal failure and the drug is not appreciably hemodialyzed, there is no need to adjust the dosage in such patients. Fifty percent of an administered dose of ceftriaxone is eliminated in the bile; the rest is eliminated renally. Ceftriaxone elimination is decreased to a small extent in end-stage renal disease; however, because the drug is normally given every 12 to 24 hours, there is little accumulation and therefore no need to adjust the dose. Ceftriaxone is not appreciably hemodialyzed.[61] Cefotaxime's

half-life increases only when creatinine clearance is less than 5 ml/min, and very little accumulation occurs.[62]

In general, third-generation cephalosporins penetrate most tissue and fluid compartments in amounts that, though variable, usually exceed the MIC for most susceptible pathogens. Sputum concentrations in the range of 0.3 to 6.0 µg/ml are attained with all the agents, and higher concentrations are found in purulent sputum. Ascitic fluid concentrations ranging from 2.4 µg/ml with ceftizoxime to greater than 60 µg/ml with cefoperazone are seen in patients with peritonitis.[63]

Concentrations in excess of the MIC for susceptible aerobic and anaerobic organisms (except for *B. fragilis*) are achieved in female genital tissue with all these agents.[64] Moxalactam achieves concentrations of 4 to 28 µg/g in the myometrium and 6 to 40 µg/g in the endometrium and has been used successfully against gynecologic infections involving *B. fragilis*. These compounds also appear to penetrate the prostate, the testes, the ureters, and renal tissue in significant amounts.[65] Therapeutic gallbladder wall concentrations can be obtained with each of these agents; they may be as high as 60 µg/g with cefoperazone. Bone-penetration studies reveal penetration with each of these agents.[66]

Clinical Utility

Many studies have compared third-generation cephalosporins in an effort to establish a superior drug or drug combination for life-threatening infections; most have found no statistically significant differences. It is important to remember that even if there is a difference in efficacy between two or more antibiotics, that difference may not be apparent if the study group is not large enough. For example, if one agent fails in 10% of patients and another in only 5%, a study group of 250 to 500 patients would be required to show a statistical difference.[67,68] Most comparative antibiotic trials, however, have reported on fewer than 60 patients and thus have not been able to pinpoint small differences in efficacy between antibiotics.[69] Many studies that find no difference between two regimens are in fact subject to this type of error.

Respiratory tract infections Nosocomial gram-negative bacillary pneumonia carries a high mortality.[70-72] It is difficult to establish a diagnosis of gram-negative pneumonia and equally difficult to assess clinical cure in a disease in which bacteria may not be eradicated because of the structural problems that predispose to development of the pneumonia. The frequency of cure with third-generation cephalosporins ranges from 65% to 100%. Two comparative trials have evaluated ceftizoxime against cefamandole in gram-negative bacillary pneumonia.[73,74] The dosages employed were 2 to 6 g/day for ceftizoxime and 4 to 8 g/day for cefamandole. The gram-negative organisms encountered were primarily *Klebsiella, E. coli, Serratia, Acinetobacter*, and *Proteus* species. The two drugs were equally effective; the few failures observed were mainly related to resistant organisms or undrained abscesses.

Cephalosporin activity against *P. aeruginosa* is extremely variable; ceftazidime and cefoperazone are the only agents that are truly effective. The activity of cephalosporins against organisms that are difficult to manage, such as *Enterobacter* species, *Citrobacter*, and *Serratia*, varies.[75] Small clinical and in vitro bacteriologic studies comparing cefotaxime, 2 g every 8 hours, with imipenem-cilastatin, 500 mg every 8 hours, have shown both drugs to have 85% efficacy.[76,77]

On theoretical grounds, the third-generation cephalosporins can be recommended as therapy for pneumonia caused by *Klebsiella, E. coli*, and *Serratia*, but they have not been unequiv-

Generic Name	Side-Chain Substituent (R)	Penicillin Structure
Penicillin G		
Oxacillin		
Nafcillin		
Ampicillin		
Carbenicillin		

Figure 1 **Various semisynthetic penicillins have been produced by modifying the structure of the side chain (R) attached to the penicillin nucleus (right). In this way, penicillins have been developed that lack some of the drawbacks of penicillin G, such as poor gastrointestinal absorption, limited spectrum of antibacterial activity, and inactivation by penicillinase-producing microorganisms; for example, oxacillin and nafcillin are resistant to inactivation by penicillinase. This bacterial enzyme (also termed β-lactamase) cleaves the β-lactam ring of penicillin to form an inactive product; the site of action of penicillinase is shown at right.**

ocally shown to be superior to combinations of a first- or second-generation cephalosporin with an aminoglycoside. They probably should not be used alone in the treatment of *P. aeruginosa* infection; if they are used at all, they should be combined with an aminoglycoside. Another extremely important consideration bearing on the use of β-lactamase–stable agents to treat pneumonia is the inoculum effect. In respiratory tract infections, inocula are often as large as 10^9 colony-forming units/ml sputum. The development of resistance in *Enterobacter* species, *P. aeruginosa*, and occasionally *S. marcescens* has followed therapy with all of the third-generation cephalosporins[78,79]; this may be attributable, at least in part, to the inoculum effect.

Urinary tract infections The third-generation cephalosporins have been widely tested for use in treatment of complicated and uncomplicated urinary tract infections; however, orally administered drugs, such as trimethoprim-sulfamethoxazole or a quinolone, are preferable because they provide effective therapy at considerably less expense.

Intra-abdominal infections A therapeutic regimen for treatment of intra-abdominal infection should include agents that are active against *S. aureus*, enteric gram-negative bacilli, and anaerobes, including *B. fragilis*. The gold-standard regimen includes an aminoglycoside to cover the enteric gram-negative organisms and clindamycin or metronidazole to cover the anaerobes. Appropriate surgical control of the source of the intra-

abdominal infection is of utmost importance in determining outcome; antibiotics play a necessary but secondary role.[80,81] The controversies regarding the pathogenicity of enterococci have been addressed by guidelines published by members of the Surgical Infection Society.[82] The third-generation cephalosporins have been proposed as candidates for single-agent therapy for infection in the abdominal cavity because their spectra of activity encompass both the aerobic gram-negative bacilli and some of the anaerobic isolates that cause infection in this region. No cephalosporin, of any generation, has been shown to have a clear advantage over an aminoglycoside-clindamycin combination in the treatment of intra-abdominal infections.

Interpretation of overall results in intra-abdominal infections is difficult because of the numerous variables involved, including the diversity of the possible infectious processes, the variable quality of the surgical technique employed, the variety of the patient characteristics observed, the possibility of one or more underlying diseases, and the differing doses of antibiotics used in individual studies.[83] Most third-generation cephalosporins do not cover anaerobes well and should be used in conjunction with an antianaerobic agent, such as clindamycin or metronidazole, for empirical therapy for serious intra-abdominal infections. A recent prospective, randomized, double-blind study[84] showed that cefoxitin was comparable in outcome (defined as survival) to imipenem; failure to cure infections was attributed to resistant organisms at the primary site in the cefoxitin arm of the trial.

Table 6 Adverse Effects of Selected Antibiotics[203]

Antibiotics	Frequency	Adverse Effects
Penicillins	Frequent	Rashes (more common with ampicillin); allergic reactions (rarely anaphylactic); diarrhea (most common with oral ampicillin)
	Occasional	Hemolytic anemia (with high parenteral doses); drug fever
	Rare	Myoclonic jerking and seizures (with high parenteral doses, especially in patients with renal insufficiency); interstitial nephritis; hemorrhagic cystitis (with methicillin); hyperkalemia with possible arrhythmias (with large doses of rapidly administered penicillin G); granulocytopenia; bleeding from platelet dysfunction (with high-dose I.V. therapy) or prolonged prothrombin time, or both; hepatitis (with semisynthetic penicillins such as oxacillin); sodium overload or hypokalemic alkalosis, or both (with high doses of carbenicillin); pseudomembranous colitis (with ampicillin)
Cephalosporins	Frequent	Thrombophlebitis with I.V. use; pain on I.M. injection; minor GI symptoms (particularly diarrhea)
	Occasional	Allergic reactions, including morbilliform and urticarial rashes, serum sickness, and anaphylaxis; drug fever and eosinophilia; reversible neutropenia and thrombocytopenia; pseudomembranous colitis; hemorrhagic diathesis (prolonged prothrombin time, primarily from moxalactam)
	Rare	Hemolytic anemia with direct Coombs'-positive reaction; transient rise in aspartate aminotransferase (AST) and alkaline phosphatase; interstitial pneumonitis; interstitial nephritis; disulfiram-like reaction with alcohol ingestion
Aminoglycosides	Occasional	Renal damage; rash (maculopapular); nausea and vomiting; ototoxicity (both auditory and vestibular to varying degrees—kanamycin effects more likely to be auditory; streptomycin and gentamicin effects more likely to be vestibular)
	Rare	Neuromuscular blockade and apnea (to be considered particularly in patients receiving succinylcholine or other blocking agents and in patients with myasthenia gravis)
Tetracyclines	Frequent	GI irritation (nausea, vomiting, diarrhea); inhibition of bone growth and discoloration and deformity of teeth in children younger than 8 yr and in neonates when the agent was administered after the first trimester of pregnancy; mucocutaneous candidiasis
	Occasional	Intestinal malabsorption; staphylococcal enterocolitis; pseudomembranous enterocolitis; photosensitivity (fever, sunburn reactions), most frequent with demeclocycline; negative nitrogen balance and increased azotemia with preexisting renal insufficiency (rarely with doxycycline); liver injury with large I.V. doses (> 1 g/day), especially when given to pregnant patients or to those with renal disease; prolongation of prothrombin time with extended use; vestibular reactions with minocycline; tooth discoloration in young adults with minocycline
	Rare	Allergic reactions; fixed drug eruptions; increased intracranial pressure (pseudotumor cerebri) in infants and extremely rarely in adults; Fanconi's syndrome after ingestion of outdated tetracycline; diabetes insipidus–like symptoms with demeclocycline
Erythromycin	Occasional	GI irritation (particularly epigastric distress); stomatitis; cholestatic hepatitis in adults treated with erythromycin estolate
	Rare	Allergic reactions with fever and rash (sometimes resembling Stevens-Johnson syndrome); reversible loss of hearing occurring after I.V. administration of 4 g/day; pseudomembranous colitis; potentiation of warfarin effect
Clindamycin	Frequent	Diarrhea; hypersensitivity reactions (maculopapular rashes)
	Occasional	Pseudomembranous colitis; nausea and vomiting
	Rare	Reversible neutropenia
Chloramphenicol	Occasional	Reversible anemia or leukopenia (dose-related toxic effect on bone marrow); gray syndrome in neonates; nausea, vomiting, diarrhea; glossitis; oropharyngeal candidiasis
	Rare	Aplastic anemia; rashes; drug fever; enterocolitis; neurotoxic reactions (with prolonged use: confusion, headache, peripheral neuritis, or optic neuritis)
Vancomycin	Occasional	Thrombophlebitis; chills and fever; ototoxicity (principally hearing loss with large doses or prolonged therapy, especially in patients with impaired renal function and in the elderly); nausea
	Rare	Nephrotoxicity; urticaria and other rashes; hypotension, which may be accompanied by paresthesias, pruritus, and upper-body rash (after rapid I.V. administration); neutropenia

ADVERSE EFFECTS

Cephalosporins are associated with a number of adverse side effects [*see Table 6*]. On the whole, however, third-generation cephalosporins are relatively nontoxic. The adverse reactions associated with their use are similar to those associated with use of other β-lactam compounds, such as local pain and irritation, hypersensitivity reactions, positive Coombs' reaction, leukopenia, thrombocytopenia, transient abnormalities in liver function enzymes, and gastrointestinal disturbances.[85,86] These reactions are usually mild and reversible, except in those rare patients who manifest life-threatening hypersensitivity reactions. Cephalosporins may be administered to most patients who are allergic to penicillin because only 5% to 15% of penicillin-allergic patients react adversely to cephalosporins.[87]

Aminoglycosides

Various aminoglycosides have been introduced into clinical practice since Waksman and colleagues discovered streptomycin more than 50 years ago. The aminoglycosides now available for clinical use worldwide are streptomycin, kanamycin, neomycin, gentamicin, tobramycin, amikacin, netilmicin, and sisomicin; dibelkacin is not available in the United States, although it is marketed in other countries. Because of the formidable nephrotoxicity and ototoxicity associated with neomycin, it is available only for topical use, for oral treatment of hepatic encephalopathy, and for preoperative decontamination of the large bowel.

Aminoglycosides are composed of two or more amino sugars bound by glycosidic linkage to a central hexose (aminocyclitol)

Table 7 Properties of Cephalosporins[203]

	Specific Agent	Trade Names	Comment*
First Generation	**Oral**		
	Cefadroxil	Duricef, Ultracef	Longer half-life
	Cephalexin	Keflex	Most experience with this agent
	Cephradine	Anspor, Velosef	Properties are similar to those of cephalexin
	Parenteral		
	Cefazolin	Ancef, Kefzol	Longer half-life; well tolerated when given I.M.
	Cephapirin	Cefadyl	Properties are similar to those of other first-generation cephalosporins
	Cephradine	Anspor, Velosef	Properties are similar to those of other first-generation cephalosporins
Second Generation	**Oral**		
	Cefaclor	Ceclor	Moderately active against *Hemophilus influenzae*
	Cefprozil	Cefzil	Active against *H. influenzae*
	Cefuroxime axetil	Ceftin	Active against *H. influenzae*
	Loracarbef	Lorabid	A carbacephem with properties and spectrum similar to those of cefuroxime
	Parenteral		
	Cefamandole	Mandol	Active against *H. influenzae*; may cause bleeding
	Cefmetazole	Zefazone	Spectrum and half-life similar to cefoxitin; may cause bleeding
	Cefonicid	Monocid	Spectrum similar to that of cefamandole
	Ceforanide	Precef	Spectrum similar to that of cefamandole
	Cefotetan	Cefotan	Spectrum similar to that of cefoxitin; longer half-life than cefoxitin; may cause bleeding
	Cefoxitin	Mefoxin	Active against *Bacteroides fragilis*, *Serratia*, *Neisseria gonorrhoeae*
	Cefuroxime	Zinacef, Kefurox	Active against *H. influenzae*; only second-generation drug approved for meningitis (selected pathogens)
Third Generation	**Oral**		
	Cefixime	Suprax	More active against gram-negative bacilli, gonococci, *Moraxella catarrhalis*, and *H. influenzae* than other oral cephalosporins but much less active against *Staphylococcus aureus*; not active against *Pseudomonas*
	Cefpodoxime	Vantin	Similar to cefixime but more active against *S. aureus*
	Ceftibuten	Cedax	Similar to cefixime but has poor activity against pneumococci and staphylococci
	Parenteral		
	Cefepime	Maxipime	Active against most gram-positive cocci (except enterococci and methicillin-resistant staphylococci), *Neisseria*, *Hemophilus*, enteric gram-negative bacilli, and *Pseudomonas*
	Cefoperazone	Cefobid	Increased activity against *Pseudomonas aeruginosa* but less against Enterobacteriaceae; may cause bleeding
	Cefotaxime	Claforan	More active against gram-positive cocci
	Ceftazidime	Fortaz, Tazidime, Tazicef	Most active against *Pseudomonas*
	Ceftizoxime	Cefizox	Properties are similar to those of cefotaxime
	Ceftriaxone	Rocephin	Longer half-life; less active against *Pseudomonas*, *B. fragilis*

Note: detailed information about the various cephalosporins is covered in the text.
*Agents are being compared with other members of the same generation of cephalosporins.

nucleus. Their highly polar, polycationic structure contributes to their poor gastrointestinal absorption and their meager ability to penetrate the blood-brain barrier. They bind irreversibly to the 30S bacterial ribosome and interfere with protein synthesis. They must, however, penetrate the cell before ribosomal binding can occur. This crucial step is energy dependent and oxygen dependent and does not occur under anaerobic conditions. The uptake of aminoglycosides is facilitated by the presence of inhibitors of cell wall synthesis, such as β-lactam antibiotics or vancomycin.[88] Aminoglycosides also disturb calcium homeostasis and induce cell death as a result of efflux of potassium, sodium, and other essential bacterial constituents. Unlike most other antimicrobial agents that inhibit protein synthesis, aminoglycosides are bactericidal. Their bactericidal capacity is now thought to be attributable to their disruptive effect on calcium homeostasis.

All aminoglycosides share certain pharmacokinetic properties. Because they are poorly absorbed when given orally, adequate serum concentrations can be obtained only through parenteral administration. Protein binding is negligible,[89] and the volume of distribution approximates the volume of the extracellular space.[90] In adults with normal renal function, the aminoglycosides have a half-life of about 2 hours, but there is considerable variation from one individual to the next.[91] In patients with deteriorating renal function, their half-life increases, often exceeding 24 hours in patients with end-stage renal disease.[92] These prolonged half-lives are substantially shortened during hemodialysis[93]; the agents are much less efficiently removed by peritoneal dialysis.[94] The aminoglycosides do not penetrate the blood-brain barrier well, even in patients with meningeal inflammation.[95,96] Drug levels in pulmonary secretions are typically 20% to 40% of serum levels. Low concentrations of aminoglycosides in purulent fluids are probably related to local inactivation caused by DNA released from leukocytes[97] and by the low regional pH.

The aminoglycosides are rapidly excreted, primarily by glomerular filtration. Urine concentrations may be 100 times the serum level in patients with normal renal function. The aminoglycosides accumulate in the renal cortex; sensitive assay techniques can detect them in urine and serum for up to 10 days after cessation of therapy.

STREPTOMYCIN

Widespread resistance among Enterobacteriaceae has limited the usefulness of streptomycin. At present, streptomycin is almost always employed in combination with other antimicrobial agents. With penicillin or vancomycin, it is used to treat infective endocarditis caused by viridans streptococci or susceptible enterococcal streptococci. It may also be given in conjunction with other antituberculous drugs to treat mycobacterial diseases and in conjunction with tetracycline to treat brucellosis. Streptomycin is used alone in the treatment of tularemia and plague.

KANAMYCIN

Because of widespread resistance among Enterobacteriaceae and *P. aeruginosa*, kanamycin is rarely used today. It is occasionally used as a second-line agent in combination with other antibiotics in the treatment of tuberculosis.

NEOMYCIN

Neomycin is used primarily in oral bowel preparations [*see IV:5 Prevention of Postoperative Infection*] and in local antiseptic ointments.

GENTAMICIN

Gentamicin continues to be the aminoglycoside of choice for serious hospital-acquired infections caused by Enterobacteriaceae and most strains of *P. aeruginosa* in institutions in which there is minimal background resistance to this agent (other *Pseudomonas* species are predictably resistant to aminoglycosides). Gentamicin is given with penicillin to treat enterococcal endocarditis and with vancomycin plus rifampin to treat prosthetic valve endocarditis caused by *S. epidermidis*. Finally, gentamicin together with antimicrobial agents active against *B. fragilis* is effective in the treatment of intra-abdominal infection.

TOBRAMYCIN

Tobramycin closely resembles gentamicin with respect to antimicrobial spectrum and pharmacokinetics. Tobramycin is more active against some strains of *Acinetobacter calcoaceticus* but less active against *S. marcescens*. Although tobramycin has slightly greater intrinsic activity against *P. aeruginosa*, most gentamicin-resistant strains of this organism are also resistant to tobramycin. The difference in nephrotoxicity between gentamicin and tobramycin is clinically insignificant.[98-100]

AMIKACIN

Amikacin is a semisynthetic derivative of kanamycin. Its major advantage is its resistance to aminoglycoside-modifying enzymes, the production of which is the principal mechanism of aminoglycoside resistance among bacteria. Amikacin may therefore be used against gentamicin-resistant organisms, and it is clearly the aminoglycoside of choice where gentamicin resistance is prevalent. Fortunately, no substantial increase in amikacin resistance has been noted, even in medical centers where it has been used extensively.[101]

NETILMICIN AND SISOMICIN

Netilmicin, a semisynthetic derivative of sisomicin, is not metabolized by most of the aminoglycoside-modifying enzymes and therefore is active against some strains of Enterobacteriaceae that are resistant to gentamicin and tobramycin; however, it is less active against *P. aeruginosa*. Animal studies suggest that netilmicin may be less nephrotoxic than other aminoglycosides,[99,102] and human studies suggest that it is somewhat less likely to exert toxic effects on cranial nerve VIII.[99] Sisomicin is more active than gentamicin against Enterobacteriaceae and *P. aeruginosa*, but the nephrotoxicity it has exhibited in animal studies exceeds that of other aminoglycosides.[103]

ADVERSE EFFECTS

Unlike β-lactam antibiotics, aminoglycosides have a narrow range between therapeutic and toxic levels and thus are prone to side effects [*see Table 6*]. Their ototoxicity is potentially more significant than their nephrotoxicity because it is often irreversible. Cochlear toxicity has been reported in 8% to 10% of patients and has been clinically evident in as many as 4% of patients treated with aminoglycosides for various infections.[104] Vestibular toxicity, as manifested by electronystagmographic changes, has been found in 5% to 10% of patients and has been clinically significant in 1% to 5%.[99] Vestibular toxicity is more frequently associated with streptomycin, gentamicin, and tobramycin, whereas auditory toxicity is more typical of kanamycin and amikacin. Ototoxicity and vestibular toxicity are difficult to monitor, particularly in hospitalized patients for whom formal audiometry and caloric testing may be cumbersome or uncomfortable. Because aminoglycoside-associated auditory toxicity generally affects the higher frequencies, early bedside detection is difficult. Toxic effects on cranial nerve VIII seem to be related to advanced age, prior aminoglycoside treatment, and excessive serum levels.

AMINOGLYCOSIDE PHARMACOKINETICS

Extremely active antibiotics, the aminoglycosides are clinically effective against many serious infections caused by gram-negative bacilli, and as patents have expired, these agents have become inexpensive. These advantages must be weighed against the potential renal and otovestibular toxicity of aminoglycosides. Peak aminoglycoside concentrations higher than 5 μg/ml are associated with improved survival in patients with gram-negative infections.[105,106] With gram-negative pulmonary infections, peak concentrations of 8 to 10 mg/ml are necessary because of poor penetration of aminoglycosides into the lungs.[107,108] It has been shown that a loading dose of gentamicin or tobramycin of 2 mg/kg lean body weight cannot guarantee adequate peak concentrations in acutely ill patients. The most likely explanation for the usually low peak serum concentrations of aminoglycosides in acutely ill patients is an expanded volume of distribution.[109-113] Dosage adjustments based on blood levels should be made as soon as possible after the beginning of therapy and after the steady state has been reached. The steady state is a level of drug accumulation in blood and tissue, after several doses have been given, at which input and output are in equilibrium. This state is reached after about five half-lives of the drug. It is essential to keep in mind that whenever the dosing regimen is changed, a new steady state is reached after about five half-lives.

Once-Daily Dosing of Aminoglycosides

Efforts to improve the toxic-to-therapeutic ratio of aminoglycosides include once-daily dose schedules and reevaluations of the recommended therapeutic ranges. In conventional administration of aminoglycosides to patients with normal renal function, divided doses are administered at 8- to 12-hour intervals. In an effort to improve efficacy and decrease toxicity and cost, once-daily regimens have been compared with conventional regimens. In most protocols, the total dose was equivalent in the single and divided-dose regimens. Two meta-analyses of such trials have concluded that once-daily dosing is as effective as divided dosing and has a lower risk of toxicity in patients with normal renal function.[114,115] Although most trials evaluated immunocompetent adults, similar trends were noted for children and for patients with febrile neutropenia. In elderly patients, however, the high peak serum concentrations that occur with once-daily dosing may increase the risk of nephrotoxicity,[116] probably because of diminished renal clearance. Once-daily dosing has not yet been studied adequately in pregnant women or in patients with renal dysfunction, burns, ascites, or endocarditis. There are several excellent reviews of the subject in the literature.[117,118]

Tetracyclines

The tetracyclines are close congeneric derivatives of the polycyclic substance naphthacenecarboxamide. They act against microorganisms by inhibiting protein synthesis; their site of action is the bacterial ribosome. At least two processes are necessary for the tetracyclines to gain access to the ribosomes of gram-negative microorganisms. The first is passive diffusion through hydrophilic pores in the outer cell membrane. The second is an energy-dependent active transport mechanism that pumps tetracyclines into the cell through the inner cytoplasmic membrane. Once inside the cell, the tetracyclines inhibit synthesis of protein by binding to the 30S ribosomes and preventing aminoacyl-transfer RNA (aminoacyl-tRNA) from gaining access to the messenger RNA–ribosome complex.

Resistance to the tetracyclines appears slowly and in a stepwise fashion and is mediated by plasmids. Plasmids impart resistance by coding for proteins that interfere with active transport of tetracycline through the cytoplasmic membrane. Microorganisms that acquire resistance to one tetracycline are usually resistant to the other tetracyclines as well.

At appropriate dosages, peak serum concentrations 1 hour after intravenous administration of tetracycline, doxycycline, or minocycline are typically 10 to 20 µg/ml. The newer semisynthetic tetracyclines—doxycycline, methacycline, and minocycline—have considerably longer serum half-lives than the older agents.

The tetracyclines bind to plasma proteins to varying degrees. Doxycycline, demeclocycline, and methacycline have the highest level of protein binding (80% to 95%). Minocycline and tetracycline exhibit an intermediate level of protein binding (65% to 75%). Oxytetracycline has the lowest level of protein binding (20% to 40%). Tetracyclines are metabolized by the liver and concentrated in the bile. Biliary concentrations of these agents are, on average, five to 10 times higher than concurrent plasma concentrations. The tetracyclines penetrate body tissues well and are capable of entering the CSF even in the absence of inflammation of the meninges. They readily cross the placental barrier, and relatively high concentrations are found in human milk.

Tetracyclines are useful in the treatment of sexually transmitted diseases, such as urethritis, endocervicitis, acute pelvic inflammatory disease, and rectal infections caused by *Chlamydia*. As a rule, doxycycline is used in combination with cefoxitin or another cephalosporin for treatment of patients with pelvic inflammatory infection. Tetracyclines are also effective for the treatment of other chlamydial infections, such as lymphogranuloma venereum, psittacosis, inclusion conjunctivitis, and trachoma. A tetracycline may also be used in the treatment of gonococcal infections in patients who are unable to tolerate penicillin G. Other sexually transmitted diseases that may be treated with tetracyclines are chancroid and granuloma inguinale.

A tetracycline or erythromycin is the agent of choice for the treatment of *Mycoplasma pneumoniae* infection. Tetracyclines are also effective against rickettsial infections, tularemia, and cholera;

in patients unable to tolerate penicillin, they may be used to treat actinomycosis. Doxycycline is useful as prophylaxis against traveler's diarrhea caused by toxicogenic strains of *E. coli*. Unfortunately, the widespread use of tetracyclines as additives to livestock feed has resulted in increasing bacterial resistance to these agents.

Adverse effects of these agents are outlined elsewhere [*see Table 6*].

Macrolides

ERYTHROMYCIN

Erythromycin is a macrolide that contains a many-membered lactone ring to which one or more deoxy sugars are attached. Erythromycin and other macrolide antibiotics inhibit protein synthesis through reversible binding to the 50S ribosomal subunits of susceptible microorganisms.

Erythromycin is well absorbed from the GI tract. The presence of food in the stomach reduces absorption of the drug, except when it is in the estolate form.[119] Peak serum concentrations 4 hours after oral administration of 500 mg of the base, stearate, or ethylsuccinate are typically 1 to 2 µg/ml. Serum concentrations 1 hour after intravenous administration of 0.5 to 1.0 g are approximately 10 to 15 µg/ml. Erythromycin is excreted primarily in the bile; only 2% to 5% of a given dose is excreted in the urine. Concentrations in the bile may be more than 10 times those in plasma. Erythromycin diffuses readily into most tissues, except for the brain and the CSF.

Erythromycin is the agent of choice for the treatment of *M. pneumoniae* and *Legionella* infections. It is also effective against infections caused by group A β-hemolytic streptococci or *S. pneumoniae*. Accordingly, it is the agent of choice for the treatment of community-acquired pneumonia in nonimmunosuppressed patients who do not require hospitalization and who are allergic to penicillin.[120] In addition, erythromycin may be used to treat gonorrhea and syphilis in patients who are unable to tolerate penicillin G or tetracycline. The incidence of serious erythromycin-related adverse effects is low [*see Table 6*].

CLARITHROMYCIN AND AZITHROMYCIN

Clarithromycin and azithromycin are new semisynthetic macrolides that are structurally related to erythromycin. They inhibit protein synthesis in susceptible organisms by binding to the 50S ribosomal subunit. Alteration in this binding site confers simultaneous resistance to all macrolides. Clarithromycin and azithromycin are well absorbed and widely distributed, with excellent cellular and tissue penetration. Both agents have a broader spectrum of activity than erythromycin does; in addition, they have fewer gastrointestinal side effects (a major obstacle to compliance with erythromycin therapy).

Clarithromycin is several times more active against gram-positive organisms in vitro than erythromycin is, whereas azithromycin is two to four times less potent than erythromycin. Azithromycin has excellent in vitro activity against *H. influenzae*; clarithromycin, although less active against *H. influenzae* according to standard in vitro testing, is metabolized into an active compound with twice the in vitro activity of the parent drug. Both azithromycin and clarithromycin are equivalent to standard oral therapies for respiratory tract and soft tissue infections caused by susceptible organisms, including *S. aureus*, *S. pneumoniae*, *S. pyogenes*, *H. influenzae*, and *M. catarrhalis*.[121] Clarithromycin is more active in vitro against the atypical respiratory pathogens (e.g., *Legionella*), although insufficient in vivo data are available to demonstrate a clinical difference between azithromycin and clarithromycin. Azithromycin and clarithromycin also are active against some unexpected pathogens (e.g., *Borrelia burgdorferi, Toxoplasma gondii, Mycobacterium avium* complex, and *M. leprae*). At present, clarithromycin appears to be the more active of the two against atypical mycobacteria, giving new hope to surgeons faced with what has become a difficult group of infections to treat.

Superior pharmacodynamic properties distinguish these new macrolides from the prototypical macrolide, erythromycin. Azithromycin has a large volume of distribution, and although serum concentrations remain low, it concentrates readily within tissues, demonstrating a tissue half-life of approximately 3 days; a 5-day course of therapy will provide therapeutic tissue concentrations for at least 10 days. These properties allow novel dosing schemes. For instance, azithromycin can be given once daily for 5 days to treat respiratory tract and soft tissue infections, and administration of a single 1 g dose of azithromycin can effectively treat *Chlamydia trachomatis* genital infections; these more convenient dosing schedules improve patient compliance. Clarithromycin has a longer serum half-life and better tissue penetration than erythromycin and thus can be given twice daily to treat most common infections.

Currently, clarithromycin and azithromycin are approved for treatment of respiratory tract infections and skin infections, but they may also be of use in mycobacterial and *Toxoplasma* infections in patients with AIDS.[122]

Clindamycin

Clindamycin is a 7-deoxy-7-chloro derivative of lincomycin that consists of an amino acid attached to a sulfur-containing octose. Clindamycin binds exclusively to the 50S subunit of bacterial ribosomes and suppresses the synthesis of protein. Clindamycin, erythromycin, and chloramphenicol all act at the same site, and the binding of one of these antibiotics to the ribosome may inhibit the binding of the others. Plasmid-mediated resistance to clindamycin has been reported in *B. fragilis*; this may be caused by methylation of bacterial RNA found in the 50S ribosomal subunit.[123] Peak serum concentrations 1 hour after intravenous administration of a 600 mg dose are approximately 10 to 12 μg/ml. Clindamycin is metabolized by the liver and excreted in an inactive form in the urine. It readily penetrates most body tissues but not the CSF.[124]

Clindamycin is active against *B. fragilis* and other anaerobic microorganisms and is useful in the treatment of patients with intra-abdominal, pelvic, and pulmonary infections. It is associated with a modest number of adverse effects [see Table 6].

Chloramphenicol

Chloramphenicol is unique among antibiotics in that it contains a nitrobenzene moiety and is a derivative of dichloroacetic acid. Like clindamycin, it inhibits bacterial protein synthesis by binding reversibly to the 50S ribosomal subunit, thus keeping the amino acid–containing end of aminoacyl-tRNA from binding to the ribosome. Resistance to chloramphenicol is caused by a specific plasmid that causes production of acetyltransferase, which inactivates the drug.[125] Chloramphenicol is rapidly and completely absorbed from the GI tract, and absorption is not impaired by concomitant ingestion of food or administration of antacids. It is inactivated in the liver by glucuronyl transferase. It and its metabolites are

excreted rapidly in the urine. About 80% to 90% of a dose is excreted in this way, about 5% to 10% of which is in the biologically active form. The drug penetrates well into all tissues, including the brain, and into the CSF and the aqueous humor.

Because of the risk of serious or fatal bone marrow toxicity, chloramphenicol should be used only against those infections for which the benefits of its use outweigh the risks of its potential toxicity. It still plays a major role in the treatment of typhoid fever, although plasmid-mediated resistance of *Salmonella typhi* to chloramphenicol has been reported. Chloramphenicol is effective therapy for bacterial meningitis and brain abscesses caused by susceptible microorganisms; in conjunction with penicillin, it is effective empirical therapy for brain abscesses. It is as effective as ampicillin against meningitis caused by susceptible strains of *H. influenzae*. It is active in vitro against most anaerobic bacteria, including *B. fragilis*. The most important toxic effect of chloramphenicol is bone marrow suppression [see Table 6].

Vancomycin

Vancomycin is a narrow-spectrum antibiotic derived from *Nocardia orientalis*. It was introduced in 1956, primarily because of its efficacy against resistant penicillinase-producing staphylococci (though it is also effective against other aerobic and anaerobic gram-positive organisms).[126,127] It became generally available before the semisynthetic bactericidal antistaphylococcal penicillins and cephalosporins were developed. These newer agents displaced vancomycin to a large extent, so that its main role became that of an alternative in situations in which the penicillins and cephalosporins could not be used.

Vancomycin exerts its bactericidal effect by inhibiting the biosynthesis of the major structural cell wall polymer, peptidoglycan, a complex glycopolypeptide with a molecular weight of about 1,500.[128] Vancomycin is about 55% protein bound. Its activity is not significantly affected by pH values between 6.5 and 8.0. It is poorly absorbed from the GI tract. Because patients invariably experience pain after intramuscular injections, parenteral administration is limited to the intravenous route. Vancomycin is primarily excreted by the kidneys; about 80% to 90% of the dose is eliminated in a 24-hour period. Its half-life is approximately 6 hours in patients with normal renal function. In anuric patients, the half-life may be prolonged to approximately 7 1/2 days.[129] Vancomycin is not removed by hemodialysis or peritoneal dialysis.

Vancomycin is mainly effective against gram-positive organisms. No cross-resistance has been demonstrated between vancomycin and other antibiotics, and resistance is uncommon. For streptococci, the MICs of vancomycin are uniformly low, but the MBCs vary: concentrations higher than 20 μg/ml are necessary for about one half of the viridans strains, and concentrations of 100 μg/ml or greater may be necessary to exert a bactericidal effect on the enterococci.

Vancomycin, given alone, is the agent of choice in the treatment of methicillin-resistant *S. aureus* infections.[130,131] Some strains of methicillin-resistant *S. aureus*, however, are resistant to vancomycin. If vancomycin therapy is ineffective against severe infections caused by such strains, the addition of an aminoglycoside, rifampin, or both should be considered. Several reports have indicated that vancomycin is not bactericidal for enterococci.[132] Vancomycin is indicated for other serious infections caused by organisms with multiple antibiotic resistance, such as

CSF shunt infections and prosthetic valve infection caused by *S. epidermidis* or *Corynebacterium diphtheriae*.[133] It is the agent of choice for infections caused by penicillin-resistant group JK corynebacteria[134] and is uniformly active against rare, multiply resistant strains of *S. pneumoniae*.[135] Given orally, vancomycin is also the agent of choice for *Clostridium difficile*–associated enterocolitis,[136] although less expensive agents, such as bacitracin[137] and metronidazole,[138] may be as effective.

The usual intravenous dosage of vancomycin in adults with normal renal function is 1 g every 12 hours; 500 mg every 6 hours is a commonly used alternative regimen. As with the aminoglycosides, therapy should be monitored carefully. The dosage of vancomycin must be decreased in patients who have impaired renal function. An initial dose of 15 mg/kg should be given regardless of the extent of renal impairment. When vancomycin is given in conjunction with an aminoglycoside, the dosage in adults should usually be no more than 0.5 g every 8 hours.

Anaphylactoid reactions to vancomycin have been reported since the earliest clinical trials. Such reactions can occur with the first dose; signs and symptoms range from mild pruritus to dramatic hypotension and cardiovascular arrest. The rapid intravenous infusion of vancomycin can cause a peculiar reaction consisting of pruritus; an erythematous or maculopapular rash involving the face, neck, and upper torso; and possible hypotension. This reaction has been referred to as the red neck or red man syndrome. It can often be prevented by slow infusion of the drug over a period of at least 60 minutes. When vancomycin is administered to patients with normal renal function or when therapy is monitored closely in patients with impaired renal function, the incidence of toxicity and side effects is low.[139] Highly purified preparations of vancomycin have been introduced,[140] but further clinical experience is necessary before it can be determined whether these new preparations cause fewer adverse reactions [*see Table 6*].

Metronidazole

Metronidazole was approved in 1959 for use as an antiparasitic agent against *Trichomonas vaginalis*; the drug later proved to be effective against the parasitic organisms *Entamoeba histolytica* and *Giardia lamblia*. In 1981, the FDA approved an intravenous preparation of metronidazole for the treatment of serious infections caused by anaerobic bacteria.[141] Orally administered metronidazole is excellent for treatment of pseudomembranous colitis caused by *C. difficile*. Metronidazole is also useful as part of preoperative prophylactic regimens for elective colorectal surgery. This agent, which appears to act by disrupting bacterial DNA and inhibiting nucleic acid synthesis,[142] is bactericidal against almost all anaerobic gram-negative bacilli, including *B. fragilis*, and against most *Clostridium* species. Although true anaerobic streptococci are generally susceptible to it, microaerophilic streptococci as well as *Actinomyces* and *Propionibacterium* species are often resistant.

Metronidazole is excellent for anaerobic infections of the abdomen and pelvis. For serious anaerobic infections, the drug is administered intravenously; a loading dose of 15 mg/kg is given, followed by 7.5 mg/kg every 6 hours until the patient is well enough to take an oral dosage of 7.5 mg/kg every 6 hours. The dosage need not be reduced in azotemic patients, but it should be reduced in patients with hepatic insufficiency. Because of its bactericidal action and excellent tissue penetration, intravenous metronidazole may be the treatment of choice

for *B. fragilis* endocarditis and central nervous system infections, both of which are uncommon. When metronidazole is administered orally, it is well absorbed and is widely distributed in body tissues, including those of the CNS.

Side effects of metronidazole include dry mouth (associated with a metallic taste) and nausea. Concurrent use of alcohol may cause a reaction similar to that produced when alcohol is ingested after taking disulfiram. Neurologic symptoms, including peripheral neuropathy and encephalopathic reactions, and neutropenia are uncommon. Pancreatitis has been reported,[143] but alternative drugs are available.

Carbapenems

The carbapenems include the thienamycins, the olivanic acids, the carpetimycins, the asparenomycins, the pluracidomycins, and other natural and semisynthetic compounds. They are unique among antibiotics in that they have an extraordinary level of activity against commonly encountered anaerobes, such as *B. fragilis* and other *Bacteroides* species, while still possessing excellent activity against aerobic gram-positive and gram-negative organisms.

Structurally, the carbapenems resemble the penicillins in that they have a nucleus containing a β-lactam ring and a five-membered thiazolidine ring. In the carbapenems, however, there is a double bond between the carbon atoms at positions 2 and 3 of the thiazolidine ring, and carbon is substituted for sulfur at position 1. The carbapenems differ from each other primarily in the configurations of the side chains at positions 2 and 6 of the β-lactam ring. They vary with respect to their in vitro spectra of activity and their ability to resist, inhibit, and induce β-lactamases. Many of the carbapenems (e.g., thienamycin) are highly unstable in solution, and some (e.g., imipenem) are degraded by mammalian dehydropeptidases in vivo. A recent review[144] compared the two clinically available carbapenems, imipenem and meropenem.

IMIPENEM-CILASTATIN

Imipenem, the *N*-formimidoyl derivative of thienamycin, was the first commercially available carbapenem antibiotic to come out of the numerous innovative studies that have been done on β-lactam synthesis of penems and carbapenems.[145] It is extensively internalized and metabolized by the renal tubular epithelium. This results in rapid clearance of the agent and absence of active antibiotic in the urine. To circumvent this problem, an inhibitor of the enzyme mediating renal metabolism of imipenem (a dehydropeptidase) was developed. This inhibitor, known as cilastatin, has no documented toxicities, and it is now added to imipenem preparations by the manufacturer.

Imipenem has a broad antibacterial spectrum that includes both aerobes and anaerobes. This spectrum has not changed in the years since the agent was first tested. Early comparative studies showed that imipenem was as effective as cefazolin in the treatment of minor infections.[146] It has also been shown to be highly effective against most bacterial species likely to be encountered in intra-abdominal infections, including *B. fragilis*, most members of the Enterobacteriaceae (including *Enterobacter* species), *P. aeruginosa*, and *S. faecalis*.[147] Theoretically, because it is active against both aerobic and anaerobic organisms, imipenem would be ideally suited to treatment of gynecologic infections. At present, however, there is no convincing evidence that it is superior to the many other available agents, and as one investigator has noted, the frequency with which *Chlamydia* is found in gynecologic infections necessitates the use of an agent such as tetracycline in addition to the β-lactam.

A study comparing imipenem with the combination of clindamycin and gentamicin demonstrated no difference in efficacy but found that the incidence of nephrotoxicity was lower in patients receiving imipenem.[148]

Because of its broad antibacterial spectrum, imipenem has been promoted by its manufacturer as empirical therapy for many life-threatening infections. There are, however, a number of clinical situations in which it is not the first agent that should be considered—namely, community-acquired pneumonia, urinary tract infection, skin structure infection, and osteomyelitis. Imipenem is a useful alternative when toxicity would be a serious problem if an aminoglycoside were used. It can replace combination therapy in mixed infections.

A well-designed, controlled, prospective, randomized trial that compared imipenem therapy with acceptable aminoglycoside-based regimens supports the use of imipenem as monotherapy for intra-abdominal infections in which an enteric mixed flora is anticipated.[149] A total of 290 patients were enrolled in the study, 162 of whom were evaluable. Logistic regression was used to analyze outcome at the abdominal site of infection and mortality. When the analysis was restricted to the residual effect of treatment assignment, a significant improvement in outcome was found in the patients receiving imipenem ($P = 0.043$). The differences in outcome were explained by a higher failure rate for gram-negative infections in the patients receiving tobramycin and clindamycin ($P = 0.018$). This failure rate was reflected in the significantly higher incidence of fasciitis that necessitated reoperation and prosthetic fascial replacement. The study supports the view that imipenem-cilastatin therapy yields better outcomes at intra-abdominal sites of infection than regimens based on conventional dosages of aminoglycosides.

A second study compared broad-spectrum imipenem-cilastatin monotherapy with an aminoglycoside-based antibiotic regimen in the management of intra-abdominal infections.[150] In this study, patients treated with imipenem had fewer febrile episodes, fewer breakthrough bacteremias, less antibiotic resistance, less need for empirical change of drug, and a significantly shorter hospital stay. Imipenem appears to be a safe and efficacious alternative broad-spectrum antibiotic in the treatment of seriously ill patients with intra-abdominal infections.

The primary adverse effect of imipenem is potentiation of seizure disorders. Idiosyncratic reactions and diarrhea are less problematic.

MEROPENEM

Meropenem possesses the exceptional profile of activity typical of the carbapenems and even appears to have some in vitro advantages over imipenem.[151] Additional carbapenems under development include ALP-201 and LJC 10,627.

Carbapenems are among the antibiotics that exert a postantibiotic effect (PAE) against certain medically important bacteria: S. aureus (two strains), P. aeruginosa (four), E. coli (one), S. marcescens (one), Morganella morganii (one), and Providencia stuartii (one). (The PAE is the phenomenon in which bacteria are killed or inhibited from growing after the antibiotic has been eliminated.) The PAE is determined by comparing the serial colony counts of cultures recovering from exposure to drug concentrations at four times the MIC for 1.5 hours with those of control cultures not exposed to the drugs.

Monobactams

The monobactams are monocyclic β-lactam antibiotics that lack the thiazolidine ring found in penicillins and the dihydrothiazine ring found in cephalosporins. Although there are several monobactams under investigation, only aztreonam has been approved for clinical use in the United States. It has been evaluated in open and comparative studies against a number of agents currently used to treat infections.[152,153] It inhibits only aerobic gram-negative species. It can be administered two or three times daily. It is a poor hapten and has been successfully administered to small numbers of patients with proven allergy to penicillins and cephalosporins.[154]

Aztreonam has been shown to be effective against bacteremia caused by E. coli, K. pneumoniae, P. mirabilis, S. marcescens, P. aeruginosa, Enterobacter species, Proteus species, and Providencia species.[155,156] It has also been used, alone or in combination with clindamycin, to treat gram-negative aspiration pneumonia, with results comparable or superior to those obtained with an aminoglycoside-clindamycin combination.[157,158]

Aztreonam has been advocated as directed therapy to obviate more toxic drugs. It seems possible that aztreonam could replace aminoglycosides in many situations in which they are combined with other agents.

β-Lactamase Inhibitors

A novel approach to antibacterial chemotherapy is the use of β-lactamase inhibitors with β-lactam agents. Clavulanate has been combined with both amoxicillin and ticarcillin. Because neither clavulanate nor sulbactam inhibits the β-lactamases that function primarily as cephalosporinases in Enterobacter, Serratia, and P. aeruginosa, addition of clavulanate or sulbactam does not enhance ticarcillin's activity against Pseudomonas. The principal use of amoxicillin-clavulanate has been in the treatment of upper respiratory tract infections caused by β-lactamase–producing H. influenzae or M. catarrhalis. Ticarcillin-clavulanate has been used to treat pneumonia caused by P. aeruginosa and mixed β-lactamase–producing flora as well as intra-abdominal infections and gynecologic infections in which the infecting organisms often possess β-lactamases. In febrile neutropenic patients, its efficacy is comparable to that of other agents, but superinfections may be a problem.[159,160] Because some strains of K. pneumoniae are not adequately inhibited by ticarcillin-clavulanate, addition of an aminoglycoside would be appropriate in neutropenic patients. Sulbactam has also been combined with ampicillin.

Clavulanate, sulbactam, and tazobactam have all been combined with piperacillin in an attempt to enhance the agent's activity against β-lactamase–producing bacteria.[161,162] Tazobactam enhances the spectrum of action and potency of piperacillin to a greater extent than sulbactam does. Although piperacillin-clavulanate is more potent than piperacillin-tazobactam, the two combinations are effective against virtually the same spectrum of resistant β-lactamase–producing gram-negative organisms. Piperacillin-tazobactam is more potent than ticarcillin-clavulanate and is effective against a wider range of gram-negative enteric organisms. Combinations of piperacillin with tazobactam or clavulanate have a broader spectrum of activity than combinations of piperacillin with sulbactam against bacteria that produce characterized plasmid-mediated enzymes of clinical significance. In particular, piperacillin-tazobactam and piperacillin-clavulanate inhibit TEM-1, TEM-2, and SHV-1 β-lactamases, but piperacillin-sulbactam does not. In mice infected with β-lactamase–producing *E. coli, K. pneumoniae, P. mirabilis,* and *S. aureus,* both tazobactam and clavulanate have provided greater enhancement of the therapeutic efficacy of piperacillin than sulbactam has. Reviews of the TEM-type β-lactamases[163] and the piperacillin-tazobactam combinations[164] have been published.

Quinolones

The quinolones are promising agents for several reasons: their antimicrobial spectrum of activity is wide, some of them can be used both orally and parenterally, and their toxicity does not appear to be excessive.[165,166] The newer quinolones—ciprofloxacin, norfloxacin, enoxacin, pefloxacin, and ofloxacin—have excellent activity against most isolates of Enterobacteriaceae, including organisms resistant to aminoglycosides and cephalosporins. Worldwide, most isolates are inhibited by concentrations of 0.002 to 2 µg/ml; these concentrations are readily achievable at the usual dosages [*see Table 5*]. All five agents are highly active against *H. influenzae, N. gonorrhoeae,* and *M. catarrhalis.* All are effective against *P. aeruginosa* at achievable urine levels. In particular, ciprofloxacin inhibits 90% of isolates at a concentration of 1 µg/ml in most of the published studies. The quinolones are also strongly active against staphylococci, including methicillin-resistant isolates: 90% of isolates are inhibited by an ofloxacin or ciprofloxacin concentration of 1 µg/ml. In addition, they possess impressive activity against important intracellular pathogens, such as *Brucella* species, *Legionella* species, *C. trachomatis, M. pneumoniae,* and *M. tuberculosis.* They readily penetrate phagocytic cells.

The species that the quinolones may not be effective against are the streptococci, including *S. pneumoniae* and *S. faecalis;* anaerobic cocci and bacilli may also pose problems, depending on which agent is used. Some newly synthesized quinolones, which have not yet been administered to humans, do inhibit these organisms.[167]

Resistance to the quinolones as a result of single-step mutations occurs in fewer than 0.0000001% of cases and is at least 300 times rarer than comparable resistance to the older quinolone nalidixic acid. Nevertheless, repeated exposure of bacteria to any of the newer quinolones can result in the selection of resistant organisms.[168] Cross-resistance to all quinolones is usually observed, and resistance may extend to other classes of antibiotics, including β-lactam agents. Bacteria resistant to the newer quinolones (most often, *P. aeruginosa, S. marcescens,* and staphylococci) have been found in the sputum of cystic fibrosis patients, in chronic wounds, and occasionally in the lesions of urinary tract infections. Whether the use of combination therapy (see below) will decrease the development of resistance remains to be established.

Additional quinolones are currently under investigation; these include lomefloxacin, temafloxacin, rufloxacin, tosufloxacin, levofloxacin, and sporfloxacin.

PHARMACOKINETICS

All of the quinolones are well absorbed from the GI tract, even in elderly, debilitated, or critically ill patients; however, ofloxacin is absorbed better than ciprofloxacin, pefloxacin, or enoxacin.[169,170] The presence of food does not decrease absorption, but it delays attainment of peak serum concentrations. The quinolones are widely distributed to body tissues and fluids: the apparent volume of distribution is 90 to 110 L. Tissue concentrations (except in the brain, saliva, and bronchial secretions) are at least as high as serum concentrations. Excellent concentrations are achieved in the lungs, the bones, the prostate, the kidneys, and macrophages and leukocytes.[171]

The quinolones are metabolized to varying degrees: only about 5% of an ofloxacin dose is converted to metabolites, whereas pefloxacin is almost entirely metabolized. The metabolites are generally less active than the parent compounds and do not accumulate in tissues. All of the quinolones are excreted renally, primarily by tubular secretion. The concentrations attained in the urine far exceed the MICs for most urinary pathogens, even in the presence of renal insufficiency.[169,172] Nonrenal clearance helps compensate for decreased excretion in patients with renal dysfunction who are receiving a quinolone (except for those receiving ofloxacin)

CLINICAL UTILITY

Urinary Tract Infections

All of the quinolones have proved to be at least as effective as the traditional regimens of amoxicillin or trimethoprim-sulfamethoxazole in the treatment of uncomplicated and complicated urinary tract infections (UTIs).[173] Because of their higher cost and the possibility that resistance will develop, they are not recommended as therapy for simple cystitis. These agents may be used to treat complicated UTIs caused by multiresistant organisms, either as an alternative to or as follow-up to parenteral therapy. Their advantage lies in the possibility of achieving high urinary and intestinal concentrations, which decrease the likelihood of resistance and of reinfection or suprainfection in bedridden patients.[169] In UTIs caused by *P. aeruginosa,* the fluoroquinolones have been proved effective, but resistant strains have emerged repeatedly.[173]

The quinolones have been used with some success in patients with renal failure[173]; however, dosages must be titrated properly. Concomitant use of antacids or phosphate binders that decrease intestinal absorption of the quinolones may adversely affect therapeutic outcome.

Acute and chronic prostatitis can also be treated with quinolones. Patients with chronic prostatitis, however, tend to relapse if the infecting organism is *P. aeruginosa* or *E. coli.* Still, the quinolones are at least as effective as the drugs used in the standard regimens.

Sexually Transmitted Diseases

All of the quinolones are effective as single-dose therapy for gonorrhea, including gonorrhea caused by penicillinase-producing strains.[174,175] They cannot, however, eradicate *Chlamydia* organisms.

Diarrheal Diseases

The quinolones are highly active against organisms that cause bacterial diarrhea: *Shigella* species, *Salmonella* species, toxicogenic *E. coli, Campylobacter* species, *Aeromonas* species, *Vibrio cholerae,* and *V. parahaemolyticus* are all eradicated by 48 hours of quinolone therapy.[169,176] *C. difficile,* however, is not inhibited and has caused colitis in rare instances. In addition, ciprofloxacin and norfloxacin have been effective in the carrier state of typhoid.

Skin and Skin Structure Infections

Many types of skin infections have been successfully treated with quinolones. Ofloxacin and ciprofloxacin are as effective as standard oral and parenteral regimens[171,177]; enoxacin appears to be somewhat less promising.[178]

Joint and Bone Infections

The main reason for testing the quinolones in joint and bone infections is that use of an oral agent eliminates the need to hospitalize patients for parenteral administration of antibiotics. Furthermore, because the quinolones have a long half-life and are well tolerated, compliance is likely to be high during the long treatment periods often necessary to cure these infections. To date, pefloxacin, ciprofloxacin, and ofloxacin have been studied.[179] The results achieved with these agents have been comparable to those achieved with parenteral regimens, but in many cases, follow-up has been too short or is still incomplete. As with skin infections, surgical intervention is often a valuable adjunct to antibiotic therapy.

Respiratory Infections

Ciprofloxacin, ofloxacin, enoxacin, and pefloxacin have been evaluated in the treatment of the acute exacerbation of chronic bronchitis.[180] Ofloxacin yields the best bacteriologic and clinical results because of its higher sputum concentration and its lower MIC for *S. pneumoniae*; ciprofloxacin yields the next best results. Even though some degree of success has been achieved with the quinolones, they remain second-line agents because of their limited activity against *S. pneumoniae*. This is true in patients with community-acquired pneumonia as well as in those with acutely exacerbated chronic bronchitis.

The problem of multiresistant organisms and the search for newer, more potent alternative treatments have led to growing interest in using quinolones as therapy for nosocomial pneumonia. Although further studies are necessary to define the potential role of the quinolones in this setting more clearly, the initial results are promising. These agents remain valid alternatives when resistance emerges or when follow-up oral therapy is indicated.[181]

The quinolones have also been used to treat pulmonary exacerbations in cystic fibrosis patients because they are highly active against the main causative organisms (*P. aeruginosa*, *S. aureus*, and *H. influenzae*) and can be given orally. The clinical improvement obtained after therapy with ciprofloxacin or ofloxacin is comparable to that obtained after parenteral antibiotic therapy.[169,171] However, *P. aeruginosa* is not eradicated from the sputum; in fact, a steady increase in MICs for this organism is a regular occurrence. This problem is also encountered with standard regimens. In either case, it can be minimized by avoiding prolonged therapy (longer than 4 to 8 weeks) and by alternating the agents used.

Intra-abdominal Infections

The fluoroquinolones currently available have modest activity against anaerobes. Newer fluoroquinolones with increased in vitro activity against anaerobes are under development. These include levofloxacin, clinafloxacin, sparfloxacin, trovafloxacin, grepafloxacin, and DU-6859[182]; trovafloxacin and grepafloxacin have been approved for clinical use in the United States. A randomized, double-blind, multicenter trial comparing ciprofloxacin-metronidazole with imipenem-cilastatin for the treatment of complicated intra-abdominal infections demonstrated the efficacy of the quinolones.[183] Patients were randomized to I.V. ciprofloxacin-metronidazole, I.V. imipenem, or I.V. ciprofloxacin-metronidazole followed by oral ciprofloxacin-metronidazole when oral feeding was resumed. The results demonstrated statistical equivalence between I.V. ciprofloxacin-metronidazole and I.V. imipenem in both the intent-to-treat and valid populations. Conversion to oral therapy with ciprofloxacin appeared to be as effective as continued I.V. therapy in patients able to tolerate oral feedings. Of the new quinolones, those with extremely broad-spectrum in vitro coverage, such as clinafloxacin and trovafloxacin, have the potential for widespread use in intra-abdominal infections pending favorable outcomes of current phase III clinical trials. The excellent oral absorption of these agents permits I.V.-to-oral stepdown therapy, a promising practice that is likely to reduce costs and improve the quality of care of patients with intra-abdominal infections.[184]

ADVERSE EFFECTS

Adverse reactions to the quinolones are estimated to occur in 4% to 8% of cases.[185] Most such reactions are not severe: cessation of therapy has been necessary in only about 1% to 2% of patients, and in all cases, the reactions have been reversible. The most common adverse effects are gastrointestinal—namely, nausea, vomiting, and diarrhea. The next most common are central nervous system effects, which include dizziness, headache, insomnia, hallucinations, agitation, and seizures. (The last three have been attributed to coadministration of enoxacin and theophylline.) Other effects include skin rash, pruritus, photosensitivity (with ofloxacin and pefloxacin), and mild alterations in hematologic and biochemical laboratory values.

Complications of Antibiotic Therapy

Widespread resistance to antimicrobials has become a problem in the United States. This is especially evident in intensive care units. Organisms frequently encountered in ICUs include *P. aeruginosa*, *S. aureus*, *H. influenzae* (particularly in trauma victims), enterococci, *K. pneumoniae*, *Enterobacter* species, *Acinetobacter baumanii*, *E. coli*, and *Stenotrophomonas* (*Xanthomonas*) *maltophilia*. Although antibiotics have played a major role in the treatment of such infections, the pathogens have responded to the antibiotic challenge, developing resistance to all available antimicrobial agents to a greater or lesser degree. Specific mechanisms of resistance are evident in the reduced permeability of cell wall membranes, changes in the target sites of antimicrobial agents, enzymatic inactivation of antibiotics, and the development of pathways bypassing antimicrobial targets.[186]

Clinically significant resistance has been associated with some of the third-generation cephalosporins, such as ceftriaxone and ceftazidime, even in preclinical trials. These observations, based on reported in vivo use rather than on in vitro predictions, are extremely disconcerting.

Colonization and superinfection have long been recognized as potential complications of antimicrobial therapy. *Suprainfection*—a more descriptive term that refers to superinfection related to antibiotic therapy—must also be distinguished from colonization. Suprainfection connotes both clinical and bacteriologic evidence of a new infection, whereas colonization refers only to bacteriologic evidence of a new infection.[187,188]

The incidence of suprainfection with cephalosporin therapy is actually quite low (less than 5%); however, the organisms encountered are often more virulent and difficult to eradicate than the original infecting pathogen.[189] Commonly seen suprainfecting pathogens include *Enterobacter* species, *P. aeruginosa*, *S. aureus*, *Acinetobacter* species, enterococci, and *Candida* species. Because these organisms are generally multiresistant, therapy with antibiotic combinations, including aminoglycosides, is usually necessary.

There appear to be no significant differences among the cephalosporins with respect to the incidence of suprainfection or the types of suprainfecting pathogens found.

The most worrisome resistance is that of vancomycin-resistant enterococci (VRE). Risk factors for bloodstream infection with VRE are an increasing APACHE II (Acute Physiology and Chronic Health Evaluation II) score, treatment with vancomycin, or a diagnosis of hematologic malignancy. Thus, severe illness, underlying disease, and use of vancomycin are major risk factors for infection of the bloodstream with VRE.[190]

In the United States, more than 90% of strains of *S. aureus,* one of the most common disease-producing organisms in humans, are resistant to penicillin and other β-lactam antibiotics.[191] Before 1987, antibiotic-resistant strains of *S. pneumoniae* (pneumococci) were relatively rare in the United States, but recent reports document an alarming increase in pneumococcal infections resistant to commonly used antibiotics.[192] According to the National Centers for Disease Control and Prevention (CDC), the incidence of vancomycin-resistant enterococci in the United States increased 20 times from January 1989 to March 1993.[193] Enterococci are the most common cause of hospital-acquired infections, and vancomycin is often the weapon of last resort against these potentially deadly microbes.

Fueling the excessive use of broad-spectrum antimicrobial drugs is the lack of reliable tests that would permit physicians to discern when antimicrobial drugs are not needed. When antimicrobial therapy is needed, improved diagnostic tests would permit better targeting and thereby reduce the widespread administration of broad-spectrum drugs. Selective pressure exerted by widespread antimicrobial use is the driving force in the development of antibiotic resistance. The association between increased rates of antimicrobial use and resistance has been documented for nosocomial infections[194] and community-acquired infections in studies associating resistance patterns with rates of drug use on a regional or national basis.[195] Case-control studies have shown that antimicrobial use is a significant risk factor for infection with a resistant pathogen.[196] In 1988, the National Academy of Sciences/Institute of Medicine estimated that nearly half of the annual production of antibiotics is directed toward use in farm animals.[197]

Resistance to antimicrobial drugs is a global problem. Multidrug-resistant pathogens travel not only locally but globally. Because of increased international travel and increased foreign trade in fresh-food products, the threat of global spread of antibiotic resistance is greater than ever. There is no national or global surveillance system for monitoring of antibiotic resistance in animals or humans. The most recent survey available, conducted in 1992, found that the United States spends less than $55,000 at the federal, state, and local levels for monitoring of antibiotic resistance in human pathogens.[198] National and international surveillance systems should be established, and basic research is needed to delineate the genetic and metabolic pathways, including essential regulatory factors, that determine virulence as well as antibiotic susceptibility or resistance in pathogens of human and veterinary importance.

The Future

In the war against bacterial disease, microbes have been on the offensive, and they can evade antibiotics in many ways. They have general pumps that remove several types of harmful compounds, including antibiotics, from the cell as well as pumps for specific antibodies. Bacteria can also produce enzymes that destroy or inactivate antibiotics, develop substitute proteins that are not targeted by the drugs, or change their cell wall proteins to keep drugs from getting in.[199] Researchers have recently reported work on nearly a dozen new antibiotics that show promise in controlling drug-resistant organisms. These antibiotics target protein synthesis (oxazolidinones, glycylcyclines, streptogramines, boxazomycins, and ketolides), cell wall formation (LY333328 and new β-lactams), or DNA replication (2-pyridone and new fluoroquinolones). Other antibiotics target tyrosine kinase inhibition[200] or lipid A.[201] More innovative approaches will use peptide antibiotics such as defensins and thionins, cepropins, indocidin, and bactenecin.[202] Most investigators working on these agents feel that the era of "classical antibiotics" is over and that novel approaches to bacterial resistance are needed if we are to win the battle of the microbes.

References

1. Jones RN: NCCLS regulatory guidelines. Antimicrobic Newsletter 1:5, 1984
2. Murray PR, Jorgensen JH: Quantitative susceptibility test methods in major United States medical centers. Antimicrob Agents Chemother 20:66, 1981
3. Reller LB: The serum bactericidal test. Rev Infect Dis 8:803, 1986
4. Weinstein MP, Stratton CW, Ackley A, et al: Multicenter collaborative evaluation of a standardized serum bactericidal test as a prognostic indicator in infective endocarditis. Am J Med 78:262, 1985
5. MacFarlane JT, Finch RG, Ward MJ, et al: Hospital study of adult community-acquired pneumonia. Lancet 2:255, 1982
6. Hausmann W, Karlish AJ: Staphylococcal pneumonias in adults. Br Med J 2:285, 1956
7. Feldman C, Kallenbach JM, Miller SD, et al: Community-acquired pneumonia due to penicillin-resistant pneumococci. N Engl J Med 313:615, 1985
8. Finegold SA: Aspiration pneumonia, lung abscess, and empyema. Respiratory Infections: Diagnosis and Management. Pennington JE, Ed. Raven Press, New York, 1983, p 191
9. Bohnan JA, Solomkin JS, Dellinger EP, et al: Guidelines for clinical care: anti-infective agents for intra-abdominal infection (a Surgical Infection Society policy statement). Arch Surg 127:83, 1992
10. Williams DN, Rehm SJ, Tice AD, et al: Practice guidelines for community-based parenteral anti-infective therapy. Clin Infect Dis 25:787, 1997
11. Tomasz A: From penicillin-binding proteins to the lysis and death of bacteria: a 1979 view. Rev Infect Dis 1:434, 1979
12. Wormer DC, Martin WJ, Nichold DR, et al: Concentrations in serum of procaine and crystalline penicillin G administered orally or parenterally. Antibiotics in Medicine 1:589, 1955
13. Gilbert DN, Sanford JP: Methicillin: critical appraisal after a decade of experience. Med Clin North Am 54:1113, 1970
14. Amoxicillin. Med Lett Drugs Ther 16:49, 1974
15. Bodey GP, Whitecar JP Jr, Middleman E, et al: Carbenicillin therapy for *Pseudomonas* infections. JAMA 218:62, 1971
16. Hoffman TA, Bullock WE: Carbenicillin therapy of *Pseudomonas* and other gram-negative bacillary infections. Ann Intern Med 73:165, 1970
17. Butler K, English AR, Ray VA, et al: Carbenicillin: chemistry and mode of action. J Infect Dis 122(suppl):S1, 1970
18. Hoffman TA, Cestero R, Bullock WE: Pharmacodynamics of carbenicillin in hepatic and renal failure. Ann Intern Med 73:173, 1970
19. Ticarcillin. Med Lett Drugs Ther 19:17, 1977
20. Tjandramaga TB, Mullie A, Verbesselt R, et al: Piperacillin: human pharmacokinetics after intravenous and intramuscular administration. Antimicrob Agents Chemother 14:829, 1978
21. Bergan T: Pharmacokinetics of mezlocillin in healthy volunteers. Antimicrob Agents Chemother 14:801, 1978
22. Bergan T, Brodwall EK, Wiik-Larsen E: Mezlocillin pharmacokinetics in patients with

normal and impaired renal functions. Antimicrob Agents Chemother 16:651, 1979

23. Gentry LO, Jemsek JG, Natelson EA: Effects of sodium piperacillin on platelet function in normal volunteers. Antimicrob Agents Chemother 19:532, 1981

24. Fu KP, Neu HC: Azlocillin and mezlocillin: new ureido penicillins. Antimicrob Agents Chemother 13:930, 1978

25. Bodey GP, Le Blanc B: Piperacillin: in vitro evaluation. Antimicrob Agents Chemother 14:78, 1978

26. White AR, Comber KR, Sutherland R: Comparative bactericidal effects of azlocillin and ticarcillin against *Pseudomonas aeruginosa*. Antimicrob Agents Chemother 18:182, 1980

27. Basker MJ, Edmondson RA, Sutherland R: Comparative antibacterial activity of azlocillin, mezlocillin, carbenicillin and ticarcillin and relative stability to beta-lactamases of *Pseudomonas aeruginosa* and *Klebsiella aerogenes*. Infection 7:67, 1979

28. Pancoast SJ, Jahre JA, Neu HC: Mezlocillin in the therapy of serious infections. Am J Med 67:747, 1979

29. Pancoast S, Prince AS, Francke EL, et al: Clinical evaluation of piperacillin therapy for infection. Arch Intern Med 141:1447, 1981

30. Winston DJ, Murphy W, Young LS, et al: Piperacillin therapy for serious bacterial infections. Am J Med 69:255, 1980

31. Ellis CJ, Geddes AM, Davey PG, et al: Mezlocillin and azlocillin: an evaluation of two new β-lactam antibiotics. J Antimicrob Chemother 5:517, 1979

32. Kunin CM, Chambers S: Responsibility of the infectious disease community for optimal use of antibiotics: views of the membership of the Infectious Diseases Society of America. Rev Infect Dis 7:547, 1985

33. Malangoni MA, Condon RE, Spiegel CA: Treatment of intra-abdominal infections is appropriate with single-agent or combination antibiotic therapy. Surgery 98:648, 1985

34. Tally FP, McGowan K, Kellum JM, et al: A randomized comparison of cefoxitin with or without amikacin and clindamycin plus amikacin in surgical sepsis. Ann Surg 193:318, 1981

35. Donowitz GR, Mandell GL: Empiric therapy for pneumonia. Rev Infect Dis 5(suppl):S40, 1983

36. Marx MA, Fant WK: Cefuroxime axetil. Drug Intell Clin Pharm 22:651, 1988

37. Cefotetan disodium (Cefotan). Med Lett Drugs Ther 28:70, 1986

38. Orr JW Jr, Varner RE, Kilgore LC, et al: Cefotetan versus cefoxitin as prophylaxis in hysterectomy. Am J Obstet Gynecol 154:960, 1986

39. McCarty JM, Renteria A: Treatment of pharyngitis and tonsillitis with cefprozil: review of three multicenter trials. Clin Infect Dis 14(suppl 2):S224, 1992

40. Doern G: In vitro activity of loracarbef and effects of susceptibility test methods. Am J Med 92:7S, 1992

41. Stefani S, Pellegrino MB, D'Amico G, et al: In vitro activity of a new broad-spectrum, beta-lactamase-stable oral cephalosporin, cefixime, in comparison with other drugs, against *Haemophilus influenzae, Haemophilus parainfluenzae, Moraxella catarrhalis* and *Streptococcus pneumoniae*. Chemotherapy 38:36, 1992

42. Wise R, Andrews JM, Ashby JP, et al: Ceftibuten: a new orally absorbed cephalosporin: in vitro activity against strains from the United Kingdom. Diagn Microbiol Infect Dis 14:45, 1991

43. Edelstein H, Chirurgi V, Oster S, et al: A randomized trial of cefepime (BMY-28142) and ceftazidime for the treatment of pneumonia. J Antimicrob Chemother 28:569, 1991

44. Reeves DS: In vitro activity of piperacillin and other microbials on 491 bacterial isolates. Arch Intern Med 142:2023, 1982

45. Hall WH, Opfer BJ, Gerding DN: Comparative activities of the oxa-β-lactam LY127935, cefotaxime, cefoperazone, cefamandole, and ticarcillin against multiply resistant gram-negative bacilli. Antimicrob Agents Chemother 17:273, 1980

46. Woolfrey BF, Fox JMK, Quall CO: Susceptibility of *Pseudomonas aeruginosa* to cefoperazone, cefotaxime, and moxalactam with special reference to isolates resistant to aminoglycosides, carbenicillin and ticarcillin. J Antimicrob Chemother 8:205, 1981

47. Magnussen CR, Sammartino MT, Ernest KD: Aminoglycoside-resistant gram-negative bacilli in a community hospital: comparative in vitro activity of cefotaxime, moxalactam, cefoperazone and piperacillin. Antimicrob Agents Chemother 22:154, 1982

48. Neu HC: The new beta-lactamase–stable cephalosporins. Ann Intern Med 97:408, 1982

49. Jones RN, Barry AL: Cefoperazone: a review of its antimicrobial spectrum, β-lactamase stability, enzyme inhibition, and other in vitro characteristics. Rev Infect Dis 5(suppl):S108, 1983

50. Carmine AA, Brogden RN, Heel RC, et al: Cefotaxime: a review of its antibacterial activity, pharmacological properties and therapeutic use. Drugs 25:223, 1983

51. Strandberg DA, Jorgensen JH, Drutz DJ: Activities of aztreonam and new cephalosporins against infrequently isolated gram-negative bacilli. Antimicrob Agents Chemother 24:282, 1983

52. Moellering RC Jr, Willey S, Eliopoulos GM: Synergism and antagonism of ceftizoxime and other new cephalosporins. J Antimicrob Chemother 10(suppl C):69, 1982

53. Watanakunakorn C: In vitro activity of ceftriaxone alone and in combination with gentamicin, tobramycin, and amikacin against *Pseudomonas aeruginosa*. Antimicrob Agents Chemother 24:305, 1983

54. Corrado ML, Landesman SH, Cherubin CE: Influence of inoculum size on activity of cefoperazone, cefotaxime, moxalactam, piperacillin, and N-formimidoyl thienamycin (MKO787) against *Pseudomonas aeruginosa*. Antimicrob Agents Chemother 18:893, 1980

55. Sanders CC, Sanders WE Jr: Emergence of resistance during therapy with the newer β-lactam antibiotics: role of inducible β-lactamases and implications for the future. Rev Infect Dis 5:639, 1983

56. Shimizu K: Cefoperazone: absorption, excretion, distribution, and metabolism. Clin Ther 3(special issue):60, 1980

57. Patel IH, Chen S, Parsonnet M, et al: Pharmacokinetics of ceftriaxone in humans. Antimicrob Agents Chemother 20:634, 1981

58. Stoeckel K, McNamara PJ, Brandt R, et al: Effects of concentration-dependent plasma protein binding on ceftriaxone kinetics. Clin Pharmacol Ther 29:650, 1981

59. Boscia JA, Korzeniowski OM, Snepar R, et al: Cefoperazone pharmacokinetics in normal subjects and patients with cirrhosis. Antimicrob Agents Chemother 23:385, 1983

60. Kemmerich B, Lode H, Borner K, et al: Biliary excretion and pharmacokinetics of cefoperazone in humans. J Antimicrob Chemother 12:27, 1983

61. Ti TY, Fortin L, Kreeft JH, et al: Kinetic disposition of intravenous ceftriaxone in normal subjects and patients with renal failure on hemodialysis or peritoneal dialysis. Antimicrob Agents Chemother 25:83, 1984

62. Wise R, Wright N, Wills PJ: Pharmacology of cefotaxime and its desacetyl metabolite in renal and hepatic disease. Antimicrob Agents Chemother 19:526, 1981

63. Wittmann DH, Schassan HH: Distribution of moxalactam in serum, bone, tissue fluid, and peritoneal fluid. Rev Infect Dis 4(suppl):S610, 1982

64. Saito Y, Kushima T, Seimori T, et al: Absorption and excretion of cefotaxime and its levels in uterine arterial blood, female internal genital organ tissue and pelvic cavity fluid. Jpn J Antibiot 34:481, 1981

65. Grabe M, Andersson KE, Forsgren A, et al: Concentrations of cefotaxime in serum, urine, and tissues of urological patients. Infection 9:154, 1981

66. Kosmidis J, Stathakis C, Mantopoulos K, et al: Clinical pharmacology of cefotaxime including penetration into bile, sputum, bone and cerebrospinal fluid. J Antimicrob Chemother 6(suppl A):147, 1980

67. Watts JM, McDonald PJ, Woods PJ: Clinical trials of antimicrobials in surgery. World J Surg 6:321, 1982

68. Solomkin JS, Meakins JL Jr, Allo MD, et al: Antibiotic trials in intra-abdominal infections: a critical evaluation of study design and outcome reporting. Ann Surg 200:29, 1984

69. Feinstein AR: Clinical Biostatistics. CV Mosby Co, St Louis, 1977

70. Phair JP, Bassaris HP, Williams JE, et al: Bacteremic pneumonia due to gram-negative bacilli. Arch Intern Med 143:2147, 1983

71. Gross PA, Neu HC, Aswapokee P, et al: Deaths from nosocomial infections: experience in a university hospital and a community hospital. Am J Med 68:219, 1980

72. Bryan CS, Reynolds KL: Bacteremic nosocomial pneumonia: analysis of 172 episodes from a single metropolitan area. Am Rev Respir Dis 129:668, 1984

73. Rodriguez J, Vazquez GJ, Bermudez RH, et al: A randomized clinical trial of ceftizoxime and cefamandole in the treatment of serious lower respiratory tract infections. J Antimicrob Chemother 10(suppl C):209, 1982

74. LeFrock JL, Molavi A, Lentnek AL, et al: Comparative study of ceftizoxime and cefamandole in the treatment of bronchopulmonary infections. J Antimicrob Chemother 10(suppl C):215, 1982

75. Neu HC: β-Lactam antibiotics: structural relationships affecting in vitro activity and pharmacologic properties. Rev Infect Dis 8(suppl 3):S237, 1986

76. Baumgartner JD, Glauser MP: Comparative study of imipenem in severe infections. J Antimicrob Chemother 12(suppl D):141, 1983

77. Stamboulian D, Argüello EA, Jasovich A, et al: Comparative clinical evaluation of imipenem/cilastatin vs. cefotaxime in treatment of severe bacterial infections. Rev Infect Dis 7:S458, 1985

78. Collatz E, Gutmann L, Williamson R, et al: Development of resistance to β-lactam antibiotics with special reference to third-generation cephalosporins. J Antimicrob Chemother 14(suppl B):13, 1984

79. Sanders CC, Sanders WE Jr: Microbial resistance to newer generation β-lactam antibiotics: clinical and laboratory implications. J Infect Dis 151:399, 1985

80. Nichols RL: Empiric antibiotic therapy for intraabdominal infections. Rev Infect Dis 5:S90, 1983

81. Lea AS, Feliciano DV, Gentry LO: Intra-abdominal infections: an update. J Antimicrob Chemother 9(suppl A):107, 1982

82. Barie PS, Christou NV, Dellinger EP, et al: Pathogenicity of the enterococcus in surgical infections. Ann Surg 212:155, 1990

83. Solomkin JS, Dellinger EP, Christou NV, et al: Design and conduct of antibiotic trials: a report of the Scientific Studies Committee of the Surgical Infection Society. Arch Surg 122:158, 1987

84. Christou NV, Turgeon P, Wassef R, et al: Management of intra-abdominal infections: the case for intra-operative cultures and comprehensive broad spectrum antibiotic coverage. Arch Surg 131:1193, 1996

85. Smith CR: Cefotaxime and cephalosporins: adverse reactions in perspective. Rev Infect Dis 4(suppl):S481, 1982

86. Parks D, Layne P, Uri J, et al: Ceftizoxime: clinical evaluation of efficacy and safety in the U.S.A. J Antimicrob Chemother 10(suppl C): 327, 1982

87. Petz LD: Immunologic cross-reactivity between penicillins and cephalosporins: a review. J Infect Dis 137:S74, 1978

88. Moellering RC Jr, Weinberg AN: Studies on antibiotic synergism against enterococci: II. Effect of various antibiotics on the uptake of ^{14}C-labeled streptomycin by enterococci. J Clin Invest 50:2580, 1971

89. Gordon RC, Regamey C, Kirby WMM: Serum protein binding of the aminoglycoside antibiotics. Antimicrob Agents Chemother 2:214, 1972

90. Siber GR, Echeverria P, Smith AL, et al: Pharmacokinetics of gentamicin in children and adults. J Infect Dis 132:637, 1975

91. Walker JM, Wise R: The pharmacokinetics of amikacin and gentamicin in volunteers: a comparison of individual differences. J Antimicrob Chemother 5:95, 1979

92. Lockwood WR, Bower JD: Tobramycin and gentamicin concentrations in the serum of normal and anephric patients. Antimicrob Agents Chemother 3:125, 1973

93. McHenry MC, Wagner JG, Hall PM, et al: Pharmacokinetics of amikacin in patients with impaired renal function. J Infect Dis 134(suppl):S343, 1976

94. Regeur L, Colding H, Jensen H, et al: Pharmacokinetics of amikacin during hemodialysis and peritoneal dialysis. Antimicrob Agents Chemother 11:214, 1977

95. Goitein K, Michel J, Sacks T: Penetration of parenterally administered gentamicin into the cerebrospinal fluid in experimental meningitis. Chemotherapy 21:181, 1975

96. Briedis DJ, Robson HG: Cerebrospinal fluid penetration of amikacin. Antimicrob Agents Chemother 13:1042, 1978

97. Vaudaux P, Waldvogel FA: Gentamicin inactivation in purulent exudates: role of cell lysis. J Infect Dis 142:586, 1980

98. Smith CR, Lipsky JJ, Laskin OL, et al: Double-blind comparison of the nephrotoxicity and auditory toxicity of gentamicin and tobramycin. N Engl J Med 302:1106, 1980

99. Kahlmeter G, Dahlager JI: Aminoglycoside toxicity: a review of clinical studies published between 1975 and 1982. J Antimicrob Chemother 13(suppl A):9, 1984

100. Kumin GD: Clinical nephrotoxicity of tobramycin and gentamicin: a prospective study. JAMA 244:1808, 1980

101. Betts RF, Valenti WM, Chapman SW, et al: Five-year surveillance of aminoglycoside usage in a university hospital. Ann Intern Med 100:219, 1984

102. Luft FC, Yum MN, Kleit SA: Comparative nephrotoxicities of netilmicin and gentamicin in rats. Antimicrob Agents Chemother 10:845, 1976

103. Robbins G, Tettenborn D: Toxicity of sisomicin in animals. Infection 4(suppl 4):S349, 1976

104. Fee WE Jr: Gentamicin and tobramycin: comparison of ototoxicity. Rev Infect Dis 5(suppl 2):S304, 1983

105. Moore RD, Smith CR, Lietman PS: The association of aminoglycoside plasma levels with mortality in patients with gram-negative bacteremia. J Infect Dis 149:443, 1984

106. Noone P, Parsons TMC, Pattison JR, et al: Experience in monitoring gentamicin therapy during treatment of serious gram-negative sepsis. Br Med J 1:477, 1974

107. Alexander MR, Schoell J, Hicklin G, et al: Bronchial secretion concentrations of tobramycin. Am Rev Respir Dis 125:208, 1982

108. Moore RD, Smith CR, Lietman PS: Association of aminoglycoside plasma levels with therapeutic outcome in gram-negative pneumonia. Am J Med 77:657, 1984

109. Zaske DE, Cipolle RJ, Strate RJ: Gentamicin dosage requirements: wide interpatient variations in 242 surgery patients with normal renal function. Surgery 87:164, 1980

110. Kaye D, Levison ME, Labovitz ED: The unpredictability of serum concentrations of gentamicin: pharmacokinetics of gentamicin in patients with normal and abnormal renal function. J Infect Dis 130:150, 1974

111. Zaske DE, Cipolle RJ, Strate RG: Increased gentamicin dosage requirements: rapid elimination in 249 gynecology patients. Am J Obstet Gynecol 139:896, 1981

112. Dasta JF, Armstrong DK: Variability in aminoglycoside pharmacokinetics in critically ill surgical patients (abstr). Crit Care Med 14:393, 1986

113. Hassan E, Ober J: Predicted and measured aminoglycoside pharmacokinetic parameters in critically ill patients (abstr). Crit Care Med 14:394, 1986

114. Hatala R, Dinh T, Cook DJ: Once-daily aminoglycoside dosing in immunocompetent adults: a meta-analysis. Ann Intern Med 124:717, 1996

115. Barza M, Loannidis JPA, Cappelleri JC, et al: Single or multiple daily doses of aminoglycosides: a meta-analysis. BMJ 321:338, 1996

116. Koo J, Tight R, Rajkumar V, et al: Comparison of once-daily versus pharmacokinetic dosing of aminoglycosides in elderly patients. Am J Med 101:177, 1996

117. Schumock GT, Raber SR, Crawford SY, et al: National survey of once-daily dosing of aminoglycoside antibiotics. Pharmacotherapy 15:201, 1995

118. Preston SL, Briceland LL: Single daily dosing of aminoglycosides. Pharmacotherapy 15:297, 1995

119. Griffith RS, Black HR: Comparison of the blood levels obtained after single and multiple doses of erythromycin estolate and erythromycin stearate. Am J Med Sci 247:69, 1964

120. Washington JA II, Wilson WR: Erythromycin: a microbial and clinical perspective after 30 years of clinical use (pt 2). Mayo Clin Proc 60:271, 1985

121. Whitman MS, Tunkel AR: Azithromycin and clarithromycin: overview and comparison with erythromycin. Infect Control Hosp Epidemiol 13:357, 1992

122. Stott GA: New macrolide antibiotics: clarithromycin and azithromycin. Am Fam Physician 46:863, 1992

123. Steigbigel NH: Erythromycin, lincomycin, and clindamycin. Principles and Practice of Infectious Diseases, 2nd ed. Mandell GL, Douglas RG Jr, Bennett JE, Eds. John Wiley & Sons, New York, 1985, p 224

124. Panzer JD, Brown DC, Epstein WL, et al: Clindamycin levels in various body tissues and fluids. J Clin Pharmacol 12:259, 1972

125. Holt R: The bacterial degradation of chloramphenicol. Lancet 1:1259, 1967

126. Geraci JE, Heilman FR, Nichols DR, et al: Some laboratory and clinical experiences with a new antibiotic, vancomycin. Proc Staff Meet Mayo Clin 31:564, 1956

127. Kucers A, Bennett NM: The Use of Antibiotics: A Comprehensive Review with Clinical Emphasis, 2nd ed. William Heinemann Medical Books, London, 1975, p 417

128. Sande MA, Mandell GL: Antimicrobial agents: tetracyclines, chloramphenicol, erythromycin, and miscellaneous antibacterial agents. Goodman and Gilman's The Pharmacological Basis of Therapeutics, 7th ed. Gilman AG, Goodman LS, Rall TW, et al, Eds. Macmillan Publishing Co, New York, 1985, p 1170

129. Moellering RC Jr: Pharmacokinetics of vancomycin. J Antimicrob Chemother 14(suppl D):43, 1984

130. Myers JP, Linnemann CC Jr: Bacteremia due to methicillin-resistant Staphylococcus aureus. J Infect Dis 145:532, 1982

131. Watanakunakorn C: Treatment of infections due to methicillin-resistant Staphylococcus aureus. Ann Intern Med 97:376, 1982

132. Harwick HJ, Kalmanson GM, Guze LB: In vitro activity of ampicillin or vancomycin combined with gentamicin or streptomycin against enterococci. Antimicrob Agents Chemother 4:383, 1973

133. Van Scoy RE, Cohen SN, Geraci JE, et al: Coryneform bacterial endocarditis: difficulties in diagnosis and treatment, presentation of three cases, and review of literature. Mayo Clin Proc 52:216, 1977

134. Riley PS, Hollis DG, Utter GB, et al: Characterization and identification of 95 diphtheroid (group JK) cultures isolated from clinical specimens. J Clin Microbiol 9:418, 1979

135. Liñares J, Perez JL, Garau J, et al: Comparative susceptibilities of penicillin-resistant pneumococci to co-trimoxazole, vancomycin, rifampicin and fourteen β-lactam antibiotics. J Antimicrob Chemother 13:353, 1984

136. Fekety R, Silva J, Armstrong J, et al: Treatment of antibiotic-associated enterocolitis with vancomycin. Rev Infect Dis 3(suppl):S237, 1981

137. Dudley MN, McLaughlin JC, Carrington G, et al: Oral bacitracin vs vancomycin therapy for Clostridium difficile–induced diarrhea: a randomized double-blind trial. Arch Intern Med 146:1101, 1986

138. Teasley DG, Gerding DN, Olson M, et al: Prospective randomised trial of metronidazole versus vancomycin for Clostridium difficile–associated diarrhoea and colitis. Lancet 2:1043, 1983

139. Appel GB, Neu HC: Nephrotoxicity of antimicrobial agents (pt 2). N Engl J Med 296:722, 1977

140. New preparations of vancomycin. Med Lett Drugs Ther 28:121, 1986

141. Metronidazole hydrochloride (Flagyl I.V.). Med Lett Drugs Ther 23:13, 1981

142. Koch-Wesser J, Goldman P: Drug therapy: metronidazole. N Engl J Med 303:1212, 1980

143. Corey WA, Doebbeling BN, Dejong KJ, et al: Metronidazole-induced acute pancreatitis (note). Rev Infect Dis 13:1213, 1990

144. Novvby SR, Faulkner KL, Newell PA: Differentiating meropenem and imipenen/cilastatin. Infect Dis Clin Prac 6:291, 1997

145. Wise R: In vitro and pharmacokinetic properties of the carbapenems. Antimicrob Agents Chemother 30:343, 1986

146. Marier RL, McCloskey RV, Dickenson G, et al: Comparative clinical trial of imipenem-cilastatin (N-formimidoyl-thienamycin-dehydropeptidase inhibitor) and cefazolin. J Antimicrob Chemother 12(suppl D):133, 1983

147. Barza M: Imipenem: first of a new class of beta-lactam antibiotics. Ann Intern Med 103:552, 1985

148. Solomkin JS, Fant WK, Rivera JO, et al: Randomized trial of imipenem/cilastatin versus gentamicin and clindamycin in mixed flora infections. Am J Med 78:85, 1985

149. Solomkin JS, Dellinger EP, Christou NV, et al: Results of a multicenter trial comparing imipenem/cilastatin to tobramycin/clindamycin for intra-abdominal infections. Ann Surg 212:581, 1990

150. Poenaru D, De Santis M, Christou NV: Imipenem vs. tobramycin—antianaerobe antibiotic therapy in intra-abdominal infections. Can J Surg 33:415, 1990

151. Neu HC, Novelli A, Chin NX: In vitro activity and beta-lactamase stability of a new carbapenem, SM-7338. Antimicrob Agents Chemother 33:1009, 1989

152. Barry AL, Thornsberry C, Jones RN, et al: Aztreonam: antibacterial activity, β-lactamase stability, and interpretive standards and quality control guidelines for disk-diffusion susceptibility tests. Rev Infect Dis 7(suppl 4):S594, 1985

153. Swabb EA: Clinical pharmacology of aztreonam in healthy recipients and patients: a review. Rev Infect Dis 7(suppl 4):S605, 1985

154. Adkinson NF Jr, Saxon A, Spence MR, et al: Cross-allergenicity and immunogenicity of aztreonam. Rev Infect Dis 7(suppl 4):S613, 1985

155. Scully BE, Henry SA: Clinical experience with aztreonam in the treatment of gram-negative bacteremia. Rev Infect Dis 7(suppl 4):S789, 1985

156. Pierard D, Boelaert J, Van Landuyt HW, et al: Aztreonam treatment of gram-negative septicemia. Antimicrob Agents Chemother 29:359, 1986

157. Rodriguez JR, Ramirez-Ronda CH, Nevárez M: Efficacy and safety of aztreonam-clindamycin versus tobramycin-clindamycin in the treatment of lower respiratory tract infections caused by aerobic gram-negative bacilli. Antimicrob Agents Chemother 27:246, 1985

158. Scully BE, Neu HC: Use of aztreonam in the treatment of serious infections due to multiresistant gram-negative organisms, including Pseudomonas aeruginosa. Am J Med 78:251, 1985

159. Meylan PR, Calandra T, Casey PA, et al: Clinical experience with Timentin in severe hospital infections. J Antimicrob Chemother 17(suppl C):127, 1986

160. Meunier F, Snoeck R, Lagast H, et al: Empirical antimicrobial therapy with Timentin plus amikacin in febrile granulocytopenic cancer patients. J Antimicrob Chemother 17(suppl C):195, 1986

161. Kuck NA, Jacobus NV, Petersen PJ, et al: Comparative in vitro and in vivo activities of piperacillin combined with the beta-lactamase inhibitors tazobactam, clavulanic acid, and sulbactam. Antimicrob Agents Chemother 33:1964, 1989

162. Fass RJ, Prior RB: Comparative in vitro activities of piperacillin-tazobactam and ticarcillin-clavulanate. Antimicrob Agents Chemother 33:1268, 1989

163. Knox J: Extended spectrum and inhibitor-resistant TEM-type β-lactamases: mutations, specificity, and three-dimensional structure. Antimicrob Agents Chemother 39:2593, 1995

164. Sanders E, Sanders C: Piperacillin/tazobactam: a critical review of the evolving clinical literature. Clin Infect Dis 22:107, 1996

165. Wolfson JS, Hooper DC: The fluoroquinolones: structures, mechanisms of action and resistance, and spectra of activity in vitro. Antimicrob Agents Chemother 28:581, 1985

166. Hooper DC, Wolfson JS: The fluoroquinolones: pharmacology, clinical uses, and toxicities in humans. Antimicrob Agents Chemother 28:716, 1985

167. Mandell W, Neu HC: In vitro activity of CI-934, a new quinolone, compared with that of other quinolones and other antimicrobial agents. Antimicrob Agents Chemother 29:852, 1986

168. Neu HC: Bacterial resistance to fluoroquinolones. Rev Infect Dis 10(suppl 1):S57, 1988

169. Neu HC: Quinolones: a new class of antimicrobial agents with wide potential uses. Med Clin North Am 72:623, 1988

170. Lode H, Hoffken G, Prinzing C, et al: Comparative pharmacokinetics of new quinolones. Drugs 34(suppl 1):21, 1987

171. LeBel M: Ciprofloxacin: chemistry, mechanism of action, resistance, antimicrobial spectrum, pharmacokinetics, clinical trials, and adverse reactions. Pharmacotherapy 8:3, 1988

172. Eliopoulos GM: New quinolones: pharmacology, pharmacokinetics, and dosing in patients with renal insufficiency. Rev Infect Dis 10(suppl 1):S102, 1988

173. Malinverni R, Glauser MP: Comparative studies of fluoroquinolones in the treatment of urinary tract infections. Rev Infect Dis 10(suppl 1):S153, 1988

174. Crider SR, Colby SD, Miller LK, et al: Treatment of penicillin-resistant Neisseria gonorrhoeae with oral norfloxacin. N Engl J Med 311:137, 1984

175. Oriel JD: Ciprofloxacin in the treatment of gonorrhea and non-gonococcal urethritis. J Antimicrob Chemother 18(suppl D):129, 1986

176. Keusch GT: Antimicrobial therapy for enteric infections and typhoid fever: state of the art. Rev Infect Dis 10(suppl 1):S199, 1988

177. Monk JP, Campoli-Richards DM: Ofloxacin: a review of its antibacterial activity, pharmacokinetic properties and therapeutic use. Drugs 33:346, 1987

178. Henwood JM, Monk JP: Enoxacin: a review of its antibacterial activity, pharmacokinetic properties and therapeutic use. Drugs 36:32, 1988

179. Desplaces N, Acar JF: New quinolones in the treatment of joint and bone infections. Rev Infect Dis 10(suppl 1):S179, 1988

180. Maesen FP, Davies BI, Geraedts WH, et al: The use of quinolones in respiratory tract infections. Drugs 34(suppl 1):74, 1987

181. Webster A, Gaya H: Quinolones in the treatment of serious infections. Rev Infect Dis 10(suppl 1):S225, 1988

182. Goldstein EJ: Possible role for the new fluoroquinolones (levofloxacin, grepafloxacin, trovafloxacin, clinafloxacin, sparfloxacin, and DU-6859a) in the treatment of anaerobic infections: review of current information on efficacy and safety. Clin Infect Dis(suppl 1):S25, 1996

183. Solomkin JS, Reinhart HH, Dellinger EP, et al: Results of a randomized trial comparing sequential intravenous/oral treatment with ciprofloxacin plus metronidazole to imipenem/cilastatin for intra-abdominal infections. Ann Surg 223:303, 1996

184. Conly JM, Low DE: Intravenous to oral antimicrobial stepdown therapy: improving the quality of care and reducing costs. Can J Infect Dis 6(suppl A):3A, 1995

185. Halkin H: Adverse effects of the fluoroquinolones. Rev Infect Dis 10(suppl 1):S258, 1988

186. Jenkins SG: Mechanisms of bacterial antibiotic resistance. New Horizons 4:321, 1996

187. Tillotson JR, Finland M: Bacterial colonization and clinical superinfection of the respiratory tract complicating antibiotic treatment of pneumonia. J Infect Dis 119:597, 1969

188. Weinstein L, Musher DM: Antibiotic-induced suprainfection. J Infect Dis 119:662, 1969

189. Moellering RC Jr: Enterococcal infections in patients treated with moxalactam. Rev Infect Dis 4(suppl):S708, 1982

190. Shay DK, Maloney SA, Montecalvo M, et al: Epidemiology and mortality risk of vancomycin-resistant enterococcal bloodstream infections. J Infect Dis 172:993, 1995

191. Panlilio AL: Methicillin-resistant Staphylococcus aureus in U.S. hospitals, 1975–1991. Infect Control Hosp Epidemiol 13:582, 1992

192. Rockfeller University Workshop: Special report: multiple-antibiotic resistant pathogenic bacteria. N Engl J Med 330:1247, 1994

193. Swartz MN: Hospital-acquired infections: diseases with increasingly limited therapies. Proc Natl Acad Sci USA 91:2420, 1994

194. McGowen JE: Antimicrobial resistance in hospital organisms and its relation to antibiotic use. Rev Infect Dis 5:1033, 1983

195. Baquero F, Martinez-Beltran J, Loza E: 1991: A review of antibiotic resistance patterns of Streptococcus pneumoniae in Europe. J Antimicrob Chemother 28(suppl C):31, 1991

196. Reichler MR, Allphin AA, Breiman RF, et al: The spread of multiply resistant Streptococcus pneumoniae at a day care center in Ohio. J Infect Dis 166:1346, 1992

197. Institute of Medicine: Human health risks with the subtherapeutic use of penicillin or tetracyclines in animal feed. National Academy Press, Washington, DC, 1989

198. Berkelman RL, Bryan RT, Osterholm MT, et al: Infectious disease surveillance: a crumbling foundation. Science 264:368, 1994

199. Marx J, Chin GJ: Resistance to antibiotics. Science 264:359, 1995

200. Levitski A, Gazit A: Tyrosine kinase inhibition: an approach to drug development. Science 267:1782, 1995

201. Vaara M: Lipid A: target for antibacterial drugs. Science 274:939, 1996

202. Hancock RE: Peptide antibiotics. Lancet 349:418, 1997

203. Simon HB: Antimicrobial chemotherapy. Scientific American® Medicine, Vol 2. Dale DC, Federman DD, Eds. WebMD Corp. (www.webmd.com), New York, 1998, Sect 7, Subsect XIV

204. Daney PG: Overview of drug interactions with the quinolunes. J Antimicrob Chemother 22(suppl C), 1988

13 EARLY POSTOPERATIVE PNEUMONIA

David W. Chang, M.D., and Robert H. Demling, M.D.

Diagnosis and Management of Nosocomial Pneumonia

Treatment of nosocomial pneumonia should focus first on making a rapid and accurate diagnosis. Diagnosis is often difficult in the critically ill patient because of the frequent presence of pulmonary infiltrates, some of which are not the result of infectious processes. Moreover, pharyngeal bacterial colonization makes it difficult to determine the source of the bacteria simply from their appearance in sputum.[1,2]

It is essential to maintain optimal pulmonary support as well as systemic tissue perfusion for maintenance of both local lung and systemic immune defenses. Measures must be initiated to prevent a recurrent or progressive pneumonic process from developing. These preventive measures are based on an understanding of the pathophysiology of the disease process [see Figure 1 and Discussion, below]. Initial antibiotic management is usually empirical: the regimen is selected according to which organisms are most likely to have caused the particular case of nosocomial pneumonia; this determination is made on the basis of Gram's stain, patient history, and clinical experience. A more specific antibiotic approach is initiated once culture and sensitivity results are available (see below).

Diagnosis of Nosocomial Pneumonia

ASSESSMENT OF CLINICAL AND X-RAY FINDINGS

Characteristic signs and symptoms of pneumonia include fever, cough, dyspnea, chest pain, and increased sputum production. Expiratory rales in one or more lobes are often noted. The presence or absence of clinical symptoms depends in large part on the extent of the pneumonic process. For example, bronchopneumonia is often preceded by bronchitis or bronchiolitis. Small airway obstruction by mucus and the resultant local consolidation block diffusion of oxygenated blood through involved areas of lung, with subsequent hypoxemia. Reactive hypoxic pulmonary vasoconstriction, which normally limits the blood flow through nonventilated areas, is hampered by pneumonia, probably as a result of the local release of inflammatory mediators that cause vasodilatation. Carbon dioxide removal is usually adequately maintained as a result of compensatory hyperventilation of uninvolved areas of lung. Additional ventilation-perfusion abnormalities caused by hypovolemia or by chest wall splinting that occurs with pain will magnify the impairment in gas exchange.

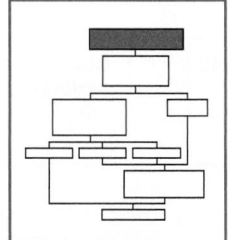

The usual criteria for diagnosing pneumonia are fever, leukocytosis, purulent sputum, new or increasing infiltrates on x-ray, and pathogens growing from the sputum[3] [see Table 1]. However, these criteria are of much less value in diagnosing pneumonia in the surgical intensive care unit or postoperative patient than in the non-ICU or preoperative patient. For example, the upper airways of approximately 75 percent of ICU patients are colonized, usually with gram-negative organisms, and purulent sputum in these patients may simply consist of aspirated pharyngeal secretions that have not as yet caused distal lung infection. Pulmonary infiltrates are also a common finding in the postoperative or ICU patient. Approximately 30 percent of new infiltrates in the surgical ICU patient prove not to be pneumonia. Thus, clinical findings alone are not sufficient for a precise diagnosis; however, if they are assessed in the context of chest x-ray findings, they can be very useful in helping to distinguish pneumonia from a noninfectious process or from nonpulmonary infection [see Table 1]. The x-ray picture of pneumonia is one of focal areas of consolidation that include inflammation and airway collapse causing focal atelectasis. (Air bronchograms that indicate a patent airway and surrounding consolidation are common in pulmonary processes, such as acute respiratory distress syndrome [ARDS], that do not start as airway obstruction.)

Figure 1 **Prevention of nosocomial pneumonia is based on an understanding of the pathogenesis.**

Diagnosis and Management of Nosocomial Pneumonia

Pneumonia is suggested by positive physical findings:
- ↑ WBC
- ↑ Temperature
- Purulent sputum
- Lung infiltrate

Findings are not diagnostic but indicate need for further workup.

Proceed to noninvasive testing

Collect sputum sample from tracheobronchial tree; submit sample for immediate plating and culture.
Rule out gross oropharyngeal contamination by microscopic inspection of sputum.
Obtain good-quality Gram's stain of smear.
Obtain blood culture.

Initiate empirical antibiotic therapy based on results of Gram's stain

Give cefazolin plus an aminoglycoside *or* oxacillin plus an aminoglycoside.
- If *Pseudomonas* is suspected, add an antipseudomonal agent or a third-generation cephalosporin.
- If methicillin-resistant *Staphylococcus aureus* is suspected, add vancomycin.
- If *Hemophilus influenzae* is suspected, add ampicillin.

Results of Gram's stain are inconclusive, or there is a significant risk with standard empirical therapy

Response to empirical antibiotics is good

Response to empirical antibiotics is poor

Culture results indicate that original specimen was inadequte

Initiate invasive diagnostic testing

Perform fiberoptic bronchoscopy by using protected specimen brush/plugged telescoping catheter technique. Transtracheal needle aspiration is another option (easier but less reliable). Lung biopsy is usually performed in an immunosuppressed patient, who is at risk for a nonbacterial process.

Initiate specific antibiotic therapy when culture and sensitivity results are available

Table 1 Clinical Diagnosis of Pneumonia

Clinical signs

Rales, rhonchi

Fever, leukocytosis, impaired lung function

New pulmonary infiltrate

New onset of purulent sputum

Differential diagnosis

Noninfectious pulmonary process (e.g., congestive heart failure, pulmonary embolism, or pulmonary infarction)

Nonpulmonary infection, tissue trauma, inflammation

Aspiration, lung contusion, postoperative atelectasis

Oropharyngeal colonization

In general, reliance on clinical signs results in overdiagnosis of pneumonia. The exception is patients with ARDS, in whom as many as 40 percent of pneumonias are missed because of the difficulty of assessing changes in the x-rays and in the clinical findings. In the absence of any new clinical findings or further lung deterioration, however, routine chest x-rays no longer appear to be indicated; in such cases, the yield of major new findings (including pneumonia) from x-ray is less than 10 percent.[3] The exception, of course, is the case in which x-ray is necessary to assess the effect of a procedure (e.g., positioning an endotracheal tube or a central venous catheter).

Types of Pulmonary Infection

Ventilator-associated pneumonia is an infection of the lung parenchyma that develops in patients who have been on a mechanical ventilator for more than 48 hours. It is characterized by a remarkably consistent spectrum of pathogenic bacteria—primarily aerobic gram-negative bacilli and to a lesser extent *Staphylococcus aureus*—which suggests unique host-bacterial interactions. This pneumonia results from repeated aspiration of secretions harboring these pathogenic organisms, which appear to be endogenously acquired.

S. aureus (coagulase-positive) lung infection is often characterized by migration of the process from one portion of the lung to another; that is, the infection tends to have a multifocal appearance. Infiltrates tend to be patchy, with rounded densities that clear as new ones appear in other lung segments. Formation of abscesses and pneumatoceles (i.e., thin-walled, spherical cysts containing air) reflects the necrotizing nature of staphylococcal pneumonia. Involvement of the pleural cavity with development of pleural effusions and empyema is also common. Copious, purulent sputum production along with evidence of a septic response is usually present; however, sputum is usually not bloody.

Klebsiella pneumoniae infection is characterized by very severe lung inflammation; clinical signs include severe systemic toxicity, pleural pain, cough, and blood-tinged sputum that has a currant-jelly appearance. Chest x-ray reveals moderately discrete areas of homogeneously increased density that may involve several lobes. Upper lobes tend to be involved more than in most other types of pneumonia, and there is a strong tendency toward abscess formation as well as development of pleural effusion and empyema.

Pseudomonas aeruginosa pneumonia does not have distinctive clinical features, although the presence of green-tinged sputum may be a helpful diagnostic clue. The process is quite variable and may involve both upper and lower lobes. The pneumonic process, as in *K. pneumoniae* infection and *S. aureus* infection, is necrotizing. The mortality associated with *P. aeruginosa* pneumonia may be as high as 85 percent. There is a high incidence of recurrent infections, defined as the development of a new infiltrate at least 48 hours after resolution of the initial pneumonia.[4]

Hemophilus influenzae pneumonia produces irregular, homogeneous densities without abscess formation, usually in the lower lobes. The organism is commonly seen with aspiration of oral secretions.

Other types of bacterial pneumonias in general have no specific characteristics and are evidenced on clinical examination and x-ray by localized infiltrates with areas of consolidation but without extensive necrosis.

Viral pneumonias are characterized by minimal physical findings and the frequent absence of large amounts of purulent sputum. Radiographic findings vary from air-space to interstitial disease, depending on the causative organism, and include patterns ranging from widespread, fine, patchy infiltrates, which are often bilateral, to peribronchial and perihilar or reticulonodular infiltrates, to frank consolidation. Confluence of the infiltrate or abscess formation is not seen unless a superinfection develops. Diagnosis is made by testing for antibody titers.

Pneumocystis carinii pneumonia is characterized by severe respiratory dysfunction but an insidious course, with a dry cough and slight or no fever. On radiography, pneumonia that is caused by *Pneumocystis* has the appearance of bilateral bronchopneumonia with the presence of interstitial edema. The infiltrate spreads from the hilum to the peripheral lung in a fanlike fashion, which can be confused with the appearance of pulmonary edema.

EXAMINATION OF SPUTUM

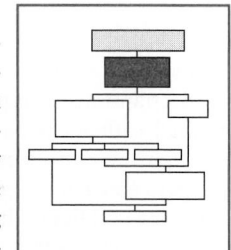

Although microscopic examination of expectorated sputum is not particularly accurate or reliable, it remains the most common method of detecting a respiratory tract infection. The sputum must be obtained by means of a deep cough, with or without the aid of aerosol provocation, or by suctioning well beyond the distal end of the endotracheal or tracheostomy tube [*see Table 2*]. A process of active infection is reflected in the presence of numerous neutrophils and mac-

Table 2 Guidelines for Sputum Analysis

Criteria for an adequate sputum sample

Sample consists of sputum expectorated after deep cough (if necessary, use aerosol provocation) or suctioned from beyond distal endotracheal or tracheostomy tube

Presence in sample of more than 25 leukocytes per low-power field

Presence in sample of only occasional squamous cells

Presence in sample of alveolar macrophages

Causes of errors in sputum analysis

Collection of saliva rather than sputum

Delay in plating sputum sample

Colonization of oropharynx

Use of antibiotics before sample was obtained

rophages along with large numbers of organisms, especially of those present in the cytoplasm of phagocytes. Usually, a dominant organism, such as a gram-positive coccus or a gram-negative rod, is present. Cultures should then be obtained from the sputum sample. This approach is reliable in approximately 50 percent of patients. In the other 50 percent, there is a discrepancy between the data from cultures of expectorated sputum and the data from cultures obtained from the lower respiratory tract via more invasive techniques [see Table 2]. The major reason for this discrepancy is contamination of sputum by organisms colonizing the oropharynx and upper airways. This contamination is most evident in ICU patients, especially those with endotracheal tubes in place. Another reason for the discrepancy relates to the handling of specimens. Some organisms, such as Streptococcus pneumoniae (pneumococcus) and H. influenzae, multiply rapidly and will overgrow a mixed culture, especially if there is a delay in plating. If the patient is receiving antibiotics, growth of the etiologic pathogen may be suppressed in culture. In addition, antibiotics will lead to altered pharyngeal colonization and specimen contamination. The presence of large numbers of squamous cells, for example, indicates that the source of the sample is more likely to be the oropharynx than the lung parenchyma.

There remains considerable interest in and controversy regarding the best method of detecting the pathogens responsible for a pneumonia. A number of methods, all involving bronchoscopy, have been studied (see below), but the ideal method has yet to be agreed upon. It is generally agreed, however, that standard expectorated sputum analysis is not the appropriate method.

EXAMINATION OF TRANSTRACHEAL, TRANSBRONCHIAL, OR BRONCHOSCOPIC ASPIRATES

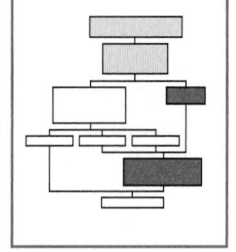

If sputum analysis has not proved diagnostic, transtracheal aspiration can be done: a small catheter is passed into the lungs through the thyroid membrane in an attempt to obtain lung secretions not contaminated by oral flora. The technique is more reliable in diagnosing true lung pathogens than is standard sputum analysis; however, it cannot be used in the intubated patient. Complications of this method, such as bleeding, are usually minor, but severe complications have been reported; hence, the method cannot be considered to be innocuous.

Bronchoscopic sampling is a more precise diagnostic method used to bypass contamination by upper airway flora.[1,5,6] However, some contamination is inevitable from passage of the bronchoscope through the upper airway. A technique of much greater sensitivity is the tube-within-a-tube technique, in which contamination of the protected specimen brush (PSB) is prevented by a distal biodegradable plug that is not ejected until the catheter reaches the deep area of the lung to be sampled. The brush is then advanced beyond the distal orifice of the scope, the sample taken, and the brush retracted back into its protective tube. This technique, known as plugged telescoping catheter (PTC), has substantially improved the sensitivity and specificity of results obtained for both sputum smear and bacteriologic evaluation. Other techniques in use include direct needle aspiration of lung secretions via a catheter passed through the endotracheal tube and sampling of bronchoalveolar lavage fluid.

Bronchoscopy, however, is not without risk. Hypoxemia and bronchospasm can occur if proper precautions are not taken. An-

other important consideration is the significant potential false negative rate. In several series, no pathogens could be identified in as many as 20 percent of samples obtained via PSB, PTC, and needle aspiration from patients likely to have pneumonia.[1,5,6] On the whole, however, the false positive rate is significantly lower with these techniques than with standard sputum analysis.

BLOOD CULTURES

If other sources of infection can be ruled out, a positive blood culture in the presence of pneumonic infiltrate can provide information as to the etiologic organism. The organism isolated from the blood in this case can be considered the organism producing the pneumonia. Bacteremia occurring in association with pneumonia, however, is not common. The incidence of bacteremia in patients with pneumonia is five to 15 percent, depending on the type of bacteria involved; with Klebsiella pneumonia, the incidence of associated bacteremia is about 15 percent.

LUNG BIOPSY

Open lung biopsy is usually not indicated to diagnose bacterial nosocomial pneumonia. It is used to detect etiologic agents that are difficult or impractical to culture, such as fungi, cytomegalovirus, or protozoa; it is generally considered the technique most likely to provide enough material for an accurate histologic and microbiological diagnosis. It is used most commonly in immunocompromised patients in whom the suspected microorganisms—that is, viruses or protozoa—cannot be readily cultured but can be diagnosed by histology. Transthoracic aspiration and transbronchial biopsy have been used to avoid upper airway contamination. Although contamination is minimized with these techniques, a high rate of complications, especially pneumothoraces, has been reported. The amount of lung material obtained by these methods is small, compared with that obtained by open lung biopsy.

OTHER DIAGNOSTIC TECHNIQUES

The finding of elastin fibers on Gram's stain is indicative of a tissue injury compatible with invasive infection.[7] Immunologic methods are commonly employed to diagnose suspected viral infection. Rising antibody titers support the diagnosis, but consecutive plasma samples are required, and the time frame necessary to observe a titer increase makes the method less practical. Advances have made possible the measurement of specific microbial antigens. Antigenemia (defined as the presence of minute amounts of circulating bacterial antigen) has been found in up to 40 percent of patients with pneumococcal pneumonias. In addition, the presence of antibody-coated bacteria in sputum is considered an indication of a reliable sputum specimen.[8]

Management

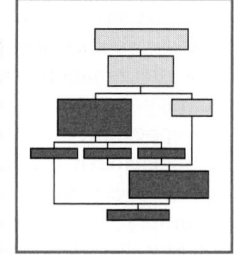

Pulmonary toilet is optimized by a strong cough and by frequent patient position changes to allow the secretions from the involved lung to drain from the distal to more proximal airways. Chest physiotherapy, with percussion and vibration followed by coughing, will greatly improve clearance of secretions. Aerosols to assist in mobilization of secretions can be given just before the chest therapy. Bronchodilator agents such as isoetharine hydrochloride (Bronkosol) and metaproterenol sulfate (Alupent) are used commonly, especially when the

Table 3 Empirical Antibiotic Regimens for Nosocomial Pneumonia

Risk Factors	Likely Causative Organisms	Therapeutic Options
Hospitalization	Core organisms: *Staphylococcus aureus, Escherichia coli, Klebsiella, Enterobacter, Proteus, Serratia marcescens, Hemophilus influenzae*	Core antibiotics: cefazolin, gentamicin, second-generation cephalosporins (e.g., cefuroxime), nonantipseudomonal third-generation cephalosporins (e.g., cefotaxime, ceftriaxone), β-lactam–β-lactamase inhibitor combination (e.g., ampicillin-sulbactam)
Gross aspiration, thoracoabdominal surgery	Core organisms and anaerobes	Core antibiotics plus clindamycin or metronidazole A β-lactam–β-lactamase inhibitor combination (e.g., ampicillin-sulbactam, ticarcillin-clavulanate)
Diabetes, coma, head injury, renal failure, previous antibiotic therapy (with possible methicillin-resistant organisms)	Core organisms and, possibly, methicillin-resistant *S. aureus*	Core antibiotics plus vancomycin (if a methicillin-resistant organism is likely)
High-dose corticosteroid therapy, cytotoxic chemotherapy (but no previous antibiotic therapy or alterations of consciousness)	Core organisms and *Legionella*	Core antibiotics plus a macrolide (e.g., erythromycin)
Multiple risk factors, including more than one of the following: previous antibiotic therapy, ICU stay, prolonged hospitalization, malnutrition, prolonged mechanical ventilation, tracheostomy, immunosuppression	Core organisms and *Pseudomonas aeruginosa*, with or without *Candida*	Combination therapy including two of the following: an antipseudomonal penicillin (e.g., piperacillin, azlocillin, mezlocillin), ceftazidime or cefoperazone, aztreonam, imipenem-cilastatin, ticarcillin-clavulanate, ciprofloxacin, an aminoglycoside; fluconazole may be added if needed

pneumonia is accompanied by an element of bronchospasm, which further impairs secretion clearance. The beta-adrenergic activity of these agents gives rise to their side effects: tachycardia, hypertension, and central nervous system irritability. There is increasing interest in early tracheostomy to improve pulmonary toilet in patients with severe lung dysfunction, especially when complicating factors, such as other infections or traumatic injuries, are present.[9] In such patients, early tracheostomy has resulted in improved pulmonary toilet, improved nursing care, and decreased sinusitis, with minimal complications. Side-to-side rotating beds have been shown to decrease the incidence of pneumonia in selected patient populations (especially neurologically impaired patients) by improving postural drainage and secretion clearance.

ANTIBIOTICS

Empirical Therapy

Because there is generally a lag of several days before the specific causative organism can be identified, empirical therapy is usually initiated on the basis of clinical impressions and the findings from Gram's stain [*see Table 3*]. A combination of two or more antibiotics is the standard recommendation for a gram-negative pneumonia, but there is increasing interest in single-drug therapy.[10] Randomized clinical trials using a variety of single agents—in particular, imipenem-cilastatin, ciprofloxacin, aztreonam, and cefoperazone—have reported these agents to be as effective as or more effective than two-drug regimens; however, subset analysis suggests that patients with risk factors for *Pseudomonas* pneumonia may benefit from a combination of antipseudomonal drugs.

Correct dosing of these agents depends on a solid understanding of antibiotic pharmacokinetics. The biologic elimination half-life and the volume of distribution for antibiotics are determined by studying healthy volunteers or minimally ill patients. Because the data obtained are used to establish dosing schedules for each antibiotic, physicians must be aware that in many circumstances—more commonly encountered by surgeons than by medical specialists—therapeutic antibiotic concentrations may be delayed or may

not be achieved at all, with poor clinical outcomes, the emergence of resistant bacteria, or both as the consequences.

Such circumstances include postoperative stress, severe infection, burns, and trauma. The septic response to injury or infection causes increased cardiac output, altered vascular permeability, increased vascular capacitance, and increased extracellular and interstitial water volume. Metabolic changes, such as hypermetabolism, protein catabolism, accelerated gluconeogenesis, and protein-mediated down-regulation of hepatic albumin synthesis, result in reduced plasma oncotic pressure, and this reduced pressure causes fluid shifts that dramatically increase the volume of distribution. A given dose of antibiotic will therefore be distributed within a much

Table 4 Common Antibiotics Used for Specific Nosocomial Pneumonias

Organism	Antibiotics	Dosage*
Staphylococcus aureus	Methicillin Oxacillin Cefazolin Vancomycin	1 g q. 4 hr 1 g q. 4–6 hr 1 g q. 6–8 hr 1 g q. 12 hr
Hemophilus influenzae	Ampicillin Cefuroxime	1–2 g q. 6 hr 2–3 g q. 8 hr
Klebsiella pneumoniae	Cefotaxime Gentamicin Tobramycin Imipenem Aztreonam	1–2 g q. 8 hr 3–5 mg/kg/day 3–5 mg/kg/day 1 g q. 8 hr 1–2 g q. 6–12 hr
Pseudomonas aeruginosa	Gentamicin Tobramycin Ceftazidime Imipenem Ciprofloxacin	3–5 mg/kg/day 3–5 mg/kg/day 1 g q. 8 hr 1 g q. 8 hr 0.5 g q. 12 hr
Escherichia coli	Gentamicin Ampicillin Ceftazidime	3–5 mg/kg/day 1–2 g q. 6 hr 1 g q. 8 hr

*Dosages are for adults with normal renal and hepatic function.

larger volume, and peak concentrations of the drug will necessarily be lower. In one study, the volume of distribution for aminoglycosides in ICU patients increased 36 to 70 percent in comparison with non-ICU patients, necessitating daily doses of 1.4 to 15.5 mg/kg rather than the recommended 3 to 5 mg/kg.[11] Other studies show similar variability in volume of distribution in the critical care setting, with the result that a number of antibiotics, including various cephalosporins, vancomycin, metronidazole, and penicillin, are often given in inadequate dosages.

An important associated concept is the compartmental volume of distribution, which determines the amount of antibiotic present at the target organ. Aminoglycosides penetrate bronchial secretions poorly: the level of the drug in these secretions is usually only 30 to 40 percent of their serum level. Moreover, because aminoglycosides are less effective in acidic environments, they are not optimal for treatment of pneumonia associated with a low endobronchial pH. Their only undisputed advantage is their synergy with β-lactam antibiotics for the treatment of *P. aeruginosa* pneumonia. Most β-lactam antibiotics achieve pulmonary concentrations that are less than 50 percent of serum concentrations[12]; however, the fluoroquinolones achieve pulmonary concentrations that are equal to or greater than serum concentrations.

Drug metabolism and excretion may affect the half-life. For example, the major enzyme system for biotransformation in the liver, cytochrome P-450, may be induced by various agents (most notably phenobarbital), and metabolism may thereby be accelerated. In other situations, biotransformation is necessary for the drug to exert its effect (e.g., clindamycin), or a metabolite of an antibiotic may have antimicrobial activity or even synergy with the parent compound (e.g., cefotaxime). These interactions are affected when competing drugs that use the same system of enzymes are being administered. Renal and hepatic clearance rates of antimicrobial agents may also be increased during hyperdynamic cardiac states.

Specific Therapy

When the specific organisms responsible for pneumonia and the sensitivities of these organisms are known, antibiotic therapy should be tailored appropriately [see Table 4]. Monotherapy is acceptable for severe nonpseudomonal nosocomial pneumonia, but a second agent should be added if isolates of *P. aeruginosa* or *Enterobacter* are obtained. *P. aeruginosa* becomes resistant to ciprofloxacin 33 percent of the time and to imipenem 53 percent of the time.[12] Given that resistance does not emerge until after at least 72 hours of treatment, single-agent therapy remains viable if serial respiratory cultures and sensitivity patterns are obtained to detect these and other, less common pathogens.

Once appropriate antibiotic therapy is initiated, a specific duration of therapy should be chosen in accordance with the clinical setting. Excessive length of treatment appears to be the most com-

Table 5 Causes of Impaired Lung Defenses

Impairment of nasopharyngeal filter system because of bypass by endotracheal tube, use of nasal tube, rhinitis, or sinusitis

Impairment of cough reflex because of decrease in state of consciousness (from anesthesia, drugs, or head injury) or decrease in necessary full inspiration followed by rapid expiration (from chest trauma, pain, muscle weakness, or use of endotracheal tube)

Impairment of mucociliary clearance because of direct mucosal damage with ciliary destruction (from inhalation of smoke, heat, or chemicals) or endobronchial obstruction (by thick mucus, tumor, or foreign body)

Impairment of alveolar macrophage function because of inhalation of smoke, hypoxia, hyperoxia, alcohol, or malnutrition

Impairment of containment process because of deficiency in cellular defenses, humoral defenses, or both (from decrease in neutrophil function, impairment of cytokine release, decrease in opsonins, decrease in antibodies), or spread of infectious focus by increase in bronchoalveolar fluid, pulmonary congestion, or high- and low-pressure edema

mon form of inappropriate antibiotic administration in current surgical practice.[13] Continuing treatment until the temperature and the white blood cell count are normal is not warranted. Fever and leukocytosis at the end of an antibiotic course often represent a sterile cytokine-mediated inflammatory response. Excessive treatment time prevents the restoration of the protective native oropharyngeal and gastrointestinal flora, increasing the risk of recurrent infection, and predisposes to the emergence of resistant pathogens. This is also true of too-lengthy surgical prophylaxis, which can lead to a higher incidence of nosocomial pneumonia.

In sum, giving antibiotics in higher dosages for shorter periods is generally preferable to giving them in lower dosages for longer periods; however, a persistent inflammatory response is an indication that one should look for other organisms and sources of infection.

MAINTENANCE OF HOST DEFENSES

The main conditions that lead to impairment of host pulmonary defenses are well known [see Table 5]. Nutrition is important for preservation of both local lung defenses and systemic immune function.

PREVENTION

The best way of managing nosocomial pneumonia is to prevent both incipient and recurrent infection. In addition to appropriate antibiotic selection and duration of therapy, attention must be paid to hand washing, evaluation of the patient's swallowing mechanism, removal of nasogastric and endotracheal tubes, elevation of the head of the bed, maintenance of gastric acidity, and implementation of preoperative and postoperative respiratory care.

Discussion

Pathophysiology of Nosocomial Pneumonia

Pneumonia is defined as inflammation of the lung parenchyma—that is, of the alveoli and terminal bronchioles. The severity of the pneumonia depends not only on the cause of the infection but also on the host immune response and other predisposing pulmonary conditions, if any.

With the exception of the early stages of an aspiration pneumonia [see VII:3 Pulmonary Dysfunction], nearly all pneumonias in surgical patients are caused by microorganisms, the majority of which are bacteria [see Table 6]. Several routes for contamination of the lung parenchyma are possible [see Table 7]. The most common route is by aspiration of bacterial organisms colonizing the pharynx. A

Table 6 Distribution of Causative Organisms of Nosocomial Pneumonia

Organism	Percent of Total
Pseudomonas aeruginosa	10–15
Proteus mirabilis	5–7
Serratia marcescens	4–6
Escherichia coli	5–8
Klebsiella pneumoniae	10–15
Staphylococcus aureus	10–15
Streptococcus pneumoniae	5–6
Enterobacter species	10
Hemophilus influenzae	8–10
Other gram-negative aerobes	5–8
Gram-negative anaerobes	1–2
Fungi	1

number of organisms can be found in the pharynx of a healthy adult, including *S. pneumoniae, H. influenzae, S. aureus,* and a large number of anaerobic organisms. Coliforms, which are uncommon in healthy adults, are present in seriously ill patients, especially ICU patients who have an endotracheal tube or tracheostomy in place, or in patients who are being treated with broad-spectrum antibiotics.

A major component of bacterial colonization appears to be an increase in the organisms' ability to adhere to the airway epithelium. This increased adherence is probably the result of a decreased secretion of immunoglobulin A (IgA), which normally inhibits the attachment of organisms (particularly gram-negative organisms) to the epithelium[7]; it may also be the result of denaturing proteases released from local inflammatory cells. In addition, any mechanical injury to the mucosa (e.g., from acid aspiration or intubation) will enhance bacterial binding through specific binding glycoproteins. Sucralfate has been reported to help decrease bacterial binding; the mechanism is currently unknown.[14]

The most significant form of pneumonia the surgeon encounters is that which develops after admission to the hospital, in a patient who had no evidence of lung infection on admission. Although other forms of nosocomial infection, such as wound and urinary tract infections, are more common, the mortality for pneumonia is much higher. Patients admitted to the ICU have the greatest risk of acquiring pneumonia; the incidence in patients admitted to the surgical ICU is 12 to 22 percent. The high incidence in this group is caused not only by the presence of virulent organisms in the ICU environment but also by the magnitude of the illness that necessitated hospital admission. Incidence of pneumonia in ARDS patients, who by definition have an acutely injured lung, exceeds

Table 7 Routes of Lung Contamination

Aspiration from naso-oropharynx
Inhalation of contaminated air
Hematogenous spread from distant focus
Direct spread from local infection

50 percent. Mortality in ICU patients in whom pneumonia develops is about 50 percent, compared with a mortality of about five percent in ICU patients without pneumonia. Mortality in patients with ARDS and pneumonia is 70 percent.[1,2]

The high mortality of pneumonia, despite the availability of potent, normally effective antimicrobial agents, reflects two problems: (1) impairment of host defenses, which are affected by a number of factors, including age, the degree of underlying systemic or pulmonary disease, nutritional status, smoking, alcohol, and the adequacy of perfusion, and (2) the difficulty of making the correct diagnosis [see Diagnosis of Nosocomial Pneumonia, *above*]. The sequence of major events occurring in the majority of nosocomial lung infections is as follows:

1. Colonization of pathogenic microorganisms in the pharynx and the proximal airways.
2. Aspiration of the tracheobronchial secretions, which are now infected.
3. Impairment of local lung defenses, particularly the ability to clear secretions, which allows the infected aspirated material to develop into a deep lung infection. (Chronic lung disease is one process that markedly impairs local defenses.)
4. Impairment of systemic immune defenses by the septic response, organ dysfunction, and malnutrition, which further increases the risk of infection. (Chronic systemic diseases such as diabetes will result in an increased risk of any infection.)

There is a very close association between the incidence of pneumonia and the duration of endotracheal intubation [see Table 8]: the duration of intubation reflects the degree of both lung and systemic diseases. The endotracheal tube also provides a potential conduit for organisms from the ICU environment to the tracheobronchial tree.

AIRWAY COLONIZATION WITH PATHOGENS

The main source of organisms that cause nosocomial pneumonia is the patient's upper respiratory tract—in particular, the oropharynx. Microorganisms are most likely to reach the lower air passages and alveoli by aspiration of pharyngeal secretions. This process occurs in up to 70 percent of sick patients with depressed consciousness and up to 25 percent of healthy individuals during sleep. The concentration of bacteria in the oropharynx frequently exceeds 10^8/ml, with anaerobes outnumbering aerobes by a factor of 10 to 1; hence, a significant bacterial inoculum may result from only 1 ml or less of aspirate.[15] This aspiration of secretions is further facilitated by the presence of an endotracheal tube.

Colonization or bacterial overgrowth of the pharynx with potential pathogens [see Figure 2], such as enteric bacteria, occurs in up to eight percent of healthy patients and about 50 percent of critically ill patients in the surgical ICU. Colonization of the oropharynx with pathogens occurs in nearly 100 percent of ICU patients with a major respiratory problem. The chance that a pneumonia will develop in a colonized patient is 75 percent, compared with a three percent chance if colonization is not present. In more than 80 percent of patients in whom nosocomial pneumonia eventually develops, evidence of colonization precedes the pneumonia. The colonization not only provides a source of infection but also makes the diagnosis of pneumonia more difficult: determining the pathogens of the pneumonia in sputum that contains oral contaminants can be very difficult. The marked increase in colonization of sick versus healthy individuals indicates an alteration in local host defenses. In healthy individuals, pathogens are rapidly cleared from

Table 8 Cumulative Incidence of Pneumonia versus Days Intubated

Number of Days Intubated	Patients Who Acquire Pneumonia (%)
1–3	8
7	21
14	32
> 14	45

the oropharynx, whereas in ill or immunocompromised patients, there is increased adherence of organisms to pharyngeal epithelium. Pathogenic colonization most commonly derives from proximate oropharyngeal sources, such as gingival and periodontal spaces, dental plaque, sinuses, or the upper GI tract. The expansion of organisms from their characteristic niche is facilitated by antibiotic therapy and altered host defenses. Prolonged prophylaxis with first-generation cephalosporins eliminates the gram-positive organisms in the normal oral flora and creates ecological pressures that en-

courage migration of endogenous gram-negative organisms. Fibronectin, found in secretions of the upper and lower respiratory tracts, is an integral component of host defense.[16] This protein mediates binding of the lipoteichoic acid–protein complex on gram-positive bacteria to buccal epithelial cells and inhibits the adherence of gram-negative bacteria. In stress states, increases in salivary protease levels lead to degradation of fibronectin, and trauma from endotracheal or nasogastric tubes denudes fibronectin-lined epithelial cells; both of these changes facilitate adherence of gram-negative bacteria. Bacterial binding to buccal mucosa is also potentiated by smoking. Moreover, the lysozyme in pulmonary secretions cleaves the peptidoglycan in bacterial cell walls, and lactoferrin deprives certain pathogens of iron, thereby killing them. Inadequate perioperative resuscitation may hinder the delivery of all these protective secretions and must therefore be avoided.

Colonization also occurs by a number of other routes [see Table 9]. Transmission of pathogens on the hands of hospital personnel to patients is a major cause. Up to 50 percent of personnel have been shown to carry either gram-negative bacilli or *S. aureus* on their hands. Frequent hand washing markedly decreases the incidence of transmission by this route. Another important route is from the patient's intestinal tract to the oropharynx—from the hand to the mouth or by retrograde movement of organisms from the stomach to the oropharynx, for example. The routine iatrogenic neutralization of gastric acidity increases the pathogen content of the stomach. This process can lead to colonization of the upper GI tract with pathogens. The presence of a nasogastric tube can contribute to the transmission of these pathogens from the stomach to the oropharynx. The need to control gastric acidity and avoid gastrointestinal distention in these patients makes this route of transmission more difficult to eliminate. However, alternative approaches to antacids and H_2-receptor blockers, such as the use of sucralfate, appear to decrease the risk of upper GI bacterial overgrowth and reduce the incidence of pneumonias in the ICU.

Another approach to decreasing airway colonization, and thereby reducing the incidence of nosocomial pneumonia, is selective gut decontamination.[17] Several combinations of agents have been used. One consists of tobramycin, polymyxin E, and amphotericin B applied to the oropharynx as a paste and administered as a suspension via a nasogastric tube. Another consists of oral gentamicin, vancomycin, and nystatin; polymyxin B is added to neutralize endotoxin. This approach has decreased the incidence of nosocomial pneumonia by more than 50 percent in a number of clinical trials. Overall mortality was not reduced in these studies, however, which indicates that the underlying disease necessitating intensive care is the primary determinant of survival.

The intensive care unit environment contains many other reservoirs of pathogenic organisms, which eventually come in contact

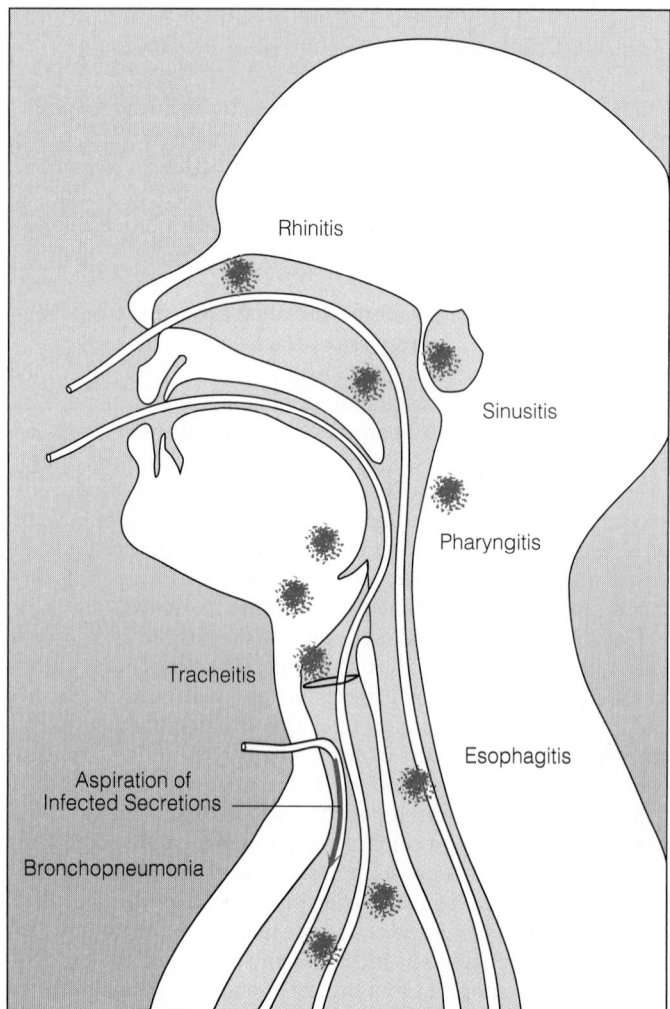

Figure 2 **Interventions associated with intensive care and impairment of normal defense mechanisms in surgical patients contribute to the development of infectious complications.**

Table 9 Causes of Colonization

Hand-to-mouth transmission of pathogens by patient and hospital personnel

Migration of GI pathogens to oropharynx potentiated by decreased acidity and nasogastric tubes

Direct contamination by aerosols, ventilators, and humidifiers

Alteration of normal flora by antibiotics

Alteration in local defenses that causes increase in bacterial adherence with the airways. Aerosol nebulizers and ventilator tubes, for example, provide moist environments for bacterial growth and are potential sources of infection. The introduction of more disposable equipment and unit-dose packaging of aerosols has decreased the incidence of contamination by these routes.

ASPIRATION OF INFECTED SECRETIONS

Aspiration of infected secretions is the next step in the development of pneumonia following pharyngeal colonization. Aspiration is potentiated by sedation or any process that impairs normal clearance of oral secretions [see Table 10], such as use of a nasogastric tube. The potential for aspiration of secretions is also markedly increased by use of an endotracheal or tracheostomy tube because the tube prevents the glottis and the cords from closing effectively, and secretions can therefore track down both inside and outside the tube. Pooled contaminated secretions present above the cuff of an endotracheal tube can readily be aspirated into the tracheobronchial tree. In one study, a radioisotopic tracer was placed in the stomachs of patients with nasogastric and endotracheal tubes; there was substantial accumulation of the tracer in the lungs within six hours when the patients were supine.[16] Endotracheal tubes provide a surface for colonizing bacteria and do not prevent gastric aspiration. Careful attention should therefore be paid to minimizing supine positioning of intubated patients.

Furthermore, the design of the endotracheal tubes currently in use encourages aspiration. The tube lumen allows the development of a biofilm containing pathogenic organisms, which are expelled centimeters beyond the endotracheal tube with each breath on positive pressure ventilation.[18] Low-pressure, high-volume cuffs cause folds in the balloon along the trachea, which facilitate translocation of secretions with respiratory motion. Nevertheless, every attempt should be made to avoid gross aspiration by suctioning the oropharynx before cuff deflation or extubation.

Other causes of bacterial inoculation include contaminated suction catheters, contaminated lavage fluid, or anything else passed through the tube during management of the patient in the operating room or during the postoperative period.

IMPAIRMENT OF HOST DEFENSES

Even with the introduction of microorganisms, the healthy host should be able to clear bacteria from the lung via normal pulmonary defenses. However, in surgical patients, the normal defense mechanisms are often impaired [see Table 5].

Impairment of the Nasopharyngeal Filter System

In the surgical patient, the nasopharyngeal filter system is frequently bypassed by means of nasogastric tubes and endotracheal tubes. Microorganisms and particulate debris that are normally filtered and trapped in the nasal passages can thereby enter the oropharynx and can then, in turn, enter the tracheobronchial tree.

Impairment of the Cough Reflex

The cough reflex, commonly impaired in the surgical patient, is normally one of the principal means by which airways are cleared of foreign material, excess secretions, and irritating stimuli (e.g., microorganisms). The larynx, the major bronchi, and the terminal bronchioles are especially sensitive to local irritation. Coughing is a reflex response initiated by means of a four-stage process that results in clearance of the irritant. First, as a reflex, the individual takes a large inspiration, usually in excess of 2 L in an adult. Second, the epiglottis closes, and the vocal cords become tightly ap-

---

Table 10 Causes of Tracheobronchial Aspiration

Pharmacological impairment of clearance of secretions by sedation, anesthesia, or paralysis

Anatomic impairment of clearance of secretions by oropharyngeal edema, trauma, nasogastric tube, endotracheal tube, or oral airway

Direct contamination of lower airways by catheters, lavage, or deflation of cuff on endotracheal tube

---

posed. Third, internal intercostal and abdominal muscles forcefully contract, pushing the diaphragm up and generating an intrathoracic pressure that usually exceeds 100 mm Hg. Fourth, the epiglottis and cords suddenly open, generating a significant force of expulsion. The rapidly moving air carries with it secretions and any other foreign material.

In the patient receiving anesthetics or postoperative narcotic analgesics, decreased consciousness markedly suppresses both the initiation of the cough reflex and the quality of the cough. Chest pain and abdominal pain, as well as residual muscle weakness if muscle paralysis was employed in general anesthesia, impair the ability to take a large inspiration, which is necessary for the cough mechanism. Pain and the instability of the chest wall mechanism in patients with chest trauma hamper the ability to generate sufficient transpulmonary pressure. The presence of an endotracheal tube decreases the ability to generate a significant propulsive force during forced expiration. The bacteria in any aspirated infected oral secretions will have the opportunity to proliferate if they are not effectively cleared.

Impairment of Mucociliary Action

In healthy individuals, airways are lined by a mucus-coated epithelium with cilia that beat toward the pharynx to assist in the continued clearance of particles and microorganisms. This mechanism for clearance is particularly useful in the smaller airways, which are less effectively cleared by coughing. Ciliary action is directly impeded by inhalation of smoke (including cigarette smoke) or of chemicals such as those found in general inhalation-type anesthetics.

A high oxygen tension also impairs mucociliary function. In a canine model,[16] tracheal mucus velocity was not affected by intubation for up to 30 hours; however, it was reduced by 84 percent at six hours in patients on 100 percent inspired oxygen and by 51 percent at 30 hours in patients on 50 percent inspired oxygen.[15]

Impairment of the cough reflex directly impinges on clearance by mucociliary action. Secretions normally coughed up eventually plug airways, thereby preventing mucociliary clearance. Obstruction by tumor and foreign bodies also impedes this clearance mechanism.

Impairment of Alveolar Macrophage Function

Bacteria and other foreign particles deposited in the alveoli are rapidly phagocytized by alveolar macrophages and either destroyed by direct killing via release of oxygen free radicals or cleared via the mucociliary system. Microorganism-laden macrophages may also migrate through the interstitium and be cleared by the lymphatics into regional lymph nodes and the systemic circulation. A large or continued exposure to organisms initiates an inflammatory response that is mediated by chemoattractants released by the macrophages. The neutrophils that are thereby attracted will later assist in the containment process. However, a number of factors hamper alveolar macrophage function in the surgical patient, thereby increasing the risk of lung infection. These factors include use of inhalation anesthetics, smoke exposure (acute and chronic), malnutrition, anemia, and hypoxia.

Impairment of Cellular Immunity

Immunosuppressed persons, such as those with human immunodeficiency virus (HIV) infection or cancer, are particularly vulnerable to pneumonia. In HIV infection, depletion and functional impairment of helper (CD4) T cells results in infection with *P. carinii* or intracellular pathogens, such as mycobacteria, cryptococci, and herpesviruses.[15] Antibody responses and vaccination are also suppressed because of disordered T cell regulation and depletion of antigen-presenting cells as well as because of direct effects on B cells. This suppression gives rise to an increased incidence of pneumococcal and *H. influenzae* infections. Coinfection with cytomegalovirus or Epstein-Barr virus may also contribute to immunosuppression.

Impairment of the Containment Process

In healthy individuals, the inflammatory process initiated by macrophages attracts other inflammatory cells to the focus of infection to assist in the process of containment. Containment refers to the process whereby a focus of infection is isolated and prevented from spreading to other portions of the lung. Immunoglobulins constitute part of this defensive process. IgA, which is normally present in the upper respiratory tract, provides protection against viral infection. IgA also decreases the ability of bacteria to attach to mucosal surfaces, thereby rendering them more easily phagocytized. IgG, which enters the lung inflammatory focus via local increases in capillary permeability, both opsonizes bacteria and activates complement, thereby promoting further neutrophil attraction. Activation of the clotting cascade results in local fibrin deposition, which further assists in the infection localization process. Neutrophil migration is assisted by chemoattractant factors released from macrophages and by opsonins and globulins released as part of the humoral system. Any impairment in these humoral and cellular defenses impairs the ability of the host to contain the infection.

The containment process is also impaired by increased amounts of lung water. Movement of edema fluid carries bacteria to uninvolved areas of lung. Edema also allows spread of infection by impairing sequestration.

Types of Pneumonia

ALVEOLAR (LOBAR) PNEUMONIA

In alveolar pneumonia, the pneumonic process involves a large portion of a lobe of a lung or an entire lobe. This process is currently much less common than in the past because of more aggressive pulmonary care. Alveolar pneumonia occurs in all age groups.

Only a few types of organisms cause most cases of lobar pneumonia. The most common type is pneumococcus. Other causative organisms are *Klebsiella, Staphylococcus, Streptococcus, H. influenzae, Pseudomonas,* and *Proteus.*

Pathology

The most common portal of entry of the bacteria that cause lobar pneumonia is the air passages, although the airways themselves remain relatively uninvolved. The causative organism, usually pneumococcus, produces an extensive exudative process that spreads among alveoli via the interconnecting pores of Kohn. The extent of the process depends on host defenses and on bacterial virulence. Segmented boundaries are not preserved, because the process can extend to the boundaries of the lobe.

The extensive suppurative consolidation of alveolar pneumonia evolves and resolves in four classic stages: (1) congestion, (2) red hepatization, (3) gray hepatization, and (4) resolution. Congestion is the initial response to infection, characterized by vascular congestion and increased alveolar fluid in the involved area. The red hepatization that follows is characterized by an intra-alveolar inflammatory exudative process during which the involved area appears airless, red, and firm. Extravasation of red blood cells causes the red color of the lung tissue. White blood cells actively engulf the invading bacteria. Gray hepatization follows, with increasing fibrin deposition and progressive lysis and removal of red blood cells producing the characteristic gray color. A more pronounced pleural reaction and, in some cases, development of empyema are evident during this period. Resolution usually begins about one week after the onset of the pneumonic process. The exudate undergoes progressive enzymatic digestion into semifluid debris, some of which is resorbed by macrophages and some coughed up as sputum.

Clinical Presentation and Course

The pneumococcal variety of alveolar pneumonia can be seen in otherwise healthy adults, whereas the gram-negative bacilli–induced process is seen in immunocompromised hosts—that is, individuals who are elderly, diabetic, alcoholic, or critically ill. The onset of lobar pneumonia is usually sudden, with fever, tachycardia, and lethargy. The cough initially produces a watery sputum indicative of the first stage, which is followed by the rusty, purulent sputum of the red hepatization stage. Chills, indicative of bacteremia, are common. Impairment of gas exchange is usually manifested by hypoxemia caused by passage of blood through nonventilated alveoli. Splinting, which occurs at the onset of any pleuritic reaction, further magnifies ventilation-perfusion mismatch.

Initial physical findings of high-pitched, end-inspiratory crackles reflect the early filling of alveoli with fluid. After two to three days, evidence of consolidation is noted, with fewer rales and dullness to percussion. During resolution, rales return, and the signs of consolidation resolve. Radiographic findings include clear evidence of consolidation, and air bronchograms indicate air-filled airways surrounded by inflammatory infiltrate. The magnitude of physical findings does not always correlate with the x-ray findings. Frequently, the patient is improving clinically before x-ray evidence of resolution. Most lobar pneumonias resolve completely, and mortality is less than 10 percent. However, septicemia can result, as can lung abscess formation. In addition, portions of the damaged lung can be replaced by fibrous tissue.

BRONCHOPNEUMONIA (LOBULAR PNEUMONIA)

The primary characteristic of bronchopneumonia is a patchy consolidation of the lung. The infection frequently represents an extension of a preexisting bronchitis or bronchiolitis caused by, for example, aspiration or smoke inhalation. Impairment of lung defenses allows the pneumonic process to progress. Patient populations that are vulnerable to development of lobular pneumonia include the very young, the very old, and the critically ill, all of whom are immunocompromised.

Any pathogen is capable of causing bronchopneumonia. The most common agents, however, are *Staphylococcus, Streptococcus,* pneumococcus, *H. influenzae, P. aeruginosa,* coliforms, and fungi (in a severely immunocompromised host).

Pathology

In bronchopneumonia, consolidated foci of suppurative inflammation extend down and around involved airways in a segmental distribution that is frequently multilobar. The involved airways become filled with purulent exudate, with subsequent extension into the alveoli. The basal portions are usually more involved as a result of gravitational migration. Confluence of multiple foci can give the appearance of lobar consolidation. Multiple abscess formation is characteristic when the causative organism is *Staphylococcus*. Frequently, bacteria are not visualized in the inflammatory focus, because they have been removed by the white blood cells. If the process resolves, a fibrous scar may persist, or there may be complete restoration of normal lung architecture.

Clinical Presentation and Course

The signs and symptoms of bronchopneumonia depend on the virulence of the invading microorganism and the extent of lung involvement. Increased temperature, productive cough, and expiratory rales are characteristic. Distribution is often patchy, and thus, there is not as much evidence of consolidation as there is with lobar pneumonia. X-rays demonstrate focal areas of consolidation with airway collapse followed by distal atelectasis and an exudative process. Air bronchograms are not characteristic, because the involved airway is usually occluded. Mortality is dependent on the status of the host, who is often elderly and immunosuppressed. When the pneumonic process is caused by organisms that are sensitive to antibiotics, infection is usually readily controlled in the absence of severe underlying systemic or pulmonary disease. Complications of bronchopneumonia include formation of abscesses, spread of infection to the chest cavity with development of empyema, and development of bacteremia.

BACTEREMIC (HEMATOGENOUS) PNEUMONIA

In bacteremic pneumonia, the pneumonic process is initiated by a bacteremia from another source. The process therefore begins in the periphery of the lung rather than in the airway. The x-ray picture is often one of a multifocal process. Abscess formation is common.

In surgical patients, the most common causative organism of bacteremic, or hematogenous, pneumonia is *S. aureus*. Increased sputum production is not an early sign of this condition in view of the lack of large airway involvement. Increased sputum is more evident with extension of the process or during resolution. The clinical signs and symptoms and the mortality are determined primarily by the underlying health of the patient and the initiating focus.

INTERSTITIAL PNEUMONIA

Interstitial pneumonia refers to an acute respiratory infection characterized by inflammatory changes in the lung, largely confined to alveolar septa and pulmonary interstitium. The process is caused by viruses such as respiratory syncytial virus, rhinoviruses, echoviruses, or coxsackieviruses. *Mycoplasma pneumoniae* is also a common cause. In the immunocompromised host, both cytomegalovirus and *P. carinii* are common causes of interstitial pneumonia. Cytomegalovirus is often detected in the lungs of transplant patients in the absence of any lung pathology; identification of cytomegalovirus is not in itself an indication for treatment.

Pathology

The pneumonic involvement may be patchy or may involve entire lobes unilaterally or bilaterally. There is no obvious consolidation. The inflammatory response is localized in the lung interstitium; mononuclear cells are the predominant cell infiltrate. The alveoli may be free of exudate or may be filled with a proteinaceous material with hyaline membranes very similar to that seen in ARDS. In fact, this process is sometimes considered a cause of ARDS.

Clinical Presentation and Course

The presentation is often subtle, with few clinical findings of lung disease except for a dry, nonproductive cough and, in extreme cases, abnormalities in gas exchange. Symptoms are quite varied. A superimposed bacterial pneumonia, usually involving *S. aureus*, is often found in the immunocompromised host, particularly the elderly patient, because local lung immune defenses are impaired by the inflammatory process. Mortality for a viral pneumonia in a relatively healthy host is less than one percent. Mortality in the compromised host is considerably higher and is dependent primarily on the immune status of the host and also on the presence of a superimposed bacterial pneumonia.

References

1. Potgieter PD, Hammond JM: Etiology and diagnosis of pneumonia requiring ICU admission. Chest 101:199, 1992
2. Scheld WM, Mandell GL: Nosocomial pneumonia: pathogenesis and recent advances in diagnosis and therapy. Rev Infect Dis 13(suppl 9):S743, 1991
3. Hall JB, White SR, Karrison T: Efficacy of daily routine chest radiographs in intubated, mechanically ventilated patients. Crit Care Med 19:689, 1991
4. Silver DR, Cohen IL, Winberg PF: Recurrent Pseudomonas aeruginosa pneumonia in an intensive care unit. Chest 101:194, 1992
5. Rodriguez deCastro F, Sole-Violan J, Lafarga-Capuz B, et al: Reliability of the bronchoscopic protected catheter brush in the diagnosis of pneumonia in mechanically ventilated patients. Crit Care Med 19:171, 1991
6. Fagon JY, Chastre J, Domart Y, et al: Nosocomial pneumonia in patients receiving continuous mechanical ventilation: prospective analysis of 52 episodes with use of a protected specimen brush and quantitative culture techniques. Am Rev Respir Dis 139:877, 1989
7. Niederman MS, Merrill WW, Polomski LM, et al: Influence of sputum IgA and elastase on tracheal cell bacterial adherence. Am Rev Respir Dis 133:255, 1986
8. Wunderink RG, Russell GB, Mezger E, et al: The diagnostic utility of the antibody-coated bacteria test in intubated patients. Chest 99:84, 1991
9. Rodriguez JL, Steinberg SM, Luchetti FA, et al: Early tracheostomy for primary airway management in the surgical critical care setting. Surgery 108:655, 1990
10. Aoun M, Klastersky J: Drug treatment of pneumonia in the hospital: what are the choices? Drugs 42:962, 1991
11. Fry DE: The importance of antibiotic pharmacokinetics in critical illness. Am J Surg 172(6A):20S, 1996
12. Niederman MS: An approach to empiric therapy of nosocomial pneumonia. Med Clin North Am 78:1123, 1994
13. Dietmar HW, Schein M: Let us shorten antibiotic prophylaxis and therapy in surgery. Am J Surg 172(6A):26S, 1996
14. Driks MR, Craven DE, Celli BR, et al: Nosocomial pneumonia in intubated patients given sucralfate as compared with antacids or histamine type 2 blockers: the role of gastric colonization. N Engl J Med 317:1376, 1987
15. Skerrett S: Host defenses against respiratory infection. Med Clin North Am 78:941, 1994
16. Estes RJ, Meduri GU: The pathogenesis of ventilator-associated pneumonia: I. Mechanisms of bacterial transcolonization and airway inoculation. Intensive Care Med 21:365, 1995
17. Stoutenbeek CP, van Saene HK, Miranda DR, et al: The effect of selective decontamination of the digestive tract on colonisation and infection rate in multiple trauma patients. Intensive Care Med 10:185, 1984
18. Koerner RJ: Contribution of endotracheal tubes to the pathogenesis of ventilator-associated pneumonia. J Hosp Infect 35:83, 1997

Acknowledgment

Figure 2 Dana Burns-Pizer.

E. Patchen Dellinger, M.D.

Approach to Postoperative Symptoms of Infection

Nosocomial infections are a potential threat to all hospitalized patients. They increase morbidity and mortality, prolong hospital stay, increase patient care costs,[1-6] and occur in almost every body site.

At any time during hospitalization, but especially postoperatively, the onset of fever or an elevated white blood cell count may signal an infectious process. Fever that begins or persists after postoperative day 4 is more likely to represent true infection. Although an infection will not develop in many febrile postoperative patients [*see* Discussion, *below*], a careful, directed examination of the patient, guided by history and operative procedure, should be undertaken, including inspection of the ears and the pharynx. Laboratory tests and x-rays are complementary. The use of empirical antibiotics or the prolonged administration of perioperative prophylactic antibiotics in the absence of a specific diagnosis is rarely efficacious. In fact, either may confuse the clinical picture and may lead to separate toxic or allergic complications. Antibiotics alone rarely constitute an adequate response to infectious complications, especially in the early postoperative period.

Respiratory infections are the most common early infection, with most wound infections presenting between postoperative days 4 and 7 and urinary tract infections occurring throughout hospitalization. However, if a high fever (temperature > 38.9° C [102° F]) develops in a patient within 48 hours of an operation, three diagnoses are most likely: atelectasis, peritonitis caused by a leaking viscus after intra-abdominal operation, and invasive wound infection. Of these, atelectasis is most often diagnosed. It is not serious if recognized and treated. It can be diagnosed on the basis of decreased breath sounds, rales, or both on physical examination and on the basis of platelike densities or volume loss on chest x-ray. Atelectasis may be accompanied by hypoxemia and usually responds to standard physical measures. However, many patients with x-ray evidence of atelectasis are not febrile, and more than one third of patients with fever and no other apparent cause have no evidence of atelectasis.[7,8]

Clues to the diagnosis of peritonitis caused by a leaking viscus are knowledge of the conduct of the operative procedure, evidence of the hemodynamic and fluid balance changes that usually accompany a leaking viscus, and findings of the abdominal examination. Technical difficulties with anastomoses, excessive operative blood loss, or multiple bowel injuries increase the risk of leak. Diffuse abdominal tenderness away from the incision, excessive fluid requirements in the early postoperative interval, and tachycardia all suggest iatrogenic peritonitis. Treatment always involves operative interven-

tion and antibiotics. The least common cause of early high postoperative fever is an invasive wound infection, either with β-hemolytic streptococci or with a *Clostridium* species. Diagnosis is made by local inspection of the wound and by Gram's stain of wound contents; treatment requires operative intervention in addition to antibiotics [*see* Infection Related to Operative Site or Injury, *below*].

Respiratory Infection

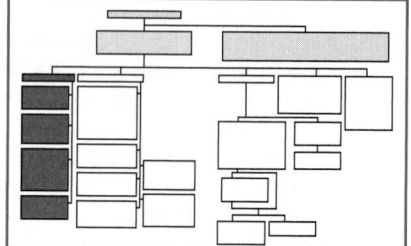

Pneumonia is the third most common nosocomial infection on surgical services[3] and is the one most commonly associated with death [*see VI:13 Early Postoperative Pneumonia*].[9] Diagnosis is not usually difficult in a patient without respiratory failure who is breathing spontaneously. In a patient with acute respiratory distress syndrome (ARDS) who is intubated and being ventilated, however, the diagnosis may be extremely difficult.[10] This is because ARDS is associated with markedly abnormal chest x-ray findings and gas exchange abnormalities and may also include an elevated temperature without infection. A number of techniques for diagnosis, including bronchoalveolar lavage both with and without a bronchoscope and protected specimen brush cultures, have been reported to increase the sensitivity and specificity of diagnosis of pneumonia in this setting but have not been widely adopted.[11,12]

The prevention of pneumonia in ventilated patients would be the best alternative, but there is not widespread agreement about the best means of prevention. Recommendations include standard infection control measures, elevation of the head of the bed, and possibly the use of endotracheal tubes that permit the aspiration of subglottic secretions.[11,13,14]

The diagnosis of pneumonitis or atelectasis (see above) is frequently entertained during the workup of postoperative fever. It is important to remember that a common cause of basilar atelectasis and pleural effusion in the postlaparotomy patient is an inflammatory process below the diaphragm.

Tracheitis or bronchitis, as indicated by purulent sputum in the absence of pulmonary infiltrate, is seen in patients in modern intensive care units, most commonly in association with an endotracheal or tracheostomy tube. Pneumonia may or may not follow. There is often a febrile response, in which case antibiotics may be appropriate on the basis of culture and sensitivity. Sorting out the cause of purulent secretions in intubated patients is important. Other causes of fever should be sought and an overall judgment rendered regarding the probable cause. If tracheitis or bronchitis is suspected, it can be treated with a brief course of antibiotics.

Paranasal sinusitis is a potentially lethal nosocomial infection, especially in ICU patients with nasogastric or nasotracheal tubes in place.[15-20] In one report, it accounted for 5% of all nosocomial infections.[15] The diagnosis of paranasal sinusitis should be considered in any febrile postoperative patient with nasal tubes or with facial fractures. Purulent nasal drainage is an important clue but may not be present. Plain films can be diagnostic but are often difficult to interpret in these patients because of superimposition of tubes, preexisting injuries, and suboptimal portable films. Fluid, air-fluid levels, and mucosal thickening are more easily detected by computed tomography. Diagnosis ultimately requires demonstration of white blood cells and bacteria on Gram's stain of sinus aspirate as well as culture for identification and sensitivity testing.

In one study of 67 patients with craniofacial injuries who underwent prospective otoscopy three times a week, 11 patients experienced either serous or purulent otitis media and were all found to have purulent paranasal sinusitis as well. Eleven of 12 patients who were ultimately diagnosed as having purulent paranasal sinusitis had coexistent otitis media.[21]

The spectrum of causative bacteria of paranasal sinusitis is similar to that of nosocomial pneumonia. Treatment includes removal of all nasal tubes and administration of decongestants and antibiotics. Occasionally, sinus irrigation or drainage, or both, may be required. If empirical therapy must be initiated before specific culture results are known, the agents chosen should be effective against bacteria known to be present in sputum. The best method of prevention is to limit the number and the duration of use of nasal tubes.

Inflammation and infection of the nasopharyngeal mucosa can be significant in an ICU patient, although it is not often identified. Eustachian tube blockage, either from tubes or from inflammation, can be associated with either serous or infective otitis media. Prudent use of tubes is the most effective preventive measure. If clinical infection is recognized, tube removal and decongestants will usually provide adequate treatment.

Infection Related to Operative Site or Injury

SURGICAL SITE INFECTION

An infection of a surgical wound—that is, an incisional surgical site infection (SSI) [see IV:5 Prevention of Postoperative Infection]—traditionally reflects on a surgeon's care and skill and is the classic surgical nosocomial infection. Such infections are diagnosed primarily on the basis of local findings. Erythema, swelling, and drainage, as well as increasing local pain and tenderness in a site at which pain should be decreasing, all suggest infection. Fever and an elevated white blood cell count may or may not be present. An incisional SSI develops most commonly in the subcutaneous layer, although animal studies fail to explain this observation.[22] In an obese patient, however, a thick, overlying layer of uninfected tissue may obscure evidence of infection and thus delay diagnosis. Presentation may also be delayed if the infection begins in anatomic layers below fascial and muscular barriers, such as after a thoracotomy or an operation on the femur.

Whether an infection will occur in a wound is probably determined within the first few hours of wounding[23,24]; efforts to prevent wound infection are probably ineffective after this period.[25-29] The incidence of SSI is reduced with appropriate use of perioperative antibiotics [see IV:5 Prevention of Postoperative Infection].[30,31] However, there is no advantage to continuing prophylactic antibiotics beyond the perioperative period in response to fever or local wound erythema in the hope of preventing an overt SSI.[32,33]

The risk that an SSI will develop in an individual patient is best described by an index defined by the Centers for Disease Control and Prevention (CDC) in its National Nosocomial Infections Surveillance (NNIS) System. The index awards one point each for an American Society of Anesthesiologists (ASA) preoperative assessment score of 3, 4, or 5; an operation classified as either contaminated or dirty-infected; and an operation duration exceeding the 75th percentile for that procedure.[34,35] The CDC definitions for SSI have been agreed to by a consensus panel representing the CDC, the Society for Hospital Epidemiology of America, the Association for Practitioners in Infection Control, and the Surgical Infection Society.[35,36]

The primary treatment of an SSI is to open the wound. When an SSI is suspected, the patient should not be given antibiotics without the wound having been opened. In most cases, the infection is confined to the incision. If the infection is of a superficial wound and if no major systemic manifestations are present, antibiotic therapy is unnecessary. If the local reaction around an infected wound is severe or extensive, administration of antibiotics is advisable until the reaction subsides. In clean wounds that are away from the perineum and that are not associated with an operation that entered the bowel, the likely pathogens are Staphylococcus aureus, streptococcal species, or both of these. In such cases, treatment with cefazolin, 1 g I.V. every 8 hours, or oxacillin, 1 g I.V. every 6 hours, is satisfactory. By contrast, SSIs in the perineum and those that occur after operations on the bowel often involve mixed aerobic and anaerobic bacterial flora. If the infection is not very serious, it can be treated with cefoxitin, 1 g I.V. every 6 hours, or with cefotetan, 1 g I.V. every 12 hours. For more aggressive infections with evidence of tissue invasion or necrosis beyond the immediate wound or with severe systemic reaction, more comprehensive antibiotic treatment is indicated—that is, a third-generation cephalosporin; a quinolone combined with clindamycin or metronidazole; aztreonam combined with clindamycin; or imipenem-cilastatin, meropenem, piperacillin-tazobactam, or trovafloxacin alone. Infection of an abdominal incision may be a superficial manifestation of an underlying intra-abdominal abscess or of peritonitis.

Occasionally, infection is invasive and necrotizing. In surgical wounds, such infection is most common after a GI procedure in which the wound was exposed to colonic microflora and in which wound closure was difficult. Necrotizing infection is also more likely in a patient who is seriously ill or who has evidence of multiple organ failure. Such infection should be suspected if there is undermining of the wound edges, extensive fascial necrosis, distant signs of infection, or a marked systemic response. It requires aggressive operative debridement and administration of antibiotics [see II:11 Soft Tissue Infection].

Clostridium species, which can cause life-threatening postoperative necrotizing SSI, can also cause routine postoperative incisional infection limited to the wound and without myonecrosis.[37] Such infection is marked by the absence of the systemic symptoms associated with clostridial myonecrosis and by the presence of intact white blood cells on Gram's stain of the wound contents. (Clostridial myonecrosis, on the other hand, is characterized by a Gram's stain that shows gram-positive rods but few or no white blood cells [see II:11 Soft Tissue Infection].)

Approach to Postoperative Symptoms of Infection

Fever or an elevated WBC develops postoperatively

Fever begins or persists after 4th postoperative day

Identify source of infection:
- Perform physical examination guided by history and prior operations.
- Inspect all intravascular devices and urinary catheters.
- Order appropriate x-rays and laboratory tests.

Respiratory Infection

Pneumonia, as suggested by ↑ WBC, ↑ temperature, purulent sputum, and lung infiltrate

Give appropriate antibiotics; provide supportive care.

Tracheitis or bronchitis, as suggested by purulent sputum, normal x-ray findings, and endotracheal or tracheostomy intubation

Give appropriate antibiotics if patient is febrile.

Paranasal sinusitis, as suggested by purulent nasal drainage, otitis media, and/or CT findings of fluid, air-fluid levels, and mucosal thickening

Identify pathogen via Gram's stain and culture of sinus aspirate. Remove all nasal tubes; administer decongestants and appropriate antibiotics. Perform sinus irrigation or drainage for unresponsive cases.

Otitis media (associated with eustachian tube blockage from nasal tubes or inflammation)

Remove nasal tube, and give decongestants.

Infection related to operative site or injury

Wound infection (incisional SSI), as suggested by erythema, swelling, drainage, and increasing local pain and tenderness

Incise and drain. For clean wounds, give cefazolin, 1 g I.V. q. 8 hr, or oxacillin, 1 g I.V. q. 6 hr. For other wounds: If infection is aggressive, give a third-generation cephalosporin; or a quinolone plus clindamycin or metronidazole; or aztreonam plus clindamycin; or imipenem-cilastatin, meropenem, piperacillin-tazobactam, or trovafloxacin alone. For less serious infections, give cefoxitin, 1 g I.V. q. 6 hr, or cefotetan, 1 g I.V. q. 12 hr. Invasive and necrotizing infection requires aggressive debridement.

Intra-abdominal infection (organ/space SSI), as suggested by fever and abdominal tenderness

Confirm diagnosis by CT or ultrasonography. Perform appropriate operative or percutaneous procedure; give antibiotics.

Sternal and mediastinal infection, as suggested by sternal instability

Debride the sternum and affected mediastinal tissues. Consider transposition of viable soft tissue for wound closure.

Osteomyelitis (suggested by nonunion of a fracture, loosening of a prosthesis, or prolonged wound drainage)

Repeated operative debridement, prolonged use of antibiotics, and fracture stabilization may be required.

Empyema, as suggested by systemic signs and pleural effusion

Examine and culture pleural fluid. Drain pleural space. Give appropriate antibiotics. If empyema fails to resolve, consider thoracoscopy, thoracotomy, and decortication.

Posttraumatic meningitis (anticipate if there is a history of CSF rhinorrhea or otorrhea)

Perform lumbar puncture for examination and culture of CSF if unexplained fever, headache, spinal pain or stiffness, or changes in mental status develop. Give appropriate antibiotics.

High fever (> 38.9° C [102.02° F]) develops within 48 hr of operation

Consider:
- Atelectasis (suggested by decreased breath sounds or rales, or both, and by platelike densities or volume loss on x-ray): Manage via standard physical measures.
- Peritonitis from a leaking viscus (suggested by hemodynamic changes, diffuse abdominal tenderness, excessive early fluid requirements, and tachycardia): Treat with operative intervention and antibiotics.
- Invasive wound infection: Inspect wound and obtain Gram's stain of wound contents; treat with operative intervention and antibiotics.

Infection related to intravascular devices

Catheter-associated urinary tract infection

Remove catheter as soon as possible.
Symptomatic bacteriuria:
Give appropriate antibiotics on the basis of culture and sensitivity results.
Asymptomatic bacteriuria: Treat with appropriate antibiotic for 1 day after catheter removal. Culture urine 1 wk later; if bacteriuria persists, give appropriate antibiotics for 7 to 10 days.

Enteric infection

Consider antibiotic-associated colitis in any patient with diarrhea.
Severe cases: Identify mucosal changes immediately via endoscopy.
All cases: Culture stool for *Clostridium difficile* and assay for *C. difficile* toxin.
Severe diarrhea with systemic manifestations: Discontinue antibiotics. Give metronidazole (500 mg p.o., t.i.d.); if unresponsive to metronidazole, give vancomycin (125 mg p.o., q.i.d.).
Mild cases: Discontinue antibiotics.

Systemic symptoms suggest catheter-related septicemia

Peripheral catheters:
Remove and culture via semiquantitative technique.
Central venous catheters:
If local signs of infection are present, remove catheter and culture insertion site and catheter.
If local infection is not present:
- Consider placing a second catheter over a guide wire.
- Culture intracutaneous segment, or the intracutaneous segment and the distal tip, of first catheter semiquantitatively.

Infection is localized

Remove catheter promptly, and culture via semiquantitative technique. Place any new catheter in a different site.

Infection progresses to septic thrombophlebitis

Correct surgically.

Culture results are not available, or empirical treatment is required

Include antibiotic effective against methicillin-resistant *Staphylococcus aureus* (e.g., vancomycin) in therapy.

Culture results are positive

Give appropriate antibiotics. Remove any second catheter placed by guide wire; place any new catheter in a different site.

Culture results are negative

Second catheter may be left in place.

1273

INTRA-ABDOMINAL INFECTION

Intra-abdominal infections—that is, organ/space SSIs—are a major cause of postoperative morbidity and mortality, particularly when diagnosis is delayed.[38,39] Suspected

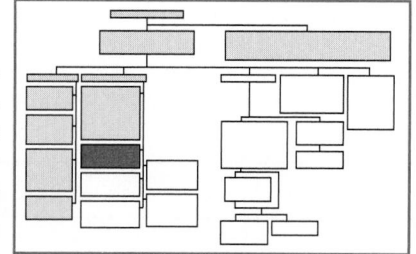

intra-abdominal organ/space SSI in a patient with fever or abdominal tenderness, or both, after an abdominal procedure or injury should not be treated with antibiotics alone; after a specific diagnosis, the appropriate operative or percutaneous procedure must be performed [see VI:15 Peritonitis and Intra-abdominal Abscesses].

EMPYEMA

Empyema, which may follow thoracotomy or chest trauma requiring tube thoracostomy, is a significant cause of post-traumatic infection.[40] Less commonly, empyema develops as a compli-

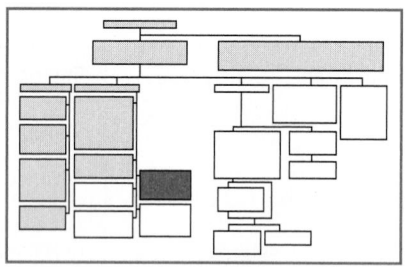

cation of pneumonia. Empyema should be suspected in any patient with systemic signs of infection, a pleural effusion, and no other obvious source of infection. Diagnosis requires thoracentesis of pleural fluid for Gram's stain and culture. The most common pathogen is *S. aureus*, although many other pathogens may be found. Initial treatment is by drainage with a chest tube and by administration of appropriate antibiotics based on the results of Gram's stain and culture. Because treatment is invasive, it should not be instituted until the diagnosis is confirmed. Cases that fail to resolve promptly and completely may ultimately require thoracoscopy or thoracotomy and decortication. Empyema after pulmonary resection or esophageal operation raises the possibility of a leaking bronchial closure or esophageal anastomosis. A leak is almost certain if an air-fluid level is present on chest x-ray. An esophageal leak requires repair or diversion.

STERNAL AND MEDIASTINAL INFECTION

Sternal and mediastinal infections are the most serious infectious complications of operations that involve a median sternotomy.[41-43] The

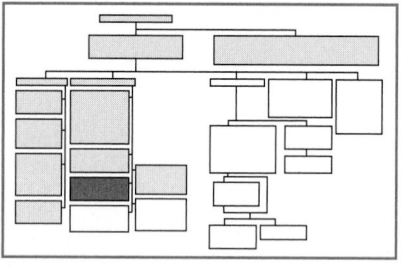

risk that a superficial infection will spread to involve the sternum and mediastinum is high because there is little soft tissue between the skin and the sternum. Infection may also start deep to the sternum without early superficial evidence. Sternal instability is an important indication of sternal infection. Computed tomography of the chest is sensitive and specific for the diagnosis of sternal osteomyelitis and mediastinitis.[44] All such infections require operative debridement of the sternum and of affected mediastinal tissues. Some wounds can then be closed. Many wounds require closure of the mediastinal space by transposition of viable soft tissue. Pectoralis or rectus muscle flaps, omental flaps, or both are commonly used.[45]

POSTTRAUMATIC MENINGITIS

A basilar skull fracture with a cerebrospinal leak increases the risk of posttraumatic meningitis.[46] The most common pathogens are *Streptococcus pneumoniae*, *S. aureus*,

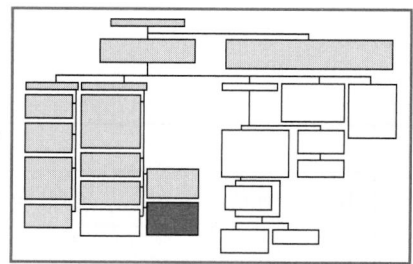

other *Streptococcus* species, and *Haemophilus influenzae*, but any oropharyngeal organism can be responsible.[47] Since the association between trauma and meningitis was first reported in 1970,[46] the appropriate use of antibiotics in these patients has been debated. Some researchers advocate prophylactic administration of antibiotics until any CSF leak ceases,[48] whereas others advocate them for an arbitrary period after injury (usually 5 days); however, controlled studies have failed to support a specific protocol.[47] Furthermore, experience in other clinical settings suggests that prophylactic antibiotics would be as likely to promote the development of resistant oropharyngeal flora and subsequent meningitis as to prevent it.[49,50]

The ideal approach to patients with CSF rhinorrhea or otorrhea is to maintain a high index of suspicion for the development of meningitis. Fever not clearly attributable to another source or not immediately responsive to specific treatment for its presumed cause should prompt a lumbar puncture for examination and culture of spinal fluid. Lumbar puncture should also be performed to investigate headache, spinal pain or stiffness, or unexplained changes in mental status. Such an approach should result in a prompt diagnosis and permit early specific treatment of the responsible pathogen if meningitis is diagnosed.

OSTEOMYELITIS

Osteomyelitis is a relatively rare complication after elective orthopedic procedures. Its diagnosis and management are similar to those of infections involving other operative sites, but because

the infection is deep and covered by muscular and fascial planes, diagnosis may be delayed. Nonunion of a fracture or loosening of a prosthesis may be the first sign of infection. Infection after open fractures is common; rates range from 5% to 50%.[51-55] The primary determinants of infection after open fracture are the degree of soft tissue damage surrounding the fracture and the surgeon's ability to stabilize the fracture fragments.[51,53,54] Other important factors include the patient's age and overall condition, the severity of other injuries, the interval between injury and definitive management, and the use of prophylactic antibiotics. Reports suggest that a brief course of perioperative antibiotics may prevent subsequent infection as effectively as a more prolonged course.[32,56]

Treatment of osteomyelitis may require repeated operative debridement, prolonged use of specific antibiotics, and fracture stabilization. Pathogens include *S. aureus* for all grades of open fracture and, increasingly, gram-negative bacteria (e.g., *Pseudomonas aeruginosa* and *Klebsiella* and *Enterobacter* species) for grade III fractures.[56]

Infection Associated with Intravascular Devices

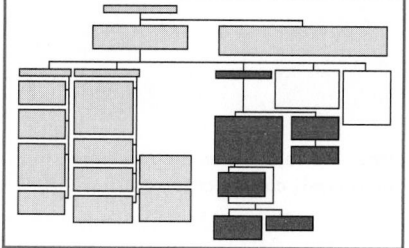

Every type and location of intravascular device has been associated with clinically significant nosocomial bloodstream infection. The incidence of infection is highest with central venous catheters used for monitoring purposes.[57,58]

It is important to specify the different definitions of catheter infection and catheter-related septicemia. Infection at the catheter site is commonly defined as the presence of lymphangitis, purulence, or at least two of the following: erythema, tenderness, increased warmth, and a palpable thrombosed vein. However, many cases of phlebitis with no evidence of bacterial infection present with erythema and with tenderness, a palpable thrombosed vein, or both.[59] Few or no premonitory signs occur before phlebitis is obvious, and the first evidence of as many as 45% of phlebitis cases appears more than 24 hours after catheter removal. If a functional catheter remains in place for 12 hours after the onset of phlebitis symptoms, the duration and severity of symptoms increase markedly.[60]

Catheter-related septicemia is characterized by (1) isolation of the same organism from the catheter and the blood, (2) clinical (or autopsy) and microbiologic data disclosing no other source of the septicemia, and (3) clinical features of bloodstream infection (e.g., fever and leukocytosis).[61] For indwelling, long-term central venous catheters (e.g., Hickman, Broviac, and Groshong), infections have been classified as exit-site and tunnel infections. Infections at the exit site are defined as the presence of erythema, tenderness, induration, or purulence within 2 cm of the skin around the exit site. They are presumably confined to the portion of the catheter external to the subcutaneous Dacron cuff. Tunnel infections are defined as the presence of the same signs along the subcutaneous tract, at a distance more than 2 cm from the tract.[62,63] The importance of this distinction is that many infections at the exit site are successfully treated with antibiotic therapy and local wound care, whereas tunnel infections usually require removal of the catheter.[62,63]

A semiquantitative technique for culturing intravascular catheters has been shown to distinguish between infection and contamination of the catheter and is more specific in the diagnosis of catheter-related septicemia than is broth culture of the catheter.[61,64,65] The catheter is removed from the patient after antiseptic cleansing of the insertion site to prevent contamination from surrounding skin. A 5 to 6 cm segment of the catheter is aseptically removed; transported to the laboratory in a dry, sterile tube; placed on the surface of an agar culture plate; and rolled at least four times across the surface of the plate [see Figure 1]. If the plate grows at least 15 colonies, the culture is positive. Most catheters associated with septicemia actually grow more than 1,000 colonies [see Figure 1]. For peripheral catheters, the entire catheter is cultured. For central catheters that are longer than 6 cm, either the intracutaneous segment or both the intracutaneous segment and the distal tip should be cultured [see Figure 2].

The most common source of bacteria involved in catheter infection is the skin around the insertion site.[66-69] When all catheter segments are studied, the intracutaneous segment almost always has a greater number of bacteria than the catheter tip.[69] Patients who have a skin colonization at the insertion site of greater than 10^3 colony-forming units per 25 cm² are 10 times more likely to have a catheter infection than those whose skin colonization was less. With the semiquantitative culture technique, 16% to 44% of catheters that have tested positive have been implicated as the source of septicemia.[61,65,70-74]

More recently, the catheter hub and lumen have been recognized as important routes of infection. These sites are not detected by roll-plate cultures but by sonication culture of catheter segments or by simultaneous cultures of blood drawn through the suspect catheter and from a distant site. Sonication cultures recovering more than 10^2 colonies, or catheter cultures more than five times the number recovered from distant sites, are sensitive and specific for catheter infection.[75-77]

For catheters that are only locally infected and not responsible for septicemia, removal is adequate treatment; the same is true for most catheters that cause septicemia. If the patient's temperature and WBC count return to normal within 24 hours after removal of the catheter and if local signs of inflammation at the catheter insertion site resolve within that period, antibiotics are not necessary.[78] However, if the patient continues to show clinical signs of bacteremia, a brief course of specific antibiotic therapy is indicated. Specific antibiotic therapy is also indicated if semiquantitative catheter

Figure 1 In a semiquantitative technique used to distinguish between infection and contamination of intravascular catheters, a 5 to 6 cm segment of the catheter is rolled at least four times across the surface of an agar culture plate (left). Typically, a positive culture grows far more than 15 colonies (right).

Figure 2 When a catheter is longer than 6 cm, either a 5 to 6 cm intracutaneous segment or both this segment and the distal 5 to 6 cm (red) can be cultured.

culture reveals a large number of *S. aureus* organisms in conjunction with systemic signs of infection. If empirical therapy for catheter-related septicemia is undertaken before culture and sensitivity results are available, the antibiotic regimen should include vancomycin or another antibiotic known to be effective against methicillin-resistant staphylococci, because coagulase-negative staphylococci are the most commonly implicated pathogens[57,78-80] and there is a high rate of methicillin resistance among these organisms. For patients with intravenous catheters and candidemia, the candidemia resolves an average of 3 days earlier if the catheters are removed at the time of diagnosis and initiation of antifungal therapy.[81]

In a small proportion of patients, local catheter-related infection may progress to a life-threatening condition characterized by the formation of microabscesses within the cannulated vein and by persistent bacteremia after catheter removal.[82,83] Septic thrombophlebitis can occur in a broad range of hospitalized patients and should be suspected when clinical signs of systemic sepsis, local signs of inflammation, and positive blood cultures persist after removal of the catheter. A surgical approach to the affected vein is required. When possible, the vein should be excised over the affected area and the wound left open. The presence of gross pus within the vein wall is not necessary for the diagnosis. The wall of the affected vein may simply appear thickened, with inflammation surrounding it and an edematous, pale thrombus enclosed within it.[83] Fungal peripheral thrombophlebitis may be especially difficult to diagnose because the local site often does not appear infected.[84] In the presence of continued candidemia without an obvious source, any palpably thrombosed vein near a site of present or previous catheterization must be suspected. Gram's stain and hematoxylin-eosin stain of the vein contents or the vein wall are relatively insensitive, whereas silver stain and culture are more sensitive.[84]

Even more rare is catheter-related septic central venous thrombosis. The diagnosis is made by the occurrence of (1) thrombosis of the internal jugular, subclavian, or brachiocephalic vein proved by venography or duplex Doppler examination; (2) central venous catheter infection with positive catheter tip culture and positive peripheral blood cultures; and (3) persistent bacteremia or candidemia after catheter removal.[85,86] Initial therapy consists of catheter removal, systemic antibiotics based on sensitivity testing and administered in a quantity and duration appropriate to treatment of endocarditis, and systemic anticoagulation during the same period. Surgical excision or drainage is reserved for failure of nonoperative measures.

Previous practice often required either complete change or exchange over a wire of both central and peripheral venous catheters at fixed intervals to reduce the risk of infection. Data from randomized, controlled, prospective trials do not demonstrate an advantage to this policy.[59,87] These trials demonstrate that the risk of infection is linear, increasing with the duration of intravenous catheterization, whether one or multiple catheters are used.

Current recommendations are to change catheters when infection is suspected, when the catheters are not working, or when they are not needed.[59,76,87-89] Clearly, any catheter that is a cause of septicemia must be removed, as should infected catheters that may not yet have caused septicemia. The practical problem is that not all in-

fected catheters show external evidence of infection. In addition, catheter culture and the subsequent clinical course confirm infection in only a small proportion of patients with central venous catheters or pulmonary artery catheters who are suspected on clinical grounds of having septicemia.[90] Changing central venous catheters over a guide wire circumvents most of the mechanical complications associated with central venous catheterization, saves time, and is more comfortable for the patient.[91] However, if a culture of the first catheter is positive, the second catheter should be removed immediately, and any new catheter should be placed in a different location.[59,76,87-90]

Recommendations for changing central venous and pulmonary artery catheters are as follows:

1. Signs of inflammation, skin irritation, or purulence at the insertion site should prompt immediate removal of the catheter. Any new catheter should be inserted in a different site. In a patient with systemic signs of infection (fever, leukocytosis, malaise), culture of the insertion site or of the catheter, or both, is indicated to identify potential pathogens and to direct therapy. In a patient without systemic signs of infection, culture is not necessary.

2. If a patient with a catheter experiences systemic signs and symptoms of infection without a readily apparent source, the catheter should be removed even in the absence of inflammation at the insertion site. In this setting, however, approximately 75% of catheters are not infected, and a new catheter can be inserted at the same site over a guide wire placed through the first catheter.[90,92-98] However, a catheter exchange places the new catheter in the old subcutaneous tunnel, which would be the most likely origin of catheter infection. The first catheter should be cultured semiquantitatively. If the culture is negative (i.e., < 15 colonies), the second catheter can be left in place. If the culture is positive (i.e., ≥ 15 colonies), the second catheter should be removed immediately, and any new catheter should be placed at a different site.

Sterile technique is always required for catheter insertion. However, most authorities advocate a surgical approach to preparation of the insertion site, with the operator wearing gown, gloves, mask, and hat for the procedure, if one or more of the following risk factors are present[99,100]: (1) the location is central, (2) catheterization will probably be long term, (3) the patient is seriously ill, or (4) parenteral nutrition is to be employed.

Traditionally, central venous catheters have been inserted most commonly via either the subclavian or the internal jugular route. There is a well-demonstrated increase in infection risk when catheters are inserted by the jugular route instead of the subclavian.[74,89,101,102] There is a prejudice against the femoral route, but published data do not demonstrate a higher incidence of either infection or thrombotic complications when the femoral route is used instead of the internal jugular route,[101] and therefore, the femoral route can be used if other access routes are not available.

A recent approach to prevention of catheter infection is antibiotic bonding of the entire catheter surface. Two trials[103,104] have reported fewer catheter and bloodstream infections in patients with antimicrobial-bonded catheters than in patients with control catheters, and one trial[105] has reported a lower infection rate with a catheter coated on both internal and external surfaces with minocycline and rifampin than with a catheter coated only on the external surface with chlorhexidine and silver sulfadiazine.

The ideal method of caring for intravascular catheters after insertion is not firmly established. Sterile dressings of gauze and tape as well as a variety of commercially available transparent dressings have been advocated. The transparent dressings appear to save nursing time and permit the insertion site to be inspected without changing the dressing, but they promote bacterial growth on the underlying skin, as compared with gauze and tape dressings.[69,106-108] Transparent dressings have also been associated with an increased number of cases of catheter infections and catheter-related septicemia in patients with central venous catheters.[109] Thus, use of transparent dressings is not recommended, at least for central lines.

In addition, there is no firm evidence that the use of polyantibiotic ointments or iodophor ointments at the insertion site prevents infection, although these ointments have not been associated with an increase in infections with resistant organisms.[99] In some hospitals, catheter teams care for all parenteral nutrition lines with excellent results. Regular inspection of insertion sites and adherence to a specific protocol for catheter care can result in acceptably low infection rates.[76,110-113]

Catheters with two or three internal lumina have become widely available and are often sold in kits that include equipment for guide-wire insertion. These catheters are more convenient when a patient requires multiple lines for monitoring and for delivery of intravenous medications and parenteral nutrition. However, these multiple-lumen lines may be associated with a higher incidence of catheter-associated septicemia than are single-lumen catheters[114,115]; the data are inconclusive.[98,116] In one small study, the insertion of two single-lumen catheters did not result in a lower complication rate than that of one double-lumen catheter.[117] A catheter with multiple infusion ports is likely to be manipulated more often than a single-lumen catheter, but it is unclear whether the extra manipulation results in a higher infection rate. In situations in which one lumen would suffice, the temptation to insert a multiple-lumen line in case additional lumina are needed later should be resisted. One study showed that 53% of all triple-lumen lines observed had only one lumen being used,[114] indicating that multiple-lumen lines are often used unnecessarily.

When long-term use of catheters is required, insertion of a Silastic catheter with a subcutaneous Dacron cuff (e.g., Broviac, Hickman, or Groshong) is associated with the lowest rate of catheter-associated infection and the longest useful catheter life.[62] In the largest reported study of these catheters, the incidence of infection was only 0.14 infection per 100 catheter-days (range, 0.0 to 0.8).[62] The study also showed that double-lumen catheters did not have a higher rate of infection than single-lumen catheters, but the rate of catheter infections was increased 10-fold in patients who had catheter-related thrombosis.[62] The mean catheter life span in this report was greater than 120 days.

Very low infection rates and long catheter life are also reported with nontunneled Silastic catheters and with peripherally inserted central catheters (PICC).[76,118] The lowest infection rates are associated with totally implantable devices with subcutaneous reservoirs.[119]

Use of warfarin to prevent thrombosis may result in a reduced rate of catheter infection. A prospective trial found a clinically and statistically significant reduction in the incidence of catheter-associated thrombosis (from 38% to 10%) over 90 days with the administration of 1 mg of warfarin daily, beginning 3 days before catheter insertion.[120] Measured prothrombin times did not increase, and no bleeding complications occurred.

Urinary Tract Infection

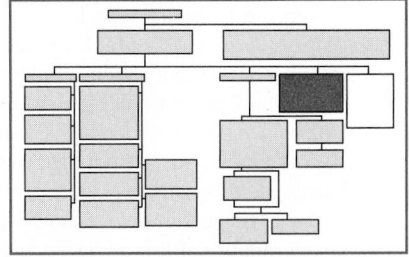

The traditional definition of urinary tract infection in patients without urinary catheters specifies the presence of at least 10^5 organisms/ml, but this criterion is probably not appropriate for catheterized patients. Research has shown that of catheterized patients who have any detectable organisms in their urine (even $< 10^2$/ml), whose catheters remain in place, and who receive no specific antimicrobial therapy, 96% have organism counts higher than 10^5/ml within 3 days.[121] (By comparison, 27% of patients with sterile urine subsequently have colony counts higher than 10^5/ml before catheter removal.)

Although a catheter-associated urinary tract infection is a significant nosocomial infection with measurable morbidity and mortality [see Discussion, below], not all cases of bacteriuria should be treated with antibiotics. If a patient with bacteriuria is symptomatic, treatment should be initiated according to culture results and sensitivity testing. Although bacteriuria can sometimes be cleared without removal of the catheter, the risk of a new episode continues while the catheter is in place.[122] Ideally, the catheter should be removed as soon as possible. In one study, only 36% of untreated women with asymptomatic bacteriuria cleared their urine within 2 weeks of catheter removal, and 17% progressed to symptomatic bacteriuria. Patients treated with a single dose of trimethoprim-sulfamethoxazole cleared their urine in 81% of cases.[123] Thus, it is prudent to obtain a culture at the time of catheter removal and to treat any bacteriuria detected.

A condom catheter is often used in male patients in place of a urethral catheter when neurologic injury or incontinence mandates long-term drainage. Data concerning the ideal care of these devices and the true infection rate associated with their use are not clear. Urinary tract infection rates as low as 0% in 79 patients managed with condom catheter drainage[124] and as high as 53%[122] to 63%[125] have been reported. Severe noninfectious local complications such as ulceration and maceration of the penis also can occur.[124,125]

Because indwelling urinary catheters are a major source of nosocomial infection, they should be employed only when necessary and removed as soon as practicable. The most effective method of reducing infections among patients with urinary catheters is to use completely closed urinary drainage systems and to limit breaks in the closed system.[126] The incidence of new infections doubles on any day in which a closed urinary drainage system is opened.[127,128] Urine samples for culture should be aspirated with a needle and syringe from the lumen of the catheter after antiseptic cleansing of the catheter sampling port. The catheter junction should not be disconnected to obtain a specimen. The use of a preconnected and sealed catheter and drainage bag system has been shown to result in a 2.7-fold reduction in the rate of catheter-associated urinary tract infections and an adjusted risk ratio for death of 0.29.[129]

Antibiotic irrigation systems do not reduce infections, but they do increase the incidence of resistant organisms.[128] Systemic antibiotics have been shown to reduce infections to a modest degree in the first 4 days of catheterization, but they do so at the expense of an increase in resistant organisms. The rate of infection is increased in females as compared with males and in patients with critical illness as compared with those without critical illness.[127] Patients with nosocomial diarrhea and an indwelling bladder catheter have a ninefold higher risk of subsequent urinary tract infection than do patients with an indwelling bladder catheter who do not have diarrhea.[130]

Although most urinary tract infections acquired by hospitalized patients are assumed to be simple bladder infections, a poor correlation exists between the location of infection and the clinical symptoms.[131,132] Many patients with upper urinary tract infections do not have flank pain, fever, or other signs of systemic infection, and patients with a bladder infection may not have dysuria or suprapubic tenderness. Many patients with upper urinary tract infections are treated without the diagnosis ever being made. Systemic infection and associated bacteremia or complications such as intrarenal or perinephric abscesses occur more commonly in immunocompromised patients, such as those with urinary tract obstruction or diabetes.[133,134] In patients with a neurogenic bladder or indwelling bladder catheters, urinary sepsis may develop without symptoms referable to the urinary tract. However, symptoms of localized flank or low back pain, along with systemic signs, such as fever, rigors, sweats, and nausea, are relatively specific indicators of renal infection.[135]

If a patient has fever and bacteriuria during the postoperative period, the surgeon should carefully evaluate the patient to determine whether he or she has pyelonephritis or a postoperative intra-abdominal infectious complication. Pyelonephritis can be treated solely with antimicrobial therapy in most cases, whereas all postoperative intra-abdominal infectious complications require surgical intervention as well as antimicrobial therapy. No simple methods are available to distinguish between these diagnoses. The operating surgeon should carefully evaluate all of the patient's clinical signs and symptoms. A hospitalized patient with pyelonephritis should usually receive antimicrobial therapy for at least 14 days. An agent demonstrated to be effective against the causative organism by in vitro sensitivity testing should be used.[135] In a patient with severe signs of systemic response to infection or in any patient who does not respond promptly to treatment, an ultrasound examination, a renal scan, or an intravenous pyelogram should be done to rule out obstruction. If obstruction is found, it must be corrected. If the patient has an indwelling bladder catheter, the catheter should be removed, appropriate therapy started, and a new, clean catheter inserted.[135]

Enteric Infection

Any organism that can cause food-borne enteric infection in the community can do so in the hospital,[136] but cultures for routine enteric pathogens are not useful for patients

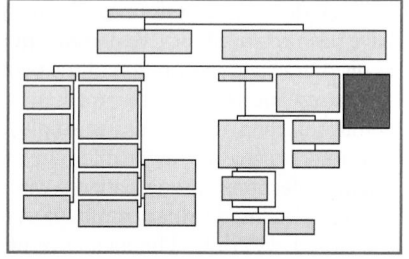

who have been hospitalized for more than 3 days.[137] The most important nosocomial enteric disease to confront most surgeons is antibiotic-associated diarrhea, which can range from trivial, self-limited episodes of diarrhea to fulminant disease with systemic signs of sepsis, collapse, and death.

The first step in diagnosis is to consider antibiotic-associated colitis in any hospitalized patient with diarrhea. Mild cases may not be associated with any systemic signs or pathologic findings in the colon, and in the majority of mild episodes, there are no identifiable pathogens. More severe cases are marked by one or more of the following signs: nonspecific hyperemia, edema, granularity, or ulceration of colonic mucosa. The most severe cases are marked by pseudomembrane formation.

The single most efficient specimen for detection of *C. difficile*–associated diarrhea is a stool sample for cytotoxin determination, with a sensitivity of 70% to 100%. Sensitivity increases slightly (to 96%) if a sample is sent for stool culture as well, but if *C. difficile* is grown, the organism must still be tested for cytotoxin production, and this

takes another day.[137,138] Rectal swab cultures, transported in anaerobic containers, are at least as sensitive as conventional stool cultures[139] but are not adequate to detect cytotoxin.[138] Although there is a potential for the development of polymerase chain reaction assays for the cytotoxin gene in stool, these are not available at present. Stool smears for detection of white blood cells are not helpful.[137,138] Endoscopy, for the detection of pseudomembranes, is indicated if the patient is seriously ill and a prompt diagnosis and initiation of specific treatment are desired. Empirical therapy until a specific pathogen is identified is appropriate in this circumstance.[138]

Severe and persistent cases of antibiotic-associated diarrhea are most commonly associated with the recovery of *C. difficile* by culture and of *C. difficile* toxin by tissue culture assay.[140,141] In more than 90% of patients who have pseudomembranous colitis, *C. difficile* toxin will be present on tissue culture assay. In antibiotic-associated diarrhea without pseudomembrane formation, positive toxin titers may be found in 70% of patients with signs of colitis and in 11% to 27% of patients without colitis.[140,142-145]

Pseudomembranes, present in about half of patients with *C. difficile*–associated diarrhea,[138] are elevated, whitish plaques that vary in size from a few millimeters to 1 to 2 cm and may coalesce and slough. Histologically, the plaques show epithelial debris, polymorphonuclear infiltrate, chronic inflammatory cells, and fibrin deposition.[141] The diagnosis of pseudomembrane formation is made by endoscopy [see Figure 3]. Most cases involve the rectum and the left colon, but as many as 25% may be missed by rigid sigmoidoscopy; by comparison, the false negative rate with flexible endoscopy is only 10%.[146] Although the great majority of cases involve only the colon, two fatal cases that primarily involved the ileum and the jejunum have been recorded.[147,148] The clinical picture of pseudomembranous colitis includes watery diarrhea in 90% to 95% of cases, with bloody diarrhea in the remaining cases. Abdominal cramps, leukocytosis, and elevated temperature are present in approximately 80% of cases.[140,141]

All commonly employed antibiotics have been implicated in cases of antibiotic-associated pseudomembranous colitis, including vancomycin[149-151] and antibiotics used for perioperative antibiotic prophylaxis, even in a single dose.[152] Treatment should include cessation of the offending antimicrobial agent, if possible, which in

Figure 3 **An endoscopic view of pseudomembrane formation is shown.**

mild cases may be all that is necessary. In 23% of such cases, resolution occurs within 2 to 3 days of stopping the antibiotic therapy.[138]

A patient with systemic symptoms should also receive one of the agents with proven efficacy against the disease. The agent with which there has been the most recorded experience is vancomycin, but it is more expensive than the alternatives. The usual dosage is 500 mg/day orally in four divided doses. Metronidazole, 500 mg three or four times daily, or bacitracin, 20,000 to 25,000 units four times daily, is also effective.[138,153-155] The current recommendation is to begin therapy with metronidazole to reduce the risk of inducing vancomycin-resistant enterococci [see Pathogens, below].[138,156]

Relapses after treatment for C. difficile colitis are common, occurring in 5% to 30% of cases, perhaps because of persistence of the organism in spore form; 92% of these cases respond to a second course of treatment without relapse.[138] However, in one report, five of 11 patients who experienced relapse had new strains of C. difficile, distinct from the original strain, as determined by restriction endonuclease analysis.[157]

A profound ileus is sometimes associated with the severe form of the disease and may prevent the delivery of oral antibiotics to the site of infection. Limited experience suggests that parenteral metronidazole may be effective in these cases.[140] However, studies have reported several cases of unsuccessful intravenous metronidazole treatment of C. difficile–associated colitis and of the development of C. difficile colitis in patients receiving intravenous metronidazole alone or together with other antibiotics.[151,158-160] In the most severe cases, the clinical evolution resembles that of toxic colitis associated with inflammatory bowel disease, and the patient may require a colectomy if the disease is unresponsive to nonoperative management.[140,161] In as many as 5% of cases, colitis may present with acute abdominal pain and tenderness and leukocytosis without diarrhea.[162,163] If colitis is suspected because of previous antibiotic administration, sigmoidoscopy may facilitate the correct diagnosis and avert unnecessary abdominal exploration. Computed tomography may show thickening of the bowel wall, but findings of operative exploration are often unimpressive.[163] Extraintestinal infections have also been reported.[164]

Transfusion-Associated Infection

The transfusion of blood would seem to be an excellent method for transmitting blood-borne diseases; however, except for posttransfusion hepatitis, transmission of disease by blood transfusion is rare.[165,166] Transfusion-associated malaria is occasionally reported in North America but occurs quite infrequently. The primary method for preventing malaria transmission is careful screening of donors by history. A handful of cases of babesiosis, Chagas' disease, trypanosomiasis, and toxoplasmosis have been reported over many years but are rare as well.[165-167] In the early years of blood collection and transfusion, cases of syphilis related to blood transfusion were reported infrequently. The practice of refrigerating blood, which kills circulating spirochetes within 1 to 2 days, is probably responsible for the absence of transfusion-associated syphilis today. The last reported case occurred in 1969.[165] Unfortunately, refrigerating blood does not kill all potential pathogens. Bacterial pathogens that can survive blood storage and cause subsequent symptomatic infection include Yersinia enterocolitica and Pseudomonas fluorescens, the two most common isolates, as well as P. putida and Campylobacter jejuni. Bacterial sepsis is estimated to cause death after only one of six million transfused units.[168] Yersinia infection occurs after approximately one in 500,000 units transfused, and some type of bacterial contamination is found in approximately one of 1,700 pooled units of platelets.[169] When transfusion-associated bacteremia or endotoxemia is suspected, the residual blood product in the bag should be examined by a hematologic stain, and the blood in the bag and samples of the recipient's blood should be cultured.[170]

The most severe and frequently occurring disease transmitted by blood transfusion in North America is viral hepatitis [see VI:19 Viral Infection]. Since the development of a specific and sensitive test for detecting hepatitis B surface antigen (HBsAg), the incidence of posttransfusion hepatitis B has dropped, from 25% to 30% of all cases of transfusion-associated hepatitis to 5% to 10%. However, serologic tests for hepatitis B have not resulted in an overall decrease in posttransfusion hepatitis (PTH), because 80% to 90% of cases of PTH were caused by hepatitis C (HCV), previously labeled non-A, non-B (NANB) hepatitis. The risk of developing NANB was estimated to be approximately 7% for recipients of volunteer blood and 28% for recipients of commercial blood.[171,172]

Molecular biologic techniques have identified HCV as the cause of most cases of NANB, and diagnostic tests for antibody to HCV have been developed to screen blood.[173] In Taiwan, 58% of patients with chronic liver disease who do not have antibodies to hepatitis B have antibodies to hepatitis C.[174]

Although most cases of hepatitis C are asymptomatic and self-limited, fulminant cases with a fatal outcome have been reported. Moreover, up to one half of hepatitis C patients may show evidence of chronic liver disease, and for some of these, there will be biopsy evidence of cirrhosis many years later.[165,171,175] Detectable anti–hepatitis C antibodies are typically found 4 weeks after transfusion of an infectious unit of blood.[173] Of the patients who seroconvert, 54% are asymptomatic, but 77% progress to have chronic elevations of alanine aminotransferase (ALT). Those who develop chronic hepatitis usually remain seropositive, but up to 27% of patients who seroconvert have no detectable antibody at 1 year.[176,177] Tests for antibody to hepatitis C have been refined and are now almost 100% sensitive. However, specificity is much lower, and additional testing is necessary, particularly in low-risk populations, to confirm the diagnosis of hepatitis C infection.[173]

The spread of AIDS [see VI:20 Acquired Immunodeficiency Syndrome] has brought a new risk of transfusion-associated viral disease. Currently, the risk of acquiring transfusion-associated HIV is extremely low. It is vastly less likely to occur and accounts for fewer deaths than posttransfusion hepatitis. However, transfusion-associated AIDS is much more frightening to most patients and physicians than PTH because of its uniformly fatal prognosis. Prevention of HIV transmission during transfusion is accomplished through screening of potential donors to eliminate those at high risk for infection[178-180] and testing of all donated units for antibody to HIV.[179,180] It has been estimated that predonation screening is 98% effective in eliminating donation of positive units and that postdonation antibody testing is more than 95% effective, for a combined effectiveness of approximately 99.9%.[179] In aggregate, posttransfusion HIV infections were reduced by 76% between 1985 and 1988, a time during which the overall prevalence of the condition was increasing.[179] The continued concern about possible HIV transmission during transfusion arises from the so-called window of seronegativity between the time at which a potential donor becomes infected and the time at which the donor's antibody test becomes positive. An analysis of available data from most United States blood banks concluded that the risk of receiving a unit of blood that contained HIV but was negative for anti-HIV antibody in 1987 was approximately one in 153,000 on the basis of an average window of 8 weeks.[179] The incidence of positive units detected through postdonation screening decreased by more than 50% between 1985 and 1987.[179] The risk of transfusing infectious seronegative blood is assumed to be proportional to the number of seropositive units detected through antibody screening.

The risk of receiving seronegative blood was also estimated by a San Francisco group, which studied seronegative blood samples from 71,800 donations by culture and polymerase chain reaction techniques before 1991. They found a point estimate of the risk of one in 61,171, with an upper limit of the 95% confidence interval of one in 10,695.[181] Because this study was conducted in a population with a high prevalence of HIV infection, the risk is probably lower in regions with a lower prevalence. A subsequent study in five blood centers across the United States tested 2,318,356 units of blood from 586,507 donors during the years 1991 through 1993. They found that the risk of acquiring an HIV infection from a unit of blood was one in 493,000. The corresponding risk for acquiring HCV was one in 103,000 and, for HBV, one in 63,000. The aggregate risk of acquiring any virus was one in 34,000, and 88% of that risk came from HBV and HCV.[182] Because of donor screening, this risk is lower than the risk among a random sample of the population. Newer and more sensitive tests have the potential to reduce the risk another 27% to 72%.[182] In comparison, the risk of experiencing a fatal hemolytic transfusion reaction is one in 100,000.[180] Thus, a transfusion recipient is more likely to die of hepatitis B or C or a hemolytic reaction than of AIDS.

The mean incubation period for transfusion-associated AIDS is 23 months, with a range from 10 to 43 months; the interval to the development of antibody is 2 to 3 months after infection.[178] The clinical progression of the disease is similar to its occurrence in the traditional high-risk groups.[183] With transfusion-associated AIDS, as with posttransfusion hepatitis, the primary preventive response of the physician should be to limit unnecessary transfusion.[184] Analysis of transfusion practices in the United States between 1982 and 1988 reveals a decrease in the number of blood, platelet, and plasma transfusions after 1986; previously, the number of these transfusions increased each year. In addition, from 1982 to 1987, the number of autologous units donated increased from 30,000 to 397,000 a year. In 1987, autologous units accounted for 3% of all blood transfused.[185]

Discussion

Postoperative Fever

Many patients experience fever in the postoperative period without infection. In a prospective study of 871 general surgery patients, 213 (24%) had a documented infection or an unexplained fever in the postoperative period.[186] The most common occurrence was unexplained fever in 81 cases (38%), followed by wound infection in 55 (26%), urinary tract infection in 44 (21%), respiratory tract infection in 27 (13%), and other infections in 6 (3%). Of all unexplained fevers, 72% occurred in the first 2 days, and of all occurrences in the first 3 days, 67 (71%) of 95 were unexplained, with only 18 (27%) representing true infection. In another study, 73 (45%) of 162 patients experienced unexplained fever after general surgical or orthopedic procedures; 25% of the unexplained fevers were at least 38.3° C (101° F).[187]

At Harborview Medical Center, 316 (98%) of 322 patients who had laparotomy for penetrating trauma experienced a temperature of at least 37.5° C (99.5° F) orally during the first 5 days after operation. Of these patients, however, only 67 (21%) actually acquired any infection during a 30-day follow-up. Even for the 80 patients whose temperatures were as high as 39° C (102.2° F) orally, only 48% actually acquired an infection before discharge. Fever that persisted or began after postoperative day 4 was more likely to represent true infection. Similarly, an elevated WBC count was nonspecific during the first 5 postoperative days: 89% of all patients had a WBC count greater than 10,000/mm^3.[188,189]

Magnitude and Significance of Nosocomial Infection

An understanding of the prevalence of nosocomial infections and of the factors predisposing to their occurrence will help in prevention, diagnosis, and treatment. Since 1970, the National Nosocomial Infections Surveillance (NNIS) system[3] has collected and analyzed data on the frequency of nosocomial infections in a voluntary sample of 51 hospitals in the United States. Although more intensive studies suggest that the NNIS underestimates the true incidence of nosocomial infections by 30% to 40%,[4,190,191] the large number of cases studied during consecutive years provides a useful description of the most frequently encountered infections, their relative incidences, and the responsible pathogens.

INCIDENCE

In the 1986 NNIS report, 33.5 patients per 1,000 discharges had acquired a nosocomial infection. The incidence ranges from 46.7 per 1,000 surgical discharges to 13.3 per 1,000 pediatric discharges. Overall, the rate of infection is highest in large teaching hospitals and lowest in nonteaching hospitals. The higher incidence of infection among surgical patients is largely attributable to SSI. Across all services, urinary tract infection is the most common infection, accounting for 38.5% of all nosocomial infections, followed by lower respiratory tract infection (17.8%), surgical wound infection (16.6%), primary bacteremia (7.5%), and cutaneous infection (5.8%). All other categories combined account for 13.8% of nosocomial infections. The total incidence of nosocomial infection from all sites on surgical services ranged from 30.8 to 59.3 per 1,000 discharges. The risk that a surgical patient will acquire any infection varies according to the type of procedure performed as well as the patient's underlying risk.[192]

A subsequent NNIS report, focusing on surgical patients, found that SSIs were the most common (37%, including 24% incisional and 13% organ/space), followed by urinary tract infections (27%), pneumonia (15%), primary bloodstream infections (7%), and all other sites combined (15%). Of the infected surgical patients, 17% had more than one nosocomial infection, and 9% of surgical patients with nosocomial infections subsequently died; nosocomial infections were reported to have caused or contributed to 60% of the deaths. Of infections related to death, 38% were pneumonia, 21% at the surgical site, and 20% primary bloodstream infections. The likelihood that a specific infection will be related to death varies with the type of infection [see Table 1].[192]

Urinary Tract Infection

With so many cases of bacteriuria occurring in catheterized patients, it would be easy to become complacent about the problem. Urinary tract catheterization is performed seven to eight million times a year in acute care hospitals in the United States.[193] Approximately 5% to 8% of catheterized, uninfected patients will acquire a urinary tract infection for each day of catheterization, leading to a cumulative infection rate of 40% to 50% after 10 days.[126,127] However, the great majority of catheterized patients with bacteriuria are asymp-

Table 1 Contribution of Nosocomial Infection to Death in Infected Surgical Patients Who Died[192]

Type of Nosocomial Infection	Probability That Infection Was Related to Death (%)
Organ/space surgical site infection	89
Primary bloodstream infection	79
Pneumonia	77
Other	48
Incisional surgical site infection	46
Urinary tract infection	22

tomatic.[115] It has been estimated that only 0.7% of catheterized patients will acquire a symptomatic infection and that 8% to 10% of patients will have bacteriuria after the catheter has been removed.[125]

In many of these patients, the bacteriuria will resolve without specific therapy after the catheter has been removed. However, a careful study of more than 1,458 patients has clearly demonstrated that mortality in catheterized patients who acquire bacteriuria is higher than in those who do not acquire it.[193] In this study, 9% of all catheterized patients acquired catheter-related urinary tract infection; this infection was associated with a threefold increase in deaths occurring during hospitalization, even after correction for other factors, such as age, severity of illness, hospital service, duration of catheterization, and renal function. In surgical patients between 50 and 70 years of age with normal renal function and without a fatal underlying disease, an increase in the death rate of 3% per patient per hospitalization was associated with the occurrence of a urinary tract infection. Of all deaths of catheterized patients, 14% were associated with a urinary tract infection.[193] By extrapolation, this mortality suggests that as many as 56,000 deaths a year in the United States may be related to catheter-acquired urinary tract infection.

Although the risk of bacteremia is small for any individual patient with bacteriuria, the large number of hospitalized patients with bacteriuria accounts for many bacteremic episodes. Urinary tract infection is the most commonly diagnosed source of gram-negative sepsis, and the rate of bacteremia secondary to urinary catheters is estimated to be between 0.7% and 2%.[194] In a case-matched study in 1978, a postoperative urinary tract infection was associated with a 2.4-day prolongation of hospital stay and an excess cost of more than $500.[195] One study revealed that 2.3% of postoperative patients with urinary tract infections were subsequently diagnosed as having a wound infection caused by the same organism responsible for the urinary tract infection. This finding accounted for 3.4% of the wound infections occurring during the study.[196]

Infection Associated with Intravascular Devices

Nosocomial infection associated with intravascular devices, which are placed for either monitoring or therapeutic purposes, assumed increasing importance during the 1970s and 1980s. As many as 8% of all venous cannulations are estimated to be complicated by catheter-related septicemia,[197] affecting approximately 23,000 patients in the United States each year.[60] Of all cases of nosocomial bacteremia occurring in NNIS hospitals between September 1984 and July 1986, 82% were associated with intravascular devices[198]: 27% were associated with parenteral nutrition catheters and 55% with other vascular access devices. With the semiquantitative culture technique for catheters, 16% to 44% of positive catheters have been implicated as the source of septicemia.[60,64,69-72] Reports from as early as

1963 called attention to the risk of serious systemic infections arising from peripheral intravenous catheters.[199-201] A study in 1971 documented the frequent occurrence of thrombophlebitis and sepsis 3 to 4 days after operation and the insertion of intravenous catheters.[202] For ICU patients with bloodstream infections associated with central venous catheters, the attributable mortality is 25% to 35%, and the excess cost for survivors is $23,000 to $33,000.[203]

In terms of infection risk, pulmonary artery catheters are no different from central venous catheters, except for their potential to cause right-sided heart lesions that could predispose to right-sided endocarditis.[204,205] Pulmonary artery catheters can be responsible for septicemia, and they require as much precaution during insertion and subsequent care as other central venous catheters.[72,204,206-210]

Arterial catheters, which are used for monitoring purposes in the ICU, have been thought to be less frequently associated with infection and septicemia than central venous catheters, but it is clear that life-threatening infections can originate with peripheral arterial lines.[211-213] In early studies of radial artery catheters in which nonquantitative culture techniques were employed, catheter contamination rates of 4% to 39% were recorded, but there were no cases of septicemia or clinical infection in 605 catheterizations.[214,215] In these studies, the majority of catheters were removed from patients within 3 days.

Two prospective studies of arterial catheters demonstrated that 18% to 35% of the lines were locally infected, as reflected in semiquantitative cultures of at least 15 colonies.[67,216] In one study, five cases of septicemia occurred, representing an overall incidence of 4% and an incidence of 23% among locally infected catheters.[216] The incidence of septicemia was increased in catheters that were inserted by cutdown rather than percutaneous puncture and in catheters with signs of local inflammation. In another, the clinical features of septicemia arising from an arterial catheter were indistinguishable from clinical features of episodes arising from a central venous line; 12% of all nosocomial bacteremias in the ICU originated from an arterial catheter. Clearly, arterial lines as well as venous lines must be considered in the examination of a patient for the source of fever or septicemia in the ICU.[72,209,213,216,217] Twelve cases of radial artery rupture after arterial line infection have been reported. All but one were associated with infection by *S. aureus*, and nearly all demonstrated systemic signs of infection for 2 or more days after catheter removal.[213] Although there is no published experience with the use of guide wires to change and culture arterial lines in relation to possible catheter-related infection, the technique can be applied with the same rationale used for central venous catheters.

PATHOGENS

In 1984, the NNIS reported on 26,965 infections. Of these cases, 64% were caused by single pathogens, 20% were caused by multiple pathogens, 6% had no pathogen identified on culture, and 10% were not cultured [see Figure 4]. Of the 84% in which a pathogen was identified, 86% were caused by aerobic bacteria, 2% by anaerobes, and 8% by fungi [see Figure 4 and Table 2]. Overall on the surgical services, the most common pathogen isolated was *Escherichia coli*, followed by *P. aeruginosa*, enterococci, *S. aureus*, *Enterobacter* species, *Klebsiella* species, coagulase-negative staphylococci, and *Proteus*, *Candida*, and *Serratia* species. These 10 types of pathogens accounted for 84% of all isolates. Gram-negative rods were most common in urinary tract infection and lower respiratory tract infection, although *S. aureus* was the second most common pathogen isolated in lower respiratory tract infection. *S. aureus* was the most common isolate from surgical wound infection, whereas coagulase-negative staphylococci, followed closely by *S. aureus*, were the pathogens most often responsible for primary bacteremia.

Nosocomial infections with resistant enterococci have become a

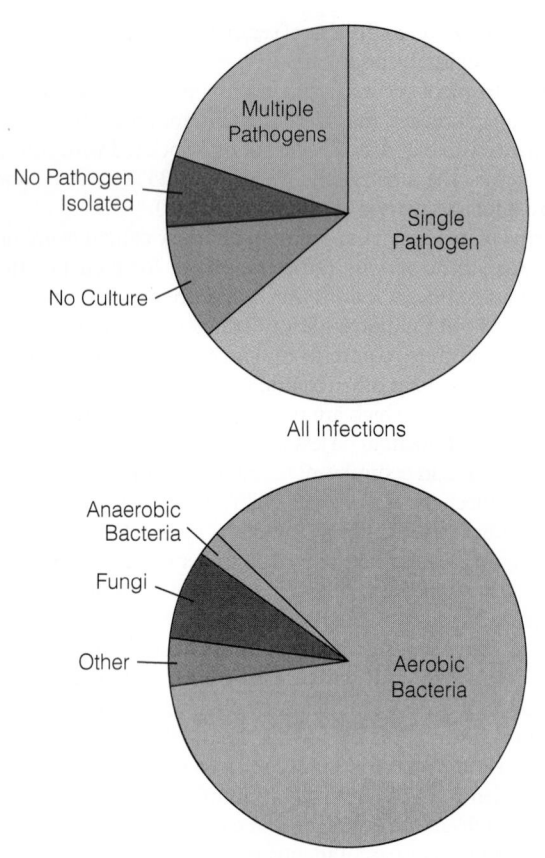

All Infections

Infections of Known Etiology

Figure 4 **Illustrated is a breakdown of the etiology of 26,965 nosocomial infections from the National Nosocomial Infections Surveillance System.[3]**

serious problem over the past 10 years. Enterococci were the third most common nosocomial bloodstream isolate reported by NNIS hospitals between 1990 and 1992.[218] The incidence of vancomycin-resistant enterococci (VRE) increased 26-fold between 1989 and 1993, from 0.3% to 7.9%, with a 34-fold rise in ICUs,[219] and the rate has continued to increase. These strains arise from endogenous flora of the patient, but nosocomial spread within the hospital environment is also an important route of spread.[219,220] The environment around infected patients is heavily contaminated with VRE, and gown and glove isolation techniques are required to stop transmission.[220] VRE are also highly resistant to other available antibiotics. Acquisition of VRE is significantly associated with prior hospitalization and with use of third-generation cephalosporins, vancomycin, or multiple antibiotics.[221,222] In one study, 16% of stool specimens submitted for testing for *C. difficile* toxin were colonized with VRE, and all surgical patients in that study had the same strain.[223]

High mortality can be associated with VRE infections. When the outcome of patients with VRE bacteremia was compared with the outcome of patients with bacteremia caused by vancomycin-sensitive enterococci (VSE), mortality was 2.3 times higher in those with VRE bacteremia, and 89% of patients with VRE bacteremia were colonized or infected with VRE at another site.[224] Prior treatment with third-generation cephalosporins is another risk factor for increased mortality.[218] Liver transplant patients with VRE bacteremia had a 92% higher mortality than comparable patients with VSE bacteremia, and those with VRE bacteremia also had a higher recurrence rate and greater need for invasive procedures.[225]

Current recommendations include decreased use, and possibly restricted use, of vancomycin as well as aggressive infection control

measures whenever VRE are isolated in a hospitalized patient.[219] In particular, vancomycin should not be used as primary treatment for *C. difficile*–associated diarrhea and should be avoided for surgical prophylaxis unless the hospital has a specific MRSA problem or the patient cannot receive other appropriate antibiotics.

ENTERIC INFECTION

C. difficile is often found in patients with severe antibiotic-associated enteric infections. In one report, 691 (2%) of 32,757 consecutive postoperative patients experienced watery diarrhea significant enough to stimulate a request for *C. difficile* toxin assay.[226] Of this number, 75 (11% of patients with diarrhea) had a positive toxin assay. All cases were associated with antibiotic administration, and 94% of the patients had received a cephalosporin either alone or in combination with other antibiotics; 29% of these responded to cessation of antibiotics and supportive measures. The remainder were treated with vancomycin, metronidazole, or bacitracin. Six (14%) of the patients who required specific therapy relapsed after initial response to treatment and were subsequently cured with one or more additional courses of treatment. Two patients died, and the overall hospital stay for the remaining patients was prolonged on average by 50%.

Most patients with mild cases of antibiotic-associated diarrhea do not have either positive cultures for *C. difficile* or positive toxin assays, and the etiologic role of *C. difficile* is unclear. Many hospitalized patients without diarrhea also have *C. difficile* in the stool, with

Table 2 Five Most Common Pathogens Isolated from Surgical Patients and Percentage of Total within Each Site[3]

Infection Site	Organism	Isolates at That Site (%)
Urinary tract infection	*Escherichia coli*	29
	Pseudomonas aeruginosa	16
	Enterococci	13
	Proteus species	7
	Klebsiella species	7
Surgical wound infection	*Staphylococcus aureus*	19
	Enterococci	12
	E. coli	12
	P. aeruginosa	10
	Coagulase-negative staphylococci	8
Lower respiratory infection	*P. aeruginosa*	17
	S. aureus	12
	Enterobacter species	11
	Klebsiella species	11
	Serratia species	7
Bacteremia	Coagulase-negative staphylococci	14
	S. aureus	10
	Enterobacter species	9
	Enterococci	9
	Klebsiella species	8
Cutaneous infections	*S. aureus*	19
	P. aeruginosa	13
	Enterococci	11
	Coagulase-negative staphylococci	10
	E. coli	8

or without toxin production,[143,144,227] and the likelihood of isolating this pathogen increases with patients' increasing length of stay.[137] A nonpathogenic yeast, *Saccharomyces boulardii*, when administered by mouth to hospitalized patients receiving antibiotics, significantly reduced the occurrence of antibiotic-associated diarrhea without affecting the rate of acquisition of *C. difficile*.[143]

Approximately 3% of asymptomatic adults carry *C. difficile* in their stools, but 30% to 40% of healthy neonates may carry the organism. The rate of carriage declines after the age of 1 to 2 years. *C. difficile* can be spread in the hospital and has been isolated from 10% of inanimate objects in the environment of patients with *C. difficile* colonization, compared with 3% in hospital areas with no known cases.[228] In one report, this organism was recovered from the hands of 13% of medical personnel working in a ward with affected patients[228]; in another, it was recovered from 60% of personnel immediately after caring for an affected patient.[229] Soap-and-water washing was ineffective in preventing acquisition, but the combination of glove use and chlorhexidine washing was effective. In another medical center, clusters of new nosocomial *C. difficile* diarrhea were prevented by screening all patients with diarrhea by active surveillance (using culture to identify *C. difficile* infection) and by instituting isolation precautions and daily disinfection of infected patients' rooms.[230]

The incidence of *C. difficile* in the environment is increased when a patient has diarrhea, compared with stool carriage without diarrhea.[228,229] In one prospectively studied cohort of patients, 21% of patients without *C. difficile* in their stools on admission acquired the organism during hospitalization, and 37% of these patients developed diarrhea. No cases of colitis occurred.[228] Diarrhea was more common in patients who received antibiotics. The rate of acquisition of *C. difficile* was 73% higher if a patient had a roommate colonized with *C. difficile*.

COST

The cost of nosocomial infections, both in dollars and in morbidity, is high. According to one estimate, 8.7 million extra hospital days and $4.5 billion in hospital charges were attributable to nosocomial infections in United States hospitals in 1976.[231] Estimates of the number of deaths caused by nosocomial infections run as high as 58,000 a year; 9,700 of these deaths and 36% of all costs attributed to nosocomial infections are due to wound infections.[231] The actual numbers may be even higher.[9] Another study found that 63 of 200 consecutive patients dying in the hospital had nosocomial infections, of which 18 (29%) were judged causal and 26 (41%) contributory. Most of the causal and contributory infections were of the lower respiratory tract, and deaths were significantly associated with invasive devices such as intra-arterial and central venous pressure monitoring devices and nasogastric tubes. Twenty-seven (47%) of 57 deaths on the surgical service were associated with nosocomial infections.

RISK

The risk of acquiring a nosocomial infection is clearly related to the reason for hospitalization as well as to underlying disease.[9,232] Patients admitted to the hospital with a fatal underlying disease have a nosocomial infection rate of 24%, compared with 10% in patients with ultimately fatal disease and 2% in those with nonfatal disease. Among 100 consecutive trauma patients admitted to the ICU at Harborview Medical Center in 1986, 42 acquired 64 nosocomial infections, including 23 lower respiratory tract infections, 17 urinary tract infections, and 6 wound infections. These 100 ICU admissions and 101 consecutive trauma admissions to the general ward were examined together. Of 153 patients admitted with injury severity scores[233] of 25 or less, nosocomial infection occurred in 32 (21%). Of 48 patients with injury severity scores higher than 25, nosocomial infection occurred in 26 (54%).[189] At the Maryland Institute for Emergency Medical Services System, the rate of nosocomial infection was 16% in 1981 and 30% in 1979.[234,235] A statewide survey of hospitals in Virginia from 1978 to 1982 found that infections in ICU patients accounted for 25% of all cases of nosocomial infections, although fewer than 10% of the beds were in ICUs.[236]

References

1. Haley RW, Schaberg DR, Crossley KB, et al: Extra charges and prolongation of stay attributable to nosocomial infections: a prospective interhospital comparison. Am J Med 70:51, 1981

2. Haley RW, Schaberg DR, Von Allmen SD, et al: Estimating the extra charges and prolongation of hospitalization due to nosocomial infections: a comparison of methods. J Infect Dis 141:248, 1980

3. Horan TC, White JW, Jarvis WR, et al: Nosocomial infection surveillance, 1984. CDC Surveillance Summaries. MMWR Morb Mortal Wkly Rep 35:17SS, 1986

4. Haley RW, Culver DH, White JW, et al: The nationwide nosocomial infection rate: a new need for vital statistics. Am J Epidemiol 121:159, 1985

5. Haley RW, White JW, Culver DH, et al: The financial incentive for hospitals to prevent nosocomial infections under the prospective payment system: an empirical determination from a nationally representative sample. JAMA 257:1611, 1987

6. Haley RW, Culver DH, Morgan WM, et al: Increased recognition of infectious diseases in US hospitals through increased use of diagnostic tests, 1970 to 1976. Am J Epidemiol 121:168, 1985

7. Roberts J, Barnes W, Pennock M, et al: Diagnostic accuracy of fever as a measure of postoperative pulmonary complications. Heart Lung 17:166, 1988

8. Engoren M: Lack of association between atelectasis and fever. Chest 107:81, 1995

9. Gross PA, Neu HC, Aswapokee P, et al: Deaths from nosocomial infections: experience in a university hospital and a community hospital. Am J Med 68:219, 1980

10. Andrews CP, Coalson JJ, Smith JD, et al: Diagnosis of nosocomial bacterial pneumonia in acute, diffuse lung injury. Chest 80:254, 1981

11. Craven DE, Steger KA: Ventilator-associated bacterial pneumonia: challenges in diagnosis, treatment, and prevention. New Horizons 6:S30, 1998

12. Croce MA, Fabian TC, Schurr MJ, et al: Using bronchoalveolar lavage to distinguish nosocomial pneumonia from systemic inflammatory response syndrome: a prospective analysis. J Trauma 39:1134, 1995

13. Valles J, Artigas A, Rello J, et al: Continuous aspiration of subglottic secretions in preventing ventilator-associated pneumonia. Ann Intern Med 122:179, 1995

14. Fernandez-Crehuet R, Diaz-Molina C, de Irala J, et al: Nosocomial infection in an intensive-care unit: identification of risk factors. Infect Control Hosp Epidemiol 18:825, 1997

15. Caplan ES, Hoyt NJ: Nosocomial sinusitis. JAMA 247:639, 1982

16. O'Reilly MJ, Reddick EJ, Black W, et al: Sepsis from sinusitis in nasotracheally intubated patients: a diagnostic dilemma. Am J Surg 147:601, 1984

17. Deutschman CS, Wilton PB, Sinow J, et al: Paranasal sinusitis: a common complication of nasotracheal intubation in neurosurgical patients. Neurosurgery 17:296, 1985

18. Kronberg FG, Goodwin WJ Jr: Sinusitis in intensive care unit patients. Laryngoscope 95:936, 1985

19. Deutschman CS, Wilton P, Sinow J, et al: Paranasal sinusitis associated with nasotracheal intubation: a frequently unrecognized and treatable source of sepsis. Crit Care Med 14:111, 1986

20. Grindlinger GA, Niehoff J, Hughes SL, et al: Acute paranasal sinusitis related to nasotracheal intubation of head-injured patients. Crit Care Med 15:214, 1987

21. Christensen L, Schaffer S, Ross SE: Otitis media in adult trauma patients: incidence and clinical significance. J Trauma 31:1543, 1991

22. Roettinger W, Edgerton MT, Kurtz LD, et al: Role of inoculation site as a determinant of infections in soft tissue wounds. Am J Surg 126:354, 1973

23. Miles AA, Milles EM, Burke J: The value and duration of defence reactions of the skin to the primary lodgement of bacteria. Br J Exp Pathol 38:79, 1957

24. Burke JF, Miles AA: The sequence of vascular events

in early infective inflammation. J Pathol Bacteriol 76: 1, 1958

25. Burke JF: The effective period of preventive antibiotic action in experimental incisions and dermal lesions. Surgery 50:161, 1961

26. Alexander JW, Altemeier WA: Penicillin prophylaxis of experimental staphylococcal wound infections. Surg Gynecol Obstet 120:243, 1965

27. Edlich RF, Smith QT, Edgerton MT: Resistance of the surgical wound to antimicrobial prophylaxis and its mechanisms of development. Am J Surg 126:583, 1973

28. McKittrick LS, Wheelock FC: The routine use of antibiotics in elective abdominal surgery. Surg Gynecol Obstet 99:376, 1954

29. Barnes J, Pace WG, Trump DS, et al: Prophylactic postoperative antibiotics: a controlled study of 1007 cases. AMA Arch Surg 79:190, 1959

30. Dellinger EP, Gross PA, Barrett TL, et al: Quality standard for antimicrobial prophylaxis in surgical procedures. Clin Infect Dis 18:422, 1994

31. Page CP, Bohnen JMA, Fletcher JR, et al: Antimicrobial prophylaxis for surgical wounds: guidelines for clinical care. Arch Surg 128:79, 1993

32. Dellinger EP: Antibiotic prophylaxis in trauma: penetrating abdominal injuries and open fractures. Rev Infect Dis 13(suppl 10):S847, 1991

33. Fabian TC, Croce MA, Payne LW, et al: Duration of antibiotic therapy for penetrating abdominal trauma: a prospective trial. Surgery 112:788, 1992

34. Culver DH, Horan TC, Gaynes RP, et al: Surgical wound infection rates by wound class, operative procedure, and patient risk index: National Nosocomial Infections Surveillance System. Am J Med 91:152S, 1991

35. Consensus paper on the surveillance of surgical wound infections. The Society for Hospital Epidemiology of America, The Association for Practitioners in Infection Control, The Centers for Disease Control, The Surgical Infection Society. Infect Control Hosp Epidemiol 13:599, 1992

36. Horan TC, Gaynes RP, Martone WJ, et al: CDC definitions of nosocomial surgical site infections, 1992: a modification of CDC definitions of surgical wound infections. Am J Infect Control 20:271, 1992

37. MacLennan JD: The histotoxic clostridial infections of man. Bacteriologic Reviews 26:177, 1962

38. Pitcher WD, Musher DM: Critical importance of early diagnosis and treatment of intra-abdominal infection. Arch Surg 117:328, 1982

39. Bohnen J, Boulanger M, Meakins JL, et al: Prognosis in generalized peritonitis: relation to cause and risk factors. Arch Surg 118:285, 1983

40. Caplan ES, Hoyt NJ, Rodriguez A, et al: Empyema occurring in the multiply traumatized patient. J Trauma 24:785, 1984

41. Rutledge R, Applebaum RE, Kim BJ: Mediastinal infection after open heart surgery. Surgery 97:88, 1985

42. Fong IW, Baker CB, McKee DC: The value of prophylactic antibiotics in aorta-coronary bypass operations: a double-blind randomized trial. J Thorac Cardiovasc Surg 78:908, 1979

43. Milano CA, Kesler K, Archibald N, et al: Mediastinitis after coronary artery bypass graft surgery: risk factors and long-term survival. Circulation 92:2245, 1995

44. Gur E, Stern D, Weiss J, et al: Clinical-radiological evaluation of poststernotomy wound infection. Plast Reconstruct Surg 101:348, 1998

45. Pairolero PC, Arnold PG, Harris JB: Long-term results of pectoralis major muscle transposition for infected sternotomy wounds. Ann Surg 213:583, 1991

46. Hand WL, Sanford JP: Posttraumatic bacterial meningitis. Ann Intern Med 72:869, 1970

47. MacGee EE, Cauthen JC, Brackett CE: Meningitis following acute traumatic cerebrospinal fluid fistula. J Neurosurg 33:312, 1970

48. Leech PJ, Paterson A: Conservative and operative management for cerebrospinal-fluid leakage after closed head injury. Lancet 1:1013, 1973

49. Davis CH: Traumatic CSF fistula: investigation and treatment. Current Controversies in Neurosurgery. Morley TP, Ed. WB Saunders Co, Philadelphia, 1976, p 572

50. Petersdorf RG, Curtin JA, Hoeprich PD, et al: A study of antibiotic prophylaxis in unconscious patients. N Engl J Med 257:1001, 1957

51. Clancey GJ, Hansen ST: Open fractures of the tibia: a review of one hundred and two cases. J Bone Joint Surg [Am] 60:118, 1978

52. Chapman MW, Mahoney M: The role of early internal fixation in the management of open fractures. Clin Orthop 138:120, 1979

53. Gustilo RB, Mendoza RM, Williams DN: Problems in the management of type III (severe) open fractures: a new classification of type III open fractures. J Trauma 24:742, 1984

54. Gustilo RB, Anderson JT: Prevention of infection in the treatment of one thousand and twenty-five open fractures of long bones: retrospective and prospective analyses. J Bone Joint Surg [Am] 58:453, 1976

55. Rittmann WW, Schibli M, Matter P, et al: Open fractures: long-term results in 200 consecutive cases. Clin Orthop 138:132, 1979

56. Dellinger EP, Miller SD, Wertz MJ, et al: Risk of infection after open fracture of the arm or leg. Arch Surg 123:1320, 1988

57. Sattler FR, Foderaro JB, Aber RC: *Staphylococcus epidermidis* bacteremia associated with vascular catheters: an important cause of febrile morbidity in hospitalized patients. Infect Control 5:279, 1984

58. Rhame FS, Maki DG, Bennett JV: Intravenous cannula-associated infections. Hospital Infections. Bennett JV, Brachman PS, Eds. Little, Brown & Co, Boston, 1979, p 433

59. Bregenzer T, Conen D, Sakmann P, et al: Is routine replacement of peripheral intravenous catheters necessary? Arch Intern Med 158:151, 1998

60. Hershey CO, Tomford JW, McLaren CE, et al: The natural history of intravenous catheter-associated phlebitis. Arch Intern Med 144:1373, 1984

61. Maki DG, Weise CE, Sarafin HW: A semiquantitative culture method for identifying intravenous-catheter-related infection. N Engl J Med 296:1305, 1977

62. Press OW, Ramsey PG, Larson EB, et al: Hickman catheter infections in patients with malignancies. Medicine (Baltimore) 63:189, 1984

63. Clarke DE, Raffin TA: Infectious complications of indwelling long-term central venous catheters. Chest 97:966, 1990

64. Band JD, Alvarado CJ, Maki DG: A semiquantitative culture technic for identifying infection due to steel needles used for intravenous therapy. American Society of Clinical Pathologists 72:980, 1979

65. Maki DG, Jarrett F, Sarafin HW: A semiquantitative culture method for identification of catheter-related infection in the burn patient. J Surg Res 22:513, 1977

66. Maki DG, Cobb L, Garman JK, et al: An attachable silver-impregnated cuff for prevention of infection with central venous catheters: a prospective randomized multicenter trial. Am J Med 85:307, 1988

67. Conly JM, Grieves K, Peters B: A prospective, randomized study comparing transparent and dry gauze dressings for central venous catheters. J Infect Dis 159:310, 1989

68. Franceschi D, Gerding RL, Phillips G, et al: Risk factors associated with intravascular catheter infections in burned patients: a prospective randomized study. J Trauma 29:81, 1989

69. Pittet D, Lew PD, Auckenthaler R, et al: Bacterial spread as a pathogenic factor in catheter-related infections (abstr No. 26). Read before the 30th Interscience Conference on Antimicrobial Agents and Chemotherapy, October 21, 1990, Atlanta. American Society for Microbiology, Washington, D.C.

70. Moyer MA, Edwards LD, Farley L: Comparative culture methods on 101 intravenous catheters: routine, semiquantitative, and blood cultures. Arch Intern Med 143:66, 1983

71. Myers ML, Austin TW, Sibbald WJ: Pulmonary artery catheter infections: a prospective study. Ann Surg 201:237, 1985

72. Cooper GL, Hopkins CC: Rapid diagnosis of intravascular catheter-associated infection by direct Gram staining of catheter segments. N Engl J Med 312: 1142, 1985

73. Singh S, Nelson N, Acosta I, et al: Catheter colonization and bacteremia with pulmonary and arterial catheters. Crit Care Med 10:736, 1982

74. Charalambos C, Swoboda SM, Dick J, et al: Risk factors and clinical impact of central line infections in the surgical intensive care unit. Arch Surg 133:1241, 1998

75. Raad I: Intravascular-catheter-related infections. Lancet 351:893, 1998

76. Guideline for prevention of intravascular device-related infections. Hospital Infection Control Practices Advisory Committee. Infect Control Hosp Epidemiol 17:438, 1996

77. Sherertz RJ, Heard SO, Raad II: Diagnosis of triple-lumen catheter infection: comparison of roll plate, sonication, and flushing methodologies. J Clin Microbiol 35:641, 1997

78. Sanders RA, Sheldon GF: Septic complications of total parenteral nutrition: a five year experience. Am J Surg 132:214, 1976

79. Freeman JB, Litton AA: Preponderance of gram-positive infections during parenteral alimentation. Surg Gynecol Obstet 139:905, 1974

80. Ponce de Leon S, Wenzel RP: Hospital-acquired bloodstream infections with *Staphylococcus epidermidis.* Am J Med 77:639, 1984

81. Rex JH, Bennett JE, Sugar AM, et al: Intravascular catheter exchange and duration of candidemia: NIAID Mycoses Study Group and the Candidemia Study Group. Clin Infect Dis 21:994, 1995

82. Stein JM, Pruitt BA: Suppurative thrombophlebitis: a lethal iatrogenic disease. N Engl J Med 282:1452, 1970

83. Munster AM: Septic thrombophlebitis: a surgical disorder. JAMA 230:1010, 1974

84. Hauser CJ, Bosco P, Davenport M, et al: Surgical management of fungal peripheral thrombophlebitis. Surgery 105:510, 1989

85. Kaufman J, Demas C, Stark K, et al: Catheter-related septic central venous thrombosis: current therapeutic options. West J Med 145:200, 1986

86. Strinden WD, Helgerson RB, Maki DG: *Candida* septic thrombosis of the great central veins associated with central catheters: clinical features and management. Ann Surg 202:653, 1985

87. Cobb DK, High KP, Sawyer RG, et al: A controlled trial of scheduled replacement of central venous and pulmonary-artery catheters. N Engl J Med 327: 1062, 1992

88. Cook D, Randolph A, Kernerman P, et al: Central venous catheter replacement strategies: a systematic review of the literature. Crit Care Med 25:1417, 1997

89. Reed CR, Sessler CN, Glauser FL, et al: Central venous catheter infections: concepts and controversies. Intens Care Med 21:177, 1995

90. Pettigrew RA, Lang SD, Haydock DA, et al: Catheter-related sepsis in patients on intravenous nutrition: a prospective study of quantitative catheter cultures and guidewire changes for suspected sepsis. Br J Surg 72:52, 1985

91. Newsome HH, Armstrong CW, Mayhall GC, et al: Mechanical complications from insertion of subclavian venous feeding catheters: comparison of de novo percutaneous venipuncture to change of catheter over guidewire. J Parenter Enteral Nutr 8:560, 1984

92. Sitzmann JV, Townsend TR, Siler MC, et al: Septic and technical complications of central venous catheterization: a prospective study of 200 consecutive patients. Ann Surg 202:766, 1985

93. Hopkins S: Diagnosing bacterial complications of temporary central venous catheters. Clinical Consultations in Nutritional Support 2:14, 1982

94. Bozzetti F, Terno G, Bonfanti G, et al: Prevention and treatment of central venous catheter sepsis by exchange via a guidewire: a prospective controlled trial. Ann Surg 198:48, 1983

95. Maher MM, Brennan MF: Central venous catheter exchange using a guidewire. J Parenter Enteral Nutr 3:515, 1979

96. Powell C, Kulich P, Mandelbaum J, et al: Effect of frequent guidewire changes on triple-lumen catheter (TLC) sepsis. J Parenter Enteral Nutr 11:15S, 1987

97. Norwood S, Jenkins G: An evaluation of triple-lumen catheter infections using a guidewire exchange technique. J Trauma 30:706, 1990

98. Norwood S, Ruby A, Civetta J, et al: Catheter-related infections and associated septicemia. Chest 99:968, 1991

99. Williams WW: Infection control during parenteral nutrition therapy. J Parenter Enteral Nutr 9:735, 1985

100. Raad II, Hohn DC, Gilbreath BJ, et al: Prevention of central venous catheter-related infections by using maximal sterile barrier precautions during insertion. Infect Control Hosp Epidemiol 15:231, 1994

101. Collignon P, Soni N, Pearson I, et al: Sepsis associated with central vein catheters in critically ill patients. Intens Care Med 14:227, 1988

102. Richet H, Hubert B, Nitemberg G, et al: Prospective multicenter study of vascular-catheter-related complications and risk factors for positive central-catheter cultures in intensive care unit patients. J Clin Microbiol 28:2520, 1990

103. Central venous catheters coated with minocycline and rifampin for the prevention of catheter-related colonization and bloodstream infections: a randomized, double-blind trial. The Texas Medical Center Catheter Study Group. Ann Intern Med 127:267, 1997

104. Maki DG, Stolz SM, Wheeler S, et al: Prevention of central venous catheter-related bloodstream infection by use of an antiseptic-impregnated catheter: a randomized, controlled trial. Ann Intern Med 127:257, 1997

105. Darouiche RO, Raad II, Heard SO, et al: A comparison of two antimicrobial-impregnated central venous catheters. N Engl J Med 340:1, 1999

106. Powell C, Regan C, Fabri PJ, et al: Evaluation of op site catheter dressings for parenteral nutrition: a prospective, randomized study. J Parenter Enteral Nutr 6:43, 1982

107. Palidar PJ, Simonowitz DA, Oreskovich MR, et al: Use of op site as an occlusive dressing for total parenteral nutrition catheters. J Parenter Enteral Nutr 6:150, 1982

108. Maki DG, Band JD: A comparative study of polyantibiotic and iodophor ointments in prevention of vascular catheter–related infection. Am J Med 70:739, 1981

109. Hoffman KK, Weber DJ, Samsa GP, et al: Transparent polyurethane film as an intravenous catheter dressing: a meta-analysis of the infection risks. JAMA 267:2072, 1992

110. Forlaw L, Torosian MH: Central venous catheter care. Rombeau JL, Caldwell MD, Eds. Clinical Nutrition, Vol 2: Parenteral Nutrition. WB Saunders Co, Philadelphia, 1986, p 316

111. Ryan JA Jr, Abel RM, Abbott WM, et al: Catheter complications in total parenteral nutrition: a prospective study of 200 consecutive patients. N Engl J Med 290:757, 1974

112. Copeland EM, MacFayden BV Jr, Dudrick SJ: Prevention of microbial catheter contamination in patients receiving parenteral hyperalimentation. South Med J 67:303, 1974

113. Padberg FT Jr, Ruggiero J, Blackburn GL, et al: Central venous catheterization for parenteral nutrition. Ann Surg 193:264, 1981

114. Hilton E, Haslett TM, Borenstein MT, et al: Central catheter infections: single- versus triple-lumen catheters: influence of guidewires on infection rates when used for replacement of catheters. Am J Med 84:667, 1988

115. Pemberton LB, Lyman B, Lander V, et al: Sepsis from triple- vs single-lumen catheters during total parenteral nutrition in surgical or critically ill patients. Arch Surg 121:591, 1986

116. Miller JJ, Venus B, Mathru M: Comparison of the sterility of long-term central venous catheterization using single lumen, triple lumen, and pulmonary artery catheters. Crit Care Med 12:634, 1984

117. Powell C, Fabri PJ, Kudsk KA: Risk of infection accompanying the use of single-lumen vs. double-lumen subclavian catheters: a prospective randomized study. J Parenter Enteral Nutr 12:127, 1988

118. Raad I, Davis S, Becker M, et al: Low infection rate and long durability of nontunneled Silastic catheters: a safe and cost-effective alternative for long-term venous access. Arch Intern Med 153:1791, 1993

119. Groeger JS, Lucas AB, Thaler HT, et al: Infectious morbidity associated with long-term use of venous access devices in patients with cancer. Ann Intern Med 119:1168, 1993

120. Bern MM, Lokich JJ, Wallach SR, et al: Very low doses of warfarin can prevent thrombosis in central venous catheters: a prospective randomized trial. Ann Intern Med 112:423, 1990

121. Stark RP, Maki DG: Bacteriuria in the catheterized patient: what quantitative level of bacteriuria is relevant? N Engl J Med 311:560, 1984

122. Kunin CM: Genitourinary infections in the patient at risk: extrinsic risk factors. Am J Med 76:131, 1984

123. Harding GK, Nicolle LE, Ronald AR, et al: How long should catheter-acquired urinary tract infection in women be treated? A randomized controlled study. Ann Intern Med 114:713, 1991

124. Hirsh DD, Fainstein V, Musher DM: Do condom catheter collecting systems cause urinary tract infection? JAMA 242:340, 1979

125. Johnson ET: The condom catheter: urinary tract infection and other complications. South Med J 76:579, 1983

126. Kunin CM: Urinary tract infections. Hospital Infection. Bennett JV, Brachman PS, Eds. Little, Brown & Co, Boston, 1979, p 239

127. Garibaldi RA, Burke JP, Dickman ML, et al: Factors predisposing to bacteriuria during indwelling urethral catheterization. N Engl J Med 291:215, 1974

128. Warren JW, Platt R, Thomas RJ, et al: Antibiotic irrigation and catheter-associated urinary tract infections. N Engl J Med 299:570, 1978

129. Platt R, Polk BF, Murdock B, et al: Reduction of mortality associated with nosocomial urinary tract infection. Lancet 1:893, 1983

130. Lima NL, Guerrant RL, Kaiser DL, et al: A retrospective cohort study of nosocomial diarrhea as a risk factor for nosocomial infection. J Infect Dis 161:948, 1990

131. Jones SR, Smith JW, Sanford JP: Localization of urinary-tract infections by detection of antibody-coated bacteria in urine sediment. N Engl J Med 290:591, 1974

132. Latham RH, Stamm WE: Role of fimbriated Escherichia coli in urinary tract infections in adult women: correlation with localization studies. J Infect Dis 149:835, 1984

133. Anderson RU: Urinary tract infections in compromised hosts. Urol Clin North Am 13:727, 1986

134. Cattell WR: Urinary infections in adults—1985. Postgrad Med J 61:907, 1985

135. Stamm WE: Approach to the patient with urinary tract infection. Infectious Disease. Gorbach SL, Bartlett JG, Blacklow NR, Eds. WB Saunders Co, Philadelphia, 1992, p 788

136. DuPont HL: Infectious gastroenteritis. Hospital Infection. Bennett JV, Brachman PS, Eds. Little, Brown & Co, Boston, 1979, p 381

137. Hines J, Nachamkin I: Effective use of the clinical microbiology laboratory for diagnosing diarrheal diseases. Clin Infect Dis 23:1292, 1996

138. Gerding DN, Johnson S, Peterson LR, et al: Clostridium difficile-associated diarrhea and colitis. Infect Control Hosp Epidemiol 16:459, 1995

139. McFarland LV, Coyle MB, Kremer WH, et al: Rectal swab cultures for Clostridium difficile surveillance studies. J Clin Microbiol 25:2241, 1987

140. Bartlett JG: Antibiotic-associated colitis. Dis Mon 30:1, 1984

141. George WL: Antimicrobial agent–associated colitis and diarrhea: historical background and clinical aspects. Rev Infect Dis 6:S208, 1984

142. Grube BJ, Heimbach DM, Marvin JA: Clostridium difficile diarrhea in critically ill burned patients. Arch Surg 122:655, 1987

143. Bartlett JG, Moon N, Chang TW, et al: Role of Clostridium difficile in antibiotic-associated pseudomembranous colitis. Gastroenterology 75:778, 1978

144. Surawicz CM, Elmer GW, Speelman P, et al: Prevention of antibiotic-associated diarrhea by Saccharomyces boulardii: a prospective study. Gastroenterology 96:981, 1989

145. McFarland LV, Surawicz CM, Stamm WE: Risk factors for Clostridium difficile carriage and C. difficile-associated diarrhea in a cohort of hospitalized patients. J Infect Dis 162:678, 1990

146. Tedesco FJ, Corless JK, Brownstein RE: Rectal sparing in antibiotic-associated pseudomembranous colitis: a prospective study. Gastroenterology 83:1259, 1982

147. Dane TE, King EG: Fatal pseudomembranous enterocolitis following clindamycin therapy. Br J Surg 63:305, 1976

148. Cheung A, Tank RE, Dellinger EP: Antibiotic-associated enterocolitis involving the small bowel. Surgical Rounds 14:821, 1991

149. Hecht JR, Olinger EJ: Clostridium difficile colitis secondary to intravenous vancomycin. Dig Dis Sci 34:148, 1989

150. Miller SN, Ringler RP: Vancomycin-induced pseudomembranous colitis (letter). J Clin Gastroenterol 9:114, 1987

151. Oliva SL, Guglielmo BJ, Jacobs R, et al: Failure of intravenous vancomycin and intravenous metronidazole to prevent or treat antibiotic-associated pseudomembranous colitis (letter). J Infect Dis 159:1154, 1989

152. Freiman JP, Graham DJ, Green L: Pseudomembranous colitis associated with single-dose cephalosporin prophylaxis (letter). JAMA 262:902, 1989

153. Bartlett JG: Treatment of Clostridium difficile colitis (editorial). Gastroenterology 89:1192, 1985

154. Bartlett JG: Treatment of antibiotic-associated pseudomembranous colitis. Rev Infect Dis 6(suppl 1):S235, 1984

155. Young GP, Ward PB, Bayley N, et al: Antibiotic-associated colitis due to Clostridium difficile: double-blind comparison of vancomycin with bacitracin. Gastroenterology 89:1038, 1985

156. Recommendations for preventing the spread of vancomycin resistance. Hospital Infection Control Practices Advisory Committee. MMWR Morb Mortal Wkly Rep 44:1, 1995

157. Johnson S, Adelmann A, Clabots CR, et al: Recurrence of Clostridium difficile diarrhea not caused by the original infecting organism. J Infect Dis 159:340, 1989

158. Guzman R, Kirkpatrick J, Forward K, et al: Failure of parenteral metronidazole in the treatment of pseudomembranous colitis (letter). J Infect Dis 158:1146, 1988

159. Johnson S, Peterson LR, Gerding DN: Intravenous metronidazole and *Clostridium difficile*–associated diarrhea or colitis (letter). J Infect Dis 160:1087, 1989

160. Gerding DN, Olson MM, Johnson S, et al: *Clostridium difficile* diarrhea and colonization after treatment with abdominal infection regimens containing clindamycin or metronidazole. Am J Surg 159:212, 1990

161. Levine B, Peskin GW, Saik RP: Drug-induced colitis as a surgical disease. Arch Surg 111:987, 1976

162. Drapkin MS, Worthington MG, Chang TW, et al: *Clostridium difficile* colitis mimicking acute peritonitis. Arch Surg 120:1321, 1985

163. Chatila W, Manthous CA: *Clostridium difficile* causing sepsis and an acute abdomen in critically ill patients. Crit Care Med 23:1146, 1995

164. Byl B, Jacobs F, Struelens MJ, et al: Extraintestinal *Clostridium difficile* infections. Clin Infect Dis 22: 712, 1996

165. Kahn RA: Diseases transmitted by blood transfusion. Hum Pathol 14:241, 1983

166. Kahn RA, Barrios SDP: Diseases transmitted by blood transfusion. Transfusion Therapy: Principles and Procedures. Rutman RC, Miller WV, Eds. Aspen Publishers, Rockville, Maryland, 1985, p 311

167. Herwaldt BL, Kjemtrup AM, Conrad PA, et al: Transfusion-transmitted babesiosis in Washington State: first reported case caused by a WA1-type parasite. J Infect Dis 175:1259, 1997

168. Wagner SJ, Friedman LI, Dodd RY: Transfusion-associated bacterial sepsis. Clin Microbiol Rev 7:290, 1994

169. Red blood cell transfusions contaminated with *Yersinia enterocolitica*—United States, 1991-1996, and initiation of a national study to detect bacteria-associated transfusion reactions. MMWR Morb Mortal Wkly Rep 46:553, 1997

170. Update: *Yersinia enterocolitica* bacteremia and endotoxin shock associated with red blood cell transfusions—United States, 1991. MMWR Morb Mortal Wkly Rep 40:176, 1991

171. Shorey J: The current status of non-A, non-B viral hepatitis. Southwestern Internal Medicine Conference. Am J Med Sci 289:251, 1985

172. Aach RD, Kahn RA: Post-transfusion hepatitis: current perspectives. Ann Intern Med 92:539, 1980

173. Iwarson S, Norkrans G, Wejstal R: Hepatitis C: natural history of a unique infection. Clin Infect Dis 20:1361, 1995

174. Chen D-S, Kuo GC, Sung J-L, et al: Hepatitis C virus infection in an area hyperendemic for hepatitis B and chronic liver disease: the Taiwan experience. J Infect Dis 162:817, 1990

175. Koretz RL, Stone O, Mousa M, et al: Non-A, non-B posttransfusion hepatitis—a decade later. Gastroenterology 88:1251, 1985

176. Esteban JI, González A, Hernández JM, et al: Evaluation of antibodies to hepatitis C virus in a study of transfusion-associated hepatitis. N Engl J Med 323: 110, 1990

177. Lee S-D, Hwang S-J, Lu R-H, et al: Antibodies to hepatitis C virus in prospectively followed patients with posttransfusion hepatitis. J Infect Dis 163:1354, 1991

178. Transfusion-associated human T-lymphotropic virus type III/lymphadenopathy-associated virus infection from a seronegative donor—Colorado. MMWR Morb Mortal Wkly Rep 35:389, 1986

179. Cumming PD, Wallace EL, Schorr JB, et al: Exposure of patients to human immunodeficiency virus through the transfusion of blood components that test antibody-negative. N Engl J Med 321:941, 1989

180. Menitove JE: Current risk of transfusion-associated human immunodeficiency virus infection. Arch Pathol Lab Med 114:330, 1990

181. Busch MP, Eble BE, Khayam-Bashi H, et al: Evaluation of screened blood donations for human immunodeficiency virus type 1 infection by culture and DNA amplification of pooled cells. N Engl J Med 325:1, 1991

182. Schreiber GB, Busch MP, Kleinman SH, et al: The risk of transfusion-transmitted viral infections: The Retrovirus Epidemiology Donor Study. N Engl J Med 334:1685, 1996

183. Curran JW, Lawrence DN, Jaffe H, et al: Acquired immunodeficiency syndrome (AIDS) associated with transfusions. N Engl J Med 310:69, 1984

184. Bove JR: Transfusion-associated AIDS—a cause for concern (editorial). N Engl J Med 310:115, 1984

185. Surgenor DMacN, Wallace EL, Hao SH: Collection and transfusion of blood in the United States, 1982–1988. N Engl J Med 322:1646, 1990

186. Garibaldi RA, Brodine S, Matsumiya S, et al: Evidence for the non-infectious etiology of early postoperative fever. Infect Control 6:273, 1985

187. Dykes MH: Unexplained postoperative fever: its value as a sign of halothane sensitization. JAMA 216: 641, 1971

188. Dellinger EP, Wertz MJ, Oreskovich MR, et al: Specificity of fever and leukocytosis after laparotomy for penetrating abdominal trauma (abstr). J Trauma 23: 633, 1983

189. Dellinger EP: Prevention and management of infections. Trauma, 2nd ed. Moore EE, Mattox KL, Feliciano DV, Eds. Appleton & Lange, Norwalk, 1988, p 231

190. Haley RW, Culver DH, White JW, et al: The efficacy of infection surveillance and control programs in preventing nosocomial infections in US hospitals. Am J Epidemiol 121:182, 1985

191. Haley RW, Hooton TM, Culver DH, et al: Nosocomial infections in US hospitals, 1975 to 1976: estimated frequency by selected characteristics of patients. Am J Med 70:947, 1981

192. Horan TC, Culver DH, Gaynes RP, et al: Nosocomial infections in surgical patients in the United States, January 1986-June 1992: National Nosocomial Infections Surveillance (NNIS) System. Infect Control Hosp Epidemiol 14:73, 1993

193. Platt R, Polk BF, Murdock B, et al: Mortality associated with nosocomial urinary tract infection. N Engl J Med 307:637, 1982

194. Stamm WE: Urinary tract infections. Hospital Infections, 4th ed. Bennett JV, Brachman PS, Eds. Lippincott-Raven, Philadelphia, 1998, p 477

195. Givens CD, Wenzel RP: Catheter-associated urinary tract infections in surgical patients: a controlled study on the excess morbidity and costs. J Urol 124:646, 1980

196. Krieger JN, Kaiser DL, Wenzel RP: Nosocomial urinary tract infections cause wound infections postoperatively in surgical patients. Surg Gynecol Obstet 156:313, 1983

197. Maki DG, Goldman A, Rhame FS: Infection control in intravenous therapy. Ann Intern Med 79:867, 1973

198. Dickinson GM, Bisno AL: Infections associated with indwelling devices: concepts of pathogenesis; infections associated with intravascular devices. Antimicrob Agents Chemother 33:597, 1989

199. Collins RN, Braun PA, Zinner SH, et al: Risk of local and systemic infections with polyethylene intravenous catheters: a prospective study of 213 catheterizations. N Engl J Med 279:340, 1968

200. Druskin MS, Siegel PD: Bacterial contamination of indwelling intravenous polyethylene catheters. JAMA 185:966, 1963

201. Bentley DW, Lepper MH: Septicemia related to indwelling venous catheter. JAMA 206:1749, 1968

202. Altemeier WA, McDonough JJ, Fullen WD: Third day surgical fever. Arch Surg 103:158, 1971

203. Pittet D, Hulliger S, Auckenthaler R: Intravascular device-related infections in critically ill patients. J Chemother 7(suppl 3):55, 1995

204. Elliott CG, Zimmerman GA, Clemmer TP: Complications of pulmonary artery catheterization in the care of critically ill patients: a prospective study. Chest 76: 647, 1979

205. Rowley KM, Clubb KS, Walker Smith GJ, et al: Right-sided infective endocarditis as a consequence of flow-directed pulmonary-artery catheterization: a clinicopathological study of 55 autopsied patients. N Engl J Med 311:1152, 1984

206. Applefeld JJ, Caruthers TE, Reno DJ, et al: Assessment of the sterility of long-term cardiac catheterization using the thermodilution Swan-Ganz catheter. Chest 74:377, 1978

207. Hudson-Civetta JA, Civetta JM, Martinez OV, et al: Risk and detection of pulmonary artery catheter–related infection in septic surgical patients. Crit Care Med 15:29, 1987

208. Prachar H, Dittel M, Jobst C, et al: Bacterial contamination of pulmonary artery catheters. Intensive Care Med 4:79, 1978

209. Pinilla JC, Ross DF, Martin T, et al: Study of the incidence of intravascular catheter infection and associated septicemia in critically ill patients. Crit Care Med 11:21, 1983

210. Michel L, Marsh HM, McMichan JC, et al: Infection of pulmonary artery catheters in critically ill patients. JAMA 245:1032, 1981

211. Rose HD: Gas gangrene and *Clostridium perfringens* septicemia associated with the use of an indwelling radial artery catheter. Can Med Assoc J 121:1595, 1979

212. Meakins JL: Infection associated with radial artery catheters (editorial). Can Med Assoc J 121:1564, 1979

213. Arnow PM, Costas CO: Delayed rupture of the radial artery caused by catheter-related sepsis. Rev Infect Dis 10:1035, 1988

214. Gardner RM, Schwartz R, Wong HC, et al: Percutaneous indwelling radial-artery catheters for monitoring cardiovascular function: prospective study of the risk of thrombosis and infection. N Engl J Med 290: 1227, 1974

215. Davis FM, Cornere B: Bacterial contamination of radial artery catheters. NZ Med J 89:128, 1979

216. Band JD, Maki DG: Infections caused by arterial catheters used for hemodynamic monitoring. Am J Med 67:735, 1979

217. Kaye W, Wheaton M, Potter-Bynoe G: Radial and pulmonary artery catheter-related sepsis (abstr). Crit Care Med 11:249, 1983

218. Stroud L, Edwards J, Danzing L, et al: Risk factors for mortality associated with enterococcal bloodstream infections. Infect Control Hosp Epidemiol 17:576, 1996

219. Recommendations for preventing the spread of vancomycin resistance: recommendations of the Hospital Infection Control Practices Advisory Committee (HICPAC). Centers for Disease Control and Prevention. MMWR Morb Mortal Wkly Rep 44(RR-12):1, 1995

220. Murray BE: What can we do about vancomycin-resistant enterococci? Clin Infect Dis 20:1134, 1995

221. Weinstein JW, Roe M, Towns M, et al: Resistant enterococci: a prospective study of prevalence, incidence, and factors associated with colonization in a university hospital. Infect Control Hosp Epidemiol 17:36, 1996

222. Tornieporth NG, Roberts RB, John J, et al: Risk factors associated with vancomycin-resistant *Enterococcus faecium* infection or colonization in 145 matched case patients and control patients. Clin Infect Dis 23: 767, 1996

223. Rafferty ME, McCormick MI, Bopp LH, et al: Vancomycin-resistant enterococci in stool specimens submitted for *Clostridium difficile* cytotoxin assay. Infect Control Hosp Epidemiol 18:342, 1997

224. Edmond MB, Ober JF, Dawson JD, et al: Vancomycin-resistant enterococcal bacteremia: natural history and attributable mortality. Clin Infect Dis 23:1234, 1996

225. Linden PK, Pasculle AW, Manez R, et al: Differences in outcomes for patients with bacteremia due to vancomycin-resistant *Enterococcus faecium* or vancomycin-susceptible *E. faecium*. Clin Infect Dis 22: 663, 1996

226. Rosenberg JM, Walker M, Welch JP, et al: *Clostridium difficile* colitis in surgical patients. Am J Surg 147: 486, 1984

227. McFarland LV, Elmer GW, Stamm WE, et al: Correlation of immunoblot type, enterotoxin production, and cytotoxin production with clinical manifestations of *Clostridium difficile* infection in a cohort of hospitalized patients. Infect Immun 59:2456, 1991

228. Fekety R, Kim KH, Brown D, et al: Epidemiology of antibiotic-associated colitis: isolation of *Clostridium difficile* from the hospital environment. Am J Med 70: 906, 1981

229. McFarland LV, Mulligan ME, Kwok RY, et al: Nosocomial acquisition of *Clostridium difficile* infection. N Engl J Med 320:204, 1989

230. Struelens MJ, Maas A, Nonhoff C, et al: Control of nosocomial transmission of *Clostridium difficile* based on sporadic case surveillance. Am J Med 91(suppl 3B):138S, 1991

231. Martone WJ, Jarvis WR, Edwards JR, et al: Incidence and nature of endemic and epidemic nosocomial infections. Hospital Infections, 4th ed. Bennett JV, Brachman PS, Eds. Lippincott-Raven, Philadelphia, 1998, p 461

232. Britt MR, Schleupner CJ, Matsumiya S: Severity of underlying disease as a predictor of nosocomial infection: utility in the control of nosocomial infection. JAMA 239:1047, 1978

233. Baker SP, O'Neill B, Haddon W Jr, et al: The injury severity score: a method for describing patients with multiple injuries and evaluating emergency care. J Trauma 14:187, 1974

234. Caplan ES, Hoyt N, Cowley RA: Changing patterns of nosocomial infections in severely traumatized patients. Am J Surg 45:204, 1979

235. Caplan ES, Hoyt N: Infection surveillance and control in the severely traumatized patient. Am J Med 70:638, 1981

236. Wenzel RP, Thompson RL, Landry SM, et al: Hospital-acquired infections in intensive care unit patients: an overview with emphasis on epidemics. Infect Control 4:371, 1983

Acknowledgments

Figures 1 and 2   Carol Donner.

Figure 4   Albert Miller.

15 PERITONITIS AND INTRA-ABDOMINAL ABSCESSES

Ori D. Rotstein, M.D., M.Sc., and Avery B. Nathens, M.D., Ph.D., M.P.H.

Approach to Peritonitis and Intra-abdominal Abscesses

There are two major manifestations of intra-abdominal infection: (1) peritonitis, or inflammation of the peritoneum, and (2) abscess formation, in which infection has become walled off from the remainder of the peritoneal cavity. Peritonitis has been classically divided into a primary form and a secondary form, which is by far the more common. In secondary peritonitis, peritoneal infection and inflammation are caused by visceral disruption that is a result of an intrinsic pathological condition or of external trauma. Because of its greater clinical importance, secondary peritonitis will receive somewhat greater emphasis than primary peritonitis.

Peritonitis

SECONDARY PERITONITIS

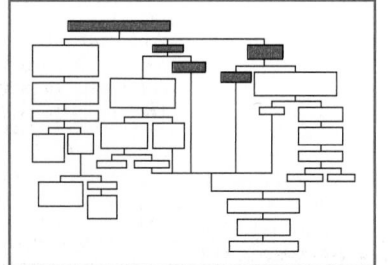

Secondary bacterial peritonitis is defined as peritoneal infection caused by perforation of a hollow viscus or transmural necrosis of the gastrointestinal tract. Excluding trauma, the common causes of generalized peritonitis include a perforated appendix, perforated duodenal ulcer, perforated sigmoid colon (caused by diverticulitis, volvulus, or cancer), strangulation obstruction of the small bowel, and postoperative peritonitis caused by anastomotic disruption.

Clinical Presentation and Diagnosis

The diagnosis of peritonitis is usually a clinical one. The predominant symptom is invariably abdominal pain. The onset of the pain may be acute or more insidious. The pain is often steady, severe, and aggravated by movement. The patient is frequently lying still in bed, either in the fetal position or supine with knees bent and head elevated. Both these maneuvers reduce the tension on the abdominal wall and thereby alleviate abdominal discomfort. Anorexia and nausea are often accompanying symptoms. Depending on the etiology of the peritonitis, a history of recent symptoms may be obtained from the patient.

The results of physical examination vary according to the cause and the extent of the peritonitis. Most patients, however, look unwell and are in acute distress. Body temperature is usually higher than 38° C (100.4° F), but in cases of severe septic shock, the patient may be hypothermic. Tachycardia and diminished pulse volume, indicative of hypovolemia, are common. Patients in septic shock may manifest high cardiac output and reduced peripheral resistance, as shown by bounding pulses with increased pulse pressure and warm extremities [*see I:4 Shock*].

Abdominal tenderness is the hallmark of peritonitis. Patients with generalized peritonitis suffer diffuse tenderness. The point of maximum tenderness frequently overlies the diseased organ. Increased abdominal tone is initially from voluntary guarding by the patient and is subsequently a result of reflex muscular spasm. The abdomen is characteristically distended, and bowel sounds are usually absent, although an occasional bowel sound may be heard.

Localized peritonitis generally produces less extreme effects in the patient. The abdomen distant from the site of maximum tenderness may be soft and nontender, and bowel sounds are frequently present. Referred rebound tenderness may accurately pinpoint the site of maximal peritoneal irritation; the rectal examination, although an essential part of the physical examination, rarely pinpoints the origin of the peritonitis.

Laboratory data, particularly the presence of a leukocytosis greater than 11,000 cells/mm³ with a shift to the left, support the clinical diagnosis of peritonitis. Leukopenia is compatible with overwhelming sepsis. Blood chemistry is generally undisturbed but in severe cases may show evidence of dehydration with elevated blood urea nitrogen levels as well as metabolic acidosis. Urinalysis is essential to rule out urinary tract diseases, such as pyelonephritis and renal colic, which may mimic peritonitis. White and red blood cells are occasionally found in the urine of patients with peritonitis, but the presence of bacteria, white blood cell casts, and large numbers of erythrocytes in the urine should suggest a urinary tract source of the pain.

Plain abdominal x-rays may show evidence of ileus, with distended loops of large and small bowel, air-fluid levels, and free fluid in the peritoneal cavity. Upright films are useful for demonstrating free air under the diaphragm, an indication of a perforated viscus. Free air is evident in 80 percent of cases of perforated duodenal ulcer but occurs much less frequently after perforation of the appendix, the small bowel, or the sigmoid colon.

Although the diagnosis of peritonitis is a clinical one, the history and physical examination may be either inconclusive with respect to the diagnosis or unreliable because of underlying patient factors, such as altered consciousness caused by head injury or toxic encephalopathy, paraplegia, the effects of immunosuppressive drugs, and, occasionally, advanced age. In these situations, several adjunctive diagnostic modalities can be helpful.

Imaging techniques may provide evidence of an inflammatory process within the peritoneal cavity. Ultrasonography is useful in equivocal cases of right lower quadrant pain, with specificity and sensitivity of 90 percent and 80 percent, respectively, for the diagnosis of appendicitis.[1] The ability of ultrasonography to detect less than 100 ml of fluid in the peritoneal cavity may support the diagnosis of peritonitis when the physical findings are equivocal.

Like ultrasonography, computed tomography is capable of detecting minute quantities of intraperitoneal fluid. In one prospective study, computed tomography provided a diagnosis in 95 percent of cases and altered the primary therapeutic strategy in 30 percent of patients.[2]

Diagnostic peritoneal lavage appears to be a safe and accurate method of determining the presence of peritonitis necessitating operation in these patients.[3,4] Several criteria for a positive lavage have been used, but the presence of more than 500 white blood cells/mm³ after a 1 L saline lavage appears to correlate best with the presence of intra-abdominal pathology. Gross pus, turbid fluid, bile, or a positive Gram's stain is a clear indication for laparotomy. In well-localized inflammatory processes or in patients who are unable to mount a significant white blood cell response, peritoneal lavage may produce false negative results. Nuclear scanning of the biliary tree with the technetium-99m–labeled iminodiacetic acid (IDA) family of compounds may also be useful for investigating right upper quadrant peritonitis in the critically ill patient in whom congestive hepatomegaly or pneumonia may mimic either calculous or acalculous cholecystitis.[5]

The laparoscope has become an important diagnostic tool, with laparoscopy providing a definitive diagnosis in more than 90 percent of cases.[6] Preoperative laparoscopy may lead to a significant modification of the therapeutic strategy in as many as 10 percent of patients.[7] The most common indication for laparoscopy is lower abdominal or pelvic pain in young women, particularly in the right iliac fossa, where the possibility of appendicitis versus tubo-ovarian processes complicates diagnosis.

In the majority of cases, the diagnosis of peritonitis is straightforward. The patient complains of abdominal pain and demonstrates evidence of peritoneal irritation on physical examination. Generally, the presence of peritonitis is an indication for early laparotomy and surgical repair. However, some disease entities, either intra-abdominal or extra-abdominal, mimic peritonitis but do not call for early surgery [see Table 1]. Many can be easily ruled out by clinical examination and laboratory tests (e.g., serum amylase level, urinalysis, electrocardiography, chest x-ray, and abdominal ultrasonography). Finally, it is worthwhile to remember a short list of diagnoses that occasionally escape consideration and can be rapidly fatal if overlooked. In patients with peritonitis, these include ruptured ectopic pregnancy and ruptured abdominal aortic aneurysm.

Table 1 Common Nonsurgical Causes of Peritonitis

INTRA-ABDOMINAL

Gastrointestinal system
  Congestive hepatomegaly
  Pancreatitis
  Acute diverticulitis
  Acute cholecystitis

Gynecologic system
  Pelvic inflammatory disease
  Ovarian pathology
    Torsion of a cyst
    Bleeding into a cyst

Urinary tract system
  Renal colic
  Pyelonephritis
  Cystitis

EXTRA-ABDOMINAL

Pulmonary system
  Basilar pneumonia
  Pulmonary embolus

Cardiac system
  Myocardial infarction
  Pericarditis

Metabolic problems
  Methanol poisoning
  Addisonian crisis
  Sickle cell disease

Management

Preoperative preparation The principal objectives in preparing patients with secondary peritonitis for operation are fluid resuscitation and the initiation of antibiotic therapy.

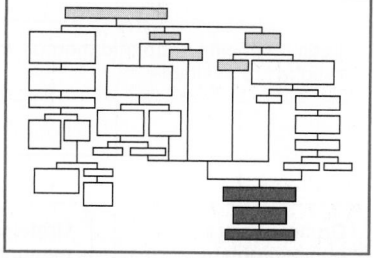

Fluid resuscitation entails the administration of fluids and the monitoring of fluid status. The extent of these measures depends very much on the patient's premorbid status and on the underlying disease process. Clearly, a teenager with acute appendicitis does not require the same preoperative resuscitation as an octogenarian with a perforated sigmoid volvulus. However, the principles are the same. All patients with peritonitis have some degree of hypovolemia. Adequate volumes of fluid should therefore be administered to restore blood volume. Adequacy of resuscitation may be assessed by monitoring blood pressure, central venous pressure, and urine output. In the elderly or critically ill patient, resuscitative measures must be directed by invasive monitoring techniques, including (1) arterial cannulation to measure blood pressure directly and to sample arterial blood for blood gas determination, (2) central venous monitoring, preferably with a Swan-Ganz catheter to measure pulmonary and left atrial pressures, and (3) measurement of urine output with an indwelling catheter. Fluid may be rapidly administered, even to elderly patients with limited cardiac reserve, if these monitoring techniques are used.

Antibiotic therapy should be initiated as soon as the clinical diagnosis of peritonitis is made, even before samples can be taken from the peritoneal cavity for aerobic and anaerobic culture. Although the initial antibiotic therapy is given on an empirical basis, the choice of antimicrobial agents should be based on the suspected offending organisms (see below) and on the ability of the antibiotics to achieve adequate levels in the peritoneal cavity. Fortunately, most antibiotics have this ability.

Approach to Peritonitis and Intra-abdominal Abscesses

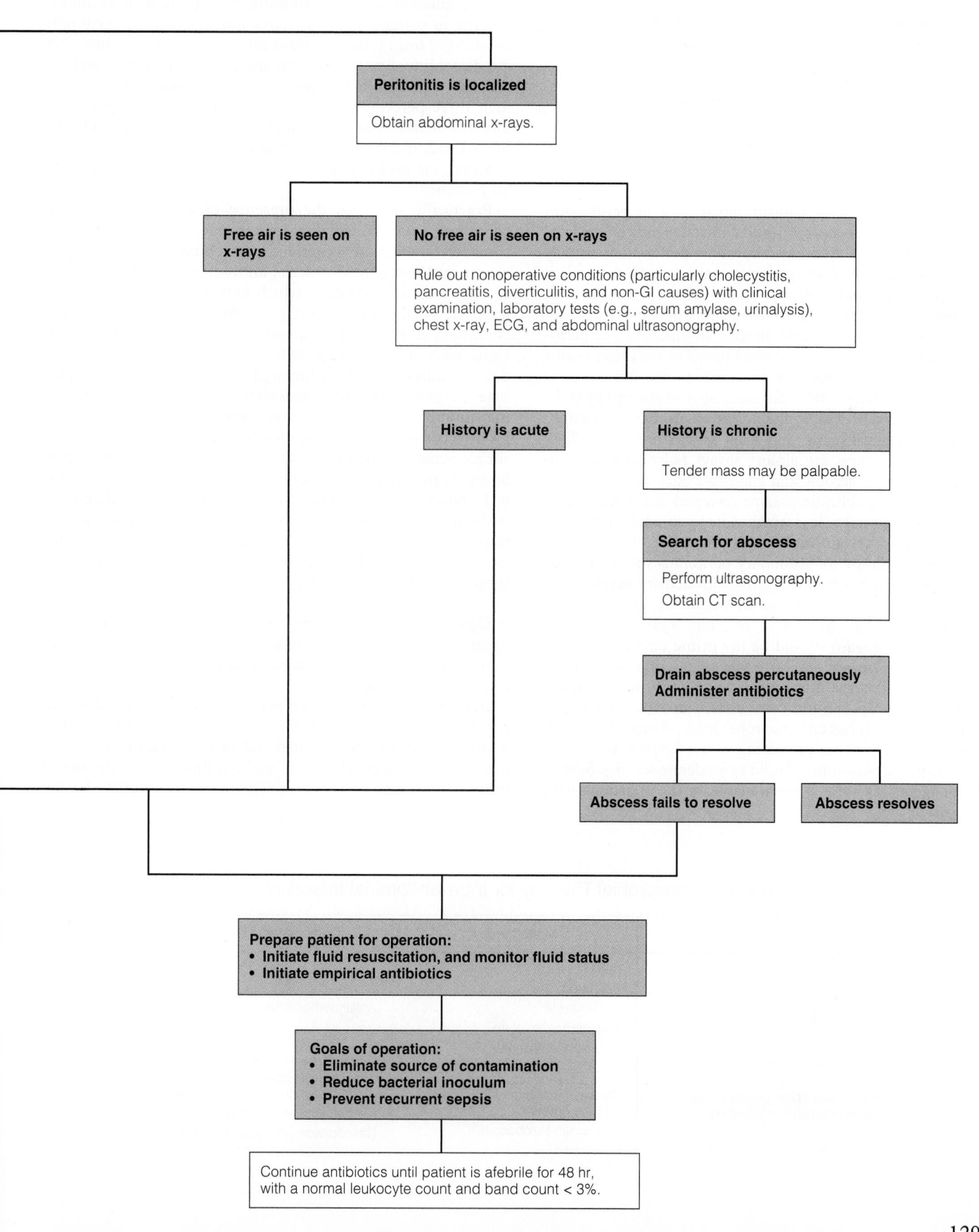

Peritonitis is localized

Obtain abdominal x-rays.

Free air is seen on x-rays

No free air is seen on x-rays

Rule out nonoperative conditions (particularly cholecystitis, pancreatitis, diverticulitis, and non-GI causes) with clinical examination, laboratory tests (e.g., serum amylase, urinalysis), chest x-ray, ECG, and abdominal ultrasonography.

History is acute

History is chronic

Tender mass may be palpable.

Search for abscess

Perform ultrasonography.
Obtain CT scan.

**Drain abscess percutaneously
Administer antibiotics**

Abscess fails to resolve

Abscess resolves

Prepare patient for operation:
• **Initiate fluid resuscitation, and monitor fluid status**
• **Initiate empirical antibiotics**

Goals of operation:
• **Eliminate source of contamination**
• **Reduce bacterial inoculum**
• **Prevent recurrent sepsis**

Continue antibiotics until patient is afebrile for 48 hr, with a normal leukocyte count and band count < 3%.

Table 2   Bacteria Causing Secondary Peritonitis

Aerobic bacteria	Anaerobic bacteria
Escherichia coli	*Bacteroides*
Streptococci	*B. fragilis*
Enterobacter, Klebsiella	Eubacteria
Enterococci	*Clostridium*
Proteus	Anaerobic streptococci

The spectrum of microorganisms inoculating the peritoneum after perforation of the gastrointestinal tract depends on the level of the perforation.[7] Upper gastrointestinal perforations usually release predominantly gram-positive organisms, which are sensitive to penicillins and cephalosporins. Patients who have been taking antacids or H_2-receptor blockers have greater numbers of facultative gram-negative bacilli in their stomachs before perforation.[8] Perforation of the distal small bowel or the colon results in the release of more than 500 bacterial species into the peritoneal cavity. It is noteworthy that many species are rapidly eliminated by host defenses or by the hostile environment. In established intraperitoneal sepsis, only a few species remain [*see Table 2*].[9-11] These infections are almost always polymicrobial, containing a mixture of aerobic and anaerobic bacteria.[9,11]

Several recent publications have reviewed antibiotic use in patients with peritonitis. It is worthwhile to summarize the recommendations for antibiotic selection [*see Table 3*].[12,13] Antimicrobial therapy for secondary peritonitis should include an agent or a combination of agents with activity against both aerobic and anaerobic bacteria. In particular, gram-negative enteric bacteria (e.g., *Escherichia coli*) and anaerobic bacteria (e.g., *Bacteroides fragilis*) should be the prime targets of antibiotic therapy. There are several single agents or combinations that fulfill these criteria. Both single-drug therapy with a broad-spectrum cephalosporin and combination therapy with agents effective against aerobes and anaerobes have proved effective for the treatment of patients presenting to the hospital with community-acquired peritonitis of mild to moderate severity. Several different agents [*see Table 3*] are available for use in patients with

postoperative peritonitis or severe physiologic derangements related to the development of peritonitis. Aminoglycosides should be used with care in elderly patients and in patients with hypotension, renal dysfunction, or both.

The guidelines for determining the duration of antibiotic therapy in patients after operative management of peritonitis are derived from retrospective studies evaluating outcome after the discontinuance of antibiotic therapy. If a patient is afebrile and has a normal leukocyte count and a band count of less than three percent, then the chance of recurrent sepsis after discontinuance of antibiotic therapy is virtually zero.[14] On the other hand, if the patient's temperature or leukocyte count is elevated, the probability of recurrent sepsis ranges from 33 to 50 percent.[15]

Practically speaking, the presence of a normal leukocyte count and a normal rectal temperature for 48 hours should be considered adequate criteria for stopping antibiotics. In a recent trial using these criteria, antibiotics were discontinued at an average of eight days, which indicated that these criteria were usually met by about day 6.[16] Antibiotics have been discontinued as early as postoperative day 4 with this approach. Conversely, if leukocytosis or fever persists after postoperative day 7, a diligent search is initiated to locate the source of persistent sepsis. There are several clinical circumstances in which the duration of antibiotic therapy approximates that used for prophylaxis rather than that used for treatment. These include simple acute appendicitis, necrotic small intestine without perforation, and traumatic enteric perforations operated on within 12 hours of injury.[12] The common feature of these diagnoses is the minimal degree of peritoneal soiling and inflammatory response present at the time of laparotomy. A preoperative dose of antibiotics followed by two doses within 24 hours of surgery is appropriate therapy for these conditions.

Operative management   The goals of operative management of peritonitis are to eliminate the source of contamination, to reduce the bacterial inoculum, and to prevent recurrent or persistent infection.

In patients with generalized peritonitis, the incision of choice is a midline vertical incision, which provides access to the entire abdomen and is readily opened and closed. When peritonitis is localized, as in appendicitis, an incision directly over the site of inflammation may be adequate. The use of laparoscopy for the

---

Table 3   Antimicrobial Therapy for Intra-abdominal Infection[13]

	Monotherapy	Combination Therapy
Community-acquired infections of mild to moderate severity	Cefoxitin Cefotetan Cefmetazole Ampicillin-sulbactam Ticarcillin-clavulanate	Antianaerobe plus aminoglycoside
Severe infections (possibly resistant gram-negative organisms)	Carbapenem imipenem-cilastatin or meropenem Piperacillin-tazobactam	Antianaerobe plus third-generation cephalosporin or aminoglycoside Clindamycin plus aztreonam Ciprofloxacin plus metronidazole

Table 4 Surgical Options for Common Causes of Peritonitis[17]

Pathology	Options	Comments
Perforated duodenal ulcer	• Omental patch • Omental patch and vagotomy plus drainage (gastrojejunostomy or pyloroplasty)	• Definitive surgery may be considered when operation is performed early, there is minimal peritoneal soiling, and there is a history of chronic peptic ulcer disease • Bypass procedure rather than simple outlet drainage may be necessary if gastric outlet is obstructed
Perforated gastric ulcer	• Gastric resection, including ulcer with Billroth I or II anastomosis • Excision of ulcer with primary closure ± patch	• Resection is preferred when perforation occurs at the site of malignancy • A patch may be considered in an elderly or unstable patient or when perforation is in a difficult area (e.g., proximal stomach)
Small bowel infarction/perforation	• Resection of small bowel with primary anastomosis • Resection of small bowel with exteriorization of ends	• The need for primary anastomosis depends on the degree of peritoneal soiling, the magnitude of the inflammatory response, and patient status
Appendicitis	Appendectomy	Perform laparoscopic appendectomy if feasible [*see text*]
Large bowel perforation	• Resection with end colostomy (ileostomy) and mucous fistula or Hartmann's procedure • Defunctioning colostomy with drainage	• Resection is preferred, but defunctioning with drainage may be used if inflammation is too intense for safe resection • Anastomosis after resection for free perforation is generally considered unsafe; when resection encompasses peridiverticular abscess, anastomosis may be considered
Postoperative peritonitis	• Depends on underlying pathology: For anastomotic dehiscence, exteriorize ends when possible; use drain ± defunction if exteriorization not possible	• Reanastomosis or closure of anastomotic dehiscence is not likely to be successful
Cholecystitis ± perforation or pericholecystic abscess	• Laparoscopic cholecystectomy • Tube cholecystostomy	• Laparoscopy is more likely to be successful if performed earlier • Use tube cholecystostomy (operative) when resection is not possible; in the critically ill, consider percutaneous cholecystostomy

diagnosis and treatment of various pathological entities, such as acute appendicitis and acute cholecystitis, has modified this approach to a significant degree. Incisions are made away from the inflamed organ to provide better visualization of the operative field and to permit manipulation of the tissues from various angles.

The operative technique used to control contamination depends on the location and the nature of the pathological condition in the gastrointestinal tract [*see Table 4*].[17] In general, continued peritoneal soiling is controlled by closing, excluding, or resecting the perforated viscus. When feasible, resection of the diseased tissue appears to be the best option, preventing continued contamination from the source. One important exception to this principle occurs when the GI tract is disrupted by trauma. In cases of hollow-viscus injury, with minimal peritoneal contamination in a patient in stable condition with a limited number of associated injuries, primary closure of the viscus is optimal.[18-20] For an inflammatory process where the disease is expected to progress in the absence of a frank perforation (e.g., acute appendicitis or small bowel necrosis), resection is clearly preferred, because the underlying disease, if left in situ, will act as a focus of ongoing infection. Occasionally, self-limited inflammatory processes are unexpectedly discovered at laparotomy.

Examples include acute Crohn's disease, an ischemic but viable loop of torsive small intestine, and acute phlegmonous pancreatitis. Under these circumstances, excision is not indicated, and treatment should address the underlying pathology.

Technical factors may also preclude resection of the diseased viscus. Perforation of extraperitoneal viscera such as the duodenum and the rectum is not routinely treated by excision, because of the technical difficulties of operating on these organs during acute inflammation. Similarly, extremely intense inflammatory changes may prevent safe excision of various organs that usually can be resected during acute inflammation. These include the gallbladder in cases of acute cholecystitis and a portion of the intraperitoneal GI tract in cases of acute perforated diverticulitis. For a pathological condition of the colon, control is usually accomplished by resecting the perforated segment of intestine, exteriorizing the proximal end as an end colostomy, and dealing with the distal end by creating a mucous fistula or oversewing it. The general principle is that a primary anastomosis in this location is at high risk for dehiscence and should be avoided.[21]

The risk associated with primary anastomosis of the small intestine after resection of a diseased segment is much lower. However, resection plus proximal and distal enterostomy may be appropriate if peritoneal soiling is particularly extensive or if the viability of the intestine is uncertain. Perforation of the duodenum because of peptic ulcer disease may be safely patched with a piece of omentum; a perforated gastric ulcer is either included in a distal gastric resection with subsequent gastroduodenal or gastrojejunal anastomosis or locally excised with primary closure. Appendicitis is treated by appendectomy.

Laparoscopy is a major advance in the diagnosis and management of the acute abdomen. Several reports demonstrate that laparoscopic cholecystectomy [see V:12 Laparoscopic Cholecystectomy] is safe for the treatment of acute cholecystitis and can reduce the length of stay. There is little morbidity in patients treated successfully by the laparoscopic approach. The principal reason for conversion is the presence of extensive adhesions or inflammation, precluding safe identification and dissection within Calot's triangle.[22,23] This is more common in patients with gangrenous cholecystitis or empyema of the gallbladder.[24,25] Compared with delayed or even interval cholecystectomy, a laparoscopic approach appears to have a higher success rate if performed early in the course of the disease.[26,27] Trocar insertion may be safer via an open technique, reducing the likelihood of hollow-viscus injury in the presence of an ileus.

Laparoscopic appendectomy, a logical extension of diagnostic laparoscopy for lower abdominal pain, appears to be safe and can be performed with a low conversion rate. Conversions are often caused by a perforated appendix or an inflammatory mass.[28] For patients with nonperforated appendicitis, the duration of hospital stay and the return to work appear to be independent of the approach (open versus laparoscopic), but hospital costs are higher for laparoscopic surgery.[29-31] For complicated appendicitis, laparoscopic removal shortens the hospital stay. Laparoscopic management of perforated gastric and duodenal ulcers, recently reported, appears to be effective.[32]

The second major goal of operative management of peritonitis is to reduce the bacterial inoculum and to prevent recurrent or persistent sepsis. At operation, gross purulent exudates should be aspirated, and loculations in the pelvis, paracolic gutters, and subphrenic regions should be gently opened and debrided. An attempt should be made to remove particulate debris, such as fecal matter or barium sulfate, if present.

Although intraoperative peritoneal lavage has become a standard procedure during operation for peritonitis, its efficacy has not been well documented. Its major roles are to reduce the quantity of bacteria and to remove adjuvant substances. The fear that this procedure may disseminate bacteria is probably unfounded; experimental studies have demonstrated that dynamics in the peritoneum cause locally applied bacteria to spread rapidly throughout the peritoneal cavity even without irrigation. The risk of leaving collections of infected fluid undrained is probably greater than the risk of spreading a small inoculum of bacteria within the peritoneal cavity. However, because the fluid itself acts as an adjuvant to infection by impairing phagocytosis and leukocyte migration, it is imperative that all fluid collections be aspirated before the abdomen is closed.

It is impossible to drain the peritoneal cavity in patients with diffuse peritonitis. Therefore, the use of drains in these patients is not indicated unless (1) the drain is to be used for postoperative lavage, (2) the drain is placed in a well-defined abscess cavity, and (3) the drain is used to establish a controlled fistula. Drains left in situ are not innocuous: they may erode into the intestine or the blood vessels or provide external bacteria with an access route into the peritoneal cavity. Researchers have demonstrated that children in whom Penrose drains were placed at operation for perforated appendicitis averaged 3.7 more hospital days than those without drains.[33]

Abdominal wall closure is accomplished with a single fascial layer of either interrupted or running monofilament suture. We routinely use Prolene, although wire or nylon is also acceptable. In the elderly, malnourished, or immunocompromised patient, full-thickness abdominal wall retention sutures are used in addition to the fascial closure. Care should be taken not to tie these sutures too tightly, because abdominal distention and abdominal wall swelling may cause pressure necrosis at suture insertion sites and lead to stitch abscesses and spreading cellulitis.

Because the risk of wound infection associated with diffuse peritonitis is 20 percent or greater, wounds should be managed by delayed primary closure of the skin and subcutaneous tissues.[34] The wound is gently packed with saline-soaked gauze during operation, and the gauze is changed every eight hours for three to four days. At that time, if the wound appears clean, with a granulating base, the skin edges can be apposed with skin tapes or fine sutures. The practice of obtaining a biopsy specimen from the subcutaneous tissue and performing quantitative bacterial counts to determine whether the wound is safe to close is somewhat impractical and is rarely undertaken.[35] If any question exists about the wound, it can be left open and allowed to close secondarily. The technique of closure of the primary wound over suction catheters irrigated with antibiotics has not reduced wound infection rates in the abdomen.[36]

PRIMARY PERITONITIS

Primary peritonitis is defined as an infection of the peritoneal cavity in which there is no obvious source, such as a perforated viscus. This type of peritonitis occurs in both children and adults.

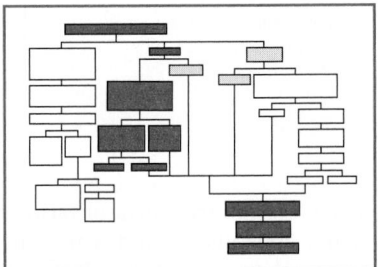

The incidence of primary peritonitis in children appears to be decreasing.[37] In the preantibiotic era, it accounted for 10 percent of acute abdominal emergencies; this incidence has been reduced to approximately one to two percent.[38,39] Children with nephrotic syndrome or postnecrotic cirrhosis appear to be at particularly high risk.[38] In adults, the presence of alcoholic cirrhosis and ascites is the most frequent underlying risk factor.[40] Primary peritonitis represents a significant source of morbidity and mortality in cirrhotic patients with ascites: it is present in 10 to 25 percent of these patients on hospital admission and accounts for as many as 30 percent of all infections in cirrhotic patients.[41,42] Cirrhotic ascites predisposes to infection because of reduced total protein and complement levels, which result in impaired bacterial opsonization.[43] Patients with systemic lupus erythematosus may also be subject to primary peritonitis or serositis; the latter mimics peritonitis and may necessitate operation.[44]

Causative organisms generally fall into two categories, depending on the patient's age. In children, the usual organisms are gram-positive cocci, such as Streptococcus pneumoniae and group A streptococci.[37,38] In cirrhotic patients, monomicrobial infections with enteric microorganisms, particularly *E. coli*, tend to predominate.[45] Anaerobes are rare, and in marked contrast to the frequency of polymicrobial infection in patients with secondary peritonitis, polymicrobial infection is present in fewer than 10 percent of cases. Immunocompromised patients are at risk for the development of primary peritonitis. In patients with the acquired immunodeficiency syndrome, *M. tuberculosis*, cytomegalovirus, and a variety of other opportunistic pathogens may cause primary peritonitis.[46]

Clinical Presentation and Diagnosis

In children, the clinical picture mimics that of secondary bacterial peritonitis with presenting signs and symptoms consisting of fever, nausea, vomiting, and abdominal pain. Abdominal examination reveals diffuse tenderness, rebound tenderness, guarding, and loss of bowel sounds. Primary peritonitis in patients with cirrhosis presents in a more subtle fashion. These patients may have a low-grade fever with minimal or no abdominal tenderness and peritonitis masked by evidence of hepatic decompensation, such as encephalopathy, hepatorenal syndrome, or increased accumulation of ascitic fluid. Tuberculous peritonitis is usually gradual in onset, with fever, night sweats, weight loss, and progressive abdominal distention. Abdominal examination may reveal some increased tone with mild diffuse discomfort on palpation. Classic signs of peritonitis are usually absent.

Primary peritonitis in children is rarely diagnosed preoperatively. Children presenting to the hospital with evidence of peritonitis usually undergo laparotomy with a provisional diagnosis of acute appendicitis. The diagnosis is made after a negative laparotomy, when gram-positive organisms are cultured from the peritoneal swabs.

In cirrhotic patients with evidence of peritonitis, a much more conservative approach is taken because of the high operative risk in these patients.[47] Two major diagnostic issues should be addressed in these patients, who frequently present with an atypical clinical picture. The first objective is to decide whether the patient has peritonitis so that treatment can be initiated. This is readily accomplished by diagnostic paracentesis. Fluid should be examined for the cell count and differential, pH, and levels of lactate, glucose, protein, and lactic dehydrogenase; Gram's stain and cultures should be performed as well. The most accurate method of culturing ascitic fluid is to inoculate 10 to 20 ml into an aerobic blood culture bottle and the same amount into an anaerobic bottle. Inoculation should be done at the bedside to enhance the sensitivity of the test.[48,49] Gram's stain of a centrifuged specimen of ascitic fluid, although helpful when positive, has a high false negative rate (60 to 80 percent).[40] Because an incubation period of 24 to 72 hours is necessary before peritonitis can be diagnosed microbiologically, it is optimal to rely on a few rapid tests to guide the initiation of therapy. In many studies,[50,51] an elevated neutrophil count ($> 250/mm^3$), a reduced pH (< 7.35), and an elevated lactate level (> 32 mg/dl) have been found to be highly predictive of the presence of peritonitis. One review of several studies concluded that evaluation of the neutrophil count in the ascitic fluid was the single best test for the detection of peritonitis and that elevation of this count was an indication for treatment.[52] An elevated neutrophil count in combination with an elevated arterial–ascitic fluid pH gradient (> 0.10) or a reduced ascitic fluid pH has a diagnostic accuracy of 91 to 97 percent.[50]

The diagnosis of peritonitis having been established, it is critical to determine whether the peritonitis is from perforation or inflammation of the gastrointestinal tract (i.e., secondary peritonitis) or spontaneous (i.e., primary peritonitis). It is difficult to distinguish these entities on the basis of clinical findings or the magnitude of the increase in the ascitic fluid neutrophil count. If the ascitic fluid is found to have a glucose level below 50 mg/dl, a lactic dehydrogenase level higher than the upper limit of the normal serum range, and a protein concentration higher than 1 g/dl, the likelihood of secondary peritonitis is significantly increased, and further investigation is warranted.[52] Plain abdominal x-rays should be taken, and Gastrografin studies should be done. Surgical intervention is indicated if (1) the ascitic fluid culture yields a mixed aerobic-anaerobic flora, (2) Gastrografin studies reveal leakage from the gastrointestinal tract, (3) free air is present on x-ray views of the abdomen, and (4) the patient fails to benefit from medical therapy. A repeat paracentesis 48 hours after initiation of therapy may be helpful because in primary peritonitis, the leukocyte count falls rapidly, whereas in secondary peritonitis, it remains stable or rises.[53] Obviously, if the fluid aspirate reveals gross feces, bile, or blood-tinged material, then a surgical course is indicated. However, this scenario is rare.

The diagnosis of tuberculous peritonitis is made by laparoscopy, with characteristic findings of a thickened peritoneum with miliary yellow-white tubercles.[54] In most cases, diagnosis can be based on the gross findings, supplemented by results of a laparoscopic peritoneal biopsy. Systemic antimicrobials directed against *M. tuberculosis* are indicated.

Management

Bacterial peritonitis caused by *S. pneumoniae* or group A streptococci should be treated with intravenous penicillin G. Single-drug therapy with cefotaxime is the preferred regimen for spontaneous bacterial peritonitis and is associated with less toxicity than aminoglycoside-containing regimens.[55] Antimicrobial therapy should be adjusted when the results of culture and sensitivity testing become available. There is no specific indication for peritoneal dialysis in these patients, because parenterally administered antibiotics achieve adequate levels in ascitic fluid.

The duration of therapy for spontaneous bacterial peritonitis is now better defined. Recurrent infection after the neutrophil count in the ascitic fluid falls below $250/mm^3$ is extremely rare.[56] In a randomized trial, five days of therapy was equal to 10 days with respect to mortality, cure rate, and recurrence rate.[57]

Prognosis Hospital mortality for cirrhotic patients in whom spontaneous bacterial peritonitis develops is approximately 50 percent[58]; most of the deaths are the result of liver failure. Furthermore, survivors of the initial episode of peritonitis are at high risk for recurrence (69 percent at one year) and have a significantly shorter survival than comparable cirrhotic patients in whom peritonitis does not develop.[59] This complication of cirrhosis may be the sign of a high-failure group that might benefit from liver transplantation.

Prevention of recurrent peritonitis may influence the outcome in this high-risk population. In one study, selective intestinal decontamination with oral norfloxacin, 400 mg a day, lowered the probability of recurrence from 68 percent to 20 percent at one year.[60] Overall mortality, however, was not altered; most patients died of liver failure and its complications. Other antimicrobials, including ciprofloxacin and trimethoprim-sulfamethoxazole, demonstrate comparable effects.[61,62] These data suggest that spontaneous bacterial peritonitis is a predictor of poor outcome caused by progressive liver failure rather than an independent cause of increased mortality.

PERITONITIS IN PERITONEAL DIALYSIS PATIENTS

Clinical Presentation and Diagnosis

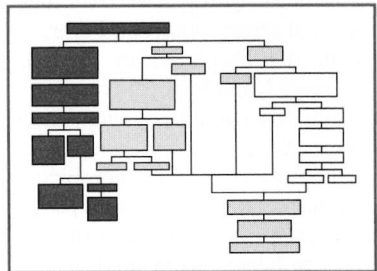

The manifestations of peritonitis in patients on peritoneal dialysis include mild abdominal pain, low-grade fever, and mild abdominal tenderness. These manifestations tend to be variable, probably because the dialysate dilutes or removes some of the products of inflammation. One definition of peritonitis includes satisfaction of at least two of the following criteria: (1) the presence of microorganisms on Gram's stain or culture of the peritoneal effluent, (2) cloudy fluid with inflammatory cells (leukocyte count > 100/mm³, with at least 50 percent neutrophils), and (3) signs and symptoms of peritoneal inflammation.[63] Occasionally, although the effluent may be contaminated with microorganisms, there are no signs of clinical infection. These findings do not constitute an episode of peritonitis, and dialysis should be continued without antibiotic therapy.

Management

Selection of antimicrobial agents In cases of peritonitis, specific antimicrobial agents must be selected before culture results are available. Thus, treatment decisions are based on the most probable causative microorganisms. Normal skin commensals are the most common causative microbes, with staphylococcal species accounting for 45 to 60 percent of all peritonitis episodes. Two thirds of these are attributable to *Staphylococcus epidermidis* and one third to *S. aureus*. Gram-negative bacteria account for 20 to 35 percent; the remainder are caused by fungi, anaerobes, and mycobacterial species.[64]

The choice of antimicrobial agent or agents should reflect the fact that gram-positive or gram-negative microorganisms cause about 90 percent of episodes, and the choice should consider sensitivity patterns within the specific institution. In our institution, we take the following approach when peritonitis is suspected. Patients are instructed to drain the fluid in the abdomen completely and to put the effluent aside for culture and cell count. The next 2 L bag, containing 1 g of cefazolin (1.5 g if body weight exceeds 50 kg) and 40 mg of tobramycin (60 mg if body weight exceeds 50 kg), is allowed to dwell for eight hours. Three more 2 L exchanges, without antibiotics, are evenly spaced over the remainder of the 24-hour period. If the aminoglycoside is given once daily, aminoglycoside levels need not be monitored. Heparin (500 to 1,000 U) is added to each bag, and a two percent lidocaine solution is included if there is significant pain. The effluent is sent daily for cell counts and every other day for culture. The selection of an antibiotic depends on whether culture results are available. In centers where methicillin-resistant staphylococci are common, the empirical regimen should include 1 g of vancomycin (2 g if body weight exceeds 50 kg) instead of a cephalosporin. Be-

cause of its long half-life in patients with renal failure and its limited clearance by dialysis, vancomycin is administered once every seven days.[65]

Within three to four days of the initiation of therapy, clinical improvement as well as a decreased cell count in the dialysate should occur. The optimal length of therapy is not well established, varying from center to center and ranging from seven to 21 days. One approach is to continue treatment for seven days after the last positive culture is obtained. For some microorganisms, such as *Pseudomonas* or *Xanthomonas* species, antibiotic treatment should be continued for at least 21 days. If clinical improvement does not occur within four to five days, antibiotic selection should be reevaluated on the basis of culture results. If severe peritonitis persists, the dialysis cannula should be removed. Rapid resolution by catheter removal helps maintain a peritoneal membrane capable of efficient exchange.

Additional issues In addition to the standard treatment protocol, a few specific issues should be addressed. The first is the management of exit-site and tunnel infections. These infections rarely cause symptoms. Exit-site infections produce local inflammation and a purulent discharge. Tunnel infections are more difficult to diagnose, particularly if there is no accompanying exit-site infection. In about 50 percent of patients, these infections can be managed by daily cleansing of the exit site with a disinfectant, together with oral administration of antibiotics.

The next issue is catheter removal and replacement. Catheters should be removed (1) when there is a persistently infected exit site or tunnel tract, (2) when there are recurrent episodes of peritonitis caused by the same organism (i.e., when the catheter may be the source), or (3) when laparotomy is required for fecal peritonitis. Occasionally, when virulent organisms, such as *Pseudomonas* species or fungi, are the causative agents, antibiotic therapy may fail, and catheter removal is required to resolve the infection.[66] Catheters removed for exit-site infections can be replaced at a new site. However, catheters removed for recurrent or fecal peritonitis should not be replaced for two to three weeks to allow the peritonitis to resolve. Dialysis can be continued during this period with a temporary catheter placed at the time of removal or with hemodialysis. One study has advocated immediate replacement of a permanent cannula, thereby obviating hemodialysis[67]; this approach may be appropriate in certain circumstances. For example, patients with recurrent bouts of peritonitis in whom the most recent bout has been adequately treated are good candidates for catheter replacement during the same operation. However, catheter replacement is probably not indicated for more complex infections, such as those caused by *Pseudomonas* species, fungi, mycobacteria, and polymicrobial fecal flora.[65]

An obvious solution to the problem of catheter-related infection is prevention. Strict aseptic technique is the most important preventive measure. The Y-system "flush-before-fill," in which the patient flushes sections of the administration set and the catheter between exchanges, has been reported to reduce the infection rate markedly.[68] Oral antimicrobial prophylaxis with cephalexin has been shown to be ineffective.[69] Nasal carriage of *S. aureus* appears to be associated with an increased risk of infection at the exit site of the catheter.[70] One study[71] suggested that intranasal mupirocin markedly reduced *S. aureus* exit-site infection and peritonitis and lessened the rate of catheter loss; the recolonization rate was frequent, however, and retreatment was required periodically.

The management of patients whose peritoneal fluid cultures reveal multiple enteric organisms or anaerobic bacteria, or both, requires comment. If organisms appear during the first 24 to 48 hours after percutaneous insertion of a temporary catheter, laparotomy should be performed for closure of the presumed perforated segment of intestine and for reinsertion of the catheter. In patients on long-term dialysis, such underlying gastrointestinal pathological conditions as appendicitis, perforated diverticulitis, or a perforated duodenal ulcer are likely to be the cause. Hypaque studies of the gastrointestinal tract may help confirm the diagnosis and the need for operation. At our institution, a laparotomy is not performed when the contrast examination is normal, the patient shows clinical improvement on dialysis, and the effluent is rendered sterile by appropriate antibiotics. In one review, 10 episodes of peritonitis with multiple enteric organisms were treated in this manner.[72] Four patients had persisting abdominal pain and required laparotomy. Significant pathological conditions were found in all four, including perforating appendicitis, gangrenous cholecystitis, perforated sigmoid diverticulitis, and perforated cecum. No postoperative sequelae were reported. Of the remaining six patients, all responded to antibiotic therapy and did not require laparotomy. Presumably, these patients had walled-off perforations of the gastrointestinal tract that were adequately controlled by local mechanisms.

Intra-abdominal Abscess

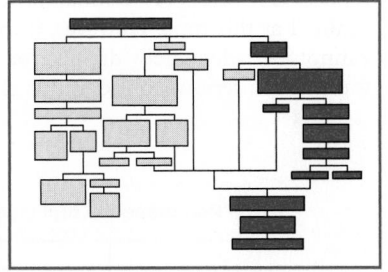

Abscesses are well-defined collections of pus that are walled off from the rest of the peritoneal cavity by inflammatory adhesions, loops of intestine and their mesentery, the greater omentum, or other abdominal viscera. Abscesses may occur in the peritoneal cavity, either within or outside of abdominal viscera, as well as in the retroperitoneum.[73] Extravisceral abscesses arise in two situations: (1) after resolution of diffuse peritonitis in which a loculated area of infection persists and evolves into an abscess and (2) after perforation of a viscus or an anastomotic breakdown that is successfully walled off by peritoneal defense mechanisms. More than 80 percent of intra-abdominal abscesses occur in the postoperative period, the majority after pancreaticobiliary or colorectal surgery [see Table 5].[74,75] This pattern may reflect the technical difficulty of anastomoses in the former and the large bacterial load in the latter. Over 30 percent of abscesses are associated with clear evidence of an anastomotic leak.[75] By contrast, intra-abdominal abscesses unassociated with previous surgery are usually attributable to inflammatory processes with a small, localized perforation, as in appendicitis, diverticulitis, and Crohn's disease.[75,76] Visceral abscesses are most commonly caused by hematogenous or lymphatic spread of bacteria to the organ. Retroperitoneal abscesses may be caused by several mechanisms, including perforation of the gastrointestinal tract into the retroperitoneum and hematogenous or lymphatic spread of bacteria to retroperitoneal organs, particularly the inflamed pancreas.

Table 5 Incidence of Postoperative Abscess Formation in Relation to Site of Initial Operation[74]

Site of Operation	Incidence of Postoperative Abscess (%)
Pancreas and biliary tract	20
Colon	15
Stomach	9
Retroperitoneum	9
Trauma laparotomy	9
Duodenum	8
Appendix	6
Kidney and adrenal gland	5
Small intestine	4
Spleen	4
Liver	4
Vascular	2
Uterus and ovary	1
Others	11

CLINICAL PRESENTATION AND DIAGNOSIS

Diagnosis is based on clinical suspicion of an abscess and radiologic confirmation of this suspicion. Patients with intra-abdominal abscesses usually have local and systemic signs of inflammation. Characteristically, mild abdominal pain and localized tenderness exist in the region of the infection. Because of the presence of adherent omentum, bowel, or adjacent viscera, it is common to feel a diffuse, rather than a discrete, mass. The patient is usually febrile and anorexic and has a leukocytosis with a shift to the left. The clinical findings associated with an intra-abdominal abscess may be masked by the administration of antibiotics to the patient. However, as previously noted, in the face of antibiotic use, the presence of a fever or a leukocytosis with a band count higher than three percent, or both, is highly indicative of persistent sepsis and should lead to more intensive investigation of the patient's condition.[14,15]

The armamentarium of radiologic techniques available for the diagnosis of intra-abdominal sepsis is quite extensive.[77] Plain abdominal x-rays, though rarely diagnostic, frequently point to the need for further investigation. These x-ray findings may document loculated extraluminal gas collections or mottled soft tissue masses, either of which is indicative of abscess formation. More subtle signs include the presence of a localized ileus, a pleural effusion, and atelectasis. A limited contrast examination may be useful, particularly when left upper quadrant abnormalities are found on x-ray examination, to differentiate the stomach from an extraluminal mass or to detect a leak. This investigation may be particularly important after splenectomy, when fluid may collect in the left upper quadrant as the result of a gastric fistula developing from the greater curvature of the stomach. Suspicion of an abscess, based on either clinical or basic radiologic findings, should indicate the necessity for imaging techniques to confirm the diagnosis and to pinpoint the location of the abscess.

Ultrasonography and computed tomographic scanning are clearly the examinations of choice; studies comparing the various techniques of imaging an abscess usually suggest CT scanning to be the superior modality.[78,79] Our general approach is to suit the imaging technique to the patient. If the potential site of infection can be localized clinically, then ultrasonography is used to confirm clinical suspicions and to direct diagnostic aspiration of the collection. If the patient appears clinically septic but the site of the infection is not obvious or if the ultrasonographic examination is unsatisfactory, then we prefer to use CT scanning of the abdomen. Nuclear medicine techniques are rarely used in this setting.

MANAGEMENT

Three basic principles guide the management of intra-abdominal abscesses: (1) general patient care, (2) antibiotic administration, and (3) drainage of the abscess.

General Patient Care

Patients with intra-abdominal abscess show a spectrum of clinical presentations: they range from the relatively well with low-grade fever and leukocytosis to those with septic shock. Clearly, the initial management of all such patients should be tailored to their clinical picture. In general, these patients have some degree of intravascular volume depletion that calls for fluid resuscitation. Resuscitation should be monitored by observing vital signs, urine output, and mental status. In the critically ill patient, Swan-Ganz catheterization and invasive arterial monitoring are essential to direct initial resuscitation, particularly if administration of inotropic agents is necessary.

Hypoxemia may be present for several reasons. Atelectasis, basilar pneumonia, and pleural effusions may exist secondary to abdominal distention with elevation of the diaphragm as well as to subphrenic infectious processes.[80] In addition, advanced sepsis may result in increased alveolar-capillary permeability and the development of adult respiratory distress syndrome in the context of the multiple organ dysfunction syndrome (MODS).[81]

Nutritional support is important in the management of patients with intra-abdominal abscess. Patients in whom abscesses develop in the postoperative period are already at a nutritional disadvantage because they have usually spent seven to 10 days without adequate caloric intake. The marked catabolic response associated with sepsis further aggravates this problem.[82] Historically, total parenteral nutrition has been preferred in patients with intra-abdominal infection. Recent evidence, however, suggests that nutritional supplementation by the enteral route may reduce the incidence of infectious complications and improve the immune status of critically ill patients.[83,84] Furthermore, enteral feeding within 24 hours of laparotomy appears to be well tolerated in most patients. This approach may be used in patients with enterocutaneous fistulas if adequate drainage prevents further contamination of the peritoneal cavity.[85] Feeding is usually accomplished by passing a tube into the upper small intestine and using an enteral pump to administer the solution. Such a technique avoids the complications of vomiting and aspiration associated with gastroparesis. In patients for whom enteral feeding is not satisfactory, parenteral nutrition should be instituted. Total caloric requirements, optimal amino acid solutions, and lipid requirements are dealt with elsewhere [*see VII:9 Nutritional Support*].

Antibiotics

Antibiotic therapy should be directed against the microorganisms most likely to be recovered from the abscess, which almost always include a combination of aerobic and anaerobic bacteria.[86] As for secondary peritonitis, administration of antibiotic combinations or single agents that are active against both aerobes and anaerobes is generally considered the gold standard for the management of intra-abdominal infection [*see Table 3*].

It should be emphasized that general patient care and antibiotic therapy serve primarily as adjuncts to drainage of the abscess cavity. Antibiotics alone are unlikely to be effective for numerous reasons, including poor penetration of antibiotics into the abscess center, inactivation of antibiotics in the microenvironment of the infection (i.e., hypoxia and acidity), and inactivity of the drug against a large bacterial inoculum. Drainage of an abscess usually reverses these adverse conditions and increases the efficacy of the antibiotics.

Drainage

Drainage, either percutaneous or surgical, is the mainstay of the management of intra-abdominal abscess. The ability to perform either technique depends on precise localization of the infection by means of CT scanning or ultrasonography.

Percutaneous drainage has made a major contribution to the management of intra-abdominal abscess. It is the treatment of choice in the management of single, well-defined intra-abdominal abscesses. The management of the patient with a well-defined abscess amenable to drainage requires close collaboration between the radiologist and the surgeon. In essence, the problem is approached from a surgical viewpoint, except that percutaneous drainage is used [*see Figure 1*]. If the patient has not improved markedly by 48 hours after initial percutaneous drainage, he or she is returned to the radiology department for a repeat CT scan. A residual abscess will be percutaneously drained at this time. However, if there is residual infection that cannot be adequately drained or if no residual collection is found, then serious consideration should be given to performing

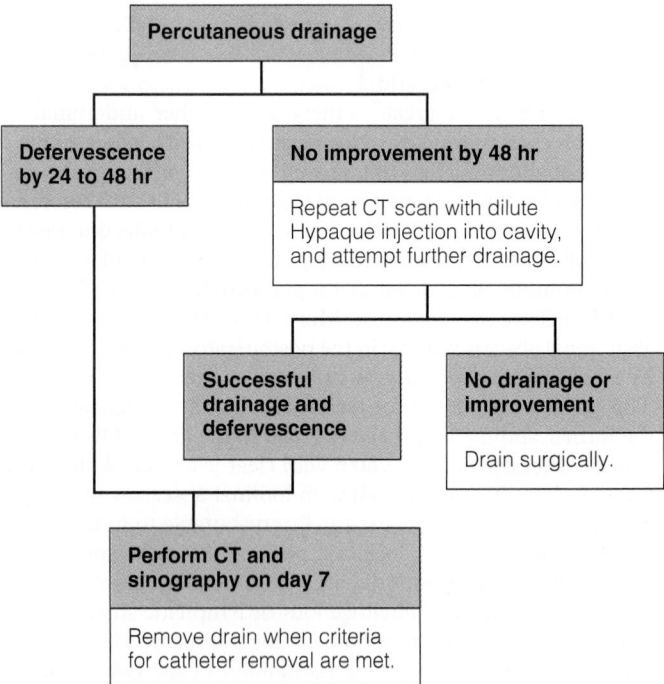

Figure 1 **Algorithm outlines the management of intra-abdominal abscess by means of percutaneous drainage.**

a formal laparotomy. Criteria for removal of the percutaneous catheter are (1) clinical resolution of sepsis as determined by the patient's well-being, temperature, and leukocyte count, (2) minimal drainage from the catheter, and (3) radiologic evidence of resolution of the abscess on sinogram or CT scan. The overall duration of drainage varies widely, ranging from four to 30 days. In general, prolonged periods of drainage are related to the presence of an enteric communication. Major complications of percutaneous drainage, which include hemorrhage, enteric fistula, and empyema, are relatively rare.

Improved localization techniques using either ultrasonography or CT scanning have also greatly simplified the surgical approach to the treatment of intra-abdominal abscess. Before the regular use of these techniques, a general abdominal explo-ration was usually performed for fear of missing multiple abscesses in the peritoneal cavity.[87] When the abscess can be located accurately by CT, a direct (often extraserous) approach to abscesses in the subphrenic, subhepatic, or pelvic region can be made, amounting to the surgical equivalent of percutaneous drainage. A general laparotomy under these circumstances is unnecessary and may lead to such complications as enteric fistula or bleeding. On the other hand, laparotomy is necessary when the abscesses are in the lesser sac or interloop or are multiple; the latter is particularly true in the early postoperative period. After evacuation of the abscess cavity, Penrose or soft sump drains should be left in situ. Criteria for removal of these drains are similar to those for removal of percutaneous drains.

Discussion

Host Response to Peritoneal Injury and Infection

LOCAL RESPONSE

After bacterial contamination of the peritoneal cavity, a complex series of events is initiated that, under ideal circumstances, effects complete eradication of invading bacteria. The three major defense mechanisms are (1) mechanical clearance of bacteria via the diaphragmatic lymphatics, (2) phagocytosis and destruction of suspended or adherent bacteria by phagocytic cells, and (3) sequestration and walling off of bacteria coupled with delayed clearance by phagocytic cells. The first two mechanisms act rapidly, usually within hours. When a pure suspension of bacteria is injected into the peritoneal cavity of an experimental animal, the bacteria begin to disappear immediately, even before the influx of phagocytic cells.[88] Bacteria can be found in the mediastinum within six minutes and in the bloodstream within 12 minutes.[89] These observations suggest that the first defense of the peritoneal cavity is physical removal, whereby bacteria are carried cephalad by the intraperitoneal circulation, absorbed into the diaphragmatic lymphatics, and then carried to the bloodstream. These blood-borne bacteria are presumably cleared by a variety of mechanisms, including the reticuloendothelial system of the liver. The escape of bacteria and their products from the peritoneal cavity probably contributes significantly to the development of the systemic response to peritonitis (see below).

The initial peritoneal response to bacterial contamination is characterized by hyperemia, exudation of fluid into the peritoneal cavity, and a marked influx of phagocytic cells. Macrophages predominate early in the infection, but the rapid influx of neutrophils after a two- to four-hour delay makes them the predominant phagocytic cell in the peritoneal cavity for the first 48 to 72 hours.[88] In essence, the response mimics a typical inflammatory reaction to bacteria. The events surrounding the development of this response have not been well studied, but many can be surmised from in vitro studies or in vivo investigations of inflammation in experimental animals. For example, in experimental peritonitis, peritoneal levels of tumor necrosis factor–α (TNF-α) and interleukin-1 (IL-1) increase rapidly after the initiation of infection.[90,91] Similarly, in humans with severe intra-abdominal infection, peritoneal levels of TNF-α,

IL-1, and IL-6 are higher than levels measured simultaneously in plasma.[92,93] Lipopolysaccharide derived from gram-negative enteric bacteria is a particularly strong stimulus for production of many of these cytokines by peritoneal macrophages. Recent studies have reported that other cell types are important in the initiation of the local peritoneal response. Peritoneal mast cells appear to release preformed tumor necrosis factor early in the genesis of peritoneal inflammation and contribute significantly to recruiting neutrophils to the peritoneal cavity. The peritoneal mesothelial cells have also been shown to be potent producers of a range of cytokines and procoagulants. Given the strategic position of both of these cell types, their role in the initiation of the local response is undoubtedly important.[94,95] The combined effects of these cytokines from various sources clearly contribute to the inflammatory response observed during peritonitis [see VII:11 Molecular and Cellular Mediators of the Inflammatory Response].[96] In addition, generation of other inflammatory mediator molecules, such as leukotriene B₄, platelet-activating factor, and components of the complement cascade (e.g., C3a and C5a), further promotes the development of local inflammation.[97-99]

Finally, fibrin deposition appears to play an important role in walling off infection, not only by incorporating large numbers of bacteria within its interstices[100] but also by causing loops of intestine to adhere to each other and the omentum, thereby creating a physical barrier against dissemination. Fibrin deposition is initiated after the exudation of protein-rich fluid containing fibrinogen into the peritoneal cavity. The conversion of fibrinogen to fibrin is promoted by the release of tissue thromboplastin from both mesothelial cells and stimulated peritoneal macrophages.[101] Furthermore, a plasminogen activator, which is responsible for the activation of fibrinolytic enzymes and is normally present in the mesothelial and submesothelial cell membranes, disappears in the face of bacterial infection.[102]

In addition to favorable effects, peritoneal defenses against bacterial soilage have seemingly paradoxical effects on the overall well-being of the host. Early mechanical clearance via diaphragmatic lymphatics reduces bacterial numbers but also results in bacteremia, which, if massive, can result in death. The influx of large amounts of protein-rich exudate into the peritoneal cavity, though important in providing opsonins and enhancing phagocyte influx, also produces massive third-space fluid shifts, which may produce hypovolemic shock. In addition, there may be significant loss of albumin into the peritoneal cavity. Locally, fluid may impair bacterial opsonization by diluting opsonins and may reduce phagocytosis both by this mechanism and by altering the neutrophils' ability to reach the bacterium.[103] Furthermore, the deposition of fibrinous exudate provides a protected sanctuary in which bacteria may proliferate and thus leads to abscess formation.[104]

In a similarly paradoxical manner, part of the objective in the management of intra-abdominal infection is to treat specific areas where peritoneal defenses have been successful (e.g., by administering antibiotics to treat systemic infection resulting from lymphatic clearance and by removing fluid and fibrinous debris from the peritoneal cavity to prevent residual intra-abdominal sepsis).

SYSTEMIC RESPONSE

The systemic response to bacterial peritonitis mimics the body's response to trauma in general and includes the rapid release of catecholamines, increased secretion of adrenocortical hormones, and secretion of aldosterone and antidiuretic hormone. Of particular note, especially with respect to the management of bacterial peritonitis, are the hemodynamic and metabolic responses to intra-abdominal infection.

The hemodynamic alterations observed in patients with intra-abdominal infection have several causes. Hypovolemia induced by peritoneal inflammation is a major contributor to the picture. Diffuse peritonitis has been likened to a total burn surface of 50 percent in terms of its effects on fluid shifts. A contracted extracellular fluid volume caused by massive fluid shifts into the peritoneal tissues and cavity produces hypovolemic shock with a reduced cardiac index, elevated peripheral vascular resistance, and increased peripheral oxygen extraction.[105] Patients with fulminant peritonitis demonstrate the more classic septic picture after fluid resuscitation[106,107]: elevated cardiac output, reduced peripheral vascular resistance, and a narrowed arteriovenous O_2 difference. Hemodynamic studies in surgical patients with peritonitis have demonstrated combined abnormalities—that is, patients initially present with evidence of hypovolemia caused by peritoneal fluid losses, and only after resuscitation do they manifest the hyperdynamic picture associated with sepsis.[107] Because survival is generally better in patients with a profile of septic shock, it appears clear that aggressive fluid resuscitation is critical in the early management period [see I:4 Shock].

As proposed for the local response to infection in the peritoneal cavity, the stimulated release of products of cells of the monocyte-macrophage lineage also appears to be responsible for the characteristic septic host response observed in patients with bacterial peritonitis. Intravenous infusion of TNF into experimental animals mimics the hemodynamic alteration and lactic acidosis that follow the administration of bacterial endotoxin.[108] Both TNF and IL-1 cause fever and neutrophilia,[108,109] and IL-6 initiates the acute-phase protein response characteristic of infection.[110]

A correlation between the magnitude of the cytokine response and outcome in infected patients has been demonstrated in several clinical studies. Higher levels of circulating TNF-α and IL-6 have been recorded in patients who later die with intra-abdominal infection.[111] Temporal analysis of this cytokine response in relation to the time of laparotomy confirms that peak TNF-α and IL-6 levels occur within two to four hours of skin incision.[112] The exaggerated cytokine response may occur as a result of mobilization of the infectious focus, with spilling of bacteria and bacterial products into the circulation. This phenomenon may account for the pronounced hemodynamic instability soon after laparotomy for intra-abdominal infection. Most recently, elevated levels of interleukin-10 have been documented in patients with intra-abdominal infection.[113] Unlike TNF-α, IL-10 has anti-inflammatory properties and may limit secretion of TNF-α by macrophages. This interleukin may provide an endogenous means to down-regulate an uncontrolled systemic inflammatory response.

The improved understanding of the cell biology of the host response to infection and inflammation has suggested potentially innovative approaches to the management of patients with intra-abdominal infection. Obviously, prevention of the adverse effects of cytokinemia would appear to represent a rational adjuvant treatment measure in these patients. In animal models, administration of anti-TNF antibody and antagonism with IL-1 receptor antagonists effectively prevents the end-organ dysfunction and the adverse hemodynamic and metabolic effects of endotoxin infusion. Before this approach is widely applied, however, consideration should be given to the beneficial effects of TNF and other cytokines in orchestrating the clearance of bacteria from the peritoneal cavity and the possible adverse effects of anticytokine therapy on this useful host response mechanism.

Management of Secondary Peritonitis—Controversies and New Concepts

ANTIBIOTICS

Research over the past three decades has created a body of knowledge forming the basis for rational recommendations for antimicrobial use in patients with intra-abdominal infection.[114-118] On the basis of this evidence, empirical antimicrobial therapy should be directed against *E. coli* and other common members of the Enterobacteriaceae as well as against the anaerobe *B. fragilis*. Guidelines have been proposed that define acceptable antimicrobial regimens for the treatment of intra-abdominal infections [see Table 3].[12,13] Decisions about a particular regimen should be tailored to the individual patient, taking into consideration the possibility of resistant organisms and the potential for adverse effects. Other considerations that may affect the choice of an antimicrobial regimen include its pharmacokinetic properties in the particular patient and its cost. The calculation of costs must include not only acquisition, which may be institution dependent, but also the costs of administration, monitoring, and management of toxicity.

Combination Regimens

The combination of an aminoglycoside and an antianaerobic agent (clindamycin or metronidazole) has, until recently, been considered the gold standard for treatment of patients with intra-abdominal infection. Aminoglycosides have broad coverage of gram-negative bacteria, are inexpensive, have a low incidence of inducing resistant microorganisms, and have been used extensively with great success in a large number of clinical trials. Aminoglycoside-based regimens have fallen into disfavor, however, because of their toxicity profiles as well as the perceived difficulty in attaining and maintaining adequate serum levels of antibiotic. High-risk groups include the elderly, patients with preexisting renal or hepatic disease, and patients with recent episodes of hypotension.[119] The efficacy of aminoglycosides may also be reduced by underdosing and the consequent inability to maintain therapeutic levels. A recent study[118] documented a four-day delay in achieving therapeutic levels of an aminoglycoside in patients with intra-abdominal infection. The inability to attain therapeutic levels may be due in part to the expanded extracellular fluid volume, and hence larger volume of distribution, in critically ill patients with intra-abdominal infection.[120] Finally, the requirement for monitoring serum aminoglycoside levels has reduced the appeal of aminoglycoside-based regimens. Despite these perceived shortcomings, the weight of the clinical evidence supports the use of aminoglycoside-based regimens for the management of intra-abdominal infection in young patients with no renal compromise or hypotension.

The problems of toxicity, dosing, and cost may potentially be overcome by changing the mode of aminoglycoside administration. Several studies have suggested that once-daily aminoglycoside administration is as efficacious as thrice-daily dosing in serious (including intra-abdominal) infections.[121,122] The high peak levels and postantibiotic effect of this mode of administration ensure efficacy, and the high peak/low trough has been associated with a reduced incidence of nephrotoxicity.[122] Monitoring of serum aminoglycoside levels is probably not required in patients receiving once-daily dosing—with the exception of patients with renal dysfunction—because high peak levels and low trough levels are almost guaranteed. The lower incidence of toxicity, the limited requirement for monitoring serum levels, and the proven efficacy of aminoglycosides suggest that aminoglycoside-based regimens using once-daily dosing may provide acceptable antimicrobial therapy.

The combination of a third-generation cephalosporin and an antianaerobic agent or the combination of aztreonam and clindamycin is a suitable alternative to aminoglycoside-based regimens if microbial resistance or nephrotoxicity is a concern.[12] A recent randomized, controlled trial has shown that the combination of metronidazole and the quinolone antibiotic ciprofloxacin is equivalent to single-agent therapy with imipenem-cilastatin.[11]

The choice of the agent to be used for antianaerobic activity in combination regimens is limited to either metronidazole or clindamycin. Both agents are effective, safe, and inexpensive, with excellent anaerobic bacterial coverage. A retrospective study comparing the incidence of *Clostridium difficile*–related disease after the use of each of these agents revealed a lower incidence of diarrhea and colonization in patients receiving metronidazole.[123] This finding is not unexpected, because metronidazole is used in the treatment of *C. difficile* colitis,[124] whereas clindamycin has been implicated in its induction.[123]

Monotherapy

These agents include the extended-spectrum cephalosporins, such as cefmetazole, cefotetan, and cefoxitin[12]; the penicillin-based regimens that contain a β-lactamase inhibitor, such as ampicillin-sulbactam, ticarcillin-clavulanate, and piperacillin-tazobactam; and the carbapenems imipenem and meropenem.[12,13] In well-controlled clinical trials, these agents

have been shown to be equivalent to aminoglycoside-based combination therapy in the treatment of intra-abdominal infections.

The choice of agent depends to a great extent on the anticipated resistance profile of organisms contaminating the peritoneal cavity. For example, resistant organisms are unlikely to be a concern in patients with community-acquired peritonitis. A second-generation cephalosporin or a combination of a penicillin and a β-lactamase inhibitor provides adequate therapy in these patients. The extended-spectrum cephalosporins (cefmetazole, cefotetan, and cefoxitin) are not recommended for hospital-acquired infections because of the risk of resistant facultative gram-negative bacteria. Resistant organisms are more likely to represent a therapeutic problem in patients with recent exposure to previous antimicrobials, those acquiring postoperative peritonitis, and immunosuppressed patients. In these situations and in patients with severe intra-abdominal infection, the empirical use of broad-spectrum antimicrobials (including piperacillin-tazobactam, carbapenems, or a combination regimen with aztreonam or a third-generation cephalosporin) is warranted. A recent study comparing cefoxitin to imipenem-cilastatin for the treatment of complex intra-abdominal infections demonstrated equivalent outcomes between groups, even though the failures in the cefoxitin group tended to have more resistant organisms.[125]

Intravenous administration of antimicrobial agents is the most reliable way of ensuring adequate serum and tissue levels. Recent studies have suggested, however, that conversion from I.V. therapy to oral treatment with ciprofloxacin plus metronidazole might be equivalent to continued I.V. treatment in patients whose gut function has returned.[16] These agents are well absorbed by the oral route and, in combination, have an antimicrobial spectrum including both gram-negative enteric bacteria and anaerobes. Clearly, this approach may have a significant impact on costs, including reduced drug acquisition costs and a reduced length of hospital stay. Studies are currently examining these issues. Whether these agents are effective in critically ill patients receiving enteral feeding remains unknown. Preliminary studies suggest limited bioavailability in critically ill trauma patients,[126] but further investigation of this subgroup of patients is under way.

Treatment of Enterococci and Candida

The need for therapy aimed at enterococci is still unclear.[127] Experimental studies have shown that they can act as significant copathogens with *E. coli*.[128] One study demonstrated that recovery of enterococcus in the initial culture was an independent predictor of treatment failure.[129] However, clinical evidence suggests that antibiotic coverage directed against coliforms and anaerobes is sufficient treatment of intra-abdominal infection and usually does not result in treatment failure or relapse caused by enterococci.[115,129] Thus, if enterococci are recovered as part of the polymicrobial flora of an intra-abdominal infection, there is no need to add antienterococcal coverage if the patient is recovering well. If, on the other hand, the patient is compromised with respect to susceptibility to opportunistic pathogens (as might be the case after major burns, trauma, or transplantation), a drug that is effective against enterococci should be included in the antibiotic regimen. Finally, enterococcal bacteremia or the recovery of enterococci from a residual or recurrent intra-abdominal infection is an indication for coverage by the appropriate antienterococcal antibiotic (i.e., ampicillin or, in penicillin-allergic patients, vancomycin).[130]

Occasionally, *Candida* species are isolated from patients with secondary peritonitis and are part of a polymicrobial infection. At present, there appears to be no indication for specific treatment of these microorganisms in patients with straightforward secondary peritonitis.

In some patients who have had a prolonged hospital stay with multiple abdominal operations and evidence of the systemic inflammatory response syndrome (SIRS) and MODS, tertiary peritonitis develops [see Persistent or Tertiary Peritonitis, *below*]. For patients with tertiary peritonitis, the usual empirical therapy is no longer valid, because the microbial flora of their infections consists of *S. epidermidis, Pseudomonas aeruginosa, Candida* species, and enterococci rather than the usual *E. coli* and *B. fragilis*.[131,132] Therapy specifically directed against these microorganisms appears most rational. However, from retrospective studies examining the efficacy of appropriate antibiotics for such infections, it appears that microbiological cure is unusual,[131,133] which is probably an indication of a general failure of host defense mechanisms rather than a failure of the antibiotics themselves.

Role of Peritoneal Cultures in Selection of Antimicrobial Agents

Inadequate use of empirical antimicrobial therapy results in an increase in infection-related adverse events, including wound infections, postoperative abscesses, reoperations, and the duration of hospital stay. If an empirical choice is inappropriate, the rate of these complications is not altered by a subsequent change of the antimicrobial regimen on the basis of culture results obtained at laparotomy.[134] These data suggest that use of intraoperative cultures to guide management is less important in overall outcome than the correct choice of an empirical antimicrobial regimen. Culture data rarely exert a positive influence on antibiotic selection in the postoperative period. The findings of cultures have resulted in an appropriate change in antibiotic therapy in fewer than 10 percent of patients.[134,135]

If they have so little effect on both management and outcome, why are intraoperative cultures taken? In a retrospective study, intra-abdominal isolates obtained at initial laparotomy were analyzed for antimicrobial resistance.[136] Analysis of the susceptibility of intraoperative isolates indicated a significant relationship between resistance to the empirical antimicrobials and the development of postoperative infection. In patients whose intra-abdominal infections resolved, 44 percent had resistant isolates; of patients with postoperative infection, 82 percent had resistant isolates. These data suggest that resistant organisms may contribute to the development of postoperative infection, but a significant number of patients are cured despite the presence of resistant organisms. It is not clear whether an expeditious change in antimicrobial therapy, based on operative site susceptibility independent of the patient's early clinical response, would reduce the incidence of postoperative infections. In the absence of such data, one can make a case for obtaining intraoperative cultures in patients at high risk for postoperative infections, particularly those who have previously taken antimicrobial agents and are more likely to harbor resistant organisms, including immunocompromised patients and patients with recurrent intra-abdominal infection. In these patients, changes in antimicrobial agents may be warranted only if an inadequate clinical response is demonstrated.

ADJUVANT SURGICAL TECHNIQUES

The addition of antibiotics and antiseptic agents to intraoperative peritoneal lavage fluid has been advocated to reduce septic complications. Available data do not unanimously support the use of antibiotics in lavage fluid as an effective means of reducing the septic complication rate below that achieved by systemic antibiotics alone.[137,138] This result is not surprising, given that systemically administered antibiotics achieve levels in the peritoneal fluid of patients with peritonitis that are comparable to serum levels.[139] Antiseptic agents, such as povidone-iodine,[140] noxythiolin,[141] and taurolin,[142] have shown some ability to reduce postoperative intra-abdominal infection. Further study using these agents may be warranted. At present, we routinely add cefazolin (1,000 mg/L) to the irrigation fluid used to lavage the peritoneal cavity at the end of the operation. We perform a vigorous lavage to remove necrotic debris and blood. Admittedly, the reason for adding antibiotics is somewhat theoretical. Cefazolin, however, is safe and inexpensive, and because local instillation achieves very high concentrations, penetration of the agent into areas of loculated infection may be enhanced.

In addition to standard techniques for care of the patient in the postoperative period, two other treatment modalities have been used to prevent recurrent intra-abdominal sepsis. These techniques, continuous postoperative peritoneal lavage and open drainage of the peritoneal cavity, are postoperative extensions of intraoperative techniques. In general, these preventive methods are similarly aimed at reducing the bacterial inoculum and removing potential adjuvants for infection. Most of the advances in the management of peritonitis have succeeded in reducing early mortality by providing adequate fluid resuscitation, hemodynamic monitoring, and broad-spectrum antibiotic coverage. The more innovative postoperative techniques may ultimately lower mortality by preventing the onset of organ failure.

The concept of continuous postoperative peritoneal lavage is not a new one, but it is receiving more attention as a means of reducing postoperative sepsis.[143-145] At the time of initial operation, peritoneal drains are left in situ, and lavage is begun in the immediate postoperative period. Lavage is performed with large exchange volumes (> 2 L) during each three-hour cycle to ensure dispersion of fluid throughout the peritoneum and to prevent fluid loculations. Antibiotic mixtures with broad coverage, as well as low-dose heparin, are usually included in the lavage fluid. Lavage is continued for 48 to 72 hours or until the effluent is clear.

Studies of this technique are somewhat difficult to evaluate because of poor experimental design. One study showed a reduction in postoperative abscess formation from 16 percent to zero percent in patients who underwent postoperative lavage with a mixture of cefamandole, erythromycin, and heparin.[143] However, the control group was not randomly selected and received no lavage at all. Whether lavage was beneficial because of mechanical debridement, antibiotic administration, or the use of heparin could not be ascertained from the study. A prospective, randomized, controlled study demonstrated that postoperative lavage containing neither antibiotics nor heparin did not benefit patients who were already receiving broad-spectrum systemic therapy.[144] However, no postoperative septic complications were noted even in the control group, which suggests that the patient group studied was not at high enough risk to warrant such aggressive therapy. This technique is extremely labor intensive, necessitates intensive care unit monitoring, and is potentially complicated by the development of enteric fistulas from erosion of the cannula. A well-performed prospective, randomized trial of postoperative peritoneal lavage in high-risk patients is required to determine the efficacy of the technique.

Over the past decade, the concept of planned relaparotomy (or staged abdominal repair [STAR]) and open management for severe peritonitis has been rejuvenated with the expectation that they might prevent recurrent intra-abdominal infection and associated morbidity. Planned relaparotomy refers to the practice of performing repeat operations at fixed intervals (usually 24 to 72 hours) regardless of the patient's clinical condition. In this way, the development of new abscesses is prevented, necrotic tissue is debrided, and enteric fistulas are recognized early. The difficulties arising from frequent exploration, with its forceful, repeated closure of the abdominal wall, have resulted in the development of the open abdomen approach, or laparostomy. Reported benefits of this technique include the conceptual advantage of treating the entire peritoneal cavity as one large abscess, with exteriorization permitting drainage. Other possible advantages include improved ventilation and renal perfusion [see Abdominal Compartment Syndrome, below]. In the open abdomen approach, the fascia is kept open with saline gauze packing. Complications of this technique include evisceration, massive fluid losses, spontaneous fistulas, and contamination of the open wound, as well as the necessity for mechanical ventilation. Moreover, an open abdomen does not necessarily eliminate the need for repeat abdominal exploration.

Complications associated with the open abdomen approach have resulted in popularization of a semiopen technique, in which temporary abdominal closure prevents evisceration yet allows easy reexploration of the peritoneal cavity. Towel clips and mesh composed of polypropylene (Marlex), polyglycolic acid (Dexon), or an expanded polytetrafluoroethylene patch (PTFE, Gore-Tex) have all been used for this purpose. One popular strategy involves the use of polypropylene with or without an insewn zipper or burr-like device (Velcro) to allow repeated and rapid access to the peritoneal cavity [see Figure 2].[146-148] Mesh prevents evisceration in the early postoperative period, reduces the risk of spontaneous fistulization, allows for drainage of fluid and pus through its interstices, and may function as an exit site for a stoma or drain. At reexploration, adhesions are lysed, and fibrinous exudates, fluid, and necrotic debris are removed. This procedure is continued daily until clinical evidence of sepsis has subsided and the abdominal cavity appears clean, as determined by the presence of healthy granulation tissue and adhesion formation. The mesh and zipper are then removed, and the wound is allowed to granulate and contract. A split-thickness skin graft may be used for coverage, although this is not absolutely necessary. Several complications have been associated with the use of mesh, including enteric fistulization, prolonged ventilation, and hernia formation.

Initial reports evaluating the use of planned relaparotomy were quite positive.

Two studies used the Acute Physiology and Chronic Health Evaluation II (APACHE II) stratification system to define underlying severity of illness.[148,149] In one, the Marlex mesh technique was applied to patients with diffuse nonlocalizing

Figure 2 A plastic zipper sewn into a Marlex mesh is opened to gain access to the peritoneal cavity for repeated laparotomies.

peritonitis.[149] The mortality in patients receiving a mesh at the time of reoperation for postoperative peritonitis was one third the rate predicted on the basis of APACHE II scores. Evaluation of the subgroups of APACHE II scores indicated that critically ill patients with scores higher than 25 had a mortality of 100 percent, whereas those with low scores already had a low mortality that was independent of treatment. These data suggest that patients with midrange APACHE II scores are the ones who may derive the greatest benefit from this approach—a finding that was confirmed in the second study mentioned.[148]

Subsequent data tempered the initial enthusiasm for planned relaparotomy. A case-control study that matched patients managed with planned relaparotomy to patients managed with relaparotomy on demand (based on APACHE II score, age, cause of infection, site of origin of peritonitis, and the ability of the surgeon to securely eliminate the source of infection) found that patients managed by planned relaparotomy had higher rates of recurrent intra-abdominal sepsis, anastomotic leaks, and septicemia as well as worse organ dysfunction than those managed by relaparotomy on demand.[150] Further, the patients in the former group had a higher rate of unplanned laparotomies than their conventionally managed controls (21 percent versus eight percent), although this difference was not statistically significant. These data suggest that planned relaparotomy may not even obviate unplanned laparotomy. A review of the literature, compiling data on 642 patients in 22 series, concluded that there was insufficient evidence to support either open management or planned relaparotomy in patients with postoperative peritonitis.[151]

Because of the limited data supporting the efficacy of planned relaparotomy in the critically ill patient with severe peritonitis, our general approach is to tailor the need for subsequent laparotomy to the patient's clinical status (i.e., relaparotomy on demand). Absence of improvement or clinical deterioration requires either abdominal imaging studies or laparotomy, or both, depending on the clinical status of the patient. In certain situations, we find that planned relaparotomy may be useful. For example, it may be practical in patients in whom there is a large segment of bowel with marginal viability. These patients may best be served with a second operation that allows the bowel to demarcate, thus minimizing the length of bowel resected. Patients with necrotizing pancreatitis may also benefit from planned relaparotomy. Complete debridement may be precluded by extensive bleeding or a lack of demarcation of necrotic tissue. Under such circumstances, we recommend multiple limited operations rather than a single attempt at complete debridement.

PROGNOSIS OF SECONDARY PERITONITIS

The morbidity and mortality of intra-abdominal infection vary widely depending on the particular study quoted. Studies examining the efficacy of antibiotics in intra-abdominal infection tend to include patients within a defined age limit, with normal organ function, and with minimally deranged physiologic parameters.[152] As a result, these studies show a very favorable outcome for intra-abdominal infection, with a mortality in the range of three to five percent. Conversely, studies specifically designed to investigate mortality associated with intra-abdominal infection have yielded rates exceeding 20 percent.[153,154] This discrepancy is consistent with the fact that intra-abdominal infection is not a homogeneous disease but rather one that poses a high risk of complications for some patients and a low risk for others. The ability to stratify patients into these risk groups is of critical importance for several reasons. First, it allows us to predict which patients are at high risk. Second, the ability to identify high-risk patients will pinpoint the subgroup in which new and innovative techniques should be tried. Finally, stratification of patients into risk groups enhances our ability to interpret the results of studies examining new treatments. A clear example for surgeons is the importance of wound classification for identifying patients who will benefit from administration of prophylactic antibiotics [see IV:5 Prevention of Postoperative Infection].

Several scoring systems are currently available for accurate assessment of patient risk. Few of these methods adequately address the risk associated with intra-abdominal infection. One study approached classification from an anatomic standpoint: risk correlated well with the organ from which the peritonitis originated.[155] Peritonitis arising from duodenal or appendiceal pathology was associated with low mortality (about 10 percent), whereas peritonitis in the postoperative period was associated with high mortality (60 percent). A discriminant function equation, based on the patient's age, immunologic function (as measured by delayed-type hypersensitivity), and nutritional status (based on albumin level), has been developed.[156] It accurately predicted mortality after major operations, including those for intra-abdominal infection.

A surgical infection stratification system has been developed for patients with intra-abdominal infection.[154] In a five-center study, 178 patients with established intra-abdominal sepsis were found to have an overall mortality of 24 percent. When risk factors were analyzed independently, it was found that the patients who died were generally older, had higher acute physiology scores (APS, which measures the degree of deviation from normal in 34 routinely measured laboratory tests or physical findings), and tended to be diabetic, malnourished, or in shock on admission. Multivariate analysis determined that APS, malnutrition, and age were the most reliable predictors of outcome. A discriminant function based on these parameters could predict survival or death with an 84 percent accuracy. The APACHE II stratification system has now supplanted APS as a useful predictive score.[157] This system is based on the evaluation of 12 acute physiology parameters as well as an assessment of the patient's general state of health.[158]

In a multicenter trial evaluating outcome in patients with severe peritonitis (APACHE II score > 10), logistic regression analysis showed that a high APACHE II score, a low serum albumin level, and high New York Heart Association cardiac function status were significantly and independently associated with death.[159] Although the APACHE II system is used most often, recent evidence suggests that the APACHE II score may underestimate mortality risk in critically ill patients with intra-abdominal infection.[160] A slight improvement in the predictive value of the APACHE II system has been demonstrated when delayed-type hypersensitivity (DTH) scores were added to the discriminant analysis, reflecting the importance of host immune function in prognosis.[161]

Persistent or Tertiary Peritonitis

In most patients, the combination of appropriate antibiotic therapy, timely surgical intervention, and normal host defense mechanisms results in complete resolution of the infection and subsequent recovery. Even when infection persists, localization of the infection with resultant abscess formation limits the magnitude of the systemic response and permits straightforward management by means of either percutaneous or directed surgical drainage. Some patients, however, are unable to localize infection because of either impaired host defenses or overwhelming infection, and these individuals may go on to manifest persistent diffuse peritonitis, also called tertiary peritonitis. The clinical picture is one of occult infection, signaled by fever, leukocytosis, hyperdynamic cardiovascular parameters, and a general hypermetabolic state. The development of progressive dysfunction of one or more organ systems is a frequent concomitant finding.[131] In this patient population, mortality has been as high as 64 percent despite aggressive surgical and antibiotic therapy.[162]

Laparotomy often reveals poorly defined serosanguineous collections instead of discrete purulent abscesses. This probably indicates the host's inability to localize an infectious process, reflecting global immune dysfunction. Additional support for this hypothesis is provided by the flora associated with tertiary peritonitis. Peritoneal cultures yield organisms markedly different from those isolated in cases of community-acquired secondary peritonitis. Organisms traditionally thought to be of low virulence, such as enterococci, Candida, S. epidermidis, and P. aeruginosa, predominate.[131,162,163] Their presence may reflect selection by antibiotic pressures or the impaired systemic and local host defenses of MODS.

Early studies of multiorgan failure in patients with peritonitis

Figure 3 **Ultrasonographic examination of the left lower quadrant demonstrates the presence of an abscess (left). An obvious mass was palpable at this site on clinical examination. Under ultrasonographic guidance, a pigtail catheter was placed percutaneously into the abscess. The cavity is well outlined after injection of a small amount of contrast material (right).**

showed a strong association between organ failure and the presence of uncontrolled residual infection in the peritoneal cavity.[81] As a result, surgeons were encouraged, for a short time, to perform so-called blind laparotomy to look for undrained abscesses. However, comparison of preoperative CT scans with operative findings showed that significant radiologically occult infectious foci were uncommon and that even when such foci were encountered, MODS persisted despite surgical drainage.[132,164-166] Laparotomy is recommended only if imaging studies, blood cultures, or a change in clinical status is consistent with the presence of an undrained infection.

Given the postulated role of the GI tract in the development and perpetuation of MODS in these patients, selective decontamination of the GI tract, enteral feeding, and avoidance of H$_2$-receptor blockade represent worthwhile management strategies [*see VII:7 Multiple Organ Dysfunction Syndrome*].

ABDOMINAL COMPARTMENT SYNDROME

Markedly increased intra-abdominal pressures may develop in critically ill patients with intra-abdominal infection as a result of visceral edema, the accumulation of peritoneal fluid, and closure of an edematous, noncompliant abdominal wall. Intra-abdominal pressures may increase to the point that systemic hemodynamics, respiratory function, and renal function are compromised. This entity, referred to as the abdominal compartment syndrome, is characterized by hypotension and low cardiac output in the presence of elevated central filling pressures, high systemic vascular resistance, elevated peak airway pressures, and oliguria.[167,168] High intra-abdominal pressure impairs venous return and increases systemic vascular resistance. Elevation of the diaphragm increases intrathoracic pressure, impairing ventilation and artificially elevating central filling pressures.[169] Renal vein compression, coupled with a reduction in cardiac output and renal blood flow, may play a role in renal dysfunction associated with the syndrome. The syndrome may account for some of the adverse consequences of laparotomy for peritonitis that have previously been attributed to the release of proinflammatory mediators. The incidence of this syndrome is difficult to ascertain because intra-abdominal pressures are rarely measured.

The diagnosis should be suspected in patients with the clinical picture described above. Intra-abdominal pressure may be evaluated indirectly by measuring urinary bladder pressure.[168] Sterile saline (50 to 100 ml) is injected into the empty bladder through a Foley catheter. Tubing for the drainage bag is connected to the catheter, and once the catheter and proximal tubing are filled with saline, a clamp is placed on the tubing of the drainage bag distal to the culture aspiration port. A 16-gauge needle is inserted into the aspiration port and connected to a pressure transducer. The zero reference point is the symphysis pubis. Normal intra-abdominal pressure approximates atmospheric pressure. Clinically significant changes in hemodynamics occur with intra-abdominal pressures above 20 mm Hg, with severe alterations occurring when pressures exceed 40 mm Hg.

Management involves decompressive laparotomy with concomitant fluid resuscitation. Laparotomy usually results in prompt resolution of the hemodynamic alterations and a brisk diuresis. The abdominal wall should be closed without tension, usually with the fascia opened and a prosthesis used to prevent evisceration. Fascial closure may be attempted after the acute process has resolved and the likelihood of repeat laparotomies is remote.

**Intra-abdominal Abscess—
Radiologic Diagnosis and Intervention**

Ultrasonography and CT scanning have become the modalities of choice for the diagnosis of intra-abdominal abscess. Each has its own advantages and disadvantages. Ultrasonography is fast and inexpensive and delivers no radiation. It is also highly accurate in the appropriate setting [*see Figure 3*].[170] Furthermore, the availability of mobile machines permits bedside and intraoperative examination. Endoluminal probes allow transvaginal and transrectal visualization and potential drainage of deep pelvic abscesses.[171,172] The major disadvantages of ultrasonography are that it is extremely operator dependent, its images may be obscured by gas, and it is difficult to study patients with open wounds or drains. The last two problems are particularly relevant for the critically ill postoperative patient who has intestinal ileus and has had multiple operative interventions.

Computed tomography is the most accurate technique available for the diagnosis of intra-abdominal abscess.[110,173] The major advantage of CT is its ability to display, independent of the operator, both intraperitoneal and retroperitoneal structures with a high degree of resolution and accuracy [see Figure 4]. In addition, the presence of ileus, as well as of drains, dressings, or stomas, does not interfere with the performance of the test. The major disadvantages of CT scanning are its nonportability and the need for the patient to be cooperative and immobile. The accuracy of the scan is reduced in those patients whose GI tract is not opacified with contrast. Under these circumstances, the scans are limited in their ability to distinguish fluid-filled bowel loops from an abscess. Interloop abscesses, which represent approximately four percent of all abscesses, are also poorly visualized on CT scan.[77]

Two other imaging techniques for intra-abdominal infections involve the use of radionuclides: granulocytes are labeled with gallium-67 citrate or indium-111. Gallium has an affinity for iron-binding proteins (e.g., lactoferrin, ferritin, and bacterial siderophores) and is incorporated into abscesses by binding to lactoferrin present in leukocytes at the site of infection and by binding to bacterial surfaces.[174] The detection of an abscess is based on increased uptake outside of expected sites. One major drawback is that gallium is excreted in the colon and therefore accumulates in the stool. An enema to clear radiolabeled stool is frequently necessary to permit interpretation of the study. Other shortcomings of this technique include the false positive imaging of neoplasms and the 24- to 72-hour delay required between injection of the radionuclide and the scanning procedure.

Indium-111 in the form of the chelate indium In 111 oxyquinoline is used to label granulocytes drawn from the patient.[175,176] After labeling, the cells are reinjected into the

Figure 4 CT scan demonstrates a left psoas abscess (arrows) in a patient with Crohn's disease (top, left). After percutaneous insertion of a pigtail catheter, CT scan shows the catheter to be situated in the abscess (bottom, left). A small amount of contrast injected via the catheter illustrates the extent of the retroperitoneal abscess cavity (right).

Table 6 Probability of Success Using Percutaneous
Drainage of Intra-abdominal Abscesses

Clinical Condition	Probability of Success		Reason for Failure
Single, well-defined bacterial abscess with no enteric communication	High	Curative	
Abscess with enteric communication (e.g., diverticular abscess or Crohn's disease abscess)	High	Palliative	Prolonged drainage or recurrence
Abscess with enteric communication	Medium	Curative	
Infected tumor mass	Medium	Palliative	Poor drainage
Fungal abscess	Low		Poor drainage
Infected hematoma	Low		Poor drainage
Early postoperative diffuse peritonitis (e.g., caused by anastomotic dehiscence or bile peritonitis)	Low		Inadequate drainage
Interloop abscess	Low		Difficult visualization using scanning techniques; inaccessibility

patient, and the patient is scanned with a gamma camera. Presumably, normal granulocytes will accumulate at the site of an acute infection. The major disadvantage of indium-111 scanning is the significant number of false negative results in patients with chronic infections, which are less likely to lead to accumulation of acute inflammatory cells.[176] In general, these two techniques do not add much to the diagnostic armamentarium for intra-abdominal infection.

The role of magnetic resonance imaging in the diagnosis of intra-abdominal abscesses requires further definition. Initial studies suggest potential advantages.[177] Surgical clips do not interfere with imaging, and intravenous contrast is not necessary to outline the abscess or distinguish it from adjacent structures. Use of the sagittal plane may provide improved anatomic definition of the pelvis. The extended time required for imaging, compared with the excellent sensitivity and specificity of computed tomography and ultrasonography, suggests only a minor role for MRI in the diagnosis of intra-abdominal infection. The use of spectroscopy to evaluate parameters such as tissue pH may ultimately help differentiate between various fluid collections, something that ultrasonography and CT cannot do.

Percutaneous drainage is now well accepted as a treatment option in the management of intra-abdominal abscess. The early studies established rigid criteria for the use of this technique, including the presence of unilocular abscess and a direct window to the collection from the skin without intervening bowel or solid viscera.[178,179] When percutaneous drainage was used in accordance with these criteria, the success rate ranged from 80 to 90 percent. As radiologists have become more skilled in the technique and surgeons more confident in its use, the indications for percutaneous drainage have expanded, albeit with a somewhat lower overall success rate.[180] Acceptable criteria now include multiple or loculated abscesses, abscesses in which there is enteric communication, and, occasionally, abscesses that are reached by traversing solid viscera (e.g., traversing the liver to

drain lesser sac abscesses).[181]

Successful percutaneous drainage has been redefined and is now divided into two categories[182]: (1) curative success—the drainage provides complete cure without the need for subsequent operation—and (2) palliative success—the drainage improves the patient's status so that operative intervention may be safely performed (e.g., an abscess with enteric communication). Palliative success also includes the patient for whom cure is impossible, such as the patient with an unresectable, infected tumor mass. For nonvisceral abscesses, clinical scenarios can be categorized according to the probability of successful drainage [*see Table 6*]. At the Toronto Hospital, percutaneous drainage is not attempted in that group in which the probability of success is low, except under unusual circumstances.

No randomized, controlled studies have been done comparing percutaneous with surgical drainage of intra-abdominal abscesses. The classic mortality figure associated with surgical drainage of intra-abdominal abscesses has been in the range of 30 percent.[153] Studies advocating the use of percutaneous drainage have quoted mortality figures between 11 and 15 percent, which suggests an advantage to the approach. However, comparisons in noncontrolled studies demonstrate no gross differences in mortality, although the percutaneously drained patient may stay in the hospital a shorter time.[183,184] The surgical patients were generally sicker, which perhaps explains this difference.[184] It is likely that the apparent improvement in survival associated with the use of percutaneous drainage is related to the use of improved imaging modalities, which can facilitate early diagnosis. One series, in which abscesses were treated surgically after location with CT scanning, reported a 12 percent mortality.[173] These results and those achieved with percutaneous drainage strongly support the concept that early diagnosis and treatment of abscesses before MODS develops are critical in reducing the overall mortality associated with such infections.

References

1. Abu-Yousef MM, Bleicher JJ, Maher JW, et al: High-resolution sonography of acute appendicitis. AJR Am J Roentgenol 149:53, 1987

2. Taourel P, Baron MP, Pradel J, et al: Acute abdomen of unknown origin: impact of CT on diagnosis and management. Gastrointestinal Radiology 17:287, 1992

3. Lobbato V, Cioroiu M, LaRaja RD, et al: Peritoneal lavage as an aid to diagnosis of peritonitis in debilitated and elderly patients. Am Surg 51:508, 1985

4. Richardson JD, Flint LM, Polk HC Jr: Peritoneal lavage: a useful diagnostic adjunct for peritonitis. Surgery 94:826, 1983

5. Fink-Bennett D, Freitas JE, Ripley SD, et al: The sensitivity of hepatobiliary imaging and real-time ultrasonography in the detection of acute cholecystitis. Arch Surg 120:904, 1985

6. Navez B, d'Udekem Y, Cambier E, et al: Laparoscopy for management of nontraumatic acute abdomen. World J Surg 19:382, 1995

7. Drasar BS, Hill MJ: Human Intestinal Flora. Academic Press, London, 1974

8. Ruddell WSJ, Axon ATR, Findlay JM, et al: Effect of cimetidine on the gastric bacterial flora. Lancet 1:672, 1980

9. Stone HH, Kolb LD, Geheber CE: Incidence and significance of intraperitoneal anaerobic bacteria. Ann Surg 181:705, 1975

10. Gorbach SL, Thadepalli H, Norsen J: Anaerobic microorganisms in intraabdominal infections. Anaerobic Bacteria: Role in Disease. Balows A, De-Hann RH, Dowell VR, et al, Eds. Charles C Thomas, Publisher, Springfield, Illinois, 1974, p 339

11. Lorber B, Swenson RM: The bacteriology of intra-abdominal infections. Surg Clin North Am 55:1349, 1975

12. Bohnen JMA, Solomkin JS, Dellinger EP, et al: Guidelines for clinical care: anti-infective agents for intra-abdominal infection—a Surgical Infection Society policy statement. Arch Surg 127:83, 1992

13. Nathens AB, Rotstein OD: Antimicrobial therapy for intra-abdominal infections. Am J Surg 172:1S, 1996

14. Stone HH, Bourneuf AA, Stinson LD: Reliability of criteria for predicting persistent or recurrent sepsis. Arch Surg 120:17, 1985

15. Lennard ES, Dellinger EP, Wertz MJ, et al: Implications of leukocytosis and fever at conclusion of antibiotic therapy for intra-abdominal sepsis. Ann Surg 195:19, 1982

16. Solomkin JS, Reinhart HH, Dellinger EP, et al: Results of a randomized trial comparing sequential intravenous/oral treatment with ciprofloxacin plus metronidazole to imipenem/cilastatin for intra-abdominal infections. Ann Surg 223:303, 1996

17. Nathens AB, Rotstein OD: Therapeutic options in peritonitis. Surg Clin North Am 74:677, 1994

18. Burch DM, Brock JC, Gevirtzman L, et al: The injured colon. Ann Surg 203:701, 1986

19. Stahl WM, Ivatury R: Small bowel injury. Common Problems in Trauma. Hurst JM, Ed. Year Book Medical Publishers, Chicago, 1987, p 314

20. George SM, Fabian TC, Mangiante EC: Colon trauma: further support for primary repair. Am J Surg 156:16, 1988

21. Shrock TR, Deveney CW, Dunphy JE: Factors contributing to leakage of colonic anastomoses. Ann Surg 177:513, 1973

22. Zucker KA, Flowers JL, Bailey RW, et al: Laparoscopic management of acute cholecystitis. Am J Surg 165:508, 1993

23. Rattner DW, Ferguson C, Warshaw AL: Factors associated with successful laparoscopic cholecystectomy for acute cholecystitis. Ann Surg 217:233, 1993

24. Cox MR, Wilson TG, Luck AJ, et al: Laparoscopic cholecystectomy for acute inflammation of the gallbladder. Ann Surg 218:630, 1993

25. Singer JA, McKeen RV: Laparoscopic cholecystectomy for acute or gangrenous cholecystitis. Am Surg 60:326, 1994

26. Koo KP, Thirlby RC: Laparoscopic surgery in acute cholecystitis. What is the optimal timing for surgery? Arch Surg 131:540, 1996

27. Lo CM, Liu CL, Lai EC, et al: Early versus delayed laparoscopic cholecystectomy for treatment of acute cholecystitis. Ann Surg 233:37, 1996

28. Scott-Conner CEH, Hall TJ, Anglin BL, et al: Laparoscopic appendectomy: initial experience in a teaching program. Ann Surg 215:660, 1992

29. McCahill LE, Pellegrini CA, Wiggins T, et al: A clinical outcome and cost analysis of laparoscopic versus open appendectomy. Am J Surg 171:533, 1996

30. Martin LC, Puente I, Sosa JL, et al: Open versus laparoscopic appendectomy: a prospective randomized comparison. Ann Surg 222:256, 1995

31. Tate JJ, Dawson JW, Chung SC, et al: Laparoscopic versus open appendectomy: prospective randomized trial. Lancet 342:633, 1993

32. Nathanson LK, Easter DW, Cuschieri A: Laparoscopic repair/peritoneal toilet of perforated duodenal ulcer. Surg Endosc 4:232, 1990

33. Haller JA Jr, Shaker IJ, Donahoo JS, et al: Peritoneal drainage versus non-drainage for generalized peritonitis from ruptured appendicitis in children. Ann Surg 177:595, 1973

34. Bernard HR, Cole WR: Wound infections following potentially contaminated operations. JAMA 184:290, 1963

35. Robson MC, Hegger JP: Delayed wound closures based on bacterial counts. J Surg Oncol 2:379, 1970

36. Farnell MB, Worthington-Self S, Mucha P Jr, et al: Closure of abdominal incisions with subcutaneous catheters: a prospective randomized trial. Arch Surg 121:641, 1986

37. Harken AH, Shochat SJ: Gram-positive peritonitis in children. Am J Surg 125:769, 1973

38. McDougal WS, Izant RJ Jr, Zollinger RM Jr: Primary peritonitis in infancy and childhood. Ann Surg 181:310, 1975

39. Golden GT, Shaw A: Primary peritonitis. Surg Gynecol Obstet 135:513, 1972

40. Conn HO, Fessel JM: Spontaneous bacterial peritonitis in cirrhosis: variations on a theme. Medicine (Baltimore) 50:161, 1971

41. Hoefs JC, Runyon BA: Spontaneous bacterial peritonitis. Dis Mon 31:1, 1985

42. Wyke RJ: Problems of bacterial infection in patients with liver disease. Gut 28:623, 1987

43. Akalin HE, Laleli Y, Telatar H: Bactericidal and opsonic activity of ascitic fluid from cirrhotic and noncirrhotic patients. J Infect Dis 147:1011, 1983

44. Shesol BF, Rosato EF, Rosato FE: Concomitant acute lupus erythematosus and primary pneumococcal peritonitis. Am J Gastroenterol 63:324, 1975

45. Correia JP, Conn HO: Spontaneous bacterial peritonitis in cirrhosis: endemic or epidemic? Med Clin North Am 59:963, 1975

46. Wilcox CM, Forsmark CE, Darragh TM, et al: Cytomegalovirus peritonitis in a patient with the acquired immunodeficiency syndrome. Dig Dis Sci 37:1288, 1992

47. Doberneck RC, Sterling WA Jr, Allison DC: Morbidity and mortality after operation in nonbleeding cirrhotic patients. Am J Surg 146:306, 1983

48. Runyon BA, Umland ET, Merlin T: Inoculation of blood culture bottles with ascitic fluid: improved detection of spontaneous bacterial peritonitis. Arch Intern Med 147:73, 1987

49. Runyon BA, Canawati HN, Akriviadis EA: Optimization of ascitic fluid culture technique. Gastroenterology 95:1351, 1988

50. Garcia-Tsao G, Conn HO, Lerner E: The diagnosis of bacterial peritonitis: comparison of pH, lactate concentration, and leukocyte count. Hepatology 5:91, 1985

51. Yang C-Y, Liaw Y-F, Chu C-M, et al: White count, pH and lactate in ascites in the diagnosis of spontaneous bacterial peritonitis. Hepatology 5:85, 1985

52. Hoefs JC: Diagnostic paracentesis: a potent clinical tool. Gastroenterology 98:230, 1990

53. Runyon BA, Hoefs JC: Spontaneous vs. secondary bacterial peritonitis: differentiation by response of ascitic fluid neutrophil count to antimicrobial therapy. Arch Intern Med 146:1563, 1986

54. Bhargava DK, Shriniwas, Chopra P, et al: Peritoneal tuberculosis: laparoscopic patterns and its diagnostic accuracy. Am J Gastroenterol 87:109, 1992

55. Felisart J, Rimola A, Arroyo V, et al: Cefotaxime is more effective than is ampicillin-tobramycin in cirrhotics with severe infections. Hepatology 5:457, 1985

56. Fong TL, Akriviadis EA, Runyon BA, et al: Polymorphonuclear cell count response and duration of antibiotic therapy in spontaneous bacterial peritonitis. Hepatology 9:423, 1989

57. Runyon BA, Antillon MR: Ascitic fluid pH and lactate: insensitive and nonspecific tests in detecting ascitic fluid infection. Hepatology 13:929, 1991

58. Gilbert JA, Kamath PS: Spontaneous bacterial peritonitis: an update. Mayo Clin Proc 70:365, 1995

59. Tito L, Rimola A, Llach J, et al: Recurrence of spontaneous bacterial peritonitis in cirrhosis: frequency and predictive factors. Hepatology 8:27, 1988

60. Gines P, Rimola A, Planas R, et al: Norfloxacin prevents spontaneous bacterial peritonitis recurrence in cirrhosis: results of a double-blind, placebo-controlled trial. Hepatology 12:716, 1990

61. Rolachon A, Cordier L, Bacq Y, et al: Ciprofloxacin and long term prevention of spontaneous bacterial peritonitis: results of a prospec-

tive controlled trial. Hepatology 22:1171, 1995

62. Singh N, Gayowski T, Yu VL, et al: Trimethoprim-sulfamethoxazole for the prevention of spontaneous bacterial peritonitis: a randomized trial. Ann Intern Med 122:595, 1995

63. Vas SI: Peritonitis during CAPD: a mixed bag. Perit Dial Bull 1:47, 1981

64. Bailie GR, Eisele G: Continuous ambulatory peritoneal dialysis: a review of its mechanics, advantages, complications, and areas of controversies. Ann Pharmacother 26:1409, 1992

65. Vas SI: Treatment of peritonitis. Perit Dial Int 14:S49, 1994

66. Bernardini J, Piraino B, Sorkin M: Analysis of continuous ambulatory peritoneal dialysis-related Pseudomonas aeruginosa infection. Am J Med 83:829, 1987

67. Paterson AD, Bishop MC, Morgan AG, et al: Removal and replacement of Tenckhoff catheter at a single operation: successful treatment of resistant peritonitis in continuous ambulatory peritoneal dialysis. Lancet 2:1245, 1986

68. Swartz R, Reynolds J, Lees P, et al: Disconnect during CAPD: retrospective experience with three different systems. Perit Dial Int 9:175, 1989

69. Low DE, Vas SI, Oreopoulos DG, et al: Prophylactic cephalexin ineffective in chronic ambulatory peritoneal dialysis (letter). Lancet 2:753, 1980

70. Luzar MA, Coles GA, Faller B, et al: Staphylococcus aureus nasal carriage and infection in patients on continuous ambulatory peritoneal dialysis. N Engl J Med 322:505, 1990

71. Perez-Fontan M, Garcia-Falcon T, Rosales M, et al: Treatment of Staphylococcus aureus nasal carriers in continuous ambulatory peritoneal dialysis with mupirocin: long-term results. Am J Kidney Dis 22:708, 1993

72. Spence PA, Mathews RE, Khanna R, et al: Indications for operation where peritonitis occurs in patients on chronic ambulatory peritoneal dialysis. Surg Gynecol Obstet 161:450, 1985

73. Altemeier WA, Culbertson WR, Shook CD: Intra-abdominal abscesses. Am J Surg 125:70, 1973

74. Levison MA, Zeigler D: Correlation of APACHE II score, drainage technique and outcome in postoperative intra-abdominal abscess. Surg Gynecol Obstet 172:89, 1991

75. Lambiase RE, Deyoe L, Cronan JJ, et al: Percutaneous drainage of 335 consecutive abscesses: results of primary drainage with 1-year follow-up. Radiology 184:167, 1992

76. Field TC, Pickleman J: Intra-abdominal abscess unassociated with prior operation. Arch Surg 120:821, 1985

77. Baker ME, Blinder RA, Rice RP: Diagnostic imaging of abdominal fluid collections and abscesses. CRC Crit Rev Diagn Imaging 25:233, 1986

78. Korobkin M, Callun PW, Filly RA, et al: Comparison of computed tomography, ultrasonography and gallium-67 scanning in the evaluation of suspected abdominal abscess. Radiology 129:89, 1978

79. Moir C, Robins RE: Role of ultrasonography, gallium scanning, and computerized tomography in the diagnosis of intraabdominal abscess. Am J Surg 143:582, 1982

80. Richardson JD, DeCamp MM, Garrison RN, et al: Pulmonary infection complicating intra-abdominal sepsis: clinical and experimental observations. Ann Surg 195:732, 1982

81. Polk HC Jr, Shields CL: Remote organ failure: a valid sign of occult intra-abdominal infection. Surgery 81:310, 1977

82. Wilmore DW, Aulick LH: Thermoregulatory responses and metabolism. Surgical Infectious Diseases. Simmons RL, Howard RJ, Eds. Appleton-Century-Crofts, East Norwalk, Connecticut, 1982, p 297

83. Moore F, Feliciano D, Andrassy R, et al: Early enteral feeding, compared with parenteral, reduces postoperative septic complications: the results of a meta-analysis. Ann Surg 216:172, 1992

84. Cerra F: Nutrient modulation of inflammatory and immune function. Am J Surg 161:230, 1991

85. Levy E, Frileux P, Cugnenc PH, et al: High-output external fistulae of the small bowel: management with continuous enteral nutrition. Br J Surg 76:676, 1989

86. Wang SMS, Wilson SE: Subphrenic abscess: the new epidemiology. Arch Surg 112:934, 1977

87. Halasz NA: Subphrenic abscesses: myths and facts. JAMA 214:724, 1970

88. Hau T, Hoffman R, Simmons RL: Mechanisms of the adjuvant effect of hemoglobin in experimental peritonitis: I. In vivo inhibition of peritoneal leukocytosis. Surgery 83:223, 1978

89. Steinberg B: Infections of the Peritoneum. Hoeber, New York, 1944

90. Bagby GJ, Plessala KJ, Wilson LA, et al: Divergent efficacy of antibody to tumor necrosis-alpha in intravascular and peritonitis models of sepsis. J Infect Dis 163:83, 1991

91. Astiz ME, Saha DC, Carpati CM, et al: Induction of endotoxin tolerance with monophosphoryl lipid A in peritonitis: importance of localized therapy. J Lab Clin Med 123:89, 1994

92. Holzheimer RE, Schein M, Wittmann DH: Inflammatory response in peritoneal exudate and plasma of patients undergoing planned relaparotomy for severe secondary peritonitis. Arch Surg 130:1314, 1995

93. Schein M, Wittmann DH, Holzheimer R, et al: Hypothesis: compartmentalization of cytokines in intra-abdominal infection. Surgery 119:694, 1996

94. Malaviya R, Ikeda T, Ross E, et al: Mast cell modulation of neutrophil influx and bacterial clearance at sites of infection through TNF-alpha. Nature 381:77, 1996

95. Topley N, Brown Z, Jorres A, et al: Human peritoneal mesothelial cells synthesize interleukin-8: synergistic induction by interleukin-1 beta and tumor necrosis factor-alpha. Am J Pathol 142:1876, 1993

96. West MA: Role of cytokines in leukocyte activation: phagocytic cells. Mechanisms of Leukocyte Activation: Current Topics in Membranes and Transport. Grinstein S, Rotstein OD, Eds. Academic Press, New York, 1990, p 537

97. Ford-Hutchinson AW: Leukotriene B$_4$ in inflammation. CRC Rev Immunol 10:1, 1990

98. Corderio RSB, Martins MA, Silva PMR: Proinflammatory activity of platelet-activating factor: pharmacological modulation and cellular involvement. Prog Biochem Pharmacol 22:156, 1988

99. Mason MJ, van Epps DE: In vivo neutrophil emigration in response to interleukin-1 and tumor necrosis factor-alpha. J Leukoc Biol 45:62, 1989

100. Dunn DL, Simmons RL: Fibrin in peritonitis: III. The mechanism of bacterial trapping by polymerizing fibrin. Surgery 92:513, 1982

101. Sinclair SB, Rotstein OD, Levy GA: Disparate mechanisms of induction of procoagulant activity by live and inactivated bacteria and viruses. Infect Immun 58:1821, 1990

102. Hau T, Payne WD, Simmons RL: Fibrinolytic activity of the peritoneum during experimental peritonitis. Surg Gynecol Obstet 148:415, 1979

103. Dunn DL, Barke RA, Ahrenholz DH, et al: The adjuvant effect of peritoneal fluid in experimental peritonitis: mechanism and clinical implications. Ann Surg 199:37, 1984

104. Ahrenholz DH, Simmons RL: Fibrin in peritonitis: I. Beneficial and adverse effects of fibrin in experimental E. coli peritonitis. Surgery 88:41, 1980

105. Beecher HK, Simeone FA, Burnett CH, et al: The internal state of the severely wounded man on entry to the most forward hospital. Surgery 22:672, 1947

106. Clowes GHA Jr, Vucinic M, Weidner MG: Circulatory and metabolic alterations associated with survival or death in peritonitis: clinical analysis of 25 cases. Ann Surg 163:866, 1966

107. MacLean LD, Mulligan WG, McLean APH, et al: Patterns of septic shock in man—a detailed study of 56 patients. Ann Surg 166:543, 1967

108. Tracey KJ, Beutler B, Lowry SF, et al: Shock and tissue injury induced by recombinant human cachectin. Science 234:470, 1986

109. Dinarello CA: Interleukin-1. Rev Infect Dis 6:51, 1984

110. Castell JV, Gomez-Lechon MJ, David M, et al: Interleukin-6 is a major regulator of acute phase protein synthesis in adult human hepatocytes. FEBS Lett 242:237, 1989

111. Holzheimer RG, Schein M, Wittmann DH: Inflammatory response in peritoneal exudate and plasma of patients undergoing planned relaparotomy for severe secondary peritonitis. Arch Surg 130:1314, 1995

112. Tang G-J, Kuo C-D, Yen T, et al: Perioperative plasma concentrations of tumor necrosis factor-alpha and interleukin-6 in infected patients. Crit Care Med 24:423, 1996

113. Galandiuk S, Gardner SA, Heinzelmann M: Constituent analysis may permit improved diagnosis of intra-abdominal abscess. Am J Surg 171:335, 1996

114. Rotstein OD, Pruett TL, Simmons RL: Mechanisms of microbial synergy in polymicrobial surgical infections. Rev Infect Dis 7:151, 1985

115. Berne TV, Yellin AW, Appleman MD, et al: Antibiotic management of surgically treated gangrenous or perforated appendicitis: comparison of gentamicin and clindamycin versus cefamandole versus cefoperazone. Am J Surg 144:8, 1982

116. Bartlett JG, Louie TJ, Gorbach SL, et al: Therapeutic efficacy of 29 antimicrobial regimens in experimental intraabdominal sepsis. Rev Infect Dis 3:535, 1981

117. Solomkin JS, Dellinger EP, Christou NV, et al: Results of a multicentre trial comparing imipenem/cilastatin to tobramycin/clindamycin for intra-abdominal infection. Ann Surg 212:581, 1990

118. Solomkin JS, Hemsell DL, Sweet R, et al: General guidelines for the evaluation of new anti-infective drugs for the treatment of intra-abdominal and pelvic infections. Clin Infect Dis 15:S33, 1992

119. Smith CR, Moore RD, Lietman PS: Studies of risk factors for aminoglycoside nephrotoxicity. Am J Kidney Dis 8:308, 1986

120. Niemiec PWJ, Allo MD, Miller CF: Effect of altered volume of distribution on aminoglycoside levels in patients in surgical intensive care. Arch Surg 122:207, 1987

121. Hollener LF, Bahnini J, De Manzini N, et al: A multicentric study of netilmicin once daily versus thrice daily in patients with appendicitis and other intra-abdominal infections. J Antimicrob Chemother 23:773, 1989

122. Prins JM, Buller HR, Kuijper EJ, et al: Once versus thrice daily gentamicin in patients with serious infections. Lancet 341:335, 1993

123. Gerding DN, Olson MM, Peterson LR, et al: Clostridium difficile-associated diarrhea and colitis in adults: a prospective case-controlled epidemiologic study. Arch Intern Med 146:95, 1986

124. Teasley DG, Gerding DN, Olson MM, et al: Prospective randomised trial of metronidazole versus vancomycin for the treatment of Clostridium-difficile-associated diarrhea and colitis. Lancet 2:1043, 1983

125. Christou NV, Turgeon P, Wassef R, et al: Management of intra-abdominal infection: the case for intraoperative cultures and comprehensive broad-spectrum antibiotic coverage. Arch Surg 131:1193, 1996

126. Cohn SM, Cohn KA, Rafferty MJ, et al: Enteric absorption of ciprofloxacin during the immediate postoperative period. J Antimicrob Chemother 36:717, 1995

127. Dougherty SH: Role of enterococcus in intraabdominal sepsis. Am J Surg 148:308, 1984

128. Fry DE, Berberich S, Garrison RN: Bacterial synergism between the enterococcus and Escherichia coli. J Surg Res 38:475, 1985

129. Fass RJ, Scholand JF, Hodges GR, et al: Clindamycin in the treatment of serious anaerobic infections. Ann Intern Med 78:853, 1973

130. Barie PS, Christou NV, Dellinger EP, et al: Pathogenicity of the enterococcus in surgical infections. Ann Surg 212:155, 1990

131. Rotstein OD, Pruett TL, Simmons RL: Microbiologic features and treatment of persistent peritonitis in patients in the intensive care unit. Can J Surg 29:247, 1986

132. Marshall JC, Christou NV, Horn R, et al: The microbiology of multiple organ failure: the proximal gastrointestinal tract as an occult reservoir of pathogens. Arch Surg 123:309, 1988

133. Solomkin JS, Dougherty SH: The role of enterococci and Candida in intraabdominal surgical infection. Topics in Intraabdominal Surgical Infection, Part 2. Simmons RL, Ed. Appleton-Century-Crofts, East Norwalk, Connecticut, 1984, p 17

134. Mosdell DM, Morris DM, Voltura A, et al: Antibiotic treatment for surgical peritonitis. Ann Surg 214:543, 1991

135. Dougherty SH, Saltzstein EC, et al: Perforated or gangrenous appendicitis treated with aminoglycosides. Arch Surg 124:1280, 1989

136. Hopkins JA, Lee JCH, Wilson SE: Susceptibility of intra-abdominal isolates at operation: a predictor of postoperative infection. Am Surg 59:791, 1993

137. Hau T, Nishikawa R, Phangsab A: Irrigation of the peritoneal cavity and local antibiotics in the treatment of peritonitis. Surg Gynecol Obstet 156:25, 1983

138. Noon GP, Beall AC Jr, Jordon GL Jr, et al: Clinical evaluation of peritoneal irrigation with antibiotic solution. Surgery 62:73, 1967

139. Gerding DN, Hall WH, Schieri EA: Antibiotic concentrations in ascitic fluid of patients with ascites and bacterial peritonitis. Ann Intern Med 86:708, 1977

140. Sindelar WF, Mason GR: Intraperitoneal irrigation with povidone-iodine solution for presentation of intra-abdominal abscesses in the bacterially contaminated abdomen. Surg Gynecol Obstet 148:409, 1979

141. Pickard RG: Treatment of peritonitis with pre- and postoperative irrigation of the peritoneal cavity with noxythiolin solution. Br J Surg 59:642, 1972

142. Browne MK, MacKenzie M, Doyle PJ: A controlled trial of taurolin in established bacterial peritonitis. Surg Gynecol Obstet 146:721, 1978

143. Washington BC, Villalba MR, Lauter CB, et al: Cefamandole-erythromycin-heparin peritoneal irrigation: an adjunct to the surgical treatment of diffuse bacterial peritonitis. Surgery 94:576, 1983

144. Hallerback B, Andersson C, Englund N, et al: A prospective randomized study of continuous peritoneal lavage postoperatively in the treatment of purulent peritonitis. Surg Gynecol Obstet 163:433, 1986

145. Stephen M, Loewenthal J: Continuing peritoneal lavage in high-risk peritonitis. Surgery 85:603, 1979

146. Wittmann DH, Aprahamian C, Bergstein JM, et al: A burr-like device to facilitate temporary abdominal closure in planned multiple laparotomies. Eur J Surg 159:75, 1993

147. Bleichrodt RP, Simmermacher RKJ, van der Lei B, et al: Expanded polytetrafluoroethylene patch versus polypropylene mesh for the repair of contaminated defects of the abdominal wall. Surg Gynecol Obstet 176:18, 1993

148. Walsh GL, Chiasson P, Hedderich G, et al: The open abdomen: the Marlex mesh and zipper technique: a method of managing intraperitoneal infection. Surg Clin North Am 68:25, 1988

149. Garcia-Sabrido JL, Tallado JM, Christou NV, et al: Treatment of severe intra-abdominal sepsis and/or necrotic foci by an "open-abdomen" approach: zipper and zipper-mesh techniques. Arch Surg 123:152, 1988

150. Hau T, Ohmann C, Wolmershauser A, et al: Planned relaparotomy vs relaparotomy on demand in the treatment of intra-abdominal infections. Arch Surg 130:1193, 1995

151. Schein M, Hirshberg A, Hashmonai M: Current surgical management of severe intra-abdominal infection. Surgery 112:489, 1992

152. Solomkin JS, Meakins JL Jr, Allo MD, et al: Antibiotic trials in intraabdominal infections: a critical evaluation of study design and outcome reporting. Ann Surg 200:29, 1984

153. Fry DE, Garrison RN, Heitsch RC, et al: Determinants of death in patients with intraabdominal abscess. Surgery 88:517, 1980

154. Dellinger EP, Wertz MJ, Meakins JL, et al: Surgical infection stratification system for intra-abdominal infection: multicenter trial. Arch Surg 120:21, 1985

155. Bohnen J, Boulanger M, Meakins JL, et al: Prognosis in generalized peritonitis: relation to cause and risk factors. Arch Surg 118:285, 1983

156. Christou NV: Predicting septic related mortality of the individual surgical patient based on admission host-defence measurements. Can J Surg 29:424, 1986

157. Bohnen JMA, Mustard RA, Oxholm SE, et al: APACHE II score and abdominal sepsis: a prospective study. Arch Surg 123:225, 1988

158. Knaus WA, Draper EA, Wagner DP, et al: APACHE II: a severity of disease classification system. Crit Care Med 13:818, 1985

159. Christou NV, Barie PS, Dellinger EP, et al: Surgical Infection Society Intra-abdominal Infection Study: prospective evaluation of management techniques and outcome. Arch Surg 128:193, 1993

160. Cerra FB, Negro F, Abrams J: APACHE II score does not predict multiple organ failure or mortality in postoperative surgical patients. Arch Surg 125:519, 1990

161. Poenaru D, Christou NV: Clinical outcome of seriously ill surgical patients with intra-abdominal infection depends on both physiologic (APACHE II score) and immunologic (DTH score) alterations. Ann Surg 213:130, 1991

162. Nathens AB, Rotstein OD, Marshall JC: Tertiary peritonitis: clinical features of a complex nosocomial infection. Crit Care Med 21(suppl):S129, 1993

163. Sawyer RG, Rosenlof LK, Adams RB, et al: Peritonitis into the 1990's: changing pathogens and changing strategies in the critically ill. Am Surg 58:82, 1992

164. Norwood SN, Civetta JM: Abdominal CT scanning in critically ill surgical patients. Ann Surg 202:166, 1985

165. Nel CJC, Pretorius DJ, DeVaal JB: Re-operation of suspected intra-abdominal sepsis in the critically ill patient. S Afr J Surg 24:60, 1986

166. Wells CL, Maddaus MA, Simmons RL: Proposed mechanisms for the translocation of intestinal bacteria. Rev Infect Dis 10:958, 1988

167. Bendahan J, Coetzee CJ, Papagianopoulos C, et al: Abdominal compartment syndrome. J Trauma 38:152, 1995

168. Schein M, Wittmann DH, Aprahamian CC, et al: The abdominal compartment syndrome: the physiologic and clinical consequences of elevated intra-abdominal pressure. J Am Coll Surg 180:745, 1995

169. Cullen DJ, Coyle JP, Teplick R, et al: Cardiovascular, pulmonary, and renal effects of massively increased intra-abdominal pressure in critically ill patients. Crit Care Med 17:118, 1989

170. Taylor KJW, Wasson JFM, De Graaff C, et al: Accuracy of grey-scale ultrasound diagnosis of abdominal and pelvic abscesses in 220 patients. Lancet 1:83, 1978

171. van Sonnenberg E, D'Agostino HB, Casola G, et al: US-guided transvaginal drainage of pelvic abscesses and fluid collections. Radiology 181:53, 1991

172. Bennett JD, Kozak RI, Taylor BM, et al: Deep pelvic abscesses: transrectal drainage with radiologic guidance. Radiology 185:825, 1992

173. Saini S, Kellum JM, O'Leary MP, et al: Improved localization and survival in patients with intraabdominal abscesses. Am J Surg 145:136, 1983

174. Hoffer P: Gallium mechanisms. J Nucl Med 21:282, 1980

175. Dutcher JP, Schiffer CA, Johnston GS: Rapid migration of 111-indium-labelled granulocytes to sites of infection. N Engl J Med 304:586, 1981

176. Knochel JQ, Koehler PR, Lee TG, et al: Diagnosis of abdominal abscesses with computed tomography, ultrasound and 111-In leukocyte scans. Radiology 137:425, 1980

177. Wall SD, Fisher MR, Amparo EG, et al: Magnetic resonance imaging in the evaluation of abscesses. Am J Radiol 144:1217, 1985

178. Gerzof SG, Robbins AH, Johnson WC, et al: Percutaneous catheter drainage of abdominal abscesses: a five year experience. N Engl J Med 305:653, 1981

179. Haaga JR, Weinstein AJ: CT-guided percutaneous aspiration and drainage of abscesses. AJR Am J Roentgenol 135:1187, 1980

180. Gerzof SG, Johnson WC, Robbins AH, et al: Expanded criteria for percutaneous abscess drainage. Arch Surg 120:227, 1985

181. Mueller PR, Ferrucci JT Jr, Simeone JF, et al: Lesser sac abscesses and fluid collections: drainage by transhepatic approach. Radiology 155:615, 1985

182. Pruett TL, Rotstein OD, Crass J, et al:

Percutaneous aspiration and drainage for suspected abdominal infection. Surgery 96:731, 1984

183. Johnson WC, Gerzof SG, Robbins AH, et al: Treatment of abdominal abscesses: comparative evaluation of operative versus percutaneous

catheter drainage guided by computed tomography or ultrasound. Ann Surg 194:510, 1981

184. Olak J, Christou NV, Stein LA, et al: Operative vs percutaneous drainage of intraabdominal abscesses: comparison of morbidity and mortality. Arch Surg 121:141, 1986

Acknowledgments

This work was supported by the Medical Research Council of Canada and the Physicians' Services Incorporated Foundation. The author wishes to thank Christina Wareham for preparation of the manuscript.

16 INFECTIONS IN THE UPPER ABDOMEN: BILIARY TRACT, PANCREAS, LIVER, AND SPLEEN

Jeffrey S. Barkun, M.D., and Ronald T. Lewis, M.B.B.S., M.Sc.

Approach to the Patient with Upper Abdominal Sepsis

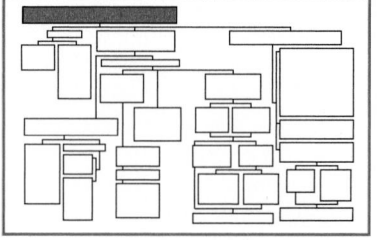

Biliary tract and pancreatic infection present as systemic sepsis or as infection localized in the upper abdomen. Typical findings include abdominal pain, a tender upper abdominal mass, fever and leukocytosis, and jaundice. Various combinations of these symptoms may occur, but it is convenient to consider three common clinical presentations; in each of these, one or two symptoms dominate: (1) upper abdominal pain and fever, (2) fever and jaundice, and (3) an upper abdominal mass and fever. These clinical findings signal the need for a battery of screening tests, which include a complete blood count; routine blood tests of liver function; determination of serum amylase level, prothrombin time, and partial thromboplastin time; blood culture; chest and abdominal x-rays; and an abdominal ultrasound examination. When considered together, the clinical findings and test results allow early differentiation of the three most common disease entities: acute cholecystitis, acute cholangitis, and acute pancreatitis.

Upper Abdominal Pain and Fever

DIAGNOSIS

The patient with upper abdominal sepsis may present with epigastric or right upper quadrant pain and fever. Only two thirds of these patients admitted with a working diagnosis of acute cholecystitis have acute biliary inflammation.[1] In some patients, nonsurgical conditions such as pneumonia, acute hepatitis, familial Mediterranean fever, herpes zoster of intercostal nerves, and gastrointestinal disease can be distinguished clinically from biliary disease. The most important screening test for acute biliary infection is the abdominal ultrasound examination: an abnormal image of the gallbladder or bile ducts supports a biliary etiology [*see Figure 1*].

Diagnosis should include differentiation of acute cholecystitis, biliary colic, acute pancreatitis, and acute cholangitis because each of these entities requires specific management [*see Table 1*]. For example, the initial management of biliary colic and mild acute pan-

creatitis is usually nonoperative, whereas severe acute cholangitis and acute cholecystitis require surgical, endoscopic, or radiologic intervention (see below). The clinical features and blood test results are helpful but may be inconclusive. The abdominal ultrasonogram may provide specific clues. Stones appear in biliary colic [*see Figure 1*]; stones and thickening of the gallbladder wall, in acute cholecystitis; gallstones and dilatation of the common bile duct, in acute cholangitis; and pancreatic enlargement and sonolucency, in pancreatitis. A radionuclide excretion scan using technetium-99m–labeled HIDA differentiates acute cholecystitis from acute biliary colic if the common bile duct, but not the gallbladder, is visualized up to 4 hours after injection of the isotope.[2]

Differentiating acute pancreatitis from acute cholecystitis may be difficult. The serum amylase level lacks specificity,[3] but if the clinical

Figure 1 **Abnormal abdominal ultrasound examination shows calculi in the gallbladder casting shadows on the underlying liver tissue.**

Table 1 Diagnostic Indicators of Upper Abdominal Pain and Fever

	Biliary Colic	Acute Cholecystitis	Acute Pancreatitis
Duration	Short: 40% < 1 hr	Persistent	Persistent
Pathogenesis	Visceral	Somatic	Retroperitoneal
Signs	Tender	Guarding and spasm	Guarding and spasm
Laboratory tests Liver function tests	Occasionally abnormal	Abnormal	Abnormal
Serum amylase	Normal	Normal or slightly increased	Increased
Leukocyte counts	Often normal	Increased	Increased

findings suggest acute pancreatitis, an elevated level of serum amylase clinches the diagnosis. In one study, the initial laboratory results in 100 patients with acute pancreatitis were compared with those in 100 patients with acute abdominal pain caused by acute cholecystitis, perforated peptic ulcer, or acute appendicitis.[4] The serum amylase concentrations were elevated in 95% of patients with acute pancreatitis but were normal in 95% of patients with acute abdominal pain of other causes. These concentrations peak within the first 48 hours and are almost always elevated in biliary pancreatitis[5]; in fact, a serum amylase concentration above 1,000 U/L strongly suggests a diagnosis of biliary pancreatitis.[6] Unless clinical findings and the results of biochemical tests and ultrasound are unequivocal, a contrast-enhanced spiral abdominal CT scan should be performed for establishment of the diagnosis and staging of acute pancreatitis. It has been suggested, however, that CT scanning should be reserved for patients with clinically suspected severe acute gallstone pancreatitis, on the grounds that the results would not change the recommended course of action in other patients.[7] Occasionally, a very mild pancreatitis may give rise to no findings on a CT scan, and the demonstration of a normal ^{99m}Tc-labeled HIDA scan may be helpful in differentiating this condition from acute cholecystitis.

Concurrent acute obstructive cholangitis must be considered in all patients with acute cholecystitis. Risk factors for acute cholangitis include advanced age, hypotension, a high serum bilirubin level, and a positive blood culture. Diagnostic indicators include a positive test for bilirubin in the urine, increased levels of the direct serum bilirubin, and increased alkaline phosphatase determinations. Positive blood cultures and a finding of dilated biliary ducts on the abdominal ultrasound examination usually confirm the diagnosis.

TREATMENT

Gallstone Pancreatitis

Standard therapy for gallstone pancreatitis includes intravenous fluids and narcotic analgesics. Nasogastric suction is useful in patients with severe pain or significant ileus but should not be used routinely.[8] The use of systemic antibiotics is controversial (see below); they are of benefit in the 10% to 34% of patients who have concomitant cholangitis.[9] Other treatments suggested previously have not proved useful when given in all cases of gallstone pancreatitis. These treatments include total parenteral nutrition and many pharmacologic agents, such as cimetidine, somatostatin, glucagon, and insulin.[10] Although continuous intraduodenal infusion of an el-

emental diet reduces exocrine pancreatic secretions in animal experiments,[11] enteral feeding is usually avoided in clinical treatment because premature feeding may cause a relapse of pancreatitis.[12]

In clinical practice, the need for further treatment depends on the severity of pancreatitis. The severity of the episode determines both the patient's risk of developing sepsis, which governs outcome, and the risk associated with early cholecystectomy [see V:11 Biliary Tract Procedures and V:12 Laparoscopic Cholecystectomy]. The clinical prognostic index developed by Ranson best defines the severity of pancreatitis [see Table 2]. In mild pancreatitis, one or two Ranson signs are present; in more severe pancreatitis, three to five signs are present; and in very severe pancreatitis, more than five signs are present. This distinction serves to stratify further treatment.

Mild pancreatitis usually subsides within 1 week of onset. Most surgeons defer cholecystectomy until then.[13] Urgent operation within 72 hours of admission may reveal acute cholecystitis in as many as 31% of patients.[14] It has also been suggested that urgent surgical decompression may prevent a relatively mild attack of pancreatitis from progressing to a lethal form.[15,16] An attack of acute gallstone pancreatitis is initiated by obstruction at the confluence of the lower end of the common bile duct and the pancreatic duct by a stone or by edema at the ampulla of Vater resulting from stone migration. These stones may be found and removed in 63% to 78% of patients who undergo operation within 72 hours of admission[14,15,17]; by contrast, they are present in only 3% to 33% of patients explored after the first week.[15,17-20] A randomized trial of the timing of surgery for gallstone pancreatitis showed that early surgery (within 48 hours after admission) was not associated with a significant increase in morbidity or mortality in patients with mild pancreatitis but did not change prognosis.[13]

Some surgeons have suggested that early endoscopic retrograde cholangiopancreatography (ERCP) and sphincterotomy [see V:6 Gastrointestinal Endoscopy] is an alternative to surgery of the common bile duct in patients with mild pancreatitis.[21] However, randomized trials comparing endoscopic treatment with conservative treatment within the first 72 hours in patients with mild pancreatitis did not find that urgent endoscopic sphincterotomy improved outcome in this group of patients.[22,23] Other studies[24,25] found that delaying surgery beyond 6 weeks may lead to a 32% to 57% risk of recurrent pancreatitis. Therefore, cholecystectomy and cholangiography should be delayed only until just before patients are discharged from the hospital 5 to 15 days after the onset of symptoms. Laparoscopic cholecystectomy has facilitated this approach without prolonging hospital stay.

Severe pancreatitis   Patients with three or more Ranson signs are at particular risk for pancreatic sepsis.[12] Repeated clinical and ra-

Table 2 Ranson's Early Objective Signs of Severity of Acute Pancreatitis[4]

On Admission	After Initial 48 Hours
Age > 55 yr Glucose > 200 mg/dl WBC > 16,000/mm^3 LDH > 350 IU/L AST > 250 Sigma Frankel U/dl	Serum Ca^{2+} < 8 mg/dl Arterial Po$_2$ < 60 mm Hg Base deficit > 4 mEq/L BUN increase > 5 mg/dl Hematocrit fall > 10% Fluid sequestration > 6,000 ml

Note: < 3 signs = mild pancreatitis; ≥ 3 signs = severe pancreatitis.
AST—aspartate aminotransferase   BUN—blood urea nitrogen   Po$_2$—oxygen tension   WBC—white blood cell

Patient presents with one or more of the following: upper abdominal pain, fever, jaundice, upper abdominal mass

Order screening tests:
- Blood tests (CBC, liver function, serum amylase, PT, PTT, culture)
- Chest and abdominal x-rays
- Abdominal ultrasonography

Normal ultrasound image

No biliary tract disease

Consider acute MI, pleuritis, pneumonia, acute hepatitis, herpes zoster, or peptic ulcer. Provide appropriate care.

Nongallstone pancreatitis

Diagnosis supported by clinical findings, ↑ serum amylase, and normal HIDA scan.
Provide supportive care (e.g., I.V. fluids, narcotic analgesics, NG suction).
Evaluate repeatedly with CT scan for septic complications of pancreatitis.
Repeat ultrasonography to verify absence of gallstones.

Abnormal ultrasound image located in biliary tract (e.g., stones; distended, thick-walled, or shrunken gallbladder; distended common bile duct)

Perform HIDA scan when feasible if diagnosis is unclear.

Gallbladder is visualized on HIDA scan, or results are equivocal

Gallstone pancreatitis

Diagnostic indicators:
- Absence of localized right upper quadrant tenderness
- ↑ Serum amylase or lipase
- ↑ WBC
- Abnormal LFTs

Biliary colic

Diagnostic indicators:
- Stones in gallbladder
- WBC often normal
- LFTs occasionally abnormal
Treatment:
- Provide analgesics and fat-free diet
- Perform elective laparoscopic cholecystectomy

Gallbladder is not visualized on HIDA scan

Diagnose acute cholecystitis, with right upper quadrant tenderness, abnormal LFTs, ? ↑ WBC, ? stones or gas in gallbladder.

Acute cholecystitis at high risk for perforation

Diagnostic indicators:
- Systemic toxicity
- Emphysematous cholecystitis
- Acalculous cholecystitis
Treatment:
- Give gentamicin and ampicillin or a single agent (e.g., piperacillin, ceftriaxone, or ciprofloxacin) for ≥ 5 days
- Perform urgent cholecystectomy
- Consider cholecystostomy

Ordinary acute cholecystitis

Good operative risk

Perform elective cholecystectomy.
Give cefazolin on call.

Poor operative risk

Give gentamicin and ampicillin or a single agent (e.g., piperacillin, ceftriaxone, or ciprofloxacin) for ≥ 5 days. If antibiotics fail, perform percutaneous transhepatic cholecystostomy oroperation.

Initiate conservative treatment

Provide I.V. fluids, narcotic analgesics, NG suction. Consider use of gentamicin and ampicillin.

Evaluate repeatedly for septic complications of pancreatitis

Consider Ranson's signs in timing of operation

< 3 Ranson's signs: Perform cholecystectomy if pancreatitis is not settling or when settled.
≥ 3 Ranson's signs: If pancreatitis is not settling, perform ERCP and sphincterotomy. When pancreatitis settles, perform cholecystectomy.

Approach to the Patient with Upper Abdominal Sepsis

Ultrasonography identifies mass not associated with biliary tree

Evaluate screening tests for WBC > 12,000/mm³, positive blood culture, and abnormal liver function

---

Liver mass

Perform serologic tests for *Entamoeba histolytica* and *Echinococcus*. Evaluate for history of travel to endemic areas. Perform GI evaluation.
Treat underlying cause:
- **Amebic abscess:** Give metronidazole for 10 days.
- **Echinococcal cyst with secondary infection:** Give gentamicin and ampicillin or single agent (e.g., ciprofloxacin). Perform definitive operation.
- **Pyogenic abscess:** Give gentamicin and metronidazole or single agent (e.g., imipenem or ticarcillin-clavulanate). Perform abdominal CT, followed by ERCP or PTC. Perform CT- or ultrasound-guided continuous percutaneous drainage or operative drainage.
- **Abscess secondary to inflammatory bowel disease:** Give gentamicin and metronidazole or single agent (e.g., imipenem or ticarcillin-clavulanate). Perform definitive operation, and drain abscess.
- **Cryptogenic abscess:** Give gentamicin and metronidazole or single agent (e.g., imipenem or ticarcillin-clavulanate). Perform continuous CT-guided closed drainage.

Acute cholangitis

Diagnostic indicators:
- Dilated biliary ducts on ultrasound
- Positive blood cultures
- Leukocytosis
- T° > 38.5° C
- Jaundice
- Abnormal LFTs

Biliary tract has undergone manipulation

Provide broad-spectrum antibiotic coverage (e.g., with imipenem or ticarcillin-clavulanate).

Biliary tract has not undergone manipulation

Give gentamicin and ampicillin. Alternatively, give a single agent (e.g., piperacillin, ceftriaxone, or ciprofloxacin).

Splenic hypoechoic mass

Confirm splenic abscess via contrast-enhanced abdominal CT scan. Give gentamicin and cloxacillin. Perform percutaneous catheter drainage; consider splenectomy.

Pancreatic mass

Give imipenem.
Differentiate pancreatic abscess and pseudocyst from phlegmon via Ranson's signs and CT findings.

Therapy is successful

Continue antibiotics for > 5 days. Perform abdominal CT scan, followed by ERCP or PTC. Perform definitive operation later.

Patient has serum bilirubin > 3 mg/dl, low BP, mental confusion, T° > 39.5° C

Perform emergency biliary decompression.

Previous cholecystectomy

Distal obstruction (dilated intrahepatic and extrahepatic biliary ducts on ultrasound):
Perform ERCP and sphincterotomy.
Proximal obstruction (dilated intrahepatic ducts):
Perform PTC and PTBD.

No previous cholecystectomy

High operative risk: Evaluate via ERCP or PTC; perform endoscopic sphincterotomy or PTBD.
Low operative risk: Perform urgent biliary exploration and appropriate drainage procedure.

< 3 Ranson's signs and category A or B on CT

Diagnose phlegmon; attempt nonoperative management first.

≥ 3 Ranson's signs and category C, D, or E on CT

Suspect pancreatic abscess or infected pseudocyst. Confirm suspicion of abscess with fine-needle aspirate yielding pus cells and bacteria.

Patients with cholangitis who remain in a septic state after biliary decompression should be evaluated for pyogenic liver abscess

Perform urgent surgical debridement and sump drainage. Alternatively, consider open drainage or marsupialization. Perform ancillary procedures as indicated.

diologic evaluation is required in these patients to ensure early detection of complications, because the outcome of an episode of pancreatitis depends on whether sepsis supervenes. When infection occurs, operative debridement and drainage are required [see Fever and Abdominal Mass, below]. Some surgeons have attempted to alter the course of severe disease by early operation. However, urgent operation is associated with a high mortality in patients with more than three Ranson signs.[13,17,19,26] To avoid the mortality associated with early operative intervention, some clinicians advocate early diagnosis by ERCP [see Figure 2] followed by biliary decompression by means of endoscopic sphincterotomy and stone extraction.[21] In a randomized trial comparing early ERCP and sphincterotomy to conservative therapy in patients with severe acute pancreatitis, ERCP and sphincterotomy decreased morbidity from 61% to 24% and lowered mortality from 18% to 4%.[22] The results of this trial, however, have been the subject of debate, and the success of this approach has been attributed by some authors to the treatment of a concomitant cholangitis rather than of the actual pancreatitis.[23] A well-conducted trial that excluded patients with concomitant cholangitis was published in 1997; unfortunately, this trial was unable to answer the question definitively, because too few patients with severe pancreatitis had been recruited.[27] Some authors have also argued that ERCP may also show pancreatic ductal disruption in some patients, and endoscopic placement of a pancreatic ductal stent may help reduce morbidity.[28]

Use of peritoneal lavage in early severe pancreatitis was advocated in one study[29] to decrease morbidity and mortality. Use of standard lavage over a 2-day period did not improve patient outcome, but use of peritoneal lavage for 7 days (long peritoneal lavage) provided some improvement in outcome.[30] Early use of antibiotics and selective decontamination have been proposed as means of reducing septic complications, but neither has convincingly or reproducibly been shown to improve prognosis.[31,32] More recently, investigators have made renewed attempts to modulate the initial systemic inflammatory response seen in early severe acute pancreatitis in such a way as to reduce the risk of subsequent infection and improve overall prognosis. Somatostatin has exhibited limited success in this regard,[33,34] but early reports on the use of lexipafant, an inhibitor of platelet-aggregating factor, have yielded promising results.[35]

Acute Cholecystitis

The standard treatment of acute cholecystitis consists of intravenous fluid administration, analgesics, and cholecystectomy. Although the timing of operation is somewhat controversial in ordinary acute cholecystitis,[36] cholecystectomy should be performed at the earliest opportunity [see V:11 Biliary Tract Procedures and V:12 Laparoscopic Cholecystectomy]. This approach has been confirmed by a randomized trial comparing early to late laparoscopic cholecystectomy.[37] The delayed-surgery group demonstrated a greater need for conversion to open cholecystectomy (23% versus 11%) as well as a longer total hospital stay and convalescence. The administration of systemic antibiotics is not required; however, single-dose antibiotic prophylaxis, such as cefazolin, 2 g I.V., can be given at the start of operation to prevent postoperative wound infection and intra-abdominal infection.[38]

Some patients with acute cholecystitis are at high risk for gangrene and perforation of the gallbladder. It is crucial to identify these patients and perform cholecystectomy promptly because delay increases morbidity and mortality. The three risk factors for gangrene and perforation of the gallbladder in patients with acute cholecystitis are marked systemic toxicity, emphysematous cholecystitis, and acute acalculous cholecystitis.

In ordinary acute cholecystitis, body temperature averages 37.8°C (100.04°F) but is normal in 20% of patients.[39] By comparison, the risk of gangrene and perforation is reportedly higher in patients with marked systemic toxicity, which is manifested by a pulse rate greater than 120 beats/min, body temperature above 39°C (102.2°F), and a shift to the left of the differential white blood cell count, showing more than 90% polymorphonuclear leukocytes.[40] Unfortunately, findings of systemic toxicity are frequently absent in elderly patients.

Emphysematous cholecystitis is an uncommon and insidious variant of acute cholecystitis; it is characterized by gas in the gallbladder lumen, wall, or pericholecystic soft tissue and biliary ducts secondary to gas-forming bacteria. The key to diagnosis is the evidence of air on abdominal x-ray[41] [see Figure 3] or ultrasound examination. Three stages of emphysematous cholecystitis have been defined: (1) gas is seen only in the lumen of the gallbladder, (2) a ring of gas is identified in the wall of the gallbladder, and (3) gas is seen in the tissues adjacent to the wall.[42] Compared with ordinary acute cholecystitis, emphysematous cholecystitis is associated with a fivefold increase in the risk of gallbladder perforation as well as a 10-fold increase in mortality in patients younger than 60 years [see Table 3].[43]

Studies from the 1960s noted an increased risk of gangrene and perforation of the acutely inflamed gallbladder in patients with diabetes mellitus.[44,45] The mortality for acute cholecystitis was shown to be five to 10 times higher in patients with diabetes than in other patients. Later studies, however, did not show an increased mortality in patients with both diabetes and acute cholecystitis.[46,47] Nevertheless, one third of patients with emphysematous cholecystitis also have diabetes. This factor plus the current tendency to perform chole-

Figure 2 Endoscopic retrograde cholangiopancreatography shows distal common bile duct stone in acute pancreatitis. The papillotome has been placed through the sphincter of Oddi in preparation for endoscopic sphincterotomy.

Figure 3 **Air outlines the gallbladder and bile ducts in emphysematous cholecystitis.**

Table 3 Comparison of Acute Cholecystitis and Emphysematous Cholecystitis

	Emphysematous Cholecystitis	Acute Cholecystitis
Gender	70% male	70% female
Stones	70%	90%
Bile culture positive	95%	66%
Clostridia found	46%	1.2%
Gangrenous gallbladder	75%	2.5%
Perforation of gallbladder	20%	4%
Mortality at age < 60 yr	15%	1.5%
Pathogenesis	Ischemia, obstruction	Obstruction

cystectomy early in most patients with acute cholecystitis may account for the disparity between previous studies and current reports.

Acute acalculous cholecystitis is another rare variant of acute cholecystitis, although its frequency increased from the 1950s through the 1990s.[48] This disease was originally described as occurring after surgical treatment of unrelated disease[49]; however, it has since been identified in patients with multiple trauma,[50] prolonged critical illness,[51] and sepsis.[52] Predisposing factors include gallbladder ischemia (in patients with shock or trauma) and biliary stasis (in prolonged fasting, hyperalimentation, and sustained narcotics therapy). In addition, focal inflammation may cause biliary colonization[51] or may activate coagulation factor XII, thereby causing severe injury to the blood vessels in the gallbladder muscularis and serosa.[48] A high index of suspicion is necessary. Acute acalculous cholecystitis should be considered in any postoperative or acutely ill patient with upper abdominal pain and fever or with unexplained fever and leukocytosis. It is particularly common 2 to 4 weeks after injury. The diagnosis is confirmed by findings on abdominal ultrasound examination [*see Figure 4*][53] and ^{99m}Tc–labeled HIDA scanning coupled with infusion of cholecystokinin and morphine.[54-56]

Patients with acute cholecystitis who demonstrate systemic toxicity, emphysematous cholecystitis, or acalculous cholecystitis are at high risk for gallbladder gangrene and perforation and therefore require prompt and aggressive treatment. Intravenous antibiotic therapy with agents such as gentamicin, 1.5 mg/kg every 8 hours, and ampicillin, 1 g every 6 hours, should be given for a period of at least 5 days. In patients exhibiting renal failure, a single agent, such as ceftriaxone, piperacillin, or a quinolone (e.g., ciprofloxacin or ofloxacin) can be used.[57,58] Early cholecystectomy is the treatment of choice.

If perforation and gangrene are not suspected but medical illness poses a high risk of mortality from operation, nonoperative supportive therapy may suffice. If this fails, another treatment option is cholecystostomy. Unfortunately, mortality may be as high as 20% to 30% with the traditional surgical approach.[59] Percutaneous transhepatic cholecystostomy has therefore been recommended for these high-risk patients,[60] particularly for those at low risk for perforation of the gallbladder.[61] To determine the risk of gallbladder perforation, a risk score can be assigned to each of seven findings that may be present on the preoperative abdominal ultrasound examination: pericholecystic fluid, 7 points; distention of the gallbladder, 4 points; intraluminal membrane, 4 points; intraluminal debris, 3 points; round gallbladder, 3 points; sonolucent zone in the gallbladder wall, 2 points; and a thick gallbladder wall (> 3.5 mm), 1 point.[61] A patient with a total risk score of 12 or more points requires urgent cholecystectomy; one with a lower score who does not respond to conservative treatment may be treated with percutaneous transhepatic cholecystostomy. A 1997 review of 59 patients exhibiting the septic response who underwent successful percutaneous radiologic cholecystostomy defined predictors of a successful clinical outcome: localized right upper quadrant tenderness and gallstones, as well as gallstones and pericholecystic fluid on ultrasound examination.[62] Patients with more equivocal findings may derive greater benefit from more invasive techniques that can simultaneously be used for diagnostic purposes (e.g., laparoscopy, which can even be performed at the ICU bedside[63]).

Figure 4 **Abnormal abdominal ultrasound examination confirms diagnosis of acute acalculous cholecystitis. When this image is compared with that in Figure 1, the thickening of the gallbladder wall and intraluminal debris are obvious.**

A few patients with acute cholecystitis will have concurrent acute cholangitis. Cholecystostomy is contraindicated in these patients because of its high mortality.[64] Adequate drainage of the common bile duct is required [see Fever and Jaundice, below].

Fever and Jaundice

DIAGNOSIS

If a patient presents with a temperature greater than 38.5°C (101.3°F) and jaundice [see II:6 Jaundice], the possibility of acute cholangitis should be investigated. If cholangitis is present, laboratory studies will reveal leukocytosis, and blood cultures will often be positive. A finding of gallstones and dilated biliary ducts on abdominal ultrasound examination supports the diagnosis. Reynolds' pentad is present in the full-blown syndrome.[65] This syndrome includes upper abdominal pain, fever and chills, jaundice, hypotension, and mental confusion.

Most of the findings associated with acute cholangitis are mimicked in empyema of the gallbladder.[66] In this condition, acute cholecystitis is complicated by suppuration within the gallbladder, which then becomes the focus of generalized sepsis. The distended gallbladder may be palpable and tender. When jaundice is present in empyema of the gallbladder, it is less likely to be obstructive than jaundice in acute cholangitis. True empyema of the gallbladder is rare. A positive ^{99m}Tc–labeled HIDA scan clinches the diagnosis. Treatment includes administration of intravenous fluids, systemic antibiotic therapy, analgesics, and early cholecystectomy.

Acute cholecystitis is occasionally manifest as an acute nonobstructive cholangitis; in this condition, systemic toxicity and low-grade obstructive jaundice are caused by a diffuse intrahepatic process transported from the acutely inflamed gallbladder to the liver through the lymphatics.[67] In some patients, the inflammatory process extends to involve the common bile duct and is most pronounced in the region of the ampulla. The obstructive edema in this area accounts for a transient mild elevation of the serum bilirubin concentration to approximately 3 mg/dl and for an increase in the serum alkaline phosphatase level to the upper limit of normal. These patients are not usually sufficiently ill to warrant immediate exploration. The ^{99m}Tc–labeled HIDA scan confirms acute cholecystitis, and blood cultures are negative. These patients are treated for acute cholecystitis.

In some patients with jaundice and inflammation, a stone impacted in the cystic duct or Hartmann's pouch of the gallbladder may suggest choledocholithiasis, but preoperative diagnosis by ERCP shows an extrinsic compression of the duct known as Mirizzi's syndrome. Two types of Mirizzi's syndrome exist. In type I Mirizzi's syndrome, a stone impacted in the cystic duct or Hartmann's pouch compresses the common hepatic duct and causes inflammation, thereby leading to jaundice. Treatment of type I Mirizzi's syndrome consists of obliteration of the cystic duct and careful partial cholecystectomy, with the neck of the gallbladder left in place. In type II Mirizzi's syndrome, protrusion of the stone into the hepatic duct erodes the septum between the cystic duct and the hepatic duct and causes a cholecystocholedochal fistula. Treatment of type II Mirizzi's syndrome involves internal biliary drainage to the wall of the cholecystocholedochal defect, usually with a choledochojejunostomy [see V:11 Biliary Tract Procedures], in addition to cholecystectomy.[68]

Patients with primary sclerosing cholangitis, especially those who have undergone internal or external biliary drainage, are at high risk

for recurrent bouts of ascending cholangitis.[69,70] Primary sclerosing cholangitis predominantly affects young males, particularly those with chronic ulcerative colitis. The diagnosis is suggested by the dominant cholestatic biochemical profile—that is, elevation of the serum bilirubin concentration, the serum alkaline phosphatase level, and aspartate aminotransferase activity. Because of the concomitant hepatic scarring, ultrasonography may not reveal the presence of dilated intrahepatic ducts [see II:6 Jaundice]. Definitive diagnosis requires visualization of the beaded appearance of the biliary tree by cholangiography. Cholangiocarcinoma and secondary sclerosing cholangitis in patients with Caroli's disease or choledochal cysts may mimic these clinical, biochemical, and radiologic features, but this is an unusual occurrence and can be distinguished by careful follow-up of patients.

Patients with oriental cholangiohepatitis present with recurrent episodes of cholangitis. Subsequent intrahepatic duct scarring will be shown by cholangiography. Irreversible extrahepatic liver damage may result because of the overwhelming propensity of these patients to form calcium bilirubinate stones.[71]

TREATMENT OF ACUTE CHOLANGITIS

Once acute cholangitis is diagnosed, resuscitation is started with intravenous fluids and a combination of antibiotics, such as gentamicin, 1.5 mg/kg I.V. every 8 hours, and ampicillin, 1 g I.V. every 6 hours. Alternatively, a single agent may be used, such as mezlocillin, cefoperazone, or piperacillin,[57,72-75] particularly in patients with marked hyperbilirubinemia, in whom treatment with aminoglycosides may contribute to renal toxicity in up to 33% of cases.[76] These antibiotics are required to deal with the various aerobic bacteria: most frequently, Escherichia coli, Klebsiella species, and enterococci. Anaerobic bacteria may be isolated in 15% to 30% of patients and are particularly likely to be present in diabetics, the elderly, or patients who have previously undergone biliary manipulation [see Discussion, Bacteriology of Acute Biliary Infection, below]. In patients with indwelling catheters, Enterobacter, Pseudomonas, and Candida organisms are now being isolated with increasing frequency. Indications of high risk include a serum bilirubin concentration greater than 3 mg/dl.

Approximately 75% of patients with acute cholangitis will respond to conservative measures,[77] and supportive treatment is continued. Subsequent investigations may include computed tomography followed by ERCP or needle percutaneous transhepatic cholangiography (PTC) to investigate proximal duct obstruction.[78,79]

For the 25% of patients who do not respond to conservative treatment, early recognition may improve their prognosis. In one study, patients who did not respond immediately to antibiotics had a mortality of 62%, compared with a mortality of 1.5% in those who improved.[80] In another study, indicators of high risk were an arterial blood pH less than 7.4, a serum bilirubin concentration above 9 mmol/L, a blood platelet count below 150×10^9/L, and a serum albumin concentration less than 30 g/L.[81] These high-risk patients will often have systemic hypotension, mental confusion, or temperature above 39°C (102.2°F) or hypothermia. Occasionally, acute cholangitis is complicated by disseminated intravascular coagulation [see I:5 Bleeding and Transfusion], which manifests itself as a tendency to bruise and bleed or merely as prolongation of the prothrombin time and the partial thromboplastin time, together with a fall in the blood platelet count. If disseminated intravascular coagulation is suspected, diagnosis should be confirmed and treatment started before biliary decompression.

Patients with refractory cholangitis who do not improve within 24 hours will require urgent biliary decompression.[82] Urgent biliary decompression has traditionally been accomplished via surgical exploration of the common bile duct and T-tube drainage [*see V:11 Biliary Tract Procedures*]. Cholecystostomy is an inadequate and often fatal option.[64,83] T-tube insertion alone may be lifesaving in the desperately ill patient,[84] but definitive internal decompression by means of an operative drainage procedure may be preferable in less urgent cases. In patients treated by choledochoduodenostomy, blood cultures and liver function returned to normal more rapidly, hospital stay was reduced, and no infection or recurrent stones developed. By contrast, 10% of patients treated with T-tube drainage had recurrent choledocholithiasis during a follow-up period that ranged from 1 to 5 years. A large common bile duct diameter is recommended for choledochoduodenostomy.[85]

Unfortunately, surgical decompression in these critically ill patients can result in a mortality of 30% to 40%.[82,86-89] Furthermore, reoperation is required in one third of survivors because important diagnostic information is not available at the initial laparotomy. As a result, nonoperative methods of biliary decompression, including percutaneous transhepatic biliary drainage (PTBD) and endoscopic sphincterotomy, have gained favor. PTBD was originally developed for preoperative management of biliary obstruction without cholangitis[90] but has not been found to be beneficial in that setting. PTBD has been associated with several minor periprocedural complications as well as major complications, such as septicemia and bleeding.[91] However, the so-called skinny Chiba needle technique and the use of a small volume of contrast material to locate catheter placement have lowered the complication rate during original catheter placement to less than 10%.[92]

Although PTBD can reduce the mortality associated with initial biliary decompression, definitive operation is still required for many patients. Consequently, endoscopic sphincterotomy [*see V:6 Gastrointestinal Endoscopy*] has been proposed as a definitive means of decompressing the biliary tree in patients with acute cholangitis [*see Figure 5*].[93] In a study of 82 patients with acute cholangitis caused by common bile duct calculi, early operation was employed in 28 patients, endoscopic sphincterotomy in 43, and antibiotic therapy alone in 11. Surgical mortality was 21% and morbidity 57%; by comparison, mortality for endoscopic sphincterotomy was 5% and morbidity 28%. A later study confirmed these findings.[81] In patients whose gallbladder is still in place, endoscopic sphincterotomy may even be a reasonable long-term option in the absence of cholecystectomy. Of 23 patients whose gallbladders were left in situ,[93] only two required cholecystectomy in the follow-up period of 1 to 7 years: one for empyema of gallbladder and one for recurrent cholangitis. The final choice of the method of nonoperative drainage will of course depend on local practice and available resources, as well as the patient's biliary anatomy.

Figure 5 Endoscopic sphincterotomy for acute biliary decompression in acute obstructive cholangitis is shown: at left, a stone is visible in the common hepatic duct, and the papillotome has been passed through the sphincter of Oddi; at right, the stone is held within a Dormia basket before extraction.

Fever and Abdominal Mass

A third group of patients who have upper abdominal sepsis present with fever and an upper abdominal mass that is identified either by clinical signs or by imaging techniques. Even if the mass is only vaguely palpable, the mass effect will be clarified by ultrasound examination of the abdomen. If the abdominal ultrasound examination is technically unsatisfactory because of intestinal gas, contrast-enhanced computed tomography of the abdomen will facilitate the diagnosis. The differential diagnosis is aided by the location of the mass. A mass that is located in the right upper quadrant usually indicates acute cholecystitis, although the presence of a liver abscess must also be considered. A mass that is located in the epigastrium or in the left upper quadrant usually signals a pancreatic infection; in rare instances, a solitary splenic abscess will be found. Patients with an intra-abdominal abscess in the subphrenic space or an interloop abscess may also present in this manner [see VI:15 Peritonitis and Intra-abdominal Abscesses].

RIGHT UPPER QUADRANT MASS

Diagnosis

In the setting of acute upper abdominal sepsis, a tender mass in the right upper quadrant is most likely an enlarged inflamed gallbladder. The diagnosis and treatment of acute cholecystitis have been discussed [see Upper Abdominal Pain and Fever, above].

Occasionally, abdominal ultrasound examination will reveal a pyogenic liver abscess. The most common cause of this abscess is biliary tract obstruction (35% of cases) caused by gallstones or malignant disorders, and the ultrasound examination may reveal both the abscess and the dilated biliary ducts. Previously, the most common cause of pyogenic liver abscess was portal pyemia caused by diverticulitis, inflammatory bowel disease, or perforated appendicitis. It now accounts for 20% of cases. Even less common is hematogenous spread via the hepatic artery. Approximately 20% of hepatic abscesses are cryptogenic. Ultrasonographic imaging of the liver may demonstrate lesions as small as 2 cm in the liver substance.[94] CT scanning, however, is superior to ultrasonography for evaluating the presence of air and abscesses as small as 0.5 cm in diameter, especially near the hemidiaphragms.[95,96] Abdominal CT is also the diagnostic modality of choice in the postoperative patient.[97] Radionuclide scanning with ^{99m}Tc sulfur colloid or gallium-67 citrate complements ultrasonography or CT scan[98,99] but cannot identify abscesses less than 2 cm in diameter. ERCP and percutaneous transhepatic cholangiography are indicated only when gallstone or biliary malignancy is the potential source of the abscess. Most liver abscesses occur in the right lobe: 40% are 1.5 to 5 cm in diameter, 40% are 5 to 8 cm in diameter, and 20% are more than 8 cm in diameter.

No imaging technique can reliably differentiate pyogenic from amebic abscesses. The best indication of a parasitic infection is a history of travel to an endemic area, such as Mexico, Central America, or Southeast Asia. However, when a hepatic abscess is detected by an imaging technique, serologic tests should be performed to rule out active amebiasis or echinococcal infection. Examination of stool for amebae is insensitive; consequently, isoenzyme analysis, *Entamoeba histolytica*–specific antigen detection, or even PCR is preferred to confirm the diagnosis of amebiasis.[100] The diagnosis of echinococcal liver abscess can be confirmed by means of elevated indirect hemagglutination (IHA) titers (> 250).[101] In the late 1980s, a combination of tests that included IHA for *Echinococcus granulosus* and enzyme-linked immunosorbent assay (ELISA) using *E. multilocularis* antigen was shown to allow an 89% species-specific diagnosis of echinococcal disease.[102] Later work indicated that IgG ELISA and IHA were the best tests for follow-up after resection of the abscess. In patients with a favorable clinical outcome, the specific IgG level decreased toward the end of the first year; in some cases, a positive serologic result persisted beyond 6 years.[103] Diagnostic aspiration is indicated when a diagnosis of pyogenic or amebic abscess is in doubt, but not in echinococcal disease. Aspiration may also be beneficial in patients with left-sided abscesses and abscesses more than 10 cm in diameter. Chest x-ray will be abnormal in up to 50% of cases of amebic abscess; the plain abdominal x-ray may show calcification of an echinococcal cyst with secondary pyogenic infection.

It is essential to differentiate infected echinococcal cysts from pyogenic abscess: special precautions are required for drainage of echinococcal cysts because of the risk of spillage and anaphylaxis. Blood cultures are positive in up to 50% of patients with pyogenic abscess, particularly in those with multiple abscesses; in fact, the presence of *Streptococcus milleri* in the blood suggests a visceral abscess.[104]

Treatment

The preferred treatment of pyogenic abscess is closed continuous percutaneous drainage guided by CT or ultrasonography, provided that the technique is technically feasible and no other indication for laparotomy exists.[105] Use of more than one catheter may be required for complete drainage. An alternative treatment is repeated percutaneous needle aspiration, the results of which have been comparable to those of continuous drainage.[106] One advantage to repeated needle aspiration is the elimination of cumbersome, painful drainage tubes, which are prone to dislodgment. Further studies, however, will be required to establish the place of this modality in the treatment of pyogenic abscess.

The abscess cavity is followed up by serial imaging until it collapses, and the catheter can usually be removed 2 to 3 weeks later. In the English literature, continuous percutaneous drainage has been associated with a complication rate of 4% and a failure rate of 15%.[107] However, operative drainage is the treatment of choice in patients with an identified intra-abdominal focus of infection and in patients in whom percutaneous drainage is not feasible or has failed.[108] Operative drainage is a highly effective treatment option that is associated with low mortality and morbidity.[109] In some patients, a limited hepatic resection may be required to eliminate multiple abscesses, particularly when an underlying intrahepatic stricture is the source.[110,111]

Treatment of pyogenic liver abscess should include systemic antibiotic therapy. Approximately 70% of pyogenic liver abscesses yield polymicrobial isolates,[112] and 25% to 45% of the organisms are anaerobic.[113] Multiple anaerobic isolates suggest the colon as a source, whereas a single isolate of *E. coli* suggests a nidus in the biliary tree. Antibiotic treatment should include initial coverage of both aerobes and anaerobes with either a single agent or multiple agents. The need to cover enterococci has been debated, but these organisms are becoming increasingly important nosocomial pathogens. Antipseudomonal treatment, on the other hand, appears to be unnecessary when antibiotic coverage is chosen empirically; thus, there is less need for an aminoglycoside as part of a dual drug treatment regimen.[114] An acceptable initial treatment regimen is gentamicin, 1.5 mg/kg, and metronidazole, 500 mg I.V. every 8 hours; alternatively, a single broad-spectrum agent (e.g., ticarcillin-clavulanate or meropenem) may be given.

The duration of antibiotic therapy is controversial[115]; according to one set of guidelines, antibiotics should be continued for 3 to 4 weeks when the abscess has been excised, 4 to 8 weeks when a solitary abscess has been drained, and 6 to 8 weeks when multiple macroscopic abscesses have been drained.[116] Multiple microscopic abscesses require that the biliary source be treated by decompression.[89] The overall prognosis for multiple small hepatic abscesses is not as good as that for solitary abscesses, and the development of a pyogenic abscess in a patient with an underlying hepatobiliary or pancreatic malignancy has been identified as a preterminal event associated with a hospital mortality of 28% and survival of less than 6 months.[117]

Medical treatment is now the standard approach to management of the patient with amebic liver abscess. Administration of the antiprotozoal agent metronidazole, 750 mg orally three times a day for 10 days, is a highly effective regimen.[118] A favorable response to treatment occurs within 4 to 5 days, and a decrease in the size of the abscess is apparent within a week on ultrasonographic examination, although a small residual cavity may persist for as long as 2 years.[119] If the patient's condition does not improve, needle aspiration and culture are indicated. Secondary infection is treated as a pyogenic abscess. Otherwise, oral emetine, 65 mg/day, is added for up to 10 days. Symptomatic or secondarily infected echinococcal cysts are best treated by means of surgical excision or marsupialization. The use of oral anthelmintics such as mebendazole has met with limited success.[120]

EPIGASTRIC OR LEFT UPPER QUADRANT MASS

Diagnosis

When the mass is in the epigastrium or left upper quadrant, a pancreatic source is most likely. Prompt and accurate diagnosis is crucial because severe pancreatic infection is fatal if untreated. The key to successful treatment is early diagnosis of infected pancreatic necrosis, infected pseudocyst, and pancreatic abscess. A high index of suspicion is required to diagnose these three infectious processes and to differentiate them from pancreatic inflammatory mass or phlegmon,[12] in which pancreatic edema and inflammation are present without necrosis or infection.

Correct diagnosis and treatment of infected pancreatic necrosis, infected pseudocyst, and pancreatic abscess requires an understanding of pathophysiology. It is generally assumed that infected pancreatic necrosis develops by a transmural, transductal, lymphatic, or hematogenous infection of a necrotic region of the pancreas. Infection develops in 40% of cases of pancreatic necrosis, usually in the second or third week of acute pancreatitis.[121] Surgical debridement is required in these cases to prevent death. Pancreatic abscesses form by liquefaction of infected necrosis. They usually occur after the fifth week of pancreatitis, when the acute phase of disease has subsided.[122] Pancreatic abscesses are associated with a lower mortality than infected pancreatic necrosis. Like pancreatic abscesses, infected pancreatic collections and pseudocysts present late in the course of pancreatitis. They are associated with a lower mortality than pancreatic abscesses. Caused by infection in 13% of localized collections resulting from ductal blowout, infected pancreatic collections and pseudocysts may occur in the pancreas, in contiguous peripancreatic tissue, or in remote (extrapancreatic) tissue.

Clinical evaluation alone is generally insufficient to diagnose pancreatic infection. A clearly defined upper abdominal mass is palpable in only 50% to 75% of cases.[12] In most patients, the screening battery of tests reveals leukocytosis with leukocyte counts greater than 15,000/mm³. Blood cultures are positive in 50% of cases. However, the common clinical indicators of sepsis (i.e., fever, leukocytosis, and toxicity) only suggest infection. CT-guided percutaneous aspiration and Gram's stain[121] and culture[123] provide the best method of diagnosing pancreatic infection. In one study of 75 patients with clinical toxicity suggestive of pancreatic sepsis, infection was confirmed in only 40%.[124] In another study of 21 patients with

pancreatic infection, only five had specific signs on abdominal CT scan.[125] The use of CT-guided diagnostic needle aspiration permitted correct diagnosis within 72 hours in two thirds of patients, and the mortality associated with operative intervention was 19%.

CT-guided needle aspiration, however, is only beneficial to the patient if pancreatic infection is suspected and if the technique is used early in the course of disease. The most important risk factors for pancreatic sepsis are clinical indicators of severe pancreatitis and findings on dynamic abdominal CT scan suggesting pancreatic necrosis.

Of the several methods of grading the severity of pancreatitis,[126-128] Ranson's method is the most widely used [see Table 2]. Pancreatic abscess occurs in 3% of patients with fewer than three signs, in 30% of patients with three to five signs, and in approximately 50% of patients with more than five signs.[12] To these criteria, Bank has added the clinical criterion of multisystem illness [see Table 4].[127] The presence of any one of these criteria indicates severe and potentially lethal disease. In patients with acute pancreatitis, shock and respiratory distress have been associated with mortalities of 88% and 71%, respectively[129]; furthermore, pancreatic abscess subsequently develops in 25% of patients with pancreatitis and shock.[130]

Comparison of these prognostic systems in acute pancreatitis shows that no system is more effective than another.[131] Their overall accuracy is 60% to 70%, but their correlation with pancreatic pathology is poor.[132] Nevertheless, it may be difficult to differentiate between pancreatic phlegmon, pseudocyst, and abscess.[130] In one study, the correct preoperative diagnosis of pancreatic abscess was made in only 44% of cases.[133]

Contrast-enhanced spiral abdominal CT scanning (dynamic pancreatography) helps to predict the severity of pancreatitis[134,135]; it has become an indispensable tool in the management of complicated pancreatitis. The finding of enhancement defects on abdominal CT distinguishes pancreatic necrosis from the inflammation and edema of pancreatic phlegmon; the site and size of major pancreatic collection or pseudocysts are clearly defined; and pancreatic abscess may be diagnosed by the presence of gas on the CT scan. CT scanning should, however, be repeated weekly in patients suspected of pancreatic infection because enhancement of the pancreas in a single examination does not rule out the presence of necrosis.[136]

Several laboratory markers of pancreatic necrosis have been investigated, such as serum methemalbumin,[137,138] serum ribonuclease,[139] and C-reactive protein.[140] Most of these markers are too insensitive for routine clinical practice. However, serum levels of

---

Table 4   Clinical Criteria for Severity of Pancreatitis[127]

Cardiac	Shock, tachycardia > 130 beats/min, arrhythmia, ECG changes
Pulmonary	Dyspnea, rales, Po₂ < 60 mm Hg, adult respiratory distress syndrome
Renal	Urine output < 50 ml/hr; rising blood urea nitrogen or creatinine, or both
Metabolic	Low or falling Ca²⁺, pH, albumin
Hematologic	Falling hematocrit, diffuse intravascular coagulation (low platelets, split products)
Hemorrhagic pancreatitis	Signs or peritoneal tap findings
Tense distention	Severe ileus, fluid

Note: positive signs in one system or more indicate severe (potentially lethal) disease.

C-reactive protein above 10 mg/dl were reported to have 95% accuracy in predicting necrosis.[141]

Currently, the best indicators of infected pancreatic necrosis or abscess are a combination of Ranson's objective prognostic signs and dynamic abdominal CT scan findings.[142] In Ranson's series, the pancreatic findings on computed tomography have been graded in five categories [see Figure 6][142,143]: (a) normal, (b) pancreatic enlargement alone, (c) inflammation of the pancreas and peripancreatic fat, (d) one peripancreatic fluid collection, and (e) two or more peripancreatic fluid collections. Only category e was associated with a high incidence (61%) of pancreatic abscess. The number of objective prognostic signs present also predicted the incidence of abscess: fewer than three signs, 12.5%; three to five signs, 31.8%; and more than five signs, 80%. However, the value of this method was limited because only five of the 83 patients evaluated had more than five prognostic signs. By combining the objective prognostic signs with positive abdominal CT findings, the investigators identified 30 patients who had three or more objective signs and were graded as either category c, d, or e on abdominal CT scan; in these patients, the incidence of pancreatic abscess was 56.7%. By contrast, no patient with fewer than three prognostic signs and graded as category a or b on abdominal CT scan had a pancreatic abscess.

Treatment

Once pancreatic infection is diagnosed, supportive measures are initiated. These include nasogastric suction, withholding of oral feeding, meticulous attention to respiratory care and fluid and electrolyte balance, systemic antibiotic therapy, and nutritional support (see below). However, the key to successful treatment is surgical, interventional radiologic, or endoscopic drainage.

Sterile pancreatic necrosis is not an indication for surgical debridement. In one prospective study, 11 patients with demonstrated sterile pancreatic necrosis were all followed successfully with conservative treatment.[144] Once infected pancreatic necrosis is confirmed by Gram's stain or culture, surgical debridement is required to remove the infected slough because radiologic or endoscopic methods are not effective.

The choice of drainage technique is controversial. Many clinicians prefer operative debridement and sump drainage.[12,145] The mortality associated with operative debridement and sump drainage may range from 30% to 40%[146]; unfortunately, this technique may be associated with a 30% to 40% reoperation rate because of sepsis or gastrointestinal complications.[12,145,147]

To reduce the frequency of reoperation and to lower mortality, some clinicians have opted for open drainage or marsupialization of the infected pancreas.[148,149] Others have modified the method further by employing Marlex mesh and a zipper to facilitate repeated reexplorations in patients with severe intra-abdominal abscess.[150] A 1991 meta-analysis of published surgical studies on infected pancreatic necrosis since 1980 found statistically better results with debridement and lavage or debridement and open packing than with conventional debridement and sump drainage.[151] However, surgical treatment should be customized for each patient. In one study, open packing was used for massive necrosis (more than 100 g removed by debridement at operation or CT evidence of at least 50% pancreatic necrosis) or for extrapancreatic necrosis, whereas conventional debridement and sump drainage were used in other cases[143]; the overall mortality in this study was only 14%. Pancreatic abscess resulting from liquefaction of necrosis is also best treated by surgical drainage because residual necrosis may cause failure of treatment by percutaneous methods.[152] On the other hand, infected pancreatic fluid collections and pseudocysts can usually be treated by nonoperative methods. In one prospective study, percutaneous

and surgical methods of drainage were equally successful in treating infected pancreatic fluid collections and pseudocysts.[153] Clinical findings rather than CT findings are the best indicators of the need for intervention, and nonoperative methods should be attempted before open surgery is planned.

In the past, debridement and sump drainage were accompanied by the triple ostomy technique, which comprises cholecystostomy, gastrostomy, and jejunostomy.[154] However, the role of these ancillary procedures is controversial. Cholecystostomy is now employed only if gallstones are detected. Evidence also suggests that intravenous hyperalimentation is preferable to jejunostomy feeding because early oral feeding appears to predispose to recrudescence of pancreatitis and eventual abscess formation, whereas prolonged restriction of oral feeding allows pancreatic inflammation to subside.[12]

Other operative procedures may be required to manage gastric or colonic complications. Gastric bleeding, gastric outlet obstruction, and gastric fistula requiring reoperation are relatively infrequent in this setting. By contrast, colonic necrosis and fistula formation are more common and occur either spontaneously or as a result of treatment. The usual site of involvement is the splenic flexure or upper descending colon. Treatment consists of colonic resection or diverting colostomy [see V:17 Colorectal Procedures].

The role of systemic antibiotic therapy in the prophylaxis of pancreatic abscess is controversial. Experimental evidence suggests that antibiotics may sometimes decrease the severity of pancreatitis,[155] and endoscopic cannulation of the pancreatic duct has now yielded bacteria in pancreatic secretions of patients with acute pancreatitis.[156] In patients with pancreatic abscess, bacteriologic cultures are usually polymicrobial. The most common organisms are *E. coli*, enterococci, *K. pneumoniae*, *P. aeruginosa*, *Staphylococcus aureus*, *B. fragilis*, and *Clostridium perfringens*. The reported incidence of anaerobic infection is low (6%). As a result, broad-spectrum antibiotic therapy, such as gentamicin, 1.5 mg/kg I.V. every 8 hours, and clindamycin, 600 mg I.V. every 6 hours, is indicated. Intravenous monotherapy, such as imipenem, ticarcillin-clavulanate, or ciprofloxacin, which are effective against most pancreatic pathogens, is becoming increasingly popular. Of late, there has been a growing trend toward early use of prophylactic antibiotics in cases of pancreatic necrosis, even though there are no data that convincingly demonstrate a clinical benefit.[31] This trend may be partly responsible for the increasing prevalence of *Candida* species in pancreatitis-related sepsis. A 1996 report stated that *Candida* infection was detected in 21% of patients.[157]

Nutritional support of the patient with pancreatic abscess usually consists of total parenteral nutrition. In these patients, the metabolic demand is high, and glucose intolerance or hyperlipidemia may occur. Still, intravenous feeding is generally well tolerated. A 10-fold increase in mortality (2.5% versus 21%) has been reported in patients in whom a positive nitrogen balance had not been achieved.[158]

Splenic Abscess

Diagnosis Splenic abscess should be considered in patients who present with fever and a left upper quadrant mass, although it is rarely the cause of these symptoms. Most abscesses encountered by the clinician are solitary. Multiple abscesses are usually covert and are found at autopsy of patients who had disseminated malignancy, collagen vascular disease, or chronic debility.[159]

Because splenic abscess is rare, correct diagnosis requires a high index of suspicion. The main clue is the clinical setting: both bacteremia and local splenic disease are required to produce splenic abscess.[160] In the preantibiotic period, this combination was seen most

Figure 6 Pancreatic findings on CT scan have been graded by Ranson into five categories: grade A—normal pancreas (*a*); grade B—diffuse enlargement of the pancreas and nonhomogeneous density of the gland (*b*); grade C—diffuse enlargement of the pancreas associated with peripancreatic inflammation (*c*); grade D—high-density fluid collection in left anterior pararenal space (only the head of the pancreas is visualized at this level) (*d*); and grade E—diffuse enlargement of the pancreas with several intrapancreatic small fluid collections and poorly defined fluid collections adjacent to the tail and head of the pancreas (*e*). In the final CT scan of this series (*f*), a pancreatic abscess is demonstrated; a partially encapsulated fluid collection containing bubbles of air represents a large abscess.

frequently in patients with bacterial endocarditis[161] and typhoid.[162] Even today, 80% of splenic abscesses occur in patients in whom an infection is already evident elsewhere in the body[163]; splenic abscesses can also occur in patients with splenic infarcts, splenic hematomas, or local splenic disease caused by hemoglobinopathies.[164,165]

The diagnosis of splenic abscess may be supported by indirect radiologic signs, such as an elevated left hemidiaphragm or the finding of a left upper quadrant air-fluid level simulating the stomach. To clinch the diagnosis, an abdominal ultrasound examination or abdominal CT scan is required. The abdominal CT scan, enhanced by intravenous or oral contrast, is preferred [*see Figure 7*].[166] This technique provides a direct image of the spleen; abscesses appear as low-density areas that may contain gas.

Treatment   Treatment of splenic abscess includes intravenous administration of antibiotics and splenectomy. The usual pathogen-

Figure 7 Abdominal CT scan, enhanced by contrast material, confirms diagnosis of splenic abscess.

ic organisms found are staphylococci and streptococci, although gram-negative bacilli and anaerobic bacteria may also be present. Cloxacillin, 1 g intravenously every 6 hours, and gentamicin, 1.5 mg/kg intravenously every 8 hours, should be given for a period of at least 5 days. When splenic abscesses are not drained, the mortality approaches 100%. In previous years, splenotomy was the preferred operative treatment of splenic abscess,[162-167] but splenectomy has since become the preferred method. Percutaneous catheter drainage is currently being performed with increasing frequency and appears to be as effective as operative drainage.[8,168-171]

Discussion

Pathophysiology of Acute Bacterial Cholangitis

Longmire's widely accepted classification of acute bacterial cholangitis consists of five categories—acute nonobstructive, acute nonsuppurative, acute suppurative, acute obstructive suppurative, and acute suppurative with intrahepatic abscess. It implies that the severity of disease parallels the degree of obstruction of biliary ducts.[171] This suggestion is well founded. In acute nonobstructive cholangitis associated with acute cholecystitis, infection ascends along the intrahepatic and extrahepatic lymphatics.[67] In obstructive cholangitis, the bile duct contains bacteria under pressure. When the pressure is at or above the normal secretion pressure (i.e., 200 mm Hg), bacteria pass into the lymphatic system. At a pressure greater than 250 mm Hg, bacteria may pass directly from the bile ductules through the spaces of Mall and Disse and into the hepatic sinusoids via cholangiovenous reflux.[172,173] One study confirmed the clinical significance of increasing ductal pressure by demonstrating a higher ductal pressure and a higher incidence of bacteremia in patients with proximal ductal obstruction, compared with those with distal malignant biliary obstruction.[174] However, no correlation exists between the degree of suppuration in the duct and the clinical or pathologic severity of obstructive cholangitis.[82,175] Therefore, the terms acute nonsuppurative cholangitis and acute suppurative cholangitis are purely descriptive and do not imply differing degrees of severity.

The source of bacteria in acute cholangitis is most often the duodenum. The ease with which organisms reflux from the duodenum is dependent on the degree of obstruction. Thus, in patients with malignant biliary obstruction, in whom obstruction is usually complete, bile culture is positive in only 10% to 15% of patients[176]; acute cholangitis is seldom spontaneous in this setting but often follows radiologic intervention.[177] By comparison, in patients with ductal stones or benign strictures, in whom biliary obstruction is often incomplete, bile cultures obtained on ERCP are positive in 64% to 87% of cases; in these patients, acute cholangitis occurs frequently, both spontaneously and after ductal manipulation.[178]

An alternative source of organisms in acute bacterial cholangitis is portal venous blood. In patients who have recurrent pyogenic cholangitis, which occurs frequently in the Far East, a 40% incidence of positive portal blood culture has been reported.[179] In studies in rats who have ligated bile ducts, bacteria were shown to be effectively transmitted to the bile ducts and liver through portal blood.[180] Finally, in nonobstructive cholangitis and acute cholecystitis, as well as in the early stages of obstructive cholangitis, infection ascends to the liver through the lymphatic system.

Bacteriology of Acute Biliary Infection

Most biliary infections are polymicrobial. The organisms most frequently cultured are *E. coli*, *Klebsiella* species, *Enterobacter* species, and enterococci.[83] Anaerobic bacteria are infrequently implicated in biliary infections. Peptostreptococci and clostridia are found occasionally; clostridia are especially common in patients with emphysematous cholecystitis.[43] Gram-negative anaerobic bacilli are rarely present in patients with biliary infection. In one study, only two of 28 patients with acute cholangitis had anaerobic bacteria in the bile; another investigator found anaerobic bacteria in 3% to 4% of cultures in similar patients.[181] However, a higher incidence of anaerobic bacteria has been reported in patients who have acute cholangitis and acute cholecystitis than in patients who have chronic cholecystitis and cholelithiasis.[182]

One investigator noted an increased incidence of anaerobic bacteria in biliary infection and suggested that *B. fragilis* may play a more important role in the polymicrobial flora of biliary tract infection than appreciated previously.[183] To date, these findings have been controversial. *Bacteroides* species are generally considered to be of limited importance in biliary tract infections, except in selected groups of patients. These patients include diabetics, the elderly,[184] and those with acute cholangitis who have previously undergone biliary operation[185,186]; in particular, malfunctioning biliary-intestinal anastomoses increase the risk of *Bacteroides* infection.[187]

References

1. Schofield PF, Hulton NR, Baildam AD: Is it acute cholecystitis? Ann R Coll Surg Engl 68:14, 1986

2. Weissmann HS, Frank MS, Bernstein LH, et al: Rapid and accurate diagnosis of acute cholecystitis with ^{99m}Tc-HIDA cholescintigraphy. AJR Am J Roentgenol 132: 523, 1979

3. Adams JT, Libertino JA, Schwartz SI: Significance of an elevated serum amylase. Surgery 63:877, 1968

4. Ranson JHC: Acute pancreatitis. Curr Probl Surg 16:1, 1979

5. Winslet M, Hall C, London NJ, et al: Relation of diagnostic serum amylase levels to etiology and severity of acute pancreatitis. Gut 33:982, 1992

6. Patti M, Pellegrini CA, Way LW: Serum amylase is useful in the differential diagnosis of acute abdominal pain. Gastroenterology 90:1580, 1986

7. Toosie A, Chang L, Renslo R, et al: Early computed tomography is rarely necessary in gallstone pancreatitis. Am Surg 63:904, 1997

8. Sarr MG, Sanfrey H, Cameron JL: Prospective, randomized trial of nasogastric suction in patients with acute pancreatitis. Surgery 100:500, 1986

9. Bradley EL III: Antibiotics in acute pancreatitis: current status and future direction. Am J Surg 158:472, 1989

10. Steinberg WM, Schlesselman SE: Treatment of acute pancreatitis: comparison of animal and human studies. Gastroenterology 93:1420, 1987

11. McArdle AH, Rosenberg M, Fried GM, et al: Pancreatic exocrine secretion in response to continuous and bolus feeding (abstr). Presented at the 19th Annual Meeting, Association for Academic Surgery, 1985, Cincinnati, Ohio

12. Ranson JH, Spencer FC: Prevention, diagnosis, and treatment of pancreatic abscess. Surgery 82:99, 1977

13. Kelly TR, Wagner DS: Gallstone pancreatitis: a prospective randomized trial of the timing of surgery. Surgery 104:600, 1988

14. Stone HH, Fabian TC, Dunlop WE: Gallstone pancreatitis: biliary tract pathology in relation to time of operation. Ann Surg 194:305, 1981

15. Acosta JM, Rossi R, Galli OMR, et al: Early surgery for acute gallstone pancreatitis: evaluation of a systematic approach. Surgery 83:367, 1978

16. Acosta JM, Pellegrini CA, Skinner DB: Etiology and pathogenesis of acute biliary pancreatitis. Surgery 88:118, 1980

17. Kelly TR: Gallstone pancreatitis: the timing of surgery. Surgery 88:345, 1980

18. Dixon JA, Hillam JD: Surgical treatment of biliary tract disease associated with acute pancreatitis. Am J Surg 120:371, 1970

19. Ranson JHC: The timing of biliary surgery in acute pancreatitis. Ann Surg 189:654, 1979

20. Paloyan D, Simonowitz D, Skinner DB: The timing of biliary tract operations in patients with pancreatitis associated with gallstones. Surg Gynecol Obstet 141:737, 1975

21. Neoptolemos JP, London N, Slater ND, et al: A prospective study of ERCP and endoscopic sphincterotomy in the diagnosis and treatment of acute pancreatitis: a rational and safe approach to management. Arch Surg 121:697, 1986

22. Neoptolemos JP, Carr-Locke DL, London NJ, et al: Controlled trial of urgent endoscopic retrograde cholangiopancreatography and endoscopic sphincterotomy versus conservative treatment for acute pancreatitis due to gallstones. Lancet 2:979, 1988

23. Fan S-T, Lai ECS, Mok FPT, et al: Early treatment of acute biliary pancreatitis by endoscopic papillotomy. N Engl J Med 328:228, 1993

24. Williamson RC: Early assessment of severity in acute pancreatitis. Gut 25:1331, 1984

25. Srinathan SK, Barkun JS, Mehta SN, et al: Evolving management of mild-to-moderate gallstone pancreatitis. J Gastrointest Surg 2:385, 1998

26. Osborne DH, Imrie CW, Carter DC: Biliary surgery in the same admission for gallstone-associated acute pancreatitis. Br J Surg 68:758, 1981

27. Foelsch UR, Nitsche R, Luedtke R, et al: Early endoscopic retrograde cholangiopancreatography was not beneficial in pancreatitis. N Engl J Med 336:237, 1997

28. Kozarek RA, Patterson DJ, Ball TJ, et al: Endoscopic placement of pancreatic stents and drains in the management of pancreatitis. Ann Surg 209:261, 1989

29. Stone HH, Fabian TC: Peritoneal dialysis in the treatment of acute alcoholic pancreatitis. Surg Gynecol Obstet 150:878, 1990

30. Ranson JHC, Berman RS: Long peritoneal lavage decreases pancreatic sepsis in acute pancreatitis. Ann Surg 211:708, 1990

31. Pedrezoli P, Bassi C, Vesentini S, et al: A randomized multicenter clinical trial of antibiotic prophylaxis of septic complications in acute necrotizing pancreatitis with imipenem. Surg Gynecol Obstet 176:483, 1993

32. Luiten EJ, Hop WC, Lange JF, et al: A controlled clinical trial of selective decontamination for the treatment of severe acute pancreatitis. Ann Surg 222:57, 1995

33. Fiedler F, Jauernig G, Keim V, et al: Octreotide treatment in patients with necrotizing pancreatitis and pulmonary failure. Intens Care Med 22:909, 1996

34. Paran H, Neufeld D, Mayo A, et al: Preliminary report of a prospective randomized study of octreotide in the treatment of severe acute pancreatitis. J Am Coll Surg 181:121, 1995

35. Kingsnorth AN, Galloway SW, Formela LJ: Randomized, double blind phase 2 trial of lexipafant, a platelet-activating factor antagonist, in human acute pancreatitis. Br J Surg 82:1414, 1995

36. Sianesi M, Ghirarduzzi A, Percudani M, et al: Cholecystectomy for acute cholecystitis: timing of operation, bacteriologic aspects, and postoperative course. Am J Surg 148:609, 1984

37. Lo CM, Liu CL, Fan ST, et al: Prospective randomized study of early versus delayed laparoscopic cholecystectomy for acute cholecystitis. Ann Surg 227:461, 1998

38. Lewis RT, Allan CM, Goodall RG, et al: A single preoperative dose of cefazolin prevents postoperative sepsis in high risk biliary surgery. Can J Surg 27:44, 1984

39. Eliason EL, Stevens LW: Acute cholecystitis. Surg Gynecol Obstet 78:98, 1944

40. Clifford WJ: Acute gangrenous cholecystitis. N Engl J Med 241:640, 1949

41. Hegner CF: Gaseous pericholecystitis with cholecystitis and cholelithiasis. Arch Surg 22:993, 1931

42. Jacob H, Appelman R, Stein HD: Emphysematous cholecystitis. Am J Gastroenterol 71:325, 1979

43. Mentzer RM, Golden GT, Chandler JG, et al: A comparative appraisal of emphysematous cholecystitis. Am J Surg 129:10, 1975

44. Turner RJ III, Becker WF, Coleman WO, et al: Acute cholecystitis in the diabetic. South Med J 62:228, 1969

45. Turrill FL, McCarron MM, Mikkelsen WP: Gallstones and diabetes: an ominous association. Am J Surg 102:184, 1961

46. Walsh DB, Eckhauser FE, Ramsburgh SR, et al: Risk associated with diabetes mellitus in patients undergoing gallbladder surgery. Surgery 91:254, 1982

47. Pickleman J: Controversies in biliary tract surgery. Can J Surg 29:429, 1986

48. Glenn F, Becker CG: Acute acalculous cholecystitis: an increasing entity. Ann Surg 195:131, 1982

49. Glenn F: Acute cholecystitis following the surgical treatment of unrelated disease. Ann Surg 126:411, 1947

50. Rice J, Williams HC, Flint LM, et al: Post-traumatic acalculous cholecystitis. South Med J 73:14, 1980

51. Long TN, Heimbach DM, Carrico CJ: Acalculous cholecystitis in critically ill patients. Am J Surg 136:31, 1978

52. Orlando R III, Gleason E, Drezner AD: Acute acalculous cholecystitis in the critically ill patient. Am J Surg 145:472, 1983

53. Deitch EA, Engel JM: Acute acalculous cholecystitis: ultrasonic diagnosis. Am J Surg 142:290, 1981

54. Weissmann HS, Berkowitz D, Fox MS, et al: The role of technetium-99m iminodiacetic acid (IDA) cholescintigraphy in acute acalculous cholecystitis. Radiology 146:177, 1983

55. Chen CC, Holder LE, Maunoury C, et al: Morphine augmentation increases gallbladder visualization in patients pretreated with cholecystokinin. J Nucl Med 38:644, 1997

56. Cabana MD, et al: Morphine-augmented hepatobiliary scintigraphy: a meta-analysis. Nucl Med Commun 16:1068, 1995

57. Karachalios GN, Nasiopoulou DD, Bourlinou PK, et al: Treatment of acute biliary tract infections with ofloxacin: a randomized, controlled clinical trial. Int J Clin Pharmacol Ther 34:555, 1996

58. Krajden S, Yaman M, Fuksa M, et al: Piperacillin versus cefazolin given perioperatively to high-risk patients who undergo open cholecystectomy: a double-blind, randomized trial. Can J Surg 36:245, 1993

59. Skillings JC, Kumal C, Hinshaw JR: Cholecystostomy: a place in modern biliary surgery? Am J Surg 139:865, 1980

60. Klimberg S, Hawkins I, Vogel SB: Percutaneous cholecystostomy for acute cholecystitis in high-risk patients. Am J Surg 153:125, 1987

61. Miyazaki K, Uchiyama A, Nakayama F: New approach to the timing of operative intervention for acute cholecystitis: use of ultrasound risk score (abstr). The 32nd World Congress of Surgery, Sydney, Australia, September 20–26, 1987

62. England RE, McDermott VG, Smith TP, et al: Percutaneous cholecystostomy: who responds? AJR Am J Roentgenol 168:1247, 1997

63. Orlando R 3rd, Crowell KL: Laparoscopy in the critically ill. Surg Endosc 11:1072, 1997

64. Gagic N, Frey CF: The results of cholecystostomy for the treatment of acute cholecystitis. Surg Gynecol Obstet 140:255, 1975

65. Reynolds BM, Dargan EL: Acute obstructive cholangitis: a distinct clinical syndrome. Ann Surg 150:299, 1959

66. DuPont HL, Spink WW: Infections due to gram-negative organisms: an analysis of 860 patients with bacteremia at the University of Minnesota Medical Center, 1958–1966. Medicine (Baltimore) 48:307, 1969

67. Glenn F: Anatomy and physiology of the liver and

biliary system and diseases of the gallbladder and bile ducts. Christopher's Textbook of Surgery, 6th ed. Davis L, Ed. WB Saunders Co, Philadelphia, 1956, p 722

68. Baer HU, Matthews JB, Schweizer WP, et al: Management of the Mirizzi syndrome and the surgical implications of cholecystocholedochal fistula. Br J Surg 77:743, 1990

69. Wiesner RH, Ludwig J, LaRusso NF, et al: Diagnosis and treatment of primary sclerosing cholangitis. Semin Liver Dis 5:241, 1985

70. Helzberg JH, Petersen JM, Boyer JL: Improved survival with primary sclerosing cholangitis: a review of clinicopathologic features and comparison of symptomatic and asymptomatic patients. Gastroenterology 92:1869, 1987

71. Nakayama F, Koga A: Hepatolithiasis: present status. World J Surg 8:9, 1984

72. Gerecht WB, Henry NK, Hoffman WW, et al: Prospective randomized comparison of mezlocillin therapy alone with combined ampicillin and gentamicin therapy for patients with cholangitis. Arch Intern Med 149:1279, 1989

73. Thompson JE Jr, Pitt HA, Doty JE, et al: Broad spectrum penicillin as an adequate therapy for acute cholangitis. Surg Gynecol Obstet 171:275, 1990

74. Thompson JN, Edwards WH, Winearls CE, et al: Renal impairment following biliary tract surgery. Br J Surg 74:843, 1987

75. Muller EL, Pitt HA, Thompson JE Jr, et al: Antibiotics in infections of the biliary tract. Surg Gynecol Obstet 165:285, 1987

76. Pitt HA, Postier RG, Cameron JL: Consequences of preoperative cholangitis and its treatment on the outcome of operation for choledocholithiasis. Surgery 94:447, 1983

77. Leung JW, Chung SC, Sung JJ, et al: Urgent endoscopic drainage for acute suppurative cholangitis. Lancet 1:1307, 1989

78. Elias E, Hamlyn AN, Jain S, et al: A randomized trial of percutaneous transhepatic cholangiography with the Chiba needle versus endoscopic retrograde cholangiography for bile duct visualization in jaundice. Gastroenterology 71:439, 1976

79. Pereiras R, Chiprut RO, Greenwald RA, et al: Percutaneous transhepatic cholangiography with the "skinny" needle: a rapid, simple, and accurate method in the diagnosis of cholestasis. Ann Intern Med 86:562, 1977

80. Gigot JF, Leese T, Derme T, et al: Acute cholangitis: multivariate analysis of risk factors. Ann Surg 209:435, 1989

81. Lai EC, Tam PC, Paterson IA, et al: Emergency surgery for severe acute cholangitis: the high risk patients. Ann Surg 211:55, 1990

82. Boey JH, Way LW: Acute cholangitis. Ann Surg 191:264, 1980

83. Saik RP, Greenburg AG, Peskin GW: Cholecystostomy hazard in acute cholangitis. JAMA 235:2412, 1976

84. Glenn F, Moody FG: Acute obstructive suppurative cholangitis. Surg Gynecol Obstet 113:265, 1961

85. Kraus MA, Wilson SD: Choledochoduodenostomy: importance of common duct size and occurrence of cholangitis. Arch Surg 115:1212, 1980

86. O'Connor MJ, Schwartz ML, McQuarrie DG, et al: Acute bacterial cholangitis: an analysis of clinical manifestation. Arch Surg 117:437, 1982

87. Thompson JE Jr, Tompkins RK, Longmire WP Jr: Factors in management of acute cholangitis. Ann Surg 195:137, 1982

88. Bismuth H, Kuntziger H, Corlette MB: Cholangitis with acute renal failure: priorities in therapeutics. Ann Surg 181:881, 1975

89. Cho SR, Turner MA: Hepatic abscesses due to suppurative cholangitis. South Med J 75:488, 1982

90. Ferrucci JT, Mueller PR, Harbin WP: Percutaneous transhepatic biliary drainage: technique, results and applications. Radiology 135:1, 1980

91. Mueller PR, vanSonnenberg E, Ferrucci JT Jr: Percutaneous biliary drainage: technical and catheter-related problems in 200 procedures. AJR 138:17, 1982

92. Gould RJ, Vogelzang RL, Neiman HL, et al: Percutaneous biliary drainage as an initial therapy in sepsis of the biliary tract. Surg Gynecol Obstet 160:523, 1985

93. Leese T, Neoptolemos JP, Baker AR, et al: Management of acute cholangitis and the impact of endoscopic sphincterotomy. Br J Surg 73:988, 1986

94. Richardson R, Norton LW, Eule J, et al: Accuracy of ultrasound in diagnosing abdominal masses. Arch Surg 110:933, 1975

95. Alfidi RJ, MacIntyre WJ, Haaga JR: The effects of biological motion on CT resolution. AJR 127:11, 1976

96. Saini S: Imaging of the hepatobiliary tract. N Engl J Med 336:1889, 1997

97. Bearcroft PW, Miles KA: Leucocyte scintigraphy or computed tomography for the febrile post-operative patient? Eur J Radiol 23:126, 1996

98. McAfee JG, Ause RG, Wagner HN: Diagnostic value of scintillation scanning of the liver: follow-up of 1,000 studies. Arch Intern Med 116:95, 1965

99. Lomas F, Dibos PE, Wagner HN: Increased specificity of liver scanning with the use of ^{67}gallium citrate. N Engl J Med 286:1323, 1972

100. Haque R, Ali JK, Akther S, et al: Comparison of PCR, isoenzyme analysis and antigen detection for diagnosis of E. histolytica infection. J Clin Microbiol 36:449, 1998

101. Moazam F, Nazir Z: Amebic liver abscess: spare the knife but save the child. J Pediatr Surg 33:119, 1998

102. Auer H, Picher O, Aspock H: Combined application of enzyme-linked immunosorbent assay (ELISA) and indirect haemagglutination test (IHA) as a useful tool for the diagnosis and post-operative surveillance of human alveolar and cystic echinococcosis. Zentralbl Bakteriol Mikrobiol Hyg 270:313, 1988

103. Force L, Torres JM, Carrillo A: Evaluation of eight serological tests in the diagnosis of human echinococcosis and follow-up. Clin Infect Dis 15:473, 1992

104. Moore-Gillon JC, Eykyn SJ, Phillips I: Microbiology of pyogenic liver abscess. Br Med J 283:819, 1981

105. Aeder MI, Wellman JL, Haaga JR, et al: Role of surgical and percutaneous drainage in the treatment of abdominal abscesses. Arch Surg 118:273, 1983

106. Ch Yu S, Hg Lo R, Kan PS: Pyogenic liver abscess: treatment with needle aspiration. Clin Radiol 52:912, 1997

107. Gerzof SG, Johnson WC, Robbins AH, et al: Intrahepatic pyogenic abscesses: treatment by percutaneous drainage. Am J Surg 149:487, 1985

108. Seeto RK, Rockey DC: Pyogenic liver abscess: changes in etiology, management, and outcome. Medicine (Baltimore) 75:99, 1996

109. Herman P, Pugliese V, Montagnini AL, et al: Pyogenic liver abscess: the role of surgical treatment. Int Surg 82:98, 1997

110. Pitt HA, Zuidema GD: Factors influencing mortality in the treatment of pyogenic hepatic abscess. Surg Gynecol Obstet 140:228, 1975

111. Klatchko BA, Schwartz SI: Diagnostic and therapeutic approaches to pyogenic abscess of the liver. Surg Gynecol Obstet 168:332, 1989

112. Gyorffy EJ, Frey CF, Silva J Jr, et al: Pyogenic liver abscess: diagnostic and therapeutic strategies. Ann Surg 206:699, 1987

113. Sabbaj J, Sutter VL, Finegold SM: Anaerobic pyogenic liver abscess. Ann Intern Med 77:629, 1972

114. Bartlett JG: Intraabdominal sepsis. Med Clin North Am 79:599, 1995

115. Schein M, Wittmann DH, Lorenz W: Duration of antibiotic treatment in surgical infections of the abdomen. Forum statement: a plea for selective and controlled postoperative antibiotic administration. Eur J Surg Suppl 576:66, 1996

116. Rubin RH, Swartz MN, Malt R: Hepatic abscess: changes in clinical, bacteriologic and therapeutic aspects. Am J Med 57:601, 1974

117. Yeh TS, Jan YY, Jeng LB: Pyogenic liver abscesses in patients with malignant disease: a report of 52 cases treated at a single institution. Arch Surg 133:242, 1998

118. Cohen HG, Reynolds TB: Comparison of metronidazole and chloroquine for the treatment of amoebic liver abscess. Gastroenterology 69:35, 1975

119. Sheen IS, Chien CS, Lin DY, et al: Resolutions of liver abscesses: comparison of pyogenic and amebic liver abscess. Am J Trop Med Hyg 40:384, 1989

120. Most H: Treatment of parasitic infections of travelers and immigrants. N Engl J Med 310:298, 1984

121. Stiles GM, Byrne TV, Thommen VD, et al: Fine needle aspiration of pancreatic fluid collections. Am Surg 56:764, 1990

122. Bittner R, Block S, Buchler M, et al: Pancreatic abscess and infected pancreatic necrosis: different local septic complications in acute pancreatitis. Dig Dis Sci 32:1082, 1987

123. Beger HG, Bittner R, Block S, et al: Bacterial contamination of pancreatic necrosis: a prospective clinical study. Gastroenterology 91:433, 1986

124. Banks PA, Gerzof SG, Chong FK, et al: Bacteriologic status of necrotic tissue in necrotizing pancreatitis. Pancreas 5:330, 1990

125. Crass RA, Meyer AA, Jeffrey RB, et al: Pancreatic abscess: impact of computerized tomography on early diagnosis and surgery. Am J Surg 150:127, 1985

126. Ranson JHC, Rifkind KM, Roses DF, et al: Prognostic signs and the role of operative management in acute pancreatitis. Surg Gynecol Obstet 139:69, 1974

127. Bank S, Wise L, Gersten M: Risk factors in acute pancreatitis. Am J Gastroenterol 78:637, 1983

128. Imrie CW, Whyte AS: A prospective study of acute pancreatitis. Br J Surg 62:490, 1975

129. Satiani B, Stone HH: Predictability of present outcome and future recurrence in acute pancreatitis. Arch Surg 114:711, 1979

130. Kune GA, King R: The late complications of acute pancreatitis: pancreatic swelling, cyst and abscess. Med J Aust 1:1241, 1973

131. Demmy TL, Burch JM, Feliciano DV: Comparison of multiple-parameter prognostic systems in acute pancreatitis. Am J Surg 156:492, 1988

132. Nordback I, Pessi T, Auvinen O, et al: Determination of necrosis in necrotizing pancreatitis. Br J Surg 72:225, 1985

133. Becker JM, Pemberton JH, DiMagno EP, et al: Prognostic factors in pancreatic abscess. Surgery 96:455, 1984

134. Balthazar EJ, Freeny PC, van Sonnenberg E: Imaging and intervention in acute pancreatitis. Radiology 193:297, 1994

135. Balthazar EJ, Robinson DL, Megibow AJ: Acute pancreatitis: value of CT in establishing prognosis. Radiology 174:331, 1990

136. Maier W: Early objective diagnosis and staging of acute pancreatitis by contrast enhanced computed tomography. Acute Pancreatitis. Beger HG, Buchler M, Eds. Springer-Verlag, Berlin, 1987, p 132

137. Northam BE, Rowe DS, Winstone NE: Methaemalbumin in the differential diagnosis of acute haemorrhagic and oedematous pancreatitis. Lancet 1:348, 1963

138. Geokas MC, Rinderknecht H, Walberg CB, et al: Methaemalbumin in the diagnosis of acute hemorrhagic pancreatitis. Ann Intern Med 81:483, 1974

139. Warshaw AL, Lee KH: Serum ribonuclease elevations and pancreatic necrosis in acute pancreatitis. Surgery 86:227, 1979

140. Wilson C, Heads A, Shenkin A, et al: C-reactive protein, antiproteases and complement factors as objective markers of severity in acute pancreatitis. Br J Surg 76:177, 1989

141. Buchler M, Malfertheiner P, Schoetensack C, et al:

Sensitivity of antiproteases, complement factors and C-reactive protein in detecting pancreatic necrosis: results of a prospective clinical study. Int J Pancreatol 1:227, 1986

142. Ranson JHC, Balthazar E, Caccavale R, et al: Computed tomography and the prediction of pancreatic abscess in acute pancreatitis. Ann Surg 201:656, 1985

143. Stanten R, Frey CF: Comprehensive management of acute necrotizing pancreatitis and pancreatic abscess. Arch Surg 125:1269, 1990

144. Bradley EL III, Allen K: A prospective longitudinal study of observation versus surgical intervention in the management of necrotizing pancreatitis. Am J Surg 161:19, 1991

145. Aranha GV, Prinz RA, Greenlee HB: Pancreatic abscess: an unresolved surgical problem. Am J Surg 144:534, 1982

146. Warshaw AL: Pancreatic abscesses. N Engl J Med 287:1234, 1972

147. Frey CF, Lindenauer SM: Pancreatic abscess. Surg Gynecol Obstet 149:722, 1979

148. Bolooki H, Jaffe B, Gliedman ML: Pancreatic abscesses and lesser omental sac collections. Surg Gynecol Obstet 126:1301, 1968

149. Davidson ED, Bradley EL III: "Marsupialization" in the treatment of pancreatic abscess. Surgery 89:252, 1981

150. Hedderich GS, Wexler MJ, McLean APH, et al: The septic abdomen: open management with Marlex mesh and a zipper. Surgery 99:399, 1986

151. D'Egidio A, Schein M: Surgical strategies in the treatment of pancreatic necrosis and infection. Br J Surg 78:133, 1991

152. Rotman N, Mathieu D, Anglade MC, et al: Failure of percutaneous drainage of pancreatic abscesses complicating severe acute pancreatitis. Surg Gynecol Obstet 174:141, 1992

153. Lang EK, Paolini RM, Pottmeyer A: The efficacy of palliative and definitive percutaneous versus surgical drainage of pancreatic abscess and pseudocysts: a prospective study of 85 patients. South Med J 84:55, 1991

154. Lawson DW, Daggett WM, Civetta JM, et al: Surgical treatment of acute necrotizing pancreatitis. Ann Surg 172:605, 1970

155. Williams LF Jr, Byrne JJ: The role of bacteria in hemorrhagic pancreatitis. Surgery 64:967, 1968

156. Gregg JA: Detection of bacterial infection of the pancreatic ducts in patients with pancreatitis and pancreatic cancer during endoscopic cannulation of the pancreatic duct. Gastroenterology 73:1005, 1977

157. Farkas G, Marton J, Mandi Y: Surgical strategy and management of infected pancreatic necrosis. Br J Surg 80:980, 1996

158. Grant JP, James S, Grabowski V, et al: Total parenteral nutrition in pancreatic disease. Ann Surg 200:627, 1984

159. Lawhorne TW Jr, Zuidema GD: Splenic abscess. Surgery 79:686, 1976

160. Caldarera E: L'ascesso acuto della milza. Ann Ital Chir 16:953, 1937

161. Blumer G: Subacute bacterial endocarditis. Medicine (Baltimore) 2:105, 1923

162. Billings AE: Abscess of the spleen. Ann Surg 88:416, 1928

163. Chulay JD, Lankerani MR: Splenic abscess: report of 10 cases and review of the literature. Am J Med 61:513, 1976

164. Pickleman JR, Paloyan E, Block GE: The surgical significance of splenic abscess. Surgery 68:287, 1970

165. Parrish RA, Sherman HC: The surgical significance of splenic abscess. Am J Surg 30:712, 1964

166. Johnson JD, Raff MJ, Drasin GF, et al: Radiology in the diagnosis of splenic abscess. Rev Infect Dis 7:10, 1985

167. Reid SE, Lang SJ: Abscess of the spleen. Am J Surg 88:912, 1954

168. Sones PJ: Percutaneous drainage of abdominal abscesses. AJR Am J Roentgenol 142:35, 1984

169. Teich S, Oliver G, Canter JW: The early diagnosis of splenic abscess. Am Surg 52:303, 1986

170. Berkman WA, Harris SA Jr, Bernardino ME: Nonsurgical drainage of splenic abscess. AJR Am J Roentgenol 141:395, 1983

171. Longmire WP: Suppurative cholangitis. Critical Surgical Illness. Hardy JD, Ed. WB Saunders Co, Philadelphia, 1971, p 400

172. Huang T, Bass JA, Williams RD: The significance of biliary pressure in cholangitis. Arch Surg 98:629, 1969

173. Stewart L, Pellegrini CA, Way LW: Cholangiovenous reflux pathways as defined by corrosion casing and scanning electron microscopy. Am J Surg 155:23, 1988

174. Lygidakis NJ, Brummelkamp WH: Bacteremia in relation to intrabiliary pressure in proximal versus distal malignant biliary obstruction. Acta Chir Scand 152:305, 1986

175. O'Connor MJ, Sumner HW, Schwartz ML: The clinical and pathologic correlations in mechanical biliary obstruction and acute cholangitis. Ann Surg 195:419, 1982

176. Flemma RJ, Flint LM, Osterhout S, et al: Bacteriologic studies of biliary tract infection. Ann Surg 166:563, 1967

177. Weissglas IS, Brown RA: Acute suppurative cholangitis secondary to malignant obstruction. Can J Surg 24:468, 1981

178. Elson CO, Hattori K, Blackstone MO: Polymicrobial sepsis following endoscopic retrograde cholangiopancreatography. Gastroenterology 69:507, 1975

179. Ong GB: A study of recurrent pyogenic cholangitis. Arch Surg 84:199, 1962

180. Jackaman FR, Triggs CM, Thomas V, et al: Experimental bacterial infection of the biliary tract. Br J Exp Pathol 61:369, 1980

181. Thompson JE, Tompkins RK, Longmire WP Jr: Factors in management of acute cholangitis. Ann Surg 195:137, 1982

182. Lewis RT, Goodall RG, Marien B, et al: Biliary bacteria, antibiotic use, and wound infection in surgery of the gallbladder and common bile duct. Arch Surg 122:44, 1987

183. Finegold SM: Anaerobes in biliary tract infection (editorial). Arch Intern Med 139:1338, 1979

184. Shimada K, Inamatsu T, Yamashiro M: Anaerobic bacteria in biliary disease in elderly patients. J Infect Dis 135:850, 1977

185. Shimada K, Noro T, Inamatsu T, et al: Bacteriology of acute obstructive suppurative cholangitis of the aged. J Clin Microbiol 14:522, 1981

186. Lee WJ, Chang KJ, Lee CS: Surgery in cholangitis: bacteriology and choice of antibiotic. Hepatogastroenterology 39:347, 1992

187. Bourgault AM, England DM, Rosenblatt JE, et al: Clinical characteristics of anaerobic bactibilia. Arch Intern Med 139:1346, 1979

Acknowledgments

Figures 2 through 5   Dr. L. Stein, Montreal, Quebec.

Figure 6   From "Computed Tomography and the Prediction of Pancreatic Abscess in Acute Pancreatitis," by J. H. C. Ranson, E. Balthazar, R. Caccavale, et al, in *Annals of Surgery* 201:656, 1985. Used by permission.

Figure 7   From "Nonsurgical Drainage of Splenic Abscess," by W. A. Berkman, S. A. Harris Jr., and M. E. Bernardino, in *American Journal of Roentgenology* 141:395, 1983. Used by permission.

17 HAND INFECTION

Thomas M. Sinclair, M.D., C.M., and H. Bruce Williams, M.D.

At the beginning of the 20th century, with the Industrial Revolution under way, hand injuries became extremely common, but most hand deformities or disabilities were still the result of minor injuries that became infected. Indeed, during the preantibiotic era, infection was responsible for 50% to 75% of hand deformities.[1] Kanavel's pioneering anatomic work on defining the fascial planes led to the development of a unique approach to the localization and proper surgical drainage of hand infections.[2] His principles of treating hand infections remain useful to this day.

Although antibiotics have greatly decreased the incidence of serious, life-threatening infections, minor hand infections are still responsible for considerable morbidity, numerous lost manpower hours, and substantial health care costs.[3] Accurate, prompt diagnosis is the first and most important step in the treatment of hand infections. The diagnosis is based on a clear understanding of the anatomy of the hand, a careful history and physical examination, a thorough knowledge of the organisms that are likely to be involved, and an informed awareness of the specific host factors that might alter the treatment plan (e.g., diabetes, intravenous drug abuse, and immunocompromised states).

Anatomy of the Hand

Almost all hand infections develop after the skin barrier has been violated in some manner. Because infectious organisms usually spread through specific anatomic fascial planes or compartments, it is often possible for the physician to predict how the infection will subsequently be disseminated throughout the hand. To this end, a

brief review of the relevant anatomic structures in the hand should prove useful.

Tendon sheaths in the hand have double walls, made up of a visceral layer (epitenon) and a parietal layer. They are hollow structures that join at their proximal and distal ends.[4] In most hands, the sheaths of the index, long, and ring fingers extend from the palm at the midpalmar crease to just proximal to the distal interphalangeal joint [*see Figure 1*]. The flexor sheath of the little finger expands radially at the level of the midpalm to envelop the tendons of the ring, long, and index fingers and continues 2 cm proximal to the volar wrist crease. This expanded proximal portion of the sheath is commonly called the ulnar bursa. The thumb flexor sheath extends from 2 cm proximal to the volar wrist crease to the distal phalanx. The proximal half of this sheath is often called the radial bursa.[5,6] In 50% to 80% of patients, there is a communication between the radial bursa and the ulnar bursa, and this communication is responsible for the appearance of the so-called horseshoe abscess as a result of suppurative tenosynovitis of the little finger or the thumb[6] [*see* Management of Specific Common Hand Infections, Suppurative Flexor Tenosynovitis, *below*].

There are two major deep potential spaces within the hand [*see Figure 1*] whose function is to protect neurovascular structures and to permit the gliding of tendons within the hand.[5,7] The first potential space is the thenar space, which lies deep to the flexor tendons and extends from the third metacarpal bone toward the thumb to occupy the area of the thenar eminence. The dorsal boundary of this space is the adductor pollicis, and the volar boundary is the flexor tendon sheath of the index finger.[5,7,8] The second potential

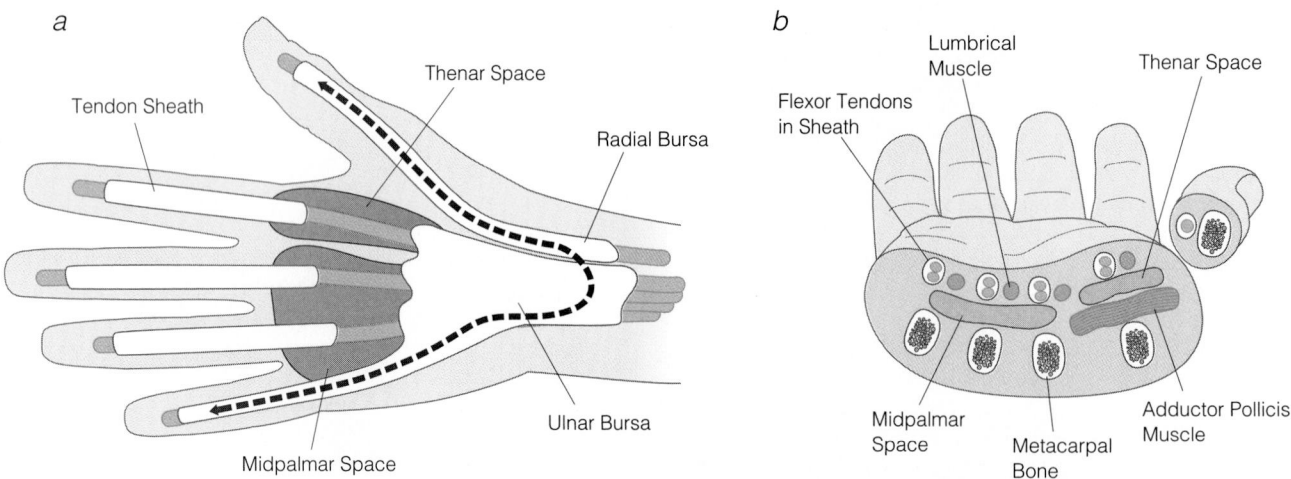

Figure 1 Depicted are the anatomic relations of the flexor sheaths, the bursae, and the deep spaces. The dashed arrow (*a*) represents the path of a horseshoe abscess, in which a communication exists between the radial bursa and the ulnar bursa. A cross-section of the hand through the palm (*b*) provides a different view of several of these structures. The midpalmar space and the thenar space are actually potential spaces in which infection can predictably spread.

Table 1 Causative Organisms and Appropriate Antibiotic Therapy for Specific Hand Infections

Infection	Causative Organisms	Antibiotic Therapy
Cellulitis/lymphangitis	Streptococci	First-generation cephalosporin or penicillin
Paronychia	*Staphylococcus aureus*	First-generation cephalosporin or penicillinase-resistant penicillin
Felon	*S. aureus*	First-generation cephalosporin or penicillinase-resistant penicillin
Suppurative flexor tenosynovitis	*S. aureus*, streptococci, gram-negative bacteria	First-generation cephalosporin and penicillin Consider aminoglycoside
Abscess in web space, thenar space, or midpalmar space	*S. aureus*, gram-negative bacteria, anaerobes	First-generation cephalosporin and penicillin Consider aminoglycoside
Human-bite wound infection	*S. aureus*, streptococci, *Eikenella corrodens*, anaerobes	First-generation cephalosporin and penicillin
Animal-bite wound infection	*Pasteurella*, *S. aureus*, viridans streptococci, anaerobes	First-generation cephalosporin and penicillin
Septic arthritis	*S. aureus*, streptococci, *Neisseria gonorrhoeae*, gram-negative bacteria	First-generation cephalosporin or penicillinase-resistant penicillin Consider aminoglycoside High-dose penicillin for gonococcal infection
Osteomyelitis	*S. aureus*, gram-negative bacteria, pseudomonads	First-generation cephalosporin or penicillinase-resistant penicillin Consider aminoglycoside Consider third-generation cephalosporin
Necrotizing fasciitis	Group A streptococci, mixed anaerobes (e.g., *Bacteroides*)	Penicillin with metronidazole and aminoglycoside Consider clindamycin and aminoglycoside

space is the midpalmar space, which extends from the third metacarpal bone to the hypothenar eminence. Its dorsal boundary consists of the metacarpal bones and the interosseous muscles, and its volar boundary is made up of the flexor tendons and the lumbrical muscles.[5,7,8]

Microorganisms usually enter these spaces either as a result of direct injury or by spreading from adjacent compartments such as tendon sheaths, joint spaces, or fascial planes. An infection that develops in one of these closed spaces can cause significant and rapid tissue necrosis; the inflammation and edema produce early venous congestion and subsequent local arterial compromise.

History and Physical Examination

The history and the physical examination are extremely important in the evaluation of a patient with a hand infection. The treating physician must remember to ask about the patient's employment history, drug abuse history, and any associated medical problems, such as diabetes or acquired immunodeficiency. Any possibility of an altercation with another human or an animal must be actively sought. Any delay between the time of injury and presentation should also be noted. Attention must be paid to the presence of puncture wounds, tenderness, erythema, edema, lymphangitic streaking, and lymphadenopathy as well as to any systemic signs of infection.

Tests should include radiographs of the hand and a complete blood count, and the exudate should undergo Gram's staining and be sent out for both aerobic and anaerobic cultures. If a patient whose tetanus immunization status is not up to date or not known has a tetanus-prone wound, appropriate tetanus prophylaxis should be provided.

Likely Pathogens

In the preantibiotic era, β-hemolytic streptococci were a common cause of rapidly spreading and often lethal hand infection.

Since the advent of antibiotics, however, the situation has changed: at present, the principal bacterial pathogen in 50% to 80% of hand infections is *Staphylococcus aureus*.[9,10] Knowledge of the likely pathogen or pathogens is essential in planning antibiotic therapy for hand infections.

The mode of injury, the presentation of the infection, and the status of the host will all help identify the most likely causative organism. Cultures of the exudate and Gram's staining (see above) should be performed routinely before empirical antibiotic treatment is begun. Preliminary antibiotic therapy should be focused on the most likely causative organism [see Table 1] for the specific infection present (see below). In most home and industrial injuries, gram-positive organisms are the predominant pathogens. Because the majority of community-acquired *S. aureus* species have become penicillin resistant, either a first-generation cephalosporin or a penicillinase-resistant penicillin is required to treat infections caused by these organisms.[11] Traumatic injuries, although usually monomicrobial, may include gram-negative organisms if the injury involves contamination from soil.[12] In such cases, an aminoglycoside should be combined with a first-generation cephalosporin and penicillin for adequate coverage.

Intravenous drug users, diabetics, and immunocompromised patients are prone to polymicrobial infections in which opportunistic pathogens play a role; consequently, an antibiotic regimen that covers gram-positive, gram-negative, and anaerobic organisms will be necessary.[13-16] In the immunocompromised patient, one should have a high degree of suspicion for fungal or atypical mycobacterial infections, especially if the infection is not responding to broad-spectrum antibiotics.[13] Tissue biopsy may be required for diagnosis.

Antibiotic regimens for bite wounds must include anaerobic coverage. *Eikenella corrodens*, an anaerobic gram-negative rod, is isolated from a large number of human-bite wounds,[17,18] and *Pasteurella multocida*, a gram-negative facultative anaerobe, is often isolated from animal-bite wounds.[19,20] Both pathogens are highly sensitive to penicillin.

General Principles of Treatment

There are four general therapeutic principles that are fundamental to the treatment of hand infections: (1) appropriate antibiotic therapy, (2) adequate debridement and surgical drainage, (3) a period of immobilization and elevation, and (4) early remobilization.[18]

Administration of antibiotics is guided by the clinical situation and the suspected organism [see Likely Pathogens, above]. If an infection is still in the cellulitic phase with no suppuration, then a period of nonoperative treatment with antibiotics is indicated [see Table 1].

If there is no improvement after 24 to 48 hours of adequate antibiotic therapy or if suppuration is evident, surgical drainage is indicated. After adequate anesthesia has been induced, the extremity is elevated but not exsanguinated, and a tourniquet is applied. Incisions should be made in parallel with the neurovascular structures whenever possible but should never cross flexion crease lines at a perpendicular angle. It is essential that debridement of infected and necrotic tissue accompany surgical drainage of closed spaces. Abscesses are drained through an incision located over the point of maximal tenderness or fluctuance. It is best to leave incisions and contaminated wounds open so that they can drain and heal secondarily. Delayed primary closure can be considered once the infection has cleared and the wound is clean.

It is important to elevate and immobilize the hand. Splinting of the hand in the so-called safe position helps prevent joint stiffness, decrease pain, and prevent further spread of infection through muscle activity [see Figure 2]. Elevation of the hand above the level of the heart promotes drainage and alleviates edema and tenderness.

It is also important, however, that hand therapy and remobilization be started early, when pain, edema, and erythema begin to resolve. Early motion helps reduce morbidity by preventing joint stiffness and encouraging the patient to become actively involved with his or her treatment.[21]

Management of Specific Common Hand Infections

CELLULITIS AND LYMPHANGITIS

Cellulitis is a nonsuppurative inflammation of the connective tissue planes that is associated with pain, erythema, edema, and warmth in the involved region. Usually, a streptococcus is the responsible pathogen, but both aerobic and anaerobic organisms have been implicated.[4,15,16,22] Treatment involves administration of antibiotics and elevation and immobilization of the hand. If there is no improvement after 48 hours of adequate antibiotic therapy, then an abscess may be present that must be drained surgically.

Figure 2 Shown is the proper hand position for splinting. The wrist is extended so that the slightly abducted thumb is in line with the axis of the radius. This safe position helps minimize joint stiffness, pain, and spread of infection.

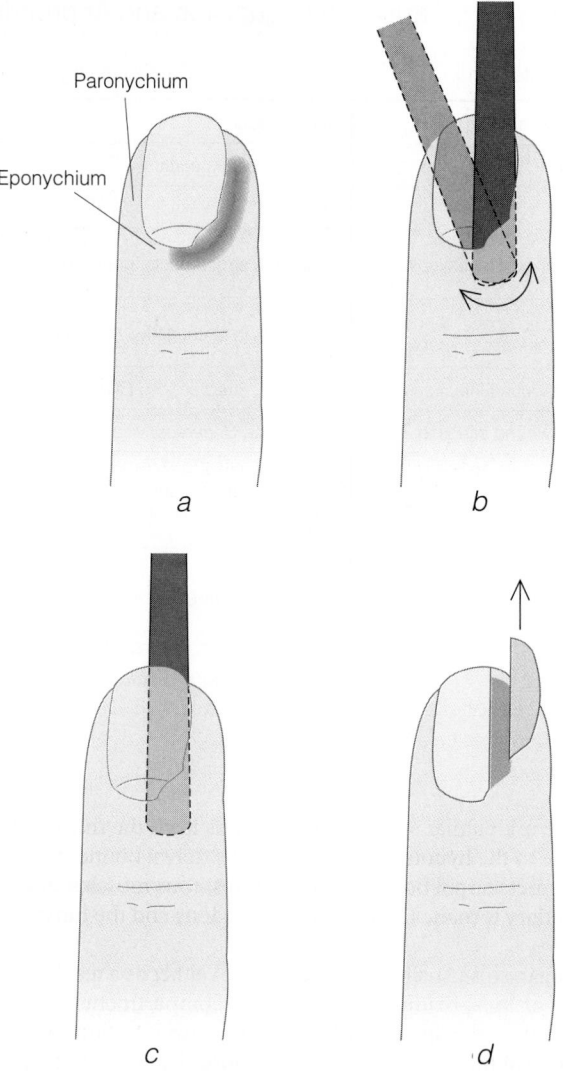

Figure 3 A paronychial infection can involve both the paronychium and the eponychium (a). The edge of a submucous elevator works well to lift the paronychium off the nail to facilitate abscess drainage (b). If the abscess has extended beneath the nail, the instrument should be gently pushed along the underside of the lateral portion of the nail to lift it off the nail bed (c). A small piece of the nail is then cut and removed to allow drainage (d).

Lymphangitis is an inflammation of the lymphatic pathways that is identified by red streaks extending along the dorsum of the hand and up the volar or dorsal aspect of the forearm. It is generally caused by streptococci. Treatment with appropriate antibiotics and elevation and splinting of the extremity usually lead to rapid improvement.[18,23]

PARONYCHIA

The thin layer of tissue extending onto the dorsum of the nail is called the paronychium laterally and the eponychium proximally [see Figure 3]. A paronychia is a subcuticular abscess in the paronychial fold. It must be distinguished from herpetic whitlow, which is a viral infection of the digit, because the two conditions are treated very differently [see Management of Specific Uncommon Hand Infections, Viral Infections, below]. A paronychia usually results from nail biting, manicures, or hangnails and is most commonly caused by S. aureus.[3,6,7,18,23] Local pain and swelling develop, but the infection may also spread proximally under the nail to involve the nail bed.

Figure 4   An improperly placed incision for drainage of a paronychia has left this patient with a notched defect in the eponychium.

If paronychia is diagnosed before pus is present, then treatment with oral antibiotics and lukewarm soaks may terminate the infection. Surgical drainage, however, is required if an abscess has formed. The drainage procedure is done simply by placing the edge of a submucous elevator or a No. 11 scalpel blade into the nail sulcus to elevate the paronychial fold, thereby decompressing the abscess [*see Figure 3*]. The tips of fine curved scissors or a mosquito hemostat may also be used. If the abscess extends beneath the nail, a portion of the nail must be removed to allow the abscess to drain. It is not necessary to incise the paronychium or eponychium; such incisions can lead to deformity [*see Figure 4*]. Continued drainage is accomplished by placing a small piece of fine gauze in the sulcus. Antistaphylococcal antibiotics should also be given.

Chronic paronychia is a different disease process and is commonly seen in persons whose hands are chronically exposed to moisture, such as cleaners, dishwashers, and swimmers. The nail fold becomes tender, swollen, and erythematous and pulls away from the nail. Repeated exacerbations are the rule and are difficult to treat.[3,7] Fungal organisms are commonly implicated in this condition. Appropriate treatment of chronic paronychia involves avoidance of chronic exposure to moisture and, sometimes, packing the nail fold with antifungal agents or surgically removing a crescent-shaped piece of skin parallel to the eponychium to promote drainage.[18]

FELON

A felon is a subcutaneous infection of the pulp space of the distal phalanx, but it is considered a closed-space infection because of the multiple septa that divide the pulp into fascial compartments[5] [*see Figure 5*]. An abscess forms in the pulp space, usually as a result of a penetrating injury. The organism most commonly implicated in the infection is *S. aureus*. The fingertip becomes painful, erythematous, and swollen. Since a felon is a closed-space infection, early treatment is advocated before increased pressure causes tissue necrosis. An untreated felon can lead to osteomyelitis of the distal phalanx, suppurative flexor tenosynovitis (see below), or skin necrosis.

Of the many incisions that have been used for drainage, the high lateral incision or the palmar longitudinal incision is recommended[3,8,24,25] [*see Figure 5*]. When the latter is used, care must be taken not to cross the flexion crease. A loose gauze packing and frequent luke-

warm soaks help keep the wound draining. The patient should be instructed to elevate the hand so as to reduce the pain and swelling. An oral antistaphylococcal antibiotic (e.g., a penicillinase-resistant penicillin or a first-generation cephalosporin) should also be given.

SUPPURATIVE FLEXOR TENOSYNOVITIS

Pyogenic flexor tenosynovitis is an infection of the closed synovial flexor tendon sheaths [*see Figure 6*]. Although pyogenic flexor tenosynovitis is not as common as it once was, it is still potentially devastating. Penetrating trauma is the usual mode of entry; *S. aureus* is the most common pathogen, followed by streptococci and pseudomonads.[6] There are four cardinal signs associated with these tendon sheath infections: (1) fusiform swelling of the entire finger, (2) semiflexed resting position of the finger, (3) excessive tenderness along the entire sheath, and (4) excruciating pain along the entire sheath on passive extension of the digit. The last sign is the most important because the first three may be seen in other finger infections that do not involve the sheaths.[25,26]

If the diagnosis is made early in the disease process, nonoperative treatment is indicated: I.V. administration of high doses of a broad-spectrum cephalosporin, immobilization, and elevation. Because ongoing infection can lead to tendon necrosis or proximal spread, surgical treatment is indicated if improvement is not seen after 24 hours of conservative management. Suppurative tenosynovitis of the little finger or thumb can develop into a horseshoe abscess if the infection spreads proximally and there is a communication between the radial bursa and the ulnar bursa[5,8,26] [*see Figure 7*]. An ulnar bursa infection should be drained through an incision along the radial aspect of the hypothenar eminence and a proximal incision on the ulnar aspect of the wrist[5,7] [*see Figure 8*]. The radial bursa is opened with both a thenar crease incision and a longitudinal incision on the proximal radial aspect of the wrist.

The closed flexor tendon sheath irrigation technique is a popular method of drainage that lacks the disadvantages associated with an extensive digital incision.[26] Incisions are made at the proximal and distal levels of the sheath [*see Figure 9*]. After the fluid is cultured, a 16- or 18-gauge catheter is placed within the proximal portion of the sheath and sutured in place. Another catheter or a small rubber drain is placed in the distal end of the sheath to form a patent irriga-

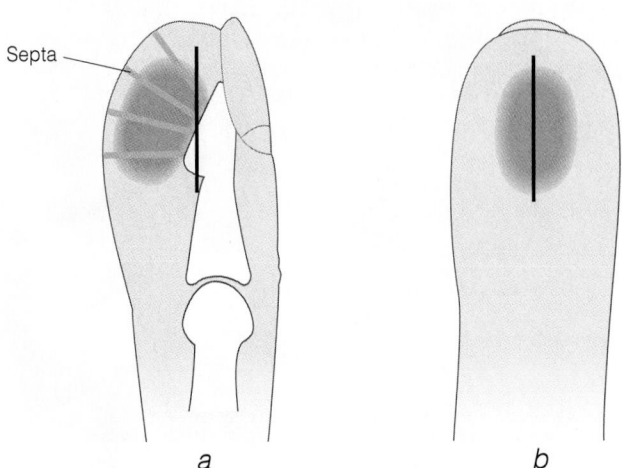

Figure 5   A felon can be drained through a high lateral incision with blunt dissection carried into the closed spaces defined by the septa in the finger pulp (*a*). An alternative method of drainage is through a palmar longitudinal incision that must not cross the distal flexion crease (*b*).

Figure 6 This patient has suppurative flexor tenosynovitis of the index finger caused by a puncture wound. Note the fusiform swelling and the classic semiflexed resting position of the finger.

tion system. The hand is then placed in a bulky dressing, and the sheath is irrigated every 2 hours with 50 ml of saline. In 48 to 72 hours, if the tenderness is gone, the catheter can be removed and hand therapy with mobilization can begin.

WEB SPACE INFECTION

A subcutaneous infection of the web between the digits is most commonly caused by a puncture or by extension of a palmar blister or callus that becomes secondarily infected.[18,27] Because the skin adheres to the underlying fascia, pus can track dorsally to produce a secondary abscess on the dorsum of the hand. An infection of this sort is called a collar button abscess because of its hourglass appearance.[27] Both a palmar and a dorsal incision are required to drain these abscesses [*see Figure 10*]. Drains should be used to keep the wound open until no more purulent material is forthcoming.

An unusual type of web space infection is that known as barber's hand. Cellulitis, an abscess, or an epithelialized fistulous tract can

Figure 7 A horseshoe abscess has developed in this 73-year-old patient with rheumatoid arthritis who is receiving long-term steroid therapy. The arrows show the abscess "pointing" over the flexor tenosynovial sheaths of the thumb and the little finger as well as over the radial bursa. Despite aggressive surgical drainage, the patient died of overwhelming sepsis.

develop between the fingers of barbers as a result of hairs that have penetrated the skin of the web space.[28] Usually, a pinpoint opening with a protruding hair is noted in the web space, and occasionally, a localized cyst may develop. Treatment primarily consists of removal of the offending hair and, if cellulitis is present, administration of antibiotics. Abscess drainage may be required. Once the cellulitis has resolved, the cyst and the fistulous tract should be excised.

THENAR SPACE INFECTION

The thenar space is vulnerable to infection resulting from puncture wounds or from contiguous spread of flexor tendon sheath infections. Clinically, thenar space infections present as a swollen thenar eminence with the thumb abducted [*see Figure 11*]. Passive adduction of the thumb causes significant pain. Pus in the thenar space can spread dorsally around the adductor pollicis to produce swelling on the dorsum of the hand.[18,27] Again, both a palmar incision and a dorsal incision may be necessary for adequate drainage of these infections. The palmar incision parallels the thenar crease, and the dorsal incision extends longitudinally along the border of the first dorsal interosseous muscle. Catheters may be left in place for irrigation with saline.

MIDPALMAR SPACE INFECTION

Like thenar space infections, midpalmar space infections result from penetrating trauma or from spread of sheath infections of the overlying long and ring fingers. Infection may spread to the dorsal subcutaneous space to cause impressive swelling. Infections in the midpalmar space can be drained through a transverse incision located near the distal palmar crease[27] [*see Figure 10*].

BITE WOUND INFECTION

Dogs and cats are responsible for the majority of bites to the human hand. Although rabies is uncommon in domestic dogs and cats, it is essential to verify the rabies immunization status of any dog or cat that bites a human; if this is impossible, the animal must be observed for signs of rabies. Both dogs and cats harbor a variety of organisms in their saliva, including *S. aureus,* viridans streptococci, and *P. multocida.*[19,23,29,30] *Pasteurella* is isolated from 50% of dog-bite wounds and 75% of cat-bite wounds.[20] Cat bites are usually more severe than dog bites because cats' sharp teeth can penetrate farther into the tissue, making the wound more difficult to clean.[29] When

Figure 8 Shown is the proper placement of incisions for drainage of infections within the flexor sheath (solid lines), infections within the ulnar bursa (dotted lines), and infections within the radial bursa (dashed lines).

A₁ Pulley

Figure 9 The closed flexor tendon sheath irrigation technique is a popular method of drainage in patients with suppurative flexor tenosynovitis. The proximal catheter enters beneath the A₁ pulley of the tendon sheath.

Figure 10 Shown is the proper placement of incisions, on palmar and dorsal aspects of the hand, for drainage of a web space abscess (solid lines), a thenar space abscess (dotted lines), and a midpalmar space abscess (dashed line).

treated early, animal-bite wounds should be cleansed, irrigated, and either left open to heal secondarily or closed loosely. The patient's tetanus immunization status should be checked, and an oral penicillin should be given for 7 days. Established infections with cellulitis and lymphangitis may initially be treated conservatively with high-dose I.V. penicillin and a first-generation cephalosporin, along with splinting and elevation. If there is no improvement within 24 to 48 hours, surgical debridement is indicated.

A human bite to the hand can be a very serious injury. To begin with, a wide variety of pathogens may be involved: human saliva is known to contain at least 42 species of bacteria, among which staphylococci, streptococci, and *E. corrodens* are predominant.[31-33] In addition, presentation is often late and treatment delayed. The most common hand injury from human bites is the full-thickness bite wound, followed by the so-called clenched fist injury[17] [*see Figure 12*]. The clenched fist injury has a higher incidence of complications because the subcutaneous, joint, and tendon sheath spaces may be involved. Patients who present less than 24 hours after injury may

Figure 11 This patient has a thenar space abscess. Note the thenar swelling and the abducted position of the thumb.

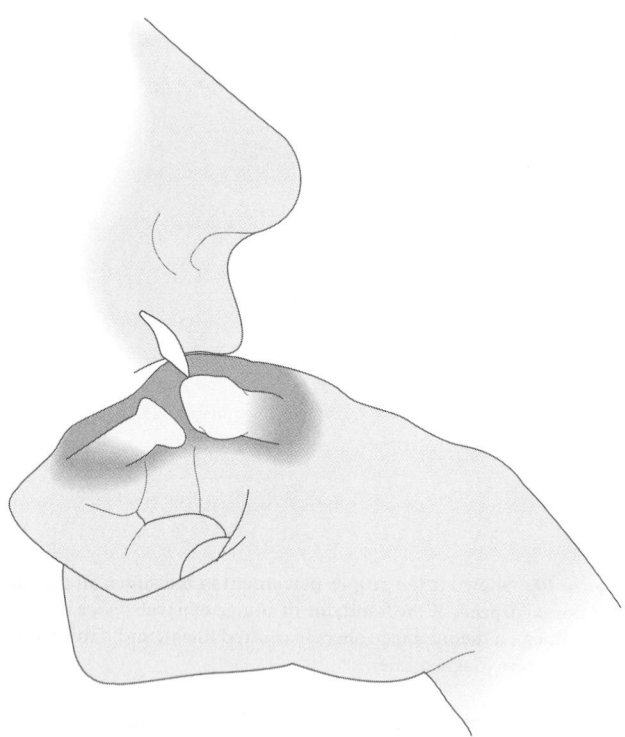

Figure 12 **The clenched fist injury classically results in a tooth puncture wound with violation of the metacarpophalangeal joint space. The joint space must be promptly opened surgically and drained to prevent septic arthritis.**

be treated with oral antibiotics on an outpatient basis, provided that the wound is cleansed and adequately explored and the metacarpal joint space is not violated.[7,17] If the joint space is involved, surgical drainage and intravenous antibiotics are necessary. Patients who present more than 24 hours after injury should be hospitalized and treated with intravenous antibiotics, splinting, and elevation. Again, surgical drainage is required if a closed space is involved or if there is no response to conservative management. The antibiotic therapy that is best suited to human-bite wound infections is a combination of a first-generation cephalosporin (to eliminate staphylococci and streptococci) and penicillin (to eliminate *Eikenella* and anaerobes). Tetanus prophylaxis should be given when indicated.

SEPTIC ARTHRITIS AND OSTEOMYELITIS

Septic arthritis is an infection within the closed space of a joint capsule and is often caused by a direct puncture of the capsule or contiguous spread from an adjacent bone or soft tissue infection.[18,34] The involved joint is swollen and extremely painful when moved, and the overlying skin is erythematous and warm. On early radiographs, no evidence of joint involvement may be apparent. Joint aspiration may facilitate the diagnosis, but if a septic joint is suspected, treatment should be prompt. As in many other hand infections, *S. aureus* is the most likely pathogen; however, nontraumatic monoarticular septic arthritis is often caused by hematogenous spread of *Neisseria gonorrhoeae*. Treatment involves intravenous antibiotics, open drainage of the joint through a dorsal or midaxial approach, and debridement of any devitalized tissue.[7,8,34] The fluid should be cultured to guide antibiotic therapy. The joint space should be left open to drain; alternatively, an irrigation catheter may be left in place.

Osteomyelitis in the hand most commonly develops from open fractures or from contiguous spread of soft tissue infections. Early di-

agnosis may be difficult; because radiographs initially appear normal, a high degree of suspicion is necessary. Combined use of technetium-99m and gallium-67 scanning may help differentiate between a soft tissue infection and osteomyelitis. Although a biopsy of the infected bone is the most effective way of identifying the pathogen, treatment still involves drainage and surgical debridement of infected bone and sequestra, along with 4 to 6 weeks of intravenous antibiotics.[34]

NECROTIZING SOFT TISSUE INFECTIONS

Despite their rarity in surgery in general and in hand surgery in particular, necrotizing soft tissue infections are important infectious complications. Underlying conditions that predispose to such infections include an impaired immune system, wound contamination, and a decreased blood supply to the involved area.

Necrotizing soft tissue infections are usually polymicrobial: organisms present may include aerobic or anaerobic gram-positive organisms (e.g., staphylococci and streptococci) as well as gram-negative enteric bacteria and anaerobes. These infections are typically synergistic, which accounts for their severity. Clostridial infections may also occur. Clinical diagnosis is based on the presence of skin discoloration or necrosis; blebs; drainage of thin, watery, grayish, foul-smelling fluid; and, often, subcutaneous crepitus.

Treatment should be prompt and should include aggressive and extensive debridement, wound tissue cultures, and broad-spectrum antibiotic support. For gram-positive organisms, penicillin, vancomycin, or a semisynthetic penicillin is given; for gram-negative organisms, an aminoglycoside or a monobactam is given. Anaerobic coverage is generally achieved by giving metronidazole or clindamycin.

Management of Specific Uncommon Hand Infections

GAS-FORMING INFECTIONS

The reported mortality from gas-forming hand infections is greater than 20% and increases if debridement is delayed.[18] *Clostridium perfringens*, a gram-positive anaerobe, is the classic causative organism, but other organisms, such as coliforms, *Bacteroides*, and anaerobic streptococci, can also produce gas-forming infections.[35] These infections are seen in areas of trauma, burns, or ischemia in which the local conditions favor anaerobic bacterial growth. Clostridial gangrene presents as a swelling and a brownish discoloration of the skin in association with pain and palpable subcutaneous crepitation.

Figure 13 **This patient has herpetic whitlow. Note the development of the vesicles, which is pathognomonic of this infection.**

The infection progresses rapidly and is usually associated with signs of systemic toxicity. Treatment involves fluid resuscitation, immediate debridement of all involved tissue, and high-dose I.V. penicillin. Hyperbaric oxygen therapy may also have a role in the treatment of these serious infections.

VIRAL INFECTIONS

The virus most commonly associated with infection of the hand is herpes simplex virus, which causes a cyclic infection of the skin.[18] The virus is spread by direct contact or autoinoculation.[36,37] In the hand, herpetic whitlow presents as a painful localized swelling of the distal phalanx coupled with the appearance of clear vesicles[38] [see Figure 13]. The most important aspect of diagnosis of this infection is to recognize it and distinguish it from a felon or paronychia; with herpetic whitlow, surgical drainage is contraindicated because it can lead to viral dissemination. The appearance of vesicles is virtually pathognomonic of a herpetic infection; however, the diagnosis can be confirmed by means of a relatively simple and rapid immunofluorescent diagnostic test. Scrapings from the bases of the vesicles are placed on a glass slide, which is then fixed with a fluorescein-labeled monoclonal antibody that is specific for the herpes simplex virus. The diagnosis is made if the preparation fluoresces when exposed to ultraviolet light.

The infection is self-limited but may take up to 4 weeks to disappear. Simple unroofing of the vesicles may help relieve the pain.[36] Over the first 2 weeks, the vesicles coalesce to form an ulcer, which gradually resolves. Acyclovir is generally not necessary except for immunocompromised patients, in whom it may decrease morbidity and may actually be needed to cure the infection.[15]

MYCOBACTERIAL INFECTIONS

Mycobacterium tuberculosis infections are rare in the hand but may be seen in immunocompromised patients[15] or in patients who live in areas where tuberculosis is very prevalent. The ubiquitous atypical mycobacteria, however, are being identified more frequently in hand infections, and in fact, approximately 75% of all atypical mycobacterial infections involve the hand. *M. marinum* is the most common pathogen.[18] This organism inhabits freshwater and saltwater environments; accordingly, inoculation is usually the result of penetrating trauma (e.g., fish bites) or scrapes from boat docks, fish tanks, or swimming pools.[39,40] Diagnosis of mycobacterial infections in the hand is difficult and depends on a high degree of suspicion. Cultures and tissue biopsy are usually required. Histologic evidence of granulomas or smears showing acid-fast bacilli also help verify the diagnosis.

Most mycobacterial skin lesions are self-limited; however, deeper infections involving the tendon sheath, the bursae, the joints, or bone call for surgical debridement and long-term administration of oral antituberculous antibiotics, such as isoniazid, ethambutol, and rifampin. Minocycline has also been shown to be effective in the treatment of *M. marinum* infections.[39,40] Antibiotic treatment usually must be continued for anywhere from 3 months to a year.

Other atypical mycobacterial organisms involved in hand infections include *M. kansasii*, *M. fortuitum*, and *M. chelonei*.

FUNGAL INFECTIONS

Fungal infections should always be considered in the differential diagnosis of chronic nail and skin lesions. *Trichophyton rubrum* is the most common pathogen, causing tinea of the skin and infections of the fingernails (onychomycosis).[41] Treatment involves removal of the nail and topical administration of fungicides.

Fungal infections involving the subcutaneous tissues or the closed spaces of the hand are relatively uncommon but are difficult to treat when present. Sporotrichosis is a lymphocutaneous infection caused by *Sporothrix schenckii*,[18,41] an organism that is found in soil and plant material. A chronic granulomatous infection develops and then ulcerates. A chain of nodules or ulcers develops and ascends the arm along the course of the lymphatic vessels. The lesions heal spontaneously but will recur unless they are treated with oral potassium iodide. Deep histoplasmosis, blastomycosis, or coccidioidomycosis can cause tenosynovitis, septic arthritis, or osteomyelitis. These conditions may be seen in immunocompromised surgical patients; surgical debridement and intravenous administration of amphotericin B are required.

Conclusion

In summary, hand infections should be treated with the utmost respect. The key to successful management of these infections is accurate diagnosis and prompt treatment. Appropriate tetanus prophylaxis must be provided, when indicated, in cases of penetrating injury. Many hand infections, if diagnosed early, can be treated with antibiotic therapy and elevation and immobilization of the hand. In the case of an established infection characterized by suppuration or involvement of a closed space, prompt surgical drainage and debridement are required in addition to the steps just mentioned. Once the infection has resolved, hand therapy and remobilization are essential. If these principles are followed, rapid and complete recovery can be achieved, with minimal morbidity.

References

1. Mock HE: Treatment of hand infections from an economic viewpoint: based on a study of 1600 cases. Surg Gynecol Obstet 21:481, 1915

2. Kanavel AB: An anatomical, experimental, and clinical study of acute phlegmons of the hand. Surg Gynecol Obstet 1:221, 1905

3. Canales FL, Newmeyer WL 3rd, Kilgore ES Jr: The treatment of felons and paronychias. Hand Clin 5:515, 1989

4. Neviaser RJ: Tenosynovitis. Hand Clin 5:525, 1989

5. Lampe EW: Surgical anatomy of the hand: with special reference to infections and trauma. Clin Symp 40(3):1, 1989

6. Siegel DB, Gelberman RH: Infections of the hand. Orthop Clin North Am 19:779, 1988

7. McGrath MH: Infections of the hand. Plastic Surgery, Vol 8: The Hand. McCarthy JG, Ed. WB Saunders Co, Philadelphia, 1990

8. Neviaser RJ: Infections. Operative Hand Surgery, 2nd ed. Green DP, Ed. Churchill Livingstone, New York, 1988, p 1027

9. Carter SJ, Mersheimer WL: Infections of the hand. Orthop Clin North Am 1:445, 1970

10. Mann RJ: Infections of the Hand. Lea & Febiger, Philadelphia, 1988

11. Spiegel JD, Szabo RM: A protocol for the treatment of severe infections of the hand. J Hand Surg 13:254, 1988

12. Fitzgerald RH Jr, Cooney WP 3rd, Washington JA 2nd, et al: Bacterial colonization of mutilating hand injuries and its treatment. J Hand Surg 2:85, 1977

13. Jones NF, Conklin WT, Albo VC: Primary invasive aspergillosis of the hand. J Hand Surg 11:425, 1986

14. Dhaliwal AS, Garnes AL: Tenosynovitis in drug addicts. J Hand Surg 7:626, 1982

15. Glickel SZ: Hand infections in patients with acquired immunodeficiency syndrome. J Hand Surg 13:770, 1988

16. Mann RJ, Peacock JM: Hand infections in patients with diabetes mellitus. J Trauma 17:376, 1977

17. Faciszewski T, Coleman DA: Human bite wounds. Hand Clin 5:561, 1989

18. Hausman MR, Lisser SP: Hand infections. Orthop Clin North Am 23:171, 1992

19. Arons MS, Fernando L, Polayes IM: *Pasteurella multocida*—the major cause of hand infections following domestic animal bites. J Hand Surg 7:47, 1982

20. Lucas GL, Bartlett DH: *Pasteurella multocida* infection in the hand. Plast Reconstr Surg 67:49, 1981

21. Mancini LH, Fort LK: Rehabilitation of the infected hand. Hand Clin 5:635, 1989

22. Burton RI: The hand. Principles of Surgery, 4th ed. Schwartz SI, Ed. McGraw-Hill, New York, 1984, p 2061

23. Kilgore ES Jr: Hand infections. J Hand Surg 8:723, 1983

24. Kilgore ES Jr, Brown LG, Newmeyer WL, et al: Treatment of felons. Am J Surg 130:194, 1975

25. American Society for Surgery of the Hand: The Hand: Primary Care of Common Problems. ASSH, Aurora, Colorado, 1985

26. Neviaser RJ: Closed tendon sheath irrigation for pyogenic flexor tenosynovitis. J Hand Surg 3:462, 1978

27. Burkhalter WE: Deep space infections. Hand Clin 5:553, 1989

28. Cahill JM: Special infections of the hand. Hand Surgery. Flynn JE, Ed. Williams & Wilkins, Baltimore, 1966, p 832

29. Snyder CC: Animal bite wounds. Hand Clin 5:571, 1989

30. Goldstein EJ, Citron DM, Wield B, et al: Bacteriology of human and animal bite wounds. J Clin Microbiol 8:667, 1978

31. Chuinard RG, D'Ambrosia RD: Human bite infections of the hand. J Bone Joint Surg [Am] 59:416, 1977

32. Mann RJ, Hoffield TA, Farmer CB: Human bites of the hand: twenty years of experience. J Hand Surg 2:97, 1977

33. Dreyfuss UY, Singer M: Human bites of the hand: a study of one hundred six patients. J Hand Surg 10:884, 1985

34. Freeland AE, Senter BS: Septic arthritis and osteomyelitis. Hand Clin 5:533, 1989

35. Schecter W, Meyer A, Schecter G, et al: Necrotizing fasciitis of the upper extremity. J Hand Surg 7:15, 1982

36. Polayes I, Arons M: The treatment of herpetic whitlow—a new surgical concept. Plast Reconstr Surg 65:811, 1980

37. Fowler JR: Viral infections. Hand Clin 5:613, 1989

38. Louis DS, Silva J Jr: Herpetic whitlow: herpetic infections of the digits. J Hand Surg 4:90, 1979

39. Hurst LC, Amadio PC, Badalamente MA, et al: *Mycobacterium marinum* infections of the hand. J Hand Surg 12:428, 1987

40. Gunther SF, Levy CS: Mycobacterial infections. Hand Clin 5:591, 1989

41. Hitchcock TF, Amadio PC: Fungal infections. Hand Clin 5:599, 1989

Recommended Reading

Burton RI, Rockwell WB: Hand. Principles of Surgery, 6th ed. Schwartz SI, Shires GT, Spencer FC, Eds. McGraw-Hill, New York, 1994, p 2001

Dunn DL: Infection. Surgery: Scientific Principles and Practice, 2nd ed. Greenfield LJ, Mulholland MW, Oldham KT, et al, Eds. Philadelphia, Lippincott-Raven Publishers, 1997, p 173

Acknowledgments

Figures 1 through 3, 5, 8 through 10, and 12   Tom Moore. Adapted from original drawings by Jennifer Morrison, Audiovisual Department, Montreal Children's Hospital.

Figures 6 and 7   Supplied by H. Brown, M.D., Division of Plastic and Reconstructive Surgery, Montreal General Hospital.

Figure 11   Supplied by C. L. Kerrigan, M.D., Division of Plastic and Reconstructive Surgery, Royal Victoria Hospital, Montreal.

Figure 13   Supplied by B. Moroz, M.D., Department of Dermatology, Montreal Children's Hospital.

18 FUNGAL INFECTION

Elias J. Anaissie, M.D., Albair B. Bishara, M.D., and Joseph S. Solomkin, M.D.

Approach to the Surgical Patient at Risk for Candidiasis

The infectious diseases that are most commonly encountered by surgeons are acute events in which fever, leukocytosis, and localized signs of inflammation develop in a reasonably healthy host. In this clinical situation, the presence of microorganisms in such normally sterile foci as blood and intra-abdominal sites indicates an infection and the need for antimicrobial chemotherapy.

The clinical setting in which *Candida* species are isolated from various body sites is generally much different. Patients harboring *Candida* infections frequently have had antecedent infections that were treated with antibacterial agents, have received therapy that suppressed their immunologic responses,[1] or have undergone extensive surgery or several operations, especially on the gastrointestinal tract. Such patients are generally long-term residents in acute care hospitals. Previous operative intervention may have left surgical wounds or drainage tracts. These circumstances favor colonization by various opportunistic pathogens, with the resultant risk of overgrowth or invasion by normal enteric microorganisms such as *Candida* species. In this setting, the elements that characterize most infectious processes (i.e., an acute change from wellness to illness and isolation of microorganisms from ordinarily sterile sites) no longer have great diagnostic value.

The problem of defining indications for administration of antifungal therapy in surgical patients is compounded by the limited data available, the difficulty of establishing a diagnosis, and the small number of effective antifungal agents. Although amphotericin B is currently the standard antifungal agent, fluconazole, a newer triazole antifungal that is generally well tolerated, appears to be effective in the treatment of serious *Candida* infections in surgical patients.

Noncandidal fungal infections, although still rare in surgical patients, may cause morbidity and mortality. Because infections such as aspergillosis and mucormycosis may be refractory to standard antifungal therapy, there is an urgent need to define the role of novel antifungal agents in surgical patients.

This chapter summarizes the current understanding of fungal infections, particularly candidiasis, in nonneutropenic surgical patients and provides recommendations for prophylaxis and therapy.

Magnitude of the Problem in the Surgical Patient

Whereas the high mortality associated with bacterial infections in surgical patients has been reduced by the early administration of antibacterial therapy, the incidence of fungal infections, particularly with *Candida* species, has dramatically increased.[2] In a 1984 nationwide survey of medical and surgical patients, *Candida* species were the eighth most common cause of nosocomial bloodstream infection.[3] In a similar survey conducted between October 1986 and December 1990, *Candida* species became the fourth leading cause of nosocomial bloodstream infection, preceded only by coagulase-negative-staphylococci, *Staphylococcus aureus*, and enterococci.[3] According to the National Nosocomial Infections Surveillance (NNIS) system, the percentage of nosocomial infections caused by *C. albicans* increased from 2% in 1980 to an average of 5% over the 4-year period from 1986 through 1989.[4] Data from NNIS hospitals also show that between 1980 and 1989, the incidence of primary bloodstream infections attributable to *Candida* species increased by 487% in large teaching hospitals and by 219% in small (< 200 bed) hospitals.[5] In addition, the NNIS system reported that the rate of nosocomial fungal infection increased from 2.0 to 3.8 infections per 1,000 patients discharged between 1980 and 1990.[6] Current data from the SCOPE (Surveillance and Control of Pathogens of Epidemiologic Importance) system confirm that *Candida* species were the fourth leading cause of bloodstream infection.[7] These data are supported by the Surveillance Network–USA, which compiles information from more than 100 laboratories in the United States. Fungi including *Candida* species were isolated from 17% of 10,038 patients included in a European study of the prevalence of infection in patients in intensive care units.[8]

The most marked increase in candidiasis occurred in surgical patients, particularly in burn and trauma patients followed by cardiac surgery patients and general surgery patients. *Candida* species now account for 78% of all nosocomial fungal infections.[6]

Nosocomial bloodstream infections caused by *Candida* species are an independent predictor of risk of mortality (38% mortality directly attributable to candidiasis) and prolonged hospital stay (30 additional days in comparison with controls).[1] In a more recent prospective study, *Candida* species were the only microorganisms that independently influenced the outcome of nosocomial primary infections of the bloodstream (odds ratio for mortality, 1.84; 95% confidence interval [CI]) and were associated with the highest mortalities (35% at 28 days and 69% at discharge).[9] In properly conducted multivariate analyses, the most important prognostic factors in patients with hematogenous candidiasis include older age, poor performance status (on Acute Physiology and Chronic Health Evaluation [APACHE] or other measures), the presence and persistence of neutropenia, and dissemination of the infection to noncontiguous organs. Central venous catheter retention appears to play a minimal role.[8,10]

Definitions of Hematogenous *Candida* Infection Syndromes

In this chapter, the general term hematogenous candidiasis is used to identify all infections involving the bloodstream. Hence,

Identify patient at risk for *Candida* infection

Major risk factors include
- Previous bacterial infection and therapy with multiple antibiotics.
- Isolation of *Candida* from ≥ 2 sites.
- Disruption of the intestinal mucosal barrier (total parenteral nutrition, severe diarrhea, colitis, major operation, trauma, or extensive burns).
- Immunosuppression (neutropenia, cancer, organ transplantation, hemodialysis, or extensive burns).

Other risk factors include
- Tunneled central venous catheters • Urinary catheters • Prematurity • Heroin addiction.

Initiate studies to diagnose candidiasis

Obtain cultures of sputum, oropharynx, stool, urine, drain sites, and blood.

Obtain 2 sets of blood cultures daily for 2 days (or longer if the patient remains febrile).

Consider serologic tests and histologic analyses (see text).

Look for findings that may signal hematogenous candidiasis:
- Endophthalmitis • Suppurative thrombophlebitis • High-grade candiduria without instrumentation of the bladder or the renal pelvis.

Exclude other possible causes of persistent fever.

Blood cultures are positive for *Candida*, or clinical or laboratory signal of potential hematogenous candidiasis is present

Patient is hemodynamically stable, does not have high-grade candidemia, and does not appear to have organ infection

Remove all venous catheters.

or

Leave venous catheter in place initially, and consider removal if clinical condition deteriorates or does not improve after 2 days of therapy.

Patient is infected or colonized by *C. albicans*, *C. tropicalis*, *C. parapsilosis*, or other germ tube–positive candidal organism

Give fluconazole, 600–800 mg/day I.V. for 2–3 days, then, if possible, lower dosage to 400 mg/day p.o.

Treat for 7–10 days (patient should be free of signs and symptoms of infection for 5 days before treatment is ended).

Patient is infected or colonized by *C. krusei*, *C. glabrata*, or *C. lusitaniae*

Give amphotericin B, 0.5–0.7mg/kg/day. (Consider adding flucytosine, 25 mg/kg/day p.o. in 2 divided doses, for *C. glabrata* and *C. lusitaniae*.)

Treat for 5–7 days (patient should be free of signs and symptoms of infection for 5 days before treatment is ended).

Approach to the Surgical Patient at Risk for Candidiasis

Blood cultures are negative for *Candida*, and no clinical or laboratory signal of potential hematogenous candidiasis is present, but *Candida* is isolated from ≥ 2 remote sites (≥ 1 site for *C. tropicalis*)

Give fluconazole, 400 mg/day I.V. for 2–3 days, then 400 mg/day p.o. If patient is colonized by *C. krusei*, *C. glabrata*, or *C. lusitaniae*, give amphotericin B, 0.5 mg/kg/day. (Consider adding flucytosine, 25 mg/kg/day p.o. in 2 divided doses, for *C. glabrata* and *C. lusitaniae*.)

Treat for 7–10 days (patient should be free of signs and symptoms of infection for 5 days before treatment is ended).

Blood cultures are negative for *Candida*, no clinical or laboratory signal of potential hematogenous candidiasis is found, and *Candida* is isolated from ≤ 1 remote site (0 sites for *C. tropicalis*)

Continue surveillance cultures weekly.

Patient is hemodynamically unstable, has high-grade candidemia, or shows evidence of organ infection

Remove all venous catheters.

Treat any associated syndromes of hematogenous candidiasis (e.g., endophthalmitis, pericarditis, suppurative thrombophlebitis, endocarditis).

Patient is infected or colonized by *C. albicans*, *C. tropicalis*, *C. parapsilosis*, or other germ tube–positive candidal organism

Give fluconazole, 800 mg/day I.V. (Consider adding flucytosine, 25 mg/kg/day p.o. in 2 divided doses. Also consider adding G-CSF, 300 µg/day.)

Treat for 10–14 days after disappearance of all signs and symptoms of infection.

Patient is infected or colonized by *C. krusei*, *C. glabrata*, or *C. lusitaniae*

Give amphotericin B, 0.7–1.0 mg/kg/day I.V. (Consider adding flucytosine, 25 mg/kg/day p.o. in 2 divided doses. Also consider adding G-CSF, 300 µg/day).

Treat for 10–14 days after disappearance of all signs and symptoms of infection.

hematogenous candidiasis refers to candidemia, disseminated candidiasis, or both.

CANDIDEMIA

Candidemia is defined as the isolation of any pathogenic species of *Candida* from at least one blood culture specimen. The recovery of *Candida* species from the bloodstream can be a significant observation in the absence of clinical signs and symptoms, especially if the patient is debilitated or uremic or is receiving adrenal corticosteroid therapy.

CATHETER-ASSOCIATED CANDIDEMIA

Catheter-associated candidemia is candidemia that occurs in a patient with an intravascular catheter and no other obvious origin of infection after careful clinical and laboratory evaluation. Several procedures have been developed to aid in the diagnosis of catheter-associated candidemia. If the catheter is removed, a quantitative culture of the tip should recover at least 15 colony-forming units (CFU) of the same *Candida* species as that found in blood culture by the roll-plate technique (or at least 100 CFU of the same *Candida* species as that found in blood culture by the sonication technique). If the catheter is not removed, a quantitative blood culture collected through a central catheter should contain at least a 10-fold greater concentration of *Candida* species than a simultaneously collected quantitative peripheral blood culture. Routine catheter tip cultures appear to be of no value.

ACUTE DISSEMINATED CANDIDIASIS

Patients who have several noncontiguous organs infected by *Candida* species have a disseminated infection acquired through hematogenous spread. For diagnosis, the organism must be identified by histologic analysis, culture of tissue samples obtained from at least one internal organ, or both; the patient should have radiographic, pathologic, or cultural evidence of infection in at least one other organ. Candidemia associated with *Candida* skin lesions or endophthalmitis consistent with a diagnosis of *Candida* infection also indicates a diagnosis of disseminated candidiasis.[11]

CHRONIC DISSEMINATED CANDIDIASIS

Chronic disseminated candidiasis, a chronic form of disseminated infection that is also known as hepatosplenic candidiasis, occurs in cancer patients who have been afflicted with protracted neutropenia.[12] This form of hematogenous candidiasis has not yet been described in the nonneutropenic surgical patient.

Characteristics of Surgical Patients at Risk for Candidiasis

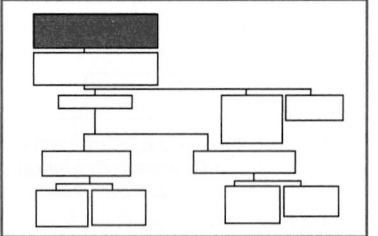

Fungal translocation that leads to hematogenous candidiasis is believed to be promoted by (1) colonization of the GI tract by *Candida* species, (2) physical disruption of the intestinal mucosal barrier, and (3) immunosuppression of the host leading to dissemination of the infection in the bloodstream and other organs [*see* Discussion, *below*].

Other important risk factors for hematogenous candidiasis include malignancies,[13] neutropenia and immunosuppressive therapy,[14] use of urinary catheters and diarrhea, prematurity,[15] heroin addiction,[16] abdominal surgery,[17] organ transplantation,[18] and extensive burns.[19]

The reported frequency of hematogenous candidiasis in burn patients ranges from 2% to 14%, depending on the reporting center and the study period.[19-21] Colonization by *Candida* species, hematogenous dissemination, and mortality caused by *Candida* infections have been found to correlate with the amount of body surface area burned and with the extent of full-thickness burn.

The pathogenesis, the incidence, and the microbial etiology of fungal infection vary in different groups of transplant recipients, depending on the organ transplanted, the donor source, the type of surgical procedure performed, and the recipient's age and general condition at the time of the procedure; other influential factors are the conditioning regimen, the type and duration of immunosuppressive therapy, and the presence or absence of organ rejection and graft versus host disease. In heart transplant recipients, for example, *Aspergillus* infection is a major problem, whereas in other organ transplant recipients, most fungal infections are attributable to *Candida*.[22] The infection is usually located at the site of the operation (e.g., an intra-abdominal abscess in liver[18] or pancreas[23] transplantation, the mediastinum or the lungs in heart[24] or heart-lung[25] transplantation, and the urinary tract in kidney[26] transplantation); however, dissemination from the primary site is common.

The central venous catheter has been reported as a risk factor in some studies but not in others,[10] particularly with *Candida parapsilosis*. This species, which may become part of the biofilm of intravascular catheters, may not respond to antifungal agents. Alternatively, *Candida* colonization of the catheter may result from gut-derived hematogenous seeding.[27,28]

Laboratory and Clinical Assessment of Candidiasis

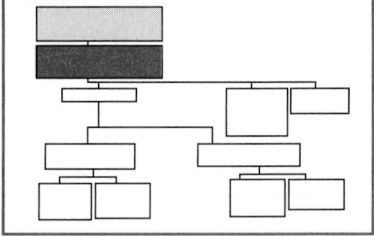

CULTURES

The workup of the surgical patient suspected of having hematogenous candidiasis begins with a complete set of cultures of sputum, oropharynx, stool, urine, all drain sites, and blood [*see* Table 1]. Candidiasis rarely develops in patients whose cultures show no evidence of *Candida* at some site. Obtaining more than six sets of blood cultures has little value, and there is no evidence to support arterial cultures.

The incidence of positive antemortem blood cultures in patients found to have candidiasis at autopsy is about 30% to 50%, possibly as a result of concomitant bacteremia, which may decrease the recovery of *Candida* species from the bloodstream. Because *Candida* species grow poorly under anaerobic conditions, venting the blood culture bottles is thought to improve the yield. The use of biphasic media also improves recovery of *Candida* species from the blood. Improved sensitivity and time to positivity of fungal blood cultures has been achieved with the development of new media, including biphasic media, automated radiometric and nonradiometric systems, and the lysis-centrifugation technique, a system that allows estimation of the number of *Candida* CFU/ml blood).[29] Commercial applications of these techniques include the BACTEC high-blood-volume fungal media system and the BacT/Alert system, both having comparable sensitivity to lysis-centrifugation. There is little evidence, however, that use of these newer methods provides a clinical advantage in the management of patients with hematogenous candidiasis. In a study by Berenguer and colleagues, the sensitivity of the lysis-centrifugation method increased with increasing numbers of involved organs but was still only 58% overall.[30]

Table 1   Clinical Presentation and Diagnostic Methods for Common Fungal Infections[139]

Host Fungus	Major Clinical Presentations	Diagnostic Methods
Normal host		
Aspergillus	Allergic bronchopulmonary	Serum IgE, precipitins
Blastomyces	Acute pneumonitis: chronic lung or skin	Culture, tissue
Candida	Vaginitis, thrush, candidemia, I.V. catheter	Culture/smear
Coccidioides	Acute pneumonitis, chronic cavitary, pulmonary nodule	Precipitins, complement fixation, culture
Cryptococcus	Pulmonary, meningitis	Culture, latex agglutination
Histoplasma	Acute pulmonary, progressive dissemination in infants and elderly, chronic cavitary in chronic airway obstruction	Culture, antigen detection
Compromised host		
Diabetes mellitus		
Candida	Disseminated, pyelonephritis, vaginitis	Culture/smear
Torulopsis	Pyelonephritis	Culture
Zygomycetes	Rhinocerebral, paranasal, pulmonary, gastrointestinal, cutaneous	Culture, tissue
Malignancy or corticosteroids		
Aspergillus	Invasive/lung, sinuses, disseminated	Culture, tissue
Candida	Fungemia, acute and chronic disseminated candidiasis	Culture, tissue
Coccidioides	Disseminated	Culture, precipitins, complement fixation
Cryptococcus	Pulmonary, meningeal, disseminated	Culture, latex agglutination, India ink preparation
Dematiaceous fungi	Lung, sinuses, brain, disseminated	Culture, tissue
Fusarium	Lung, sinuses, cellulitis at site of onychomycosis, disseminated	Culture, tissue
Histoplasma	Progressive disseminated	Culture, antigen detection
Torulopsis	Disseminated	Culture, tissue
Trichosporon	Disseminated	Culture, tissue
Zygomycetes	Rhinocerebral, paranasal, pulmonary, gastrointestinal, cutaneous, disseminated	Culture, tissue
Extensive surgery and previous antibiotic therapy		
Candida	Vaginitis, thrush, esophagitis, disseminated	Culture, tissue
Torulopsis	Disseminated	Culture

A rapid and inexpensive test is the germ tube test that can distinguish *C. albicans* (positive test) from other *Candida* species. More than 90% of *C. albicans* isolates produce germ tubes when incubated in serum for 2 to 3 hours at 37° C.

Several newer culture media allow the rapid identification of *C. albicans*. These include Albicans ID (bioMerieux, France), CandiSelect (Sanofi Diagnostics Pasteur, France), CHROMagar *Candida* (Becton Dickinson, USA), Fluoroplate *Candida* (Merck, Germany), Fongiscreen 4H (Sanofi Diagnostics Pasteur), and Murex *Candida albicans* (Murex Diagnostics, USA). CHROMagar and Fongiscreen 4H are also used for detection of other *Candida* species, including *C. glabrata, C. tropicalis,* and *C. krusei.* A recent study of 485 isolates (350 of *C. albicans* and 135 of other candidal species) evaluated the presumptive identification of *C. albicans* by comparing results of the germ-tube test to results of these six commercial tests. For *C. albicans,* the sensitivity and specificity of all six tests were greater than 97%. The sensitivity and specificity of the two tests that allow presumptive identification of other candidal species (CHROMagar *Candida* and Fongiscreen 4H) were lower, especially for *C. glabrata* and *C. tropicalis.*

Positive cultures from nonsterile sites (sputum, urine, and wound drainage) need to be interpreted with caution because of the frequent occurrence of *Candida* as a normal commensal of humans. Such cultures are useful mainly as an indication of colonization and, consequently, of the risk of infection in the appropriate setting.

ANTIBODY DETECTION

Previous studies have reported the use of incompletely characterized antigenic extracts of *C. albicans* to detect anticandidal antibodies in human sera. Difficulties with consistent production of uniform materials[31] have limited the usefulness of these tests. A variety of detection technologies (enzyme-linked immunosorbent assay [ELISA], immunodiffusion, and latex agglutination) have been used in attempts to detect antibodies directed toward defined purified antigen, but the sensitivity and specificity of these methods are low.[32] Methods using newly described antigens appear more promising.[33]

ANTIGEN DETECTION AND POLYMERASE CHAIN REACTION

Mannan, a polysaccharide component of the *Candida* cell wall, has the disadvantages of a short serum half-life and binding by antimannan antibody.[34] Although mannan can be detected by several methods,[35] complicated techniques are required to dissociate the mannan-antibody complex.[36] The sensitivity of mannan detection is approximately 70%.

A simple test available commercially (CAND-TEC *Candida* detection system, manufactured by Ramco Laboratories, USA) relies on the detection of a heat-labile antigen; however, its low sensitivity (as low as 19%) and specificity have limited its clinical use.[37] An antigen studied more recently is an immunodominant 48 kd cytoplasmic protein, *Candida* enolase. Because it is thought that cytoplasmic antigens are released during invasive infection, detection of this antigen may be able to distinguish between colonization and invasive infection.[33] A sensitivity of 54% was demonstrated in a study of 24 patients with invasive candidiasis,[38] but the sensitivity increases to 75% with the use of multiple samples. A sensitivity of 65% and a specificity of 97% were shown in a study assessing multiple samples.[39] Unfortunately, this test is not commercially available.

A commercial kit (Bichro-latex albicans) using monoclonal antibodies against cell wall extracts of *C. albicans* mannoprotein appears to have high sensitivity and specificity for *C. albicans*.[40]

Another antigen studied is (1-3)-β-D-glucan, an important cell wall constituent of fungi that is not shared with bacteria. Studies of this assay, which indicates the presence of fungi but does not identify the genus causing infection, have been promising in patients with fungal colonization. In these patients, its concentration remains lower than 20 pg/ml.

Amplification of the DNA of *Candida* species appears to be a quick and specific diagnostic tool. Although multiple approaches have been pursued,[41-43] several limitations need to be overcome before this method can be used routinely.[44]

METABOLITES

Systems based on the detection of D-arabinitol and mannose release by the fungus have been proposed,[45] but only those detecting D-arabinitol have been extensively developed. D-Arabinitol, a pentose produced by all of the major *Candida* species except *C. krusei* and *C. glabrata,* is excreted by the kidneys in the same rate as creatinine, and the ratio of D-arabinitol to creatinine must be used to interpret any observed concentration of D-arabinitol. Gas-liquid chromatographic as well as enzymatic methods are available for the detection of D-arabinitol, but gas-liquid chromatography is both technically demanding and expensive; it has been replaced by the recently developed enzymatic assay system. The sensitivity of the serum D-arabinitol–creatinine ratio for the diagnosis of invasive candidiasis, reported in the range of 40% to 83%, rises with repeated sampling.[46] Sensitivity is highest in patients with fungemia (74% to 83%) and lowest in patients with tissue-invasive *Candida* infections (40% to 44%). The magnitude of the D-arabinitol–creatinine ratio is strongly related to the degree of tissue invasion.[28,46] Although this assay may produce false positive results in some patients, it offers the promise of earlier detection of invasive candidiasis.[46]

Mannose, the other metabolite of *Candida* species that has been studied, can be detected only by a complicated gas-liquid chromatographic system. Initial estimates of its sensitivity (39%) have limited interest in this technique.[45]

HISTOLOGIC ANALYSES

Fungal smears are relatively insensitive methods of diagnosing candidiasis in otherwise sterile sites (e.g., joint fluid, peritoneal fluid, vitreous humor, or cerebrospinal fluid). Centrifugation of these fluids and examination of the sediment may improve the diagnostic yield. Conventional fungal stains, such as hematoxylin-eosin, periodic acid–Schiff (PAS), and Gomori methenamine-silver (GMS), are useful. The most sensitive stain is calcofluor white, but unfortunately, it requires fluorescent microscopy. Deep tissue biopsy provides a definitive diagnosis of candidiasis.

CLINICAL DIAGNOSIS

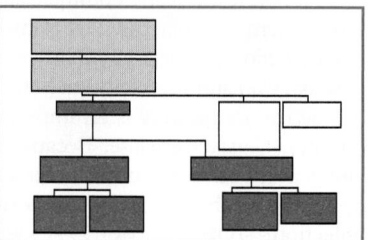

Hematogenous candidiasis has no characteristic clinical picture. Three clinical findings that may lead to an early diagnosis of hematogenous candidiasis in the surgical patient are candidal endophthalmitis, suppurative phlebitis, and candiduria in the absence of bladder instrumentation. A careful eye examination to identify the presence of candidal infection should be performed while the results of cultures of various sites are being awaited, and a repeat examination should be performed after therapy for proven candidemia. Candidal endophthalmitis may remain asymptomatic until late in the course of infection.

The presence of peripheral suppurative phlebitis that fails to yield bacteria or does not respond to antibacterial agents may be an early clue to the presence of hematogenous candidiasis. Gentle squeezing of the venous catheter exit site may express pus that yields *Candida* species on a smear or culture. Surgical excision of the infected vein usually reveals *Candida* infection in its lumen.

The presence of high-grade candiduria in surgical patients who have not had instrumentation of the renal pelvis or the bladder suggests hematogenous candidiasis and should prompt a workup for this infection. In this setting, candiduria may result from seeding of or filtering through the kidney.

Fever may be the only sign of infection but may be absent in patients who are receiving corticosteroids. Occasionally, a patient with hematogenous candidiasis presents with the systemic inflammatory response syndrome (SIRS) or septic shock. The diagnosis should be seriously considered in high-risk patients who are persistently febrile. Because of the high mortality associated with this infection, empirical antifungal therapy is recommended for early treatment of a clinical occult fungal infection or for the prevention of new fungal infections.

Management of Hematogenous Candidiasis

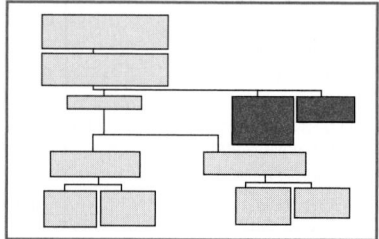

CANDIDEMIA AND ACUTE DISSEMINATED CANDIDIASIS

During the 1960s and the 1970s, the standard approach to managing candidemia was to classify patients according to degree of risk of disseminated candidiasis and to withhold antifungal treatment from those in whom dissemination appeared to be unlikely. This approach was based on unawareness of the magnitude of the problem in surgical patients and on acute awareness of the toxicities of amphotericin B, which was the only systemic antifungal agent available at the time; eventually, this type of management was found to be associated with a substantial mortality and a high incidence of long-term sequelae (e.g., deep-seated candidiasis presenting with endophthalmitis or other organ infection).[1] Consequently, it is now common practice to treat all candidemic patients except those who are afebrile, asymptomatic, or at low risk for disseminated candidiasis [*see Table 2*].

Candidates for empirical antifungal therapy are at high risk for candidiasis, colonized by *Candida* species (at one or more sites for *C. tropicalis* or at two or more for other candidal species), and unresponsive to broad-spectrum antibiotics in the absence of any other cause for their fever. Unresponsive patients may be characterized by rapid clinical deterioration, particularly if there is evidence of physical disruption of the intestinal mucosal barrier or immunosuppression.

The role of amphotericin B in the treatment of hematogenous candidiasis in surgical patients has been difficult to determine—first, because most of the studies that evaluated amphotericin B were retrospective trials with small sample sizes, and second, because few of the studies defined hematogenous candidiasis in the same way. In one study, treatment with amphotericin B had no effect on overall outcome in a mixed population of patients; however, the timing of therapy and the dose administered were not clearly stated.[47] In general, mortality was lower in patients who re-

Table 2 Antimicrobial Agents of Choice for Candidal Infections*

Infection	Agent of Choice	Alternative Agents	Comments
Hematogenous			
Candidemia and acute disseminated candidiasis	Fluconazole, or amphotericin B ± flucytosine	Lipid formulations of amphotericin B	Fluconazole should be given for *C. albicans,* amphotericin for all other *Candida* species; a 2-drug regimen should be given to hemodynamically unstable patients with persistent high-grade fungemia
Candida endophthalmitis	Fluconazole	Amphotericin B + flucytosine	Patients with vitral involvement require vitrectomy in addition to antifungal therapy
Suppurative phlebitis	Fluconazole + flucytosine	Amphotericin B + flucytosine	The central venous catheter should be removed and the infected vein excised
Endocarditis	Amphotericin B + flucytosine	—	Surgical replacement or repair of valves is essential to prevent death from embolization or cardiac failure; oral fluconazole should be given after successful completion of a prolonged course of amphotericin B therapy
Pericarditis	Amphotericin B	Fluconazole	
Prosthetic device–related infection	Fluconazole or amphotericin B	—	Removal of device is required for successful therapy
Arthritis	Fluconazole	—	—
Osteomyelitis	Amphotericin B	Fluconazole	Surgical drainage of pus is required
Meningitis	Amphotericin B + flucytosine	Fluconazole + flucytosine	—
Nonhematogenous			
Oropharyngeal			
Otherwise normal host	Nystatin	Ketoconazole, fluconazole, clotrimazole troches	—
Patients at risk for hematogenous infection (e.g., cancer patients, surgical patients)	Fluconazole	Ketoconazole	
Deep candidiasis			
Esophagitis and GI candidiasis	Fluconazole	Amphotericin B	Amphotericin B should be reserved for cases of fluconazole failure without endoscopic evidence of other causes of disease
Peritonitis and intra-abdominal	Fluconazole	Amphotericin B	—
Wound	Fluconazole	Amphotericin B	Antifungal therapy should be given to patients who do not respond to antibacterial therapy
Urinary tract			
Cystitis	Fluconazole	Amphotericin B	Fluconazole is preferable because of its high drug concentration in urine and because it is better tolerated
Pyelitis			
Without papillitis	Fluconazole	—	—
With papillitis	Fluconazole + flucytosine	Amphotericin B	—
Pyelonephritis	Fluconazole + flucytosine	Amphotericin B	—

*Therapy is individualized on the basis of the patient's clinical condition and the infecting species.

ceived amphotericin B than in those who did not.[48] Significant amphotericin B–related nephrotoxicity may occur.

The discovery of the azole antifungal agents has changed the management of *Candida* infections. The first two azoles, clotrimazole and miconazole, were not, however, suitable for systemic use. As for ketoconazole, the lack of a parenteral formulation and the erratic bioavailability of the drug in patients receiving H_2 receptor blockers or antacids have limited its use in the treatment of hematogenous candidiasis in surgical patients.

Fluconazole is a well-tolerated triazole with good activity in hematogenous candidiasis. Data available from several clinical trials suggest that the drug is as effective as and better tolerated than amphotericin B. Overall, four comparative studies have been completed in various patient populations. Two were randomized,[49,50] one was prospective observational,[51] and one used matched cohorts.[50] Fluconazole dosages ranged from 200 to 800 mg/day, given orally or intravenously, while intravenous amphotericin B was given at doses of 0.3 to 1.2 mg/kg.

The first prospective, randomized study of fluconazole included 40 surgical patients with hematogenous candidiasis, of whom 20 received 300 mg/day of fluconazole and 20 received 0.5 mg/kg/day of amphotericin B plus flucytosine.[52] There were no significant differences in outcome between the two study groups.

A matched-pair study compared the outcomes of 45 candidemic cancer patients who were treated with fluconazole with the outcomes of 45 candidemic cancer patients who were treated with amphotericin B[53]; in several of the 90 patients, hematogenous candidiasis had developed after operation. This study demonstrated that fluconazole was as effective as and better tolerated than amphotericin B. In one prospective, randomized multicenter study, 164 patients with documented or presumed invasive candidiasis received either amphotericin B, 0.7 mg/kg/day, or fluconazole, 400 mg/day.[50] The response rate for fluconazole (62%) was virtually identical to that for amphotericin B (63%), and fluconazole was better tolerated. In another prospective, randomized multicenter study, 206 nonimmunocompromised candidemic patients received either amphotericin B or fluconazole.[49] Once again, the two drugs were comparable in their efficacy, and fluconazole had a better safety profile.

Newer therapeutic options have now become available with the advent of the lipid-associated formulations of amphotericin B, which are less nephrotoxic than the parent compound.[54] Thus far, three lipid products of amphotericin B have been marketed in Europe or the United States: Abelcet (amphotericin B lipid complex), Amphocil (amphotericin B colloidal dispersion), and AmBisome (liposomal amphotericin B). A prospective, randomized trial has shown that Abelcet is as efficacious as conventional amphotericin B in hematogenous candidiasis.[55]

All patients with candidemia should receive antifungal therapy. We recommend the administration of fluconazole, 600 to 800 mg/day I.V. for 3 days, particularly if the infecting organism is known to be or is likely to be *C. albicans*. If the patient responds rapidly to this regimen, the dosage may be decreased to 400 mg/day and administered orally. For patients with hematogenous candidiasis who are known to be colonized by *C. glabrata*, *C. krusei*, or *C. lusitaniae*, amphotericin B, 0.5 to 0.7 mg/kg/day, should remain the treatment of choice. For patients who are hemodynamically unstable and for those who have high-grade persistent fungemia, we recommend a two-drug antifungal regimen: the combination of fluconazole and flucytosine or the combination of amphotericin B and flucytosine, depending on the infecting strain.

Clinical data on the effect of itraconazole in hematogenous candidiasis are scant. Given that itraconazole has limited bioavailability in the presence of antacids and H_2 receptor blockers, it should not be used to treat hematogenous candidiasis in the critically ill. However, an I.V. formulation of itraconazole is now available, and it is possible that this formulation may prove effective in patients with hematogenous candidiasis.

Liposomal formulations of amphotericin B offer new therapeutic alternatives. Their substantial cost limits their routine use, but they are appropriate if the patient has renal failure and is infected with an azole-resistant strain. Of the three available formulations, AmBisome is the best tolerated and yields the highest blood levels of amphotericin B.

The duration of therapy depends on the extent and severity of the infection. Therapy can be limited to 7 to 10 days for patients with low-grade fungemia and no evidence of organ involvement or hemodynamic instability. Patients with high-grade fungemia and evidence of organ involvement or hemodynamic instability need to receive antifungal therapy for 10 to 14 days after resolution of all signs and symptoms of infection.

Catheter Management

Controversy remains concerning the role of central venous lines in patients' outcome in hematogenous candidiasis. According to Nguyen and colleagues,[51] patients with catheter-related candidemia had a more favorable prognosis than patients with candidemia from other sources, but the prognosis was worse in patients whose catheters were retained. In contrast, studies by Carroll and colleagues, Nucci and coworkers,[56] and Anaissie and associates[10] failed to show a major role for retention of central venous catheters in the outcome of hematogenous candidiasis. The study by Anaissie and associates[10] examined the impact of catheter management on outcome in 416 cancer patients with candidemia who had an indwelling catheter at the time of candidal infection. Catheter exchange within 0, 2, or 4 days of the first positive blood culture had no significant effect on outcome. A second analysis, performed in a subset of 363 patients who had a central venous catheter in place and received antifungal therapy, revealed that catheter exchange was associated with improved outcome (80% versus 54%; $P < 0.001$). However, the subset in which the catheter was not exchanged had higher APACHE III scores and were more likely to be neutropenic. By multivariate analysis, catheter retention was not found to significantly affect outcome.

In one study in noncancer patients, Rex and colleagues[57] showed that replacement of all vascular catheters shortened the duration of candidemia from 5.6 days to 2.6 days. This finding suggests that catheters may play a role in perpetuating infection in nonneutropenic patients. In neutropenic patients, however, the primary source of candidemia is usually the GI tract, not the intravenous catheter, and other factors (e.g., the severity of disease, visceral dissemination, and neutrophil recovery) appear to have more impact on the outcome of neutropenic patients with candidemia.

Given the available data, we recommend that physicians consider the removal of all intravascular catheters in inpatients who have candidemia with persistent fever, persistent or high-grade fungemia, or *C. parapsilosis* (which is more likely to be catheter related than infection with other *Candida* species).

Cytokine Therapy for Opportunistic Infections

Polymorphonuclear leukocytes and macrophages are the predominant host defense against candidal infections. Candidal antigens induce lymphocyte proliferation and cytokine synthesis (interferon gamma and tumor necrosis factor); tumor necrosis factor enhances the candidacidal activity of phagocytes,[58] probably through increased production of reactive oxygen radicals. Another mechanism by which interferon gamma may augment host defenses against candidal infections is modulation of endothelial cell phagocytosis of *C. albicans*.[59] Granulocyte colony-stimulating factor (G-CSF) and granulocyte-macrophage colony-stimulating factor (GM-CSF) activate phagocytic cells to restrict the growth of *C. albicans*.[60]

Recently, a multicenter, double-blind, randomized phase II trial examined the activity of G-CSF in combination with fluconazole for treatment of hematogenous candidiasis in nonneutropenic patients. Preliminary analysis (Kullberg BJ and associates, unpublished report, 2000) indicated that an increase in the number of circulating neutrophils strongly correlates with accelerated clearance of bloodstream infection and reduced mortality. Additional data are needed to confirm these findings.

Antifungal Prophylaxis

Prophylaxis may be considered in surgical patients at high risk for invasive candidiasis. To date, there have been few trials of antifungal prophylaxis, whether as part of selective bowel decontamination[61] or in the form of low-dose amphotericin B[62] or liposomal formulations of amphotericin B in surgical transplant recipients.[63]

Fluconazole prophylaxis has been shown to reduce the rate of superficial and systemic fungal infections in cancer patients undergoing chemotherapy (with or without bone marrow transplantation)[64,65] and oropharyngeal and esophageal candidiasis in patients infected with HIV.[66] A recent double-blind randomized trial showed that intravenous fluconazole prophylaxis was effective in preventing candidal colonization and invasive intra-abdominal candidal infections in high-risk surgical patients.[67]

A retrospective study in burn patients reported that topical nystatin in the wound dressing was associated with a significant decrease in yeast acquisitions in burn wounds and fungemia but with an increase in colonization and fungemia caused by nystatin-resistant, amphotericin B–susceptible *C. rugosa*.[68]

Invasive fungal infection is one of the most important causes of mortality in organ transplant recipients.[69] Antifungal prophylaxis has been recommended in organ transplant recipients undergoing immunosuppressive therapy, but there is controversy about which drug is most effective and least toxic. Some physicians use fluconazole prophylactically in organ transplant recipients, but others recommend itraconazole or liposomal amphotericin B.[1,70,71]

ORGAN INFECTIONS

Candida *Endophthalmitis*

The diagnosis of candidal endophthalmitis usually implies hematogenous spread to multiple organs and the need for systemic antifungal therapy. Patients with chorioretinitis alone respond better to drug therapy alone than do those with vitreal involvement. Because antifungal drugs do not penetrate the vitreous body as well as the other ocular compartments,[72] patients with vitreal involvement require early vitrectomy in addition to antifungal therapy. Fluconazole is currently the drug of choice because of its proven efficacy and its higher concentration (20% to 70% of the corresponding plasma level) in ocular tissue, including the vitreous body.[73] Thus, we recommend 800 mg/day of fluconazole until a major response is observed, at which time it may be possible to reduce the dose to 400 mg/day. Although endophthalmitis due to *C. albicans* is commonly seen, recent series have reported on the importance of endophthalmitis caused by other candidal species. If the infecting organism (especially *C. krusei*) is potentially resistant to fluconazole, the recommended therapy is amphotericin B, 0.7 to 1.0 mg/kg/day I.V., preferably in conjunction with flucytosine.[74] Intravitreal injection of amphotericin B is recommended for vitreal infections.

The optimal duration of therapy for endogenous endophthalmitis is unknown, but we recommend that treatment be continued for at least 10 to 14 days after complete resolution of all signs and symptoms of infection. Ophthalmologic consultation is critical in establishing the diagnosis, assessing the patient's response to therapy, detecting complications, and determining whether early vitrectomy is indicated to prevent loss of sight.[75]

Suppurative Thrombophlebitis

A rare but serious consequence of hematogenous candidemia is suppurative thrombophlebitis, which results from infection of a vessel traumatized by prolonged catheterization. Endothelial disruption exposes the basement membrane and leads to thrombus formation and propagation. Suppurative thrombophlebitis is particularly serious because intravascular infection results in a persistent high-density fungemia. Management of this disease consists of high-dose antifungal therapy, removal of the central venous catheter, and excision of the infected vein, when possible.[76] Typically, blood cultures remain positive for several days; sometimes, they remain positive for as long as 3 to 4 weeks despite appropriate antifungal therapy, if the infected vein is not excised.

Endocarditis

Hematogenous candidiasis may also lead to the establishment of endocarditis, particularly in patients with a prosthetic heart valve or with a previously damaged native valve. Intravenous drug abuse and central intravenous catheterization appear to be predisposing factors. Candidal endocarditis after permanent pacemaker implantation has also been reported. The clinical picture is similar in many respects to that of bacterial endocarditis, although embolic phenomena have been more commonly associated with fungal endocarditis. Transesophageal echocardiography is more sensitive than transthoracic echocardiography in detecting candidal vegetation. Mortality due to *Candida* prosthetic valve endocarditis (PVE) is high, especially when complicated by congestive heart failure and persistent fungemia. For uncomplicated PVE, the mortality for patients receiving antifungal therapy alone (40%) is no worse than that for patients receiving combined medical and surgical therapy (33%).

Candidal endocarditis is very difficult to treat. Surgical replacement or repair of valves is essential to prevent death from embolization or cardiac failure in patients with complicated PVE. Ampho-

tericin B, with or without flucytosine, has been the therapy of choice; however, neither the optimal dosage nor the optimal duration of therapy has been determined. There is anecdotal information on the successful use of fluconazole in this setting, primarily as long-term suppressive therapy after the initial administration of amphotericin B.[73,77] Because of the high risk of late relapse, long-term maintenance therapy with oral fluconazole should be begun after successful completion of a prolonged course of amphotericin B.

Pericarditis

Candidal pericarditis is a very rare complication of hematogenous candidiasis. The surgical patients at risk for purulent pericarditis caused by *Candida* species are those who have undergone a cardiac operation, those who have a malignancy and whose host defenses are impaired, and those who have a debilitating chronic disease.[78] High-dose amphotericin B therapy, with or without surgical drainage, is recommended in these cases.

Arthritis

Joint infections with *Candida* species have resulted from hematogenous spread from inadvertent direct inoculation during joint procedures or intra-articular injection of corticosteroids. These infections typically involve a single joint, most frequently the knee, and tend to occur in patients with rheumatoid arthritis or prosthetic joint devices.[79] Local symptoms of pain on weight bearing or on full extension may be present. Diagnosis is best achieved by visualizing or growing the organisms from the joint fluid. Early diagnosis and systemic antifungal therapy are important to prevent destruction of the cartilage or loosening of the prosthesis. Successful treatment with fluconazole has been reported in several patients with fungal arthritis.[80] We recommend a dose of 400 to 800 mg/day for 6 months. Fluconazole can be used in acute therapy, alone or in combination with surgery, as well as in long-term suppressive therapy in patients at risk for recurrence or those who cannot undergo surgical debridement.

Osteomyelitis

Except for sternal infections complicating median sternotomy, most cases of candidal osteomyelitis have followed hematogenous spread. Vertebral body involvement is common. Back pain and fever may be followed by radiculopathy. Surgical drainage of pus is essential for a good response; however, surgical debridement of bony lesions may not be needed. Although amphotericin B has been the standard drug of choice, fluconazole offers an alternative in the treatment of these cases.[81]

Meningitis

Candidal meningitis may follow hematogenous spread or be a complication of neurosurgery or the implantation of ventriculoperitoneal shunts.[82] The infection is insidious and may remain undiagnosed. Most patients have recently received antibacterial agents, and half have had antecedent bacterial meningitis. The overall mortality is around 10%. The standard therapy is amphotericin B with flucytosine. The combination of high-dose fluconazole (800 mg/day) and flucytosine (50 mg/kg/day) is a particularly attractive approach because of the high CSF concentrations achieved with both agents. Removal of the infected shunts is recommended when possible.[51,82] The duration of treatment should be based on clinical response and culture results.

Nonhematogenous Candidiasis

SUPERFICIAL INFECTION

Oral candidiasis (thrush) appears as a whitish, patchy pseudomembrane covering an inflamed oropharynx and commonly involves the tongue, the hard and soft palates, and the tonsillar pillars. Controlled trials have documented the efficacy of nystatin suspension, clotrimazole troches, oral ketoconazole, fluconazole, or itraconazole in eradicating the clinical symptoms of oral candidiasis.[83,84]

Nystatin should be given as a 10 to 30 ml suspension five times daily, and the patient should be instructed to swish it around the mouth before swallowing; alternatively, the patient may take one or two troches five times daily. Clotrimazole troches are given five times daily as a 10 mg troche that should be held in the mouth until dissolved. In surgical patients at risk for hematogenous infection, systemic therapy with ketoconazole (200 to 400 mg once daily), itraconazole (100 to 200 mg/day), or fluconazole (100 mg once daily) is preferred.[85] Antifungal therapy should be administered for 1 week, except for fluconazole therapy, which is likely to be effective when given for 2 or 3 days.

DEEP CANDIDIASIS

Esophagitis and Gastrointestinal Candidiasis

Superficial candidiasis involving only mucosal surfaces used to be a common finding at autopsy in surgical patients who had a protracted hospital stay characterized by recurrent sepsis. Such lesions may arise at any site in the GI tract but appear most commonly in the esophagus and the small bowel and may progress to hematogenous infection [see Figure 1].

In a minority of patients, the pathology of infection of the lower GI tract by Candida species may change from diarrhea without demonstrable tissue invasion to direct penetration into the submucosa, which eventually leads to pseudomembranous enterocolitis. Direct vascular invasion through the bowel wall has been reported only in patients receiving immunosuppressive chemotherapy.[86] These patients may have extensive involvement of the GI tract from mouth to anus. Nonneutropenic surgical patients exhibit more localized involvement.

The preferred therapy for esophageal candidiasis is fluconazole or itraconazole, 200 mg daily. In patients who remain symptomatic after 5 days of therapy, endoscopy is needed to rule out other causes of esophagitis. If endoscopy proves that esophagitis is caused by candidal infection, low-dose amphotericin B (0.4 mg/kg/day) should be administered. Therapy for esophageal candidiasis should be continued for at least 4 days after symptoms resolve; immunosuppressed patients generally require more extended therapy to prevent relapse.

Because stool cultures do not differentiate between colonization and infection, candidiasis in the lower gastrointestinal tract is usually a postmortem diagnosis; hence, there are no reliable criteria governing when and how to treat this condition. It has been reported, however, that patients who have diarrhea that can only be caused by heavy colonization with Candida species may respond dramatically to 2 to 4 days of nystatin therapy.[87]

Peritonitis and Intra-abdominal Abscess

Perhaps the most controversial aspect of Candida infectious syndromes in surgical patients is whether specific systemic therapy is required to eradicate the infection within intra-abdominal abscesses, peritoneal fluid, or fistula drainage. Candida is frequently cultured from intra-abdominal infectious foci but should be considered a serious threat only in high-risk patients. Four risk factors for intra-abdominal candidiasis are gastrointestinal perforations, anastomotic leakage, surgery for acute pancreatitis, and splenectomy.[88]

Patients with peritonitis and intra-abdominal abscesses should receive systemic antifungal therapy, usually in combination with antibacterial therapy, given that these infections are almost always polymicrobial in origin. The risk of dissemination is increased by

Figure 1 **Superficial candidiasis may be found at all levels of the GI tract. Here, the esophagus of a patient found at autopsy to have disseminated candidiasis shows disrupted epithelium, submucosal inflammation, and the presence of yeast in the submucosa.**

both the recurrence of intra-abdominal infections and the presence of extensive areas of communication between the abdominal cavity and the external environment via either fistulas or drain tracts.

On rare occasions, candidal peritonitis occurs after long-term ambulatory peritoneal dialysis. In such cases, the infection tends to remain localized and to manifest with low-grade fever and abdominal pain and tenderness. The peritoneal dialysate is usually cloudy and contains more than 100 neutrophils/mm^3. Therapy consists of systemic antifungal therapy and removal of the peritoneal catheter. The abdominal pain caused by the addition of amphotericin B to the dialysate has raised concern that chemical peritonitis might give rise to adhesions and thus impair the efficacy of dialysis.

Because fluconazole is very safe and is capable of reaching high concentrations in peritoneal fluid, it is likely to be useful in the management of candidal peritonitis.[89] Fluconazole should be given at a dosage of 100 to 200 mg/day orally for 2 to 6 weeks. Immediate removal of the peritoneal catheter has been recommended. In one study, however, seven of nine patients treated with oral flucytosine responded to therapy without catheter removal.[90]

A prospective, randomized study in patients on continuous ambulatory dialysis found that successful prophylaxis for Candida peritonitis was achieved with oral nystatin (tablets containing 500,000 units given four times a day).[91]

Occasionally, Candida species may cause cholangitis, biliary tract disease, pancreatic abscess, or liver abscess. This problem is increasingly found in patients with percutaneously placed drainage catheters for malignancy. Such patients must be given systemic therapy for clinical evidence of infection, including candidemia, and the drainage catheter must be changed. Diverticulitis complicated by candidal pylephlebitis has also been reported.

Wound Infections

The diagnosis and treatment of candidal wound infections are problematic. Recovering Candida species from drains and wounds does not necessarily mean that this organism is causing tissue infection. Colonization of wounds by Candida species should not compel physicians to use systemic antifungal therapy. However, such therapy should be administered to those patients whose wound infections do not respond to appropriate antibacterial therapy, particularly if one Candida species is repeatedly isolated from the site and the patient is at high risk for hematogenous infection. Antifungal therapy should be administered to prevent the establishment of *Candida* osteomyelitis when sternal wound cultures obtained after coronary artery bypass surgery yield *Candida* species.

Urinary Tract and Genital Candidiasis

The recovery of *Candida* species from the urinary tract most commonly results from contamination from the perirectal or the genital area or from colonization of the bladder, which is usually seen in patients who have undergone prolonged catheterization or who have diabetes mellitus or another disease that leads to incomplete bladder emptying. In addition, *Candida* species usually colonize ileal conduits. Persistent candiduria in the surgical intensive care unit may, however, be an early marker of disseminated infection in critically ill high-risk patients.[92] In a study of 91 pediatric ICU patients who were clinically suspected of having disseminated candidiasis, the isolation of candidal species other than *C. albicans* from the urine was a better indicator of candidemia than was isolation of *C. albicans;* 60% of the patients whose urine contained candidal species other than *C. albicans* had candidemia, versus 33.3% of the patients whose urine contained *C. albicans.*[93]

Alkalization of the urine with oral potassium-sodium hydrogen citrate is a simple and effective method of treating candiduria in patients with an indwelling catheter.[94] Replacing or removing the bladder catheter is preferable. If *Candida* colonization persists, particularly if the patient has a risk factor for cystitis (e.g., diabetes mellitus or a disease that leads to incomplete bladder emptying) or for hematogenous dissemination (e.g., immunosuppression or manipulation of the genitourinary system), antifungal therapy should be considered. Amphotericin B bladder irrigation provides only temporary clearance of funguria, and systemic agents (a single I.V. dose of amphotericin B or a 5-day course of oral fluconazole) are usually needed.

The spectrum of urinary tract infection by *Candida* species includes cystitis, pyelitis (i.e., infection of the renal pelvis), fungus ball of the ureter, and renal abscesses. The diagnosis of cystitis is based on the presence of symptoms of cystitis, diffuse erythema or fungal plaques on cystoscopy, candiduria, and pyuria. *Candida* cystitis warrants therapy. If a triple-lumen catheter is in place, bladder irrigation with amphotericin B, 50 mg/L/day for 2 days, may be tried. Fluconazole, 200 mg once daily, is a more attractive approach because of the convenience, lower cost, and very high drug concentrations achieved in the urine.[95] Flucytosine is excreted in the urine in high concentrations and may be particularly useful against *C. glabrata* infection.

The management of pyelitis depends on whether the renal papillae are invaded or the ureter is obstructed with a fungus ball. Patients with no papillitis and an open ureter usually respond to irrigation with amphotericin B through a ureteral or percutaneous catheter. If papillitis is present, systemic antifungal therapy with fluconazole, 400 mg daily, is recommended. If fungus balls are present, surgical removal should be considered in addition to treatment with antifungal agents.

Hematogenous infections of the kidneys leading to multiple renal abscesses are treated as instances of hematogenous candidiasis. However, because both fluconazole and flucytosine are well tolerated, have good tissue diffusion, and are excreted in the urine in high concentrations, it is reasonable to assume that the combination of these two agents represents the therapy of choice for candidiasis that involves renal parenchyma.

Surgical patients are also at risk for vulvovaginal candidiasis. The diagnosis is based on the clinical findings and on the presence of pseudohyphae on a fungal smear. Various antifungal agents, including oral azoles and topical medications (suppositories, creams, and vaginal tablets) are effective in more than 80% of uncomplicated infections. Oral agents include fluconazole (150 mg in a single dose), ketoconazole (400 mg daily for 5 days), and itraconazole (200 mg in a single dose). However, women with four or more episodes of vulvovaginal candidiasis during a 12-month period and women with acute severe attacks of candidal vaginitis are less likely to respond to conventional therapy. Preventive measures include control of host factors such as diabetes mellitus, antifungal prophylaxis during the use of antibiotics and under other high-risk conditions, and the avoidance of systematic corticosteroids, oral contraceptives, and antibiotics if possible. Therapy with oral fluconazole, itraconazole, or ketoconazole is recommended for approximately 14 days to ensure clinical remission and negative fungal culture, followed by a maintenance regimen of fluconazole (150 mg once weekly for 6 months). Recurrence of vulvovaginal candidiasis is common, occurring in 30% to 40% of patients after cessation of the maintenance regime.[96]

Other Fungal Infections

ASPERGILLOSIS

Aspergillosis, a rare infection in the surgical patient, usually occurs in those who are markedly immunosuppressed after undergoing chemotherapy with cytotoxic agents or adrenal corticosteroids. Most cases of nosocomial aspergillosis are acquired via airborne transmission.[13,97] Colonization of the respiratory tract is followed by invasive disease if these predisposing factors are present. Sources of airborne fungi in microepidemics frequently are associated with construction within the hospital or at adjacent sites. Other modes of transmission of aspergillosis have been reported, including infections associated with foreign bodies, catheters, and bandages.

Acute invasive pulmonary aspergillosis is the most common form of *Aspergillus* infection in immunocompromised surgical patients. The organisms tend to invade blood vessels and cause thrombosis and infarction of the surrounding tissues. The infection may manifest itself in the form of acute vascular events such as pulmonary embolus or, more rarely, myocardial infarction, cerebral hemorrhage, or Budd-Chiari syndrome. Pulmonary *Aspergillus* infections include necrotizing bronchopneumonia and hemorrhagic pulmonary infarction, each accounting for about one third of these infections. Pulmonary aspergillosis may extend to contiguous organs or be disseminated. The rhinocerebral form of aspergillosis occurs less often than pulmonary infection. It originates in the sinuses and progresses through soft tissues, cartilage, and bone, causing lesions in the palate and the nose. Occasionally, the infection progresses through the base of the skull and involves the brain.

Diagnosis of *Aspergillus* infection is difficult and relies on identifying the organism in culture or histopathologic specimens.[13] The recovery of *Aspergillus* species from the respiratory tract culture of a surgical patient should be considered to represent contamination or colonization unless the patient is symptomatic and severely immunosuppressed. The standard therapy is high-dose amphotericin B (1 mg/kg/day) for a minimum of 2 g.[98] The addition of flucytosine may be useful. Liposomal formulations of amphotericin B and itraconazole offer additional treatment alternatives; at present, however, clinical experience with these new antifungal agents in patients with aspergillosis is limited.

ZYGOMYCOSIS (MUCORMYCOSIS)

Agents of zygomycosis have caused nosocomial infections in the surgical patient. The reservoir, the mode of transmission, the pathogenesis, and the clinical presentations are similar to those of *Aspergillus* species. In the surgical patient, the major risk factors include diabetic ketoacidosis, immunosuppression after cytotoxic chemotherapy, adrenocorticosteroid therapy, organ transplantation, skin damage (e.g., from adhesive tape, an arm board, or severe burns), and a prolonged postoperative stay.[99] Zygomycotic infections include rhinocerebral, paranasal, pulmonary, gastrointestinal, cutaneous, and, very rarely, disseminated disease.

Appropriate management of zygomycosis consists of extensive surgical debridement of infected areas, rapid correction of the underlying disease, and high-dose amphotericin B therapy up to a total dose of 2 to 3 g.

EMERGING PATHOGENS

Fungi such as *Fusarium* species, *Curvularia* species, *Alternaria* species, and *Trichosporon beigelii* were once thought to represent contamination or harmless colonization when isolated from tissue specimens. These and other newly recognized fungi have since been clearly shown to be potentially serious pathogens in immunosuppressed surgical patients.[100] In such patients, the recovery of any fungus from any site should prompt an evaluation by an infectious disease specialist to determine the clinical significance of the isolate.

Systemic Antifungal Agents

AMPHOTERICIN B

Amphotericin B is structurally similar to membrane sterols, and its major mechanism of action is believed to be through interaction with membrane sterols and creation of pores in the fungal outer membrane. The clinical usefulness of amphotericin B is believed to be attributable to the greater affinity of amphotericin B for ergosterol (found in fungal cell membranes) than for cholesterol (the principal sterol found in mammalian cell membranes). Oxidation-dependent amphotericin B-induced stimulation of macrophages is another proposed mechanism of action.[101] Most species of fungi that cause human infections are susceptible to amphotericin B.

Amphotericin B is supplied as a sterile lyophilized powder in vials containing 50 mg of amphotericin B, deoxycholate, and buffer. The contents are then diluted in 5% dextrose in water at a concentration of 10 mg/dl. Less precipitation occurs in saline solutions. The agent is stable at room temperature for 24 hours and is not sensitive to light. An acute infusion-related reaction, consisting of fever, hypotension, and tachycardia, occurs in about 20% of patients.[90] Premedication with acetaminophen may blunt this response. If this approach is unsuccessful, premedication with meperidine (25 to 50 mg I.V.) or hydrocortisone (25 to 50 mg I.V.) is recommended. Hypotension, hypertension, hypothermia, and bradycardia are other reported infusion-related toxic effects of amphotericin B deoxycholate. Ventricular arrhythmias have been associated with rapid infusion of amphotericin B deoxycholate and with administration of the agent to patients with severe hypokalemia or renal failure. Through inhibition of erythropoietic production secondary to nephrotoxicity, amphotericin B suppresses the production of red blood cells, causing a normocytic, normochromic anemia.

Common practice is to give a 1 mg test dose and observe the patient for 1 hour in the hope of identifying patients at risk for severe acute reactions. The full dose of the drug (0.6 to 1 mg/kg/day) is then infused over a period of 4 to 6 hours, although there is evidence to suggest that much shorter infusion times (e.g., 1 hour in patients with adequate cardiopulmonary and renal function) may be acceptable. The total dose depends on the extent of the infec-

tion and the patient's condition. Patients must be monitored carefully during the first day of therapy. The infusion should be discontinued if the patient becomes hemodynamically unstable.

If acute reactions limit the amount of drug that can be infused, patients are premedicated with hydrocortisone, 25 to 50 mg I.V., either alone or in combination with meperidine, 25 to 50 mg I.V., 30 minutes before amphotericin B infusion is begun.

The distribution of the drug after I.V. infusion does not directly correlate with the daily dose. This finding is consistent with the unusual pharmacokinetics of amphotericin B. The initial serum half-life of the drug is about 24 hours, and the terminal half-life is about 15 days.

Renal toxicity and hypokalemia are the primary toxicities of amphotericin B [*see Table 3*]. Amphotericin B-induced nephrotoxicity may be glomerular, characterized by a decrease in glomerular filtration rate and renal blood flow, or tubular, with urinary casts, hypokalemia, hypomagnesemia, renal tubular acidosis, and nephrocalcinosis).[102] All of these abnormalities occur to varying degrees in almost all patients receiving the drug. In most patients, renal dysfunction gradually resolves after discontinuance of therapy. Amphotericin B nephrotoxicity may be minimized by avoiding other agents with synergistic nephrotoxicity (e.g., aminoglycosides, vancomycin, cisplatin, and cyclosporine) and by the administration of sodium supplementation. The latter approach consists of I.V. infusion of 500 ml of 0.9% saline solution 30 minutes before the administration of amphotericin B and a second infusion of the same amount of saline after the amphotericin B infusion is completed.

If the serum creatinine level exceeds 3.5 mg/dl, amphotericin B should be discontinued and the serum creatinine level monitored twice weekly. Administration of amphotericin B may be resumed at 50% to 75% of the original dosage when the serum creatinine level falls below 3 mg/dl.

The combined use of amphotericin B deoxycholate and other nephrotoxic agents, such as cyclosporine, aminoglycosides, and foscarnet, may result in synergistic nephrotoxicity.[103] Less nephrotoxic lipid formulations of amphotericin B include amphotericin B lipid complex (Abelcet), amphotericin B colloidal dispersion (Amphotec), and liposomal amphotericin B (AmBisome). These preparations differ in the amount of amphotericin B and the type of lipid used as well as in the physical form, pharmacokinetics, and toxicities. Of the three formulations, AmBisome is the one that is best tolerated.

FLUCYTOSINE

Flucytosine can be useful for the treatment of hematogenous candidiasis; however, a high failure rate and secondary emergence of resistance have been reported when flucytosine was used alone, and serious concerns exist regarding its myelosuppressive potential. A review of the literature on the activity of flucytosine in acute disseminated candidiasis and candidemia indicates a good response rate.

The standard dosage for flucytosine is 37.5 mg/kg every 6 hours. On the basis of the pharmacokinetics of flucytosine and the in vitro susceptibility of *Candida* species to the drug, much lower dosages of flucytosine (e.g., 12.5 mg/kg every 12 hours) would probably maintain serum and tissue levels significantly above the minimal inhibitory concentration (MIC) needed for most susceptible strains throughout therapy. For example, giving 25 mg/kg/day at 12-hour intervals would result in peak and trough serum levels of about 25 and 5 μg/ml, respectively, given a steady state and normal kidney function in a 70 kg patient. Because the MIC of flucytosine for most susceptible *Candida* species is usually 1 μg/ml or less, such a dosage schedule will constitute

Table 3 Antifungal Chemotherapy[140]

Drug	Indications	Route of Administration	Major Side Effects
Amphotericin B	Hematogenous and deep-seated candidiasis; aspergillosis; blasto-mycosis; coccidioidomycosis; histoplasmosis; cryptococcosis	Intravenous, intrathecal	Anemia, headache, chills, fever, nausea, renal dysfunction, hypotension, tachypnea, hypokalemia, phlebitis
Clotrimazole	Oropharyngeal candidiasis	Oral	—
Flucytosine	Candidiasis (septicemia, endocarditis, and urinary tract infections); cryptococcosis	Oral	Leukopenia, thrombocytopenia, liver dysfunction, diarrhea
Fluconazole	Oropharyngeal and esophageal candidiasis; hematogenous candidal infection; other candidal infections (e.g., urinary tract infections, peritonitis); meningeal coccidioidomycosis; cryptococcosis	Oral, intravenous	Nausea and vomiting, skin rash, liver dysfunction
Itraconazole	Histoplasmosis; blastomycosis; aspergillosis	Oral	Nausea, vomiting, liver dysfunction
Ketoconazole	Candidiasis (chronic mucocutaneous candidiasis or oropharyngeal candidiasis); candiduria; blastomycosis; coccidioidomycosis; histoplasmosis; chromomycosis; paracoccidioidomycosis	Oral	Hepatotoxicity, nausea or vomiting, occasional suppression of adrenal function

appropriate therapy, given that the drug is used in combination with other antifungals. This approach may decrease the myelosuppressive potential that the drug usually exhibits at levels of 100 μg/ml, and it may lead to the drug's wider use.

Peak serum concentrations should be monitored and the dosage adjusted so as to maintain a peak level of about 25 μg/ml. Flucytosine is removed by hemodialysis and peritoneal dialysis. Patients undergoing hemodialysis should receive a 37.5 mg/kg dose of flucytosine after each dialysis session unless their initial peak serum concentration is higher than 25 μg/ml or their postdialysis concentration is higher than 10 μg/ml. Patients undergoing peritoneal dialysis should receive a single 37.5 mg/kg dose daily.

FLUCONAZOLE

The mechanism of action of fluconazole is preferential inhibition of cytochrome P-450 enzymes in fungal organisms. Fluconazole is active against several *Candida* species, including *C. tropicalis. C. krusei*, however, is highly resistant to this agent.[90] Fluconazole also does not appear to have good clinical activity against *Aspergillus* species. Fluconazole is available in either an oral form or an I.V. form, both of which are rapidly and almost completely absorbed from the GI tract. The serum concentrations after oral administration are almost identical to those achieved when the drug is administered intravenously. A major advantage of fluconazole over ketoconazole is its high degree of GI absorption, which is not affected by gastric acidity or the presence of food. Steady-state serum concentrations of fluconazole are obtained within 5 to 10 days. An initial loading dose that is twice the usual daily dose is recommended. Fluconazole is distributed evenly in body tissues, penetrates into the vitreous humor and the aqueous humor of the eye, and crosses the blood-brain barrier. The drug is excreted largely unchanged in the urine, with only minimal liver metabolism. Consequently, dosage schedules must be adjusted in patients with renal impairment. Hemodialysis significantly reduces the serum concentrations, and the drug appears also to be removed by peritoneal dialysis. A standard dose should be given after each course of dialysis.

The toxicities of fluconazole are similar to those of other azoles and include nausea and vomiting in about 2% of patients, as well as headache, fatigue, abdominal pain, and diarrhea[104]; exfoliative dermatitis also occurs, but very rarely. Transient abnormalities of liver function have been observed in 3% of patients receiving fluconazole. In addition, fatal hepatic necrosis developed in two patients who were receiving fluconazole, but it was unclear whether the agent played a causal role in this event. No significant hormonal abnormalities have been reported after administration of fluconazole.

Because fluconazole interacts with warfarin, phenytoin, and cyclosporine when given in a daily dose of 200 mg or more,[104] serum concentrations of these agents should be monitored.

ITRACONAZOLE

Itraconazole is the only available azole that has substantial activity against *Aspergillus* species. It exists in an oral capsule formulation, the bioavailability of which is approximately 55%. Absorption is enhanced by the presence of food in the stomach but is significantly reduced by the presence of antacids or H$_2$ receptor blockers. A new solution, which has significantly higher bioavailability, may not be well tolerated by patients. When erratic absorption is of concern, use of the I.V. formulation is recommended. The serum elimination half-life, 15 to 25 hours, increases to 34 to 42 hours after weeks of administration and with increasing itraconazole doses.

Metabolized by the liver, itraconazole is excreted as metabolites primarily in the feces (54%) and urine (35%). A hepatic metabolite, hydroxyitraconazole, has an antifungal spectrum similar to that of the parent compound. Because itraconazole is metabolized to a large degree in the liver, the dosage must be adjusted in patients with hepatic failure; however, its pharmacokinetics are not affected by renal impairment or hemodialysis. Serum concentrations of digoxin may increase when this agent is given with itraconazole,[105] and the metabolism of itraconazole may be accelerated when drugs that induce hepatic enzymes are given simultaneously.[106] Serum concentrations of itraconazole should therefore be measured in patients with invasive infections.

Itraconazole is generally well tolerated in dosages of up to 400 mg/day. The most common side effects are nausea, vomiting, diarrhea, and abdominal discomfort. Headaches, rash, pruritus, and dizziness occasionally occur. At higher doses, a mineralocorticoid excess syndrome (hypokalemia, hypertension, and edema) has been described, and hypokalemia develops in as many as 6% of patients who take 400 mg/day for several months.[107]

Itraconazole is available in 100 mg capsules and oral suspension (10 mg/ml). Because itraconazole may be teratogenic, it should be avoided in pregnant patients. A large number of drug interactions occur with itraconazole, many related to inhibition of the cytochrome P-450 enzyme system. Care should be taken in prescribing itraconazole with these agents. Itraconazole is currently approved for the treatment of blastomycosis, histoplasmosis, and aspergillosis but is also effective for the treatment of candidiasis and cryptococcosis.

KETOCONAZOLE

Ketoconazole is effective against yeast infections of the skin and the mucous membranes; however, it should not be used to treat hemato-

Table 4 Characteristics of Currently Available Azoles*[139]

	Ketoconazole	Fluconazole	Itraconazole
Spectrum	Narrow	Expanded	Expanded
Route(s) of administration	Oral	Oral, intravenous	Oral
Bioavailability	Erratic, requires gastric acidity	Excellent	Erratic, requires gastric acidity
Plasma half-life (hr)	6–9	30	20–40
Hepatotoxicity	Occasional	Occasional	Occasional
Gastrointestinal intolerance	Frequent	Occasional	Occasional
CSF penetration	No	Yes	No
Renal excretion	No	Yes	No
Interaction with other drugs	Frequent	Occasional	Frequent

*Intravenous miconazole is also available but offers no advantage over the currently available azoles.

genous candidiasis. Ketoconazole is not available in an intravenous form, and the serum levels it is capable of reaching depend largely on gastric acidity [see Table 4]. The same adverse events and drug-drug interactions observed with itraconazole occur with ketoconazole.

SPECIAL CONSIDERATIONS IN ORGAN TRANSPLANT RECIPIENTS

Intravenous amphotericin B (0.4 to 0.8 mg/kg/day) has been the mainstay of treatment in organ transplant recipients, but concerns have been expressed about increased nephrotoxicity, particularly in patients receiving cyclosporine or tacrolimus. The lipid formulations of amphotericin B (1 to 3 mg/kg/day) are less nephrotoxic, particularly liposomal amphotericin B (AmBisome). Fluconazole has a minimal effect on hepatic microsomal enzymes in comparison with ketoconazole and itraconazole and therefore is the drug of choice in organ transplant recipients who have candidiasis caused by fluconazole-susceptible strains.

Conclusion

Continued progress in supportive care, including the development of antibiotics with increasingly broad spectra of activity, has resulted in an increased incidence of fungal infections, particularly candidiasis. Because of the inadequacy of the available knowledge base, we do not fully understand the pathophysiology of these infections in surgical patients, nor can we be certain precisely when prophylaxis and therapy should be administered.

Despite these limitations, there is now sufficient information available to justify an aggressive therapeutic approach to suspected *Candida* infections. Now that less toxic agents are available (the newer triazoles, particularly fluconazole, and the lipid formulations of amphotericin B), the clinical approach to presumed fungal infections in surgical patients has been made far simpler.

Discussion

Microbiologic Characteristics of Pathogenic *Candida* Species

Candida species multiply by producing buds from ovoid yeast cells. They are differentiated from other yeasts (e.g., *Saccharomyces* species) by their ability to produce pseudohyphae on certain media and, in the case of *C. albicans*, true hyphae in serum [see Figure 2].

VIRULENCE FACTORS

Four virulence factors have been demonstrated for *Candida* species: adherence to mucosal epithelial cells; secretion of proteinases, which degrade connective tissue proteins, thereby allowing yeast to enter beyond connective tissue barriers; ambient pH[108]; and resistance to oxidative killing by neutrophils.

For *Candida* species to disseminate, the organisms must be able to adhere to the vascular system (i.e., endothelium, the basement membrane, or both), an ability that is probably receptor mediated.[109] In vitro, however, *Candida* adheres more avidly to the subendothelial extracellular matrix than to endothelial cells. This finding

may explain the increased risk of hematogenous candidiasis in patients receiving cytotoxic chemotherapy. Such therapy causes denudation of endothelium and consequent exposure of the basement membrane, to which *Candida* then readily adheres.

Genetic studies have evaluated the role of various virulence factors for *Candida* species, including ambient pH,[108] adherence mechanisms, and enzyme production. Mechanisms by which *Candida* species lose virulence include the following: gene dysregulation, stopping the switch from budding yeast to filamentous form; disruption of a gene that results in decreased hyphal growth, adherence, and virulence[110]; deficiency of *C. albicans* in mannosyl transferase, resulting in decreased adherence and virulence; and deletion of the gene that encodes the production of phospholipase leading to decreased cell wall penetration.

CHANGING MICROBIOLOGIC SPECTRUM OF *CANDIDA*

Although there are more than 100 described species of *Candida*, only four are commonly associated with infection: *C. albicans, C. tropi-*

Figure 2 *Candida* takes several forms as it grows. A blastospore is a unicellular form (*a*). Blastospores divide by budding, a process in which new cellular material grows from a site on the blastospore (*b*). Nuclear division then occurs, and a septum forms between the two new cells. A hypha is a long tube of several cells divided by septa (*c*). A mycelium is a cellular aggregate that includes a hypha and its branches (*d*). A pseudohypha differs from a true hypha in that it is composed of morphologically distinct, elongated blastospores.

calis, *C. parapsilosis*, and *C. glabrata*.[10] Of these, *C. albicans* has been isolated from more than 60% of candidal infections; the other three major species are seen at rates varying from 5% to 20%. Mucosal colonization by *C. tropicalis*, a virulent organism, frequently leads to invasive infection. *C. glabrata* and *C. parapsilosis* appear to be relatively less virulent,[111] and the latter typically causes infection in association with prosthetic materials (e.g., catheters) or glucose-rich intravenous solutions.[10] Finally, *C. krusei* and *C. lusitaniae* rarely cause disease, being isolated from fewer than 1% of cultures.[10] The epidemiology of candidiasis has changed, with reduced rates of *C. albicans* in favor of other candidal species—in particular, *C. glabrata* and *C. krusei*.[112] This change is important because *C. krusei* and several strains of *C. glabrata* are highly resistant to the triazoles such as fluconazole and itraconazole.[10,112]

A study by the NNIS group evaluated 1,579 bloodstream isolates of *Candida* species obtained from more than 50 hospitals in the United States over a 7-year period (1992–1998) to detect trends in species distribution and susceptibility to fluconazole. *C. albicans* accounted for 52% of isolates, followed by *C. glabrata* (18%), *C. parapsilosis* (15%), *C. tropicalis* (11%), and *C. krusei* (2%). Since 1995, *C. glabrata* has been more prevalent than *C. parapsilosis*. The susceptibility of all *Candida* species to fluconazole has remained stable.[113]

Pathogenesis of Candidiasis in the Surgical Patient

COLONIZATION OF THE GUT BY *CANDIDA* SPECIES

That colonization is a necessary prelude to infection is supported by studies demonstrating (1) that 95% of neutropenic patients and 84% of nonneutropenic patients were infected with the same strains that had previously colonized them and (2) that infection was significantly less likely to develop in patients who were not colonized.[114,115] In a study investigating the sequence of colonization and candidemia in nonneutropenic patients, Voss and colleagues[114] found that the strains recovered from the initial colonized or infected site and from

the bloodstream were identical in patients with disseminated candidiasis; furthermore, nearly every patient was infected with a distinct or unique *Candida* strain. In another study, positive surveillance cultures were found to be highly predictive of systemic infection, whereas negative surveillance cultures correlated with a low risk of candidal dissemination.[116] Clinical studies of antifungal prophylaxis in neutropenic cancer patients have also suggested that antifungal regimens effectively prevent hematogenous infection when they can eliminate or reduce colonization by *Candida*.[117]

The density of colonization appears to be predictive of the risk of hematogenous candidiasis. In two large series of neutropenic cancer patients, hematogenous candidiasis almost never developed in noncolonized patients, compared with an infection rate of more than 30% in patients with multiple colonized sites.[115,118] In a study of patients with acute lymphocytic leukemia, a relatively high concentration of *Candida* organisms in the stools was found to be a significant risk factor for hematogenous candidiasis.[119] In 40 infants of very low birth weight, a value of 8×10^6 *Candida* CFU/g stool was established as a threshold, beyond which GI symptoms (attributed to *Candida*) developed in 50% of the infants and a systemic septic response in 28.5% during 1 to 3 weeks of heavy colonization.[120] In a prospective study of patients admitted to surgical and neonatal intensive care units, Pittet and coworkers demonstrated that the intensity of *Candida* colonization (as determined by a *Candida* colonization index) was significantly higher in patients who subsequently became infected than in those who did not.[121] Other case-control studies have demonstrated that colonization by *Candida* species at various body sites and exposure to several antibiotics were independent risk factors for candidemia.[122]

The normal endogenous intestinal flora inhibits GI colonization and overgrowth by potentially pathogenic bacteria and fungi by forming what may be thought of as living wallpaper in the large intestine. Suppression of endogenous microflora as a consequence of antimicrobial administration[123] may permit overgrowth of pathogenic strains in the GI tract and selection of resistant strains, which may result in enterocolitis, systemic infection, or the septic response.

PHYSICAL DISRUPTION OF THE INTESTINAL MUCOSAL BARRIER

In humans, as well as in animals, the GI tract is considered to be the most important portal of entry for microorganisms, including yeasts, into the bloodstream. The passage of endogenous fungi from the GI tract to extraintestinal sites can be referred to as fungal translocation (by analogy with bacterial translocation).

Although yeast cells have no intrinsic motility, they are able to translocate from the intestinal lumen within a few hours of ingestion. In a study conducted in the 1960s, two nonpathogenic yeasts were surgically instilled into the rat duodenum and were recovered from the cisterna chyli within 4 hours.[124] Even in the absence of disease, any marked increase in the intestinal population of *Candida* can lead to fungal translocation and subsequent hematogenous infection. That candidal species can translocate from the gut to the bloodstream was demonstrated in a study in which signs and symptoms of sepsis developed in a healthy volunteer 2 hours after ingestion of a suspension containing 10^{12} *C. albicans* organisms, and blood cultures taken 3 and 6 hours after ingestion were positive for *Candida*.[125] In addition, autopsy studies conducted in patients with hematogenous candidiasis found involvement of the GI tract and submucosal invasion in almost all patients.[86]

Microbial translocation has been demonstrated in several animal models and has been shown to be enhanced by several factors, including fasting, which induces complex changes in host defenses, and protein deficiency, which results in intestinal microbial overgrowth, increased intestinal absorption of intact proteins, and decreased intracellular killing of bacteria and fungi. In one study involving *C. albicans*, volatile fatty acids and secondary bile salts

Figure 3 *Candida* endophthalmitis is common in patients with persistent fungemia. On funduscopy, a characteristic white, cotton-wool–like exudate can be seen (*a*). Cut section of an eye shows *Candida* retinitis (*b*). A microscopic view of *Candida* chorioretinitis is also provided (*c*).[138]

reduced fungal adhesion to the mucosa, colonization, and dissemination in mice by causing the formation of a dense layer of bacteria in the mucus gel; these bacteria successfully competed with the yeast cells for the same adhesion sites and produced various substances that inhibited fungal growth.[126] In another animal model, bile duct ligation resulted in bacterial translocation.[127] In yet another, splanchnic ischemia in guinea pigs increased fungal translocation.[128] Similar results were obtained in guinea pigs and rats that had burns covering 50% of their total body surface area. After the yeast cells penetrated the lamina propria, the cells were found either free in the lymphatic vessels and in the blood vessels or engulfed by macrophages.[129]

Microbial translocation has been shown to be clinically relevant in humans. Surveillance cultures from patients with leukemia have demonstrated an association between the bacterial biotype or serotype that was most prevalent in the patient's feces and the bacterial biotype or serotype that subsequently caused septicemia. Significant microbial translocation has been demonstrated in patients who underwent operation for colorectal carcinoma, intestinal obstruction, or Crohn disease. In addition, translocation is thought to occur as a result of flattening of the intestinal villi that results from the administration of total parenteral nutrition.[130]

Immunosuppression Leading to Dissemination of Candidiasis

Host defenses against *Candida* infections include T cell immunity, to prevent colonization and superficial invasion, and phagocytic immunity, to prevent deeper tissue invasion and hematogenous dissemination. Any condition that suppresses any of these arms of the immune system puts the patient at increased risk for candidiasis. Phagocytes ingest intestinal microbes. In a patient whose immune system has been compromised, these phagocytes transport microbes out of the intestine, fail to kill them, and finally liberate them in extraintestinal sites. Examples of immunosuppression include hematologic malignancy, bone marrow or organ transplantation, and immunosuppressive therapy such as cancer chemotherapy and corticosteroid therapy. Total parenteral nutrition (TPN) may result in immunosuppression. Transient hyperglycemia in patients receiving TPN causes an acceleration in the nonenzymatic glycosylation of immunoglobulin G, leading to its inactivation and impairment of complement fixation.[131] In a randomized, prospective study,[132] long-chain triglycerides in TPN significantly decreased the ratio of helper B cells to suppressor T cells. There is evidence that fat emulsions may impair polymorphonuclear and macrophage function.[133] In animal models, TPN induced macrophage suppression with decreased peritoneal macrophage superoxide production and *Candida* phagocytosis, associated with bacterial translocation to mesenteric lymph nodes.[134]

Pathology of *Candida* Colonization and Infectious Syndromes

The evolution of *Candida* microabscesses after hematogenous distribution has been studied in animal models. After intravenous infusion in nonneutropenic animals, the liver, the kidneys, the heart, the eyes, the brain, and the skin show a pattern of intracapillary fungi (yeasts and pseudohyphae) with an accumulation of neutrophils. In time, focal areas of necrosis occur, resulting in organ dysfunction that ultimately leads to death.

In nonneutropenic patients who are dying of candidiasis, a similar histologic picture and a similar pattern of organ involvement are seen. The organs most frequently involved are the brain, the heart, the kidneys, and the eyes. *Candida* produces microabscesses and, frequently, noncaseating granulomas. The histologic picture suggests that blood-borne fungi are lodged in the microvasculature, resulting in vasculitis. This multifocal microscopic disease explains the absence of localizing findings despite the progressive cerebral, renal, and cardiac dysfunction seen in infected persons.

The high incidence of cerebral involvement has been underscored by findings in an autopsy study of 41 nonneutropenic patients with tissue-verified deep candidiasis, of whom 26 (63%) had undergone major operations.[135] Nineteen (46%) were found to have cerebral candidal infections; all 19 individuals had antecedent proven or suspected gram-negative sepsis and had been treated with appropriate antibiotic therapy. In every patient studied, *Candida* organisms were identified at sites outside the brain, including the kidneys (90%) and the heart (80%). Candidiasis produced intracerebral microabscesses and noncaseating granulomas without diffuse leptomeningitis.

In a nearly identical autopsy series, 18 patients with disseminated candidiasis were found to have myocardial involvement.[136] This mycosis was characterized by myocardial microabscesses with yeasts and pseudohyphal elements. Noncaseating granulomas were seen in only one patient. Eight patients had recognized conduction disturbances, including alterations in both heart rate and heart rhythm.

As in the animal models, ocular involvement is a common finding in patients with disseminated candidiasis and by itself is an indication for systemic therapy. The eye pathology is a chorioretinitis with microabscess formation. Funduscopic examination, mandatory in patients suspected of having systemic *Candida* infection, reveals patchy, wool-like tufts [*see Figure 3*].

Despite the frequent finding of *Candida* in sputum cultures, primary *Candida* pneumonitis is extremely uncommon[137]; when it occurs, it usually follows aspiration of oropharyngeal contents. However, pulmonary involvement resulting from hematogenous seeding is common.

References

1. Wey SB, Mori M, Pfaller MA, et al: Hospital-acquired candidemia: the attributable mortality and excess length of stay. Arch Intern Med 148:2642, 1988

2. Pfaller M, Wenzel R: Impact of the changing epidemiology of fungal infections in the 1990s. Eur J Clin Microbiol Infect Dis 11:287, 1992

3. Jarvis WR, Martone WJ: Predominant pathogens in hospital infections. J Antimicrob Chemother 29:19, 1992

4. Schaberg DR, Culver DH, Gaynes RP: Major trends in the microbial etiology of nosocomial infection. Am J Med 91:72S, 1991

5. Banerjee SN, Emori TG, Culver DH, et al: Secular trends in nosocomial primary bloodstream infections in the United States, 1980–1989. National Nosocomial Infections Surveillance System. Am J Med 91(3B):86S, 1991

6. Beck-Sagué C, Jarvis WR: Secular trends in the epidemiology of nosocomial fungal infections in the United States, 1980-1990. National Nosocomial Infections Surveillance System. J Infect Dis 167:1247, 1993

7. Pfaller MA, Jones RN, Messer SA, et al: National surveillance of nosocomial blood stream infection due to Candida albicans: frequency of occurrence and antifungal susceptibility in the SCOPE Program. Diagn Microbiol Infect Dis 31:327, 1998

8. Vincent JL, Anaissie E, Bruining H, et al: Epidemiology, diagnosis and treatment of systemic Candida infection in surgical patients under intensive care. Intens Care Med 24:206, 1998

9. Pittet D, Li N, Woolson RF, et al: Microbiological factors influencing the outcome of nosocomial bloodstream infections: a 6-year validated, population-based model. Clin Infect Dis 24:1068, 1997

10. Anaissie EJ, Rex JH, Uzun O, et al: Predictors of adverse outcome in cancer patients with candidemia. Am J Med 104:238, 1998

11. Bodey GP, Luna M: Skin lesions associated with disseminated candidiasis. JAMA 229:1466, 1974

12. Anaissie E, Bodey GP, Kantarjian H, et al: Fluconazole therapy for chronic disseminated candidiasis in patients with leukemia and prior amphotericin B therapy. Am J Med 91:142, 1991

13. Anaissie E: Opportunistic mycoses in the immunocompromised host: experience at a cancer center and review. Clin Infect Dis 14:S43, 1992

14. Meunier F, Aoun M, Bitar N: Candidemia in immunocompromised patients. Clin Infect Dis 14:S120, 1992

15. Baley JE, Annable WL, Klegman RM: Candida endophthalmitis in the premature infant. J Pediatr 98:458, 1981

16. Dupont B, Drouhet E: Cutaneous, ocular, and osteoarticular candidiasis in heroin addicts: new clinical and therapeutic aspects in 38 patients. J Infect Dis 152:577, 1985

17. Eubanks PJ, de Virgilio C, Klein S, et al: Candida sepsis in surgical patients. Am J Surg 166:617, 1993

18. Castaldo P, Stratta RJ, Wood RP, et al: Clinical spectrum of fungal infections after orthotopic liver transplantation. Arch Surg 126:149, 1991

19. Prasad JK, Feller I, Thomson PD: A ten-year review of Candida sepsis and mortality in burn patients. Surgery 101:213, 1987

20. Desai MH, Rutan RL, Heggers JP, et al: Candida infection with and without nystatin prophylaxis: an 11-year experience with patients with burn injury. Arch Surg 127:159, 1992

21. Desai MH, Herndon DN: Eradication of Candida burn wound septicemia in massively burned patients. J Trauma 28:140, 1988

22. Paya CV: Fungal infections in solid-organ transplantation. Clin Infect Dis 16:677, 1993

23. Hesse UJ, Sutherland DE, Simmons RL, et al: Intra-abdominal infections in pancreas transplant recipients. Ann Surg 203:153, 1986

24. Hofflin JM, Potasman I, Baldwin JC, et al: Infectious complications in heart transplant recipients receiving cyclosporine and corticosteroids. Ann Intern Med 106:209, 1987

25. Brooks RG, Hofflin JM, Jamieson SW, et al: Infectious complications in heart-lung transplant recipients. Am J Med 79:412, 1985

26. Ramsey DE, Finch WT, Birtch AG: Urinary tract infections in kidney transplant recipients. Arch Surg 114:1022, 1979

27. Anaissie E, Samonis G, Kontoyiannis D, et al: Role of catheter colonization and infrequent hematogenous seeding in catheter-related infections. Eur J Clin Microbiol Infect Dis 14:134, 1995

28. Walsh TJ, Lee JW, Sien T, et al: Serum D-arabinitol measured by automated quantitative enzymatic assay for detection and therapeutic monitoring of experimental disseminated candidiasis: correlation with tissue concentrations of Candida albicans. J Med Vet Mycol 32:205, 1994

29. Brannon P, Kiehn TE: Large-scale clinical comparison of the lysis-centrifugation and radiometric systems for blood culture. J Clin Microbiol 22:951, 1985

30. Berenguer J, Buck M, Witebski F, et al: Lysis-centrifugation blood cultures in the detection of tissue-proven invasive candidiasis: disseminated versus single-organ infection. Diagn Microbiol Infect Dis 17:103, 1993

31. Ho YM, Ng MH, Teoh-Chan CH, et al: Indirect immunofluorescence assay for antibody to germ tube of Candida albicans—a new diagnostic test. J Clin Pathol 29:1007, 1976

32. Greenfield RA, Stephens JL, Bussey MJ, et al: Quantitation of antibody to Candida mannan by enzyme-linked immunosorbent assay. J Lab Clin Med 101:758, 1983

33. van Deventer AJM, van Vlient HJA, Hop WCJ, et al: Diagnostic value of anti-Candida enolase antibodies. J Clin Microbiol 32:17, 1994

34. Jones JM: Quantitation of antibody against cell wall mannan and a major cytoplasmic antigen of Candida in rabbits, mice, and humans. Infect Immun 30:78, 1980

35. Weiner MH, Coats-Stephen M: Immunodiagnosis of systemic candidiasis: mannan antigenemia detected by radioimmunoassay in experimental and human infections. J Infect Dis 140:989, 1979

36. Bailey JW, Sada E, Brass C, et al: Diagnosis of systemic candidiasis by latex agglutination for serum antigen. J Clin Microbiol 21:749, 1985

37. Fung JC, Donta ST, Tilton RC: Candida detection system (CAND-TEC) to differentiate between Candida albicans colonizations and disease. J Clin Microbiol 24:542, 1986

38. Walsh TJ, Hathorn JW, Sobel JD, et al: Detection of circulating Candida enolase by immunoassay in patients with cancer and invasive candidiasis. N Engl J Med 324:1026, 1991

39. Gutiérrez J, Maroto C, Piédrorla G, et al: Circulating Candida antigens and antibodies: useful markers of candidemia. J Clin Microbiol 31:2550, 1993

40. Freydiere AM, Buchaille L, Guinet R, et al: Evaluation of latex reagents for rapid identification of Candida albicans and C. krusei colonies. J Clin Microbiol 35:877, 1997

41. Fujita S-I, Lasker BA, Lott TJ, et al: Microtitration plate enzyme immunoassay to detect PCR-amplified DNA from Candida species in blood. J Clin Microbiol 33:962, 1995

42. Sandhu GS, Kline BC, Stockman L, et al: Molecular probes for diagnosis of fungal infections. J Clin Microbiol 33:2913, 1995

43. Walsh TJ, Francesconi A, Kasai M, et al: PCR and single-strand conformational polymorphism for recognition of medically important opportunistic fungi. J Clin Microbiol 33:3216, 1995

44. Reiss E, Morrison CJ: Nonculture methods for diagnosis of disseminated candidiasis. Clin Microbiol Rev 6:311, 1993

45. de Repentigny L, Marr LD, Keller JW, et al: Comparison of enzyme immunoassay and gas-liquid chromatography for the rapid diagnosis of invasive candidiasis in cancer patients. J Clin Microbiol 21:972, 1985

46. Walsh TJ, Merz WG, Lee JW, et al: Diagnosis and therapeutic monitoring of invasive candidiasis by rapid enzymatic detection of serum D-arabinitol. Am J Med 99:164, 1995

47. Dyess DL, Garrison N, Fry DE: Candida sepsis: implications of polymicrobial blood-borne infection. Arch Surg 120:345, 1985

48. Rantala A, Niinikoski J, Lehtonen OP: Yeasts in blood cultures: impact of early therapy. Scand J Infect Dis 21:557, 1989

49. Rex JH, Bennett JE, Sugar AM, et al: A randomized trial comparing fluconazole with amphotericin B for the treatment of candidemia in patients without neutropenia. Candidemia Study Group and the National Institute. N Engl J Med 331:1325, 1994

50. Anaissie EJ, Vartivarian SE, Abi-Said D, et al: Fluconazole versus amphotericin B in the treatment of hematogenous candidiasis: a matched cohort study. Am J Med 101:170, 1996

51. Nguyen MH, Peacock JE Jr, Tanner DC, et al: Therapeutic approaches in patients with candidemia: evaluation in a multicenter, prospective, observational study. Arch Intern Med 155:2429, 1995

52. Kujath P, Lerch K, Kochendorfer P, et al: Comparative study of the efficacy of fluconazole versus amphotericin B/flucytosine in surgical patients with systemic mycoses. Infection 21:376, 1993

53. Van't Wout JW, Mattie H, van Furth R: A prospective study of the efficacy of fluconazole (UK-49,858) against deep-seated fungal infections. J Antimicrob Chemother 21:665, 1988

54. de Marie S, Janknegt R, Bakker-Woudenberg IA: Clinical use of liposomal and lipid-complexed amphotericin B. J Antimicrob Chemother 33:907, 1994

55. Walsh TJ, Hiemenz JW, Seibel NL, et al: Amphotericin B lipid complex for invasive fungal infections: analysis of safety and efficacy in 556 cases. Clin Infect Dis 26:1383, 1998

56. Nucci M, Colombo AL, Silveira F, et al: Risk factors for death in patients with candidemia. Infect Control Hosp Epidemiol 19:846, 1998

57. Rex JH, Bennett JE, Sugar AM, et al: Intravascular catheter exchange and duration of candidemia: NIAID Mycoses Study Group and the Candidemia Study Group. Clin Infect Dis 21:994, 1995

58. Stevenhagen A, van Furth R: Interferon-gamma activates the oxidative killing of Candida albicans by human granulocytes. Clin Exp Immunol 91:170, 1993

59. Fratti RA, Ghannoum MA, Edwards JE Jr, et al: Gamma interferon protects endothelial cells from damage by Candida albicans by inhibiting endothelial cell phagocytosis. Infect Immun 64:4714, 1996

60. Gaviria JM, van Burik JA, Dale DC, et al: Comparison of interferon-gamma, granulocyte colony-stimulating factor, and granulocyte-macrophage colony-stimulating factor for priming leukocyte-mediated hyphal damage of opportunistic fungal pathogens. J Infect Dis 179:1038, 1999

61. Gorensek MJ, Carey WD, Washington JA 2nd, et al: Selective bowel decontamination with quinolones and nystatin reduces gram-negative and fungal infections in orthotopic liver transplant recipients. Cleve Clin J Med 60:139, 1993

62. Mora NP, Cofer JB, Solomon H, et al: Analysis of severe infections (INF) after 180 consecutive liver transplants: the impact of amphotericin B prophylaxis for reducing the incidence and severity of fungal infections. Transplant Proc 23:1528, 1991

63. Tollemar J, Ringden O, Andersson S, et al: Randomized double-blind study of liposomal amphotericin B (AmBisome) prophylaxis of invasive fungal infections in bone marrow transplant recipients. Bone Marrow Transplant 12:577, 1993

64. Slavin MA, Osborne B, Adams R, et al: Efficacy and safety of fluconazole prophylaxis for fungal infections after bone marrow transplantation—a prospective, randomized, double-blind study. J Infect Dis 171:1545, 1995

65. Rotstein C, Bow EJ, Laverdiere M, et al: Randomized placebo-controlled trial of fluconazole prophylaxis for neutropenic cancer patients: benefit based on purpose and intensity of cytotoxic therapy. The Canadian Fluconazole Prophylaxis Study Group. Clin Infect Dis 28:331, 1999

66. Powderly WG, Finkelstein D, Feinberg J, et al: A randomized trial comparing fluconazole with clotrimazole troches for the prevention of fungal infections in patients with advanced human immunodeficiency virus infection. NIAID AIDS Clinical Trials Group. N Engl J Med 332:700, 1995

67. Eggimann P, Francioli P, Bille J, et al: Fluconazole prophylaxis prevents intra-abdominal candidiasis in high-risk surgical patients. Crit Care Med 27:1066, 1999

68. Dube MP, Heseltine PN, Rinaldi MG, et al: Fungemia and colonization with nystatin-resistant Candida rugosa in a burn unit. Clin Infect Dis 18:77, 1994

69. Torbenson M, Wang J, Nichols L, et al: Causes of death in autopsied liver transplantation patients. Mod Pathol 11:37, 1998

70. Lumbreras C, Cuervas-Mons V, Jara P, et al: Randomized trial of fluconazole versus nystatin for the prophylaxis of Candida infection following liver transplantation. J Infect Dis 174:583, 1996

71. Lorf T, Braun F, Ruchel R, et al: Systemic mycoses during prophylactical use of liposomal amphotericin B (AmBisome) after liver transplantation. Mycoses 42:47, 1999

72. Savani DV, Perfect JR, Cobo LM, et al: Penetration of new azole compounds into the eye and efficacy in experimental Candida endophthalmitis. Antimicrob Agents Chemother 31:6, 1987

73. Venditti M, De Bernardis F, Micozzi A, et al: Fluconazole treatment of catheter-related right-sided endocarditis caused by Candida albicans and associated with endophthalmitis and folliculitis. Clin Infect Dis 14:422, 1992

74. Moyer DV, Edwards JE Jr: Candida endophthalmitis and central nervous system infection. Candidiasis: Pathogenesis, Diagnosis, and Treatment. Bodey GP, Ed. Raven Press, New York, 1993, p 331

75. Martinez-Vazquez C, Fernandez-Ulloa J, Bordon J, et al: Candida albicans endophthalmitis in brown heroin addicts: response to early vitrectomy preceded and followed by antifungal therapy. Clin Infect Dis 27:1130, 1998

76. Yackee JM, Topiel MS, Simon GL: Septic phlebitis caused by Candida albicans and diagnosed by needle aspiration. South Med J 78:1262, 1985

77. Czwerwiec FS, Bilsker MS, Kamerman ML, et al: Long-term survival after fluconazole therapy of candidal prosthetic valve endocarditis. Am J Med 94:545, 1993

78. Kraus WE, Valenstein PN, Corey GR: Purulent pericarditis caused by Candida: report of three cases and identification of high-risk populations as an aid to early diagnosis. Rev Infect Dis 10:34, 1988

79. Cuende E, Barbadillo C, E-Mazzuchelli R, et al: Candida arthritis in adult patients who are not intravenous drug addicts: report of three cases and review of the literature. Semin Arthritis Rheum 22:224, 1993

80. Penk A, Pittrow L: [Status of fluconazole in the therapy of endogenous Candida endophthalmitis]. Mycoses 41(suppl 2):41, 1998

81. Tang C: Successful treatment of Candida albicans osteomyelitis with fluconazole. J Infect 26:89, 1993

82. Shapiro S, Javed T, Mealey J Jr: Candida albicans shunt infection. Pediatr Neurosci 15:125, 1989

83. Mascarenas CA, Hardin TC, Pennick GJ, et al: Treatment of thrush with itraconazole solution: evidence for topical effect. Clin Infect Dis 26:1242, 1998

84. Crutchfield CE 3rd, Lewis EJ: The successful treatment of oral candidiasis (thrush) in a pediatric patient using itraconazole (letter). Pediatr Dermatol 14:246, 1997

85. Tunkel AR, Thomas CY, Wispelwey B: Candida prosthetic arthritis: report of a case treated with fluconazole and review of the literature. Am J Med 94:100, 1993

86. Walsh TJ, Merz WG: Pathologic features in the human alimentary tract associated with invasiveness of Candida tropicalis. Am J Clin Pathol 85:498, 1986

87. Gupta TP, Ehrinpreis MN: Candida-associated diarrhea in hospitalized patients. Gastroenterology 98:780, 1990

88. Calandra T, Bille J, Schneider R, et al: Clinical significance of Candida isolated from peritoneum in surgical patients. Lancet 2:1437, 1989

89. Corbella X, Sirvent JM, Carratala J: Fluconazole treatment without catheter removal in Candida albicans peritonitis complicating peritoneal dialysis. Am J Med 90:277, 1991

90. Eisenberg ES, Leviton I, Soeiro R: Fungal peritonitis in patients receiving peritoneal dialysis: experience with 11 patients and review of the literature [published erratum appears in Rev Infect Dis 8:839, 1986]. Rev Infect Dis 8:309, 1986

91. Lo WK, Chan CY, Cheng SW, et al: A prospective randomized control study of oral nystatin prophylaxis for Candida peritonitis complicating continuous ambulatory peritoneal dialysis. Am J Kidney Dis 28:549, 1996

92. Huang CT, Leu HS: Candiduria as an early marker of disseminated infection in critically ill surgical patients (letter; comment). J Trauma 39:616, 1995

93. Chakrabarti A, Reddy TC, Singhi S: Does candiduria predict candidaemia? Ind J Med Res 106:513, 1997

94. Strassner C, Friesen A: [Therapy of candiduria by alkalinization of urine: oral treatment with potassium-sodium-hydrogen citrate]. Fortschr Med 113:359, 1995

95. Tacker JR: Successful use of fluconazole for treatment of urinary tract fungal infections. J Urol 148:1917, 1992

96. Sobel JD: Recurrent vulvovaginal candidiasis: a prospective study of the efficacy of maintenance ketoconazole therapy. N Engl J Med 315:1455, 1986

97. Walsh TJ, Dixon DM: Nosocomial aspergillosis, environmental microbiology, hospital epidemiology, diagnosis and treatment. Eur J Epidemiol 5:131, 1989

98. Denning DW, Stevens DA: Antifungal and surgical treatment of invasive aspergillosis: review of 2,121 published cases [published erratum appears in Rev Infect Dis 13:345, 1991]. Rev Infect Dis 12:1147, 1990

99. Anaissie E, Bodey GP: Nosocomial fungal infections: old problems and new challenges. Infect Dis Clin North Am 3:867, 1989

100. Anaissie E, Bodey GP, Kantarjian H, et al: New spectrum of fungal infections in patients with cancer. Rev Infect Dis 11:369, 1989

101. Sokol-Anderson ML, Brajtburg J, Medoff G: Amphotericin B-induced oxidative damage and killing of Candida albicans. J Infect Dis 154:76, 1986

102. Burgess JL, Birchall R: Nephrotoxicity of amphotericin B, with emphasis on changes in tubular function. Am J Med 53:77, 1972

103. Kennedy MS, Deeg HJ, Siegel M, et al: Acute renal toxicity with combined use of amphotericin B and cyclosporine after marrow transplantation. Transplantation 35:211, 1983

104. Zervos M, Meunier F: Fluconazole (Diflucan): a review. Int J Antimicrob Agents 3:147, 1993

105. McClean KL, Sheehan GJ: Interaction between itraconazole and digoxin (letter; comment). Clin Infect Dis 18:259, 1994

106. Drayton J, Dickinson G, Rinaldi MG: Coadministration of rifampin and itraconazole leads to undetectable levels of serum itraconazole (letter). Clin Infect Dis 18:266, 1994

107. Tucker RM, Haq Y, Denning DW, et al: Adverse events associated with itraconazole in 189 patients on chronic therapy. J Antimicrob Chemother 26:561, 1990

108. De Bernardis F, Muhlschlegel FA, Cassone A, et al: The pH of the host niche controls gene expression in and virulence of Candida albicans. Infect Immun 66:3317, 1998

109. Klotz SA: Fungal adherence to the vascular compartment: a critical step in the pathogenesis of disseminated candidiasis. Clin Infect Dis 14:340, 1992

110. Gale CA, Bendel CM, McClellan M, et al: Linkage of adhesion, filamentous growth, and virulence in Candida albicans to a single gene, INT1. Science 279:1355, 1998

111. Lecciones JA, Lee JW, Navarro EE, et al: Vascular catheter-associated fungemia in patients with cancer: analysis of 155 episodes. Clin Infect Dis 14:875, 1992

112. Abi-Said D, Anaissie E, Uzun O, et al: The epidemiology of hematogenous candidiasis caused by different Candida species [published erratum appears in Clin Infect Dis 25:352, 1997]. Clin Infect Dis 24:1122, 1997

113. Pfaller MA, Messer SA, Hollis RJ, et al: Trends in species distribution and susceptibility to fluconazole among blood stream isolates of Candida species in the United States. Diagn Microbiol Infect Dis 33:217, 1999

114. Voss A, Hollis RJ, Pfaller MA, et al: Investigation of the sequence of colonization and candidemia in nonneutropenic patients. J Clin Microbiol 32:975, 1994

115. Martino P, Girmenia C, Venditti M, et al: Candida colonization and systemic infection in neutropenic patients: a retrospective study. Cancer 64:2030, 1989

116. Pfaller M, Cabezudo I, Koontz F, et al: Predictive value of surveillance cultures for systemic infection due to Candida species. Eur J Clin Microbiol Infect Dis 6:628, 1987

117. Uzun O, Anaissie EJ: Antifungal prophylaxis in patients with hematologic malignancies: a reappraisal. Blood 86:2063, 1995

118. Martino P, Girmenia C, Micozzi A, et al: Fungemia in patients with leukemia. Am J Med Sci 306:225, 1993

119. Richet HM, Andremont A, Tancrede C, et al: Risk factors for candidemia in patients with acute lymphocytic leukemia. Rev Infect Dis 13:211, 1991

120. Pappu-Katikaneni LD, Rao KP, Banister E: Gastrointestinal colonization with yeast species and Candida septicemia in very low birth weight infants.

Mycoses 33:20, 1990

121. Pittet D, Monod M, Suter PM, et al: Candida colonization and subsequent infections in critically ill surgical patients. Ann Surg 220:751, 1994

122. Wey SB, Mori M, Pfaller MA, et al: Risk factors for hospital-acquired candidemia: a matched case-control study. Arch Intern Med 149:2349, 1989

123. Giuliano M, Barza M, Jacobus NV, et al: Effect of broad-spectrum parenteral antibiotics on composition of intestinal microflora of humans. Antimicrob Agents Chemother 31:202, 1987

124. Wolochow H, Hildebrand GJ, Lamanna C: Translocation of microorganisms across the intestinal wall of the rat: effect of microbial size and concentration. J Infect Dis 116:523, 1966

125. Krause W, Matheis H, Wulf K: Fungaemia and funguria after oral administration of Candida albicans. Lancet 1:598, 1969

126. Kennedy MJ, Volz PA: Ecology of Candida albicans gut colonization: inhibition of Candida adhesion, colonization, and dissemination from the gastrointestinal tract by bacterial antagonism. Infect Immun

49:654, 1985

127. Deitch EA, Sittig K, Li M, et al: Obstructive jaundice promotes bacterial translocation from the gut. Am J Surg 159:79, 1990

128. Gianotti L, Alexander JW, Fukushima R, et al: Translocation of Candida albicans is related to the blood flow of individual intestinal villi. Circ Shock 40:250, 1993

129. Alexander JW, Boyce ST, Babcock JF, et al: The process of microbial translocation. Ann Surg 212:496, 1990

130. Pappo I, Polacheck I, Zmora O, et al: Altered gut barrier function to Candida during parenteral nutrition. Nutrition 10:151, 1994

131. Hennessey PJ, Black CT, Andrassy RJ: Nonenzymatic glycosylation of immunoglobulin G impairs complement fixation. JPEN J Parenter Enteral Nutr 15:60, 1991

132. Gogos CA, Kalfarentzos FE, Zoumbos NC: Effect of different types of total parenteral nutrition on T-lymphocyte subpopulations and NK cells. Am J Clin Nutr 51:119, 1990

133. Gogos CA, Kalfarentzos F: Total parenteral nutrition and immune system activity: a review. Nutrition 11:339, 1995

134. Shou J, Lappin J, Minnard EA, et al: Total parenteral nutrition, bacterial translocation, and host immune function. Am J Surg 167:145, 1994

135. Parker JC Jr, McCloskey JJ, Lee RS: Human cerebral candidosis—a postmortem evaluation of 19 patients. Hum Pathol 12:23, 1981

136. Parker JC Jr: The potentially lethal problem of cardiac candidosis. Am J Clin Pathol 73:356, 1980

137. Haron E, Vartivarian S, Anaissie E, et al: Primary Candida pneumonia: experience at a large cancer center and review of the literature. Medicine (Baltimore) 72:137, 1993

138. Gaines JD, Remington JS: Disseminated candidiasis in the surgical patient. Surgery 72:730, 1972

139. Greenburg SB: Fungal and viral infections. Critical Care, 2nd ed. Civetta JM, Taylor RW, Kirby RR, Eds. JB Lippincott Co, Philadelphia, 1993, p 1055

140. Medoff G, Kobayashi GS: Systemic fungal infections: an overview. Hosp Pract 26(2):41, 1991

19 VIRAL INFECTION

Jennifer W. Janelle, M.D., and Richard J. Howard, M.D., Ph.D.

Approach to Viral Exposure

Compared with primary care physicians, such as internists, family physicians, and pediatricians, surgeons are seldom called on to treat viral infections. Viral infections nonetheless deserve the attention of surgeons because these infections can cause illness in patients after operation, albeit infrequently, and can spread to the hospital staff. Some viral infections (e.g., infections with the hepatitis viruses, HIV, and cytomegalovirus [CMV]) can result from administration of blood or blood products or can be transmitted to hospital personnel through needle-stick injury. Viral infections can also result from organ transplantation or trauma (e.g., rabies, which is transmitted by the bite of an infected animal). Some viruses, especially the herpesviruses, frequently infect immunosuppressed patients, in whom the viruses can cause severe illness and even death. In many surgical practices, there are increasing numbers of immunosuppressed patients, including organ transplant recipients; patients with cancer; patients receiving cancer chemotherapy, steroids, and other immunosuppressive drugs; the elderly; and the malnourished. Some viral infections can cause neoplastic disease for which operation may become necessary. Examples are hepatitis B virus (HBV) and hepatitis C virus (HCV), which are implicated in the etiology of hepatocellular carcinoma; Epstein-Barr virus (EBV), which can cause a lethal lymphoproliferative disorder in immunosuppressed patients; and human T cell lymphotropic virus type I (HTLV-I), which can induce a T cell leukemia. Viral infections very likely can cause other neoplasms as well.

Prevention of Transmission of HIV, Hepatitis B Virus, and Hepatitis C Virus

TRANSMISSION FROM PATIENTS TO HEALTH CARE WORKERS

The Centers for Disease Control and Prevention (CDC) has published extensive recommendations for preventing transmission of HIV, the etiologic agent of AIDS.[1-5] Applicable to clinical and laboratory staffs,[3,4] to workers in health care settings [see Table 1][1] and in other occupational settings,[1] and to health care workers performing invasive procedures,[1-5] these precautions are appropriate for preventing transmission not only of HIV but also of other blood-borne viruses, including HBV and HCV. The recommendations share the objective of minimizing exposure of personnel to blood and body secretions from infected patients, whether through needle-stick injury or through contamination of mucous membranes or open cuts.

Despite the apparently low risk of such exposure, the CDC recommends enforcement of these as well as other standard infection control precautions, regardless of whether health care workers or patients are known to be infected with HIV or HBV. The CDC has taken the position that blood and body fluid precautions should be used consistently for all patients because medical history and physical examination cannot reliably identify all patients infected with HIV or other blood-borne pathogens and because in emergencies there may be no time for serologic testing. If these universal precautions are implemented, as the CDC recommends,[1-5] no additional precautions should be necessary for patients known to be infected with HIV.

The CDC does not recommend routine HIV serologic testing for all patients.[1-5] HIV serologic testing of patients is recommended for management of health care workers who sustain parenteral or mucous membrane exposure to blood or other body fluids, for patient diagnosis and treatment, and for counseling associated with efforts to prevent and control HIV transmission in the community.[1-5]

Nevertheless, some hospitals and physicians are likely to perform serologic testing of patients if it is possible that health care workers will be exposed to the patients' blood or other body fluids, as would be the case with patients undergoing major operative procedures or receiving treatment in intensive care units. Those who favor routine preoperative testing of patients undergoing invasive procedures maintain that precautions are more likely to be followed and additional steps taken to lower the likelihood of virus transmission from patients to health care workers when it is known which patients are HIV positive.[6,7] If such policies are adopted, the CDC advocates certain principles: (1) obtain consent for testing, (2) inform patients of results and provide counseling to seropositive patients, (3) ensure confidentiality, (4) ensure that seropositive patients will not receive compromised care, and (5) prospectively evaluate the efficacy of the program in reducing the incidence of exposure of health care workers to blood or body fluids of patients who are infected with HIV.

Although possible acquisition of HIV infection is the major concern for any health care worker who is exposed to blood products in the workplace, acquisition of viral hepatitis is actually much more likely. From a single needle-stick exposure, the estimated average risk of HIV transmission is 0.3%, whereas that of HCV transmission ranges from 0% to 10%.[8] The risk that HBV will be transmitted from a single needle-stick exposure varies according to the hepatitis B e antigen (HBeAg) status of the source patient, ranging from 1% to 6% for HBeAg-negative patients to 22% to 40% for HBeAg-positive patients.[9-11] That health care workers are at increased risk for hepatitis B is indicated by the seroprevalence of HBV in this population, which is two to four times that in the general United States population (6% to 15% versus < 5%).[9,12] This seroprevalence is expected to decrease with the availability of the hepatitis B vaccine and the mandate from the Occupational Safety

1356

Table 1   Precautions to Prevent Transmission of HIV[1]

Universal Precautions

1. All health care workers should use appropriate barrier precautions routinely to prevent skin and mucous membrane exposure when contact with blood or other body fluids of any patient is anticipated. Gloves should be worn for touching blood and body fluids, mucous membranes, or nonintact skin of all patients; for handling items or surfaces soiled with blood or body fluids; and for performing venipuncture and other vascular-access procedures. Gloves should be changed after contact with each patient. During procedures that are likely to generate aerosolized droplets of blood or other body fluids, masks and protective eyewear or face shields should be worn to prevent exposure of mucous membranes of the mouth, nose, and eyes. Gowns or aprons should be worn during procedures that are likely to generate splashes of blood or other body fluids.

2. Hands and other skin surfaces should be washed immediately and thoroughly if contaminated with blood or other body fluids. Hands should be washed immediately after gloves are removed.

3. All health care workers should take precautions to prevent injuries caused by needles, scalpels, and other sharp instruments or devices during procedures; when cleaning used instruments; during disposal of used needles; and when handling sharp instruments after procedures. To prevent needle-stick injuries, needles should not be recapped, purposely bent or broken by hand, removed from disposable syringes, or otherwise manipulated by hand. After they are used, disposable syringes and needles, scalpel blades, and other sharp items should be placed in puncture-resistant containers for disposal; the puncture-resistant containers should be located as close as practical to the area of use. Large-bore reusable needles should be placed in a puncture-resistant container for transport to the reprocessing area.

4. Although saliva has not been implicated in HIV transmission, to minimize the need for emergency mouth-to-mouth resuscitation, mouthpieces, resuscitation bags, or other ventilation devices should be available for use in areas in which the need for resuscitation is predictable.

5. Health care workers who have exudative lesions or weeping dermatitis should refrain from all direct patient care and from handling patient care equipment until the condition resolves.

6. Pregnant health care workers are not known to be at greater risk for contracting HIV infection than health care workers who are not pregnant; however, if a health care worker acquires HIV infection during pregnancy, the infant is at risk for infection resulting from perinatal transmission. Because of this risk, pregnant health care workers should be especially familiar with and strictly adhere to precautions to minimize the risk of HIV transmission.

Additional Precautions for Invasive Procedures

1. All health care workers who participate in invasive procedures must use appropriate barrier precautions routinely to prevent skin and mucous membrane contact with blood and other body fluids of all patients. Gloves and surgical masks must be worn for all invasive procedures. Protective eyewear or face shields should be worn for procedures that commonly result in the generation of aerosolized droplets, splashing of blood or other body fluids, or the generation of bone chips. Gowns or aprons made of materials that provide an effective barrier should be worn during invasive procedures that are likely to result in the splashing of blood or other body fluids. All health care workers who perform or assist in vaginal or cesarean deliveries should wear gloves and gowns when handling the placenta or the infant until blood and amniotic fluid have been removed from the infant's skin and should wear gloves during postdelivery care of the umbilical cord.

2. If a glove is torn or a needle-stick or other injury occurs, the glove should be removed and a new glove used as promptly as patient safety permits; the needle or instrument involved in the incident should also be removed from the sterile field. In the event of an injury, postexposure evaluation should be sought as soon as possible.

& Health Administration (OSHA) directing that all health care workers potentially exposed to blood or other potentially infectious material either be offered hepatitis B vaccine free of charge, demonstrate immunity to hepatitis B, or formally decline vaccination.[13] That vaccination has been effective in decreasing the incidence of hepatitis B in health care workers is shown by the decrease in infection rates from 174/100,000 in 1982 to 17/100,000 in 1995.[14] Most series have not found the seroprevalence of HCV to be higher in health care worker groups at risk than in the general population.[14] That hepatitis B and hepatitis C are much more common than HIV in health care workers is a strong argument for using universal precautions in all patients.

One reason why hepatitis B is so much more transmissible than HIV is the greater number of virus particles in the blood of hepatitis B carriers. These persons have blood concentrations of 10^8 to 10^9 virus particles/ml, compared with 10^2 to 10^4/ml for persons with HIV infection and 10^6/ml for persons with HCV infection.

The extensive guidelines that have been established by the CDC for the care of patients with HBV infection[4,15-17] also apply to patients with HIV infection. Patients known to have hepatitis B, hepatitis C, or AIDS need not be put in a private room unless they are fecally incontinent or are shedding virus in body fluids. Health care workers should wear gloves and gowns when they have contact with or may have contact with a patient's blood, feces, or other body fluids. Needles used for drawing blood should be disposed of with special care: they must not be reused, recapped, or removed from the syringe. Hands must be washed before and after direct contact with the patient or with items that have been in contact with the patient's blood, feces, or body fluids.

Published recommendations also provide guidelines for health care workers who are not directly involved in patient care (e.g., housekeeping personnel, kitchen staff, and laundry workers).[1-7] No additional precautions are necessary for these individuals because their risk of acquiring HIV, HCV, or HBV is so low; in fact, transmission to them has not been documented. However, staff should be educated about appropriate procedures. Workers should wear gloves when handling blood and body fluids of all patients and should wear masks in areas where blood may spatter (e.g., the dialysis unit or the obstetrics unit).

TRANSMISSION FROM HEALTH CARE WORKERS TO PATIENTS

To date, there have been only two reports of HIV transmission from infected health care workers to patients. In one report, DNA sequence analysis linked a Florida dentist with AIDS to HIV infection in six of his patients.[18] In the other, an orthopedic surgeon in France may have transmitted HIV to one of his patients in the course of an operation.[19] Despite extensive investigation, no break in infection control precautions was documented in either case, nor was any clear-cut means of transmission identified.

HBV transmission from health care workers to patients is known to occur. Nineteen case reports have documented physician-to-patient transmission.[20-32] Eighteen of the 19 physicians were surgeons; seven of the surgeons were gynecologists, three were cardiac surgeons, and one was an orthopedic surgeon. All of the physicians were positive for HBeAg. Three of the gynecologists made a practice of handling needle tips. Of the 135 patients studied, 121 had clinical hepatitis B, and 14 had only serologic evidence of infection. Forty-one of the 135 patients were accounted for by the only nonsurgeon, a family practitioner from rural Switzerland. There are many additional cases of HBV having been transmitted by dentists and oral surgeons. In addition, three patients' relatives, two members of a surgeon's family, and one laboratory technician became infected.

Human immunodeficiency virus (HIV)

Health care worker is exposed to any patient's blood or body secretions by a needle stick or by a splash in the eye or mouth

The health care worker should be counseled about the risk of HIV infection and should follow U.S. Public Health Service recommendations for preventing HIV transmission.

Patient is judged on clinical and epidemiologic grounds to be a likely source of HIV infection

Ask the patient to consent to serologic testing for HIV.

Patient refuses to be tested

Follow state and local laws regarding testing for a nonconsenting patient's HIV source status.

Patient is seropositive

Evaluate the health care worker for clinical or serologic evidence of HIV infection as soon as possible after the exposure. Consider prophylaxis:
Low to moderate risk: AZT plus 3TC.
High risk: AZT plus 3TC plus indinavir.

Patient is seronegative and has no other evidence of HIV infection

No further follow-up of the health care worker is necessary.

Patient is seronegative but has engaged in high-risk behavoirs

Perform baseline HIV testing of the health care worker. Repeat test 3 months and 6 months after exposure.

Health care worker is seronegative

Repeat serologic testing 6 wk and 3, 6, 12 mo after exposure.

Rabies

All bites and wounds should be immediately and thoroughly cleansed with soap and water.

Bite of domestic animal (dog or cat)

Animal is healthy at time of attack

Observe the animal for 10 days. If the animal shows signs of rabies, proceed with treatment.

Animal shows signs of rabies

Animal escapes

Consult with public health officials to determine need for treatment.

Bite of wild animal (skunk, bat, fox, coyote, raccoon, bobcat, or other carnivore)

Regard as rabid unless proved negative by laboratory tests.

Bite of another animal (e.g., livestock)

Consult with public health officials to determine need for treatment.

Give the exposed person RIG (20 IU/kg). If anatomically feasible, infiltrate the full dose around the wounds. Infiltrate any remaining RIG I.M. at a site distant from that of vaccine administration. Also, administer 1.0 ml of HDCV into the deltoid muscle or, in children, the upper thigh on days 0, 3, 7, 14, and 28. If the animal is available, kill it and immediately examine its brain tissue for the presence of rabies by using fluorescent antibody tests. If the tests are negative, discontinue HDCV.

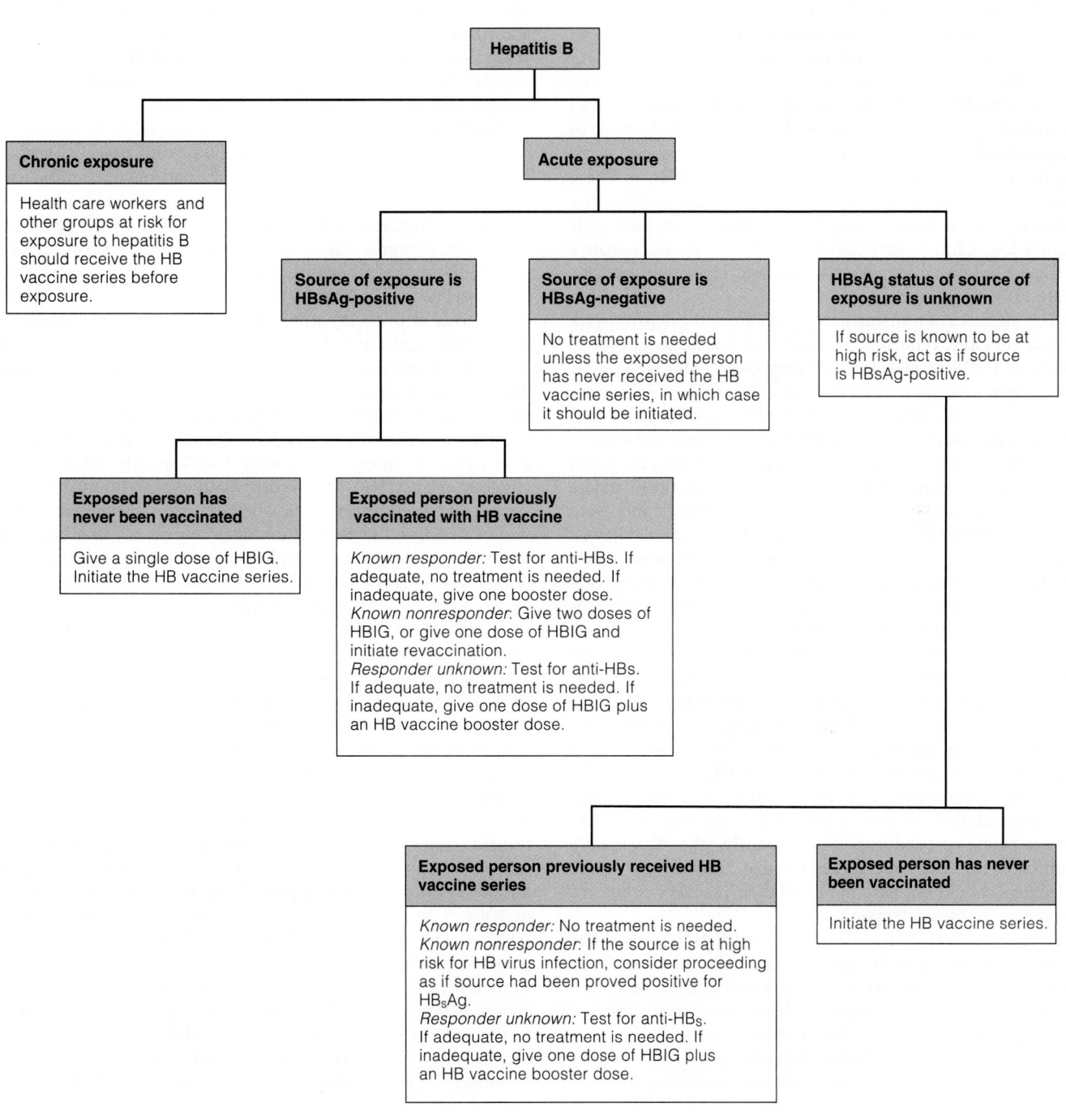

Hepatitis B

Chronic exposure

Health care workers and other groups at risk for exposure to hepatitis B should receive the HB vaccine series before exposure.

Acute exposure

Source of exposure is HBsAg-positive

Source of exposure is HBsAg-negative

No treatment is needed unless the exposed person has never received the HB vaccine series, in which case it should be initiated.

HBsAg status of source of exposure is unknown

If source is known to be at high risk, act as if source is HBsAg-positive.

Exposed person has never been vaccinated

Give a single dose of HBIG. Initiate the HB vaccine series.

Exposed person previously vaccinated with HB vaccine

Known responder: Test for anti-HBs. If adequate, no treatment is needed. If inadequate, give one booster dose.
Known nonresponder: Give two doses of HBIG, or give one dose of HBIG and initiate revaccination.
Responder unknown: Test for anti-HBs. If adequate, no treatment is needed. If inadequate, give one dose of HBIG plus an HB vaccine booster dose.

Exposed person previously received HB vaccine series

Known responder: No treatment is needed.
Known nonresponder: If the source is at high risk for HB virus infection, consider proceeding as if source had been proved positive for HBsAg.
Responder unknown: Test for anti-HBs. If adequate, no treatment is needed. If inadequate, give one dose of HBIG plus an HB vaccine booster dose.

Exposed person has never been vaccinated

Initiate the HB vaccine series.

Approach to Viral Exposure

Hepatitis C

Perform serologic testing for ALT and HCV antibody at time of exposure and again at 6 months. If anti-HCV is detected, confirmatory testing with recombinant immunoblot is indicated. HCV immunoglobulin is no longer recommended.

In five studies, patients of 16 health care workers (including two surgeons) who were positive for hepatitis B surface antigen (HBsAg) were prospectively followed for evidence of hepatitis.[33-37] A total of 784 patients were followed and were compared with 656 patients cared for by health care workers who were HBsAg negative. None of the patients acquired overt hepatitis or became seropositive for HBsAg. Eight (1.02%) of the 784 patients cared for by HBsAg-positive health care workers developed antibody to HBsAg (anti-HBs), but so did six (0.91%) of the 656 patients cared for by health care workers who were negative for HBsAg. These reports suggest that the likelihood of infected surgeons' or other health care workers' transmitting HIV or HBV to their patients is extremely low. Chronic carriers of HBsAg who are seronegative for HBeAg are much less likely to transmit HBV than persons who are HBeAg positive.

Before the cases of transmission of HIV from the dentist to six of his patients were reported, the CDC had not taken a position on whether HBV- or HIV-infected surgeons should be allowed to continue practicing medicine. After these cases were reported, the CDC held meetings of health care professionals and other interested parties and published its recommendations on July 12, 1991.[38] These recommendations called for physicians not to perform "exposure-prone invasive procedures" unless they sought counsel from an expert review panel and were advised under what circumstances, if any, they might be allowed to continue to perform these procedures. Physicians would have to notify prospective patients of their seropositivity. These recommendations were strongly resisted by the medical community because at that time, only one health care worker, the dentist, had been implicated in transmitting HIV to his patients, no mechanism of transmission had been elucidated, no other patients had HIV transmitted by a health care worker, and invasive procedures that were "exposure prone" (exposing the patient to blood of the health care worker) were impossible to define. After subsequent meetings, the CDC abandoned its attempts to define exposure-prone procedures but did not alter its recommendations. Rather, it left it up to the states to define exposure-prone procedures. Subsequently, the President's Commission on AIDS recommended that HIV-infected health care workers should not have to curtail their practices or inform their patients of their infection.

Transmission of HCV from health care workers to patients has been reported. In one such case, a cardiac surgeon transmitted HCV to at least five patients during valve replacement surgery.[39] In another, an anesthesiologist in Spain may have infected more than 217 patients by first injecting himself with narcotics, then giving the remainder of the drugs to his patients.[40] At present, no recommendations exist for restricting the professional activities of health care workers with HCV infection.

Management of Viral Exposure

HIV

The CDC has issued recommendations for the management of potential exposure of health care workers to HIV.[1,4,41] If a health care worker is exposed by a needle stick or by a splash in the eye or mouth to any patient's blood or other body fluids, and the HIV serostatus of the patient is unknown, the patient should

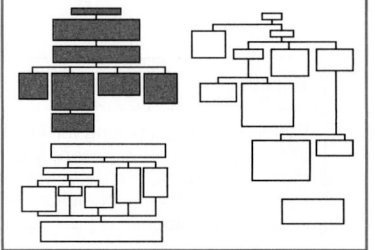

be informed of the incident and, if consent is obtained, tested for serologic evidence of HIV infection. If consent cannot be obtained, procedures for testing the patient should be followed in accordance with state and local laws. Testing of needles or other sharp instruments associated with exposure to HIV is not recommended, because it is unclear whether the test results would be reliable and how they should be interpreted.[41]

Health care workers exposed to HIV should be evaluated for susceptibility to blood-borne infection with baseline testing, including testing for HIV antibody. If the patient who is the source of exposure is seronegative and exhibits no clinical evidence of AIDS or symptoms of HIV infection, further follow-up of the health care worker is usually unnecessary.[41] If the source patient is seropositive or is seronegative but has engaged in high-risk behaviors, baseline and follow-up HIV-antibody testing of the health care worker at 6 weeks, 3 months, and 6 months after exposure should be considered.[41] Seroconversion usually occurs within 6 to 12 weeks of exposure; infrequently, it occurs considerably later. Three cases of delayed HIV seroconversion among health care workers have been reported.[42-44] In all three patients, an HIV antibody test yielded negative results at 6 months but positive results at some point during the following 1 to 7 months. In two cases, coinfection with HCV had occurred and took an unusually severe course. At present, it is unclear whether coinfection with these two viruses directly influences the timing or severity of either infection, but most experts recommend close monitoring for up to 1 year for health care workers exposed to both viruses in whom serologic evidence of HCV infection develops.

Treatment of the exposed health care worker should begin with careful washing of the exposure site with soap and water. Mucous membranes should be flushed with water. There is no evidence that either expressing fluid by squeezing the wound or applying antiseptics is beneficial, though antiseptics are not contraindicated. The use of caustic agents (e.g., bleach) is not recommended.

Any health care worker concerned about exposure to HIV should receive follow-up counseling regarding the risk of HIV transmission, postexposure testing, and medical evaluation, regardless of whether postexposure prophylaxis is given. HIV antibody testing should be performed at specified intervals for at least 6 months after the exposure (e.g., at 6 weeks, 3 months, and 6 months). The risk of HIV transmission is believed to depend on several factors: how much blood is involved in the exposure, whether the blood came from a source patient with terminal AIDS (thought to be attributable to the presence of large quantities of HIV), whether any host factors are present that might affect transmissibility (e.g., abnormal CD4 receptors for HIV), and whether the source patient carries any aggressive HIV viral mutants (e.g., syncytia-inducing strains). Factors indicating exposure to a large quantity of the source patient's blood (and thus a high risk of HIV transmission) include a device visibly contaminated with the patient's blood, a procedure that involved a needle placed directly in a vein or artery, and a deep injury.[45]

During the follow-up period, especially the first 6 to 12 weeks, exposed health care workers should follow the U.S. Public Health Service recommendations for preventing further transmission of HIV.[1-4] These recommendations include refraining from blood, semen, or organ donation and either abstaining from sexual intercourse or using measures to prevent HIV transmission during intercourse.[46]

The circumstances of the exposure should be recorded in the worker's confidential medical record and should include the following:

Table 2 Recommendations for Hepatitis B Prophylaxis after Percutaneous or Permucosal Exposure[15]

Hepatitis B Vaccination Status of Exposed Person	HBsAg Status of Source of Exposure		
	HBsAg-Positive	HBsAg-Negative	Untested or Unknown
Unvaccinated	Give single dose of HBIG Initiate HB vaccine series	Initiate HB vaccine series	Initiate HB vaccine series
Previously vaccinated Known responder	Test exposed person for anti-HBs If anti-HBs levels are adequate,* no treatment is needed; if they are inadequate, give an HB vaccine booster dose	No treatment is needed	No treatment is needed
Known nonresponder	*No response to three-dose vaccine series:* give two doses of HBIG or one dose of HBIG plus revaccination *No response to three-dose vaccine series plus revaccination:* give one dose of HBIG as soon as possible and a second dose 1 mo later	No treatment is needed	If source is at high risk for hepatitis B infection, consider proceeding as if source had been demonstrated to be HBsAg-positive
Response unknown	Test exposed person for anti-HBs If anti-HBs levels are adequate,* no treatment is needed; if they are inadequate, give one dose of HBIG plus an HB vaccine booster dose	No treatment is needed	Test exposed person for anti-HBs If anti-HBs levels are adequate,* no treatment is needed; if they are inadequate, initiate revaccination

*An adequate anti-HBs level is ≥ 10 mIU/ml, which is approximately equivalent to 10 sample ratio units (SRU) on radioimmunoassay or a positive result on enzyme immunoassay.

1. The date and time of the exposure.
2. Details of the exposure, including (a) where and how the exposure occurred, (b) the type and amount of fluid or other material involved, and (c) the severity of the exposure (for a percutaneous exposure, this would include the depth of injury and whether fluid was injected; for a skin or mucous membrane exposure, it would include the extent and duration of contact and the condition of the skin—chapped, abraded, or intact).
3. A description of the source of the exposure, including (if known) whether the source material contained HIV or other blood-borne pathogens, whether the source was HIV positive, the stages of any diseases present, whether the patient had previously received antiretroviral therapy, and the viral load.
4. Details about counseling, postexposure management, and follow-up.[41]

The data currently available on primary HIV infection indicate that systemic infection does not occur immediately. There may be a brief window of opportunity during which postexposure antiretroviral therapy may modify viral replication. Findings from animal and human studies provide indirect evidence of the efficacy of antiretroviral drugs in postexposure prophylaxis. The majority of these studies included zidovudine (AZT); consequently, all postexposure prophylaxis regimens now in use include AZT. Combination treatment regimens using nucleoside reverse transcriptase inhibitors and protease inhibitors have proved effective. Accordingly, most experts now recommend dual therapy with two nucleosides (zidovudine and lamivudine) for low- to moderate-risk exposures. For high-risk exposures, most experts would add a protease inhibitor (usually either indinavir or nelfinavir) to the two nucleoside reverse transcriptase inhibitors. These medications should be started as soon as possible after the exposure (within hours rather than days) and should be continued for 4 weeks.

An important component of postexposure care is encouraging and facilitating compliance with the lengthy course of medication. Therefore, careful consideration must be given to the toxicity profiles of the antiretroviral agents chosen. All of these agents have been associated with side effects, include GI (e.g., nausea or diarrhea), hematologic, endocrine (e.g., diabetes), and urologic effects (e.g., nephrolithiasis with indinavir). According to some early data, 50% to 90% of health care workers receiving combination regimens for postexposure prophylaxis (e.g., zidovudine plus 3TC, with or without a protease inhibitor) reported one or more subjective side effects that were substantial enough to cause 24% to 36% of the workers to discontinue postexposure prophylaxis.[47-49]

Whether antiretroviral agents should be chosen for postexposure prophylaxis on the basis of the resistance patterns of the source patient's HIV remains unclear. Transmission of resistant strains has been reported[50-52]; however, in the perinatal clinical trial that studied vertical transmission of HIV, zidovudine prevented perinatal transmission despite genotypic resistance of HIV to zidovudine in the mother.[53] Further study of the significance of genotypic resistance is necessary before definitive recommendations can be made.

HEPATITIS B

Both passive immunization with hepatitis B immune globulin (HBIG) and active immunization with hepatitis B vaccine (HB vaccine) are currently available for prophylaxis against hepatitis B [*see Table 2*].

Passive Immunoprophylaxis

HBIG is prepared by Cohn ethanol fractionation from plasma selected to contain a high titer of anti-HBs; this process inactivates and eliminates HIV from the final product. In the United States, HBIG has an anti-HBs titer of at least 1:100,000 by radioimmunoassay.[54] HBIG provides temporary, passive protection. It is indicated after low-volume percutaneous or mucous membrane exposure to HBV; it is not effective for high-

Table 3 Candidates for Hepatitis B Vaccine[15]

Preexposure vaccination	Persons with occupational risk (e.g., health care workers, public safety workers)
	Clients and staffs of institutions for the developmentally disabled
	Hemodialysis patients
	Sexually active homosexual men
	Users of illicit injectable drugs
	Recipients of certain blood products (e.g., patients with clotting disorders who receive clotting factor concentrates)
	Household and sexual contacts of HBV carriers
	Adoptees from countries of high HBV endemicity
	Other contacts of HBV carriers (vaccination is usually not required unless there are special circumstances, such as biting or scratching, or medical conditions, such as severe skin disease, that facilitate transmission)
	Populations with high endemicity of HBV infection (e.g., Alaskan natives, Pacific islanders, and refugees from HBV-endemic areas)
	Inmates of long-term correctional facilities
	Sexually active heterosexual persons with multiple sexual partners
	International travelers who spend more than 6 mo in HBV-endemic areas and have close contact with the local population
	All infants born in the United States
	Adolescents 11 to 12 years old who have not previously been vaccinated
Postexposure vaccination	Perinatal exposure (infants born to HBsAg-positive mothers)
	Acute exposure to blood that contains (or might contain) HBsAg
	Sexual partners of persons with acute HBV infections
	Household contacts of persons with acute HBV infections (infants and older persons who have had identifiable blood exposure to the index patient)

volume exposure (e.g., blood transfusion). The recommended dose of HBIG for adults is 0.06 ml/kg I.M. Passive prophylaxis with HBIG should begin as soon as possible after exposure—ideally, within 24 hours.[54]

Active Immunoprophylaxis

Two types of HB vaccine are currently licensed in the United States, plasma-derived vaccine (Heptavax-B) and recombinant vaccine (Recombivax HB and Engerix-B). Heptavax-B contains alum-adsorbed 22 nm HBsAg particles purified from human plasma and processed to inactivate the infectivity of HBV and other viruses. Plasma-derived vaccine is no longer being produced in the United States, but similar vaccines are produced and used in China and other countries. In the United States, use of Heptavax-B is limited to persons allergic to yeast. Recombivax HB and Engerix-B are prepared by recombinant DNA technology in common baker's (or brewer's) yeast, Saccharomyces cerevisiae.

For primary vaccination, three I.M. injections (into the deltoid muscle in adults and children and into the anterolateral thigh muscle in infants and neonates) are given, with the second and third doses 1 and 6 months after the first dose.[54] The dose for Heptavax-B and Engerix-B is 20 µg (volume, 1.0 ml) for persons older than 11 years, and that for Recombivax HB is 10 µg (1.0 ml) for persons

older than 19 years and 5 µg (0.5 ml) for persons 11 to 18 years of age. For immunologically impaired patients, including hemodialysis patients, the dose is 40 µg for all three vaccines. For postexposure prophylaxis with Engerix-B, a regimen of four doses given soon after exposure and 1, 2, and 12 months afterward has been approved.

HB vaccine is more than 90% effective at preventing infection or clinical hepatitis in susceptible persons. Protection is virtually complete in persons who develop adequate antibody. Routine testing for immunity after vaccination is not recommended, but testing should be considered for persons at occupational risk who require postexposure prophylaxis for needle-stick exposure.

Between 30% and 50% of persons who have been vaccinated will cease to have detectable antibody levels within 7 years, but protection against infection and clinical disease appears to persist.[54,55] The need for booster doses has not been established. Revaccination of individuals who do not respond to the primary series will produce adequate antibody in 15% to 25% of cases after one additional dose and in 30% to 50% after three additional doses.[56]

Although effective HB vaccines have been available since 1982, the incidence of hepatitis B in the United States continued to increase in the first decade of HB vaccine use. In 1991, the Advisory Committee for Immunization Practices (ACIP), citing the safety of the vaccine and the evidence of continuing spread of HBV, recommended universal vaccination of all infants born in the United States.[57]

Recommendations for Exposure to Blood That Contains (or May Contain) HBsAg

Acute exposure The U.S. Public Health Service has provided recommendations for hepatitis B prophylaxis after accidental percutaneous, mucous membrane, or ocular exposure to blood that contains (or may contain) HBsAg [see Table 2].[43] These recommendations are based on consideration of several factors: (1) whether the source of the blood is available, (2) the HBsAg status of the source, and (3) the hepatitis B vaccination and vaccination-response status of the exposed person. After exposure, a blood sample should be obtained from the person who was the source of the exposure and should be tested for HBsAg. The hepatitis B vaccination status and the anti-HBs response status (if known) of the exposed person should be reviewed. Because passive administration of antibody with HBIG does not inhibit the active antibody response to HB vaccine, the two can be given simultaneously.

Chronic exposure The U.S. Public Health Service recommends that persons who are at risk for exposure to HBV receive the HB vaccine series [see Table 3].[54] Health care workers who are at increased risk for acquiring hepatitis B include all physicians (especially surgeons), dentists, and laboratory and support personnel, such as nurses and technicians who work in the operating room or who have contact with infected patients, blood or blood products, or excreta. Because of their frequent exposure to blood and their high risk of hepatitis B, all surgeons should receive HB vaccine. As of 1994, however, only 50% of surgeons had been vaccinated, despite the proven efficacy and safety of the vaccine and surgeons' increased risk of exposure.[58] Hospital personnel who do not have frequent contact with blood or blood products (e.g., the janitorial, laundry, and kitchen staffs) need not be vaccinated.

Screening of personnel and patients for anti-HBs before vaccination is indicated only for individuals in high-risk groups; it has not been found to be cost-effective outside these groups.

HEPATITIS C

The only tests currently approved by the U.S. Food and Drug Administration for diagnosis of hepatitis C are those that measure antibody to HCV. These tests detect anti-HCV in at least 97% of infected patients, but they cannot distinguish between acute, chronic, and resolved infection.[59] The positive predictive value of enzyme immunoassay (EIA) for anti-HCV varies depending on the prevalence of the infection in the population. Therefore, supplemental testing of a specimen with a positive EIA result with a more specific assay (e.g., the recombinant immunoblot assay [RIBA]) may detect false positives, especially when asymptomatic persons are being tested. Qualitative polymerase chain reaction (PCR) testing for HCV RNA can also be used to identify HCV. This test can detect HCV at concentrations as low as 100 to 1,000 viral genome copies/ml, and it can detect HCV RNA in serum or plasma within 1 to 2 weeks after viral exposure and weeks before alanine aminotransferase (ALT) levels rise or anti-HCV appears.[59] Under optimal conditions, the reverse transcriptase PCR assay for HCV can identify 75% to 85% of persons who are anti-HCV–positive and more than 95% of persons with acute or chronic hepatitis C.[59] Quantitative assays for measuring HCV RNA are also available but are less sensitive and should not be used as primary tests for confirming or excluding the diagnosis of HCV infection or monitoring the end point of treatment.[59] The data currently available on prevention of HCV infection with immune globulin (IG) indicate that this approach is not effective as postexposure prophylaxis for HCV infection.[59] Interferon may have a role in the treatment of acute hepatitis C: several studies have shown that interferon may delay or prevent the onset of chronic hepatitis C in patients treated early in the course of acute HCV infection.[60-62]

RABIES

The CDC has made recommendations for the prevention of rabies in people bitten by animals [see Table 4].[63] Bite wounds should always be thoroughly scrubbed with soap and 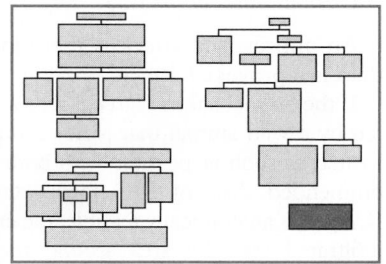 water. Postexposure antirabies treatment includes both rabies immune globulin (RIG) and human diploid cell (rabies) vaccine (HDCV). The decision to administer such treatment should be based on the following considerations.

Species and Availability of Biting Animal

In the United States, rabies is most commonly transmitted by skunks, raccoons, foxes, and bats. Livestock occasionally transmit the virus, but rodents and lagomorphs (i.e., rabbits and hares) are rarely infected.[64] In different parts of the country, different animals predominate in the transmission of the virus. The likelihood that domestic cats or dogs in the United States will be infected varies from region to region. The chances of rabies transmission by a domestic animal that has been properly immunized are minimal.

Whether an animal is available for observation after biting someone also influences the need for antirabies prophylaxis. In certain cases, an animal that bites a person must be killed and tissue from its brain checked for the presence of rabies by fluorescent antibody tests as soon as possible [see Table 4].

Type of Exposure

Infected animals transmit rabies primarily by biting, although licking may introduce the virus into open cuts in skin or mucous membranes. Transmission occasionally occurs as a result of aerosol exposure: the virus may be excreted in the urine and feces of infected bats, aerosolized during urination and defecation, and then inhaled, for example, by spelunkers exploring caves.

Table 4 Rabies Postexposure Prophylaxis[63]

	Animal Species	Condition of Animal at Time of Attack	Treatment of Exposed Person*
Domestic	Dog, cat	Healthy and available for 10 days of observation	None, unless animal develops rabies†
		Rabid or suspected rabid	RIG (20 IU/kg)‡ and HDCV§ (five 1.0 ml doses intramuscularly, on days 0, 3, 7, 14, and 28)
		Unknown (escaped)	Consult public health officials. If treatment is indicated, give RIG‡ and HDCV
Wild	Skunk, bat, fox, coyote, bobcat, raccoon, other carnivores	Regard as rabid unless proved negative by laboratory tests‖	RIG (20 IU/kg)‡ and HDCV (five 1.0 ml doses intramuscularly, on days 0, 3, 7, 14, and 28)
Other	Livestock, rodents, lagomorphs (rabbits and hares)	Consider individually. Local and state public health officials should be consulted on questions about the need for rabies prophylaxis. Bites of squirrels, hamsters, guinea pigs, chipmunks, gerbils, rats, mice, other rodents, and lagomorphs almost never call for antirabies prophylaxis.	

*All bites and wounds should immediately be thoroughly cleansed with soap and water. If antirabies treatment is indicated, both rabies immune globulin (RIG) and human diploid cell rabies vaccine (HDCV) should be given as soon as possible, regardless of the interval from exposure. (The administration of RIG is the more urgent procedure. If HDCV is not immediately available, start RIG and give HDCV as soon as it is obtained.) Local reactions to vaccines are common and do not contraindicate continuing treatment. Discontinue vaccine if fluorescent antibody tests of the animal are negative.

†During the usual holding period of 10 days, begin treatment with RIG and HDCV at first sign of rabies in a dog or cat that has bitten someone. The symptomatic animal should be killed immediately and tested.

‡The full dose should be infiltrated around the wounds; any remaining RIG should be given I.M. at a site distant from that of vaccine administration. If RIG is not available, use antirabies serum, equine (ARS). Do not use more than the recommended dosage of RIG or ARS.

§HDCV should be administered into the deltoid (not the gluteus) muscle in adults and adolescents. In children, it may be administered into the upper thigh.

‖The animal should be killed and tested as soon as possible. Holding for observation is not recommended.

Circumstances of the Bite

An unprovoked attack is more indicative of a rabid animal than is a provoked attack.

If the animal shows signs of rabies or the patient has been bitten by a wild animal that is not captured, the patient should be treated as soon as possible with both RIG and HDCV. The recommended dose of RIG for postexposure prophylaxis is 20 IU/kg.[63] If anatomically feasible, the entire dose of RIG should be infiltrated into the area around the wound.[65,66] Postexposure HDCV should be given I.M. in five 1.0 ml doses on days 0, 3, 7, 14, and 28.[63] Those with adequate preexposure immunization should receive two 1.0 ml doses of HDCV I.M. on days 0 and 3 but should receive no RIG. For adults, the vaccine should be administered in the deltoid area. For children, the anterolateral aspect of the thigh is also acceptable. The gluteal area should never be used for HDCV injections, because administration in this area results in lower neutralizing antibody titers.[63] HDCV must not be given in the same region as RIG.

The CDC recommends that preexposure immunization be considered for high-risk groups, such as animal handlers, certain laboratory workers and field personnel, and persons planning to stay for more than 1 month in areas where canine rabies is highly prevalent and access to appropriate medical care is limited. The recommended preexposure regimen is 0.1 ml of HDCV on days 0, 7, and 21 or 28.[67] Testing for adequate antibody response is not necessary for persons at low risk for exposure, but administration of booster doses every 2 to 3 years is recommended for those at high risk for exposure. Postexposure treatment for persons who have received preexposure immunization consists of 1 ml HDCV on days 0 and 3 only, without RIG.[68]

Although only a few cases of clinical rabies occur each year in the United States, approximately 30,000 persons a year are given postexposure prophylaxis. In 1992, 49 states, the District of Columbia, and Puerto Rico collectively reported 8,644 cases of animal rabies and one case of human rabies to the CDC.[69] The total expense associated with one rabid dog in California was $105,790, even though no human contracted rabies.[70] This amount represents the costs of human antirabies treatment, vaccination of other animals, and animal-containment programs.

Discussion

Size and Structure of Viruses

Viruses are among the smallest and simplest of microorganisms. Human viruses can be as small as 18 to 26 nm in diameter (parvoviruses) or as long as 300 nm (vaccinia virus), slightly longer than *Chlamydia* (a bacterium). Viruses do not have the complex enzyme systems required for synthesis of nucleic acid precursors, they lack ribosomes for protein synthesis, and they have no energy-generating mechanism. Consequently, they cannot replicate outside cells.

The core of a virus is made of either RNA or DNA, but never both. The nucleic acid can be either single stranded or double stranded. This nucleic acid core is surrounded by the capsid, which is a protein coat made up of capsomers, repetitive subunits consisting of one protein or at most a few. Because the viral nucleic acid must code for coat proteins, a limitation in the number of capsid proteins conserves viral nucleic acid. The capsid protects the nucleic acid from nucleases in the environment, serves as its vehicle of transmission from one host to another, and plays a role in the attachment of the virus to the receptor sites on susceptible cells. The complete nucleic acid–protein coat complex is termed the nucleocapsid. For many viruses, the nucleocapsid is the complete virus particle, the virion. Other viruses, such as herpesviruses, may acquire an envelope, an additional lipid-containing membrane coat around the nucleocapsid, by budding through a membrane of the host cell [*see Figure 1*]. Some viruses may also have an enzyme associated with their core that replicates the nucleic acid. Examples are the DNA polymerase of the HBV and the reverse transcriptase of retroviruses.

Classification of Viruses

Viruses, like other organisms, are classified into families, genera, and species, but most viral species do not have formal names and in practice are referred to by common names (e.g., cytomegalovirus, coxsackievirus, Norwalk virus, and varicella-zoster virus). Viruses can also be classified by chemical characteristics and by structural characteristics determined from electron microscopy (e.g., dimensions and site of assembly). Viruses are categorized into two broad groups depending on whether their nucleic acid is RNA or DNA. These two groups can be subdivided first according to whether the nucleic acid is single stranded or double stranded and then according to the presence or absence of an envelope. Single-stranded RNA viruses that replicate by means of a DNA step (i.e., retroviruses) are grouped separately from those that do not.

Identification of Viruses

Viruses can be identified by means of (1) serologic tests, (2) isolation of virus, (3) histologic examination, (4) detection of viral antigens, (5) detection of viral nucleic acid, and (6) electron microscopy. One or more of these techniques may be applicable to a given viral infection.

Specimens must be handled properly to maximize the likelihood of identifying the virus. If isolation of the virus is desired, blood and tissue samples should be taken promptly to the virology laboratory and inoculated onto the appropriate cell line. Samples obtained at night or on weekends can be placed in a balanced salt solution or tissue culture medium and kept in a refrigerator until taken to the laboratory. If microscopic identification of the virus is planned, specimens must be preserved appropriately. Routine preservation in formalin, for example, permits visualization of viral inclusions by routine staining and light microscopy. For identification of viral antigens by immunofluorescence techniques, the tissue specimen should be immediately frozen, preferably in liquid nitrogen. Specimens to be examined by electron microscopy must be placed in glutaraldehyde or another appropriate fixative.

SEROLOGIC TESTS

The antibody response to viral antigens can be detected in the serum of patients with viral infections. An IgM response usually indicates recent exposure to the virus, whereas the presence of IgG reflects past exposure.

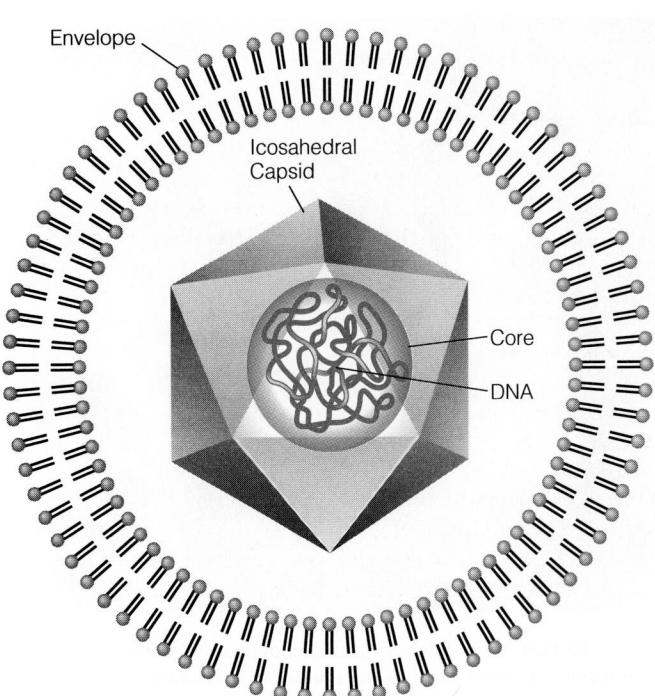

Envelope

Icosahedral
Capsid

Core

DNA

Figure 1 **The capsomers and the irregularly shaped surrounding envelope of a cytomegalovirus are highlighted by negative staining with uranyl acetate (above). A typical herpesvirus (right) consists of a central core containing DNA; an icosahedral capsid, a surrounding layer of protein made up of 162 individual capsomers; and an envelope, a membrane coat acquired when the virus buds from the nuclear membrane of the host cell.**

For most acute primary infections, serum obtained during late recovery or after recovery (convalescent serum) has an increased antibody titer, compared with serum obtained early in the course of the disease (acute serum). Most tests are performed on an initial serum dilution of 1:2 or 1:10 and on serial twofold dilutions thereafter. A fourfold increase in titer (indicated by reactivity of a two-tube dilution) usually represents a significant increase in antibody response and is considered to constitute seroconversion. An immunocompromised host may occasionally fail to mount an antibody response.

Some viruses are so common that patients may already have antibody titers when the disease is first suspected. Herpesviruses are ubiquitous and are present in many healthy people in latent form. At the onset of herpesvirus infections, patients may already have the corresponding antibody. Nevertheless, their antibody titer will almost always increase significantly after recovery.

A variety of serologic tests are available in the clinical laboratory: complement fixation, radioimmunoassay, enzyme-linked immunosorbent assay (ELISA), immunofluorescence, immune precipitation, immune blotting, latex agglutination, virus neutralization, indirect hemagglutination, immune adherence hemagglutination, and hemagglutination inhibition. None of these serologic tests is appropriate for identification of all viruses.

ISOLATION OF VIRUS

The isolation of virus requires appropriate specimen collection and inoculation into animals or onto appropriate cell lines. Blood sent for virus isolation should be unclotted because some viruses, such as herpesviruses, are found primarily in lymphocytes. If cell-associated viruses are suspected, lymphocytes should be inoculated directly onto target cells. Several types of cells are available for growing viruses, and no single cell line is appropriate for all of them. Therefore, it is helpful to the laboratory to know which virus the clinician suspects.

Viruses that grow in cell monolayers in tissue culture have cytopathic effects that can be recognized under the microscope (e.g., rounding, transformation, or death) [see *Figure 2*]. Some viruses, such as rubella, produce no direct cytopathic effects but can be detected because they inhibit the cytopathic effects of a second test virus. This phenomenon is called viral interference. Other viruses (e.g., myxoviruses) cause changes in the cell membrane so that red blood cells adhere to the cell surface (hemadsorption). The identity of isolated viruses can be confirmed by use of specific antisera that are known to inhibit viral growth.

Tissue suspected of containing an encephalitis or other neurotropic virus can be minced and the extract injected intracerebrally into an infant mouse. If the mouse dies and bacteria cannot be cultured from the brain, the injected material presumably contained such a virus. If antiserum of known specificity neutralizes the virus, the specificity of the antiserum indicates the specific identity of the virus. The criterion for neutralization is that inoculation of neutralized virus will not kill the mouse.

Figure 2 **Cells infected with cytomegalovirus become large and round (arrows). Note the uniform appearance of adjacent uninfected cells.**

Figure 3 **Kidney biopsy shows cytomegalovirus-infected tubular epithelial cells (arrows). In such cells, a dark intranuclear inclusion is surrounded by a clear halo. Inclusions usually indicate sites of previous or current viral replication.**

HISTOLOGIC EXAMINATION

Histologic examination of biopsy and autopsy tissues may demonstrate changes that are typical of certain viruses. Members of the herpesvirus group can be characterized by intranuclear inclusions surrounded by a clear halo [*see Figure 3*]. RNA viruses usually produce inclusions in the cytoplasm; for instance, dark-staining intracytoplasmic inclusions in the brain tissue of animals or patients are diagnostic of rabies infection and are called Negri bodies. Inclusion bodies are either masses of closely packed virus particles or remnants of prior virus replication.

DETECTION OF VIRAL ANTIGENS

Viral antigens can be detected in tissues by techniques employing their corresponding antibodies. If virus is present, these antigens may be visible microscopically under ultraviolet light either by direct immunofluorescence (i.e., in tissue sections stained with fluorescein-labeled antiviral antibody) or by indirect immunofluorescence (i.e., in tissue sections exposed first to antiviral antibody and then to fluorescein-labeled anti–γ-globulin antibody). Fluorescence microscopy requires specimens that are fresh frozen (preferably in liquid nitrogen). Immunofluorescence staining of cells in tissue culture can detect viral antigens before cytopathic effects are evident. Viral antigens in formalin-fixed tissue can be identified by immunohistochemical microscopy (e.g., using peroxidase-labeled antibodies).

DETECTION OF VIRAL NUCLEIC ACID

Viral nucleic acids can be detected in body fluids and tissues at virus concentrations too low to be detected by other means. The PCR permits amplification of even a small number of copies of viral nucleic acid. In theory, even a single copy of a specific DNA can be detected by PCR. Before PCR is performed, DNA can be synthesized from viral RNA by means of reverse transcriptase. The PCR product can be detected by gel electrophoresis and compared with known viral DNA. This test is currently being used to diagnose CMV infection and is more sensitive than current serologic testing for HCV. Nucleic acid hybridization can detect viral nucleic acid in tissue specimens. Epstein-Barr virus genomes

can be detected in this way in EBV-related cancers and lymphoproliferative disorders.

ELECTRON MICROSCOPY

Although seldom used routinely, electron microscopy allows rapid identification (in a matter of hours) of viruses in body fluids, tissues, and tissue extracts. Identification of viruses in body fluids and tissue extracts by this method is easier if the samples are first concentrated by ultracentrifugation, evaporation, or ultrafiltration. HBV has been observed in specimens from hepatitis patients only after ultracentrifugation.

Epidemiology of Viral Infections of Interest to Surgeons

Viral infections are spread to humans via several patterns of transmission: (1) direct transmission from humans with symptomatic infection (e.g., HBV, HCV herpesviruses, and HIV), (2) transmission from asymptomatic human carriers (e.g., HBV, HCV, HIV, and varicella-zoster virus), (3) transmission from arthropods (e.g., encephalitis and dengue viruses), and (4) transmission from other animals (e.g., rabies virus).

Viral infections are common in immunosuppressed patients in general and especially in recipients of organ transplants, who must take immunosuppressive drugs to prevent rejection. The overwhelming majority of these infections are caused by members of the herpesvirus family (e.g., CMV, herpes simplex viruses, varicella-zoster virus, and EBV); infections with HBV and with papovaviruses (e.g., human papillomavirus, which causes warts, and BK virus) are also frequent.

Because surgical patients are frequently given transfusions of blood or blood products and because hospital staff often incur accidental needle-stick injury, viruses that can be transmitted by these routes are of prime interest to surgeons and their patients. Examples of such viruses are HBV, hepatitis D, HCV, HIV, HTLV-I, and the herpesviruses, including EBV and CMV. These viruses can also be transmitted by organ transplantation either from the cells of the organ itself (e.g., HBV in liver cells or CMV in kidney cells) or from blood that has not been completely removed from the organ. Changes in donor acceptance and screening policies over time have increased the safety of the blood supply and should continue to do so in the future [*see Table 5*].[71]

HIV

Two serotypes of HIV, HIV-1 and HIV-2, have been identified. Both can cause AIDS. HIV-1 accounts for virtually all cases of AIDS in the United States and equatorial Africa. HIV-2 is found almost exclusively in West Africa; only a few cases of HIV-2 infection have occurred in the United States.

Because AIDS patients are immunodepressed, they are susceptible to opportunistic infections and neoplasms, especially non-Hodgkin lymphoma, *Pneumocystis carinii* pneumonia, and Kaposi sarcoma. AIDS is most prevalent in the United States among male homosexuals, abusers of I.V. drugs, and hemophiliacs. Since the implementation of testing for blood-borne HIV and the near-elimination of HIV from blood products, the incidence of HIV infection in the hemophiliac population has diminished markedly; however, in recent years, the incidence in the heterosexual population has been increasing rapidly.

HIV can be transmitted by transfusion of whole blood, packed red cells, plasma, factor VIII concentrates, factor IX concentrates, and platelets. The likelihood that a person will become infected with HIV after receiving a single-donor blood product that tests

Table 5 Changes in Donor Acceptance and Screening Policies Instituted to Reduce the Risk of Transmitting Infectious Diseases[71]

Policy	Implementation Date
Screening for HBsAg	July 1972
Voluntary exclusion of persons at high risk for AIDS	March 1983
Redefinition of high-risk behavior to include men who have had sex with more than one man since 1979	December 1984
Testing for antibody to HIV-1	Spring 1985
Redefinition of high-risk behavior to include any man who has had sex with another man since 1977	September 1985
Implementation of a mechanism to allow donors to indicate confidentially that their donations should not be used for transfusion	October 1986
Testing for alanine aminotransferase (ALT, formerly SGPT)	Winter 1986–1987
Testing for anti-HBc	Spring 1987
Testing for antibody to HTLV-1	January 1990
Testing for antibody to HCV	May 1990
Testing for antibody to HIV-2	April 1992
Testing for HIV-1 antigen	March 1996

positive for HIV approaches 100%.[72-73] Before the advent of serologic testing for HIV in 1985, 0.04% of 1,200,000 blood donations in the United States were estimated to be HIV positive.[74] AIDS has developed in more than 8,500 recipients of blood transfusions, blood components, or transplanted organs or tissue.

Federal regulations now require that all prospective blood and plasma donors be screened for antibody to HIV by ELISA. Because this test yields a low rate of false positive results, assay by the more sensitive Western blot electrophoresis is always used to confirm positive ELISA results. Routine testing of blood donors has greatly reduced HIV transmission via blood transfusions, but infection can still occur if the donor has been infected with HIV but has not yet developed antibody.[75] The risk of HIV transmission via transfusion of screened blood that is negative for HIV is estimated to be one in 200,000 to one in 2,000,000 per unit transfused in the United States.[76] Antibody to HIV usually develops within 4 weeks to 6 months of HIV infection.[77] From the time of infection until the appearance of antibody, infected individuals will test negative by ELISA or Western blot, and their blood might still be used for transfusion.

HIV and AIDS can also be transmitted by organ transplantation.[78] So far, only a small number of patients have been found to be infected in this way, but more will undoubtedly be reported. These patients received transplants before HIV testing of potential donors became possible. All prospective organ and tissue donors now should be tested for HIV infection and other blood-borne viral infections.

HIV infection is also a potential problem in health care workers, who are exposed to a large and growing population of AIDS patients. In the United States, an estimated 1.0 to 1.5 million people are infected with HIV but as yet have no symptoms. HIV transmission from blood, tissue, or other body fluids can occur in the health care setting as a result of percutaneous injury (e.g., from needles or other sharp objects), contamination of mucous membranes or nonintact skin (e.g., skin that is chapped, abraded, or affected by dermatitis), prolonged contact with intact skin, or contamination involving an extensive area.[79] HIV infection may be contracted through a variety of sources including blood, semen, vaginal secretions, visibly bloody fluids, and a number of other fluids for which the precise risk of transmission is undetermined (e.g., cerebrospinal, synovial, pleural, peritoneal, pericardial, and amniotic fluid). Infection may also be contracted from concentrated HIV used in research settings.[79] The results of multiple prospective studies quantifying transmission risk associated with a discrete occupational HIV exposure indicate that the average risk of HIV transmission associated with needle punctures or similar percutaneous injuries is approximately 0.3%. The estimated risk of transmission from mucocutaneous exposure to HIV-contaminated material is 0.03%. As of December 1999, the CDC had received reports of 56 U.S. health care workers in whom documented HIV seroconversion was temporally related to occupational HIV exposure. Of these 56, 48 had percutaneous exposures, five mucocutaneous exposures, two both percutaneous and mucous membrane exposures, and one an unknown route of exposure.[80] Another 138 possible cases of occupational HIV transmission—six involving surgeons—have been reported in persons with no risk factors for HIV transmission other than workplace exposure; however, seroconversion after a specific exposure was not documented. There may be other health care workers who also have acquired HIV infection from needle-stick or mucous membrane exposure but have not been reported, either because they and their patients have not been tested or because they have other risk factors for HIV infection

The concentration of virus in the blood or serum of antigen-positive individuals is several orders of magnitude less for HIV than for HBV. The number of needle-stick exposures to HIV that have actually led to a positive test result for HIV has been extremely small, whereas hepatitis B occurs in as many as 40% of health care workers exposed to the virus by needle-stick injury. Despite this relatively low infectiousness, AIDS is much more feared than hepatitis B because AIDS is often fatal. Although hepatitis B is usually not fatal and is often of short duration, several health care workers die of hospital-acquired hepatitis B and hepatitis C each year.

Hepatitis

Several viruses can cause hepatitis. Hepatitis A virus (HAV) and HBV cause what were formerly known as infectious hepatitis and serum hepatitis, respectively. HCV is the major cause of parenterally transmitted non-A, non-B hepatitis. Hepatitis E virus is a common cause of epidemic non-A, non-B hepatitis, which is chiefly found in developing countries in Africa and Asia. Hepatitis D virus (HDV, formerly called the delta agent) is defective or incomplete and is pathogenic only in the presence of HBV. The hepatitis viruses are the most common infectious agents to which hospital personnel may be exposed. Herpesviruses can also cause serious and sometimes fatal hepatitis, especially in severely immunocompromised patients, such as recipients of organ or bone marrow transplants and patients receiving intensive chemotherapy for cancer.

HEPATITIS A

HAV is a small (27 nm), single-stranded RNA virus belonging to the enterovirus subgroup of picornaviruses. Its almost exclusive transmission by the fecal-oral route is enhanced by poor personal hygiene, poor sanitary conditions, and crowding. Transmission can be contained by careful hand washing and the isolation of excretions. Unlike other types of viral hepatitis, hepatitis A is rarely transmitted by blood, blood products, or needle sticks and is rarely transmitted among hemodialysis patients, health care workers, and I.V. drug abusers. The infrequent parenteral transmission of HAV is attributed in part to its lack of an asymptomatic carrier state. Hepatitis A can be transmitted percutaneously only during a brief period of viremia before the onset of symptoms and jaundice. The chance that an infected person will donate blood during this short period is small; also, patients are usually outside the hospital during this period.

HEPATITIS B

HBV is a member of the Hepadnaviridae family of DNA viruses. It is most prevalent in the Far East, the Middle East, Africa, and parts of South America, where as many as 15% of the general population are chronic carriers. Worldwide, the most common mode of transmission is from mother to child during the perinatal period. In the United States, however, sexual or parenteral transmission has been implicated in most infections. The high-risk groups for chronic HBV infection in the United States include I.V. drug users, men who have sex with men, other individuals with multiple sexual partners, household contacts and sexual partners of HBV carriers, health care workers, patients on long-term hemodialysis, and organ transplant recipients.[81]

Clinical Course

The clinical course of hepatitis B is extremely variable: infection ranges from the completely asymptomatic to the rapidly fatal. The incubation period averages 75 days but can last from 40 to 180 days. Exposure to HBV has five potential outcomes: (1) no infection occurs; (2) acute hepatitis develops, followed by clearance of infection; (3) acute fulminant infection develops, leading to hepatic necrosis and death; (4) acute hepatitis develops without clearance of infection, and a chronic carrier state ensues; and (5) no acute illness develops, but a chronic carrier state ensues.

Approximately 55% of adults infected with HBV have no symptoms despite serologic documentation of infection (see below), which explains why blood donors who seem to be in good health are capable of transmitting the virus. Other individuals infected with HBV may have such mild symptoms (e.g., slight malaise, fatigability, and loss of appetite) that they do not seek medical attention.

Approximately 45% of people infected with HBV experience typical acute, icteric hepatitis, which is characterized by fatigue, anorexia, nausea, vomiting, and hepatomegaly. In approximately 1% of adults infected with HBV, acute fulminant hepatitis develops. This condition is characterized by progressive hepatocellular destruction, encephalopathy, and deepening coma. Fulminant hepatitis causes death in approximately 80% of affected adults and 30% of affected children.

In approximately 5% to 10% of hepatitis B cases, the infection becomes chronic. Patients with chronic hepatitis may be asymptomatic or may have clinical and histologic evidence of the disease, as well as persistently elevated levels of serum aminotransferases [see Figure 4]. With time, many patients pass to an asymptomatic carrier state, and serum aminotransferase levels fall. The duration of the asymptomatic carrier state appears to be indefinite. Chronic HBV infection can result in hepatocellular carcinoma, which is especially common in China, Southeast Asia, and sub-Saharan Africa.

Because most patients remain asymptomatic until the development of end-stage liver disease, there are no specific clinical findings that are indicative of chronic HBV infection. There are, however, several clinical syndromes linked to HBV infection that may provide a clue to the presence of chronic HBV infection. These syndromes include polyarteritis nodosa, membranous or membranoproliferative glomerulonephritis, leukocytoclastic vasculitis, erythema nodosum, arthritis, and serum sickness.

Antigens

HBV has a diameter of 42 nm and contains circular, double-stranded DNA. The protein coat on its outer surface is termed hepatitis B surface antigen. HBsAg is made in quantities greatly exceeding the amount required to coat the nucleic acid. The excess surface antigen appears in the serum as spheres 22 nm in diameter or tubules of the same diameter and of varying length. These spheres and tubules contain no nucleic acid and hence are not infectious. They may persist in the serum for prolonged periods, even for life, and in great quantities, up to 10^{12} to 10^{14} surface antigen particles (500 μg protein) per milliliter.[82]

The hepatitis B virus also has a nucleocapsid core, the outside of which contains the hepatitis B core antigen (HBcAg). HBcAg is not detected in hepatitis B during acute infection, because its antigenic determinants are hidden by the outer surface antigen of the intact virion.

Inside the hepatitis B nucleocapsid is a DNA-dependent DNA polymerase and the hepatitis B e antigen, which is thought to be either an internal component or a degradation product of the core antigen. HBeAg is found only in the serum of individuals whose serum also contains HBsAg, and it appears in the serum of virtually all patients early in the course of HBV infection. The presence of HBeAg in serum is indicative of the presence of large numbers of circulating intact virions: serum containing HBeAg is estimated to be one million times more infectious than serum containing HBsAg but not HBeAg.

Serology

HBsAg can be detected in the serum within a few weeks of viral exposure [see Figure 5]. It usually persists throughout the symptomatic period and does not disappear until after recovery. Anti-HBs appears shortly after the disappearance of HBsAg [see Table 6]. During this window period, neither HBsAg nor anti-HBs is detectable [see Table 7]. Anti-HBs persists for years and is associated with immunity to reinfection. HBV can be differentiated into eight serotypes on the basis of determinants of the surface antigen.

Hepatitis B core antigen (HBcAg) is not found free in the serum, but antibody to HBcAg (anti-HBc) becomes detectable at an early stage in the course of acute infections, 1 to 2 weeks after the appearance of HBsAg. Titers of anti-HBc fall after the disappearance of HBsAg but persist for life. In patients with chronic hepatitis B, HBsAg remains detectable indefinitely, and titers of anti-HBc remain high. Years after infection, titers of anti-HBs may have fallen to undetectable levels, and anti-HBc may be the only marker of previous infection. HBeAg is detectable immediately after the appearance of HBsAg. Antibody to HBeAg (anti-HBe) appears just after HBeAg becomes undetectable (usually before the disappearance of HBsAg) and persists for 1 to 2 years [see Figure 5].

HEPATITIS D

HDV is a defective, 35 to 37 nm RNA virus that can infect only persons who are also infected with HBV, because it uses HBsAg for its structural protein shell. HDV is found worldwide and is especially prevalent in the Amazon basin, central Africa, southern Italy, and the Middle East.[83] HDV infection is less common in the United States and Western Europe, where it is generally associat-

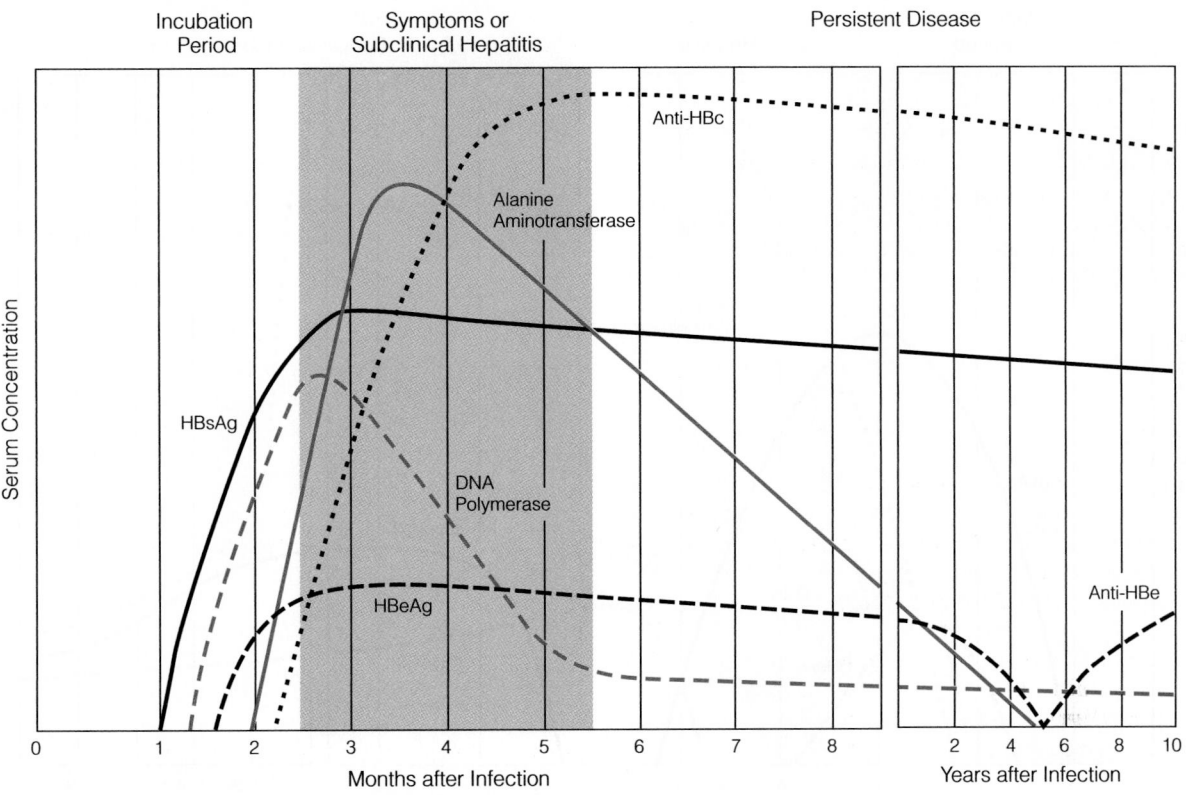

Figure 4 Schematic shows virologic, clinical, and serologic events of a hepatitis B infection that becomes persistent.

ed with parenteral blood exposure, typically in the setting of I.V. drug abuse or multiple transfusions.

Clinically, hepatitis D is found only in association with acute or chronic hepatitis B, and it cannot last longer than hepatitis B does. Depending on the state of the HBV infection, HDV infection appears either as a coinfection or a superinfection. Coinfection occurs when acute HDV infection and acute HBV infection are present simultaneously; superinfection occurs when acute HDV infection is superimposed on chronic HBV infection. Coinfection with HDV is associated with fulminant hepatitis and a mortality of 2% to 20%.[84] Fewer than 5% of cases of coinfection progress to chronic hepatitis D. In contrast, superinfection with HDV results in chronic HDV hepatitis, often with cirrhosis, in more than 70% of cases. The clinical and biochemical features of HDV infection resemble those of HBV infection alone. Chronic active hepatitis B progresses faster when hepatitis D is also present. Chronic HDV infection is more likely to result in severe morbidity and mortality than chronic HBV or HCV infection alone.

Diagnosis of acute HDV infection may be difficult: HDAg appears in the circulation only briefly and often goes undetected. Antibody to HDAg (anti-HD) of the IgM class subsequently appears in serum in low titers. Because no anti-HD IgG response occurs, no serologic marker of previous HDV infection may remain after recovery. Chronic HDV infection is easier to diagnose: high titers of anti-HD in the serum indicate ongoing HDV infection, and HDV antigen is detectable in the liver by means of immunohistochemical techniques. Moreover, IgM anti-HD remains detectable in serum.[83]

NON-A, NON-B HEPATITIS: HEPATITIS E AND HEPATITIS C

Non-A, non-B hepatitis is divided into two varieties, an epidemic form (hepatitis E) and a parenterally transmitted form (hepatitis C).[85] Hepatitis E is an acute, self-limited disease whose clinical features are similar to those of other types of hepatitis. Hepatitis E virus (HEV) is prevalent in the developing world, where it is spread by the fecal-oral route and has been associated with large outbreaks as well as sporadic cases. Outbreaks have been linked to contaminated water supplies. No cases of HEV infection acquired in the United States have been reported to date, but HEV acquisition has been reported in international travelers.

Hepatitis C is the most common cause of nonalcoholic liver disease in the United States. HCV is an RNA virus of the flavivirus family. It can be transmitted through parenteral exposure (usually in the setting of I.V. drug abuse), sexual contact, or the sharing of a household with an HCV-infected person; however, some persons with HCV infection have none of these risk factors, and there may be other means of transmission that have yet to be elucidated. Before the advent of antibody testing, HCV infection accounted for the majority (75% to 95%) of cases of posttransfusion hepatitis.[83] Since the spring of 1990, when a serologic test for HCV became available, all transfused blood has been screened for HCV, and the incidence of transfusion-associated hepatitis C has fallen precipitously. At present, however, I.V. drug use still accounts for a large proportion (60%) of HCV transmission in the United States.[59]

The presence of anti-HCV IgG appears not to be protective: blood donors with anti-HCV antibody can transmit hepatitis.[62] Surveys of HCV seropositivity indicate that 0.2% to 0.6% of volunteer blood donors carry anti-HCV IgG,[83] and the prevalence may be much higher among high-risk populations (e.g., residents of large inner-city communities). The prevalence of anti-HCV IgG is high among I.V. drug users, hemodialysis patients, and hemophiliacs.

Clinical Manifestations

The incubation period of hepatitis C averages 7 to 8 weeks in length but may be as short as 2 weeks or as long as 15. The clini-

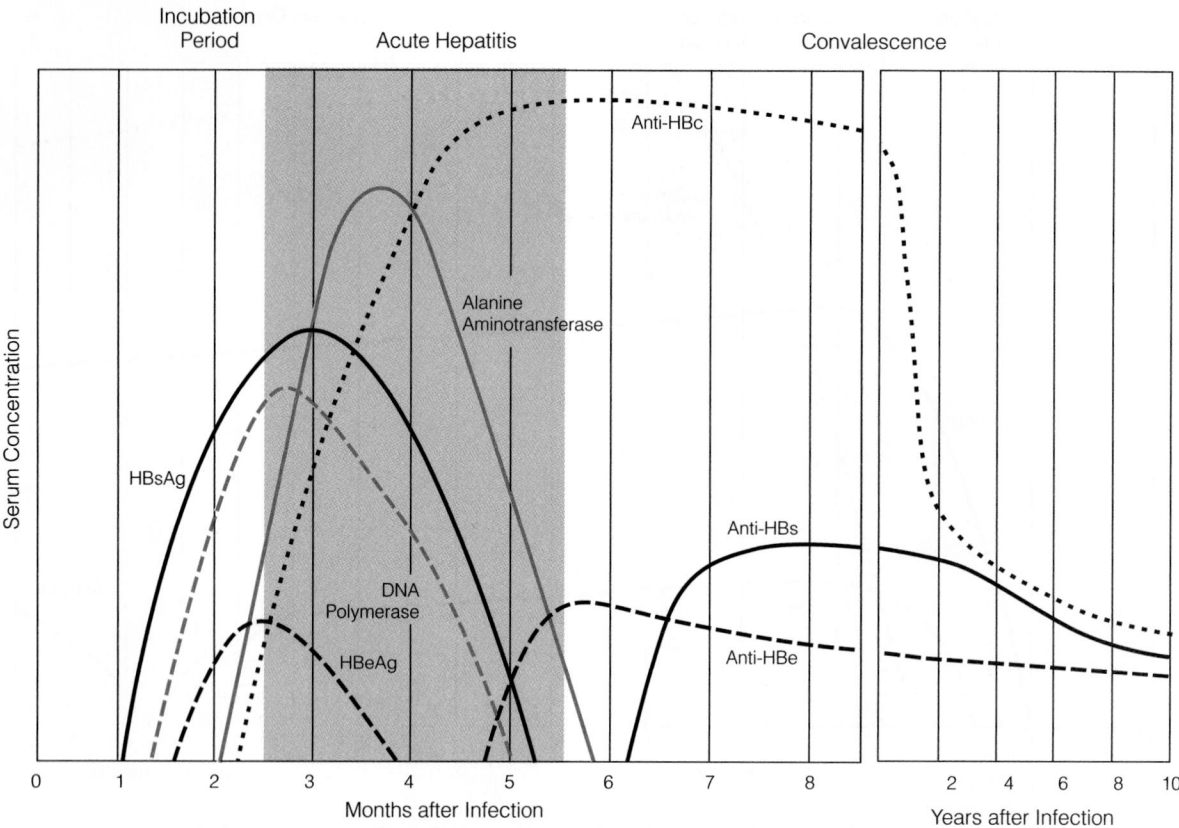

Figure 5 Schematic shows virologic, clinical, and serologic events during acute hepatitis B infection.

cal manifestations and biochemical alterations associated with acute hepatitis C are similar to but milder than those associated with hepatitis B. Serum aminotransferase levels can fluctuate widely; the peak levels are lower than those seen in hepatitis B (10 to 20 times normal as opposed to 20 to 50 times normal). Only about 25% of cases of acute HCV infection are icteric, and the mortality for acute infection is about 1%. Most patients have no acute illness suggestive of HCV infection. Antibody is not always present early in infection, and there are no clinically available assays for detecting IgM antibody to HCV. Thanks to improvements in the immunodetection of HCV, however, the interval before anti-HCV can be detected has decreased from the 6 to 12 months required with the first-generation tests to 8 to 12 weeks with the second-generation assays.[83]

The most striking feature of HCV infection is its tendency to become chronic in as many as 50% to 75% of cases. One study found that even among the 1% to 10% of individuals with HCV whose bloodstreams had been cleared of HCV according to RT-PCR assay, as many as 90% still had HCV in the liver.[86] It is estimated that in the United States, nearly four million people are seropositive for HCV, and more than 30% of liver transplantations are performed to treat end-stage liver disease related to chronic HCV infection. The presence of anti-HCV IgG does not distinguish acute from chronic hepatitis. Within 10 years, cirrhosis may develop in as many as 20% to 25% of patients with active hepatitis[87]; accordingly, these patients must be followed up carefully.

Chronic active hepatitis is characterized by elevated serum aminotransferase levels; however, other test results remain normal, and the patient is usually asymptomatic until end-stage liver disease develops. Liver biopsy shows inflammation around the portal triads. Recombinant interferons have been used to treat

chronic HCV infection, with mixed results: frequently, there is little response to treatment, or viremia returns after treatment. The combination of interferon with ribavirin has shown promise, however. Interferon treatment is generally reserved for patients who have chronic HCV infection and show evidence of active necroinflammatory liver disease with persistent ALT elevations.

HEPATITIS IN HOSPITAL PERSONNEL

Patients with hepatitis can infect hospital personnel with the

Table 6 Serologic Markers of Hepatitis B Infection

HBsAg	Present in acute and chronic infection Indicator that person is infectious
Anti-HBs	Appears 2 to 16 wk after HBsAg disappears from the serum Persists for years Confers immunity
HBcAg	Not present in the serum Found in the hepatocyte
Anti-HBc	Appears in serum with or shortly after HBsAg Persists for years May be only indicator of hepatitis B infection
HBeAg	Appears in the early acute phase Indicates serum is highly infectious Persistence beyond 10 wk suggests progression to chronic carrier state
Anti-HBe	Good prognosis for resolution of infection

virus via needle-stick injuries and other forms of accidental exposure. Conversely, physicians who are chronic carriers of HBV or HCV can infect their patients. According to a nationwide seroepidemiologic survey reported in 1978, approximately 19% of physicians have anti-HBs, compared with 3.5% of healthy volunteer blood donors [*see Table 8*].[88] Anti-HBs was found in 28% of surgeons, the highest prevalence in any medical specialty. For physicians, the likelihood of being positive for anti-HBs correlates with age and the number of years in practice. The risk of hepatitis is greatest among medical staff members in renal dialysis units, oncology units, and the clinical laboratory. Since 1978, when these data were reported, HBV vaccination has made it impossible to perform similar, more recent studies, because vaccination rather than previous infection would be responsible for the presence of antibodies.

Physicians and other staff members who care for hemodialysis patients with end-stage renal disease are at greater risk for acquiring HBV because of the high prevalence of hepatitis in such patients [*see Table 9*].[89,90] Transmission of HBV decreases in dialysis centers when close attention is paid to hygienic technique. Isolation of patients who are carriers of HBsAg also reduces the incidence of HBV in hemodialysis patients and staff.[91]

From 0.28% to 9.3% of health care workers have antibody to HCV.[92-94] In one study from Connecticut, five (12.5%) of 40 surgeons had antibody to HCV.[92] In another study, from New York City, eight (1.75%) of 456 dentists had anti-HCV antibody.[93] The highest prevalence among dentists was found to occur in oral surgeons (9.3%). As use of vaccines for HBV becomes more widespread [*see* Management of Viral Exposure, Hepatitis B, *above*], HCV may come to predominate over HBV as the cause of the rare cases of hepatitis transmitted from hospital personnel to patients.

EPIDEMIOLOGY OF POSTTRANSFUSION HEPATITIS

Both HBV and HCV can be transmitted by percutaneous and other routes.[89] Rare cases of hepatitis have been attributed to the infusion of immune globulin, although its preparation by ethanol fractionation normally destroys hepatitis virus (as well as HIV). Albumin is pasteurized by heating at 60° C for 10 hours, which destroys hepatitis virus.

Because of the current criteria for acceptable blood donors, elimination of payment for blood donation, and serologic testing for HBV and HCV, the risk of contracting hepatitis B from a blood transfusion is now much lower than it once was. In the United States, it is now rare for either HBV or HCV to be transmitted via blood transfusion. According to the latest estimates available, the risk of HCV transmission via this route is approximately 1/103,000 (95% CI, 28,000 to 288,000), and that of HBV transmission is 1/63,000 (95% CI, 31,000 to 147,000).[95]

HDV can also be passed by transfusion. In a study of 262 patients who had posttransfusion hepatitis and whose serum was positive for HBsAg, anti-HD was found in nine patients.[96] HDV can be detected in 24% of HBsAg-positive drug abusers and in approximately 50% of HBsAg-positive hemophiliacs.

LONG-TERM EFFECTS OF CHRONIC HEPATITIS

Chronic hepatitis can lead to problems requiring surgical intervention. It can cause cirrhosis, which in turn can cause portal hypertension and bleeding varices that necessitate portal systemic shunting. In addition, HBV and HCV predispose to hepatocellular carcinoma, the most prevalent visceral cancer in the world. The condition is especially prevalent in China, Southeast Asia, and sub-Saharan Africa. It is estimated that 25% of chronically infected persons die of cirrhosis or hepatocellular carcinoma.[97] HBV coinfec-

Table 7   Serologic Patterns of Hepatitis B Infection

HBsAg	Anti-HBs	Anti-HBe	Interpretation
+	–	–	Early acute hepatitis B
+	–	+	Late acute hepatitis B
–	–	+	Window period between disappearance of HBsAg and appearance of anti-HBs *or* Chronic carrier with low HBsAg level *or* Infection in the remote past
–	+	+	Past hepatitis B infection
–	+	–	Infection in the remote past *or* Immunization with hepatitis B vaccine *or* HBIG received within the past 1 to 2 mo

+ = detectable   – = not detectable

tion appears to increase the risk of hepatocellular carcinoma in HCV-infected persons. A widespread program of vaccination against HBV could greatly decrease the incidence of hepatocellular carcinoma. Epidemiology, molecular biology, and comparative pathology provide strong circumstantial evidence that hepatitis B is a significant factor in the etiology of hepatocellular carcinoma. The risk of primary hepatocellular carcinoma is more than 250 times greater in carriers of HBV than in noncarriers. HBV markers can be found in 80% to 90% of patients with hepatocellular carcinoma. Perhaps the best epidemiologic data indicating that hepatitis B precedes hepatocellular carcinoma were obtained in Taiwan from male civil servants between 40 and 60 years of age.[98] Approximately 3,500 HBsAg carriers were matched by age and place of birth (either mainland China or Taiwan) to 3,000 HBsAg-negative men, who served as control subjects. An additional group of 16,000 HBsAg-negative men between 40 and 60 years of age served as unmatched control subjects. After subjects were followed for 2 to 4 years, 50 cases of hepatocellular carcinoma were found, all but one of which occurred in chronic HBsAg carriers.

HCV is also associated with chronic infection in a high percentage (approximately 50%) of cases. In many countries, chronic HBV infection remains the leading factor in the development of hepatocellular carcinoma, whereas in Japan, Korea, and southern Europe, 50% to 75% of cases of hepatocellular carcinoma are

Table 8   Frequency of Antibody to Hepatitis B Surface Antigen (Anti-HBs) by Physician Specialty[88]

Specialty	Number of Patients Tested	Positive Results (%)
Surgery	176	50 (28)
Pathology	37	10 (27)
Pediatrics	63	13 (21)
Internal medicine	259	46 (18)
Anesthesiology	59	10 (17)
Obstetrics-gynecology	63	10 (16)
Family practice	341	54 (16)
Nonpatient care	25	1 (4)
All others combined	169	26 (15)
Total	1,192	220 (18.5)

Table 9 Prevalence of Hepatitis B Virus (HBV) Serologic Markers in Various Populations[90]

Population		Prevalence of Serologic Markers of HBV Infection (%)	
		HBsAg	All Markers
High risk	Immigrants or refugees from areas where HBV is highly endemic	13	70–85
	Clients in institutions for the mentally retarded	10–20	35–80
	Users of illicit parenteral drugs	7	60–80
	Homosexually active men	6	35–80
	Household contacts of HBV carriers	3–6	30–60
	Hemodialysis patients	3–10	20–80
Intermediate risk	Health care workers with frequent blood contact	1–2	15–30
	Prisoners (male)	1–8	10–80
	Staffs of institutions for the mentally retarded	1	10–25
Low risk	Health care workers with no or infrequent blood contact	0.3	3–10
	Healthy adults (first-time volunteer blood donors)	0.3	3–5

associated with chronic HCV infection.[99] In Japan, mortality from hepatocellular carcinoma increased approximately twofold in the 1980s, a change that may be attributable to a higher incidence of HCV-associated liver cancer.[100]

Herpesviruses

CYTOMEGALOVIRUS

CMV is a member of the B herpesvirus family and is the largest virus known to infect humans. In some U.S. cities, the seroprevalence of CMV is 60% to 70%. Like other members of the herpesvirus family, CMV is capable of remaining within its host in a latent state, probably by down-regulating cell surface markers (e.g., HLA-1) and thus avoiding immune destruction. Latent CMV has been found in circulating mononuclear cells, polymorphonuclear cells, vascular endothelium, renal epithelial tissue, and pulmonary secretions. The virus may become reactivated in the setting of immunodeficiency, such as may arise with HIV infection, transplantation, or significant stress from operations or injuries. In nonimmunocompromised patients, CMV typically causes a self-limited mononucleosis-like syndrome characterized by fever and mild hepatic transaminase abnormalities. In immunocompromised patients, however, CMV infection can be much more severe and even potentially life threatening, causing myelosuppression, pneumonitis, colitis, and retinopathy.

Posttransfusion Cytomegalovirus Infection (Posttransfusion or Postperfusion Syndrome)

The transmission of CMV by extracorporeal perfusion is responsible for the occasional development of a syndrome similar to mononucleosis in patients who have undergone open-heart operation. The syndrome characteristically appears 3 to 5 weeks after operation; its features are splenomegaly, fever, atypical lymphocytosis, and, occasionally, hepatomegaly, erythematous rash, and eosinophilia.[89] CMV can be isolated from the blood of virtually all patients with the typi-

cal posttransfusion syndrome and from the urine of half of these patients.[89] The condition is nonfatal and self-limited, but it may result in prolonged hospitalization and a long, expensive search for the source of fever. Although uncommon in adults 30 years of age and older, the syndrome can occur in as many as 10% of susceptible children and adults younger than 30 years.

This syndrome can also occur in patients who receive transfusions but who do not undergo open-heart operation. Occasional cases that develop postoperatively in patients who did not receive transfusions are thought to be the result of reactivation of latent infection. EBV can sometimes cause the syndrome.

The incidence of posttransfusion CMV infection is related to the kind of blood or blood product transfused. CMV is highly cell associated and is transmitted with leukocytes, which may be present in transfusions of packed red blood cells, platelets, or white blood cells; transmission from transfusion of fresh frozen plasma or cryoprecipitate has not been documented.[14] Therefore, efforts to decrease the number of white blood cells in the transfused blood would be expected to decrease the rate of transfusion-associated CMV infection. Approximately 50% of patients who receive whole blood seroconvert to CMV, whereas only 10% of those who receive washed packed red blood cells seroconvert. The risk of seroconversion to CMV is between 12% and 100% when whole blood, either fresh or stored, is transfused.[101] In one study, transfusion of frozen deglycerolized red blood cells resulted in seroconversion in only 3% of patients,[89] whereas in another, seroconversion occurred in 58% of 36 leukemic patients transfused with lymphocytes.[102]

The risk of posttransfusion CMV infection is also related to the volume of blood received. In one study, 7% of patients receiving a single unit of whole blood seroconverted, whereas anti-CMV antibody titers rose in 21% of patients receiving more than one unit.[103] The risk of infection per unit of blood transfused is estimated to range between 2.7% and 12%.[104]

Preexisting antibody to CMV does not protect transfusion recipients against reinfection. After transfusion of whole blood, titers of antibody to CMV will increase in 10% of recipients (an indication of reinfection) and in 19% of patients who did not have antibody to CMV before transfusion (an indication of infection). Whereas a seronegative recipient of CMV-positive blood has a 21% chance of seroconversion, the risk of seroconversion from the receipt of one unit of CMV-negative blood is only 2%.[89] However, the sensitivity of the serologic test for CMV is such that even when blood that tests seronegative is used, there is still a residual 0% to 6% risk of CMV transmission.[105]

Because so many patients receive blood transfusions during operation, it is understandable that evidence of posttransfusion CMV infection has been found in many patients postoperatively (e.g., after gynecologic surgery, cholecystectomy, appendectomy, lumbosacral fusion, splenectomy, and transplantation). It has also been found in surgical patients who are victims of trauma or burns.

However, it is surprising that infection with CMV, a ubiquitous virus, does not occur more frequently after transfusion. Between 30% and 54% of the adult population in the United States have antibody to CMV, an indication of previous infection.[89] Because infection with the virus is probably lifelong, a significant proportion of blood donors harbor the virus. The prevalence of antibody to CMV is 25% in units of blood from donors between 18 and 23 years of age and increases to 89% in blood from donors older than 60 years. The overall prevalence of seropositive blood donors is between 30% and 70%.

Cytomegalovirus in Transplant Recipients

CMV infection occurs not only in patients who have received blood transfusions but also in those who have suffered trauma, those receiving immunosuppressive therapy, and those with neoplastic disease. The groups at highest risk for CMV infection are probably recipients of organ transplants and of bone marrow transplants.[106-108] Numerous studies have documented the high incidence of CMV infection after organ transplantation: the rates range from 26% to 100%.[89,109,110] Primary CMV infection occurs in patients who do not have antibody to CMV before receiving transplants. Infections are considered to be reactivated if they occur in patients who did have antibody to CMV before receiving transplants. Rates of infection in patients receiving cardiac or bone marrow transplants are similar to those in patients receiving kidney transplants.

The high incidence of CMV infections after transplantation was recognized in the early days of such procedures. At autopsy of patients who died after renal transplantation, the intranuclear inclusions typical of CMV were found in tissue from the lungs, the parotid glands, the lymph nodes, the liver, the pancreas, the parathyroid, and the brain. CMV has been cultured repeatedly from the urine of transplant recipients, and the frequency of seroconversion among them has been high.

Likely sources of the virus are blood, because fresh blood can transmit CMV, and the organ transplant itself, because CMV can grow in renal tubular epithelial cells and can be transmitted as a latent virus. In several studies, recipients of kidney transplants had a much higher incidence of CMV infection when the donors had antibody to CMV than when the donors did not. In one study, 57% of recipients of kidneys from seropositive donors acquired CMV infection after transplantation, compared with 8% of recipients of kidneys from seronegative donors.[111] Even patients who have antibody to CMV can acquire new CMV infections as a result of transfusion or transplantation because there is more than one antigenic variety of the virus. Also, CMV that is latent in many patients who have antibody before transplantation may be reactivated after transplantation by host versus graft reactions, corticosteroids, or other immunosuppressive drugs. Hospital personnel, family members, and the environment play very small roles in transmission of CMV to transplant recipients.

Several systematic studies have demonstrated that CMV causes clinical illness in renal transplant recipients. In four studies, clinical illness developed in 83% of 76 patients with primary infection, compared with 44% of 268 patients with reactivation of a previous infection.[89,109,110]

Recipients of renal transplants in whom CMV causes clinical illness most commonly present with fever. Fever occurs in 95% of patients with CMV infection and may be prolonged. Patients with CMV infection also frequently present with anorexia, arthralgias, and leukopenia. Other clinical features of the disease are diffuse pulmonary infiltrates, pancreatitis, transplant malfunction, and systemic bacterial and fungal superinfections. Invasion of the GI tract by CMV may cause gastritis and ulcers in both the duodenum and the colon, which in turn may lead to hemorrhage and perforation. Biopsies demonstrate CMV inclusions at the base of the ulcers. The virus appears to invade the vascular endothelium, and bleeding is possibly a result of vascular occlusion and ischemic necrosis of the overlying tissue.

Lethal CMV disease is characterized by the presence of most of the features listed above. Liver dysfunction is found in 100% of patients with lethal disease but in only 50% to 75% of patients with mild or moderate infection, and CMV viremia occurs in 46% to 48% of patients with severe CMV infection but in only 26% to 28% of patients with mild to moderate infection. Leukopenia and the presence of atypical leukocytes also correlate with the severity of the disease. CMV infection after renal transplantation is also associated with pneumonia, hepatitis, encephalitis, and retinitis.

Whether or not CMV infection causes or leads to graft rejection is uncertain. Both the highest incidence of CMV infection (> 80%)[89,109,110] and the highest incidence of graft rejection occur within the first 3 months after transplantation. In several studies, young patients and recipients of second kidney transplants were at higher risk for graft loss if they had CMV than if they did not.[89,109,110] In most studies, however, it is extremely difficult to demonstrate a relation between CMV infection and graft rejection.

Of the multiple factors affecting the risk of CMV infection in transplant recipients, the most important are (1) the familial relation and HLA matching between the kidney donor and the recipient and (2) the CMV serology of both the donor and the recipient. The presence of antibody in transplant recipients before transplantation seems to offer a small amount of protection against fever caused by CMV but does not protect against more serious consequences of the infection, such as leukopenia, graft failure, and death.

CMV infection is also a major problem in liver, heart, and bone marrow transplant recipients.[106,108] In liver transplant recipients, CMV is a cause of hepatitis and liver dysfunction that can be confused with rejection or other causes of liver malfunction,[106] and it can lead to lethal infection. CMV pneumonitis in bone marrow transplant recipients is the most common life-threatening infectious complication after transplantation. The severity of infection in bone marrow transplant recipients may be attributable to the higher incidence of host versus graft disease in patients with CMV pneumonitis (82%) than in those without CMV pneumonitis (27%).[112]

Prevention and Treatment of Cytomegalovirus Infection

Several methods have been proposed to reduce the incidence of CMV infection after transfusion or transplantation. One method is to eliminate as many white blood cells as possible from transfused blood because CMV is almost certainly transmitted solely through these cells. From 90% to 100% of viable leukocytes in blood have been removed from frozen deglycerolized erythrocytes. In one study, transfusion of 24 hemodialyzed patients with leukocyte-free red blood cells from frozen deglycerolized blood prevented subsequent CMV infection.[104]

Another approach is to transfuse blood only from CMV-negative donors. Because the majority of posttransfusion CMV infections are asymptomatic, however, the increased cost of performing serologic tests on all donated units might be difficult to justify.

Storage of blood to reduce infectiousness of CMV is another approach, but storage from 48 to 72 hours does not significantly reduce transmission of CMV infection. Irradiating the blood to render the CMV noninfectious is unacceptable because it causes cell transformation in vitro. Furthermore, in one study, administration of leukocytes previously exposed to 1,500 cGy (1,500 rads) of gamma radiation resulted in an increased incidence of CMV infection among recipients of these cells.[102]

Because the incidence of CMV infection is higher in patients who receive kidney transplants from seropositive donors, some centers do not transplant kidneys from seropositive donors into seronegative recipients. However, no published reports indicate that this practice leads to a significant alteration in the outcome of renal transplantation with respect to graft rejection. Moreover, excluding kidneys from seropositive donors makes it more difficult to find kidneys for seronegative recipients.

Many attempts have been made to develop a CMV vaccine for administration before viral exposure by multiple passages of the virus in tissue culture. Two such vaccines have been used in clinical trials, one prepared from the AD169 strain and the other from the Towne 125 strain of the virus. Immunization with these vaccines can elicit both serum antibody and cell-mediated immunity. In one trial, the vaccine prepared from the Towne 125 strain lowered the incidence of clinical disease but not of infection, and the disease tended to be less severe in vaccinated patients than in control subjects who received placebo.[113]

Human IG has been administered after transfusion or transplantation in attempts to prevent associated CMV infection. In one study, it reduced life-threatening infection to a less severe form in most patients, but in other studies, not surprisingly, it provided no consistent benefit.[114-117] In patients who are already seropositive, the virus is latent inside their cells, where it is probably not accessible to serum antibody. Patients with primary infections may not benefit from antibody treatment, because herpesviruses seem to transfer from cell to cell without ever existing free in serum. Even CMV hyperimmune globulin has no clear benefit in patients with clinical CMV infection.[118] It may, however, help control severe infections, such as those seen in bone marrow transplant recipients.

Several antiviral agents have been used in attempts to reduce the incidence or lessen the effect of CMV infection. Among these agents are interferon, transfer factor, immune globulin, and nucleoside derivatives, such as cytarabine, vidarabine, and acyclovir (see below). Immune globulins, acyclovir, and ganciclovir are effective at preventing CMV infection in transplant recipients.[109,110,114,119,120] Ganciclovir and foscarnet are active against CMV in vitro. Ganciclovir is currently being used to treat CMV and is the most effective agent in organ transplant recipients (see below).[109,110,119-121]

EPSTEIN-BARR VIRUS

EBV is the herpesvirus responsible for infectious mononucleosis. It can be found in B cells in peripheral blood of infected patients and in tumor cells of patients with Burkitt lymphoma and nasopharyngeal carcinoma. It remains in a latent form in an infected host for years, probably for life. Most posttransfusion EBV infections are asymptomatic. Seroconversion to EBV will develop in approximately 8% of recipients transfused with between two and 14 units of blood. In as many as 5% of patients with preexisting antibody to EBV, significant elevations of antibody titers may develop, beginning

2 weeks after transfusion. These elevations indicate either reinfection or reactivation of a latent infection.[89] Because EBV is associated with cells and does not exist free in serum to any great extent, antibody to EBV in either donors or recipients is unlikely to provide substantial protection against infection resulting from blood transfusions or organ transplants. Among transfused patients who do not have preexisting antibody to EBV, the prevalence of EBV infection can reach 33% to 46%. In these patients, the absence of preexisting antibody presumably rules out reactivation of latent EBV infection as the source of infection.

EBV occurs worldwide. In the United States, nearly all adults and as many as 65% of persons of all ages have antibody to EBV. Infection is thought to occur in infancy, and as many as 17% of infants have antibody to EBV. By 5 years of age, 72% of children have antibody to EBV, and the prevalence in adults is similar.[122] Thus, the majority of blood donors in the United States have been previously infected with EBV and probably have latent virus in their leukocytes. Although it is clear that EBV can be transmitted by blood when the transfusion occurs within 3 days of donation, it is not known whether blood stored for longer periods can transmit the virus. Because EBV is predominantly intracellular, plasma and its derivatives do not transmit the virus.

The diagnosis of EBV infection is made serologically. Tests both for IgM antibody to capsid antigens and for IgG antibody to the early antigens of EBV or tests of serial samples for IgG antibody to capsid antigens must be used. The heterophil antibody test (the Paul-Bunnell test) and a rapid slide test that is equivalent (the monospot test) are also used in most clinical studies to screen for EBV infection before more specific diagnostic tests are performed.

In cases of posttransfusion infection, IgG antibody to EBV can be detected at least 10 days before the onset of symptoms, and EBV can be cultured from circulating lymphocytes 11 days before the onset of symptoms. In patients with acute infection, EBV is found in approximately three of every 10^4 peripheral blood lymphocytes.[123] In contrast, all recovered persons with antibodies to EBV are thought to have the virus in one of every 10^7 circulating lymphocytes.

EBV is strongly implicated in the etiology of a posttransplantation lymphoproliferative disorder (PTLD).[89,124,125] EBV has been isolated from the tissues of most cases of PTLD, but not all.[126,127] Non–EBV-related cases of PTLD typically occur later after transplantation, and their etiology has not been elucidated.

PTLD comprises three general clinical presentations: (1) a mononucleosis-like syndrome involving the tonsils and the peripheral lymph nodes, (2) a diffuse polymorphous B-cell infiltration in many visceral organs, and (3) localized extranodal tumors in the GI tract, the neck, the thorax, or other parts of the body. Patients whose disease is limited to a single organ or to lymph nodes often respond to a reduction in immunosuppression or antiviral therapy; however, once the infection becomes widespread, the disease progresses rapidly and is fatal in more than 75% of cases.[128] In solid organ transplant recipients, PTLD may be limited to the allograft. There is some evidence to suggest that PTLD may have organ-specific features that promote lymphoproliferation: allograft involvement has been reported in 17% of renal transplant recipients, 8.6% of liver transplant recipients, and as many as 60% to 80% of lung or intestinal transplant recipients.[128]

The persons at highest risk for PTLD are EBV-seronegative persons receiving EBV-positive organs or bone marrow. Most infections occur within the first 4 months after transplantation.[129] Several specific risk factors for the development of PTLD have been identified: a seropositive graft in a seronegative recipient, certain types of organ allografts (with intestinal transplants carrying the highest risk), any type of immunosuppression that blunts cellular immunity to EBV (with risk increasing as immunosuppression becomes more pronounced), and the presence of other infections (CMV in particular).

The optimal treatment of lymphoproliferative disorders remains unclear. Some early EBV-associated lymphoproliferative disorders in solid organ transplant recipients have regressed completely after reduction of immunosuppression.[130,131] Early PTLD may respond to antiviral therapy with acyclovir or ganciclovir, which may prevent infection of resting B cells, but such therapy is less likely to be effective in the face of high concentrations of latently infected circulating or tissue-invasive B cells. Some investigators also report resolution of PTLD after treatment with interferon alfa.[132,133]

Transmission of EBV can occur simultaneously with transmission of CMV or hepatitis virus. Although hepatitis accompanies EBV infections in sporadic cases, EBV alone has not been documented as a cause of posttransfusion hepatitis.

HERPES SIMPLEX VIRUS

Infection or reactivation of infection with herpes simplex virus type 1 (HSV-1) follows renal transplantation in 50% to 75% of patients, most often within 30 days after transplantation. Reactivation of infection is more common than primary infection: only 14% of patients who are seronegative before transplantation become infected, but infection is reactivated in 64% of patients who were already seropositive before transplantation.

Most cases of HSV-1 infection after transplantation are clinically inapparent and are indicated only by a significant rise in titer of antibody to the virus. The most prevalent clinical manifestation is herpes labialis, that is, fever blisters affecting not only the lips but also the mucous membranes of the oral cavity and the skin of the head and neck. Although these lesions are painful and may make eating, drinking, and taking oral medications difficult, they are usually self-limited and heal without treatment or reduction of immunosuppression. However, HSV-1 infection can take a much more malignant course, disseminating to cause pneumonitis, fulminant hepatitis, upper GI hemorrhage, encephalitis, aseptic meningitis, and death.

VARICELLA-ZOSTER VIRUS

Varicella-zoster virus (VZV), another herpesvirus, is the etiologic agent of herpes zoster and chicken pox. This virus resides in the dorsal root ganglia of adults who had primary varicella infection in childhood. Herpes zoster is more common in organ transplant recipients, in patients with cancer (especially those who have leukemia or lymphomas), in burn patients, and in patients receiving immunosuppressive drugs. Serologic evidence of VZV infection occurs in 8% to 16% of renal transplant recipients. The lesions of herpes zoster become evident 12 to 511 days after organ transplantation.

In children or adults who have not already had chicken pox and occasionally even in children who have, VZV can cause disseminated chicken pox in many organs, which may be fatal.

AGENTS EFFECTIVE AGAINST HERPESVIRUSES

Because the essential synthetic activities of viruses depend on the metabolic machinery of their host, it has been difficult to devise specific antiviral agents that interfere with viral replication but are not harmful to host cells.[134,135] Many antiviral agents are too toxic to be used clinically. In contrast, antibacterial agents that are both toxic to bacteria and safe for human cells are easier to design because the structure and metabolic machinery of bacteria are distinct from those of host cells.

Although intracellular processes unique to viral replication have

been identified and specifically targeted for chemotherapeutic attack, very few agents have been effective against human viruses. Among these is amantadine, which is used for both prophylaxis and treatment of influenza A. Agents that were found to be effective for prophylaxis against smallpox, such as methisazone, now have no use, because the disease has been eradicated.

There are few effective chemotherapeutic agents for hepatitis or most of the other major viral diseases that concern surgeons, but several agents have been used for the treatment of herpesvirus infections, especially in immunosuppressed patients [*see Table 10*]. These agents, derivatives of purines and pyrimidines, interfere with viral nucleic acid synthesis.

Acyclovir and Valacyclovir

Acyclovir (acycloguanosine) is a nucleoside derivative that is used to treat herpesvirus infections, especially herpes simplex and varicella-zoster infections in immunocompromised hosts. Valacyclovir is the L-valyl ester prodrug of acyclovir. In cases of mucocutaneous herpes simplex and herpes zoster, acyclovir can shorten the period of virus shedding, decrease pain, and promote more rapid scabbing and healing of lesions. Acyclovir is also the drug of choice for encephalitis caused by herpes simplex, but it is not effective in patients with established neurologic damage resulting from herpes simplex or varicella-zoster infections or in patients infected with CMV. Acyclovir inhibits the replication of EBV in actively replicating cells but does not affect latent or persistent infection.

The total daily dose of acyclovir is 10 to 25 mg/kg, given by I.V. infusion lasting 60 minutes. The recommended length of parenteral acyclovir therapy ranges from 5 to 10 days, depending on the indication. A major side effect of such therapy is phlebitis at the injection site; rash, leukopenia, and neurotoxicity may also occur. Acyclovir applied topically as a 5% ointment is effective in immunocompromised patients for the treatment of limited cutaneous herpes infections and in patients with normal immunity for the treatment of initial episodes (but not recurrent episodes) of genital herpes simplex infection. Oral acyclovir seems to be effective as prophylaxis against reactivated herpes simplex infection in recipients of bone marrow transplants and in patients immunosuppressed as a result of HIV infection.

Penciclovir and Famciclovir

Penciclovir is a nucleoside analogue that is similar to acyclovir with respect to spectrum of activity and potency against herpesviruses. Famciclovir is the diacetyl ester of penciclovir. Penciclovir requires thymidine kinase (TK) for phosphorylation and thus is inactive against thymidine kinase–deficient strains of HSV or VZV; however, it may be active against some TK-altered or polymerase mutants that are resistant to acyclovir as well as against some foscarnet-resistant HSV isolates. In experimental settings, topical, parenteral, and oral penciclovir and oral famciclovir have been effective against HSV infection.

Vidarabine

Vidarabine (ara-A) is effective against herpes simplex and varicella-zoster viruses as well as poxviruses, oncornaviruses, and rhabdoviruses. It is used mostly to combat herpesvirus infections in immunosuppressed patients. In these patients, vidarabine accelerates healing of cutaneous herpes zoster, decreases its rates of cutaneous dissemination and of visceral complications, and shortens the duration of postherpetic neuralgia. For systemic use, a daily dose of 10 to 15 mg/kg of vidarabine is administered I.V. over a period of 12 hours. The duration of therapy for herpes zoster is

Table 10   Antiviral Therapy of Clinical Benefit

Virus	Condition	Regimen
Herpes simplex virus	Keratitis	3% Acyclovir ointment *or* 1% Trifluridine solution *or* 3% Vidarabine ointment *or* 0.5% IDU ointment or 0.1% IDU drops
	Herpes labialis	Treatment usually not indicated; may use 1% penciclovir cream or topical acyclovir q. 2 hr while patient is awake for 4 days
	Genital herpes Primary	Acyclovir, 200 mg p.o. 5 times daily or 400 mg p.o., t.i.d., for 10 days, *or* Valacyclovir, 500 mg–1 g p.o., b.i.d., for 10–14 days, *or* Famciclovir, 250 mg p.o., t.i.d., for 10 days*
	Recurrent	Acyclovir, 200 mg p.o. 5 times daily or 400 mg p.o., t.i.d., for 5 days, *or* Valacyclovir, 500 mg p.o., b.i.d., for 5 days, *or* Famciclovir, 125 mg p.o., b.i.d., for 5 days
	Prophylaxis	Acyclovir, 400 mg p.o., b.i.d., *or* Valacyclovir, 500 mg–1 g p.o., q.d., *or* Famciclovir, 250 mg p.o., b.i.d.
	Encephalitis	Acyclovir, 10 mg/kg t.i.d. I.V. for 14–21 days
	Neonatal HSV	Acyclovir, 10 mg/kg I.V. q. 8 hr for 10–21 days (20 mg/kg I.V. q. 8 hr if neonate is premature)
	Immunocompromised host	Acyclovir, 5 mg/kg I.V. q. 8 hr for 7 days or 400 mg p.o. 5 times daily for 14–21 days, *or* Famciclovir, 500 mg p.o., b.i.d., for 7 days,* *or* Valacyclovir, 1 g p.o., t.i.d., for 7 days*

Varicella-zoster virus	Immunocompetent host
	   Eye infections
	   Shingles
		3% Acyclovir ointment
		 Acyclovir, 800 mg p.o. 5 times daily for 7–10 days, *or*
		 Valacyclovir, 1 g p.o., t.i.d., for 7–10 days, *or*
		 Famciclovir, 500 mg p.o., t.i.d., for 7–10 days

	Immunocompromised host	Acyclovir, 10–12 mg/kg I.V. q. 8 hr for 7 days (500 mg/m²)
Cytomegalovirus	Immunocompromised host Retinitis	Ganciclovir, 5 mg/kg I.V. q. 12 hr for 14–21 days,† *or* Foscarnet, 90 mg/kg (adjusted for renal function) I.V. q. 12 hr for 14–21 days, *or* Cidofovir, 5 mg/kg I.V. weekly for 2 weeks, then every other week
	CMV pneumonia	Ganciclovir, 2.5 mg/kg I.V. q.d. for 20 days

*Not approved by the FDA for this indication.
†An intraocular insert is also available.

5 days. Side effects include anorexia, weight loss, nausea, vomiting, weakness, anemia, leukopenia, thrombocytopenia, tremors, and thrombophlebitis at the site of administration.

Idoxuridine

Idoxuridine (5-iodo-2′-deoxyuridine) (IUdR, IDU) was the first clinically effective antiviral nucleoside. It is a halogenated pyrimidine that resembles thymidine in structure. Topical application of either a 0.1% solution or a 0.5% ointment of idoxuridine is effective treatment of herpes simplex keratitis but not of recurrent herpes labialis or localized zoster. In the United States, IDU is approved only for topical treatment of HSV keratitis. When combined with dimethyl sulfoxide (DMSO), IDU is active against herpes zoster and recurrent or primary genital HSV infection. In Europe, IDU is available in combination with DMSO for the treatment of herpes labialis, herpes genitalis, and herpes zoster.

Ganciclovir

Ganciclovir (DHPG, 2′-NDG, or BIOLF-62) is an acyclic nucleoside structurally related to acyclovir but with greater activity against CMV in vitro and in vivo. It is effective in treating CMV disease in transplant recipients and AIDS patients. The usual total daily dose of ganciclovir is 7.5 to 10 mg/kg, given in two or three divided doses. The dosage should be adjusted if the patient has decreased renal function. Myelosuppression is the principal dose-limiting toxic side effect.

Foscarnet

Foscarnet (trisodium phosphonoformate) is a pyrophosphate derivative that inhibits herpesvirus DNA polymerases and retroviral reverse transcriptases.[134-136] In the United States, it has been used for the prevention and treatment of CMV retinitis in patients with AIDS. For patients who have received renal or bone marrow transplants, foscarnet is given in a bolus injection of 9 mg/kg followed by infusion of 0.015 to 0.090 mg/kg/min I.V. for 7 days. Foscarnet is also used to treat acyclovir-resistant HSV infection. The major toxicity associated with foscarnet is nephrotoxicity; CNS side effects (e.g., headache, tremor, irritability, and seizures) can also occur.

Viral Infections from Animal and Human Bites

Surgeons are frequently called on to treat patients who have been bitten by either an animal or another person. Such bites can transmit several viruses and other infections. Certainly, rabies is the most feared viral infection transmitted in this way. Viruses that are found in saliva, such as HBV, herpesviruses, and possibly HIV, can be transmitted by a human bite, although such cases are most likely rare.

From zero to five cases of human rabies occur each year in the United States. Animal rabies is widespread and is found in every state except Hawaii. In 1992, more than 8,600 cases of animal rabies were reported to the CDC by 49 states, the District of Columbia, and Puerto Rico. The great majority of cases occur in wild animals.[69] Before 1950, more than 8,000 cases of rabies in dogs were reported each year in the United States; the number is now fewer than 150 a year.

Rabies proceeds from a prodrome of fever, malaise, and headache, to hyperactivity and diffuse cerebral dysfunction, and then to coma and death. From 5% to 20% of patients may also show progressive paralysis. Occasionally, there is no history of an animal bite. Diagnosis can be confirmed by culture of saliva, cerebrospinal fluid, or brain tissue; demonstration of rabies antigen in the cornea or skin; or measurement of serum antibody to rabies virus. At postmortem examination, typical intracytoplasmic inclusions (Negri bodies) can be seen in the brain cells.

Although the number of cases of human rabies is small, the disease is an important problem because of the large number of animal bites that occur each year. Surgeons may have to consider rabies prophylaxis in patients whom they treat for bite injuries [see Management of Viral Exposure, Rabies, above, and I:8 Acute Wound Care]. Also, two fatal cases of rabies have occurred in recipients of corneal transplants from a patient whose cause of death was later found to be rabies.[137]

References

1. Recommendations for prevention of HIV transmission in health-care settings. MMWR Morb Mortal Wkly Rep 36(suppl 2):1S, 1987
2. Recommendations for preventing transmission of infection with human T-lymphocyte type III/lymphadenopathy-associated virus in the workplace. MMWR Morb Mortal Wkly Rep 34:681, 1985
3. Update: universal precautions for prevention of transmission of human immunodeficiency virus, hepatitis B virus, and other blood-borne pathogens in health-care settings. MMWR Morb Mortal Wkly Rep 37:377, 1988
4. Guidelines for prevention of transmission of human immunodeficiency virus and hepatitis B virus to health-care and public-safety workers. MMWR Morb Mortal Wkly Rep 38(suppl 6):1, 1989
5. Recommendations for HIV testing services for inpatients and outpatients in acute-care hospital settings and technical guidance on HIV counseling. MMWR Morb Mortal Wkly Rep 42(RR-2):1, 1993
6. Rhame F, Maki D: The case for wider use of testing for HIV infection. N Engl J Med 320:1248, 1989
7. Telford GL, Quebbeman EJ, Condon RE: A protocol to reduce risk of contracting AIDS and other blood-borne disease in the OR. Surg Rounds 10:30, 1987
8. Recommendations for follow up of health care workers after occupational exposure to hepatitis C. MMWR Morb Mortal Wkly Rep 46:603, 1997
9. Mast EE, Alter MJ: Prevention of hepatitis B virus infection among health-care workers. Hepatitis B Vaccines in Clinical Practice. Ellis RW, Ed. Marcel Dekker, New York, 1993, p 295
10. Werner BG, Grady GF: Accidental hepatitis B-surface-antigen-positive inoculations: use of e antigen to estimate infectivity. Ann Intern Med 97:367, 1982
11. Gerberding JL: Management of occupational exposures to blood-borne viruses. N Engl J Med 125:917, 1996
12. Sepkowitz KA: Occupationally acquired infections in health care workers (part II). Ann Intern Med 125:917, 1996
13. Department of Labor, OSHA: Occupational exposure to blood-borne pathogens. Final rule. Fed Regist 56:64175, 1991
14. Sepkowitz KA: Nosocomial hepatitis and other infections transmitted by blood and blood products. Principles and Practice of Infectious Disease, 5th ed. Mandell GL, Bennet JE, Dolin R, Eds. Churchill Livingstone, Philadelphia, 2000, p 3039
15. Protection against viral hepatitis: recommendations of the Immunization Practices Advisory Committee (ACIP). MMWR Morb Mortal Wkly Rep 39 (RR-2):1, 1990
16. Syndman DR, Bryan JA, Dixon RE: Prevention of nosocomial viral hepatitis, type B (hepatitis B). Ann Intern Med 83:838, 1975
17. Favero MS, Maynard JE, Leger RT, et al: Guidelines for the care of patients hospitalized with viral hepatitis. Ann Intern Med 91:872, 1979
18. Ciesielski C, Marianos D, Ou C-Y, et al: Transmission of human immunodeficiency virus in a dental practice. Ann Intern Med 116:798, 1992
19. Lot F, Seguier J, Fegeux S, et al: Probable transmission of HIV from an orthopedic surgeon to a patient in France. Ann Intern Med 130:1, 1999
20. Welch J, Webster M, Tilzey A, et al: Hepatitis B infections after gynecological surgery. Lancet 1:205, 1989
21. Lettau LA, Smith JD, Williams D, et al: Transmission of hepatitis B with resultant restriction of surgical practice. JAMA 255:934, 1986
22. Communicable Disease Surveillance Centre: Acute hepatitis B associated with gynaecological surgery. Lancet 1:1, 1980
23. Carl M, Frances DP, Blakey DL, et al: Interruption of hepatitis B transmission by modification of a gynaecologist's surgical technique. Lancet 1:731, 1982
24. Coutinho RA, Albrecht-van Lent P, Stoutjesdijk L, et al: Hepatitis B from doctors (letter). Lancet 1:345, 1982
25. Grob PJ, Bischof B, Naeff F: Cluster of hepatitis B transmitted by a physician. Lancet 2:1218, 1981
26. Meyers JD, Stamm WE, Kerr MM, et al: Lack of transmission of hepatitis B after surgical exposure. JAMA 240:1725, 1978
27. Haerem JW, Siebke JC, Ulstrup J, et al: HBsAg transmission from a cardiac surgeon incubating hepatitis B resulting in chronic antigenemia in four patients. Acta Med Scand 210:389, 1981
28. Acute hepatitis B following gynecological surgery. J Hosp Infect 9:34, 1987
29. Polakoff S: Acute hepatitis B in patients in Britain related to previous operations and dental treatment. Br J Med 293:33, 1986
30. Heptonstall J: Outbreaks of hepatitis B virus infection associated with infected surgical staff. Communicable Disease Report 1:R81, 1991
31. Surgeons who are hepatitis B carriers. BMJ 303:184, 1991
32. Jones D: Hepatitis leaves Halifax surgeon an operating room outcast. Can Med Assoc J 145:1345, 1991
33. Alter HJ, Chalmers TC, Freeman BM, et al: Health-care workers positive for hepatitis B surface antigen: are their contacts at risk? N Engl J Med 292:454, 1975
34. Williams SV, Pattison CP, Berquist KR: Dental infection with hepatitis B. JAMA 232:1231, 1975
35. Gerber MA, Lewin EB, Gerety RJ, et al: The lack of nurse-infant transmission of type B hepatitis in a special care nursery. J Pediatr 91:120, 1977
36. LaBrecque DR, Dhand AK: The risk of hepatitis B transmission from staff to patients in hemodialysis units—an overrated problem? Hepatology 1:398, 1981
37. LaBrecque DR, Muhs JM, Lutwick LI, et al: The risk of hepatitis B transmission from health care workers to patients in a hospital setting—a prospective study. Hepatology 6:205, 1986
38. Recommendations for preventing transmission of human immunodeficiency virus and hepatitis B virus to patients during exposure-prone invasive procedures. MMWR Morb Mortal Wkly Rep 40(RR-8), 1991
39. Esteban JI, Gomez J, Martell M, et al: Transmission of hepatitis C by a cardiac surgeon. N Engl J Med 334:555, 1996
40. Bosch H: Hepatitis C outbreak astounds Spain. Lancet 352:1415, 1998
41. Public Health Service guidelines for the management of health-care worker exposures to HIV and recommendations for post-exposure prophylaxis. MMWR Morb Mortal Wkly Rep 47:1, 1998
42. Chiarello LA, Gerberding JL: Human immunodeficiency virus in health care settings. Principles and Practice of Infectious Disease, 5th ed. Mandell GL, Bennett JE, Dolin R, Eds. Churchill Livingstone, Philadelphia, 2000, p 3052
43. Ciesielski CA, Metler RP: Duration of time between exposure and seroconversion in healthcare workers

with occupationally acquired infection with human immunodeficiency virus. Am J Med 102(suppl 5B): S115, 1997

44. Busch MP, Satten GA: Time course of viremia and antibody seroconversion following human immunodeficiency virus exposure. Am J Med 102(suppl 5B):S117, 1997

45. Cardo DM, Culver DH, Ciesielski CA, et al: A case-control study of HIV seroconversion in healthcare workers after percutaneous exposure. N Engl J Med 337:1485, 1997

46. Public Health Service Statement on management of occupational exposure to human immunodeficiency virus, including considerations regarding zidovudine postexposure use. MMWR Morb Mortal Wkly Rep 39 (RR-1):1, 1990

47. Wang SA, the HIV PEP Registry Group: Human immunodeficiency virus (HIV) postexposure prophylaxis (PEP) following occupational HIV exposure: findings from the HIV PEP Registry (abstract 482). Program and abstracts of the 35th Annual Meeting of the Infectious Diseases Society of America, Alexandria, Virginia, Sept 13–16, 1997, p 161

48. Steger KA, Swotinsky R, Snyder S, et al: Recent experience with post-exposure prophylaxis (PEP) with combination antiretrovirals for occupational exposure (OE) to HIV (abstract 480). Program and abstracts of the 35th Annual Meeting of the Infectious Diseases Society of America, Alexandria, Virginia, Sept 13–16, 1997, p 161

49. Beekmann R, Fahrner R, Nelson L, et al: Combination post-exposure prophylaxis (PEP): a prospective study of HIV-exposed health care workers (HCW) (abstract 481). Program and abstracts of the 35th Annual Meeting of the Infectious Diseases Society of America, Alexandria, Virginia, Sept 13–16, 1997, p 161

50. Imrie A, Beveridge A, Genn W, et al: Transmission of human immunodeficiency virus type 1 resistant to nevirapine and zidovudine. J Infect Dis 175:1502, 1997

51. Veenstra J, Schuurman R, Cornelissen M, et al: Transmission of zidovudine-resistant human immunodeficiency virus type 1 variants following deliberate injection of blood from a patient with AIDS: characteristics and natural history of the virus. Clin Infect Dis 21:556-60, 1995

52. Fitzgibbon JE, Gaur S, Frenkel LD, et al: Transmission from one child to another of human immunodeficiency virus type 1 with a zidovudine-resistance mutation. N Engl J Med 329:1835, 1993

53. Coombs RW, Shapiro DE, Eastman PS, et al: Maternal viral genotypic zidovudine (ZDV) resistance and infrequent failure of ZDV therapy to prevent perinatal transmission (abstract 17). Program and abstracts of the 35th Annual Meeting of the Infectious Diseases Society of America, Alexandria, Virginia, Sept 13–16, 1997, p 74

54. Protection against viral hepatitis. Recommendations of the Immunization Practices Advisory Committee (ACIP). MMWR Morb Mortal Wkly Rep 39(RR-2):1, 1990

55. Hadler SC: Are booster doses of hepatitis B vaccine necessary? Ann Intern Med 108:457, 1988

56. Hadler SC, Francis DP, Maynard JE, et al: Long-term immunogenicity and efficacy of hepatitis B vaccine in homosexual men. N Engl J Med 315:209, 1986

57. Hepatitis B virus: A comprehensive strategy for eliminating transmission in the United States through universal childhood vaccination. Advisory Committee for Immunization Practices. MMWR Morb Mortal Wkly Rep 40:PR-13, 1991

58. Barie PS, Dellinger EP, Dougherty SH, et al: Assessment of hepatitis B virus immunization status among North American surgeons. Arch Surg 129:27, 1994

59. Recommendations for prevention and control of hepatitis C virus (HCV) infection and HCV-related chronic disease. MMWR Morb Mortal Wkly Rep 47(RR-19):1, 1998

60. Noguchi S, Sata M, Suzuki H, et al: Early therapy with interferon for acute hepatitis C acquired through the needlestick. Clin Infect Dis 24:992, 1997

61. Vogen W, Graziadei I, Umlauft F, et al: High-dose interferon-α_{2b} treatment prevents chronicity in acute hepatitis C: a pilot study. Dig Dis Sci 41(suppl 12):81S, 1996

62. Ohnishi K, Nomura F, Nakano M: Interferon therapy for acute posttransfusion non-A, non-B hepatitis: response with respect to anti-hepatitis C virus antibody status. Am J Gastroenterol 86:1041, 1991

63. Rabies prevention—United States, 1991: recommendations of the Immunization Practices Advisory Committee (ACIP). MMWR Morb Mortal Wkly Rep 40:1, 1991

64. Fishbein DB, Robinson LE: Rabies. N Engl J Med 329:1632, 1993

65. Rabies prevention—United States, 1999: recommendations of the Immunization Practices Advisory Committee (ACIP). MMWR Morb Mortal Wkly Rep 48(RR-1):1, 1999

66. WHO Recommendations on Rabies Post-exposure Treatment and the Correct Technique of Intradermal Immunization against Rabies. World Health Organization, Geneva, 1997

67. Rabies prevention: supplementary statement on the preexposure use of human diploid cell rabies vaccine by the intradermal route. MMWR Morb Mortal Wkly Rep 35:767, 1986

68. Bleck TP, Rupprecht CE: Rabies virus. Principles and Practice of Infectious Disease, 5th ed. Mandell GL, Bennett JE, Dolin R, Eds. Churchill Livingstone, Philadelphia, 2000, p 1811

69. Krebs JW, Strine TW, Childs JF: Rabies surveillance in the United States during 1992. J Am Vet Med Assoc 203:1718, 1993

70. The cost of one rabid dog—California. MMWR Morb Mortal Wkly Rep 30:527, 1981

71. Bove JR: Transfusion-associated hepatitis and AIDS: what is the risk? N Engl J Med 317:242, 1987

72. Donegan E, Stuart M, Niland JC, et al: Infection with the human immunodeficiency virus type 1 (HIV1) among recipients of antibody-positive blood donations. Ann Intern Med 113:733, 1990

73. Ward JW, Deppe DA, Samson S, et al: Risk of human immunodeficiency virus infection from blood donors who later developed the acquired immunodeficiency syndrome. Ann Intern Med 106:61, 1987

74. Ward JW, Grindon AJ, Feorino PM, et al: Laboratory and epidemiologic evaluation of an enzyme immunoassay for antibodies to HTLV-III. JAMA 256:357, 1986

75. Ward JW, Holmberg AD, Allen JR, et al: Transmission of human immunodeficiency virus (HIV) by blood transfusions screened as negative for HIV antibody. N Engl J Med 318:473, 1988

76. Schreiber GB, Bush MP, Kleinman SH, et al: The risk of transfusion-transmitted viral infections: the retrovirus epidemiology donor study. N Engl J Med 334:1685, 1996

77. Horsburgh BR Jr, Ou C-Y, Jason J, et al: Duration of human immunodeficiency virus infection before detection of antibody. Lancet 2:637, 1989

78. Erice A, Rhame FS, Heussner RC, et al: Human immunodeficiency virus infection in patients with solid-organ transplants: report of five cases and review. Rev Infect Dis 13:537, 1991

79. Public Health Service guidelines for the management of health-care worker exposures to HIV and recommendations for post-exposure prophylaxis. MMWR Morb Mortal Wkly Rep 47:1, 1998

80. Guidelines for national human immunodeficiency virus case surveillance, including monitoring for human immunodeficiency virus infection and acquired immunodeficiency syndrome. MMWR Morb Mortal Wkly Rep 48(RR-13):1, 1999

81. Alter M, Mast E: The epidemiology of hepatitis in the United States. Gastroenterol Clin North Am 23:437, 1994

82. Kim CY, Tilles JG: Purification and biophysical characterization of the hepatitis B antigen. J Clin Invest 52:1176, 1973

83. Kawai H, Feinstone SM: Acute viral hepatitis. Principles and Practice of Infectious Diseases, 5th ed. Mandell GL, Bennett JE, Dolin R, Eds. Churchill Livingstone, Philadelphia, 2000, p 1279

84. Omata M: Treatment of chronic hepatitis B infection. N Engl J Med 339:114, 1998

85. Kuo G, Choo Q-L, Alter HJ, et al: An assay for circulating antibodies to a major etiologic virus of non-A, non-B hepatitis. Science 244:362, 1989

86. Hayden GH, Jarvis LM, Blair CS, et al: Clinical significance of intrahepatic hepatitis C virus levels in patients with chronic HCV infection. Gut 42:570, 1998

87. Koretz RL, Stone O, Gitnick GL: The long-term course of non-A, non-B post-transfusion hepatitis. Gastroenterology 79:893, 1980

88. Denes AE, Smith JL, Maynard JE, et al: Hepatitis B infections in physicians: results of a nationwide sero-epidemiologic survey. JAMA 239:210, 1978

89. Howard RJ: Viral infections in surgery. Problems in General Surgery 1:522, 1984

90. Recommendations for protection against viral hepatitis. MMWR Morb Mortal Wkly Rep 34:313, 1985

91. Valent WM, Wehrle PP: Selected viruses of nosocomial importance. Hospital Infections, 2nd ed. Bennett JV, Brachman PS, Eds. Little, Brown & Company, Boston, 1986, p 531

92. Cooper BW, Krusell A, Tilton RC, et al: Seroprevalence of antibodies to hepatitis C virus in high-risk hospital personnel. Infect Control Hosp Epidemiol 13:82, 1992

93. Klein RS, Freeman K, Taylor PE, et al: Occupational risk for hepatitis C virus infection among New York City dentists. Lancet 338:1539, 1991

94. Zuckerman J, Clewley G, Griffiths P, et al: Prevalence of hepatitis C antibodies in clinical health-care workers. Lancet 343:1618, 1994

95. Schreiber GB, Busch MP, Kleinman SH, et al: The risk of transfusion-transmitted viral infections. N Engl J Med 334:1685, 1996

96. Rosina F, Saracco G, Rizzetto M: Risk of posttransfusion infection with hepatitis delta virus: a multicenter study. N Engl J Med 312:1488, 1985

97. Friedman LS, Dienstag JL: Recent developments in viral hepatitis. Dis Mon 32:320, 1986

98. Beasley PR, Lin CC: Hepatoma risk among HBsAg carriers. Am J Epidemiol 108:247, 1978

99. Edamoto Y, Tani M, Durata T, et al: Hepatitis C and B virus infections in hepatocellular carcinoma—analysis of direct detection of viral genome in paraffin embedded tissues. Cancer 77:1787, 1996

100. Kiyosawa K, Furuta S: Hepatitis C virus and hepatocellular carcinoma. Curr Stud Hematol Blood Transfus 61:98, 1994

101. Rook AH, Quinnan GV Jr: Cytomegalovirus infections following blood transfusions. Infectious Complications of Blood Transfusion. Tabor E, Ed. Academic Press, San Diego, 1982, p 45

102. Winston DJ, Ho WG, Howell CL, et al: Cytomegalovirus infections associated with leukocyte transfusions. Ann Intern Med 93:671, 1980

103. Prince AM, Szmuness W, Millins SJ, et al: A serological study of cytomegalovirus infections associated with blood transfusions. N Engl J Med 284:1125, 1971

104. Tolkoff-Rubin NE, Rubin RH, Keller EE, et al: Cytomegalovirus infection in dialysis patients and personnel. Ann Intern Med 89:625, 1978

105. Bowden RA: Transfusion-transmitted cytomegalovirus infection. Hematol Oncol Clin North Am 9:155, 1995

106. Paya CV, Hermans PE, Wiesner RH, et al: Cytomegalovirus hepatitis in liver transplantation: prospective analysis of 93 consecutive orthotopic liver transplantations. J Infect Dis 160:752, 1988

107. Barkholt LM, Ericzon BG, Ehrnst A, et al: Cytomegalovirus infections in liver transplant patients: incidence and outcome. Transplant Proc 22:235, 1990

108. Englehard D, Or R, Strauss N, et al: Cytomegalovirus infection and disease after T cell depleted allogeneic bone marrow transplantation for malignant hematologic disease. Transplant Proc 21:3101, 1989

109. Griffiths PD: Current management of cytomegalovirus disease. J Med Virol (suppl 1):106, 1993

110. Farrusia E, Schwab TR: Management and prevention of cytomegalovirus infection after renal transplantation. Mayo Clin Proc 67:879, 1992

111. Ho M, Suwansirikul S, Dowling JN, et al: The transplanted kidney as a source of cytomegalovirus infection. N Engl J Med 293:1109, 1975

112. Myers JD, Fluornoy N, Thomas ED: Risk factors for cytomegalovirus infection after human marrow transplantation. J Infect Dis 153:478, 1986

113. Balfour HH Jr, Sachs GW, Welo P, et al: Cytomegalovirus vaccine in renal transplant candidates: progress report of a randomized, placebo-controlled, double-blind trial. Birth Defects 20:289, 1984

114. Snydman DR, Werner BG, Heinze-Lacey B, et al: Use of cytomegalovirus immune globulin to prevent cytomegalovirus disease in renal-transplant recipients. N Engl J Med 317:1049, 1987

115. Martin M: Antiviral prophylaxis for CMV infection in liver transplantation. Transplant Proc 25(suppl 4):10, 1993

116. Steinmuller DR, Novick AC, Streem SB, et al: Intravenous immunoglobulin infusions for the prophylaxis of secondary cytomegalovirus infection. Transplant 49:68, 1990

117. Kasiske BL, Heim-Duthoy KL, Tortorice KL: Polyvalent immune globulin and cytomegalovirus infection after renal transplantation. Arch Intern Med 149:2733, 1989

118. Lautenschlager I, Ahonen J, Eklund B, et al: Hyperimmune globulin therapy of clinical cytomegalovirus infection in renal allograft recipients. Scand J Infect Dis 21:139, 1989

119. Balfour HH Jr: Prevention of cytomegalovirus disease in renal allograft recipients. Scand J Infect Dis Suppl 80:88, 1991

120. Snydman DR, Rubin RH, Werner BG: New developments in cytomegalovirus prevention and management. Am J Kidney Dis 21:217, 1993

121. Emanuel D: Treatment of cytomegalovirus disease. Semin Hematol 27(suppl 1):22, 1990

122. Tabor E: Epstein-Barr virus and blood transfusion. Infectious Complications of Blood Transfusion. Tabor E, Ed. Academic Press, San Diego, 1982, p 65

123. Rocchi G, de Felici A, Ragona G, et al: Quantitative evaluation of Epstein-Barr-virus-infected mononuclear peripheral blood leukocytes in infectious mononucleosis. N Engl J Med 296:132, 1977

124. Armitage JM, Kormos RL, Stuart RS, et al: Posttransplant lymphoproliferative disease in thoracic organ transplant patients: ten years of cyclosporine-based immunosuppression. J Heart Lung Transplant 10:877, 1991

125. Lager DJ, Burgart LJ, Slagel DD: Epstein-Barr virus detection in sequential biopsies from patients with a posttransplant lymphoproliferative disorder. Mod Pathol 6:42, 1993

126. Dotti G, Fiocchi R, Motta T, et al: Epstein-Barr virus-negative lymphoproliferative disorders in long-term survivors after heart, kidney, and liver transplant. Transplantation 69:827, 2000

127. Leblond V, Davi F, Charlotte F, et al: Posttransplant lymphoproliferative disorders not associated with Epstein-Barr virus: a distinct entity? J Clin Oncol 16:2052, 1998

128. Preiksaitis JK, Cockfield AM: Epstein-Barr virus and lymphoproliferative disorders after transplantation. Transplant Infections. Bowden RA, Ljungman P, Paya CV, Eds. Lippincott-Raven Publishers, Philadelphia, 1998, p 245

129. Breinig MK, Zitelli B, Ho M: Epstein-Barr virus, cytomegalovirus and other viral infections in children after liver transplantation. J Infect Dis 156:273, 1987

130. Starzl TE, Porter KA, Iwatsuki SK, et al: Reversibility of lymphomas and lymphoproliferative lesions developing under cyclosporine-steroid therapy. Lancet 1:583, 1984

131. Hanto DW, Frizzera G, Gajl-Peczalska KJ, et al: Epstein-Barr virus, immunodeficiency, and B cell lymphoproliferation. Transplantation 39:461, 1985

132. Shapiro RS, McClain K, Frizzera G, et al: Epstein-Barr virus associated B cell lymphoproliferative disorders following bone marrow transplantation. Blood 71:1234, 1988

133. Benkerru M, Durandy A, Fischer A: Therapy for transplant-related lymphoproliferative diseases. Hematol Oncol Clin North Am 7:467, 1993

134. Keating MR: Antiviral agents. Mayo Clin Proc 67:160, 1992

135. de Clercq E: Antivirals for the treatment of herpesvirus infections. J Antimicrob Chemother 32(suppl A):121, 1993

136. Oberg B: Antiviral effects of phosphonoformate (PFA, foscarnet sodium). Pharmacol Ther 40:213, 1989

137. Houff SA, Burton RC, Wilson RW, et al: Human-to-human transmission of rabies virus by corneal transplant. N Engl J Med 300:603, 1979

Acknowledgments

Figure 1 Micrograph courtesy of F. K. Lee, A. J. Nahmias, and S. Stagno, Emory University. Drawing by George V. Kelvin.

Figures 4 and 5 Albert Miller.

20 ACQUIRED IMMUNODEFICIENCY SYNDROME

John Mihran Davis, M.D.

Approach to Human Immunodeficiency Virus Infection

No immediate end to the epidemic of acquired immunodeficiency syndrome (AIDS) is in sight. Because surgeons will be increasingly involved with AIDS patients, it is important for them to become familiar with the basic principles of the disease process. All operating room personnel need to take great care in handling tissue, all sharp instruments, and body secretions. Although it is hoped that a cure for human immunodeficiency virus (HIV) infection will be found soon, the likelihood of this is small.

CDC Classification of HIV Infection

The Centers for Disease Control and Prevention (CDC) has devised a classification system that includes all individuals with HIV infection, the cause of AIDS.[1] Four groups are defined. They are mutually exclusive and hierarchical in that patients classified into a particular group should not 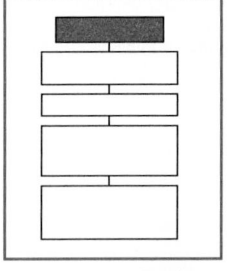 be reclassified into a preceding group if clinical findings resolve. A given patient does not necessarily pass through all four groups. This classification is based on data accumulated during the clinical application of serum antibody testing for HIV. Before the availability of such antibody testing, national reporting was considered appropriate only for patients with AIDS (i.e., severely immunosuppressed patients with opportunistic infection or secondary malignancy).[2] It is now evident that AIDS patients represent only a fraction of a larger group of HIV-infected individuals [*see Figure 1*], although the fraction has increased over the past decade and is expected to increase further.

Within most groups considered to be at risk for infection, the incidence of HIV positivity is quite high but varies depending on the region of the country. The HIV seropositivity rate in homosexual and bisexual men ranges from 10 to 70 percent and averages 25 percent. Among intravenous drug abusers in New York, northern New Jersey, and Puerto Rico, the rate of seropositivity approaches 60 percent. In contrast, in other areas of the United States, the rate of seropositivity for intravenous drug abusers is about five percent. Among hemophiliacs, the HIV seropositivity rate varies depending on the patient's need for blood products: 35 percent of hemophiliacs with the less severe hemophilia B are seropositive for HIV, whereas 70 percent of

those with hemophilia A are seropositive. Sexual partners of intravenous drug abusers, bisexuals, and hemophiliacs have an HIV-positive rate of approximately five percent.[3]

Although the natural history of AIDS has been well studied during the past several years, the prognosis for HIV-infected patients who do not have opportunistic infections or secondary cancers is still not well defined. The availability and widespread use of antibody testing should allow further understanding of the natural history of HIV infection.

GROUP I—THE ACUTE SYNDROME

The acute syndrome that occurs in some patients after HIV infection is an acute viral illness, similar in nature to an episode of mononucleosis.[4] Patients in this group are reclassified into one of the other three groups (see below) once their acute symptoms resolve. For surgeons and other health care workers, the major 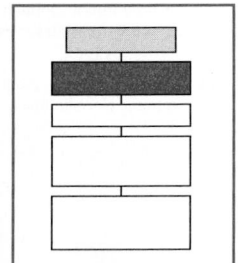 significance of patients with the acute syndrome is the risk these patients pose of transmitting HIV infection. Although some studies document that the antibody response to HIV may not appear for more than one year after exposure to the virus, detectable antibodies usually appear in six to eight weeks.[5-7] It is during the initial six weeks of infection that a patient with a negative antibody may unknowingly transmit the virus.

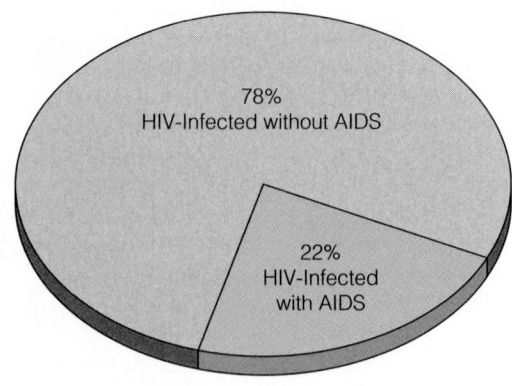

Figure 1 **Shown is the percent of HIV-infected individuals in the United States with AIDS in 1992.[85]**

Approach to Human Immunodeficiency Virus Infection

CDC classification of HIV infection

The four groups defined are mutually exclusive and hierarchical in that patients classified into a particular group should not be reclassified into a preceding group if clinical findings resolve. A given patient does not necessarily pass through all four groups.

Group I—the acute syndrome

In some individuals, HIV infection may cause an acute viral illness similar to mononucleosis. Such patients may not have detectable serum antibodies to HIV. Test symptomatic individuals who belong to one of the AIDS risk groups for HIV antibodies at the onset of symptoms and then every 3 mo for a year or until seroconversion. To detect HIV antibodies, first test serum by enzyme-linked immunosorbent assay; positive results must be confirmed by Western blot assay.

Group I patients are reclassified into one of the other three groups once their acute symptoms resolve.

Group II—the asymptomatic carrier

A large number of asymptomatic carriers are expected to undergo operation unrelated to their HIV infection. Screening of all potential surgical patients is controversial; adoption of universal precautions against HIV transmission is more appropriate.

Group III—persistent generalized lymphadenopathy

Definition is palpable lymphadenopathy > 1 cm in diameter in at least two extrainguinal sites persisting for longer than 3 mo.

Lymph node biopsy provides prognostic information:
- Explosive follicular hyperplasia, either alone or in a mixed pattern with follicular involution, suggests a prolonged clinical course, even in the presence of Kaposi's sarcoma
- Follicular involution alone is associated with opportunistic infection, Kaposi's sarcoma, lymphoma, and survival time < 1 yr
- Lymphocyte depletion represents end-stage disease

Prognosis is also closely correlated with the number of circulating helper T cells. Currently, the only indication for lymph node biopsy is to rule out a *treatable* lymphoma; however, it may be used to confirm the presence of ongoing infection.

Group IV—other human immunodeficiency virus diseases

Included are patients meeting the CDC definition of AIDS:
- Patients with at least one of 12 specified secondary infections (e.g., *Pneumocystis carinii* pneumonia) with no explanation other than HIV infection
- Patients with at least one of three secondary cancers known to be associated with HIV infection (e.g., Kaposi's sarcoma)

Surgical interventions that may be suitable for possible complications of AIDS are
- Biliary surgery for acute cholecystitis or acute cholangitis
- Resection, bypass, or colostomy for acute GI perforation or obstruction
- Splenectomy for splenomegaly or thrombocytopenia
- Indwelling central venous catheterization for drug therapy or venous access

Protect the patient from other infections by proper sterilization or disinfection of instruments and equipment.

Because acute HIV infection is possible in any symptomatic patient who is involved in high-risk behavior, antibody testing should be done at the onset of symptoms, at six weeks, and then every three months for a year or until the patient sero-converts.

Since the outbreak of the AIDS virus, the composition of AIDS patients has gradually shifted. In 1986, 90 percent of patients with AIDS were homosexual men, bisexual men, or intravenous drug abusers. The remaining 10 percent included hemophiliacs, recipients of HIV-contaminated blood, and sex partners of persons in high-risk groups. By 1995, the percentage of AIDS patients who were homosexual men had declined significantly, from 65 percent to 45 percent, and the incidence of perinatal and heterosexual transmission of HIV had increased from one percent to 11 percent.[8,9] A significant number of instances of heterosexual transmission occur among young inner-city adults and are related to the use of crack cocaine, which seems to promote high-risk sexual behavior.[10]

Detection of HIV Infection

Two tests for determining if a patient is infected with HIV are commercially available: the enzyme-linked immunosorbent assay (ELISA) and the Western blot assay. Both tests are designed to detect the presence of HIV antibody in serum. The ELISA test uses antigenic material that is adsorbed onto wells in plastic dishes. The wells are then exposed to serum from the patient who is being tested. After the test serum has reacted with the antigen, the wells are washed and then incubated with an antibody to human immunoglobulin. Before application to the wells, the antibody is linked to an enzyme that can be detected by a colorimetric reaction when exposed to the appropriate substrate. The intensity of color that is ultimately produced is directly related to the concentration of HIV antibody in the patient's blood. The ELISA test is considered very sensitive (i.e., its false negative rate is low), but its false positive rate is high. The weakness of the ELISA test is that some individuals have antibodies that react with HIV antigens but are not specific for HIV.

The Western blot assay is considered a more specific test but has a high false negative rate. It is therefore used most effectively in confirming ELISA results; it is not a good screening test. In Western blotting, antigenic HIV particles are separated by electrophoresis and then allowed to react with serum from the patient. Antigen-antibody complexes form and are subsequently identified by tagging with radiolabeled staphylococcal A protein, which has a high affinity for antigen-antibody complexes. This test is almost 100 percent positive in HIV-infected patients whose blood shows a positive ELISA reaction. Results of both the ELISA test and the Western blot assay must be positive in an individual before HIV infection can be confirmed. However, most blood banks will not use blood that has demonstrated a positive ELISA reaction, even if HIV antibody was not detected by Western blotting.[11]

On August 8, 1995, the Food and Drug Administration recommended that all blood donated for transfusion be screened for the p24 antigen (the core structural protein of HIV) to reduce the risk of administering HIV-contaminated blood.[12] With the current test for HIV, there is a so-called window period of 25 days between infection and seroconversion. It has been estimated that since 1985, when all banked blood was tested for HIV, 35 patients have contracted HIV infection

because the donor blood was collected from an HIV-infected individual during this window period.[13,14]

The p24 antigen is present in blood as soon as the virus begins to replicate, typically about two to three weeks after infection. Thus, the window period can be reduced by six days if the assay for this antigen is added to routine screening for HIV antibody. As the host begins to make virus-specific antibody to HIV, the p24 antigen is either cleared or neutralized, so that in an HIV-infected patient, the assay eventually yields negative results. For this reason, the p24 antigen assay is useful primarily as a screening test for blood, and it must be combined with a neutralization assay. In selected patients, the p24 antigen assay may be a helpful clinical tool. Additional laboratory tests that may help in the diagnosis of patients who are believed to have HIV infection but in whom HIV antibody screening yields negative results include DNA polymerase chain reaction (PCR), antigen testing after immune complex disruption, and reverse transcriptase PCR.[14]

GROUP II— THE ASYMPTOMATIC CARRIER

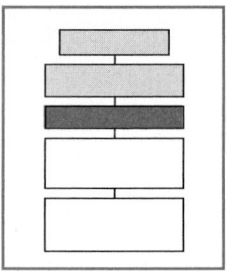

The asymptomatic carrier is the second major category of patients with HIV infection. The growing numbers of patients with heterosexually or perinatally transmitted disease [see Figure 2] has been well established by continued CDC monitoring. The evidence that military recruits and candidates for the Job Corps have HIV seroprevalence rates similar to the national average is significant because these groups are composed primarily of heterosexual sexually active teenagers.[15,16] Although the need for educational programs to reach this group of potential AIDS victims is clear, the approach has been controversial.

A 1992 analysis of hospitalized patients revealed an even higher incidence of HIV seroprevalence in this patient population (4.7 percent) than in the population at large. Because only one third of those patients with HIV seroreactivity were aware of their condition, a large population of patients were unable to benefit from antiretroviral therapy.[17] These data stress the need for routine voluntary testing and emphasize the importance of the use of universal precautions for protecting all health workers in the hospital environment.

GROUP III—PERSISTENT GENERALIZED LYMPHADENOPATHY

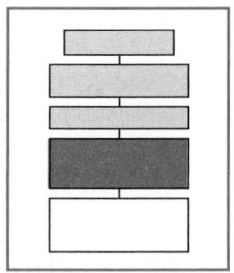

Another group of HIV-infected patients defined by the CDC comprises those with persistent generalized lymphadenopathy, that is, palpable lymphadenopathy measuring greater than 1 cm in diameter in at least two extrainguinal sites and persisting for longer than three months. Before the availability of HIV antibody testing, the relation of this lymphadenopathy to systemic manifestations of immunosuppression (systemic symptoms, neurologic symptoms, secondary infections, or cancers) was not known. It is now clear that lymphadenopathy is part of the general clinical spectrum associated with HIV infection, and opportunistic infection, Kaposi's sarcoma, or large cell lymphoma will develop in some, if not all, lymphadenopathy

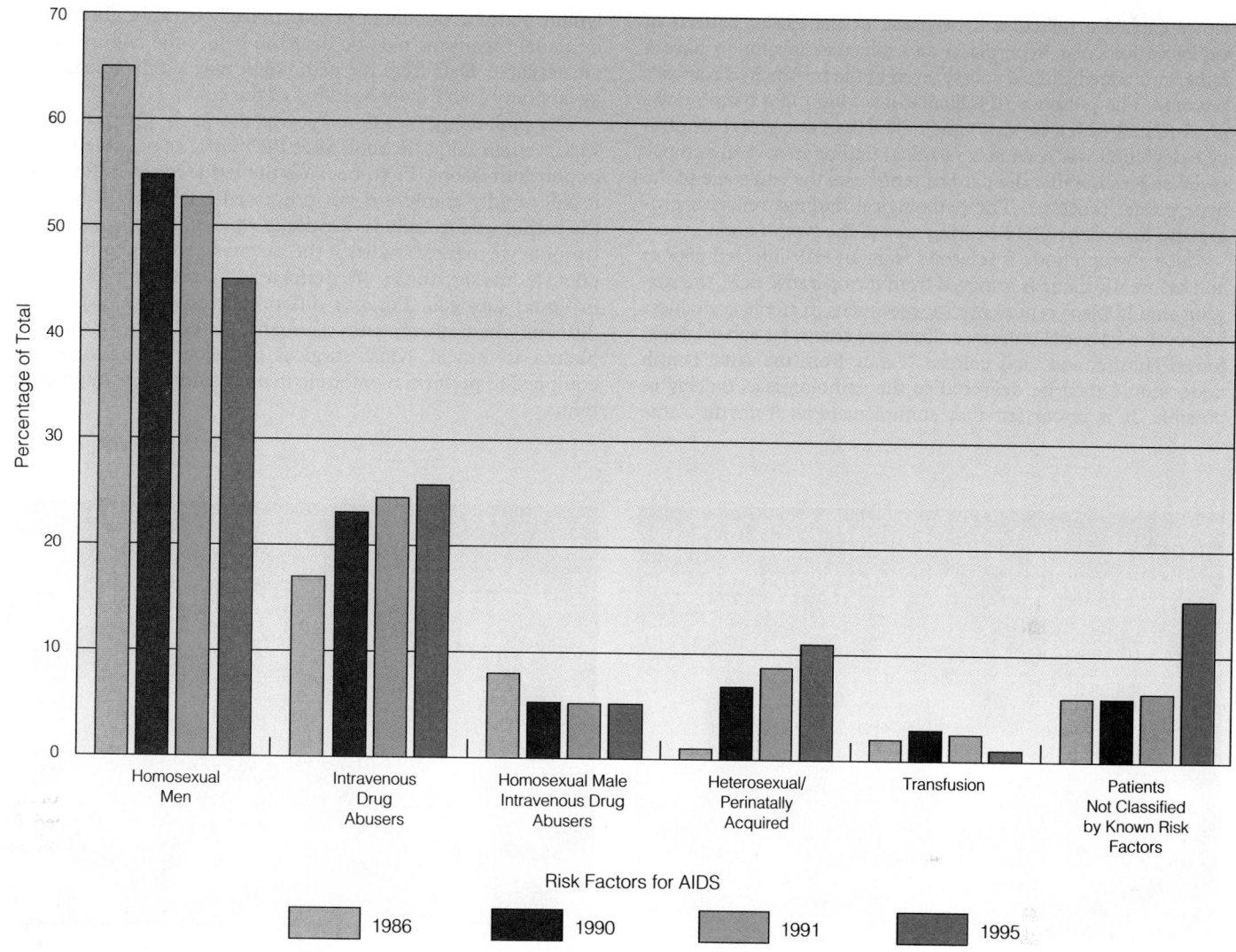

Figure 2 **Major risk groups for AIDS in 1986, 1990, 1991, and 1995 are shown as percentages of the total population of AIDS patients.**[9,86]

patients. The precise reason why lymphadenopathy occurs in some but not all patients who acquire HIV infection is not known.

The role of lymph node biopsy in these patients is currently of academic interest only since the development of serologic tests to diagnose HIV infection.[18] The histologic appearance of a clinically enlarged lymph node has prognostic value (see below); however, when the decision whether to perform a lymph node biopsy is being made, the value of the biopsy findings must be weighed against the value of the information that can be obtained by means of clinical staging with lymphocyte helper:suppressor T cell ratios and total lymphocyte counts. The total number of helper T cells in the circulation has been correlated with the risk of AIDS in patients with generalized lymphadenopathy[19-22]; the Walter Reed classification provides the most detailed clinical staging system.[21,22] The chance that an opportunistic organism will be present nowhere in the body but in the nodes is extremely low. Currently, the only compelling reason to perform a lymph node biopsy in an HIV-infected patient without AIDS is to diagnose lymphoma, because such a patient would be a candidate for chemotherapy.[18,23]

Four basic histologic patterns have been described and have been correlated with prognoses. Explosive follicular hyperplasia describes a pattern of enlarged confluent follicles with disruption of the medullary zone of the lymph node [*see Figure 3*]. Follicular involution is associated with a hypocellular, frequently hyalinized follicle and with hyperplasia of the paracortical areas [*see Figure 4*]. The mixed pattern contains explosive follicular hyperplasia and follicular involution in the same lymph node [*see Figure 5*]. Finally, the lymphocyte-depleted pattern is characterized by the total absence of follicular and paracortical areas. The loss of lymphocytes in the lymph node is associated with the predominance of histiocytes and plasma cells [*see Figure 6*].

The presence of enlarged follicles is associated with a good immunologic response and slower progression of disease, whereas the presence of involuted, hyalinized follicles is more frequently associated with opportunistic infections, Kaposi's sarcoma, and lymphoma. Evidence suggests that patients with either explosive follicular hyperplasia or the mixed pattern of explosive follicular hyperplasia and follicular involution have a rather prolonged clinical course, even in the presence of Kaposi's sarcoma. The presence of follicular involution in a lymph node is associated with a survival time of less than one year. Lymphocyte depletion was seen as a terminal finding in several autopsy cases, suggesting that the pattern represents the end stage of the hyperplastic process.[24] The pathological findings reflect a progressive loss of the CD4-bearing area of the lymph node.

Once a lymph node is removed from an HIV-infected patient and before the tissue is removed from the operative field, the surgeon should place representative specimens in sterile containers for routine bacterial culture, culture and smear for tuberculosis, fungal culture, and viral culture. Tissue from the same lymph node should then be delivered to the pathologist as quickly as possible. It is important that culture material from the same

lymph node be examined microscopically because granulomas or actual organisms may be detected before the culture results are available. Data from the pathologist may aid the microbiology laboratory staff in its handling of the cultures.

The pathologist needs to receive the fresh, gently handled specimen, in saline, as soon after the biopsy as possible for two important reasons. First, because the tissue is not in formalin, it will rapidly autolyze if not processed immediately. Second, the pathologist must have the tissue when it is fresh to perform lymphocyte marker studies if the diagnosis is lymphoma. Lymphocyte marker studies are performed on tissue rapidly frozen in liquid nitrogen. Because different lymphomas respond to different chemotherapeutic regimens, the cell type of the lymphoma is critical. Most surgical pathology laboratories are equipped to perform membrane marker studies on lymph node tissue.

Figure 3 Lymph node under low power exhibits explosive follicular hyperplasia.

Figure 4 Lymph node under low power exhibits follicular involution.

Figure 5 Lymph node under low power exhibits a mixed pattern of both explosive follicular hyperplasia and follicular involution.

Figure 6 Lymph node under low power exhibits a pattern of lymphocyte depletion.

GROUP IV—OTHER HIV DISEASES

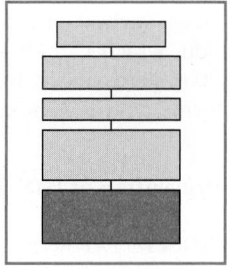

Patients whose clinical problems place them in group IV have more generalized and serious symptoms than patients in the first three disease groups. Not all patients in this group, however, fulfill the current definition of AIDS as used by the CDC for national reporting. Only those patients in category C-1 and subgroup D are classified as AIDS patients. The subgroups and categories of group IV are defined as follows[1]:

Subgroup A—constitutional disease. One or more of the following with no explanation other than HIV infection: fever persisting for more than one month, involuntary weight loss amounting to more than 10 percent of baseline weight, and diarrhea persisting for more than one month.

Subgroup B—neurologic disease. One or more of the following with no explanation other than HIV infection: dementia, myelopathy, and peripheral neuropathy.

Subgroup C—secondary infectious disease. An opportunistic infection that indicates a defect in cell-mediated immunity with no explanation other than HIV infection. These infectious diseases are subdivided into two categories. Category C-1 includes patients with symptomatic or invasive disease stemming from one or more of the 12 specified secondary infectious diseases listed in the CDC surveillance definition of AIDS: *Pneumocystis carinii* pneumonia (PCP), chronic cryptosporidiosis, toxoplasmosis, extraintestinal strongyloidiasis, isosporiasis, candidiasis (esophageal, bronchial, or pulmonary), cryptococcosis, histoplasmosis, mycobacterial infection with *Mycobacterium avium-intracellulare* or *M. kansasii*, cytomegalovirus infection, chronic mucocutaneous or disseminated herpes simplex virus infection, and progressive multifocal leukoencephalopathy. Category C-2 includes patients with symptomatic or invasive disease arising from six other specified secondary infectious diseases: oral hairy leukoplakia, multidermatomal herpes zoster, recurrent *Salmonella* bacteremia, nocardiosis, tuberculosis, and oral candidiasis (thrush).

Subgroup D—secondary cancers. The diagnosis of one or more of the kinds of cancers known to be associated with HIV infection and included as part of the CDC surveillance definition of AIDS: Kaposi's sarcoma, non-Hodgkin's lymphoma (small noncleaved cell lymphoma or immunoblastic sarcoma), and primary lymphoma of the brain.

Subgroup E—other conditions in HIV infection. The presence of unclassifiable clinical findings or diseases, such as chronic lymphoid interstitial pneumonitis, that may be attributed to HIV infection or may indicate a defect in cell-mediated immunity. Also included are those patients whose signs or symptoms could be attributed either to HIV infection or to another coexisting disease not classified elsewhere and those patients with other clinical illnesses, the course or management of which may be complicated or altered by HIV infection.

Surgical Interventions

The treatment of patients with AIDS involves multimodality therapy and consultation with oncology and infectious disease specialists. It is beyond the scope of this discussion to describe the specific therapeutic approaches to the complications of HIV infections; however, three principal problems must be addressed when a cure for these infections is considered. First, the opportunistic infection or secondary malignant disorder must be treated; second, the underlying immunodeficiency must be corrected; and finally, the cause of the problem, the HIV infection, must be eradicated from the host. Although there has been some progress in treating patients with HIV infections, no fast or simple cures are expected in the near future. The role of surgeons in the management of these chronically ill, and sometimes critically ill, patients includes performing diagnostic biopsies, giving supportive care, and managing complications of malignant or infectious processes. These complications include a number of nonsurgical gastrointestinal problems, such as so-called gay bowel syndrome, gonococcal proctitis, and a fulminant watery diarrhea caused by *Cryptosporidium*.[25,26] A growing number of studies have documented the strange surgical complications caused by the opportunistic infections and secondary cancers that plague the AIDS patient.

Cryptosporidiosis and cytomegalovirus infection of the biliary tree have been reported to cause acute cholecystitis and acute cholangitis, necessitating emergency surgical intervention.[27] It is suggested that choledochoenteric bypass provides the best palliation in these patients. It is not known, however, whether the biliary tree is ever cleared of the infectious pathogens. *Candida* infection and Kaposi's sarcoma have also caused cholangitis, necessitating bypass operation.[28]

Acute perforations of the gastrointestinal tract from cytomegalovirus infection, cryptosporidiosis, and candidiasis, as well as from necrotic lymphoma, have been reported.[18,29,30] Obstruction of the gastrointestinal tract caused by Kaposi's sarcoma or lymphoma may also be an indication for resection, bypass, or colostomy. One study of AIDS patients who required abdominal operation described four distinct clinical syndromes that called for surgical intervention: (1) peritonitis secondary to cytomegalovirus enterocolitis and perforation, (2) non-Hodgkin's lymphoma of the gastrointestinal tract (usually the terminal ileum), presenting as obstruction or bleeding, (3) Kaposi's sarcoma of the gastrointestinal tract, and (4) mycobacterial infection of the retroperitoneum or the spleen.[31]

The role of splenectomy in patients with marked splenomegaly or with thrombocytopenia must be individualized. Thrombocytopenia occurs in AIDS patients as a result of the circulating immune complex deposition on platelets rather than as a result of a specific antiplatelet antibody.[32,33] Splenectomy has been a very successful means of managing some of these patients. Occasionally, patients in subgroup A (see above) who have debilitating fevers associated with significantly enlarged spleens experience dramatic palliation after splenectomy. In patients with massive splenomegaly and fever, simple splenomegaly is sometimes difficult to distinguish from abscess or parenchymal necrosis. In addition, splenectomy may be indicated in instances in which there is merely a likelihood of injury and in those in which a large spleen compresses the stomach, thereby contributing to the patient's malnutrition.

A request frequently directed to the general surgeon from the primary care physician, the infectious disease consultant, or the hematologist caring for an AIDS patient is for placement of an indwelling central catheter. Long-term venous access for treating fungal infections or, occasionally, for nutritional support in patients with debilitating diarrheal syndromes can significantly enhance the delivery of care to these patients. However, line placement often occurs when the patient is febrile, as a result of either the underlying infectious problem or treatment with amphotericin B. Therefore, the surgeon should keep a close watch postoperatively to ensure that fevers are not related to an infected catheter [see VI:14 Nosocomial Infection].

Protection from Common Infections

Although AIDS patients with general surgical complications are quite ill, morbidity and mortality from surgical intervention usually result from progression of the disease rather than from common pathogenic bacteria: infectious complications in AIDS patients are usually caused by opportunistic organisms associated with severe immunosuppression. The incidence of the perioperative infections seen in the general population as complications of abdominal operation, such as infections with gram-negative anaerobes and aerobes, is not increased in the AIDS patient postoperatively.[26-29] A study that prospectively evaluated infection rates in almost 100 AIDS patients who had clean operative procedures (lymph node biopsies) found that bacterial infection occurred at a rate approaching one percent.[34] This rate is comparable to that in the population at large. Additional clinical studies have confirmed these findings.[28] These data support research showing little or no change in neutrophil function despite significant alterations in lymphocyte and macrophage responsiveness.

It is also quite evident that the organisms that often infect an AIDS patient have, in the past, not been very contagious. A key question for surgeons, operating room committees, infection control committees, and clinicians involved with endoscopy is how to effectively clean instruments, equipment, or other inanimate objects to be used with AIDS patients. Agents that are effective against mycobacteria, the most resistant group of organisms, are also the agents considered most effective against other bacterial and viral pathogens.[35] (A complete list of agents and their efficacies can be obtained from the Disinfectants Branch, Office of Pesticides, United States Environmental Protection Agency, 401 M Street, S.W., Washington, DC 20460.)

Agents are classified according to whether they are to be used for sterilization, disinfection, or antisepsis.[36] Agents that sterilize inanimate objects kill all microbial organisms as well as bacterial endospores. Disinfectants are not quite as effective in that they are not capable of killing bacterial spores. In many cases, an agent may serve as a disinfectant when placed in contact for a short time with the object requiring cleansing. The same agent may be capable of sterilizing surgical instruments when exposed to them for longer periods. Disinfectants are subclassified as having high-level, intermediate-level, and low-level germicidal activity. High-level agents are effective against bacterial spores. Intermediate-level disinfectants are less effective against spores but are mycobactericidal. Low-level disinfectants do not kill mycobacteria and some fungi. Antiseptic agents are used on tissue and therefore must be less toxic than sterilants or disinfectants.

According to the current recommendations from the CDC, agents classified by the United States Environmental Protection Agency as sterilants can be used for sterilization or high-level disinfection, depending on contact time. All instruments entering the bloodstream or other sterile tissues should be sterilized before use. Instruments that contact mucosal surfaces, such as endoscopes, should receive high-level disinfection, which can be achieved with solutions of glutaraldehyde (two percent), hydrogen peroxide (three to six percent), or formaldehyde (one to eight percent).

Prevention of HIV Transmission

RISKS TO PATIENTS

Transfusions

All fresh whole blood, packed red blood cells, platelets, plasma (not Plasmanate), cryoprecipitate, and leukocytes can carry HIV. In addition, clotting factor concentrates may also carry the virus. Some preparations of γ-globulin can temporarily cause a false positive ELISA test for HIV, but they do not contain the virus or transmit it to recipients. Albumin and plasma extracts (Plasmanate), although prepared from whole blood, do not carry HIV, hepatitis B virus (HBV), or hepatitis C virus, because the process by which they are purified inactivates the virus particles. Since adequate antibody testing has become available, the incidence of undetected HIV in transfused blood has been extremely low.

To minimize the risk of HIV being transmitted by transfusion, patients have increasingly requested the use of predeposited autologous blood or blood donated by family members or friends. Although this approach was originally discouraged by some blood bank administrators,[37] both directed donations and predeposited autologous blood storage have become widely accepted [see I:5 Bleeding and Transfusion]. Analysis of the incidence of HIV seropositivity in directed donation programs has not established that these programs pose any greater risk of transmitting HIV; however, directed donations are more costly.

Intraoperative blood salvage in trauma or emergency cases is a reasonable alternative to blood transfusion. At present, however, such collection methods are very costly because of the need to maintain trained personnel to run the equipment.

Transplantation

Because it has been shown that HIV can be present in semen, blood, urine, tears, breast milk, cerebrospinal fluid, and saliva and because it is suspected that HIV can be present in all secretions and excretions as well as all body tissues,[38] potential donors of tissue for transplantation must be tested for serum antibodies to HIV to prevent inadvertent transfer of the virus. (The risk of transmitting the virus by artificial insemination has also been documented and should be considered whenever artificial insemination is planned.[39])

Transmission from Surgical Personnel

Whenever a surgeon who is an asymptomatic carrier of the human immunodeficiency virus performs an operation, there is a risk that he or she will transmit the virus to the patient. This risk is well known to the public and consequently has become a potential medicolegal issue.[40] The question of whether HIV-infected surgeons should cease operating is surrounded by controversy. Because there have been no documented instances of transmission of the virus from a surgeon to a patient, the Centers for Disease Control and Prevention has not recommended that surgeons who are seropositive for human immunodeficiency virus refrain from performing surgery.[41] The report from a few years ago of HIV transmission to five patients from an HIV-positive dentist rekindled debate and prompted the CDC to reassess its policy. Recent court decisions have further confused the situation. In New York State, a case was brought by an HIV-positive pharmacist against a hospital that denied him a job because it feared he could possibly spread HIV while preparing intravenous solutions. After a year of testimony and 17 expert witnesses, the court found that the pharmacist should not be restrained from performing his clinical duties. In neighboring New Jersey, a hospital permitted an ENT surgeon who had AIDS to continue to practice, provided that he inform his patients of his disease. The doctor sued his hospital for discrimination. In this case, the judge ruled that patients have the right to know whether their doctor is HIV positive. What impact these decisions may have on national policy is currently unclear.

The issue of HBV transmission provides a noteworthy counterpoint. In a well-documented report involving a nonimmunized cardiac surgeon who acquired HBV infection in the workplace, transmission of the virus occurred in 19 (13 percent) of 122 patients on whom the surgeon operated over a 12-month period.[42] The surgeon was positive for hepatitis B e antigen (HB$_e$Ag), and sweat from inside his glove was found to contain both the antigen and HBV DNA. No deficiencies were found in the surgeon's infection control practice by the CDC, which suggested that the virus may have spread through microperforations in his gloves. This case did not receive the same publicity that cases of HIV transmission have received in the lay press. However, its significance is clear: contact between health care workers who are HBV (HB$_e$Ag) positive and patients should be restricted.

RISKS TO HEALTH CARE WORKERS

Asymptomatic HIV carriers present a potential threat to health care workers, especially to surgeons who may be operating on them. Such carriers may not know that they have the virus or have been exposed to it. The number of asymptomatic HIV carriers in the United States is estimated to be between one million and two million. For this reason, surgeons in the operating room as well as all others in the hospital environment should exercise extreme caution to prevent injury by sharp instruments. The threat of HIV transmission is significant because it results in a uniformly fatal outcome for all individuals in whom an opportunistic infection or secondary malignant disorder develops.

Although the risk of transmission of HIV in the operating room is very low, the documented incidence of tuberculosis in AIDS patients is of great concern, especially to health care workers involved in the care of AIDS patients.[43] After a 30-year decline in the incidence of tuberculosis, the incidence has steadily risen approximately 20 percent a year since 1984. This increase is thought to be due in part to the AIDS epidemic. Of greater concern is the very high percentage of patients who have multiple drug–resistant tuberculosis (MDR-Tb). Approximately 30 percent of AIDS patients infected with tuberculosis have MDR-Tb, and these patients require prolonged antitubercular therapy and have an extremely high case mortality. A significant risk of transmission to health care workers has clearly been established.[44] AIDS patients, the homeless, prison inmates, and

Table 1 Preventable Exposures to HIV among Health Care Workers*[49]

Circumstances of Preventable Exposure	Number of Health Care Workers (% of 938 Exposed Health Care Workers)
Recapping of needle	152 (16%)
Injury from improper disposal of needle or sharp object	119 (13%)
Contamination of open wound	93 (10%)
Use of needle-cutting device	9 (1%)
Total preventable exposures	373 (40%)

*The total sample under surveillance consisted of 938 health care workers exposed to blood or other body fluids of a patient with AIDS or an AIDS-related illness.

indigent patient populations with pulmonary symptoms need to be adequately screened, especially before undergoing surgery.

The CDC now recommends that all precautions to prevent HIV transmission be taken with all patients, not only those known to be infected with HIV or at high risk for such infection [see VI:19 Viral Infection].[45-48] It is important that any hospital personnel who come in contact with patients, with their tissues, or with their blood, body fluids, or excreta know of the potential risk in handling materials from these patients and take appropriate precautions. Patients in high-risk groups should be placed on enteric precautions to protect health care workers not only from HIV infection but also from hepatitis B infection (up to 80 percent of such patients are hepatitis B carriers). As part of any operative procedure on HIV-infected patients, all operating room, nursing, and anesthesia personnel, as well as employees of surgical pathology laboratories and any other laboratories, should employ universal precautions. Employees in ancillary areas, such as housekeeping and dietary services, and the venipuncture team need to be trained in the use of universal precautions.

Exposure to the virus in the workplace is considered to be preventable in many cases.[49] Most injuries result from carelessness in handling sharp objects, such as needles [see Table 1]. Self-inflicted puncture incurred in the course of recapping used needles is the most common cause of inadvertent exposure to the human immunodeficiency virus. Consequently, the most important rule to follow when handling used needles is to discard them—uncapped—in a container that is large enough to accommodate the attached syringe. Tissue specimens, wastes, soiled linen, blood samples, and sharp objects (e.g., surgical instruments, needles, and glassware) must be handled with extreme care. Dressings and other disposable materials should be discarded in specially marked containers and not with the regular hospital refuse.

The use of double gloves has been shown to minimize the possibility of contact with patient blood through small defects in the gloves, and it reduces the likelihood of blood contact with skin when a glove puncture occurs.[50,51]

The following are some additional precautions health care workers should take when handling any potentially infectious materials.

1. Wear gloves when handling body fluids.
2. Wear a gown to prevent contamination of clothing.
3. Wash hands after contact with body fluids.
4. Place fluid from a potentially contaminated host in two impervious containers.
5. Clean spills with either a 1:10 dilution of 5.25 percent sodium hypochlorite in water or with some other type of sterilant.
6. Wear masks and protective eyeglasses when there is a possibility of aerosolization of material.

Even health care workers who do not have exfoliative dermatitis or an open wound should wear gloves during patient care. Evidence suggests that the affinity of HIV for Langerhans cells may permit the virus to invade a host through intact skin or mucous membranes.[52]

Discussion

Epidemiology

AIDS

In June 1981, the CDC published a report of *P. carinii* pneumonia in a unique cohort of five previously healthy homosexual males living in Los Angeles.[53] At that time, the CDC was the sole distributor of pentamidine, the only treatment for this rare pulmonary infection. PCP traditionally was seen only in severely immunosuppressed patients who were receiving chemotherapy for disseminated cancer. Even in this select group, PCP was rare, and *P. carinii* was not considered pathogenic in otherwise healthy adults. The sudden increased demand for pentamidine in one geographic area raised the prospect of a new disease process. In July 1981, the CDC reported a group of young homosexual males with Kaposi's sarcoma.[54] Kaposi's sarcoma, like PCP, was a rare lesion not commonly seen in young, healthy adults. Many of these patients also had severe infections caused by organisms associated with immunodeficiency (PCP, toxoplasmosis, candidiasis, cryptococcosis, and cytomegalovirus infections). These two accounts represent the first recognition that AIDS was a new disease complex, although it is believed that infection by the causative agent must have occurred at least three to four years earlier. The cause of the severely depressed immune function in these individuals, who were not otherwise at risk for opportunistic infection, was controversial until late 1983 and early 1984, when two independent laboratories isolated similar retroviruses in patients with the syndrome of acquired immunodeficiency.[55,56] These retroviruses, formerly known as human T cell lymphotropic virus type III (HTLV-III) and lymphadenopathy-associated virus (LAV), are now recognized to be the same virus, which has been renamed human immunodeficiency virus.

Since 1981, the number of AIDS victims has increased. All individuals in whom clinical manifestations of the disease, such as Kaposi's sarcoma, lymphoma, or opportunistic infections, have developed either have died or are expected to die as a result.[57] In September 1987, the definition of AIDS was expanded to include symptomatic, HIV-infected patients who were suspected of having an opportunistic infection. This new definition precipitated a misleading sudden increase in the number of new cases.[58]

Since 1986, the percentage of homosexual or bisexual AIDS patients has steadily declined, and the percentage of AIDS patients who are intravenous drug abusers or heterosexual has increased [*see Figure 2*].

TRANSFUSION-ASSOCIATED HIV TRANSMISSION

Although currently administered blood transfusions are very safe, a vast number of patients who received blood between 1977 and April 1985 may have received HIV-infected blood. This eight-year period is when blood was most likely to have been unknowingly contaminated. The New York Blood Center studied stored blood samples from a group of 600,000 individuals who received blood transfusions during this eight-year period and who consequently were at risk for receiving HIV-contaminated blood. It was estimated that only 418 of these former patients received infected transfusions. On the basis of these data, the risk of any one unit of blood being HIV-infected was 0.01 percent during the years 1977 to 1980, 0.02 percent for 1981 to 1982, and 0.03 percent for 1984 to 1985. The risk of becoming infected equals the number of units transfused multiplied by the risk for each time period. Thus, it is evident that even during the maximal risk period, blood transfusions were remarkably safe.

Since May 1985, all blood for clinical use has been screened for antibody to HIV, and only anecdotal cases of contaminated blood have since been reported to the CDC. It is currently estimated that the risk of receiving a unit of blood that is contaminated with HIV is one in 150,000 (< 0.0007 percent).[59]

The first transmission of HIV from a blood donor since antibody testing became available for use in blood banking occurred when a seronegative but recently infected victim donated blood.[60] In two patients—one receiving a unit of platelet-poor packed red blood cells and the other a unit of platelets, both of which were isolated from the infected donor—positive titers of HIV antibodies developed after transfusion. The new p24 antigen assay (see above) should help detect such donors.

Pathogenesis of HIV Infection

HIV is an oncovirus belonging to the retrovirus family. The potential of retroviruses to cause neoplasia was first recognized in 1911 by the American pathologist Rous, who associated them with certain malignant disorders in animals.[61] Human T cell lymphotropic virus type I (HTLV-I), which is a retrovirus that is related to HIV, has been identified as causing leukemia in humans.[62]

One of the characteristic features of retroviruses such as HIV is the presence of an enzyme called reverse transcriptase. This enzyme allows the virus to transcribe viral RNA to DNA. The virus can synthesize double-stranded DNA from single-stranded DNA that has been liberated from the RNA-DNA hybrid. This double-stranded DNA inserts itself into the host's nucleus and serves as a template for viral replication. Thus, whenever the infected host cell divides, new HIV particles are also reproduced. HIV has been isolated in many cell types, but it is thought that the helper T cell is the cell that is most frequently infected. The virus resides in the nucleus of these cells, and it is believed that when the cell is activated by some secondary infection, the virus is replicated, resulting in the dissemination of mature virions. During this process, the virus also kills the cell in which it was residing. The length of time between HIV infection and the development of AIDS (i.e., the manifestation of opportunistic infections or secondary cancers) is not known, but data from patients in the risk groups for AIDS suggest that the latency period is approximately five years.

This estimate of latency period is probably misleading because patients in the high-risk groups are more frequently exposed to other infectious challenges, and exposure to various microbes activates the T cells that harbor HIV. Frequent and repetitive activation of the immune system disseminates the virus throughout the host and significantly impairs cellular immunity. Thus, the latency period of HIV infection will probably be longer in members of the general population than has been previously documented in members of high-risk groups. The reason is the lower incidence of concomitant infectious problems in members of the general population.

Risks to Surgeons

HIV TRANSMISSION

The risk to a surgeon of acquiring an HIV infection while treating a patient who has undetected AIDS is quite low.[41,49] The CDC initially evaluated nearly 1,500 health care workers who cared for AIDS victims. Serum samples were taken from these workers when they first began to work with immunocompromised patients and were stored in anticipation of a test for HIV. Of these workers, 666 were exposed to HIV through needle sticks or through cuts from sharp instruments. When tests were performed on these exposed individuals, none were found to have seroconverted after their exposure to HIV. However, two health care workers who had had no baseline blood sample drawn did show a positive antibody test after an injury. Because they did not belong to a known risk group for AIDS, they were believed to have generated antibody to HIV as a result of exposure in the workplace. On the basis of this study, the risk to a health care worker of acquiring HIV infection after an accidental needle-stick exposure was concluded to be 2 divided by 666, or 0.3 percent. A follow-up study found the rate of infection to be 0.5 percent.[63] Subsequent surveillance of health care workers identified 151 individuals who acquired HIV infection in the workplace [see Table 2]; 49 had proven seroconversion and 102 were HIV-positive, with no HIV-negative baseline serum sample.

A serosurvey of 770 surgeons practicing in two inner-city areas, where more than 3,000 cases of AIDS have been reported, was conducted by the CDC.[64] Accompanying the assay for HIV, HBV, and HCV was a questionnaire designed to elucidate the various practice patterns of the surgeons tested. One (0.13 percent) of the 770 surgeons was HIV positive; he had practiced for more than 25 years and performed more than 300 operations in the past year. The study did not specify how the surgeon

Table 2 Health Care Workers with Documented or Suspected HIV Infection[9]

	Number of Health Care Workers	
	With Documented HIV (%)*	With Suspected HIV (%)†
Dental	0	7 (7%)
Mortician	0	3 (3%)
Emergency medical team/paramedic	0	9 (9%)
Health aide	1 (2%)	12 (12%)
Housekeeper	1 (2%)	7 (7%)
Laboratory technician	18 (37%)	15 (15%)
Nurse	19 (39%)	24 (24%)
Physician		
Surgeon	0	4 (4%)
Nonsurgeon	6 (12%)	10 (10%)
Respiratory therapist	1 (2%)	2 (2%)
Surgical technician	2 (4%)	1 (1%)
Other	1 (2%)	8 (8%)
Total	49	102

*Evidence of seroconversion after occupational exposure to HIV.
†HIV seropositivity in health care workers with occupational exposure to HIV who do not have behavioral or transfusion risks for HIV infection.

acquired HIV, except to note that he did not participate in high-risk behavior. To date, there has been no documented seroconversion in OR personnel after a solid-bore needle injury in the operating room.

Transmission via skin contact with body fluids was documented in the case of a woman whose infant had received multiple transfusions, one of which was from an HIV-infected donor. The baby had received the contaminated transfusion at three months of age. The presence of HIV antibody in the mother was not determined until one year later, at which time an ELISA result was positive. The mother was closely involved with the baby's care and took no precautions against contact with the child's blood and body fluids. Seventeen months after the child received the infected blood transfusion, the mother seroconverted. No other risk factors accounted for the change in the mother's HIV antibody titer.[65]

Exposure to blood in the operating room has been of great concern to all operating room personnel since the AIDS epidemic began. The average practicing surgeon has 30 parenteral exposures to blood a year.[66] The fact that hollow-bore needles carry more blood than solid-bore needles may be the reason transmission in the operating room has not yet occurred. Four studies from the early 1990s established a blood-skin exposure rate of approximately 20 percent and a parenteral exposure rate of approximately four percent.[51,67-69] Long operative procedures requiring transfusions are most likely to be associated with blood exposure. Procedures that pose a high risk of exposure to blood are cardiac surgery; obstetrics, especially cesarean sections; trauma surgery; and emergency surgery. Special care must be taken to minimize exposure in these procedures; eye protection and use of double gloves are two barrier precaution measures that can reduce the likelihood of surgeon-patient blood contact.

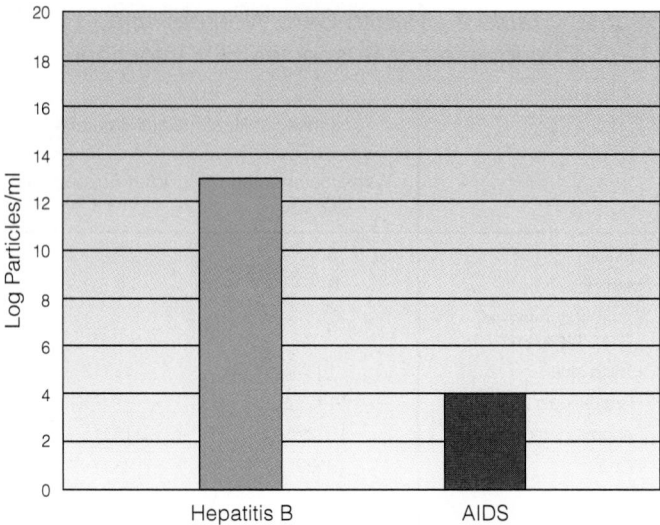

Figure 7 **The numbers of infectious viral particles per milliliter of blood in patients with active hepatitis B infections and in AIDS patients are compared.**[70]

Transmission of HIV to hospital workers is uncommon when compared with transmission of hepatitis B virus because of the relatively low concentration of HIV in the blood of AIDS patients [*see Figure 7*]. The concentration of virus particles is estimated to be 10^4 particles/ml in an AIDS patient, whereas it is 10^{13} particles/ml in a patient who has an active hepatitis B infection.[70]

Although HIV transmission is uncommon in the hospital environment, the risk to surgeons is very real. Unprotected anal intercourse is considered to be high-risk behavior, with a transmission rate of 0.4 percent (one in 250), and is discouraged by health officials.[71] The 0.5 percent (one in 200) risk of acquiring HIV infection through a needle stick is comparable.[72] Three independent factors are important in determining a surgeon's

risk of acquiring HIV infection: (1) the number of needle sticks or punctures contaminated with the patient's body fluids, (2) the percent of HIV-infected patients in the surgeon's patient population, and (3) the number of years a surgeon is at risk for acquiring an HIV infection. If the risk of HIV transmission by a contaminated needle is 0.5 percent, the HIV-infected population is 10 percent, the number of needle sticks averages 30 a year, and a practicing surgeon has 40 years of exposure, then the lifetime risk of acquiring AIDS is 60 percent![73]

If a health care worker is injured by a sharp object contaminated by exposure to fluid or tissue from an HIV-positive patient, a series of blood samples should be drawn at the time of injury and again at six weeks, three months, six months, and 12 months after the injury to determine whether HIV infection has occurred.

Although administration of antiretroviral therapy is recommended,[74] to date no prospective trials have been performed to confirm its effectiveness in humans. In 1996, a retrospective case-control study was published that supported the use of zidovudine.[75] The current recommendations for prophylaxis after a needle-stick injury are based on the amount of blood in the inoculum and on the likelihood that the source patient has a high HIV titer.[76] (In general, terminally ill HIV-infected patients have high HIV titers because the virus is rapidly replicating and destroying host cells.) The injuries associated with the highest degree of risk are those in which a health care worker is injured by a hollow-bore needle containing blood from a terminally ill HIV-infected patient. The injuries associated with the next highest degree of risk are those involving *either* a large inoculum (e.g., from a hollow-bore needle) *or* parenteral exposure to blood from a patient with a high HIV titer (e.g., a terminally ill HIV-infected patient). For all of these high-risk injuries, the recommended approach is a four-week course of treatment with a combination of zidovudine, lamivudine (3TC), and indinavir (IND). If the injury was from a solid-bore needle or the source patient is asymptomatic, zidovudine alone is offered. In these lower-risk situations, the risk of drug

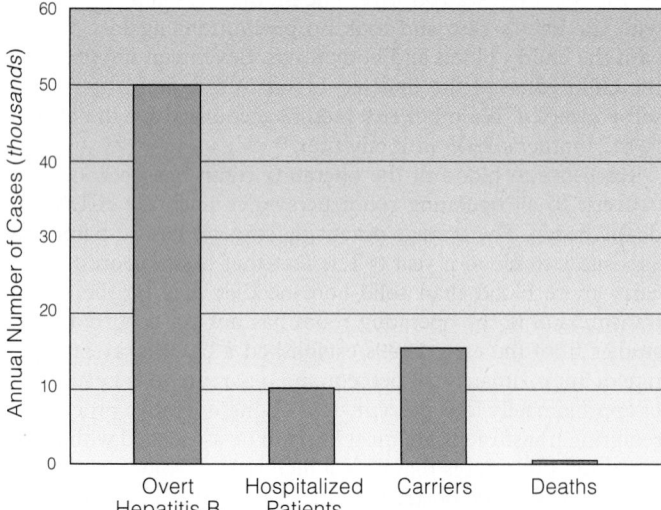

Figure 8 **The annual incidence of hepatitis B infection in the United States is 200,000 cases. Various subgroups of hepatitis B patients are shown.**[77]

Table 3 Prevalence of Hepatitis B Virus (HBV) Serologic Markers in Various Populations[87]

Population	Maximum Expected Prevalence of Serologic Markers of HBV Infection (%)
High risk	
Immigrants or refugees from areas where HBV is highly endemic	85
Clients in institutions for the mentally retarded	80
Users of illicit parenteral drugs	80
Homosexually or bisexually active men	80
Individuals who have household contact with HBV carriers	60
Hemodialysis patients	80
Intermediate risk	
Staff of institutions for the mentally retarded	25
Health care workers who have frequent contact with blood	30

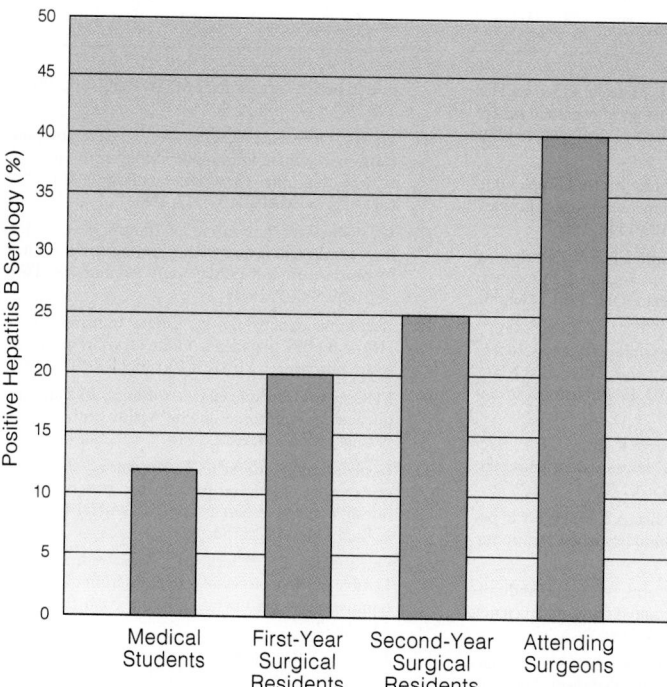

Figure 9 **The prevalence of positive serology for hepatitis B increases among individuals in successive stages of a surgical career.**[83]

toxicity must be carefully weighed against the benefits of protection against HIV transmission.

HEPATITIS TRANSMISSION

The primary health risk to surgeons caring for immunocompromised patients is that of acquiring hepatitis B or hepatitis C (non-A, non-B hepatitis). The epidemiology of hepatitis B has been well studied because there are numerous antigen and antibody markers of the virus in the blood of chronic carriers. On the basis of data from assays of these markers, it is estimated that more than 200,000 Americans acquire new hepatitis B infections each year.[77] Of these individuals, 25 percent will have symptoms of hepatitis. Five percent of the 200,000 will require hospitalization for their acute illness, and fulminant hepatitis that is fatal will develop in one to two percent of these hospitalized patients [*see Figure 8*]. The hepatitis D virus has been identified as causing an additional risk of death in patients with acute hepatitis, and individuals who are infected with both hepatitis B virus and hepatitis D virus have a higher mortality.[78]

Between five and 10 percent of patients infected with hepatitis become chronic carriers—that is, they do not effectively clear the antigen from their systems, and they have a subclinical hepatic infection for prolonged periods. This group of patients is at risk for cirrhosis with subsequent hepatic failure or hepatoma. Patients who are chronic carriers are frequently unable to clear the viral infection because they are immunosuppressed as a result of another disease process, such as advanced HIV infection (AIDS). The AIDS patient is very likely to have had a hepatitis B infection and to be a chronic carrier. HIV-infected patients are also less likely to manifest an inflammatory response to hepatic infection.[79] The epidemiology of hepatitis in patient populations frequently associated with AIDS has been evaluated by the CDC.[80] It is estimated that as many as 80 percent of the population of homosexual males, intravenous drug users, mentally retarded individuals, and hemodialysis patients have serologic markers indicating a prior hepatitis B infection. Household contact or sexual relations with these high-risk individuals also involves a significant risk of acquiring hepatitis B virus infection [*see Table 3*]. It is estimated that up to 60 percent of these contacts have positive serology for the hepatitis B virus.

Exposure to hepatitis carriers is a risk for health care workers, particularly for those who work with blood products [*see VI:19 Viral Infection*]. Physicians involved with direct patient care are at especially high risk.[81] Those in administrative situations who do not have clinical contact with patients have a relatively low risk of acquiring hepatitis, whereas surgeons, particularly cardiac surgeons and transplant surgeons, are at especially high risk. The risk of hepatitis infection also increases with age.[82,83] The incidence of positive hepatitis serology is between 12 and 13 percent in students in their last year of medical school, nearly 20 percent in surgical residents at the end of their first year, and about 25 percent in surgical residents after the second year. During the course of a senior surgeon's career, the risk of having hepatitis approaches 50 percent [*see Figure 9*]. These risks are exceedingly high and emphasize the importance of widespread use of the hepatitis B vaccine [*see VI:19 Viral Infection*].

At least two studies showed that there are numerous nonimmunized practicing surgeons who had finished medical school, training, or both before the hepatitis vaccine first became available.[64,84] These surgeons are at substantial risk for HBV infection and consequently need to be immunized. Those who have not been immunized for five years or more should have their titers checked; if titers are low, a booster is advisable.

References

1. Classification system for human T-lymphotropic virus type III/lymphadenopathy-associated virus infections. MMWR 35:335, 1986

2. Update on Kaposi's sarcoma and opportunistic infections in previously healthy persons—United States. MMWR 31:294, 1982

3. Human immunodeficiency virus infection in the United States: a review of current knowledge. MMWR 36(suppl 6):1, 1987

4. Ho DD, Sarngadharan MG, Resnick L, et al: Primary human T-lymphotropic virus type III infection. Ann Intern Med 103:880, 1985

5. Wantzin GR, Lindhardt BO, Weismann K, et al: Acute HTLV III infection associated with exanthema, diagnosed by seroconversion. Br J Dermatol 115:601, 1986

6 Marlink RG, Allan JS, McLane MF, et al: Low sensitivity of ELISA testing in early HIV infection. N Engl J Med 315:1549, 1986

7. Imagawa DT, Lee MH, Wolinsky SM, et al: Human immunodeficiency virus type 1 infection in homosexual men who remain seronegative for prolonged periods. N Engl J Med 320:1458, 1989

8. Update: acquired immunodeficiency syndrome—U.S. MMWR 35:17, 1986

9. HIV/AIDS Surveillance Report, volume 7, No. 2, year-end edition 1995. US Department of Health and Human Services, Public Health Service, Centers for Disease Control and Prevention, National Center for HIV, STD, TB

10. Brown BR, Irwin KL, Faruque S, et al: Intersecting epidemics—crack cocaine use and HIV infection among inner city young adults. N Engl J Med 331:1422, 1994

11. Barnes DM: Keeping the AIDS virus out of blood supply. Science 233:514, 1986

12. Recommendations for donor screening with a licensed test for HIV-1 antigen. US Department of Health and Human Services, Public Health Service, Food and Drug Administration, Center for Biologics Evaluation and Research, Rockville, Maryland, 1995

13. US Public Health Service guidelines for testing and counseling blood and plasma donors for human immunodeficiency virus type I antigen. MMWR 45(R-22):1, 1996

14. Persistent lack of detectable HIV-1 antibody in a person with HIV infections—Utah, 1995. MMWR 45:182, 1996

15. Human T-lymphotropic virus type III/lymphadenopathy-associated virus antibody prevalence in U.S. military recruit applicants. MMWR 35:421, 1986

16. St. Louis ME, Conway GA, Hayman CR, et al: Human immunodeficiency virus infection in disadvantaged adolescents: findings from the US Job Corps. JAMA 266:2387, 1991

17. Janssen RS, St. Louis ME, Satten GA, et al: HIV infection among patients in U.S. acute care hospitals: strategies for the counseling and testing of the hospital patients. N Engl J Med 327:445, 1992

18. Nugent P, O'Connell TX: The surgeon's role in treating acquired immunodeficiency syndrome. Arch Surg 121:1117, 1986

19. Kaplan JE, Spira TJ, Fishbein DB, et al: Lymphadenopathy syndrome in homosexual men: evidence for continuing risk of developing the acquired immunodeficiency syndrome. JAMA 257:335, 1987

20. Goedert JJ, Biggar RJ, Melbye M, et al: Effect of T4 count and cofactors on the incidence of AIDS in homosexual men infected with human immunodeficiency virus. JAMA 257:331, 1987

21. Redfield RR, Burke DS: HIV infection: the clinical picture. Sci Am 259(October):90, 1988

22. Redfield RR, Wright DC, Tramont EC: The Walter Reed staging classification for HTLV-III/LAV infection. N Engl J Med 314:131, 1986

23. Fernandez R, Mouradian J, Metroka C, et al: The prognostic value of histopathology in persistent generalized lymphadenopathy in homosexual men. N Engl J Med 309:185, 1983

24. Davis JM, Chadburn A, Mouradian JA: Lymph node biopsy in patients with human immunodeficiency virus infections. Arch Surg 123:1349, 1988

25. Rubin RH: Acquired immunodeficiency syndrome. Scientific American Medicine, Section 7, Subsection XI. Rubenstein E, Federman DD, Eds. Scientific American, Inc, New York, 1990

26. Karchmer AW: Sexually transmitted diseases. Scientific American Medicine, Section 7, Subsection XXII. Rubenstein E, Federman DD, Eds. Scientific American, Inc, New York, 1990

27. Margulis SJ, Honig CL, Soave R, et al: Biliary tract obstruction in the acquired immunodeficiency syndrome. Ann Intern Med 105:207, 1986

28. Robinson G, Wilson SE, Williams RA: Surgery in patients with acquired immunodeficiency syndrome. Arch Surg 122:170, 1987

29. Barone JE, Gingold BS, Arvantis ML, et al: Abdominal pain in patients with acquired immunodeficiency syndrome. Ann Surg 204:619, 1986

30. Potter DA, Danforth DN, Macher AM, et al: Evaluation of abdominal pain in the AIDS patient. Ann Surg 199:332, 1984

31. Wilson SE, Robinson G, Williams RA, et al: Acquired immune deficiency syndrome (AIDS): indications for abdominal surgery, pathology, and outcome. Ann Surg 210:428, 1989

32. Morris L, Distenfeld A, Amorosi E, et al: Autoimmune thrombocytopenic purpura in homosexual men. Ann Intern Med 96:714, 1982

33. Walsh CM, Nardi MA, Karpatkin S: On the mechanism of thrombocytopenic purpura in sexually active homosexual men. N Engl J Med 311:635, 1984

34. Davis JM, Mouradian J, Fernandez R, et al: Acquired immune deficiency syndrome—a surgical perspective. Arch Surg 119:90, 1984

35. Favero MS: Sterilization, disinfection, and antisepsis in the hospital. Manual of Clinical Microbiology, 4th ed. Lenette EH, Balows A, Hausler W, et al, Eds. American Society for Microbiology, Washington, DC, 1985, p 129

36. Jawetz E, Melnick JL, Adelberg EA: Antimicrobial chemotherapy. Review of Medical Microbiology, 15th ed. Lange Medical Publications, Los Altos, California, 1982, p 117

37. Moore SB: AIDS, blood transfusions, and directed donations. N Engl J Med 314:1454, 1986

38. Ho DD, Byington RE, Schooley RT, et al: Infrequency of isolation of HTLV-III virus from saliva in AIDS. N Engl J Med 313:1606, 1985

39. Morgan J, Nolan J: Risks of AIDS with artificial insemination. N Engl J Med 314:386, 1986

40. Gerbert B, Maguire BT, Hulley SB, et al: Physicians and acquired immunodeficiency syndrome: what patients think about human immunodeficiency virus in medical practice. JAMA 262:1969, 1989

41. Summary: recommendations for preventing transmission of infection with human T-lymphotropic virus type III/lymphadenopathy-associated virus in the workplace. MMWR 34:681, 1985

42. Harpaz R, Von Seidlein L, Averhoff FM, et al: Transmission of hepatitis B virus to multiple patients from a surgeon without evidence of inadequate infection control. N Engl J Med 334:549, 1996

43. National action plan to combat multidrug-resistant tuberculosis. MMWR 41(RR-11):1, 1992

44. Beck-Sague C, Dooley SW, Hutton MD, et al: Hospital outbreak of multidrug-resistant *Mycobacterium tuberculosis* infections. JAMA 268:1280, 1992

45. Recommendations for prevention of HIV transmission in health-care settings. MMWR 36(suppl 2S):1, 1987

46. Update: Universal precautions for prevention of transmission of human immunodeficiency virus, hepatitis B virus, and other bloodborne pathogens in health-care settings. MMWR 37:377, 1988

47. Guidelines for prevention of transmission of human immunodeficiency virus and hepatitis B virus to health-care and public-safety workers. MMWR 38(suppl S-6):1, 1989

48. Recommendations for preventing transmission of HIV and HBV to patients during exposure-prone invasive procedures. MMWR 40(suppl RR-8):1, 1991

49. McCray E: Occupational risk of the acquired immunodeficiency syndrome among health care workers. N Engl J Med 314:1127, 1986

50. Genberding JL, Littel C, Tarkington A, et al: Risk of exposure of surgical personnel to patients' blood during surgery at San Francisco General Hospital. N Engl J Med 322:1788, 1990

51. Quebbeman EJ, Telford GL, Wadsworth K, et al: Double gloving: protecting surgeons from blood contamination in the operating room. Arch Surg 127:213, 1992

52. Braathen LR, Ramirez G, Kunze RO, et al: Langerhans cells as primary target cells for HIV infection (letter). Lancet 2:1094, 1987

53. *Pneumocystis* pneumonia—Los Angeles. MMWR 30:250, 1981

54. Kaposi's sarcoma and *Pneumocystis* pneumonia among homosexual men—New York City and California. MMWR 30:305, 1981

55. Barré-Sinoussi F, Chermann JC, Rey F, et al: Isolation of a T-lymphotropic retrovirus from a patient at risk for acquired immune deficiency syndrome (AIDS). Science 220:868, 1983

56. Popovic M, Sarngadharan MG, Reed E, et al: Detection, isolation, and continuous production of cytopathic retroviruses (HTLV-III) from patients with AIDS and pre-AIDS. Science 224:497, 1984

57. Institute of Medicine & National Academy of Sciences: Mobilizing against AIDS: The Unfinished Story of a Virus. Harvard University Press, Cambridge, Massachusetts, 1986

58. Update: acquired immunodeficiency syndrome—United States, 1981–1988. MMWR 38:229, 1989

59. Cumming PD, Wallace EL, Schorr JB, et al: Exposure of patients to human immunodeficiency virus through the transfusion of blood components that test antibody-negative. N Engl J Med 321:941, 1989

60. Transfusion-associated human T-lymphotropic virus type III/lymphadenopathy-associated virus infection from a seronegative donor—Colorado. MMWR 35:389, 1986

61. Rous T: Transmission of a malignant growth by means of a cell-free filtrate. JAMA 56:198, 1911

62. Robert-Guroff M, Nakao Y, Notake K, et al: Natural antibodies to human retrovirus HTLV in a cluster of Japanese patients with adult T-cell leukemia. Science 215:975, 1982

63. Marcus R, The CDC Cooperative Needlestick Surveillance Group: Surveillance of health care workers exposed to blood from patients infected with the human immunodeficiency virus. N Engl J Med 319:1118, 1988

64. Panlilio AL, Shapiro CN, Schable CA: Serosurvey of HIV, HBV, HCV infection among hospital-based surgeons. J Am Coll Surg 180:16, 1995

65. Apparent transmission of human T-lymphotropic virus type III/lymphadenopathy-associated virus from a child to a mother providing health care. MMWR 35:76, 1986

66. Howard RJ: Human immunodeficiency virus testing and the risk to the surgeon of acquiring HIV. Surg Gynecol Obstet 171:22, 1990

67. Popejoy SL, Fry DE: Blood contact and exposure in the operating room. Surg Gynecol Obstet 172:480, 1991

68. Panlilio AL, Foy DR, Edwards JR, et al: Blood contacts during surgical procedures. JAMA 265:1533, 1991

69. Tokars JI, Bell DM, Culver DH: Percutaneous injuries during surgical procedures. JAMA 267:2899, 1992

70. Levy JA, Kaminsky LS, Morrow JW, et al: Infection by the retrovirus associated with the acquired immunodeficiency syndrome: clinical, biological, and molecular features. Ann Intern Med 103:694, 1985

71. Lorian V: AIDS, anal sex, and heterosexuals (letter). Lancet 1:1111, 1988

72. Update: acquired immunodeficiency syndrome and human immunodeficiency virus infection among health-care workers. MMWR 37:229, 1988

73. Hagen MD, Meyer KB, Kopelman RI, et al: Human immunodeficiency virus infection in health care workers: a method for estimating individual occupational risk. Arch Intern Med 149:1541, 1989

74. Henderson DK, Gerberding JL: Prophylactic zidovudine after occupational exposure to the human immunodeficiency virus: an interim analysis. J Infect Dis 160:321, 1989

75. Case-control study of HIV seroconversion in health-care workers after percutaneous exposure to HIV-infected blood—France, United Kingdom, and United States, January 1988–August 1994. MMWR 44:929, 1996

76. Update: provisional Public Health Service recommendations for chemoprophylaxis after occupational exposure to HIV. MMWR 45:468, 1996

77. Alter HJ: The evolution, implications, and applications of the hepatitis B vaccine (editorial). JAMA 247:2272, 1982

78. Govindarajan S, Chin KP, Redeker AG, et al: Fulminant B virus hepatitis: role of delta agent. Gastroenterology 86:1417, 1984

79. Perrillo RB, Regenstein FG, Roodman ST: Chronic hepatitis B in asymptomatic homosexual men with antibody to human immunodeficiency virus. Ann Intern Med 105:382, 1986

80. Recommendation of the Immunization Practices Advisory Committee (ACIP): Recommendations for protection against viral hepatitis. MMWR 34:313, 1985

81. Denes AE, Smith JL, Maynard JE, et al: Hepatitis B infection in physicians: results of a nationwide sero-epidemiologic survey. JAMA 239:210, 1978

82. Lemmer JH: Hepatitis B as an occupational disease of surgeons. Surg Gynecol Obstet 159:91, 1984

83. Parry MF, Brown AE, Dobbs LG: The epidemiology of hepatitis B infection in housestaff. Infection 6:204, 1978

84. Barie PS, Dellinger P, Dougherty SH, et al: Assessment of HBV immunization status among North American surgeons. Arch Surg 129:27, 1994

85. Mann J, Tarontola D, Netter T: AIDS in the World. Harvard University Press, Cambridge, Mass, 1992.

86. Update: acquired immunodeficiency syndrome—United States, 1991. MMWR 41:463, 1992

87. Surveillance for occupationally acquired HIV infection—United States, 1981–1992. MMWR 41:823, 1992.

Acknowledgments

Figures 1 and 2   Tom Moore.

Figures 3 through 6   Micrographs courtesy of Dr. Janet Mouradian, Department of Pathology, Cornell University Medical College, New York.

Figures 7 through 9   Albert Miller.

VII CARE IN THE ICU

1 CARDIOPULMONARY MONITORING

James W. Holcroft, M.D.

Indications for and Uses of ICU Monitoring Equipment

Monitoring of cardiopulmonary variables is frequently necessary in critically ill surgical patients. Specific indications for each of the monitoring devices are discussed elsewhere in the text. This discussion will concentrate on how to insert and use monitoring devices and how to interpret data obtained from them. Not all of the measurements available from these devices are provided in continuous readouts; some of the measurements made possible by the technology, such as blood gas analysis or determination of cardiac indices, require interventions or calculations by nurses or physicians [*see Table 1*]. Newer devices, such as pulse oximeters, are capable not only of providing information noninvasively but of doing so continuously. These sorts of devices will be used more and more as problems with calibration and reliability are solved.

Systemic Arterial Catheters

INDICATIONS
FOR INSERTION

The information obtained from systemic arterial catheters includes measurements of systemic arterial pressure and blood gases [*see Sidebar* Insertion of Systemic Arterial Catheters]. Indications for insertion of such a catheter include the need for frequent or continuous monitoring of these parameters. Recognition of these needs requires clinical judgment. In general, if it is necessary to measure blood gases more often than three times a day, it is best to insert a catheter. Additionally, the possibility of sudden hemorrhage, the presence of sepsis, the need for titration of vasoactive drugs, or the need for administration of cardiotonic agents each dictates that such a catheter be inserted.

COMPLICATIONS ASSOCIATED
WITH SYSTEMIC ARTERIAL CATHETERS

Line sepsis is probably the single most serious problem associated with any indwelling vascular device.[1] Infection rates with systemic arterial catheters are much lower than those with central venous or pulmonary arterial catheters, but even systemic arterial catheters must be protected from possible contamination. Diagnosis and treatment of infection arising from

such catheters are described elsewhere [*see VI:11 Blood Cultures and Infection in the Patient with the Septic Response and VI:14 Nosocomial Infection*].

Thrombosis associated with insertion and maintenance of indwelling arterial catheters can lead to ischemia and even necrosis distal to the site of insertion. The risk of thrombosis is minimized by inserting the catheter in arteries with abundant collateral circulation. Thus, the radial artery is safer to use than the brachial artery, and the dorsalis pedis is safer than the femoral artery. The risk of thrombosis can also be reduced by continuous infusion of a dilute heparin solution through the catheter. If concern about heparin-induced thrombocytopenia arises, the heparin can be removed with only a minimal increase in the likelihood of catheter thrombosis. Flushing of the catheter must be done carefully with volumes of fluid no larger than 2 ml. Rapid infusion of large amounts of solution through radial artery catheters in particular can lead to retrograde flow and embolization to the brain of particulate matter or air.

MEASUREMENT OF SYSTEMIC ARTERIAL PRESSURE

Pressures obtained from systemic arterial catheters include the systolic, diastolic, and mean pressures. The mean pressure can be approximated as the diastolic pressure plus one third of the pulse pressure, the pulse pressure being defined as the systolic pressure minus the diastolic. Exact measurements of the mean pressure require computer analysis of the pressure waveform. Many pressure monitors perform such analysis, and the mean pressure can be taken from the digital readout on the oscilloscope screen. The mean pressure is the most accurate of the systemic arterial pressures obtained from the catheter and should be used for governing patient decisions [*see Figure 1*].

There are three reasons why the mean pressure should be used.[2] First, the systolic and diastolic pressures measured at the transducer will frequently be different from the systolic and diastolic pressures in the artery itself because the stiffness and resistance of the catheter and the rest of the measuring system can differ substantially from the stiffness and resistance of the vascular system. Second, movement of the catheter within the vessel can produce transient falls in measured hydrostatic pressures. Third, the systolic and diastolic pressures in the radial artery or in any distal artery will be higher and lower, respectively, than the systolic and diastolic pressures in the ascending aorta. The mean pressures in the distal artery and the ascending aorta will be the same, however.

Indications for and Uses of ICU Monitoring Equipment

Monitoring of cardiopulmonary parameters is required to optimize O₂ consumption, nitrogen balance, and metabolic status

Systemic arterial catheters

Indications:
- Need for frequent or continuous monitoring of systemic arterial pressure and blood gases
- Possibility of sudden hemorrhage
- Presence of sepsis
- Need for titration of vasoactive drugs
- Need for administration of cardiotonic agents

Central venous catheters

Useful for monitoring only when it is certain that the cardiovascular abnormality is confined to the right side of the heart.

Systemic arterial pressures

Mean pressure taken from the monitor's digital readout is more accurate than systolic or diastolic pressure.

Consider effects of the following:
- Mismatch between measuring system and patient's vasculature
- Catheter whip
- Distance of measuring site from the heart

Systemic arterial blood gases

Values that may be obtained include the following:
- Partial pressure of O_2
- Partial pressure of CO_2
- Hydrogen ion concentration (pH)
- O_2 saturation
- O_2 content

Central venous pressure

Pulmonary arterial pressure

Monitoring of cardiopulmonary parameters is required to optimize O₂ consumption, nitrogen balance, and metabolic status

Values that may be derived from measurements obtained by monitoring devices include cardiac output, stroke volume, left ventricular and right ventricular end-diastolic volumes, left ventricular and right ventricular end-systolic volumes, left ventricular and right ventricular end-systolic unstressed volumes, left ventricular and right ventricular end-systolic pressures, vascular resistances, aortic root and pulmonary arterial end-systolic pressure-volume relations, left ventricular and right ventricular end-systolic pressure-volume relations, power, O₂ transport, O₂ return, O₂ consumption, sodium bicarbonate concentration, shunt fractions, and A-aDo₂ gradients

Pulmonary arterial catheters

Indicated to monitor central venous pressure, pulmonary arterial pressure, PAWP, cardiac output, right ventricular end-diastolic volume, and mixed venous gases in the following:
- Patients with severe cardiopulmonary derangements
- Patients at high risk for intraoperative or postoperative development of cardiopulmonary problems
- Patients undergoing procedures associated with large volume requirements or fluid shifts

Other monitoring techniques

It is possible to monitor the following values continuously:
- Arterial O_2 saturation (by means of pulse oximetry)
- P_aO_2 (by means of transcutaneous or conjunctival devices)
- Perfusion (by means of devices that measure skin temperature)
- Mixed venous O_2 saturation (by means of special pulmonary arterial catheters)
- End-expiratory CO_2 tension (by means of ventilatory monitoring devices)

Pulmonary arterial wedge pressure

PAWP correlates well with mean left atrial pressure and reflects pulmonary microvascular hydrostatic pressure. In the absence of mitral valve disease, PAWP correlates with LVEDP.

Cardiac output

Value is obtained by making 3 injections of cool solution at a consistent point in the ventilatory cycle. The thermistor in the catheter measures the T° drop in the pulmonary artery as the cool blood flows past; the monitor provides a digital readout.

Right ventricular end-diastolic volume

Measurement requires use of a cold injectate and a fast-response thermistor. Level is accurate if patient has a regular heart rate <140 beats/min. Echocardiography can determine if end-diastolic volume in the right ventricle is similar to that in the left.

Mixed venous blood gases

Use P_{CO_2} level to confirm a good specimen.

O_2 saturation is the most reliable measurement obtained from mixed venous blood.

Table 1   Normal Values Obtained from Commonly Used Monitors*

Parameters	Sources for Measurement or Calculations	Values Not Indexed or Indexed to Body Surface Area	Values in Subjects of Different Weights†					Units
			Formulas Used to Calculate Values‡	Subject Weight				
				45 kg	60 kg	75 kg	90 kg	
Heart rate (HR)§	Electrocardiogram	60 beats/min	$167 \div wt^{0.25}$	64	60	57	54	beats/min
Cardiac output (CO)	Swan-Ganz catheter	$3.5\ L \cdot min^{-1} \cdot m^{-2}$	$0.28 \cdot wt^{0.75}$	4.9	6.0	7.1	8.2	L/min
Stroke volume (SV)§	CO ÷ HR	59 ml/m²	$1.67 \cdot wt$	75	100	125	150	ml
Left ventricular end-diastolic volume (LVEDV)	See text	88 ml/m²	$2.50 \cdot wt$	113	150	188	225	ml
Right ventricular end-diastolic volume (RVEDV)	Swan-Ganz catheter	88 ml/m²	$2.50 \cdot wt$	113	150	188	225	ml
Left ventricular end-systolic volume (LVESV)§	LVEDV – SV	29 ml/m²	$0.83 \cdot wt$	37	50	62	75	ml
Right ventricular end-systolic volume (RVESV)	RVEDV – SV	29 ml/m²	$0.83 \cdot wt$	37	50	62	75	ml
Left ventricular end-systolic unstressed volume (LV V_0)	See text	4 ml/m²	$0.10 \cdot wt$	5	6	8	9	ml
Right ventricular end-systolic unstressed volume (RV V_0)	See text	4 ml/m²	$0.10 \cdot wt$	5	6	8	9	ml
Mean systemic arterial pressure (MAP)	Arterial catheter	90 mm Hg	—	90	90	90	90	mm Hg
Mean pulmonary arterial pressure (MPAP)	Swan-Ganz catheter	15 mm Hg	—	15	15	15	15	mm Hg
Left ventricular end-systolic pressure (LVESP)	See text	100 mm Hg	—	100	100	100	100	mm Hg
Right ventricular end-systolic pressure (RVESP)	See text	20 mm Hg	—	20	20	20	20	mm Hg
Pulmonary arterial wedge pressure (PAWP)	Swan-Ganz catheter	5 mm Hg	—	5	5	5	5	mm Hg
Central venous pressure (CVP)	Swan-Ganz catheter	2 mm Hg	—	2	2	2	2	mm Hg
Systemic vascular resistance	(MAP – CVP) ÷ CO	$25\ mm\ Hg \cdot L^{-1} \cdot min \cdot m^2$	$314 \div wt^{0.75}$	18.1	14.6	12.3	10.7	$mm\ Hg \cdot L^{-1} \cdot min$
Pulmonary vascular resistance	(MPAP – PAWP) ÷ CO	$2.9\ mm\ Hg \cdot L^{-1} \cdot min \cdot m^2$	$35.7 \div wt^{0.75}$	2.1	1.7	1.4	1.2	$mm\ Hg \cdot L^{-1} \cdot min$
Aortic root end-systolic pressure-volume relation§	LVESP ÷ SV	$1.7\ mm\ Hg \cdot ml^{-1} \cdot m^2$	$59.9 \div wt$	1.3	1.0	0.8	0.7	mm Hg/ml
Pulmonary arterial end-systolic pressure volume relation§	RVESP ÷ SV	$0.34\ mm\ Hg \cdot ml^{-1} \cdot m^2$	$12 \div wt$	0.27	0.20	0.16	0.13	mm Hg/ml
Left ventricular end-systolic pressure-volume relation	LVESP ÷ (LVESV – V_0)	$4.0\ mm\ Hg \cdot ml^{-1} \cdot m^2$	$137 \div wt$	3.0	2.3	1.8	1.5	mm Hg/ml

(continued)

Table 1 (continued)

Parameters	Sources for Measurement or Calculations	Values Not Indexed or Indexed to Body Surface Area	Values in Subjects of Different Weights[†]					Units
			Formulas Used to Calculate Values[‡]	Subject Weight				
				45 kg	60 kg	75 kg	90 kg	
Right ventricular end-systolic pressure-volume relation	$RVESP \div (RVESV - V_0)$	0.24 mm Hg $\cdot$ ml^{-1} $\cdot$ m^2	$27.4 \div$ wt	0.61	0.46	0.37	0.30	mm Hg/ml
Total power delivered into aorta	$LVESP \cdot CO$	350 mm Hg $\cdot$ L $\cdot$ ml^{-1} $\cdot$ m^{-2}	$28 \cdot$ wt$^{0.75}$	490	600	710	820	mm Hg $\cdot$ L $\cdot$ min^{-1}
Steady-flow aortic power	$MAP \cdot CO$	315 mm Hg $\cdot$ L $\cdot$ ml^{-1} $\cdot$ m^{-2}	$25.2 \cdot$ wt$^{0.75}$	440	540	640	740	mm Hg $\cdot$ L $\cdot$ min^{-1}
Power dissipated in microvasculature	$(MAP - CVP) \cdot CO$	308 mm Hg $\cdot$ L $\cdot$ ml^{-1} $\cdot$ m^{-2}	$24.6 \cdot$ wt$^{0.75}$	427	530	627	719	mm Hg $\cdot$ L $\cdot$ min^{-1}
Power used to fill right heart	$CVP \cdot CO$	7 mm Hg $\cdot$ L $\cdot$ ml^{-1} $\cdot$ m^{-2}	$0.56 \cdot$ wt$^{0.75}$	10	12	14	16	mm Hg $\cdot$ L $\cdot$ min^{-1}
Oscillatory power	$(LVESP - MAP) \cdot CO$	35 mm Hg $\cdot$ L $\cdot$ ml^{-1} $\cdot$ m^{-2}	$2.80 \cdot$ wt$^{0.75}$	49	60	71	82	mm Hg $\cdot$ L $\cdot$ min^{-1}
Total power delivered into pulmonary artery	$RVESP \cdot CO$	70 mm Hg $\cdot$ L $\cdot$ ml^{-1} $\cdot$ m^{-2}	$5.6 \cdot$ wt$^{0.75}$	97	121	143	164	mm Hg $\cdot$ L $\cdot$ min^{-1}
Steady-flow pulmonary arterial power	$MPAP \cdot CO$	53 mm Hg $\cdot$ L $\cdot$ ml^{-1} $\cdot$ m^{-2}	$4.2 \cdot$ wt$^{0.75}$	73	91	107	123	mm Hg $\cdot$ L $\cdot$ min^{-1}
Power dissipated in microvasculature	$(MPAP - PAWP) \cdot CO$	35 mm Hg $\cdot$ L $\cdot$ ml^{-1} $\cdot$ m^{-2}	$2.8 \cdot$ wt$^{0.75}$	49	60	71	82	mm Hg $\cdot$ L $\cdot$ min^{-1}
Power used to fill left heart	$PAWP \cdot CO$	18 mm Hg $\cdot$ L $\cdot$ ml^{-1} $\cdot$ m^{-2}	$1.4 \cdot$ wt$^{0.75}$	24	30	36	41	mm Hg $\cdot$ L $\cdot$ min^{-1}
Oscillatory power	$(RVESP - MPAP) \cdot CO$	18 mm Hg $\cdot$ L $\cdot$ ml^{-1} $\cdot$ m^{-2}	$1.4 \cdot$ wt$^{0.75}$	24	30	36	41	mm Hg $\cdot$ L $\cdot$ min^{-1}
Systemic arterial O_2 tension (P_aO_2)[‖]	O_2 electrode	70–97 mm Hg	—	70–97	70–97	70–97	70–97	mm Hg
Mixed venous O_2 tension ($P_{mv}O_2$)[¶]	O_2 electrode	37–47 mm Hg	—	37–47	37–47	37–47	37–47	mm Hg
Arterial O_2 saturation (S_aO_2)[‖]	Co-oximeter	93%–97%	—	93%–97%	93%–97%	93%–97%	93%–97%	—
Mixed venous O_2 tension ($S_{mv}O_2$)[¶]	Co-oximeter	73%–80%	—	73%–80%	73%–80%	73%–80%	73%–80%	—
Arterial CO_2 tension	CO_2 electrode	40 mm Hg	—	40	40	40	40	mm Hg
Mixed venous CO_2 tension	CO_2 electrode	45 mm Hg	—	45	45	45	45	mm Hg
Arterial pH	pH electrode	7.40	—	7.40	7.40	7.40	7.40	—
Mixed venous pH	pH electrode	7.35	—	7.35	7.35	7.35	7.35	—
Arterial venous O_2 content difference	$1.39 \cdot [Hb] \cdot (S_aO_2 - S_{mv}O_2)$	3.6 ml O_2/dl	—	3.6	3.6	3.6	3.6	ml O_2/dl
O_2 consumption	$1.39 \cdot [Hb] \cdot (S_aO_2 - S_{mv}O_2) \cdot CO$	126 ml O_2 $\cdot$ min^{-1} $\cdot$ m^{-2}	$10 \cdot$ wt$^{0.75}$	174	216	255	292	ml O_2/min

*Mean values in young 60 kg subject in good condition, height 169 cm, body surface area 1.70 m², in a supine position, fasting, and breathing spontaneously; thermoneutral environment. Range of normal, approximately ± 25% of values listed.

[†]Values for subjects of different weights calculated taking into account fractal distributions of nutrient blood vessels and minimization of energy distribution to metabolizing organs.[29]

[‡]All weights in kg.

[§]Resting HR in a poorly conditioned subject is faster than that in a well-conditioned subject by a factor of approximately 1.2; however, resting CO is the same. As a consequence, resting SV is smaller and parameters that depend on SV differ from those in a well-conditioned person.

[‖]P_aO_2 and S_aO_2 decrease with age: 98 mm Hg (97% saturation) is normal for a person 20 yr of age, and 75 mm Hg (95% saturation) for a person 70 yr of age.

[¶]$P_{mv}O_2$ and $S_{mv}O_2$ depend on [Hb], arterial O_2 content, cardiac output, and O_2 consumption. For a 60 kg person with an arterial saturation of 97%, a cardiac output of 6 L/min, and an O_2 consumption of 216 ml O_2/min, [Hb] of 11, 13, and 15 g/dl will result in $S_{mv}O_2$ of 73% (37 mm Hg), 77% (43 mm Hg), and 80% (47 mm Hg), respectively.

Matching the Measuring System to the Patient's Vasculature

The systolic and diastolic pressures depend not only on the true pressures in the patient's vascular system but also on the nature of the equipment used to measure those pressures.[2,3] If the catheter-tubing-transducer system is excessively stiff in comparison with the stiffness of the vasculature, the systolic and diastolic pressures will be exaggerated: the systolic pressure at the transducer will be higher than the true systolic pressure, and the diastolic pressure will be lower than the true diastolic pressure. Conversely, if the measuring system is more compliant than the patient's vasculature, the systolic and diastolic pressures will be damped: the systolic pressure measured at the transducer will be lower than the true systolic, and the diastolic pressure will be greater than the true diastolic. Damping will also be introduced if the vascular catheter is obstructed by a blood clot or if the tube is too narrow or too long or has a kink in it.

The accuracy of systolic and diastolic pressures at the transducer can be assessed by the so-called snap test [*see Figure 2*].[3] This test consists of infusing a square wave of pressure into the catheter-tubing-transducer system by pulling on the tab that allows influx of fluid from the high-pressure bag used to keep the tubing-catheter system patent. The tab is then snapped shut, and the pressure in the system returns abruptly to baseline levels. If the catheter-tubing-transducer system is adequately matched to the patient's vasculature, this abrupt return to baseline pressures will occur smoothly and with no interruption of the arterial pressure tracing.

Insertion of Systemic Arterial Catheters

Systemic arterial lines are generally placed in one of four major vessels: radial artery, brachial artery, femoral artery, or dorsalis pedis artery.

When using the radial artery, the clinician should perform an Allen test before catheter placement. In the Allen test, the fist is clenched or the arm elevated to drain blood from the hand. Both the ulnar and radial arteries are compressed by the clinician. The fist is released or the arm lowered, and the ulnar artery is released. A blush of the hand indicates a patent palmar arch that is supplied by the ulnar artery. If occlusion of the radial artery were to occur, the ulnar artery should then be able to provide adequate blood supply to the hand. Although very few patients have inadequate palmar arch collateral, some groups are at risk for necrosis of the hand if the radial artery is occluded. These patients include those with arteritis, diabetes, low-flow states, and hypercoagulable states. Once evidence of ulnar flow through the palmar arch is established, the area is prepared with antiseptic solution and draped in sterile fashion. The catheter is then placed into the arterial lumen percutaneously, using sterile technique. The dorsalis pedis artery may be used as an alternative to the radial artery.

Use of the brachial artery is associated with a higher likelihood of complication. The brachial artery lies between the bicipital tendon and median nerve at the antecubital fossa. Nerve injury as the result of catheter placement is more likely. If thrombosis occurs, circulation to the hand and arm may be severely compromised; in patients with diabetes, upper extremity vascular disease may be sufficiently advanced that partial loss of the hand may occur.

In patients who are restricted to bed, femoral arterial lines have a low complication rate and may be the most satisfactory choice. The femoral artery is usually superficial and easy to palpate. Disadvantages of the femoral site include difficulty in controlling bleeding near the genital region should such bleeding occur, impairment of mobility, and vascular compromise caused by thrombosis of the femoral artery or embolization from the catheter.

If the measuring system is too stiff, the snap will result in hyperresonance and overshooting of the pressure recording on the oscilloscope screen. If the measuring system is too compliant or if the catheter or tubing is obstructed, sudden release of the tab will lead to a slow and slurred descent toward the baseline.

The catheter-tubing-transducer system should be set up so that it is hyperresonant. The stiffest possible tubing should be obtained from the manufacturer, and the tubing should be kept at the shortest length consonant with patient care. If the system introduces excessive resonance, it can be damped with commercially available devices. It is not possible to compensate for systems that are too compliant.

Systolic and diastolic pressure measurements from the transducer cannot be relied on unless the snap test indicates that the measuring system and the patient's vasculature are adequately matched.

Catheter Whip

Systolic and diastolic pressures are also not to be trusted if the intravascular catheter moves around in the vascular lumen as the heart beats[2] [*see Figure 3*]. This movement, called catheter whip or catheter fling, is usually not a problem if the systemic arterial pressure is being measured by a catheter in the radial artery—such catheters cannot move around very much. When measurements are made by catheters in larger arteries, however, such as the femoral, catheter whip can introduce errors of 20 mm Hg or more in measurements of arterial pressures. Again, mean measurements are more accurate than systolic or diastolic measurements. Often, distortion introduced by a hyperresonant measuring system looks very much like catheter whip, and the two causes of distortion cannot be distinguished from each other. If this is the case, a device can be added to the catheter-tubing-transducer system to eliminate hyperresonance. Distortions that remain must be the result of catheter whip.

Pressure Differences at Varying Distances from the Heart

Systolic and, to a lesser extent, diastolic pressures in distal arteries are usually exaggerated with respect to central arterial or aortic pressures.[2,4] Systolic pressures in the radial artery tend to be higher than those in the brachial, which in turn tend to be higher than those in the aorta. The diastolic pressures tend to be slightly lower in the radial artery. These effects are caused by pulse wave reflection[5] [*see Figure 4*]. In normal persons younger than 50 years, the peak systolic pressure in the aortic root is approximately 20 mm Hg less than the systolic pressure in the radial artery; in normal persons 50 years of age and older, the peak systolic pressure in the aortic root is approximately 10 mm Hg less than the systolic pressure in the radial artery.[4] Once again, however, the mean pressures in the smaller arteries are close to the mean pressures in the larger ones.

Thus, measurements of systolic and diastolic pressures, even by catheter-transducer systems, can be suspect for three reasons: mismatched measuring systems, catheter whip, and true differences in systolic and diastolic pressures in arteries at different distances from the heart. It is always safe to use the mean pressure. With appropriate precautions—such as performing the snap test and making allowances for pulse wave amplification as the pressure wave advances distally—it is possible to use the systolic pressure in a peripheral artery to calculate back to the systolic pressure in the aortic root.

Figure 1 The mean pressure is defined as the area under a pressure tracing over an entire cycle divided by the time needed to produce that cycle. A pressure wave in the ascending aorta with a blood pressure of 120/80 mm Hg will have the same mean pressure as a pressure wave in the radial artery of the same patient, even though the radial artery pressure might be 140/75 mm Hg, because the systolic pressure in the radial artery is usually inscribed more rapidly than the systolic pressure in the aorta. The areas underneath the aortic pressure and radial artery pressure curves are identical. A useful but not infallible approximation of the mean pressure is to take the diastolic pressure plus one third of the difference between the systolic and diastolic pressures. In these examples, this formula would not work. The mean aortic pressure would be approximated at 93 mm Hg, whereas the mean radial artery pressure would be approximated at 97 mm Hg. Such results would be impossible: if the mean pressure in the radial artery actually were greater than the mean pressure in the aorta, blood would flow backward. This confusion is avoided by actually measuring the area under the curve and calculating the mean pressure exactly. Computer circuits in most pressure-monitoring systems make exact calculations of the mean pressure. Thus, the mean pressure taken from the digital readout of the pressure monitor is the single most accurate indicator of the actual pressure being measured and should be used for measurements of systemic arterial pressure.

MEASUREMENTS OBTAINED FROM SYSTEMIC ARTERIAL BLOOD

An indwelling systemic arterial catheter allows measurement of systemic arterial blood gases (i.e., the partial pressures of both oxygen [Po_2] and carbon dioxide [Pco_2] and the hydrogen ion concentration, which is expressed as the pH), oxygen saturation, and oxygen content. The partial pressure of oxygen or CO_2 refers to the pressure exerted by those gases dissolved in the plasma. Partial pressures are relatively easy and inexpensive to measure, and they are the most commonly used measurements of oxygen and CO_2 levels in the blood.

The partial pressure of oxygen may not provide sufficient information, however, because it is not linearly proportional to the total amount of oxygen in the blood: most of the blood's oxygen is not dissolved in the plasma but is combined with hemoglobin molecules and exerts no pressure whatsoever.[1] Of more consequence is the oxygen saturation. This term refers to the fraction of hemoglobin occupied by oxygen. The saturation can be approximated from measurements of blood Po_2, pH, Pco_2, and temperature. These calculations are typically made by computer in the blood gas laboratory, and the approximated saturation value is returned by the laboratory along with the measured values of partial pressures and pH. Oxygen saturation can also be measured directly through use of a co-oximeter. This device is simple to use and inexpensive, and it gives a more

accurate value because it makes a direct measure of the saturation. It does require another several milliliters of blood, however, and therefore adds to the amount of blood required of the patient.

But the greatest significance of the oxygen saturation measurement lies in its role in yielding values for oxygen content. The content shows the concentration of oxygen in the blood, and it is this value that counts. It literally refers to the amount of oxygen contained in a given volume of blood and is typically expressed as a volume percent or as milliliters of oxygen dissolved in 100 ml of blood. The oxygen content is a measure of all the oxygen in the blood, including oxygen attached to the hemoglobin molecule and oxygen dissolved in the plasma.

The amount of oxygen dissolved in plasma is small compared with the amount that is bound to hemoglobin. As long as the Po_2 is less than about 100 mm Hg, the contribution of the oxygen in the plasma to the total oxygen content need not be considered, assuming that the hemoglobin concentration is at least 7 g/dl. Neglecting to count the oxygen dissolved in the plasma makes calculation of oxygen content simple: the oxygen content is approximately 1.39 multiplied by the hemoglobin concentration multiplied by the oxygen saturation (So_2):

$$O_2 \text{ content} = 1.39 \times [Hb] \times So_2$$

Figure 2 **The snap test will indicate if the pressure measured at the transducer is the same as the pressure measured at the tip of the catheter in the vasculature. A pressure of 250 mm Hg is superimposed on the pressure-measuring system by opening the flow-controlling device of the Intraflow equipment. The pressure is abruptly removed from the transducer system by snapping the valve closed. If the catheter-tubing-transducer system is well matched to the patient's vasculature, a normal arterial tracing (left) should resume promptly. If the catheter-tubing-transducer system is excessively compliant or obstructed by a clot in the catheter or by a kink in the tubing, sudden closure of the valve between the pressure bag and the transducer system leads to a slurred, hyporesonant response (center). When the measuring system is excessively stiff in comparison with the patient's vasculature, sudden closure of the flow-controlling device with abrupt removal of the high pressure produces a hyperresonant arterial tracing (right), as manifested by an overshoot of the pressure to levels even below 0.**

WELL MATCHED

HYPORESONANT

HYPERRESONANT

Pressure *(mm Hg)*

240
180
120
60
0

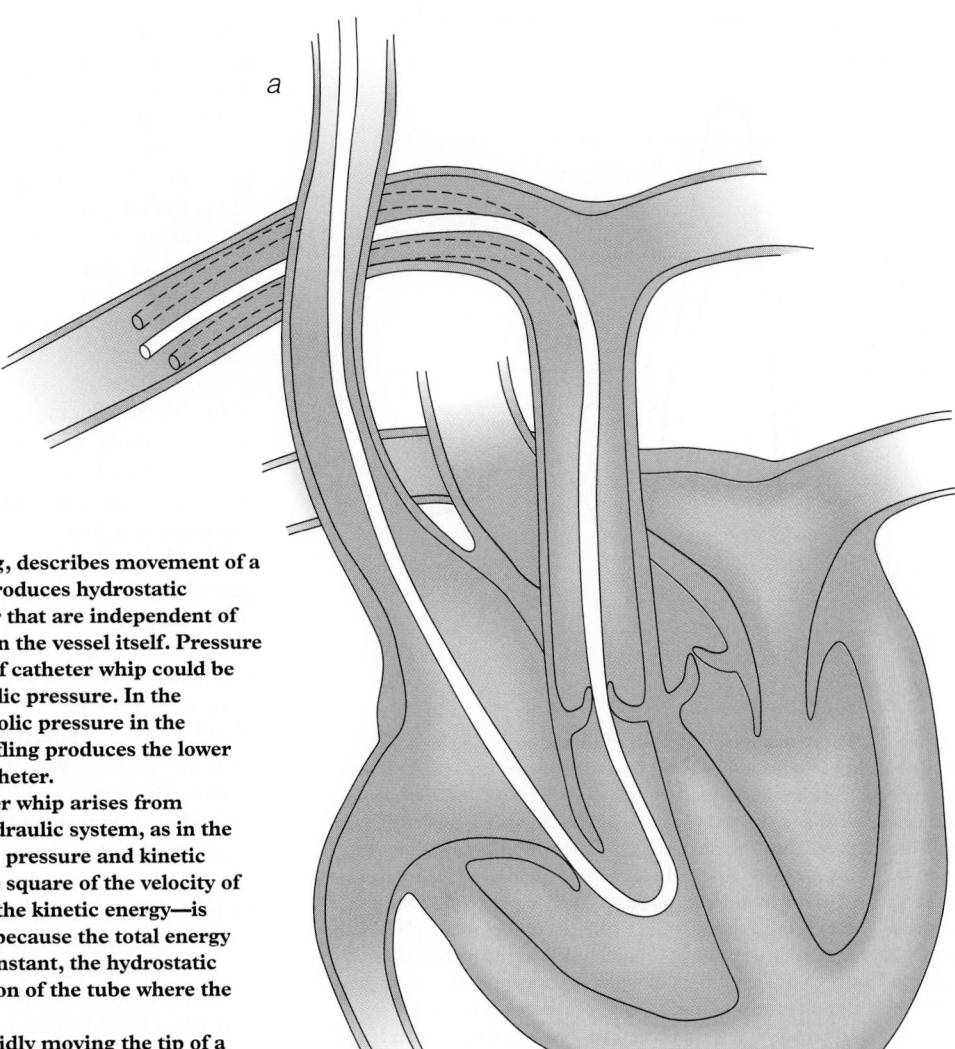

Figure 3 Catheter whip, or catheter fling, describes movement of a catheter within the vasculature (*a*) that produces hydrostatic pressure changes at the tip of the catheter that are independent of any changes in hydrostatic pressure within the vessel itself. Pressure drops during diastole that are the result of catheter whip could be falsely interpreted as true vascular diastolic pressure. In the pressure tracing shown (*b*), the true diastolic pressure in the pulmonary artery is 24 mm Hg; catheter fling produces the lower pressure of 12 mm Hg at the tip of the catheter.

The pressure drop produced by catheter whip arises from Bernoulli's principle: total energy in a hydraulic system, as in the vascular system, is the sum of hydrostatic pressure and kinetic energy. The kinetic energy depends on the square of the velocity of the fluid. Because the velocity—and thus the kinetic energy—is greater the narrower the system (*c*), and because the total energy measured at any point in the system is constant, the hydrostatic pressure must be less in the narrow portion of the tube where the velocity of flow is higher.

Catheter whip can be simulated by rapidly moving the tip of a fluid-filled catheter through a water bath at a constant depth beneath the surface. If the catheter were held immobile, the hydrostatic pressure would be seen to be constant at a given depth in the bath. The kinetic energy, however, increases as the catheter moves through the water because the more rapidly the catheter moves, the greater is the velocity of the fluid past the tip and the greater the kinetic energy component; the greater the kinetic energy, the lower the hydrostatic pressure as measured at the tip. Similarly, if a femoral or pulmonary arterial catheter moves within the vasculature as the heart beats, the velocity of blood across its orifice will increase; as the velocity increases and the kinetic energy increases, the hydrostatic pressure as measured at the tip will fall. This transient decrease in hydrostatic pressure at the tip of the catheter (as seen in the tracing) does not reflect the true hydrostatic pressure in the artery.

The radial artery catheter is best for determining the total energy in the blood flow. The catheter will not whip, because the artery is small and the catheter has no room to move about, and there will be no kinetic energy component in the blood, because the radial artery catheter is end-on (i.e., it faces into the direction of the flow) and thus the velocity of the blood as it runs into the end of the catheter is zero. Therefore, the hydrostatic pressure will represent the total energy of the blood at that point of the vasculature. A catheter placed in the ascending aorta will be buffeted by the rapidly accelerating blood in the aorta, and catheter whip will be introduced. A pulmonary arterial catheter potentially has both the problem of catheter whip and the problem that it measures pressure in the direction of flow rather than end-on.

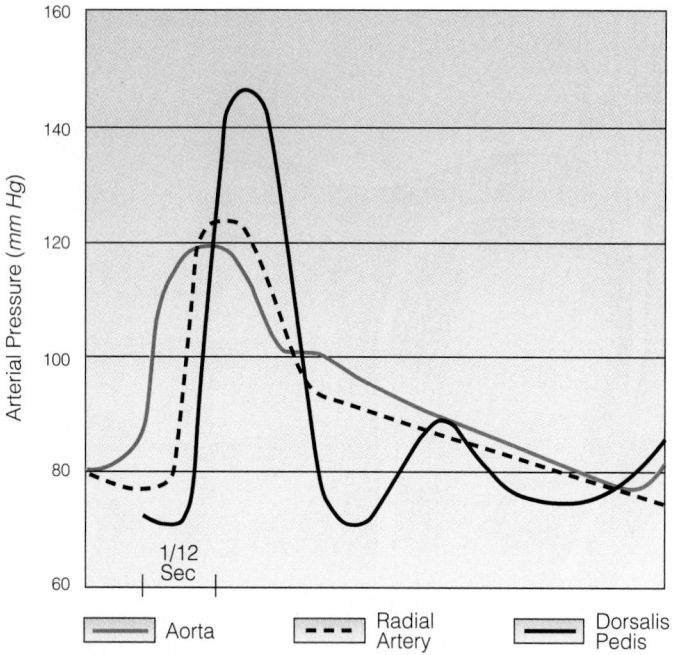

Figure 4 There are true differences in systolic and diastolic pressures in arteries at different distances from the heart. These differences result when pressure waves reflected from distal arteriolar sites are superimposed onto the forward-traveling pressure waves from the aorta. As the measuring point (i.e., the catheter) moves closer to the distal reflecting site, systolic pressures increase and diastolic pressures decrease because the reflected pressure waves from the periphery return sooner to a catheter that is placed distally. The result of this in-phase superimposition of reflected waves onto anterograde waves is augmentation of systolic pressures and diminution of diastolic pressures. The systolic pressure in the radial artery, therefore, can be 10 to 20 mm Hg higher than the systolic pressure in the ascending aorta, leading to confusion. Furthermore, the pressure tracing at the root of the aorta is wider than the pressure tracing in the radial artery because reflected waves are returning from the periphery at different times; their effect is thus distributed over a larger portion of the cardiac cycle, and the pressure wave in the aorta is broad. The pressure wave in the radial artery is narrow because the reflected waves tend to be superimposed on the forward-traveling waves, in phase. The mean pressures, however, will be almost the same in both vessels, with the mean pressure in the radial artery being just slightly less than the mean pressure in the ascending aorta. Use of the mean pressure will eliminate inaccuracies introduced by catheter-vascular mismatching and confusion introduced by pulse wave reflection; inspection of the tracing will usually reveal aberrations introduced by catheter whip.

Thus, if the hemoglobin concentration is 12.5 and the oxygen saturation is 97 percent, the oxygen content of the blood will be 16.9 ml/dl. This value is normal for a person with a hematocrit of 38 to 39 percent. The normal value for mixed venous blood rests on the finding that mixed venous oxygen saturation ($S_{mv}O_2$) for such a person is normally 75 percent. Therefore, the oxygen content of pulmonary arterial blood in this example is 1.39 × 12.5 × 75 percent, or 13 ml/dl. Although 1.39 is probably the most accurate figure available for calculating the oxygen content of blood, other values—some as low as 1.33—have also been reported. Thus, for purposes of simplification, one may use a value of 4/3 instead of 1.39. The value of 4/3 makes calculations easier to perform.

The partial pressure of carbon dioxide indicates the amount of CO_2 dissolved in the plasma. Carbon dioxide content can be calculated, but it seldom is because within physiologic ranges of P_{CO_2}, the CO_2 in the blood is almost linearly related to the partial pressure.[6] Thus, measurements of carbon dioxide are easier to deal with than measurements of oxygen levels.

Hydrogen ion concentration is usually expressed as pH and is obtained by direct measurement with ion-sensitive electrodes. Measurements of serum lactate can also be used to identify and quantitate acidosis. The arterial blood reflects whole body metabolism. Normal lactate concentrations are less than 2 mmol/L. In hypermetabolic critically ill patients, lactate concentrations can be elevated to 3 mmol/L or greater; values greater than 8 mmol/L indicate severe metabolic acidosis. Normal lactate-to-pyruvate ratios are less than 20.

Blood that is drawn for blood gas determinations should be placed immediately on ice to inhibit oxygen consumption by the neutrophils in the specimen. The blood, when measured in the blood gas apparatus, will be rewarmed to 37° C by a heating element in the cuvette. Thus, values for partial pressure of oxygen and for pH will be obtained by the laboratory with the blood at 37° C. The patient's blood may be warmer or colder than 37° C, however. If the patient's blood is 35° C when it is drawn, for example, some of the oxygen will come out of solution when it is warmed up to 37° C. Thus, the partial pressure measured by the apparatus will be higher than the partial pressure of the gas in the blood when it was circulating in the patient at the lower temperature. One way to remember this concept is to imagine a glass of cool beer as it gradually warms up to the surrounding room temperature. As the beer warms, carbon dioxide dissolved in the liquid will come out of solution and form bubbles; that is, as the liquid warms up, the partial pressure exerted by the gas will increase.

The physician and nurse caring for the patient need not make this temperature correction themselves. The blood gas laboratory typically will report temperature-corrected values for the partial pressures and pH if the patient's temperature is supplied to the laboratory along with the specimen.[7]

An increasing number of clinicians, however, no longer make temperature corrections for blood gases.[8] This technique has been termed the alpha-stat method for managing blood gas abnormalities in hypothermic or hyperthermic patients. It is thought to induce fewer abnormalities in acid-base balance when the patient's temperature returns to normal [see I:7 Life-Threatening Acid-Base Disorders].

Central Venous Catheters

INDICATIONS FOR INSERTION

There are several indications for placement of central venous catheters[1] [see Sidebar Insertion of Central Venous Catheters]. Administration of parenteral nutrition requires a suitably placed central venous catheter [*see VII:9 Nutritional Support*]. In addition, prolonged administration of antibiotics or chemotherapeutic regimens may require central venous access. Central venous pressure (CVP), or right atrial pressure, is used to aid in the assessment of right-sided heart function. When combined with variables obtained from placement of a pulmonary arterial catheter, the measurement of right atrial pressure can be used to calculate pulmonary vascular

SPONTANEOUS VENTILATION

Expiration | Inspiration

MECHANICAL VENTILATION

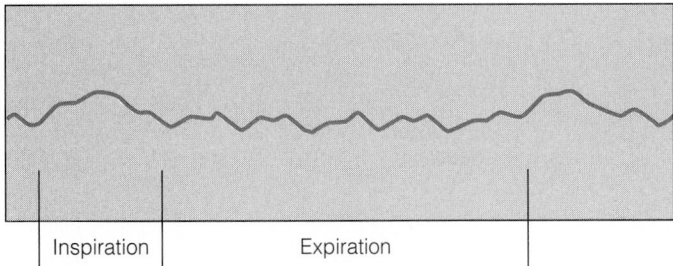

Inspiration | Expiration

INTERMITTENT MANDATORY VENTILATION

IMV Inspiration | Expiration | Two Spontaneous Inspirations | IMV Inspiration

Figure 5 **End-expiratory pressure is relatively independent of the patient's ventilatory status and thus is most representative of the patient's vascular volume. For example, in a patient breathing spontaneously (top), central venous pressure (or, equivalently, right atrial pressure) falls as the lungs pull away from the intrathoracic great veins and right atrium. In these patients, the end-expiratory pressure is the highest pressure measured during the ventilatory cycle. During mechanical ventilation (middle), the lungs are pushed against the outside of the heart and great veins; intracavitary and intravascular pressures are thereby increased during inspiration, and the end-expiratory pressure is the lowest pressure measured during the ventilatory cycle. During intermittent mandatory ventilation (bottom), the machine-generated breaths produce increases in the CVP and spontaneous breaths produce decreases; the end-expiratory pressure is the plateau pressure between the two extremes.**

Insertion of Central Venous Catheters

Several sites of central venous access are commonly used: internal jugular [*see Figure 6*], subclavian, and external jugular veins and subcutaneous veins in the antecubital fossa or arm. A determination of whether to use the internal jugular or the subclavian approach must take several considerations into account. The right internal jugular has the lowest overall complication rate. The right side also provides a straight course to the right atrium. When the internal jugular approach is used, injury to the carotid artery is possible, but the carotid artery is also more easily palpated than the subclavian artery. On the left side, the thoracic duct is at risk for injury. The potential for nerve damage is greater with use of the internal jugular vein. The subclavian approach is generally more comfortable for the patient.

When the subclavian approach is used, the patient is placed in the supine position and Trendelenburg's position. The subclavicular area is prepared and draped in sterile fashion. Local anesthesia is obtained along the inferior portion of the clavicle. A 21-gauge needle is used to locate the subclavian vein. The needle is directed perpendicular to the sagittal plane and parallel to the coronal plane. The skin is entered, and the clavicle is followed inferiorly. Contact with the underside of the clavicle is essential. The subclavian vein is between the clavicle and first rib. When blood is aspirated, a guide wire is placed through the needle. The needle is then removed and the catheter placed over the guide wire. A chest x-ray is obtained to verify satisfactory positioning of the catheter. The subclavian approach to central venous catheterization is illustrated elsewhere [*see 97 Nutritional Support*].

The external jugular approach is associated with a risk of subclavian vein injury when a relatively stiff catheter is used. Catheters placed in the external jugular vein are more frequently used as peripheral lines than as central venous lines.

The long arm approach has a high incidence of thrombophlebitis but may be satisfactory for 48 to 72 hours. In the long arm approach, the antecubital fossa is prepared and draped in sterile fashion. The basilic vein is percutaneously entered and the catheter advanced. On average, 50 cm of catheter must be inserted from the left antecubital vein to reach the right atrium [*see Table 2*]. A chest x-ray is obtained to verify satisfactory placement of the catheter.

resistance. Right-sided heart function, especially in critically ill patients, is a poor predictor of left-sided heart function.

COMPLICATIONS ASSOCIATED
WITH CENTRAL VENOUS CATHETERS

Percutaneous puncture of central veins, through either a jugular or a subclavian approach, can lead to several complications, some of which are immediately life threatening.[1] Penetration of the parietal pleura can produce a pneumothorax. This complication occurs in approximately six percent of cases. Puncture of the subclavian artery can lead to exsanguination into the pleural cavity. Intrapleural infusion of administered hyperalimentation can occur with improper catheter placement. The brachial plexus lies near the large veins that are commonly catheterized. Puncture of one of the major trunks or divisions can permanently impair the extremity. Puncture of the trachea, esophagus, or lung during catheter insertion can lead to subcutaneous emphysema. Puncture of the internal jugular vein on the left side can damage the thoracic duct and lead to a chylothorax. Improper use of the introducing needle can result in shearing of the catheter and catheter emboli. These complications will occur occasionally no matter how experienced the person performing the procedure; the goal is to keep the incidence of such complications to a minimum. All are results of technical errors, and as with all technical errors associated with procedures, prevention requires knowledge of anatomy and gentleness in performing the procedure.

MEASUREMENT OF CENTRAL VENOUS PRESSURE

Ideally, central venous pressures are measured with a transducer rather than with a manometer. It may be necessary to use manometers while waiting for the required equipment to be set up or when working in areas of the hospital where monitors are not available. It is preferable, however, to place the patient in a unit with the appropriate monitoring devices.

Central venous pressure measurements are usually made at end-expiration and are best obtained by direct observation of the pressure tracing on the oscilloscope screen. In some monitoring systems, digital readouts of the central venous pressure represent the mean pressure averaged over several ventilatory cycles; in other monitoring units, the digital readouts make an attempt to give the end-expiratory values. In the case of arterial pressures, mean pressure averaging is desirable [see Systemic Arterial Catheters, Measurement of Systemic Arterial Pressure, above]; in the case of central venous pressures, however, such averaging will usually result in values that are higher than those attained at end-expiration.

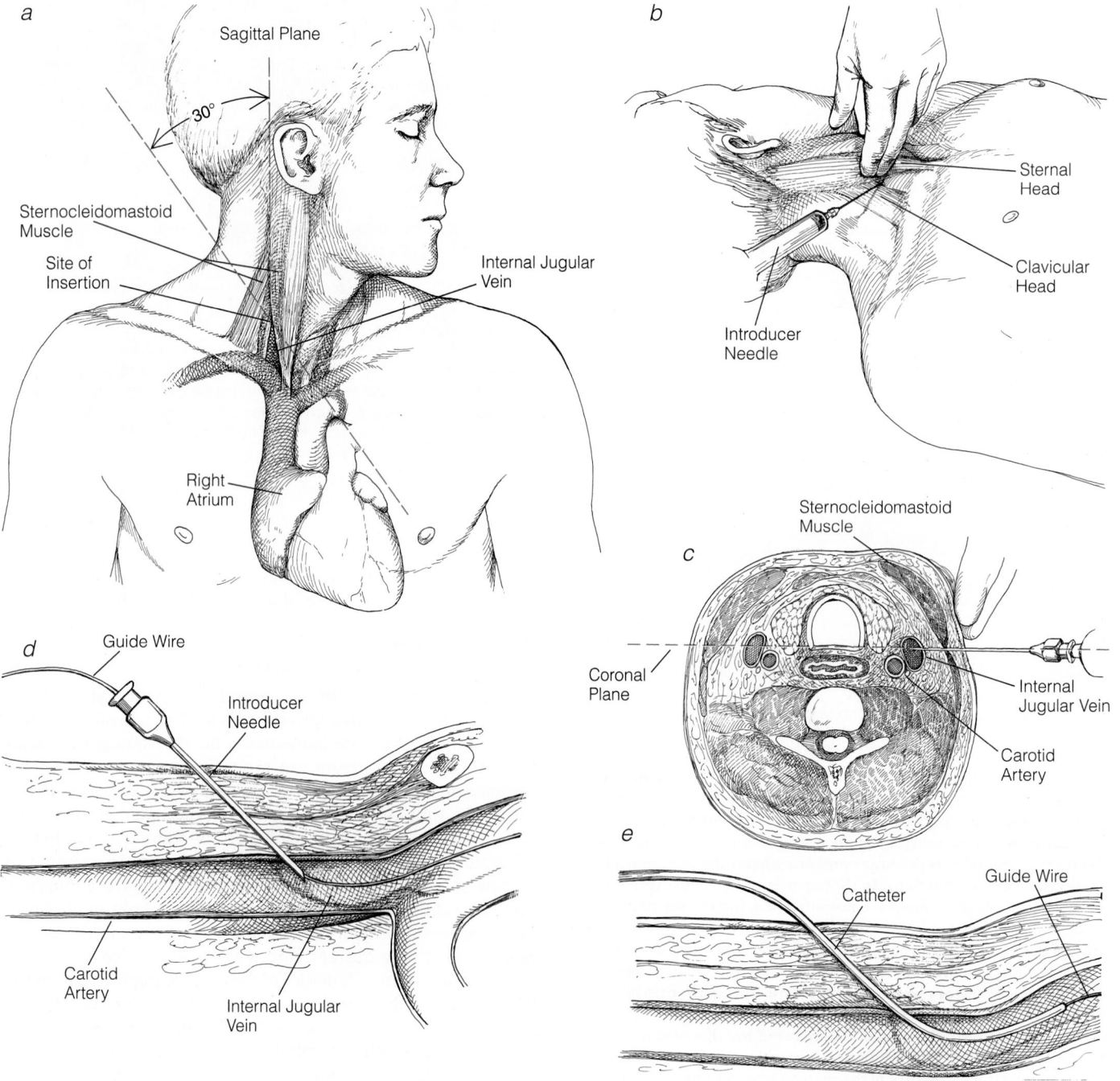

The end-expiratory pressure is often the most representative of the patient's vascular volume because it is relatively independent of the patient's ventilatory status. During spontaneous inspiration, as the lungs pull away from the great veins and cardiac chambers, the intracardiac pressures fall. Thus, the end-expiratory pressure is typically the highest pressure recorded on the oscilloscope. In contrast, during mechanical ventilation, insufflation of the lungs compresses the cardiac chambers, thereby increasing intracardiac pressures, and the end-expiratory pressure is typically the lowest pressure recorded. Intermittent mandatory ventilation produces both augmented vascular pressures when the ventilator gives a mechanical breath and lowered intracardiac pressures when the patient takes a spontaneous breath. In this case, the end-expiratory pressure is typically the plateau that develops between the two extremes [see Figure 5].

During inspiration, large tidal volumes or rapid inspiratory flow rates can produce peak intracardiac pressures that exceed end-expiratory values by as much as 10 mm Hg. If end-expiratory values are used, these effects are eliminated. Some physicians try to minimize the effects of positive-pressure ventilation on interpretation of pressure tracings by taking the patient off the ventilator while making the measurements. This maneuver makes it easier to interpret the pressures, but it has the disadvantage that the most significant pressures are those that exist when the patient is being ventilated. Removing the critically ill patient from the ventilator produces a condition that no longer represents accurate values.

Although most physicians use the end-expiratory pressures with the patient on the ventilator as the values on which to base clinical decisions, some physicians have switched to the use of digital readouts. The advantage of the digital readouts is that the readings are independent of the nurse or physician. Attempting to read end-expiratory pressure tracings can sometimes be difficult even for the most experienced clinician or nurse,[9,10] and digital readouts eliminate this element of potential variability.

Zeroing of the transducer or manometer must be done precisely. Small errors in positioning of the transducer can lead to large errors in measurement. Most intensive care units use the midaxillary line as the zero level for vascular pressures.

Figure 6 For central venous access via the internal jugular vein, first place the patient in the supine position. Clear all objects from the head of the bed, pull the bed away from the wall to gain access to the head of the bed, and remove the headboard. Adjust the bed to a comfortable height for working, and place the patient in Trendelenburg's position (10° to 20°) to prevent air emboli and to produce venous distention. Have the patient turn his or her head 90° away from the side of venipuncture. The right side is preferred for two reasons: first, because it provides direct access to the superior vena cava, and second, because injury to the thoracic duct is avoided. Put on mask and hat, wash hands, and put on gown and gloves. Prep and drape the patient.

Identify the triangle formed by the two heads of the sternocleidomastoid muscle. The apex of the triangle is more apparent if the patient is able to lift his or her head. Infiltrate local anesthetic into the skin and underlying soft tissue along the proposed path of the introducer needle. Generally, this path will run from the apex of the triangle to the nipple of the opposite breast. Aspirate before infiltration to avoid intravascular injection.

The internal jugular vein is then located in the coronal plane posterior to the sternocleidomastoid and above the first rib insertion of the scalenus anticus muscle. Either the lateral or the central approach should be used. The initial efforts at finding the internal jugular vein should be done parallel to the coronal plane, with the needle directed toward the nipple of the opposite breast, and at an angle of 30° to the sagittal plane (a, b, and c). All attempts at finding the internal jugular vein should be made with an 18-gauge or smaller needle. The operator should be aware of the carotid artery, which is located medially to the vein.

Once the vein is located, enlarge the skin wound at the puncture site. If the finder needle is of a diameter too small for the guide wire, one must use the appropriate size introducer needle to cannulate the internal jugular vein. The finder needle may be left in place to serve as a guide, or it may be removed. Once the internal jugular vein is cannulated, insert the guide wire (d). The guide wire must thread easily. When the guide wire has been inserted a generous length, remove the introducer needle, holding the guide wire in place. Insert a dilator and then the catheter (e). Firm pressure can be maintained on these objects during insertion as long as the guide wire maintains free movement in the lumen. Insert the catheter to an appropriate length. Remove the wire and the dilator. Aspirate blood, flush the catheter with heparinized saline, and place Luer-lock caps on all ports. Suture the catheter in place, and apply sterile dressings. A chest x-ray should be obtained to verify placement and to rule out pneumothorax.

Pulmonary Arterial Catheters

INDICATIONS FOR INSERTION

Use of pulmonary arterial catheters (Swan-Ganz catheters) is indicated in patients with any severe cardiopulmonary derangement[11] [see Sidebar Insertion of Pulmonary Arterial Catheters]. For example, when myocardial function is compromised in myocardial failure or myocardial infarction, the catheter can provide crucial information on the efficacy of pharmacological support and can aid in the diagnosis of abnormalities such as pericardial tamponade and acute mitral regurgitation.

Hypovolemic shock that does not respond readily to volume administration is another indication for insertion of a pulmonary arterial catheter; the catheter may reveal abnormalities of myocardial function or of the pulmonary or systemic vasculature that require specific interventions in addition to volume loading. Similarly, pulmonary arterial monitoring is frequently required in patients with sepsis who have inadequate urine output or who are hypotensive; the information provided by the catheter about the adequacy of oxygen consumption and of pharmacological support is of great value.

Pulmonary disorders, especially those that carry a high risk of associated myocardial dysfunction, are another indication. For example, pulmonary edema may be caused by elevated left atrial and pulmonary microvascular hydrostatic pressures or by endothelial disruption, which in turn may reflect inadequately resuscitated shock. (In the first example, treatment of the pulmonary failure would require diuresis; in the case of increased microvascular permeability, the treatment may require more aggressive fluid resuscitation.)

Pressure *(mm Hg)*

RIGHT ATRIUM

Inspiration | Expiration

RIGHT VENTRICLE

Inspiration | Expiration

PULMONARY ARTERY

Inspiration | Expiration

PULMONARY ARTERIAL WEDGE

Inspiration | Expiration

Figure 7 **Illustrated here are pressure tracings in the right atrium, right ventricle, pulmonary artery, and pulmonary arterial wedge positions for a patient on mechanical ventilation. Note the gradually increasing pressure during diastole and the low mean diastolic pressure in the right ventricle. The pulmonary arterial tracing is characterized by a relatively high mean diastolic pressure and decreasing pressures during diastole. The pressure in the pulmonary arterial wedge position is characterized by a damped waveform, compared with the pulmonary arterial pressure. More important, the wedge pressure is easily converted to a pulmonary arterial pressure by deflation of the balloon.**

Pulmonary arterial catheters may also be indicated for patients with good cardiopulmonary function who are undergoing procedures associated with large volume requirements and fluid shifts (e.g., procedures on the abdominal aorta), as well as for patients who will undergo elective procedures and who either have underlying myocardial or pulmonary disease or are at high risk for intraoperative or postoperative development of cardiopulmonary problems. A pulmonary arterial catheter is indicated if the patient has failure of two organs that might have different priorities with respect to fluid administration: a patient with both pulmonary failure and oliguria might benefit from fluid restriction, to reduce pulmonary microvascular hydrostatic pressures; on the other hand, that patient's kidneys might require fluid administration. A patient with a head injury and oliguria poses the same problem. The catheter, by giving precise information

about the cardiovascular system, can greatly simplify the management of such complicated patients.

COMPLICATIONS ASSOCIATED WITH SWAN-GANZ CATHETERS

Complications of Swan-Ganz catheter insertion include those associated with central venous puncture [*see* Central Venous Catheters, Complications Associated with Central Venous Catheters, *above*] and others that are unique to the long intra-

---

Insertion of Pulmonary Arterial Catheters

Sites of access that are commonly used for insertion of a Swan-Ganz catheter include the right internal jugular and the subclavian veins. Before the catheter is placed, all lines are flushed and the balloon is tested and verified to be functional. Swan-Ganz catheters are typically placed without fluoroscopic equipment; passage relies on correct interpretation of pressures as the catheter passes through the cardiac chambers and into the pulmonary artery. The catheter is placed through an introducer and advanced under constant pressure monitoring [*see Figure 7*]. When respiratory excursion is seen, the balloon is inflated, and the catheter is advanced until a right atrial tracing is encountered. The catheter is then advanced to the right ventricle. Entry into the right ventricle is usually obvious because right ventricular pressure tracings show pressure excursions that far exceed any seen in tracings from the superior vena cava or the right atrium. The right ventricular pressure tracing is also characterized by an increase in pressure during diastole. The catheter should then be drawn gently back into the right atrium with the balloon inflated. The balloon will be felt to tug on the tricuspid valve as the catheter passes between the two chambers. The precise position of the tricuspid valve then becomes known, and the catheter should be reinserted into the right ventricle and advanced into the pulmonary artery with the insertion of only a few more centimeters of catheter. The pulmonary arterial tracing is characterized by a gradually decreasing pressure during diastole and by a mean diastolic pressure that is greater than the mean right ventricular diastolic pressure. Once entry into the pulmonary artery is confirmed, the catheter should be advanced until a wedge tracing is obtained; the wedge tracing is usually easily recognized by damping of the pressure tracing. The balloon should then be deflated; deflation should produce a full pulmonary arterial excursion. Reinflation of the balloon should reproduce the wedge reading.

Mechanical ventilation exerts an influence on pressure tracings that can lead to misinterpretations. In patients on mechanical ventilation, the right ventricular diastolic pressure may be higher than the pulmonary arterial diastolic pressure during expiration. Looking only at a diastolic pressure, without coordinating the reading with the phase of the ventilator cycle, can be very confusing [*see Figure 8*].

One of the difficulties that may be encountered during insertion of a pulmonary arterial catheter is curling of the catheter in the right atrium. It is important to remember that once the catheter passes the tricuspid valve, it should enter the pulmonary artery with passage of just a few more centimeters [*see Table 2*]. If a pulmonary arterial tracing is not obtained with insertion of an additional 10 cm of catheter, the catheter must be curling in the right ventricle. Another difficulty is entrapment of the end of the catheter in the muscular trabeculae of the right ventricle; the resultant damped tracing can closely resemble a pulmonary arterial wedge tracing [*see Figure 9*]. Entrapment can be avoided by verifying that the catheter has entered the pulmonary artery before advancing more tubing. Lastly, arrhythmias can develop during passage of the pulmonary arterial catheter, particularly while the end of the catheter is in the right ventricle. The risk of arrhythmias is minimized by keeping the balloon inflated as the catheter passes through the ventricle and, when appropriate, with administration of prophylactic doses of lidocaine during insertion.

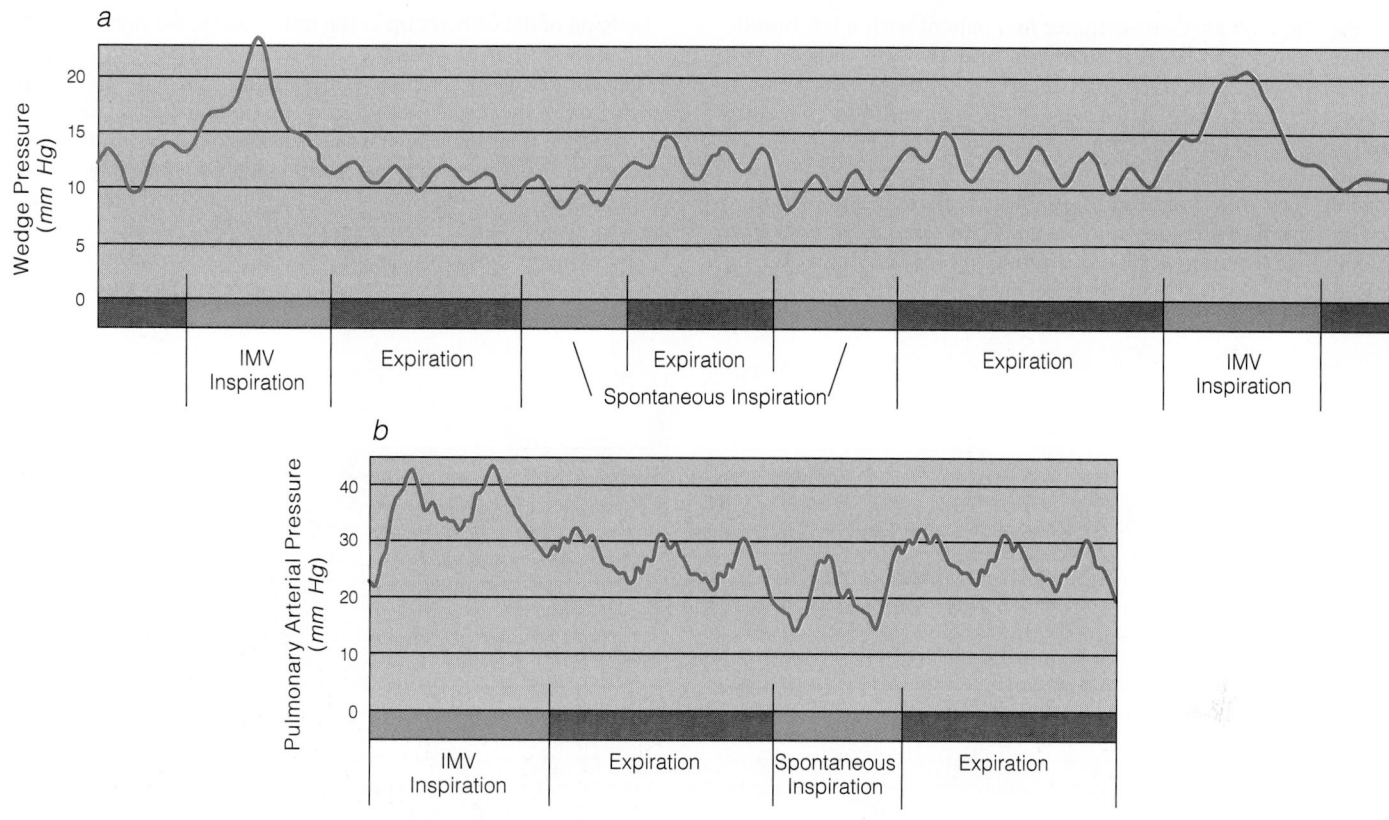

Figure 8 Mechanical ventilation can generate wide swings in pressure and make it difficult to assign a value to wedge or pulmonary arterial pressures. When the wedge tracing shown here (*a*) was obtained, the patient was on intermittent mandatory ventilation (IMV). The mechanical breaths generated pressure peaks of more than 20 mm Hg; spontaneous inspiratory efforts by the patient developed trough pressure readings of 8 mm Hg. The correct value, which should be taken at the plateau between the machine and spontaneous breaths, in this patient is 12 mm Hg. Similar difficulties arise with interpretation of pulmonary arterial pressure (*b*). Wide swings in pressure between systole and diastole in the pulmonary artery compound the problem even more. The mean pressure is somewhere between the two extremes; during the IMV inspiration shown here, the mean pressure is between 32 and 43 mm Hg. Approximating the mean pressure as the diastolic pressure plus one third of the pulse pressure would give a value of 36 mm Hg. During the spontaneous inspiration, the mean pressure is between 15 and 28 mm Hg; approximating the mean pressure would give a value of 19 mm Hg. The ideal is to read the mean pressure during expiration, toward the end of the expiratory cycle, but this can be a challenge for even the most experienced ICU nurse. Here, the mean pressure during expiration is between 23 and 31 mm Hg; the approximated mean pressure is 26 mm Hg.

vascular device.[1] These complications include ventricular arrhythmias, ventricular rupture, valvular damage on the right side of the heart, intracardiac knotting of the catheter, and pulmonary infarction induced by permanent wedging of the catheter in the distal pulmonary vasculature. It is necessary that pressures be interpreted correctly as the catheter passes through the cardiac chambers [*see Figure 7*].

Ventricular arrhythmias are relatively common during passage of the catheter, particularly in patients who have suffered recent myocardial infarctions and in those with an irritable myocardium as indicated by a preexisting arrhythmia or conduction defect. Some of these patients are best served by prophylactic administration of lidocaine. In rare instances, aggressive treatment of such arrhythmias may be required. Usually, the arrhythmia will subside when the end of the catheter finally passes through the ventricle and enters the pulmonary artery; sometimes, however, the arrhythmia can be ablated only by completely removing the

catheter. The balloon on the end of the catheter should be kept inflated during passage to cushion the tip and minimize myocardial irritability.

Table 2 Distances between Catheter Insertion Sites and the Right Atrium

Insertion Site	Distance to Right Atrium*
Internal jugular subclavian vein	15 cm
Right antecubital vein	40 cm
Left antecubital vein	50 cm
Femoral vein	30 cm

*Add 15 cm to obtain distance to main pulmonary artery.

Passing a Swan-Ganz catheter in a patient with a left bundle branch block can be particularly hazardous. The catheter can eliminate conduction through the right ventricle, producing a complete heart block. Treatment of such a condition (if it does not resolve on prompt withdrawal of the catheter) may require insertion of a transvenous pacemaker or the use of external pacing. The time required to establish a rhythm, however, may be so long that a fatality may result. Therefore, in patients with a left bundle branch block, Swan-Ganz catheters should be placed only when absolutely necessary.

Lodging of the catheter tip in the trabeculae of the right ventricle is a common problem when the catheter is being passed [see Figure 9]. The end of the catheter can puncture the right ventricular wall, but this rarely occurs. Puncture may not be immediately obvious. On occasion, the puncture site seals by itself; it is far more likely, however, to lead to pericardial tamponade and, possibly, death. Measurements from the Swan-Ganz catheter will indicate pericardial tamponade, which mandates emergency operation.

The catheter can damage the tricuspid and pulmonic valves as it passes through them, especially if it is roughly pulled back

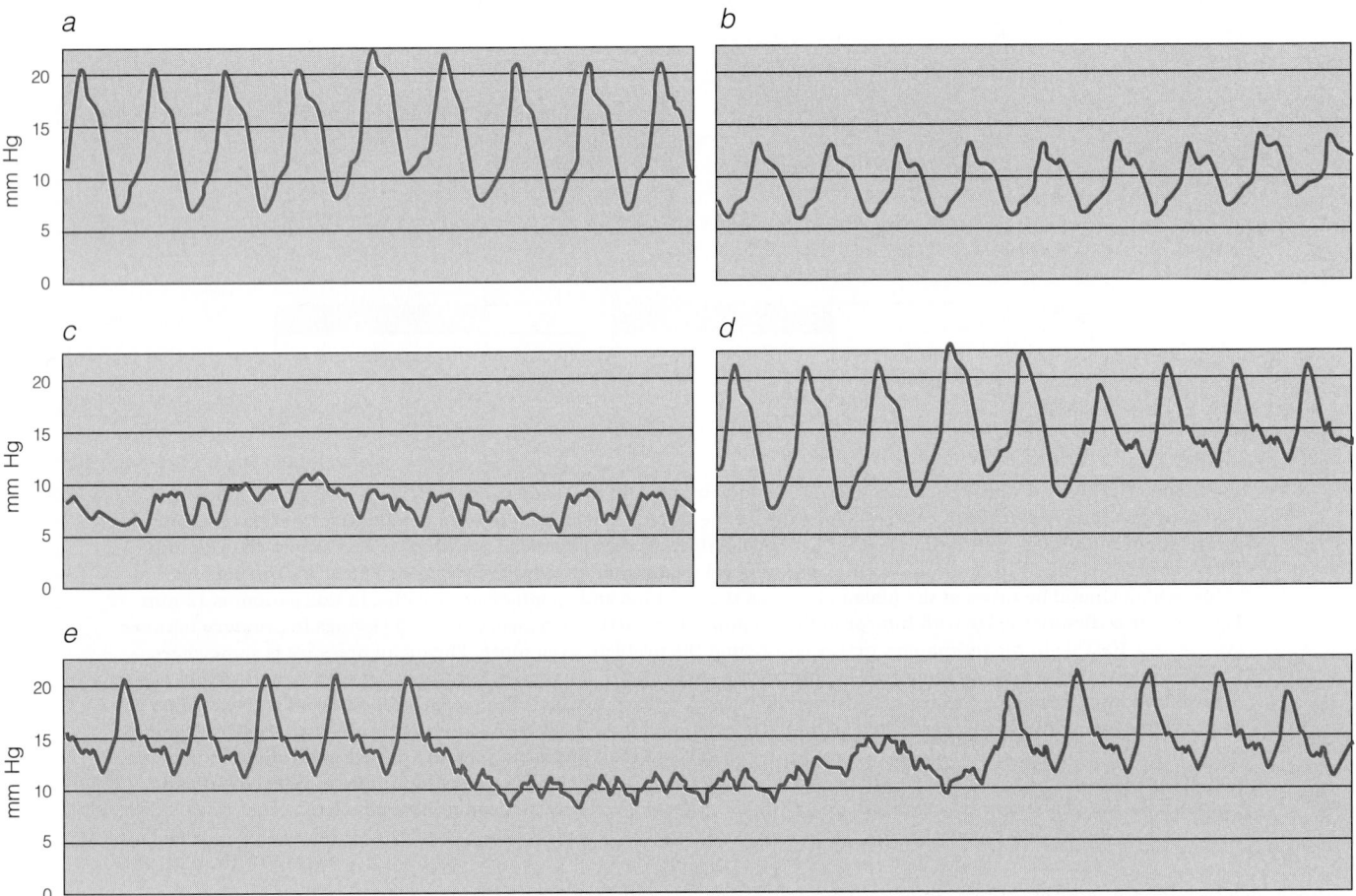

Figure 9 Lodging of the catheter tip in the trabeculae of the right ventricle is a common problem when a Swan-Ganz catheter is passed. Right ventricular tracings (*a*) are characterized by dramatic pressure excursions and pressure increases during diastole. If the tip of the catheter becomes caught in the ventricular trabeculae (*b*), a smaller pulse pressure is generated. The tracing obtained is different from the right ventricular tracing and could be misinterpreted: at first glance, it could be a tracing from the pulmonary artery. Closer analysis, however, shows that the pressure during diastole increases and that diastolic and systolic pressures are both decreased. A pulmonary arterial tracing would have a decreasing pressure as diastole progresses, and the mean diastolic pressure should be greater than the mean ventricular diastolic pressure. Further advancement of the catheter (*c*) produces further damping and confusion. The tracing could be interpreted as a wedge pressure. Pulling back on the catheter, however, and sequential deflation and inflation of the balloon do not produce a reproducible alternation between a pulmonary arterial tracing and a wedge tracing. This inability to generate such a reproducible alternation makes the tracing suspicious. Further manipulation of the catheter (*d*) gives a clear transition into a pulmonary arterial tracing. The pressure decreases during diastole, and the mean pulmonary arterial diastolic pressure is greater than the mean right ventricular diastolic pressure. The position of the catheter in the pulmonary artery (*e*) is confirmed by balloon inflation, which produces a wedge reading, and balloon deflation, which produces the return of a normal pulmonary arterial tracing.

through those valves in a retrograde manner with the balloon inflated. Gentleness is important in this regard. In addition, if the catheter is left in place for more than a few days, valvular damage may result. Little can be done to prevent this damage other than minimizing long-term use of the catheters.

Another problem unique to the Swan-Ganz catheter is intra-cardiac knotting, which is most likely to develop when the catheter is being placed. The knot can occasionally be untied by manipulation of the catheter under fluoroscopy. A J-wire passed into the right side of the heart from the groin is also useful in untying the knot. Otherwise, the catheter will have to be withdrawn to the site of entry and then removed, usually under direct surgical control.

Swan-Ganz catheters that are left in place for more than a few days can migrate distally and cut off the blood supply to the pulmonary parenchyma, resulting in pulmonary infarction. This situation is best prevented by continuous monitoring of the pulmonary arterial waveform. Development of a permanently wedged pattern on the oscilloscope is an indication that the catheter should immediately be withdrawn far enough to reestablish a normal pulmonary arterial tracing.

The pulmonary arterial catheter can, on rare occasions, perforate the pulmonary artery. This event typically presents with hemoptysis; it may present with acute cardiopulmonary collapse during or immediately after measurement of a wedge pressure. Advanced age, pulmonary arterial hypertension, anticoagulation with warfarin, clotting deficiencies, migration of the catheter distally into the pulmonary vasculature, and balloon overinflation can all contribute to the risk of pulmonary arterial rupture. Patients who have tumors surrounding the pulmonary artery are also at increased risk for such rupture. The balloon itself may directly disrupt the pulmonary artery, or inflation of the balloon may force the tip of the catheter through the vessel wall. Prevention (which, as always, is better than attempted cure) consists of continuous monitoring of pulmonary arterial pressure tracings. The catheter location should be confirmed by chest x-ray at least once daily. Wedge pressures should be measured only when needed. The degree of balloon inflation necessary to obtain a wedge tracing should be noted, and overinflation should be avoided. The balloon inflation port should be identified so that unintentional infusion is not directed into the balloon. The catheter should never be left in the wedge position. Rupture associated with only mild hemoptysis can be treated by removing the catheter. Rupture associated with cardiovascular collapse will require lobectomy or pneumonectomy, which occasionally permits patient salvage.

MEASUREMENT OF CENTRAL VENOUS PRESSURE

Pressures in the right atrium, which are equivalent to pressures in the superior vena cava, can be accurately measured with a pulmonary arterial catheter; of all the pressures measured by the catheter, the right atrial pressure is the most reproducible. Most clinicians measure the pressure at end-expiration. Pressures are typically low, on the order of 5 to 15 mm Hg. Care should be taken to ensure that the transducer system is adequately zeroed.

MEASUREMENT OF PULMONARY ARTERIAL PRESSURE

The end-expiratory pulmonary arterial pressure can be approximated by measuring the mean of the systolic and diastolic pressures toward the end of the expiratory cycle on the oscillo-

scope screen. These two values are then used to calculate the mean pulmonary arterial pressure, taken as the pressure one third of the way between the diastolic and systolic pressures. As with other central pressure measurements, the monitoring equipment does not recognize the difference between spontaneous breaths and mechanical breaths [see Central Venous Catheters, Measurement of Central Venous Pressure, above]. The end-expiratory mean pressure can be quite difficult to interpret, however. Thus, some clinicians use the digital readout, even though they realize that the readout will not be giving the end-expiratory value.

Distortions introduced by measuring systems that are too stiff or too compliant produce inaccuracies [see Systemic Arterial Catheters, Measurement of Systemic Arterial Pressure, above]. The Swan-Ganz catheter frequently is quite stiff compared with the patient's vasculature, and sometimes the exaggerations produced by this stiffness can generate inaccuracies of 10 to 20 mm Hg. Catheter whip can also introduce inaccuracies [see Figure 3]. Thus, it is best not to rely on measurements of pulmonary arterial systolic and diastolic pressures unless a snap test confirms that these pressures are accurate [see Figure 2]. The mean pressure, however, will remain accurate no matter what the characteristics of the measuring system are, and thus, it is the best single measurement to use for pulmonary arterial pressure.

The pulmonary arterial diastolic pressure sometimes correlates quite well with the pulmonary arterial wedge pressure (PAWP). In some cases, this correlation occurs more by chance than by physiology because the diastolic pressure measured at the transducer depends so much on the measuring system itself. If it is known that the diastolic pressure tracks the wedge pressure well, it can sometimes be used to estimate wedge pressure if the balloon on the Swan-Ganz catheter breaks (until another catheter can be inserted). However, pulmonary arterial diastolic pressure cannot be used to track wedge pressures, even briefly, in certain situations, including obstructive pulmonary disease, adult respiratory distress syndrome, and heart rate greater than 125 beats/min. Increased pulmonary interstitial pressure, mitral valve disease, reduced left ventricular compliance, and constriction of pulmonary veins also militate against good correlation of pulmonary arterial wedge pressure and pulmonary arterial diastolic pressure. For the most part, it is best to avoid relying greatly on the pulmonary arterial diastolic pressure. The mean pulmonary arterial pressure and the wedge pressure, either measured at end-expiration or taken from the digital readout of the monitoring equipment, will give the necessary physiologic information.

MEASUREMENT OF PULMONARY ARTERIAL WEDGE PRESSURE

The pulmonary arterial wedge pressure is one of the most influential variables measured by the pulmonary arterial catheter. Because there are no valves between the left atrium and the pulmonary arteries, the pressure obtained with inflation of the balloon on the Swan-Ganz catheter and occlusion of proximal flow will reflect the pressure in the left atrium [see Figure 10].[12,13] The fundamental assumption in making this measurement is that there is an unbroken, unmoving column of fluid between the tip of the catheter and the left atrium. If this condition is met and there is no significant mitral valvular disease, PAWP will closely approximate left ventricular end-diastolic pressure (LVEDP).

The wedge pressure indirectly gives information about the pulmonary capillary or microvascular pressure. The microvascular pressure is between the mean pulmonary arterial pressure and the left atrial (or wedge) pressure. If the wedge pressure is high, the pulmonary microvascular pressure must also be high. A high PAWP (≥ 25 mm Hg) will always be associated with microvascular pressures that will generate at least some interstitial pulmonary edema, even if the microvascular endothelium is intact. If the endothelium is disrupted, as in sepsis, pulmonary edema can be produced even with wedge pressures in the mid-teens. In this setting, the pulmonary microvascular leak is the result of injury to the microvasculature rather than of ventricular dysfunction and high left atrial pressures.

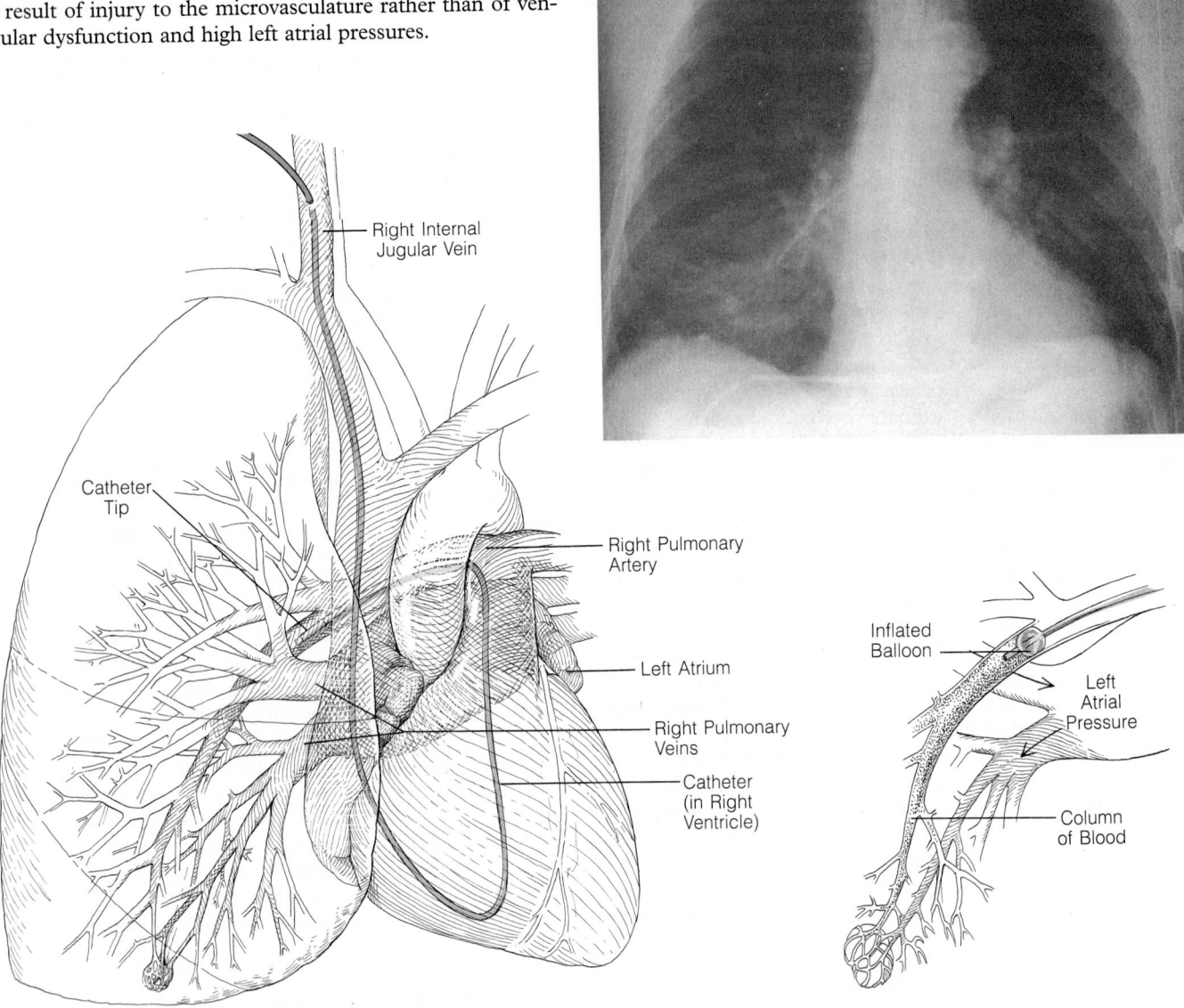

Figure 10 The pulmonary arterial catheter measures pressure in the pulmonary artery when the balloon is deflated. Because flow in the vascular system generates a pressure drop as the blood passes through the microvasculature, the pressure from the pulmonary artery to the left atrium gradually falls. When the balloon is inflated, flow in the vasculature distal to the tip is eliminated; therefore, there is no pressure drop. Because there is no pressure drop and because there are no valves between the left atrium and the pulmonary artery, the pressure in the pulmonary artery distal to the point of occlusion must equal the pressure in the left atrium, provided that there is an open column of blood between the end of the catheter and the left atrium. That is, pulmonary arterial wedge pressure will equal left atrial pressure as long as the catheter is in a dependent portion of the lung with a vasculature that remains open during ventilation. Because the catheter is flow directed, it usually will end up in such a dependent, well-perfused area. This is not a certainty, however. If inflated alveoli occlude the microvasculature, wedge pressure will equal alveolar pressure. This inaccuracy cannot be easily detected. Verification that the catheter is in the dependent portion of the lung requires a cross-table lateral chest x-ray. We do not routinely obtain these x-rays unless the wedge pressures are absolutely critical for treatment and unless the reliability of the wedge pressure tracing is suspect. Suspicion usually arises when excessively wide pressure swings are evident as the lungs are inflated and deflated.

Although the wedge pressure gives indirect information about the microvascular pressure, the two pressures are not the same. The term pulmonary capillary wedge pressure is misleading and should probably be discarded.

Cardiac output is affected by preload, which can be quantified as left ventricular end-diastolic volume (LVEDV), as reflected by the Frank-Starling curve or by pressure-volume loops. Changes in preload are reflected by changes in LVEDV. It is frequently assumed that PAWP, which reflects changes in left ventricular end-diastolic pressure, is also a reliable monitor of LVEDV and that PAWP can be used to judge the adequacy of preload and to make the diagnosis of cardiac failure and volume overload. Pressure is not equivalent to volume. Starling's law of the heart states that ventricular contraction depends on the myocardial fiber length that precedes the next contraction. That length is determined largely by LVEDV. Measurement of pressure (e.g., PAWP or right atrial pressure) does not necessarily reflect end-diastolic volume, because of diastolic ventricular compliance. A high intracavitary pressure in a ventricle with small diastolic compliance may be associated with a small end-diastolic volume. Similarly, a low intracavitary pressure in a ventricle with a large diastolic compliance may be associated with a large end-diastolic volume.

Because of the pressure-volume relation, in many clinical settings PAWP may not differentiate changes or problems in left ventricular contractility from those in left ventricular compliance.[12] A bedside echocardiogram may contribute to more effective management of the patient in these settings. As an index of blood volume, the PAWP may be neither very sensitive nor very specific. Ventricular compliance can be estimated at the bedside by administering a fluid bolus, usually 250 ml, and monitoring the rate of change of filling pressure [see I:4 Shock]. A rapid increase suggests that there is a stiff ventricle during diastole. Diastolic myocardial compliance is reduced by ischemia, septic or hypovolemic shock, pericardial effusion, inotropic support, and positive end-expiratory pressure (PEEP).[14-16] On the other hand, afterload reduction, cardiomyopathy, malnutrition, and a reduction of inotropic support usually increase myocardial compliance.

If the catheter is located in lung zones where alveolar pressure is greater than arterial pressure (zone I) or venous pressure (zones I and II), PAWP may reflect airway pressure and not left atrial pressure (LAP). In this situation, the fundamental assumption of PAWP measurement is not met.

In zone III (the dependent portion of the lung), in which both arterial and venous pressures exceed alveolar pressure, there is continuous flow, and PAWP correlates with LAP. Most of the lung enters zone III when the patient is supine, and most pulmonary arterial catheters will preferentially float into zone III. It has been shown that if the tip of the catheter is at or below the level of the left atrium, the conditions in zone III exist even if positive end-expiratory pressures are as high as 30 cm H_2O, provided that there is no embolic obstruction. On occasion, if accuracy of left atrial pressure measurement is absolutely essential for patient care, a cross-table lateral film should be obtained to confirm the location of the catheter tip relative to the left atrium [see Figure 10]. If the tip is above the atrium, the catheter should be repositioned. A damped tracing, the need for balloon overinflation to produce a wedged reading, and wide pressure changes on respiration should all call into question the reliability of the measurement.

MEASUREMENT OF CARDIAC OUTPUT

Today, pulmonary arterial catheters are almost always equipped to measure cardiac output by means of thermodilution. The outputs are obtained by injecting a solution that is colder than blood through the right atrial port of the catheter and measuring the resultant temperature drop in the pulmonary artery as the cool blood flows past the thermistor. Commercially available computers calculate the cardiac output on the basis of indicator dilution theory [see Figure 11]. Flow into the cardiovascular system is calculated on the basis of the amount of cold solution injected proximally, the temperature of that solution compared with the baseline temperature of the blood, the physical characteristics of the solution that determine its cold capacity, and the area inscribed under the thermodilution curve. Cardiac output computers allow calibration for varying amounts and temperatures of injectates. The computer finds the area under the thermodilution curve and gives a digital readout of the cardiac output, usually in liters per minute. Either room-temperature or ice-cold solutions may be used as the thermal indicators. The important point is to know the exact temperature of the injectate because the temperature is necessary for accurate computer calculation of output. The advantages of room-temperature injections include simplicity and little variation in the injectate temperature. Ice-cold injections generate a large signal-to-noise ratio because the magnitude of the pulmonary arterial temperature changes increases as the temperature of the injectate decreases. Ventilation affects flow into and out of the right ventricle, and the pulmonary arterial temperature changes as a function of insufflation of the lungs. Therefore, three injections should be made for each determination of cardiac output. The injections should be made at a consistent point in the ventilatory cycle, typically at end-expiration.[17] The three values should be within 15 percent of one another; otherwise, the series should be repeated.

Methods have been developed to measure cardiac output without placement of invasive pulmonary arterial catheters. The direct Fick method is best used in awake, alert patients.[18] Transthoracic electrical impedance requires placement of electrodes, which may interfere with surgical procedures.[19] Doppler ultrasonography probes have been placed at the suprasternal notch and the esophagus for continuous cardiac output determination.[20,21] The suprasternal notch probe requires an estimate of the diameter of the ascending aorta. The esophageal Doppler probe measures the blood velocity in the descending aorta distal to the origins of the aortic arch vessels. Measurement of cardiac output in the descending aorta requires ascending aortic velocity calibration, which is obtained by a suprasternal notch probe. Expired gas analysis has also been used to obtain cardiac output. These methods are currently under clinical evaluation.[22-24]

MEASUREMENT OF RIGHT VENTRICULAR END-DIASTOLIC VOLUME

The introduction of fast-response thermistors has allowed development of thermodilution pulmonary arterial catheters for measurement of right ventricular end-diastolic volume.[25,26] Such measurements require use of a cold injectant. They have proved to be accurate as long as the patient has a

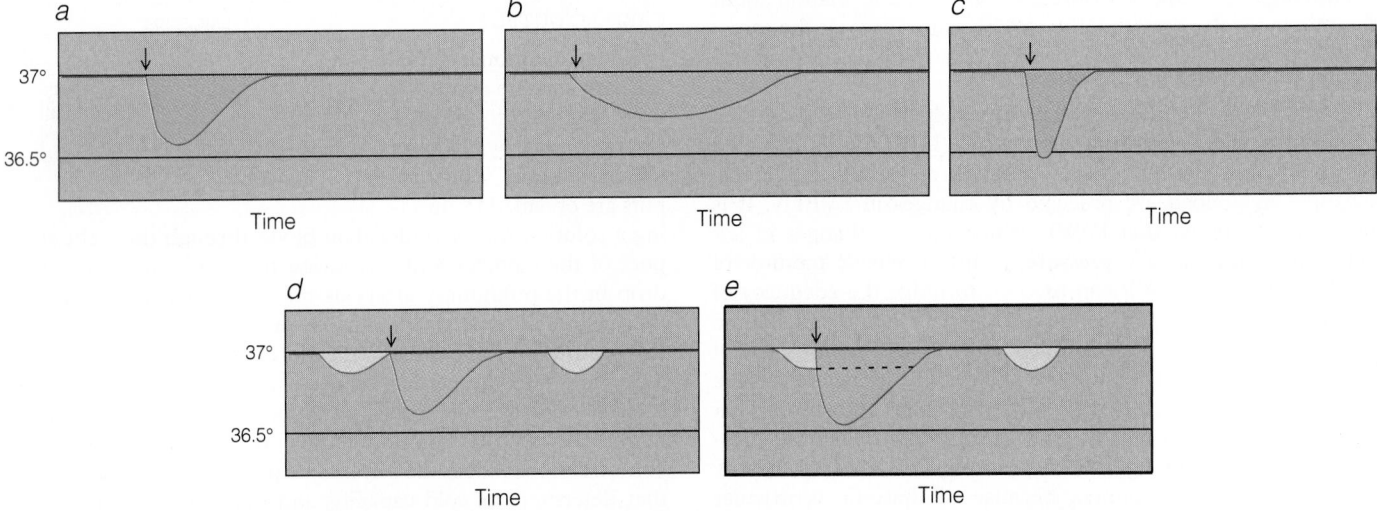

Figure 11 In the normal thermodilution curve shown here (*a*), the baseline pulmonary arterial temperature is 37° C; when a cold solution is injected to measure cardiac output (arrow), the temperature may fall to a low of 36.6° C as the cooled blood flows past the thermistor. When cardiac output is low (*b*), the cooled blood flows sluggishly past the end of the thermistor. The temperature drop in the blood might be to 36.7° C, but the cooled blood stagnates near the thermistor, and the blood at that portion of the pulmonary artery remains cool for a long time. Because the cardiac output is calculated as the inverse of the area, the output is recorded as a smaller number. By contrast, a supranormal cardiac output (*c*) pushes the pulse of cool blood rapidly past the thermistor. The result is a transiently low pulmonary arterial temperature. The area under the curve, however, is smaller than normal because the fall in temperature is brief; this small area leads to a calculation of a high cardiac output. These examples assume a stable temperature for pulmonary arterial blood, however, which is usually not the case. Pulmonary arterial blood temperature can vary during the ventilatory cycle by as much as several hundredths of a degree as a result of sequential and cyclic return of blood from different parts of the body. (The cyclic dips in temperature are represented here by the lightly shaded areas in *d* and *e*.) During inspiration, elastic recoil in the venules and small veins of the nonsplanchnic part of the body pushes the cool blood from the extremities back to the right atrium; relatively little blood returns from the hepatic veins as the diaphragm pushes down on the liver and kinks those vessels. During expiration, the diaphragm and liver rise, and the accumulated warm blood in the liver is discharged into the inferior vena cava as the hepatic veins open up and the liver reassumes its normal anatomic position. This cyclic return of blood to the right atrium leads to temperature changes in the blood in that chamber. This fact becomes important in the timing of the three injections for cardiac output determinations. If an injection is superimposed onto the baseline high temperature (*d*), the computer will detect a relatively small area under the curve. If an injection is superimposed onto a dip in the pulmonary arterial temperature (*e*), however, the computer will detect a larger area because it will be using the temperature of 37° C for its baseline. (The excess area is that above the broken line.) The only way to eliminate the variability introduced by ventilation-dependent changes in baseline pulmonary arterial temperature is to make each of the three injections at the same point in the ventilatory cycle. We make all of our injections at end-expiration.

regular heart rate of less than 140 beats/min. Right ventricular end-diastolic volume does not necessarily reflect left ventricular end-diastolic volume, but transesophageal or transthoracic echocardiography can determine whether the end-diastolic volume in the ventricles is similar. If so, measurement of the right ventricular volume can be used for estimates of the left.

The availability of the right ventricular end-diastolic volume can be very useful for patient management. Many patients with severe lung disease induced by critical illness have right-sided ventricular dysfunction. Knowledge of the end-diastolic volume can facilitate decisions about whether to volume load or diurese, whether to attempt pulmonary vasodilatation, or whether to use inotropic agents.

MEASUREMENT OF MIXED VENOUS GASES

Mixed venous, or pulmonary arterial, blood can be obtained from the end of the Swan-Ganz catheter for measurement of mixed venous gases. Mixed venous blood, by definition, is blood that represents a mixture of all blood returned from all organs of the body. Venous blood from the heart is returned to the right atrium through the coronary sinus. This blood is markedly desaturated (the heart, after all, is a working muscle). Blood in the right ventricle or in the pulmonary artery will be truly mixed venous blood because it includes the blood from the heart as well as the blood from the rest of the body. Measurements of gases in blood from the superior vena cava may be falsely elevated because that sample will not include the blood from the heart. Measurements of gases in blood obtained from the right atrium may be falsely low if the catheter tip is placed near the coronary sinus.

The residual blood in the catheter should be removed before the specimen is obtained for measurements of mixed venous gases. If the blood sample is withdrawn too forcefully, the pulmonary artery may collapse around the end of the catheter, and the blood will have been drawn in a retrograde manner past ventilated alveoli [*see Figure 12*]. The result, a specimen with very high oxygen levels, does not reflect desaturated pulmonary arterial blood. The possibility that blood has been drawn in a retrograde fashion can be checked by measuring the P_{CO_2} in the specimen. The P_{CO_2} in true pulmonary arterial blood is typically 5 mm Hg higher than the P_{CO_2} in a simultaneously drawn specimen of systemic arterial blood.[6] Blood drawn back past ventilated alveoli will have a very low P_{CO_2}. If the P_{CO_2} in the specimen is equal to or less than that in systemic arterial blood, the specimen should be discarded. Another specimen should be obtained by drawing back on the syringe more slowly. One should rely on measurements of oxygen saturation of the specimen (by co-oximetry) rather than on the P_{O_2}. The mixed venous partial pressure of oxygen and the oxygen saturation lie on the steep portion of the oxyhemoglobin dissociation curve. A minor error in measurement of partial pressure can result in a major error in calculation of the saturation [see I:7 Life-Threatening Acid-Base Disorders].

In certain situations, it may be worthwhile to monitor $S_{mv}O_2$ continuously with a specially equipped pulmonary arterial catheter. An oximeter attached to the tip of a pulmonary arterial catheter can measure the $S_{mv}O_2$ by means of spectrophotometry. Continuous measurement of this variable is useful because abrupt drops in $S_{mv}O_2$ usually indicate that something is amiss. The heart extracts much of the oxygen delivered to it. If the blood returning from the heart and the rest of the body is markedly desaturated, it is likely that not enough blood is being transported to the heart. The $S_{mv}O_2$ falls if the heart suddenly delivers less oxygen to the tissues (e.g., if the cardiac index decreases rapidly or if the hemoglobin concentration or arterial oxygen saturation [S_aO_2] drops rapidly) or if the body suddenly demands increased amounts of oxygen (as with the onset of a hypermetabolic septic state or with the onset of shivering).

However, although a low $S_{mv}O_2$ is a warning signal, a normal or high value provides no assurances, because normal or high values do not necessarily reflect satisfactory cardiopulmonary status or adequate oxygen for metabolic demands. In low-output septic shock, for example, well-oxygenated blood is returned to the heart because blood is functionally shunted away from the tissues. High $S_{mv}O_2$ in patients with low-output sepsis do not

 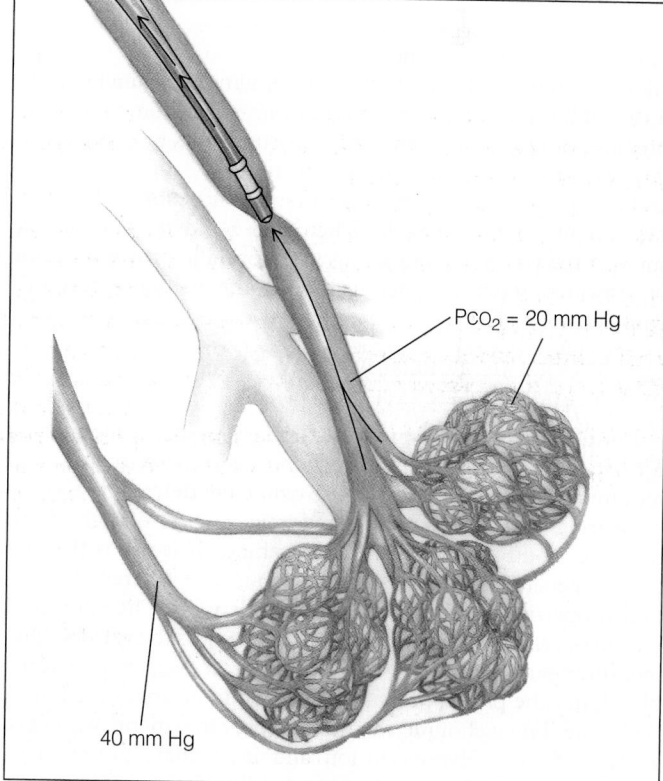

Figure 12 **The Swan-Ganz catheter allows collection of mixed venous blood for measurement of mixed venous oxygen saturation and content (left). If blood from the pulmonary artery is withdrawn through the catheter too forcefully, however, arterial walls can collapse around the tip of the catheter (right). The blood that is withdrawn for sampling will in that case consist of blood from the distal pulmonary vasculature that has been pulled back past ventilated alveoli. To determine whether pullback of blood through the catheter has led to retrograde flow (right), the partial pressure of carbon dioxide in the sample can be checked. P_{CO_2} in mixed venous blood is typically about 5 mm Hg greater than P_{CO_2} in systemic arterial blood. If the arterial walls have collapsed around the catheter, the sample will consist of blood from which much of the CO_2 will already have been excreted into the ventilated alveoli, and the recovered blood will have a P_{CO_2} that may be as much as 20 mm Hg lower than that of simultaneously obtained arterial blood. Specimens of this sort should be discarded and new specimens obtained.**

indicate that these patients' metabolic needs are being met; rather, the high values result from deranged peripheral metabolic processes with futile metabolic cycling. Cirrhotic patients, who have functional arteriovenous shunts, are another group in whom $S_{mv}O_2$ is generated in the presence of inadequate metabolic activity.

Catheters are available for continuous measurement of $S_{mv}O_2$. They can be difficult to keep calibrated and require some nursing time for maintenance. Nevertheless, they can be useful in selected patients if physicians or nurses are familiar with the potential drift of the calibration. If the $S_{mv}O_2$ drops, measurements should be made of the cardiac index, hemoglobin concentration, systemic S_aO_2, oxygen consumption, and other indicators of overall cardiopulmonary function. Therapy should be directed as indicated by these measurements.

Continuous Monitoring Techniques

In addition to continuous measurement of $S_{mv}O_2$ with a specially equipped pulmonary arterial catheter (see above), other techniques are available that allow continuous monitoring of cardiopulmonary function. The S_aO_2 can be continuously monitored with pulse oximetry, partial pressure of arterial oxygen with transcutaneous or conjunctival devices, perfusion with devices that measure skin temperature, and P_aCO_2 with devices that measure the end-expiratory partial pressure of carbon dioxide. There are no data, however, to support the view that continuous monitoring improves outcome or provides better or safer care than the methods currently employed.

CONTINUOUS MEASUREMENT OF ARTERIAL OXYGEN SATURATION

Pulse oximeters have proved extremely useful in monitoring S_aO_2 in ICU patients. They are noninvasive, easy to use, and require minimal calibration. Pulse oximeters determine S_aO_2 by measuring absorption of selected wavelengths of light from pulsatile blood flow. The principle behind their use is the fact that oxygenated and reduced hemoglobin have different absorption properties for light of known wavelengths. The sites used for measurement are the nail bed on a finger or the earlobe. The measurement obtained is the saturation of oxygen in arterial blood, not the partial pressure of oxygen in arterial blood or in the tissue. The technique can be used only in patients who have good perfusion. Hypoperfusion and inadequate pulsation of blood in the arterioles make it impossible for the oximeter to distinguish between arteriolar and venular blood.

CONTINUOUS MEASUREMENT OF TISSUE OXYGEN TENSION

P_O_2 in the tissues can be determined by monitoring conjunctival or cutaneous tissues. Conjunctival oxygen tension is measured by a small oxygen sensor placed directly on the conjunctiva. The device is safe, and it does reflect changes in oxygen delivery to the tissue. It is not commonly used in most ICUs. Transcutaneous oxygen tension can be determined by placing a polarographic surface oxygen electrode directly on heated skin (heating the skin results in arterialized cutaneous tissue); tissue oxygen tension is measured beneath this surface electrode. This value correlates well with P_aO_2 if local tissue perfusion is good.

A decrease in S_aO_2 measured by pulse oximetry or a decrease in tissue oxygen tension measured by conjunctival or transcutaneous devices should prompt a search for evidence of cardiac or pulmonary impairment, such as decreases in cardiac index, hemoglobin concentration, and S_aO_2 or increases in peripheral oxygen consumption.

CONTINUOUS MEASUREMENT OF SKIN TEMPERATURE

Skin temperature can be monitored on the toe or thumb with noninvasive devices, but accurate measurements are difficult to obtain unless there is good control of ambient temperatures in the ICU. Skin temperature, however, is a sensitive indicator of poor perfusion: a gradient of less than 2° C between the skin temperature and the ambient temperature indicates critically low perfusion. Fluid loading or pharmacological support should increase skin perfusion and increase the gradient, so that the skin is substantially warmer than the environment.

CONTINUOUS MEASUREMENT OF END-EXPIRATORY CARBON DIOXIDE TENSION

Continuous measurement of end-expiratory carbon dioxide tension gives information about the P_{CO_2} in the systemic arterial blood. The monitoring devices are typically inserted into the ventilator circuit between the end of the endotracheal tube and the Y connector to the ventilator. Credible readings must show a smooth curve of P_{CO_2} that begins at zero during inspiration and then rises exponentially to a plateau at end-expiration. A long plateau indicates that the alveoli are probably emptying at a regular rate, in which case the value can be used to detect trends in the P_aCO_2. Values obtained at end-expiration depend not only on the P_aCO_2 but also on dead-space ventilation. Thus, the devices are best used for detecting trends rather than as indicators of the absolute value of the arterial carbon dioxide.

Noninvasive Monitoring of Blood Pressure

All patients in intensive care units will require blood pressure measurement by sphygmomanometry at times. The principles behind blood pressure measurement by cuff are simple. The cuff is applied to the upper arm and inflated to a pressure that occludes the underlying brachial artery. The cuff is then deflated, and resumption of blood flow in the brachial artery distal to the cuff is detected by listening for turbulence in the vessel with a stethoscope or with a Doppler flowmeter.

These measurements are usually easy to obtain and pose no risk to the patient, but they can be misleading. Systolic blood pressure measurements obtained by this technique are accurate as long as the pressure in the cuff equals the pressure applied to the inside of the artery. These pressures will usually be equal, except in diabetic patients who have calcified brachial arteries and in obese patients, in whom the subcutaneous fat between the cuff and the artery can dissipate any pressure applied externally, especially if the cuff is narrow with respect to the diameter of the arm. In both diabetic and obese patients, the systolic pressure indicated by the cuff method will be higher than the true intravascular systolic pressure. In all patients, measurement of diastolic pressures by the cuff method poses even greater problems. As the cuff is deflated, the sounds change character and then cease altogether. The diastolic pressure is now taken at the level at which the sound disappears. The sounds, however, can be so hard to detect that it becomes difficult to make this determination accurately.

The measurements obtained by this method reflect the pressure in the portion of the arterial system that is underneath the cuff. Using a Doppler device over the radial artery with the cuff over the brachial artery gives a measure of systolic pressure in the arm, not at the wrist.

Doppler devices give no measure of diastolic pressures; they can help only with measurements of systolic pressure in patients who have soft sounds in their brachial arteries that are difficult to hear with the stethoscope. Other devices that facilitate the measurement of blood pressure by cuff suffer from similar limitations. Some of these devices have Doppler probes incorporated into the cuff apparatus. These can automatically record systolic pressures, but they have the same limitations as hand-held Doppler devices. Other automatic devices sense pulsatility in volume changes in the arm as the cuff is deflated. These can work well in euvolemic patients, but they frequently fail in the presence of hypovolemia.

The inability to measure any pressures accurately in obese patients or in patients with calcified vessels, the uncertainty associated with measurements of diastolic pressure in all patients, and the inability of Doppler measurements to give any indication of diastolic pressures under any circumstances all make cuff measurements of arterial pressure less than ideal in critically ill patients. Most patients in an intensive care unit will benefit from the use of intra-arterial catheters for measurement of blood pressure, at least for some of their time in the ICU.

Derived Values

The measurements obtained from the devices described above allow calculation of derived values, which include cardiac output, stroke volume, left ventricular and right ventricular end-diastolic volumes, 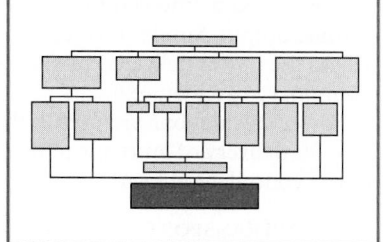 left ventricular and right ventricular end-systolic volumes, left ventricular and right ventricular end-systolic unstressed volumes, left ventricular and right ventricular end-systolic pressures, vascular resistances, aortic root and pulmonary arterial end-systolic pressure-volume relations, left ventricular and right ventricular end-systolic pressure-volume relations, power, oxygen transport, oxygen return, oxygen consumption, and bicarbonate concentration [see Table 1]. Values can also be derived for shunt fractions and alveolar-arterial oxygen gradients, both of which are discussed elsewhere [see VII:3 Pulmonary Dysfunction].

CARDIAC OUTPUT

The cardiac output computers that are used with thermodilution Swan-Ganz catheters typically report flow in terms of liters per minute. This value is important because it indicates the absolute volume flow, but it can be misleading unless the patient's size is taken into account. This problem can be overcome by dividing output by body surface area to calculate the cardiac index (CI), which is expressed in terms of liters per minute per square meter, or by dividing output by the patient's weight, which gives the output as milliliters of blood flow per kilogram per minute.

Body surface area is typically calculated from a nomogram.[27] The weight used in the nomogram can be the patient's weight at the time

of cardiac output measurements, premorbid weight, or ideal weight. The patient's weight during the critical illness is the least representative of the patient's metabolically active mass as a result of illness-associated water accumulation. The premorbid weight has an advantage in that it avoids the problem of water accumulation. The ideal weight has the added advantage that it emphasizes the portion of the body that is most metabolically active and deemphasizes the role played by fat.[28]

Alternatively, one can use values that take into account the fractal distribution of the nutritive arterial network and the consequences of minimizing the energy requirements of the cardiovascular system.[29] The values for a 60 kg well-conditioned woman are easy to remember and can be adjusted to subjects of different weights [see Table 1].

STROKE VOLUME

The stroke volume is calculated by dividing the cardiac output by the heart rate. The value can be expressed as milliliters, or it can be indexed to the body surface area or to the patient's weight [see Table 1].

LEFT VENTRICULAR AND RIGHT VENTRICULAR END-DIASTOLIC VOLUMES

The ventricular end-diastolic volumes can be estimated from the filling pressures, though one must take into account that filling pressures reflect only intracavitary pressures. A pulmonary arterial catheter equipped to measure right ventricular end-diastolic volume can be very useful in patients who are thought to have decreased diastolic compliance or compression of the heart caused by mechanical ventilation or a raised diaphragm.[30] The left ventricular end-diastolic volume can be estimated by means of transesophageal echocardiography. These values can be indexed either to the body surface area or to the body weight [see Table 1].

LEFT VENTRICULAR AND RIGHT VENTRICULAR END-SYSTOLIC VOLUMES

End-systolic volumes can be obtained by subtracting the stroke volume from the end-diastolic volumes [see Table 1].

LEFT VENTRICULAR AND RIGHT VENTRICULAR END-SYSTOLIC UNSTRESSED VOLUMES

The term end-systolic unstressed volume refers to the volume that a ventricle would assume if all of its blood were removed with the ventricle in a fully contracted state.[31] These unstressed volumes cannot be measured routinely in the ICU. For the great majority of patients, unstressed volumes are quite small, on the order of 5 ml/m². In severe congestive heart failure, however, values can increase to as much as 40 ml/m².[32]

LEFT VENTRICULAR AND RIGHT VENTRICULAR END-SYSTOLIC PRESSURES

The left ventricular end-systolic pressure can be estimated by multiplying the aortic root systolic pressure by 0.9.[33] The aortic root systolic pressure can be obtained in patients younger than 50 years by subtracting 20 mm Hg from the radial artery systolic pressure and in patients 50 years of age or older by subtracting 10 mm Hg from the radial artery systolic pressure.[34] The right ventricular end-systolic pressure can be obtained by multiplying the pulmonary arterial systolic pressure by 0.9.

For calculation of both the left ventricular and right ventricular end-systolic pressures, it is important that measurements of the arterial pressure be as accurate as possible. A snap test should be performed to ensure that the stiffness and resistance of the measuring system reasonably approximate the stiffness and resistance of the vasculature being interrogated.

VASCULAR RESISTANCES

Pressure across a resistance equals the flow across the resistance multiplied by the resistance itself. This equation can be used to solve for the systemic vascular resistance: the cardiac index (representing the flow) is divided into the difference between the mean aortic pressure and the right atrial pressure. Pulmonary vascular resistance equals the CI divided into the difference between the mean pulmonary arterial and pulmonary arterial wedge pressures.

The advantage of dividing by cardiac indices rather than by cardiac outputs is that the values obtained are relatively independent of the patient's size.[5] For example, small and large patients tend to have equivalent pressures throughout their vascular spaces. Dividing by the CI will give equivalent values for the vascular resistances. If cardiac outputs are used as the denominator, quite different values will be obtained for the resistances, complicating assessment of individual values.

Units used for expression of vascular resistances vary from hospital to hospital. It is simplest, and also perfectly acceptable scientifically, to express the resistances in arbitrary units. We prefer $mm\ Hg \cdot L^{-1} \cdot min \cdot m^2$. That is, we divide the difference in pressure by the CI, using the body surface area calculated on the basis of the patient's ideal weight, and use the number so obtained without making any further corrections [see Table 1]. Some prefer to multiply this raw number by 80 to convert the resistances to units in the centimeter-gram-second (CGS) system.

The pulmonary vascular resistance index is more difficult to measure than the systemic vascular resistance index. It is also more likely to change under different conditions. The pulmonary vascular resistance depends on the difference between two relatively small numbers: the mean pulmonary arterial pressure and the PAWP. A slight error in the measurement of either of these pressures can result in a large error in the calculated resistance. Furthermore, the pulmonary arterial pressure and, to a lesser extent, the wedge pressure vary tremendously with phases of ventilation. In patients on mechanical ventilation, swings in pulmonary arterial pressure can exceed 20 mm Hg. It can be difficult for even the most experienced ICU nurse to obtain accurate end-expiration measurements of these pressures. Furthermore, the mode of ventilation can substantially affect the pulmonary vascular resistance index. Hyperinflation of the lungs with mechanical ventilation can compress the intra-alveolar vasculature and increase the pulmonary vascular resistance index.

The variability of the pulmonary vascular resistance makes it difficult to state a specific normal value. Consequently, although we rely heavily on systemic vascular resistance indices to govern care of the patient, pulmonary vascular resistance is less heavily weighted.

AORTIC ROOT AND PULMONARY ARTERIAL END-SYSTOLIC PRESSURE-VOLUME RELATIONS

The aortic root end-systolic pressure-volume relation can be calculated by dividing the left ventricular end-systolic pressure by the stroke volume.[35] The pulmonary arterial end-systolic pressure-volume relation can be determined by dividing the right

ventricular end-systolic pressure by the stroke volume. This relation gives a good approximation of the input impedance [see Table 1]. Input impedance reflects the total hindrance that a ventricle faces when it ejects its pulsatile load into a vasculature that has both compliant and resistive elements.[5,36,37]

LEFT VENTRICULAR AND RIGHT VENTRICULAR END-SYSTOLIC PRESSURE-VOLUME RELATIONS

The left ventricular end-systolic pressure-volume relation can be determined by subtracting the left ventricular end-systolic unstressed volume from the left ventricular end-systolic volume and dividing the difference into the left ventricular end-systolic pressure [see Table 1].[30,31] The right ventricular end-systolic pressure-volume relation can be determined in a similar manner. These relations give a good indication of the contractile state of the ventricles.

POWER

The total power delivered into the aorta can be calculated as the left ventricular end-systolic pressure multiplied by the cardiac output, indexed appropriately.[32] The steady-flow aortic power is the mean arterial pressure multiplied by the cardiac output. The oscillatory power is the difference between the total power and the steady-flow power. Of the steady-flow power, a great majority is dissipated as heat in the microvasculature; the amount of heat dissipated can be calculated as the mean arterial pressure minus the central venous pressure multiplied by the cardiac output. The remainder of the steady-flow power fills the right atrium and right ventricle during diastole; this value can be calculated as the central venous pressure multiplied by the cardiac output. Similar formulas [see Table 1] can be used to calculate the power delivered by the right side of the heart into the pulmonary vasculature.

Power calculations are useful; they quantify the energy available for delivery of nutrients to tissues and for delivery of energy to the contralateral heart.

OXYGEN TRANSPORT

Oxygen transport—the amount of oxygen delivered by the heart to the tissues—is calculated by multiplying the cardiac index by the systemic arterial oxygen content (C_aO_2).[1] The calculation is simple, although care must be taken to obtain the correct units. Cardiac indices are typically expressed as liters of $blood \cdot min^{-1} \cdot m^{-2}$. Oxygen content is usually expressed as ml O_2/100 ml of blood. Multiplying liters of $blood \cdot min^{-1} \cdot m^{-2}$ by milliliters of $blood \cdot min^{-1}$ introduces a factor of 10 (from division of the unit of 100 ml of blood used for expression of oxygen content into the liters of blood used for expression of CI).

For example, in a patient with a normal CI of $3.6\ L \cdot min^{-1} \cdot m^{-2}$, a normal hemoglobin concentration of 12.5 g/dl, and a normal S_aO_2 of close to 100 percent, normal oxygen transport is $607\ ml\ O_2 \cdot min^{-1} \cdot m^{-2}$.

$$
\begin{aligned}
O_2\ transport &= cardiac\ index \times arterial\ O_2\ content \\
&= 36\ dl\ blood \cdot min^{-1} \cdot m^{-2} \times 1.39 \times 12.5 \times 97\% \\
&= 36\ dl\ blood \cdot min^{-1} \cdot m^{-2} \times 16.9\ ml\ O_2/dl\ blood \\
&= 607\ ml\ O_2 \cdot min^{-1} \cdot m^{-2}
\end{aligned}
$$

A decrease in CI, the hemoglobin concentration, or S_aO_2 will decrease oxygen transport.

OXYGEN RETURN

The amount of oxygen returned to the heart can be calculated by multiplying the CI by the mixed venous oxygen content ($C_{mv}O_2$). For a normal CI of 3.6 L · min^{-1} · m^{-2}, with a hemoglobin concentration of 12.5 g/dl and an $S_{mv}O_2$ of 75 percent (for a $C_{mv}O_2$ of 13.0 ml/dl), the oxygen return to the heart will be 470 ml O_2 · min^{-1} · m^{-2}.

OXYGEN CONSUMPTION

Oxygen consumption is the difference between oxygen delivered by the heart and oxygen returned to the heart. The formula thus becomes CI multiplied by the difference between the oxygen content in the systemic arterial blood and the oxygen content in the mixed venous blood.

$$\text{Oxygen consumption} = CI \times (C_aO_2 - C_{mv}O_2)$$

Normal oxygen consumption, then, is 140 ml O_2 · min^{-1} · m^{-2} because

$$36 \text{ dl blood} \cdot \text{min}^{-1} \cdot \text{m}^{-2} \times (16.9 - 13.0) \text{ ml } O_2/\text{dl blood}$$
$$= 140 \text{ ml } O_2 \cdot \text{min}^{-1} \cdot \text{m}^{-2}$$

The values given in the examples above are average values only. It is probably easiest to memorize a single normal value, however, rather than ranges of values. As long as the physician recognizes that, for example, an oxygen consumption calculated to be 120 ml · min^{-1} · m^{-2} is close to the average of 140, no harm will be done. An oxygen consumption of 100 ml · min^{-1} · m^{-2}, however, is clearly abnormally low. A value this low should prompt investigation to detect a low CI, a low hemoglobin concentration, or a low C_aO_2 and to correct the abnormality.

BICARBONATE CONCENTRATION

The calculated value for bicarbonate concentration is obtained from measurements of the P_{CO_2} and the hydrogen ion concentration of the blood by using the Henderson-Hasselbalch equation [see I:7 Life-Threatening Acid-Base Disorders]. The advantage of this equation is its familiarity; its disadvantage is that it involves the use of logarithms.

It is possible, however, to estimate bicarbonate concentration without using logarithms. The formula is as follows:

$$[HCO_3^-] = 24 \times P_{CO_2} \div [H^+]$$

The formula will give a value for bicarbonate concentration in mmol/L. The P_{CO_2} should be expressed as mm Hg; the hydrogen ion concentration, however, has to be expressed as nmol/L [see Table 3]. Note that most of the values can be obtained by multiplying the preceding value by 0.8. A pH of 7.0 corresponds to a hydrogen ion concentration of 100 nmol/L; a pH of 7.1 corresponds to a hydrogen ion concentration of 80 nmol/L.

Thus, for example, if the P_{CO_2} is 40 mm Hg and the hydrogen ion concentration is 80 nmol/L, the bicarbonate concentration is 12 mmol/L. This bicarbonate concentration closely approximates the actual concentration of bicarbonate in the arterial blood. The value obtained from the clinical laboratories for a venous blood specimen includes all of the compounds involved with dissociation of carbonic acid, including carbonic acid itself,

Table 3 Conversion of pH to Hydrogen Ion Concentration

pH		Hydrogen Ion Concentration (nmol/L)
7.0		100
7.1	100 x 0.8 =	80
7.2	80 x 0.8 =	64
7.3	63 x 0.8 ≈	50
7.4	50 x 0.8 =	40
7.5	40 x 0.8 =	32
7.6	32 x 0.8 ≈	25

Note: values not indicated in the table can be derived by interpolation. For example, a pH of 7.35 corresponds to a hydrogen ion concentration of approximately 45.

bicarbonate, and carbon dioxide. Thus, the bicarbonate calculated from the blood gases gives a value for a specific compound and is usually of more use than values obtained from the laboratories for a venous specimen.

INFLUENCE OF AGE AND OTHER VARIABLES

The values given in the example [see Table 1] are for a young patient in normal cardiovascular condition under resting circumstances in a supine position. However, several variables can affect these values, including the patient's age, cardiovascular condition, positioning, consumption of a large meal, mechanical ventilation, and thermal stress.

Age does not affect the resting heart rate, cardiac output, stroke volume, or ventricular end-diastolic volumes [see VI:7 The Elderly Surgical Patient]. Increased age is associated, however, with increases in ventricular end-systolic pressure and mean and systolic pressures in both the pulmonary and systemic arterial circulations.[38]

The achieving of good cardiovascular condition results in a slower resting heart rate, a larger stroke volume, and larger ventricular end-diastolic volumes.[39] Conditioning does not influence the resting cardiac output or, in an otherwise normal individual, the resting blood pressures.

Assumption of an upright position does not affect the resting heart rate, but it does decrease the cardiac output and the stroke volume by approximately 25 percent.[40]

Consumption of a large meal can slightly increase the cardiac output and oxygen consumption values. Institution of mechanical ventilation can decrease the oxygen consumption by approximately 10 percent. The effects of mechanical ventilation on the other parameters vary depending on the intravascular volume status of the patient. As a rule, mechanical ventilation with tidal volumes of 10 ml/kg decreases the ventricular end-diastolic volumes, the stroke volume, and the cardiac output. These effects can be partially reversed by the infusion of fluid to return the ventricular end-diastolic volumes back toward normal.

Any environment that poses a thermal stress on the patient can influence the values obtained. If the environment is cold enough to produce shivering, oxygen consumption and cardiac output can rise to levels several times greater than those of a normal person. Hypothermia in the absence of shivering decreases the oxygen consumption and the cardiac output. Extreme hypothermia can decrease these values to as low as one fourth of normothermic values. Hyperthermia or systemic inflammation can increase oxygen consumption and cardiac output to values as high as twice those of a normothermic or uninjured or noninfected person, but no higher [see VII:8 Metabolic Response to Critical Illness].

References

1. Cerra FB: Manual of Critical Care. CV Mosby Co, St Louis, 1987

2. Kofke WA, Levy JH: Postoperative Critical Care Procedures of the Massachusetts General Hospital. Little, Brown & Co, Boston, 1986

3. Gardner RM: Direct blood pressure measurement—dynamic response requirements. Anesthesiology 54:227, 1981

4. Karamanoglu M, O'Rourke MF, Avolio AP, et al: An analysis of the relationship between central aortic and peripheral upper limb pressure waves in man. Eur Heart J 14:160, 1993

5. O'Rourke MF: Vascular impedance in studies of arterial and cardiac function. Physiol Rev 62:570, 1982

6. Klocke RA: Carbon dioxide transport. Handbook of Physiology, Sect 3, Vol 4. American Physiological Society, Bethesda, Maryland, 1987, p 173

7. Andritsch RF, Muravchick S, Gold MI: Temperature correction of arterial blood-gas parameters: a comparative review of methodology. Anesthesiology 55:311, 1981

8. Swain JA: Hypothermia and blood pH: a review. Arch Intern Med 148:1643, 1988

9. Morris AH, Chapman RH, Gardner RM: Frequency of wedge pressure errors in the ICU. Crit Care Med 13:705, 1985

10. Komadina KH, Schenk DA, LaVeau P, et al: Interobserver variability in the interpretation of pulmonary artery catheter pressure tracings. Chest 100:1647, 1991

11. Celoria G, Steingrub JS, Vickers-Lahti M, et al: Clinical assessment of hemodynamic values in two surgical intensive care units. Arch Surg 125:1036, 1990

12. O'Quin R, Marini JJ: Pulmonary artery occlusion pressure: clinical physiology, measurement, and interpretation. Am Rev Respir Dis 128:319, 1983

13. Raper R, Sibbald WJ: Misled by the wedge? the Swan-Ganz catheter and left ventricular preload. Chest 89:427, 1986

14. Alyono D, Ring WS, Chao RYN, et al: Characteristics of ventricular function in severe hemorrhagic shock. Surgery 94:250, 1983

15. Grossman W: Diastolic dysfunction in congestive heart failure. N Engl J Med 325:1557, 1991

16. Natanson C, Fink MP, Ballantyne HK, et al: Gram-negative bacteremia produces both severe systolic and diastolic cardiac dysfunction in a canine model that simulates human septic shock. J Clin Invest 78:259, 1986

17. Stevens JH, Raffin TA, Mihm FG, et al: Thermodilution cardiac output measurement: effects of the respiratory cycle on its reproducibility. JAMA 253:2240, 1985

18. Selzer A, Sudrann RB: Reliability of the determination of cardiac output in man by means of the Fick principle. Circ Res 6:485, 1958

19. Porter JM, Swain ID: Measurement of cardiac output by electrical impedance plethysmography. J Biomed Eng 9:222, 1987

20. Huntsman LL, Stewart DK, Barnes SR, et al: Noninvasive Doppler determination of cardiac output in man. Circulation 67:593, 1983

21. Mark JB, Steinbrook RA, Gugino LD, et al: Continuous noninvasive monitoring of cardiac output with esophageal Doppler ultrasound during cardiac surgery. Anesth Analg 65:1013, 1986

22. Kety SS: Theory and applications of the exchange of inert gas in the lungs and tissues. Pharmacol Rev 3:1, 1951

23. Homer LD, Denysyk B: Estimation of cardiac output by analysis of respiratory gas exchange. J Appl Physiol 39:159, 1975

24. Capek JM, Roy RJ: Noninvasive measurement of cardiac output using partial CO_2 rebreathing. IEEE Trans Biomed Eng 35:633, 1988

25. Diebel LN, Wilson RF, Tagett MG, et al: End-diastolic volume: a better indicator of preload in the critically ill. Arch Surg 127:817, 1992

26. Diebel L, Wilson RF, Heins J, et al: End-diastolic volume versus pulmonary artery wedge pressure in evaluating cardiac preload in trauma patients. J Trauma 37:950, 1994

27. Du Bois EF: The estimation of the surface area of the body. Basal Metabolism in Health and Disease, 3rd ed. Lea & Febiger, Philadelphia, 1936, p 125

28. Feldschuh J, Enson Y: Prediction of the normal blood volume: relation of blood volume to body habitus. Circulation 56:605, 1977

29. West GB, Brown JH, Enquist BJ: A general model for the origin of allometric scaling laws in biology. Science 276(5309):122, 1997

30. Guazzi M, Polese A, Magrini F, et al: Negative influences of ascites on the cardiac function of cirrhotic patients. Am J Med 59:165, 1975

31. Sagawa K: The end-systolic pressure-volume relation of the ventricle: definition, modifications and clinical use (editorial). Circulation 63:1223, 1981

32. Asanoi H, Sasayama S, Kameyama T: Ventriculoarterial coupling in normal and failing heart in humans. Circ Res 65:483, 1989

33. Kelly R, Fitchett D: Noninvasive determination of aortic input impedance and external left ventricular power output: a validation and repeatability study of a new technique. J Am Coll Cardiol 20:952, 1992

34. Kelly R, Hayward C, Avolio A, et al: Noninvasive determination of age-related changes in the human arterial pulse. Circulation 80:1652, 1989

35. Kelly RP, Ting C-T, Yang T-M, et al: Effective arterial elastance as index of arterial vascular load in humans. Circulation 86:513, 1992

36. O'Rourke MF, Kelly RP: Wave reflection in the systemic circulation and its implications in ventricular function. J Hypertens 11:327, 1993

37. Piene H: Pulmonary arterial impedance and right ventricular function. Physiol Rev 66:606, 1986

38. Avolio AP, Chen S-G, Wang R-P, et al: Effects of aging on changing arterial compliance and left ventricular load in a northern Chinese urban community. Circulation 68:50, 1983

39. Ogawa T, Spina RJ, Martin WH III, et al: Effects of aging, sex, and physical training on cardiovascular responses to exercise. Circulation 86:494, 1992

40. Bevegård S, Holmgren A, Jonsson B: The effect of body position on the circulation at rest and during exercise, with special reference to the influence on the stroke volume. Acta Physiol Scand 49:279, 1960

Acknowledgments

Figure 1   Albert Miller.

Figure 2   Top, Dana Burns-Pizer; bottom, Albert Miller.

Figure 3   Top and bottom, Dana Burns-Pizer; center, Albert Miller.

Figures 4 and 5   Albert Miller.

Figure 6   Carol Donner.

Figures 7 through 9   Albert Miller.

Figure 10   Carol Donner.

Figure 11   Albert Miller.

Figure 12   Dana Burns-Pizer.

2 SUPPORT OF THE FAILING HEART

Charles L. Rice, M.D., and R. John Solaro, Ph.D.

Approach to the Failing Heart

The sole purpose of the heart's electrical and mechanical activity is to provide adequate organ perfusion. When there is evidence of inadequate perfusion of more than one organ, cardiac function must be evaluated. The classic manifestations of shock, which are discussed elsewhere [see I:4 Shock], are one indication of inadequate perfusion. The failing heart may also show evidence of left-sided heart failure (pulmonary edema), right-sided heart failure (peripheral edema, hepatic congestion, and distended neck veins), or both.

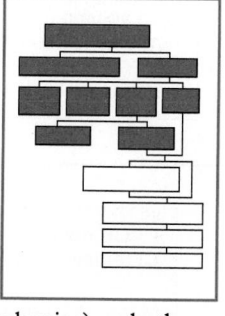

The principal determinants of cardiac output are preload (the volume presented to the heart), afterload (the resistance against which the heart must pump), and the inotropic state (the extent to which cells can contract against the preload). When a patient with circulatory instability is encountered, the first step must always be to verify that the patient's intravascular volume is adequate [see 4 Shock]. Measurement of the central venous pressure (CVP) is useful for this determination. If the CVP is low and the patient is hypotensive, volume replacement is the therapy of choice. If the CVP is high and the patient is hypotensive, insertion of a thermodilution Swan-Ganz catheter and measurement of the pulmonary arterial occlusion pressure (PAOP) and cardiac output are crucial [see VII:1 Cardiopulmonary Monitoring].

If the PAOP and the cardiac index are both elevated, the patient has most likely been overresuscitated. Volume infusion should be dramatically slowed. Patients who have pulmonary edema should also receive furosemide in a dose of 20 to 40 mg intravenously. Although there is a temptation to provide catecholamines (e.g., norepinephrine) to profoundly hypotensive patients in this situation, there is no evidence that this therapy is beneficial.

If the PAOP is low but the cardiac index is high, consider as underlying causes sepsis, anaphylaxis, and hepatic or autonomic dysfunction.

If the pulmonary arterial occlusion pressure and the cardiac index are both low, administer lactated Ringer's solution to raise the occlusion pressure by 3 to 5 mm Hg. Remeasure the cardiac index; if it is improving, continue volume resuscitation until the patient stabilizes.

If the PAOP is high and the cardiac index is low, the decision whether to administer an inotropic agent or an afterload-reducing agent is based on the adequacy of systemic arterial pressure. If the patient is normotensive, systemic vascular resistance is elevated, and afterload reduction can be employed.

There is no single, all-purpose cardiotonic agent that will meet every clinical situation. It is possible, however, to choose an agent or, occasionally, a combination of agents that best meets the patient's needs.

Afterload-Reducing Agents

SODIUM NITROPRUSSIDE

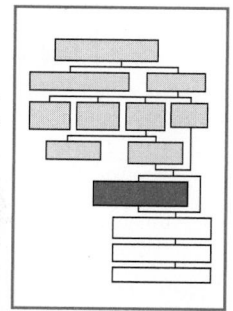

Sodium nitroprusside is valuable for reducing afterload. It is usually prepared by adding a 50 mg vial to 500 ml of five percent dextrose in water, for a final concentration of 100 µg/ml. Sodium nitroprusside's onset of action is rapid (usually one to two minutes), and its effect disappears almost immediately once the infusion is stopped. Resistance, tolerance, and tachyphylaxis are rare.[1] The infusion is begun at 0.5 µg/kg/min and titrated in 0.5 µg increments until the desired effect is achieved. Ideally, the reduction in systemic vascular resistance should result in improved cardiac output, so that the net effect on systemic arterial pressure should be minimal. It is advisable, however, to prevent the systolic blood pressure from falling below 80 mm Hg. Sodium nitroprusside administration also causes venous pooling, which, along with the unloading of the left ventricle, generally results in a lowered PAOP.

When sodium nitroprusside, which contains ferrous ion, reacts with sulfhydryl-containing compounds in erythrocytes, cyanide is produced. In the liver, cyanide is converted to less toxic thiocyanate, which is then excreted by the kidneys. Toxicity is caused by poisoning of the cytochrome system and occurs when the rate of cyanide production exceeds the rate of conversion to thiocyanate. Toxic reactions most often occur when the rate of sodium nitroprusside infusion exceeds 10 µg/kg/min or when administration is continued at lower rates for several days. The first manifestation of cyanide toxicity is usually a reduction in oxygen consumption over the course of a few hours. Although

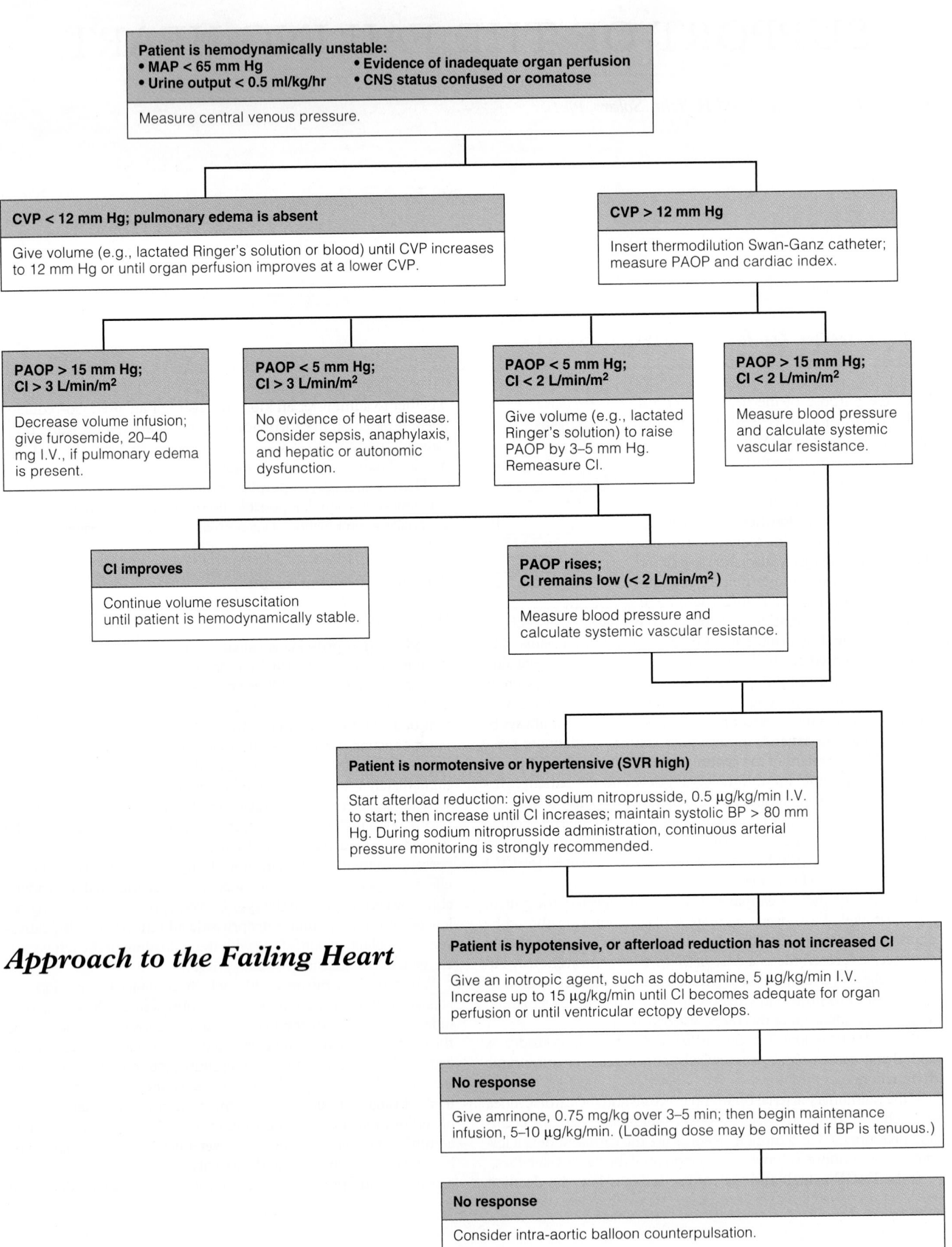

Patient is hemodynamically unstable:
- MAP < 65 mm Hg
- Urine output < 0.5 ml/kg/hr
- Evidence of inadequate organ perfusion
- CNS status confused or comatose

Measure central venous pressure.

CVP < 12 mm Hg; pulmonary edema is absent

Give volume (e.g., lactated Ringer's solution or blood) until CVP increases to 12 mm Hg or until organ perfusion improves at a lower CVP.

CVP > 12 mm Hg

Insert thermodilution Swan-Ganz catheter; measure PAOP and cardiac index.

PAOP > 15 mm Hg; CI > 3 L/min/m²

Decrease volume infusion; give furosemide, 20–40 mg I.V., if pulmonary edema is present.

PAOP < 5 mm Hg; CI > 3 L/min/m²

No evidence of heart disease. Consider sepsis, anaphylaxis, and hepatic or autonomic dysfunction.

PAOP < 5 mm Hg; CI < 2 L/min/m²

Give volume (e.g., lactated Ringer's solution) to raise PAOP by 3–5 mm Hg. Remeasure CI.

PAOP > 15 mm Hg; CI < 2 L/min/m²

Measure blood pressure and calculate systemic vascular resistance.

CI improves

Continue volume resuscitation until patient is hemodynamically stable.

PAOP rises; CI remains low (< 2 L/min/m²)

Measure blood pressure and calculate systemic vascular resistance.

Patient is normotensive or hypertensive (SVR high)

Start afterload reduction: give sodium nitroprusside, 0.5 µg/kg/min I.V. to start; then increase until CI increases; maintain systolic BP > 80 mm Hg. During sodium nitroprusside administration, continuous arterial pressure monitoring is strongly recommended.

Approach to the Failing Heart

Patient is hypotensive, or afterload reduction has not increased CI

Give an inotropic agent, such as dobutamine, 5 µg/kg/min I.V. Increase up to 15 µg/kg/min until CI becomes adequate for organ perfusion or until ventricular ectopy develops.

No response

Give amrinone, 0.75 mg/kg over 3–5 min; then begin maintenance infusion, 5–10 µg/kg/min. (Loading dose may be omitted if BP is tenuous.)

No response

Consider intra-aortic balloon counterpulsation.

1424

this reduction in oxygen consumption is not clinically apparent, it may be signaled by an otherwise unexplained rise in mixed venous oxygen tension or saturation or by a decrease in the calculated oxygen consumption. Treatment must be rapid to be effective and consists of administration of sodium nitrite (10 ml of a three percent solution). Sodium nitrite converts hemoglobin to methemoglobin, and the ferric ion in methemoglobin competes with the ferric ion in cytochrome for the cyanide ion. Methemoglobin is then reduced by the prompt administration (after administration of sodium nitrite) of methylene blue (1 mg/kg over five minutes), which induces the enzyme methemoglobin reductase. Thiocyanate is generally well tolerated up to levels of 10 mg/dl, but higher levels of thiiocyanate may necessitate hemodialysis.

NITROGLYCERIN

In patients in whom both preload and afterload are elevated (and especially in those with accompanying pulmonary edema), consideration should be given to the administration of nitroglycerin, a potent dilator of arteriolar and venous smooth muscle.[2] At lower concentrations (5 to 15 µg/min), the venous effect predominates, so that the principal effect is on preload. Infusion should be started at 5 µg/min and titrated to effect. The maximum rate is generally about 300 µg/min. Because nitroglycerin (like sodium nitroprusside) is a potent vasodilator, intravenous use requires monitoring of filling pressures, arterial pressure, and cardiac output; the principal adverse effects of administration are related to a too rapid reduction in these parameters. Should adverse effects occur, a reduction in dosage (or a temporary cessation of the infusion) results in rapid reversal.

GANGLIONIC BLOCKING AGENTS

Arterial pressure can be reduced by blockade of the autonomic ganglia responsible for maintenance of arteriolar tone.[3] The most important ganglionic blocking agent is trimethaphan camsylate. Although this drug has been used for rapid reduction in arterial pressure, it also reduces myocardial contractility. This property makes it useful for the control of hypertension in patients with acute aortic dissection but limits its value in the management of a failing heart. An additional disadvantage is the abrupt onset of tachyphylaxis. Trimethaphan may occasionally be useful, however, in those few patients who are resistant to sodium nitroprusside. It is generally administered at a rate of 0.3 to 3.0 mg/min.

ANGIOTENSIN-CONVERTING ENZYME INHIBITORS

Angiotensin-converting enzyme (ACE) is responsible for the conversion of angiotensin I to angiotensin II. Angiotensin II is a potent vasoconstrictor; in addition, it stimulates aldosterone secretion by the adrenal cortex. In a patient with congestive heart failure, therefore, inhibition of ACE has therapeutic benefit.

A recent study in patients with severe congestive heart failure and mitral regurgitation examined the effect of enalaprilat.[4] Afterload reduction was prompt and sustained, with improved cardiac index and decreased mitral regurgitation in the most severely ill patients. Enalaprilat is administered in a dosage of 1.25 mg I.V. every six hours (the dosage is lowered in patients with renal failure). Hypotension may occasionally result but is usually mild and self-limited.

ACE inhibitors are now an important adjunct in the management of patients with congestive heart failure, and initiation of treatment in the intensive care unit appears to be both safe and effective.

Inotropic Agents

If the patient is hypotensive or if afterload reduction has not resulted in increased cardiac output, an inotropic agent should be administered. This class of agents has been the subject of intense research activity during the 1980s and 1990s, with the development of a number of new agents and a better understanding of some of the older ones.[5,6]

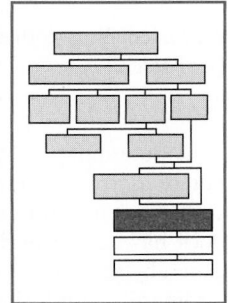

CATECHOLAMINES

Catecholamines act on the heart by stimulating beta receptors; they act on the peripheral vasculature by activating alpha$_1$- and beta$_2$-adrenergic receptors, as well as D_1 and D_2 dopamine receptors [see Table 1]. The effects of these adrenergic agonists

Table 1 Cardiovascular Effects of Adrenergic Stimulation

Receptor Site	Heart	Systemic Arteries	Pulmonary Arteries	Veins
Alpha$_1$	0	↑Constriction (+ + +)*	↑Constriction (+)	↑Constriction (+ +)
Beta$_1$	↑Rate (+ +) ↑Contractility (+ + +) ↑Atrioventricular conduction (+ + +)	0	Constriction†	0
Beta$_2$	?↑Rate ?↑Contractility	Dilatation (+ +)	Dilatation (+)	Dilatation (+ +)
D_1 dopamine	0	Dilatation (+ +)	Dilatation (+ +)	0
D_2 dopamine	↓Rate‡	Dilatation†	?	?

*Plus symbols (+) indicate relative potency of effect.
†Indirect effect: mediated by increased renin secretion in the kidneys.
‡Indirect effect: inhibition of norepinephrine.

Table 2 Receptor Types Stimulated by Adrenergic Agonists

Agonist	Alpha$_1$	Beta$_1$	Beta$_2$	D$_1$ Dopamine	D$_2$ Dopamine
Epinephrine	++++*	+++	++	0	0
Norepinephrine	+++	+++	0	0	0
Isoproterenol	0	++++	++++	0	0
Dopamine†	++	+++	0	++++	++++
Dobutamine	0	++++	++	0	0
Ibopamine	+	+	+	++	++
Fenoldopam	0	0	0	++	0
Dopexamine	0	+	++++	+++	+++
Propylbutyldopamine	+	0	0	++	++++

*Plus symbols (+) indicate relative degree of stimulation.
†The action of dopamine is dose dependent.

vary according to their relative selectivity for specific receptors [*see Table 2*].

Dobutamine

Dobutamine, a synthetic sympathomimetic amine, is a potent inotropic agent that has less tendency to produce tachycardia or arrhythmias than does dopamine.[7,8] Dobutamine does have some peripheral vasodilating effects, but they are generally seen only at higher infusion rates (> 20 µg/kg/min). Ordinarily, an infusion rate of 5 to 15 µg/kg/min is sufficient to achieve the maximum inotropic effect. Infusion rates in excess of 15 µg/kg/min are likely to be accompanied by arrhythmias because of increased myocardial oxygen consumption.[9]

Dopamine

Dopamine is a naturally occurring precursor of epinephrine and norepinephrine that has several pharmacological effects, including increased heart rate, increased contractility, and peripheral vasoconstriction. Its effect on renal perfusion is controversial.[10] In general, it is of greatest use in those situations in which arterial pressure is insufficient to perfuse the brain, heart, or kidneys. It is given by continuous infusion; rates lower than 8 µg/kg/min are associated with maximum inotropic effect. At higher infusion rates, the peripheral vasoconstrictive effect predominates, increasing afterload and myocardial oxygen consumption. Dopamine is therefore less useful at these high doses when the predominant effect sought is inotropic support.

Dopexamine

Dopexamine, another synthetic inotropic agent, stimulates beta$_2$-adrenergic receptors and D$_1$ and D$_2$ dopamine receptors, producing both inotropic and vasodilating effects. Unlike dopamine, dopexamine does not stimulate alpha$_1$ receptors. In a study from Europe of patients who had undergone coronary artery bypass surgery, administration of dopexamine resulted in

increased cardiac output (as a consequence of increased heart rate rather than increased stroke volume).[11] Systemic vascular resistance was unchanged. This study and others suggest that dosages higher than 5 µg/kg/min offer no additional benefit. Dopexamine for this use has not yet been approved by the Food and Drug Administration.

Epinephrine

Epinephrine was discovered in 1895. It is a naturally occurring, extremely potent alpha- and beta-adrenergic agonist. When administered intravenously, it produces a dose-dependent increase in both systolic and diastolic blood pressure, although systolic pressure is generally increased more than diastolic pressure. These increases in pressure are caused by the increases in heart rate and myocardial contractility (beta$_1$ effects) and an increase in peripheral vasoconstriction (an alpha$_1$ effect). Because of these increases in both peripheral vasoconstriction and heart rate, myocardial oxygen consumption is dramatically increased, and arrhythmias are common, limiting the usefulness of epinephrine for supporting the failing heart. If the patient is unresponsive to more selective agents, however, and particularly if the patient has profound hypotension, epinephrine may be of some limited value. It is titrated intravenously at a rate of 0.01 mg/kg/min, but the clinician must be alert to the development of malignant ventricular arrhythmias and severe hypertension (which will be short-lived).

Norepinephrine

Norepinephrine, also known as levarterenol, is a potent alpha$_1$- and beta$_1$-adrenergic agonist but a much weaker beta$_2$ agonist. Thus, its most pronounced effects are on peripheral vascular resistance. Norepinephrine may elevate blood pressure, but it usually causes cardiac output to fall. Its primary value, therefore, is in support of mean arterial pressure in a patient whose cardiac output is increased but whose blood pressure is too low to perfuse the pressure-dependent vascular beds in the heart, brain, and kidneys. Such situations are uncommon.

Isoproterenol

Isoproterenol is a powerful beta agonist that has virtually no effect on alpha receptors. When administered intravenously, therefore, it produces both peripheral vasodilatation (a beta$_2$ effect) and increases in heart rate and myocardial contractility (beta$_1$ effects). Although it is of some immediate benefit for complete heart block, its usefulness as an inotropic agent is outweighed by its arrhythmogenic potential; arrhythmia results from increased myocardial oxygen consumption that greatly exceeds increased cardiac output.

Mephentermine, Metaraminol, and Phenylephrine

Mephentermine, metaraminol, and phenylephrine all primarily produce peripheral vasoconstriction. None has any useful role in support of the failing heart, and all have potential for greatly increasing myocardial ischemia because of their effect on afterload.

PHOSPHODIESTERASE INHIBITORS

Amrinone

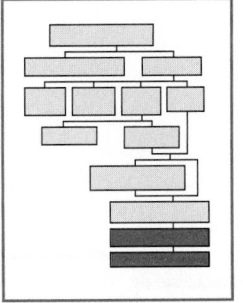

Amrinone is representative of a class of agents known as phosphodiesterase inhibitors.[12] Although its mechanism of action is not yet fully understood, it appears to inhibit the breakdown of intracellular cyclic adenosine monophosphate (cAMP).[13] Given intravenously, amrinone increases cardiac output and reduces afterload and preload.[14] It does not usually cause tachycardia or arrhythmias except when administered at higher doses. For these reasons, it is extremely useful in the acute management of refractory congestive heart failure. The recommended loading dose of amrinone is 0.75 mg/kg over three to five minutes, followed by continuous maintenance infusion of 5 to 10 μg/kg/min. Care must be taken when therapy with amrinone is initiated, however, because it is a potent vasodilator and patients frequently become profoundly hypotensive. In our experience, merely beginning with the maintenance infusion and titrating to effect appears to yield satisfactory results. Because the half-life of the drug is brief, stopping the infusion in the event of profound hypotension usually results in a return of blood pressure to preinfusion levels. Administration can then be resumed if the loading dose is omitted and the infusion rate is decreased. Amrinone is less useful for long-term therapy because of gastrointestinal side effects and thrombocytopenia. A few patients appear to benefit from the combination of dobutamine and amrinone.

Milrinone

Milrinone is related to amrinone, and its mechanism of action is similar.[15] It is approximately 20 times more potent in its inotropic effects than amrinone and has fewer side effects. Milrinone also has arteriolar and venous dilator activity. It is administered in an initial loading dose of 50 μg/kg over 10 minutes, followed by a maintenance infusion of 0.375 to 0.75 μg/kg/min. In one study comparing milrinone with dobutamine

in patients with severe congestive heart failure, milrinone produced a sustained decline in PAOP and a prolonged improvement in stroke volume.[16] Dobutamine, on the other hand, resulted in tachycardia in 25 percent of patients, and increases in stroke volume disappeared after about 12 hours. This study suggests that milrinone may be of value in some patients with severe congestive heart failure who are unresponsive to or intolerant of dobutamine.

Enoximone

Enoximone is another phosphodiesterase inhibitor, with actions similar to those of milrinone and amrinone, although at least one study suggests that it may be a more potent inotropic agent.[17] A study that evaluated the combination therapy of moderate-dose dobutamine and enoximone in patients with severe congestive heart failure demonstrated that such therapy produced synergistic effects that outweighed the benefits of either drug used alone.[18] Enoximone has not yet been approved by the FDA for clinical use.

CALCIUM SENSITIZERS

Another class of inotropic agents, calcium sensitizers, or inodilators, both inhibits phosphodiesterase activity and acts directly on the cardiac myofilaments to increase their responsiveness to calcium.[19] The phosphodiesterase inhibitory activity is associated with smooth muscle relaxation. One example of this class of agents is pimobendan, which is in clinical use in Japan and is undergoing clinical trials in the United States. Another example is MCI-154, an agent being developed in Japan. Both of these agents increase cardiac contraction to the same extent as isoproterenol, but they cause only a minimal increase in the amount of calcium released during a cardiac cycle. Pimobendan and MCI-154 also increase the calcium-binding affinity of troponin C, the myofilament calcium receptor, and both are thought to reduce the energy cost of nonmechanical work.

COLFORSIN

Another agent under study is colforsin (forskolin), which directly activates the catalytic unit of adenylate cyclase. It also reduces cardiac afterload and produces venous pooling, thereby decreasing preload. In one study comparing colforsin with dobutamine and sodium nitroprusside in patients with severe congestive cardiomyopathy, patients treated with colforsin demonstrated a 70 percent increase in stroke volume—greater than the increases seen with either dobutamine or nitroprusside.[20] The drug has not yet been approved for this use by the FDA, but further studies are under way.[21]

CALCIUM

The calcium ion plays a central role in the development of contractile force in all muscles, including the heart. Although calcium administration has been widely employed for inadequate myocardial function, clinical improvement is relatively rare.[22] Moreover, because calcium administration increases arteriolar vasoconstriction, local ischemia and increased afterload may result from its use. In addition, excessive influx of calcium into myocardial cells results in muscle necrosis.[23] Routine administration of calcium in cardiopulmonary resuscitation is therefore no longer recommended.[24]

CARDIAC GLYCOSIDES

Although the cardiac glycosides, such as digitalis, are the oldest and most widely used inotropic agents,[25] they are far more useful for the management of chronic congestive heart failure than for acute failure, primarily because of their slow onset of action, relatively low potency, and narrow therapeutic index. Digitalis (in its various forms) is now used in the acute setting only for the control of cardiac rhythm.

Intra-aortic Balloon Counterpulsation

Intra-aortic balloon counterpulsation is indicated when pharmacological methods have been ineffective and when myocardial failure has an underlying cause that can be surgically corrected, such as high-grade coronary artery stenosis, acute mitral regurgitation, or intraventricular septal defect.[26] Although this intervention has occasionally been used for other conditions, no study has yet been performed to demonstrate its benefit. Intra-aortic balloon counterpulsation is unlikely to be of permanent value in most patients in the absence of an anatomic cardiac problem.

The theoretical advantage that intra-aortic balloon counterpulsation offers is its ability to maintain a relatively high diastolic pressure, which increases coronary blood flow, while reducing afterload and thereby diminishing myocardial oxygen consumption. The balloon catheter is inserted into the femoral artery by means of the modified Seldinger technique; it is then advanced to the proximal descending aorta, just distal to the origin of the left subclavian artery. The catheter is then connected to a device that alternately inflates and deflates the balloon in synchrony with the electrocardiogram. During inflation, which occurs during cardiac diastole, the balloon displaces approximately 40 ml of blood, both retrograde (into the coronary arteries) and antegrade (into the descending aorta and its branches). At the beginning of systole, the balloon is abruptly deflated, which assists the left ventricle in ejecting its stroke volume.

One of the most thorough analyses of the long-term results of intra-aortic balloon counterpulsation is a study by Naunheim and coworkers, who analyzed 580 patients in whom an intra-aortic balloon had been inserted before, during, or after a cardiac surgical procedure.[27] As expected, mortality was high (44 percent). The data indicate that the mortality has changed little over the past decade and that the increase in cardiac output achievable with intra-aortic balloon counterpulsation (10 to 15 percent) rarely permits reduction in the dosage of inotropic agents.

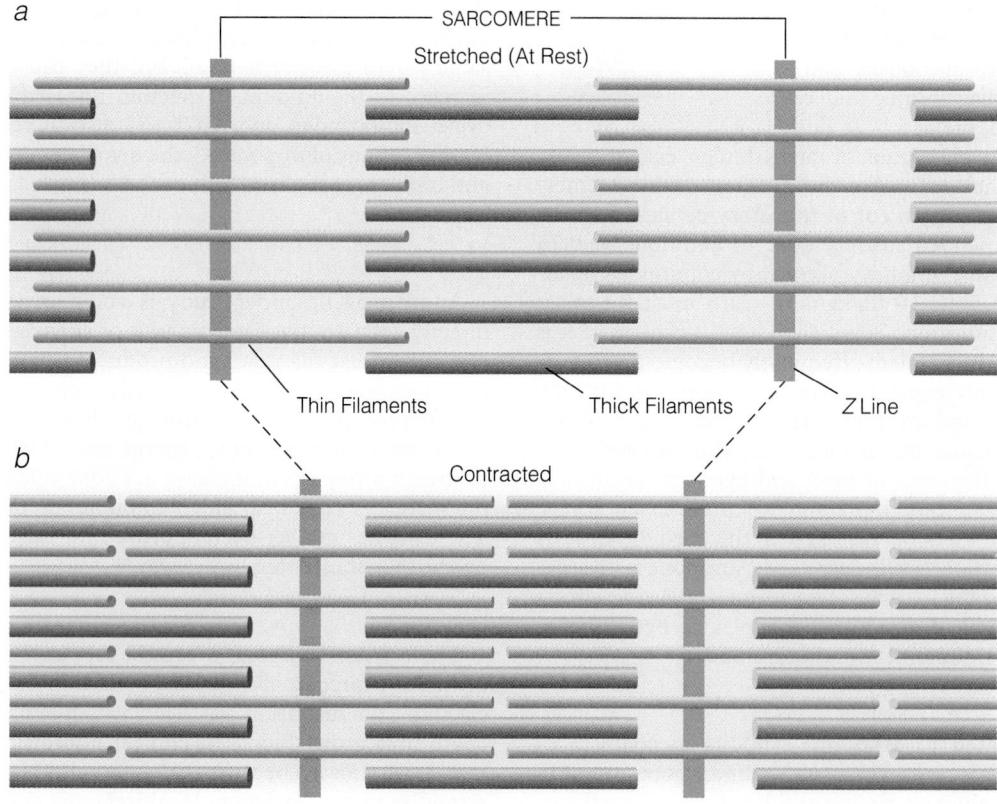

Figure 1 **Thick and thin filaments in the sarcomere (the unit of muscle fiber between the Z lines) are shown both stretched, during diastole (*a*), and contracted, during systole (*b*). Contractile force is produced by the shortening of the sarcomere, which results from the movement of the thin filaments toward the center of the sarcomere.**

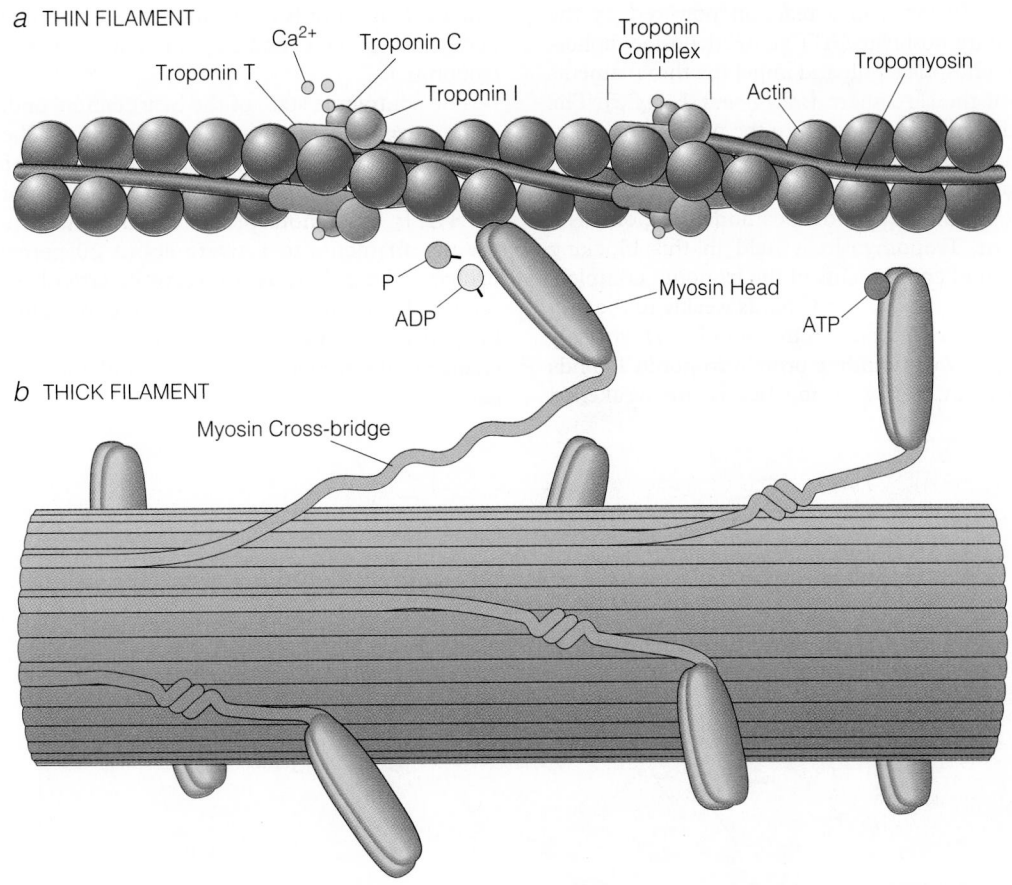

a THIN FILAMENT

b THICK FILAMENT

Figure 2 Schematized is the detailed structure of a single thin filament and its associated thick filament. During diastole, the reaction between actin and the myosin cross-bridge is inhibited by tropomyosin and the troponin complex in the absence of calcium. During systole, calcium binds to troponin C, releasing the thin filament from inhibition. The myosin cross-bridges then react with actin and swivel, moving the thin filament toward the center of the sarcomere, which results in contraction of the muscle fiber. Each cross-bridge cycle involves the splitting of one adenosine triphosphate molecule into adenosine diphosphate and inorganic phosphate.

Discussion

Oxygen Delivery

The primary function of the heart is to deliver oxygenated blood to tissues. An understanding of the determinants of oxygen consumption, oxygen delivery, and the relation between the two (the oxygen extraction ratio) is essential for successful management of the critically ill patient [*see VII:3 Pulmonary Dysfunction and VII:4 Use of the Mechanical Ventilator*].

The oxygen extraction ratio is normally 0.25. Empirical observations and experimental data suggest that myocardial decompensation occurs at an oxygen extraction ratio of 0.5 or greater. Efforts to lower the oxygen extraction ratio, either by augmenting oxygen delivery or by reducing oxygen consumption (e.g., through fever reduction or through the use of paralytic agents), are essential.

It is also important to decrease myocardial oxygen utilization by decreasing heart rate and preload (while maintaining adequate cardiac output) and by reducing afterload to the lowest level at which adequate perfusion of the pressure-dependent beds (e.g., heart, brain, and kidney) can be maintained. The latter effect helps account for the primacy of ACE inhibition in the management of chronic congestive heart failure.

The Physiology of Myocardial Contraction

Like other types of muscle cells, myocardial muscle cells generate force as a result of a reaction between actin of the thin filaments and myosin of the thick filaments. The heads of the myosin molecules, the cross-bridges, extend from the thick filaments, bind to actin, and, in a reaction powered by the splitting of adenosine triphosphate (ATP) into adenosine diphosphate and inorganic phosphage, tilt and impel the thin filaments toward the center of the sarcomere [*see Figures 1 and 2*]. The force generated is directly proportional to the number of cross-bridges reacting with the thin filaments.

In diastole, intracellular calcium is very low, and the actin cross-bridge reaction is blocked by the position of tropomyosin on the thin filament. Tropomyosin is held in this blocking position by the action of components of the troponin complex. When no calcium is bound, troponin C binds weakly to the thin filament, whereas the inhibitory protein troponin I binds strongly to actin and the tropomyosin-binding protein troponin T binds strongly to tropomyosin. These strong bonds are weakened when calcium binds to troponin C to promote a tight binding between troponin C and troponin I and between troponin C and troponin T.

The contractile state of the heart can be understood in terms of the myofilament activation by calcium. The binding of calcium to troponin C activates one functional unit that consists of a cross-bridge, actin, tropomyosin, and troponin in a ratio of 1:7:1:1. In basal inotropic states, enough calcium is released to the myofilaments to activate about 20 percent of the cross-bridges. Thus, there is a reserve of cross-bridges that can be recruited to participate in the contraction. This recruitment can happen in two ways: by the release of more calcium or by a change in the responsiveness of myofilaments to a given level of calcium.

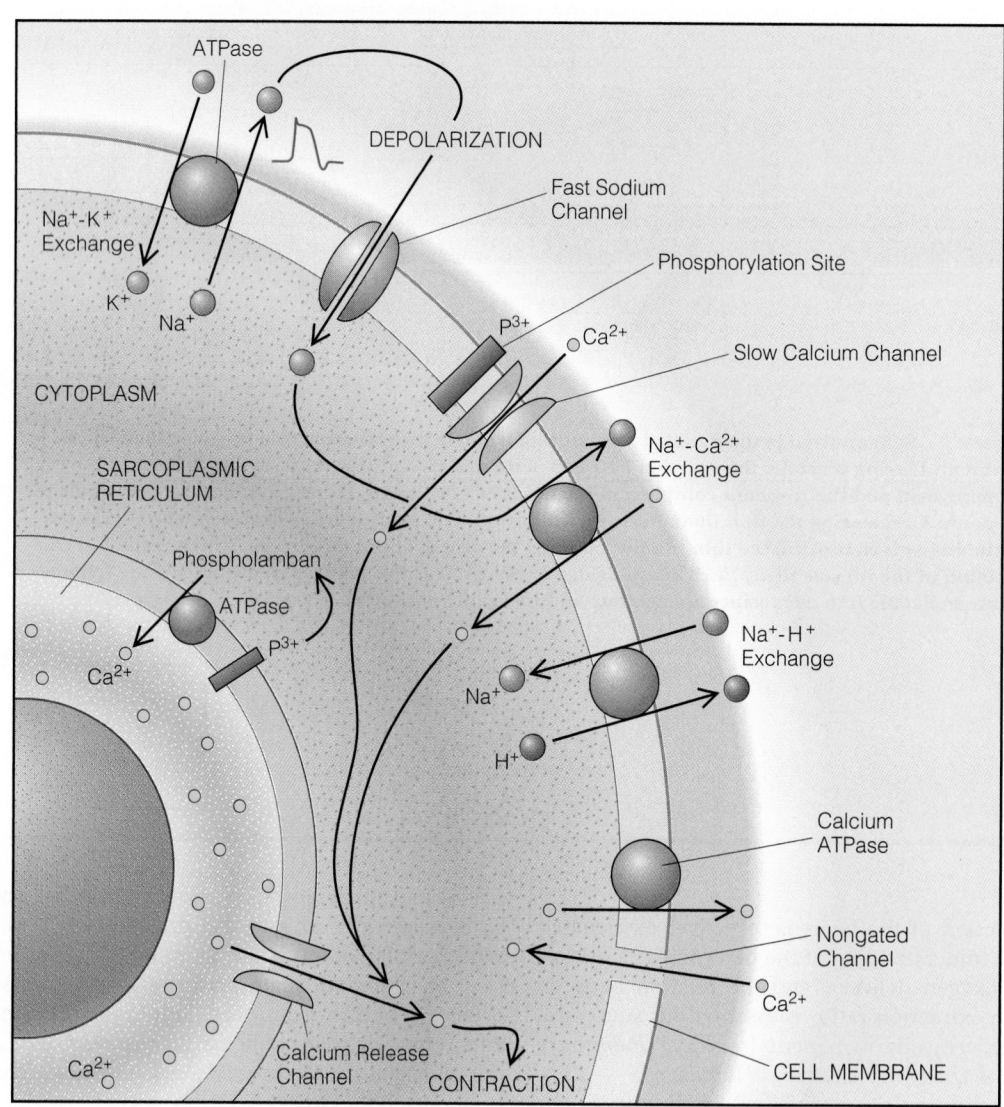

Figure 3 Ionic flux occurs via several pathways across the cell membrane and from within the sarcoplasmic reticulum. When the cell membrane is depolarized, calcium and sodium move into the cytoplasm. Sodium is exchanged for calcium, and additional calcium is released into the myofilament space from the sarcoplasmic reticulum, which provides ample amounts of calcium for binding with troponin. During repolarization, the process is reversed.

Calcium entry into and exit from the myofilaments occur across the cell surface membrane and across an internal, enclosed membrane network, the sarcoplasmic reticulum [see Figure 3]. During systole, calcium entry into the myofilament space from the interstitial space occurs via (1) voltage-sensitive channels (L-type channels), (2) a voltage-sensitive sodium-calcium exchange protein, and (3) nongated calcium channels. Calcium entry into the myofilament space from storage sites in the sarcoplasmic reticulum compartment occurs through a calcium-release channel that is gated by calcium. Depolarization of myocardial cells results in the opening of fast sodium channels. As the cell depolarizes, calcium channels open, the sodium-calcium exchanger reverses, and there is a relatively small and rapid net movement of calcium into the cell. These calcium ions gate the calcium-release channels of the sarcoplasmic reticulum, resulting in a relatively large release of calcium, which binds to troponin C and activates the myofilaments. Extrusion of calcium from the myofilament space during relaxation occurs primarily via a calcium–adenosine triphosphatase (ATPase) pump in the sarcoplasmic reticulum membrane but also through the sodium-calcium exchanger and through a surface-membrane calcium-ATPase pump.

Transmembrane ionic channels governing sodium movement play an important, albeit indirect, role in calcium homeostasis; these channels are (1) the fast sodium channel, (2) the Na^+-K^+-ATPase pump, which exchanges intracellular sodium for extracellular potassium, and (3) a sodium-hydrogen exchange protein. Thus, one of the more important mechanisms for increasing intracellular calcium is linked to the concentration of intracellular sodium. It follows that any process that increases intracellular sodium will act indirectly to increase intracellular calcium.

Cyclic adenosine monophosphate is a critically important intracellular regulator of calcium transport.[28] It is generated by the enzyme adenylate cyclase,[29] which is located in the cell membrane, and it is metabolized by a variety of phosphodiesterases. Increases in the intracellular level of cAMP result in enhanced movement of calcium through the slow channels and an increase in calcium that is stored in the sarcoplasmic reticulum.

INOTROPIC AGENTS

It should be apparent from this sequence of events that three of the most important variables governing myocardial contraction are the availability of intracellular calcium (to permit actin-myosin interaction), the response of the myofilaments to calcium, and the availability of ATP (to provide energy for both contraction and relaxation). Inotropic agents exert their actions primarily by increasing the intracellular calcium concentration.[5] This increase may result from an inhibition of Na^+-K^+ ATPase, which increases the level of intracellular sodium and, hence, exchange for calcium. Most investigators think that this mechanism underlies the activity of the cardiac glycosides.[25] This indirect effect of cardiac glycosides on the calcium level may explain their relative lack of potency.

A second mechanism that increases the intracellular calcium level is the stimulation of cAMP production by beta agonists. Agents such as isoproterenol, epinephrine, dopamine, and dobutamine bind to the $beta_1$ receptor, which is coupled to adenylate cyclase, an enzyme that mediates cAMP production. Levels of cAMP rise to activate kinases that phosphorylate the calcium channels (promoting their open state) and phospholamban, a protein that regulates calcium pumping by the sarcoplasmic reticulum ATPase. Both of these phosphorylations increase calcium entry into the myofilament space.

A third mechanism that increases intracellular calcium concentration is inhibition of phosphodiesterase, which degrades cAMP. Like adenylate cyclase stimulation, phosphodiesterase inhibition increases the intracellular calcium level and, hence, results in increased contractile force. This mechanism is thought to underlie the action of newer inotropic agents, such as amrinone, milrinone, and enoximone. Some of these agents may also enhance myofilament response to calcium.

PRELOAD

Within limits, the contractility of the myocardium varies directly with resting muscle length. In the intact heart, resting length is primarily dependent on end-diastolic volume, which is generally related to end-diastolic pressure. The relation between resting muscle length and the tension developed by contracting heart muscle is referred to as the Frank-Starling relation and is widely employed in clinical practice. When using this relation, however, it is essential to remember that measurement of left ventricular end-diastolic volume (LVEDV) is difficult and that the most widely used index—PAOP—is subject to a number of assumptions and confounding factors.[1] Notable among these factors are the influences of increased airway pressure, myocardial ischemia, and mitral valve disease on PAOP measurement and interpretation. These conditions may make PAOP high when LVEDV is low. Hence, in clinical practice, Frank-Starling curves must be interpreted with great caution.[30]

AFTERLOAD

The resistance against which the ventricle must pump is reflected primarily by the mean arterial pressure. Laplace's law states that the wall tension of a cylinder is directly proportional to the radius and to the pressure supported by the wall. Hence, left ventricular afterload increases with enlargement of the left ventricle (which increases the radius) and with increasing mean arterial pressure. Because wall tension, along with heart rate, is a prime determinant of myocardial oxygen consumption, it follows that reduction in afterload will beneficially decrease work done by the ischemic heart. This provides the rationale for afterload-reduction therapy for both acute and chronic heart failure.

References

1. Rudd P, Blaschke TF: Anti-hypertensive agents and the drug therapy of hypertension. The Pharmacologic Basis of Therapeutics, 7th ed. Gilman AG, Goodman LS, Roll TW, et al, Eds. Macmillan Publishing Co, New York, 1985, p 784

2. Leier CV, Bambach D, Thompson MJ, et al: Central and regional hemodynamic effects of intravenous isosorbide dinitrate, nitroglycerin and nitroprusside in patients with congestive heart failure. Am J Cardiol 48:1115, 1981

3. Salem MR: Therapeutic uses of ganglionic blocking drugs. Int Anesthesiol Clin 16:171, 1978

4. Varriale P, David W, Chryssos BE: Hemodynamic response to intravenous enalaprilat in patients with severe congestive heart failure and mitral regurgitation. Clin Cardiol 16:235, 1993

5. Colluci WS, Wright RF, Braunwald E: New positive inotropic agents in the treatment of congestive heart failure: mechanisms of action and recent clinical development (pt 1). N Engl J Med 314:290, 1986

6. Leier CV: General overview and update of positive inotropic therapy. Am J Med 81(suppl 4C):40, 1986

7. Leier CV, Unverferth DV: Drugs five years later: dobutamine. Ann Intern Med 99:490, 1983

8. Gray R, Shah PK, Singh B, et al: Low cardiac output states after open heart surgery: comparative effects of dobutamine, dopamine, and norepinephrine plus phentolamine. Chest 80:16, 1981

9. Monrad ES, Baim DS, Smith HS, et al: Milrinone, dobutamine, and nitroprusside: comparative effects on hemodynamics and myocardial energetics in patients with severe congestive heart failure. Circulation 73(suppl 3):168, 1986

10. Goldberg LI: Dopamine: clinical uses of an endogenous catecholamine. N Engl J Med 291:707, 1974

11. Friedel N, Wenzel R, Matheis G, et al: Haemodynamic effects of different doses of dopexamine hydrochloride in low cardiac output states following cardiac surgery. Eur Heart J 13:1271, 1992

12. Benotti JR, Grossman W, Braunwald E, et al: Hemodynamic assessment of amrinone: a new inotropic agent. N Engl J Med 299:1373, 1978

13. Endoh M, Yamashita S, Taira N: Positive inotropic effect of amrinone in relation to cyclic nucleotide metabolism in the canine ventricular muscle. J Pharmacol Exp Ther 221:775, 1982

14. Silke B, Verma SP, Midtbo KA, et al: Comparative hemodynamic dose-response effects of dobutamine and amrinone in left ventricular failure complicating acute myocardial infarction. J Cardiovasc Pharmacol 9:19, 1987

15. Earl CQ, Linden J, Weglicki WB: Biochemical mechanisms for the inotropic effect of the cardiotonic drug milrinone. J Cardiovasc Pharmacol 8:864, 1986

16. Mager G, Klocke RK, Kux A, et al: Phosphodiesterase III inhibition or adrenoreceptor stimulation: milrinone as an alternative to dobutamine in the treatment of severe heart failure. Am Heart J 121:1974, 1991

17. Installe E, De Coster P, Gonzalez M, et al: Comparison between the positive inotropic effects of enoximone, a cardiac phosphodiesterase III inhibitor, and dobutamine in patients with moderate to severe congestive heart failure. Eur Heart J 12:985, 1991

18. Thuillez C, Richard C, Teboul JL, et al: Arterial hemodynamics and cardiac effects of enoximone, dobutamine, and their combination in severe heart failure. Am Heart J 125:799, 1993

19. Rüegg JC, Solaro RJ: Calcium-sensitizing positive inotropic drugs. Heart Failure: Basic and Clinical Aspects. Gwathmey JK, Briggs GM, Allen PD, Eds. Marcel Dekker, New York, 1993, p 457

20. Baumann G, Felix S, Sattelberger U, et al: Cardiovascular effects of forskolin (HL 362) in patients with idiopathic congestive cardiomyopathy: a comparative study with dobutamine and sodium nitroprusside. J Cardiovasc Pharmacol 16:93, 1990

21. Mulieri LA, Leavitt BJ, Martin BJ, et al: Myocardial force-frequency defect in mitral regurgitation heart failure is reversed by forskolin. Circulation 88:2700, 1993

22. Hughes WG, Ruedy JR: Should calcium be used in cardiac arrest? Am J Med 81:285, 1986

23. Winegar CD, White BC: Physiology of resuscitation. Emerg Med Clin North Am 1:479, 1983

24. National Conference on Cardiopulmonary Resuscitation (CPR) and Emergency Cardiac Care (ECC) standards and guidelines for cardiopulmonary resuscitation (CPR) and emergency cardiac care (ECC): III. Adult advanced cardiac life support. JAMA 255:2933, 1986

25. Noble D: Mechanism of action of therapeutic levels of cardiac glycosides. Cardiovasc Res 14:495, 1980

26. Bregman D, Kaskel P: Intra-aortic balloon counterpulsation in refractory shock. Trauma: Emergency Surgery and Critical Care. Siegel JH, Ed. Churchill Livingstone, New York, 1987, p 331

27. Naunheim KS, Swartz MT, Pennington DG, et al: Intraaortic balloon pumping in patients requiring cardiac operations: risk analysis and long-term follow-up. J Thorac Cardiovasc Surg 104:1654, 1992

28. Osterrieder W, Brum G, Hescheler J, et al: Injection of subunits of cyclic AMP–dependent protein kinase into cardiac myocytes modulates Ca^{2+} current. Nature 298:576, 1982

29. Katz AM: Cyclic adenosine monophosphate effects on the myocardium: a man who blows hot and cold with one breath. J Am Coll Cardiol 2:143, 1983

30. Hansen RM, Viquerat CE, Matthay MA, et al: Poor correlation between pulmonary arterial wedge pressure and left ventricular end-diastolic volume after coronary artery bypass graft surgery. Anesthesiology 64:764, 1986

Acknowledgment

Figures 1, 2, and 3   Tom Moore.

3 PULMONARY DYSFUNCTION

Robert H. Demling, M.D.

Approach to Management of Pulmonary Dysfunction

Respiratory injury in surgical patients is usually acute in onset and is associated with a number of different primary diseases. Although some surgical patients with respiratory dysfunction have a

history of chronic lung disease, most had normal pulmonary function before the onset of the surgical disease. The initial etiology of respiratory injury varies according to the disease involved, but the final physiologic and clinical manifestations are remarkably constant. Treatment modalities for a wide variety of respiratory syndromes are also relatively constant.

Each of the disease states that will be described can induce moderate to severe pulmonary dysfunction. The diagnosis of acute respiratory failure, which by definition usually necessitates mechanical ventilatory support, is based on the magnitude of the pulmonary abnormalities. Certain diagnostic criteria have been established [*see Table 1*]. It is not necessary, however, that all the criteria be met before the diagnosis is made or before endotracheal intubation and mechanical ventilation are instituted.

Initial Support Measures

ENDOTRACHEAL INTUBATION

There are four indications for controlling the airway by endotracheal intubation (the so-called rule of four P's): (1) impaired airway patency, (2) inadequate airway protection, (3) inadequate pulmonary toilet, and (4) requirement for positive pressure ventilation. Each of these is an absolute indication for intubation. Current and anticipated problems that may affect airway patency must be considered; for example, with direct injury from trauma or burns, one must anticipate mucosal edema or external compression by edema or hemorrhage. The objective is to secure the airway before the anticipated problem occurs. The adequacy of airway protection—in particular, protection from aspiration—depends on neurologic status as well as on the structural integrity of the larynx and the ability of the epiglottis to protect the airway. Pulmonary toilet is the clearance of secretions to avoid airway obstruction, atelectasis, and infection. If coughing is inadequate, direct airway access must be obtained for suctioning. Patients with an adequate cough but with voluminous secretions (e.g., those with inhalation injury) may also require intubation to avoid the fatigue attendant on the increased work of breathing. The tube select-

ed should be of sufficient size (7 mm internal diameter or wider) to allow adequate suctioning while minimizing airflow resistance; the larger the diameter of the tube, the less the resistance to airflow. Positive pressure ventilation, which is indicated when spontaneous ventilation is inadequate, can be provided by continuous positive airway pressure (CPAP) with spontaneous breathing or by mechanical ventilation with or without positive end-expiratory pressure (PEEP).

Choice of Intubation Route

The choice of intubation route depends on the presence or absence of spontaneous breathing, on the skill of the physician, and on circumstances that may favor a particular approach [*see Table 2*]. In general, the initial choice is between nasal and oral routes. Endotracheal tubes provide adequate airway access and can be safely left in place for three to four weeks, after which patients requiring continued airway access should undergo tracheostomy. Patients with facial and neck injuries and those with copious airway secretions and large particulate debris (as seen in severe necrotizing inhalation injury) do better when

Table 1 Criteria for Diagnosis of Acute Respiratory Failure

Parameter	Normal Range	Respiratory Failure
Respiratory rate	12–20	> 35
Vital capacity (ml/kg body wt)*	65–75	< 15
FEV_1 (ml/kg body wt)*	50–60	≤ 10
Inspiratory force (cm H_2O)	–(75–100)	≥ –25
Compliance (ml/cm H_2O)	100	< 20
P_aO_2 (mm Hg)	80–95 (room air)	< 70
A-aDO_2 (mm Hg) (F_iO_2 = 1.0)	25–65	> 450
$\dot{Q}_S/\dot{Q}_T$ (%)	5–8	> 20
P_aCO_2 (mm Hg)	35–45	> 55†
V_D/V_T	0.2–0.3	> 0.60

*Ideal body weight should be used.
†Chronic lung disease constitutes the exception.

FEV_1—forced expiratory volume in one second P_aO_2—partial pressure of oxygen in arterial blood   A-aDO_2—alveolar-arterial oxygen gradient F_iO_2—fraction of inspired oxygen $\dot{Q}_S/\dot{Q}_T$—shunt fraction P_aCO_2—partial pressure of carbon dioxide in arterial blood V_D/V_T—ratio of dead space to tidal volume

Approach to Management of Pulmonary Dysfunction

Clinical symptoms of pulmonary dysfunction include
- Dyspnea
- Tachypnea
- Cyanosis
- Suprasternal and intercostal retractions
- Altered mental state
- Tachycardia and hypotension or hypertension

Order pulmonary function studies

Clinical and laboratory evaluation includes
- Measurement of arterial blood gases
- Chest x-rays
- Bronchoscopy
- Ventilation-perfusion scans
- Pulmonary function tests
- Microbial surveillance

Absolute indications for intubation are
- Impaired airway patency
- Inadequate airway protection
- Inadequate pulmonary toilet
- Requirement for positive pressure ventilation

Cardiogenic pulmonary edema

Treat hypoxemia.
Measure pulmonary arterial pressures and cardiac output.
Administer dopamine or dobutamine if cardiac output is low.
Consider administration of furosemide.
Consider sodium nitroprusside for afterload reduction.

ARDS

Treat hypoxemia and hypercapnia.
Measure pulmonary arterial pressures and cardiac output.
Maintain PAWP below 15–18 mm Hg with infusion of crystalloid or red blood cells, if possible.
Give dopamine or dobutamine to maintain cardiac output.

Atelectasis

Treat hypoxemia.
Maintain airway toilet, with tracheal suctioning.
Order incentive spirometry.
Ensure airway humidification.
Relieve chest wall pain.
Evacuate pleural cavity.

Pulmonary embolism

Treat hypoxemia and hypercapnia.
If ventilation-perfusion lung scan shows defects, confirm with pulmonary angiogram.
Administer heparin in an initial bolus of 10,000 U, followed by 1,000 U/hr to maintain PTT at 1.5 times normal.
Consider caval interruption in selected patients.

Acid aspiration

Treat hypoxemia.
Perform laryngoscopy or
bronchoscopy, or both, for
verification and removal of
aspirated contents.
Maintenance of intravascular
volume may require pulmonary
arterial monitoring.
Administer bronchodilators for
small airway obstruction.

Lung contusion

Treat hypoxemia.
Careful fluid management is
indicated.
Relieve chest wall pain.
Monitor arterial blood gases to
assess need for ventilatory
support.

Bacterial pneumonia

Treat hypoxemia.
Order Gram's stain of sputum and
antibiotic susceptibility testing.
Maintain meticulous pulmonary
toilet.
Guide antibiotic therapy by
surveillance and diagnostic
cultures.

Impaired neuromuscular function

Treat hypoxemia.
Control pain from rib or muscle injury. Bilateral multiple
fractures call for ventilatory assistance.
Maintain some degree of muscle work to prevent atrophy,
taking care not to fatigue patient.
Optimize nutritional status.
Avoid overinflation of lung and distention of abdomen.
Avoid prolonged neuromuscular blockade.

Table 2 Choice of Intubation Route

Route	Advantages	Disadvantages
Nasotracheal	Tube can be inserted blindly Can be performed with the neck in neutral position More comfortable Easily secured Allows better oral hygiene	Spontaneous breathing required for placement Diameter of tube limited by size of nares Longer tube required Pulmonary toilet diminished Nasal hemorrhage or sinusitis possible Tracheal damage possible
Orotracheal	Tube more easily inserted by less experienced personnel Tube can be wider and shorter, thereby allowing better pulmonary toilet	Neck hyperextension usually required Less comfortable Less easily secured Tracheal damage possible
Tracheotomy (cricothyrotomy)	Wide, short tube allows better pulmonary toilet More comfortable Tube can remain inserted for a very long time	Operative complications More experienced personnel required for safe and expedient placement Tracheal damage possible

tracheostomy is performed sooner [*see I:3 Burn Care in the Immediate Resuscitation Period, III:3 Injuries to the Face and Jaw, and III:4 Injuries to the Neck*].

DEFINING MECHANICAL VENTILATION

Mechanical ventilation is largely defined as positive pressure ventilation. Positive pressure increases intra-alveolar pressure relative to pleural pressure, leading to lung expansion and in turn to expansion of the chest wall.[1] This approach makes possible adequate ventilation in the presence of major impairments in ventilatory mechanics involving either the lung or the chest wall. Lung volume can be maintained despite increased airway resistance and decreased lung compliance. Collapsed lung tissue can be reexpanded,

Table 3 Nonpulmonary Side Effects of Mechanical Ventilation[25]

Cardiac effects

Impairment of preload attributable to decrease in venous return

Increase in right ventricle size and decrease in left ventricle size as a result of right-to-left septal shift

Support of the failing ventricle by the surrounding positive pressure and by reduction of preload and afterload

Decrease in systemic oxygen demand through decreased work of breathing and increased sedation

Renal effects

Decrease in renal blood flow comparable to overall decrease in cardiac output

Redistribution of blood flow from cortical to medullary areas (thought to be the result of increased renal vein pressure), leading to decreased filtration rate and urine output

Increase in antidiuretic hormone resulting from increased intrathoracic pressure and a neural reflex initiated by the pressure-distorted atrial wall

Increase in plasma renin activity

which decreases the shunt fraction and improves arterial oxygen tension (P_aO_2).

The necessary increase in mean airway pressure can also produce complications [*see Table 3*]. The normal ventilation-to-perfusion ratio of spontaneous breathing can be disrupted, which leads to overexpansion and resultant regional hypoperfusion. Transmission of positive airway pressure to mediastinal structures and the pulmonary vasculature can cause a decrease in venous return and an increase in pulmonary vascular resistance, both of which can impair cardiac output and oxygen delivery.[2] The more compliant the lung or the less compliant the chest wall, the greater will be the transmission of the positive airway pressure to the mediastinum. The concomitant decrease in cardiac output can in large part be overcome by volume loading. Barotrauma will occur from high airway pressure, with the potential for alveolar disruption.

Ventilators can be classified as pressure cycled or volume cycled. With a pressure-cycled ventilator, inspiration is determined by a preset inspiratory pressure. With a volume-cycled ventilator, the inspiratory volume is preset. Volume-cycled ventilators are generally preferred in the intensive care unit because they maintain a relatively constant tidal volume and minute ventilation when changes in compliance or resistance occur. Procedures for initiating and maintaining positive pressure ventilation are described in detail elsewhere [*see VII:4 Use of the Mechanical Ventilator*].

Clinical Recognition of Pulmonary Dysfunction

CARDIOGENIC PULMONARY EDEMA

Cardiogenic, or high-pressure, pulmonary edema can be detected clinically through measurement of arterial blood gas pressures and invasive hemodynamic monitoring.[3] The interstitial edema that

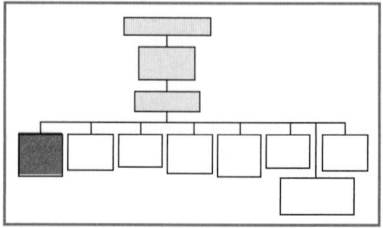

precedes any alveolar edema is generally manifested by dyspnea, tachypnea, mild hypoxemia, diffuse bilateral rhonchi, and wheezing (cardiac asthma). Signs of hypervolemia or congestive failure, such as distended neck veins and peripheral edema, are evident. Pulmonary arterial wedge pressure (PAWP) is usually high, about 25 mm Hg.[4] Radiographic signs of cardiogenic pulmonary edema include bronchovascular fluid cuffs (reflecting the interstitial edema), redistribution of blood flow to nondependent areas, cardiomegaly, and pleural effusions [see Table 4].[5]

Alveolar flooding, which ensues if interstitial edema progresses, dramatically accentuates lung dysfunction and hypoxemia. Diffuse rales become evident, and lung compliance and functional residual capacity (FRC) decrease. X-ray findings include evidence of interstitial edema followed by diffuse parenchymal involvement (usually greater in the bases).

The primary causes of interstitial edema are volume overload and left-sided heart failure resulting from myocardial ischemia or infarction. Frequently, elements of both causes are responsible, because a normal heart and normal kidneys can usually compensate for excessive fluid administration. Elevated pulmonary capillary hydrostatic pressure (P_{cap}) leads to increased fluid transport from the capillaries to the lung interstitium because of an imbalance of Starling forces. If the pumping capability of the lymphatics is overwhelmed, the excess fluid migrates beyond the lymphatic openings in the peripheral lung toward the loose interstitium around the larger airways and vessels. A decrease in the oncotic gradient between plasma and interstitium resulting from severe hypoproteinemia accentuates the edema.

Interstitial edema leads to external compression of the bronchovascular structures in the loose interstitial space, increasing airway resistance and vascular resistance. Increased vascular resistance redistributes blood flow away from areas of edema, resulting in ventilation-perfusion ($\dot{V}/\dot{Q}$) mismatch.

Alveolar flooding occurs when the interstitial space, including the septum, has expanded and interstitial pressure has increased to such a degree that alveolar cell apposition is disrupted and edema fluid enters the alveolar compartment. Each alveolus fills completely, and surfactant action is impaired. A fluid-filled alveolus is incapable of gas exchange, even when the fraction of inspired oxygen (F_IO_2) is increased. Positive end-expiratory pressure redistributes the contained water in a layer along the alveolus and allows oxygen to cross, although the alveolar-arterial oxygen gradient (A-aDo_2) is still significantly increased. A diffusion abnormality, however, is much more easily managed in this situation than is a complete shunt of blood past a totally fluid-filled alveolus, because the former can be partly corrected by administering oxygen to increase alveolar oxygen tension.

Cardiogenic edema resolves relatively rapidly once volume overload is corrected and capillary hydrostatic pressure decreases. Typically, there is improvement within 24 hours. Water is transported back into the interstitium and also is cleared through the airway. Edema fluid is a transudate rather than an exudate, so there is relatively little protein to remove. Excess water in the loose interstitium around the hilum has less effect on lung function, but it takes as long as several days to clear because its reabsorption rate is fairly slow. Consequently, chest films will continue to show evidence of interstitial edema for 24 to 48 hours after correction of the etiologic process and restoration of adequate gas exchange.

Table 4 Radiographic Manifestations of Pulmonary Edema[25]

Cardiogenic (High-Pressure) Pulmonary Edema	Low-Pressure Pulmonary Edema (as Seen in ARDS)
Redistribution of blood flow away from dependent lung	Normal vascular pattern
Bronchovascular fluid cuffs	Few to no fluid cuffs, but frequent air bronchograms
Increased septal (Kerley B) lines	Absence of septal lines
Cardiomegaly	Normal heart size
Pleural effusions	Infrequent effusions

ARDS—acute respiratory distress syndrome

Treatment

Young patients with high-pressure pulmonary edema caused by obvious fluid overload can be treated safely with only fluid restriction, diuretic therapy, or both. In surgical patients with underlying cardiopulmonary or renal disease, flow-directed pulmonary arterial catheters [see VII:1 Cardiopulmonary Monitoring] are necessary to distinguish high-pressure from low-pressure pulmonary edema; high-pressure edema is confirmed by PAWP greater than 20 to 25 mm Hg. Hypoxemia and hypercapnia are treated with oxygen administration or ventilatory support [see VII:4 Use of the Mechanical Ventilator]. Low cardiac output is restored to normal by administration of dopamine or dobutamine, beginning at 3 to 5 μg/kg/min and increasing as needed. Dobutamine is preferred in patients with a PAWP in excess of 20 mm Hg, tachycardia, or high systemic vascular resistance. Left atrial pressure is reduced by administration of a loop diuretic; furosemide is the drug of choice because it induces immediate venodilation in addition to diuresis. Low-dose dopamine (1 to 3 μg/kg/min) can be added to higher dosages of dobutamine to improve renal blood flow selectively and allow a more effective diuresis. In patients with high systemic vascular resistance, afterload should be reduced by administration of sodium nitroprusside. Patients who have coronary insufficiency and a high PAWP may benefit from intravenous nitroglycerin. Fluid administration must be appropriately monitored to avoid hypervolemia.

ACUTE RESPIRATORY DISTRESS SYNDROME

The term acute respiratory distress syndrome (ARDS) refers to the clinical manifestations of a number of indirect lung injury states characterized by dyspnea, severe hypoxemia, decreased lung compliance, and radiographic evidence of diffuse bilateral pulmonary infiltrates.[6,7] Pulmonary edema in the presence of a normal PAWP (i.e., low-pressure pulmonary edema) is also characteristic [see Table 5]. The lung damage is the result

Table 5 Identifying Characteristics of Cardiogenic and Low-Pressure Pulmonary Edema[25]

Cardiogenic (High-Pressure) Pulmonary Edema	Low-Pressure Pulmonary Edema
Initiated by local process: increased pulmonary capillary hydrostatic pressure	Initiated by distant focus, usually inflammation or infection
PAWP > 25 mm Hg	PAWP normal, usually 10–15 mm Hg
Low-protein edema	High-protein edema
Good correlation between increased water and increased shunt	Poor correlation between increased water and increased shunt: an indication other factors involved in shunt
Parenchymal involvement a later finding; interstitium involved first	Parenchymal involvement an early finding
Rapid resolution (24–48 hr)	Slow resolution (4–7 days)

of a systemic process, such as tissue damage, infection, or inflammation, rather than of a direct lung injury [*see Table 6*]. There are probably several distinct ARDS states, each with a different cause. The common practice of referring to ARDS as a single entity has probably been more confusing than helpful.

Although the various pathophysiologies are complex and the etiologies numerous, the presenting signs and symptoms for the ARDS states are nearly identical. They can be divided into three phases [*see Table 7*].

The first phase is characterized by dyspnea, tachypnea, relatively normal $P_{a}O_2$, and hyperventilation-induced respiratory alkalosis. Physical and x-ray examination reveal no significant lung findings. This prodrome is mediator induced.

The second phase usually begins within 12 to 24 hours of the onset of the early symptoms and is characterized by physiologic and pathological evidence of lung injury. Hypoxemia, accompanied by continuing dyspnea, is evident. The hypoxemia is typically refractory to an increase in F_IO_2, which indicates increased shunting. The degree of the shunt, however, is not directly correlated with the extent of the increase in alveolar and interstitial water content, as it is in cardiogenic edema. Auscultatory findings consist mostly of signs of early patchy consolidation rather than the rales heard with a strictly water-induced process. Radiographic evidence of scattered and heterogeneous early infiltrates appears initially in dependent lung fields; there is little evidence of loose interstitial fluid collection (i.e., cuffing) unless high-pressure edema is also present. Pathological changes include bilateral interstitial inflammation, with some intra-alveolar exudate containing water, protein, and blood. The interstitial and alveolar changes lead to a restrictive type of lung dysfunction that progressively impairs lung expansion; in this phase, modest decreases in dynamic and static compliance and FRC occur. A significant portion of the ventilatory impairment is unrelated to water; mediator-induced bronchoconstriction is the probable cause. In many cases, ARDS resolves in this phase if the initiating condition is controlled.

Progression to the third phase is manifested by the onset of acute respiratory failure necessitating mechanical ventilation. The lungs become more diffusely involved and stiffer. The shunt fraction increases as a result of patchy atelectasis and focal alveolar consolidation. The increasing thickness of the alveolar capillary membrane contributes to impaired diffusion. Redistribution of blood flow, together with vascular occlusion by microemboli or local thromboses, brings about an increase in physiologic dead space, which reduces alveolar ventilation and leads to a slow rise in arterial carbon dioxide tension ($P_{a}CO_2$) if a compensatory increase in minute ventilation is not initiated. Pulmonary arterial hypertension is usually seen. It is mediator induced; the likely agents are cytokines that activate the vasoconstrictors thromboxane A_2, leukotrienes C_4 and D_4, and serotonin.[8] These agents are produced and released by white cells and platelets. Thromboxane is also produced by the lung tissue itself. The hypertension can be exacerbated by hypoxic pulmonary vasoconstriction or by increased pulmonary blood flow, as is seen in systemic inflammatory response syndrome (SIRS). A hyperdynamic state frequently evolves: cardiac output is increased, but lactic acidosis develops because the tissues are unable to increase extraction of oxygen from hemoglobin in response to increased oxygen requirements. This impairment is characteristic of the septic syndrome of ARDS and may be related to impaired metabolic function of the lung, which normally removes vasodilating agents from the blood. These agents may cause the decrease in systemic vascular resistance (SVR) that occurs, producing maldistribution of blood flow to the tissues. The increasing cardiac output required to maintain adequate tissue oxygenation may accentuate the degree of pulmonary hypertension and the magnitude of the shunt.

If ARDS persists for more than seven days, the pathological manifestations begin to change from those typical of acute inflammation to those typical of mononuclear cell infiltration with interstitial fibrosis. In addition, areas of lung infection become evident as a result of impaired bacterial clearance or the presence of an endotracheal tube. The physiologic response consists of a gradual, progressive impairment of both gas exchange and ventilation. At this point, the process is no longer easily reversible. Areas of the lung become relatively acellular and are replaced by fibrous tissue.

The mechanism of the acute injury process has not been completely defined, but the initiating event is an injury to the circulatory side of the alveolar capillary membrane. Increased pulmonary vascular permeability is characteristic. The result is that protein-rich fluid crosses into the interstitial space. The

Table 6 Causes of ARDS

Disseminated intravascular coagulation

CNS injury (neurogenic pulmonary edema)

Drug reaction

Septic response

Fat embolism

Massive blood transfusion

Oxygen toxicity

Splanchnic ischemia

Tissue trauma

Barotrauma

Pancreatitis

mechanism of injury appears to be neutrophil margination in the lung vessels, followed by activation and release of a number of neutrophil-derived factors (e.g., oxygen radicals and proteases) toxic to the endothelial cells, the alveolar cells, and the interstitium. Intracapillary accumulation of neutrophils, platelets, and fibrin is evident at an early stage of the disease, and biochemical changes appear in lung tissue that are compatible with damage by neutrophil-derived factors.

An interstitial inflammatory reaction, accompanied by neutrophil and macrophage infiltration, is also evident. There is early accumulation of fluid and exudate in the alveoli without any preceding fluid filling of the perihilar loose interstitial space. These findings indicate that an alteration in the interstitium itself—probably involving basement membrane fibronectin and gel components, especially hyaluronic acid—disrupts this normal protective mechanism and facilitates fluid accumulation in the lung parenchyma.

The alveoli are found to contain not only fluid but also inspissated protein in the form of hyaline membranes. The increased protein must be cleared by macrophages. Surfactant production is altered, and there is an increased tendency toward alveolar collapse. Initially, this process of alveolar fluid collection and collapse appears to affect the dependent areas of the lung. The presence of alveolar protein, coupled with the initial neutrophil sequestration and activation, produces an inflammatory process in the lung that can lead to further inflammation and lung injury as chemotactic agents are released from injured tissue. Macrophages are a likely source of the mediators that exacerbate the inflammation. In addition, macrophage-derived factors can enhance the growth of the local fibroblast population and collagen deposition, resulting in an injury that is not readily reversible.

Treatment

Initial treatment of ARDS is aimed at removing the source of the lung injury. Overhydration should be avoided because it accentuates the edema. In the second phase, there is evidence of hypoxia. The hemoglobin oxygen saturation should be kept above 90 percent with supplementary oxygen.

If ARDS progresses rapidly toward acute respiratory failure, endotracheal intubation and positive pressure ventilation are needed.[1] Continued readjustment of ventilatory support is required to minimize the risks of oxygen toxicity and barotrauma. An F_IO_2 of 0.5 or less is preferred. Tidal volume may have to be decreased if the need for PEEP increases, to avoid marked increases in peak inspiratory and mean airway pressures.

Blood volume and electrolyte balance should be carefully maintained with blood, colloid, and crystalloid to replace losses. Early placement of a pulmonary arterial catheter is advantageous; clinical assessment of volume status is often misleading. Even small increases in capillary hydrostatic pressure can produce rapid progression of the edema because the permeability of lung capillaries is increased. Aggressive diuresis may improve P_aO_2 but can decrease tissue perfusion, producing inadequate oxygen delivery and lactic acidosis. Factors that increase oxygen demand—which include pain, anxiety, excessive muscle activity, and hyperthermia—should be minimized. Inotropic support may be needed to meet tissue oxygen demands. The beta agonists dopamine and dobutamine are the agents of choice.

Adequate nutritional support is also essential to meet the increased metabolic demands, which include increased work of

Table 7 Clinical Presentation of ARDS

Prodrome
  Tachypnea
  Dyspnea, but no cyanosis
  Auscultation normal
  Chest x-ray usually normal
Onset of parenchymal changes
  Tachypnea
  Dyspnea
  Tachycardia
  Mild cyanosis
  Auscultation: few coarse rales
  Chest x-ray: early patchy infiltrates, usually in lower lung fields
Progression to respiratory failure
  Tachypnea
  Tachycardia
  Cyanosis
  Auscultation: diffuse rhonchi, signs of consolidation
  Chest x-ray: diffuse parenchymal infiltrates, air bronchograms, decreased lung volumes

breathing. On the basis of animal studies, the provision of increased quantities of antioxidants—vitamin C, 1 g/day; vitamin E, 500 to 1,000 IU/day; and glutamine, 30 g/day—has been recommended even though there are few hard data on the efficacy of this practice in humans. Close monitoring for nosocomial pneumonia is necessary because local lung and systemic immune defenses are impaired in ARDS. Appropriate antibiotic therapy for any lung infection must be initiated early to avoid progression of acute ARDS to chronic inflammation and fibrosis. In selected cases, instillation of nitric oxide through the ventilator has decreased pulmonary arterial hypertension to some extent: aerosolized surfactant has not been proved to be of benefit in adults with ARDS, as it has in infants.

ATELECTASIS

Atelectasis is the collapse of previously inflated lung tissue and the consequent collapse of alveoli [see Table 8]. If infection supervenes, inflammatory exudate and necrotic debris may obstruct larger bronchi, causing significant parenchymal collapse and consolidation.

Atelectasis in surgical patients is most often associated with a recent surgical procedure that results in a pain-induced decrease in respiratory excursion or with direct lung injury. As with any variety of pulmonary dysfunction, dyspnea, tachypnea, and tachycardia are prominent clinical features of alveolar collapse, especially when it occurs acutely. The response appears to be mediated in part by vagal stretch receptors in the lung. This mechanism may be responsible for the cough associated with atelectasis, which is usually nonproductive. Fever is almost always present and is often unrelated to concomitant infection. When the collapsed lung tissue reinflates, the fever promptly

Table 8 Types and Causes of Atelectasis[25]

Obstructive atelectasis
  Excessive mucus
  Airway edema
  Infection
  Impaired mucociliary clearance (from smoking or anesthesia)
  Bronchial neoplasms
  Foreign bodies
Compressive atelectasis
  Pneumothorax
  Hemothorax
  Hydrothorax
  Excessive elevation of diaphragm
Contraction atelectasis
  Local inflammatory or fibrotic process
  Abscess
  Prior infection with scar formation
Patchy atelectasis
  Surfactant denaturation
  ARDS

disappears. If large portions of lung are atelectatic, clinical examination may reveal dullness to percussion, decreased breath sounds, and elevation of the diaphragm. Tracheal deviation signals massive lung collapse and is most often observed in association with pneumothorax. The extent of alveolar collapse and right-to-left shunt is reflected in arterial blood gas pressures. Hypoxemia of variable severity is typical and is initially accompanied by mild hypocapnia. As the atelectasis becomes more severe, hypercapnia and impending respiratory failure supervene.

Chest films are valuable diagnostic tools. Microatelectasis after operation may appear as tiny platelike linear densities, usually located bilaterally in the lung bases. However, the only clue on x-ray examination may be a decrease in lung volume as manifested by elevation of the diaphragm. Obstructions of major lobar bronchi with distal collapse of the involved lobe appear as triangular densities. These abnormalities are most easily seen on lateral chest films. If the entire lung collapses, the contralateral lung is hyperinflated, and the mediastinum is shifted toward the collapsed lung. Segmented lesions produce horizontal lines or plate atelectasis on x-ray as a result of the increased compactness of the collapsed lung tissue. Areas of lung hyperinflation are frequently seen in the adjacent lung.

Atelectasis is most deleterious when perfusion through the collapsed lung persists, increasing the shunt. Moreover, the collapsed lung tissue becomes more prone to infection because bacterial clearance is impaired. Mucus plugging of the involved lung is common; it is not only a cause but also a result of the local collapse and failure of mucus clearance. The transpulmonary pressure necessary to reexpand the areas of atelectasis exceeds that required simply to maintain alveolar volume because surface tension forces, which must be overcome, are greatest when alveolar volume is low. Increases in pressure, such as those that occur with coughing or bagging, are usually necessary; unfortunately, they may cause barotrauma.

Treatment

Management of atelectasis should be aggressive, with frequent clinical assessment. It is essential to identify and alleviate the underlying disease process, even if this requires invasive techniques. Significant amounts of air or fluid in the pleural space should be removed. Meticulous airway toilet and maintenance of airway patency are of paramount importance in the management of all forms of atelectasis.

Pain associated with a chest wall injury or a recent surgical procedure in the torso predisposes to shallow breathing and is the major cause of postoperative atelectasis. Intraoperative infiltration of the surgical incision with a local anesthetic or continual epidural anesthesia to the involved area in the postoperative period relieves the pain and permits increased ventilatory effort without discomfort.

Tracheal suction, deep breathing maneuvers, and airway humidification are also indicated for prevention and treatment of postoperative atelectasis. Incentive spirometry is useful to prevent small airway collapse; the patient initiates an inspiration with increased tidal volume followed by a forced expiration. Bronchoscopy is valuable to remove debris from larger airways, especially if a lobe or an entire lung is collapsed. In addition, this procedure yields definitive material for bacterial culture. Use of bronchodilators, either aerosolized or administered systemically, is beneficial if a component of reactive airway disease is present. Administration of aerosolized or systemic corticosteroids may be required in refractory cases.

An unusual but well-recognized complication of rapid lung reexpansion after lung collapse from air or fluid in the intrapleural space is unilateral pulmonary edema in the affected lung. The postexpansion chest film may be the only initial indication of this complication. In most cases, it is not an entire lung that is involved but only certain lobes or segments.

PULMONARY EMBOLISM

Pulmonary embolism is a major source of mortality and morbidity in surgical patients[9,10] [*see VI:2 Thromboembolic Problems*]. Pulmonary emboli can be classified as large emboli, 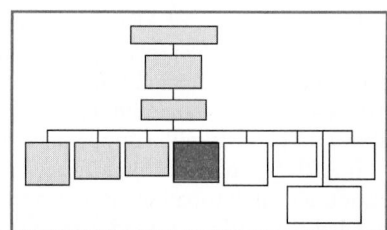 moderate-sized emboli, or microemboli. Moderate-sized to large emboli result chiefly from venous thrombi that break loose and circulate to the lung. They are often big enough to occlude moderate- to large-diameter pulmonary arteries, which may result in sudden death. This occurs when the portion of the pulmonary circulation occluded by clot is sufficient to reduce blood flow to the left side of the heart and limit cardiac output. The likelihood of a clinically significant pulmonary embolism in the general surgical population at high risk exceeds two to three percent, whereas the risk of a fatal embolism approaches one percent. Risk factors include age greater than 45 years, malignant disease, obesity, history of thrombosis, and any process that leads to venous stasis. The incidence of fatal pulmonary embolism in orthopedic patients undergoing a hip or knee procedure approaches three percent.

Most pulmonary emboli are asymptomatic. Symptomatic emboli are often those that fragment and embolize distally (thereby contributing to infarction) or those large enough to occlude a substantial portion of the pulmonary circulation.

Table 9 Clinical, Radiographic, and Laboratory Features of Moderate-Sized to Large Pulmonary Emboli[25]

Clinical Findings (% of Cases)	Radiographic (Chest X-ray) Findings (% of Cases)
Tachypnea (97)	Pulmonary infarction (48)
Dyspnea (70)	Hemidiaphragm elevation (36)
Pleuritic pain (50)	Pleural effusion (36)
Hemoptysis (30)	Atelectasis (22)
Syncope (15)	Focal blood flow loss (20)
Shock (14)	Pulmonary hypertension (20)

Laboratory Findings
Arterial blood gas levels: changes not reliable except with the most severe embolism
Electrocardiogram: of diagnostic benefit in 25% of cases; changes most prominent with massive embolism
Serum enzyme levels: lactic dehydrogenase (LDH) increases in only 40% of cases; both LDH and bilirubin increase in only 5%

The clinical presentation of very large obstructing emboli depends on the physiologic consequences [*see Table 9*]. Dyspnea and tachypnea are the most common symptoms, apparently occurring as reflex responses to the local lung changes. Also noted are tachycardia and hypotension, the severity of which correlates with the degree of vascular obstruction. The usual CNS effect of both hypoxemia and reduced blood flow is obtundation; pain is relatively rare unless infarction has occurred. Transient, dull substernal pain caused by the acute distention of the proximal pulmonary vessels is occasionally present. Mild to moderate hypoxemia, accompanied by normocapnia or hypocapnia, is common if hyperventilation is present. The increased ventilation can usually compensate at least temporarily for the increased dead space that results from ventilation of poorly perfused lung tissue. Severe hypoxemia and hypercapnia occur in cases of massive embolism with shock. In some lung areas, blood flow is excessive in relation to ventilation. When cardiac output is reduced, the deleterious effect of the low $\dot{V}/\dot{Q}$ ratio becomes more evident, and hypoxemia results. In addition, the inadequate clearance of CO_2 becomes more evident. Pulmonary hypertension and increased capillary hydrostatic pressure in the overperfused areas may produce local lung edema. Alveolar edema and obstructive atelectasis caused by splinting or bronchospasm both accentuate the shunt fraction, thereby further impairing gas exchange.

Physical examination of the chest is often normal except for tachypnea. Cardiac examination may reveal evidence of right-sided heart strain with a loud pulmonary second sound. Chest x-rays usually show normal aeration and may show a focal decrease in pulmonary blood flow. A ventilation-perfusion scan, followed by pulmonary angiography if a perfusion defect is noted, is the most accurate method of ascertaining the presence of large pulmonary emboli. Local fibrinolytic activity partially dissolves the emboli over several days; about 50 percent of the clots are gone seven days after the emboli lodge in the lung.

Moderate-sized emboli are either fragments of larger emboli or blood clots released from smaller veins such as those in the pelvis. As with large emboli, dyspnea and tachypnea are the most common symptoms. Hypotension and impairment of cardiac output are less dramatic with moderate-sized emboli. Pain occurs in 50 percent of cases as a result of the inflammation that develops in devitalized lung tissue; the onset of pain is delayed for many hours or days after the embolic event. A pleural friction rub may be evident, but again, the onset is delayed until an inflammatory response develops. Blood gas levels are often normal in patients who have moderate-sized pulmonary emboli without complications. The degree of hypoxemia reflects the extent of lung parenchymal damage as well as secondary complications such as atelectasis and edema.

Bronchoconstriction, mediated mainly by platelet-derived serotonin, occurs and results in decreased lung compliance, decreased FRC, and a predisposition to atelectasis. Pain-induced splinting of the chest wall caused by infarction-induced pleuritis results in hypoventilation, further atelectasis, and an increase in shunt fraction. Pulmonary hypertension results from impaired blood flow and the release of vasoconstrictors from platelets.

The finding of a wedge-shaped infiltrate on a chest film or of a pleural effusion is helpful in making the diagnosis of pulmonary infarction. A ventilation-perfusion scan is also useful. If the results are positive (i.e., if it reveals areas that are ventilated but not perfused), the scan should be followed by a pulmonary angiogram, which is the most accurate study for diagnosing pulmonary embolism.

Treatment

The patient must first be resuscitated, particularly after a large embolism. Cardiopulmonary resuscitation may be necessary. Oxygen should be administered, and peripheral perfusion should be supported with fluid loading. The patient should be supine so as to optimize right ventricular function. Morphine, diuretics, vasodilators, and any other agents that decrease cardiac output are contraindicated. Inotropic support may be necessary, but alpha-adrenergic agonists or other agents that increase afterload should be avoided.

The diagnosis must then be established. A ventilation-perfusion scan should be done promptly, followed by an angiogram. If these studies cannot be performed promptly and the index of suspicion for pulmonary embolism is high, a bolus of heparin (5,000 to 10,000 units I.V.) can be given. Heparin prevents further clotting and antagonizes serotonin; consequently, it may correct much of the early bronchoconstriction and vasoconstriction. When the diagnosis is established, heparin is given in a loading dose of 5,000 to 10,000 units I.V., followed by continuous I.V. infusion of about 1,000 units/hr to maintain the partial thromboplastin time at about 150 percent of the normal value for seven to 10 days. After this period, heparin is replaced with an oral anticoagulant for three to six months.

If pulmonary embolism recurs during anticoagulant therapy, a filter should be placed in the inferior vena cava. Filters should be used immediately in patients for whom anticoagulation is contraindicated, including those who have had a head injury or craniotomy. A recommendation regarding the use of thrombolytic agents must await adequate definition of their role in pulmonary embolism.

ACID ASPIRATION

Aspiration of gastric contents is a major cause of pulmonary problems and subsequent mortality in surgical patients. About 50 percent of patients who aspirate gastric 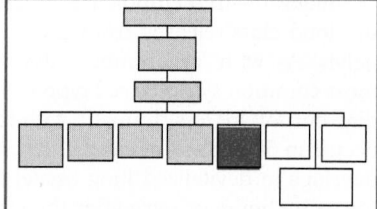 contents acquire pneumonia, and half of these die.[11,12] The volume and character of the aspirate dictate the degree of injury. Large particulate debris causes initial airway obstruction. However, a more important determinant of the magnitude of injury is the gastric pH. A pH of less than 3 induces the most severe injuries.

There are three main causes of aspiration [see Table 10]. The most common cause is impairment of laryngeal competence and glottic closure. This is usually caused by neurologic dysfunction, resulting either from drug use or from primary neurologic disease. The second major cause is increased gastric fluid volume or pressure, such as results from gastric outlet obstruction or poorly tolerated tube feedings. The third major cause is increased ease of passage of gastric contents up the esophagus, such as results from hiatal hernia.

The clinical presentation and pathogenesis of the acid aspiration syndrome can be divided into four sequential processes [see Table 11]. The first process is airway obstruction caused by particulate debris in the aspiration fluid. Immediately after aspiration, conscious, alert patients usually cough and expel particulate material; more obtunded patients begin to show symptoms of major airway obstruction. If the aspirated material is liquid, the acute incident may pass unnoticed. If the obstruction is extensive, however, it can itself be fatal. Obstruction atelectasis, accompanied by shunt formation and hypoxemia, occurs if the debris is not rapidly removed. Hypoventilation and hypercapnia can also ensue.

The second process in the acid aspiration syndrome is the direct airway injury caused by the acid. Within several hours after aspiration, the acid aspirate produces a chemical burn in the airway. Dyspnea, wheezing, and rhonchi are present, as

Table 10 Causes of Acid Aspiration[25]

Impaired laryngeal competence (glottic closure)
  Neurologic impairment (e.g., head injury)
  Drugs (e.g., narcotics, alcohol, sedatives)
  Anesthesia
  Laryngeal fracture
  Laryngeal burn
Increased gastric fluid volume or pressure
  Bowel obstruction
  Gastric atony
  Recent meal
  Poorly tolerated tube feedings
Increased regurgitation
  Impaired gastroesophageal junction
  Hiatal hernia
  Large-bore nasogastric tube

Table 11 Clinical Presentation of Acid Aspiration

Mechanical effects of aspirate (immediately after aspiration)
  Dyspnea
  Tachypnea
  Cyanosis (sometimes)
  Chest wall retractions
  Noisy respirations
  Evidence of gastric aspiration in oropharynx
  X-ray: progressing local infiltrate
Response to chemical injury (within first several hours)
  Continued dyspnea
  Increasing sputum production
  Wheezing, rhonchi on involved side
  X-ray: progressing local infiltrate
Response to inflammatory reaction (within first few days)
  Increased dyspnea
  Increased tachycardia
  Evidence of decreased blood volume
  More diffuse wheezing, rhonchi, rales
  X-ray: beginning consolidation; extension of infiltrate beyond point seen on initial x-rays
Infection (potential complication)
  Clinical course of bacterial pneumonia

with other types of burns. There is fluid loss (often massive) into the injured areas that leads to hypovolemia and compromised peripheral perfusion. The airway is severely irritated, and bronchoconstriction and bronchorrhea become apparent. In addition, the mucociliary activity of the airways is markedly impaired, which slows clearance of particles and mucus. The alveoli may also suffer direct injury if exposed to large volumes of a low-pH aspirate; edema and patchy atelectasis are the immediate results, and mortality is particularly high if this occurs. Dynamic compliance, static compliance, and functional residual capacity fall, and work of breathing and $\dot{V}/\dot{Q}$ mismatch increase.

The third process in the acid aspiration syndrome, which develops over the next 18 to 24 hours, is an inflammatory reaction to the chemical injury. Beginning several hours after aspiration, an intense leukocyte and platelet infiltration into the microvessels and airways of the injured lung is accompanied by increased release of vasoactive prostaglandins and leukotrienes. Platelets in the pulmonary vasculature release serotonin. Oxygen radicals and lysosomal enzymes from inflammatory cells promote thromboses and increase the permeability of the microvessels to protein. Degeneration of the alveolar epithelium leads to decreased surfactant production, and oxygen radicals alter the surfactant already formed, promoting alveolar collapse and flooding. Pulmonary edema and atelectasis result in increased shunting and hypoxemia, whereas microvascular thrombosis and vasoconstriction increase physiologic dead space and impair removal of carbon dioxide. The work of breathing is markedly raised as a consequence of decreased dynamic compliance (caused by increased airway resistance), decreased static compliance (caused by lung edema), and surfactant denaturation. Hypovolemia may occur as a result of loss of protein-rich fluid into the lung. This increases the physiologic dead space further because more of the lung is underperfused.

The fourth process in the acid aspiration syndrome is infection, which causes additional inflammation and tissue damage. The clinical course is that of bacterial pneumonia. The entire spectrum of bacterial infection may be found, depending on whether the normal flora has been eliminated early with prophylactic antibiotics and whether the more resistant hospital strains of bacteria have colonized the injury site.

Treatment

Treatment of the early phase of aspiration consists of rapid removal of any mechanical debris or gastric fluid from the upper airway. Endotracheal intubation is indicated if the patient cannot protect the airway. A nasogastric tube should be placed and the stomach evacuated to prevent a subsequent episode. Gas exchange is restored with oxygen administration and correction of hypoventilation.

Treatment during the next few hours consists of pulmonary support. Blood gas monitoring is necessary. A chest x-ray should be obtained to assess distal airway obstruction. If obstruction is evident, fiberoptic bronchoscopy is indicated to remove the obstructive debris. In the early stage, bronchospasm contributes to airway resistance; thus, bronchodilators can improve ventilatory function. Steroids have not proved advantageous.

If the injury progresses to an intense inflammatory process, treatment becomes that of acute respiratory failure, which includes positive pressure ventilation. The combined loss of fluid and protein into the lung can lead to hypovolemia, and it is essential to maintain normal volume status. Because hypervolemia will accentuate the lung edema, a pulmonary arterial catheter is indicated to optimize volume replacement. Inotropic support, preferably with a beta agonist, can help maintain tissue perfusion and oxygen delivery while minimizing edema-induced complications [*see VII:2 Support of the Failing Heart*]. The lung infection stage should be managed in the same way as nosocomial pneumonia would be.

PULMONARY INJURY FROM
BLUNT CHEST TRAUMA
(LUNG CONTUSION)

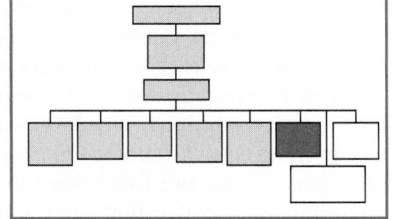

Blunt chest trauma is a common cause of pulmonary injury. There are often at least two components to the injury: impaired chest wall function and direct parenchymal disruption, or lung contusion.[13]

The clinical presentation ranges from modest tachypnea with blood-tinged secretions to labored respiration, cyanosis, and hemoptysis. Diffuse coarse rales are most marked in the areas of injury. In more severe injuries, evidence of consolidation is present. Some symptoms of impaired lung function are often present initially. Symptoms often worsen during the following 48 hours, particularly if there is an element of volume overload during resuscitation, which aggravates extravasation of fluid. The initial chest x-ray usually demonstrates localized parenchymal infiltrates that become progressively more opaque during the following 24 to 48 hours. Computed tomographic scanning of the chest can better define the magnitude of injury. Compared

with chest x-ray, CT scanning has a higher degree of sensitivity in assessing the extent of lung parenchymal injury.

A major mechanism of trauma-induced lung dysfunction is direct damage to the underlying lung tissue. Disruption of alveolar capillary integrity results in local bronchoalveolar hemorrhage. The extent to which gas exchange is impaired depends on the amount of lung parenchyma involved and on the degree of concomitant chest wall injury. Progression of tissue damage during the first 24 to 48 hours usually stems initially from continued parenchymal bleeding and later from lysis of red cells and proteins. Bronchiolar plugging with blood initially elevates the shunt fraction and gives rise to significant hypoxemia; the disrupted parenchyma remains partially perfused. With the lysis of the localized parenchymal hemorrhage and the onset of inflammation in the damaged parenchyma, a more dense consolidation develops, and neighboring lung tissue becomes involved. Lung compliance decreases, further reducing the FRC and exacerbating the atelectasis. This process increases shunting and hypoxemia. Redistribution of ventilation and blood flow increases the $\dot{V}/\dot{Q}$ mismatch. Compliance continues to decrease, and the work of breathing increases.

An intrapleural process such as hemothorax can produce compressive atelectasis on the involved side. This compression is readily corrected by the removal of blood.

Disruption of chest wall function ranges from flail chest to chest wall splinting resulting from a single rib fracture. Much of the lung dysfunction that follows chest wall injury results from hypoventilation induced by pain. The main exception is severe flail chest, in which it is impossible to generate sufficient transpulmonary pressure for lung expansion. Inability to expand the chest wall—whether from pain or from flail chest—results in hypoventilation, decreased FRC, focal alveolar collapse, and, finally, hypoxemia with hypercapnia. In addition, the inability to clear mucus and bacteria with an effective cough leads to obstruction of airways and secondary infection. Mortality is correlated with the amount of lung directly damaged and the magnitude of the associated injuries.

Treatment

Initial treatment of chest trauma during resuscitation consists of correction or control of immediately life-threatening problems such as airway obstruction, tension pneumothorax, hemothorax, hypovolemia, myocardial contusion, and flail chest [*see III:1 Emergency Department Evaluation of the Patient with Multiple Injuries*]. In addition, sufficient analgesia to permit an adequate respiratory effort and coughing is necessary. Positive pressure ventilation may be needed early if the chest wall is too unstable to maintain alveolar ventilation. A moderate flail segment can usually be managed without mechanical positive pressure ventilation. Continuous positive airway pressure can be delivered by mask if positive pressure is required. Initial fluid resuscitation must be carefully monitored to prevent overhydration, in particular administration of excessive crystalloid. Pulmonary arterial and peripheral arterial catheters are indicated in potentially severe cases.

Adequate treatment after resuscitation is critical to prevent acute respiratory failure. Good pulmonary toilet, including maintenance of an adequate cough, and avoidance of overhydration are crucial. During this period, lung compliance continues to decrease as contused and neighboring lung areas become inflamed. The increased work of breathing often augments the chest wall pain. Pain control is essential to pulmonary toilet. Regional anesthesia using rib blocks successfully restores a good respiratory effort when only a few ribs are involved. For severe chest wall injury, continuous epidural infusion of a narcotic agent combined with a local anesthetic agent is the analgesic method of choice.

Endotracheal intubation, positive pressure ventilation, and PEEP may be necessary if progressive respiratory dysfunction develops. Early treatment of lung infection is necessary because the contused lung is very susceptible to infection. However, prophylactic antibiotics are not indicated.

IMPAIRED NEUROMUSCU-LAR FUNCTION

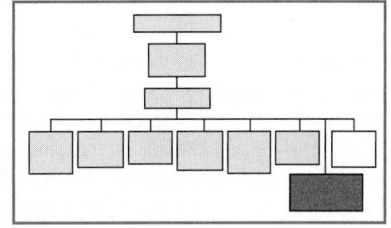

A large number of disease- and drug-related processes can alter the mechanical action of respiration and result in lung dysfunction. These processes can be loosely categorized as related either to muscles or to nerves.[14-18]

The most common muscle-related lung dysfunction arises from a failure to reverse drug-induced muscle paralysis. The next most common early problem is impaired muscle function as a result of pain, especially from rib fractures. Muscle atrophy as a consequence of long-term malnutrition or disease atrophy results in inadequate respiratory excursion. Impaired muscle function occurs if the lung is hyperinflated during ventilatory assistance. In addition, an adequate amount of oxygen must be delivered to the respiratory muscles to allow for adequate function; any reduction in cardiac output leading to impaired oxygen delivery will cause muscle fatigue.

Neurologic dysfunctions of the lung include the common failure to reverse the effects of paralyzing agents. Although uncommon, a prolonged neurologic block can develop, especially if the paralyzing agent is a steroid derivative and has been used for several days. Another neurologic cause of lung dysfunction is a disease process, now more frequently recognized but poorly understood, termed multineuropathy of critical illness. This process leads to profound weakness but seems to resolve along with the underlying illness.

Treatment

Treatment of muscle dysfunctions consists mainly of prevention and support. The use of nerve blocks, such as epidural agents, markedly diminishes pain, improves muscle function, and prevents muscle atrophy. The use of a pressure-support mode on the ventilator also prevents atrophy by providing patients with some ongoing muscle exercise. Early institution of optimal nutrition after injury or during critical illness is essential to prevent excessive muscle breakdown. Maintenance of adequate oxygen delivery for aerobic metabolism is also essential.

It is important to recognize whether muscle mechanics have become optimized. A hyperinflated lung and chest wall, excess tidal volume, underlying asthma, and increased auto-PEEP can all lead to stretched muscles and impaired muscle contraction—common causes of weaning failure.

Neurologic abnormalities related to incomplete reversal of paralysis are easily treated. Prolonged neuromuscular blockade, however, is not easily treated; at present, this and the general neuropathy of critical illness have no effective treatment but time.

BACTERIAL PNEUMONIA

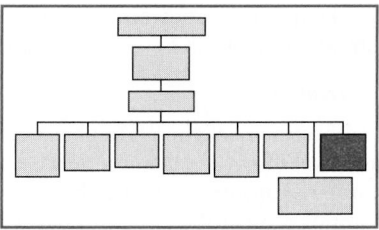

Bacterial pneumonia is a common form of direct lung injury in surgical patients [see VI:13 Early Postoperative Pneumonia]. The term pneumonia refers to an exudative consolidation of lung tissue in response to bacterial invasion. The mortality associated with treated pneumonia caused by antibiotic-sensitive organisms is about 10 percent. The superimposition of pneumonia on another form of acute lung injury substantially increases lung dysfunction and mortality: death rates exceed 60 percent in many series.

The clinical presentation begins with a high fever and the production of thick, purulent sputum. Dyspnea, tachypnea, and cyanosis may occur if more than one lobe is involved. Decreased breath sounds or bronchial breath sounds reflecting consolidation are heard. Rales and rhonchi appear as the consolidation forms and resolves.

Impairment of the lung's defense mechanisms against bacterial invasion predisposes to local infection. Pulmonary congestion and edema impair defenses, possibly by allowing bacteria to spread beyond a local area and escape the local phagocytic defenses. Increased production or decreased removal of mucus leads to small-airway obstruction, which further impairs the clearance of bacteria.

Bronchopneumonia, which is particularly common in the elderly, results in pathway consolidation of the lung, which is morphologically characterized by areas of acute suppurative inflammation. Neutrophils are the dominant cell type. The shunt fraction rises because the involved areas continue to be perfused. Compliance in the involved lung decreases, and the work of breathing increases. A hyperdynamic sepsis state, in which total-body oxygen consumption is increased, also ensues.

Lobar pneumonia is an infection-induced consolidation of a large portion of a lobe. This large consolidation is attributable to a more extensive exudative reaction, usually to encapsulated organisms. There are four stages in the development of lobar pneumonia: (1) congestion and the onset of inflammation (0 to 24 hours); (2) red hepatization, characterized by neutrophil, red cell, and fibrin deposition in the alveolus (days 4 to 7); (3) gray hepatization, characterized by increased fibrin deposition and disintegration of neutrophils and red cells; and, if bacteria are controlled, (4) resolution (days 7 to 10), in which the exudate is enzymatically digested by macrophage proteases and cleared via the airway.

Treatment

Treatment of bacterial pneumonia is discussed elsewhere [see VI:13 Early Postoperative Pneumonia].

Discussion

Basic Pulmonary Physiology

Accurate assessment of pulmonary status in surgical patients requires an understanding of seven major aspects of lung function: (1) tissue oxygenation, (2) oxygen exchange, (3) carbon dioxide removal, (4) mechanics of ventilation, (5) pulmonary circulatory function, (6) pulmonary defense mechanisms, and (7) pulmonary metabolic function. Failure of the lung to perform one or more of these functions properly is a major cause of morbidity and mortality in surgical patients.[19-24]

TISSUE OXYGENATION

Oxygenation is the process whereby molecular oxygen is extracted from inspired air and delivered to cells. The demand for oxygen by the tissues stems from their metabolic activity. Inadequate oxygenation, even for brief periods, drastically alters cell function. Anaerobic glycolysis only partially corrects for an oxygen shortage, and the resulting generation of lactic acid can lead to cell injury.

Oxygenation has three distinct components: (1) oxygen uptake by the lung from the environment, (2) oxygen delivery to the tissues, and (3) oxygen utilization or consumption by the cell. Specific terms, defined below, describe the process of oxygenation [see Table 12].

Oxygen demand is the amount of oxygen required to satisfy metabolic requirements.

Oxygen saturation (S_O_2) is the percentage of the oxygen-carrying capacity of hemoglobin that is saturated with oxygen (more than 95 percent of oxygen in the blood is carried by hemoglobin).

Oxygen content (C_O_2) is the amount of oxygen in arterial (C_aO_2) or mixed venous ($C_{mv}O_2$) blood. Oxygen content depends on hemoglobin content, on oxygen saturation in arterial (S_aO_2) and mixed venous ($S_{mv}O_2$) blood, and on the partial pressure of oxygen dissolved in plasma in arterial (P_aO_2) and mixed venous ($P_{mv}O_2$) blood. The oxygen content is computed as follows:

$$C_aO_2 \text{ (ml/dl)} = 1.34 \times Hb \text{ (g/dl)} \times S_aO_2 \text{ (\%)} + [0.003 \times P_aO_2 \text{ (mm Hg)}]$$

$$C_{mv}O_2 \text{ (ml/dl)} = 1.34 \times Hb \text{ (g/dl)} \times S_{mv}O_2 \text{ (\%)} + [0.003 \times P_{mv}O_2 \text{ (mm Hg)}]$$

Oxygen extraction ($C_{a-v}O_2$) is defined as the difference between C_aO_2 and $C_{mv}O_2$. Under normal conditions, in which $S_{mv}O_2$ is about 75 percent and $P_{mv}O_2$ about 40 mm Hg, 4 to 5.5 ml of oxygen is extracted per deciliter of arterial blood. The ability of tissues to increase oxygen extraction serves to protect them from hypoxia. Any impairment in the increased extraction process eliminates this safety valve and makes oxygen consumption totally dependent on the delivery system.

Oxygen delivery ($\dot{D}O_2$) is a measure of the amount of oxygen being delivered to the tissues. It is calculated from C_aO_2 and cardiac output (CO):

$$\dot{D}O_2 = C_aO_2 \times CO$$

Cardiac output is usually expressed as cardiac index (CI), which is the cardiac output divided by body surface area in m^2.

Oxygen consumption ($\dot{V}O_2$) is a measure of the amount of oxygen used by the body. It is calculated from cardiac index and oxygen extraction:

$$\dot{V}O_2 = C_{a-v}O_2 \times CI$$

When insufficient oxygen is available, aerobic metabolism is diminished; pyruvate cannot enter the Krebs cycle but is converted to lactate instead.

Carbon dioxide production ($\dot{V}CO_2$), the total volume of carbon dioxide generated by tissue metabolism per minute, is measured directly in expired air.

OXYGEN EXCHANGE

The ability of the lung to exchange sufficient oxygen to saturate hemoglobin is the consequence of (1) the excellent solubility of oxygen in tissue; (2) the extreme thinness of the alveolar capillary membrane; and (3) the extensive alveolar and capillary surface area.

Table 12 Tissue Oxygenation Parameters

Parameter	Abbreviation	Derivation	Mean Normal Value*
Arterial oxygen content	C_aO_2	$1.34 \times Hb \times S_aO_2 + (0.003 \times P_aO_2)$	20 ml/dl
Mixed venous oxygen content	$C_{mv}O_2$	$1.34 \times Hb \times S_{mv}O_2 + (0.003 \times P_{mv}O_2)$	15 ml/dl
Oxygen extraction	$C_{a-v}O_2$	$C_aO_2 - C_{mv}O_2$	5 ml/dl
Fractional oxygen extraction	—	$(C_aO_2 - C_{mv}O_2)/C_aO_2$	0.25
Cardiac index	CI	Cardiac output/m^2 surface area	3 L/min/m^2
Oxygen delivery	$\dot{D}O_2$	$C_aO_2 \times CI$	600 ml/min/m^2
Oxygen consumption	$\dot{V}O_2$	$C_{a-v}O_2 \times CI$	150 ml/min/m^2
Carbon dioxide production	$\dot{V}CO_2$	Direct measurement	120 ml/min/m^2
Respiratory quotient	R	$\dot{V}CO_2/\dot{V}O_2$	0.8

*Variability about mean normal values is about ± 25%. Values given assume a blood hemoglobin concentration of 15 g/dl.

Hb—blood hemoglobin concentration S_aO_2 and $S_{mv}O_2$—oxygen saturation of hemoglobin in arterial and mixed venous blood, respectively
P_aO_2 and $P_{mv}O_2$—partial pressure of oxygen in arterial and mixed venous blood, respectively

Table 13 Gas Exchange Parameters

Parameter	Abbreviation	Derivation	Normal Value
Partial pressure of oxygen in arterial blood	P_aO_2	Direct measurement	Varies with age: 80–95 mm Hg (room air)
Partial pressure of carbon dioxide in the alveolus	P_ACO_2	Direct measurement	40 mm Hg
Partial pressure of carbon dioxide in arterial blood	P_aCO_2	Direct measurement	35–45 mm Hg
Partial pressure of oxygen in mixed venous blood	$P_{mv}O_2$	Direct measurement	Varies with $\dot{V}O_2$: 40–45 mm Hg
Partial pressure of carbon dioxide in mixed venous blood	$P_{mv}CO_2$	Direct measurement	44–51 mm Hg
Partial pressure of oxygen in the alveolus	P_AO_2	$[P_B - P_{H_2O} \times F_IO_2] - \dfrac{P_aCO_2}{0.8}$	Depends on P_B and F_IO_2: 95–110 mm Hg (room air), 630–670 mm Hg ($F_IO_2 = 1.0$)
Alveolar-arterial oxygen gradient	A-aDO$_2$	$P_AO_2 - P_aO_2$	25–65 mm Hg ($F_IO_2 = 1.0$)
Oxygen saturation of arterial hemoglobin	S_aO_2	Direct measurement	94%–95% (room air)
Oxygen saturation of mixed venous hemoglobin	$S_{mv}O_2$	Direct measurement	Varies with $\dot{V}O_2$: 75% by oximeter (room air)
Shunt fraction	$\dot{Q}_S/\dot{Q}_T$	$\dfrac{C_cO_2 - C_aO_2}{C_cO_2 - C_{mv}O_2}$	5%–8%

P_B—barometric pressure P_{H_2O}—water vapor pressure F_IO_2—fraction of inspired oxygen C_cO_2—oxygen content of pulmonary capillary blood $\dot{V}O_2$—oxygen consumption

Several of the terms used to describe oxygen exchange are discussed below [*see Table 13*].

P_aO_2 is a measure of the amount of oxygen dissolved in plasma; it is expressed in mm Hg. Because supplementary oxygen is often given to surgical patients, P_aO_2 by itself often is not a sensitive indicator of the adequacy of oxygen exchange.

Alveolar oxygen tension (P_AO_2) is the amount of oxygen in the alveolus. It is calculated by the alveolar air equation:

$$P_AO_2 = [(P_B - P_{H_2O}) \times F_IO_2] - \frac{P_aCO_2}{0.8}$$

where P_B is barometric pressure and P_{H_2O} is the partial pressure of water vapor (normally 45 to 48 mm Hg). The transfer of oxygen from inspired alveolar air across the alveolar capillary membrane to blood occurs by simple passive diffusion down a concentration gradient; no active mechanism is involved. P_AO_2 is normally 95 to 110 mm Hg, and P_aO_2 is normally 80 to 95 mm Hg.

A-aDO$_2$ is the average oxygen gradient across the alveolar capillary membrane. The higher the gradient necessary for adequate transfer of oxygen, the more abnormal the exchange process is. The gradient is typically 10 to 25 mm Hg.

Hemoglobin, with its high affinity for oxygen, acts as a sponge for the oxygen crossing from the alveolus. Normally, this process is in equilibrium with the P_aO_2; a P_aO_2 of 90 mm Hg yields an S_aO_2 of over 95 percent.

The P_{50} is the oxygen tension at which 50 percent of the hemoglobin is saturated with oxygen. At a pH of 7.4 and a temperature of 37°C, the P_{50} is 26 ± 2 mm Hg. The P_{50} increases—that is, the oxygen-hemoglobin dissociation curve shifts to the right—with a decrease in pH, an increase in temperature, or an increase in 2,3-diphosphoglycerate (2,3-DPG). This shift is advantageous to cells in need of additional oxygen because it increases oxygen unloading at the tissue level. A decrease in P_{50}—that is, a left shift—occurs with alkalosis, decreased temperature, or decreased 2,3-DPG. Less oxygen is unloaded from the hemoglobin at a given Po_2, which can be detrimental if oxygen delivery is marginal.

Pulmonary shunt fraction ($\dot{Q}_S/\dot{Q}_T$) is defined as the portion of the cardiac output ($\dot{Q}_T$) that perfuses unventilated alveoli ($\dot{Q}_S$). It measures the percentage of the cardiac output that returns to the left side of the heart unoxygenated. This process is also referred to as pulmonary venous admixture. Normal anatomic shunt flow through bronchial vessels and thebesian veins is about three to five percent of total pulmonary blood flow.

The shunt fraction can be measured with the patient breathing either 100 percent oxygen or a lesser concentration. Although an F_IO_2 of 1.0 simplifies the calculation, it is essential to recognize that an F_IO_2 of 1.0 can lead to absorption atelectasis and may itself impair oxygen exchange.

The shunt fraction is calculated as follows:

$$\dot{Q}_S/\dot{Q}_T = \frac{C_cO_2 - C_aO_2}{C_cO_2 - C_{mv}O_2}$$

where C_cO_2 is the oxygen content of pulmonary capillary blood. Because pulmonary capillary blood is inaccessible to direct measurement, C_cO_2 is assumed to be the oxygen content that arterial blood would have if it were fully equilibrated with alveolar air. The P_AO_2 in patients receiving 100 percent oxygen is always greater than 150 mm Hg; consequently, the pulmonary capillary blood can be assumed to be fully saturated.

CARBON DIOXIDE REMOVAL

Carbon dioxide production depends on the metabolic activity of the cells. It averages about 200 ml/min (120 ml/min/m^2) in a healthy adult. Carbon dioxide is highly soluble and readily diffuses across cell membranes and into fluid compartments. It is removed by the same process of diffusion that governs oxygen exchange and by the weak buffer system. Carbon dioxide exists in a so-called open system: it is continually produced at the cellular level and removed via the lungs. A carbon dioxide gradient is maintained between the cell and plasma. As carbon dioxide enters the plasma, most of it (70 to 90 percent) is soaked up by red cells in the form of bicarbonate and then combines with hemoglobin or forms carbamino compounds.

Bound carbon dioxide equilibrates with a small amount of the gas dissolved in plasma at a given partial pressure (P_{CO_2}). The dissolved amount is calculated as follows:

$$CO_2 \text{ dissolved in plasma} = 0.03 \times P_{CO_2}$$

A second gradient exists between plasma and alveolar gas space, because ambient air contains essentially no carbon dioxide. This gradient drives carbon dioxide from the blood until the mixed venous P_{CO_2} equilibrates with the alveolar P_{CO_2}. As plasma P_{CO_2} falls, carbon dioxide unloads from red cells. The mixed venous carbon dioxide tension, which is usually 44 to 51 mm Hg, equilibrates with the alveolar carbon dioxide tension to reach a pressure of about 40 mm Hg at end inspiration (end-tidal P_{ACO_2}). If the P_{ACO_2} is either lower or higher than 40 mm Hg, the P_aCO_2 equilibrates with this new value, which results in hypocapnia or hypercapnia. Thus, the adequacy of ventilatory mechanisms for removal of carbon dioxide dictates the plasma content of the gas. Approximately 24,000 mEq of acid is cleared daily through the lung in the form of carbon dioxide. Any impairment of carbon dioxide removal will have major effects on blood and tissue pH.

Carbon dioxide removal is dependent on adequate exchange of alveolar air [see Mechanics of Ventilation, below]. Elevation of P_aCO_2 indicates inadequate ventilation. Sometimes, a normal P_aCO_2 can be maintained by compensatory hyperventilation, even in the presence of significant lung failure. This is possible because blood from hyperventilated areas low in carbon dioxide mixes with blood from hypoventilated areas high in carbon dioxide. In contrast, low oxygen content in a hypoventilated area cannot be compensated for by regional hyperventilation.

Normal arterial pH is between 7.37 and 7.43. If the pH is less than 7.37, the patient has an acidosis. If the pH is greater than 7.43, the patient has an alkalosis. The normal P_aCO_2 is 37 to 43 mm Hg. If P_aCO_2 is greater than 43 mm Hg, there is a respiratory acidosis. If P_aCO_2 is less than 37 mm Hg, there is a respiratory alkalosis. The normal bicarbonate (measured as CO_2 content) is 22 to 28 mEq/L. If the bicarbonate is less than 22 mEq/L, there is a metabolic acidosis. If the bicarbonate is greater than 28 mEq/L, there is a metabolic alkalosis.

MECHANICS OF VENTILATION

Movement of air into and out of the lungs, or ventilation, involves three main processes: (1) the stimulus to breathe, (2) maintenance of open alveoli, and (3) mechanical motion of the lungs.

The Stimulus to Breathe

The stimuli for maintaining adequate alveolar ventilation ($\dot{V}_A$) are the P_aO_2 detected by chemoreceptors in the carotid body and aortic arch and the pH sensed by the central chemoreceptors in the brain stem. The pH is altered by dissolved carbon dioxide, which rapidly crosses the blood-brain barrier, whereas plasma buffers such as bicarbonate cannot. Small changes in blood carbon dioxide levels, therefore, yield significant changes in pH at the receptors. A decrease in pH (caused by increased carbon dioxide levels) is a strong stimulus to increase ventilation; conversely, an increase in pH sharply decreases the ventilatory drive. A decrease in P_aO_2 initiates a comparable increase in alveolar ventilation via the carotid body and aortic arch chemoreceptors. In the case of combined hypoxemia and hypercapnia, which occurs in some chronic forms of lung dysfunction, hypoxemia becomes the dominant stimulus.

Maintenance of Open Alveoli

The lung has a continual tendency to collapse, for two reasons. First, the elasticity of the interstitial connective tissue helps to deflate the lung. Interstitial elasticity accounts for about one third of the lung's total elastic recoil. Second, there is considerable surface tension in the thin fluid layer that lines the alveolar walls and protects alveolar cells from direct contact with air. The intermolecular forces in the surface fluid tend to reduce the surface area of the alveoli, and these forces increase as the radius of curvature, or the alveolar volume, decreases.

Surfactant—a mixture of phospholipids—reduces surface tension more effectively as alveolar size decreases, which helps counteract the increased surface tension at low lung volumes. Because surfactant has a half-life of about 48 hours, impairment of its production by type II alveolar cells may not be evident for several days after an injury. If surfactant is denatured, however—as may occur in alveolar edema or with local release of inflammatory mediators—alveoli become immediately unstable. Alveolar surface tension accounts for about two thirds of the lung's total elastic recoil.

Lung Movement

In the face of the tendency of the lungs to collapse, active chest wall work is needed to inflate the lungs. Muscle activity must expand the chest wall and contract the diaphragm to expand the lung effectively during spontaneous ventilation.

Several important terms used to describe the mechanics of ventilation are discussed below [see Table 14].

Physiologic dead space (V_D) is that portion of the tidal volume (V_T) that is not involved in exchanging gas with pulmonary blood. A portion of the V_D is anatomic dead space, made up of structures such as the trachea and the large airways; it amounts to about 150 ml in adults. The remainder, which is called alveolar dead space, is made up of nonperfused ventilated alveoli, such as result from embolic occlusion. The ratio of dead space to tidal volume (V_D/V_T) is normally 0.2 to 0.3. It is calculated as follows:

$$V_D/V_T = \frac{P_aCO_2 - P_ECO_2}{P_aCO_2}$$

where P_ECO_2 is the mean expired carbon dioxide tension. The V_D/V_T ratio varies with changes in either anatomic or alveolar dead space or in tidal volume; however, because it measures only total dead space, it does not distinguish changes in anatomic V_D from changes in alveolar V_D.

Minute ventilation ($\dot{V}_E$) is simply the amount of air moved into or out of the lungs in a minute. The normal resting value is usually about 5 to 8 L/min. This value includes ventilation of alveoli and dead space.

Alveolar minute ventilation ($\dot{V}_A$) is a measure of the amount of air being exchanged in the alveoli. It is determined by subtracting the calculated V_D from the V_T and multiplying the result by the respiratory rate.

Inspiratory force (IF) is the transpulmonary pressure generated during an inspiratory effort. The maximum inspiratory pressure is measured again st a completely occluded airway over about 10 seconds. This measurement does not require the cooperation of the patient and thus is particularly useful in unconscious or anesthetized patients. The inspiratory force usually required to generate a vital capacity of 15 ml/kg is at least −25 cm H_2O.

Vital capacity (V_C) is defined as the lung volume generated by a maximal expiration after a maximal inspiration. It is nor-

Table 14 Ventilation Parameters

Parameter	Abbreviation	Derivation	Normal Value
Tidal volume	V_T	Direct measurement	4–5 ml/kg
Vital capacity	V_C	Direct measurement	65–75 ml/kg
Functional residual capacity	FRC	Direct measurement	2,000–2,600 ml
Inspiratory force	IF	Direct measurement	$-(75$–$100)$ cm H_2O
Dead space to tidal volume ratio	V_D/V_T	$\dfrac{P_aCO_2 - P_ECO_2}{P_aCO_2}$	0.2–0.3
Effective dynamic compliance	C_{dyn}	$V_T/(PIP - PEEP)$	Mechanical ventilation: 60–80 ml/cm H_2O
Static compliance	C_{stat}	$V_T/(\text{plateau pressure} - PEEP)$	Mechanical ventilation: 80–100 ml/cm H_2O

P_ECO_2—mean expired carbon dioxide tension   PIP—peak inspiratory pressure   PEEP—positive end-expiratory pressure

mally about 65 to 75 ml/kg. A vital capacity of less than 15 ml/kg is an indication for mechanical ventilatory assistance; at this level, alveolar volume is insufficient to prevent collapse.

Functional residual capacity (FRC) is the volume of gas left in the lung after normal expiration, which, in conjunction with surfactant, helps keep alveoli patent. FRC is decreased in patients with pulmonary insufficiency, resulting in atelectasis and impaired gas exchange. PEEP increases FRC.

Lung compliance is defined as the change in lung volume per unit of transpulmonary pressure. Lung compliance actually measures the combined performance of the lung parenchyma and the chest wall. During spontaneous ventilation, it is normally about 200 ml/cm H_2O. During mechanical ventilation, compliance is normally closer to 60 to 80 ml/cm H_2O, because the chest wall is expanded by the lung inflation rather than actively assisting in this process.

Dynamic compliance (C_{dyn}) refers to lung expansibility during air movement. It is measured during inspiration at the peak transpulmonary pressure. It is determined as follows:

$$C_{dyn} = V_T/\text{peak transpulmonary pressure}$$

When mechanical ventilation is employed, C_{dyn} is calculated differently:

$$C_{dyn} = V_T/PIP - PEEP$$

where PIP is peak inspiratory pressure. The C_{dyn} reflects lung and chest wall expansibility in addition to resistance to airflow in the airway, including ventilator tubing.

Static compliance (C_{stat}) is a measure of the recoil properties of the lung and chest wall or the ability of the system to stay inflated. C_{stat} is measured when there is no flow, at the end of inspiration. The inspiratory volume is held in the lung by an end-inspiratory pause or plateau; the transpulmonary pressure measured at this point is the plateau pressure. The C_{stat} is calculated as follows:

$$C_{stat} = V_T/\text{plateau pressure} - PEEP$$

Decreased static compliance can reflect alveolar collapse, as occurs with surfactant denaturation or pulmonary edema.

Work of breathing is an important parameter in ventilation. Normally, less than five percent of total oxygen consumption is used for the work of breathing. An increase in dead space or shunt or a decrease in compliance can markedly increase the work load. If the increased oxygen demand cannot be met or

muscle fatigue occurs, respiratory distress will ensue. Work of breathing can be assessed by monitoring changes in oxygen consumption that result from changes in ventilatory effort, such as are seen in the process of weaning.

PULMONARY CIRCULATORY FUNCTION

The integrity of pulmonary circulatory function is essential to adequate gas exchange and tissue oxygenation. This function can be described in terms of (1) pulmonary blood flow, (2) blood volume and surface area, (3) vascular pressure and resistance, and (4) vascular permeability properties.

Pulmonary Blood Flow

Blood flow, or cardiac output, is a major component of lung oxygen exchange and systemic oxygen delivery. Low blood flow through ventilated lungs may actually improve the arterial oxygen tension and saturation because the increased lung transit time allows more oxygen loading; however, oxygen delivery will be inadequate. This illustrates the importance of assessing lung oxygen exchange and systemic oxygen delivery when evaluating a patient's physiologic status.

Blood flow must be present if gas exchange is to occur. Pulmonary blood flow can be divided into three lung zones as follows:

Zone I: alveolar pressure > mean PAP > venous pressure
Zone II: mean PAP > alveolar pressure > venous pressure
Zone III: mean PAP > venous pressure > alveolar pressure

where PAP is pulmonary arterial pressure. In zone I, alveolar pressure exceeds vascular pressure, resulting in cessation of flow and creation of dead space. In zone III, both PAP and pulmonary venous pressure exceed alveolar pressure, resulting in continual pulmonary blood flow. This zone accounts for most of a healthy lung.

Blood Volume and Surface Area

Blood volume in the pulmonary capillary bed depends on total body blood volume and vascular pressures and resistances. Capillary volume determines the vascular surface area available for gas exchange.

Vascular Pressure and Resistance

PAP is monitored through a Swan-Ganz catheter. A normal mean PAP is 12 to 16 mm Hg. Acute increases in PAP can be caused by several disease processes, including (1) an increase in pulmonary venous pressure, (2) increased pulmonary vascular tone caused by circulating mediators (for instance, in SIRS), (3) pulmonary emboli, with obstruction of flow, (4) hypoxia-induced vasoconstriction, and (5) positive airway pressure.

Pulmonary vascular tone is regulated by the autonomic nervous system and by many inflammatory vasoconstrictors and vasodilators. An elevated PAP increases the afterload to the right side of the heart, thereby increasing right-sided heart work. An acute increase in mean PAP to greater than 30 mm Hg can lead to right-sided heart dilatation, right-to-left shift of the ventricular septum, and subsequent impairment of left-sided heart function. The increased PAP may have little effect on capillary hydrostatic pressure if arterial resistance is increased as a result of smooth muscle constriction. This process can protect the lung from pulmonary edema.

Monitoring of capillary hydrostatic pressure is important because a significant increase can lead to pulmonary congestion and edema as a result of an imbalance of Starling forces. When the PAWP is about 20 mm Hg, there is usually radiographic evidence of pulmonary congestion, hilar engorgement, and other abnormalities. When PAWP exceeds 30 mm Hg, pulmonary edema is usually present.

Vascular Permeability

The rate at which fluid crosses the capillary membrane from plasma to interstitium is dictated by the Starling equation:

$$\dot{Q}_f = K_f[(P_{cap} - P_i) - \sigma (COP_{cap} - COP_i)]$$

where $\dot{Q}_f$ is the rate of fluid filtration, K_f is the filtration coefficient describing the ease of water transfer across the capillary membrane and through the interstitium, P_i is interstitial hydrostatic pressure, σ is the reflection coefficient describing the ability of the capillary membrane and interstitium to prevent protein crossing, and COP_{cap} and COP_i are the capillary and interstitial colloid osmotic (oncotic) pressures generated by proteins. The importance of oncotic pressure is reflected in the difference between plasma and interstitial values, which favors intravascular fluid retention. Interstitial protein content is normally about half that of plasma. Changes in the interstitial oncotic pressure can partially compensate for acute changes in the plasma forces. This compensatory capacity, however, depends on the ability of the pulmonary lymphatics to remove any increased fluid and protein from the interstitium and on the presence of relatively normal capillary permeability. An increase in capillary hydrostatic pressure forces more fluid but not more protein across the membrane; the result is a decrease in COP_i and an increase in the difference between COP_{cap} and COP_i. The increase in the oncotic gradient, which enhances intravascular fluid retention, counteracts the increase in P_{cap} pressure and minimizes the net increase in the rate of fluid filtration.

A decrease in plasma oncotic pressure, such as may occur in hypoproteinemia, transiently decreases the oncotic gradient. The COP_i also falls, however, and this compensatory mechanism can restore the oncotic gradient for decreases in plasma protein of as much as 40 percent. Greater decreases narrow the oncotic gradient because COP_i, normally about 15 mm Hg, can only decrease to 3 to 5 mm Hg.

The intact alveolar membrane is completely impermeable to protein. Under normal circumstances, water also cannot cross into the alveolus because of the surface tension properties of the alveolar membrane. Disruption of this membrane leads to alveolar flooding.

PULMONARY DEFENSE MECHANISMS

The normal lung is kept free of bacteria by a highly efficient system of bacterial and particle clearance. Alveolar clearance is provided by alveolar macrophages, which ingest the particles and either digest them or carry them along the ciliated bronchioles to the oropharynx. Particles or bacteria that are not eliminated, either because the macrophage defenses have been overwhelmed or because ciliary clearance has been impaired, initiate an inflammatory response that is signaled by the migration of neutrophils into the area. Tracheobronchial clearance is accomplished through the mucociliary action of the lining cells. The continued beating motion of the cilia moves a film of mucus containing entrapped particles, bacteria, and white cells from bronchioles to the oropharynx.

Impairment of clearance predisposes to pulmonary infection, particularly if organisms gain access to the lungs by way of a foreign body (e.g., a suction catheter or an endotracheal tube) or, less commonly, by the hematogenous route. Airway collapse impairs clearance of bacteria and mucus from the distal segments of the lung. Increased mucus production or impaired mucus clearance further aggravates the obstructing process. Increased alveolar or interstitial fluid allows an infectious process to spread more rapidly by impairing the walling off and clearance of the organisms by local defenses.

PULMONARY METABOLIC FUNCTION

Pulmonary endothelial cells are active in metabolizing biogenic amines, peptides, and prostaglandins. The lung is an important site for degradation of serotonin and, to a lesser degree, of norepinephrine. Metabolism of serotonin occurs in all pulmonary vessels. This function is impaired after hyperbaric oxygen injury, which results in increasing levels of serotonin in the blood.

Of greater importance is the role of the lung in peptide metabolism, in particular the degradation of bradykinin and the conversion of angiotensin I to angiotensin II. A single enzyme system in the lung is the major site of both these activities. Thus, extraction of the most potent vasodilator in the body, bradykinin, and activation of the most potent vasoconstrictor, angiotensin II, both take place in the lung. Patients with ARDS have decreased levels of angiotensin-converting enzyme; this may explain the systemic hypotension that can accompany ARDS. Cardiopulmonary bypass, in which the lung is excluded from the circulation, increases levels of endogenous bradykinin, providing further evidence of the nonrespiratory function of the lung. The lung is the major site of breakdown of prostaglandins of the E and F series as well as a major site of synthesis of these prostaglandins and prostacyclin. Alterations in this system may potentiate respiratory failure and failure of other organ systems.

General Pulmonary Abnormalities in Surgical Patients

Eight common pathophysiological mechanisms impair gas exchange and ventilation: (1) impaired diffusion, (2) $\dot{V}/\dot{Q}$ mismatch, (3) alveolar hypoventilation, (4) increased pulmonary shunt, (5) decreased oxygen delivery, (6) pulmonary hypertension, (7) decreased hypoxic pulmonary vasoconstriction, and (8) atelectasis. The last of these has already been discussed from a

Table 15   Causes of Hypoxia

Decreased oxygen tension in arterial blood (hypoxemia)
   Impaired diffusion
   $\dot{V}/\dot{Q}$ mismatch
   Alveolar hypoventilation
   Increased pulmonary shunt
Decreased oxygen content in arterial blood
   Decreased hemoglobin content
   Decreased arterial oxygen tension
   Carbon monoxide poisoning
   Methemoglobinemia
Decreased cardiac output
   Myocardial depression
   Decreased coronary perfusion
   Increased peripheral vascular resistance
   Increased pulmonary vascular resistance
   Cardiac arrhythmia
   Decreased circulating blood volume

clinical standpoint [*see* Clinical Recognition of Pulmonary Dysfunction, Atelectasis, *above*].

The end results of impaired gas exchange are hypoxia and hypercapnia. Hypoxia is the delivery of a less than adequate amount of oxygen to the tissues; hypercapnia is an excess of carbon dioxide in the blood. Hypoxemia is a lower than normal P_aO_2, which alters the amount of oxygen carried on hemoglobin. The components of oxygen delivery include S_aO_2, hemoglobin content, and cardiac output. Of these, the lung is directly responsible only for the first. The other two components are the responsibility of the vascular system [*see Table 15*]. The first four pathophysiological mechanisms discussed below—impaired diffusion, $\dot{V}/\dot{Q}$ mismatch, alveolar hypoventilation, and increased pulmonary shunt—constitute the principal abnormalities in the pulmonary component of oxygen delivery.

IMPAIRED DIFFUSION

Diffusion capacity refers to the volume of a gas that crosses a membrane per unit time per unit of partial pressure gradient. Diffusion capacity is determined by three variables: (1) the solubility of the gas in the membrane, (2) the surface area of the membrane, and (3) the thickness of the membrane. In the lung, both oxygen and carbon dioxide are readily soluble in the barrier that separates blood from alveolar air, and they rapidly equilibrate across this membrane. Thus, any changes in their diffusion capacity stem from changes in membrane surface area or thickness.

Diffusion abnormalities increase the alveolar-arterial oxygen gradient. If P_aO_2 falls below 70 mm Hg, arterial oxygen saturation and oxygen content decrease significantly. A modest diffusion impairment may not be clearly evident when the blood transit time through the lung is normal or even somewhat slower than normal, because oxygen readily crosses the membrane. The same diffusion abnormality becomes more evident, however, as cardiac output increases and the time available for oxygen exchange decreases, as occurs in the hyperdynamic septic state or during exercise. Increasing F_IO_2 raises P_aO_2 when the problem is abnormal membrane thickness. Hypoxemia induced by diffu-

sion impairment is, therefore, correctable through the use of exogenous oxygen. Pulmonary function tests for diffusion capacity cannot, however, distinguish increased membrane thickness from decreased surface area.

VENTILATION-PERFUSION MISMATCH

Gas exchange would be optimal if ventilation and perfusion (capillary blood flow) were perfectly matched and completely uniform—that is, if the $\dot{V}/\dot{Q}$ ratio were 1.0. In the normal lung, however, there is some mismatch, and the average $\dot{V}/\dot{Q}$ ratio is about 0.8. There are several reasons for this. The shape of the thoracic cavity and the descent of the diaphragm result in greater lung expansion in the lower lobes than in the upper lobes. Blood flow is also more prominent in the dependent lung during spontaneous ventilation; this area is in zone III, in which both PAP and venous pressure exceed alveolar pressure. Blood flow also varies with body position and with changes in ventilatory volume.

When positive pressure ventilation is used, some lung areas may be overexpanded while obstructed or stiff areas remain hypoventilated. An increase in alveolar pressure can substantially alter blood flow by changing an area of the lung from zone III to zone I or II. In addition, local blood flow through hyperinflated areas of lung is retarded by compression of the loose interstitium through which the blood vessels travel on their way to forming the capillary bed; local pulmonary vascular resistance increases, and blood flow is redistributed to hypoventilated areas, where resistance is lower.

Pathological conditions can substantially increase $\dot{V}/\dot{Q}$ mismatch and severely impair gas exchange. An acute reduction in blood flow resulting from embolic occlusion or more chronic obliteration of the lung vasculature by processes such as emphysema yields a $\dot{V}/\dot{Q}$ ratio greater than 1.0. The relative increase in $\dot{V}/\dot{Q}$ ratio does not, however, improve S_aO_2 if oxygen exchange is already reasonably good. Much of the ventilation is therefore wasted. A ventilated area through which there is no perfusion contributes to dead space [*see Table 16*].

Alternatively, ventilation may be reduced in areas with normal or increased perfusion. This occurs in conditions such as focal atelectasis and edema and in chronic processes that destroy the alveolar architecture (e.g., emphysema). The result is a very low $\dot{V}/\dot{Q}$ ratio. Not enough alveolar oxygen is available to oxygenate the excessive amount of blood perfusing the area, especially if the patient is breathing room air. Consequently, S_aO_2 and P_aO_2 are reduced. This impairment cannot be compensated for by an increased $\dot{V}/\dot{Q}$ ratio in another part of the same lung. As with diffusion abnormalities, however, much of the impaired oxygen exchange in a low $\dot{V}/\dot{Q}$ area can be corrected by increasing F_IO_2, which makes

Table 16   Causes of Increased Dead Space[25]

Vascular destruction
Vascular obstruction by emboli or thrombi
Hypovolemia leading to impaired perfusion in nondependent lung areas
Regional lung hypoperfusion resulting from increased airway pressure

additional alveolar oxygen available. If an alveolus has no ventilation, no gas exchange will occur, regardless of the F_IO_2 [*see* Increased Shunt, *below*].

Carbon dioxide is removed in proportion to the degree of alveolar ventilation. The carbon dioxide dissociation curve is linear, and unlike the oxygen-hemoglobin dissociation curve, it does not plateau. Therefore, the greater the ventilation of perfused areas, the greater the removal of carbon dioxide. Actually, hyperventilation, which often follows hypoxemia, can increase elimination of carbon dioxide and give rise to hypocapnia.

The lung normally compensates for acute decreases in regional ventilation by decreasing pulmonary blood flow to these areas. The active vasoconstriction initiated by local alveolar hypoxia is known as hypoxic pulmonary vasoconstriction [*see* Decreased Hypoxic Pulmonary Vasoconstriction, *below*]. This protective mechanism is impaired by vasodilators given exogenously or produced locally by inflammation or by the septic response. Moreover, it may begin to fail if it is chronically activated, as it is in emphysema. The failure of hypoxic pulmonary vasoconstriction increases both $\dot{V}/\dot{Q}$ mismatch and the shunt fraction. If both alveoli and capillaries are destroyed—as, for example, in necrotizing pneumonia—total ventilation-perfusion matching remains relatively normal; gas exchange is impaired only if a large portion of the alveolar capillary exchange system is destroyed.

ALVEOLAR HYPOVENTILATION

Alveolar hypoventilation, or decreased alveolar minute ventilation, can be considered a specific form of alveolar minute ventilation mismatch. It is caused by impairment of CNS respiratory center activity or by physical impairment of ventilation [*see* Table 17]. Alveolar hypoventilation produces hypoxia and hypercapnia because neither gas is adequately exchanged. In alveoli with at least some ventilation, exogenous administration of oxygen increases the P_AO_2 and may maintain sufficient oxygen content and gas exchange. The P_ACO_2, however, will increase relatively rapidly, resulting in a concomitant increase in P_aCO_2, or respiratory acidosis. The P_aCO_2 in blood leaving an alveolus is equal to the end-inspiratory P_ACO_2 of that alveolus.

Total minute ventilation is often normal, but alveolar ventilation may decrease if the V_D/V_T ratio is greater than its normal value of 0.2 to 0.3. This can occur even in the absence of lung parenchymal injury. The ratio increases with shallow breathing because the anatomic dead space stays constant (100 to 150 ml) while the V_T decreases. When V_T is inadequate, FRC is reduced as well. Airway collapse and atelectasis result if FRC falls below the closing volume.

Physical Impairment

Upper airway obstruction A significant impairment in upper airway patency as a result of anatomic distortion—e.g., posterior tongue displacement or oropharyngeal edema—will lead to hypoventilation. Depression of CNS activity increases the potential for anatomic distortion and airway obstruction.

Impaired respiratory muscle function Considerable inspiratory force, in excess of −25 cm H_2O, is needed to produce an adequate spontaneous tidal volume and vital capacity. Any impairment of chest wall or diaphragmatic muscle function that prevents the generation of an adequate transpulmonary pressure will result in hypoventilation. A number of drugs, including muscle relaxants used intraoperatively and antibi-

Table 17 Causes of Hypoventilation[25]

Impairment of CNS respiratory center activity
  Cerebral trauma
  Anesthesia, narcotics, sedatives
  Excessively high P_aCO_2
Physical impairment of ventilation (impaired lung expansion)
  Upper airway obstruction
  Muscular impairment: neuromuscular disease, drug-induced weakness, abdominal distention, pain
  Chest wall instability: rib fractures, flail chest
  Stiff lung parenchyma: edema, fibrosis, ARDS

otics such as neomycin, can produce such an impairment. Neurologic disorders that alter neuromuscular function or abdominal distention that limits excursion of the diaphragm will also impair respiratory activity.

Temporary paralysis caused by spinal anesthetic or more prolonged paralysis caused by trauma are additional causes of hypoventilation. Pain, either from direct muscle trauma, pleural irritation, or neuralgia, is a major cause of impaired respiratory muscle function in surgical patients.

Chest wall instability Multiple rib fractures, particularly those in more than one place that give rise to a flail segment, can substantially impair chest wall activity. Much of the impairment is the result of pain. With bilateral flail chest, ventilatory assistance is usually necessary.

Stiff lung Impaired lung expansion can result from a restrictive lung process, such as pneumonia, edema, or interstitial fibrosis (which causes decreased static compliance) or severe bronchospasm (which causes decreased dynamic compliance). Even very high transpulmonary pressures may be insufficient to expand a lung with poor compliance. A moderate impairment in compliance, as occurs with lung edema, may produce hypoventilation if the increased work of breathing causes oxygen demand to exceed oxygen transport to the respiratory muscles, resulting in fatigue [*see* Table 18].

INCREASED SHUNT

An increase in the shunt fraction lowers arterial oxygen tension and saturation because nonoxygenated blood from the shunt mixes with oxygenated blood from ventilated lung regions. Because the oxygen saturation of oxygenated blood normally approaches 100 percent, no satisfactory compensation can be made for the low oxygen saturation of the shunted blood. Raising the F_IO_2 will not improve oxygen exchange in the shunt area, because there is no ventilation. A shunt fraction of 15 percent or greater produces severe hypoxemia and tissue hypoxia. An increased anatomic shunt can result from a traumatic pulmonary arteriovenous fistula or a large vascular intrapulmonary tumor; however, this is rarely the case. Most often, increased venous admixture stems from functional or physiologic shunts created by alveolar collapse, edema, or consolidation.

DECREASED OXYGEN DELIVERY

A decrease in oxygen delivery, the product of cardiac output and arterial oxygen content, results in tissue hypoxia, even if

Table 18 Causes of Decreased Ventilatory Compliance[25]

	Decreased Dynamic Compliance	Decreased Static Compliance
Lung	Bronchospasm	Increased tone in small airways
	Pneumothorax	Surfactant impairment
	Stiff lung parenchyma (e.g., edema, fibrosis, ARDS)	Atelectasis
		Edema
		Pneumonia
		ARDS
Chest	Edema	Edema
	Muscle spasm	Muscle spasm
	Rib fractures	Rib fractures

Table 19 Common Causes of Pulmonary Hypertension[25]

Vascular obstruction
  Thromboemboli
  Fat emboli
  Fibrin-platelet emboli
  Microemboli
Release of vasoactive inflammatory mediators
  Thromboxane
  Leukotriene C_4 and D_4
  Serotonin
External vascular compression
  Interstitial and obstructive lung disease
Hypoxic pulmonary vasoconstriction
Increased left atrial pressure
  Heart failure
  Volume overload
  Valvular disease

10 percent for every 1° F increase in body temperature. Also, processes such as the septic response and traumatic injury will increase oxygen consumption by more than 50 percent. Attempts to minimize oxygen consumption may be preferable to further manipulation of lung function.

PULMONARY HYPERTENSION

The pulmonary circulation is a low-resistance circuit: normal PAP is only about one eighth that of systemic arterial pressure. The thin-walled right ventricle is not accustomed to pumping against high resistance. Pulmonary hypertension is caused by an increase in pulmonary vascular resistance. Pulmonary arteries, arterioles, capillaries, and venules all contribute to pulmonary vascular resistance. The normal values for systolic and diastolic PAP are 18 to 25 mm Hg and 6 to 10 mm Hg, respectively, with a mean value of 12 to 15 mm Hg.

There are five common causes of pulmonary hypertension [see Table 19]. The first is obstruction of a significant portion of the pulmonary circulation by macroemboli or microemboli. The second is release of vasoactive mediators—such as thromboxane, leukotrienes (released in ARDS), and serotonin (released after an embolic episode)—in the course of a lung disease process. These mediators act primarily on the arterial circulation. The third is external vascular compression by interstitial disease processes, as occurs in edema, acute ARDS, fibrosis, and chronic obstructive disease. The fourth is reflex pulmonary artery vasoconstriction caused by alveolar hypoxia. The fifth is elevated left atrial pressure, as is seen in left-sided heart failure, valvular heart disease, or severe volume overload.

Acute pulmonary hypertension is readily reversible when the stimulus is eliminated. Persistent hypertension that lasts for several weeks or longer results in anatomic changes in the vessels. Progressive thickening of the intima and media converts large arteries into small arterioles. This form of pulmonary hypertension, often seen in chronic lung disease, is much more difficult to reverse, and chronic cor pulmonale typically ensues.

DECREASED HYPOXIC PULMONARY VASOCONSTRICTION

Hypoxic pulmonary vasoconstriction is an important component of lung function: it helps to match ventilation and perfusion, thereby maintaining arterial oxygen tension and saturation. Precapillary pulmonary arterioles constrict in response to a local alveolar hypoxia, increasing local pulmo-

gas exchange in the lung is adequate. Arterial oxygen-carrying capacity is reduced by a decreased hemoglobin level or by a diminished affinity of oxygen for hemoglobin, as occurs in carbon monoxide poisoning. Under both of these circumstances, oxygen transport can be markedly impaired while P_aO_2 remains normal. A decrease in cardiac output also can hinder delivery of oxygen to tissues in the presence of normal lung function.

Any manipulation that is aimed at improving lung oxygen exchange must be considered in light of its potential effect on the other components of oxygen delivery, particularly cardiac output. Moreover, a correction of tissue hypoxia may not require a major alteration in lung physiology; such a correction can often be achieved by correcting the hemoglobin content or cardiac output.

The adequacy of oxygen delivery also depends significantly on oxygen demand. Increased demand, which occurs in hypermetabolic states, may make a relatively normal delivery system inadequate. Oxygen consumption increases by about eight to

Table 20 Factors That Impair Hypoxic Pulmonary Vasoconstriction[25]

Disease states	Drugs
ARDS	Phentolamine
Pneumonia	Sodium nitroprusside
Alkalosis	Nitroglycerin
Pulmonary hypertension	Aminophylline
Elevated left atrial pressure	Terbutaline
Liver cirrhosis	Nitrous oxide
	Methoxyflurane
	Nifedipine
	Verapamil

nary vascular resistance and diverting blood flow to other areas. The precise location and nature of the oxygen sensor have not been defined. Leukotrienes are believed to be involved. The response is most evident with lung collapse and atelectasis. Generalized alveolar hypoxia produces generalized vasoconstriction and pulmonary hypertension.

The status of hypoxic pulmonary vasoconstriction significantly affects the degree of hypoxemia associated with a given lung injury. Acidosis potentiates this process; alkalosis and vasodilator agents, such as prostacyclin, hinder it, as do a number of other conditions [see Table 20]. Local release of vasodilators triggered by inflammation in the lung may explain why the pulmonary shunt can be so severe in ARDS. The protective effects of hypoxic pulmonary vasoconstriction are also less evident in pneumonia.

A number of drugs and anesthetic agents impair hypoxic vasoconstriction. Vasodilators and bronchodilators must be used cautiously in the presence of a lung injury in which further $\dot{V}/\dot{Q}$ mismatch could be extremely deleterious.

References

1. Cherniack RM: Pulmonary Function Testing. WB Saunders Co, Philadelphia, 1977
2. Macklem PT: New tests to assess lung function. N Engl J Med 293:339, 1975
3. Demling RH, LaLonde C, Ikegami K: Pulmonary edema: pathophysiology, methods of measurement, and clinical importance in acute respiratory failure. New Horizons 1:371, 1993
4. Mitchell J, Schuller P, Calandrino F, et al: Improved outcome based on fluid management in critically ill patients requiring pulmonary artery catheterization. Am Rev Respir Dis 145:990, 1992
5. Ilne E, Pistoleser M, Minestic M: The radiologic distinction of cardiogenic and noncardiogenic edema. Am J Radiol 144:1, 1985
6. Demling R: Current concepts on the adult respiratory distress syndrome. Circulatory Shock 30:297, 1990
7. Montgomery AB, Stager MA, Carrico CJ, et al: Causes of mortality in patients with adult respiratory syndrome. Am Rev Respir Dis 132:485, 1985
8. Roten R, Markret M, Feihl F, et al: Plasma levels of tumor necrosis factor in the adult respiratory distress syndrome. Am Rev Respir Dis 143:590, 1991
9. Bell WR, Simon TL: Current status of pulmonary thromboembolism disease: pathophysiology, diagnosis, prevention, and treatment. Am Heart J 103:239, 1982
10. Hayes SP, Bone RC: Pulmonary emboli with respiratory failure. Med Clin North Am 67:1179, 1983
11. Bone D, Davis L: Aspiration pneumonia: prevention of aspiration in patients with tracheostomies. Ann Surg 18:30, 1974
12. Britto J, Demling RH: Aspiration lung injury. New Horizons 1:435, 1993
13. Demling RH, Pomfret EA: Blunt chest trauma. New Horizons 1:402, 1993
14. Anderson W, Zavecy J: The chest wall, diaphragm, and mediastinum. Pulmonary and Critical Care Medicine. Bone R, Ed. Mosby–Year Book, St. Louis, 1990, p 1
15. Rochester DR: Respiratory muscles and ventilatory failure: 1993 perspective. Am J Med Sci 305:394, 1993
16. Roussos C, Macklem PT: The respiratory muscles. N Engl J Med 307:786, 1982
17. Roussos C, Fixley M, Gross D, et al: Fatigue of inspiratory muscles and their synergic behavior. J Appl Physiol 46:897, 1979
18. Klessig HT, Geiger HJ, Murray MJ, et al: A national survey on the practice patterns of anesthesiologist intensivists in the use of muscle relaxants. Crit Care Med 20:1341, 1992
19. Marini J: New approaches to the ventilatory management of the adult respiratory distress syndrome. J Crit Care 7:256, 1992
20. Dreyfuss D, Sauman G: Lung overinflation. Adult Respiratory Distress Syndrome. Zapul N, Ed. Marcel Dekker, New York, 1991, p 433
21. Taylor AE, Granger DN: Exchange of neuromolecules across the neurocirculation. Physiology Handbook. Renken EM, Ed. American Physiologic Society, Bethesda, Maryland, 1985, p 462
22. West JB: Respiratory Physiology: The Essentials, 2nd ed. Williams & Wilkins, Baltimore, 1979
23. Rossi A, Gottfried SB, Zocchi L, et al: Measurement of static compliance of the total respiratory system in patients with acute respiratory failure during mechanical ventilation: the effect of intrinsic positive end-expiratory pressure. Am Rev Respir Dis 131:672, 1985
24. Tobin MJ: Respiratory monitoring in the intensive care unit. Am Rev Respir Dis 138:1625, 1988
25. Demling RH: Decision Making in Surgical Critical Care. Brian Decker, Burlington, Ontario, 1988

4 USE OF THE MECHANICAL VENTILATOR

Robert H. Bartlett, M.D.

Approach to Mechanical Ventilation

An essential concept in mechanical ventilation is the distinction between two key processes, ventilation and oxygenation. The primary purpose of ventilation is to excrete carbon dioxide. The minute ventilation ($\dot{V}_E$) is the total amount of gas exhaled per minute, computed as the product of the rate and the tidal volume (V_T). Approximately two thirds of the minute ventilation reaches the alveoli and promotes gas exchange (alveolar ventilation, or $\dot{V}_A$); the remaining third moves in and out of the conducting airways and nonperfused alveoli (the dead space ventilation, or $\dot{V}_D$). Thus, the ratio of dead space to tidal volume (V_D/V_T) is normally 0.33. The efficiency of carbon dioxide excretion is directly related to the amount of alveolar ventilation. During spontaneous breathing, the minute ventilation is regulated by the respiratory center; during mechanical ventilation, the operator uses a mechanical ventilator to excrete enough CO_2 to maintain the partial arterial pressure of CO_2 (P_aCO_2) at 40 mm Hg. Ventilation is monitored by measuring P_aCO_2.

Oxygenation, on the other hand, refers to the equilibrium of oxygen in the pulmonary capillary blood and oxygen in inflated alveoli. The partial pressure of oxygen (Po_2) gradient between alveolus and capillary favors transfer of oxygen into blood because alveolar Po_2 is maintained by ventilation or by provision of supplemental oxygen to the airway. Hence, oxygenation depends less on good alveolar ventilation than on the appropriate matching of pulmonary blood flow to well-inflated alveoli, a process that can be affected by patient position, altered airway pressure, pulmonary parenchymal disease, or small airway disease. The efficiency of this ventilation-perfusion matching, and therefore of oxygenation, can be evaluated by measuring the Po_2 in arterial blood (P_aO_2) at a known value for the fraction, or concentration, of inspired oxygen (F_IO_2).

Mechanical ventilators are designed to provide ventilation by regulating tidal volume, rate, and inspiratory flow, thereby controlling CO_2 excretion. Because they can also regulate airway pressure and F_IO_2, they offer some control over oxygenation as well. In either case, proper use of a mechanical ventilator necessitates a solid understanding of normal and abnormal pulmonary mechanics, gas exchange, and the relation between systemic oxygen delivery and consumption. Most mechanical ventilators allow the operator to monitor at least some of these variables. In practice, a mechanical ventilator is employed differently depending on whether the main goal is adequate ventilation or adequate oxygenation. Therefore, these two aspects of ventilator use will be discussed separately.

Basic Mechanical Ventilation

VENTILATION

For basic mechanical ventilation, the rate should initially be set at 10/min and the tidal volume at 10 ml/kg, provided that the inspiratory plateau pressure (P_{plat}) is

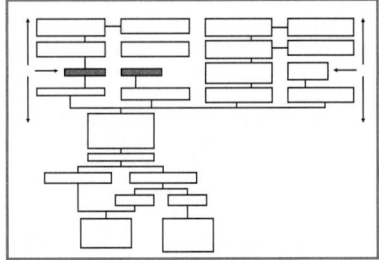

less than 30 cm H_2O; if P_{plat} is higher than 30 cm H_2O, smaller tidal volumes, such as 6 ml/kg, are appropriate. This setting will yield a minute ventilation of 100 ml/kg/min. If the V_D/V_T ratio is nearly normal, the alveolar ventilation produced (approximately 4 L/min) will be sufficient to eliminate all the metabolically produced CO_2 and to maintain the P_aCO_2 at about 40 mm Hg. If the patient's brain stem function is normal, the mechanical ventilator should be set on the assist mode, which allows the patient to adjust his or her own respiratory rate to keep the P_aCO_2 within normal limits. As a safeguard, a controlled backup rate is set below the patient's assist rate in case spontaneous effort ceases.

OXYGENATION

For basic oxygenation, the F_IO_2 should initially be set at 0.5. This level is not damaging to the alveoli and does not deplete nitrogen levels from the alveoli. If the pulmonary parenchyma and ventilation-perfusion relations are normal, P_aO_2 will

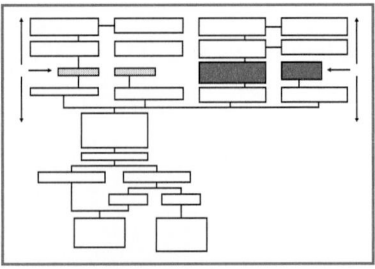

be unnecessarily elevated, and the F_IO_2 should be turned down until the saturation and Po_2 are in the normal range. The positive end-expiratory pressure (PEEP) should be set at +5 cm H_2O. This value is high enough to maintain inflation of some alveoli that would close at end expiration at lower pressures yet low enough not to induce any deleterious effects. The peak inspiratory pressure (PIP), which is always measured after a short inspiratory hold or plateau, is determined by the tidal volume, inspiratory gas flow, and compliance of the lung. If the compliance is relatively normal, the ventilator settings described will lead to a P_{plat} of 20 cm H_2O. The high airway pressure cutoff and alarm should be set at 40 cm H_2O. These settings will result in a mean airway pressure of between 5 and 10 cm H_2O, with the exact lev-

Figure 1 Shown are measurements for determining the optimal PEEP. The objective is to maximize the oxygen delivery:oxygen consumption ratio, which is measured by mixed venous saturation. Here, the best PEEP is 10 cm H_2O, even though the P_aO_2 and the arterial oxygen content are higher at higher levels of PEEP.

el depending on the respiratory rate, the inspiratory gas flow rate, and the amount of spontaneous inspiratory effort generated by the patient. The patient's inspiratory effort will appear as negative pressure measured at the airway, but such effort is beneficial rather than deleterious.

After the patient has been started on a course of mechanical ventilation, ventilation and oxygenation must be assessed, usually by measuring P_aCO_2 and P_aO_2. Adjustments are then made on the basis of this assessment [*see Figure 1*]. If P_aCO_2 and P_aO_2 are normal and if the patient is to remain on mechanical ventilation for pulmonary prophylaxis or because of CNS depression, these settings are maintained until it is time to wean the patient from ventilation [*see* Weaning from Mechanical Ventilation, *below*]. If the settings do not provide adequate gas exchange or if the patient's condition worsens, further adjustments are required.

Worsening Respiratory Status

VENTILATION

If the P_aCO_2 is elevated despite a minute ventilation of 100 ml/kg/ min, either the metabolically produced carbon dioxide is inappropriately high or the alveolar

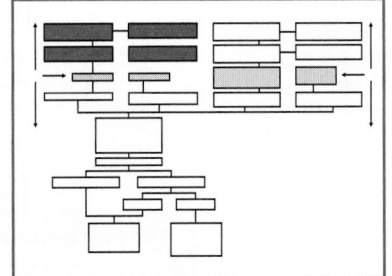

ventilation is an inappropriately low percentage of the tidal volume, or both. To increase ventilation, the first step should be to increase the respiratory rate (stepwise) to 20/min. (Increasing the respiratory rate raises the mean airway pressure and may necessitate administration of fluid volume to maintain hemodynamic stability; however, because increasing the tidal volume elevates the P_{plat}, possibly lead-

ing to barotrauma, the respiratory rate must be changed first.) The volume of CO_2 excreted is easily measured by collecting and analyzing exhaled gas. If it is greater than normal (130 ml/m²/min), CO_2 production can be decreased by reducing muscular activity or seizures, controlling hypermetabolic states (if possible), and minimizing the exogenous carbohydrate load.

If the P_aCO_2 has still not returned to normal after these measures have been taken, the respiratory rate can be increased to 25/min or higher, although it should be kept in mind that the efficiency of ventilation decreases as the respiratory rate increases (i.e., the percentage of minute ventilation that becomes alveolar ventilation decreases as the respiratory rate increases because there may be inadequate time for alveolar emptying during expiration and because the dead space remains unchanged). A tidal volume greater than 15 ml/kg is rarely necessary unless there is a major air leak. A minute ventilation higher than 300 ml/kg/min indicates major metabolic or respiratory dysfunction. The pressures required to generate this amount of ventilation are harmful to the lungs and adversely affect hemodynamic status. If the P_aCO_2 is higher than 40 mm Hg despite a respiratory rate of 20 to 25/min, a P_{plat} of 35 cm H_2O, and a minute ventilation of 250 to 300 ml/kg/min, alternatives should be seriously considered, such as allowing the patient to equilibrate at an abnormally high P_aCO_2, inducing paralysis to decrease muscular activity and CO_2 production, or instituting extracorporeal circulation through a membrane oxygenator to remove CO_2 [*see* Fighting the Ventilator, Permissive Hypercapnia, *and* Extracorporeal Life Support, *below*].

OXYGENATION

If the initial ventilator settings are not adequate to oxygenate the patient's arterial blood, then some areas in the lung are perfused but not inflated (i.e., right-to-left shunting). To enhance oxygenation, the first step is to raise the PEEP to 10 cm

H_2O, in the hope of maintaining or improving alveolar inflation. It is wise to decrease tidal volume and to increase the respiratory rate at the same time, to avoid raising the P_{plat}. The P_{plat} should not exceed 45 cm H_2O. Even with these changes in ventilation, the mean airway pressure may increase to the point at which it interferes with venous return. Whenever the PEEP is raised above 5 cm H_2O, the balance between systemic oxygen delivery and oxygen consumption should be evaluated because increasing the mean airway pressure may raise the P_{O_2} but may actually decrease systemic oxygen delivery by decreasing cardiac output.

Several measurements are necessary for determining the optimal PEEP level [*see Figure 1*]. Effective lung compliance is the simplest measurement, but optimal lung compliance does not always correlate with optimal oxygen delivery. The best measurement is that of venous oxygen content, which is approximated as mixed venous oxyhemoglobin saturation. This measurement requires samples of blood from the pulmonary artery or, better yet, a continuous indwelling catheter to monitor venous saturation. Obviously, therefore, a pulmonary arterial catheter should be inserted whenever PEEP levels higher than 5 cm H_2O are necessary for ensuring adequate oxygenation. Venous saturation measures the ratio of systemic oxygen delivery to oxygen consumption. This ratio is normally 4, which corresponds to a mixed venous saturation of 75%, when arterial saturation is near 100%. (That is, normally 25% of the oxygen delivered to tissues is extracted and utilized.) Consequently, PEEP testing is best done by gradually increasing the

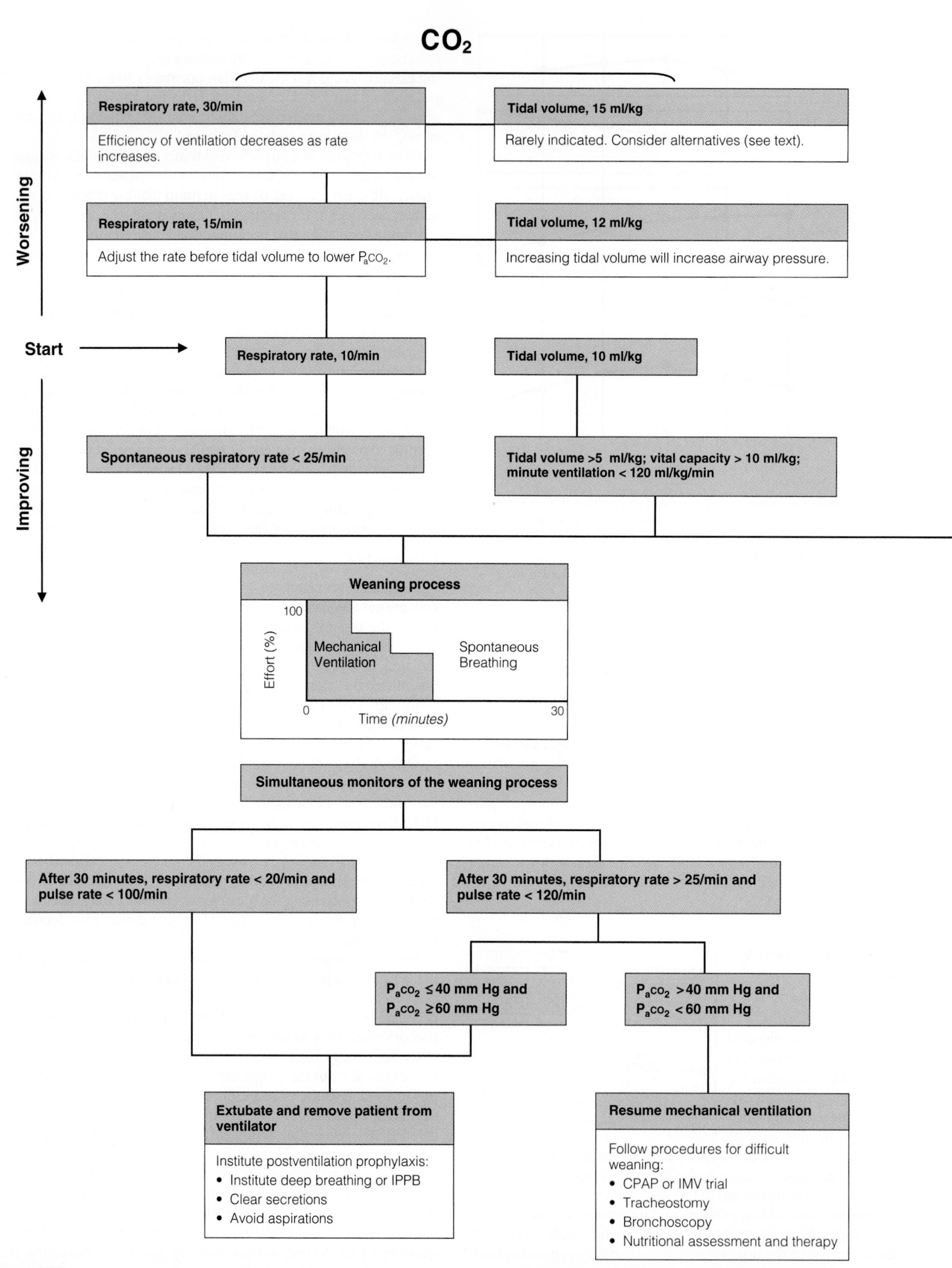

CO₂

Respiratory rate, 30/min	Tidal volume, 15 ml/kg
Efficiency of ventilation decreases as rate increases.	Rarely indicated. Consider alternatives (see text).

Worsening

Respiratory rate, 15/min	Tidal volume, 12 ml/kg
Adjust the rate before tidal volume to lower P_aCO_2.	Increasing tidal volume will increase airway pressure.

Start →

Respiratory rate, 10/min	Tidal volume, 10 ml/kg

Improving

Spontaneous respiratory rate < 25/min	Tidal volume >5 ml/kg; vital capacity > 10 ml/kg; minute ventilation < 120 ml/kg/min

Weaning process

Effort (%)
100
Mechanical Ventilation — Spontaneous Breathing
0 — Time (*minutes*) — 30

Simultaneous monitors of the weaning process

After 30 minutes, respiratory rate < 20/min and pulse rate < 100/min	After 30 minutes, respiratory rate > 25/min and pulse rate < 120/min

P_aCO_2 ≤ 40 mm Hg and P_aCO_2 ≥ 60 mm Hg	P_aCO_2 > 40 mm Hg and P_aCO_2 < 60 mm Hg

Extubate and remove patient from ventilator

Institute postventilation prophylaxis:
- Institute deep breathing or IPPB
- Clear secretions
- Avoid aspirations

Resume mechanical ventilation

Follow procedures for difficult weaning:
- CPAP or IMV trial
- Tracheostomy
- Bronchoscopy
- Nutritional assessment and therapy

1456

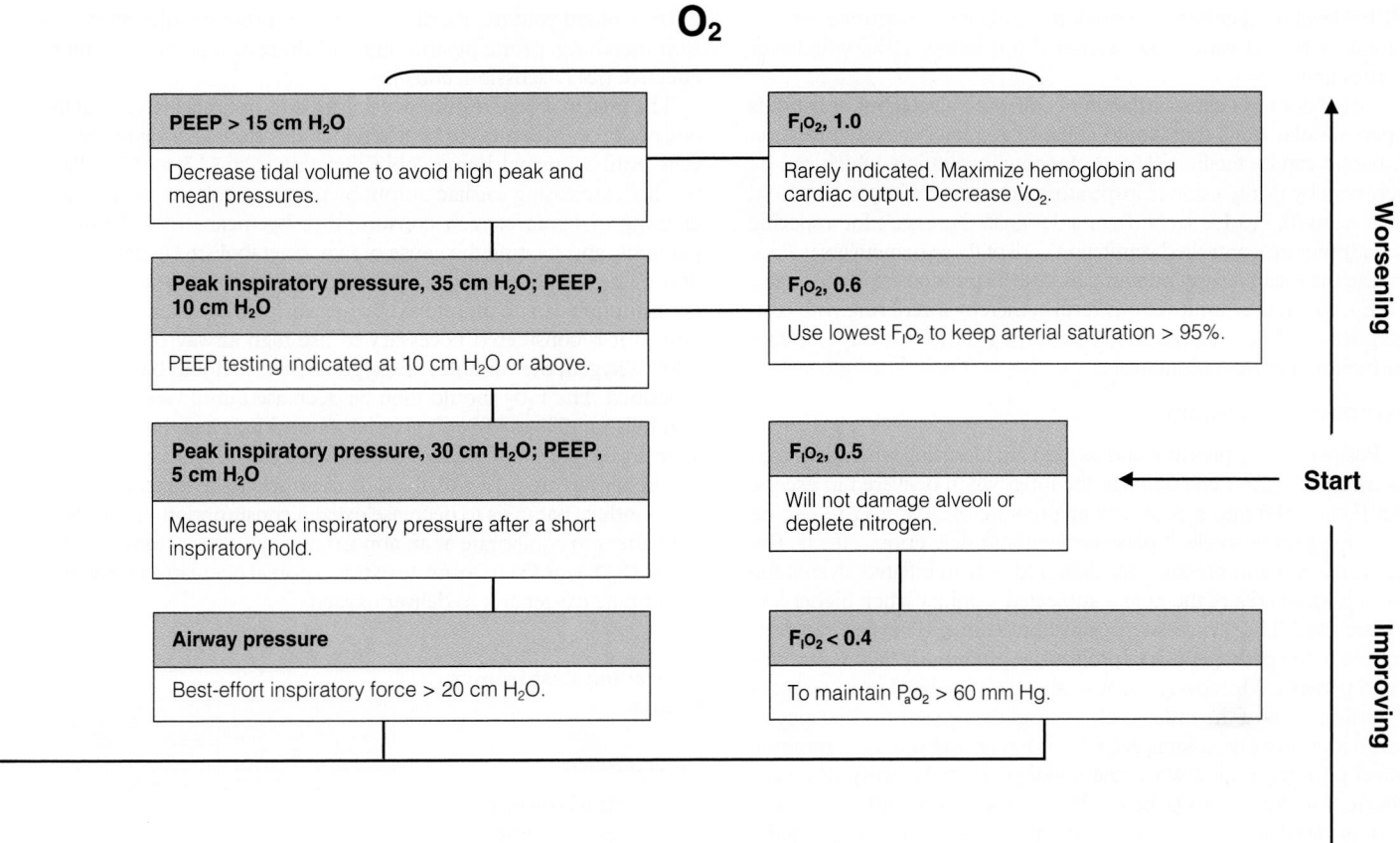

Approach to Mechanical Ventilation

PEEP level until either oxygenation is sufficient to saturate arterial blood or mixed venous saturation drops below 70%, whichever comes first.

PEEP does not cause inflation of collapsed alveoli but only holds open alveolar units that would collapse at a lower airway pressure. Inflation can be facilitated by prolonging inspiration, which can be achieved by using a slower inspiratory flow rate, an inspiratory hold or plateau (0.5 to 1.0 second), or a designated pressure for a specific time (pressure-controlled ventilation). All of these maneuvers will increase the mean airway pressure and the inspiration-expiration ratio (I/E), which may limit venous return, thereby interfering with oxygen delivery. Venous saturation monitoring is the best way to titrate inspiratory pressure maneuvers.

AVOIDING LUNG INJURY

Positive airway pressure and oxygen are lifesaving when delivered in moderation but can damage the lungs when delivered in excess. An F_IO_2 of 0.6 and a peak airway pressure of 30 cm H_2O can be used for days or weeks if necessary without deleterious effects. Because oxygen and pressure are delivered only to inflated alveoli, the most normal area of the lung is subjected to injury when higher levels are used. Thus, excessive positive pressure and oxygen can contribute to the pathogenesis of progressive pulmonary failure in ventilated patients. Moreover, pressure above 40 cm H_2O simply causes overdistention of the inflated alveoli and decreases the efficiency of ventilation [see Discussion, below]. An F_IO_2 above 0.6 has a minimal effect on oxygenation when the major problem is transpulmonary shunt. For these reasons, before P_{plat} is raised above 40 cm H_2O or F_IO_2 is raised above 0.6, all other variables of systemic oxygen delivery should be considered [see Table 1].

If oxygenation remains inadequate at these higher airway pressures, then F_IO_2 can be increased to 0.6 or higher, although it should be noted that if the problem is a major transpulmonary shunt, major increases in F_IO_2 will have little effect on P_aO_2. High concentrations of oxygen in the airway should generally be avoided, primarily because of the resultant depletion of nitrogen, which helps maintain inflation of the alveoli. Only very rarely is it necessary to raise F_IO_2 above 0.6; usually, it is preferable to increase the PEEP instead while progressively decreasing tidal volume and sup-

porting blood volume. PEEP is used to improve ventilation-perfusion matching; prone positioning and diuresis may be even more effective [see Discussion, below].

The goal in severe respiratory failure is to optimize oxygen delivery, not P_aO_2. Measures to be taken include administering red blood cells until a normal hemoglobin concentration (13 to 15 g/dl) is reached, increasing cardiac output by means of volume loading, decreasing systemic oxygen consumption by means of sedation or paralysis, and treating the cause of hypermetabolism (usually infection). The relation between systemic oxygen delivery and oxygen consumption can be monitored by measuring mixed venous saturation. If it is considered necessary to use high airway pressure and 100% oxygen, the variables of oxygen delivery should be set as just described. The F_IO_2 should then be decreased until venous saturation falls to 65% to 70%. If arterial saturation is less than 90% despite an F_IO_2 of 1.0, PEEP of more than 10 cm H_2O, and a hemoglobin of more than 13 g/dl, the next measures to be taken should be (1) to induce paralysis to decrease oxygen consumption, (2) to allow the patient to equilibrate at an abnormally low arterial oxygen saturation (S_aO_2), or (3) to institute extracorporeal circulation through a membrane oxygenator to deliver oxygen.

Improving Respiratory Status

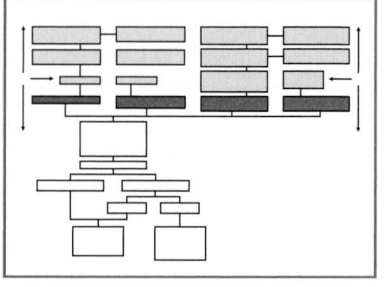

VENTILATION

Patients whose respiratory status is improving should be alert enough to regulate their own respiratory rate with the ventilator in the assist mode. Tidal volume is maintained at 10 ml/kg until the patient is ready for weaning. (As noted, if P_{plat} is greater than 30 cm H_2O, a smaller tidal volume is appropriate.) When respiratory status is improving, the ventilator should remain in the assist mode rather than in the controlled mechanical ventilation (CMV) mode because the patient can adjust his or her respiratory rate to maintain a normal P_aCO_2.

Table 1 Interventions to Optimize the Ratio of Oxygen Delivery to Oxygen Consumption in Patients with Impaired Oxygenation

Intervention	Benefits	Risk
Increase O₂ content		
↑ F₁O₂ to above 0.6	0.3 ml O₂/dl for each 100 mm Hg P$_a$O₂ after full saturation	O₂ toxicity to lung Less nitrogen in alveoli
↑ Hemoglobin (Hb) to normal	1.36 ml O₂/dl for each g HbO₂/dl	Transfusion risk (viral infection)
Increase cardiac output		
↑ Blood volume to pulmonary capillary wedge pressure of 15–20 mm Hg	200 ml Ḋo₂ increase for each L/min increase in cardiac output*	Transfusion risk ↑ Pulmonary hydrostatic pressure
Administer inotropic drugs to achieve S$_{\bar v}$O₂ 75%–80%	200 ml Ḋo₂ increase for each L/min increase in cardiac output*	Increased V̇o₂ and V̇co₂ with catecholamines Tachycardia
Administer vasodilator drugs to achieve S$_{\bar v}$O₂ 75%–80%	200 ml Ḋo₂ increase for each L/min increase in cardiac output*	Hypotension Variable regional blood flow
Decrease O₂ consumption		
Drain and treat infection	Eliminate stimulus to metabolism	None
Patient paralysis	10%–15% decrease in V̇o₂ and V̇co₂	Weakness, atrophy, need for positional changes, difficult patient examination
↓ Body temperature	7% decrease in V̇o₂ and V̇co₂ for each 1° C increase in body temperature	Requires patient paralysis, coagulopathy

*Hb = 15 g/dl; S$_a$O₂ = 100%.

OXYGENATION

The F_IO_2 should be decreased to a concentration (0.4 or 0.3) that ensures an arterial saturation higher than 90% (equivalent to a P_aO_2 higher than 60 mm Hg). Keeping the F_IO_2 in this range will lead to increased arterial oxygenation, which serves as a slight safety buffer during suctioning or disconnection. The PEEP can be reduced to 0, although there is a theoretical advantage to maintaining a low level of PEEP as long as the patient is intubated.

WEANING PARAMETERS

When the patient can maintain satisfactory gas exchange at the ventilator settings just given, the next step is to determine whether the patient is ready for extubation. Accordingly, the patient's ability to ventilate is measured during spontaneous breathing a few minutes after the removal of mechanical support. The findings that generally indicate that weaning and extubation can be carried out successfully are (1) a spontaneous respiratory rate lower than 25/min, (2) a tidal volume greater than 5 ml/kg, (3) a vital capacity greater than 10 ml/kg, (4) a minute ventilation less than 120 ml/kg/min, and (5) an inspiratory pressure that is more negative than –20 cm H_2O. If the patient meets these parameters and if arterial oxygenation is satisfactory at an F_IO_2 of 0.4 or less, then pulmonary mechanics and gas exchange are probably close enough to normal to permit extubation and spontaneous breathing. It should be kept in mind that these measurements are made while the patient is breathing through a long, narrow endotracheal or tracheostomy tube, which causes significant resistance and increases the work of breathing. Therefore, the results will be even better when the patient is extubated and breathing through his or her own airway. If metabolic alkalosis is present, it should be corrected before weaning is attempted. The one variable that cannot be measured with this amount of testing is the endurance of the patient's respiratory efforts. Measurement of endurance is, in essence, the weaning process.

Weaning from Mechanical Ventilation

In the weaning process, the work of breathing that had been the task of the mechanical ventilator is reassumed by the respiratory muscles of the patient. When the results of respiratory testing indicate that the patient 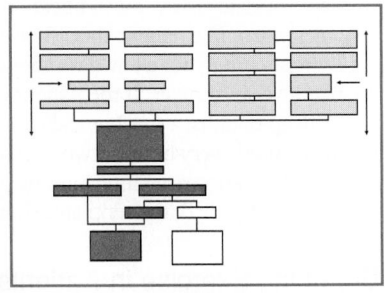 can be weaned from the ventilator, a trial of spontaneous breathing is indicated. During this trial, supplemental humidified oxygen is supplied by way of the endotracheal tube. The balloon is deflated to allow some breathing around the tube and to minimize airway resistance. The patient should be sitting upright. The transition from mechanical support to spontaneous breathing should be swift: the mechanical ventilator should be either turned down rapidly or simply disconnected [see Figure 2]. In addition, the gas supply to the endotracheal tube must be free-flowing; at no point in the trial should the patient have to trigger a demand valve on the ventilator. Most ventilators do not supply a free flow of gas in the continuous positive airway pressure (CPAP) or intermittent mandatory ventilation (IMV) mode but require patient effort to trigger gas flow. The purpose of the spontaneous breathing trial is to determine the endurance of the patient. If it is obvious that the patient can make a strong respiratory effort and is fully alert and awake, he or she can be extubated without further testing after a few minutes of spontaneous breathing.

The simplest way to monitor a spontaneous breathing trial is to watch respiratory rate and pulse rate. If, after 5 to 30 minutes of spontaneous breathing, the respiratory rate is lower than 25/min, the patient will probably be able to sustain an adequate minute ventilation when extubated. If the pulse rate is less than 120/min, the work of breathing is probably not excessive. If the respiratory rate is lower than 20/min and the pulse rate less than 100/min, the patient can be extubated without any further measurements being made. If, however, the pulse rate and respiratory rate are moderately elevated, the P_aCO_2 and P_aO_2 should be measured; if the P_aCO_2 is 40 mm Hg or lower and the P_aO_2 is 60 mm Hg or higher, the patient may be extubated. Postventilation prophylactic maneuvers, to be discussed later [see Postventilation Prophylaxis, below], are indicated. If the results of these four measurements indicate that the trial of spontaneous breathing has failed, mechanical ventilation is resumed to improve the patient's respiratory status before weaning is tried again.

The weaning process should never take more than an hour. If the indicators for weaning are present, the trial of spontaneous breathing is usually successful, and the patient should be extubated. If the indicators are not present, mechanical support should not be gradually decreased—for example, over a period of hours or days—except under strictly controlled conditions.

Difficult Weaning

There are a number of reasons why patients may remain ventilator dependent. If the patient has chronic lung disease that predated the acute event, it may be necessary to wean from the ventilator at a level of P_aCO_2 corresponding to compensated 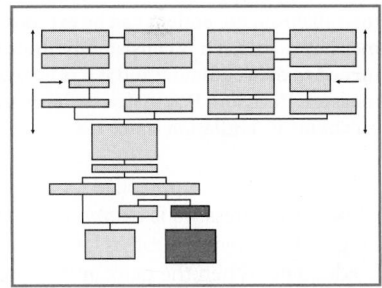 respiratory acidosis. If chronic bronchitis, acute resolving pneumonitis, or injury to the respiratory epithelium is present, bronchoscopy is indicated to examine the airway and clear any inspissated secretions. If the patient has lower-lobe infiltrates (as is commonly the case following a prolonged period of ventilation and supine position), vigorous chest physical therapy and postural drainage are indicated.

VENTILATION

Hypoventilation with gradual CO_2 accumulation is the most common finding in patients who are difficult to wean from mechanical ventilation. Hypermetabolism with increased CO_2 load is a common cause of this problem. Patients who have barely enough respiratory endurance to excrete a normal amount of carbon dioxide cannot maintain the extra ventilation necessary for sustained hyperventilation. Often, muscular weakness is the problem, particularly when compliance is decreased by the acute lung disease that requires extra work with every breath.

In addition to the general measures listed (see above), the first step in a patient in whom attempts at weaning have failed is to do a tracheostomy. This procedure not only minimizes the rebreathing space but also eliminates the urgency and potential risk of extubation, thereby greatly facilitating the weaning process. When the tracheostomy is in place and all the general measures have been carried out, progressive breathing exercises are begun. The type of progressive breathing exercise depends to some extent on the type of mechanical ventilator available. The tidal volume should remain greater than 5 ml/kg while the inspiratory work gradually shifts from the ventilator to the patient. The pressure-support mode on newer ventilators is ideal for this purpose, or a pressure-controlled mode can be

Figure 2 **For most patients, ventilator weaning consists of a brief trial of spontaneous breathing in which pulse and respiratory rates are measured. Mechanical support is decreased until the patient can breathe spontaneously (with or without continuous positive airway pressure [CPAP]), and the respiratory rate is measured every few minutes to determine whether the patient can be extubated. If the respiratory rate is consistently below 20/min and the pulse rate is less than 100/min, the patient can be extubated without the need for further measurements; if it is consistently above 30/min, the patient must be returned to the ventilator; and if it is between 25/min and 30/min, measure P_{CO_2} and P_{O_2} to determine whether another trial of mechanical ventilation is needed.**

used. In pressure-controlled or pressure-support ventilation, the peak airway pressure is decreased (typically, 2 cm H_2O/15 min) as long as the respiratory rate is lower than 25/min and the tidal volume is adequate. When the peak airway pressure is 5 to 10 cm H_2O for several hours, the patient can be extubated or can be managed with only humidified air to the tracheostomy [*see Table 2*].

Some volume ventilators do not allow pressure-controlled weaning and instead decrease the rate of volume-controlled breaths. The patient is expected to sustain normal minute ventilation by spontaneous nonassisted breaths. This so-called intermittent mandatory ventilation weaning technique often leads to rapid, shallow breathing and exhaustion in patients [*see Table 2*]. Periods of totally spontaneous breathing should be alternated with assist-mode volume ventilation if pressure-controlled weaning is not possible.

OXYGENATION

Oxygenation is rarely a problem with the hard-to-wean patient because supplemental inspired oxygen (30% to 40%) can counter the hypoventilation that makes weaning difficult. As mentioned earlier [*see* Worsening Respiratory Status, Oxygenation, *above*], other components of the oxygen delivery system (hemoglobin and cardiac output) should be optimized because the patient may have to be weaned at a lower than normal P_aO_2.

NUTRITION AND METABOLISM

A common cause of weaning failure is hypermetabolism caused by occult infection, which manifests itself as increased oxygen consumption ($\dot{V}O_2$) and CO_2 production ($\dot{V}CO_2$). The underlying cause should be treated before weaning is attempted again. Good nutrition is essential for respiratory muscle strength and endurance [*see VII:9 Nutritional Support*]. If a patient is chronically nutritionally depleted, enteral or parenteral feeding to improve muscular strength may be necessary before the patient can be weaned from the ventilator. On the other hand, if carbohydrates are given in amounts exceeding energy expenditure, lipogenesis occurs, which leads to excess CO_2 production. The appropriate nutritional manipulations to avoid this problem depend on direct measurement of $\dot{V}O_2$ and $\dot{V}CO_2$ and calculation of the respiratory quotient. As mentioned earlier [*see* Improving Respiratory Status, Weaning Parameters, *above*], it is important to correct metabolic alkalosis.

Postventilation Prophylaxis

The recently extubated patient is at risk for respiratory failure and consequently should be watched carefully. Airway secretions, stimulated by the chronic indwelling tube, may be thick and difficult to clear. The airway should be carefully lavaged and suctioned before the tube is removed. Direct endotracheal suctioning should be avoided in the period just after removal of the tube because of the risk of hypoxia, vagal stimulation, and vocal cord edema. Postural drainage combined with appropriate airway humidification is a better way of draining airway secretions. The patient should be encouraged to do deep breathing exercises hourly for a few days after extubation, aided, if desired, by an incentive spirometer. If the patient cannot or will not take spontaneous deep breaths, a mechanical ventilator fitted with a mouthpiece should be used every hour or two to ensure periodic maximal inflation (a procedure known as intermittent positive pressure breathing, or IPPB). During IPPB, the ventilator should be used as described in this

Table 2 Methods of Progressive Breathing Exercise in Patients
Who Are Difficult to Wean from Mechanical Ventilation

Method	Benefit	Risk
Intermittent mandatory ventilation (IMV)	Commonly available Assisted breath V_T not dependent on compliance	Rapid, shallow breaths may be exhausting Unassisted breaths may require demand valve trigger
Pressure-controlled ventilation	Commonly available V_T supported during each breath	V_T varies with compliance
Pressure support (flow-controlled)	Best support of V_T during each breath	V_T varies with compliance Not commonly available
Pressure support with IMV	V_T supported during each breath IMV not dependent on compliance	IMV may slow the weaning process Not commonly available
Spontaneous-breathing trials	Easy to quantitate status and progress Not dependent on demand valve trigger Universally available	Rapid, shallow breaths may be exhausting

chapter, except that periodic maximal inflation (to a PIP of 30 to 40 cm H_2O) is used to ensure maximal alveolar filling. Even if only a few assisted deep breaths are taken every few hours, inflation will be sufficient to prevent atelectasis. Another option is the use of continuous positive airway pressure by mask or nasal catheter.

The vocal cords will be edematous and may be chronically damaged or dislocated. Aerosolized racemic epinephrine helps to mini-mize upper airway edema. If the voice is abnormal or there is any sign of upper airway obstruction, laryngoscopy should be done to determine the condition of the glottis. Aspiration of oral contents is common in the early postextubation period, particularly if an endotracheal tube has been in position for several days. Thick liquids are easier to swallow than clear liquids. The patient should be observed very carefully during the first few feedings.

Discussion

Pulmonary Physiology and Mechanical Ventilation

PULMONARY MECHANICS

The interrelations of gas volumes and pressures that are an integral part of ventilation are collectively referred to as pulmonary mechanics and are more fully described elsewhere [see VII:3 Pulmonary Dysfunction]. The use of a mechanical ventilator is an exercise in pulmonary mechanics, which may be illustrated by comparing the compliance curve for a normal lung with that for an atelectatic or edematous lung [see Figure 3]. The standard compliance, or volume-pressure, curve is obtained by measuring volume and pressure at stages of lung deflation after total inflation. Total lung compliance, normalized for patient size, is approximately 1 ml/cm H_2O/kg. A comparison of volume-pressure curves for normal lungs from three different patients shows the effect of patient size [see Figure 3, left]. In fact, the curves would be the same if normalized for patient size. If the lung volume is decreased by half (as a result of pneumonectomy or main bronchus occlusion, for example), the com-

pliance is decreased by half (to 0.5 ml/cm H_2O/kg). Although the lung is said to be stiffer, it is actually only smaller [see Figure 3, right]. Volume, pressure, and flow are related in time [see Figure 4]. During a normal volume-controlled mechanical breath, the ventilator generates gas flow until the desired volume is reached. The pressure is then simply measured. In this example [see Figure 4], a short 1-second inspiratory hold is applied to show the difference between plateau pressure, which is equilibrated with alveoli, and peak inspiratory pressure, which is slightly higher because of airflow resistance in the tubing.

In acute respiratory failure, the cause of decreased compliance is almost always associated with a decrease in the functional residual capacity (FRC). In the example cited earlier [see Figure 3, right], normal tidal breathing from volume A to volume B would result with 10 cm of inflating pressure. During atelectasis, the decreased FRC (point C) represents the lost alveoli that are either collapsed or filled with fluid but are still perfused with blood. Tidal breathing (to volume D) requires higher pressure. Because the compliance curve is

Figure 3 Depicted are pulmonary mechanics involved in mechanical ventilation. At left are compliance curves for a child weighing 20 kg, an adult weighing 40 kg, and an adult weighing 80 kg, all with normal lungs. The dotted line identifies FRC for the person weighing 80 kg. Functional residual capacity (FRC), total lung capacity, and compliance, which are proportional to patient size, must be normalized to patient weight to permit comparisons with other normal persons and between patients. At right are compliance curves for a patient weighing 80 kg who has normal lungs (upper curve) (compliance, 1 ml/cm H_2O/kg) and the same patient with major atelectasis (lower curve). The mechanics are altered in atelectasis because a smaller lung volume is available for inflation.

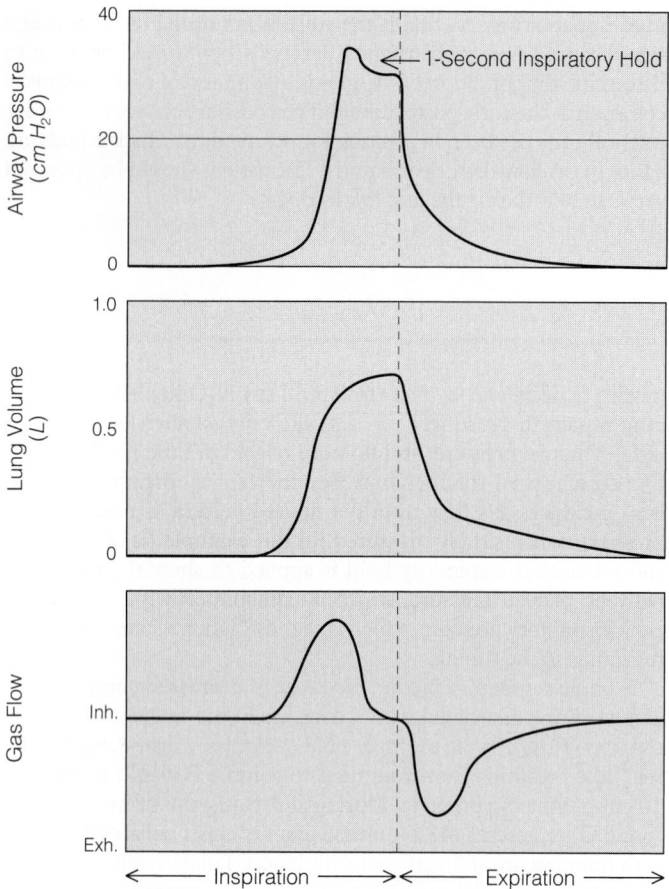

Figure 4 Shown are airway pressure, lung volume, and gas flow during a normal volume-controlled mechanical breath. The ventilator generates gas flow until the desired lung volume is reached, and the airway pressure is simply measured. A 1-second inspiratory hold shows the difference between peak inspiratory and plateau pressures. Dotted line separates inspiration from expiration.

Figure 5 In a patient with normal lungs (black line), the inspiratory volume/pressure curve is very close to the expiratory curve. In a patient with severe parenchymal disease (red line), the inspiratory volume/pressure curve may be nearly flat until enough pressure is exerted to open edematous and collapsed airways and alveoli. As illustrated here, this event (identified as P_{flex}) occurs at 10 cm H_2O. The functional lung is fully inflated at 40 cm H_2O (the curve becomes flat at P_{max}). There is a substantial gap between the deflation curve and the inflation curve.

shifted to the right, much higher pressures are required to achieve the same level of inflation. To inflate the lung to point E, for example, a pressure of 40 cm H_2O would be necessary.

The best way of managing ventilation in these circumstances is to maintain positive end-expiratory pressure at 10 cm H_2O (point C^1 in Figure 3, right) and ventilate to point D with tidal breathing. The PEEP is set at this level to maintain the inflation of alveoli that might close at lower end-expiratory pressures; the volume of pressure used for tidal ventilation is safe and adequate for normal gas exchange.

In normal lungs, the inspiratory limb of the volume/pressure curve is almost the same as the expiratory limb. In severe respiratory failure, variable inspiratory inflation of the lung results in a significant difference between the inflation and deflation limbs, which can be useful in ventilation management [*see Figure 5*]. Collapsed small airways "pop" open at a critical inflating pressure, resulting in an inflation point early in inhalation (P_{flex}). The volume plateaus when all available alveoli are inflated (P_{max}). The P_{flex} and P_{max} are not always well defined, but when they are, it is reasonable to set PEEP above P_{flex} and to set P_{plat} at P_{max}.

Several measurements must be taken to determine whether positive airway pressure is recruiting collapsed alveoli or simply distending normal alveoli [*see Figure 6*]. The signs that collapsed alveoli are being reinflated are (1) improved normalized compliance, (2) decreased dead space ventilation, (3) unaffected cardiac output, and (4) improved oxygenation and decreased shunt at the same ventila-

tor settings. These signs must be kept in mind during management of a patient on a mechanical ventilator.

The effect of the abdominal viscera on pulmonary mechanics is significant. Most data on patients and normal subjects were obtained from individuals in the sitting position, yet most patients on mechanical ventilation are in the supine position. Even in normal subjects, the functional residual capacity is decreased by 25% when measured with the subjects in the supine position. This effect is exaggerated in

Distention	Positive Airway Pressure	Recruitment
↓ Compliance		↑ Compliance
↑ V_D/V_T		↓ V_D/V_T
↓ Cardiac Output		→ Cardiac Output
→ Shunt		↓↓ Shunt
↑ Air Leak		→ Air Leak

Figure 6 The results of serial measurements of compliance, dead space ventilation, cardiac output, oxygenation, shunting, and air-leak risks indicate whether positive airway pressure is recruiting collapsed alveoli or simply distending normal alveoli.

patients with ascites or abdominal distention and is exacerbated by a weak inspiratory effort. The reason is that the weight of the viscera literally pulls down on the diaphragm when patients are in the upright position, creates slight negative (inflating) pressure in the pleural space, and facilitates inspiration. These beneficial effects on lung inflation are even greater in the prone position, if the abdomen is free to expand. When patients are in the supine position, the weight of the viscera pushes against the diaphragm, which decreases alveolar volume and makes inspiration more difficult.[1]

These principles apply to mechanical ventilation as well as spontaneous breathing. Unless unstable hemodynamics make the supine position necessary, patients who are on ventilators (or are being weaned from ventilators) should be placed in a sitting position most of the time. This positioning is particularly important during spontaneous-breathing trials.

Because high airway pressure can cause lung damage, overdistention [see Figure 6] is not merely inefficient but actually detrimental.[2-4] Even in diffuse pulmonary disease, some areas of lung are not inflated and some are nearly normal.[5] The most normal areas of lung have the best compliance and therefore are the areas most vulnerable to overdistention, which may contribute to the steady progression of lung dysfunction in ventilated patients.[6]

The deleterious effects of alveolar overdistention on the lung itself have been demonstrated in many laboratory studies.[2,4] It has been suggested that the resulting lung injury can trigger the multiple organ dysfunction syndrome. Recent prospective randomized clinical studies by Amato and associates[7] and the Acute Respiratory Distress Syndrome Network of the National Institutes of Health[8] confirm the risks of overdistention injury; moreover, these studies report improved survival and decreased organ failure when overdistention is avoided during either pressure-limited[7] or volume-limited[8] modes of mechanical ventilation. The point at which inflation becomes overdistention has not been precisely determined; however, using end-inspiratory P_{plat} as an indicator of alveolar distention, one would be wise to keep P_{plat} below 40 cm H_2O (some would say 30 cm H_2O) during any mode of mechanical ventilation.[9] In patients with decreased FRC and diminished compliance, limiting P_{plat} in this fashion will result in hypoventilation, which in turn will result in hypercapnia. The physiologic risks of respiratory acidosis are minimal in comparison with the risks of alveolar overdistention. Therefore, it is safer to avoid overdistention injury and tolerate respiratory acidosis (so-called permissive hypercapnia[10]).

OXYGEN KINETICS

Oxygen consumption ($\dot{V}O_2$) is normally 3 ml/kg/min (120 ml/m²/min) at rest and is moderately elevated (as high as 6 ml/kg/min) by catecholamines or sepsis. $\dot{V}O_2$, the measure of metabolic rate, is converted to resting energy expenditure expressed in calories through the arithmetic of indirect calorimetry (5 cal for each liter of $\dot{V}O_2$). $\dot{V}O_2$ at rest stays constant from hour to hour, even in critically ill patients. Oxygen delivery ($\dot{D}O_2$) is normally 12 to 15 ml/kg/min (480 to 600 ml/m²/min) at rest. $\dot{D}O_2$ is measured as cardiac output in deciliters per minute times oxygen content (milliliters of oxygen per deciliter). Oxygen content is a function of the saturation and amount of hemoglobin; each gram of fully saturated hemoglobin carries 1.36 ml of oxygen. A very small amount of oxygen is dissolved in plasma, which is measured as P_aO_2.

In patients on a mechanical ventilator, F_IO_2 and pressure are manipulated to optimize oxygen content and delivery without causing injury to the lung. When $\dot{V}O_2$ is increased, as in sepsis or hypermetabolism, $\dot{D}O_2$ increases through an automatic increase in cardiac output until the ratio between $\dot{D}O_2$ and $\dot{V}O_2$ ($\dot{D}O_2/\dot{V}O_2$) is reestablished at 5:1 [see Figure 7]. A compensatory increase in cardiac out-

Figure 7 In mechanical ventilation, F_IO_2 and airway pressure are manipulated to optimize oxygen content and $\dot{D}O_2$ so that the lung is not injured. $\dot{D}O_2$ is normally five times greater than $\dot{V}O_2$. Shown are the relationships between the $\dot{D}O_2/\dot{V}O_2$ ratio, the O_2 extraction (Ext.) ratio, and the $S_{\bar{v}}O_2$ when arterial blood is 100% saturated. Gas volumes are standard temperature (0° C) and pressure (760 mm Hg), dry. N indicates values in a normal person at rest; the red line represents hypermetabolism.

put also occurs during anemia or hypoxia to maintain a normal $\dot{D}O_2/\dot{V}O_2$. When $\dot{D}O_2$ changes, no corresponding change in $\dot{V}O_2$ occurs unless $\dot{D}O_2/\dot{V}O_2$ is severely decreased to less than 2:1. When $\dot{D}O_2$ is less than twice $\dot{V}O_2$, anaerobic metabolism occurs, $\dot{V}O_2$ falls, and hemodynamic instability results. These changes occur at both normal and elevated metabolic rates [see Figure 7].[11,12] Although it has been reported that pathologic supply dependency occurs in patients with the acute respiratory distress syndrome,[13,14] this is an artifact,[15] and normal oxygen kinetics exist, even in hypermetabolic conditions.[16] $\dot{D}O_2$ is optimal when it is four to five times greater than $\dot{V}O_2$. Although this point could be determined by repeated measurements of $\dot{V}O_2$, oxygen content, and cardiac output, a simpler way exists.

When arterial blood is nearly 100% saturated, the mixed venous oxygen saturation ($S_{\bar{v}}O_2$) directly reflects $\dot{D}O_2/\dot{V}O_2$, regardless of the metabolic rate. For example, if $\dot{D}O_2$ is three times $\dot{V}O_2$, the $S_{\bar{v}}O_2$ will be 66% [see Figure 7]. This variable can be measured in samples of pulmonary arterial blood or by continuous use of a fiberoptic catheter.[17,18] When $\dot{D}O_2$ is adequate, $\dot{V}O_2$ at rest stays constant. Thus, any change in $S_{\bar{v}}O_2$ over minutes or hours directly reflects changes in $\dot{D}O_2$. This phenomenon is used to adjust F_IO_2, PEEP, I/E, and mean airway pressure, in addition to inotropic drug dosages, blood volume, and blood transfusion. The ventilator should be set at the lowest settings that maintain $S_{\bar{v}}O_2$ above 70%.

$S_{\bar{v}}O_2$ does not show the cause of a problem, only whether $\dot{D}O_2/\dot{V}O_2$ is abnormal. If $S_{\bar{v}}O_2$ is abnormally high, the delivery may be higher than necessary (e.g., as in the case of arteriovenous shunt), or the $\dot{V}O_2$ may be decreased at the cellular level (e.g., as in the case of endotoxin affecting cellular enzymes). If $S_{\bar{v}}O_2$ is abnormally low, the delivery might be lower than necessary (e.g., low cardiac output), or the $\dot{V}O_2$ might be elevated above the level at which delivery can compensate (e.g., exercise in a patient with a fixed-rate pacemaker). All of these factors must be taken into account when using $S_{\bar{v}}O_2$ to regulate the mechanical ventilator. The principles of the physiology of oxygen kinetics become particularly important in patients with severe respiratory failure when their pressure and F_IO_2 requirements approach the limits of safety. When $\dot{D}O_2/\dot{V}O_2$ is low, it is better to raise oxygen content by transfusion or decrease $\dot{V}O_2$ by sedation than to use 100% oxygen or very high pressure [see Table 1].

VENTILATION-PERFUSION MATCHING

In surgical patients with pulmonary failure, the lung is usually characterized by areas of congestion and atelectasis (low ventilation-perfusion matching [$\dot{V}/\dot{Q}$], or a shuntlike effect) and areas of normal inflation (high $\dot{V}/\dot{Q}$). When blood shunts through lung areas with low $\dot{V}/\dot{Q}$, arterial hypoxemia and hypercapnia result. Hyperventilation of lung areas with high $\dot{V}/\dot{Q}$ will normalize P_aCO_2 but will not improve oxygenation. Improving oxygenation depends on matching blood flow to inflated ventilated alveoli. This matching can be done in three ways: (1) reinflating alveoli by positive airway pressure, (2) reinflating alveoli by decreasing pulmonary interstitial edema, or (3) diverting blood flow to lung areas with high $\dot{V}/\dot{Q}$. The role of peak inspiratory pressure in opening alveoli and of PEEP in holding alveoli open has been discussed [see Pulmonary Mechanics, above]. Decreasing lung extravascular water is accomplished by diuresis, reduction of left atrial pressure, and postural drainage. The edematous lung is heavy, and dependent alveoli are compressed by the weight of the lung, which is why consolidation occurs in dependent areas in acute respiratory distress syndrome.[19] Decreasing edema minimizes compression, which results in improved lung function[20] and improved survival in patients with the acute respiratory distress syndrome.[21]

Turning the patient so that lung areas with high $\dot{V}/\dot{Q}$ are dependent (usually the prone position) usually improves oxygenation immediately by diverting blood flow to the inflated lung areas and decreasing the blood flow in the consolidated lung areas.[22] When patients are in the prone position for several hours, the effects of lung weight are reversed, so that consolidated areas of the lung may become reinflated, resulting in improved oxygenation even when the patient is returned to the supine position.[23] Of these three maneuvers, diuresis and positioning are usually safer and more effective than airway pressure manipulation.

Types and Features of Mechanical Ventilators

At least 20 makes and models of mechanical ventilators are used in North America today. Almost all the ventilators used in operating rooms, recovery rooms, and intensive care units are volume-controlled ventilators. With a device of this type, the operator sets the tidal volume, the respiratory rate, and the inspiratory gas flow, and the ventilator will keep delivering the set volume of gas regardless of the airway pressure (unless a pressure cutoff is set). In a pressure-controlled ventilator, however, the operator selects the respiratory rate, the inspiratory gas flow, and the peak airway pressure, and the ventilator delivers inspired gas until the desired pressure is reached. The tidal volume is measured. Most ICU ventilators can be used in the volume- or pressure-controlled mode or in combinations of the two.

Ventilators come with an extensive array of knobs, gauges, controls, electronic microprocessors, digital displays, and instruction books. Although the features and accoutrements of mechanical ventilators can be intimidating, the functions and controls are actually quite simple. All ventilators have certain basic controls and monitors [see Table 3]. They all are capable of delivering gas of known composition and volume at a given flow rate and of measuring and controlling the pressure at various phases of the respiratory cycle.

Different ventilators accomplish gas delivery in different ways, such as by employing a motor-driven piston, by metering in a quantity of gas supplied to the ventilator under very high pressure, or by keeping a constant reservoir of gas under moderate pressure. Measurement of airway pressure, gas volume, inspiratory effort, F_IO_2, and other parameters is also accomplished in a variety of different ways. A surgeon caring for ventilator patients should know what ventilator is used in his or her hospital and how these variables are controlled in that specific ventilator. Circuit diagrams and descriptions of how

each make and model of ventilator functions are available from the hospital respiratory therapy department, from the manufacturer, and in the literature. Extensive and excellent descriptions of specific mechanical ventilators have been published by Mushin and Rendell-Baker,[24] Kirby and colleagues,[25] and Burton and associates.[26] Surgeons should familiarize themselves with the available documentation and descriptions so that they can better understand the limitations of the equipment they use as well as alert themselves and others to possible malfunctions.

The primary controls for tidal volume, rate, and F_IO_2 are straightforward. The end-expiratory airway pressure control, or PEEP control, provides graduated occlusion of the expiratory system, thereby regulating positive end-expiratory pressure. There is also a primary control for maximum inspiratory pressure, which is set by the operator. If this pressure is reached, an alarm sounds and inflation stops, so that the preset volume is not reached. These simple primary controls allow regulation of all the components of routine mechanical ventilation.

There is also a set of secondary controls for fine-tuning the mechanical ventilator. These controls vary the flow (and therefore the pressure) during the inflation phase of the ventilator. The most important of them is the inspiratory flow rate control. If the tidal volume is delivered at a low flow rate, the time of inspiration will be long, the pressure accumulation will be gradual and minimal, and ventilation will be smoother, but the patient may feel dyspneic. If the flow rate of gas is high, however, the inspiratory time will be short, the peak inspiratory pressure will be reached abruptly, the mean airway pressure will be increased, the high-pressure cutoff will be reached more often, and the blast of ventilating gas may stimulate coughing. Because the respiratory rate is set per minute, a higher inspiratory flow rate will shorten inspiration and result in a lower I/E. A short inspiratory phase with a low I/E favors expiration and CO_2

Table 3 Controls and Monitors on a Volume-Controlled Ventilator

Controls	Monitors and Alarms
Primary controls	
F_IO_2	
Tidal volume (minute volume)	Tidal volume
Respiratory rate	Respiratory rate
Positive end-expiratory pressure (PEEP)	PEEP
Maximum inspiratory pressure	PIP
	Mean airway pressure
	Apnea or disconnect
Secondary controls	
Inspiratory flow rate	
Inspiratory flow wave pattern	Inspiratory time, I/E
Inspiratory hold	
Sigh rate, volume, and maximum pressure	Sigh PIP
Trigger sensitivity for assist and IMV models	

Modes of Ventilation

Controlled mechanical ventilation (CMV)
Assist control (AC)
Intermittent mandatory ventilation (IMV)
Synchronized IMV
Continuous positive airway pressure (CPAP)
Pressure-controlled ventilation (PCV)
Pressure-controlled inverse-ratio ventilation (PC-IRV)
Pressure support (PS)

excretion, whereas a long inspiration with a high I/E favors inflation and oxygenation. When a patient with normal lungs is undergoing mechanical ventilation, the inspiratory flow rate should be adjusted so that the patient is comfortable and I/E is close to normal (1:3). This is best done by examining the patient while adjusting the inspiratory flow rate. Often, high mean airway pressures can be decreased significantly simply by decreasing the inspiratory flow rate. When a patient with poor oxygenation is undergoing mechanical ventilation, the time spent during inflation should be increased. I/E can be increased until CO_2 excretion is inadequate. This unusual pattern of breathing is uncomfortable and often requires sedation.

Most ventilators provide an inspiratory flow wave pattern control, which varies the pattern of gas flow from sine wave to square wave to various combinations of waves. The normal inspiratory flow pattern is essentially a sine wave, which is usually the best pattern for mechanical ventilation. Most modern ventilators also provide a control for timed inspiratory hold, or plateau pressure. This setting occludes the expiratory circuit for 1 or 2 seconds. There are two reasons for using the inspiratory hold control: (1) to allow pressures throughout the system to equilibrate so that effective compliance (exhaled volume divided by plateau pressure as measured on the ventilator gauge) can be measured and (2) to simulate a forced sustained inspiration to reinflate collapsed alveoli (a procedure to be distinguished from an automatic sigh [see Modes of Ventilation, below]). As a rule, ventilators deliver gas only during the inflation phase of the respiratory cycle,

but some provide continuous gas flow, which is a significant advantage in the CPAP and IMV modes of ventilation.

Humidification is an essential part of mechanical ventilation. The inspired gas is usually humidified by passing it over water warmed to 37° C. A chamber for nebulizing drugs may be included in the inspiratory circuit; it is powered by a gas line separate from the ventilator.

Modes of Ventilation

Ventilators always have at least two and sometimes as many as six modes of ventilation. Each mode of ventilation is characterized by what starts the gas flow (time- or effort-triggered) and what stops the gas flow (volume-controlled, pressure-time–controlled, or flow-controlled; or volume-limited, pressure-time–limited, or flow-limited) [see Figure 8]. In the controlled mechanical ventilation mode, the ventilator is time-triggered and either volume-limited or pressure-limited, and it functions exactly as determined by the primary controls, regardless of what the patient does. This mode is appropriate for a patient who is under anesthesia, paralyzed, heavily sedated, or suffering from brain stem injury.

In the assist-control mode, the ventilator is effort-triggered and either volume-controlled or pressure-controlled and delivers the V_T and F_IO_2 determined by the primary controls whenever the patient initiates a spontaneous breath. A control or backup rate is specified so that the ventilator will automatically deliver the tidal volume if the pa-

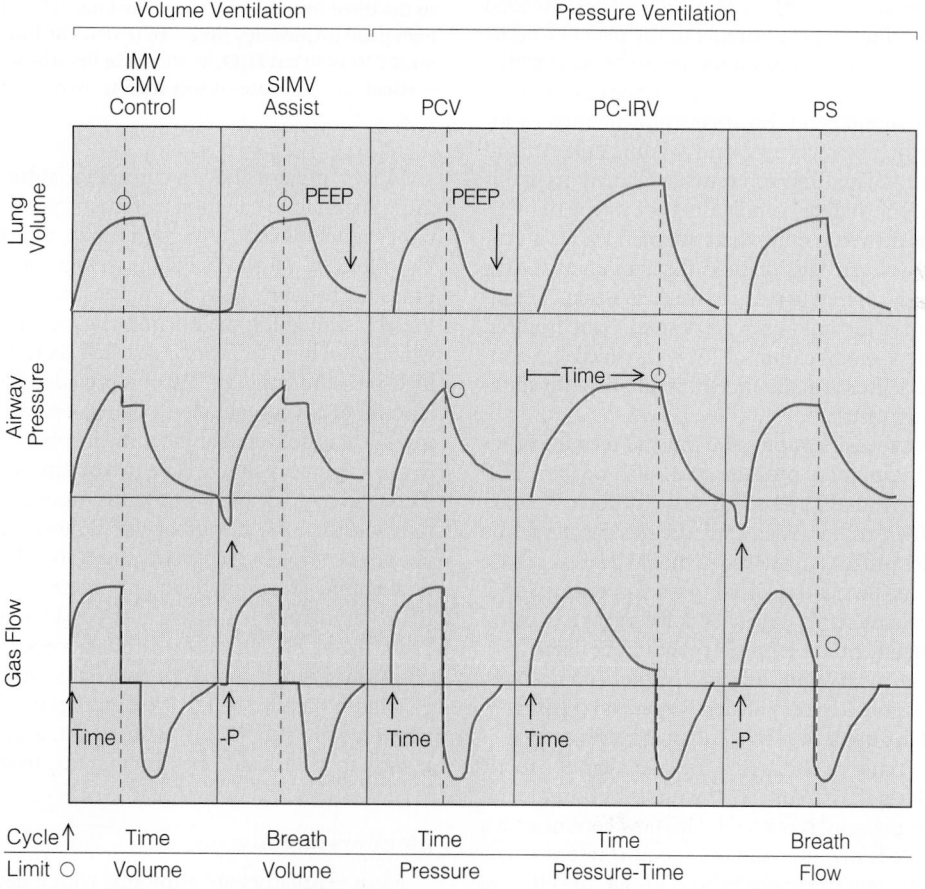

Figure 8 Shown are lung volume, airway pressure, gas flow, and the inspiration-expiration ratio (I/E) during commonly used modes of mechanical ventilation. The event that starts the gas flow is the cycle (↑), and the event that stops the gas flow is the limiting factor (○). The cessation of gas flow is shown by the dotted lines. Time and negative pressure (-P) may be responsible for cycling or limiting gas flow, as indicated. PEEP is shown in two modes of ventilation as examples of the effect of that maneuver.

tient does not initiate a spontaneous breath within an appropriate period. The control rate is usually set at approximately half the spontaneous rate. The ventilator is triggered to deliver an assisted breath when the pressure in the airway is decreased by the patient's inspiratory effort. When the assist-control mode is used, the sensitivity of this trigger mechanism should be adjusted. If the setting is too sensitive, a ventilator inflation may be triggered simply by the pressure drop during expiration. If the adjustment is not sensitive enough, the patient may be unable to generate enough pressure to trigger the ventilator.

Because of the relatively poor pressure transmission through the gas in the system, the negative deflection on the ventilator pressure gauge is not nearly as great as the negative pressure actually generated in the pleural space by inspiratory effort. Whenever possible, therefore, the patient's inspiratory pressure should be measured at the airway. The sensitivity control should be adjusted so that the mechanical breath is delivered with the minimum of effort by the patient. It must be readjusted whenever the PEEP level is changed. The assist mode greatly simplifies the monitoring and management of mechanical ventilation. It is the preferred mode in any patient with a normally functioning brain stem and respiratory center.

In the intermittent mandatory ventilation mode, time-triggered controlled mechanical ventilation occurs at the rate and volume determined by the primary controls (time-triggered and either volume-limited or pressure-limited), and additional inspired gas is made available if the patient generates a spontaneous inspiration. (The latter feature distinguishes IMV from CMV, in which no gas flows if the patient makes an inspiratory effort.) The volume of gas provided during the spontaneous effort is proportional to the patient's effort and is usually small. IMV was originally designed to be used with a continuous high-volume gas flow and PEEP (requiring minimal effort by the patient for spontaneous breaths) supplemented by intermittent mechanical breaths at a rate and volume sufficient to maintain CO_2 clearance.[27] The Emerson ventilator functions in this fashion, but most other mechanical ventilators have a type of pseudo-IMV, in which gas is delivered only when a demand valve is activated by the inspiratory effort. This method requires considerable work by the patient[28] and can lead to progressive exhaustion of respiratory muscles rather than the mild exercise desired. Synchronized IMV (SIMV) is simply a modification of IMV in which the controlled ventilation V_T is delivered at the time of spontaneous inspiratory effort (i.e., effort-triggered).

In the continuous positive airway pressure mode, breathing is entirely spontaneous, with expiratory pressure controlled by the PEEP control [see Figure 9]. This mode corresponds to the period of spontaneous breathing with IMV as described earlier and is subject to the same variables and criticisms. The CPAP mode should be used in conjunction with a continuous-flow and reservoir system. Because in most ventilators the CPAP mode requires the patient to trigger a demand valve during inspiration rather than supplying continuous flow of gas, this mode may at times be more exhausting than helpful. A variation of CPAP is so-called pressure-release ventilation, in which CPAP is applied and then released to a controlled PEEP level at intervals.

Pressure support is a time- or effort-triggered, flow-limited mode of ventilation.[29] Rapid gas flow is initiated by effort or a timer and continues until a preset pressure is reached. Gas flow continues at a slower rate, and pressure is maintained until the flow rate is only a fraction of the initial flow rate (typically 25%). This has the effect of an inspiratory hold but continues to supply gas during the inspiratory hold, which results in a relatively large tidal volume at moderate pressure. If the patient generates inspiratory effort during the pressure-support breath, an even higher tidal volume will result, making pressure support a valuable method of weaning. The same principle applies to the pressure-limited mode, without the inspiratory hold.

Figure 9 Shown is the effect of positive end-expiratory pressure (PEEP) during five breaths. PEEP is added after the second breath, so the third breath, with the same lung volume, results in unacceptably high peak inspiratory pressure (PIP). The lung volume is decreased until PIP is 40 cm H_2O, as shown in breaths four and five. The dotted vertical line separates inspiration from expiration.

Most ventilators have a control for automatic sighs. (It would be more accurate to call these automatic yawns because sighs are expiratory maneuvers.) In the sigh mode, the ventilator delivers a large V_T (typically 15 to 25 ml/kg) at regular intervals (usually several times each hour). This setting ensures regular maximal inflation, thereby simulating the normal physiologic pattern of breathing, in which total lung capacity is reached six times each hour. A separate high-pressure limit and alarm is provided for the sighs. Although the amount of gas contained in a sigh is considerably larger than the normal V_T, it is delivered at the same inspiratory flow rate; consequently, the inspiratory time will be two or three times longer than normal. This system is a more effective means of achieving maximal alveolar inflation than the inspiratory hold described earlier [see Types and Features of Mechanical Ventilators, *above*], in which a normal-sized tidal volume is simply held at pressure for a second or two. When PEEP is maintained above 5 cm H_2O and P_{plat} is close to 30 cm H_2O, the sigh mechanism is not necessary and may even lead to dangerously high airway pressures; however, when PEEP is 5 cm H_2O or lower and the tidal volume is controlled in the normal range, periodic sighs should be used to maintain alveolar inflation. Overdistention may be avoided by limiting P_{plat} to 40 cm H_2O or lower.

Monitors and Alarms

Most ventilators are equipped with a device to measure exhaled volume, usually by integrating a measurement of flow with time. The exhaled volume can be displayed either breath by breath or as minute ventilation. It should correspond to the preset inspired volume; if it does not, an air leak exists, and the volume of the leak can be calculated by simple subtraction. It should be remembered that a considerable part of the exhaled volume is gas that was compressed in the tubing and in the patient's lungs and that therefore did not enter into the alveolar ventilation. This compression volume in the ventilator and tubing can be measured by capping the airway and measuring the volume exhaled over a range of pressures. In some ventilators, the tubing compression volume is automatically subtracted in the final volume display. This compressed gas will appear as V_D when V_D/V_T is calculated from arterial and mixed expired CO_2. The appearance of compression volume as $\dot{V}_D$ makes it seem as if a patient with poor compliance has a large anatomic or physiologic dead space, but it is nothing more than a measurement artifact.

The apnea or disconnect alarm on most ventilators is triggered by an abnormally low expired volume measurement. Pressure limits and alarms can be set for PIP in all ventilators, PEEP in some, and mean airway pressure in others. The PIP and the PEEP can be displayed either on a gauge or on a digital readout in all ventilators. Some ventilators can display the mean airway pressure as well—a desirable feature because the mean airway pressure affects venous return. The F_IO_2 is displayed on most ventilators, but this display usually reflects the setting made by the operator rather than the actual F_IO_2 value. There can be considerable variation between the desired and the actual F_IO_2, so some device must be used to measure F_IO_2 if the ventilator cannot measure it.

In the process of adjusting the respiratory rate, tidal volume, and inspiratory flow rate, it is possible to arrive at unreasonable settings. Most ventilators have an alarm system to notify the operator. Usually, this alarm system will be triggered if I/E exceeds 2:1.

Some of the newer ventilators can calculate and display effective compliance, flow-volume loops, or volume-pressure curves. In the near future, mechanical ventilators will include apparatus to measure oxygen consumption, CO_2 production, respiratory quotient, and work of breathing. These measurements, combined with measurements of arterial and venous oxyhemoglobin saturation, will allow ventilators to display oxygen delivery-consumption ratios, cardiac output, and other hemodynamic variables, as well as energy expenditure expressed in calories. The same generation of ventilators will be able to regulate minute ventilation on the basis of CO_2 load and to regulate airway pressure and F_IO_2 on the basis of oxygenation. These devices will appear to be even more complex than today's ventilators, but they will have the same basic functions and features.

In addition to monitors built into the ventilator, some other patient monitors are used to manage mechanical ventilation. The use of the pulmonary arterial catheter and mixed venous oximetry has already been discussed [see Worsening Respiratory Status, Oxygenation, above]. An arterial catheter is helpful because of the frequency of arterial blood gas measurement. Pulse oximeters measure arterial saturation in capillary blood by ignoring the nonpulsatile venous phase. These instruments have become invaluable for both safety and management monitoring. Transcutaneous, corneal, and tissue gas sensors have not gained general acceptance, because they drift and require frequent recalibration. End-tidal CO_2 monitoring at the airway generally corresponds to P_aCO_2. End-tidal CO_2 is the same as P_aCO_2 when lung function is normal, and it is less than P_aCO_2 when real or apparent dead space (compression volume) is elevated. End-tidal CO_2 is particularly helpful during weaning.

Learning to Use a Mechanical Ventilator

Every surgeon who is responsible for ventilator patients should understand the mechanical ventilators at his or her hospital and should be able to set all the controls and make any necessary adjustments, even if such tasks are traditionally done by nurses or respiratory therapists. The best way for a surgeon to learn to use a mechan-

ical ventilator is first to regulate the primary control settings by using a rubber-bag test lung, then to regulate the secondary controls and select the modes of ventilation while acting as the patient (easily accomplished by attaching a mouthpiece to the ventilator tubing and applying a noseclip). Whenever a new ventilator is introduced into the ICU, each surgeon who will use the ventilator should go through a detailed self-instruction routine [see Table 4]. It is well worth the cost of an extra set of sterile ventilator tubing.

Writing Ventilator Orders

Mechanical ventilators are generally operated by nurses and respiratory therapists under a set of orders from the responsible physician [see Table 5]. These orders may range from very specific directions to broad guidelines, depending on the experience and ability of the ICU personnel; however, the orders should always include a statement of the goals of mechanical ventilation and specify the system to be used to determine how well those goals have been achieved. For example, in an ICU in which ventilators are routinely used, it may be sufficient merely to say: "Measure arterial saturation and P_aCO_2 every 4 hours. Maintain P_aCO_2 between 35 and 45 mm Hg with rate and tidal volume, and maintain arterial saturation of more than 95% by using F_IO_2 less than 0.6 and PEEP less than 6." Conversely, if mechanical ventilators are not used routinely, or if a nurse or respiratory therapist on a given shift is not comfortable with such responsibility, it is advisable to specify the exact mode, the primary control and secondary control settings, and the monitoring alarm systems that are to be used.

Related Topics

FIGHTING THE VENTILATOR

Fighting the ventilator means that the patient is dyspneic and trying to breathe out while the ventilator is inflating. Usually, this situation can be handled by placing the ventilator in the assist mode

---

Table 4 Self-Instruction Routine for Ventilator Training

1. Set: F_IO_2, V_T, rate, PEEP, PIP.
2. Set mode: CMV.
3. Set ranges for alarms: V_T, rate, PIP, PEEP.
4. Attach test lung (rubber bag), and ventilate.
5. Measure: V_T, rate, minute volume, PIP, PEEP, effective compliance.
6. Limit the bag to simulate poor compliance. Readjust ventilator, and repeat measurements.
7. Set primary controls to ventilate yourself. Rate = 16/min.
8. With a mouthpiece and a noseclip, ventilate yourself. Relax until you are on controlled ventilation. Then, adjust V_T (5–20 ml/kg) and PEEP (0–10 cm H_2O) to get the feel, and observe the measurements. Try the sigh mode.
9. At baseline settings, resist inspiration, cough, and try to hyperventilate. How does it feel? Do the monitors and alarms work?
10. At baseline settings, turn to the AC mode. Rate = 0/min. Adjust the sensitivity from low to high.
11. In the AC mode, adjust the inspiratory flow rate and pattern. Which I/E feels comfortable?
12. Reset mode to IMV, then CPAP. How much work does it take to initiate a breath?
13. Repeat steps 10–12, but using an endotracheal tube instead of a mouthpiece in your mouth. What are the effects of the added resistance?

Table 5 Sample Orders for Ventilator Patients

1. Objectives (range of acceptable values)
   A. Arterial blood oxygenation
   Hemoglobin saturation _____ to _____
   or
   P_aO_2 _____ to _____
   B. Arterial carbon dioxide (P_aCO_2) _____ to _____
2. Standard respiratory care for all ventilator patients
   A. Alternating lateral and sitting positions, never supine.
   B. 100% airway humidity at 35°–37° C.
   C. Airway irrigation and suctioning every 8 hours, more frequently as required.
   D. Percussion and chest physical therapy every 8 hours, more frequently as required.
   E. Deflation of cuffed tubes every 8 hours (before suctioning) and reinflation with the minimum volume necessary to achieve the required peak inspiratory pressure.
   F. Continuous monitoring of V_T and airway pressure.
   G. Mouth care every other hour (for patients with endotracheal tubes).
   H. Tracheal stoma care every other hour for patients with tracheostomy tubes.
3. Ventilator settings: Mode _____
   F_IO_2 _____
   V_T or PIP _____ Rate _____ PEEP _____
   Alarm limits: V_T _____ Rate _____ P_{plat} _____
   Other: _____
4. Monitoring frequency
   Arterial blood gases _____
   Venous blood gases _____
   Compliance _____
   Weaning parameters _____
   Chest x-ray _____

---

and increasing the inspiratory flow and tidal volume until respiratory alkalosis occurs and breathing slows, and then backing off to more comfortable settings. Mild sedation of the patient may be necessary, particularly if he or she is disoriented or extremely anxious. Almost never is it necessary or indicated to paralyze a patient to achieve mechanical ventilation. (There are, however, some specific indications for paralysis, such as tetanus, seizures, delirium tremens, and major ventilatory failure [see Worsening Respiratory Status, above].)

VENTILATION OF INFANTS AND CHILDREN

Although this discussion has been concerned solely with mechanical ventilation for adults, the principles underlying pulmonary mechanics, gas exchange, monitoring and alarms, and modes of ventilation all apply to pediatric patients as well. In children older than 2 years, volume-controlled ventilators can be used according to the guidelines given here for adults. Pressure-limited continuous-flow ventilators are generally preferred in infants. Techniques for neonatal ventilation are well described in standard texts [see VI:8 The Pediatric Surgical Patient].[30,31]

INTERMITTENT POSITIVE PRESSURE BREATHING

Intermittent positive pressure breathing is nothing more than mechanical ventilation through a mouthpiece rather than through direct tracheal access. All of the relevant variables can be monitored and controlled when a mouthpiece rather than an endotracheal tube is used, and any of the modes can be selected. Intermittent positive pressure breathing is a useful technique in patients who have border-

line pulmonary function or minimal reserve.[32] When it is employed, the ventilator is placed at the bedside and set in the assist mode with a backup rate of zero, and all the primary and secondary controls are adjusted to the appropriate settings. The patient is taught to use the ventilator and is allowed to pick up the mouthpiece for mechanical assistance at will. He or she is encouraged to use the ventilator at least every hour while awake, to prevent or treat atelectasis.[33] This variety of mechanical ventilation differs considerably from intermittent positive pressure breathing provided by a nurse or respiratory therapist every 6 or 8 hours, which is useful for delivering nebulized drugs and for encouraging the patient to think about deep breathing but is usually ineffective unless the mechanical support is provided more frequently.

BRONCHOSCOPY

Bronchoscopy with flexible fiberoptic instruments is an essential adjunct to the management of mechanical ventilation. Introducing the instrument through a sphincter adapter allows bronchoscopy to be performed during ventilation but increases the resistance to gas flow through the airway. Therefore, ventilator adjustments are necessary to maintain adequate gas exchange. The inspiratory flow rate and peak inspiratory pressure must be increased significantly to maintain inspired tidal volume. This clinical setting is the one exception to the PIP limit of 40 cm H_2O; an inspiratory pressure of 50 to 80 cm H_2O may be required. This pressure level, required to overcome airway resistance, is not injurious to the lung. Distal pressure is low, and overdistention will not occur. Expiration is also limited by the increased resistance. More time will be required for exhalation, and PEEP should be decreased. Without these changes, exhalation of each breath will be incomplete, resulting in auto-PEEP [see Auto-PEEP, below] and CO_2 retention. Obviously, ventilator settings must be adjusted carefully to facilitate bronchoscopy.

Conversely, bronchoscopy is used to facilitate mechanical ventilation. Airway placement and positioning, evaluation of tracheal injury and bronchial patency, identification of sources of bleeding and mucus production, tissue level diagnoses, and selective lobar study and treatment all require bronchoscopy. A surgeon who is managing mechanical ventilation should be proficient in performing this procedure.[34]

AUTO-PEEP

When exhalation is incomplete, the functional residual capacity is increased, airway pressure increases, and alveoli are more inflated than they would be if exhalation continued to the point of equilibration with atmospheric pressure. This phenomenon can be exploited by using PEEP to limit exhalation and maintain alveolar inflation. If bronchial or prosthetic airway resistance is increased or if the time for exhalation is short, incomplete exhalation can occur regardless of externally regulated PEEP. If this process continues during many breaths, alveolar volume increases in association with increased alveolar pressure; this process has been referred to as auto-PEEP.[35] This phenomenon also occurs in asthma, with the same physiologic consequences of CO_2 retention and capillary obstruction. Auto-PEEP occurs during mechanical ventilation as a result of the ventilator settings, sometimes combined with bronchospasm. It can be measured by placement of a catheter-transducer system into the trachea or esophagus. Auto-PEEP should be suspected if CO_2 clearance is impaired and is paradoxically worsened by increasing respiratory rate (i.e., shortening exhalation time). If auto-PEEP is suspected, the respiratory rate or tidal volume, or both, should be decreased. If CO_2 clearance is enhanced by this maneuver, ventilator settings are readjusted to permit full exhalation or to control exhalation solely by the external PEEP valve.

Special Techniques for Patients with Severe Respiratory Failure

When the principles outlined above are used, most surgical patients can be managed without difficulty. However, a small percentage of patients with pneumonitis, aspiration, contusion, or the acute respiratory distress syndrome will develop such a large shunt, air leak, or alveolar damage that conventional mechanical ventilation is inadequate. The mortality associated with severe respiratory failure, defined as a shunt persistently over 30% despite and after all appropriate therapy, is 60% to 90%.[36-39] The following innovative approaches have been recommended for these patients.

NONVENTILATORY TREATMENT

Oxygenation can often be improved by placing the patient in the full lateral or prone position.[40] This positioning diverts blood flow to the anterior lung, which is usually the most inflated part of the lung, and promotes reinflation of the posterior lung. Oxygen delivery should be optimized by use of transfusion to achieve a normal hematocrit[41] and administration of inotropes (with the caveat that catecholamines increase $\dot{V}O_2$ and $\dot{V}CO_2$).[42] When the hematocrit and cardiac output are normal, an arterial saturation of 80% to 90% is well tolerated.

PERMISSIVE HYPERCAPNIA

Even in patients with severe lung disease, a normal P_aCO_2 can be maintained at 40 mm Hg by hyperventilation. Indeed, in patients with atelectasis and consolidation, a small portion of the lung is hyperventilated to maintain normocapnia while hypoxia is treated with attempted reinflation. However, because this intervention causes overdistention and induced tissue alkalosis in the most normal and compliant area of the lung, it can damage the lung in a very short time.[43] The risk of hypercapnia is minimal, particularly when it is compared with the risk of hyperventilation-induced lung damage. Therefore, ventilation should be limited to safe levels (plateau pressure below 40 cm) to avoid lung injury. This limitation may result in a P_aCO_2 as high as 80 mm Hg, but the resulting acidosis can be buffered with bicarbonate or TRIS buffer and no deleterious effects result. This approach has been used for many years in the management of asthma[44] and neonatal respiratory failure[45] but has rarely been used in acute adult respiratory failure. Recommendations to strictly limit peak airway pressure[46,47] were generally ignored in favor of normocapnia. In the early 1990s, this approach, named permissive hypercapnia, was advocated in patients with adult respiratory failure.[10] Critical care practitioners recognized the dangers of hyperventilation and began regulating mechanical ventilator peak pressure. Although transient hypercapnia may result, that is a small price to pay for ultimate lung recovery.

PRESSURE-LIMITATION (LOW-STRETCH) VENTILATION

The rationale for limiting overdistention (high pressure, high volume, or high stretch) was defined by Gattinoni and colleagues[5] and demonstrated by Hickling and coworkers.[6,10] Several recent prospective, randomized studies have shown a significant survival advantage to so-called low-stretch modes of ventilation.[7,8] Other studies have shown no advantage,[48] but the differences can be explained by the number of patients in the various treatment groups who were actually ventilated with damaging pressure. Ranieri and colleagues demonstrated that high-stretch ventilation was associated with increased plasma levels of inflammatory cytokines.[49] Amato and coworkers[7] advocate that the high-stretch limit be combined with PEEP adjustment based on P_{flex} (the so-called open-lung approach), a combination providing survival advantage.

HIGH-FREQUENCY OR OSCILLATION VENTILATION

High-frequency ventilation (HFV) is an intriguing technique in which oxygenation is achieved by continuous positive airway pressure with supplemental oxygen, and ventilation is achieved by shaking the airway—that is, by supplying a very small tidal volume (≤ 100 ml) at a very rapid rate (200 to 2,000/min) by means of a jet of gas, a piston, or a loudspeaker. This unusual airway pressure manipulation enhances CO_2 diffusion and induces excretion of a normal metabolic load of CO_2 without conventional tidal ventilation. Reports on HFV in adults indicate that the mean airway pressure is lower than with CMV and that barotrauma and air leaks are less frequent, but the duration of ventilation and the outcome in ventilated patients are about the same.[50,51] There are, however, anecdotal cases of spectacular recovery with HFV despite the apparent failure of conventional mechanical ventilation, suggesting that the development of this technique should be watched carefully.

PRESSURE-CONTROLLED INVERSE-RATIO VENTILATION

If one objective of mechanical ventilation is to inflate collapsed alveoli, inspiration can be prolonged until I/E (normally 1:3 or 1:4) reaches or, in certain cases, exceeds 1:1 (inverse). As long as there is adequate time during expiration for CO_2 clearance and as long as the effects of elevated mean airway pressure are taken into account, pressure-controlled inverse-ratio ventilation is an effective mode of mechanical ventilation. Because it requires total control of the breathing patterns, the patient must be heavily sedated. Pressure-controlled ventilation and pressure-controlled inverse-ratio ventilation are standard techniques in neonatal ventilation.

TRACHEAL INSUFFLATION

During mechanical ventilation, the major bronchi, trachea, and endotracheal airway make up the anatomic dead space. At the end of exhalation, this dead space is filled with alveolar gas that contains carbon dioxide. Under normal conditions, this CO_2 is rapidly diluted with fresh air, which creates a suitable gradient for CO_2 excretion. However, when V_D/V_T is more than 50%, reequilibration at a higher level of blood CO_2 may ultimately occur. This effect is not necessarily deleterious [see Permissive Hypercapnia, above]. However, preferably, a normal P_aCO_2 should be maintained as long as hyperventilation is avoided. CO_2 clearance can be facilitated by the insufflation of ventilating gas near the level of the carina through a small catheter. This maneuver, known as tracheal insufflation, removes CO_2 from the major airway. This removal lowers V_D/V_T and allows CO_2 clearance without overdistention and hyperventilation. When the gas flow is mechanically directed out of the airway, a Bernoulli effect results, which facilitates CO_2 clearance from the distal airways and alveoli.[52] This technique has been studied in detail by Kolobow, who refers to it as intratracheal pulmonary ventilation. This technique can be used in conjunction with conventional mechanical ventilation or as the sole source of ventilating gas. Of course, intratracheal pulmonary ventilation holds the greatest promise for patients whose conducting airways constitute a large fraction of the tidal volume, specifically newborn infants. This technique is now entering clinical trials.[53]

EXTRACORPOREAL LIFE SUPPORT

Extracorporeal membrane oxygenation (ECMO) is the use of a modified heart-lung machine for days or weeks to support gas exchange while resting the diseased lung.[54] This technique has the advantage of avoiding the oxygen toxicity and barotrauma that may accompany mechanical ventilation in severe respiratory failure. It has become standard treatment in the management of severe respiratory failure in newborn infants [*see VI:8 The Pediatric Surgical Patient*].[55] In patients with adult respiratory failure considered moribund, 50% survival with extracorporeal life support (ECLS) has been reported from several centers.[56,57] In adult patients, venovenous blood access is generally used for patients with adequate cardiovascular function; venoarterial access is used when cardiac failure coexists.

ECLS might be considered when the risk of mortality with continuing conventional ventilation is more than 90% and the primary process is reversible. Thus, the specific indications in most ECMO centers are a transpulmonary shunt over 30% and compliance less than 0.5 ml/cm H_2O/kg after and despite optimal therapy. The contraindications to ECLS are advanced age, malignancy or brain damage, and mechanical ventilation longer than 5 to 7 days. ECLS can play a significant role in the management of severe respiratory failure in adults.[58] However, ECLS is complex and requires a well-trained team.

Summary

Management of mechanical ventilation is an exercise in applied pulmonary mechanics, just as the management of respiratory failure is an exercise in the full spectrum of applied pulmonary physiology. CO_2 clearance and oxygenation should be considered and managed as distinctly separate processes, although they are obviously interrelated. CO_2 clearance is the result of breathing and is thus the goal in mechanical ventilation. Although it is almost always possible to maintain normal P_aCO_2 by hyperventilation, a peak airway pressure greater than 40 cm H_2O injures the lung and should be avoided. Maintaining and improving oxygenation is a process of matching pulmonary blood flow to inflated alveoli, which should be done by positioning, diuresis, and optimization of hemoglobin concentration and cardiac output. Although oxygenation can be facilitated by increased F_IO_2 and PEEP, these methods of treatment, like hyperventilation, do more harm than good when applied in excess. The goal of mechanical ventilation is to provide adequate gas exchange without damaging the lung.

References

1. Agostoni E, Mead J: Statics of the respiratory system. Handbook of Physiology, Vol 1. American Physiological Society, Washington, DC, 1964, Sect 3, p 387

2. Kolobow T, Moretti MP, Fumagalli R, et al: Severe impairment in lung function induced by high peak airway pressure during mechanical ventilation. Am Rev Respir Dis 135:312, 1987

3. Bowton DL, Kong DL: High tidal volume ventilation produces increased lung water in oleic acid–injured rabbit lungs. Crit Care Med 17:908, 1989

4. Dreyfuss D, Soler P, Basset G, et al: High inflation pressure pulmonary edema: respective effects of high airway pressure, high tidal volume, and positive endexpiratory pressure. Am Rev Respir Dis 137:1159, 1988

5. Gattinoni L, Pesenti A, Torresin A, et al: Adult respiratory distress syndrome profiles by computed tomography. J Thorac Imaging 1:25, 1986

6. Hickling KG: Ventilatory management of ARDS: can it affect the outcome? Intensive Care Med 16:219, 1990

7. Amato MB, Barbas CS, Medeiros DM, et al: Effect of a protective-ventilation strategy on mortality in the acute respiratory distress syndrome. N Engl J Med 338:347, 1998

8. Ventilation with lower tidal volumes as compared with traditional tidal volumes for acute lung injury and the acute respiratory distress syndrome. The Acute Respiratory Distress Syndrome Network. N Engl J Med 342:1301, 2000

9. Lee PC, Helsmoortel CM, Cohn SM, et al: Are low tidal volumes safe? Chest 97:430, 1990

10. Hickling KG, Henderson SJ, Jackson R: Low mortality associated with low volume pressure limited ventilation with permissive hypercapnia in severe adult respiratory distress syndrome. Intensive Care Med 16: 372, 1990

11. Cilley RE, Polley TZ Jr, Zwischenberger JB, et al: Independent measurement of oxygen consumption and oxygen delivery. J Surg Res 47:242, 1989

12. Hirschl RB, Heiss KF, Cilley RE, et al: Oxygen kinetics in experimental sepsis. Surgery 112:37, 1992

13. Danek SJ, Lynch JP, Weg JG, et al: The dependence of oxygen uptake on oxygen delivery in the adult respiratory distress syndrome. Am Rev Respir Dis 122:387, 1980

14. Gutierrez G, Pohil RJ: Oxygen consumption is linearly related to O_2 supply in critically ill patients. J Crit Care 1:45, 1986

15. Bartlett RH, Dechert RE: Oxygen kinetics: pitfalls in clinical research (editorial). J Crit Care 5:77, 1990

16. Vermeij CG, Feenstra BW, Bruining HA: Oxygen delivery and oxygen uptake in postoperative and septic patients. Chest 98:415, 1990

17. Zwischenberger JB, Cilley RE, Kirsh MM, et al: Does continuous monitoring of mixed venous oxygen saturation accurately reflect oxygen delivery and oxygen consumption following coronary artery bypass grafting? Surg Forum 37:66, 1986

18. Rashkin MC, Bosken C, Baughman RP: Oxygen delivery in critically ill patients: relationship to blood lactate and survival. Chest 87:580, 1985

19. Gattinoni L, Mascheroni D, Turresin A, et al: Morphological response to positive end expiratory pressure in acute respiratory failure: computerized tomography study. Intensive Care Med 12:137, 1986

20. Ali J, Duke K: Colloid osmotic pressure in pulmonary edema clearance with furosemide. Chest 92:540, 1987

21. Simmons RS, Berdine GG, Seidenfeld JJ, et al: Fluid balance and the adult respiratory distress syndrome. Am Rev Respir Dis 135:924, 1987

22. Langer M, Mascheroni D, Marcolin R, et al: The prone position in ARDS patients. Chest 94:103, 1988

23. Gattinoni L, Presenti A: Computed tomography scanning in acute respiratory failure. Adult Respiratory Distress Syndrome. Zapol WM, Lemaire F, Eds. Marcel Dekker, New York, 1991, p 199

24. Mushin WW, Rendell-Baker L, Thompson DW, et al: Automatic Ventilation of the Lungs. Blackwell Scientific Publishers, Oxford, 1980

25. Kirby RR, Smith RA, Desautels DA: Mechanical Ventilation. Churchill Livingstone, New York, 1985

26. Burton GG, Hodgkin JE, Ward JJ: Respiratory Care, 3rd ed. JB Lippincott Co, Philadelphia, 1991

27. Downs JB, Mitchell LA: Intermittent mandatory ventilation following cardiopulmonary bypass (abstr). Crit Care Med 2:39, 1974

28. Marini JJ, Rodriguez RM, Lamb V: The inspiratory workload of patient-initiated mechanical ventilation. Am Rev Respir Dis 134:902, 1986

29. MacIntyre N, Nishimura M, Usada Y, et al: The Nagoya conference on system design and patient-ventilator interactions during pressure support ventilation. Chest 97:1463, 1990

30. Gille JP: Neonatal and Adult Respiratory Failure. Elsevier, Paris, 1989

31. Levin DL, Moriss FC: Essentials of Pediatric Intensive Care. Quality Medical Publishing, St. Louis, 1990

32. Anderson HL III, Bartlett RH: Respiratory Care of the Surgical Patient. Respiratory Care, 3rd ed. JB Lippincott Co, Philadelphia, 1991, p 821

33. Bartlett RH: Respiratory therapy to prevent postoperative pulmonary complications. Respiratory Intensive Care. Pierson DJ, Ed. Daedalus Enterprises, Dallas, 1986, p 369

34. Bartlett RH: Bronchoscopy in surgical patients. Surgical Endoscopy. Dent TL, Strodel WE, Turcotte JG, Eds. Year Book Medical Publishers, Inc, Chicago, 1985

35. Blanch L, Fernandez R, Artigas A: The effect of autopositive end-expiratory pressure on the arterial endtidal carbon dioxide gradient and expired carbon dioxide slope in critically ill patients during total ventilatory support. J Crit Care 6:202, 1991

36. Zapol WM, Snider MT, Hill JD, et al: Extracorporeal membrane oxygenation in severe acute respiratory failure: a randomized prospective study. JAMA 242: 2193, 1979

37. Bartlett RH, Morris AH, Fairley HB, et al: A prospective study of acute hypoxic respiratory failure. Chest 89:684, 1986

38. Gillespie DJ, Marsh HMM, Divertie MB, et al: Clinical outcome of respiratory failure in patients requiring prolonged (> 24 hours) mechanical ventilation. Chest 90:364, 1986

39. Zapol WM, Frikker MJ, Pontoppidan H, et al: The adult respiratory distress syndrome at Massachusetts General Hospital. Adult Respiratory Distress Syndrome. Zapol WM, Lemaire F, Eds. Marcel Dekker, New York, 1991

40. Maunder RJ, Shuman UP, McHugh JW, et al: Preservation of normal lung regions in the adult respiratory distress syndrome: analysis by computed tomography. JAMA 255:2463, 1986

41. Bryan-Brown CW, Gutierrez G: O_2 transport and tissue oxygenation in the critically ill. Clinical Aspects of O_2 Transport and Tissue Oxygenation. Rinhart K, Eyrich K, Eds. Springer-Verlag, Berlin, 1989

42. Ruttimann Y, Chiolero R, Jequier E, et al: Effects of dopamine on total oxygen consumption and oxygen delivery in healthy men. Am J Physiol 257:E541, 1989

43. Gattinoni L, Mascheroni D, Basilico E, et al: Volume/pressure curve of total respiratory system in paralyzed

patients: artefacts and correction factors. Intensive Care Med 13:19, 1987

44. Williams TJ, Tuxen DV, Scheinkestel CD, et al: Risk factors for morbidity in mechanically ventilated patients with acute severe asthma. Am Rev Respir Dis 146:607, 1992

45. Wung JT, James LS, Kilchevsky E, et al: Management of infants with severe respiratory failure and persistence of the fetal circulation, without hyperventilation. Pediatrics 76:488, 1985

46. Eriksen J, Andersen J, Rasmussen JP, et al: Effects of ventilation with large tidal volumes or positive end-expiratory pressure on cardiorespiratory function in anesthetized obese patients. Acta Anaesthesiol Scand 22:241, 1978

47. Bendixen HH, Hedley-White J, Laver MB: Impaired oxygenation in surgical patients during general anesthesia with controlled ventilation. N Engl J Med 269:991, 1963

48. Stewart TE, Meade MO, Cook DJ, et al: Evaluation of a ventilation strategy to prevent barotrauma in patients at high risk for acute respiratory distress syndrome. N Engl J Med 338:355, 1998

49. Ranieri VM, Suter PM, Tortorella C, et al: Effect of mechanical ventilation on inflammatory mediators in patients with acute respiratory distress syndrome: a randomized controlled trial. JAMA 282:54, 1999

50. Hurst JM, Branson RD, Davis K Jr, et al: Comparison of conventional mechanical ventilation and high-frequency ventilation: a prospective, randomized trial in patients with respiratory failure. Ann Surg 211:486, 1990

51. Carlon GC, Guy Y, Groeger JS, et al: Early prediction of outcome of respiratory failure: comparison of high-frequency jet ventilation and volume-cycled ventilation. Chest 86:194, 1984

52. Lehnert BE, Oberdorster G, Slutsky AS: Constant-flow ventilation of apneic dogs. J Appl Physiol 53:483, 1982

53. Wilson JM, Thompson JR, Schnitzer JJ, et al: Intratracheal pulmonary ventilation: human case report. Presented at 3rd Annual Extracorporeal Life Support Organization Meeting, Ann Arbor, Michigan, September 1991

54. Gattinoni L, Pesenti A, Mascheroni D, et al: Low-frequency positive-pressure ventilation with extracorporeal CO_2 removal in severe acute respiratory failure. JAMA 256:881, 1986

55. Stolar CJ, Snedecor SM, Bartlett RH: Extracorporeal membrane oxygenation and neonatal respiratory failure: experience from the extracorporeal life support organization. J Pediatr Surg 26:563, 1991

56. Kolla S, Awad SA, Rich PB, et al: Extracorporeal life support for 100 adult patients with severe respiratory failure. Ann Surg 226:544, 1997

57. Lewandowski K, Lewandowski M, Pappert D, et al: Outcome and follow-up of adults following extracorporeal life support. ECMO: Extracorporeal Cardiopulmonary Support in Critical Care. Zwischenberger JB, Bartlett RH, Eds. ELSO, Ann Arbor, Michigan, 1995

58. Bartlett RH: Management of ECLS in adult respiratory failure. ECMO: Extracorporeal Cardiopulmonary Support in Critical Care. Zwischenberger JB, Bartlett RH, Eds. ELSO, Ann Arbor, Michigan, 1995

Acknowledgments

Figure 1 Albert Miller.

Figures 2, 4, and 7 through 9 Talar Agasyan.

Figures 3 and 5 Marcia Kammerer.

Figure 6 Dana Burns-Pizer.

5 RENAL FAILURE

Renae E. Stafford, M.D., Bruce A. Cairns, M.D., and Anthony A. Meyer, M.D., Ph.D.

Approach to the Patient with Renal Failure

Normal renal function provides a mechanism for eliminating toxic metabolites and maintaining homeostasis of fluid and electrolytes. Loss of normal function results in alterations in volume and electrolyte homeostasis and inadequate excretion of metabolic wastes. Acute renal failure (ARF) has been defined as a sudden and sustained decline in glomerular filtration rate (GFR) that is usually associated with azotemia and a fall in urine output.[1] This presents clinically as oliguria or anuria and results in a rise in serum creatinine and blood urea nitrogen (BUN). Fortunately, most patients in whom acute renal dysfunction develops do not progress to acute renal failure. However, ARF remains a complex problem associated with a high mortality in surgical patients. Most of the renal failure encountered in contemporary surgical care is not single-organ failure; rather, it occurs in the context of the simultaneous dysfunction or failure of several organ systems.

The annual incidence of ARF is approximately 50 to 100 cases per million population. Among hospitalized patients, ARF is particularly prevalent in the intensive care unit.[2] Risk factors for the development of ARF include hypotension and shock; sepsis and the systemic inflammatory response syndrome; trauma[3]; nephrotoxic agents such as ionic contrast agents,[4,5] aminoglycosides, vancomycin, and cyclosporine; atheroembolic events[6]; abdominal compartment syndrome[7]; and preexisting renal insufficiency. Those factors tend to have an additive effect, particularly in patients whose renal function is already compromised. The mortality of ARF is greater than 50%.[8] Hence, prevention and early recognition of acute renal dysfunction are of paramount importance.

Recognition of Acute Renal Dysfunction

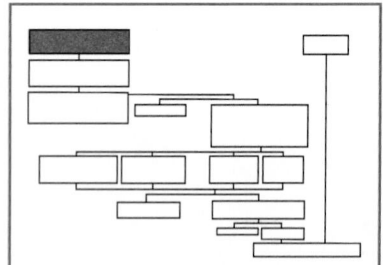

Acute renal dysfunction is approached clinically from the presenting problems of oliguria or rising serum creatinine levels. Evaluation of renal dysfunction generally takes into account prerenal, renal parenchymal, and postrenal mechanisms of dysfunction [see Table 1]. In some patients, more than one cause of renal dysfunction may be present, and it is important to consider all possible mechanisms. The goals in management of ARF are prevention and early diagnosis to limit renal damage and to maintain adequate residual function.

The clinical manifestations of renal dysfunction vary. Patients with acutely deteriorating renal function become symptomatic earlier than those with acute-on-chronic renal failure.[9] In the early stages, patients may be asymptomatic. As the renal dysfunction progresses, they may become oliguric or anuric and develop edema or cardiopulmonary compromise as a result of volume overload. Patients with uremia (creatinine clearance < 10 ml/min) may present with nausea, pruritus, malaise, weakness, and mental status changes.[10-12] Laboratory manifestations include a rising creatinine level and a fall in the serum bicarbonate level. BUN levels usually rise, but they may be normal. Although laboratory values are useful adjuncts for recognizing acute renal dysfunction, they cannot be used to predict outcome in ARF [see Discussion, Perspective on Acute Renal Failure, *below*].

ACUTE OLIGURIA

Acute renal dysfunction may be signaled by the acute onset of oliguria. This is defined as a urine output of less than 0.5 ml/kg/hr or 400 ml/24 hr in an adult and less than 1.0 ml/kg/hr in a child weighing less than 10 kg.[13-16] Patients may progress to or even present with anuria, defined as a urine output of less than 100 ml/24 hr. Acutely decreased urine output most often is the result of a fall in renal perfusion from diminished circulating blood volume [see Initial Clinical Assessment, *below*]. A Foley catheter should be placed in acutely oliguric patients to follow urine output closely and to evaluate the effects of treatment. Efforts should be made to determine the cause of the oliguria and to reestablish adequate urine output. Oliguria has many causes, and most patients who present with oliguria do not have ARF.

INCREASED SERUM CREATININE

Creatinine, a product of amino acid metabolism, is cleared by the kidneys. This is done principally by glomerular filtration, although a limited amount of creatinine is secreted into the tubular fluid.[17] A serum creatinine level of 1.2 mg/dl or less is considered normal. The rate of creatinine production is relatively constant and depends primarily on muscle mass. Among patients with renal dysfunction, therefore, smaller rises in creatinine may be seen in small women than in large, muscular men. In addition, GFR decreases with age, as do creatinine production and muscle mass.[18] Therefore, a normal creatinine level in an elderly patient does not represent the same GFR as the same creatinine level would in a younger patient. A rising serum creatinine level implies decreased renal clearance; an increase of 1 mg/dl over normal or baseline levels indicates a 50% decrease in the GFR. The serum creatinine level can rise acutely even with normal urine output, such as with aminoglycoside-induced acute tubular necrosis (ATN)[19] and thus is another marker of acute renal dysfunction. Not all elevated creatinine levels represent renal insufficiency, however. The presence of ketones[20] or some cephalosporins[21] may produce a factitiously elevated creatinine level by interfering with its assay. Other drugs, such as trimethoprim-sulfamethoxazole[22] and

Table 1 Classification of Acute Renal Failure

Prerenal (50%–90% of Total Cases)

Volume depletion

  Dehydration (i.e., from cutaneous or gastrointestinal losses or renal losses in adrenal insufficiency)

  Hemorrhage (i.e., from trauma, surgery, childbirth, or GI lesions)

  Fluid redistribution (e.g., from trauma, crush injury, burns, pancreatitis, peritonitis, sepsis, or hypoalbuminemia)

Cardiac failure

  Myocardial or valvular dysfunction, arrhythmia, or tamponade

Systemic vasodilatation

  Sepsis, anaphylaxis, neurogenic shock, anesthesia, or antihypertensive medications

Renovascular obstructive disease

  Arterial (e.g., arteriosclerosis, embolism, dissection, fibromuscular dysplasia, vasculitis, or disease related to aortic or any retroperitoneal operation)

  Venous (e.g., renal vein thrombosis)

Renal Parenchymal (10%–30% of Total Cases)

Acute tubular necrosis

  Ischemia

  Nephrotoxins

    Endogenous: pigments (myoglobin and hemoglobin), crystals (uric acid, calcium phosphate, and oxalate), or tumors (tumor lysis syndrome and myeloma)

    Exogenous: antibiotics (aminoglycosides, cephalosporins, sulfonamides, and amphotericin B), anesthetics (methoxyflurane and enflurane), chemotherapeutic and immunosuppressive agents (e.g., cisplatin and cyclosporine), contrast media, organic solvents (heavy metals, poisons, or other chemicals), and dextran

Glomerulonephritis

  Postinfectious (e.g., associated with streptococcal, pneumococcal, viral, and shunt infections and abdominal abscesses)

  Membranoproliferative

  Rapidly progressive (e.g., associated with lupus erythematosus, Goodpasture syndrome, polyarteritis nodosa, Wegener granulomatosis, Schönlein-Henoch purpura)

  Serum sickness

  Thrombotic microangiopathy (e.g., hemolytic-uremic syndrome or thrombotic-thrombocytopenic purpura) and other microvascular diseases (e.g., scleroderma, malignant hypertension, radiation, and disseminated intravascular coagulation)

Vasculitides

  Polyarteritis nodosa, hypersensitivity angiitides, scleroderma, hemolytic-uremic syndrome, coagulopathy, radiation, diffuse intravascular coagulation, eclampsia, malignant hypertension, or thrombotic-thrombocytopenic purpura

Interstitial nephritis

  Drugs (e.g., penicillin, cephalosporins, sulfonamides, rifampin, nonsteroidal anti-inflammatory drugs, thiazides, cimetidine, and interferon)

  Infection

    Direct invasion (e.g., by *Staphylococcus,* viruses, or fungi)

    Indirect effects (e.g., of streptococcal or pneumococcal infection, typhoid, or diphtheria)

  Infiltration (lymphoma, leukemia, or sarcoidosis)

  Idiopathic

Papillary necrosis (e.g., associated with analgesics, infection, obstruction, or diabetes)

Acute cortical necrosis (e.g., profound shock, often associated with complicated pregnancy or septic abortion)

Atheroembolic syndrome (renal failure with lower extremity ischemia)

SIADH

Intrarenal shunting

  Systemic infection, SIRS, hepatorenal syndrome

Postrenal (1%–15% of Total Cases)

Obstructive uropathy

  Renal pelvis and ureters (i.e., from calculus, tumor, clot, papillae, infection, trauma, or retroperitoneal fibrosis)

Bladder and urethra (i.e., from calculus, bladder or prostatic tumor, clot, trauma, benign prostatic hypertrophy, neuropathic bladder, obstructed bladder catheter, or phimosis)

Extravasation (i.e., from trauma)

---

cimetidine,[23] inhibit the tubular secretion of creatinine and may cause an elevated serum creatinine level in a patient with normal renal function.

As with oliguria, most patients who present with a rising serum creatinine level do not have acute renal failure. However, an increase of more than 1 mg/dl above normal or baseline levels should be investigated and appropriate preventive and therapeutic measures taken. An increase of more than 2 mg/dl/day, even in the presence of anuria, suggests a rapid rate of protein breakdown, such as might occur in the presence of ischemic muscle or a resolving hematoma.[24] Furthermore, a BUN-to-creatinine ratio higher than 40:1 suggests that volume depletion is the cause of the rising creatinine.[25]

INCREASED BLOOD UREA NITROGEN

The BUN measurement depends on many variables, which include GFR and rates of urea production and tubular reabsorption. In addition, extrarenal factors such as blood in the GI tract, a high-protein diet, the administration of glucocorticoid hormones, protein catabolism, and sepsis can increase BUN.[25] Therefore, a high BUN cannot be equated with a low GFR.

Initial Clinical Assessment

The first step in evaluating acute renal dysfunction, as manifested by acute oliguria or a rising serum creatinine, is physical examination. Laboratory tests and imaging procedures should not be used as surrogates. A clinical examination is necessary to assess the patient's perfusion status and to rule out urinary tract obstruction as a cause of renal dysfunction. Signs

Patient presents with signs of acute renal dysfunction

- *Oliguria:* urine output < 0.5 ml/kg/hr or < 1.0 ml/kg/hr in child < 10 kg.
- *Rising creatinine level:* ≥ 1.0 mg/dl increase.
- *Worsening of preexisting renal insufficiency.*
- *Note:* these manifestations may have nonrenal causes, which should be excluded.

Clinical assessment

Perform physical examination to look for signs of hypovolemia, CHF, poor perfusion, and urinary tract obstruction.
- Estimate intravascular volume and peripheral perfusion, and consider possible causes of impaired renal perfusion (cardiac disease, renovascular disease, renal artery injury, abdominal compartment syndrome). If renal artery is injured, consider renal perfusion scan.
- Identify and treat any urinary tract obstruction.

Initial treatment measures

Administer I.V. fluid challenge (~10% of circulating volume, more in hypovolemic patients), preferably isotonic crystalloid bolus. Give blood if patient has acute blood loss or is anemic. Do not administer fluid challenge to patients who have CHF or other primary cardiorespiratory conditions until more extensive evaluation of cause of renal dysfunction has been done. Maintain urine volume. Consider diuresis with mannitol or loop diuretic only in selected cases.

Renal dysfunction resolves

Continue monitoring. Avoid hypovolemia and use of nephrotoxic agents.

Prerenal dysfunction (U$_{Na}$ < 20 mEq/L or FE$_{Na}$ < 1)

Expand intravascular volume if necessary. Improve renal blood flow; if intravascular volume is adequate, consider dopamine, 2–5 μg/kg/min. Monitor CVP, PAWP, or RVEDVI. Decompress abdomen if abdominal compartment pressure remains elevated. If acute renal arterial problems are present, emergency operation and revascularization may be necessary.

Renal parenchymal dysfunction (no obstruction; U$_{Na}$ > 40 mEq/L or FE$_{Na}$ > 3)

Stop nephrotoxic drugs if possible. Avoid using contrast agents if possible. Maintain renal perfusion. Assess tubular function. Consider loop diuretics or mannitol. Evaluate for SIADH and hepatorenal syndrome.

Renal function returns to normal

Continue monitoring. Avoid hypovolemia and use of nephrotoxic agents.

Approach to the Patient with Renal Failure

Patient has chronic renal failure

Evaluate renal function.
Assess patient for symptoms
[*see Table 4*].

Renal dysfunction does not resolve

Initiate more extensive evaluation of renal function. Attempt to identify potentially reversible prerenal, renal parenchymal, and postrenal causes.
Evaluate
• Intravascular volume (CVP, PAWP).
• Perfusion (cardiac output, mixed venous O_2 saturation).
• Tubular function (urine and plasma electrolytes, urinalysis). Calculate FE_{Na}.
• Collecting system (US, IVP).
Review medications. Stop nephrotoxic drugs if possible, and adjust all dosages as necessary.
Consider miscellaneous causes (e.g., abdominal compartment syndrome and damage to renal artery).

Mixed prerenal and renal parenchymal dysfunction (U_{Na} > 20 mEq/L but < 40 mEq/L and FE_{Na} > 1 but < 3)

Expand intravascular volume. Stop nephrotoxic drugs if possible. Monitor CVP, PAWP, RVEDVI, and urine electrolyte concentrations.

Postrenal dysfunction (obstruction of urinary system)

Drain obstructed area.
• *Bladder:* use Foley catheter or suprapubic tube.
• *Ureter:* use nephrostomy tube or stent.

Renal dysfunction continues or progresses

Monitor and adjust medications and fluids. Maintain general supportive care. Provide renal replacement therapy via CVVHD/CAVHD, intermittent hemodialysis, peritoneal dialysis, or hemofiltration.

Renal deterioration stops or slows

Chronic renal failure ensues

Continue renal replacement therapy.

Measure and correct fluid, electrolyte, and metabolic abnormalities as needed. Monitor patient for other chronic complications of renal failure, including hypertension, anemia, and platelet dysfunction. Monitor and adjust medications.

of hypovolemia, congestive heart failure, poor peripheral perfusion, and urinary tract obstruction should be sought.

Decreased renal perfusion is the most common cause of acute renal dysfunction in surgical patients[25-28] and is usually the result of decreased intravascular volume, as signaled by flat neck veins, tachycardia, diminished jugular pulse, and other signs of hypovolemia [see I:4 Shock]. Perfusion can be estimated clinically on the basis of skin color, temperature, and capillary refill. It is important to remember, however, that although patients who have systemic infections, exhibit the systemic inflammatory response syndrome (SIRS), have been burned, or have recently undergone a major surgical procedure or sustained a serious injury may have liters of excess body fluid, their intravascular volume may still be depleted. These patients may have associated systemic vasodilatation that contributes to the poor perfusion. In such patients, tissue edema and weight change may be of limited help in estimating intravascular volume.

Another cause of acute renal dysfunction is diminished peripheral perfusion secondary to poor myocardial function. This should be considered if the patient has a history of cardiac disease or evidence of acute myocardial ischemia.

Obstructive renovascular disease and acute renal artery injury also lead to diminished renal perfusion. The patient with obstructive renovascular disease and acute renal dysfunction may be oliguric and tachycardic but will be hypertensive. Patients who have sustained trauma or have undergone retroperitoneal or invasive vascular procedures may have a renal artery injury. If such injury is thought to be present, a renal perfusion scan should be considered.

Impaired renal perfusion and subsequent ARF have been documented in patients with abdominal compartment syndrome.[7,29] If the abdomen is extremely rigid, abdominal pressure can be measured through a Foley catheter. If the pressure is higher than 30 to 40 cm H_2O and there is a decrease in urine output that cannot be attributed to other causes, decompression should be considered, although this is not without risk.

A similar mechanism accounts for the decreased urine output that is sometimes seen after laparoscopic surgery. Insufflation of the abdominal cavity with gas during laparoscopy causes an increase in intra-abdominal pressure, which can decrease renal function and urine output. The decrease is transient and resolves after release of the pneumoperitoneum.[30]

Urinary tract obstruction causes up to 10% of ARF. Bladder outlet obstruction from prostatic enlargement or a plugged Foley catheter may be missed without a physical examination. Placement of a Foley catheter, or irrigation of the catheter if one is already present, will help eliminate outlet obstruction as a cause of acute renal dysfunction. Obstruction of the upper collecting system is generally unilateral and rarely accounts for acute renal dysfunction. However, patients who experience acute renal dysfunction after surgical procedures in which the ureters could potentially be injured or ligated should be evaluated for ureteral obstruction or injury. Acute dysfunction that is caused solely by obstruction of the upper or lower collecting system should resolve when the obstruction is corrected.[31]

Assessment of the patient with acute renal dysfunction is not a one-time event. Reevaluating the patient after tests and monitoring the patient's response to treatment with measures such as daily weights, total fluid input and output, and hourly urine output are essential to minimize renal injury and prevent progression to frank renal failure.

Initial Treatment Measures

I.V. FLUID CHALLENGE

Because acute oliguria or increased serum creatinine levels in surgical patients are usually the result of decreased renal perfusion, treatment should begin with administration of an intravenous fluid bolus to expand intravascular volume. The bolus should be approximately 10% of the estimated circulating volume if it is to produce a significant increase in perfusion. Under the assumption that blood makes up 7% of body weight, a bolus for an 80 kg patient should be calculated as follows:

$$80 \text{ kg} \times 0.07 \text{ L/kg} = 5.6 \text{ L}$$
$$5.6 \text{ L} \times 0.10 = 560 \text{ ml}$$

An even larger bolus may be appropriate if severe hypovolemia is present. If the patient has suffered acute blood loss or is significantly anemic, blood will be required to expand vascular volume effectively. Otherwise, isotonic salt-containing crystalloid solutions, such as normal saline or lactated Ringer solution, are the most effective volume expanders. Colloid solutions may be used in some patients, such as those with significant burns or liver disease, but they have not been proved to be more effective than crystalloid solutions. In fact, they may be detrimental.[32] Use of hypertonic saline may produce dramatic physiologic effects, but these solutions are not routinely given for management of acute renal dysfunction. The intravenous fluid bolus should improve hypovolemia and should at least partially correct acute renal dysfunction.

Volume infusion should also benefit patients in whom decreased renal perfusion is caused by myocardial dysfunction. Increasing preload will usually improve left ventricular performance. Although in rare cases an intravenous fluid bolus may be harmful to such patients, the renal injury may be worsened if fluid therapy is withheld to prevent the unlikely possibility of congestive heart failure. Patients who are normovolemic will not suffer cardiorespiratory complications as the result of such a fluid challenge, because 65% to 75% of infused fluid leaves the vascular compartment within 30 minutes.

Patients with congestive heart failure or other primary cardiorespiratory conditions, on the other hand, should not receive a fluid bolus until a more extensive evaluation of the cause of their renal dysfunction has been performed [see Evaluation to Determine Cause of Renal Failure, below].

MAINTENANCE OF URINE OUTPUT

Maintenance of urine output during a period of renal injury may have a significant influence on survival. Oliguric renal failure has been shown to have a mortality twice as high as that for nonoliguric failure and has higher morbidity.[33] Prompt fluid therapy may be all that is necessary to handle the problem. Diuretics or osmotic agents have not been shown to prevent or reverse ARF[34] or to decrease mortality from renal failure. However, if prerenal and postrenal causes of oliguria have been corrected, a trial of mannitol[35] or a loop diuretic[33,36] may convert oliguric to nonoliguric renal failure.[19,33] Diuretics may be appropriate in patients with high intravascular volume or who have been taking diuretics for long periods of time and are dependent on them. Critically ill patients who are refractory to intermittent dosing of loop diuretics or have severe fluid overload may have improved diuresis with continuous infusion.[37] This type of dosing is more commonly used in patients with heart failure and in kidney transplant recipients. Mannitol may be used in patients who can tolerate the osmotic load and may be particularly helpful for renal dysfunction caused by rhabdomyolysis.[3] In general, loop and osmotic diuretics should be avoided because their administration will abrogate the use of urine volume and electrolyte levels as useful tests of renal function for approximately 24 hours. In addition, diuretic agents may cause further renal injury in patients who are intravascularly depleted.[38]

Evaluation to Determine Cause of Renal Failure

Patients who fail to respond to a fluid challenge or to correction of urinary obstruction, those who require repeat fluid boluses, and those with complicating and severe acute and chronic medical problems require more extensive evaluation to determine the cause or causes of their renal failure before appropriate treatment can be initiated. Potentially reversible prerenal, renal parenchymal, and postrenal causes must be considered. Prerenal causes involve decreased perfusion of the kidney; renal parenchymal causes include ischemia and toxic injury; and postrenal causes involve obstruction of the ureters, bladder, or urethra. Acute renal dysfunction from renal parenchymal causes is usually diagnosed by excluding prerenal and postrenal causes, rather than by specific diagnosis.

In the critically ill patient, maintenance of urine output is an inadequate indicator of renal perfusion.[39] Instead, specific measurements can be made that will help determine the cause of renal dysfunction [see Table 2]. Hemodynamic monitoring will allow assessment of intravascular volume as well as cardiac function. Intravascular volume can be estimated clinically on the basis of the jugular pulse and physiologically on the basis of the central venous pressure (CVP) or the pulmonary arterial wedge pressure (PAWP). Physiologic measures of perfusion are usually derived from measurement of cardiac output by

means of a thermodilution pulmonary arterial catheter or measurement of mixed venous oxygen saturation by means of a Swan-Ganz catheter, though other methods of measuring cardiac performance and perfusion can also be used [see VII:1 Cardiopulmonary Monitoring]. These measurements are useful in diagnosing prerenal causes of renal failure (e.g., hypovolemia and decreased perfusion), but they do not reflect renal function itself.

Water and solute dynamics are good measures of renal function. Prerenal causes of renal failure can be distinguished from renal parenchymal or postrenal causes through measurement of the urine sodium level (U_{Na}) on a spot urine sample: a urine sodium level lower than 20 mEq/L indicates a prerenal cause, whereas a level higher than 40 mEq/L indicates a renal parenchymal or postrenal cause. The levels of sodium and creatinine in the urine or plasma (P) can be used to calculate the fractional excretion of sodium (FE_{Na}),[40-42] which represents the fraction of the sodium filtered by the glomeruli that is excreted in the urine. FE_{Na} is expressed as a percentage:

$$FE_{Na} = [(U_{Na} / P_{Na})/(U_{Cr} / P_{Cr})] \times 100$$

An FE_{Na} lower than 1 indicates that the cause of dysfunction is prerenal, whereas an FE_{Na} higher than 3 suggests a renal parenchymal or postrenal cause. Urine sodium measurements of 20 to 40 mEq/L and an FE_{Na} between 1 and 3 have been shown to be nonspecific.[43]

It is essential to review all present and recent medications and treatments, looking for nephrotoxic agents that may be responsible for the acute renal dysfunction or failure. Nonsteroidal anti-inflammatory drugs, cyclosporine and tacrolimus, and the combination of angiotensin-converting enzyme (ACE) inhibitors with diuretics may all precipitate prerenal azotemia.[44] The administration of any such agents that are not absolutely necessary should be limited or stopped. Even if these agents are not the cause of the renal dysfunction, they can exacerbate it substantially. Patients who are to receive nephrotoxic agents, such as intravenous contrast dye, aminoglycosides, or antineoplastic agents, should be adequately hydrated beforehand in an attempt to prevent renal dysfunction or worsening of preexisting renal dysfunction.[5,45] A new dopaminergic agonist, fenoldopam, may prove useful in the prevention of renal toxicity associated with intravenous contrast agents.[46,47] The antioxidant acetylcysteine has been shown to prevent radio-

Table 2 Findings in Acute Renal Dysfunction

Assessment	Findings			
	Prerenal	Renal Parenchymal	Mixed Prerenal and Renal Parenchymal	Postrenal
Intravascular volume (measure central venous pressure or pulmonary arterial occlusion pressure)	Decreased	Normal	Decreased	Normal
Perfusion (measure cardiac output or mixed venous O_2 saturation)	Decreased	Normal	Decreased	Normal
Urine sodium	< 20 mEq/L	> 40 mEq/L	> 20 but < 40 mEq/L	Usually > 40 mEq/L
Fractional excretion of sodium (FE_{Na})	< 1	> 3	> 1 but < 3	Usually > 3
Collecting system (perform sonography or intravenous pyelography)	Normal	Normal	Normal	Dilated
Tubular function (measure urine and plasma electrolytes; perform urinalysis)	Specific gravity > 1.020, pH < 6	Red cell and white cell casts, tubular cells	Red cell and white cell casts, tubular cells	Specific gravity < 1.015, pH > 6

graphic contrast–induced decreases in renal function in patients with chronic renal insufficiency.[48] In addition, dosages of all medications should be adjusted as necessary.

Diagnosis of urinary outlet obstruction in patients with renal dysfunction can usually be made by means of ultrasonography or intravenous pyelography. Ultrasonography can be performed on critically ill patients in the ICU without jeopardizing them by transport to x-ray facilities and can identify urinary tract obstruction in the kidneys or in the bladder. A dilated collecting system indicates a postrenal cause of renal dysfunction. In the acute setting, this may be relieved by percutaneous nephrostomy or retrograde cystoscopy.

Urinalysis can identify urine of high specific gravity and low pH; both findings indicate a prerenal cause. Microscopic urine examination may reveal tubular casts indicative of renal parenchymal dysfunction; hemoglobinuria as a result of transfusion reaction, parenchymal injury, rhabdomyolysis, or vasculitic disease; eosinophilia associated with interstitial nephritis; or myoglobinuria from muscle ischemia or crush injury.[3,49] Relatively benign urinary sediments are often seen in hepatorenal syndrome.

These assessments and measurements can help distinguish the causes of acute renal dysfunction and failure but are of somewhat limited use in elderly patients and in those with pre-existing renal disease. They are of little or no use in patients who have received diuretics or osmotic agents in the previous 24 hours. In some patients, results may be difficult to interpret and clinical and laboratory evidence will have to be used to determine the most likely cause. If the specific cause remains uncertain, the condition may have several causes. Further workup and management will depend on whether the problem has a prerenal, renal parenchymal, or postrenal origin. In addition, although urinalysis and determination of urine sodium concentration and the fractional excretion of sodium can help identify the cause of acute renal failure, they do not indicate its severity. These studies can be supplemented by periodic measurements of creatinine clearance, which can be used to estimate the severity of acute renal failure and to assess the patient's clinical course. Normal creatinine clearance is greater than 100 ml/min; however, this value decreases by nearly half by 70 years of age.

Management

ACUTE DYSFUNCTION FROM PRERENAL CAUSES

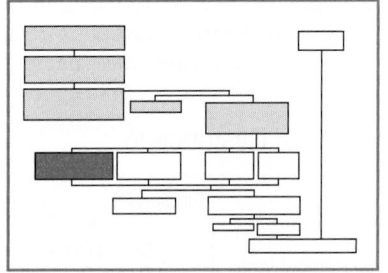

Prerenal causes of acute renal dysfunction include those that diminish blood flow; hence, management is designed to improve renal blood flow. Prerenal azotemia is reversed with treatment of the underlying cause. Intravascular volume is expanded to guarantee adequate preload. CVP, PAWP, or right ventricular end-diastolic volume index (RVEDVI) should be monitored to avoid excess fluid administration. In addition, blood pressure should be controlled adequately, because severe hypertension may worsen preexisting disease. In patients with renovascular disease, however, overcorrection of hypertension may decrease renal blood flow and worsen renal dysfunction.[19,50]

If cardiac dysfunction is present, inotropic support may be useful. It is important not to use agents with alpha-adrenergic activity. Although these agents increase blood pressure, when they are used in high doses their vasoconstrictive effect on

renal arteries leads to reduced renal blood flow.[51,52] Selective renal artery dilation and subsequent diuresis can be achieved with low dosages of dopamine (2 to 5 µg/kg/min).[51,53,54] The contribution of this effect may be trivial or very significant, depending on the patient and coexisting problems. It may also be arrhythmogenic. Administration of dopamine can be useful adjunctive therapy, however, and may be tried in patients who do not respond to simple fluid boluses [see Discussion, Treatment of Developing Acute Renal Failure, below].

If acute renal arterial problems are present, emergency operation and revascularization may be required. Renal artery disease should also be evaluated in the patient undergoing abdominal aortic aneurysm repair, because reimplantation, endarterectomy, or both may be indicated.[55] In cases of documented abdominal compartment syndrome, the abdomen may have to be reapproximated with a prosthetic patch in the fascia to reduce the transmission of external pressure to the kidneys.

Even if prerenal mechanisms do not appear to be the cause of acute renal dysfunction, it is nevertheless important to maintain adequate renal blood flow to minimize injury and facilitate recovery.

ACUTE DYSFUNCTION FROM RENAL PARENCHYMAL CAUSES

Renal parenchyma can be affected or damaged by many substances and mechanisms. Initial attention in patients with renal parenchymal disorders should be directed at stopping the injury. The most common cause of ARF in surgical patients is ATN from systemic infection, ischemia, or exposure to nephrotoxins.[56] Nephrotoxic drugs, such as aminoglycosides, other antibiotics, and nonsteroidal anti-inflammatory drugs, should be discontinued and nonnephrotoxic drugs substituted where possible. The use of radiographic contrast agents should be avoided. Radiologic studies that do not require intravenous contrast, such as magnetic resonance and carbon dioxide imaging, should be selected where possible. If this is not possible, a nonionic agent should be used. It is also important to limit the amount of contrast medium given, because multiple doses have been associated with an increased risk of contrast-induced nephropathy, and to ensure that the patient's intravascular volume is adequate before administration begins.[5] Clearance of circulating myoglobin and hemoglobin should be increased by encouraging diuresis with crystalloid solution infusion. Osmotic agents and urine alkalinization have been used to treat myoglobinuria,[3,57] but they are no substitute for diuresis of at least 100 ml/hr until the urine is clear. Again, maintenance of renal perfusion is essential.

In patients whose serum creatinine level is normal but whose urine sodium level is greater than 40 mEq/L and whose serum sodium level is normal or low, oliguria may reflect the syndrome of inappropriate antidiuretic hormone secretion (SIADH). SIADH is treated by water restriction and, if necessary, administration of diuretics. In patients who have a history of chronic or acute liver disorders, the combination of persistent oliguria, rising serum creatinine levels, low urine sodium levels, low serum sodium levels, and normal intravascular volume should suggest the hepatorenal syndrome [see VII:6 Hepatic Failure]. There are two findings by which this syndrome can be distinguished from prerenal causes of renal failure: (1) urine output does not increase in response to fluid challenge and (2) the ratio of urine creatinine to plasma creatinine is higher than 30:1 (this ratio is lower than 30:1 when prerenal causes are present).[58] There is no proven treatment for hepatorenal syndrome. Peritoneovenous shunts have been used but are of unproven efficacy. Liver transplantation is sometimes lifesaving.[58] Many patients require dialysis until transplantation or resolution of renal dysfunction.[59]

Renal dysfunction from parenchymal causes often takes longer to resolve and has a less predictable course than renal dysfunction from prerenal or postrenal causes.[6] Identification of the specific injurious agent may not be possible. Any patient who is receiving nephrotoxic substances or who has been exposed to such substances should be monitored closely to limit damage. Daily measurement of serum levels of nephrotoxic drugs and adjustment of dosage are indicated in patients in whom these drugs cannot be substituted.

ACUTE DYSFUNCTION FROM A MIXTURE OF PRERENAL AND RENAL PARENCHYMAL CAUSES

Some patients exhibit a mixed pattern of renal dysfunction, in which the mechanism is not obviously prerenal or renal parenchymal. Such patients typically have oliguria or an elevated serum creatinine concentration. The urine sodium concentration is usually between 20 and 40 mEq/L, and the FE_{Na} is usually between 1 and 3. Several potential causes of dysfunction may be present, including diminished renal perfusion and exposure to nephrotoxic agents. These may be superimposed on some degree of baseline renal dysfunction. The administration of diuretics or osmotic agents in this situation may also lead to this mixed pattern through their effects on renal electrolytes.

Treatment of renal dysfunction of mixed origin is generally based on increasing intravascular volume. Unless the patient is known to have intravascular fluid overload, a fluid bolus should be given, and the I.V. fluid infusion rate should be increased. Edema in itself is not a sufficient reason to withhold further fluid challenge: it may be extravascular, rendering the patient paradoxically hypovolemic. Again, all nephrotoxic drugs should be discontinued to prevent any further injury to the renal parenchyma. The patient's CVP, PAWP, or RVEDVI should be monitored to ensure that intravascular volume is not pushed to a high level. Continued monitoring of urine electrolyte concentrations should be undertaken to detect any further deterioration of renal function.

ACUTE DYSFUNCTION FROM POSTRENAL CAUES

Treatment of obstructive lesions that produce acute renal dysfunction is relatively straightforward. Decompression of the obstructed area will usually correct the problem and permit return of all or some degree of renal function. Obstructing lesions that are

complicated by urosepsis may be associated with more prolonged renal dysfunction. These patients often have prerenal dysfunction as a result of the sepsis, and a Swan-Ganz catheter may be necessary to guide therapy. Similar assessment of cardiac output, using a somewhat less invasive method than pulmonary artery catheterization, may be accomplished by the use of continuous cardiac output arterial thermodilution calibrated pulse contour analysis.[60]

The bladder can be drained by means of a Foley or suprapubic catheter. Continued monitoring of urine output is then possible. If ureteral obstruction is present, ureteral stents or nephrostomy tubes can be placed to relieve the obstruction.

Return to Normal Renal Function

Successful management of acute renal dysfunction will correct oliguria and serum creatinine levels. However, monitoring of renal function must be continued until there appears to be no further risk, particularly if other medical problems necessitate ongoing treatment. Documentation of the acute renal dysfunction is important because it may help prevent recurrent problems in the future. Drug selection should be carefully reviewed with an eye to avoiding nephrotoxic agents, if possible. If nephrotoxic drugs must be used, the serum levels of the drugs and parameters of renal function, such as serum creatinine, must be followed closely.

Progressive Renal Dysfunction

Attempts to maintain renal blood flow and preserve urine output are important even in the presence of advancing renal failure.[61] Nonoliguric renal failure has a better prognosis than oliguric or anuric renal failure.[33] Adequate hydration remains the principal method for sustaining urine output. Inotropic agents may have a positive influence in some patients but are not recommended as routine treatment. Attempts to preserve urine output and convert oliguric to nonoliguric renal failure by administering diuretics[62,63] have been largely unsuccessful; these attempts appear only to identify patients with the least severe renal dysfunction (i.e., those with enough residual renal function to respond to the diuretics).[33] Furthermore, diuretics confer no long-term benefit in the treatment of ARF.

If renal function deteriorates, medication doses and dosing intervals must be adjusted. Adjustments for drugs should be based on product information from the manufacturer or on the recommendations of a pharmacologist. The principles to be considered in adjustment of drug dosage in patients with renal failure are (1) the desired concentration, (2) the volume of distribution of the drug, and (3) the mechanism and rate of metabolism or excretion. Drug levels should be checked frequently as renal function changes; fluid and electrolyte therapy should also be adjusted. Drug dosages should be adjusted downward in elderly patients because of their age-related decline in renal function.[64]

Comorbid conditions also require attention. Urinary tract infections should be aggressively treated to prevent further deterioration of renal function. Uncontrolled hypertension should be treated.[65]

Adequate nutrition appears to be important for recovery from renal failure,[66,67] but nutritional support in the patient with ARF can be complicated.[68] Patients who are critically ill are hypercatabolic, with an increased energy expenditure and increased protein turnover with negative nitrogen balance. They often have comorbid disease processes that impair their nutritional status. Although renal failure decreases energy expenditure, dialysis may increase energy expenditure, so it would seem appropriate to increase protein and caloric intake in these patients. However, in some patients, decreasing the dietary protein intake will decrease glomerular hyperfiltration and may slow the progression of renal failure.[69,70] Measurement of nitrogen balance, along with more sophisticated techniques such as metabolic cart measurements, will help guide nutritional support.

RENAL REPLACEMENT THERAPY

Patients who have symptomatic fluid overload associated with congestive heart failure, encephalopathy, or acid-base and electrolyte disorders may require some degree of artificial renal support. Dialysis is necessary to correct encephalopathy or severe metabolic disorders. Other criteria for initiating renal replacement therapy (RRT) in the critically ill ICU patient have been proposed: these include azotemia, uremic pericarditis, neuropathy and myopathy, acute respiratory distress syndrome, and sepsis.[71,72] Elevated absolute values of BUN and creatinine are not indicators for dialysis.

If dialysis is indicated, it should be initiated promptly. Early dialysis in ARF is associated with improved survival.[14,73,74]

There are many options for providing RRT in the hospital setting, and each has advantages and disadvantages [see Table 3]. RRT can be done with an intermittent or a continuous technique.[75] Standard intermittent techniques include peritoneal dialysis and intermittent hemodialysis. These are typically used in patients with established renal failure who are already receiving some form of RRT and are undergoing an elective procedure. Continuous therapy is most commonly employed in critically ill ICU patients.

Along with the clinical setting, the indications for replacement therapy guide the selection of the appropriate method of RRT. Therapy may be required to remove fluid, metabolic wastes, or both. These management decisions are made in conjunction with nephrologists to provide optimal care to the patient requiring RRT.

Acute continuous hemodiafiltration is an excellent option in critically ill patients, who often are too hemodynamically labile to tolerate standard hemodialysis.[76-79] The most commonly employed method is continuous venovenohemodialysis (CVVHD). This method of dialysis is usually performed via a temporary double-lumen central venous dialysis catheter, which is placed percutaneously in the subclavian, internal jugular, or femoral vein. Blood is pumped by a peristaltic pump through a filter against the flow of peritoneal dialysate, which is pumped into the nonblood portion of the filter in the opposite direction. The machine is programmed and various concentrations of dialysate are chosen to effect the desired removal

Table 3 Comparison of Renal Replacement Therapy Options[147]

	Advantages	Disadvantages
Intermittent hemodialysis	Efficient fluid, filtrate, and solute removal	Hemodynamic instability; resource and personnel intensive
Continuous renal replacement therapy (CVVH/D, CAVH/D, hemofiltration)	Hemodynamic stability; multiple filtration options; relative ease of use	Inefficient fluid and filtrate removal; requires immobilization and continuous anticoagulation
Peritoneal dialysis	No vascular access, hemodynamic stability, minimal equipment	Contraindicated in abdominal surgery patients; peritonitis

of fluid and wastes.[2,79] Continous arteriovenous hemodiafiltration (CAVHD) is performed in the same way but requires large-bore arterial access or a Scribner shunt in addition to venous access. This method allows for slow but continuous removal of fluid and clearance of toxic wastes. Compared with intermittent hemodialysis, continuous RRT provides better hemodynamic stability, maintenance of cerebral perfusion, and control of fluid balance. It is therefore indicated in patients with renal failure and critical illness and may be the treatment of choice for ARF in this patient population.[2,72,80]

Patients who have fluid overload as evidenced by cardiopulmonary congestive failure but no other need for dialysis can be treated with continuous hemofiltration, which permits clearance of fluid and plasma solutes.[2,81,82] Continuous hemofiltration can be performed in patients who are hemodynamically unstable and can be done using the same machine and vascular access as that used for CVVHD. This process may be particularly useful in patients with severe cardiac failure and sepsis, in whom the ability to remove proinflammatory mediators may improve the clinical course.[2]

Treatment of patients requiring dialysis or other RRT should be directed at returning renal function to normal levels, or at least to levels that eliminate the need for renal support. Free water clearance or creatinine clearance should be monitored. Improvement in these urinary clearance measurements may signal a return to normal or baseline renal function. It is important to remember that baseline renal function in the elderly is usually less than normal.

For patients who do progress to renal failure, recovery depends on age, cause of renal failure, and urine output during the time of renal dysfunction. Young patients and those who maintain adequate urine output despite ARF have a significantly better prognosis.[33,83] Mortality in patients with severe ARF has remained unchanged despite improved dialysis and other advances[8]; it ranges from 30% to 80% and varies with comorbid factors. It is highest in patients with multiorgan failure from infection or SIRS. Of patients who survive ARF, most can discontinue dialysis after recovery of renal function.[84]

Death related to renal failure is most often caused by infectious complications. Pneumonia is the most common fatal infection, although peritonitis and urinary infection may lead to sepsis and death. Bleeding complications may occur as a result of platelet dysfunction caused by uremia and heparin anticoagulation during dialysis; this may also contribute to death in these patients.[85-87]

Chronic Renal Failure

Chronic renal failure (CRF), which is irreversible, may be caused by a number of factors. Diabetes mellitus, hypertension, glomerular diseases, obstructive disease with chronic pyelonephritis, congenital hypoplasia or aplasia, tubulointerstitial diseases, and polycystic disease are the most common causes of CRF.[88] These patients will have varying degrees of renal insufficiency, and as in patients with acute renal failure, a good history and physical examination are critical in their evaluation in the perioperative period [see Table 4]. Particular attention should be paid to the baseline status of the patient whenever possible. This includes attention to baseline blood pressure and cardiac function; urine output; medications that may affect blood pressure, renal blood flow, and cardiac output; and any history of preexisting renal disease or signs and symptoms of obstruction and urinary tract infection.

Perioperative Management of Patients with Renal Failure

Elective and emergency operations can be performed safely in patients with renal failure. Many patients will experience some complication. The most common complication is hyperkalemia; others include volume overload, bleeding, and infection.[89] However, most of these complications can be prevented or managed with both preoperative and postoperative dialysis, judicious use of appropriate perioperative antibiotics, choice of anesthetic agents, and meticulous surgical technique and hemostasis. Attention should be paid to maintaining blood pressure and volume homeostasis before, during, and after surgery. In addition, attention to operative planning, exposure, blood loss, and the use of renal protective measures where possible becomes important.[46,55] In patients with a hemodialysis access graft, hospital staff should also be cautioned to avoid measurement of blood pressures and placement of I.V. access in the arm with the graft.

The patient with stable renal failure requires standard preoperative evaluation before elective surgery. Particular attention is paid to fluid and electrolyte status. In patients on chronic dialysis who are stable, dialysis is usually performed the day before and the day after the procedure, and more often as necessary.[9] Patients on peritoneal dialysis who are to have an intra-abdominal procedure will require vascular access for hemodialysis. In the patient with acute or acute-on-chronic renal failure who has volume overload or severe metabolic imbalance, dialysis should be performed early and should be aggressive.[11,90] Patients with hepatorenal syndrome may be dialyzed throughout liver transplantation surgery to deal with the large fluid volumes often required for the procedure.

Patients who require emergency surgery and cannot be dialyzed may become hyperkalemic and require medical management. Calcium (e.g., 5 to 10 ml of 10% calcium chloride solution I.V. over 2 minutes) will stabilize cardiac membranes. Subsequently, the intravenous administration of sodium bicarbonate (44 mEq over 5 minutes) and insulin (e.g., 10 to 25 U over 30 minutes) will drive potassium into the cells; those are given along with glucose (e.g., 250 ml of 20% dextrose) to counterbalance the hypoglycemic effects of the insulin. Sodium polystyrene sulfonate (Kayexalate), an orally or rectally administered exchange resin, will bind potassium. However, this agent takes hours to work.

The actions of some neuromuscular blockers and anticholinesterases are affected by renal failure.[91,92] Their use can potentiate acidosis and hyperkalemia. In particular, the use of succinylcholine, which causes a transient hyperkalemia in normal persons, is controversial in the anesthetic management of the patient with renal failure.[93]

Intraoperative hypotension should be avoided. This is particularly true in patients with chronic renal insufficiency but without end-stage disease requiring dialysis, who are at greatest risk for ARF and for the development of toxic nephropathies in the postoperative period.[94] In addition, hypotension may lead to dialysis graft thrombosis.

Postoperatively, patients with renal failure should be managed as any other patient. However, special consideration must be given to fluid and electrolyte management and acid-base balance. Dialysis should be instituted early to prevent complications.[9] Wound healing may be delayed in renal failure patients.[94] In addition, these patients may be protein malnourished, which will also affect wound healing.[68] Appropriate nutritional support is essential in these patients (see above). Nutritional support should be provided as early as possible postoperatively, and the enteral route is preferred.[66] Drug dosages should be modified for those drugs that are excreted renally or are dialyzable.[95]

Patients who have prolonged bleeding times as a result of renal failure are managed with dialysis. Those with clinically evident bleeding may require cryoprecipitate, vasopressin (DDAVP), and conjugated estrogens to correct bleeding disorders.[96]

Table 4 Findings Suggestive of Chronic Rather Than Acute Renal Failure

History
- Symptoms of uremia (e.g., nausea, pruritus, malaise, weakness, mental status changes, weight loss, edema)
- Hypertension
- Hematuria or proteinuria
- Abnormal blood chemistry values (elevated urea nitrogen or creatinine levels)

Physical examination
- Debility
- Alopecia
- Excoriations and yellow pallor of skin
- Peripheral neuropathy
- Conjunctival calcification
- Band keratopathy
- Gynecomastia, testicular atrophy, or both

Laboratory examination*
- Anemia on presentation (only if there is no history of acute blood loss)
- Low urinary sodium level or high urine osmolarity (either suggests prerenal azotemia)

X-rays or ultrasonography
- Bilateral small kidneys
- Other evidence of long-standing renal dysfunction (e.g., chronic obstruction, pyelonephritis, or polycystic kidney disease)
- Bone changes of secondary hyperparathyroidism (e.g., osteitis fibrosa cystica, osteomalacia, or osteosclerosis)

*Serum chemistry values are not helpful, because they may be altered in both acute and chronic renal failure.

Figure 1 The rate of red cell production in the marrow is determined by erythropoietin elaboration in the kidneys. In normal kidneys, as shown here, endothelial cells in the tubules or peritubular capillaries are thought to produce most of the renal erythropoietin. Synthesis is stimulated by renal hypoxemia. (The hypoxemia would not necessarily be caused by anemia. It could, for example, be the result of dwelling at high altitudes.) In the marrow, the erythropoietin binds to erythroid progenitors, stimulating their differentiation and proliferation. In patients with renal failure, decreased production of erythropoietin by the diseased kidneys impairs erythropoiesis in the marrow. Red cell morphology is unaffected, however.

Many patients on chronic hemodialysis are anemic because of decreased endogenous erythropoietin levels [*see Figure 1*] and blood losses during dialysis, as well as depletion of iron stores. Blood transfusions were commonly used to treat anemia in these patients until the 1990s, when recombinant erythropoietin became available. This agent has largely eliminated the need for transfusions and their associated morbidity; it also corrects clotting abnormalities associated with decreased platelet function and improves quality of life.[97-101] Blood transfusion remains necessary, however, in the setting of acute blood loss with hemodynamic compromise.

Discussion

Perspective on Acute Renal Failure

The incidence of ARF has decreased since the mid-1940s; however, mortality among patients who have renal failure severe enough to necessitate dialysis has not been improved.[8,44] This lack of improvement appears to be related to the increasing percentage of patients who experience acute renal failure as one manifestation of multiorgan failure. Mortality from ARF without multiorgan dysfunction is 8% to 30%, whereas mortality from renal failure that is associated with sepsis or multiorgan failure is 70% to 80%.[8,39,44]

Groups of patients at risk for acute renal failure can be identified, but the specific degree of risk for an individual patient cannot be calculated. Patients with burns, severe injury, prolonged periods of hypoperfusion, or cardiopulmonary bypass are at significantly higher risk for ARF than routine surgical patients.[25,102-104] Other than relative amount of injury or ischemia, the variables that correlate with renal failure are older age and a history of limited renal function.[44] Tests to predict renal failure and outcome of renal failure have proved elusive.[42,105]

It is well accepted that the fundamental goal in the management of ARF is prevention, or at least limitation of its severity. Attention to the cause or causes of acute renal dysfunction and to the mechanisms involved often permits correction of the problem before progression to actual renal failure occurs. If acute renal dysfunction and failure are to be managed by prevention, early diagnosis, and correction, it is necessary to understand renal pathophysiology.

Normal Renal Physiology

Understanding of both normal and altered renal physiology is greatly aided by familiarity with the anatomy of the nephron and with the sites of action of the hormones essential to normal renal function [*see Figure 2*]. Anatomic or functional injury to a sufficient number of nephrons can lead to measurable renal dysfunction and ultimately to renal failure. Renal function can be analyzed in terms of blood flow, glomerular filtration, and tubular reabsorption and secretion.

Blood flow to the kidneys is determined by cardiac output and renal vascular resistance. Renal vascular resistance is principally controlled at the arteriolar level. When renal perfusion pressure falls, the efferent arterioles constrict to maintain glomerular filtration pressure despite the decreased flow. If the systemic systolic pressure drops below 70 mm Hg, however, this mechanism fails and the afferent arterioles constrict, leading to a rapid decrease in glomerular filtration and consequently to a decrease in urine output.

This system is controlled by several hormonal and mediator systems that act at various sites in the nephron. The renin-angiotensin mechanism is important for the control of arteriolar resistance.[106,107] When renal perfusion pressure falls, secretion of renin by the juxtaglomerular apparatus increases. This leads to increased production of angiotensin I, which is converted to angiotensin II. Angiotensin II is a powerful vasoconstrictor that increases peripheral vascular resistance.

Nitric oxide and prostaglandins have been found to be important mediators of blood flow to different areas of the kidney[1,108] and may exert some control over renin release through a feedback mechanism. Catecholamines, ATP-$MgCl_2$, and calcium[109,110] have also been found to participate in the control of renal blood flow. Adequate blood flow largely controls glomerular filtration and is essential for normal renal function.

Glomerular filtration is determined by the hydrostatic pressure in the afferent arteriole and by the filtration coefficient, K_f. The glomerular filtration rate is an important variable but is not easily measured[111]; it is usually approximated by calculations based on creatinine clearance (C_{Cr}) and free water clearance (C_{H_2O}). These clearance values (expressed in ml/min) can be calculated by the following formulas:

$$C_{Cr} = V \times (U_{Cr}/P_{Cr})$$
$$C_{H_2O} = V - C_{osm} = V - [V \times (U_{osm}/P_{osm})]$$

in which V is urine volume (ml/min), C_{osm} is osmolar clearance, U_{osm} is urine osmolality (mOsm/L), and P_{osm} is plasma osmolality (mOsm/L).

These calculations are usually indexed to a standard patient size (1.73 m^2 body surface area) by multiplying each calculated clearance by 1.73/patient's estimated body surface area. The creatinine clearance provides a good estimate of the glomerular filtration rate. A positive C_{H_2O} measures net water excretion; a negative C_{H_2O} measures water retention. A change in free water clearance into the range of ± 0.15 ml/min precedes a rise in creatinine by 24 to 48 hours. Free water clearance is not routinely measured, however, and does not usually establish the diagnosis of renal dysfunction. Rather, renal dysfunction is signaled clinically by the onset of oliguria or a rising serum creatinine level.

Most physicians use the serum creatinine level as an indicator of GFR because it is the simplest to determine. However, a small fraction of creatinine is secreted into the renal tubular fluid. The serum creatinine level becomes a less accurate measure of GFR as the relative component of creatinine clearance from GFR decreases.[112] Furthermore, medications such as cimetidine and the cephalosporin antibiotics can be measured as creatinine in laboratory tests and thus can give a falsely decreased measure of GFR.[20-23] Despite its limitations, however, measurement of serum creatinine levels continues to be the mainstay of the initial assessment of GFR and renal clearance.

The principal functions of the renal tubules are reabsorption of sodium and water.[113] Sodium reabsorption occurs in the distal tubule and is controlled primarily by aldosterone.[114] Water reabsorption occurs predominantly in the collecting tubule and is regulated by antidiuretic hormone (ADH), which is also known as vasopressin.[115] In addition, atrial natriuretic factor appears to affect tubular cells and the renal vasculature.[116] Hypovolemia and hypotension cause increased production of these hormones, which act to increase tubular reabsorption in an attempt to maintain intravascular volume.

Pathophysiology of Acute Renal Failure: Cellular and Molecular Changes

PRERENAL PATHOPHYSIOLOGY

Prerenal causes of acute renal failure are principally associated with inadequate blood flow and altered hemodynamics[117] and account for 50% to 90% of ARF, with the exact distribution somewhat varied.[118,119] Impaired blood flow to the kidneys is the result of hypovolemia in most cases and of depressed myocardial function in a small percentage of patients with an acute cardiac insult or chronic cardiac dysfunction. Renal injury from inadequate perfusion can be exacerbated if low arterial oxygen saturation further impairs oxygen delivery.[120]

The decreased arterial and arteriolar pressures associated with hypovolemia cause production of ADH and aldosterone to increase; the reabsorption of sodium and water is thereby increased as well. If the systemic systolic pressure falls below 70 mm Hg, afferent arterioles constrict, decreasing the GFR further.[121] This decrease in glomerular filtration leads to increased sodium reabsorption and concentrated urine, eventually resulting in the urine characteristics associated with a prerenal cause of renal dysfunction—namely, low urine sodium levels, low fractional excretion of sodium, and high urine specific gravity.

Renal blood flow can also be impaired by high intra-abdominal pressure, which seems to decrease renal blood flow.[7,30,122,123] Prompt reduction of increased intra-abdominal pressure appears to correct developing renal failure, possibly because of improved renal blood flow.

RENAL PARENCHYMAL PATHOPHYSIOLOGY

Redistribution of blood flow inside the kidneys can occur as a result of systemic infection, SIRS, or the hepatorenal syndrome,[58,59] causing glomerular filtration to decrease. The changes in small renal vessel impedance that mediate intrarenal blood flow distribution are probably controlled by local release of prostaglandins and nitric oxide.[108,124] The use of prostaglandin inhibitors or inhibitors of inducible nitric oxide synthase, however, has not been shown to alter function or outcome in patients with systemic infection, SIRS, or the hepatorenal syndrome.

Pathophysiologic changes associated with parenchymal injury depend on the specific cause of renal injury. Several such changes

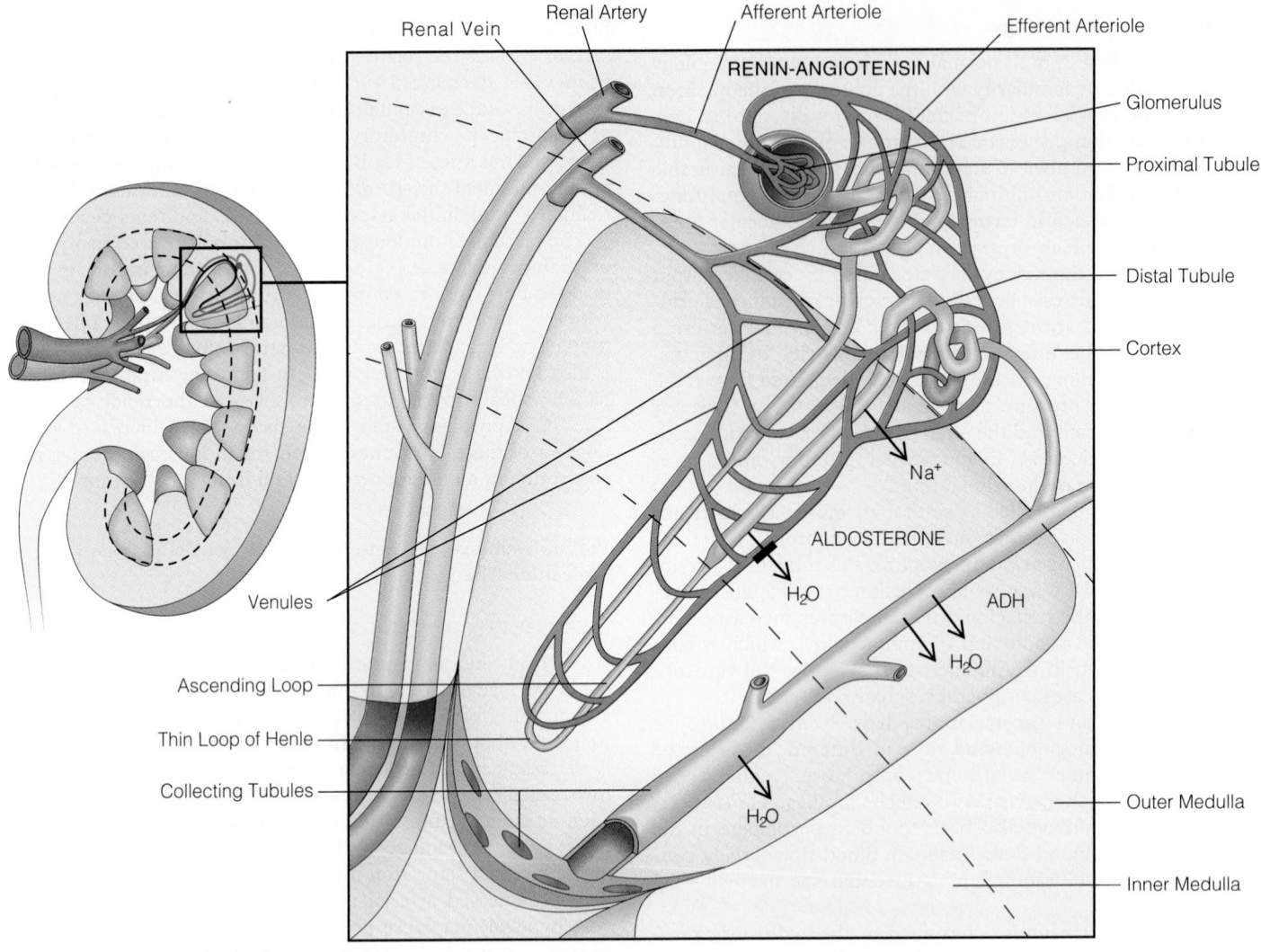

Figure 2   **Depicted are the major anatomic features of a juxtamedullary nephron, its blood supply, and the sites of action of the renin-angiotensin system, aldosterone, and ADH. The renin-angiotensin system controls resistance in the renal arterioles, primarily the efferent arteriole. By constricting the efferent arteriole, angiotensin can increase the glomerular pressure, thereby helping to maintain a relatively constant glomerular filtration rate even in the face of low arterial pressure. Aldosterone affects sodium reabsorption in the late distal tubule and the collecting duct. When aldosterone is present in large amounts, virtually all of the sodium is reabsorbed, and almost none is excreted. In the absence of aldosterone, however, substantial quantities of sodium are not reabsorbed and are excreted in the urine. ADH affects the permeability of the epithelium of the collecting duct. When ADH is absent, the collecting duct is almost totally impermeable to water. When it is present in substantial concentrations, however, the collecting duct becomes highly permeable to water; this increased permeability, coupled with the hyperosmolality of the medullary interstitial fluid, results in rapid reabsorption of water from the collecting duct.**

may occur concomitantly. Impairment of tubular function by ischemia, toxic substances, or increased intraluminal pressure may alter the normal polarity between the luminal and basal surfaces of the cell membranes of the tubular cells. This loss of polarity alters membrane function, disrupts the microfilaments in the cells, and causes intercellular tight junctions to open, thereby affecting transport of sodium and potassium and inducing fluid shifts.[125] Progression of tubular functional impairment eventually leads to alterations in ultrafiltrate flow by several mechanisms. Swelling of tubular cells or increased back pressure from distal obstruction raises tubular luminal pressure, thereby decreasing glomerular filtration. Simultaneously, the loss of integrity of the tubular cell junctions leads to back-leakage of fluid into the renal interstitium.[126,127] Tubular glomerular feedback may also occur, in

which the relatively high sodium concentration at the distal tubule near the macula densa leads to reflex vasoconstriction of the afferent arterioles and consequently a further decrease in glomerular filtration.[128] Renal blood flow may be further affected by the shunting of blood from the cortex to the medulla, probably in association with increased nitric oxide production.

There are two major parenchymal causes of ARF. The first is ischemia, which is a common cause of tubular injury. The medullary thick ascending limb of the loop of Henle and the pars recta of the proximal tubule are the segments of the nephron most sensitive to ischemia.[129] Tubular cells can be identified in the urine of patients with this form of renal injury, which is sometimes called acute tubular necrosis. The term is not an accurate pathologic description of this form of renal injury but continues to be used, frequently to describe any renal parenchymal cause of ARF.

Toxic injury to renal cells is the other major parenchymal cause of acute renal failure. Many compounds are toxic to renal tissue; the most commonly encountered are aminoglycosides, ionic radiographic contrast media, myoglobin, hemoglobin, cyclosporine,[130] and nonsteroidal anti-inflammatory drugs. Aminoglycosides appear to have toxic effects on tubular cells, with the extent of toxicity related primarily to their trough levels. Close monitoring of levels of these drugs is essential, especially in burn patients, in whom clearance of aminoglycosides and other drugs is increased and who therefore require higher doses to achieve therapeutic levels.[131] Aminoglycosides also appear to decrease renal blood flow independently of cardiac output.[132]

Intravenous ionic radiographic contrast media have been demonstrated to cause acute renal parenchymal injury. The toxicity is potentiated by decreased renal perfusion. Nonionic contrast material appears to have less renal toxicity and may be an alternative for patients with borderline renal function. Pretreatment with half-normal saline has been shown to be more effective than mannitol or furosemide in preventing renal dysfunction associated with contrast media.[63] Use of the dopaminergic agonist fenoldopam or the nitric oxide scavenger acetylcysteine along with hydration may further lessen the effects of contrast agents on renal function.[47,48]

ARF from myoglobinuria was first described in trauma victims with crush injury and myonecrosis. Myoglobin is an 18 kd protein that filters easily through the glomeruli and causes more damage than hemoglobin, a 67 kd protein. Myoglobin appears to cause tubular injury through direct toxicity as well as through obstruction resulting from precipitation in the tubule.[3]

Many other toxins may play a role in ARF and should be considered if parenchymal renal failure develops without an apparent cause.[126]

Inflammatory and vasculitic causes of ARF are uncommon in surgical patients. These disease processes usually present as medical problems associated with autoimmune or postinfectious states. Still, appropriate workup is required to rule out other contributing causes or processes. Identification of red cell or white cell casts and proteinuria is useful in diagnosing inflammation.

SYNDROME OF INAPPROPRIATE ANTIDIURETIC HORMONE SECRETION

The diagnosis of SIADH is made by excluding other causes of oliguria. Patients with SIADH have low urine output, high urine sodium levels, and low serum sodium levels. Furthermore, serum creatinine levels do not usually rise in these patients, despite prolonged borderline oliguria. Treatment consists of water restriction, although some patients require diuretics.[133] Hypertonic saline is infused only if the patient appears to be symptomatic from hyponatremia. SIADH usually resolves spontaneously with no injurious consequences to the kidneys.

Treatment of Developing Acute Renal Failure

If prevention fails, treatment of developing acute renal failure is directed at preserving remaining renal function and limiting further damage by increasing blood flow and urine output and decreasing tubular cell injury. Adequate renal blood flow is essential in treating renal injury from all causes and is usual-

ly successfully achieved by volume infusion. In patients with normal cardiac and respiratory function, fluid administration can probably be guided with only a central venous line. Although inotropes can increase cardiac output and low-dose dopamine can increase renal blood flow, use of these agents has not been shown to affect the incidence or outcome of acute renal failure.[134] Even the combination of inotropes and diuretics has not been shown to have any effect.[135] Despite this lack of proven efficacy, dopamine (2 to 5 mg/kg/min) should be considered if urine output does not respond to intravascular volume expansion.

Urine output should be maintained in patients with developing ARF to ensure filtration; in addition, adequate urine output implies adequate blood flow. Nonoliguric renal failure has a much better prognosis than renal failure associated with oliguria. Many physicians will attempt to convert oliguric to nonoliguric renal failure. It is unclear whether the increase in urine output upon treatment is an actual conversion or simply a means of identifying the patients with the most residual renal function. Attempts to increase urine output in ARF have often involved administration of diuretics. Studies have found that diuretics do increase GFR and urine output.[33] There have been no differences in outcome, however, between patients who received diuretics and those who did not; this result is most notable in prospective, randomized trials.[136] Response to furosemide appears to have only prognostic value in ARF.[33,136] There are also potential problems with high-dose diuretics, including ototoxicity, arrhythmias, and hypokalemia.[37] Nevertheless, diuretics still are commonly used to treat developing ARF.[37,38,44]

Decreasing tubular injury is an attractive concept. Mannitol has been found to shrink tubular cells, but like diuretics, it does not affect patient outcome.[137] The use of calcium channel blockers to limit tubular cell damage may have some clinical benefit.[138-140] ACE inhibitors may limit injury in patients with diabetic renal disease because of the drugs' ability to decrease arteriolar and glomerular capillary pressures.[141] The use of agents that modify nitric oxide production may provide a means of treating evolving renal failure. Other molecular therapies for renal failure, including the use of epidermal growth factor, are under investigation.[141] Elimination of nephrotoxic substances and maintenance of perfusion are currently the only effective methods for decreasing tubular injury.

Differential Diagnosis of Acute Renal Failure

Because prevention and limitation of renal injury are the goals in the management of ARF, early diagnosis is essential. However, determination of which patients with oliguria or elevated serum creatinine levels will progress to ARF and differentiation among the causes of their renal dysfunction remain difficult.

A measurable change in free water clearance into the range of $\pm$ 0.17 ml/min/1.73 m^2 body surface area or a creatinine clearance of 30 ml/min/1.73 m^2 body surface area indicates ARF.[41] These calculated clearances do not identify the cause of ARF, however. Identification of the cause is best accomplished through physical examination, review of the history and treatment, urinalysis, and measurement of urine and plasma sodium and creatinine levels. The most reliable means of differentiating prerenal from other causes of ARF are measurement of urine sodium levels and calculation of the fractional excretion of sodium.[43] The renal failure index (RFI) is another means of distinguishing prerenal causes and is defined as follows:

$$RFI = [U_{Na}/(U_{Cr}/P_{Cr})] \times 100$$

This formula is similar to that for the fractional excretion of sodium:

$$FE_{Na} = [(U_{Na}/P_{Na})/(U_{Cr}/P_{Cr})] \times 100$$

Although the RFI is used by some nephrologists, it is not superior to FE_{Na} in discriminating between prerenal and renal parenchymal causes of ARF.[119] The usefulness of FE_{Na} for diagnosing ARF has been challenged in some reports[142,143]; however, these reports failed to measure FE_{Na} at the same period in the course of acute renal failure.[144] Furthermore, complaints that FE_{Na} is not predictive are not well founded, because the calculation is not intended to be a predictor but rather a tool for distinguishing prerenal from renal parenchymal causes of ARF.[14,40,145,146]

Other tests to distinguish the causes of ARF are of limited value, except in identifying possible parenchymal disorders. The presence of red cell and white cell casts may indicate vasculitic or inflammatory causes. Identification of tubular cells in the urine, either microscopically or by detection of surface antigen, suggests a postischemic cause, but these markers are not specific.

Measurement of urine electrolyte concentrations (e.g., chloride and bicarbonate), measurement of the products of inflammation (e.g., complement components), and renal biopsy are useful in assessing chronic renal problems; however, these determinations add little to the diagnosis and treatment of ARF.

References

1. Nissenson AR: Acute renal failure: Definition and pathogenesis. Kidney Int 53 (suppl 66):S-7, 1998

2. Ronco C, Barbacini S, Digito A, et al: Achievements and new directions in continuous renal replacement therapies. New Horizons 3:708, 1995

3. Slater MS, Mullins RJ: Rhabdomyolysis and myoglobinuric renal failure in trauma and surgical patients: a review. J Am Coll Surg 186:695, 1998

4. Quader MA, Sawmiller C, Sumpio BA: Contrast-induced nephropathy: review of incidence and pathophysiology. Ann Vasc Surg 12:612, 1998

5. Tublin ME, Murphy ME, Tessler FN: Current concepts in contrast media induced nephropathy. AJR Am J Roentgenol 171:933, 1998

6. Thadani RI, Camargo CA, Xavier RJ, et al: Atheroembolic renal failure after invasive procedures. Natural history based on 52 histologically proven cases. Medicine (Baltimore) 74:350, 1995

7. Tan IK, Kua JS: Abdominal compartment syndrome and acute anuria. Nephrol Dial Transplant 13:2651, 1998

8. Alkhunaizi AM, Schrier RW: Management of acute renal failure: new perspectives. Am J Kidney Dis 28:315, 1996

9. Lazarus JM, Morgan AP, Tilney NL: Patients with chronic renal failure: general management and acute surgical illness. Surgical Care of the Patient with Renal Failure. Tilney NL, Lazarus JM, Eds. WB Saunders Co, Philadelphia, 1982, p 1

10. Vincent F: Preoperative and postoperative care: renal disease. Handbook of Surgery. Schrock TR, Ed. Jones Medical Publications, Greenbrae, California, 1985, p 47

11. Bellomo R, Parkin G, Love J, et al: A prospective comparative study of continuous arteriovenous hemodiafiltration and continuous venovenous hemodiafiltration in critically ill patients. Am J Kidney Dis 21:400, 1993

12. Rosen T: Uremic pruritus: a review. Cutis 23:790, 1979

13. Engle WD: Evaluation of renal function and acute renal failure in the neonate. Pediatr Clin North Am 33:129, 1986

14. Tilney NL, Lazarus JM: Acute renal failure in surgical patients: causes, clinical patterns, and care. Surg Clin North Am 63:357, 1983

15. Narayanan S: Renal biochemistry and physiology: pathophysiology and analytical perspectives. Adv Clin Chem 29:121, 1992

16. Espinel CH: Diagnosis of acute and chronic renal failure. Clin Lab Med 13:89, 1993

17. Bjornsson TD: Use of serum creatinine concentrations to determine renal function. Clin Pharmacokinet 4:200, 1979

18. Rowe JW: Clinical research on aging: strategies and directions. N Engl J Med 297:1332, 1977

19. Lieberthal W, Levinsky NG: Treatment of acute tubular necrosis. Semin Nephrol 10:571, 1990

20. Nanji AA, Campbell DJ: Falsely elevated serum creatinine values in diabetic ketoacidosis: clinical implications. Clin Biochem 14:91, 1981

21. Guay DR, Meatherall RC, Macauley PA: Interference of selected second and third generation cephalosporins with creatinine determination. Am J Hosp Pharm 40:435, 1983

22. Shouval D, Ligumsky M, Ben-Ishay D: Effects of co-trimoxazole on normal creatinine clearance. Lancet 1:244, 1978

23. Larsson R, Bodemar G, Kagedal B, et al: The effects of cimetidine (Tagamet) on renal function in patients with renal failure. Acta Med Scand 208:27, 1980

24. Baek SM, Makabali GG, Shoemaker WC: Clinical determinants of survival from postoperative renal failure. Surg Gynecol Obstet 140:685, 1975

25. Kellerman PS: Perioperative care of the renal patient. Arch Intern Med 154:1674, 1994

26. Finn WF, Arendshorst WJ, Gottschalk CW: Pathogenesis of oliguria in acute renal failure. Circ Res 36:675, 1975

27. Burnier M, Schrier RW: Pathogenesis of acute renal failure. Adv Exp Med Biol 212:3, 1987

28. Fishchereder M, Trick W, Nath KA: Therapeutic strategies in the prevention of acute renal failure. Semin Nephrol 14:41, 1994

29. Sugrue M: Prospective study of intra-abdominal hypertension and renal function after laparotomy. Br J Surg 82:235, 1995

30. Dunn MD, McDougall EM: Renal physiology. Laparoscopic considerations. Urol Clin North Am 27:609, 2000

31. Link D, Leff RG, Hildel J, et al: The use of percutaneous nephrostomy in 42 patients. J Urol 122:9, 1979

32. Bunn F, Lefebvre C, Li Wan Po A, et al: Human albumin solution for resuscitation and volume expansion in critically ill patients. The Cochrane Database of Systematic Reviews 2:CD 001208, 2000

33. Anderson RJ, Linas SL, Berns AS, et al: Nonoliguric acute renal failure. N Engl J Med 296:1134, 1977

34. Aurora RN: Preventing renal failure in critically ill patients. Crit Care Med 27:2044, 1999

35. Bonventre JV, Weinberg JM: Kidney preservation ex vivo for transplantation. Annu Rev Med 43:523, 1992

36. Cantarovich F, Galli C, Benedetti L, et al: High dose frusemide in established acute renal failure. Br Med J 4:449, 1973

37. Martin SJ, Danziger LH: Continous infusion of loop diuretics in the critically ill: a review of the literature. Crit Care Med 22:1323, 1994

38. Kellum JA: Use of diuretics in the acute care setting. Kidney Int 53(suppl 66):S67, 1998

39. DuBose TD, Warnock DG, Mehta R, et al: Acute renal failure in the 21st century: recommendations for management and outcomes assessment. Am J Kidney Dis 29:793, 1997.

40. Farber MD, Kupin WL, Krishna GG, et al: The differential diagnosis of acute renal failure. Acute Renal Failure, 3rd ed. Lazarus JM, Brenner BM, Eds. WB Saunders Co, Philadelphia, 1993, p 133

41. Brown R, Babcock R, Talbert J, et al: Renal function in critically ill postoperative patients: sequential assessment of creatinine osmolar and free water clearance. Crit Care Med 8:68, 1980

42. Kellen M, Aronson S, Roizen MF, et al: Predictive and diagnostic tests of renal failure: a review. Anesth Analg 78:134, 1994

43. Miller TR, Anderson RJ, Linas SL: Urinary diagnostic indices in acute renal failure: a prospective study. Ann Intern Med 89:47, 1978

44. Thadani R, Pascual M, Bonventre JV: Acute renal failure. N Engl J Med 334:1448, 1996

45. Belzberg H, Cornwell EE, Berne TV: The critical care of the severely injured patient: pulmonary and renal support. Surg Clin North Am 76:971, 1996

46. Garwood S: New pharmacologic options for renal preservation. Anesth Clin North Am 18:753, 2000

47. Mathur VS, Swan SK, Lambrecht LJ, et al: The effects of fenoldopam, a selective dopamine receptor agonist, on systemic and renal hemodynamics in normotensive subjects. Crit Care Med 27:1832, 1999

48. Tepel M, Van der Giet M, Schwarzfeld C, et al: Prevention of radiographic-contrast induced reductions in renal function by acetylcysteine. N Engl J Med 343:180, 2000

49. Flamenbaum W, Gehr M, Gross M, et al: Acute renal failure associated with myoglobinemia and hemoglobinemia. Acute Renal Failure. Brenner BM, Lazarus JM, Eds. WB Saunders Co, Philadelphia, 1983, p 269

50. Mattern WD, Sommers SC, Kassirer JP: Oliguric acute renal failure in malignant hypertension. Am J Med 52:187, 1972

51. Goldberg LI: Cardiovascular and renal actions of dopamine: potential clinical applications. Pharmacol Rev 24:1, 1972

52. Bellomo R, Cole L, Ronco C: Hemodynamic support and the role of dopamine. Kidney Int 53:(suppl 66):S71, 1998

53. Davis RF, Lappas DG, Kirklin JK, et al: Acute oliguria after cardiopulmonary bypass: renal functional improvement with low-dose dopamine infu-

sion. Crit Care Med 10:852, 1982

54. Pavoni V, Verri M, Volta CA, et al: Plasma dopamine concentration and effects of low dopamine doses on urinary output after major vascular surgery. Kidney Int 53(suppl 66):S75, 1998

55. Allen BT, Anderson CB, Rubin BG, et al: Preservation of renal function in juxtarenal and suprarenal abdominal aortic aneurysm repair. J Vasc Surg 17:948, 1993

56. Pascual J, Liano F, Ortuno J: The elderly patient with acute renal failure. J Am Soc Nephrol 6:144, 1995

57. Braun SR, Weiss FR, Keller AI, et al: Evaluation of the renal toxicity of heme proteins and their derivatives: a role in the genesis of acute tubular necrosis. J Exp Med 131:443, 1970

58. Laffi G, LaVilla G, Gentilini P: Pathogenesis and management of the hepatorenal syndrome. Semin Liver Dis 14:71, 1994

59. Keller F, Heinze H, Jochimsen F, et al: Risk factors and outcome of 107 patients with decompensated liver disease and acute renal failure: the role of hemodialysis. Renal Failure 17:135, 1995

60. Goedje O, Koeke K, Lichtwarck-Aschoff M, et al: Continuous cardiac output by femoral arterial thermodilution calibrated pulse contour analysis: comparison with pulmonary arterial thermodilution. Crit Care Med 27:2407, 1999

61. Finn WF: Enhanced recovery from postischemic acute renal failure: micropuncture studies in the rat. Circ Res 46:440, 1980

62. Russo D, Memoli B, Andreucci VE: The place of loop diuretics in the treatment of acute and chronic renal failure. Clin Nephrol 28(suppl 1):S69, 1992

63. Solomon R, Werner C, Mann D, et al: Effects of saline, mannitol and furosemide on acute decreases in renal function induced by radiocontrast agents. N Engl J Med 331:1416, 1994

64. Rowe JW, Andres R, Tobin JD, et al: The effect of age on creatinine clearance in men: a cross sectional and longitudinal study. J Gerontol 31:155, 1976

65. Shimamura T, Morrison AB: A progressive glomerulosclerosis occurring in partial five-sixths nephrectomized rats. Am J Pathol 79:95, 1975

66. Compher C, Mullen JL, Barker CF: Nutritional support in renal failure. Surg Clin North Am 71:597, 1991

67. Abel RM: Nutritional support in the patient with acute renal failure. J Am Coll Nutr 2:33, 1983

68. Leverve X, Barnoud D: Stress metabolism and nutritional support in acute renal failure. Kidney Int 53(suppl 66):S62, 1998

69. Maschio G, Oldrizzi L, Tessitore N, et al: Effects of dietary protein and phosphorus restriction on the progression of early renal failure. Kidney Int 22:371, 1982

70. Abel RM, Beck CH Jr, Abbott WM, et al: Improved survival from acute renal failure after treatment with intravenous essential L-amino acids and glucose: results of a prospective double blind study. N Engl J Med 288:695, 1973

71. Bellomo R, Ronco C: Indications and criteria for initiating renal replacement therapy in the intensive care unit. Kidney Int 53(suppl 66):S106, 1998

72. Schetz MR: Classical and alternative indications for continuous renal replacement therapy. Kidney Int 53:(suppl 66):S129, 1998

73. Conger JD: Management of acute renal failure. Principles and Practice of Nephrology. Jacobson HR, Striker GE, Klahr S, Eds. BC Decker, Philadelphia, 1991, p 666

74. Gettings LG, Reynolds HN, Scalea T: Outcome in post-traumatic acute renal failure when continuous renal replacement therapy is applied

75. Bellomo R, Ronco C: Continuous versus intermittent renal replacement therapy in the intensive care unit. Kidney Int 53(suppl 66):S125, 1998

76. Bellomo R, Boyce N: Acute continuous hemodiafiltration: a prospective study of 110 patients and a review of the literature. Am J Kidney Dis 21:508, 1993

77. Kierdorf H: Continuous versus intermittent treatment: clinical results in acute renal failure. Contrib Nephrol 93:1, 1991

78. Ronco C: Continuous renal replacement therapies for the treatment of acute renal failure in intensive care patients. Clin Nephrol 40:187, 1993

79. Bellomo R, Farmer M, Boyce N: The outcome of critically ill elderly patients with severe acute renal failure treated by continuous hemodiafiltration. Int J Artif Organs 17:466, 1994

80. Silvester W: Outcome studies of continuous renal replacement therapy in the intensive care unit. Kidney Int 53(suppl 66):S138, 1998

81. Reichow W, Koehler H, Dietrich K, et al: Continuous arterio-venous hemofiltration for the treatment of acute renal failure in septic shock. Prog Clin Biol Res 236B:235, 1987

82. Golper TA: Continuous arteriovenous hemofiltration in acute renal failure. Am J Kidney Dis 6:373, 1985

83. Cioffi WG, Ashikaga T, Gamelli RL: Probability of surviving postoperative acute renal failure: development of a prognostic index. Ann Surg 200:205, 1984

84. Briglia A: Acute renal failure in the intensive care unit. Clin Chest Med 20:347, 1999

85. Guild WR, Bray G, Merrill JP: Hemopericardium with cardiac tamponade in chronic uremia. N Engl J Med 257:230, 1957

86. Talalla A, Halbrook H, Barbour BH, et al: Subdural hematoma associated with long-term hemodialysis for chronic renal disease. JAMA 212:1847, 1970

87. Galen MA, Steinberg SM, Lowrie EG, et al: Hemorrhagic pleural effusion in patients undergoing chronic hemodialysis. Ann Intern Med 82:359, 1975

88. Wineman RJ: Endstage renal disease. Dial Transplant 7:1034, 1978

89. Schreiber SS, Korzets A, Powsner E, et al: Surgery in chronic dialysis patients. Isr J Med Sci 31:479, 1995

90. Gillum DM, Dixon BS, Yanover MJ, et al: The role of intensive dialysis in acute renal failure. Clin Nephrol 25:249, 1986

91. Booij LH: Neuromuscular transmission and its pharmacological blockade. Pharm World Science 19:35, 1997

92. Williams AR, Bailey M, Joye T, et al: Marked prolongation of the succinylcholine effect two hours after neostigmine reversal of neuromuscular blockade in a patient with renal insufficiency. South Med J 92:77, 1999

93. Thapa S, Sorin J: Succinylcholine–induced hyperkalemia in patients with renal failure: an old question revisited. Anesth Analg 91:237, 2000

94. Nayman J: Effect of renal failure on wound healing in dogs: response to hemodialysis following uremia induced by uranium nitrate. Ann Surg 164:227, 1966

95. Bennett WM: Altering drug dosage in patients with diseases of the kidney and liver. Clinical Uses of Drugs in Patients with Kidney and Liver Disease. Anderson RJ, Schrier RW, Eds. WB Saunders Co, Philadelphia, 1981, p 16

96. Schetz MR: Coagulation disorders in acute renal failure. Kidney Int 53(suppl 66):S96, 1998

97. Eschbach JW: The anemia of chronic renal fail-

ure: pathophysiology and the effects of recombinant erythropoietin. Kidney Int 35:134, 1989

98. Lim VS, DeGowin RL, Zavala D, et al: Recombinant human erythropoietin treatment in predialysis patients: a double-blind placebo-controlled trial. Ann Intern Med 110:108, 1989

99. Tang WW, Stead RA, Goodkin DA: Effects of epoetin alfa on hemostasis in chronic renal failure. Am J Nephrol 18:263, 1998

100. Macdougall IC: Quality of life and anemia: the nephrology experience. Semin Oncol 25(suppl 7):39, 1998

101. McMahon LP, McKenna MJ, Sangkabutra T, et al: Physical performance and associated electrolyte changes after haemoglobin normalization: a comparative study in haemodialysis patients. Nephrol Dial Transplant 14:1182, 1999

102. Tilney NL, Bailey GL, Morgan AP: Sequential system failure after rupture of abdominal aortic aneurysms: an unsolved problem in postoperative care. Ann Surg 178:117, 1973

103. Abel RM, Buckley MJ, Austen WG, et al: Etiology, incidence, and prognosis of renal failure following cardiac operations: results of a prospective analysis of 500 consecutive patients. J Thorac Cardiovasc Surg 71:323, 1976

104. Kron IL, Joob AW, Van Meter C: Acute renal failure in the cardiovascular surgical patient. Ann Thorac Surg 39:590, 1985

105. Durakovic Z, Durakovic A, Durakovic S, et al: The lack of clinical value of laboratory parameters in predicting outcome in acute renal failure. Ren Fail 11:213, 1989

106. Wilkes BM, Mailloux LU: Acute renal failure: pathogenesis and prevention. Am J Med 80:1129, 1986

107. Henrich WL, Anderson RJ, Berns AS, et al: The role of renal nerves and prostaglandins in control of renal hemodynamics and plasma renin activity during hypotensive hemorrhage in the dog. J Clin Invest 61:744, 1978

108. Garrison RN, Wilson MA, Matheson PJ, et al: Nitric oxide mediates redistribution of intrarenal blood flow during bacteremia. J Trauma 39:90, 1995

109. Humes HD: Role of calcium in pathogenesis of acute renal failure. Am J Physiol 250:F579, 1986

110. Rasmussen H, Kojima I, Apfeldorf W, et al: Cellular mechanism of hormone action in the kidney: messenger function of calcium and cyclic AMP. Kidney Int 29:90, 1986

111. Gates GF: Glomerular filtration rate: estimation from fractional renal accumulation of 99mTc-DTPA (stannous). AJR Am J Roentgenol 138:565, 1982

112. Carrie BJ, Golbetz HV, Michaels AS, et al: Creatinine: an inadequate filtration marker in glomerular diseases. Am J Med 69:177, 1980

113. Cronin RE, de Torrente A, Miller PD, et al: Pathogenic mechanisms in early norepinephrine-induced acute renal failure: functional and histological correlates of protection. Kidney Int 14:115, 1978

114. Morel F, Doucet A: Hormonal control of kidney functions at the cell level. Physiol Rev 66:377, 1986

115. Jard S, Butlen D, Cantau B, et al: The mechanisms of action of antidiuretic hormone. Adv Nephrol 13:163, 1984

116. Capasso G, Anastasio P, Giordano D, et al: Atrial natriuretic factor increases glomerular filtration rate in the experimental acute renal failure induced by cisplatin. Adv Exp Med Biol 212:285, 1987

117. Myers BD, Moran SM: Hemodynamically mediated acute renal failure. N Engl J Med 314:97, 1986

118. Levinsky NG: Pathophysiology of acute renal

failure. N Engl J Med 296:1453, 1977

119. Oken DE: On the differential diagnosis of acute renal failure. Am J Med 71:916, 1981

120. Jones DP: Renal metabolism during normoxia, hypoxia, and ischemic injury. Annu Rev Physiol 48:33, 1986

121. Adams PL, Adams FF, Bell PD, et al: Impaired renal blood flow autoregulation in ischemic acute renal failure. Kidney Int 18:68, 1980

122. Harman PK, Kron IL, McLachlan HD, et al: Elevated intra-abdominal pressure and renal function. Ann Surg 196:594, 1982

123. Kron IL, Harman PK, Nolan SP: The measurement of intra-abdominal pressure as a criterion for abdominal re-exploration. Ann Surg 199:28, 1984

124. Epstein M, Lifschitz M, Ramachandran M, et al: Characterization of renal prostaglandin E responsiveness in decompensated cirrhosis: implications for renal sodium handling. Clin Sci 63:555, 1982

125. Molitoris BA: New insights into the cell biology of ischemic acute renal failure. J Am Soc Nephrol 1:1263, 1991

126. Stein JH: Acute renal failure: lessons from pathophysiology. West J Med 156:176, 1992

127. Hohenfellner M, Thuroff JW, Thurau K: Cellular changes in acute renal failure: functional and therapeutic consequences. Eur Urol 22:265, 1992

128. Braam B, Mitchell KD, Koomans HA, et al: Relevance of the tubuloglomerular feedback mechanism in pathophysiology. J Am Soc Nephrol 4:1257, 1993

129. Brezis M, Rosen S, Silva P, et al: Renal ischemia: a new perspective. Kidney Int 26:375, 1984

130. Myers BD: Cyclosporine nephrotoxicity. Kidney Int 30:964, 1986

131. Loirat P, Rohan J, Baillet A, et al: Increased glomerular filtration rate in patients with major burns and its effect on the pharmacokinetics of tobramycin. N Engl J Med 299:915, 1978

132. Bayliss C: The mechanism of the decline in glomerular filtration rate in agent induced acute renal failure in the rat. J Antimicrob Chemother 6:381, 1980

133. Rose BD: Syndrome of inappropriate ADH (SIADH). Clinical Physiology of Acid-Base and Electrolyte Disorders, 2nd ed. McGraw-Hill Book Co, New York, 1984

134. Duke GJ, Bensten AD: Dopamine and renal salvage in the critically ill patient. Anaesth Intensive Care 20:277, 1992

135. Graziani G, Cantaluppi A, Casati S, et al: Dopamine and frusemide in oliguric acute renal failure. Nephron 37:39, 1984

136. Brown CB, Ogg CS, Cameron JS: High dose frusemide in acute renal failure: a controlled clinical trial. Clin Nephrol 15:90, 1981

137. Warren SE, Blantz RC: Mannitol. Arch Intern Med 141:493, 1981

138. Schrier RW: Role of calcium channel blockers in protection against experimental renal injury. Am J Med 90:21S, 1991

139. Wetzels JF, Burker JF, Schrier RW: Calcium channel blockers: protective effects in ischemic acute renal failure. Renal Failure 14:327, 1992

140. Conger JD: Interventions in clinical acute renal failure: what are the data? Am J Kidney Dis 26:565, 1995

141. Humes HD: Potential molecular therapy for acute renal failure. Cleve Clin J Med 60:166, 1993

142. Pru C, Kjellstrand CM: The FENa test is of no value in acute renal failure. Nephron 36:20, 1984

143. Saha H, Mustonen J, Helin H, et al: Limited value of the fractional excretion of sodium test in the diagnosis of acute renal failure. Nephrol Dial Transplant 2:79, 1987

144. Brosius FC, Lau K: Fractional excretion of sodium in acute renal failure: role of timing of the test and ischemia. Am J Nephrol 6:450, 1986

145. Danielson RA: Differential diagnosis and treatment of oliguria in post-traumatic and post-operative patients. Surg Clin North Am 55:697, 1975

146. Lucas CE: The renal response to acute injury and sepsis. Surg Clin North Am 56:953, 1976

147. Schetz M: Renal replacement therapy in patients with chronic renal failure and acute illness in ESRD. Critical Care Nephrology. Ronco C, Bellomo R, Eds. Kluwer, Dordrecht, Netherlands, 1998, p 1139

Acknowledgment

The authors would like to acknowledge the work of Drs. Nicholas L. Tilney, Julian L. Seifter, and Robert J. Rizzo in a chapter entitled "Renal Dysfunction," which appeared in previous versions of *ACS Surgery: Principles & Practice*. Some of their work was incorporated into this chapter.

Figure 2   Dana Burns.

6 HEPATIC FAILURE

Walid S. Arnaout, M.D., and Achilles A. Demetriou, M.D., Ph.D.

Approach to the Patient with Liver Failure

Hepatic failure and cirrhosis continue to be major causes of morbidity and mortality among critically ill patients. Since the beginning of the 1980s, several advances have been made in the management of hepatic failure. Newer diagnostic techniques and therapeutic modalities have been introduced that have led to significantly better overall outcomes. In addition to improved medical therapy, liver transplantation has proved to be effective in treating end-stage liver disease and liver failure, regardless of etiology.

In what follows, we outline general management guidelines for hepatic failure and its complications. We also discuss the role of artificial liver support and its potential use in managing hepatic failure.

Patient Evaluation

RISK FACTORS AND WORKUP

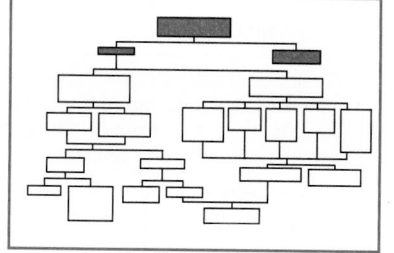

Liver disease is usually suspected on the basis of several risk factors, including a history of alcohol or I.V. drug abuse. Receipt of a blood transfusion before 1992 raises the index of suspicion for viral hepatitis, hepatitis C virus (HCV) infection in particular.[1-3] Other risk factors for liver disease are tattoos, sexual promiscuity, and snorting cocaine. Rare risk factors include a family history of certain liver diseases and exposure to various toxins and chemicals (e.g., aflatoxin and carbon tetrachloride).

Evaluation of patients with suspected liver disease is often complex and typically requires an extensive workup—including a detailed history and physical examination as well as various diagnostic studies—to establish the diagnosis and confirm the underlying cause. The laboratory data usually required include a complete blood count, a platelet count, liver function tests, a prothrombin time (PT), and serum albumin and cholesterol levels. In addition, imaging studies (e.g., abdominal ultrasonography, computed tomography, or magnetic resonance imaging) may be indicated. These studies usually demonstrate anatomic and structural abnormalities in the liver parenchyma, the biliary tree, or the vascular system. Occasionally, a liver biopsy is required to establish or confirm the diagnosis of liver disease.

Liver disease commonly gives rise to several manifestations that are easily recognized by most health care workers: jaundice [*see II:6 Jaundice*], muscle wasting, malnutrition, ascites, lower-extremity edema, and varying degrees of hepatic encephalopathy. Common findings on physical examination of patients with liver disease include bitemporal muscle wasting, vascular spiders, abdominal wall collaterals, caput medusae, palmar erythema, and clubbing. Umbilical and inguinal hernias are frequently noted in patients with tense ascites. Bilateral gynecomastia and testicular atrophy are often seen in male patients.

PRIMARY VERSUS SECONDARY HEPATIC FAILURE

Hepatic failure is generally classified as either primary or secondary, depending on the underlying cause. Primary hepatic failure derives from underlying liver disease, whereas secondary hepatic failure is caused by various underlying conditions unrelated to the liver. Most patients with primary hepatic failure have a history of preexisting liver disease and possibly of cirrhosis, generally presenting with one or more complications of chronic liver disease (e.g., GI bleeding, hepatic encephalopathy, spontaneous bacterial peritonitis, or renal failure). A subgroup of patients, however, exhibit hepatic failure secondary to acute exacerbation of the preexisting liver disease (e.g., acute reactivation of hepatitis B, acute decompensated Wilson disease, or autoimmune hepatitis). In another subgroup, primary hepatic failure develops acutely among patients who have no preexisting liver disease and no known risk factors (so-called acute or fulminant hepatic failure). These patients present with massive liver necrosis, jaundice, and profound coagulopathy and often go on to experience deep coma and cerebral edema, which may lead to irreversible brain damage and death. Acute liver failure can be associated with severe multisystem organ involvement, as in the acute respiratory distress syndrome (ARDS) or the multiple organ dysfunction syndrome (MODS), which makes diagnosis difficult. (This may also be the case with chronic liver disease, but to a lesser degree.)

Secondary liver failure is seen among critically ill patients admitted to the ICU for management of a non–liver-related illness. It is usually manifested by cholestatic jaundice, impaired synthetic activity, varying degrees of hepatocellular damage, and altered mental status. Hepatic insufficiency is common in patients with life-threatening injuries, severe systemic infection, or ARDS. These patients usually have no preexisting liver disease: their liver dysfunction is simply a reflection of their overall critical condition. The extent of the liver dysfunction in such cases usually depends on the severity of the underlying nonhepatic disease; in general, it tends to lessen as the causative problem is controlled or resolved. Failure to control the primary underlying condition leads to progressive MODS and death.

Management of secondary hepatic failure typically involves treating underlying nonhepatic disorders. Accordingly, we focus here on management of acute and chronic primary hepatic failure, which by definition involves treating hepatic disease and its associated complications.

Approach to the Patient with Liver Failure

Patient has signs of liver disease or known risk factors

Perform extensive workup: history, physical examination, laboratory tests, and imaging studies as needed. Liver biopsy is occasionally required.

Distinguish primary from secondary hepatic failure.

Primary hepatic failure

Acute liver failure

Determine etiology—viral, drug-induced, toxin-induced, or other—and treat accordingly.

Begin medical management of complications.

Concurrently, assess prognosis by means of King's College criteria.

Cerebral edema

Initiate invasive ICP monitoring.

Manage elevated ICP.

Extrahepatic complications

Treat fluid, electrolyte, and nutritional abnormalities; renal failure; pulmonary complications; infectious complications; and coagulopathy and bleeding.

Good prognosis with medical management

Continue medical therapy.

Poor prognosis with medical management

Medical management succeeds

Medical management fails

Consider emergency OLT if not contraindicated.

Treat toxic liver syndrome with total hepatectomy and end-to-side portacaval shunt, followed by OLT.

Consider use of BAL support system.

Transplantation is contraindicated

Manage medically.

No contraindications to transplantation are present

Secondary hepatic failure

Treat underlying nonhepatic cause.

Chronic liver disease

Determine etiology [*see Table 4*], and treat accordingly.
Begin medical management of complications.

Portal hypertension

Treat complications of PHT:
- Variceal bleeding
- Ascites: restrict sodium and give diuretics. If medical management fails, perform LVP or use a shunt (peritoneovenous or TIPS).

Hepatic encephalopathy

Control precipitating factors, and control ammonia levels with lactulose or antibiotics.

Renal failure

Treat HRS, ATN, RTA, and drug-induced interstitial nephritis.
Correct underlying causes. Manage fluids and electrolytes carefully.

Malnutrition

GIve glucose with fat emulsion.
Use enteral feeding unless contraindicated.

Coagulopathy and bleeding

Identify hemostatic defect.
Give FFP, cryoprecipitate, prothrombin complex concentrates, platelets, AT-III concentrate, or antifibrinolytic agents as appropriate.

Medical management is unsatisfactory, and no contraindications to transplantation are present

Medical management is satisfactory, or transplantation is contraindicated

Manage medically.

Perform OLT when donor organ is available.
Consider use of BAL support system while awaiting organ.

Acute Liver Failure

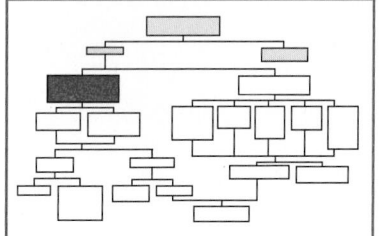

In the United States, acute liver failure (ALF) affects approximately 5,000 persons each year. The definition of ALF depends on the temporal relation between the initial onset of illness and the manifestation of jaundice, encephalopathy, and coagulopathy. The classic definition of Trey and Davidson is based on massive liver necrosis associated with encephalopathy developing within 8 weeks of the onset of illness.[4] In most cases, however, it is difficult to determine the precise time of onset of the disease process and thus the exact time elapsed before the establishment of hepatic failure. Recognizing that clinical findings and prognosis varied depending on the interval between onset of jaundice and encephalopathy, Bernuau and coworkers defined fulminant hepatic failure (FHF) as ALF complicated by encephalopathy developing within 2 weeks of the onset of jaundice and defined subfulminant hepatic failure (SFHF) as ALF complicated by encephalopathy developing 2 to 12 weeks after onset of jaundice.[5]

Differences in nomenclature and classification notwithstanding, the defining characteristic of ALF is the absence of known preexisting liver disease. We use the term FHF more or less interchangeably with ALF as defined by Trey and Davidson.

ETIOLOGY

The causes of FHF may be classified into four major groups: viral, drug-induced, toxin-induced, and miscellaneous. In one multicenter study, acetaminophen-induced FHF toxicity was found to be the most common variety (20%), followed by FHF of indeterminate etiology (15%).[6]

Viral Hepatitis

Hepatitis A   The incidence of FHF and SFHF in hepatitis A virus (HAV) infection is very low (< 0.01%).[5] Young patients with HAV infection rarely manifest FHF, and their chances of survival with medical therapy are relatively good (40% to 60%). About 10% of patients experience relapses, usually within 2 to 3 months after an initial clinical improvement. Relapse is signaled by an increase in serum transaminase and bilirubin levels and the reappearance of virus in the stool. If encephalopathy occurs during this period, the outcome is poor.[7]

Hepatitis B   ALF related to hepatitis B virus (HBV) accounts for fewer than 1% of HBV infections but is the most common form of viral-induced FHF.[6,8] Like HAV infection, HBV infection leads to FHF more often than to SFHF. Hepatitis B surface antigen (HBsAg) and HBV DNA may be absent in some cases of FHF secondary to HBV infection.[9] These findings indicate that in certain FHF patients, an enhanced immune response prevents further HBV replication and results in more rapid clearance of HBsAg. The survival rate for patients who are HBsAg-positive on presentation (17%) is much lower than that for patients who are HBsAg-negative (47%).[5] Clearance of HBsAg and HBV DNA results in better survival rates as well as lower recurrence rates after emergency liver transplantation.[10]

Hepatitis D   Hepatitis D virus (HDV, also referred to as the delta agent) is a defective virus that uses HBsAg as its envelope protein. HDV RNA is detected in only 10% of patients with fulminant hepatitis D.[11] HDV infection can be either a coinfection, in conjunction with HBV infection, or a superinfection in patients with previous HBV infection [see VI:19 Viral Infection].[12] Among patients with FHF,

HDV coinfection is more common than superinfection; however, HDV superinfection is associated with a higher mortality than HDV coinfection (72% versus 52%) and more often predisposes to chronic liver disease (54% versus 31%).[13]

Hepatitis C and hepatitis of indeterminate etiology   Previously, FHF of indeterminate etiology was attributed to non-A, non-B viral hepatitis. It is now clear that some such cases are caused by hepatitis C virus (HCV) infection, though the precise extent to which HCV infection contributes to this indeterminate group is unclear. Unlike HAV and HBV infection, HCV infection is more likely to cause SFHF than FHF. Despite the availability of advanced serologic testing, there are still many cases of FHF and SFHF whose cause cannot be determined.[14,15] These patients are placed into a non-A, non-B, non-C (NANBNC) category, implying a viral etiology. A more accurate designation for this category would be "of indeterminate etiology," in that the true cause is unknown and may not, in fact, be undiagnosed viral hepatitis.

Drugs

Drug toxicity accounts for 35% of all cases of FHF and SFHF and usually runs a subfulminant course.[6] Drug ingestion causes hepatic injury in fewer than 1% of patients, about 20% of whom manifest FHF or SFHF. Increasing the total drug dose, simultaneously ingesting other drugs that induce or inhibit hepatic enzymes, and continuing drug administration after the onset of liver disease all increase the risk of hepatic failure.[5] Acetaminophen toxicity is the most common cause of drug-induced hepatic failure. The prognosis for FHF caused by acetaminophen is usually better than that for FHF caused by other drugs (e.g., isoniazid, psychotropic drugs, antihistamines, and nonsteroidal anti-inflammatory drugs [NSAIDs]).[16] Halothane-induced FHF occurs within 2 weeks of general anesthesia and carries a high mortality.[17]

Toxins

Most cases of toxin-induced FHF involve mushroom poisoning or exposure to industrial hydrocarbons. In mushroom poisoning, the active agents are heat-stable and are not destroyed by cooking. Liver damage from mushroom toxins is delayed and is usually preceded by several days of vomiting and diarrhea. Mortality is high: up to 22% in one series.[18] Emergency liver transplantation is sometimes successful.[19]

Industrial hydrocarbons (e.g., carbon tetrachloride and trichloroethylene) are rare causes of FHF. In developing nations, aflatoxin and herbal medicines have been implicated as causes of FHF.

Miscellaneous Conditions

Wilson disease may present as FHF or SFHF with intravascular hemolysis and renal failure.[20,21] A family history of hepatic and neurologic disease, the presence of Kayser-Fleischer rings, and low serum ceruloplasmin levels help establish the diagnosis. Acute decompensated Wilson disease carries a high mortality and is therefore an indication for emergency liver transplantation.[22]

Acute fatty liver of pregnancy is a rare cause of FHF that carries a high mortality for both mother and infant. Delivery of the fetus results in regression of the microvesicular steatosis and abnormal liver test results for the mother. The risk of FHF is increased with misdiagnosis and continuation of pregnancy. Liver transplantation has been successfully performed.[23]

Several other conditions and disease processes are known to cause ALF in both adults and children [see Table 1].

ASSESSMENT OF PROGNOSIS

Several prognostic criteria and indicators have been proposed for

Table 1 Etiology of Acute Liver Failure

Infectious
Viral: hepatitis A, B, C, D, and E and hepatitis of indeterminate etiology; infection by herpes simplex virus, cytomegalovirus, Epstein-Barr virus, or adenovirus
Bacterial: Q fever
Parasitic: amebiasis

Drugs

Toxins
Mushrooms: *Amanita phalloides, verna,* and *virosa; Lepiota* species
Bacillus cereus
Hydrocarbons: carbon tetrachloride, trichloroethylene, 2-nitropropane, chloroform
Copper
Aflatoxin
Yellow phosphorus

Miscellaneous conditions
Wilson disease
Acute fatty liver of pregnancy
Reye syndrome
Hypoxic liver cell necrosis
Hypothermia or hyperthermia
Budd-Chiari syndrome
Veno-occlusive disease of the liver
Autoimmune hepatitis
Massive malignant infiltration of the liver
Partial hepatectomy
Liver transplantation
Postjejunoileal bypass
Galactosemia
Hereditary fructose intolerance
Tyrosinemia
Erythropoietic protoporphyria
Irradiation
α_1-Antitrypsin deficiency
Niemann-Pick disease
Neonatal hemochromatosis
Cardiac tamponade
Right ventricular failure
Circulatory shock
Tuberculosis

predicting outcome after optimal medical management of FHF. The two main factors determining the likelihood of survival are (1) the extent of liver necrosis and (2) the potential for hepatocyte regeneration. In a 1989 study, investigators at King's College Hospital in London compiled a set of indicators for predicting a poor outcome after medical therapy and hence the need for emergency liver transplantation.[24] Underlying etiology was the single most important predictive variable. Therefore, patients were divided into two groups, one comprising all cases of acetaminophen-induced FHF and the other all cases of FHF from other causes. Age, degree of encephalopathy, serum pH, PT, interval to onset of encephalopathy, and admission serum creatinine and bilirubin levels also proved to be significant variables [see Table 2]. Patients who met the criteria in either group had a 95% chance of dying with medical therapy alone and were identified as candidates for emergency liver transplantation.

The major strength of the King's College study is that it based patient assessment on parameters that are easily obtained within a few hours of admission to the emergency department. This approach to assessment facilitates early referral of patients with a poor prognosis to a specialized liver unit for evaluation for transplanta-

tion. In another study, plasma factor V level and age were found to be independent predictors of survival.[25] The criteria for liver transplantation were the presence of hepatic encephalopathy (stage III or IV) and a factor V level either less than 20% of normal in patients younger than 30 years or less than 30% of normal in patients older than 30 years.

In addition to biochemical and synthetic activities, assessment of the residual functional reserve of the liver has been studied as an indicator of prognosis. The ratio of acetoacetate to β-hydroxybutyrate in an arterial blood sample (also known as the arterial ketone body ratio [AKBR]) is thought to reflect hepatic energy status.[26] Galactose clearance reflects both residual liver mass and hepatic blood flow.[27] This test has long been considered a standard test of liver functional reserve, and newer tests are routinely compared to it. At present, functional assessment tools are not routinely used in patient assessment.

The wide variety of potential prognostic indicators for FHF notwithstanding, the King's College criteria are still the most widely used. These criteria have been validated in several large series and are currently considered the gold standard for predicting outcome in FHF patients undergoing medical management.

At our center, we apply the King's College criteria at admission to predict the likely outcome with medical therapy. Once the initial assessment is completed, the decision for or against emergency evaluation for liver transplantation is made. Evaluation, if indicated, is usually completed within 12 to 24 hours. The evaluation is similar to that of patients with chronic liver disease [see Chronic Liver Disease, below], with a few exceptions. In particular, patients with FHF usually do not have preexisting liver disease; thus, it is vital that the evaluation [see Table 3] reveal the probable cause of liver failure. Unlike chronic liver disease, FHF is associated with cerebral edema and elevated intracranial pressure (ICP), which is the leading cause of death among these patients. Therefore, an extensive neurologic evaluation should be completed before a patient is listed for transplantation. Serial neurologic assessment is necessary to rule out irreversible brain damage and brain-stem herniation; however, previous sedation often makes this step very difficult.

Table 2 King's College Hospital Prognostic Criteria Predicting Poor Outcome for Patients with FHF

Acetaminophen-induced FHF	pH < 7.30 (irrespective of grade of encephalopathy) *or* All of the following: PT > 100 sec (INR > 6.5) Serum creatinine > 3.4 g/dl Stage III or IV hepatic encephalopathy
Non–acetaminophen-induced FHF	PT > 100 sec (INR > 6.5) (irrespective of grade of encephalopathy) *or* Any three of the following (irrespective of grade of encephalopathy): Age < 10 or > 40 yr Etiology: non-A, non-B hepatitis, halothane hepatitis, drug toxicity Duration of jaundice to encephalopathy > 7 days PT 50 sec (INR > 3.5) Serum bilirubin > 17.5 g/dl

FHF—fulminant hepatic failure   INR—international normalized ratio
PT—prothrombin time

TREATMENT
OF COMPLICATIONS

Cerebral Edema

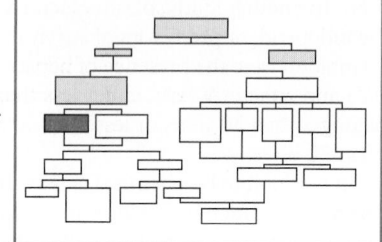

Cerebral edema is one of the hallmarks of FHF, and its presence significantly influences management and outcome. Autopsy studies indicate that cerebral edema is present in 80% of patients who die of FHF.[28,29] It occurs in advanced stages of FHF and can be recognized by clinical, radiologic, or invasive means. Clinical findings include decerebrate posturing, myoclonus, spastic rigidity, seizure activity, systemic hypertension, bradycardia, hyperventilation, and mydriasis with diminished pupillary response. These findings initially are paroxysmal but later become persistent. Papilledema is a late finding and often does not occur at all, even in the advanced stages of the disease.[30] Noninvasive diagnostic modalities (e.g., CT scanning, electroencephalographic monitoring, and transcranial Doppler flow measurement) have not proved helpful for early detection and management of cerebral edema.[31,32] CT scanning of the brain is not a sensitive test for detecting early cerebral edema: 25% to 30% of patients with high ICP exhibit no radiographic changes.[33] It is, however, useful for ruling out intracranial bleeding.

Currently, ICP monitoring is the best means of monitoring intracranial hypertension and is recommended for guiding treatment in patients with stage III or IV encephalopathy. ICP can be measured by using epidural, subdural, or intraventricular catheters. Although epidural catheters are slightly less sensitive to ICP changes, they have the lowest complication rate (3.8%) and lowest rate of fatal hemorrhage (1%).[34] Despite a slightly higher complication rate, we prefer subdural catheters: in our view, they offer more reliable ICP monitoring. Institution of ICP monitoring necessitates aggressive treatment of any concomitant coagulopathy. Fresh frozen plasma (FFP) infusions are given to bring the PT below 25 seconds, and platelet transfusions are indicated if the patient has severe thrombocytopenia (platelet count < 50,000/mm³). Once ICP monitoring is established, bolus administration of FFP is repeated as needed to keep the prothrombin time low (international normalized ratio [INR] ≤ 5) so as to reduce the risk of intracranial bleeding.

The goal of invasive monitoring is to keep ICP below 15 mm Hg while keeping cerebral perfusion pressure (CPP), which is a better predictor of outcome, above 50 mm Hg. CPP is calculated by subtracting ICP from mean arterial pressure (MAP) [see I:9 Coma, Seizures, Cognitive Impairment, and Brain Death]. ICP monitoring allows early detection of cerebral edema and hence early introduction of aggressive management. To date, no randomized, controlled trials have addressed the effect of either high ICP or low CPP on outcome after liver transplantation; however, it appears that the persistence of either an ICP higher than 25 mm Hg or a CPP lower than 40 mm Hg for more than 2 hours is associated with an increased risk of irreversible brain damage and a poor outcome.[35,36]

Management of elevated ICP involves hyperventilation, minimization of external stimuli, deep sedation, elevation of the head, maintenance of hemodynamic stability, and infusion of mannitol. Patients are usually sedated with a short-acting agent (e.g., fentanyl) in small boluses before operation, nasotracheal suction, venipuncture, or line placement. Mechanical hyperventilation lowers ICP by lowering arterial carbon dioxide tension (P_aCO_2) to 25 to 30 mm Hg, thereby maximizing cerebral vascular constriction and reducing blood flow. This vascular effect diminishes progressively after 6 hours of therapy, though a clinical response is apparent for days. As many as 80% of patients without renal failure respond to mannitol infusions.[37] Serum

osmolality should be measured frequently and maintained at 300 to 320 mOsm/L. Mannitol should be withheld if osmolality reaches or exceeds 320 mOsm/L, if renal failure occurs, or if oliguria and rising serum osmolality develop simultaneously. Repeated administration of mannitol may reverse the osmotic gradient. Mannitol should be discontinued if ICP does not respond after the first few boluses.

Patients who do not respond to conventional therapy may be placed in a barbiturate coma. Thiopental infusion decreases cerebral metabolic activity, lowers CNS oxygen demand, and protects the brain from ischemic injury secondary to decreased cerebral blood flow. In one retrospective, nonrandomized study, it lowered ICP and reduced mortality from FHF.[38] In our experience, however, the effect of thiopental infusion on ICP is transient and unpredictable.

Other Complications

In addition to cerebral edema and increased ICP, MODS and a variety of life-threatening complications are associated with FHF. Most of these complications are similar to those seen in chronic liver disease

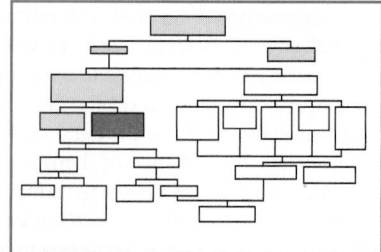

[see Chronic Liver Disease, Treatment of Complications, below]; however, the following complications are seen with particular frequency in FHF.

Table 3 Liver Transplant Evaluation and Workup for FHF Patients

Laboratory workup
  CBC and differential count
  Chemistry panel
  Coagulation profile
  24-hr creatinine clearance
  Urinalysis
  Arterial blood gases
  ANA, AMA, ceruloplasmin, urinary copper, α_1-antitrypsin
  AFP
  RPR
  Thyroid function tests
  Alcohol and drug toxicology screen

Viral serologies
  Hepatitis A virus (IgM, IgG)
  Hepatitis B virus (HBsAg, HBcAb, HBeAg, HBV DNA)
  Hepatitis C virus (HCV antibody, HCV RNA-PCR)
  Cytomegalovirus
  Epstein-Barr virus
  HIV

Cultures
  Bacterial, fungal, and viral cultures
  Blood
  Sputum
  Urine
  Ascites

12-lead ECG

Chest x-ray

Pulmonary function tests

Abdominal Doppler ultrasonography

CT scans of head

AFP—α-fetoprotein AMA—antimitochondrial antibody ANA—antinuclear antibody RPR—rapid plasma reagent

Fluid, electrolyte, and nutritional abnormalities Euvolemia must be maintained to prevent fluid overload, pulmonary edema, and dehydration; extreme fluid shifts should be avoided. The presence of cerebral edema and intracranial hypertension calls for careful fluid administration so as not to expand the intravascular space or exacerbate the edema. Electrolyte and acid-base imbalances are frequent in FHF patients and should be managed appropriately. Hyperkalemia may be multifactorial; usually, it is secondary to liver necrosis, massive transfusion, acid-base imbalance, or renal failure. Acidosis results from increased lactic acid production and decreased handling of lactate by the failing liver. Compensatory respiratory alkalosis develops initially, but if encephalopathy progresses, respiratory acidosis may result. Sodium or potassium bicarbonate infusions should be administered in cases of severe acidosis. Acetate provides twice the bicarbonate load and is metabolized outside the liver; thus, if sodium and potassium intake is severely restricted, continuous infusion of acetate salts may be useful.

Initially, amino acids should be withheld to prevent excessive nitrogen loading; later, limited nitrogen supplementation (70 to 80 g protein/day) may be provided. Most patients present with severe hypoglycemia, which can be fatal and warrants aggressive therapy. Hypoglycemia should be corrected rapidly by infusion of a 50% dextrose solution, followed by continuous infusion of a more dilute solution at a rate of 4 mg/kg/min. A 10% solution is usually adequate; however, higher concentrations should be considered in patients whose hypoglycemia persists or whose fluid intake is restricted. Caloric supplementation has not been extensively studied in FHF.

Renal failure Renal failure occurs in as many as 55% of FHF patients. Functional renal failure is the most common cause of renal failure in this population. However, acute tubular necrosis is more common in these patients than in those with chronic liver disease and cirrhosis.[39] This is especially true in patients who have not been resuscitated adequately, who have experienced prolonged hypotension, or who have ingested hepatotoxins that are also nephrotoxic (e.g., acetaminophen).

Adequate urine volume can be maintained by means of judicious volume expansion, administration of loop diuretics, or both, along with infusion of renal doses of dopamine. Depleted intravascular volume may be managed by giving blood products, volume expanders, or both. Because the plasma albumin level is invariably low, salt-poor albumin solutions may be preferable to carbohydrate-based volume expanders. If oliguria is present—especially if mannitol is administered to treat ICP—hemodialysis or hemofiltration may be needed to maintain optimal fluid volume.

Pulmonary complications Pulmonary complications—especially pulmonary edema, aspiration pneumonia, and ARDS—are common in FHF patients.[40] Pulmonary edema is seen in as many as 40% of cases. Supplemental oxygen and mechanical ventilation are always indicated. Sedative and paralytic agents may be required to ensure tolerance of ventilation; however, they should be used sparingly because they may hinder neurologic evaluation. Aspiration pneumonia should be treated aggressively because it is a potential contraindication to transplantation.

Infectious complications Infection poses a serious threat to FHF patients both by placing them at risk for sepsis and by constituting a contraindication to liver transplantation. Immunologic defects observed in this setting include impaired opsonization, impaired chemotaxis, impaired neutrophil and Kupffer cell function, and complement deficiency.[41,42] Bacterial infection, usually deriving from the respiratory or urinary tract or from a central venous catheter, occurs in more than 80% of cases. In one study, bacteremia was documented in

25% of patients, with staphylococci, streptococci, and gram-negative rods the most common pathogens.[43] Because most FHF patients have percutaneous lines and indwelling catheters in place, iatrogenic sources must always be considered. Fungal infection is less common than bacterial infection in this setting; however, one series found a significant incidence of fungal infections, with *Candida albicans* cultured in 33% of the patients studied.[44] The majority of these patients had renal failure and had been treated with antibiotics for longer than 5 days.

The high prevalence of infection notwithstanding, we do not advocate antibiotic prophylaxis in this population unless there is a strong suspicion of active infection or an ICP monitor is in place. However, our decision threshold for starting antibiotics is low, given that the usual clinical presentations (e.g., fever and leukocytosis) may be absent in as many as 30% of FHF patients.[43] Surveillance cultures for bacteria and fungi must be obtained at frequent intervals from blood (peripheral and central lines), urine, sputum, and open wounds. If ascites is present, the ascitic fluid should be cultured. In addition, chest x-rays should be obtained to identify developing infiltrates. Administration of broad-spectrum antibiotics should be initiated at the first sign of infection; as soon as an organism is identified, coverage may be focused more narrowly. Initiation of antifungal therapy with either amphotericin B or another agent should be considered either if fungal culture is positive or if fever persists beyond 5 days while the patient is receiving antibiotics—especially if renal failure is present. The duration of antimicrobial therapy should be individualized for each patient. Follow-up cultures are recommended if a specific organism is isolated.

Coagulopathy and bleeding Bleeding is a frequent complication of FHF, typically resulting from massive liver necrosis, impaired hepatic synthesis of clotting factors, and platelet dysfunction. All clotting factors synthesized by the liver (i.e., factors II, V, VII, IX, and X) exhibit depressed plasma activity in FHF. Factor II, with a half-life of 2 hours, is the first to be depleted with hepatocellular dysfunction and also the first to be repleted with hepatocellular recovery. The PT is invariably prolonged, reflecting a generalized clotting factor deficiency; it is used as one of the criteria for determining the chances of spontaneous recovery. At some centers, FFP transfusion is withheld and the PT is followed carefully to determine upward or downward trends in the course of the disease and hence the likelihood of spontaneous recovery or need for transplantation (unless the PT > 25 seconds or the INR > 5, especially if an ICP monitor is in place). Intracranial bleeding and its neurologic sequelae are the most devastating complications of coagulopathy in FHF patients.

Thrombocytopenia and abnormalities of platelet function are also common in FHF. Acute splenomegaly, consumptive coagulopathy, and bone marrow suppression all contribute to the development of thrombocytopenia. Conversely, clearance of older platelets from the blood by the reticuloendothelial system is hindered, which results in an older, less effective platelet pool. In one study, a mean platelet count of 50,000/mm³ was associated with a higher incidence of GI hemorrhage.[45] Our current practice is to give platelets to patients who either are thrombocytopenic (platelet count < 50,000/mm³) or are actively bleeding.

OUTCOME OF MEDICAL THERAPY

Because of the complexity of the underlying disease, medical management of FHF requires a multidisciplinary approach. Hemodynamic and respiratory support and prevention and

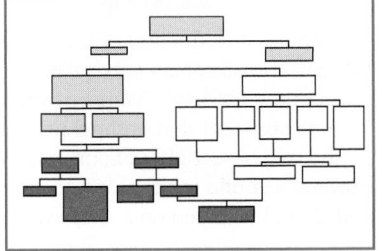

treatment of cerebral edema are major goals. Complications of liver failure must be treated aggressively to prevent sepsis, ARDS, and MODS, which is the second most common cause of death in these patients if they survive the first few days. As noted [see Assessment of Prognosis, above], liver transplant evaluation must be carried out simultaneously with aggressive ICU care, and the patient's chances of spontaneous recovery must be assessed. In addition to determining the King's College prognostic score at admission, we follow the general trend in the clinical course with respect to the development of encephalopathy, ICP elevation, coagulopathy, metabolic acidosis, and renal failure. The decision whether to continue with medical therapy or to perform liver transplantation must be made whenever a donor liver becomes available. In general, patients who appear to be deteriorating rapidly and who have no contraindications to liver transplantation should undergo emergency liver transplantation. Similarly, patients whose synthetic function does not improve within the first 48 to 72 hours should be considered for liver transplantation: the risk of complications and death from MODS if transplantation is not done outweighs the risk attendant on the procedure.

Toxic Liver Syndrome

Even with a multidisciplinary, comprehensive approach to therapy, a few patients with FHF go on to manifest the so-called toxic liver syndrome, characterized by severe intracranial hypertension, profound lactic acidosis, hemodynamic instability, and MODS. It has been suggested that removal of the necrotic liver might improve the hemodynamic status of these patients and lower their ICP. In such extreme cases, a two-stage procedure has been performed: total hepatectomy with an end-to-side portacaval shunt, followed by liver transplantation when an allograft becomes available. In one large series,[46,47] 32 adult patients with toxic liver syndrome underwent total hepatectomy with a portacaval shunt. The patients were anhepatic for several hours (range, 6.5 to 41.4). Whereas 13 patients showed no signs of improvement after hepatectomy and soon died of MODS, 19 became more stable and underwent the full procedure. Only seven patients were alive at 46 months.

In the early 1990s, we used this approach to treat an 18-year-old female patient with uncontrollable cerebral edema secondary to FHF; she underwent total hepatectomy with a portacaval shunt, followed by orthotopic liver transplantation (OLT) 14 hours later.[48] During the anhepatic period, she was supported with the help of a bioartificial liver (BAL) [see Discussion, Bioartifical Liver Support System, below]. With artificial liver support, the severe neurologic dysfunction was reversed, ICP was normalized, and the serum ammonia level was reduced. The patient recovered completely, with no neurologic deficits. We subsequently used the same approach with another FHF patient in our unit, also successfully (unpublished data). It appears that for highly selected patients exhibiting severe toxic metabolic derangement and uncontrollable intracranial hypertension, total hepatectomy with a portacaval shunt—preferably accompanied by some form of artificial liver support—followed by OLT may be considered as a desperate salvage measure.

LIVER TRANSPLANTATION

With the introduction of OLT as a treatment modality for FHF patients, overall patient survival has improved from less than 20% to greater than 60%.[49,50] As more experience was gained with OLT, it became apparent that optimal patient selection is essential for successful outcome. FHF patients must be considered for OLT before irreversible brain injury, MODS, and sepsis develop. Patient selection should be based on a clear understanding of the natural history of the disease as well as of the underlying etiology and the likelihood of spontaneous recovery without transplantation. One of the most difficult aspects of the management of these patients is the lack of reliable prognostic indicators or criteria predicting outcome. In our experience, the King's College criteria are less sensitive and specific in determining prognosis for patients with acetaminophen-induced FHF than for patients with FHF from other causes (71% and 78% versus 96% and 100%).[51]

As a result of these imperfectly reliable criteria, a small number of patients who either might have recovered spontaneously or might have sustained irreversible brain damage undergo unnecessary or unwarranted liver transplantation. Given the severe shortage of organ donors as well as the cost and medical consequences of liver transplantation and a commitment to lifelong immunosuppression, this is a significant problem.

Chronic Liver Disease

Chronic liver disease usually develops as a result of long-standing, ongoing injury to one or more components of the liver, including the liver parenchyma, the biliary tree, and the hepatic and biliary blood vessels. 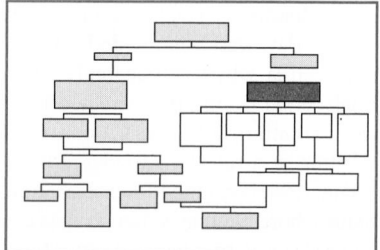 The repeated injury and the ensuing repair usually result in deposition of excessive amount of extracellular matrix (ECM), with or without accompanying inflammation. As the disease process progresses, excess ECM forms connective tissue bridges linking portal and central areas (so-called bridging fibrosis), which eventually lead to the formation of dense collagen bands enclosing nodules of hepatocytes—that is, to cirrhosis. Cirrhosis is an irreversible state that gives rise to significant physiologic impairment, including poor exchange of nutrients and metabolites between sinusoidal blood and hepatocytes. Eventually, the lobular architecture becomes distorted and blood flow altered, leading to portal hypertension and its numerous complications. In addition to portal hypertension, repeated parenchymal injury results in the loss of a large number of functioning hepatocytes and subsequently in hepatic failure.

ETIOLOGY

Like ALF, chronic liver disease is usually classified into various categories on the basis of the underlying causative process [see Table 4].

TREATMENT OF COMPLICATIONS

Chronic liver disease may be associated with a variety of complications, depending on the nature and extent of hepatocyte injury and regeneration. Most patients with chronic liver disease and possible cirrhosis are well compensated, maintain a relatively normal functional status, and remain essentially undiagnosed; however, a small percentage eventually become symptomatic. Hepatic failure secondary to cirrhosis is not an all-or-none phenomenon: patients may lose one or more specific liver functions while retaining the remainder. In addition to the hepatic effects, cirrhosis and hepatic failure can exert a wide range of extrahepatic effects that involve virtually every organ system, leading to MODS and death in most cases if appropriate therapy is not instituted promptly. Consequently, treatment of cirrhosis and chronic hepatic failure must focus on treating both the underlying primary disease and all of its extrahepatic manifestations and complications.

Table 4 Etiology of Chronic Liver Disease

Alcoholic liver disease (exclude acute alcoholic hepatitis)
Viral hepatitis
  Hepatitis B virus
  Hepatitis C virus
Biliary cirrhosis
  Primary biliary cirrhosis
  Primary sclerosing cholangitis
  Secondary sclerosing cholangitis
  Biliary atresia
Autoimmune hepatitis
Metabolic abnormalities
  Wilson disease
  α_1-Antitrypsin deficiency
  Hemochromatosis
  Inborn errors of metabolism
Cryptogenic cirrhosis
Miscellaneous
  Vascular anomalies (Budd-Chiari syndrome)
  Toxin- or drug-induced
  Inborn errors of metabolism
  Other

Portal Hypertension

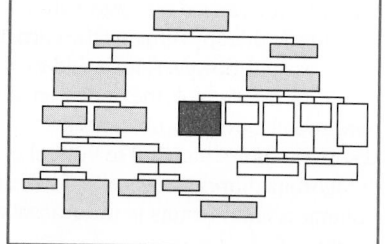

In the majority of patients with chronic liver disease and cirrhosis, portal hypertension (PHT) develops as a result of increased resistance to portal venous blood flow within the liver. PHT is defined as portal venous pressure higher than 12 mm Hg or a hepatic wedge venous pressure that exceeds the inferior vena cava pressure by more than 5 mm Hg. It is classified as prehepatic, hepatic, or posthepatic according to the anatomic site of increased portal venous resistance [see Table 5]. Hepatic PHT is further classified according to the functional relationship to the hepatic sinusoids. Sinusoidal obstruction is more frequently seen with postnecrotic cirrhosis (e.g., from HCV and HBV infection), whereas postsinusoidal obstruction is more common with alcoholic cirrhosis. Prehepatic and posthepatic causes of PHT are less often encountered in patients with cirrhosis; however, efforts should always be made to rule out such causes, because these conditions all require different therapeutic approaches.

PHT is associated with numerous complications, most of which are life-threatening if not diagnosed and treated promptly [see Table 6]. Generally, these complications result from adaptive physiologic responses to elevated portal venous pressure, which lead to the development of collateral vessels or shunts to decompress the portal venous system. The absence of valves within the portal venous system allows retrograde portal blood flow into the splenic and mesenteric circulation and rerouting of blood into the systemic circulation through newly formed collaterals. Several portosystemic venous collateral networks have been identified within the GI tract, the peritoneal cavity, the chest, the retroperitoneum, and subcutaneous tissue. Patients with cirrhosis frequently have one or more areas of collateral formation.

Variceal bleeding The most dramatic and catastrophic complication of PHT is bleeding from esophageal and gastric varices.

Prompt diagnosis and management are vital. Since the early 1990s, management of variceal bleeding has evolved significantly, thanks to the advent of novel endoscopic therapies and nonoperative portosystemic shunt procedures.

Although the esophagus and the stomach are the most common sites of bleeding varices, other sites within the GI tract may be involved as well, including the duodenum, the jejunum, the rectum, and ileostomy and colostomy sites [see Table 7]. The diagnosis and management of gastrointestinal bleeding associated with varices are discussed in more detail elsewhere in this text [see II:8 Upper Gastrointestinal Bleeding].

Ascites Ascites—that is, leakage of lymph fluid into the peritoneal cavity—is one of the principal clinical manifestations of cirrhosis and PHT. Its appearance is indicative of advanced liver disease and is associated with a poor prognosis.[52] It is believed that increased hepatic sinusoidal pressure results in increased formation of lymph and causes hepatic lymph to weep from Glisson's capsule into the peritoneal cavity. As ascitic fluid accumulates, patients exhibit increasing abdominal distention, which causes abdominal pain, decreased appetite, dyspnea, and, occasionally, pleural effusion (so-called hepatic hydrothorax). Umbilical and inguinal hernias are common in patients with tense ascites.

Evaluation. Hepatic ascites should be distinguished from other types of ascites (e.g., chylous, malignant, or cardiac). All patients with ascites should undergo diagnostic paracentesis to characterize the fluid and rule out bacterial peritonitis (see below). In addition, therapeutic large-volume paracentesis (LVP) is indicated for patients who are symptomatic as a result of the large volume of ascitic fluid.

Ascitic fluid analysis should include a white blood cell count and a differential count, Gram stain and cultures, and measurement of total protein, albumin, glucose, lactic dehydrogenase (LDH), and

Table 5 Etiology of Portal Hypertension

Prehepatic obstruction
  Splenic vein thrombosis
  Portal vein thrombosis
  Partial nodular transformation
Hepatic obstruction
  Presinusoidal
    Idiopathic portal hypertension
    Schistosomiasis
    Congenital hepatic fibrosis
    Sarcoidosis
  Sinusoidal
    Nodular regenerative hyperplasia
    Most forms of cirrhosis
    Viral hepatitis
    Acute alcoholic hepatitis
  Postsinusoidal
    Alcoholic cirrhosis
    Veno-occlusive disease
Posthepatic obstruction
  Budd-Chiari syndrome
  IVC web
  Right-sided congestive heart failure/tricuspid valve insufficiency
  Constrictive pericarditis

IVC—inferior vena cava

Table 6 Complications of Portal Hypertension

Variceal bleeding
Portal hypertensive gastropathy
Ascites
    Spontaneous bacterial peritonitis
Spontaneous shunts
Encephalopathy
Hypersplenism

---

amylase concentrations. In addition, the serum albumin level should be measured at the same time so that the serum-ascites albumin gradient (SAAG) may be determined; this value has been shown to correlate directly with portal pressure.[53,54] Portal hypertensive ascitic fluid is characterized by a low albumin content, with a SAAG greater than 1.1 g/dl; non–portal hypertensive ascites fluid is characterized by a SAAG less than 1.1 g/dl.[55]

Spontaneous bacterial peritonitis. An elevated WBC count in the ascitic fluid provides immediate information about possible bacterial infection. Cell counts higher than 500/mm³ suggest bacterial peritonitis, especially when the absolute neutrophil count exceeds 250/mm³.[56] More than 20% of cirrhotic patients with ascites eventually manifest bacterial peritonitis—an occurrence known as spontaneous bacterial peritonitis (SBP). Patients with a low total protein level in their ascitic fluid (< 1.5 g/dl) appear to be at highest risk as a result of the reduced complement level and opsonic activity in the fluid. SBP should be considered in any cirrhotic patient with fever, abdominal pain, or worsening encephalopathy or renal function. Ascitic fluid analysis [*see Table 8*] allows SBP to be distinguished from secondary bacterial peritonitis, which develops as a consequence of an intra-abdominal abscess or a perforated viscus.

Once the diagnosis is made, empirical antibiotic therapy is employed until the final culture result becomes available. At present, cefotaxime (or a similar third-generation cephalosporin) is considered the treatment of choice. A dosage of 1 to 2 g I.V. every 6 to 8 hours (depending on renal function) is optimal. Therapy is continued for 14 days. The response to therapy should be monitored by repeating the paracentesis within 48 hours. Ciprofloxacin, either 200 mg I.V. every 12 hours for 7 days or 200 mg I.V. every 12 hours for 2 days followed by 500 mg orally every 12 hours for 5 days, has been shown to be effective as well.[57]

Currently, it is recommended that antibiotic prophylaxis for SBP (norfloxacin, 400 mg/day) be given only to patients with active GI bleeding and low protein levels in their ascitic fluid or to those who have had SBP before and are awaiting liver transplantation.[58] There is no good evidence to support antibiotic prophylaxis in patients whose ascitic fluid protein levels are low and who have never had SBP. Like ascites, SBP carries a grave prognosis: estimated 1-year survival is less than 50% without liver transplantation.[59,60]

Table 7 Ectopic Sites for Variceal Bleeding

Site	Frequency
Duodenum	17%
Jejunum and ileum	18%
Colon	15%
Rectum	9%
Ileostomy or colostomy	27%
Miscellaneous	14%

Medical management. Sodium retention is the pathophysiologic hallmark of ascites in cirrhotic patients, and the rate of fluid accumulation is directly related to the amount of sodium retained. Many patients excrete sodium at rates lower than 10 mmol/day, in which case even a modest sodium intake results in a positive sodium balance and continued accumulation of ascitic fluid. Therefore, to achieve effective control of ascites, dietary intake of sodium should be restricted to 1 to 2 g/day (43 to 87 mmol/day). With simple bed rest and salt restriction, ascites can be controlled in about 20% of patients.[61]

In addition to salt retention, patients with cirrhosis exhibit impaired free water excretion, which may cause hyponatremia. This state appears to be partially attributable to excessive secretion of antidiuretic hormone (ADH) caused by a reduced effective plasma volume. Water intake need not be restricted in all patients with ascites, because many will not become seriously hyponatremic. Water intake should be restricted (to 1.0 to 1.5 L/day) only in patients who become hyponatremic (serum sodium level < 130 mmol/L) and in those who continue to gain weight despite severe sodium restriction and diuretic therapy. Hyponatremia is associated with a variety of neurologic symptoms resembling those of hepatic encephalopathy. Severe hyponatremia (serum sodium < 120 mmol/L), on the other hand, is associated with seizure activity and should be corrected judiciously. Given the risk of the development of demyelinating lesions associated with rapid changes in the serum sodium concentration, it is recommended that correction of serum sodium—mainly by free water restriction to a serum sodium level between 120 and 130 mmol/L—be carried out gradually.

Diuretic therapy remains the cornerstone of management of cirrhotic ascites; however, it should be monitored carefully to ensure that intravascular volume depletion, development of prerenal azotemia, and electrolyte imbalances do not occur. The peritoneum can absorb no more than 700 to 900 ml of ascitic fluid a day; accordingly, vigorous diuresis in excess of this amount (in the absence of peripheral edema) results in intravascular volume depletion and renal failure.

The two groups of diuretic agents most commonly used to treat ascites are distal tubular–acting agents (e.g., spironolactone) and loop diuretics (e.g., furosemide). Spironolactone inhibits sodium reabsorption in the distal tubules by blocking the effect of serum aldosterone, which is usually elevated in patients with cirrhosis. A spironolactone dosage of 150 to 300 mg/day is sufficient for achieving effective natriuresis in many patients; however, larger dosages (up to 500 to 600 mg/day) may be preferable in certain patients with markedly elevated serum aldosterone concentrations. Adverse effects of spironolactone therapy include hyperkalemia and hyperchloremic acidosis. Tender gynecomastia is also an important side effect; if gynecomastia occurs, amiloride (20 to 40 mg/day) is a good alternative to spironolactone.

Furosemide therapy is usually started if the desired diuresis is not achieved with spironolactone or if the urinary sodium-potassium ratio is less than 1. A typical starting dosage is 40 to 80 mg/day, which is gradually increased until adequate diuresis is achieved. Because furosemide causes loss of urinary sodium and potassium, its use may lead to hypokalemia and metabolic alkalosis.

Surgical management. Despite large doses of diuretics, some patients become refractory to medical therapy and manifest tense ascites. Abdominal paracentesis is a safe and effective alternative to diuretic therapy and is currently used in patients with poor renal function who cannot tolerate aggressive diuresis and intravascular volume depletion. Most patients tolerate removal of large amounts of ascitic fluid (5 to 10 L) without significant adverse hemodynamic effects.[62] Albumin replacement (7 to 9 g/L) with LVP has been asso-

Table 8 Differentiation of Spontaneous Bacterial Peritonitis from Secondary Bacterial Peritonitis through Analysis of Ascitic Fluid

Fluid Assay	Spontaneous Bacterial Peritonitis	Secondary Bacterial Peritonitis
WBC (cells/mm³)	> 500	> 500
Total protein (g/dl)	< 1.0	> 1.0
Glucose (mg/dl)	> 50	< 50
Lactic dehydrogenase (U/L)	< 225	> 225
Gram stain	Monomicrobial	Polymicrobial

ciated with a significantly lower rate of complications (e.g., hyponatremia, encephalopathy, and renal insufficiency) and is recommended when repeated LVP is indicated.[63]

In performing paracentesis, one should avoid surgical scars and obvious large subcutaneous collaterals. In general, a point 1 to 2 cm below the umbilicus along the midline is an optimal site in patients with no previous surgical incisions. Ultrasonographic guidance is usually necessary for localization when the amount of fluid present is small and when the fluid is loculated because of earlier episodes of peritonitis or previous surgical procedures.

The most common complications of LVP are bleeding, peritonitis, perforated viscus, and intra-abdominal abscess. Other complications (e.g., renal failure and cardiovascular instability) are less common and can usually be prevented by means of albumin and colloid replacement and intravascular volume expansion.

A few patients with ascites either become refractory to medical therapy or have contraindications to diuretic therapy or LVP. The usual practice has been to treat these patients with a peritoneovenous shunt through which the ascitic fluid can be reinfused into the systemic circulation, so that effective plasma volume is not reduced. The early enthusiasm for these shunts and their potential advantages notwithstanding, it is clear that there are a number of major complications limiting their use—in particular, early shunt occlusion, disseminated intravascular coagulation (DIC), sepsis, and central venous thrombosis. These complications occur with widely varying degrees of frequency; overall, however, it is estimated that about half of all shunted patients die within 1 year of the operation.[64,65]

If ascites develops as a result of PHT, it is logical to assume that reduction of the portal pressure might relieve the stimulus for ascites and control its formation. Earlier experience with the side-to-side portacaval shunt showed that this approach effectively controlled ascites; however, about one third of the patients died of postoperative complications and liver failure.[66] More recently, the transjugular intrahepatic portosystemic shunt (TIPS) has proved effective in correcting portal hypertension and controlling acute variceal bleeding while carrying low morbidity and mortality.[67]

These results have led to increasing use of TIPS to manage refractory ascites. In most patients, ascites can be completely or partially controlled with TIPS.[68,69] Approximately two thirds of patients with refractory ascites exhibit significantly reduced fluid accumulation and improved renal function. There are, however, a number of complications. Some of these complications are technical (e.g., bleeding from the liver capsule caused by inadvertent puncture, hemobilia, contrast-induced renal failure, and stent malposition or migration). The most significant nontechnical complications associated with the use of TIPS are an increased incidence of encephalopathy

(seen in about 25% to 30% of patients),[70,71] hemolysis, and worsening jaundice.[72]

Stenosis or occlusion of the shunt that necessitates shunt revision is so frequent that it is considered the norm rather than a complication: in most series, 1-year patency rates range from 27% to 57%.[73] No long-term follow-up data are available; however, in one study, the overall survival rate was lower among patients who underwent TIPS placement than among those who received repeated LVP.[74] These data suggest that whereas TIPS is superior to LVP in controlling refractory ascites, it confers no survival advantage, and most patients will die of other complications of cirrhosis.

Hepatic Encephalopathy

Hepatic encephalopathy is a complex neuropsychiatric syndrome that arises in patients with severe hepatic insufficiency and cirrhosis. It is characterized by progressive alteration of cognitive function and coordination 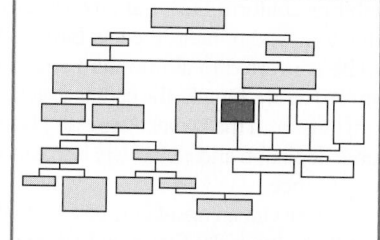 and depression of consciousness, leading to deep coma. Hepatic encephalopathy takes two main forms: (1) acute encephalopathy associated with FHF and (2) portosystemic encephalopathy (PSE) associated with cirrhosis and portosystemic shunts. It is classified into four stages according to the severity and extent of CNS impairment [*see Table 9*].

For accurate diagnosis of hepatic encephalopathy, all other disorders that affect cerebral function—including fluid and electrolyte abnormalities, hypoglycemia, azotemia, metabolic acidosis or alkalosis, hypoxia, and plasma hyperosmolality—must be recognized and corrected. Sedatives and paralytic agents should be avoided during the initial assessment period if possible; if sedation or paralysis is required, the combination of poor hepatic function with the shunting of blood away from the liver may greatly lengthen drug elimination, thereby complicating patient assessment.

Management of PSE begins with treatment and reversal of all potential precipitating factors: sedatives and other drugs with CNS effects should be discontinued, fluid and electrolyte abnormalities should be corrected, GI bleeding should be controlled, and underlying infectious states (especially SBP) should be treated. Early elective tracheal intubation and airway protection may be necessary in patients with stage III or IV encephalopathy because of the high risk of aspiration and subsequent pneumonia.

The classic therapeutic objectives in the management of hepatic

Table 9 Grading of Hepatic Encephalopathy

Encephalopathy Stage	Neurologic Changes
Stage I	Mild confusion, euphoria or depression, decreased attention span, slowing of ability to perform mental tasks, irritability, disorder of sleep pattern
Stage II	Drowsiness, lethargy, gross deficit in ability to perform mental tasks, obvious personality changes, inappropriate behavior, intermittent and short-lived disorientation
Stage III	Somnolent but arousable, unable to perform mental tasks, disorientation with respect to time or place, marked confusion, amnesia, occasional fits of rage, speech present but incomprehensible
Stage IV	Coma

encephalopathy are (1) to minimize ammonia formation and (2) to augment ammonia elimination [*see* Discussion, Mechanism of Hepatic Encephalopathy, *below*]. Lactulose and certain antibiotics are commonly employed to achieve these ends. Lactulose is a synthetic disaccharide cathartic that can be delivered orally, through a nasogastric tube, or via a high enema and can be administered early in the course of the disease. The dosage should begin at 25 g/day and then be titrated to a level at which the patient can produce three or four loose bowel movements a day. Lactulose is neither absorbed nor metabolized in the upper GI tract. When it reaches the colon, the ensuing bacterial degradation acidifies the luminal contents and causes an intraluminal osmotic shift. The more acid environment that results inhibits coliform bacterial growth, thereby reducing ammonia production. Additionally, the low intraluminal gut pH causes ammonia to be converted to ammonium ions, which do not enter the bloodstream easily. Finally, the cathartic action of lactulose clears ammonium ions from the bowel. Aggressive lactulose therapy may induce volume depletion and electrolyte imbalances; metabolic acidosis is a rare occurrence.

Neomycin, an agent commonly used for bowel preparation, alters gut flora, especially *Escherichia coli* and other urease-producing organisms, and thereby causes production of ammonia to fall. Only about 1% of a neomycin dose is absorbed systemically; because of possible ototoxicity and nephrotoxicity, special care should be taken if it is administered on a continuous basis.[75] Other oral antibiotics used to treat hepatic encephalopathy are polymyxin B, metronidazole, and vancomycin; they affect gut flora in much the same fashion as neomycin.

Aromatic amino acids (AAAs) are known neurotransmitter precursors, and it has been suggested that their products interfere with the activity of true neurotransmitters. It has also been shown that the ratio of branched-chain amino acids (BCAAs) to AAAs in plasma decreases steeply with encephalopathy. Because AAAs and BCAAs compete for the same blood-brain barrier carrier transport sites, the relative paucity of BCAAs leads to increased cerebral uptake of AAAs, which in turn promotes synthesis of false neurotransmitters that then compete with the endogenous transmitters dopamine and norepinephrine.[76] Parenteral administration of BCAA-enriched formulas to patients with hepatic encephalopathy has been advocated, but it has not proved beneficial in comparison with administration of conventional parenteral amino acid solutions.[77]

Renal Failure

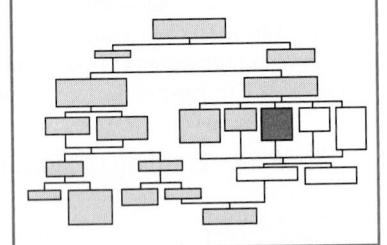

Liver disease and cirrhosis are commonly associated with functional renal failure—that is, impaired renal function in the absence of significant underlying renal pathology. The most common functional renal abnormality in cirrhotic patients is a condition known as hepatorenal syndrome (HRS). HRS is defined as a reversible state of renal failure characterized by azotemia, oliguria (< 500 ml/day), low urinary sodium excretion (< 10 mEq/L), and an increased urine-plasma osmolality ratio (U/P > 1.0) in the absence of urinary sedimentation. HRS occurs in 18% to 55% of cirrhotic patients with ascites and is characterized by intense renal vasoconstriction, a decreased glomerular filtration rate (GFR), preserved tubular function, and normal renal histology.[39,78] Although the exact etiology of HRS is not known, the evidence currently available suggests that it is multifactorial, involving systemic vasodilatation and reduced effective plasma volume along with increased activity of the renin-angiotensin-aldosterone system, which causes further reduction of the GFR. On clinical grounds,

Table 10   Differentiation of Hepatorenal Syndrome from Acute Tubular Necrosis

Criteria	Hepatorenal Syndrome	Acute Tubular Necrosis
Underlying liver disease	Advanced liver damage with jaundice and impaired synthetic function	Mild or severe liver disease
Precipitant	GI bleeding, diuretics, paracentesis, sepsis, or none	Shock, nephrotoxins, sepsis
Onset	Days to weeks	Hours to days
Urinalysis	Renal epithelial cells with or without pigmented granular cells	Pigmented granular casts with or without RBCs, WBCs
Urinary sodium concentration	< 10 mEq/L	> 10 mEq/L
Urinary osmolarity	> Serum osmolarity	Isotonic
Urinary volume	Oliguric	Variable
Course	Progressive, unremitting	Deterioration followed by improved renal function

HRS has been classified into two types: (1) type 1 HRS, in which renal failure is rapidly progressive, as defined by a doubling of the initial serum creatinine level to a value higher than 2.5 mg/dl or a 50% reduction in the initial creatinine clearance to a value lower than 20 ml/min in less than 2 weeks; and (2) type 2 HRS, in which renal failure takes a slower, more gradual course.

The prognosis for patients with HRS is poor: to date, all therapeutic approaches have proved unsuccessful. Pharmacologic therapy has consisted of correcting effective volume status and attempting to reverse renal vasoconstriction through I.V. administration of vasodilators (e.g., dopamine, misoprostol, and aminophylline) or drugs that inhibit the synthesis or the effects of endogenous vasoconstrictors (e.g., captopril and thromboxane inhibitors). These approaches have not yielded any effective and reproducible improvements in renal hemodynamics and renal function. Several investigators, however, have reported improved renal function after OLT.[79]

Subsequently, a newer approach to the management of HRS was introduced that aimed at correcting the primary underlying defect (i.e., systemic vasodilatation) instead of the secondary renal vasoconstriction. Two classes of drugs have been investigated, either individually or in various combinations: (1) agents that inhibit the effects of endogenous systemic vasodilators (e.g., prostacyclin, nitric oxide, and glucagon) and (2) agents that cause systemic vasoconstriction (e.g., ornipressin and terlipressin). In one small series of patients with type 1 HRS, a combination of an oral β-adrenergic drug with midodrine and octreotide led to improved renal function and better long-term outcome.[80]

Besides functional renal failure, various types of nonfunctional, or organic, renal failure (e.g., acute tubular necrosis [ATN], renal tubular acidosis [RTA], and drug-induced interstitial nephritis) may occur in patients with cirrhosis. ATN is especially common among patients with chronic liver disease or FHF and is usually seen in patients who are poorly resuscitated, have experienced prolonged hypotension, have undergone severe septic episodes, or have ingested hepatotoxins that are also nephrotoxic (e.g., acetaminophen). ATN is characterized by an abrupt rise in blood urea nitrogen (BUN) and serum creatinine levels accompanied by oliguria or anuria. Unlike HRS, ATN leads to impairment of the concentrating ability of the tubular system and to excessive urinary sodium excretion; accordingly, a urine sodium concentration higher than 10 mEq/L has been proposed as a diagnostic criterion for ATN in cirrhotic patients [*see Table 10*]. RTA is commonly seen in patients with primary biliary cirrhosis (PBC), autoimmune liver disease, and alcoholic cirrhosis. It is characterized by an inability of the renal tubules to acidify the urine in the presence of a normal GFR.

Management of renal failure is usually aimed at correcting the underlying precipitating causes. In patients with ascites, who experience ongoing loss of fluid and protein into the peritoneum, it is important to maintain an adequate intravascular volume. If intravascular volume is depleted, blood components, volume expanders, or both should be given. Given that the plasma albumin level is invariably low in these patients, salt-poor albumin solutions may be preferable to carbohydrate-based volume expanders. Albumin replacement has been effectively used for volume expansion after LVP.[63]

Because of the complex interaction between the liver and the kidneys, fluid and electrolyte management often proves exceptionally challenging. In particular, it is difficult to estimate the actual intravascular volume, which is depleted in most cirrhotic patients even though total body fluid volume is higher than normal. Sodium retention and free water retention are the two most common abnormalities of renal function that lead to ascites and dilutional hyponatremia. Typically, sodium retention is an early manifestation, whereas water retention and renal failure are late findings. Nephrotoxic drugs and I.V. contrast agents should be avoided, and dosages of antibiotics and other medications should be adjusted appropriately.

Hypernatremia and metabolic acidosis can develop secondary to excessive lactulose therapy and dehydration and cause renal function to deteriorate. Hypokalemia is also common; it develops secondary to increased serum aldosterone concentration, which leads to excessive excretion of potassium in exchange for sodium. Once renal failure develops, hyperkalemia, hypercalcemia, and hyperphosphatemia become significant problems, often necessitating dialysis.

Malnutrition

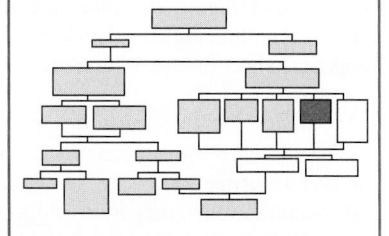

Most cirrhotic patients present with depleted glycogen stores, severe protein-calorie malnutrition, and wasting. Impaired hepatic synthetic activity, causing a deficiency of both visceral and structural proteins, is one of the hallmarks of advanced liver disease. In addition, poor appetite, tense ascites, abdominal pain, and excessive loss of protein through repeated LVP and overall increased energy expenditure tend to exacerbate malnutrition.

Excessive protein administration can induce hepatic encephalopathy; accordingly, protein intake should be limited to 1 to 1.2 g/kg/day. Glucose is the main energy source given to malnourished cirrhotic patients; however, its use is not without complications, in that these patients typically exhibit glucose intolerance. Lipid emulsion can be safely administered to most patients with liver failure and should be withheld only from patients with overt coma.[81] It is generally agreed that the ideal energy source should consist of a mixture of glucose and fat emulsion. Approximately 30% to 40% of all nonprotein calories can be provided in the form of fat. The total energy requirement should be in the range of 25 to 35 kcal/kg/day.

As noted [*see Hepatic Encephalopathy, above*], although AAAs have been implicated in the pathogenesis of hepatic encephalopathy,

administration of BCAA solutions has not proved helpful, and the evidence does not support their routine use.[77,82]

In general, the potential risks and complications associated with total parenteral nutrition (TPN) outweigh the benefits in patients with a functioning GI tract. When properly administered, enteral nutrition is safer, more physiologically correct, and significantly more cost-effective than TPN. It should therefore be considered the first choice for nutritional support in most patients with chronic liver disease unless a contraindication to enteral feeding is present.

Coagulopathy and Nonvariceal Bleeding

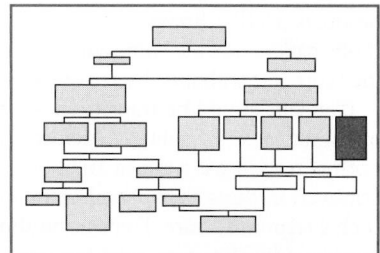

The spectrum of coagulation disorders in patients with liver disease varies from minor localized bleeding to massive life-threatening hemorrhage. Abnormal bleeding may be spontaneous in some patients, but it is more often the result of a hemostatic challenge (e.g., surgical wounds or procedures, gastritis, portal hypertensive gastropathy, gastric or duodenal ulcers, or ruptured varices). The underlying anatomic lesion is believed to be as responsible for bleeding as the hemostatic defect is; accordingly, therapy should be directed at correcting both.

Although most bleeding episodes are secondary to decreased synthesis of clotting factors, other causes of bleeding (e.g., defective or dysfunctional factor synthesis and increased consumption of clotting components) must always be ruled out [*see I:5 Bleeding and Transfusion*]. In most patients, the decreased levels of clotting factors parallel the progressive loss of parenchymal cell function. Usually, the levels of the vitamin K–dependent factors (i.e., prothrombin, factor VII, factor IX, factor X, protein S, and protein C) fall first, followed by the levels of other factors as cirrhosis progresses. Factor V is synthesized independently of vitamin K availability, and its concentration is of special interest because the plasma factor V level seems to be a predictor of the extent of liver cell damage. Impaired synthesis of coagulation proteins also has an impact on antithrombin III (AT-III), protein C inhibitor, plasminogen, and α_2-antiplasmin as well as on several other inhibitors and activators of both the extrinsic coagulation pathway and the intrinsic pathway. The combination of decreased factor levels and impaired synthesis of coagulation proteins explains the prolongation of the PT, the activated partial thromboplastin time (aPTT), and the thrombin clotting time (TCT) in these patients.[83,84]

Given the complexity of hemostasis in cirrhotic patients, accurate diagnosis of a bleeding disorder is often hard to achieve. Several disorders and abnormalities may be present simultaneously, and one or more parameters of hemostasis and coagulation may be impaired. Therefore, any effective treatment approach should be broad-based and aimed at correcting several deficiencies or abnormalities at once. FFP contains all of the components of the clotting and fibrinolytic systems but lacks platelets. In most cases, transfusion of 6 to 8 units of FFP suffices to correct severe clotting factor defects; however, the excess volume may not be well tolerated. Cryoprecipitate, the precipitate formed when FFP is thawed at 4°C, is rich in factor VIII, von Willebrand factor, and fibrinogen but lacks the vitamin K–dependent factors. Therefore, it should be given only when the fibrinogen level is lower than 100 mg/dl. Prothrombin complex concentrates contain only the vitamin K–dependent factors and proteins, and their use can provoke serious thromboembolic complications, including disseminated intravascular coagulation (DIC). Therefore, their potential utility must be weighed carefully against the risk that thrombotic events may develop.[85]

Other major disorders of hemostasis in patients with chronic liver disease and cirrhosis involve platelets and are manifested as thrombocytopenia, abnormal platelet function (thrombocytopathy), or both. In most cases, thrombocytopenia is related to splenomegaly and hypersplenism (a common feature of PHT). Abnormal platelet function is attributed to many causes, including intrinsic platelet defects and abnormal interaction among platelets, endothelial surfaces, and clotting factors. It is manifested by a prolonged bleeding time, impaired platelet aggregation, and reduced adhesiveness. Some authorities attribute the inhibition of platelet aggregation to fibrin degradation products (FDPs); however, the FDP levels noted in the plasma of cirrhotic patients are not sufficient to impair platelet aggregation, nor do they correlate with the observed reductions in platelet aggregation.[86]

Platelets should be transfused whenever a patient with either a quantitative or a qualitative defect experiences active bleeding. A normal response is a rise of 10,000/mm^3 with each unit transfused; however, in cases of hypersplenism and accelerated consumption, such a response is rare. Transfusion should be continued until all serious bleeding has ceased, with the therapeutic goal being the maintenance of a platelet count near 50,000/mm^3. Platelet transfusion is also indicated before any surgical or invasive procedure (e.g., paracentesis or liver biopsy). Indications for prophylactic platelet transfusion are less clear, and any potential gains must be balanced against potential side effects and development of antibodies. Most patients with advanced cirrhosis and liver failure have platelet counts lower than 100,000/mm^3; however, prophylactic platelet transfusion is usually not recommended until the count falls below 15,000 to 20,000/mm^3, at which point the risk of spontaneous bleeding is considerably increased.

Another feature of severe liver disease is increased fibrinolytic activity, which may be either primary or secondary to DIC.[87] The exact causes of primary fibrinolysis and DIC remain unclear. Primary fibrinolysis appears to derive from increased activity of tissue plasminogen activator and decreased levels of α_2-antiplasmin.[88] DIC is believed to be triggered by the release of thromboplastic substances into the circulation as a consequence of liver cell damage or necrosis and by poor clearance of circulating activated tissue and clotting factors and FDPs by a defective reticuloendothelial system. Accelerated fibrinolysis is manifested by reductions in the whole blood clot lysis time and the euglobulin clot lysis time as well as by elevated levels of fibrinolysis products (e.g., FDPs and D-dimer). Although enhanced fibrinolysis is relatively common in patients with cirrhosis,

Table 11 Contraindications to Liver Transplantation

Absolute contraindications	Severe, irreversible brain damage
	HIV infection
	Extrahepatic malignancy
	Uncontrolled sepsis
	Severe pulmonary hypertension and advanced cardiopulmonary disease
	Active substance abuse or major psychosocial problems
	Extrahepatic portal vein thrombosis in patients with hepatocellular carcinoma
Relative contraindications	Elevated ICP or reduced CPP (in patients with FHF)
	Multiple organ dysfunction syndrome
	Hemodynamic instability
	Advanced age
	Portal vein thrombosis (except when secondary to hepatocellular carcinoma)

CPP—cerebral perfusion pressure   ICP—intracranial pressure

Table 12 Child-Turcotte-Pugh Scoring System

Points	1	2	3
Encephalopathy	None	Stage I or II	Stage III or IV
Ascites	Absent	Slight (or controlled by diuretics)	Moderate despite diuretic treatment
Bilirubin (mg/dl)	< 2	2–3	> 3
Patients with PBC or PSC	< 4	4–6	> 6
Albumin (g/L)	> 3.5	2.8–3.5	< 2.8
PT (prolonged sec)	< 4	4–6	> 6
INR	< 1.7	1.7–2.3	> 2.3

PBC—primary biliary cirrhosis   PSC—primary sclerosing cholangitis

most of the characteristic abnormalities can occur after many types of physiologic stress and are not necessarily accompanied by a bleeding tendency.

At present, no satisfactory method of managing DIC is available. An extensive workup must be completed to rule out underlying causes (e.g., sepsis, ARDS, and MODS). FFP, platelet concentrates, and, possibly, low-dose heparin (200 to 800 U/hr) may be given. AT-III concentrate has been used in an attempt to inhibit the action of thrombin, thereby decreasing procoagulant consumption, restoring normal levels of factors, and improving hemostasis. Clinical experience with AT-III therapy in this setting has been limited to a few case reports and a few small series; however, there is some evidence to suggest that AT-III may reduce the hemostatic abnormalities and help control bleeding.[89]

Antifibrinolytic agents (e.g., ε-aminocaproic acid and tranexamic acid) impede fibrinolysis and thus may be useful for treating bleeding in patients who have liver disease and show evidence of fibrinolysis.[90] In patients with DIC, however, administration of antifibrinolytic agents is contraindicated because of the potential for thrombotic complications. D-dimer levels should be determined to rule out DIC before use of these medications is considered. Because DIC is difficult to rule out in patients with liver disease, the use of antifibrinolytic agents in liver disease is limited.

LIVER TRANSPLANTATION

The standard indications for liver transplantation are well documented[91]: they include PHT, poor hepatic synthetic function, hepatic encephalopathy, progressive jaundice, severe malnutrition, and excessive fatigue. 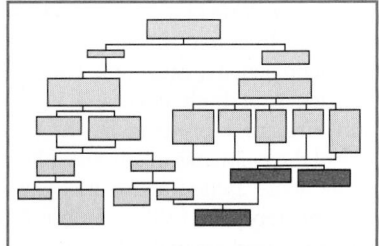 As noted [see Treatment of Complications, above], PHT is manifested by variceal bleeding, hypersplenism, thrombocytopenia, ascites, hepatic hydrothorax, and SBP. Poor synthetic function is usually manifested by a prolonged PT and low serum albumin and cholesterol levels. In general, any concurrent medical or psychosocial condition that prohibits a major surgical procedure or subsequent immunosuppression constitutes a contraindication to liver transplantation [see Table 11].

The United Network for Organ Sharing (UNOS) currently regulates organ allocation to transplant candidates. In January 1988, minimal listing criteria for liver transplantation were implemented.[92] These criteria are based on the Child-Turcotte-Pugh (CTP) scoring system [see Table 12], which includes five parameters: serum albumin and bilirubin levels, PT, ascites, and hepatic encephalopathy. To be listed for liver transplantation, a patient must have a CTP score of 7 or higher. In addition to the general listing criteria, various disease-specific criteria were developed for patients with alcoholic liver disease, patients with cholestatic liver disease (e.g., PBC or primary sclerosing cholangitis), and patients with hepatocellular carcinoma.

Discussion

Mechanisms of Hepatic Encephalopathy

The association between liver disease and altered mental status and consciousness has been recognized for centuries, but the exact underlying mechanisms remain unknown. It appears that this syndrome has a multifactorial etiology and is associated with a number of complex changes, which are manifested collectively as hepatic encephalopathy. It is generally believed that hepatocerebral dysfunction is caused by accumulation of cerebral toxins as a result of low hepatic clearance.[93]

Of all the physiologic factors thought to contribute to the development of encephalopathy, the best known is ammonia. Arterial ammonia levels are frequently elevated in persons with hepatic encephalopathy; however, the clinical severity of hepatic encephalopathy correlates poorly with the degree to which the ammonia level is elevated.[94] The precise contribution of ammonia to hepatic encephalopathy remains unclear; however, ammonia is known to inhibit the uptake of glutamate into the astrocytes, thereby causing a rise in the extracellular glutamate level that appears to downregulate the postsynaptic glutamate receptors, resulting in decreased neuronal excitation.[95]

Endogenous or exogenously ingested benzodiazepines may also play a role in the etiology of acute and chronic hepatic encephalopathy by interacting with the high-affinity γ-aminobutyric acid (GABA)–benzodiazepine receptor complexes. These substances are known to enhance inhibitory GABA-ergic tone. Animal studies suggest that the gut flora may contribute benzodiazepine ligand activity[96] as well as increased benzodiazepine receptor agonist activity.[97] Clinical studies of FHF patients show increased benzodiazepine receptor ligands with enhanced GABA-ergic tone in all stages of encephalopathy.[98] Ammonia-induced activation of peripheral-type benzodiazepine receptors on astrocytes may cause the release of neurosteroids that enhance GABA-ergic neurotransmission. Hence, neurosteroids may potentate the inhibitory actions of GABA at the receptor level as well as lengthen the period during which the GABA ligand remains in the synaptic cleft. Ammonia also acts directly to potentiate GABA-ergic tone by enhancing the affinity of GABA for GABA-A receptors.[99]

Despite these seemingly compelling findings, there is no apparent correlation between benzodiazepine ligand activity and clinical stage of encephalopathy, nor is ligand elevation a consistent finding in all patients. Furthermore, clinical and animal studies in which a benzodiazepine receptor antagonist has been administered have not shown consistent effects. The anecdotal success of flumazenil, the principal benzodiazepine antagonist, has been ascribed to the antagonism of benzodiazepines ingested by patients. Support for the concept of so-called endogenous benzodiazepines arising from the intestine can be found in a number of sources, including studies of dogs with congenital portacaval shunts, which document ligand activity in stool samples.[100] Whether there is a causal relation to hepatic encephalopathy or whether this is merely a case of associated phenomena remains to be determined. Whatever the contribution of benzodiazepines to the pathophysiology of acute hepatic encephalopathy and cerebral edema, it appears likely that other mechanisms are involved.

Bioartificial Liver Support System

Despite the best management efforts, the morbidity and mortality associated with ALF remain exceptionally high. For most severe cases, liver transplantation is still the only effective therapeutic modality. Unfortunately, because of the severe organ donor shortage, the waiting period for transplantation is long, and patients consequently are at risk for the development of irreversible complications or contraindications to liver transplantation while awaiting a donor. In an effort to mitigate this problem, investigators have studied various artificial liver support systems designed to provide full metabolic, hemodynamic, and physiologic support until either the native liver regenerates or a liver becomes available for transplantation. From the 1970s to the 1990s, most therapeutic attempts focused primarily on detoxifying plasma. All such attempts either failed or had no significant impact on survival.[101]

The ongoing severe organ shortage has led several investigators to develop and test a number of xenogeneic-based liver support systems employing whole-organ perfusion or isolated hepatocytes. At our institution, we developed and tested a hybrid bioartificial liver (BAL) support system employing isolated porcine hepatocytes in an extracorporeal perfusion circuit. We subsequently initiated a clinical trial addressing the use of this system in patients with severe ALF as a bridge to either transplantation or spontaneous recovery.[102-104]

CLINICAL TRIAL

Study Design

Hepatocytes Methods of porcine hepatocyte isolation, purification, attachment to a collagen-coated matrix, cryopreservation,

Table 13 Neurologic Effects of BAL Treatment

Study Group	Results		
	Pre-BAL	Post-BAL	P
Group I			
ICP (mm Hg)	17.0 ± 1.5	10.9 ± 1.0	< 0.0002
CPP (mm Hg)	70 ± 2	75 ± 2	< 0.04
GCS	6.8 ± 0.4	7.4 ± 0.4	< 0.01
CLOCS	24.7 ± 1.2	32.0 ± 1.1	< 0.000001
Group II			
GCS	5.0 ± 1.1	7.0 ± 1.4	< 0.2
CLOCS	29.7 ± 7.4	31.7 ± 7.9	< 0.5
Group III			
ICP (mm Hg)	12.3 ± 0.9	14.0 ± 1.5	< 0.4
CPP (mm Hg)	85 ± 1	98 ± 8	< 0.3
GCS	8.2 ± 0.7	8.4 ± 0.7	< 0.4
CLOCS	29.7 ± 2.3	34.0 ± 1.7	< 0.001

BAL—bioartificial liver   CLOCS—Comprehensive Level of Consciousness score
CPP—cerebral perfusion pressure   GCS—Glasgow Coma Scale   ICP—intracranial pressure

Table 14 Metabolic Effects of BAL Treatment

Study Group	Results		
	Pre-BAL	Post-BAL	*P*
Group I			
AST (U/L)	1,255 ± 261	879 ± 148	< 0.002
ALT (U/L)	1,075 ± 184	674 ± 120	< 0.000005
Total bilirubin (mg/dl)	17.9 ± 1.5	14.6 ± 1.2	< 0.000001
Glucose (mg/dl)	126 ± 5	175 ± 7	< 0.0000006
Ammonia (μmol/L)	160 ± 8	134 ± 6	< 0.0002
Lactate (mmol/L)	4.4 ± 0.7	4.2 ± 0.6	< 0.2
Albumin (g/dl)	3.12 ± 0.08	2.6 ± 0.1	< 0.0000006
Creatinine (mg/dl)	1.5 ± 0.2	1.1 ± 0.1	< 0.000001
Group II			
AST (U/L)	5,661 ± 2,613	2,821 ± 1,291	< 0.1
ALT (U/L)	2,139 ± 704	1,633 ± 544	< 0.05
Total bilirubin (mg/dl)	19.1 ± 2.2	14.7 ± 1.7	< 0.009
Glucose (mg/dl)	117 ± 26	144 ± 24	< 0.06
Ammonia (μmol/L)	81 ± 9	91 ± 13	< 0.03
Lactate (mmol/L)	13.1 ± 2.9	13.2 ± 2.2	< 0.9
Albumin (g/dl)	3.7 ± 0.3	2.7 ± 0.1	< 0.01
Creatinine (mg/dl)	1.6 ± 0.3	1.6 ± 0.3	< 1.0
Group III			
AST (U/L)	692 ± 374	723 ± 409	< 0.5
ALT (U/L)	349 ± 126	281 ± 114	< 0.06
Total bilirubin (mg/dl)	26.0 ± 2.7	21.6 ± 2.2	< 0.000003
Glucose (mg/dl)	141 ± 9	171 ± 11	< 0.001
Ammonia (μmol/L)	173 ± 31	131 ± 15	< 0.08
Lactate (mmol/L)	5.7 ± 1.1	5.6 ± 0.9	< 0.9
Albumin (g/dl)	3.0 ± 0.1	2.6 ± 0.1	< 0.00003
Creatinine (mg/dl)	2.8 ± 0.3	2.2 ± 0.2	< 0.00002

ALT—alanine aminotransferase   AST—aspartate aminotransferase   BAL—bioartificial liver

and storage were developed. Five to seven billion fresh or cryopreserved hepatocytes (70% to 90% viability) were used for each patient treatment.[103,104]

System characteristics   The system was standardized and subsequently modified and is currently manufactured as the HepatAssist 2000 (Circe Biomedical, Inc., Lexington, Massachusetts). The main components are (1) a plasmapheresis unit, (2) an activated cellulose-coated charcoal column, (3) an oxygenator, (4) a blood warmer, and (5) a hollow-fiber module containing isolated microcarrier-attached porcine hepatocytes. The module consists of (a) an intracapillary chamber made of several porous, hollow 0.2 μm fibers through which plasma flows and (b) an extracapillary chamber surrounding the hollow fibers, where the microcarrier-attached hepatocytes are suspended. Plasma circulates through the fibers at a rate of 400 ml/min, with free exchange of macromolecules across the surface of the fibers driven by a transmembrane pressure gradient. When plasma and blood

cells return from the BAL, they are reconstituted and returned to the patient via the double-lumen venous dialysis catheter.

Patient population   Three groups of patients were enrolled in the phase 1 trial. Group I patients (N = 24) had no previous history of liver disease, fulfilled all the diagnostic criteria of FHF, and were candidates for OLT at the time of admission. Group II patients (N = 3) had undergone OLT and exhibited primary nonfunction (PNF) of the transplanted liver in the immediate postoperative period with rapid deterioration. Group III patients (N = 10) presented with acute exacerbation of known underlying chronic liver disease and were not candidates for OLT at the time of study enrollment. Patients were enrolled in the study when stage III or IV encephalopathy developed in the course of optimal standard medical therapy.

Results

Of the 24 group I patients, 18 were candidates for OLT. Five additional patients with FHF secondary to acetaminophen toxicity who were treated with the BAL support system recovered fully without the need for liver transplantation. One patient with FHF secondary to heatstroke received BAL treatment while awaiting OLT; he died as a result of MODS after 21 days. All 18 OLT candidates in group I and all three patients in group II were successfully bridged to transplantation, experienced full neurologic and functional recovery, and were discharged from the hospital. Patients in group III experienced transient clinical improvement after BAL treatment. Two patients recovered enough native liver function to survive; they subsequently became candidates for OLT and underwent the procedure successfully. The remaining eight patients died 1 to 21 days (mean, 7.1 days) after their last BAL treatment as a result of variceal bleeding, sepsis, or MODS.

Treatment with the BAL support system gave rise to several neurologic and metabolic effects that were seen in all three groups of patients. Of these, the neurologic changes were the most dramatic. Patients with FHF (group I) exhibited remarkable neurologic improvement after BAL treatment, with the reversal of decerebrate posturing states, anisocoria, and sluggish pupillary reflexes. Both responsiveness to external stimuli and brain-stem function improved, as shown by a higher comprehensive level of consciousness score. There was a significant reduction in ICP with a concomitant increase in CPP; these changes were most dramatic in patients with ICP levels higher than 25 mm Hg [*see Table 13*]. In patients with PNF (group II), the impact of BAL treatment on neurologic status was difficult to assess because heavy sedation was used in the postanesthetic period; however, transient neurologic improvements were noted after BAL treatment, manifested primarily by increased responsiveness.

Additional metabolic effects of BAL treatment on liver function included improvements in renal function and hematologic and coagulation parameters [*see Table 14*]. There was a significant (*P* < 0.01) increase in the plasma BCAA-AAA ratio in plasma, which may be one of many possible reasons for the observed mitigation of encephalopathy. This increase was primarily due to a reduction in AAA levels.

References

1. Kotwal GJ, Baroudy BM, Kuramoto IK, et al: Detection of acute hepatitis C virus infection by ELISA using a synthetic peptide comprising a structural epitope. Proc Natl Acad Sci USA 89:4486, 1992

2. Polito AJ, DiNello RK, Quan S, et al: New generation RIBA hepatitis C strip immunoblot assays. Ann Biol Clin (Paris) 50:329, 1992

3. Bukh J, Purcell RH, Miller RH: Importance of primer selection for the detection of hepatitis C virus RNA with the polymerase chain reaction assay. Proc Natl Acad Sci USA 89:187, 1992

4. Trey C, Davidson CS: The management of fulminant hepatic failure. Prog Liver Dis 3:282, 1970

5. Bernuau J, Rueff B, Benhamou JP: Fulminant and

subfulminant liver failure: definitions and causes. Semin Liver Dis 6:97, 1986

6. Schiodt FV, Atillasoy E, Shakil AO, et al: Etiology and outcome for 295 patients with acute liver failure in the United States. Liver Transpl Surg 5:29, 1999

7. Ritt DJ, Whelan G, Werner DJ, et al: Acute hepatic

necrosis with stupor or coma: an analysis of thirty-one patients. Medicine (Baltimore) 48:151, 1969

8. Lettau LA, McCarthy JG, Smith MH, et al: Outbreak of severe hepatitis due to delta and hepatitis B viruses in parenteral drug abusers and their contacts. N Engl J Med 317:1256, 1987

9. Gimson AE, Tedder RS, White YS, et al: Serological markers in fulminant hepatitis B. Gut 24:615, 1983

10. Samuel D, Bismuth A, Mathieu D, et al: Passive immunoprophylaxis after liver transplantation in HBsAg-positive patients. Lancet 337:813, 1991

11. Govindarajan S, Chin KP, Redeker AG, et al: Fulminant B viral hepatitis: role of delta agent. Gastroenterology 86:1417, 1984

12. Smedile A, Farci P, Verme G, et al: Influence of delta infection on severity of hepatitis B. Lancet 2:945, 1982

13. Lichtenstein DR, Makadon HJ, Chopra S: Fulminant hepatitis B and delta virus coinfection in AIDS. Am J Gastroenterol 87:1643, 1992

14. Rakela J, Lange SM, Ludwig J, et al: Fulminant hepatitis: Mayo Clinic experience with 34 cases. Mayo Clin Proc 60:289, 1985

15. Castells A, Salmeron JM, Navasa M, et al: Liver transplantation for acute liver failure: analysis of applicability. Gastroenterology 105:532, 1993

16. Zimmerman HJ: Update of hepatotoxicity due to classes of drugs in common clinical use: non-steroidal drugs, anti-inflammatory drugs, antibiotics, antihypertensives, and cardiac and psychotropic agents. Semin Liver Dis 10:322, 1990

17. Carney FM, Van Dyke RA: Halothane hepatitis: a critical review. Anesth Analg 51:135, 1972

18. Floersheim GL: Treatment of human amatoxin mushroom poisoning. Myths and advances in therapy. Med Toxicol 2:1, 1987

19. Klein AS, Hart J, Brems JJ, et al: Amanita poisoning: treatment and the role of liver transplantation. Am J Med 86:187, 1989

20. Rector WG Jr, Uchida T, Kanel GC, et al: Fulminant hepatic and renal failure complicating Wilson's disease. Liver 4:341, 1984

21. McCullough AJ, Fleming CR, Thistle JL, et al: Diagnosis of Wilson's disease presenting as fulminant hepatic failure. Gastroenterology 84:161, 1983

22. Stremmel W, Meyerrose KW, Niederau C, et al: Wilson disease: clinical presentation, treatment, and survival. Ann Intern Med 115:720, 1991

23. Amon E, Allen SR, Petrie RH, et al: Acute fatty liver of pregnancy associated with preeclampsia: management of hepatic failure with postpartum liver transplantation. Am J Perinatol 8:278, 1991

24. O'Grady JG, Alexander GJ, Hayllar KM, et al: Early indicators of prognosis in fulminant hepatic failure. Gastroenterology 97:439, 1989

25. Bernuau J, Goudeau A, Poynard T, et al: Multivariate analysis of prognostic factors in fulminant hepatitis B. Hepatology 6:648, 1986

26. Saibara T, Onishi S, Sone J, et al: Arterial ketone body ratio as a possible indicator for liver transplantation in fulminant hepatic failure. Transplantation 51:782, 1991

27. Ranek L, Andreasen PB, Tygstrup N: Galactose elimination capacity as a prognostic index in patients with fulminant liver failure. Gut 17:959, 1976

28. Ware AJ, D'Agostino AN, Combes B: Cerebral edema: a major complication of massive hepatic necrosis. Gastroenterology 61:877, 1971

29. Silk DB, Trewby PN, Chase RA, et al: Treatment of fulminant hepatic failure by polyacrylonitrile-membrane haemodialysis. Lancet 2:1, 1977

30. Lidofsky SD: Fulminant hepatic failure. Crit Care Clin 11:415, 1995

31. Wijdicks EF, Plevak DJ, Rakela J, et al: Clinical and radiologic features of cerebral edema in fulminant hepatic failure. Mayo Clin Proc 70:119, 1995

32. Sidi A, Mahla ME: Noninvasive monitoring of cerebral perfusion by transcranial Doppler during fulminant hepatic failure and liver transplantation. Anesth Analg 80:194, 1995

33. Munoz SJ, Robinson M, Northrup B, et al: Elevated intracranial pressure and computed tomography of the brain in fulminant hepatocellular failure. Hepatology 13:209, 1991

34. Blei AT, Olafsson S, Webster S, et al: Complications of intracranial pressure monitoring in fulminant hepatic failure. Lancet 341:157, 1993

35. Aldersley MA, Juniper M, Richardson P, et al: Inability of intracranial pressure monitoring to select patients with acute liver failure for transplantation (abstract). Hepatology 22:208A, 1995

36. Davies MH, Mutimer D, Lowes J, et al: Recovery despite impaired cerebral perfusion in fulminant hepatic failure. Lancet 343:1329, 1994

37. Canalese J, Gimson AE, Davis C, et al: Controlled trial of dexamethasone and mannitol for the cerebral oedema of fulminant hepatic failure. Gut 23:625, 1982

38. Forbes A, Alexander GJ, O'Grady JG, et al: Thiopental infusion in the treatment of intracranial hypertension complicating fulminant hepatic failure. Hepatology 10:306, 1989

39. Ring-Larsen H, Palazzo U: Renal failure in fulminant hepatic failure and terminal cirrhosis: a comparison between incidence, types, and prognosis. Gut 22:585, 1981

40. Trewby PN, Warren R, Contini S, et al: Incidence and pathophysiology of pulmonary edema in fulminant hepatic failure. Gastroenterology 74(5 pt 1):859, 1978

41. Bailey RJ, Woolf IL, Cullens H, et al: Metabolic inhibition of polymorphonuclear leucocytes in fulminant hepatic failure. Lancet 1:1162, 1976

42. Imawari M, Hughes RD, Gove CD, et al: Fibronectin and Kupffer cell function in fulminant hepatic failure. Dig Dis Sci 30:1028, 1985

43. Rolando N, Harvey F, Brahm J, et al: Prospective study of bacterial infection in acute liver failure: an analysis of fifty patients. Hepatology 11:49, 1990

44. Rolando N, Harvey F, Brahm J, et al: Fungal infection: a common, unrecognised complication of acute liver failure. J Hepatol 12:1, 1991

45. O'Grady JG, Langley PG, Isola LM, et al: Coagulopathy of fulminant hepatic failure. Semin Liver Dis 6:159, 1986

46. Ringe B, Pichlmayr R, Lubbe N, et al: Total hepatectomy as temporary approach to acute hepatic or primary graft failure. Transplant Proc 20(1 suppl 1):552, 1988

47. Ringe B, Lubbe N, Kuse E, et al: Management of emergencies before and after liver transplantation by early total hepatectomy. Transplant Proc 25(1 pt 2): 1090, 1993

48. Rozga J, Podesta L, LePage E, et al: Control of cerebral oedema by total hepatectomy and extracorporeal liver support in fulminant hepatic failure. Lancet 342: 898, 1993

49. Ascher NL, Lake JR, Emond JC, et al: Liver transplantation for fulminant hepatic failure. Arch Surg 128:677, 1993

50. Emond JC, Aran PP, Whitington PF, et al: Liver transplantation in the management of fulminant hepatic failure. Gastroenterology 96:1583, 1989

51. Choi W-C, Arnaout WS, Villamil FG, et al: Comparison of the applicability of two prognostic indicator scores in patients with fulminant hepatic failure (abstract). Gastroenterology 118(suppl 2, pt 1):A896, 2000

52. Powell WJ, Jr., Klatskin G: Duration of survival in patients with Laennec's cirrhosis: influence of alcohol withdrawal, and possible effects of recent changes in general management of the disease. Am J Med 44: 406, 1968

53. Pare P, Talbot J, Hoefs JC: Serum-ascites albumin concentration gradient: a physiologic approach to the differential diagnosis of ascites. Gastroenterology 85: 240, 1983

54. Runyon BA: Paracentesis and ascitic fluid analysis. Textbook of Gastroenterology. Yamada T, Alpers D, Owyang C, et al, Eds. JB Lippincott Co, New York, 1991, p 2455

55. Runyon BA, Montano AA, Akriviadis EA, et al: The serum-ascites albumin gradient is superior to the exudate-transudate concept in the differential diagnosis of ascites. Ann Intern Med 117:215, 1992

56. Akriviadis EA, Runyon BA: Utility of an algorithm in differentiating spontaneous from secondary bacterial peritonitis. Gastroenterology 98:127, 1990

57. Terg R, Cobas S, Fassio E, et al: Oral ciprofloxacin after a short course of intravenous ciprofloxacin in the treatment of spontaneous bacterial peritonitis: results of a multicenter, randomized study. J Hepatol 33:504, 2000

58. Gines P, Rimola A, Planas R, et al: Norfloxacin prevents spontaneous bacterial peritonitis recurrence in cirrhosis: results of a double-blind, placebo-controlled trial. Hepatology 12(4 pt 1):716, 1990

59. Hoefs JC, Canawati HN, Sapico FL, et al: Spontaneous bacterial peritonitis. Hepatology 2:399, 1982

60. Mihas AA, Toussaint J, Hsu HS, et al: Spontaneous bacterial peritonitis in cirrhosis: clinical and laboratory features, survival and prognostic indicators. Hepatogastroenterology 39:520, 1992

61. Gregory PB, Broekelschen PH, Hill MD, et al: Complications of diuresis in the alcoholic patient with ascites: a controlled trial. Gastroenterology 73:534, 1977

62. Tito L, Gines P, Arroyo V, et al: Total paracentesis associated with intravenous albumin management of patients with cirrhosis and ascites. Gastroenterology 98:146, 1990

63. Gines P, Tito L, Arroyo V, et al: Randomized comparative study of therapeutic paracentesis with and without intravenous albumin in cirrhosis. Gastroenterology 94:1493, 1988

64. Bernhoft RA, Pellegrini CA, Way LW: Peritoneovenous shunt for refractory ascites: operative complications and long-term results. Arch Surg 117:631, 1982

65. Greig PD, Langer B, Blendis LM, et al: Complications after peritoneovenous shunting for ascites. Am J Surg 139:125, 1980

66. Welch HF: Prognosis after surgical treatment of ascites: results of side-to-side shunt in 40 patients. Surgery 56:75, 1964;

67. Burroughs AK, Patch D: Transjugular intrahepatic portosystemic shunt. Semin Liver Dis 19:457, 1999

68. Ochs A, Rossle M, Haag K, et al: The transjugular intrahepatic portosystemic stent-shunt procedure for refractory ascites [published erratum appears in N Engl J Med 332:1587, 1995]. N Engl J Med 332: 1192, 1995

69. Trotter JF, Suhocki PV, Rockey DC: Transjugular intrahepatic portosystemic shunt (TIPS) in patients with refractory ascites: effect on body weight and Child-Pugh score. Am J Gastroenterol 93:1891, 1998

70. Rossle M: [Transjugular intrahepatic portasystemic shunt (TIPS)—indications and outcome]. Z Gastroenterol 35:505, 1997

71. Jalan R, Forrest EH, Stanley AJ, et al: A randomized trial comparing transjugular intrahepatic portosystemic stent-shunt with variceal band ligation in the prevention of rebleeding from esophageal varices. Hepatology 26:1115, 1997

72. Rouillard SS, Bass NM, Roberts JP, et al: Severe hyperbilirubinemia after creation of transjugular intrahepatic portosystemic shunts: natural history and predictors of outcome. Ann Intern Med 128:374, 1998

73. Sterling KM, Darcy MD: Stenosis of transjugular intrahepatic portosystemic shunts: presentation and management. AJR Am J Roentgenol 168:239, 1997

74. Lebrec D, Giuily N, Hadengue A, et al: Transjugular intrahepatic portosystemic shunts: comparison with paracentesis in patients with cirrhosis and refractory ascites: a randomized trial. French Group of Clinicians and a Group of Biologists. J Hepatol 25:135, 1996

75. Berk DP, Chalmers T: Deafness complicating antibiotic therapy of hepatic encephalopathy. Ann Intern Med 73:393, 1970

76. Soeters PB, Fischer JE: Insulin, glucagon, aminoacid imbalance, and hepatic encephalopathy. Lancet 2:880, 1976

77. DerSimonian R: Parenteral nutrition with branched-chain amino acids in hepatic encephalopathy: meta analysis. Hepatology 11:1083, 1990

78. Gines A, Escorsell A, Gines P, et al: Incidence, predictive factors, and prognosis of the hepatorenal syndrome in cirrhosis with ascites. Gastroenterology 105:229, 1993

79. Gonwa TA, Goldstein M, Holman M, et al: Orthotopic liver transplantation and renal function: outcome of hepatorenal syndrome and trial of verapamil for renal protection in nonhepatorenal syndrome. Transplant Proc 25:1891, 1993

80. Angeli P, Volpin R, Gerunda G, et al: Reversal of type 1 hepatorenal syndrome with the administration of midodrine and octreotide. Hepatology 29:1690, 1999

81. Nagayama M, Takai T, Okuno M, et al: Fat emulsion in surgical patients with liver disorders. J Surg Res 47:59, 1989

82. Gluud C: Branched-chain amino acids for hepatic encephalopathy? Hepatology 13:812, 1991

83. Mammen EF: Coagulopathies of liver disease. Clin Lab Med 14:769, 1994

84. Mammen EF: Coagulation defects in liver disease. Med Clin North Am 78:545, 1994

85. Mannucci PM, Franchi F, Dioguardi N: Correction of abnormal coagulation in chronic liver disease by combined use of fresh-frozen plasma and prothrombin complex concentrates. Lancet 2:542, 1976

86. Ballard HS, Marcus AJ: Platelet aggregation in portal cirrhosis. Arch Intern Med 136:316, 1976

87. Brophy MT, Fiore L, Deykin D: Hemostasis. Hepatology: A Textbook of Liver Disease. Zakim D, Boyer T, Eds. WB Saunders Co, Philadelphia, 1996, p 691

88. Hersch SL, Kunelis T, Francis RB Jr: The pathogenesis of accelerated fibrinolysis in liver cirrhosis: a critical role for tissue plasminogen activator inhibitor. Blood 69:1315, 1987

89. Riewald M, Riess H: Treatment options for clinically recognized disseminated intravascular coagulation. Semin Thromb Hemost 24:53, 1998

90. Bismuth H, Samuel D, Castaing D, et al: Liver transplantation in Europe for patients with acute liver failure. Semin Liver Dis 16:415, 1996

91. Rosen HR, Shackleton CR, Martin P: Indications for and timing of liver transplantation. Med Clin North Am 80:1069, 1996

92. Lucey MR, Brown KA, Everson GT, et al: Minimal criteria for placement of adults on the liver transplant waiting list: a report of a national conference organized by the American Society of Transplant Physicians and the American Association for the Study of Liver Diseases. Liver Transpl Surg 3:628, 1997

93. Butterworth RF: The neurobiology of hepatic encephalopathy. Semin Liver Dis 16:235, 1996

94. Ferenci P, Puspok A, Steindl P: Current concepts in the pathophysiology of hepatic encephalopathy. Eur J Clin Invest 22:573, 1992

95. Maddison JE, Watson WE, Dodd PR, et al: Alterations in cortical [3H]kainate and alpha-[3H]amino-3-hydroxy-5-methyl-4-isoxazolepropionic acid binding in a spontaneous canine model of chronic hepatic encephalopathy. J Neurochem 56:1881, 1991

96. Yurdaydin C, Walsh TJ, Engler HD, et al: Gut bacteria provide precursors of benzodiazepine receptor ligands in a rat model of hepatic encephalopathy. Brain Res 679:42, 1995

97. Jones EA, Basile AS, Skolnick P: Hepatic encephalopathy, GABA-ergic neurotransmission and benzodiazepine receptor ligands. Adv Exp Med Biol 272:121, 1990

98. Basile AS, Harrison PM, Hughes RD, et al: Relationship between plasma benzodiazepine receptor ligand concentrations and severity of hepatic encephalopathy. Hepatology 19:112, 1994

99. Takahashi K, Kameda H, Kataoka M, et al: Ammonia potentiates GABAA response in dissociated rat cortical neurons. Neurosci Lett 151:51, 1993

100. Aronson LR, Gacad RC, Kaminsky-Russ K, et al: Endogenous benzodiazepine activity in the peripheral and portal blood of dogs with congenital portosystemic shunts. Vet Surg 26:189, 1997

101. Demetriou AA, Watanabe F: Support of the Acutely Failing Liver, 2nd ed. RG Landes Co, Austin, Texas, 2000.

102. Rozga J, Holzman MD, Ro MS, et al: Development of a hybrid bioartificial liver. Ann Surg 217:502, 1993

103. Watanabe FD, Mullon CJ, Hewitt WR, et al: Clinical experience with a bioartificial liver in the treatment of severe liver failure: a phase I clinical trial. Ann Surg 225:484, 1997

104. Watanabe FD, Arnaout WS, Ting P, et al: Artificial liver. Transplant Proc 31:373, 1999

7 MULTIPLE ORGAN DYSFUNCTION SYNDROME

John C. Marshall, M.D., and Avery B. Nathens, M.D., Ph.D., M.P.H.

Approach to Multiple Organ Dysfunction Syndrome

Recognition of the Susceptible Patient

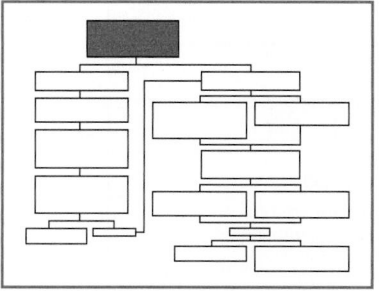

The phenomenon of multiple organ dysfunction syndrome (MODS) is characterized by the progressive but potentially reversible physiologic dysfunction of two or more organs or organ systems that arises after resuscitation from an acute life-threatening event. Formerly known as progressive systems failure,[1] multiple organ failure,[2] and multiple organ systems failure,[3] the phenomenon was designated multiple organ dysfunction syndrome by a 1991 consensus conference of the American College of Chest Physicians (ACCP) and the Society of Critical Care Medicine (SCCM). This designation is meant to emphasize that certain dynamic alterations in physiologic function in the critically ill patient may constitute a clinical syndrome with common pathophysiological underpinnings.[4] However, MODS may be less a syndrome than a paradigm—an approach to the care of the critically ill patient that emphasizes intensive monitoring and support of organ system function, specific therapies for isolated disease processes, and prevention or minimization of physiologic derangements resulting from ICU interventions.

MODS evolves in the wake of a profound disruption of systemic homeostasis.[5] Classic MODS is seen in patients with overwhelming infection, multiple injuries, or massive ischemia, but the syndrome has a number of risk factors, some of which overlap [see Table 1].

The hallmark of MODS is the involvement of organs or organ systems remote from the site of the original insult in a dynamic process that ranges in severity from mild, transient dysfunction to frank, irreversible organ system failure. Disruption of normal homeostasis causes altered patterns of organ system interaction; the fundamental problem in the clinical approach to MODS is that attempts to support one organ or organ system may aggravate dysfunction in another. Although preexisting abnormalities of organ system function—such as those that occur in diabetes, chronic renal failure, and hepatic failure—also contribute to adverse outcomes in critical illness, MODS is considered to be an acute and potentially reversible process rather than a manifestation of chronic and irreversible disease.

Prevention

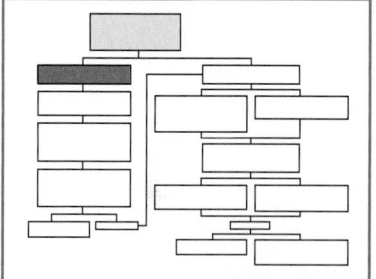

Any patient with acute physiologic instability from a variety of diagnoses [see Table 1] is at risk for MODS. Varying degrees of organ system dysfunction may be present at the time of ICU admission—depending on the severity of the process and the duration of its evolution—and these derangements have an important impact on prognosis.[6] The cornerstone of care for ICU patients with minimal organ dysfunction is the prevention of MODS through the support of optimal systemic physiologic function in circumstances in which an acute insult has altered patterns of normal homeostasis. In general, such prevention consists of the provision of the highest-quality clinical care. This objective has three discrete elements: hemodynamic support, metabolic support, and immunologic support. In each case, optimal care involves both physiologic intervention and appropriate monitoring to direct that intervention.

HEMODYNAMIC SUPPORT

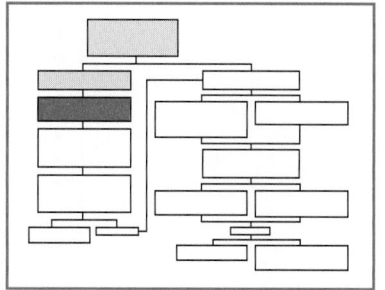

Optimal hemodynamic homeostasis is achieved when oxygen delivery to tissues and use of oxygen by tissues are maximized and when anaerobic metabolism is prevented.

Oxygen delivery ($\dot{D}o_2$) is a function of three variables: the hemoglobin level, the oxygen saturation, and the cardiac output. In cases of mild or moderate surgical stress, oxygen demands are not substantially altered, myocardial function remains intact, and microvascular permeability remains normal. Adequate $\dot{D}o_2$ can thus be assumed if the pulse rate, blood pressure, urine output, and central venous pressure (CVP) remain normal.

In a normal person, oxygen consumption (calculated as the product of the cardiac output and the arteriovenous gradient in oxygen content) remains constant despite changes in $\dot{D}o_2$, until oxygen delivery reaches a critically low level, at which point oxygen consumption is said to be supply dependent. In a patient at

Recognize the susceptible patient

Patients at high risk for multiple organ dysfunction syndrome (MODS) are those who have experienced a profound disruption of systemic homeostasis resulting from one or more of the following:

- Overwhelming infection
- Sterile inflammation
- Massive injury
- Massive ischemia
- Immune system activation
- Intoxication
- Iatrogenic factors
- Idiopathic factors

Minimal organ dysfunction

Prevent progression to MODS by optimizing support of hemodynamic, metabolic, and immunologic function.

Hemodynamic support

Maximize O_2 delivery to tissues by the following measures:

- Fluid replacement therapy
- Inotropic agents
- Vasoactive agents
- Mechanical ventilation

Metabolic support

Reverse catabolic state with early, definitive surgical therapy, including the following:

- Debridement of devitalized tissue
- Burn wound excision and grafting
- Rigid fixation of long bone fractures

Provide early, aggressive nutritional support, by the enteral route if possible. If gut function is inadequate, total parenteral nutrition should be employed until gut function returns.

Immunologic support

Prevent nosocomial infection, eradicate established infection, and minimize the effects of injurious host defense responses by such measures as the following:

- Timely and appropriate surgical intervention
- Limiting the breach of mucosal defenses
- Avoidance of antacids for stress ulcer prophylaxis
- Selective, targeted use of systemic antibiotics

Organ function is restored

Patient survives. Discharge patient from ICU.

Organ function deteriorates

Approach to Multiple Organ Dysfunction Syndrome

Significant organ dysfunction

Characterize the physiologic derangement and institute supportive therapy.

Single organ dysfunction

Search for correctable causes, including the following:
- Exacerbation of preexisting chronic disease
- Complications from invasive devices and medications
- Local complications (e.g., fluid overload, pneumothorax, biliary tract obstruction)
- Local pathology (e.g., myocardial infarction, pulmonary embolism, pneumonia)

Multiple organ dysfunction

Search for correctable causes, including the following:
- Occult infection
- Missed injuries
- Adverse effects of medical therapy (e.g., transfusions, total parenteral nutrition)

Modify supportive care

Minimize adverse consequences of supportive care through the use of techniques such as pressure-limited ventilation and continuous hemodialysis. Manage infectious complications with local measures and sparing use of antimicrobial agents. Evaluate need for antibiotic therapy or surgical intervention.

Antibiotic therapy

- Sparing use of empirical antibiotic therapy
- Microbiological diagnosis can almost always be made in MODS
- If organism cannot be isolated, discontinue antibiotics and repeat cultures

Surgical intervention

Prepare the patient for operation through the following measures:
- Preoperative optimization of physiologic function
- Safe, well-organized transport to the operating room
- Surgical intervention in the ICU when appropriate and feasible

Reevaluate clinical status

MODS resolves, and patient's condition improves

Transfer patient from ICU.

MODS persists, and patient's condition deteriorates or fails to improve despite support and in the absence of correctable underlying disease

Probability of death is overwhelming. Consider withdrawal of life support.

Table 1   Risk Factors for MODS

Infection	Peritonitis and intra-abdominal infections
	Pneumonia
	Necrotizing soft tissue infections
	Group A streptococcal infections
	Endocarditis
	Meningitis
	Candidiasis
Inflammation	Pancreatitis
Injury	Multiple trauma
	Burn injury
Ischemia	Ruptured aneurysm
	Hypovolemic shock
	Aortic occlusion
	Mesenteric vascular occlusion
Immune Reactions	Autoimmune disease
	Transplant rejection
	Graft versus host disease
	Administration of interleukin-2
Iatrogenic Factors	Delayed or missed injury
	Blood transfusion
	Total parenteral nutrition
Intoxication	Drug reactions
	Salicylate intoxication
	Arsenic intoxication
	Acetaminophen overdose
Idiopathic Factors	Thrombotic thrombocytopenic purpura
	HELLP syndrome
	Pheochromocytoma

HELLP—hemolysis, elevated liver enzymes, and a low platelet count

risk for MODS, increasing $\dot{D}o_2$ results in a progressive increase in oxygen consumption, producing a state that has been termed pathological supply dependency. It remains controversial whether the phenomenon of pathological supply dependency is a true physiologic abnormality[7] or an artifact resulting from the incorporation of shared mathematical variables into the equations for $\dot{D}o_2$ and oxygen consumption.[8] Whichever the case may be, many authors view this abnormal relation as evidence of occult tissue hypoxia and as justification for strategies to increase $\dot{D}o_2$ to supraphysiologic values.[9]

In the patient at risk for MODS, a variety of acute changes in hemodynamic homeostasis make the optimization of tissue oxygenation particularly challenging. Acute lung injury may impair pulmonary gas exchange as a consequence of increased interstitial edema (from both the original injury and the effects of resuscitation) and may result in ventilation-perfusion ($\dot{V}/\dot{Q}$) mismatch. Myocardial depression resulting from circulating depressant factors[10] and the loss of peripheral vascular tone (likely from increased nitric oxide release[11]) lead to alterations in regional blood flow and $\dot{D}o_2$. Increases in tissue edema[12,13] and impairment of red cell deformability[14] hinder $\dot{D}o_2$ at the microcirculatory level.

Hemodynamic optimization of critically ill patients begins with volume replacement, guided by values for urine output, CVP, pulmonary arterial wedge pressure (PAWP), and cardiac index [see VII:1 Cardiopulmonary Monitoring]. Fluid replacement is best monitored by physiologic responses to therapy rather than by targeting an arbitrary ideal value for urine output or PAWP. In general, the appropriate volume of fluid is that which optimizes cardiac output and mixed venous oxygen saturation ($S_{mv}O_2$) without impairing pulmonary gas exchange and that which typically results in a PAWP of 12 to 16 mm Hg. No benefit has been proved for the use of colloids over crystalloids in fluid resuscitation; any theoretical benefit of colloids in increasing oncotic pressure is offset by increased vascular permeability and increased extravasation into the tissues.[15]

Beyond a certain point, the beneficial effects of fluid administration are outweighed by the detrimental effects—namely, an increase in pulmonary edema (resulting in worsening gas exchange) and in cerebral edema (resulting in deterioration of the level of consciousness). Oxygen delivery can be further augmented by the use of inotropic agents, such as dopamine and dobutamine, and vasoactive medications. Inotropic drugs augment $\dot{D}o_2$ through a direct action on myocardial contractility but have differential peripheral effects; for example, dopamine increases vascular resistance, whereas dobutamine reduces it. When the calculated peripheral vascular resistance is low, the addition of a vasopressor agent, such as norepinephrine, may prove beneficial in increasing mean arterial pressure and cardiac output. Conversely, when peripheral vascular resistance is abnormally high and stroke volume is reduced, the use of a selective vasodilator, such as sodium nitroprusside, may increase $\dot{D}o_2$. A combination of agents is often required to optimize physiologic benefits.

Therapy for hemodynamic optimization is generally individualized by titrating agents, guided by the results obtained through invasive monitoring [see VI:1 Cardiopulmonary Monitoring]. Use of a pulmonary arterial catheter permits the calculation of $\dot{D}o_2$ and the indirect measurement of oxygen consumption. Measurement of the $S_{mv}O_2$ provides a rapid and sensitive measure of oxygen uptake in the tissues. In a normal person, approximately 30 percent of the oxygen carried to the tissues in arterial blood is extracted, so that the hemoglobin returning to the heart in mixed venous blood has an oxygen saturation of approximately 70 percent. A reduction in the oxygen extraction ratio is a characteristic finding during the hemodynamic alterations associated with a septic response, and the $S_{mv}O_2$ is correspondingly higher—often in the range of 80 percent. When oxygen delivery to the tissues is impaired, oxygen extraction by the tissues increases, and the $S_{mv}O_2$ decreases. Lactic acid is produced as a result of anaerobic metabolism in the tissues, and elevated serum lactate levels reflect ongoing anaerobic metabolism[16]; however, lactate levels are relatively insensitive to minor degrees of tissue hypoxia. An indirect evaluation of the adequacy of oxygen delivery to the gut can be made using a gastric tonometer, a modified nasogastric tube with a semipermeable balloon reservoir at its tip. Because carbon dioxide in the gastric wall diffuses freely into the reservoir, tonometric measurement of the carbon dioxide tension (Pco_2) and simultaneous measurement of arterial pH and the arterial carbon dioxide tension (P_aCO_2) permit calculation of gastric intramural pH using the Henderson-Hasselbalch equation [see I:7 Life-Threatening Acid-Base Disorders].[17] Although several reports suggest that gastric tonometry can provide information of greater potential therapeutic usefulness than information obtained through more conventional monitoring techniques,[18,19] the benefits of tonometry are controversial[20] and the device must still be considered experimental.

METABOLIC SUPPORT

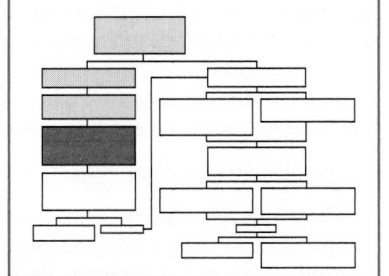

The acute response to stress and injury is a complex, coordinated process characterized by increases in levels of catecholamines, glucocorticoids, antidiuretic hormone, and hormones that regulate intermediary metabolism, including insulin, glucagon, and growth hormone[21] [see VII:8 Metabolic Response to Critical Illness]. The activation of this response results in a predictable series of metabolic alterations, including retention of salt and water, increased production of glucose, enhanced lipolysis,[22] increased protein catabolism,[23] an altered pattern of hepatic protein synthesis known as the acute-phase response,[24] and a reduction in ketone body ratios.[25]

Metabolic prophylaxis of MODS is directed toward the reversal of stimuli responsible for the catabolic hormonal milieu and toward the provision of adequate biochemical substrates at a time of increased metabolic demand. Early definitive surgical therapy in the form of debridement of devitalized tissue,[26] burn wound excision and grafting,[27,28] and rigid fixation of long bone fractures[29,30] can attenuate the postinjury hypermetabolic state and minimize the subsequent development of MODS.[31] Conversely, a delay in definitive therapy is a risk factor for MODS.[32]

Nutritional support should be provided by the enteral route if possible.[33] In many cases, the gastrointestinal tract can be used even in the face of significant physiologic derangement[34]; however, if enteral feeding is not feasible, total parenteral nutrition (TPN) should be initiated until gut function returns. The primary objective of nutritional support is not the administration of calories but the provision of the substrates required for the biologic processes of inflammation and healing. Optimal formulations are yet to be established. Parenteral solutions enriched in branched-chain amino acids have not proved beneficial in the prevention of MODS.[35] Because of the critical importance of glutamine in the maintenance of the mucosa of the GI tract, there is considerable interest in the use of glutamine-enriched formulations[36]; preliminary clinical studies suggest that glutamine supplementation can prevent intestinal atrophy and maintain normal gut barrier function.[37] Supplementation of enteral nutrition with arginine, nucleotides, and fish oils appears to have a beneficial effect on both length of ICU stay and infectious morbidity.[38] However, beyond the evolving practice of beginning enteral nutritional support early in the high-risk patient and ensuring adequate substrate delivery by supplementing enteral with parenteral feeds as needed, there are as yet no compelling reasons to recommend any specific formulation of parenteral or enteral nutrition. Approaches to nutritional support of the surgical patient are discussed in detail elsewhere [see VII:9 Nutritional Support].

IMMUNOLOGIC SUPPORT

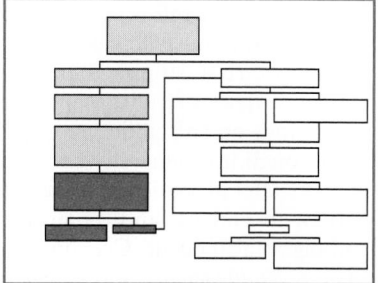

Immunologic support of critically ill surgical patients has two objectives: to prevent nosocomial infection and to eradicate established infection while attenuating any potentially injurious host defense responses. Infection is an important risk factor for MODS, but the converse is equally true—the patient with MODS is at substantially increased risk for the development of infection. This risk arises for two reasons: impairment of normal host defense mechanisms and colonization with potentially infectious nosocomial pathogens.[39,40]

Although numerous discrete immunologic derangements have been described in critical illness,[41] impairment of mucosal defenses is probably the most important and certainly the most readily preventable. Normal mucosal defenses are physically breached by surgical incisions and by invasive devices, including intravascular catheters, urinary catheters, and endotracheal and nasogastric tubes. Limiting the number of such devices[42] and paying rigorous attention to their proper insertion and maintenance[43] are important in minimizing rates of nosocomial infection. Gastric acidity plays a primary role in the normal mucosal defenses of the stomach. Antacids ablate this aspect of defense and are a well-established risk factor for nosocomial pneumonia[44]; they should probably not be used for stress ulcer prophylaxis. A striking decline in the incidence of clinically significant stress bleeding in the contemporary ICU suggests that such prophylaxis should be limited only to those patients at high risk for stress ulcer.[45] Whether cytoprotective agents have any benefit over H_2-receptor antagonists or proton pump blockers is controversial[46]; definitive recommendations regarding the safest mode of stress ulcer prophylaxis await the results of larger, better-designed clinical trials.

Popular in European ICUs is an alternative approach to the prevention of pathological colonization—namely, the topical use of nonabsorbable antibiotics specifically targeted at aerobic gram-negative bacteria and fungi, along with a short course of systemic antimicrobial therapy. This technique is known as selective decontamination of the digestive tract (SDD). SDD has been evaluated in a large number of studies of varying methodological quality. The results of a meta-analysis of these studies demonstrate that the technique can significantly reduce rates of nosocomial pneumonia but that it has only a marginally beneficial effect on ICU survival, and even then only when both topical and systemic agents are used.[47] The expense of the topical agents and the unpleasant taste of the topical paste have limited the popularity of SDD in North America. Nonetheless, SDD does show promise as a prophylactic measure, particularly in trauma patients and transplant recipients.

Early institution of enteral nutrition also appears to have salutary consequences for the prevention of infection.[48] It has been suggested that acidification of the feeding formulation may result in greater benefit,[49] but the utility of this approach remains unproved.

Systemic antibiotics suppress the indigenous flora of mucosal surfaces, promoting pathological colonization with resistant organisms.[50] Therefore, use of antimicrobial agents in critically ill patients must be selective and targeted, and the use of broad-spectrum empirical therapy should be minimized by regular reviews of culture and sensitivity results and through restrictions on antibiotic prescription practices.

Although it is generally believed that nosocomial infections in critically ill patients arise from endogenous reservoirs, patient-to-patient and environment-to-patient spreads of pathogens also occur. Certain organisms—particularly *Acinetobacter*, *Xanthomonas*, and *Legionella*—are transmitted through aqueous sources in the ICU, and the isolation of such organisms from critically ill patients is evidence of a potential problem in environmental infection control. Hand washing is an important but underutilized mode of infection prevention in the ICU. There is no clear evidence that protective isolation of critically ill patients warrants the increased costs and increased demands on nursing staff.

Untreated infection is both a cause of impaired immunologic responsiveness and a potent stimulus of the inflammatory and cytokine responses that figure centrally in the pathogenesis of MODS. Early fixation of fractures not only attenuates hypermetabolism but also reduces infectious complications.[30]

The role of immunomodulation in the prevention of MODS is undefined. Nonspecific immunomodulatory techniques have aroused considerable theoretical interest; however, there are as yet no convincing data to support the use of these techniques in clinical situations. Moreover, attempts to enhance host immunity by pharmacological means may actually augment morbidity by amplifying the detrimental consequences of the cytokine response.[51] To date, studies of immunomodulation using specific immunotherapy directed against endotoxin[52-54] and other strategies designed to moderate the proinflammatory cytokine response[55,56] have yielded generally disappointing results. Although improved techniques for identifying the patient populations that may benefit from such interventions will likely establish a role for these strategies, it is clear that timely and appropriate surgical intervention remains the most potent form of immunotherapy currently available to the surgeon.[57]

Definitions of Organ System Dysfunctions

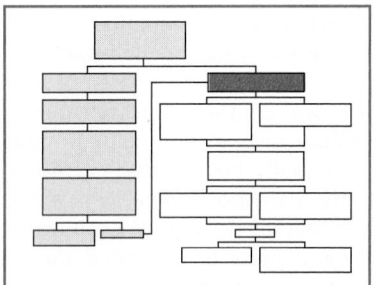

No consensus has yet been reached on how best to characterize MODS according to the dysfunctioning organ systems, the descriptors that optimally reflect dysfunction within a given organ system, or the degree of abnormality that constitutes the dysfunction or failure of a particular organ system. Nonetheless, it would appear that such a consensus may not be far off.

A systematic review of the published literature from 1969 through 1993 identified 30 clinical studies of 20 or more patients with MODS that provided explicit criteria for organ failure or dysfunction.[58] Although criteria varied significantly among the studies, seven organ systems were cited in over half

of the published reports: the respiratory system (all 30 reports), the renal system (29 reports), the hepatic system (27 reports), the cardiovascular system (25 reports), the hematologic system (23 reports), the GI system (22 reports), and the central nervous system (18 reports). Both a recent European consensus conference and two North American collaborations[59] define MODS by the above systems, eliminating the GI system because of the declining incidence of stress-related upper GI bleeding and the lack of satisfactory descriptors of GI dysfunction. The available scoring systems have many similarities [*see Table 2*], and it is likely that a wider consensus on the description of clinical MODS will emerge over the next few years.

RESPIRATORY DYSFUNCTION

The adult respiratory distress syndrome (ARDS) is the prototypical expression of respiratory dysfunction in MODS.[60] In its mildest form, respiratory dysfunction is characterized by tachypnea, hypocapnia, and hypoxemia. As the injury evolves, a combination of worsening hypoxemia and an increase in the work of breathing necessitates mechanical ventilatory support [*see VII:3 Pulmonary Dysfunction and VII:4 Use of the Mechanical Ventilator*].

Increased capillary permeability is the earliest pathological event in ARDS.[61] Respiratory impairment is reflected in a reduction in functional lung capacity and results from both the increased distance across which oxygen must pass from the alveolus to the capillaries and the decreased compliance of the edematous lung.[62] As the acute inflammatory process resolves, further lung injury results from the process of repair, which involves fibrosis and deposition of hyaline material.[63]

Lung involvement in ARDS is inhomogeneous: areas of functional and aerated alveoli are interspersed between areas of nonfunctional alveoli.[64] Pathological examination of an involved lung reveals injury to alveolar epithelial cells and capillary endothelial cells, with plugging of the alveoli by proteinaceous fluid containing inflammatory cells and cell fragments. Deposition of hyaline material is seen in the alveolar ducts.[65] The aerated lung units that remain appear to have normal gas-tissue ratios and well-preserved mechanical and gas-exchanging properties.

Physiologic impairment of the respiratory system is reflected by a reduced arterial oxygen tension (P_aO_2). Normalization of the P_aO_2 often requires the institution of mechanical ventilation with an adequate value for the fraction of inspired oxygen (F_IO_2) [*see VII:4 Use of the Mechanical Ventilator*]. The ratio of P_aO_2 to F_IO_2 is an objective measurement of the degree to which oxygenation is impaired and is probably the best available measurement of respiratory dysfunction.[66]

RENAL DYSFUNCTION

Acute renal failure emerged as a significant clinical problem during World War II, but supportive therapy, in the form of dialysis, did not become available until the 1950s. Clinical or subclinical evidence of renal dysfunction is common in MODS. Early-onset renal dysfunction typically results from hypotension. The etiology of late-onset renal failure is multifactorial and includes both prerenal factors (e.g., decreased cardiac output, hypovolemia) and the cumulative effects of nephrotoxic agents, such as medications and radiocontrast

Table 2 Recognition and Assessment of Organ System Dysfunctions[59,179,264,285,286]

Organ System	Indicators of Dysfunction	Degree of Dysfunction				
		None (0)*	Minimal (1)*	Mild (2)*	Moderate (3)*	Severe (4)*
Respiratory	P$_a$O$_2$/F$_i$O$_2$ ratio	> 300[†] > 400[‡]	226–300[†] 300–400[‡]	151–225[†] 200–300[‡]	76–150[†] 100–200[‡]	≤ 75[†] < 100[‡]
	Duration of mechanical ventilation	—	—	> 48 hr	> 72 hr	> 72 hr (PEEP > 10 or F$_i$O$_2$ > 0.50)
Renal	Creatinine level	≤ 100 μmol/L	101–200 μmol/L	201–350 μmol/L	351–500 μmol/L	> 500 μmol/L
	Urine output	—	—	—	< 500 ml/day	< 200 ml/day
	Need for dialysis	—	—	—	—	Dialysis
Neurologic	Glasgow Coma Scale score	Glasgow Coma Scale score, 15	Glasgow Coma Scale score, 13–14	Glasgow Coma Scale score, 10–12	Glasgow Coma Scale score, 7–9	Glasgow Coma Scale score, ≤ 6
Hepatic	Bilirubin	≤ 20 μmol/L[†] < 20 μmol/L[‡]	21–60 μmol/L[†] 20–32 μmol/L[‡]	61–120 μmol/L[†] 33–101 μmol/L[‡]	121–240 μmol/L[†] 162–204 μmol/L[‡]	> 240 μmol/L[†] > 204 μmol/L[‡]
	Albumin	—	—	< 28 mg/dl	< 23 mg/dl	< 19 mg/dl
	AST	—	< 25 U/L	—	25–50 U/L	> 50 U/L
Cardiovascular	Systolic blood pressure	> 90 mm Hg	71–90 mm Hg (fluid responsive)	61–70 mm Hg (not fluid responsive)	51–60 mm Hg	≤ 50 mm Hg
	pH	—	—	—	≤ 7.3	≤ 7.2
	Inotropic agent dosages	—	—	Dopamine < 5 μg/kg/min *or* Any dose of dobutamine	Dopamine > 5 μg/kg/min *or* Epinephrine < 0.1 μg/kg/min *or* Norepinephrine < 0.1 μg/kg/min	Dopamine > 15 μg/kg/min *or* Epinephrine > 0.1 μg/kg/min *or* Norepinephrine > 0.1 μg/kg/min
	$\dfrac{\text{Heart rate} \times \text{CVP}}{\text{MAP}}$	< 10.0	10.1–15.0	15.1–20.0	20.1–30.0	> 30.0
Hematologic	Platelet count	> 120,000/mm³	81,000–120,000/mm³	51,000–80,000/mm³	21,000–50,000/mm³	≤ 20,000/mm³
	Leukocyte count	—	—	—	> 30,000/mm³	> 60,000/mm³ *or* < 2,500/mm³
Gastrointestinal	Enteral nutrition	—	—	Mild intolerance	Moderate intolerance	Severe intolerance
	Stress ulcer bleeding	None	None	None	Stress bleeding	> 2 U/day
Metabolic	Insulin requirements	None	None	> 1 U/hr	2–4 U/hr	> 4 U/hr

*Multiple organ dysfunction syndrome (MODS) score.
[†]Data from reference 59.
[‡]Data from references 285 and 286.
AST—aspartate aminotransferase F$_i$O$_2$—fraction of inspired oxygen MAP—mean systemic arterial pressure P$_a$O$_2$—arterial oxygen tension
PEEP—positive end-expiratory pressure CVP—central venous pressure

material.[67] Histologic studies show acute tubular necrosis with disruption of the basement membrane, patchy necrosis of the tubules, interstitial edema, and tubular casts; these changes correlate poorly with functional impairment[68] [*see VII:5 Renal Failure*].

Renal dysfunction in the multiple organ dysfunction syndrome is reflected biochemically by an increasing serum creatinine level. The creatinine clearance provides a sensitive reflection of early subclinical renal dysfunction[69] but is probably too sensitive to be of use in the evaluation of established dysfunction.

HEPATIC DYSFUNCTION

Hepatic dysfunction in critical illness was first described during World War II[70] and occurs in up to 54 percent of patients admitted to an ICU[71] [*see VII:6 Hepatic Failure*]. Two clinical syndromes have been described: ischemic hepatitis and ICU jaundice. Ischemic hepatitis, or shock liver, characteristically follows an episode of hypotension. Early elevations of aminotransferase levels are striking and may be associated with an increased prothrombin time and hypoglycemia; centrilobular necrosis is evident histologically. Successful resuscitation of the shock state results in rapid normalization of the biochemical abnormalities.[71] ICU jaundice, which is more common than ischemic hepatitis, typically evolves many days after the inciting physiologic insult. Conjugated hyperbilirubinemia is a prominent feature, whereas elevation of aminotransferase levels and prothrombin time are less pronounced.[72] Histologic features include intrahepatic cholestasis, steatosis, and Kupffer cell hyperplasia.[73] The pathogenesis is multifactorial and includes ongoing hepatic ischemia, TPN-induced cholestasis, and drug toxicity.

CARDIOVASCULAR DYSFUNCTION

Both peripheral vascular and myocardial function are altered in MODS. Characteristic changes in the peripheral vasculature include a reduction in vascular resistance and an increase in microvascular permeability, resulting in a hyperdynamic circulatory profile and peripheral edema. The reduction in systemic vascular resistance results in an increase in cardiac index; however, this increase may be insufficient to maintain an adequate mean arterial pressure because of intrinsic impairment of myocardial contractility. Cardiovascular dysfunction in MODS is evident clinically as hypotension that is refractory to volume challenge (necessitating inotropic and vasopressor support), tachydysrhythmias, and peripheral edema. Biventricular dilatation with a reduction in right and left ventricular ejection fractions is apparent.[74] Right ventricular dysfunction is particularly prominent, perhaps as a consequence of increased pulmonary vascular resistance secondary to concomitant lung injury.[75,76]

The mechanisms of altered myocardial function in MODS are incompletely characterized, though the myocardial depressant effects of circulating cytokines,[77] potentially mediated through the local release of nitric oxide,[78] appear to play an important role.

NEUROLOGIC DYSFUNCTION

Abnormalities of both central and peripheral nervous system function have been described in critical illness. CNS dysfunction occurs in up to 70 percent of critically ill patients, typically presenting as alterations in level of consciousness without localizing signs.[79] Its pathophysiology is poorly understood; postulated mechanisms include the direct effects of proinflammatory mediators on cerebral function, the development of vasogenic cerebral edema, areas of infarction related to hypotension, and alterations in the blood-brain barrier that result in changes in the composition of the interstitial fluid.[80] The electroencephalogram typically shows one of four patterns indicating increasingly abnormal activity: diffuse theta wave rhythms, intermittent rhythmic delta waves, triphasic delta waves, and suppression or burst-suppression patterns.[80]

The peripheral nervous system dysfunction of MODS, also known as critical illness polyneuropathy, affects up to 70 percent of critically ill patients.[81] The clinical presentation of peripheral neuropathy in the critically ill patient is subtle. It may present as failure to wean a patient from mechanical ventilation.[82] Other manifestations include weakness of the limbs or absent deep tendon reflexes, with relative sparing of the cranial nerves, resulting in weak or absent limb movements with preservation of facial grimacing in response to painful stimuli. Like the encephalopathy of MODS, the pathophysiology of peripheral neuropathy remains speculative; however, endoneural edema and axonal hypoxia have been implicated.[83]

HEMATOLOGIC DYSFUNCTION

The most common hematologic abnormality of critical illness is thrombocytopenia, which occurs in approximately 20 percent of ICU admissions.[84] Causes include increased consumption, intravascular sequestration, and impaired thrombopoiesis secondary to suppression of bone marrow function.[85] In addition, heparin-induced thrombocytopenia resulting from antibodies to complexes of heparin and platelet factor 4 develops in up to 10 percent of patients receiving heparin.[86] Prolongation of the prothrombin time and the partial thromboplastin time occurs less frequently. The most fulminant expression of hematologic dysfunction in MODS is disseminated intravascular coagulation (DIC), which is characterized by derangements in platelet numbers and clotting times and the presence in plasma of fibrin degradation products.[87]

Anemia is common in critical illness and arises not only as a result of diagnostic blood draws but also as a manifestation of the acute-phase response mediated in part by interleukin-1 (IL-1).[88] Transient leukopenia is a classic manifestation of early endotoxemia[89]; more commonly, the leukocyte count in MODS is elevated as a manifestation of a systemic septic response. Lymphopenia is common, though the cause is unknown.

GASTROINTESTINAL DYSFUNCTION

Upper GI hemorrhage after burn injury was first described by Curling in 1842.[90] Until recently, stress GI bleeding was a common problem, occurring in up to a quarter of all ICU admissions.[91] Improved techniques of resuscitation and hemodynamic support, earlier diagnosis of infection, and the widespread use of stress ulcer prophylaxis have contributed to a reduction in the frequency of this complication; through such measures, rates of clinically important bleeding in the contemporary ICU have dropped below four percent.[45] Other manifestations of GI dysfunction in MODS include ileus and intolerance of enteral feeding,[92] pancreatitis,[93] and acalculous cholecystitis.[94] Splanchnic hypoperfusion with mucosal acidosis is a pathological feature common to all of these.[95]

OTHER ORGAN SYSTEM DYSFUNCTION

Hyperglycemia with insulin resistance is the most common manifestation of endocrine dysfunction in critical illness.[96] The sick euthyroid syndrome, which is characterized by reductions in serum T_3 with or without an increase in reverse T_3 levels and a normal T_4 level, is another expression of endocrine dysfunction in the critically ill; thyrotropin levels are reduced, and the magnitude of the reduction correlates with the severity of illness.[97] Abnormalities of adrenal function have also been reported.[98,99]

Immunologic dysfunction can be evaluated by means of delayed hypersensitivity skin-testing[100]; responses of critically ill patients are characteristically suppressed.[101,102] Documentation of the full spectrum of immune derangements in critical illness requires more complex technology than is available in the average ICU; however, the development of ICU-acquired infection with endemic ICU pathogens of low intrinsic virulence, such as *Candida*, coagulase-negative staphylococci, and enterococci, can be considered a surrogate marker of immune dysfunction in MODS.[102]

Abnormalities of wound healing represent an expression of MODS. Common manifestations of impaired wound healing include the failure of an open wound to develop satisfactory granulation tissue and the development of decubitus ulcers.

Evaluation of the Patient with Organ Dysfunction

SINGLE-ORGAN DYSFUNCTION

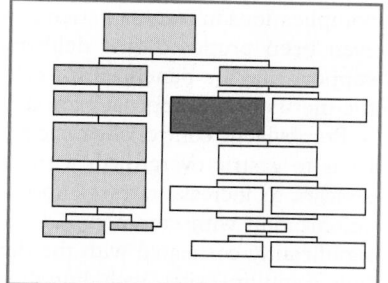

Single-organ dysfunction strongly suggests local pathology and should trigger a search for potentially correctable causes in the affected organ system. Isolated organ dysfunction may arise as a result of preexisting chronic disease or may reflect a local problem, such as fluid overload, atelectasis, biliary tract obstruction, or increased intracranial pressure. Complications related to invasive devices and adverse effects of medication are common causes of single-organ dysfunction; the diagnosis is often presumptive, established on the basis of improvement after discontinuance of the agent or removal of the device. Finally, single organ dysfunction may indicate acute organ injury such as a myocardial infarction, pulmonary embolism, or pneumonia. Because the prognosis of single-organ dysfunction is relatively good—even in cases of profound functional deficit—consideration of heroic supportive measures is justified.[103]

Search for Correctable Causes

Deteriorating function in a single organ system should prompt an evaluation to detect potentially reversible problems. Respiratory dysfunction may occur as a result of complications such as fluid overload, pneumonia, pleural effusion, pneumothorax, or pulmonary embolism. Hypotension can be caused by hypovolemia or overly aggressive diuresis. Central venous and pulmonary arterial catheters may induce tachyarrhythmias as a result of mechanical irritation of the conducting system. Renal dysfunction may reflect inadequate intravascular volume or the nephrotoxic effects of medications (e.g., acute tubular necrosis caused by aminoglycosides and interstitial nephritis caused by penicillins and cephalosporins). Occasionally, renal dysfunction arises from a postrenal cause, such as ureteral obstruction or blockage of a Foley catheter.

Medications are important causes of liver dysfunction in the critically ill patient. Erythromycin, ketoconazole, and haloperidol can induce cholestatic liver injury.[104] Thrombocytopenia is an important adverse effect of a number of medications, including heparin flushes used to maintain the patency of arterial lines.[105] A decreased level of consciousness is usually the result of the poorly characterized metabolic encephalopathy of critical illness; however, it is necessary to rule out other causes, such as meningitis, encephalitis, brain abscess, and subdural empyema. Excessive or prolonged use of narcotics or sedative-hypnotics may lead to prolonged alterations in level of consciousness, particularly when hepatic or renal function is impaired. Nondepolarizing muscle relaxants, such as vecuronium, may cause prolonged neuromuscular blockade and persistent peripheral nerve dysfunction.[106]

MULTIPLE ORGAN DYSFUNCTION

Some authors have described a characteristic temporal sequence to the evolution of MODS[3,59] [see Table 3]; however, the clinical course tends to be highly variable. The specific pattern of dysfunction is much less important than the course of the evolving syndrome. Resolution of dysfunction suggests an appropriate response to specific and supportive therapy. Worsening of dysfunction, on the other hand, should prompt a search for potentially correctable causes and a reevaluation of the specific methods of supportive care being used. Not infrequently, a readily treatable cause of evolving MODS is found; often, however, no cause will be evident. In cases with an unknown cause, the objective of therapy is to optimize supportive measures to limit iatrogenic injury until the patient recovers or, alternatively, until a considered decision is made regarding the futility of continued active care.

Search for Correctable Causes

Occult infection Uncontrolled infection, particularly that arising in the abdomen, is an important risk factor for MODS[2,3,107,108]; the development of otherwise unexplained organ dysfunction should trigger a careful search for an occult intra-abdominal focus.[109] However, MODS also develops in patients with pneumonia[109] and other life-threatening infections, and it can evolve in patients in whom no significant focus of infection can be identified.[102,110]

When MODS develops in the postoperative surgical patient, a careful search for infection must be undertaken, concentrating in particular on the operative site. With appropriate attention to the clinical possibilities, aided by ultrasonography and CT scanning, the presence or absence of significant intra-abdominal pathology can usually be established. Local wound exploration can suggest the possibility of occult intra-abdominal injury through the demonstration of impaired wound heal-

Table 3   Temporal Evolution of MODS[3,59]

System	Time from ICU Admission to Onset of Significant Dysfunction (days)
Respiratory	2
Hematologic	3
Central Nervous	4
Cardiovascular	4
Hepatic	5–6
Renal	4–11
Gastrointestinal	10

ing or fascial dehiscence or through the isolation of typical intestinal microflora from a wound infection. The diagnosis of pneumonia in intubated ICU patients is notoriously difficult[111]; however, the use of quantitative techniques, such as protected specimen brush bronchoscopy[112] and bronchoalveolar lavage,[113] can establish or rule out this diagnosis with confidence in most cases.[114]

Urinary tract infections or device-related bacteremias are rarely the cause of MODS, though they commonly develop in patients with significant organ dysfunction.[102] Disseminated candidiasis, however, may present as deteriorating organ dysfunction in critically ill patients.

Iatrogenic factors MODS can be considered the quintessential iatrogenic disorder, reflecting both the successes and the shortcomings of contemporary ICU practice. MODS has developed only because advances in supportive care have permitted the prolonged survival of critically ill patients who once would have died; however, several iatrogenic factors that figure prominently in its expression are potentially avoidable.[21]

Technical and judgmental errors often set the stage for the development of MODS.[32,115,116] Whenever a patient manifests unexplained organ failure in the postoperative period, the surgeon must consider the possibility of an iatrogenic complication—for example, a missed intestinal perforation in a trauma victim, a leak from a tenuous anastomosis, or left colon ischemia after aneurysmectomy.

Many of the therapeutic interventions that are mainstays of ICU care have the potential to induce organ dysfunction. Oxygen in high concentrations can produce pulmonary damage, probably as a result of the generation of toxic oxygen intermediates,[117] and mechanical ventilation can induce barotrauma, particularly when high peak airway pressures are generated[118] [see VII:4 Use of the Mechanical Ventilator]. Ventilatory strategies designed to limit airway pressure and maintain F_IO_2 at the lowest level compatible with an adequate arterial oxygen saturation are preferable in the management of patients with acute lung injury.

Blood transfusion has been implicated in the development of organ dysfunction, an effect that occurs independent of the effects of shock, blood loss, and fluid resuscitation.[119] Both to reduce the risk of blood-borne diseases and to minimize the potential for aggravating organ dysfunction, transfusion should probably be withheld if the hemoglobin level is greater than 8 g/dl unless a critical need for enhanced oxygen delivery exists. The optimal target for transfusion of critically ill patients is unknown.[120] The age of the blood administered may be an underappreciated factor in defining optimal transfusion strategies: Marik and Sibbald demonstrated in 1993 that the effects of blood transfusion on splanchnic blood flow as measured by a gastric tonometer depended on the age of the blood administered and that the use of blood more than 12 days old had an adverse impact on oxygen delivery.[121]

Total parenteral nutrition can also contribute to organ dysfunction. TPN-associated alterations in hepatic function with intrahepatic cholestasis and fatty infiltration are relatively common and are manifested by elevated aminotransferase and alkaline phosphatase levels.[122] TPN may also give rise to glucose intolerance and can aggravate ventilatory impairment because of increased CO_2 production. In patients with border-

line pulmonary function, this additional CO_2 production may prevent weaning from ventilatory support.[123] Animal studies demonstrate that TPN is associated with a loss of gut barrier function and increased rates of bacterial translocation[124]—an observation that may explain the increased risk of infectious complications in trauma patients maintained on TPN.[125] It has even been proposed that deliberate limitation of nutritional support may be beneficial for critically ill patients,[126] though the merits of this approach are unproved.

Prophylactic control of gastric pH to prevent stress ulceration leads to gastric overgrowth with gram-negative organisms and appears to increase rates of nosocomial pneumonia.[46] Gastric colonization with common ICU pathogens is frequent and is significantly correlated with the development of invasive infection at multiple sites, including the lungs, the urinary tract, and the blood.[127] Whether the severity of MODS can be reduced through suppression of pathological colonization with topical antibiotics,[47] acidification of enteral feeds,[49] or the use of cytoprotective agents for stress ulcer prophylaxis[128] remains unresolved. A recent epidemiological study suggests that stress ulcer prophylaxis can be safely omitted from the regimen of most ICU patients[45] [see Prevention, Immunologic Support, above].

Support of the Patient with MODS

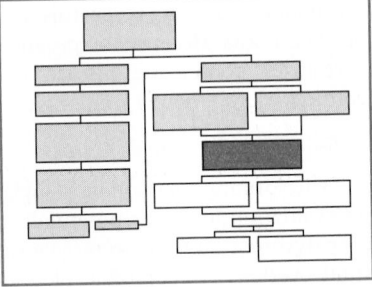

MODS is a complication to be prevented rather than a disease to be treated. Unfortunately, even with optimal attention to preventive measures and a careful search for treatable complications, progressive and refractory MODS presents the intensivist with a significant challenge: to support the patient during a period of otherwise lethal organ system dysfunction without causing further injury in the process. Detailed approaches to organ-specific supportive care are outlined elsewhere in this text. Selected approaches to supportive care that may minimize some of the adverse consequences of MODS are discussed below.

RESPIRATORY SUPPORT

In patients with MODS, the immediate challenge of respiratory support is to maintain an adequate arterial oxygen saturation and allow for the elimination of CO_2—particularly in the patient with renal dysfunction—without inducing lung injury from hyperoxia or barotrauma. Oxygenation can be optimized through the judicious use of positive end-expiratory pressure, a maneuver that may in addition decrease accumulation of interstitial fluid and minimize ventilator-associated lung injury.[118] Ventilation with large tidal volumes and high peak inspiratory pressures contributes to lung injury, and as a result, ventilatory strategies that limit airway pressures are being used more widely. Pressure-controlled ventilatory techniques limit peak airway pressures to a maximum predetermined level, optimizing gas exchange by inverting the inspiration:expiration (I:E) ratio (i.e., reducing the I:E ratio from a normal value of 1:2 to a value of 1:1 or less) and by changing the shape of the inspiratory flow curve (normally square) to one in which flow is initially rapid, then decelerates[129] [see VII:4 Use of the Mechanical Ventilator]. Peak airway pressure can also be limited by the use of low tidal volumes. Although oxygenation can be maintained with low tidal volumes, ventilation is jeopardized and CO_2 levels rise; as a result, this approach is known as permissive hypercapnia. As long as renal compensatory mechanisms are intact, acidosis is usually not life-threatening, despite levels of P_aCO_2 in excess of 100 mm Hg, and mortality may be improved, even in patients with established organ failure.[130] Another strategy developed to optimize ventilation while minimizing both peak airway pressures and the hemodynamic consequences of positive pressure ventilation is the technique of airway pressure–release ventilation, in which airway pressures are maintained at a continuous positive baseline level and intermittently decreased or released to permit gas exchange in the lung.[131]

Inhaled nitric oxide, a potent vasodilator, is selectively delivered to ventilated lung segments and has shown some preliminary promise as a means of reducing pulmonary arterial pressures and $\dot{V}/\dot{Q}$ mismatch in patients with acute lung injury.[132] The benefits of nitric oxide administration are still largely anecdotal, and properly designed clinical trials will be needed to define its role in the management of ARDS. Extracorporeal lung support by means of extracorporeal membrane oxygenation or extracorporeal CO_2 removal can be lifesaving in patients with isolated severe respiratory failure that has been refractory to all other forms of respiratory support.[103] However, these techniques are resource intensive and have not been shown to improve outcome in clinical trials comparing them with conventional mechanical ventilation.[133,134]

CARDIOVASCULAR SUPPORT

Recent reports suggest that after ICU admission, a patient's prognosis is improved if $\dot{D}o_2$ is increased to supraphysiologic levels (in excess of 600 ml/min/m², compared with a normal value of approximately 450 ml/min/m²).[9,135,136] However, a cautionary note has been sounded by the results of a recent prospective, randomized study that demonstrated an increase in mortality and a worsening of organ dysfunction when attempts were made to drive $\dot{D}o_2$ to supranormal levels with dobutamine[137]; therefore, an alternative interpretation has been offered—that the ability to raise $\dot{D}o_2$ to supranormal levels identifies a subgroup of patients with a more favorable prognosis.[135,138]

Fluid administration is the mainstay of cardiovascular support of the critically ill. However, it too carries a potential cost in aggravating the dysfunction of other organ systems, and a recent randomized study has suggested that intentional under-resuscitation of patients with penetrating chest trauma may improve outcome.[139] The potential reasons for this are speculative. The critically ill patient receives massive volumes of fluid as a result of a generalized reduction in peripheral vascular resistance, an increase in vascular permeability, and an increase in the level of preload required for optimal cardiac function. Excessive interstitial fluid contributes to impairment of pulmonary gas exchange and increases the distance across which oxygen must diffuse in the tissues. Cerebral edema may contribute to worsening of injury in head-injured patients and to alterations in neurologic function in critically ill patients.

RENAL SUPPORT

Dopamine is commonly employed at low dosages (1 to 3 µg/kg/min) to minimize renal dysfunction. Dopamine increases renal blood flow directly via effects on D_1 and D_2 dopamine receptors in the renal vasculature[140,141] and, indirectly, by increasing the cardiac index. In addition, diuresis may occur as a result of a direct renal tubular effect.[142] However, a recent clinical trial questioned the role of dopamine as a renal protective agent and suggested that dobutamine has a greater beneficial effect on creatinine clearance, with a lower incidence of side effects, especially tachyarrhythmias.[143]

Conventional intermittent hemodialysis is difficult when cardiovascular instability is present. Continuous renal replacement therapies—in particular, continuous arteriovenous hemodialysis (CAVHD) and continuous venovenous hemodialysis—have proved valuable in the management of these patients and may improve clinical outcomes.[144,145] Complications result from the need for vascular access; such complications include limb ischemia, hemorrhage, and arteriovenous fistula formation.[146] In addition to the conventional benefits of such therapy, hemodialysis may increase the elimination of a number of low-molecular-weight proinflammatory mediators.[147,148]

SUPPORT OF OTHER ORGANS

Techniques for support of hepatic and GI function are not well defined. Early enteral nutritional support is desirable and has been associated with a reduction in infectious complications after multiple trauma.[125,149,150] At least one report, however, suggests that enteral nutrition does not prevent the development of organ dysfunction in patients with persistent hypermetabolism.[151] Techniques for bioartificial liver support have been developed but remain experimental.[152]

Support of hematologic function is largely confined to replacement of cellular elements (e.g., red blood cells and platelets) and coagulation factors (using plasma or concentrates such as cryoprecipitate). Neurologic support is limited to the correction of metabolic abnormalities.

MODS AND ICU-ACQUIRED INFECTION

Just as uncontrolled infection is an important predisposing factor for the development of MODS, so is the reverse equally true. Patients with MODS are at significantly increased risk for the development of ICU-acquired infection, and the incidence increases as the severity of MODS increases.[102] Several series have documented a shift in the most common infecting species of microbial flora in ICU-acquired infection from enteric gram-negative organisms to Staphylococcus epidermidis, Candida, Pseudomonas, and enterococci.[102,153] There are two important reasons for this: (1) these organisms are the most common causes of proximal gastrointestinal colonization in critically ill patients[127] and (2) they are resistant to the antibiotics commonly used in the empirical treatment of nosocomial infection.

ICU-acquired infections develop in those patients at greatest risk for ICU mortality; however, it is unclear the extent to which the infections themselves contribute to that risk.[154-156] ICU-acquired infections are rarely true disseminated infections; more often, they are localized processes occurring as a consequence of a contaminated intravenous line or urinary catheter, in which case removal of the contaminated device is the appropriate therapy, rather than administration of systemic antibiotics.

CRITICAL DECISIONS IN THERAPY

Progression of MODS in a patient who is receiving apparently optimal ICU support is a relatively common occurrence that presents the clinician with a series of diagnostic and therapeutic dilemmas.

Infection is a common trigger of MODS, and the temptation to initiate empirical anti-infectious therapy is great, but as a rule, such an approach should be resisted. Antibiotics are a double-edged sword in critically ill patients with MODS. Although antibiotics eliminate susceptible microorganisms, they disrupt the normal indigenous flora and set the stage for superinfection with resistant microorganisms. Empirical broad-spectrum antibiotic therapy for suspected nosocomial infection has never been demonstrated to improve outcome; indeed, there are grounds for concluding that this practice may be harmful. Previous broad-spectrum antimicrobial therapy is an independent risk factor for death from nosocomial pneumonia[157] and for nosocomial infection with *Candida*.[158] Clinical manifestations of sepsis in critically ill patients frequently arise from noninfectious causes.[154,159] With techniques currently available, a microbiological diagnosis can almost always be made when an infection severe enough to induce organ dysfunction is present. When an organism cannot be isolated, it is safer to discontinue antibiotics and repeat cultures than to escalate empirical antibiotic therapy.

Empirical therapy with corticosteroids is less common today than it once was, largely as a result of two well-designed clinical trials that failed to demonstrate benefit for the use of high-dose corticosteroid therapy in patients with septic shock.[160,161]

The association of organ dysfunction with occult intra-abdominal infection[109,110] stimulated a period of enthusiasm for the practice of blind laparotomy, or laparotomy undertaken to identify and treat an intra-abdominal infectious focus in the absence of radiographic evidence that such a focus is present.[162,163] However, the role of blind, or nondirected, laparotomy in the ICU patient with worsening organ dysfunction has been controversial. Proponents of nondirected laparotomy have argued that the rate of positive findings may be as high as 60 percent,[164] whereas skeptics point out that even when correctable pathology is encountered, the ultimate prognosis remains poor.[165,166] We believe that evolving organ dysfunction in itself is rarely an indication for abdominal exploration and that the decision to operate must be made on the basis of careful analysis of the clinical circumstances, guided by appropriate radiologic investigations. With improvements in ultrasonography and CT scanning, missed intra-abdominal abscesses have become distinctly uncommon. Ultrasonography and CT scanning are less reliable for the diagnosis of anastomotic leaks with minimal spillage or of gut ischemia. Anastomotic leaks can frequently be delineated using water-soluble contrast studies; however, if the clinical concern is

ischemic bowel, an aggressive surgical approach is indicated. Diagnostic peritoneal lavage may have a role to play in the abdominal evaluation of critically ill patients, yielding purulent fluid or bowel contents in cases of GI perforation and bloody fluid in cases of advanced gut ischemia [see I:2 Trauma Resuscitation]. It goes without saying that conventional physical findings of peritonitis—particularly in the nonoperated abdomen—may be the sole indication for surgical exploration. Moreover, in the case of the complicated postoperative patient transferred from another institution because of worsening organ dysfunction, we have adopted the philosophy that laparotomy is a legitimate component of the admission physical examination.

Preparation of the Critically Ill Patient for Operation

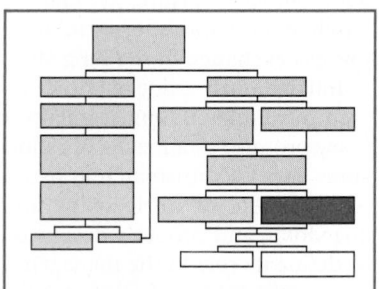

Operative intervention is frequently required in the critically ill surgical patient: in our surgical ICU, approximately 10 percent of patients undergo an operative procedure during their ICU stay. Immediate operative intervention is occasionally required to control life-threatening hemorrhage or hemodynamic instability. More typically, however, intervention is undertaken either urgently (e.g., to drain an abscess or resect an ischemic bowel) or electively (e.g., to create a tracheostomy or feeding jejunostomy).[167] The logistical challenges involved in preparing critically ill patients for operation and transporting them to the operating room can be significant (see below). The decision to operate, however, is not synonymous with the decision to transport; it has become increasingly appropriate to consider the ICU as an extension of the operating room and to perform procedures of moderate complexity within the ICU setting.

OPTIMIZATION OF THE PATIENT

Operative intervention carries the risk of transient deterioration, and it is therefore critical that physiologic function be optimized before the surgical procedure. Intraoperative gas exchange may deteriorate as a result of inhibition of hypoxic pulmonary vasoconstriction—an effect of many volatile anesthetics.[168] Cardiac output may be jeopardized by the vasodilatory and myocardial depressant effects of anesthesia—effects that may be compounded by intraoperative blood and fluid loss. Moreover, evaluation of the patient while under operative drapes can be difficult, and the diagnosis of potentially life-threatening complications may be delayed. For this reason, it may be prudent to perform bilateral tube thoracostomies to prevent the development of tension pneumothorax when the patient requires high ventilatory pressures. Preoperative correction of electrolyte abnormalities and coagulopathies will also render the operative procedure safer [see I:6 Life-Threatening Electrolyte Abnormalities].

TRANSPORT TO THE OPERATING ROOM

Transport between the ICU and the operating room is potentially dangerous for critically ill patients: significant per-

Table 4 Prognosis in MODS[3,6,177,178]

Number of Failing Systems	Mortality (%)
0	3
1	30
2	50–60
3	85–100
4	72–100
5	100

turbations in cardiovascular and respiratory status occur in more than 10 percent of such transports.[169,170] The most common problems are hypoxemia, hypotension, and arrhythmias, often as a result of migration of the endotracheal tube and mishaps associated with drug infusion pumps. Such problems are generally preventable if the transport is adequately planned and organized.

Placement of monitoring devices, such as arterial lines and pulmonary arterial catheters, should be undertaken in the ICU before transport both to facilitate monitoring during the transport phase and to permit optimization of preoperative therapy. Portable monitors permit a continuous display of heart rate, blood pressure, and So_2 during transport and should be used routinely. Planning of the transport must take into account the unexpected. For example, it is always wise to bring an extra tank of oxygen in the event of an elevator malfunction as well as adequate fluids and drugs to cover an unanticipated delay between the ICU and the operating theater. Battery-operated devices must be adequately charged to ensure uninterrupted operation.

Transfers of the patient from the ICU bed to a transport stretcher and from the stretcher to the operating room table carry the risk of inadvertent dislodgment of endotracheal tubes and vascular lines. One member of the operating team—usually the anesthetist—must assume responsibility for the integrity of these devices while the patient is being moved.

SURGICAL INTERVENTIONS IN THE ICU

The risks associated with patient transport and the delays in arranging timely intervention can be eliminated by performing certain surgical procedures in the intensive care unit. The operating room has the advantage of better lighting and equipment and the availability of skilled anesthetic and nursing support; however, it is often possible to duplicate these conditions in the intensive care unit. The advantages of the operating room environment from an infection control perspective are negligible.

Tracheostomy is readily performed at the bedside in the ICU, with complication rates comparable to those in the operating room.[171-173] A greater risk of complications exists for patients with preexisting coagulopathy, morbidly obese persons, nonintubated patients, and patients with abnormal neck anatomy (e.g., those in whom the cricoid cartilage is not palpable above the sternal notch during neck extension); such patients are probably managed more safely in the operating room setting.[171] Loss of control of the airway in critically ill patients can be fatal; thus, elective bedside tracheostomies should be performed only by skilled personnel capable of deal-

ing with any such complications. Several reports have documented the ease and relative safety of bedside percutaneous tracheostomy, though the risks and contraindications remain to be defined.[174,175] Zipper laparotomy for poorly controlled intra-abdominal infection is readily performed in the ICU,[176] as are gastrostomy, jejunostomy, open-lung biopsy, and exploratory laparotomy.

Prognosis of MODS

The prognosis of MODS is directly related to the severity of the underlying organ dysfunction, which can be expressed either as the number of failing systems[3,6,177,178] [*see Table 4*] or as the global severity of dysfunction as determined by an organ dysfunction score[59,179] [*see Figure 1*]. It must be emphasized, 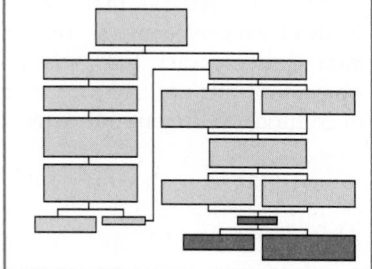 however, that prognostic indicators reflect the expected outcome for a group of patients and are of limited use in making decisions about the care of an individual patient. Moreover, these indicators reflect standards of critical care prevalent at a particular time and in a particular clinical setting. For instance, although in 1976 patients with pancreatitis and six or more positive indicators (according to Ranson's criteria[180]) had a mortality of 100 percent, a significant

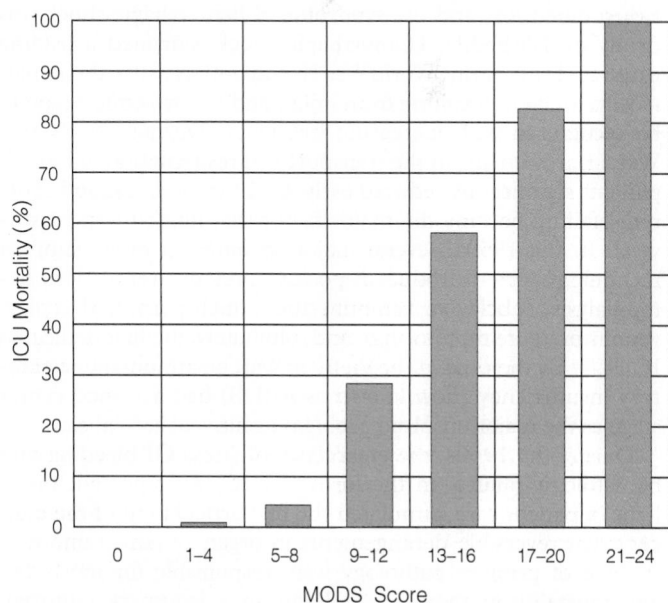

Figure 1 **Mortality increases as the overall degree of organ system dysfunction, reflected in the MODS score, increases. To calculate a MODS score, dysfunction in each of six different organ systems (renal, hematologic, cardiovascular, hepatic, respiratory, and central nervous systems) is first separately assigned a score from 0 to 4 [*see Table 2*]. The worst scores for each of the six systems over the length of the ICU stay are then totaled to produce the MODS score.[59]**

number of such patients now survive.[181]

Organ dysfunction in MODS is potentially recoverable when the factors responsible for the persistence or progression of the syndrome can be reversed. Identifying these factors, treating them appropriately, and providing optimal physiologic support can prove a daunting challenge, and it is often advisable to consider seeking independent advice or transporting the patient to a center that has the clinical expertise and facilities to manage the multidisciplinary problems faced by patients with MODS. Given that MODS not uncommonly evolves as a consequence of medical misadventure, early consultation or referral may be a sound philosophy from a medicolegal perspective as well. On the other hand, it is a common contemporary ICU scenario that MODS evolves and worsens despite optimal care, necessitating a decision whether to continue or discontinue active care.

WITHDRAWAL OF LIFE SUPPORT

The most common mode of death for the patient with advanced MODS is the limiting or withdrawal of life support in the face of a persistent failure to respond to full, aggressive ICU care. Such decisions are complex, and it is clear that there is considerable divergence of professional approach regarding the decision to withdraw life support.[182] Factors that must be taken into consideration include the nature of the underlying disease, the premorbid health of the patient, the wishes of the patient and family regarding long-term ICU care, the ultimate prospects for independent existence, and the presence of active problems amenable to medical therapy. Although such deliberations are difficult for medical staff and family alike, proper consideration for the expectations of all involved can facilitate a decision to discontinue active therapy in an atmosphere that is dignified and humane rather than adversarial.

Discussion

Evolution of MODS

The evolution of MODS has been an inevitable consequence of advances in the management of multiply traumatized and critically ill patients.[1] Prolongation of survival of the most severely ill patients has led to the emergence of a new spectrum of problems resulting not from the underlying disease process itself but from the host response to that process and from the measures required to sustain vital organ system function.

Blood transfusions were first used extensively during World War I[183]; however, it was not until 1930 that the connection between blood loss and the syndrome of hemorrhagic shock was firmly established.[184] Hemorrhagic shock remained a leading cause of death during World War II, and both renal[185] and hepatic[70] dysfunction resulting from injury and hypovolemia began to be recognized with increasing frequency. During the Korean War, improvements in the transport and resuscitation of injured patients significantly reduced early deaths from shock, and acute renal failure became the major factor that limited patient survival. In the 1950s, several major advances in organ-support technology were introduced: positive pressure ventilation, hemodialysis, subclavian venipuncture (which permitted central venous pressure monitoring), and, ultimately, the first dedicated ICUs.[186] By the time of the Vietnam War, posttraumatic respiratory insufficiency (now known as ARDS) had assumed center stage as the major unsolved problem in surgical critical care.

During the 1960s, the emergence of stress GI bleeding and hematologic failure (in the form of DIC) as important problems in patient care stimulated the first articulation of the concept that reversible derangements in organ systems remote to the site of primary pathology were responsible for morbidity and mortality in the ICU.[187] Baue, in a landmark editorial, coined the term "multiple, progressive, or sequential systems failure"[1] and established this as the dominant paradigm of critical care. Clinical reports used a variety of terms to describe this new syndrome: multiple organ failure,[2] multiple system organ failure,[3] multiple organ system failure,[93] nonbacteremic clinical sepsis,[107] and the hypermetabolism organ failure complex.[188] The 1991 ACCP-SCCM consensus conference proposed the designation MODS to reflect the contemporary view that it is a clinical syndrome with common pathological and prognostic implications.[4]

Changes in microbial ecology and in the clinical management of infection in hospitalized patients paralleled advances in ICU therapy. In the 1940s and 1950s, the widespread use of antibiotics in hospitalized patients produced a shift in the cause of microbial infections from primarily exogenous to primarily endogenous species. However, the overall prevalence of infection remained unchanged.[189] By the 1960s, gram-negative species replaced pneumococci and streptococci as the leading causes of lethal bacterial infection.[190] Studies of the systemic effects of gram-negative bacteremia gave rise to important advances in the hemodynamic management of critically ill patients, with the result that florid septic shock is seen less frequently today. In its place has emerged a more indolent syndrome of recurrent infection with organisms of relatively low pathogenicity: S. epidermidis, Candida, and enterococci.

As MODS has evolved, awareness has grown of the central role played by endogenous host factors in the syndrome's pathogenesis. Studies of host defenses in critical illness demonstrate that immune responses are altered and suggest that the critically ill patient should be considered an immunocompromised host.[101,191] More recently, it has been suggested that overactivity, rather than failure, of host defense is responsible for the morbidity of critical illness.[154,192] These notions are by no means contradictory; both, in fact, reflect the complexities of the interactions of infection and the host inflammatory response.

Evolving Terminology

The earliest descriptions of MODS emphasized its intimate association with infection[3,108,109,187] and uncontrolled inflammation.[179] Advances in the understanding of the biology of the host inflammatory response have rendered obsolete much of the terminology classically used to describe these processes[193] and have triggered a vigorous debate on optimal phraseology.[194,195] These debates are much more than semantic quibbles, for terminology reflects a model of biology for the guidance of therapy. Moreover, the inflammatory response is clearly a biologic double-edged sword, with the potential both to benefit and to harm the host; therefore, it is critical that therapeutic decisions be based on an adequate evaluation of the precise nature of the physiologic process.

In an attempt to reconcile terminology with a contemporary understanding of biology, the 1991 ACCP-SCCM consensus conference proposed that a new term, the systemic inflammatory response syndrome (SIRS), should be used to describe the clinical syndrome of disseminated inflammation, independent of its cause [see VI:10 Clinical and Laboratory Diagnosis of Infection]. SIRS is a clinical syndrome whose differential diagnosis includes autoimmune disease, drug reactions, sterile inflammation in pancreatitis, and a variety of other disorders associated with activation of an inflammatory response. Under the new definitions, sepsis describes the development of SIRS as a consequence of infection, whereas infection denotes the invasion of normally sterile tissues by bacteria or their toxins, independent of the response evoked in the host.

By this model, MODS develops not because of uncontrolled infection but as a consequence of SIRS. In other words, if SIRS represents an appropriate adaptive response to disruptions of homeostasis, MODS is the maladaptive consequence of that systemic response.

Theories of Pathogenesis

Although the epidemiological association between organ dysfunction and SIRS is strong, no compelling pathogenetic model has yet been determined to account for the evolution of MODS, nor is it even known whether the clinical syndrome reflects a single pathological process. A number of overlapping theories have been advanced,[196] the most compelling of which interpret MODS as a dynamic process—the outcome of the interaction between an acute stimulus and the host response to that stimulus.

INFECTION AND THE HOST SEPTIC RESPONSE

Cellular Mechanisms

Activated host immune cells—particularly neutrophils and macrophages—have been shown to produce tissue injury similar to that produced by MODS in both clinical studies and animal models.

Neutrophils are critical effectors of local inflammatory responses, and it is postulated that they play a role in the pathological organ injury of MODS.[197-200] Experimental studies demonstrate a critical role for neutrophils in acute injury to the lung,[201,202] gut,[203,204] and liver,[205,206] as well as in the pathogenesis of increased vascular permeability in a variety of acute models of injury and infection.[207-209] Descriptive clinical studies have shown neutrophils from patients with SIRS to be activated[210-212] and, more specifically, have shown increased activation of neutrophils that have passed through the lung in patients with acute lung injury.[213] Similarly, experimental interventions to deplete neutrophils or to block their interactions with endothelial cells have resulted in attenuation of organ injury.[199,201,209] It has been recognized, however, that neutrophils alone cannot account for the development of clinical MODS, because although neutrophil depletion has reduced lung injury in a variety of experimental models, the phenomenon of ARDS is still seen in neutropenic patients.[214]

Circulating monocytes and fixed-tissue macrophages are also recognized to be key cellular mediators of tissue injury,[215] largely on the basis of their ability to release virtually all of the endogenous mediator molecules that have been implicated in tissue injury in acute injury and infection.[216] Macrophages exert an important regulatory influence, modulating the expression of lymphocyte-mediated immunity[217] and releasing substances, such as IL-8, that serve as potent chemoattractants for neutrophils.[218] Through the expression of cellular procoagulants, activated macrophages can initiate intravascular coagulation and fibrin deposition.[219] Endotoxin-activated hepatic Kupffer cells modulate hepatocyte protein synthesis in vitro[220]; activation of these cells in vivo can reproduce the hypermetabolic state[221] and immunologic abnormalities[222] characteristic of critical illness. In experimental animals, Kupffer cell blockade reduces mortality in endotoxemia[223] but increases mortality in peritonitis induced by cecal ligation and puncture.[224]

Humoral Mediators

A large number of inflammatory mediators of host origin can reproduce manifestations of MODS when administered to experimental animals. Tumor necrosis factor (TNF),[225,226] IL-1,[227,228] and platelet-activating factor (PAF)[229] are among the most extensively studied of these, and strategies to alter their activities have undergone clinical trials (see below). Experimental studies have shown that diffuse organ injury can be induced not only by the excess activation of proinflammatory mediators but also by the deficiency of counterinflammatory mediators, such as transforming growth factor–β (TGF-β)[230] and IL-10.[231] These and other host-derived mediators are discussed in greater detail elsewhere [see VII:11 Molecular and Cellular Mediators of the Inflammatory Response].

Cytokines and other inflammatory mediators exert their most important activities locally within the microenvironment of inflammation, and there is considerable variability in circulating cytokine levels from one patient to the next.[232,233] Levels of inflammatory mediators in the systemic circulation correlate poorly with clinical status and outcome. IL-6[234,235] and IL-8[236-238] appear to be the most reliable markers of the activation of a systemic inflammatory response.

THE MICROVASCULATURE

Microvascular Injury

Autopsies of MODS patients show diffuse microvascular thrombosis with neutrophil sequestration,[239] pointing to a pathogenetic role for the microvasculature. Neutrophils and monocytes accumulate in sites of inflammation through a series of interactions with microvascular endothelial cells. These interactions are mediated by complementary adhesion molecules expressed on the circulating inflammatory cells and on the endothelium.[240,241] Bacterial products and host inflammatory cytokines up-regulate endothelial adhesion molecules. Moreover, activated endothelial cells lose their anticoagulant properties and express tissue factors, and as a consequence, the extrinsic coagulation pathway is activated.[242] Tissue injury results from both the local release of cytodestructive products from neutrophils and monocytes and ischemia secondary to

Table 5 Divergent Effects of Cytokine Manipulation in Animal Models

Mediator	Administration Augments Survival	Blockade Augments Survival
Tumor necrosis factor	Pretreatment before cecal ligation and puncture *Listeria* infection	Endotoxemia Gram-negative bacteremia *Staphylococcus aureus* enterotoxin administration
Interleukin-1 (IL-1)	*Escherichia coli* peritonitis *Klebsiella* infection	*E. coli* bacteremia *Klebsiella* (when IL-1 is given at low dose for short course)
Interleukin-10	Endotoxemia	*Candida albicans* infection *Listeria* infection
Interferon gamma	*Listeria* infection	Endotoxemia

microvascular thrombosis. Animal studies have demonstrated that remote organ injury both in thermal injury[243] and in gram-negative infection[244] can be attenuated by pretreatment with monoclonal antibodies directed against adhesion molecules.

Reperfusion Injury

After short, nonlethal periods of ischemia, tissue injury evolves as a result of events that occur during reperfusion—in particular, the generation of reactive oxygen species.[245] Free radical–mediated tissue injury results from damage to the plasma membrane, oxidation of critical intracellular proteins, adenosine triphosphate depletion, and DNA strand breakage[246]; in addition, oxidative stress can induce programmed cell death, or apoptosis.[247] Oxygen free radicals contribute to further local injury by triggering the expression of endothelial adhesion molecules[248,249] and the release of the neutrophil chemoattractant PAF.[250] This local injury results in intravascular thrombosis and increased capillary permeability. In addition, ischemia-reperfusion injury to the intestine or to a limb can induce remote organ injury in the lung.[203,251]

THE GUT HYPOTHESIS

MODS sometimes evolves in patients in whom no obvious focus of infection or ischemia is clinically evident[102] and persists despite apparently adequate management of identifiable foci.[166] It was for this reason that a number of authors, building on concepts articulated nearly a half century ago,[252,253] proposed that the GI tract may sometimes serve as an unseen motor of MODS.[36,151,198,254] This involvement of the GI tract may arise from the gut's role as both an occult microbial reservoir and a potent immunoregulatory organ whose normal function is to maintain a tonic counterinflammatory influence on immunologic activation.

The normal GI tract harbors in excess of 400 discrete microbial species whose ecological balance is maintained by competition for nutrients and mucosal binding sites.[255] Pathological colonization of the oropharynx[256] and the proximal GI tract[127,257,258] develops rapidly in the critically ill patient and predisposes to nosocomial infection with the same organism.[127] Such infections may develop as a result of subclinical aspiration[44,259] but may also arise as a consequence of the passage of viable bacteria through the wall of the gut, a phenomenon termed bacterial translocation. Bacterial translocation is

readily observed in the experimental animal in response to the same insults that predispose to MODS: trauma, hemorrhage, burn injury, pancreatitis, intra-abdominal infection, and endotoxemia.[260] Evidence that translocation occurs as a clinically relevant phenomenon in humans is largely circumstantial[261-263] and occasionally contradictory.[264] Endotoxin presumably of gut origin has been detected in the plasma of patients after thermal injury[265] and repair of ruptured aortic aneurysms[266]; however, its significance, too, is controversial.

Under normal circumstances, the extensive immunologic tissues of the gut and liver blunt the expression of the immune response[267]; this influence may be impaired in critical illness, permitting the expression of a systemic inflammatory response. Intestinal epithelial cells dampen the release of TNF by macrophages in response to endotoxin, but they lose this suppressive activity in a hypoxic environment.[268] Levels of TNF and IL-6 are elevated in portal venous blood from animals subjected to hemorrhagic shock,[269] and elevated systemic TNF levels are observed within minutes of intestinal reperfusion after an ischemic insult.[270] Elevated portal venous levels of TNF have been seen in humans after aortic aneurysm repair.[271] Portal endotoxemia with resultant Kupffer cell activation triggers the release of potent immunosuppressive activity from alveolar and splenic macrophages[272]; conversely, Kupffer cell blockade lessens the clinical manifestations and reduces the mortality of systemic inflammation.[273]

THE TWO-HIT HYPOTHESIS

A complementary hypothesis of MODS pathogenesis suggests that an acute insult, such as infection or trauma, serves to prime the host in such a way that a second, relatively trivial, insult produces a markedly exaggerated host response.[197,274] Such a model would explain the apparent differences between MODS that develops early after trauma and MODS that occurs later[178]; like other theories of MODS, however, this hypothesis remains unproved.

Experimental Therapies

MANIPULATION OF INFLAMMATORY MEDIATORS

The administration or blockade of a number of the putative mediators of the systemic inflammatory response can improve survival in a variety of animal models of acute infectious challenge [see VII:11 Molecular and Cellular Mediators of the Inflammatory Response]. However, attempts to apply insights derived from these studies to the care of critically ill patients have proved disappointing.

Nonspecific blockade of systemic inflammation with the use of high-dose corticosteroids has been evaluated in two clinical trials, both of which failed to demonstrate clinical efficacy.[161,162] A phase II clinical study of IL-1 receptor antagonist, a naturally occurring antagonist of IL-1, showed great promise,[275] but this promise failed to be realized in a subsequent double-blind, multicenter trial.[55] A number of phase II trials evaluating monoclonal antibodies to TNF have been undertaken; however, clinical benefit has been evident primarily in retrospective subgroup analyses, and a trial employing soluble TNF receptors has suggested that experimental manipulation may actually increase mortality.[56] At least two large phase III studies of anti-TNF monoclonal antibodies are in progress. Finally, one phase III trial of an antagonist to PAF has shown a significant reduction in mortality in a subgroup of patients with gram-negative infection and shock.[276]

Although efficacy has been suggested in retrospective subgroup analyses, no overall benefit has yet been documented in the use of mediator-targeted therapy in the management of critically ill patients at risk for MODS. There are many potential explanations for the apparent failure of these strategies. Entry criteria defined for the original corticosteroid trials identify a group of patients at significant risk for mortality,[277] but this population is highly heterogeneous with regard to the underlying clinical diagnoses and mediator profiles, and a significant percentage of these patients ultimately prove to be uninfected.[234] Moreover, the population is also heterogeneous in regard to its risk of ICU mortality.[278,279] Dosing intervals have been arbitrary, and the validity of using 28-day mortality as an outcome measure has been questioned.[280] Finally, animal studies demonstrate striking differences in the effects of antagonism of specific mediators, depending on the model used [see Table 5]. In general, strategies that improve survival in animal endotoxemia models have the opposite effect in models in which the problem is uncontrolled infection. Which model is most relevant to the critically ill patient with MODS is unknown, and at present, the potential for harm appears to be as great as the potential for benefit.

EXTRACORPOREAL TECHNIQUES

Another experimental strategy for the management of MODS has been to attempt to remove circulating mediators without identifying which ones may be present. Preliminary studies have suggested that CAVHD may remove mediators such as PAF.[148] Similarly, case reports have demonstrated the potential utility of plasma exchange in the management of patients with MODS.[281-283] Another experimental strategy has been the extracorporeal adsorption of circulating endotoxin to polymyxin B–coated filters.[284] Evaluation of potential roles for these approaches awaits the results of larger clinical trials.

Conclusion

MODS is a complex phenomenon, the course of which is determined by the dynamic interplay of the inciting event, the host response to that stimulus, and the consequences of ICU supportive care. As an outcome in critical illness, MODS is a relatively homogeneous process, with predictable patterns of organ dysfunction and characteristic patterns of organ injury; however, the disease processes leading to this outcome are highly heterogeneous. Considerable progress has been made in understanding the pathogenesis of the syndrome; increasingly, it appears that the mediators of MODS are endogenous products of the host response rather than the exogenous stimuli that evoke that response. At present, however, it is unclear whether MODS is the outcome of a single process of mediator activation or whether there are multiple pathways to the same outcome. Indeed, it remains to be determined whether the final outcome reflects variable expression of a single pathogenetic process or similar expression of a number of biologically diverse processes.

An increased understanding of the role of cytokines has stimulated research interest in the potential benefits of mediator manipulation therapies. However, there are as yet no data to justify the use of cytokine modulators outside of the context of clinical trials.

Ultimately, the most successful approaches to the multiple organ dysfunction syndrome have been those focusing on prevention by the application of time-honored surgical principles: aggressive resuscitation, timely operative intervention, adequate drainage of infection and debridement of devitalized tissue, and sound surgical judgment.

References

1. Baue AE: Multiple, progressive, or sequential systems failure: a syndrome of the 1970s. Arch Surg 110:779, 1975

2. Eiseman B, Beart R, Norton L: Multiple organ failure. Surg Gynecol Obstet 144:323, 1977

3. Fry DE, Pearlstein L, Fulton RL, et al: Multiple system organ failure: the role of uncontrolled infection. Arch Surg 115:136, 1980

4. Bone RC, Balk RA, Cerra FB, et al: Definitions for sepsis and organ failure and guidelines for the use of innovative therapies in sepsis. Chest 101:1644, 1992

5. Tran DD, Cuesta MA, Van Leeuwen PAM, et al: Risk factors for multiple organ system failure and death in critically injured patients. Surgery 114:21, 1993

6. Knaus WA, Draper EA, Wagner DP, et al: Prognosis in acute organ-system failure. Ann Surg 202:685, 1985

7. Shoemaker WC: Relation of oxygen transport patterns to the pathophysiology and therapy of shock states. Intensive Care Med 13:230, 1987

8. Phang PT, Cunningham KF, Ronco JJ, et al: Mathematical coupling explains dependence of oxygen consumption on oxygen delivery in ARDS. Am J Respir Crit Care Med 150:318, 1994

9. Shoemaker WC, Appel PL, Kram HB, et al: Prospective trial of supranormal values of survivors as therapeutic goals in high risk surgical patients. Chest 94:1176, 1988

10. Parrillo JE, Parker MM, Natanson C, et al: Septic shock in humans: advances in the understanding of pathogenesis, cardiovascular dysfunction, and therapy. Ann Intern Med 113:227, 1990

11. Moncada S, Higgs A: The L-arginine nitric oxide pathway. N Engl J Med 329:2002, 1994

12. Kreuzfelder E, Joka T, Keinecke H, et al: Adult respiratory distress syndrome as a specific manifestation of a general permeability defect in trauma patients. Am Rev Respir Dis 137:95, 1988

13. Fleck A, Hawker F, Wallace PI, et al: Increased vascular permeability: a major cause of hypoalbuminaemia in disease and injury. Lancet 1:781, 1985

14. Hurd TC, Dasmahpatra KS, Rush BF: Red cell deformability in human end experimental sepsis. Arch Surg 123:217, 1988

15. Astiz ME, Galera-Santiago A, Rackow EC: Intravascular volume and fluid therapy for severe sepsis. New Horiz 1:127, 1993

16. Mizock BA, Falk JL: Lactic acidosis in critical illness. Crit Care Med 20:80, 1992

17. Antonsson JB, Boyle CC III, Kruithoff KL, et al: Validation of tonometric measurement of gut intramural pH during endotoxemia and mesenteric occlusion in pigs. Am J Physiol Gastrointest Liver Physiol 259:G519, 1990

18. Gutierrez G, Palizas F, Doglio G, et al: Gastric intramucosal pH as a therapeutic index of tissue oxygenation in critically ill patients. Lancet 339:195, 1992

19. Marik PE: Gastric intramucosal pH: a better predictor of multiorgan dysfunction syndrome and death than oxygen-derived variables in patients with sepsis. Chest 104:225, 1993

20. Boyd O, MacKay CJ, Lamb G, et al: Comparison of clinical information gained from routine blood gas analysis and from gastric tonometry for intramural pH. Lancet 341:142, 1993

21. Beal AL, Cerra FB: Multiple organ failure syndrome in the 1990's: systemic inflammatory response and organ dysfunction. JAMA 271:226, 1994

22. Beylot M, Chassard D, Chambrier C, et al: Metabolic effects of a D-beta-hydroxybutyrate infusion in septic patients: inhibition of lipolysis and glucose production but not leucine oxidation. Crit Care Med 22:1091, 1994

23. Bessey PQ, Lowe KA: Early hormonal changes affect the catabolic response to trauma. Ann Surg 218:476, 1993

24. Sganga G, Siegel JH, Brown G, et al: Reprioritization of hepatic plasma protein release in trauma and sepsis. Arch Surg 120:187, 1985

25. Ozawa K, Aoyama H, Yasuda K, et al: Metabolic abnormalities associated with postoperative organ failure: a redox theory. Arch Surg 118:1245, 1983

26. Heideman M, Saravis C, Clowes GHA: Effect of nonviable tissue and abscesses on complement depletion and the development of bacteremia. J Trauma 22:527, 1982

27. Herndon DN, Barrow RE, Rutan RL, et al: A comparison of conservative versus early excisional therapy in severe burn patients. Ann Surg 209:547, 1989

28. Cryer HG, Anigian GM, Miller FB, et al: Effects of early tangential excision and grafting on survival after burn injury. Surg Gynecol Obstet 173:449, 1991

29. Johnson KD, Cadambi A, Seibert B: Incidence of adult respiratory distress syndrome in patients with multiple musculoskeletal injuries: effect of early operative stabilization of fractures. J Trauma 25:375, 1985

30. Seibel R, LaDuca J, Hassett JM, et al: Blunt multiple trauma (ISS 36), femur traction, and the pulmonary failure-septic state. Ann Surg 202:283, 1985

31. Goris RJA: Prevention of ARDS and MOF by prophylactic mechanical ventilation and early fracture stabilization. Prog Clin Biol Res 236B:163, 1987

32. Henao FJ, Daes JE, Dennis RJ: Risk factors for multiorgan failure: a case control study. J Trauma 31:74, 1991

33. Moore FA, Feliciano DV, Andrassy RJ, et al: Early enteral feeding, compared with parenteral, reduces postoperative septic complications: the results of a meta-analysis. Ann Surg 216:172, 1992

34. Cerra FB, Shronts EP, Konstantinides NN, et al: Enteral feeding in sepsis: a prospective, randomized, double-blind trial. Surgery 98:632, 1985

35. Bower RH, Muggia-Sullam M, Vallgren S, et al: Branched chain amino acid–enriched solutions in the septic patient: a randomized prospective trial. Ann Surg 203:13, 1985

36. Wilmore DW, Smith RJ, O'Dwyer ST, et al: The gut: a central organ after surgical stress. Surgery 104:917, 1988

37. Tremel H, Kienle B, Weilemann LS, et al: Glutamine dipeptide-supplemented parenteral nutrition maintains intestinal function in the critically ill. Gastroenterology 107:1595, 1994

38. Bower RH, Cerra FB, Bershadsky B, et al: Early enteral administration of a formula supplemented with arginine, nucleotides, and fish oil in intensive care patients: results of a multicentre prospective, randomized, clinical trial. Crit Care Med 23:436, 1995

39. Nathens AB, Chu PTY, Marshall JC: Nosocomial infection in the surgical intensive care unit. Infect Dis Clin North Am 6:657, 1992

40. Craven DE, Kunches LM, Lichtenberg DA, et al: Nosocomial infection and fatality in medical and surgical intensive care unit patients. Arch Intern Med 148:1161, 1988

41. Nishijima MK, Takezawa J, Hosotsubo KK, et al: Serial changes in cellular immunity of septic patients with multiple organ-system failure. Crit Care Med 14:87, 1986

42. Maki DG: Risk factors for nosocomial infection in intensive care: devices vs nature and goals for the next decade. Arch Intern Med 149:30, 1989

43. Maki DG, Ringer M, Alvarado CJ: Prospective randomized trial of povidone iodine, alcohol, and chlorhexidine for prevention of infection associated with central venous and arterial catheters. Lancet 338:339, 1991

44. Du Moulin GC, Paterson DG, Hedley-Whyte J, et al: Aspiration of gastric bacteria in antacid-treated patients: a frequent cause of postoperative colonisation of the airway. Lancet 1:242, 1982

45. Cook DJ, Fuller H, Guyatt GH, et al: Risk factors for gastrointestinal bleeding in critically ill patients. N Engl J Med 330:377, 1994

46. Cook DJ, Laine LA, Guyatt GH, et al: Nosocomial pneumonia and the role of gastric pH: a meta-analysis. Chest 100:7, 1991

47. Meta-analysis of randomised controlled trials of selective decontamination of the digestive tract. Selective Decontamination of the Digestive Tract Trialists' Collaborative Group. BMJ 307:525, 1993

48. Meagher LC, Savill JS, Baker A, et al: Phagocytosis of apoptotic neutrophils does not induce macrophage release of thromboxane B_2. J Leukocyte Biol 52:269, 1992

49. Heyland D, Bradley C, Mandell LA: Effect of acidified enteral feedings on gastric colonization in the critically ill patient. Crit Care Med 20:1388, 1992

50. Van Der Waaij D: The ecology of the human intestine and its consequences for overgrowth by pathogens such as Clostridium difficile. Annu Rev Microbiol 43:69, 1989

51. Natanson C, Hoffman WD, Suffredini AF, et al: Selected treatment strategies for septic shock based on proposed mechanisms of pathogenesis. Ann Intern Med 120:771, 1994

52. Greenman RL, Schein RMH, Martin MA, et al: A controlled clinical trial of E5 murine monoclonal IgM antibody to endotoxin in the treatment of gram-negative sepsis. JAMA 266:1097, 1991

53. Ziegler EJ, Fisher CJ Jr, Sprung CL, et al: Treatment of gram-negative bacteremia and septic shock with HA-1A human monoclonal antibody against endotoxin: a randomized, double-blind, placebo-controlled trial. N Engl J Med 324:429, 1991

54. McCloskey RV, Straube RC, Sanders C, et al: Treatment of septic shock with human monoclonal antibody HA-1A: a randomized double-blind, placebo-controlled trial. Ann Intern Med 121:1, 1994

55. Fisher CJ, Dhainaut J-FA, Opal SM, et al: Recombinant human interleukin 1 receptor antagonist in the treatment of patients with sepsis syndrome: results from a randomized, double-blind, placebo-controlled trial. JAMA 271:1836, 1994

56. Dhainaut JF, Mira JP, Brunet F: Investigational therapy of sepsis: anti-TNF, IL-1ra, anti-PAF, and G-CSF. Clinical Trials for the Treatment of Sepsis. Sibbald WJ, Vincent J-L, Eds. Springer-Verlag, New York, 1995, p 267

57. Meakins JL: Surgeons, surgery, and immunomodulation. Arch Surg 126:494, 1991

58. Marshall JC: Multiple organ dysfunction syndrome (MODS). Clinical Trials for the Treatment of Sepsis. Sibbald WJ, Vincent J-L, Eds. Springer-Verlag, New York, 1995, p 122

59. Marshall JC, Cook DJ, Christou NV, et al: The multiple organ dysfunction score: a reliable descriptor of a complex clinical outcome. Crit Care Med 23:1638, 1995

60. Bone RC, Balk R, Slotman G, et al: Adult respiratory distress syndrome: sequence and importance of development of multiple organ failure. Chest 101:320, 1992

61. Sibbald WJ, Short AK, Warshawski FJ, et al: Thermal dye measurements of extravascular lung water in critically ill patients: intravascular Starling forces and extravascular lung water in the adult respiratory distress syndrome. Chest 87:585, 1985

62. Marini JJ: New options for the ventilatory management of acute lung injury. New Horiz 1:489, 1993

63. Clark RA: The commonality of cutaneous wound repair and lung injury. Chest 99(suppl):57S, 1991

64. Gattinoni L, Pesenti A, Bombino M: Relationships between lung computed tomographic density, gas exchange, and PEEP in acute respiratory failure. Anesthesiology 69:824, 1988

65. Pietra GG, Ruttner JR, Wust W, et al: The lung after trauma and shock: fine structure of the alveolar capillary barrier in 23 autopsies. J Trauma 21:454, 1981

66. Murray JF, Matthay MA, Luce JM, et al: An expanded definition of the adult respiratory distress syndrome. Am Rev Respir Dis 138:720, 1988

67. Morris JA Jr, Mucha P Jr, Ross SE, et al: Acute posttraumatic renal failure: a multicenter perspective. J Trauma 31:1584, 1991

68. Tilney NL, Lazarus JM: Acute renal failure in surgical patients: causes, clinical patterns and care. Surg Clin North Am 63:357, 1983

69. Wilson RF, Soullier G, Antonenko D: Creatinine clearance in critically ill surgical patients. Arch Surg 114:461, 1979

70. Bywaters EGL: Anatomical changes in the liver after trauma. Clin Sci 6:19, 1946

71. Hawker F: Liver dysfunction in critical illness. Anaesth Intens Care 19:165, 1991

72. Schwartz DB, Bone RC, Balk RA, et al: Hepatic dysfunction in the adult respiratory distress syn-

drome. Chest 95:871, 1989

73. Nunes G, Blaisdell FW, Margaretten W: Mechanism of hepatic dysfunction following shock and trauma. Arch Surg 100:546, 1970

74. Parker MM, Shelhamer JH, Bacharach SL, et al: Profound but reversible myocardial depression in patients with septic shock. Ann Intern Med 100:483, 1984

75. Redl G, Germann P, Plattner H, et al: Right ventricular function in early septic shock states. Intensive Care Med 19:3, 1993

76. Vincent JL, Gris P, Coffernils M, et al: Myocardial depression characterizes the fatal course of septic shock. Surgery 111:660, 1992

77. Vincent J, Bakker J, Marecaux G, et al: Administration of anti-TNF antibody improves left ventricular function in septic shock patients. Chest 101:810, 1992

78. Finkel MS, Oddis CV, Jacob TD, et al: Negative inotropic effect of cytokines on the heart mediated by nitric oxide. Science 257:387, 1992

79. Young GB, Bolton CF, Austin TW, et al: The encephalopathy associated with septic illness. Clin Invest Med 13:297, 1990

80. Bolton CF, Young GB, Zochodne DW: The neurological complications of sepsis. Ann Neurol 33:94, 1993

81. Witt NJ, Zochodne DW, Bolton CF, et al: Peripheral nerve function in sepsis and multiple organ failure. Chest 99:176, 1991

82. Coronel B, Mercatello A, Couturier J-C, et al: Polyneuropathy: potential cause of difficult weaning. Crit Care Med 18:486, 1990

83. Bolton CF: Neuromuscular complications of sepsis. Intensive Care Med 19(suppl 2):S58, 1993

84. Baughmann RP, Lower EE, Flessa HC, et al: Thrombocytopenia in the intensive care unit. Chest 104:1243, 1993

85. Sigurdsson G, Christenson J, El-Rakshy M, et al: Intestinal platelet trapping after traumatic and septic shock: an early sign of sepsis and multiorgan failure in critically ill patients? Crit Care Med 20:458, 1992

86. Aster RH: Heparin-induced thrombocytopenia and thrombosis. N Engl J Med 332:1374, 1995

87. Ten Cate H, Brandjes DP, Wolters HJ, et al: Disseminated intravascular coagulation: pathophysiology, diagnosis, and treatment. New Horiz 1:312, 1993

88. Dinarello CA: Interleukin-1 and the pathogenesis of the acute phase response. N Engl J Med 311:1413, 1984

89. Suffredini AF: Endotoxin administration to humans: a model of inflammatory responses relevant to sepsis. Mediators of Sepsis. Lamy M, Thijs LG, Eds. Springer-Verlag, New York, 1992, p 13

90. Curling TB: On acute ulceration of the duodenum in cases of burns. Medical-Chirurgical Transactions of London 25:260, 1842

91. Cook DJ, Witt LG, Cook RJ, et al: Stress ulcer prophylaxis in the critically ill: a meta-analysis. Am J Med 91:519, 1991

92. Chang RWS, Jacobs S, Lee B: Gastrointestinal dysfunction among intensive care unit patients. Crit Care Med 15:909, 1987

93. Bell RC, Coalson JJ, Smith JD, et al: Multiple organ system failure and infection in adult respiratory distress syndrome. Ann Intern Med 99:293, 1983

94. Glenn F, Becker CG: Acute acalculous cholecystitis: an increasing entity. Ann Surg 195:131, 1982

95. Fiddian-Green RG: Should measurements of tissue pH and Po_2 be included in the routine monitoring of intensive care unit patients? Crit Care Med 19:141, 1991

96. Black PR, Brooks DC, Bessey PQ, et al: Mechanisms of insulin resistance following injury. Ann Surg 196:420, 1982

97. Rothwell PM, Udwadia ZF, Lawler PG: Thyrotropin concentration predicts outcome in critical illness. Anaesthesia 48:373, 1993

98. Rothwell PM, Lawler PG: Prediction of outcome in intensive care patients using endocrine parameters. Crit Care Med 23:78, 1995

99. Baldwin WA, Allo M: Occult hypoadrenalism in critically ill patients. Arch Surg 128:673, 1993

100. Christou NV, Boisvert G, Broadhead M, et al: Two techniques of measurement of the delayed hypersensitivity skin test response for the assessment of host resistance. World J Surg 9:798, 1985

101. Meakins JL, Pietsch JB, Bubenick O, et al: Delayed hypersensitivity: indicator of acquired failure of host defenses in sepsis and trauma. Ann Surg 186:241, 1977

102. Marshall JC, Christou NV, Horn R, et al: The microbiology of multiple organ failure: the proximal GI tract as an occult reservoir of pathogens. Arch Surg 123:309, 1988

103. Egan TM, Duffin J, Glynn MFX, et al: Ten-year experience with extracorporeal membrane oxygenation for severe respiratory failure. Chest 94:681, 1988

104. Zimmerman HJ, Maddrey WC: Toxic and drug-induced hepatitis. Diseases of the Liver. Schiff L, Schiff ER, Eds. JB Lippincott, Philadelphia, 1987, p 591

105. Cines DB, Kaywin P, Bina M, et al: Heparin-associated thrombocytopenia. N Engl J Med 303:788, 1980

106. Segredo V, Caldwell JE, Matthay MA, et al: Persistent paralysis in critically ill patients after long-term administration of vecuronium. N Engl J Med 327:524, 1992

107. Fry DE, Garrison RN, Heitsch RC, et al: Determinants of death in patients with intraabdominal abscess. Surgery 88:517, 1980

108. Skillman JJ, Bushnell LS, Goldman H, et al: Respiratory failure, hypotension, sepsis, and jaundice: a clinical syndrome associated with lethal hemorrhage and acute stress ulceration in the stomach. Am J Surg 117:523, 1969

109. Polk HC, Shields CL: Remote organ failure: a valid sign of occult intraabdominal infection. Surgery 81:310, 1977

110. Meakins JL, Wicklund B, Forse RA, et al: The surgical intensive care unit: current concepts in infection. Surg Clin North Am 60:117, 1980

111. Tobin MJ, Grenvik A: Nosocomial lung infection and its diagnosis. Crit Care Med 12:191, 1984

112. Chastre J, Fagon JY, Soler P, et al: Diagnosis of nosocomial bacterial pneumonia in intubated patients undergoing ventilation: comparison of the usefulness of bronchoalveolar lavage and protected specimen brush. Am J Med 85:499, 1988

113. Johanson WG, Seidenfeld JJ, Gomez P, et al: Bacteriologic diagnosis of nosocomial pneumonia following prolonged mechanical ventilation. Am Rev Respir Dis 137:259, 1988

114. Meduri GU, Chastre J: The standardization of bronchoscopic techniques for ventilator-associated pneumonia. Chest 102:557S, 1992

115. Muckart DJ, Thomson SR: Undetected injuries: a preventable cause of increased morbidity and mortality. Am J Surg 162:457, 1991

116. Davis JW, Hoyt DB, McArdle MS, et al: The significance of critical care errors in causing preventable death in trauma patients in a trauma system. J Trauma 31:813, 1991

117. Deneke SM, Fanburg BL: Normobaric oxygen toxicity of the lung. N Engl J Med 303:76, 1980

118. Parker JC, Hernandez LA, Peevy KJ: Mechanisms of ventilator induced lung injury. Crit Care Med 21:131, 1993

119. Maetani S, Nishikawa T, Tobe T, et al: Role of blood transfusion in organ system failure following major abdominal surgery. Ann Surg 203:275, 1986

120. Hebert PC, Wells G, Marshall J, et al: Transfusion requirements in critical care: a pilot study. JAMA 273:1439, 1995

121. Marik PE, Sibbald WJ: Effect of stored blood transfusion on oxygen delivery in patients with sepsis. JAMA 269:3024, 1993

122. Grant JP, Cox CE, Kleinman LM, et al: Serum hepatic enzyme and bilirubin elevations during parenteral nutrition. Surg Gynecol Obstet 145:2398, 1977

123. Askanazi J, Rosenbaum SH, Hyman AI, et al: Respiratory changes induced by the large glucose loads of total parenteral nutrition. JAMA 243:1444, 1980

124. Alverdy JC, Aoys E, Moss GS: Total parenteral nutrition promotes bacterial translocation from the gut. Surgery 104:185, 1988

125. Moore FA, Moore EE, Jones TN, et al: TEN versus TPN following major abdominal trauma—reduced septic morbidity. J Trauma 29:916, 1989

126. Zaloga GP, Roberts P: Permissive underfeeding. New Horiz 2:257, 1994

127. Marshall JC, Christou NV, Meakins JL: The gastrointestinal tract: the "undrained abscess" of multiple organ failure. Ann Surg 218:111, 1993

128. Driks MR, Craven DE, Celli BR, et al: Nosocomial pneumonia in intubated patients given sucralfate as compared with antacids or histamine type 2 blockers: the role of gastric colonization. N Engl J Med 317:1376, 1987

129. Munoz J, Guerrero JE, Escalante JL, et al: Pressure-controlled ventilation versus controlled mechanical ventilation with decelerating inspiratory flow. Crit Care Med 21:1143, 1993

130. Hickling KG, Walsh J, Henderson S, et al: Low mortality rate in adult respiratory distress syndrome using low-volume, pressure-limited ventilation with permissive hypercapnia: a prospective study. Crit Care Med 22:1568, 1994

131. Räsänen J, Cane RD, Downs JB, et al: Airway pressure release ventilation during acute lung injury: a prospective multicenter trial. Crit Care Med 19:1234, 1991

132. Rossaint R, Falke KJ, Lopez F, et al: Inhaled nitric oxide for the adult respiratory distress syndrome. N Engl J Med 328:399, 1993

133. Zapol WM, Snider MT, Hill JD, et al: Extracorporeal membrane oxygenation in severe acute respiratory failure. JAMA 242:2193, 1979

134. Morris AH, Wallace CJ, Menlovet RL, et al: Randomized clinical trial of pressure-controlled inverse ratio ventilation and extracorporeal CO_2 removal for adult respiratory distress syndrome. Am J Respir Crit Care Med 149:295, 1994

135. Yu M, Levy MM, Smith P, et al: Effect of maximizing oxygen delivery on morbidity and mortality rates in critically ill patients: a prospective, randomized, controlled study. Crit Care Med 21:830, 1993

136. Tuchschmidt J, Fried J, Astiz M, et al: Elevation of cardiac output and oxygen delivery improves

137. Hayes MA, Timmins AC, Yau EHS, et al: Elevation of systemic oxygen delivery in the treatment of critically ill patients. N Engl J Med 330:1717, 1994

138. Hayes MA, Yau EHS, Timmins AC, et al: Response of critically ill patients to treatment aimed at achieving supranormal oxygen delivery and consumption: relationship to outcome. Chest 103:886, 1993

139. Bickell WH, Wall MJ Jr, Pepe PE, et al: Immediate versus delayed fluid resuscitation for hypotensive patients with penetrating torso injuries. N Engl J Med 331:1105, 1994

140. McDonald RH, Goldberg LI, McNay JL, et al: Effects of dopamine in man: augmentation of sodium excretion, glomerular filtration rate, and renal plasma flow. J Clin Invest 45:733, 1973

141. Duke GJ, Bersten AD: Dopamine and renal salvage in the critically ill patient. Anaesth Intens Care 20:277, 1992

142. Krishna GG, Danivitch GM, Beck FWJ, et al: Dopaminergic mediation of the natriuretic response to volume expansion. J Lab Clin Med 105:214, 1985

143. Duke GJ, Briedis JH, Weaver RA: Renal support in critically ill patients: low dose dopamine or low dose dobutamine. Crit Care Med 22:1919, 1994

144. Hirasawa H, Sugai T, Ohtake Y, et al: Continuous hemofiltration and hemodiafiltration in the management of multiple organ failure. Contrib Nephrol 93:42, 1991

145. McDonald BR, Mehta RL: Decreased mortality in patients with acute renal failure undergoing continuous arteriovenous hemodialysis. Contrib Nephrol 93:51, 1991

146. Ronco C: Continuous renal replacement therapies for the treatment of acute renal failure in intensive care patients. Clin Nephrol 40:187, 1993

147. Tonneson E, Hansen MB, Hohndorf K, et al: Cytokines in plasma and ultrafiltrate during continuous arteriovenous haemofiltration. Anaesth Intens Care 21:752, 1993

148. Ronco C, Tetta C, Lupi A, et al: Removal of platelet-activating factor in experimental continuous arteriovenous hemofiltration. Crit Care Med 23:99, 1995

149. Kudsk KA, Croce MA, Fabian TC, et al: Enteral versus parenteral feeding. Ann Surg 215:503, 1992

150. Border JR, Hassett J, LaDuca J, et al: The gut origin septic states in blunt multiple trauma (ISS = 40) in the ICU. Ann Surg 206:427, 1985

151. Cerra FB, McPherson JP, Konstantinides FN, et al: Enteral nutrition does not prevent multiple organ failure syndrome (MOFS) after sepsis. Surgery 104:727, 1988

152. Rozga J, Podesta L, LePage E, et al: A bioartificial liver to treat severe acute liver failure. Ann Surg 219:538, 1994

153. Rotstein OD, Pruett TL, Simmons RL: Microbiologic features and treatment of persistent peritonitis in patients in the intensive care unit. Can J Surg 29:247, 1986

154. Marshall JC, Sweeney D: Microbial infection and the septic response in critical surgical illness: sepsis, not infection, determines outcome. Arch Surg 125:17, 1990

155. Poole GV, Muakkassa FF, Griswold JA: Pneumonia, selective decontamination, and multiple organ failure. Surgery 111:1, 1992

156. Poole GV, Muakkassa FF, Griswold JA: The role of infection in outcome of multiple organ failure. Am Surg 59:727, 1993

157. Rello J, Ausina V, Ricart M, et al: Impact of previous antimicrobial therapy on the etiology and outcome of ventilator associated pneumonia. Chest 104:1230, 1993

158. Wey SB, Mori M, Pfaller MA, et al: Risk factors for hospital acquired *Candidemia*: a matched case control study. Arch Intern Med 149:2349, 1989

159. Rangel-Frausto MS, Pittet D, Costigan M, et al: The natural history of the systemic inflammatory response syndrome. JAMA 273:117, 1995

160. Bone RC, Fisher CJ, Clemmer TP, et al: A controlled clinical trial of high dose methylprednisolone in the treatment of severe sepsis and septic shock. N Engl J Med 317:654, 1987

161. Effect of high dose glucocorticoid therapy on mortality in patients with clinical signs of systemic sepsis. The Veterans Administration Systemic Sepsis Cooperative Study Group. N Engl J Med 317:659, 1987

162. Ferraris VA: Exploratory laparotomy for potential abdominal sepsis in patients with multiple organ failure. Arch Surg 118:1130, 1983

163. Hinsdale JG, Jaffe BM: Re-operation for intra-abdominal sepsis: indications and results in modern critical care setting. Ann Surg 199:31, 1984

164. Sutherland RF, Temple WJ, Snodgrass T, et al: Predicting the outcome of exploratory laparotomy in the ICU patients with sepsis or organ failure. J Trauma 29:152, 1989

165. Norton LW: Does drainage of intraabdominal pus reverse multiple organ failure? Am J Surg 149:347, 1985

166. Bunt TJ: Non-directed relaparotomy for intraabdominal sepsis: a futile procedure. Am Surg 52:294, 1986

167. Wolfe BM, Moore PG: Preparation of the intensive care patient for major surgery. World J Surg 17:184, 1993

168. Marshall C, Lindgren L, Marshall BE: Effects of halothane, enflurane, and isoflurane on hypoxic pulmonary vasoconstriction in rat lungs in vitro. Anesthesiology 60:304, 1984

169. Venkataraman ST, Orr RA: Intrahospital transport of critically ill patients. Crit Care Clin 8:525, 1992

170. Insel J, Weissman C, Kemper M, et al: Cardiovascular changes during transport of critically ill and postoperative patients. Crit Care Med 14:539, 1986

171. Futren ND, Dutcher PO, Roberst JK: The safety and efficacy of bedside tracheotomy. Otolaryngol Head Neck Surg 109:707, 1993

172. Goldstein SI, Breda SD, Schneider KL: Surgical complications of bedside tracheotomy in an otolaryngology residency program. Laryngoscope 97:1407, 1987

173. Dayal VS, el Masri W: Tracheotomy in the intensive care setting. Laryngoscope 96:58, 1986

174. Friedman Y, Mayer AD: Bedside tracheotomy in critically ill patients. Chest 104:532, 1993

175. Moore FA, Haenel JB, Moore EE, et al: Percutaneous tracheostomy after trauma and critical illness. J Trauma 32:133, 1992

176. Garcia-Sabrido JL, Tellado JM, Christou NV, et al: Treatment of severe intra-abdominal sepsis and/or necrotic foci by an "open abdomen" approach. Arch Surg 123:152, 1988

177. Faist E, Baue AE, Dittmer H, et al: Multiple organ failure in polytrauma patients. J Trauma 23:775, 1983

178. Pine RW, Wertz MJ, Lennard ES, et al: Determinants of organ malfunction or death in patients with intra-abdominal sepsis: a discriminant analysis. Arch Surg 118:242, 1983

179. Goris RJ, te Boekhorst TP, Nuytinck JK, et al: Multiple-organ failure: generalized autodestructive inflammation? Arch Surg 120:1109, 1985

180. Ranson JHC, Rifkind KM, Turner JW: Prognostic signs and nonoperative peritoneal lavage in acute pancreatitis. Surg Gynecol Obstet 143:209, 1976

181. Ranson JHC, Berman RS: Long peritoneal lavage decreases pancreatic sepsis in acute pancreatitis. Ann Surg 211:708, 1990

182. Cook DJ, Guyatt GH, Jaeschke R, et al: Determinants in Canadian health care workers of the decision to withdraw life support from the critically ill. JAMA 273:703, 1995

183. The Rise of Surgery: From Empiric Craft to Scientific Discipline. Wangensteen OH, Wangensteen SD. University of Minnesota Press, Minneapolis, 1979

184. Blalock A: Experimental shock: the cause of the low blood pressure produced by muscle injury. Arch Surg 20:959, 1930

185. Bywaters EGL, Beall O: Crush injuries with impairment of renal function. Br Med J 1:427, 1941

186. Safar P, DeKornfeld T, Pearson J, et al: Intensive care unit. Anesthesia 16:275, 1961

187. Burke JF, Pontoppidan H, Welch CE: High output respiratory failure: an important cause of death ascribed to peritonitis or ileus. Ann Surg 158:581, 1963

188. Cerra FB: The hypermetabolism organ failure complex. World J Surg 11:173, 1987

189. Rogers DE: The changing pattern of life-threatening microbial disease. N Engl J Med 261:677, 1959

190. McCabe WR, Jackson GG: Gram negative bacteremia: I. Etiology and ecology. Arch Intern Med 110:847, 1962

191. MacLean LD, Meakins JL, Taguchi K, et al: Host resistance in sepsis and trauma. Ann Surg 182:207, 1975

192. Tellado JM, Giannias B, Kapadia B, et al: Anergic patients before elective surgery have enhanced nonspecific host-defense capacity. Arch Surg 125:49, 1990

193. Bone RC: Let's agree on terminology: definitions of sepsis. Crit Care Med 19:973, 1991

194. Sibbald WJ, Marshall JC, Christou NV, et al: "Sepsis"—clarity of existing terminology . . . or more confusion? Crit Care Med 19:996, 1991

195. Sprung CL: Definitions of sepsis: have we reached a consensus? Crit Care Med 19:849, 1991

196. Deitch EA: Multiple organ failure: pathophysiology and potential future therapy. Ann Surg 216:117, 1992

197. Carrico CJ, Meakins JL, Marshall JC, et al: Multiple-organ–failure syndrome. Arch Surg 121:196, 1986

198. Anderson BO, Brown JM, Harken AH: Mechanisms of neutrophil-mediated tissue injury. J Surg Res 51:170, 1991

199. Bone RC: Inhibitors of complement and neutrophils: a critical evaluation of their role in the treatment of sepsis. Crit Care Med 20:891, 1992

200. Smith JA: Neutrophils, host defense, and inflammation: a double-edged sword. J Leukocyte Biol 56:672, 1994

201. Mallick AA, Ishizaka A, Stephens KE, et al: Multiple organ damage caused by tumor necrosis factor and prevented by prior neutrophil depletion. Chest 95:1114, 1989

202. Schmeling DJ, Caty MG, Oldham KT, et al:

Evidence for neutrophil-related acute lung injury after intestinal ischemia reperfusion. Surgery 106:195, 1989

203. Schoenberg MH, Poch B, Younes M, et al: Involvement of neutrophils in postischaemic damage to the small intestine. Gut 32:905, 1991

204. Simpson R, Alon R, Kobzik L, et al: Neutrophil and nonneutrophil mediated injury in intestinal ischemia reperfusion. Ann Surg 218:444, 1993

205. Holman JM, Saba TM: Hepatocyte injury during postopertive sepsis: activated neutrophils as potential mediators. J Leukocyte Biol 43:193, 1988

206. Langdale LA, Flaherty LC, Liggitt HD, et al: Neutrophils contribute to hepatic ischemia reperfusion injury by a CD18 independent mechanism. J Leukocyte Biol 53:511, 1993

207. Sekiya S, Yamashita T, Sendo F: Suppression of late phase enhanced vascular permeability in rats by selective depletion of neutrophils with a monoclonal antibody. J Leukocyte Biol 48:258, 1990

208. Welbourn R, Goldman G, Kobzik L, et al: Interleukin-2 induces early multisystem organ edema mediated by neutrophils. Ann Surg 214:181, 1991

209. Mileski WJ, Winn RK, Vedder NB, et al: Inhibition of CD18-dependent neutrophil adherence reduces organ injury after hemorrhagic shock in primates. Surgery 108:206, 1990

210. Trautinger F, Hammerle AF, Pöschl HG, et al: Respiratory burst capability of polymorphonuclear neutrophils and TNF: serum levels in relationship to the development of septic syndrome in critically ill patients. J Leukocyte Biol 49:449, 1991

211. Tellado JM, Christou NV: Critically ill anergic patients demonstrate polymorphonuclear neutrophil activation in the intravascular compartment with decreased cell delivery to inflammatory foci. J Leukocyte Biol 50:547, 1991

212. Fasano MB, Cousart S, Neal S, et al: Increased expression of the interleukin 1 receptor on blood neutrophils of humans with the sepsis syndrome. J Clin Invest 88:1452, 1991

213. Nahum A, Chamberlin W, Sznajder JI: Differential activation of mixed venous and arterial neutrophils in patients with sepsis syndrome and acute lung injury. Am Rev Respir Dis 143:1083, 1991

214. Ognibene FP, Martin SE, Parker MM: Adult respiratory distress syndrome in patients with severe neutropenia. N Engl J Med 315:547, 1986

215. Border JR: Hypothesis: sepsis, multiple organ failure, and the macrophage. Arch Surg 123:285, 1988

216. Nathan CF: Secretory products of macrophages. J Clin Invest 79:319, 1987

217. Pierce CW: Macrophages: modulators of immunity. Am J Pathol 98:10, 1980

218. Rankin JA, Sylvester I, Smith S, et al: Macrophages cultured in vitro release leukotriene B₄ and neutrophil attractant/activation protein (interleukin 8) sequentially in response to stimulation with lipopolysaccharide and zymosan. J Clin Invest 86:1556, 1990

219. Kucey DS, Kubicki EI, Rotstein OD: Platelet activating factor primes endotoxin stimulated macrophage procoagulant activity. J Surg Res 50:436, 1991

220. Keller GA, West MA, Cerra FB, et al: Macrophage mediated modulation of hepatic failure in multiple system failure. J Surg Res 39:555, 1985

221. Arita H, Ogle CK, Alexander JW, et al: Induction of hypermetabolism in guinea pigs by endotoxin infused through the portal vein. Arch Surg 123:1420, 1988

222. Marshall JC, Lee C, Meakins JL, et al: Kupffer cell modulation of the systemic immune response. Arch Surg 122:191, 1987

223. Iimuro Y, Yamamoto M, Kohno H, et al: Blockade of liver macrophages by gadolinium chloride reduces lethality in endotoxemic rats: analysis of mechanisms of lethality in endotoxemia. J Leukocyte Biol 55:723, 1994

224. Callery MP, Kamei T, Flye MW: Kupffer cell blockade increases mortality during intra-abdominal sepsis despite improving systemic immunity. Arch Surg 125:36, 1990

225. Tracey KJ, Fong Y, Hesse DG, et al: Anti-cachectin/TNF monoclonal antibodies prevent septic shock during lethal bacteraemia. Nature 330:662, 1987

226. Beutler B, Cerami A: Cachectin: more than a tumor necrosis factor. N Engl J Med 316:379, 1987

227. Okusawa S, Gelfand JA, Ikejima T, et al: Interleukin 1 induces a shock-like state in rabbits: synergism with tumour necrosis factor and the effect of cyclooxygenase inhibition. J Clin Invest 81:1162, 1988

228. Arend WP: Interleukin-1 receptor antagonist: a new member of the interleukin-1 family. J Clin Invest 88:1445, 1991

229. Anderson BO, Bensard DD, Harken AH: The role of platelet activating factor and its antagonists in shock, sepsis, and multiple organ failure. Surg Gynecol Obstet 172:415, 1991

230. Rabinovici R, Yue T, Farhat M, et al: Platelet activating factor (PAF) and tumor necrosis factor-α (TNF-α) interactions in endotoxemic shock: studies with BN 50739, a novel (PAF) antagonist. J Pharmacol Exp Ther 255:256, 1990

231. Kuhn R, Lohler J, Rennick D, et al: Interleukin-10 deficient mice develop chronic enterocolitis. Cell 75:263, 1993

232. Donnelly TJ, Meade P, Jagels M, et al: Cytokine, complement, and endotoxin profiles associated with the development of the adult respiratory distress syndrome after severe injury. Crit Care Med 22:768, 1994

233. Casey LC, Balk RA, Bone RC: Plasma cytokines and endotoxin levels correlate with survival in patients with the sepsis syndrome. Ann Intern Med 119:771, 1993

234. Hack CE, De Groot E, Felt-Bersma RJF, et al: Increased plasma levels of interleukin-6 in sepsis. Blood 74:1704, 1989

235. Damas P, Ledoux D, Nys M, et al: Cytokine serum level during severe sepsis in human IL-6 as a marker of severity. Ann Surg 215:356, 1992

236. Hack CE, Hart M, Strack van Schijndel RJM, et al: Interleukin-8 in sepsis: relation to shock and inflammatory mediators. Infect Immun 60:2835, 1992

237. Chollet-Martin S, Montravers P, Gibert C, et al: High levels of interleukin-8 in the blood and alveolar spaces of patients with pneumonia and adult respiratory distress syndrome. Infect Immun 61:4553, 1993

238. Marty C, Misset B, Tamion F, et al: Circulating interleukin-8 concentrations in patients with multiple organ failure of septic and nonseptic origin. Crit Care Med 22:673, 1994

239. Nuytinck HKS, Offermans X, Kubat K, et al: Whole-body inflammation in trauma patients. Arch Surg 123:1519, 1988

240. Carlos TM, Harlan JM: Leukocyte-endothelial adhesion molecules. Blood 84:2068, 1995

241. Talbott GA, Sharar SR, Harlan JM, et al: Leukocyte-endothelial interactions and organ injury: the role of adhesion molecules. New Horiz 2:545, 1994

242. Pober JS, Cotran RS: Cytokines and endothelial cell biology. Physiol Rev 70:427, 1990

243. Mulligan MS, Till GO, Smith CW, et al: Role of leukocyte adhesion molecules in lung and dermal vascular injury after thermal trauma of skin. Am J Pathol 144:1008, 1994

244. Walsh CJ, Carey PD, Cook DJ, et al: Anti-CD18 antibody attenuates neutropenia and alveolar capillary-membrane injury during gram-negative sepsis. Surgery 110:205, 1991

245. Weixiong H, Aneman A, Nilsson U, et al: Quantification of tissue damage in the feline small intestine during ischemia-reperfusion: the importance of free radicals. Acta Physiol Scand 150:241, 1994

246. Kehrer JP: Free radicals as mediators of tissue injury and disease. Crit Rev Toxicol 23:21, 1993

247. Buttke TM, Sandstrom PA: Oxidative stress as a mediator of apoptosis. Immunol Today 15:7, 1994

248. Patel KD, Zimmerman GA, Prescott SM, et al: Oxygen radicals induce human endothelial cells to express GMP-140 and bind neutrophils. J Cell Biol 112:749, 1991

249. Lo SK, Janakidevi K, Lai L, et al: Hydrogen peroxide-induced increase in endothelial adhesiveness is dependent on ICAM-1 activation. Am J Physiol 264:L406, 1993

250. Lewis MS, Whatley P, Cain TM, et al: Hydrogen peroxide stimulates the synthesis of platelet-activating factor by endothelium and induces endothelial cell–dependent neutrophil adhesion. J Clin Invest 82:2045, 1988

251. Anner H, Kaufman RP, Kobzik L, et al: Pulmonary hypertension and leukosequestration after lower torso ischemia. Ann Surg 206:642, 1987

252. Lillehei RC: The intestinal factor in irreversible hemorrhagic shock. Surgery 42:1043, 1957

253. Fine J, Frank ED, Ravin HA, et al: The bacterial factor in traumatic shock. N Engl J Med 260:214, 1959

254. Deitch EA: The role of intestinal barrier failure and bacterial translocation in the development of systemic infection and multiple organ failure. Arch Surg 125:403, 1990

255. Lee A: Neglected niches: the microbial ecology of the gastrointestinal tract. Adv Microbial Ecol 8:115, 1985

256. Johanson WG, Pierce AK, Sanford JP: Changing pharyngeal bacterial flora of hospitalized patients. N Engl J Med 281:1137, 1969

257. Garvey BM, McCambley JA, Tuxen DV: Effects of gastric alkalization on bacterial colonization in critically ill patients. Crit Care Med 17:211, 1989

258. Hillman KM, Riordan T, O'Farrell SM, et al: Colonization of the gastric contents in critically ill patients. Crit Care Med 10:444, 1982

259. Craven DE, Driks MR: Nosocomial pneumonia in the intubated patient. Semin Respir Infect 2:20, 1987

260. Wells CL, Maddaus MA, Simmons RL: Proposed mechanisms for the translocation of intestinal bacteria. Rev Infect Dis 10:958, 1988

261. Krause W, Matheis H, Wulf K: Fungaemia and funguria after oral administration of Candida albicans. Lancet 1:598, 1969

262. Fiddian-Green RG, Gantz NM: Transient episodes of sigmoid ischemia and their relation to infection from intestinal organisms after

abdominal aortic operations. Crit Care Med 15:835, 1987

263. Levy J, Van Laethem Y, Verhaegen G, et al: Contaminated enteral nutrition solutions as a cause of nosocomial bloodstream infection: a study using plasmid fingerprinting. J Parenter Enteral Nutr 13:228, 1989

264. Moore FA, Moore EE, Poggetti R, et al: Gut bacterial translocation via the portal vein: a clinical perspective with major torso trauma. J Trauma 31:629, 1991

265. Winchurch RA, Thupari JN, Munster AM: Endotoxemia in burn patients: levels of circulating endotoxins are related to burn size. Surgery 102:808, 1987

266. Roumen RM, Hendriks T, van der Jongekrijg J, et al: Cytokine patterns in patients after major vascular surgery, hemorrhagic shock, and severe blunt trauma: relation with subsequent adult respiratory distress syndrome and multiple organ failure. Ann Surg 218:769, 1993

267. Tomasi TB: Oral tolerance. Transplantation 29:353, 1980

268. Nathens AB, Rotstein OD, Dackiw A, et al: Intestinal epithelial cells downregulate macrophage TNF production: a mechanism for immune regulation in the gut-associated lymphoid tissues. Surgery 118:343, 1995

269. Deitch EA, Xu D, Franko L, et al: Evidence favoring the role of the gut as a cytokine generating organ in rats subjected to hemorrhagic shock. Shock 1:141, 1994

270. Caty MG, Guice KS, Oldham KT, et al: Evidence for tumor necrosis factor induced pulmonary microvascular injury after intestinal ischemia-reperfusion injury. Ann Surg 212:694, 1990

271. Cabie A, Farkas JC, Fitting C, et al: High levels of portal TNF-alpha during abdominal aortic surgery in man. Cytokine 5:448, 1993

272. Marshall JC, Ribeiro MB, Chu PTY, et al: Portal endotoxemia stimulates the release of an immunosuppressive factor from alveolar and splenic macrophages. J Surg Res 55:14, 1993

273. Nieuwenhuijzen GAP, Haskel Y, Lu Q, et al: Macrophage elimination increases bacterial translocation and gut origin septicemia but attenuates symptoms and mortality rate in a model of systemic inflammation. Ann Surg 218:791, 1993

274. Moore FA, Moore EE: Evolving concepts in the pathogenesis of postinjury multiple organ failure. Surg Clin North Am 75:257, 1995

275. Fisher CJ, Slotman GJ, Opal SM, et al: Initial evaluation of human recombinant interleukin-1 receptor antagonist in the treatment of sepsis syndrome: a randomized, open-label, placebo-controlled multicenter trial. Crit Care Med 22:12, 1994

276. Dhainaut J-FA, Tenaillon A, Le Tulzo Y, et al: Platelet-activating factor receptor antagonist BN 52021 in the treatment of severe sepsis: a randomized, double-blind, placebo-controlled, multicenter clinical trial. Crit Care Med 22:1720, 1994

277. Bone RC, Fisher CJ, Clemmer TP, et al: Sepsis syndrome: a valid clinical entity. Crit Care Med 17:389, 1989

278. Knaus WA, Harrell F, Fisher CJ, et al: The clinical evaluation of new drugs for sepsis: a prospective study design based on survival analysis. JAMA 270:1233, 1993

279. Le Gall J-R, Lemeshow S, Leleu G, et al: Customized probability models for early severe sepsis in adult intensive care patients. JAMA 273:644, 1995

280. Petros AJ, Marshall JC, van Saene HKF: Should morbidity replace mortality as an endpoint for clinical trials in intensive care? Lancet 345:369, 1995

281. McClelland P, Williams PS, Yaqoob M, et al: Multiple organ failure: role for plasma exchange? Intensive Care Med 16:100, 1990

282. Ahren B, Evander A, Hammarstrom L-E, et al: Plasmapheresis and hemodialysis in a case of septic cholangitis complicated by hepatic and renal failure. Acta Chir Scand 154:157, 1988

283. Barzilay E, Kessler D, Berlot G, et al: Use of extracorporeal supportive techniques as additional treatment for septic-induced multiple organ failure patients. Crit Care Med 17:634, 1989

284. Aoki H, Kodama M, Tani T, et al: Treatment of sepsis by extracorporeal elimination of endotoxin using polymyxin B-immobilized fiber. Am J Surg 167:412, 1994

285. Vincent J-L, Moreno R, Takala J, et al: The SOFA (sepsis-related organ failure assessment) score to describe organ dysfunction/failure. Intensive Care Med 22:707, 1996

286. Bernard GR, Doig BG, Hudson G, et al: Quantification of organ failure for clinical trials and clinical practice. Am J Respir Crit Care Med 151:A323, 1995

Acknowledgment

Figure 1 Marcia Kammerer.

8 METABOLIC RESPONSE TO CRITICAL ILLNESS

Palmer Q. Bessey, M.D.

Metabolic Responses in Surgical Patients

Debility commonly accompanies surgical illness. It occurs in varying degrees after elective operations, major trauma, burns, infections, and other critical illnesses. Debility is caused by a variety of factors, including specific biochemical and physiologic alterations that usually occur in response to injury and disease, especially those that persist for a long time. Some aspects of surgical care that are common to almost all patients can also cause debility. This discussion will review these clinical factors and metabolic responses in critically ill surgical patients and will indicate how the clinician can manage them so as to minimize patient debility.

The metabolic responses to critical illness have been studied in a variety of critically ill patients, especially those with trauma, burns, or sepsis. The responses are often grouped into phases on the basis of their temporal relation to the injury or insult. The so-called ebb phase, which is the early phase of the injury response, is characterized by (1) an elevated blood glucose level, (2) normal glucose production, (3) elevated free fatty acid levels, (4) a low insulin concentration, (5) elevated levels of catecholamines and glucagon, (6) an elevated blood lactate level, (7) depressed oxygen consumption, (8) below-normal cardiac output, and (9) below-normal core temperature.[1] The subsequent phase, the so-called flow phase, is characterized by (1) a normal or slightly elevated blood glucose level, (2) increased glucose production, (3) normal or slightly elevated free fatty acid levels, with flux increased, (4) a normal or elevated insulin concentration, (5) high normal or elevated levels of catecholamine and an elevated glucagon level, (6) a normal blood lactate level, (7) elevated oxygen consumption, (8) increased cardiac output, and (9) elevated core temperature.[1]

The ebb phase is dominated by cardiovascular instability, alterations in circulating blood volume, impairment of oxygen transport, and heightened autonomic activity. Emergency support of cardiopulmonary performance is the paramount therapeutic concern. Shock [see I:4 Shock] is the prototypical clinical manifestation of the ebb phase. After effective resuscitation has been accomplished and restoration of satisfactory oxygen transport has been achieved, the flow phase comes into play. These responses are marked by hyperdynamic circulatory changes, signs of inflammation, glucose intolerance, and muscle wasting. Surgical patients in the ICU usually exhibit these clinical features; these patients and the clinical challenge they pose are the focus of this chapter.

When wounds are closed and infection has resolved, repletion of lean tissue and fat stores and restoration of strength and stamina can begin. This final, anabolic phase often begins near the time of hospital discharge and may persist for months before the patient fully recovers.

Features of Critical Illness That Can Cause Debility

THE WOUND

The surgical wound is not only a site of tissue disruption but also a site of inflammation and repair [see I:8 Acute Wound Care]. After resuscitation, the surgeon's principal task is to expedite and promote wound healing and restore tissue integrity. Because the wound is often the proximate cause of patient debility, providing optimal wound care amounts to providing the best patient care.

Wounds with necrotic or devitalized tissue (e.g., from ischemic necrosis, gangrene, or burns), foreign debris, or grossly contaminated material do not heal readily, if they heal at all. Necrotic tissue and eschar (slough) must be debrided, usually surgically, although application of enzymatic agents to wounds has also been effective in some cases. Foreign material must be removed by either hydrotherapy or debridement. Pus must be drained or removed by irrigation and dressing changes. Contaminated wounds are left open so that they can be repeatedly examined and further necrotic material can be removed. Open wounds should be covered with a dressing to prevent drying (i.e., tissue oxidation) and further tissue slough, to reduce bacterial contamination, and to prevent further mechanical injury. Unfortunately, none of the currently available dressing materials achieve all of these goals. Once it becomes apparent that the wound tissues are viable and uninfected, the wound should be closed primarily if possible or with a skin graft.

The cellular processes involved in wound healing are critically dependent on adequate perfusion and delivery of oxygen, glucose, and other essential nutrients. Inadequate perfusion may result in relative tissue ischemia and delay wound healing. A principal responsibility of the clinician is therefore to ensure adequate tissue perfusion during the entire period of wound healing. For instance, resuscitation from shock should be continued after blood pressure is stabilized and until there is clinical evidence of adequate flow—usually associated with warm extremities, pink nail beds, brisk capillary refilling, full peripheral pulses, urine output greater than 0.5 ml/kg/hr (50 to 70 ml/hr in adults), clear sensorium, and improving metabolic acidosis. Adequate oxygenation must also be ensured. Occasionally, invasive monitoring of cardiopulmonary performance and tissue oxygenation as well as pharmacologic support may be required to ensure adequate perfusion and oxygen delivery.

Contused tissue, fractures, tissues surrounding an abscess or site

Patient problems that lead to debility

Wound

Debride necrotic tissue and foreign debris.
Drain pus.
Avoid drying of tissues.
Maintain satisfactory cardiopulmonary performance to optimize oxygen delivery.
Expedite wound closure.
For clean surgical wounds:
- Handle tissues gently.
- Use precise surgical technique and hemostasis.
Avoid contamination.
Use primary closure when possible.

Pain

Use systemic analgesics judiciously.
Consider patient-controlled analgesia.
Consider regional (epidural) anesthesia.

Inflammation

Fever
- If < 38.5° C (101.3° F), usually no treatment or evaluation is necessary.
- If ≥ 38.5° C (101.3° F), survey for source of infection; consider administering antipyretics.
- If > 41° C (105.8° F), increase antipyretics; consider use of cooling blankets, ice packs, etc.
Altered thermoregulation
- Maintain warm environment (26°–33° C [78.8°–91.4° F]) to achieve thermal comfort.
Anorexia
- Limit period of fasting to 3–4 days.
Immunosuppression
- Sterile technique for all procedures, including intravenous line manipulations, suctioning, etc.
- Universal precautions; change gloves, wash hands between patients.

Metabolic response to critical illness

Hyperdynamic or hypermetabolic state

Expect
- Tachycardia
- Widened pulse pressure
- Increased cardiac output
- Increased O_2 consumption
- Increased minute ventilation
- Increased energy expenditure
- Fever
- Sodium and water retention
Provide
- Volume and pharmacologic support of cardiovascular performance as appropriate
- Warm environment (26°–33° C)
- Increased water intake
- Increased caloric intake
- Judicious sedation and analgesia

Muscle wasting

Expect
- Rapid wasting of muscle and loss of strength and endurance
- Increased osmotic load filtered by kidney
- Increased formation and urinary loss of urea
- Increased urinary loss of potassium, phosphorus, and magnesium
Provide
- Increased protein or amino acid intake to 15%–20% of total energy
- Increased intake of potassium, phosphorus, and magnesium
- Massage, active and passive exercise, and early mobilization

Glucose intolerance

Expect
- Hyperglycemia that is aggravated by glucose intake, infection, and other stressors
- Relative insensitivity to insulin, which improves with recovery
Provide
- Glucose control
- Human insulin I.V. to maintain blood glucose in a target range of 110–160 mg/dl
- Maintenance nutritional support
- Glucose as 60%–75% of total energy (5–7 mg/kg/min or 7–10 g/kg/day)
- Lipid as 25%–40% of total energy

Infection	Hospital treatment
Initially diagnose by abrupt changes in fever, leukocytosis, hyperglycemia, pulmonary function, or pulse and blood pressure. Culture appropriately to establish micro-biologic diagnosis. Administer broad-spectrum antibiotics empirically to cover likely pathogens if signs of organ system dysfunction and of sepsis develop. Debride necrotic tissue. Establish drainage; remove catheters. Prevent contamination of different sites on same patient. Prevent cross-contamination between patients.	Bed rest: • Encourage frequent turning, coughing, and deep breathing. • Encourage active, assisted exercise in bed when feasible. • Move to chair as soon as possible. • Use incentive spirometer or similar device. • Practice good hygiene and skin care, and provide massage. Food deprivation: • Limit period of fasting to 3–4 days. • Begin nutritional support as soon as needed. • Provide enteral feeding when possible. Invasive devices: • Remove as soon as no longer required. • Remove I.V. lines placed under suboptimal conditions as soon as feasible. • Consider changing I.V. lines or rotating site every 2 or 4 days. • Change I.V. site if redness or inflammation develops. Sleep deprivation: • Reduce lighting and noise in ICU periodically, especially at night. • Orient patient frequently to time of day and situation. • Use sedation judiciously.

Metabolic Responses in Surgical Patients

of infection, inflammatory sites such as the pancreas in pancreatitis or the lung in acute respiratory distress syndrome (ARDS)—in fact, any mass of inflammatory tissue—can be considered to constitute the patient's wound because resolution of those focal sites of inflammation depends on the same basic cellular processes as does healing of an external wound.

Patients with a large total mass of inflammatory tissue—large wounds—usually are critically ill and clearly manifest most of the metabolic responses associated with critical illness [see Metabolic Responses That Can Cause Debility, below]. In contrast, patients with small wounds do not appear critically ill and are not significantly debilitated. Although elective operations result in wounds, the incisions are made under sterile, controlled conditions; there is minimal direct tissue injury, little contamination, no shock, and limited net loss of blood and fluid. The incisions are closed primarily and most often heal expeditiously. With the proliferation of minimally invasive surgical techniques in the past several years, operative incisions are now even more limited, patients recover more rapidly, and the resultant debility is minimal—often little more than a transient indisposition.

PAIN

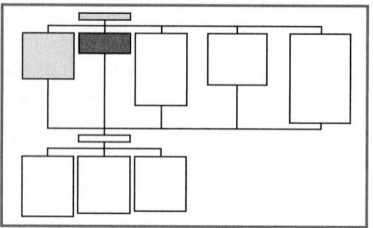

Virtually all surgical patients experience some pain. Pain usually occurs in association with an incision or with a wound resulting from fracture, burn, contusion, or another type of injury. In addition to creating an unpleasant subjective experience, pain often limits physical activities, such as turning in bed, deep breathing, coughing, and walking, and thereby directly interferes with recovery. A variety of techniques are available for pain management. However, each approach has side effects, the potential for abuse, or other features that limit its application.

Acute pain has traditionally been managed by intermittent parenteral administration of narcotic analgesics when requested by the patient or when the nurse perceives the patient to be in pain. The intravenous route is now preferred, because it does not require a painful injection and avoids potential uptake abnormalities. Intravenous analgesics have a short duration of action and must be given frequently to maintain good, sustained pain control; the dose also must be relatively small to minimize the side effects of sedation and impaired gastric motility. Thus, this approach to pain control is relatively labor intensive. Theoretically, this approach can prevent overuse of narcotics; in practice, it often results in inconsistent pain control and underdosing.

Continuous infusion of narcotic analgesics provides more consistent pain control and is common in the ICU. The dose should be adjusted upward before painful procedures but otherwise should be kept as low as possible to avoid ileus and prolonged sedation. Patient-controlled analgesia (PCA) is an extension of this approach. The patient controls a pump that administers a prescribed dose of the agent when activated; the clinician determines the amount of drug in each dose and the total dose permissible in a given period. This technique has been well accepted by patients who are awake and alert and are capable of controlling the system. One benefit is that the total amount of drug administered for pain relief is usually less than is given in a conventional as-needed dosing schedule.[2]

Administration of local anesthetics or narcotics into the epidural space may provide effective local pain relief without the sedating effects of parenteral narcotics. In addition, epidural anesthetics (but not opioids) reduce postoperative ileus.[3] Effective epidural analgesia can be maintained for several days and may have a beneficial effect on pulmonary function in patients with rib fractures or truncal wounds.[4] This technique requires placement of a catheter in the epidural space.

Patients must be monitored closely, and the dosage schedule must be individualized. This technique is best suited to patients who will be relatively inactive for 24 to 36 hours postoperatively and who can be observed closely, such as patients in the ICU.

INFLAMMATION

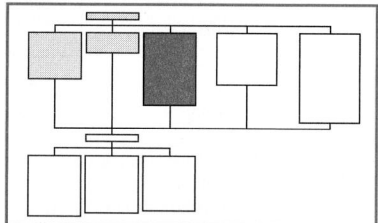

Elevation of body temperature above normal, leukocytosis, and other signs of inflammation are common features of critical surgical illness and should be expected. The extent of temperature elevation is generally proportional to the severity of illness. In a patient with a major burn—an extreme example of critical surgical illness—body temperature may be as high as 39° C (102.2° F). The leukocyte count is also typically elevated and may be as high as 20,000 cells/ mm³ during satisfactory recovery. A normal or subnormal body temperature or white blood cell count is atypical and may indicate sepsis, drug-induced leukopenia, or limited physiologic reserve. For example, a critically ill elderly patient with a major injury or infection may be afebrile and have a white blood cell count in the normal range.

Fever, however, is also a cardinal sign of infection. It may be difficult to distinguish between a typical postoperative or posttraumatic fever and a fever caused by invasive infection. An acute elevation in rectal temperature of 1.0° to 1.5° C (1.8° to 2.7° F) that occurs within a short period or a rectal temperature higher than 38.5° C (101.3° F) should be considered indicative of infection and should be investigated thoroughly. Sputum, urine, and blood cultures should be obtained, and all wounds should be inspected carefully for signs of inflammation or infection. Devices commonly associated with nosocomial infection—intravenous cannulas, urinary catheters, and endotracheal tubes—should be removed as soon as feasible or else changed (see below).

Because inflammation is such a prominent feature of all critical illness, including that in patients with serious infectious complications of chronic diseases, several clinical syndromes have been defined in an effort to stratify patients according to the severity of their inflammatory responses [see Table 1].[5] These syndromes are associated with increased mortality, even in the absence of documented infection.[6] In the remainder of this chapter, I will refer repeatedly to the metabolic responses to critical illness; this term incorporates these inflammatory syndromes and more besides, and its use permits a more comprehensive discussion.

Mild elevation of body temperature is usually well tolerated and requires no specific treatment. However, a higher fever may impose significant stress on the patient, as indicated by pronounced tachycardia, tachypnea, malaise, and, occasionally, restlessness. Thus, a body temperature higher than 39° C (102.2° F) is usually treated with antipyretics (acetaminophen, aspirin, indomethacin, or ibuprofen).

The fever experienced by critically ill patients is an upward adjustment of the thermoregulatory center in the brain, the central thermostat [see VII:10 Fever, Hyperpyrexia, and Hypothermia]. A consequence of this adjustment is that the patient usually prefers a warmer environmental temperature than do normal individuals. An ambient temperature in the hospital that is comfortable for the staff is often perceived as cool by the patient, who must generate extra heat to maintain the adjusted body temperature. Thus, patient areas of the

Table 1 Components of Inflammatory Syndromes[5]

Systemic inflammatory response syndrome (SIRS)—two or more of the following are required:
  Temperature > 38° C (100.4° F) or < 36° C (96.8° F)
  Heart rate > 90 beats/min
  Respirations > 20/min
  WBC > 12,000/mm³, < 4,000 mm³, or > 10% bands

Sepsis
  SIRS
  Clinically likely source of infection (does not require bacteriologic confirmation)

Severe sepsis
  Sepsis
  Impaired cardiovascular performance necessitating fluid resuscitation

Septic shock
  Severe sepsis
  Impaired cardiovascular performance necessitating inotropic support

hospital should be kept warm, usually in the range of 26° to 33° C (78.8° to 91.4° F). This temperature range will promote patient comfort and reduce the physiologic demands of cold stress. When moved into the operating room, radiology suite, or other typically cool environments, patients should be insulated, or the room should be warmed.

Attempts to treat a patient with fever by surface cooling (ice packs, alcohol rubs, cooling blankets) are not uncommon. Rather than addressing the altered physiology underlying the fever, however, surface cooling imposes a marked cold stress on an already critically ill and stressed patient. Except in the presence of hyperpyrexia (temperature ≥ 41° C [105.8° F]), surface cooling should be avoided; antipyretics should be administered first to reduce body temperature.

During acute surgical illness, patients typically have a poor appetite. Even when able to eat, they often do not consume sufficient nutrients even to approximate their needs. Accordingly, the clinician should initiate exogenous nutritional support early in the patient's course, especially if it is likely to be prolonged by the need for additional reparative procedures, such as fracture fixation or delayed wound closure.

Some degree of immunosuppression is also a common feature of inflammation. Thus, critically ill patients are more susceptible than normal to colonization and infection with a variety of microorganisms. Special attention to sterile technique during bedside procedures, the use of universal precautions, and hand washing after each patient encounter by all care providers should help reduce the risk of nosocomial infection.

INFECTION

Infections in hospitalized patients fall into two categories: they may be directly related to the patient's primary disease or injury (e.g., invasive burn wound sepsis, gangrene of an ischemic limb, or intra-abdominal abscess after perforated diverticulosis), or they may develop as a complication of physiologic support (e.g., pneumonia after prolonged mechanical ventilatory support).

Early diagnosis and treatment of infection in surgical patients can

minimize debility. Most critically ill surgical patients experience fever, leukocytosis, tachycardia, widened pulse pressure (reduced vascular resistance), glucose intolerance, fluid retention, some impairment of oxygenation, and other signs associated with the septic response. The challenge for the clinician is to distinguish patients in whom this response is caused by established infection from those in whom it is not the result of an infectious focus. A temperature higher than 38.5° C (101.3° F) or an acute increase in temperature accompanied by an abrupt change in the white blood cell count should prompt investigation for a developing infection [*see Figure 1*], which would include appropriate cultures and other diagnostic studies. Other signs that suggest underlying infection include relative hypothermia, leukopenia, thrombocytopenia, abrupt elevation or depression of the blood glucose level, restlessness, lassitude, hyperpnea, and failure to progress as expected.

If the presence of infection is suggested by the clinical setting, the magnitude of fever, or any other systemic signs (such as renal or respiratory dysfunction, marked hyperglycemia or hypoglycemia, hypothermia, or hypotension), broad-spectrum antibiotic coverage should be instituted empirically before culture results are available. Specific antimicrobial therapy should be begun once the presence of infection has been confirmed and the microbiologic diagnosis has been established. Other therapeutic measures may also be necessary to treat the infection. Draining an abscess, debriding or excising necrotic tissue, removing indwelling catheters and placing new ones at other sites, performing therapeutic bronchoscopy to ensure drainage of major airways, or creating a tracheostomy in the patient who requires an airway for improved bedside pulmonary toilet may also be advisable.

Because all critically ill patients are at risk for infection, efforts directed at prevention are worthwhile. Medical and nursing personnel can prevent the transmission of organisms from one patient to another by effective hand washing between patient contacts. Gloves

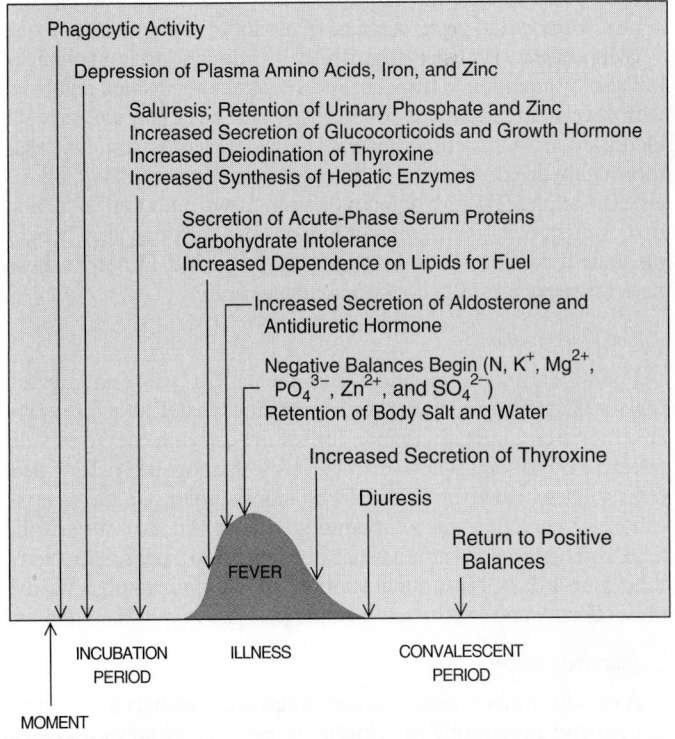

Figure 1 **Illustrated is the time course of events that constitute the classic response to bacterial infection.[231]**

used by health care workers for their own protection whenever they have contact with patients must be changed between patients. Of course, sterile techniques should be used during invasive procedures. Sites of insertion of intravascular cannulas should be inspected regularly, and the catheters should be moved to a new site if the skin becomes reddened or if pus is observed. Antibiotic-impregnated central venous catheters may reduce the incidence of catheter-related infection and thereby lower the frequency with which lines must be replaced.[7] The prophylactic use of antibiotics in the ICU is controversial[8-10] and cannot be encouraged at present.

IATROGENIC FACTORS

Bed Rest

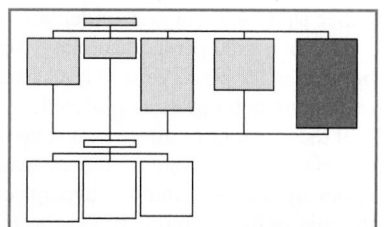

Bed rest and inactivity both contribute to loss of muscle mass and strength. Immobility may result in progressive atelectasis, respiratory insufficiency, and pulmonary sepsis. If immobility is prolonged, open pressure sores may develop over bony prominences. Thus, patients should be turned frequently, and their position should be changed often. Patients who are able to participate actively in repositioning themselves should be encouraged to do so by helping to turn or lift themselves. They should be urged to take deep breaths and cough. An incentive spirometer is inexpensive and is often helpful in this regard. When patients are hemodynamically stable, they should be moved to a chair, provided that no musculoskeletal contraindications are present. This position improves ventilation and helps preserve postural reflexes. Patients should assist in sitting up as much as is feasible. Even simple actions such as standing in place or bearing weight during the transfer may be beneficial. Active and passive range-of-motion exercises can help maintain joint function. Proper positioning of the extremities may be necessary to prevent contractures and to preserve range of motion.

Skin integrity is preserved not only by frequent position changes but also by attention to hygiene. Patients should be bathed regularly, with special attention paid to intertriginous areas. Any soilage with blood, stool, urine, or other material should be removed and the skin thoroughly dried. Massage and application of moisturizing lotions are also helpful. The use of foam or air mattress pads that distribute body weight over a large area or low-air-loss beds may also benefit the patient confined to bed for a prolonged period. However, these devices are no substitute for good nursing care.

Food Deprivation

Food is commonly withheld from the patient before and during various diagnostic and therapeutic procedures as well as before operations or after injury. Starvation for several days appears to be well tolerated by patients who were relatively well nourished before their critical illness. However, if food deprivation is prolonged, the complications of starvation will compound the effects of critical surgical illness. Total starvation should usually be limited to a period no longer than 3 or 4 days. Nutritional support should be instituted via the most effective and safest route possible [see VII:9 Nutritional Support].

Invasive Devices

A variety of tubes, catheters, and drains are essential for the proper care and monitoring of critically ill patients. However, each of these devices transgresses a normal barrier to infection, and each is associated with infectious risks and other complications. An invasive device should be removed as soon as it is no longer required. Intra-

venous lines placed in the emergency room or under less than ideal conditions (e.g., at the scene of an accident or while the patient is en route to the hospital) should be removed as soon as possible and replaced, if necessary, with new devices by means of appropriate sterile technique. Such lines should also be changed if the puncture site is red, inflamed, or purulent. With most of these devices, the risk of infectious complications increases after 3 or 4 days.[11] Regular replacement is commonly practiced, especially if the patient becomes febrile. Catheters impregnated with antibiotics appear not to require such frequent exchanges and may be safely used for longer periods.[7]

Sleep Deprivation

Normal sleep patterns are disturbed in ICU patients, in part because of the constant light and noise in the ICU and because of repetitive stimulation by the ICU staff. Such disturbances, in combination with other stresses associated with illness, often result in confusion, disorientation, anxiety, and, occasionally, frank psychosis. As many efforts as possible should be made to orient the patient, including the use of wall calendars, clocks, and other methods that serve as normal day-night indicators (e.g., turning the lights down at night). Even the personal activities of daily living, such as bathing and shaving, can serve as time cues. Patients should be reassured and reminded about the date, the time, their location, and the reason for their hospitalization. Sedatives and hypnotics may be useful in critically ill patients but occasionally have a paradoxically excitatory effect.

Metabolic Responses That Can Cause Debility

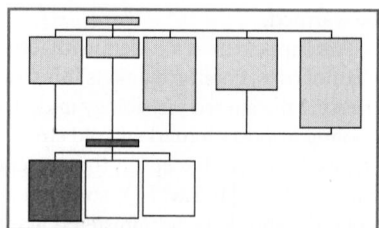

All of the clinical factors of surgical care contribute to or affect various physiologic and biochemical alterations that occur in response to critical illness; these physiologic and biochemical alterations collectively constitute the metabolic response to critical illness. The intensity and duration of this response determine debility. Current critical care management generally supports rather than modifies the response. Three major features of the metabolic response to critical illness affect clinical care: the hyperdynamic or hypermetabolic state, muscle wasting, and glucose intolerance.

HYPERDYNAMIC OR HYPERMETABOLIC STATE

In recovery from critical illness, several organ systems function at an accelerated pace. Principal among these is the cardiovascular system. Tachycardia and a widened pulse pressure are typically present and reflect cardiac output greater than that expected in a resting, healthy individual. The increased blood flow is distributed to most vascular beds, especially to inflammatory tissue or the wound, and supports increased cellular activity in the healing wound. In the kidneys, increased flow is associated with an elevated glomerular filtration rate. Thus, drug excretion may be accelerated, and increased dosages may be required to maintain therapeutic plasma concentrations.

Accompanying the increases in cardiac output and regional blood flow is an increase in oxygen delivery (transport) to the microcirculation. This increase in oxygen delivery supports the enhanced oxygen requirements of several organ systems. Total body oxygen consumption ($\dot{V}o_2$) is greater than normal because of the increased oxidation of body fuels—carbohydrates, fats, and amino acids—needed to provide the energy to drive the cellular machinery at this accelerated pace [see Figure 2]. These reactions produce heat. Heat production, also referred to as energy expenditure or metabolic rate, is increased in critically ill patients, who thus are said to be hypermetabolic.

The increase in $\dot{V}O_2$ is paralleled by increased carbon dioxide production ($\dot{V}CO_2$), which, under normal conditions, stimulates breathing and augments minute ventilation. For patients who require ventilatory assistance, the ventilator should be set to deliver a minute ventilation that is greater than normal.

As discussed earlier, critically ill patients typically have a fever and prefer warmer ambient temperatures than normal individuals. In these patients, metabolic rates increase in part to maintain a higher than normal core temperature. A warm environment may help blunt the patient's increased heat production and energy needs.

Associated with the hyperdynamic state of critical illness is expansion of the extracellular fluid (ECF) compartment. Total body water and total body sodium are increased. This expansion occurs perioperatively or with resuscitation after injury. Short-term changes in body weight reflect alterations in body water and in lean tissue mass. Slow, persistent expansion of the ECF may mask loss of tissue mass. Conversely, spontaneous diuresis of sodium and water during recovery may lead to pronounced weight loss in a patient who otherwise appears to be progressing well.

During critical illness, the daily loss of body water is increased in several ways. Fever accelerates insensible loss of body water, and renal loss may be greater than normal because of the increased osmotic load caused by the breakdown of lean tissue (see below). If there are open wounds, evaporative water loss is markedly increased, in proportion to the size of the open wound. Thus, maintenance water requirements may be greater than normal. It is often necessary to monitor both the intravascular fluid volume, using values for central venous or pulmonary arterial wedge pressures, and the ECF composition or tonicity, as indicated by changes in serum sodium concentrations.

The clinician should provide not only volume and possible pharmacologic support to maintain a hyperdynamic circulation but also an increased amount of calories to meet the patient's elevated energy needs. These needs can often be reliably estimated on the basis of the patient's age, sex, body size, and critical illness. Occasionally, it may be helpful to measure the patient's $\dot{V}O_2$ and $\dot{V}CO_2$ and to use these values to calculate daily caloric requirements.

In addition to providing cardiopulmonary and nutritional support to critically ill, hyperdynamic patients, the clinician should try to neutralize factors that may augment the hyperdynamic response to critical illness. Judicious analgesia and sedation provide metabolic benefits and relieve pain and anxiety. Providing a warm environment mitigates the hyperdynamic response by reducing cold stress. Antipyretics reduce the heart rate during periods of extreme fever.

MUSCLE WASTING

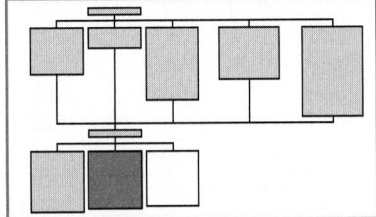

The distinguishing feature of the debility of critical illness is marked muscle wasting and weakness. Wasting is in part a consequence of accelerated muscle protein breakdown, which is generally related to the severity of illness [see Figure 2]. The increased protein breakdown presumably serves to mobilize amino acids for synthesis of new protein in wounds; for proliferation of phagocytes, macrophages, and other cellular components involved in wound healing; and for synthesis of acute-phase proteins and glucose in the liver. The increased synthetic work and processing of amino acids in the liver result in increased production of urea, which is filtered and

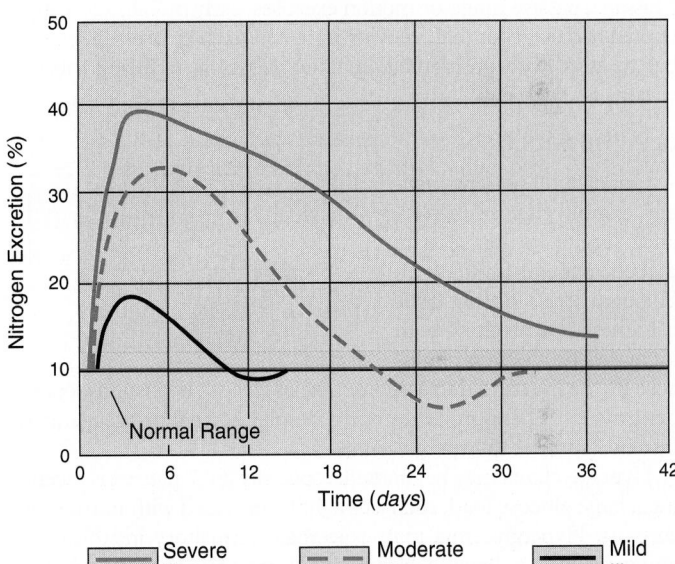

Severe Illness — Moderate Illness — Mild Illness

Figure 2 Increased resting metabolic activity (hypermetabolism) and increased nitrogen loss are closely related during critical surgical illness. Both correlate with the severity of illness and return to normal as the patient recovers. Patients with severe illness are represented by the solid red line, those with moderate illness by the broken red line, and those with mild illness by the solid black line; the normal range is shown by the light-red bar.

excreted by the kidneys. In the presence of renal dysfunction, blood urea nitrogen (BUN) may rise rapidly.

To reduce muscle wasting, additional exogenous protein or amino acids are provided through nutritional support. In general, protein needs increase in proportion to caloric requirements. However, for the critically ill surgical patient, it may be beneficial to provide at least 20% to 25% of total calories as protein or amino acids. BUN may be higher than normal (at least 20 to 30 mg/dl) with this level of amino acid intake, even if renal function is normal.

In addition to amino acids, other intracellular constituents are released by these catabolic processes and subsequently excreted. Thus, metabolic alkalosis often develops, associated with mild hypochloremia and with reduction in total body potassium and magnesium. Re-

Table 2 Blood Glucose and Insulin Concentrations in Burn Patients[1]

Group	N	Burn Size (% TBS)	Postburn Day Studied	Fasting Blood Glucose		Basal Insulin (µU/ml)
				(mmol/L)	(mg/dl)	
Control subjects	12	—	—	3.88 ± 0.11	69.8 ± 1.9	22 ± 3
Resuscitated burn patients	4	71	1	7.77 ± 0.61	139.9 ± 10.9	20 ± 6
Hypermetabolic burn patients	17	42	9	6.27 ± 0.28	112.9 ± 5.0	22 ± 2
Convalescing burn patients	5	56.5	69	4.05 ± 0.33	72.9 ± 5.9	14 ± 1
Septic burn patients	15	71	10	6.43 ± 0.55	115.8 ± 9.9	22 ± 4
Treated septic burn patients	4	72	11	6.11 ± 0.83	110.0 ± 15.9	12 ± 3

pletion with potassium chloride and magnesium sulfate is usually effective. During nutritional support, generous amounts of potassium (≥ 100 mEq/day), magnesium (≥ 30 mEq/day), phosphate (20 to 30 mmol/day), and trace minerals should be provided to promote synthesis and restoration of intracellular proteins and other constituents.

Muscle mass is also lost as a result of disuse. The critically ill patient is usually confined to bed and may be further immobilized because of traction, monitoring devices, mechanical ventilation, and sedation. Massage, passive range-of-motion exercises, early mobilization, and limited bed exercises (e.g., moving from bed to chair, use of a trapeze bar to assist with positioning) may be helpful in reducing muscle wasting and debility.

GLUCOSE INTOLERANCE

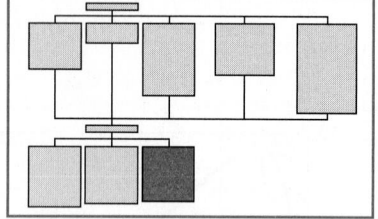

Critically ill patients usually exhibit glucose intolerance similar to that seen in diabetic patients [*see Table 2*]. Hyperglycemia during critical illness is a result of both increased production of glucose by the liver and decreased uptake of glucose by insulin-dependent tissues. These processes occur despite normal or exaggerated insulin responses to hyperglycemia.

Hyperglycemia may be marked, especially if the patient is receiving a large glucose load, such as might be provided with nutritional support. Hyperglycemia may exacerbate ventilatory insufficiency and contribute to hepatic dysfunction. It may also provoke osmotic diuresis, dehydration, and a hyperosmolar state. Vigorous attempts should therefore be made to control the blood glucose concentration, maintaining it at least below the renal threshold value of approximately 180 mg/dl (10 mmol/L).

The provision of safe amounts of glucose and the administration of exogenous recombinant human insulin are the mainstays of therapy for glucose control. Because insulin resistance is present in patients with critical illness, relatively large quantities of insulin may be required to control the blood glucose level. Intravenous administration of insulin provides rapid control and prevents unpredictable subcutaneous uptake caused by variations in blood flow. Because of its short half-life, intravenous insulin must be administered either in frequent intermittent doses or by continuous infusion. Either technique can be effective, and both provide a reasonable margin of safety. Blood glucose levels may be determined rapidly by using a portable glucose analyzer at the bedside on a small blood sample drawn every 1 or 2 hours. On the basis of the blood glucose value, a predetermined insulin dose may be administered, or the infusion rate may be regulated (a so-called sliding scale). The doses should be adjusted as required to maintain blood glucose in a target range of approximately 110 to 160 mg/dl.[12] One half to two thirds of the total insulin dose required to maintain blood glucose in this target range in a 24-hour period may be added to the intravenous feeding regimen on the next day. In this way, the blood glucose level is ultimately maintained in an acceptable range.

The degree of glucose intolerance will vary over the course of the critical illness. Therefore, regular monitoring of blood glucose concentrations is advisable, even after adequate control has been achieved. Further episodes of stress-inducing conditions, especially infection, may exacerbate glucose intolerance; an abrupt rise in blood glucose concentration may be the first indication of impending sepsis. As the patient recovers, glucose tolerance improves and the requirement for insulin decreases. When the patient is transferred from intravenous nutrition to enteral nutrition, insulin requirements often decrease despite similar nutrient intake.

Glucose remains an important fuel during critical illness, especially for healing wounds. However, the ability to utilize glucose effectively appears to be limited. Most of the total energy administered in nutritional support should be provided by glucose (60% to 75% of total calories). The dose of glucose should, however, be limited if marked hyperglycemia cannot be readily controlled with insulin. The remaining calories can be provided by fat emulsion.

Discussion

The clinical features of all critical illnesses are similar, regardless of the type of insult sustained, be it injury, operation, or infection. Similar responses can be seen in a wide variety of animals that have been injured or challenged by invasive infection.[13,14] These responses to critical illness presumably evolved because they confer an advantage with respect to survival. In fact, it seems indisputable that when an individual organism acquires an enhanced ability to recover from an injury or infection, the species is thereby benefited. Accordingly, the metabolic responses to critical illness are often considered to be adaptive reactions that serve to promote recovery.

There is a cost for this benefit, however, and that is debility. In addition, the metabolic responses to critical illness can lead to organ system dysfunction. Critically ill patients also typically have immunologic abnormalities that may make them more susceptible to invasive infection by a variety of microorganisms, including those that are not usually pathogenic [*see VI:6 Non-AIDS Immunosuppres-*

sion]. The syndrome of multiorgan failure and sepsis that may develop in association with the metabolic responses to critical illness is often the final route to death [*see VII:7 Multiple Organ Dysfunction Syndrome*]. Thus, in some ways, certain metabolic responses seem maladaptive in that they retard recovery and lead to organ failure and death.

An improved understanding of the metabolic responses to critical illness may benefit patients in two ways. First, it may facilitate the development of improved supportive therapies. Much of current critical care practice is based on our understanding of these processes and has been designed to support them. Second, a better understanding of the mechanisms underlying the metabolic responses to critical illness may lead to strategies for altering the responses in such a way that those features that are beneficial and promote recovery are stimulated and those features that are debilitating or lead to organ system dysfunction are suppressed or limited.

Integrated Metabolic Response to Critical Illness

The metabolic responses to injury and critical illness occur simultaneously. They primarily involve the liver, skeletal muscle, the gut, the kidneys, and the wound or focus of inflammation [*see Figure 3*]. The heart also plays a major role by providing the motive force for the high rate of blood flow that is required to support increased exchange of nutrients and other substances between organs. The central and autonomic nervous systems and endocrine tissues are mainly involved in regulation of the responses.

The wound, which may include one or more foci of infection and other sites of inflammation in addition to external injuries, plays a principal role. It acts as a large arteriovenous shunt, robbing the host of blood supply and demanding increased cardiovascular work. The wound also induces and controls profound metabolic changes, which subside as the wound heals. Tissues are broken down, presumably to provide substrates for a variety of synthetic and energy-producing processes. The cost to the patient is increased metabolic work, elevated energy requirements, erosion of lean body tissue, and debility.

The healing wound is a site of intense metabolic activity. Dissolution and removal of necrotic tissue, containment and killing of bacteria, collagen synthesis and wound repair, cellular proliferation, and restoration of tissue integrity occur, often simultaneously. These processes require energy and a variety of substrates, particularly amino acids for protein synthesis. The microenvironment of a wound is often relatively hypoxic. However, inflammatory cells have a marked capacity for glycolytic metabolism,[15] in which adenosine triphosphate (ATP) can be generated without the consumption of oxygen. This capacity persists even when oxygen delivery is sufficient. Glucose is thus the principal fuel for the healing wound. It is metabolized to lactate, which is then released into the circulation for transport to the liver.

The liver produces the additional glucose that is required by the wound. It is capable of manufacturing glucose from lactate. In this manner, glucose is recycled between the liver and the wound, and there is no net gain or loss of carbon atoms. The liver also synthesizes glucose from amino acids, principally alanine, which comes from both skeletal muscle and the gut. This mechanism is termed gluconeogenesis. The nitrogen contained in the amino acids is converted to urea and excreted. The liver also synthesizes a variety of circulating proteins in response to inflammation and infection (so-called acutephase proteins). All of these synthetic processes require energy, produced in part by fat oxidation, and therefore contribute to a general increase in energy utilization, heat production, and metabolic rate.

Skeletal muscle protein breaks down at an accelerated rate after injury and critical illness, releasing a variety of substances into the circulation, including creatine and creatinine, 3-methylhistidine, potassium, magnesium, and amino acids. The amino acids serve as precursors for protein synthesis in the wound and in the liver. The released amino acids do not reflect a simple dissolution of protein. Rather, alanine and glutamine are disproportionately released. Alanine can be readily converted to glucose in the liver. Glutamine serves both as a fuel—especially for the gut and for rapidly proliferating cells, including inflammatory cells and fibroblasts—and as a precursor for renal ammonia production, which is an important mechanism for neutralizing excreted acid loads.

Although muscle tissue in healthy persons is usually quite sensitive to insulin and commonly serves as a site of glucose storage, muscle is resistant to insulin after injury or critical illness, and its capacity for glucose storage is reduced significantly. This response contributes to glucose intolerance and helps direct glucose to the healing wound.

The gut was long considered to be essentially inactive during convalescence, but it now appears to play a central role in the metabolic response to critical illness [*see VII:9 Nutritional Support*]. During critical illness, the gut utilizes glutamine as its principal fuel, converting glutamine to alanine, which is transported to the liver by the portal circulation. More important, perhaps, the gut can be a portal of entry for bacteria and bacterial toxins, which can worsen or perpetuate critical illness [*see VI:15 Peritonitis and Intra-abdominal Abscesses and VII:7 Multiple Organ Dysfunction Syndrome*].

The kidneys also contribute to the generalized increase in physiologic work and energy requirements that accompanies critical illness. The kidneys must excrete an increased solute load consisting of urea, potassium, magnesium, weak acids, and other intracellular constituents. In addition, many drugs and their metabolites depend on renal excretion. Production of ammonia from glutamine may be increased to neutralize acid loads. Many of these processes require energy.

All of these regional metabolic processes occur simultaneously. The net integrated metabolic response is evident clinically as increased energy expenditure and heat production, fever, accelerated nitrogen excretion and muscle wasting, and glucose intolerance. The wound appears to exert a controlling influence on the intensity and duration of the responses to critical illness or injury: the intensity is proportional to the size of the wound or the mass of inflammatory tissue. The larger the wound, the more intense the metabolic responses. As the wound heals and as inflammation subsides, the heightened metabolic demands abate. Expeditious wound closure and definitive treatment of infection are the most effective forms of anticatabolic therapy.

Hypermetabolism

Because humans maintain fairly constant body temperature, the heat generated by the body is equal to the heat lost in biochemical and physiologic processes and is an indicator of overall metabolic activity. This heat ultimately results from the oxidation of organic fuels. The rate of heat production, or metabolic rate (MR), is therefore related to $\dot{V}_{O_2}$ and $\dot{V}_{CO_2}$. It may be measured directly by means of direct calorimetry, or it may be calculated from measurements of $\dot{V}_{O_2}$, $\dot{V}_{CO_2}$, and body surface area (BSA) by means of indirect calorimetry:

$$MR \ (kcal/m^2/hr) = \frac{[(3.9 \times \dot{V}_{O_2} \ [L/min]) + (1.1 \times \dot{V}_{CO_2} \ [L/min])] \times 60 \ (min/hr)}{BSA \ (m^2)}$$

A third term, $-3.3 \times$ urea nitrogen loss (g/time), is sometimes added to account for the heat produced by urea formation. However, it is usually a small factor, adjusting MR by only 2% to 3%.[16]

Values determined by direct and indirect calorimetry under steady-

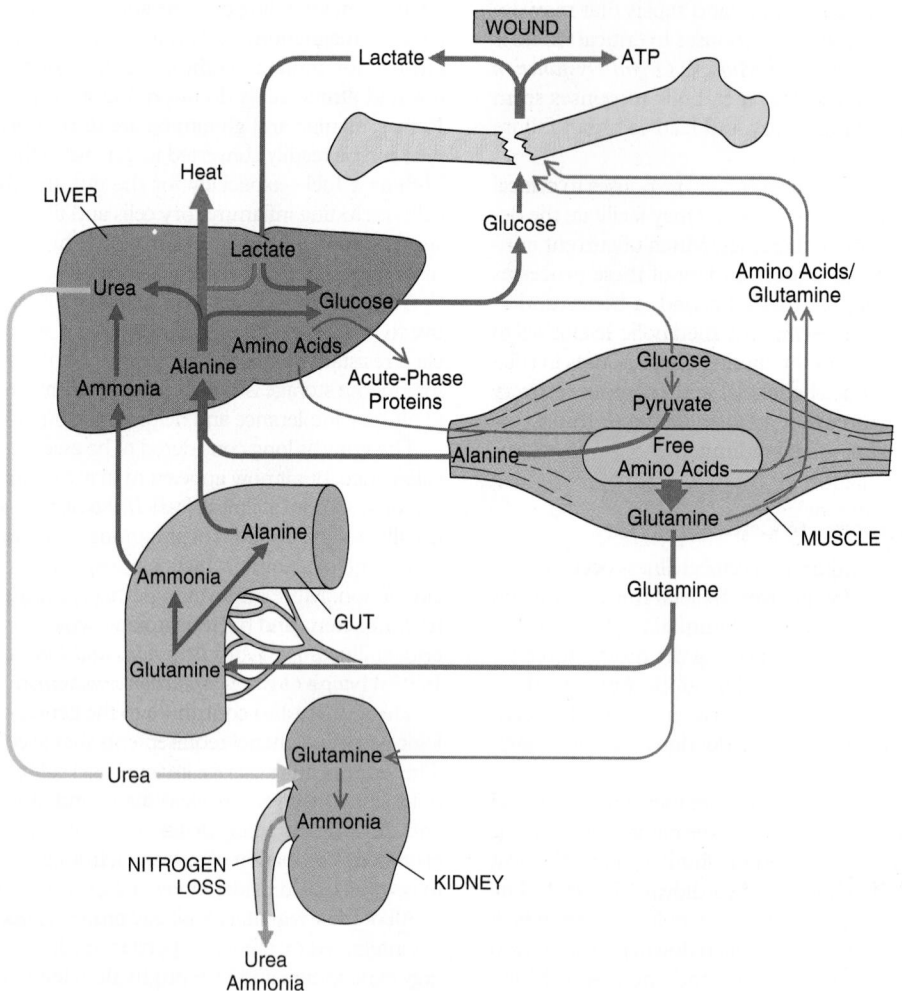

Figure 3 The metabolic response to critical illness includes characteristic alterations in the exchange of substrates between organs. Presumably, these responses occur in support of the healing wound and are facilitated by a hyperdynamic circulation. The wound requires glucose (and probably glutamine) as a primary respiratory fuel. Glucose is converted to lactate; this conversion can occur in an aerobic environment. Lactate is transported to the liver for conversion back into glucose. The recycling of lactate to glucose is a major pathway that requires the input of energy and thereby contributes to increased energy utilization. Most of the glucose required for the healing wound (i.e., inflammatory tissue) is produced by the liver, not only from lactate but also from alanine and other glucogenic amino acids. These reactions require energy and also result in the formation of urea. Muscle is the major source of amino acids, which are used for protein synthesis both in the wound and in the liver. The most abundant amino acids released from muscle are alanine and glutamine. Glutamine serves as a primary fuel for the gut, producing ammonia and other products (e.g., alanine) that are processed by the liver. In addition, glutamine may help buffer filtered acid loads in the kidneys by the formation of ammonia. These metabolic processes contribute to the hypermetabolism, hyperdynamic circulation, increased nitrogen loss, and glucose intolerance that are clinically evident in critically ill patients.

state conditions are comparable.[17] When metabolic rates of normal individuals are determined under controlled basal conditions, the values are reproducible and predictable (± 12%) on the basis of age, sex, and body size.[18] When metabolic rates of critically ill patients with satisfactory hemodynamic function are determined under similar conditions, the rates are greater than predicted. Thus, patients are said to be hypermetabolic.

The degree of hypermetabolism is proportional to the severity of illness. This phenomenon was most dramatically demonstrated in careful studies of burn patients performed in the 1970s.[19] The increase in resting metabolic rate was proportional to the extent of tissue injury—that is, to the amount of the BSA that was burned. Hypermetabolism has

also been demonstrated in a variety of other critically ill patients, but it has usually been less severe than that seen in patients with major burns.[20] In the burn patients, moreover, there was a limit to the hypermetabolism: metabolic rates of patients with extensive burns were little different from those of patients with burns covering 50% to 60% of BSA.

These observations suggest that there is a limit to the metabolic activity that patients can support in response to critical illness. The difference between this limit and the magnitude of the patient's actual responses defines physiologic reserve [*see Figure 4*]. Physiologic reserve is presumably also affected by the patient's age and state of health before the critical illness. It reflects the patient's ability to meet additional complicating stresses, such as infection, volume loss, pain, anxiety, and cold ambient temperatures. For example, when patients are exposed to progressively colder ambient temperatures, the metabolic rate generally increases. However, when a group of patients with very large burns were exposed to cold temperatures, their already high metabolic rates did not increase but actually fell.[19] None of these patients survived the injury, presumably because of inability to respond to new stresses. In another group of burn patients, the inability to increase metabolic rate to facilitate rewarming after skin grafting procedures also identified nonsurvivors.[21] When patients are cared for in a warm environment, hypermetabolism is reduced and physiologic reserve is increased.

Hypermetabolism refers to an increase in total body oxidative metabolism that is manifested by increases in total body $\dot{V}O_2$, cardiac output, and MR. Regional $\dot{V}O_2$ is generally increased throughout most tissue beds, but regional blood flow is not. The additional total body flow is directed largely to the wound or site of inflammation and to the splanchnic circulation, and it appears to supply the wound with increased amounts of glucose and other nutrients. In studies of patients who had sustained a large burn on one leg and no burn on the other, Wilmore and colleagues found that $\dot{V}O_2$ of both limbs was increased in proportion to the total BSA burned and represented a fairly constant 6% of total body $\dot{V}O_2$.[22] However, blood flow to the injured extremity was approximately twice that to the uninjured limb. Blood flow was proportional to the extent of the local injury and was directed to the surface wound.[23]

Oxygen consumption by the splanchnic and renal circulations also increases in proportion to total body $\dot{V}O_2$ and hence in proportion to total body injury.[24] Splanchnic flow increases in proportion to total body flow (cardiac output), and together with the blood flow to the wound, it accounts for a large part of the increase in cardiac output in critically ill patients.[25] The increase in renal blood flow correlates with solute load rather than with $\dot{V}O_2$. From these and other studies, it is possible to calculate how oxygen consumption and cardiac output are partitioned among different vascular beds.[26]

Altered Temperature Regulation

Body temperature is determined by the balance between heat production and heat loss [see VII:10 Fever, Hyperpyrexia, and Hypothermia]. It is normally closely regulated and maintained within a narrow range. Critically ill patients typically have an elevated body temperature, even in the absence of clinical infection.[27] Heat production, as measured by metabolic rate, is increased in the critically ill patient. Heat loss may also be elevated in these patients.

It was once thought that increased evaporative heat loss was the driving force for hypermetabolism, at least in burn patients.[28,29] Barr and associates tested this assumption.[30] Although patients treated in warm, dry air showed substantially increased evaporation of water from the burn wound and more rapid drying of the wound surfaces than did patients exposed to normal ward conditions, they had reduced hypermetabolism and a smaller degree of weight loss.

Several other studies have examined the relation between thermoregulatory factors (evaporative heat loss and ambient temperature) and hypermetabolism. For example, the metabolic rates of burn patients were determined at several ambient temperatures, ranging from 19° to 33° C (66.2° to 91.4° F) [see Table 3].[31] Metabolic rate decreased as ambient temperature was increased, but core temperature remained elevated at all ambient temperatures, indicating that thermoregulation in these patients occurred in relation to an elevated central reference temperature. When febrile burn patients in another study were allowed to set the ambient temperature to achieve thermal comfort, they invariably preferred higher than normal tem-

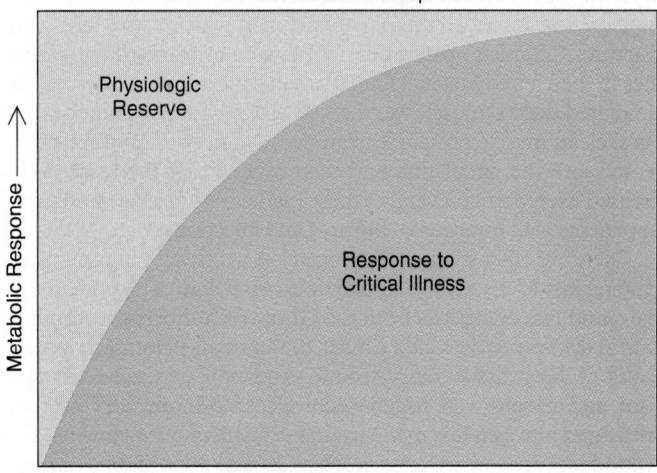

Figure 4 **The intensity of the metabolic response to critical surgical illness increases as a function of the severity of illness. In patients with extremely severe critical illness (e.g., patients with burns covering 60% of the body surface area), responses are near maximal, and physiologic reserves, with which patients respond to additional stressors (e.g., infection, hemorrhage, or cold exposure), are limited. Patients may also have limited physiologic reserves because of preexisting disease, starvation, or advanced age. Therapies that attenuate the stressors of critical surgical illness improve physiologic reserve.**

peratures, in the range of 30° to 33° C (86.0° to 91.4° F).[32] The patients' unburned skin remained relatively vasoconstricted at the higher temperatures as an additional way of maintaining the febrile state. However, even under these conditions of thermal comfort, the patients continued to maintain elevated metabolic rates. Thus, although thermoregulatory factors may influence hypermetabolism, the increased rate of heat production appears to be determined primarily by metabolic factors. Hypermetabolism is temperature sensitive but not temperature dependent.

Altered Protein Metabolism

MUSCLE WASTING, NITROGEN LOSS, AND ACCELERATED PROTEIN BREAKDOWN

One of the most striking features of the metabolic response to critical illness is the marked degree of muscle wasting. This atrophy is as-

Table 3 Effect of Ambient Temperature on Metabolic Rate and on Core and Skin Temperatures

Ambient Temperature (°C)	N	Core Temperature (°C)	Skin Temperature (°C)	Metabolic Rate (kcal/m²/hr)
Normal subjects				
21	3	36.7	30.0	41.2
25	4	36.8	31.4	35.6
33	4	36.8	34.2	36.3
Burn patients (45% TBS)				
21	9	38.1	32.1	83.7
25	20	38.5	33.1	63.5
33	20	38.0	36.2	62.0

sociated with increased urinary excretion of nitrogen. Sir David Cuthbertson first described this phenomenon in patients with long-bone fractures.[27] Similar observations were made by Howard and associates in the United States.[33] Cuthbertson concluded that injured and uninjured skeletal muscle was the source of the excreted nitrogen.[34,35] As skeletal muscle protein is degraded, a variety of markers are released into the circulation and then excreted by the kidneys. Increased excretion of several of these markers[36,37] has been observed in patients with trauma,[36,38] burns,[39] and infections.[40]

There are other sources of nitrogen loss in critically ill patients, including loss of tissue from slough or excision, loss of blood and exudate, and loss of mucosa from the GI tract. Cuthbertson estimated that in the first 10 days after a burn, the amounts of nitrogen lost as a result of direct tissue injury, wound exudation, generalized catabolism, and atrophy were roughly equivalent.[41] Moore and coworkers measured nitrogen loss in the wound exudate of burn patients. This wound loss accounted for as much as 20% to 30% of total nitrogen loss during the early postburn period.[42]

The time course of nitrogen excretion during critical illness is distinctive. Cuthbertson observed that nitrogen excretion peaked several days after injury and gradually returned to normal during a period of several weeks.[34] The pattern was similar to that of increased oxygen consumption. Thus, both hypermetabolism and muscle proteolysis peak shortly after the onset of critical illness and gradually return to normal as recovery proceeds. This too appears to be a characteristic feature of the metabolic responses to critical illness [see Figure 2].[43-45]

Protein turnover is an indicator of overall protein metabolic activity. It is determined through use of tracers. Both extracellular and intracellular amino acids are considered part of a free amino acid pool. Nitrogen is added to this pool by nitrogen intake (diet) and by protein breakdown. Nitrogen is removed by protein synthesis and by conversion to urea. When a small quantity of a labeled amino acid is infused, the rate of appearance of nitrogen in the free amino acid pool can be determined. Under steady-state conditions, this appearance rate represents protein turnover and matches protein disappearance.[46] During critical illness, protein turnover is increased.[47] When nitrogen turnover data are combined with measurements of nitrogen intake and loss, rates of total body protein synthesis and catabolism can be estimated. These estimates indicate that protein catabolism is increased in critically ill patients.[48] Synthesis rates remain normal during fasting but increase to approach or match catabolic rates when feeding is adequate. Thus, the increase in net nitrogen loss during critical illness appears to result from an increase in protein breakdown. Decreased protein synthesis is less of a factor as long as nutritional intake is satisfactory [see Table 4].

ALTERED AMINO ACID METABOLISM

Protein synthesis and breakdown are processes that occur in cells and involve intracellular amino acids. It has been estimated that skeletal muscle contains as much as 80% of the free amino acid pool.[49] Intracellular concentrations of free amino acids in skeletal muscle are approximately 30 times greater than plasma concentrations of free amino acids.[50] Thus, the total muscle mass of a 70 kg man contains approximately 87 g of free amino acids in the intracellular water, whereas the extracellular pool contains only 1.2 g.

The relative amounts of individual free amino acids in cells differ from the proportions found in protein. Glutamine, a nonessential amino acid, accounts for only about 5% to 6% of protein, but it is the most abundant intracellular free amino acid, accounting for about 60% of the total intracellular free amino acid pool. In contrast, the eight essential amino acids together account for only 8.4% of the intracellu-

Table 4 Alterations in Rates of Protein Synthesis and Catabolism That May Affect Hospitalized Patients

	Synthesis	Catabolism
Normal—starvation	↓	0
Normal—fed, bed rest	↓	0
Elective surgical procedure	↓	0
Injury/sepsis—I.V. dextrose	↑↑	↑↑↑
Injury/sepsis—fed	↑↑↑	↑↑↑

↓—decrease   ↑—increase   0—no change

lar pool. The intracellular concentration of glutamine decreases under many catabolic conditions, including starvation, inactivity,[51] elective operation,[52] trauma,[53] and sepsis.[54] This decrease occurs early in the course of the acute illness, persists until late in convalescence, and appears to be related to the severity of illness.[55,56] The intracellular concentrations of phenylalanine, tyrosine, alanine, and the branched-chain amino acids (BCAAs)—leucine, isoleucine, and valine—typically increase after trauma and infection.[51,54] These levels return to normal during convalescence, usually before glutamine levels do.

Plasma concentrations of free amino acids generally decrease after operation, injury, or infection, largely because of a fall in the concentrations of the nonessential amino acids. Changes in extracellular concentrations of specific amino acids have been inconsistent between studies, presumably as a reflection of differences in patient selection, analytic methods, or treatment.[54]

The ECF compartment is important for amino acid transport between organs and between regions of the body. Aulick and Wilmore calculated amino acid release rates from peripheral tissues of burn patients on the basis of measurements of leg blood flow and of femoral arterial and venous plasma concentrations of 10 amino acids.[57] The net release of amino acid nitrogen was five times greater in burn patients than in control subjects. Alanine was the only amino acid whose release rate was significantly elevated (glutamine concentration was not determined). Alanine release was related to total burn size (injury severity) and to total body $\dot{V}O_2$. In related studies, the accelerated peripheral amino acid release was matched by increased uptake across the splanchnic bed.[24] Alanine uptake was three to four times control values. This increased release of amino acids from the periphery and transport to splanchnic tissues appears to be another characteristic metabolic response to critical burn injury.

Garber and colleagues observed that glutamine and alanine together constituted as much as 70% of the amino acids released from skeletal muscle in vitro.[58] Furthermore, the release rates of alanine and glutamine reflected the net rates of formation from other amino acids.[59] Thus, during critical illness, skeletal muscle protein is broken down into amino acids that are largely converted to glutamine and alanine, which are then released into the ECF for transport. Although all amino acids are required for protein synthesis at remote locations, glutamine and alanine are the major nitrogen carriers from muscle. These two amino acids have other roles as well. Alanine is a precursor of glucose production in the liver. In that process, urea is also formed and subsequently excreted by the kidneys. Although there may be some minor recycling of urea nitrogen under certain conditions,[60] formation of urea is the final step in the loss of body protein, representing an irreversible loss of nitrogen.

Glutamine is a precursor for production of ammonia in the kidneys, an important buffering mechanism for excreted acid loads. Increased breakdown of intracellular constituents could result in such an acid load, and ammonia excretion is often increased after injury.

Intracellular skeletal muscle glutamine may be an important determinant of net skeletal muscle protein breakdown.[61,62] After a standard operation in an animal model, net amino acid efflux from the hindquarter was increased as the glutamine concentration fell. However, if the intracellular glutamine concentration was maintained by the provision of exogenous glutamine, net efflux was reduced.

Glutamine also appears to be an important respiratory fuel for rapidly dividing cells. Glutamine can be converted to glutamate and then to α-ketoglutarate for participation in the citric acid cycle. The nitrogen of glutamine is used to form ammonia, alanine, and citrulline.[63] This process occurs in colonocytes, enterocytes, fibroblasts, and, possibly, inflammatory cells such as macrophages. Phagocytic cells are found in fixed locations in the GI tract, such as Peyer's patches and other regions containing Kupffer's cells, as well as in the wound, at other sites of inflammation, and in the bone marrow. Windmueller measured the nutrient requirements of the rat intestine using an isolated, perfused segment of small bowel.[63] The intestinal segment extracted large amounts of glutamine from the recirculated perfusate. Souba and Wilmore measured amino acid uptake by the gut in conscious animals and demonstrated that the consumption of glutamine by the gut was significantly increased after celiotomy, even though the circulating glutamine concentration was reduced (i.e., glutamine was actively taken up by the intestine).[64]

Dissolution of skeletal muscle protein during critical illness seems to serve many purposes. First, it provides amino acids to support protein synthesis at remote sites such as the wound, other inflammatory foci, and the liver. Proteolysis also provides amino acid precursors for glucose production by the liver and for production of ammonia in the kidneys. Finally, it provides glutamine, which appears to be a specific fuel for the gut and possibly for other tissues with rapid cell turnover, such as the wound, bone marrow, and fixed macrophages of the GI tract. This mobilization of amino acids from muscle protein, however, leads to an irretrievable loss of nitrogen in the form of urea, ammonia, creatinine, uric acid, and other compounds. The cost to the patient is rapid erosion of muscle mass and debility.

Altered Carbohydrate Metabolism

ACCELERATED ENDOGENOUS GLUCOSE PRODUCTION

The liver normally produces sufficient glucose to permit maintenance of the blood glucose concentration within narrow limits, even during periods of fasting. During critical illness, the rate of endogenous glucose production is increased.[24,65,66] Increased basal glucose production is matched by an increase in glucose uptake, so that glucose levels remain relatively stable. Thus, the mass flow, or turnover, of glucose is increased. In studies of patients with burns, glucose turnover was related to total body $\dot{V}O_2$ and thus to the size of the burn (i.e., to injury severity).[67] Regional uptake was closely related to regional blood flow and regional lactate release but not to regional $\dot{V}O_2$. Thus, glucose was directed by the circulation to the wound, where it was taken up and converted via glycolysis to lactate, even in the presence of adequate or increased oxygen delivery.

The liver produces glucose by a variety of mechanisms. Hydrolysis of hepatic glycogen mobilizes glucose rapidly to serve as an energy source in times of acute need. This mechanism is most important immediately after injury and during acute stress states, such as shock, fever, pain, and anxiety (ebb-phase responses). Glycogen reserves are limited, however, and glycogen is not the major source of hepatic glucose production during recovery from critical illness.

Glucose can also be formed from lactate and from alanine.[68] The conversion of lactate to glucose occurs via the Cori cycle in the liver.

Lactate is formed from pyruvate, which is the end product of glycolysis. In critically ill patients with adequate oxygen delivery, the wound is a major source of lactate. Adenosine triphosphate (ATP) is formed during glycolysis and provides energy for the wound, but ATP is required to convert lactate back to glucose. The increased mass flow of glucose serves as a fuel for the healing wound. It may also reflect an inefficient biochemical cycle that requires energy but in which there is no net gain or loss of substrate. Accelerated glucose cycling has been documented both in burn patients and in blunt trauma patients.[69,70] The purpose of these so-called futile cycles is not clear. Because they result in the net generation of heat, they presumably contribute to hypermetabolism. That overall conversion requires net input of ATP and is thus another energy drain for the patient.

GLUCOSE INTOLERANCE AND INSULIN RESISTANCE

When glucose is administered to critically ill patients, hyperglycemia is often the result. Glucose tolerance tests typically yield abnormal results after injury.[71] During shock, immediately after injury or operation, and in the course of ebb-phase responses, the insulin response to hyperglycemia may be blunted. During the flow phase, however, after resuscitation and stabilization, the insulin response to glucose is normal or even exaggerated.[72,73] Both glucose and insulin levels are greater in trauma patients than in control subjects [see Table 5], and the increase in the insulin level is proportionally greater than the rise in glucose.

Black and associates maintained a fixed level of hyperglycemia in patients recovering from trauma by adjusting a glucose infusion on the basis of bedside glucose readings and a negative-feedback algorithm.[74] Because the glucose concentration was at steady state, the glucose infusion rate reflected the rate of total body glucose uptake or disposal. Control subjects demonstrated continuously increasing glucose disposal over time; the glucose infusion rate was increased repeatedly to maintain fixed hyperglycemia. Glucose disposal was closely related to insulin concentration, which increased steadily during the 2-hour study. In contrast, glucose disposal in trauma patients was markedly lower than in control subjects, and it did not increase appreciably over time. The insulin concentrations did, however, increase throughout the study and were always greater than corresponding control values. The trauma patients were therefore less responsive (i.e., were resistant) to insulin.

These investigators also infused insulin into trauma patients and control subjects to maintain specific fixed levels of hyperinsulinemia. During these infusions, the glucose concentration was maintained at basal values (i.e., euglycemia). The glucose infusion rate again reflected total body glucose disposal, which was a function of tissue responsiveness to the insulin level. At all insulin levels, glucose disposal was lower in trauma patients than in control subjects. These studies quantitated posttraumatic insulin resistance and suggested that this response was caused by a postreceptor defect. In similar conditions, Brooks and associates demonstrated reduced forearm glucose uptake, indicating that peripheral tissue—principally skeletal muscle—was a major site of insulin resistance[75] [see Table 6].

Table 5   Basal Glucose and Insulin Concentrations*

	N	Plasma Glucose (mg/dl)	Serum Insulin (μU/ml)
Normal subjects	49	98 ± 1	12 ± 1
Trauma patients	19	104 ± 2	17 ± 2
P		< 0.02	< 0.01

*Mean ± SEM.

ALTERED FUEL METABOLISM

The studies by Black and associates[74] demonstrated that in recovering trauma patients, there is an upper limit to glucose disposal of 5 to 6 mg/kg/min, despite hyperglycemia and hyperinsulinemia. Additional studies have confirmed that critically ill patients are limited in their ability to utilize glucose as a fuel. Long and coworkers studied the effect of increasing carbohydrate intake on net nitrogen loss in recovering burn patients.[76] They found that nitrogen loss was reduced as carbohydrate was increased to 60% to 70% of total caloric needs (also approximately 5 to 6 mg/kg/min). Very little additional reduction in nitrogen loss was observed with higher carbohydrate levels. Wolfe and associates used isotope-labeled glucose to measure glucose oxidation in postoperative[77] and burn patients[66,78] and found that both groups exhibited an upper limit of glucose oxidation. These studies also suggested that maximum glucose oxidation is inversely related to injury severity.

Lipid metabolism is also affected by critical illness. In an elegant series of kinetic studies performed in blunt trauma patients, Shaw and Wolfe[70] documented a greater than twofold increase in glycerol turnover, reflecting an accelerated rate of triglyceride hydrolysis to form free fatty acid (FFA) and glycerol. They also demonstrated a doubling of FFA oxidation rate; however, the measured turnover of FFA was only 30% greater than the control value, which suggested that some of the FFA released from triglyceride was oxidized in the cell and did not enter the circulating pool. These studies further demonstrated a high rate of FFA recycling, a phenomenon also described in burn patients.[69]

Askanazi and associates studied the metabolic effects of hypercaloric, glucose-based total parenteral nutrition (TPN) on starved patients.[79] Patients who were nutritionally depleted but were not critically ill showed an increase in $\dot{V}CO_2$ and an increase in the respiratory quotient (RQ, the ratio of $\dot{V}CO_2$ to $\dot{V}O_2$) to 1.0 or greater. These findings indicated that these patients were able to meet all of their energy needs with glucose and that fat oxidation was suppressed. Patients who were depleted and also manifested hypermetabolic responses showed an increase not only in $\dot{V}CO_2$ but also in $\dot{V}O_2$, and the RQ remained below 1.0; therefore, these critically ill patients could not meet all of their energy needs by oxidation of glucose. Not only was there a limit to the ability of these critically ill patients to use glucose as a metabolic fuel, but the high glucose load intensified hypermetabolism as well. Thus, overfeeding with glucose can aggravate critical illness. The mechanisms of this phenomenon are not clear, but they may involve the futile cycling of glucose via fructose 1,6-diphosphate and its associated heat generation.[69]

In addition to protein, nutritional support of critically ill patients often consists of a mixture of carbohydrate and fat to meet energy requirements. In such a system, exogenous carbohydrate is oxidized directly, but exogenous lipid is added to body fat stores.[80] Lipid is mobilized from these endogenous stores for oxidation. Such a mixed-fuel preparation should provide sufficient glucose for those tissues that require it (i.e., central nervous system, renal medulla, hematopoietic cells, and inflammatory cells), prevent excessive hyperglycemia, stimulate insulin elaboration, and approach nitrogen equilibrium.

Systemic Mediators

It was once generally thought that the metabolic alterations associated with injury and critical illness were derived from some harmful substance (e.g., a toxin) or dysfunctional process (e.g., a deranged endocrine mechanism). We now appreciate that the regulatory mechanisms affecting these processes are intricate and highly complex and depend on the actions of a myriad of mediators that influence the proliferation, development, and behavior of cells. It is hard to judge which, if any, of these mediators is maladaptive or harmful: those that seem to have harmful effects that exacerbate debility and organ dysfunction in some settings often promote healing and recovery in others.

These mediators may be synthesized by one or many cell types. Some mediators may affect the cell that made them, thus exerting an autocrine effect. Others may affect cells in close proximity, thus exerting a paracrine effect. If they gain access to the ECF, they can be transported via the circulation and affect cells far removed from their site of origin, thus exerting an endocrine effect. Most interact with a specific receptor, usually on the surface of the target cell. This molecular interaction can influence the cell's biology in a number of ways. First, it may alter the cell membrane, affecting its permeability to certain substances or changing the availability or affinity of other receptors for interaction with their specific mediators. Second, it may alter the structural organization of the cell, making certain intracellular constituents more or less available to exert their effects on cell behavior. Finally, it may initiate one of several intracellular molecular mechanisms that ultimately affect the nucleus, thereby altering gene expression for protein synthesis or DNA replication and cell proliferation.

These mediators have been categorized as endocrine hormones, inflammatory mediators, and growth factors. But as our knowledge about them has grown, it has become apparent that the distinctions are not always clear-cut, and some mediators can fit in more than one category. For example, the hormone insulin exerts definite endocrine metabolic effects, but it is also an important growth factor. Insulin receptors have been identified in embryos and in plants, and insulin is an important constituent of many cell culture media.[81]

The metabolic response to critical illness is a clinical phenomenon that dominates the clinical presentation and course of critically ill patients. It involves alterations that affect either the whole body or specific organ systems. In what follows, I discuss several ways in which these clinical events may be regulated.

HORMONES

During critical illness, the concentrations of several hormones are altered. The levels of the counterregulatory or so-called stress hor-

Table 6 Glucose Disposal and Forearm Glucose Uptake during Hyperinsulinemia and Euglycemia

Target Dose	N	Plasma Glucose Concentration (mg/dl)	Serum Insulin Concentration (μU/ml)	Glucose Disposal Rate (mg/kg/min)	Arterial–Deep Venous Glucose Difference (mg/dl)	Forearm Glucose Uptake (mg/dl/min)
Normal subjects						
100 μU/ml	7	92 ± 2	106 ± 6	9.32 ± 1.04	21 ± 3	0.76 ± 0.12
200 μU/ml	6	92 ± 2	183 ± 19	8.91 ± 0.78	26 ± 4	1.10 ± 0.11
Injured patients						
200 μU/ml	4	97 ± 1	145 ± 11	5.29 ± 0.80	8 ± 4	0.36 ± 18
500 μU/ml	1	117	506	5.79	2	0.20

mones—cortisol, glucagon, and the catecholamines epinephrine and norepinephrine—are typically increased. These hormones have several direct and indirect effects and appear to function as important regulating signals in the response to critical illness.

The sympathetic-adrenal axis is one of the major systems by which the body initiates responses to critical illness. It also modifies the elaboration and effects of other hormones and thus serves as a link between the central nervous system and the endocrinologic organs. Many of the changes in vital signs observed during critical illness, such as tachycardia, tachypnea, and widened pulse pressure, are ascribed to adrenergic and catecholamine effects; in addition, many of the signs of shock indicate autonomic overactivity. The catecholamine levels are increased in proportion to the severity of injury.[82] During the flow phase of critical illness, concentrations of the catecholamines may be persistently elevated; catecholamine turnover after burn injury is markedly increased.[44,83] $\dot{V}O_2$ and metabolic rate have been directly related to the excretion of catecholamines. In one study, alpha- and beta-adrenergic blockade significantly reduced the metabolic rate in burn patients, although the rate did not return to control levels.[19] This effect was not produced by alpha-adrenergic blockade alone, which indicates that beta-adrenergic stimulation predominates in the flow phase of the response to critical illness.

The sympathetic-adrenal axis also affects the endocrine pancreas. Porte and Robertson determined that the insulin response to glucose in normal individuals was reduced substantially with alpha-adrenergic stimulation but was enhanced with beta-adrenergic stimulation.[84] Catecholamines may also modulate the peripheral action of insulin. When epinephrine was infused into normal individuals at doses low enough to allow beta-adrenergic effects to predominate, insulin resistance was observed in uninjured forearm tissue.[85] Despite its apparent catabolic effects on metabolic rate and insulin resistance, epinephrine alone reduces the release of amino acid from skeletal muscle in vitro.[86]

Cortisol[87] and glucagon[88] levels are elevated after major injury and during critical illness. The degree of elevation appears to be related to the extent or severity of the injury. An increased cortisol level is associated with glucose intolerance.[89] Patients with Cushing's syndrome manifest reduced muscle mass and loss of protein from the skin. Owen and Cahill administered hydrocortisone to starved obese patients.[90] Although they observed an increase in ammonia excretion and a decrease in urea excretion, there was no net change in total nitrogen loss. Glucagon promotes gluconeogenesis.[91] This effect may be overcome by increased concentrations of insulin.[92] Wolfe and colleagues administered glucagon to fasting normal individuals and observed a slight increase in nitrogen excretion, primarily as urea.[93] However, net nitrogen loss from peripheral tissues did not increase.

Although injury and critical illness clearly affect hormone levels, it has not been possible to ascribe all of the physiologic responses observed in patients to the known actions of individual hormones. A number of studies, however, have identified interacting effects by altering more than one hormone level simultaneously. For example, when Shamoon and coworkers infused a combination of hydrocortisone, glucagon, and epinephrine, they observed a synergistic effect on glucose production.[94]

Bessey and associates extended these observations.[95] In an attempt to simulate the endocrine environment of injured patients, they infused the same combination of hormones for 3 days in normal individuals. The infusion maintained elevated catabolic hormone levels, similar to those observed in patients with mild to moderate injury. The investigators monitored a variety of metabolic parameters and compared these results with measurements obtained in a control study of the same individuals, in which the patients received an infusion of saline. The alteration in the hormonal environment increased the resting heart and respiratory rates, widened the pulse pressure, and slightly elevated the rectal temperature. In addition, hypermetabolism, a negative potassium balance, increased endogenous glucose production, insulin resistance, sodium retention, and leukocytosis were observed [see Table 7]. During the control study, the individuals maintained nitrogen equilibrium, but during the triple-hormone infusion, they were in persistently negative nitrogen balance, even though nutritional intake was identical in the two studies. Whole body protein turnover, as measured by ^{15}N kinetics, was increased in the subjects who received the hormone infusion because of an increase in protein catabolism. These changes, which are typically seen in critically ill patients, occurred in the absence of a wound or inflammatory focus.

The negative nitrogen balance and increased turnover of whole body protein observed during the triple-hormone infusion were also associated with a significant decrease in total intracellular amino acid nitrogen in skeletal muscle.[96] This decrease was caused primarily by a fall in the intracellular glutamine level. Although these changes suggest that the posttraumatic hormonal environment plays a causative role in increasing net muscle proteolysis, the triple-hormone infusion did not appreciably alter either whole blood amino acid concentrations or amino acid efflux from the forearm. A potential explanation for these findings is that the triple-hormone infusion, particularly the glucagon component, may have affected processing of amino acid by the liver, thereby reducing the net retention of dietary amino acids.[97]

The endocrine environment in critically ill patients, however, is not static. Although catabolic hormone levels may be persistently elevated, insulin is often suppressed during the early phases of critical illness but elevated later, during the flow phase. Bessey and Lowe attempted to simulate this changing hormonal environment in normal subjects by administering a somatostatin analogue during the first 24 hours of a 3-day infusion of catabolic hormones so as to inhibit the elaboration of insulin in response to hyperglycemia.[98] They compared the findings to those obtained from studies of the same individuals during triple-hormone infusion, when insulin levels were allowed to rise unchecked. Early whole body nitrogen loss was increased in the studies with the somatostatin analogue, but there was no difference in forearm nitrogen release at 24 hours; however, 2 days later, when glucose and insulin concentrations were similar in the two studies, total body nitrogen loss was equivalent, but forearm nitrogen release was increased in the patients receiving the somatostatin analogue. Coadministration of exogenous insulin with somatostatin prevented this acceleration of net muscle protein breakdown (P. Q. Bessey, K. A.

Table 7 Effect of Infusion of Cortisol, Glucagon, and Epinephrine on Metabolism

	Saline	Hormones*
Metabolic rate (kcal/m²/hr)	32.24 ± 1.05	38.42 ± 1.31
Nitrogen balance (g/day)	−0.2 ± 0.4	−3.2 ± 0.4
Protein catabolic rate (g nitrogen/day)	38.4 ± 1.9	46.5 ± 2.5
Plasma glucose (mg/dl)	94 ± 2	133 ± 4
Serum insulin (μU/ml)	8 ± 1	22 ± 3
Glucose production rate (mg/kg/min)	2.08 ± 0.06	2.55 ± 0.06
Insulin-mediated glucose disposal (mg/kg/min)	8.62 ± 0.51	3.22 ± 0.51
Insulin-mediated forearm glucose uptake (mg/dl/min)	1.03 ± 0.09	0.48 ± 0.12

*All significantly different from control values.

Lowe, D. C. Blake; unpublished data). Thus, the interacting effects of multiple hormones and the changing relationships among them over time appear to be capable of inducing, at least qualitatively, most of the metabolic responses to critical illness.

Several investigators have attempted to modulate the catabolic responses of critical illness by altering the endocrine environment. For example, Hulton and colleagues monitored hind-leg amino acid efflux after abdominal operation in an animal model.[99] The accelerated efflux of skeletal muscle amino acids observed postoperatively was attenuated by complete alpha- and beta-adrenergic blockade or by thoracic epidural anesthesia. Both pharmacologic techniques are known to attenuate the hormonal response to operative stress. Brandt and coworkers measured hormonal and protein catabolic responses after abdominal hysterectomy.[100] In the patients who underwent epidural anesthesia, concentrations of cortisol and catecholamines were lower and nitrogen loss was less than in patients who received general anesthesia alone. Tsuji and associates reported similar findings.[101] Subsequent studies have shown that perioperative management of patients with high thoracic epidural analgesia and intravenous somatostatin and etomidate to inhibit elaboration of glucagon and cortisol prevents the typical postoperative increases in amino acid clearance and urea synthesis.[102]

In summary, the altered endocrine environment characteristically associated with critical illness appears to play a major role in mediating the metabolic responses observed in critically ill surgical patients. Simple alteration of the hormonal environment in healthy individuals is capable of inducing many of these metabolic changes; however, the magnitude of these changes is generally less than that observed in critically ill patients. Blunting of the hormonal changes after operation or injury can modulate the catabolic responses.

CYTOKINES

A number of cell types appear in a healing wound soon after injury.[103] These cells are actively involved in angiogenesis, production and remodeling of collagen, scavenging of necrotic debris, and engulfment and killing of bacteria. Many of them release substances that influence cellular proliferation, development, and function and so regulate local inflammation and wound healing. These substances, collectively known as cytokines, can be produced by and interact with a wide variety of cells in addition to inflammatory cells and appear to be major mediators of multiple cellular responses to injury and infection [see VII:11 Molecular and Cellular Mediators of the Inflammatory Response].

Certain of the cytokines primarily stimulate inflammatory responses; these are known as proinflammatory cytokines. There are also anti-inflammatory cytokines, which retard inflammatory processes. In addition, specific receptor antagonists have been identified that interfere with the interaction between a cytokine and its cellular receptor. Finally, there are specific soluble receptors, unassociated with a cell, that can effectively neutralize the cytokine before it interacts with a target cell. Both proinflammatory and anti-inflammatory mechanisms may be stimulated together in acute illness.[104] The balance and interactions between them determine the course of the inflammatory process.

The major proinflammatory cytokines, tumor necrosis factor (TNF), interleukin-1 (IL-1), and IL-6, are closely related in that they are elaborated in a characteristic pattern (or cascade) in response to an inflammatory stimulus, such as trauma[105] or endotoxin.[106] TNF appears first, followed by IL-1 and then IL-6. The elaboration of TNF and IL-1 is relatively brief, but IL-6 persists longer.

Cytokines appear to play a dominant role in regulating cell recruitment, proliferation, development, and other cellular events that occur in the wound, but how and to what extent they exert systemic effects and modulate the metabolic responses to critical illness is less clear. One conceptual model proposes that when local cytokine production is particularly abundant, owing to extensive wounds or uncontrolled infection, certain cytokines spill over into the circulation and then affect tissues at distant sites [see Figure 5]. Although elevated circulating cytokine levels have been detected in critically ill patients, only IL-6 has been consistently associated with severe illness and outcome.[107,108]

Several investigations have sought to determine the metabolic effect of the proinflammatory cytokines. TNF can initiate the cytokine cascade, ultimately producing fever, leukocytosis, and other signs and symptoms of critical illness.[109] To characterize the role of TNF in proteolysis associated with endotoxin or sepsis, Michie and coworkers analyzed the responses of both animals and humans during prolonged infusions of TNF.[110] Negative nitrogen balance was related to the onset of anorexia and reduced food intake and not to the development of hypermetabolism. Mealy and associates performed adrenalectomies and abrogated the increase in nitrogen loss associated with TNF infusion.[111] Hall-Angeras and colleagues found that a steroid antagonist prevented the increase in myofibrillar protein breakdown usually seen in an animal model of intra-abdominal sepsis.[112] These observations suggest that even though TNF may be a major initiating signal for a variety of cellular events in critical illness, other mediators are required for the full development of the metabolic responses to injury and infection.

IL-1 was one of the first fever-producing cytokines, or pyrogens, to be identified.[113,114] Early in vitro studies appeared to present conflicting findings,[115-117] but the preponderance of the data currently available indicate that IL-1 can increase proteolysis, especially in intact animals. For example, Zamir and colleagues measured increased muscle protein breakdown in vitro after administration of IL-1 to intact animals.[118] In another study, they were able to reduce but not prevent the increased proteolysis that followed endotoxin administration by pretreating animals with IL-1 receptor antagonist (IL-1ra).[119]

To characterize the metabolic effects of IL-1 in vivo, Watters and associates gave daily intramuscular injections of etiocholanolone to normal individuals.[120] (This steroid stimulates the development of an inflammatory focus and the production of IL-1.) The subjects manifested an acute-phase response: fever, leukocytosis, increased concentrations of acute-phase proteins, and hypoferremia. They were not hypermetabolic, however, and they remained in nitrogen equilibrium when fed a standard diet. The concentrations of catabolic hormones were not affected by this treatment. When hydrocortisone, glucagon, and epinephrine were administered in conjunction with etiocholanolone, however, both inflammatory and metabolic responses were observed.[121] These healthy subjects exhibited the same clinical features as did patients with infection. These findings suggested that both endocrine and cytokine mechanisms influence the responses to critical illness.

IL-6 can induce many of the components of the acute-phase response[122] and may be measured in the blood of patients experiencing trauma,[123] sepsis,[124] pancreatitis,[125] or other critical illnesses (e.g., myocardial infarction).[126] Mateo and associates identified IL-6 in wound fluid from both animals and humans, and they found that the capacity of wound macrophages to produce IL-6 increased with time.[127] Thus, IL-6 might be one mechanism by which the wound influences critical illness. Persistent measurable levels of IL-6 have been related to mortality in both trauma[107] and burn[108] patients.

Stouthard and associates infused recombinant IL-6 (rIL-6) into uninjured cancer patients for 4 hours, then measured glucose and lipid kinetics, metabolic rate, and hormonal profiles during the infusion and during a saline control infusion.[128] IL-6–induced hypermetabolism and energy expenditure increased by 25%. Glucose production, lipolysis, and fatty acid oxidation also increased. Glucose clearance was also increased; serum glucose concentrations were not significantly affected by IL-6 infusion. Tsigos and colleagues administered increasing doses of IL-6 subcutaneously to healthy subjects and demonstrated a dose-response relationship between IL-6 dose and circulating level and glucose concentration.[129] In both of these studies, IL-6 also induced elevations in circulating stress hormone levels.

IL-6 also affects protein metabolism. Transgenic mice that overexpress IL-6 exhibit retarded growth and muscle atrophy. These observations have been correlated with reduced circulating concentrations of insulinlike growth factor–1 (IGF-1).[130] In another report, a specific IL-6 receptor antibody administered to the young IL-6 transgenic mice restored muscle growth to normal.[131] The muscle atrophy in these studies was associated with an increase in the synthesis and activity of several enzymes that catalyze muscle protein breakdown, and these changes too were blocked by IL-6 receptor antibody. The effects of IL-6 on long-term protein accretion in humans have not yet been elucidated, but severely burned children who survive after a long period of critical illness often experience growth retardation.[132]

Both endocrine and inflammatory mediators affect metabolic responses in critically ill patients. In fact, the two systems are closely linked—perhaps inseparably—and probably influence each other.[121] For example, Bornstein and colleagues identified IL-6 messenger RNA (mRNA) expression in the steroid-producing cells of the adrenal gland, which were located not only in the cortex but also in the medulla, adjacent to catecholamine-producing cells.[133] In a subsequent study, they detected IL-6 and IL-6 receptor expression in adrenal cell cultures, both with macrophages present and with macrophages absent.[134] They also found that IL-6 stimulated release of steroid hormones, aldosterone, cortisol, and androgens in vitro in a dose-dependent manner; however, these effects developed over a period of 24 hours. These findings indicate not only that IL-6 exerts autocrine and paracrine effects on adrenal cellular synthetic function but also that it is probably involved in the long-term regulation of adrenal steroidogenesis rather than being responsible for acute changes in adrenal function.

On the other hand, glucocorticoids have long been known to exert anti-inflammatory effects. They interfere with the proliferation and function of leukocytes and other immune cells, and they inhibit the synthesis and cellular action of cytokines and other molecules important for cellular responses.[135] In a clinical study, Barber and colleagues demonstrated that glucocorticoid administration led to a dose- and time-dependent reduction in TNF production and symptoms in response to endotoxin.[136]

Cytokines and hormones may also affect metabolic responses at the end-organ level via different mechanisms. For example, skeletal muscle protein breakdown can occur via any of at least four intracellular proteolytic systems.[137] One of the major pathways affecting myofibrillar proteins is energy dependent (i.e., ATP-dependent) and involves the cytosolic peptide cofactor ubiquitin. In animals, glucocorticoids stimulate an ATP-dependent proteolytic system and increase the expression of ubiquitin.[138] Zamir and colleagues administered a glucocorticoid antagonist to rats with intraperitoneal sepsis and demonstrated that it reduced but did not eliminate the increased muscle proteolysis.[118] In a subsequent study, they induced accelerated skeletal muscle proteolysis by injecting IL-1 intraperitoneally.[119] Previous adrenalectomy, which eliminated glucocorticoid elaboration, had little effect on the proteolysis observed.[139] These observations suggest that both glucocorticoid-dependent and glucocorticoid-independent proteolytic mechanisms can be activated during critical illness.

Role of the Central Nervous System

The CNS plays a major role in the regulation of the metabolic response to critical illness. Hume and Egdahl were among the first to demonstrate its role in mediating early responses to injury.[140] They measured the rise in 17-hydroxycorticosteroids in adrenal venous

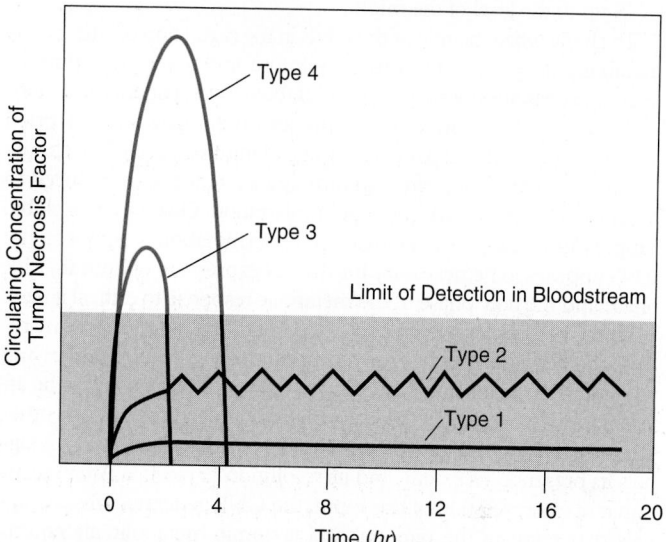

Figure 5 Different infectious states are likely to be associated with different patterns of cytokine release into the circulation.[232] Type 1 in this figure could be considered to represent localized cellulitis, such as might be present at an infected intravenous catheter infusion site. Generation of tumor necrosis factor (TNF) and other cytokines occurs locally to produce local responses that aid host defense and tissue repair. Overspill into the circulation is minimal.

The second type might represent the responses ensuing from appendiceal abscess. There is local generation of cytokines, and as bacteria or their endotoxins leak into the circulation, circulating mononuclear cells also elaborate cytokines and give rise to moderate systemic responses. The low level of persistent endotoxemia is reflected in the cytokine response. Because only a small number of cytokine-producing cells are stimulated at any one time, the responses of these cells, although of long duration, are not strong enough to be detectable in the bloodstream. However, this signal is sufficient to generate systemic manifestations of the localized infection.

A third type of infection might be one that follows manipulation of a catheter in the biliary tree or urinary bladder to resolve an obstruction. A few cytokine-producing cells simultaneously elaborate TNF to produce a high-amplitude signal. Because the endotoxemia is transient, both the signal and the host responses are short-lived. Clinical features include a brief episode of hyperpyrexia with rigors and severe symptoms, but the cytokine response is too short and of insufficient amplitude to give rise to life-threatening, irreversible host alterations.

A fourth type of infection might be precipitated by sudden dehiscence of a colonic anastomosis or by meningococcal septicemia. An acute, massive entry of endotoxins into the circulation stimulates virtually every cytokine-producing cell in the body. A very high amplitude signal occurs, but its duration is short, despite the host's continuing exposure to endotoxin. The short duration of the strong signal is caused by the quick disappearance of cytokines from the circulation; their half-life is short, and the cytokine-producing cells become refractory after their simultaneous explosive response to the initial, lethal signal. This high-amplitude signal is misinterpreted by the host, causing the entire body to behave as if it were a massive wound. The entire vascular tree shows increased permeability and vasodilatation, resulting in the clinical state of irreversible shock. These situations have been reversed or prevented by the use of TNF antibodies in animals and occasionally by the use of plasmapheresis in humans.

blood in response to a burn to the lower limb of an animal under anesthesia. The limb was almost completely separated from the body, so that the only connections between the limb and the rest of the animal were the femoral vessels and the sciatic nerve. The prompt rise in the venous adrenocorticoid concentration after the burn could be prevented by sectioning of the sciatic nerve or of any portion of the CNS up to the level of the midbrain.

To characterize the role of the CNS in the regulation of later hypermetabolic flow-phase responses, Wilmore and associates administered inert gas anesthesia to hypermetabolic burn patients and demonstrated reduced core temperature and metabolic rates.[141] Fried and coworkers studied patients with head injuries during barbiturate coma.[142,143] Metabolic rate and nitrogen excretion were reduced to basal values during barbiturate administration. Given that its global suppression reduces the intensity of hypermetabolic responses, the CNS appears to be necessary for the full expression of both the ebb phase and the flow phase of the metabolic response to critical illness.

The CNS has long been considered part of a neuroendocrine reflex arc,[144] a view that has proved useful for explicating underlying regulatory mechanisms. According to this concept, there must be afferent input whereby (1) the body is alerted to an injury or any other threat to its integrity and (2) the wound or inflammatory focus signals its presence, its extent, and its resolution or closure. After reception and interpretation of this input, the CNS generates efferent signals that regulate the regional and systemic metabolic alterations observed clinically. This model is most obviously relevant to the early phase of the response to critical illness (the ebb phase). The hypothalamus, the peripheral and spinal neural pathways, and the adrenals all participate in the classic fright-fight-flight syndrome. Pain, hypovolemia, acidosis, and hypoxia stimulate neural afferent signals to the CNS. The importance of these neural pathways in transmitting afferent signals to the CNS during hypermetabolism is less clear. For example, when lidocaine was applied to burn wounds to anesthetize them, no decrease in hypermetabolism was observed.[145]

Recent investigations have begun to elucidate the role the CNS may play in a variety of immunologic and inflammatory responses.[146] Early studies demonstrated that a small amount of IL-1 injected intrathecally elicited the same increase in body temperature as a much larger dose administered intravenously. This suggested that IL-1 could act centrally and that it might function as an afferent signal from the wound to the CNS.[147] Demonstration of IL-1 immunoreactivity in the hypothalamus of humans lent weight to this suggestion.[148] Later studies, however, showed that astrocytes and microglia could express cytokines and cytokine receptors themselves.[149,150] In addition, these cells increased expression of IL-1 and IL-6 in vitro in response to hypoxia or endotoxin in vitro,[151,152] and systemic administration of endotoxin to intact animals increased cytokine expression in the CNS.[153,154]

Hill and colleagues used an animal model to assess the metabolic effects of IL-1 continuously infused either subcutaneously or into the lateral ventricle for 6 days.[155] Subcutaneous IL-1 was given in different doses, which induced fever, anorexia, increased protein catabolism, and weight loss in a dose-dependent manner. Intracerebroventricular (ICV) IL-1 evoked qualitatively similar responses. Subcutaneous IL-1, however, resulted in a greater leukocytosis and a more pronounced acute-phase response than did ICV IL-1, even though the other systemic alterations were quantitatively similar. Thus, IL-1 produced in the CNS may not have the same physiologic consequences as IL-1 produced in other anatomic sites.

In another study, Hill and colleagues pair-fed control animals with animals receiving ICV IL-1.[156] They observed that the pair-fed animals also lost weight, but the weight loss was significantly less severe than in the animals receiving ICV IL-1. Long-term ICV IL-1 infu-

sion also caused increased adrenal gland weight and corticosteroid levels in comparison with values in both pair-fed and chow-fed controls. The ICV IL-1–induced catabolic changes were not, however, attenuated by previous adrenalectomy. This finding indicates that the protein-catabolic effects induced by ICV IL-1 may involve not only glucocorticoid-dependent ATP-ubiquitin proteolysis but also systems that are independent of glucocorticoids. Such a conclusion is consistent with the finding by Zamir and associates that intraperitoneal IL-1 increased total and myofibrillar proteolysis in both adrenalectomized animals and sham controls.[139] Thus, the CNS may be able to influence metabolic responses via both endocrine pathways and other mechanisms that do not involve endocrine activation.

Elaboration of IL-6 typically follows elaboration of IL-1, and IL-6 is a potent activator of corticosteroid synthesis and release.[106,157] Long-term IL-1 infusion leads to increased muscle protein breakdown and nitrogen loss over and above what is attributable to reduced food intake, and it results in elevated circulating levels of IL-6.[158] When Hill and associates infused IL-6 into the CSF of rats, it had no effect, unlike ICV IL-1.[156] Reyes and Coe followed the appearance of IL-6 in CSF in primates after intravenous injection of IL-1α, IL-1β, and IL-6.[159] All three cytokines raised the circulating levels of IL-6, IL-1ra, and cortisol, but only IL-1β raised the CSF level of IL-6. Furthermore, IL-6 appeared in CSF from the lumbar region 2 hours after it peaked in CSF from the cervical region. These data suggest that the IL-6 in the CSF after the appearance of IL-1 in the periphery is elaborated by the brain.

Romero and colleagues gave an ICV injection of IL-1β to rats and measured IL-6 concentrations in CSF and in blood from the superior sagittal sinus and the aorta.[160] IL-6 was elevated in all three compartments, and the concentration gradient between the sagittal sinus and the aorta was widened in comparison with the control value. Both adrenergic pathways and adrenal activation are known to be stimulated by IL-1 administration; but the changes observed were not affected by sympathetic blockade, and ICV corticotropin-releasing hormone did not result in alterations in IL-6 levels in CSF or in blood. The investigators concluded that the IL-6 that appeared in both the CSF and the blood was derived from the brain.

Recent neurophysiologic research is also providing insights into the effects of injury and inflammation on nerve function. Numerous compounds elaborated by platelets, neutrophils, and other inflammatory cells can alter the phenotype of neurons, affecting their growth, function, and electrical properties[161]; IL-6 is one of these. The complex of IL-6 and its receptor can activate specific neuronal signal transduction systems on sensory neurons and so affect gene expression and protein synthesis.[162] Sensory nerve injury induces the expression of IL-6 and IL-6 receptor in more central neurons, and this seems to promote nerve repair.[163] Niijima gave varying doses of IL-1β to rats by portal vein injection.[164] He observed a dose-dependent increase in the afferent activity of the haptic branch of the vagus nerve. He also detected efferent signals in autonomic nerves to the spleen and thymus after intraportal administration of IL-1. Because these signals were eliminated by vagotomy, they appeared to be the result of reflex activation. These findings suggest that there are sensors in the hepatoportal system that can detect IL-1 and other inflammatory mediators and generate neural afferent activity, stimulating the brain to generate signals that affect host defense and other responses.

Thus, the CNS is intimately involved in the regulation of the metabolic response to critical illness. Not only pain, acidosis, hypoxia, and hypovolemia but also cytokines and other substances produced by inflammatory cells may generate afferent signals to the CNS through a variety of mechanisms. Some signals may elicit a rapid effector response, whereas others appear to induce mechanisms that result in delayed and more prolonged end-organ functional alterations. The CNS affects both metabolic and inflammatory processes, and it may do so in multiple complementary but largely independent ways. Activation of the hypothalamic-pituitary-adrenal axis is one of these mechanisms, but the CNS also appears to be able to induce catabolic responses without this intervention. The CNS may even be a source of mediators that are released into the circulation for systemic distribution, thus acting as an endocrine organ.

An early theory of how cytokines produced in wounds or other sites of inflammation might affect metabolic responses was that they spilled over into the circulation to be transported to other organs, including the brain, where they constituted an afferent signal. Some of the data now available suggest that there may also be much more direct lines of communication between a wound and the CNS, so that cytokines and other substances in the wound environment might stimulate specific neural afferent activity that could then elicit highly specific effector signals and end-organ responses. By this view, the CNS may support multiple streams of information and thus regulate physiologic processes in several coordinated and comprehensive ways. We have long tended to think of the nervous system as little more than a number of telegraph lines and a central switching station; however, a better metaphor might be a fiberoptic cable network, which is capable of transmitting television programming, computer data, and telephone and fax transmissions to and from multiple users simultaneously.

Role of the Gut

Although the idea that endotoxin absorbed from the gut lumen during shock states might result in irreversible critical illness was first proposed nearly 40 years ago,[165,166] most clinicians continued to think that the gut was inert after operation and injury until relatively recently. Now, however, it is generally recognized that the gut plays an important role in augmenting or perpetuating the response to critical illness.[167]

Gram-negative pathogens are the predominant infectious organisms in the ICU, and the gut appears to be a major source of contamination. The gut lumen forms a large reservoir for gram-negative enteric bacteria, but the normal GI mucosa protects the host from intraluminal bacteria and their toxins. The maintenance of tight intracellular junctions between epithelial cells prevents the transepithelial migration of bacteria.[168] The GI tract is also richly supplied with macrophages and fixed immune cells. The elaboration of surface immunoglobulins (e.g., IgA) aids in the recognition of foreign antigens.[169] Finally, the liver and the spleen serve as backup systems for trapping bacteria and neutralizing absorbed toxins. The combination of an intact gut mucosa and a normally functioning immune system provides maximal barrier function. Even in immunosuppressed states, the mucosa can still maintain an effective barrier to infection. This suggests that cell-mediated immunity is secondary in importance to an intact intestinal epithelial lining.

When the barrier function of the GI epithelium is impaired, intraluminal bacteria and toxins can invade the host. In one set of experiments in rabbits, fatal endotoxic shock was observed after temporary occlusion of the superior mesenteric artery or a 30% scald burn[170]; however, if the enteric flora was reduced, the animals did not die. Endotoxemia has been observed in patients with a variety of critical illnesses.[166] Wellmann and associates reported that whole gut lavage with saline reduced the concentration of circulating endotoxin and improved the clinical outcome in a large group of patients with inflammatory bowel disease that was unresponsive to medical therapy.[171] Moreover, bacteremia in portal blood has been observed at the time of operation in as many as 30% of patients with noninflammato-

ry bowel disease.[172] Ambrose and associates cultured both intestinal serosa and mesenteric lymph nodes during abdominal operation.[173] In patients without inflammatory bowel disease, the incidence of positive cultures was low, but in patients with Crohn's disease, the incidence increased markedly, to approximately 30%.

Bacterial translocation is the migration of bacteria across the bowel wall to invade the host. In a review of the available animal and human data on this process, Berg identified three conditions that appear to promote translocation: altered permeability of the intestinal mucosa, decreased host defenses, and an increased number of bacteria within the intestinal lumen.[174] Deitch and colleagues observed this phenomenon in animals after a variety of insults, including burns,[175] hemorrhagic shock,[176] and endotoxin administration.[170] Malnutrition alone did not lead to translocation, but it made the gut barrier more susceptible to endotoxin.[177]

The extent of bacterial translocation in critically ill patients is not well defined. Moore and colleagues obtained both portal venous and systemic venous blood cultures in patients at risk for multiorgan failure after laparotomy for severe trauma.[178] Only 2% of cultures were positive in the first 5 days, which suggests that translocation of bacteria in sufficient quantities to cause portal vein bacteremia is not a major determinant of organ failure soon after injury.

More recent studies have focused on the gut as a source of cytokines. Even the normal gut contains a large number of intestinal lymphocytes that elaborate proinflammatory cytokines, and these are counteracted by expression of anti-inflammatory cytokines in a state of so-called controlled inflammation.[179] Guy-Grand and colleagues detected measurable levels of TNF, IL-6, and interferon gamma in proximal small bowel secretions in humans.[180] The presence of bacterial overgrowth, especially colonic-type bacteria, however, was associated with increased IL-6 concentrations. Wyble and associates investigated the cytokine response to intestinal ischemia-reperfusion in ex vivo perfused segments of human intestine.[181] Concentrations of TNF and IL-1 increased in the venous effluent after reperfusion. The investigators subsequently exposed cultured human endothelial cells to physiologic concentrations of TNF and IL-1 that were lower than those observed after ischemia-reperfusion. The cytokines up-regulated expression of E-selectin and intercellular adhesion molecule–1 (ICAM-1), which are thought to mediate the adhesion of neutrophils in the microcirculation and their transmigration across the capillary membrane into tissue, thus initiating tissue inflammation.

Mainous and colleagues produced sterile peritonitis with both a nonlethal and a median lethal dose (LD_{50}) of zymosan.[182] They detected increased IL-6 and TNF in both blood and lymph, but these changes did not correlate with zymosan dose or with bacterial translocation. Thus, the gut appears capable of producing cytokines in response to an inflammatory insult, and this may occur even in the absence of bacterial translocation.

Mochizuki and associates were among the first to demonstrate the importance of enteral feedings in maintaining gut mucosal integrity and modulating catabolic responses in critical illness.[183] They measured intestinal mucosal weight and several metabolic parameters in experimental animals after a standard burn injury. In one group of animals, feedings were delivered through a gastrostomy tube and were begun soon after the burn injury, whereas in a second group, feedings were oral and were begun after a 72-hour fast. Mucosal weight was preserved in the first group but reduced in the second group. In the animals that fasted, postburn hypermetabolism developed, but this response was attenuated in the ones that received early enteral feedings. Intravenous feeding did not preserve mucosal mass or modify postburn metabolic responses.[184] In an early clinical study, Alexander and colleagues documented improved survival in children with burns who were nourished enterally.[185] Furthermore, Border and associates found that the provision of enteral protein was one of only two factors statistically associated with improved survival in a large group of severely injured patients.[186]

Ogle and colleagues extended these observations by comparing intestinal and splenic cytokine expression in animals nourished by parenteral nutrition but allowed no oral intake with cytokine expression in control animals allowed food ad libitum.[187] After 7 days of infusion, mRNA expression for IL-1, IL-6, and TNF was increased in the intestine and decreased in the spleen. Lyoumi and associates also reported that protein malnutrition alone enhances intestinal IL-6 expression and acute-phase responses.[188] These findings suggest that augmented intestinal cytokine production is responsible, in part, for the earlier clinical observations that bowel rest or inadequate enteral protein amplifies the responses to critical illness and may adversely affect outcome.

The presence of food in the gut lumen is known to be a major stimulus for mucosal cell growth. Mucosal atrophy is observed in the absence of enteral nutrition (as occurs during starvation[189] or periods of parenteral nutrition[190]) and in defunctionalized intestinal segments.[191] Enteral feeding not only provides nutrients but also stimulates the elaboration of trophic hormones for the intestinal mucosa.[192,193] In addition to luminal bulk, specific nutrients (e.g., glutamine and butyrate) are important for the growth of gut mucosa. Glutamine is a major respiratory fuel for the gut, especially during critical illness (see above). Colonocytes also utilize butyrate, a short-chain fatty acid that is produced by bacterial fermentation of polysaccharides in the colonic lumen. In solution, glutamine decomposes into toxic substances; it is therefore not included in any commercially available parenteral amino acid solutions or in most enteral nutrition products. When glutamine was added to parenteral nutrition in place of other nonessential amino acids, however, increased mucosal cellularity was observed in the jejunum, ileum, and colon in an animal model.[194,195] In other studies, the toxic effects of methotrexate were alleviated and mucosal cellularity and nitrogen balance improved when parenteral solutions containing glutamine were used.[196]

If these study results correlate with any specific clinical situation, it might be that of a patient with abdominal and skeletal trauma in the ICU who is recovering from shock and is on bowel rest. Bowel rest frequently is associated with intraluminal bacterial overgrowth. This association, coupled with reperfusion of the gut during resuscitation and the presence of peritoneal inflammation, could contribute to increased intestinal production of proinflammatory cytokines. The gut may function, therefore, as an additional inflammatory focus and, in conjunction with the peripheral wounds, may act to stimulate systemic responses. The release of glutamine from muscle can support epithelial proliferation. If the initial injuries are limited, normal GI function soon returns, with the result that the intensity of the systemic inflammatory responses is reduced and the patient recovers. If, however, the insult is massive, if there is a prolonged period of reduced enteral nutrition, or if the supply of glutamine is insufficient to support mucosal cell growth, then recovery of mucosal integrity may be delayed, and the gut could continue to be an inflammatory focus, exacerbating and perpetuating the patient's catabolic responses.

Endotoxin, Bacteria, Inflammation, and Organ Failure

Endotoxin is a lipopolysaccharide component of bacterial cell walls that can reproduce the syndrome of sepsis and shock when given to animals or humans.[197] The presence of endotoxin is considered a major determinant of the clinical sequelae of bacterial infection. A low continuous dose of endotoxin in animals produces a hypermetabolic state that exhibits all of the features of the response to critical illness.[198]

Revhaug and associates administered *Escherichia coli* endotoxin to normal individuals under controlled conditions of activity and diet and compared the metabolic responses with those of subjects given only saline.[199] About 2 to 4 hours after administration of endotoxin, the subjects experienced headache, chills, malaise, nausea, fever, tachycardia, and an increased respiratory rate. In these and subsequent studies, endotoxin injection was also associated with leukocytosis, mild glucose intolerance, an increased metabolic rate, and elevated concentrations of adrenocorticotropic hormone, cortisol, catecholamines, and growth hormone.

Michie and colleagues found that the symptoms that followed a single dose of endotoxin in normal subjects were preceded by an abrupt and transient rise in circulating TNF concentration.[200] The symptoms developing after endotoxin injection were similar to those developing during TNF infusion, but they appeared 60 to 90 minutes after injection, in contrast with the appearance of symptoms 30 minutes after the start of TNF infusion.[109] In these studies, IL-1 was not detected, but Fong and associates detected both a peak rise in TNF and a later peak of IL-1 after administration of a lethal dose of bacteria in primates.[201] In those studies, death was prevented by an anti-TNF antibody. Thus, TNF is the first in a characteristic cascade of cytokines that mediate the physiologic responses to endotoxin.

Circulating endotoxin can be detected in patients who have experienced trauma[107] or burns[108] and even in those who have undergone cardiopulmonary bypass.[202] In healthy persons, repeated doses of endotoxin result in tolerance. In injured or critically ill patients, however, the responses to sustained or repeated doses of endotoxin have not been well characterized.

O'Dwyer and associates measured intestinal permeability in healthy human volunteers after a single dose of *E. coli* endotoxin or saline.[203] Lactulose and mannitol were administered orally as markers of intestinal permeability. (Lactulose is not absorbed to any significant extent under normal conditions.) After endotoxin administration, the urinary excretion of lactulose was increased almost twofold, which indicated that intestinal permeability was markedly altered. This change was closely associated with increases in norepinephrine and cortisol levels, which suggested that these hormonal changes or other systemic responses induced by endotoxin were responsible for the change in permeability. If alteration of the gut barrier led to increased absorption of endotoxin, that could be another mechanism by which the systemic responses to critical illness were amplified and perpetuated.

Patients with infectious disease (e.g., typhoid fever or malaria)[204,205] manifest many of the clinical features observed in critically ill surgical patients; however, these phenomena are less intense in patients with infectious disease. Surgical patients with uninfected wounds also usually manifest relatively mild responses to injury; those with infected wounds exhibit the most intense metabolic alterations. The infection may be associated with the wound (e.g., surgical site infection, mature abscess, or ARDS and pulmonary sepsis), or it may be remote (e.g., pneumonia in a patient with multiple fractures). Peak catabolic responses in surgical patients often occur several days after operation or injury. This period corresponds to the development of the cellular phase of wound healing[103] and to colonization of the wound or another site.

Aulick and colleagues examined the possible contribution of bacteria or bacterial products to the metabolic response to injury in animals.[206] They measured $\dot{V}o_2$ and core temperature in animals for up to 3 weeks after a standard scald burn. Some of the wounds were seeded with bacteria (virulent and nonvirulent *Pseudomonas aeruginosa* and *Staphylococcus epidermidis*), and some of the infected wounds were treated with topical antibacterial agents. The use of topical antibiotics was associated with a reduction in hypermetabolism. In addition, in animals that became bacteremic, the degree of hypermetabolism was at least twice that in nonbacteremic animals. The metabolic effects of infection thus appear to be proportional to the severity and invasiveness of the infection. In analogous studies, Wilmore and associates examined burn patients with and without bacteremia.[24] Although total body $\dot{V}O_2$ and cardiac index were already elevated, the onset of bacteremia resulted in further increases in these parameters. In addition, hepatic glucose production and splanchnic uptake of lactate and alanine were significantly increased in patients with systemic infection. Hypermetabolism decreased, however, once organ failure occurred.

Bacteria are ubiquitous in both health and critical illness. The mechanisms by which bacteria become infective and invade host tissues and produce physiologic responses are only beginning to be elucidated. In part, these involve intracellular regulatory systems that respond to complex reciprocal interactions with the host and that can modify bacterial virulence. Guo and associates investigated the dual peptide system PhoP-PhoQ in *Salmonella*.[207] PhoP-PhoQ regulates genes required for the synthesis of lipid A, the active component of endotoxin. It is capable of modifying the structure of lipid A, and this structurally modified lipid A can affect the expression both of adhesion molecules by host endothelial cells and of TNF by neighboring monocytes. This capability may be a mechanism by which bacteria can not only increase their chances of survival in host tissues but also affect the character or intensity of host inflammatory responses to the infection. PhoP-PhoQ and other intracellular systems respond to characteristics of the host environment, such as pH, PO_2, and ionic composition.[208] Thus, the condition of the patient may influence the virulence characteristics of resident bacteria, and these characteristics, in turn, may modulate the patient's responses to critical illness.

The cellular response to localized injury or other inflammatory stimuli initially consists of the recruitment and proliferation of neutrophils. This process appears to be mediated in part by the expression of adhesion molecules by endothelial cells. These molecules capture passing circulating neutrophils and facilitate their passage through the capillary wall.[209] Neutrophils, macrophages, and other inflammatory cells have the capacity to engulf and dispose of necrotic debris and to kill bacteria. These same properties also make them potentially toxic to normal cells. Neutrophil infiltration of specific organs, such as the lung, appears to be a first step in the development of organ failure after shock, endotoxin, and other insults.[210] This finding suggests that neutrophils activated by potent inflammatory stimuli can invade unaffected tissues and so contribute to organ dysfunction in critically ill patients.

Not surprisingly, anti-inflammatory mechanisms exist to limit the intensity and toxicity of inflammatory processes. One such mechanism is apoptosis, or programmed cell death, which is thought to participate in the clearing of inflammatory cells as the wound heals and the inflammatory process subsides. Biffl and colleagues demonstrated that IL-6 inhibited apoptosis in human neutrophils in vitro.[211] They proposed that circulating IL-6 in critically ill patients retarded neutrophil apoptosis and thus enhanced and prolonged the toxic effects of the neutrophils. This could be another mechanism by which the responses to critical illness could be prolonged and lead to worsening organ failure and death.

Manipulating the Response to Critical Illness

The metabolic response to critical illness has survival value. Young patients are able to mount more intense hypermetabolic responses than elderly persons and in general have higher survival rates. However, these responses are debilitating in all patients and may be associated with organ failure and death. Many have sought to develop

therapeutic strategies that would reduce the debilitating aspects of these responses, accelerate recovery, or both.

The endocrine response to injury or operation has been attenuated by adrenergic blockade or regional anesthesia (see above). These maneuvers are associated with an improved postoperative nitrogen balance[100,101] and decreased muscle protein breakdown.[99] Herndon and colleagues reported that continuous administration of propranolol to children with burns reduced cardiac work without adversely affecting mortality, postburn course, or wound healing.[212] This technique may benefit elderly, critically ill patients with limited cardiovascular reserve.

Several studies have evaluated the effectiveness of combined neural and humoral blockade in inhibiting the metabolic responses to operative injury. Schulze and associates compared the responses of patients receiving morphine and acetaminophen for pain control after colonic surgery with those of patients managed with methylprednisolone pretreatment, thoracic epidural analgesia, intrathecal anesthesia, and intravenous indomethacin.[213] In the patients receiving combined therapy, postoperative pain and fever were prevented, pulmonary function was improved, and fatigue was reduced. Synthesis of acute-phase proteins and IL-6 was reduced. Similarly, Heindorff and coworkers prevented the typical increases in amino acid clearance and urea synthesis with a combination of intravenous somatostatin and etomidate (to inhibit the elevation of glucagon and cortisol levels) and high thoracic epidural analgesia (to provide neural blockade).[102]

Advances in cell and molecular biology have led to an extraordinary expansion of knowledge about the mechanisms involved in the many local and systemic responses to injury, sepsis, and other critical illness. Developments in technology have also led to the formulation of novel strategies for inhibiting various components of these responses that were thought to be particularly deleterious. Thus, antibodies to endotoxin, IL-1, and TNF were developed and studied in clinical trials, along with receptor antagonists and other compounds designed to interfere with systemic inflammatory responses. None of these demonstrated clinical benefit in controlled trials.[214] Given that the regulatory mechanisms are highly complex and that the same ones that may be harmful in some cases promote recovery in others, it is not surprising that blockade of one component of the response might offer no net benefit.

An alternative strategic approach is to enhance or accelerate those components of the response to critical illness that seem to be primarily restorative and lead to wound healing and recovery.

Nutritional support of critically ill patients is important both for promoting protein synthesis and other anabolic processes essential to recovery and for reducing the net drain on the patient's fuel and protein stores. Enteral nutrition is preferred, but the availability of effective intravenous techniques allows the clinician to provide appropriate nutrition to virtually all patients. Exercise and mobility have clear anticatabolic effects and should be initiated as early as is practicable.

Previously, provision of glutamine to critically ill patients had not been possible; glutamine had not been included in most commercial nutrient preparations because of its instability in aqueous solutions. When added to standard TPN, however, glutamine can promote nitrogen retention in postoperative patients.[215] Ziegler and associates demonstrated that glutamine-supplemented TPN improved nitrogen balance, diminished clinical infection, and shortened hospital stay in a group of critically ill patients recovering from bone marrow transplantation.[216] Enteral preparations enriched with glutamine are now commercially available.

Kudsk and associates randomly selected patients with moderately severe injuries to receive either an enteral formulation enriched with glutamine, arginine, omega-3 fatty acids, and nucleotides or a standard formula that provided an isonitrogenous, isocaloric diet.[217] In both cases, protein content was moderately high (2 g/kg/day). Infectious complications in patients surviving to recovery were less frequent in those receiving the enhanced formula than in those receiving the standard diet.

Growth hormone is an anabolic hormone capable of improving nitrogen balance. Human growth hormone can be synthesized with recombinant technology, and recombinant growth hormone is safer and more readily available than an animal preparation. When administered to normal subjects, growth hormone improves nitrogen balance, even if caloric intake is less than energy expenditure.[218] Jiang and associates administered growth hormone and hypocaloric parenteral nutrition perioperatively to patients undergoing elective abdominal operations.[219] They monitored a variety of metabolic parameters and compared the results with those from a control group of patients receiving parenteral nutrition alone. Growth hormone markedly reduced cumulative nitrogen loss. Although both groups of patients lost weight, those receiving growth hormone lost less. Bioelectric impedance data indicated that most of the weight lost by patients receiving growth hormone came from fat mass and not from the muscle compartment. Growth hormone also preserved muscle strength.

Herndon and colleagues administered growth hormone to severely burned children in a randomized trial.[220] Growth hormone accelerated donor site healing, allowing earlier reharvesting of skin. As a result, the time between skin graft procedures and the total length of time required for the children's recovery were both reduced. Knox and associates gave growth hormone to a group of severely burned adults and compared their outcome with that of a similar group of patients cared for without growth hormone in the immediately preceding years[221]; mortality was lower in the growth hormone group.

Two large multi-institutional randomized trials were recently conducted in Europe in which the efficacy of growth hormone was evaluated in a variety of critically ill patients, including trauma patients, patients who had undergone cardiac procedures, and patients with other acute surgical illnesses. In all, more than 500 patients were enrolled. The two studies obtained very similar results. The combined mortality of the patients receiving growth hormone was 42%, more than twice the 18% mortality in the control subjects. Although the reasons for this adverse outcome have not yet been elucidated, the manufacturer of the recombinant product issued a safety statement recommending that recombinant growth hormone not be used in catabolic patients.[222]

Although there has been good experience with growth hormone in burn patients and other surgical patients in some centers, the widespread use of growth hormone cannot be recommended at present. Certain anabolic steroids, such as oxandrolone, are available and have a good margin of safety. These may also promote nitrogen retention and accelerate recovery. Oxandrolone, combined with a high-protein diet (2 mg/kg/day), promoted weight gain and functional improvement in a randomized study of burn patients who had recovered sufficiently to enter a rehabilitation program.[223] Controlled data in critically ill patients, however, are not yet available.

Insulin attenuates cortisol-induced breakdown of skeletal muscle protein in vitro.[224] Inculet and associates demonstrated improved nitrogen utilization in patients receiving TPN and insulin after operation.[225] The apparent mild beneficial effects of TPN enriched with branched-chain amino acids may be caused by increased insulin elaboration.[226] Bessey and Lowe induced accelerated skeletal muscle protein catabolism in normal subjects by blocking insulin elaboration during the first day of a 3-day infusion of stress hormones,[98] thereby simulating the typical hormonal profiles of injured patients. When insulin elaboration was allowed to rise unchecked or when exogenous insulin was administered to limit the rise of blood glucose, net muscle protein breakdown did not increase.

Table 8 Factors Affecting Metabolic Response to Critical Illness and Patient Outcome

Factors that *cannot* be directly controlled or influenced at present
  Patient's genetic makeup and premorbid state of health
  Gene transcription and translation
  Expression of hormones, cytokines, and growth factors
  Expression of hormone, cytokine, growth factor, and other specific cell receptors
  Expression of secondary messengers
  Generation of nitric oxide and other reactive oxygen intermediates
  Signal transduction mechanisms
  Intracellular transporters and other regulatory peptides and organelles
  CNS neural pathway traffic and cytokine expression
  Futile cycles
  Enzymes controlling protein synthesis and breakdown
  Bacterial virulence factors
  Expression of adhesion molecules
  Inflammatory and noninflammatory cell proliferation
  Apoptosis
  Wound-healing biology

Factors that *can* be directly controlled or influenced at present
  Whole-body oxygenation
  Whole-body perfusion
  Pain, anxiety
  Body temperature
  Acid-base balance
  ECF electrolyte composition and balance
  Nutrient supply
  Glucose concentration
  Anabolic factors
  Gut mucosal integrity
  Focal infection and bacteremia
  Wound repair and closure

Although some degree of hyperglycemia may facilitate glucose uptake by the inflammatory cells in the wound, excessive elevations—in excess of 10 mmol/L (180 mg/dl)—have been associated with a variety of adverse effects, including impaired phagocytosis and immune function, increased CO_2 production and ventilatory requirements, increased vascular tone and reduction of regional blood flow, and altered collagen formation.[12] Close control of blood glucose concentration (110 to 160 mg/dl) with insulin therapy may not only prevent these effects but also exert a beneficial effect on net protein loss. The insulin resistance in critically ill patients blunts the hypoglycemic effects of insulin, so that it may be administered continuously and regulated safely at the bedside by means of a standardized algorithm (sliding scale).[227]

One of the most effective means of manipulating the metabolic response to critical surgical illness, however, remains excellent surgical care. Such care is directed toward reducing, limiting, preventing, or neutralizing the signals that initiate these debilitating responses. Aggressive and prompt resuscitation, restoration of tissue oxygenation, debridement of necrotic tissue, drainage of pus, and wound repair all should have a high priority in the early management of a critically ill patient. Maintenance of effective cardiopulmonary function and tissue oxygenation, provision of a warm environment, preservation of GI tract integrity, and control of infection are clinical objectives of later management.

Over the course of the past few decades, close attention to these details has resulted in improved outcome for critically ill patients. For example, Pruitt and Mason analyzed a population of over 8,000 burn patients treated at the US Army Burn Unit from 1950 through 1991.[228] Since the mid-1970s, the burn size associated with a 50% mortality steadily rose from 57% of BSA to 77%. Similarly, Milberg and colleagues demonstrated a reduction in ARDS-related mortality from nearly 70% to 30% between 1983 and 1993.[229]

In a 1995 study, Kelleman and colleagues determined the effect of burn size on resting energy expenditure.[230] This study reproduced that of Wilmore done at the same institution almost 20 years before. In the earlier study, the resting metabolic rate increased steadily with burn size and plateaued at about twice the basal level with burns larger than 50% of BSA. Kelleman found that energy expenditure plateaued at only 1.5 times the basal level with burns of about 25% of BSA or more. This dramatic change in the relationship between burn size (injury severity) and metabolic activity (hypermetabolism) probably reflects the combined effects of improvements in all aspects of burn care, including resuscitation, cardiopulmonary and metabolic support, wound care, nursing practice, occupational and physical therapy, and reduced time to excision and grafting and wound closure. Improvements in care have thus reduced the metabolic cost of critical surgical illness.

Conclusion

The physiologic impact of major trauma, burns, intra-abdominal catastrophe, sepsis, or other critical illness reverberates throughout the body and affects all organ systems. Knowledge about the mechanisms that regulate this comprehensive and commanding response is growing at an exponential rate. These mechanisms are intricate, interrelated, and redundant. Where we once looked for a simple, direct answer, we now see dizzying complexity. The critically ill patient is a true example of controlled inflammation, suspended between anabolic and catabolic forces and between inflammatory and anti-inflammatory forces.

Unfortunately, our ability to apply our improved understanding to the care of critically ill patients still lags far behind. When the patient is not progressing well, we lack the ability to make a specific bedside diagnosis that will pinpoint the part of the system that is out of balance. Even if we could make such a diagnosis, however, we still lack the accurately targeted therapies that would allow us to intervene precisely.

Thus, a wide variety of factors and processes, with both beneficial and adverse effects, appear to be involved in the metabolic response to critical illness, but we are unable to affect many of them directly with the means currently available [see Table 8]. We can remove necrotic tissue, repair wounds, and drain pus. We can also usually ensure excellent cardiovascular performance and maintain extracellular electrolyte and nutrient composition and acid-base balance. We can often suppress bacteremia and can treat some infections effectively with antibiotics. We can prevent many additional insults to and stresses on our patients. These measures may seem unsophisticated and clumsy in the light of our contemporary understanding of the biology of convalescence, but they clearly are capable of nudging the metabolic response to critical illness toward a successful outcome. At present, such measures constitute the essentials of excellent comprehensive care of critically ill patients, and they give these patients their best hope for recovery.

References

1. Wilmore DW: Metabolic Management of the Critically Ill. Plenum Press, New York, 1980

2. Patient-controlled analgesia (editorial). Lancet 1:289, 1980

3. Kehlet H: Multimodal approach to control postoperative pathophysiology and rehabilitation. Br J Anaesth 78:606, 1997

4. MacKersie RC, Shackford SR, Hoyt DB, et al: Continuous epidural fentanyl analgesia: ventilatory function improvement with routine use in treatment of blunt chest injury. J Trauma 27:1207, 1987

5. Bone RC, Balk RA, Cerra FB, et al: Definitions for sepsis and organ failure and guidelines for the use of innovative therapies in sepsis. Chest 101:1644, 1992

6. Rangel-Frausto MS, Pittet D, Costigan M, et al: The natural history of the systemic inflammatory response syndrome (SIRS): a prospective study. JAMA 273:117, 1995

7. Civetta JM, Hudson-Civetta J, Bell S: Decreasing catheter-related infection and hospital costs by continuous quality improvement. Crit Care Med 24:1660, 1996

8. Mandal AK, Monturo J, Thadepelli H: Prophylactic antibiotics and no antibiotics compared in penetrating chest trauma. J Trauma 25:639, 1985

9. Stoutenbeek CP, van Saene HKF, Miranda DR, et al: The effect of oropharyngeal decontamination using topical nonabsorbable antibiotics on the incidence of nosocomial respiratory tract infections in multiple trauma patients. J Trauma 27:357, 1987

10. Goldman DA, Weinstein RA, Wenzel RP, et al: Strategies to prevent and control the emergence and spread of antimicrobial-resistant microorganisms in hospitals: a challenge to hospital leadership. JAMA 275:234, 1996

11. Sise MJ, Hollingsworth P, Brimm JC, et al: Complications of the flow-directed pulmonary artery catheter. Crit Care Med 8:272, 1980

12. Bessey PQ, Watters JM: Glucose metabolism following trauma or sepsis. Trauma, Sepsis, and Shock: The Physiological Basis of Therapy. Burke PA, Forse RA, Eds. Marcel Dekker, New York (in press)

13. Cuthbertson DP: Surgical metabolism: historical and evolutionary aspects. Metabolism and the Response to Injury. Wilkinson AW, Cuthbertson DP, Eds. Year Book Medical Publishers, Chicago, 1977, p 1

14. Thomas L: The Lives of a Cell. Viking Press, New York, 1974, p 75

15. Im MJC, Hoopes JE: Energy metabolism in healing skin wounds. J Surg Res 10:459, 1970

16. Ben-Porat M, Sideman S, Bursztein S: Energy metabolism rate equation for fasting and postabsorptive subjects. Am J Physiol 244:R764, 1983

17. Atwater WO, Benedict FG: Experiments on the metabolism of matter and energy in the human body. US Department of Agriculture Office of Experimental Stations Bulletin, publication No. 136, 1903

18. Dubois EF: Basal Metabolism in Health and Disease. Lea & Febiger, Philadelphia, 1936, p 163

19. Wilmore DW, Long JM, Mason AD Jr, et al: Catecholamines: mediator of the hypermetabolic response to thermal injury. Ann Surg 180:653, 1974

20. Wilmore DW: Metabolic Management of the Critically Ill. Plenum Medical, New York, 1977, p 33

21. Shiozaki T, Kishikawa M, Hiraide A, et al: Recovery from postoperative hypothermia predicts survival in extensively burned patients. Am J Surg 165:326, 1993

22. Wilmore DW, Aulick LH, Mason AD, et al: Influence of the burn wound on local and systemic responses to injury. Ann Surg 186:444, 1977

23. Aulick LH, Wilmore DW, Mason AD Jr, et al: Muscle blood flow following thermal injury. Ann Surg 188:778, 1978

24. Wilmore DW, Goodwin CW, Aulick LH, et al: Effect of injury and infection on visceral metabolism and circulation. Ann Surg 192:491, 1980

25. Aulick LH, Goodwin CW Jr, Becker RA, et al: Visceral blood flow following thermal injury. Ann Surg 193:112, 1981

26. Wilmore DW, Aulick LH: Metabolic changes in burned patients. Surg Clin North Am 58:1173, 1978

27. Cuthbertson DP: The disturbance of metabolism produced by bony and non-bony injury, with notes on certain abnormal conditions of bone. Biochem J 24:1244, 1930

28. Monafo WW: Wound care: physiologic concepts. Treatment of Burns: Principles and Practice. Monafo WW, Pappalardo C, Eds. Warren H Green, Inc, St Louis, 1971, p 111

29. Caldwell FT Jr, Osterholm JL, Sower ND, et al: Metabolic response to thermal trauma of normal and thyroprivic rats at three environmental temperatures. Ann Surg 150:976, 1959

30. Barr PO, Birke G, Liljedahl SO, et al: Oxygen consumption and water loss during treatment of burns with warm dry air. Lancet 1:164, 1968

31. Wilmore DW, Mason AD Jr, Johnson DW, et al: Effect of ambient temperature on heat production and heat loss in burn patients. J Appl Physiol 38:593, 1975

32. Wilmore DW, Orcutt TW, Mason AD Jr, et al: Alterations in hypothalamic function following thermal injury. J Trauma 15:697, 1975

33. Howard JE, Parson W, Stein KE, et al: Studies on fracture convalescence: I. Nitrogen metabolism after fracture and skeletal operations in healthy males. Johns Hopkins Hospital Bulletin 75:156, 1944

34. Cuthbertson DP: Observations on disturbance of metabolism produced by injury to the limbs. Q J Med 25:233, 1932

35. Cuthbertson DP, McGirr JL, Robertson JSM: The effect of fracture of bone on the metabolism of the

rat. Quarterly Journal of Experimental Physiology 29:13, 1939

36. Threlfall CJ, Stoner HB, Galasko CSB: Patterns in the excretion of muscle markers after trauma and orthopedic surgery. J Trauma 21:140, 1981

37. Young VR, Munro HN: N$^\gamma$-methylhistidine (3-methylhistidine) and muscle protein turnover: an overview. Federal Proceedings 37:2291, 1978

38. Williamson DH, Farrell R, Kerr A, et al: Muscle protein catabolism after injury in man as measured by urinary excretion of 3-methylhistidine. Clin Sci Molec Med 52:527, 1977

39. Bilmazes C, Kien CL, Rohrbaugh DK, et al: Quantitative contribution by skeletal muscle to elevated rates of whole-body protein breakdown in burned children as measured by N$^\gamma$-methylhistidine output. Metabolism 27:671, 1978

40. Long CL, Schiller WR, Blakemore WS, et al: Muscle protein catabolism in the septic patient as measured by 3-methylhistidine excretion. Am J Clin Nutr 30:1349, 1977

41. Cuthbertson DP: The physiology of convalescence after injury. Br Med Bull 3:96, 1945

42. Moore FD, Langohr JL, Ingebretsen M, et al: The role of exudate losses in the protein and electrolyte imbalance of burned patients. Ann Surg 132:1, 1950

43. Soroff HS, Pearson E, Artz CP: An estimation of the nitrogen requirements for equilibrium in burned patients. Surg Gynecol Obstet 112:150, 1961

44. Wilmore DW: Nutrition and metabolism following thermal injury. Clin Plast Surg 1:603, 1974

45. Kinney JM: Energy deficits in acute illness and injury. Proceedings of a Conference on Energy Metabolism and Body Fuel Utilization. Morgan AP, Ed. Harvard University Press, Cambridge, Massachusetts, 1966, p 174

46. Picou D, Taylor-Roberts T: The measurement of total protein synthesis and catabolism and nitrogen turnover in infants on different amounts of dietary protein. Clin Sci 36:283, 1969

47. Birkhahn RH, Long CL, Fitkin D, et al: Effects of major skeletal trauma on whole body protein turnover in man measured by L-[1,^{14}C]-leucine. Surgery 88:294, 1980

48. Kien CL, Young VR, Rohrbaugh DK, et al: Increased rates of whole body protein synthesis and breakdown in children recovering from burns. Ann Surg 187:383, 1978

49. Munro HN: Free amino acid pools and their role in regulation. Mammalian Protein Metabolism, Vol 4. Munro HN, Ed. Academic Press, New York, 1970, p 299

50. Bergström J, Fürst P, Noree L-O, et al: Intracellular free amino acid concentration in human muscle tissue. J Appl Physiol 36:693, 1974

51. Askanazi J, Elwyn DH, Kinney JM, et al: Muscle and plasma amino acids after injury: the role of inactivity. Ann Surg 188:797, 1978

52. Vinnars E, Bergström J, Fürst P: Influence of the postoperative state on the intracellular free amino acids in human muscle tissue. Ann Surg 182:665, 1975

53. Fürst P, Bergström J, Chao L, et al: Influence of amino acid supply on nitrogen and amino acid metabolism in severe trauma. Acta Chir Scand 494(suppl):136, 1979

54. Askanazi J, Carpentier YA, Michelson CB, et al: Muscle and plasma amino acids following injury: influence of intercurrent infection. Ann Surg 192:78, 1980

55. Askanazi J, Fürst P, Michelsen CB, et al: Muscle and plasma amino acids after injury: hypocaloric glucose vs. amino acid infusion. Ann Surg 191:465, 1980

56. Wilmore DW, Black PR, Muhlbacher F: Injured man: trauma and sepsis. Nutritional Support of the Seriously Ill Patient. Winters RW, Greene HL, Eds. Academic Press, New York, 1983, p 33

57. Aulick LH, Wilmore DW: Increased peripheral amino acid release following burn injury. Surgery 85:560, 1979

58. Garber AJ, Karl IE, Kipnis DM: Alanine and glutamine synthesis and release from skeletal muscle: I. Glycolysis and amino acid release. J Biol Chem 251:826, 1976

59. Garber AJ, Karl IE, Kipnis DM: Alanine and glutamine synthesis and release from skeletal muscle: II. The precursor role of amino acids in alanine and glutamine synthesis. J Biol Chem 251:836, 1976

60. Close JH: The use of amino acid precursors in nitrogen-accumulation diseases. N Engl J Med 290:663, 1974

61. Johnson DJ, Jiang ZM, Colpoys M, et al: Branched chain amino acid uptake and muscle free amino acid concentrations predict postoperative muscle nitrogen balance. Ann Surg 204:513, 1986

62. Rennie MJ, Hundal HS, Babij P, et al: Characteristics of a glutamine carrier in skeletal muscle have important consequences for nitrogen loss in injury, infection, and chronic disease. Lancet 2:1008, 1986

63. Windmueller HG: Glutamine utilization by the small intestine. Adv Enzymol 53:201, 1982

64. Souba WW, Wilmore DW: Postoperative alteration of arteriovenous exchange of amino acids across the gastrointestinal tract. Surgery 94:342, 1983

65. Long CL, Spencer JL, Kinney JM, et al: Carbohydrate metabolism in man: effect of elective operations and major injury. J Appl Physiol 31:110, 1971

66. Wolfe RR, Durkot MJ, Allsop JR, et al: Glucose metabolism in severely burned patients. Metabolism 28:1031, 1979

67. Wilmore DW, Mason AD, Pruitt BA Jr: Alterations in glucose kinetics following thermal injury. Forum on Fundamental Surgical Problems 26:81, 1975

68. Ruderman MB: Muscle amino acid metabolism and gluconeogenesis. Annu Rev Med 26:245, 1975

69. Wolfe RR, Herndon DN, Jahoor F, et al: Effect of severe burn injury on substrate cycling by glucose and fatty acids. N Engl J Med 317:403, 1987

70. Shaw JHF, Wolfe RR: An integrated analysis of glucose, fat, and protein metabolism in severely traumatized patients: studies in the basal state and the response to total parenteral nutrition. Ann Surg 209:63, 1989

71. Howard JM: Studies of the absorption and metabolism of glucose following injury: the systemic response to injury. Ann Surg 141:311, 1955

72. Allison SP, Hinton P, Chamberlain MJ: Intravenous glucose-tolerance, insulin, and free–fatty-acid levels in burned patients. Lancet 2:1113, 1968

73. Wilmore DW, Mason AD Jr, Pruitt BA Jr: Insulin response to glucose in hypermetabolic burn patients. Ann Surg 183:314, 1978

74. Black PR, Brooks DC, Bessey PQ, et al: Mechanisms of insulin resistance following injury. Ann Surg 196:420, 1982

75. Brooks DC, Bessey PQ, Black PR, et al: Post-traumatic insulin resistance in uninjured forearm tissue. J Surg Res 37:100, 1984

76. Long JM III, Wilmore DW, Mason AD Jr, et al: Effect of carbohydrate and fat intake on nitrogen excretion during total intravenous feeding. Ann Surg 185:417, 1977

77. Wolfe RR, O'Donnell TF Jr, Stone MD, et al: Investigation of factors determining optimal glucose infusion rate in total parenteral nutrition. Metabolism 29:892, 1980

78. Burke JF, Wolfe RR, Mullany CJ, et al: Glucose requirements following burn injury: parameters of optimal glucose infusion and possible hepatic and respiratory abnormalities following excessive glucose intake. Ann Surg 190:274, 1979

79. Askanazi J, Carpentier YA, Elwyn DH, et al: Influence of total parenteral nutrition on fuel utilization in injury and sepsis. Ann Surg 191:40, 1980

80. Goodenough RD, Wolfe RR: Effect of total parenteral nutrition on free fatty acid metabolism in burned patients. JPEN J Parenter Enteral Nutr 8:357, 1984

81. Roth J, LeRoith D, Lesniak MA, et al: Molecules of intercellular communication in vertebrates, invertebrates, and microbes: do they share common origins? Prog Brain Res 68:71, 1986

82. Davies CL, Newman RJ, Molyneux SG, et al: The relationship between plasma catecholamines and severity of injury in man. J Trauma 24:99, 1984

83. Harrison TS, Seaton JF, Feller I: Relationship of increased oxygen consumption to catecholamine excretion in thermal burns. Ann Surg 165:169, 1967

84. Porte D Jr, Robertson RP: Control of insulin secretion by catecholamines, stress, and the sympathetic nervous system. Fed Proc 32:1792, 1973

85. Bessey PQ, Brooks DC, Black PR, et al: Epinephrine acutely mediates skeletal muscle insulin resistance. Surgery 94:172, 1983

86. Garber AJ, Karl JE, Kipnis DM: Alanine and glutamine synthesis and release from skeletal muscle: IV. β-Adrenergic inhibition of amino acid release. J Biol Chem 251:851, 1976

87. Vaughan GM, Becker RA, Allan JP, et al: Cortisol and corticotrophin in burned patients. J Trauma 22:263, 1982

88. Wilmore DW, Lindsey CA, Moylan JA, et al: Hyperglucagonaemia after burns. Lancet 1:73, 1974

89. Baxter JD, Forsham PH: Tissue effects of glucocorticoids. Am J Med 53:573, 1972

90. Owen OE, Cahill GF Jr: Metabolic effects of exogenous glucocorticoids in fasted man. J Clin Invest 52:2596, 1973

91. Felig P, Wahren J, Hendler R: Influence of physiologic hyperglucagonemia on basal and insulin-inhibited splanchnic glucose output in normal man. J Clin Invest 58:761, 1976

92. Ferrannini E, DeFronze RA, Sherwin RS: Transient hepatic response to glucagon in man: role of insulin and hyperglycemia. Am J Physiol 242:E73, 1982

93. Wolfe BM, Culebras JM, Aoki TT, et al: The effects of glucagon on protein metabolism in normal man. Surgery 86:248, 1979

94. Shamoon HM, Hendler R, Sherwin RS: Synergistic interactions among anti-insulin hormones in the pathogenesis of stress hypoglycemia in humans. J Clin Endocrinol Metab 52:1235, 1981

95. Bessey PQ, Watters JM, Aoki TT, et al: Combined hormonal infusion simulates the metabolic response to injury. Ann Surg 200:264, 1984

96. Bessey PQ, Jiang Z-M, Johnson DJ, et al: Post-traumatic skeletal muscle proteolysis: the role of the hormonal environment. World J Surg 13:465, 1989

97. Vilstrup H, Hansen BA, Aldal T: Glucagon enhances hepatic efficacy for urea production. Clinical Nutrition 7(suppl):35, 1988

98. Bessey PQ, Lowe KA: Early hormonal changes affect the catabolic response to trauma. Ann Surg 218:476, 1993

99. Hulton N, Johnson DJ, Smith RJ, et al: Hormonal blockade modifies post-traumatic protein catabolism. J Surg Res 39:310, 1985

100. Brandt MR, Fernandes A, Mordhorst R, et al: Epidural analgesia improves postoperative nitrogen balance. Br Med J 1:1106, 1978

101. Tsuji H, Shirasaka C, Asoh T, et al: Effects of epidural administration of local anaesthetics or morphine on postoperative nitrogen loss and catabolic hormones. Br J Surg 74:421, 1987

102. Heindorff H, Schulze S, Morgensen T, et al: Hormonal and neural blockade prevents the postoperative increase in amino acid clearance and urea synthesis. Surgery 111:543, 1992

103. Hunt TK: Physiology of wound healing. Trauma, Sepsis, and Shock: The Physiological Basis of Therapy. Clowes GHA Jr, Ed. Marcel Dekker, New York, 1988, p 443

104. Dinarello CA: Proinflammatory and anti-inflammatory cytokines as mediators in the pathogenesis of septic shock. Chest 112:321S, 1997

105. Cinat M, Waxman K, Vaziri ND, et al: Soluble cytokine receptors and receptor antagonists are sequentially released after trauma. J Trauma 39:112, 1995

106. Akira S, Hirano T, Taga T, et al: Biology of multifunctional cytokines: IL-6 and related molecules (IL-1 and TNF). FASEB J 4:2860, 1990

107. Jiang JX, Tian KL, Chen HS, et al: Plasma cytokines and endotoxin levels in patients with severe injury and their relationship with organ damage. Injury 28:509, 1997

108. Drosst AC, Burleson DG, Cioffi WG Jr, et al: Plasma cytokines following thermal injury and their relationship with patient mortality, burn size, and time post-burn. J Trauma 35:335, 1993

109. Michie HR, Spriggs DR, Manogue KR, et al: Tumor necrosis factor and endotoxin induce similar metabolic responses in human beings. Surgery 104:280, 1988

110. Michie HR, Sherman ML, Spriggs DR, et al: Chronic TNF infusion causes anorexia but not accelerated nitrogen loss. Ann Surg 209:19, 1989

111. Mealy K, van Lanschot JJB, Robinson BG, et al: Are the catabolic effects of tumor necrosis factor mediated by glucocorticoids? Arch Surg 125:42, 1990

112. Hall-Angeras M, Angeras U, Zamir O, et al: Effect of the glucocorticoid receptor antagonist RU 38486 on muscle protein breakdown in sepsis. Surgery 109:468, 1991

113. Dinarello CA: Interleukin-1. Rev Infect Dis 6:51, 1984

114. Dinarello CA: An update on human interleukin-1: from molecular biology to clinical relevance. J Clin Immunol 5:287, 1985

115. Baracos V, Rodemann HP, Dinarello CA, et al: Stimulation of muscle protein degradation and prostaglandin E_2 release by leukocytic pyrogen (interleukin-1): a mechanism for the increased degradation of muscle proteins during fever. N Engl J Med 308:553, 1983

116. Sobrado JL, Moldawer LL, Dinarello CA, et al: Effect of ibuprofen on fever and metabolic changes induced by leukocytic pyrogen (interleukin-1) and endotoxin. Infect Immun 42:997, 1983

117. Moldawer LL, Svaninger G, Gelin J, et al: Interleukin-1 and tumor necrosis factor do not regulate protein balance in skeletal muscle. Am J Physiol 253:C766, 1987

118. Zamir O, Hasselgren P-O, von Allmen D, et al: The effect of interleukin-1 alpha and the glucocorticoid receptor blocker RU 38486 on total and myofibrillar protein breakdown in skeletal muscle. J Surg Res 50:579, 1991

119. Zamir O, Hasselgren P-O, O'Brien WO, et al: Muscle protein breakdown during endotoxemia in rats and after treatment with interleukin-1 receptor antagonist (IL-1ra). Ann Surg 216:381, 1992

120. Watters JM, Bessey PQ, Dinarello CA, et al: The induction of interleukin-1 in humans and its metabolic effects. Surgery 98:298, 1985

121. Watters JM, Bessey PQ, Dinarello CA, et al: Both inflammatory and endocrine mediators stimulate host responses to sepsis. Arch Surg 121:179, 1986

122. Koj A: The role of interleukin-6 as the hepatic stimulating factor in the network of inflammatory cytokines. Ann NY Acad Sci 557:1, 1989

123. Biffl WL, Moore EE, Moore FA, et al: Interleukin-6 in the injured patient: marker of injury or mediator of inflammation? Ann Surg 224:647, 1996

124. Casey LC, Balk RA, Bone RC: Plasma cytokines and endotoxin levels correlate with survival in patients with the sepsis syndrome. Ann Intern Med 119:771, 1993

125. de Beaux AC, Ross JA, Maingay JP, et al: Proinflammatory cytokine release by peripheral blood mononuclear cells from patients with acute pancreatitis. Br J Surg 83:1071, 1996

126. Guillen I, Blaines M, Gomez-Lechon MJ, et al: Cytokine signaling during myocardial infarction: sequential appearance of IL-1β and IL-6. Am J Physiol 269:R229, 1995

127. Mateo RB, Reichner JS, Albina JE: Interleukin-6 activity in wounds. Am J Physiol 266:R1840, 1994

128. Stouthard JM, Romijn JA, van der Poll T, et al: Endocrinologic and metabolic effects of interleukin-6 in humans. Am J Physiol 268:E813, 1995

129. Tsigos C, Papanicolaou DA, Kyrou I, et al: Dose-dependent effects of recombinant human interleukin-6 on glucose regulation. J Clin Endocrinol Metab 82:4167, 1997

130. De Benedetti F, Alonzi T, Moretta A, et al: Interleukin-6 causes growth impairment in transgenic mice through a decrease in insulin-like growth factor–1. J Clin Invest 99:643, 1997

131. Tsujinaka T, Fujita J, Ebisui C, et al: Interleukin-6 receptor antibody inhibits muscle atrophy and modulates proteolytic systems in interleukin-6 transgenic mice. J Clin Invest 97:244, 1996

132. Rutan RL, Herndon DN: Growth delay in postburn pediatric patients. Arch Surg 125:392, 1990

133. Gonzalez-Hernandez JA, Bornstein SR, Ehrhart-Bornstein M, et al: Interleukin-6 messenger ribonucleic acid expression in human adrenal gland in vivo: new clue to a paracrine or autocrine regulation of adrenal function. J Clin Endocrinol Metab 79:1492, 1994

134. Path G, Bornstein SR, Ehrhart-Bornstein M, et al: Interleukin-6 and the interleukin-6 receptor in the human adrenal gland: expression and effects on steroidogenesis. J Clin Endocrinol Metab 82:2343, 1997

135. Bone RC, Fisher CJ, Clemmer TP, et al: A controlled clinical trial of high-dose methylprednisolone in the treatment of severe sepsis and septic shock. N Engl J Med 317:653, 1987

136. Barber AE, Coyle SM, Maranao MA, et al: Glucocorticoid therapy alters hormonal and cytokine responses to endotoxin in man. J Immunol 150:1999, 1993

137. Hasselgren P-O: Protein Metabolism in Sepsis. RG Landes Co, Austin, Texas, 1993, p 82

138. Wing SS, Goldberg AL: Glucocorticoids activate the ATP-ubiquitin–dependent proteolytic system in skeletal muscle during fasting. Am J Physiol 264:E668, 1993

139. Zamir O, Hasselgren P-O, von Allmen D, et al: In vivo administration of interleukin-1α induces muscle proteolysis in normal and adrenalectomized rats. Metabolism 42:204, 1993

140. Hume DM, Egdahl RH: The importance of the brain in the endocrine response to injury. Ann Surg 150:697, 1959

141. Taylor JW, Hander EW, Skreen R, et al: The effect of central nervous system narcosis on the sympathetic response to stress. J Surg Res 20:313, 1976

142. Dempsey DT, Guenter P, Crosby LO, et al: Barbiturate therapy and energy expenditure in head trauma. Presented at the 42nd Annual Meeting of the American Association for the Surgery of Trauma, Colorado Springs, 1982

143. Fried R, Dempsey D, Guenter P: Barbiturates improve nitrogen balance in patients with severe head trauma (abstr) JPEN J Parenter Enteral Nutr 4:86, 1984

144. Wilmore DW, Long JM, Mason AD, et al: Stress in surgical patients as a neurophysiologic reflex response. Surg Gynecol Obstet 142:257, 1976

145. Wilmore DW, Taylor JW, Handler EW, et al: Central nervous system function following thermal injury. Metabolism and the Response to Injury. Wilkinson AW, Cuthbertson DP, Eds. Year Book Medical Publishers, Chicago, 1977, p 274

146. Chrousos GP: The hypothalamic-pituitary-adrenal axis and immune-mediated inflammation. N Engl J Med 332:1351, 1995

147. Turchik JB, Bornstein DL: Role of the central nervous system in acute-phase responses to leukocyte pyrogen. Infect Immun 30:439, 1980

148. Breder CD, Dinarello CA, Saper CB: Interleukin-1 immunoreactive innervation of the human hypothalamus. Science 240:321, 1988

149. Cunningham ET, Wada E, Carter DB, et al: In situ localization of type I interleukin-1 receptor messenger RNA in the central nervous system, pituitary, and adrenal gland of the mouse. J Neurosci 12:1101, 1991

150. Schöbitz R, DeKloet ER, Sutanto W, et al: Cellular localization of interleukin-6 mRNA and interleukin-6 receptor RNA in rat brain. Eur J Neurosci 5:1426, 1993

151. Lieberman AP, Pitha PM, Shin HS, et al: Production of tumor necrosis factor and other cytokines by astrocytes stimulated with lipopolysaccharide or a neurotrophic virus. Proc Natl Acad Sci USA 86:6348, 1989

152. Maeda Y, Matsumoto M, Hori O, et al: Hypoxia/reoxygenation-mediated induction of astrocyte interleukin-6: a paracrine mechanism potentially enhancing neuron survival. J Exp Med 180:2297, 1994

153. Klir JJ, McClellan JL, Kluger MJ: Interleukin-1β causes the increase in anterior hypothalamic interleukin-6 during LPS-induced fever in rats. Am J Physiol 266:R1845, 1994

154. Nakamori T, Morimoto A, Yamaguchi K, et al: Interleukin-1β production in the rabbit brain during endotoxin-induced fever. J Physiol Lond 476:177, 1994

155. Hill AG, Hiegel J, Rounds J, et al: Metabolic responses to interleukin-1: centrally and peripherally mediated. Ann Surg 225:246, 1997

156. Hill AG, Jacobson L, Gonzalez J, et al: Chronic central nervous system exposure to interleukin-1β causes catabolism in the rat. Am J Physiol 271:R1142, 1996

157. Mastorakos G, Chrousos GP, Weber JS: Recombinant interleukin-6 activates the hypothalamic-pituitary-adrenal axis in humans. J Clin Endocrinol Metab 77:1690, 1993

158. Ling PR, Schwartz JH, Jeevanandam M, et al: Metabolic changes in rats during a continuous infusion of recombinant interleukin-1. Am J Physiol 270:E305, 1996

159. Reyes TM, Coe CL: The proinflammatory cytokine network: interactions in the CNS and blood of rhesus monkeys. Am J Physiol 274:R139, 1998

160. Romero LI, Kakucska I, Lechan RM, et al: Interleukin-6 (IL-6) is secreted from the brain after intercerebroventricular injection of IL-1β in rats. Am J Physiol 270:R518, 1996

161. Senba E, Kashiba K: Sensory afferent processing in multi-responsive DRG neurons. Prog Brain Res 113:387, 1996

162. Thompson SW, Priestley JV, Southall A: gp130 cytokines, leukemia inhibitory factor, and interleukin-6 induce neuropeptide expression in intact adult rat sensory neurons in vivo: time-course, specificity, and comparison with sciatic nerve axotomy. Neuroscience 84:1247, 1998

163. Hirota H, Kiyama H, Kishimoto T, et al: Accelerated nerve regeneration in mice by upregulated expression of interleukin (IL) 6 and IL-6 receptor after trauma. J Exp Med 183:2627, 1996

164. Niijima A: The afferent discharges from sensors for interleukin-1β in the hepatoportal system in the anesthetized rat. J Autonom Nerv Sys 61:287, 1996

165. Ravin HA, Rowley D, Jenkins C, et al: On the absorption of bacterial endotoxin from the gastro-intestinal tract of the normal and shocked animal. J Exp Med 112:783, 1960

166. Caridis DT, Reinhold RB, Woodruff PW, et al: Endotoxaemia in man. Lancet 1:1381, 1972

167. Wilmore DW, Smith RJ, O'Dwyer ST, et al: The gut: a central organ after surgical stress. Surgery 104:917, 1988

168. Marin ML, Greenstein AJ, Geller SA, et al: A freeze fracture study of Crohn's disease of the terminal ileum: changes in epithelial tight junction organization. Am J Gastroenterol 78:537, 1983

169. Dobbins WO III: Gut immunophysiology: a gastroenterologist's view with emphasis on pathophysiology. Am J Physiol 242:G1, 1982

170. Deitch EA, Berg R, Specian R: Endotoxin promotes the translocation of bacteria from the gut. Arch Surg 122:185, 1987

171. Wellmann W, Fink PC, Schmidt FW: Whole-gut irrigation as antiendotoxinaemic therapy in inflammatory bowel disease. Hepatogastroenterology 31:91, 1984

172. Schatten WE, Desprez JD, Holden WD: A bacteriologic study of portal-vein blood in man. Arch Surg 71:404, 1955

173. Ambrose NS, Johnson M, Burdon DW, et al: Incidence of pathogenic bacteria from mesenteric lymph nodes and ileal serosa during Crohn's disease surgery. Br J Surg 71:623, 1984

174. Berg RD: Translocation of indigenous bacteria from the intestinal tract. Human Intestinal Microflora in Health and Disease. Hentges DJ, Ed. Academic Press, New York, 1983

175. Deitch EA, Winterton J, Berg R: Thermal injury promotes bacterial translocation from the gastrointestinal tract in mice with impaired T-cell–mediated immunity. Arch Surg 121:97, 1986

176. Baker JW, Deitch EA, Li M, et al: Hemorrhagic shock induces bacterial translocation from the gut. J Trauma 28:896, 1988

177. Deitch EA, Winterton J, Li M, et al: The gut as a portal of entry for bacteremia: role of protein malnutrition. Ann Surg 205:681, 1987

178. Moore FA, Moore EE, Poggetti R, et al: Gut bacterial translocation via the portal vein: a clinical perspective with major torso trauma. J Trauma 31:629, 1991

179. O'Farrely C: Just how inflamed is the normal gut? Gut 42:603, 1998

180. Guy-Grand E, DiSanto JP, Henchoz P, et al: Small bowel enteropathy: role of intraepithelial lymphocytes and of cytokines (IL-12, IFN-γ, TNF) in the induction of epithelial cell death and renewal. Eur J Immunol 28:730, 1998

181. Wyble CW, Desai TR, Clark ET, et al: Physiologic concentrations of TNFα and IL-1β released from reperfused human intestine upregulate E-selectin and ICAM-1. J Surg Res 63:333, 1996

182. Mainous MR, Ertel W, Chaudry IH, et al: The gut: a cytokine-generating organ in systemic inflammation? Shock 4:193, 1995

183. Mochizuki H, Trocki O, Dominioni L: Mechanism of prevention of postburn hypermetabolism and catabolism by early enteral feeding. Ann Surg 200:297, 1984

184. Saito H, Trocki O, Alexander JW: The effect of route of nutrient administration on the nutritional state, catabolic hormone secretion, and gut mucosal integrity after burn injury. JPEN J Parenter Enteral Nutr 11:1, 1987

185. Alexander JW, MacMillan BG, Stinnett JD: Beneficial effects of aggressive protein feeding in severely burned children. Ann Surg 192:505, 1980

186. Border JR, Hassett J, La Duca J: The gut origin septic states in blunt multiple trauma (ISS = 40) in the ICU. Ann Surg 206:427, 1987

187. Ogle CK, Zuo L, Mao JX, et al: Differential expression of intestinal and splenic cytokines after parenteral nutrition. Arch Surg 130:1301, 1995

188. Lyoumi S, Tamion F, Petit J, et al: Induction and modulation of acute-phase response by protein malnutrition in rats: comparative effect of systemic and localized inflammation on interleukin-6 and acute-phase protein synthesis. J Nutr 128:166, 1998

189. Steiner M, Bourges HR, Freedman LS, et al: Effect of starvation on the tissue composition of the small intestine in the rat. Am J Physiol 215:75, 1968

190. Clarke RM: Evidence for both luminal and systemic factors in the control of rat intestinal epithelial replacement. Clin Sci Mol Med 50:139, 1976

191. Gleeson MH, Dowling RH, Peters TJ: Biochemical changes in intestinal mucosa after experimental small bowel by-pass in the rat. Clin Sci 43:743, 1972

192. Johnson LR, Lichtenberger LM, Copeland EM, et al: Action of gastrin on gastrointestinal structure and function. Gastroenterology 68:1184, 1975

193. Sagor GR, Ghatei MA, Al-Mukhtar MYT, et al: Evidence for a humoral mechanism after small intestinal resection: exclusion of gastrin but not enteroglucagon. Gastroenterology 84:902, 1983

194. Hwang TL, O'Dwyer ST, Smith RJ, et al: Preservation of small bowel mucosa using glutamine-enriched parenteral nutrition. Forum on Fundamental Surgical Problems 37:56, 1986

195. Jacobs DO, Evans DA, O'Dwyer ST, et al: Trophic effects of glutamine-enriched parenteral nutrition on colonic mucosa. JPEN J Parenter Enteral Nutr 12 (suppl):6S, 1988

196. O'Dwyer ST, Smith RJ, Scott T: Glutamine enriched nutrition decreases intestinal injury and increases nitrogen retention. Br J Surg 74:1162, 1987

197. Young LS, Stevens P, Kaijser B: Gram-negative pathogens in septicaemic infections. Scand J Infect Dis 31(suppl):78, 1982

198. Fish RE, Spitzer JA: Continuous infusion of endotoxin from an osmotic pump in the conscious, unrestrained rat: a unique model of chronic endotoxemia. Circ Shock 12:135, 1984

199. Revhaug A, Michie HR, Manson JM, et al: Inhibition of cyclooxygenase attenuates the metabolic response to endotoxin in humans. Arch Surg 123:162, 1988

200. Michie HR, Manogue KR, Spriggs DR, et al: Detection of circulating tumor necrosis factor after endotoxin administration. N Engl J Med 318:1481, 1988

201. Fong Y, Tracey KJ, Moldawer LL, et al: Antibodies to cachectin/tumor necrosis factor reduce interleukin 1β and interleukin 6 appearance during lethal bacteremia. J Exp Med 170:1627, 1989

202. Riddington DW, Venkatesh B, Boivin CM, et al: Intestinal permeability, gastric intramucosal pH, and systemic endotoxemia in patients undergoing cardiopulmonary bypass. JAMA 275:1007, 1996

203. O'Dwyer ST, Michie HR, Ziegler TR, et al: A single dose of endotoxin increases intestinal permeability in healthy humans. Arch Surg 123:1459, 1988

204. Coleman W, DuBois EF: Calorimetric observations on the metabolism of typhoid patients with and without food. Arch Intern Med 15:887, 1915

205. Beisel WR, Sawyer WD, Ryll ED, et al: Metabolic effects of intracellular infections in man. Ann Intern Med 67:744, 1967

206. Aulick LH, McManus AT, Mason AD Jr, et al: Effects of infection on oxygen consumption and core temperature in experimental thermal injury. Ann Surg 204:48, 1986

207. Guo L, Lim KB, Gunn JS, et al: Regulation of lipid A modifications by Salmonella typhimurium virulence genes phoP-phoQ. Science 276:250, 1997

208. Mekalanos JJ: Environmental signals controlling expression of virulence determinants in bacteria. J Bacteriol 174:1, 1992

209. Springer TA: Traffic signals for lymphocyte recirculation and leukocyte emigration: the multistep paradigm. Cell 76:301, 1994

210. Demling RH: Adult respiratory distress syndrome: current concepts. New Horizons 1:388, 1993

211. Biffl WL, Moore EE, Moore FA, et al: Interleukin-6 delays neutrophil apoptosis via a mechanism involving platelet-activating factor. J Trauma 40:575, 1996

212. Herndon DN, Barrow RE, Rutan TC, et al: Effect of propranolol administration on hemodynamic and metabolic responses of burned pediatric patients. Ann Surg 208:484, 1988

213. Schulze A, Sommer P, Bigler D, et al: Effect of combined prednisolone, epidural analgesia, and indomethacin on the systemic response after colonic surgery. Arch Surg 127:325, 1992

214. Vincent J-L: New therapies in sepsis. Chest 112:330S, 1997

215. Hammarqvist F, Wernerman J, Ali R, et al: Addition of glutamine to total parenteral nutrition after elective abdominal surgery spares free glutamine in muscle, counteracts the fall in muscle protein synthesis, and improves nitrogen balance. Ann Surg 209:455, 1989

216. Ziegler TR, Young LS, Benfell K, et al: Clinical and metabolic efficacy of glutamine-supplemented parenteral nutrition after bone marrow transplantation: a randomized, double blind, controlled study. Ann Intern Med 116: 821, 1992

217. Kudsk KA, Minard G, Croce MA, et al: A randomized trial of isonitrogenous enteral diets after severe trauma: an immune-enhancing diet reduces septic complications. Ann Surg 224:531, 1996

218. Manson JM, Wilmore DW: Positive nitrogen balance with human growth hormone and hypocaloric intravenous feeding. Surgery 100:188, 1986

219. Jiang Z-M, He G-Z, Zhang S-Y, et al: Low dose growth hormone and hypocaloric nutrition attenuate the protein-catabolic response following major operation. Ann Surg 210:513, 1989

220. Herndon DN, Barrow RE, Kunkel KR, et al: Effects of recombinant human growth hormone on donorsite healing in severely burned children. Ann Surg 212:424, 1990

221. Knox J, Demling R, Wilmore D, et al: Increased survival after major thermal injury: the effect of growth hormone therapy in adults. J Trauma 39:526, 1995

222. Pharmacia & Upjohn: Safety statement from Pharmacia & Upjohn regarding the use of recombinant somatropin (Genotropin/Genotonorm) for treatment of acute catabolism in critically ill patients. Kalamazoo, Michigan, 1997

223. Demling RH, DeSanti L: Oxandrolone, an anabolic steroid, significantly increases the rate of weight gain in the recovery phase after major burns. J Trauma 43:47, 1997

224. Tishler ME, Leng E, Al-Kanhal M, et al: Metabolic response of muscle to trauma: altered control of protein turnover. Clinical Nutrition and Metabolic Research: Proceedings of the 7th Congress of ESPEN, Munich 1985. Dietze D, Grünert A, Kleinberger G, et al, Eds. S Karger, Basel, 1986, p 40

225. Inculet RI, Finley RI, Duff JH, et al: Insulin decreases muscle protein loss after operative trauma in man. Surgery 99:752, 1986

226. Bower RH, Muggia-Sullam M, Vallgren S, et al: Branched chain amino acid–enriched solutions in the septic patient: a randomized prospective trial. Ann Surg 203:13, 1986

227. Cole M, Lipp J, Bessey PQ: Effective glucose control in the critically ill using a bedside, algorithm controlled insulin infusion (in preparation).

228. Pruitt BA Jr, Mason AD Jr: Epidemiological, demographic and outcome characteristics of burn injury. Total Burn Care. Herndon, DN. WB Saunders Co, London, 1996, p 5

229. Milberg JA, Davis DR, Steinberg KP, et al: Improved survival of patients with acute respiratory distress syndrome (ARDS) 1983–1993. JAMA 273:306, 1995

230. Kelleman JJ 3rd, Cioffi WG Jr, Mason AD Jr, et al: Effect of ambient temperature on metabolic rate after thermal injury. Ann Surg 223:406, 1996

231. Beisel WR: Magnitude of host nutritional responses to infection. Am J Clin Nutr 30:1237, 1977

232. Michie HR, Wilmore DW: Sepsis, signals, and surgical sequelae. Arch Surg 125:531, 1990

Acknowledgments

Figures 1 and 5   Al Miller.

Figure 3   Nancy Lou Makris.

9 NUTRITIONAL SUPPORT

John L. Rombeau, M.D., Rolando H. Rolandelli, M.D., Douglas W. Wilmore, M.D., and John M. Daly, M.D.

Nutritional Management of Hospitalized Patients

Evaluation of the Need for Nutritional Support

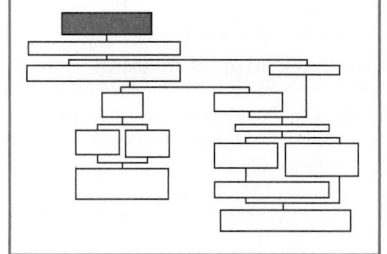

INDICATIONS FOR NUTRITIONAL INTERVENTION

In general, nutritional support should be considered in the following circumstances:

1. The patient has been without nutrition for 5 to 7 days. In a well-nourished individual, body stores are generally adequate to provide nutrients during shorter periods of stress without compromising physiologic functions, altering resistance to infection, or impairing wound healing. Patients who are unable to ingest nutrients orally usually receive intravenous solutions containing 5% dextrose, which provides some energy (approximately 170 kcal/L) and reduces, to varying degrees, protein breakdown. The provision of nutrients becomes more important as body stores become eroded because of inadequate food intake and accelerated catabolism. In general, deficits occur in surgical patients after 7 to 10 days of partial starvation; nutritional intervention should be initiated before this time.

2. The duration of illness is anticipated to be more than 10 days. In patients whose illness is known to have a moderately prolonged course, nutritional support should be considered essential care. Thus, individuals with severe peritonitis or pancreatitis, major injury (injury severity score > 15), or extensive burns (> 20% total body surface area) are candidates for nutritional support because of the known duration of their illness. (The duration of illness in chronically malnourished patients also would be expected to exceed 10 days.)

3. The patient is malnourished (loss of > 15% of usual body weight over 3 months). In general, the degree of weight loss can be used as an index of nutritional deficiency, and recovery may be compromised in patients who do not have adequate body nutrient stores because of an existing nutritional deficit [*see Figure 1*]. The patient should receive nutritional support when the weight loss approaches or exceeds 15% of usual body weight:

$$\% \text{ Weight loss} = \frac{\text{Usual weight} - \text{Present weight}}{\text{Usual weight}} \times 100$$

Patients who do not meet one of these three general indications should be reassessed after 7 days to identify individuals in whom complications develop after admission to the hospital and who require nutritional support. Serum proteins with a short half-life, such as prealbumin, transferrin, or retinol-binding protein, are useful markers for serial assessments.

PRIORITY OF CARDIOPULMONARY FUNCTION

Intensive care unit patients are frequently candidates for nutritional support but often have a number of complex medical and surgical problems that may take precedence. In decreasing order of importance, the priorities are maintenance of airway, breathing, circulation, tissue oxygenation, acid-base neutrality, normal electrolyte concentrations, and adequate nutrition. The six functions that take priority over nutrition are usually impaired by acute and potentially life-threatening disorders that are often correctable over the short term. To optimize nutrient metabolism, circulation and tissue oxygenation must be adequate. In addition, hydrogen ion and electrolyte concentrations should be near normal in the extracellular fluid compartment, as reflected by blood or serum measurements.

If cardiopulmonary function is abnormal, nutrient administration may potentiate the abnormalities and create additional problems. For example, in a patient with respiratory insufficiency, infusion of moderate quantities of carbohydrate could increase carbon dioxide tension (P_{CO_2}) and lower serum potassium concentration. These changes could initiate a life-threatening cardiac

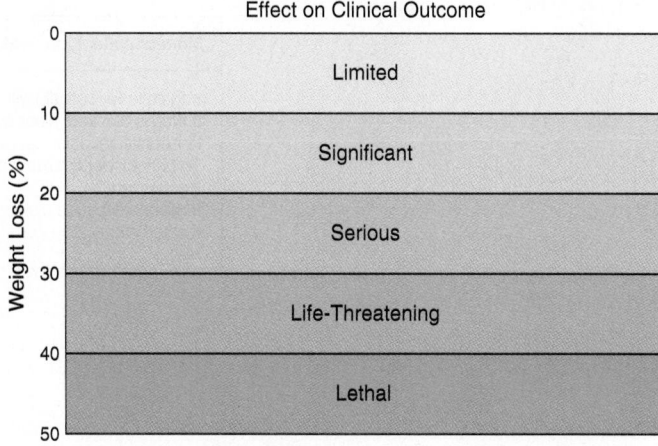

Figure 1 The magnitude of weight loss is a rough predictor of its effect on clinical outcome.

Give nutritional support if any of the following conditions is present:
- **Patient has been without nutrition for 7–10 days**
- **Expected duration of illness > 10 days**
- **Patient is malnourished (weight loss > 15% of usual weight)**

If nutritional intervention is not indicated initially, reassess patient after 5 days.

Initiate nutritional support only if tissue perfusion is adequate and Po$_2$, Pco$_2$, electrolyte concentrations, and acid-base balance are near normal

Estimate requirements for fluid, calories, protein, minerals, trace elements, and vitamins according to BMR, disease state, and activity level.

Abdominal distention, diarrhea, massive GI hemorrhage, obstruction, and hemodynamic instability are absent

Use existing nasogastric tube for enteral nutrition. Verify location of NG tube by aspiration of GI contents or by x-ray. Select balanced or disease-specific diet; deliver 30 ml/hr continuously at isotonicity for 24 hr. Elevate head during and after feeding to prevent regurgitation. Assess feeding tolerance.

Enteral feeding is tolerated

Assess risk for aspiration. Risk factors include depressed sensorium, gastroesophageal reflux, and history of aspiration or regurgitation.

Risk for aspiration is low

Give continuous gastric feedings of an isotonic formula at 30 ml/hr. Increase rate daily by 30 ml/hr. Increase tonicity after increasing volume.

Risk for aspiration is high

Pass feeding tube into jejunum; verify tube location by x-ray. Give formulas of 300 mOsm/kg at an initial rate of 30 ml/hr. Increase rate daily by 30 ml/hr. Increase tonicity after volume is fully increased.

Monitor patient; prevent and treat complications as necessary

Irrigate tube routinely with 20–25 ml normal saline or water.
If tube is blocked, clear by injection of a small volume of carbonated beverage.
For persistent diarrhea, give kaolin-pectin, 30 ml q. 3 hr.
To prevent peptic ulcers and bleeding, titrate gastric pH to 4.5–6.5 with antacids if necessary.
If nasoenteric tube dislodgment is recurrent, consider tube enterostomy.
If enterostomy tube leaks persistently, replace with tube of larger diameter.

Nutritional Management of Hospitalized Patients

Abdominal distention, diarrhea, massive GI hemorrhage, obstruction, or hemodynamic instability is present

Enteral feeding not tolerated

Symptoms of intolerance include increased gastric residuum, worsening of diarrhea, emesis, severe abdominal cramping, and abdominal distention.

Administer parenteral nutrition into central or peripheral vein

Initiate central venous infusion

Indications include
- Duration of I.V. feeding > 10 days
- Increased energy needs (≥ 2,200 kcal/day) but normal or limited fluid requirements (< 2.5 L/day)
- Organ failure

Initiate peripheral venous infusion

Indications include
- Duration of I.V. feeding 5–10 days
- Patient is nondepleted, can tolerate 2.5–3.0 L fluid/day, and has near-basal energy requirements
- Central venous catheterization is contraindicated or impossible, or central line is used for other purposes
- Enteral feedings are inadequate and must be supplemented with peripheral infusions

Insert central line (preferably a percutaneously inserted central catheter [PICC]), and order nutrient mix

Use chest x-ray to confirm placement in superior vena cava. Adjust solution for organ failure. Reserve catheter or lumen exclusively for nutrient administration.

Monitor patient

If body weight falls gradually for 2 wk or longer, calculate metabolic rate and increase calorie intake to match.
Give sufficient protein to avoid negative nitrogen balance.
Treat hyperglycemia with insulin; if glucose intolerance is severe, decrease glucose and increase fat emulsion administered.
Ensure catheter asepsis.

Table 1 Alterations in Metabolic Rate

Patient Condition	Basal Metabolic Rate
No postoperative complications Fistula without infection	Normal
Mild peritonitis Long-bone fracture or mild to moderate injury	25% above normal
Severe injury or infection in ICU patient Multiorgan failure	50% above normal
Burn of 40%–100% of TBS	100% above normal

arrhythmia. The need for nutritional support in the ICU patient should always be evaluated with respect to other care problems; acute disorders of cardiorespiratory function, disturbed acid-base status, and altered electrolyte concentrations should generally be corrected before nutritional support is initiated.

NUTRIENT REQUIREMENTS

The energy requirements of an individual are primarily related to body size, age, gender, and energy expenditure of activity (muscular work). In hospitalized patients who are generally inactive, the basal metabolic rate (BMR) accounts for the greatest amount of energy expenditure. The BMR can be calculated according to the Harris-Benedict formulas[1]:

Males: BMR (kcal/day) = 66 + [13.7 × weight (kg)] + [5 × height (cm)] – [6.8 × age (yr)]

Females: BMR (kcal/day) = 665 + [9.6 × weight (kg)] + [1.7 × height (cm)] – [4.7 × age (yr)]

The BMR is influenced by the disease process; hypermetab-

olism occurs in surgical patients with moderate to severe infection or injury. In these individuals, the magnitude of the increase in the BMR depends on the extent of injury or infection. Patients generally fall into one of four categories according to their metabolic requirements [see Table 1].

Estimates that are based on normal basal metabolic requirements and adjusted only for the disease state of the patient should reflect the energy needs of patients requiring mechanical ventilation or those at bed rest. However, further adjustments are necessary for individuals who are out of bed and physically active: they should receive additional calories. To meet the energy needs of physically active patients, who are in a nonbasal state, calculated requirements should be increased an additional 15% to 20%. The metabolic response to stress and critical illness is complex and is mediated by interactions between the neuroendocrine system and circulating cytokines. This interaction produces a metabolic milieu in which the body cannot utilize supranormal amounts of nutritional substrates (i.e., hyperalimentation). In fact, administering excessive nutrients with the purported goal of acutely correcting nutrient deficits is often harmful, leading to an abnormal accumulation of hepatic glycogen, enhancing total energy expenditure, and causing increased urea production and elevation of the blood urea nitrogen (BUN).

Weight gain usually should not be a priority for ICU patients. Complications of nutrient delivery are minimized and nutrient metabolism is generally optimized if the ICU patient receives only the energy necessary for weight maintenance throughout a complex and complicated clinical course. (This quantity of energy rarely exceeds 35 total calories/kg body weight/day in most general surgical patients who are admitted to the ICU for non–trauma-related care.) With resolution of the disease process, the hormonal environment is altered to favor anabolism. In addition, increases in spontaneous activity and in planned exercise stimulate rebuilding of lean body mass.

Table 2 Vitamin Requirements

Vitamin	Units	Recommended Dietary Allowance (RDA) for Daily Oral Intake[134]	Daily Requirement of the Moderately Injured	Daily Requirement of the Severely Injured	Amount Provided by One Vitamin Pill	Daily Amount Provided by Standard Intravenous Preparations[135]
Vitamin A (retinol)	IU	1,760 (females)–3,300 (males)	5,000	5,000	10,000	3,300 (retinal)
Vitamin D (ergocalciferol)	IU	200	400	400	400	200
Vitamin E (tocopherol)	mg TE	8–10	unknown	unknown	15	10 IU*
Vitamin K (phylloquinone)	μg	20–40†	20	20	0	0‡
Vitamin C (ascorbic acid)	mg	60	75	300	100	100
Thiamine (vitamin B_1)	mg	1.0–1.5	2	10	10	3.0
Riboflavin (vitamin B_2)	mg	1.2–1.7	2	10	10	3.6
Niacin	mg	13–19	20	100	100	40
Pyridoxine (vitamin B_6)	mg	2.0–2.2	2	40	5	4.0
Pantothenic acid	mg	4–7 (adults)†	18	40	20	15
Folic acid	mg	0.4	1.5	2.5	0	0.4
Vitamin B_{12}	μg	3.0	2	4	5	5
Biotin	μg	100–200†	unknown	unknown	0	60

*Equivalent to RDA. †Estimated to be safe and adequate dietary intakes. ‡Must be supplemented in peripheral venous solutions.

Table 3 Trace Mineral Requirements

Mineral	Recommended Dietary Allowance (RDA) for Daily Oral Intake (mg)	Suggested Daily Intravenous Intake[136] (mg)	Daily Amount Provided by a Commercially Available Mixture (mg)
Zinc	15	2.5–5.0*	5.0
Copper	2–3†	0.5–1.5	1.0
Manganese	2.5–5.0†	0.15–0.8	0.5
Chromium	0.05–0.2†	0.01–0.015	0.1
Iron	10 (males)–18 (females)	3	—

*Burn patients require an additional 2 mg. †Estimated to be safe and adequate dietary intakes.

Protein

After energy requirements are determined, protein needs are calculated. The protein requirement for most individuals is 0.8 g/kg body weight/day (about 60 to 70 g protein/day). Critically ill patients may need 1.5 to 2.0 g protein/kg/day. Most standard enteral and parenteral feeding mixtures provide this increased quantity of protein if sufficient volume of formula is delivered to meet the increased caloric requirements of these patients. The nitrogen-to-calorie ratio for most feeding formulas prepared for surgical patients is 1:150 (i.e., 1 g of nitrogen for every 150 kcal).

The contraindications to this increased quantity of protein (a daily amount of 100 to 150 g, which is equivalent to the amount of protein in a lean 16 oz steak) are renal failure before dialysis (BUN > 40 mg/dl) and hepatic encephalopathy. Patients with systemic inflammatory response syndrome often require increased quantities of dietary protein [see VII:7 Multiple Organ Dysfunction Syndrome]. Nutritional support reduces net nitrogen losses in such patients, but positive or even neutral nitrogen balance is generally not achieved because of the disturbance in metabolism and reduced intake of dietary protein.

Vitamins and Minerals

The requirements for vitamins, minerals, and trace elements are usually met when adequate volumes of balanced nutrient formulas are provided [see Tables 2 and 3]. The requirements for most of the major minerals (sodium, potassium, chloride, phosphorus, magnesium, and zinc) are satisfied by monitoring serum concentrations of these elements and adjusting intake to maintain levels within the normal range. Some minerals and electrolytes are restricted in patients with renal failure. Although serum concentrations may not directly reflect total body deficits, sufficient quantities of these nutrients are available to support normal cellular functions if adequate blood concentrations are maintained. Most premixed enteral formulas provide adequate quantities of these substances if caloric needs are met. Vitamins and trace elements must be added to parenteral solutions.

Pharmacologic Recommendations for Stress in Surgical Patients

The doses of vitamins given are often not the recommended dietary allowance (RDA) but rather some multiple of the RDA; for example, stressed patients usually receive three to 10 times the RDA for normal persons.

The prescription of vitamins and minerals for therapeutic use should be based on the patient's nutritional history as well as on estimated requirements for the current disease state. These considerations are particularly important in prescription of the fat-soluble vitamins, which are stored in body fat and thus may become toxic at high levels. Current recommendations stipulate that therapeutic dosages of vitamins not exceed 10 times the recommended dietary allowance.[2] However, it has been suggested that some vitamins may be safe if given at dosages 50 to 100 times the RDA[3] [see Table 4]. Vitamins and minerals are sometimes given in large dosages to exert antioxidant effects. Vitamins A, C, and E and the minerals zinc and selenium can attenuate the tissue-damaging effects of free radicals. Many physicians are giving these vitamins and minerals as supplements to injured and infected patients[4]; supplementation with glutamine should also be considered because of its ability to enhance intracellular glutathione stores, which also play a major antioxidant role [see Discussion, below].

Enteral Nutrition

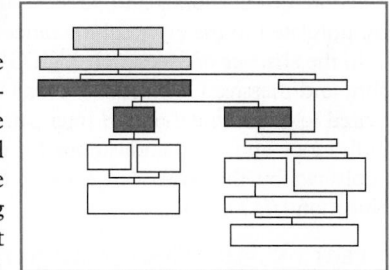

Enteral nutrition is the provision of liquid-formula diets by mouth or tube into the gastrointestinal tract. The GI tract is the preferred site for feeding the critically ill patient. It cannot be used safely, however, in patients who are hemodynamically unstable or who have abdominal distention, intestinal obstruction, or massive GI bleeding. For patients who are able to receive enteral nutrition, either a balanced or a modified diet is selected on the basis of diagnosis and nutritional requirements. An isotonic (approximately 300 mOsm/kg) diet is given continuously for a trial period of 24 hours. If the patient tolerates this regimen but is at increased risk for aspiration, feeding is delivered into the jejunum rather than into the stomach. A standard protocol is helpful in reducing complications.

SAFE USE OF THE GASTROINTESTINAL TRACT FOR FEEDING

Enteral nutrition should be prescribed only if safety and a low complication rate can be ensured. To determine whether the critically ill patient can be fed safely via the GI tract, a clinical assessment of intestinal function is performed. A good determinant of safe tolerance of enteral nutrition is a GI output of less than 600 ml/24 hr. For the purpose of these guidelines, GI output is defined as the volume of effluent from a nasogastric tube, ostomy, or rectal tube. Examples of conditions in critically ill patients that produce excessively high (> 600 ml/24 hr) GI outputs and therefore preclude the use of enteral nutrition are gastroparesis, intestinal obstruction, paralytic ileus, high-output enteric fistulas, antibiotic-

Table 4 Safety Levels of Vitamins[3]

Safety Level	Vitamin
At least 50 to 100 times RDA	Vitamin B$_1$ Vitamin B$_2$ Niacin Vitamin C Vitamin E Biotin Folic acid Pantothenic acid
10 times RDA	Vitamin A Vitamin B$_6$ Vitamin D Vitamin K

induced colitis, severe idiopathic diarrhea, and the initial phase of short bowel syndrome. Selected patients with enteric losses exceeding 600 ml/24 hr may receive enteral nutrition, however, if carefully monitored by an experienced team.

Another major cause of increased GI output is massive GI bleeding. Conditions that produce bleeding of this magnitude include peptic ulcer disease, esophageal varices, diverticulosis, and angiodysplasia of the colon. Mild bleeding such as that produced by stress gastritis may actually resolve with the delivery of enteral nutrition into the stomach because the liquid diet buffers gastric acid.[5] Enteral nutrition does not exacerbate mild lower intestinal bleeding.

Although commonly used at bedside as indicators of intestinal function, bowel sounds and passage of flatus are nonspecific and are unrelated to the eventual tolerance of enteral nutrition.

In the absence of excessively high GI output, abdominal distention, and massive GI bleeding, a trial of enteral nutrition is warranted to determine if the GI tract can be used safely for feeding.[6] Indications and contraindications for enteral nutrition have been published by the American Society for Parenteral and Enteral Nutrition [*see Table 5*].[7]

SELECTION OF DIET AND STARTING THE DELIVERY

Before delivery of enteral nutrition, the appropriate diet must be selected on the basis of the patient's nutrient requirements [*see Indications for Nutritional Intervention, above*]. Most liquid-formula diets consist of either a balanced or a modified formula.

Balanced diets contain carbohydrates, proteins, and fats in complex (polymeric) forms in proportions similar to those of a regular Western diet. Frequently, however, the fat content is reduced to 10% to 15% of total calories, and the carbohydrate content is increased. Carbohydrates are present as oligosaccharides, polysaccharides, or maltodextrins; fats consist of medium- or long-chain triglycerides. The nitrogen source is a natural protein, which may be either intact or partially hydrolyzed. In general, balanced diets are isotonic, lactose free, and available in ready-to-use, liquid form. Flavored balanced diets can be used for oral supplementation as well as for enteral tube feeding.

Selection of a balanced diet is based on nutrient and fluid requirements. The caloric density of balanced diets can be 1.0, 1.5, or 2.0 kcal/ml. The largest number of commercially available diets provide 1.0 kcal/ml. The nonprotein caloric content of these diets is derived from either carbohydrates or lipids. Balanced diets formulated with carbohydrates as the main caloric source have higher osmolarity than isocaloric diets containing lipids. These carbohydrate-based diets are well tolerated when adminis-

tered directly into the stomach and may be helpful for patients with steatorrhea. Balanced diets that are fat based may be more appropriate for patients who have diarrhea caused by diet hyperosmolarity, especially when feedings are infused directly into the small intestine. However, fat malabsorption is common in critically ill patients when the fat content of the diet exceeds 30% of total calories. In modified formulas, the proportions and types of nutrients differ from those of a regular Western diet. Manufacturers of enteral diets have introduced these modifications to meet the special nutrient needs of patients with renal failure or short bowel syndrome.

Modified diets are also known as elemental diets or chemically defined diets. These diets contain crystalline amino acids or short peptides in compositions that differ from the reference composition of proteins of high biologic value, such as egg albumin. The fat-to-carbohydrate ratio of these modified diets varies depending on the purpose of the modification. The source of carbohydrate is either dextrose or oligosaccharides; fats are usually in the form of medium-chain triglycerides, essential fatty acids, or both. Because they are not palatable, modified diets are rarely used as oral supplements. Modified diets are further characterized according to the conditions for which they are formulated: stress, immunomodulation, and hepatic, renal, respiratory, or GI dysfunction [*see Table 6*].

Hepatic formulas are indicated for patients with hepatic failure who are hypercatabolic and encephalopathic. When such patients

Table 5 Indications for Enteral Nutrition (Partial Listing)

Considered Routine Care in the Following:
  Protein-calorie malnutrition with inadequate oral intake of nutrients for the previous 5–7 days
  Normal nutritional status but < 50% of required oral intake of nutrients for the previous 7–10 days
  Severe dysphagia
  Major full-thickness burns
  Low-output enterocutaneous fistulas
  Major trauma

Usually Helpful in the Following:
  Radiation therapy
  Mild chemotherapy
  Liver failure and severe renal dysfunction
  Massive small bowel resection (> 50%) in combination with administration of total parenteral nutrition

Of Limited or Undetermined Value in the Following:
  Intensive chemotherapy
  Immediate postoperative period or poststress period
  Acute enteritis
  > 90% resection of small bowel

Contraindicated in the Following:
  Complete mechanical intestinal obstruction
  Abdominal distention
  Ileus or intestinal hypomotility
  Severe diarrhea
  Severe GI bleeding
  High-output external fistulas
  Severe, acute pancreatitis
  Shock
  Case of aggressive nutritional support not desired by the patient or legal guardian and respect of such wish being in accordance with hospital policy and existing law
  Prognosis not warranting aggressive nutritional support

receive standard protein sources, neurologic symptoms may be aggravated. Hepatic formulas contain increased amounts of branched-chain amino acids (BCAAs) and decreased quantities of aromatic amino acids (i.e., phenylalanine, tyrosine, and tryptophan) and of the sulfur-containing amino acid methionine. These formulas were initially developed for parenteral nutrition to reduce the availability of aromatic amino acids, which are precursors of neurotransmitters synthesized in excess during the development of hepatic encephalopathy.[8]

Renal formulas contain all essential amino acids, including histidine, but lack the nonessential amino acids. These formulas promote the reuse of urea nitrogen associated with hepatic transamination, which is one step in the synthesis of nonessential amino acids.[9,10] Renal diets are indicated for patients with renal failure who do not need dialysis and are not receiving broad-spectrum antibiotics, which reduce urea recycling by colonic bacteria.

The composition of enteral diets can also be altered to reduce carbon dioxide production in ventilator-dependent patients.[11] This reduction is accomplished by increasing the ratio of fat to carbohydrate in the formula. This approach has been shown to be effective when nutrients are given intravenously[12]; however, controlled clinical trials are needed in enterally fed patients.

Diets for patients with GI dysfunction have modified nitrogen and fat composition. Transport of dietary nitrogen across the intestinal mucosa is enhanced when nitrogen is provided in the form of short peptides rather than free amino acids. It is also well documented that the small bowel mucosa utilizes glutamine as the preferred fuel [see Discussion, below]. Consequently, some modified diets contain nitrogen in the form of short peptides, whereas others have an extra amount of glutamine. Medium-chain triglycerides (MCTs) are more easily absorbed and metabolized than long-chain triglycerides (LCTs). Diets modified for improved absorption contain a higher proportion of MCT oil. These diets may be efficacious when used during the transition phase after a period of prolonged bowel rest or when the intestine is inflamed. Controlled trials are necessary to verify their clinical efficacy. Stress formulas are indicated for hypercatabolic patients whose nitrogen balance continues to be negative despite increased intake of a balanced diet. Stress formulas are often enriched with BCAAs (e.g., leucine, valine, and isoleucine) in an attempt to improve nitrogen balance by providing precursors for synthesis of muscle protein.[13] Little evidence supports the use of diets that provide BCAAs in concentrations higher than 20% to 25% of total amino acid content for stressed patients.

The fat sources used for enteral diets are primarily omega-6 fatty acids—the arachidonic acid family. Ongoing research suggests that supplementation with omega-3 fatty acids—the eicosapentaenoic acid family—results in the synthesis of eicosanoids (prostaglandins, leukotrienes, and thromboxanes) that enhance the immune response [see Discussion, below]. The immune response can also be improved by supplemental arginine and glutamine; diets formulated for immunomodulation are enriched with these nutrients. The administration of one of these diets, which also contained RNA, is reported to have reduced postoperative complications and hospital stay after surgery for GI malignancies and trauma.[14]

ASSESSMENT OF FEEDING TOLERANCE

The selected formula is started at isotonicity and delivered continuously at 30 ml/hr for 24 hours. During this initial trial,

the formula is delivered via a previously inserted Salem sump or rubber nasogastric (Levin) tube. If a nasogastric tube is not already in place, a soft tube made of either silicone rubber or polyurethane is inserted (see below).

Feeding tolerance is assessed for the first 24 hours. Poor tolerance is indicated by vomiting and severe abdominal cramps, gastric residuum greater than 50% of the volume administered during the previous 4-hour period of feeding, increased abdominal distention (a particularly important factor to assess in comatose patients and individuals being mechanically ventilated), and worsening of diarrhea. If any one of these conditions is present, parenteral nutrition is recommended. If there is no evidence of feeding intolerance, the patient is assessed for the risk for aspiration.

ASSESSMENT OF RISK FOR ASPIRATION

Aspiration is a major complication in patients receiving enteral nutrition.[15] The propensity to aspirate enteral feedings is often related to the patient's primary disease and neurologic status as well as to the site of GI access and the method of delivery.

Important factors in assessing risk for aspiration include depressed sensorium, increased gastroesophageal reflux, and history of previously documented episodes of aspiration. Depressed sensorium in the critical care setting is secondary to organic lesions of the central nervous system, metabolic encephalopathies, or medications. Head trauma, hypoxemia, hepatic and septic encephalopathies, and the use of H_2 receptor blockers are common causes of depressed sensorium in critically ill patients. Increased gastroesophageal reflux may be present in individuals with reduced lower esophageal sphincter pressure and increased intragastric pressure. Many medications used in the ICU, such as theophylline, anticholinergics, calcium channel blocking agents, beta-adrenergic agonists, and alpha-adrenergic antagonists, cause a reduction in lower esophageal sphincter pressure.[16] Finally, a history of aspiration places the patient at increased risk for recurrent episodes.

For most enterally fed patients, safety demands that the head be elevated at feeding time and for some period thereafter to prevent regurgitation. If elevating the patient's head is not possible, an alternative site of nutrient delivery should be considered. Nasogastric intubation, in particular, requires elevation of the head because the tube may render the upper and lower esophageal sphincters incompetent and liable to reflux. Even the presence of a tracheostomy or endotracheal tube does not ensure that regurgitated gastric contents will not be aspirated. Liquid filling the pharynx will inevitably trickle past even an overinflated endotracheal tube cuff and into the lung. Aspiration of liquid formulas can be verified if a bit of food coloring or methylene blue is included in the feeding mixture and subsequently detected in pharyngeal and tracheal secretions.[17]

ACCESS FOR FEEDING

In most general and thoracic surgical patients, access for feeding is most commonly obtained via the stomach or jejunum. Methods of access for intragastric feedings include nasogastric tubes and feeding gastrostomies placed through a laparotomy or percutaneously with the aid of endoscopy, fluoroscopy, or laparoscopy.

Table 6 Composition of Modified Diets

Formula	Protein (g/L)	Carbohydrate (g/L)	Fat (g/L)	Ratio of Nitrogen (g) to Nonprotein Calories (kcal)	Caloric Density (kcal/ml)	Product* (Manufacturer)
Elemental	50	127	34	1:100	1.0	Subdue (Mead Johnson Nutritionals)
	40	127	39	1:131	1.0	Peptamen (Nestlé Clinical Nutrition)
Stress	56	130	28	1:71	1.0	Impact (Novartis)
	66	177	37	1:97	1.3	Perative (Ross Laboratories)
Hepatic	44	168	36	1:148	1.2	Hepatic Aid II (B. Braun Medical Inc.)
Renal	19	365	46	1:800	2.0	Amin-Aid (R&D Laboratories)

*Partial listing.

Nasogastric tubes provide the most common method of access for gastric feeding. Tubes made of polyurethane or silicone rubber are preferred because they are soft, nonreactive, and well tolerated by most patients. They are also less corrosive to the nasopharynx than tubes made of rubber or polyvinyl chloride. The soft consistency of these tubes often makes insertion into critically ill patients difficult and precludes the checking of gastric residuum. Difficulties of tube passage into the stomach are increased when thin, floppy tubes are inserted into obtunded patients. Useful aids include stylets, judicious use of gravity and positioning, and designation of especially experienced and certified nursing personnel to assist in this task [*see Table 7*].

Passage of a tube through the pylorus into the jejunum may be necessary if the patient is at increased risk for aspiration (see above). Our practice is to place the tube into the stomach, to position the patient on the right side for several hours once or twice in the next 24 hours, and then to obtain an abdominal roentgenogram. If the tube has not passed, 10 mg of metoclopramide is given intravenously while the patient is still in the radiology department, and the roentgenogram is repeated. If the location of the feeding tube is still not evident, a small amount of contrast material can be given through the tube to verify the position.

If the tube still has not passed through the pylorus, the aid of the fluoroscopist is enlisted. (Interventional radiologists take justifiable pride in their ability to cannulate almost any internal orifice.) Finally, if all else has failed and no alternative route for nutrition is appropriate, the GI endoscopist can capture the tube tip in the stomach with the biopsy forceps of the flexible endoscope (aided by a suture through the tube end) and guide the tube through the pylorus.[18]

When any type of nasoenteric tube is placed to administer enteral nutrition, verification of tube location before starting feedings is mandatory. The simplest means of assessing proper tube placement in the GI tract is by the aspiration of gastric contents, the source of which can be confirmed by measuring the pH of the aspirate. Because small-bore, soft tubes tend to collapse under high negative pressure, a small syringe should be used to aspirate gastric contents. If gastric contents cannot be aspirated through the tube, radiographic confirmation of tube location is mandatory before enteral feedings are started. Because feeding tubes are often radiopaque, a simple plain film of the abdomen may be adequate. If the exact location of the tube is still in doubt, a small amount of contrast material can be injected through the tube. Placement of the distal tip of the tube in the duodenum is usually confirmed by abdominal roentgenogram before transpyloric

feedings are started. The tube should be inserted to a length sufficient to permit migration into the proximal jejunum.

Simple insufflation of air into the tube is not sufficient to verify the position of the tube. Auscultation over the stomach can detect sound transmitted through a tube that has been inadvertently passed into the bronchial tree. Many of these tubes are small enough to pass through the glottis and the trachea without markedly interfering with phonation or respiration. Enteral formulas delivered into the bronchial tree through a misplaced tube can cause severe pneumonitis and death.

The development of percutaneous techniques for the placement of gastrostomies has been a major contribution to enteral nutrition. Percutaneous endoscopic gastrostomy (PEG) [*see V:6 Gastrointestinal Endoscopy*] is the gold standard for gastric feeding in the United States. Compared with operative gastrostomy, PEG is less expensive and is associated with fewer complications. Operative gastrostomies are most commonly created for long-term use (i.e., for more than 4 weeks of feeding) when either a nasoenteric tube cannot be inserted or severe intolerance of the

---

Table 7 Procedure for Inserting Nasoenteric Tubes

Provide privacy.

Explain procedure and its purpose.

Place patient in sitting position with neck flexed slightly and head of bed elevated to 45°.

Lubricate stylet and insert into feeding tube.

Inspect nares and determine optimal patency by having the patient breathe through one nostril while the other is temporarily occluded.

Estimate the length of tubing required to reach into the stomach by measuring the distance from the tip of the nose to the earlobe and then from the earlobe to the xiphoid process. Add 25 cm to this length for nasoduodenal intubation.

If the patient seems uncooperative, instill generous amounts of lidocaine jelly into the nares and nasopharynx before tube insertion. Lubricate the end of the tube and pass it posteriorly. Ask a cooperative patient to swallow water to facilitate passage of the tube.

Once the tube is beyond the nasopharynx, allow the patient to rest.

Have the patient continue neck flexion and swallowing while the tube is advanced.

If the patient begins to cough, withdraw the tube into the nasopharynx and then reattempt passage.

Confirm passage into the stomach by obtaining an abdominal x-ray.

Remove stylet.

Secure tube to bridge of nose or upper lip with nonallergenic tape and prevent undue pressure on external nares.

tube occurs. The Stamm [see V:9 Gastric Procedures] and Witzel techniques for these procedures are well documented.[19] Operative methods of access into the jejunum include the Witzel and Delaney techniques of tube placement.[19]

Concurrent decompression of the stomach and feeding into the small intestine have been used to reduce the risk of aspiration in critically ill patients. This combination of procedures requires either the insertion of a multilumen nasojejunal tube,[20] the surgical placement of combined gastrojejunal tubes,[19] modification of PEG,[21] or insertion of a nasogastric tube in conjunction with a surgical jejunostomy. Such access to the GI tract also provides a route for the delivery of crushed medications and the option to provide cyclic nocturnal enteral nutrition with gastric decompression (i.e., the patient receives nutrients by mouth during the day).

FEEDING REGIMENS

If the patient tolerates the initial trial of enteral nutrition, then the delivery site for future feeding is chosen according to the risk of aspiration, and the feeding regimen is gradually intensified. If the risk of aspiration is minimal, intragastric feedings are preferred. These feedings are better tolerated physiologically, easier to administer, and less restrictive for the patient than continuous feeding into the small intestine. Patients fed into the stomach receive an isotonic formula delivered continuously at a rate of 30 ml/hr. The delivery is advanced each day by 30 ml/hr [see Table 8]. If the risk of aspiration is increased, feedings are delivered via nasoduodenal or nasojejunal tubes. Patients fed into either the duodenum or the jejunum receive formulas of 300 mOsm/kg delivered at an initial rate of 30 ml/hr with the aid of a peristaltic pump. The rate is increased daily by 30 ml/hr [see Table 8].

MONITORING AND PREVENTION OF COMPLICATIONS

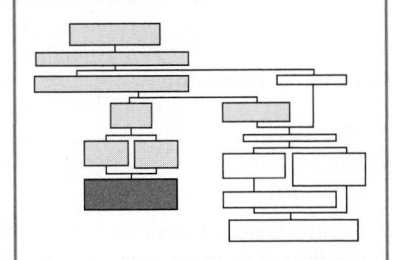

Patients who receive enteral nutrition require careful monitoring that is similar to that performed in patients who receive parenteral nutrition. Particular attention is directed to the patient's metabolic status and fluid and electrolyte balance. A protocol should be established and followed to ensure that nutritional goals are met and complications minimized. A standard checklist is helpful in starting and maintaining enteral nutrition and prevents omission of important details [see Table 9].

Four types of complications are related to enteral nutrition: gastrointestinal, mechanical, metabolic, and infectious.[22] The two most common types are gastrointestinal and mechanical complications.

The most frequent GI complication is diarrhea, which may occur in as many as 75% of critically ill patients receiving enteral nutrition. Diarrhea is best defined as stool weight greater than 300 g/24 hr or volume greater than 300 ml/24 hr; however, these measurements are impractical and difficult to obtain. A more practical definition of diarrhea is more than three loose bowel movements during a period of 24 hours. There are many causes of diarrhea in critically ill patients receiving enteral nutrition [see Figure 2]. The desired therapeutic approach is to adjust the enteral nutrition regimen accordingly rather than to discontinue it completely. Only one variable of the feeding regimen (i.e., osmolality, volume, rate, or type of diet) should be altered at a time. In our experience, critically ill patients tolerate a continuous feeding regimen better than intermittent feeding. If the patient still has diarrhea when receiv-

Table 8 Suggested Starter and Advancement Regimens for Intragastric and Intrajejunal Feeding

Feeding Regimen	Days			
	1	2	3	4
Intragastric				
mOsm/kg	300	300	300	480
ml/hr	30	60	90	90
Intrajejunal				
mOsm/kg	300	300	300	300
ml/hr	30	60	90	90

ing feeding at a rate of 30 ml/hr and at a concentration of 150 to 300 mOsm/kg, antidiarrheal treatment is indicated.

In many instances, antidiarrheal medication is given without a definite diagnosis; therefore, it is essential to select medications with both a wide therapeutic range and a low incidence of side effects. For these reasons, we prefer kaolin-pectin over opiates such as paregoric. Every 3 hours, 30 ml of kaolin-pectin solution is given through the feeding tube and followed by 25 ml of normal saline for irrigation. If this regimen is unsuccessful after 48 hours and opiates are not contraindicated, paregoric is added at a dose of 1 ml/100 ml of formula [see Figure 2]. Opiates act by slowing intestinal motility, which may promote greater bacterial overgrowth. In addition, opiates are respiratory depressants and are also contraindicated in patients with infectious diarrhea.

Several diagnostic methods may help in identifying the cause of diarrhea associated with enteral nutrition. These include the assay of stool for *Clostridium difficile* enterotoxin, analysis of stool for fat malabsorption, the D-xylose test for carbohydrate malabsorption, and breath H_2 analysis for bacterial overgrowth. The D-xylose test and the breath H_2 analysis are more commonly used in non–critically ill patients with diarrhea associated with enteral feeding.

Table 9 Standard Orders for Enteral Nutrition

Obtain abdominal x-ray to confirm tube location before feeding.

Elevate head of bed 45° when feeding into the stomach.

Record type and strength of diet and rate of infusion.

Check gastric residuum every 4 hr in patients receiving gastric feedings. Withhold feedings for 4 hr if residuum is 50% greater than ordered volume. Notify physician if two consecutive measurements detect excessive residuum.

Check for abdominal distention. Check frequency, consistency, and volume of stool output.

Weigh patient on Monday, Wednesday, and Friday. Record weight on graph.

Record intake and output daily. For every shift, chart volume of formula administered separately from water or other oral intake.

Change administration tubing and cleanse feeding bag daily.

Irrigate feeding tube with 20 ml of water at the completion of each intermittent feeding, when tube is disconnected, after the delivery of crushed medications, of if feeding is stopped for any reason.

When patient is ingesting oral nutrients, ask the dietitian to provide calorie counts daily for 5 days, then weekly thereafter.

On a weekly basis, obtain complete blood count with red blood cell indices, SMA-12, serum iron, and serum magnesium.

Obtain SMA-6 every Monday and Thursday.

Once a week, collect urine for 24 hours, starting at 8:00 A.M., and analyze for urea nitrogen.

To prevent peptic ulcerations and bleeding, gastric acidity is controlled with H_2 receptor blockers in critically ill patients. Although these drugs help control hyperacidity, which is a cause of diarrhea, they also lead to bacterial overgrowth in the intestine.[23] Therefore, the use of H_2 receptor blockers should be avoided in patients who receive feedings into the stomach, because the presence of the liquid formula in the stomach already provides a physiologic means of buffering acid. If necessary, antacids rather than H_2 receptor blockers should be used to titrate gastric pH to 4.5 to 6.5. The amino acid glutamine is also utilized to prevent or treat ulceration of the upper GI tract.

The most common mechanical complications that are related to enteral nutrition are tube dislodgment, clogging of the tube, and leakage of enteric contents around the exit site of the tube onto the skin.[24] Tube dislodgment occurs more frequently in agitated patients and hypoxic patients. Inadvertent removal of the tube is usually prevented by adequate taping of the nasoenteric tube or, in agitated patients, by suturing the tube or using a Velcro abdominal wall binder.

Clogging or plugging of the tube often results from the failure to use saline irrigations after intermittent feedings or the inadvertent delivery of crushed medications through a small-bore tube. This complication is reduced by routine irrigations of 20 to 25 ml of normal saline or water after each intermittent feeding. Liquid medications may also help prevent this complication, although these medications are frequently hyperosmolar and may produce discomfort and diarrhea when delivered rapidly into the jejunum. The injection of a small volume of a carbonated beverage into a plugged tube will often clear the blockage. Occasionally, a guide wire and the help of the interventional radiologist will be needed.

Another mechanical complication is the leakage of enteric contents onto the skin around the exit site of a tube enterostomy. Leakage is often uncomfortable for the patient and may produce a moderate amount of skin irritation. One cause of such leakage is an excessively large incision in the skin at the exit site of the enterostomy tube. Leakage around a tube is prevented by creating the exit site so as to be almost identical in diameter to the tube. A larger tube may also be inserted through the exit site if leakage continues. The enterostomal therapist and the use of products such as karaya gum, zinc oxide, Stomahesive, and locally applied antacid are often helpful. Also problematic is the inappropriate use of urinary catheters for enteral access; these devices were not designed to function as gastrostomy or enterostomy tubes. The catheters currently preferred for these purposes are made of either silicone rubber or polyurethane and include a system to prevent migration of the tube into the stomach.

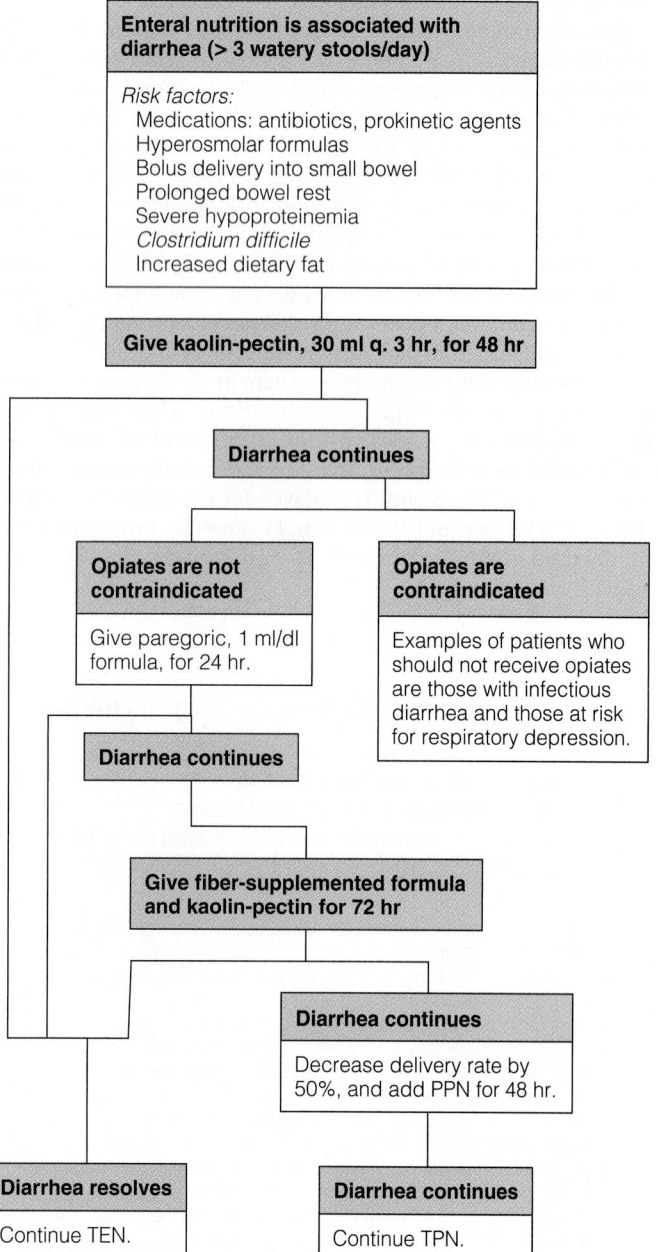

Figure 2 The decision-making approach for pharmacologic and dietary treatment of diarrhea associated with enteral nutrition is shown.

Parenteral Nutrition

CENTRAL VENOUS VERSUS PERIPHERAL VENOUS INFUSIONS

Central venous infusions are indicated in most critically ill patients who receive parenteral nutrition, because (1) patients in the intensive care unit often require increased quantities of energy and cannot tolerate large fluid volumes and (2) solutions of much greater caloric density and tonicity can be infused into central veins than can be infused into peripheral veins. Nonetheless, peripheral venous infusions may be indicated in certain situations [see Table 10]; peripheral venous infusions will be discussed in detail below.

CENTRAL VENOUS NUTRIENT INFUSION

Hypertonic nutrient solutions are infused into a large-bore central vein. These solutions are rapidly diluted, and the nutrients are delivered throughout the body by the bloodstream. Usually, the hypertonic nutrient solutions contain hypertonic glucose (25%), amino acids (5%), and other essential nutrients. The tonicity of the hypertonic nutrient solutions is so great (> 1,900 mOsm/kg) that administration of the mixture into peripheral veins would cause severe thrombophlebitis and venous sclerosis. If the solution is continuously infused at a constant rate into the superior vena cava, however, the nutrient mixture is rapidly diluted to near-iso-

---

Table 10 Indications for Central Venous
or Peripheral Venous Infusions

Central Venous Infusions

To provide adequate intravenous nutritional support for 10 days or more

To satisfy nutrient requirements in patients with increased energy needs and normal or decreased fluid requirements

To support the patient with single- or multiple-organ failure by infusing modified nutrient solutions in a limited fluid volume

Peripheral Venous Infusions

To provide initial feeding (< 5 days) before catheter insertion in a patient who will require central venous feedings

To infuse less concentrated solutions via a multiuse central catheter (i.e., a line for blood drawing, medication, and nutrients) into an individual in whom other venous access cannot be easily or safely obtained

To supplement enteral feedings that are inadequate because of gastrointestinal dysfunction

To satisfy energy requirements that are near basal (1,500–1,800 kcal/day) in a nondepleted patient who can tolerate 2.5–3.0 L I.V. solution each day

---

tonic concentrations, and the nutrients are cleared from the bloodstream by body tissues. The hypertonic nutrient solutions contain at least 1 kcal/ml, and thus, infusion of 2.0 to 2.5 L/day provides 2,000 to 2,500 kcal of energy and all essential nutrients. This calorie load is sufficient to meet energy requirements in more than 90% of surgical patients.

Once positioned, the catheter is used exclusively for administration of the hypertonic nutrient solution. Drawing blood, monitoring central venous pressure, and administering medication through this dedicated lumen are prohibited. Multiple-lumen central venous catheters are now available; manufacturers suggest that at least one port be devoted to the infusion of hypertonic nutrient solutions and additional ports be used for drawing blood, monitoring pressure, and infusing medications. Reports suggest that the rates of catheter sepsis associated with use of these lines are greater than the rates associated with single-lumen feeding catheters.[25,26] In our experience, the infection rate associated with multiple-lumen catheters was similar to that observed with single-lumen catheters (3.3% versus 1.0%, NS), but the multiple-lumen catheters were in place for a shorter period than the single-lumen catheters (7 versus 14 days).[27] Removal of the multiple-lumen catheters was indicated when multiple central access ports were no longer required or when one of the lumens became clotted or malfunctioned. It appears that multiple-lumen catheters can be used in the ICU for central venous nutrient infusions if strict protocols are maintained to ensure that one lumen is dedicated to nutrient infusion, that other lumens are handled safely, and that the catheters are removed when they are no longer required.

Occasionally, a patient may require the infusion of a hypertonic nutrient solution, when percutaneous puncture of central veins is impossible or contraindicated. In these individuals, catheterization of an antecubital vein and insertion of a peripherally inserted central catheter (PICC) with the tip positioned in the superior vena cava should be considered. These catheters are readily inserted by the interventional radiologist, and they eliminate the complications associated with infraclavicular and supraclavicular catheter insertion. The PICC line has become the primary route of central venous access in many institutions.

Newer types of catheters made of Silastic have been safely kept in place for extended periods and provide an additional option for care of patients who require central venous infusions. Catheterization of the femoral vein may provide a route for central venous access in some situations. Because of the high density of skin pathogens in the groin area, these catheters should be replaced every 2 to 3 days. If the catheter tip is positioned in the iliac vein or the inferior vena cava, the concentration of solution infused through the catheter should not exceed 15%. Strict care of the entrance site should be maintained because of the high complication rate associated with lines placed in the groin.[28]

Central Venous Solutions

Central venous solutions are formulated in the hospital pharmacy. These solutions are commonly combinations of 500 ml of 50% dextrose and 500 ml of a 10% amino acid mixture [*see Table 11*] to which electrolytes, vitamins, and trace elements are added (see below). Each day, 2 L of the solution can be infused. Administration of fat emulsion (500 ml, 20%) 1 day each week meets essential fatty acid requirements. Alternatively, the three major nutrients may be mixed together in a 3 L bag (triple mix or three-in-one) and the entire contents of the single bag infused during the 24-hour period [*see Table 11*]. Another innovation is the use of an automated mixing device (Auto-mix, Travenol Laboratories) that compounds various proportions of 70% glucose, 10% amino acids, and 20% fat emulsions into 3 L bags. This device allows the hospital pharmacy to manufacture a variety of nutrient combinations with minimal effort. More concentrated solutions can be made, and the computer will generate a label for the bag that allows nurses to verify the order.

Electrolytes and minerals are added to the base formula as required [*see Table 12*]. Sodium and potassium salts are added as chloride or acetate, depending on the acid-base status of the patient. The solution should usually consist of approximately equal quantities of chloride and acetate. If chloride losses from the body are increased, as in a patient who requires nasogastric decompression, most salts should be administered as chloride. Sodium bicarbonate is incompatible with the nutrient solutions, and acetate is administered when additional base is required (when metabolized, acetate generates bicarbonate). Phosphate is usually given as the potassium salt; sodium phos-

Table 11 Composition of Central Venous Solutions

	Standard Solution	Triple-Mix Solution
Volume		
Amino acids 10% (ml)	500	1,000
Dextrose 50% (ml)	500	1,000
Fat emulsion 20% (ml)	—	250
Total (ml)	1,000	2,250
Contents		
Amino acids (g)	50	100
Dextrose (g)	250 (25%)	500
Total nitrogen (g)	8.4	16.8
Total calories (kcal)	1,050	2,600
Ratio of nitrogen to calories	1:125	1:154
Caloric density (kcal/ml)	1.0	1.15
Osmolarity (mOsm/kg)	≈1,970	≈1,900

phate is used when potassium is contraindicated. Phosphate is also present in fat emulsions.

Commercially available preparations of vitamins, minerals, and trace elements are also added to the nutrient mix for daily administration unless they are contraindicated. A solution containing both fat- and water-soluble vitamins should be added. Vitamin K_1 (phytonadione), 10 mg, is given once a week but is contraindicated in patients receiving warfarin.

Trace elements are given daily. Usual requirements are satisfied by the addition of commercially available mixtures either to 1 L of standard solution or to the triple-mix bag each day. Trace elements are indicated for all patients receiving central venous nutrient solutions, except those with chronic renal failure or severe liver disease. At especially high risk for zinc deficiency are alcoholics and patients with pancreatic insufficiency with malabsorption, massive small bowel resection, renal failure with dialysis, or nephrotic syndrome; at high risk for copper deficiency are patients with short bowel syndrome, jejunoileal bypass, malabsorptive conditions with severe diarrhea, or nephrotic syndrome. Copper and manganese are excreted primarily via the biliary tract. Therefore, in patients with biliary tract obstruction, excess retention of copper and manganese should be avoided by decreasing intake of these ions, monitoring blood levels, or both. Although the main excretory route for zinc and chromium is via the feces, renal excretion will minimize dangers from modest excesses of these elements. In patients with renal insufficiency, however, daily zinc and chromium administration may be contraindicated. ICU patients usually do not require iron. Iron is contraindicated in patients with sepsis because iron supports bacterial growth. Iron may be required to treat iron deficiency anemia, particularly during convalescence from this condition. Rarely does the anemia that is associated with chronic disease and inflammation respond to iron therapy during the active stages of disease.

Like other invasive therapies, total parenteral nutrition (TPN) is associated with potential complications deriving either from central venous access or from the composition of the formula given. Most such complications are preventable with appropriate attention to detail [*see Table 13*].

PERIPHERAL VENOUS SOLUTIONS

Slightly hypertonic nutrient solutions (approximately 600 to 900 mOsm/kg) can be prepared for peripheral venous infusions from commercially available amino acid mixtures (5%), dextrose solutions (10%), and fat emulsions (20%). These nutrient mixtures have a low caloric density (approximately 0.3 to 0.6 kcal/ml) and thus provide only 1,200 to 2,300 kcal in 2,000 to 3,500 ml of solution. Large volumes of fluid are required.

These dilute nutrient mixtures can be infused through plastic cannulas placed in large-bore peripheral veins. The catheter insertion site and surrounding tissue should be inspected periodically for signs of phlebitis or infiltration, and the infusion site should be rotated every 48 to 72 hours to prevent thrombophlebitis. Only fat emulsion should be administered simultaneously through the same I.V. site as a peripheral venous solution. The nutrient solution should be temporarily stopped if the catheter is used for administration of antibiotics, chemotherapeutic agents, blood, or blood products. The infusion line should then be flushed with saline and infusion of the nutrient solution resumed.

If the fat emulsion is infused in a piggyback manner, administration should be performed during a period of 8 to 12 hours and concluded in the early morning (3:00 A.M.) to allow clearance of the emulsion from the bloodstream. Blood sampling should be avoided during short-term periods of fat infusion because the associat-

Table 12 Electrolytes Added to Central Venous Solutions

	Usual Electrolyte Concentration	Usual Range of Electrolyte Concentration
Sodium (mEq/L)	30	0–150
Potassium (mEq/L)	30	0–80
Phosphate (mmol/L)	15	0–20
Magnesium (mEq/L)	5	0–15
Calcium* (mEq/L)	4.7	0–10
Chloride (mEq/L)	50	0–150
Acetate (mEq/L)	70	70–220

*As gluconate.

ed hypertriglyceridemia will interfere with many of the serum measurements. In patients who are receiving peripheral venous solutions by triple mix, hypertriglyceridemia is rare because the rate of infusion has been reduced and infusion extended over a 24-hour period.

Patients receiving peripheral venous feedings should be monitored as suggested for individuals receiving central venous feedings (see below). Mechanical and septic complications are uncommon. Fluid imbalances and alterations in serum electrolyte concentrations are similar to those seen in standard I.V. support, and corrections are made by altering the volume of the infusion or adding or omitting electrolytes. Hyperglycemia and glycosuria are rarely observed unless the patient is diabetic.

MONITORING THE PATIENT: OPTIMIZING NUTRITIONAL SUPPORT, PREVENTING COMPLICATIONS, AND RESOLVING COMMON PROBLEMS

General Measures

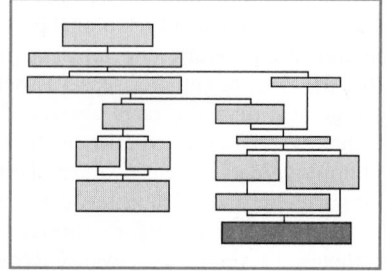

Patients receiving central venous feedings should be weighed daily, and accurate intake and output records should be maintained. Urinary glucose should be monitored daily. Persistent glucosuria indicates hyperglycemia and may be associated with a concomitant osmotic diuresis and dehydration. If such glucosuria occurs, a more stringent schedule of monitoring blood glucose should be instituted and specific therapy initiated (see below).

The quantity of energy administered to most ICU patients should maintain lean body mass and adipose tissues. Thus, variations in body weight usually reflect alterations in fluid balance. If sustained weight loss occurs (as characterized by a gradual fall in body weight during a period of 2 weeks or more), caloric intake may be inadequate. Additional calories (500 to 1,000 kcal/day) should be administered to maintain weight. Alternatively, the metabolic rate could be calculated from the volume of oxygen consumed per minute ($\dot{V}O_2$) and calorie intake then matched to equal energy expenditure:

$$\text{Metabolic rate (kcal/hr)} = \dot{V}O_2 \text{ (ml/min)} \times 60 \text{ min/hr} \times 1 \text{ L}/1{,}000 \text{ ml} \times 4.83 \text{ kcal/L}$$

This calculation is required in only 5% of our patients.

Table 13 Diagnosis, Treatment, and Prevention of Potential Mechanical and Metabolic Complications Associated with Total Parenteral Nutrition

	Complications	Diagnosis	Treatment	Prevention
Mechanical	Pneumothorax	Dyspnea, chest x-ray	Tube thoracostomy Observation	Avoid emergency procedures Trendelenburg's position
	Hemothorax	Dyspnea, chest x-ray	Remove catheter Observation	Insert catheter using appropriate technique
	Venous thrombosis	Inability to cannulate	Remove catheter Heparin therapy	Use silicone catheters Add heparin to solution
	Air embolism	Dyspnea, cyanosis, hypotension, tachycardia, precordial murmur	Trendelenburg's position Left lateral decubitus position	Trendelenburg's position Valsalva maneuver Tape intravenous connections
	Catheter embolism	Sheared catheter	Fluoroscopic retrieval	Never withdraw catheter through needle
	Arrhythmias	Catheter tip in right atrium	Withdraw catheter to superior vena cava	Estimate distance to SVC before insertion; confirm position with x-ray
	Subclavian artery injury	Pulsatile red blood	Remove needle Apply pressure Chest x-ray	Review anatomy
	Catheter tip misplacement	Chest x-ray	Redirect with a guide wire	Direct bevel of needle caudally
Metabolic	Hyperglycemic, hyperosmolar, nonketotic coma	Dehydration with osmotic diuresis, disorientation, lethargy, stupor, convulsions, coma, glucose 1,000 mg/dl, osmolarity 350 mOsm/kg	Discontinue TPN; infuse D5 in 0.45% S at 250 ml/hr Insulin 10–20 U/hr Bicarbonate Monitor glucose, potassium, pH	Monitor glucose
	Hypoglycemia	Headache, sweating, thirst, convulsions, disorientation, paresthesias	D50W I.V.	Taper TPN by 1/2 for 12 hr; then 12 hr of D5W at 100 ml/hr
	CO_2 retention	Ventilator dependence, high respiratory quotient	Taper glucose	Provide 30%–40% of calories with fat
	Azotemia	Dehydration, elevated BUN	Increase nonprotein calories	Monitor fluid balance
	Hyperammonemia	Lethargy, malaise, coma, seizures	Discontinue amino acid infusions Infuse arginine	Avoid casein or fibrin hydrolysate
	Essential fatty acid deficiency	Xerosis, hepatomegaly, impaired healing, bone changes	Fat administration	Provide 25–200 mg/kg/day of essential fatty acids
	Hypophosphatemia	Lethargy, anorexia, weakness	Supplemental phosphate	Treat causative factors: alkalosis, gram-negative sepsis, vomiting, malabsorption Provide 20 mEq/kcal
	Abnormal liver enzymes	Fatty infiltrate in liver	Evaluate for other causes	Provide balanced TPN solution
	Hypomagnesemia	Weakness, nausea, vomiting, tremors, depression, hyporeflexia	Infuse 10% $MgSO_4$	Supply 0.35–0.45 mEq/kg/day
	Hypermagnesemia	Drowsiness, nausea, vomiting, coma, arrhythmia	Dialysis Infuse calcium gluconate	Monitor serum levels

In non–ventilator-dependent patients, oxygen consumption and, in turn, the metabolic rate can be derived from measurements of respiratory gas exchange. Equipment (e.g., the Metabolic Measuring Cart) is commercially available to make these measurements at bedside. In a patient with a Swan-Ganz catheter in place, oxygen consumption can be calculated from cardiac output determinations and simultaneous measurements of mixed venous oxygen content ($C_{mv}O_2$) and arterial oxygen content (C_aO_2):

$$\dot{V}O_2 \text{ (ml/min)} = \text{cardiac output (L/min)} \times (C_aO_2 \text{ [ml/L]} - C_{mv}O_2 \text{ [ml/L]}) \times 1 \text{ L/10 dl}$$

Another objective of nutritional support in the ICU patient is the maintenance of lean body mass, which is reflected by nitrogen equilibration or positive nitrogen balance. Although complete nitrogen balance determination is a complex and sophisticated study, nitrogen equilibration can be estimated by using common analytic procedures. To estimate nitrogen balance, total nitrogen loss is subtracted from total nitrogen intake [*see Sidebar* Sample Calculation of Nitrogen Balance]. Calculation of total nitrogen loss requires several steps. The urine urea nitrogen (UUN) concentration is multiplied by the total volume of urine output during a given day to yield the 24-hour UUN, that is, the total amount of urea excreted during that period. Because urea accounts for only approximately 80% of the nitrogen excreted in the urine, the value for the 24-hour UUN must be increased by an additional 20%. This quantity and an additional 2 g/day are added to the value for the 24-hour UUN to account for nonurea nitrogen, stool, and integumentary losses:

$$24\text{-hour UUN (g/day)} = \text{UUN (mg/dl)}$$
$$\times \text{urine output (ml/day)} \times 1 \text{ g/1,000 mg} \times 1 \text{ dl/100 ml}$$

$$\text{Total nitrogen loss (g/day)} = 24\text{-hour UUN (g/day)}$$
$$+ (0.20 \times 24\text{-hour UUN [g/day]}) + 2 \text{ g/day}$$

Metabolic Monitoring

A wide variety of metabolic complications may occur during parenteral feeding [see Table 14]. They are minimized by frequent monitoring [see Table 15] and appropriate adjustment of nutrients in the infusion.

The most common metabolic problems occurring in ICU patients are hyperglycemia and glucosuria. Initially, elevated levels of blood glucose should be treated by the administration of subcutaneous insulin (5.0 units every 4 to 6 hours for glucose 200 to 250 mg/dl; 7.5 units for 250 to 300 mg/dl; 10.0 units for 300 to 350 mg/dl). When the nutritional solution is ordered for the next 24-hour period, half the quantity of insulin administered subcutaneously is added to the bag. At least 10 units of regular insulin per liter of solution should be used as the initial dose, and in some cases, as much as 40 U/L may be required. If larger doses of insulin are needed (> 100 U/day), a separate insulin infusion or drip should be used. Blood glucose levels can be monitored at the bedside by using a small refractometer or other similar devices, and the insulin infusion can be adjusted hourly, if necessary, to control the blood glucose concentration.

In most patients with severe glucose intolerance, the rate of glucose administered should not exceed 5 mg/kg/min (approximately 500 g/day).[29] Additional calories should be administered as fat emulsion. The commercially available fat emulsions are all generally well tolerated by critically ill patients. Triglyceride levels should be monitored, and the rate of administration of the emulsion should be decreased or the emulsion temporarily discontinued if levels exceed 500 mg/dl. Fat emulsion should be used with caution in patients with known hypertriglyceridemia or in those with gram-negative septicemia that is associated with hyperlipidemia.

The infusion of excess glucose or lipid energy may alter pulmonary function and in some patients prevent weaning from a mechanical ventilator. Excessive carbohydrate loads (usually > 500 g/day) increase CO_2 production. If the quantity of CO_2 produced exceeds the ability of the lungs to excrete this oxidative end product, hypercapnia results. CO_2 production can be greatly reduced by diminishing the carbohydrate load; if the patient receives less than 5 mg/kg/min of carbohydrate and cannot be weaned from the ventilator, one approach is to administer only 5% glucose solution overnight and then to attempt weaning the next morning. If the patient can be removed from the ventilator, parenteral feedings may be gradually reinstituted.

Fat emulsion may also interfere with diffusion of gas across the alveolar membranes. This interference is generally related to the concentration of the emulsion in the bloodstream; hence, monitoring triglyceride levels and preventing hypertriglyceridemia will minimize this complication.

Catheter Care and Catheter Sepsis

The most serious problem associated with central venous feedings is catheter sepsis [see VI:14 Nosocomial Infection]. Primary catheter sepsis is defined as the signs and symptoms of infection

---

Sample Calculation of Nitrogen Balance

A 65-year-old man with an infected aortic graft and ileus is receiving 2.2 L triple-mix solution containing 16.8 g nitrogen each day. His UUN is 500 mg/dl, and his urine output is 2,000 ml/day. Is he receiving adequate nitrogen?

24-hour UUN = 500 mg/dl × 2,000 ml/day × 1 g/1,000 mg
　　　　　　× 1 dl/100 ml
　　　　　= 10 g/day

Nitrogen output
　　　　= 24-hr UUN + (0.20 × 24-hr UUN) + 2 g/day
　　　　= 10 g/day + (0.20 × 10 g/day) + 2 g/day
　　　　= 14 g/day

Nitrogen balance
　　　　= 16.8 g/day (N intake) – 14 g/day (N output)
　　　　= 2.8 g/day

The patient is in positive nitrogen balance, retaining approximately 2 to 3 g nitrogen/day. If positive nitrogen balance had not been achieved, his protein and caloric intake would have had to be increased and the nitrogen balance recalculated.

(usually a febrile episode), with the indwelling catheter being the only anatomic focus of sepsis. After removal of the catheter, the symptoms usually attenuate. Cultures of the catheter tip with semiquantitative techniques yield at least 10^3 organisms.[30] The organisms are the same as those recovered from cultures of blood drawn from a peripheral vein during the initial evaluation of the infection.

Secondary catheter infection, in contrast to primary catheter sepsis, is associated with a second infectious focus that causes bacteremia and thus seeds or contaminates the catheter. The microorganisms cultured from the catheter tip are similar to those cultured from the primary source. The infection clears after specific treatment of the primary infection.

Primary catheter sepsis is prevented or at least greatly reduced by following strict protocols to govern the use and manipulation of the central venous feeding catheter and by employing a systematic method of care and surveillance of the catheter entrance site. Usually, catheter care and its supervision and certification are performed by a nurse with expertise in maintenance of long-term intravenous access (the nurse may be assigned to the nutrition support service or may be experienced in I.V. access or infection control). Every 48 to 72 hours, the dressing that covers the entrance site of the catheter is removed, the site inspected, the area around the entrance site cleaned, a topical antibiotic or antiseptic ointment applied, and the site redressed with a new sterile dressing. This procedure is documented in the clinical record; if drainage or crusting appears at the entrance site, appropriate cultures are taken. In addition, the dressing is changed if it becomes wet or soiled or no longer remains intact. In individuals who have either draining wounds in close proximity to the catheter entrance site or tracheostomies, the entire dressing should be covered with a transparent barrier drape to minimize contamination.

If signs and symptoms of infection develop in a recipient of central venous parenteral nutrition, a history should be taken and a physical examination performed [see Figure 3]. Appropriate tests (e.g., complete blood count and urinalysis) and diagnostic studies (including roentgenogram) should also be performed. If blood cultures are needed, they should be drawn from a peripheral vein. If trained nurses have maintained the catheter and no evidence of infection at the exit site has been noted, the catheter dressing should not be removed, and the catheter should not be manipulated. Blood cultures should

Table 14 Metabolic Complications of Total Parenteral Nutrition

Problems	Possible Causes	Solutions
Glucose		
Hyperglycemia, glycosuria, osmotic diuresis, hyperosmolar nonketotic dehydration and coma	Excessive total dose or rate of infusion of glucose; inadequate endogenous insulin; increased glucocorticoids; sepsis	Reduce amount of glucose infused; increase insulin; administer a portion of calories as fat emulsion
Ketoacidosis in diabetes mellitus	Inadequate endogenous insulin response; inadequate exogenous insulin therapy	Give insulin; reduce glucose input
Postinfusion (rebound) hypoglycemia	Persistence of endogenous insulin production secondary to prolonged stimulation of islet cells by high-carbohydrate infusion	Administer 5%–10% glucose before infusate is discontinued
Fat		
Pyrogenic reaction	Fat emulsion, other solutions	Exclude other causes of fever
Altered coagulation	Hyperlipidemia	Restudy after fat has cleared bloodstream
Hypertriglyceridemia	Rapid infusion, decreased clearance	Decrease rate of infusion; allow clearance before blood tests
Impaired liver function	May be caused by fat emulsion or by an underlying disease process	Exclude other causes of hepatic dysfunction
Cyanosis	Altered pulmonary diffusion capacity	Discontinue fat infusion
Essential fatty acid deficiency	Inadequate essential fatty acid administration	Administer essential fatty acids in the form of one 500 ml bottle of fat emulsion every 2–3 days
Amino Acids		
Hyperchloremic metabolic acidosis	Excessive chloride and monohydrochloride content of crystalline amino acid solutions	Administer Na^+ and K^+ as acetate salts
Serum amino acid imbalance	Unphysiologic amino acid profile of the nutrient solution; differential amino acid utilization with various disorders	Use experimental solutions if indicated
Hyperammonemia	Excessive ammonia in protein hydrolysate solutions; deficiency of arginine, ornithine, aspartic acid, or glutamic acid, or a combination of these deficiencies in amino acid solutions; primary hepatic disorder	Reduce amino acid intake
Prerenal azotemia	Excessive amino acid infusion with inadequate calorie administration; inadequate free water intake, dehydration	Reduce amino acid intake; increase glucose calories; increase intake of free water
Calcium and Phosphorus		
Hypophosphatemia	Inadequate phosphorus administration; redistribution of serum phosphorus into cells or bones, or both	Administer phosphorous ($\geq$ 20 mEq potassium dihydrogen phosphate/1,000 I.V. calories); evaluate antacid or calcium administration, or both
Hypocalcemia	Inadequate calcium administration; reciprocal response to phosphorus repletion without simultaneous calcium infusion; hypoalbuminemia	Administer calcium
Hypercalcemia	Excessive calcium administration with or without high doses of albumin; excessive vitamin D administration	Decrease calcium or vitamin D
Vitamin D deficiency; hypervitaminosis D	Inadequate or excessive vitamin D	Alter vitamin D administration
Miscellaneous		
Hypokalemia	Potassium intake inadequate relative to increased requirements for protein anabolism; diuresis	Alter nutrient administration
Hyperkalemia	Excessive potassium administration, especially in metabolic acidosis; renal failure	Alter nutrient administration
Hypomagnesemia	Inadequate magnesium administration relative to increased requirements for protein anabolism and glucose metabolism; diuresis; cisplatin administration	Alter nutrient administration
Hypermagnesemia	Excessive magnesium administration; renal failure	Alter nutrient administration
Anemia	Iron deficiency; folic acid deficiency; vitamin B_{12} deficiency; copper deficiency; other deficiencies	Alter nutrient administration
Bleeding	Vitamin K deficiency	Alter nutrient administration
Hypervitaminosis A	Excessive vitamin A administration	Alter nutrient administration
Elevations in AST (formerly SGOT), ALT (formerly SGPT), and serum alkaline phosphatase	Enzyme induction secondary to amino acid imbalance or to excessive deposition of glycogen or fat, or both, in the liver	Reevaluate status of patient

never be taken through the catheter. The one possible exception to this rule is the case in which the initial presentation of infection is characterized by marked hyperpyrexia or hypotension, or both. (In this case, contamination of the catheter is immaterial because the catheter will be removed.) If no other focus of sepsis is identified, the physician may elect to remove all indwelling lines, including the feeding catheter. In addition, either drainage around the catheter or a previous positive culture from the catheter exit site may also indicate immediate removal. If another primary source of the infection is diagnosed, then specific therapy should be instituted, and the parenteral nutrition should be continued. If no source of infection is identified, the catheter should be removed and the catheter tip cultured.

A dilemma arises if another source of infection is identified and if signs and symptoms of infection persist despite what appears to be appropriate therapy. If blood cultures are positive, we favor removal of the catheter to avoid the complications that are associated with a contaminated indwelling catheter (e.g., septic emboli and endocarditis). If, however, peripheral blood cultures are negative, the catheter can be changed over a guide wire and the

Table 15 Variables to Be Monitored during Intravenous Alimentation and Suggested Frequency of Monitoring

Variables	Suggested Monitoring Frequency	
	First Week	Later
Energy Balance		
Weight	Daily	Daily
Metabolic Variables		
Blood measurements		
Plasma electrolytes (Na⁺, K⁺, Cl⁻)	Daily	3 × weekly
Blood urea nitrogen	3 × weekly	2 × weekly
Plasma osmolarity*	Daily	3 × weekly
Plasma total calcium and inorganic phosphorus	3 × weekly	2 × weekly
Blood glucose	Daily	3 × weekly
Plasma transaminases	3 × weekly	2 × weekly
Plasma total protein and fractions	2 × weekly	Weekly
Blood acid-base status	As indicated	As indicated
Hemoglobin	Weekly	Weekly
Ammonia	As indicated	As indicated
Magnesium	2 × weekly	Weekly
Triglycerides	Weekly	Weekly
Urine measurements		
Glucose	Daily	Daily
Specific gravity or osmolarity	Daily	Daily
General measurements		
Volume of infusate	Daily	Daily
Oral intake (if any)	Daily	Daily
Urinary output	Daily	Daily
Prevention and Detection of Infection		
Clinical observations (activity, temperature, symptoms)	Daily	Daily
WBC and differential counts	As indicated	As indicated
Cultures	As indicated	As indicated

*May be predicted from 2 × Na concentration (mEq/L) + [blood glucose (mg/dl) ÷ 18].

catheter tip cultured to confirm that catheter infection does not exist. Central venous feeding can be continued during this interval. If the cultured catheter tip is positive ($\geq 10^5$ organisms), the catheter should be removed.

Changing the central venous catheter over a guide wire can aid in the diagnosis of primary catheter infection.[31] Because most ICU patients have multiple potential sources for infection, this technique allows culture of the catheter tip but minimizes the risks associated with reinsertion of a new central catheter. Strict aseptic technique is used. The area surrounding the catheter entrance site is sterilized, the I.V. tubing is disconnected from the catheter, a guide wire is passed into the catheter, and the catheter is removed over the guide wire. A new catheter is inserted over the wire and sutured in place. The tip of the old catheter is cut, placed in a transfer vessel, and taken to the microbiology laboratory for semiquantitative culture. With strict care of catheters, the incidence of catheter sepsis should be less than 6%.[32] Septicemia is most commonly caused by growth and invasion of organisms along the catheter tract. Occasionally, bacteria are infused through the catheter because of a breach in sterility during care of the infusion apparatus. The most common bacterial organisms causing catheter sepsis are the skin contaminants *Staphylococcus epidermidis*, *S. aureus*, *Klebsiella pneumoniae*, and *Candida albicans*. In some rare cases, the intravenous solutions may be contaminated.

Moreover, most patients requiring central venous alimentation are immunocompromised hosts; their resistance is lowered further by disease, severe malnutrition, or treatment or by some combination of these factors. Coexisting conditions such as urinary tract infection, abscess, pneumonia, or mucositis secondary to chemotherapy predispose these patients to bacteremia, which may contaminate the central venous catheter.

Immunosuppressed critically ill patients receiving multiple broad-spectrum antibiotics are also at risk for *Candida* septicemia. Blood cultures positive for *C. albicans* in an ICU patient are an indication for catheter removal and treatment with fluconazole. An ophthalmologist should examine the eyegrounds of patients with proven candidemia to exclude the possibility of metastatic *Candida* ophthalmitis [*see VI:18 Fungal Infection*].

Home Nutritional Support

Home parenteral nutrition is indicated for patients who are unable to eat and absorb enough nutrients for maintenance.[33] Most of the adult surgical patients who require home parenteral nutrition suffer from short-bowel syndrome caused by (1) extensive Crohn's disease, (2) mesenteric infarction, or (3) severe abdominal trauma. Pseudo-obstruction, radiation enteritis, carcinomatosis, necrotizing enterocolitis, and intestinal fistulas are other indications for home nutritional support. Patients with these conditions cannot receive adequate nutrition enterally, although in some cases compensatory mucosal growth occurs that may either reduce or eventually eliminate the need for continued home parenteral nutrition.

To be eligible for home parenteral nutrition, patients must (1) have an appropriate level of intelligence, (2) be highly motivated, and (3) have adequate support from their families. Patients must receive extensive evaluation, teaching, and training during hospitalization if home parenteral nutrition is to prove successful. These services should be provided by a team consisting of a physician, a a nurse, a dietitian, a pharmacist, and a social worker. The team's instructions should be thorough and wide-ranging, covering the basic principles of parenteral nutrition as well as providing mechanical guidelines for catheter care, asepsis, and use of infusion pumps. Patients should be objectively evaluated before being discharged from the hospital to ensure that they have both an adequate understanding of the principles of intravenous nutrition and the technical ability to carry out home parenteral nutrition properly.

A patient who is judged by the nutrition support team to be a candidate for home TPN requires placement of a Silastic catheter designed for more permanent use than the central venous catheter employed during hospitalization.[34] The catheter is typically 90 cm long, with a thin 55 cm intravascular segment that is inserted either by venous cutdown into the internal or external jugular vein or the cephalic vein or directly into the subclavian vein by means of venipuncture. The intravascular portion of the catheter is cut so that its tip will lie at the junction of the superior vena cava and the right atrium. Placement of the catheter is carried out in the operating room by using local anesthesia (1% lidocaine) and adequate sedation. The catheter is tunneled subcutaneously from a small incision lateral to the sternum to the site of venous insertion. The catheter exit site is chosen on the basis of the patient's gender, physique, and hand dominance. In women, lower paraxiphoid or upper abdominal exit sites permit a more natural appearance. If the patient's coagulation status is abnormal, the cephalic vein is isolated in the deltapectoral groove and tied distally, and the catheter is inserted proximally by means of venotomy. Otherwise, a percutaneous approach to the subclavian vein is taken. The pa-

Figure 3 Evaluation of a febrile patient receiving central venous parenteral nutrition is shown.

tient is placed in Trendelenburg's position, and a needle is inserted into the subclavian vein while negative pressure is applied to the attached syringe. Once a flashback of venous blood is obtained, a J-wire is introduced through the needle into the superior vena cava. A large introducer (e.g., a No. 10 tube) that has an internal obturator and an external cannula is then inserted over the guide wire to dilate the tract. After the catheter has been cut to the appropriate length and flushed with heparinized saline, it is inserted into the cannula, which is then peeled away and removed. Proper positioning of the catheter is confirmed by fluoroscopy, and the incisions are closed with absorbable sutures. The catheter is sutured to the skin exit site, and the sutures are left attached for at least 2 weeks while tissue ingrowth into the Dacron velour cuff takes place. After the sutures are placed, sterile dressings are applied.

Calorie, protein, and fluid needs are carefully estimated for each patient, and the administration schedule is arranged so that the total volume may be infused nocturnally over 10 to 12 hours. Electrolytes, micronutrients, and trace minerals are added as indicated. Fat emulsions may be given either separately or admixed with glucose and protein and are used to reduce the requirement for dextrose calories and to prevent essential fatty acid deficiency.

The complications of home TPN are much the same as those of in-hospital TPN. They may be divided into four categories: mechanical, infectious, metabolic, and psychosocial. Mechanical complications, which are generally easy to remedy, include catheter oc-

clusion and dislodgment and damage to the external portion of the catheter. Infectious complications that are superficial to the Dacron cuff usually respond well to antibiotics. Infections of the intravascular catheter may necessitate removal of the catheter after the diagnosis is confirmed by blood cultures obtained through the catheter, but the usual therapeutic approach is to initiate a trial of parenteral antibiotics. Metabolic complications related to individual nutrient deficiencies may be corrected by addition of the appropriate substance to the solution. The role of serum levels of trace minerals and micronutrients in the delineation of nutrient deficiency states remains unclear. In patients receiving insulin, hyperinsulinemia after infusion may be prevented by reducing the rate of administration gradually over the last hour of infusion. Psychosocial complications may vary from slight depression to suicidal tendencies, which must be treated with appropriate counseling.

The costs of a home TPN program may also be divided into four categories: patient training, equipment, supplies, and follow-up. It has been estimated that the average annual cost of home TPN is 70% less than that of in-hospital TPN. The growth of private companies that deliver equipment and supplies to the home, maintain inventory, bill patients, and help with insurance problems has considerably facilitated home care.

Home enteral nutrition is frequently utilized, either as the sole source or as a partial source of nutritional support. It is the preferred method when GI tract function is adequate. In patients undergoing surgery of the aerodigestive tract for cancer, jejunostomy feedings can supplement oral feedings, especially during periods of adjuvant chemotherapy and radiation treatment. Patients are taught to cycle the feedings over 12-hour periods, using an enteral pump system to provide 20 to 30 kcal/kg/day. Use of an appropriate feeding tube and immediate flushing of the tube after use reduce the incidence of clogging at home. If blockage occurs, proteases or carbonated beverages can be introduced into the tube in an attempt to open it. Jejunostomy feedings reduce the risk of aspiration and help maintain nutritional status during periods of inadequate oral intake. Use of inexpensive nutritionally complete commercial formulas is encouraged. For patients who have more permanent disabilities that prevent adequate oral intake, a gastrostomy (either PEG [see V:6 Gastrointestinal Endoscopy] or a surgically placed Stamm gastrostomy [see V:9 Gastric Procedures]) may be preferable. It reduces the GI complications of feeding by making use of the reservoir and admixing functions of the stomach.

Debilitated patients have been fed for many years through enteral feeding tubes. The advantages of home enteral nutrition parallel those of in-hospital programs: low cost, ease of administration, and fewer complications.

Discussion

Nutrition and the Gastrointestinal Tract

INFLUENCE OF NUTRITION ON INTESTINAL METABOLISM AND FUNCTION

The small intestine undergoes both morphologic and functional changes when enteral nutrition is absent, even in the face of optimal parenteral nutrition [see Figure 4]. Villous height and cellular mass decrease, and the activity of brush border enzymes is reduced.[35] These abnormalities may result in decreased nutrient absorption, as evidenced by the frequent intolerance to enteral feedings in critically ill patients.

Another potential problem associated with the absence of enteral nutrition during critical illness is disruption of the mucosal barrier. This disruption allows increased translocation of bacteria and absorption of endotoxin from the gut lumen.[36] Bacterial translocation is the process of bacterial migration (or invasion) across the mucosal barrier into mesenteric lymph nodes and the portal bloodstream. Factors that are associated with increased bacterial translocation include alterations in the GI microflora, impaired host immunity, and physical disruption of the mucosal barrier.[37]

Bacterial translocation has been studied most extensively in animal models, and it is not known whether much of this information is applicable in humans. For example, the translocation of indigenous enteric bacteria to mesenteric lymph nodes occurred in rats after scald burns of 40% of total body surface area.[38] Because translocation was not associated with increased numbers of bacteria within the intestinal tract, it was thought that the egress of bacteria was caused by a breakdown in the barrier function of the gut associated with the thermal injury. In another model, abscesses were created by intraperitoneal implantation of a fibrin clot contaminated with nonenteric organisms. When cultured at a later time, enteric organisms were present that had presumably translocated from the bowel lumen into the abscess.[39]

More than 40 years ago, intraoperative bacteriologic cultures of the portal venous bloodstream in a heterogeneous group of patients with noninflammatory lesions of the GI tract were performed. Eight of 25 patients had positive portal venous cultures, demonstrating that bacteria pass from the GI tract to the liver via the portal vein.[40] Life-threatening infections from gut-associated bacteria and fungi have been documented in patients with multiorgan failure[36] (now known as multiple organ dysfunction syndrome), in those with cancer who have had chemotherapy[41] or bone marrow transplants,[39] and in those with major burns.[42] These patients are immunocompromised, do not receive adequate enteral nutrition, and are given antibiotics, H_2 receptor blockers, and other therapies that alter the intestinal mucosa and microflora. In spite of this strong association, however, therapy aimed at reducing or diminishing bacterial flora, such as the administration of intestinal antibiotics, has not reduced the incidence of infectious complications in such patients.

In addition to the movement of bacteria from the gut lumen, bacterial endotoxin may be absorbed across abnormal gut mucosa. Current evidence suggests that small amounts of endotoxin are frequently absorbed into the portal bloodstream but are rapidly detoxified by hepatic Kupffer's cells, which act as a barrier to these toxins.[43] Studies were done on rabbits with one of three different injuries: a single dose of endotoxin, temporary occlusion of the superior mesenteric artery, or a 30% scald burn. All three injuries produced fatal endotoxic shock within 12 hours.[44] When gram-negative bacteria were either absent from or present in reduced amounts in the intestinal tract of similar animals, these injuries were not lethal.

Studies in mice reveal that endotoxin given intraperitoneally promotes bacterial translocation from the gut to the mesenteric lymph nodes in a dose-dependent manner.[45] The incidence and magnitude of endotoxin-induced bacterial translocation in endotoxin-resistant mice were similar to those in nonresistant mice, indicating that bacterial translocation was not prevented by genetic resistance to endotoxin. Finally, these same investigators examined the combined effects of malnutrition and endotoxemia on promoting bacterial translocation.[46] This combination was associated with a significantly higher number of translocated bacteria to systemic organs than was seen in normally nourished mice receiving endotoxin.

In clinical studies, circulating endotoxin was found in the blood of individuals with chronic inflammatory bowel disease that progressed despite standard medical treatment.[47] Whole gut lavage with normal saline reduced the levels of endotoxins; as a result, the condition of all patients improved, plasma endotoxin levels dropped rapidly, and abnormal elevations of body temperature were reduced.

The intestinal mucosa is also disrupted in critically ill patients after cardiovascular instability and hypotension. Hypovolemic shock produces sloughing of intestinal mucosal cells and a cessation of mucus production,[48] patchy or diffuse areas of superficial necrosis, openings of tight junctions between epithelial cells, and mucosal edema.[49] These combined effects lead to increased mucosal permeability of the colon and bowel wall edema, process-

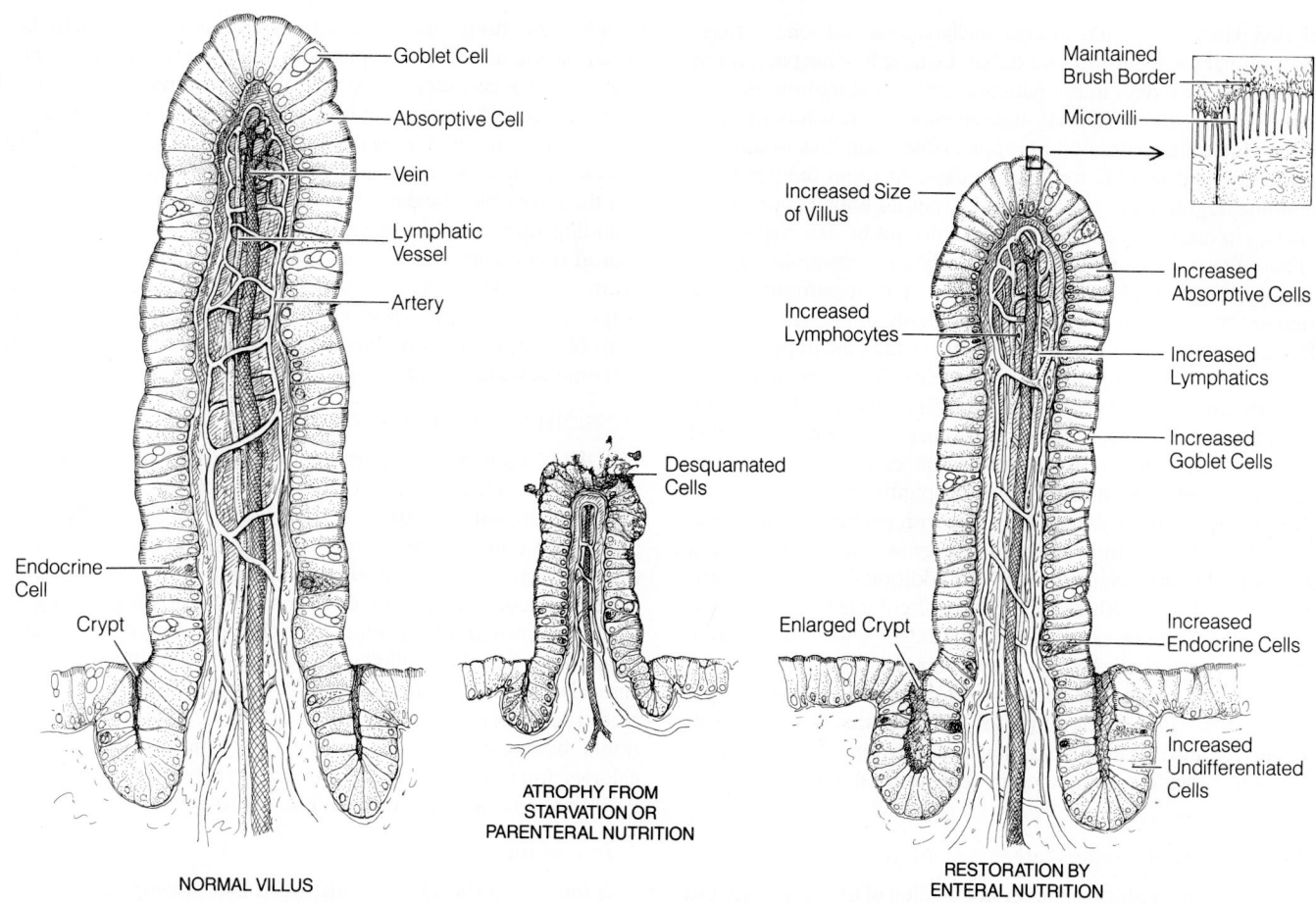

Figure 4 Enteral nutrition maintains and restores intestinal epithelium, whereas starvation or parenteral nutrition causes villous atrophy.

es that have been attenuated by creating a proximal, diverting ileostomy or administering a hydrolyzed chemical diet.[50]

In summary, during critical illness, the GI tract is altered in such a way that the protective barrier function of the gut is lost. This loss allows enteric bacteria to cross the gut wall or accommodates the absorption of endotoxins into the body, or both. Because most patients with critical illness cannot receive enteral feedings and because parenteral nutrition results in gut atrophy, current techniques of nutritional support neither facilitate repair of the intestinal mucosa nor maintain its barrier function.

NUTRITIONAL SUPPORT FOR THE INTESTINAL TRACT

Enteral feedings are the best method of maintaining the integrity of the GI mucosa. The provision of these feedings may have profound effects on the reduction of systemic manifestations of critical illness. For example, early enteral feedings in a 30% burn model not only protected against mucosal atrophy in the GI tract but also decreased the overall elaboration of stress hormones and minimized the catabolic response to this injury.[51]

Glutamine is a nutrient that supports intestinal cell replication and growth and may be useful as specific therapy for the support of the intestinal mucosa. Glutamine is absent from all standard parenteral nutrient solutions unless a specific request is made to provide glutamine-supplemented parenteral nutrition. Glutamine is present in insufficient amounts in most enteral formulas, although there are at least two modified diets that contain adequate glutamine. Glutamine may also be provided as a supplement to standard enteral feedings and is usually given as 0.5 g/kg/day in

divided doses. When animals or humans are maintained on parenteral nutrition, atrophy of the intestinal mucosa is observed. When glutamine is added to the parenteral nutrition, this response is greatly attenuated, both in animals[52] and in humans.[53] The effect of this specific bowel nutrient on GI organs has been studied under a variety of conditions in both animals and humans. For example, when rats were treated with the chemotherapeutic agents methotrexate or fluorouracil, growth arrest and GI mucosal atrophy occurred. The addition of glutamine to an enteral diet promoted recovery of the mucosa of the small bowel and colon in animals receiving this diet as compared with animals receiving standard but glutamine-free diets.[54,55] Glutamine solutions also attenuate the pancreatic atrophy and hepatic steatosis associated with standard intravenous formulas. A series of detailed clinical studies have described unique clinical advantages associated with glutamine-supplemented solutions. Glutamine-supplemented solutions were given to postoperative cholecystectomy patients,[56] and parenteral solutions supplemented with the dipeptide of glutamine and alanine were administered to patients after cancer surgery.[57] Glutamine-treated patients in both groups showed improved nitrogen balance as compared with control subjects, who received I.V. feedings. Two randomized, blind, prospective trials have been performed in patients undergoing bone marrow transplantation. In the first study, 45 patients with hematologic malignancies were randomized to receive standard or glutamine-containing I.V. feedings. The patients receiving glutamine feedings had less accumulation of extracellular water,[58] a reduced rate of infection, and a 7-day reduction in the length of hospital stay.[59] The second study, which included patients with hematologic malignancies and solid tumors, used a similar protocol and found that the length of hospitalization was reduced by 6 days in the patients receiving glutamine.[60]

Studies of solution stability demonstrated that solutions containing glutamine generated no appreciable quantities of ammonia when stored at 4° C for 7 to 30 days. At room temperature, glutamine degradation was about 0.1% per 24 hours; appreciable increases in ammonia concentration could not be detected.[61]

The efficacy of glutamine may be related to its ability to enhance proliferation of the GI mucosa,[53] to enhance immunologic function,[62,63] or to aid synthesis of the highly important intracellular antioxidant glutathione.[64,65] Further studies are in progress to evaluate the efficacy of glutamine in patients with severe infection, burns, trauma, other states associated with injury or inflammation, and inflammatory bowel disease and other conditions associated with bowel injury. It appears that glutamine can modulate disease, decreasing morbidity and shortening hospitalization.

Supplementation of enteral formulas with pectin, a fermentable fiber polysaccharide, improved mucosal growth and function in a model of intestinal adaptation.[66,67] In additional studies, pectin-supplemented diets reduced the effects of colonic injury and improved recovery from experimental colitis.[68,69] Other studies have demonstrated metabolic benefits of exogenously administered growth hormone and epidermal growth factor on bowel growth and nutrient use.[70] The development of therapies that combine both appropriate nutrient administration and hormonal growth stimulation may provide optimal therapy for intestinal mucosal growth.

Clinical Trials of Perioperative Nutrition

Increasing medical costs, the pervasive influx of managed care, and the paucity of confirmatory clinical data have all contributed to a decreased use of perioperative nutritional support since the mid-1990s. It is now recognized that only the most critically ill and severely malnourished patients will benefit from perioperative nutritional support. The characteristics of these patients include (1) loss of at least 15% of usual body weight, (2) significant hypoalbuminemia, (3) major organ dysfunction, and (4) projected inability to eat for 7 to 10 days. Patients most apt to benefit from perioperative nutritional support include the injured, the critically ill, and those in need of major upper GI surgery. Among those who do require perioperative nutrition, enteral feeding by tube is increasingly common. In comparison with parenteral nutrition, enteral feeding is less costly, obviates central venous catheterization and its associated risks, and probably stimulates restoration of GI structure and function to a greater degree.

The association between malnutrition and a poor clinical outcome suggests that providing nutritional support to malnourished patients undergoing surgery ought to have therapeutic benefits. The degree of malnutrition, however, is often associated with the severity of disease, and thus, malnourished patients usually have a poor prognosis simply because they are sicker than patients who are well nourished. Consequently, in some instances, nutritional therapy may not improve clinical outcome unless the presence of malnutrition is itself an independent contributor to postoperative complications.

Surgeons are now being asked to provide objective documentation, based on controlled clinical trials, to justify the use of expensive adjuvant therapies such as TPN. The quality of the data adduced to support any given treatment must be carefully examined. The gold standard is usually the prospective, randomized, controlled trial (PRCT); however, such studies are extremely expensive and often require large numbers of patients to meet the rigid demands of statistical analysis. Moreover, there are circumstances in which such

trials have not been conducted and will never be conducted. In these instances, the next level of evidence—data from well-designed non-randomized or case cohort–control studies—is considered. Finally, if even this level of data is lacking, the least compelling form of evidence—uncontrolled experiences, case reports, or the opinion of experts in the field—is considered. Every effort should be made to obtain the most objective data available on any major form of therapy, including nutritional support; however, there are many accepted clinical treatments that are not supported by data from PRCTs. From an ethical perspective, patients should not be denied nutritional support simply because evidence from the most objective form of clinical trial is not yet available—especially given that the outcome of withholding feeding is starvation.

CONSENSUS CONFERENCE REPORT

A 1997 conference report jointly published by the National Institutes of Health, the American Society for Parenteral and Enteral Nutrition, and the American Society of Clinical Nutrition provided a critical review of the current evidence concerning the value of perioperative nutritional support, with an emphasis on patient selection, criteria for entry, timing of initiating feeding, the route and content of nutritional supplementation, outcome criteria, and the length of follow-up necessary to identify an effect on clinical outcome.[71] The committee reviewed PRCTs that met specific criteria: in particular, it addressed only studies in which nutritional therapy was given for at least 5 days and provided sufficient calories and nitrogen to meet daily requirements. In all, more than 2,500 patients were included in the studies reviewed.

Preoperative TPN

A total of 13 PRCTs were identified that investigated the use of preoperative TPN.[71] These studies contained mostly patients with GI cancer who were considered to be at least moderately malnourished on the basis of weight loss, decreased plasma protein levels, or abnormal prognostic indices. A pooled analysis of the data showed that patients who received preoperative TPN had 10% fewer postoperative complications than the control group did (i.e., the complication rate dropped from approximately 40% to 30%); in five studies these differences reached statistical significance. The pooled analysis found no significant difference in mortality between the TPN groups and the control groups.

Postoperative TPN

Use of TPN in the immediate postoperative period without preoperative TPN was evaluated in nine PRCTs.[71] These studies included mostly patients with GI cancer who were considered to be at least moderately malnourished on the basis of weight loss, decreased plasma protein levels, or abnormal prognostic indices. In contrast to the pooled analysis of the preoperative data, a pooled analysis of the postoperative data showed that patients who received TPN after operation had an approximately 10% higher risk of ensuing complications (i.e., the complication rate rose from approximately 30% to 40%).

Perioperative Enteral Nutrition

Only seven PRCTs, involving a relatively small number of patients, were identified that evaluated perioperative enteral nutrition.[71] Two studies compared preoperative enteral with an ad libitum oral diet,[72,73] and in one,[73] postoperative complications were significantly lower in patients who received enteral tube feeding. Four PRCTs compared early postoperative jejunal tube feeding with a standard oral diet that was advanced as tolerated.[74-77] No consistent differences in postoperative morbidity or mortality were identified. One study evaluated the use of postoperative jejunostomy tube feeding with a special formula enriched with arginine, ribonucleic acids, and omega-3 fatty acids after operation for upper GI tract cancer.[78] When all patients were included in the analysis, no statistically significant differences were found; however, when only patients who were successfully fed were evaluated, those who received the enriched formula had fewer complications and a shorter hospital stay than those who received the standard formula.

Patients with Hip Fractures

In two studies, the effect of supplementary postoperative feeding was evaluated in elderly underweight women after surgical repair of a femoral neck fracture.[79,80] These studies found that weight bearing and independent mobility were possible at an earlier date, there were fewer complications, and patients were discharged from the hospital earlier in the groups who received postoperative oral supplementation or nighttime tube feedings than in the groups who received a normal diet.

Conclusions

The consensus conference report reached four main conclusions. First, TPN given to malnourished patients (defined on the basis of weight loss, decreased plasma protein levels, or abnormal prognostic indices) with GI cancer for 7 to 10 days before surgery decreases postoperative complications by approximately 10%. Second, routine use of early postoperative TPN in malnourished general surgical patients (defined in the same fashion) who did not receive preoperative TPN increases postoperative complications by approximately 10%; however, postoperative nutritional support is necessary to prevent the adverse effects of starvation in patients who are unable to eat for long periods after operation. Third, in the majority of currently published PRCTs evaluating the use of perioperative TPN, the quantity and type of substrates given were not optimal by current standards; therefore, it is possible that nutritional support may have a greater therapeutic effect if given according to our current understanding of caloric needs and other metabolic requirements. Fourth, postoperative enteral feeding given to underweight elderly women after operation for hip fracture speeds recovery of mobility, decreases postoperative complications, and shortens hospital stay.

MORE RECENT CLINICAL TRIALS

Since 1994, several additional PRCTs have made important contributions to our understanding of the use of nutritional support in the surgical patient. In what follows, we review some of the most significant of these.

Cancer Patients

PRCTs addressing perioperative nutritional support have been conducted in patients undergoing surgery for pancreatic, hepatocellular, and upper GI malignancies. In one, patients undergoing major pancreatic resection were randomly assigned either to a group that received TPN on postoperative day 1 or to a non-TPN group.[81] No significant benefit from the use of adjuvant TPN could be demonstrated, and the incidence of complications (primarily those associated with infection) was significantly greater in the TPN group. It was concluded that routine use of postoperative TPN in patients undergoing major pancreatic resection for malignancy cannot be recommended; moreover, the investigators stated that further studies should be performed to determine why infectious complications were more common in these patients.

A PRCT from the Netherlands examined the effects of cyclic versus continuous enteral nutrition on postoperative gastric function after pylorus-preserving pancreaticoduodenectomy.[82] Patients were evaluated with respect to gastric emptying, resumption of normal diet, and length of hospital stay. It was hypothesized that enteral infusions of fat and protein would activate a neurohumoral feedback and therefore potentiate impaired gastric emptying, which occurs in approximately 30% of these patients. Nasogastric intubation was maintained for a shorter period in the enterally fed group than in the control group (6.7 days versus 9.1 days, NS). The first day of normal diet came earlier for the enterally fed group (12.2 days after operation versus 15.7 days, $P < 0.05$). Hospital stay was shorter in the cyclic enterally fed group (17.5 days versus 21.4 days, $P < 0.05$). It was concluded that cyclic enteral nutrition was clinically efficacious in this selected group of patients.

Resection of hepatocellular carcinoma is associated with high rates of morbidity and mortality. Studies using experimental models have shown that nutritional support reduces the catabolic response, improves protein synthesis, and enhances liver regeneration. In a prospective study from Hong Kong, perioperative nutritional support was investigated in patients undergoing hepatectomy for hepatocellular carcinoma.[83] A total of 64 patients were randomly selected to receive perioperative intravenous support in addition to their oral diet, and 60 patients (33 with cirrhosis, 12 with chronic active hepatitis, and 15 with no associated liver disease) were randomly assigned to a control group. The perioperative nutritional therapy consisted of a solution enriched with 35% BCAAs, dextrose, and a lipid emulsion (50% MCTs) given intravenously for 14 days perioperatively. The overall postoperative morbidity rate was reduced in the perioperative nutrition group (34% versus 55%), mainly because the rate of infection-related complications was lower (17% versus 37%, $P = 0.02$). These benefits were seen predominantly in patients with underlying cirrhosis who underwent major hepatectomy. It was concluded that perioperative nutritional support can reduce complications after major hepatectomy for hepatocellular carcinoma associated with cirrhosis.

Early Postoperative Enteral Nutrition

At present, there is considerable interest in the early postoperative use of enteral nutrition. Experiments in humans demonstrate normal small bowel absorptive capacity in the early postoperative period. Moreover, investigations in animal models show reduced energy expenditure with early enteral feeding. A nonrandomized, uncontrolled study of 38 patients who underwent colorectal surgery over a 3-month period found that 31 patients were able to tolerate an early feeding regimen.[84] Patients who tolerated early feeding had shorter postoperative stays[6] (5.7 versus 10.6 days); those who did not had longer operative procedures and lost more blood intraoperatively. (Longer operative time and increased intraoperative blood loss may indicate a more difficult operation, which may in turn result in prolongation of recovery and decreased tolerance to early enteral feeding.) The investigators concluded (1) that early postoperative feeding is safe and is tolerated by the majority of patients and (2) that if early feeding is tolerated, it shortens hospital stay and may decrease health care costs.

The current emphasis on early access for long-term enteral feeding has led to increased use of early postoperative feeding through PEG. A randomized, prospective study evaluated 41 patients in the Veterans Affairs Medical Center in Dayton, Ohio.[85] One patient group received tube feedings 3 hours postoperatively, and the other received similar feedings 24 hours after PEG placement. All patients received an iso-osmolar formula. There were no significant differences in postoperative morbidity between the two groups. It was concluded that early PEG tube feeding (3 hours after tube placement) is as safe as next-day feeding in selected elderly patients.

A 1997 PRCT included 28 patients undergoing esophagectomy or pancreaticoduodenectomy who received either immediate postoperative enteral feeding via jejunostomy (N =13) or no feedings during the first 6 days after operation (N =15).[86] Hand-grip strength, vital capacity, forced expiratory volume in 1 second (FEV$_1$), and maximal inspiratory pressure were measured before operation and on postoperative days 2, 4, and 6. Postoperative vital capacity ($P < 0.05$) and FEV$_1$ ($P = 0.07$) were consistently lower in the fed group than in the unfed group, whereas there were no significant differences in grip strength and maximal inspiratory pressure. Postoperative mobility was lower in the fed group, and these patients tended to recover less rapidly. There were no significant differences in fatigue or vigor between the two groups. The investigators concluded that immediate postoperative jejunal feeding is associated with impaired respiratory mechanics and postoperative mobility and does not influence the loss of muscle strength or the increase in fatigue occurring after major surgery; they further concluded that immediate postoperative enteral feeding should not be routine in well-nourished patients who are at low risk for nutrition-related complications. This PRCT is noteworthy not only for its intriguing, unanticipated results but also for its inclusion of an unfed control group, a decision that underscores the importance of such groups in the design of these clinical investigations. Heretofore, many institutional review boards, on ethical grounds, have not permitted investigation of unfed control groups.

Another 1997 PRCT evaluated early enteral feeding after resection of upper GI malignancies.[87] The purpose of the study was to determine whether early postoperative enteral feeding with an immune-enhancing formula could decrease morbidity, mortality, and length of hospital stay. A total of 195 patients with upper GI cancer were randomly selected to receive either the immune-enhancing formula (supplemented with arginine, RNA, and omega-3 fatty acids) via jejunostomy or standard I.V. crystalloid solutions. There were no significant differences between the two groups with respect to the number of minor, major, or infectious wound complications; the length of the hospital stay; or mortality. The two main strengths of this study were (1) its inclusion of an "intent to treat" analysis and (2) the large number of subjects enrolled. It is noteworthy that even though all of the patients had upper GI cancer, the average postoperative weight loss was only 5% to 6%, and serum albumin levels were normal in both groups.

A 1998 report investigated the effects of early postoperative enteral feeding in 43 patients with nontraumatic intestinal perforation and peritonitis.[88] After laparotomy, patients were randomly assigned to either a control group (N = 22) or a study group (N = 21). The study group received a feeding jejunostomy, and enteral feeding was started 12 hours after operation. The mortality rate was high in both groups (18% for the control group versus 19% for the study group). The control group had more septic complications than the study group (22 versus 8, $P < 0.05$).

Complications of Enteral Nutrition

A number of reports have examined the complications of enteral nutrition in different settings. Needle-catheter jejunostomy (NCJ) is the jejunal access method of choice in many centers. Some reports have suggested that this feeding route may be associated with a high rate of complications.[89] In a retrospective review of 2,022 NCJs performed in 1,938 patients, 34 NCJ-related complications occurred in 29 patients (1.5%).[90] The most common com-

plication was premature loss of the catheter from occlusion or dislodgment (N = 15 [0.7%]), and the most serious was bowel necrosis (N = 3 [0.15%]). The investigators concluded that NCJ is associated with low complication rates and that most of the complications that occur can be prevented through greater attention to detail and better monitoring of the physical examination of patients with marginal gut function. Another retrospective review of jejunal feeding was performed in 1,359 patients over a period of 6 years.[91] Small bowel necrosis occurred in 14 patients, and 12 succumbed to this complication. The mechanism of small bowel necrosis was unclear but was thought to be associated with increased intraluminal pressure arising from severe abdominal distention.

As noted, PEG has become the gold standard for the delivery of enteral nutrition into the stomach. Compared with surgical gastrostomy, it is associated with significantly reduced morbidity and cost. Despite the increased use of this technique, however, overall survival remains poor because of the frequent placement of PEGs in patients with terminal disease. A 1997 study reviewed 64 patients consecutively referred for PEGs with the aim of examining possible predictive postoperative variables.[92] Of the 64, 43 survived at least 30 days after tube placement; only one death was directly attributable to tube placement. The 30-day survival correlated directly with the serum albumin concentration and inversely with the serum creatinine concentration. After multivariable logistic regression analysis, only albumin could be identified as an independent predictor of 30-day survival ($P = 0.04$): 83% of patients with a serum albumin level higher than 3.0 g/dl survived for 30 days, compared with 58% of patients with an albumin level lower than 3.0 g/dl. The investigators concluded that serum albumin concentration appeared to be a predictor of early survival in patients undergoing PEG placement.

Conclusions

Parenteral and enteral nutritional support is a valuable adjunctive—and sometimes life-saving—therapy in the management of selective types of surgical patients. It is generally agreed that patients who are unable to ingest adequate nutrients for a prolonged period require nutritional therapy to prevent the adverse effects of malnutrition. It is not entirely clear, however, precisely how "adequate" and "prolonged" should be defined. In practice, the definitions are likely to vary from patient to patient, depending on the amount of body energy stores and lean body mass, the presence or absence of preexisting medical illnesses, the number and severity of postoperative complications, and the nature of the surgical procedure. Summation of the data from the PRCTs suggests that giving nutritional support for 7 days before operation decreases postoperative complications. Severely malnourished patients (defined on the basis of percentage of body weight lost or nutritional risk index score) may derive greater clinical benefit from preoperative nutritional support, but this conclusion is based largely on retrospective analysis of prospective data. In addition, there are subsets of patients who may derive particular benefit from nutritional support, such as patients undergoing hepatic resection for hepatocellular carcinoma and elderly patients with hip fractures. The increased rate of complications in patients given postoperative TPN and the case reports of small bowel necrosis in patients who receive early postoperative enteral nutrition are evidence that nutritional support has risks and should not be given indiscriminately. Future studies are needed for better identification of specific subsets of patients who may benefit from perioperative nutritional therapy, particularly enteral nutrition. Such studies must consider the effect of nutritional therapy on both short-term and long-term outcome.

Nutrition Pharmacotherapy

The role of nutrient administration to surgical patients has evolved from the maintenance of a positive energy and nitrogen balance to the use of nutrients to modulate tissue metabolism and organ system function. This new role is referred to as nutrition pharmacotherapy. Like other forms of adjuvant therapy, nutrition pharmacotherapy is usually a multitargeted therapeutic modality. For instance, one form of nutrition pharmacotherapy, immuno-nutrition, makes use of combinations of specific amino acids, fatty acids, and, in some enteral formulas, nucleotides. Another form, so-called bowel rehabilitation, uses an amino acid (glutamine) in combination with growth hormone and a modified diet. Inclusion of a specific nutrient as part of a plan of nutrition pharmacotherapy is based either on clinical studies or, more often, on extrapolations from experimental observations.

In what follows, we discuss each of the nutrients used, or proposed for use, in nutrition pharmacotherapy, with emphasis on chemical characteristics, physiologic effects, available forms for exogenous administration, and, if available, clinical data supporting its use for this purpose.

BRANCHED-CHAIN AMINO ACIDS

The BCAAs—leucine, isoleucine, and valine—are unique among amino acids in that they undergo very little, if any, metabolism by the liver. Instead, most absorbed BCAAs remain intact until they reach muscle tissue, where they increase protein synthesis by 50% and decrease protein degradation by 25%.[93] These effects are attributable more to leucine (and its metabolite α-ketoisocaproate) than to isoleucine or valine. These effects reach physiologic significance only during stress or injury, which is why most of the studies that show BCAAs to have beneficial effects have been conducted in animals or patients manifesting the septic response.

In experimental primate models of sepsis, induced by administration of *Salmonella typhimurium* or *Streptococcus pneumoniae,* a positive nitrogen balance can be achieved only by giving high-dose glucose (85 kcal/kg/day) when the nitrogen source is a balanced mixture of amino acids (containing 24% BCAAs). If, however, the formula is enriched to 48% BCAAs, the same amount of nitrogen retention is achieved at a much lower intake of glucose (32 kcal/kg/day). Given the usual glucose intolerance seen in patients with the septic response, this is a highly desirable effect.

In 1986, several clinical studies reported in the late 1970s and early 1980s were reviewed by a panel of experts in a research workshop sponsored by the American Society of Parenteral and Enteral Nutrition.[93] The panel's main conclusion was that whereas some positive parameters of nitrogen metabolism had been noted using BCAA-enriched solutions in the most severely ill patients, a major effect on outcome was not demonstrated.

An entire decade elapsed before a subsequent study attempted to address this issue. In a prospective, randomized, multicenter study conducted in ICUs in Spain, 69 patients with the septic response were randomly selected to receive amino acids in dosages of 1.5 g/kg/day with 23% BCAAs, 1.5 g/kg/day with 45% BCAAs, or 1.1 g/kg/day with 45% BCAAs. Compared with patients who received the standard 23% BCAA solution, patients who received the 45% BCAA solution, at either nitrogen intake, exhibited significantly increased prealbumin and retinol-binding protein levels as well as a lower mortality.[94]

Thus, there are data to support the use of BCAAs in clinical practice, but the indications are very specific. First, the only patients who seem to benefit from BCAA supplementation are those who are in a septic state and critically ill; however, most such patients can be successfully treated either with conventional nutritional

therapy or with no nutritional therapy at all. Therefore, a second indication should be a clear need for nutritional therapy, as outlined earlier (see above), coupled with unsuccessful use of conventional amino acid formulations, as demonstrated by persistently low levels of short-lived serum proteins and a negative nitrogen balance.

GLUTAMINE

Glutamine is the most abundant amino acid in the body and appears to be the most versatile. Most free glutamine is synthesized and stored in skeletal muscle, where its concentration is 30 times greater than it is in plasma.[95] Skeletal muscle releases net glutamine for transport to the gut, immune cells, and the kidneys. The cells of the gut and those of the immune system proliferate rapidly, and glutamine acts as the main source of fuel and as a biosynthetic precursor. One of the compounds derived from glutamine is glutathione, a tripeptide (glutamate-cysteineglycine) with potent antioxidant effects. Finally, glutamine participates in acid-base regulation via the release of ammonia, which combines with H^+ to form NH_4^+ and is lost in urine.

Catabolism induced by major injury, surgery, sepsis, or burns results in increased release of glutamine from skeletal muscle.[96] This output of glutamine into the circulation is associated with increased uptake and consumption by the gut, the immune system, the liver, and the kidneys. The net effect is a profound fall in intracellular muscle stores of glutamine. This deficit exceeds all other amino acid deficits and persists even when stores of all other amino acids have already been replenished.[97]

Standard amino acid formulations have always included all of the essential amino acids and most of the nonessential ones. For a long time, glutamine was excluded from parenteral formulations because of its instability in aqueous solutions. In the early formulations, glutamine that had remained in solution for an extended period would undergo spontaneous transformation into a cyclic compound called pyroglutamate, which can cause neurotoxicity. As more knowledge of the potential benefits of glutamine became available, the pharmaceutical industry began to develop ways of keeping glutamine stable in an aqueous solution. For instance, Glamin (Pharmacia & Upjohn, Sweden), an amino acid formulation that is already commercially available in Europe, includes the dipeptide glycyl-L-glutamine, which is readily hydrolyzed to free glutamine in plasma and tissues.

Several clinical studies of supplementation of parenteral formulas with glutamine have been published. The most striking results have been reported in patients undergoing bone marrow transplantation and in patients with short-bowel syndrome. The first randomized, double-blind, controlled study to investigate the effects of glutamine on metabolic parameters and clinical outcome in patients undergoing bone marrow transplantation was published in 1992.[98] A total of 45 adults receiving allogeneic bone marrow transplants for hematologic malignancies were randomly selected to receive L-glutamine, 0.57 g/kg/day, or a standard glutamine-free isonitrogenous formula for an average of 4 weeks after operation. The patients who received the glutamine-supplemented formula had a better nitrogen balance than the control group (−1.4 g/day versus −4.2 g/day); more important, they also had a lower incidence of microbial colonization and clinical infection and a shorter hospital stay. Subsequently, these findings were confirmed by a study performed by a different group of investigators.[99]

One of the most challenging pathologic conditions for surgeons is the short-bowel syndrome that develops after massive small bowel resection. Fortunately, the advent of parenteral nutrition has improved survival for many patients with this condition who previously would have died of dehydration and malnutrition; however, it has also created a dependency on this therapy, which in the long term can have life-threatening complications. For this reason, many surgical scientists have searched for ways of augmenting these patients' intestinal absorption capacity so that their need for parenteral nutrition can be eliminated or at least greatly reduced. Having achieved a better understanding of the roles of glutamine, dietary fiber, short-chain fatty acids, and growth factors in the process of intestinal adaptation, investigators designed clinical trials with the aim of evaluating the effects of supplementation of these substances on patients with short-bowel syndrome.

After a pilot study involving eight patients with short-bowel syndrome, one group of investigators performed a controlled study in which recombinant human growth hormone, 0.14 mg/kg/day; glutamine, 0.45 to 0.63 g/kg/day; and a high-carbohydrate, low-fat diet were given to 31 patients with this syndrome.[100,101] The criteria for inclusion were (1) either the entire colon present with a minimum of 50 cm of small bowel remaining or the colon absent with a minimum of 100 cm of small bowel remaining and (2) previous need for long-term parenteral nutrition. By the end of a 3-week treatment period, there was a significant improvement in nutrient and fluid absorption, and as a result, parenteral nutrition was discontinued in 40% of patients. After an extended follow-up period (6 years) and the inclusion of more patients (87), this bowel rehabilitation regimen led to the discontinuance of parenteral nutrition in 52% of patients and to reduced requirements for parenteral nutrition in an additional 38%.[102] Another group of investigators using a similar protocol found only a modest improvement in electrolyte assimilation and no improvement in gut morphology or nutrient absorption.[103] Although these studies do not settle the issue of how effective the bowel rehabilitation regimen is, they do raise important questions—in particular, how administration of these substances should be timed and whether a multi-institutional study is needed.[104]

All of the studies just cited were conducted according to research protocols that used L-glutamine, which is not practical for I.V. use. As noted, glutamine is now commercially available (in Europe) in a dipeptide form that is stable in an aqueous solution. A 1998 study evaluated the use of the dipeptide glycyl-L-glutamine, 0.3 g/kg/day, in 28 patients who underwent elective abdominal surgery.[105] Over a 5-day period, the mean cumulative nitrogen balance was significantly better with glutamine supplementation than without it (−7 g/day versus −23 g/day). Immune function, as determined by lymphocyte counts and generation of cysteinyl leukotrienes by polymorphonuclear neutrophils, was also improved. In addition, the hospital stay was 6.2 days shorter for the glutamine group. The investigators concluded that glutamine administered as the dipeptide glycyl-L-glutamine appears to be safe and effective.

The precise indications for glutamine supplementation remain to be determined. There is no question regarding the benefits of glutamine administration after bone marrow transplantation. We believe it is safe to assume that glutamine supplementation, when available, is beneficial to stressed surgical patients, particularly those who are immunosuppressed. Further research is needed before its widespread use to augment intestinal absorption can be recommended.

ARGININE

Arginine is a nitrogen-dense amino acid that is considered a semiessential amino acid because it is required for growth.[106] The effect of arginine on growth seems to be mediated by its role in polyamine and nucleic acid synthesis. In addition, arginine is a potent secretagogue of growth hormone, insulin, glucagon, prolactin, and somatostatin.[107-109] When the secretagogue effect of arginine is abolished by hypophysectomy, the stimulatory effect on

wound healing is lost.[110] Supplemental dietary arginine has thymotrophic effects and enhances the responsiveness of thymic lymphocytes to mitogens in rats.[111] A similar response occurs in peripheral blood mononuclear cells of healthy human volunteers[112] and postoperative patients,[113] as evidenced by an enhanced response to concanavalin A and phytohemagglutinin.

Arginine enhances cellular immunity, as demonstrated by an increased delayed hypersensitivity response in animals with burns.[51] Dietary supplementation with arginine improves the response to dinitrofluorobenzene (DNFB) and enhances the survival of guinea pigs with 30% body surface burns. However, in a model of acute peritonitis in guinea pigs, supplemental arginine did not improve DNFB response or survival.[114]

Supplemental arginine also has antitumor properties.[115] The inhibition of tumor growth induced by supplemental arginine is associated with increased tumor cyclic adenosine monophosphate levels and decreased ornithine decarboxylase activity.[116] The exact mechanism of action of arginine on tumor growth is not known, but it seems to be twofold: nonspecific immunomodulation and augmentation of the response to immunoregulatory lymphokines. In accordance with this hypothesis, supplemental arginine has been investigated as an immunotherapeutic agent to enhance the effect of interleukin-2 (IL-2).[117] When compared with a glycine-treated group, arginine reduced tumor engraftment and growth and prolonged survival in a model of murine neuroblastoma treated with IL-2.

The experimental evidence currently available demonstrates a physiologic role in growing animals and a therapeutic benefit in posttraumatic states, burns, and cancer. A new enteral formula that includes arginine in combination with fish oil and RNA is now available in the United States (see Fatty Acids, below).

NUCLEOTIDES

Purines and pyrimidines are precursors of DNA and RNA, which are essential for cell proliferation. Purines and pyrimidines are synthesized by the liver de novo from amino acids and reutilized by salvage pathways. Reduction of dietary nucleotides results in suppression of cellular immune responses and prolongation of allograft survival.[118] The mechanism of immunosuppression associated with nucleotide restriction seems to be an inability of T cells to undergo blastogenesis. Dietary supplements containing RNA or uracil (but not adenine) maintain resistance to infection by C. albicans or S. aureus in rodents.[119,120] However, the immune response is not enhanced when compared with a standard control diet.

On the basis of the immunosuppressive effect of dietary restriction of nucleotides, it has been postulated that nucleotide supplementation could provide an immunostimulant effect. This postulate has been tested in studies of the RNA–fish oil–arginine formula now available [see Fatty Acids, below].

FATTY ACIDS

Fatty acids in the systemic circulation can be used in two forms: as fuels to be stored and oxidized as needed by the organism and as precursors for other essential compounds, such as eicosanoids (prostaglandins, leukotrienes, and thromboxanes). The eicosanoids are 20-carbon compounds derived from the essential fatty acids. They function as regulatory compounds in various physiologic processes, such as the immune response. Although organisms can oxidize other compounds to meet caloric needs, fatty acids in minimal amounts are essential as precursors for the synthesis of eicosanoids.

Fatty acids are classified in many different ways. One classification is based on chain length: short (two to five carbons), medium (six to 11 carbons), and long (12 to 26 carbons). Another classification is based on the presence of double bonds in the carbon chain: those with double bonds are called unsaturated and are further classified as either monounsaturated fatty acids or polyunsaturated fatty acids (PUFAs), depending on the number of double bonds. Another classification that has gained popularity is the omega classification, which indicates where the first double bond is located when the carbons are counted from the noncarboxyl end of the chain (e.g., omega-3, omega-6, omega-9).

Humans can synthesize only fatty acids with double bonds at position 7 (counting from the noncarboxyl end toward the carboxyl end). Therefore, fatty acids with double bonds at position 6 or position 3 must be supplied exogenously. Because humans can elongate and desaturate linoleic acid and α-linolenic acid to produce the remaining omega-6 and omega-3 PUFAs, these are considered the essential fatty acids. The requirements for omega-6 PUFAs exceed the requirements for omega-3 PUFAs by a ratio of approximately 5:1.

PUFAs of the omega-6 series are abundant in vegetable oils, such as corn oil and soybean oil, and PUFAs of the omega-3 series are abundant in fish oils, such as menhaden oil. Other oils rich in omega-3 PUFAs are seed oils, such as black currant oil and canola oil (canola oil is derived from rape seeds and genetically modified to optimize the fatty acid composition).

The availability of 20-carbon PUFAs—arachidonic acid in the omega-6 series and eicosapentaenoic acid in the omega-3 series—is the determining factor for the synthesis of eicosanoids [see VII:11 *Molecular and Cellular Mediators of the Inflammatory Response*]. There are two major metabolic pathways for the synthesis of eicosanoids. The cyclooxygenase pathway results in the production of prostanoids. Inasmuch as prostanoids contain two double bonds in the carbon side chain, they are also called di-enoic products, or the two series. These include prostaglandin E_2 (PGE_2), prostaglandin D_2 (PGD_2), prostaglandin F_2 (PGF_2), prostaglandin I_2 (PGI_2, also called prostacyclin), and thromboxane A_2 (TXA_2). The lipoxygenase pathway yields trienoic products (three double bonds in the carbon side chain), such as thromboxane A_3 (TXA_3) and prostaglandin I_3 (PGI_3). All nucleated cells, with the exception of lymphocytes, can synthesize eicosanoids. Platelets are the major sources of thromboxanes, and the leukocytes mainly produce leukotrienes. Prostaglandins have various effects on the tone of blood vessels and the aggregation of platelets. Leukotrienes promote leukocyte migration (chemotaxis) and degranulation, release of lysosomal enzymes, and superoxide production.

Cells obtain arachidonic acid and eicosapentaenoic acid from degradation of phospholipids by phospholipase A_2 and phospholipase C or by elongation and desaturation of linoleic acid and α-linolenic acid. Mature immune cells, such as monocytes, macrophages, lymphocytes, and polymorphonuclear cells, lack δ-6 desaturase, the critical rate-limiting enzyme for transformation of 18-carbon PUFAs into 20-carbon PUFAs.[121] Therefore, the availability of precursors for eicosanoid synthesis in immune cells is largely dependent on their lipid composition. Because lipid intake influences the lipid composition of immune cells, the type of PUFAs ingested can influence the immune response.[122,123] Eicosanoids, especially PGE_2 and the lipoxygenase products leukotriene B_4 (LTB_4), 5-hydroxyeicosatetraenoic acid (5-HETE), and 15-hydroxyeicosatetraenoic acid (15-HETE) are immunomodulatory; when produced in excess (as in posttraumatic states), they are generally immunosuppressive.[124] Dietary supplementation with omega-3 PUFAs has improved survival of endotoxic shock in guinea pigs.[125] The reduced intake of omega-6 PUFAs seems to be as important as the enrichment with omega-3 PUFAs. When animals are made deficient in linoleic acid, they have only a 24% mortality after endotoxin challenge. However, the mortality reaches 100% when arachidonic acid is given 2 days before endotoxin challenge.[126] Similar results have been reported in guinea pigs recovering from flame burns covering 30% of body surface area.[127] When compared with animals fed dietary safflower oil (74% linoleic acid) or linoleic acid alone, animals fed fish oil had less weight loss, better skeletal muscle mass, lower resting metabolic expenditure, better cell-mediated immune responses, better opsonic indices, higher splenic weight, lower adrenal weight, higher serum transferrin levels, and lower serum C3 levels.

In conclusion, high intake of omega-6 PUFAs (e.g., linoleic acid) is associated with increased synthesis of PGE_2, which is immunosuppressive. A reduction in the intake of omega-6 PUFAs appears prudent in patients who are immunocompromised or in posttraumatic states. Dietary supplements with omega-3 PUFAs are associated with incorporation of eicosapentaenoic acid into leukocytes and with concurrent decreases in the incorporation of arachidonic acid. When these cells are challenged, there is a significantly lower production of LTB_4, which exacerbates undesirable immune responses such as those seen in trauma and autoimmune diseases. Formulas for nutritional support should include omega-3 PUFAs, although the exact amount of omega-3 PUFAs and the precise ratio of omega-6 PUFAs to omega-3 PUFAs remain to be determined.

The fat emulsions currently available for I.V. use in the United States are made with long-chain triglycerides derived either from soybean oil alone or from soybean oil and safflower oil. All of the fatty acids in LCTs are in the form of PUFAs, which include the essential fatty acids (i.e., linoleic and linolenic acids). As noted (see above), an excess of omega-6 PUFAs can have an immunosuppressive effect. Intravenously administered LCT emulsions are cleared in part through the reticuloendothelial system (RES).[128] When such emulsions are used as a calorie source, they may impair the ability of the RES to clear bacteria if given too rapidly or in excessively large amounts.

Moreover, the PUFAs in LCT emulsions require carnitine-mediated transport to cross the mitochondrial membrane for oxidation. Carnitine is a quaternary amine derived from two essential amino acids, lysine and methionine. During sepsis, urinary excretion of free carnitine rises significantly, and the plasma acylcarnitine level falls.[129] One way of circumventing these problems is to use emulsions that contain MCTs.

MCT-containing emulsions have long been used in enteral nutrition for their absorptive advantage over LCT-containing emulsions: whereas LCTs are absorbed via lacteals and the lymphatic system, MCTs are absorbed via the portal system. MCTs are obtained from coconut oil and contain saturated fatty acids (with octanoic acids predominating). Because MCTs are smaller than LCTs, they are more water soluble; they are also poorly bound to albumin and diffuse more easily across body compartments.

Several reports on the use of intravenously administered MCT fat emulsions have been published. One study evaluated the effect of a 75% MCT/ 25% LCT emulsion on RES function as demonstrated by ^{99m}Tc-sulfur colloid (Tc-SC) clearance. Clearance of Tc-SC was significantly higher after 3 days of MCT/LCT administration than after 3 days of LCT administration.[130] Another study investigated the metabolic effects of MCT-containing emulsions on surgical patients.[131] The main finding of this study was the appearance of β-hydroxybutyrate in association with infusion of the MCT emulsion, which was indicative of a ketogenic effect. A tendency toward improved nitrogen balance was also observed, but it was not statistically significant.

Another feature of fat emulsions that is exploited in surgical patients is the salutary effect of omega-3 fatty acids on the immune response. A diet is now commercially available in the United States that contains fish oil in addition to arginine and RNA. This diet was tested in a 1993 study of postoperative patients who underwent surgery for upper GI malignancies.[132] A total of 85 patients were randomly selected to receive either the experimental diet or a standard formula. The patients who received the experimental diet had better nitrogen balance (–2.2 g/day versus –6.6 g/day) and improved in vitro lymphocyte mitogenesis. Infection and wound complication rates were also lower in the experimental group (11% versus 37%), and hospital stay was shorter (15.8 days versus 20.2 days).

This experimental diet was subsequently tested in a randomized, double-blind study in which 325 patients from eight different hospitals were enrolled.[133] The inclusion criteria were (1) admission to the ICU as a result of trauma, operation, or sepsis and (2) an APACHE II score of 10 or higher or a Therapeutic Intervention Scoring System score of 20 or higher. Patients started tube feedings within 48 hours of admission with either the experimental formula (N = 68) or a standard tube-feeding formula (N = 15). Patients receiving the experimental formula had significantly higher plasma levels of arginine, ornithine, eicosapentaenoic acid, and docosahexaenoic acid, with a concomitant decrease in linoleic acid levels. Hospital stay was significantly shorter in several subgroups (including patients who received more than a certain amount of formula and patients in a septic state) in association with a significant reduction in the incidence of acquired infections.

In summary, specific fatty acids have significant potential for use in nutrition pharmacotherapy. Omega-6 fatty acids are potential immunosuppressants, whereas omega-3 fatty acids are potential immunostimulants. In the United States, the only emulsions commercially available for I.V. use at present are made of LCTs containing omega-6 fatty acids. MCTs offer some metabolic advantages over LCTs and obviate the side effects resulting from an excess of omega-6 fatty acids. Enteral diets containing omega-3 fatty acids appear to benefit stressed surgical patients, particularly those who are immunosuppressed as a result of therapy for cancer.

References

1. Wilmore DW: Metabolic Management of the Critically Ill. Plenum Publishing Corp, New York, 1977

2. Vitamin preparations as dietary supplements and as therapeutic agents. Council on Scientific Affairs. JAMA 257:1929, 1987

3. Marks J: The safety of vitamins: an overview. Int J Vitam Nutr Res 30(suppl):12, 1989

4. Demling R, LaLonde C, Saldinger P, et al: Multiple-organ dysfunction in the surgical patient: pathophysiology, prevention, and treatment. Curr Probl Surg 30:345, 1993

5. Pingleton SK, Hadzima SK: Enteral alimentation and gastrointestinal bleeding in mechanically ventilated patients. Crit Care Med 11:13, 1983

6. Koruda MJ, Guenter P, Rombeau JL: Enteral nutrition in the critically ill. Critical Care Clinics 3:133, 1987

7. Guidelines for the use of parenteral and enteral nutrition in adult and pediatric patients. JPEN J Parenter Enteral Nutr 17(4 suppl):1SA, 1993

8. Fischer JE, Rosen HM, Ebeid AM, et al: The effect of normalization of plasma amino acids on hepatic encephalopathy in man. Surgery 80:77, 1976

9. Abel RM: Parenteral nutrition in the treatment of renal failure. Total Parenteral Nutrition. Fischer JE, Ed. Little, Brown & Co, Inc, Boston, 1976, p 143

10. Steffee WP, Anderson CF: Enteral nutrition and renal disease. Clinical Nutrition, Vol 1: Enteral and Tube Feeding. Rombeau JL, Caldwell MD, Eds. WB Saunders Co, Philadelphia, 1984, p 363

11. Heymsfield SB, Head CA, McManus CB III, et al: Respiratory, cardiovascular, and metabolic effects of enteral hyperalimentation: influence of formula dose and composition. Am J Clin Nutr 40:116, 1984

12. Askanazi J, Weissman C, Rosenbaum SH, et al: Nutrition and the respiratory system. Crit Care Med 10:163, 1982

13. Cobb LM, Cartmill AM, Barry M, et al: A tube for enteral nutrition of patients with aphagopraxia and patients with ventilator assistance. Surg Gynecol Obstet 155:81, 1982

14. Daly JM, Lieberman MD, Goldfine J, et al: Enteral nutrition with supplemental arginine, RNA, and omega-3 fatty acids in patients after operation: immunologic, metabolic, and clinical outcome. Surgery 112:56, 1992

15. Winterbauer RH, Durning RB Jr, Barron E, et al: Aspirated nasogastric feeding solution detected by glucose strips. Ann Intern Med 95:67, 1981

16. Rolandelli RH, Rombeau JL: Liquid defined formula diets. Current Therapy in Gastroenterology and Liver Disease. Bayless TM, Ed. BC Decker Inc, Toronto, 1986, p 206

17. Treolar DM, Stechmiller J: Pulmonary aspiration in tube-fed patients with artificial airways. Heart Lung 13:667, 1984

18. McLean GK: Radiologic techniques of gastrointestinal intubation. Clinical Nutrition, Vol 1: Enteral and Tube Feeding. Rombeau JL, Caldwell MD, Eds. WB Saunders Co, Philadelphia, 1984, p 240

19. Rombeau JL, Barot LR, Low DW, et al: Feeding by tube enterostomy. Clinical Nutrition, Vol 1: Enteral and Tube Feeding. Rombeau JL, Caldwell MD, Eds. WB Saunders Co, Philadelphia, 1984, p 275

20. Moss G: Early enteral feeding after abdominal surgery. Nutrition in Clinical Surgery, 2nd ed. Deitel M, Ed. Williams & Wilkins Co, Baltimore, 1985, p 220

21. Ponsky JL, Gauderer MW, Stellato TA, et al: Percutaneous approaches to enteral alimentation. Am J Surg 149:102, 1985

22. Cataldi-Betcher EL, Seltzer MH, Blocum BA, et al: Complications occurring during enteral nutrition support: a prospective study. JPEN J Parenter Enteral Nutr 7:546, 1983

23. Du Moulin GC, Paterson DJ, Hedley-White J, et al: Aspiration of gastric bacteria in antacid-treated patients: a frequent cause of postoperative colonization of the airway. Lancet 1:242, 1982

24. Forlaw L, Chernoff R: Enteral delivery systems. Clinical Nutrition, Vol 1: Enteral and Tube Feeding. Rombeau JL, Caldwell MD, Eds. WB Saunders Co, Philadelphia, 1984, p 228

25. Pemberton LB, Lyman B, Lander V, et al: Sepsis from triple- vs single-lumen catheters during total parenteral nutrition in surgical or critically ill patients. Arch Surg 121:591, 1986

26. Miller JJ, Venus B, Mathru M: Comparison of the sterility of long-term central venous catheterization using single lumen, triple lumen, and pulmonary artery catheters. Crit Care Med 12:634, 1984

27. Belliveau K: Catheter infection rate using multiple lumen catheters. Read before the National Intravenous Therapy Association, New Orleans, April 1986

28. Moncrief JA: Femoral catheters. Ann Surg 147:166, 1958

29. Black PR, Brooks DC, Bessey PQ, et al: Mechanisms of insulin resistance following injury. Ann Surg 196:420, 1982

30. Maki DG, Weise CE, Sarafin HW: A semiquantitative culture method for identifying intravenous-catheter–related infection. N Engl J Med 296:1305, 1977

31. Pettigrew RA, Lang SDR, Haydock DA, et al: Catheter-related sepsis in patients on intravenous nutrition: a prospective study of quantitative catheter cultures and guidewire changes for suspected sepsis. Br J Surg 72:52, 1985

32. Williams WW: Infection control during parenteral nutrition therapy. JPEN J Parenter Enteral Nutr 9:735, 1985

33. Grundfest S, Steiger E: Home parenteral nutrition. JAMA 244:1701, 1980

34. Broviac JW, Scribner BH: Prolonged parenteral nutrition in the home. Surg Gynecol Obstet 139:24, 1974

35. Levine GM, Deren JJ, Steiger E, et al: Role of oral intake in maintenance of gut mass and disaccharidase activity. Gastroenterology 67:975, 1974

36. Border JR: Trauma and sepsis. Principles and Practice of Trauma Care. Worth MH, Ed. Williams & Wilkins Co, Baltimore, 1982, p 330

37. Udall JN, Walker WA: Mucosal defense mechanisms. Immunopathology of the Small Intestine. Marsh MN, Ed. John Wiley & Sons, Inc, New York, 1986, p 3

38. Deitch EA, Maejima K, Berg R: Effect of oral antibiotics and bacterial overgrowth on the translocation of the GI tract microflora in burned rats. J Trauma 25:385, 1985

39. Wells CL, Rotstein OD, Pruett TL, et al: Intestinal bacteria translocate into experimental intraabdominal abscesses. Arch Surg 121:102, 1986

40. Schatten WE, Desprez JD, Holden WD: A bacteriologic study of portal-vein blood in man. Arch Surg 71:404, 1955

41. Bodey GP: Antibiotic prophylaxis in cancer patients: regimens of oral, nonabsorbable antibiotics for prevention of infection during induction of remission. Rev Infect Dis 3(suppl):S259, 1981

42. Jarrett F, Balish L, Moylan JA, et al: Clinical experience with prophylactic antibiotic bowel suppression in burn patients. Surgery 83:523, 1978

43. Keller GA, West MA, Cerra FB, et al: Multiple systems organ failure: modulation of hepatocyte protein synthesis by endotoxin activated Kupffer cells. Ann Surg 201:87, 1985

44. Hammer-Hodges D, Woodruff P, Cuevas P, et al: Role of the intraintestinal gram negative bacterial flora in response to major injury. Surg Gynecol Obstet 138:599, 1974

45. Deitch EA, Berg R, Specian R: Endotoxin promotes the translocation of bacteria from the gut. Arch Surg 122:185, 1987

46. Deitch EA, Winterton J, Li M, et al: The gut as a portal of entry for bacteremia: role of protein malnutrition. Ann Surg 205:681, 1987

47. Wellmann W, Fink PC, Schmidt FW: Whole-gut irrigation as antiendotoxinaemic therapy in inflammatory bowel disease. Hepatogastroenterology 31:91, 1984

48. Bounous G: Acute necrosis of the intestinal mucosa. Gastroenterology 82:1457, 1982

49. Rhodes RS, Depalma RG, Robinson AV: Intestinal barrier function in hemorrhagic shock. J Surg Res 14:305, 1973

50. Bounous G, Cronin RFP, Gurd FN: Dietary prevention of experimental shock lesions. Arch Surg 94:46, 1967

51. Saito H, Trocki O, Alexander JW, et al: The effect of route of nutrient administration on the nutritional state, catabolic hormone secretion, and gut mucosal integrity after burn injury. JPEN J Parenter Enteral Nutr 11:1, 1987

52. Hwang TL, O'Dwyer ST, Smith RJ, et al: Preservation of small-bowel mucosa using glutamine enriched parenteral nutrition. Forum on Fundamental Surgical Problems 37:56, 1986

53. van der Hulst RRWJ, van Kreel BK, von Meyenfeldt MF, et al: Glutamine and the preservation of gut integrity. Lancet 341:1363, 1993

54. Jacobs DO, Evans A, O'Dwyer ST, et al: Disparate effects of 5-fluorouracil on ileum and colon of enterally fed rats with protection by dietary glutamine. Forum on Fundamental Surgical Problems 38:45, 1987

55. Fox AD, Kripke SA, Berman JM, et al: Reduction of the severity of enterocolitis by glutamine-supplemented enteral diets. Forum on Fundamental Surgical Problems 38:43, 1987

56. Hammarqvist F, Wernerman J, Ali R, et al: Addition of glutamine to total parenteral nutrition after elective abdominal surgery spares free glutamine in muscle, counteracts the fall in muscle protein synthesis, and improves nitrogen balance. Ann Surg 209:455, 1989

57. Stehle P, Zander J, Mertes N, et al: Effect of parenteral glutamine peptide supplements on muscle glutamine loss and nitrogen balance after major surgery. Lancet 1:231, 1989

58. Scheltinga MR, Young LS, Benfell K, et al: Glutamine-enriched intravenous feedings attenuate extracellular fluid expansion after a standard stress. Ann Surg 214:385, 1991

59. Ziegler TR, Young LS, Benfell K, et al: Clinical and metabolic efficacy of glutamine-supplemented parenteral nutrition after bone marrow transplantation: a randomized, double-blind, controlled study. Ann Intern Med 116:821, 1992

60. Schloerb PR, Amare M: Total parenteral nutrition with glutamine in bone marrow transplantation and other clinical applications (a randomized, double-blind study). JPEN J Parenter Enteral Nutr 17:407, 1993

61. Hardy G, Bevan SJ, McElroy B, et al: Stability of glutamine in parenteral feeding solutions (letter). Lancet 342:186, 1993

62. Parry-Billings M, Evans J, Calder PC, et al: Does glutamine contribute to immunosuppression after major burns? Lancet 336:523, 1990

63. Jensen GL, Miller RH, Talabiska D, et al: A double-blind prospective randomized study of glutamine-enriched versus standard peptide-based feeding in critically ill. JPEN J Parenter Enteral Nutr 17(suppl):33S, 1993

64. Hong RW, Rounds JD, Helton WS, et al: Glutamine preserves liver glutathione after lethal hepatic injury. Ann Surg 215:114, 1992

65. Welbourne TC, King AB, Horton K: Enteral glutamine supports hepatic glutathione efflux during inflammation. J Nutr Biochem 4:236, 1993

66. Koruda MJ, Rolandelli RH, Settle RG, et al: The effect of a pectin-supplemented elemental diet on intestinal adaptation to massive small-bowel resection. JPEN J Parenter Enteral Nutr 10:343, 1986

67. Koruda MJ, Rolandelli RH, Settle RG, et al: Small bowel disaccharidase activity in the rat as affected by intestinal resection and pectin feeding. Am J Clin Nutr 47:448, 1988

68. Rolandelli RH, Koruda MJ, Settle RG, et al: The effect of enteral feedings supplemented with pectin on the healing of colonic anastomosis in the rat. Surgery 99:703, 1986

69. Rolandelli RH, Saul SH, Settle RG, et al: Comparison of parenteral nutrition and enteral feeding with pectin in experimental colitis in the rat. Am J Clin Nutr 47:715, 1988

70. Jacobs DO, Evans DA, Smith RJ, et al: Combined effects of glutamine and epidermal growth factor on the rat intestine. Surgery 104:358, 1988

71. Klein S, Kinney J, Jeejeebhoy K, et al: Nutrition support in clinical practice: review of published data and recommendations for further research directions. JPEN J Parenter Enteral Nutr 21:133, 1997

72. von Meyenfeldt MF, Meijrink WJHJ, Rouflart MMJ, et al: Perioperative nutritional support: a randomized clinical trial. Clin Nutr 11:180, 1992

73. Shukla HS, Rao RR, Banu N, et al: Enteral hyperalimentation in malnourished surgical patients. Ind J Med Res 80:339, 1984

74. Sagar S, Harland P, Shields R: Early postoperative feeding with elemental diet. Br Med J 1:293, 1979

75. Ryan JA, Page CP, Babcock L: Early postoperative jejunal feeding of elemental diet in gastrointestinal surgery. Am Surg 47:393, 1981

76. Smith RC, Hartemink RJ, Holinshead JW, et al: Fine bore jejunostomy feeding following major abdominal trauma: a controlled randomized clinical trial. Br J Surg 72:458, 1985

77. Tovinelli G, Marsili I, Varrassi G: Nutrition support after total laryngectomy. JPEN J Parenter Enteral Nutr 17:445, 1993

78. Daly JM, Lieberman MD, Goldfine J, et al: Enteral nutrition with supplemental arginine, RNA and omega-3 fatty acids in patients after operation: immunologic, metabolic and clinical outcome. Surgery 112:56, 1992

79. Bastow MD, Rawlings J, Allison S: Benefits of supplementary tube feeding after fractured neck of femur: a randomized controlled trial. Br Med J 187:1589, 1983

80. Delmi M, Rapin CH, Bengoa JM, et al: Dietary supplementation in elderly patients with fractured neck of the femur. Lancet 335:1013, 1990

81. Brennan MF, Pisters PW, Posner M, et al: A prospective randomized trial of total parenteral nutrition after major pancreatic resection for malignancy. Am Surg 220:436, 1994

82. van Berge Henegowen M, Akkermans L, van Gulik T, et al: Prospective, randomized trial on the effect of cyclic versus continuous enteral nutrition on postoperative gastric function after pylorus-preserving pancreatoduodenectomy. Ann Surg 226:677, 1997

83. Fan ST, Lo CM, Lai E, et al: Perioperative nutritional support in patients undergoing hepatectomy for hepatocellular carcinoma. N Engl J Med 331:1547, 1994

84. Bufo A, Feldman S, Daniels G, et al: Early postoperative feeding. Dis Col Rect 37:1260, 1994

85. Choudhry U, Barde C, Markert R, et al: Percutaneous endoscopic gastrostomy: a randomized prospective comparison of early and delayed feeding. Gastrointest Endosc 44:164, 1996

86. Watters JM, Kirkpatrick SM, Norris SB, et al: Immediate postoperative enteral feeding results in impaired respiratory mechanics and decreased mobility. Ann Surg 226:369, 1997

87. Heslin MJ, Latkany L, Leung D, et al: A prospective, randomized trial of early enteral feeding after resection of upper gastrointestinal malignancy. Ann Surg 226:567, 1997

88. Singh G, Ram RP, Khanna SK: Early postoperative enteral feeding in patients with non-traumatic intestinal perforation and peritonitis. J Am Coll Surg 187:142, 1998

89. Smith-Choban P, Max MH: Feeding jejunomy: a small bowel stress test? Am J Surg 155:112, 1988

90. Myers JG, Page CP, Stewart RM, et al: Complications of needle catheter jejunostomy in 2,022 consecutive applications. Am J Surg 170:547, 1995

91. Schunn CD, Daly JM: Small bowel necrosis associated with postoperative jejunal tube feeding. J Am Coll Surg 180:410, 1995

92. Friedenberg F, Jensen, G, Gujral N, et al: Serum albumin is predictive of 30-day survival after percutaneous endoscopic gastrostomy. JPEN J Parenter Enteral Nutr 21:72, 1997

93. Brennan MF, Cerra F, Daly JM, et al: Report of a research workshop: branched-chain amino acids in stress and injury. JPEN J Parenter Enteral Nutr 10:446, 1986

94. Garcia-de-Lorenzo A, Ortiz-Leyba C, Planas M, et al: Parenteral administration of different amounts of branch-chain amino acids in septic patients: clinical and metabolic aspects. Crit Care Med 25:418, 1997

95. Souba WW, Herskowitz K, Augstgen TR, et al: Glutamine nutrition: theoretical considerations and therapeutic impact. JPEN J Parenter Enteral Nutr 14: 237S, 1990

96. Furst P, Albers S, Stehle P: Stress-induced intracellular glutamine depletion. Contr Infusion Ther Clin Nutr 17:117, 1987

97. Lacey JM, Wilmore DW: Is glutamine a conditionally essential amino acid? Nutr Rev 48:297, 1990

98. Ziegler TR, Young LS, Benfell K, et al: Clinical and metabolic efficacy of glutamine-supplemented parenteral nutrition after bone marrow transplantation. Ann Intern Med 116:821, l992

99. Schloerb PR, Amare M: Total parenteral nutrition with glutamine in bone marrow transplantation and other clinical applications. JPEN J Parenter Enteral Nutr 17:407, 1993

100. Byrne TA, Morrissey T, Naltakom T, et al: Growth hormone, glutamine and a modified diet enhance nutrient absorption in patients with severe short bowel syndrome. JPEN J Parenter Enteral Nutr 19:296, 1995

101. Byrne TA, Persinger RC, Young LS, et al: A new treatment for patients with short bowel syndrome. Ann Surg 222:243, 1995

102. Wilmore DW, Byrne TA, Persinger RL: Short bowel syndrome: new therapeutic approaches. Curr Probl Surg 34:398, 1997

103. Scolapio JS, Camilleri M, Fleming R, et al:

Effect of growth hormone, glutamine, and diet on adaptation in short bowel syndrome: a randomized, controlled study. Gastroenterology 113:1074, 1997

104. Thompson JS: Can the intestine adapt to a changing environment? Gastroenterology 113:1402, 1997

105. Morlion BJ, Stehle P, Wachtler P, et al: Total parenteral nutrition with glutamine dipeptide after major abdominal surgery: a randomized, double blind, controlled study. Ann Surg 227:302, l998

106. Barbul A: Arginine and immune function. Nutrition 6:53, 1990

107. Rakoff JS, Siler TM, Sinha YN, et al: Prolactin and growth hormone release in response to sequential stimulation by arginine and synthetic TRF. J Clin Endocrinol Metab 37:641, 1973

108. Palmer JP, Walter RM, Ensinck JW: Arginine-stimulated acute phase of insulin and glucagon secretion: I. In normal man. Diabetes 24:735, 1975

109. Utsumi M, Makimura H, Ishihara K, et al: Determination of immunoreactive somatostatin in rat plasma and responses to arginine, glucose and glucagon infusion. Diabetologia 17:319, 1979

110. Barbul A, Rettura G, Levenson SM, et al: Wound healing and thymotropic effects of arginine: a pituitary mechanism of action. Am J Clin Nutr 37:786, 1983

111. Barbul A, Wasserkrug HL, Seifter E, et al: Immunostimulatory effects of arginine in normal and injured rats. J Surg Res 29:228, 1980

112. Barbul A, Sisto DA, Wasserkrug HL, et al: Arginine stimulates lymphocyte immune response in healthy human beings. Surgery 90:244, 1981

113. Daly JM, Reynolds J, Thom A, et al: Immune and metabolic effects of arginine in the surgical patient. Ann Surg 208:512, 1988

114. Gonce SJ, Peck MD, Alexander JW, et al: Arginine supplementation and its effect on established peritonitis in guinea pigs. JPEN J Parenter Enteral Nutr 14:237, 1990

115. Daly JM, Reynolds J, Sigal RK, et al: Effect of dietary protein and amino acids on immune function. Crit Care Med 18(suppl):S86, 1990

116. Cho-Chung YS, Clair T, Bodwin JS, et al: Arrest of mammary tumor growth in vivo by L-arginine: stimulation of NAD-dependent activation of adenylate cyclase. Biochem Biophys Res Commun 95:1306, 1980

117. Lieberman MD, Nishioka K, Redmond HP, et al: Enhancement of interleukin-2 immunotherapy with L-arginine. Ann Surg 215:157, 1992

118. Van Buren CT, Kim E, Kulkarni AD, et al: Nucleotide-free diet and suppression of immune response. Transplant Proc 19:57, 1987

119. Fanslow WC, Kulkarni AD, Van Buren CT, et al: Effect of nucleotide restriction and supplementation on resistance to experimental murine candidiasis. JPEN J Parenter Enteral Nutr 12:49, 1988

120. Kulkarni AD, Fanslow WC, Drath DB, et al: Influence of dietary nucleotide restriction on bacterial sepsis and phagocytic cell function in mice. Arch Surg 121:169, 1986

121. Chapkin RS, Somers SD, Erickson KL: Inability of murine peritoneal macrophages to convert linoleic acid into arachidonic acid. J Immunol 140:2350, 1988

122. Johnston DV, Marshall LA: Dietary fat, prostaglandins and the immune response. Prog Food Nutr Sci 8:3, 1984

123. Meade CJ, Mertin J: Fatty acids and immunity. Adv Lip Res 16:127, 1978

124. Kinsella JE, Lokesh B: Dietary lipids, eicosanoids, and the immune system. Crit Care Med 18(suppl):S94, 1990

125. Mascioli E, Leader L, Flores E, et al: Enhanced survival to endotoxin in guinea pigs fed IV fish oil emulsions. Lipids 23:623, 1988

126. Cook JA, Wise WC, Knapp DR, et al: Essential fatty acid deficient rats: a new model for evaluating arachidonate metabolism in shock. Adv Shock Res 6:93, 1981

127. Alexander JW, Saito H, Trocki O, et al: The importance of lipid type in the diet after burn injury. Ann Surg 204:1, 1986

128. Seidner DL, Mascioli EA, Istfan NW, et al: Effects of long-chain triglyceride emulsions on reticuloendothelial system function in humans. JPEN J Parenter Enteral Nutr 13:614, 1989

129. Nanni C, Pittiruti M, Giovannini I, et al: Plasma carnitine levels and urinary carnitine excretion during sepsis. JPEN J Parenter Enteral Nutr 9:483, 1985

130. Jonsen GL, Mascioli EA, Seidner DL, et al: Parenteral infusion of long- and medium-chain triglycerides and reticuloendothelial system function in man. JPEN J Parenter Enteral Nutr 14:467, 1990

131. Jiang Z, Zhang S, Wang X, et al: A comparison of medium-chain and long-chain triglycerides in surgical patients. Ann Surg 217:175, 1993

132. Daly JM, Lieberman MD, Goldfine J, et al: Enteral nutrition with supplemental arginine, RNA, and omega-3 fatty acids in patients after operation: immunologic, metabolic, and clinical outcome. Surgery 112:56, 1992

133. Bower RH, Cerra FB, Bershadsky B, et al: Early enteral administration of a formula (impact) supplemented with arginine, nucleotides, and fish oil in intensive care unit patients: results of a multicenter, prospective, randomized, clinical trial. Crit Care Med 24:173, 1995

134. Food and Nutrition Board: Recommended Dietary Allowances, 9th ed. National Academy of Sciences, Washington DC, 1980

135. Multivitamin preparations for parenteral use: a statement by the Nutrition Advisory Group, American Medical Association Department of Foods and Nutrition, 1975. JPEN J Parenter Enteral Nutr 3:258, 1979

136. Guidelines for essential trace element preparations for parenteral use: a statement by an expert panel, AMA Department of Foods and Nutrition. JAMA 241: 2951, 1979

Acknowledgments

Figure 2   Talar Agasyan.
Figure 4   Carol Donner.

10 FEVER, HYPERPYREXIA, AND HYPOTHERMIA

Douglas W. Wilmore, M.D.

Emergency Management of Life-Threatening Temperature Derangements

Management of Life-Threatening Fever and Hyperpyrexia

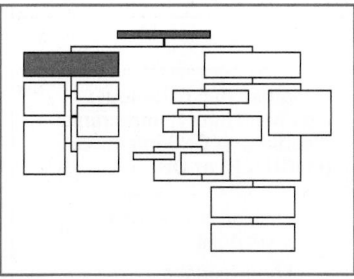

INITIAL CARE

When the physician learns (usually from a member of the nursing staff or an associate) of a dramatic elevation in a patient's temperature, his or her initial response should be to check that the temperature was measured in the rectum, not in the mouth or the axilla. The only situation in which a rectal measurement is unnecessary is when a patient's body temperature must be obtained in the operating room. In this situation, monitoring with an esophageal, nasopharyngeal, or tympanic probe yields acceptable results.

The first step in addressing the problem of life-threatening elevations in body temperature (≥ 40° C [104° F]) [*see Figure 1*] always is to evaluate the adequacy of the cardiorespiratory system and circulation. If the patient is already intubated and receiving ventilatory support, inspired oxygen should be delivered in generous concentrations; if not, the indications for intubation should be reviewed [*see VII:4 Use of the Mechanical Ventilator*]. If ventilatory support is not required, oxygen should be administered by face mask. Finally, if the patient is dehydrated, fluids should be administered intravenously. These measures ensure that sufficient oxygen is delivered to essential organs that have increased metabolic requirements because of the temperature elevation; they also help maintain skin perfusion, which is necessary to offload body heat.

The next step is to institute measures to reduce the patient's temperature. Clothing, bedcovers, and, if possible, operative drapes should be removed to facilitate heat loss from the body surface to the environment. If life-threatening hyperpyrexia is present in an individual who has been exercising and has sustained severe heatstroke, rapid cooling can be achieved by placing the person in an ice bath; this measure, together with rehydration, will lower body temperature dramatically. In extreme situations, uncontrolled malignant hyperthermia in a patient who is undergoing operation may be managed through partial cardiopulmonary bypass with a heat exchanger, an approach that can rapidly offload heat and reduce body temperature [*see* Treatment of Fever and Hyperpyrexia, Malignant Hyperthermia, *below*].

Finally, the cause of the temperature elevation should be determined, if it is not already apparent. Because elevation in body temperature is a response to a disease process, returning the temperature to normal can reduce morbidity and potential mortality considerably. However, the underlying disease process that is causing the temperature elevation also requires treatment because in

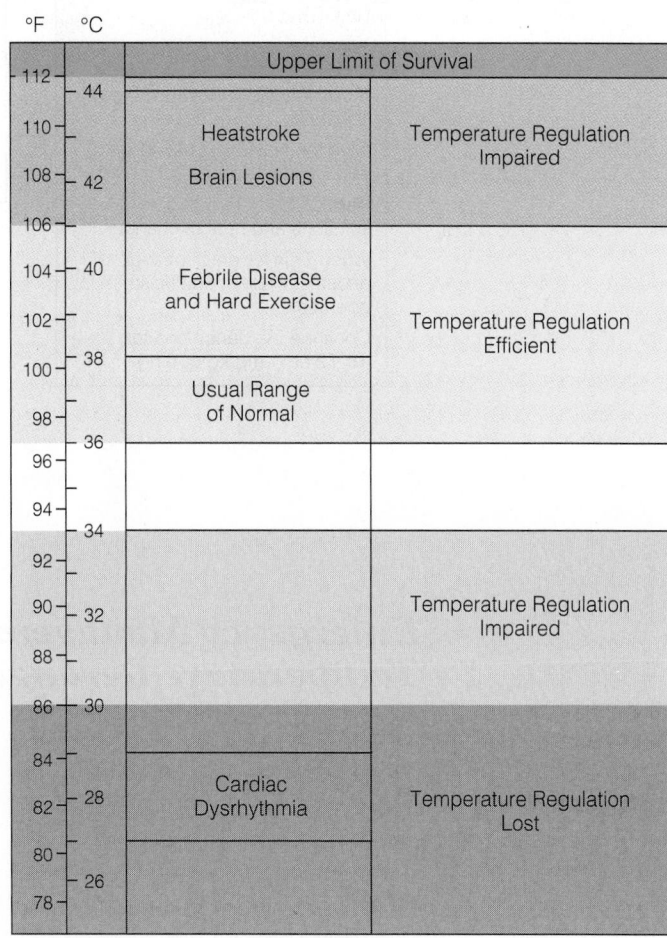

Figure 1 **Extreme variations in body temperature are associated with morbidity and mortality.**[14]

Patient's core T° is outside normal range of 36° to 38° C (96.8° to 100.4° F)

Rectal T° ≥ 40° C (104° F); fever or hyperpyrexia is life-threatening

Institute appropriate cardiorespiratory support.

Reduce body T° (e.g., remove clothes, bathe skin with cool H_2O).

Establish diagnosis (may depend to an extent on whether patient is seen in the ER, ICU, or OR), and institute specific therapy.

Infection/inflammation (in ICU, ER, or OR)

Give aspirin or NSAIDs to lower set point.

Cool body surface.

Provide hydration and metabolic support.

Diagnose and treat infection.

Heatstroke (in ER)

Cool the patient.

Rehydrate.

Hypothalamic pathology: e.g., head injury, intracranial bleeding, or CNS infection (in ICU, ER, or OR)

Give aspirin or NSAIDs to lower set point.

Cool body surface.
Treat underlying disease.

Malignant hyperthermia (in OR)

Stop operation.

Stop inhalation anesthesia; give 100% O_2.

Give I.V. $NaHCO_3$ (1–2 mEq/kg) and I.V. dantrolene (2.5 mg/kg).

Reduce body T° with cold solutions and heat exchanger.

When T° is lowered, change anesthetic agent and finish operation.

Continue I.V. dantrolene for 48–72 hr (1 mg/kg q. 6 hr).

Endocrine excess: hyperthyroidism or pheochromocytoma (in OR or ICU)

Cool body surface.

Use appropriate drugs to block end-organ endocrine response.

Emergency Management of Life-Threatening Temperature Derangements

Life-threatening hypothermia: rectal T° ≤ 35° C (95° F) as measured with low-reading thermometer, *not* standard clinical-grade thermometer

Ensure adequate oxygenation and circulation. Establish I.V. access. (Remember: monitoring may be difficult; manipulation may initiate arrhythmias.)

Consider whether hypothermia is primary (caused by exposure to cold or immersion in water) or secondary to concomitant conditions.

Circulatory collapse has not occurred or has been resolved

Patient is breathing spontaneously.

Circulatory collapse:
- **Cold, asystolic, apparently dead patient**
- **Ventricular fibrillation**
- **Marked hypotension**

Resuscitate; intubate and initiate external cardiac massage.

Rewarm using cardiopulmonary bypass with heat exchanger or peritoneal dialysis.

Use pharmacologic therapy or countershock *only with extreme caution*.

DO NOT TERMINATE resuscitative efforts until T° > 30° C (86° F) but vital signs remain absent.

Core T° is ≥ 28° C (82.4° F), and cardiovascular function is stable

Core T° is < 28° C (82.4° F) (patients are usually unconscious at this T°); cardiovascular function is unstable or at risk

Patient is extremely susceptible to arrhythmias. Monitor carefully and prepare for ventricular fibrillation or asystole.

Patient is conscious

Patient is unconscious

Unconsciousness in patients with core T° > 28° C (82.4° F) is rare and suggests underlying disease process.

Distinguish between primary hypothermia and secondary hypothermia (if not already done), and manage accordingly

In secondary hypothermia, initiate evaluation and treatment of life-threatening conditions that may alter consciousness: e.g.,
- Head injury — reduction of intracranial pressure
- Drug overdose — dialysis, naloxone
- Alcohol abuse — dialysis, thiamine
- Hypoglycemia — glucose administration

Rewarm the patient gently

Wrap patient in warm blankets.

Maintain ambient T° at 32° C (89.6° F).

Administer warm fluid (40° C; 104° F) I.V. in conjunction with hot, humidified, O₂-enriched air by face mask.

Consider microwave diathermy to increase body heat.

Table 1 Pathophysiology and Treatment of Common Causes of Elevated Body Temperature

Diagnosis	Pathophysiology	Treatment
Infection and inflammation	Activated macrophages liberate pyrogens (IL-1, TNF, and interferon) to reset the thermoregulatory center in the hypothalamus. This set-point alteration mediates increased heat production and decreased heat loss.	Give drugs that lower the set point: aspirin, acetaminophen, ibuprofen. Cool the body surface and provide general supportive measures. Provide hydration and metabolic support. Diagnose and treat infection or cause of inflammation.
Malignant hyperthermia	Certain inhalation agents or muscle relaxants stimulate abnormal metabolic reactions, particularly in skeletal muscle, that produce increased heat, acidosis, hyperkalemia, skeletal muscle rigidity, alterations in coagulation, and circulatory collapse.	Interrupt the operation. Stop inhalation anesthetics; give 100% O_2. Give I.V. $NaHCO_3$ (1–2 mEq/kg) and I.V. dantrolene (2.5 mg/kg). Reduce body temperature with cold solutions and heat exchanger. When temperature is lowered, change anesthetic agents and complete the operation. Continue dantrolene for 48 to 72 hr (1 mg/kg q. 6 hr).
Heatstroke	Heatstroke usually occurs in healthy individuals exercising on hot days (e.g., runners, football players). Subjects become dehydrated and lose less heat while continuing to produce heat through exercise.	Cool the patient. Rehydrate.
Hypothalamic pathology (head injury, intracranial bleeding, CNS tumors, encephalitis)	Intracerebral pyrogens cause resetting of thermoregulatory set point, or the hypothalamus is directly altered by the disease process.	Give drugs to lower the set point. Cool the body surface and provide general supportive measures. Treat the underlying disease process.
Endocrine excess (pheochromocytoma, hyperthyroidism)	Excess of hormones results in increased heat production.	Cool the body surface and provide general supportive measures. Block the effects of hormones: for pheochromocytoma, use alpha- and beta-adrenergic blockade; for hyperthyroidism, use beta-adrenergic blockade. Consider glucocorticoid administration.

most instances the disease, not the fever, causes mortality. It is essential to diagnose the underlying disease process accurately because each of the many physiologic processes that may be involved requires specific therapy [*see Table 1*]. The most common cause of fever is infection or inflammation (accounting for the majority of marked temperature elevations in hospitalized adults).[1] Other causes of extreme pyrexia include heatstroke, malignant hyperthermia, hypothalamic pathology, and endocrine excess.

Treatment of Fever and Hyperpyrexia

INFECTION AND INFLAMMATION

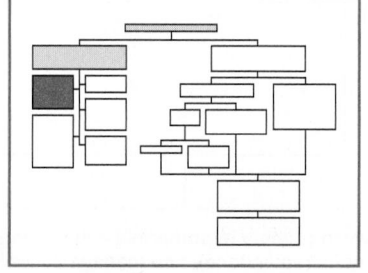

The inflammatory response activates cytokines that are released locally within the brain or into the bloodstream and act on the hypothalamus. These molecules are pyrogens: they cause an upward resetting of the thermoregulatory apparatus. This shift triggers two physiologic mechanisms for increasing body temperature: vasoconstriction, which limits heat loss from the body, and increased heat production, which is manifested by shivering. These two processes in combination increase body temperature until it reaches the level that is required by the new set point in the hypothalamus [*see Figure 2*].

The treatment of set-point elevation should begin with administration of a drug that blocks the actions of the pyrogens in the hypothalamus and allows body temperature to return to normal. Aspirin, acetaminophen, and ibuprofen have all been frequently used to reduce fever; they act by blocking the formation of prostaglandins (i.e., PGE_2) in the hypothalamus. Other drugs, including morphine, general anesthetics, chlorpromazine, and certain tranquilizers, have

a nonspecific depressive effect on the central nervous system and therefore are capable of decreasing body temperature when used in the ICU or the operating room.

Surface cooling should be started only after administration of the antipyretic because unless the central set point is first pharmacologically reduced, cooling the surface only stimulates additional vasoconstriction and heat production in the form of shivering. Shivering, in turn, increases oxygen consumption dramatically and places additional demands on an already stimulated and possibly overstressed

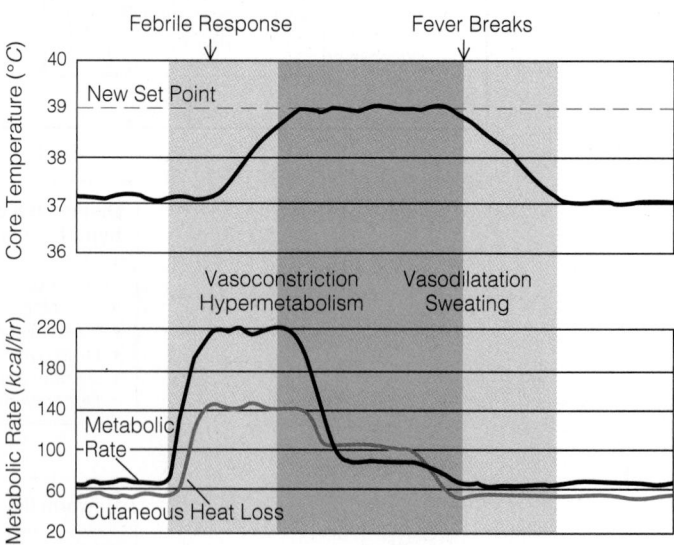

Figure 2 **A pyrogenic stimulus to the hypothalamus results in an elevated set point for body temperature. Changes in body temperature reflect the shifting relation between metabolic rate and cutaneous heat loss.[15]**

cardiovascular system. Once the antipyretics have been administered and have begun to act, a number of common techniques can be implemented, such as removing bed clothing, lowering the room temperature, sponging the patient with tepid water, increasing airflow over the patient, and applying refrigeration blankets. A 1997 study, however, found that the use of hypothermia blankets was no more effective in reducing core temperature than other cooling methods and was associated with more temperature fluctuations and more episodes of rebound hypothermia.[2] These methods of surface cooling should be used only as long as they do not induce shivering.

Other general measures should also be considered, such as correction of dehydration and electrolyte imbalance and provision of adequate quantities of glucose, a substrate that the body may consume at increased rates when hyperpyrexia is present. A careful physical examination should be performed, and tests should be ordered to diagnose the source of the infection. Antimicrobial therapy should be initiated if indicated, and definitive surgical therapy, such as drainage, extirpation, or debridement, should be considered.

MALIGNANT HYPERTHERMIA

Early diagnosis of malignant hyperthermia is difficult but nevertheless essential for effective therapy. The usual signs are an unexplained tachycardia and an increase in core temperature (i.e., rectal or esophageal temperature), which ordinarily falls in anesthetized patients. Cardiac arrhythmias that are related to acute acidosis or hyperkalemia, excessive bleeding, a rise in end-tidal carbon dioxide concentration, and marked hyperpyrexia are common developments as the syndrome progresses.[3,4]

If this symptom complex is recognized early in the course of an operation—or if its presence is even suspected—administration of the inhalation agent should be stopped, and 100% oxygen should be given instead. The operation should be halted. To promote heat loss, as many drapes as possible should be removed from the patient without compromising sterility. Sodium bicarbonate, 1 to 2 mEq/kg I.V., should be given to buffer the metabolic acidosis, along with dantrolene sodium, 2.5 mg/kg I.V. Administration of dantrolene should be repeated every 5 to 10 minutes if necessary. Serum electrolytes should be measured. Glucose and insulin therapy may also be required to correct the marked hyperkalemia that may follow. If necessary, body heat can be offloaded by means of partial cardiopulmonary bypass using a heat exchanger.

HEATSTROKE

Acute hyperpyrexia, or heatstroke, often develops in persons who are working or exercising strenuously in a hot, humid environment. Typical victims are marathon runners, members of military units taken on a forced march, and football players practicing and playing in late summer. However, heatstroke may occur without being precipitated by strenuous effort. For instance,

elderly persons with circulatory impairment or other chronic diseases often sustain marked increases in body temperature when exposed to high environmental temperatures, such as during a heat wave.[5]

Whatever the cause of the heatstroke, the initial steps in treatment must be to draw heat from the body and to support circulation. The heat overload syndromes, of which heatstroke is the most severe, represent a spectrum of physiologic disturbances that range from mild effects, such as heat cramps, to more severe symptoms, such as headache, vomiting, tachycardia, and hypotension associated with moderate dehydration.[6] The milder manifestations of heat overload generally do not qualify as emergencies; however, heatstroke—diagnosed on the basis of a core temperature greater than 40° C (104° F) coupled with hot, dry skin—can be life-threatening, and thus emergency measures must be taken. Rapid cooling can be achieved by placing the patient in an ice bath, which provides accelerated removal of heat through inductive cooling. The bath also improves venous return and thus enhances cardiac output by initiating venoconstriction in the skin and displacing blood back to the heart to increase ventricular end-diastolic volumes; in addition, it constricts the arterioles and increases the blood pressure. The core temperature of the patient should be reduced at a rate of 0.1 to 0.2° C/min so that it will be below 38° C (100.4° F) within 30 minutes. The patient can then be removed from the ice bath, but core temperature should be monitored frequently to ensure that rebound hyperthermia does not occur.

When treating a previously healthy, exercising person with heatstroke, it is advisable to remove the patient's clothing and to place the patient in a cool room. Further cooling can be achieved by using a fan to circulate air over the body or, if the elevation in body temperature is particularly severe, by packing the patient in ice or even placing him or her in an ice bath. All these techniques accelerate heat removal and minimize damage to vital tissues, particularly those of the central nervous system. Cautious administration of a balanced salt solution replenishes fluid and electrolyte deficits, supports circulation, and enhances blood flow to the skin, thereby further facilitating body heat loss. It is rare that more than 1.5 L of intravenous fluid is required during the first 4 hours.

When treating elderly, nonexercising persons, similar measures—that is, heat unloading and fluid replacement—should be taken; however, because of the relative impairment of physiologic function in the elderly, a more gentle approach to body cooling and fluid resuscitation should be followed.

In all heatstroke patients, inotropic support should be initiated if hypotension persists after volume loading or if heart failure occurs [see VII:2 Support of the Failing Heart]. Other complications of heatstroke include damage to the CNS, rhabdomyolysis, acute renal failure, disseminated intravascular coagulation, and hepatic and myocardial necrosis. Mannitol administration may be advisable to promote urine output and to prevent acute tubular necrosis in the presence of myoglobinuria. An initial loading dose of 25 g is given, and 12.5 g of mannitol is added to each liter of intravenous fluid. Systemic heparinization is effective for disseminated intravascular coagulation [see I:5 Bleeding and Transfusion]. Ventilatory support should be provided if indicated. Appropriate laboratory studies should be performed to evaluate any complications that occur.

Mortality from heatstroke ranges from 10% to 80% and is directly related to the duration and intensity of the hyperthermia, to the length of time that elapses before initiation of therapy, and to the effectiveness of the treatment.

HYPOTHALAMIC PATHOLOGY

A variety of central nervous system disorders can cause fever, including meningitis, brain abscesses, blood present in the subarachnoid space as a consequence of trauma or intracranial hemorrhage, postoperative responses to neurosurgical procedures, and disturbances of the hypothalamus or brain stem, such as those associated with transtentorial (uncal) herniation or localized tumors or those that occur after encephalitic disorders. Although the fever is often mild and indolent, occasionally the temperature may reach a life-threatening level. In the case of more generalized infection of the central nervous system or subarachnoid bleeding, signs of meningismus (e.g., headache, neck guarding, and back pain) accompany the fever; in other disorders, nonspecific or localizing neurologic signs and symptoms may be present. In all cases in which hypothalamic pathology is suspected, a spinal tap should be performed. The fluid should be examined for cells, and the concentrations of protein and glucose should be biochemically determined. Bloody fluid confirms the diagnosis of intracranial hemorrhage, whereas the presence of white cells or frank pus confirms the presence of infection; what specific type of infection is present and which antibiotics should therefore be prescribed are determined on the basis of culture results.

In most patients, general measures aimed at reducing fever should be employed. In patients who have undergone neurosurgery and in those with significant head injuries, the fever may be severe enough to warrant paralysis, ventilation, and heat unloading by means of a cooling blanket. Although the inflammatory response following intracranial injury may be the cause of the elevated temperature, it is still essential to inspect the surgical wounds and to search vigilantly for other sources of infection, particularly in the urinary tract and lungs.

ENDOCRINE EXCESS

Thyrotoxic Crisis

Thyrotoxic crisis, or so-called thyroid storm, is the acute accentuation of thyrotoxicosis. It is an infrequently observed but serious complication of Graves' disease. It may occur after subtotal thyroidectomy or may be precipitated by infection, trauma, a surgical emergency, thyroiditis, or parturition.

The clinical picture is dominated by the signs of acute hyperthyroidism. Fever may be severe and persistent, and sweating may be profuse. A marked tachycardia is frequently associated with congestive heart failure and pulmonary edema. Nausea, vomiting, abdominal pain, delirium, and psychosis may be observed as well.

The goals of treatment are to correct the severe thyrotoxicosis and to provide supportive therapy. The patient should be sedated, cooled, and given oxygen by face mask. Adequate hydration should be maintained with glucose-containing fluids to ensure sufficient exogenous substrate.

The excess thyroid hormone should be counteracted with large doses of an antithyroid agent (propylthiouracil, 200 mg orally every 4 to 6 hours), iodine (five drops of a saturated solution of potassium iodide orally every 6 hours or I.V. infusion of 0.5 g of sodi-

um iodide every 12 hours), and glucocorticoids (dexamethasone, 2 mg orally, or hydrocortisone sodium succinate [Solu-Cortef], 100 mg I.V.). If there is no cardiac insufficiency, an adrenergic blocking drug should be given (propranolol, 40 to 80 mg orally every 6 hours, or up to 2 mg I.V., administered in conjunction with ECG monitoring and repeated when the pulse increases). If heart failure is present, digitalis and diuretics should be administered.

Pheochromocytoma

Occasionally, pheochromocytomas are associated with hyperpyrexia. These endocrine tumors secrete catecholamines that produce a variety of physiologic effects, including an increased metabolic rate. Such an increase is frequently manifested by an increased respiratory rate and weight loss. Tachycardia, hypertension, psychosis, and tremulousness are associated symptoms. Pheochromocytomas should be treated with adrenergic blocking agents such as phentolamine, 1 to 5 mg intravenously, and propranolol, 40 to 80 mg orally every 6 hours or 2 mg I.V. General supportive measures should also be instituted.

Management of Accidental Hypothermia

Life-threatening hypothermia (rectal temperature ≤ 35° C [95° F]) is frequently encountered in the emergency room. In temperate areas, it is most common during the winter, but in regions with cold climates, it is seen throughout the year. Certain patients, such as those who are either very young or very old, those who are mentally ill, those who have a disabling physical illness, and those who are unconscious because of drug overdose or alcohol abuse, appear to be predisposed to hypothermia; lack of adequate housing, homelessness, malnutrition, and low levels of fitness are also contributing factors.[7] Even healthy young persons experience hypothermia after immersion in cold water, after injury and prolonged exposure to cold, or after mild to moderate exertion in a cold environment.

INITIAL CARE

The first step in the treatment of hypothermic patients is to ensure adequate oxygenation and tissue perfusion by following the ABCs of resuscitation [see I:1 Initial Emergency Management of Noninjured Patients: Cardiopulmonary Resuscitation and Correction of Acute Dysrhythmias and I:2 Trauma Resuscitation]. Conscious patients may require I.V. fluid resuscitation to counteract fluid losses associated with injury, cold diuresis, or internal fluid shifts. As a rule, the preferred fluid is a 5% solution of dextrose in saline, without added potassium. The fluids can be either warmed before infusion or administered through a blood-warming apparatus. Comatose patients with a detectable heartbeat who are breathing spontaneously, no matter how slowly, should be handled with extreme care. Ventricular fibrillation or asystole may be initiated by intubation, chest compression, insertion of a central line or a Swan-Ganz catheter, or extreme movements (e.g., transferring the patient from a bed to a litter); the reason is that a cold, bradycardic heart is extremely sensitive to potentially arrhythmogenic stimuli [see Figure 1]. If circulatory collapse occurs or is present on admission, resuscitation should be instituted (see below).

If the patient is unconscious but has cardiac activity, measures

Table 2 Clinical Manifestations, Treatment, and Outcome of Varying Degrees of Hypothermia

Core Temperature	Clinical Findings	Treatment	Outcome
32°–35° C (90°–95° F)	Cold to touch; confused, disoriented; cardiovascular function stable	Active heating with top and bottom warming blankets	Usually uneventful
28°–32° C (82°–90° F)	Bradycardia, atrial fibrillation, but stable cardiovascular function; muscle rigidity; blood pressure difficult to detect; pupils dilated	Rewarm slowly but actively with blankets, I.V. fluids, heated oxygen, etc.	Depends on underlying disease
< 28° C (< 82° F)	Hypotensive; ventricular fibrillation or cardiac instability; appearing clinically dead (apnea and asystole)	Rewarm with cardiopulmonary bypass or peritoneal dialysis	Mortality high (50%)

should be initiated to evaluate and treat conditions that may underlie a life-threatening coma [*see I:9 Coma, Seizures, Cognitive Impairment, and Brain Death*]. These conditions include hypoglycemia, which is treated by intravenous administration of glucose; narcotics overdose, which is treated by administration of naloxone; and cardiovascular collapse, which is treated by resolution of the problems associated with airway obstruction, hypovolemia, or severe arrhythmias.

The next step in initial care of a hypothermic patient is to determine the patient's actual temperature. Proper measurement of core temperature is vital because both the choice of treatment and the therapeutic outcome are linked with the extent of the hypothermia [*see Table 2*]. Because most clinical-grade mercury thermometers read only as low as 34° C (93.2° F), it is possible that when the physician is told that the patient has a rectal temperature of 34° C (93.2° F), the patient's actual temperature is considerably lower. Therefore, in these instances, the physician should remeasure the rectal temperature with either a low-reading thermometer or a thermistor probe attached to a temperature-monitoring device, such as those commonly used in the OR or the ICU.

The final step, to be taken either during or after initial care, is to make an attempt to diagnose the cause of the hypothermia. The fundamental distinction to be made is between primary hypothermia that occurs in an otherwise healthy person and hypothermia that is secondary to an associated disease that alters heat balance or thermoregulation [*see Table 3*]. The distinction between primary and secondary hypothermia is an essential one because hypothermia associated with another disease process may necessitate additional therapy or some modification of the approach that is taken for treatment of primary hypothermia, or both.

PATIENTS WITH HYPOTHERMIC CARDIAC ARREST

The most seriously ill hypothermic patients are those who present with circulatory collapse and rectal temperature of less than 28° C (82.4° F). The chances of resuscitating such patients by conventional methods are slight or nonexistent. However, even though young persons suffering from sudden, severe hypothermia because of cold exposure may appear dead, resuscitation should be attempted. Clinical experience demonstrates that such patients often survive with little or no cerebral impairment.[8] (As a rule, a patient should not be pronounced dead until the rectal temperature is greater than 30° C [86° F] but all signs of life remain absent.) The patient should be intubated, intravenous lines should be inserted, and resuscitation should be initiated.

Unfortunately, the cold heart is relatively insensitive to atropine, electrical pacing, countershock, and most antiarrhythmic drugs and

pressor agents. Moreover, the hypothermic liver cannot detoxify or conjugate drugs in a normal manner. Pharmacologic therapy must therefore be used with extreme caution in these patients. If ventricular fibrillation is present, it may be appropriate to try countershock once or twice; however, if this measure is unsuccessful, cardiopulmonary resuscitation should be continued until the patient can be placed on cardiopulmonary bypass with a heat exchanger. The core temperature can then be raised to a level above which the arrhythmia can be successfully treated. An alternative but less successful method is to maintain external cardiac massage and to attempt to rewarm the patient using external means and peritoneal dialysis with warm fluid. Thoracotomy and mediastinal lavage with warm fluid should be reserved for persons with persistent ventricular fibrillation or asystole.

HYPOTHERMIC PATIENTS WITH CARDIAC ACTIVITY

Treatment of the hypothermic patient with cardiac activity is determined by the patient's state of consciousness, the clinical findings, and the severity of the hypothermia.

Conscious Patients

Hypothermia in a conscious patient with stable cardiovascular function and rectal temperature of 28° to 30° C (82.4° to 86° F) or higher is relatively easy to manage. The patient's clothing should be removed, and he or she should be dried off and wrapped in warm blankets. The room in which the patient is placed should be warmed to at least 32° C (89.6° F). Warm fluids should be given intravenously, in conjunction with hot, humidified, oxygen-enriched air administered by face mask. Microwave diathermy can also be used to increase body heat.

Table 3 Causes of Hypothermia

Primary hypothermia
Exposure to a cold environment
Immersion in cold water

Secondary hypothermia
Drugs: narcotics, tranquilizers, anesthetics, beta blockers
Metabolic disorders: myxedema, hypopituitarism, hypoadrenalism, diabetes mellitus, hypoglycemia, protein-calorie malnutrition
Impaired thermoregulation as a result of CNS disorders
Impaired muscular activity as a result of paralysis, dementia, or injury
Increased heat loss as a result of burns

Blood tests should be performed to evaluate blood count, electrolyte concentrations, and renal and liver function. Blood culture should also be obtained, and a chest x-ray is imperative. It may also be advisable to screen the blood for toxic substances.

Unconscious Patients

If the patient is unconscious but has stable cardiovascular function and rectal temperature of 28° to 30° C (82.4° to 86° F) or higher, treatment should proceed as outlined above, except that additional measures should be taken to diagnose and treat the altered state of consciousness. Although hypothermia is associated with disorientation and confusion, unconsciousness is rare at body temperatures greater than 28° C (82.4° F); its presence suggests that central nervous system dysfunction may underlie the hypothermia. Because mortality and morbidity are usually linked not with hypothermia but with associated conditions, every effort should be made to diagnose and treat the pathologic state that induced the altered state of consciousness. Drug and alcohol overdose can be treated by dialysis, head injury by operative decompression or standard measures to reduce cerebral edema, and hypoglycemia by glucose administration.

Once a preliminary diagnosis has been reached, it must be confirmed with appropriate tests. Blood test results must be carefully interpreted in hypothermic patients because changes in body temperature have a direct effect on blood chemical values. For example, the initial laboratory findings in a hypothermic patient may include a high hematocrit, an elevated potassium level, a low pH, and altered blood gas tensions. Therefore, the laboratory should correct the blood gas determinations for the altered temperature. When allowances for actual core temperature are made, most hypothermic patients are found to be alkalemic. Blood glucose levels are often elevated, and ketones may be present in blood and urine. However, hypothermic patients are extremely resistant to the hypoglycemic effects of insulin; if the glucose level can be kept below 400 mg/dl, exogenous insulin is seldom indicated.

Every effort should be made to treat hypothermic patients with extreme care. Gradual rewarming will minimize complications. Overhydration and hyperventilation are frequently associated with lethal complications.

A more severe form of hypothermia causes unconsciousness and cardiac instability in patients who retain adequate perfusion but whose rectal temperature is less than 28° C (82.4° F). Such patients are extremely susceptible to cardiac arrhythmias. The cornerstones of management are gentle rewarming, careful monitoring, and preparation for the possibility of ventricular fibrillation or asystole.

Discussion

Thermoregulation in the Hospital Environment

Fever is an upward resetting of the thermoregulatory set point. Hyperpyrexia is an elevation of the core temperature above the body's set point. Patients become febrile as a result of the actions of pyrogens [*see Figure 2*]. When patients are febrile, their central thermoregulatory mechanism works both to minimize heat loss and to accelerate heat production (by adjusting the flow of metabolic substrate) so that body temperature is raised to the level demanded by the new central nervous system set point and is maintained there.

Many of the adaptive mechanisms that respond to alterations in body or environmental temperature are closely linked with behavioral changes. For example, during a febrile episode, a patient may curl up in bed under layers of blankets, as if cold. The reason for this behavior is that the patient's temperature is below the elevated thermoregulatory set point, even though it is above normal. Removing the bedcovers from such patients in an effort to reduce body temperature brings not relief but heightened stress; the preferred approach is to administer an antipyretic at an adequate dosage. The patient will start to sweat and remove the blankets as soon as the set point has been readjusted downward (i.e., as soon as the fever has broken).

Behavioral adaptation allows patients to establish the environmental temperature most comfortable for them. This temperature is called thermal neutrality. Achievement of thermal neutrality can be facilitated by making thermostats available in patients' rooms to allow each person to select the ambient temperature he or she prefers. Studies have demonstrated that certain groups of patients tend to select an ambient temperature that is much warmer than that preferred by the hospital staff.[9] In one study, for example, when burn patients without known infection (but with burn wound colonization) were placed in an environmentally controlled chamber and allowed to regulate the ambient temperature by means of a bedside remote control unit, the mean ambient temperature they selected as most comfortable was significantly higher than the temperature selected by normal individuals [*see Table 4*].[9] Furthermore, when comfortable, the burn patients had significantly higher core and mean skin temperatures than did the normal subjects. These results indicate that in burn patients, the thermoregulatory set point is reset upward because of the pyrogens that are produced during the inflammatory process that is associated with the injury. In these patients, the minimal level of environmental stress is achieved at warmer ambient temperatures (30° to 32° C [86° to 89.6° F]) than in normal subjects, and these conditions are associated with comfort.

Other classes of hospitalized patients also feel cold at temperatures that normal persons consider comfortable: persons with large wounds, peritonitis, pancreatitis, sepsis, and the multiple organ dysfunction syndrome (MODS) all have an elevated central set point. Moreover, very old and very young patients are known to be especially vulnerable to the effects of a cool ambient environment, and the prevailing ambient temperature in a modern air-conditioned hospital may cause them considerable discomfort and additional cold stress. It is clear that ambient temperatures of 23° to 25° C (73.4° to 77° F) are too cold for most patients, particularly those in intensive care areas. In the operating room, temperatures

Table 4 Ambient Temperatures of Comfort[9]

Subjects (N)	Room Comfort Temperature (° C)	Skin Temperature (° C)	Core Temperature (° C)
Control subjects (5)	27.8 ± 0.6	33.4 ± 0.6	36.9 ± 0.1
Burn patients* (9)	30.4 ± 0.7 $P < 0.05$	35.2 ± 0.4 $P < 0.05$	38.4 ± 0.3 $P < 0.01$

Note: mean ± SE.
*Mean burn size was 39% TBS.

Figure 3 **Depicted are the effects of various warming methods on body temperature.**[10]

of 21° to 23° C (69.8° to 73.4° F) may induce marked hypothermia in certain critically ill patients: those with burns or sepsis, elderly persons with organ system failure, and infants.

With routine perioperative care, mild hypothermia (a 1° C fall in core temperature) develops in about one half of surgical patients in the OR, and frank hypothermia (a 2° C or greater fall in core temperature) develops in approximately one third. Perioperative cooling occurs because almost all forms of anesthesia impair thermoregulation and because cold ORs accelerate heat loss (open body cavities are exposed to the relatively cold air, and cold I.V. fluids and blood products are frequently administered).

Perioperative hypothermia carries a high morbidity in terms of patient discomfort, shivering, bleeding, nitrogen loss, surgical site infection rate, incidence of morbid cardiac events, and length of hospital stay.[10] A major reason for this morbidity is that even mild hypothermia triggers the dramatic elaboration of catecholamines and other counterregulatory hormones,[11] which is associated with a sequence of cardiovascular events that includes hypertension, systemic vasoconstriction, tachycardia, and cardiac arrhythmias. Accordingly, investigators have recently begun to focus on ways of resolving mild perioperative hypothermia.

One approach is to improve environmental conditions in the OR so as to keep the patient's core temperature at or near normal. Raising the room temperature can achieve this goal, but even an ambient temperature of 25° C (77° F) is uncomfortable for a gowned surgical team. Blankets and heated I.V. solutions appear to be beneficial to an extent [*see Figure 3*], but in most patients under-

going prolonged procedures (i.e., operations lasting longer than 2 hours), active warming is necessary. Forced-air warming can usually keep the patient's core temperature above 37° C (98.6° F) and seems, on the whole, to be the most effective available method.

Two important studies have examined the use of supplemental warming in the perioperative period. A 1997 study performed at the Johns Hopkins Hospital examined 300 patients undergoing abdominal, thoracic, or vascular surgical procedures who were at high risk for untoward cardiac events.[12] The group was randomized so that one half of the patients received routine thermal care and the other half received supplemental warming via a forced-air warming system. The patients who received standard thermal support had lower core temperatures than those who received supplemental warming; in addition, they experienced many more perioperative morbid cardiac events and showed a higher incidence of postoperative ventricular tachycardia.

Another large study addressed the question of whether perioperative normothermia might reduce the surgical site infection rate.[13] The investigators speculated that perioperative hypothermia, by causing vasoconstriction and reduced tissue oxygen content, could impair host defense and hinder wound healing. A group of 200 patients undergoing colorectal procedures were randomized so that 96 received routine care and 104 received additional warming. As in the Johns Hopkins study, those who received standard care had lower temperatures than those who received additional warming. The hypothermic patients had a higher incidence of surgical site infection than the normothermic patients, as well as a longer average duration of hospitalization.

These two studies demonstrate that the maintenance of near-normothermia in patients during the perioperative period can greatly reduce mortality, morbidity, length of hospital stay, and overall cost. Those who would benefit from supplemental warming include the very young, the very old, those with MODS, burn patients, trauma patients, and all patients undergoing operative procedures that last longer than 2 hours.

Unlike hospitalized critically ill patients, hyperpyrexic heatstroke victims seen in the emergency room feel warm and seek to cool themselves off; they prefer to be in a cool room and drink cold liquids. If adequately hydrated, patients sweat noticeably—a sign that the body temperature is above the set point and that the patients are trying to offload heat. Restoration of blood volume and cessation of exercise lead to markedly increased skin perfusion, which is associated with profuse sweating. Restoration of normal body temperature follows shortly thereafter.

References

1. Sioson PB, Brown RB: Hyperpyrexia among patients in a large community hospital: causes, features, and outcomes. South Med J 86:773, 1993

2. O'Donnell J, Axelrod P, Fisher C, et al: Use and effectiveness of hypothermia blankets for febrile patients in the intensive care unit. Clin Infect Dis 24:1208, 1997

3. Gronert GA: Malignant hyperthermia. Anesthesia. Milla RD, Ed. Churchill Livingstone, New York, 1986, p 1971

4. Meier-Hellman A, Romer M, Hannemann L, et al: Early recognition of malignant hyperthermia using capnometry. Anaesthetist 39:41, 1990

5. Jones TS, Liang AP, Kilbourne EM, et al: Morbidity and mortality associated with the July 1980 heat wave in St. Louis and Kansas City, Mo. JAMA 247:3327, 1982

6. Amundson DE: The spectrum of heat related injury

with compartment syndrome. Milit Med 154:450, 1989

7. Hypothermia-related deaths—Suffolk County, New York, January 1999–March 2000, and United States, 1979–1998. MMWR 50:53, 2000

8. Walpoth BH, Walpoth-Aslan BN, Mattle HP, et al: Outcome of survivors of accidental deep hypothermia and circulatory arrest treated with extracorporeal blood warming. N Engl J Med 337:1500, 1997

9. Wilmore DW, Orcutt TW, Mason AD Jr, et al: Alterations in hypothalamic function following thermal injury. J Trauma 15:697, 1975

10. Sessler DI: Mild perioperative hypothermia. N Engl J Med 336:1730, 1997

11. Frank SM, Higgins MS, Breslow MJ, et al: The catecholamine, cortisol, and hemodynamic response to mild perioperative hypothermia. Anesthesiology 82:83, 1995

12. Frank SM, Fleischer LA, Breslow MJ, et al: Perioperative maintenance of normothermia reduces the incidence of morbid cardiac events. JAMA 227:1127, 1997

13. Kurz A, Sessler DI, Lenhardt R, et al: Perioperative normothermia to reduce the incidence of surgical wound infection and shorten hospitalization. N Engl J Med 334:1209, 1996

14. DuBois EF: Fever and the Resolution of Body Temperature. Charles C Thomas, Springfield, Ill., 1948, p 9

15. Wilmore DW: Metabolic Management of the Critically Ill. Plenum Press, New York, 1977, p 70

Acknowledgment

Figures 1 and 2   Albert Miller.

11 MOLECULAR AND CELLULAR MEDIATORS OF THE INFLAMMATORY RESPONSE

Vivienne M. Gough, M.B., CH.B., Constantinos Kyriakides, M.D., and Herbert B. Hechtman, M.D.

The Inflammatory Response

The inflammatory response to injury is complex, involving not only the area of injury but also systemic tissues. The four cardinal signs of acute inflammation—calor (heat), rubor (redness), dolor (pain), and tumor (swelling)—were first described by Celsus in the first century A.D. Subsequent descriptions added a fifth sign, functio laesa (loss of function). Although the descriptive features of acute inflammation have long been known, there is still no single satisfactory definition of this phenomenon. It is commonly considered to be the reaction of living tissues to all forms of injury and involves vascular, neurogenic, humoral, and cellular responses.

The vascular events associated with inflammation typically involve changes in blood flow and alterations in permeability. In 1924, Lewis first described the so-called triple response, in which drawing a blunt instrument across the skin induced a flush, a flare, and a wheal. Thus, directly after injury, local arteriolar dilatation, preceded by a fleeting interval of vasoconstriction, is the dominant vascular response. Precapillary sphincters dilate, leading to increased flow in already active capillaries as well as to the opening of inactive capillary beds. At the same time, postcapillary venules dilate to cope with the increased flow of blood. The rise in hydrostatic pressure is followed by fluid exudation through the vascular bed, leading to edema (wheal). As the edema increases, the wheal turns pale as a result of the increased interstitial pressure compressing the capillaries. The changes observed in the skin after mechanical trauma are typical of those seen in other organs after various injuries.

In what follows, we focus on humoral and cellular responses to injury, making use of several types of clinically important events (e.g., ischemia-reperfusion and sepsis) to illustrate important inflammatory pathways.

Neutrophil

That leukocytes are involved in inflammation was first demonstrated in 1887 by Metchnikoff, who found that rose thorns inserted into the body of starfish resulted in the local accumulation of leukocytes within hours.[1] Metchnikoff also documented the existence of different types of leukocytes and the ability of these cells to kill and digest bacteria, and he was the first to suggest that products released by white blood cells could damage vessel walls. In 1960, Marchesi and Florey, using electron microscopy to follow the movement of neutrophils across blood vessel walls in rat mesentery, found that neutrophils penetrated vascular endothelium at or near cell junctions and that after their diapedesis, no sign of a passageway could be seen.[2] Furthermore, they demonstrated that the site at which such diapedesis occurred was the postcapillary venule.

MECHANISM OF NEUTROPHIL-MEDIATED INJURY

Once it was established that neutrophils were invariably present during an acute inflammatory reaction, efforts were launched to explore their role in mediating this response. In the 1960s and 1970s it became clear that during inflammation, neutrophils actively secreted products that were injurious[3,4]; these products included reactive oxygen metabolites (ROMs) as well as proteases such as elastase and collagenase. The importance of the neutrophil in mediating inflammation was further underscored by the finding that the increased permeability resulting from an injection of the eicosanoid leukotriene B_4 (LTB_4), the complement fragment C5a, or the formylated bacterial peptide formyl-methionyl-leucyl-phenylalanine (fMLP) into the skin was prevented by previous neutrophil depletion. That neutrophil depletion did not affect the release of serotonin, histamine, and bradykinin from mast cells in response to these stimuli suggested that these mast cell–derived agents did not play a major role in mediating permeability.[5]

In the early 1980s, it was shown that neutrophils stimulated with phorbol myristate acetate damaged endothelial cells via a mechanism that could be interrupted by catalase, a hydrogen peroxide scavenger.[6] Subsequent investigations demonstrated that neutrophil-mediated endothelial damage was also caused by elastase.[7] The mechanism of injury required further clarification, given that normal plasma was known to contain potent protease inhibitors and superoxide dismutase (SOD), which inactivate circulating proteases and ROMs, respectively. Furthermore, a better understanding of how neutrophils were selectively activated was needed, given that indiscriminate release of proteases and ROMs would clearly be both inefficient and dangerous.

The mechanism by which the neutrophil is currently thought to produce its injurious effects on target cells involves the formation of a protected environment in which there is close contact between cells. This concept, though not proved, has some evidence to support it. Neutrophils lyse substrate protein only when in close contact.[8] Phorbol myristate acetate–induced lung injury occurs only when neutrophils are in direct contact with the endothelium.[9] When neutrophils are stimulated with fMLP,[7] C5a, or endotoxin,[10] they must adhere to the endothelium to cause vascular injury, which is governed by molecules expressed on the surfaces of both cell types.

The normal immune action of the neutrophil is to phagocytose its target cell. This process results in the creation within the neutrophil of a protected microenvironment known as a phagosome, which contains the targets for destruction [see Figure 1]. When the phagosome has been established, the neutrophil releases large quantities of ROMs and proteases into it. Any plasma protease inhibitors gaining access to this restricted space are themselves inhibited by the neutrophil secretory products hydrogen peroxide

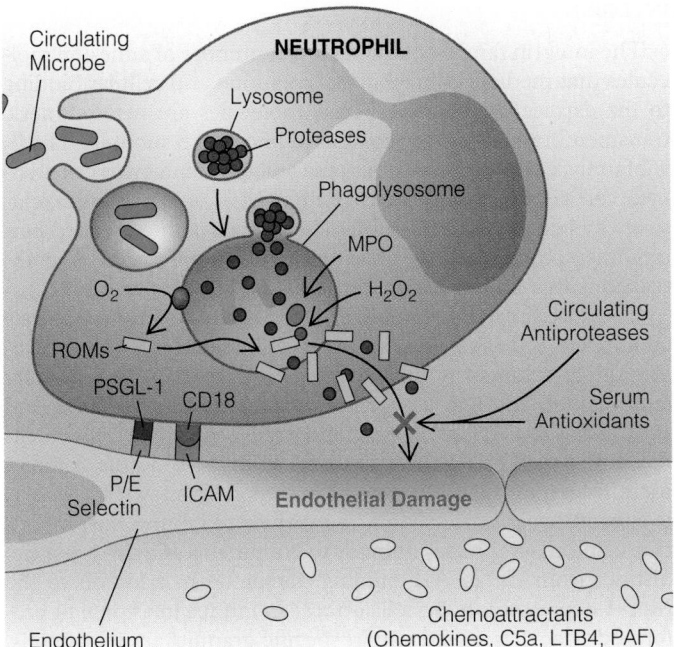

Figure 1 **Proteases and ROMs are stored in intracellular lysosomes. These fuse with microbe-containing phagosomes, forming
phagolysosmes that initiate destruction of the microbes. Antiproteases that gain entry to this area, such as serum α_1-anti-
trypsin, are inhibited by hydrogen peroxide and myeloperoxidase
secreted by neutrophils. The same neutrophil products that cause
microbial destruction may also damage surrounding endothelial
tissue. Tissue damage is somewhat reduced by natural protective
mechanisms, such as ROM scavenging by SOD, catalase, and α_1-
antitrypsin.**

and myeloperoxidase, either of which is capable of neutralizing
α_1-antitrypsin, the major protease inhibitor.[11,12] Furthermore,
myeloperoxidase activates other neutrophil proteases, such as
collagenase and gelatinase.[4] Thus, ROMs and proteases act in
synergy to digest phagocytosed matter.

In cases of strong neutrophil activation, the cells may release
their toxic products in concentrations that overwhelm the body's
regulatory defenses, causing substantial damage to surrounding
tissues through excess vascular permeability and parenchymal
injury.

ROLE IN REPERFUSION INJURY

The importance of neutrophils in the generation of reperfusion injury was first demonstrated in the context of myocardial
ischemia.[13] Histologically, the injury was characterized by an
extensive early accumulation of extravasated neutrophils, thus
resembling an acute inflammatory process. Depletion of neutrophils by means of an antiserum led to a significant reduction
in the size of myocardial infarction after temporary occlusion of
the left circumflex coronary artery.[13] Restoration of blood flow
to ischemic skeletal muscle was also associated with significant
leukocyte infiltration,[14] whereas leukocyte depletion attenuated
the associated increase in microvascular permeability and vascular resistance.[15]

Besides enhancing permeability, neutrophils were shown to
cause skeletal myocyte injury after ischemia, as evidenced by
membrane dysfunction. Such dysfunction was indicated by
depolarization of resting skeletal muscle that persisted after
restoration of blood flow despite repletion of intracellular high-

energy phosphates; in contrast, such depolarization was limited
during hindlimb reperfusion in neutropenic animals.[16]

Neutrophils have also been implicated as mediators of the
remote lung injury observed to occur as a consequence of skeletal muscle ischemia. Investigators documented leukosequestration and increased lung permeability during reperfusion after
hindlimb tourniquet ischemia.[17] Neutropenia, however, was
protective in this setting, maintaining normal microvascular permeability and lung histology.

Adhesion Molecules

To patrol the body effectively for infectious organisms and to
repair injuries in disparate regions of the body, neutrophils must
be able both to circulate as nonadherent particles in blood and
lymph and to adhere to and migrate through specific tissues sites
where they are needed. Evidence from the past 20 years indicates that inflammatory sites emit signals that activate the adjacent endothelium and circulating phagocytes. Inflammatory
events also trigger release of circulating mediators such as
cytokines, which produce more generalized activation of
endothelial cells and leukocytes, thereby rendering one or both
cell types more adhesive.[18] Circulating phagocytes then adhere
to endothelium; in response to a chemical chemoattractant gradient across the microvessel, they undergo diapedesis between
the junctions of endothelial cells, migrate through the subendothelial matrix, and participate in the parenchymal inflammatory reaction. This phagocyte adherence, though essential to the
immune response and the repair of injury, may induce pathologic consequences.

For the first few hours of the inflammatory response, the neutrophil is the predominant leukocyte at inflammatory sites.[19]
After 12 to 24 hours, mononuclear phagocytes predominate.[20]
When injury is extensive and the inflammatory response robust,
this second phase may be accompanied by immunomodulation
and increased susceptibility to infection.

The importance of leukocyte adhesion to the endothelium in
maintaining host defenses against infection is illustrated by the
example of patients with a congenital deficiency of CD11/CD18,
a family of adhesion-promoting leukocyte surface proteins.[21] This
condition, known as leukocyte adhesion deficiency I (LAD I),
results in a profound defect in phagocyte accumulation because
the leukocytes, though stimulated, cannot adhere and migrate to
extravascular sites.[7] Patients with LAD I have little or no pus at
bacterial infection sites and suffer recurrent life-threatening bacterial infections.[21] On the other hand, unmoderated leukocyte
adhesion to the endothelium can also have pathologic consequences, such as lung failure (i.e., the acute respiratory distress
syndrome [ARDS]) or organ transplant rejection.[22,23] Thus, a better understanding of the mechanism of adhesion may lead to better therapy for a number of disease states. Such therapy will have
to balance the benefit of reducing tissue damage caused by leukocyte adhesion against the possible increased risk of infection.

Adhesion molecules on endothelial cells and neutrophils may
be classified into three groups: selectins, integrins, and
immunoglobulins [*see Table 1*].

SELECTINS

The selectins are expressed only on cells within the vasculature or the lymphatic system. To date, three selectins have been
identified: L-selectin, P-selectin, and E-selectin, or endothelial
leukocyte adhesion molecule–1 (ELAM-1). These molecules are
also collectively referred to as lectin cell adhesion molecules

Table 1 Adhesion Molecules Involved in Adherence of Leukocytes to Endothelium

Family	Members
Selectins	L-selectin (LAM-1, Mel-14, Leu-8, LECCAM-1) E-selectin (ELAM-1) P-selectin (CD62, GMP-140, PADGEM)
Integrins	LFA-1 (CD11a/CD18) Mac-1 (CD11b/CD18, Mo-1, CR3) gp 150,95 (CD11c/CD18)
Immunoglobulins	ICAM-1 ICAM-2 VCAM-1

(LEC-CAMs). In general, the selectins are responsible for the earliest interaction of circulating cells, setting the stage for integrin-mediated firm adherence. All three help regulate the initial leukocyte rolling on activated endothelium. Without selectins, leukocytes interact poorly with endothelium. Leukocyte adhesion deficiency II (LAD II), a genetic deficiency of glucosyltransferase, prevents formation of sialyl Lewis^x (sLe^x), the key selectin counterreceptor, thereby increasing the risk of infection.

L-selectin, the smallest member of the selectin family, is present on the surface of neutrophils, monocytes, and lymphocytes and binds both constitutive and inducible carbohydrate ligands on the endothelial cell surface. The migration of neutrophils into certain inflammatory sites is significantly attenuated by L-selectin blockade[24]; however, other molecules play a greater role in neutrophil adhesion than L-selectin does. Where L-selectin plays a dominant role in cell trafficking is in the lymphocyte: L-selectin–deficient knockout mice have small, poorly formed lymph nodes and defective T cell function.[25]

P-selectin, the largest member of the family, plays a key part in leukocyte rolling.[26,27] It is constitutively associated with the α-granules of platelets[28] and the cytoplasmic Weibel-Palade bodies of endothelial cells[29] and is rapidly translocated to the endothelial cell surface after stimulation by histamine or thrombin.[29] Expression of P-selectin may also be induced by exposure of the vascular endothelium to free radicals (particularly superoxide),[30] C5a, the complement membrane attack complex (C5b-C9),[31] and tumor necrosis factor–α (TNF-α).[32] The extracellular N-terminal domain of the molecule binds to its carbohydrate ligand, sLe^x. An additional P-selectin mechanism of neutrophil-endothelial interaction involves platelets. By adhering to endothelial surfaces, platelets provide a rich surface of exposed P-selectin to which neutrophils can bind. Platelet-endothelial binding may occur via fibrinogen attachment to endothelial intercellular adhesion molecule–1 (ICAM-1) and to platelet GPIIb/IIIa. Platelet endothelial cell adhesion molecule–1 (PECAM-1) can also mediate attachment.

E-selectin, the third member of the selectin family, is a glycoprotein found exclusively on the surface of endothelial cells. Although not expressed on resting endothelium, E-selectin is markedly upregulated in response to the cytokines interleukin-1 (IL-1) and TNF-α as well as to lipopolysaccharide (LPS). E-selectin plays an important role in slightly later leukocyte adhesion to the microvascular endothelium.[33]

For all three selectins, P-selectin glycoprotein ligand–1 (PSGL-1), which is rich in sLe^x moieties, is the principal counterreceptor; it is located on the surface of circulating leukocytes and participates in the earliest inflammatory responses.

INTEGRINS

The integrin family comprises a vast number of adhesion molecules that mediate intercellular recognition and cellular binding to the extracellular matrix. These molecules are heterodimeric transmembrane receptors composed of α and β subunits. The β$_2$ subfamily, collectively known as the leukocyte integrins or leukocyte cell adhesion molecules (LeuCAMs), is expressed exclusively by leukocytes. This subfamily comprises three related heterodimers, each made up of a common β subunit (CD18) complexed with a unique α subunit (CD11a, CD11b, or CD11c).

CD11a/CD18, also known as lymphocyte function–associated antigen–1 (LFA-1), is expressed on all leukocytes and mediates the attachment of unstimulated neutrophils to the vascular endothelium through a specific interaction with ICAM-1 and ICAM-2. CD11b/CD18, previously referred to as complement receptor type 3 (CR3) because of its ability to bind the complement fragment iC3b but now more generally known as Mac-1, is constitutively expressed on the surface of neutrophils, monocytes, and macrophages. It binds to endothelial ICAM-1 at a site distinct from the LFA-1 binding domain.[34] In addition to the Mac-1 expressed on the cell surface, an intracellular pool of preformed Mac-1 is stored within specific granules in neutrophils. Translocation of Mac-1 from intracellular pools to the neutrophil surface via granule fusion with the plasma membrane is stimulated by chemotaxins, including C5a, LTB$_4$, IL-8, and platelet-activating factor (PAF).[35] Unlike the adhesive interactions between LFA-1 and ICAM-1, which can be demonstrated in both stimulated and unstimulated cells, Mac-1–mediated adherence to endothelial ICAM-1 requires chemotactic activation.[36] CD11c/CD18, also referred to as gp150,95, has been identified on the surfaces of neutrophils and monocytes and is believed to play its primary role in monocyte adhesion.

IMMUNOGLOBULINS

Leukocyte integrins bind to endothelial surface receptors belonging to the immunoglobulin supergene family. Members of this superfamily, which includes major histocompatibility complex (MHC) antigens I and II, T cell receptors, ICAM-1, and ICAM-2, share an immunoglobulin domain composed of 90 to 100 amino acids arranged in two sheets of antiparallel β strands stabilized at the center with a disulfide bond. Although constitutively expressed, copies of ICAM-1 are increased after stimulation by TNF-α, IL-1, LPS, lymphotoxin, or interferon gamma (IFN-γ). IL-1–induced upregulation can be observed 30 minutes after incubation, after which time it increases steadily, reaching a peak after 24 hours.[37] ICAM-1 is the counterreceptor for CD11a and CD11b.

STUDIES USING ANTIBODIES TO ADHESION MOLECULES

The development of monoclonal antibodies (mAbs) that bind to the functional epitopes of adhesion molecules has yielded useful data on adhesion mechanisms. In addition, a number of studies have aroused clinical interest.

In two trials, survival was significantly increased in rabbits and baboons treated with a CD18 mAb after hemorrhagic shock.[38,39] In a canine model of myocardial ischemia-reperfusion, treatment with a CD11b mAb led to reduced infarct size and neutrophil sequestration.[40] In a murine model of liver cell injury induced by LPS and galactosamine, a CD11b mAb reduced liver cell injury by more than 90% (as determined by assessment of alanine aminotransferase levels) but reduced neutrophil sequestration by only 40%.[41] In this setting, it is likely that neutrophils were bound to a large extent by CD11a, which may explain the discrepancy between the degree of protection afforded by the antibody and the reduction in neutrophil sequestration. The beneficial effects of CD11b antibodies may well be related more to the inhibition of neutrophil signaling and function than to sequestration per se.

In another study, treatment with a mAb to ICAM-1 led to a reduction in phorbol myristate acetate–stimulated neutrophil accumulation in rabbit lungs.[42] This mAb also reduced lymphocyte sequestration and acute graft rejection after renal transplantation in primates.[23] Attempts to modify acute allograft rejection in humans have met with little success. It must be kept in mind, however, that our understanding of the effects of antibodies to adhesion molecules on the immune system is still in its infancy. This rapidly developing field promises to offer powerful tools that may well prove applicable to the control of inflammatory and immunologic reactions.

Cytokines

The term cytokine refers to a diverse group of polypeptides and glycoproteins that are important mediators of inflammation. They are produced by numerous cell types but primarily by leukocytes. Cytokines are potent intercellular messengers that exert most of their actions on immune and inflammatory cells. Taken separately, they have a wide range of effects; considered as a group, their principal functions are to coordinate the immune response to foreign antigens by acting as growth factors and cellular activators and also to moderate this response via various feedback mechanisms.

Cytokines are not stored intracellularly: upon antigenic stimulus of the cell, they are synthesized rapidly by novel mRNA transcription, then quickly released. For example, LPS from bacterial cell walls causes macrophage activation and induces TNF release. The mRNA encoded during this process tends to be unstable, which ensures that cytokine synthesis after cell activation will be brief and self-limiting. Cytokines exert their effects through very high-affinity binding to various receptors on target cells. Thus, as a rule, very small amounts of cytokines suffice to produce their biologic effects. External signals increase the number of receptors on a cell, thereby enhancing the cellular response to a particular cytokine. For example, antigenic stimulation of lymphocytes leads to increased cytokine receptor expression. The cytokine itself can also stimulate cytokine receptor upregulation via a positive feedback mechanism.

Cytokines usually act on cells locally in an autocrine and paracrine fashion, thereby ensuring that the inflammatory response is evoked at the site of infection or injury. When they are produced in very large quantities, they can enter the circulation and exert significant systemic effects. On one hand, a single cytokine may act on more than one cell type, causing a number of different consequences (pleiotropism); on the other, several different cytokines may produce the same functional effects (redundancy). This relative nonspecificity of action limits the clinical usefulness of exogenously administered cytokines: the likelihood is high that such agents will either have unwanted side effects or be functionally useless as a result of compensation by other cytokines.[43] Another common feature of cytokines is that they often act in a cascade, with one cytokine leading to the production of another. They may also act synergistically or may antagonize the actions of other cytokines.

Discussion of cytokines is complicated by the often confusing nomenclature. Several of the earliest identified cytokines were

Table 2 General Classification of Cytokines by Primary Activity

Proinflammatory Cytokines	Anti-inflammatory Cytokines
TNF	IL-10
IL-1	IL-4
Chemokines	IL-13
Interferons	TGF-β
IL-2	
CSFs	
IL-6	

discovered in a variety of different settings and consequently bear several different names associated with specific functions. For example, TNF, initially named for its ability to cause tumor necrosis, is also known as cachectin because of its association with cachexia. Current cytokine nomenclature follows a more consistent naming system, in which the term interleukin (IL), referring to a substance that acts between leukocytes, is used in conjunction with a number (e.g., IL-10); however, many of the cytokines are still commonly referred to by their historical (and frequently misleading) names.

The cytokines we address in the following discussion do not constitute an exhaustive list. Such a list would be beyond the scope of this chapter; furthermore, given the rate at which new cytokines are being found and classified, it would be out of date before it was published. Accordingly, we focus on the better-known and more thoroughly studied cytokines.

To facilitate understanding of cytokine function, it may be helpful to classify them on the basis of their primary actions. Various classification systems have been proposed; however, none have proved entirely satisfactory, because these agents, being pleiotropic by nature, often have conflicting actions. In our view, the most useful approach is to categorize the cytokines according to whether they exert primarily proinflammatory or primarily anti-inflammatory effects [see Table 2]. Admittedly, the boundary between the two categories is frequently blurred.

PROINFLAMMATORY CYTOKINES

The general distinction between proinflammatory and anti-inflammatory cytokines is based on the observation that certain cytokines—principally TNF, IL-1, and IL-8—promote the inflammatory response by upregulating expression of genes encoding phospholipase A_2, cyclooxygenase-2 (COX-2), or inducible nitric oxide (NO) synthase, thereby increasing production of the corresponding proinflammatory mediators (PAF, eicosanoids, and NO, respectively). In addition, proinflammatory cytokines mediate neutrophil action, acting as chemoattractants, upregulating expression of leukocyte-endothelial adhesion molecules, causing cell migration into the tissues, and activating neutrophil degranulation—all of which lead to tissue damage.

Tumor Necrosis Factor and Interleukin-1

Although TNF and IL-1 are structurally dissimilar, their functions overlap considerably, and they are known to act synergistically. Originally discovered as a substance causing ischemic necrosis of tumors in rabbits treated with endotoxin, TNF is produced principally by monocytes and macrophages but also by various other immune and endothelial cells. The most potent stimulus for its production is LPS (endotoxin) from gram-nega-

Table 3 Systemic Actions of TNF

Fever

Acute-phase protein synthesis

Cachexia

Myocardial depression

Disseminated intravascular coagulation (DIC)

Hypoglycemia

tive bacteria, but other stressors (e.g., infection, trauma, ischemia, and toxins) can also induce its release.

In small concentrations, TNF acts in an autocrine and paracrine fashion, causing increased expression of endothelial E-selectin and leukocyte integrins and promoting leukocyte adhesion to the endothelium. TNF causes neutrophils to be attracted first, followed by monocytes and lymphocytes, thereby helping to regulate the inflammatory response. It also stimulates endothelial cells to produce a cytokine subset known as the chemokines (e.g., IL-8), which promote leukocyte migration into the tissues, and induces mononuclear phagocytes to produce IL-1. Finally, TNF can cause apoptosis in some cell types, an event that is of unknown physiologic significance.[43]

In large concentrations, TNF mediates a number of physiologic effects that are well-recognized components of infection. It acts on the hypothalamus via prostaglandin synthesis to cause fever [*see Table 3*]. It also induces hepatocyte production of some of the acute-phase proteins, the best known of which are C-reactive protein, fibrinogen, serum amyloid A, and α_1-antitrypsin. Prolonged TNF production also leads to cachexia, probably by reducing appetite. Massive doses of TNF produce the classic symptoms of septic shock. Hypotension results from reduced vascular smooth muscle tone and myocardial depression; disseminated intravascular coagulation (DIC) results from endothelial expression of tissue factor and inhibition of throm-bomodulin; and profound hypoglycemia results from tissue overutilization of glucose and impaired liver function.[43]

Like TNF, IL-1 is produced primarily by macrophages and to a lesser extent by other leukocytes and endothelial cells. IL-1 is a primary responder in the inflammatory cascade, and its actions are very similar to those of TNF. It mediates local inflammatory responses at low concentrations and exerts adverse systemic effects at higher concentrations. Unlike TNF, it cannot induce apoptosis. IL-1 also minimizes the perception of posttraumatic pain by causing the release of β-endorphins from the pituitary gland and increasing the number of central opioid receptors. TNF and IL-1 act synergistically to produce the acute innate immune response to invading microorganisms, manifested by neutrophil activation and release of other cytokines that promote further immune activity.

Chemokines

The chemokines are a group of cytokines that regulate migration of leukocytes from blood to other tissues. Chemokines bind to heparan sulfate proteoglycans on endothelium, thus presenting themselves to white blood cells that have become loosely attached to endothelial cells via the action of selectins and that roll along the endothelium. When a white cell interacts with a chemokine, its shape changes rapidly, becoming flatter and more motile. At the same time, surface integrins are exposed, allowing firmer attachment to the endothelium. Chemokines also induce rhythmic contraction of cellular actin filaments, causing cellular migration from the blood vessel at an interendothelial cell junction across a chemokine concentration gradient to the region of tissue injury [*see Figure 2*].

For the purposes of this discussion, chemokines may be classified into two main subsets, CC and CXC, depending on whether their two terminal cysteine residues are adjacent (CC) or separated (CXC). The CXC group, which includes IL-8 (probably the best known of the chemokines), acts mainly on neutrophils, whereas the CC chemokines act on monocytes, eosinophils, and lymphocytes. Both subsets are produced by leukocytes, endothelial cells, and fibroblasts in response to

Figure 2 Leukocytes bind loosely to the endothelium via low-affinity interaction between selectins and their ligands. Once loosely bound, they begin rolling slowly along the endothelium. Chemokines cause a conformational change in the leukocyte, exposing the leukocyte integrins that bind to endothelial ICAM-1 and VCAM-1 and thus inducing firm adherence. The leukocyte then undergoes diapedesis into tissues along the chemokine gradient.

Figure 3 **The function of T helper cells is to secrete cytokines in response to antigenic stimulation; these cytokines then act to regulate an appropriate immune response by triggering proliferation and stimulation of T cells, B cells, and other leukocytes. There are two distinct subsets of T helper cells—Th1 and Th2—which are descended from the same precursors, namely, naive CD4+ T cells. The development of Th1 and Th2 subsets occurs in response to naïve T cell stimulation by different cytokines. In turn, each subset secretes a distinct set of cytokines. IL-12 is the major stimulant for Th1 subset development. This subset assists in phagocyte-mediated responses, with IL-12 being produced by phagocytes in response to a variety of antigens (most of which are intracellular). Th1 cells secrete the proinflammatory cytokines, mainly IFN-γ, IL-2, and TNF. IL-2 acts in an autocrine fashion, stimulating further growth of this subset. Th2 cell growth is stimulated by the anti-inflammatory cytokine IL-4. This subset produces the anti-inflammatory cytokines IL-4, Il-5, IL-13, and IL-10, with IL-4 acting as an autocrine growth factor through a positive feedback mechanism. These cytokines also mediate the immune response to helminths and allergens.**

stimulation by either antigens or other cytokines (e.g., TNF and IL-1). Some are also produced constitutionally by lymphocytes to regulate the flow of these cells through the lymphatic system.

Interleukin-12

When activated by intracellular microbes (e.g., viruses, *Listeria*, and mycobacteria), mononuclear phagocytes and dendritic cells (professional antigen-presenting cells [APCs] located in lymph nodes) produce IL-12, the essential action of which is to mediate the early immune response. The most important single action of IL-12 is to stimulate synthesis and release of IFN-γ by T cells and natural killer (NK) cells (see below).

Interferon Gamma

IFN-γ is produced by T cells and NK cells in response to antigen, an event greatly enhanced by IL-12. It activates macrophages, inducing them to kill microbes by activating enzymes that trigger synthesis of ROMs and NO. In addition, by increasing IL-12 release from the macrophages it activates, IFN-γ increases differentiation of T helper cells into the Th1 cell subset that produces it while inhibiting proliferation of the Th2 subset, which produces anti-inflammatory cytokines [*see Figure 3*].

Interleukin-6

It is probably most accurate to think of IL-6 as a mixed proinflammatory/anti-inflammatory cytokine. IL-6 is produced by mononuclear phagocytes as well as by endothelial cells and fibroblasts. It acts in a proinflammatory manner by providing a potent stimulus for hepatocyte synthesis of acute-phase proteins. It is also involved in promoting T cell differentiation and maturation and immunoglobulin production and in enhancing NK cell activity.[44] However, IL-6 also has important anti-inflammatory effects. It has been shown to inhibit production of TNF and IL-1 by mononuclear cells and to reduce release of TNF secondary to endotoxin challenge.[45] Furthermore, IL-6 leads to reduced plasma concentrations of soluble TNF receptors and IL-1 receptor antagonist (IL-1Ra), which are naturally occurring anticytokines.[46]

Interferon Alfa and Interferon Beta (Type I Interferons)

IFN-α and IFN-β are two functionally similar cytokines that are often jointly referred to as the type I interferons; they are also known as the antiviral interferons because they are produced by antigen-stimulated T cells in response to viral infection. They act in a paracrine fashion to inhibit viral replication, preventing infection of neighboring cells and putting cells into an antiviral state. IFN-α and IFN-β also increase the efficiency of cytotoxic T cell–mediated cell lysis by upregulating expression of MHC class 1 molecules on infected cells. They are frequently used in the clinical setting: IFN-α seems to be effective therapy for viral hepatitis, and INF-β has been used, with some success, to treat multiple sclerosis.

Interleukin-2

Unlike the cytokines already mentioned, which exert most of their effects via the innate immune system, IL-2 mediates acquired immunity—that is, the proliferation and differentiation of lymphocytes after antigen recognition. Originally known as T cell growth factor, IL-2 acts in an autocrine manner on the T cells that produce it (i.e., T helper cells), upregulating IL-2 receptors and thereby causing preferential proliferation of T cells specific for the stimulating antigen.[43] It also promotes growth and differentiation of NK cells.

IL-2 has an immunomodulatory function as well, in that it potentiates apoptosis of antigen-stimulated T cells. This action appears to limit immune responses. It is noteworthy that IL-2 knockout mice experience overproduction of lymphocytes with hyperplasia of lymphoid organs and the development of autoimmune diseases (most strikingly, autoimmune hemolytic anemia and inflammatory bowel disease). These events are probably attributable to loss of the regulatory apoptosis function.

Hematopoietic Cytokines

The hematopoietic cytokines—including the colony-stimulating factors (CSFs), IL-7, and IL-3—are, strictly speaking, proinflammatory, in that they induce the growth and differentiation of bone marrow progenitor cells; however, this is a normal component of bone marrow hematopoiesis. CSFs are produced by bone marrow stromal cells and act to stimulate the formation of bone marrow cell colonies. There are several different varieties, named according to the type of cell line they promote (e.g., granulocytes [G-CSF], monocytes [M-CSF], or both [GM-CSF]). IL-7 is synthesized by fibroblasts and bone marrow cells and induces the differentiation of B and T cells. IL-3 is also known as multilineage colony-stimulating factor (multi-CSF) because its actions promote the differentiation of bone marrow precursors into all known mature cell types.

ANTI-INFLAMMATORY CYTOKINES

The anti-inflammatory cytokines exert their effects by inhibiting the production of proinflammatory cytokines, countering their actions, or both. In so doing, they reduce gene expression of agents such as TNF, IL-1, and the chemokines, thereby mitigating or preventing their subsequent inflammatory effects.

Interleukin-10

IL-10 is important in the homeostatic control of both innate and acquired immunity. It is produced by activated macrophages and is a potent inhibitor of these cells, regulating them via negative feedback; it is also produced by Th2 cells and B cells. IL-10 antagonizes a broad range of immune functions: it inhibits IL-12 production by activated macrophages, thereby reducing IFN-γ release and, consequently, decreasing macrophage activation. It also inhibits Th1 cells, thereby reducing production of proinflammatory cytokines (e.g., TNF, IFN-γ, and IL-2). However, IL-10 also has proinflammatory effects, stimulating B cell function and enhancing the development of cytotoxic T cells.[47]

The importance of IL-10 in normal regulation of the immune response is demonstrated by studies of IL-10 knockout mice, which experience fatal inflammatory bowel disease and show markedly increased levels of TNF in response to endotoxin challenge.[48] Administration of recombinant IL-10 before lethal doses of endotoxin reduces TNF release and prevents death.[49] In humans, it prevents fever, proinflammatory cytokine release, and clotting cascade activation during endotoxin challenge.

Interleukin-4 and Interleukin-13

IL-4 and IL-13 are structurally similar, and both are produced by Th2 cells as well as by mast cells and basophils. They are considered anti-inflammatory cytokines by virtue of their ability to antagonize INF-γ and thereby reduce macrophage activation. Because INF-γ is the major promoter of Th1 cells, these two agents indirectly suppress cytokine production by Th1 cells in much the same way that IL-10 does.

IL-4 is the principal growth factor for Th2 cells, which, in addition to their immune suppressor functions, mediate the immune response to helminths and are responsible for allergic reactions. It is also the major stimulus for production of IgE by B cells.

Transforming Growth Factor–β

Transforming growth factor–β (TGF-β) is produced by a large variety of cells, including activated T cells, phagocytes, and endothelial cells. It has potent anti-inflammatory effects, inhibiting T cell differentiation and proliferation and macrophage activation. It also counteracts the effects of proinflammatory cytokines, causing downregulation of endothelial intercellular adhesion molecules,[50] downregulation of TNF endothelial receptor expression, and inhibition of chemokine action. TGF-β

knockout mice acquire multifocal inflammatory disease, particularly involving the heart and the lungs.[51]

THERAPEUTIC IMPLICATIONS

Interleukin-1 Receptor Antagonist

A naturally occurring cytokine inhibitor is the endogenously secreted protein IL-1Ra, which competitively binds the IL-1 receptor without signaling. IL-1Ra is secreted by mononuclear phagocytes and has nearly the same affinity for the IL-1 receptor as IL-1 itself does.[52] IL-1Ra is present in high concentrations in the serum of patients with a variety of diseases, often in much higher concentrations than IL-1.[53] In patients with sepsis, juvenile rheumatoid arthritis, and inflammatory bowel disease, IL-1Ra levels have been found to correlate with disease severity; presumably, IL-1Ra acts as a natural negative feedback mechanism in inflammatory states. Unfortunately, the results of clinical trials evaluating recombinant IL-1Ra in the setting of septic shock have been largely disappointing.[54]

TNF Antagonists

There are two cell surface receptors for TNF, p55 and p75. These are normally shed after activation and are found in the circulation. In the presence of disease and in response to endotoxin challenge, they circulate in much higher concentrations.[55] It is thought that p55 and p75 act as carriers for TNF, thereby reducing the amount of TNF available to act on cells. TNF itself induces the production of its soluble receptors. Elevated levels of TNF receptors have been recorded in cancer patients, and these levels correlate well with tumor burden and the extent of metastasis.[56] Elevated TNF receptor levels in blood or joint fluid have also been recorded in patients with a variety of autoimmune and inflammatory diseases.

In response to such observations, commercial anti-TNF drugs began to be developed. The first such drug to be approved was etanercept, in 1998. This agent, a recombinant TNF p75 receptor, has proved to be effective in treating rheumatoid arthritis and spondyloarthropathies. Infliximab, approved in 1999, is a genetically engineered anti-TNF mAb that is capable of binding to both cell-bound and soluble TNF. It causes lysis of TNF-producing cells via complement- and antibody-dependant cytotoxicity.[57] Infliximab is approved for use in patients with Crohn disease, in whom it can induce and maintain remissions, bring about endoscopically and histologically demonstrable mucosal healing, reduce the number of perianal fistulae, and decrease inflammation in ileoanal pouches.[58] Infliximab also shows great promise in the treatment of rheumatoid arthritis, ankylosing spondylitis, and psoriatic arthritis.

Modulation of Cytokine Activity in Sepsis, SIRS, and CARS

Key terms and concepts associated with the systemic activation of the body's inflammatory mechanisms—systemic inflammatory response syndrome (SIRS), sepsis, septic shock, and multiple organ dysfunction syndrome (MODS)—are defined and discussed more fully elsewhere [see VI:10 Clinical and Laboratory Diagnosis of Infection, VI:11 Blood Cultures and Infection in the Patient with the Septic Response, and VII:7 Multiple Organ Dysfunction Syndrome].[59] The general understanding is that systemic inflammatory activity (i.e., SIRS), which may occur in response to either infectious or noninfectious stimuli, is the fundamental phenomenon; in this view, sepsis may be understood as SIRS occurring specifically in response to microbial invasion. This whole-body inflammatory response can lead ultimately to MODS, which is associated with mortalities higher than 50%.

The role of cytokines in the pathophysiology of SIRS and sepsis was first appreciated when experimental studies demonstrated that antibodies to TNF reduced mortality in animals to which endotoxin had been administered.[60,61] Further research revealed that the proinflammatory cytokines TNF and IL-1 were both able to evoke a clinical picture mimicking that of sepsis (i.e., hypotension and fever). In addition, TNF activated the coagulation cascade.[54] Accordingly, it was postulated that SIRS and sepsis were attributable to an overwhelming proinflammatory immune response mediated by TNF and other cytokines. A great deal of research on sepsis has now been carried out in animal and clinical trials, mostly using TNF mAbs and soluble TNF receptors. The initial results were positive, in that TNF amelioration led to increased survival in endotoxin-sensitized animals. Subsequently, however, these findings were countered by the observation that TNF had no significant effect in animal sepsis models of cecal ligation and puncture (which would be more relevant to clinical application in humans). Large-scale clinical trials employing TNF mAbs and receptors or IL-1 ablation with IL-1Ra have met with little success.[62]

The disappointing clinical results from proinflammatory cytokine ablation have brought into question the thesis that sepsis is entirely understandable in terms of persistent and uncontrolled inflammation. Another view—which is not incompatible with the basic concept of sepsis as a systemic inflammatory response—is that the body also mounts a countering anti-inflammatory reaction to an insult, which then can lead to what is referred to as the compensatory anti-inflammatory response syndrome (CARS).[63] According to this hypothesis, when the proinflammatory response to an insult predominates, SIRS and shock result, and when the anti-inflammatory response predominates, CARS, immunosuppression, and increased susceptibility to infection ensue. Homeostasis and return to health reflect a state in which the two responses are in balance. It is likely that in cases of trauma or infection, the body's first response is proinflammatory, and the resulting SIRS is responsible for early mortality. This initial response is followed by an anti-inflammatory response, and the resulting CARS is responsible for late mortality secondary to immunodepression.[62]

Numerous studies have measured cytokine concentrations in the peripheral vasculature in an effort to identify markers of sepsis, predictors of mortality, and possible clinical interventions. Perhaps surprisingly, levels of the proinflammatory cytokines (TNF, IL-1, IL-12, and IFN-γ) are not consistently correlated with either disease severity or mortality in patients with septic shock. This finding provides some evidence for the CARS hypothesis. It must be remembered, however, that systemic blood sampling is not indicative of tissue cytokine dynamics. In patients with pneumonia, for example, concentrations of TNF, IL-1, and IL-12 were found to be markedly higher in bronchial lavage samples than in serum.[64] The cytokine for which peripheral blood levels seem to correlate best with disease severity is IL-6; it is unclear why this is so, given that IL-6 certainly does not produce shock. A 1994 study found that circulating levels of the anti-inflammatory cytokine IL-10, which are normally unmeasurable, were detectable in more than 80% of patients with severe sepsis.[65] A so-called refractory immunologic state developing after infection or trauma has also been described,[47] characterized by reduced proinflammatory cytokine production by mononuclear cells but increased synthesis of IL-1Ra (which correlates with CARS).

Several studies have examined therapies aimed at promoting cytokines that enhance the proinflammatory response and there-

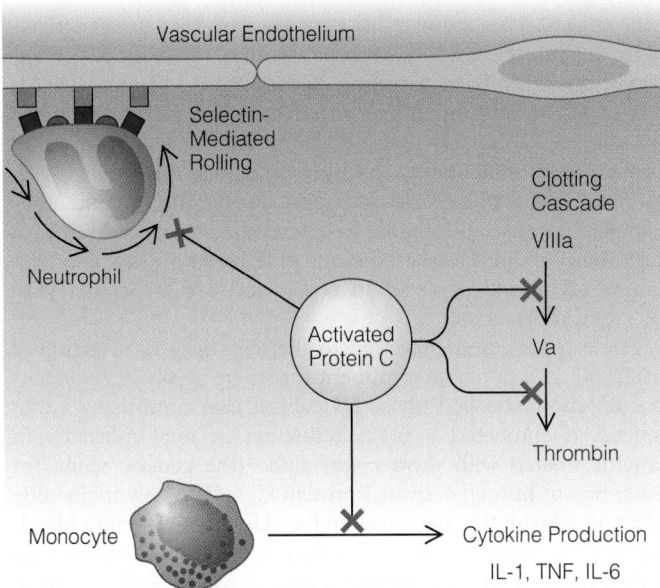

Figure 4 **Activated protein C has both anti-inflammatory and antithrombotic actions that make it a valuable antisepsis drug. It reduces cytokine release by mononuclear phagocytes, reduces leukocyte adhesion to the vascular endothelium, and inhibits thrombin formation.**

by presumably combat CARS. In one, administration of G-CSF to patients with community-acquired pneumonia resulted in reduced rates of systemic complications and sepsis.[62] INF-γ was employed in a small clinical study of patients with sepsis and later in a multicenter study of burn patients,[66] the rationale being that monocyte function had been found to be depressed in severely ill patients. In these settings, the goal of restoring monocyte activity, as defined by HLA-DR expression, was achieved, though no clinical benefit was noted with regard to mortality or incidence of infectious complications.

It is clear that the role of cytokines in sepsis is a complex one: both hypoinflammation and hyperinflammation occur, and both are major determinants of clinical outcome. To date, no therapy has been found that reliably regulates cytokine activity and reduces sepsis-related mortality. It may be that future treatments will be chosen and given on a patient-to-patient basis, with markers of immune competence (e.g., HLA-DR, IL-6, and TNF) indicating whether a proinflammatory approach or an anti-inflammatory approach is preferable in a specific instance.

Activated Protein C

It has long been recognized that the clotting system plays a major role in inflammation and in the response to invading organisms; DIC is one of the cardinal signs of sepsis. The proinflammatory cytokines TNF, IL-1, and IL-6 are known to trigger activation of the clotting cascade by stimulating the release of tissue factor from monocytes and endothelium, leading to thrombin formation and a fibrin clot. These cytokines also inhibit endogenous fibrinolytic mechanisms by stimulating the release of plasminogen-activator inhibitor–1 (PAI-1) from platelets and endothelium. At the same time, thrombin stimulates many inflammatory pathways and suppresses natural anticoagulant response by activating thrombin-activatable fibrinolysis inhibitor (TAFI).[67] This procoagulant response leads to microvascular thrombosis and is implicated in the multiple organ failure associated with sepsis.

Protein C is an endogenous anticoagulant that, when activated by thrombin bound to thrombomodulin, reduces the generation of thrombin by inactivating clotting factors Va and VIIIa. It also exerts an anti-inflammatory effect by inhibiting monocyte production of TNF, IL-1, and IL-6 and limiting leukocyte adhesion to endothelium by binding selectins[68] [see Figure 4]. Activation of protein C is impaired during the inflammatory response because endothelial injury results in reduced levels of thrombomodulin. Decreased circulating levels of activated protein C are usually present in sepsis and are associated with increased mortality.[69]

These observations have led to the investigation of activated protein C as a potential treatment for severe sepsis. A multicenter, placebo-controlled phase III clinical trial comprising 1,690 patients documented a 6.1% reduction in total mortality in patients treated with drotrecogin alpha (the generic name for recombinant human activated protein C).[67] The only major side effect noted with this agent was an increased risk of serious bleeding: 3.5%, compared with 2% in the placebo group. Drotrecogin is thus the first therapy to have shown a real clinical benefit in sepsis trials, and high hopes are held for its future therapeutic use. The United States Food and Drug Administration has recently approved this agent for treament of sepsis, and further clinical trials are planned. It is marketed under the brand name Xigris.

Reactive Oxygen Metabolites

Oxygen and its metabolites [see Table 4] are often very toxic, and this toxicity seems to have influenced the early evolution of metabolic pathways to detoxify oxygen and make life possible in an aerobic environment.[70] Although aerobic organisms are capable of exploiting oxygen's high reactivity for cellular energy, this reactivity also poses a continual assault on living tissues. Whenever the rate of endogenous oxidant generation exceeds the body's endogenous antioxidant capacity, tissue injury ensues. This occurrence is known as oxidative stress.

Free radicals and other ROMs have been implicated in a diverse array of human disease processes, including reperfusion injury, ischemic hepatitis and pancreatitis, inflammatory bowel disease, and ARDS. The common pathway for the tissue injury in these illnesses is the action of free radicals.

CHEMICAL STRUCTURE

The high reactivity of free radicals is a consequence of their chemical structure. Free radicals are molecules that contain one or more unpaired electrons in their outer orbits. As a result, they possess higher energy levels than molecules with full outer orbits and, accordingly, are less stable and more reactive.

The most abundant radical in the biologic system is molecular oxygen itself (O_2), which has two unpaired electrons in its outer orbit. In this ground (i.e., low-energy) state, the two electrons have parallel spins, rendering the molecule relatively unreactive. When the electrons have antiparallel spins, the radical—termed singlet oxygen ($^1O_2$)—is much more reactive. Various oxygen-centered free radicals and ROMs are believed to play important roles in tissue injury. The superoxide anion ($O_2^{\bullet-}$) and the hydroxyl radical (OH•) each have one unpaired electron in the outer orbit. The latter is particularly unstable: it reacts within 10^{-6} seconds of its formation and within a distance of 15 nm. Consequently, the hydroxyl radical is not only highly toxic but also very difficult to scavenge effectively.

Some ROMs, technically speaking, are not true radicals but are still quite toxic. For example, much of superoxide's tissue toxicity is actually mediated by its oxidant reduction products.

Table 4 Reactive Oxygen Metabolites and Other Free Radicals

Radicals and Metabolites	Chemical Symbol	Comments
Oxygen-centered free radicals		
Molecular oxygen		
Ground state (triplet) oxygen	$^3O_2$	Constitutes 20% of the atmosphere
Singlet oxygen	$^1O_2$	Much more reactive than $^3O_2$
Superoxide radical	$O_2^{\bullet-}$	Initial product of respiratory burst of neutrophils
Hydroxyl radical	OH•	Highly unstable; extremely toxic
Alkoxy radical	RO•	Important toxic intermediate of free radical chain reactions
Peroxy radical	ROO•	Important mediator of DNA damage
Lipoxy radical	LOO•	Important toxic metabolite of lipid peroxidation
Non–oxygen-centered free radicals		
Nitrogen centered		
Nitric oxide	NO•	Neurotransmitter
Peroxynitrite	OONO•	Important endogenous toxin
Carbon centered		
Lipid radical	L•	Important toxic metabolite of lipid peroxidation
Sulfur centered		
Thiyl	R-S•	Metabolites of cysteine and D-penicillamine
Hydrogen centered		
Hydrogen atom	H•	—
Iron centered		
Perferryl radical	Fe^{3+}-O_2-Fe^{2+}	Important final mediator of tissue injury (along with OH•)
Non–free radical reactive metabolites		
Ozone	O_3	Major air pollutant
Hydroperoxides		
Hydrogen peroxide	H_2O_2	Important endogenous tissue toxin
Lipid peroxide	LOOH	Intermediate lipid peroxidation
Hypochlorous acid	HOCl	Important mediator of neutrophil toxicity
Chloramines	R'RNCl	Important final mediator of neutrophil toxicity

The hydroperoxides constitute an important class of toxic ROMs, with hydrogen peroxide (H_2O_2) playing a particularly important part. Much of the superoxide-initiated tissue damage caused by neutrophils and macrophages can be attributed to halogenated oxidants (e.g., hypochlorous acid [HOCl]) and chloramines, which are formed by the secondary reaction of halogenated radical species with nitrogen compounds. This production of toxic ROMs as redox products substantially amplifies the toxicity of free radicals.

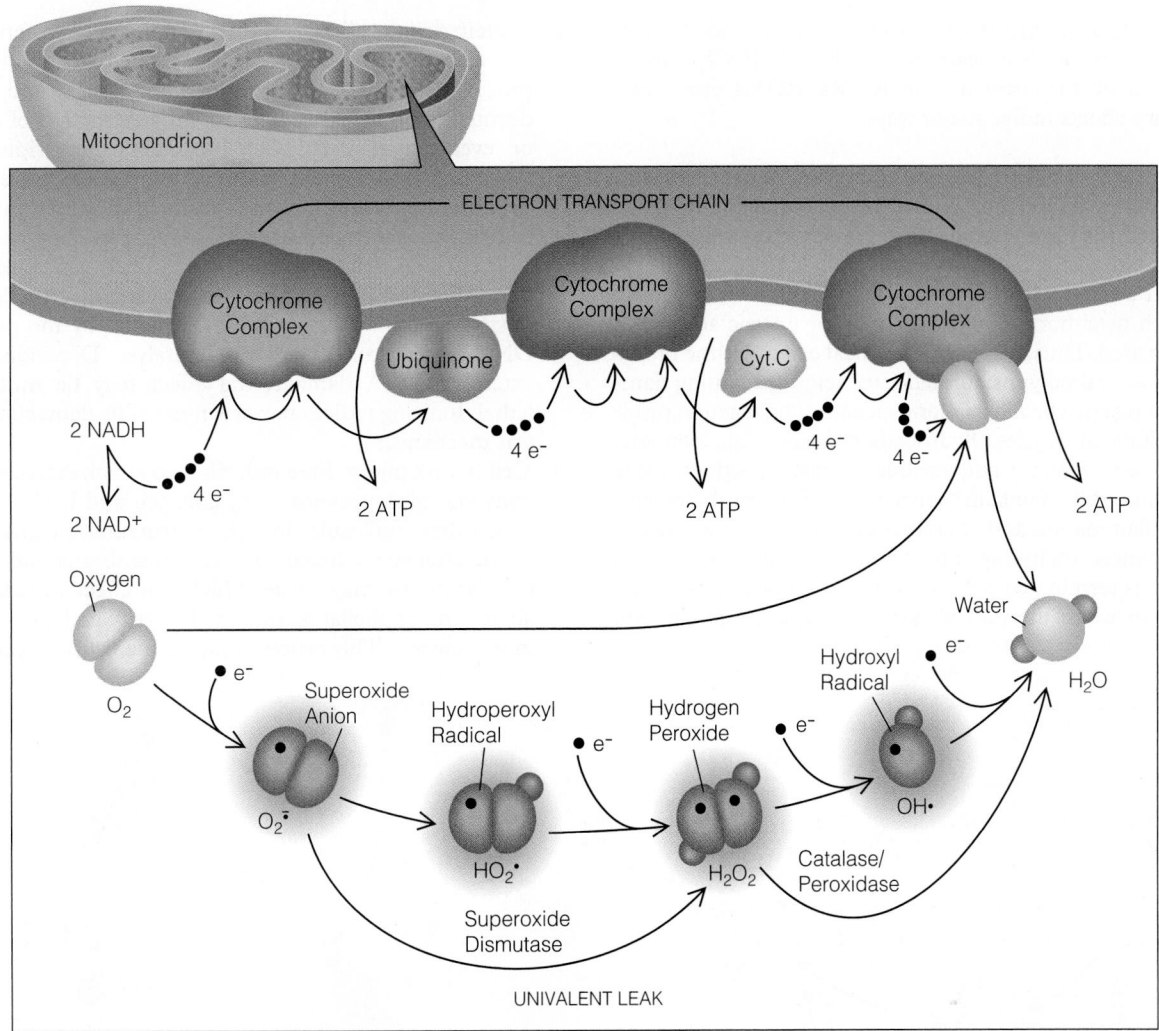

Figure 5 **The mitochondrial cytochrome oxidase complex reduces molecular oxygen by the essentially simultaneous addition of four electrons, producing water and generating adenosine triphosphate (ATP) without the production of free reactive oxygen intermediates. However, 1% to 5% of oxygen leaks from this pathway and undergoes stepwise, univalent reduction. The one-electron reduction of molecular oxygen generates the superoxide free radical (superoxide anion). This can subsequently be reduced to hydrogen peroxide (H_2O_2), most commonly in a dismutation reaction catalyzed by SOD. Hydrogen peroxide can be directly reduced to water (by a catalase- or peroxidase-catalyzed reduction), or it can be reduced to the hydroxyl radical ($OH^{\cdot}$) (usually in an iron-catalyzed reaction). The highly reactive hydroxyl radical can subsequently abstract a hydrogen atom to reduce itself to water. Normally, protective biochemical mechanisms detoxify the toxic intermediates generated by this so-called univalent leak. When increased concentrations of oxygen generate excessive amounts of reactive oxygen metabolites, however, protective mechanisms may be overwhelmed and tissue injury may result.**

FORMATION

All cells continuously generate ROMs as normal by-products of metabolism. During oxidative phosphorylation, mitochondrial cytochromes couple the production of adenosine triphosphate (ATP) to the tetravalent reduction of molecular oxygen to water [*see Figure 5*]. In the course of this process, all four electrons are effectively added to the oxygen molecule at once. No intermediaries are formed, and thus no free radicals are generated. However, about 1% to 5% of the oxygen reduced to water within the mitochondria leaks from this pathway and undergoes a stepwise, noncatalyzed reduction—the so-called univalent leak—that produces a series of toxic intermediaries. These ROMs must then be detoxified by endogenous antioxidants to prevent tissue injury.

ROMs are also formed in many other circumstances. Certain cellular oxidases (e.g., cytochrome P-450, mixed-function oxidase,

and peroxidases) can generate ROMs.[71] The arachidonic acid cascade, which produces eicosanoids [*see Eicosanoids, below*], also generates peroxy compounds and hydroxyl radicals as by-products.

In inflammatory cells, ROMs are the primary product of a highly specialized NADPH-dependent oxidant system. When activated, they cause reduction of oxygen to the superoxide anion. This process, known as the respiratory burst, may account for more than 90% of the oxygen consumption of an activated neutrophil [*see Figure 6*].[72] It is followed by formation of the major toxic product, HOCl, catalyzed by an enzyme (myeloperoxidase [MPO]) that is unique to phagocytes.

MECHANISM OF TISSUE DAMAGE

All biochemical cell components are potentially subject to attack by free radicals; however, lipids, proteins, and nucleic acids are particularly vulnerable. It should also be noted that the toxic and mutagenic effects of ionizing radiation and those of many toxic chemicals (e.g., carbon tetrachloride [CCl_4]) are in fact mediated by the formation of ROMs. ROMs exert their inflammatory effects in five major ways.

1. Lipid peroxidation. Because ROMs are so reactive, they generally react with the first molecule encountered, which is often a cell membrane lipid. By removing a hydrogen atom from the carbon chain of a polyunsaturated fatty acid, a ROM can form a fatty acid radical ($LOO^\bullet$), which is then able to react with neighboring lipids, proteins, or nucleic acids, in a chain reaction. Thus, a single free radical can cause the breakdown of several polyunsaturated fatty acids, generating damaged and reactive products along its path. The reaction products include aldehydes, hydrocarbon gases (e.g., pentane, methane, and ethane) and various chemical residues; these agents cause cell edema, influence vascular permeability, give rise to inflammation and chemotaxis, and alter the activity of cell enzymes, including phospholipase. This destructive sequence is terminated only when two of these radicals react together or when the radicals are scavenged by an electron acceptor.

2. Protein denaturation. Both structural and enzymatic proteins are vulnerable to free radical–mediated denaturation. This process can lead to loss of membrane fluidity and structural disintegration, which can cause the destruction of organelles or even entire cells. Calcium adenosine triphosphatase (ATPase) is particularly susceptible to oxidative damage; denaturation of this enzyme results in increased intracellular calcium concentration with subsequent swelling and injury.

3. Nucleic acid denaturation. Free radicals can attack nucleic acids directly, causing base hydroxylation, cross-linking, or scission. Such attacks may be facilitated by the presence of DNA-bound iron acting as a catalyst. Depending on the extent of DNA damage, the effect may be mutagenic or lethal. Ionizing radiation exerts most of its damaging effect by this mechanism.

4. Cell matrix injury. Free radicals also attack extracellular proteins and glycoproteins (e.g., collagen and hyaluronic acid). When these molecules lose their structural integrity, damage to the connective tissue basement membrane and the extracellular matrix may ensue, which can affect vascular permeability and epithelial membrane integrity and can even result in petechiae.[73] This process may be the cause of certain con-

Figure 6 **Neutrophils and other phagocytes generate the superoxide radical via the membrane-integrated enzyme NADPH oxidase. On stimulation, more than 90% of the oxygen used by the neutrophil is consumed in this respiratory burst. Although the superoxide radical itself is toxic to many invading microorganisms, the secondary generation of HOCl from hydrogen peroxide and chloride ions, catalyzed by the neutrophil-generated enzyme myeloperoxidase, substantially increases the bactericidal potential of the neutrophil.**

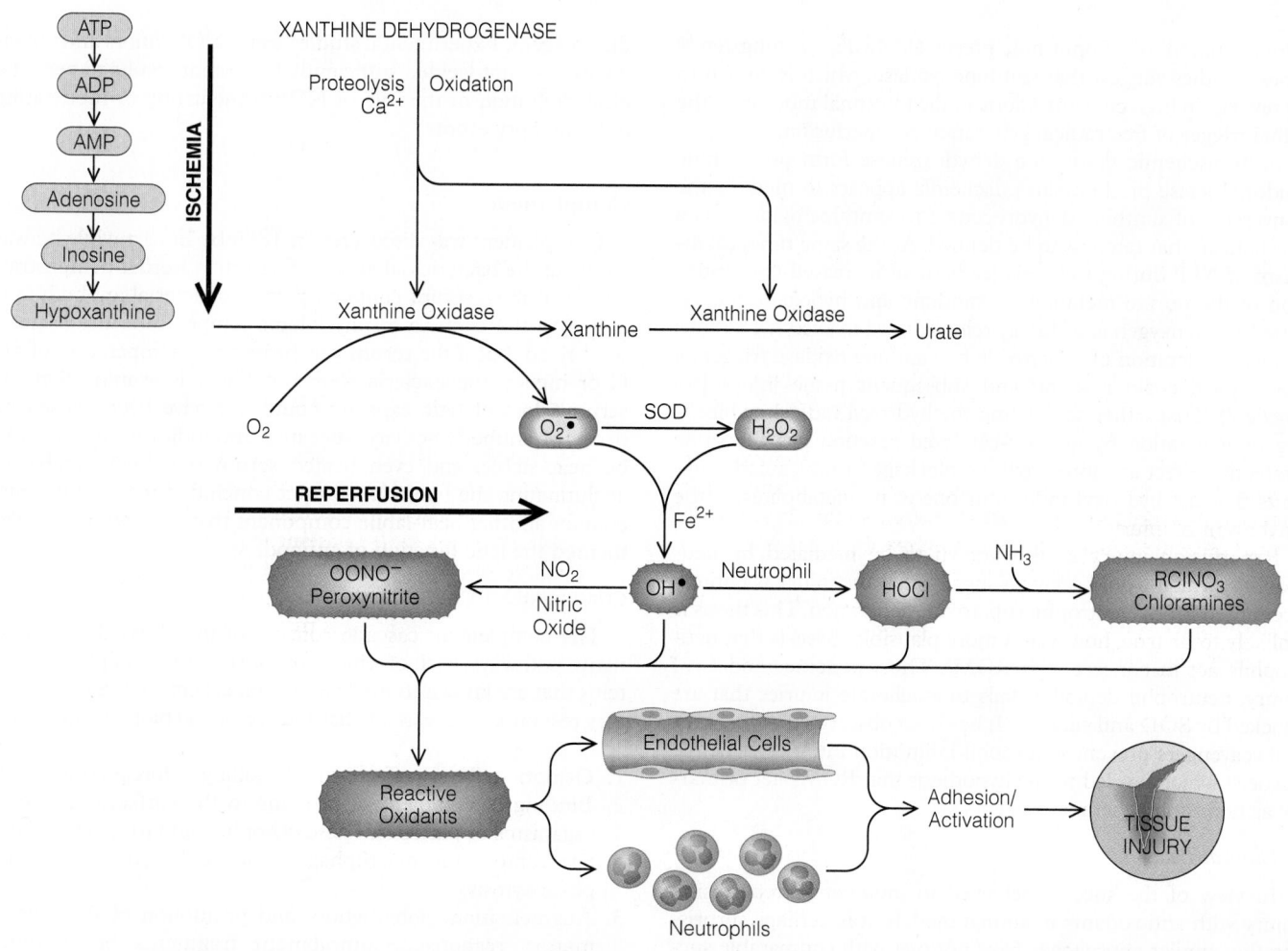

Figure 7 **Xanthine oxidase may serve as the initial source of free radical generation in postischemic reperfusion injury. With the onset of ischemia, ATP is degraded to its purine bases (e.g., hypoxanthine), the concentration of which increases. Simultaneously, xanthine dehydrogenase is converted by ischemia to xanthine oxidase. Although the concentrations of substrate and enzyme are high during ischemia, the absence of oxygen prevents purine oxidation until reperfusion. At reperfusion, oxygen becomes available, suddenly and in excess, and the oxidation of hypoxanthine (and xanthine) proceeds rapidly, generating a burst of superoxide radicals as a by-product, probably at or near the endothelial cell surface.**

nective tissue diseases (e.g., osteoarthritis and rheumatoid arthritis), with inflammatory cells serving as the source of ROMs.

5. Apoptosis. Apoptosis, a genetic mechanism that regulates cell numbers, is characterized by cell shrinkage (pyknosis), in contrast with the cell swelling and rupture typical of necrosis. Pyknotic cells are cleared by macrophages with minimal inflammation. Apoptosis is induced by ROMs, acting via diverse mechanisms.

ANTIOXIDANT DEFENSE MECHANISMS

Various endogenous mechanisms have evolved to limit or counteract the tissue damage caused by ROMs. An example is the production and release of enzymatic and nonenzymatic antioxidants such as vitamin E, vitamin C, provitamin A, glutathione, superoxide dismutase (SOD), and glutathione peroxidase, which act by scavenging ROMs. The enzymatic antioxidants require trace metals as cofactors for maximal effect: selenium for glutathione peroxidase; copper, zinc, or manganese for SOD; and iron for catalase.

These endogenous antioxidants are generally present at sites where free radicals are produced, which ensures that scavenging can occur immediately after formation—a critical point, in view of the short radii of the antioxidants' activity. For example, SOD is located almost exclusively in the mitochondrial matrix, where it scavenges superoxide radicals formed via the univalent leak, and vitamins A and E are found in cell membranes, where they inhibit lipid peroxidation.

ROLE IN REPERFUSION INJURY

Postischemic reperfusion disease provides the classic example of free radical–mediated tissue injury. This phenomenon was first demonstrated in 1981 in the feline small intestine, where administration of SOD near the end of the ischemic period but before reperfusion largely prevented the microvascular and epithelial injury seen after periods of partial ischemia.[74] Since that initial study, SOD has been shown to attenuate reperfusion injury in many organs, including skeletal muscle[75] and the heart.[76] In similar models, injury was ameliorated by (1) scavenging of hydrogen peroxide by catalase,[77] (2) scavenging of hydroxyl radicals by dimethyl sulfoxide or mannitol,[78] or (3) prevention of radical formation by chelating iron with transferrin or deferoxamine.[79] Equivalent protection was provided by inhibiting generation of superoxide by xanthine oxidase through administration of allopurinol, pterin aldehyde, or tungsten.[80] These studies suggest that xanthine oxidase, which is known to be present in high concentrations in the intestinal mucosa, is the initial trigger of free radical generation at reperfusion.

In nonischemic tissue, the dehydrogenase form of xanthine oxidoreductase predominates. Ischemia appears to mediate the conversion of xanthine dehydrogenase to xanthine oxidase via a mechanism that remains to be defined. At the same time, catabolism of ATP during ischemia leads to an increased concentration of the purine metabolites, xanthine and hypoxanthine. At reperfusion, oxygen is suddenly reintroduced in excess. The subsequent generation of superoxide by xanthine oxidase triggers a free radical chain reaction and subsequent tissue injury [see Figure 7]. That either scavenging the hydroxyl radical or blocking its generation by an iron-catalyzed reaction has the same protective effect as more proximal blockage of the cascade suggests that the hydroxyl radical, or one of its metabolites, is the final agent of injury.[77]

Reperfusion injury is also known to be mediated by neutrophils, which would seem to suggest that the injury is entirely accounted for by neutrophil superoxide generation. This thesis is unlikely to be true, however: a more plausible thesis is that neutrophils act in concert with ROMs. Thus, in some models of injury, neutrophil depletion fails to ameliorate injuries that are blocked by SOD and catalase. It has been observed that free radical scavengers prevent neutrophil infiltration into postischemic tissue,[81] which has led to the hypothesis that ROMs act primarily as neutrophil chemoattractants.

Clinical Trials

In view of the success achieved in moderating reperfusion injury with antioxidants in animal models, it is perhaps surprising that similar approaches have not met with comparable success in humans. A 1989 study using human recombinant SOD to treat myocardial ischemia-reperfusion injury after angioplasty and renal ischemia failed to demonstrate any benefit.[82] However, a renal transplant study in which SOD was infused immediately before reperfusion reported reduced rates of acute renal failure in graft recipients who underwent cold ischemia for longer than 30 hours[83]; graft survival was longer as well.

In general, ROM scavengers are partially effective at best. Despite the enormous amount of data that has been collected, the precise relationship between ROM generation and tissue injury remains unclear.

Nitric Oxide

NO• is produced in a variety of tissues (e.g., endothelial cells and platelets) by either a constitutive or an inducible form of NO• synthase. In the setting of inflammation, the inducible enzyme is activated by cytokines such as TNF. NO• is a potent inhibitor of leukocyte and platelet adhesion, exerting its effects via activation of soluble guanylcyclase and generation of cyclic guanosine monophosphate (cGMP).[84] With regard to platelets, NO• has been shown to inhibit the binding of fibrinogen to GPIIb/IIIa and to limit the expression of P-selectin.[85] Another important anti-inflammatory role of NO• is its ability to scavenge superoxide at least as fast as SOD does. Finally, inhaled NO• moderately reduces the pulmonary hypertension seen with ARDS; however, it does not increase cardiac output or reduce mortality in these patients.

Moreover, NO• acts as a source of potent free radicals when it interacts with superoxide to form peroxynitrite, a strong oxidizing agent. Experimental studies using NO• donors and antagonists have not yielded sufficiently consistent results to permit a clear definition of the role of NO• in mediating or moderating inflammatory events.

Complement

Complement was discovered in 1889 by Bordet while he was studying the bactericidal action of serum.[86] Bordet demonstrated that if fresh serum containing an antibacterial antibody was added to the bacteria at physiologic temperature, the bacteria were lysed, but if the serum was heated to a temperature of 56° C or higher, the bacteria were not lysed. Reasoning that the serum's loss of lytic capacity could not have been caused by decay of antibody activity—because antibodies were known to be heat stable, and even heated serum remained capable of agglutinating the bacteria—Bordet concluded that serum must contain another heat-labile component that assisted or complemented the lytic function of antibodies.

COMPLEMENT CASCADE

The complement cascade consists of the classical and alternative pathways, each of which comprises a series of plasma proteins that are known to mediate several aspects of the inflammatory response. This cascade has four principal biologic functions:

1. Osmotic cell lysis, effective in the killing of foreign organisms.
2. Binding of complement proteins to the surfaces of foreign organisms or particles. These opsonins bind to specific counterreceptors on macrophages and leukocytes, facilitating phagocytosis.
3. Augmentation, potentiation, and promotion of the inflammatory response. Complement fragments bring about chemotaxis of inflammatory cells. In addition, C3a and C5a stimulate a neutrophil oxidative burst and mast cell degranulation, which potentiate the inflammatory response.
4. Clearance of immune complexes from the circulation.

The classical pathway and the alternative pathway have different activating mechanisms; however, both result in the formation of the membrane attack complex C5b-C9, which leads to the creation of pores in the cell membrane and consequently to abnormal ion transport, impaired signaling, and potential lysis, particularly of nonnucleated cells. Activation of either pathway leads to production of the biologically active anaphylatoxins C3a and C5a. These peptides are generated via cleavage of native C3 and C5 complement components by C3 convertase and C5 convertase, which are formed at intermediate steps in the process of complement activation. C3a and C5a exert a variety of physiologic effects, including vasodilatation and increased vascular permeability. The effects on neutrophils include chemotaxis, diapedesis, degranulation, and free radical production as well as translocation of intracellular complement receptors to the neutrophil-plasma membrane. In addition, the complement fragments C3b and C4b serve as opsonins, thus facilitating phagocytosis of particles to which they have attached. Inactive C3b (iC3b) is a counterreceptor for the neutrophil CD11b/CD18 (Mac-1) receptor and thus has the ability to enhance neutrophil binding and signaling in response to complement-coated molecules, thereby facilitating their phagocytosis.

The complement cascade has specific features that make it an important effector mechanism in the inflammatory response. Many of its components, once activated, possess enzymatic activity. As the cascade proceeds, these activated components cause substantial amplifications at each step. In addition to this important positive feedback loop, there are multiple levels at which inhibitory proteins can intervene in the cascade to prevent its accidental or inappropriate generalized activation. Another important property of the complement cascade is that it has both specific and nonspecific activators. Once a specific antibody and antigen have reacted, the classical pathway can be activated by several closely spaced IgG molecules or by a single IgM pentamer. The alternative pathway is triggered by direct binding of components to the surface of foreign organisms. In this way, the alternative pathway participates in nonspecific immunity.

Classical Pathway

The classical pathway [see Figure 8] is usually initiated by interaction between C1 and an antigen-antibody complex. It may also be activated by infectious organisms (e.g., *Mycoplasma*) or certain molecules (e.g., DNA, heparin, and chondroitin sulfate).[87]

C1 does not interact with IgG or IgM until the antibody has bound its specific antigen. The subunit of C1 that binds is C1q. C1q attaches either to the C_H3 domain of IgM or to the C_H2 domain of IgG, both of which reside in the Fc portion of the antibody. A single C1q molecule must bind to at least two Fc portions of an immunoglobulin. Because IgM is secreted as a pentamer containing five separate Fc portions, a single molecule is an efficient activator of complement. Because IgG is secreted as a monomer, C1q must bind to two or more adjacent IgG molecules to be activated. C1q is uniquely able to bind these different Fc regions of immunoglobulins because it consists of six identical subunits, each of which has a projecting head.

Once C1q is bound to an immune complex, the other components of C1—C1r and C1s—become operative. A tetramer consisting of two C1r and two C1s molecules is formed and bonded with C1q. This process results in a serum esterase–type enzyme that acts on the next two components in the cascade, C4 and C2. C4, like several other complement proteins, has an internal thioester bond. C4 is split into two parts, C4a and C4b, with the former diffusing away. Generation of C4b results in a reactive molecule called metastable C4b, which possesses an internal thioester. Many C4b molecules react with water at the site of the internal thioester, thereby inactivating the C4 complex; alternatively, some of the C4b thioesters may esterify to cell surface proteins or carbohydrates, thereby stabilizing the C4 complex.

In the presence of magnesium, C2 binds to C4b molecules that in turn are bound to cell surface proteins or carbohydrates. A C1s molecule splits C2, generating C2a and C2b. The latter may diffuse away, whereas the C2a fragment remains complexed with C4b, resulting in C4b2a, which is the C3 convertase of the classical pathway [see Figure 8]. In the presence of calcium and magnesium, this C3 convertase binds C3 and cleaves it into C3a and C3b. Like C4b, C3b has an internal thioester, and this thioester may form a covalent bond with C4b2a or be inactivated by reacting with water. The addition of C3b to the preexisting C4b2a complex yields C4b2a3b, which is the C5 convertase of the classical pathway. This C5 convertase cleaves C5 and initiates the common terminal sequence of the complement cascade, which results in the formation of C5b-C9, the membrane attack complex.

Alternative Pathway

The alternative pathway [see Figure 8] was so named because it was discovered after the classical pathway was described, but it seems actually to have evolved before the classical pathway. Both pathways require the production of C3 and C5 convertases to generate the terminal sequence leading to generation of the membrane attack complex; however, each uses a different series of activators and proteins to produce these convertases.

The alternative pathway is in a constant state of low-level activation as a result of spontaneous hydrolysis of the internal thioester bond in the α chain of C3 (the so-called tickover of C3), a process that is believed to be ongoing at a low intensity in the circulation at all times. This hydrolysis leads to the unstable intermediate C3b. (The classical pathway may also initiate the alternative pathway by serving as the source of the first C3b molecules.) C3b is usually hydrolysed by water, but sometimes it reacts with amino or hydroxyl groups of cell surface proteins or polysaccharides to form stable amide or ester bonds. The cell-bound C3b then attaches to factor B, which in turn is proteolytically cleaved by factor D to form C3bBb, the solid-phase alternative pathway C3 convertase, which requires properdin for stabilization.

The C3 convertase then acts on additional C3b to form the C3bBbC3b complex, which is the C5 convertase of the alternative pathway. This C5 convertase initiates hydrolysis of C5, which, as in the classical pathway, eventually results in the formation of the membrane attack complex.

Membrane Attack Complex

Both of the C5 convertases cleave C5 into C5a and C5b. The C5b component binds to C6 and C7, and the resulting C5b67 complex is then inserted into the lipid bilayer of the plasma membrane. Once in place in the membrane, this molecule becomes a receptor for and binds to C8, at which point pore formation, ionic movement, and cell lysis may begin. The C5b678 complex undergoes hydrophilic association within the plasma membrane, weakening it and causing the formation of transmembrane channels. This process may lead to cell death by osmotic lysis because of the cell's inability to maintain critical intra- and extracellular concentration gradients. Because of the amplification mechanisms involved in both pathways, as many as 12 to 15 C9 molecules may be added to the C5b678 complex, resulting in the formation of C5b-C9, the membrane attack complex. Scanning electron microscopy suggests that the membrane attack complex acts as a pore within the cell membrane, allowing the collapse of ionic and osmotic gradients.

Regulation

To prevent inappropriate activation and damage to the host, the complement cascade must be tightly regulated. There are a number of circulating soluble factors that inactivate various aspects of the complement cascade, including C1 inhibitor, C4-binding protein, factor H, and factor I. Molecules that inhibit membrane attack complex formation include homologous restriction factor and the membrane inhibitor of reactive lysis, both of which are thought to play a key role in protecting normal surrounding cells in adjacent areas where complement activation and cell lysis are taking place.

In addition, there are several regulatory proteins that are found within the membranes of most cells of the myeloid line as well as those of platelets and mast cells; these include complement receptor type 1 (CR1), membrane cofactor protein, and decay-accelerating factor. CR1 is present on erythrocytes and in smaller quantities on neutrophils, monocytes, macrophages, eosinophils, and lymphocytes. It has at least three important functions: (1) it can inhibit C3 convertase activity, (2) it enhances the ability of leukocytes to ingest C3b- or C4b-coated

CLASSICAL PATHWAY   **ALTERNATIVE PATHWAY**

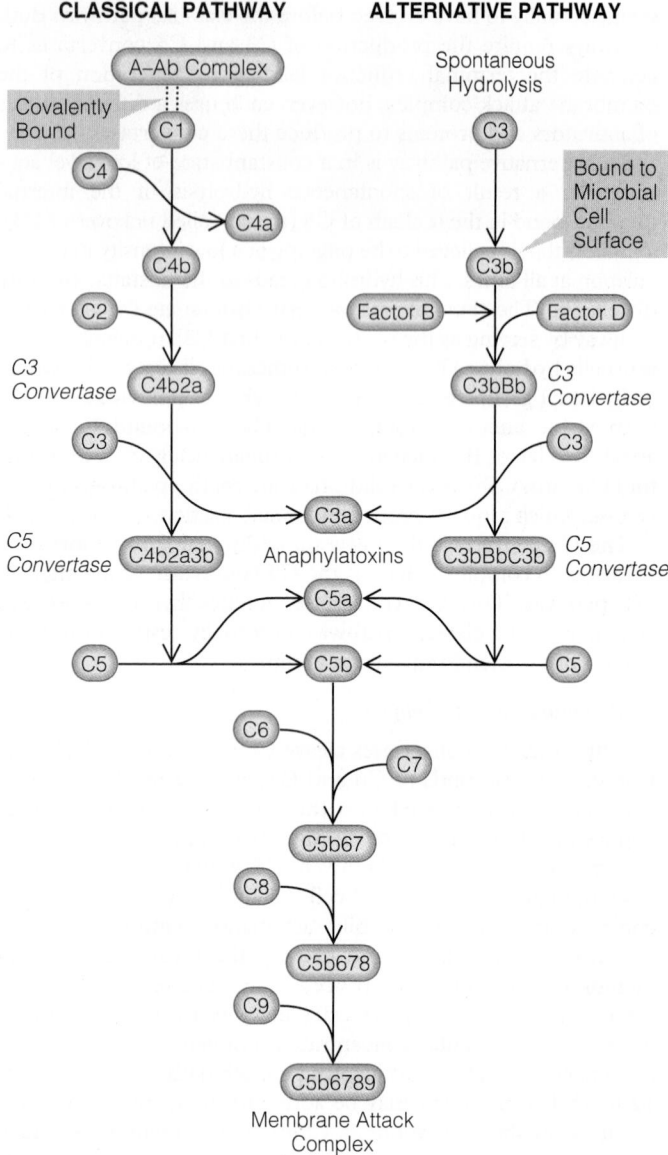

Figure 8 **Shown are the classical and alternative pathways of the complement cascade.**

particles, and (3) it facilitates clearance of immune complexes from the circulation. CR1 also inhibits the activity of C4b and thus is capable of preventing activation of the classical pathway. This powerful inhibitor of both complement pathways is currently the subject of much attention among researchers. A soluble form of CR1 that lacks the cytoplasmic and transmembrane domains has been engineered from human erythrocytes. This human soluble complement receptor type 1 (sCR1) retains the C3b- and C4b-binding activities of membrane-associated CR1.

ROLE IN REPERFUSION INJURY

The first evidence that complement might play a role in the pathogenesis of ischemia-reperfusion injury was the finding that myocardial ischemia induced complement activation.[88] It was also reported that mitochondrial fragments in cardiac lymph activated both classical and alternative complement pathways. Later studies using cobra venom factor to deplete complement by triggering its activation demonstrated reductions in myocardial necrosis after coronary artery occlusion.[89] Researchers

examining therapeutic use of sCR1 in animals documented significant reductions in myocardial infarct size and dramatic reductions in the number of neutrophils sequestered in the myocardium.[90] Moreover, treatment with sCR1 did not appear to impair healing of the infarcted area. Immunoperoxidase staining for the membrane attack complex demonstrated little or no myocardial deposition of C5b-C9 in the sCR1-treated group in comparison with untreated animals.

Several studies have examined the role of complement in skeletal muscle ischemia-reperfusion injury. In one, concentrations of C3a and C5a were elevated in patients with ischemic limbs.[91] Levels of these anaphylatoxins returned to normal after amputation, which suggested that complement was activated by acute limb ischemia. In another study, there was a significant dose-dependent reduction in muscle permeability with sCR1 treatment after hindlimb ischemia-reperfusion.[92] Subsequently, it was found that during reperfusion, skeletal muscle permeability was dependent on the presence of IgM natural antibody and on activation of the classical complement pathway. These investigations lend strong support to the thesis that complement is a significant mediator of skeletal muscle injury after ischemia-reperfusion.

In further studies, it was postulated that ischemic injury led to expression or unmasking of a neoantigen. Immunohistochemistry demonstrated colocalization of IgM and C3, indicating the formation of an immune complex in conjunction with complement activation (shown by other techniques to involve the classical pathway). Animals genetically depleted of immunoglobulins—specifically, IgM—were protected from reperfusion injury.

Mast Cell

Although mast cells were first identified more than a century ago, only comparatively recently have major advances been made in understanding their biology. All mast cells are derived from progenitors present in the bone marrow, which migrate to peripheral tissues as immature cells and undergo differentiation in situ. Thus, unlike neutrophils, mature mast cells are not found in the circulation but are located throughout the body near blood vessels and nerves, beneath epithelia, and in lymphoid organs.

STRUCTURE AND TYPOLOGY

Mast cells have (1) a mononuclear nucleus, (2) numerous cytoplasmic granules containing mediators (including peptides, proteins, proteoglycans, and amines, and (3) a plicated cell membrane. The cell membrane contains a number of receptors for important regulatory compounds, such as growth factors, activators of secretion (e.g., receptors for the Fc portion of the IgE molecule), and receptors for adhesive molecules that enable the mast cell to attach to certain sites.

Mast cells can be differentiated into two types, those found in mucosa and those found in connective tissue. These two phenotypes are relatively easy to distinguish in rodents because they stain differently, differ in size, and are found in different tissues. GI mucosal mast cells have chondroitin sulfate as their major granule proteoglycan and contain little histamine. In contrast, connective tissue mast cells (found in the lungs and in the serosa of body cavities) have heparin as their major granule proteoglycan and produce large quantities of histamine.

Two techniques have enabled researchers to distinguish between the two types of mast cells in humans. One uses electron microscopy to examine the completeness of the scroll or whorl structure of the granule (only connective tissue mast cells have a complete scroll). The other uses mAbs to identify mast cell subtypes on the basis of their constituent protease enzymes. All human mast cells contain tryptase, but only connective tissue mast cells contain chymase. Furthermore, there are a number of chymase isotypes that are unique to particular organs, which suggests that the pattern of mediators produced by mast cells might vary with anatomic location.

ACTIVATION

In diseases associated with mast cell activation, increases in the total number of mast cells and variations in the relative abundance of mast cell phenotypes occur at different tissue sites. The best understood immunologic stimulus of mast cell activation is an immune IgE complex. Other important immunologic triggers are cytokines and various histamine-releasing factors generated by neutrophils, platelets, mononuclear leukocytes, and macrophages as a consequence of the immune response.

Numerous nonimmunologic stimuli are also important in mast cell activation associated with wheal-and-flare reactions. Such stimuli include the complement fragments C3a, C4a, and C5a; various neuropeptides, including calcitonin gene–related peptide; substance P; neurotransmitters; and drugs. These nonimmunologic activators are generally more effective on connective tissue mast cells than on mucosal mast cells.

When mast cells are activated, their granules move to the surface, dissolve, and release their contents. Some of these products (e.g., histamine and other low-molecular-weight components) are freely soluble; others (e.g., proteoglycans, enzymes, and larger proteins) are poorly soluble. Differential release of these materials may have a bearing on the mast cell's role in disease.

ROLE IN ACUTE LUNG INJURY

The central role played by mast cells in the immediate hypersensitivity reaction has long been known. In the lung, this reaction is typically manifested either by an asthma attack or by a more generalized systemic hypersensitivity reaction (i.e., anaphylactic shock).

Asthma is characterized by paroxysms of bronchial constriction and increased production of thick mucus, which leads to bronchial obstruction and exacerbation of respiratory distress. The smooth muscle in the airway is often hypertrophied and hyperreactive to constricting stimuli. Anaphylactic shock is characterized by vasodilation and exudation of plasma in vascular beds throughout the body, usually resulting from the presence of a triggering antigen that gains systemic access via injection, an insect sting, or absorption across an epithelial surface (e.g., skin or GI mucosa). The decrease in vascular tone and leakage of plasma lead to a fall in blood pressure that may be fatal. The cardiovascular effects are complicated by constriction of the musculature surrounding the upper and lower airways, increased mucosal reactivity with outpouring of mucus in the gut and the respiratory tract, and urticarial lesions on the skin.

In both asthma and anaphylaxis, mast cell activation takes place in response to an immunologic trigger. Specifically, IgE antibody insertion on mast cell surface Fcε receptors leads to the production and release of inflammatory mediators. Mast cell–derived leukotrienes and PAF are thought to be major mediators of acute airway constriction. In addition, mast cell–derived cytokines (e.g., TNF-α, IL-4, and IL-5) are thought to be the major factors causing sustained airway inflammation via the recruitment of eosinophils and basophils.

Nonimmunologic mechanisms may also play a part in mast cell–mediated lung injury. In one study, when pulmonary alveolar mast cells were exposed to hypoxia, they released their granules, thereby causing lung injury.[93] Perivascular mast cells from the hypoxic lungs showed none of the morphologic changes associated with IgE-mediated mast cell degranulation, such as granule swelling, fusion, and exocytosis.

In a murine model of hindlimb ischemia-reperfusion that made use of two congenic animal strains, one mast cell–sufficient and the other mast cell–deficient, it was demonstrated that pulmonary mast cells mediated neutrophil sequestration and pulmonary edema, probably through the production and release of leukotrienes.[94] Vagal efferent nerves appeared to play an important role in the induction of remote lung injury after hindlimb ischemia; in this setting, bilateral cervical vagotomy limited mast cell degranulation and associated lung injury.[95]

Vagal mechanisms also appear to play a key role in mast cell activation in a murine model of acid aspiration.[96] Blocking substance P, a neuropeptide released at the end of C-fibers located near mast cells, modified the lung injury; the C-fibers travel with vagal nerves. A similar benefit was obtained by using the chymase antagonist chymostatin, which blocked the effect of a key mast cell secretory product. The reduction in injury achieved with these two approaches was the same as the injury reduction observed in mast cell knockout mice.[96] This similarity suggested that the final common pathway of lung damage in aspiration was activation of the alternative complement pathway. These data indicate that vagal stimulation with release of substance P leads to release of mast cell–derived chymase that triggers activation of the alternative complement pathway, thereby causing aspiration lung injury.

Eicosanoids

Eicosanoids are vasoactive and immunomodulatory derivatives of membrane fatty acids that can be produced by virtually all cells in the body. They may be divided into three major subgroups: prostaglandins, thromboxanes, and leukotrienes. These agents are not stored but are rapidly synthesized in response to signaling stimuli. After release, they act in an autocrine and paracrine fashion. They have very short half-lives (largely because of their susceptibility to spontaneous hydrolysis or active enzymatic conversion to inactive metabolites) and thus rarely act as circulating hormones.

Prostaglandins were discovered in the 1930s by von Euler when a substance in human semen was found to cause myometrial contraction. The active agent, an acidic lipid, was thought to be a product of the prostate gland and hence was named prostaglandin. The next major observation was the description of the slow-reacting substance of anaphylaxis (SRS-A) in the early 1940s. Thromboxanes were discovered in 1975 and leukotrienes in 1979. In 1980, SRS-A was identified as a combination of the three cysteinyl leukotrienes: LTC_4, LTD_4, and LTE_4.

FORMATION

Liberation of Arachidonic Acid

Arachidonic acid (eicosatetraenoic acid), the major substrate for eicosanoid synthesis, is a long-chain polyunsaturated fatty acid that is incorporated into the phospholipid mammalian cell membrane. It is also present in plasma, but it is tightly bound to plasma proteins and therefore biologically unavailable. The first step in eicosanoid synthesis is liberation of arachidonic acid from the cell membrane. An agonist binds to the membrane receptor, causing activation of the enzyme phospholipase C, which generates

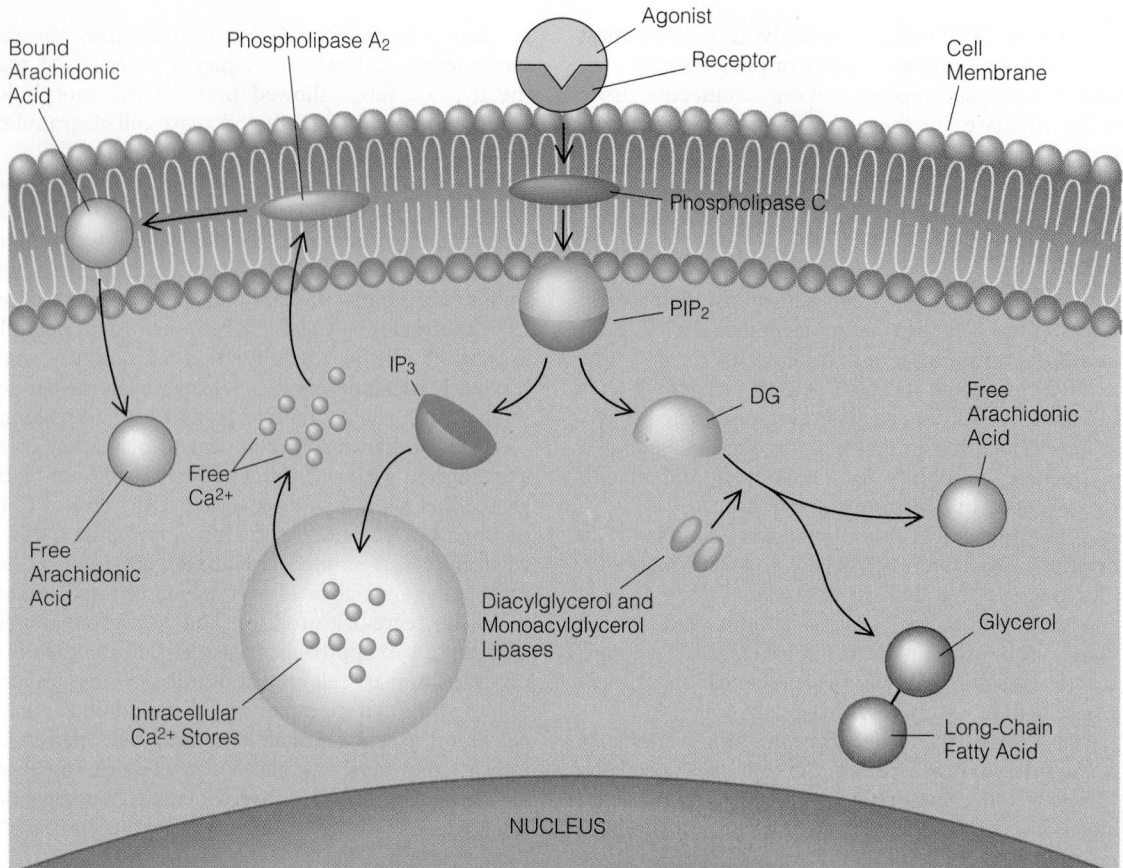

Figure 9 **Shown is the production of free arachidonic acid in the cytosol. The binding of an agonist to a receptor activates phospholipase C, which hydrolyzes phosphatidylinositol 4,5-bisphosphate (PIP$_2$) to inositol 1,4,5-trisphosphate (IP$_3$) and diacylglycerol (DG). From this point, free arachidonic acid can be generated in two ways. First, IP$_3$, by increasing the intracellular calcium ion concentration, activates phospholipase A$_2$, which then liberates arachidonic acid from the cell membrane. Second, DG is broken down enzymatically into several products, one of which is arachidonic acid.**

free arachidonic acid via the production of the intracellular second messengers inositol triphosphate and diacylglycerol. These messengers, in turn, activate phospholipase A$_2$ [*see Figure 9*].

Phospholipase activation is a crucial step in arachidonic acid liberation; in fact, it serves as the rate-limiting step in all eicosanoid production. Once freed, arachidonic acid is metabolized via two pathways. The cyclooxygenase pathway produces prostaglandins and thromboxanes (collectively referred to as prostanoids), and the lipoxygenase pathway, present in cells of myeloid origin, produces leukotrienes.

Cyclooxygenase Pathway

All cells except nonnucleated red cells are capable of generating cyclooxygenase products. Two related but distinct cyclooxygenase isozymes have now been identified, COX-1 and COX-2. COX-1 is constitutively present in cells, and its products are considered to have housekeeping functions (e.g., gastric mucosal protection). COX-2 is an inducible enzyme that is rapidly upregulated in response to various immune and inflammatory mediators (e.g., cytokines, growth factors, and tumor promoters), and its products play a more inflammatory role [*see Figure 10*]. Admittedly, this polarized view of the functions of COX-1 and COX-2 products is somewhat oversimplified; nevertheless, we believe it is useful for the purposes of general discussion.

Both COX-1 and COX-2 convert arachidonic acid into an endoperoxide, prostaglandin G$_2$ (PGG$_2$), which in turn is con-verted to PGH$_2$. PGH$_2$ is then metabolized by different pathways to prostaglandins, prostacyclin (PGI$_2$), and thromboxanes [*see Figure 11*].

Cells typically synthesize one or two COX products, depending on the enzymes they express. Platelets, for example, produce thromboxane A$_2$ (TXA$_2$) through the action of thromboxane synthetase, whereas endothelial cells primarily produce PGI$_2$ through the action of prostacyclin synthetase.

Six cyclooxygenase products are currently in widespread use in clinical settings. Alprostadil (PGE$_1$) is used for its smooth muscle–relaxing effects; misoprostol, a synthetic analogue of PGE$_1$, is used for gastric cytoprotection; PGE$_2$ and latanoprost (PGF$_{2\alpha}$) are used in obstetrics and gynecology; latanoprost is used in ophthalmology, and PGI$_2$ is used for its properties as a potent vasodilator and a moderate inhibitor of platelet aggregation. At present, however, greater clinical importance is attached to inhibition of the synthesis of cyclooxygenase products by means of nonsteroidal anti-inflammatory drugs (NSAIDs) and selective COX-2 inhibitors, which act as anti-inflammatory and analgesic compounds [*see* Therapeutic Implications, Cyclooxygenase Inhibition with NSAIDs and COX-2 Antagonists, *below*].

Lipoxygenase Pathway

There are several differences between the cyclooxygenase and lipoxygenase pathways. Unlike cyclooxygenase, which is ubiquitous, lipoxygenase is present only in inflammatory cells.

HOUSEKEEPING FUNCTIONS

Platelets

Kidney

Stomach

Endothelium

INFLAMMATORY FUNCTION

Tissue Macrophages

Leukocytes

Endothelium

Free Arachidonic Acid

COX-1

COX-2

TXA_2
PGI_2
PGE_2

Eicosanoid Products

PGI_2
PGE_2

GI Mucosal Integrity
Renal System Homeostasis
Platelet Aggregation

Inflammation
Mitogenesis
Bone Formation

Figure 10 **The products of COX-1 tend to have so-called housekeeping functions. This enzyme is constitutively present in cells. In contrast, the COX-2 enzyme is induced in cells in response to inflammatory stimuli. The products of both enzymes tend to cause inflammation.**

Furthermore, whereas cyclooxygenase is always active, requiring only the presence of arachidonic acid for endoperoxidase production, lipoxygenase is quiescent and must be activated for leukotriene synthesis to occur. Activating stimuli for the lipoxygenase pathway include GM-CSF, C5a, and fMLP.

In the lipoxygenase pathway, liberated arachidonic acid is converted to 5-hydroperoxyeicosatetraenoic acid (5-HPETE) by 5-lipoxygenase (5-LO). This same enzyme then converts 5-HPETE into LTA_4, which then is either metabolized by LTA_4 hydrolase to LTB_4 or conjugated by LTC_4 synthetase with reduced glutathione to form LTC_4. LTC_4, in turn, is converted into LTD_4 and LTE_4 [*see Figure 11*].

LTA_4 may diffuse extracellularly and be taken up by cells that possess LTA_4 hydrolase and LTC_4 synthetase (e.g., erythrocytes and endothelium), with the result that leukotrienes may be produced by nonmyeloid cell lines that do not possess 5-LO and thus do not ordinarily generate leukotrienes. This process can amplify the inflammatory response.

PROSTAGLANDINS

There are nine prostaglandin groups: A, B, C, D, E, F, G, H, and I. With some prostaglandins (e.g., PGA_2), the letter refers to the chemical structure of its five-member ring. With others, however, the letter means something else: for example, E originally stood for "ether" and F for "phosphate buffer," which were the substances in which PGE and PGF were most readily soluble. Within a prostaglandin group, the subscript numerals 1, 2, and 3 are used to indicate the number of unsaturated double bonds present in the two side chains. Finally, the subscript Greek letters α and β are used to indicate the spatial orientation of the hydroxyl groups on the side chains in relation to the ring.

Prostaglandins primarily exert their effects on the smooth muscle of the GI tract, the airways, the vasculature, and the reproductive tract; however, they also play important roles in platelet regulation and in the nervous system. Their main biologic actions may be summarized as follows:

1. Effects on the vasculature. PGI_2 is a vasodilator that is synthesized by both smooth muscle and endothelial cells in response to agents such as bradykinin, thrombin, serotonin, platelet-derived growth factor, and IL-1. Its actions are essentially antagonistic to those of TXA_2: it causes vasodilatation, inhibits platelet aggregation, and is thought to control the release of tissue plasminogen activator. In contrast, $PGF_{2\alpha}$ is a potent vasoconstrictor.

2. Effects on the nervous system. PGE_1 and PGE_2 are responsible for the increase in body temperature associated with inflammation. Their synthesis in the hypothalamus is promoted by TNF and IL-1 (also known as endogenous pyrogen), which are released by phagocytes in response to viruses, bacteria, fungi, endotoxin, and antigen-antibody complexes. PGE_2 also exerts a strong hyperalgesic effect: it increases sensitivity to a variety of mechanical and chemical pain stimuli, with additive effects occurring over time and with increasing concentration. At high concentrations, PGE_2 can even stimulate nociperceptive nerve endings directly.

3. Effects on the renal system. PGE_1, PGE_2, and PGI_2 increase the glomerular filtration rate and moderate renal blood flow by means of local vasodilatation. They also increase sodium and water excretion, though the mechanisms by which they do so are unclear.

4. Effects on the GI tract. Prostaglandins play a central role in gastric epithelial defense and repair and are produced in large amounts by the gastric mucosa. Most of them induce contraction of GI smooth muscle. Specifically, PGE_2 and $PGF_{2\alpha}$ contract longitudinal smooth muscle, whereas PGI_2 and

$PGF_{2\alpha}$ contract circular smooth muscle. Administration of these agents causes colicky abdominal pain.

5. Effects on the respiratory tract. PGE_1, PGE_2, and PGI_2 relax respiratory smooth muscle, and $PGF_{2\alpha}$ contracts it.
6. Effects on the reproductive system. Prostaglandins have potent effects on the uterus and the cervix, moderating uterine contraction during delivery. Although they were originally discovered in semen, their function there remains unknown.

THROMBOXANES

TXA_2, originally called rabbit aortic contracting substance, was identified in 1975 as an agent that contracted vascular smooth muscle and caused platelet aggregation.[97] In picogram amounts, it exerts five major biologic effects.

1. Vasoconstriction. TXA_2 is one of the most potent naturally occurring constrictors of smooth muscle. It acts on virtually all vascular beds, but its effects are particularly prominent in small arteries and arterioles.
2. Bronchoconstriction. TXA_2 exerts a marked spastic effect on tracheal rings and pulmonary parenchymal strips and causes bronchoconstriction in intact animals.
3. Enhanced platelet aggregation. TXA_2 activates platelets, inducing aggregation with subsequent stimulation to synthesize and release more TXA_2. This autocrine action leads to further platelet activation.
4. Increased membrane permeability. TXA_2 increases vascular endothelial permeability, possibly via restructuring of the endothelial cytoskeleton. It also causes the breakdown of actin microfilaments, leading to increases in intercellular junction size and loss of microvascular barrier function.
5. Neutrophil activation. TXA_2 is both a chemoattractant and chemoactivator of neutrophils; accordingly, it increases neutrophil oxidative activity and diapedesis.

TXA_2 is usually produced at low baseline concentrations; however, there are a number of triggers that can rapidly increase its synthesis and release from platelets or white blood cells. The presence of thrombin or contact with collagen can stimulate release of TXA_2 from platelets, and cytokines, complement fragments, and PAF all can directly stimulate release of TXA_2 from white blood cells. Thus, clinical situations associated with increased thromboxane production include vascular injury; arteriosclerosis; conditions associated with complement activation, such as sepsis, dialysis, and ischemia; and cytokine production.

TXB_2 is the metabolite of TXA_2, produced via nonenzymatic hydrolysis. Although it is only one tenth as potent as TXA_2, it does have some degree of biologic activity (e.g., enhancement of endothelial permeability, activation of neutrophils, and promotion of neutrophil diapedesis).

LEUKOTRIENES

Leukotrienes derive their name from their origin and their chemical structure: they are products of leukocytes that have a conjugated triene as their common structural feature. They can be divided into two classes on the basis of differing biologic actions: (1) LTB_4 and (2) the cysteinyl leukotrienes (LTC_4, LTD_4, and LTE_4). The most important actions of the leukotrienes have to do with their central role in allergic and inflammatory diseases.

The primary effects of LTB_4 are neutrophil chemotaxis and activation. Neutrophils activated by LTB_4 exhibit increased oxidative activity, granule release, and enhanced integrin expression. LTB_4 is also weakly chemotactic for eosinophils. The primary effects of the cysteinyl leukotrienes are bronchoconstriction and stimulation of mucus secretion. LTC_4 and LTD_4 are 1,000 times more potent than histamine at causing smooth muscle contraction in human bronchi. LTE_4 also causes bronchoconstriction, but it is less potent. All of the cysteinyl leukotrienes are potent mucus secretagogues. They also contribute to plasma extravasation and tissue edema by increasing vascular permeability.

Figure 11 **Arachidonic acid is metabolized by two different enzymes, cyclooxygenase (including both COX-1 and COX-2 variants) and lipoxygenase. The products of cyclooxygenase are the prostaglandins and the thromboxanes; the products of lipoxygenase are the leukotrienes.**

THERAPEUTIC IMPLICATIONS

Antileukotrienes in Asthma

It is now recognized that the pathogenesis of asthma is more complicated than was previously realized: airway smooth muscle contraction in response to an irritant is only part of a larger overall picture. Asthma has been defined as "a chronic inflammatory disease of the airways,"[98] in which many cells and cellular elements are involved, particularly mast cells, eosinophils, T cells, neutrophils, and epithelial cells.

Leukotrienes have been shown to play a major role in asthma, producing the characteristic pathophysiologic signs (bronchoconstriction, mucus, airway edema, and cellular infiltration). The clinical manifestations of asthma can be reproduced by administering leukotrienes. Furthermore, increases in bronchoalveolar lavage and urinary leukotriene concentrations have been documented in patients with asthma.[99]

These findings have led to the development of a new class of antiasthma drugs, the antileukotrienes. Two types of antileukotrienes are now in clinical use. The first type, currently exemplified by zafirlukast and montelukast, acts through competitive antagonism of the cysteinyl leukotriene receptor, thereby blocking the action of LTC_4, LTD_4, and LTE_4. The second type, of which zileuton is the only example currently available, competitively inhibits 5-LO, thereby blocking all leukotriene synthesis. Both types are highly effective at moderating asthma: their use leads to improved airway function, less frequent nighttime awakenings, fewer episodes of asthma exacerbation necessitating steroid therapy, and lower required dosages of inhaled steroids. An additional benefit of the antileukotrienes is their ease of use: they are orally administered, are well tolerated, and need be taken only once or twice daily.[100] Routine use of these agents is now recommended as part of the multitiered pharmacologic approach to asthma management.

Whether the antileukotrienes might also be useful in the management of other inflammatory disease states is currently under investigation. Preliminary reports suggest that they might someday play a part in the management of rheumatoid arthritis, systemic lupus erythematosus, urticaria, and atopic dermatitis.

Exogenous Prostaglandins in Obstetric and Gynecologic Settings

Prostaglandins are potent stimulators of myometrial smooth muscle contractility, as are other prostanoids (e.g., TXA_2 and eicosatetraenoic acid). These mediators are thought to play an important—though not yet fully explained—role in normal fetal delivery. Concentrations of certain prostanoids and their metabolites are known to increase before the onset of spontaneous labor and continue to increase during birth. NSAIDs, which inhibit prostanoid synthesis, are known to reduce myometrial contractions and delay or even prevent labor.[101] PGE_2 and PGF_2 also induce the cervical ripening that must occur before normal delivery.

Prostaglandin receptors are present on myometrial tissue throughout gestation, unlike many other receptors, such as those for oxytocin, which are only induced in the latter phase of pregnancy. Consequently, therapy with prostaglandins is possible throughout pregnancy. Gemeprost (the methyl ester of PGE_1) and dinoprostone (PGE_2) are currently approved for cervical ripening and labor induction. When given vaginally, they are safe and effective, posing no risk to the fetus even though they cross the placental barrier. These agents are safe in promoting first- and second-trimester terminations, whether used alone or given in combination with mifepristone or methotrexate; moreover, they are effective for inducing cervical softening before surgical termination of pregnancy.

Cyclooxygenase Inhibition with NSAIDs and COX-2 Antagonists

Management of inflammation Histologically, acute inflammation is characterized by vasodilatation, edema, and early neutrophil accumulation. Production of eicosanoids at the inflammatory site by damaged vessels, leukocytes, and platelets leads to vasodilatation (caused by PGI_2 and PGE_2), increased vascular permeability (caused by TXA_2 and leukotrienes), and neutrophil recruitment and activation (caused by LTB_4 and TXA_2). In addition, LTB_4 is a potent stimulus for production of the proinflammatory cytokines IL-1 and TNF, and PGE_2 gives rise to pain. Eicosanoids have been implicated in the pathophysiology of many inflammatory diseases, including rheumatoid arthritis, ulcerative colitis, Crohn disease, and asthma.

The use of NSAIDs to treat the symptoms of inflammation is a long-standing practice. NSAIDs counteract inflammation by inhibiting cyclooxygenase, thereby decreasing the synthesis of all prostanoids and exerting antipyretic and analgesic effects. NSAIDs are routinely used in the management of chronic inflammatory diseases such as rheumatoid arthritis and are among the most widely prescribed drugs for musculoskeletal conditions and pain. By inhibiting cyclooxygenase, NSAIDs may also effectively redirect arachidonic acid into the lipoxygenase pathway, thus indirectly increasing leukotriene synthesis. This redirection is hypothesized to be the mechanism by which aspirin can trigger asthma in susceptible individuals.

Regulation of blood flow Eicosanoids modulate blood flow to organs and tissues by adjusting local balances between production of vasodilators and production of vasoconstricting components. Loss of these controls, such as occurs when age, diabetes, or atherosclerosis decreases the capacity of the vascular endothelium for PGI_2 production, may impair normal regulatory mechanisms. For example, in occlusive vascular disease, ischemia may cause elevated TXA_2 levels by stimulating the synthesis of TXA_2 by neutrophils and platelets. This would explain why output of TXA_2 is significantly elevated in the clinical settings of unstable angina and acute myocardial infarction and variably elevated after cerebrovascular accidents. Without enhanced PGI_2 production, the resulting vasoconstriction and platelet aggregation may exacerbate ischemia in these settings.

Aspirin, alone among the NSAIDs, causes irreversible methylation of COX-1 and COX-2. It is 50 to 100 times more potent at the COX-1 site than at the COX-2 site. Accordingly, it is capable of permanently eliminating platelets' ability to produce TXA_2 even when given only once daily in low doses; however, to antagonize COX-2, which is largely responsible for inflammation, much higher and more frequent doses are necessary. Platelets, being nonnucleated, are unable to resynthesize COX-1 and COX-2. Because somewhat less than 10% of the platelet population is turned over each day, it takes several days for platelet production of prostanoids to return to normal levels. Nucleated cells, on the other hand, rapidly resynthesize COX-1 and COX-2 enzymes and thus can resume producing prostaglandins a few hours after aspirin administration.

Aspirin, therefore, is antithrombotic when given in small amounts and at wide intervals. When so used, it permits synthesis of vasodilating, antithrombotic prostaglandins while inhibiting platelet synthesis of thromboxane. Accordingly, aspirin has been widely applied to the management of atherosclerotic disease. One large international trial reported that in patients who took a single 162.5 mg tablet of aspirin daily, starting within 24 hours of a suspected myocardial infarction and continuing for 5 weeks, mortality was reduced by 23%, the incidence of nonfatal reinfarction by 49%, and the incidence of nonfatal stroke by 46%, with no increase in the incidence of either GI bleeding or hemorrhagic stroke.[102] It is now believed that long-term low-dose (75 to 180 mg/day) aspirin therapy may benefit all persons who have unstable angina, have a history of myocardial infarction, or are at risk for ischemic stroke, as well as many other persons at high risk for atherosclerotic events.

Prostaglandins also play an essential role in regulating neonatal circulatory changes. Very soon after birth, the fetal ductus arteriosus starts to contract, thereby reducing the size of the large vascular shunt present in the fetus, which diverts 90% of right ventricular output away from the lungs and into the aorta. In approximately 20% of full-term infants, the ductus arteriosus is functionally closed at 24 hours post partum, and in all, the ductus is closed at 96 hours. The ductus is extremely sensitive to the vasodilatory action of PGE_2. Normally, the high circulating fetal concentration of this prostaglandin decreases after birth; however, in preterm, low-birth-weight infants, this decrease does not occur, and thus the ductus does not close. In these instances, administration of indomethacin is a safe and effective way of promoting duct closure.[103]

There are, however, two groups of patients in whom maintenance of a patent ductus arteriosus is necessary: (1) newborns whose systemic blood flow depends on shunting from the pulmonary artery to the aorta (e.g., those who have an interrupted aortic arch) and (2) newborns whose pulmonary blood flow depends on shunting from the aorta to the pulmonary artery (e.g., those who have pulmonary valve atresia). For both groups, infusions of PGE_1 have proved highly beneficial, enabling resuscitation and stabilization even in the face of major respiratory and electrolyte disturbances.

Prevention of tumors An exciting new potential therapeutic use of NSAIDs derives from epidemiologic studies that document a reduced incidence of colorectal carcinoma in subjects taking aspirin. Of the more than 90 rodent studies of carcinogen-induced and genetically induced colorectal tumors carried out to date, the majority showed definite decreases at all stages of tumorigenesis with NSAID therapy.[104] The results from observational human studies suggest that NSAID therapy is associated with approximately a 40% relative risk reduction with respect to the incidence of colorectal carcinoma. This issue should be clarified further when the results of three ongoing phase III clinical trials of aspirin in colorectal carcinoma prevention become available. COX-2 antagonists have been less well studied, but there is some evidence suggesting that such agents may modify the growth of bladder tumors.

Precisely how NSAIDs exert their antitumor effects is not yet fully understood. Colorectal carcinomas are known to overexpress COX-2 and PGE_2,[105] and it is possible that these agents act to promote cellular proliferation and inhibit cell apoptosis, thereby giving rise to cancer. PGE_2, the eicosanoid most prevalent in GI tissue, has immunosuppressive effects that may reduce tumor surveillance.

Side effects of NSAIDs and development of COX-2 inhibitors The ability of aspirin to cause gastric ulceration and bleeding, originally documented in the first half of the 20th century, is now understood to be attributable to prostaglandin

inhibition. Endogenous prostaglandins play a central role in maintenance of the gastroduodenal mucosal defense barrier by regulating mucosal bicarbonate production, stimulating mucosal blood flow, and modulating epithelial cell proliferation. Oral therapy with misoprostol has proved effective in healing both gastric and duodenal ulcers.

The coxibs, of which rofecoxib and celecoxib are the best-known examples, were developed specifically with the aim of overcoming the ulcerogenic side effects of COX-1 antagonists. The coxibs selectively inhibit COX-2 and thus should be capable of exerting anti-inflammatory effects without interfering with the gastric protection afforded by COX-1 products. To date, they have been at least partially successful in achieving the desired aim. The coxibs are as effective as conventional NSAIDs at treating rheumatoid arthritis and osteoarthritis and reducing pain.[106] In addition, patients receiving coxibs show significantly lower rates of gastric ulceration than patients receiving conventional NSAIDs.[107] Use of coxibs is not, however, without drawbacks. These agents are associated with dyspepsia, though to a lesser degree than conventional NSAIDs are. Moreover, they exert the same delaying effect on ulcer healing that NSAIDs do; this is because both COX-1 products and COX-2 products are necessary for angiogenesis.

Another important side effect of NSAIDs is their nephrotoxicity, which results from interference with prostaglandin-mediated control of local renal vascular flow. PGE_2, PGI_2, and TXA_2 play important roles in regulating the glomerular filtration rate, especially in disease states such as shock, cirrhosis, and congestive heart failure. In these settings, there is a compensatory increase in renal PGE_2 production, leading to improved blood flow. Administration of NSAIDs may cause fluid retention. In addition, NSAIDs are responsible for 20% of cases of drug-induced acute renal failure. To date, the coxibs have not been shown to possess substantial advantages over NSAIDs in regard to nephrotoxicity: they appear to produce the same degree of fluid retention as conventional NSAIDs do, though it is possible that their effect on the glomerular filtration rate is less damaging.

Because TXA_2 is a COX-1 product, the coxibs do not inhibit thromboxane-mediated platelet aggregation. Therefore, it is unlikely that they will be able to reduce the thrombotic complications of vascular disease, as NSAIDs do. Indeed, a recent clinical report indicated that COX-2 inhibitors were associated with a slight but significant increase in myocardial infarction.

Dietary Fatty Acids

The long-chain polyunsaturated fatty acids that are the precursors of eicosanoids cannot be synthesized in the human body and must therefore be supplied through diet. In North America and western Europe, the primary dietary source for eicosanoid synthesis is linoleic acid, the precursor of arachidonic acid. Linoleic acid is found predominantly in vegetable oils. It and its derivatives are termed omega-6 fatty acids because the last of their four double bonds occurs at the sixth carbon atom from the methyl end of the chain. α-Linolenic acid, found in marine fish and to a lesser extent in green vegetables, is the precursor of eicosapentaenoic acid (EPA) and docosahexaenoic acid (DHA), which are also eicosanoid precursors. These substances are termed omega-3 fatty acids because their last double bond occurs at the third carbon atom from the methyl end of the chain.

The relative prevalence of the various fatty acid precursors has important clinical implications, in that higher proportions of one precursor or another will affect which eicosanoid products are generated. For example, when EPA is the substrate for cyclooxygenase, TXA_3, which is biologically inactive, is produced; EPA also competitively binds cyclooxygenase, thereby reducing TXA_2 synthesis. However, PGI_3 synthesized from omega-3 fatty acids is fully active. In this setting, therefore, with thromboxane activity reduced but prostacyclin activity maintained, the overall effects are to increase platelet survival, to reduce platelet aggregation, and to increase bleeding time.

Interest in the possible clinical use of dietary omega-3 fatty acids came from the observation that Greenland Eskimos had a low incidence of myocardial infarction despite eating a high-fat diet.[108] Their plasma and platelet lipids were found to contain a high proportion of omega-3 long-chain polyunsaturated fatty acids. Furthermore, they had hypoaggregable platelets and increased bleeding times. The same effects were noted in other populations who were fed dietary supplements containing omega-3 fatty acids. The potential long-term benefits of increased omega-3 fatty acid intake were suggested by epidemiologic studies in the Netherlands and Japan that showed a reduced incidence of coronary artery disease in men whose diet contained a large amount of fish supplements.[109,110] Subsequent randomized, controlled clinical trials demonstrated that dietary supplementation with either fish or fish oil conferred significant benefits on men who had recently had myocardial infarctions, reducing the risk of death and especially of sudden cardiac death. In particular, increased dietary intake of omega-3 fatty acids had a potent antidysrhythmic effect, apparently because incorporation of these substances into the myocyte cell membrane increased the stability and lengthened the refractory period of these cells.

Although the precise mechanisms underlying the protective effect associated with dietary omega-3 fatty acids have not been determined, it is likely that reduced TXA_2 production is a major contributor. Altered leukotriene biochemistry may also play a role: the main leukotriene synthesized from omega-3 fatty acids is LTB_5, which is less active than LTB_4. Reduced synthesis of LTB_4 by neutrophils may underlie the observation that fish supplements reduce symptom severity in patients with rheumatoid arthritis. It has also been noted that fewer low-birth-weight children are born in northern European populations, who typically consume substantial amounts of fish, than in non–fish-eating populations. In animal studies, experimental subjects that either are deficient in omega-6 fatty acids or have been fed diets high in omega-3 fatty acid exhibit decreased prostaglandin synthesis and longer gestation periods.

It is believed that early hominids evolved on a diet containing roughly equal proportions of omega-3 and omega-6 fatty acids. In contrast, the typical diet in North America and western Europe today, which is high in dairy, meat, and fried foods, contains 10 to 25 times more omega-6 than omega-3 fatty acids. This relative deficiency of omega-3 fatty acids may be a major cause of the high rates of cardiac and inflammatory diseases recorded in the more developed areas of the world.

Conclusion

Inflammation is a highly complex process that involves many interacting systems, which may complement each other, antagonize each other, or both. A degree of redundancy is built in, so that antagonism of one pathway may lead to augmentation of another alternative inflammatory mechanism. Furthermore, simultaneous or sequential production of both proinflammatory and anti-inflammatory signals often occurs. Accordingly, the success of a therapeutic intervention depends not only on the type of injury or insult present but also on the timing of the intervention. Unfortunately, the clinical trials done to date, evaluating a host of anti-inflammatory agents of different classes, have been largely disappointing. For more successful therapies to be developed, much more information regarding the fundamental mechanisms of the inflammatory response will be needed.

References

1. Metchnikoff ME: Sur la des cellules de l'organisme contre l'invasion des microbes. Ann Inst Pasteur 7:321, 1887

2. Marchesi VT, Florey HW: Electron micrographic observations on the emigration of leukocytes. Q J Exp Physiol 45:334, 1960

3. Harlan JM, Schwartz BR, Reidy MA, et al: Activated neutrophils disrupt endothelial monolayer integrity by an oxygen radical-independent mechanism. Lab Invest 52:141, 1985

4. Weiss SJ: Tissue destruction by neutrophils. N Engl J Med 320:365, 1989

5. Wedmore CV, Williams TJ: Control of vascular permeability by polymorphonuclear leukocytes in inflammation. Nature 289:646, 1981

6. Weiss SJ, Young J, LoBuglio AF, et al: Role of hydrogen peroxidase in neutrophil-mediated destruction of cultured endothelial cells. J Clin Invest 68:714, 1981

7. Harlan JM: Leukocyte-endothelial interactions. Blood 65:513, 1985

8. Campbell EJ, Senior RM, McDonald JA, et al: Proteolysis by neutrophils: relative importance of cell-substrate contact and oxidative inactivation of proteinase inhibitors in vitro. J Clin Invest 70:845, 1982

9. Shasby DM, Shasby SS, Peach MJ: Granulocytes and phorbol myristate acetate increase permeability to albumin of cultured endothelial monolayers and isolated perfused lungs: role of oxygen radicals and granulocyte adherence. Am Rev Respir Dis 127:72, 1983

10. Smedly LA, Tonnenson MG, Sandhaus RA, et al: Neutrophil mediated injury to endothelial cells: enhancement by endotoxin and essential role of neutrophil elastase. J Clin Invest 77:1233, 1986

11. Carp H, Janoff A: In vitro suppression of serum elastase-inhibitory capacity by reactive oxygen species generated by phagocytosing polymorphonuclear leukocytes. J Clin Invest 63:793, 1979

12. Ossanna PJ, Test ST, Matheson NR, et al: Oxidative regulation of neutrophil elastase-alpha-1-proteinase inhibitor interactions. J Clin Invest 77:1939, 1986

13. Romson JK, Hook BG, Kunkel SL, et al: Reduction of the extent of acute myocardial injury by neutrophil depletion in the dog. Circulation 67:1016, 1983

14. Dahlbäck L, Rais O: Morphologic changes in striated muscle following ischemia: immediate postischemic phase. Acta Chir Scand 131:430, 1966

15. Korthuis RJ, Grisham MB, Granger DN: Leukocyte depletion attenuates vascular injury in postischemic skeletal muscle. Am J Physiol 254:H823, 1988

16. Yokota J, Minei JP, Fantini GA, et al: Role of leukocytes in reperfusion injury of skeletal muscle after partial ischaemia. Am J Physiol 257:H1068, 1989

17. Klausner JM, Paterson IS, Valeri CR, et al: Limb ischemia-induced increase in permeability is mediated by leukocytes and leukotrienes. Ann Surg 208:755, 1988a

18. Argenbright LW: Inflammatory mediators, cytokines and leukocyte adhesion in postcapillary venules. Physiology and Pathophysiology of Leukocyte Adhesion. Granger DN, Schmid-Schönbein GW, Eds. Oxford University Press, Oxford, 1995, p 171

19. Issekutz AC, Movat HZ: The in vivo quantitation and kinetics of rabbit neutrophil leukocyte accumulation in the skin in response to chemotactic agents and Escherichia coli. Lab Invest 42:310, 1980

20. Issekutz TB, Issekutz AC, Movat HZ: The in vivo quantitation and kinetics of monocyte migration into acute inflammatory tissue. Am J Pathol 103:47, 1981

21. Anderson DC, Schalmsteig FC, Finegold MJ, et al: The severe and moderate phenotypes of heritable Mac-1, LFA-1 deficiency: their quantitative definition and relation to leukocyte dysfunction and clinical features. J Infect Dis 152:668, 1985

22. Repine JE, Beehler CJ: Neutrophils and adult respiratory distress syndrome: two interlocking per-

spectives in 1991. Am Res Respir Dis 144:251, 1991

23. Cosimi AB, Geoffrion C, Anderson T, et al: Immunosuppression of cynomolgus recipients of renal allografts by R6.5, a monoclonal antibody to intercellular adhesion molecule-1. Leukocyte Adhesion Molecules. Springer TA, Anderson DA, Rosenthal AS, et al, Eds. Springer-Verlag, New York, 1990, p 274

24. Jutila MA, Rott L, Berg EL, et al: Function and regulation of the neutrophil MEL-14 antigen in vivo: comparison with LFA-1 and Mac-1. J Immunol 143:3318, 1989

25. Steeber DA, Green NE, Sato S, et al: Lyphocyte migration in L-selectin-deficient mice: altered subset migration and aging of the immune system. J Immunol 157:1096, 1996

26. Lawrence MB, Springer TA: Leukocytes roll on a selectin at physiologic flow rates: distinction from and prerequisite for adhesion through integrins. Cell 65:859, 1991

27. Doré M, Korthuis RJ, Granger DN, et al: P-selectin mediates spontaneous leukocyte rolling in vivo. Blood 82:1308, 1993

28. Hsu-Lin S, Berman CL, Furie BC, et al: A platelet membrane protein expressed during platelet activation and secretion: studies using a monoclonal antibody specific for thrombin-activated platelets. J Biol Chem 259:9121, 1984

29. McEver RP, Beckstead JH, Moore KL, et al: GMP-140, a platelet alpha-granule membrane protein, is also synthesized by vascular endothelial cells and is located in Weibel-Palade bodies. J Clin Invest 84:92, 1989

30. Patel KD, Zimmerman GA, Prescott SM, et al: Oxygen radicals induce human endothelial cells to express GMP-140 and bind neutrophils. J Cell Biol 112:749, 1991

31. Hattori R, Hamilton KK, Fugate RD, et al: Stimulated secretion of endothelial von Willebrand factor is accompanied by rapid redistribution to the cell surface of the intracellular granule membrane protein GMP-140. J Biol Chem 264:7768, 1989

32. Weller A, Isenmann S, Vestweber D: Cloning of the mouse endothelial selectins: expression of both E- and P-selectin is inducible by tumor necrosis factor. J Biol Chem 267:15176, 1992

33. Bevilacqua MP, Pober JS, Mendrick DL, et al: Identification of an inducible endothelial-leukocyte adhesion molecule. Proc Natl Acad Sci USA 84:9238, 1987

34. Diamond MS, Staunton DE, de Fougerolles AR, et al: ICAM-1 (CD54): a counter-receptor for Mac-1 (CD1b/CD18). J Cell Biol 111:3129, 1990

35. Sengelov H, Kjeldsen L, Diamond MS, et al: Subcellular localization and dynamics of Mac-1 ($\alpha_m\beta_2$) in human neutrophils. J Clin Invest 92:1467, 1993

36. Smith CW, Marlin SD, Rothlein R, et al: Cooperative interactions of LFA-1 and Mac-1 with intercellular adhesion molecule-1 in facilitating adherence and transendothelial migration of human neutrophils in vitro. J Clin Invest 83:2008, 1989

37. Luscinskas FW, Brock AF, Arnaout MA, et al: Endothelial-leukocyte adhesion molecule-1-dependent and leukocyte (CD11/CD18)-independent mechanisms contribute to polymorphonuclear leukocyte adhesion to cytokine-activated human vascular endothelium. J Immunol 142:2257, 1989

38. Vedder NB, Winn RK, Rice CL, et al: A monoclonal antibody to the adherence-promoting leukocyte glycoprotein, CD18, reduces organ injury and improves survival from hemorrhagic shock and resuscitation in rabbits. J Clin Invest 81:939, 1988a

39. Mileski WJ, Winn RK, Vedder NB, et al: Inhibition of CD18-dependent neutrophil adherence reduces organ injury after hemorrhagic shock in primates. Surgery 108:206, 1990

40. Simpson PJ, Todd RF, Fantone JC, et al: Reduction of experimental canine myocardial reperfusion injury by a monoclonal antibody (anti-Mol, anti-CD11b) that inhibits leukocyte adhesion. J Clin Invest 81:624, 1988

41. Jaeschke H, Farhood A: Neutrophil and Kupffer cell-induced oxidant stress and ischemia-reperfusion injury in rat liver. Am J Physiol 260:G355, 1991

42. Barton RW, Rothlein R, Ksiazek J, et al: The effect of anti-intercellular adhesion molecule-1 on phorbol ester-induced rabbit lung inflammation. J Immunol 143:1278, 1989

43. Abbas AK: Cellular and Molecular Immunology, 4th ed. WB Saunders Co, Philadelphia, 2000

44. Kishimoto T, Akira S, Narazaki M, et al: Interleukin-6 family of cytokines and gp130. Blood 86:1243, 1985

45. Acton RD, Dahlberg PS, Uknis ME, et al: IL-6 inhibits lipopolysaccharide-induced tumor necrosis factor production in cultured human monocytes, U937 cells and in mice. J Immunol 143:3517, 1989

46. Tilg H, Trehu E, Atkins MB, et al: Interleukin-6 as an antiinflammatory cytokine: induction of circulating IL-1 receptor antagonist and soluble tumor necrosis factor receptor p55. Blood 83:113, 1994

47. van der Poll T, van Deventer S: Cytokines and anticytokines in the pathogenesis of sepsis. Infect Dis Clin North Am 13:413, 1999

48. Berg DH, Kuhn R, Rajewsky K, et al: Interleukin-10 is a central regulator in the response to LPS in murine models of endotoxic shock and the Shwartzman reaction but not endotoxin tolerance. J Clin Invest 96:2339, 1995

49. Gerard C, Bruyns C, Marchant A, et al: Interleukin-10 reduces the release of tumor necrosis factor and prevents lethality in experimental endotoxemia. J Exp Med 177:547, 1993

50. DiChiara MR, Kiely JM, Lee ME, et al: Inhibition of E-selectin gene expression by transforming growth factor β in endothelial cells involves coactivator integration of Smad and nuclear factor κB mediated signals. J Exp Med 192:695, 2000

51. Shull MM, Ormsby I, Kier AB, et al: Targeted disruption of the mouse transforming growth factor-β 1 gene results in multifocal inflammatory disease. Nature 359:693, 1992

52. Hannun CH, Wilcox CJ, Arend WP, et al: Interleukin-1 receptor antagonist activity of a human interleukin-1 inhibitor. Nature 434:336, 1990

53. Granowitz EV, Santos A, Poutsiaka DD, et al: Circulating interleukin-1 receptor antagonist levels during experimental endotoxemia in humans. Lancet 338:1423, 1991

54. Dinarello C: Proinflammatory and anti-inflammatory cytokines as mediators in the pathogenesis of septic shock. Chest 112(suppl 6):S321, 1997

55. Shapiro L, Clark BD, Orencole SF, et al: Detection of tumor necrosis factor soluble receptor p55 in blood samples from healthy and endotoxemic humans. J Infect Dis 167:1344, 1993

56. Aderka D, Englemann H, Hornik V, et al: Increased levels of soluble receptors for tumor necrosis in cancer patients. Cancer Res 51:5602, 1991

57. Keystone E: Tumor necrosis factor-α blockade in the treatment of rheumatoid arthritis. Rheum Dis Clin North Am 27:427, 2001

58. Blam M, Stein R, Lichtenstein G: Integrating anti-tumor necrosis factor therapy in inflammatory bowel disease: current and future perspectives. Am J Gastroenterol 96:1977, 2001

59. American College of Chest Physicians/ Society of Critical Care Medicine Consensus Conference Committee: Definitions for sepsis and multiple organ failure and guidelines for the use of innovative therapies in sepsis. Crit Care Med 20:864, 1992

60. Beutler B, Milsark IW, Cerami A: Passive immunization against cachectin/tumor necrosis factor protects mice from lethal effects of endotoxin. Science 229:869, 1985

61. Tracey K, Fong Y, Hesse DG, et al: Anti cachectin/TNF monoclonal antibodies prevent septic shock during lethal bacteremia. Nature 330:662, 1987

62. Kox WJ, Volk T, Kox SN, et al: Immunomodulatory therapies in sepsis. Intens Care Med 26:S124, 2000

63. Bone RC: Sir Isaac Newton, sepsis, SIRS and CARS. Crit Care Med 24:1125, 1996

64. Dehoux MS, Boutten A, Ostinelli J, et al: Compartmentalized cytokine production within the human lung in unilateral pneumonia. Am J Respir Crit Care Med 150:710, 1994

65. Marchant A, Deviere J, Byl B, et al: Interleukin-10 production during septicaemia. Lancet 343:707, 1994

66. Dries DJ, Jurkovich GJ, Maier RV, et al: Effect of interferon-gamma on infection-related death in patients with severe injuries. Arch Surg 129:1031, 1994

67. Bernard GR, Vincent JL, Laterre PF, et al: Efficacy and safety of recombinant human activated protein C for severe sepsis. N Engl J Med 344:699, 2001

68. Grinnell BW, Hermann RB, Yan SB: Human protein C inhibits selectin-mediated cell adhesion: role of unique glucosylated oligosaccharide. Glycobiology 4:221, 1994

69. Lorente JA, Garcia-Frade LJ, Landin L, et al: Time course of hemostatic abnormalities in sepsis and its relation to outcome. Chest 101:816, 1992

70. Gilbert DL: Speculation on the relationship between organic and atmospheric evolution. Perspect Biol Med 4:58, 1960

71. Raukman EJ, Rosen GM, Kitchell BB: Superoxide radical as an intermediate in the oxidation of hydroxylamines by mixed function amine oxidases. Mol Pharmacol 15:131, 1979

72. Klebanoff SJ: Oxygen metabolism and the toxic properties of phagocytes. Ann Intern Med 93:480, 1980

73. Bjork J, Del Maestro RF, Arfors KE: Evidence for participation of hydroxyl radical in increased microvascular permeability. Agents Actions Suppl 7:208, 1980

74. Granger DN, Rutili G, McCord JM: Superoxide radicals in feline intestinal ischemia. Gastroenterology 81:22, 1981

75. Korthuis RJ, Granger DN, Townsley M, et al: The role of oxygen derived free radicals in ischemia-induced increases in canine skeletal muscle vascular permeability. Circ Res 57:599, 1985

76. Simpson PJ, Mickelson JK, Lucchesi BR: Free radical scavengers in myocardial ischemia. Fed Proc 46:2422, 1987

77. Granger DN, Hollwarth ME, Parks DA: Ischemia-reperfusion injury: role of oxygen derived free radicals. Acta Physiol Scand 548:47, 1986

78. Hernandez LA, Grisham MB, Granger DN: A role for iron in oxidant-mediated ischemic injury to intestinal microvasculature. Am J Physiol 253:G49, 1987

79. Babior BM: Oxygen-dependent microbial killing by phagocytes (pts 1 & 2). N Engl J Med 93:480, 1978

80. Granger DN: Role of xanthine oxidase and granulocytes in ischemia-reperfusion injury. Am J

Physiol 255:H1269, 1988

81. Grisham MB, Hernandez LD, Granger DN: Xanthine oxidase and neutrophil infiltration in intestinal ischemia. Am J Physiol 251:G567, 1986

82. Werns S, Brinker J, Gruber J, et al: A randomised, double-blind trial of recombinant human superoxide dismutase (SOD) in patients undergoing PTCA for acute MI. Circulation 80(suppl):A113, 1989

83. Land W, Schneeberger H, Schleibner S, et al: The beneficial effect of human recombinant superoxide dismutase on acute and chronic rejection events in recipients of cadaveric renal transplants. Transplantation 57:211, 1994

84. Radomski MW, Vallance P, Whitley G, et al: Platelet adhesion in human vascular endothelium by constitutive and cytokine-induced nitric oxide. Cardiovasc Res 27:1380, 1993

85. Gries A, Bode C, Peter K, et al: Inhaled nitric oxide inhibits human platelet aggregation, P-selectin expression, and fibrinogen binding in vitro and in vivo. Circulation 97:1481, 1998

86. Bordet J, Gengou O: Sur l'existences de substance sensibilisations. Ann Inst Pasteur 15:290, 1901

87. Müller-Eberhard HJ: Molecular organization and function of the complement system. Annu Rev Biochem 57:321, 1988

88. Hill JH, Ward PA: The phlogistic role of C3 leukocyte fragment in myocardial infarct of rats. J Exp Med 133:885, 1971

89. Maroko PR, Carpender CD, Chiariello M, et al: Reduction by cobra venom factor of myocardial necrosis after coronary artery occlusion. J Clin Invest 61:661, 1978

90. Weisman HF, Bartow T, Leppo MK, et al: Soluble human complement receptor type 1: in vivo inhibitor of complement suppressing post-ischemic myocardial inflammation and necrosis. Science 249:146, 1991

91. Bengtson A, Holmberg P, Heideman M: The ischaemic leg as a source of complement activation. Br J Surg 74:697, 1987

92. Lindsay TF, Hill J, Ortiz F, et al: Blockade of complement activation prevents local and pulmonary albumin leak after lower torso ischemia-reperfusion. Ann Surg 216:677, 1992

93. Nadziejko CE, Loud AV, Kikkawa Y: Effect of alveolar hypoxia on pulmonary mast cells in vivo. Am Rev Respir Dis 140:743, 1989

94. Goldman G, Welbourn R, Klausner JM, et al: Mast cells and leukotrienes mediate neutrophil sequestration and lung edema after remote ischemia in rodents. Surgery 112:578, 1992

95. Mukundan C, Friend D, Hechtman H: Vagotomy limits mast cell activation in ischemia/reperfusion injury. Surgical Forum LII, 2001

96. Kyriakides C, Austen W, Wang Y, et al: Mast cells mediate complement activation after acid aspiration. Shock 16:21, 2001

97. Hamberg M, Svensson J, Samuelson B: Thromboxanes: a new group of biologically active compounds derived from prostaglandin endoperoxidase. Proc Natl Acad Sci USA 72:2884, 1977

98. National Asthma Education and Prevention Program: Expert Panel Report 2: Guidelines for the Diagnosis and Management of Asthma. NIH Publication No. 97-4051A. National Institutes of Health, Bethesda, Maryland, 1997

99. Wenzel SE: Anti-leukotriene drugs in the management of asthma. JAMA 20:2068, 1998

100. Korenblat P, for the anti-leukotriene working group: The role of anti-leukotrienes in the treatment of asthma. Ann Allergy Asthma Immunol 86(suppl):31, 2001

101. Lewis RB, Schulman J: Influence of acetylsalicylic acid, an inhibitor of prostaglandin synthesis, on the duration of human gestation and labour. Lancet 2:45, 1973

102. Baigent C, Collins R, Appleby P, et al: ISIS-2: 10 year survival among patients with suspected acute myocardial infarction in randomised comparison of intravenous streptokinase, oral aspirin, both, or neither. The ISIS-2 (Second International Study of Infarct Survival) Collaborative Group. BMJ 316:1337, 1998

103. Gersony WM, Peckham GJ, Ellison RC, et al: Effects of indomethacin in premature infants with patent ductus arteriosus: results of a national collaborative study. J Pediatr 102:895, 1983

104. Hawk ET, Viner JL, Limburg PJ: Cancer of the
colorectum: epidemiology and prevention of colorectal cancer. The Principles and Practice of Gastrointestinal Oncology. Evans D, Willett C, Hamilton S, et al, Eds. Oxford University Press, New York, 2001

105. Eberhart CE, Coffey RJ, Radhika A, et al: Up-regulation of cyclooxygenase 2 gene expression in human colorectal adenomas and adenocarcinomas. Gastroenterology 107:1183, 1994

106. Schnitzer T, Truitt R, Fleischmann R, et al: The safety profile, tolerability and effective dose range of rofecoxib in the treatment of rheumatoid arthritis. Phase II Rofecoxib Rheumatoid Arthritis Study Group. Clin Ther 21:1688, 1999

107. Bombardier C, Laine L, Reicin A, et al: Comparison of upper gastrointestinal toxicity of rofecoxib and naproxen in patients with rheumatoid arthritis. N Engl J Med 343:1520, 2000

108. Bang HO, Dyerberg J, Sinclair HM: The composition of the Eskimo food in northwestern Greenland. Am J Clin Nutr 33:2657, 1980

109. Kromhout D, Bosschieter EB, de Lezenne-Coulander C: The inverse relationship between fish consumption and 20 year mortality from coronary artery disease. N Engl J Med 312:1205, 1985

110. Kagawa Y, Nishizawa M, Suzuki M, et al: Eicosapolyenoic acids of serum lipids of Japanese islanders with low incidence of cardiovascular diseases. J Nutr Sci Vitaminol (Tokyo) 28:441, 1982

Acknowledgments

Figures 1 through 4 and 8 through 10   Seward Hung.

Figures 5 and 6   Dana Burns-Pizer.

Figures 7 and 11   Tom Moore.

The authors would like to acknowledge the work of Drs. Patrick M. Reilly, Susan A. Kelly, Henry J. Schiller, and Gregory B. Bulkley in a chapter entitled "Reactive Oxygen Metabolites," which appeared in previous versions of *ACS Surgery: Principles and Practice*. Some of their work served as the basis for the ROM section of the present chapter.

VIII POSTOPERATIVE MANAGEMENT

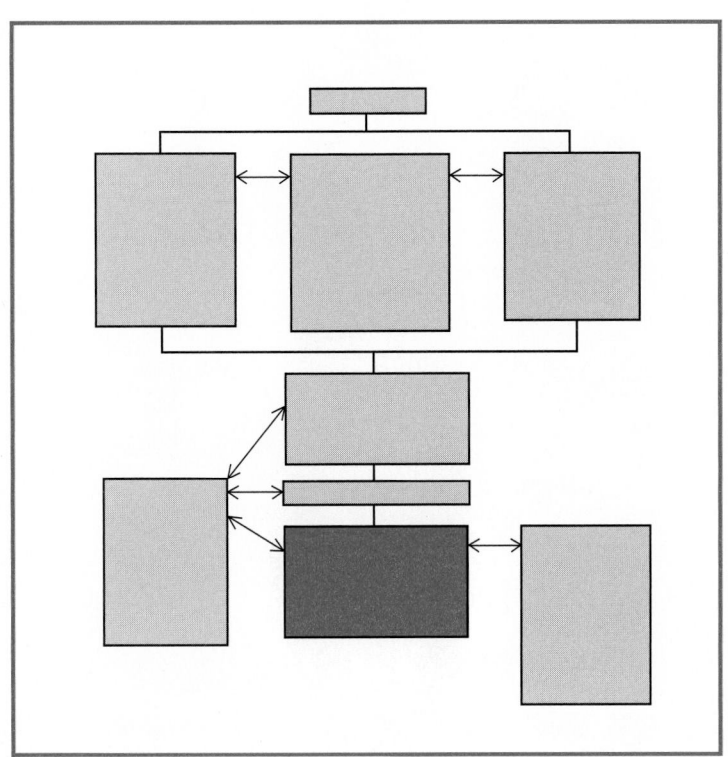

1 POSTOPERATIVE MANAGEMENT

Samir M. Fakhry, M.D., Edmund J. Rutherford, M.D., and George F. Sheldon, M.D.

Postoperative care is an integral part of complete surgical management. For a patient undergoing an elective operation, such care should be thought of within the context of perioperative care: that is, it should be considered as part of a continuum that ranges from evaluating and preparing the patient for a surgical procedure to minimizing the stress of the procedure to promoting a return to health after the procedure.

As a result of ongoing surgical and anesthetic advances and the growing application of minimally invasive surgical techniques, many procedures that once necessitated hospitalization are now commonly performed in day surgical units [see IV:3 Outpatient Surgery]. Other procedures are proving to be amenable to a fast track surgical approach [see IV:4 Fast Track Surgery], in which postoperative care focuses on minimizing postoperative pain, enhancing mobility and exercise capacity, and encouraging enteral intake. Such programs typically reduce the length of stay after a major procedure to 1 to 4 days.

In what follows, we focus on postoperative management of more seriously ill patients undergoing major operations, for whom outpatient and fast track approaches generally are not well suited. Such patients may include those with comorbid conditions that prolong recovery, those who have sustained intraoperative complications, and those who are undergoing emergency operations. These patients are heavy users of hospital resources but benefit greatly from medical care available in the modern hospital setting (e.g., ventilatory support, continuous monitoring, and an extensive pharmacopoeia). A portion of this care is provided in the recovery room or the intensive care unit, and its efficient delivery depends on collaboration among physicians from several different disciplines. The surgeon brings balanced surgical judgment to this setting and interacts frequently with the patient and the family.

Postoperative Orders

The direction that postoperative management of a seriously ill patient will take is outlined in the surgeon's postoperative orders [see Sidebar Sample Postoperative Orders]. Through this document, the nursing staff is informed of (1) the diagnosis, (2) the operation performed, and (3) the patient's condition. Monitoring measures are listed, and the therapeutic measures to be employed (analgesia, antibiotics, wound care, I.V. fluid administration, and the handling of tubes, catheters, and drains) are detailed. Evidence-based analyses indicate that certain common therapies are indeed valuable (e.g., inhaled oxygen[1,2]), whereas others either are not of proven benefit (e.g., intermittent positive-pressure breathing [IPPB] and room humidification) or are indicated only in selected situations (e.g., prophylaxis for gastritis, which is appropriate only in patients who are undergoing mechanical ventilation or who have coagulopathies[3]).

Some uniformity in the postoperative orders is valuable because it allows a decrease in the floor stock of medications and increases the nursing staff's experience with specific medications and procedures. Physicians should become acquainted with the costs of the various treatments and medications at their institution. Choices made on the basis of both efficacy and expense will become increasingly common as hospital systems adapt to the changing health care environment.

Postoperative Monitoring

In the postoperative period, many patients return to the same room they occupied preoperatively. Some, however, require more advanced monitoring and care and will require admission to a monitored telemetry bed, an intermediate care unit, or a surgical critical care unit.

The selection of postoperative monitoring is guided by a thorough understanding of the patient's preoperative status and medical history, the diagnosis that led to the operation, the operation performed, and the circumstances of the operative procedure. The vital signs that are commonly monitored on a surgical ward include temperature, pulse rate, blood pressure, respiratory rate, urine output (hourly or at some other interval), weight (daily), and fluid intake and output. These can generally be obtained at intervals of 2 to 4 hours. If more frequent monitoring or nursing care (e.g., frequent suctioning) is required, admission to an intermediate care unit may be advisable. On a telemetry ward, continuous cardiac monitoring can be provided for patients who have significant cardiopulmonary disease or for those at risk for perioperative myocardial infarction or dysrhythmia. In a CCU, additional monitoring is provided, including both noninvasive and invasive monitoring with arterial lines, continuous monitoring of central venous pressure (CVP) and right-sided pulmonary arterial pressures via Swan-Ganz catheterization, continuous monitoring of arterial oxygen saturation via pulse oximetry, measurement of end-tidal carbon dioxide tension, and electrocardiographic monitoring [see VII:1 Cardiopulmonary Monitoring]. Recommended criteria for ICU admission and discharge have been formulated.[4] When resources are limited, such guidelines may be useful in resolving triage difficulties, but each institution and each unit will have to develop its own approach to this sometimes thorny problem.

Controversy continues regarding what level of monitoring is most appropriate for each patient. In many hospitals, requests for ICU beds exceed the number of available critical care beds, and triage of patients is necessary. This sometimes means moving patients from the ICU before their primary physician feels they are ready for transfer, canceling or delaying operative procedures, and providing less than the requested level of postoperative monitoring for some patients. The increased use of intermediate or step-down units has provided some relief in these difficult situations, but appropriate allocation of resources continues to be a major issue in postoperative bed selection. It has been argued that in some clinical circumstances, our ability to monitor disease

Sample Postoperative Orders

An otherwise healthy 50-year-old, 70 kg man was recently diagnosed with a cecal carcinoma. He has type 2 (adult-onset) diabetes, for which he takes an oral hypoglycemic. He has arrived in the postanesthesia care unit (PACU) in stable condition after an uneventful right hemicolectomy and primary reanastomosis of 2 hours' duration under general anesthesia. Intraoperative blood loss is estimated at 100 ml, fluid replacement was 2,500 ml of lactated Ringer solution, and urine output totaled 250 ml.

[Date and Time]

1. Admit to PACU; Service: surgery H; Attending: Sheldon; Resident: Fakhry
2. Diagnosis: colon cancer; status: post right hemicolectomy
3. Condition: stable
4. Vital signs per PACU routine, then every 4 hours on ward × 24 hours, then every shift
5. Activity: out of bed to chair three times a day, beginning this evening; walk hall three times a day
6. Diet: nothing by mouth, but may have sips of ice chips and hard candy
7. Allergies: no known drug allergies
8. [Daily weight]
9. Accurate intake and output
10. Foley catheter to gravity
11. Fluids: 5% dextrose in lactated Ringer solution at 125 ml/hr
12. Antithrombosis prophylaxis
13. Medications:
    patient-controlled analgesia (if indicated): morphine sulfate, 1 to 2 mg I.V. every 10 minutes on demand
    other medications as indicated (e.g., pain medication, acetaminophen, preoperative medications)
14. Insulin sliding scale (for diabetic patients): finger-stick glucose every 6 hours and cover as follows:
    < 60 ----------------- call physician
    60–180 ------------ no coverage
    180–240 ---------- 5 units subcutaneous regular insulin
    240–300 ----------- 10 units subcutaneous regular insulin
    > 300 -------------- 15 units subcutaneous regular insulin, and call physician
15. Morning laboratory tests: complete blood count and electrolyte panel (if indicated)
16. Call physician for
    systolic blood pressure > 180 mm Hg or < 90 mm Hg
    diastolic blood pressure > 100 mm Hg
    heart rate > 120 or < 60 a minute
    respirations > 32 or < 12 a minute
    temperature > 38.5° C (101.3° F)
    urine output < 200 ml every 4 hours

---

may have outpaced our ability to intervene therapeutically.[5] A consensus conference sponsored by the National Institutes of Health in 1983 concluded that although the care provided in ICUs appears beneficial, the only area in which improved outcome could be documented was coronary care.[6] Acceptable indications for admission to CCUs and invasive monitoring with arterial lines and pulmonary arterial catheters have been proposed; they include myocardial infarction, shock, drug overdose, major cardiovascular surgery, acute respiratory distress syndrome (ARDS), and other forms of respiratory failure that call for mechanical ventilation [see VII:1 Cardiopulmonary Monitoring].[7]

The laboratory tests that are often obtained postoperatively may be thought of as another form of postoperative monitoring. Although such tests can be valuable, they are infrequently used to make important clinical judgments. Technological developments have made it possible for the nursing staff to monitor blood gas pressures, pH, and other biochemical indices at the bedside. For example, finger-stick blood glucose measurements are indicated in insulin-resistant patients and should be obtained every 6 hours (see below). Hematocrits should be obtained postoperatively only if serious bleeding is suspected. The white blood cell count routinely increases after the stress of operation and is therefore of little diagnostic value during the first few days after operation. Thrombocytopenia routinely accompanies major trauma, massive transfusion, and major operative procedures (e.g., cardiac bypass operation); platelet counts are necessary only if the patient shows evidence of bleeding.

In healthy individuals with normal renal function, serum electrolyte levels are usually well maintained despite major stress. In these patients, infrequent measurements of serum electrolytes are appropriate (every 2 or 3 days). By contrast, in patients with an underlying chronic disease, such as renal or hepatic disease or an illness that routinely results in electrolyte derangement, frequent measurements of electrolytes are indicated. The electrolyte abnormalities that are the most serious and potentially the most immediately life threatening are hypokalemia and hyperkalemia. These abnormalities must be corrected rapidly; multiple potassium measurements to confirm this correction are required. Abnormal levels of sodium and chloride should be corrected over a period of days.

Serum calcium measurements reflect total serum calcium. Only the ionized fraction of serum calcium is active, however, and thus, total serum calcium levels are not reliable indicators of the need for calcium administration.[8] However, after parathyroid operation, measurements of calcium levels are valuable because the other factors that affect the level of ionized calcium are usually unchanged.

Coagulation studies are overused preoperatively and are unnecessary postoperatively, except to monitor anticoagulation therapy or to evaluate the bleeding patient. Arterial blood gas measurements are useful in ventilated or hypoxic patients but should be used judiciously.

Postoperative Pain Relief

Despite the considerable progress that has been made in understanding the pathophysiology of pain,[9] routine pain management is often unsatisfactory.[10] Many hospitals have established pain services that improve quality of care and optimize relief of pain,[11,12] which is a prerequisite for optimal recovery.[13]

Treatment of postoperative pain actually begins before the procedure, as the health care team educates the patient about the events that will occur before, during, and after the procedure. Classic studies demonstrated that such an educational approach reduced patients' requirements for analgesics and diminished their perception of pain.[14]

Preemptive anesthesia reduces the sensation of pain before the creation of the incision, thereby significantly decreasing pain per-

Table 1   Suggested Dosing of Opioid and Nonopioid Analgesics

Class	Drug	Oral Dosage	Parenteral Dosage	Comments
Opioid agonists	Morphine	10–30 mg q. 4 hr	0.05–0.1 mg/kg I.V. (maximum, 15 mg), followed by 4–6 mg/hr I.V. 5–20 mg I.M. q. 4 hr	—
	Heroin	—	—	Not available in United States
	Fentanyl	—	1–2 μg/kg I.V., followed by 1–2 μg/kg/hr I.V.	Transdermal patches available in 25, 50, 75, and 100 μg/hr release
	Sufentanil	—	0.2–0.6 μg/kg I.V., followed by 0.01–0.05 μg/kg/min I.V.	—
	Alfentanil	—	10–25 μg/kg I.V., followed by 0.5–3.0 μg/kg/min I.V.	Safe in renal insufficiency
	Remifentanil	—	0.0125–0.025 μg/kg/min I.V.	—
	Hydromorphone	2–4 mg q. 4–6 hr	0.5–2 mg I.V. q. 1–2 hr	—
	Oxymorphone	—	1–1.5 mg S.C. or I.M. q. 4–6 hr 0.5 mg I.V.	—
	Levorphanol	2–3 mg q. 4 hr	2–3 mg S.C. q. 4–6 hr	Optimal I.V. dose has not been established
	Methadone	5–20 mg q. 3–4 hr	2.5–10.0 mg S.C., I.M., or I.V. q. 3–4 hr	Excellent I.V.-to-oral bioavailability, 1:2 mg
	Meperidine	50–150 mg q. 3–4 hr	25–100 mg I.V. q. 3–4 hr	Generally not recommended, because of oral effectiveness and active metabolites; increased bioavailability in liver failure exacerbates action of the normeperidine metabolite
	Oxycodone	5–10 mg q. 4–6 hr	—	Certain preparations contain acetaminophen
	Hydrocodone	5–10 mg q. 4–6 hr	—	—
	Acetaminophen with codeine	15–60 mg q. 3–6 hr	15–60 mg S.C., I.M., or I.V. q. 4 hr	—
	Propoxyphene	32–65 mg q. 4 hr	—	—
Opioid agonist antagonists	Buprenorphine	—	0.3 mg I.M. or I.V. q. 6 hr	—
	Pentazocine	25 mg t.i.d.–q.i.d.	30 mg S.C., I.M., or I.V. q. 3–4 hr	—
	Nalbuphine	—	10 mg S.C., I.M., or I.V. q. 3–6 hr	Often used with epidural narcotics to decrease side-effect profile of itching and hypotension
	Butorphanol	—	1 mg I.V. q. 3–4 hr 2 mg I.M. q. 3–4 hr	—
	Dezocine	—	5–20 mg I.M. q. 3–6 hr 2.5–10.0 mg I.V. q. 2–4 hr	—
	Tramadol	50–100 mg q. 4–6 hr	—	—

COX—cyclooxygenase   OA—osteoarthritis   PDA—patent ductus arteriosus   RA—rheumatoid arthritis

(continued)

ception in the postoperative period. Techniques utilizing epidural anesthesia[15] or major field block[16] achieve a greater reduction in perceived pain than general anesthesia does, and they greatly reduce the need for postoperative analgesics while enhancing postdischarge activity. Epidural anesthesia and other regional techniques are being applied more frequently, now that a number of trials have found them to be superior to general anesthesia.[17] In the case of epidural anesthesia, the catheter can be used to provide sustained pain relief for several days after operation. This approach is particularly useful in patients who have undergone operations on the lower abdomen or the lower extremities: it can lead to earlier mobilization and return of bowel function after operation, thereby shortening hospital stay.[18]

Systemic medications used for postoperative pain relief include opioids, nonsteroidal anti-inflammatory drugs (NSAIDs), and other nonnarcotic agents [see Table 1]. Surgeons are currently moving away from systemic opioids: in addition to their well-recognized capacity for inducing respiratory depression, opioids prolong ileus and increase nausea and vomiting. Regional anesthesia coupled with NSAID administration appears to yield better results in terms of patient recovery.[18]

On occasion, however, systemically administered narcotics are still the best available choice. Studies addressing postoperative pain have shown that most cases of severe pain are not uniformly relieved by the current practice of narcotic prescription. According to one study, physicians prescribe inadequate doses of

Table 1   Suggested Dosing of Opioid and Nonopioid Analgesics (*continued*)

Class	Drug	Oral Dosage	Parenteral Dosage	Comments
Nonopioid analgesics	Acetaminophen	325–650 mg q. 4 hr	—	Maximum, 4 g/day
	Acetylated salicylate Aspirin	325–650 mg q. 4 hr	—	—
	Nonacetylated salicylates Diflunisal	Loading dose, 1,000 mg, then 500–1,000 mg/day	—	FDA indications: pain, OA, and RA
	Salsalate	1,500 mg b.i.d.	—	FDA indications: RA and OA
	Choline magnesium trisalicylate	1,000–2,000 mg b.i.d.	—	FDA indications: OA, RA, and acute painful shoulder
	Propionic acids Ibuprofen	400–800 mg t.i.d.–q.i.d.	—	FDA indications: RA, OA, pain, and dysmenorrhea
	Fenoprofen	200 mg q. 4–6 hr	—	FDA indications: RA, OA, and pain
	Ketoprofen	50–75 mg t.i.d. or q.i.d.	—	FDA indications: RA, OA, pain, and dysmenorrhea
	Naproxen	500 mg, followed by 250 mg q. 6 hr	—	FDA indications: pain, RA, OA, dysmenorrhea, juvenile arthritis, ankylosing spondylitis, tendinitis, bursitis, and gout
	Flurbiprofen	50–100 mg b.i.d. or t.i.d.	—	FDA indications: RA and OA
	Oxaprozin	1,200 mg q. day	—	FDA indications: OA and RA
	Acetic acids Indomethacin	25 mg b.i.d. or t.i.d.	I.V. used to close PDA	FDA indications: RA, OA, ankylosing spondylitis, acute painful shoulder, and gout
	Sulindac	200 mg b.i.d.	—	FDA indications: OA, RA, ankylosing spondylitis, acute painful shoulder, and gout
	Tolmetin	400 mg t.i.d.	—	FDA indications: RA and OA
	Diclofenac	50 mg t.i.d.	—	FDA indications: RA, OA, and ankylosing spondylitis
	Etodolac	200–400 mg q. 6–8 hr, to maximum of 1,200 mg/day	—	FDA indications: OA and pain
	Nabumetone	1,000 mg/day	—	FDA indications: OA and RA
	Ketorolac	10 mg q. 4 hr	30 mg I.V., followed by 15–30 mg I.V. q. 6 hr 60 mg deep I.M., followed by 30 mg I.V. q. 6 hr	Maximum, 120 mg/day
	Oxicam Piroxicam	20 mg/day	—	FDA indications: OA and RA
	Fenamates Meclofenamate	50 mg q. 4 hr	—	FDA indications: pain, dysmenorrhea, RA, and OA
	Mefenamic acid	500 mg, followed by 250 mg q. 6 hr	—	FDA indications: pain and dysmenorrhea
	COX-2 inhibitors Rofecoxib	12.5–25.0 mg/day	—	FDA indications: OA, pain, and dysmenorrhea
	Celecoxib	100–200 mg q. 12–24 hr	—	FDA indications: OA, RA, and familial adenomatous polyposis

narcotic analgesics for patients with moderate or severe pain, and nurses give only 40% to 50% of the amount prescribed.[19] In this study, the effective dose of narcotic required for pain relief was underestimated, the fear of respiratory depression was high, the duration of action was overestimated, and the danger of addic-

tion was exaggerated. (Addiction usually does not develop unless narcotics are prescribed regularly for more than 2 weeks.)

NSAIDs, though safer than narcotics, have side effects of their own. In particular, they inhibit prostaglandin synthesis, thereby decreasing inflammation. This prostaglandin inhibition may

Table 2 Guidelines for I.V. Patient-Controlled Analgesia

Drug (Concentration)	Basal Dosage	Demand Dosage	Lockout Interval
Morphine (1–2 mg/ml)	0–0.5 mg/hr	0.5–3.0 mg	5–12 min
Meperidine (10 mg/ml)	0–5 mg/hr	5–30 mg	5–12 min
Fentanyl (10–20 µg/ml)	0–5 µg/hr	10–20 µg	5–10 min
Hydromorphone (0.2–0.5 mg/ml)	0–0.1 mg/hr	0.1–0.5 mg	5–10 min
Oxymorphone (0.25 mg/ml)	—	0.2–0.4 mg	8–10 min
Methadone (1 mg/ml)	0–0.5 mg/hr	0.5–2.5 mg	8–20 min
Nalbuphine (1 mg/ml)	—	1–5 mg	5–10 min

exacerbate renal insufficiency; for this reason, NSAIDs should be used with caution in patients with preexisting renal dysfunction. Other side effects include GI bleeding, inhibition of platelet aggregation, and prolonged bleeding time.

Patient-controlled analgesia (PCA) represents an important advance in pain management [*see VIII:2 Postoperative Pain*].[20-22] This modality has gained widespread acceptance because it provides improved pain control and greater patient satisfaction, which are attributable both to more expedient administration of the drug and to more consistent plasma levels. PCA generally takes the form of intermittent drug doses administered on demand, with a minimal required interval between doses (the lockout interval). A constant background infusion (basal dosage) may be given to supplement the intermittent dose, but it should be used cautiously so as not to induce respiratory depression. The narcotics most commonly used for PCA are morphine, meperidine, and fentanyl. Methadone is rarely given in this setting because of its slow onset and long duration of action [*see Table 2*]. Nalbuphine, though possessing narcotic analgesic properties of its own, is generally used for its antagonist properties, which act against side effects such as pruritus. Other side effects seen with patient-controlled analgesia are nausea, vomiting, sweating, and the aforementioned respiratory depression.

Management of Fluid Imbalance, Electrolyte Abnormalities, and Acid-Base Disorders

Postoperative fluid therapy is guided by the patient's overall preoperative condition, the preoperative diagnosis, and the circumstances of the operative procedure. The presence of cardiac, pulmonary, renal, or hepatic disease will affect the type and rate of fluid required postoperatively. Similarly, peritonitis, the septic response, or other conditions that affect the patient's volume status and peripheral capillary permeability will influence the approach to fluid therapy. In an adequately hydrated patient who has undergone a minor procedure with minimal blood loss and for whom the postoperative recovery period is expected to be short, maintenance fluid administration alone is adequate. Maintenance requirements for a 70 kg patient are normally about 100 ml/hr of 5% dextrose in one-half normal saline, with approximately 20 mEq/L of potassium added. By contrast, in a patient with bowel obstruction, small bowel infarction, and bowel perforation, maintenance fluid administration alone is inadequate. In these patients, reequilibration and fluid loss from the intravascular space continue for many hours after operation; consequently, resuscitation must be continued postoperatively, and as much as 7 to 10 L of crystalloid may have to be given over 24 hours to maintain adequate perfusion.

In patients who require continued postoperative volume resuscitation, hypotonic fluids, even at an increased rate, are not appropriate. Isotonic fluid is required to maintain adequate intravascular volume. Administration of 5% dextrose in lactated Ringer solution at the rate of 150 ml/hr provides about six times as much intravascular volume resuscitation as the usual maintenance regimen. Adjustments in volume should be guided by careful monitoring of urine output, pulse rate, and BP. A common error in postoperative fluid therapy is to order hypotonic fluids at an increased rate of administration (i.e., 150 ml/hr of 5% dextrose in 0.5 N saline) after determining, on the basis of physical examination findings (i.e., tachycardia, decreased BP, and decreased urine output in the appropriate clinical situation), that a patient is relatively hypovolemic. Because fluid losses into the interstitium are isotonic, isotonic fluid replacement is indicated.

In addition, the use of isotonic fluids is important because of the presence of elevated levels of antidiuretic hormone (ADH) and other counterregulatory hormones. In a normal, unstressed person, free-water loading (e.g., the drinking of several glasses of water) results in a fall in ADH levels and excretion of very dilute urine by the kidney, thus allowing the serum sodium and osmolality to return to normal. Various stressful stimuli, including operative procedures, result in an inability to lower ADH levels and an inability to excrete free water.[23-25] The administration of hypotonic fluid, with its free-water content, can lead to hyponatremia in postoperative patients and others with elevated levels of counterregulatory stress hormones. The resultant hyponatremia may cause significant morbidity and mortality.[26,27] The use of isotonic fluid prevents this problem. In uncomplicated elective procedures of brief duration (e.g., hernia repair, cholecystectomy, and uncomplicated bowel surgery), the stress response is short-lived and the patient can be switched to maintenance fluids 24 hours after operation. Patients who undergo operation under local anesthesia do not experience a stress response and generally need little, if any, fluid.

Once recovery from a major insult has begun, the capillary leak closes and fluid is mobilized from the periphery into the vascular space. At this point, the fluid orders should be changed to maintenance rates or lower and from isotonic resuscitation fluid to hypotonic saline. An important sign that the capillary leak has reversed is the return of a brisk urine output. Such spontaneous diuresis is a significant marker of the patient's recovery. It is associated with a fall in levels of ADH, aldosterone, steroids, catecholamines, and other counterregulatory hormones and with a rise in atrial natriuretic factor.[28,29] The use of diuretics in an attempt to "diurese off" excess fluid masks this physiologic response; therefore, diuretics should be reserved for use in patients who have inadequate renal or cardiac function and should be administered only after the capillary leak has reversed, so as not to cause intravascular volume depletion.

Several I.V. fluids are commonly employed for maintenance and resuscitation [*see Table 3*]. Crystalloids are the fluids of choice for perioperative fluid replacement. The use of colloid solutions offers no clear advantages in perioperative care, and their very high cost makes it difficult to justify their use in the majority of surgical patients.[30-32] A meta-analysis of 30 randomized, controlled trials comparing albumin to either no albumin or crystalloid in critically ill patients with hypovolemia, burns, or hypoalbuminemia found strong evidence suggesting that use of albumin may increase mortality.[33]

In the first 24 hours after operation, potassium supplementation is unnecessary in most patients. Potassium levels in I.V. fluids should be adjusted according to serum potassium levels.

Unfortunately, the serum potassium level provides an extremely inaccurate estimate of total body potassium. A profound depletion may exist despite serum potassium levels in the low to normal range. The long-term use of diuretics such as furosemide and the thiazides is commonly associated with low body stores of potassium. Patients undergoing nutritional repletion will also tend to have low serum potassium levels. If the patient has questionable renal function, potassium should be withheld until a serum level is available. If renal function is normal and urine output is not compromised, we add 20 mEq/L of potassium to the I.V. fluids after the first 24 postoperative hours.

FLUID IMBALANCE

Patients who undergo uncomplicated elective procedures usually experience relatively inconsequential abnormalities of their intravascular volume. However, patients who undergo lengthy or complicated procedures or have abnormalities of intravascular volume preoperatively are more likely to manifest abnormalities of circulating volume and should be evaluated carefully in the postoperative period to assess their intravascular volume status and tissue perfusion.

Hypovolemia

Hypovolemia is a decrease in the effective intravascular volume, caused by losses incurred either externally (e.g., hemorrhage or loss of transcellular fluid) or internally (e.g., transcapillary leakage of fluid into traumatized tissue). Oxygen delivery and tissue perfusion are dependent on the ability to generate an adequate cardiac output in the presence of hemoglobin that is sufficiently saturated (arterial oxygen saturation [S_aO_2] more than 90%, arterial oxygen tension [P_aO_2] more than 60 mm Hg). An inadequate intravascular volume can lead to poor perfusion either because of a lowered preload that results in a depressed cardiac output or because of a low hemoglobin concentration (e.g., from bleeding). Younger patients usually tolerate a lowered hemoglobin

concentration by increasing cardiac output, provided that intravascular volume is adequate. Older patients with coronary artery disease are more likely to suffer deleterious effects if their intravascular volume, their hemoglobin concentration, or both are low, because such patients have a limited ability to augment cardiac output under these circumstances.

Standard monitoring of volume status includes vital signs, mental status, and urine output. Because of the effects of general anesthesia, unrecognized intravascular volume depletion may develop. If a Foley catheter has been inserted, a decrease in the urine output can be an early sign of such depletion. Hypovolemia with depletion of the intravascular compartment should not be confused with changes in total body water, which may or may not occur in hypovolemia. If body weight is used to assess total body water content, it is possible to assume that a patient is "fluid overloaded" because of an elevated body weight, though in fact the intravascular volume has been depleted and the patient is underperfused and hypovolemic. This is a common scenario in patients who have sustained significant losses of intravascular volume and blood with resulting shock, capillary leakage, and fluid accumulation in the interstitium and the intracellular compartment.[34]

It has been demonstrated that the volume status of an individual patient, especially if he or she has unstable vital signs or is critically ill in the ICU, cannot be easily estimated by means of clinical assessment alone.[35,36] The use of invasive monitoring is therefore important in determining the status of the intravascular compartment and the ability of the body to maintain tissue perfusion. The use of a pulmonary arterial catheter to determine cardiac filling pressures and cardiac output usually allows a more accurate assessment of the patient's intravascular volume status. In patients who are relatively stable hemodynamically but manifest signs of a contracted intravascular volume (e.g., low urine output, increased heart rate, low or borderline blood pressure, depressed mental status, poor capillary refill), an isotonic fluid challenge should be administered. At least 500 and preferably 1,000 ml of lactated Ringer solution or normal

Table 3 Commonly Used I.V. Fluids

Solution	Plasma Osmolality (mOsm/L)	pH	Na+ (mEq/L)	Cl− (mEq/L)	K+ (mEq/L)	Ca2+ (mEq/L)	Other Components	Cost* ($)	Comments
D5LR (1,000 ml)	525	5	130	109	4	3	Lactate 28 mEq/L, 50 g dextrose	6	Fluid of choice for initial resuscitation and postoperative replacement
D5NS (1,000 ml)	560	4	154	154	0	0	50 g dextrose	6	Alternative to D5LR, but large amounts may cause metabolic acidosis
D5½NS (1,000 ml)	406	4	77	77	0	0	50 g dextrose	6	Hypotonic maintenance fluid
D5¼NS (1,000 ml)	321	4	34	34	0	0	50 g dextrose	6	Hypotonic maintenance fluid
D5W (1,000 ml)	321	4.5	0	0	0	0	50 g dextrose	6	Free-water source, no role in resuscitation
25% Albumin (100 ml)	Equal to plasma	Equal to plasma	145	0	0	0	25 g albumin	67	Colloid, expensive
5% Plasma protein fraction (250 ml)	Equal to plasma	Equal to plasma	145	0	< 2	0	12.5 g protein	33	Colloid, expensive
6% Hetastarch in 0.9% NaCl (500 ml)	310	3.5–7.0	154	154	0	0	30 g hydroxyethyl starch	42	Use limited volume (500–1,000 ml); coagulation abnormalities with larger volumes

*Reflects sample cost to pharmacy at the University of North Carolina at Chapel Hill School of Medicine. Actual cost to the patient is likely to be significantly higher.
D5LR—5% dextrose in lactated Ringer solution   D5NS—5% dextrose in normal saline solution   D5½NS—5% dextrose in one-half normal saline solution   D5¼NS—5% dextrose in one-quarter saline solution   D5W—5% dextrose in water

saline solution should be given rapidly and the patient's response evaluated. If the vital signs normalize and the urine output rises, the patient is assumed to be responding to volume loading. Further observation will determine whether the patient requires more isotonic fluid administration. If the patient does not respond to the initial bolus of fluid or has significant renal or cardiopulmonary dysfunction, it is generally more prudent to employ invasive monitoring with a pulmonary arterial catheter to determine the status of the intravascular compartment. The use of diuretics in this setting should be limited to patients who have known severe cardiopulmonary dysfunction or advanced renal disease with a known dependency on diuretics. The administration of a diuretic to a patient with intravascular volume depletion can result in further depletion of the intravascular volume despite the production of urine.

Other techniques useful in the assessment of a patient's volume status include measurement of sodium in the urine sediment, cardiac echocardiography, and the determination of serum lactate levels. None of these techniques is entirely accurate or practical. The response to a fluid bolus remains a practical means of assessing the status of the intravascular compartment. Failure to respond to one or more fluid boluses should prompt further evaluation, including invasive monitoring if indicated.

Fluid Overload

Fluid overload in the postoperative surgical patient is reported to occur with varying frequency and has been associated with inferior outcomes.[37] The degree to which a patient may become "overloaded" with fluid is determined by the patient's preoperative status, age, and existing cardiopulmonary, renal, or hepatic disorders; the length of the operative procedure; the fluids administered; and the presence or absence of infection and inflammatory mediators. Although it is generally accepted that patients who require large amounts of fluid and who gain weight in the postoperative period are likely to have a less favorable outcome, it is difficult to separate the effect of large-volume resuscitation from the circumstances that prompt such therapy, most commonly shock, a septic response, or both.

Judicious use of fluids in the perioperative period and the application of the principles of invasive monitoring outlined above generally allow appropriate volume resuscitation without precipitating pulmonary edema or congestive heart failure. It should be recognized, however, that in patients who sustain shock or manifest a septic response (with or without bacterial infection), fluid will leak from the intravascular compartments and total body anasarca will develop. The resultant increase in body weight associated with an increased requirement for fluid infusion will give the impression that the patient is receiving excessive amounts of fluid. Although this may be the case, it is generally difficult to determine intravascular volume status in more seriously ill patients through simple observation alone.[35,36] The value of invasive monitoring in the ICU should again be emphasized. Patients suspected of being "fluid overloaded" should be carefully evaluated by an experienced clinician, and if they do not respond to preliminary measures to correct their volume status, they should undergo invasive monitoring.

ELECTROLYTE ABNORMALITIES

Disorders of Sodium Concentration

Hyponatremia Hyponatremia is caused by excess free water in the intravascular space [see I:6 Life-Threatening Electrolyte Abnormalities]. The serum sodium concentration is not an accurate measure of total body sodium but rather reflects the concentration of sodium relative to the amount of free water in the intravascular compartment. The serum sodium concentration is not related to the volume state of the intravascular compartment. Patients may be normovolemic, hypovolemic, or hypervolemic in the presence of hyponatremia.

In the postoperative setting, hyponatremia usually results from an excess of free water. This occurs when hypotonic fluid is administered to patients whose ADH levels cannot fall because of the stress of operation or injury. In these patients, the free water administered as hypotonic fluid cannot be eliminated through the kidney, and hyponatremia results. In most cases, the stress subsides in 24 to 48 hours and the ADH levels fall, which allows the kidney to correct the free-water excess. Patients who continue to be ill or under stress and those who have poor renal function may experience difficulty in correcting the free-water excess. Significant morbidity and mortality can occur if the serum sodium concentration falls below 120 mEq/L.[26,27] Hyponatremia in the postoperative setting is best avoided by means of appropriate I.V. fluid management, including the use of isotonic fluid in the immediate postoperative period.

The treatment of hyponatremia depends on the serum sodium concentration and how long it took serum sodium to reach that level. Intravascular volume deficits, if present, should be corrected first. Patients who have chronically depressed serum sodium concentrations will tolerate slow correction with isotonic fluid (e.g., lactated Ringer solution or normal saline solution). Patients who experience an acute, rapid falloff of their serum sodium concentration or those who are symptomatic require correction with hypertonic (3%) saline over 24 to 48 hours.

Hypernatremia Hypernatremia reflects a relative deficiency of free water compared with sodium. Under normal circumstances, hypernatremia stimulates thirst, and the intake of free water returns the serum sodium concentration to normal. Hypernatremia may develop in patients who are unable to regulate their fluid intake (e.g., obtunded patients) or do not have their fluids replaced appropriately. This is especially likely in patients with large free-water losses such as sweat and insensible losses. Patients with diabetes insipidus (e.g., as a result of head injury) develop hypernatremia because of large (> 10 L/day) losses of very dilute urine.

Treatment of hypernatremia consists of providing adequate volumes of free water to correct the deficit. Serum sodium concentration is a good indicator of the adequacy of replacement. In the case of diabetes insipidus, treatment with desmopressin acetate, either parenterally or by the nasal route, in concert with careful fluid management will generally alleviate the hypernatremia.

Disorders of Potassium Concentration

Hypokalemia Hypokalemia may have a number of causes in the postoperative patient. Chronic use of diuretics, poor nutrition with total body potassium depletion, and GI losses are all associated with varying degrees of hypokalemia. Among the most common causes is alkalosis, which brings about a shift of potassium into the intracellular compartment.

Since the serum potassium level does not accurately reflect the total body potassium pool, hypokalemia at levels of 3 mEq/L or less is associated with severe total body potassium depletion (usually in excess of 100 mEq). Such patients may require ECG monitoring and should receive I.V. potassium and have levels measured frequently to monitor their progress. Correction of the underlying cause of the problem is important. Potassium should be given only if there is reliable urine flow, however, as dangerously high potassium levels may result in anuric patients. Our practice is to deliver three doses of 10 mEq of potassium chloride in 50 to 100 ml of saline solution and then check serum levels.

Hyperkalemia Hyperkalemia is among the most dangerous of electrolyte abnormalities. It is especially likely to occur in patients with renal dysfunction but can also result from crush injury, hemolysis, myonecrosis, and acidosis. Hyperkalemia can also occur in malignant hyperthermia and after the administration of succinylcholine to patients with spinal cord injury, burns, or neurologic disorders secondary to severe muscle contractions.

The most serious manifestations of hyperkalemia are cardiac in nature and include high-peaked T waves, absent P waves, widened QRS complexes, ventricular arrhythmias, and cardiac arrest (in diastole). Heart block can also occur. Cardiac effects begin at serum potassium levels of around 6.5 mEq/L; serious risk of death is associated with levels exceeding 8 mEq/L. Patients with serum levels above 6.5 mEq/L should be strongly considered for cardiac monitoring until their serum potassium level is under control.

Treatment consists of discontinuance of any exogenous potassium. If acidosis is present, sodium bicarbonate (50 mEq/L I.V.) should be administered. This dose can be repeated after 10 to 15 minutes. Since sodium bicarbonate is hypertonic saline, caution should be exercised in its use if hypernatremia or fluid overload is present. Calcium, 5 mmol I.V. over 5 minutes, will transiently depress the membrane threshold potential and antagonize the effect of potassium on the myocardium. Infusion of glucose and insulin will lower the serum potassium level by driving potassium into the cell. An ampule (50 ml) of 50% dextrose is administered intravenously along with 10 units of regular insulin. Administration of furosemide with or without a bolus of saline in patients with reasonable kidney function will also decrease potassium levels. The administration of cation-exchange resins (e.g., sodium polystyrene sulfonate) either orally or by enema will decrease potassium levels more slowly by binding to ions in the GI tract. If other measures fail, dialysis is highly effective in reducing potassium levels.

ACID-BASE DISORDERS

Respiratory Acidosis

Homeostatic mechanisms maintain arterial carbon dioxide tension (P_aCO_2) and serum pH within the normal range through the central regulation of minute ventilation (tidal volume × respiratory rate). Respiratory acidosis results when the ability to eliminate the produced CO_2 is exceeded [see I:7 Life-Threatening Acid-Base Disorders]. A variety of causes of respiratory acidosis have been identified. They include central causes (e.g., excess sedation and neuromuscular disorders) as well as disorders of ventilation associated with respiratory failure and ventilatory malfunction. Patients with acute respiratory acidosis characteristically have an elevation in their P_aCO_2 associated with a decreased pH. Acute compensation is relatively limited; it is not until the respiratory acidosis has persisted for at least 12 to 24 hours that renal compensatory mechanisms are activated. Serum bicarbonate gradually rises over a period of several days and drives the pH back (but not completely) toward normal. It is thus possible to differentiate between patients with acute respiratory acidosis and those with chronic respiratory acidosis by the assessment of their serum bicarbonate level and pH. Patients should be assessed for potentially reversible factors. Those on mechanical ventilation should have an immediate increase in minute ventilation. If respiratory acidosis fails to resolve in a spontaneously breathing patient and respiratory distress develops, intubation and mechanical ventilation are necessary.

Respiratory Alkalosis

Respiratory alkalosis occurs when CO_2 elimination exceeds CO_2 production. This is usually caused by an increase in minute ventilation with a decrease in P_aCO_2 and an elevation of pH. Only small changes in the serum bicarbonate level occur in the acute form. If respiratory alkalosis persists, renal compensation will lead to a lowering of the serum bicarbonate level and a return of serum pH almost to normal. Patients with respiratory alkalosis generally have mild hypokalemia and hyperchloremia. The hypokalemia is related to the exchange of potassium for hydrogen ions between the intracellular and extracellular compartments in compensation for the alkalemia. In addition, potassium wasting occurs in the kidney. Hyperchloremia results from the renal retention of chloride to offset the gradually falling levels of serum bicarbonate.

The compensation that occurs in the first week of respiratory alkalosis is generally insufficient to return the pH to normal. More chronic forms of alkalosis will ultimately result in a normalization of the serum pH.

Metabolic Acidosis

Metabolic acidosis in the postoperative surgical patient is always worrisome. It occurs when there is either an increase in the production of H^+ or a significant loss of bicarbonate. Increased production of hydrogen ions is generally associated with underperfusion of tissues and the development of lactic acidosis. Although other conditions can result in metabolic acidosis, hypovolemia and poor tissue perfusion must be ruled out in the postoperative patient.

The initial compensatory response to metabolic acidosis in the spontaneously breathing patient is an increase in minute ventilation. Lactic acidosis exhibits a greater increase in minute ventilation than that seen in other forms of metabolic acidosis. If a patient is sedated or mechanically ventilated, this compensation may not occur, in which case the patient will continue to manifest a low serum pH. A pH of 7.2 or greater has not been associated with significant detrimental effects. Once the patient is known to have metabolic acidosis, assessment of the intravascular volume status should be undertaken immediately. If the metabolic acidosis does not resolve with preliminary maneuvers such as fluid bolus therapy, then invasive monitoring should be undertaken to establish the status of the intravascular circulation and the cardiopulmonary system. Persistent acidosis may signal myocardial ischemia, ischemic bowel, sepsis syndrome, or inadequate volume resuscitation in an injured or critically ill patient.

Determination of the anion gap [see I:7 Life-Threatening Acid-Base Disorders], the base deficit, and the serum lactate level can be helpful in determining the cause of the metabolic acidosis. Besides poor tissue perfusion, causes may include renal failure, ketoacidosis, lactic acidosis, and poisoning (all associated with an increased anion gap) as well as renal tubular acidosis, diarrhea, ureteral diversion, and a variety of other conditions (all associated with a normal anion gap).

The base deficit has been shown to be a function of oxygen debt,[38] to correlate with mortality,[39,40] and to be a valuable guide to resuscitation.[40,41] In that the base deficit is a function of all unmeasured cations, it can also arise from types of acidosis other than lactic acidosis. The most common causes of a base deficit besides lactic acidosis are hyperchloremic acidosis and renal insufficiency.

The serum lactate level is a useful indicator of anaerobic metabolism. Clearance of lactate within 24 hours has been shown to correlate with survival.[42] Inadequate perfusion is a major cause of lactic acidosis, but other causes also exist that do not involve perfusion abnormalities. The administration of I.V. bicarbonate generally does not materially affect the outcome of patients who have metabolic acidosis related to inadequate tissue perfusion; the net effect of this measure is a temporary elevation of serum pH associated with an increase of CO_2 production. Bicarbonate combines with hydrogen ions to form carbonic acid and, subsequently, water and CO_2. It should be noted that this increased CO_2 production can result in a worsening of intracellular acidosis if minute ventilation is not increased to allow elimination of the excess CO_2. Furthermore, exogenous bicarbonate eliminates the utility of measuring the base deficit and may worsen oxygen delivery by causing an adverse shift in the oxygen dissociation curve.

Metabolic Alkalosis

Metabolic alkalosis is most often caused by a loss of hydrogen ions from the GI tract (e.g., through vomiting or nasogastric suction) or in the urine (e.g., as a result of diuretic therapy). The loss of hydrogen ions is associated with the liberation of bicarbonate, as shown in the following equation:

$$CO_2 + H_2O \rightarrow H_2CO_3 \rightarrow H^+ + HCO_3^-$$

Hypokalemia can result in metabolic alkalosis by causing a shift of hydrogen ions into the cell in exchange for potassium. Although perceived as extracellular metabolic alkalosis, this is in fact an intracellular metabolic acidosis because of the hydrogen ion shift. Prompt repletion of potassium in the hypokalemic patient can minimize the effect of these changes. Metabolic alkalosis can also result from contraction of the extracellular volume. This contraction alkalosis occurs when the lost fluid contains chloride but little or no bicarbonate, as occurs with diuretic therapy.

Of particular significance in the postoperative period is the development of hypokalemic, hypochloremic metabolic alkalosis associated with the loss of significant amounts of gastric secretions. This can occur either through nasogastric suction or with repeated vomiting. Patients develop intravascular volume contraction in addition to alkalosis and hypochloremia as they lose volume and HCl. This development is associated with an increase in sodium and water retention in the kidney, mediated by ADH and aldosterone. The volume deficit, hypochloremia, and hypokalemia all result in increased bicarbonate absorption by the kidney. Paradoxical aciduria will result as bicarbonate reabsorption, together with sodium and potassium retention, leads to an increased hydrogen ion concentration in the urine. Treatment of hypokalemic, hypochloremic metabolic alkalosis is directed at decreasing the fluid losses, if possible, and providing significant amounts of volume, potassium, and chloride.

Chloride repletion is important because chloride is the only reabsorbable anion in this setting. If adequate chloride is not given, electroneutrality in the distal nephron can be maintained only by the excretion of hydrogen ions. Since the patient is volume contracted, no excess sodium ions are available for excretion, and hypokalemia precludes the excretion of potassium ions. Bicarbonate is being reabsorbed avidly at this time. Thus, as sodium is reabsorbed in the hypovolemic state, hydrogen ions will of necessity be excreted in the urine. If chloride is provided in adequate amounts, it will be reabsorbed with sodium, thus obviating excretion of hydrogen ion (or potassium ions if they are available) to maintain electroneutrality.

Metabolic alkalosis can be divided into two varieties: saline responsive and saline resistant. Saline-responsive metabolic alkalosis is generally caused by GI losses or by diuresis, whereas saline-resistant metabolic alkalosis is usually a consequence of either severe hypokalemia or an edematous state such as cirrhosis. Patients with the saline-responsive variety generally respond well to volume expansion with sodium chloride.

Management of Tubes and Drains

Guidelines for the perioperative use of tubes and drains should be developed on the basis of scientific data. For the most part, current practices in this regard are not rigorously formulated and tested but are simply passed on to surgical trainees on little basis other than surgical tradition. With the development of evidence-based medicine, these approaches are being evaluated and challenged. As a result, this aspect of surgical care is evolving.

NASOGASTRIC TUBES

Traditionally, nasogastric tubes were routinely used in all patients undergoing GI surgery. In the past decade, however, the value of this routine practice for elective surgical patients has been questioned. A 1995 meta-analysis of 26 trials that included 3,964 patients concluded that nasogastric tubes are unnecessary in elective surgical patients and may even add to debility [see Table 4].[43] Nasogastric decompression is appropriate on a selective basis for any patient in whom severe nausea, vomiting, or gastric distention develops [see Figure 1]. Moreover, it is indicated in patients with intestinal obstruction or those with severe prolonged ileus, usually related to intra-abdominal sepsis.

FINE, PLIABLE FEEDING TUBES

The introduction of the Dobbhoff tube by Dobbie and Hoffmeister allowed routine intubation past the pylorus for feeding.[44] The Dobbhoff tube is a highly flexible No. 8 polyurethane tube with two distal side holes and a mercury-weighted tip. A steel wire is used to stent the tube during placement and is removed after the tube is positioned. The Dobbhoff tube and the Entriflex tube (a similar tube with a thin, elongated distal segment) are placed in a manner similar to that of a nasogastric tube [see Figure 1]. Once in the stomach, the tube can be advanced under fluoroscopic guidance into the duodenum. Alternatively, the tube can be allowed to pass spontaneously through the pylorus by placing the patient in the right lateral decubitus position and allowing enough slack externally. The use of metoclopramide can sometimes facilitate passage into the duodenum. A radiograph should always be obtained before the initiation of feedings through a nasoenteric small-bore catheter [see Figure 2]. These tubes can pass easily into the trachea even in intubated patients and can cause a pneumothorax or a pneumonic process if feedings are given without radiographic confirmation that the location of the tip is correct.[45,46]

LONG INTESTINAL TUBES

Long intestinal tubes (e.g., the Cantor tube and the Miller-Abbott tube) are occasionally used in patients with partial small-bowel obstruction early after operation, although mechanical bowel obstruction usually necessitates early operation. Use of long intestinal tubes should be reserved for selected patients who are not candidates for early reoperation. Because movement distally is dependent on peristalsis, these tubes are of little value in patients with paralytic ileus. The Cantor tube is made of silicone-coated polyvinyl chloride and has a small balloon tip. The tip is filled with mercury, passed through the nose, and allowed to advance into the small intestine either passively or under fluoroscopic guidance; there, it will aspirate fluid and gas. Removal of the tube is accomplished by pulling approximately 30 cm of tube out of the nose every 1 or 2 hours and either taping or clamping it to prevent slippage.

BILIARY DRAINAGE CATHETERS

Biliary tract drains include cholecystostomy tubes, percutaneous drains of the biliary tract placed under fluoroscopic control, T tubes, and endoscopically placed nasobiliary tubes. Cholecystostomy tubes may be placed with the help of local anesthesia in patients with advanced medical problems who cannot tolerate general anesthesia and formal cholecystectomy. Patients in whom dissection would be technically difficult and associated with a high risk of complications can also be treated by cholecystostomy tube placement. Ultrasonographically guided percutaneous cholecystostomy tube placement has gained acceptance for patients who are not considered good candidates for operation.

The use of T tubes is generally limited to operative exploration or repair of the common bile duct (CBD). In most cases, the CBD is explored for the presence of stones. The duct is then closed around the T-shaped end of the tube to stent the duct. The long end of the T tube is then brought out of an incision, sutured to the skin, and attached to a drainage bag. The exit site should be chosen to allow direct percutaneous access into the distal CBD should this become necessary for later stone extraction or duct manipulation. A T tube usually drains most of the bile produced (600 to 700 ml daily) initially. A decrease in the volume of bile drained indicates patency of the distal duct and free flow into the duodenum. At 7 to 10 days after the operation, a cholangiogram is obtained to assess the patency of the CBD and look for stones. I.V. antibiotics should be administered during cholangiography. A normal cholangiogram shows no stones; a patent, nondilated CBD without leakage; and free flow of contrast medium into the duodenum. The tube can be removed by gentle withdrawal; alternatively, the tube is clamped, and if the patient continues to do well, it is removed on an outpatient basis after 1 to 2 weeks. If the cholangiogram is abnormal, the T tube should be left to drain and the problem addressed either through the tract of the T tube or by means of endoscopic retrograde cholangiopancreatography.

Nasobiliary tubes are placed at the time of endoscopic evaluation of the biliary tree, usually to alleviate CBD obstruction. These tubes are left to drain by gravity and can otherwise be managed in much the same fashion as nasoenteric tubes.

DRAINS

Various tubes and associated devices have been used to drain purulent materials, blood, or serum from body cavities. These include Penrose drains (very soft rubber tubes with a gauze wick), closed suction drains (e.g., Jackson-Pratt or Hemovac drains), and sump drains (multiple-lumen tubes that draw air into one interior lumen and fluid from a companion tube). Controlled clinical trials in elective surgical patients indicate that routine use of drains does not improve outcome for patients undergoing cholecystectomy,[47] laminectomy,[48] colon surgery,[49]

Table 4 Meta-analysis of 26 Clinical Trials of Selective versus Routine Nasogastric Decompression[43]

	Selective Decompression	Routine Decompression	*P*
Total no. of patients	1,986	1,978	—
Patients with complications	833	1,084	< 0.03
Patients with pneumonia	53	119	< 0.0001
Patients with atelectasis	44	94	0.001
Patients with fever	108	212	0.02
Time to oral feeding (days)	3.53	4.59	0.04

or thyroid surgery.[50] Postoperative drainage does, however, reduce serum formation and other wound problems after mastectomy.[51] Postmastectomy wound drainage can be managed on an outpatient basis and thus need not hinder or delay discharge.

FOLEY CATHETERS

Foley catheters are routinely used after operation to drain the urinary bladder [see Figure 3]. Bladder catheterization alleviates the patient's discomfort and allows precise monitoring of urine output. When interpreted in the appropriate clinical situation, few measurements are more valuable than urine output. However, placement of a Foley catheter can lead to a number of complications, the most common of which is urinary tract infection.

Among general surgery patients, the overall infection rate is 10%, and 26% of these infections occur secondary to urinary tract infections[52]; for example, 49% of orthopedic infections and 75% of urologic and medical infections are related to urinary tract infections. The distal urethra is usually colonized with bacteria. Even one catheterization of the bladder will result in urinary tract infection in 1% of ambulatory patients.[52] Infection will develop within 3 to 4 days of catheterization in 95% of patients managed with indwelling catheters and open drainage systems.[52] A variety of organisms can cause urinary tract infection. *Escherichia coli* is by far the most common pathogen, although other Enterobacteriaceae are also common. Staphylococci, streptococci, and enterococci also frequently cause urinary tract infection. Dysuria can be a symptom of urinary tract infection; however, infection may often present only as fever or a septic response. Diagnosis is based on microscopic examination of the urine and urine culture [see VI:14 Nosocomial Infection]. Urinary tract infection can be prevented by (1) avoiding nonessential catheterization, (2) allowing only trained personnel to insert catheters, (3) using meticulous aseptic technique to avoid introduction of bacteria, (4) adequately securing the catheter after insertion so it does not move in and out of the urethra and the bladder, (5) maintaining proper drainage, and (6) removing the catheter at the earliest possible opportunity.

Few controlled studies have been published that address the optimal duration of bladder catheter drainage. One study suggests that such drainage should be limited to about 3 days after a major low-rectal operation and to about 1 day after other types of colon operations.[53] Epidural drug administration in the postoperative period should not be an indication for bladder drainage beyond 24 hours.[54]

Antinausea Prophylaxis

Postoperative nausea and vomiting are common problems and are best treated pharmacologically [see IV:4 Fast Track Surgery] unless intestinal obstruction or severe ileus exists. For example, H_2-receptor antagonists and dexamethasone have been shown to be effective if given perioperatively. Droperidol may also be effective, and a 1999 randomized trial suggested that supplemental oxygen may also reduce nausea and vomiting.[2]

The use of local and regional anesthetic techniques reduces patient exposure to agents such as nitrous oxide, which predisposes to nausea. Administration of NSAIDs instead of a narcotic also reduces the incidence of this complication.

Ambulation and Nutrition

Traditional postoperative care generally included bed rest, which is now considered undesirable in that it increases muscle

a

b

c

Figure 1 (*a*) The nasogastric tube (generally a No. 18 sump catheter) is passed through the nose to the posterior pharynx, at which point it must make a nearly 90° turn into the esophagus—a maneuver that should be executed gently and with extreme caution. Ideally, the patient should be in a sitting position with head forward and should be sipping liquids, which will help ease the progress of the tube into the stomach. The position of the tube is confirmed by rapid injection of 10 to 20 ml of air into the tube and auscultation over the gastric area of the abdomen. The exterior portion of the tube is gently secured with adhesive tape, preferably to the upper lip or to the nose, without tension or deviation of the alae or septum. If intubation does not drain fluid regularly, the tube may have to be irrigated or repositioned. If the position of the tube is in doubt, a radiograph should be taken (*b*) before feeding is initiated. Examples of inappropriate positioning include passage into the prevertebral fascia, which can cause mediastinitis, or into the lung, which can lead to pneumothorax (*c*) or pneumonia after feeding. At removal, the nasogastric tube is disconnected from the suction tubing and the adhesive tape removed. The patient is instructed to hold his or her breath, and the tube is then withdrawn gently but quickly. After removal, the tube is discarded.

Long intestinal tubes, most commonly a Cantor or Miller-Abbott tube, are passed through the nose and into the stomach in a manner similar to that of a nasogastric tube. Weighted by a balloon tip filled with 5 to 8 ml of mercury, the tube continues on through the stomach and into the small intestine either passively or with assistance under fluoroscopy. Once in the small intestine, it will aspirate fluid and gas as it proceeds. Removal of a long intestinal tube is accomplished gradually; approximately 30 cm of tubing is pulled out through the nose once every 1 or 2 hours and then taped or clamped to prevent slippage.

loss and weakness, impairs pulmonary function and tissue oxygenation, and predisposes to thromboembolic and pulmonary complications and orthostatic intolerance.[55,56] Every effort should be made to enforce postoperative mobilization, which is possible in most cases if effective pain relief is provided.

Oral intake is frequently limited in the postoperative period. When enteral feedings are provided, they are frequently given as

Figure 2 **Abdominal radiograph shows that the small-caliber feeding tube was passed into the stomach with its tip advanced into the duodenum, confirming that the tip of the feeding tube is safely positioned, so that feedings can be initiated.**

a dietary progression, starting with liquids and proceeding to soft food and finally to solid food. There is no scientific basis for this practice; in fact, several studies have shown that early oral feedings are safe in elective surgical patients even after colon procedures involving bowel anastomoses.[57] If nausea, vomiting, or ileus is present, pharmacologic treatment should be considered and feeding initiated. If a prolonged delay in initiating enteral nutrition is expected, parenteral nutrition should be considered [*see VII:9 Nutritional Support*]

Postoperative Complications

POSTOPERATIVE FEVER

A number of studies[58,59] have shown that postoperative fever is common. In one study, 72% of 153 postoperative patients had a temperature greater than 37° C (98.6° F), and 41% had a temperature greater than 38° C (100.4° F).[58] Postoperative fever usually is not associated with significant infection (only four of 256 febrile patients in one series had an infectious process[59]). Fever associated with infection usually occurs later than fever of noninfectious origin (2.7 versus 1.6 days after operation in one study[59]); fever associated with infection also lasts longer (5.4 versus 3.4 days). The absence of fever does not rule out infection; fever was experienced by only 50% of patients in whom an infection subsequently developed.[59]

Although fever is occasionally caused by serious underlying infection, the practice of routinely ordering a battery of expensive laboratory tests (e.g., chest x-ray, blood cultures, complete blood count, sputum culture, urinalysis, and urine culture) when fever is present should be avoided. The best way of differentiating between patients who have an infectious process and the vast majority who do not is via physical examination. The indiscriminate use of laboratory studies is costly and usually not diagnostic; by comparison, laboratory studies directed by physical examination are frequently valuable.

Factors that increase the risk of fever developing in the postoperative period include an operation more than 2 hours long, intraoperative transfusion, preexisting infection, and preoperative antibiotic prophylaxis (which implies contamination or potential operative contamination). Common causes of fever include atelectasis, pneumonia, urinary tract infection, septic and nonseptic phlebitis, drug allergies, wound infection, and other deep infections. Postoperative fever occurs more commonly in patients who have drains in place, even though infection may not subsequently develop.[60,61] Unusual causes of fever include delayed hemolytic reaction to transfusion (i.e., fever and anemia in a patient with a history of blood transfusion)[62] and other inflammatory disease processes such as systemic lupus erythematosus, rheumatoid arthritis, and gout. Other rare causes include hepatic toxicity resulting from anesthetic agents (e.g., halothane or enflurane[63]) or viral infections (e.g., cytomegalovirus or Epstein-Barr virus[64]). These complications generally occur late after the surgical procedure.

If the fever does reflect a serious underlying infection, the patient is at risk for multiple organ dysfunction syndrome (MODS). Various interventions aimed at preventing MODS by interrupting the cytokine cascade proved unsuccessful. In 2001, however, an international multicenter prospective, randomized, double-blind, placebo-controlled trial showed that activated protein C (drotrecogin alfa) caused a decrease in mortality (30.8% in the placebo group versus 24.7% in the treatment group.)[65]

HYPOTHERMIA

Mild hypothermia, a common postoperative complication, results from blockage of normal autoregulatory processes by the anesthetic agent, heat loss through the open abdomen or chest cavity, and the administration of cold fluids. Mild hypothermia is generally well tolerated and, except for the slight increase in peripheral vascular resistance and the decrease in total-body oxygen consumption that it causes, is of little concern. However, more marked hypothermia can cause a variety of serious complications, including marked elevation of peripheral vascular resistance, decreases in cardiac contractility and cardiac output, depressed neurologic status, and a coagulopathy with clotting system enzyme dysfunction. Profound hypothermia is frequently associated with major operations, particularly those performed after multiple trauma or those involving massive transfusion of cold stored blood and cold crystalloid [*see VII:10 Fever, Hypothermia, and Hyperpyrexia*].[66-70]

CARDIAC COMPLICATIONS

A variety of cardiovascular complications are commonly associated with general surgical procedures. These include dysrhythmias, myocardial infarction, ventricular failure, and hypertension.[71,72] As the average age of patients undergoing general surgical procedures has increased, so too has the incidence of significant heart disease in this population. Ideally, selective management to prevent significant cardiovascular complications is initiated preoperatively and is continued both intraoperatively and postoperatively. Specific measures should be taken to control congestive heart failure; such measures may include aggressive management with careful volume management as well as appropriate use of diuretics, digoxin, afterload reduction therapy, and oxygen therapy. There is a growing body of data supporting the use of prophylactic beta blockade in high-risk patients undergoing noncardiac surgery [*see IV:2 Risk Stratification, Operative Planning, and Preoperative Testing*]. Factors indicative of elevated risk include ischemic heart disease, congestive heart failure, major surgery (intraperitoneal, intrathoracic, and suprainguinal vascular procedures), diabetes mellitus, renal insufficiency, and poor functional

a Straight Catheter

Coudé Catheter

Foley Catheter

b

c

Figure 3 The Foley catheter is the primary type of catheter utilized for long-term bladder catheterization (*a*). If the bladder is to be catheterized a single time, however, a straight catheter without a balloon is used. When difficulty is encountered in passing a Foley catheter (often in men with an enlarged prostate gland), a curved-tip catheter, or coudé catheter, can often be passed by experienced personnel. The smallest-diameter catheter that will accomplish the task should be selected (16 French to 24 French for adult men, 16 French to 26 French for adult women). Before insertion, the balloon at the end of the Foley catheter should be tested, the patient's genital area cleansed, and the tip of the catheter well lubricated. In men, the penis should be held erect and the catheter inserted into the meatus and advanced gently until urine returns (*b*). In women, the labia should be gently spread, the urethral meatus located, and the catheter gently inserted until urine returns. In both men and women, once urine returns, the catheter is then advanced a little farther to ensure that the balloon does not lie in the urethra. The balloon is inflated by the injection of 5 to 10 ml of saline solution through the balloon port. After insertion is completed, the exterior portion of the catheter is taped to the patient's thigh (*c*). Once it is no longer necessary, the catheter should be removed. Removal consists of deflating the balloon and then withdrawing the catheter as gently as possible.

status.[73] The surgeon should be alert for the presence of angina, cardiac valve disease, and arrhythmias, including heart block, ventricular arrhythmias, and supraventricular tachycardia.[74,75]

Hypertension in the postoperative period frequently occurs secondary to pain or hypoxia. Initial treatment, therefore, consists of administering adequate analgesia to control pain and ensuring adequate oxygenation. Once pain is alleviated and hypoxia corrected, drug treatment may be considered. A variety of agents are available for the treatment of hypertension [*see Table 5*].[76,77] The physician should generally become familiar with one or two medications and use them with confidence rather than try to master a large number of them.

RESPIRATORY COMPLICATIONS

Pulmonary complications are common after operative procedures. In one study, dependent atelectasis (3.4% of lung volume) developed in 100% of patients 5 to 10 minutes after administration of anesthesia[78]; 1 hour later, atelectasis was present in 90% of the patients, and 24 hours after operation, it was present in 50%. Up to 40% of obese patients show evidence of basal pulmonary atelectasis on initial postoperative x-ray.[79]

Postoperative respiratory complications include atelectasis, aspiration pneumonia, and other pneumonias. A variety of factors contribute to the development of these complications, and various approaches have been used to prevent and treat them. For example, abdominal incisions cause pain, which limits the patient's activity and shifts predominantly abdominal breathing to chest wall breathing. Fluoroscopy of the diaphragm after operation has demonstrated reduced diaphragmatic movement, with a shift from abdominal to rib cage breathing.[80] This shift begins to reverse after 24 hours. However, the placement of the incision can influence the risk of postoperative respiratory compromise. For example, lower abdominal and transverse incisions are associated with a lower rate of com-

Table 5 Drugs Used in Urgent and Emergency Treatment of Hypertension

Drug	Administration	Onset of Action	Mechanism of Action	Side Effects	Indications/Contraindications
Sodium nitroprusside	Prepare 50–100 mg/500 ml 5% dextrose in water; administer at rate of 25–50 μg/min and titrate (solution is light sensitive and should be covered with aluminum foil) Patient needs constant monitoring	Immediate	Vasodilatation	Nausea, restlessness, disorientation, severe hypotension, thiocyanate toxicity (check blood levels every 48 hr; discontinue if levels exceed 10 mg/dl), hypothyroidism or methemoglobinemia (rare), ↓ platelet adhesiveness, intracranial hypertension	Especially useful in patients with ischemic heart disease, aortic dissection (combined with a beta blocker), or intracranial hemorrhage
Trimethaphan	Prepare 500 mg/500 ml 5% dextrose in water; administer 1 mg/min initially and titrate Patient needs constant monitoring	Immediate	Ganglionic blockade	Severe hypotension, tachyphylaxis, orthostatic effect, sympathetic blockade (urinary retention, constipation, ileus, pupillary dilatation), respiratory arrest (> 5 mg/min)	Second-choice agent in patients with aortic dissection, intracranial hemorrhage, or ischemic heart disease when sodium nitroprusside cannot be used
Nifedipine	Administer 10–20 mg sublingually or orally as a broken or chewed capsule	5–30 min	Calcium channel blocker	Hypotension, tachycardia, flushing	Drug of choice for hypertensive emergencies when invasive monitoring is not required; contraindicated in patients with aortic dissection
Labetalol	Administer 20–80 mg I.V. at 10-min intervals (maximum cumulative dose 300 mg)	Immediate	Nonselective beta blocker and alpha₁ blocker	Pressor response after previous beta-blocker treatment, nausea, paresthesia, headache, hypotension, bradycardia, bronchospasm, urinary retention, ? congestive heart failure	Experience limited; contraindicated for patients with asthma, heart failure, heart block greater than first degree, or bradycardia
Diazoxide	Give 150–300 mg rapid I.V. push or 50–150 mg I.V. every 5 min; to minimize overshoot hypotension, use 7.5–30 mg/min constant I.V. infusion instead Each dose after the first 300 mg should be preceded by furosemide, 40 mg I.V.	Immediate	Vasodilatation	↑ CO, ↑ HR, ↑ blood glucose, ↑ uric acid, Na⁺ retention; may precipitate angina and cardiac ischemia, nausea, postural hypotension, painful extravasation	Hypertensive encephalopathy, accelerated hypertension, eclampsia; not to be given to patients with ischemic heart disease, intracranial hemorrhage, or aortic dissection
Nicardipine	Administer 5 mg/hr by I.V. infusion and increase by 1–2 mg/hr every 15 min up to 15 mg/hr	1–5 min	Calcium channel blocker	Hypotension, headache, tachycardia, nausea, and vomiting	Similar to other calcium channel blockers; preferential vasodilatory effects; useful in patients who require careful detrition for the control of hypertension
Phentolamine mesylate	Administer 5–20 mg by I.V. bolus or 10–20 mg by I.M. injection	Immediate	Alpha blocker	Hypotension, tachycardia, vomiting, angina, nausea	Drug of choice in patients with pheochromocytoma and monoamine oxidase inhibitor–tyramine interaction; also useful for patients in whom severe hypertension develops after discontinuance of clonidine; short duration of action may require repeated boluses; can precipitate angina and myocardial ischemia in patients at risk
Hydralazine	Administer 5–10 mg I.V. or I.M.	15–30 min	Direct arteriolar vasodilatation	Tachycardia, flushing, angina	Associated with undesirable reflex tachycardia, which may be especially worrisome in patients with coronary artery disease; current usage restricted mostly to patients with renal insufficiency and toxemia
Clonidine	Initial dose 0.2 mg, then 0.1 mg every hr to a maximum of 0.7 mg	30–60 min	Central alpha-adrenergic agonist	Hypotension, sedation, dry mouth; blood pressure should be monitored for 4 hr after last dose	Especially useful in patients with severe hypertension (especially diastolic) without end-organ damage; useful in the emergency department and on the ward

CO—cardiac output   HR—heart rate

plications and a lower rate of respiratory compromise than longitudinal or midline incisions.[81] Other factors that increase the risk of postoperative pulmonary complications include age, underlying disease, malnutrition, and chronic obstructive pulmonary disease with subsequent colonization.[82,83]

A variety of preoperative, intraoperative, and postoperative respiratory treatments are available that may be valuable in preventing serious postoperative pulmonary complications. Preoperative treatment with incentive spirometry and chest physical therapy has been studied and appears to be of some value in improving patients' overall pulmonary status in preparation for operation.[84] Smoking should be discontinued, and underlying pulmonary infection such as bronchitis or pneumonia should always be treated and operation delayed if possible because the ciliary paralysis that occurs with the use of anesthetics has the potential for causing a severe pneumonia after operation.

Routine respiratory therapy is frequently used postoperatively to prevent pulmonary complications. Routine therapeutic measures include administration of bronchodilator aerosol or ultrasonic mist aerosol, IPPB, incentive spirometry, and oxygen therapy. However, some studies have questioned the value of many of these respiratory treatments.[85,86] One study demonstrated that a hospital-wide effort to reduce the use of specific respiratory therapy services did not adversely affect patient outcome.[87] For example, administration of beta agonists was successfully switched from air-driven aerosols to handheld nebulizers. The use of IPPB was almost completely eliminated, and treatment by incentive spirometry was reduced by 55%. The decrease in the use of incentive spirometry occurred in the late postoperative period, when, studies suggest, it is no longer of value. In patients at high risk, such as those undergoing upper abdominal operation, respiratory therapy is most beneficial when performed in the immediate postoperative period. Patients treated with incentive spirometry return more rapidly to preoperative pulmonary lung volumes than do untreated patients.[84] In this study, use of ultrasonic nebulization was also decreased markedly, whereas oxygen therapy was retained at about the same level.[87] Aerosol ultrasonic nebulization and mist aerosol are of little or no value.

Early mobilization after operation is believed to improve the patient's overall respiratory status. In several studies, early mobilization appeared to be as effective in improving overall respiratory status as chest physical therapy.[88,89] Early mobilization (i.e., turning every 2 hours) in coronary artery bypass patients was shown to decrease the incidence of atelectasis and pneumonia significantly. In high-risk patients, routine postoperative prophylactic chest physical therapy has been shown to decrease the frequency of pulmonary infection significantly.[90] However, in a study of children undergoing cardiac procedures, chest physical therapy had no effect on the development of pulmonary atelectasis.[91]

Atelectasis indicates pulmonary dysfunction and may also presage pneumonia. Postoperative pneumonia is an extremely serious complication and is a major cause of mortality on surgical services. Factors that increase the risk of postoperative pneumonia include advanced age, gram-negative bacterial infection, emergency operation, use of a ventilator, and postoperative peritonitis.

THROMBOEMBOLISM

Pulmonary Embolism

Pulmonary embolism is the most common fatal acute pulmonary disorder in hospitalized patients [*see VI:2 Thromboembolic Problems*]. In the United States, pulmonary embolism occurs in more than 250,00 patients each year[92]; mortality ranges from 8%

to 23%.[93] Approximately one third of deaths occur in the first hour after embolism; however, as many as 90% of patients survive long enough to be evaluated and for therapeutic intervention to be considered. Aggressive early anticoagulation therapy is associated with 90% survival. Up to 95% of pulmonary emboli originate in the deep veins of the leg; a small percentage originate in pelvic veins and at other sites. There have been reports of pulmonary emboli originating in veins of the upper extremities, but such cases are exceedingly uncommon.

Dyspnea is the most common symptom of pulmonary embolism and is usually of sudden onset. Dyspnea can be transient. The most common physical finding is tachypnea. Rales are present in 50% of cases. Circulatory collapse characterized by shock or syncope occurs in 20% of patients with pulmonary embolism and correlates with larger emboli. Although most patients with pulmonary embolism are hypoxemic, a P_aO_2 greater than 80 mm Hg was found in 10% of patients in the urokinase-streptokinase pulmonary embolus trial. The chest x-ray, although it may be abnormal, is commonly nondiagnostic. The most common abnormalities evident on the electrocardiogram are T wave inversion, nonspecific ST segment elevation or depression, and sinus tachycardia. Ventilation-perfusion scans are frequently valuable in ruling out pulmonary embolism in a patient with a clear chest x-ray, but some data cast doubt on the utility of a ventilation-perfusion scan result of low or intermediate probability.[93,94] If the lung scan is equivocal, pulmonary angiography should be performed. Pulmonary arterial pressures are routinely elevated in patients with significant pulmonary embolism. The role of spiral CT in the detection of pulmonary embolism has not yet been fully defined; its specificity is good, but its sensitivity is poor as a consequence of its inability to detect subsegmental emboli.[95]

Treatment of pulmonary embolism is supportive and includes administration of oxygen, adequate maintenance of fluid resuscitation, and rapid I.V. anticoagulation. If heparin is used, it is given in an 80 U/kg bolus, then infused at a rate of 18 U/kg/hr.[96] The partial thromboplastin time (PTT) is then adjusted according to a nomogram.[97] Low-molecular-weight heparin can be used for prophylaxis and treatment of both deep vein thrombosis (DVT) and pulmonary embolism.[98] Patients who cannot receive heparin[99] or other forms of prophylaxis or who exhibit continued or recurrent signs and symptoms of pulmonary embolus should be strongly considered for vena caval filter placement.[100] Some patients may benefit from thrombolytic therapy administered early, but this option is generally not available for postoperative patients.[101]

Deep Vein Thrombosis

Some degree of DVT develops in approximately 30% of patients after abdominal or thoracic procedures and in up to 80% of patients after hip procedures [*see VI:2 Thromboembolic Problems*]. Some reviews suggest that routine prophylaxis is justified in all surgical patients who are at high risk for DVT (e.g., those older than 40 years, obese patients, patients with malignant disease, patients with prior DVT or pulmonary embolism, or patients undergoing long, complicated operative procedures). Low-dose unfractionated heparin (5,000 units subcutaneously every 12 hours) should be given until the patient is ambulatory. Increasing the frequency of administration does not decrease the incidence of emboli but does increase the risk of hemorrhagic complications. The addition of dihydroergotamine to heparin may improve efficacy, but the risk associated with its vasoconstrictor effects may outweigh its potential benefits. Dextran in an initial dose of 10 ml/kg appears to be equally effective in decreasing the risk of pulmonary embolism but is more expensive.

Dextran 70 and dextran 40 appear to be equally efficacious. External pneumatic compression and gradient elastic stockings can also be employed to prevent DVT.

Findings from several reviews suggest that mortality from pulmonary embolism is decreasing and that effective prophylaxis with either subcutaneous heparin or pneumatic compression devices can decrease the risk of DVT and pulmonary embolism.[102-104] To achieve optimal results, prophylaxis must be started before the operative procedure begins.

CENTRAL VENOUS CATHETER COMPLICATIONS

Central venous catheters, arterial catheters, and triple-lumen catheters may be associated with such complications as perforation of the vascular system, thrombi, and infection. In one study, complications related to initial catheter placement occurred in 5.7% of patients, sepsis occurred in 6.5%, and mechanical complications occurred in 9%.[105,106] Complications of catheter placement are hemorrhage and pneumothorax. The most common late mechanical complications are major venous thrombosis and nursing mishaps. Central venous thrombophlebitis and sepsis usually necessitate immediate removal of the central venous catheter and antibiotic therapy. In some patients with Silastic catheters, treatment with I.V. antibiotics and anticoagulants and careful monitoring for potential exploration and drainage of perivascular infection or vein excision may be indicated.[105] Other studies have shown that administration of antibiotics through the indwelling catheter is effective. In one study of catheter-associated infections, 18 patients (86%) were cured without removal of the catheter. Absolute indications for catheter removal are lack of defervescence and continued positive blood cultures despite antibiotic therapy.[106] An effective method of assessing catheter contamination in patients with central lines in place is routine catheter exchange and culture [see VI:14 Nosocomial Infection]. Studies have shown a direct link between catheter infection and contamination of the site. To avoid mechanical complications, an x-ray should be obtained after insertion of any central line to document its position. The catheter should be evaluated every 2 to 7 days to ensure that it has not migrated or been displaced.

UPPER GASTROINTESTINAL BLEEDING

Before the advent of routine administration of antacids, life-threatening upper GI bleeding was a common problem in patients undergoing major stress, particularly in those with head injury, burns, or multiple trauma. A number of agents have been used for prophylaxis, including antacids, sucralfate, H_2 receptor antagonists, and proton pump inhibitors. The antacid regimen for bleeding prophylaxis is 30 to 60 ml by nasogastric tube every 1 to 2 hours to maintain gastric pH above 4. According to one study, sucralfate may also be effective for bleeding prophylaxis.[107] By comparison, H_2 receptor antagonists have not proved to be more effective than antacids in preventing major upper GI bleeding.[108,109] Agents that elevate gastric pH may increase the risk of nosocomial pneumonia by favoring gastric colonization.[110] Proton pump inhibitors significantly reduce rebleeding rates and offer an alternative to H_2 receptor antagonists.[111] With adequate prophylaxis, the incidence of massive upper GI bleeding is essentially zero.

POSTOPERATIVE TRANSFUSION AND ANEMIA

A decreased hematocrit and relative anemia occur very commonly after major operative procedures. In patients with these conditions, blood transfusion is often considered [see I:5 Bleeding and Transfusion]. It is important, however, to avoid unnecessary transfusions because of the potential for transfusion-associated complications, which include hemolytic transfusion reactions, nonhemolytic transfusion reactions, and transmission of infection (e.g., hepatitis, AIDS, cytomegalovirus, and herpesvirus). In addition, blood transfusion itself may be a significant immunodepressant.[112-115] In the past, it was typically considered reasonable to order a blood transfusion when the hematocrit measured 30% or less. Today, however, there are few, if any, situations in which this practice should be followed. For example, in a young healthy patient who has no other disease and is expected to continue to improve, hematocrits in the low to middle 20s are acceptable. This restrictive approach to red blood cell transfusion is as effective as, and possibly superior to, a liberal transfusion approach in ICU patients.[116] In addition, patients with a variety of other chronic diseases that lead to persistently low hematocrits (e.g., chronic renal insufficiency) have been safely observed at relatively low hematocrit levels without transfusion.

Alternatives to transfusion include autologous donation, hemodilution, cell-saving techniques, oxygen-carrying solutions (both perfluorocarbon-based and hemoglobin-based), and recombinant erythropoietin. Autologous donation, hemodilution, and cell saver techniques require considerable advanced planning and are not cost-effective for widespread use. Perfluorocarbon-based and hemoglobin-based oxygen-carrying solutions are, at present, still investigational.[117] Recombinant erythropoietin has been used in anemic medical patients since 1989 and in surgical patients since 1997.[118] The indications and end points for its use have not yet been fully defined.

DIABETES MELLITUS

The diabetic patient presents a series of management problems in the postoperative period. Careful management of blood glucose levels is necessary to avoid hypoglycemia or hyperglycemia with associated complications such as diabetic ketoacidosis and dehydration secondary to glycosuria. Diabetes has a significant negative impact on wound healing. For patients whose disease is managed by diet alone, additional measures are usually unnecessary. In the postoperative period, careful monitoring, including finger-stick glucose measurements every 6 hours, is appropriate, with a sliding scale of regular insulin administered as needed. In patients who are receiving oral hypoglycemic agents, the medication should be discontinued on the day before operation, and insulin should be given as needed for hyperglycemia. Patients who require insulin should be given a dextrose infusion and one half of the total daily dose of insulin as regular insulin the morning of the operation. Glucose is administered throughout the operation, as guided by measured glucose levels. In patients who require major operations and massive fluid administration, blood glucose should be measured frequently during operation, and insulin should be given I.V. as needed. Postoperatively, glucose levels in some patients will be well controlled by administration of insulin on a sliding scale based on finger-stick glucose monitoring.

Shock, major trauma, or extremely prolonged operations can lead to hypoperfusion of the skin and subcutaneous tissue. In these patients, subcutaneous administration of insulin is inappropriate and dangerous. Instead, monitoring in the ICU, with frequent glucose measurements, and treatment with I.V. insulin should be undertaken. Dextrose should be included in postoperative administration of fluids.

OTHER ENDOCRINE COMPLICATIONS

Another postoperative endocrine complication is hypothyroidism, which usually occurs in the elderly. Hypothyroidism is frequently associated with (1) a low temperature and (2) a low blood pressure that does not respond to fluid management or pressors. The elderly are also at risk for hyponatremia, hypoventilation, and hypoglycemia. In these cases, thyroid levels should be measured and intravenous thyroxine (200 to 500 µg) given. This dose should provide adequate thyroid levels for several days.

Postoperative hypoadrenocorticism occurs in patients who have been receiving oral or parenteral steroids. The stress of operation necessitates replacement with hydrocortisone (300 to 400 mg/day) or its equivalent. The suggested regimen is 100 mg I.V. every 8 hours on postoperative day 1 or 2, which should be rapidly tapered if the level of stress and the length of preoperative therapy allow it. In patients who are treated with steroids, the wound healing process is slowed. This deleterious effect can be reversed by administration of vitamin A (25,000 units orally or by nasogastric tube).

Discharge from Hospital and Follow-up Care

Discharge from the hospital is an important milestone in the postoperative care of a patient. For many patients who return home after their hospitalization, discharge represents a marker of major improvement. For other patients who have more complex problems and require significant care after hospital discharge, it is the beginning of a long and often difficult journey through a rehabilitation system or a skilled nursing facility.

The vast majority of patients admitted for elective surgery and most patients admitted for emergency surgery are discharged from the hospital back to their preoperative domicile. Patients with complex injuries (especially head injury), advanced malignancy, or significant disabilities or elderly patients may require placement in a facility rather than being sent home. In some cases, support from agencies in their community, such as home health care groups, may obviate placement in a nursing facility. There is evidence to suggest that well-developed family networks contribute significantly to a decreased risk of institutionalization.[119] A continuum of care services exists but may vary from one community to another [see Table 6]. A qualified medical social worker or discharge planner is invaluable in providing access to the various available options in each particular locale.

Most patients are discharged once the physician determines that they have met certain criteria: they must be medically stable and afebrile, tolerant of oral intake, ambulatory, and reasonably comfortable, and they must have wounds or drains that require only minimal care. The physician should then write discharge orders in the hospital chart to notify the nursing staff and the hospital administration [see Sidebar Sample Discharge Orders]. The discharge summary, written or dictated by the physician, should

---

Sample Discharge Orders

[Date and Time]
1. Discharge patient home.
2. Return to clinic in 1 wk to see Dr. Smith. Patient may call 919-555-4343 for questions or problems.
3. Prescriptions for discharge medications on the chart.
4. Instructions regarding wound care or care of drains: as indicated.
5. Activity: ambulatory.
6. Patient may bathe or shower.
7. Diet: regular as tolerated.
8. Work status: to be determined at follow-up appointment.
9. Discharge summary dictated.
[Physician's signature and ID number]

---

include information from the patient's history; data from physical examinations, laboratory tests, and radiographs; details of the hospital course; and full discharge plans. A copy of the discharge summary may be sent to the referring or family physician, or a personal letter can be forwarded to inform the physician of the patient's progress and plans for follow-up.

Certain patients, however, require significantly more sophisticated discharge planning. These include patients with severe multiple injuries (especially head injury), elderly patients with limited ability to care for themselves, patients with significant disabilities and functional impairment, patients with advanced malignancy, and patients with one or more significant socioeconomic difficulties, including homelessness, a history of substance abuse, or AIDS. Such patients will require either significant levels of support at home or placement in a care facility [see Table 7]. Discharge planning for these patients should begin as soon as possible after admission. Once such a patient is identified, the physician should notify a medical social worker or other hospital employee with experience in discharge planning and placement. Such early notification will permit planning for discharge and placement to proceed more efficiently. This is especially relevant for patients with complex needs, such as those requiring placement into a rehabilitation facility or those who have no insurance and who can perhaps be enrolled in Medicaid to provide them with financial support for placement.

DISCHARGE PLANNING

With today's emphasis on decreasing the length of hospitalizations, discharge planning has become a crucial part of the management of patient care in the inpatient setting. Even for the most complicated patient, the issue of a patient's disposition can be addressed from the moment of admission. Comprehensive discharge planning can reduce readmissions, lengthen the interval between discharge and readmission, and decrease the cost of providing health care.[120]

Early in a patient's admission, discharge planning primarily takes the form of assessment. All health care workers involved in the patient's care may provide input based on their interactions with patient and family. How a patient and family cope initially in a crisis and throughout the course of recovery can indicate the strength or weakness of the existing support system. Once a patient progresses beyond the initial crisis, more concrete information pertaining to the patient's financial resources, living situation, physical and emotional supports, and family dynamics is essential. This information is most often obtained by a social worker or trained discharge planner. Once the complete picture of the numerous facets of a patient's life outside of the hospital

---

Table 6 Care Services

In-home services	Community services
Telephone reassurance	Congregate meals
Emergency response systems	Senior centers
Home-delivered meals	Day care
Respite care	Retirement communities
Housekeeping/shopping services	Institutional services
Congregate housing	Family care home
Home health care	Rest home
Hospice care	Nursing home
	Intermediate care facility
	Skilled nursing facility

comes into focus, it can be compared with the new limitations and needs that may have resulted from the illness or injury that necessitated the hospitalization. One should always remember that functioning well in the hospital setting and being independent at home, work, or school can be dramatically different.

A number of options are available for acute care placement for those patients who have special care needs after discharge [see Table 7]. They fall into two categories: in-home care and extended care facilities.

In-Home Care

In-home care consists of home health services, private duty nurses, and community resources such as Meals on Wheels and transportation services. For patients who can be discharged home but require assistance or support, home health services represent an excellent alternative to continued hospitalization. Home health agencies can provide skilled nursing care, assistance in the home (homemakers or aides), physical therapy services, speech therapy services, occupational therapy services, and medical social worker support [see Table 8]. These patients must be otherwise independent, as home health agencies do not provide long periods of custodial care. Patients who require greater assistance must therefore either hire private duty nurses or consider an extended care facility as an alternative after discharge.

Home health agencies charge per service per visit. Charges for skilled therapies, such as skilled nursing, occupational therapy, and physical therapy, may cost up to $100 a visit or an hour. These fees are comparable to those charged in acute care facilities. Charges for nonskilled assistance range from a few dollars an hour to as high as $15 an hour. Services offered through home health providers are time limited under Medicare and Medicaid rules.

The use of home health services has increased dramatically over the past decade. Medicare data indicate that $2.1 billion was spent in 1988, compared with $15 billion in 1999. Between 1980 and 1997, home health care costs increased from $842/recipient to $6,595/recipient.[121]

Extended Care Facilities

Extended care facilities, such as rest homes, nursing homes, and rehabilitation centers, are often very successful in maximizing a patient's potential for independence. They offer more intensive skilled therapies than are offered by home health agencies and provide supervision and assistance with activities of daily living that can be difficult for working family members to provide. Rehabilitation facilities are distinguished from skilled nursing facilities primarily by the amount of activity an individual patient can endure. The standard amount of activity for a rehabilitation center is 3 to 4 hours a day, though this need not be constant activity. Physical therapists, occupational therapists, and speech therapists can assist in making judgments about a patient's endurance, potential, and goals for independence.

Patients who require assistance with convalescence that cannot be provided in their home setting are most often referred to a rest home facility. This is a relatively cost-effective alternative and is generally an intermediate step before the patient returns to a home setting.

Patients who require a higher level of care than that provided in either a rest home or through home health care require admission to a nursing home. A nursing home is either an intermediate care facility or a skilled nursing facility. At an intermediate care facility, registered nurses or licensed practical nurses are on duty for at least 4 hours a day to tend to patients' special medical needs; additional care is provided full time by trained staff who are not registered or practical nurses. Patients who require round-the-clock care from either a registered nurse or a licensed practical nurse must be admitted to a skilled nursing facility. Such patients include those who are potentially unstable or who may have a special need such

Table 7   Options for Acute Care after Hospital Discharge

Facility	Approximate Daily Cost ($)	Insurance Coverage	Services Offered
Rest home	40–60*	Medicaid Private payment plans	Convalescent care
Intermediate care facility	85–135*	Medicaid Private payment plans Medicare will cover skilled services but not room and board	Skilled nursing, 4 hr a day Other skilled services (e.g., physical and occupational therapy) only on contractual basis
Skilled nursing facility	100–150*	Medicaid Medicare (for 100 days) Some insurance plans Private payment plans	Skilled nursing, 24 hr a day Other skilled services (e.g., physical and occupational therapy) only on contractual basis; some provide in-house physical therapy
Subacute care facility	400–600	Medicare (for 100 days) Medicaid Some insurance plans Private payment plans	Skilled nursing, 24 hr a day Other skilled services often provided in-house Specialize in complex wound care and ventilator-dependent patients
Rehabilitation facility	800–1,000	Medicare Medicaid Some insurance plans Private payment plans	All skilled services (physical, occupational, and speech therapy) provided in-house Intensive therapy provided 3–5 hr a day
Acute care facility	1,000+	All current payor sources	Therapies provided on less frequent basis and for shorter duration than at rehabilitation facilities

*Includes only room and board; additional fees required for therapies and medications.
Prices reflect average cost in 1998 based on semiprivate room rates.

Table 8 Services Offered by Home Health Professionals

Skilled nursing
Injections
Ostomy care
Dressing changes
Catheter care
Observation
Instruction in medication/disease process
In-home management training
Hospice care
Respiratory care
Tracheotomy
Post–cataract surgery care
Instruction in diabetes care and monitoring

Home health aide/homemaker
Bathing
Meal assistance
Personal grooming
Ambulation assistance

Physical therapy
Muscle strengthening
Gait or prosthesis training
Training in ambulation and transfer techniques (e.g., bed to wheelchair)
Pulmonary exercises
Ultrasound treatments

Speech therapy
Retraining speech and language function
Developing alternative communication skills
Swallowing therapy

Occupational therapy
Preparation for independence in activities of daily living
Motor coordination improvement
Increase in upper extremity function

Medical social services
Disability assistance
Coordination of community resources

team provides care in a structured, graded fashion. Most rehabilitation centers will send a member of their team to assess a patient while the patient is still in the hospital to determine whether he or she is a candidate for admission. In general, for admission to a rehabilitation facility, the following criteria must be met:

1. Patients must be medically stable.
2. Patients must require an intensive rehabilitation program as offered by the multidisciplinary team. An intensive rehabilitation program is one in which the patient has a demonstrated need for round-the-clock nursing care and is capable of receiving 3 to 4 hours of physical, occupational, or speech therapy.
3. Patients must be able to participate actively in the rehabilitation process and should be able to follow at least simple commands, except in cases of severe brain injury or stroke.
4. The patient must have the potential for attaining significant functional improvement, with the expectation that he or she will return to an acceptable level of functional recovery.

Current trends in posthospital care focus on providing patient care at home and on shortening the length of acute hospital stays. Some skilled nursing facilities are able to provide complex care without the high cost associated with a stay in an acute care hospital. Services provided include ventilator support, I.V. drug therapy, care of advanced decubitus ulcers, total parenteral nutrition, tracheostomy care, and dialysis. These advanced care facilities are often referred to as subacute facilities. If a patient has relatively complex needs, such as ongoing wound care or a need for mechanical ventilation, then admission to a subacute facility would be required. Medicare will cover up to 100 days at such a facility, as will some insurance companies. Because of the generally sophisticated level of care, these facilities tend to have long waiting lists, as do many nursing homes. It is therefore crucial to begin seeking placement for such patients as early as possible in their hospital course to ensure bed availability.

Other Options

Hospice programs provide care for patients who are no longer seeking a cure but rather require care near the end of life. The majority of patients admitted to hospices have terminal illnesses as a result of disseminated malignancy. Hospice care provides the opportunity for patients to gain greater control over decisions regarding their care and allows the family to become more closely involved with the day-to-day progress of the patient. Hospices offer such specialized services as pain management and grief counseling. They are designed to allow patients in the last phase of an incurable illness to live at home or in equally comfortable surroundings for as long as possible. The program strives to keep patients as active as possible and provides them outlets for expressing their feelings in a supportive environment. The hospice team includes members of the family, nurses, social workers, physicians, clergy, and volunteers. Help is available to the patient on a continuous basis. Many of the services provided through the hospice system are covered under Medicare as long as the patient's physician and the hospice medical director certify that the patient is terminally ill, with a life expectancy of less than 6 months, and the hospice providing care is certified by Medicare. Physician services unrelated to hospice care continue to be provided for under standard Medicare Part B coverage.

Some pharmaceutical companies and home health agencies combine skills and efforts to provide I.V. drug therapies at home for patients who are otherwise independent and have adequate family support and assistance. For patients who require more aggressive physical therapy than can be provided at home, outpa-

as I.V. fluid administration or oxygen therapy. In addition, such patients may require advanced comprehensive support services such as physical and occupational therapy. Although physical and occupational therapy and related services can be provided at an intermediate care facility, a skilled nursing facility provides a more comprehensive approach to such needs. Both intermediate care and skilled nursing facilities require physician involvement for admission evaluation and supervision of subsequent care. Payment arrangements may vary among different settings, and such information should be obtained with the assistance of a social worker or other discharge planner. In general, Medicare will cover nursing home costs for a period of up to 100 days.

Rehabilitation facilities are ideally suited for patients who have complex problems that require comprehensive care and graded rehabilitation. They offer nursing services as well as physical, occupational, and speech therapy. They can also provide complex care services in addition to general rehabilitation, and many specialize in areas such as head injury, spinal cord injury, respiratory rehabilitation, stroke, burns, or advanced neurologic disorders. The goal of such centers is to allow patients to attain their maximum level of independence and reintegration into society. An interdisciplinary tient physical therapy at a local hospital or clinic may be a good option to enable the patient to live at home. This option, however, requires extensive family support to provide transportation to therapy and care in the home.

Services for Indigent Patients

Patients without insurance and with no available financial resources can present a difficult problem for discharge planners. Most home health agencies are mandated to set aside funds for indigent clients, but the services provided tend to be the bare minimum. Nursing homes and rehabilitation facilities have no such mandate, however. They set aside a limited number of beds for Medicare and Medicaid patients, but these tend to be in high demand and may represent a resource drain for these facilities. Patients who are not eligible for Medicare can sometimes be enrolled in Medicaid programs. Patients who are not eligible for Medicaid assistance will have to spend their private funds until they qualify for Medicaid. In general, adults are eligible for Medicaid if they are disabled, have dependent children, or have inadequate financial resources.

References

1. Greif R, Akca O, Horn EP, et al: Supplemental perioperative oxygen to reduce the incidence of surgical wound infection. N Engl J Med 342:161, 2000
2. Greif P, Lucing S, Rapf B, et al: Supplemental oxygen reduces the incidence of nausea and vomiting. Anesthesiology 91:1246, 1999
3. Cook DJ, Fuller HD, Guyatt GH, et al: Risk factors for gastrointestinal bleeding in critically ill patients. N Engl J Med 330:377, 1994
4. Recommendations for intensive care unit admission and discharge criteria. Task Force on Guidelines, Society of Critical Care Medicine. Crit Care Med 16:807, 1988
5. Wiedemann HP, Matthay MA, Matthay RA: Cardiovascular-pulmonary monitoring in the intensive care unit (pt 1). Chest 85:537, 1984
6. Critical care medicine. NIH Consensus Conference. JAMA 250:798, 1983
7. Wiedemann HP, Matthay MA, Matthay RA: Cardiovascular-pulmonary monitoring in the intensive care unit (pt 2). Chest 85:656, 1984
8. Burchard KW, Gann DS, Colliton J, et al: Ionized calcium, parathormone, and mortality in critically ill surgical patients. Ann Surg 212:543, 1990
9. Carr DB, Goudas LC: Acute pain. Lancet 353:2051, 1999
10. McQuay HJ, Moore RA, Justins D: Treating acute pain in hospital. BMJ 314:1531, 1997
11. Warfield CA, Kahn CH: Acute pain management: programs in US hospitals and experiences and attitudes among US adults. Anesthesiology 83:1090, 1995
12. American Pain Society Quality of Care Committee: Quality improvement guidelines for the treatment of acute pain and cancer pain. JAMA 274:1874, 1995
13. Kehlet H: Acute pain control and accelerated postoperative surgical recovery. Surg Clin North Am 79:431, 1999
14. Egbert LD, Battit GE, Welch CE, et al: Reduction of postoperative pain by encouragement and instruction of patients: a study of doctor-patient rapport. N Engl J Med 270:825, 1964
15. Gottschalk A, Smith DS, Jobes DR, et al: Preemptive epidural analgesia and recovery from radical prostatectomy: a randomized controlled trial. JAMA 279:1076, 1998
16. Kato J, Ogawa S, Katz J, et al: Effects of presurgical local infiltration of bupivacaine in the surgical field on postsurgical wound pain in laparoscopic gynecologic examinations: a possible preemptive analgesic effect. Clin J Pain 16:12, 2000
17. Rogers A, Walker N, Schug S, et al: Reduction of post-operative mortality and morbidity with epidural or spinal anesthesia: results from an overview of randomized trials. BMJ 321:1, 2000
18. Kehlet H: Acute pain control and accelerated postoperative surgical recovery. Surg Clin Nutr Am 79:431, 1999
19. Marks RM, Sachar EJ: Undertreatment of medical inpatients with narcotic analgesics. Ann Intern Med 78:173, 1973
20. Bollish SJ, Collins CL, Kirking DM, et al: Efficacy of patient-controlled versus conventional analgesia for postoperative pain. Clin Pharm 4:48, 1985
21. Graves DA, Foster TS, Batenhorst RL, et al: Patient controlled analgesia. Ann Intern Med 99:360, 1983
22. Bennett RL, Batenhorst RL, Bivins BA, et al: Patient-controlled analgesia: a new concept of postoperative pain relief. Ann Surg 195:700, 1982
23. Moore FD: Common patterns of water and electrolyte change in injury, surgery and disease. N Engl J Med 258:277, 1958
24. Moran WH Jr, Miltenberger FW, Shuayb WA, et al: Relationship of antidiuretic hormone secretion to surgical stress. Surgery 56:99, 1964
25. Ukai M, Moran WH Jr, Zimmerman B: The role of visceral afferent pathways on vasopressin secretion and urinary excretory patterns during surgical stress. Ann Surg 168:16, 1968
26. Ayus JC, Krothapalli RK, Arieff AI: Treatment of symptomatic hyponatremia and its relation to brain damage. N Engl J Med 317:1190, 1987
27. Arieff AI: Hyponatremia, convulsions, respiratory arrest, and permanent brain damage after elective surgery in healthy women. N Engl J Med 314:1529, 1986
28. Needleman P, Greenwald JE: Atriopeptin: a cardiac hormone intimately involved in fluid, electrolyte, and blood-pressure homeostasis. N Engl J Med 314:828, 1986
29. Putensen C, Mutz N, Pomaroli A, et al: Atrial natriuretic factor release during hypovolemia and after volume replacement. Crit Care Med 20:984, 1992
30. Virgilio RW, Rice CL, Smith DE, et al: Crystalloid vs. colloid resuscitation: is one better? Surgery 85:129, 1979
31. Foley EF, Borlase BC, Dzik WH, et al: Albumin supplementation in the critically ill. Arch Surg 125:739, 1990
32. Golub R, Sorrento JJ Jr, Cantu R Jr, et al: Efficacy of albumin supplementation in the surgical intensive care unit: a prospective, randomized study. Crit Care Med 22:613, 1994
33. Cochrane Injuries Group Albumin Reviewers: Human albumin administration in critically ill patients: systematic review of randomized controlled trials. BMJ 317:235, 1998
34. Shires GT, Canizaro PC: Fluid resuscitation in the severely injured. Surg Clin North Am 53:1341, 1973
35. Eisenberg PR, Jaffe AS, Schuster DP: Clinical evaluation compared to pulmonary artery catheterization in the hemodynamic assessment of critically ill patients. Crit Care Med 12:549, 1984
36. Connors AF, McCaffree DR, Gray BA: Evaluation of right-heart catheterization in the critically ill patient without acute myocardial infarction. N Engl J Med 308:263, 1983
37. Lobo DN, Bostock KA, Neal KR, et al: Effect of salt and water balance on recovery of gastrointestinal function after elective colonic resection: a randomised controlled trial. Lancet 359:1812, 2002
38. Dunham CM, Siegel JH, Weireter L, et al: Oxygen debt and metabolic acidemia as quantitative predictors of mortality and the severity of the ischemic insult in hemorrhagic shock. Crit Care Med 19:231, 1991
39. Siegel JH, Rivkind AI, Dalal S, et al: Early physiologic predictors of injury severity and death in blunt multiple trauma. Arch Surg 125:498, 1990
40. Rutherford EJ, Morris Jr JA, Reed GW, et al: Base deficit stratifies mortality and determines therapy. J Trauma 33:417, 1992
41. Davis JW, Shachford SR, MacKersie RC, et al: Base deficit as a guide to volume resuscitation. J Trauma 28:1464, 1988
42. Abramson D, Scalea TM, Hitchcock R, et al: Lactate clearance and survival following injury. J Trauma 35:584, 1993
43. Cheatham ML, Chapman WC, Key SP, et al: A meta-analysis of selective versus routine nasogastric decompression after elective laparotomy. Ann Surg 221:469, 1995
44. Dobbie RP, Hoffmeister JA: Continuous pump-tube enteric hyperalimentation. Surg Gynecol Obstet 143:273, 1976
45. Roubenoff R, Ravich WJ: Pneumothorax due to nasogastric feeding tubes: report of four cases, review of the literature, and recommendations for prevention. Arch Intern Med 149:184, 1989
46. Harris MR, Huseby JS: Pulmonary complications from nasoenteral feeding tube insertion in an intensive care unit: incidence and prevention. Crit Care Med 17:917, 1989
47. Trowbridge PE: A randomized study of cholecystectomy with and without drainage. Surg Gynecol Obstet 155:171, 1982
48. Payne DH, Fischgrund JS, Herkowitz HN, et al: Efficacy of closed wound suction drainage after single-level lumbar laminectomy. J Spinal Disord 9:401, 1996
49. Urbach DR, Kennedy ED, Cohen MM: Colon and rectal anastomosis do not require rectal drainage: a systematic review and meta-analysis. Ann Surg 229:174, 1999
50. Wihlborg O, Bergljung L, Martensson H: To drain or not to drain in thyroid surgery: a controlled clinical study. Arch Surg 123:40, 1988
51. Somers RG, Jablon LK, Kaplan MJ, et al: The use of closed suction drainage after lumpectomy and axillary node dissection for breast cancer: a prospective randomized trial. Ann Surg 215:146, 1992

52. Sobel JD, Kaye D: Urinary tract infections. Principles and Practice of Infectious Diseases, 2nd ed. Mandell GL, Douglas RG Jr, Bennett JE, Eds. John Wiley & Sons, New York, 1985

53. Benoist S, Panis Y, Denet C, et al: Optimal duration of urinary drainage after rectal resection: a randomized controlled trial. Surgery 125:135, 1999

54. Basse L, Werner M, Kehlet H: Is urinary drainage necessary during continuous epidural analgesia after colon resection? Reg Anesth Pain Med 25:498, 2000

55. Kovacevich GJ, Gaich SA, Lavin JP, et al: The prevalence of thromboembolic events among women with extended bed rest prescribed as part of the treatment for premature labor or preterm premature rupture of membranes. Am J Obstet Gynecol 182:1089, 2000

56. Convertino VA, Goldwater DJ, Sandler H: Effects of orthostatic stress on exercise performance after bedrest. Aviat Space Environ Med 53:652, 1982

57. Kehlet H, Mogensen T: Hospital stay of 2 days after open sigmoidectomy with a multimodal program. Br J Surg 86:227, 1999

58. Yeung RS, Buck JR, Filler RM: The significance of fever following operations in children. J Pediatr Surg 17:347, 1982

59. Galicier C, Richet H: A prospective study of postoperative fever in a general surgery department. Infect Control 6:487, 1985

60. Locker D, Norwood SH, Torma MJ, et al: A prospective randomized study of drained and undrained cholecystectomies. Am Surg 49:528, 1983

61. Trowbridge PE: A randomized study of cholecystectomy with and without drainage. Surg Gynecol Obstet 155:171, 1982

62. Soper DE: Delayed hemolytic transfusion reaction: a cause of late postoperative fever. Am J Obstet Gynecol 153:227, 1985

63. Lewis JH, Zimmerman HJ, Ishak KG, et al: Enflurane hepatotoxicity: a clinicopathologic study of 24 cases. Ann Intern Med 98:984, 1983

64. Siegman-Igra Y: Late postoperative fever-viral infection following multiple blood transfusion. Isr J Med Sci 19:267, 1983

65. Bernard GR, Vincent JL, Laterre PF, et al: Efficacy and safety of recombinant human activated protein C for severe sepsis. N Engl J Med 344:699, 2001

66. Slotman GJ, Jed EH, Burchard KW: Adverse effects of hypothermia in postoperative patients. Am J Surg 149:495, 1985

67. Valeri CR, Cassidy G, Khuri S, et al: Hypothermia-induced reversible platelet dysfunction. Ann Surg 205:175, 1987

68. Luna GK, Maier RV, Pavlin EG, et al: Incidence and effect of hypothermia in seriously injured patients. J Trauma 27:1014, 1987

69. Rutherford EJ, Fusco MA, Nunn CR, et al: Hypothermia in critically ill trauma patients. Injury 29:605, 1998

70. Ku J, Brasel KJ, Baker CC, et al: Triangle of death: hypothermia, acidosis, and coagulopathy. N Horizons 7:61, 1999

71. Lee TH, Marcantonio ER, Mangione CM, et al: Derivation and prospective validation of a simple index for prediction of cardiac risk of major noncardiac surgery. Circulation 100:1043, 1999

72. O'Kelly B, Browner WS, Massie B, et al: Ventricular arrhythmias in patients undergoing noncardiac surgery. JAMA 268:217, 1992

73. Fleisher LA, Eagle KA: Lowering cardiac risk in noncardiac surgery. N Engl J Med 345:1677, 2001

74. Pritchett ELC: Management of atrial fibrillation. N Engl J Med 326:1264, 1992

75. Salerno DM, Anderson B, Sharkey P, et al: Intravenous verapamil for treatment of multifocal atrial tachycardia with and without calcium pretreatment. Ann Intern Med 107:623, 1987

76. Calhoun DA, Oparil S: Treatment of hypertensive crisis. N Engl J Med 323:1177, 1990

77. Halpern NA, Goldberg M, Neely C, et al: Postoperative hypertension: a multicenter, prospective, randomized comparison between intravenous nicardipine and sodium nitroprusside. Crit Care Med 20:1637, 1992

78. Strandberg A, Tokics L, Brismar B, et al: Atelectasis during anaesthesia and in the postoperative period. Acta Anaesthesiol Scand 30:154, 1986

79. Ramsey-Stewart G: The perioperative management of morbidly obese patients (a surgeon's perspective). Anaesth Intensive Care 13:399, 1985

80. Ford GT, Whitelaw WA, Rosenal TW, et al: Diaphragm function after upper abdominal surgery in humans. Am Rev Respir Dis 127:431, 1983

81. Becquemin JP, Piquet J, Becquemin MH, et al: Pulmonary function after transverse or midline incision in patients with obstructive pulmonary disease. Intensive Care Med 11:247, 1985

82. Lawrence VA, Dhanda R, Hilsenbeck SG, et al: Risk of pulmonary complications after elective abdominal surgery. Chest 110:744, 1996

83. Mitchell CK, Smoger SH, Pfeifer MP, et al: Multivariate analysis of factors associated with postoperative pulmonary complications following general elective surgery. Arch Surg 133:194, 1998

84. Minschaert M, Vincent JL, Ros AM, et al: Influence of incentive spirometry on pulmonary volumes after laparotomy. Acta Anaesthesiol Belg 33:203, 1982

85. O'Donohue WJ Jr: National survey of the usage of lung expansion modalities for the prevention and treatment of postoperative atelectasis following abdominal and thoracic surgery. Chest 87:76, 1985

86. Pontoppidan H: Mechanical aids to lung expansion in non-intubated surgical patients. Am Rev Respir Dis 122:109, 1980

87. Zibrak JD, Rossetti P, Wood E: Effect of reductions in respiratory therapy on patient outcome. N Engl J Med 315:292, 1986

88. Morran CG, Finlay IG, Mathieson M, et al: Randomized controlled trial of physiotherapy for postoperative pulmonary complications. Br J Anaesth 55:1113, 1983

89. Castillo R, Haas A: Chest physical therapy: comparative efficacy of preoperative and postoperative in the elderly. Arch Phys Med Rehabil 66:376, 1985

90. Connors AF Jr, Hammon WE, Martin RJ, et al: Chest physical therapy: the immediate effect on oxygenation in acutely ill patients. Chest 78:559, 1980

91. Reines HD, Sade RM, Bradford BF, et al: Chest physiotherapy fails to prevent postoperative atelectasis in children after cardiac surgery. Ann Surg 195:451, 1982

92. Goldhaber SZ: Pulmonary embolism. N Engl J Med 339:93, 1998

93. Douketis JD, Kearon C, Bates S, et al: Risk of fatal pulmonary embolism in patients with treated venous thromboembolism. JAMA 279:458, 1998

94. Bone RC: Ventilation/perfusion scan in pulmonary embolism: "the emperor is incompletely attired" (editorial). JAMA 263:2794, 1990

95. Garg K: CT of pulmonary thromboembolic disease. Radiol Clin North Am 40:111, 2002

96. Hirsh J, Warkentin TE, Raschke R, et al: Heparin and low-molecular-weight heparin: mechanisms of action, pharmacokinetics, dosing considerations, monitoring, efficacy, and safety. Chest 114:489S, 1998

97. de Groot MR, Buller HR, ten Cate JW, et al: Use of a heparin nomogram for treatment of patients with venous thromboembolism in a community hospital. Thromb Haemost 80:70, 1998

98. Hirsh J, Warkentin TE, Shaughnessy SG, et al: Heparin and low-molecular-weight heparin: mechanisms of action, pharmacokinetics, dosing, monitoring, efficacy, and safety. Chest 119:64S, 2001

99. Laster J, Cikrit D, Walker N, et al: The heparin-induced thrombocytopenia syndrome: an update. Surgery 102:763, 1987

100. Greenfield LJ, Peyton R, Crute S, et al: Greenfield vena caval filter experience. Arch Surg 116:1451, 1981

101. Molina JE, Hunter DW, Yedlicka JW, et al: Thrombolytic therapy for postoperative pulmonary embolism. Am J Surg 163:375, 1992

102. Collins R, Scrimgeour A, Yusuf S, et al: Reduction in fatal pulmonary embolism and venous thrombosis by perioperative administration of subcutaneous heparin. N Engl J Med 318:1162, 1988

103. Clagett GP, Reisch JS: Prevention of venous thromboembolism in general surgical patients: a meta-analysis. Ann Surg 208:227, 1988

104. Geerts WH, Heit JA, Clagett GP, et al: Prevention of venous thromboembolism. Chest 119(1 suppl):132S, 2001

105. Wang EE, Prober CG, Ford-Jones L, et al: The management of central intravenous catheter infections. Pediatr Infect Dis 3:110, 1984

106. Verghese A, Widrich WC, Arbeit RD: Central venous septic thrombophlebitis—the role of medical therapy. Medicine (Baltimore) 64:394, 1985

107. Borrero E, Ciervo J, Chang JB: Antacid vs sucralfate in preventing acute gastrointestinal tract bleeding in abdominal aortic surgery: a randomized trial in 50 patients. Arch Surg 121:810, 1986

108. Shuman RB, Schuster DP, Zuckerman GR: Prophylactic therapy for stress ulcer bleeding: a reappraisal. Ann Intern Med 106:562, 1987

109. Cheung LY: Pathogenesis, prophylaxis, and treatment of stress gastritis. Am J Surg 156:437, 1988

110. Driks MR, Craven DE, Celli BR, et al: Nosocomial pneumonia in intubated patients given sucralfate as compared with antacids or histamine type 2 blockers. N Engl J Med 317:1376, 1987

111. Morgan D: Intravenous proton pump inhibitors in the critical care setting. Crit Care Med 30:S369, 2002

112. Opelz G, Terasaki PI: Dominant effect of transfusions on kidney graft survival. Transplantation 29:153, 1980

113. Blumberg N, Heal JM: Transfusion and host defenses against cancer recurrence and infection. Transfusion 29:236, 1989

114. Busch OR, Hop WC, Hoynck van Papendrecht MA, et al: Blood transfusions and prognosis in colorectal cancer. N Engl J Med 328:1372, 1993

115. Fong Y, Karpeh M, Mayer K, et al: Association of perioperative transfusions with poor outcome in resection of gastric adenocarcinoma. Am J Surg 167:256, 1994

116. Hebert PC, Wells G, Blajchman MA, et al: A multicenter, randomized, controlled clinical trial of transfusion requirements in critical care. N Engl J Med 340:409, 1999

117. Goodnough LT, Brecher ME, Kanter MH, et al: Transfusion medicine: blood conservation. N Engl J Med 340:525, 1999

118. Goodnough LT: Erythropoietin therapy versus red cell transfusion. Curr Opin Hematol 8:405, 2001

119. Freedman VA, Berkman LF, Rapp SR, et al: Family networks: predictors of nursing home entry. Am J Public Health 84:843, 1994

120. Naylor MD, Brooten D, Campbell R, et al: Comprehensive discharge planning and home follow-up of hospitalized elders: a randomized clinical trial. JAMA 281:613, 1999

121. Social Security Bulletin. Annual statistical supplement, 1997. Annu Stat Suppl Soc Secur Bull, Dec 1997, p 1

Acknowledgments

Figures 1a, 3 Tom Moore.
Figures 1b, 1c, 2 Courtesy Samir M. Fakhry, M.D.
The authors wish to thank Ms. Eva Powell, M.S.W., for her invaluable contributions to the section on hospital discharge planning.

2 POSTOPERATIVE PAIN

Henrik Kehlet, Prof. M.D., Ph.D., and F. Michael Ferrante, M.D.

Approach to the Patient with Postoperative Pain

Pain may usefully be classified into two varieties: acute and chronic. As a rule, postoperative pain is considered a form of acute pain, although it may become chronic if it is not effectively treated.

Postoperative pain consists of a constellation of unpleasant sensory, emotional, and mental experiences associated with autonomic, psychological, and behavioral responses precipitated by the surgical injury. Despite the considerable progress that has been made in medicine during the past few decades, the apparently simple problem of how to provide total or near total relief of postoperative pain remains largely unsolved. Pain management does not occupy an important place in academic surgery. However, government agencies have recently attempted to foster improved postoperative pain relief.[1,2]

Postoperative pain relief has two practical aims. The first is provision of subjective comfort, which is desirable for humanitarian reasons. The second is inhibition of trauma-induced nociceptive impulses to blunt autonomic and somatic reflex responses to pain and to enhance subsequent restoration of function by allowing the patient to breathe, cough, and move more easily. Because these effects reduce pulmonary, cardiovascular, thromboembolic, and other complications, they may lead secondarily to improved postoperative outcome.

Inadequate Treatment of Pain

A common misconception is that pain, no matter how severe, can always be effectively relieved by opioid analgesics. It has repeatedly been demonstrated, however, that in a high proportion of postoperative patients, pain is inadequately treated. This discrepancy between what is possible and what is practiced can be attributed to a variety of causes [see Table 1], which to some extent can be ameliorated by increased teaching efforts. In general, however, the scientific approach to postoperative pain relief has not been a great help to surgical patients in the general ward, where intensive surveillance facilities are not available.

Guidelines for Postoperative Pain Treatment

The recommendations provided below are aimed at surgeons working on the general surgical ward; superior regimens have been constructed by specialized groups interested in postoperative pain research, but these regimens are not currently applicable to the general surgical population, unless an acute pain service is available. Consideration is given to the efficiency of each analgesic technique, its safety versus its side effects, and the cost-efficiency problems arising from the need for intensive surveillance. For many of the recommendations, there are not sufficient data in the literature to form a valid scientific data base; accordingly, these recommendations are made on empirical grounds only.

THORACIC PROCEDURES

Pain after thoracotomy is severe, and pain therapy should therefore include a combination regimen, preferably of epidural local anesthetics and opioids plus systemic nonsteroidal anti-inflammatory drugs (NSAIDs). If the epidural regimen is not available, NSAIDs and systemic opioids should be given to obtain the documented synergistic-additive effect. Finally, cryoanalgesia is recommended because it is moderately effective, easy, and without side effects or considerable cost.

Pain after cardiac operation with sternotomy is less severe, and systemic opioids plus NSAIDs are recommended. The combined regimen of epidural local anesthetics and opioids is recommended when more effective pain relief is necessary.

ABDOMINAL PROCEDURES

Pain after major and upper abdominal operations is severe, and a combined regimen of epidural local anesthetics and opioids plus systemic NSAIDs is recommended because it has proved to be very effective and to have few and acceptable side effects. Furthermore, the epidural regimen will reduce postoperative pulmonary complications, as compared with treatment

---

Table 1 Contributing Causes of Inadequate Pain Treatment

Insufficient knowledge of drug pharmacology among surgeons and nurses

Uniform (p.r.n.) prescriptions

Lack of concern for optimal pain relief

Failure to give prescribed analgesics

Fear of side effects

Fear of addiction

---

with systemic opioids. Intrapleural local anesthetics may have some analgesic effect in unilateral procedures, but the combined epidural local anesthetic–opioid regimens are more effective.

After gynecologic operations, systemic opioids with NSAIDs are recommended except in patients in whom more effective pain relief is desirable. In such patients, the combined regimen of epidural local anesthetics and opioids is preferable, possibly in combination with systemic NSAIDs.

Pain following prostatectomy is usually not severe and may be treated with systemic opioids. However, blood loss and thromboembolic complications are reduced when epidural local anesthetics are administered. This method is therefore recommended intraoperatively and continued for pain relief after open prostatectomy and in selected high-risk patients undergoing transurethral resection. In other transurethral resection patients, systemic opioids, NSAIDs, or both provide postoperative pain alleviation.

PERIPHERAL PROCEDURES

After vascular procedures, postoperative pain control is probably best achieved with epidural local anesthetic–opioid mixtures, possibly combined with systemic NSAIDs. This regimen will be effective, and the increase in peripheral blood flow that is documented to occur with epidural local anesthetics may lower the risk of graft thrombosis.

Pain relief after major joint procedures (e.g., hip and knee operations) should also involve an epidural regimen because of the documented reduction in thromboembolic complications and in intraoperative blood loss. The severe pain after knee replacement is probably best treated with epidural local anesthetics combined with opioids. If epidural regimens are not available, combined treatment with systemic opioids and NSAIDs may provide moderately effective pain relief. After arthroscopic joint procedures, instillation of a local anesthetic and an opioid analgesic (e.g., morphine) provides effective early postoperative pain relief.

During superficial procedures, the use of systemic opioids combined with NSAIDs is sufficient. Transcutaneous electrical nerve stimulation (TENS) may have an additional effect during soft tissue procedures but cannot alone alleviate pain very effectively.

Treatment Modalities

PSYCHOLOGICAL INTERVENTIONS

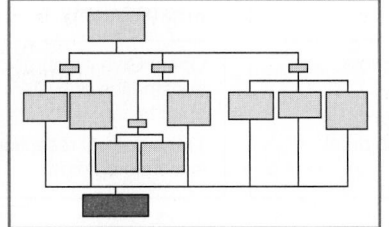

Individuals differ considerably in how they respond to noxious stimuli; much of this variance is accounted for by psychological factors. Cognitive, behavioral, or social interventions should be used in combination with pharmacological therapies to prevent or control acute pain, with the goal of such interventions being to guide the patient toward partial or complete self-control of pain.[3,4] Sophisticated psychological techniques, such as biofeedback and hypnosis therapy, are not applicable to a busy surgical unit, but simple psychological techniques are a valuable part of good medical practice.

Psychological preparation in patients with postoperative pain has been demonstrated to shorten hospital stay and to reduce postoperative narcotic use [see Table 2].[5] Psychological

Table 2 Psychological Preparation of Surgical Patients

Procedural information Give a careful and relevant description of what will take place

Sensory information Describe the sensations that will be experienced either during or after the operation

Pain treatment information Outline the plan for administering sedative and analgesic medication, and encourage patients to communicate concerns and discomforts

Instructional information Teach patients postoperative exercises, such as leg exercises, and show them how to turn in bed or move so that pain is minimal

Reassurance Reassure those who are mentally, emotionally, or physically unable to cooperate that they are not expected to take an active role in coping with pain and will still receive sufficient analgesic treatment

techniques should be combined with pharmacological or other interventions, but care must be taken to ensure that the pharmacological treatment does not compromise the mental function necessary for the success of the planned psychological intervention.

SYSTEMIC OPIOIDS

The terminology associated with the pharmacology of the opioids is confusing, to say the least. Opiate is an appropriate term for any alkaloid derived from the juice of the poppy plant (i.e., from opium). The proper term for the class of agents, whether exogenous, endogenous, natural, or synthetic, is opioid.

Mechanisms of Action

When administered for pain relief, opioids produce analgesia and other physiologic effects by binding to specific receptors in the central nervous system. These receptors normally bind a number of endogenous substances called opioid peptides. These receptor-binding interactions mediate a wide array of physiologic effects [see Table 3]. Five types of opioid receptors and their subtypes have been discovered: mu, delta, kappa, epsilon, and sigma receptors [see Table 3]. Most commonly used opioids bind to mu receptors. The mu_1 receptor is responsible for the production of opioid-induced analgesia, whereas the mu_2 receptor is responsible for the production of respiratory depression, cardiovascular effects, and the inhibition of the gastrointestinal motility commonly seen with the opioids.

The relation between receptor binding and the intensity of the resultant physiologic effect is known as the intrinsic activity of an opioid. Most of the commonly used opioid analgesics are agonists. An agonist produces a maximal biologic response by binding to its receptor. Other opioids, such as naloxone, are termed antagonists because they compete with agonists for opioid receptor binding sites. Still other opioids are partial agonists because they produce a submaximal response after binding to the receptor. (An excellent example of a submaximal response produced by partial agonists is buprenorphine's action at the mu receptor.)

Drugs such as nalbuphine, butorphanol, and pentazocine are known as agonist-antagonists or mixed agonist-antagonists.[6] These opioids simultaneously act at different receptor

Approach to the Patient with Postoperative Pain

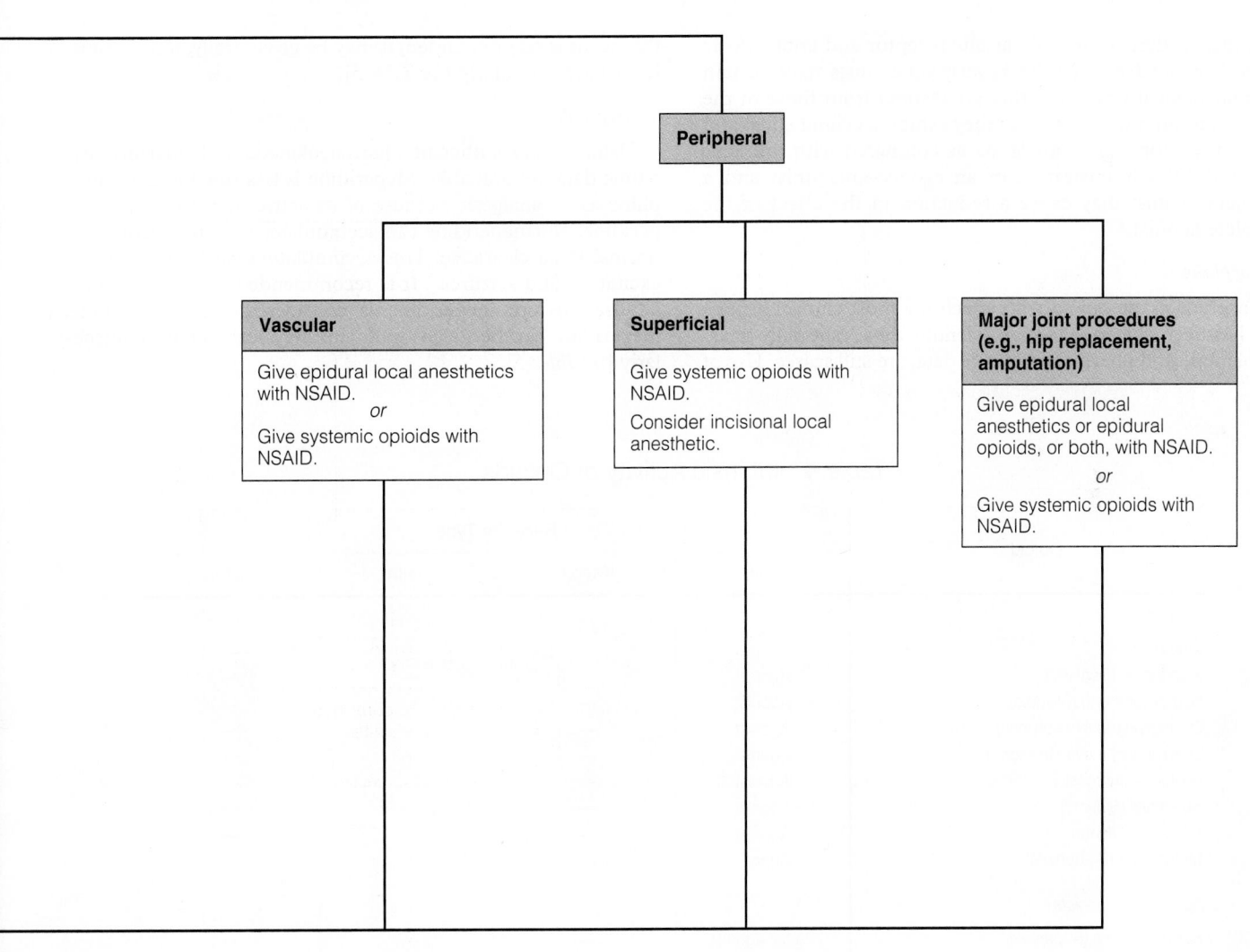

Table 3 Opioid Receptor Types and Physiologic Actions

Receptor Type	Prototypical Ligand		Physiologic Actions
	Endogenous	Exogenous	
Mu$_1$	β-Endorphin	Morphine	Supraspinal analgesia
Mu$_2$	β-Endorphin	Morphine	Respiratory depression
Delta	Enkephalin	—	Spinal analgesia
Kappa	Dynorphin	Ketocyclazocine	Spinal analgesia, sedation
Epsilon	β-Endorphin	—	Hormone?
Sigma	—	N-Allylnormetazocine	Psychotomimetic effect, dysphoria

sites; their action is agonistic at one receptor and antagonistic at another [*see Table 4*]. The agonist-antagonists have certain pharmacological properties that are distinct from those of the more common mu agonists: (1) they exhibit a ceiling effect and cause only submaximal analgesia as compared with mu agonists and (2) administration of an agonist-antagonist and a complete agonist may cause a reduction in the effect of the complete agonist.[6]

Morphine

Morphine is the opioid with which the most clinical experience has been gained, although scientific data, especially pharmacokinetic and pharmacodynamic data, are still scarce. Use of this agent is recommended; it may be given orally, intravenously, or intramuscularly [*see Table 5*].

Meperidine

Detailed and sufficient pharmacokinetic and pharmacodynamic data are available. Meperidine is less suitable than morphine as an analgesic because of its active metabolite, normeperidine. Normeperidine can accumulate, even in patients with normal renal clearance. This accumulation can result in CNS excitation and seizures.[7] It is recommended that other agents be used before meperidine is considered.[2] Like morphine, meperidine can be given orally, intravenously, or intramuscularly [*see Table 5*].

Table 4 Intrinsic Activity of Opioids

Opioid	Receptor Type			
	Mu	Kappa	Delta	Sigma
Agonists				
Morphine	Agonist	—	—	—
Meperidine (Demerol)	Agonist	—	—	—
Hydromorphone (Dilaudid)	Agonist	—	—	—
Oxymorphone (Numorphan)	Agonist	—	—	—
Levorphanol (Levo-Dromoran)	Agonist	—	—	—
Fentanyl (Duragesic)	Agonist	—	—	—
Sufentanil (Sufenta)	Agonist	—	—	—
Alfentanil (Alfenta)	Agonist	—	—	—
Methadone (Dolophine)	Agonist	—	—	—
Agonist-Antagonists				
Buprenorphine (Buprenex)	Partial agonist	—	—	—
Butorphanol (Stadol)	Antagonist	Agonist	Agonist	—
Nalbuphine (Nubain)	Antagonist	Partial agonist	Agonist	—
Pentazocine (Talwin)	Antagonist	Agonist	Agonist	—
Dezocine (Dalgan)	Partial agonist	—	—	Agonist
Antagonists				
Naloxone (Narcan)	Antagonist	Antagonist	Antagonist	Antagonist

Table 5 Suggested Regimens for
Systemic Opioid Administration

Intermittent Administration (Suggested Initial Dose)*				
	p.o.	I.M.	I.V.	Duration (hr)
Morphine	30–50 mg	10 mg	5–10 mg	3–4
Meperidine	300 mg	75–100 mg	25–50 mg	2–4
Buprenorphine	0.4 mg (sublingual)	0.3 mg	0.3 mg	6–8

Continuous I.V. Infusion†	
Morphine	$\approx$ 3 mg/hr (loading dose: 5–10 mg)
Meperidine	$\approx$ 25 mg/hr (loading dose: $\approx$ 25–50 mg)

*Number of doses to be given is calculated with the following formula:

$$\frac{24\ hr}{actual\ duration\ of\ single\ effective\ dose\ (hr)}$$

Single doses should be given at calculated fixed intervals approximately 30 min before expected recurrence of pain. Single dose should be readjusted daily. Elderly patients may be more susceptible to opioids.

†Dose should be adjusted according to effect and side effects.

Methadone

Methadone has a half-life of about 35 hours, and it relieves pain for a comparably long period. Because one dose is effective for so long, there is an increased risk of accumulation if further doses are given. This risk notwithstanding, a single 20 mg dose of methadone may be useful after relatively minor procedures that result in fairly short periods of postoperative pain.[8]

Buprenorphine

Buprenorphine is a mixed agonist-antagonist analgesic with a longer duration of action than morphine.[9] Unlike morphine, it is only partially antagonized by naloxone; however, doxapram, 1.0 to 1.5 mg/kg I.V., is effective. Sublingual and injectable preparations are available [*see Table 5*].[10] Buprenorphine may lead to respiratory depression with repetitive dosing.

Side Effects

By depressing or stimulating the CNS, opioids cause a number of physiologic effects in addition to analgesia. The depressant effects of opioids include analgesia and altered respiration and mood. The excitatory effects of opioids include nausea, vomiting, and miosis.

All mu agonists produce a dose-dependent decrease in the responsiveness of brain stem respiratory centers to increased carbon dioxide tension (PCO_2).[11] This is clinically manifested as an increase in resting PCO_2 and a shift in the CO_2 response curve. Agonist-antagonist opioids have a limited effect on the brain stem and appear to elicit a ceiling effect on increases in PCO_2.[6,12]

Opioids also have effects on the gastrointestinal tract. Nausea and vomiting are caused by stimulation of the chemoreceptor trigger zone of the medulla. Opioids enhance sphincteric tone and reduce peristaltic contraction. Delayed gastric emptying is caused by decreased motility, increased antral tone, and increased tone in the first part of the duodenum. Delay in passage of intestinal contents because of decreased peristalsis and increased sphincteric tone leads to greater absorption of water, increased viscosity, and desiccation of bowel contents, which cause constipation. Opioids also increase biliary tract pressure.[12,13]

EPIDURAL AND SUBARACHNOID OPIOIDS

Opioids were first used in the epidural and subarachnoid space in 1979. Since that time, they have become the mainstay of postoperative pain management. Epidural opioids may be administered in a single bolus or in continuous infusions. They are usually combined with local anesthetic in a continuous epidural infusion.

Mechanisms of Action

Opioids injected into the epidural or subarachnoid space cause segmental (i.e., selective, spinally mediated) analgesia by binding to opioid receptors in the dorsal horn of the spinal cord. The lipid solubility of an opioid, described by its partition coefficient, predicts its behavior when administered to the epidural or subarachnoid space. Opioids with low lipid solubility (i.e., hydrophilic opioids) have a slow onset of action and a long duration of action. Opioids with high lipid solubility (i.e., lipophilic opioids) have a quick onset of action but a short duration of action [*see Table 6*]. Thus, the lipid solubility of an opioid determines its access to the dorsal horn via (1) diffusion through the arachnoid granulations and (2) diffusion into spinal radicular artery blood flow.[14-16]

Subarachnoid opioids should be used when the required duration of analgesia after surgery is relatively short. When protracted analgesia is required, epidural administration is preferred; repeated injections may be given through epidural catheters, or continuous infusions may be used. Smaller doses of subarachnoid opioids are generally required to produce analgesia. Ordinarily, no more than 0.25 to 0.50 mg of morphine should be used. This range provides reliable pain relief with few side effects. These doses are about one tenth to one fifth that of effective epidural morphine doses. Fentanyl has also been extensively used in the subarachnoid space in a dose range of 6.25 to 50 μg. Pain relief after administration of subarachnoid fentanyl is as potent but not as prolonged as analgesia after administration of morphine.[15]

Regimens for Acute Pain Relief

Most studies agree that at least 2 mg of epidural morphine is needed to achieve a significant analgesic response [see Table 6], but the criteria used to assess this response have varied greatly in reported studies, and no firm conclusion can be derived from them.[16,17] Epidural opioids are less efficient in the earliest stages of the acute pain state than on subsequent days; moreover, they appear to be more successful at alleviating pain after procedures in the lower half of the body than at alleviating upper abdominal and thoracic pain.[16] In general, 2 to 4 mg of morphine epidurally is sufficient after minor procedures, whereas about 4 mg is needed after vascular and gynecologic procedures and about 4 to 6 mg after major upper abdominal and thoracic procedures.[17-19] On the first postoperative day, however, such a regimen, even when repeated as many as three times, relieves pain completely in fewer than 50 percent of patients in contrast to an increased success rate on subsequent days. Its efficiency will be lowest after major procedures.

Information now suggests that use of continuous epidural morphine in low dosages (0.1 to 0.3 mg/hr) may lower the risk of late respiratory depression and may be more efficient than intermittent higher dosages of morphine.[20-22] It is therefore recommended.

Side Effects

The chief side effects associated with epidural and subarachnoid opioids are respiratory depression, nausea and vomiting, pruritus, and urinary retention.[14-16,23,24] The poor lipid solubility of morphine is responsible for its protracted duration of action but also allows morphine to undergo cephalad migration in the cerebrospinal fluid. This migration can cause delayed respiratory depression with a peak incidence three to 10 hours after an injection.[16,23,24] The high lipid solubility of lipophilic opioids such as fentanyl allows them to be absorbed into lipids close to the site of administration. Consequently, the lipophilic opioids do not migrate rostrally in the CSF and cannot cause delayed respiratory depression. Of course, the high lipid solubility of lipophilic opioids allows them to be absorbed into blood vessels, which may cause early respiratory depression, as is commonly seen with systemic administration of opioids.[14-16]

Naloxone reverses the depressive respiratory effects of spinal opioids. In an apneic patient, 0.4 mg administered intravenously will usually restore ventilation. If a patient has a depressed respiratory rate but is still breathing (i.e., one to four breaths a minute), small aliquots of naloxone (0.04 mg) can be given until the respiratory rate returns to normal. Because naloxone has a short half-life, it is best to start a continuous infusion of naloxone at a rate of 5 mg/kg/hr to prevent respiratory depression from recurring.[15]

Nausea and vomiting are caused by transport of opioids to the vomiting center and the chemoreceptor trigger zone in the medulla via CSF flow or systemic circulation.[15] Nausea can usually be treated with antiemetics, naloxone (small increments of 0.04 to 0.10 mg followed by infusion of 1 mg/kg/hr I.V.), and agonist-antagonist opioids (e.g., butorphanol, 0.25 to 0.50 mg, or nalbuphine 2.5 to 5.0 mg).[15]

Pruritus is probably the most common side effect of the spinal opioids. Histamine is released by certain opioids, but this mechanism probably plays a negligible role in the genesis of itching. The production of spinal opioid–induced pruritus is probably caused by changes in the electrophysiology of neurons of the dorsal horn.[23] The treatment of pruritus is similar to that of nausea.

The mechanism of spinal opioid–induced urinary retention involves inhibition of volume-induced bladder contractions and blockade of the vesical reflex.[24] Naloxone administration is the treatment of choice, though bladder catheterization is sometimes required.

EPIDURAL LOCAL ANESTHETICS AND OTHER REGIONAL BLOCKS

Local anesthetics have gained increasing popularity because of the growing familiarity with the techniques of both epidural catheterization and regional nerve blocks.[17,25] In addition, there is a great deal of experimental evidence that documents the benefits of blocking noxious impulses.[26,27] Local anesthetic neural blockade is unique among available analgesic techniques in that it may offer complete afferent neural blockade, resulting in relief of pain; inhibition of the stress response; reduction in the cardiorespiratory effects of severe pain; avoidance of sedation, respiratory depression, and nausea; and, finally, efferent sympathetic blockade resulting in increased blood flow to the region

Table 6 Dosage Regimens for Epidural Opioids

Drug	Lipid Solubility*	Bolus Dose	Onset (min)	Duration (hr)	Comments
Morphine	1	2–5 mg	30–60	6–24	Because of spread in CSF, preferred when incisions are extensive and injection site is distant from source of pain
Diamorphine	10	4–6 mg	5	10–12	
Meperidine (Demerol)	30	35–50 mg	5–10	6–8	
Methadone (Dolophine)	100	1–10 mg	10	6–10	May accumulate in blood with repeated dosing
Fentanyl (Duragesic)	800	50–100 μg	5	4–6	Not recommended when incision is extensive or injection site is distant from source of pain
Sufentanil (Sufenta)	1,500	10–60 μg	5	2–4	Higher doses may produce excessive sedation or ventilatory depression, presumably because of vascular uptake

*Octanol/pH 7.4 buffer partition coefficient relative to morphine.

of neural blockade.[25-27] Despite the considerable scientific data documenting these beneficial effects, the place of epidural local anesthesia as a method of pain relief remains somewhat controversial in comparison with that of other analgesic techniques; side effects, such as hypotension, urinary retention, and motor blockade, combined with the need for trained staff for surveillance, argue against its use. However, the risk of these side effects can be reduced by use of combination regimens (see below).

Mechanism of Action

Local anesthetic neural blockade is a nondepolarizing block that reduces the permeability of cell membranes to sodium ions.[28] Whether different local anesthetics have different effects on different nerve fibers is debatable.

Choice of Drug

For optimal management of postoperative pain, the anesthetic agent should provide excellent analgesia of rapid onset and long duration without inducing motor blockade. The various local anesthetic agents all meet one or more of these criteria, but it is bupivacaine that comes closest to meeting all of them. This should not preclude the use of other agents, because their efficacy has also been demonstrated.

Continuous Epidural Analgesia

No regimen has been found that provides complete analgesia in all patients all of the time, and it is unlikely that one ever will be found. As a rule, the block should be limited to the area in which pain is felt. Care should be taken to avoid motor blockade and to spare autonomic function to the urinary bladder, as well as to formulate a regimen that requires only minimal attention from staff members and carries no significant toxicity. Given these requirements, continuous infusion is more effective and reliable than intermittent injection [*see Table 7*]. Whether low hourly volume and high concentration approaches are preferable

Table 8 Procedures for Maintenance of Epidural Anesthesia for Longer Than 24 Hours

1. Administer appropriate drug in appropriate dosage at selected infusion rate as determined by physician.
2. Nurse evaluates vital signs and intake and output as required for a postoperative patient.
3. Nurse checks infusion pump hourly to ensure that it is functioning properly, that infusion rate is proper, and that alarm is on.
4. Nurse also assesses
   - Bladder—for distention, if patient is not catheterized
   - Lower extremities—for status of motor function
   - CNS—for signs of toxicity or respiratory depression
   - Relief of pain (drug dosage may require modification)
   - Skin integrity on back (breakdown may occur if motor function is not present)
   - Tubing and dressing (disconnection of tubing or dislodgment of catheter may occur)
5. Every 48 hr, the catheter dressing should be removed, the catheter entrance site cleaned, and topical antibiotic applied (much as in care of a central venous catheter)

to high hourly volume and low concentration approaches remains to be determined. The weaker solutions may produce less motor blockade while continuing to block smaller C and A-delta pain fibers and are recommended in lumbar epidural analgesia as a means of reducing the risk of orthostatic hypotension and lower extremity motor blockade.[25]

Specific indications for continuous epidural analgesia that are supported by data from controlled morbidity studies include (1) pain relief and reduction of deep venous thrombosis and of pulmonary embolism and hypoxemia after total hip replacement and prostatectomy; (2) pain relief, facilitation of coughing, and reduction of chest infections after thoracic, abdominal, and orthopedic procedures; (3) pain relief, control of hypertension, and enhancement of graft flow after major vascular operations; and (4) pain relief and reduction of paralytic ileus after abdominal procedures.[27,29]

Side Effects

The main side effects of epidural local anesthesia are hypotension caused by sympathetic blockade, vagal overactivity, and decreased cardiac function (during a high thoracic block). Under no circumstances should epidural local anesthetics be used before a preexisting hypovolemic condition is treated. Hypotension may be treated with ephedrine, 10 to 15 mg I.V., and fluids, with the patient tilted in a head-down position. Atropine, 0.5 to 1.0 mg I.V., may be effective during vagal overactivity.

Urinary retention occurs in 20 to 100 percent of patients. Fortunately, urinary catheterization for only 24 hours in the course of a high-dose regimen probably has no important side effects, and many patients for whom epidural analgesia is indicated need an indwelling catheter for other reasons in any case. The incidence of urinary retention is below 10 percent when epidural local anesthetics are used in weak solutions [*see Table 8*]. Motor blockade may delay mobilization; however, its incidence can be reduced by using the weakest concentration of local anesthetic that is compatible with adequate sensory blockade. Cerebral and cardiovascular toxicity are seldom encountered, and epidural hematoma

Table 7 Regimen for Pain Relief with Continuous Epidural Bupivacaine during the Initial 24 Postoperative Hours

Type of Operation	Interspace for Catheter Insertion	Concentration (%)	Volume (ml/hr)
Thoracic procedures	T4–6	0.250–0.125	5–10
Upper laparotomy	T7–8	0.250–0.125	4–12
Gynecologic laparotomy	T10–12	0.250–0.125	4–10
Hip procedures	L2	0.125–0.0625	4–8
Vascular procedures	T10–12	0.250–0.125	4–10

Note: indications for postoperative epidural bupivacaine may be strengthened if this method is also indicated for intraoperative analgesia. Dosage requirements may vary and should be assessed 3 hr after the start of treatment, every 6 hr thereafter on the first day, and then every 12 hr (more often if pain occurs). The duration of treatment is 1–4 days, depending on the intensity of the pain. The concentration of bupivacaine employed should be the lowest possible and should be decreased with time postoperatively. Some patients, especially those who have undergone major upper abdominal operation, require 0.5 percent bupivacaine initially.

and abscess are extremely rare. Epidural analgesia should not be employed in patients already receiving anticoagulant therapy, but it may be started with catheter insertion before vascular or other procedures in which controlled heparin therapy is used. Epidural analgesia has been used in patients receiving thromboembolic prophylaxis with low-dose heparin or low-molecular-weight heparin without significantly increased risk.[30,31] The complications associated with the epidural catheter are minimal when proper nursing protocols are followed [see Table 8]. The decision to employ epidural local anesthetics in such patients should be made only after the risks are carefully compared with the documented advantages of such anesthetics.[25-27]

Other Nerve Blocks

The popularity of single-dose intercostal block and intrapleural regional analgesia has decreased in comparison with that of continuous epidural treatment. Intermittent or continuous administration of bupivacaine through a catheter inserted into the intercostal space seems to be a promising approach to providing anesthesia after abdominal procedures, but further data are needed.[32] Intravenous and intraperitoneal administration of local anesthetics cannot be recommended, because they are not efficacious. Intraincisional administration of bupivacaine, which has negligible side effects and demands little or no surveillance, is recommended in shorter procedures[33] but should receive additional study. More detailed information on special blocks can be found in the anesthesiology literature.

In general, despite its disadvantages, neural blockade with local anesthetics is recommended for relief of postoperative pain because of the advantageous physiologic effects it exerts and the reduction in postoperative morbidity it brings about.

NONSTEROIDAL ANTI-INFLAMMATORY DRUGS

NSAIDs are minor analgesics that, because of their anti-inflammatory effect, may be suitable for management of postoperative pain associated with a significant degree of inflammation, such as bone or soft tissue damage. However, they may also have central analgesic effects and may therefore have analgesic efficacy after all kinds of operations. Only a few of them may be given parenterally. The data now available on the use of NSAIDs for postoperative pain are insufficient to allow definitive recommendation of any agent or agents over the others, and selection may therefore depend on convenience of delivery, duration, and cost.[34,35] It is clear, however, that they may play a valuable role as adjuvants to other analgesics—in particular because of their ability to reduce platelet adhesion. All the NSAIDs, except acetaminophen, have a potentially serious side effect: gastrointestinal hemorrhage. Fortunately, this effect is probably of minor importance during short-term postoperative treatment,[35] and it may be further minimized by intravenous, intramuscular, or rectal administration.

The NSAIDs exert their anti-inflammatory effect by inhibiting prostaglandin synthesis at the wound site (and probably also in the CNS), thereby decreasing the release of local inflammatory agents. Because prostaglandins are important for regulation of water and mineral homeostasis by the kidneys[36] in the dehydrated patient, perioperative treatment with NSAIDs may lead to postoperative renal failure. Although little systematic evaluation has been done, extensive clinical experience with these drugs suggests that this risk is not substantial.[34,35] Nonetheless, NSAIDs should be used with caution in patients who have preexisting renal dysfunction.

Although NSAIDs may also prolong bleeding time and inhibit platelet aggregation, increased bleeding does not seem to be a clinically significant risk.[34,35] However, in procedures where strict hemostasis is critical (e.g., cosmetic surgery and eye surgery), these drugs should be given with caution.

Despite the gaps in our current understanding of the workings of NSAIDs, what is known is sufficiently encouraging to suggest that NSAIDs probably should be recommended for baseline analgesic treatment after most operative procedures, except in the earliest part of the postoperative period immediately after heparinization during cardiovascular procedures [see Table 9]. NSAIDs are a valuable component of multimodal pain treatment (see below) and may be of special value in patients undergoing short operations (e.g., laparoscopic procedures) in whom opioid-sparing effects may reduce postoperative nausea and vomiting. Until further data can be obtained on safety and efficacy, four of the available NSAIDs are recommended: acetylsalicylic acid, acetaminophen, indomethacin, and ibuprofen.

CRYOANALGESIA

Cryoanalgesia is the application of low temperatures (−20° to −29° C) to peripheral nerves with the goal of producing axonal degeneration and thus analgesia [see Figure 1].[37] Axonal regeneration takes place at a rate of 1 to 3 mm/day, which means that analgesia after intercostal blocks lasts about 30 days. Cryoanalgesia has no cardiac, respiratory, or cerebral side effects, and local side effects (e.g., neuroma formation) are extremely rare. However, it can be used only on sensory nerves or on nerves supplying muscles of no clinical importance. At present, no information is available on the use of cryoanalgesia in operative procedures other than thoracotomy and herniotomy. Whereas the significance of the data on inguinal nerve cryoanalgesia after herniotomy is debatable, the data on postthoracotomy cryoanalgesia indicate improved pain alleviation and a concomitant reduction in the need for narcotics.[38-41] Furthermore, combining cryoanalgesia with administration of indomethacin may yield an additive analgesic effect after thoracotomy.[42]

The positive results after thoracotomy, together with the simplicity and low cost of the modality and the absence of side effects, present a strong argument for more extensive use of cryoanalgesia.

TRANSCUTANEOUS ELECTRICAL NERVE STIMULATION

Transcutaneous electrical nerve stimulation is the application of a mild electrical current through the skin surface to a specific area, such as a surgical wound, to achieve pain relief; the exact mechanism whereby it achieves this effect is yet to

Table 9 Recommended Dosages of Nonsteroidal Anti-inflammatory Drugs (NSAIDs) for Relief of Postoperative Pain

NSAID	Dosage
Acetylsalicylic acid	500–1,000 mg q. 4–6 hr
Acetaminophen	500–1,000 mg q. 4–6 hr
Indomethacin	50–100 mg q. 6–8 hr
Ibuprofen	200–400 mg q. 4–6 hr
Ketorolac	30 mg q. 4–6 hr

be explained. Many TENS devices are available for clinical use, but the specific value and the proper use of the various stimulation frequencies, waveforms, and current intensities have not been determined; however, most would agree that a high-frequency (50 to 100 Hz), low-intensity (12 to 20 mA at 1,000 Ω) current with an asymmetric biphasic waveform is the most effective current.[43] Whereas TENS has been shown to be effective in reducing postoperative pain and narcotic requirements after knee, hip, and low-back operations,[43] results after abdominal, herniotomy, and thoracic procedures are inconclusive. The effect of TENS on acute pain is too small to warrant a recommendation for routine use.

PATIENT-CONTROLLED ANALGESIA

Patient-controlled administration of opioids has experienced a dramatic increase in use. This increased use may be attributed to (1) awareness of the inadequacy of traditional I.M. opioid regimens, (2) the development of effective and safe biotechnology, and (3) the widespread patient satisfaction with patient-controlled analgesia (PCA).[44-46]

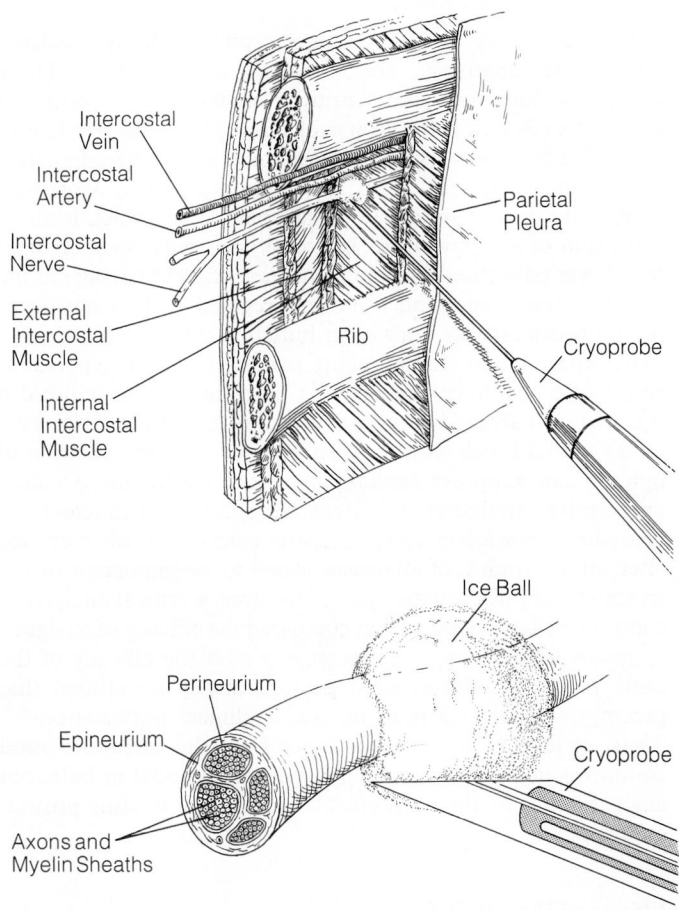

Figure 1 **Illustrated is the procedure for performing cryoanalgesia in a thoracotomy. The intercostal nerve in the thoracotomy space is isolated, together with the two intercostal nerves above the space and the two below it, and the cryoprobe is applied to the nerves for 45 seconds. The probe is then defrosted and reapplied to the nerves for 45 seconds. The analgesia obtained lasts about 30 days.**

Table 10 Prescription Guidelines for Intravenous Patient-Controlled Analgesia

Drug (Concentration)	Demand Dose	Lockout Interval (min)
Morphine (1 mg/ml)	0.5–3.0 mg	5–12
Meperdine (10mg/ml)	5–30 mg	5–12
Fentanyl (10 µg/ml)	10–20 µg	5–10
Hydromorphone (0.2 mg/ml)	0.1–0.5 mg	5–10
Oxymorphone (0.25 mg/ml)	0.2–0.4 mg	8–10
Methadone (1 mg/ml)	0.5–2.5 mg	8–20
Nalbuphine (1 mg/ml)	1–5 mg	5–10

Mechanism of Action

Traditional I.M. dosing of opioids does not result in consistent blood levels,[47,48] because opioids are absorbed at a variable rate from the vascular bed of muscle. Moreover, administration of traditional I.M. regimens results in opioid concentrations that exceed the concentrations required to produce analgesia only 35 percent of the time during any four-hour dosing interval. PCA avoids these pitfalls by allowing repeated dosing on demand. PCA provides more constant and consistent plasma opioid levels and therefore better analgesia.[47,48]

Modes of Administration and Dosing Parameters

Several modes can be used to administer opioids under patient control. Intermittent delivery of a fixed dose is known as demand dosing. Background infusions may be used to supplement patient-administered doses, but this increases the risk of respiratory depression.[49]

There are several basic prescription parameters for PCA: loading dose, demand dose, lockout interval, background infusion rate, and four-hour limits [*see Table 10*].[49] When PCA is used for postoperative care, it is usually instituted in the recovery room. The patient is made comfortable by administration of as much opioid as needed (i.e., loading dose). When the patient is sufficiently recovered from the anesthetic, he or she may begin to use the infuser.

Side Effects

Minor side effects associated with PCA include nausea, vomiting, sweating, and pruritus. Clinically significant respiratory depression with PCA is rare. There is no evidence to suggest that PCA is associated with a higher incidence of side effects than are other routes of systemic administration of opioids.[50] Side effects are the result of the pharmacological properties of opioids, not the method of administration.[44,45] One fatality has been reported with PCA.[46]

COMBINATION REGIMENS

Because no single pain treatment modality is optimal, combination regimens (e.g., balanced analgesia or multimodal treatment) offer major advantages over single-modality regimens, whether by maintaining or improving analgesia, by reducing side effects, or by doing both. Combinations of epidural local anesthetics and morphine[51,52] and of NSAIDs and opioids[34,35,52] or cryoanalgesia[43] have been reported to have additive effects, but detailed recommendations must await the results of further studies.

Discussion

Physiologic Mechanisms of Acute Pain

The basic mechanisms of acute pain are (1) afferent transmission of nociceptive stimuli through the peripheral nervous system after tissue damage, (2) modulation of these injury signals by control systems in the dorsal horn, and (3) modulation of the ascending transmission of pain stimuli by a descending control system originating in the brain [see Figure 2].[53-56]

PERIPHERAL PAIN RECEPTORS AND NEURAL TRANSMISSION TO THE SPINAL CORD

Peripheral pain receptors (nociceptors) can be identified by function but cannot be distinguished anatomically. The responsiveness of peripheral pain receptors may be enhanced by endogenous analgesic substances (e.g., prostaglandins, serotonin, bradykinin, and histamine) as well as by increased efferent sympathetic activity.[55] Antidromic release of substance P may amplify the inflammatory response and thereby increase pain transmission. The peripheral mechanisms of visceral pain still are not well understood[57]—for example, no one has yet explained why cutting or burning may provoke pain in the skin but not in visceral organs. Peripheral opioid receptors have been demonstrated to appear in inflammation on the peripheral nerve terminals.[58] Preliminary clinical studies have demonstrated analgesic effects from peripheral opioid administration during arthroscopic knee surgery.[59]

Somatic nociceptive input is transmitted to the CNS through A-delta and C fibers, which are small in diameter and either unmyelinated or thinly myelinated. Visceral pain is transmitted through afferent sympathetic pathways; the evidence that afferent parasympathetic pathways play a role in visceral nociception is inconclusive.[60]

DORSAL HORN CONTROL SYSTEMS AND MODULATION OF INCOMING SIGNALS

All incoming nociceptive traffic synapses in the gray matter of the dorsal horn (Rexed's laminae I to VI). Several substances may be involved in primary afferent transmission of nociceptive stimuli in the dorsal horn: substance P, enkephalins, somatostatin, neurotensin, γ-aminobutyric acid (GABA), glutamic acid, angiotensin II, vasoactive intestinal polypeptide (VIP), and cholecystokinin octapeptide (CCK-8).[54-56] From the dorsal horn, nociceptive information is transmitted through the spinothalamic tracts to the hypothalamus, through spinoreticular systems to the brain stem and reticular formation, and finally to the cerebral cortex.

DESCENDING PAIN CONTROL SYSTEM

A descending control system for sensory input exists that originates in the brain stem and reticular formation and in certain higher brain areas. The main neurotransmitters in this system are norepinephrine, serotonin, and enkephalins. Epidural-in-trathecal administration of alpha-adrenergic agonists (e.g., clonidine) may therefore provide pain relief.[58]

SPINAL REFLEXES

Nociperception may be enhanced by spinal reflexes that affect the environment of the nociceptive nerve endings. Thus, tissue damage may provoke an afferent reflex that causes muscle spasm in the vicinity of the injury, thereby increasing nociperception. Similarly, sympathetic reflexes may cause decreased microcirculation in injured tissue, thereby generating smooth muscle spasm, which amplifies the sensation of pain.

POSTINJURY CHANGES IN PERIPHERAL AND CENTRAL NERVOUS SYSTEMS

After an injury, the afferent nociceptive pathways undergo physiologic, anatomic, and chemical changes.[53,55,61] These changes include increased sensitivity on the part of peripheral nociceptors as well as the growth of sprouts from damaged nerve fibers that become sensitive to mechanical and alpha-adrenergic stimuli and eventually begin to fire spontaneously. Moreover, excitability may be increased in the spinal cord, which leads to expansion of receptive fields in dorsal horn cells. Such changes may lower pain thresholds, may increase afferent barrage in the late postinjury state, and, if normal regression does not occur during convalescence, may contribute to a chronic pain state.

In experimental studies, acute pain behavior or hyperexcitability of dorsal horn neurons may be eliminated or reduced if the afferent barrage is prevented from reaching the CNS. Preinjury neural block with local anesthetics or administration of opioids can suppress excitability of the CNS; this is called preemptive analgesia.[53,55] Because similar antinociceptive procedures were less effective in experimental studies when applied after injury, timing of analgesia seems to be important in the treatment of postoperative pain. However, a critical analysis of controlled clinical studies that compared the efficacy of analgesic regimens administered preoperatively with the efficacy of the same regimens administered postoperatively concluded that preemptive analgesia is of no major clinical importance.[62,63] Thus, as long as the afferent input from the surgical wound continues, continuous treatment with multimodal or balanced analgesia may be the most effective method of treating postoperative pain.

Effects of Pain Relief

METABOLIC RESPONSE TO OPERATION

It has not been generally appreciated that acute pain in the postoperative period or after hospitalization for accidental injury not only serves no useful function but also may actually exert harmful physiologic and psychological effects. Therefore,

Perception of Pain

To the Limbic System

Descending Inhibitory Pathway

Neurotransmitters at
Dorsal Horn Level:
Norepinephrine
Serotonin
Enkephalins

Spinothalamic Tract

Primary Afferent
Neurotransmitter
Candidates
Substance P
L-Glutamate
GABA
VIP
CCK-8
Somatostatin

Sensory Nerve

Trauma

Capillary

Release of:
Substance P
Histamine
Serotonin
Bradykinin
Prostaglandins

Release of:
Norepinephrine

Muscle

Motor of Other Efferent Nerve

Segmental Reflexes:
Increased Skeletal Muscle Tension
Decreased Chest Compliance
More Nociceptive Input
Increased Sympathetic Tone
Decreased Gastric Mobility
Ileus, Nausea, Vomiting

Figure 2 **Shown are the major neural pathways involved in nociperception. Nociceptive input is transmitted from the periphery to the dorsal horn via A-delta and C fibers (for somatic pain) or via afferent sympathetic pathways (for visceral pain). It is then modulated by control systems in the dorsal horn and sent via the spinothalamic tracts and spinoreticular systems to the hypothalamus, to the brain stem and reticular formation, and eventually to the cerebral cortex. Ascending transmission of nociceptive input is also modulated by descending inhibitory pathways originating in the brain and terminating in the dorsal horn. Nociperception may be enhanced by reflex responses that affect the environment of the nociceptors, such as smooth muscle spasm.**

except in the initial stage in acutely injured hypovolemic patients for whom increased sympathetic activity may provide cardiovascular support, the pain-induced reflex responses that may adversely affect respiratory function, increase cardiac demands, decrease intestinal motility, and initiate skeletal muscle spasm (thereby impairing mobilization) should be counteracted by all available means.

The traditional view of the physiologic role of the stress response to surgical injury is that it is a homeostatic defense mechanism that helps the body heal tissue and adapt to injury. However, the necessity for the stress response in modern anesthesiology and surgery has been questioned.[26] Thus, concern about the detrimental effects of operative procedures, such as myocardial infarction, pulmonary complications, and thromboembolism—which cannot be attributed solely to imperfections in surgical technique—has led to the hypothesis that the injury response may instead be a maladaptive response that erodes body mass and physiologic reserve.[26,27] Because neural stimuli play an important role in releasing the stress response to surgical injury, pain relief may modify this response, but this modulation is dependent on the mechanism of action of the pain treatment modality employed.[26,27,63]

Alleviation of pain by antagonism of peripheral pain mediators (i.e., through use of NSAIDs) has no important modifying effect on the response to operation.[34] The effects of blockade of afferent and efferent transmission of pain stimuli by means of regional anesthesia have been studied in detail.[26,27] Spinal or epidural analgesia with local anesthetics prevents the greater part of the classic endocrine metabolic response to operative procedures in the lower region of the body (e.g., gynecologic and urologic procedures and orthopedic procedures in the lower limbs). However, this effect is considerably weaker in major abdominal and thoracic procedures, probably because of insufficient afferent neural blockade. The modifying effect of epidural analgesia on the stress response is most pronounced if the neural blockade takes effect before the surgical insult. The optimal duration of neural blockade for attenuating the hypermetabolic response has not been established, but it probably should include the initial 24 to 48 hours.

Alleviation of postoperative pain by administration of epidural-intrathecal opioids has a smaller modifying effect on the surgical stress response, in comparison with the degree of pain relief it provides[26,27]; furthermore, it does not provide efferent sympathetic blockade. Systemic administration of opioids, either according to a fixed administration regimen or according to a demand-based regimen, has no important modifying effect on the stress response.[26,27] The effects of pain relief by cryoanalgesia or TENS on the stress response are not known.

POSTOPERATIVE MORBIDITY

The effects of nociceptive blockade and pain relief on postoperative morbidity have not been adequately studied, except with respect to epidural local anesthetics, about which the following conclusions can be made[26,27,29,64,65]:

1. Intraoperative blood loss is reduced by about 30 percent after hip replacement, prostatectomy, and other lower body procedures.
2. Thromboembolic complications are reduced by about 30 to 50 percent after hip replacement, knee replacement, and prostatectomy.

3. Pulmonary infectious complications appear to be reduced by about 40 percent, but as yet, too few patients have been studied to permit a firm conclusion.
4. The duration of postoperative ileus after colonic operation is reduced.

At present, it is impossible to determine whether a short-term neural blockade that lasts throughout the operation and shortly thereafter has a more beneficial effect on postoperative morbidity than a prolonged continuous epidural blockade that lasts several days postoperatively.

Controlled studies on the effect of epidural morphine or epidural morphine–bupivacaine combinations on morbidity after abdominal or thoracic operation have yielded inconclusive results,[66-70] although ambulation, cardiovascular and pulmonary complications, and hospital stay were improved in some studies.[67,69,70]

Controlled studies comparing the improved pain relief obtained by patient-controlled opioid analgesia with conventional intermittent opioid treatment have not demonstrated clinically important advantages in outcome.[71-74] The most plausible explanation for the lack of improvement in outcome associated with improved postoperative analgesia is that general postoperative care has not adapted to make optimum use of the postoperative pain-free state. Thus, recent observations suggest that a combination of improved pain relief, enhanced early mobilization, oral feeding, and reinforced psychological preparation of the patient may lead to major improvements in postoperative morbidity, including reduction in fatigue and hospital stay. This level of care is probably best implemented in a postoperative rehabilitation unit.

TOLERANCE, PHYSICAL DEPENDENCE, AND ADDICTION

Continued exposure of an opioid receptor to high concentrations of opioid will cause tolerance. Tolerance is the progressive decline in potency of an opioid with continued use; higher and higher concentrations of the drug are required to cause the same analgesic effect. Physical dependence refers to the production of an abstinence syndrome when an opioid is withdrawn. It is defined by the World Health Organization as follows:

> A state, psychic or sometimes also physical, resulting from interactions between a living organism and a drug, characterized by behavioral and other responses that always include a compulsion to take the drug on a continuous or periodic basis in order to experience its psychic effects, and sometimes to avoid discomfort from its absence.[75]

This definition is very close to the popular conception of addiction. However, it is important to distinguish addiction (implying compulsive behavior and psychological dependence) from tolerance (a pharmacological property) and from physical dependence (a characteristic physiologic effect of a group of drugs). Physical dependence does not imply addiction. Moreover, tolerance can occur without physical dependence; the converse does not appear to be true.

The possibility that the medical administration of opioids could result in a patient's becoming addicted has generated much debate about the use of opioids. In a prospective study of 12,000 hospitalized patients receiving at least one strong opioid for a protracted period of time, there were only four reasonably well documented cases of subsequent addiction.[76] (None of these patients had a prior history of substance abuse.) Thus, the iatrogenic production of opioid addiction may be very rare.

Conclusion

The choice of therapeutic intervention for acute postoperative pain is determined largely by the nature of the patient's problem, the resources available, the efficacy of the various treatment techniques, the risks attendant on the procedures under consideration, and the cost to the patient. It appears that whereas trauma has been the subject of intensive research, the mechanisms of pain associated with trauma and surgical injury and the optimal methods of relieving such pain have received comparatively little attention. The exciting new data on basic pain mechanisms and therapy now being collected, combined with promising data supporting the idea that adequate inhibition of surgically induced nociceptive stimuli may reduce postoperative morbidity, will probably stimulate surgeons to turn their attention to this area. Effective control of postoperative pain, combined with a high degree of surgical expertise and judicious use of other perioperative therapeutic interventions, is certain to improve surgical outcome.

References

1. Report of a working party of the commission on the provision of surgical services. Pain after Surgery. The Royal College of Surgeons of England and the College of Anaesthetists, London, 1990

2. Agency for Health Care Policy and Research: Acute Pain Management and Trauma: Operative or Medical Procedures. Publication No 92-0032. U.S. Department of Health and Human Services, Rockville, Maryland, 1992

3. Chapman CR: Psychological factors in postoperative pain. Acute Pain. Smith G, Covino BG, Eds. Butterworth Publishers, Stoneham, Massachusetts, 1985, p 22

4. Peck CL: Psychological factors in acute pain management. Acute Pain Management. Cousins MJ, Phillips GD, Eds. Churchill Livingstone, Inc, New York, 1986, p 251

5. Egbert LD, Battit GE, Welch CE, et al: Reduction of postoperative pain by encouragement and instruction of patients: a study of doctor-patient rapport. N Engl J Med 270:825, 1964

6. Freye E: Opioid Agonists Antagonists and Mixed Narcotic Analgesics: Theoretical Background and Considerations for Practical Use. Springer-Verlag, Berlin, 1987

7. Kaiko RF, Foley KM, Grabinski PY, et al: Central nervous system excitatory effects of meperidine in cancer patients. Ann Neurol 13:180, 1983

8. Gourlay GK, Cousins MJ: Strong analgesics in severe pain. Drugs 28:79, 1984

9. Rosow CE: Newer synthetic opioid analgesics. Acute Pain. Smith G, Covino BG, Eds. Butterworth Publishers, Stoneham, Massachusetts, 1985, p 68

10. Shah MV, Jones DI, Rosen M: "Patient demand" postoperative analgesia with buprenorphine: comparison between sublingual and I.M. administration. Br J Anaesth 58:508, 1986

11. Bellville JW, Seed JC: The effect of drugs on the respiratory response to carbon dioxide. Anesthesiology 21:727, 1960

12. Ferrante FM: Opioids. Postoperative Pain Management. Ferrante FM, VadeBoncouer TR, Eds. Churchill Livingstone, Inc, New York, 1993, p 145

13. McCammon RL, Stoelting RK, Madura JA: Effects of butorphanol, nalbuphine, and fentanyl on intrabiliary tract dynamics. Anesth Analg 63:139, 1984

14. Cousins MJ, Cherry DA, Gourlay GK: Acute and chronic pain: use of spinal opioids. Neural Blockade in Clinical Anesthesia and Management of Pain, 2nd ed. Cousins MJ, Bridenbaugh PO, Eds. JB Lippincott Co, Philadelphia, 1988, p 955

15. VadeBoncouer TR, Ferrante FM: Epidural and subarachnoid opioids. Postoperative Pain Management. Ferrante FM, VadeBoncouer TR, Eds. Churchill Livingstone, Inc, New York, 1993, p 279

16. Cousins MJ, Mather LE: Intrathecal and epidural administration of opioids. Anesthesiology 61:276, 1984

17. Staren ED, Cullen ML: Epidural catheter analgesia for the management of postoperative pain. Surg Gynecol Obstet 162:389, 1986

18. Allen PD, Walman T, Concepcion M, et al: Epidural morphine provides postoperative pain relief in peripheral vascular and orthopedic surgical patients. Anesth Analg 65:165, 1986

19. Rawal N, Sjöstrand UH, Dahlström B, et al: Epidural morphine for postoperative pain relief: a comparative study with intramuscular narcotic and intercostal nerve block. Anesth Analg 61:93, 1982

20. El-Baz NMI, Faber LP, Jensik RJ: Continuous epidural infusion of morphine for treatment of pain after thoracic surgery: a new technique. Anesth Analg 63:757, 1984

21. Cullen ML, Staren ED, El-Ganzouri A, et al: Continuous epidural infusion for analgesia after major abdominal operations: a randomized, prospective, double-blind study. Surgery 98:718, 1985

22. Chrubasik J, Wiemers K: Continuous-plus-on-demand epidural infusion of morphine for postoperative pain relief by means of a small, externally worn infusion device. Anesthesiology 62:263, 1985

23. Ballantyne JC, Loach AB, Carr DB: Itching after epidural and spinal opiates. Pain 33:149, 1988

24. Durant PA, Yaksh TL: Drug effects on urinary bladder tone during spinal morphine-induced inhibition of the micturition reflex in unanesthetized rats. Anesthesiology 68:325, 1988

25. Bowler GMR, Wildsmith JA, Scott DB: Epidural administration of local anesthetics. Acute Pain Management. Cousins MJ, Phillips GD, Eds. Churchill Livingstone, Inc, New York, 1986, p 187

26. Kehlet H: Modification of responses to surgery and anesthesia by neural blockade. Neural Blockade in Clinical Anesthesia and Management of Pain. Cousins MJ, Bridenbaugh PO, Eds. JB Lippincott Co, Philadelphia, 1987, p 145

27. Kehlet H: General vs. regional anesthesia. Principles and Practice of Anesthesiology, Vol 2. Rogers MC, Tinker JH, Covino BG, et al, Eds. Mosby–Year Book, St. Louis, 1993, p 1218

28. Butterworth JF IV, Strichartz GR: Molecular mechanisms of local anesthesia: a review. Anesthesiology 72:711, 1990

29. Scott NB, Kehlet H: Regional anaesthesia reduces surgical morbidity. Br J Surg 75:299, 1988

30. Wille-Jørgensen P, Jørgensen LN, Rasmussen LS: Lumbar regional anaesthesia and prophylactic anticoagulant therapy: is the combination safe? Anaesthesia 46:623, 1991

31. Bergqvist D, Lindblad B, Mätzsch T: Low molecular weight heparin for thromboprophylaxis and epidural/spinal anaesthesia—is there a risk? Acta Anaesthesiol Scand 36:605, 1992

32. Murphy DF: Continuous intercostal nerve blockade: an anatomical study to elucidate its mode of action. Br J Anaesth 56:627, 1984

33. Dahl JB, Møniche S, Kehlet H: Wound infiltration with local anaesthetics for postoperative pain relief. Acta Anaesthesiol Scand 38:7, 1993

34. Dahl JB, Kehlet H: Non-steroidal anti-inflammatory drugs: rationale for use in severe postoperative pain. Br J Anaesth 66:703, 1991

35. Kehlet H, Mather LE, Eds: The value of NSAIDs in the management of postoperative pain. Drugs 44(suppl 5):1, 1992

36. Harris K: The role of prostaglandins in the control of renal function (editorial). Br J Anaesth 69:233, 1992

37. Cryoanalgesia (editorial). Lancet 1:779, 1982

38. Orr IA, Keenan DJM, Dundee JW: Improved pain relief after thoracotomy: use of cryoprobe and morphine infusion. Br Med J 283:945, 1981

39. Joucken K, Michel L, Schoevaerdts JC, et al: Cryoanalgesia for post-thoracotomy pain. Acta Anaesthesiol Belg 38:179, 1987

40. Roberts D, Pizzarelli G, Lepore V, et al: Reduction of post-thoracotomy pain by cryotherapy of intercostal nerves. Scand J Thor Cardiovasc Surg 22:127, 1988

41. Gough JD, Williams AB, Vaughan RS: The control of post-thoracotomy pain: a comparative evaluation of thoracic epidural fentanyl infusions and cryo-analgesia. Anaesthesia 43:780, 1988

42. Keenan DJM, Cave K, Langdon L, et al: Comparative trial of rectal indomethacin and cryoanalgesia for control of early postthoracotomy pain. Br Med J 287:1335, 1983

43. Tyler E, Caldwell C, Ghia JN: Transcutaneous electrical nerve stimulation: an alternative approach to the management of postoperative pain. Anesth Analg 61:449, 1982

44. Bahar M, Rosen M, Vickers MD: Self-administered nalbuphine, morphine and pethidine: comparison, by intravenous route, following cholecystectomy. Anaesthesia 40:529, 1985

45. Bollish SJ, Collins CL, Kirking DM, et al: Efficacy of patient-controlled versus conventional analgesia for postoperative pain. Clin Pharm 4:48, 1985

46. Grey TC, Sweeney ES: Patient-controlled analgesia (letter). JAMA 259:2240, 1988

47. Austin KL, Stapleton JV, Mather LE: Multiple intramuscular injections: a major source of variability in analgesic response to meperidine. Pain 8:47, 1980

48. Austin KL, Stapleton JV, Mather LE: Relationship between blood meperidine concentrations and analgesic response: a preliminary report. Anesthesiology 53:460, 1980

49. Ferrante FM: Patient-controlled analgesia: a conceptual framework for analgesic administration. Postoperative Pain Management. Ferrante FM, VadeBoncouer TR, Eds. Churchill Livingstone, Inc, New York, 1993, p 255

50. Mather LE, Owen H: The pharmacology of patient-administered opioids. Patient-Controlled Analgesia. Ferrante FM, Ostheimer GW, Covino BG, Eds. Blackwell Scientific Publications, Boston, 1990, p 27

51. Dahl JB, Rosenberg J, Hansen BL, et al: Differential analgesic effects of low-dose epidural morphine and morphine-bupivacaine at rest and during mobilization after major abdominal surgery. Anesth Analg 74:362, 1992

52. Kehlet H, Dahl JB: The value of "multi-modal" or "balanced analgesia" in postoperative pain treatment. Anesth Analg 77:1048, 1993

53. Woolf CJ: Central mechanisms of acute pain. Proceedings of the VIth World Congress on Pain. Bond MR, Charlton JE, Woolf CJ, Eds. Elsevier Science Publishers, Amsterdam, 1991, p 25

54. Raja SN, Meyer RA, Campbell JN: Peripheral mechanisms of somatic pain. Anesthesiology 68:571, 1988

55. Hyperalgesia and Allodynia. Willis WD Jr, Ed. The Bristol-Myers Squibb Symposium on Pain Research. Raven Press, New York, 1992

56. Fields HL, Heinricher MM, Mason P: Neurotransmitters in nociceptive modulatory circuits. Annu Rev Neurosci 14:219, 1991

57. Ness TJ, Gebhart GF: Visceral pain: a review of experimental studies. Pain 41:167, 1990

58. Maze M, Tranquilli W: Alpha-2 adrenoceptor agonists: defining the role in clinical anesthesia. Anesthesiology 74:581, 1991

59. Stein C: Peripheral mechanisms of opioid analgesia. Anesth Analg 76:182, 1993

60. Randich A, Gebhart GF: Vagal afferent modulation of nociception. Brain Res Rev 17:77, 1992

61. Treede R-D, Meyer RA, Raja SN, et al: Peripheral and central mechanisms of cutaneous hyperalgesia. Prog Neurobiol 38:397, 1992

62. McQuay HJ: Pre-emptive analgesia (editorial). Br J Anaesth 69:1, 1992

63. Dahl JB, Kehlet H: The value of pre-emptive analgesia in the treatment of postoperative pain. Br J Anaesth 70:434, 1993

64. Kehlet H: Surgical stress: the role of pain and analgesia. Br J Anaesth 63:189, 1989

65. Sorenson RM, Pace NL: Anesthetic techniques during surgical repair of femoral neck fractures: a meta-analysis. Anesthesiology 77:1095, 1992

66. Rawal N, Sjöstrand U, Christoffersson E, et al: Comparison of intramuscular and epidural morphine for postoperative analgesia in the grossly obese: influence on postoperative ambulation and pulmonary function. Anesth Analg 63:583, 1984

67. Hjortsø N-C, Neumann P, Frøsig F, et al: A controlled study on the effect of epidural analgesia with local anaesthetics and morphine on morbidity after abdominal surgery. Acta Anaesthesiol Scand 29:790, 1985

68. Yeager MP, Glass DD, Neff RK, et al: Epidural anesthesia and analgesia in high-risk surgical patients. Anesthesiology 66:729, 1987

69. Tuman KJ, McCarthy RJ, March RJ, et al: Effects of epidural anesthesia and analgesia on coagulation and outcome after major vascular surgery. Anesth Analg 73:696, 1991

70. Seeling W, Bruckmooser K-P, Hüfner C, et al: No reduction in postoperative complications by the use of catheterized epidural analgesia following major abdominal surgery. Anaesthesist 39:33, 1990

71. Jackson D: A study of pain management: patient controlled analgesia versus intramuscular analgesia. Journal of Intravenous Nursing 12:42, 1989

72. Wasylak TJ, Abbott FV, English MJM, et al: Reduction of post-operative morbidity following patient-controlled morphine. Can J Anaesth 37:726, 1990

73. Egbert AM, Parks LH, Short LM, et al: Randomized trial of postoperative patient-controlled analgesia vs intramuscular narcotics in frail elderly men. Arch Intern Med 150:1897, 1990

74. Kenady DE, Wilson JF, Schwartz RW, et al: A randomized comparison of patient-controlled versus standard analgesic requirements in patients undergoing cholecystectomy. Surg Gynecol Obstet 174:216, 1992

75. World Health Organization: Expert committee on drug dependence, 16th report. Technical Report Series No 407. World Health Organization, Geneva, 1969

76. Porter J, Jick H: Addiction rare in patients treated with narcotics (letter). N Engl J Med 302:123, 1980

Acknowledgments

Figure 1   Carol Donner.

Figure 2   Dana Burns Pizer.

3 STOMAL CARE

M. Joyce Rosenthal, R.N., M.S., C.E.T.N., and Daniel Rosenthal, M.D.

Approach to Perioperative Stomal Care

Preoperative Counseling

Once a surgeon decides that the creation of a stoma is essential to the cure or alleviation of a patient's disease, the next task is to convince the patient that the cure is not worse than the disease. It must be emphasized to the patient that although the stoma will be an inconvenience, the chances are excellent that he or she will go on to live a fruitful life after recovery from operation. Elderly patients or patients with an advanced stage of cancer may not be as receptive to these words of comfort as a younger or healthier patient would be. In such instances, strong emotional support from the entire health care team and from the patient's family is crucial.

Certain specific topics should always be discussed with the patient preoperatively:

1. The procedure itself. The normal intestinal anatomy, the patient's specific disease process, and the planned rerouting of the bowel should be outlined with the help of simple sketches or preprinted diagrams. Common complications associated with the intended operation should be candidly reviewed. Whether the stoma will be temporary or permanent and whether a pouch will have to be worn at all times should also be discussed. Finally, there should be a brief discussion addressing how long the operation is likely to take; what the postoperative recovery room routine will be; when the patient is likely to be able to return to the hospital room; how the nasogastric tube and the urinary catheter are used and how long they are likely to be needed; how soon after the operation the family will be able to visit the patient; and how soon after the operation the patient will be able to eat. These points have no bearing on the actual procedure, but addressing them instills in the patient and the family some sense of participation in the event and provides some answers they can use when questioned by relatives or friends. Such discussion may seem trivial to the surgeon, but it is of great importance for bolstering patient and family morale.

2. Stoma appliances. The stoma appliances currently available should be described to the patient, with special emphasis placed on their inconspicuousness and ability to contain odor completely. An easy-to-use pouch (probably a one-piece appliance) should be selected and shown to the patient and the family, who should be told that in the postoperative period they will receive detailed instruction in its use. The patient should also be made aware that at some future date, whether because of a change in body habitus or out of a desire to try another type of

appliance more suitable to a particular lifestyle, he or she may switch to another pouch system. If time permits, the pouch may be worn before the procedure to yield a better idea of the suitability of the stoma site.

3. Bathing and showering. Soap and water do not hurt a stoma: ostomates can bathe or shower, with or without their pouch, as often as they wish. If circumstances permit and the patient is physically able, he or she should take a shower in the hospital after the operation with the pouch off, then reapply the pouch just as would be the routine at home. In so doing, the patient gains confidence in his or her ability to return to normal daily activities. Good hygiene is crucial to the care of the peristomal skin. Soaps with creams or oils may prevent the pouch from adhering properly and thus should not be used in the peristomal area. Often, patients want to use strong lye-based or antimicrobial soaps to sterilize the peristomal skin. This practice should be discouraged because such soaps may cause local irritation and alter the normal skin flora. The use of alcohol to clean the peristomal skin should also be discouraged.

4. Employment and physical activities. Once patients have recovered from their operation, they can generally go back to their former occupations with few or no physical limitations; however, heavy lifting or straining should be avoided because the presence of a stoma predisposes to the development of a peristomal hernia.

5. Diet. After the operation, the patient should be fed in the same manner as any other patient who has undergone a major GI operation (whether conventionally or laparoscopically performed), progressing from sips of water to clear liquids to full liquids and then to a soft, low-roughage, low-fat diet. Moving directly to a regular diet after a full-liquid diet often results in premature exposure to high-fat, gas-forming, high-roughage items. Very often, new ostomates cannot tolerate such a diet and may start vomiting or experience ileus.

In our practice, the Dietary Department is involved in coordinating the foods offered after the patient has shown the ability to tolerate a fluid diet. An "ostomy diet" order on the chart alerts the dietitian to the presence of a newly created stoma, which necessitates adjustments to the patient's diet. An ostomy diet should include three small meals supplemented by between-meal snacks. A soft or regular diet should be changed to a low-residue, low-fat, and low-lactose diet for about 2 days. Snacks should be offered at midmorning, midafternoon, and bedtime. Provided that the hospital course has been uneventful, a sample menu for postoperative day 1 might be as follows:

- Breakfast: orange juice, cream of wheat, scrambled egg, white toast, and coffee, tea, or water.

1655

Approach to Perioperative Stomal Care

Stoma with external pouch

In operating room

Mature the stoma and apply disposable pouch, allowing for 3 mm postoperative swelling. If necessary, trim adhesive area to avoid drains or retention sutures. Support loop colostomy with bridge (e.g., segment of No. 16 rubber catheter with ends folded) inside stoma pouch. If opening of digestive stoma is delayed, cover exteriorized bowel segment with petrolatum gauze and sterile dressing.

First postoperative day

Do not change pouch if it is not leaking and stoma color is good. If stoma color cannot be determined, remove pouch, gently wipe off stoma with wet gauze, and inspect. If stoma appears healthy, apply new disposable pouch.

Start involving patient's family in care. If patient is alert, begin teaching process.

Subsequent days

48 hr after operation: Remove entire pouch system, and clean peristomal skin. Select and apply long-term pouch system. Demonstrate working of clamp or spigot, and gradually increase patient involvement.

- Digestive stoma: During next 48 to 72 hr, whenever pouch is one half to two thirds full, remove clamp, empty pouch, and rinse, using water-filled bulb syringe.
- Urinary stoma: Once a day, rinse pouch through spigot with 20 to 30 ml vinegar; reconnect to drainage.

Change pouch system every other day (unless leakage occurs): carefully detach portion adhering to abdomen with help of moist gauze or washcloth, and gently wipe stoma and peristomal skin clean.

Teach patient to fit adhesive wafer snugly around stoma, connect wafer and pouch, and position appliance over stoma and to recognize potential local skin problems.

Consider use of nonadhesive reusable pouch system (VPI).

In preparation for discharge from hospital

If necessary, ensure assistance of relative, friend, or social worker. Advise patient and caretaker of available social and medical support systems.

Patient or caretaker should be familiar with one type of pouch system, including the following:
- Emptying pouch and cleansing closure tail
- Detaching adhesive portion of pouch
- Caring for peristomal skin
- Measuring stoma and cutting hole of correct size in adhesive portion of pouch
- Applying pouch
- Recognizing, preventing, and correcting peristomal skin problems

Early postoperative skin problems include allergic contact dermatitis, folliculitis, and irritant dermatitis; problems that may arise later include radiation reactions, parastomal abscesses and ulcers, pseudoepithelial hyperplasia, and pyoderma gangrenosum.

Do not change pouch as long as wafer is securely fixed to and protecting peristomal skin. Wearing time generally ranges from 3 to 6 days; if patient has problems, consult enterostomal therapist and consider changing systems.

Counsel patient and family preoperatively

Discuss:
- Procedure itself
- Stoma appliances
- Bathing and showering

- Employment and physical activities
- Diet

- Sports and travel
- Sexual activity
- Reproduction and pregnancy

- Availability of home health care and financial support
- Importance of family support system
- Ostomate Bill of Rights

Enlist services of enterostomal therapist and trained ostomy visitor.
For emergency procedures, explain briefly and clearly what a stoma is and why its creation may be unavoidable.

Select and mark stoma site

Site must be visible to the patient and surrounded by a radius of 5 cm of flat, unencumbered skin; flexing thigh, standing, sitting, or lying should not interfere. Avoid iliac crest, costal margins, umbilicus, symphysis pubis, and folds, grooves, or scars in skin.
Proper sites tend to fall in right or left lower quadrant, below beltline, over body of rectus muscle, and 5 cm lateral to and below umbilicus.

Special considerations in site selection:
- Transverse colostomy or continent stoma
- Multiple stomas

- Abdominal shape in obese patient, newborn, or infant; unusual lower abdominal skin folds; abdominal scars

- Handicaps and prostheses
- Anticipated need for or history of radiation therapy
- Laparoscopic creation of a stoma

To mark stoma site, the preferred technique is intradermal injection of methylene blue. Superficial scratch marks are sometimes used.

Continent stoma (Kock pouch)

Intubate with No. 30 Silastic catheter.
Mark correct position of tube with silk tie at stomal level.
Affix tube securely to skin. Leave in place for 10 days, and allow intestinal pouch to empty by gravity.
Irrigate tube with 30 ml normal saline q. 6 hr.

10 days after operation: Teach patient to extubate and intubate intestinal pouch. Do not keep tube out of pouch for > 30 min at a time.

4 wk after operation: Have patient extubate and reintubate stoma at gradually increasing intervals.

1657

a

Figure 1 (*a*) **Specially designed underwear that includes a pocket for the pouch helps ostomates feel more at ease. Such underwear is available in female (*b*) and male (*c*) versions.**

- Lunch: baked chicken, mashed potatoes, boiled carrots, roll, and coffee, tea, or water.
- Dinner: turkey, cup of soup, canned fruit, and coffee, tea, or water.
- Snacks: midmorning, crackers and canned fruit; midafternoon, vanilla wafers with juice; and bedtime, low-fat flavored yogurt with tea or coffee.

Specific instructions are needed for the first week or two at home as more roughage and fats are introduced into the diet. Any lactose-intolerance problems should also be taken into account as milk products are slowly reintroduced into the diet. Patients with an ileostomy should have more fluids in their diet to make up for increased stomal water loss. Patients with cardiac or renal disease should be closely monitored by their physicians so that fluid overload may be prevented.

A sample menu plan for week 1 at home might be as follows:

- Breakfast: orange juice, cream of wheat, toast with jam, and milk, coffee, or tea.
- Lunch: pureed soup, turkey sandwich with reduced mayonnaise, canned fruit, and milk, coffee, or tea.
- Dinner: tomato juice; boneless, skinless chicken breast; white rice; cooked carrots; roll with margarine; and coffee or tea.
- Snacks: midmorning, half a banana and four or five graham crackers with water or juice; midafternoon, applesauce and three or four vanilla wafers with water or juice; and bedtime, low-fat flavored yogurt with milk, coffee, or tea.

Beyond the postoperative period, the diet of an ostomate, except for whatever individual modifications are necessary, can be relatively unrestricted. Overall, there is no specific ostomy diet. Any dietary restrictions adhered to are generally voluntary, and their main purpose is the prevention and relief of gas, diarrhea, constipation, or unusual odor. If any of these problems persist for more than 24 hours, the patient should notify a physician. Most difficulties can be averted if patients follow a few simple instructions, which should be emphasized to the patient before discharge:

- Avoid foods that were troublesome preoperatively. (Often, patients know which foods do not agree with them.)
- Chew foods well to break down bulk and fiber. (Failure to chew adequately may lead to stomal obstruction.)
- Eat slowly to minimize swallowing of air. (Eating fast may also result in stomal obstruction.)
- For the first few weeks after operation, avoid high-residue foods, such as fresh fruits and vegetables and whole-grain breads and cereals.
- About 6 weeks after operation, reintroduce high-residue foods into the diet, one at a time. If any food causes problems, try it again at a later date.
- If you have diarrhea, do not restrict fluid intake; instead, drink beverages that contain salt, such as Gatorade or bouillon.
- Keep well hydrated: drink four to six extra glasses of fluid a day.
- If you wish to drink alcoholic beverages, practice moderation.

Some patients with ileostomies tend to pass enteric-coated tablets or time-release capsules before the medication can be absorbed. In such cases, these products should be avoided. If a liquid form of the medication is available, it should be given instead; alternatively, a similar product that is available as a liquid may be substituted.

6. Sports and travel. Contact sports may injure the stoma and should therefore be avoided. Otherwise, ostomates may enjoy a wide range of sports activities, including swimming, as their general state of health allows. They need not avoid Jacuzzis or hot tubs, and they pose no health threat to themselves or to others if they use community pools. Any fears of possible pouch leakage may be allayed by "picture-framing" the stoma appliance with waterproof tape (i.e., placing tape on all four sides of the wafer).

Ostomates should feel free to travel, although they should be careful not to place all of their stoma supplies in their checked luggage when traveling by air. In areas where it is not safe to drink the water, they should use bottled water to irrigate their colostomies.

7. Sexual activity. Sexual activity will be a paramount consideration to some future ostomates, although probably not to all.

Figure 2 **Shown are three different pouch covers: a commercially available cover (ConvaTec), a lace cover, and a plain handmade cover.**

This matter is of such importance that it should be candidly discussed not only in the preoperative period but during follow-up visits as well. The surgeon should not hesitate to offer any patient the opportunity to voice his or her concerns about this matter. Male patients should be made aware that the amount of erectile or ejaculatory dysfunction that occurs after pelvic surgery or the removal of the rectum is related to the extent of the pelvic dissection necessary to eradicate the disease as well as to the degree of sexual vigor present before operation. Those male patients who are interested in having children may be advised to bank their sperm for future use; a certain number of patients will have permanent ejaculatory dysfunction in spite of the most careful pelvic surgery.[1] Female patients should be told that loss of the rectum and the presence of a stoma do not preclude sexual activity, even though dyspareunia, increased vaginal discharge, and altered orgasmic response are common complications of total rectal excision in women.[2-4] The use of specially designed underwear [*see Figure 1*] or pouch covers [*see Figure 2*] may help patients feel more at ease with their sexuality by enhancing the feeling of normality during intimacy.

8. Reproduction and pregnancy. Women in their reproductive years should be reassured that a stoma is not incompatible with pregnancy and that many female ostomates do in fact become pregnant and undergo normal vaginal delivery. For pregnant women who have an ileal pouch after a proctocolectomy for inflammatory bowel disease, cesarean section may be preferable to vaginal delivery at term, given that anal sphincter damage would be catastrophic in their case. Pregnant women undergoing stoma surgery for Crohn disease should be made aware that recurrent disease and some of the medications required to treat such recurrence may be detrimental to the fetus.[5] As a rule, a pregnant woman undergoing an ostomy procedure should be managed exactly as a nonpregnant woman would be. Major reconstructive procedures, however, should probably be deferred until after delivery. Closer to term, uterine enlargement may preclude even a conventional proctectomy, in which case a staged operation that spares the rectum is appropriate.[6] In our practice, we have seen 11 cases in which pregnant ostomates came to term with normal babies. A few were followed for the entire 9 months of gestation, whereas others were seen only during the last month or two for support and reassurance. We have seen both vaginal deliveries and cesarean sections in patients with ileostomies, colostomies, or ileal conduits; however,

we have not been involved in the care of any pregnant patients with Kock or J ileal pouches. One women who had undergone a total colectomy and an ileostomy for Crohn disease and who had a vaginal fistula became pregnant and gave birth to a normal baby girl via cesarean section. These women are some of the best ostomy visitors we know of—living proof that life goes on despite a stoma.

9. Home health care needs. After an ostomy, some patients may require additional nursing care at home or a period of recuperation in a convalescent center.

10. Financial support. The expense of stoma equipment, along with that of home health care needs, may place a heavy financial burden on patients and their families. Surgeons should anticipate such problems preoperatively and should not hesitate to inquire into patients' insurance coverage. Patients who are 65 years of age or older should be made aware that Medicare covers, to some extent, posthospital nursing care facilities, home health care, and stoma appliance expenses. Because Medicare and Medicaid benefits and deductible expenses tend to vary annually, medical personnel may wish to update their knowledge by obtaining new schedules of Medicare and Medicaid benefits. Handbooks listing Medicare Part B benefits are reviewed annually and are available at Medicare state headquarters; their locations can be obtained by calling 800-442-2620. Pamphlets describing Medicaid benefits can be obtained by calling the individual state's department of human services. The help of a hospital social worker familiar with these problems is frequently invaluable. Retired military personnel and military dependents who are not eligible for Medicare or Medicaid should consult an adviser from the Civilian Help and Medical Program of the Uniformed Services (CHAMPUS) to determine the extent of the benefits available to them.

11. Family support system. It is vital that the surgeon keep a relative or friend of the patient informed of the upcoming operation and its consequences. Well-informed relatives who are involved in the patient's care and demonstrate by words and deeds that they will continue to offer love and concern, regardless of the outcome of the procedure, can exert a positive influence on the patient's recovery.

12. The Ostomate Bill of Rights. According to this manifesto, developed by the United Ostomy Association (UOA), the ostomate shall have the following:

- Preoperative counseling.
- An appropriately positioned stoma site.
- A well-constructed stoma.
- Skilled postoperative nursing care.
- Emotional support.
- Individual instruction.
- Information on the availability of supplies.
- Information on community resources.
- Posthospital follow-up and lifelong supervision.
- Team efforts of health care professionals.

The process of counseling can be greatly aided by the publications for patients available from the UOA [*see Table 1*], 19772 MacArthur Boulevard, Suite 200, Irvine, CA 92612-2405 (800-826-0826; http://www.uoa.org; e-mail uoa@deltanet.com); Crohn's and Colitis Foundation of America, Inc., 386 Park Avenue South, New York, NY 10016-8804 (800-932-2423; http://www.ccfa.org; e-mail info@ccfa.org); and the Wound, Ostomy and Continence Nurses Society, 1550 South Coast Highway, Suite 201, Laguna Beach, CA 92651 (888-224-WOCN [9626]; http://www.wocn.org; e-mail maria@wocn.org).

Table 1 Selected Publications for Patients, Available from the United Ostomy Association

The Ostomy Handbook
Colostomies: A Guide
Transverse Colostomies: A Guide
Ileostomy: A Guide
The Continent Ileostomy
Urostomy: A Guide
My Child Has an Ostomy
All about Jimmy and His Friend
Sex and the Female Ostomate
Sex and the Male Ostomate
Sex, Courtship, and the Single Ostomate
Pregnancy and the Woman with an Ostomy
Employment of the Ostomate
Handicapped Ostomate

CONSULTING AN ENTEROSTOMAL THERAPIST

Before operation, the surgeon may wish to consult an enterostomal therapy (ET) nurse. (In the United States, most enterostomal therapists are registered nurses; however, there are a few very able ones who are not.) By training and experience, ET nurses are ideally suited to the physical and emotional preparation of ostomy candidates for surgery. Reassurance aimed at dispelling any lingering apprehensions about the upcoming operation often allows the ET nurse to establish a good rapport with the patient and his or her family. To alleviate the patient's fears further, the ET nurse may display a sample pouch, which can even be worn by the candidate if desired. The ET nurse can also explain how one cares for the pouch and how one lives comfortably wearing it, provided that the patient is able and willing to assimilate this information. The patient should be assured that he or she will be taught how to take care of the stoma before leaving the hospital. This point should be reinforced by telling the patient that the ET nurse will be caring for the patient's stoma and the peristomal skin after the operation and will be slowly teaching the patient and any other personal care provider how to provide this care.

If the patient is not opposed, the ET nurse may bring in a well-adjusted ostomate of the same gender as the patient, preferably a trained ostomy visitor. This approach can reassure the patient considerably, especially if the visitor appears self-confident, is well dressed, and is about the same age as the patient. It is helpful, but not necessary, for the visitor to have the same type of stoma as the patient. Ostomy visitors are usually quite eager to help; they can generally be contacted through the local chapters of the UOA or the American Cancer Society. Local telephone directories list numbers for both agencies. In communities where no local chapters are present, the location of the nearest facility can be obtained by calling the national headquarters of either organization. The headquarters of the American Cancer Society is located at 1599 Clifton Road N.E., Atlanta, GA 30329 (800-ACS[227]-2345; http://www.cancer.org).

EMERGENCY COUNSELING

When creation of an intestinal stoma is being planned or considered under emergency conditions, the time available for counseling may be short. This time is best used in briefly but clearly explaining to the patient and the family what a stoma is and why its creation may be unavoidable in this case. Emergency stomas must be constructed according to the same basic principles of stoma construction that govern nonemergency stomas.

Preoperative Selection and Marking of the Stoma Site

The selection and marking of the stoma site directly affect the likelihood of complications associated with the creation of the stoma.[7,8] Proper location of a stoma can mean the difference between an active, independent life and one of social isolation. Poorly placed stomas are hard to pouch and tend to leak. Accidental pouch leaks are a nuisance and a source of considerable embarrassment to ostomates. Many, in fact, avoid social contacts out of fear of such accidents.

GENERAL CONSIDERATIONS FOR SITE SELECTION

There are several general considerations for site selection that the surgeon must take into account. Proper placement of the stoma may prevent parastomal hernia, prolapse, and leakage (which can lead to skin problems and consequent patient anxiety). Stomas should be placed away from the iliac crest, the costal margins, the umbilicus, the symphysis pubis, and any folds, grooves, or scars in the skin [*see Figure 3*]. There must be a radius of about 5 cm of flat, unencumbered skin around the stoma site if an appliance is to fit well. Flexing the ipsilateral thigh should not interfere with the wearing of the appliance. The stoma site should also be visible to the patient and, ideally, should not interfere with the beltline. If the stoma site is to be placed above the beltline, care should be taken to ensure that pendulous breasts are not hanging over it. In this situation, not only would the patient find it difficult to see the stoma, but the weight of the breast would apply pressure on the appliance wafer, causing it to loosen and thus resulting in leakage.

Because the shape of the abdomen tends to change as an individual stands, sits, or lies down, it is imperative that the stoma site selected be suitable for the wearing of an appliance in all three positions—

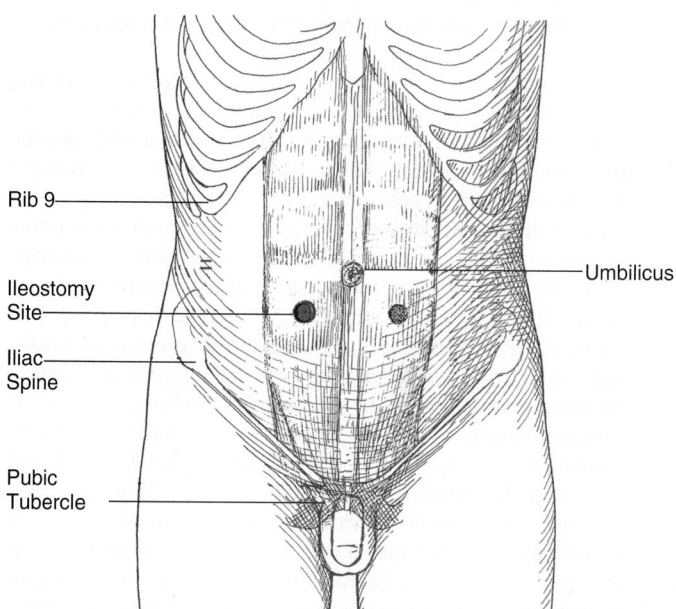

Figure 3 Shown is a stoma site selected for a conventional ileostomy. A site located in the same spot on the left side of the abdomen would be ideally suited for a sigmoid colostomy.

Figure 4 A 5 cm marking disk is used to select the proper stoma site with the patient lying down (*above*) and sitting up (*below*).

especially the sitting position, because it is sitting that brings about the greatest changes in abdominal contours. Often, a lower stoma site is selected so that the patient can wear the beltline low; however, a low site may lead to kinks in the appliance when the patient sits, which could result in overfilling of the upper part of the appliance. The use of a skin barrier wafer or a marking disk [*see Figure 4*] is invaluable for determining the adequacy of the stoma site selection.

The right and left lower quadrants of the abdomen are still the most common locations for digestive and urinary stomas. Properly selected stoma sites in these areas tend to fall below the beltline, over the body of the rectus muscle, about 5 cm lateral to and below the umbilicus. In our experience, creation of the stoma through the rectus sheath and muscle is associated with a lower incidence of peristomal hernia.

SPECIAL CONSIDERATIONS FOR SITE SELECTION

Besides these general considerations, the surgeon must also take into account five special considerations: (1) the type of stoma to be created, (2) whether more than one stoma is to be constructed, (3) the shape of the patient's abdomen, (4) whether the patient is handicapped or wears special prosthetic equipment, and (5) whether future radiation therapy to the abdomen is likely to be necessary.

Type of Stoma

In transverse colostomies, the stoma is generally placed in the right

or left upper quadrant of the abdomen, away from the costal margins and the umbilicus. It should also be brought through the rectus sheath and muscle [*see Figure 5*] to minimize the chances of peristomal herniation. Transverse loop colostomies have a tendency to prolapse, particularly if they are created close to the hepatic flexure.

Because with a continent stoma (e.g., Kock pouch or reservoir) there is no need to wear an external pouch, the stoma can be created below the bikini line, in an inconspicuous yet accessible and visible area of the abdomen. A location about 2.5 cm above the pubic hairline over the right rectus sheath area is generally a suitable site.

Multiple Stomas

Unless there is no alternative, two functioning stomas should not be placed on the same side of the abdomen. To do so would greatly reduce the area of peristomal skin available for affixing the appliances and would complicate the emptying of the individual pouches. In addition, the weight of each pouch impinges on the other and makes the wearing of a belt very difficult for the patient. If both a urinary stoma and a digestive stoma are to be created, the stoma that is more likely to necessitate the use of a belt (i.e., the urinary stoma) should be placed somewhat higher than the other. If both stomas were placed at the same level, a belt would interfere with the second one.

Abdominal Shape

A patient must be able to see a stoma to be able to care for it [*see Figure 6*]. As a rule, therefore, a stoma cannot be placed over the lower abdomen in obese patients or patients with unusual lower abdominal skin folds [*see Figure 7*]. The deep skin creases associated with obesity also render the lower abdomen unsuitable for the placement of an appliance. In such patients, the stoma should be placed higher on the abdomen (generally above the belt line), brought through the rectus muscle, and located where it is visible and can easily be pouched [*see Figure 8*]. In a patient with a distended abdomen, the stoma site chosen should be where the stoma is to sit once the abdomen has regained its normal contour.

The general principles of stoma site selection on the abdomen apply to newborns and infants. Because their abdominal walls are more rounded and their hips are usually flexed, however, their abdominal stomas should be placed somewhat higher than is usual in adults. A diaper should not be used instead of a pouch to contain bowel efflux or urine. Many companies make stoma pouches specif-

Figure 5 Shown is a properly placed loop colostomy in the right upper quadrant.

Figure 6 This poorly placed stoma is in a deep skin fold, on top of the iliac crest; it is invisible to the patient.

Figure 7 These multiple skin folds make the use of a leakproof pouch system very difficult.

Figure 8 In this massively obese patient about to undergo an abdominoperineal proctectomy, the colostomy site selected (black dot) is above the belt line. The arrow points to the umbilicus.

Figure 9 Shown are three pouches that are suitable for infant and newborn ostomates: a one-piece opaque pouch, a two-piece urinary pouch, and a one-piece clear infant pouch (Hollister).

ically for infants and newborns. These pouches not only are smaller but also have skin barriers that are gentler to and safer for newborns' skin [*see Figure 9*].

If the creation of a stoma in the vicinity of a scar is unavoidable, use of easily molded paste or wafers made of pectin, gelatin, and cellulose (e.g., Stomahesive or Hollihesive) can minimize, to some extent, the fitting problems such skin irregularities present.

Stomas for Handicapped Patients

In patients who wear orthopedic braces, are confined to wheelchairs, or are restricted by other handicaps, the stoma may have to be placed in an unconventional location. A surgeon must select a stoma site for such a patient with particular care, taking into consideration both the patient's infirmity and the position in which the patient plans to be when caring for the stoma. Accordingly, it may be advisable to choose the stoma site with the patient sitting in a wheelchair or wearing braces.

Often, with bedridden patients, the surgeon does not select a specific stoma site preoperatively. This is a mistake: when the patient is repositioned, especially into a sitting position, an appliance covering a stoma that was placed in a skin fold or a deep crease, too close to a scar, under a sagging breast, or too close to a feeding tube will tend to loosen and spill its contents. To minimize such problems, the surgeon need only spend a few minutes looking at the patient lying in bed in the usual position and then examine the abdomen for scars, deep folds, feeding tube sites, and other physical features that might impinge on the stoma. This simple step will save the surgeon many calls asking for a revision or a relocation of the stoma.

Stomas and Radiation Therapy

When it is anticipated that radiation therapy through lower abdominal portals will be necessary after operation, the stoma site should be located outside the radiation field, if possible.

When a patient has already undergone irradiation, the stoma should be placed outside the treated area to prevent skin breakdown and delayed healing.

MARKING THE STOMA SITE

It is essential that skin marks placed at the selected stoma site not fade away when the patient showers preoperatively or when his or her abdomen is washed in the operating room. Because truly indelible skin markers are unavailable, the preferred technique for identifying the selected stoma site is intradermal injection of methylene blue. Placement of superficial scratch marks, unless done immediately before operation, can cause local cellulitis that may contribute to postoperative problems with the stoma.

THE LAPAROSCOPICALLY CREATED STOMA

Because the only major difference between laparoscopic and conventional surgery is the access to the operative site,[9] stomal care is, for the most part, the same in patients who have undergone laparoscopic procedures as in those who have undergone open procedures. Creating a stoma laparoscopically involves pulling a segment of intestine through a trocar site and then enlarging the site to deliver the bowel onto the abdomen. Too often, either by necessity or by lack of foresight, the trocar site is not where the stoma site ideally should be. Additional thought must be given to trocar placement when one plans to create a stoma; a good site for the stoma must be selected and marked, even if this means inserting an additional port devoted exclusively to pulling out the stoma. The common practice of enlarging the trocar site by simply incising the adjacent skin is not to be recommended: it causes the stoma to be slit-shaped, with poor projection and a tendency to retract. Instead, the trocar orifice should be enlarged by excising a circular button of skin around the trocar site.

Postoperative Care

The following discussion is on general principles of stomal care. We do not address care of the various types of stoma separately, because the basic principles governing care are essentially the same for all types, except for some details that will be noted. Care of a continent pouch will be described separately.

IN THE OPERATING ROOM

Provided that the general principles of stoma construction are clearly followed (i.e., that the bowel is brought through the abdominal wall to the skin without tension, is brought through the rectus muscle with a good blood supply, and is everted and sutured primarily to the skin away from the incision, drains, and retention sutures), all electively created stomas, with very few exceptions, are matured and are ready for pouching at the end of the operation. Stomas created under emergency conditions should also be matured. The advantages of maturing the stoma (i.e., the immediate decompression of the bowel and the ease of caring for a matured stoma) far outweigh the disadvantages (i.e., the additional operating time needed to mature the stoma and the theoretical possibility of contaminating the peritoneal cavity with bowel contents). When a surgeon decides to delay the opening of a digestive stoma, the exteriorized bowel segment can simply be covered with a piece of petrolatum gauze and a sterile dressing. The gaseous distention, serositis, and bowel wall edema that eventually develop in such cases often make pouching and caring for these stomas after their opening a challenge.

The pouch used in the operating room should be transparent, drainable, disposable, and of one- or two-piece construction [see Figure 10]. A pouch system is available for digestive stomas that is simple and inexpensive yet fully adequate for the purpose. Before applying the pouch, the surgeon should cut a hole in the adhesive backing about 3 mm larger than the stoma to allow for postoperative swelling. Whereas digestive stoma pouches are closed by means of a clamp, urinary stoma pouches are connected to a drainage system.

Once a segment of bowel (i.e., the future stoma) has been exteri-

Figure 10 **Four different types of pouch are shown: a one-piece urinary system (United) (*a*), a two-piece urinary system (ConvaTec) (*b*), a one-piece digestive pouch system (Hollister) (*c*), and a two-piece digestive pouch system (Coloplast) (*d*).**

orized, the surgeon should exert his or her utmost efforts to avoid impinging on the peristomal skin necessary for securing the appliance. All too often, one sees retention sutures, drains, and feeding catheters placed carelessly in close proximity to a stoma. Such carelessness makes pouching difficult at best and frequently leads to leaks and the attendant skin problems. The problem of insufficient peristomal skin area can be circumvented to some degree by cutting and reshaping the adhesive area; however, this loss of adhesive surface may reduce the stability of the appliance.

Rigid bridges of various designs are available for support of loop colostomies [see Figure 11]. These bridges should fit inside the stoma pouch; however, many do not. In addition, if these rigid bridges are sewn to the skin, the pouch opening will not fit adequately around the stoma. The peristomal skin will be bathed by stomal efflux, and the stitch holes create an avenue by which urine or stool can infect the skin. We recommend using a segment of No. 16 rubber catheter with its ends folded [see Figure 12]; this will serve the same purpose and can easily be inserted completely into the pouch. If a supporting bridge cannot be accommodated within the pouch, it is difficult

Figure 11 **Rigid colostomy bridges that can fit inside a pouch system are used to support loop colostomies. They come in one- and two-piece forms.**

Figure 12 **Use of a segment of No. 16 catheter is an easy and practical way to support a loop colostomy (*left*). The rubber bridge shown at left fits into the pouch (*right*).**

to make the pouch system leakproof, unless some adhesive paste is used to fill the gap created by the rod between the skin and the adhesive wafer. The bulky plastic rods with rubber tubing that are traditionally used to hold a loop colostomy are out of place in modern stomal care.

FIRST POSTOPERATIVE DAY

If the pouch is not leaking and the stoma color is good, there is little to be gained by changing the pouch. If a stoma is smeared with stool or its color cannot be determined, the pouch should be removed and the stoma gently wiped off with wet gauze and inspected. If the stoma appears to be healthy, a new disposable pouch should be applied; if not, the surgeon should be notified. The patient should be reassured and told that in the next few days he or she will be thoroughly instructed in the care of the stoma. Given the pressure for accelerated discharges imposed by managed care, it is necessary to begin involving the family in the care of the patient on the day after the operation, even if the patient is still somewhat obtunded. If the patient is alert at this time, the ET nurse or the staff nurse can start the postoperative education process by showing the patient how the pouch is changed and doing it for him or her. On the next day, the ET nurse or the staff nurse helps the patient change the pouch, and by the third day (or at least the third teaching session), the patient should be able to change the pouch unassisted under the guidance of the ET nurse or the staff nurse.

Whereas urinary stomas drain immediately, ileostomies generally begin to function within the first 48 postoperative hours, and colostomies take about twice that long. Stomas created under emergency conditions to relieve bowel obstruction may start to discharge promptly.

SUBSEQUENT DAYS

About 48 hours after operation, the entire pouch system should be removed and the peristomal skin cleaned. If any discoloration, retraction, or mucocutaneous separation is noted or, in a urinary stoma, if any of the stents seem displaced, these problems should be promptly reported to the surgeon. Mucocutaneous separation at the base of the stoma may be caused either by the breaking or untying of the sutures uniting the intestine to the skin or by the sutures having cut through the tissues. If such a separation is noted, one must apply a minimum of pressure at the base of the stoma when pouching to prevent further separation. If the separation is superficial, the area can be covered with a coating of Stomahesive powder. If the separation is wider and deeper, it should be filled with Stomahesive paste to protect the area, keep it moist, and promote granulation. The pouch wafer should cover the filled site to protect the subcutaneous tissue from the stoma efflux.

The pouch system with which the patient is to become familiar is then selected. The patient should be shown how the clamp or the spigot at the bottom of the pouch works. If the system is a two-piece one, the pouch and adhesive wafer are connected and then applied over the stoma as a unit, with care taken not to put pressure on the newly created stoma and the sutures fixing it to the skin. The patient should then be invited to place and close the clamp or to connect the spigot to drainage on the newly applied pouch; in this way, he or she is coaxed into looking at the stoma and touching the pouch. Further involvement of the patient in the care of the stoma should progress gradually, under the gentle and patient supervision of a member of the health care team.

During the next 48 to 72 hours, whenever the pouch of a diges-

Figure 13 Shown is the VPI nonadhesive pouch system for intestinal and urinary stomas. The urinary appliance is the larger of the two.

tive stoma is one half to two thirds full, the pouch clamp should be removed and the pouch emptied and rinsed out rather than replaced. Rinsing is easily accomplished by means of a bulb syringe filled with tap water. The pouch should not be allowed to fill to the point where its sheer weight pulls it away from the patient's skin.

Once a day, the pouch of a urinary stoma should be rinsed through its spigot with 20 to 30 ml of vinegar to break up mucous plugs and to acidify the pouch wall so as to prevent bacterial proliferation and

1/2 in (12 mm)

3/4 (19 mm)

1 1/8 in (29 mm) 1 1/4 in (32 mm) 1 1/2 in (38 mm)

7/8 (22 mm)

1 in (25 mm)

2 in (50 mm)

1 3/4 in (45 mm)

2 1/2 in (64 mm) 3 in (76 mm)

Figure 14 Patients must learn to measure their stomas with the help of measuring guides, such as this one, provided by the manufacturers of stoma appliances.

the formation of uric acid crystals. The pouch should then be reconnected to drainage.

At this stage, the pouch system should be changed every other day, unless leakage occurs. This schedule allows the staff to teach the patient how to care for the stoma. When the patient's appliance is changed, the portion adhering to the patient's abdomen should be carefully detached with the help of a cloth (either a piece of gauze or a washcloth) moistened with tap water; it should never be pulled off. The stoma and the peristomal skin should then be gently wiped clean with a moist cloth. We do not use permanent appliances that are cemented to the skin in the postoperative period. If such appliances are used, it must be remembered that skin cement solvent rather than water is needed to detach them from the skin. Currently, with the large assortment of disposable pouch systems available, the use of cement and rigid faceplates is seldom, if ever, indicated.

A reusable pouch system (the VPI system) [*see Figure 13*] has been developed that uses no adhesive and consists of a Silastic ring held in place with a belt. This system is favored by patients who have problems with adhesive pouch systems or who wish to change their pouch frequently. In particular, it is attractive to active people and to persons in wheelchairs, who appreciate the large capacity of the pouch and the fact that they can easily and atraumatically change their pouch system frequently. All of the components of the system—the belt, the Silastic ring, and the large-capacity pouch—are reusable and easy to clean and care for.

The patient should learn to measure the stoma with a measuring guide [*see Figure 14*] and cut out a properly sized hole in the appliance wafer so that the edge of the wafer is approximately $1/8$ in. away from the stomal mucosa; this allows for expansion. The wafer and the pouch should be connected and the appliance positioned as one piece over the stoma. The importance of a well-fitting stoma appliance to protect the peristomal skin cannot be overemphasized. The patient should be told about some of the potential local skin problems associated with the type of stoma selected and taught how to recognize them. The instructor must stress that most of these skin problems can be prevented by (1) proper fitting of the pouch system, (2) using the least irritating products at the stoma site, and (3) avoiding physical trauma to the skin in the region around the stoma. When a stoma is being pouched, additional support for the appliance can be provided by use of a belt or by framing the adhesive wafer with adhesive tape. Waterproof Perma Type tape can be used by patients planning to swim.

DISCHARGE OBJECTIVES

The psychosocial aspects of care discussed earlier [*see* Preoperative Counseling, *above*] should be reemphasized and elaborated on throughout the postoperative period. If the patient did not see or refused to see an ostomy visitor preoperatively, it may be appropriate to ask if he or she wants to see one at this time. If the patient is willing, a relative may learn to help him or her look after the stoma. If infirmity or age prevents a patient from attending to the stoma, a relative or friend must be called in. If relatives and friends are unavailable or are unable or unwilling to help, the services of a social worker must be obtained as soon as possible. In fact, this need for postdischarge assistance should have been anticipated preoperatively, and steps should have been taken to provide the patient with adequate support. Patients and caretakers should be made aware of the social and medical support systems available to them [*see Table 2*]. Either the surgeon or

Table 2 Social and Medical Support Systems Available to Ostomates and Caretakers

Social Resources	Medical Resources
Hospital social worker	Surgeon
Medicare or CHAMPUS advisers	Enterostomal therapy (ET) nurse
Local chapter of the United Ostomy Association	Family physician
United Ostomy Association ostomy visitor	Psychologist
American Cancer Society	Dietitian

the ET nurse should provide the patient with written instructions, supplies, and lists of suppliers (including phone numbers).

Before discharge, a patient or caretaker should be familiar with one type of pouch system. He or she should be able to (1) empty the pouch and cleanse the closure tail [*see Figure 15*], (2) detach the adhesive portion of the pouch system properly, (3) care for the peristomal skin, (4) measure the stoma and cut a hole of the correct size in the adhesive portion of the system, (5) apply the pouch system properly, and (6) be aware of the telltale signs of peristomal skin problems and know how to prevent and correct them.

Peristomal Skin Care

As noted, many skin problems can be prevented by taking a few simple precautions. Fungal infections (most commonly caused by *Candida*) often occur under a wafer because of body heat. These infections respond rapidly to topical antifungal powders such as Mycostatin. Fungal overgrowth can also occur where the warm plastic appliance presses over the abdomen. This problem can often be prevented by using a pouch cover, wearing bikini underpants under the pouch, or wearing specially designed underwear [*see Figure 1*] to keep the plastic away from the skin.

The following three conditions can arise soon after surgery and demand immediate attention if they do:

1. Allergic contact dermatitis. The skin appears erythematous, weepy, or eroded in a pattern exactly corresponding to the shape of the offending product (e.g., tape or a skin barrier). Before a change is made to another skin barrier, a skin-barrier wipe or a transparent dressing should be used on the damaged skin in the interim so that a pouch can be secured. Patch test-

Figure 16 Shown are three convex pouches: a one-piece precut urostomy pouch (ConvaTec), an open-end bowel pouch (ConvaTec), and a one-piece bowel stoma pouch (NuHope).

a

b

Figure 17 Shown are selected (*a*) two-piece pouches (Coloplast open-end, ConvaTec urinary, and Cymed open-end) and (*b*) closed-end pouches (ConvaTec, Dansac, United, and Hollister).

Figure 15 Once an open-end pouch is emptied, the closure tail must be cleansed.

ing of another pouch system can be done by cutting a small piece of the new barrier wafer and tape and placing them on the opposite side of the patient's abdomen, forearm, or back for 24 hours and checking for any reaction.

2. Folliculitis (i.e., inflammation or infection of hair follicles). This condition usually arises when the abdominal hairs have grown back in the peristomal area and are forcibly pulled out with each pouch change. The patient should be instructed to remove the pouch using a wet piece of gauze or washcloth in a push-pull motion. When the folliculitis has healed, the patient should use an electric razor to shave the area and apply a skin sealant to protect the skin during pouch removal. Safety razors may cause small skin cuts that lead to skin infections. Application of an antimicrobial powder after the skin has been cleaned and dried is also helpful.

3. Irritant dermatitis. Either efflux from the stoma or the use of harsh cleansers may cause chemical burns. The skin appears erythematous, weepy, and painful, and the irritation may be restricted to a specific area of leakage. Treatment consists of (1) gently cleansing all of the peristomal skin, (2) dusting with Stomahesive powder, and (3) correcting any pouching problems that may have caused the leak.

Besides these three conditions, all of which may appear in the early postoperative period, there are a number of complications that may arise later, such as radiation reactions, parastomal abscesses, caput medusae, pseudoepithelial hyperplasia, pyoderma gangrenosum, and parastomal ulcers.

The patient should be seen for stomal and pouch evaluation 3 months after the operation and subsequently on an annual basis or as necessary for management of complications. Either weight gain or weight loss may necessitate changing the pouch system. In either event, the use of convex pouches may prove helpful [*see Figure 16*].

The patient must be aware that as long as the wafer is protecting the peristomal skin and is securely fixed to it, there is no compelling reason to change it. Wearing time generally ranges from 3 to 6 days and depends on both the individual and the pouch system used. If a patient has problems with the appliance, he or she should consult the surgeon or an ET nurse, who may recommend a change in the pouching steps or, if necessary, a change of pouch systems. Improvements are constantly being made in the design and manufacture of stoma equipment; some of the newer systems may fit or be worn more comfortably. There are several makers of high-quality equipment whose products [*see Figure 17*] we use regularly [*see Table 3*].

Written Patient Information

Most ostomy patients are under such intense stress after the op-

a

b

Figure 18 Illustrated are (*a*) the standard method of emptying a pouch and (*b*) an alternative emptying method that may be necessary after abdominoperineal resection or extensive rectal surgery. (For patients who have undergone lower GI surgery of this type, sitting beside the commode can be more comfortable than sitting on it, placing less stress on the perineal wound or the suture line.)

Table 4   Selected Companies Selling Stoma Appliances through Mail-Order Catalogues

AOS—American Ostomy Supply Guide, P.O. Box 13396, Milwaukee, WI 53213-9906; 800-858-5858

Edgepark Surgical, Inc., 1810 Summit Commerce Park, Twinsburg, OH 44087-9931; 800-321-0591

MED EXPRESS, P.O. Box 49850, Minneapolis, MN 55449-9908; 877-409-1234

Parthenon Co., 3311 W. 2400 Street, Salt Lake City, UT 84119; 800-453-8898

eration and the creation of the stoma that they cannot absorb all the oral instructions they receive. For this reason, it is important to give them some written information, preferably in a folder; they may or may not read this material while in the hospital, but they will have it at home to use as a reference after discharge. The patient information folder should contain the following components:

1. General stomal care instructions [*see Figure 18*].
2. Specific instructions on caring for their particular type of stoma.
3. Specific directions for applying and caring for their particular pouch system.
4. A list of the steps involved in changing the pouch.
5. Some general dietary instructions, along with explanations of what a stoma blockage is, how to prevent it, and what to do before calling the physician.
6. A guide to recognizing signs of urinary infection (for patients with ileal conduits).
7. A number where the ET can be reached for answers to questions and for discussion of any stoma or pouch problems that may arise, along with the date of the 3-month return visit to the ET for evaluation of the stoma and the pouch system.
8. A referral to local ostomy support group meetings. Ideally, the patient will have seen an ostomy visitor while in the hospital.

Figure 19   **This patient is about to insert an irrigating cone into his stoma. Note the presence of the irrigation sleeve and the retaining belt.**

9. Information on where and how to obtain stoma appliances and a reminder to check with the insurance company to see whether supplies must be purchased from a specific vendor. A list of local pharmacies or medical suppliers should be included, along with, if needed or desired, a mail-order catalogue [*see Table 4*].

POSTOPERATIVE CARE OF PATIENTS WITH CONTINENT STOMAS

A patient with a continent stoma does not use an external pouch, and hence, certain aspects of his or her care are different. Nevertheless, a patient with a continent stoma also requires the expert planning, counseling, and care that other ostomates require.

After the construction of a continent ileostomy, the surgeon intubates the intestinal pouch with a No. 30 Silastic catheter. A silk tie is placed around the catheter at the level of the stoma to mark the correct position of the tube. The tube is then affixed securely to the skin. It is left in place for about 10 days, and the intestinal pouch is allowed to empty by gravity. The tube must be irrigated with 30 ml of normal saline solution every 6 hours or so to ensure that it remains patent. As soon as the patient expresses interest, he or she may participate in the irrigation of the intestinal pouch and in the washing of the stoma and the surrounding skin. About 10 days after operation, the patient should be taught how to extubate and intubate the intestinal pouch. At this point, the tube should not be kept out of the pouch for more than 30 minutes at a time. Drainage through the catheter is facilitated by saline irrigations.

About 4 weeks after the operation, the patient will extubate and reintubate the stoma at preset times separated by gradually longer intervals, which allows the intestinal pouch to distend progressively.

A similar postoperative approach is required after the creation of a urinary continent pouch, such as the so-called Indiana pouch.[10]

COLOSTOMY IRRIGATION

Colostomy irrigation is not essential to the good functioning of a stoma.[11] It is time consuming and should be performed only for the convenience of the patient. Stomas proximal to the splenic flexure should not be irrigated because of the liquid stools present in that portion of the bowel. In most cases, the teaching of colostomy self-irrigation [*see Sidebar* Recommended Procedures for Irrigation *and Figure 19*] should be deferred for several weeks, until the patient has recuperated from the operation and has gained some familiarity with the stoma. Another reason for deferring instruction in self-irrigation is that the colon may need several weeks to recover from the operation and return to its previous pattern of motility. When deciding who should be taught self-irrigation, the surgeon must take into consideration the patient's age and general state of health, the availability of reasonable bathroom facilities, and the patient's motivation and ability to put up with the inconvenience (and, at times, the variable results) of self-irrigation.

If a patient is to receive chemotherapy postoperatively, instruction in self-irrigation should be postponed. If the patient is already irrigating when placed on chemotherapy, irrigation should be discontinued. All too often, a patient receiving chemotherapy is too tired to perform an adequate irrigation; moreover, the diarrhea that frequently accompanies chemotherapy will render irrigation ineffectual. Irrigation can be resumed, if desired, after chemotherapy is completed.

Recommended Procedures for Irrigation

If irrigation is to be performed, the following instructions for the patient are recommended.

Supplies

Irrigation bag with long tube and cone; sleeve with belt.

Water

Tepid tap water, 1,000–1,500 ml.

Procedure

1. Fill the irrigation bag with tepid water, remove air in the tube by allowing water to run through it and into the sink, close the clamp, hang up the irrigation bag at a height that will allow the bottom of the bag to be at the level of your shoulder when you are seated.

2. Sit on the toilet or a chair beside the toilet (if the perineum is still sore).

3. Remove the colostomy appliance.

4. Center the opening of the irrigation sleeve over the stoma, and place the end of the sleeve in the toilet bowl. To avoid splashing, the sleeve need only be long enough to touch the water. If it is too long, it may be cut. Tighten the irrigation sleeve belt to prevent leakage.

5. Lubricate the end of the cone with water or a water-soluble lubricant. Insert the cone tip gently through the top of the open sleeve and into the stoma, and rotate the cone until the water flows in freely. (If the water does not flow in freely, do not push the cone in further; instead, pull the cone back and rotate it because usually the cause of the limited water flow is that the opening of the cone is against the bowel wall.)

6. Press the cone firmly and gently against the stoma to prevent leakage.

7. The water must flow in slowly. It takes about 5 minutes to instill a quart. Stop the flow of water if you become uncomfortable or experience cramps, but do not remove the cone, because removal would allow the water to return too soon.

8. When all the water has been emptied from the irrigation bag and tube, remove the cone from the stoma. Close the top of the irrigation sleeve with clips or ties.

9. Allow about 15 to 20 minutes for the bowel to empty, with the sleeve end remaining in the toilet.

10. Rinse the sleeve with water, and clamp the end closed. You may leave the bathroom and do what you wish for the next 30 to 45 minutes. During this time, additional water and stool may be expelled.

11. Return to the bathroom, unclamp the sleeve, empty any effluence, and rinse the sleeve. With time, you will know when evacuation is completed. Unsnap the belt, and remove the sleeve.

12. Wash the peristomal skin with warm water, rinse well, pat dry, and replace your appliance.

13. Clean the sleeve with detergent and water, rinse it well, and allow it to air-dry. Let any remaining fluid in the irrigation bag and tubing drain out. Wash, rinse, and dry off the cone.

The entire procedure should take about 1 hour.

General Pointers

1. For the first irrigations you perform, write down the amount of water used, the amount of time for the procedure, and the amount and character of the water and stool expelled. If you record this information for the first few irrigations, you will learn how long to wait for a total evacuation, how much fluid to use, and how often you need to irrigate.

2. Good results are obtained by performing the procedure at about the same time each day. Some individuals need to irrigate only every other day.

3. Because you do not eat the same type or amount of food daily, the amount of elimination will vary from day to day. Persons who are dehydrated may at times need extra irrigation fluid because some of that fluid will be quickly absorbed by the colon.

4. Try to relax when performing irrigation. If you are nervous or upset, often this method will not work for you. If you are ill or experiencing diarrhea, you should temporarily discontinue irrigation.

5. Remember: to irrigate or not to irrigate is your choice.

References

1. Rothman CP: Sperm banking. Common Problems in Infertility and Impotence. Rajfer J, Ed. Year Book Medical Publishers, Chicago, 1990, p 200

2. Metcalf AM, Dozois RR, Kelly KA: Sexual function in women after proctocolectomy. Ann Surg 204:624, 1986

3. Emblem R, Stray Pedersen S, Bergan A, et al: Female complaints after proctocolectomy. Proceedings of the Seventh Biennial Congress of the World Council of Enterostomal Therapists. Palex International SA, 1990, p 20

4. Gloeckner MR, Starling JR: Providing sexual information to ostomy patients. Dis Colon Rectum 25:575, 1982

5. Physician's Desk Reference, 51st ed. Medical Economics, Montvale, New Jersey, 1997, pp 1103, 1677, 2588

6. Fazio VW, Erwin-Toth P: Enterostomal therapy. Colon and Rectal Surgery, 4th ed. Corman ML, Ed. Lippincott-Raven, Philadelphia, 1998

7. Ohmura Y: Evaluation of preoperative stoma site marking. Proceedings of the Seventh Biennial Congress of the World Council of Enterostomal Therapists. Palex International SA, 1990, p 27

8. Bass EM, Pino AD, Tan A, et al: Does preoperative stoma marking and education by the enterostomal therapist affect outcome? Dis Colon Rectum 40:440, 1997

9. Milsom JW, Bohm B: Laparoscopic Colorectal Surgery. Springer, New York, 1995

10. Rowland RG, Mitchell ME, Bihrie R, et al: Indiana continent urinary reservoir. J Urol 137:1136, 1986

11. Laucks SS 2nd, Mazier WP, Milsom JW, et al: An assessment of colostomy irrigation. Dis Colon Rectum 31:279, 1988

Reviews

Broadwell DC, Jackson BS: Principles of Ostomy Care. CV Mosby Co, St. Louis, 1982

Celestin LR: Color Atlas of the Surgery and Management of Intestinal Stomas. Year Book Medical Publishers, Chicago, 1987

Dozois R: Alternatives to Conventional Ileostomy. Year Book Medical Publishers, Chicago, 1985

Goldstein BG, Jackson BS: Principles of Ostomy Care. CV Mosby Co, St. Louis, 1982

Gordon PH, Nivatvong S: Colon, Rectum, and Anus. Quality Medical Publishers, St. Louis, 1999

Jeter K: These Special Children: The Ostomy Book for Parents of Children with Colostomies, Ileostomies, and Urostomies. Bull Publishing Co, Palo Alto, 1982

McDougal WS: Use of intestinal segments and urinary diversions. Campbell's Urology, vol 3. Walsh PC, Retik AB, Vaughan ED, et al, Eds. WB Saunders Co, Philadelphia, 1998, p 3121

Smith DB, Johnson DE: Ostomy Care and the Cancer Patient: Surgical and Clinical Considerations. Grune & Stratton, Orlando, Florida, 1986

Acknowledgments

Figures 1, 15, and 18   Tom Moore.

Figure 3 and Sidebar illustrations   Carol Donner.

4 REHABILITATION OF THE BURN PATIENT

Robert H. Demling, M.D.

Return to Normal Function after a Burn

Rehabilitation is the return to normal function. This process is particularly difficult in burn patients because healing is a long-term process and burn scars are permanent.

Rehabilitation begins on the day of admission, with the objectives of restoring cardiopulmonary stability and minimizing musculoskeletal dysfunction. Long-term objectives are the maintenance or restoration of function in affected areas, the control of scarring and wound contractures, the restoration of the whole patient to functional activity, and the adjustment to cosmetic and functional abnormalities. Rehabilitation efforts include the following six components aimed at minimizing disability: early wound closure; exercise, positioning, and splinting; skin care; thermoregulation; psychological support; and restoration of function. Each component requires special expertise, making an integrated team approach essential.

Components of Rehabilitation

EARLY WOUND CLOSURE

Early wound excision can minimize functional loss by removing the nonpliable eschar and eliminating wound pain [*see III:12 Burn Care in the Early Postresuscitation Period*]. Even with deep burns, pain develops after eschar separation, which begins approximately 1 week after the burn. A split-thickness skin graft, although more elastic than eschar, does not have normal elasticity, and wound stiffness has to be counterbalanced with aggressive therapy and splinting.

Early grafting can hamper general function in two ways. First, pain at the sites of donor skin can limit the range of motion, often interfering with ambulation. The use of skin substitutes can decrease pain at donor sites and improve mobility. Second, grafted areas must be immobilized to permit neovascularization. From 3 to 5 days of immobilization is usually adequate if the grafts are placed on residual dermis or fascia, but grafts on fatty tissue take 5 to 7 days to revascularize. The use of temporary skin substitutes on superficial second-degree burns and donor sites improves function by decreasing pain and increasing flexibility.

EXERCISE

As soon as feasible, the burn areas should be evaluated for estimates of current and future limitations of motion. This evaluation should be made in the first 24 hours after a small to moderate burn and during the first 24 to 48 hours after a large burn. Supervised motion of burned areas should begin as soon as possible. The goals of exercise are to maintain normal joint range, maintain strength and endurance, and promote functional independence. Although functional independence is the long-range goal, progressive independence is needed throughout rehabilitation. Proper positioning and splinting must be used to maintain the positive effects of exercise.

The selection of exercise techniques depends on the extent of injury and the patient's progress in recovery. In active exercises, the patient achieves a greater range of motion, resistance is increased as the patient progresses, and eventually the patient exercises independently. In active assistive exercise, the patient receives assistance from weights, pulleys, and other devices that permit stretching that exceeds the patient's strength. Passive exercises are used in critically ill patients, often with anesthesia, to increase the range of motion. Passive resistive exercise relies on weights and other mechanical means to increase strength and endurance. Stretching, which can be a component of either active or passive exercise, gradually increases force to increase the range of motion and restore position; stretching is used in conjunction with splints. Any of these active and passive techniques can be used in combination with a stationary bicycle or other means of developing endurance. Ambulation improves the patient's range of motion, strength, endurance, and independence.

Active and passive motion are assisted by the use of hydrotherapy, which relaxes the patient as well as affected muscles. A daily hydrotherapy session is ideal to begin movement in previously immobilized joints. A 3- to 5-minute period of muscle activity every few hours helps maintain joint motion; longer periods of muscle activity (25 to 30 minutes twice daily) help improve muscle strength. With increased muscle action, tissue edema resolves more rapidly, the appetite is stimulated, and the patient's self-image improves with evidence of progress. Between 2 and 3 weeks after injury, weight lifting and isometric exercise can be added to standard exercises to extend the range of motion.

Early exercise for the hand should emphasize finger range of motion, particularly flexion of the metacarpophalangeal joints, extension of the interphalangeal joints, and thumb abduction and opposition. Wrist exercises should emphasize extension and ulnar deviation because flexion and radial deviation are the most common abnormalities. Forearm supination and pronation are performed with the elbow close to the side to keep the shoulder from assuming the motion of the forearm. Elbow extension, shoulder abduction, and external rotation should be emphasized. Riding a stationary bicycle is an excellent means of strengthening the lower extremities while improving cardiopulmonary reserve. Consistent activity is an essential component of care, even in patients with massive burns. The success of the activity program depends on control of pain and anxiety and on motivation. Premedication before exercise is important, and biofeedback techniques are benefi-

Table 1   Positioning of Burn Areas during Rest

Area	Position
Neck	Extended by pillow or rolled towel placed under neck
Arm	Shoulder abducted 80° to 90°, elbow fully extended, wrists extended 30° to 40° by use of pillows and bedside tables
Hand	Elevated, with metacarpophalangeal joint in 90° flexion; fingers separated, with interphalangeal joints in midflexion; and thumb in midabduction
Trunk/hip	Hip abducted 20°, with knee extended; for short periods, prone position promotes hip extension
Foot	Neutral ankle position, with padding for heel

cial, although difficult to learn. A successful exercise program requires a team effort, with the involvement of all care providers.

The criteria of pulse, blood pressure, respiration, fatigue, pain, and electrocardiography are used to monitor exercise tolerance. Pain is probably the most difficult criterion to monitor because it is the most subjective. All components of the exercise plan are essential and must be integrated into other daily activities, especially burn care, sleep, and nutrition. Exercise and nutrition can be combined, for example, by fabricating simple devices that allow the patient to feed himself or herself. This approach increases independence and improves the patient's self-image. Evidence of progress maintains the patient's cooperation and enthusiasm. Simple techniques, such as marking the floor where the last attempt at ambulation stopped or the wall at the height of the last stretch, show progress and establish new goals.

Careful supervision is required if a joint has been immobilized for a long period or muscle atrophy has eliminated joint protection by muscle tone. Heterotopic calcification is particularly difficult to treat because movement is extremely painful and forced movement may exaggerate the local inflammatory process. Early mobilization of injured areas and early ambulation can prevent heterotopic calcification.

POSITIONING AND SPLINTING

Although exercise is effective in preventing loss of function, patients invariably resume the position of comfort between exercise sessions. This position then leads to contractures. For this reason, exercise, positioning [*see Table 1*], and splinting are closely linked, all being essential to rehabilitation. Splints maintain position in areas not amenable to positioning techniques or, after grafting, allow revascularization. Splints and positioning are often needed for burns of the neck, especially at night or when fatigue develops. Splints are often needed for elbows [*see Figure 1*], but the area most likely to require splinting is the burned wrist and hand. Wrist flexion is a common abnormality, affecting hand and finger function. If the wrist requires a splint, it should be placed over the wound dressing, from the proximal forearm to the palmar crease, extending the wrist 20° to 40°. The burned hand requires a splint that maintains wrist extension and keeps the metacarpophalangeal joint at 80° to 90° flexion and the interphalangeal joint fully extended. The thumb should be abducted and opposed. Splints may be needed to maintain the foot in neutral, overcoming the powerful pull of the extensors.

Thermoplastic materials used in many splints become pliable in hot water (at 160° to 170° F) and cool rapidly at room temperature, making it possible to mold and readjust them as edema resolves or

other gains are made. Splints should be worn at night and during other periods of extended inactivity. Dynamic splinting, with the addition of a pull, adds a component of exercise. Such splinting techniques require a well-trained therapist because improper splints can result in serious complications.

PRESSURE GARMENTS AND SKIN CARE

Constant pressure of 25 to 30 mm Hg on the hypertrophic scar reduces its size and hyperemia. The initial reduction reflects decreased edema and blood flow in the wound. The long-term reduction appears to be caused by decreases in collagen and ground substance deposition, also reflecting decreased blood flow and a decrease in available tissue oxygen. After several weeks of pressure for 22 to 23 hours daily, there is a measurable reduction in wound chondroitin sulfate and myofibroblasts. Pressure garments also improve venous return, which is particularly important if the venous system was compromised by a deep burn or excision to fascia. Because of their contours, areas such as the eyes, nose, mouth, and anterior chest usually do not receive adequate pressure. For these areas, a mold of the contour can be fitted and a garment placed over the mold, providing pressure [*see Figure 2*]. Custom-made pressure inserts can fit any area. Once the wound is closed, garments are used; at first, they are worn for only a few hours a day, but gradually, the period of use is increased to about 22 hours daily. The pressure has to be applied until the scar matures, as is evident from lack of hyperemia, a process taking 12 to 18 months. Problems can occur if the fitting is not perfect or if rapid weight gain makes the fit too tight. Wound erosions can develop, necessitating removal of the garments until the wounds heal.

The skin must also be constantly lubricated to prevent drying and cracking. Skin moisturizers, usually lanolin based, need to be applied several times a day [*see Table 2*]. Patients who wear pressure garments need to use a special lubricant that does not harm the fabric. Prolonged exposure to direct sunlight should be avoided until the scar has matured or the skin has thickened. Temperature and humidity extremes must be avoided, especially by patients with large burns. If sweat glands have been destroyed, increased humidity is poorly tolerated in the summer, often requiring the use of an air conditioner and dehumidifier in the home or at work. In cold weather, the dry air often leads to rapid drying of skin, necessitating use of a humidifier in the home. Many of these early problems resolve in 12 to 24 months.

Figure 1   **Shown is an elbow splint being molded to hold the joint in the proper position.**

Figure 2 **Shown is a compression garment applied to a healed or grafted burn to decrease scar formation.**

PSYCHOSOCIAL SUPPORT

Members of the treatment team must be aware of potential problems and be able to recognize them if they occur. Some emotional problems can be prevented or minimized if the staff communicates adequately with patients, preparing them for procedures and discussing their likely outcome. Because patients may regress and be-

come dependent, they must be strongly encouraged, if not required, to be as independent as possible. Patients' independence must be maintained by their families as well. A key to this independence is a structured plan for daily activities, allowing each patient a measure of control.

Thus, psychosocial support requires independence, good communication, avoidance of unnecessary anxiety (caused by fear of the unknown), adequate sedation and analgesia, an organized daily plan, adequate sleep, and psychosocial assistance for patients, their families, and staff.

Patients should have some input in the scheduling of daily activities. Initially, staff members may need to establish goals. Because of the close interaction of patients and staff over a long period of time, it is often difficult for staff to remain objective. In addition, patients' family members suffer stress because of the magnitude of injury as well as the time required for healing. A psychiatrist or psychologist and a social worker are key members of the burn team. They must become involved early in the course of treatment and not be called in only when serious difficulties arise, because preventive measures may be much more effective than treatment of psychological problems.

Table 2 Skin Care in Burn Rehabilitation

Problem	Treatment
Skin surface blistering and breakdown	Avoid poorly fitted compression garments, splints, and clothing
	Use lubricating lotions
	Use nonadherent dressings
	Use mild soaps
Pigmentation	Wear pressure garments
	Avoid direct sunlight until scar matures and skin is thickened
Itching	Consider using antihistamines or hydrocortisone cream
	Use nonirritating skin lubricants
	Avoid temperature extremes that induce sweating
Impaired thermoregulation	Avoid temperature extremes
	Wear loose-fitting clothing appropriate for the season

Discussion

Pathophysiology

BURN EDEMA AND ESCHAR RIGIDITY

The massive edema that develops beneath the eschar and the nonpliable nature of the eschar seriously impair muscle and joint motion. The edema-induced stiffness lasts 7 to 10 days, long enough for a contracture to develop if the correct position is not maintained. Compared with normal skin, the burn eschar is extremely noncompliant, shrunken by the loss of water and cell substances. Muscle and joint motion depends on the stretching of contiguous nonburned or more superficially burned skin. The eschar may remain in place for extended periods, depending on the approach to grafting and the availability of donor sites. It is important to recognize functional limitations, such as joint stiffness and muscle atrophy.

FUNCTIONAL IMPAIRMENT

Stretching of a burn wound is painful, the comfortable position being the one that minimizes stretch. Continued flexion or adduction at large joints, as well as hyperextension of the metacarpophalangeal joints, often develops. A particularly disabling process with a third-degree hand burn is pressure necrosis of the central slip of the digital extensor tendon at the proximal interphalangeal joint. This is caused by exaggerated flexion when the metacarpophalangeal joint is hyperextended. The most common position abnormalities are adduction of shoulders; flexion at the elbows, wrists, neck, or interphalangeal joints; and hyperextension of the feet.

The patient's motion is limited not only by pain but also by monitoring devices, ventilator tubing, and other equipment. The forced immobility may be necessary if the patient is in a life-threatening situation with cardiopulmonary instability. More often, however, the lack of motion is for the convenience of both patient and medical care providers. In nonburned patients, inactivity is often well tolerated with few, if any, permanent sequelae; in burn patients, immobility may mean losing the battle against the contracting wound. What begins as voluntary immobility rapidly evolves into an intrinsic defect. Another form of restraint occurs after early skin grafting (and later reconstructive procedures). Although it would be ideal to immobilize the graft for 7 to 10 days, as in a nonburned patient, the result in a burn patient would be significant tissue rigidity and muscle atrophy, seriously restricting motion.

Three pathophysiologic processes—contracture and hypertrophic scar formation, muscle loss, and heterotopic calcification and ossification—are potentiated by lack of motion.

CONTRACTURE AND HYPERTROPHIC SCAR FORMATION

The natural course of a wound that remains open for more than 3 weeks is the deposition of dense scar. Complete epithelialization before 3 weeks usually leads to only minimal scarring, but some patients produce incredible amounts of scar despite relatively superficial injuries. Wound contraction is produced by contractile myofibroblasts and the deposition of ground substance and collagen. A shortened noncompliant wound at a joint results in a contracture, the most common contractures being identical to the most common position abnormalities (resulting from inadequate motion). These are flexion contractures (of the elbows, wrists, neck, and interphalangeal joints), adduction contractures of the shoulders, and extension contractures of the feet and metacarpophalangeal joints.

Hypertrophic scarring occurs after continued scar deposition in the reepithelialized wound. The scar is a raised, hyperemic, pruritic wound—a serious physical blemish as well as a cause of rigidity and pain, impairing function. Pain associated with movement limits activity, and continued itching leads to scratching, skin breakdown, and the risk of superficial infection. Exercise may cause the scar to split, especially if the scar becomes dry, increasing pain and the risk of infection. Keloid formation is the exaggerated form of this process, which is more likely to occur if there is any delay in wound closure. Wounds requiring more than 4 weeks to heal, such as deep dermal burns that heal spontaneously, are most likely to produce hypertrophic scars. Grafted wounds produce much less hypertrophic scarring. Both contracture and hypertrophic scarring peak from 3 to 6 months after injury and partially resolve at 12 to 18 months.

Care providers must recognize the delayed onset of hypertrophic scarring so that precautionary measures can be taken. As the inflammatory process diminishes and the rate of collagen lysis exceeds the rate of collagen deposition, the hypertrophic scar decreases in size. Between 12 and 18 months, the scar becomes softer and flatter and less hyperemic. Any hyperemia indicates active scar turnover, but the lack of hyperemia is a good sign that the scar is mature. Although the scar may relax, the underlying tissues can become permanently foreshortened, resulting in joint ankylosis.

MUSCLE LOSS

Inactivity of muscle leads to rapid atrophy, as is evident after a fracture is placed in a cast or, on a more general level, after head or spinal cord injury. The muscle catabolism in burn patients accentuates muscle loss caused by inactivity. The first muscles to decrease in size and strength are the proximal thigh muscles, which are essential for ambulation. Restoration of muscle mass, requiring a continuing increase in work load, is seriously hampered by any contractures or hypertrophic scarring. It is clearly more efficient to maintain muscle mass than to attempt to rebuild muscle, especially in elderly patients who lack the cardiopulmonary reserve needed for an increased work load.

HETEROTOPIC CALCIFICATION AND OSSIFICATION

The earliest sign of calcification, usually appearing 3 to 6 months after injury, is loss of range of motion or increased pain on attempted motion. X-ray evidence of calcium deposition usually postdates initial symptoms by at least 1 week. Calcium and phosphate may be deposited in soft tissue (heterotopic calcification) in 1% to 3% of burn patients, generally patients with major burns involving a joint. Calcium and phosphate deposits may produce bone (ossification), a process that can occur in the ligaments and capsule around a joint or in tissues distant from the joint. The joint most often involved is the elbow, followed by the shoulder. Bone scanning is the most reliable method for monitoring ossification.

Immobility appears to correlate directly with the amount of calcium deposited, although there are usually no measurable changes in serum levels of calcium, phosphorus, or alkaline phosphatase. The mechanism remains unknown, but immobility and hypermetabolism, with rapid tissue turnover, are clearly involved. Both *Staphylococcus aureus* and β-hemolytic streptococci are often found in the wound, but infection does not appear to be a prerequisite. With forceful range-of-motion exercise, there may be bleeding into the joint.

TEMPERATURE REGULATION

Compared with normal skin, thin grafted or healed skin is more prone to heat loss for years after injury. The loss is greatest when there is increased blood flow to the wound. As the scar matures, blood flow to the wound decreases, as does the potential for heat loss. Autoregulation of the microcirculation is impaired, especially for the first few months after injury, limiting the ability to vasoconstrict and vasodilate in response to changes in environmental temperature. Large, deep burns also destroy sweat glands, impairing an important mechanism for eliminating heat generated by pyrogens or exercise. Sensitivity to temperature extremes is a long-term problem in patients who have had burns over large areas of the body.

Recommended Reading

Abdullah A, Herndon D, Robson M: Visible scars and self esteem in pediatric patients with burns. J Burn Care Rehabil 15:164, 1994

Bernstein N, O'Connell K, Chedekel D: Patterns of burn adjustment. J Burn Care Rehabil 13:4, 1992

Evans E: Prevention and correction of deformity after severe burns. Surg Clin North Am 50:1361, 1970

Hallock G: A systematic approach to flap selection for the axillary burn contracture. J Burn Care Rehabil 14:343, 1993

Kealy G, Jensen K, Laubenthal K: Prospective randomized comparison of two types of pressure therapy garments. J Burn Care Rehabil 11:334, 1990

Leivis W, San K: Hypertrophic scar: a genetic hypothesis. Burns 16:176, 1990

Long R, Cope O: Emotional problems of burned children. N Engl J Med 264:1121, 1961

Mann R, Yeong EK, Moore M, et al: Do custom-fitted pressure garments provide adequate pressure? J Burn Care Rehabil 18:247, 1997

Powers P, Crase W: Post traumatic stress disorder in patients with burns. J Burn Care Rehabil 15:147, 1994

Richard R, Staley M, Miller S, et al: To splint or not to splint—past philosophy and practice: part III. J Burn Care Rehabil 18:251, 1997

Robison MC: Prevention and treatment of post burn scars and contracture. World J Surg 16:87, 1992

Rosenberg D, Nelson M: Rehabilitation concerns in electrical burn patients. J Trauma 28:808, 1988

INDEX

A

Aaron sign, 233t
Abdomen, great vessels of, traumatic
  injury to, 432-442
  AAST injury scale for, 432, 433t
  aortic compression device for,
    434, 434f
  celiac axis in, 435
  complications of, 442
  damage-control laparotomy in, 442
  iliac artery in, 440-441, 435t,
    440f
  iliac vein in, 441, 437t
  inferior vena cava in, 436-438,
    437t, 438f
  inframesocolic, 436-438
  infrarenal aorta in, 436, 438f,
    435t
  intra-abdominal hematoma in, 432,
    432f-433f
  left medial visceral rotation for,
    432-433, 434f
  perirenal hematoma in, 438-439,
    438f-439f
  porta hepatis in, 441, 441f
  proximal renal artery in, 435-436,
    435t
  PTFE prosthetic graft for, 434-
    435, 435f
  renal artery in, 438-440, 439f,
    435t
  renal vein in, 438-440, 437t
  retrohepatic area in, 441-442
  superior mesenteric artery in,
    435, 436f-437f, 435t
  superior mesenteric vein in, 436,
    437t
  supramesocolic, 432-436
  survival rate after, 435, 435t
  zone 1, 432-438
  zone 2, 438-440
  zone 3, 440-441
Abdominal compartment syndrome
  in acute renal failure, 1476
  in peritonitis, persistent or
    tertiary, 1305
Abdominal defect(s), flaps for, 1015
Abdominal infection. See also Acute
  abdominal pain; Intra-abdominal
  infection; Upper abdominal
  infection
Abdominal injury, 400-407
  blunt, nonoperative management of,
    417-418
  bowel in, damaged or devitalized,
    404-405
  closure in, 406-407

general technique for, 406-407
open fascial closure in, 406,
  405f
"quick outs" and damage control
  in, 406-407, 406f
skin closure in, 406
contamination in, control of, 403
hemorrhage control in, 403, 404f
incision in, 400
initial exploration in, 400-401
management of, priorities in, 403-
  406
operative exposure in, 401-403
  for aorta, 401, 402f
  for biliary tract, 403
  for duodenum, 403
  for pancreas, 403
  for vena cava, 401-403, 402f,
    404f
patient preparation in, 400
retroperitoneal hematoma in, 401,
  401f
retroperitoneal injury repair in,
  405-406
vascular repair in, 403-404
Abdominal mass, 238-247
  angiography in, 243
  barium studies, 243
  biopsy in, 245-246
    image-guided percutaneous, 245-
      246, 245f
    laparoscopic, 246
  clinical history in, 238-239
  computed tomography in, 244, 244f
  differential diagnosis in, 239
  evaluation of, *Algorithm,* 240-241
  excretory urography in, 243
  exploratory laparotomy in, 246
  investigative studies in, 242-246
  laboratory studies in, 242
  magnetic resonance imaging in, 243
  physical examination in, 239-242
  plain abdominal radiography in,
    243
  radiographic studies in, 242-244,
    243f-244f
  radionucleotide scan in, 243
  ultrasonography in, 243-244
  working diagnosis in, 242
Abdominal pain
  acute. See Acute abdominal pain
  in children, 1165
  in elderly patient, 1152
  in pregnancy. See Pregnancy,
    abdominal pain in
  upper. See Upper abdominal
    infection
Abdominal radiography
  in abdominal mass, 243

in intestinal obstruction, 265-
  266, 266f-269f
Abdominal wall hernia(s). See also
  under Femoral hernia(s);
  Inguinal hernia(s)
  open repair of, 864-882
Abdominoperineal resection, 841-843
  complications of, 842-843
  operative planning in, 841
  operative technique in, 841-842,
    842f
  outcome in, 843
Abrasion, in extremity trauma, 472
Abscess
  anal. See Anal abscess
  breast, 212
  cerebral, coma in, 149
    treatment of, 154-155
  cutaneous
    confined, 311
    pathogens in, 322
  hepatic, 1320-1321
  intra-abdominal. See Intra-
    abdominal abscess
  pericholecystic, surgical options
    for, 1293t
  rectal, in neutropenia, 1116
  renal, candidal, 1347
  retroperitoneal, 1297
  splenic, 1322-1324, 1324f
Accident(s). See also Trauma
  motorcycle, acute wound management
    after, 123
  motor vehicle, elderly patient
    and, 1152
Acetabular fracture, 466-467
Acetaminophen. See also Nonsteroidal
  anti-inflammatory drug(s)
  (NSAIDs)
  suggested dosing for, 1622t
  toxicity, in acute hepatic
    failure, 1492
Acetaminophen with codeine,
  suggested dosing for, 1621t
Acetic acid, contraindicated in
  acute wound care, 126
Acetylsalicylic acid. See Aspirin;
  Nonsteroidal anti-inflammatory
  drug(s) (NSAIDs)
Achalasia, esophageal, reoperation
  for, 718-719
Acid(s), causing chemical burns, 49t
Acid aspiration. See Aspiration,
  acid
Acid-base disorder(s)
  arterial blood samples for
    temperature correction for, 105
    venous *vs.,* 105
  bicarbonate concentration in,

measured *vs.* calculated, 105
in cardiac arrest, sodium
  bicarbonate and, 22
definitions and measurement issues
  in, 105
discussion of, 117-118
evaluation of, *Algorithm,* 106-107
in infants and neonates, 1165-1166
life-threatening, 105-118
mixed, 115-116
  classification of, 115t
  computers in analysis of, 116
  pH in, 115, 116f
  primary *vs.,* 105-108
postoperative, 1626-1627
primary. *See also* Metabolic
  acidosis; Metabolic alkalosis;
  Respiratory acidosis;
  Respiratory alkalosis
  expected compensation for, 108,
    108t
in trauma patient, sodium
  bicarbonate and, 45
Acidosis. *See* Acid-base disorder(s)
  lactic. *See* Lactic acidosis
  metabolic. *See* Metabolic acidosis
  respiratory. *See* Respiratory
    acidosis
Acinetobacter infection,
  antimicrobial agents for, 1236t
Acquired immunodeficiency syndrome
  (AIDS), 1380-1393. *See also*
  Human immunodeficiency virus
  (HIV) infection
  central venous catheterization in,
    1385-1386
  choledochoenteric bypass in, 1385
  common infections in, protection
    from, 1386
  epidemiology of, 1388
  lower GI bleeding in, 297
  lymph node biopsy in, 1383, 1384f
  major risk groups for, 1383f, 1382
  peritonitis in, 1295
  splenectomy in, 1385
  sterilization of surgical
    equipment in, 1386
  surgical interventions in, 1385-
    1386
ACTH stimulation test, 1097, 1097t,
  1126
Actinomyces israelii infection,
  antimicrobial agents for, 1237t
Action potential(s), Purkinje
  (ventricular muscle), 24-25, 25f
Activated charcoal, for emergency
  management, of substance abuse,
  171
Activities of daily living (ADL),

pressure, 355

Barium studies, in abdominal mass, 243

Bartonella henselae infection, antimicrobial agents for, 1236t

Basal cell carcinoma, 302-303, 302f
of neck, 190
nodular, 302-303, 302f
sclerosing (morpheaform), 302, 302f
ulceration and pigmentation in, 302, 302f

Basal metabolic rate. *See* Metabolic rate

Bassini hernioplasty, 866-869, 867f-868f

Bassler sign, 233t

Battered child syndrome, 1179

B cell deficiency, 1121, 1121t

B cell function, in surgical patients, 1112

Bed rest. *See* Immobilization

Beevor sign, 233t

Beta$_1$ agonist(s), 1426t

Beta$_2$ agonist(s), 1426t

Betamethasone, glucocorticoid and mineralocorticoid activities of, 1096f

Beta$_1$ receptor(s), cardiovascular effects of, 1425t

Beta$_2$ receptor(s), cardiovascular effects of, 1425t

Bicarbonate. *See also* Sodium bicarbonate
concentration
calculation of, 1421, 1421t
Henderson-Hasselbalch equation for, 105
loss, metabolic acidosis in, 111-112

Bile, normal volume and composition of, 101t

Bile duct
common. *See* Common bile duct
resection of, for tumor, 757-760
assessment of resectability in, 758, 759f
basic principles of, 757
closure and postoperative care in, 760
complications of, 760
division of common bile duct in, 758, 759f
location of tumor in, 757, 758f
operative technique in, 758-760, 759f-762f
proximal dissection in, 758-759, 759f-762f
reconstruction in, 759-760
trauma to, 415

Biliary anastomosis, guidelines for, 747-748, 748f-750f

Biliary colic, abdominal pain and fever in, 1312-1313, 1312f, 1313t

Biliary drainage catheter(s), postoperative management of, 1627-1628

Biliary stricture, malignant, ERCP for, 677, 678f

Biliary tract
infection of, enterococcal bacteremia due to, 1218
obstruction of, management of, prior to biliary tract procedures, 746
operative exposure of, in abdominal injury, 403
procedures for, 746-763. *See also*

specific procedures, e.g., Cholecystectomy
anastomosis for, 747-748, 748f-750f
exposure of subhepatic field for, 747
imaging studies in, 746
positioning for, 746-747
postoperative care in, 762
preoperative evaluation for, 746
Roux loop for, 748-749

Biliary tract disease. *See* Cholangitis; Cholecystitis

Bilirubin, unconjugated, 248. *See also* Jaundice

Billroth I reconstruction, 726-727, 726f

Billroth II reconstruction, 727, 727f

Biopsy. *See also* Laboratory method(s)
of abdominal mass
image-guided percutaneous, 245-246, 245f
laparoscopic, 246
of breast, 210, 606-611. *See also* Breast, biopsy of
of burn wound, technique for, 480
of lung, for nosocomial pneumonia, 1262
of lymph node. *See* Lymphatic mapping and sentinel node biopsy
in HIV infection, 1383, 1384f
of neck mass, 186-187
of skin, 300
in melanoma, 307

Biotin, requirements for, in ICU patient, 1558t

Birth trauma, 1179

Bite(s)
animal
antibiotic prophylaxis for, 122
antibiotic regimens for, 1329
of hand, 1332-1334, 1334f
infection after, 319-320
rabies prophylaxis for, 124, 320, 329
viral infections from, 1377
black widow spider, 125
brown recluse spider, 125
cat
antibiotic prophylaxis in, 122
of hand, 1332-1334, 1334f
coral snake, 125
dog
antibiotic prophylaxis in, 122
of hand, 1332-1334, 1334f
hand infection in, 1332-1334, 1334f
human
antibiotic prophylaxis in, 119, 122
antibiotic regimens for, 1329
of hand, 1332-1334, 1334f
infection after, 320
viral infections from, 1377
pit viper, 124-125

Black widow spider bite(s), 125

Bladder. *See also entries under* Urinary
exstrophy of, in infants and neonates, emergency surgery in, 1167
infection. *See* Urinary tract infection
trauma to, 449-450
initial evaluation of, 449, 449f-450f

pelvic fracture and, 449

Blastomyces dermatitidis infection, antimicrobial agents for, 1237t

Blastomycosis, clinical presentation and diagnosis of, 1341t

Bleeding disorder(s). *See* Coagulation disorder(s)

Bleeding (hemorrhage), 75-88. *See also* Coagulation disorder(s); Hemostasis
in abdominal injury, 403, 404f
in acute wound, timing of closure for, 123
adrenal, heparin-induced, 1070
after hemorrhoid surgery, 854
Algorithm, 76-77
anemia in, 81-82, 81f, 82t
approach to patient with, 75-82
coagulation parameters in, 78-81
exclusion of technical bleeding in, 75
increased INR
normal aPTT and, 79, 80t
prolonged aPTT and, 80-81, 80t
normal INR
normal aPTT and, 78
prolonged aPTT and, 78, 79t
in chest trauma, 397
in chronic hepatic disease, 1501-1502
esophageal variceal. *See* Esophageal varices
gastrointestinal. *See* Gastrointestinal bleeding; Lower gastrointestinal bleeding; Upper gastrointestinal bleeding
laboratory assessment of, 86-87, 86f, 87t
maxillofacial, 367
shock in, 67
transfusion in, 81

Blood
arterial. *See under* Arterial blood
fecal occult. *See* Fecal examination
substitutes for, 82, 82t
venous. *See under* Venous blood

Blood culture(s), 1214-1228. *See also* Bacteremia
Algorithm, 1215
for candidiasis, 1340-1341
negative, with infection, 1222-1223
evaluation and management of, 1222-1223, 1222t
reasons for, 1222
for nosocomial pneumonia, 1262
positive
with infection, 1214-1220, 1216f
anaerobes in, 1219-1220
fungi in, 1220, 1221t
gram-negative Enterobacteriaceae in, 1218-1219, 1219t
gram-positive cocci in, 1214-1218
staphylococci in, 1214-1217, 1217t, 1217f
streptococci in, 1217-1218
without infection, 1220-1222
gut barrier function and, 1221
microbial translocation and, 1221-1222

Blood donor(s), acceptance policy for, 1366, 1367t

Blood flow. *See also* Circulation
eicosanoids in, 1611-1612

Blood gas(es)

arterial. *See* Arterial blood gas(es)
venous. *See* Venous blood gas(es)

Blood pressure. *See also* Hypertension; Hypotension; Pulmonary arterial pressure; Systemic arterial pressure
cuff method for, 1418-1419
Doppler devices for, 1419
in infants and neonates, 1159, 1159t
noninvasive monitoring of, 1418-1419
in obese patients, 1419

Blood transfusion. *See* Transfusion therapy

Blood urea nitrogen (BUN)
in acute renal failure, 1473
in burn patient, 56

Blumberg sign, 233t

Blunt trauma, need for operation in, 421-422

Body composition, of elderly patients, 1148-1149, 1145f

Body stuffing or packing, in substance abuse, 171

Body temperature. *See* Fever and hyperpyrexia; Temperature

Body water
in hyperdynamic state of critical illness, 1535
total, 99
body weight for, 1624
in infants and neonates, 1162, 1164f

Body water compartment(s), 99
infants and neonates, 1160, 1162, 1164f

Body weight. *See* Weight, body

Bone infection, quinolone for, 1254

Borrelia burgdorferi infection, antimicrobial agents for, 1237t

Borrelia recurrentis infection, antimicrobial agents for, 1237t

Bowel
large. *See* Colon
small. *See* Small bowel

Bowel irrigation, whole, for emergency management, of substance abuse, 170-171

Bowel preparation, 561, 569t, 570-571, 572t-573t, 577-578

Bowel resections, intestinal anastomosis for, 817-818

Bowen disease, 304

Brachial artery, for systemic arterial catheterization, 1402

Brachial plexus injury, in birth trauma, 1179

Bradycardia, in shock, 65

Bradykinin, pulmonary metabolism of, 1449

Brain death, 161-162
in children, 162
clinical criteria for, 995
confirmatory tests for, 162
guidelines for determination of, 161-162, 160f, 161t

Brain herniation syndromes, 162-163
central (axial), 163
lateral (uncal), 162-163
posterior (tectal), 163
subfalcial (cingulate), 162
tonsillar, 163

Brain injury. *See* Head injury

Brain protection, in head injury. *See* Intracranial pressure, reduction of

Branchial cleft cyst, 188

O

oxygen content and, 1445
tissue, measurement of,
continuous, 1418
transcutaneous ($P_{tc}O_2$),
measurement of, continuous,
1418
Oxygen therapy
for burn patients, in immediate
resuscitation period, 53
in multiple organ dysfunction
syndrome, complications of,
1516
postoperative, in pulmonary
insufficiency, 1050
Oxygen transport
calculation of, 1420
in elderly patients, 1149-1151,
1150f
Oxyhemoglobin dissociation curve, in
metabolic acidosis, 108, 108f
Oxymorphone
for patient-controlled analgesia,
1649t
suggested dosing for, 1621t
Oxytetracycline, for bacterial
infections, 1242t-1243t

P

Pacemaker(s)
for asystole, 11
troubleshooting for, 16-17
ventricular capture and, 17
ventricular sensing and, 17
Pain
abdominal
acute. See Acute abdominal pain
in elderly patient, 1152
in pregnancy. See Pregnancy
upper. See Upper abdominal
infection
acute
descending pain control system
in, 1650
dorsal horn control systems and
modulation of incoming
signals in, 1650
epidural analgesia for, 1532
narcotic analgesics for, 1532
patient-controlled analgesia
for, 1532
peripheral receptors and neural
transmission to spinal cord
in, 1650
physiologic mechanisms of, 1650,
1651f
postinjury changes in peripheral
and central nervous systems
in, 1650
spinal reflexes in, 1650
breast, 211-212
burn, 483, 483t
drug therapy for, 58
in infection, 1206
in metabolic response to critical
illness, 1532
phantom, after below-the-knee
amputation, 970-971
postoperative, 1620-1623, 1640-1654
1621t-1623t
in abdominal procedures, 1640-
1641
after outpatient surgery, 549
Algorithm, 1642-1643
combination regimens for, 1649-
1650

cryoanalgesia for, 1648, 1649f
in elderly patient, 1142-1143
epidural anesthetics for, 1621,
1646-1648, 1647t
epidural opioids for, 1645-1646,
1646t
in fast track surgery, 555
guidelines for, 1640-1641
inadequate treatment of, 1640,
1640t
nerve blocks for, 1648
nonsteroidal anti-inflammatory
drugs for, 1648, 1648t
opioids for, systemic, 1621-1622,
1641-1645, 1621t-1622t,
1644t-1645t
patient-controlled analgesia
for, 1649, 1903, 1623t,
1649t
in peripheral procedures, 1641
psychological interventions for,
1641, 1641t
subarachnoid opioids for, 1645-
1646
in thoracic procedures, 1640
transcutaneous electrical nerve
stimulation for, 1648-1649
treatment of, 1620-1623, 1640-
1650, 1621t-1623t. See also
under specific drugs and
procedures
Pain relief
effects of, 1650-1653
on metabolic response to
operation, 1650, 1652
on postoperative morbidity, 1652
postoperative. See Pain,
postoperative
Pain threshold, in elderly patient,
1151-1152
Pancreas
as donor organ, technique for,
1003, 1003f-1004f
injuries to, 424-428, 421t, 423f-
426f
grade I, 424-425, 421t, 423f
grade II, 424, 423f
grade III, 425, 423f
grade IV, 427-428, 423f, 426f
grade V, 428, 423f
operative exposure of, in
abdominal injury, 403
Pancreas transplantation, in
diabetes mellitus, 1091
Pancreatectomy, distal, for chronic
pancreatitis, 788-789, 789f-790f
Pancreatic abscess, 1321-1322
treatment of, 1322
antibiotics for, 1322
drainage for, 1322
nutritional support for, 1322
Pancreatic carcinoma
jaundice in, 254-255. See also
Jaundice, in malignant
obstruction
unresectable, palliative bypass
for, 793-795, 794f-795f
Pancreatic juice, normal volume and
composition of, 101t
Pancreatic necrosis, infected, 1321-
1322
Pancreaticoduodenectomy (Whipple
procedure), pylorus-preserving,
785-788, 785f-788f
Pancreaticojejunostomy, longitudinal
(Puestow procedure), 789-791,
790f-791f
Pancreatic procedure(s), 785-796
distal pancreatectomy for chronic

pancreatitis, 788-789, 789f-
790f
drainage of pancreatic pseudocyst
into Roux-en-Y jejunal loop,
791-792, 792f
drainage of pancreatic pseudocyst
into stomach, 792-793, 793f
longitudinal
pancreaticojejunostomy
(Puestow procedure), 789-791,
790f-791f
palliative bypass for unresectable
pancreatic cancer, 793-795,
794f-795f
pylorus-preserving
pancreaticoduodenectomy
(Whipple procedure), 785-788,
785f-788f
Pancreatic pseudocyst
drainage of
into Roux-en-Y jejunal loop, 791-
792, 792f
into stomach, 792-793, 793f
infected, 1321-1322
Pancreatitis
acute
abdominal pain and fever in,
1312-1313, 1313t
septic response in, 1223
chronic, distal pancreatectomy
for, 788-789, 789f-790f
clinical criteria for severity of,
1321, 1321t
gallstone
cholecystectomy for, 1313-1316
ERCP sphincterotomy for, 1316,
1316f
Ranson clinical prognostic index
in, 1313, 1313t, 1323f
treatment of, 1313-1316, 1313t,
1316f
in pregnancy, 1191
Ranson clinical prognostic index
in, 1313, 1313t, 1323f
p24 antigen testing, for blood
donations, for HIV screening,
1382
Pantothenic acid, requirements for,
in ICU patient, 1558t
Paraldehyde intoxication, metabolic
acidosis in, 111
Paramedic(s), in prehospital trauma
resuscitation, 41-42
Paranasal sinusitis, nosocomial,
1271
Paraplegia, in chest trauma, 398
Parastomal hernia(s), 879-880
Parathyroidectomy, 604-605
complications in, 605
hypocalcemia after, 98
operative planning in, 604
operative technique in, 604-605
outcome evaluation in, 605
Paronychia, 1330-1331, 1330f-1331f
Parotid duct injury, 369
Parotitis, clinical and laboratory
diagnosis of, 1211
Partial thromboplastin time (PTT),
in burn patient, 56
Pasteurella multocida
in animal-bite wound, 122, 320
antimicrobial agents for, 1236t
Patellar fracture, 469
Patient-controlled analgesia (PCA)
for acute pain, 1532
mechanism of action of, 1649
modes of administration and dosing
parameters for, 1649, 1649t
for postoperative pain, 1649,

1903, 1623t, 1649t
side effects of, 1649
Patient education
in fast track surgery, 554
surgical risk and, 533
PCP, abuse of, emergency management
of, 174
in acute exposure, 174
in chronic use, 174
in withdrawal, 174
Pectin, enteral, intestinal mucosal
effects of, 1574
Pediatric surgical patient, 1159-
1181. See also Children; Infants
and neonates
Pediatric trauma score, 1176, 1177t
Pelvic examination, in acute
abdominal pain, 232
Pelvic fracture
in children, 1178
emergency department management
of, 40, 42f
Pelvic hernia(s), 879
Pelvis fracture, bladder rupture in,
449
Penciclovir, for herpesvirus
infections, 1375
Penicillin(s), 1230, 1232-1234, 1238
adverse effects of, 1246t
for Enterobacteriaceae bacteremia,
1219t
for nosocomial gram-negative
bacteremia, 1219t
penicillinase-resistant, 1233-1234
semisynthetic, 1245f
in vivo drug interactions with,
1232t
Penicillin G
aqueous crystalline, 1232-1233
for bacterial infections, 1240t-
1241t
benzathine, 1233
for bacterial infections, 1240t-
1241t
procaine, 1233
for bacterial infections, 1240t-
1241t
Penicillin V, 1233
for bacterial infections, 1240t-
1241t
Penrose drain(s), postoperative
management of, 1628
Pentazocine, suggested dosing for,
1621t
Peptic ulcer
in enteral nutrition, prevention
of, 1564
in immunosuppressed patient,
1119, 1114t
in pregnancy, 1191
Peptide(s), pulmonary metabolism of,
1449
Peptococcal bacteremia, 1220
Peptostreptococcal bacteremia, 1220
Peptostreptococcal infection,
antimicrobial agents for, 1235t
Pefloxacin, for bacterial
infections, 1242t-1243t
Perianal ulceration, in
immunosuppressed patient,
prevention of, 1114t
Pericardial effusion, in chest
trauma, 398
Pericardial tamponade
pulseless electrical activity in,
12t
shock in, 66
traumatic, emergency management
of, 36-37, 38f-39f